NEONATOLOGY

Pathophysiology and Management of the Newborn

Fifth Edition

NEONATOLOGY
Pathophysiology and Management of the Newborn

Fifth Edition

Edited by

GORDON B. AVERY, M.D., PH.D.
Emeritus Professor of Pediatrics
The George Washington University School of Medicine and Health Sciences; and
Scholar in Residence
Children's Research Institute
Children's National Medical Center
Washington, D.C.

MARY ANN FLETCHER, M.D.
Clinical Professor of Pediatrics
The George Washington University School of Medicine and Health Sciences
Washington, D.C.; and
Staff Neonatologist and Director
Newborn Follow-Up Program
Shady Grove Adventist Hospital
Rockville, Maryland

MHAIRI G. MACDONALD, M.B.CH.B., F.R.C.P.(E), D.C.H.
Clinical Professor of Pediatrics
The George Washington University School of Medicine and Health Sciences
Washington, D.C.; and
Director, Neonatology Services
Loudoun Hospital Center
Leesburg, Virginia

WITH 111 CONTRIBUTORS

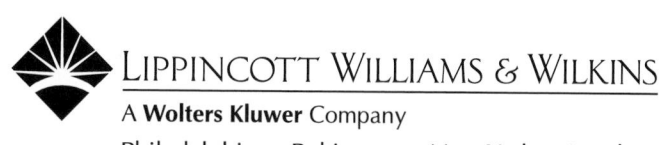

LIPPINCOTT WILLIAMS & WILKINS
A **Wolters Kluwer** Company
Philadelphia · Baltimore · New York · London
Buenos Aires · Hong Kong · Sydney · Tokyo

Acquisitions Editor: Paula Callaghan
Developmental Editor: Michelle LaPlante
Manufacturing Manager: Tim Reynolds
Production Manager: Liane Carita
Production Editor: Jeffrey Gruenglas
Cover Designer: Christine Jenny
Indexer: Mary Kidd
Compositor: Lippincott Williams & Wilkins Desktop Division
Printer: Courier Westford

Printed in the United States of America

9 8 7 6 5 4 3

Library of Congress Cataloging-in-Publication Data
Neonatology: pathophysiology and management of the newborn / edited by Gordon B. Avery, Mary Ann
    Fletcher, Mhairi G. MacDonald; with 111 contributors. —5th ed.
        p.   cm.
    Includes bibliographical references and index.
    ISBN 0-7817-1210-6
    1. Infants (Newborn)—Diseases. 2. Neonatology. I. Avery, Gordon B. II. Fletcher, Mary Ann.
III. MacDonald, Mhairi G.
    [DNLM: 1. Infant, Newborn, Diseases—physiopathology. 2. Infant, Newborn,
Diseases—therapy. 3. Prenatal Diagnosis.   WS 421N439 1999]
RJ254.N46   1999
618.92′01—dc21
DNLM/DLC
For Library of Congress   98-42248
                                                                            CIP

Contents

Part Three: Transition and Stabilization

Part Four: The Low-Birth-Weight Infant

Part Five: The Newborn Infant

Contributors

Thomas E. Adrian, Ph.D., F.R.C.Path.
Professor
Department of Biomedical Sciences
Creighton University School of Medicine
Omaha, Nebraska

Marianne S. Anderson, M.D.
Fellow, Neonatal-Perinatal Medicine
Department of Pediatrics
University of Colorado Health Sciences Center
Denver, Colorado

Robert J. Arceci, M.D.
Division of Hematology and Oncology
Children's Hospital Medical Center
Cincinnati, Ohio; and
Massachusetts General Hospital
Boston, Massachusetts

John H. Arnold, M.D.
Assistant Professor
Department of Anaesthesia (Pediatrics)
Harvard Medical School; and
Associate Director
Multidisciplinary Intensive Care Unit
Children's Hospital
Boston, Massachusetts

Gordon B. Avery, M.D., Ph.D.
Emeritus Professor of Pediatrics
The George Washington University School of
*   Medicine and Health Sciences; and*
Scholar in Residence
Children's Research Institute
Children's National Medical Center
Washington, D.C.

Claudette L. Bardin, Ph.D., M.D., F.A.A.P.
Assistant Professor
Department of Pediatrics
McGill University; and
Assistant Director, Neonatology
Department of Pediatrics and Neonatology
SMBD-Jewish General Hospital
Montreal, Quebec
Canada

Stephen Baumgart, M.D.
Professor and Vice Chairman
Department of Pediatrics
Thomas Jefferson University
Jefferson Medical College; and
Senior Staff Physician
Department of Pediatrics
Thomas Jefferson University Hospital
Philadelphia, Pennsylvania

David A. Beckman, Ph.D.
Associate Professor
Department of Pediatrics
Thomas Jefferson University; and
Nemours Research Programs
Alfred I. duPont Hospital for Children
Wilmington, Delaware

Edward F. Bell, M.D.
Professor
Department of Pediatrics
University of Iowa; and
Director
Divison of Neonatology
Children's Hospital of Iowa
Iowa City, Iowa

Joseph A. Bellanti, M.D.
Professor
Department of Pediatrics and Microbiology-
*   Immunology*
Georgetown University Medical Center
Washington, D.C.

Forrest C. Bennett, M.D.
Professor
Department of Pediatrics
University of Washington
Seattle, Washington

Judy C. Bernbaum, M.D.
Professor
Department of Pediatrics
University of Pennsylvania School of Medicine;
*   and*
Director, Neonatal Follow-Up Program
The Children's Hospital of Philadelphia
Philadelphia, Pennsylvania

Victor Blanchette, M.D., M.R.C.P.
Chief
Division of Hematology/Oncology
The Hospital for Sick Children; and
Professor
Department of Pediatrics
University of Toronto
Toronto, Ontario
Canada

Carl L. Bose, M.D.
Professor
Department of Pediatrics
University of North Carolina at
*   Chapel Hill; and*
Chief
Division of Neonatal-Perinatal Medicine
UNC Hospitals
Chapel Hill, North Carolina

Michael J. Boyajian, M.D.
Assistant Professor
Department of Surgery and Pediatrics
The George Washington University
*   School of Medicine; and*
Chief
Department of Plastic Surgery
Children's National Medical Center
Washington, D.C.

T. Berry Brazelton, M.D.
Professor Emeritus
Department of Pediatrics
Harvard Medical School
Cambridge; and
Professor Emeritus
Department of Pediatrics
Children's Hospital
Boston, Massachusetts

Robert L. Brent, M.D., Ph.D., D.Sc.
Distinguished Professor of Pediatrics,
*   Radiology, and Pathology*
Department of Pediatrics
Jefferson Medical College
Philadelphia, Pennsylvania; and
Division of Research
duPont Hospital for Children
Wilmington, Delaware

Luc P. Brion, M.D.
Professor
Department of Pediatrics
Albert Einstein College of Medicine and
*   Jack D. Weiler Hospital of the Montefiore*
*   Medical Center*
Bronx, New York

Richard L. Bucciarelli, M.D.
Professor and Associate Chair
Department of Pediatrics
University of Florida
Gainesville, Florida

Dorothy I. Bulas, M.D.
Associate Professor
Departments of Radiology and Pediatrics
The George Washington University
*   Medical Center; and*
Staff Radiologist
Department of Diagnostic Imaging
Children's National Medical Center
Washington, D.C.

Barbara K. Burton, M.D.
Professor and Head
Division of Genetics and Metabolism
Department of Pediatrics
University of Illinois College of Medicine;
*   and*
Director, Center for Medical and
*   Reproductive Genetics*
Michael Reese Hospital
Chicago, Illinois

Anthony J. Camerota, M.D.
Department of Critical Care Medicine
Naval Regional Center
Portsmith, Virginia

Sukgi S. Choi, M.D.
Associate Professor
Department of Otolaryngology and
*   Pediatrics*
The George Washington University
*   School of Medicine; and*
Vice Chairman
Department of Otolaryngology
Children's National Medical Center
Washington, D.C.

Jonathan M. Davis, M.D.
Professor
Department of Pediatrics
State University of New York at Stony Brook
*   School of Medicine*
Stony Brook;
Director, Neonatology and Newborn Medicine;
*   and*
Director, Cardiopulmonary Research
*   Institute*
Department of Pediatrics
Winthrop-University Hospital
Mineola, New York

John J. Doyle, M.D.
Assistant Professor
Division of Hematology/Oncology
The Hospital for Sick Children; and
Department of Pediatrics
University of Toronto
Toronto, Ontario
Canada

Arie Drugan, M.D.
Associate Professor
Department of Obstetrics and Gynecology
Wayne State University
Hutzel Hospital
Detroit, Michigan; and
Vice-Chairman
Department of Obstetrics and Gynecology
Rambam Medical Center
Haifa, Israel

Chester M. Edelmann, Jr., M.D.
Professor and Senior Associate Dean
Department of Pediatrics
Albert Einstein College of Medicine
Bronx, New York

Martin R. Eichelberger, M.D.
Professor
Department of Surgery and Pediatrics
The George Washington University
*   School of Medicine; and*
Director, Emergency Trauma Services
Children's National Medical Center
Washington, D.C.

Beryl Epstein, B.S., R.N.
Intensive Care Nursery
Children's Hospital
Oakland, California

Mark I. Evans, M.D.
Charlotte B. Failing Professor, Vice-Chairman,
*   and Vice-Chief of Obstetrics and Gynecology;*
Professor of Molecular Medicine and Genetics;
Professor of Pathology;
Director, Division of Reproductive Genetics;
*   Director, Center for Fetal Diagnosis and*
*   Therapy; and*
Director, Human Genetics Program
Hutzel Hospital/Wayne State University
Detroit, Michigan

Baruch Feldman, M.D., Ph.D.
Clinical Fellow
Division of Reproductive Genetics
Department of Obstetrics/Gynecology
Hutzel Hospital
Wayne State University
Detroit, Michigan

Michael F. Flanagan, M.D.
Department of Pediatrics
Section of Pediatric Cardiology
Dartmouth Medical School; and
Dartmouth–Hitchcock Medical Center
Lebanon, New Hampshire

Alan W. Flake, M.D.
Department of Pediatric Surgery
Children's Hospital of Philadelphia
Philadelphia, Pennsylvania

Mary Ann Fletcher, M.D.
Clinical Professor of Pediatrics
The George Washington University
*   School of Medicine and Health Sciences*
Washington, D.C.; and
Staff Neonatologist and Director
Newborn Follow-Up Program
Shady Grove Adventist Hospital
Rockville, Maryland

Bishara J. Freij, M.D.
Chief
Division of Infectious Diseases
Department of Pediatrics
William Beaumont Hospital
Royal Oak; and
Clinical Associate Professor
Department of Pediatrics
Wayne State University
*   School of Medicine*
Detroit, Michigan

David M. Frim, M.D., Ph.D.
Assistant Professor
Department of Surgery and Pediatrics
The University of Chicago; and
Chief
Section of Pediatric Neurosurgery
The University of Chicago
*   Children's Hospital*
Chicago, Illinois

Michael K. Georgieff, M.D.
Professor
Department of Pediatrics
University of Minnesota; and
Staff Neonatologist
Department of Pediatrics
Fairview-University Medical Center
Minneapolis, Minnesota

Harold M. Ginzburg, M.D., J.D., M.P.H.
Clinical Professor
Departments of Psychiatry and Neurology
Tulane Medical Center
New Orleans, Louisiana

Penny Glass, Ph.D.
Associate Professor of Pediatrics
Department of Neonatology
Children's National Medical Center
Washington, D.C.

Stanley N. Graven, M.D.
Professor
Community and Family Health
Department of Pediatrics
University of South Florida; and
Staff Physician
Department of Pediatrics
Tampa General Hospital
Tampa, Florida

Paul P. Griffin, M.D.
Professor Emeritus
Department of Orthopaedic Surgery
Medical University of South Carolina; and
Orthopaedic Surgeon
Department of Orthopaedic Surgery
University Hospital
Charleston, South Carolina

Michael R. Harrison, M.D.
Department of Pediatric Surgery
University of California, San Francisco
San Francisco, California

Susan C. Harrsch, R.N., M.S.N., C.R.N.P.
Neonatal Nurse Practitioner
Division of Neonatology
Thomas Jefferson University
Jefferson Medical College
Philadelphia, Pennsylvania

Gary E. Hartman, M.D.
Professor of Surgery and Pediatrics
Department of Surgery
The George Washington University School of Medicine; and
Chairman
Department of Pediatric Surgery
Children's National Medical Center
Washington, D.C.

William W. Hay, Jr., M.D.
Professor and Director
Neonatal-Perinatal Medicine Training Program; and
Director, Neonatal Clinical Research Center
Department of Pediatrics
University of Colorado Health Sciences Center
Denver, Colorado

Alan Hill, M.D., Ph.D.
Professor
Department of Pediatrics
University of British Columbia; and
Head, Division of Neurology
Department of Pediatrics
British Columbia's Children's Hospital
Vancouver, British Columbia
Canada

W. Alan Hodson, M.D.
Department of Pediatrics
University of Washington
Seattle, Washington

Wolfgang Holzgreve, Professor Dr. Med
University of Basel
Basel
Switzerland

Carl E. Hunt, M.D.
Department of Pediatrics
Medical College of Ohio
Toledo, Ohio

Nelson B. Isada, M.D.
Alaska Perinatology Associates
Anchorage, Alaska; and
Assistant Professor
Divisions of Reproductive Genetics and Maternal-Fetal Medicine
Department of Obstetrics and Gynecology
Wayne State University
Hutzel Hospital
Detroit, Michigan

Sherwin J. Isenberg, M.D.
Lantz Professor of Pediatric Ophthalmology and Vice-Chairman
Department of Ophthalmology
Jules Stein Eye Institute
Harbor–UCLA School of Medicine
Los Angeles, California

Mark Paul Johnson, M.D.
Associate Professor
Departments of Obstetrics/Gynecology, Pathology, Molecular Medicine, and Genetics
Wayne State University; and
Associate Director, Reproductive Genetics
Department of Obstetrics and Gynecology
Hutzel Hospital/The Detroit Medical Center
Detroit, Michigan

Lauren A. Johnson-Robbins, M.D.
Assistant Professor
Department of Pediatrics
Albany Medical College; and
Attending Neonatologist
Albany Medical Center
Albany, New York

George W. Kaplan, M.D., M.S., F.A.A.P.,
F.A.C.S.
Clinical Professor
Department of Surgery and Pediatrics
School of Medicine
University of California, San Diego; and
Chairman
Division of Urology
Children's Hospital
San Diego, California

Joan McGregor Kelly, M.D.
Physician
Division of Neonatology
Holy Cross Hospital
Silver Spring, Maryland

Winston W. K. Koo, M.B.B.S.
Professor
Department of Pediatrics
Wayne State University; and
Neonatologist
Department of Pediatrics
Hutzel Hospital
Detroit, Michigan

Helain J. Landy, M.D.
Associate Professor
Division of Maternal-Fetal Medicine
Department of Obstetrics and Gynecology
Georgetown University Medical Center
Washington, D.C.

Ralph A. Lugo, M.D.
Assistant Professor
College of Pharmacy; and
Adjunct Assistant Professor
Department of Pediatrics
University of Utah
Salt Lake City, Utah

Carolyn Houska Lund, R.N., M.S.N, F.A.A.N.
Intensive Care Nursery
Children's Hospital
Oakland, California

George H. McCracken, Jr., M.D.
Professor
The Sarah M. and Charles E. Seay Chair
in Pediatric Infectious Diseases
Department of Pediatrics
University of Texas
Southwestern Medical Center; and
Attending Physician
Children's Medical Center
Dallas, Texas

Mhairi G. MacDonald, M.B., Ch.B.,
F.R.C.P.(E), D.C.H.
Clinical Professor of Pediatrics
The George Washington University
School of Medicine and Health Sciences
Washington, D.C.; and
Director, Neonatology Services
Loudoun Hospital Center
Leesburg, Virginia

Joseph R. Madsen, M.D.
Assistant Professor
Department of Surgery
Harvard Medical School; and
Associate Professor
Department of Neurosurgery
Children's Hospital
Boston, Massachusetts

M. Jeffrey Maisels, M.B., B.Ch.
Clinical Professor of Pediatrics
Wayne State University School of Medicine
University of Michigan Medical Center;
and
Chairman, Department of Pediatrics
William Beaumont Hospital
Royal Oak, Michigan

Andrew M. Margileth, M.D.
Clinical Professor
Department of Pediatrics
Mercer University School of Medicine
Hilton Head, South Carolina; and
Director, Pediatrics and Dermatology
Department of Pediatrics
Backus Children's Hospital
Savannah, Georgia

Bradley S. Marino, M.D., M.P.P.
Fellow, Division of Cardiology
The Cardiac Center
The Children's Hospital of Philadelphia
Philadelphia, Pennsylvania

Gilbert I. Martin, M.D.
Clinical Professor
Department of Pediatrics
University of California, Irvine
Irvine; and
Director, Neonatal Intensive Care Unit
Citrus Valley Medical Center
West Covina, California

Laura S. Martin, M.D.
Department of Pediatrics
Madigan Army Medical Center
Tacoma, Washington

Irene M. McAleer, M.D.
Department of Surgery
School of Medicine
University of California, San Diego; and
Division of Urology
Children's Hospital
San Diego, California

Scott D. McLean, M.D.
Chief, Medical Genetics
Department of Pediatrics
Wilford Hall Medical Center
Lackland Air Force Base, Texas

Thomas Moshang, Jr., M.D.
Professor
Department of Pediatrics
University of Pennsylvania; and
Chief
Department of Pediatrics
Children's Hospital of Philadelphia
Philadelphia, Pennsylvania

Nicholas M. Nelson, M.D.
Professor
Division of General Pediatrics
Department of Pediatrics
The Milton S. Hershey Medical Center
Hershey, Pennsylvania

Kurt D. Newman, M.D.
Professor
Department of Surgery
The George Washington University
*   School of Medicine; and*
Vice-Chairman
Department of Pediatric Surgery
Children's National Medical Center
Washington, D.C.

Edward S. Ogata, M.D., M.M.
Professor
Department of Pediatrics
Northwestern University Medical School; and
Chief Medical Officer
Children's Memorial Hospital
Chicago, Illinois

William Oh, M.D.
Department of Pediatrics
Brown University School of Medicine
Providence, Rhode Island

Enrique M. Ostrea, Jr., M.D.
Professor
Department of Pediatrics
Wayne State University School of Medicine; and
Chief
Department of Pediatrics
Hutzel Hospital
Detroit, Michigan

Apostolos Papageorgiou, M.D., F.R.C.P.C.,
**   F.A.A.P.**
Professor
Departments of Pediatrics and of
*   Obstetrics and Gynecology*
McGill University; and
Chief, Department of Pediatrics and
*   Neonatology*
SMBD-Jewish General Hospital
Montreal, Quebec
Canada

Roderic H. Phibbs, M.D.
Department of Pediatrics
University of California, San Francisco
San Francisco, California

J. Edgar C. Posecion, M.D.
Division of Neonatal–Perinatal Medicine
Department of Pediatrics
Wayne State University School of Medicine
Hutzel Hospital; and
Children's Hospital of Michigan
Detroit, Michigan

David Mann Powell, M.D.
Assistant Professor
Department of Surgery
The George Washington University
*   School of Medicine; and*
Attending Surgeon
Department of Pediatric Surgery
Children's National Medical Center
Washington, D.C.

Gabriella Pridjian, M.D.
Human Genetics Program
The Hayward Genetics Center
New Orleans, Louisiana

Gloria S. Pryhuber, M.D.
Department of Pediatrics
University of Rochester
Rochester, New York

Yung-Hao Pung, M.D., M.P.H.
Assistant Professor
Department of Pediatrics
Georgetown University School of Medicine
Washington, D.C.

Mary E. Revenis, M.D.
Assistant Professor of Pediatrics
Department of Neonatology
The George Washington University School of
*   Medicine and Health Sciences; and*
Children's National Medical Center
Washington, D.C.

Ward R. Rice, M.D, Ph.D.
Associate Professor of Pediatrics
University of Cincinnati College of Medicine
Children's Hospital Medical Center
Cincinnati, Ohio

William W. Robertson, Jr., M.D.
Professor
Departments of Orthopaedic Surgery and
*   Pediatrics*
The George Washington University
*   School of Medicine; and*
Chairman
Departments of Pediatric and
*   Orthopaedic Surgery*
Children's National Medical Center
Wahington, D.C.

Mark A. Rosen, M.D.
Professor and Vice-Chairman
Department of Anesthesia and
*   Perioperative Care;*
Professor
Department of Obstetrics, Gynecology and
*   Reproductive Sciences; and*
Director, Obstetrical Anesthesia
Moffitt-Long Island Hospital
University of California, San Francisco
San Francisco, California

Warren N. Rosenfeld, M.D.
Professor
Department of Pediatrics
State University of New York at Stony Brook
*   School of Medicine*
Stony Brook; and
Chairman
Department of Pediatrics
Winthrop-University Hospital
Mineola, New York

Lisa M. Satlin, M.D.
Assistant Professor
Division of Pediatric Nephrology
Department of Pediatrics
Mount Sinai School of Medicine
New York, New York

Barbara Schmidt, M.D., M.Sc.
Staff Neonatologist
Chedoke McMaster Hospital; and
Professor
Department of Pediatrics
McMaster University
Hamilton, Ontario
Canada

John L. Sever, M.D., Ph.D.
Professor
Departments of Pediatrics,
*   Obstetrics and Gynecology,*
*   Microbiology, and Immunology*
The George Washington University
*   School of Medicine*
Children's National Medical Center
Washington, D.C.

Billie Lou Short, M.D.
Professor of Pediatrics
Department of Neonatology
Children's National Medical Center
Washington, D.C.

Paul S. Thornton, M.B., B.Ch., M.R.C.P.I.
Director
National Metabolic Unit
The Children's Hospital
Dublin
Ireland

Suzanne M. Touch, M.D.
Research Fellow
Division of Neonatology
Thomas Jefferson University
Jefferson Medical College
Philadelphia, Pennsylvania

William E. Truog, M.D.
Department of Pediatrics
Children's Mercy Hospital
Kansas City, Missouri

Reginald C. Tsang, M.D.
Division of Neonatology
Department of Pediatrics
University of Cincinnati Medical Center
Cincinnati, Ohio

Jon A. Vanderhoof, M.D.
Professor of Pediatrics and Director
Joint Section of Pediatric Gastroenterology
*   and Nutrition*
University of Nebraska Medical Center
Omaha, Nebraska

Maria Esterlita T. Villanueva, M.D.
Division of Neonatal–Perinatal Medicine
Department of Pediatrics
Wayne State University School of Medicine
Hutzel Hospital; and
Children's Hospital of Michigan
Detroit, Michigan

Joseph J. Volpe, M.D.
Bronson Crothers Professor of Neurology
Harvard Medical School; and
Neurologist-in-Chief
Children's Hospital
Boston, Massachusetts

Robert M. Ward, M.D.
Professor
Department of Pediatrics
University of Utah
Salt Lake City, Utah

Barbara B. Warner, M.D.
William Cooper Proctor Research Scholar
University of Cincinnati College of Medicine
Children's Hospital Medical Center
Cincinnati, Ohio

Steven N. Weindling, M.D.
Department of Pediatrics
Section of Pediatric Cardiology
Dartmouth Medical School; and
Dartmouth–Hitchcock Medical Center
Lebanon, New Hampshire

Howard J. Weinstein, M.D.
Associate Professor
Division of Hematology and Oncology
Children's Hospital Medical Center
Cincinnati, Ohio; and
Massachusetts General Hospital
Boston, Massachusetts

Gil Wernovsky, M.D.
Associate Professor
Department of Pediatrics
University of Pennsylvania
*   School of Medicine; and*
Director, Cardiac Intensive Care Unit
The Children's Hospital of Pennsylvania
Philadelphia, Pennsylvania

Susan E. Wert, Ph.D.
Research Associate
Divisions of Neonatology and
*   Pulmonary Biology*
Department of Pediatrics;
Research Scholar
University of Cincinnati
*   College of Medicine; and*
Director, Morphology Care
Division of Pulmonary Biology
Children's Hospital Research Foundation
Cincinnati, Ohio

Robert D. White, M.D.
Clinical Assistant Professor
Department of Pediatrics
Indiana University School of Medicine
Indianapolis; and
Director, Regional Newborn Program
Memorial Hospital
South Bend, Indiana

Jeffrey A. Whitsett, M.D.
Professor
Department of Pediatrics
University of Cincinnati
*   College of Medicine; and*
Director
Division of Pulmonary Biology
Children's Hospital Medical Center
Cincinnati, Ohio

Betty Anne (Chaze) Wilkins,
**   R.N., B.S.N., M.S.N.**
Risk Management Operations Manager
Risk & Insurance Management
Inova Health Systems
Falls Church, Virginia

Scott B. Yeager, M.D.
Associate Professor
Department of Pediatrics
University of Vermont; and
Chief
Division of Pediatric
*   Cardiology*
Medical Center Hospital of
*   Vermont*
Burlington, Vermont

Terence L. Zach, M.D.
Associate Professor
Department of Pediatrics
Creighton University
Omaha, Nebraska

Barbara J. Zeligs
Research Associate
Department of Pediatrics
Georgetown University School of Medicine; and
International Center for Interdisciplinary
*   Studies of Immunology*
Washington, D.C.

Alvin Zipursky, M.D.
Professor Emeritus
Division of Hematology/Oncology
The Hospital for Sick Children; and
Professor Emeritus
Department of Pediatrics
University of Toronto
Toronto, Ontario
Canada

Preface

Twenty-five years have elapsed between the publication of the first and the fifth editions of *Nenatology: Pathophysiology and Management of the Newborn*. During those years there have been striking changes in our understanding of human biology as it applies to the conditions and diseases of the newborn infant. In addition, the structure of the health care system in the United States has changed drastically. Thus, both the *pathophysiology* and the *management* have changed materially and have neccessitated regular new editions of the book. With co-editors Mhairi G. MacDonald, M.B.Ch.B., F.R.C.P.(E), D.C.H., and Mary Ann Fletcher, M.D., we have rethought the book in light of today's knowledge. The book's broad structure has been retained, but many chapters have been replaced and others fundamentally rewritten.

A central focus of neonatal intensive care unit (NICU) care is the premature infant. This emphasis derives from the large number of prematures born annually, the staggering cost of their care, the importance of their long-term outcomes, and the markedly improved survival of what is often termed "the micro-premie": the infant of less than 1,000 grams birth weight. The LD50 for prematurity during this period has changed from 1,500 grams to 500–800 grams. Contributing to this dramatic result are advances in every aspect of care: provision of thermoneutral environment, nutritional and metabolic support, intravenous alimentation, administration of exogenous surfactant, ventilatory support, continuous monitoring, management of infection, microlaboratory determinations, avoidance of trauma, and understanding of the developmental needs of the extrauterine fetus. New science has included biophysical devices, better understandings of cell and organ differentiation, delineation of neurotransmitters, cell signaling, gene regulation, and a host of cytokines and growth factors. It is significant that three scientists were awarded the Nobel Prize for Medicine in 1998 for describing the role of nitric oxide in vasodilation, just as inhaled NO has been featured as a treatment for persistent pulmonary hypertension in the neonate.

The scope of neonatology has been far broader than care of the premature infant, however. Management of the infant with congenital anomalies, perinatal infections, genetic syndromes and errors of metabolism, hypoxic-ischemic encephalopathy, surgical problems, and a host of other conditions, has kept neonatology in the forefront as the largest specialty within pediatrics. This is reflected by the significant number of neonatology months required in the basic pediatric residency, the number of active neonatologists nationally, and the proportion of papers in research journals which address problems of the newborn infant. A June, 1998 report of the Section on Perinatal Pediatrics of the American Academy of Pediatrics supplied the following manpower figures: Board Certified and Eligible Neonatologists, 3,688; actively practicing neonatology, 92%; practicing neonatology >75% time and effort, 70%; active training programs nationwide, 102; active neonatology fellows in training, 150; and neonatal nurse practitioners (NNP), 1,700. This report estimates that upwards of 300 neonatologists and an equal number of NNPs will be required in the next year.

What can I say about managed care and health care funding? In the United States we have a highly regulated but almost totally unplanned health care system. Neonatology, more so than most specialties, is a systems-dependent series of transactions. It is a complex team which actually gives around-the-clock care. The de-regionalization of neonatology, coupled with the proliferation of small NICUs providing level III care in community hospitals, has seemingly increased the cost and decreased the efficiency of neonatal care.

In this edition, fourteen chapters are new, and nearly all have been extensively rewritten. There has been increased emphasis on the new molecular biology and on ultrasonography and other imaging techniques, as they impinge on the practice of neonatology. A new chapter has been devoted to Sudden

Infant Death Syndrome. Innovative techniques of infant ventilation have been described. New chapters discuss the extremely-low-birth-weight infant, and the small-for-gestational-age infant. The nursing roles in the NICU have been treated in a completely new chapter. Likewise, both nursery design and Law, Risk Management, and the Practice of Neonatology are entirely new chapters which reflect the needs of the health care provider entering the new millenium. Further developments in neonatal neurology and the outcomes on follow-up of neonatal care have been detailed. In response to the increasing incidence of corrective cardiac surgery in the neonatal period, the chapter on cardiac surgery has been fundamentally revised to provide detailed information on pre- and postsurgical care.

Even as I write this, new science, new therapies, and new health systems changes are coming into being. This textbook hopes to achieve what a textbook is best at: assembling current best thinking across a broad array of subtopics to help the health professional integrate what otherwise is a disorganized blizzard of fragmented information. It remains for professional journals, research meetings—and now, electronic media and the Internet—to bring in the news flashes. If this book helps in the broad understanding of the biology of the human neonate and the care of neonatal diseases and conditions, our efforts will have been amply rewarded.

Gordon B. Avery, M.D., Ph.D.

Preface to the First Edition

Neonatology means knowledge of the human newborn. The term was coined by Alexander Schaffer, whose book on the subject, *Diseases of the Newborn*, was first published in 1960. This book, together with Clement Smith's *Physiology of the Newborn Infant,* formed cornerstones of the developing field. In the past fifteen years, neonatology has grown from the preoccupation of a handful of pioneers to a major subspecialty of pediatrics. Knowledge in this area has so expanded that it now seems important to collect this material into a multiauthor reference work.

Although the perinatal mortality rate has declined over the past fifty years, the best presently attainable survival rates have not been achieved throughout the world, and indeed the United States lags behind fifteen other countries, despite its vast resources. New knowledge and improvement in the coordination of services for mother and child are needed to drive down perinatal mortality further. And finally, far greater emphasis must be placed on morbidity, so that surviving infants can lead full and productive lives. One hopes that in the future the yardstick of success will be the quality of life and not the mere fact of life itself.

In this past decade, neonatology, as a recognized subspeciality of pediatrics, has come into being around the intensive care–premature nursery. Needless to say, the problems of prematurity are far from solved. But neonatology is ripe for a broadening-out from its prematurity–hyaline membrane disease beginnings. The newborn is heir to so many problems, and his or her physiology is so unique and rapidly changing that all conditions of the newborn should come within the concern of the new and expanding discipline of neonatology. It has long since become standard practice to admit to premature nurseries other high-risk infants such as those of diabetic or toxemic mothers. Here the criterion is the need for intensive care. However, the neonatologist's specialized knowledge should give him a significant role in the care of other infants in the first two to three months of life, whether they require intensive care and whether they are readmitted for problems unrelated to prematurity and birth itself. Detailed knowledge of newborn physiology can assist in the management of congenital anomalies, surgical conditions of the neonate, failure to thrive, nutritional problems, genetic, neurologic, and biochemical diseases, and a host of conditions involving delayed maturation. Thus one can conceive of a subspecialty sharply limited in age to early infancy but broad in its study of the interaction of normal physiology and disease processes.

Neonatology must also grow in its relationship to obstetrics and fetal biology. In the best centers, an active partnership has developed between obstetrics and pediatrics around the management of high-risk pregnancies and newborns. Sometimes training has been cooperative, but in only a few instances have basic scientists concerned with fetal biology been brought into this effort. Important beginnings have been made in studying the fetomaternal unit, such as the endocrine studies of Egon Diczfalusy, the cardiopulmonary studies of Geoffrey Dawes, and the immunologic studies of Arther Silverstein. But fundamental processes such as the controls of fetal growth and the onset of labor are not understood at this time. Centers or institutes bringing together workers of diverse points of view are needed to wrestle with the profound problems of fetal biology. At the clinical level, the interdependence of obstetrics and neonatology is obvious. As an ultimate development, these two specialties may one day be joined as a new entity—perinatology—at least at the level of training and certification. In the meantime, far greater mutual understanding and daily interaction are needed for the optimal care of mothers and their infants.

This book is organized around problems as they occur, as well as by organ systems. It hopes to achieve a balance between presentation of the basic science on which rational management must rest, and the advice concerning patient care which experts in each subarea are qualified to give. Individual chapter authors have approached their subjects in various ways, and no attempt has been made to achieve a completely uniform format. In some instances, there is overlap of subject material, but the somewhat different viewpoints presented, and the desire to spare the reader from hopscotching through the book after cross references, have persuaded me to leave small overlaps undisturbed.

It is appreciated that no volume such as this can have more than a finite useful lifetime. Yet while its currency lasts, I hope it will serve as a practical guide to therapy and an aid in the understanding of pathophysiology for those active in the care of newborns.

Gordon B. Avery, M.D., Ph.D.

PART ONE

General Considerations

CHAPTER 1

Neonatology: Perspective at the End of the Twentieth Century

Gordon B. Avery

Rapid change has characterized neonatology since the name was coined in 1960 by Alexander Schaffer. Structurally, it can be compared with a tree (Fig. 1–1). Its "roots"—obstetrics, pediatrics, and physiology—began at the turn of the century. A sturdy "trunk" has developed in the intensive care nurseries (ICNs) scattered across the United States and around the world. The "branches" have spread so widely that it is difficult for a single person to be expert in all the areas of activity required for a tertiary neonatology service. Important interactions have gone beyond allied disciplines such as obstetrics, anesthesiology, cardiology, radiology, and surgery. Neonatologists today struggle with hospital administrators, pediatric training program directors, legislatures, Congress, the courts, the federal government, malpractice lawyers, right-to-life groups, and ethicists in an effort to determine their proper roles and limits. Caught in a cross-fire between strenuous cost-containment measures and regulations mandating the vigorous treatment of all newborns regardless of prognosis, many neonatologists wonder when a stable situation will be reached. Yet stimulating growth has occurred—mainly since 1960.

THE ROOTS

One of the main roots from which neonatology grew was supplied by obstetricians such as Pierre Budin and Sir Dugald Baird, who were interested in the babies they delivered and not merely in the immediate welfare of the mother. It may be a serious oversimplification to imply that, in former times, obstetricians were content if the baby was liveborn. Childbirth, however, was the cause of

a significant number of maternal deaths and for many was a fearful experience. Premature infants were expected to die, as were most neonates with malformations. There was a feeling that natural selection should be allowed to discard the "runt of the litter," as suggested by the designation of prematures as "weaklings." It was Budin and his pupil Couney who pioneered incubator care of premature infants and thus helped change some of the early, pessimistic attitudes toward these babies.

Another significant root of neonatology can be found in the "quiet premature nursery," such as that run by Julius Hess and Evelyn Lundeen in Chicago in the early 1900s (1). Only premature infants were admitted to these nurseries, and gentleness with minimal intervention was the policy. To prevent infection, staff wore gowns, caps, and masks and set up a scrub routine that excluded parents and minimized traffic in the area. Feedings of breast milk by eyedropper were delayed for up to 72 hours, and the infants were handled as little as possible. Yet the supportive conditions needed to allow the body to recover, as described by Florence Nightingale, were present: "warmth, rest, diet, quiet, sanitation, space, and others" (2). Perhaps some of the high-tech nurseries of today could benefit from an infusion of this superb nurturing orientation.

Physiology is a tap root of neonatology. Advances in neonatal care rest directly on descriptions of the changing body processes of the newborn infant. Men such as Barcroft and Dawes began delineation of fetal circulation and placental function. These studies in turn led to the establishment of the fetal lamb model, which subsequently was widely exploited. Neonatal metabolic, gastrointestinal, respiratory, and central nervous system functions were studied by Levine, Smith, Peiper, and others. The 1945 publication of the first edition of Clement Smith's textbook, *The Physiology of the Newborn Infant*, was a

G. B. Avery: Children's Research Institute, Children's National Medical Center; and Department of Pediatrics, George Washington University School of Medicine and Health Sciences, Washington, D.C.

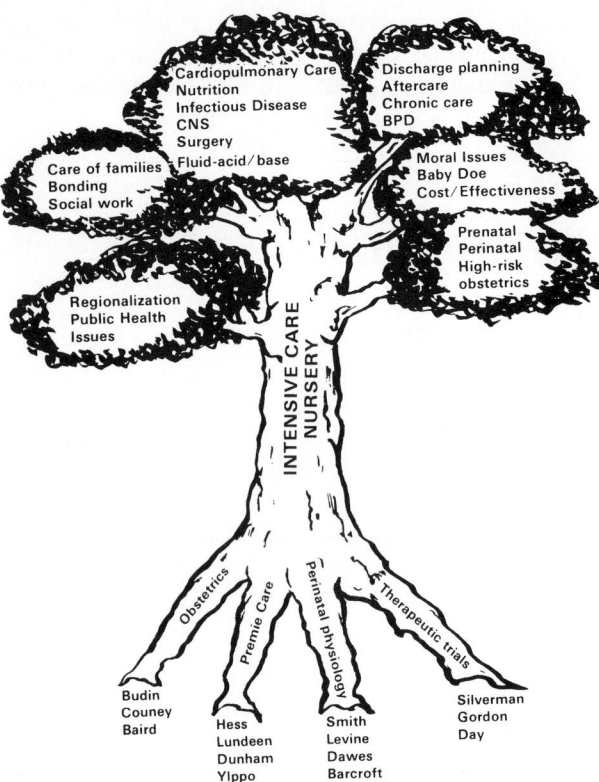

FIG. 1–1. The neonatal–perinatal tree shows the roots, trunk, and branches of the specialty.

signal event in our evolving ability to care for sick newborns in a rational manner (3).

A final anchoring root of neonatology is the therapeutic trial. Innumerable traditional teachings about premature infants eventually have been proved false. Without scientific testing as a guide, neonatologists would constantly be off course. As it is, several dangerous misadventures have been averted by clinical trials. An example is prophylactic sulfonamide treatment of premature infants, which was found to cause increased kernicterus (4). Silverman, Gordon, and Day were pioneers who insisted on rigor in such trials.

THE TRUNK

The ICN is the institution that forms the sturdy trunk of endeavors in neonatology. The ICN is a therapeutic environment, a collection of equipment, and a multidisciplinary team that is guided by dedicated leadership, by a group of specific protocols, and by a body of relevant scientific knowledge. It is the ICN as an integrated organism, rather than any single person or collection of people, that takes care of the sick neonate—in a sense, this is holistic medicine turned inside out. The ICN has proved very effective in the care of desperately ill babies, but its rationale remains difficult to explain to hospital administrators, insurance companies, and congressmen.

Over the years, there has been a steady increase in the intensity of illness observed in the ICN. With this rise has come an increase in the number and variety of personnel and the amount of technically sophisticated equipment. In the 1950s, premature care was a major concern. The principal interventions were resuscitation, thermoregulation, careful feeding, simple and exchange transfusion, and supportive care of respiratory distress. By the 1960s, electronic monitors came into use, and blood gases began to be measured. Feedings were aided by nasogastric tubes, and increased laboratory monitoring became possible. Antibiotics became available for treatment of neonatal sepsis.

By the 1970s, the use of umbilical catheters and arterial pressure transducers was routine, and respirator therapy of hyaline membrane disease began to succeed. Nutritional support for sick infants was aided by transpyloric feeding tubes and finally by complete intravenous alimentation. Microchemistry tests for most necessary parameters became widely available. Neonatal surgery was shown to be feasible for many congenital abnormalities, including serious cardiac defects. With the 1980s came the advent of computed tomography and ultrasonography. Significant concern centered around ventricular hemorrhages and consequent posthemorrhagic hydrocephalus in small premature infants. Transcutaneous electrodes became available first for measurement of oxygen and then for carbon dioxide. Pulse oximetry increasingly has been used for continuous physiologic monitoring. Nutritional and metabolic supports were significantly refined. Surfactant replacement has reduced the severity of lung disease in premature infants. Extracorporeal membrane oxygenation permitted the survival of some previously unsalvageable infants. In the 1990s, magnetic resonance imaging improved visualization of lesions, and positron emission tomography and magnetic resonance spectroscopy promise to reveal the physiology of the intact brain. As survival has become common for infants who weigh as little as 600 g at birth, increased attention has swung to assuring intact survival, and the 1990s have been dubbed the decade of the brain.

THE BRANCHES

Perinatalology

A body of specialized knowledge, a group of subspecialized professionals, the advent of technically advanced equipment, and the formation of special care units all contributed to the development of neonatology. In obstetrics, these same elements came together about 10 years later and resulted in the specialty of maternofetal medicine. Perinatologists developed high-risk prenatal clinics and special delivery facilities for unstable patients. A steadily growing body of literature from animal and clinical investigations allowed improved management of pregnancy complications and monitoring of fetal status. Ultrasonography allowed the detection of fetal abnormalities and determination of fetal size, anatomy, activity, breathing, and response to stress. For the first time, mothers were given drugs designed to treat fetal conditions, and intrauterine transfusions were performed in cases of threatened hydrops. Fetal surgery has yet to find its proper place, but prenatal shunts have been inserted for hydrocephalus, obstructed urinary tracts have been drained, and repair of diaphragmatic hernia has been attempted.

In many major teaching hospitals, perinatal obstetric and neonatal services have joined forces to form perinatal centers. Often with codirectors from the two disciplines, these centers fostered cooperation in the best interests of the high-risk patient. Integrated planning and management in optimal cases consisted of a high-risk prenatal clinic, timing and management of labor and delivery, resuscitation, and intensive care in the nursery. Statistics on morbidity and mortality, reviewed in periodic joint conferences, permit constant refinement of policy and technique. These centers have been the locations of training programs in both perinatology and neonatology and the sources of important research. They have demonstrated the best survival rates for small prematures and other categories of infants at highest risk, and they provide the standard by which perinatal care is judged.

The natural alliance between perinatal obstetrics and neonatology is so great that some have suggested that it receive department status within the medical complex. In some ways, the perinatal center accomplishes this on an *ad hoc* basis. But perinatologists and neonatologists are parts of traditional departments of obstetrics and pediatrics, with surgical and medical orientations, respectively. Allocation of resources and ranking of faculty occur predominantly through the parent departments, where the priorities of the chairmen are paramount.

Regional Connections

The medical community found that to optimize function of the perinatal center, it was necessary to form complex relationships among hospitals and community resources (see Chap. 3). First neonatal and then maternal transport services were developed to move patients safely and efficiently to the center and back. Hot lines were established to provide consultation and bed allocation, which could be coordinated through a single phone number. Affiliations for continuing education were formed, and standard protocols for referral were worked out. In some instances, exchange of personnel and joint review of statistics helped cement the connection.

Government agencies extended a helping hand in this networking. Some state legislatures were convinced early of the public health advantage of regional systems. The government began to award grants to perinatal centers to underwrite some of the cost of outreach and system activities. Training and research grants from the federal government often were given to the same perinatal centers and served to buttress the resources of these centers. With passage of the National Health Planning and Resources Development Act (Public Law 93-641) in 1974, the federal government mandated regional planning of expensive resources in the interest of efficiency and economy. Designation of care levels I, II, and III was adopted, and publication of regional plans for perinatal care became widespread.

Unfortunately, during the 1980s, regionalization suffered striking reversals. The mandated state health planning mechanisms were emasculated. Hospitals became increasingly competitive and wished to offer full services to prepaid health plans. Large numbers of neonatologists moved into suburban hospitals and set up level II nurseries. The result was a decentralization of perinatal high-risk care, with loss of efficiency and economy of scale.

Finally, I wish to call attention to the involvement of neonatologists in a mixture of educational, administrative, and political activities that have been very taxing and time consuming. Although neonatology training has emphasized bedside care, a business school or public health degree would be directly useful to today's neonatologist. A thorough training in counseling, group dynamics, and law also would be invaluable.

Ethics

During the newborn period, babies with congenital malformations, asphyxia, and extreme immaturity are seen. Modern powerful life-support systems provide the technology for relatively prolonged continuation of futile care. These circumstances have thrust neonatologists into the center of a national debate on medical ethics. In the midst of all this, neonatologists must keep their heads and care for babies and their families as best they can. Chapter 2 deals extensively with the moral issues raised by neonatal intensive care.

Care of the Family

In general, there has been striking improvement in care of the distressed families of critically ill newborn infants. Formerly excluded from the ICN because of fear of infection, parents are brought to the bedside and encouraged to touch their babies. Limited sibling visitation often is permitted. Nurses help parents get used to intrusive medical equipment and, as soon as possible, parents perform simple caretaking procedures with their child. Social workers, parent support groups, chaplains, and literature for parents have become increasingly available. Starting with the work of Klaus and Kennell, a growing body of publications has appeared that suggests that bonding of parents to the newborn infant is important to later functioning of the family unit. The change of the title of Klaus and Kennell's monograph from *Maternal–Infant Bonding* in 1976 to *Parent–Infant Bonding* in 1982 reflects recognition of the role of fathers in the parenting of neonates (5,6).

Home Care

The aftercare of discharged high-risk newborns has become an increasingly important area of concern for neonatologists. Although many problems are resolved quickly and require only routine follow-up, a significant number of babies with chronic problems are taken home from the ICN. As a small premature infant approaches discharge, it becomes clear that parent instruction, sleep apnea testing, cardiopulmonary resuscitation training, concern with feeding and growth, schedules for testing sight, hearing, and speech, physical medicine, and developmental psychology foreshadow a first year of life crowded with clinic visits and special needs. Infants with chronic lung disease not uncommonly go home on oxygen therapy, multiple medications, and special feeding regimens. During the first year or two of life, intercurrent infections may require several readmissions. The best outcomes have been achieved with early diagnosis of developmental difficulties and the mobilization of community resources. All this necessitates input from a physician with appreciation of the stormy neonatal period and an understanding of the continuing problems of infants born prematurely with other perinatal insults. Often, a multidisciplinary team at the tertiary center collaborates with the family's pediatrician to provide this special care. Although oriented to neonatal intensive care, neonatologists have begun to assume responsibility in this aftercare.

The Intensive Care Nursery as a Space Station

The quiet, simple, gentle premature nursery of 50 years ago has been transformed into a bustling space station. Suspended halfway up a tall building, too often it is drenched in bright light and alive with activity throughout the night. The tiny baby in the incubator is dwarfed by a procedure light, a respirator, a multichannel monitor, four intravenous pumps, and a transcutaneous oxygen module. The baby's chest is covered with electrodes, and tubes lead into and out of his or her body at several points. Eight to twelve electrical cords, two oxygen lines, and a suction catheter attach to the bedside console. Medications and flush solutions are drawn up in syringes close at hand. A resuscitation bag is at the head of the baby's bed in case he or she should stop breathing. Alarms sound, knots of people move busily about, and large machines are pushed among the incubators. Ultrasonographic elements are touched to the infant's head, chest, and abdomen. Images flash on a screen and are recorded on tape for later analysis. House officers speak rapidly in an acronymic code barely intelligible to residents who graduated 2 years previously. Hess and Lundeen, coming some morning for a visit, might wonder if they had missed the address and arrived on the wrong planet!

At such a bedside, today's neonatologist must cope with a constantly enlarging body of new literature on cardiopulmonary physiology, nutritional and metabolic support, new antibiotics and infectious disease conditions, ventricular hemorrhage and asphyxial syndromes, and surgical, genetic, and cardiac problems. It is no longer possible for a physician to read all the new publications, even when restricted to the area of neonatology. New therapeutic approaches are proposed much faster than they can be tested in an orderly way; many such theories never will be tested.

IMPLICATIONS FOR THE FUTURE

The field of neonatology will never again return to the quiet premature nursery of Hess and Lundeen, but we must conserve some of the gentleness and nurturing qualities of that era.

Neonatology is now, and hereafter will be, a team activity. We must therefore care for our teams with skill and make them effective instruments.

The ICN is embedded in a community to which it must be related in an efficient and systematic way. We can ill afford to begrudge the time it takes to maintain regional systems.

The government is involved with neonatal intensive care more than with most other areas of medicine. Regional systems, Medicaid regulations, Baby Doe regulations, cost-containment measures, and maternal and child health programs all bring neonatologists in contact with government agencies. Neonatologists will need to become diligent and skillful advocates, negotiators, and lobbyists.

Within medical centers, relationships among the hospital, the medical school, and the neonatologists as a practice group are changing. A satisfactory support base must be developed for activities split among patient care, teaching, administration, research, and advocacy.

Some specialization within neonatology is inevitable. No one person can be at the forefront in all the branches of the field.

Neonatology training programs should include opportunities to gain knowledge and skill in the business aspects of nursery and practice management, in administrative and negotiating techniques, and in public health and regional planning.

Despite all this complexity, the final need is for calm and simplicity. Within health care systems, in the last analysis, we meet others one by one. Patient care can never be better than the quality of individual human encounters. Today, our ideal role model could still be Evelyn Lundeen putting tiny hats on premature infants to keep their heads warm.

REFERENCES

1. Hess JH, Lundeen EC. *The premature infant:* its medical and nursing care. Philadelphia: JB Lippincott Co., 1941.
2. Nightingale F. *Notes on nursing:* what it is and what it is not. (A facsimile of the first edition printed in London, 1859, with a foreword by Annie W. Goodrich.) Philadelphia: JB Lippincott Co., 1969.
3. Smith CA. *The physiology of the newborn infant.* Springfield, IL: Charles C. Thomas, 1945.
4. Silverman WA, Anderson DH, Blanc WA, Crozier DN. A difference in mortality rate and incidence of kernicterus among premature infants allotted to two prophylactic antibiotic regimens. *Pediatrics* 1956;18:614.
5. Klaus MH, Kennell JH. *Maternal–infant bonding.* St. Louis: CV Mosby, 1976.
6. Klaus MH, Kennell JH. *Parent–infant bonding.* St. Louis: CV Mosby, 1982.

CHAPTER 2

Futility Considerations in the Neonatal Intensive Care Unit[1]

Gordon B. Avery

PHYSICIAN JUDGMENT

Judgments made by treating physicians played the dominant role in determining which treatments would be offered to critically ill newborn infants (until the Baby Doe regulations in 1983). The responsible physician tried to avoid inherently futile therapy and at times advised the withdrawal of treatments deemed unlikely to produce a satisfactory outcome.

In all of medicine, the physician traditionally has both diagnosed diseases and decided what therapies were *indicated.* The decision about what is indicated has two steps. The first is a consideration of the disease and an inventory of remedies that conceivably might be beneficial. The second step is to weigh the advantages of a treatment against its side effects and toxicity. A therapeutic goal must be in place against which the treatment can be judged. The goal may be cure of the disease, relief of major symptoms, or merely comfort of the patient. Where multiple disease processes and multiple treatments are simultaneous, the physician also must consider their interactions, the general direction of the patient's progress, and the overall prognosis for a satisfactory outcome. All these steps occur whether the issue is a shot of penicillin for a streptococcal pharyngitis or prolonged intravenous alimentation for an infant with only 20 cm of bowel remaining after necrotizing enterocolitis.

These duties are central to the practice of medicine. Additional duties include discussion with the patient and striving for understanding and concurrence; in a team situation, discussion and consultation with team members;

putting in motion the procedures to implement the chosen treatments; and documentation of the rationale and outcome. These duties are required of all treating physicians, and failure to perform them is potential grounds for malpractice litigation.

It is interesting that in the controversies about decision making in regard to intensive care of the newborn infant, neither parents nor governmental proxies for the community, nor even medical insurance payers, explicitly try to take over the practice of medicine. In all relevant legislation, the prohibition is against withholding or withdrawing *indicated treatment.* Thus, the question of what treatment is indicated still holds a central place. Whether a treatment is likely to be efficacious or futile or perhaps harmful is inherently a medical question as well as a legal or ethical one.

Neonatologists considered the duty to recommend indicated therapy to be inherent in their practice of medicine. As treatment became more highly technical, the

G. B. Avery: Children's Research Institute, Children's National Medical Center; and Department of Pediatrics, George Washington University School of Medicine and Health Sciences, Washington, D.C.

[1]The purpose of this article is to summarize and comment upon the history of medical decision making in the neonatal intensive care nursery, emphasizing considerations of futility. Several epochs will be described, with shifting roles of health care providers, the infant's family, and proxies for society at large. Futility has been an issue in the intensive care of newborn infants throughout the last 35 years. Long before the Baby Doe regulations and the formation of ethics committees, neonatologists tried to determine which care measures were indicated. Given the frequency of severe malformations, birth asphyxia, and extreme prematurity, it has been a common event for the responsible physician to ask himself or herself: will this treatment be beneficial or merely futile? As the therapeutic armamentarium became more powerful and complex, the choices from among a possible array of interventions became increasingly difficult. The autonomy of parents as decision makers was increasingly affirmed. In the 1980s, the federal government, the courts, and frequent malpractice suits set boundaries on medical decision making. In the 1990s, third party payers became increasingly assertive in limiting resource expenditure. These legal and societal mandates are frequently at variance with one another. Thus, the issue of medical futility, as it applies to neonates in the United States, must be considered unresolved.

need to form judgments on behalf of babies and their families seemed increasingly compelling. With the high mortality in certain conditions, there frequently loomed the issue of futility. Physicians held with families discussions that varied in depth and detail, depending upon the apparent ability of the family to understand, the family's aggressiveness in seeking to be actively involved, and the penchant of the individual neonatologist. Individual practice patterns developed, which varied from aggressive "commandos" who used maximum treatment until there were unequivocal indications of death, to those who took into consideration quality of life in the event of recovery, pain, and suffering of the infant, the wishes of parents, and even resource consumption.

All these interventions initially were being made in the context of medical practice, without broad public discussion or the provision of boundaries or guidelines. Physicians might be said to have been paternalistic, making most of the decisions on the basis of what they deemed best for the baby and baby's family. The neonatology literature dealt with outcomes of the various conditions, but said little about decisions to withhold or withdraw treatment.

In this situation, the milestone 1973 paper of Duff and Campbell (1) sounded an alarm bell. These authors studied the practice at the Yale–New Haven Hospital, where a well-established neonatal intensive care unit (NICU) had been in operation for several years. They determined that, of 299 consecutive deaths in the period 1970 to 1972, 43 (14%) were the immediate result of withdrawing life-support systems. The major diagnoses were multiple anomalies, trisomy, and two cases of short gut. Prognosis was poor for "meaningful life"; thus, the treatments were considered essentially futile. The existence of "passive euthanasia" on a significant scale had been documented.

There followed reverberations in which concern for the sanctity of life was set against the judgment of treating physicians (2,3). Neonatologists were accused of playing God when they discontinued critical life-support measures. In this debate, quality of life was accepted as a factor in decisions to terminate or withhold treatment. A distinction began to emerge between *ordinary* or usual measures, and drastic or *heroic* treatment. The assumption was that ordinary treatment always should be given, but that heroic treatment, with its presumed marginal utility, could be the subject of judgment by the family and the responsible physician. It was in these discussions that the role of the family assumed greater prominence.

AUTONOMY AND THE INCREASED ROLE OF FAMILIES

The ethical principle of autonomy, applied to decisions to limit medical care, suggests that the patient cannot be forced to receive undesired treatment. In the case of the newborn infant, the principle has been extended to include the parents, as proxies for the baby. In some instances, the parents' decision may appear so inappropriate that an alternate proxy for the infant is designated. A familiar example is the Jehovah's Witness family, which refuses life-saving transfusion therapy for their baby. In other cases, the parents are unavailable or incompetent, and here again an alternate *guardian ad litem* must be appointed. Thus, in deciding whether apparently futile care should be delivered, the family would seem to be the default decision makers.

During these same years (1970 to 1985), activism of patients in general, *vis-á-vis*, their physicians, was on the rise. The emphasis on detailed informed consent is an example of the more direct role of patients in choosing their own care. In the arena of neonatal intensive care, parents increasingly wanted details of the contemplated treatment and consent for individual treatment phases rather than blanket consent for the entire hospitalization. In a 1973 commentary in the *New England Journal of Medicine*, Shaw (4) highlighted the ambiguities of informed consent in the NICU. Can parents understand the medical complexities well enough to consent meaningfully? Does the right to consent include the right to refuse indicated treatment of their child? The author suggests individualized decisions, which include the possibility of withholding surgical rescue of infants who are severely deformed or retarded. Rivers (5) adds the point that parents must be given time to come to terms with the situation and to make an unhurried decision.

The demand for parental involvement in decision making was reenforced by malpractice suits, more common in obstetrics but a feature of intensive care generally. In 1987, Lantos (6) suggested that neonatologists were considerably restricted in the latitude of their decision making regarding the critically ill newborn infant. Given that deaths in the NICU may be 10% of admissions, the active participation of families, and the documentation of informed consent, became important considerations. Parents could consent to the care measures, or their withdrawal, but could not order care that was not indicated medically over the objection of the medical providers. As we will see, this latter issue is now in contention.

Baby Doe, the index case of the Baby Doe Regulations (see below), was an infant with Down syndrome and intestinal obstruction. The physicians and parents decided not to repair the obstruction in light of the Down Syndrome and expected mental retardation. Thus, the prognosis for surgical intervention was not hopeless or futile. Rather, quality-of-life considerations predominated.

Finally, the case of Baby Jane Doe set up some additional presumptions of parental autonomy and privacy

(7). The parents, physicians, and hospital agreed to withhold surgery for a child with spina bifida. A third party lawyer, who had never met either the family or the child, actively appealed to the courts to intervene, because of the presumed failure to give indicated treatment. The lower courts and ultimately the United States Supreme Court failed to uphold his contentions on the grounds that the lawyer offered no evidence of improper care. The hospital, in turn, refused access to the child's records without the parents' consent, on the grounds of privacy and the confidentiality of medical records.

GOVERNMENT INTERVENTIONS: THE BABY DOE REGULATIONS

The United States Department of Health and Human Services threw a bombshell into this debate with the famous "Baby Doe" regulations of 1983 to 1984 (8). Infants with critical illnesses were described as handicapped and entitled to protection against discrimination under the United States Rehabilitation Act. Discrimination here meant the withholding of indicated treatment on the basis of handicap. The regulations were promulgated by the Reagan administration in response to political pressure from individuals, who were concerned that neonatologists and parents were failing to give life-saving treatment to babies on the basis of anticipated poor quality of life. The law instituted placards placed in NICUs, which suggested that care perhaps was being denied illegally. An anonymous hot line was created, wherein anybody could call in a tip that would be investigated promptly. The hot line, during its existence, failed to yield any instances of illegal withholding of care. It was challenged in court and ultimately set aside by the United States Supreme Court. A useful commentary was written in 1988 by Kopelman et al. (9).

A successor to the Baby Doe Regulations was a 1985 amendment to the Child Abuse laws, which also forbade the withholding of indicated treatment, but allowed some discretion for judgment by the family and physicians (10). The law did not require merely prolonging the act of dying, or giving care that was futile, or giving care that was virtually futile and under the circumstances inhumane. Thus, determination of what care could be considered futile again was brought to center stage.

Individuals having cause to believe that care was being withheld illegally could appeal through local child protection agencies. Although relatively few cases have been brought by this route, the government has, by this legislation, placed some legal boundaries on medical decision making. Undoubtedly, medical practice has been affected.

ETHICS COMMITTEES

One of the suggestions of the 1985 Child Abuse legislation was that institutions develop ethics committees to advise on troublesome cases involving neonates. In many cases these came to be called Infant Care Review Committees (ICRCs). They were not mandated by the law, but by 1984, a survey of 710 hospitals revealed that 56.6% of those with level 2 and level 3 nurseries had ICRCs. Using a 1986 survey, Fleming et al. noted that teaching institutions were more likely to have ethics committees, in contrast to for-profit hospitals and government-run institutions. The committees review only a portion of the difficult cases, but generate precedents within the institution that help shape other cases (11). Michaels and Oliver (12), from the University of Pittsburgh, report that, in Pittsburgh, a consultation team initially addresses the case and then reports to the full Human Rights Committee. Consultations are advisory and optional, but they help to resolve differences and apparently are well received. The very ambiguities of the Child Abuse legislation seem to invite broader consultations to assist families and health provider teams.

Efforts to apply classic ethical principles to infant cases frequently lead to conflict. In a classic review article, Pelligrino (13) cites the frequent dissonance between beneficence (best outcome for the patient), nonmaleficence (not doing harm), autonomy (allowing the family to decide), and distributive justice (fair allocation of limited resources). The law mandates the first three, but it gives little guidance on how to resolve conflicts in duty.

THE RIGHT OF PROVIDERS TO REFUSE TREATMENT

The normal equation of medical therapy is "Doctor recommends; patient agrees; treatment occurs." We have discussed the issue of the patient's right to refuse recommended treatment and the requirement for informed consent. But what if the patient wants treatment that the doctor opposes? As a public trust, physicians have custody over dangerous drugs, harmful irradiation, and potentially mutilating surgery. The Hippocratic oath requires us to do no harm (nonmaleficence). Certainly a patient cannot arrive at the office and demand morphine, or that his leg be cut off. Hence, an understanding has developed that physicians are not required to give treatment that is against their conscience.

In the gray zone of neonatal intensive care, the courts have ruled on both sides of this issue. The perception of futility is central to this inconsistency. Persisting with painful and expensive treatment that is futile can be seen as causing harm. Frequently, it seems so to the health provider team in the case of irreversible coma, multiple organ failure, and massive brain damage. Troug et al. (14) point out that futility is a relative term. In their words, one "could prolong the dying of almost any patient." The likelihood of success must be set against a goal. This goal could be recovery from the disease, long-term survival, short-term survival, reasonable quality of life, palliation of symptoms, or merely improvement of physiologic parameters. In the view of these authors, futility is a probability statement.

On the other hand, parents may view even one chance in a million as a chance worth taking. They may believe that a miracle will happen for their particular child. Whereas the law would like to regard futility as an absolute, physicians often say that treatment is futile because a good outcome is extremely unlikely. In this setting, the burden of the illness looms large. Caregivers at the bedside may hear echoes of the words of the Child Abuse legislation: "Virtually futile, and under the circumstances inhumane." Thus, it is understandable that parents and health team members might disagree about futility, and that courts would long for an unambiguous definition of the term.

Paris et al. (15,16) report two cases in which the health team refused to provide care that was deemed futile and under the circumstances inhumane. In the first, a 5-year-old boy with severe respiratory failure was placed on extracorporeal membrane oxygenation (ECMO) as a 2-week trial to buy time for spontaneous improvement. He did not improve, and on return to conventional ventilation could not be maintained. The parents wanted indefinite continuation on ECMO, whereas the care team said this was merely prolonging the dying and, therefore, was futile. Hospital counsel said there was no duty to give inappropriate treatment, and the ethics committee agreed, citing a physician's right to refuse treatment that he or she professionally and morally opposes. The ECMO was discontinued and the baby died.

The second case was Baby L, a 2-year-old infant with severe brain damage who was in a chronic vegetative state (16). The baby suffered from recurrent pneumonia, and the mother desired that the child be put back on the respirator. The care team opposed this, and the ethics committee suggested that the respirator not be provided, considering it as being futile and under the circumstances inhumane. The mother insisted on the respirator. The court appointed a *guardian ad litem*, who sided with the mother. The hospital—Children's Hospital of Boston— backed its physicians in refusing to give care that they opposed, even if ordered by the court. The denouement was that the child was transferred to another facility, but there was no prosecution of the physicians or the hospital.

These two cases appeared to establish some right of conscience for physicians, who could not be compelled to give care that they deemed inappropriate. This, however, reckons without Baby K. The incredible ruling in this lat-

ter case appears to authorize parents to demand and get for their infants any treatment, no matter how futile, how expensive, or how contrary to recommendations by physicians, ethics committees, or even national professional bodies. If extrapolated to all NICU cases, the Baby K judgment would seem to obviate the need for any thought processes whatsoever and would mandate uniform maximum treatment until cessation of heartbeat, provided the parents wish it.

Baby K was an anencephalic infant girl born in 1992 to a deeply religious mother, who insisted against all protestations that everything should be done to keep the baby alive (17). As a consequence, the baby was in and out of the hospital repeatedly and several times was placed on a ventilator for respiratory failure. Eventually the mother found arrayed against her the father, all the doctors in the case, the ethics board, the hospital, and the relevant professional medical societies: the American Academy of Pediatrics and the Society of Critical Care Medicine. The mother hoped that a miracle would occur, but in any case felt that God should decide the time of her child's death. The physicians argued that the child was without cerebral cortex, irreversibly in a coma, incapable of self-awareness, and with a hopeless prognosis. The hospital, in its frustration at being compelled to give unindicated care, went to court and asked for permission to withdraw respirator support, citing futility and the standard of care for anencephalic infants.

The court found for the mother and ordered respirator care continued. The hospital appealed, and a panel of three judges of the Fourth Circuit Court of Appeals upheld the original decision. There was a split vote. Two judges argued that respiratory failure was the relevant diagnosis, and therefore it could be treated, and a respirator was effective therapy. The third judge held that anencephaly was the fundamental diagnosis, and that it was untreatable. Further, the standard of medical care for anencephaly did not include ventilator support.

The judgment was on a narrow point of law. Baby K was brought to the emergency room and there was put on the respirator. The Emergency Medical Treatment and Labor Act (EMTALA) requires initial stabilization in emergency rooms. It has been called the antidumping law, as it forbids the nontreatment of undesirable patients. It was this law that was used to require the initial ventilator treatment. The matter ultimately was appealed to the United States Supreme Court. The Supreme Court upheld the lower courts, but narrowly on the grounds of the EMLATA law.

A number of authors have commented on the apparently unlimited authority this ruling appears to give parents to demand care that goes beyond the standard of medical practice and that is opposed by the responsible physicians (18,19). However, the ruling may be too narrow to give parents *carte blanche* in the NICU. In fact, Annas (17) chides physicians for involving the courts needlessly, rather than acting on their own convictions:

> To avoid these scenarios, physicians must work toward a third, in which they not only set standards for medical practice, but also follow them. Physicians cannot expect parents, trial judges, insurance companies, or government regulators to take practice standards more seriously than they do themselves. If physicians cannot set standards for the care of anencephalic infants and adhere to them, standard-setting by physicians is a dead issue.

DISTRIBUTIVE JUSTICE AND THE RATIONING OF CARE

We are living in the era of managed care. Women are sent home the day after delivery, 2 days after mastectomy. The use of laboratory tests is curtailed. Certain categories of care are unavailable under medical insurance or health maintenance organization plans, unless the individual has private funds to pay for them. Consultations require the permission of a gatekeeper. Medicare and Medicaid are being cut back. In plain English: care is being rationed.

It is in this context that we must note that enormously expensive care is being mandated, although it is apparently futile and is given over the objections of the responsible physicians. In the case of Baby L, the unpaid bill was estimated to be $1 million dollars. "In a civil suit against Brigham and Women's Hospital and the delivering obstetrician, Danielle Hall's [Baby L] attorney presented evidence that her lifetime medical cost will be $10 million. The jury awarded $20 million to the family. A settlement for an undeclared sum was made in the case" (16). Some of the care undertaken in the wake of the Baby Doe legislation is likewise very expensive.

The state of Oregon undertook to spread its limited funds more equitably by removing coverage of certain procedures, such as liver transplantation, on the grounds of marginal utility (20). Marginal utility looks at the end of the cost–benefit spectrum where lots of bucks bring a small, uncertain bang. Figure 2–1 is a cost–benefit diagram, which gives a quantitative representation to marginal utility. In effect, futility is extreme marginal utility. The Oregon policy matches that of many countries with universal health coverage, such as Canada and England. Limiting care with marginal utility fits into the scheme of fair allocation of scarce resources, or distributive justice. It is curious that, as a society, we can leave children medically uninsured and can underfund immunizations, while we mandate futile care in some of our neonates.

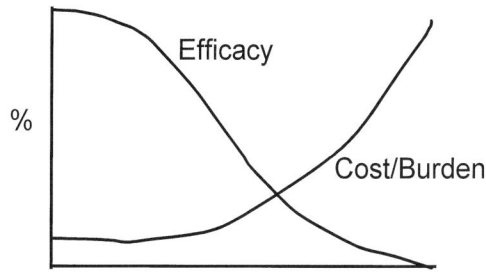

FIG. 2–1. A cost–benefit diagram is depicted, with declining efficacy of treatment simultaneous with rising cost and burden of the therapy. Marginal utility is defined by the *right half* of the figure, in which efficacy is very low and cost and burden of care are high. Futility might be seen as the limit, where benefit is almost nil and cost and burden are extreme.

YESTERDAY, TODAY, AND TOMORROW: WHAT IS FUTILITY?

Where have we gone since Duff and Campbell (1) reported in 1973 that 14% of deaths in the Yale NICU were associated with withholding or withdrawing life-support therapy? Neonatologists still recommend treatment that they think is indicated. They also still suggest withdrawing care that appears futile, or virtually futile, and under the circumstances inhumane. Parents, as proxies for their infants, still consider the benefits. They advise and consent, often taking strong positions of advocacy. ICRCs still weigh and consider the issues in troubling cases and make Solomon-like recommendations. The government still defines boundaries within which discretion can be exercised. And the courts continue to confuse the issues by making seemingly contradictory rulings, which often ignore the realities of care in the intensive care nursery.

It is clear that neonatologists and families step in and declare a halt even more frequently today than in Duff and Campbell's time. Wall and Partridge (21) reported on discharges from the NICU at the University of California, San Francisco between 1989 and 1992. During that period, 165 deaths occurred among 1,609 babies (10.3%). Of those who died, 108 of 165 were associated with withdrawal of support and 13 of 165 followed withholding of treatments, leaving only 44 of 165 (26.7%) who died while maximum therapy continued. Quality-of-life considerations were stated in 51% of these cases and were the major issue in 23%. Death was considered imminent and care futile in 75% of those in whom care was withdrawn. Withdrawal or withholding of treatments occurred in 29% of infants with extremely low birth weight, 35% with major intracranial hemorrhage, 23% with necrotizing enterocolitis, 12% with respiratory failure, and 16% with major congenital anomalies.

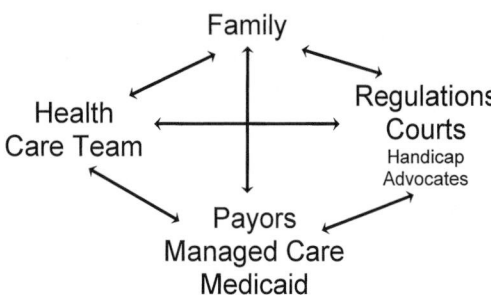

FIG. 2–2. Decision makers regarding the neonatal intensive care unit are depicted, with complex interactions between and among them. No one member of the complex is always in charge.

We are left with a welter of conflicts and unresolved issues when we consider medical futility in the NICU. The decision makers are legion, and no one of them is clearly in charge (Fig. 2–2). Finally, ethical principles are in tension—perhaps necessarily so (Fig. 2–3).

The conclusion of Paris and Schreiber's article (22) is worth quoting as a summation:

Sanctity of Life

Burden of Illness

Beneficence

Autonomy   Distributive Justice

Quality of Life

Non-maleficence

FIG. 2–3. The major ethical principles in neonatal intensive care unit decisions are shown. Each has a prominent influence and a legitimate claim to recognition, yet conflict among these principles is frequent. For example, unqualified reverence for the sanctity of life may fail to acknowledge the requirement to do no harm, the burden of illness, or issues related to quality of life.

. . . There is a long and continuing tradition, summed up in the Society for Critical Care Medicine's consensus report (23), that "treatments that offer no benefit and serve to prolong the dying process should not be employed." With both professional and societal support being given to that tradition, it is now time for physicians to reassert the role of clinical judgment in treatment decisions.

REFERENCES

1. Duff RS, Campbell AGM. Moral and ethical dilemmas in the special-care nursery. *N Engl J Med* 1973;289:890.
2. Robertson JA. Involuntary euthanasia of defective newborns: a legal analysis. *Stanford Law Rev* 1975;27:213.
3. Horan DJ, Delahoyde M, eds. *Infanticide and the handicapped newborn.* Provo, UT: Brigham Young University Press, 1982.
4. Shaw A. Dilemmas of "informed consent" in children. *N Engl J Med* 1973;289:885.
5. Rivers RP. Decision making in neonatal intensive care environment. *Br Med Bull* 1996;52:238.
6. Lantos J. Baby Doe five years after: implications for child health. *N Engl J Med* 1987;317:444.
7. *United States v University Hospital, State University of New York*, 729 F2d 144, 1984.
8. Department of Health and Human Services. Non-discrimination on the basis of handicap relating to health care for handicapped infants. *Federal Register* 1984;49:1622.
9. Kopelman LM, Irons TG, Kopelman AE. Neonatologists judge the "Baby Doe" regulations. *N Engl J Med* 1988;318:677.
10. Department of Health and Human Services. Child abuse and treatment program. *Federal Register* 1985;50:14878.
11. Fleming GV, Hudd SS, Le Bailly SA, et al. Infant care review committees: the response to federal guidelines. *Am J Dis Child* 1990;144:778.
12. Michaels RH, Oliver TK Jr. Human rights consultation: a 12-year experience of a pediatric bioethics committee. *Pediatrics* 1986;78:566.
13. Pelligrino ED. The metamorphosis of medical ethics. *JAMA* 1991;266:1158.
14. Troug RD, Brett AS, Frader J. The problem of futility. *N Engl J Med* 1992;326:1560.
15. Paris JJ, Schreiber MD, Statter M, et al. Beyond autonomy—physicians' refusal to use life-prolonging extracorporeal membrane oxygenation. *N Engl J Med* 1993;329:354.
16. Paris JJ, Crone RK, Reardon F. Physicians' refusal of requested treatment: the case of Baby L. *N Engl J Med* 1990;322:1012.
17. Annas GJ. Asking the courts to set the standard of emergency care—the case of Baby K. *N Engl J Med* 1994;331:1383.
18. Biesecker LG: The case of Baby K. *N Engl J Med* 1994;331:1383.
19. Paris JJ. Guidelines on the care of anencephalic infants: a response to Baby K. *J Perinatol* 1995;15:318.
20. Eddy DM. What's going on in Oregon? *JAMA* 1991;266:417.
21. Wall SN, Partridge JC. Death in the intensive care nursery: physician practice of withdrawing and withholding life support. *Pediatrics* 1997;99:64.
22. Paris JJ, Schreiber MD. Physicians refusal to provide life-prolonging medical interventions. *Clin Perinatol* 1996;23:563.
23. Task Force on Ethics of the Society of Critical Care Medicine. Consensus report on the ethics of foregoing life-sustaining treatments in the critically ill. *Crit Care Med* 1990;18:1435.

CHAPTER 3

Neonatology in the United States: Scope and Organization

Richard L. Bucciarelli

The practice of neonatal and perinatal medicine has changed enormously since its recognition as a distinct subspecialty in 1975. The development of technologies as complex as extracorporeal membrane oxygenation and as simple as the administration of exogenous surfactant has resulted in the survival of many infants who would have succumbed to their illnesses a few years ago.

Unfortunately, these and other technological advances of the 1980s have been countered by trends in American society that have diminished the impact of this progress. During the early 1990s, the United States tragically discovered that it lagged further behind many less wealthy countries in measurements of perinatal outcome than it did 20 years earlier. Record numbers of women and children were living in poverty. Despite targeted local, state, and federal programs, significant barriers to access to prenatal care existed, and teen pregnancies reached an all-time high as record numbers of children were born to children. Epidemics of perinatally acquired immune deficiency syndrome and perinatal exposure to crack cocaine led to a new type of perinatal morbidity, which presented significant challenges to our communities. These and other societal problems prevented our nation from achieving its goals of lowering the incidence of low birth weight (LBW) deliveries and preventing the morbidities associated with prematurity.

The poor performance of the United States compared with other nations was not because of an unwillingness to commit significant financial and human resources to perinatal care. In 1985, expenditures for obstetric and neonatal care approached $15 billion. By the end of 1995, the figure exceeded $28 billion. In addition to these huge expenditures, the United States continued to invest vast

amounts of capital in neonatal intensive care units (NICUs) as almost every hospital in the nation joined the race to care for infants with special needs. Fellowship programs in neonatal and perinatal medicine continued to produce physicians with the expertise to care for the most complex patients and with the vision to develop new technologies for the future. Entire new professions, such as neonatal nurse practitioners (NNPs) and neonatal developmental interventionists, grew out of the increased neonatal workforce demands in acute and long-term care settings.

Despite these levels of commitment to perinatal care, the United States continues to have an LBW rate that has not decreased significantly in over a decade and one that exceeds that of 29 other nations. Recent declines in infant mortality have not kept pace with other nations, leaving the United States ranked twenty-first, with an infant mortality rate (IMR) twice that of Sweden, Finland, and Japan.

The apparent incongruity between investment and performance diminishes with the realization that past efforts have concentrated on developing the world's most sophisticated high-tech neonatal care without investing equal time and effort in attempting to understand the societal issues responsible for producing high-risk infants. Our nation has developed a superb ability to care for the individual high-risk infant after delivery, but it has failed to develop systems that integrate resources to provide efficient, cost-effective prenatal care that could prevent significant human suffering and conserve vast economic resources.

Even with these concerns, there are reasons to be optimistic. The perinatal treatment of women who test positive for human immunodeficiency virus has decreased significantly the vertical spread of infection (1).

The teen birth rate has declined for a fourth year in a row, and the incidence of LBW is beginning to decrease

R.L. Bucciarelli: Department of Pediatrics, University of Florida, Gainesville, Florida

in high-risk populations (2). Recent federal legislation has given the states the opportunity to expand prenatal care access to more pregnant women and to provide health insurance for neonates after they leave the intensive care center (3). Both providers and payers are beginning to realize that perinatal care can be delivered more efficiently by developing integrated systems of care (4,5). In parallel with this focus on conserving resources, we must develop methods to hold these new systems accountable for delivering the highest quality of perinatal care possible (6).

In this chapter, the current size and scope of the practice of neonatology in the United States is reviewed, with emphasis on how resources are used to deliver neonatal care. Recent changes in the financing of health care and their potential impact on perinatal outcome are discussed.

SIZE AND SCOPE OF NEONATOLOGY IN THE UNITED STATES

Neonatal Hospital Capacity

Because there is no national database defining or inventorying special care neonatal beds, the exact capacity for the provision of NICU services in the United States is unknown. One of the most complete discussions of this topic was published by National Perinatal Information Center in 1996 (7). This study utilized data tapes from the American Hospital Association annual hospital surveys for 1983, 1987, and 1991 to assess the supply and demand for obstetric and neonatal special care beds in the United States. While the number of hospitals reporting obstetric services declined by 17%, the number of hospitals operating NICUs increased by 46%, and those operating neonatal intermediate care beds increased by 47%.

The change in availability of obstetric services appears to have been the result of a consolidation of services from rural to metropolitan areas, with 75% of the decrease in services occurring in rural hospitals. As a result, the average number of births per hospital increased by 37%, whereas the average length of stay (LOS) decreased by 29% (Table 3–1).

On the other hand, the total number of hospitals operating neonatal special care beds increased by 64% from 551 in 1983 to 902 in 1991, resulting in almost one-third of all hospitals with obstetric services also operating a neonatal special care unit (Table 3–2). There also was a dramatic increase in the number of neonatal special care beds, from 3 of 1,000 live births in 1983 to 4.3 of 1,000 live births in 1991 (43%). Assuming an optimal occupancy rate of 85%, the available neonatal special care bed-days increased from 3.2 million to 5.3 million. When this capacity was compared to the American Academy of Pediatrics estimates of neonatal bed demand, Schwartz (7) observed that the 1991 supply of neonatal special care beds exceeded the demand by 300,000 bed-days (Table 3–3). Further analysis by region revealed a nonuniform distribution of services, with 6 of 9 regions showing significant surpluses and 3 of 9 showing significant calculated deficits. These variations seemed to be independent of populations trends, the number of births, or perinatal outcomes.

This study and others suggest that the supply of neonatal special care services exceed the calculated demand by a factor between 2 and 3 (8,9). Further, when one adds to the equation the potential effects of managed care and the pressures to reduce costs and utilization of resources, the excess capacity in the system increases even more dramatically, raising concerns about financial viability and the quality of care delivered in many of our neonatal special care units (10).

TABLE 3–1. *Overview of births and hospitals with births, 1983 to 1991*

	All hospitals				Metropolitan				Nonmetropolitan			
	1983	1987	1991	Change (%)	1983	1987	1991	Change (%)	1983	1987	1991	Change (%)
U.S. births (NCHS) (millions)	3.6	3.8	4.1	+11	—	—	—	—	—	—	—	—
AHA births (millions)[a]	3.5	3.6	4.0	+15	2.8	3.0	3.3	+19.3	0.7	0.6	0.7	—
No. of hospitals with >5 births	4,651	4,259	3,874	−17	2,185	2,069	1,991	−9	2,466	2,190	1,883	−23
Average no. of births per hospital	752	845	1,032	+37	1,281	1,449	1,657	+29	283	273	371	+31
Average LOS per birth	3.4	2.9	2.4	−29	3.5	2.9	2.4	−30	3.1	2.8	2.4	−25

[a]Those births included in the present analysis.
Metropolitan refers to hospitals within the standard metropolitan statistical area (SMSA); nonmetropolitan hospitals are defined as those outside the SMSA.
AHA; American Hospital Association; LOS, length of stay; NCHS, National Center for Health Statistics.
From ref. 7.

TABLE 3–2. *Supply of neonatal special care in the United States, 1983 to 1991*

	All hospitals				Metropolitan				Nonmetropolitan			
	1983	1987	1991	Change (%)	1983	1987	1991	Change (%)	1983	1987	1991	Change (%)
Hospitals with special care bed needs												
NICU	487	596	712	46	427	536	641	50	60	58	71	18.30
NINT	222	353	386	74	202	309	341	69	20	44	45	125
NICU or NINT	709	949	1,098	59.20	629	847	982	61	80	102	116	44
Special care bed trends in the U.S.												
NICU	6,893	8,956	11,518	67	6,457	8,510	10,868	68	414	446	660	57
NINT	2,547	3,898	4,366	71	2,422	3,660	4,087	69	125	238	279	123
NICU and NINT	9,440	12,854	15,884	68	8,879	12,170	14,955	68	539	684	939	72
Special care beds per 10,000 births												
NICU	20	25	29	45	23	28	32	41	6	7	9	60
NINT	7	11	11	49	9	12	12	41	2	4	4	128
NICU and NINT	27	36	40	46	32	40	44	41	8	11	13	41

Metropolitan refers to hospitals within the standard metropolitan statistical area (SMSA); nonmetropolitan hospitals are defined as those outside the SMSA.
NICU, neonatal intensive care unit; NINT, neonatal intermediate treatment.
From ref. 7.

Neonatal Workforce: Needs and Assessment

Neonatologist

In 1975, 355 physicians were certified by the American Board of Pediatrics' Sub-Board of Neonatal and Perinatal Medicine as the first neonatologists in the United States. Since then, an average of 280 new neonatologists have been certified each time the certification examination has been given (Fig. 3–1) (11). As of 1995, 3,069 neonatologists were certified, and the attrition rate, once thought to be high, has been only 1% to 2% during a 5- to 10-year period. It is estimated that there are 1,533 physicians actively engaged in the practice of neonatology as board-eligible physicians who have not successfully completed sub-board certification requirements or as pediatricians with special training in neonatology who concentrate their efforts on caring for neonates with special needs (12). The total number of physicians providing care to high-risk neonates is estimated to be 4,603. These data suggest that the physician workforce capacity for providing level II and level III NICU care has more than tripled since 1985 (13).

In 1982, the Residency Review Committee of the Accreditation Council for Graduate Medical Education of the American Medical Association (ACGME) began certifying fellowship training programs in neonatology. Certified programs require 3 years of training in an environment that fosters the development of clinical and research skills and exposes the neonatal fellow to other important aspects of neonatal care, including transport, long-term follow-up, and the organization of perinatal care (14). Initially, 114 programs submitted applications for review. From this group, approximately 90 were approved. There are currently 100 approved training pro-

TABLE 3–3. *Supply and demand for special care bed-days*

	No. (in millions)		
	1983	1987	1991
Supply NINT and NICU bed-days	3.5	4.7	5.8
Supply children's hospital bed-days	0.37	0.43	0.50
Total bed-day supply	3.8	5.1	6.3
Supply at 85% occupancy	3.2	4.4	5.3
Bed-day demand based on American Academy of Pediatrics estimates	4.3	4.6	5.0

NICU, neonatal intensive care unit; NINT,
From ref. 7.

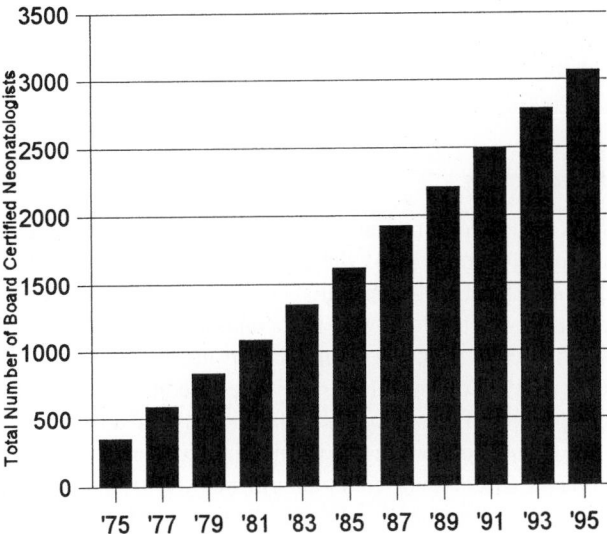

FIG. 3–1. Cumulative total of neonatologists who successfully completed certification by the American Board of Pediatrics Sub-Board of Neonatal and Perinatal Medicine (personal communication, December 1997).

grams in neonatal and perinatal medicine, with 404 fellows in training (15).

The concerns about physician workforce devoted to neonatology, its distribution, and the effect on regionalization has been raised several times. In its 1985 statement on neonatal workforce, the American Academy of Pediatrics Committee on the Fetus and Newborn (COFN) estimated that 1,479 neonatologists were needed to provide special care services for a population of 3.8 million live births (i.e., neonatologists:live births = 1:2,569) (16). In 1983, Merenstein et al. (13) conducted an extensive national telephone survey of the numbers and distribution of practicing neonatologists and found the average ratio of neonatologists to live births in the United States was 1:2,547, a figure close to the estimated needs. Although the distribution of neonatologists varied greatly among regions (i.e., from a high of 1:1,860 in the mid-Atlantic states of New York, New Jersey, and Pennsylvania to a low of 1:3,217 in the mountain states of Idaho, Wyoming, Colorodo, New Mexico, Arizona, Utah, and Nebraska), the actual infant mortality in each region was similar, suggesting that neonatal outcome may be the result of factors other than the availability of specialized neonatal care. These data, combined with the increasing number of positions available for neonatologists, led the COFN to conclude that "trends in the recruitment of neonatologists appeared to be based more on institutional entrepreneurial efforts than on patient need, were not consistent with the concept of regionalization, and would result in the fragmentation of perinatal care" (16).

Using currently available data, the ratio of neonatologists to live births is 1:847, implying that the supply of neonatologists is more than three times the number necessary to care for the needs of the 3.8 millions live births in 1996. This excess in neonatal physician workforce, in combination with the excess in NICU bed capacity and the economic pressures associated with managed care, magnifies the potential for competition and enhances the probability of the unnecessary use of resources.

Pediatricians

Providers other than neonatologists have emerged as important members of the neonatal care team. The role and supply of these specialists must be considered in any discussion of manpower in neonatology, because they undoubtedly affect the projection of needs.

The ACGME requires a certified pediatric residency program to offer a minimum of 4 months and a maximum of 6 months of training in neonatal intensive care (14). It appears that pediatricians should be well trained in the practice of neonatology, and data suggest that many would like to have the opportunity to practice those skills after completion of their training. This concept is supported by the original recommendations of the Committee on Perinatal Health, the American Academy of Pedi-

atrics, the American College of Obstetricians and Gynecologists, and others (4,9,17,18). Although the role and level of activity of pediatricians in the care of sick neonates varies from region to region, most agree that pediatricians should be considered a key resource in the delivery of normal newborn care and in level II units, providing stabilization and acute care to the newly born infant and participating in the long-term care and follow-up of NICU graduates. Involvement of the local pediatrician in the continuing care of convalescing infants reserves level III resources for more acutely ill patients and may be more cost-effective (19).

The role of the pediatrician in NICU care and in the delivery room has been significantly restricted for many reasons, including medical liability and the need for maintaining special skills. Many programs are reassessing the time committed to neonatal training as part of the general pediatric residency. Any reduction in time devoted to training in neonatal care may cause the pediatrician to feel less qualified to treat critically ill neonates and withdraw further from neonatology, resulting in more positions for neonatologists in community hospitals and more residents entering neonatal fellowship programs.

Neonatal Nurse Clinicians and Nurse Practitioners

The neonatal nurse clinician (NNC) and the neonatal nurse practitioner (NNP) are additional valuable members of the neonatal care team. These extended care givers have proven to be of considerable benefit in providing acute and long-term neonatal care under the supervision of a neonatologist or, in some level II units, under the supervision of a pediatrician (20). Nationwide, there are approximately 1,700 licensed NNCs and NNPs. These professionals have been effective in providing continuity of care to some of the more complex, chronically ill patients and their families. In many instances, their roles are evolving from the practice of acute-care inpatient neonatology into case management and long-term follow-up after discharge.

Because most NNCs and NNPs function as neonatologist extenders rather than as nurses, their impact on neonatal practice raises many questions (21). However, they are well established as members of the neonatal care team, and future reductions in the availability of residents in the NICU will make these professionals even more valuable to the level III centers. Their presence affects neonatal physician requirements, adds to existing excess provider capacity, and should be considered as part of health care planning.

Neonatal Respiratory Therapists

Special care nurseries depend on respiratory therapists for assistance with the ventilation and the respiratory support of its patients. These specialists have the responsibility for monitoring and maintaining ventilators and administering inhaled medications. In some units, they perform blood gas determinations. They are often valued members of the neonatal transport team, assisting in the stabilization and treatment of the critically ill neonate before and during transport.

Neonatal Intensive Care Unit Nurses

The duties of NICU nurses vary from unit to unit and region to region. Most units use their talents in roles considerably broader than those of nurses 25 years ago. In addition to traditional bedside nursing, the NICU nurse is responsible for continuous monitoring and assessment of the patient and has the responsibility to initiate resuscitative efforts in emergencies. The NICU nurse is the main communication link between the patient and parents and often a major source of strength and support. Like respiratory therapists, NICU nurses have proven their value as key members of neonatal transport teams. The development of regional level III centers could not have occurred without the creation of neonatal transport teams and the unique contributions of NICU nurses.

Neonatal Social Workers

The admission of any infant to the NICU produces anxiety and stress for the parents and family. Neonatal social workers provide the emotional support necessary to allow these families to survive the roller coaster atmosphere of the NICU. Because many infants are transported great distances and families are separated during the hospitalization of the neonate, social workers provide the support needed to keep families together emotionally. More NICU social workers are becoming responsible for coordinating discharge planning, serving as case managers for the family after discharge, and providing assistance with the transition from the hospital to the home.

Neonatal Developmental Interventional Specialists

Several studies indicate the benefit of developmental intervention on the long-term outcome of NICU graduates (22–24). The long-term developmental needs of the extremely-low-birth-weight (ELBW) infant often require a mixture of expertise in dealing with sensory and motor deficits. Ideally, these needs are supplied by persons trained in early childhood development with an understanding of occupational and physical therapy and expertise in teaching infants and children with hearing and visual impairment. Few formal training programs exist. Most developmental specialists receive on-the-job multidisciplinary training as members of the neonatal developmental follow-up team. In many cases, they can supply previously unavailable developmental services and can serve as valuable case managers for infants with special needs and their families after discharge. Caution must be used so that they do not replace the need for pediatric follow-up, further isolating the pediatrician from participating in the care of the NICU graduate and adding to the existing excess capacity in this field.

Other Members of the Neonatal Care Team

In addition to the direct members of the NICU team, many other ancillary services are needed to care for the high-risk infant in level II and level III care units. These services include the need for a broad spectrum of imaging services (e.g., radiology, ultrasound, magnetic resonance imaging), microlaboratory techniques, nutritional consultation, and pharmacokinetics support. Ideally, each of these programs should include someone with special training or interest in the needs of critically ill neonates. Level III NICU capabilities should have full pediatric subspecialty support, including pediatric cardiology, surgery, and neurology and neurosurgery (9).

The delivery of neonatal intensive care requires more than just hospital beds and a neonatologist. It requires a complete team made up of many highly skilled professionals dedicated to the care of the critically ill neonate and his or her family during the hospital stay and for years after discharge.

HIGH-TECH NEONATAL CARE

Acute Care Costs

Estimates suggest that the 1995 expenditures for perinatal care will approach $28 billion or $6,850 per mother–infant pair (4). This represents 4.5% of personal health care spending by all Americans and 7% of health care spending by the population less than age 65. Most of these resources are spent on acute high-tech care of the critically ill neonate, with daily charges easily reaching $1,000 to $1,500 for hospital services and an additional $250 to $300 each day for physician services (25).

Actual expenditures are difficult to determine, because there is no national database containing information on total public, private, and out-of-pocket payments for hospital and physician services. Most published data are limited to inpatient expenses and reflect individual hospital, state, or regional experiences. In may instances, estimates of disease- and patient-specific expenditures are based on small samples, resulting in wide variations within and between studies. Expenditure comparisons are complicated further by regional variations in costs, charges, standards of care, differences in patient population demographics, and intensity of illness. Further, much of the available information is derived from urban level III NICUs or state-funded perinatal programs, which include a high percentage of publicly funded patients. Because these patients often represent the highest perinatal risks, disease-specific expenditures may be skewed by overrepresentation of the most complex patients in the database, resulting in higher cost estimates when compared to private sector spending.

In a recent series from the United Kingdom, Stevenson et al. (26) determined that the mean cost per LBW infant, born at less than 1,500 g and surviving without major disability, was 13 times greater than that of an infant weighing between 1,501 and 2,000 g, and the cost per infant weighing less than 1,000 g at birth was 55 times control. Further, LBW infants continued to utilize hospital and practioner services at a greater rate than control until age 8 to 9.

In an attempt to control payments, both private and public payers have begun to move away from direct fee-for-service reimbursement and toward prospective payment methodologies that pass on a portion of the financial risk to the providers. In order to be successful, these systems must be based on large, comprehensive datasets and must contain sensitive indicators that adjust for the

intensity of the case mix. Two such systems have been applied to the experience of Florida's ten regional perinatal intensive care centers (RPICCs) and appear to accurately reflect true expenditures of resources.

The RPICC prospective payment system, implemented in 1985, uses 15 neonatal care groups (NCGs) as a basis for determining reimbursement for services rendered by hospitals and physicians to the state's Medicaid-sponsored patients (Fig. 3–2) (27–30). These state-approved reimbursement categories appear to be reasonable proxies for true costs, because, unlike charges, they are free of hospital and physician pricing practices (e.g., cost shifting due to uncompensated care and differences in accounting practices), they are based on clinical conditions, and they are calculated against a state standard. Total expenditures for fiscal year (FY) 1996 exceeded $84 million serving 2,161 patients and accounting for 76,418 inpatient days (Table 3–4) (31). While total program expenditures decreased as a result of changes in

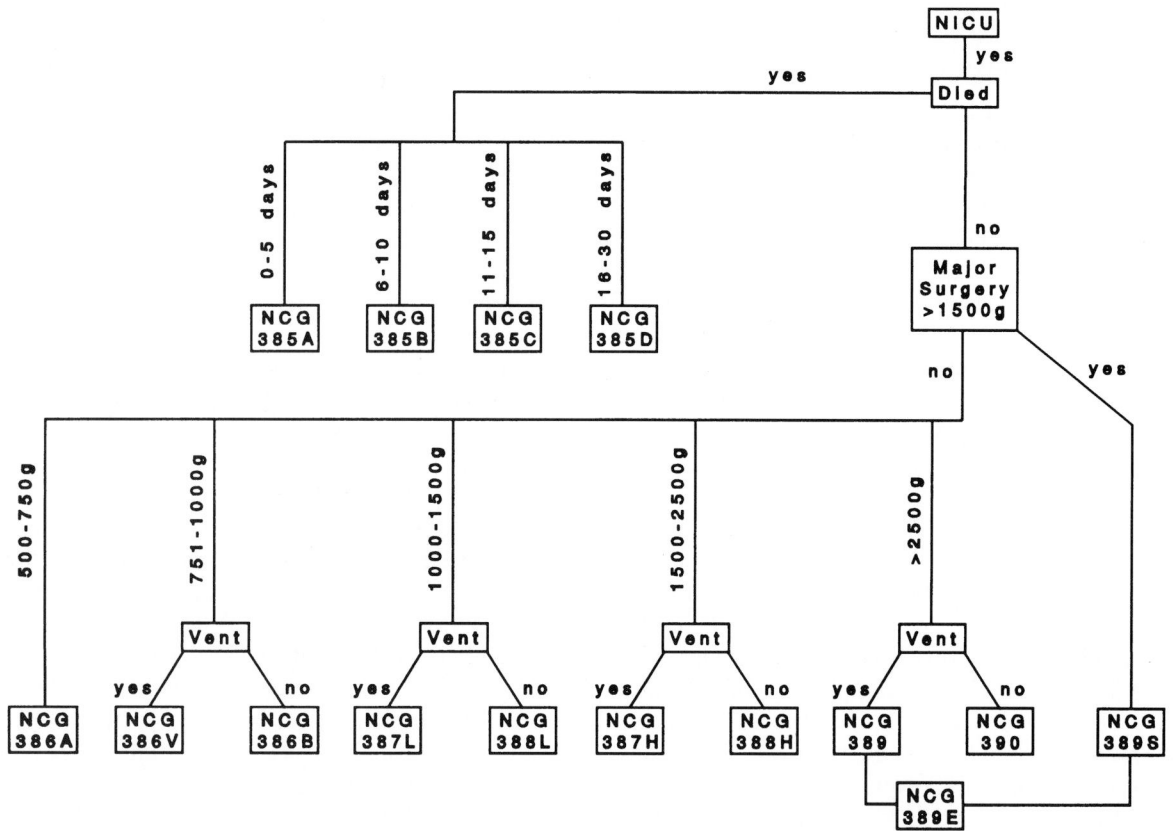

FIG. 3–2. Florida neonatal care groups (NCGs). Categories are based on diagnostic-related groups and subdivided into cells according to birth weight. Neonatal groups serve as a basis for reimbursement for neonatal physicians only. Consultative subspecialty care is reimbursed independent of NCG. Neonatal care groups served as a basis for hospital reimbursement from 1987 to 1990. NCG 385: Death (A, 0–5 days; B, 6–10 days; C, 11–15 days; D, 16–30 days); NCG 387L: 1,000- to 1,500-g birth weight; NCG 387H: 1,500- to 2,500-g birth weight; NCG 386A: 500- to 750-g birth weight; NCG 386B: 751- to 1,000-g birth weight; NCG 389: less than 2,500-g birth weight. E, extracorporeal membrane oxygenation; NICU, neonatal intensive care unit; S, surgery; V, ventilated. (From State of Florida Department of Health and Rehabilitative Services. Children's Medical Services regional perinatal intensive care center (RPICC) program handbook. Tallahassee: State of Florida Department of Health and Rehabilitative Services, 1991.)

TABLE 3–4. *State of Florida Approved Neonatal Care Group Payments for Regional Perinatal Intensive Care Centers, Fiscal Year 1995 to 1996*

	Fiscal year 1990	Fiscal year 1996	Percent change
Total program expenditures[a]	$117,900,000	$84,600,000	–33%
No. of patients served[a]	5,016	2,161	–57%
RPICC approved average reimbursement per patient			
Hospital	$19,657	$33,365	+70%
Physician	$1,345	$5,542	+75%

[a]Reduction in total expenditure and numbers of patients served are a result of Medicaid expansions, Medicaid health maintenance organization coverage, and changes in program eligibility.

RPICC, regional perinatal intensive care center.

From ref. 31.

program eligibility, the average approved reimbursement per patient increased for both the hospital and physician components, from $19,657 (hospital) and $1,345 (physician) in FY 1990 to $33,365 (hospital) and $5,542 (physician) in FY 1996. The highest levels of approved reimbursement in the NCG system continue to be for the ELBW infant less than 1,000 g, who has respiratory distress syndrome and requires mechanical ventilation. Payment for inpatient services for these infants exceeds $150,000 per surviving infant (32). These data are supported by similar relative expenditures and trends reported by other authors, although the actual dollar amounts vary among studies (33,34).

In February 1996, the Florida Agency for Health Care Administration issued its first report card on the performance of Florida hospitals, comparing costs and average LOSs for specific diagnosis-related group (DRG) categories. The gross data collected suggested that the RPICCs were considerably more expensive and had a significantly greater average LOS than non-RPICC institutions. However, when the All-Patient Refined Diagnosis-Related Groups (APR-DRGs v 12.0) methodology was applied, the differences became minimal with observed average charges and LOS closely approximating the expected (35). The APR-DRG methodology includes several adjustors for case-mix intensity and other proxy variables for socioeconomic status, resulting in a more accurate estimate of appropriate reimbursement.

In addition to these two systems, others have been proposed. All recognize the importance of case-mix adjustment in predicting true costs and adequate levels of reimbursement (36–38). As more competitive models of care are developed, public comparisons between institutions are made, and competitive contracts for reimbursement are developed, these adjustments for severity of illness become critical.

Costs after Discharge

Because the ELBW infant is at high risk for long-term sequelae, the resources dedicated to providing acute care must be supplemented with the continued investment of resources for long-term follow-up. With the realization that the long-term outcome of the ELBW infant is enhanced by developmental follow-up, including multidisciplinary intervention programs, postdischarge costs per NICU graduate have become substantial (22). Shankaran et al. (39) reported 1988 expenditures for NICU graduates with no disabilities to be in the range of $31.00 per month, predominantly for primary health care but also for limited occupational and physical therapy, as well as neurologic and ophthalmologic follow-up. These expenditures increase to $86.50 per month for infants with mild developmental or physical residuals and to $108.90 per month for infants with severe disabilities receiving care in the home (Table 3–5). In both cases, additional costs were related to the need for extensive occupational and physical therapy. The costs of neuro-

TABLE 3–5. *Outpatient costs after neonatal intensive care unit discharge*

Cost components	Group A (n = 23)	Group B (n = 15)	Group C (n = 22)	F value	Significant comparisons
Total outpatient costs	31.2 (22.9)	86.5 (93.4)	108.9 (58.7)	9.8	A < B[b]; A < C[c]
Specialized services	10.7	9.1	9.3	0.3	NS
Primary health care	(8.9)	(5.7)	(6.3)		
Occupational or physical therapy	0.7 (2.4)	14.1 (15.8)	18.9 (21.9)	8.2	A < B[b]; A < C[c]
Neurology	0.5 (1.4)	4.1 (9.1)	6.6 (8.7)	4.4	A < C[b]
Ophthalmology	3.6 (7.4)	4.8 (5.7)	5.6 (1.7)	0.6	NS
Emergency room	1.1 (2.9)	0.8 (1.5)	1.7 (2.8)	0.5	NS

Group A children had no developmental disabilities; group B children were mildly developmentally disabled; and group C children were moderately or severely developmentally disabled. Results are mean dollars per infant per month with standard deviations in parenthesis. Analyses of variance by groups were done for outpatient costs.

Significant comparisons: [a]p < 0.5, [b]p < 0.01, [c]p < 0.001, Scheffe tests were performed on pairwise comparisons.

From ref. 39.

logic follow-up were less, but they were significantly greater for severely damaged infants than for normal infants. The cost of institutional care for an NICU graduate up to 3 years of age exceeded $1,200 per month ($43,200 per 36 months). Although this study attempted to identify total postdischarge costs, out-of-pocket expenses were not estimated. A recent survey indicates that these expenses for children with special health care needs can exceed 15% of annual family income (40).

The increased survival of ELBW infants presents several challenges to our educational system. Stevenson et al. (41) report that 52% of the long-term expenditures related to LBW are related to special education needs. In an attempt to define more specifically the long-term educational needs of these infants, Walker et al. (42) estimated the 1982 costs of early intervention (i.e., from 0 to 3 years of age) and transitional education (i.e., from 3 to 5 years of age) for mild or moderately handicapped ELBW infants (i.e., Bayley development quotient of 80 to 85 for mild and 65 to 80 for moderate) to be $13,800 per year for each survivor, with a 1982 total lifetime cost of $24,177 (Table 3–6). The educational costs of the severely handicapped exceed $22,000 per year and $192,000 at 1982 value of lifetime costs (42).

Cost-Effectiveness of Neonatal Care

When long-term cost–benefit ratios were calculated in the 1970s and early 1980s, provision of neonatal care appeared extremely cost-effective. This is still true, because high-quality neonatal care decreases the inci-

dence of significant morbidity in almost all weight groups. However, the increased number of surviving ELBW infants with their financial, social, and educational impacts has led several researchers to raise significant ethical and moral questions about future directions in therapy. Two studies designed to address the cost–benefit ratio of neonatal care showed significant savings for infants with birth weights greater than 1,000 g. The treatment of neonates between 500 and 999 g showed a loss, questioning the economic value of treating this group of patients (43,44).

Although the cost–benefit ratio for ELBW infants is of concern, ethical and moral decisions about the treatment of the extremely premature infant have not kept pace with technology. Our nation has only recently been willing to admit that even the richest country in the world cannot afford to buy all that science has to offer. Some states are beginning to respond to this reality and make prospective decisions based on economics and on ethical and social considerations (45). Prioritizing therapies and rationing resources will be discussed more in years to come.

Missed Opportunities

One cannot consider the magnitude of these costs and the amount of human suffering involved in the delivery of a high-risk infant without wondering why America continues to expend enormous resources on postnatal care when one-half of the number of ELBW deliveries could be avoided with early prenatal care (46). The benefit of $1,000 of prenatal care instead of $150,000 for each surviving LBW infant is obvious. In 1985, the Institute of Medicine reported that for every $1.00 spent on prenatal care, $3.00 were saved in the first year and $10.00 more saved over a lifetime (47).

Recent expansions in Medicaid eligibility have made 85% of women eligible to receive prenatal care, with 82% receiving care within the first trimester (Fig. 3–3) (2). Financial access to care, combined with comprehensive prepregnancy and prenatal programs, including good nutrition and avoidance of high-risk lifestyles, have been identified as key in our attempts to reduce LBW with its attendant costs and human loss (4). Of major concern are the remaining economic and noneconomic barriers confronting African-Americans, resulting in an early prenatal care rate that is 20% less than for Caucasians.

Major Payers for Neonatal Care

One study identified four groups of major payers for neonatal care: private health insurance (52%), public programs including Medicaid and other state and local programs (27%), special perinatal demonstration projects both public and private (7%), and uninsured, self-paying (14%) (Fig. 3–4) (4). None of the major payers completely cover the costs of high-risk obstetric and neonatal

TABLE 3–6. *Long-term educational needs of neonatal intensive care unit graduates weighing less than 1,000g at birth*

	Moderately handicapped		Severely handicapped	
	Annual costs/ survivor	1982 value	Annual costs/ survivor	1982 value
Early intervention (0–3 yr)	$1,800	$4,902	$1,800	$4,902
Transitional (3–5 y)	$12,000	$19,275		
Meeting Street School (3–21 yr)			$12,000	$121,175
Group home residence (21 yr to death)			$10,000	$66,193
1982 value of total lifetime costs		$24,177		$192,270

From ref. 42.

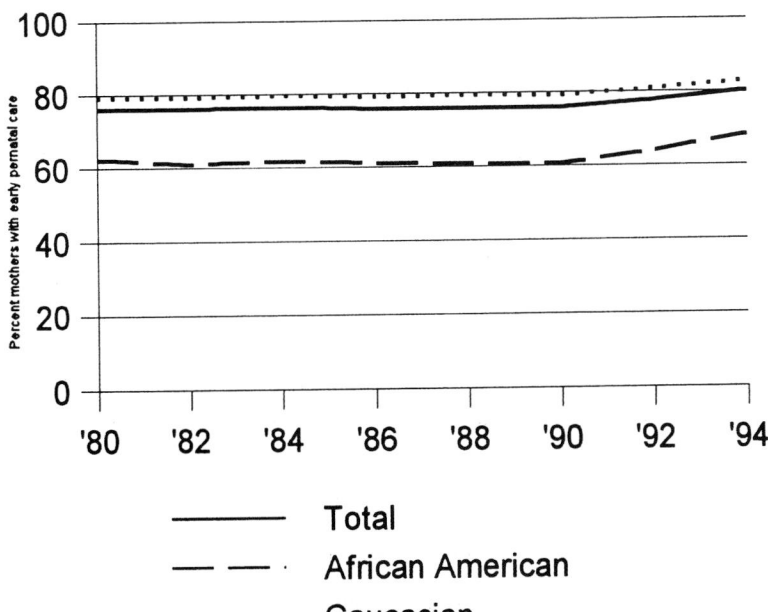

FIG. 3–3. Trends in prenatal care from 1980 to 1994 by race of mother. Early prenatal care is defined as care begun within the first 3 months of pregnancy. (Derived from ref. 2.)

care, especially for the complicated ELBW infant. A significant portion of this uncompensated care is shifted to other subscribers in the form of increased charges. One study suggested that as much as 27% of total costs of NICU care in the state of Florida is shifted to paying patients who are responsible for generating 60% of total revenues while accounting for only 33% of costs (48). In recent years, as payments under fee-for-service plans are replaced by managed care and discounted payments for bundled services, the ability for cost shifting has been significantly diminished, placing many of the NICUs in financial jeopardy.

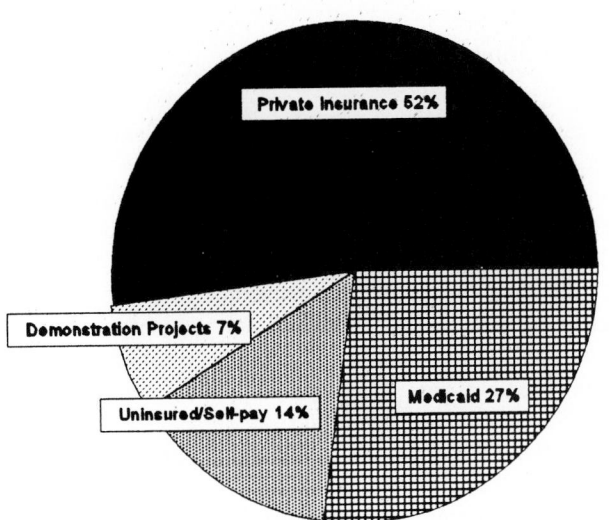

FIG. 3–4. Primary sources of payment for perinatal care. Total expenditures were estimated at $28 billion. (Drawn from refs. 55 and 57.)

Private Health Insurance

Although private health insurance is the financial foundation of the health care system in the United States, coverage for pregnant women and their neonates is more limited than for any other segment of the population and is being continually eroded. Only 67% of civilian women of child-bearing age and only 61% of the 3.9 million infants less than 1 year of age are insured privately (49). These rates are well below the 85% to 87% coverage for the general population. More than one-half of women covered under group insurance policies received coverage as a dependent of their employed husband. This is of major concern, because employer-based coverage of dependents has decreased by almost 20% during the last decade, leaving many working families totally uncovered for prenatal care and for all types of neonatal care, preventive and catastrophic (50). Even among policies that include dependent coverage, few cover the prenatal and newborn costs related to the 500,000 annual deliveries of teenage pregnancies (51). Neglecting this segment of the population produces significant financial barriers to care and increases the chance of high-risk delivery.

To counter escalating costs, most insurers have introduced substantial cost-sharing requirements (e.g., deductibles, copayments), leaving even the insured family directly responsible for a significant portion of the costs of their infant's care. In the case of high-risk neonatal care, obligation for copayments can be financially devastating. For example, a 20% copayment responsibility on a combined hospital and physician bill for an LBW infant of $125,000 results in a family responsibility of $25,000, an amount that would be impossible for most families to pay.

In an attempt to counter the erosion of prenatal coverage, many states have passed mandates requiring obstetric and neonatal benefits for families and for teens living at home. Despite being cognizant of the long-term benefits of prenatal care, many insurance companies and employers see mandated coverage for dependents, particularly the high-risk neonate, as adding significantly to the cost of insurance, making it unaffordable to employers and middle-class Americans. Instead of recognizing the long-term benefits of access to prenatal care and the financial burden of neonatal intensive care, they are opting for short-term reductions in premiums by attempting to overturn these and other state mandates (52). If these attempts are successful, coverage will be further eroded, increasing the number of uninsured and placing more financial pressure on other payers.

Medicaid

The largest public program for the financing of prenatal and neonatal care is Medicaid. Authorized as Title XIX of the Social Security Act in 1965, Medicaid is a federal–state public partnership that finances care for 35 million low-income persons who are elderly, blind, disabled, or members of families with children (53—55). During the past several years, the federal–state match has remained relatively constant, with federal funds accounting for an average of 56.9% of total FY 1989 program expenditures. The exact level of federal funding is determined from a formula reflecting the state's per capita income and varies between 50% and 80% of the state's total Medicaid expenditures (53).

In 1997, 57% of the targeted population consisted of pregnant women and children; however, only 23% of the $120 billion in total program expenditures were directed toward them (56). Until recently, pregnant women and children received less than 5% of total federal spending, 20% of the amount spent on the population older than 65 years of age (55). The more than 3.9 million children younger than 1 year of age did worse, receiving only 4.2% of all Medicaid spending for an average of $1,174 per infant (57). Approximately 15% of all Medicaid-sponsored deliveries require NICU care, a rate three times those with other sources of payment (30).

With the exception of the matching requirements for federal funds and the required compliance with specific federal mandates, each state has the responsibility for developing and administering its own Medicaid program. This includes setting eligibility and coverage standards within broad federal guidelines. As a result, there is considerable variation among states in eligibility, range of services offered, limitations on services, and reimbursement policies.

Over the past several years, Congress has been successful in extending Medicaid eligibility to more women and children in need. Beginning in 1989, all states were required to cover pregnant women and children younger than 6 years of age with family incomes below 133% of the federal poverty level (FPL) (1997 FPL for a family of four, $16,050.00) and had the option of extending benefits to pregnant women and infants younger than 1 year of age with family incomes below 185% of FPL. The new State Children's Health Insurance Program under Title XXI of the Social Security Act gives states new latitude in identifying eligible patients and allows states to expand coverage for children up to 200% of the FPL, with some states utilizing additional funds to reach 300% FPL (3). These higher levels of eligibility could provide coverage for many of our nation's working poor, who are employed in small business or hold part-time jobs and who do not receive health insurance through their employer.

In 1995, Medicaid was the source of payment for 1,383,425 births, 39% of the nation's deliveries, ranging from a low of 16% in Hawaii (the first state with universal health coverage) to a high of 56% of all births in Mississippi (55). With expansions of coverage available through Title XXI, Medicaid could be responsible for providing coverage for the majority of newborns in our nation. This fact becomes a concern when one considers the low level of reimbursement provided to hospitals and physicians to care for Medicaid patients. In some instances, reimbursement is less than 55% of total obstetric and neonatal hospital costs, resulting in enormous losses for hospitals that provide high-tech neonatal intensive care (58). Because most Medicaid-sponsored pregnant women and their infants are cared for in large urban hospitals or teaching centers, increased volume and intensity combined with low reimbursement are placing an increasingly disproportional load on these centers, threatening their very existence.

Title V Maternal and Child Health Block Grant Program

Located within the Health Resources and Services Administration (HRSA) of the Department of Health and Human Services (HHS), the Maternal and Child Health (MCH) Block Grant Program was authorized by Title V of the Social Security Act to provide grants to states for a variety of preventive and primary care services to women and children, including prenatal care, immunizations, and rehabilitative services for children with special needs. Although FY 1998 funding for this program exceeded $630 million, it accounts for less than 1% of the HHS budget (59). Current funding levels allow less than one-half of eligible women access to prenatal care under the program. As Title XXI expands access to health care for women and children, the future of programs in the MCH program could be seriously threatened.

Community Health Centers, Migrant Health Centers, and the National Health Service Corps

As part of HRSA, $826 million for community health centers, migrant health centers, and programs of the National Health Service Corps are directed toward providing primary preventive care, including prenatal and well-child care for those served in urban community health centers and in rural areas of the United States (59). Chronically underfunded, these programs have seen little increase in funding in the last few years and have been targets for reduction or elimination of programs.

Special Demonstration Projects

Because early prenatal care can positively effect perinatal outcome, many public (e.g., state, county, and municipal governments) and private (e.g., March of Dimes, Robert Wood Johnson, Pew Foundation) organizations have dedicated significant resources to study how to reach high-risk populations more effectively to reduce the mortality and morbidity related to premature deliveries. Although most of these projects are small and contribute little to covering the total costs of perinatal care, many are highly successful and result in significant overall savings for individual patients. A major problem with these projects is that targeted patients are highly selected, making it difficult to apply program results to larger populations. Many programs are funded for a limited time, creating the problem of how to continue to provide services after funding has expired.

Uninsured, Self-Paying Patients

Most of the uninsured, self-paying patients cannot afford to pay for any type of medical care. They contribute little to the financing of perinatal care used by themselves and their families. Being uninsured is the greatest barrier to receiving prenatal care, and it results in the highest risk for delivering an LBW infant, approximately three times the rate for women with even minimal prenatal care (60). In 1990, an estimated 8.4 million women of child-bearing age had no health insurance coverage, public or private, and an additional 5 million women had private, employer-based coverage without maternity benefits (4). Coverage for maternity benefits appears to be even worse than these figures suggest, because it is estimated that as many as 20 million women have their insurance interrupted for at least 2 months over a 24-month period. Data indicate that 26% of women are uninsured when they conceive, and 15% are uninsured when they deliver, leaving an estimated 800,000 pregnant women with no maternity coverage and more than 70,000 births without the benefit of any prenatal care (60).

MAJOR MEASURES OF OUTCOME

Infant Mortality Rate

The IMR is defined by the National Center for Health Statistics and by the World Health Organization as the number of deaths occurring within the first year of life per 1,000 live births. Infant mortality can be divided further into neonatal mortality (i.e., death before 29 days of age) and postneonatal mortality (i.e., death between 29 days and 1 year of age). Neonatal mortality generally is the result of factors related to pregnancy and birth, and postneonatal mortality generally is the result of environmental factors (e.g., trauma, infection, nutrition, sudden infant death syndrome) (61).

Infant mortality in the United States has declined by greater than 60% since 1970 (Fig. 3–5). Initially, the largest declines were seen in the neonatal mortality rate (NMR), but in the last 10 years these advances have been matched by similar declines in the postneonatal mortality rate (PNMR). Between 1988 and 1992, the IMR dropped 17% (from 9.9 deaths per 1,000 live births to 8.5 deaths per 1,000 live births), with a 14% drop in the NMR (62). This drop is coincident with the release of commercially available artificial surfactant for the treatment of respiratory distress syndrome and may be reflective of the use of this new treatment modality. The projected 1996 IMR of 7.2 deaths per 1,000 live births would be 5% lower than the final 1995 rate of 7.6 deaths per 1,000 live births and could be the lowest ever recorded in the United States. If this trend continues, the overall United States IMR will be 6.2 per 1,000 live births in the year 2000 and will surpass the goal of 7.0 per 1,000 live births (Table 3–7) (63). Despite these achievements, it is sobering to realize that the United States ranks twenty-first in the world among countries with a population of at least 2.5 million (64).

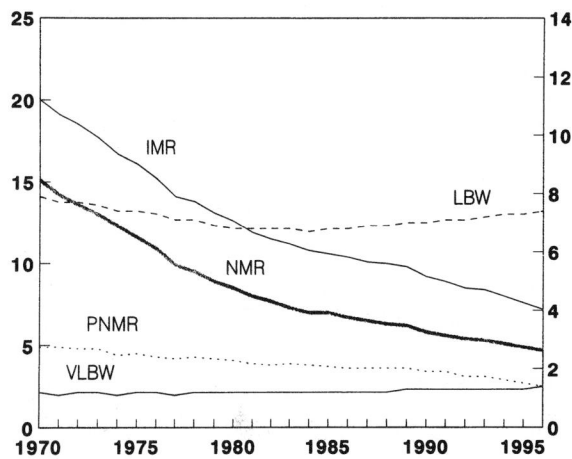

FIG. 3–5. Infant, neonatal, and postnatal mortality, and low and very low birth weight in the United States from 1970 to 1995. IMR, infant mortality rate; LBW, low birth weight (less than 2,500 g); NMR, neonatal mortality rate; VLBW, very low birth weight (less than 1,500 g). (From ref. 62.)

TABLE 3–7. *Progress toward meeting the U.S. Surgeon General's maternal and child health goals for the year 2000*

Indicator	Race	1991 rate	1994 rate	2000 goal	Projected 2000 rate	Projected year goal reached
Infant mortality	Overall	8.9 infant deaths per 1,000 live births	8.0	7.0	6.2	1998
	Black	17.6	15.8	11.0	12.2	2002
Early prenatal care	Overall	76.2% of all birth	80.2%	90%	88.2%	2002
	Black	61.9%	68.3%	90%	81.1%	2005
	Hispanic	61.0%	68.9%	90%	84.7%	2002
Low birth weight	Overall	7.1% of all births	7.3%	5%	7.7%	Never
	Black	13.6%	13.2%	9%	12.4%	2026

For Hispanics, the Surgeon General articulated a distinct goal only for early prenatal care. To project future numbers, this chart assumes a continuation of 1991 to 1994 trends.
From ref. 63.

Of major concern is the persistent disparity in the IMR between Caucasian and African-American infants. Although all race groups have seen a decrease in IMR, the difference in rate between Caucasian and African-American infants has increased. Provisional 1996 rates show an IMR for Caucasian infants at 6.0 per 1,000 lives births, whereas that of African-American infants is expected to be 14.2 deaths per 1,000 live births, a ratio of 2.4:1 (Fig. 3–6). At this rate, the year 2000 IMR for African-Americans will be 12.2 death per 1,000 live births and exceed the goal of 11.0 per 1,000 live births (63).

Neonatal Mortality Rate

Although IMR reflects the general health of a community, separate examination of early and late infant deaths can further pinpoint problems. The NMR equals the number of deaths occurring at less than 29 days after birth per 1,000 live births (61). These account for about 67% of all infant deaths. One-half of all neonatal deaths can be attributed to four leading causes: (i) LBW, (ii) acute perinatal asphyxia, (iii) congenital anomalies, and (iv) perinatal infections.

Between 1988 and 1996, both the NMR and the PNMR declined by almost 30%. The 1996 provisional rates of 4.7 deaths per 1,000 live births and 2.5 deaths per 1,000 live births are thought to be a reflection of the marked improvement in death related to acute perinatal conditions as well as those related to late neonatal deaths (deaths occurring after 28 days of age). In 1995, 63% of all infants deaths were related to LBW. African-Americans and other minority NMRs parallel the IMR and are considerably higher than Caucasian NMRs, with a African-American:Caucasian ratio for NMR of 2.3:1 compared to an IMR African-American:Caucasian ratio of 2.4:1 (Fig. 3–7). These differences appear to be primarily due to the higher incidence of LBW (less than 2,500 g) and very-low-birth-weight (VLBW; less than 1,500 g) infants born to African-American women and are reduced when one considers birth weight-specific IMRs (62).

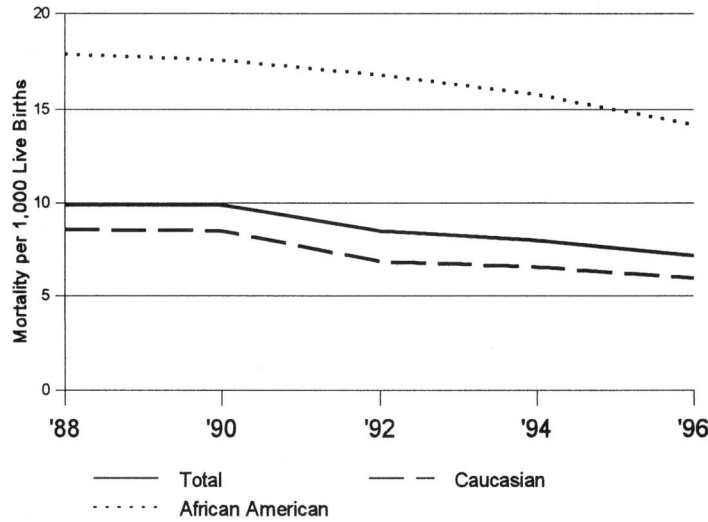

FIG. 3–6. Infant mortality in the United States from 1988 to 1996 by race. Infant mortality constitutes deaths that occur before 1 year of age. (Modified from refs. 61 and 62.)

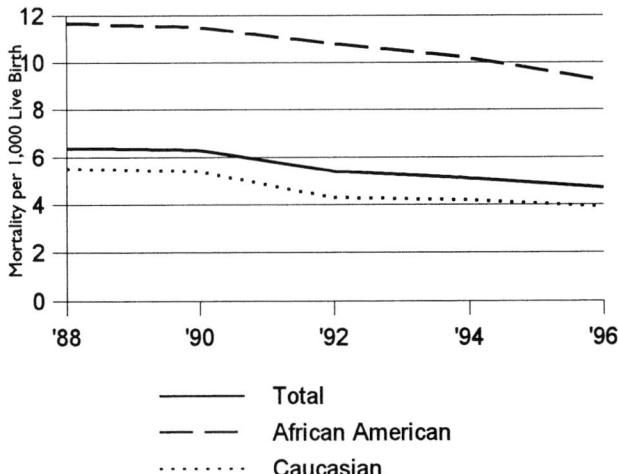

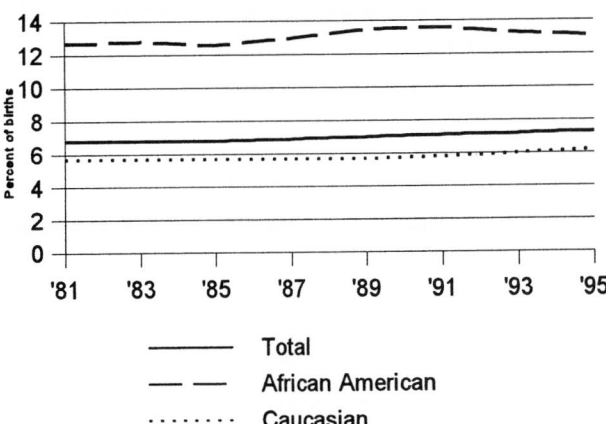

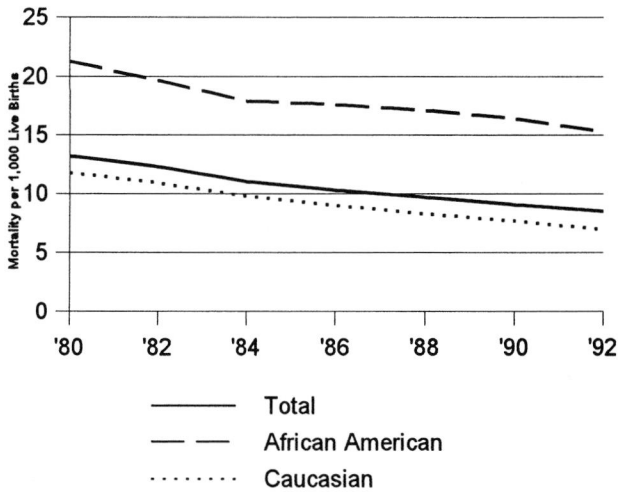

FIG. 3–7. Neonatal mortality in the United States from 1988 to 1996 by race. Neonatal mortality constitutes deaths that occur before 28 days of age. (Modified from refs. 61 and 62.)

Perinatal Mortality Rate

The perinatal mortality rate (PMR) is defined by the National Center for Health Statistics as the number of late fetal deaths (i.e., fetal deaths of 28 weeks or more gestation) plus early neonatal deaths (i.e., deaths of infants 0 to 6 days of age) per 1,000 live births (65). Because there is no uniform international definition of fetal deaths, international comparisons of PMR are difficult to interpret.

Most fetal deaths are a result of chronic asphyxia (60% to 70%); congenital malformations (20% to 25%); superimposed complications of pregnancy, such as placental abruption, diabetes mellitus, intrauterine infection (5% to 10%); and unexplained deaths (5% to 10%) (66). Although the incidence of congenital malformations has

remained relatively constant over the last few years, improvements in the management of pregnancy-related complications, combined with improved early neonatal survival, has resulted in a significant decrease in PMR to 9.1 deaths per 1,000 live births for 1990. Race variations in PMR are identical to those seen in IMR and NMR (Fig. 3–8). PMR in African Americans is in excess of twice that of Caucasians (17.1 deaths per 1,000 live births compared to 8.3 deaths per 1,000 live births) (55).

MAJOR MORBIDITIES

Low Birth Weight

LBW is responsible for 63% of the United States IMR and carries a 40-fold increased risk of death in the first month of life and a two- to threefold increase in the chance of long-term disability (62,67). Considering these realities, the prevention of LBW has been one of the nation's top priorities in its effort to reduce infant mortality and morbidity. Despite this focus, no progress has been made in reducing the incidence of LBW over the last decade. In fact, the 1996 LBW rate of 7.4% is higher than that of the 1988 rate of 6.9% and places us twenty-fifth among the world's largest countries (64). Currently, the LBW rate among African-Americans is in excess of twice that of Caucasians. Examination of annual LBW statistics reveals a slow but continued increase in the overall numbers of infants born at LBW since 1984 (Fig. 3–9) (2). The greatest rise in LBW occurred between 1985 and 1992 in African-Americans, increasing from 12.6% to 13.6%. At the same time, the number of births to teens increased dramatically, reaching an all-time high of 118 births per 1,000 girls aged 15 to 19 years (Fig. 3–10). More recent data show a reversal of both of these trends, with decreases in each of the last 4 years. This association is not surprising when one realizes that teen pregnancy carries a very significant increase in the risk of

FIG. 3–8. Perinatal mortality in the United States from 1980 to 1992 by race. Perinatal mortality constitutes fetal death before 28 weeks of gestation plus infant deaths at 0 to 6 days of age. (Modified from ref. 65.)

FIG. 3–9. Trends in low-birth-weight births (less than 2,500 g) by race as a percentage of all births. (Modified from ref. 2.)

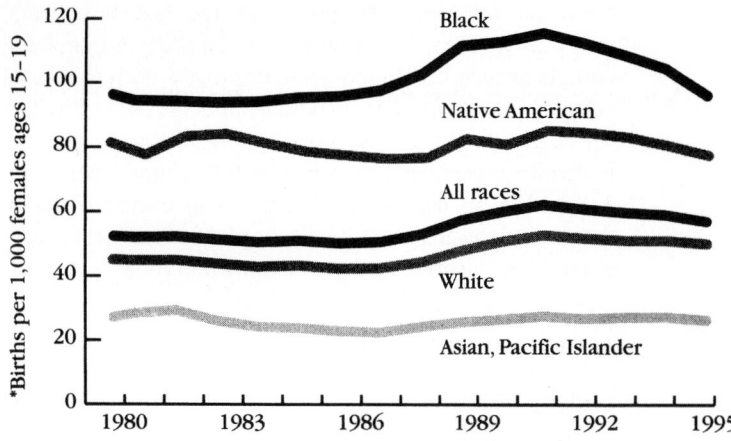

FIG. 3–10. Trends in teen birth rates* from 1980 to 1995 by race of mother. (From ref. 2.)

having an LBW infant. On the other hand, LBW among Caucasians has continued to increase to a 1995 level of 6.2%, whereas teen pregnancies have remained constant for the past 5 years. Some of this increase in LBW infants may be related to the greater prevalence of multiple births among Caucasians, but other factors appear to be contributing to this trend (62).

Like other measures of perinatal outcome, LBW rates are disproportionately higher in large cities and in the urban African-American population (68). In 1987, cities with populations of 100,000 or more accounted for 33% of all LBW births nationally, but they were responsible for only 14.4% of all United States births.

The birth weight of United States infants is related to several important maternal demographic characteristics (Fig. 3–11). The lowest incidence of LBW is seen in married Caucasian women between 25 and 29 years of age, who completed at least 16 years of school and who

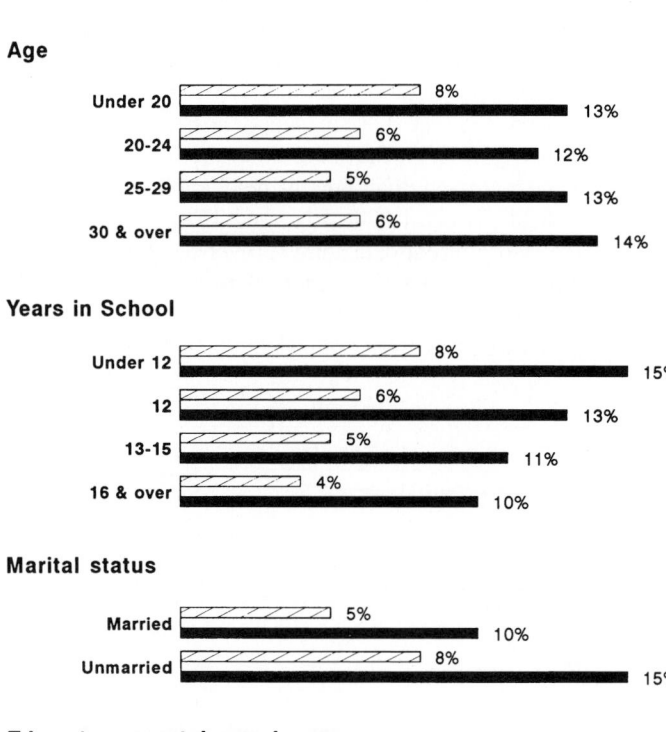

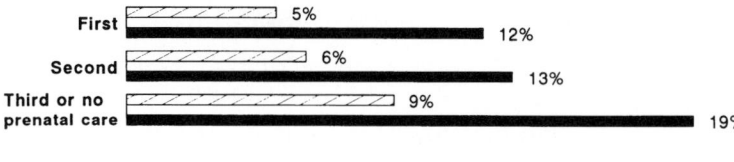

FIG. 3–11. Low-birth-weight rates in 1988 by race for selected maternal characteristics. *Open bars*, Caucasians; *solid bars*, African-Americans. (From ref. 69.)

received prenatal care starting in the first trimester. The highest risks occur in unmarried African-American women who attended school for fewer than 12 years and received late or no prenatal care. Although maternal age was not a factor in LBW rates among African-Americans, the LBW rate for Caucasians younger than 20 years of age was almost twice the rate for women 25 to 29 years of age (69). Given the complex interaction of physical, demographic, and societal factors contributing to the LBW rate, it is not surprising to discover that our current rate of LBW far exceeds the year 2000 goal of 5% and, if current trends continue, will reach 7.7%, a rate 50% higher than target (63).

The benefit of early prenatal care is seen in both Caucasians and African-Americans, with the incidence of LBW decreasing for each group when prenatal care is initiated in the first trimester, rather than late or not at all. Data from western Europe, where early prenatal care is available and is used by most women, suggest that the United States LBW rate could be halved with a minimal investment in prenatal care (70,71).

Lifestyle Choices: Cigarette Smoking, Alcohol, and Illicit Drugs

Some of the perinatal risk factors associated with LBW and poor perinatal outcome are not within a pregnant woman's immediate control. However, many of the factors associated with lifestyle choices are. Very little is known about the exact number of women who use drugs while pregnant, or their pattern and intensity of use. Data from anonymous urine toxicology analysis combined with self-reporting suggests the incidence ranges between 7.5% and 15%, with a high incidence of women using multiple drugs (Fig. 3–12) (72).

Cigarette smoking during pregnancy is the single largest modifiable risk factor for LBW and infant mortality and accounts for up to 20% of LBW. Babies born to mothers who smoke are, on average, 8 oz lighter than those born to mothers who do not smoke. Because most of these infants are term and near-term LBW infants, their prognosis is good and their medical costs are only moderate. Nonetheless, reduction of smoking during pregnancy can decrease the incidence of LBW and improve perinatal outcome (72).

The use of alcohol during pregnancy has been associated with both short- and long-term morbidity. Fetal alcohol syndrome is a well-recognized consequence of excessive consumption of alcohol during pregnancy. However, several studies report an increase in LBW in babies born to women who consume between one and three drinks per day, resulting in an average decrease in birth weight of between 1 and 8 oz (73–75).

The exact incidence of illicit drug use during pregnancy is unknown, but several researchers report perinatal cocaine exposure rates between 0.4% and 27%, depending on the region of the country and population demographics (76–80). Recent evidence suggests that although the overall use of drugs during pregnancy has remained unchanged, the number of new drug users appears to be declining (81).

A myriad of neonatal complications have been reported as a result of cocaine exposure, ranging from none to antenatal cerebral infarction (Table 3–8). The long-term neurodevelopmental effects of perinatal illicit drug exposure are just now being studied carefully. In addition to these physical and social implications of perinatal cocaine abuse, the direct fiscal costs to the health care system are enormous. One report estimated the short-term initial hospitalization costs of treating infants of cocaine-exposed pregnancies at $5,110 per patient and a total yearly cost of $1,057,921, more than twice the costs for control infants (82). A recent analysis shows that most of these costs are related to LBW, admission to the NICU, and a longer lengths of stay as a result of complex social and family situations that delay discharge. Prenatal identification of these issues could lead to significant cost reduction and better outcomes (83).

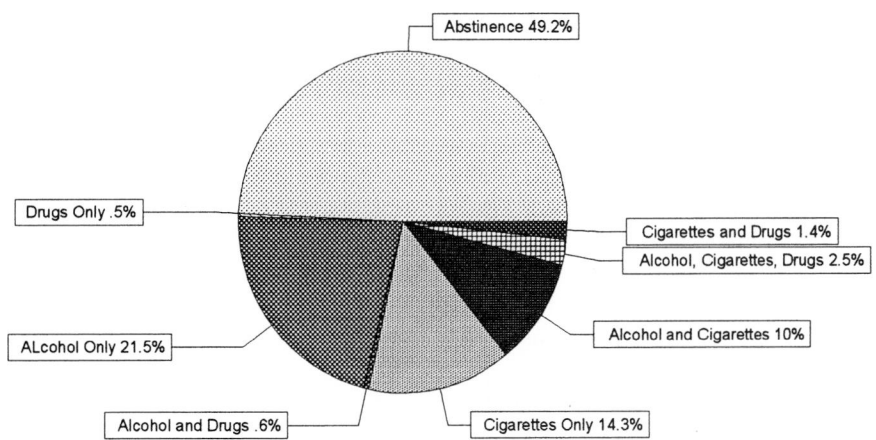

FIG. 3–12. Profile of substance abuse during pregnancy. (From ref. 72.)

TABLE 3–8. *Effects of cocaine on the neonate*

Common complications	Rare problems
Intrauterine growth retardation	Antenatal cerebral
Microcephaly	infarction
Prematurity	Birth defects secondary
Infections, especially STDs	to vasoconstriction
Neurobehavioral abnormalities	Myocardial infarction,
Neurophysiologic abnormalities	ischemic changes
Poor feeding	Necrotizing enterocolitis
Small CNS bleeds	

CNS, central nervous system; STD, sexually transmitted disease.
From ref. 79.

Neurodevelopmental Sequelae

With survival rates approaching 95% for premature infants weighing between 1,200 and 2,500 g and 60% for those between 500 and 750 g, the incidence and magnitude of the neurodevelopmental sequelae related to the treatment of premature and critically ill neonates has become increasingly important (see also Chaps. 26 and 59) (84). Although abnormalities vary with gestational age, population demographics, and length of follow-up, most sequelae are seen in the smallest infants, often those weighing less than 1,250 g. Caution must be used in interpreting short-term NICU follow-up data, because minor neuromuscular abnormalities seen in the immediate neonatal period may not persist, and significant abnormalities in cognitive function may not be detectable until the infant is older and more sophisticated testing can be performed. Grogaard and associates reported an 18% incidence of major handicaps in VLBW infants (infants less than 1,500 g) at 18 months' follow-up (85). Cerebral palsy was found in 7.6%, and 6.5% were mentally retarded with development quotients of less than 70. Severe retinopathy of prematurity existed in 5.5%, with neurosensory hearing loss occurring at a similar frequency of 5.4%. Further analysis of the data from two treatment periods (1976 to 1980 and 1981 to 1985) showed that the incidence of major handicaps were reduced to less than one-half: 12.1% of the infants treated during the later period demonstrated major sequelae compared with 27.2% of those treated between 1976 and 1980. Similar improvements were seen in ELBW infants, with a 37.3% incidence of major sequelae between 1976 and 1980 decreasing to 15.9% between 1981 and 1985. However, the absolute number of VLBW and ELBW infants with major sequelae has increased, as proportionally more VLBW and ELBW infants are surviving intact. Teplin et al. (86) found an 18% incidence of moderate or severe handicaps in infants weighing less that 1,001 g at 6 years of follow-up, but 46% had no functional disability, and 36% had only mild residua.

Certain sociodemographic variables (e.g., race, family income, mother's marital status, age, educational level) have a significant effect on the mental development of NICU survivors. In a study of 6,281 NICU graduates followed for as long as 48 to 60 months, Resnick et al. (87) found that developmental performance decreased significantly between first testing at 12 months and second testing at 24 months. The greatest decrease was seen in non-Caucasian populations, and although Caucasian infants stabilized or improved between 24 and 48 to 60 months, non-Caucasians continued to decline four additional development quotient points. Multivariant analysis showed these declines were more closely related to the maternal sociodemographic factors than to birth weight or NICU course (87). When this analysis was extended to 457 NICU graduates attending public school, strong correlations among poverty, race, and academic school performance were evident. The NICU medical course and treatment correlated with school performance only for those graduates with significant sensory (e.g., blind, hearing impaired) or motor (e.g., cerebral palsy) handicaps (88).

Although the absolute number of NICU graduates with severe sensory and motor handicaps is small, their need for special education can have a significant impact on the educational system. Resnick et al. (89) utilized the Florida statewide database to assess the educational disabilities of a cohort of 9,943 NICU graduates born between 1980 and 1987 and located in kindergarten through third grade. More than 73% of children were in mainstream education. Severe disabilities (placement into categories of physically impaired, sensory impaired, profoundly mentally handicapped, trainable mentally handicapped, educable mentally handicapped) were closely associated with perinatal events and accounted for only 9% of the sample. Seventeen percent of the sample fell into the categories of emotionally handicapped, specific learning disabilities, and speech and language impaired. Long-term outcome for these children was more directly related to sociodemorgraphic indicators than to perinatal history, illustrating the influence of postnatal societal factors on the long-term investment and outcome of NICU graduates (89).

REGIONALIZATION: A CONCEPT IN EVOLUTION

Regionalization of perinatal care has been lauded by many as the single most important factor influencing the birth weight-specific neonatal mortality. Outlined in 1977 by the Committee on Perinatal Health (COPH) of the National Foundation of the March of Dimes in its landmark report, *Toward Improving the Outcome of Pregnancy: Recommendations for the Regional Development of Maternal and Perinatal Health Services*, this concept served as the guide for the development of perinatal services for the last two decades (90). The Committee's concept of regionalization was based on the geographic concentration of neonatal intensive care services supported by cooperative arrangements among hospitals within a region to provide, as a network, the necessary levels of care defined in the document as level I, II, and III services.

Although quite intuitive and logical, this concept of cooperation is rather foreign to the American health care system, which is built on the philosophy of free market, free enterprise, and competition. The level of planning and cooperation necessary to make regionalization work often is resisted by all levels of health care providers.

Then, how did regionalization take hold? Many observers think that it came at the right time, when knowledge of high-risk mothers and neonates was advancing rapidly. It came when the transfer of technology was confined to larger urban teaching hospitals and academic centers. It came at a time when other hospital services were running at near capacity.

Under the plan, regions were not defined strictly by geography, but by tradition and the organizational skills of the early leaders in neonatology. This informal approach to the organization of perinatal care worked well as long as cooperation was seen as mutually beneficial to all involved. In the late 1970s and early 1980s, the health care environment began to change significantly. Driven by dramatic changes in the public financing of health care, the fragile alliance built on cooperation was being replaced by a drive for competition (91).

Medicare's replacement of fee-for-service reimbursement with a prospective payment system caused hospital inpatient census to drop as adult care was shifted to the outpatient clinics and ambulatory surgical centers. Declining hospital margins with excess capacity in the form of empty beds began to drive competition. The diffusion of technology into the community in conjunction with increased numbers of available neonatologists made competition for neonatal patients a possibility. Managed care plans captured an increasing share of the traditional indemnity plan markets and required hospitals to be full-service providers, making competition a reality. Obstetric and newborn services, once seen as avoidable losses, became a requirement of participation in health plans.

In some parts of the country, other factors hastened the move to competition. The medical liability crisis of the 1980s and the huge legal awards for poor neonatal outcome, particularly in the southern United States, increased the desire to have a neonatologist present at almost every delivery. At the same time, the presence of a hospital-based neonatologist presented the opportunity and the necessity to expand neonatal services beyond the delivery room into newly acquired NICU beds in an attempt to cover the costs of the neonatologist and to present appropriate clinical challenges to him or her and the nursery staff. In other regions, the overcrowding of level III units and the need to back transport convalescing neonates provided additional opportunity for community hospitals to begin neonatal programs. The differences in the levels of care, as defined by the COPH and by the American Academy of Pediatrics, became blurred. A comprehensive study of regionalization revealed a general weakening of structures and relationships, with many hospitals and physicians working outside the designed networks (91). As a result, the COPH was reconvened in 1990 to respond to the changing health care environment and to make recommendations for the regionalization of perinatal care in the 1990s and beyond.

The COPH's report reinforced the concept of regionalization of perinatal services, emphasizing the need for developing systems that integrate all levels of care within the region into a matrix with specific mechanisms for quality review and accountability between and among the various components. To facilitate this integration, the COPH suggested the formation of state and regional perinatal boards with the authority and responsibility for providing or coordinating regional planning, monitoring access, data collection, and providing education (4). The plan's foundation appeared to be very regulatory in nature at a time when competition and the market were still very strong. As a result, very little progress has been made on the implementation of its recommendations.

Managed Care and Regionalization of Perinatal Services

The market forces responsible for the evolution of the practice of neonatology in the 1980s and early 1990s are intensifying as payers attempt to cut costs even further. Because reproductive health and perinatal services represent 25% to 40% of all non-Medicare health maintenance organization expenses, insurance companies and managed care organizations are negotiating tighter contracts with hospitals and physicians (92). Reduced reimbursement is forcing providers to also cut costs. In areas where competition is most intense, the pressure to cut costs is translated into a reduction in LOS for both obstetric and neonatal patients (93). The lower LOS results in empty beds in a system that already appears to contain excess capacity. Ultimately, a critical point is reached when it is no longer profitable to offer the service, and consolidation of providers occurs. Using a managed care model that predicts bed utilization, National Perinatal Information Center (NPIC) estimates that by the year 2000, the need for level II and III NICU beds will be between 41% and 56% less than the 17,630 existing beds in 1996 (Fig. 3–13) (92). These levels of excess capacity will result in consolidations and mergers as the market attempts to concentrate high-tech services in a few strategically placed centers. Many have been concerned that quality of care will suffer in a health care delivery system driven by market forces (10). Balancing this concern is the realization that managed care organizations are required to internally monitor quality and state agencies are beginning to report rough outcome and satisfaction data to payers and plan members. In areas of the country

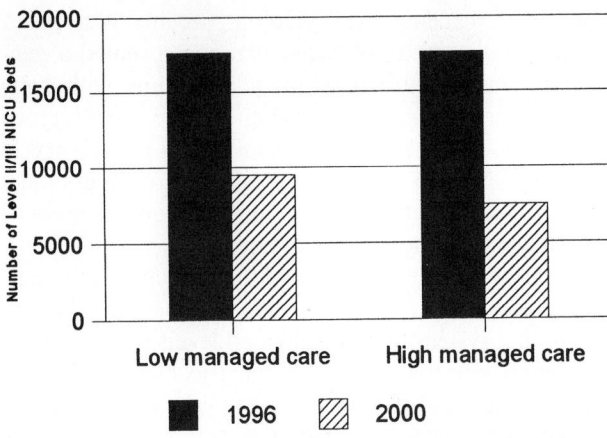

FIG. 3–13. Decline in the required number of level II and III NICU beds in the United States between 1996 and 2000. If managed care has a low penetration rate in 2000, the model predicts a 41% decline in needed NICU beds. If managed care has a high penetration rate in 2000, the model predicts a 56% decline in needed NICU beds. (From ref. 92.)

most affected by the managed care movement, regionalization is returning and quality of care is being preserved (94,95). If this trend continues, the competitive market perhaps may be able to accomplish what the COPH could not. Regionalization could be based on forces that appear to be responsive to change in levels of need, rather than on tradition and cooperation.

REFERENCES

1. Goodman RA, ed. Morbidity and mortality weekly report. Zidovudine for the prevention of HIV transmission from mother to infant. Washington: US Department of Health and Human Services/Public Health Services, 1994:43.
2. Clevenger SS, ed. *CDF reports.* Children's Defense Fund 1997;8:1.
3. State Child Health Insurance Program (SCHIP). Amendments to the Social Security Act, Title XXI, Balanced Budget Act of 1997. P.L. 105-33.
4. Committee on Perinatal Health. *Toward improving the outcome of pregnancy:* the 90's and beyond. White Plains, NY: The National Foundation-March of Dimes, 1993.
5. Pediatric Excellence in Health Delivery Systems. National Association of Children's Hospitals and Related Institutions, Alexandria, VA, 1996.
6. Stahlman MT. Improving health care provision to neonates in the United States. *American Journal of Diseases of Childhood AJDC* 1993; 147:516.
7. Schwartz RM. Supply and demand for neonatal intensive care: trends and implications. *J Perinatol* 1996;16:483.
8. Jung AL, Streeter NS. Total population estimate of newborn special care needs. *Pediatrics* 1985;75:993.
9. Hurth JC, Merenstein GB, eds. *Guidelines for perinatal care,* 4th ed. Elk Grove, IL: American Academy of Pediatrics and American College of Obstetrics and Gynecology, 1997.
10. Bowen FW. Neonatology in a managed care environment. *J Perinatol* 1995;15:403.
11. American Board of Pediatrics. Sub-board of neonatal and perinatal medicine. *Personal communication,* November 1997.
12. Bhatt DR, Escobedo M, Kattwinkel J, et al. *1996 United States Neonatologists Directory.* Elk Grove, IL: Section on Perinatal Pediatrics, American Academy of Pediatrics, 1996.
13. Merenstein GB, Rhodes PG, Little GA. Personnel in neonatal pediatrics: assessment of numbers and distribution. *Pediatrics* 1985;76:454.
14. Accreditation Council for Graduate Medical Education. *1996–97 direc-tory of graduate medical education programs.* Chicago, IL: American Medical Association, 1997.
15. Dunn MR, Miller RS. U.S. Graduate Medical Education, 1996–97. *JAMA* 1997;278:750.
16. American Academy of Pediatrics Committee on Fetus and Newborn. Manpower needs in neonatal pediatrics. *Pediatrics* 1985;76:312.
17. Merenstein GB. The pediatrician s role in the level II nursery. *Pediatr Ann* 1988;17:453.
18. Avery GB. The pediatrician and neonatology today. *Pediatr Ann* 1988; 17:7.
19. Bose CL, La Pine TR, Jung AL. Neonatal back-transport cost-effectiveness. *Med Care* 1985;23:14.
20. Martin RG, Fenton LJ, Leonardson G, Reid TJ. Consistency of care in an intensive care nursery staffed by nurse clinicians. *Am J Dis Child* 1985;139:169.
21. Cassidy G. Through the looking glass—or look before you leap. *Pediatrics* 1982:70:1001.
22. Resnick MB, Eyler FD, Nelson RM, Eitzman DV, Bucciarelli RL. Developmental intervention for low birth weight infants: improved early developmental outcome. *Pediatrics* 1987;80:68.
23. Leib SA, Benfield G, Guidubaldi J. Effects of early intervention and stimulation on the preterm infant. *Pediatrics* 1980;66:83.
24. Achenbach TM, Phares V, Howell CT, Rauh VA, Nurcombe B. Seven-year outcome of the Vermont Intervention Program for low birth weight infants. *Child Dev* 1990;61:1672.
25. Resnick MB, Eitzman DV, Dickman H, et al. Data base management for Children's Medical Services Regional Perinatal Intensive Care Centers program. *J Fla Med Assoc* 1983;70:718.
26. Stevenson RC, McCabe CJ, Pharoah OD, Cooke RW. Cost of care for a geographically determined population of low birth weight infants to age 8-9 years. I. Children without disability. *Arch Dis Child* 1996;74: 114.
27. Resnick MB, Ariet M, Carter RL, et al. Prospective pricing system by diagnosis-related groups: comparison of federal diagnosis-related groups with high-risk obstetric care groups. *Am J Obstet Gynecol* 1987; 156:567.
28. Resnick MB, Ariet M, Carter RL, et al. Prospective pricing system for tertiary neonatal intensive care. *Pediatrics* 1986;78:820.
29. Resnick MB, Ariet M, Carter RL, et al. Prospective pricing model for neonatologists and obstetricians in tertiary care centers. *Pediatrics* 1988;82:442.
30. State of Florida Department of Health and Rehabilitative Services. *Children's Medical Services regional perinatal intensive care center program handbook.* Tallahassee: State of Florida Department of Health and Rehabilitative Services, 1987.
31. Regional Perinatal Intensive Care Program. *Florida Department of Health, Children's Medical Services annual report FY 1995–96.* Tallahassee: Florida Department of Health, 1996.
32. Regional Perinatal Intensive Care Program. *Department of Health and Rehabilitative Services, Children's Medical Services annual report FY 1996–97.* Tallahassee: Florida Department of Health and Rehabilitative Services, 1998.
33. Walker DB, Vohr BR, Oh W. Economic analysis of regionalized neonatal care for very low-birth-weight infants in the state of Rhode Island. *Pediatrics* 1985;76:69.
34. Boyle MH, Torrance GO, Sinclair J, Horwood SP. Economic evaluation of neonatal intensive care of very-low-birth-weight infants. *N Engl J Med* 1983;308:1330.
35. Muldoon J. Florida profiles its hospitals. In: *Today.* Alexandria, VA: National Association of Children's Hospitals and Related Institutions, 1996;Summer:10.
36. Khoshnood B, Lee K, Corpuz M, et al. Models for determining cost of care and length of stay in neonatal intensive care units. *Int J Tech Assess Health Care* 1996;12:62.
37. Berk SE, Schneier NB. Frequency and cost of DRG outliers among newborns. *Pediatrics* 1987;79:874.
38. Lichtig LK, Knauf RA, Bartoletti A, et al. Revising diagnosis-related groups for neonates. *Pediatrics* 1989;84:49.
39. Shankaran S, Cohen SN, Linver M, Zonia S. Medical care costs of high-risk infants after neonatal intensive care: a controlled study. *Pediatrics* 1988;81:372.
40. Committee on Children, Health Insurance, and Access to Care. *Health insurance and access to care for children.* Washington: Institute of Medicine, 1998.

41. Stevenson RC, Pharoah PO, Stevenson CJ, et al. Cost of care for a geographically determined population of low birthweight infants to age 8–9 years. II Children with disability. *Arch Dis Child* 1996;74:117.

42. Walker DB, Feldman A, Vhor BR, Oh W. Cost–benefit analysis of neonatal intensive care for infants weighing less than 1000 grams at birth. *Pediatrics* 1984;74:20.

43. US Congress, Office of Technology Assessment. Neonatal intensive care for low birth weight infants: cost and effectiveness. Health technology case study 38. Washington: US Government Printing Office, 1987.

44. Hack M, Horbar JD, Malloy MH, et al. Very low-birthweight outcomes of the National Institute of Child Health and Human Development Neonatal Network. *Pediatrics* 1991;87:587.

45. Kitzhaber JA. The Oregon model. In: *The Richard and Linda Rosenthal lectures. Improving access to affordable health care.* Washington: Institute of Medicine, 1990:69.

46. Developmental Disabilities Planning Council State of Florida. *Florida's children, their future is in our hands:* the report of the Task Force for Prevention of Developmental Handicaps. Tallahassee: The Florida Developmental Disabilities Planning Council, 1991:11.

47. Committee to Study the Prevention of Low Birth Weight. *Preventing low birthweight.* Washington: National Academy Press, 1985.

48. Imershein AW, Turner C, Wells JG, Pearman A. Covering the costs of care in neonatal intensive care units. *Pediatrics* 1992;89:56.

49. Foley JD, Employee Benefit Research Institute. *Uninsured in the United States:* the nonelderly population without health insurance—analysis of the March 1990 current population survey. Special Report SR-10. Washington: Employee Research Institute, 1991.

50. American Academy of Pediatrics. *Children first:* a legislative proposal. Washington: American Academy of Pediatrics, Department of Governmental Relations, 1991.

51. Children's Defense Fund. *S.O.S. America! A children's defense budget.* Washington: The Children's Defense Fund, 1990:160.

52. Gabel JR, Jensen GA. The price of state mandated benefits. *Inquiry* 1989;26:419.

53. Ford M. Medicaid: FY 1991 budget and child health initiatives. CRS issue brief. Washington: Library of Congress, 1991.

54. American Academy of Pediatrics. *Medicaid state reports, FY 1989.* Washington: American Academy of Pediatrics, Department of Research, 1991.

55. American Academy of Pediatrics. *Medicaid state reports, FY 1995.* Washington: American Academy of Pediatrics, Department of Research, 1996.

56. American Academy of Pediatrics. *Children and health insurance, 1997.* Elk Grove Village, IL: American Academy of Pediatrics, 1997.

57. Hewlett SA. *When the bough breaks.* New York: Basic Books, 1991:169.

58. Kenny AM, Torres A, Ditts W, Macias J. Medicaid expenditures for maternity and newborn care in America. *Fam Plann Perspect* 1986;18:103.

59. US Congress, Department of Labor, Health and Human Services and Education and Related Agencies for FY Ending 9/98. PL 105-78 Conference agreement. Washington: US Government Printing Office.

60. National Commission on Children. *Beyond rhetoric: a new American agenda for children and families.* Washington: National Commission on Children, 1991:122.

61. Wegman M. Annual summary of vital statistics. *Pediatrics* 1991;88:108.

62. Guyer B, Martin JA, MacDorman MF, et al. Annual summary of vital statistics. *Pediatrics* 1996;100:905.

63. *The State of America's Children's 1997.* Washington: Children's Defense Fund, 1997.

64. *The State of the World's Children 1998.* United Nation Children's Fund. New York: Oxford University Press, 1998:94.

65. Hogart DL. Perinatal mortality in the United States, 1985–91. National Center for Health Statistics. *Vital Health Statistics* 1995:20.

66. Gabbe SG, Niebye JN, Simpson JL, eds. *Obstetrics:* normal and problem pregnancies. New York: Churchill Livingstone, 1986:271.

67. Committee to Study the Prevention of Low Birth Weight. *Preventing low birth weight.* Washington: National Academy Press, 1985.

68. Children's Defense Fund. *Maternal and child health in America.* Special report three. Washington: Children's Defense Fund, 1991:20.

69. Robert Wood Johnson Foundation. *Challenges in health care:* perspective 1991. Princeton: RWJ Foundation 1991:35.

70. US Congress, Office of Technology Assessment. Neonatal intensive care for low birth weight infants: cost and effectiveness. Health technology case study 38. Washington: US Government Printing Office, 1987.

71. Shiono PH, Behrman RE. Low birth weight analysis and recommendation. *The Future of Children* 1995;5:4.

72. Chomitz VR, Cheung L, Lieberman E. The role of lifestyle in preventing low birth weight. The David and Lucile Packard Foundation. *The Future of Children* 1995;5:121.

73. Mills JL, Gravard BJ, Hanley EE, et al. Maternal alcohol consumption and birth weight: how much drinking during pregnancy is safe? *JAMA* 1994;252:1875.

74. Larroque B, Kaminski M, Lelory N, et al. Effects on birth weight of alcohol and caffeine consumption during pregnancy. *Am J Epidemiology* 1993;137:941.

75. Halmesmaki E, Raivio R, Ylikoukale O. Patterns of alcohol consumption during pregnancy. *Obstet Gynecol* 1987;69:594.

76. Chasnoff IJ, Burns WJ, Schnoll SH, Burns KA. Cocaine use in pregnancy. *N Engl J Med* 1985;313:666.

77. Chasnoff IJ. Drug use in women, establishing standard of care. *Ann N Y Acad Sci* 1989;562:208.

78. Frank DA, Zuckerman BS, Amaro H, et al. Cocaine use during pregnancy: prevalence and correlates. *Pediatrics* 1988;82:888.

79. Dixon SD, Bresnahan K, Zuckerman B. Cocaine babies: meeting the challenge of management. *Contemp Pediatr* 1990;7:70.

80. Chasnoff IJ, Bussey ME, Savich R, Stack CM. Clinical and laboratory observations. *J Pediatr* 1986;108:456.

81. NIDA Notes. National Institute on Drug Abuse. 1995;10:6.

82. Chiu TTW, Vaughn AJ, Carzoli RP. Hospital costs for cocaine-exposed infants. *J Fla Med Assoc* 1990;77:897.

83. Behnke ML, Eyler FD, Conlin M, Casanova OQ, Woods NS. How fetal cocaine exposure insures neonatal hospital costs. *Pediatrics* 1997;99:204.

84. Roth J, Resnick MB, Ariet M, et al. Changes in survival patterns of very low birth weight infants from 1980 to 1993. *Arch Pediatr Adolesc Med* 1995;149:1311.

85. Grogaard JB, Lindstrom DP, Parker RA, Culley B, Stahlman MT. Increased survival rate in very low birth weight infants (1500 grams or less): no association with increased incidence of handicaps. *J Pediatr* 1990;117:139.

86. Teplin SW, Burchinal M, Johnson-Martin N, Humphry RA, Kraybill EN. Neurodevelopmental, health, and growth status at age 6 years of children with birth weights less than 1001 grams. *J Pediatr* 1991;118:768.

87. Resnick MB, Stralka K, Carter RL, et al. Effects of birth weight and sociodemographic variables on mental development of neonatal intensive care unit survivors. *Am J Obstet Gynecol* 1990;162:374.

88. Resnick MB, Roth J, Ariet, M, et al. Educational outcome of neonatal intensive care graduates. *Pediatrics* 1992;89:373.

89. Resnick MB, Gomatam SV, Carter RL, et al. Educational disabilities of neonatal intensive care graduates. *Pediatrics* 1998 (*in press*).

90. Committee on Perinatal Health. *Toward improving the outcome of pregnancy.* White Plains: The National Foundation March of Dimes, 1977, pp 7–34.

91. Gagnon DE, Allison-Cook S, Schwartz RM. Perinatal care: the threat of re-regionalization. *Pediatr Ann* 1988:17:447.

92. Smulian D, Campbell D, Gagnon DE. Managed care's impact on perinatal services. The Medici Report. *Medici Healthcare Consulting* 1996;2:35.

93. Marbella AM, Chetty VK, Layde PM. Neonatal hospital lengths of stay, readmissions, and charges. *Pediatrics* 1998;101:32.

94. Richardson DK, Reed K, Cutler C, et al. Perinatal regionalization versus hospital competition: the Harford example. *Pediatrics* 1995;96:417.

95. Wirtschafter DD. Perinatal services in the era of managed care: A Kaiser Permanente physician's perspective. *J Perinatol* 1995;15:414.

CHAPTER 4

Neonatal Transport

Carl L. Bose

In 1900, the development of the first mobile incubator for the care of "weakly and prematurely born infants" was described by Dr. Joseph DeLee, of the Chicago Lying-In Hospital (1). This incubator was used to transport "these delicate infants from distant parts of the city and suburbs" (1). The development of this device represented a recognition of the need to create a controlled environment for the transport of infants that simulated the inpatient environment. The first report of an organized transport program in the United States appeared in 1950 (2). This program was sponsored by the New York Department of Health in conjunction with area hospitals. This remarkable system, created long before the evolution of neonatal intensive care, incorporated many of the features of modern neonatal transport programs. These included around-the-clock staffing by specially trained nurses, dedicated vehicles, a clerk to receive referral calls, and equipment designed specifically for neonatal transport. During a 2-year period, this program transported 1,209 patients, of whom 194 weighed less than 1,000 g (3).

Except at a few major medical centers, organized transport programs were not available until the late 1970s, when perinatal care was regionalized in many areas. Regionalization had two effects on transport. First, the number of infants requiring transport was minimized by shifting the hospital of birth to a center capable of delivering neonatal intensive care. Second, the responsibility for transporting infants shifted to tertiary centers. For example, in 1976 in North Carolina, fewer than 40% of very-low-birth-weight (VLBW) infants were delivered in level III hospitals; approximately 30% were delivered in level I hospitals (Fig. 4–1). By 1982, after the evolution of an organized program of regionalized perinatal care, more than 70% of VLBW infants were delivered in level

III hospitals. The remainder, however, continued to be delivered in community hospitals ill-equipped to manage high-risk infants. During the remainder of the 1980s, the percentage of VLBW infants delivered in level III centers changed little. Since the late 1980s, patterns of referral dictated by schemes of regionalization have deteriorated in many areas (4). The percentage of VLBW infants born in small community hospitals with limited resources remains small. However, a significant number of larger hospitals without subspecialists and limited support services now deliver infants of VLBW and extreme prematurity.

The impact on transport programs of regionalization and, more recently, deregionalization has been significant. The continued delivery of VLBW infants in hospitals incapable of providing for all of the needs of neonatal patients is inevitable, because of either a conscious choice on the part of obstetric caretakers or unpredictable, emergent events. Even in areas where regionalized perinatal care persists and prenatal risk assessment is routine, neonatal transport of some VLBW infants is still necessary. The impact of community-based neonatal intensive care has been the more frequent need to transport infants at a critical time in their illness, occasionally while receiving therapies that are not easily portable, e.g., high-frequency ventilation. It is clear that neonatal transport remains a necessity and may now require greater expertise and sophistication.

Neonatal transport can be performed by either the community hospital referring the patient (one-way transport) or by the tertiary center receiving the patient (two-way transport). In most perinatal regions, two-way transport is preferable for economic and other reasons (5). Two-way transport also may result in improved survival (6,7). For these reasons, the responsibility of tertiary centers to provide two-way neonatal transport generally has been accepted and is recommended by the American Academy of Pediatrics (8).

C. L. Bose: Department of Pediatrics, University of North Carolina at Chapel Hill; and Division of Neonatal-Perinatal Medicine, UNC Hospitals, Chapel Hill, North Carolina

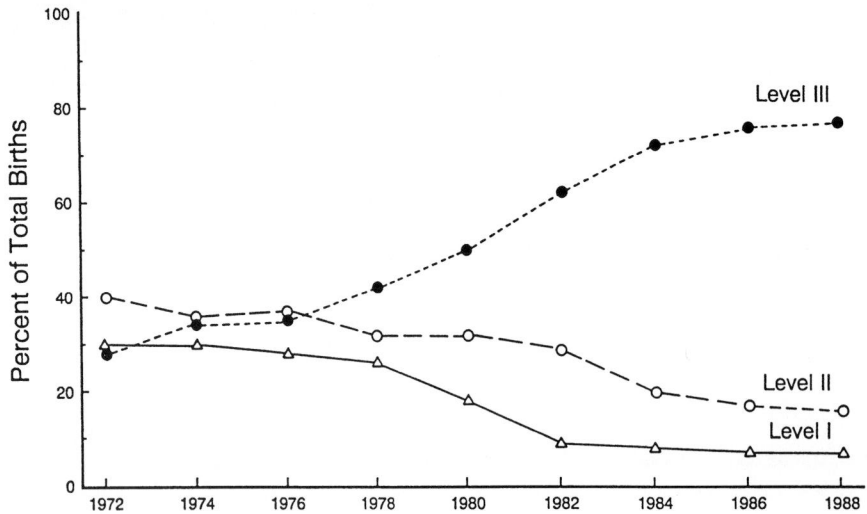

FIG. 4–1. Percentage of live births of infants with birth weights less than 1,500 g born in level I, II, and III hospitals in North Carolina from 1972 to 1988. (R. Nugent, *personal communication,* 1989.)

ORGANIZATION AND ADMINISTRATION

Administrative Personnel

Transport programs have components that generally can be categorized into those related to medical care and those related to transportation, communications, and finances, the nonmedical components. The medical components of a transport program must fall under the direction of a physician who is credentialed to supervise the patients served by the program. Direction of the non-medical components of the program often is the responsibility of a member of the hospital administration (Fig. 4–2). This division of responsibility may create problems when the interests of various components compete; in practice, however, the division is rarely this precise. Rather, a collaborative effort exists that takes advantage of the availability and expertise of professionals in all

disciplines (9). A brief discussion of each of the potential contributors to the administration of a transport program follows.

Hospital Administrator

A hospital administrator generally is responsible for those aspects of the program that are not directly related to patient care. Many decisions on the operation of a program require an analysis of costs and benefits. Whereas medical personnel generally are relied on to provide an estimate of benefit, the hospital administrator must assess financial impact. Therefore, the hospital administrator should be prepared to receive advice from medical personnel and develop the nonmedical components of the program in consideration of the financial resources of the institution.

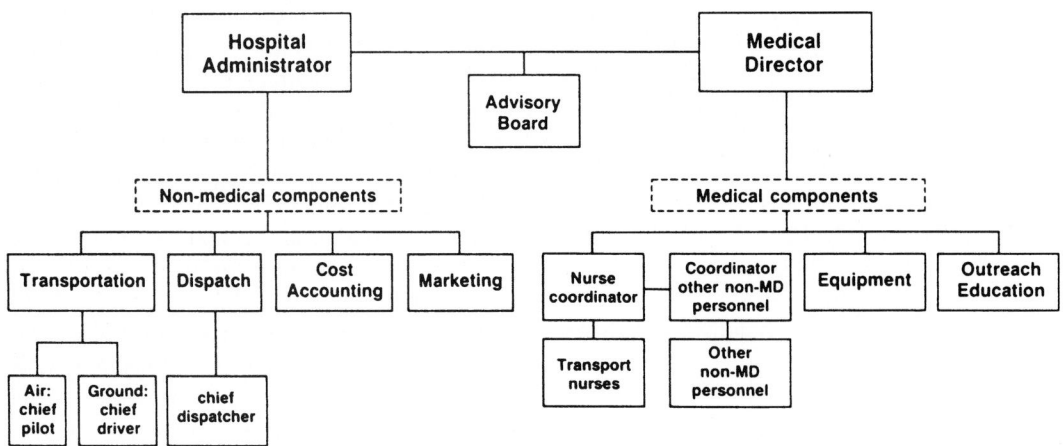

FIG. 4–2. The administrative structure of a typical neonatal transport program.

Medical Director

The medical director of a neonatal transport program usually is a neonatologist who has expertise or a special interest in transport. The medical director is ultimately responsible for the quality of care provided by the transport team; this is particularly true if physicians do not participate directly in transport. The medical director is responsible for developing training programs and treatment protocols. The medical director, in conjunction with the coordinator of nonphysician personnel, must ensure that all personnel have completed training requirements successfully and have satisfied the regulations of the agencies that govern the various professional groups. The director also must develop and maintain a system for reviewing the quality of care provided during transport.

Coordinator of Nonphysician Personnel

Each group of professionals (e.g., nurses and respiratory therapists) on the transport team should have a person who is designated as the coordinator of that group. The coordinator should supervise the selection and training of personnel and develop a system of peer review. This person should be responsible for scheduling and identifying the needs of team members. It also is advisable to designate a single person to coordinate team activities who will interface closely with the medical director. Most often, this person will be the nurse coordinator of the team.

Consulting Neonatalogists and Other Subspecialists

During the transport of a patient, it is important, and often mandated by law, that a physician provide consultation to the transport team. The logical person to provide such consultation is the one who will receive the patient on return to the tertiary center. This person often already has discussed the patient's care with the referring physician and made suggestions about interim care. Given this broad consultative role to both the referring physician and to the transport team, the consultant should be a person with extensive training, at a level in excess of that available in the community hospital. For this reason, the consultant usually should be a neonatologist or comparably trained subspecialist, or a postdoctoral fellow. In addition, the consultant must be aware of the handicaps and hazards imposed by the transport environment and must be familiar with the operational aspects of the program.

The Advisory Board

A transport program should be considered an extension of the inpatient unit to which it delivers patients. Therefore, the operation of the program should be reviewed periodically by representatives of all of the services that interface with the inpatient unit. These representatives might include the following:

- Medical Director of the Neonatal Intensive Care Unit (NICU)
- Director of the Neonatal Division
- Respiratory Therapy Administrator
- Nursing Administrator
- Outreach Education Coordinator
- Director of Public Relations
- Representatives of other hospitals to which patients are transported.

Advice should be solicited from this group about all major changes in the program because of the impact these changes may have on their respective services.

The Transport Team

A variety of personnel participate in the inpatient care of infants; all should be considered candidates for caretakers during neonatal transport. These personnel include the following:

- Neonatologists
- Neonatal fellows
- Pediatric housestaff
- Nurse practitioners
- Transport nurses
- NICU staff nurses
- Respiratory therapists.

The selection of the type of personnel used by each program usually is based on the unique aspects of that program; however, some general principles apply that determine the relative desirability of various professionals. As the number of transports increases, it becomes less practical to send physicians on transport. Neonatologists rarely have sufficient time to devote to frequent transports, and reimbursement usually is not adequate to support a neonatologist's professional effort. Although participation in transport can be very educational, in high-volume programs, time spent on transport by housestaff and fellows often competes with other aspects of training. In addition, the interest in participation and expertise may vary considerably among trainees. This is a particular problem when participation is mandated. If pediatric residents participate in transport, they should be senior-level trainees and be supervised closely.

Most high-volume programs have chosen to use nonphysician personnel as attendants during transport. The use of neonatal nurse practitioners offers an attractive alternative to physician attendance (10). Nurse practitioners generally are highly skilled and provide a consistency of expertise not usually encountered in other professional groups. They are licensed in most states to perform all the diagnostic and therapeutic procedures required during transport. The greatest disadvantage to the use of neonatal nurse practitioners in some regions is their scarcity and their relatively high salaries. Also, they are rarely trained, or willing, to transport patients other than neonates.

As an alternative to nurse practitioners, many centers have chosen to train NICU staff nurses to participate in transport. This often is a very practical alternative, because salaries of staff nurses are less than those of practitioners, and they generally are more available. In addition, in most states, they are permitted to perform invasive procedures as an extension of their inpatient nursing role under guidelines and protocols approved by the boards of nursing. Therefore, they can be trained to provide all the care required by a critically ill neonate during transport. This training often is extensive, however, because most staff nurses lack the cognitive knowledge necessary to diagnose problems and the experience in performing invasive procedures. This extensive training must be considered when estimating the cost of using staff nurses compared to nurse practitioners. The requirement of training is particularly burdensome when the turnover rate of personnel is high.

Most patients transported to NICUs either have respiratory failure requiring mechanical ventilation or are receiving supplemental oxygen. For this reason, respiratory therapists should be considered when selecting transport personnel. Their expertise in the use and maintenance of respiratory care equipment is extremely valuable. Physicians and nurses rarely have acquired this expertise. The therapists' ability to adapt this equipment to the unique environment of transport can be life-saving, particularly in circumstances when unexpected events occur. The only disadvantage of using therapists is the narrow focus of their usual training. They rarely are prepared to assist with aspects of care beyond respiratory therapies. This disadvantage can be minimized by cross-training them to perform tasks generally assigned to physicians and nurses.

Eliminating physicians from attendance during transport can create problems that must be anticipated. Advisory personnel at the tertiary center, particularly physicians, often are unwilling to endorse a patient care program that does not mandate initial evaluation by a physician. This resistance usually stems from a concern for the well-being of the patient and can be overcome by the selection and training of competent nonphysician personnel. The support and endorsement of an involved medical director also may be critical. A similar attitude may prevail in community hospitals. Referring physicians may find it unacceptable to relinquish care of a critically ill patient to nonphysician personnel. In an environment in which tertiary centers compete for patients, this may be a motivation for maintaining physician attendance during transport. Most referring physicians, however, are concerned only with transferring their patients in a safe and timely fashion. Anecdotal experience and

one controlled study suggest that properly selected and trained nurses provide a satisfactory level of care during transport (11,12). Once a nonphysician team demonstrates its competence and efficiency, the concerns of most referring physicians will vanish. Because the use of specially trained nonphysician personnel represents both a safe and economic alternative to physician participation in neonatal transport, most programs now rely on nonphysician personnel for patient care.

Transport personnel must be proficient in cognitive knowledge of neonatal diseases, principles of management of acute problems, and technical skills. The method and extent of training necessary to reach proficiency will depend on the type of personnel; however, the pattern of preparation will be similar for all professionals (13). Cognitive knowledge is best provided in didactic sessions in conjunction with self-study exercises. Management principles also may be taught in a didactic setting, but refinement of these skills usually requires repeated experiences in the inpatient setting. Laboratory simulation of technical skills, such as intubation, umbilical catheterization, and thoracostomy tube placement, provide a good introduction to these procedures. These skills then can be refined in the inpatient setting under supervision. Demonstration of proficiency in these areas should be ensured by examination or observation by a qualified supervisor. After this initial preparation, a period of training should be provided, during which the trainee accompanies a more experienced team member on transport. Final certification of competence should be awarded by both the medical director and the coordinator for the trainee's professional group.

Communication

The success or failure of many transport programs depends on the quality of the communication system that supports the program (14). The communication system serves two basic functions: to provide a point of access for the physician referring a patient, and to coordinate the activities of the transport team. A single call by the referring physician should provide access to all of the services of the tertiary center related to neonatal care. The use of a toll-free hot line often associated with a memorable acronym is favored by some centers (15). An alternative is to request that referring physicians call the NICU directly. If consultation is requested, the referring physician should be connected in a timely fashion with a consultant of appropriate training. If transfer is requested and deemed appropriate, an available bed in the NICU of the tertiary center, or an alternate center if necessary, should be identified. Without further calls by the referring physician, the transport team should be dispatched.

In some parts of the country, locating an available and appropriate site of care is difficult because of a shortage of NICU beds or the lack of availability of subspecialty support in some centers. These regions often benefit from an organized system of identifying available resources. Several such programs exist and are of two varieties. In some areas, sophisticated computerized communications networks linking neighboring centers have been developed (16). An alternative is the use an operator-assisted central referral or bed locator system. These systems speed the referral of patients and relieve both referring physicians and the physician at the tertiary center of the burden of placing numerous calls to locate a bed.

Once a bed has been located and the decision has been made to transport the patient, the role of the communications system shifts to that of dispatching the team and disseminating information about the transport. In this role, the system is best served by a communication center that is staffed and equipped for emergency medical service functions. The referring hospital should be informed of the estimated time of arrival and of any necessary preparations for the arrival of the vehicle. The receiving unit should be notified and be provided with any information necessary for admission of the patient.

During the conduct of the transport, periodic communication between the dispatch center and the vehicle operator is advisable. In so doing, unexpected delays or mishaps are identified promptly and appropriate action taken. When the transport team does not include a physician, the team should have the capability of communicating directly with the consulting physician at all times. This level of communication is mandated by the nurse practice acts in some states. This is a trivial problem while the team is in the referring hospital, but it can present a challenge during transit. This problem usually can be solved by the acquisition of telecommunications equipment. The use of cellular phones is ideal during ground transport because of the broad coverage in most areas and the general familiarity with this type of communication. The use of VHF and UHF radios with patching devices to phone lines is an alternative during flight.

Many communication centers are equipped with automated devices that record all communications. Although not essential, the recordings made by these devices may be valuable educational tools and often are critical if a medicolegal question arises.

Financial Considerations

Subjecting a transport program to periodic cost–benefit analyses is a critical aspect of the program's operation. The following elements should be included in the cost of operation:

- Medical components
- Nonphysician personnel salaries
- Salary support of the medical director
- Equipment and supplies
- Medication

- Expenses related to education of personnel
- Nonmedical components
- Administrative overhead
- Vehicle operation and maintenance
- Communications
- Educational and marketing material.

Identifying the costs associated with the program may be difficult if its operation is financially integrated into the operation of the NICU. For example, personnel costs often are difficult to quantify because, except in very high-volume programs, transport personnel usually contribute to inpatient services during transport duty time. Therefore, the cost assigned to the transport program should be discounted based on this contribution. The proportion of time devoted by the medical director is even more difficult to quantify and often is ignored in the financial analysis. The cost of equipment is most easily separated from the cost of inpatient services because transport equipment rarely is used for purposes other than transport. Included in estimates of equipment costs should be allowances for depreciation and maintenance.

The nonmedical components of a program often are more costly than the medical components because of expenses related to transportation. This is particularly true when air transportation is used. The expense of transportation can be minimized by sharing resources with other hospitals or agencies. Ground ambulances may be shared with local emergency medical service agencies or be used for convalescent transport. Aircraft sometimes can be used by a consortium of hospitals. The major disadvantage of this approach is the possibility of a vehicle being unavailable at the time of a request for transport; however, the potential for this occasional conflict may be far outweighed by the cost reductions.

The net costs of a program are determined by subtracting costs from revenues, which come from three general sources: reimbursement, support from governmental agencies, and support from other extramural organizations (17). Support from government and charitable organizations is now unusual. Hospitals are increasingly dependent on reimbursement to support transport programs. Unfortunately, the costs of a transport program nearly always exceed the revenues. Subsistence of the program therefore depends on subsidy by the sponsor hospital.

The decision to fund a transport program usually is based on a favorable cost–benefit analysis, and benefit is extremely difficult to define. Medical personnel typically define benefit in terms of medical outcomes, morbidity, and mortality. Although there has been a number of studies that support the use of hospital-based transport programs for adult patients based on improved morbidity and mortality, these studies are not necessarily applicable to neonates (18,19). In an attempt to quantify the benefits of a neonatal transport program, the most prudent approach may be to scrutinize carefully the type of patients being transported to ensure that they are likely to benefit from transport. These benefits should be combined with nonmedical benefits to the institution, such as improved public relations and recruitment of new patients. Unfortunately, managed care may have diminished the traditional benefit of transport programs as services that help recruit patients. As a greater portion of a potential population is covered by managed care, particularly capitated contracts, transport programs are more likely to be considered merely resource consumptive. Under these circumstances, transport programs will have to justify their expenses based on the provision of a critical service, one that improves a significant outcome, e.g., decreased length of stay.

A potential economy may be to combine services, either within a program or between programs. An example of the former would be to cross-train members of specialty transport teams, e.g., pediatric, neonatal, and adult, such that the total number of personnel can be reduced. This strategy invariably results in some loss of expertise but may be necessary to ensure financial viability. Collaboration between programs may include the sharing of vehicles or teams. Smaller institutions may benefit from outsourcing entirely, that is, contracting with larger medical centers for the provision of all transport services.

TECHNICAL ASPECTS

The Transport Environment

The principles of care provided during transport are not different from the principles of inpatient care. Any differences in practices arise from the unique features of the transport environment (20). The following features may distinguish the environment in transport vehicles from the inpatient environment:

- Excessive noise
- Vibration
- Improper lighting
- Variable ambient temperature and humidity
- Changes in barometric pressure
- Confined space
- Limited support services.

High sound levels are already inherent to the NICU; although dependent on the type of vehicle, levels recorded during transport are significantly higher (21,22). Brief exposure to these levels probably has little long-term effect on the caretakers; however, repeated exposure over time may result in hearing loss. High-frequency range hearing loss is a well-recognized occupational hazard of pilots. Personnel should protect themselves from exposure by using sound-attenuating devices. The effects of exposure to high sound levels on the neonate are not known. The possibility of physiologic changes, however, is suggested by studies of hospitalized infants (23). Probably the most significant problem resulting from high sound levels is the inability to use auscultation to assess the patient. This handicap must be recognized before transport. Alternative methods for assessing heart rate and respiratory sufficiency must be available during transport.

Exposure to vibration is a problem unique to the transport environment (24). The physiologic consequences of this exposure are not known. Animal studies and investigation using healthy adults suggest that effects on the autonomic and central nervous system may occur (25,26). Whether these effects are a hazard to a critically ill patient is unknown. The effects on personnel may be less profound but are potentially more important. For example, a typical helicopter transport results in vibration exposure associated with reduced efficiency (27). The overt symptoms of motion sickness resulting from low-frequency vibration may be incapacitating. A more subtle manifestation of motion sickness, termed the sopite syndrome, also may affect personnel (28). The symptoms associated with this syndrome include drowsiness, inability to concentrate, and disinclination to communicate with others. The sopite syndrome is common among personnel during transport, regardless of the mode of transportation (29). The impact on patient care is poorly understood but may be significant.

The effect of vibration on equipment also constitutes a major problem. Monitor artifact is a common phenomenon. Personnel should be familiar with monitor artifact and with the use of alternative monitoring techniques. The selection of equipment should be made in consideration of resistance to the effects of vibration. Premature failure of equipment should be anticipated, and preventive maintenance should be on an accelerated schedule. The problem of early obsolescence should be anticipated when transport budgets are developed.

An appreciation of the problems created by the transport environment and plans to minimize these problems are essential for safe transport. Some general principles include the following:

Prepare the transport vehicle. The vehicle should be retrofitted to simulate the inpatient environment as much as is possible and practical. This generally requires that supplemental lighting, sound insulation, and a regulated heating–cooling system be added.

Assess and stabilize the patient extensively before transport. Most neonates have problems that can be managed adequately by the transport team. Rarely is there urgency in returning to the tertiary center. Therefore, time spent in the community hospital preparing the patient for transport is not time wasted. This stabilization will prepare the patient for the most risky period of transport, the time in transit between hospitals.

Monitor electronically all possible physiologic parameters. Because of the dynamic nature of the diseases in most transported patients and the inability to assess patients by physical examination, electronic monitoring is critical to the identification of significant changes in physiology.

Anticipate deterioration. All possible forms of deterioration should be anticipated before transport; strategies to support the patient in the event of deterioration should be planned. Application of this principle often results in the performance of procedures or therapies that may not be necessary in the inpatient setting. For example, intubation and ventilation may not be necessary for mild degrees of respiratory failure or apnea in the hospitalized patient, but may be advisable before transport because of the difficulty of intubation during transport.

Equipment

Before the 1970s, transport equipment generally was fabricated from equipment acquired from the NICU. Although this equipment often was designed with great ingenuity, failures or inadequacies often occurred. In the past two decades, considerable effort has been devoted to the development of devices specifically for neonatal transport, resulting in greater safety. The following is a list of the major pieces of equipment used during transport:

Essential equipment
  Portable incubator
  Mechanical ventilator
  Cardiorespiratory monitor
  Blood pressure transducer
  Transcutaneous O_2 monitor or pulse oximeter
  Intravascular infusion pumps
  Air–oxygen blender
  Suction apparatus
Desirable equipment
  Body temperature monitor
  Transcutaneous CO_2 or end-tidal CO_2 monitor
  Noninvasive blood pressure monitor
  Airway humidification system.

Although these devices can be purchased individually and either carried separately or attached to the incubator, it usually is advisable, and often more economic, to purchase a modular incubator that includes many of the devices listed. Modular transport incubators have been designed to minimize space and weight. They also use a common battery power supply for most devices. Several of these incubators are commercially available. The logical choice for each program often depends on the size, weight, and heating capability of the unit.

Accessory equipment and supplies can be divided into respiratory care supplies and medical–nursing supplies. These supplies can be divided in this manner and carried in packs or equipment bags (Tables 4–1 through 4–4). They should be organized in a recognized and reproducible fashion. This technique will aid in rapidly locating a needed item and assist in restocking after use. It also is helpful to separate medications into an accessory pack.

Transport Vehicles

An essential component of neonatal transport is rapid, safe transportation. The types of vehicles in use include standard ambulances, specially prepared ground ambulances, helicopters, and fixed-wing aircraft. The selection of one or more of these vehicles to support a neonatal transport program usually is based on resources, geography, and practical issues, such as the use of the vehicle by other hospital-based services (30,31).

Ambulances are the least costly and most available; however, they generally require modest retrofitting to make them acceptable for neonatal transport. Extensive retrofitting, including the addition of radiant heat and a blood gas analyzer, improves patient care capabilities but dramatically increases costs and decreases the vehicle's usefulness for other services. The major disadvantage of ground ambulance transport is the long travel time compared to air transport. This disadvantage can be prohibitive if frequent long transports are anticipated.

Helicopters minimize transit time and, for distances between hospitals of up to 150 miles, usually provide the fastest service. The major disadvantages of helicopter transportation are the constraints of the patient care environment (e.g., limited space, high noise and vibration) and the high cost of operation. Although the impact of the former can be minimized, the cost of helicopter transportation usually cannot be justified unless the vehicle can be shared by other emergency medical services.

Fixed-wing aircraft are less costly, roomier, less noisy, and faster than helicopters. Because they must travel between airports, however, at least two additional transfers are required. These shuttles between the hospital and airport often are troublesome and may increase the likelihood of mishap. For these reasons, transportation by fixed-wing aircraft usually is advantageous only for distances between hospitals in excess of 150 miles.

Record Keeping

Transport programs traditionally have developed record-keeping systems that are unique and distinct from the inpatient record. The accurate, thorough record of each transport is essential for several reasons. As a part of the medical record, it provides permanent documentation of the care rendered. As such, it should adhere to the standards of record keeping of the sponsor institution. The record also is a valuable tool for quality assurance and

TABLE 4–1. *Neonatal nursing pack*

Equipment	Amount	Equipment	Amount
Procedure tray, sterile	1	Disposable transducer	2
Omphalocele bag, sterile	1	Scissors	1
Dextrostix bottle	1	Hemostat	1
Sterile lancets	5	Tape measure	1
Blood culture bottle	1	K-Y jelly	2
Angiocath		Disposable blood pressure cuffs	
18 gauge	2	Sizes 2, 3, 4, and 5	1 each
22 gauge	2	Pacificier	1
24 gauge	9	Bulb syringe	1
Intraosseous needles	2	Sterile gauze	2
IV limb board	2	Stopcocks	2
Rubber bands	6	Extension tubing	1
Safety pins	6	Thoracostomy tubes	
Tape		10 Fr	2
Silk	1 roll	12 Fr	2
Dermaclear	1 roll	Digital thermometer	1
Stethoscope	1	Umbilical catheters	
IV fluids		3.5 Fr	2
$D_{10}W$	1 500-mL bag	5.0 Fr	2
D_5W	1 500-mL bag	Heimlich valves	2
NS	1 100-mL bag	Alcohol and Betadine swabs	10 each
Masks	2	IV extension T-connectors	2
Syringes		Butterfly needles	
20-mL Luer Lok	2	19 gauge	2
60-mL Luer Lok	4	23 gauge	2
Transilluminator	1	25 gauge	3
Gloves, sterile		Syringes	
Size 6½	2 pairs	10 mL	3
Size 7½	2 pairs	3 mL	9
Suction catheters, sterile		1 mL	9
Size 6 Fr	2	60-cc catheter tip syringe	1
Size 8 Fr	2	60-cc Luer Lok syringe	4
Stockinette for caps	2	Needles, 19 gauge	10
Cotton balls	4	Purple adapters, blunt needles	2
Feeding tubes		Replogle, 10 Fr	2
8 Fr	2	Tubing	
5 Fr	2	Mini-volume extension	1
Gowns	2	Low-volume extension	4
Blood gas syringe	2	Blood component and filter set	1
Tegaderm	1	IV extension double "T"-connector	1

education. The critical components of a typical transport record include the following:

- Consultation–referral form
- Transport record
- Parental consent form
- Billing slip.

Quality Assurance

Review of the performance of a transport program should be a continual process and involve two strategies. First, all activities of the program should be reviewed periodically to ensure that standard operating procedures are being observed. These reviews are best conducted by people directly related to program activities. Second, the medical care provided by the team should be scrutinized to determine if quality care is being rendered. It is not adequate merely to demonstrate that medical care protocols are being executed properly. An equally important issue is whether the appropriate protocol was selected. For nonphysician teams, this level of review should be conducted by the medical director or a physician designate.

Periodic reviews should include seven critical aspects of the program (32):

- Safety
- Expediency
- Resource allocation
- Triage
- Appropriateness of care
- Interface with receiving facility
- Data collection.

TABLE 4–2. *Neonatal respiratory therapy pack*

Equipment	Amount	Equipment	Amount
Exterior Pockets		O₂ flowmeter nipple	2
Oxygen tubing	3	One-way valve	1
Infant nasal cannula	1	Set of ECG lead wires	2
Complete ventilator setup with exhalation valve (plus one in isolette)	1	32-gauge and 25-gauge ½-inch butterfly	3 each
Spare exhalation valve	1	Breath Tracker	1
Face tent	1	Albuterol	1
Treatment setup	1	Racemic epinephrine	1
Space blanket	1	Tape measure	1
Thermal hats	2	Infant MVB bag with O₂ tubing (plus one in isolette) and PEEP valve	1
Pulse oximeter sensors (N-25 and I-20)	2 each		
Suction catheters		Infant oral airway	2
6 Fr, 8 Fr, 10 Fr	3 each	Normal saline	4 vials
NCPAP prongs	1	Silk tape	1 roll
Luekens trap	1	Oxygen connectors	2
Interior of Bag		Hemostat	1
Airway supplies		Briggs T-adapters	2
Laerdal masks		15-mm adapter	2
No. 0	2	O₂ connectors (NCG, OES, P-B)	1 each
No. 1	2	Air connectors (NCG, P-B)	1 each
No. 2	1	ECG lead pads	3
Infant McGill forceps	1	Three-way stopcock	2
Laryngoscope handle with no. 0 and no. 1 Miller blades	1 each	E-Z Heat hot packs	4
		Stethoscope	1
Other equipment		1-mL and 3-mL syringe	3 each
Benzion applicators	6	ABG kit	3
Alcohol preps	4	Low-volume extension tubing	4
Adjustable wrench	1	Full set Mini-Med Tubing	1
E-tank wrench	1	Endotracheal tubes	
Cable ties	10	2.5 mm	3
Scissors	1	3.0 mm	3
9-volt battery	1	3.5 mm	3
Assorted laryngoscope bulbs	4	4.0 mm	3
Adjustable venturi	2	4.5 mm	3
Silicone adapter	2	Pedi-cap detector	2

ECG, electrocardiogram; MVB, manual ventilation bag; NCPAP, nasal continuous positive airway pressure; PEEP, positive end-expiratory pressure; ABG, arterial blood gas.

TABLE 4–3. *Neonatal medicine pack*

Drug	Amount	Drug	Amount
Isotonic saline vials, 20 mL	4	Lasix	1
Heparin	1	Lacrilube	1
Sodium chloride (2%)	1	Lidocaine 1%	1
Dilantin	2	Digoxin	1
Narcan	2	Clindamycin	1
Regitine	1	Aminophylline	1
Epinephrine 1:1,000, 1 mL	1	Dopamine	1
Epinephrine 1:1,000, 30 mL	1	Pavulon	1
Ampicillin	2	Sodium bicarbonate	1
Gentamicin	1	Cardiac lidocaine Bristojet	1
Acyclovir	1	Albumin 25%	2
Cefotaxime	1	Vitamin K	1
Romazicon	1	**Neonatal Narcotic Pack**	
Calcium gluconate	1	Morphine	2
Dobutamine	1	Chloral hydrate supplement	1
Norcuron	1	Versed	1
D₅₀W	1	Phenobarbital	3
Calcium chloride Bristojet	1	Valium	1
Atropine Bristojet	1	Fentanyl	1
Tubex	1	Ativan	1
Exosurf	2	**For Personal Use**	
Sterile water vials, 20 mL	4	Aspirin	12
Heparin lock flush	2	Tylenol	12
KCl	1	Antivert	6
Decadron	1	Scopolamine discs	6

TABLE 4–4. *Back transport pack*

Equipment or drug	Amount	Equipment or drug	Amount
Equipment		Mini-volume extension	1
Dextrostix bottle	1	Oximeter probes	2
Lancets, sterile	5	Monitor electrodes	6
Stethoscope	1	K-Y jelly	1
Syringes		Hot packs	
1 mL	3	Small	2
3 mL	3	Large	2
10 mL	3	Silver thermal hats	
20 mL	1	Small	2
60 mL	1	Large	2
Needles, 19 gauge	10	IV tubing	1
Nonsterile gloves	4 pairs	IV arm board	1
Bulb syringe	1	Rubber bandsy	6
Feeding tubes		Intraosseous needle	1
5 Fr	1	BP cuffs of various sizes	1 each
8 Fr	1	Scissors	1
Butterfly needles		Hemostat	1
23 gauge	2	T-connector	2
25 gauge	2	Angiocath, 24 gauge	4
ET tubes, 2.5 through 5.0	2 of each	Safety pins	6
Stylettes	4	Tape	2 rolls
Larygnoscope and blades	1	Benzoin	1
Face masks, assorted sizes	3	Sterile gloves	
Face tent	1	Size 6½	1
Manual ventilation bag	1	Size 7½	1
Nebulizer setup	1	Diapers	3
Venturi tubing	2	Pacifiers oxygen tubing	1
Nasal canula	4	**Medications**	
IV fluid, D_5W	1 100-mL bag	Isotonic saline	2
Alcohol and Betadine swabs	10 each	Heparin flush	2
Thermometers		Sodium bicarbonate	1
Suction catheters		Epinephrine 1:10,000 Bristojet	1
6 Fr	2	Atropine Bristojet	1
8 Fr	2	Sterile water	2
10 Fr	1	Dextrose 50%	1
Yankauer	1	Calcium gluconate	1
Three-way stopcock	2	D_5W, 100 cc	1
IV tubing		D_5, 0.5NS, 250 cc	1
Low-volume extension	2	Aminophylline	1

BP, blood pressure; ET, endotracheal.

Quality assurance activities should be closely linked to education and research. Review of individual transport records can be an extremely valuable method of identifying transport personnel in need of further education and training. The compilation of reviews and the monitoring of patient outcomes provide an assessment of the efficacy of existing protocols and procedures and may identify a need to alter program activities. In addition, new therapies and equipment can be evaluated using existing quality assurance techniques.

Although transport programs traditionally have not been closely scrutinized by regulatory agencies, as the number of programs increases and standards become better defined, review by these agencies is inevitable. Guidelines for developing quality assurance programs, not specific to transport, have been published (33,34). A more helpful guide has been produced by the Association of Air Medical Services (35). An external review can be conducted by the Commission on Accreditation of Medical Transport Systems (36).

PSYCHOSOCIAL CONSIDERATIONS

Psychological Impact on the Family

There is virtually no way to eliminate the parental anxiety associated with neonatal transport. However, there are a few techniques that may help families in coping with this anxiety. The transport team should provide the family with as much information as possible on the nature of their child's illness, the therapies and equipment that will be used, the NICU to which the infant will be transported, and the professionals who will provide care. A member of the referring hospital staff should be in attendance during this discussion to prepare them for dealing with questions that arise after the departure of the transport team (37). This information should be provided both verbally and in written form. Audiovisual aids also may assist in the dissemination of this information. The transport team of the University of North Carolina Hospitals distributes a videotape to community hospitals in their area, which is made available to families of transported infants. It describes and pictures the NICU, providing a more comprehensive view of the NICU milieu compared to the information provided at the time of transport. This technique is particularly effective with illiterate parents, or those with little understanding of the hospital environment.

It is almost always advisable to arrange contact between parents and infant before departure from the referring hospital. Visitation should be encouraged even during the transport of a critically ill infant or when parents are reluctant to view their child. A photograph of the infant should be left with the family. Immediately on arrival in the receiving hospital, the transport team should call the family to reassure them that their child has arrived safely. The transport team should alert the NICU staff to any unusual problems with the parents' preparedness to cope with their child's illness.

Relationships with Referring Hospital Personnel

Transporting a neonate from a community hospital to a tertiary center has the potential to improve dramatically the relationship between institutions or to cause irreparable damage to the relationship. Each transport represents an opportunity for success or failure. To ensure success, referring personnel must have easy access to the service. The team should respond in a reasonable period of time. Rapidity of response often is critical from a public relations standpoint, even when the infant's medical condition does not mandate speed. All reasonable efforts should be made to minimize the time between the request and arrival in the referring hospital.

Even the most responsive service will fail to satisfy personnel in the referring hospital if the team does not conduct itself appropriately. The team must understand the psychological milieu surrounding a transport. The event often is emotionally charged because of the acute nature of the infant's illness. Emotions may be fragile because of feelings of inadequacy on the part of referring hospital personnel. These feelings seem to arise even when excellent, comprehensive care is provided. Referring hospital personnel may be very sensitive to criticism; any critique of care, unless requested, should be deferred until a later time. The team should appreciate the contribution made by the referring staff. They should seek information about the history and condition of the infant before their arrival. They should ask for assistance when practical. The team should explain the

need for performing all procedures. This is particularly important when referring personnel have made the decision not to perform a procedure because of their lack of understanding of the transport environment. Nonphysician teams must avoid conflicts with referring physicians over the need for therapies or procedures. Any disagreements should be resolved through discussion between the referring physician and the consultant in the tertiary center.

Communication should not end with the departure of the transport team from the referring hospital. It is incumbent on the tertiary center staff to provide comprehensive follow-up to the referring hospital caretakers. Failure to provide follow-up is one of the most common criticisms of tertiary centers. There are several critical points in time at which information should be provided. A call should be made by the receiving physician within 24 hours of the transport. Plans for further follow-up can be established at that time. Referring hospital personnel should be notified immediately on the death of a patient. Failure to fulfill this obligation may result in embarrassment and anger toward the tertiary center. It also is imperative that the referring physician be contacted in advance of discharge of the patient.

LEGAL CONSIDERATIONS

The medicolegal climate in which perinatal medicine is practiced has changed dramatically in the past several decades. Litigation of malpractice suits involving perinatal caretakers is common. Transport personnel, by contrast, usually have avoided legal entanglements. It is unlikely, however, that this trend will continue. Neonatal transport is more closely associated with inpatient intensive care and less likely to be considered an emergency service providing extraordinary care under adverse conditions. A standard of care is expected by other medical professionals; a good outcome usually is expected by families.

Although there are few regulations and little case law defining legal obligations of transport services, understanding the principles that are likely to govern legal decision-making will help guide programs in establishing sound practices, those that are most likely to limit risk of litigation (38). The principles of respondent superior define the hospital as the party responsible for governing the protocols and procedures followed by its personnel (39). These principles, no doubt, apply to mobile services as well as inpatient care. Therefore, the hospital that sponsors a transport program is responsible for selecting and training the personnel and defining their scope or practice. Logically, the medical director, as the medical professional delegated to ensure the quality of care, also is liable for the governance of the team. Team members assume personal liability only if they perform outside their enfranchised scope of practice.

The method used for selecting, training, and certifying personnel should be documented. Similarly, protocols and procedures should be recorded and approved by the medical director. Activities of nonphysician personnel that exceed their usual scope of practice in the inpatient setting should be approved by the respective governing bodies (e.g., board of nursing). All documentation should be kept on permanent file.

During the conduct of a transport, the team should adhere to established protocols and procedures unless the patient's needs dictate an abridgement of usual standards (40). In this situation, advice from a consulting physician should be sought. Recommendations by this person should be noted in the patient record.

Referring hospitals have both ethical and legal responsibilities, the latter outlined primarily in the Consolidated Omnibus Budget Reconciliation Act of 1985 (41). This federal legislation assigns to the referring hospital the responsibility to stabilize adequately the patient prior to transport. The referring hospital also must establish an agreement from a hospital to receive the patient and must ensure that the receiving hospital is capable of providing for the predicted needs of the patient. Amendment of this act in 1989 added the requirement that referring hospitals make an effort to obtain written consent from parents prior to transport. Failure to comply with these requirements is considered medical abandonment.

Special problems arise during interstate transport when medical professionals are not licensed in the state of the referring or receiving hospital (42). Although some neighboring states have established reciprocal relationships regarding licensure, this is not routine. Unfortunately, there is no simple solution to this problem.

NEONATAL BACK TRANSPORT

Overcrowding of tertiary centers remains a problem in some regions of the country. One strategy for managing this problem has been to transport convalescing infants to community hospitals before discharge home. This strategy often is referred to as back transport. The benefits of back transport include the following:

- Reserves level III center resources for critically ill patients (43)
- Improves use of level I and level II center resources and helps prepare their personnel for the care of acutely ill patients
- Familiarizes primary care physicians with infants before discharge home
- Improves relationships between level III and level I and II hospitals
- Improves family visitation and promotes family–infant bonding (44)
- Reduces the total cost of medical care (45,46).

There also are potential disadvantages associated with back transport, including the following:

- Parental anxiety and loss of continuity of care caused by the change of caretakers (47)
- Hazards and cost of transport
- Lack of reimbursement by third party payers for the transport (46)
- Occasional requirement for readmission to the level III center
- Loss of the opportunity by level III personnel to participate in convalescent care.

Back transport should be considered an option for all infants who no longer require the unique resources of the level III center and for whom the level III center is not the site of primary care (47).

REFERENCES

1. Cone TE. *History of the care and feeding of the premature infant.* Boston: Little, Brown and Company, 1985:46.
2. Losty MA, Orlofsky I, Wallace H. A transport service for premature babies. *Am J Nurs* 1950;50:10.
3. Wallace HM, Losty MA, Baumgartner L. Report of two years experience in the transportation of premature infants in New York City. *Pediatrics* 1952;22:439.
4. Richardson DK, Reed K, Cutler C, et al. Perinatal regionalization versus hospital competition: the Hartford experience *Pediatrics* 1995;96:417.
5. Bose CL. Organization and administration of a perinatal transport service. In: MacDonald MG, Miller MK, eds. *Emergency transport of the perinatal patient.* Boston: Little, Brown and Company, 1989:43.
6. Hood JL, Cross A, Hulka B, et al. Effectiveness of the neonatal transport team. *Crit Care Med* 1983;11:419.
7. Chance GW, Matthew JD, Gash J, et al. Neonatal transport: a controlled study of skilled assistance. *J Pediatr* 1978;93:662.
8. American Academy of Pediatrics, Committee on Fetus and Newborn, and American College of Obstetricians and Gynecologists, Committee on Obstetrics. *Maternal and fetal medicine:* guidelines for perinatal care. Evanston, IL: American Academy of Pediatrics and American College of Obstetricians and Gynecologists, 1997:51.
9. Brimhall D. Developing administrative support for the transport system. In: McCloskey K, Orr R, eds. *Pediatric transport medicine.* St. Louis: Mosby, 1995:56.
10. Mitchell A, Watts J, Whyte R, et al. Evaluation of graduating neonatal nurse practitioners. *Pediatrics* 1991;88:789.
11. Pettett G, Merenstein GB, Battaglia FC, et al. An analysis of air transport results in the sick newborn infant: part I. The transport team. *Pediatrics* 1975;55:774.
12. Thompson TR. Neonatal transport nurses: an analysis of their role in the transport of newborn infants. *Pediatrics* 1980;65:887.
13. American Academy of Pediatrics, Task Force on Interhospital Transport. *Guidelines for air and ground transport of neonatal and pediatric patients.* Elk Grove Village, IL: American Academy of Pediatrics, 1993:33.
14. Conn AKT, Bowen CY. The communications network for perinatal transport. In: MacDonald MG, Miller MK, eds. *Emergency transport of the perinatal patient.* Boston: Little, Brown and Company, 1989:92.
15. Perlstein PH, Edwards NK, Sutherland JM. Neonatal hot line telephone network. *Pediatrics* 1979;64:419.
16. Bostick JS, Hsiao HS, Lawson EE. A minicomputer-based perinatal/neonatal telecommunication network. *Pediatrics* 1983;71:272.
17. Risemberg HM. Financing a perinatal transport program in the United States. In: MacDonald MG, Miller MK, eds. *Emergency transport in the perinatal patient.* Boston: Little, Brown and Company, 1989:85.

18. Baxt WG, Moody P. The impact of rotorcraft aeromedicine emergency care service on transport mortality. *JAMA* 1983;249:3047.

19. Elliot JP, O'Keeffe DF, Freeman RK. Helicopter transportation of patients with obstetric emergencies in an urban area. *Am J Obstet Gynecol* 1982;143:157.

20. Bose CL. The transport environment. In: MacDonald MG, Miller MK, eds. *Emergency transport of the perinatal patient.* Boston: Little, Brown and Company, 1989:194.

21. Shenai J. Sound levels for neonates in transit. *J Pediatr* 1977;90:811.

22. Campbell AN, Lightstone AD, Smith JM, et al. Mechanical vibration and sound levels experienced in neonatal transport. *Am J Dis Child* 1984;138:967.

23. Gadeke R, Doring B, Keller R, et al. The noise level in a children's hospital and the wake-up threshold in infants. *Acta Paediatr Scand* 1969;58:164.

24. Shenai JP, Johnson GE, Varney RV. Mechanical vibration in neonatal transport. *Pediatrics* 1981;68:55.

25. Floyd WN, Broderson AB, Goodno JF. Effects of whole body vibration on peripheral nerve conduction time in the rhesus monkey. *Aerospace Med* 1973;44:281.

26. Clark JG, Williams JD, Hood WB, et al. Initial cardiovascular response to low frequency whole body vibration in humans and animals. *Aerospace Med* 1967;38:464.

27. Adey WR, Winters WD, Kado RT, et al. EEG in simulated stresses of space flight with special reference to problems of vibration. *Electroencephalogr Clin Neurophysiol* 1963;15:305.

28. Graybiel A, Knepton J. Sopite syndrome: a sometimes sole manifestation of motion sickness. *Aviat Space Environ Med* 1976;47:873.

29. Wright MS, Bose CL, Stiles AD. The incidence and effects of motion sickness among medical attendants during transport. *J Emerg Med* 1995;13:15.

30. Schneider C, Gomez M, Lee R. Evaluation of ground ambulance, rotorwing, and fixed-wing aircraft services. *Crit Care Clin* 1992;8:533.

31. Brink LW, Neuman B, Wynn J. Air transport. *Pediatr Clin North Am* 1993;40:439.

32. American Academy of Pediatrics, Task Force on Interhospital Transport. *Guidelines for air and ground transport of neonatal and pediatric patients.* Elk Grove Village, IL: American Academy of Pediatrics, 1993:49.

33. Council on Medical Services. Guide for quality assurance. *JAMA* 1988;259:2572.

34. Joint Commission on the Accreditation of Hospitals and Health Organizations. *Examples of monitoring and evaluation in emergency services.* Chicago: JCAHHO, 1988:13.

35. Eastes L, Jacobson J, eds. *Quality assurance in air medical transport.* Orem, UT: WordPerfect Publishers, 1990.

36. *Accreditation Standards of the Commission on Accreditation of Medical Transport Systems,* 3rd ed. Anderson, SC: Commission on Accredition of Medical Transport Systems, 1997.

37. McBurney B. The role of the community hospital nurse in supporting parents of transported infants. *Neonat Network* 1988;6:60.

38. Ginzburg HM. Legal issues in medical transport. In: MacDonald MG, Miller MK, eds. *Emergency transport of the perinatal patient.* Boston: Little, Brown and Company, 1989:152.

39. Tonsic v Wagner, 458 Pa 246, 329 A2d 497, 1974.

40. American Academy of Pediatrics, Task Force on Interhospital Transport. *Guidelines for air and ground transport of neonatal and pediatric patients.* Elk Grove Village, IL: American Academy of Pediatrics, 1993:16.

41. Bolte R. Responsibilities of the referring physician and referring hospital. In: McCloskey K, Orr R, eds. *Pediatric transport medicine.* St. Louis: Mosby, 1995:33.

42. Brimhall DC. The hospital administrator's perspective. In: MacDonald MG, Miller MK, eds. *Emergency transport of the perinatal patient.* Boston: Little, Brown and Company, 1989:147.

43. Jung AL, Bose CL. Back transport of neonates: improved efficiency of tertiary nursery bed utilization. *Pediatrics* 1983;71:918.

44. Meyer CL, Mahan CK, Schreiner RL. Retransfer of newborns to community hospitals: questionnaire survey of parents' feelings. *Perinatol Neonatol* 1982;6:75.

45. Bose CL, LaPine TR, Jung AL. Neonatal back transport: cost effectiveness. *Med Care* 1985;23:14.

46. Phibbs CS, Mortensen L. Back transporting infants from neonatal intensive care units to community hospitals for recovery care: effect on total hospital charges. *Pediatrics* 1992;90:22.

47. Lynch TM, Jung AL, Bose CL. Neonatal back transport: clinical outcome. *Pediatrics* 1988;82:845.

CHAPTER 5

Newborn Intensive Care Unit Design: Scientific and Practical Considerations

Robert D. White, Gilbert I. Martin, and Stanley N. Graven

DEVELOPING A MISSION STATEMENT

The first step in any successful newborn intensive care unit (NICU) design project is the development of a shared vision among NICU, hospital, and community leaders. The construction of a new unit or redesign of an existing facility should successfully address key problems in the current system of neonatal care. For an existing, stable unit wishing to modernize its facility, these problems may be primarily internal, e.g., the need for more space, computerization, and family support. For an entirely new facility, these issues will be predominantly external: who are the existing providers, and what niche will this new unit most appropriately fill? A careful, thoughtful appraisal of medical care trends anticipated within the community over the next 20 years, especially with regard to obstetric and intensive care services, should precede any decision on a mission statement intended to guide NICU construction and operation. Whether a hospital is the only provider of NICU services in its area or one of several, it is crucial that it understand its niche and the responsibilities inherent to that role, so that appropriate physical facilities can be constructed to fulfill its mission.

A mission statement that might provide a framework for most NICUs is as follows:

"The Newborn Intensive Care Unit will provide a state-of-the-art integrated, family-centered approach to neonatal care. This interdisciplinary program will strive to give patients, families, and payers high quality and compassionate care through the provision of:

- Care that honors the racial, ethnic, cultural, religious, and socioeconomic diversity of family and staff.
- Education, information, and emotional support.
- Access to the most current effective therapies.
- Integrated treatment plans emphasizing coordination throughout the continuum of care.
- Encouragement of family support and involvement."

When consensus is reached on a mission statement, specific goals and objectives can be defined, which apply this mission to the local realities of demographics, care practices, and competition. Defining these goals will be the first step toward decisions on the bed capacity, types of equipment needed, and changes in care practices that might be considered, all of which then can be explored in depth by the teams described below. These goals and objectives should be measurable (e.g., survival and morbidity rates compared to regional and national standards, staff experience and turnover, parental satisfaction ratings, cost per patient day) and realistic, so that the overall value of the project can be ascertained at the time cost projections are available, and on an ongoing basis after construction is complete.

CREATING THE TEAMS

Once a decision has been made to proceed with the development of either a new or renovated NICU, it is important to form specialized teams with well-defined goals. Although these groups will interact throughout the process, a senior neonatologist should attend every planning meeting. In many hospitals, several persons will serve on two or more teams. Each team should have access to the several excellent reference materials available to assist in the design of an NICU (1–5).

R.D. White: Department of Pediatrics, Indiana University School of Medicine, Indianapolis; and Regional Newborn Program, Memorial Hospital, South Bend, Indiana

G.I. Martin: Department of Pediatrics, University of California, Irvine, Irvine; and Neonatal Intensive Care Unit, Citrus Valley Medical Center, West Covina, California

S.N. Graven: Community and Family Health, Department of Pediatrics, University of South Florida; and Department of Pediatrics, Tampa General Hospital, Tampa, Florida

The Strategic Planning Team

This team will continue to develop the vision and goals that led to the decision to pursue new construction. It should include, at a minimum, an administrator, a neonatologist, and a nursing director. This group will be responsible for reviewing utilization and demographic information (available from state and local planning and health agencies, the insurance industry, and the Census Bureau) in order to define the NICU's service area and appropriate number of beds. Some general guidelines in this area include estimates that about 5% of all newborns will need intensive care at the time of birth and 1.5% will need ventilator care. Total NICU days for a defined region will approximate 1.25 patient-days per live birth, i.e., if a region has 10,000 live births per year, it will generate about 12,500 NICU patient-days, or an average census of about 34 babies, with an average length of stay of about 20 days. These numbers will be influenced considerably by the level of care provided by a particular NICU, referral and back transport patterns, admission and discharge criteria, and competing NICUs serving the same region. Because of fluctuations in census, a unit should have sufficient bed positions to care for 40% to 50% more babies than the average census calculations, so a region with 10,000 deliveries per year will need approximately 50 NICU beds. Most areas currently exceed this number by a sizable proportion because of serving a particularly high-risk population, or because of inefficiencies inherent in multiple NICUs serving a single region.

The strategic planning team also should make some basic calculations regarding staffing patterns, if this is to be a new service for the hospital. Depending on patient mix, overall staffing patterns may require four to six nurses and two support staff (inclusive of nursing administration, respiratory therapy, developmental therapy, social work, ward clerk, and housekeeping staff) for every ten babies. A unit with an average census of 20 babies, for example, would require 8 to 12 nurses on each shift, or 40 to 65 full-time equivalents (FTEs), with an additional 20 to 25 FTEs for support staff. One neonatologist is needed for each six to eight babies (average census); this is one area, among several, where units with an average census of less than 20 infants encounter certain inefficiencies because of their size. Large units (more than 40 beds or so) also are difficult to design and manage efficiently, so some hospitals have addressed this issue by breaking their NICU into intensive care and continuing care, or stepdown areas. Some units will also need to plan staffing for transport team or nurse practitioner coverage. Six to seven full-time positions are required for 24-hour coverage of each position for these services. A transport team with two nurses and a respiratory therapist, for example, would require at least 12 nurses and six therapists to provide full-time, in-house coverage.

Next, the strategic planning team also will need to assess the impact of the new or renovated NICU on other hospital departments, especially obstetric, maintenance, and supply services. When these issues are clear, the team will proceed to interview and engage an architect. The timing of this step is important—the architectural firm should be involved before any design decisions are made, but after the strategic planning team has articulated a clear set of goals for the process. Several architectural firms can be asked to make formal presentations of their general concepts for the project, as well as present examples of other projects that they have designed. The architectural firm chosen should have complete engineering and interior design specialists on staff: an equipment representative and a neonatal nurse planner. The entire architectural team should be familiar with the latest trends in NICU design and the scientific principles behind the design process. Once chosen, the architectural group and the strategic planning team then can develop a time table for planning and construction of the new facility.

The Financial Planning Team

This group is composed of the hospital's chief financial and operational officers, nursing management, and any other individuals representing areas of the hospital whose budgets will be significantly affected by the new construction. Consultants, such as those helpful in the equipment selection process (see following), also may be asked to join the team. The one-time costs for the project will include architectural fees, the physical plant, and new equipment. Ongoing costs will include increased staffing for direct patient care, housekeeping, and maintenance functions. These costs should be clearly identified early in the planning sequence, with the assistance of the care practices team (see following). This team should continue to meet intermittently throughout the planning process, because some unanticipated expenses will undoubtedly surface as the design takes shape.

The Care Practices Team

This is the largest group, made up of caregivers in the NICU. At a minimum, the following disciplines should be represented: neonatology, nursing management and staff, respiratory therapy, social work, pharmacy, laboratory, radiology, nutrition, housekeeping, and parents. Depending on local care practices, surgery, obstetrics, and clinical research may be appropriate additions to this list. As each individual provides information on his or her own specialty to enhance care for babies, families, and staff, the team should be encouraged to look beyond existing practices and view the new construction as an opportunity to change the way things are done. In particular, most NICUs will need to reevaluate their care practices with respect to parental access and developmentally supportive care, which may have been severely restricted under their previous NICU design. They should consider environmental design features that will provide the most optimal living conditions for babies, working conditions for staff, and integration of families, and they should begin to address some of the conflicts inherent in these ideals. As a team, this group then can identify general space, equipment, staffing, and maintenance and cleaning requirements, which can be reported to the financial and design teams for determination of feasibility.

The Design Team

When the strategic planning, financial planning, and care practice teams have agreed on the general scope of the project, including goals, approximate size and cost, major changes in care practices, and an architectural firm, the design team can begin its work. Members of this team should include the architectural group, the hospital's project manager, neonatology, nursing, respiratory therapy, parents, and the equipment consultant. After creating a functional plan that addresses all the needs identified by the care practices team, this group should visit new or updated NICUs to get additional ideas, learn how to avoid pitfalls, and solicit suggestions on their functional plan. This team then will meet regularly over several months as blueprints are developed to reconcile all these concepts into a working unit. Detailed minutes should be kept and reviewed at the beginning of each meeting.

SPECIFIC DESIGN ISSUES

Floor Space Requirements

NICUs have historically been undersized, with insufficient room for storage, parental access, and offices, even when accurate estimates are made for the number of babies to be cared for. Change has been incremental, as administrators, architects, and NICU staff gradually expand their horizons to accommodate new practices, particularly increased parental access. There are few, if any, NICUs currently in operation where the staff feel they have space adequate for their needs and those of the babies' families.

Given this historical perspective and extrapolating from floor space requirements in adult and pediatric intensive care units (ICU), it is likely that an NICU design should allow 600 gross square feet per bed to meet the needs of the babies, staff, and families. This figure includes office, storage, and support space as well as the patient care areas; gross square footage estimates also include space required for hallways, ductwork, restrooms, and the like. This figure is an average; teaching hospitals with active clinical research programs, for example, might require more than 600 gross square feet per bed, whereas a community NICU might require somewhat

less. Any design that provides less than 500 gross square feet per bed, however, will inevitably demand compromises and limit flexibility for the future, when parental access desires and length of stays (due to increasing survival of extremely low-birth-weight infants) may be even greater than they are today.

Previous estimates of floor space requirements often recommended square footage per bed position (e.g., 100 square feet per intensive care bed position), and some state codes still use this convention. If this method is used, an additional 30 square feet of storage space must be planned outside of the patient care area, as well as 24 cubic feet of cabinet storage at each bedside, at a minimum.

Location within the Hospital

The NICU should be immediately adjacent to the high-risk delivery rooms whenever possible. There are few, if any, NICUs that are more than a few hundred feet from a high-risk delivery service that do not consider their location as the source of certain risks to optimal care. In some circumstances, especially very large hospital complexes or freestanding childrens' hospitals, this ideal may be impossible to achieve. In the former situation, a resuscitation area within the delivery room complex or in each delivery suite, always valuable, becomes crucial; in the latter case, all infants are accepted as transfers, and proximity to the ambulance entrance and heliport becomes particularly significant. When the NICU is on a different floor from the delivery suites, as often occurs in larger hospitals, dedicated elevator access between these two areas is essential.

Many NICUs, particularly in small or medium-sized hospitals, share staff and responsibilities with the well-baby nursery or pediatric ICU. When these areas are contiguous, much of the support space (e.g., family lounge, staff lockers, equipment storage) can be shared, and the opportunities for staff to assist one another are enhanced.

Traffic patterns for infants who will leave the NICU for procedures should be identified and private hallways created wherever possible, so that ill infants and their attendants will not need to utilize public areas.

Security Considerations

As family access to the NICU has become more prevalent, so have security considerations. Most NICUs now permit continuous access to families, so traffic in and out of the NICU is commonplace. Certain design features are necessary in this setting to protect babies and staff. First, the NICU should be designed with only a single public entrance. Other entrance and exits (e.g., to the delivery suite, the clean utility room, and the staff lockers) may be desirable, but these should be less apparent to the public (except as fire exits) and within constant observation of the staff, because one would never expect the public to utilize these exits.

The public entrance to the NICU needs to be designed with the security of all major parties (babies, families, and staff) in mind. Families and staff need a secure locker area to store valuables (even overcoats or jackets can easily disappear!). This area should be large enough to allow more than one family to enter or leave at a time and should be under constant observation. Electronic detection systems increasingly are being utilized in newborn nursery areas to prevent kidnapping; these are uncommon in NICU settings, but worthy of consideration if constant visual monitoring of all exits from the NICU is not feasible.

Fire exits should be carefully planned in the initial design, and clearly marked, as should the location of fire extinguishers. The fire marshal should be given the first draft of the design documents, so that any problems can be corrected early.

Reception Area

In most NICUs, the reception area is part of, or near, the public entrance. This area also may encompass the family lounge and the ward clerk's workspace. The size and layout of this space is highly dependent on the size of the NICU, and its "culture" or typical practices.

The family lounge should always be large enough to accommodate at least two families comfortably, with appropriate seating, i.e., comfortable, but not too conducive to overnight sleeping. Lockers for valuables, a coffee pot, a television set, reading material (including informational and educational literature for families of NICU babies), and a toy box for children are items found in many such areas; public restrooms and telephones should be close by.

Families and the public need to be able to immediately reach an NICU staff member from the reception area. In some larger units, this might be a full-time ward clerk; in others, it might be a hot line or direct visual contact into the patient care area. In any case, this function should be carefully thought out so that those who should be encouraged to enter (i.e., families) find themselves feeling welcomed, whereas those who should be discouraged (e.g., curious folks wandering through the hospital) leave unfulfilled.

Direct Patient Care

As might be expected, the greatest design effort is spent creating the patient care area. The first and major decision to be made is the extent to which individualized environments are desirable. The goal to provide each baby with a space that is not impinged upon by noise, bright lights, and commotion from an adjacent bed position, and that has enough space to accommodate staff, family, and bedside equipment and storage seems intuitive and is certainly the norm for adult ICUs, but has not historically been the pattern for NICUs, for several reasons.

NICUs in the 1970s and 1980s were routinely designed as large, open wards. These permitted care of the largest number of babies in a given space and allowed direct visibility of each baby by the staff, and of staff members by one another. Babies (and staff) were not thought to be adversely affected by the noise and bright lighting that were the norm for such designs. New practices and equipment (as long as they did not require much additional space) could be incorporated easily into this design, and highly variable census patterns also could be accommodated more easily than in the older premature nursery design of several smaller rooms. Parents were allowed, or expected, to visit for only short periods, so very little space at the bedside was allotted to them.

In recent years, many of these assumptions have changed. Direct, continuous observation of most babies no longer is considered necessary, thanks to improved monitoring systems (especially noninvasive, automated oximetry, and blood pressure monitoring), and certainly is no longer practiced except for the sickest babies, even in units where it is still physically possible. Babies clearly are affected by excessive, noxious levels of light and noise, and their response to these environmental hazards varies with their gestational age and medical condition (see Chap. 8 for a thorough discussion of these issues). Extensive adult studies in workplace settings also have established that staff needs and responses can be quite different from those of babies (6). Perhaps most dramatically, family expectations have changed. Many families now wish access to their babies on a continuous basis and want to be able to stay at the bedside, without interfering with the ability of staff to care for their baby, in any but the most extraordinary circumstances.

Designing an NICU that takes these newer realities into consideration requires establishing a local philosophy on individualized environments. In some units, private or semiprivate rooms for at least some of the infants will be considered desirable and feasible; in others, space, staffing, or philosophical considerations will lead the design team in a different direction. Often, a combination of "pods" (one, two, or four beds), with a larger room for recovering neonates, has been the design of choice. In any NICU, however, the need for each baby to be protected as much as possible from the noise, light, and activity generated at other bed positions and the differing needs of babies from staff need to be discussed and integrated into the design process at the outset.

Certain principles can be established for any direct patient care area plan, regardless of whether a single large room, multiple smaller rooms, or private rooms are chosen as the model. First, each bed position must have sufficient space for families to stay for extended periods without interfering with staff duties. Second, each bed position must have individualized lighting, data entry, and communications systems (each of these will be discussed in more detail below). Third, traffic patterns must be well planned, with sufficient aisle widths to accommodate diagnostic equipment and personnel; generally, this will require aisles of at least 5 feet in width. Nursing functions should be separated from the bedside whenever possible. For babies, the NICU is perhaps ideally visualized as a bedroom for a sick infant; for staff, it is a workplace, where both work-related and social communication occurs. These concepts are often in conflict, yet the NICU design must accommodate both to the greatest extent possible. Therefore, the design team should (again, within the local culture and practices) separate those nursing functions that do not involve direct patient care (e.g., most charting, giving report, receiving and making most phone calls) from the bedside to the greatest extent possible, especially if those activities require different lighting levels or create noise that would disturb the baby. This is done by providing adequate space for these functions away from the bedside, yet sufficiently proximate to allow appropriate response to the unpredictable needs of the baby. Finally, in any plan that utilizes modules or individual rooms, staffing patterns should be considered. In general, enough babies should be clustered together to justify staffing with at least three nurses. Designing smaller clusters creates significant staffing issues during those times when at least one nurse must leave the area.

When these considerations are adequately debated and decided, the general layout of the patient care area can proceed. Each bed position can be identified, as well as nursing work areas (charting, medication preparation, etc.), sinks, and traffic flow patterns. At this point, an infectious disease specialist also should be consulted, to assure that the design is conducive to good infection control practices. This individual also will be interested in air flow considerations and in floor, wall, and ceiling finishes (discussed below). Proximity to other important support areas also will begin to take shape at this stage; specific design features for each of these areas will be discussed in the next section.

The design team then can spend considerable time planning the layout of a typical bed position. Perhaps most important in this regard is the headwall, including monitoring and communication systems. Construction of a full-size mockup of an individual bed position, complete with headwall, monitors, and communications systems is well worth the effort and expense to be sure the ergonomics of the design have been adequately thought out. Many members of the design team will be unable to fully visualize the layout from a blueprint, and it would be rare that a new NICU would resemble an existing design closely enough to bypass this step. Most NICUs will want to include one or more special care areas for isolation, treatment rooms, parent rooming in, or breastfeeding. In most units, some of these functions can be combined, and many will choose to eliminate one or more of these due to local practice patterns. The need for each should be carefully considered in new designs, however, and if not served by a dedicated space, at least clearly accommodated at some appropriate location in the NICU.

General Support Space

Clean utility, soiled utility, and general storage are functions that each require a dedicated space. In some units, a satellite pharmacy, clinical laboratory, and x-ray processing also are given designated areas, although technological advances have made the need less clear for the latter in the future. The layout of these rooms is straightforward; errors in design usually are made by allowing too little space or placing these rooms in an inconvenient position away from the direct patient care area. Ideally, these areas also should be accessible from an outside corridor so that restocking can take place without unnecessary traffic through the NICU, but this must be designed in accordance with security precautions discussed previously. Storage areas should have a generous supply of electrical outlets and shelving so that battery-powered devices can be recharged. Additional specific considerations are outlined in each state's code documents and in several published guidelines (1,2).

Staff Support Space

As noted previously, some charting space, especially for the nursing and respiratory therapy staff, needs to be allocated within the direct patient care area. Additional space, especially for physician and nurse practitioner charting and discussion, should be provided adjacent to the patient care area, so that the noise and activity generated there does not impinge on the babies' bedsides. The communications systems (phone, computer terminal, printer) that link the NICU with the hospital laboratory, pharmacy, and central supply generally will be situated in this area as well, which therefore will benefit from being centrally located.

The staff lounge and locker room should be adjacent to the NICU, with restroom facilities integral or nearby. The lounge should be large enough to accommodate at least one-third of all NICU staff (nurses, therapists, physicians, and other support staff) at one time and be accessible to the NICU by phone or intercom.

Several disciplines should have office space immediately adjacent to the NICU, including social work, medical and nursing administration, and developmental and respiratory therapy. When parent support or research staff are actively involved in a unit' activities, they also will need nearby office space. On-call rooms and a conference room should be situated within this complex, with phone and computer links, including digital x-ray transmission, and restrooms with showers.

Family Support Space

In addition to generous provision of space at the bedside and in the family lounge, parents need space to stay overnight, to meet in private with staff to discuss their baby or to grieve, and to breast-feed. Again, depending on the size of the NICU and its local practices, some of these functions can be combined, but none can be ignored.

Rooming in, even with critically ill patients, is provided (indeed, encouraged) in all areas of a typical hospital except for the NICU, where this practice usually is limited to those infants close to discharge. We are unaware of any documented factors other than tradition that justify the exclusion of parents from rooming in with NICU patients from immediately after birth, however, and suggest that future designs should anticipate that this practice will become more prevalent as families come to request and expect this opportunity. To be sure, many families will not choose or will be unable to room in with their ill newborn, so an ideal design need not anticipate that all babies will need space for rooming in at all times, but it should allow most parents who desire this privilege the opportunity to do so.

Breast-feeding of premature or ill infants also is poorly accommodated in existing NICUs, because of space and privacy considerations. Mothers should be able to breast-feed babies at the bedside without compromising their privacy or being asked to wait until the baby is stable enough to be transferred to an area where these problems do not exist. Alternatives in this regard include private rooms for those babies whose mothers plan to room in and/or breast-feed, or moveable partitions. Breast-feeding rooms are also a good alternative for babies who are healthy enough to be moved and can be utilized by mothers who need to use a breast pump. These rooms should be designed with most of the capabilities of a headwall (e.g., oxygen, suction, monitor, electrical outlets, and direct communication to the NICU staff), yet be as much like home as possible.

Room for parent education and counseling should be available within the NICU complex. This is particularly important when private discussions need to occur with families of critically ill infants.

The location and content of signs often are overlooked when planning an NICU. Some thought should be given to traffic patterns for families and the public from the hospital entrance(s), however, and how signage will be used to direct them clearly to the NICU. Information on signs should be phrased warmly, in a way that will make families feel welcome, rather than sternly, in a way that could make them feel like outsiders and intruders.

Lighting

Planning appropriate lighting for the NICU requires consideration of the disparate needs of both the babies and staff. In general, babies need very little light, and the high levels of lighting previously common in NICUs may be dangerous to very immature premature babies (see Chap. 8).

Staff need moderate levels of illumination at the bedside to evaluate babies and to perform paperwork and manual tasks. At times, intense levels of illumination are necessary to perform procedures and are used for phototherapy of hyperbilirubinemia. It is doubtful that babies need natural lighting, but studies of adult office workers and hospital patients document the benefit of windows for staff and families (7).

Consideration of these disparate needs should lead the design team to plan a multilevel lighting scheme. At the bedside, a very low level of ambient lighting (200 lux [20 footcandles] or less) is desirable, so the baby is not exposed to a continuous bright light source. Task lighting, both for the bed surface and the nursing work surface(s), should be highly focused ("framed"), and rheostatically controlled, so that only the amount of light needed is provided, and only to the specific location desired. This may require multiple light sources at the bedside. The ideal task light would be adjustable to an infinite variety of positions, yet be able to recess fully into the wall or ceiling. It would have a beam of adjustable width and intensity and be free of shadowing effects.

At nursing work areas and traffic circulation areas elsewhere in the patient care area, moderate lighting levels (200 to 1,000 lux) are suitable. The light sources utilized should avoid glare, especially on work surfaces and computer terminals, and should have multiple switches or rheostatic controls to allow flexibility in lighting levels. A single master switch may be useful, however, if a darkened room is desired for transillumination. All fixtures should have filters or shields that block ultraviolet radiation and minimize the risk to babies and staff if a bulb should shatter.

Provision of natural lighting is highly dependent on the NICU locale. Ideally, each room where adults spend several hours at a time would have a window with an attractive view, allowing the eye to escape and orient to external conditions. In the northern hemisphere, windows that face north are optimal, because they will not transmit glare or heat gain. Windows facing other directions should be appropriately shaded, either with an external overhang or with internal louvers. If the ability to completely darken the room is desired, internal (within a triple-glazed window unit) electrically operated louvers are essential. Because even well-insulated external windows allow some heat gain or loss, these should be situated several feet away from any baby's bed position.

Noise Abatement

The initial design issue in making an NICU as quiet as possible is to eliminate or reduce as many sources of background noise as possible. Some NICUs are situated in noisy communities, which requires extra insulation in the external walls to minimize the impingement of outside sounds into the NICU. Air flow through the heating and cooling ducts also can produce considerable background noise in an NICU, but this can be reduced through appropriate sizing and baffling of the ducts. These issues must be addressed in the design process, because it is prohibitively expensive to correct a poor design after construction begins.

Traffic patterns also play a role in determining the level of noise to which babies and staff are exposed. To the greatest extent possible, traffic flow should be designed so that an echocardiogram, ultrasound, x-ray, or electroencephalographic technician can get to each baby's bedside as directly as possible, without wheeling the equipment past several other bed positions. As noted previously, support areas should be designed so that restocking functions can be accomplished without creating unnecessary bedside traffic.

Noise production also should be a prime consideration in design of the monitoring and communication systems and in the selection of equipment. The hum of fluorescent lights and the repetitive whoosh of a ventilator are examples of equipment sounds that vary from one manufacturer to another and should, therefore, be evaluated as part of the design and selection process. Incubators also have great variance in noise production by their internal motors; as a major determinant of environmental background noise for many neonates, these should be chosen with background noise levels as an important selection criterion. Whenever possible, equipment should be selected with a noise criterion rating of less than 40. Based on available data for sound levels that do not interfere with newborn sleep or adult conversation, overall background noise levels in the NICU should be maintained below 55 decibels on the A-weighted slow response scale, with peak levels not in excess of 70 dB.

Once all unnecessary sources of sound are minimized, the next design consideration is the abatement of unavoidable sound, e.g., voices, equipment noise, anything that might disturb a sleeping baby. Here, there is no substitute for adequate space, and another cogent argument for individualized environments becomes apparent. Increasing the distance between beds will diminish noise transfer from one baby's bedside to another, as will higher ceilings, especially those that are angled to reflect sound laterally rather than directly back to the bedside. Obviously, floor, wall, and ceiling materials are crucial in this regard and will be discussed in the next section.

Finally, care practices should be reevaluated as part of the design process to see whether many sources of noise produced by the staff can be diminished or eliminated. Radios, pagers, rounds, and report are examples of care practices that are considerable sources of noise at the bedside, which can be modified or eliminated.

Surface Finishes

In the past, selection of surface finishes was given little attention in NICU design, which focused primarily on integration of the newest technology. The choice of wall, ceiling, and floor finishes is important, however, for reasons of aesthetics, noise abatement, and infection control.

Perhaps the most controversial design issue in this regard is the choice between carpet and hard flooring. Hard flooring (usually a vinyl composite) is easily cleaned, durable, and provides little resistance to wheeled equipment. Carpeting provides noise abatement and may be more attractive and more comfortable to those who are on their feet for several hours a day. The differences between these two choices have started to blur in recent years, as carpet has become more durable and cleanable, and hard flooring has become more resilient and sound absorbent. It seems clear that vinyl flooring is the ideal for isolation, procedure, and clean and soiled utility areas and around sinks. Carpeting may be desirable for other areas; the direct patient care area is where this question remains most controversial. Carpet, however, has a significantly higher replacement factor and the hospital administration must demonstrate a commitment to the greater maintenance required to keep it clean.

Wall finishes are increasingly utilizing quilts or soft sculpture to provide aesthetic and sound-absorbent qualities. Even curtains separating NICU beds can have baffles added, which will decrease the amount of noise transmitted. Extensive use of highly durable railings or moldings is necessary throughout the NICU, as walls are easily damaged by portable equipment.

Ceiling and wall materials should be designated with a noise reduction coefficient of at least 0.60. Many states are now allowing the use of certain types of nonfriable acoustical ceiling tile, which will help with noise abatement. The method of cleaning the ceiling and changing lights should be considered in the design process so that this can be accomplished with minimal disruption to patient care.

Infection Control Considerations

As noted previously, an infection control practitioner will be an important member of the design team during the discussion of the layout of the NICU and the choice of surface finishes. In addition, they will be helpful in discussing air quality issues in design of the heating and cooling system. They also will be very interested in the location and design of hand-washing areas.

Sinks should be readily accessible throughout the NICU. They should be within a few steps of any bedside and given several feet of wall space, so that splatter will not fall on any patient care areas. The sinks themselves should be large and deep, so that a full surgical scrub can be performed with minimal splatter, and the walls and floor surrounding them should be covered with easily cleanable surfaces. Porcelain sinks generally are more attractive and quieter in use than stainless steel. Faucets should operate hands-free; mechanical devices such as foot pedals currently seem more reliable than electronic sensors. Soap, hand-drying supplies, and large trash receptacles should be easily accessible. These should be designed to avoid cross-contamination, to be easily cleanable, and to minimize noise production. At least some sinks should be provided for children and handicapped individuals. Signage above each sink should contain written and pictorial hand-washing instructions.

Headwalls

The area surrounding the baby's bedside, containing service outlets, shelving, and bedside storage, is commonly referred to as the "headwall." It is the focal point for creating a self-contained workstation at each bedside. This area must be easily adaptable to changes in census and acuity and to future changes in care practices. It must support and provide easy access to necessary equipment and supplies, as well as to the baby. The headwall design also should contain a comfortable working area for the staff and provide space for the family to personalize the baby's surroundings. There are several vendors that supply headwall systems, or these can be built on site, using either moveable or fixed-rail systems that can be customized for local equipment and practices.

A complete headwall system might include the following items and capabilities:

- Dimmer (rheostat) controlled task lighting
- Two gas manifolds
- Three to six oxygen ports
- Three to six compressed air ports
- Four to eight vacuum ports
- Twenty to thirty electrical outlets, with a common ground
- Telephone jack
- Computer terminal jack.

Consideration also should be given to allowing space for future needs, such as a nitric oxide port.

All electrical, vacuum, and gas outlets need to be simultaneously and conveniently accessible, that is, usage of one outlet cannot obstruct other outlets, even when equipment contains oversized plugs. Some electrical outlets should provide normal power, whereas others should be on emergency power, because either system could be temporarily incapacitated.

A fixed or moveable shelf to contain monitoring equipment should be located as near to eye level as possible and within easy reach. A countertop should be provided as a work surface, with at least 24 cubic feet of cabinet space below to hold supplies. Raceways within this cabinetry to hold wiring and gas lines can minimize the danger and unattractiveness of a clutter of cords, but should be easily accessible for repairs or modifications. Support beams should be placed to avoid visual obstruction or access problems. A ledge at the base of the headwall will prevent moveable equipment, such as incubators or warmers, from damaging the wall.

Heating and Cooling Systems

Heating, ventilation, and air conditioning (HVAC) is perhaps the most mundane segment of NICU design, and the one in which the majority of the design team feels they have the least expertise, yet it is important to consider for several reasons. We have discussed previously the contribution HVAC makes to background noise in the NICU, a problem that is amenable to some design considerations. The number of air changes per hour needs to be specified for the patient care area in general, and for the isolation and procedure areas in particular; minimums usually are dictated by state code. In the case of the isolation area(s) and soiled utility room, a negative air pressure design, with 100% of the air exhausted to the outside, is imperative. If protective isolation is desired, a reversal of this flow will be needed. In all cases, a high-efficiency filtering system is needed to remove particulate matter from the air.

Control of temperature and humidity is particularly important when designing the HVAC system for an NICU. The system should be able to maintain ambient temperature in the NICU between 72 and 78 degrees Fahrenheit throughout the year, even at the extremes of outside temperatures for that particular locale. A relative humidity of 30% to 60% should be maintained as well, again, even at local extremes externally. Maintaining temperature and humidity within these guidelines will minimize heat and water loss for the babies and discomfort for the staff.

Delivery of air flow into the unit requires considerable forethought. Return ducts should be situated near the floor so that particulate matter is not carried upward. Supply ducts should be located where drafts will not be a problem and should be generous in number, so that high-velocity air flow is avoided. Placement of supply ducts near external walls and windows should be carefully planned to avoid condensation and to minimize convective heat loss or gain to the babies nearby. The fresh air intake into the hospital HVAC system should be planned carefully to avoid areas that will contain exhaust fumes from vehicles, nearby buildings, or from the hospital itself.

Communications Systems

This is perhaps the segment of NICU design that requires the greatest anticipation of future developments. It is likely that communication patterns among NICU staff, and between the NICU and other support areas of the hospital such as laboratory, radiology, and pharmacy, will change dramatically in the next decade. Likewise, information transfer among infant monitoring devices, the staff, and the medical record will accelerate rapidly in the same time frame. Because unit design and construction typically takes several years, lack of foresight in this area can be inconvenient at best and often quite expensive.

Those planning an NICU for the twenty-first century should anticipate digital transfer of virtually all information and at least a tenfold increase in the volume of information transferred currently. Thus, the NICU should be wired and designed accordingly. It is likely that the entire medical record will be computerized, and work areas within the patient care area should be designed accordingly, with adequate space to add terminals. Ergonomics and lighting should be considered, so that staff can work at these terminals with minimal strain. Monitoring systems will be interfaced with all the equipment supporting the baby, such as the incubator, ventilator, and intravenous pumps, and then with the patient chart. This will allow the obvious benefit of making data acquisition faster and more accurate, and it will provide new alternatives for patient alarm systems. At present, most NICUs depend on audible alarms to alert staff that a baby needs attention, but, in the future, these alarms can be transmitted digitally to the staff via headsets, pagers, or other devices that will not add to the noise of the unit.

Telephone and intercom systems also will change drastically with newer technology. Much of the noise generated in the NICU is due to these devices, but alternatives already exist, e.g., wireless headsets, which allow communication to occur very efficiently without adding to noise levels. These systems also will facilitate communication among staff in the multiple room arrangement utilized in most NICUs currently being constructed. Another recent development is the availability of speech recognition and text-to-speech software, which will provide rapid, hands-free input to, and data retrieval from, clinical information systems. Because utilizing these systems requires a considerable adjustment in the local culture of the NICU, the design process should include discussion with end users so that the system chosen will address their needs and concerns.

Maintenance Issues

Many NICU designs that looked good in the blueprint stage required major revisions soon after construction because maintenance issues were not considered adequately. The choice of carpeting, lighting systems, HVAC design, computer devices, and bedside equipment should not be finalized until maintenance problems are identified fully with those who will be responsible for their upkeep. Many of these devices or systems cost more to maintain than to buy, so the economic perspective also should be considered carefully over the anticipated 10- to 20-year lifespan of the NICU, as well as the extent to which routine or unanticipated maintenance will interfere with patient care.

Designing for Renovations

Unless the pace of change slows dramatically, all NICUs will be faced with the desire to upgrade their facility every few years. Many of the suggestions listed previously are practical to implement without a major building program (e.g., reduced ambient lighting, some noise control measures, better, more welcoming signage). Others can be accomplished through a renovation-in-place project (e.g., adding carpeting, wall hangings, acoustical tile; providing more rooming-in space for families), but some will be impossible without new construction and significant increases in available floor space. In the course of a new construction project, it will be impossible to anticipate all the changes that might occur in neonatal care and technology over the next 20 years, but a couple of general principles should be kept in mind.

First, there is no substitute for adequate space. The square footage needed for state-of-the-art NICU care has increased relentlessly, yet is still less, per patient, than that allotted to pediatric or adult ICUs in virtually all hospitals. Most NICU new construction projects completed in the last 20 years have been forced to accept reductions in floor space from the ideal for fiscal considerations, which often proved to be short sighted, as renovations were required only a few years later. It is hard to imagine new developments that would reduce the floor space requirements for NICUs, but it is easy to suggest those that might increase them, such as increased parental access and continued development of new technology to improve monitoring, diagnosis, and thereby survival and outcome of extremely-low-birth-weight infants.

Second, we are in the midst of a dramatic transition from the NICU as a high-tech, sterile (in every sense of the word) environment, to one that resembles a baby's bedroom, with all the implications that carries for parental access. This does not mean technology will disappear, or that many bedsides will not continue to resemble an operating room setup. It does suggest that this latter situation should be the exception, and that NICU design teams therefore will need to consider the norm to be an area where each baby is surrounded by its family and a nurturing environment.

EQUIPMENT SELECTION

Equipment selection is an integral part of the planning process, whether for renovation or new construction. It is important to recognize that equipment features change rapidly and that, with the advance of technology, specific plans for space allocation and cost must be easily modifiable. Categories of equipment that will need to be specified include environmental (e.g., incubators, radiant warmers), life support (ventilators, extracorporeal membrane oxygenation, nitric oxide systems), monitors, diagnostic (x-ray, ultrasound, electronic scales), treatment (infusion pumps, phototherapy, suction, chest percussion), communications (telephone, computer terminals, and printers), and general support (breast milk and pharmacy refrigerators). All users, as well as consultants familiar with the process of equipment inventory, planning, procurement, and installation, and with maintenance of the equipment, should be part of the planning team.

The first step of the equipment selection process involves preparing a list of all fixed and portable equipment that will be needed. Next, existing equipment should be evaluated to determine which items can be utilized in the newly constructed NICU. At this point, dimensions and general space and equipment mounting requirements should be transmitted to the design team so that design of the patient care and storage areas can proceed while decisions are being made regarding purchase of new equipment.

The choice and procurement of new equipment is itself a several-step process. After deciding exactly what equipment will be needed and the budget available, the selection team should familiarize themselves with options available in the market. If a considerable amount of new equipment is anticipated, it is wise to organize an exhibitors' day where all the major vendors can demonstrate their products to the largest number of staff possible (a list of all vendors is published annually by *Perinatology/Neonatology* journal). Alternatively, most large medical and nursing conferences have displays by the major vendors.

When evaluating a new product, considerations should include ease of use, durability, ease of maintenance, the ability to interface easily with computer and monitor systems, hazards such as noise and electromagnetic radiation, size and portability, ability to upgrade, and cost. After all this information is gathered, the equipment consultant should organize it into a report, which can be given to all interested parties (users, maintenance, and procurement staff) for comment. Procurement then can proceed with a request for bids, and a final purchasing decision can be made when these are available. A delivery schedule should be developed in coordination with the design and construction teams so that equipment will arrive in sufficient time to be assembled, tested, and installed prior to opening of the NICU, but not so far in advance that upgrades and modifications in the technology occur while the equipment is sitting in storage.

After selecting the equipment, the financial planning team will need to consider decisions regarding purchase or lease, and service contracts on each item. Although many hospitals have standing policies for such decisions, certain factors may still be worth reviewing. If a piece of equipment is a newer model of an item from a manufacturer with which the hospital has had considerable experience, the biomedical maintenance department may feel quite comfortable with assuming the responsibility for repair without the benefit of a service contract, and purchase of the item usually will be less expensive than leasing in the long run (although the chief financial officer should confirm this based on the specific terms offered). On the other hand, if the piece of equipment is an entirely new device and only one or two are being acquired, lease or purchase with a service contract has considerable value in that repairs will be made by experienced technicians, and faulty equipment may be replaced more readily. In either case, the hospital should have a very clear understanding of how quickly service will be available, and whether replacement items will be immediately available if repairs cannot be made promptly, especially if the equipment is crucial to the management of a critically ill child. These commitments should be obtained in writing, and their reliability confirmed by calling other units currently using similar equipment from each manufacturer.

Before installation occurs, the equipment consultant should review architectural, mechanical, electrical, and plumbing drawings to ensure that all specifications are current and compatible with the equipment that has been selected. There is nothing more frustrating than trying to install a piece of equipment that does not fit or has inadequate electrical or plumbing support. There are also many human dynamics that are crucial to this process, and the equipment consultant must be able to work with each of the specialists involved and organize a process that will be well structured and successfully implemented. Again, the construction of a full-sized, functional mockup of a patient care area should be considered as part of this process before final approval of the blueprints.

REVIEW AND APPROVAL PROCESS

After several months of planning, the architects will review the completed plans with the design team for final comment and approval. The hospital administration will be asked to sign off on a series of construction documents, prior to submitting them to contractors for bids. Although it is common knowledge to architects and construction managers, many members of the design team may be unaware that changes after this time usually are expensive and sometimes impossible. A design that has considerable flexibility built in will become an obvious benefit, so that interim changes in care practices or equipment can be accommodated easily. When bids on the project are received, however, some major changes may still be required, because financial projections by the architects are, of necessity in such one-of-a-kind projects, only rough estimates. Sometimes compromises are fairly straightforward; if aisles were generously sized, for example, a reduction in all aisle widths by 1 foot might save tens of thousands of dollars; bed positions might be reduced in number or size, or offices and conference areas might be reduced in size, shared with adjacent units, or redesigned as flexible-use spaces. The mission statement developed at the beginning of the planning process provides an important point of reference here. If compromises appear to be required that would make accomplishing that mission and the accompanying goals and objectives difficult or impossible, it may be more appropriate to revise the budget rather than the design or (particularly in areas that already have high-quality neonatal providers) to reconsider the project's feasibility altogether.

Before finalizing the blueprints, the design team should spend one more session exploring all the possible opportunities for Murphy's law to manifest itself. Any device or system that could break or malfunction should be reevaluated to see if any change in the design would minimize the impact of such an event. For example, is there anything in, or attached to, the ceiling that could break or come loose and fall on a baby? Is there any wiring, plumbing, or ductwork hidden in a wall for which access might be very difficult or disruptive? Is there any passageway that might be obstructed by a piece of equipment just when a resuscitation became necessary? Architects cannot anticipate all of these events, which usually are not discussed in the planning process, and staff have difficulty visualizing the impact of such events from looking at blueprints, so this process usually is best done with several members of each discipline committed to brainstorming together for several hours. This is another reason visits to other NICUs can be particularly valuable to one who is as interested in the flaws as well as the positive features of the design.

After a bid is accepted (a process that, like the choice of an architect, should be based not only on cost but on the extent and quality of the contractor's previous experience), a meeting should be held with the contractor and members of all the planning teams to be sure the construction team has "caught the vision" so carefully thought out over the previous months. Far from being simply contractors, the construction team can offer many helpful suggestions along the way if they understand the planning teams desires, especially with regard to specifics such as easily accessible wiring, minimizing noise generation from HVAC and plumbing supplies, and so forth. Walkthroughs should be performed on a regular basis throughout the construction process, as multiple fine-tuning issues that were not anticipated in advance undoubtedly will occur. Any resulting changes from the architectural drawings should be documented carefully on "as is" drawings, so that future renovations are not hampered by unpleasant surprises.

HUMAN DYNAMICS CRUCIAL TO A SUCCESSFUL MOVE

In renovation projects, construction often must proceed in stages, while patient care continues to be provided in the existing unit. With either new construction or renovation, the implementation of new equipment and care practices can be both exciting and stressful, and it is not unusual for turnover of staff to increase around the time of the move. There are two contrasting strategies that have been utilized to ease the transition to a new unit. One school of thought suggests that introducing new equipment and practices to the greatest extent possible before the move is valuable to minimize the culture shock of transition. An alternative strategy is based on the concept that acceptance of new practices is most successful when undertaken wholesale, especially if some issues that are

anxiety provoking (e.g., increased access for families) are balanced by others about which the staff will be excited (more space, better equipment). In practice, the transition period requires utilization of both philosophies, because some changes may not be possible until the new unit is built (e.g., rooming in for parents), whereas others will be desirable to implement as soon as possible (e.g., a new ventilator).

Certainly the most important strategy in this regard is to integrate the staff as fully as possible into the planning, design, and construction process. The staff must understand and buy into the conceptual changes intended by the mission statement and around which the design process proceeded. Attendance at committee meetings and posting blueprints are helpful in this regard, especially if comments are encouraged and utilized, but working with a full-scale mockup of a patient care area and occasional visits to the construction site are very helpful to those who have difficulty visualizing two-dimensional renderings.

CHANGE-IN-PLACE

The final step of any NICU construction is a commitment to "change-in-place." We are just beginning to understand the biological effects of the environment on premature infants, especially the positive and negative effects of light, sound, touch, movement, and smell at each gestation stage. Likewise, a better recognition of the role of parents and staff in the care and nurture of their babies will lead to improved care practices, and technological improvements are sure to continue. Each of these trends will influence our concept of the optimal NICU design and should be incorporated to the greatest extent possible on an ongoing basis within an existing structure, rather than waiting until new construction again becomes feasible. An agreement by all members of the planning process that the NICU will be considered a work in progress, rather than a finished edifice, will enhance the readiness of all disciplines to implement change when the need becomes apparent and will drive the design teams to build in as much flexibility as possible.

REFERENCES

1. Hauth JC, Merenstein GB, eds. *Guidelines for perinatal care*, 4th ed. Elk Grove Village, IL: American Academy of Pediatrics, 1997.
2. *Recommended standards for newborn ICU design. Report of the Third Consensus Committee.* 1996. URL: http://www.nd.edu/~kkolberg/DesignStandards.htm.
3. Hall JH, Johnson BH. *Family centered care.* Bethesda, MD: Institute for Family-Centered Care, 1997.
4. White RD. Enhanced neonatal intensive care design: a physiological approach. *J Perinatol* 1996;16:381.
5. Guidelines for intensive care unit design. *Crit Care Med* 1995;23:582.
6. Bullough J, Rea MS. Lighting for neonatal intensive care units: some critical information for design. *Lighting Res Technol* 1996;28:189.
7. Rea MS, ed. *Lighting handbook*, 8th ed. New York: Illuminating Engineering Society of North America, 1993.

CHAPTER 6

Neonatal Nursing: The Organization of Care and Quality Assurance in the NICU

Carolyn Houska Lund and Beryl Epstein

Providing current, research-based care to critically ill newborns requires the collaboration of highly skilled, dedicated, and motivated caregivers from a variety of disciplines. Professional nurses, physicians, respiratory therapists, social workers, developmental care specialists, pharmacists, clinical dieticians, and occupational and physical therapists have roles to play in planning, implementing, and evaluating the care for infants and their families in the neonatal intensive care unit (NICU). In this chapter the role of neonatal nurses in the direct care of high-risk newborns is described, as well as the necessary knowledge and skills that are needed in order to assure competency. Organizational structures of nursing leadership in the NICU are discussed, and other nursing roles are defined.

Systems to monitor and improve the quality of care in the NICU, involving all professional disciplines, are integral in providing care to high-risk infants. Components of a practical and useful quality assurance program are outlined, including developing unit-based, written documents such as standards of care, organizational structures, clinical practice guidelines, critical pathways, algorithms, protocols, and procedures. Practice committees that evaluate the delivery of care are also a part of this system and are included in the discussion.

ROLE OF NURSING IN NICU PATIENT CARE

The keystone of care delivery to the neonatal patient and family is the nurse assigned to the hour-by-hour care of each patient in the NICU. Neonatal nursing is a challenging and changing specialty. The experienced NICU nurse serves as the infant's link to a new and sometimes hostile environment. Education and experience give nurses the tools to serve as interpreter for the infant, using intuition and assessment of physiologic data and behavior to discern the infant's response to treatment and environment.

Factors that combine to make neonatal nursing practice so important and difficult include the frequent introduction of new treatment modalities, absence of verbal communication with the newborn patient, narrow margin between safe and adverse responses to therapy, lack of specific responses because of immature organ development, and extreme vulnerability, particularly in the most premature or critically ill infants. The small size of these patients places them at increased risk of injury from even minute mistakes and presents difficulties when delivering complex technical treatments and procedures.

Further complicating the care of the high-risk newborn who is premature or has complex medical or surgical conditions is the unknown, and at times adverse, effects of the disease process on organs that are still in the process of development. Newborns lack extensive history to determine baselines for diagnoses and physiologic parameters. The process of development that occurs alongside the process of healing means that the normal baseline also keeps changing. The nurse must be cognizant of the changing baseline of each infant as he or she progresses from a 24-week infant to a 32-, 34-, or 36-week infant. This often changes the interpretation of data and modifies what are appropriate interventions. There is also a gradual appearance of individual and often unique reactions to stimuli and caregiving procedures in specific infants in addition to the developmental differences noted.

Because the nurse's scope of responsibility is limited to a small number of patients at any given time (generally

C. H. Lund and B. Epstein: Intensive Care Nursery, Children's Hospital, Oakland, California

two or three), and because of the need to be in constant proximity to the bedside of their patients, the observations and evaluations made by nurses often guide interventions by the health care team. Observations by nurses may stimulate further scrutiny by the medical team including lab work and other diagnostic evaluations.

Finally, because newborns are in the earliest stages of their relationship to their families, parents may not be fully able to understand their infant's behaviors and reactions. Thus, they may not be able to communicate their infant's unique traits and responses to the nurse. The nurse may need to assist parents in learning to identify and interpret their infant's signals so that the parents can successfully assume their parental roles and advocate for their infant. Often the family's own special needs are a major focus for nursing intervention. Helping families cope with crisis, adjusting to altered perceptions of parenting, and learning skills necessary to become caregivers for their newborns are other facets of neonatal nursing care.

In summary, the nurse at the bedside plays a major role as protector, advocate, and nurturer to the infant in an NICU. Nurses provide a vital link between the patient and the rest of the multidisciplinary team because of their knowledge, proximity to the patient, and skill at interpretation of physiologic, behavioral, and technical information.

Nursing Assessment

Nurses assess their patients during their admission to the NICU and at regular intervals each day throughout the course of hospitalization. This includes evaluation of physical characteristics such as color, neuromuscular tone, skin integrity, vascular perfusion, and edema. Organ systems are assessed using chest auscultation, heart sounds, palpation of pulses, urine output, bowel sounds, and presence of neurologic reflexes. Level of neurobehavioral and developmental activity is determined, including assessment of pain and discomfort in relation to treatments administered and other environmental stimuli.

The technology that surrounds the infant is another important aspect of assessment. This includes patency and functioning of all intravascular devices, security of endotracheal tubes, and evaluation of all other invasive tubes and lines. The presence and appropriate functioning of all respiratory equipment, monitoring devices, intravenous pumps, thermoregulatory devices, and emergency equipment such as bag and mask and suctioning equipment is confirmed.

Assessment of the family is an important and shared responsibility with social workers and physicians. Nurses evaluate families in direct contact with their infants and thus can identify behaviors that are commonly seem versus those with significant concern for later attachment difficulties or needing crisis resolution. They also assess how well the family is able to assume caregiving tasks and how learning is progressing regarding any special needs the infant may have. This should be accomplished before discharge to home becomes near.

Technical Skills

Psychomotor skills are necessary components of competence in neonatal nursing. These include an exhaustive list of procedures (Table 6–1). However, Table 6–1 remains a partial list; the type of patient population and level of care may necessitate many others. Nurses also assist physicians and advanced-practice nurses in the following procedures: chest tube insertion, endotracheal intubation, umbilical catheter insertion, lumbar puncture, central line insertion, and exchange transfusion. In some NICUs nurses are certified to perform some of these advanced practice procedures under the direction of physicians.

Safe use of medical devices is also a necessity in the NICU (Table 6–1). Competency with medical devices is extremely important to assure patient safety, especially with the current standard of ten to 12 devices in use for each patient in an NICU. Many disposable supplies are also in use, such as intravenous tubing, stopcocks, catheters, and tubes that carry risks of cracking, breaking, or malfunction. The neonatal nurse is responsible for using these items with a level of expertise that allows for recognition and identification of problems before enlisting the appropriate support services such as biomedical engineers, respiratory therapists, or other technical specialists.

Daily Care Practices

Certain practices form the foundation for the daily care that nurses provide in the NICU. These include assessment and monitoring, thermoregulation, skin care and basic hygiene, assisted ventilation and oxygen therapy, nutrition, intravenous access and fluid provision, administration of medications, pain relief, comfort, and developmental care.

Assessment and monitoring include evaluating the cardiovascular, respiratory, gastrointestinal, genitourinary, neurologic, musculoskeletal, and integumentary system at least once every shift. Disease process monitoring includes measuring abdominal girth and observing discoloration, gastric residuals, and frank or occult blood in stools to identify necrotizing enterolcolitis or gastrointestinal perforation. Symptoms of sepsis involve assessment of hypo- or hyperthermia, hypoglycemia, above-baseline apnea and bradycardia episodes, lethargy, hypotonia, and poor feeding. Other assessment activities include measuring weights, intake and output measurements, temperatures of infant and environment, heart

TABLE 6–1. *Competency list of technical skills for procedures and medical devices*

Procedures	Medical devices
Gavage and gastrostomy feeding	Providing thermoregulation via radiant warmers, incubators
Placement of naso-, orogastric, transpyloric, and gastrostomy tubes	Cardiorespiratory monitors
Administration of fluids, electrolytes, parenteral nutrition	Pulse oximeters
Administration of blood and blood products	Noninvasive blood pressure monitoring devices
Establishing vascular access via peripheral venous catheters	Transcutaneous oxygen and carbon dioxide monitors
Maintaining and monitoring central venous and umbilical catheters, chest tubes	Phototherapy lights and blankets
Invasive blood pressure monitoring	Infusion pumps
Obtaining blood samples via venipuncture, arterial puncture, heelstick, umbilical lines	Scales
Monitoring and maintaining oxygen delivery via nasal cannulas, hoods	Defibrillators
Monitoring and maintaining assisted ventilation via nasal CPAP, conventional and high-frequency ventilators	Breast pumps
Suctioning and securing ETTs	Blood warmers
Suctioning and reinserting tracheostomy tubes	Point-of-care testing for glucose, hemoglobin measurements
Ostomy care	
Urinary catheterization	
Isolation procedures	
Administration of intravenous, intramuscular, and oral medications	
Administration of intravenous drug drips	

rate, respiratory rate and quality, blood pressure and perfusion, as well as oxygen saturation monitoring.

Thermoregulation goals include attaining a normal core temperature utilizing thermoregulatory techniques that result in minimal energy expenditure and water loss through evaporative processes. Strategies in providing this thermally neutral environment include techniques that reduce heat losses as well as providing heat sources. Incubators and radiant warmers are used with a variety of modifications including servocontrol skin temperature monitoring, supplemental conductive heating mattresses, warmed humidity, and heat shields and plastic tents to reduce evaporative heat losses. Insulation techniques such as knit caps, clothing, blankets, and buntings are also used to reduce heat losses. Axillary temperatures are measured every 2 to 4 hours along with continuous skin temperatures in servocontrolled devices. These are evaluated by comparison to environmental temperatures and changes in baseline readings over time in order to determine if hypo- or hyperthermia is present.

Skin care practices should be focused on reducing trauma, protecting immature barrier function (especially in prematures), and minimizing exposure to topical agents that can be absorbed. This includes using soaps, cleansers, emollients, and other topical agents sparingly and selecting products with minimal perfumes, dyes, preservatives, and chemicals. Emollients are used to promote skin integrity, especially in small premature infants and when the skin surface is dry, cracking, or fissured. Skin disinfection solutions such as povidone iodine or chlorhexidine are applied before invasive procedures such as venipuncture, umbilical catheter insertion, and

chest tube placement. These agents should be completely removed after use to minimize exposure to readily absorbed chemicals. Adhesive application and removal often causes trauma to skin integrity; minimal use of adhesives is optimal, with removal done carefully and without chemical solvents.

Because many of the disease processes necessitating admission to the NICU involve the respiratory system, assisted ventilation and oxygen delivery are essential components of nursing care. Maintaining a patent airway requires adherence to suctioning practices that minimize airway trauma while effectively removing secretions. Security of endotracheal tubes, nasal CPAP devices, and oxygen cannulas is established and evaluated frequently. Monitoring of ventilation equipment, oxygen delivery systems, and patient oxygenation requires ongoing activity, much of it a shared responsibility with respiratory therapists in the NICU.

Nutrition is an important aspect of care that involves monitoring, delivery of nutrients, and evaluation of nutrient adequacy by observing patient growth. Patients are weighed regularly, and caloric intake determinations are calculated daily to assess adequacy of intake; these activities are often shared among nursing, medical staff, and dieticians. When introducing enteral nutrients, the nurse observes the absorption and utilization of intake by monitoring stooling frequency and type, distension, gastric residuals, and emesis. Promoting healthy patterns of breast-feeding or bottle feeding is a final goal of nutritional care and involves the nurse in conjunction with the parents.

Intravenous access and fluid administration are important in the delivery of care and involve technical skills of peripheral intravenous device placement and the use of pumps to deliver fluids accurately. Nurses should determine if the ordered fluid intake is appropriate for specific patients and monitor urine output and electrolyte determinations to assess patient response. Central venous lines are often used in the NICU, and security of these devices, infection control practices, and problem solving if occlusions occur are ongoing concerns that are addressed during daily nursing care.

Medication administration is a very frequent activity in the NICU. Patients receive a multitude of medication doses every day, including antibiotics, corticosteroids, vitamins and mineral supplements, anticonvulsants, analgesics, and sedatives, and many others. Accurate calculation of doses, appropriate administration techniques and monitoring side effects are among the many activities performed by nurses to assure safe medication use in the NICU.

Developmental care is necessary to protect the delicate central nervous system and promote optimal neurodevelopmental outcome in NICU patients. This includes reducing harsh and at times unrelenting sensory stimuli such as excessive noise, light, and unnecessary handling. Careful observation and interpretation of an individual infant's reactions and behaviors are important to create an environment that is responsive to each infant's unique needs. Providing analgesia and sedation during unavoidable painful procedures, along with adequate postoperative pain relief, are essential for patients in the NICU.

Safety and Emergency Situations

Neonatal nurses provide a safe and secure environment for patients and families. This includes strict adherence to infection control measures, electrical safety, equipment maintenance, transport policies, and visitor controls. It also means timely and accurate reporting of errors, "unusual occurrences," and parental complaints.

Medical emergencies are often averted through early and accurate assessment of changes in an individual infant's baseline patterns that is communicated to other team members. However, the complicated and severe medical problems of NICU patients coupled with the number of treatments, devices, and medications in use can result in deterioration and medical emergencies. Nurses must be prepared to initiate cardiopulmonary resuscitation and to assist in emergency measures such as establishing intravenous access, mixing and administering resuscitation medications such as drug drips or single-bolus infusions, and administering volume replacement and blood products.

Other emergency situations that require anticipation by the NICU staff include fire, disaster, and other conditions necessitating evacuation. Policies must be in place giving explicit instructions, planning meetings, providing evacuation supplies including oxygen tanks for each patient, and holding evacuation drills (1,2).

Documentation

Accurate and thorough, yet concise, written or computerized documentation is another necessary component of nursing practice. Vital signs, patterns of apnea and bradycardia, breath sounds, and suctioning results as well as laboratory information such as blood gases, bedside testing of glucose, and hemoglobin are displayed in graphic or table form. Accurate hourly confirmation of fluid intake, drug drips, and urine output is also documented. The record of all medications administered, including route, time, and patient response, is written. Baseline assessments of all organ systems as well as the physical characteristics of the patient are documented by the nurse at the beginning of each shift of care. Assessment of the physical environment, including all thermoregulatory and monitoring devices as well as emergency equipment, is written in this assessment. Problem-oriented charting at the end of each shift of care includes the symptoms noted, intervention, and evaluation of the effect of intervention. In addition, any changes noted from the initial baseline assessment made at the beginning of the shift are documented. If protocols or practice guidelines are in effect, evaluation of that particular patient in the context of the noted protocol is recorded. Communication with parents is recorded with specific attention to completion of parent education goals.

Knowledge Base for Neonatal Nursing

There is a large body of knowledge that is necessary for neonatal nursing to achieve the goal of safe, effective, family-centered care for high-risk newborns. Associated risk factors, including genetics, critical periods of development, and social risk factors such as substance abuse and poverty, are areas of knowledge needed by the neonatal nurse. Principles of nutrition, infection control, pharmacology, ventilation, and thermoregulation comprise the foundation for many neonatal care practices and must be thoroughly understood. Developmental care is essential and involves knowledge about the impact of development on behavioral reactions, the effect of environmental stimuli on the immature central nervous system, and an appreciation for the individual differences among infants in the NICU.

A thorough understanding of normal physiology as well as the pathophysiology of disease processes is imperative. Understanding the effects of disease processes on the developing organ systems of the premature and term newborn is necessary to interpret the responses of the individual infant at any point on the gestational progression.

Knowledge of recent nursing and medical research that addresses clinical issues and current standards used in maintaining the level of care is necessary for neonatal nurses to apply these in the delivery of care. This includes hospital policies and procedures as well as national standards adopted by the NICU so that care is maintained according to these standards.

Neonatal nurses need to utilize appropriate written resources including current medical and nursing textbooks and journals specific to the care of high-risk newborns. Attending unit-based in-service education is expected, and participating in regional or national neonatal nursing conferences is promoted to further enhance knowledge about current practices and to encourage networking with other neonatal nurses.

ROLE OF NURSING IN FAMILY-CENTERED CARE

The initial phase of hospitalization for high-risk infants results in significant disequilibrium for families, and the neonatal nurse often helps them in their adjustment. The expected outcome for their pregnancy has been changed from a healthy, full-term newborn to a newborn who is premature or has significant medical or surgical problems. With prenatal detection of problems, as well as perinatal care for premature labor, the families may have some idea of the situation they are facing. Yet, many have not faced a crisis of such importance and may need help in developing coping skills, understanding complicated medical information, and identifying how to be an advocate for their infant. Nurses utilize therapeutic communication, crisis intervention, and supportive techniques to assist families during this time (3).

Because many families may have additional social risk factors, including language or cultural differences, poverty, chronic illness, or substance abuse, knowledge about the impact of these factors on coping with crises and parenting is needed. The importance of early intervention cannot be emphasized strongly enough, and interventions by neonatal nurses along with NICU social workers and neonatologists can have considerable positive effects for high-risk families during this time of disequilibrium.

Family-centered care is both a philosophy and an approach to care that can enhance the potential of families to cope with the crisis and experience a positive outcome. Principles for family-centered neonatal care include open and honest communication on both medical and ethical considerations as well as in-depth medical information in terms that are meaningful and providing access to other parents who have had infants in similar circumstances. Information is provided to families early if prenatal diagnosis about neonatal problems becomes apparent. Parents are allowed the right to make decisions for their infants about aggressive treatments once they are fully informed with adequate medical knowledge. Additional areas addressed in family-centered care are alleviation of pain, ensuring an appropriate environment, pro-

viding safe and effective treatments, and policies and programs that promote parenting skills and maximum involvement of families with their infant in the NICU (4–6). Key elements of family-centered care are outlined in Table 6–2.

Parent and family education are necessary throughout the hospitalization in the NICU. Initially, parents need information about their infant's medical condition, what it means and what the prognosis is, as well as an orientation to the NICU in terms of the personnel they will encounter ("who does what"). Pamphlets and booklets about premature infants or specific disease conditions may be helpful. There are also several books written by parents or NICU professionals that contain detailed information, illustrations, and accounts of other parents' reactions to the experience in the NICU (7,8). The Internet is another source of information for parents. Each unit would wisely evaluate which resources on the Internet contain the most up-to-date, factual, nonbiased information about specific conditions and post these resources

TABLE 6–2. *The key elements of family-centered care[a]*

- Incorporating into policy and practice the recognition that the family is the constant in a child's life while the service systems and support personnel within those systems fluctuate.
- Facilitating family/professional collaboration at all levels of hospital, home, and community care:
  Care of an individual child
  Program development, implementation, evaluation, and evolution
  Policy formation
- Exchanging complete and unbiased information between families and professionals in a supportive manner at all times.
- Incorporating into policy and practice the recognition and honoring of cultural diversity, strengths, and individuality within and across all families, including ethnic, racial, spiritual, social, economic, educational, and geographic diversity.
- Recognizing and respecting different methods of coping and implementing comprehensive policies and programs that provide developmental, educational, emotional, environmental, and financial supports to meet the diverse needs of families.
- Encouraging and facilitating family-to-family support and networking.
- Ensuring that hospital, home, and community service and support systems for children needing specialized health and developmental care and their families are flexible, accessible, and comprehensive in responding to diverse family-identified needs.
- Appreciating families as families and children as children, recognizing that they possess a wide range of strengths, concerns, emotions, and aspirations beyond their need for specialized health and developmental services and support.

[a]Reprinted with permission from Shelton TL, Stepanek JS. *Family-centered care for children needing specialized health and development services.* Bethesda: Association for the Care of Children's Health, 1994.

for parents to access if they wish. Although written information is valuable, this is not a substitution for parent conferences and verbal interchange with parents, focused not only on what the professional staff think they need to hear but also on what the parents are concerned about, as well as their feelings and reactions to what is happening to them and to their infant.

The environment surrounding the infant must be explained, including the type of monitors, special beds, and other equipment that is used in the care of their infant. Nurses can help parents become involved in the physical care of their infant by showing them the things they can do such as comfort measures, bathing, skin care or mouth care, changing the diaper, taking the temperature, holding as soon as their infant is stable on the ventilator or in oxygen (Fig. 6–1), and providing breast milk.

Nurses plan and orchestrate discharge teaching. This includes well-baby care with knowledge about specific patterns of feeding, sleeping, urination, stooling, breathing, and skin care for their baby. Medication administration, including the purpose, method of administration, side effects, as well as where to obtain the medications, is essential. Special needs are described and skills taught, including gavage or gastrostomy feeding, oxygen administration, ostomy care, tracheostomy care, cardiorespiratory monitors, and others. Different disease processes or conditions are identified for parents, such as bronchopulmonary dysplasia, short-bowel syndrome, and hydrocephalus, and symptoms are identified for parents so they can assess and seek medical care appropriately after the infant is home (9,10).

Nurses can help families in their adaptation and resolution of crisis by providing consistency in the delivery of daily nursing care. Infants are regularly assigned to a nurse or a group of nurses on admission or shortly thereafter, and consistent care is delivered by this primary nurse or primary team throughout the hospital course.

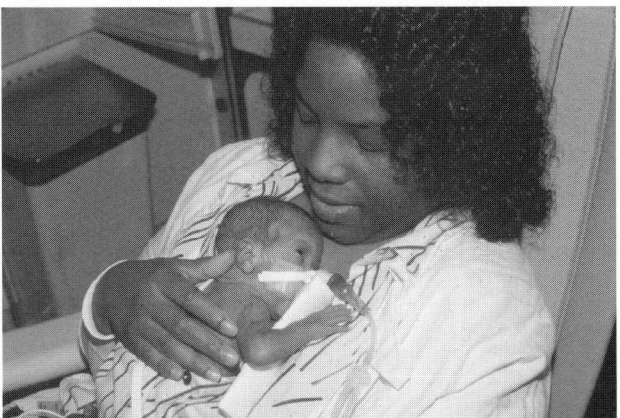

FIG. 6–1. Photo of a mother holding her ventilated premie skin to skin.

Primary nurses provide direct patient care, organize and write individual care plans, and collaborate with the neonatologist, social worker, and advanced practice nurse to facilitate the smooth transition of the infant throughout the hospital stay and discharge from the NICU. They have extensive knowledge about the individual responses of patients they care for on a daily basis and are invaluable to the neonatologist and other team members because of their knowledge of the infant over a period of time. Primary nursing care lends itself well to developmental care that is specific in both assessment and interventions aimed at the individual needs and unique characteristics of neonatal patients.

Primary nursing is highly valued by families of infants in the NICU. Seeing the same person caring for their infant is comforting and establishes trust during this period of crisis and disequilibrium for families. Families often will share their feelings and reactions best with someone they come to know and trust; this is often the primary nurse.

NURSING LEADERSHIP AND OTHER NURSING ROLES

The organization of care in the NICU is a collaboration among the medical staff, nursing, and other departments involved in the care of patients in the NICU. Decisions about delivery of care, unit philosophy, and future directions are best the result of this collaborative process rather than any one department or discipline operating in a vacuum.

However, most NICUs are organized structurally and financially around the nursing component. The organization and functioning of an NICU is dependent on nursing leadership that can provide knowledgeable support and nursing input for the following functions: strategic planning, budget development and implementation, staff development, education, quality assurance and improvement, interdepartmental collaboration, and clinical standards development.

Nursing leadership can be provided by nurses with advanced education, training, and experience in the following roles: Nurse Manager, Clinical Nurse Specialist, Neonatal Nurse Practitioner, Nurse Educator, Transport or ECMO Coordinator, and Case Manager. Depending on the size and complexity of the NICU, some of these roles may be combined.

Emotional support is necessary for caregivers who work in the NICU because of the high stress and sensitive nature of their work with critically ill infants and families. The nursing leadership group seeks out stressful situations and provides support to staff through stress debriefing and staff case conferences. Referrals to hospital ethics committees and to appropriate professionals such as psychologists, psychiatric nurse liaisons, chaplains, and employee assistance programs should be made early to assist staff when needed.

Nurse Manager

The nurse manager has overall responsibility for the day-to-day operation of the NICU and for coordinating and collaborating with the medical staff, other department directors, and nursing managers from other units. The manager is usually expected to plan and implement both capital and operations budgets. Further, the manager collaborates with the nursing leadership team to assure that education, ongoing development, and competency of the nursing staff are attained. The nursing leadership group, in collaboration with the medical team and ancillary disciplines, is also responsible for assuring that the quality of care delivered in the NICU is safe and appropriate, meets regulatory standards, and demonstrates a commitment to ongoing quality improvement.

Although the nurse manager and nursing leadership group are accountable for the care delivered in the NICU, the staff nurses are, again, the keystone of care delivery. Therefore, facilitating staff participation at every level of decision making is critical to the success of any unit operations. In some units, this collaboration may be formalized through a system of shared governance in which staff nurses are empowered to govern many aspects of unit operations. However, even in more traditional organizational structures, participation by staff is critical to the successful operation of the unit.

Advanced Practice Nurses

The clinical nurse specialist (CNS) is a master's-prepared advanced practice practitioner in a nonline position in the nursing structure. This generally means that the CNS has no direct authority over other staff. The CNS role involves direct clinical care, consultation to nursing staff and other professionals, and education of staff and parents. Research is a component of the CNS role, and this is accomplished by keeping abreast of current research applicable to care, implementing research-based practices, supporting and facilitating research efforts in the NICU, and participating in research as primary investigator or coinvestigator. Maintaining quality of care is another aspect of CNS practice; monitoring care practices, identifying problems, and participating in the NICU multidisciplinary practice committee are essential aspects of the CNS role and its effective implementation in the NICU (11).

Many units are involving the CNS in performing case management functions. Case management, a model of care delivery, focuses on multidisciplinary care throughout hospitalization to achieve desired patient outcomes in an expected time frame and with efficient use of resources (12,13). Within this model, the CNS follows a caseload of patients throughout their length of stay in the NICU, consulting with nursing staff, physicians, and other team members about the patients' expected course and any variations that occur. The CNS coordinates the interdisciplinary model by holding weekly interdisciplinary rounds to discuss medical and social aspects of care for each infant in the NICU and to identify needed interventions, procedures, or family communication. The CNS may identify a need for individual patient care conferences, for staff and consultants or for families with the medical and nursing staff, to discuss a complicated patient and identify reasonable goals with evaluation criteria to determine the efficacy of the plan.

The neonatal nurse practitioner (NNP) has formal education and certification in the medical management of high-risk newborns. The NNPs generally carry a caseload of neonatal patients with consultation, collaboration, and supervision from a neonatologist. With an extensive knowledge of physiology, pathophysiology, and pharmacology, the NNP functions both independently and interdependently with physicians, in the assessment, diagnosis, and implementation of specific medical practices and procedures. Other responsibilities can include delivery room resuscitation, stabilization and transport either within the hospital or to other facilities, education, consultation, and research at varying levels (11,14,15).

Other nursing roles that are present as distinct entities or included in the previously mentioned titles include neonatal clinical educators, outreach educators, transport nurses, discharge planners, nursing shift coordinators, and extracorporeal membrane oxygenation (ECMO) specialists.

The role of the charge nurse in the NICU is an important leadership position in the daily operations of the unit. Charge nurses may be nurse managers, shift coordinators, or experienced staff nurses responsible for the smooth functioning of the unit during each shift in a 24-hour day. This involves evaluating the number and level of acuity of all infants in order to determine the number of nursing and support staff required and communicating the assignments of patients and staff.

Charge nurses also arrange incoming and outgoing transports and may in some settings attend high-risk deliveries. They are often the "extra pair of hands" needed during emergency situations or special procedures, are consulted by other nurses in problem situations and conflict resolution, and become involved in crisis intervention with families. Astute assessment and problem-solving skills, along with excellent communication abilities, are necessary in the successful implementation of the charge nurse role and the daily running of the NICU.

These nursing roles provide a structure around which to organize care delivery in the NICU. However, to move beyond day-to-day care delivery and address issues of quality of care, or improvement of care delivery, a multidisciplinary group provides the perspective needed to arrive at a consensus that can change patient care directly and improve ultimate outcome.

IMPROVING THE QUALITY OF CARE IN THE NICU

When Hippocrates intoned "First, do no harm," he set the first standard in medical practice. During the intervening centuries, we have progressed from standards designed to prevent harm (or iatrogenic events) to standards that attempt to improve the quality of health care delivered to the patient.

As the delivery of medical care moved from the home to hospital in the late 19th century, the need to set standards of practice for these institutions arose, and the concept of standards development for health professions evolved. For example, in her classic *Notes on Nursing* (16), published in 1859, Florence Nightingale described standards of nursing practice that were aimed at improving the care and long-term outcomes of patients in hospitals. She based her standards and recommendations for change on data she collected and analyzed, setting the groundwork for quality assurance practices that we know today.

In the early 1900s, Dr. Ernest Codman, a prominent surgeon at Massachusetts General Hospital in Boston, described a process for surgeons to look at the outcomes for patients by systematically gathering information about surgical procedures and care and to make this information publically known to future patients. With his colleague, Edward Martin, the American College of Surgeons was created, and the Hospital Standardization Program was formed. This program, which imposed a self-measurement mandate on hospitals, was the antecedent of the Joint Commission on Accreditation of Healthcare Organizations (JCAHO) (17).

The JCAHO, formed in 1951, initially developed standards for hospitals and evaluated compliance to these standards, hypothesizing that compliance with these standards would correlate with quality care and good outcomes for patients in hospitals. Despite this somewhat reassuring model, the usefulness of monitoring standards in hospitals did not address basic questions about clinical care as it was delivered in hospitals that received accreditation. Other issues that needed evaluation were the systems for management of hospitals and other health care organizations, utilization of resources, and, most importantly, what actually were the patient outcomes that were produced. Interest and concern about these aspects of care delivery were stimulated in part by the escalation of health care costs, the lack of reliable outcome reporting, and the dramatic organizational changes that occurred in the health care system in the 1980s and is continuing into the 21st century.

As a result of these changes, quality in health care settings is evaluated by monitoring adherence to accepted standards and measurement of outcome. Standards are derived from a variety of sources, including governmental (via regulatory agencies, at both the federal and state levels) as well as professional and community-based standards of practice.

For the NICU, governmental regulations may describe environmental standards, such as the number of square feet per patient bed space, minimum equipment requirements, infection control practices, equipment maintenance, etc. In some states government standards require certain staffing levels or patterns, the type of licensure required for staff who deliver patient care (based on acuity or degree of illness), as well as ancillary and support staff required for appropriate multidisciplinary practice.

Other standards that are used by the NICU may include those determined by professional societies such as the American Academy of Pediatrics (AAP), the American Medical Association (AMA), or the Association of Women's Health, Obstetrics and Neonatal Nursing (AWHONN). Public sector agencies such as the National Institutes of Health Office of Medical Applications and Research, Centers for Disease Control and Prevention (CDC), or the Agency for Health Care Policy and Research (AHCPR) also establish standards or guidelines that utilize current research to better define a plan of care.

The Institute of Medicine, a branch of the AHCPR, defines clinical practice guidelines as "systematically developed statements to assist practitioner and patient decisions about appropriate health care for specific clinical circumstances" (18). There is currently great interest in reducing variability in health care treatments and interventions associated with changes in health care delivery and reimbursement structures; there is also research demonstrating wide variations in resource utilization and hospital costs with no difference in outcome (19). A number of factors are motivating this trend, including a desire to reduce variations in practice that delay patient care, prolong hospital stays, and increase use of resources leading to increased costs; providing a consistent plan of care that all members of an increasingly complex health care team are aware of and can use to communicate with each other; and having a plan that can be communicated to patients and families so that they can anticipate the day-to-day progress and know their own responsibilities in regard to health care outcome (18,20,21).

Standards and guidelines are also being developed by individual hospitals, health care insurers, and health maintenance organizations. Terms that describe these standards and guidelines include clinical practice guidelines, practice policies, care maps, critical pathways, algorithms, and protocols. Definitions for these terms vary, and they are sometimes used interchangeably. In many settings, however, clinical practice guidelines, pathways, and care maps refer to a time-based sequencing of events for a particular diagnosis or procedure leading to an ideal plan of care, whereas algorithms and protocols involve a series of decisions and actions to be taken for a specific treatment, medication, or activity (22).

There is an ongoing discussion about the validity and appropriateness of practice guidelines as well as doubts about their contribution toward improving patient outcomes (23,24). A concern is raised about the lack of congruency between two stated purposes of guidelines: the improvement of quality and the reduction of costs. This is because it is difficult to agree on quality standards, and it is easier to measure cost than quality. Therefore, financial concerns may dominate in the evaluation of effectiveness of guidelines. There are other concerns as well: the possibility of the courts upholding a practice guideline as definitive of the standard of care in a clinical area is noted, as well as the potential for increasing health care costs if practitioners are unwilling to vary practices from the guideline even when their clinical judgment determines that another intervention is more appropriate for an individual patient (23).

However, in developing practice guidelines for individual units, there are important benefits in the process of reaching consensus among a varied multidisciplinary staff and in discussing the pros and cons of different practices in the context of current research findings. Critical pathways or practice guidelines can be extremely valuable in communication with parents by providing a road map of the usual course for infants with a specific disease or level of prematurity and gives parents a sense of what to expect through a sometimes lengthy hospitalization. The guidelines can also include a section specifically for parents' roles and responsibilities including adding their infant to their health plan, applying for government-sponsored programs where applicable, preparing their home for bringing their infant home, and learning the care of the infant before his or her release from the hospital. These benefits may ultimately establish practice guidelines as a way to improve quality, and they may also prove useful in reducing health care costs (25–27). Figure 6–2 shows a time-based critical pathway designed to monitor the progression of care in premature infants according to gestational and postconceptional age.

Process of Quality Monitoring and Improvement

Quality assurance has become the process of monitoring and improving the quality of care. The Joint Commission on Accreditation of Healthcare Organizations (JCAHO) uses standards that address the following hospital functions: care-of-patient functions, including assessment, direct care activities such as medication use and nutritional care, education, and providing continuity of care from entry to discharge; and organizational functions such as leadership, management of information, the environment of care, infection control, and organizational improvement. Both the processes (what are the steps) and

the outcomes (what happens as a result of the steps being followed) are priorities when measuring the quality of care (28). There is an emphasis on efficient and cost effective use of resources in all aspects of care delivery.

Theories and methodologies utilized under the JCAHO mandate include total quality management (TQM) and continuous quality improvement (CQI). These have evolved from systems theory: an organization is a system with individual parts that must work well together if performance, patient outcomes, quality, and cost effectiveness are to be attained.

Measuring quality of care involves selecting indicators that describe the process or the outcome of care. Terminology used to define indicators is common to research methodology: indicators should be quantitative (expressed in units of measurement), valid (identifying events that are important enough to merit review), and reliable (accurately and thoroughly identifying events and occurrences) (17).

Examples of indicators in the NICU setting are listed in Table 6–3. Some indicators reflect aggregate data related to an abundance of similar cases or routine processes in the NICU. Other indicators may reflect sentinel events or situations that are infrequent but extremely undesirable.

It is important not only to collect information that accurately reflects measures of quality of care in the NICU but also to be able to compare or evaluate the meaning of the measurements. Comparisons can be made from information compiled from one period of time to another within the same NICU, or from one unit in a hospital to another. The term "benchmarking" is used to describe the process of comparing data from one hospital to a national standard of care (17). There is a great deal of interest in compiling benchmarking measurements utilizing national collaborative data bases and sources such as the Vermont–Oxford Neonatal Database (29) or the National Institute of Child Health and Human Development Neonatal Research Network (30).

Quality monitoring in the NICU also involves the ongoing evaluation of staff performance. For nurses this includes establishing a list of competencies necessary to provide safe and effective care and ongoing competency assessment for both high-risk and new technologies (31). Through peer evaluation and performance review by managers, staff competence can be documented and used to develop individual performance improvement plans. Physicians in the NICU may establish a process of peer review and compile statistics regarding mortality and morbidity for specific patient groups. This process is referred to as "physician profiling."

Multidisciplinary Process for Quality Improvement in the NICU

The process and structure for quality monitoring and improvement in the NICU, although in part determined

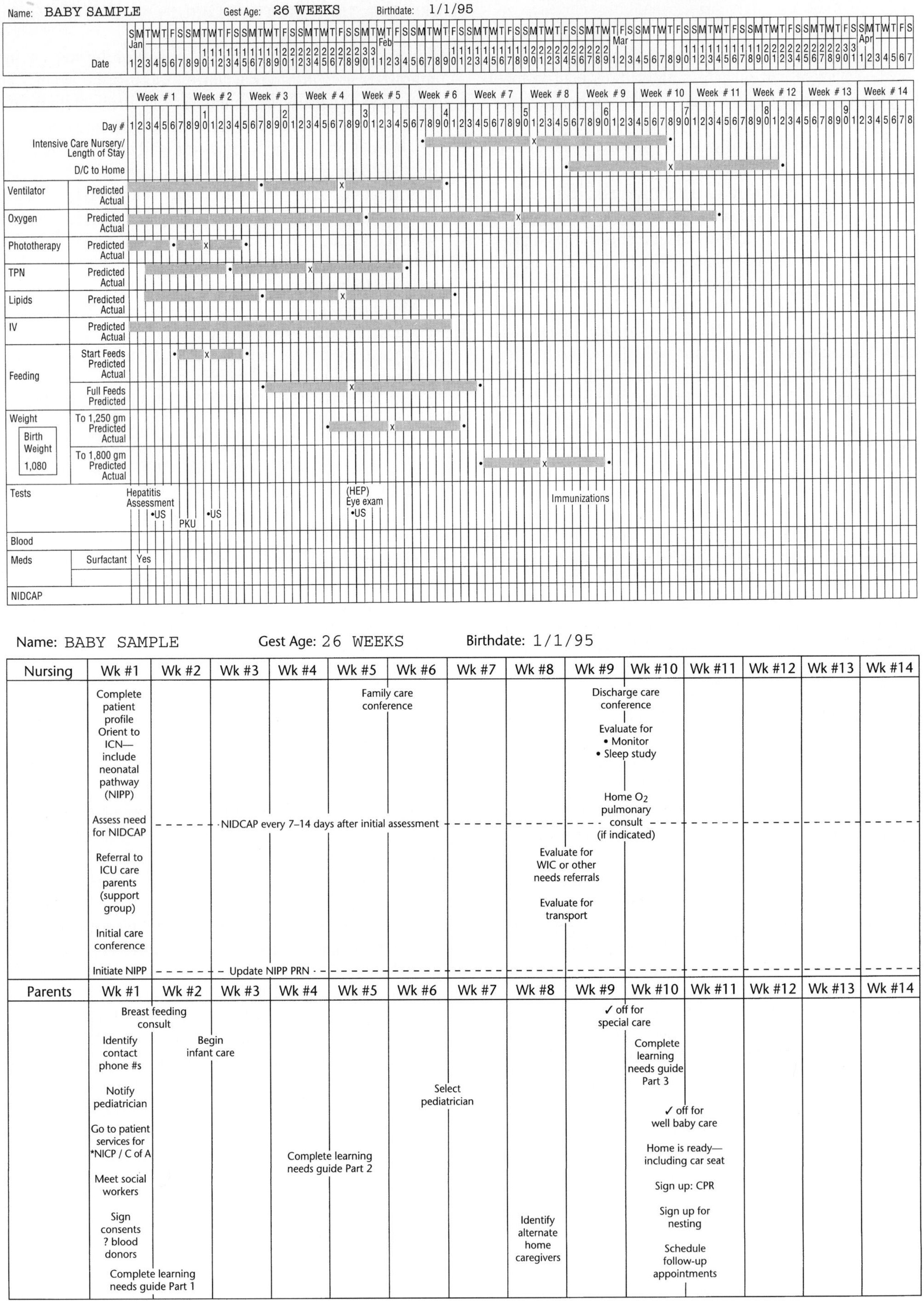

Name: BABY SAMPLE   Gest Age: 26 WEEKS   Birthdate: 1/1/95

Top chart (date/calendar grid with weeks #1–#14):

	Week #1	Week #2	Week #3	Week #4	Week #5	Week #6	Week #7	Week #8	Week #9	Week #10	Week #11	Week #12	Week #13	Week #14
Day #	1234567890	1234567890	1234567890	1234567890	1234567890	1234567890	1234567890	1234567890	1234567890	1234567890	1234567890	1234567890	1234567890	12345678

Intensive Care Nursery/Length of Stay
D/C to Home

Ventilator — Predicted / Actual
Oxygen — Predicted / Actual
Phototherapy — Predicted / Actual
TPN — Predicted / Actual
Lipids — Predicted / Actual
IV — Predicted / Actual
Feeding — Start Feeds Predicted / Actual; Full Feeds Predicted
Weight — Birth Weight 1,080 — To 1,250 gm Predicted / Actual; To 1,800 gm Predicted / Actual
Tests — Hepatitis Assessment •US   PKU   •US   (HEP) Eye exam •US   Immunizations
Blood
Meds — Surfactant Yes
NIDCAP

Name: BABY SAMPLE   Gest Age: 26 WEEKS   Birthdate: 1/1/95

Nursing	Wk #1	Wk #2	Wk #3	Wk #4	Wk #5	Wk #6	Wk #7	Wk #8	Wk #9	Wk #10	Wk #11	Wk #12	Wk #13	Wk #14
	Complete patient profile; Orient to ICN—include neonatal pathway (NIPP); Assess need for NIDCAP; Referral to ICU care parents (support group); Initial care conference; Initiate NIPP		— Update NIPP PRN · —		Family care conference				Discharge care conference; Evaluate for • Monitor • Sleep study; Home O₂ pulmonary consult (if indicated); Evaluate for WIC or other needs referrals; Evaluate for transport					

·NIDCAP every 7–14 days after initial assessment·

Parents	Wk #1	Wk #2	Wk #3	Wk #4	Wk #5	Wk #6	Wk #7	Wk #8	Wk #9	Wk #10	Wk #11	Wk #12	Wk #13	Wk #14
	Breast feeding consult; Identify contact phone #s; Notify pediatrician; Go to patient services for *NICP / C of A; Meet social workers; Sign consents ? blood donors; Complete learning needs guide Part 1		Begin infant care	Complete learning needs guide Part 2		Select pediatrician		Identify alternate home caregivers	✓ off for special care; Complete learning needs guide Part 3; ✓ off for well baby care; Home is ready—including car seat; Sign up: CPR; Sign up for nesting; Schedule follow-up appointments					

FIG. 6–2. Sample of a critical pathway based on gestational age. (From ref. 27. Copyright Phoenix Children's Hospital, with permission.)

TABLE 6–3. *Examples of quality indicators for the NICU*

	Process indicator	Outcome indicator
Practice improvement		
Standardized skin care protocol	Nurse's knowledge of skin care practices that cause trauma increased as evidenced by competency testing	Decreased incidence of visible skin trauma on inspection at 5 days postadmission
Safe suctioning protocol	Compliance w/ protocol assessed by visual observation of suctioning technique	Physical evidence of decreased airway trauma
Promote early parent involvement with VLBW ventilated infants	Facilitation of early parent holding of ventilated infants as evidenced by increased incidence of holding within first 2 weeks of life	Improved incidence of parent visiting patterns, phone contact, and involvement with direct physical care of infant
Practice problem		
Breast milk handling	All breast milk labeled and stored per protocol by audit	No further events of "wrong breast milk to wrong patient"
Quality maintenance		
Percutaneous line management	All percutaneous lines are: Documented per protocol in the medical and nursing record Secured and dressed per protocol	Decreased incidence of line-related problems: Infiltration Unplanned removal Inappropriate fluids for tip location

by state health department standards and JCAHO standards, are constructed by the individual unit. The following is an example of the components of a quality improvement plan in the NICU.

The NICU multidisciplinary team is comprised of representatives from the following disciplines: neonatology, nursing, pharmacy, respiratory therapy, social services, clinical nutrition, occupational therapy/physical therapy, and audiology. Other subspecialists and consultants who are involved in NICU patient care or processes are invited to participate on an "as needed" basis as indicated by the scope of a problem or performance issue under discussion.

The members of this multidisciplinary team develop and implement written care delivery tools such as clinical practice guidelines, algorithms, patient care protocols, standards of care, procedures, and references such as a medication reference book specific to that NICU. Although there are published practice guidelines and other documents, it may be more valuable for individual NICUs to develop their own because it is in the process of evaluating pertinent research and identifying institutional resources and constraints that a consensus of best practice is reached. This consensus means that the individuals representing different disciplines feel a sense of ownership and will be more effective in the implementation of each guideline, algorithm, or procedure.

The team identifies and prioritizes opportunities for improvement by the discussion generated in developing guidelines, by reviewing sentinel events, and by keeping abreast of current research in the field. They may identify excessive variation of measured outcomes compared to previously measured baseline data or benchmark data from outside sources. Organized patient and family satisfaction surveys also assist the team in identifying areas

for improvement. Smaller subcommittees are often formed to solve identified problems through process improvement methods, followed by both an initial evaluation and ongoing monitoring of improvement.

Sentinel events and incidents including medication errors, patient/parent complaints, and injuries involving patients or staff are reviewed by the appropriate members of the team and reported to the hospital quality assurance and risk management committees. Trends or multiple events may lead to a more formal CQI team process including gathering baseline information, forming hypotheses about causes, determining changes in practice that can improve the outcome, implementing the changes, and evaluating whether this was effective in reducing the pattern observed.

Regular assessment of the routine functioning of the NICU can include impact rounds that look at maintaining certain standard duties such as checking emergency carts, determining that licensures are current, and quality monitoring of point-of-care laboratory tests such as blood glucose monitoring and hemoglobin determinations. Medication use is reviewed by means of chart review, staff interviews regarding knowledge of medicines, and quantifying medication errors over a denominator of medication doses given. Parent or family interviews are utilized to see if families understand the plan of care for their infant, know the names of the physician and nurse members of the team caring for their infants, and have contact with a member of the social services team within a prescribed time frame, such as 72 hours. Length of stay is monitored monthly and compared to historic data for the specific NICU.

Performance improvement activities are decided on and then discussed by team members. They can include such activities as adherence to standardized endotracheal suctioning practices that are designed to reduce injury to airway, transport indicators such as time to respond to referrals and respiratory status on return from transports, and review of special programs such as extracorporeal membrane oxygenation (ECMO) patient outcomes. An important aspect of quality monitoring is the incidence of nosocomial infections, and historic data as well as benchmark data from other institutions are utilized. Drug utilization evaluations (DUE) are suggested for medications commonly used (or misused) in the NICU to determine if appropriate prescribing and monitoring techniques are being followed. Hospital-wide indicators are also reviewed, which often includes evaluating cardiac arrests, iatrogenic complications, delays in care, and mortalities.

In conclusion, the delivery of nursing care in the NICU is dependent on neonatal nurses with a high level of knowledge, skills, and commitment, on a nursing structure that can plan and organize the delivery of care efficiently to motivate and support the nursing staff, and on a multidisciplinary process for quality improvement that combines the efforts of medicine, nursing, and other professionals in the ongoing monitoring and delivery of care leading to optimal outcomes for high-risk infants and their families.

REFERENCES

1. Franck L, Epstein B, Adams S. Disaster preparedness for the ICN: evolution and testing of one unit's plan. *Pediatr Nurs* 1993;19:122–127.
2. Mulligan K, Webb LZ. Developing an evacuation procedure for a nursery complex. *Neonat Netw* 1988;6:47–52.
3. Kenner C. Caring for the NICU parent. *J Perinat Neonat Nurs* 1990;4:78–87.
4. Harrison H. The principles for family-centered neonatal care. *Pediatrics* 1993;82:643.
5. Johnson BH, Jeppson ES, Redburn L. *Caring for children and families: Guidelines for hospitals, 1st ed.* Bethesda: Association for the Care of Children's Health, 1992.
6. Stepanek JS. *Moving beyond the medical/technical: analysis and discussion of psychosocial practices in pediatric hospitals,* 1st ed. Bethesda: Association for the Care of Children's Health, 1995.
7. Zaichkin J. *Newborn intensive care: what every parent needs to know.* Petaluma, CA: NICU INK Book Publishers, 1996.
8. Harrison H. *The premature baby book.* New York: St. Martin's Press, 1983.
9. Kenner C, Bagwell GA. Assessment and management in the transition to home. In Kenner C, Lott JW, Flandermeyer AA, eds. *Comprehensive neonatal nursing: A physiologic perspective.* Philadelphia: WB Saunders, 1998.
10. Hall L. Home care. In Kenner C, Lott JW, Flandermeyer AA, eds. *Comprehensive neonatal nursing: A physiologic perspective.* Philadelphia: WB Saunders, 1998.
11. Stafford M, Appleyard JA. Clinical nurse specialists and nurse practitioners: Who are they, what do they do, and what challenges do they face? In McCloskey J, Grace HK, eds. *Current issues in nursing.* St Louis: Mosby-Year Book, 1994.
12. Elizondo A. Nursing case management in the neonatal intensive care unit. Part 1: Pioneering new territory. *Neonat Netw* 1994;13:9–12.
13. Strong A. Case management and the CNS. *Clin Nurse Specialist* 1992;6:64–69.
14. Farah AL, Bieda A, Shiao SY. The history of the neonatal nurse practitioner in the United States. *Neonat Netw* 1996;15:11–20.
15. Buus-Frank ME, Conner-Bronson J, Mullaney D, McNamara LM, Laurizio VA, Edwards WH. Evaluation of the neonatal nurse practitioner role: the next frontier. *Neonat Netw* 1996;15:31–40.
16. Nightingale F. *Notes on nursing: What it is, and what it is not,* 1st ed. Philadelphia: JB Lippincott, 1859 (reissued as commemorative edition 1992).
17. Organizations. JCoAoH. *The measurement mandate: On the road to performance improvement in health care.* Oakbrook Terrace, IL: Joint Commission on Accreditation of Healthcare Organizations, 1993.
18. Field M, Lohr KN, eds. *Guidelines for clinical practice: from development to use.* Washington DC: National Academy Press, Institute of Medicine, 1992.
19. Wennberg J. Outcomes research, cost containment, and the fear of health care rationing. *N Engl J Med* 1990;323:1202–1204.
20. Coffey R, Richards JS, Remmert CS, LeRoy SS, Schoville RR, Baldwin PJ. An introduction to critical paths. *Qual Manage Health Care* 1992;1:45–54.
21. Thompson D, Maringer M. Using case management to improve care delivery in the NICU. *Am J Matern Child Nurs* 1995;20:257–260.
22. Schriefer J. The synergy of pathways and algorithms: two tools work better than one. *J Qual Improve* 1994;20:485–499.
23. Merritt T, Palmer D, Bergman DA, Shiono PH. Clinical practice guidelines in pediatric and newborn medicine: implications for their use in practice. *Pediatrics* 1997;99:100–114.
24. Grimshaw J, Russell IT. Effect of clinical guidelines on medical practice: a systematic review of rigorous evaluations. *Lancet* 1993;342:1317–1322.
25. Thompson D. Critical pathways in the intensive care and intermediate care nurseries. *Am J Matern Child Nurs* 1994;19:29–32.
26. Tobin CR, Sabatte E, Sandhu AS, Penafiel E. A neonatal care map based on gestational age. *Neonat Netw* 1998;17:41–51.
27. Vecchi C, Vasquez L, Radin T, Johnson P. Neonatal individualized predictive pathway (NIPP): a discharge planning tool for parents. *Neonat Netw* 1996;15:7–13.
28. Organizations. JCoAoh. *Framework for improving performance: From principles to practice.* Oakbrook Terrace, IL: Joint Commission on Accreditation of healthcare Organizations, 1994.
29. Investigators, V-OTNDP. The Vermont–Oxford Trials Network. Very low birth weight outcomes for 1990. *Pediatrics* 1993;91:540–545.
30. Hack M, Horbar JD, Malloy MH, et al. Very low birth weight outcomes of the National Institute of Child Health and Human Development Neonatal Network. *Pediatrics* 1991;87:587–597.
31. Yocom C. Validating clinical competence. In McCloskey J, Grace HK, eds. *Current issues in nursing.* St Louis: Mosby-Year Book, 1994.

CHAPTER 7

Law, Risk Management, and the Practice of Neonatology

Harold M. Ginzburg, Betty Ann (Chaze) Wilkins, and Mhairi G. MacDonald

Health care professionals have always been subject to punishment should their medical skills or judgment fall below a community standard. Reports from the middle ages, in England, indicate that compensation was paid when patients were injured. In other nations during the middle ages, the health care provider, if found responsible for poor medical care, was deformed in the same manner as the injury that he caused. Physicians were not motivated to be innovative or take risks. They were not motivated to treat patients with complicated illnesses unless the patient and his or her extended family clearly understood that treatment would be palliative. Although litigation has replaced amputation in modern western societies, health care providers and health care institutions still practice under the specter of retribution and public criticism.

Litigation can be initiated when negligence has occurred or is perceived to have occurred. A lack of good communication skills and empathy can be as self-destructive as a faulty knowledge base, performing unacceptably or functioning in an impaired manner. A thorough knowledge and understanding of one's medical subspecialty is insufficient to prevent involvement in malpractice litigation. Institutional and individual behaviors often precipitate a lawsuit. The failure to communicate and document patient and health care system interactions may place a health care system or health care provider in an untenable position when his or her actions are reviewed in an arbitration, mediation, or courtroom environment.

H.M. Ginzburg: Departments of Psychiatry and Neurology, Tulane University Medical Center, New Orleans, Louisiana

B.A. Wilkins: Risk & Insurance Management, Inova Health Systems, Falls Church, Virginia

M.G. MacDonald: The George Washington University School of Medicine and Health Sciences, Washington, D.C.; and Neonatology Services, Loudoun Hospital Center, Leesburg, Virginia

The mundane aspects of medical care and treatment, such as scheduling of appointments, documentation of procedures, and an understanding of the federal, state, and local guidelines, procedures, policies, regulations, and laws, are frequently the basis for confrontations between members of the medical and legal professions.

The vast majority of medical education pertains to understanding basic sciences and providing clinical services. Little formal attention is given to the myriad of governmental policies, procedures, and regulations that control all aspects of health care delivery.

Medical care is a contract between the health care professional and the patient. In almost all instances, if the patient is unable, because of age or illness, to render informed educated consent, then others must provide such consent. Thus, as a patient is examined or interviewed, law and medicine become intertwined.

The basic legal considerations relating the care and treatment of a neonate flow from the following four concepts:

1. The duty to act. When does the health care professional–patient or health care facility–patient relationship commence?
2. Knowledge and application of hospital policies and local, state, and federal mandates. What resources are available to facilitate information transfer to health care facilities and health care service providers?
3. Responsibility and accountability of the health care provider (individual or organization) to provide adequate care and treatment. Who is responsible for the decisions made in the provision of health care? Who monitors the quality of the services provided? Who ensures that the services provided are consistent with hospital policies and local, state, and federal mandates?
4. Information transfer to patients and their families or guardians. Who obtains educated informed consent, in what manner, and with what documentation? Who

is responsible for providing ongoing medical information to the families or guardians of neonates and ensuring that the information, and the implications of the information, are understood?

Defensive medicine has become a medical term of art. However, it can connote a thoughtful systematic approach to health care rather than the excessive ordering of investigatory studies because of anticipatory fear of litigation for malpractice. Medical malpractice lawsuits are based on the principle of negligence. Negligence implies some wrongful act of commission or omission (1). The essence of negligence is unreasonableness.

Due care is simply reasonable conduct (2). In order for negligence to be demonstrated in a courtroom, the injured person-plaintiff must demonstrate that (i) there was a legal duty owed to him, (ii) there was a breach of that duty (a deviation from the accepted standard of care), (iii) as a result of the duty and the breach thereof, damages or an injury occurred, and (iv) the damages or injury can be determined to have been caused by, or shown to have flowed from, the care or lack of care provided by the health care provider and or the health care organization responsible for the environment in which the health care was provided.

RESPONSIBILITY AND LIABILITY

"The duty to act—Determination of when the health care professional or health care organization–patient relationship commences."

A "duty" is a legal and ethical responsibility (3). There is no legal duty, under most circumstances, for a health care provider or health care institution to accept a patient for care unless they hold themselves out as providing emergency care or they are required to do so by law, regulation, or contract. If a medical center, hospital, or physician represents itself to the public as a source of emergency medical care and the community has come to expect such care, then a patient cannot be arbitrarily denied such services (4). Once a health care service is initiated, a health care provider/institution– patient relationship exists, a duty is created, and there is then a legal and moral obligation not to abandon the patient. Further, the care that is being provided must be adequate care under the circumstances. A moral and legal obligation attaches, which precludes abandonment or "dumping" of the patient (5). A referring hospital transferring an infant to another institution for further care is not perceived as abandoning the patient, as long as the reason for transfer is medical and not financial. The senior medical person responsible for the transport, whether stationed at a hospital or directly providing patient care during transport, is deemed to be supervising the health care until the transport team transfers care to the clinical staff at the receiving referral medical facility. The transport team's legal and ethical duty to the patient exceeds that of other parties, such as the referring or the referral hospital.

The complexity of health care responsibility and liability has been increasing rapidly during this century. Public health care facilities have existed since the middle ages. Commencing in the 13th century, the Hotel Dieu, in Paris, provided indigent care for many centuries. In the United States (U.S.), city, municipal, state, and federal public hospitals provided care for those unable to obtain it elsewhere, and the physicians and hospitals were not held liable for the patient outcome of care that was provided free of charge. The doctrine of charitable immunity protected hospitals from legal liability if medical negligence occurred within their boundaries. However, an individual's inability to pay for medical care no longer affects his or her ability to demand and receive services that are commensurate with those provided to patients who pay for their care directly or through third party payment systems. Thus, providing care to patients who are unable to pay no longer protects a health care provider or medical institution from liability for negligence or malpractice. Physicians, other health providers, suppliers, and manufacturers of equipment, medical devices, and medicines can now all be sued for negligence and be held individually or jointly liable, that is, for their own actions, those that they supervise, and those that are performed by members of their health care team.

Licensure—Interstate Practice

In the U.S., health care providers (physicians, nurses, emergency medical technicians, etc.) may be licensed in more than one state. They must be licensed in the state in which they maintain their primary office or place of employment. The authorities in most states are not concerned about whether a health care provider who enters the state solely to transport a patient to another health care facility is licensed in that state; however, they are concerned that the individuals involved in the transport are competent to perform their job.

An individual who enters a state, regardless of the reason, will be subject to that state's laws. If a driver is involved in an accident, he or she is subject to the laws of the state in which the accident occurred, not to those of the state that issued the driving license; this legal principal also applies to medical transport vehicle operators (6). Failure to obtain informed consent may result in litigation in the state in which it was inadequately obtained or in the state to which the patient was transferred.

Recent advances in telephone-linked care (TLC) or "telemedicine" have initiated new questions regarding the practice of medicine across state lines (7). TLC has been applied as a supplement to direct patient care, to monitor patient progress, and as a service expander for specialized medical expertise and technology (for example, the interpretation of neonatal radiologic or cardiologic films and tracings). Landwehr et al. (8) demonstrated the feasibility of telesonography for the interpretation of fetal anatomic scans from a remote location. Lewis and Moir (9) in Scotland and Landquist (10) in Finland demonstrated that telemedicine is an international technology.

TLC has been practiced for more than 30 years (in its simplest form, it includes giving advice over the telephone). In 1996, the U.S. Congress passed the Telecommunications Reform Act, which required a study of patient safety, efficacy, and the quality of services (11). The neonatologist has the opportunity to engage in "telehealth," which includes consultation, transportation, and interpretation of radiographic, cardiologic, and other data, as well as professional education, community health education, public health, and administration of health services. The American Medical Association (AMA) and the American Telemedicine Association (ATA) have urged medical specialty societies to develop appropriate practice standards. Managed care organizations have begun to embrace telemedicine. Louisiana recently passed a law dealing with telemedicine reimbursement that specifies a certain reimbursement rate for physicians at the originating site and includes language prohibiting insurance carriers from discriminating against telemedicine as a medium for delivering health care services. At the present time, issues relating to cross-state licensure are perceived to be potential barriers to the expansion of telemedicine, especially now that reimbursement is possible. States license physicians and other health care providers within their boundaries, but the federal government has the authority to prepare national licensure standards as they relate to national programs such as Medicaid and Medicare. In the future, there may be alternative approaches to licensure (12). Regardless of the end result of the issues surrounding telemedicine, neonatologists increasingly cross state and even internationl boundaries and need to appreciate that the laws of political jurisdictions other than their home state may significantly impact the manner in which they practice.

Patients and their guardians may initiate medical malpractice litigation in the state in which they reside, the state in which the alleged negligence occurred, the state in which the hospital is located, or the state in which the physician resides. If the patient-plaintiff can show that his or her residence is in a different state from that of the defendant-hospital and defendant-health care provider, then the plaintiff can commence the litigation in a federal court, because the matter involves diversity of jurisdiction, that is, residents of two or more states. The defendant can request that the matter be removed to the federal court system for a similar reason (13). Most plaintiffs prefer state courts, especially if the defendant is from a different state. Some state courts are known for their large awards to plaintiffs, whereas others are known to be more sympathetic to defendant-health care providers.

Medical Torts and Contracts

The legal system is divided into two broad areas. Civil litigation is based on the need to correct or remedy a wrong between one individual (corporation or partnership) and another. Criminal prosecution is instituted to correct a wrong against the community. In a civil litigation matter (or case), the plaintiff is the party bringing the lawsuit and alleging the wrong; it is filed against the party (defendant) who is accused of causing the damage. In a criminal prosecution, the plaintiff is the government (local, state, federal) alleging that the community has been harmed by the action or inaction of a party (also known as the defendant).

Civil matters resulting in litigation generally are either contract disputes or torts. A contract dispute occurs when two or more parties have entered into an agreement and one or more parties believes that the terms and conditions of the agreement, either an oral or written contract, have not been met. It is important to appreciate that, in a court, most oral contracts have the same weight as written contracts.

A personal tort is an injury to a person or his or her reputation or feelings that directly results from a violation of a duty owed to the plaintiff (in medical malpractice cases, this is usually the patient) and produces a damage. The remedy in any civil matter, after the nature and extent of the damages have been proved to the court (a judge, with or without a jury) by a preponderance of the evidence (more than 50.01%), is usually the award of monetary damages.

Battery

Battery is a tort; it is an intentional and volitional act, without consent, which results in touching that causes harm (e.g., the touching of a patient's body without consent). A technical battery can occur when there is no actual harm but touching occurred without consent. Patient care, even with a beneficial outcome but without informed consent, may be considered battery.

Plaintiffs may sue for an injury that occurred as a result of negligence or a tort (physical or mental harm), or both. Because the criminal court usually will not award monetary damages to the victim of a crime, and because the standard of proof for conviction is "beyond a reasonable doubt" (quantitatively, this can be conceptualized as at least 95% certain), plaintiffs usually will prefer to sue for injuries from a tort in civil court. In civil litigation, monetary damages may be awarded and, if the injury was determined to be egregious, punitive damages also can be assessed against the defendant. The standard of proof in civil litigation is the "preponderance of the evidence" or the "more likely than not" standard; it is a "superiority of weight" test that requires that for the plaintiff to be successful, 50.01% of the evidence must weigh in his or her favor (14). Thus, the preponderance of the evidence rule is a threshold test (15). In general, either the plaintiff proves that the damages were more likely to have been caused by the defendant agent than by any other source and is, therefore, entitled to full compensation, or he or she fails to meet the burden of proof and is entitled to nothing (16).

Professional Negligence

Negligence is "conduct, and not a state of mind" (17); it "involves an unreasonably great risk of causing damage" (17); and is "conduct which falls below the standard established by the law for the protection of others against unreasonable risk of harm" (18,19).

Professional negligence, or medical malpractice, is a special instance of negligence. The medical profession is held to a specific minimum level of performance based on the possession, or claim of possession, of "special knowledge or skills" that have been accrued through specialized education and training.

Ely et al. (20) found that when family physicians recalled memorable errors, the majority fell into the following categories: physician distractors (hurried or overburdened), process of care factors (premature closure of the diagnostic process), patient-related factors (misleading normal results), and physician factors (lack of knowledge, inadequately aggressive patient management). Understanding the common causes of errors alerts the practitioner to situations when errors are most likely to occur.

THE ELEMENTS OF A MALPRACTICE CASE

To establish a *prima facie* medical malpractice case (one that still appears obvious after reviewing the medical evidence), the patient-plaintiff must demonstrate (Fig.

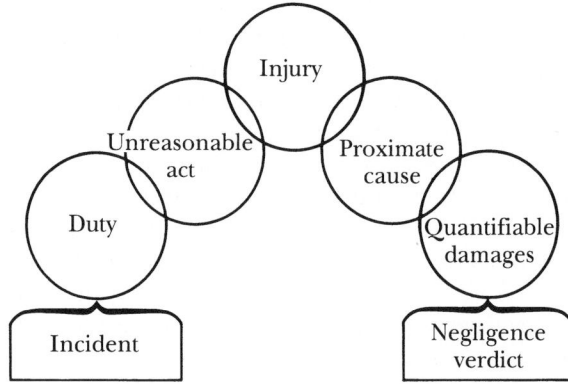

FIG. 7–1. The elements of negligence. There must be an unbroken chain for successful litigation. If any link is not proved, the plaintiff will lose the case. (From Ginzburg HM. Legal issues in patient transport. In: MacDonald MG (ed.), Miller MK (assoc. ed.). *Emergency transport of the perinatal patient.* Philadelphia: Little, Brown and Company, 1989, p 163.)

7–1): that (i) there is a *duty* on the part of the defendant-health care provider and/or defendant-health care facility to the patient-plaintiff, (ii) the defendant failed to conform his or her conduct to the requisite *standard of care* required by the relationship, and (iii) an *injury* to that patient-plaintiff resulted from that failure (21).

Generally, in order for the plaintiff to establish a claim of medical malpractice, the plaintiff must establish by medical expert testimony (i) what the applicable *standard of care* is, (ii) how the defendant breached or violated that standard of care, and (iii) that the breach or violation (also referred to as the negligence) was the proximate cause of the injury.

A medical malpractice action can only proceed if the court determines that there is a genuine issue of material fact and if damages are quantifiable (e.g., the future costs of treatment, economic lost value of productive activities, etc.).

The most difficult element to prove is whether or not the standard of care was adequate. The plaintiff usually must provide expert witnesses to establish what a prudent health care provider in similar circumstances might have done. A "conspiracy of silence" may have existed in prior years, but today there are many "experts" willing to testify anywhere about anything.

More than 100 years ago, in Massachusetts, it was held that a physician in a small town is bound to have only the skill that physicians of ordinary ability and skill in similar localities possess. The court believed that a small town physician should not be expected to have the skill of surgeons practicing a specialty in a large city (22). It was also held that a physician is required to use only ordinary skill and diligence, the average of that possessed by the profession as a body, and not by the thoroughly educated (23). However, a physician is not excused for failing to keep himself or herself informed of medical progress. State requirements for continuing education and the effects of telemedicine consultations and educational programs essentially have removed clinicians' ability to say that they are too busy or so geographically inaccessible as to be precluded from keeping current with new treatments and new understanding of the illnesses that affect their patients.

Courts admit medical evidence based upon rules of evidence. In 1993, the Supreme Court, in *Daubert v Merrill Dow Pharmaceuticals, Inc.* ruled that the Federal Rules of Evidence standards for acceptance of evidence would be used (24). This was an attempt to remove junk science from distracting the jury. The court held that scientific (medical) evidence had to be grounded in relevant scientific principles. Publication in a peer-reviewed or peer-refereed journal was not the only qualification for acceptance of evidence in a courtroom. The district (trial) court judges have the latitude to permit or exclude experts, based on the perceived scientific merit of the information they intend to provide to the court and, thus, to the jury. The fundamental issue for a clinician is not an understanding of the rules of evidence and the workings of the civil justice system but practicing medicine and acting in a professional manner, as documented in a patient's medical record.

Many states have medical peer-review panels in place. In these states, before a medical malpractice case may be heard in a court, the facts of the case are presented to the panel (which usually consists of an equal number of lawyers and physicians) on behalf of both the plaintiff and defendant. The facts often are buttressed by the opinions of retained medical experts. Even when there is a finding for the defendant by the medical review panel, the plaintiff may continue litigation in the local court. However, the findings of the medical review panel are admissible on behalf of the defendants.

Res ipsa Loquitur

There are circumstances in which no expert witness is required to corroborate the findings of negligence. The doctrine of *res ipsa loquitur* essentially means that the thing speaks for itself. Under such circumstances, the negligence is inferred from the act itself, that is, proof from circumstantial evidence. In the classic case, *Ybarra v Spangard*, a patient was well prior to being anesthetized for an appendectomy, and when he woke up he had an injury to his arm (25). Clearly, he could not determine how his arm was injured; the operating room and recovery room staff either could not or would not explain the etiology of the injury. The court found for the injured plaintiff, without the introduction of any expert witnesses, because (i) the plaintiff had not done anything that in any way could have contributed to the injury, (ii) the injury could not have occurred unless someone was negligent, and (iii) the instrumentalities (hospital staff and physicians) that allegedly caused the injury were at all times under the control of the defendant hospital.

Informed Consent

Informed consent requires that sound, reasonable, comprehensible, and relevant information be provided by a health care professional to a competent individual (patient or guardian) for the purpose of eliciting a voluntary and educated decision by that patient (or guardian) about the advisability of permitting one course of clinical action as opposed to another (18). Physicians and other health care providers are held to have a fiduciary duty to their patients. Such a duty exists when one individual relies on another because of the unequal possession of information. The failure to obtain proper informed consent may result in the defendant-physician or defendant-hospital being sued for battery in some states, or for negligence in others.

According to the battery theory, the defendant is to be held liable if any deliberate (not careless or accidental) action resulted in physical contact. The contact must have occurred under circumstances in which the plaintiff-patient did not provide either express or implied permission and the defendant-health care provider knew or should have known that the action was unauthorized. If the scope of consent obtained from the patient is exceeded, a claim of battery is proper. The plaintiff in *Mohr v Williams* consented to have her right ear operated on (26). During the procedure, the surgeon determined that the right ear was not sufficiently diseased to require surgery, but the left ear required surgery. Because the patient was already anesthetized, the surgeon performed the operation. The operation was a success, but the patient successfully sued for battery. The court held that there was no informed consent for an operation to the left ear. Thus, it is not necessary for injury to occur for damages to be awarded; demonstration that there was unpermitted touching is sufficient. In this instance, the court found that there was no medical emergency that would threaten the plaintiff-patient if the surgery were not immediately commenced. If there were evidence of a medical emergency, the court's decision might have been significantly different.

Failure to specifically identify the risks that accompany a surgical procedure also can result in a successful claim of battery. In *Canterbury v Spence*, the plaintiff-patient successfully proved that he was not informed of the risks attendant to the surgical procedure and that had he known them he would not have given permission (27). The court held that the physician has a duty to disclose all reasonable risks of a surgical procedure, and because he failed to perform that duty, the court held him liable for damages to the patient. The court noted that the concept of informed consent may be more appropriately replaced with the concept of educated consent. The court also articulated an objective standard that could be used in legal cases involving informed consent. This objective standard is based on what a reasonable person in circumstances similar to that of the patient would have decided if he or she had been provided with an adequate amount of information. Therefore, the central issue in a medical battery is whether an educated, effective, or valid consent was given for the procedure that actually was performed.

A physician is not required to disclose every possible risk to a patient for fear of being guilty of battery (28). The court in *Cooper v Roberts* held that "[t]he physician is bound to disclose only those risks which a reasonable man would consider material to his decision whether or not to undergo treatment" (29). Thus, the court stated that such a standard creates no unreasonable burden for the physician. However, the physician must disclose risks that are material and feasible alternatives that are available. The information should be provided in a language and a manner that reflects the emotional and educational status of the patient or, when the patient is a neonate, the parents. In *Davis v Wyeth*, the court held that any medical complication or risk that has a probability of greater than 1:1,000 should be included in the informed consent (30).

When a therapeutic procedure is for the benefit of a minor, the decision to proceed usually belongs to the parent or legal guardian. The failure of the parent to consent to blood transfusions (even if the refusal is based on sincere religious convictions) or other now routine procedures, for a small child, that are clearly medically indicated and required for the maintenance of life can be overridden by the physician and/or hospital petitioning the court for the appointment of a temporary legal guardian (31).

The unavailability of a parent in a life-threatening circumstance should not preclude therapeutic action. Just as informed consent is imputed to an unconscious accident victim who has a life-threatening condition that requires surgery, such rational behavior can be imputed to the absent parent in the case of a sick neonate. However, in such circumstances, if time permits, detailed documentation and consultation with the hospital administration is recommended.

Informed consent in neonatal-perinatal medicine is not an empty gesture to reduce liability, but, rather, an interaction with the physician that helps parents to become full partners in decision-making. This is intended to support them in their choices, rather than to merely have them ratify decisions already made (32). The informed consent process can be extremely complex, with several legal "gray areas." For example, are maternal rights any more definitive in making critical decisions for a fetus or neonate than paternal rights? Conflicts can arise even when the putative or alleged father is not the legal spouse of the mother. Emergency hearings, in front of local judges, may be required to resolve conflicting opinions, especially when the decision of one parent may lead, to a medical degree of certainty [more likely than not], to the death of the infant.

It is one of the ironies of the law, in most states, that a unwed teenage mother has the ultimate legal responsibility for the care of her child, unless the court is petitioned to appoint an alternative guardian. In many states, the live birth of a child, regardless of the age of the mother, results in the mother being declared an emancipated minor. In contrast, a nonpregnant teenager, living at home and attending school, does not have the legal right to make decisions about many aspects of her own medical care.

The disclosure of risks in the informed consent process tends to underscore a parent's sense of helplessness and to portray the physician as somewhat helpless as well. The powerlessness of the parents and their wish that the physician be omnipotent creates unrealistic expectations of the outcomes of procedures and treatment. Gutheil et al. (33) suggest that the physician acknowledge the parent's wish for certainty and substitute the mystical with a physician–parent alliance in which uncertainty is accepted.

Medical Records

Medical records are legal documents. They are designed to be a contemporaneous record of the available clinical information and the medical and other decisions that flow from the clinical information and interactions with the patient's significant others. Records provide an opportunity for adequate documentation. Documentation is the key to management of patients, especially those with difficult and complex clinical presentation. The course of treatment and the meeting or failure to meet therapeutic goals should be noted in the hospital chart. Treatment options, including the option of no treatment, should be explained to the patient's family and, if necessary, others potentially involved in the decision-making process. The patient's family's understanding, or lack thereof, of the various treatment options also should be noted, especially if there are divergent views among family members. Ultimately, one family member or guardian has to be acknowledged by the family and the health care providers as the decision-maker. Identifying such an individual, in the medical record, will facilitate treatment decisions and posthospital treatment care and management.

Adequate medical records will document that the risks of a given procedure have been shared with the patient's decision-makers. A record that indicates that specific known adverse side effects, or rare but serious untoward events, were discussed with a patient's family members or guardians helps protect the clinician should one of these untoward events actually occur. No medical procedure is risk-free, and although families may be informed of the relative risks of the various procedures and pharmacologic interventions, the stress of the moment may shorten their attention span, concentration, and recall. Medical record documentation at least provides a contemporaneous record of what information actually was provided.

Medical records provide the basis for reimbursement of the costs for patient care and treatment. The severity of a condition, justification for laboratory and other investigations, the need for consultations, and the manner in which the consultative advice is incorporated into patient care should be present within a patient's medical record. In the spring of 1998, the U.S. Justice Department announced the hiring of 250 Federal Bureau of Investigation agents for the purpose of investigating Medicare and Medicaid fraud. Recently, the U.S. federal government has paid increasing attention to the issue of fraudulent billing for health care services. Adequate documentation facilitates medical audit, permits those who prepare invoices for reimbursement, or payment to justify the categories or International Classification of Diseases (ICD) codes placed on the universal billing forms (sometimes identified as HCFA-1500 forms), and prevents errors that may result in the appearance of fraud (34).

MEDICAL CONFIDENTIALITY OF ORAL AND WRITTEN COMMUNICATIONS

The Hippocratic oath states, in part, "Whatever, in connection with my professional practice or not in connection with it, I see or hear, in the life of men, which ought not to be spoken of abroad, I will not divulge, as reckoning that all should be kept secret" (35). This oath, taken by many physicians upon graduating from medical school, has been codified by state and federal law. The confidentiality of the information obtained by the physician is considered to be "privileged" (36). The privilege, however, belongs to the patient or his or her guardian; it does not belong to the physician or other health care provider. A court may order a health care provider to breach medical confidentiality; legislation may require it.

As the delivery of medical care becomes more complex, individuals not generally thought of as direct health care providers are requiring access to confidential medical information. The legitimate needs, for example, of physical therapists, occupational therapists, hospital administrative personnel, and medical insurance personnel may appear to conflict with the principle that medical information is confidential and should be restricted only to physicians. The ethical basis for confidentiality derives from the concept that assurance of confidentiality encourages patients to seek the medical care that they require and to be candid with their health care providers. The legal basis for confidentiality is derived from statutes which have been enacted in essentially all states within the U.S.

There is a significant variation, among the states, as to what classes of health care providers (doctors, nurses, social workers, etc.) can assert that they cannot share medical information provided to them without the patient's express permission or a court order directing them to do so.

Legislatures create state disease-reporting requirements that require medical confidentiality to be breached as, historically, the courts have found that the state has a compelling need to protect its citizens from certain infectious diseases (37). Certain behaviors, such as dangerousness, also have resulted in reporting requirements that compel a health care professional to notify authorities when a patient has made an explicit threat against a known individual (38) or even an unknown but identifiable group of individuals (39).

Medical records also are protected by state and federal legislation. The U.S. Public Health Service Act provides for the explicit protection of medical records dealing with treatment for drug (40) and alcohol abuse (41). However, even the contents of substance abuse treatment records may be released "to medical personnel to the extent necessary to meet a bona fide medical emergency "(42,43). If release of the medical records is authorized by a court order, then appropriate safeguards need to be put into place to preclude unauthorized disclosure.

The courts recognize that they must balance the public interest and the need for disclosure against injury to the patient, to the physician–patient relationship, and to the treatment services (44,45).

"A hospital medical record is the property of the hospital, but it is kept for the benefit of the patient, the physician and the hospital" (35). A patient's medical record is preserved to document events, in a contemporaneous manner, for later use. Later use includes further medical care and treatment, documentation for financial payment by third party payers, and defense of medical malpractice claims.

The medical record librarian becomes the custodian of the medical records. The American Association of Medical Record Librarians has a code that is similar to the Hippocratic oath taken by physicians. Hospital policies and procedures, consistent with state and federal statutes and regulations, prevent a medical record from being released without either a patient release or a court order. Under certain defined circumstances, medical records can be admitted as evidence in a court of law. They can be authenticated as business records. They also can be used to refresh a doctor's memory and document his or her actions.

The American Hospital Association, the Joint Commission on Accreditation of Healthcare Organizations (JCAHO), and other professional organizations have asserted that a patient's medical records are to be protected from unauthorized and unnecessary access. Hematology, blood chemistry, urinalyses, and radiographic, sonographic, and electrodiagnostic findings are all considered a part of a patient's authorization or court order. Third party payers, as a condition of their insuring the patient, almost invariably are given access to patient medical records, as are state and federal auditors.

The privilege of medical confidentiality does not extend to third parties present who are not part of the health care being delivered. That is, police officers present during an evaluation or treatment cannot be prevented from sharing with other law enforcement personnel or the courts any information that they obtained under such circumstances. When an individual engages in litigation in which his or her physical or mental status is an issue, that individual cannot assert the privilege to prevent unfavorable information from reaching the ear of the court. Thus, in a lawsuit for malpractice, the patient-plaintiff has waived his or her right to medical confidentiality of any oral, written, or electronic communication concerning his or her medical history, diagnosis, treatment, or prognosis. Medical confidentiality statutes were and are designed to protect a patient's privacy and to encourage treatment for conditions that may bear social or other stigmas. The laws were not made to give the moving party, the patient-plaintiff in a medical malpractice case, an unfair advantage by allowing the individual to select only those records considered testimony favorable to his or her case. A medical record cannot be used as both a sword and a shield.

In 1991, the Institute of Medicine (IOM) advocated the adoption of the computer-based patient record as standard medical practice in the U.S. (46). A computer-based record is perceived as a continuous chronological history of a patient's medical care. The medical care record can be linked to various aids, including reminders and alerts to clinicians and clinical decision-making instruments. However, a computer-based record increases access to a patient's record and increases the array of data maintained in a single record (47). The more information compressed into an easily accessible single location, the greater the precautions needed to prevent misuse. As Annas (48) notes, in a setting of private practice, medical information that identifies a patient is supposed to be transferred from physician to physician only with the patient's written informed consent. In contrast, he explains, within a medical institution, information is generally passed around on a perceived, usually self-designated, "need to know basis," without first obtaining a patient's informed consent. Individuals who receive their medical care through managed care facilities and integrated health care delivery systems that have multiple treatment sites and use computer-based patient records can anticipate that the traditional standards of medical confidentiality will be diminished. Even a minor error, such as dialing an incorrect telecopier number and sending an electronic report to an unintended recipient, can result in damage to the patient and ultimately cost to the individual who authorized the report to be transmitted in error.

A release of medical information request can be general or it can be rather specific, depending on the clinical and social circumstances, the needs of the treating health care providers, and the instructions of the patient or guardian. In general, medical information is released upon written instruction; however, oral instructions frequently are sufficient or necessary. This may be the case in a medical emergency. Documentation of oral permission for release of medical information is recommended.

Local health departments usually are delegated the task of collecting vital statistics that include birth, death, and marriage information. These documents generally are protected to some degree. Autopsy reports usually are not released beyond the treating physician and/or coroner/medical examiner, unless there is authorization to do so. Civil or criminal courts can order the contents of an autopsy revealed if it will assist a party in asserting his or her civil claim, criminal prosecution, or defense from prosecution, or in asserting a civil claim.

LEGAL ISSUES SPECIFIC TO MANAGED CARE

Although the incidence of malpractice litigation against health professionals has increased exponentially in the U.S. since the 1970s (49), it is not a recent phenomenon. Documented medical professional liability cases date to 1374, when a surgeon in England was sued for negligent treatment of a wound (50). However, a hybrid of lawsuits against health care providers, focusing on managed care issues, is new. Profit is the bottom line in today's health care system (51). Managed care developed in response to a perception on the part of both government and society in general that there was unnecessary medical procedures being performed, an associated overutilization of medical resources and services, and an unrestrained lack of uniformity of cost in health care. Managed care filled a vacuum; it was developed and marketed because of a perceived need to control by those who paid costs (the employers) and those who managed health care dollars (health care insurance companies). Health care providers did little to inform their constituencies of the potential problems associated with managed care.

Managed care may be defined as "any entity capable of negotiating to deliver health care to a group of recipients at a predetermined rate on a per capita basis" (51). The American Association of Health Plans claims that 150 million Americans were enrolled in health maintenance organizations (HMOs) or other managed care entities in 1995 (52). Almost 75% of those who receive health insurance through their employers are covered by some type of managed care plan (53).

Managed care has become "big business," with the administrative costs and profit deriving in major part from cost savings and efficiencies (54). The focus of the decision-maker to authorize or perform a service or procedure or order a medication now has an aspect of a real or perceived profit motive. There has been considerable media coverage of managed care programs that firmly control costs to the detriment of those paying premiums and expecting the best services available. In many cases, unqualified personnel are placed in a position of second-guessing and overruling physician decision-making responsibilities and obligations. Delays in receiving permission for expensive procedures, or outright denials for critical but costly procedures, occur. In some instances, so-called "gag" orders are inserted in physicians' contracts, which effectively prohibit physicians from disclosing expensive alternatives to their patients (51). However, in February 1997, President Clinton requested that the Department of Health and Human Services (DHHS) send a letter to all state Medicaid directors informing them that "gag rules" are prohibited for Medicaid HMOs. He also supported national legislation to ban gag rules for all managed care organizations within the U.S. Approximately half the states in the U.S. have enacted or introduced their own laws regulating "gag rule" provisions in medical care policies. In *Moore v Regents of the University of California,* the California Supreme Court held that the concept of informed consent is broad enough to include the physicians' duty to inform their patients that they have an economic interest that might affect that physician's professional judgment (55).

Although managed care attempts to reduce costs by creating economies of scale and coordinating care among health care providers and health care resources, they also attempt to reduce costs by eliminating unnecessary care, as they define it. In some instances, a managed care program's criteria for emergency or extensive and expensive care may conflict with those held by the physician. The physician's contract may have a provision in which a percentage of fees is paid only if utilization goals are met. The physician's contract also may have a capitation provision, which means that the physician is provided a fixed amount, regardless of the level of service provided to each patient. In the latter circumstances, the physicians essentially become coinsurers and may have a perceived conflict of interest in the manner and degree to which they provide services to their patients.

The most unique feature of an HMO is that an enrolled patient pays a prepaid, fixed fee for medical services. This is in contrast to "fee-for-services," in which the patient pays a separate fee for each service rendered by the independent physician. Preferred provider organizations (PPOs) differ from HMOs in that a PPO is an organized group of health care providers offering their services at a discount. Services are provided on a predetermined fee-for-service basis. Members may choose their physicians regardless of whether they are in "their" plan, but receive "discounts" only from the plan. PPO physicians have relatively minimal financial incentive to limit services, and physicians practicing under such an arrangement would appear to have greater control of their practice and of their potential liability.

The HMO may contract directly with physicians and pay them a salary (staff model), or they may contract with a group of physicians. The physician group may or may not devote a majority of its time to serving the needs of a specific HMO. It may offer a mixture of financial arrangements to its patients, including fee for service. The HMO may contract with an individual practice association (IPA), usually a partnership or corporation of physicians, to provide health care services to the HMO membership. The IPA then contracts with its physicians to provide services to the HMO. The fundamental difference between the IPA and the staff and group physician arrangements is that the IPA physicians usually work in their own facilities, use their own equipment, and keep their own records. The HMO pays the IPA a capitation fee (a specific amount per enrollee or subscriber); the IPA pays the treating physicians on a fee-for-services basis (56).

Physicians and their managed care carriers are being sued jointly. Allegations of malpractice now are joined with allegations of bad faith, and contract theories of liability are being added to the more traditional negligence/medical malpractice theories of liability (57). Under the doctrine of *respondeat superior*, HMOs have been found responsible for the alleged negligence of their employee-physicians (58). The doctrine of *respondeat superior* states that an employer is vicariously liable for the negligence of an employee acting within the scope of his employment (59). The doctrine does not apply if the negligent party is a true independent contractor (60). The distinction between an employee and an independent contractor is control or independence, that is, an employee is subject to the immediate direction and control of the employer, and independent contractors use their own judgment and are not subject to direct control. In some instances, an HMO can be held vicariously liable for the negligence of a consultant requested by the HMO's physician (61). This issue may be decided on the wording in the promotional material provided to subscribers.

Regardless of the employment status of the health care provider, the hospital has an obligation to oversee the quality of patient care and services (62). Ultimately, however, the courts have held that it is the physician's responsibility to uphold good medical practice in the face of improper or incorrect cost-containment procedures put forth by HMOs or other managed care organizations. The California Court of Appeals has held that, "while we recognize, realistically, that cost consciousness has become a permanent feature of the health care system, it is essential that cost limitation programs are not permitted to corrupt medical judgment" (63). The court found for the plaintiff, because the physician did not protest the health insurer's determination that a prolonged hospitalization for his patient was not necessary, with severe negative consequences for the patient (63).

The Employees Retirement Income Security Act of 1974 (ERISA) (64) "supersedes any and all state laws insofar as they may now or hereafter relate to any employee benefit" (65). In *Shea v Esensten*, a federal court found that ERISA requires HMOs to disclose to their enrollees the compensation agreement between the HMO and its physicians (66). That is, there is an affirmative duty, by the HMOs, to inform their subscribers of any financial incentives that the health care providers may receive as they manage their patients' care. These financial "incentives must be disclosed and the failure to do so is a breach of ERISA's fiduciary duties" (66). Physicians who have challenged managed care decisions about patient care have been removed from the HMO panels. Suits, for reinstatement on the grounds that they were removed from the panel without good cause, and in violation of public policy, and the implied covenant of good faith and fair dealing traditionally read into contracts have had mixed results (67,68). Just as medicine has evolved significantly during the past several decades, so too has the law. Both will continue to change, and their progress, conflicts, and resolutions will be documented in the media, the professional journals, the legislature, and the courts.

PHYSICIAN LIABILITY ARISING FROM NON-PHYSICIAN PROVIDERS

Liability exposure arising from the use of non-physician providers (NPPs) (e.g., Neonatal Nurse Practitioner, Clinical Nurse Specialist, Physician Assistant) is rela-

TABLE 7–1. *Liability risk and risk reduction for neonatologists working with NPPs*

Areas of risk	Risk reduction

• Inadequate supervision by physician
• NPPs working beyond their scope
• Parent unhappy about access to their newborn's physician
• Physician viewed as "deep pocket" by plaintiff's bar
• Apparent physician delay in seeing critical patient
	• Check NPP credentials before hiring, and maintain documentation
	• Establish, and review at least annually, written policies, protocols, and procedures for:
	  • patient examination
	  • treatment
	  • delegation
	  • supervision
	  • patient's/parent's right of access to physician
	• Instruct NPP to adhere as closely as possible to patient care protocols, utilizing physician input when significant deviation may be required; the rationale for deviations should be documented
	• Document completion of skills inventory check
	• Document current competency and establish a quality monitoring system
	• Educate other staff about the role and limits of the NPP
	• Understand and keep current regarding statutory requirements for NPPs
	• Use name tags to identify the professional status of the NPP
	• Introduce NPP to parents and explain role
	• Review NPP's charts on a regular basis and cosign orders in a timely fashion
	• Establish protocol for physician to see patient and parents at set intervals
	• Obtain adequate liability insurance for NPP; physician's liability insurer should be informed that they are supervising NPPs
	• Ensure that NPP complies with hospital credentialling requirements and has sufficient time allotted for continuing professional education; require that copies of licensure renewal and certification of continuing education are kept on file
	• Inform physicians covering call of NPP's role

tively new. It can be assumed, however, that as NPPs increase their roles, there will be a concommittant increase in malpractice allegations against NPPs and the physicians working with them, based upon the fact that the NPP is acting as an agent for the physician.

To the extent that NPPs exercise control over their professional activities, they will be held responsible for their negligent acts. Under the old "Captain of the ship" *(respondeat superior)* doctrine, the physician was presumed to be responsible for the activities of all the non-physicians working with the physician. Contemporary courts have moved away from this theory and have placed responsibility on those professionals exercising control. However, this does not eliminate the liability risk for the supervising physician.

Potential areas of risk for neonatologists working with NPPs, and methods for reducing risk, are listed in Table 7–1.

THE NATIONAL DATA BANK

Some malpractice insurance carriers retain the right to settle lawsuits independent of the wishes or sentiments of the health care provider. The federally mandated and operated National Practitioner Data Bank contains information, available to hospitals and individuals, and lists settled medical malpractice claims (69). General medical malpractice carriers may not always be knowledgeable regarding the specific nuances of specialty practice.

Health professionals should do more than comparison shop the price of a malpractice policy. They need to determine the financial soundness of the malpractice carrier and their own rights to control settlement and to determine the sophistication and knowledge of the legal representation provided by their insurance carrier.

ESTABLISHING A RISK MANAGEMENT PROGRAM

The Growth of Risk Management

In the U.S., risk management programs grew out of changes in the medical malpractice insurance market (insurance became more difficult and more expensive to obtain) and accelerated malpractice claims in the 1970s (49). As the cost of liability insurance increased, the establishment of risk management programs made health care facilities more attractive to insurance underwriters. When institutions formed their own self-insurance trust funds, risk management programs provided some assurances to hospital board members that the financial liability of the institution would be limited to the greatest extent possible by their own risk managers. Health care errors rarely are due to a mistake made by an individual; they are usually an indication of the failure of a health care system (70). System issues are referred by risk management to staff trained in quality improvement and to the hospital administration.

Risk and Risk Management

Risk is the possibility of harm, the uncertainty of danger, and the probability of loss. The essence of risk management lies in maximizing the areas where there is some control over the outcome, while minimizing the areas where there is absolutely no control over the outcome (71). The existence of risk does not imply that there are always alternatives. Risk management is a process of examining any potential alternatives and thereby influencing the level of risk to which patients, health care providers, and institutions are exposed. An outcome of managing risk is the identification of a level of harm, danger, or loss that can be tolerated. In the health care setting, harm or danger expressed in human terms pertains to the safety of patients, visitors, and employees and to health care delivery practices. The losses can be expressed in financial terms, such as losses in settlements, jury verdicts, legal expenses, and insurance premiums. Thus, Risk management is a means of appropriately protecting the financial assets of an organization against losses from legal liability.

Risk management is achieved using a process that involves investigating, evaluating, planning, organizing, and implementing procedures. These processes are applied to all disciplines in an organization in order to minimize the adverse effects of accidental loss. The resulting benefit of risk management is improved quality and understanding of patient care. There is financial benefit to the institution and personal benefit to the clinician when there are fewer claims made and fewer lawsuits brought against the health care providers (72). Financial and psychological benefits also are realized when malpractice cases are dismissed or settled for reduced amounts, based on the strength of the defense.

Health Care Risk Management

The level of risk exposure in the health care environment is inversely proportional to the control maintained by the health care service providers. Total control is not possible in the face of complex disease processes, and complex care and treatment managed in complex patient care delivery systems. In the critical care environment, the risk manager must establish a program that anticipates, identifies, and responds to risk. The risk manager then plans the implementation of this program and promotes its ongoing use by health care providers. Where it is possible in the process of delivering care to patients, failsafe systems are established to prevent errors from affecting the patient.

The elements of a risk management program reflect the health care organization's attempt to define, describe, and limit liability. Functional definitions of health care executives, and their roles and responsibilities for supervising and administering health care activities, enable the health care providers to identify chains of management decision-making and accountability. Health care providers need to understand who supervises each administrative component of a health care facility so that complaints, comments, and recommendations reach those who are in a position to respond affirmatively. The chain of responsibility for developing, implementing, supporting, monitoring, and evaluating a risk management program reflects interdisciplinary health and management activities. Risk management must be recognized as a reactive (responding to an incident) and proactive (preventing future similar incidents) system of intervention to protect the institution, the clinician, and the patient. Although assignment of responsibility does occur in a either a proactive or reactive risk assessment, responsibility is not to be perceived as the same as negligence. For example, there is no negligence in a situation in which a physician orders a specific dose of medication, the nurse responsible administers the proper dosage, and there is a resultant catastrophic effect on the patient. In many instances, either the risk was known and shared with the parents or the patient, or the adverse consequences could not reasonably have been foreseeable.

Risk management programs strive to reduce risk to the greatest extent possible and to manage the remaining risk. Quality improvement committees, safety committees, and specialized subcommittees provide the administrative and management structure to review the various aspects of clinical care and support and provide constructive guidance and assistance. The outcome of this effort is improved quality of care, within the context of the goals of the health care team and the patient's family.

Risk financing, the partner to risk control, involves the financial arrangement (insurance) made for the payment for losses that inevitably do occur. The liability insurance program may be coordinated by the risk management department. The risk manager notifies the insurance carrier of reportable events, claims, and lawsuits. Members of the health care team have a shared responsibility to report adverse events, to contribute to the data that will track these events, and to alert the malpractice insurance carrier to potential financial loss. The risk manager may select defense counsel and assist counsel in the defense of the institution and/or health care providers. In addition to contributing to the quality of patient care, the risk manager, under the direction of counsel, contributes to the quality of the defense of the health care provider in a claim or suit (73). Conflicts of interest between the institution and the health care provider need to be identified and addressed as soon as possible. Separate counsel may be required when there are divergent legal and personal interests. To achieve the goals of risk management, the following activities must take place:

- Systematic and continuous investigation of risk loss exposures—Risk management must be made aware of potential exposures and actual exposures (adverse events) as they occur, and of system changes that may affect exposure to risk. To achieve this level of awareness, it is necessary for risk managers to establish a communication network that provides real-time feedback. The risk manager utilizes the knowledge, impressions, and experience of the health care team to investigate events that have occurred and to identify events that might occur in the future. Methods of communication to risk management include incident reports, risk management presence on committees, and ready accessibility by electronic means.

- Evaluation of risk loss exposure—An examination of the nature, frequency, severity of risk, and potential impact on the organization. This evaluation detects patterns in recurrent events, which can be used to predict their recurrence. For example, if medication errors are observed to occur just before a change of shift, examination of the human dynamics that contribute to these errors and breaking the pattern can lead to correction of an error-producing systems flaw. Administration and clinical staff are called upon to identify potential risk areas for evaluation.

- Planning and organization of appropriate risk avoidance and prevention techniques to efficiently minimize loss to the organization—Currently in the U.S., order, stability, and consistency are not the hallmarks of a successful health care organization. Risk managers must establish an information-gathering network, which identifies emerging organizational changes. Areas of risk can be identified as projects are developed. The monitoring of system changes after implementation is used to detect any negative impact on patient care. Recommendations then can be made to adjust system changes. Anticipation is one of the most important considerations. Identifying pertinent questions regarding the level of risk for potential adverse events and those who should be involved in evaluating a system helps the direct service providers avoid some significant errors (74).

- Implementation of risk reduction—Because clinical staff are being flexible, innovative, and creative, the risk manager is constantly aware of the potential for an adverse event to emerge from new technology or treatment modalities. Simplifying the organization or health care practices to gain control is not a realistic goal in today's complex health systems. By using reporting and communication connections within and outside the organization and analyzing data from the investigation of adverse events, the risk manager identifies areas of greatest risk. The information about potential risk is communicated to committees or individuals who then put in place mechanisms to reduce the risk to the patient and to the institution. That the risk cannot be controlled completely should be communicated to the parents or guardian.

The Risk Management Plan

The activities of risk management are outlined in a program description. Such a document provides clear and concise information about the risk management program, which is available to all those in the institution.

Staff Education

Risk managers are educators. Every committee meeting, exchange with a staff member, or participation in orientation is an opportunity to dispel misinformation and increase understanding of the risk management process.

The fundamentals of risk management are not highlighted in medical and nursing schools, but are necessary to prepare future health care providers for risk issues that arise in the clinical setting. The development of a risk management curriculum gives structure to educational efforts and provides a framework to cover essential topics, ranging from the orientation of new employees and residents to seminars for advanced practitioners, department chairpersons, and administrators.

As an outcome of a core curriculum in risk management, all individuals in health care should be able to:

- Define risk
- Describe what a risk manager does and why
- Understand what events need to be communicated to risk management
- Describe how to access risk management for reporting and receiving information
- Describe what relationship risk management has with professional liability insurance.

Grupp-Phelan et al. (75) reported that pediatric residents were named in 26% of malpractice suits. All health care providers, including nurses, NPPs, residents, house staff, and ancillary staff such as respiratory therapists and clinical nutritionists, should know what kind of process a risk management investigation will follow (Fig. 7–2).

Health care professionals should not keep personal notes about clinical events. Objective clinical impressions belong in a patient's medical record. Physicians, nurses, and other health care professionals should understand that investigations take time, and the findings may be very different from the initial views of the staff. Speculation about the causes of adverse events or discussions of the events outside the peer-review/quality improvement areas should be discouraged.

With an understanding of the fundamentals of risk management, the health care provider can move on to identify systems and processes in his or her care that can be examined for safety and effectiveness. The risk manager analyzes the frequency or severity of adverse events or unexpected outcomes and the findings during the course of discovery in lawsuits, and then identifies topics that can be presented in an advanced risk management curriculum. These include: retroactive peer review (e.,g. clinicopathologic review, regular review of perinatal-neonatal patient care statistics), documentation, communication, supervision, monitoring and assessment, coordination of care, medication administration, system

The Risk Management Investigation Process

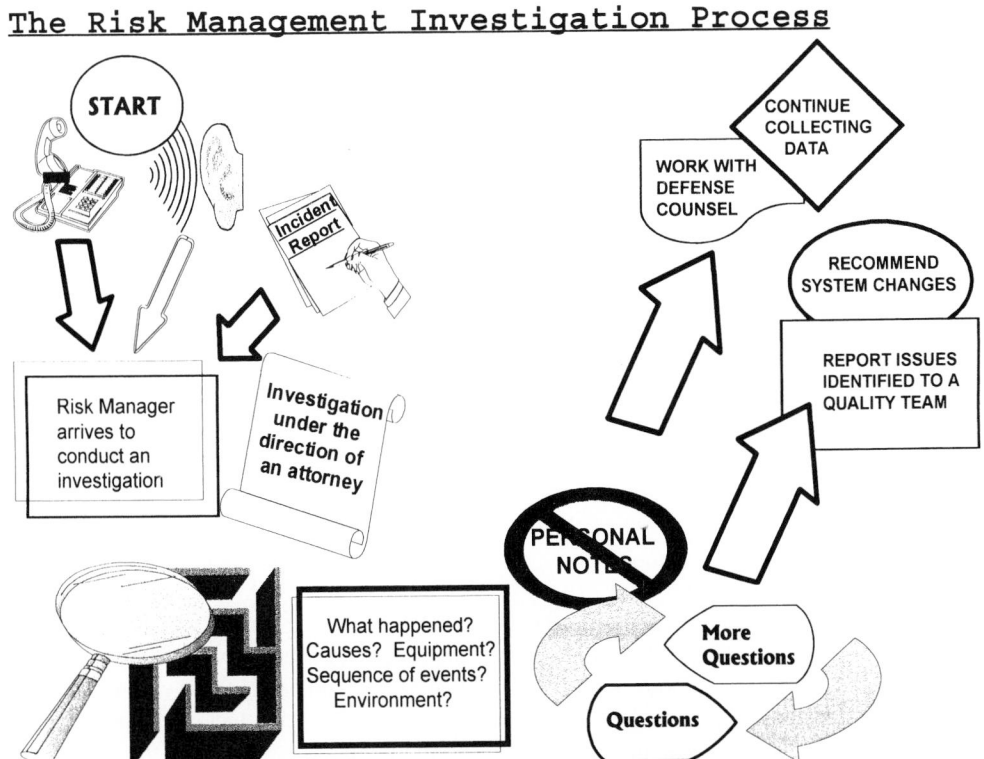

FIG. 7–2. The risk management investigation process begins with the receipt of notice that an adverse event has occurred. An attorney directs some investigations in jurisdictions where the risk management activities are not protected from discovery in litigation. The personal notes of health care providers are not protected from discovery. After many rounds of questions, opportunities for improvement are reported to quality improvement councils. In a separate activity, the results of investigation directed by the defense attorney are sent to him or her.

failure(s) and human error, and changes in local, state, or national regulations or laws.

Adverse Events

Adverse sentinel events were defined by the JCAHO in 1996 as unexpected occurrences involving death or serious physical or psychological injury or risk thereof. The term "sentinel" is used because the event should sound a warning that requires immediate attention. A root cause analysis is recommended by the JCAHO as the format for an intensive assessment to reduce the variation and prevent the event in the future. This type of analysis addresses these questions: what happened, why did it happen, and what processes were involved when it happened? The analysis can be used to piece together the reasons why a mistake or complication occurred. If the system worked previously, what elements have changed to produce the potential for error? (76).

In some instances, it is not possible to sort out the exact sequence of events. Interruptions in the system of care delivery that are identified should be repaired or redesigned to prevent further breakdowns. Because serious occurrences do not occur very often, it is necessary to optimize the lessons learned from each event, including an application of those potential events that did not

occur. Adverse, unexpected, or poor patient outcomes do not necessarily indicate that a mistake has been made. It is important not to make this assumption within the health care team, nor to accuse or to place blame. When there is an unexpected outcome, the risk manager is called upon to perform the long process of identifying the possible contributing factors.

Receiving an incident report and investigating problems that have occurred or potentially might occur is viewed by the risk manager as an opportunity for improvement in the system of care delivery. This positive outlook may not be shared by the staff. The stigma of punishment or retaliation in relation to incident reports exists and is a deterrent to obtaining the information on which to base a recommendation for change and improvement in health care delivery.

Accountability versus Blame

System and practice patterns are the focus of a risk management investigation. Investigations may reveal systems and patterns that do not provide sufficient or effective safety checks to prevent human error or miscommunication. In addition to identifying the flaws in systems or processes that potentiate mistakes, adverse event investigations, studied in the aggregate, identify the types of patients most likely to be effected. Andrews et al. (77) found that more patients with a serious illness had an initial adverse event, and that the likelihood of an adverse event increased 6% for each additional hospital day. The analysis of event databases provides the health care team with information that they can use to modify practice or alert other practitioners, thereby improving care and reducing the likelihood of lawsuits.

Reported predictors of successful pediatric litigation have included severity of resulting disability (78), defensibility of the case (79), and parental anger (80) (often exacerbated by a perception that communication with health care providers was less than satisfactory). The importance of patient or parental anger was demonstrated by Andrews et al. (77), who found that of 1,047 patients with serious injury, 17.7% experienced serious adverse events that led to longer hospital stays, but only in 1% to 2% of these adverse events was a legal claim made for compensation.

Pichert et al. (80) studied 43 closed claims, covering 8 years, involving children. A significant portion of the claims was associated with high-risk medical conditions (37%) and problems associated with intravenous therapies, central lines, and catheters (21%). In 9% of the claims, physicians relied on faulty information, and in 19% the parent(s) became particularly enraged by an injury (66).

Conventional wisdom holds the view that human beings are intrinsically unreliable. From this it follows that when something goes wrong, someone must have erred. It is assumed that mistakes such as these are the result of inattention, carelessness, and negligence. The remedies invoked to prevent further lapses include finding the culprit, assigning blame, and acting to correct future misdeeds. The truth is that the errors people make often are traceable to extrinsic factors that predispose an individual to fail. Whenever human error is suspected, it is a sound policy to trace the error to its root causes. To assign blame to an individual who makes an error is no assurance that the same error will not be made again by that individual or another (81).

The health care provider should not assume that he or she or another member of the team is responsible or liable for an unexpected outcome. Frequently, the first impression regarding the cause of poor patient outcomes is significantly different from the cause(s) recorded at the conclusion of an investigation. There is also a possibility that a cause may never be found. There should be no speculation by those directly or peripherally involved as to the cause of the event. A defensive position in response to the family's accusations should be avoided, as should the assignation of blame to other disciplines, departments, and/or systems.

The analysis of a single event and the analysis of event trends provide the health care team with information that they can use to modify practice or alert other practitioners, thereby improving care and reducing the likelihood of repeated errors.

COMMUNICATION

With Parents and Guardians

Many factors that lead to medical malpractice lawsuits are perceptual and qualitative in nature. In many cases, lawsuits are not the result of malpractice, but are instituted because the patient or patient's family feels that information was withheld from them or that they were not told the truth. Effective communication skills used in data collection, developing relationships, and dealing with parents' emotions help to prevent anger and possible malpractice litigation (82).

The perception by the family of the competency of the physician, nurses, and other health care team members are drawn from interaction. Ideally, this contact with the family inspires trust, confidence, and openness. Positive contact with the family of a neonate is based upon the fundamentals of communication: body language that conveys attention to the family and infant; taking time to answer questions; asking for input from the family regarding their impressions of the baby's progress; and speaking in terms that can be understood by the family represent good defensive medicine techniques. It is important to convey that the team members taking care of the infant are communicating with each other, are fully aware of the treatment plan, and are coordinated in their approach to the care of the infant. Judgments and preconceived opinions about the family should be avoided, regardless of their lifestyle or behavior toward the health care team. A study by Cuttini et al. (83) concluded that parents generally are satisfied about the information received, although some complained about the style of communication and especially the need to ask repeatedly in order to be informed. The latter complaint may be more common in teaching hospitals, because of the greater complexity of the health care hierarchy produced by the presence of medical students, interns, residents, and attending physicians who may change each month. No matter how large the team caring for a neonate, the attending physician should be known to the parents and guardians and readily accessible.

Those who provide health care need to understand how parents may respond to information that is conveyed or withheld. Unexpected or even negative expected changes in an infant's condition not only are upsetting to parents but may damage their confidence in the health care team. For example, when physicians or parents assume an initial diagnosis to be an absolute, undesirable outcomes may occur (84).

For the family of a critically ill neonate, the distinction is unclear between a bad outcome due to disease progression and unfortunate circumstances or errors of negligence. Anxiety over the uncertainty inherent in the care of the seriously ill may evoke feelings of helplessness. Outcomes that are expected by the physician may be a shock for the family. This nonconcurrence in expected outcomes leaves the parents feeling that a mistake has been made. Families who experience disappointments in clinical outcomes may take out their grief and despair on the health care provider. The health provider may be unprepared for the parents' anger and distrust.

If an adverse event occurs, the honest, sincere, and compassionate response of the health care team to the family will reduce the family's view that there is a need to bring a lawsuit. Without burdening the family with personal feelings of inadequacy, regret, or vague misgivings, it is helpful to show concern and to express empathy regarding the patient outcome. Silverman (85) offers insight into how parents of infants blinded by retrolental fibroplasia (retinopathy of prematurity) view the health professional who fails to convey appropriate concern.

As compared with conversations with RLF-blind young adults, discussion with parents, singly and in groups, were much more difficult for me (and for them). Most of the parents were still bitterly angry at the medical profession, but not for the reason I imagined. They understood and accepted the fact of limited knowledge at the time their children were born. Most were convinced that physicians had rendered excellent care and had used supplemental oxygen liberally in well-meant efforts to improve the chances of the small babies for intact survival. But, almost without exception, parents recalled (with rancor) that once the diagnosis of RLF was made, a chill in relationships developed. At the very time when they needed support and advice, their physicians became distant and defensive, the parents recalled. Most blamed their doctors for failing to maintain interest and concern, not for the failure of clairvoyance! The parents said it was anger at personal, not professional, behavior of physicians which prompted many of the RLF legal suits charging malpractice which burgeoned in this country.

A member of the health care team should be designated the primary communicator, to share with the family the treatment plans that have been formulated in response to the adverse event. At the request of the family, extended family and other support may be included in family conferences and discussion of the causes or possible causes of the event. Maintenance of a coordinated and ongoing communication with the family may be difficult in the face of the family's anger and despair. However, the goal of the health care team must remain the support and treatment of the patient and family.

Communication with and within the Health Care Team

From the significant number of dangerous errors that occur in the intensive care unit, Donchin et al. (86) found many were attributed to problems of communication between physicians and nurses (86). They suggest that studying the weak points of a unit may reduce errors, and that errors should not be considered an incurable disease but rather a preventable phenomenon. Clear oral communication is vital in a newborn intensive care unit; the medical record alone cannot be relied upon to adequately convey urgent information between members of a health care team (e.g., stat orders).

The medical record should be designed to achieve clear communication with and among the members of the health care team. Clinical information is focused on the patient and family, and it derives from repeated assessments, analyses, judgments, and actions aimed at achieving specific goals. Documentation in the patient record allows ongoing evaluation of patient progress and review of the clinical management plan. The individual contributions of the members of the health care team are recorded and used by other team members as a basis for planning each new step in patient care. This documentation of the exchange of information among the team and the recording of the outcome of each team member's analysis of the information also helps to support the team's choices and judgments. Documenting patient care, contemporaneous with the events, provides the clinical picture that will be utilized in the defense of the care provided should an adverse event occur. If the clinical record has the appearance of being a battle ground for warring or defensive factions of the team, the record will reflect a lack of team cohesion and direction that is difficult to defend. The record should contain the facts of the event, assessments of the patient, the decision-making processes, and the interventions undertaken.

Any documentation of an abnormality in the medical record should be accompanied by the reassuring factors that support the overall interpretation of the clinical findings. All factors that explain decisions made in the face of abnormal finding(s) should be recorded. In fact, documentation of reassuring factors should accompany the recording of abnormal factors (87).

It is very important not to draw conclusions or relate events to outcomes that are speculative in nature. Avoid placing an inappropriate medical diagnosis as a label to clinical findings. The members of the team will erroneously draw upon speculative casual relationships and refer to them further in the record as absolute. Applying an outcome diagnosis or finding with incomplete data does not lessen the impact of such a premature diagnosis during the course of either treatment or litigation, for example, concluding, based on insufficient data, that encephalopathy found on computed tomographic scan is *hypoxic* encephalopathy, or going even further and speculating that the hypoxic encephalopathy is related to a specific hypotensive episode.

Clinical findings, if possible, are best graded using numeric values. Modifiers such as the words "extreme," "severe," or "massive" do not provide objective information and will feed into the drama of a courtroom presentation. Contributors to the evaluation and care of the patient must avoid inflammatory language, markings, or punctuation that attempt to draw attention to the writer and imply that the team may be inattentive to the remarks otherwise.

It is possible that an infant's condition is changing so rapidly that thorough, contemporaneous notes in the medical record cannot be made. Although "not documented, not done" (88) is a well-known legal motto, there is much that occurs that cannot be documented in the patient record at the time of a critical event. It is often hindsight that focuses the care provider on events not recorded in contemporaneous records. A decision must be made as to whether an addendum to the medical record would contribute to patient care, or whether the additional information relates to system issues and should be conveyed to the risk manager by completing an incident report. An incident report is a confidential document and provides a means to communicate system issues. References to the completion of the incident report or discussions with the risk manager are not appropriate for, and should not appear in, the medical record. An incident report relates to an adverse event; the patient's record reflects care and treatment delivered, the patient's response, and further plan of care.

When additional information, identified after an adverse event, is necessary to the care of the patient, communication of this information is achieved in an addendum in the medical record. Such entries must include the date and time that they were written. Under no circumstances should an attempt be made to make this entry appear contemporaneous with the adverse event. The addendum must be placed sequentially in the medical record in the next available space, not on a separate page and never inserted into the text of previous entries. The purpose of an addendum is not to provide a defense or to make excuses. The medical record should never be destroyed, obliterated, or altered.

With Consultants

The "curbside" consult between colleagues is becoming a thing of the past. This type of consultation tends to be documented poorly, if at all, and can lead to damaging finger-pointing in a court of law. Guidelines for the consultation process are shown in Table 7–2.

TABLE 7–2. *Steps in the consultation process*

- Identify when it is appropriate to obtain consultation
- Choose the type of consultant (sequencing of a variety of consultants)
- Share the purpose of the consultation with the family
- Decide what information is necessary to provide to the consultant, including the purpose of the consultation and provide as a written consultation request
- Arrange a formal consultation or designate this responsibility to a specific individual
- Give a time frame within which the consultation is to be done
- Agree with the consultant on how the consultation will be reported and who will discuss the findings with the family/parent(s)
- Share the outcome of the consultation with the family
- Tell the family what will be done with the resulting information
- Document in the medical record the reasons for requesting a consultation, discussions with the family, and the plan of treatment, including the reasons why the recommendations of the consultant will or will not be followed

When a consultant is contacted for a specific patient with a formal request for evaluation and/or management, both the primary physician and the consultant should interact in such a way as to limit unnecessary risk for both (89).

CONCLUSION

In the final analysis, the determination of whether a lawsuit will be filed against a health care provider and a medical institution is based on one or more of the following issues:

1. Whether the patient or his or her legal guardians or parents were dissatisfied with the medical care
2. Whether the patient was injured, had an untoward medical event, or was led to believe that the outcome would be better than that achieved
3. Whether the medical records are complete and adequately and factually document all events.

REFERENCES

1. *Eckert v Long Island R.R.*, 43 NY 502 (1871).
2. *Kambat v St. Francis Hospital,* 89 NY2d 489, 678 NE2d 456, NYS2d 844 (1997).
3. Keeton WP. *Prosser and Keeton on the Law Torts,* 356 (5th ed 1984).
4. Manchini M, Gale A. *Emergency Care and the Law* 50 (1981).
5. Frew SA, Roush WR, LaGreca K. COBRA: implications for emergency medicine. *Ann Emerg Med* 1988;17:835.
6. *Hess v Paulowski,* 279 US 352 (1927).
7. Friedman RH, Stollerman JE, Mahoney DM, Rozenblyum L. The Virtual visit: using telecommunications technology to take care of patients. *J Am Inform Assoc* 1997;4:413.
8. Landwehr JB Jr, Zador IE, Wolf HM, et al. Telemedicine and fetal ultrasonography: assessment of technical performance and clinical feasibility. *Am J Obstet Gynecol* 1997;177:846.
9. Lewis M, Moir AT. Medical telematics and telemedicine; an agenda for research evaluation in Scotland. *Health Bull (Edinb)* 1995;53:129.
10. Landquist A. Finland is a leading country when it comes to telemedicine. *Lakartidningen* 1996;93:7.
11. S. 652. 104th Congress, 1st Session (1996). Telecommunications Reform Act (Section 709).
12. Telemedicine Report to Congress, January 31, 1997. Legal Issues Licensure and Telemedicine. Http://www.ntia.doe.gov/reports/telemed/execsum.htm
13. 28 USC 1332.
14. *Jackson v Johns-Mansville Sales Corp.,* 727 F2d 506,516 (5th Cir 1984).
15. McCormick C. *McCormick on Evidence,* Section 339 (2nd ed 1972).
16. Morgan E. *Basic Problems of Evidence,* 24 (4th ed. 1963).
17. Terry. *Negligence,* 29 Harv L Rev 40 (1915).
18. *Zebarth v Swedish Hospital Medical Center,* 81 Wash 2d 12 499 P2d 1 (1972).
19. *Second Restatement of Torts,* Section 282.
20. Ely JW, Levinson W, Elder EC, et al. Perceived causes of family physicians errors. *J Fam Pract* 1995;40:337.
21. *Oelling v Rao,* Ind 593 NE2d 189 (1992).
22. *Small v Howard,* 128 Mass 131.
23. *Peck v Hurchinson,* 88 Iowa 320, 55 NW 511.
24. *Daubert v Merill Dow Pharmaceuticals, Inc.* 509 US 579 (1993).
25. *Ybarra v Spangard,* 25 Cal App 2d 486, 154 P2d 687 (1944).
26. *Mohr v Williams,* 104 NW 12 (S Ct 1905).
27. *Cantebury v Spence,* 464 F2d 772 (DC Cir 1972), *cert denied,* 409 US 1064 (1972).
28. *Getchell v Mansfield,* 260 Or, 174,489 P2d, 953 (1971).
29. *Cooper v Roberts,* 286 A2d 647,650 (1971).
30. *Davis v Wyeth,* 399 F2d 121 (9th Cir 1968).
31. *Application of President of Georgetown College, Inc.,* 331 F2d 1000 (DC Cir), *cert denied,* 377 US 978 (1964).

32. King N. Transparency in neonatal intensive care. *Hastings Center Report* 1992;22:18.

33. Gutheil TG, Burszatjn H, Brodsky A. Malpractice prevention through the sharing of uncertainty. *N Engl J Med* 1984;311:49.

34. Federal crackdown puts risk managers in hot seat [Editorial]. *Health Care Risk Management* 1997;19:49.

35. Hayt E, Hayt LR, eds. *Law of hospital, physician, and patient,* 2nd ed. New York: Hospital Textbook Co., 1952:637.

36. Beck JC, ed. *Confidentiality versus the duty to protect.* Washington, DC: American Psychiatric Press, 1990.

37. *Reisner v Regents of the University of California et al.,* 31 Cal App 4th 1195, 37 Cal Rptr 2d 518 (1995).

38. *Tarasoff v Regents of University of California et al.,* 108 Cal Rptr 878 (Cal App 1973), superseded by *Tarasoff v Regents of University of California et al.,* 13 Cal 3d 177, 118 Cal Rptr 129,529 P2d 553 (1974), subsequent op on reh *Tarasoff v Regents of University of California et al.,* 17 Cal 3d 425, 131 Cal Rptr 14,551 P2d 334 (1976).

39. *Lipari v Sears Roebuck & Co.,* 497 F Supp 185 (D Neb 1980).

40. 42 USC 290ee-3.

41. 42 USC 290dd-3.

42. 42 USC 290ee-3(b)(2)(A).

43. 42 USC 290dd-3(b)(2)(A).

44. 42 USC 290ee-3(b)(2)(C).

45. 42 USC 290dd-3(b)(2)(C).

46. Dick RS, Steen EB, eds. *The computer-based patient record:* an essential technology for health care. Washington, DC: National Academy Press, 1991.

47. Kassirer JP. Sounding board. The computer-based patient record and confidentiality. *N Engl J Med* 1995;333:1419.

48. Annas GJ. *The rights of patients:* the basic UCLU guide to patient rights, 2nd ed. Carbondale: Southern Illinois University Press, 1989:178.

49. Balsalmo RR, Brown MD. Risk management. In: Sanbar SS, ed. *Legal medicine, American Colleges of Legal Medicine.* St. Louis: Mosby 1995:237.

50. Kramer C. Medical Malpractice 5 (1976), citing *History of Reported Medical Professional Liability Cases,* 30 Temple LQ 367 (1957).

51. Malone TW, Thaler DH. Managed health care: a plaintiff's perspective. *Tort Insurance Law J* 1996;32:123.

52. Clifford RA. Physician's liability in a managed care environment. *Health Lawyer* 1997;10:5.

53. Bodenheimer J. The HMO backlash—righteous or reactionary? *N Engl J Med* 1997;336:1329.

54. Blum JL, ed. *Monograph 5, achieving quality care:* the role of the law. Health Law Section of the American Bar Association, Loyola University, Chicago, June 1997.

55. *Moore v Regents of the University of California,* 793 P2d 479, 51 Cal 2d 120 (1990).

56. Kanute M. *Evolving Theories of Malpractice Liability in HMOs,* 20 Loy. Univ. Of Chic. L Rev. 841-73 (1989).

57. *Fox v Health-Net,* Civ No 21962 (Riverside County Super Ct, Cal, Dec 28, 1993).

58. *Sloan v Metropolitan Health Council,* 516 NE2d 1104 (Ind Ct App 1987).

59. Restatement (second) of Agency paragraph sign 216 (1958).

60. Restatement (second) of Agency paragraph sign 250 (1958).

61. *Schleier v Kaiser Foundation Health Plan,* 876 F2d 174 (DC Cir 1989).

62. *Darling v Charleston Community Memorial Hospital,* 211 NE2d 253 (1965), *cert denied,* 383 US 946 (1966).

63. *Wickline v State,* 192 Cal App 3d 1630, 239 Cal Rptr 810 (1986).

64. 29 USC Sections 1001–1461.

65. 29 USC Section 1144 (a).

66. *Shea v Esensten,* 107 F3d 625 (8th Cir 1997).

67. *Harper v Healthsource New Hampshire,* 674 A2d 962 (NH 1996).

68. *Texas Medical Association v Aetna Life Insurance Co.,* 80 F3d 153 (5th Cir 1996).

69. 42 USCA 11131–11137 (West Supp 1995).

70. Belkin L. How can we save the next victim? *The New York Times Magazine,* June 18, 1997.

71. Bernstein P.L. *Against the gods:* the remarkable story of risk. New York: John Wiley and Sons, 1996:197.

72. Morlock LL, Malitz FE. Do hospital risk management programs make a difference: relationships between risk management program activities and hospital malpractice claims experience. *Law Contemp Probl* 1991;54:133.

73. Acerbo-Avalone N, Kremer K. *Medical malpractice claims investigation:* a step-by-step approach. Gaithersburg, MD: Aspen, 1997:xv.

74. Stelovich S. Framework for handling adverse events. *Forum* 1997;18:5.

75. Grupp-Phelan J, Reynolds S, Lingl LL. Professional liability of residents in a children's hospital. *Arch Pediatr Adolesc Med* 1996;150:87.

76. Joint Commission on Accreditation of Healthcare Organizations. *Conducting a root cause analysis in response to a sentinel event.* Oakbrook Terrace, IL: JCAHO, 1996.

77. Andrews LB, Stocking C, Krizek T, et al. An alternative strategy for studying adverse events in medical care. *Lancet* 1997;349:309.

78. Brennan TA, Sox CM, Burstin HR. Relation between negligently adverse events and the outcomes of medical-malpractice litigation. *N Engl J Med* 1996;335:1963.

79. Taragrin MI, Willet LR, Wilczek AP, et al. The influence of standard of care and severity of injury on the resolution of malpractice claims. *Ann Intern Med* 1992;117:780.

80. Pichert JW, Hickson GB, Bledsoe S, et al. Understanding the ethiology of serious medical events involving children: implications for pediatricians and their risk managers. *Pediatr Annu* 1997;26:162.

81. Vancott H. Human errors: their causes and reduction. In: Bogner MS, ed. *Human error in medicine.* Bethesda MD: US Drug Administration, 1994:153.

82. Levison W. Doctor–patient communication and medical malpractice: implications for pediatricians. *Pediatr Annu* 1997;26:186.

83. Cuttini M, Romito P, Del Santo M, et al. Communications in the neonatal intensive therapy unit: the opinions of parents and of medical personnel compared. *Pediatr Med Chir* 1994;16:325.

84. Epstein AL. The inevitability of narrow diagnostic focus and trust. *Forum* 1997;5 and 6, winter:17.

85. Silverman WA. *Retrolental fibroplasia:* a modern parable. New York: Grune and Straton 1980:83.

86. Donchin Y, Gopher D, Olin M. A look into the nature and causes of human errors in the intensive care unit. *Crit Care Med* 1995;23:244.

87. Chilton JH, Shimmel TR. Inappropriate word choice in the medical record. In: Donn SM, Fisher CW, eds. *Risk management techniques in perinatal and neonatal practice.* Arrmonk, NY: Futura Publishing Co., 1996:603.

88. Abbott DA. Truth and justice: dispelling the myths of medical malpractice. *J Healthcare Risk Management* 1996;16:19.

89. Hartline JV, Smith CG. Risk management in medical consultation. In: Donn SM, Fisher CW, eds. *Risk management techniques in perinatal and neonatal practice.* Armonk, NY: Futura Publishing Co., 1996:617.

CHAPTER 8

The Vulnerable Neonate and the Neonatal Intensive Care Environment

Penny Glass

Environmental factors in the neonatal intensive care unit (NICU) have major implications for the care of the sick newborn infant. Advances in medical technology during the last three decades are credited with dramatic reductions in mortality, with the point of 50% survival decreasing from birth weight of 1,500 g in 1970 to less than 700 g in 1990. Morbidity among survivors, however, is a problem of increasing proportions. The rate of major morbidity has remained fairly stable, around 10%, and yet this focus on major morbidity has overlooked the much larger number of children born prematurely who have learning disabilities at school age. Broad evidence implicates the environment in the NICU as a factor in neonatal morbidity. Abnormal sensory input can be a source of potentially overwhelming stress and, at a sensitive period during development, can modify the developing brain. The NICU environment therefore assumes a crucial role in the care of the sick newborn infant.

Preterm birth is the most common single risk factor for developmental problems in childhood, and learning disability is the most pervasive developmental problem. This is a catch-all term, but includes children of low average or otherwise normal intelligence who have deficits in language, visual perception, or visuomotor integration, deficiencies in attention span, hyperactivity, or social immaturity. Such children require either special services to function in a regular classroom or placement in a special class. Reports of school-age children who were of very low birth weight indicate that as many as one-half have learning disabilities (1–8). Such deficits may originate from overt damage to the brain or from a more general disturbance in brain organization.

Throughout infancy, both behavioral and neurologic differences exist between full-term and preterm infants, even when matched for conceptional age. The latter often exhibit manifestations of altered brain organization, including disrupted sleep, difficult temperament, both hyperresponsivity and hyporesponsivity to sensory input, prolonged attention to redundant information, inattention to novel stimuli, and poor quality of motor function (9–15). These precursors of learning problems in school are not fully explained by either the severity of illness among the preterm infants or by later conditions in the home environment (10).

The sensory environment in the NICU is different in virtually every respect, both from the environment of a fetus *in utero* and from that of a full-term newborn at home. The NICU experience contains frequent aversive procedures, excess handling, disturbance of rest, noxious oral medications, noise, and bright light. These conditions are sources of stress and anomalous sensory stimulation, both of which may affect morbidity.

The immediate effects of stress are autonomic instability, apnea/bradycardia, vasoconstriction, and decreased gastric motility. Cortisol, adrenaline, and catecholamines are secreted during stress as part of an intricate hypothalamic–pituitary–adrenocortical system (16,17). High levels of these hormones interfere with tissue healing. Noxious stimuli disrupt sleep and can have biological consequences for the neonate. Even medical complications commonly associated with prematurity per se, such as bronchopulmonary dysplasia and necrotizing enterocolitis, may be, in part, stress-related diseases (18).

Sensory input is essential during maturation. Most of the cortex is part of one of the sensory systems. Abnormal experience, both depriving and overstimulating, can modify the developing brain. The most vulnerable period occurs during rapid brain growth and neuronal differenti-

P. Glass: Department of Neonatology, Children's National Medical Center, Washington, D.C.

ation (19,20). The timing of these events for the human fetus corresponds to 28 to 40 weeks of gestation (21). It is assumed that, for the fetus, the optimal sensory environment is experienced within the womb. One of the more striking aspects of this environment is the bidirectional contingency between mother and fetus.

The potential impact of the anomalous NICU environment on the vulnerable newborn infant has raised unabated concerns for nearly two decades (22–28). A more optimal NICU environment might reduce iatrogenic morbidity and improve the outcome of sick neonates; however, the parameters are not yet well defined. This chapter summarizes the maturation of each sensory system during late fetal development, with particular reference to evidence for the prenatal onset of function, compares the intrauterine and NICU sensory experience, and critiques techniques of developmental intervention.

NEONATAL SENSORY SYSTEMS: DEVELOPMENT, DISORDERS, ENVIRONMENT, AND INTERVENTION

Maturation of all the sensory systems begins during the latter part of embryogenesis; however, the process is neither unitary nor fixed. Within each system some reciprocity between structure and function probably exists. To some extent, sensory input drives maturation (29). In addition, the rate of maturation of each sensory system varies, with the onset of function generally in the following order: tactile, vestibular, gustatory–olfactory, auditory, and visual (30). These sensory systems also are interrelated in a hierarchical manner—stimulation of early-maturing senses (e.g., tactile, vestibular) has a positive influence on development of later-maturing ones (e.g., visual) (31). Recent research also indicates that untimely stimulation within this sequence (e.g., visual) may disrupt the normal maturational process of another sensory system (e.g., auditory) (32).

This hierarchical organization and integration of sensory function is well supported and lends two guiding principles for developmental intervention in the NICU: stimulation of the senses should begin with the most mature; and the optimal form of stimulation for initial postnatal development resembles the sources naturally available to the fetus and infant—those that come from the mother.

Tactile System

The cutaneous system includes sensation of pressure, pain, and temperature. Only pressure will be discussed here; pain is discussed in Chapter 57. Receptors in the skin respond to pressure and then transmit impulses to the spinal cord through the dorsal root, ascending in the posterior tract and terminating in the gray matter of the cord. At this point, connecting fibers decussate and continue in the ventral spinothalamic tract to the medulla and the thalamus, terminating in the postcentral gyrus of the cortex. Representation here is somatotopic and contralateral to the stimulated side. Increased stimulation to an area of the body or loss of a limb can alter the pattern of representation in the somatosensory cortex.

Development

Like the vestibular system, the tactile sense develops early in fetal life and is thought to play a particularly pervasive role in the early development of the organism. Receptor cells are present in the perioral region in the fetus by the eighth week of gestation and spread to all skin and mucosal surfaces by the twentieth week. The cortical pathway is intact by 20 to 24 weeks of gestation, and some myelin is already present. Response to tactile stimulation has been observed by ultrasound as early as 8 weeks of conceptional age (33,34). Response to stroking in the lip region occurs first, followed by a response to stimulation of the palms. Most of the body is sensitive to touch by 15 weeks (35).

Tactile threshold is very low in the preterm infant. It is more related to postconceptional age (PCA) than to natal age but increases by term. Infants younger than 30 weeks PCA respond by an unequivocal leg withdrawal to pressure of a 0.50-g von Frey hair applied to the plantar surface of the foot compared to 1.7-g pressure by 38 weeks PCA (36). A qualitative shift occurs around 32 weeks PCA. Infants less than 32 weeks PCA respond to repeated stimulation with sensitization and a diffuse behavioral response. In contrast, infants after this age show habituation to the same stimuli.

Classic studies by Harlow and Harlow (37) demonstrated the profound importance of contact comfort for normal development. In a parallel fashion, even preterm infants will seek and maintain contact with a physical object within their incubator and even more so if the tactile source contains rhythmic stimulation (38). These findings provide strong support for intervention in the tactile modality.

Disturbances

Tactile hypersensitivity, or tactile defensive behavior, is contained in clinical reports of children with developmental delay, many of whom were born preterm. It also is seen in infants and children who otherwise appear normal. The behavior frequently is said to be a manifestation of sensory integration deficit and thought to have its origins in the prenatal or perinatal period. It appears as an infant's overreaction to touch, generally the hands or oral/facial regions. With oral hypersensitivity, the infant may withdraw, gag, or retch when touched even around the outside of the mouth. Some infants are intolerant of food with texture and resist transition from liquids or very smooth puree. Infants also may be hypersensitive to touch on their extremities, with prolonged palmar/mental reflex, exaggerated hand and toe grasp, or leg withdrawal. An extreme case was a 2-month-old (corrected-age) infant who, when supine, arched his buttocks off the table surface in response to his legs being grasped. Additional manifestations of tactile sensitivity may appear as an intolerance for grasping toys or handling play materials of certain textures. In another extreme example, a 1-year-old infant would gag when his hand was placed in dry macaroni. Some children are intolerant of normal clothing and even may avoid body contact. Such aversion adversely affects parent–infant bonding. The link between early tactile disturbances and learning disabilities at school age is unlikely to be a causal one, but may be related to a similar mechanism of brain dysfunction.

Intrauterine Experience

The fetus is housed in a thermoneutral, fluid-filled space that is a source of cutaneous input throughout the body surface. Fetal movement provides tactile self-stimulation. Perhaps even more important, fetal movement often evokes a contingent maternal response. As term approaches and the intrauterine space becomes more constraining, the normal posture of flexion evokes hand-to-mouth, skin-to-skin, and body-on-body tactile feedback. The effect is progressive throughout the gestation.

After a normal term birth, a ventral–ventral position is preferred by both mother and infant, with touch followed by slow stroking (39). Traditionally, the infant is then swaddled and held. As before birth, human proximity produces contingent touch.

Touch and Handling in the Neonatal Intensive Care Unit

After premature birth, tactile input is radically altered. The extrauterine fetus is frequently nursed naked, with the exception of maybe a diaper and a hat. The surface of the mattress generally is unyielding. She or he is exposed to air currents, cold stress, tape, instruments, handling by caregivers, and painful stimuli. Pressure is not uniform.

The type and frequency of tactile stimulation imposed on a preterm newborn in the NICU would be overwhelming even for a healthy adult. Over a 2-week period, a sick neonate may be handled by more than ten different nurses, in addition to physicians, occupational or physical therapists, laboratory and x-ray technicians, and finally the parent (40).

Handling occurs more often among the sickest infants, typically is related to procedures, generally is disturbing, and often is painful. In spite of wide attention in the literature over the last decade to the consequences of excess handling in the NICU, the amount has not decreased from 1976 to 1990, even among the more severely ill infants

(41). On the average, sick preterm newborns are handled more than 150 times a day, with less than 10 minutes of consecutive uninterrupted rest (26). Disturbance of sleep has biologic and immunologic consequences (42,43). Secretion of cortisol and adrenaline normally is inhibited during sleep. Growth hormone, which is released during quiet sleep, increases protein synthesis and mobilization of free fatty acids for energy use. Thus, sleep facilitates healing.

Excess handling has other significant physiologic consequences for the sick neonate. Blood pressure changes, alterations in cerebral blood flow, and episodes of oxygen desaturation are associated with noxious procedures, handling, or crying (44–48). Fluctuations in blood pressure may contribute to intracranial hemorrhage in the unstable preterm infant (49). Importantly, when caretakers monitor the infant's level of oxygenation during procedures, the severity of hypoxemic episodes can be reduced significantly (44). Thus, the amount and type of handling may have direct detrimental consequences for the vulnerable neonate.

In addition to the hemodynamic impact of obviously noxious procedures described earlier, more benign manipulations, such as those that occur during neurodevelopmental assessment, also may adversely affect the preterm infant (25,48). Decreased plasma growth hormone has been reported after administration of the Brazelton Neonatal Behavioral Assessment Scale to preterm infants at 36 weeks PCA (50). Even at the time of discharge, the evaluation was associated with elevated cortisol levels (17,51). It is not clear whether these effects were from the neurodevelopmental assessment or from the stress associated with crying, which normally occurs during administration of the Neonatal Behavioral Assessment Scale. Handling could be stressful even for stable preterm infants.

Tactile Intervention in the Neonatal Intensive Care Unit

The two general approaches to tactile intervention in the NICU provide either reduction of general handling or provision of planned touch experiences. Touch may be pressure alone or may include stroking. The neonates may be acutely ill or medically stable. These distinctions are important.

As part of an individualized approach to developmental care for acutely ill preterm infants, Als et al. (52) provided "minimal handling" and clustering of routine procedures, as well as positive tactile input and containment from bunting, rolls, positioning, and the like. Short- and long-term outcomes were improved for her intervention group compared to a nonintervention group. This technique has had a major impact on developmental intervention as a whole. Although it is not possible to isolate which aspect of this multimodal approach was effective, a significant change was made in the role of the nurse/caregiver.

More specific to the tactile modality, Jay (53) evaluated the effects of planned, gentle, touch for 12-minute periods four times a day for acutely ill preterm infants. This intervention, which consisted of hands-on contact but not stroking or manipulating, was associated with a lower fraction of inspired oxygen (FiO_2) after 5 days compared to a similar nonintervention group.

In apparent contrast, Field et al. (54) and Scafidi et al. (55) initiated a touch intervention that differed from that of Jay (53) and Als et al. (52) in important respects: the infants were recruited when "stable and growing" rather than during an acute period; the treatment provided three 15-minute periods a day of massage (i.e., stroking and passive limb movement) for a 10-day treatment period. The massaged infants showed a greater weight gain, even though the groups did not differ in formula intake. These early effects on growth are thought to be mediated by induction of catecholamine release (50). The massaged infants also spent more time awake, showed better performance on the Brazelton neonatal assessment, were discharged home 6 days sooner, and had better performance on developmental assessment at 8 months past term.

Although overall effects of the tactile intervention have been positive, the response of individual infants is variable and deserves attention. For example, an increase in periods of oxygen desaturation during parent touch, compared to baseline, has been reported (56). A number of infants have responded with apnea and bradycardia to the type of intervention described by Field et al. (54) and Scafidi et al. (55). This physiologic response may occur after the intervention. It is not clear whether the intervention itself was excessive or whether the abrupt shift after the cessation of tactile input leads to an unexpected physiologic response. Individual differences exist among caregivers that also affect the infants' response to the stimulation. Finally, the distinction between touch, stroking, and massage is probably important.

All of these issues advise against standardized protocols of stroking or massage for all preterm infants. When any form of tactile and kinesthetic intervention is applied, the caregiver should continue to monitor the infant's physiologic and behavioral responses before onset, during, and after the cessation of the intervention. Consistency of contact across caregivers would help.

Soft swaddling or clothing may provide tactile input in a more sustained fashion than periodic hands-on contact. Arguments that this obscures the view of the infant and interferes with temperature regulation by servocontrol simply argue against servocontrol rather than against covers. Clothing or swaddling actually could dampen the fluctuations in temperature that occur during incubator care and inhibit exaggerated movement or agitation, which in itself may be stabilizing. Creative swaddling with crisscrossed strips and Velcro could allow for more

visualization of the infant. The use of swaddling in the NICU is necessary if the parent is to have that option at home as a means of calming and supporting sleep.

Thus, the amount and type of stimulation are important and change with acuity, maturation, and the response of the infant. Parents need specific guidance and modeling from the beginning. The general order of tactile intervention might be: *if acutely ill,* minimal handling, containment (e.g., swaddling, rolls), gentle touch (e.g., warm hand) without stroking; *when medically stable,* holding, rocking gently, and stroking. Minimal handling protocols have a definite place in the NICU, but not as the end point. It also is important during the hospital stay to help the infant develop increased tolerance for social contact and gentle handling, especially as discharge approaches. Systematic desensitization may even be necessary in cases of chronically ill infants.

Nonnutritive Sucking

Nonnutritive sucking in the neonate represents an early endogenous rhythm and a manifestation of sensorimotor integration (57). It is reported in the fetus (58) and observed in the preterm newborn at least by 28 weeks of gestation. Increase in the number of sucks per burst occurs with maturation. Duration of the burst appears fairly stable across ages. Nonnutritive sucking is an important oral/tactile intervention that supports both feeding and early behavioral regulation.

Nipples used for nonnutritive sucking abound, varying in size, configuration, consistency, and utility. A feeding nipple is not designed for nonnutritive sucking and is inappropriate. It readily collapses; the infant experiences little resistance to his or her suck and may loll the device. Gauze inserted in the nipple may absorb oral secretions and breed bacteria. In larger infants, the nipple is unsafe because of possible aspiration. A variety of commercially available pacifiers should be available in any NICU to suit the individual needs of each infant. Some neonates who are hypersensitive to touch in the perioral region often respond positively to contact (and perhaps smell) from their own hands.

Nonnutritive sucking experience may facilitate important physiologic and behavioral mechanisms and potentially reduce cost of care. Infants provided with nonnutritive sucking during gavage feeding showed significantly improved gastrointestinal transit time, greater suck pressure, more sucks per burst, and fewer sporadic sucks. They initiated bottle feeding earlier, showed better weight gain, and thereby had shorter hospital stays (59,60). Having a pacifier continuously available, however, may not be beneficial and may, in fact, encourage inappropriate sucking patterns, particularly in the chronically ill neonate.

Nonnutritive sucking also acts as a behavioral organizer or facilitator. It has been shown to decrease motor activity and increase quiet states in stable preterm infants (61). It dampens an infant's behavioral response after a painful procedure such as circumcision or heelstick (62,63). although it does not appear to dampen the cortisol response (17). It is noteworthy that sucking on a pacifier before the onset of repeated painful procedures, such as heelsticks, may be inappropriate, because simple aversive conditioning to the pacifier could occur.

Vestibular System

The vestibular system responds to movement as well as directional changes in gravity and is situated in the nonauditory labyrinth of the inner ear. The three fluid-filled semicircular canals lie at right angles to each other, one for each major plane of the body. The ampulla, located at the end of each canal, contains hair fibers in a sac or cupula. Motion of the body or head causes pressure changes that move the cupula, which stimulates the hair cells and transmits an impulse along the vestibular portion of the eighth cranial nerve to the vestibular nuclei of the medulla. The vestibular organs consist of the utricle and saccule, which respond to changes of head position involving linear motion. The macula, a thickening in the wall of the utricle and saccule, contains hair cells sensitive to position of the head. Impulses from the macula transmit along the vestibular nerve to the medulla and cerebellum. From there, information is transmitted to motor fibers going to the neck, eye, trunk, and limb muscles. There are no connections to the cortex (64). Vestibular stimulation affects level of alertness. Slow, rhythmic, continuous movement induces sleep. Periodic or higher amplitude swing increases arousal.

Development

Initial vestibular development is concurrent with auditory development, emanating from the same otocyst early in gestation. The three semicircular canals begin to form before 8 weeks of gestation, reaching morphologic maturity by 14 weeks, and full size by week 20 (29). The vestibular sacs probably develop at the same time. Response to vestibular stimulation has been observed by 25 weeks of gestation (35). The traditional vertex presentation of the fetus at term gestation is thought to occur from fetal activity in response to vestibular input.

Disturbances

Considerable research with animals has demonstrated the importance of both tactile and vestibular input (37,65). Lack of normal vestibular stimulation in the developing organism is thought to affect general neurobehavioral organization (31). Children who were born preterm are reported to have deficits in balance at preschool age (8), but this is not necessarily a vestibular problem.

Intrauterine Experience

The fetus experiences both contingent and noncontingent vestibular stimulation that varies during gestation. From the beginning of embryonic life, the fluid environment of the womb provides periodic oscillations and movements that emanate from normal movements of the mother as well as activity of the fetus itself. Reports by mothers of fetal movement occur around 16 weeks. After 28 weeks of gestation, there is a decrease in the relative amount of amniotic fluid, and, thus, the movement of the fetus becomes partially constrained by the more limited physical space. Vestibular experience is then less contingent on self-activation and more related to normal maternal activity and position change, which often occurs in response to fetal activity. In general, maternal activity level slows as parturition approaches.

After birth, the infant is held normally. Movement is slow from maternal breathing and shifting. Change of position is gradual. Vestibular stimulation is used to affect state—moving to upright or laying down increases arousal; monotonous side-to-side rocking and walking in the form of parental pacing reduce the level of arousal.

Vestibular Experience in the Neonatal Intensive Care Unit

Vestibular stimulation after preterm birth is limited to efficient manipulation or turning of the neonate by the caregiver. It clearly lacks any of the temporal qualities or contingencies that the maternal environment may have provided. Spontaneous limb movement generally is diffuse, often unrestricted, and typically disorganizing in its effect.

Intervention in the Neonatal Intensive Care Unit

Like the tactile sense, the early development of the vestibular system provides a theoretical basis for primary intervention with preterm neonates. More than three decades ago, Neal (66) demonstrated that daily rocking facilitated the development of preterm infants. Subsequent research simulated the intrauterine environment and provided compensatory vestibular stimulation. An oscillating waterbed was devised, which moved with the rhythm of maternal respirations but with an amplitude less than 2.5 mm at the surface of the unoccupied waterbed. The safety of this paradigm, as well as efficacy in reduction in apnea of prematurity, have been well demonstrated (67). In addition, the infants on waterbeds demonstrated more organized sleep state and motor behavior, decreased irritability, enhanced visual alertness, and improved somatic growth (67–70).

Difficulty in nursing sick infants on an oscillating surface may have precluded more widespread adoption of the waterbed. An infant's own movement also can induce more than optimal movement of the surface, as, for example, an infant with gastroesophageal reflux; however, some babies still are likely to benefit. At the least, it would seem prudent to provide a trial on a waterbed for a nonventilated infant with apnea of prematurity, before introduction of pharmacologic intervention.

Other sources of vestibular stimulation, such as rocking chairs, swings, and hammocks, have not been investigated formally. Rocking chairs probably belong in any nursery. Swings are questionable, given the excessive upright position of the baby and the standard rate of oscillation (i.e., too fast). A crib has been devised that provides controlled motion similar to a woman walking; the duration of motion may be individually controlled and proportionally reduced over time (71), but the rate of ocillation appears too rapid for a preterm infant. The device appears to be effective in modulating fussiness in full-term infants and is in used with preterm infants. The infants are well swaddled and further contained on each side by rolls.

Positioning

The physical position of an infant is part of the NICU tactile–vestibular experience. Nursing sick preterm infants routinely has been with the infant in supine and exposed, which may simplify management but may not be advantageous for the infant. Prone positioning in the NICU has been strongly supported physiologically. The current NICU dilemma is that the prone sleep position is contrary to the recommendation by the Academy of Pediatrics (AAP), which now supports supine positioning because epidemiologic data associate supine positioning with a lower rate of sudden infant death syndrome. The optimal position of the infant needs to address anatomic and physiologic consequences. Positioning for optimal care in the NICU needs to take account of the AAP recommendation before the infant is ready for discharge home.

Yu (72) demonstrated that gastric emptying was facilitated in either the prone or right lateral position compared to the supine or left lateral position. This was particularly significant for the sick preterm who already showed a delay in gastric emptying. Prone position, compared to supine, is associated with more quiet sleep and less active sleep or crying. Quiet sleep, in turn, is associated with improved lung volume, more stable respiration, less apnea, and improved PaO_2 (73,74). Finally, prone position compared to supine is associated with a higher PaO_2 among healthy preterm infants and, even more significantly, in those with respiratory distress syndrome (74,75). The evidence suggests that, when possible, the sick infant should be nursed in a prone or right lateral position.

Parents of preterm infants often complain that their baby's feet turn out. In fact, the legs more often are externally rotated at the hip. Grenier (76) described hip deformities seen on roentgenograms of preterm infants after prolonged nursing in a frog-leg position. The bulk of the diaper in extremely preterm infants exacerbates the problem. Winging of the scapula also is frequent in the preterm infant. Proper support of the trunk and limbs in prone or supine position lessens this extreme rotation and may diminish orthopedic or neuromuscular complications.

In prone position, placing the infant on a small folded strip from shoulder to hip could allow more physiologic flexion and adduction. In side lying, it may be easier to position the infant in soft flexion. Gentle containment of the limbs usually can be managed with strips of soft cloth across the upper arm and thigh. Some movement should be allowed within a controlled range. A posture of physiologic flexion and adduction in supine position would require swaddling. Maintenance of postures can be facilitated by nesting the infant in soft rolls, but the rolls must not reach above the level of the shoulder. Each posture should facilitate the infant bringing hands to mouth.

For older, more medically stable preterm infants, infant seats are used as an alternative to continuous lying in bed. The infant should be swaddled and nested, the angle probably should be no more than 30 degrees, and the length of time should be limited. Oxygen desaturation has been reported in stable preterm infants placed in car seats.

Kangaroo Care

Kangaroo care is a technique that evolved primarily in South America (77). Traditionally, the infant is clad only in a diaper and placed under the mother's clothing between her breasts, remaining there according to the mother's comfort, and feeding on demand. The technique provides fairly sustained multimodal stimulation: tactile, vestibular, proprioceptive, olfactory, and auditory. It appears to be safe for larger preterm infants or those who are medically stable. Temperature regulation in the infant does not appear to be a problem, but needs to be carefully monitored on an individual basis. It seems to have the greatest benefit in terms of facilitating and maintaining lactation and enhancing maternal sense of competency for these infants. The studies, however, are of insufficient sample size to evaluate whether morbidity, such as intracranial hemorrhage, is increased. More data are needed among medically stable infants before kangaroo care should be attempted prior to 32 weeks conceptional age or with infants requiring mechanical ventilation. The increased tactile stimulation and additional handling easily could be overly stressful for the immature or sick infant.

Chemical Senses

The chemoreceptors include taste and olfaction. Taste receptors are in the taste buds, which are located primarily in the papillae of the tongue but also are found on the soft palate and epiglottis (29,78). Taste stimuli (i.e., sweet, sour, bitter, salt) transmit to the brainstem with a primary branch to the hypothalamus. Cortical regions are involved in learned taste preferences. The olfactory receptors are located in the lining of the olfactory epithelium in the posterior portion of the nasal passage. The afferent pathway has no cortical projection area, but is direct to the limbic system. Olfaction plays an important part in gustatory experiences. Olfaction also is an integral part of infant attachment to caregiver and may even be mutual (79).

Development of Taste

The chemoreceptors are well developed within the first trimester (29,78). Taste buds appear around 8 to 9 weeks of gestation. The receptors are present at least by the sixteenth week of gestation, and increase by term to adult levels. During the second one-half of gestation, morphologic changes occur that continue after term. By term, taste is sufficiently sensitive to detect a 0.1 mol/L concentration of NaCl in water (80). Stimulation of taste receptors has important implications for early feeding. Smotherman and Robinson (81) hypothesized that tastes of milk activate a centrally mediated endogeneous opioid system in newborn term infants, consistent with that shown in the animal model. This would suggest that, in normal development, the mechanism to support early feeding extends beyond maintenance of chemical or caloric balance and becomes feeding to thrive.

Taste discrimination has been measured by differential consumption, autonomic responses, and facial expressions. Full-term neonates as well as anencephalic infants demonstrate differential behavioral responses to sweet, bitter, sour, and salt (82). Plain water evokes an aversive response, which may be a biologically based protective mechanism. In a behavior described as "savoring," normal newborns discriminate between different concentrations of sucrose and even among various sugars (80). Similarly, preterm infants (30 to 36 weeks of gestation) show stronger sucking in response to glucose compared to plain water (83) and characteristic behavioral expression in response to sour or bitter solutions (82). Behavioral response to formula, or breast milk, administered to the tip of the tongue has been documented in preterm infants prior to 28 weeks of gestation (84).

Taste preferences and sensitivity change with postnatal development, including the endogeneous opioid response, which is no longer elicited in the human infant after 6 weeks of age (85).

Stimulation of taste receptors may have applications beyond basic feeding. Recent studies in the fetal rat model demonstrated that intraoral infusion of milk stimulates the endogenous opioid systems and raises the threshold to noxious tactile stimuli, whereas intragastric infusions do not (86). Parallel research with human infants has a similar effect (87).

Taste receptors are functional before birth. It is well known that the human fetus swallows amniotic fluid. Injection of distinct tastes into the amniotic fluid of pregnant women between 34 and 39 weeks of gestation altered fetal swallowing behavior, which increased with the sweeter taste and decreased with bitter (29). The preterm infant also will exhibit characteristic facial expressions when tasting a sour or sweet substance (82).

Development of Olfaction

The olfactory epithelium is evident around 5 weeks in the lining of the posterior nasal passage. Nerve fibers and cells form the olfactory nerve, which extends from the epithelium to the ventral wall of the forebrain. At that time, the olfactory bulb develops (29). No information exists about the functional onset of human olfaction, but it is presumed to be present prenatally, having been demonstrated in a rat model. Rat fetuses exposed to citral in the amniotic fluid will selectively attach postnatally to a nipple of the same scent (88).

Prenatal olfactory function also is inferred from the sophistication present by term, including behavioral discrimination, preference, and conditioning to olfactory stimuli. For example, 1-week-old infants will reliably turn their heads away from a noxious smell (89). In response to a series of pleasant or aversive odors, infants less than 12 hours old will exhibit different facial expressions that are discriminable by adults (82). Infants under 1 week of age reliably prefer the odor of their mother's breast pad to the breast pad of another mother (90). Neonates who were given a period of familiarization to a novel odor subsequently demonstrated a preference for that odor, whereas infants exposed to it for the first time did not (79). Finally, classic conditioning to a novel olfactory stimulus has been demonstrated empirically within the first 48 hours after term birth (91). Given ten 30-second pairings of citrus odor with stroking, neonates the following day showed increased activity and head turning in the presence of the citrus but not to a novel odor.

Disorders

Feeding disorders are reported commonly among preterm infants, particularly those with chronic lung disease. The infant may even respond aversively to the introduction of food in the mouth. The cause generally is attributed to frequent stressful procedures around the mouth as well as poor coordination of suck/swallow. Abrupt changes in formula composition and concentration, not to mention temperature, nipple type, flow rate, and caregiver's style, also play a part. An additional consideration is the restriction of oral feeding, which is standard prior to 32 weeks of gestation, because of immature coordination of the feeding/breathing mechanism. This orogustatory deprivation significantly alters the sensory environment. Feeding disorders also are common among neonates who have sustained brain damage. No studies have attempted to identify whether deficits in taste or smell are present in infants with feeding disorders. Certainly in adults, loss of the sense of smell radically affects eating habits.

Intrauterine Experience

The amniotic fluid is a complex solution of suspended particulate and dissolved odorants that changes in volume and chemical composition during pregnancy (29,86). The fluid is swallowed by the fetus, bathing taste and olfactory receptors. The fetus contributes to the chemical status through urination, oral mucosa, and lung secretions, and the mother contributes to the chemical status through hormones and perhaps even the types of food consumed. These chemical fluctuations coupled with the normal episodic closing of the mouth probably change the oral environment sufficiently to stimulate the receptor cells (29).

Experience in the Neonatal Intensive Care Unit

The environment in the NICU has not been described previously in terms of gustatory or olfactory content, but it clearly is not well adapted here. Stimulation of taste receptors in sick as well as extremely premature neonates is absent. Oral feeding is not initiated until the preterm infant has a reasonably coordinated suck/swallow reflex, usually not until 32 weeks of gestation. The chemical composition of the breast milk or formula that is offered is different from amniotic fluid or colostrum. The addition of oral medications, electrolyte supplements, as well as common changes in formula composition and concentration, introduce wide variability. Noxious-tasting medication and electrolytes repeatedly administered orally and temporally associated with feeding could lead to aversive conditioning. More research in this area would be clinically productive. Quite obviously, avoiding aversive experiences would likely benefit feeding behavior. Finally, in contrast to the healthy full-term neonate, preterm infants in the NICU lack a stable olfactory source that would be provided by sustained body contact of a consistent caretaker.

Intervention in the Neonatal Intensive Care Unit

Stimulation of the chemoreceptors has significant implications for enhancing care in the NICU. A period of familiarization with the odor of breast milk or formula, prior to the oral introduction of food, can facilitate acquisition of oral feeding skills (79). For a medically fragile infant, the mother's breast pad can be placed nearby. Small tastes of formula or breast milk before the introduction of the nipple may foster behavioral organization and facilitate the onset of feeding (86). Most babies who are restricted from oral feeds can safely tolerate a small drop of formula or breast milk on the tongue or lips. Finally, like breast milk from the source, bottle feeding ideally should be at body temperature rather than the typical room temperature.

From another standpoint, familiarization to the odor of medications before ingestion could make the medication less aversive by the process of habituation. Sucrose solution has been used to decrease the pain response to a heel-stick procedure or even to circumcision in healthy term infants (87,92). However, repeated use is unwarranted, potentially creating an aversive reaction to the induction of sucrose or even milk.

The limited research available suggests that gut priming in the extremely preterm or sick full-term infant probably should not bypass the mouth entirely. Finally, based on the animal model, surfactant and colostrum may have unsuspected roles in initiation of human feeding (81).

Auditory System

The auditory system is composed of both peripheral and central components (93–95). Sound waves are conducted through the auditory canal and physically displace the tympanic membrane. Movement of the membrane is amplified by the ossicles in the middle ear and transmitted to the oval window. This action displaces fluid in the cochlea. A mechanical disturbance differentially displaces hair cells at a specific place on the basilar membrane of the cochlea, as a function of both frequency and intensity of the sound. The hair cells are organized tonotopically, so that those that respond to high-frequency sounds are near the oval window and those that respond to low-frequency sounds are at the apex of the cochlea. The complex neural impulse thus generated proceeds to the auditory cortex via the cochlear nucleus, superior olivary nucleus, inferior colliculus, and medial geniculate body. The primary cortical reception area is the Herschl gyrus in the temporal region. Approximately 60% of the nerve fibers from each ear transmit to the contralateral hemisphere. The tonotopic organization is repeated in the cortical structures. The initial development of the central component of the auditory system is independent of peripheral maturation; however, once the auditory pathway is complete, the absence of auditory stimulation will cause cortical neuronal degeneration (95).

Development

Development of the auditory system begins around 3 to 6 weeks of gestation (95,96). Although the adult dimensions of the external auditory canal, tympanic membrane, and middle ear cavity will not be attained until 1 year after birth, all the major structures of the ear are essentially in place by 25 weeks of gestation. The ossicles have evolved from a thickening of mesenchymal tissue and are of adult proportions, although residual mesenchyme may diminish auditory thresholds. The cochlear nucleus has reached adult proportions and differentiated sufficiently to be functional by this time, although microscopically the cochlea still is not mature even at term. The hair cells are fully present and in a process of differentiation. The frequency-specific place on the basilar membrane is shifting systematically during this period of development (95). The afferent pathway from the cochlea to the auditory cortex is complete, and even myelination of the auditory pathway is present.

With regard to function, both cortical auditory evoked responses and brainstem auditory evoked responses can be elicited by 25 to 28 weeks (97,98). The morphology is different from the full-term infant's, and the latency is prolonged. A blink response to vibroacoustic stimulation has been obtained in human fetuses of 24 to 25 weeks of gestational age. A more complex behavioral response to sound occurs at least by 28 weeks, but readily fatigues. The maximum rate of electrophysiologic change occurs in the cortical auditory evoked response and brainstem auditory evoked response between 28 and 34 weeks of gestation. Orienting behavior to soft sound can be elicited by this time.

Maturation of the fetal auditory system is marked by an increase in spectral sensitivity, in both lower and higher frequencies, and a decrease in auditory threshold (93–95). The range of auditory sensitivity initially is fairly restricted: from 500 to 1,000 Hz in the third trimester compared to around 500 to 4,000 Hz at term and an adult range of 30 to 20,000 Hz. Changes in auditory threshold are related to maturation of both peripheral and central components. Auditory thresholds in a preterm infant at 25 weeks of gestation have been obtained with a 65-dB stimulus compared to 25 dB at term.

Evidence for a functional auditory system in the fetus is strong. Specific anatomic sites are present in the cortex that are responsible for processing complex sounds, such as language. A biological predisposition to respond to the specific acoustic patterns of speech is present in full-term neonates. For example, they have lower thresholds for sound within the most important range for speech perception (i.e., 500 to 3,000 Hz) (99). Within this frequency range, they respond differently to speech and nonspeech stimuli. There are even hemispheric differences in auditory evoked potentials that support this language sensitivity (100). Finally, healthy full-term neonates demonstrate a preference for sound they were exposed to *in utero*. Research has shown that 2- to 4-day-old neonates prefer their mother's voice compared to another female voice and a recording of a story read by their mother prenatally to a recording of a story read by their mother that was not read prenatally (101–105).

Deficits

Preterm infants are at increased risk for sensorineural hearing loss and developmental language disorders (20). Language disorders may be receptive or expressive dysfunctions. Receptive language disorders often are referred to as auditory processing deficits. These deficits include primarily phonemic-based disorders that involve discrimination between speech sounds, such as ba/ versus pa/, short-term memory deficits, and difficulty in interpreting the meaning of words implied by grammatical structure. Expressive language problems may include disorders of speech (as in articulation or fluency), word finding difficulty, and deficient or disordered sentence structure (grammar). Language disorders can result from direct damage to central structures as well as incidental to more general brain dysfunction. They occur in children with normal hearing thresholds and otherwise normal intelligence. They occur more commonly among children who were born preterm (106).

Intrauterine Experience

Development of the auditory system during fetal life occurs within a uterine environment that contains rhythmic, structured, and patterned sound emanating predominantly from the mother. Internal sounds include maternal respirations, borborygmi, placental and heart rhythms, and the like. Maternal speech transmits both externally and internally. Prosody (i.e., intonation, rhythm, stress) is probably the most salient aspect of speech available to the fetus. The intensity of internally recorded sound within the amniotic fluid is approximately 70 to 85 dB, with a predominance of low frequency (Fig. 8–1) (107). External sound also is transmitted to the fetus, but is attenuated by the time it reaches the intrauterine cavity, more so at higher frequencies (i.e., 70 dB at 4000 Hz) than lower frequencies (i.e., 20 dB at 50 Hz) (108). Given these considerations, the fetus probably is minimally exposed to frequencies above 1,000 dB (109). The available frequencies *in utero* also parallel cochlear development (102).

The auditory environment in the womb likely provides the most appropriate substrate for normal development of the sensory system, but defining the acoustic properties of the sound actually transmitted to the inner ear of the intrauterine fetus is problematic. The fluid-filled womb would alter the conductive property of the middle ear; data are unavailable. The best guess generally is that fetal hearing is limited to bone conduction. Hearing thresholds are elevated in the prematurely born infant, but no unequivocal data are available on the actual hearing thresholds of the fetus *in utero*.

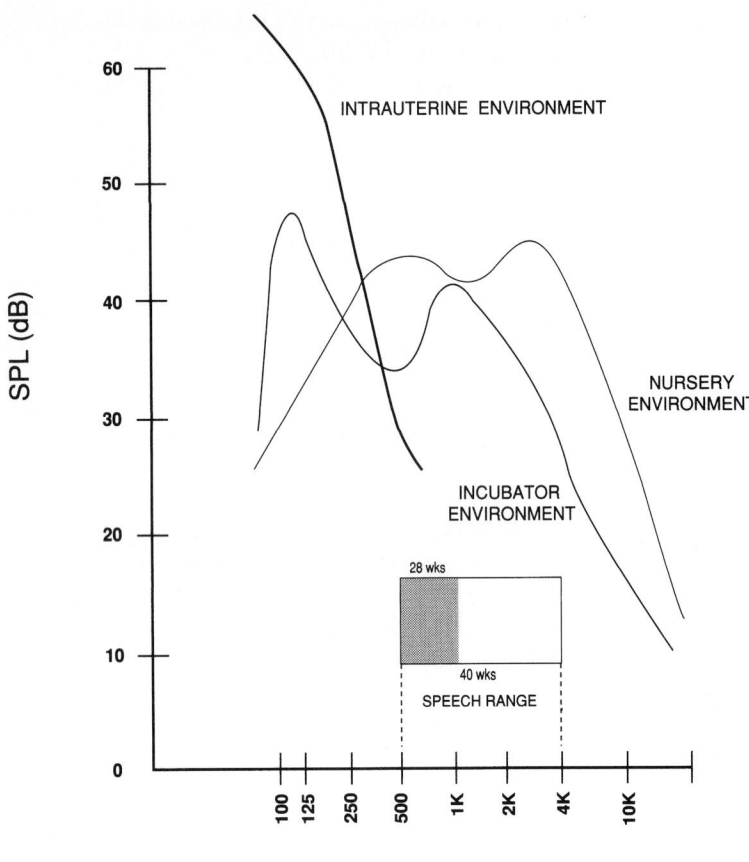

FIG. 8–1. Comparison of the frequency-specific auditory environment of the fetus *in utero* and the preterm infant in the neonatal intensive care unit. SPL, sound pressure level. (Data from ref. 109, with permission; and Otho Boone, *personal communication,* December 1992.)

After a normal full-term birth, the auditory environment is quiet by contrast. This may serve to increase the salience of the human voice. Early speech directed to the neonate is subdued and generally contingent on the infant's response.

Neonatal Intensive Care Unit Environment

The acoustic environment in the NICU differs from the intrauterine environment in peak intensity, spectral characteristics, and pattern (see Fig. 8–1). Ambient noise is generated by motors, fans, ventilator equipment, personnel, telephones, alarms, handwashing areas, trash lids, pagers, intercoms, and carts, to name a few. The intensity of background noise is around 50 to 60 dB and, therefore, not louder than *in utero,* although episodic bursts of higher intensity (i.e., less than 100 dB) occur. It would appear (see Fig. 8–1) that speech input for the neonate is selectively masked by the NICU auditory environment.

The auditory environment is different for babies nursed in open beds or in incubators. To some degree, the incubator may partially attenuate high-frequency room noise (see Fig. 8–1), but produces its own background noise level for the baby within (i.e., 50 to 70 dB). In addition, the infant in an incubator may be subjected to the closing of porthole doors, an object being placed on the top surface, or rapping on the incubator to stimulate an infant who is apneic or bradycardic, which may peak over 100 dB.

Effect of the Neonatal Intensive Care Unit Environment

Exposure to aberrant noise levels in the NICU may cause sensorineural damage, induce stress, and contribute to language or auditory processing disorders in the preterm neonate. Schulte et al. (20) reported nearly 12% hearing loss in a follow-up of preterm infants. Damage to the outer hair cells of the cochlea of neonatal guinea pigs has been reported after exposure to noise of similar intensities and frequencies found in the NICU (110). These researchers found no correlation between hearing loss and duration of exposure to incubator noise, but did report an association between hearing loss and a measure of severity of illness. Although not stated, more severely ill neonates may be exposed to increased NICU noise compared to healthy preterm infants. In other research, the combination of noise and ototoxic drugs commonly given to sick preterm infants (e.g., aminoglycosides, diuretics) was found to have a potentiating effect on hearing loss (111–113). The data further suggest that the immature cochlea may be more susceptible to damage than the mature one. Increased susceptibility is coincident with the final stages of anatomic development and differentiation of the cochlea (113). Given these data, incubator manufacturers have lessened the noise level emitted by the incubator motor, but limits on the environmental source of noise in the NICU itself are few.

In addition to possible sensory nerve damage, loud noise could have physiologic consequences in the newborn preterm infant in the form of stress, leading to alterations in corticosteroid levels and autonomic changes. Decreases in oxygen tension recorded by transcutaneous monitors as well as increases in intracranial pressure and in peripheral vasoconstriction are reported in preterm infants after exposure to sudden noise (114). Finally, sleep is disrupted by intermittent noise in the NICU.

The abnormal NICU auditory environment could contribute to language problems in preterm children. The normal auditory habituation pattern was impaired in chicks reared in a NICU-sound environment (115). Delayed cortical auditory evoked response among healthy preterm infants have been reported, as well as deficits in brainstem response when linguistic stimuli were used (106,116). The NICU environment, like the fetal environment, has an important role in the normal development of the auditory system.

Intervention in the Neonatal Intensive Care Unit

Auditory intervention in the NICU includes efforts both to reduce ambient noise and to induce patterned auditory input. Personnel in the NICU generally have made focused efforts to lower the level of noise in the environment. Quiet times during each shift are prevailing and radios are less constant. Evidence would suggest the value of caring for the smallest and sickest preterm infants inside an incubator, as a shield against environmental noise. The steady incubator noise may induce sleep in the preterm (117). At some point, however, the continuous white noise in the incubator masks more socially relevant auditory stimuli. Prolonged housing in this environment becomes disadvantagous at some point, but the timing is unknown.

Another approach to decreasing the level of ambient noise reaching the infant has been occluding the infant's ears. Zahr and de Traversay (118), using a within-subjects design, found increased quiet sleep and fewer state changes during the two observation periods. Caution here is warranted. Auditory input could be particularly critical for hearing-impaired infants. Preterm infants' auditory thresholds generally are not tested until near the time of discharge. Thus, if attenuation is practiced, the safer device would model that provided by the womb, where higher frequencies are selectively attenuated. Without a more selective approach, speech sounds also would be dampened. The strategy is therefore potentially harmful. On the other hand, short-term occlusion might be appropriate during a brief, acute phase of illness. Research is needed, with both short- and long-term consequences carefully evaluated, including speech stimuli and hearing thresholds as outcome measures.

Auditory stimulation, as a single modality, has been studied in the preterm infant. Schmidt et al. (117) reported that auditory stimulation, in the form of a heartbeat, lengthened the duration of the first quiet sleep period; quiet sleep is a more stabilized state that reflects central nervous system maturity. Some NICUs have urged using sound as a protective window for the infant—when music is played, the infant will not be disturbed. This approach responds to the potential for conditioning in the preterm infant. Soothing sound is soft, simple, repetitive, and harmonic, with a limited dynamic range. Nonetheless, speech and nonspeech stimuli differentially stimulate the cerebral hemispheres (100). Availability of speech sounds may be more critical. In one of the earliest studies, Katz (119) reported using auditory stimulation in the form of recorded maternal speech, played to healthy preterm infants of 28 to 32 weeks of gestation, until each reached 36 weeks PCA. Compared to controls, the intervention group showed better neuromotor development and improved auditory and visual responses. This study highlights once more that the effects of an intervention may not be limited to the stimulated sense. Even so, recorded speech still lacks the contingency associated with normal human speech.

Visual System

The visual system is the most extensively studied sensory system; therefore, the mechanisms are better understood. The eye is like a window to the brain, as it contains two-thirds of the afferent nerve fibers in the central nervous system. Light energy is transmitted through the cornea, pupil, lens, and optic media to the retina. There it bypasses the retinal blood vessels, a layer of ganglion cells, and a layer of bipolar cells, before it finally reaches the outer segments of the photoreceptors (i.e., rods and cones). Light is absorbed by the photoreceptors in a photochemical response that converts the radiant energy to an electrical impulse. The amount of light energy necessary to stimulate a single photoreceptor cell is extremely small—one quantum (120). In the absence of a light stimulus, retinal firing still occurs in the form of a tonic discharge. Some processing occurs even at the level of the retina (120). From the photoreceptors, the impulse travels to the ganglion cells, the optic nerve, and through the lateral geniculate nucleus to the occipital cortex. Fibers from the medial portion of each retina decussate, whereas those from the lateral one-half do not. Thus, information from either the left or right visual field will fall on the contralateral portion of each retina and be transmitted to the same hemisphere of the brain. Representation in the cortex is topographic, but upside down and reversed.

Development

The eye is an outgrowth of the brain from the early embryonic stage. By 24 weeks of gestation, gross anatomic structures are in place and the visual pathway is complete. As shown in Table 8–1, the visual system is undergoing extensive maturation and differentiation between 24 and 40 weeks of gestation. Corresponding functional visual responses have been elicited in the preterm infant (10,121–127).

As early as 24 to 28 weeks of gestation, a visual evoked response to bright light can be obtained, but it consists of a long-latency negative wave that readily fatigues. A behavioral response to bright light consists of lid tightening, but the response also fatigues quickly. The refractive error is about -5 diopters. The optic media is cloudy. Important functional changes occur between 30 to 34 weeks of gestation. The morphology of the visual evoked response becomes more complex, with the addition of a positive wave, and the latency decreases. The pupillary reflex is more efficient. A bright light will cause immediate lid closure, and the response sustains. The optic media has often cleared. The eyes may open spontaneously, and the infant may even briefly fixate. This has been described as the beginning of "attention" (121). Attention as such may be best elicited with a large, high-contrast form held closer to the eyes than would be necessary at term, and under conditions of low illumination (i.e., 5 foot-candles [ftc]). By 36 weeks, the visual evoked response resembles that of a full-term infant, but the latency is still longer for the preterm infant and remains so. Spontaneous eye opening, even *in utero*, has been observed on ultrasound. Although alertness still is less sustained than at term, the preterm infant now shows a spontaneous orientation toward a soft light and can track an object horizontally and vertically. Additionally, the infant prefers a pattern to a nonpatterned surface, in a manner similar to a full-term infant. The refractive error is near zero.

Relative to the other sensory systems, the visual system is the least mature by term birth, with considerable development continuing over the next 6 months (128). Having less dense optic media and less macular pigmentation than an adult, the eye of the newborn infant transmits more short-wavelength light than an adult by a factor of four (80). Newborns are photophobic; thus, visual attention is facilitated under low illumination (i.e., approximately 5 ftc). Acuity estimates are in the range of 20/200 Snellen equivalents. The refractive error is normally slightly hyperopic (i.e., +1 diopter).

The newborn can attend to form, object, and face. Specifically, he or she can fixate a high-contrast form (i.e., 1/16-inch wide line at a distance of 1 foot) as well as show preference for patterns along dimensions of brightness and complexity. She or he will track a bright object horizontally across midline and vertically. Attention to the human face by a neonate can been explained as a predisposition to respond to contrast (e.g., eyes, open mouth) or to edge (e.g., hairline), to slow movement (e.g., nodding), and to contingent stimulation (e.g., adult's voice). In any event, this behavior is powerfully adaptive.

Deficits

It generally is agreed that the visual system of the preterm infant is particularly susceptible to insult. The most well-known visual problem is retinopathy of prematurity (ROP), which is a proliferative vascular disease of multifactorial origin. ROP has been linked to oxygen toxicity, but it occurs in preterm infants with cyanotic heart disease who have never been hyperoxic. ROP is most

TABLE 8–1. *Maturation of the fetal eye in the third trimester*

Fetal eye components	26–28 weeks of gestation	30–32 weeks of gestation	34–36 weeks of gestation
Eyelid	Fused early in development, now reopens	Less translucent	
Pupil	Tunica vasculosa lentis begins to atrophy	Fully atrophied by end of period	Few remnants
	No reflex present	Sluggish reflex	Complete reflex
Lens	Second of four-layer nucleus forming	Second complete, third begins	
Media	Cloudy	Clears	
	Hyaloid system begins to regress	Hyaloid almost disappeared	Some remnants may still be present
Retina	Rod differentiation begins	Complete except for fovea, cone differentiation begins	Cone number in fovea increases
	Vascularization just beginning	Nasal portion nearly complete	Temporal region nearly fully vascularized
Visual cortex	Rapid dendritic growth and differentiation	Marked development of dendritic spines and synapses	Morphologically now similar to full term

strongly associated with degree of immaturity of the retina (129–132). Visual disorders other than ROP also commonly are associated with prematurity, including thicker lenses, poorer visual acuity, higher incidence of astigmatism, high myopia, strabismus, anisometropia, and color deficits (blue–yellow) (133–135). For example, among a sample of 5-year-old, low-birth-weight children, 35% lacked stereopsis and 25% had less than 20/20 corrected acuity in both eyes (134). Visual disorders occurred at a higher frequency (60%) among the children who weighed less than 1,500 g at birth.

In addition to these visual problems, the preterm infant also has difficulty processing visual information at a more cognitive level. Performance on tests of visual attention, visual pattern discrimination, visual recognition memory, and visuomotor integration repeatedly indicates particular vulnerability for the preterm infant (9,12,13,136,137).

Intrauterine Environment

The womb generally is dark, but under certain conditions light can transmit to the fetus. A behavioral response by a fetus to light has been described (138). Transmission through all the tissue is limited to small amounts of red, or long-wavelength, light. Probably only 2% of incident light reaches the uterus (D. Sliney, *personal communication,* June 1992). In later pregnancy, the head of the human fetus is in the vertex position, the neck is flexed, and the face is posterior, thereby diminishing exposure. It is unlikely that light exposure is a necessary condition for the fetus, or that periodic exposure to low levels of long-wavelength light is harmful. Aspects of the light–dark cycle that reach the fetus probably are mediated more by maternal sources such as rest–activity cycles and hormones than by light directly.

After birth, ambient light increases markedly, although typically the room is kept dim and cycled with dark to some extent. In dim light, the newborn is more likely to open his or her eyes. A prolonged wake period linked to catecholamine release occurs during this transition to extrauterine life.

Neonatal Intensive Care Unit Environment

Modern intensive care nurseries are brightly lit environments with ambient light in excess of standard office lighting for adults (Fig. 8–2). The general range reported has been 30 to 150 ftc, with peaks over 1,500 ftc from sunlight (139,140). The intensity of ambient illumination for any individual infant is determined by the location of the crib in a room, the number of overhead light units, the size, location, and compass direction of windows, the season of the year, and even the prevailing weather conditions (i.e., sunny vs. hazy). The duration of exposure generally is 24 hours a day over the length of hospital stay, which is a function of degree of immaturity and medical complications. Thus, light exposure is greater for those most vulnerable to visual problems.

In addition to ambient light, preterm infants routinely are exposed to supplementary sources, such as the bililight, the heat lamp, and the indirect ophthalmoscope. The standard double-bank phototherapy unit produces 300 to 400 ftc of illumination. The mini bili-lite has an intense beam, estimated at over 10,000 ftc. Infants' eyes are routinely patched under phototherapy; however, in some cases the eye pads are inadequate or may slip off. A commonly used heat lamp consists of one or two infrared bulbs that produce an intensity over 300 ftc at an infant's face. Exposure time varies, but typically is longer for younger and sicker infants. The eyes of infants typically are not covered while they are under the heat lamp.

Finally, an indirect ophthalmoscope is used for the routine eye examinations to rule out ROP. Exposure for 2 minutes, which is the approximate time of retinal examination, at maximum power has been estimated as equivalent to

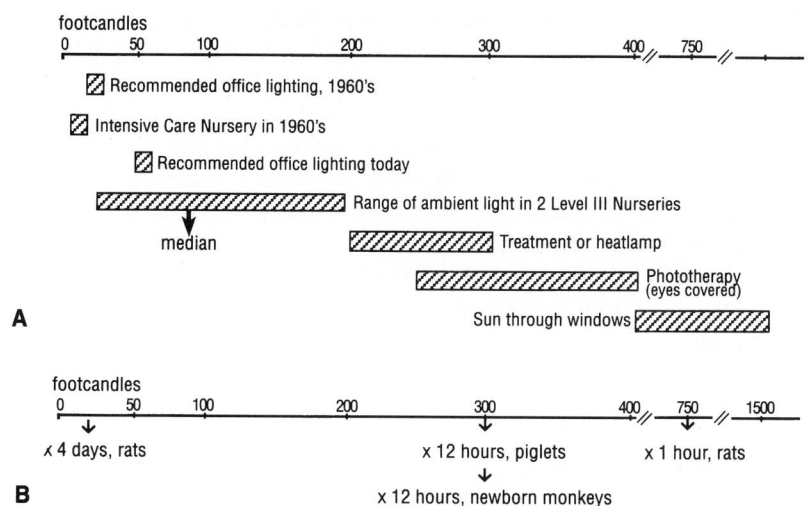

FIG. 8–2. A: Levels of light exposure in the intensive care nursery. **B:** Light exposure and retinal damage in animals. (From ref. 150.)

exposure at 2,000 ftc for 3 hours (141). Extra precautions for protecting the infant's dilated eyes from ambient or supplementary sources of light before and after the eye examination are not routine. For the smallest infants, the addition of a heat lamp during the examination often is necessary to maintain the baby's temperature.

Phototoxicity in Animals

Animals exposed to similar levels of light have sustained damage to their photoreceptors, pigment epithelium, and choroid (141,142). Phototoxicity is a consequence of a photochemical effect, but may be exacerbated by heat. The effectiveness of light in producing retinal damage is proportional to its efficiency in bleaching rhodopsin. A level of 100 ftc bleaches rhodopsin to 80% in approximately 10 minutes. Continuous illumination is more potent than cyclic, but intermittent exposure may be cumulative.

Factors that enhance photochemical damage to the animal retina strikingly parallel the perinatal course of the preterm infant (139). Retinal damage in animals is facilitated by maintenance of the animal in constant dark before light exposure, an increase in body temperature, conditions of hyperoxia, hypoxia, or ischemia, and retinal disease. Finally, light and oxygen may have a synergistic adverse effect on ROP (143). In spite of all these considerations, safety standards have not yet been determined.

Photobiological Effects of Light in the Neonatal Intensive Care Unit

Mounting data indicate that light has potent biological effects that are not considered routinely in standard NICU care. An association between light and ROP was first suggested by Terry (144) in 1946. Potential mechanisms to account for phototoxicity as one of the contributing factors in ROP have been proposed and are consistent with the oxygen toxicity hypotheses: damage to endothelial cells, alteration of normal retinal metabolism, disruption of the normal regenerative process of the retina, and generation of free radicals (139,143,145–148).

There is no evidence that light is a necessary condition for ROP or that maintaining a preterm infant in the dark will completely prevent it. Seiberth et al. (149) found no difference in incidence of ROP for preterm infants (birthweight less than 1,250 g) who had opaque eye patches day and night from birth to 35 weeks of gestation compared to an unpatched control group. The daytime ambient light levels were already low (30 to 40 lux), and the control group had cycled lighting at night.

Three converging lines of evidence lend empirical support to an association between light and ROP. In a prospective but nonrandomized study, preterm infants for whom the light levels were reduced for the duration of their hospital stay had a lower incidence of ROP compared to a similar group of preterm infants exposed to standard bright

levels of nursery light (150). The same effect was found in both NICUs studied. Similar findings were reported by Hommura et al. (151). Reynolds et al. (152) reported no difference in incidence of ROP for preterm infants who wore light-reducing goggles compared to infants who did not; however, the goggles were discontinued at 31 weeks of gestation. In a separate study, increased ROP was identified in the region of the retina more exposed to light—specifically, more in the regions around 3 o'clock and 9 o'clock compared to the superior and inferior regions (153). In addition, preterm infants with a higher degree of retinal pigment are less likely to develop ROP than infants with less retinal pigment (154,155). Retinal pigment is protective against phototoxicity.

Photobiological effects are not limited to the retina. Elevated room light or phototherapy may cause degradation of riboflavin and vitamin A, which are common components of total parenteral nutrition (156). Solutions containing these vitamins may be covered at the source, but tubing often is not shielded. Light in the visible spectrum penetrates the skin and thereby may alter more than the bilirubin concentration in the blood. Riboflavin levels were reduced *in vivo* in infants undergoing phototherapy (157). Thrombocytopenia (i.e., platelets less than $150,000/mm^3$) was more than tripled among preterm infants exposed to phototherapy light (158). *In vitro* experiments demonstrated inhibition in the normal constriction of immature lamb ductal rings exposed to ambient laboratory light (159). Subsequently, Rosenfeld et al. (160) found a significant reduction in the occurrence of patent ductus arteriosus among preterm infants whose chests were shielded from exposure to phototherapy light.

Light and Behavior

Bright light in an infant's face is a source of stress (161). Even routine ambient light level affects sleep and wake states in preterm infants. Lower ambient light is associated with significantly less active rapid eye movement sleep and significantly more quiet sleep among preterm infants at 35 to 36 weeks PCA (162). Rapid eye movement is a more destabilized state, with greater fluctuations of oxygen saturation and more frequent occurrence of apnea/bradycardia. Lower ambient light also is associated with increased eye opening and awake periods. Light level influences an infant's response to sound. Under bright light, an infant shows an aversive response to a tone, whereas under a dim light the same tone elicits an orienting response (163). Dimming the light has a quieting effect on caregivers, who are apt to behave as though someone were sleeping.

Intervention in the Neonatal Intensive Care Unit

The optimal level of NICU lighting has not been determined; however, no study supports the safety of current bright light levels. Therefore, tt would be prudent to limit ambient nursery light to necessary levels and shield the infant's eyes and chest from ambient as well as supplementary sources. Shading does not mean occluding. Evidence does not suggest that infants' eyes should be patched beyond what is necessary for phototherapy. Prolonged patching may be detrimental, both in terms of stimulus deprivation and possible effects on corneal growth.

Opportunities for spontaneous eye opening under dim (i.e., 5 ftc) or dark conditions should be provided. Visual attention is facilitated under these conditions. Animal studies suggest that dim–dark cycling may be beneficial for regeneration after retinal damage.

A day–night cycling regimen in the intermediate care nursery before hospital discharge affects behavior (164). Infants in the cycled nursery showed improved sleep patterns both in the hospital and after discharge, spent less time feeding, and gained more weight; however, light, noise, and handling all were reduced at night in the experimental unit. That does not negate the effect, but the necessity of entrainment of preterm infants to light–dark cycles is not supported. Rest–activity cycles may be more potent. Biological rhythms are much more complex (165,166).

The question then becomes whether to provide patterned stimulation. An infant's ability to respond to a level of stimulation does not necessarily mean that he or she should be stimulated at that level. For example, infants are more likely to respond to a louder sound, yet psychologists do not recommend higher-intensity noise just because the baby hears it better. Likewise, babies attend more to high-contrast black-and-white stimuli than to pastels, but that does not necessarily mean that the baby should be stimulated with the stronger visual pattern either. Prolonged or obligatory visual attention is not a preferred behavior. Given that the visual system is the least mature, the most parsimonious approach would be to provide stimulation of the other senses first. Then the most appropriate visual stimulus to begin with is probably the human face, which bears no resemblance to strong black-and-white patterns.

GENERAL PRINCIPLES

A central issue in developmental intervention is whether to conceptualize the preterm infant as an extrauterine fetus and therefore attempt to reproduce the intrauterine environment, or whether by dint of being born, the system now requires other forms of stimulation to foster the unique development of the preterm infant. To some extent this is a nonissue: abrupt change to extrauterine life in altricial species most always has been modulated by the mother. The aversive conditions found in the NICU would not be conducive to development for even the healthiest full-term infant. Further research is not

necessary to determine whether excess handling, noise, and bright light ought to be reduced. The NICU environment is a potential source of stress and overt damage to the preterm brain. Research is needed to establish safety limits, rather than to study whether or not aversive conditions do harm.

Sensory deprivation also can affect development. Research still is necessary to determine the optimal type, timing, duration, and level of stimuli; however, basic guiding principles for developmental intervention do exist:

Preterm infants are not a homogeneous group. Thus, determining the appropriate level of stimulation is based on an understanding of developmental neurophysiology and evaluation of an individual infant's medical status, neurologic maturation, physiologic stability, and social and physical needs.

Sensory development is not a simple unitary process. The hierarchical organization and integration of function among the sensory systems provides the conceptual framework for developmental intervention. Thus, intervention should begin with the most mature system, should support the normal maturational process, and should not attempt to accelerate development.

The model of optimal stimulation for early development lies in the sources naturally available to the fetus and infant (i.e., the mother). The optimal NICU model thus would begin with the intrauterine conditions, then parallel and extend the transition period that occurs immediately after a normal term birth.

A general algorithm therefore seems possible:

For any infant, provide protective care, minimal handling, undisturbed rest, dim, and quiet. Provide for stabilization of autonomic, state, and motor processes through positioning and containment. Model supportive touch.

Consider the role of olfaction and taste.

If the infant is medically stable, introduce graded tactile–vestibular and auditory input before visual input. Introduce stimulation at lower intensity first, and only if no major medical changes are occurring simultaneously. Avoid any attempt to "accelerate" development.

Monitor and modify the program.

Decreasing aversive conditions such as bright light, noise, and handling in the NICU, as well as enhancing comfort through touch, holding, positioning, and containment, benefit the infant and communicate directly to parents.

ACKNOWLEDGMENTS

I thank Cara Coffman, M.A., and Susan Lydick, M.A., for substantial contributions to this chapter by providing research, suggestions, and encouragement, and R.D. Walk, Ph.D., my mentor.

REFERENCES

1. Hack M, Breslau N, Weissman B, et al. Effect of very low birth weight and subnormal head size on cognitive abilities at school age. *N Engl J Med* 1991;325:231.
2. Hunt J, Cooper BA, Tooley WH. Very low birth weight infants at 8 and 11 years of age: role of neonatal illness and family status. *Pediatrics* 1988;82:596.
3. McCormick MC, Gortmaker SL, Sobol AM. Very low birth weight children: behavior problems and school difficulty in a national sample. *J Pediatr* 1990;117:687.
4. Klein N, Hack M, Gallaher J, et al. Preschool performance of children with normal intelligence who were very low birth weight infants. *Pediatrics* 1985;75:531.
5. Ross G, Lipper EG, Auld PAM. Educational status and school-related abilities of very low birth weight premature children. *Pediatrics* 1991; 88:1125.
6. Vohr BR, Garcia Coll CT. Neurodevelopmental and school performance of very low birthweight infants: a seven-year longitudinal study. *Pediatrics* 1985;76:345.
7. Volpe JJ. Cognitive deficits in premature infants. *N Engl J Med* 1991; 325:276.
8. Sostek AM. Prematurity as well as IVH influence development outcome at five years. In: Friedman S, Sigman M, eds. *The psychological development of low birth weight children.* New York: Academic Press, 1992:259.
9. Kopp C, Sigman M, Parmelee A, et al. Neurological organization and visual fixation in infants at 40 weeks conceptional age. *Dev Psychobiol* 1975;8:165.
10. Parmelee AH, Sigman M. Development of visual behavior and neurological organization in preterm and fullterm infants. In: *Minnesota symposium on child psychology,* vol. 10. Minnesota: University of Minnesota Press, 1976:119.
11. Sostek AM, Quinn PO, Davitt MX. Behavior, development and neurologic status of premature and full-term infants with varying medical complications. In: Field TM, Sostek A, Goldberg S, et al, eds. *Infants born at risk.* New York: Spectrum, 1979:281.
12. Caron A, Caron R. Processing of relational information as an index of infant risk. In: Friedman S, Sigman M, eds. *Preterm birth and psychological development.* New York: Academic Press, 1981:219.
13. Rose SA. Enhancing visual recognition memory in preterm infants. *Dev Psychol* 1980;16:85.
14. Garcia-Coll C. Behavioral responsivity in preterm infants. *Clin Perinatol* 1990;17:113.
15. Sigman M. Early development of preterm and fullterm infants: exploratory behavior in eight-month olds. *Child Dev* 1976;47:606.
16. Gunnar M, Hertsgaard L, Larson M, et al. Cortisol and behavioral responses to repeated stressors in the human newborn. *Dev Psychobiol* 1991;24:487.
17. Gunnar MR. Reactivity of the hypothalmic-pituitary-adrenocortical system to stressors in normal infants and children. *Pediatrics* 1992;90:491.
18. Gorski PA. Developmental intervention during neonatal hospitalization. *Pediatr Clin North Am* 1991;38:1469.
19. Weisel TN, Hubel DH. Single cell response in striate cortex of kittens deprived of vision in one eye. *J Neurophysiol* 1963;26:1003.
20. Schulte FJ, Stennert E, Wulbrand H, et al. The ontogeny of sensory perception in preterm infants. *Eur J Pediatr* 1977;126:211.
21. Dobbing J. Later development of the brain and its vulnerability. In: Davis JA, Dobbing J, eds. *Scientific foundations of paediatrics.* London: Heinemann, 1974:565.
22. Field T. Supplemental stimulation of preterm infants. *Early Hum Dev* 1980;4:301.
23. Cornell EH, Gottfried AW. Intervention with premature human infants. *Child Dev* 1976;47:32.
24. Lawson KR, Daum C, Turkewitz G. Environmental characteristics of the neonatal intensive care unit. *Child Dev* 1977;48:1633.
25. Gorski PA. Premature infant behavioral and physiological responses to caregiving interventions in the intensive care nursery. In: Call JD, Galenson E, Tyson RL, eds. *Frontiers of infant psychiatry.* New York: Basic Books, 1983:256.
26. Korones S. Iatrogenic problems in intensive care. In: Moore TD, ed. *Report of the sixty-ninth Ross conference on pediatric research.* Columbus, OH: Ross Laboratories, 1976:94.
27. Korner AF. Preventive intervention with high-risk newborns: theoretical, conceptual, and methodological perspectives. In: Osofsky JD, ed. *Handbook of infant development,* 2nd ed. New York: John Wiley and Sons, 1987:1006.
28. Avery GB, Glass P. The gentle nursery: developmental intervention in the NICU. *J Perinatol* 1989;9:204.
29. Bradley RM, Mistretta CM. Fetal sensory receptors. *Physiol Rev* 1975;55:352.
30. Gottlieb G. The psychobiological approach to developmental issues. In: Mussen PH, ed. *Handbook of child psychology,* vol. II, 2nd ed. New York: John Wiley and Sons, 1983:1.
31. Turkewitz G, Kenny PA. The role of developmental limitations of sensory input on sensory/perceptual organization. *J Dev Behav Pediatr* 1985;6:302.
32. Philbin MK. *Personal communication,* 1998.
33. Humphrey T. Correlation between appearance of human fetal reflexes and development of the nervous system. *Prog Brain Res* 1964;4:93.
34. Birnholtz JC, Farrell EE. Ultrasound images of human fetal development. *Am Sci* 1984;72:608.
35. Hooker D. *The prenatal origin of behavior.* New York: Hafner, 1969.
36. Fitzgerald M, Shaw A, MacIntosh N. Postnatal development of the cutaneous flexor reflex: comparative study of preterm infants and newborn rat pups. *Dev Med Child Neurol* 1988;30:520.
37. Harlow H, Harlow M. The effects of rearing conditions on behavior. *Bull Menninger Clin* 1962;26:213.
38. Thoman EB, Ingersoll EW, Acebo C. Premature infants seek rhythmic stimulation, and the experience facilitates neurobehavioral development. *J Dev Behav Pediatr* 1991;12:11.
39. Klaus MH, Kennell JH. *Maternal–infant bonding.* St. Louis: CV Mosby, 1976.
40. Tribotti SJ. Effects of gentle touch on the premature infant. In: Gunzenhauser N, ed. *Advances in touch:* new implications in human development. Skillman, NJ: Johnson & Johnson Consumer Products, 1990:80.
41. Eyler FD, Woods NS, Behnke M, et al. Changes over a decade: adult-infant interaction in the NICU, 1992 *(unpublished manuscript).*
42. Adam K, Oswald I. Sleep helps healing. *Br Med J* 1984;289:1400.
43. Sassin JF, Parker DC, Mace JW, et al. Human growth hormone release: relation to slow-wave sleep and sleep-waking cycles. *Science* 1969;165:513.
44. Long JG, Philip AGS, Lucey JF. Excessive handling as a cause of hypoxemia. *Pediatrics* 1980;65:203.
45. Murdoch DR, Darlow BA. Handling during neonatal intensive care. *Arch Dis Child* 1984;59:957.
46. Peabody JL, Lewis K. Consequences of newborn intensive care. In: Gottfried AW, Gaiter JL, eds. *Infant stress under intensive care:* environmental neonatology. Baltimore: University Park Press, 1985:201.
47. Perlman JM, Volpe JJ. Suctioning in the preterm infant: effects on cerebral blood flow velocity, intracranial pressure, and arterial blood pressure. *Pediatrics* 1983;72:329.
48. Speidel BD. Adverse effects of routine procedures on preterm infants. *Lancet* 1978;2:864.
49. Volpe JJ. Intraventricular hemorrhage and brain injury in the premature infant: diagnosis, prognosis, and prevention. *Clin Perinatol* 1989; 16:387.
50. Schanberg S, Field T. Maternal deprivation and supplemental stimulation. In: Field T, McCabe P, Schneiderman N, eds. *Stress and coping across development.* Hillsdale, NJ: Erlbaum, 1988:3.
51. Kuhn CM, Schanberg SM, Field T, et al. Tactile-kinesthetic stimulation effects on sympathetic and adrenocortical function in preterm infants. *J Pediatr* 1991;119:434.
52. Als H, Lawhon G, Brown E, et al. Individualized behavioral and environmental care for the very low birth weight preterm infant at high risk for bronchopulmonary dysplasia: neonatal intensive care unit and developmental outcome. *Pediatrics* 1986;78:1123.
53. Jay S. *The effects of gentle human touch on mechanically ventilated very short gestation infants.* Ph.D. Thesis, University of Pittsburgh, Pittsburgh, PA, 1982.
54. Field TM, Schanberg SM, Scafidi F, et al. Tactile/kinesthetic stimulation effects on preterm neonates. *Pediatrics* 1986;77:654.
55. Scafidi FA, Field TM, Schanberg SM, et al. Massage stimulates growth in preterm infants: a replication. *Infant Behav Dev* 1990;13:167.
56. Harrison LL, Leeper JD, Yoon M. Effects of early parent touch on preterm infants' heart rates and arterial oxygen saturation levels. *J Adv Nurs* 1990;15:877.

57. Hack M, Estabecek M, Robertson S. Development of sucking rhythm in preterm infants. *Early Hum Dev* 1985;11:133.

58. Birnholz J, Stephens J, Faria M. Fetal movement patterns: a possible means of defining neurologic developmental milestones in utero. *AJR* 1978;130:537.

59. Bernbaum JC, Pereira GR, Watkins JB, et al. Nonnutritive sucking during gavage feeding enhances growth and maturation in premature infants. *Pediatrics* 1983;71:41.

60. Field T, Ignatoff E, Stringer S, et al. Nonnutritive sucking during tube feedings: effects on preterm neonates in an intensive care unit. *Pediatrics* 1982;70:381.

61. Woodson R, Drinkwin J, Hamilton C. Effects of nonnutritive sucking on state and activity: term-preterm comparisons. *Infant Behav Dev* 1985;8:435.

62. Dixon S, Syder J, Holve R, et al. Behavioral effects of circumcision with and without anesthesia. *J Dev Behav Pediatr* 1984;5:246.

63. Field T, Goldson E. Pacifying effects of nonnutritive sucking on term and preterm neonates during heelstick procedures. *Pediatrics* 1984;74:1012.

64. Geldard FA. *The human senses.* New York: John Wiley and Sons, 1967.

65. Mason WA. Wanting and knowing: a biological perspective on maternal deprivation. In: Thoman EB, ed. Origins of infant's social response. Hillsdale, NJ: Erlbaum, 1979:225.

66. Neal MV. Vestibular stimulation and developmental behavior of the small premature infant. *Nurs Res Rep* 1968;3:1.

67. Korner AF. The use of waterbeds in the care of preterm infants. *J Perinatol* 1986;6:142.

68. Cordero L, Clark DL, Schott L. Effects of vestibular stimulation on sleep states in premature infants. *Am J Perinatol* 1986;3:319.

69. Kramer LI, Pierpont ME. Rocking waterbeds and auditory stimuli to enhance growth of preterm infants. *J Pediatr* 1976;88:297.

70. Pelletier JM, Short MA, Nelson DL. Immediate effects of waterbed flotation on approach and avoidance behaviors of premature infants. In: Ottenbacher KJ, Short-DeGraff MA, eds. *Vestibular processing dysfunction in children.* Binghamton, NY: Haworth Press, 1985:81.

71. Gatts J, Winchester S, Fisle K. The safety of part intrauterine analog transition environment: a literature review and discussion. *Neonat Intens Care* 1992;5:51.

72. Yu VYH. Effect of body position on gastric emptying in the neonate. *Arch Dis Child* 1975;50:500.

73. Henderson-Smart DJ, Read DJ. Depression of intercostal and abdominal muscle activity and vulnerability to asphyxia during active sleep in the newborn. In: Guilleminault C, Dement W, eds. *Sleep apnea syndromes.* New York: Alan R. Liss, 1978:93.

74. Martin RJ, Herrell N, Rubin D, et al. Effect of supine and prone positions on arterial oxygen tension in the preterm infant. *Pediatrics* 1979;63:528.

75. Wagaman MJ, Shutack JG, Moomijian AS, et al. The effects of different body positions on pulmonary function in neonates recovering from respiratory disease. *Pediatr Res* 1978;12:571(abst).

76. Grenier A. Prévention des déformations précoces de hanche chez les nouveau-nés à cerveau lésé: maladie de Little sans ciseaux? *Ann Pediatr (Paris)* 1988;35:423.

77. Anderson GC. Current knowledge about skin–skin (kangaroo) care for preterm infants. *Perinatology* 1991;11:216.

78. Mistretta CM, Bradley RM. Development of the sense of taste. In: Blass EM, ed. *Handbook of behavioral neurobiology, vol. 8:* developmental psychobiology and developmental neurobiology. New York: Plenum Press, 1986:205.

79. Porter RH, Balogh RD, Makin JW. Olfactory influences on mother–infant interaction. In: Rovee-Collier C, Lipsitt LP, eds. *Advances in infancy research.* Camden, NJ: LP Ablex Publication, 1988:39.

80. Werner JS, Lipsitt LP. The infancy of human sensory systems. In: Gollin ES, ed. *Developmental plasticity:* behavioral and biological aspects of variations in development. New York: Academic Press, 1981:35.

81. Smotherman WP, Robinson SR. Milk as the proximal mechanism for behavioral change in the newborn. *Acta Paediatr Suppl* 1994;397:64.

82. Steiner JE. Human facial expressions in response to taste and smell stimulation. *Adv Child Dev Behav* 1979;13:257.

83. Tatzer E, Schubert MT, Timischl W, et al. Discrimination of taste and preference for sweet in premature babies. *Early Hum Dev* 1985;12:23.

84. Zorc L. Unpublished doctoral dissertation.

85. Barr RG, Quek VS, Cousineau D, et al. Effects of intra-oral sucrose on crying, mouthing and hand-mouth contact in newborn and six-week-old infants. *Dev Med Child Neurol* 1994;36:608.

86. Smotherman WP, Robinson SR. Dimensions of fetal investigation. In: Smotherman WP, Robinson SR, eds. *Behavior of the fetus.* Caldwell, NJ: Telford, 1988:19.

87. Blass EM, Hoffmeyer LB. Sucrose as an analgesic for newborn infants. *Pediatrics* 1991;87:215.

88. Pedersen PE, Greer CA, Shepherd GM. Early development of olfactory function. In: Blass EM, ed. *Handbook of behavioral neurobiology. vol. 8:* developmental psychobiology and developmental neurobiology. New York: Plenum Press, 1986:163.

89. Rieser J, Yonas A, Wikner K. Radial localization of odors by human newborns. *Child Dev* 1976;47:856.

90. Macfarlane JA. Olfaction in the development of social preferences in the human neonate. In: *Parent–infant interaction:* Ciba Foundation Symposium 33. Amsterdam: Elsevier, 1975:103.

91. Sullivan RM, Taborsky-Barba S, Mendoza R, et al. Olfactory classical conditioning in neonates. *Pediatrics* 1991;87:511.

92. Blass EM, Shah A. Pain-reducing properties of sucrose in human newborns. *Chem Senses* 1995;20:29.

93. Aslin RN, Pisoni DB, Jusczyk PW. Auditory development and speech perception in infancy. In: Mussen PH, ed. *Handbook of child psychology*, vol. II, 2nd ed. New York: John Wiley and Sons, 1983:573.

94. Hecox K. Electrophysiological correlates of human auditory development. In: Cohen LB, Salapatek P, eds. *Infant perception:* from sensation to cognition. *Perception of space, speech, and sound,* vol. II. New York: Academic Press, 1975:151.

95. Rubel EW. Auditory system development. In: Gottlieb G, Krasnegor N, eds. *Measurement of audition and vision in the first year of postnatal life:* a methodological overview. Camden, NJ: Ablex Publishing, 1985:53.

96. Parmelee HP, Sigman MD. Perinatal brain development and behavior. In: Mussen PH, ed. *Handbook of child psychology*, vol. II, 2nd ed. New York: John Wiley and Sons, 1983:95.

97. Birnholz JC, Benacerraf BR. The development of human fetal hearing. *Science* 1983;222:516.

98. Querleu D, Renard X, Boutteville C, et al. Hearing by the human fetus? *Semin Perinatol* 1989;13:409.

99. Berg, KM, Smith M. Behavioral thresholds for tones during infancy. *J Exp Child Psychol* 1983;35:409.

100. Molfese D, Freeman R, Palermo D. Ontogeny of brain lateralization for speech and non-speech stimuli. *Brain Lang* 1975;2:356.

101. Fifer W, Moon C. Psychobiology of newborn auditory preferences. *Semin Perinatol* 1989;13:430.

102. Fifer WP, Moon C. Auditory experience in the fetus. In: Smotherman WP, Robinson SR, eds. *Behavior of the fetus.* Caldwell, NJ: Telford Press, 1988:175.

103. DeCasper AJ, Fifer WP. Of human bonding: newborns prefer their mothers' voices. *Science* 1980;208:1174.

104. DeCasper AJ, Spence MJ. Prenatal maternal speech influences on newborn's perception of speech sounds. *Infant Behav Dev* 1986;9:133.

105. Spence M, DeCasper A. Newborns prefer a familiar story over an unfamiliar one. *Infant Behav Dev* 1987;10:133.

106. Kurtzberg D, Stapells DR, Wallace IF. Event-related potential assessment of auditory system integrity: implications for language development. In: Vietze PM, Vaughan HG, eds. *Early identification of infants with developmental disabilities.* Philadelphia: Grune & Stratton, 1988:160.

107. Gerherdt K. Characteristics of the fetal sheep sound environment. *Semin Perinatol* 1989;13:362.

108. Armitage SE, Baldwin BA, Vince MA. The fetal sound of sheep. *Science* 1980;208:1174.

109. Walker D, Grimwade J, Wood C. Intrauterine noise: a component of the fetal environment. *Am J Obstet Gynecol* 1970;109:91.

110. Douek E, Dodson HC, Bannister LH, et al. Effects of incubator noise on the cochlea of the newborn. *Lancet* 1976;2:1110.

111. Falk SA. Combined effects of noise and ototoxic drug. *Environ Health Perspect* 1972;2:5.

112. Walton JP, Hendricks-Munoz K. Profile and stability of sensorineural hearing loss in persistent pulmonary hypertension of the newborn. *J Speech Hear Res* 1991;34:1362.

113. Carlier E, Pujol R. Supra-normal sensitivity to ototoxic antibiotic of the developing rat cochlea. *Arch Otorhinolaryngol* 1980;226:129.

114. Long JG, Lucey JF, Philip AGS. Noise and hypoxemia in the intensive care nursery. *Pediatrics* 1980;65:143.

115. Philbin MK, Ballweg DD, Gray L. The effect of an intensive care unit sound environment on the development of habituation in healthy avian neonates. *Dev Psychobiol* 1994;27:11.

116. Salamy A, Mendelson T, Tooley WH, et al. Differential development of brainstem potentials in healthy and high-risk infants. *Science* 1980;210:553.

117. Schmidt K, Rose SA, Bridger WH. Effect of heartbeat sound on the cardiac and behavioral responsiveness to tactual stimulation in sleeping preterm infants. *Dev Psychol* 1980;16:175.

118. Zahr LK, de Traversay J. Premature infant responses to noise reduction by earmuffs: effects on behavioral and physiologic measures. *J Perinatol* 1995;15:448.

119. Katz V. Auditory stimulation and developmental behavior of the premature infant. *Nurs Res* 1971;20:196.

120. Gregory RL. *Eye and brain:* the psychology of seeing, 4th ed. Princeton: Princeton University Press, 1990.

121. Hack M, Mostow A, Miranda S. Development of attention in preterm infants. *Pediatrics* 1976;58:669.

122. Dreyfus-Brisac C. Neurophysiological studies in human premature and fullterm newborns. *Biol Psychiatry* 1975;10:485.

123. Mann I. *Development of the human eye.* New York: Grune & Stratton, 1964.

124. Purpura DP. Morphogenesis of visual cortex in the preterm infant. In: Brazier MAB, ed. *Growth and development of the brain: nutritional, genetic, and environmental factors. International Brain Research Organization Monograph Series.* New York: Raven Press, 1975:1.

125. Dubowitz LM, Dubowitz V, Morante A, et al. Visual function in the preterm and fullterm newborn infant. *Dev Med Child Neurol* 1980;22:465.

126. Miranda SB. Visual abilities and pattern preferences of premature infants and full-term neonates. *J Exp Child Psychol* 1970;10:189.

127. Senecal J, Defawe G, Roussey M, et al. Le comportement visuel du premature. *Arch Fr Pediatr* 1979;36:454.

128. Abramov I, Gordon J, Hendrickson A, et al. Light and the developing visual system. In: Marshall J, ed. *Vision and visual dysfunction.* Boca Raton, FL: CRC Press, 1991.

129. James L, Lanman J. History of oxygen therapy and retrolental fibroplasia. *Pediatrics* 1976;57:590.

130. Lucey J, Dangman B. A reexamination of the role of oxygen in retrolental fibroplasia. *Pediatrics* 1984;73:82.

131. Johns KJ, Johns JA, Feman SS, et al. Reinopathy of prematurity in infants with cyanotic congenital heart disease. *Am J Dis Child* 1991;145:200.

132. Inder TE, Clemett, RS, Austin NC, et al. High iron status in very low birth weight infants is associated with an increased risk of retinopathy of prematurity. *J Pediatr* 1997;131:541.

133. Fledelius T. Prematurity and the eye. *Acta Ophthalmol* 1976;128:3.

134. Hoyt C. Long-term visual effects of short-term binocular occlusion of at-risk neonates. *Arch Ophthalmol* 1980;98:1967.

135. Dobson V, Quinn GE, Abramov I, et al. Color vision measured with pseudoisochromatic plates at five-and-a-half-years in eyes of children from the CRYO-ROP study. *Invest Ophthalmol Vis Sci* 1996;37:2467.

136. Sigman M, Parmelee A. Visual preferences of four month old premature and fulltern infants. *Child Dev* 1974;45:959.

137. Siegel L. The prediction of possible learning disabilities in preterm and fullterm children. In: Field T, Sostek A, eds. *Infants born at risk: physiological, perceptual, and cognitive processes.* New York: Grune & Stratton, 1983:295.

138. Brazelton TB, Field TM. Introduction. In: Gunzenhauser N, ed. *Advances in touch: new implications in human development.* Skillman, NJ: Johnson & Johnson Consumer Products, 1990:xiii.

139. Glass P. Light and the developing retina. *Doc Ophthalmol* 1990;74:195.

140. Landry RJ, Scheidt PC, Hammond RW. Ambient light and phototherapy conditions of eight neonatal care units: a summary report. *Pediatrics* 1985;75:434.

141. Lanum J. The damaging effects of light on the retina: empirical findings, theoretical and practical implications. *Surv Ophthalmol* 1978;22:221.

142. Williams TP, Baker BN, eds. *The effects of constant light on visual processes.* New York: Plenum Press, 1980.

143. Ham WT, Mueller HA, Ruffolo JJ. Mechanisms underlying the production of photochemical lesions in the mammalian retina. *Curr Eye Res* 1984;3:165.

144. Terry L. Retrolental fibroplasia. *J Pediatr* 1946;29:770.

145. Dorey CK, Delori FC, Akeo K. Growth of cultured RPE and endothelial cells is inhibited by blue light but not green or red light. *Curr Eye Res* 1990;9:549.

146. Riley PA, Slater TF. Pathogenesis of retrolental fibroplasia. *Lancet* 1969;2:265.

147. Stefansson E, Wolbarsht ML, Landers MB. In vivo O₂ consumption in rhesus monkeys in light and dark. *Exp Eye Res* 1983;37:251.

148. Zuckerman R, Weiter JJ. Oxygen transport in the bullfrog retina. *Exp Eye Res* 1980;30:117.

149. Seiberth V, Linderkamp O, Knorz MC, et al. A controlled clinical trial of light and retinopathy of prematurity. *Am J Ophthalmol* 1994;118:492.

150. Glass P, Avery GB, Subramanian KN, et al. Effect of bright light in the hospital nursery on the incidence of retinopathy of prematurity. *N Engl J Med* 1985;313:401.

151. Hommura S, Usuki Y, Takei K, et al. Ophthalmic care of very low birthweight infants, report 4: clinical studies of the influence of light on the incidence of ROP. *Nippon Ganka Gakkai Zasshi* 1988;92:456.

152. Reynolds JD, Hardy RJ, Kennedy KA, et al. Lack of efficacy of light reduction in preventing retinopathy of prematurity. *N Engl J Med* 1998;338:1572.

153. Fielder AR, Robinson J, Shaw DE, et al. Light and retinopathy of prematurity: does retinal location offer a clue? *Pediatrics* 1992;89:648.

154. Monos T, Rosen SD, Karplus M, et al. Fundus pigmentation in retinopathy of prematurity. *Pediatrics* 1996;97:343.

155. Schaffer D, Palmer E, Plotsky D, et al, on behalf of the CRYO-ROP Cooperative Group. Prognostic factors in the natural course of retinopathy of prematurity. *Ophthalmology* 1993;100:230.

156. Bhatia J, Mims L, Roesel R. The effect of phototherapy on amino acid solutions containing multivitamins. *J Pediatr* 1980;96:284.

157. Sisson T. Advances in phototherapy of neonatal hyperbilirubinemia. In: Helene C, Charlier M, Montenay-Garestier T, et al, eds. *Trends in photobiology.* New York: Plenum Press, 1982:339.

158. Maurer H, Fratkin M, McWilliams N, et al. Effects of phototherapy on platelet counts in lowbirthweight infants and on platelet production and life span in rabbits. *Pediatrics* 1976;57:506.

159. Clyman RI, Rudolph AM. Patent ductus arteriosus: a new light on an old problem. *Pediatr Res* 1978:12:92.

160. Rosenfeld W, Sadhev S, Brunot V, et al. Phototherapy effect on the incidence of patent ductus arteriosus in premature infants: prevention with chest shielding. *Pediatrics* 1986;78:10.

161. Shogan MG, Schumann LL. The effect of environmental lighting on the oxygen saturation of preterm infants in the NICU. *Neonat Netw* 1993;12:7.

162. Glass P, Sostek A. Sleep organization in preterm infants: the effect of nursery illumination. Presented at the International Conference of Infancy Studies, New York, New York, April 21, 1984 (poster session).

163. Haith MM. *Rules that babies look by.* Hillsdale, NJ: Erlbaum, 1980.

164. Mann NP, Haddow R, Stokes L, et al. Effect of night and day on preterm infants in a newborn nursery: randomised trial. *Br Med J* 1986;293:1265.

165. Glotzbach SF, Rowlett EA, Edgar DM, et al. Light in the newborn nursery: chronobiologic issues. *Sleep Res* 1991;20:457.

166. Mirmiran M, Kok JH. Circadian rhythms in early human development. *Early Hum Dev* 1991;26:121.

PART TWO

The Fetal Patient

CHAPTER 9

Prenatal Diagnosis in the Molecular Age

Nelson B. Isada, Laura S. Martin, and Mark I. Evans

The modern era of molecular and biochemical genetics commenced with the observations of Sir Archibald Garrod (1) at the turn of the twentieth century. He proposed that four diseases, namely, alkaptonuria, albinism, cystinuria, and pentosuria, resulted from inherited disorders of chemical metabolism. He also suggested that these disorders, which he called "inborn errors of metabolism," represented only a small fraction of every human's "chemical individuality" that had gone awry (1).

Advances in biochemistry have confirmed Garrod's concepts by characterizing the structural protein abnormality or enzymatic defect of many disorders. Other advances in molecular genetics have allowed precise identification of the defect in the deoxyribonucleic acid (DNA) message, sometimes before the protein defect itself is known (2). This knowledge has direct and immediate applications in the field of prenatal diagnosis (3).

This chapter will discuss gene organization, mutations and polymorphism analysis, molecular diagnostic techniques, DNA cloning, an approach to disorders diagnosable by molecular genetics, biochemical disorders not amenable to DNA technology or better studied by protein chemistry techniques, and carrier screening.

GENE ORGANIZATION

The Watson–Crick double-helix model of DNA organization is well known (4). DNA conveys information

encoded by a series of four nucleotides: adenine (A), thymine (T), cytosine (C), and guanine (G), connected sequentially on two strands. The two strands are complementary to each other, with nucleotide base pairs (bp) being formed by hydrogen bonding between adenine–thymine and guanine–cytosine. Eukaryotic DNA is located in the nucleus and organized into structures called chromosomes. During interphase, chromosomes are not visible by light microscopy. They become visible only when the genetic content has doubled, and the chromosomes have condensed before mitosis. Chromosomal material is organized into euchromatin and heterochromatin. The former is vigorously transcribed into ribonucleic acid (RNA). Heterochromatin is relatively inactive. An example of heterochromatin is the inactivated X chromosome.

An unexpected discovery made in the 1970s was that some regions of the eukaryotic chromosome do not code for any known protein (5). Specifically, these noncoding regions (i.e., introns), were noted to be interspersed within coding regions (i.e., exons) (Fig. 9–1) (6,7). Exons carry information to direct the assembly of amino acids into a protein, whereas introns do not. Messenger RNA (mRNA) acts as an intermediate molecule to convey information encoded by the DNA by a process called translation. Posttranslational modification of mRNA takes place such that introns are removed. After additional biochemical modifications, the mRNA passes out of the nucleus into the cytoplasm, where protein-synthesizing organelles are located.

About 60% of the human genome comprises regions of unique nucleotide sequences that presumably code for proteins (8). It is estimated that there are 50,000 to 100,000 expressed genes and proteins active in humans; however, expressed genes make up less than 10% of total genomic DNA. A significant portion of the human genome, perhaps about 40%, contains repetitive DNA sequences (9). Various terms are used for the different

N. B. Isada: Alaska Perinatology Associates, Anchorage, Alaska; and Divisions of Reproductive Genetics and Maternal-Fetal Medicine, Department of Obstetrics and Gynecology, Wayne State University, Hutzel Hospital, Detroit, Michigan

L. S. Martin: Department of Pediatrics, Madigan Army Medical Center, Tacoma, Washington

M. I. Evans: Division of Reproductive Genetics; Center for Fetal Diagnosis and Therapy; and Human Genetics Program, Hutzel Hospital/Wayne State University, Detroit, Michigan

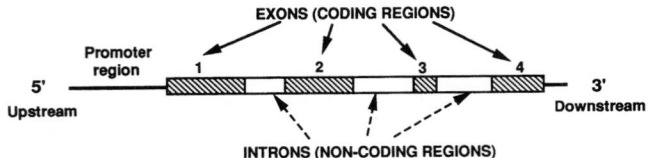

FIG. 9–1. An idealized representation of mammalian gene structure shows the promotor region, exons, and introns.

classes of repetitive DNA sequences found in humans. Highly repetitive sequences are found in the chromosome region adjacent to centromere. These are simple sequences repeated thousands of times, present in more than 10^4 copies and comprising about 20% of the genome. These repeating simple sequences have compositions unlike most of the organism's DNA, are several hundred bp long, and are separated easily by centrifuging slightly fragmented DNA through a cesium chloride density gradient. DNA separated by this process is called satellite DNA, because the centrifuged DNA forms a main band and several satellite bands above and below the main band. In humans, four satellite bands comprise about 6% of the total DNA, with each band representing tandem repeat sequences. Blocks of satellite DNA are readily localized to regions around the centromeres of metaphase chromosomes by *in situ* hybridization. Satellite DNA should not be confused with satellites, a cytogenetic term referring to the segment of an acrocentric chromosome distal to short arm, separated by a constriction. Other classes of repetitive DNA, which may overlap, are moderately repetitive DNA, which are gene sized in length, repeated about 10 to 1,000 times, and comprise about 20% of genome (i.e., one-half of the 40% that is repetitive DNA); a variable number of tandem repeat sequences, which are stretches of DNA in which a short nucleotide sequence is tandemly repeated 20 to 100 times, the exact number varying from person to person; alphoid DNA, which are chromosome-specific, repeated monomeric 170-bp units located in centromeric regions; and *Alu* sequences, which are highly repetitive sequences not clustered around centromeres, but instead more evenly distributed throughout the genome and interspersed within longer stretches of unique or moderately repetitive DNA. In humans, most such 300-bp sequences belong to a single group called the *Alu* family. Most contain a single cleavage site near the middle for the restriction enzyme *Alu* I, derived from the bacterium *Arthrobacter luteus* (see Restriction Fragment Length Polymorphism Analysis, below). Almost one million *Alu* sequences are present in the human genome, accounting for 3% to 6% of the total DNA. Each individual human has a unique amount of repetitive DNA. This genetic fingerprint has been used for paternity testing and forensic analysis.

A discovery involving repeat sequences has demonstrated an association between triplet repeat mutations and human disease. In this situation, a sequence of three repeated nucleotides has been found in normal individuals; when these sequences are found to be significantly increased, there is a marked tendency toward clinical morbidity. This was first described in the fragile X syndrome, a common form of heritable male mental retardation, where a polymorphic sequence of -CGG- repeats on the X chromosome is increased from a mean of 29 repeats to more than 200 repeats in affected males. Triplet expansion of -GCT- has been found in association with congenital myotonic dystrophy; triplet expansion of -CAG- has been found in spinal–bulbar muscular atrophy (i.e., Cannaday disease), spinocerebellar ataxia, and Huntington disease (10–12).

Regulation of gene expression occurs at many levels. Substrate concentrations have been shown both to enhance and repress specific enzymes, especially in bacteria. In eukaryotes and prokaryotes, a region separate from a given gene but still involved in regulation of expression is called a promoter, which binds RNA polymerase and initiates transcription (see Fig. 9–1). Similar functional areas have been found that bind a large group of transcription factors. In eukaryotes, such an area or box contains a common or consensus nucleotide sequence, CAAT, and is called a CAAT box. A conserved area associated with RNA polymerase positioning contains repeated sequences of the nucleotides thymine and adenine, and is called a TATA box.

Extranuclear DNA found in mitochondria (mtDNA) is inherited independently of nuclear DNA, is 16.5 kb in length, contains no introns, and is organized as a double-stranded circle. mtDNA is subject to a relatively high rate of mutation compared to nuclear DNA and is inherited maternally, the paternal spermatic mitochondria being excluded from the oocyte at the time of fertilization. A variety of neonatal and pediatric disorders, predominantly neuromuscular, have been associated with mtDNA deletions. The high rate of mutation and maternal inheritance of mtDNA have enhanced the studies of potential human origins and migration (13–15).

MUTATIONS AND POLYMORPHISMS

Many types of mutations can affect a gene. The DNA within a gene contains information for the final sequence of a protein and signals for the correct expression and processing of mRNA. If the actual coding region is altered, then the resultant protein may be changed. These alterations can be in the form of deletions that may be many kilobases or as small as a single base, inversions or translocations that produce no net nucleotide changes but potential or actual protein changes, or single-base changes. Even a change at the junction of a coding and noncoding region can result in abnormal mRNA formation. Defects in the promoter region may result in too little or too much expression of mRNA, which will be reflected in abnormal protein synthesis. A deletion of all or part of the gene will result almost always in the disruption of normal gene expression. Two examples of molecular pathology can be seen in Tay–Sachs disease and Gaucher disease in the Ashkenazi Jewish population (16,17). In the severe infantile type of Tay–Sachs disease, a mutation at an exon–intron splice site in the alpha-subunit has been identified (i.e., G to C transversion); another mutation is a four-base insertion in exon 11 of the alpha-subunit causing a frameshift mutation and marked reduction in mRNA (18,19). Another example is the identification of the mutation most commonly found in cystic fibrosis (CF) in people of northern European ancestry. There is a phenylalanine deletion in the CF transmembrane regulator (CFTR) protein at a critical adenosine triphosphate binding site, arising from a deletion of three amino acids, two of which code for phenylalanine. This is called the ΔF508 mutation and accounts for approximately 70% of CF mutations in people of northern European ancestry, with the remaining 30% being a heterogeneous assortment of other mutations (20–22). Commercial testing is available for 70 of the more than 500 known mutations at this site and can detect 90% of mutations in the northern European populations (23). However, other ethnic groups carry their own particular repertoire of mutations, such as Jews of different ethnic or geographic origins (24).

Mutations are possible for practically all loci. Genes not found associated with mutations *in vivo* include those whose products are so vital that any change would probably result in lethality early in development (i.e., housekeeping genes). Possible examples of this type include enzymes coded by nuclear or possibly mtDNA that catalyze critical steps in aerobic metabolism. Genes not associated with clinical mutation include those whose protein products are coded by repetitive DNA, whereby the remaining DNA can compensate. For example, ribosomal RNA (rRNA) genes are so abundant that the deletion that occurs when acrocentric chromosomes fuse, as in a robertsonian translocation, has no phenotypic effect. Other mutations unassociated with clinical disease can occur in noncoding areas such as introns, or in other unexpressed areas of the genome such as pseudogenes, which are duplicated sequences similar to normally expressed genes, but contain no introns.

A variety of approaches have been used to detect mutations. Optimally, determination of DNA structure and sequence, followed by elucidation of gene structure and organization in the normal allele, are completed before beginning a search for specific defects. Only about 5% to 10% of clinically significant mutations, however, are due to gross alterations in gene structure detectable by Southern blot analysis of genomic DNA, leaving unknown the remaining 90%. The problem is compounded by normal variation in the nucleotide sequence (i.e., polymorphisms). Thus, when variations from the normal sequence are found, additional analysis is required before these changes can be construed as being a disease-causing mutation.

Linkage Analysis

Linkage analysis is a very powerful technique that can be used to follow genetic disorders throughout a family and to localize specific genes by closer mapping of linked markers to a putative disease gene (25). Linkage analysis can be used for genetic diagnosis when the precise nucleotide mutations are not known. As mentioned previously, there is a variety of genetic differences among individuals for a given trait, called polymorphisms, spread throughout the entire human genome. The functions of these polymorphisms are not always known. Many are associated with bacterial endonuclease cleavage sites, described later. Linkage analysis has proven and continues to be an extremely powerful tool in mapping the human genome (26–30).

A standard principle of classic mendelian inheritance states that inherited traits sort independently. This is not always the case, however; some traits or characteristics associate more frequently than can be accounted for by chance. With the discovery of chromosomes, the idea arose that multiple traits could be carried on one chromosome. This implied that the closer together two genetic traits were on a chromosome, the more likely they would be to segregate together during meiosis and the less likely crossing over would occur between them. When genes are in such close proximity that crossing over rarely occurs, such as for hemophilia A and color blindness, the two sites are said to be linked (31). Any polymorphism that is found to be linked with the trait of interest is termed informative. Unfortunately, family studies are not always informative, because molecular or clinical polymorphisms are not always present.

The degree of linkage can be described mathematically by a number called the logarithm of the odds (LOD) score, developed in 1955 by Morton (32). The LOD can be thought of as the likelihood that two given traits are linked. It can be derived from recombinations observed between clinical or biochemical traits from pedigree analysis, or from molecular polymorphisms (33). The probability of recombination during meiosis between two loci is quantified by a term called the recombination fraction (i.e., theta or q), the maximum being 0.5. The LOD score is derived from various values of q. Viewed simplistically, the higher the LOD score, the higher the likelihood of linkage. Because this number is used on a logarithmic scale, each integer increase reflects a tenfold increase in likelihood of linkage. A LOD score of 4 suggests that there is linkage between two polymorphisms, the odds of random association being 10,000 to 1. A LOD score of zero suggests there is no linkage and that the two traits are on different chromosomes or are far apart on the same chromosome. Tight linkage indicates little or no recombination and suggests an actual physical proximity of two polymorphisms, measured in physical map distances, with the common unit of genetic distance reported as centimorgans. Linkage disequilibrium describes closely linked genes that occur more frequently than would be expected from random distribution, suggesting nonrandom or nonequilibrium mating, or some survival advantage from natural selection. Examples of linkage disequilibrium include the carrier states for sickle-cell disease and thalassemia, where those affected have increased resistance to certain types of malarial infections.

Restriction Fragment Length Polymorphism Analysis

Bacteria possess enzymes that recognize and cleave DNA at specific sites. Presumably, these enzymes evolved as a defense against hostile invading DNA, as might occur with bacteriophages. Because these cleavage sites are quite specific, that is, are restricted to specific palindromic sequences four to ten nucleotides in length, these enzymes are called restriction endonucleases. When these enzymes are added to eukaryotic DNA, the resultant mixture contains a variety of DNA fragments of different sizes, which can be separated by gel electrophoresis and transferred for analysis by Southern blotting. Each enzyme cuts an individual's DNA according to the positions of the cleavage sites, with every person having his or her own unique pattern of cleaved DNA fragments. Thus, people are polymorphic for the resulting lengths of DNA fragments, which vary between which of the different restrictor enzymes are used and the distribution of cleavage sites. Many of these recognition site polymorphisms are neutral and represent normal inherited variability. These characteristics have given rise to the term restriction fragment length polymorphisms (RFLPs), which refer to the polymorphic patterns observed in specific nucleotide sequences that are cleaved by bacterial restriction enzymes (Fig. 9–2). The resultant mixture of DNA fragments can be separated and further characterized by gel electrophoresis, Southern blotting, and oligonucleotide probes (34).

DNA alterations that affect an RFLP site either by creating a new site for endonuclease cleavage or eliminating a previously existing one can be detected on Southern blot as a result of changes in the size of the DNA fragment associated with this site (35). If, by chance, either a mutation or normal sequence corresponds to an RFLP site, this situation can be exploited for allele identification using linkage analysis. An initial use of such mapping involved the Huntington disease locus, as yet undefined (36). Another early application was for prenatal identification of the sickle-cell mutation in the beta chain of hemoglobin (37–40). For example, the restriction enzyme *Dde* I,

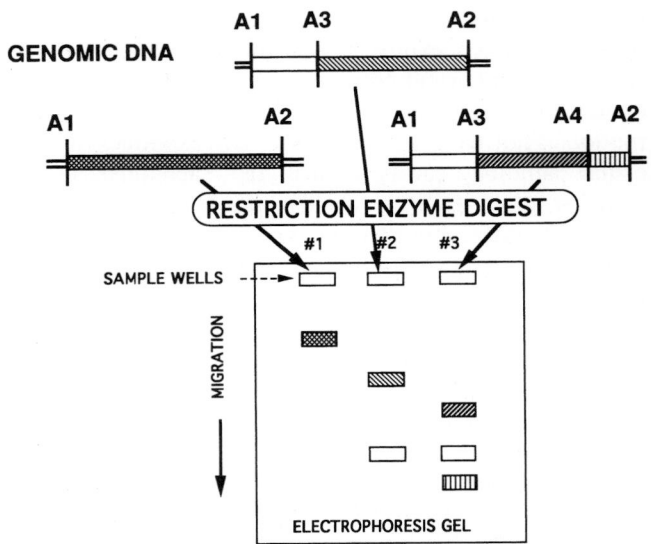

FIG. 9–2. Restriction fragment length polymorphisms. Lane 1, A1 and A2 present; lane 2, A1–A3 present; lane 3, A1–A4 present; A1–A5, hypothetical polymorphisms.

derived from the bacterium *Desulfovibrio desulfuricans*, recognizes the nucleotide sequence -CTNAG- (where N indicates that any nucleotide may occupy that position) that occurs within the hemoglobin A (-CTGAG-) and hemoglobin C (-CTAAG-) gene, but not within hemoglobin S (-CTG*T*G-). In hemoglobin S, the nucleotide thymine is substituted for adenine, which is not recognized and thus not cleaved by *Dde* I. This results in a much larger RFLP fragment that can be recognized on Southern blot. Initially, this technology used unamplified DNA and Southern blot transfer. Target gene sequences can now be preamplified a millionfold by polymerase chain reaction (PCR) (see later) and cut by restriction endonucleases, which greatly facilitates target sequence recognition. This approach is potentially useful in prenatal diagnosis, particularly when the quantity of clinical material is limited.

MOLECULAR DIAGNOSTIC TECHNIQUES

Because DNA is present in each cell nucleus, any nucleated cell theoretically is suitable for DNA analysis, regardless of whether the gene in question is being transcribed and expressed. Thus, leukocytes, amniocytes, and chorionic villi all are candidate cells for DNA analysis. RFLP analysis was described earlier. Several other methods also are used for DNA diagnosis (i.e., Southern blot, oligonucleotide probe, PCR). Northern blotting is used for RNA analysis.

Southern Blot

Southern blot is a standard method for DNA analysis in both the clinical and basic science settings. In the Southern blot technique, named after the investigator Edwin Southern, double-stranded DNA is digested by a restriction endonuclease (see later) chosen because of its ability to detect a DNA polymorphism that may or may not have any clinical significance (41). After endonuclease digestion, the resulting DNA fragments are separated using gel electrophoresis. The DNA in the gel is denatured to generate single-stranded DNA molecules. DNA fragments are transferred from the gel to nylon filter paper (i.e., blotting), and specific filter-bound DNA fragments then can be detected by hybridization. A radiolabeled DNA or RNA probe is used that has sequence homology to the DNA fragment of interest, usually 200 to 2,000 bases long. Subsequent autoradiography produces a radiographic film with banding patterns that indicate the hybridization locations on the filter that reflect the fragment sizes of the DNA sequences homologous to that particular probe (Fig. 9–3).

Oligonucleotide Probe Analysis

Oligonucleotide probe analysis is similar to Southern blot analysis in that DNA is digested and electrophoresed in a gel. It differs in that a shorter probe, known as an

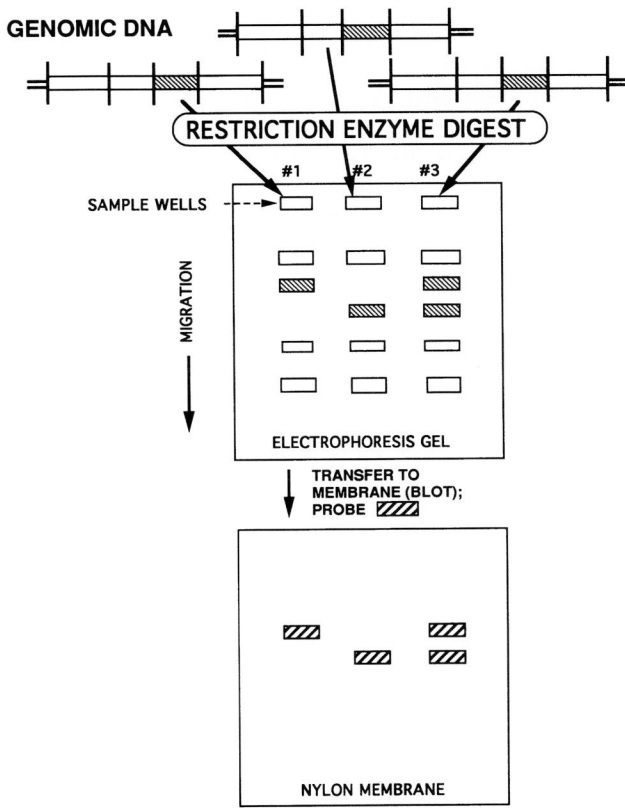

FIG. 9–3. Southern blot for a hypothetical autosomal recessive disorder. Lane 1, unaffected; lane 2, affected; lane 3, carrier.

oligonucleotide probe, is used for hybridization. Each oligonucleotide probe is biochemically synthesized and is about 20 bases in length. Because of their short length, they will not hybridize to genomic DNA sequences that differ by even a single nucleotide from the probe sequence. Thus, these probes are useful because they can detect very subtle variations in genomic sequences, but only if the specific nucleotide alterations in genomic DNA are known.

This approach for mutation detection involves direct DNA analysis using sequence-specific oligonucleotides. These specific oligonucleotides were first used for detection of the single-base mutations found in sickle-cell disease, the first "molecular disease" described (42–44). For the purposes of routine mutation screening, this method is useful only if the gene for the disorder under consideration has been sequenced and involves a small number of mutant alleles. This is important because the oligonucleotides that are complementary and specific for the mutation in question must be synthesized before testing. These nucleotide sequences can be synthesized to recognize the normal gene sequence, or ones that have specific nucleotide changes. Therefore, if a normal oligonucleotide sequence fails to recognize and hybridize to the gene in question, then a change in its sequence must be present. In contrast, if the oligonucleotide probe is constructed to complement a specific mutation, then recognition and hybridization of this probe implies that the mutation is present in that gene. Some diseases that can be detected in this manner include sickle-cell disease, CF, beta-thalassemias, Tay–Sachs disease, and Gaucher disease, where the nucleotide abnormalities for the more commonly occurring mutations are already known.

Polymerase Chain Reaction

PCR has revolutionized the field of molecular genetics (45–48). This procedure allows *in vitro* amplification of minute amounts of DNA to generate sufficient quantities of signal to make detection by more traditional methods possible. This procedure makes use of a relatively heat-stable bacterial enzyme, *Taq* I, derived from a thermoacidophilic bacterium, *Thermus aquaticus*. If the target nucleotide sequence is known, a specific set of oligonucleotides, called primers, can be synthesized to encompass the target sequence. The target DNA, oligonucleotide primers, *Taq* I polymerase, and free nucleotides are placed in solution. This reaction mixture is further heated to allow already denatured DNA to anneal with the oligonucleotides, between which the polymerase synthesizes complementary strands (Fig. 9–4). Repeated cycles of heating and cooling result in cyclic primer sequence synthesis, leading to annealing and amplification of the target sequence, because each set of DNA strands gives rise to two additional sets of sequence templates in each cycle of the reaction. This process can be

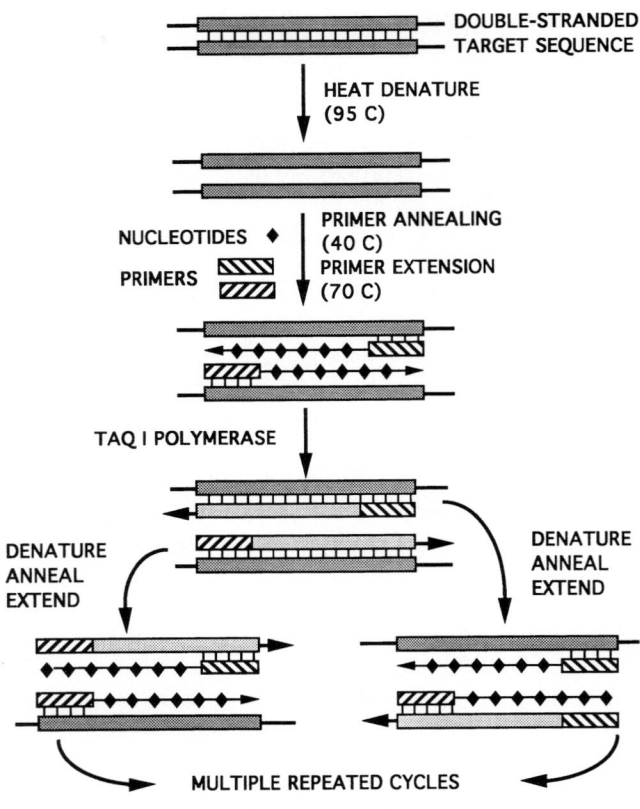

FIG. 9–4. Polymerase chain reaction.

automated to allow 20 to 30 cycles, which can produce more than a millionfold duplication of the target sequence within hours. Modifications of this process can be performed to allow the following:

• Analysis of RNA
• Analysis of multiple DNA areas (i.e., multiplex PCR)
• Selective amplification of one strand instead of both (i.e., asymmetric PCR)
• Simultaneous use of one primer set within another to increase specificity (i.e., nested PCR)
• Simultaneous use of two different primer sets, one of which selects for a normal sequence and the other for a mutant sequence (i.e., competitive oligonucleotide priming)
• Simultaneous use of a known amount of a second, easily identified target DNA to measure the amount of original DNA (i.e., semiquantitative PCR).

Many technical difficulties must be addressed to eliminate both false-positive and false-negative results. Problems with reagent or reactant contamination can lead to false-positive results and require that appropriate control methods be performed simultaneously to verify positive PCR results. Other problems such as primer instead of target amplification and nonspecific amplification must be recognized and eliminated.

Multiplex Polymerase Chain Reaction

PCR technology allows us to amplify multiple exons simultaneously. This method is known as "multiplex PCR." It combines the rapidity and sensitivity of the PCR process, and it allows us to use small or poor quality samples, i.e., those that might not be sufficient for Southern blot analysis. It requires the development of specific oligonucleotide primer sets unique to each region of the gene of interest, special amplification conditions, and the creation of amplified product of varying length for easy interpretation. This technique as been applied to the Duchenne muscular dystrophy/Becker muscular dystrophy (DMD/BMD) gene, whereby the large (nearly 2,400 kb with approximately 70 exons and 329 deletions) gene may be scanned for deletions in those patients and fetuses at risk for DMD/BMD, with detection of more than 97% of deletions in DMD and all those with BMD (49).

Northern Blot

Northern blotting is used for RNA analysis. The general principles of the technique are similar to those for Southern blotting. RNA analysis requires prompt specimen processing and committed laboratory reagents and instruments because of ubiquitous ribonucleases, present even on finger surfaces. Examination of the size and amount of a mRNA transcript is a useful initial step in evaluating mutations of genes that are expressed in cells or tissues, especially those that are expressed clinically. Fibroblasts and lymphocytes are good sources of mRNA. Hepatic or muscle tissue is useful, if available. Placental tissue can be used if maternal cell contamination can be avoided. Of the cell's total RNA, only 1% to 2% is mRNA, which is highly unstable at room temperature because of tissue RNases. The remainder of the RNA is mainly rRNA and transfer RNA (tRNA). Once isolated, the mRNA is denatured, separated by agarose gel electrophoresis, transferred to a membrane filter, and analyzed by hybridization of a specific fluorescent or radio-labeled probe.

For most diseases studied at the molecular level, about 5% to 10% of patients have no detectable mRNA for the gene product in question; 10% to 20% have reduced but detectable amounts of normal mRNA; and about 5% have some alteration in mRNA size. The approximately 50% remaining have normal amounts of normal-sized mRNA. Given this information, it is possible to deduce the general type of mutation at the DNA level, such as large or total gene deletions, which are suggested by a total absence of mRNA; mutations in promoter regions, which are suggested by reduced amounts of normal mRNA; mutations at exon–intron junctions, which are suggested by changes in mRNA size; or point mutations, which are suggested by normal-sized mRNA but abnormally functioning proteins. In some instances, the quantity of RNA is insufficient to be detected in this manner; thus, reverse transcriptase PCR methodology permits the scientist to identify and isolate these small quantities of mRNA and thereby analyze genes in a more fastidious manner. Grompe et al. (50) were unable to detect the mRNA in an ornithine transcarbamoylase–deficient patient by Northern analysis. Nonetheless, the mRNA was isolated and successfully amplified (after synthesis of a single-stranded cDNA by the utilization of the RNA-directed DNA polymerase, reverse transcriptase) and the mutation responsible for the disease was identified. This technique also allows one to isolate the shorter cDNA fragments corresponding to the coding region of the gene of interest. As in Menkes' (kinky hair) disease, a neurodegenerative disorder associated with a disturbance of copper metabolism, exon splicing is the characteristic result of the splice junction mutations seen in this rather large gene (51). Thus, by utilizing reverse transcriptase PCR, one can discern which exons are lacking by the size of fragment seen on agarose gel or by sequence analysis.

RESTRICTION ENDONUCLEASE ALLELE RECOGNITION

Hemoglobinopathies are the qualitative or quantitative disorders of the globin chains: alpha or beta. Sickle-cell anemia is the most common disease among these disorders. In the American black population, the frequency of the heterozygous state is 8%, whereas 1 in 500 individuals has the disease. The diagnosis can be readily made on examination of a peripheral blood smear. To confirm this diagnosis one must perform a hemoglobin electrophoresis. The beta-globin gene is located on chromosome 11. The only mutation responsible is an A to T transition in the second nucleotide of the sixth codon, substituting a valine for glutamic acid. Allelic heterogeneity does not exist for this disease. This alteration of DNA obliterates a sequence that the enzyme *Dde* I recognizes, CTNAG, which is present in the normal A, CTGAG, and hemoglobin C, CTAAG, allele but not in the S allele, CTGTG, and thus enables one to make the prenatal diagnosis of sickle-cell disease or trait by utilizing restriction endonuclease site analysis.

DEOXYRIBONUCLEIC ACID CLONING

The initial step in the study of a gene is now the isolation of a DNA molecule complementary to its mRNA, called cDNA. cDNA contains no intronic sequences. Using cDNA, many molecular investigations of the corresponding gene become possible. The first step in cDNA cloning is the isolation of mRNA from a particular cell or tissue that contains a significant amount of the desired mRNA. A retroviral enzyme, reverse transcriptase, is used to synthesize cDNA from the mRNA. Because the cell or tissue mRNA contains transcripts of many genes,

the resultant pool of cDNAs will be heterogeneous and must be sorted out. The cDNAs are inserted into a vector to form what is called a cDNA library. A second type of chromosome library, called a genomic library, is composed of fragments of native genomic DNA and contains introns and other noncoding regions. Vectors include viruses that can replicate within bacteria, such as bacteriophage lambda, or autonomous, self-replicating, circular DNA molecules found in bacteria called plasmids. Another vector that combines properties of plasmids and bacteriophage lambda are called cosmids. Cosmids are plasmid vectors into which larger fragments of DNA can be cloned. The term cosmid is derived from the presence of internal *co*hesive end *s*ites (cos) that have been inserted into a plasmid. Cos are nucleotide sequences from bacteriophage lambda between which DNA sequences are normally expressed as capsule proteins. In cosmids, these sequences can be replaced with other nucleotide sequences, which then can be expressed and concentrated *in vitro*.

An alternative approach to cDNA cloning uses mRNA itself instead of cDNA. Using mRNA is advantageous because the mRNA pool, although heterogeneous, is not nearly so complex as a corresponding pool of genomic DNA fragments that contains a mixture of introns, non-expressed genes, and DNA from noncoding regions. Methods of cDNA cloning to detect the presence of a specific cDNA segment include screening a cDNA library with synthetic oligonucleotide probes and screening a bacteriophage lambda library with antibodies directed against the protein of interest. Using the first approach, a set of radiolabeled oligonucleotide probes is synthesized with sequences complementary to those predicted for the mRNA from the amino acid sequence found in the protein. These oligonucleotides are used to probe a cDNA library that contains bacterial colonies infected with bacteriophage lambda. With the second approach, antibodies against the protein of interest are used to detect a corresponding protein expressed by cDNAs inserted into bacteriophage lambda.

cDNAs for many genes have been cloned using these approaches. Nucleotide sequencing is the first step in the analysis of a cDNA. With this information, the investigator can identify potential sites of restriction endonuclease cleavage, examine the deduced amino acid sequence to verify correspondence with the protein of interest, and identify regions of homology with other proteins, which can suggest evolutionary relationships and previously unrecognized functions. In addition to providing nucleotide and amino acid sequence information, these cDNAs can be used as hybridization probes to characterize and quantitate corresponding mRNA in cells and tissues from patients with a variety of diseases.

This process by which DNA analysis leads to an identifiable protein abnormality has been called "reverse genetics," or, more recently, "positional cloning"(52,53).

Several hundred genes associated with human disease have been identified. In some, the protein defect has been identified, such as with CF, and the triple-nucleotide/single–amino-acid deletion in the CFTR protein has been identified. For some diseases, the gene and protein are better characterized, such as for neurofibromatosis type 1 (54).

ALLELE-SPECIFIC OLIGONUCLEOTIDE HYBRIDIZATION

Allele-specific oligonucleotide hybridization has proven to be a valuable technique that measures the specific binding of short (18-20-mer), radioactively or nonradioactively labeled oligonucleotide probes that either match the wild type, normal, DNA sequences exactly or the mutant sequence containing a single base pair substitution under stringent washing conditions. Only the probes that exactly complement the immobilized DNA will remain bound and thus generate a signal seen on autoradiography. This technique was originally described by Conner et al. (55) in 1983 for the detection of sickle cell β^s-globin allele without the luxury of PCR amplification of genomic DNA. This technique greatly facilitates the evaluation of genetic disorders in which the gene has to be screened for numerous mutations such as thalassemia or CF, or in those where a restriction site is neither created nor obliterated.

PRENATAL DIAGNOSIS

Molecular Biology

Prenatal diagnosis has been accomplished successfully by analysis of fetal DNA extracted from a variety of samples (56). In the initial cases, the fetus was at risk for having a hemoglobinopathy, such as sickle-cell anemia or thalassemia (38,57–59), in which the specific protein, mRNA, and DNA defects were known. Since that time, the number of genetic disorders in which DNA technology can be applied to prenatal diagnosis continues to grow geometrically. In addition to the hemoglobinopathies, a partial list of other potentially prenatally diagnosable defects that can be evaluated by molecular genetic techniques include DMD (60–63), CF, fragile X syndrome (10,11), infantile myotonic dystrophy, hemophilias A and B (64,65), congenital adrenal hyperplasia (66), Tay–Sachs disease (67), neurofibromatosis type 1 (68,69), ornithine transcarbamylase deficiency (70,71), phenylketonuria (72,73), and Smith–Lemli–Opitz syndrome (74).

If the molecular abnormality of the abnormal gene is known, RFLP analysis or oligonucleotide probes can be used. PCR also can be used to amplify known regions and the resultant product analyzed by Southern blot. PCR is especially useful when using milligram amounts of clinical material obtained at the time of chorionic villus sampling, amniocentesis tissue culture, or cordocentesis. If the exact gene abnormality and location is not known, linkage analysis with RFLPs can be performed as an indirect method if family members are informative, i.e., affected family members must be available and willing to be tested. Occasionally, a patient may have a previously undescribed molecular pathologic condition, and the standard probes and markers are not helpful. This situation invariably lengthens the time to diagnosis. Other difficult situations arise when a disease appears in a family of a particular ethnic group where the molecular pathologic condition differs from that in other ethnic groups with a known molecular pathologic condition. An example of this situation is an African–American or Asian couple who have a child with CF, in whom studies for the delta F 508 mutation, most commonly found in northern Europeans, are negative. Despite these problems, as more genes are cloned and more chromosomal markers identified, this approach to prenatal diagnosis will become more common. The further applications of invasive fetal diagnostic modalities are discussed in Chapter 12.

Biochemistry

Biochemical assays remain an important aspect of prenatal diagnostic testing, even with the tremendous advances in molecular genetics. These assays include assessment of gene products such as enzymes, receptors, and transport proteins, and metabolites such as amino acids, organic acids, vitamins, and hormones. Prenatal diagnosis of biochemical defects may be made by assay of fetal tissue, fetal cells, or tissue culture supernatant if the particular product is produced solely or primarily by the gene in question, and the product already is known to be expressed in the fetal specimen to be analyzed. Enzyme assays can be performed using tissue, extracts from cultured fetal cells, or from live cells kept in tissue culture. Biochemical tests for the diagnosis of metabolic disorders consist of identification of abnormal metabolites or abnormal levels of metabolites that reflect a metabolic block. Ultimately, the goal is identification, quantitation, and characterization of the defective or deficient gene product that is responsible for the metabolic block. When the underlying biochemical defect is known and is expressed in accessible fetal tissue (e.g., chorionic villi, fetal muscle, liver) or cells (e.g., trophoblasts, amniocytes, fetal erythrocytes and leukocytes), prenatal diagnosis can be approached by analysis of the enzyme or other protein product that has been shown to be primarily involved.

Definitive biochemical diagnosis of an inherited metabolic disorder must be based on a clear-cut distinction between the values of affected and unaffected fetuses. In genetic disorders, there is potential for overlap between the normal and heterozygous ranges of enzyme activities.

This arises mainly as a result of the wide variation found in the activity of almost any biological enzyme in the normal population. Because variability due to different mutations and different genomic backgrounds exists among families, additional testing of leukocytes or cultured skin fibroblasts from presumably unaffected parents and siblings can provide valuable information. In addition to the benefit in interpretation of prenatal results, such studies may provide a reliable means for identification of other carriers among members of the extended family.

The fetus also can be assessed indirectly by determination of maternal serum enzyme activities during pregnancy. For example, the normal increase in serum hexosaminidase A seen in pregnancy appears to be of fetal origin (75,76). Therefore, unchanged levels in pregnant women at risk for Tay–Sachs disease may indicate an affected fetus. However, a pseudodeficiency allele has been found in non-Jewish individuals biochemically identified as Tay–Sachs carriers, in whom biochemical screening cannot differentiate between true Tay–Sachs carriers and pseudocarriers (both tests are positive); additional genetic testing is required (77).

For many inherited metabolic disorders or inborn errors of metabolism, biochemical means of prenatal diagnosis are available or theoretically are possible. For an autosomal recessive disease, the assay used should discriminate among homozygous affected, heterozygous unaffected, and homozygous normal fetuses. Assays for detection of autosomal dominant diseases, such as some of the porphyrias, usually are capable of identifying affected homozygotes, but sometimes fail to differentiate conclusively affected heterozygotes from unaffected fetuses. X-linked disorders present unique difficulties in heterozygote detection, which arise because of random X inactivation. Depending on the ratio of an active mutant X to normal X in tissues involved in the pathogenesis of the disease, a female heterozygous for an X-linked disorder may be clinically normal, or may have mild or even severe disease manifestations (78). To complicate matters further, measured enzymatic activities also vary depending on the ratio of mutant to normal X chromosomes that are active in the analyzed specimen—chorionic villi, for example. Occasionally, the activity levels in chorionic villi may not correlate with clinical expression. Males, on the other hand, have only one X chromosome, and are either hemizygous affected with deficient enzyme activity or hemizygous normal with activity in the normal range. Thus, prenatal biochemical assessment of X-linked disorders is less complicated if the fetus is male.

Fluorescence *In Situ* Hybridization

The use of fluorescence *in situ* hybridization (FISH) is a valuable adjunct to standard cytogenetics (79). With this technique, chromosome-specific repetitive DNA, unique sequence regions, or site-specific cosmids are identified by fluorescent probes in uncultured cells. Fetal cells obtained at the time of amniocentesis or chorionic villus sampling can be analyzed for chromosomes 21, 18, 13, X, and Y. Provided the sample is not contaminated or too small, monosomies or trisomies can be identified reliably in the majority of cases (73%), providing an informative result (80). This testing, coupled with real-time ultrasound imaging, can suggest a cytogenetic diagnosis in 48 to 72 hours. In addition, FISH analysis can be used to identify microdeletions in which standard cytogenetics may be normal. FISH analysis can be used to identify microdeletions that may be found in Prader–Willi, Angelman, Williams, DiGeorge/velocardiofacial, or Smith–Magenis syndrome (81). It must be emphasized that FISH is an adjunct to standard cytogenetics and does not detect or identify some cases of mosaicism, translocations, marker chromosomes, or other rare aneuploidies; standard cytogenetics must still be performed.

Fetal Samples and Tissue Processing

The use of direct and cultured fetal specimens for prenatal evaluation of metabolic disorders ideally requires the availability of normal control preparations. This applies to readily obtainable specimens, such as chorionic villus tissue, cultured trophoblasts, cultured amniotic fluid cells, and amniotic fluid supernatant, as well as to those obtained by more invasive procedures, such as fetal blood sampling and fetal liver and muscle biopsies. Except for trophoblasts and amniotic fluid cells that can be maintained in culture, availability of fresh controls is often a problem, and in most instances long-term frozen controls with partial loss of activity must be used. There are other potential pitfalls that seem specific for each of these tissue, cell, and fluid types. All samples should be analyzed as soon as possible, except those requiring initial tissue culture. Chorionic villi, fetal tissue biopsies, cell pellets, amniotic fluid supernatant, and fetal serum or plasma that are not used for tissue culture can be kept frozen and shipped on dry ice. Cell cultures and tissue for cell culture, however, should be shipped at room temperature or wet ice, depending on the circumstances. Whenever possible, appropriate controls matched by gestational age should accompany the samples to be analyzed.

Extraction and analysis of labile enzymes is especially difficult, because test results are very sensitive with respect to the duration of homogenization or sonication. Using fresh chorionic villi or amniocytes or freshly harvested trophoblasts helps preserve the activity of such labile enzymes (82).

Elevated concentrations of amino acids and organic acids in amniotic fluid serve as preliminary indications for several inherited disorders, such as amino and organic acidopathies and urea cycle defects. In most cases, however, final diagnosis is made by measuring the actual gene products responsible for the metabolic block. Identification and quantitation of amino acids and organic acids in physiologic fluids and in reaction mixtures are performed by an amino acid analyzer and gas chromatography, respectively. Quantities are determined by the ratio between the peak area found in the sample compared to known controls. Organic acids also must be extracted before their subsequent separation and quantitation by gas chromatography.

In the case of chorionic villus sampling, it is crucial to obtain samples that are of fetal origin only and in which maternal cells are either completely absent or extremely rare. The use of frozen controls may adversely affect the interpretation of results by causing false-negative diagnoses, especially when the enzyme in question is very labile, such as sialidase in sialidosis, or when the normal activity levels in chorionic villi are extremely low, as for alpha-iduronidase in mucopolysaccharidosis I. Specific problems also may be encountered because of different distribution of enzymes and isozymes (83). The characteristic presence of high levels of arylsulfatase-C activity in chorionic villi hampers the differential detection of arylsulfatase-A in metachromatic leukodystrophy and arylsulfatase-B in mucopolysaccharidosis VI when villi are used.

For most first-trimester prenatal tests, the recommended practice is to use fresh chorionic villi for preliminary evaluation followed by subsequent analysis of cultured trophoblasts for confirmation of the diagnosis. One exception is with nonketotic hyperglycinemia. Although the glycine-to-serine ratio in amniotic fluid is elevated in this disease, there is a significant overlap with normal values. The potential for prenatal diagnosis of this disorder would rely exclusively on the results obtained in fresh chorionic villi, because the glycine cleavage system is not expressed in amniotic fluid cells or trophoblasts, but is detectable in fresh tissue (84,85).

Amniotic fluid supernatants should be aliquoted into multiple vials to avoid the loss of activity that occurs with repeated freezing and thawing. Determinations of amniotic fluid concentrations of specific metabolites, as well as enzymes and other proteins, usually serve as supporting evidence in prenatal diagnoses. The final diagnosis should rely preferably on demonstration of the underlying biochemical defect in fetal cells or tissue. The variability in enzyme activities or in the levels of other proteins and metabolites frequently observed in cultured amniotic fluid cells and trophoblasts can be minimized by a careful choice of control cells.

Fetal blood sampling and fetal liver and muscle biopsy should be considered only in the absence of other alternatives because of the higher risk for pregnancy loss with these invasive procedures. Fetal blood sampling by cordocentesis has a wide variety of potential applications because both fetal cells and serum can be obtained. Fetal muscle biopsy has been used in rare cases of DMD, when molecular analysis of trophoblasts, amniocytes, or fetal leukocytes is nondiagnostic and family studies are uninformative. An *in utero* fetal muscle biopsy can be performed in the middle of the second trimester to assess dystrophin levels in myoblasts by *in situ* hybridization. Absence of dystrophin suggests an affected fetus. Fetal liver biopsy also can be performed for certain rare enzyme deficiencies. For example, in one type of glycogenosis, glucose-6-phosphatase is decreased; this enzyme is expressed only in fetal liver and kidney. In the absence of direct DNA techniques, the only option available for prenatal diagnosis is fetal liver biopsy in which glucose-6-phosphatase activity can be measured. Fetal liver biopsy also is applicable in rare cases of ornithine transcarbamylase deficiency where family studies are uninformative and known deletions cannot be detected (70).

MOLECULAR AND BIOCHEMICAL TESTING FOR CARRIER SCREENING

Carrier screening usually is limited to populations or ethnic groups at increased risk for a diagnosable disease. The ultimate benefit of carrier detection programs is the identification of couples at risk before they have an affected child, empowering them with reproductive choices. For example, carrier detection for Tay–Sachs disease is offered routinely to all people of Ashkenazi Jewish descent, in whom the combined frequency for the two common mutations in the alpha-subunit gene of hexosaminidase is 1 in 31 (86). Hexosaminidase A levels can be assayed enzymatically in serum, plasma, or leukocytes, and compared to a constant value of thermostable hexosaminidase B. Pregnant women should have only the leukocyte assay performed, because of problems with false-negative or indeterminate results in serum or plasma (75). Screening also is offered to people of French–Canadian background, in whom the clinical disease is similar and the carrier frequency high, but the mutation different (i.e., 7.6-kb deletion in the alpha subunit). As previously noted, caution must be utilized in non-Jewish individuals who test positive by biochemical screening because of the possibility of a pseudodeficiency allele (77).

In people of African descent, sickle-cell screening can be offered. Sickle-cell screening usually is performed by a biochemical assay assessing hemoglobin solubility; positive results are followed up by electrophoresis to characterize the hemoglobin type. In unusual cases, the exact nucleotide defect can be characterized using techniques described earlier.

Biochemical screening programs for Tay–Sachs disease and sickle-cell disease, when coupled with appropriate counseling, generally are well received by patients. In contrast, the recent molecular and biochemical characterization of the molecular defect causing CF has not resulted in widespread implementation of screening programs, even though CF is a common genetic disease (1 in 2,000–3,000) with a relatively high heterozygote frequency in American Caucasians (1 in 25). The controversy surrounding widespread implementation of CF screening arises because of a variety of factors (87–89). First, only about 70% of northern European carriers are positive for the most common mutation (i.e., delta F 508). As a result, this requires screening for multiple mutations, which is performed with PCR and oligonucleotide probes specific for known CF mutations. Using probes for 12 mutations, about 85% of carriers can be identified; with 70 mutations, about 90% of carriers can be identified (19). If screening is implemented, the following practices have been recommended by a National Institutes of Health consensus panel: (a) individuals with a family history of CF and partners of those with CF should be offered testing; (b) CF testing should be offered to the prenatal population and couples currently planning a pregnancy, particularly those in high-risk populations; and (c) CF testing for the general population is not advocated (90). Other options include testing the fetus at the time of genetic testing for other indications or testing if prenatal sonographic findings are suggestive of CF (see following). Another factor affecting implementation of screening programs is the clinical variability of the disorder. In contrast to the infantile form of Tay–Sachs disease, CF morbidity can range from debilitating pulmonary disease and death in childhood to minimal symptomatology and survival into adulthood, which correlates with the type and magnitude of the molecular defect (20,23). A final objection is the potential counseling difficulty arising when the fetus is found to have only one positive allele for a known CF mutation, and linkage analysis cannot be applied because there is no index case. Although the likelihood of an affected fetus is low, the possibility cannot be entirely ruled out, and the parents are left with an ambiguous result (78).

Paternity Testing

Small but increasing numbers of prenatal tests are performed to confirm or exclude paternity. Such testing may be performed on cord blood obtained prenatally or postnatally, cultured amniocytes, or chorionic villi. A variety of molecular techniques are available for this purpose, such as identifying *Alu* sequences, RFLP sites, or size-specific minisatellite DNA segments of the fetus and parents. This latter technique and its variations have been called DNA fingerprinting or DNA profiling (91,92).

Real-Time Targeted Imaging

The use of targeted imaging has resulted in the marriage of molecular biology to ultrasound (92). The clinician can now identify certain sonographic features associated with aneuploidy. In the first and early-second trimesters, nuchal translucency has been associated with trisomy 21 (and a variety of other disorders, such as congenital heart disease or Smith–Lemli–Opitz syndrome) (74,93–95). In the second trimester, increased nuchal thickness may indicate Turner syndrome or Down syndrome. A variety of sonographic features have been variably associated with trisomy 21 (96). Ultrasound findings, coupled with FISH analysis, can strongly suggest a diagnosis of aneuploidy. Skeletal dysplasias identified prenatally also can be characterized at the molecular level (97). A diagnosis of fetal CF can be considered in the presence of markedly echogenic fetal bowel or dilated bowel loops suggestive of meconium ileus (98).

THE FUTURE OF MOLECULAR BIOLOGY

The knowledge explosion in molecular biology has revolutionized medical practice. Prenatal diagnosis has benefited enormously, because bench discoveries rapidly result in clinical applications. Development of PCR, increasingly sophisticated electrophoretic methods, positional cloning (52), recognition of new genetic causes of human disease such as triplet repeats (10,11), uniparental disomy (99,100), genetic imprinting (101,102), and microsegmental aneusomy (81,103), all have had direct and immediate impact on the practice of reproductive genetics. As previously noted, advances in chromosome painting and *in situ* hybridization potentially allow cytogenetic diagnoses within 24 to 48 hours (79–81). Fetal cells and DNA have been identified in maternal serum as early as 7 weeks of gestation and may be useful in screening for aneuploid pregnancies (104–106). There is increased use of antenatal genetic screening as more disease-causing genes are cloned and sequenced, and their function is characterized. Finally, the prospect of embryonic or fetal gene diagnosis and therapy, along with the *in utero* creation of a transgenic human, may not be as far in the future as many believe or fear (107,108). Immunologic reconstitution by *in utero* paternal bone marrow transplantation in X-linked combined immunodeficiency syndrome recently has been described; the fetus was identified at 12 weeks as being affected by a mutation in the interleukin-2 receptor by DNA analysis of chorionic villus tissue. The fetus was given intraperitoneal injections of enriched paternal bone marrow tissue at 16, 17.5, and 18.5 weeks of gestation. Functional paternal engraftment appears to be successful at 11 months of age (109,110). The medical community must address the applications of these technologies and the attendant myriad social, legal, and ethical issues (111,112).

REFERENCES

1. Garrod AE. The Croonian lectures. *Lancet* 1908;2:1.
2. Caskey CT. Disease diagnosis by recombinant DNA methods. *Science* 1987;236:1223.

3. King CR. Prenatal diagnosis of genetic disease with molecular genetic technology. *Obstet Gynecol Surv* 1988;43:493.
4. Watson JD, Crick FHC. Molecular structure of nucleic acids: a structure for deoxyribose nucleic acid. *Nature* 1953;171:737.
5. Berget SM, Moore C, Sharp PA. Spliced RNA segments at the 5[T407]8-terminus of late adenovirus 2 m RNA. *Proc Natl Acad Sci USA* 1977;74:3171.
6. Gilbert W. Why genes in pieces? *Nature* 1978;271:501.
7. Gilbert W. Genes-in-pieces revisited. *Science* 1985;228:823.
8. Cooper DN, Smith BA, Cooke HJ, et al. An estimate of unique DNA sequence heterozygosity in the human genome. *Hum Genet* 1985;69:201.
9. Miller DA, Choi YC, Miller OJ. Chromosome localization of highly repetitive human DNAs and amplified ribosomal DNA with restriction enzymes. *Science* 1983;219:395.
10. Caskey CT, Pizzuti A, Ying-Hui Fu, et al. Triplet repeat mutations in human disease. *Science* 1992;256:784.
11. Richards RI, Sutherland GR. Heritable unstable DNA sequences. *Nat Genet* 1992;1:7.
12. ACMG/ASHG Statement. Laboratory guidelines for Huntington disease genetic testing. *Am J Hum Genet* 1998;62:1243.
13. Cann RL, Stoneking M, Wilson AC. Mitochondrial DNA and human evolution. *Nature* 1987;325:31.
14. Schoffner JM, Wallace DC. Mitochondrial genetics: principles and practice [Invited Editorial]. *Am J Hum Genet* 1992;51:1179.
15. Shields GF, Schmiechen AM, Frazier BL, et al. MtDNA sequences suggest a recent evolutionary divergence for Beringian and northern North American populations. *Am J Hum Genet* 1993;53:549.
16. Petersen GM, Rotter JI, Cantor RM, et al. The Tay–Sachs disease gene in North American Jewish populations: geographic variation and origin. *Am J Hum Genet* 1983;35:1258.
17. Grabowski GA. Gaucher disease: gene frequencies and genotype/phenotype correlation. *Genet Testing* 1997;1:5.
18. Myerowitz R, Costigan C. The major defect in Ashkenazi Jews with Tay–Sachs disease is an insertion in the gene for the alpha-chain for beta-hexosaminidase. *J Biol Chem* 1988;263:18587.
19. Ohno K, Suzuki K. A splicing defect due to an exon–intron junctional mutation results in abnormal beta-hexosaminidase X-chain in RNAs in Ashkenazi Jewish patients with Tay–Sachs disease. *Biochem Biophys Res Commun* 1988;153:463.
20. Cutting GR, Kasch LM, Rosenstein BJ, et al. Two cystic fibrosis patients with mild pulmonary disease and nonsense mutations in each CFTR gene. *N Engl J Med* 1990;323:1685.
21. Cutting GR, Kasch LM, Rosenstein BJ, et al. A cluster of cystic fibrosis mutations in the first nucleotide-binding fold of the cystic fibrosis conductance regulator protein. *Nature* 1990;346:366.
22. Kerem E, Corez M, Kerem BS, et al. The relationship between genotype and phenotype in cystic fibrosis: analysis of the most common mutation (delta F508). *N Engl J Med* 1990;323:1517.
23. Stern RC. The diagnosis of cystic fibrosis. *N Engl J Med* 1997;336:487.
24. Kerem B, Chiba-Falek O, Kerem E. Cystic fibrosis in Jews: frequency and mutation distribution. *Genet Testing* 1997;1:35.
25. Smith CAB. The development of human linkage analysis. *Ann Hum Genet* 1986;50:293.
26. Botstein D. 1989 William Allen Award address. *Am J Hum Genet* 1990;47:887.
27. Botstein D, White RL, Skolnick M, et al. Construction of a genetic linkage map using restriction fragment length polymorphisms. *Am J Hum Genet* 1980;32:314.
28. Cavalli-Sforza LL, King MC. Detecting linkage for genetically heterogeneous diseases and detecting heterogeneity with linkage data. *Am J Hum Genet* 1986;38:599.
29. White R, Lalouel J-M. Sets of linked genetic markers for human chromosomes. *Ann Rev Genet* 1988;27:259.
30. White R. 1989 William Allen Award address. *Am J Hum Genet* 1990;47:892.
31. Haldane JBS, Smith CAB. A new estimate of the linkage between the genes for color-blindness and hemophilia in man. *Ann Genet Eugen* 1947;14:10.
32. Morton NE. Sequential tests for the detection of linkage. *Am J Hum Genet* 1955;7:277.
33. Risch N. Genetic linkage: interpreting LOD scores. *Science* 1992;255:803.
34. Antonarakis SE, Phillips JA III, Kazazian HH Jr. Genetic diseases: diagnosis by restriction endonuclease analysis. *J Pediatr* 1982;100:845.
35. Gusella JF. DNA polymorphism and human disease. *Ann Rev Biochem* 1986;55:831.
36. Gusella JF, Wexler NS, Conneally PM, et al. A polymorphic DNA marker genetically linked to Huntington disease. *Nature* 1983;306:234.
37. Antonarakis SE, Kazazian HH Jr, Orkin SH. DNA polymorphism and molecular pathology of the human globin gene clusters. *Hum Genet* 1985;60:1.
38. Boehm CD, Antonarakis SE, Phillips JA, et al. Prenatal diagnosis using DNA polymorphisms: report on 95 pregnancies at risk for sickle-cell disease or beta thalassemia. *N Engl J Med* 1983;308:1054.
39. Embury SH, Scharf SJ, Saiki RK, et al. Rapid prenatal diagnosis of sickle cell anemia by a new method of DNA analysis. *N Engl J Med* 1987;316:656.
40. Weatherall DJ, Old JM, Thein SL. Prenatal diagnosis of the common haemoglobin disorders. *J Med Genet* 1985;22:422.
41. Southern EM. Detection of specific sequences among DNA fragments separated by electrophoresis. *J Mol Biol* 1975;98:503.
42. Pauling L, Itano HA, Singer SJ, et al. Sickle cell anemia, a molecular disease. *Science* 1949;110:543.
43. Rossiter BJF, Caskey CT. Molecular scanning methods of mutation detection. *J Biol Chem* 1990;265:12753.
44. Saiki RK, Chang CA, Levenson CH, et al. Diagnosis of sickle cell anemia and beta thalassemia with enzymatically amplified DNA and non-radioactive allele-specific oligonucleotide probes. *N Engl J Med* 1988;319:537.
45. Ehrlich HA, Gelfand D, Sninsky JJ. Recent advances in the polymerase chain reaction. *Science* 1991;252:1643.
46. Mullis KB, Falloona FA. Specific synthesis of DNA in vitro via a polymerase-catalyzed chain reaction. *Methods Enzymol* 1987;155:335.
47. Saiki RK, Gelfand DH, Stoffel S, et al. Primer-directed enzymatic amplification of DNA with a thermostable DNA polymerase. *Science* 1988;239:487.
48. Scharf SJ, Horn GT, Erlich HA. Direct cloning and sequence analysis of enzymatically amplified genomic sequences. *Science* 1986;233:1076.
49. Beggs AH, Koenig M, Boyce FM, Kunkel LM. Detection of 98% of DMD/BMD gene deletions by polymerase chain reaction. *Hum Genet* 1990;86:45.
50. Grompe M, Muzny DM, Caskey CT. Scanning detection of mutations in human ornithine transcarbamoylase by chemical mismatch cleavage. *Proc Natl Acad Sci USA* 1989;86:5888.
51. Das S, Levinson B, Shitney S, Vulpe C, Packman S, Gitschier J. Diverse mutations in patients with Menkes disease often lead to exon skipping. *Am J Hum Genet* 1994;55:883.
52. Collins FS. Positional cloning: let's not call it reverse anymore. *Nat Genet* 1992;1:3.
53. Ruddle FH. The William Allan Memorial Award address: reverse genetics and beyond. *Am J Hum Genet* 1984;36:944.
54. Xu G, O'Connell P, Viskochil D, et al. The neurofibromatosis type 1 gene encodes a protein related to GAP. *Cell* 1990;62:599.
55. Conner BJ, Reyes AA, Morin C, Itakura K, Teplitz RL, Wallace RB. Detection of sickle cell β^S-globin allele by hybridization with synthetic oligonucleotides. *Proc Natl Acad Sci USA* 1983;80:278.
56. Antonarakis SE. Diagnosis of genetic disorders at the DNA level. *N Engl J Med* 1989;320:153.
57. Kan YW. The William Allan Memorial Award address: thalassemia: molecular mechanism and detection. *Am J Hum Genet* 1986;38:4.
58. Kazazian HH Jr, Boehm CD. Molecular basis and prenatal diagnosis of beta-thalassemia. *Blood* 1988;72:1107.
59. Saiki RK, Scharf S, Faloona F, et al. Enzymatic amplification of beta-globin genomic sequences and restriction site analysis for diagnosis of sickle cell anemia. *Science* 1985;230:1350.
60. Gillard EF, Chamberlain JS, Murphy EG, et al. Molecular and phenotypic analysis of patients with deletions within the deletion-rich region of the Duchenne muscular dystrophy (DMD) gene. *Am J Hum Genet* 1989;45:507.
61. Hoffman EP, Fischbeck KH, Brown RH, et al. Characterization of dystrophin in muscle-biopsy specimens from patients with Duchenne's or Becker's muscular dystrophy. *N Engl J Med* 1988;318:1363.
62. Kunkel LM. Analysis of deletions in DNA from patents with Becker and Duchenne muscular dystrophy. *Nature* 1986;322:73.

63. Multicenter Study Group. Diagnosis of Duchenne and Becker muscular dystrophies by polymerase chain reaction: a multicenter study. *JAMA* 1992;267:2609.

64. Antonarakis SE. Molecular genetics of hemophilia A and B. *Adv Hum Genet* 1988;17:27.

65. Kogan SC, Doherty M, Gitschier J. An improved method for prenatal diagnosis of genetic diseases by analysis of amplified DNA sequences: application to hemophilia A. *N Engl J Med* 1987;317:985.

66. Pang S, Pollack MS, Marshall RN, et al. Prenatal treatment of congenital adrenal hyperplasia due to 21-hydroxylase deficiency. *N Engl J Med* 1990;322:111.

67. Grabowski GA, Kruse VR, Goldberg JE, et al. First-trimester prenatal diagnosis of Tay–Sachs disease. *Am J Hum Genet* 1984;36:1369.

68. Cawthon RM, Weiss R, Yu G, et al. A major segment of the neurofibromatosis type 1 gene: a DNA sequence, genomic structure, and point mutations. *Cell* 1990;62:193.

69. Viskochil D, Buchberg AM, Yu G, et al. Deletions and a translocation interrupt a cloned gene at the neurofibromatosis type 1 locus. *Cell* 1990;62:187.

70. Holzgreve W, Golbus MS. Prenatal diagnosis of ornithine transcarbamylase deficiency utilizing fetal liver biopsy. *Am J Hum Genet* 1984;36:320.

71. Nussbaum RL, Boggs BA, Beaudet AL, et al. New mutation and prenatal diagnosis in ornithine transcarbamylase deficiency. *Am J Hum Genet* 1986;38:149.

72. Kwok SCM, Ledley FD, Dilella AG, et al. Nucleotide sequence of a full-length complementary DNA clone and amino acid sequence of human phenylalanine hydroxylase. *Biochemistry* 1985;24:556.

73. Woo SLC, Lidsky AS, Guttler F, et al. Cloned human phenylalanine hydroxylase gene allows prenatal diagnosis and carrier detection of classical phenylketonuria. *Nature* 1983;306:151.

74. Kelley RI. RSH/Smith–Lemli–Opitz syndrome: mutations and metabolic morphogenesis [Invited Editorial]. *Am J Hum Genet* 1998;63:322.

75. Ben-Yoseph Y, Pack BA, Thomas PM, et al. Maternal serum hexosaminidase A in pregnancy: effects of gestational age and fetal genotype. *Am J Med Genet* 1988;29:891.

76. Navon R, Leibokowicz I, Adam A. Fetal hexosaminidase A in mother's serum: pitfalls in carrier detection and prospects for prenatal diagnosis of GM 2 gangliosidoses. *Am J Hum Genet* 1987;40:60.

77. Triggs-Raine BL, Mules EH, Kaback MM, et al. A pseudodeficiency allele common in non-Jewish Tay–Sachs carriers: implications of carrier screening. *Am J Hum Genet* 1992;51:793.

78. Puck JM, Willard HF. X inactivation in females with X-linked disease [Editorial]. *N Engl J Med* 1998;338:325.

79. Schwartz S. Efficacy and applicability of interphase fluorescent in situ hybridization for prenatal diagnosis [Invited Editorial]. *Am J Hum Genet* 1993;52:851.

80. Ward BE, Gersen SL, Carelli MP, et al. Rapid prenatal diagnosis of chromosomal aneuploidies by fluorescent in situ hybridization: clinical experience with 4,500 specimens. *Am J Hum Genet* 1993;52:854.

81. Ligon AH, Beaudet AL, Sheffer LG. Simultaneous multilocus FISH analysis for detection of microdeletions in the diagnostic evaluation of developmental delay and mental retardation. *Am J Hum Genet* 1997;61:51.

82. Ben-Yoseph Y, Evans MI, Bottoms SF, et al. Lysosomal enzyme activities in fresh and frozen chorionic villi and in cultured trophoblasts. *Clin Chim Acta* 1986;161:307.

83. Giles L, Cooper A, Fowler B, et al. Aryl sulphatase isozymes of chorionic villi: implications for prenatal diagnosis. *Prenat Diagn* 1987;7:245.

84. Applegarth DA, Levy HL, Shih VE, et al. Prenatal diagnosis of nonketotic hyperglycinemia. *Prenat Diagn* 1986;6:257.

85. Hayasaka K, Tada K, Fueki N, et al. Feasibility of prenatal diagnosis of nonketotic hyperglycinemia: existence of the glycine cleavage system in placenta. *J Pediatr* 1987;110:124.

86. Triggs-Raine BL, Feigenbaum ASJ, Natowicz M, et al. Screening for carriers of Tay–Sachs diseases among Ashkenazi Jews. *N Engl J Med* 1990;323:6.

87. Caskey CT, Kaback MM, Beaudet AL. The American Society of Human Genetics statement on cystic fibrosis screening. *Am J Hum Genet* 1990;46:393.

88. Wilfond BS, Fost N. The cystic fibrosis gene: medical and social implications for heterozygote detection. *JAMA* 1990;263:2777.

89. Motulsky AG. Screening for genetic disease [Editorial]. *N Engl J Med* 1997;336:1314.

90. Genetic testing for cystic fibrosis. NIH Consensus Statement 1997;15:1.

91. Beaudet AL, Feldman GL, Fernback SD, et al. Linkage disequilibrium, cystic fibrosis, and genetic counseling. *Am J Hum Genet* 1989;44:319.

92. Jeffreys AJ. 1992 William Allen Award Address. *Am J Hum Genet* 1993;53:1.

93. Holzgreve W. Will ultrasound-screening and ultrasound-guided procedures be replaced by non invasive techniques for the diagnosis of fetal chromosome abnormalities [Editorial]? *Ultrasound Obstet Gynecol* 1997;9:217.

94. Taipale P, Hiilesmaa V, Salonen R, et al. Increased nuchal translucency as a marker for fetal chromosomal defects. *N Engl J Med* 1997;337:1654.

95. Souka AP, Snijders RJM, Novakov A, et al. Defects and syndromes in chromosomally normal fetuses with increased nuchal translucency thickness at 10–14 weeks gestation. *Ultrasound Obstet Gynecol* 1998:11:391.

96. Benacerraf BR. The second-trimester fetus with Down syndrome: detection using sonographic features. *Ultrasound Obstet Gynecol* 1996;7:147.

97. Horton WA. Molecular genetics of human chondrodysplasias. *Growth Genet Hormones* 1997;13:49.

98. Slotnick RN, Abuhamad AZ. Prognostic implications of fetal echogenic bowel. *Lancet* 1996;347:85.

99. Knoll JH, Nichols RD, Magenis RE, et al. Angelman and Prader–Willi syndromes share a common chromosome 15 deletion but differ in parental origin of the deletion. *Am J Med Genet* 1989;32:285.

100. Spence JE, Perciaccante RG, Greig GM, et al. Uniparental disomy as a mechanism for human genetic disease. *Am J Hum Genet* 1988;42:217.

101. Nicholls RD, Knoll JH, Butle MG, et al. Genetic imprinting suggested by maternal heterodisomy in nondeletion Prader–Willi syndrome. *Nature* 1989;342:281.

102. Reck W. Genomic imprinting and genetic disorders in man. *Trends Genet* 1989;5:331.

103. Schmickel RD. Contiguous gene syndromes: a component of recognizable syndromes. *J Pediatr* 1986;109:231.

104. Goldberg JD. Fetal cells in maternal circulation: progress in analysis of a rare event [Invited Editorial]. *Am J Hum Genet* 1997;61:806.

105. Bianchi DW, Williams JW, Sullivan LM, et al. PCR quantitation of fetal cells in maternal blood in normal and aneuploid pregnancies. *Am J Hum Genet* 1997;61:822.

106. Lo YMD, Tein MSC, Lau TK, et al. Quantitative analysis of fetal DNA in maternal plasma and serum: implications for non-invasive prenatal diagnosis. *Am J Hum Genet* 1998;62:768.

107. Gordon JW. Micromanipulation of embryos and germ cells: an approach to gene therapy? *Am J Med Genet* 1990;35:206.

108. Handyside AH, Kontogianni EH, Hardy K, et al. Pregnancies from biopsied human preimplantation embryos sexed by Y-specific DNA amplification. *Nature* 1990;344:768.

109. Gluckman E. The therapeutic potential of fetal and neonatal hematopoietic stem cells [Editorial]. *N Engl J Med* 1996;335:1839.

110. Flake AL, Roncarolo M-G, Puck JM, et al. Brief report: treatment of X-linked severe combined immunodeficiency by in utero transplantation of paternal bone marrow. *N Engl J Med* 1996;335:1806.

111. Bernhardt B. Empirical evidence that genetic counseling is directive: where do we go from here [Invited Editorial]? *Am J Hum Genet* 1997;60:17.

112. Michie S, Bron F, Bobrow M, et al. Non-directive genetic counseling: an empirical study. *Am J Hum Genet* 1997;60:40.

CHAPTER 10

Feto-Maternal Interactions: Placental Physiology and Its Role as a Go-Between

Gabriella Pridjian

Far from the primitive exchange organ in lower animals, the human placenta has evolved into a highly sophisticated interface between mother and fetus. As the gatekeeper for maternofetal interactions, its functions are diverse and essential.

HUMAN PLACENTATION

Based on the modified classification of Grosser, which separates placentas by the numbers of layers interfacing the maternal and fetal circulations, the human placenta is hemomonochorial, with only the syncytiotrophoblast, fetal connective tissue, and fetal capillary endothelium forming the barrier between the two circulations (Fig. 10–1) (1). The human placenta, with this most intimate interface, is similar to that of the guinea pig and the monkey.

Placentation in other animals is different, and there is great variation in mammalian placentation. For example, the ovine placenta is epitheliochorial. The maternal blood in the sheep does not directly bathe the syncytiotrophoblast, but is delivered to that cell by maternal capillaries. Between maternal and fetal circulations is the maternal capillary endothelium, maternal connective tissue, syncytiotrophoblast, fetal connective tissue, and fetal capillary endothelium. Although the sheep is an excellent model to study certain aspects of maternofetal physiology, ovine placental transport data, especially of diffusional substances, is not applicable to the human. For example, the ovine placenta is almost impermeable to diffusional transfer of the ketone body β-hydroxybutyrate, but human placenta is permeable to this ketone body, which has been implicated with the fetal distress accom-

G. Pridjian: Human Genetics Program, The Hayward Genetics Center, New Orleans, Louisiana

panying diabetic ketoacidosis (2). Unless otherwise specified, the discussion that follows pertains to human placentation.

The human placenta is discoid and made up of eight to ten cotyledons. Fetal blood is supplied to the placenta by two umbilical arteries and drained by one umbilical vein. On the fetal surface of the placenta, the umbilical arteries, crossing over fetal veins, decrease in caliber and increase in divisions as they travel toward the placental edges and dive deeply into the placental disc to supply individual cotyledons. Within the substance of the placenta, the caliber of the arteries decreases until only fetal capillaries exist at the level of the terminal villi. The fetal capillaries are dilated, providing a broad surface area for maternofetal transfer. The maternal blood supply to the placenta originates from the uterine artery, which divides into spiral arteries and percolates through the intervillous space, bathing the terminal villi.

PLACENTAL TRANSFER

The fetus depends almost exclusively on the placenta for nutritional, respiratory, and excretory functions. The placenta, growing steadily as gestation progresses, parallels fetal growth. Studies of placental growth and physiology in disease states suggest that placental growth and size are determined by the fetus and modulated by maternal factors. Normal placental:fetal weight ratios are approximately 1:6. As the placenta grows, villous processes increase in number as fetal vasculature expands, and by the third trimester, a large surface area is available to the maternal and fetal circulations.

Most placental transport is transcellular. Although the placenta often is thought of as a "separating membrane," it is actually a series of membranes. The most efficient areas for maternofetal exchange are the epithelial plates,

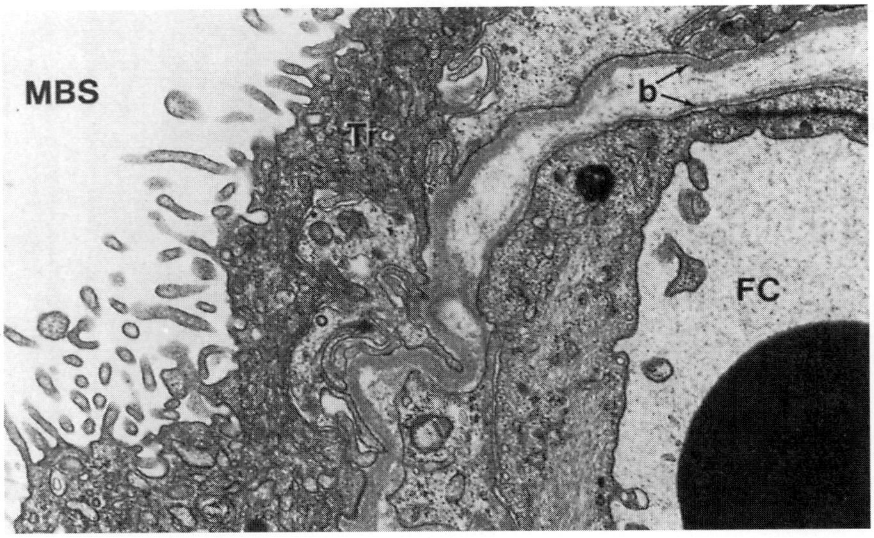

FIG. 10–1. Electron micrograph of the placental barrier of the human hemo-monochorial full-term placenta. Notice the numerous endocytotic vesicles in various stages of formation located on the maternal-side brush border membrane of the syncytiotrophoblast. b, basement membrane; FC, fetal capillary; MBS, maternal blood space or intervillous space; Tr, syncytiotrophoblast with microvillous brush border membrane. Bar = 0.5 μm. (From Thornberg KL, Faber JJ. *Placental physiology.* New York: Raven Press, 1983:19.)

which consist of thinly stretched, attenuated villous tissue separating maternal blood in the intervillous space from fetal blood in the fetal sinusoids. To cross epithelial plates from the maternal to the fetal side, a substance must traverse the brush border membrane of the syncytiotrophoblast, the cellular plasma of this cell, the basement membrane of the syncytiotrophoblast, the maternal side of the fetal capillary endothelial cell, and the fetal side of the same endothelial cell. The microvillous brush border membrane of the syncytiotrophoblast appears to be the membrane most involved in regulation of transport, especially of active or carrier mediated transport. Although there is considerable knowledge of transport mechanisms at the microvillous brush border of the syncytiotrophoblast (i.e., maternal side), less is known about transport through the basal membrane of that cell (i.e., fetal side) or through the fetal capillary endothelial cell. Certain diffusible substances traverse the trophoblast and endothelial cell intact for release on the fetal side, some substances may be partially or completely metabolized by the placenta, and others may be involved in intricate transport systems (Fig. 10–2).

Simple Diffusion

Many nutrients, metabolites, and excretory products cross the placenta by diffusion. Diffusion of substances in the placenta depends on multiple factors; these are summarized in Table 10–1.

The amount of a nutrient delivered to the placenta is directly proportional to its concentration in the maternal blood stream, which depends on nutritional intake and gastrointestinal absorption. Famine, maternal gastrointestinal diseases that interfere with absorption, or maternal pulmonary diseases that interfere with alveolar exchange may significantly affect blood concentrations

and transfer and accrual of fetal fuels. A lack of fetal fuels produces fetal and placental growth restriction. Abnormalities in maternal homeostatic mechanisms may produce either an insufficiency or an abundance of nutrients. For example, in poorly controlled diabetes, maternal hyperglycemia, hyperaminoacidemia, and hypertriglyceridemia allow unrestrained nutrient delivery to the fetus with excessive growth of fetal organs, body fat, and the placenta (3).

Delivery of a nutrient to the placenta is directly proportional to blood flow in the intervillous space. Maternal blood volume gradually increases to 30% to 40% above prepregnancy volume, with 40% directed to the uterus and placenta. Maternal cardiac disease with lower cardiac output may result in fetal and placental growth restriction.

Even in healthy women, maternal position influences blood flow to the uterus. Normal pregnant women have an 18% lower cardiac output in the standing position compared with lying on their sides, perhaps explaining why women who stand at work throughout their pregnancy have newborns of lower birth weight.

Fetal factors influencing diffusion are those that affect nutrient delivery to the fetal side of the placenta. The concentration of a substance in the umbilical artery depends on the amount of prior placental transfer, absorption from swallowed amniotic fluid, and fetal metabolism. Fetal blood flow to the uterus depends on fetal cardiac output and placental vascular tone. Normally, fetal vessels on the chorionic plate are maximally dilated, providing the least resistance to flow.

Numerous placental factors influence diffusion. The number of branching structures of the placental villus and amount of dilatation of the fetal capillaries regulate transfer surface area. Overall, transfer is governed by the quantity of epithelial plates, the specialized regions of

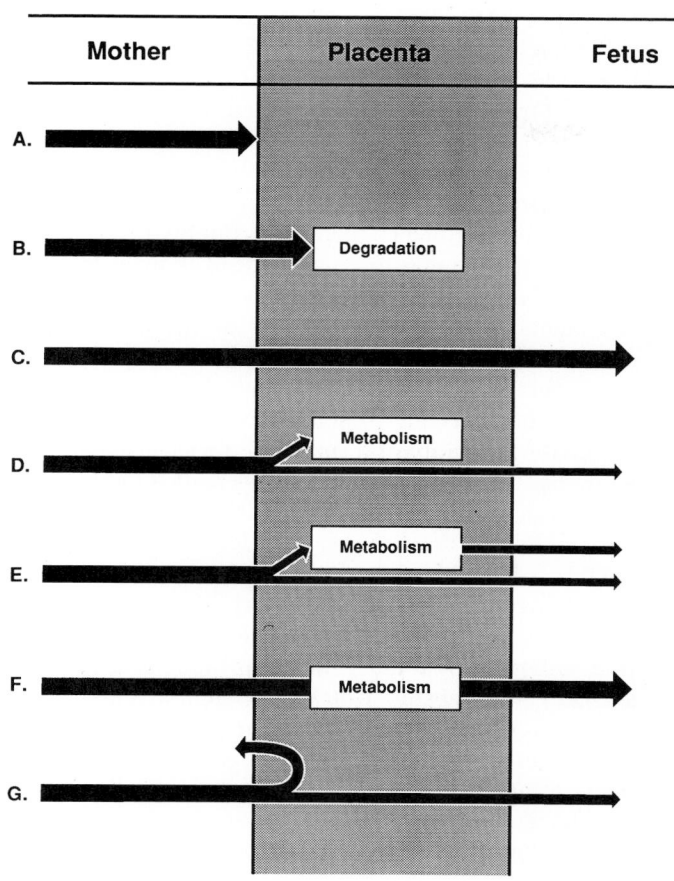

FIG. 10–2. Patterns of maternofetal transport. **A:** Minimal or no placental uptake and no fetal transfer (e.g., succinylcholine, highly charged quaternary ammonium compounds). **B:** Placental uptake, degradation, and no fetal transfer (e.g., insulin). **C:** Placental uptake and transfer predominantly unmodified to the fetus (e.g., betahydroxybutyrate, bilirubin). **D:** Placental uptake, partial use, and transfer to the fetus (e.g., oxygen, glucose, amino acids, free fatty acids). **E:** Uptake, partial metabolism, and transfer to the fetus (e.g., cyclosporine). **F:** Uptake, modification, and transfer to the fetus (e.g., 25-hydroxyvitamin D_3, of which most undergoes 1α-hydroxylation in the placenta to form 1,25-dihydroxyvitamin D_3). **G:** Carrier-coupled uptake with release of the ligand to the fetal side and regeneration of the carrier on the maternal side (e.g., transferrin–iron complex).

enhanced diffusion where the interhemal barrier is less than a few micrometers. The geometric interrelation of the maternal and fetal placental blood circulations influences diffusion.

The most efficient pattern of blood flow for exchange is countercurrent flow; the direction of flow in the maternal vessels is the reverse of that in the fetal vessels, as seen in the guinea pig placenta or human kidneys. A concurrent flow pattern is the least efficient for transfer. The human placenta has an intervillous pool flow system in which fetal capillaries in terminal villi are bathed in a maternal blood reservoir continuously filled by arteries and drained by veins (Fig. 10–3). Concurrent and countercurrent flows exist in areas of uneven distribution of flow (i.e., shunting), where a portion of the villus is well supplied by maternal blood but poorly supplied by fetal blood; in other areas, the opposite occurs.

TABLE 10–1. *Factors affecting the placental transfer of a diffusible substance*

Maternal factors	Placental factors	Fetal factor
Amount Delivered to the Intervillous Space	**Transfer Physiology**	**Amount Delivered to the Fetal Capillaries**
Blood concentration	Area of diffusing membrane(s)	Blood concentration
Exogenous and endogenous supplies	Diffusion resistance	Fetal metabolic production or gastrointestinal absorption
Homeostatic mechanisms	Characteristics of transferred material (size, charge, polarity, shape)	Prior placental transfer
Arteriovenous mixing in the intervillous space	Characteristics of membrane (physiochemical composition, fluidity)	Flow rate in the fetal capillaries
Flow rate in intervillous space	Diffusion pressure across each placental cell membrane	Hemodynamic factors in fetus
Hemodynamic factors in mother	Maternofetal concentration gradients	Local circulatory factors
Local circulatory factors	Placental cellular production or use	Shunting
Shunting	Maternofetal blood flow characteristics; intervillous flow	

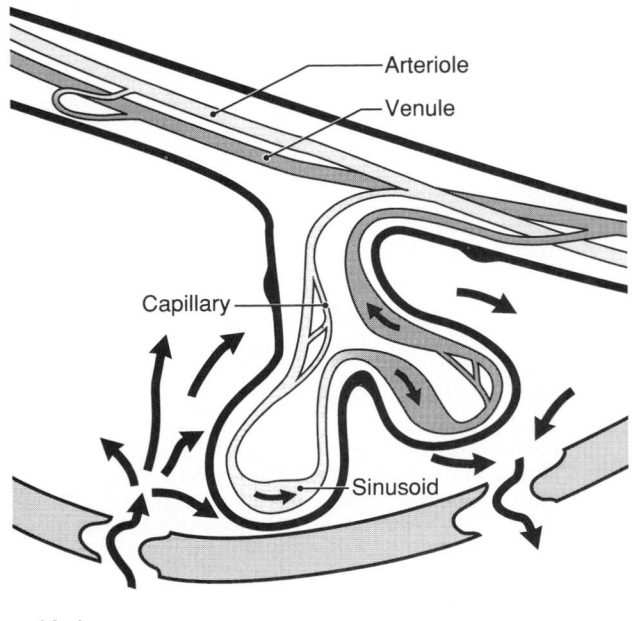

Mother

FIG. 10–3. Areas of concurrent and countercurrent flow exist in the intervillous pool flow system of the human placenta.

Stereochemical characteristics of a substance are major factors in transferability. Small, compact, nonpolar, lipophilic substances are transferred most efficiently. The placenta is relatively impermeable to large, polar molecules that do not have specific transport systems or carrier proteins or are unable to take advantage of an analogous transport system to aid in their transfer. For example, because succinylcholine is a highly charged molecule, there is minimal placental uptake and transfer to the fetus. However, cyclosporine, a lipophilic drug, is readily taken up by the placenta, partially metabolized, and quickly transferred to the fetus, producing fetal cyclosporine levels of about 50% of maternal levels (4). Bioactive cyclosporine metabolites in cord blood supersede maternal levels.

Alpha-fetoprotein (AFP), a 70-kd fetal protein, does not transfer to the maternal side in appreciable amounts despite large quantities in fetal blood. Maternal AFP is derived from transplacental transfer from fetal blood and transmembrane (i.e., chorioamnion) transfer from amniotic fluid. The fetal blood AFP level at 17 weeks of gestation is approximately 3 mg/mL when the maternal blood level is about 0.1 μg/mL, resulting in a fetomaternal gradient of about 30,000:1. The low level of fetomaternal transplacental transfer allows detection of elevated maternal serum levels from transmembrane (i.e., amniochorion) transfer of abnormally high amniotic fluid AFP, which provides the basis of maternal serum AFP screening for neural tube defects. False-positive elevations of maternal serum AFP (i.e., high maternal serum value

with a structurally normal fetus) suggest placental microabruptions or loss of integrity of the maternofetal barrier and forecast a higher rate of fetal morbidity.

Membrane characteristics regulate transport. The fluidity of the membrane, determined by the degree and character of membrane-incorporated phospholipids, influences transfer of certain substances. Diseases, such as diabetes, may influence membrane fluidity (5).

The major driving force in favor of transfer by diffusion is the concentration gradient across the placenta; the resistance to diffusion is dictated by the nature of the molecule. The principles of diffusion of molecules that are generally applicable to biological membranes hold true in the placenta, although specifics remain to be defined. Availability of a substance for diffusional transfer across the placenta is not always related to blood levels of that substance, because many metabolites, nutrients, and drugs that are poorly water soluble are protein bound.

Although proteins aid in delivery of these substances to the placenta, they may actually hinder transfer. It is the free, unbound, or soluble fraction of a substance that is available for transfer. Conversely, high-affinity carrier proteins on the receiving side of the placenta drive diffusional transfer to their side by decreasing a ligand's free fraction and increasing its maternofetal gradient. Oxygen, for example, is 98% bound to hemoglobin. It is the transplacental difference in the partial pressure (PO_2) of dissolved oxygen that determines the diffusion pressure. The more oxygen-avid fetal hemoglobin counterbalances the resistance to transfer from the maternal circulation. The O_2 content (i.e., dissolved and hemoglobin-bound O_2) of the blood on each side of the placental membrane is determined principally by different affinities of maternal and fetal hemoglobin for oxygen. In humans, the fetal oxyhemoglobin dissociation curve is displaced leftward of the maternal curve, facilitating a much greater uptake of oxygen by fetal blood at the placental capillary level than would be possible otherwise. At any given PO_2, a much higher O_2 content is achieved in fetal blood than in maternal blood. The O_2 content in the umbilical vein (14.5 mL/dL) is as high as that of the uterine artery (15.8 mL/dL) despite an umbilical venous PO_2 of only 27 mm Hg (Table 10–2). Relatively high fetal blood O_2 content confers on the fetus the ability to deliver sufficient oxygen to peripheral tissue despite low PO_2. Low PO_2 may be essential to fetal physiologic adaptation to maintain high pulmonary vascular resistance and to keep the ductus arteriosus open.

The excretion of bilirubin provides an example of fetomaternal interaction using specific permeability properties of the placenta to accomplish a given objective (6). Before birth, elimination of bilirubin from the fetus is by diffusional transfer through the placenta to the mother. The placenta is extremely permeable to unconjugated bilirubin but relatively impermeable to bilirubin–

TABLE 10–2. *Normal oxygen values in maternal and fetal blood*

Oxygen measurements	Uterine artery	Uterine vein	Umbilical vein	Umbilical artery
PO$_2$ (torr)	95	40	27	15
Hemoglobin O$_2$ saturation (%)	98	76	68	30
O$_2$ content (mL/dL)	15.8	12.2	14.5	6.4
Hemoglobin (g/dL)	12.0	12.0	16.0	16.0

Adapted from Longo L. Disorders of placental transfer. In: Assali NS, ed. *Pathophysiology of gestation.* New York: Academic Press, 1972;2:11.

glucuronide (i.e., conjugated bilirubin). In the fetus, because of minimal bilirubin glucuronyltransferase, hepatic conjugation of bilirubin is suppressed. Because fetal bilirubin is predominantly unconjugated and highly lipid soluble, it diffuses freely from the fetal to the maternal side. After transfer to the mother, it is efficiently conjugated and excreted (Fig. 10–4).

In mothers with erythrocyte hemolysis and unconjugated hyperbilirubinemia, there may be elevated bilirubin in amniotic fluid due to diffusional transfer of maternal bilirubin to the fetal compartment. The falsely elevated amniotic fluid Δ-OD450 may incorrectly suggest fetal erythrocyte hemolysis.

Facilitated Diffusion

Most substances cross the placenta by simple diffusion. Maternal glucose, the principal substrate for oxidative metabolism in the fetus, is a water-soluble, polar molecule that crosses the placenta by facilitated diffusion, which is a gradient-dependent, receptor-mediated, saturable process. Transfer of glucose by facilitated diffusion is supported by guinea pig (i.e., hemomonochorial) and human placental studies in which glucose transports more readily than other carbohydrates (e.g., fructose), even though the physiochemical properties of these carbohydrates predict equal transfer by simple diffusion. In

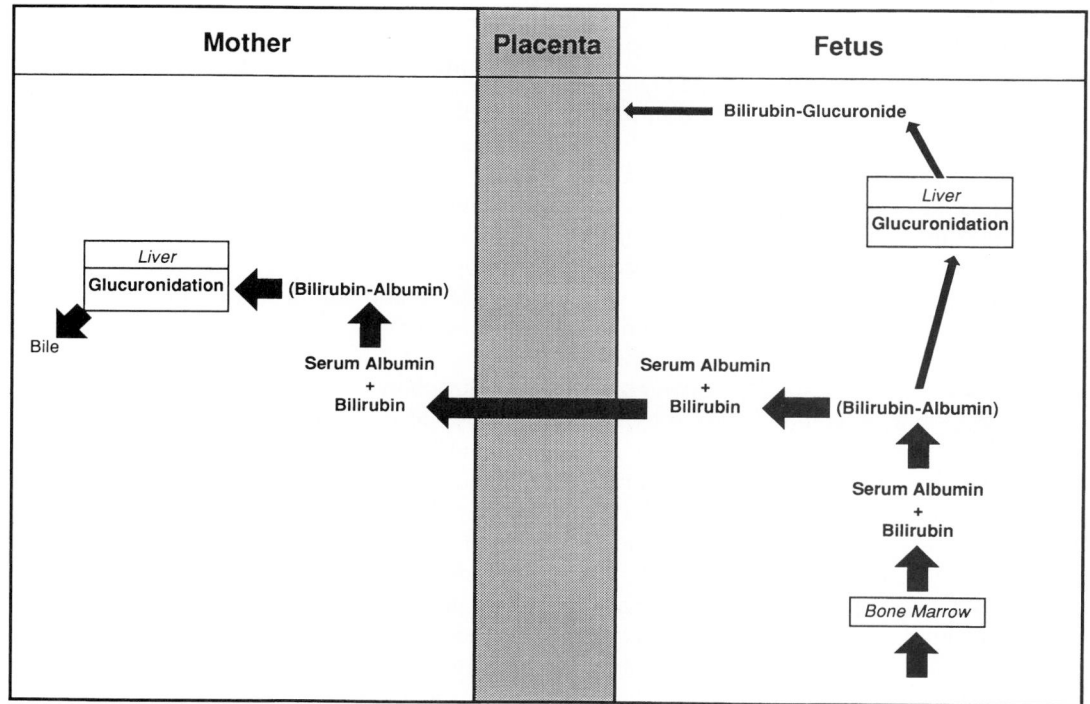

FIG. 10–4. Antepartum excretion of bilirubin. Fetal bilirubin is transferred from fetal serum albumin through the placenta to maternal serum. It then is conjugated with glucuronic acid by the maternal liver and excreted into the bile. Fetal glucuronidation is suppressed. The placenta is relatively impermeable to the glucuronide.

the human placenta, preferential transfer of D-glucose (over L-glucose) exists. Transfer stereospecificity implies a carrier-mediated process that provides the fetus with the appropriate isomer for metabolism. The presence of glucose transporter genes in the placenta that code for glucose transporter proteins confirms indirect experimental evidence for the existence of a membrane-bound D-glucose carrier protein (7,8). Under physiologic and pathologic human conditions, the carrier protein for glucose is not saturated, and the amount transferred to the fetus is directly related to the amount supplied to the placenta. Using vesicles made from the microvillous membrane of the human syncytiotrophoblast, Johnson and Smith (9) showed maternofetal-facilitated glucose transport with a K_m six times higher than the maternal blood glucose concentration.

Active Transport

To provide appropriate fuels for fetal growth, specific energy-requiring transport mechanisms in the microvillous surface aid in transfer of substances that are not readily lipid soluble and are required in large amounts by the fetus.

Most amino acids cross the placenta by an active transport mechanism (10–12). Active amino acid uptake has two major purposes: transfer to the fetus and placental production of peptide hormones.

Transfer from maternal to fetal circulation is especially important for the essential amino acids required for fetal growth, including the adult essential amino acids histidine, isoleucine, leucine, lysine, methionine, phenylalanine, threonine, tryptophan, and valine; and the proposed fetal essential amino acids cysteine, tyrosine, histidine, and taurine. Early in development, before maturation of fetal metabolic systems, all amino acids are essential to the fetus. Fetal amino acid levels are 1.5- to 5-fold higher than maternal levels, confirming a transport process against a concentration gradient.

Placental transfer of amino acids is stereospecific, with the natural L-form preferred. Transport of amino acids by animal cells is mediated by specific carrier systems that have overlapping substrate reactivities. In human villous tissue fragments, three carrier systems exist for neutral amino acids (13). System A is sodium dependent, reversible at low pH, and most reactive with amino acids that have short, polar, or linear side chains (e.g., alanine, glycine). System L is sodium independent and most reactive with large, apolar, branched-chain, and aromatic amino acids (e.g., leucine, isoleucine, tyrosine, tryptophan, valine, phenylalanine, methionine, glutamine). The ASC system is sodium dependent and is involved in transport of alanine and cysteine. Evidence suggests that a B system exists in placenta for taurine transport (14). Taurine, although produced by the maternal liver from cysteine and methionine, is essential for

fetal neurologic development but is not produced by the fetus.

Certain drugs cross the placenta by active transport. Zidovudine (formerly called azidothymidine [AZT]), which is used for treating human immunodeficiency virus (HIV), has been found in the perfused human placental model to cross from the maternal to the fetal side by energy-dependent transport (15). Because zidovudine is a thymidine analog, it may take advantage of placental thymidine transport systems. Zidovudine levels are higher in cord blood than in maternal blood, suggesting transport against a concentration gradient and an active transport mechanism. Maternal administration of zidovudine has become accepted therapy in HIV-positive mothers for prevention of vertical transmission to the fetus. In a collaborative, prospective study of pregnant, HIV-seropositive women, zidouvidine administered orally in the prenatal period and intravenously during labor was shown to decrease the vertical transmission to the fetus from 25.5% to 8.3% (16). Erythrocyte aplasia, a potential side effect of zidovudine therapy, leading to fetal hydrops due to severe fetal anemia, was not noted.

Iodide, calcium, and phosphorus are transported to the fetal side of the placenta by an energy-requiring process. Binding proteins within the trophoblast may be involved in calcium transport. Maternofetal transport of ascorbic acid is accomplished more efficiently than expected if by simple diffusion, and fetal levels are at least three times maternal levels, suggesting an active transport mechanism.

Receptor-Mediated Endocytosis

Although many large protein molecules cross the placenta by pinocytosis in extremely small quantities, specific receptor-mediated processes expedite transfer of certain larger substances that are required by the fetus. The receptor-rich microvillous brush border of the syncytiotrophoblast and the numerous coated micropinocytotic vesicles found just beneath it provide anatomic evidence for receptor-mediated endocytosis (17). The receptors involved in this process, found on the surface of the syncytiotrophoblast, are thought to extend through the glycocalyx layer of the cell membrane and bind to the protein clathrin to form a membrane complex. After the ligands are bound to their receptors, aggregation and internalization occur to form a cytoplasmic-coated vesicle (Fig. 10–5). Destiny of the contents of the vesicles depends on the ligand.

Maternal immunoglobulins are transferred to the fetus by receptor-mediated endocytosis. IgG subclasses 1 and 3 and IgA are known to cross the placenta. Once internalized, the intact immunoglobulin molecules within the vesicles are delivered from the cytoplasm of syncytiotrophoblast through the capillary endothelial cell and into the fetal circulation (18,19). Antenatal fetal transfer of maternal IgG antibodies may interfere with antibody-

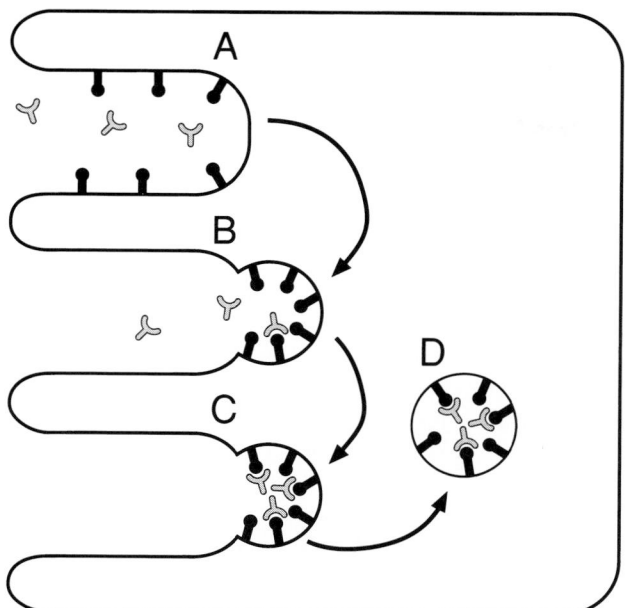

FIG. 10–5. Receptor-mediated endocytosis. The placental syncytiotrophoblast with the microvillous maternal border (see Fig. 10–1)has **(A)** specific receptors, located in the microvillous projections **(B)** clustering in intervening pits on exposure to specific ligand in the maternal blood stream. Endocytosis occurs. **C:** The receptor–ligand complexes and associated cell wall invert to form **(D)** an endocytic vesicle that is internalized. The destiny of the vesicle depends on the ligand.

based diagnostic testing in the fetus, necessitating analysis of fetal-specific IgM antibody. Developmentally, the transfer of maternal IgG to the fetus is probably protective and beneficial, but this transfer backfires in some situations, such as immune fetal hydrops (i.e., erythroblastosis fetalis) and alloimmune fetal thrombocytopenia. By receptor-mediated endocytosis, anti-D or another blood group antibody crosses the placenta to cause fetal hemolytic anemia, and anti-Pl^{A1} crosses the placenta to cause fetal thrombocytopenia (20).

Transfer of transferrin–iron complex into the placental syncytiotrophoblast occurs through receptor-mediated endocytosis. Brush border membrane transferrin-specific receptors on the maternal side of the syncytiotrophoblast bind transferrin–iron complex, and aggregate and internalize it to form vesicles of transferrin–iron complexes. In the cytoplasm, the complexes dissociate to form apotransferrin and ferrous iron. Apotransferrin is recycled to the maternal circulation, and ferrous iron is stored transiently as ferritin and released to the fetal circulation to be made into a complex with fetal transferrin. No maternal transferrin or placental ferritin is transferred to the fetus (21). Maternofetal iron transport is independent of maternal levels.

Uptake of low-density lipoprotein (LDL) cholesterol from maternal blood for progesterone synthesis by the placental trophoblast is accomplished through receptor-mediated endocytosis. Specific receptors that have a high affinity for LDL but not for high-density lipoprotein (HDL) are located on the microvillous brush border of the syncytiotrophoblast. LDL binds to its receptor and is actively internalized. Within the cytoplasm, LDL vesicles fuse with lysosomes, where enzyme hydrolysis of cholesterol esters releases cholesterol for mitochondrial synthesis of progesterone.

Other Mechanisms of Transfer

A variety of other mechanisms of transfer probably are functional in the human placenta. Large protein molecules may cross the placental membranes by a slow, non–receptor-mediated process of pinocytosis. Ions may cross placental membranes with the aid of ion pumps. Evidence suggests that small molecules and ions may cross through intercellular channels.

PLACENTAL METABOLISM

The placenta is a highly metabolic organ. Oxygen is consumed at a rate of 10 mL/min/kg, representing the amount of maternal oxygen needed to supply the placenta and fetus for metabolic functions. Approximately 20% of placental oxygen uptake is used by the placenta; the remainder diffuses to the fetus. Glucose, the principle metabolic carbon source of the placenta, is converted to lactate or oxidized to CO_2. Placental tissue requires energy for maintenance of active transfer systems, hormone production, and substrate metabolism.

PLACENTA AS AN ENDOCRINE ORGAN

It is the placenta that maintains the maternal milieu most favorable for pregnancy by elaboration of large amounts of steroid and peptide hormones, which are required to maintain the fetoplacental unit. Generally, placentally produced steroid hormones, but not peptide hormones, cross to the fetal side.

Human Chorionic Gonadotropin

Sensitive techniques demonstrate that the secretion of human chorionic gonadotropin (hCG) begins during implantation, when the cytotrophoblast differentiates into the syncytiotrophoblast. Although the messenger RNA for hCG can be found in the cytotrophoblast, this cell is thought not to be the origin of this peptide hormone, but only gains the ability to secrete hCG after it differentiates into a syncytiotrophoblast. The maternal plasma hCG level rises after implantation, peaks by 10 menstrual weeks of pregnancy, and declines to a nadir in the second trimester, after which levels remain low (Fig. 10–6).

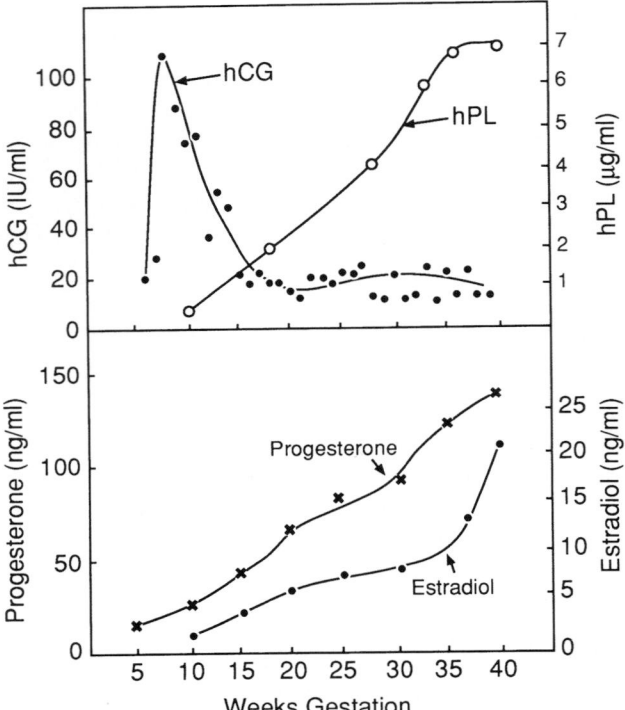

FIG. 10–6. Maternal blood levels of the major hormones produced by the placenta throughout pregnancy. (Data from Ashitaka Y, Nishimura R, Takemori M, Tojo S. Production and secretion of hCG and hCG subunits by trophoblastic tissue. In: Segal S, ed. *Chorionic gonadotropins.* New York: Plenum Press, 1980:151; Selenkow HA, Varma K, Younger D, White P, Emerson K Jr. Patterns of serum immunoreactive human placental lactogen and chorionic gonodotropin in diabetic pregnancy. *Diabetes* 1971;20:696; and Speroff L, Glass RH, Kase NG. *Clinical gynecologic endocrinology and infertility,* 4th ed. Baltimore: Williams & Wilkins, 1989.)

The only well-established role of hCG is continued stimulation of the ovarian corpus luteum to produce 17-hydroxyprogesterone for maintenance of pregnancy. Although placental production of progesterone occurs early in gestation, the transition to placental autonomy from the ovary occurs between 10 and 12 menstrual weeks. Before this transition, loss of the corpus luteum results in loss of the pregnancy unless exogenous progesterone is administered. Primary control of trophoblastic hCG production has not been determined, but hormonal modulation is apparent (22). There may be a role for hCG in the autocrine and paracrine control of production of other placental hormones. Proposed roles for hCG include the immunologic protection of the trophoblast and regulation of placental progesterone production. Falling levels of hCG before 10 menstrual weeks heralds pregnancy loss and is associated with miscarriage or ectopic gestation. Higher than normal hCG levels are seen with multiple gestations, hydatidiform mole, chori-

ocarcinoma, fetal triploidy when associated with molar changes of the placenta, and Down syndrome (23).

Human Placental Lactogen

Human placental lactogen (hPL) is a single-chain polypeptide that has about 85% similarity to human growth hormone. The quantity of hPL synthesized by the placental syncytiotrophoblast parallels placental mass, reaching its peak at term and falling dramatically after delivery of the placenta.

Functionally, hPL can be considered a fetal growth hormone, because it maintains the maternal metabolic milieu optimal for delivery of nutrients to the fetus. Despite its name, hPL has not been demonstrated conclusively to exert a lactogenic effect in humans. The physiologic role of hPL appears to be in shifting the pattern of maternal energy metabolism during pregnancy from carbohydrate to one that depends on fat. The hormone promotes adipolysis and increases free fatty acid availability for maternal metabolism, saving glucose and amino acids for transfer to the fetus. Free fatty acids do not cross the placenta as readily as amino acids and glucose.

Human placental lactogen has antiinsulin effects thought to be mediated by the elevated free fatty acids, which promote peripheral tissue resistance to insulin. The subsequent increased pancreatic production of insulin leads to down regulation of peripheral insulin receptors.

Maternal blood levels of hPL correlate with placental function. It was once thought that low hPL levels could predict pregnancies with deteriorating placental function and those with fetal compromise (24). Unfortunately, hPL levels are not as clinically useful as other methods. Similarly, elevated maternal hPL levels were thought to be predictive of gestational diabetes or outcome in preexisting diabetes, but large biological variations in maternal levels preclude its use in prediction or diagnosis. There are no clinical applications for hPL levels at this time.

Estrogen

Estrogen production by the syncytiotrophoblast requires an elaborate concerted effort by the mother, fetus, and placenta (Fig. 10–7). Because there is no activity of 17-hydroxylase and 17,20-desmolase in the human placenta, estrogen precursors must be obtained from the fetal adrenal gland. The placenta produces three major estrogens—estradiol (E2), estriol (E3), and estrone—which are secreted predominantly into the maternal circulation. Maternal estrogen levels increase with gestational age.

Little is known about the specific functions of estrogen during pregnancy. Estrogens effect many general changes in the mother to prepare for and maintain pregnancy. The uterine myometrium responds exquisitely with increased protein synthesis and cellular hypertrophy. Estrogens cause

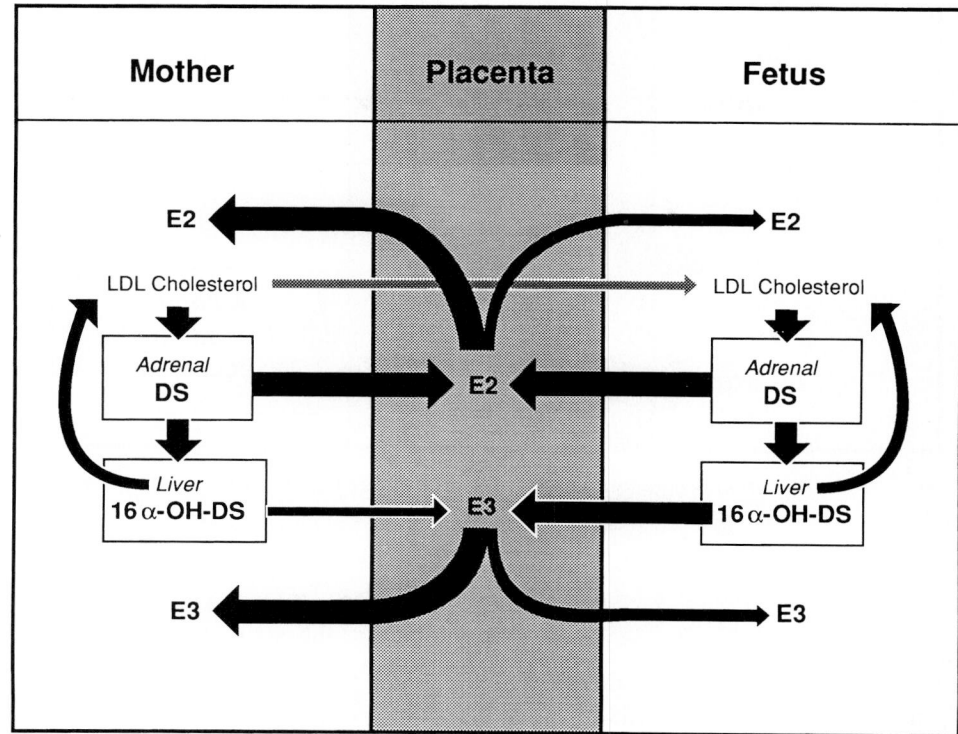

FIG. 10–7. Placental estrogen synthesis from fetal and maternal precursors. After 20 weeks of gestation, the fetal compartment supplies most steroid precursors for placental estrogen production. The fetal adrenal uses low-density lipoprotein cholesterol, produced by the fetal liver or transferred from the maternal compartment, to synthesize dehydroepiandrosterone sulfate (DS). Dehydroepiandrosterone sulfate is converted to 16 α-OH-DS in the fetal liver. Dehydroepiandrosterone sulfate and 16 α-OH-DS undergo placental metabolism to estradiol (E2) and estriol (E3), respectively, which are released predominantly on the maternal side.

vascular relaxation and increased blood flow to the uterus. Uterine contractility is increased by estrogens, supporting a role in the onset of parturition. Placental sulfatase deficiency, an X-linked fetal disorder, is associated with low estrogen levels. Except for dysfunctional labor, women with these fetuses have normal pregnancies. Fetuses with this disorder may develop ichthyosis later in life.

A specific role for estrogens in the fetus has not been determined. The fetal liver can metabolize E3 to estetrol (E4), which binds to fetal estrogen receptors but has no estrogenic activity, protecting fetal tissue from massive amounts of free estrogen.

Progesterone

The placental syncytiotrophoblast produces progesterone from maternally derived LDL cholesterol (Fig. 10–8). Fetal contribution to progesterone synthesis is minimal. Maternal progesterone levels increase with gestational age. The major role of progesterone is to maintain the pregnancy. Early production of progesterone is by the ovarian corpus luteum. After a transition period of shared function between 6 and 12 weeks of gestation, the placenta becomes the dominant producer of progesterone, and the pregnancy continues even if the corpus luteum is removed. Low levels of progesterone may be associated with first-trimester pregnancy loss.

The most important role of progesterone may be that of principal substrate for fetal adrenal gland production of glucocorticoids and mineralocorticoids. Progesterone may have a role in parturition and in suppressing the maternal immunologic response to fetal antigens.

Other Hormones

The placenta secretes a large number of proteins and peptide hormones into the maternal circulation, including human chorionic thyrotropin, chorionic adrenocorticotropic hormone, gonadotropin-releasing hormone, thyroid-releasing factor, corticotropin-releasing factor, and somatostatin. The exact functions of these hormones are unknown. Investigators have suggested that corticotropin-releasing factor may be involved in the onset of labor (25).

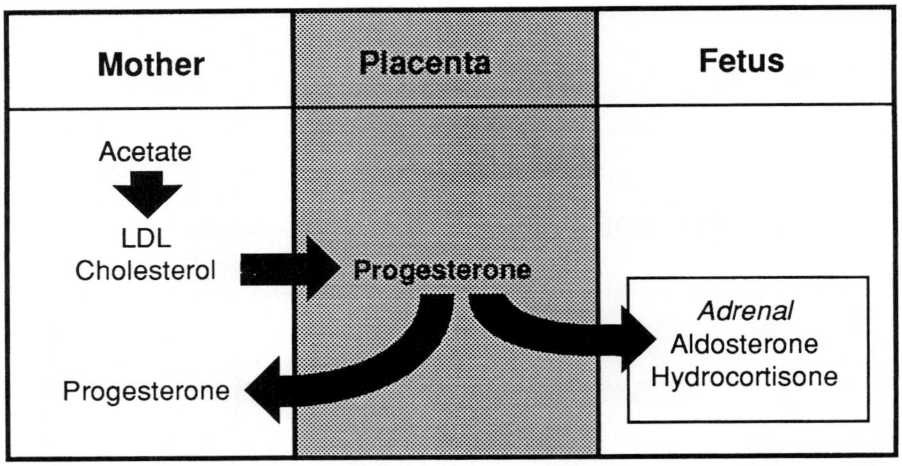

FIG. 10–8. Placental progesterone synthesis depends only on maternal precursors.

AMNIOTIC FLUID

Formation and circulation of the amniotic fluid reflect intimate and dynamic maternal and fetal interactions. Amniotic fluid is ultimately derived from maternal water. Very early in pregnancy, amniotic fluid is cellular transudate with the same tonicity but lower protein content than maternal plasma. By at least 8 gestational weeks, when the maternal and fetal blood circulations are well established, most amniotic fluid water is thought to be derived from maternal plasma water by direct transfer from the maternal circulation to fetal capillaries in response to osmotic and hydrostatic forces. Once circulating in the fetus, water is filtered and excreted by the urinary system into the amniotic cavity. By 8 gestational weeks, the urethra is patent, and the fetal kidneys begin to form urine; by 10 to 11 weeks, a fetal bladder can be seen ultrasonographically. Concurrently, the fetus begins to swallow. Swallowed amniotic fluid is reabsorbed into the fetal circulation to be reexcreted by the kidneys or transferred across the placenta to the mother. By the end of the first trimester, the amniotic fluid circulation has been established. Before fetal skin keratinization at 22 weeks, additional water transfer can occur directly through the highly permeable fetal skin.

Prolactin, produced by the decidualized endometrial cells, enters the amniotic cavity in large amounts by direct transport across the fetal membranes. Although undefined, amniotic fluid prolactin may have a role in regulating amniotic fluid volume (26).

The content of amniotic fluid changes over gestation. The early electrolyte content is similar to that of extracellular fluid. As the kidneys become functional, fetal urine electrolytes and excretory products become major components. As gestation progresses, the fetal kidneys mature and are better able to retain electrolytes and produce more dilute urine. At 20 weeks, the sodium content of amniotic fluid is 136 mEq/L and the osmolality is 276 mOsm/L; at 40 weeks, the sodium content is 124 mEq/L and the osmolality is 258 mOsm/L.

Amniotic fluid contains excretory products of the fetus and maternal products that can diffuse directly across the fetal membranes from the maternal compartment. In addition to electrolytes and proteins, amniotic fluid contains carbohydrates, amino acids, urea, creatinine, lactate, pyruvate, lipids, enzymes, hormones, and various other metabolites reflective of the fetal milieu. Their presence and the presence of desquamated fetal cells allow diagnosis of many fetal abnormalities by biochemical and genetic analysis of amniotic fluid. Amniotic fluid also contains fetal pulmonary fluid. The usefulness of the lecithin–sphingomyelin ratio in predicting maturity of the fetal lungs has its basis in contributions from this fluid. In fetal sheep, there is constant outpouring of pulmonary fluid into the trachea (27).

Although the range of normal amounts of amniotic fluid varies and depends on gestational age, abnormal volumes often herald fetal structural or growth abnormality. Maternal factors can affect amniotic fluid volume. Maternal plasma volume correlates with amniotic fluid volume. In hypovolemic mothers, expansion of plasma volume with albumin increases amniotic fluid volume (28). Maternal use of diuretics may influence amniotic fluid volume indirectly by decreasing maternal intravascular volume and directly by increasing fetal micturition after transplacental passage.

FETAL MEMBRANES

The fetal amnion and chorion, although simple in anatomic design, are intricately involved in fetomaternal interactions. The thin, avascular layer of epithelial cells that makes up the amnion arises from fetal ectodermal cells, and the chorion, several layers thick, arises from extraembryonic somatic mesoderm and a trophoblast layer. The trophoblast layer in the area of the chorion that is destined to be the fetal surface of the term placenta undergoes rapid proliferation and branching into villi. By 8 menstrual weeks, the trophoblast layer of the remaining chorion becomes compressed, attenuated, and microscopic. These microscopic cells are intimately intermingled with the outermost maternal layer, the decidua or gestational endometrium, to allow paracrine interaction of these cells.

Paracrine interactions of the fetal chorionic cells with maternal decidual cells may be involved in the control of maternal production of prolactin and amniotic fluid volume regulation. In 1977, Riddick and Kusmik (29) reported that decidua, an exclusively maternal cell line, synthesized and secreted a biologically active prolactin similar to pituitary prolactin. These investigators were able to show that decidually produced prolactin crossed the amniochorion and entered the amniotic cavity intact. Prolactin receptors have been found in the chorion but not in amnion. Transport studies with tritiated water suggest that the net transport of water by the chorioamnion with adherent decidua is greatest in the fetomaternal direction, suggesting a net outflow of water from the amniotic fluid compartment to maternal circulation (30). Lower osmolality in the amniotic fluid compartment favors movement of water from the amniotic cavity to the maternal compartment. Amniotic fluid prolactin decreases the permeability of the chorioamnion to water. Decidual prolactin production may be under amnion-derived prostaglandin control.

Indomethacin was shown to inhibit decidual prolactin production (31). Clinically, indomethacin has been associated with oligohydramnios and has been used to treat polyhydramnios (32). The cells of the amnion, rich in esterified arachidonic acid, are active in prostaglandin metabolism and are at least indirectly involved in cervical ripening and the onset or maintenance of labor. Initiation of human labor may involve autocrine and paracrine mechanisms within the fetal membranes and possibly maternal decidua, resulting in amnion cell production of prostaglandin E_2 (PGE_2), a potent cervical-ripening and uterotonic agent (33). Although amnion cell production of PGE_2 has been associated with initiation and maintenance of labor, control of its production is less well understood.

The role of the amnion in the onset of preterm labor is of interest. In preterm labor associated with intraamniotic infection, significant amounts of interleukin-1 activity has been found in the amniotic fluid (34,35). Interleukin-1, of monocyte–macrophage origin, functions as a mediator of fever and has a central role in the acute-phase response to infection and tissue injury. Interleukin-1 can stimulate PGE_2 biosynthesis by human amnion and may serve as the signal for initiation of labor in cases of intrauterine or systemic infection (36). Investigators suggest that other cytokines, in particular, interleukin-6 and interleukin-8, play a role affecting the common pathway of amnion cell production of PGE_2 and subsequent labor (37,38).

The chorioamnion produces a variety of other hormone products, including prorenin and renin, E2, progesterone, and hCG, although the rate of production of these hormones is less than that of their renal and placental counterparts. Neither the primary signals regulating secretion of these substances from the chorioamnion nor their specific targets have been elucidated.

UMBILICAL CORD

The umbilical cord contains one fetal vein and two fetal arteries, which are supported and protected by Wharton jelly, a gel-like connective tissue composed of a ground substance of open-chain polysaccharides in a network of collagen and microfibrils (39). Externally, the cord is covered by amnionic but no chorionic epithelium. The length of the umbilical cord ranges from 30 to 100 cm (mean 55 cm) with reported extremes from 0 to 155 cm. Fetuses with no umbilical cords have a severe, fatal abdominal wall defect due to failure of formation of the body stalk. The association of short cords and low IQ raises the question of whether the length of the cord is determined by fetal movement mediated by antenatal neurologic function. Fetuses with long cords are more likely to have cord entanglement. Short cords are more likely to stretch and avulse during descent of the fetus, resulting in signs of fetal distress during expulsion or hemorrhage at birth.

The normal umbilical cord increases in circumference with gestation until term, when the average circumference is 3.8 cm (40). Although excessive Wharton jelly (i.e., thick cords) has not been associated with fetal abnormalities, lack of this connective tissue has. Thin cords frequently are seen with growth-retarded fetuses and may be associated with cord strictures, umbilical vessel rupture, or thrombi (41). Thin cords are more likely to allow symptomatic external compression, stretch, or occlusion of umbilical vessels. Resolution of umbilical venous bleeding after percutaneous umbilical blood sampling is facilitated by Wharton jelly surrounding the vessel.

PLACENTAL PHYSIOLOGY IN DISEASE STATES

Preeclampsia and Hypertensive Disorders of Pregnancy

Preeclampsia, a hypertensive disease unique to pregnancy, has its genesis in the placenta. It is more common in women with multiple-gestation (i.e., multiple placentas) and molar pregnancies (i.e., excessive trophoblastic tissue), and it abates after delivery of the placenta. Altered placentation may be responsible for maternal vasospasm, the basic physiologic abnormality in preeclampsia. Vascular constriction in most maternal organs results in hypoperfusion of the uterus and placenta, making the fetus at risk for intrauterine growth restriction, placental abruption, and fetal death.

Placentas of preeclamptic women have a significantly lower total volume and volume of parenchymal and villous surface area than placentas of normal controls (42). There is a greater proportion of centrally located, infarcted areas due to poor intervillous maternal circulation. Histologically, cellular degenerative changes are found (43). An abundance of syncytial budding is common in histologic sections and teased preparations of villi. Budding, or knotting of the placental syncytiotrophoblasts, consists of bunching of the cytoplasm of these cells with aggregation of nuclei, a histologic finding suggestive of perfusional compromise.

The maternal vascular response to placentation is inadequate in women who develop preeclampsia (44). Normally, with trophoblastic invasion, spiral arteries of the placental bed lose their muscular and elastic components, which are replaced by a fibrinoid layer of irregular thickness. The uteroplacental arteries become sinusoidally distended from their origin in the myometrium through the decidua into the intervillous space, allowing optimal blood flow for maternofetal exchange. In preeclamptic pregnancies, the myometrial segments and some of the decidual segment of spiral arteries show no evidence of trophoblast-induced physiologic distention. Some spiral arteries show absence of physiologic changes throughout the entire length, suggesting a complete lack of invasion by trophoblasts (Fig. 10–9). Invasive trophoblasts from preeclamptic placentas have disorganized expression of adhesion molecules (45). In particular, preeclamptic tro-

phoblasts lack normal expression of integrin, a surface molecule important in trophoblast adherence and invasion into the endometrium. Disorganized trophoblastic integrin formation may be responsible for the poor endometrial and myometrial invasion seen in preeclampsia.

Certain spiral arterioles at the implantation site undergo acute atherosis. Initially, fibrinoid degeneration and mural thrombosis of decidual vessels occurs. The vessel wall then becomes replaced by fibrin, and the intima is replaced by cholesterol-laden macrophages. Eventually, fibrinoid necrosis and total obstruction of the lumen lead to loss of maternal blood flow, which is likely responsible for placental infarcts (46).

There are no microscopic or macroscopic placental changes that are pathognomonic for preeclampsia. The pathologic changes in placentas of preeclamptic women that suggest the disease are indistinguishable from those of women with lupus anticoagulant syndrome, suggesting a shared physiology. In the lupus anticoagulant syndrome, autoimmune antiphospholipid antibodies, detectable in the maternal blood stream, are associated with maternal arterial and venous thrombosis, recurrent miscarriage, early-onset preeclampsia, placental and fetal growth restriction, and fetal death. Placentas from these women, whether or not they show signs of overt preeclampsia, have infarctions, fibrosis, a decrease in vasculosyncytial membranes, and an increase in syncytial knots (47).

Preeclampsia is a disease resulting from abnormal maternoplacental interaction. The cause of preeclampsia is unknown. One of the most attractive pathogenetic mechanisms is that of an immune-mediated disease, supported by similarities with the lupus anticoagulant syndrome. However, in preeclampsia, neither the exact antigenic stimulus nor the antibody response has been defined, although the former probably is derived from trophoblasts.

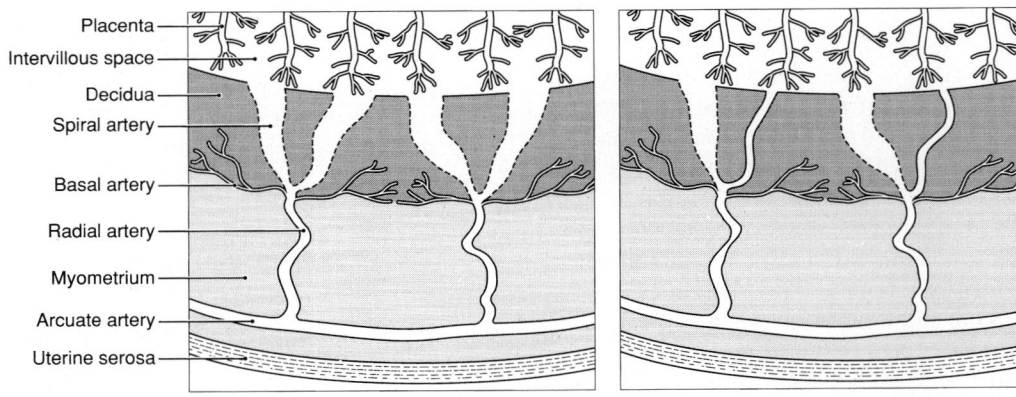

FIG. 10–9. Maternal blood supply to the placenta in normal pregnancy **(left)** and preeclampsia **(right)**. Notice the lack of normal physiologic dilation of radial arteries and of some decidual segments of spiral arteries in preeclampsia. (Adapted from ref. 44.)

Preeclampsia may be caused by placental production of a circulating humoral factor, perhaps immunologic, which affects prostaglandin homeostasis. Prostaglandins are involved in normal vasodilation of pregnancy. Prostacyclin (PGI_2), because of its potent effect in relaxing vascular smooth muscle and lowering systemic arterial pressure, is thought to be most involved. Prostacyclin is produced in vascular endothelial cells and is thought to exert its effect on vascular smooth muscle in a paracrine fashion. Prostacyclin is an inhibitor of platelet aggregation and an inhibitor of uterine contractility. The combined effects of this prostaglandin prevent maternal hypertension, prevent platelet aggregation, and promote uteroplacental blood flow. Thromboxane, produced predominantly by platelets, is a powerful vasoconstrictor, stimulator of platelet aggregation, and stimulator of uterine contractility, favoring maternal hypertension, decreased uteroplacental blood flow, and intrauterine growth restriction.

Abnormal prostaglandin homeostasis has been found in preeclampsia (48). Excessive placental production of thromboxane and insufficient production of PGI_2 result in an abnormally high ratio of thromboxane to PGI_2. Prostacyclin production is decreased in umbilical arteries, placental veins, and uterine vessels. Thromboxane production is increased in placental tissue and in circulating platelets from preeclamptic women with infants who are small for gestational age (49).

Higher thromboxane-to-PGI_2 ratios in the uterine vessels may be responsible for the abnormal maternal vascular response to placentation. Thromboxane in relative excess may decrease fetal blood flow to the placenta and cause shunting in the cotyledons; the umbilical arteries respond to these prostaglandins (50). Antiprostaglandin therapy in the form of low-dose aspirin for prevention or treatment of preeclampsia is based on aspirin's selective inhibition of thromboxane production. Initial clinical trials using low-dose aspirin have been successful (51).

Compared with normal placentas, placental findings in women with chronic or essential hypertension vary from lower total volume, lower parenchymal tissue, and infarcts to normal volumes and large, villous surface areas. Findings differ with various degrees of severity of disease and lack of differentiation between chronic hypertension and chronic hypertension with superimposed preeclampsia.

Diabetes

Just as the infant of a diabetic mother can be macrosomic, growth restricted, or normally grown, the diabetic placenta can have various findings. Some investigators have associated these findings with severity of maternal diabetes, especially the duration and complications of the disease, and others with degree of glycemic control.

Placentas of diabetic mothers without significant vascular disease (i.e., White's classes A–D) differ from normal by having more parenchymal and villous tissue, a higher cellular content, and a larger surface area of exchange between mother and fetus in terms of peripheral villous and capillary surface areas and intervillous space volume (52–54). These larger placentas are able adequately to support growth of large fetuses. Placentas of diabetic mothers with appropriate-for-gestational-age newborns are morphologically closer to control, nondiabetic placentas. It is the placentas of macrosomic infants that are heavier, predominantly due to a significant accumulation of nonparenchymal and parenchymal tissue. These placentas have retarded maturation of surface areas of terminal villi. Grossly, they appear large, thick, and plethoric. Microscopically, focal immaturity (i.e., dysmaturity) and villous edema are found.

The excessive growth and dysmaturity of these placentas suggest an accelerated growth process or a loss of the normal growth process that occurs in placentas of healthy women. Because the placenta is essentially a fetal organ different from other fetal organs only in that it is subject to more direct maternal modulation, it is not surprising that macrosomic fetuses have large placentas. The major mechanism for organ enlargement or macrosomia in the fetus of a diabetic mother involves anabolic metabolism of excess glucose and its deposition as glycogen and fat. The placenta of a macrosomic infant of a diabetic mother has neither excessive fat nor glycogen, suggesting a different mechanism by which the fetus (or mother) increases placental size and surface areas of terminal villi to maintain fetal nutrition, understanding that the size of the placenta and quality and topography of the transfer surface regulate nutrient availability to the fetus.

Placental cells respond to maternally or fetally produced hormones directly by alterations in growth and indirectly by elaboration of certain substances that control their own growth. Insulin and its associated family of growth-promoting peptide hormones, such as insulin-like growth factor I (IGF-I) and insulin-like growth factor II (IGF-II), have been implicated in affecting placental function in endocrine, autocrine, and paracrine fashion. These growth factors may be involved in excessive placental growth in the diabetic placenta.

Insulin receptors have been localized to the apical brush border of the syncytiotrophoblast (bathed in maternal blood) (55). Maternal insulin binds to these receptors, is internalized, and eventually degraded by this cell. Investigators using the *in vitro* perfused human placental cotyledon model have shown that placental facilitated uptake and metabolism of glucose does not appear to be regulated by insulin (56). The lack of insulin regulation of glucose transport in the intact placenta correlates with glucose transporter genes in placenta, *GLUT1* and *GLUT3,* both thought to code for insulin-unresponsive glucose transporter proteins (7,8). Why then is there active insulin uptake by the placental syncytiotrophoblast? Insulin, more likely fetal but possibly maternal, may have growth-promoting activity in the placenta and thereby effect placental size.

The placental trophoblast microvillous brush border membrane contains specific heterotetrameric IGF-I receptors that have been found in trophoblasts as early as 6 weeks of gestation (57). This somatomedin has been measured in placental explant cultures and placental fibroblast culture fluid and is thought to be involved in control of placental growth (58). Maternal serum IGF-I levels and the ratio of cord serum IGF-I to its binding protein correlate with birth weight (59). Cord serum IGF-II levels are 50% higher in infants of diabetic than in those of nondiabetic mothers. Because fetal macrosomia in diabetic pregnancies cannot always be prevented despite excellent maternal blood glucose control, attention has been turned to excessive placental transfer of fetal fuels other than glucose. Some investigators suggest a greater diffusional transfer of free fatty acids in diabetic pregnancies, probably related to greater maternal availability (e.g., maternal hyperlipidemia in diabetic pregnancies) and greater placental transfer surface (60). Excessive placental transfer of insulin-secretagogue amino acids (e.g., arginine) also may be responsible for fetal hyperinsulinemia and macrosomia.

Placentas of diabetic women with vascular complications (e.g., nephropathy, retinopathy, heart disease, White's class F, R, or H) frequently have infarcts and are associated with growth-retarded fetuses. The weights of the placentas of these diabetic women are lower than normal gestational age-matched placentas. There have been no specific placental findings to explain the higher stillborn rate in macrosomic fetuses of diabetic mothers.

Erythroblastosis

Erythroblastosis fetalis, or hemolytic disease of the newborn, is a condition in which specific IgG antibodies formed by the mother against erythrocyte antigens of the fetus cross the placenta by receptor-mediated endocytosis and coat fetal erythrocytes, causing their splenic sequestration, intravascular hemolysis, anemia, and unconjugated hyperbilirubinemia. Unconjugated bilirubin is transported easily to the maternal side, conjugated, and excreted by the mother. Anemia stimulates fetal hematopoiesis, especially in the liver and spleen, resulting in release of immature erythrocyte precursors into fetal blood. Severe fetal anemia causes fetal and placental hydrops, and often hypoproteinemia and thrombocytopenia. The placenta of newborns with erythroblastosis fetalis is pale and enlarged, displaying villous immaturity, edema, and an increase in Hofbauer cells (i.e., macrophages). Erythrocyte precursors are found in the vascular spaces. The severity of placental changes parallels the severity of fetal disease. There is ultrasonographic

evidence of reversal of placental thickening and edema as fetal hydrops improves with treatment.

Placental changes are secondary to the disease process and do not contribute to its formation. Hydropic placentas from fetuses with erythroblastosis fetalis are indistinguishable from those with other causes. In placentas of newborns with erythroblastosis fetalis, compensatory placental hematopoiesis, specifically in the villous stroma, is suggested because numerous erythrocyte precursors are found packed in fetal villous sinusoids mimicking de novo erythrocyte synthesis in the placenta. No specific erythrocyte synthesis occurs in the placenta.

Hydropic placentas produce elevated titers of hCG. Serum levels of this hormone are significantly above normal in women with hydropic fetuses and placentas (61). It is unclear whether this is due to overproduction of the hormone or normal production by larger placental cell mass. Other placental hormones, including hPL, are found in elevated quantities in serum of women with hydropic placentas.

Preeclampsia occurs frequently in mothers with fetal and placental hydrops. Reversal of preeclamptic signs and symptoms has been observed after fetal and placental hydrops resolved spontaneously or was reversed by fetal transfusion (62). Because hydropic placentas release greater amounts of placental hormones into the maternal circulation, this finding gives credence to a humoral placental product theory for the cause of preeclampsia.

Twin-to-Twin Transfusion Syndrome

Abnormal placental physiology due to congenital placental vascular malformations in monozygotic twins is the basis of twin-to-twin transfusion syndrome.

Although dizygotic twinning always involves separate placentas and membranes (i.e., diamnionic dichorionic), monozygotic twinning results in separation ranging from complete separation of the placentas and membranes (i.e., diamnionic dichorionic) to shared placentas and chorion (i.e., diamnionic monochorionic) to shared placentas, chorion, and amniotic cavity (i.e., monoamnionic monochorionic) to shared fetal tissues (i.e., monoamnionic conjoined).

Twin-to-twin transfusion syndrome is a disease of monochorionic twins. Extraembryonic somatic mesoderm lining the extraembryonic cavity of the developing embryo gives rise to the chorion and to the mesenchymal core of the placental villus and associated fetal vessels. Monozygotic twins who share chorions (i.e., monochorionic) also share fetal circulations by vascular connections. Fetal vascular anastomoses almost never are found on placentas of dichorionic twins, but they are usually found on those of monochorionic twins (63).

In monochorionic twin placentas, the normal 1:1 ratio between the artery supplying and the vein draining a cotyledon is lost. Haphazard vascular patterns exist

(Fig. 10–10). Certain cotyledons are supplied from a single or anastomotic artery from both twins and are drained by one or two veins. Others are supplied by an artery of one fetus and drained by a vein of the other. Drainage by the vein of the opposite fetus may not be obvious when capillaries join the venous system in a neighboring cotyledon before surfacing as a contralateral fetal vessel. An intertwin arteriovenous shunt should be suspected when an artery diving into a cotyledon is not accompanied by an adjacent emerging vein.

The most common fetal vascular anastomosis on the surface of the placenta is artery to artery, occurring in two-thirds of monochorionic placentas (64). Vein-to-vein anastomoses are the least common, occurring in only 1 of 20 monochorionic placentas. Arteriovenous anastomosis, or arterial supply with contralateral fetal venous drainage of a cotyledon, which occurs in about two-thirds of monochorionic placentas, is thought to be the most common placental lesion leading to inequality of blood flow and twin transfusion syndrome. Placental injection studies using contrast have been performed to ascertain vascular anastomosis, but injection studies only demonstrate the presence of anastomosis and do not establish overall inequality of flow.

In twin-to-twin transfusion syndrome, blood from the donor twin flows to the recipient co-twin through intertwin placental vascular connections. Remaining anastomoses are insufficient to allow return of the lost blood volume, and an imbalance of blood flow exists. The donor twin becomes hypovolemic, anemic, malnourished, growth restricted, and responds with oliguria (i.e., oligohydramnios) and, in severe cases, anuria (i.e., ahydramnios). The recipient twin becomes hypervolemic and plethoric, develops cardiomegaly and polyuria (i.e., polyhydramnios), and, if severe, develops cardiac failure and

hydrops fetalis. Grossly, the placental portion of the donor twin is anemic, pale, and usually smaller than that of the co-twin. If hydrops has not yet occurred, the recipient twin's placental portion is red, thick, and congested. After hydrops ensues, the placenta becomes pale from villous edema. Microscopically, anemia and villous immaturity are found in the donor's placental portion and polycythemia and congestion in that of the recipient.

Despite the high frequency of cross-placental vascular anastomoses in monochorionic placentas, the incidence of clinically evident twin-to-twin transfusion syndrome is only 5% to 10%. In some twin pairs, intertwin vascular connections may produce a chronic twin transfusion syndrome in which the larger twin responds with cardiac hyperplasia and hypertrophy (65). Cardiac hyperplasia may be compensatory, and certain sets of monochorionic twins may withstand the vascular inequalities throughout gestation (i.e., subclinical twin-to-twin transfusion syndrome). In others, the pumping capabilities of the enlarged heart are exceeded, and cardiac failure occurs. It is tempting to speculate that as the heart enlarges and fails, delicate pressure–flow characteristics in the placental vasculature are disrupted, exacerbating shunting to the recipient twin.

Twin-to-twin transfusion syndrome is a condition that begins early in embryonic vascular development. Benirschke (66) described the youngest example, a pair of aborted twin embryos measuring 7 and 8 cm (10 weeks of gestation) in which the heart of the donor twin was one-half the size of that of the recipient. Intertwin vascular distribution established early in the embryonic period may control intertwin placental mass distribution. Inequality in placental mass distribution may have an early, direct effect on fetal growth, causing significant growth restriction in one fetus. Antenatal ultrasono-

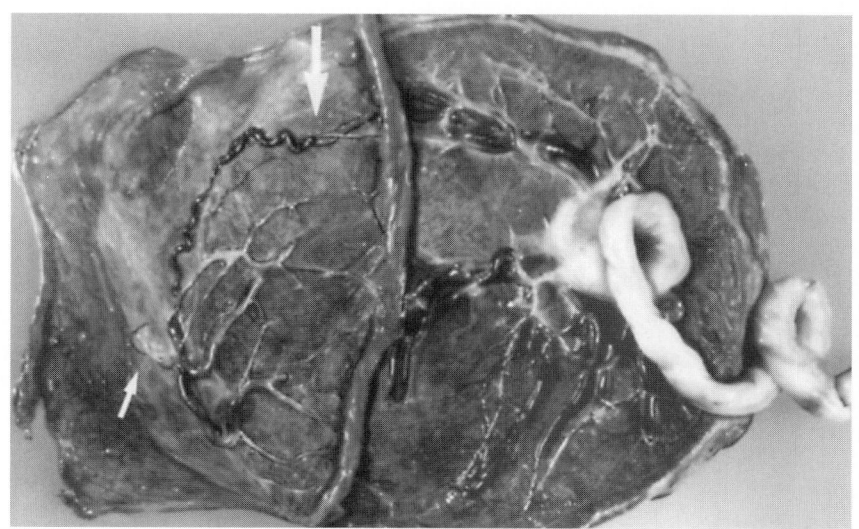

FIG. 10–10. Diamnionic, monochorionic twin placenta, with the intervening amnion rolled in the center. Notice the haphazard vascularization *(large arrow)*. The velamentous cord insertion *(small arrow)* of the smaller twin of this discordant pair is not an unusual finding in monochorionic twins.

graphic evaluation of the number of layers in intervening membranes has allowed diagnosis of chorionicity with high sensitivity and positive predictive value (67). The obstetrician can confirm chorionicity and assess placental vascular patterns immediately after delivery of the twin placenta and should impart this information to the pediatrician.

Some antenatal treatment approaches for twin transfusion syndrome attempt to reverse the abnormal placental physiology. Selective termination of one fetus, usually the donor, prevents further transfusion to the recipient. This treatment introduces risks to the living twin from passage of emboli from the dead twin through anastomotic channels (i.e., twin embolization syndrome). Serial amniocentesis to decompress the polyhydramniotic sac of the recipient twin has reversed twin-to-twin transfusion syndrome in a few cases (68). Loss of amniotic fluid pressure on a large placental vascular anastomosis allows changes in fetal blood flow. After amniotic fluid decompression of severe polyhydramnios, ultrasonographically observed placentas appear thickened and less stretched. Fetoscopic laser occlusion of placental vessels, reported by De Lia et al. (69) may prove to be the most logical therapy, because treatment is directed at the cause of the problem. At the time of delivery, the placenta is two discs, separated by an area of infarcted cotyledons previously supplied by the coagulated vessels.

Acute transplacental fetus-to-fetus bleeding can occur in monochorionic twins and is distinct from twin transfusion syndrome. Acute fetus-to-fetus bleeding occurs in placentas with medium- or large-caliber vascular anastomosis when loss of established pressure–flow relations occurs. For example, the death of one twin of a monochorionic pair may allow large shifts of blood from the living twin to the deceased co-twin. Shifts may be sufficient to cause anemia and hydrops fetalis in the surviving twin. If the deceased co-twin was the growth-retarded donor of a twin-to-twin transfusion pair, paradoxical plethora of the donor twin may occur.

Acute transplacental fetal bleeding may occur at the time of labor. For example, during the uterine contractions, umbilical cord compression may occur to a sufficient degree that it diminishes umbilical venous return but not arterial perfusion. The resulting higher resistance in the placental venous system of the cord-compressed twin favors return of blood to the co-twin. Acute intraplacental fetal bleeding may occur after delivery of the first fetus. Loss of established placental pressure–flow relations after clamping of the umbilical cord favors intraplacental pooling of the second twin's blood through anastomoses, resulting in hypovolemia. Acute transplacental fetal bleeding can create disparate newborn hematocrits that do not reflect hematocrit levels during fetal life.

REFERENCES

1. Ramsey EM. *The placenta:* human and animal. New York: Praeger Publishers, 1982:9.
2. Pridjian G, Moawad AH, Whitington PF. Handling of beta-hydroxybutyrate in the human placenta. In: *Scientific program and abstracts.* St Louis: Society for Gynecologic Investigation, 1990:230(abst).
3. Lind T, Aspillaga M. Metabolic changes during normal and diabetic pregnancies. In: Reece EA, Coustan DR, eds. *Diabetes mellitus in pregnancy:* principles and practice. New York: Churchill Livingstone, 1988: 75.
4. Venkataramanan R, Koneru B, Wang CCP, Burckart GJ, Caritis SN, Starzl TE. Cyclosporine and its metabolites in mother and baby. *Transplantation* 1988;46:468.
5. Neufeld ND, Corbo L. Increased fetal insulin receptors and changes in membrane fluidity and lipid composition. *Am J Physiol* 1982;243:E246.
6. Dancis J. Aspects of bilirubin metabolism before and after birth. *Pediatrics* 1959;24:980.
7. Kayano T, Fukumoto H, Eddy RL, et al. Evidence for a family of human glucose transporter-like proteins. *J Biol Chem* 1988;263:15245.
8. Tadakoro C, Yoshimoto Y, Sakata M, et al. Localization of human placental glucose transporter 1 during pregnancy. An immunohistochemical study. *Histol Histopathol* 1996;11:673.
9. Johnson LW, Smith CH. Monosaccharide transport across microvillous membrane of human placenta. *Am J Physiol* 1980;238:C160.
10. Yudelivech DL, Sweiry JH. Transport of amino acids in the placenta. *Biochem Biophys Acta* 1985;822:169.
11. Miller RK, Berndt WO. Characterization of neutral amino acid accumulation by human term placental slices. *Am J Physiol* 1974;227:1236.
12. Schneider H, Mohlen KH, Dancis J. Transfer of amino acids across the in vitro perfused human placenta. *Pediatr Res* 1979;13:236.
13. Enders RH, Judd RM, Donohue TM, Smith C. Placental amino acid uptake. III. Transport systems for neutral amino acids. *Am J Physiol* 1976;230:706.
14. Hibbard JU, Pridjian G, Whitington PF, Moawad AH. Taurine transport in the in vitro perfused human placenta. *Pediatr Res* 1990;27:80.
15. Fortunato SJ, Bawdon RE, Swan KF, Sobhi S. Transfer of azidothymidine (AZT) across the in vitro perfused human placenta. In: *Scientific program and abstracts.* San Diego: Society for Gynecologic Investigation, 1989:82(abst).
16. Connor EM, Sperlin RS, Gelber R, et al. Reduction of maternal–infant transmission of human immunodeficiency virus type 1 with zidovudine treatment. *N Engl J Med* 1994;331:1173.
17. Ockleford CD, Whyte A. Differentiated regions of human placental cell surface associated with the exchange of materials between maternal and fetal blood. The structure, distribution, ultrastructural cytochemistry and biochemical composition of coated vesicles. *J Cell Sci* 1977; 25:293.
18. McNabb T, Koh TY, Dorrington KJ, Painter RH. Structure and function of immunoglobulin domains V. Binding of immunoglobulin G and fragments to placental membrane preparations. *J Immunol* 1976;117:182.
19. Niezgodka M, Mikulska J, Ugorski M, Boratynski J, Lisowski J. Human placental membrane receptor for IgG-1. Studies on the properties and solubilization of the receptor. *Mol Immunol* 1981;18:163.
20. Bussel JB, Zabusky MR, Berkowitz RL, McFarland JG. Fetal alloimmune thrombocytopenia. *N Engl J Med* 1997;337:22.
21. Okuyama T, Tawada MD, Furuya H, Villee CA. The role of transferrin and ferritin in the fetal-maternal-placental unit. *Am J Obstet Gynecol* 1985;152:344.
22. Ringler GE, Kallen CB, Strauss JF. Regulation of human trophoblast function by glucocorticoids: dexamethasone promotes increased secretion of chorionic gonadotropin. *Endocrinology* 1989;124:1625.
23. Eldar-Geva T, Hochberg A, deGroot N, Weinstein D. High maternal serum chorionic gonadotropin level in Downs' syndrome pregnancies is caused by elevation of both subunits messenger ribonucleic acid level in trophoblasts. *J Clin Endocrinol Metab* 1995;80:3528.
24. Cohen M, Haour F, Dumont M, Bertrand J. Prognostic value of human chorionic somatomammotropin plasma levels in diabetic patients. *Am J Obstet Gynecol* 1973;115:202.
25. Riley SC, Walton JC, Herlick JM, Challis JRG. The localization and distribution of corticotropin-releasing hormone in the human placenta and fetal membranes throughout gestation. *J Clin Endocrinol Metab* 1991;72:1001.

26. Ross MG, Ervin MG, Leake RD, Oakes G, Hobel C, Fisher DA. Bulk flow of amniotic fluid water in response to maternal osmotic challenge. *Obstet Gynecol* 1983;147:697.

27. Adams FH, Fujiwara T. Surfactant in fetal lab tracheal fluid. *J Pediatr* 1963;63:537.

28. Goodlin RC, Anderson JC, Gallagher TF. Relationship between amniotic fluid volume and maternal plasma volume expansion. *Am J Obstet Gynecol* 1983;146:505.

29. Riddick DH, Kusmik WF. Decidua: a possible source of amniotic fluid prolactin. *Am J Obstet Gynecol* 1977;127:187.

30. McCoshen JA. Associations between prolactin, prostaglandin E₂ and fetal membrane function in human gestation. In: Mitchell BF, ed. *The physiology and biochemistry of human fetal membranes.* Ithaca, NY: Perinatology Press, 1988:117.

31. Maslar I, Rosenberg S, Riddick D. Diminished prolactin production by human endometrium exposed to drugs which inhibit prostaglandin synthetase. In: *Scientific program and abstracts.* Denver: Society for Gynecologic Investigation, 1980:277(abst).

32. Mamopoulos M, Assimakopoulos E, Reece EA, Andreou A, Zheng XZ, Mantalenakis S. Maternal indomethacin therapy in the treatment of polyhydramnios. *Am J Obstet Gynecol* 1990;162:1225.

33. Okazaki T, Casey ML, Okita JR, MacDonald PC, Johnston JM. Initiation of human parturition, XII. Biosynthesis and metabolism of prostaglandins in human fetal membranes and uterine decidua. *Am J Obstet Gynecol* 1981;139:373.

34. Keelan JA, Sato T, Mitchell MD. Interleukin (IL)-6 and IL-8 by human amnion: regulation by cytokines, growth factors, glucocorticoids, phorbol esters, and bacterial lipopolysaccharide. *Biol Reprod* 1997;57:1438.

35. Romero R, Mazor M. Infection and preterm labor. *Clin Obstet Gynecol* 1988;31:553.

36. Romero R, Brody DT, Oyarzun E, et al. Infection and labor III. Interleukin-1: a signal for the onset of parturition. *Am J Obstet Gynecol* 1989;160:1117.

37. Romero R, Duram S, Dinarello C, Oyarzun E, Hobbins JC, Mitchell MD. Interleukin-1 stimulates prostaglandin biosynthesis by human amnion. *Prostaglandins* 1989;37:13.

38. Romero R, Avila C, Santhanam U, Sehgal PB. Amniotic fluid interleukin 6 in preterm labor: association with infection. *J Clin Invest* 1990;85:1392.

39. Benirschke K, Kaufmann P. *Pathology of the human placenta,* 2nd ed. New York: Springer-Verlag, 1990:182.

40. Silver RK, Dooley SL, Tamura RK, Depp R. Umbilical cord size and amniotic fluid volume in prolonged pregnancy. *Am J Obstet Gynecol* 1987;157:716.

41. Robertson RD, Rubinstein LM, Wolfson WL, et al. Constriction of the umbilical cord as a cause of fetal demise following midtrimester amniocentesis. *J Reprod Med* 1981;26:325.

42. Boyd PA, Scott A. Quantitative structural studies on human placentas associated with preeclampsia, essential hypertension and intrauterine growth retardation. *Br J Obstet Gynaecol* 1985;92:714.

43. Cibils LA. The placenta and newborn infant in hypertensive conditions. *Am J Obstet Gynecol* 1974;118:256.

44. Khong TY, De Wolf F, Robertson WB, Brosens I. Inadequate maternal vascular response to placentation in pregnancies complicated by preeclampsia and by small for gestational age infants. *Br J Obstet Gynaecol* 1986;93:1049.

45. Zhou Y, Damsky CH, Chiu K, Roberts JM, Fisher SJ. Preeclampsia is associated with abnormal expression of adhesion molecules by invasive cytotrophoblasts. *J Clin Invest* 1993;91:950.

46. Zeek PM, Assali NS. Vascular changes in the decidua associated with eclamptogenic toxemia of pregnancy. *Am J Clin Pathol* 1950;20:1099.

47. Out HJ, Kooijman CD, Bruinse HW, Derksen RH. Histopathological findings in placentae from patients with intrauterine fetal death and antiphospholipid antibodies. *Eur J Obstet Gynecol Reprod Biol* 1991;41:179.

48. Walsh SW. Preeclampsia: an imbalance in placental prostacyclin and thromboxane production. *Am J Obstet Gynecol* 1985;152:335.

49. Wallenburg HC, Rotmans N. Enhanced reactivity of the platelet thromboxane pathway in normotensive and hypertensive pregnancies with insufficient fetal growth. *Am J Obstet Gynecol* 1982;144:523.

50. Tuvemo T. Role of prostaglandins, prostacyclin, and thromboxanes in the control of the umbilical-placental circulation. *Semin Perinatol* 1980;4:91.

51. Schiff E, Peleg E, Goldenberg M, et al. The use of aspirin to prevent pregnancy-induced hypertension and lower the ratio of thromboxane A2 to prostacyclin in relatively high risk pregnancies. *N Engl J Med* 1989;321:351.

52. Teasdale F. Histomorphometry of the placenta of the diabetic woman. Class A diabetes mellitus. *Placenta* 1981;2:241.

53. Teasdale F. Histomorphometry of the human placenta in class B diabetes mellitus. *Placenta* 1983;4:1.

54. Teasdale F. Histomorphometry of the human placenta in class C diabetes mellitus. *Placenta* 1985;6:69.

55. Deal CL, Guyda HJ. Insulin receptors of human term placental cells and choriocarcinoma (JEG-3) cells: characteristics and regulation. *Endocrinology* 1983;112:1512.

56. Challier JC, Hauguel S, Desmaizieres V. Effect of insulin on glucose uptake and metabolism in the human placenta. *J Clin Endocrinol Metab* 1986;62:803.

57. Grizzard JD, D'Ercole AJ, Wilkins JR, Moats-Staats, Williams JR. Affinity-labeled somatomedin-C receptors and binding proteins from the human fetus. *J Clin Endocrinol Metab* 1984;58:535.

58. Fant M, Monro H, Moses AC. An autocrine/paracrine role for insulin-like growth factors in the regulation of human placental growth. *J Clin Endocrinol Metab* 1986;63:499.

59. Hall K, Hansson U, Lundin G, et al. Serum levels of somatomedins and somatomedin-binding protein in pregnant women with type I or gestational diabetes and their infants. *J Clin Endocrinol Metab* 1986;63:1300.

60. Thomas CR. Placental transfer of non-esterified fatty acids in normal and diabetic pregnancy. *Biol Neonate* 1987;51:94.

61. Hatjis CG. Nonimmunologic fetal hydrops associated with hyperreactio luteinalis. *Obstet Gynecol* 1985;65[Suppl]:11.

62. Pryde PG, Nugent CE, Pridjian G, Barr Jr M, Faix RG. Spontaneous resolution of nonimmune hydrops fetalis secondary to parvovirus B19 infection. *Obstet Gynecol* 1992;79:869.

63. Robertson EG, Neer KJ. Placental injection studies in twin gestation. *Am J Obstet Gynecol* 1983;147:170.

64. Benirschke K, Kaufmann P. *Pathology of the human placenta,* 2nd ed. New York: Springer-Verlag, 1990:658.

65. Pridjian G, Nugent CE, Barr M. Twin gestation: influence of placentation on fetal growth. *Am J Obstet Gynecol* 1991;165:1394.

66. Benirschke K. Prenatal cardiovascular adaptation, comparative pathophysiology of circulatory disturbances. In: Bloor CM, ed. *Advances in experimental medicine and biology.* New York: Plenum Press, 1972:3.

67. D'Alton ME, Dudley DK. The ultrasonographic prediction of chorionicity in twin gestation. *Am J Obstet Gynecol* 1989;160:557.

68. Elliott JP, Urig MA, Clewell WH. Aggressive therapeutic amniocentesis for treatment of twin-twin transfusion syndrome. *Obstet Gynecol* 1991;77:537.

69. De Lia JE, Cruikshank DP, Keye WR. Fetoscopic neodymium:YAG laser occlusion of placental vessels in severe twin-twin transfusion syndrome. *Obstet Gynecol* 1990;75:1046.

CHAPTER 11

Fetal Ultrasonography

Dorothy I. Bulas

Improvement in high-resolution sonographic imaging has provided exquisite detail regarding the fetus and intrauterine environment. The ability to assess the health of the fetus and identify anomalies has changed the practice of both obstetrics and neonatology. By identifying the fetus at risk for intrauterine compromise, management can be guided by appropriate specialists with resultant improved outcome.

ASSESSMENT OF FETAL AGE, GROWTH, AND MATURITY

Accurate assessment of fetal age is crucial for perinatal management. Overestimating the age of a fetus can result in the delivery of a premature infant, whereas underestimating the age of a growth-retarded fetus can result in a fetal death.

Fetal age can be determined based on obstetric history and clinical data, but estimations can be inaccurate in up to 40% of patients (1). The use of ultrasound has provided a method of significantly improving the accuracy of gestational age determination. Measurements used to assess age have been chosen on the basis of their relationship with gestational age as well as for ease in obtaining the measurements and for reproducibility. The fetal biparietal diameter (BPD) measurement was the first measurement used because the cranium was the most easily visualized body part (2). As resolution improved, additional fetal measurements became available. There are currently many tables and nomograms that describe the normal growth of various fetal organs. Most predictions of gestational age are based on the 50th percentile measurement with a wide range of normal values. At the various gestational ages, each fetal dimension differs in how easily and

reliably it can be measured. Thus, a combination of measurements is superior to a single measurement, and there is computer software that permits instantaneous calculation of fetal age and weight estimates as well as plotting of growth curves. Functional studies of the fetus, such as breathing patterns, are also being evaluated to aid in the determination of gestational age.

Determining Fetal Age

First-Trimester Assessment

In the first trimester, fetal imaging using a transabdominal approach is often difficult because the uterus is low within the maternal pelvis and may be obscured by overlying gas. Transvaginal ultrasound transducers have greatly improved fetal visualization in early pregnancy. The probe is placed into the maternal vagina in close proximity to the uterus and fetus. High-resolution fetal images can thus be obtained for accurate assessment of fetal morphology. By use of transvaginal scanning, a gestational sac can be seen by 5 weeks menstrual age, and fetal heart activity by 6 weeks menstrual age. With abdominal scanning, these findings are first identified reliably a week later, at 6 and 7 weeks, respectively.

Crown–rump length is the most accurate dimension for assessing gestational age in the first trimester, with a 95% confidence interval of ±2–3.5 days (3–5). Measurement of the gestational sac diameter can also be used to estimate age, although it is not as accurate as the crown–rump length because of variability in the shape of the sac. Fetal biparietal diameter and abdominal circumference are also relatively good predictors of menstrual age in the first trimester but add little to the age estimate based on the crown–rump length (6).

Second- and Third-Trimester Assessment

After 12 weeks of gestation, the crown–rump length is difficult to obtain accurately. In the second and third

---

D. I. Bulas: Departments of Radiology and Pediatrics, The George Washington University Medical Center; and Department of Diagnostic Imaging, Children's National Medical Center, Washington, D.C.

trimesters, the main parameters of fetal age are the biparietal diameter (BPD), head circumference, abdominal circumference, and femoral length (Table 11–1).

The fetal BPD is quick, reliable, and easy to obtain. It measures the transverse diameter of the upper midbrain at the level of the thalamic nuclei and cavum septum pellucidum from the external surface of one proximal parietal bone to the inner surface of the contralateral parietal bone (Fig. 11–1) (7). The earlier the gestational age, the greater the predictive accuracy of the measurement.

Inaccuracies in measurements of the BPD may result from improper selection of the measurement plane (8). In late pregnancy, the fetal head may be too low in the pelvis to measure. Cranial molding, either from fetal position or oligohydramnios, may result in BPD measurements that do not accurately reflect true gestational age (Fig. 11–2). The cephalic index, which measures the relationship between the short and long axes of the fetal head, should be measured if the head shape appears abnormal. If this index is below 70 or above 86, the biparietal diameter should not be used in the age and weight estimates (9). The accuracy of BPD measurements decreases with advancing gestational age. In the second trimester, a BPD measurement carries a predictive accuracy of ±7 days, whereas in the late third trimester it carries a predictive accuracy of ±3 weeks (9). Serial measurements of BPD can improve the predictive accuracy (10). The fetal head circumference is obtained from the same axial image used for the BPD. This measurement is more accurate than the BPD in the third trimester, as it is less affected by shape (9).

The measurement of the fetal abdominal circumference is made from an axial image of the abdomen at the level of the portal vein. The circumference of the head is typically larger than the abdominal circumference up to 34 weeks of gestation, and the abdomen becomes larger thereafter. In the presence of intrauterine growth retardation (IUGR), head size tends to be preserved compared to abdominal size.

Femur length is defined as the distance between the greater trochanter and the distal end of the femur (Fig. 11–3) (11). Gestational age prediction from femur length is subject to error either from measurement difficulties caused by difficulty in visualizing the ends of the bone or

TABLE 11–1. *Relationships among selected fetal indices as measured by ultrasound and gestational age as determined by menstrual weeks*

Menstrual age (wk)	Biparietal diameter (cm)	Head circumference (cm)	Abdominal circumference (cm)	Femur length (cm)
12	2	7.1	5.6	0.8
13	2.3	8.4	6.9	1.1
14	2.7	9.8	8.1	1.5
15	3	11.1	9.3	1.8
16	3.3	12.4	10.5	2.1
17	3.7	13.7	11.7	2.4
18	4	15	12.9	2.7
19	4.3	16.3	14.1	3
20	4.6	17.5	15.2	3.3
21	5	18.7	16.4	3.6
22	5.3	19.9	17.5	3.9
23	5.6	21	18.6	4.2
24	5.8	22.1	19.7	4.4
25	6.1	23.2	20.8	4.7
26	6.4	24.2	21.9	4.9
27	6.7	25.2	22.9	5.2
28	7	26.2	24	5.4
29	7.2	27.1	25	5.6
30	7.5	28	26	5.8
31	7.7	28.9	27	6.1
32	7.9	29.7	28	6.3
33	8.2	30.4	29	6.5
34	8.4	31.2	30	6.6
35	8.6	31.8	30.9	6.8
36	8.8	32.5	31.8	7
37	9	33.1	32.7	7.2
38	9.1	33.6	33.6	7.3
39	9.3	34.1	34.5	7.5
40	9.5	34.5	35.4	7.6

From ref. 12.

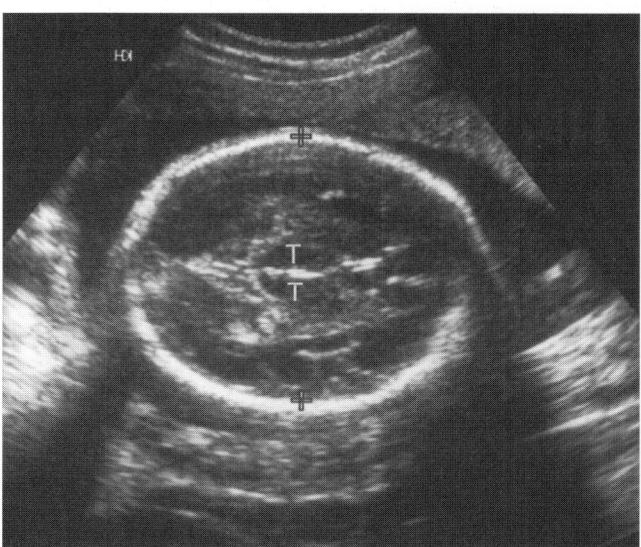

FIG. 11–1. Fetal biparietal diameter (BPD). Axial scan of the head at the standardized level for BPD measurement shows the thalami. Measurement of 6.9 cm is consistent with a 28-week gestation.

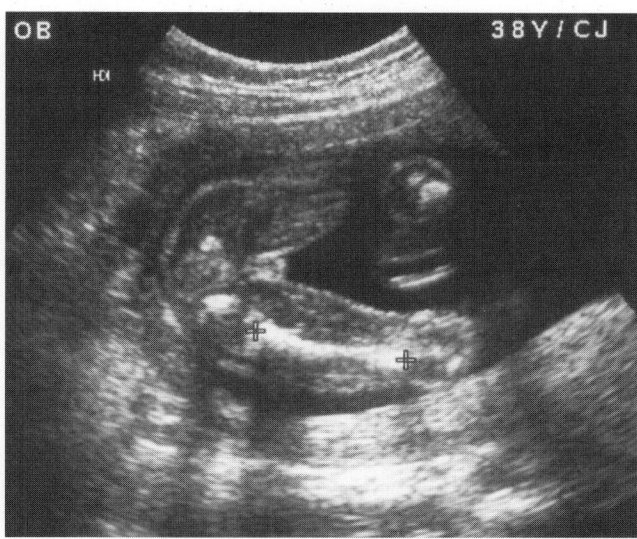

FIG. 11–3. Longitudinal scan of the fetal thigh demonstrates a femur length of 3.5 cm consistent with a 21-week gestation. Measurement is from the greater trochanter to the distal end of the femur.

from biological variation. The predictive accuracy of femur length ranges from ±1 week at 12 weeks of gestation to ±3 weeks at 36 weeks of gestation (12).

Estimation of fetal age is best accomplished using a composite assessment of multiple fetal measurements. A combination of head size (BPD or head circumference), femur length, and abdominal circumference is most commonly used. Estimates have an error of ±1.46 weeks between 24 and 30 weeks of gestation and increase to 2.3 weeks at 36 weeks of gestation (13). Individual measurements should not be used for assessing gestational age when they are affected by a pathologic process; for example, head measurements in a hydrocephalic fetus or long

bone measurements in the fetus with a bone dysplasia. After 22 weeks, age-independent fetal body ratios are useful in identifying asymmetric measurements. If the cephalic index is normal, the ratio of femur length to BPD can be measured, with normal results ranging between 71 and 87. The ratio of femur length to abdominal circumference should range between 20 and 24 (14).

Fetal Weight Estimates

It would be helpful in the assessment of fetal age, growth, and maturity if an accurate, reproducible method of determining fetal weight were available. Ultrasonographic estimates of fetal weight have been derived from single measurements such as BPD or abdominal circumference (15,16) as well as by a combination of measurements such as abdominal circumference and BPD (17). All ultrasonographic methods for fetal weight estimations, however, contain inherent error. Measurement of abdominal circumference yields an average error of 18.2% (16). The BPD and abdominal circumference yield a similar error (20%) (18). The absolute estimated error decreases as birth weight decreases.

The use of multiple parameters, especially head, abdomen, and femur measurements, provides the most accurate measurements of fetal weight. However, it is still not accurate in extremely low- or high-birth-weight fetuses. Because fetal weight estimates remain imprecise, estimation of fetal age based solely on estimates of fetal weight should not be used. Incremental fetal weight change can be determined with serial ultrasounds and is one way of detecting abnormal fetal growth (12). In the

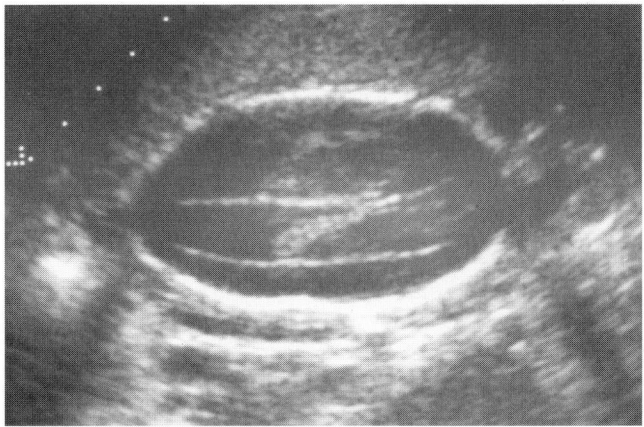

FIG. 11–2. Transverse image of the brain of a 23-week fetus with severe oligohydramnios demonstrates a narrow and elongated skull. Cephalic index was abnormally low.

future, three-dimensional reconstruction and volume estimates may improve the accuracy of fetal weight determination.

Assessment of Fetal Growth

Fetal growth abnormalities are often associated with increased risk of perinatal morbidity and mortality. The rate of growth in the normal fetus varies with gestational age, with an increasing exponential curve in the first trimester, a linear curve in the second and most of the third trimester, and a decreasing exponential curve after 36 weeks of gestation (19,20). Serial ultrasonographic measurements can be plotted to evaluate fetal growth and may include weight estimates derived from a combination of these variables.

Intrauterine Growth Retardation

The infant whose birth weight is below the tenth percentile for gestational age is considered small for gestational age (SGA). The population of SGA infants whose weight falls below the tenth percentile is heterogeneous. Normal but small fetuses represent up to 60% of the SGA group, fetuses with congenital anomalies account for up to 15%, and fetuses with true intrauterine growth retardation (IUGR) account for 25% (21). Management varies among these groups. The normal but small fetus is not at increased risk and does not require intervention. The small fetus with true growth restriction may be at high morbidity or mortality risk and may require immediate intervention. The small infant with congenital abnormalities may or may not require intervention. It can be difficult determining which group an SGA fetus falls into, particularly when the true gestational age is unknown.

Ultrasound's ability to identify the truly IUGR fetus is variable and is most successful when the disease state is severe. A slowing of the rate of head and femur growth is apparent with severe IUGR (22–24) but is more difficult to identify when the retardation is mild or early. Growth-adjusted sonographic age determination based on BPD or abdominal circumference (8,25) uses serial ultrasonographic measurements. This method assumes that fetal growth should remain within a narrow percentile band and that deviation from this may be an early sign of growth disorders (26). Because of the inherent errors, serial estimation of fetal weight identifies only the most severe growth disturbances. Asymmetric growth suggests IUGR. Abnormal ratios of head circumference to abdominal circumference, as a result of loss of liver mass with normal head growth, can be seen in severe IUGR but may not be present in milder cases (27,28).

Secondary signs aid in assessing the presence and severity of IUGR. Oligohydramnios often develops dur-ing episodes of uteroplacental insufficiency, most likely because of decreased fetal urine production and pulmonary fluid during episodes of fetal hypoxemia (29). Amniotic fluid volume may be assessed subjectively or by the semiquantitative method of measuring the vertical diameter of the largest visible pocket of amniotic fluid. Phelan, in 1987, introduced the technique termed the amniotic fluid index (AFI). The AFI is calculated by adding the vertical depths of the largest pocket in each of four equal uterine quadrants (30). Oligohydramnios has been defined by the absence of identifiable amniotic fluid pockets or when the maximum vertical pocket measures less than 2 cm in two perpendicular planes or when the amniotic fluid index measures less than 5 cm. Oligohydramnios as defined by any one of the methods is predictive of increased peripartum morbidity and mortality (30–32). Milder cases of IUGR, however, may not be associated with oligohydramnios (33).

Assessing fetal condition using the biophysical profile score (BPS) is another useful adjunct in the diagnosis of IUGR (see below) (34). If a fetus who is being followed for IUGR has no signs of asphyxial compromise, continued observation rather than intervention may be reasonable.

Macrosomia

The infant whose birth weight is above the 90th percentile for gestational age is labeled large for dates (LGA) or macrosomic. This group of large infants is heterogeneous, composed of normal but large infants as well as infants with abnormally increased growth. Macrosomia is usually associated with maternal glucose abnormalities. Macrosomia may lead to obstetric complications such as shoulder dystocia, and maternal diabetes may cause neonatal complications such as hypoglycemia, polycythemia, and cardiac abnormalities. Detection of macrosomia sonographically includes serial assessment of growth and the relationship of the variables. The ratio of abdominal circumference to head circumference is particularly useful in identifying an enlarging abdomen indicative of excessive weight gain. Other measurements have been proposed to aid in the diagnosis of macrosomia, including soft tissue thickness of the humerus or femur and cheek-to-cheek diameter (35).

Fetal Maturity

The sonographic assessment of fetal maturity is useful in the optimal timing of perinatal management. The perinatologist must maintain a balance between the risk of fetal death and the risk of neonatal death based on an estimate of whether a fetus has reached an age and weight at which lung maturity is possible. Fetal age and weight determinations, evaluation of placental architecture, and the biophysical profile have been used to assess fetal maturity. Studies on elective deliveries based on BPD, or weight estimates based on BPD and abdominal circumference, have shown good results (36–38). The grading of placental maturity sonographically, however, has not been shown to be as accurate as the lecithin/sphingomyelin (L/S) ratio in assessing lung maturity (39).

FETAL ANATOMY

Congenital anomalies are present in 2% to 5% of newborns and account for 20% to 30% of perinatal deaths (21). High-resolution ultrasonography has produced significant changes in the diagnosis and management of these anomalies, including the potential for therapeutic intervention. Factors to be considered in the counseling of these cases include gestational age, effect on maternal outcome, and neonatal prognosis with or without therapy.

A comprehensive review of the fetus should be performed, followed by evaluation of amniotic fluid volume, cord structure, and the placenta. A functional review of the fetus including hand clenching and swallowing is informative. Because some anomalies may not become evident until later in gestation (i.e., progressive hydrocephalus, congenital diaphragmatic hernia), follow-up evaluation of the fetus at risk is important. Transvaginal sonography and three-dimensional sonographic imaging have provided a means of improved visualization of fetal anomalies, particularly of the face and brain. Magnetic resonance imaging (MRI) may be used for complex cases that require confirmation of findings (40,41). Amniocentesis should be considered in cases at risk for a chromo-somal anomaly. Appropriate specialists can aid in the counseling of families when difficult decisions must be made with regard to early and potentially invasive intervention. The neonatologist can be an important consultant in the planning of optimal timing and location of delivery.

Fetal Central Nervous System Abnormalities

Fetal CNS abnormalities may be detected in the first trimester in severe cases such as anencephaly. The most favorable time to evaluate the fetal neural axis, however, is 18 to 24 weeks of gestation, when resolution is sufficient to identify most structures including the spine. Abnormal measurements of BPD and head circumference may be the first suggestion of a CNS abnormality. Structural evaluation includes the shape and size of the head, ventricles, and posterior fossa as well as an evaluation of the spine. If a CNS anomaly is identified, careful evaluation for other anomalies, especially of the face, heart, and kidneys, follows.

The ventricular diameter normally measures less than 10 mm throughout the second and third trimesters (42,43). Other criteria of ventriculomegaly include separation of choroid plexus from the medial ventricular wall. If the diagnosis of ventriculomegaly is established, a search for its etiology should be made. A differential diagnosis ranges from cerebral atrophy (hydranencephaly, porencephaly (Fig. 11–4), dysgenesis (holoprosencephaly, agenesis of the corpus callosum), to true hydrocephalus.

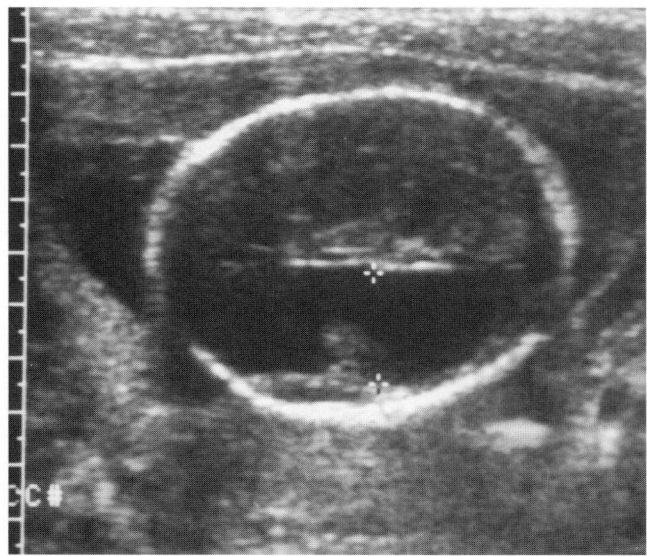
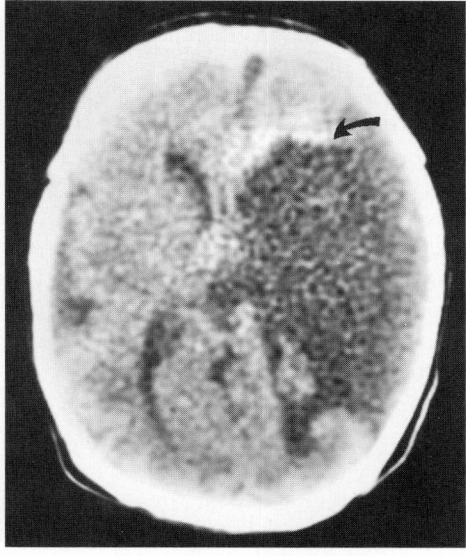

FIG. 11–4. A: Axial sonogram of the brain at 29 weeks of gestation demonstrates unilateral dilatation of the left lateral ventricle *(cursers).* **B:** Follow-up CT scan at birth confirms the finding of left hemispheric porencephaly *(arrow).*

Hydrocephalus

Hydrocephalus can be caused by an increased rate of CSF formation as in choroid plexus papilloma, decreased resorption of CSF after hemorrhage, or obstruction of CSF flow as a result of tumor or aqueductal stenosis (44). In many cases, the etiology of hydrocephalus remains unknown. Up to 85% of cases are associated with other neurologic, cardiac, renal, gastrointestinal, or skeletal anomalies. Up to 10% are associated with chromosomal abnormalities (45). Fetuses with other anatomic or chromosomal abnormalities have a grim prognosis for long-term development. When ventriculomegaly is mild, and no associated abnormalities are identified, outcome is less severe. Up to 20% of these cases, however, may demonstrate neurologic abnormalities later in life (46,47).

Neural Tube Defects

The most common condition leading to ventriculomegaly is spina bifida. Evaluation of the fetal spine and cerebellum allows prenatal identification of over 95% of fetuses with meningomyeloceles. Screening programs using maternal serum alpha-fetoprotein identify pregnancies at risk for neural tube or ventral wall defects. Sonographic findings of meningomyelocele include splaying of pedicles, presence of a cystic collection posterior to the fetal spine with absent skin covering, and scoliosis. Because of the difficulty in identifying small spinal defects prenatally, the association of cranial abnormalities is useful in evaluating cases at risk. The Arnold-Chiari malformation, which often accompanies spina bifida, results in the herniation of the cerebellum through the foramen magnum into the upper cervical spinal canal. Cranial sonographic findings of this malformation include frontal bone scalloping (lemon sign), abnormal curvature of the cerebellum (banana sign), and obliteration of the cisterna magna (48,49).

Cranial defects involving brain and meninges (encephalocele) or meninges (meningocele) may present with ventriculomegaly. Typically on ultrasonography there is a posterior paracranial mass that is cystic or solid. It is important to identify a true skull defect because the diagnosis can be confused with scalp edema, cystic hygroma, or scalp hemangiomas, which carry a better prognosis (50). Because encephalocele is a feature of other syndromes including Meckel-Gruber, additional anomalies should be excluded (51–53).

Fetal Chest Abnormalities

Most major intrathoracic structures can be identified sonographically by the second trimester. A small chest circumference suggests pulmonary hypoplasia in the presence of oligohydramnios or skeletal dysplasia (54). Pleural effusions appear as fluid collections surrounding collapsed echogenic lung (Fig. 11–5). Effusions may be primary in chylothorax or secondary in nonimmune hydrops. In the presence of effusions, prognosis is variable, with 15% mortality if an effusion is isolated but up to 95% mortality if it is associated with severe hydrops (55,56).

The normal fetal mediastinum lies in the center of the chest, anterior to the spine, with the cardiac interventricular septum forming a 45-degree angle with the midline. Deviation of this axis or shift of the heart suggests a mass effect or cardiac pathology.

Fetal lung parenchyma should be homogeneously echogenic. If it is heterogenous and/or there is shift of midline structures, a chest mass is likely. Sonographic findings will vary depending on the type of chest mass. Cystic adenomatoid malformations (CCAM) type 1 are the most common and appear as a single or multiple macrocysts. Type 2 CCAM contain small cysts less than 1 cm in size and are often associated with other anomalies. Type 3 CCAM contain multiple microcysts that appear sonographically as a homogeneously echogenic mass (57,58). Sequestrations are intralobar or extralobar masses of pulmonary tissue that lack a tracheobronchial communication and have a vascular supply from the aorta. They present as a solid or mixed solid and cystic mass in the inferior portion of the chest (59). Up to 25% have a CCAM component that may be cystic. With color Doppler, a vessel can often be seen coursing from the aorta to feed the mass, confirming the diagnosis. Bronchogenic cysts typically present as a simple mediastinal or lower lobe cyst without a feeding vessel (60).

Prognosis depends on the size of the intrathoracic mass because marked lung compression during fetal development leads to hypoplastic lungs. Polyhydramnios, ascites, and hydrops are likely secondary to compression of the

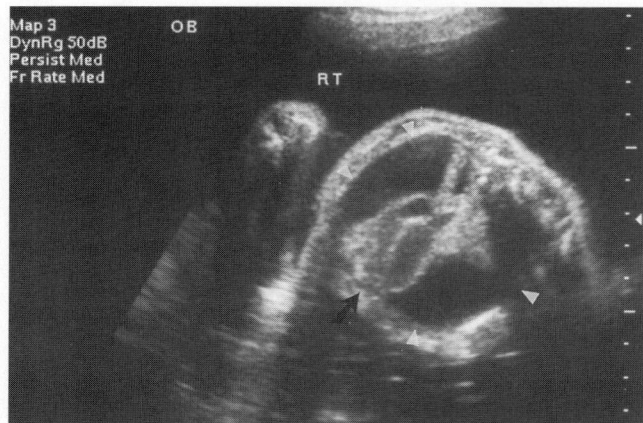

FIG. 11–5. Transverse image through the chest of a 25-week fetus demonstrates bilateral large pleural effusions (white arrowheads). The heart (black arrow) is slightly deviated to the right.

esophagus and vena cava and correlate with poor outcome (57). Type 3 CCAM tend to have the worst prognosis. The prenatal placement of shunts in cysts or pleura has resulted in some success in lung reexpansion (61). Spontaneous resolution of pleural effusions and pulmonary masses *in utero* has been reported (Fig. 11–6) (56–58). Prenatal therapy is reserved for those cases at highest risk for poor outcome (i.e., hydrops) (57,61–63). A fetus with a lung mass has an excellent prognosis if there is no hydrops and only minimal pulmonary hypoplasia (63).

Congenital Diaphragmatic Hernia

When a fetal thoracic mass is identified, the differential diagnosis includes congenital diaphragmatic hernia. This defect results from incomplete fusion of the pleuroperitoneal membranes during the seventh week of gestation. Passage of bowel and liver may occur into the thorax at any time during pregnancy. Sonographic findings include contralateral mediastinal shift and fluid-filled loops of bowel within the chest that mimic pulmonary "cystic" masses (Fig. 11–7). Findings specific to CDH include absence of an intraabdominal stomach bubble or loops of bowel within the chest. Doppler flow studies demonstrating mesenteric vessels extending into the hemithorax confirm the diagnosis. Bowing of the umbilical portion of the portal vein suggests liver herniation. Associated anomalies often present include cardiac, genitourinary, CNS, and gastrointestinal. Other conditions associated with congenital diaphragmatic hernia are Fryns' syndrome with nuchal thickening and limb anomalies and Pallister Killian syndrome (64).

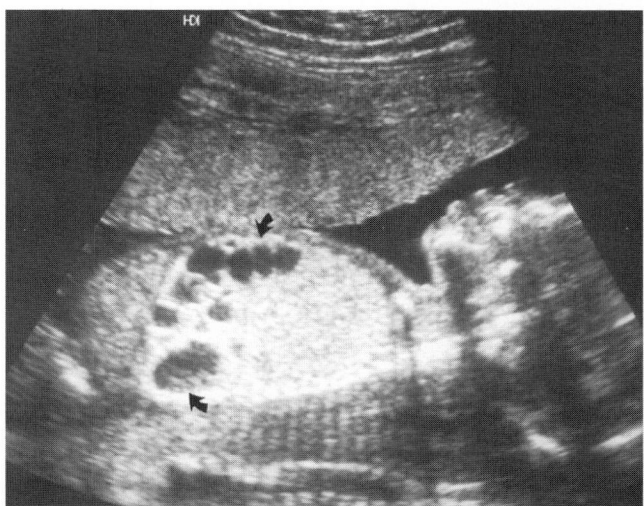

FIG. 11–6. Cystic adenomatoid malformation. Sagittal image of the left fetal chest at 26 weeks of gestation demonstrates multiple cysts *(arrows)* within the left hemithorax dispersed between unusually echogenic lung parenchyma.

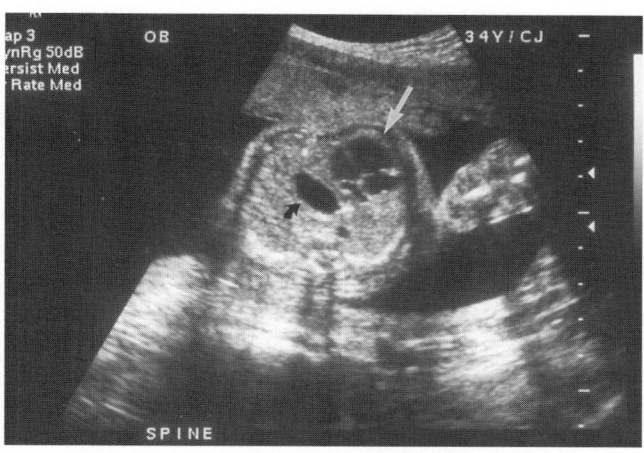

FIG. 11–7. Congenital diaphragmatic hernia. Transverse image through the chest of a 23-week fetus demonstrates the heart *(white arrow)* to be shifted to the right by a herniated fluid-filled stomach *(black arrow)*.

Further evaluation includes fetal chromosomal analysis and fetal echocardiograms. Serial sonograms every 2 to 4 weeks are useful because up to 75% of cases develop polyhydramnios, and all are at risk for IUGR (65). The mortality rate for infants with diaphragmatic hernia is variable. Cases with multiple anomalies, particularly cardiac, are likely to be lethal. Less clear is whether sonographic findings such as marked mediastinal shift, IUGR, hydrops, and polyhydramnios predict uniformly poor outcome (65,66). Ratios of right lung area to head circumference and the presence of liver in the chest appear most useful in identifying which cases carry the poorest prognosis (67–69). An MRI examination can confirm the location of the liver within the chest (40).

Congenital Heart Disease

Congenital heart disease is one of the most commonly recognized birth defects with a reported frequency of 0.8%. Any woman with a risk factor for a cardiac anomaly should undergo a detailed ultrasound examination of the fetal heart. Risk factors include nonimmune hydrops, suspected abnormality by screening sonogram, teratogen exposure, parental or sibling heart defect, aneuploidy, extracardiac anomalies, maternal diabetes, and fetal arrhythmia (70).

Detailed cardiac evaluation is difficult before 18 weeks of gestation. Examination includes visualization of the four chambers and outflow tracts. A dedicated fetal echocardiogram requires additional cross-sectional views to demonstrate fetal heart integrity. M-mode echocardiography measures chamber size, wall thickness, and wall motion and facilitates cardiac rhythm assessment. Pulsed Doppler and color flow Doppler are useful to define blood flow. Sensitivity in detecting anomalies is dependent on fetal position, maternal size, and amniotic fluid volume as well as equipment and expertise. Ventricular septal defects, anomalous pulmonary venous return, and aortic or pulmonic stenosis are especially difficult to diagnose. Ott, in 1995, reported a 14% sensitivity for detection of congenital heart disease in a low-risk population compared with a 63% sensitivity in the high-risk group (71). Heart disease diagnosed prenatally is often severe and associated with a poor long-term prognosis with chromosomal or extracardiac structural defects often present (72).

Fetal Gastrointestinal Tract

The ultrasound appearance of fetal bowel varies, with significant overlap between normal and abnormal patterns (73). The stomach is first visualized at 13 to 16 weeks of gestation. If it is not identified by 16 weeks, especially in the presence of polyhydramnios, an abnormality such as esophageal atresia or congenital diaphragmatic hernia should be suspected (74). The esophagus is typically collapsed and not visualized by US, but the absence of a fluid-filled stomach and presence of polyhydramnios and a dilated proximal pouch are findings suggestive of esophageal atresia. In cases of tracheoesophageal fistula, 70% have a fluid-filled stomach, with polyhydramnios developing in only 60% of cases. Thus, sonographic detection of TEF in unlikely (75).

When an enlarged fluid-filled duodenum and stomach are identified, duodenal obstruction is present. Duodenal atresia is the most common cause, but the differential diagnosis includes annular pancreas, duodenal stenosis, or Ladd's bands. Up to 30% of fetuses with isolated duodenal atresia have trisomy 21, so chromosome analysis and fetal echocardiography are indicated. Serial sonograms will indicate development of polyhydramnios or IUGR.

In a normal fetus, small bowel is only occasionally visualized, and loops measuring over 7 mm in diameter are considered abnormal and suggestive of obstruction (76) (Fig. 11–8). Differential diagnosis includes a duplication cyst, mesenteric cyst, ovarian cyst, and hydroure-

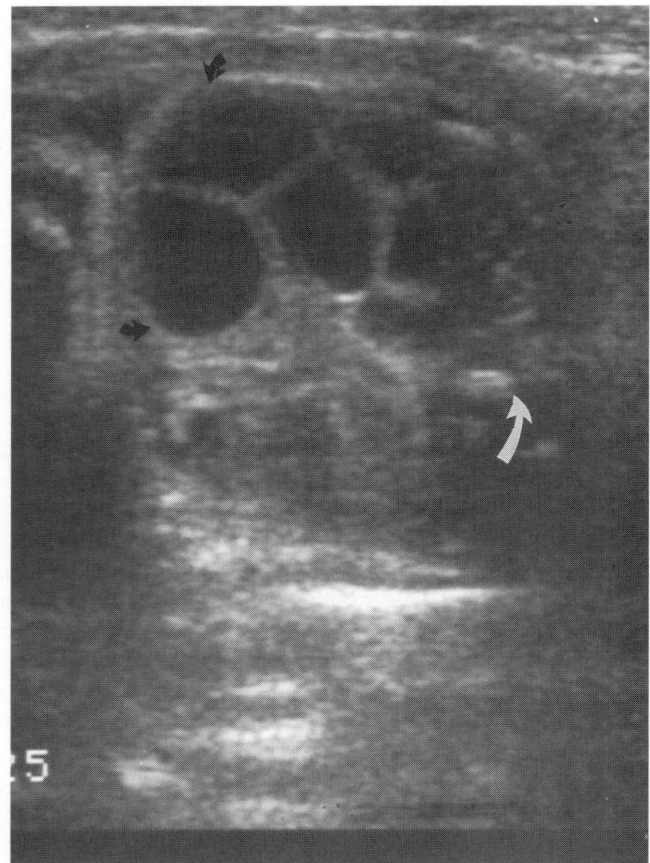 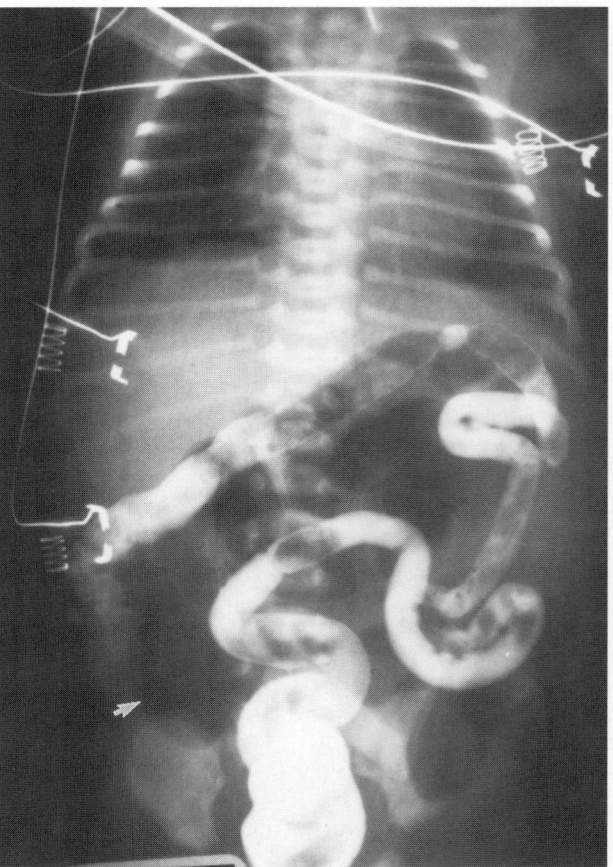

A   B

FIG. 11–8. A: Transverse image of a 33-week gestation fetal abdomen demonstrates multiple dilated loops of bowel *(black arrowheads)*. Echogenic focus *(white arrow)* is consistent with a peritoneal calcification. **B:** Following delivery at term, a water-soluble enema demonstrates a normal-caliber colon with dilated air-filled small bowel loops *(arrow)*. Jejunal atresia was found at surgery.

ter. Polyhydramnios is not always present and depends on the site of obstruction. Because a fetus with a large bowel obstruction or anal atresia typically does not develop polyhydramnios or dilated bowel, these entities are less readily diagnosed *in utero*. At times, bowel obstruction is associated with perforation and meconium spilling into the peritoneum, otherwise known as meconium peritonitis. Sonographic findings include fetal ascites, peritoneal calcifications, and meconium pseudocysts (77). The most common cause of small bowel obstruction is atresia felt to be secondary to an *in utero* vascular infarct. Fifteen percent of infants with cystic fibrosis present with meconium ileus and sonographic findings similar to those of bowel atresia. Echogenic bowel, meconium peritonitis, and pseudocyst formation occur in both meconium ileus and isolated bowel atresia. Echogenic bowel has also been associated with cytomegalovirus (CMV) and with chromosomal abnormalities such as trisomy 21 (78). Amniocentesis allows for karyotyping, CMV cultures, and analysis of amniocytes for the common CF mutations. In cases of suspected bowel abnormalities, serial sonograms will detect new onset of polyhydramnios and meconium peritonitis.

Ventral Abdominal Wall Defects

The most common abdominal wall defects identified sonographically include omphalocele and gastroschisis (79). Through maternal serum alpha-fetoprotein screening, these defects can be diagnosed early in pregnancy. Omphaloceles result from failure of intestines to return to the abdomen during the tenth week of gestation with herniation of bowel or liver into the umbilical cord. A surrounding peritoneal membrane is present, and the cord insertion is central (Fig. 11–9). Gastroschisis, on the other hand, is a paraumbilical defect located to the right of the umbilicus and is a full-thickness abdominal wall defect without a covering membrane. It is important to distinguish between the two entities for associated diagnosis and prognosis. Gastroschisis is classically an isolated entity felt to be caused by a vascular event and is not associated with chromosomal anomalies but is complicated by bowel fibrosis (80). Omphaloceles, although not as likely to have bowel fibrosis, are more at risk for associated chromosomal abnormalities (30% to 50%) as well as syndromes such as Beckwith-Wiedemann syndrome (macroglossia, organomegaly) and pentalogy of Cantrell (ectopia cordis) (81).

Normal fetal bowel migrates into the base of the cord by 12 menstrual weeks. Thus, the sonographic diagnosis of abdominal wall defects should be made only with caution before the second trimester. Chromosomal analysis and fetal echocardiography should be offered, and consultation with a pediatric surgeon is helpful. Serial sonograms will diagnose the development of polyhydramnios and IUGR (82,83).

Genitourinary Tract

Many asymptomatic genitourinary abnormalities are now being identified prenatally by sonography. Most renal lesions that are identified are cystic or obstructive. Increased detection and earlier diagnosis aid in minimizing the risk of further renal damage after birth. Detection of the fetus with irreversible or lethal renal disease also assists in obstetric and perinatal management. Renal anomalies that can be diagnosed prenatally include renal agenesis, dilated obstructed or nonobstructed collecting systems, renal cystic disease, and tumors. In a series of 17,000 women screened prospectively at 16 to 18 weeks, renal anomalies were identified in 313 cases, 55 of which were significant. Upper tract dilation was the most common finding (298 cases), but it was transient in two-thirds of these cases. Obstruction was noted in 23 infants on follow-up, with 15 of these requiring surgery. Eight infants had unilateral multicystic kidney disease, and three had posterior urethral valves (84).

A systematic approach to urinary tract abnormalities includes an assessment of amniotic fluid, characterization of the urinary tract abnormality, and a search for additional abnormalities. The kidneys contribute little amniotic fluid until 16 weeks of gestation, making it difficult to assess renal function before the second trimester. The presence of oligohydramnios secondary to a urinary abnormality carries a poor prognosis. Rarely, polyhydramnios may be present in a fetus with a mesoblastic nephroma, incomplete UPJ obstruction, or associated cranial or gastrointestinal abnormalities.

Fetal kidneys can be visualized as early as 14 weeks of gestation. Standard renal measurements include length [age in weeks = fetal kidney length (mm)], AP diameter,

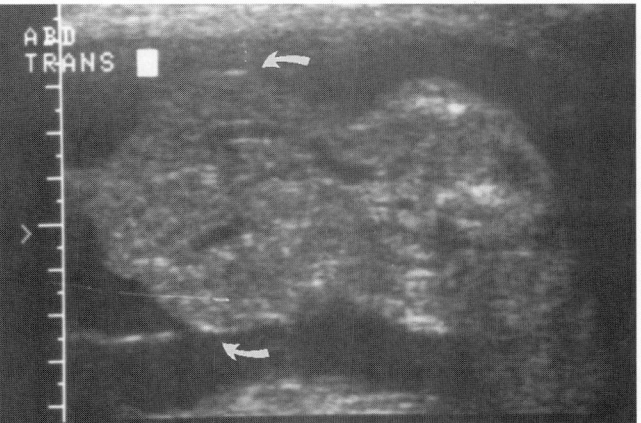

FIG. 11–9. Omphalocele. Transverse image at the level of the umbilical cord insertion demonstrates a large outpouching *(arrows)* with a covering membrane containing liver and bowel.

and renal circumference to abdominal circumference ratio (0.27 to 0.33). If a fetal renal pelvis is dilated and fluid-filled, one must determine if it is physiologic, obstructive, secondary to reflux, or simply nonobstructive megacystis. In most cases, if the pelvic diameter measures less than 1 cm, the finding is nonpathologic. When the pelvic diameter measures over 1 cm, the ratio of pelvic diameter to renal diameter measures greater than 0.5, or caliectasis or hydroureter is present, a pathologic process is likely (85).

Obstructive Uropathy

The most common cause of fetal pyelectasis is uteropelvic junction (UPJ) obstruction (84). Differential includes extrarenal pelvis, vesicoureteral reflux, or a multicystic dysplastic kidney. When bilateral, the severity of obstruction is usually asymmetric. Rarely, dysplasia, urinoma, or urine ascites develops. If associated nonrenal anomalies are identified, chromosome analysis is indicated. The frequency of follow-up sonograms depends on whether both kidneys are involved and the severity of obstruction. Outcome is variable, with 10% increasing in dilation, 50% remaining stable, and 40% improving (86).

Bladder Outlet Obstruction

If hydroureter and pyelectasis are bilateral, the differential diagnosis includes urethral obstruction, bilateral reflux, or bilateral megacystis. In the male fetus, the differential also includes posterior urethral valves and prune belly syndrome. Accurate diagnosis of posterior valves includes the finding of a dilated, thick bladder with keyhole posterior urethral expansion, dilated tortuous ureters, and caliectasis. Urinary ascites may be present (Fig. 11–10). Findings that suggest a poor outcome

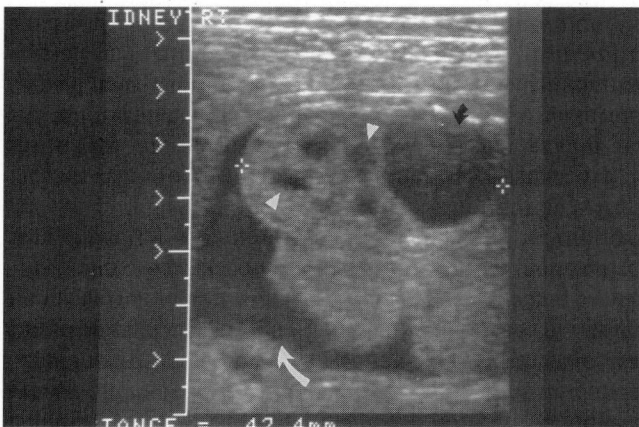

FIG. 11–10. Longitudinal image of a right kidney in a 23-week gestation male fetus with posterior urethral valves demonstrates a kidney with a large upper pole cortical cyst *(black arrow)*, caliectasis *(arrowheads)*, and urinary ascites *(white arrow)*.

include dysplastic echogenic renal parenchyma and oligohydramnios (87). If fetal bladder aspirate demonstrates elevated fetal urine electrolytes and elevated osmolarity, a poor outcome is also suggested.

Frequent sonograms will detect progressive oligohydramnios and IUGR. If severe oligohydramnios is present, up to 95% die from pulmonary hypoplasia. Those who survive require an emergency voiding cystourethrogram to confirm the diagnosis and valvuloplasty or cystostomy to relieve the obstruction. Up to 40% of survivors may develop renal failure at a later date.

Cystic Renal Disease

Cystic changes of the fetal kidneys may be secondary to hereditary diseases (autosomal recessive infantile polycystic kidneys), dysmorphology (multicystic dysplastic kidney disease), or severe obstruction (Potter type II). Differentiating the various diagnoses, at times, may be difficult. When renal cystic disease is identified, the most important factors to evaluate are amniotic fluid volume and whether one or both kidneys are affected. If the cysts are unilateral and amniotic fluid is normal, prognosis typically is good.

Multicystic dysplastic kidneys are felt to be an early error in development of mesonephric blastema or early obstructive uropathy. Up to 75% of multicystic dysplastic kidneys are associated with other renal abnormalities in the contralateral kidney, especially UPJ obstruction and vesicoureteral reflux. Sonographically, multiple cysts are identified in various sizes that do not connect to a renal pelvis. No normal renal parenchymal tissue is seen. Following delivery, the diagnosis is confirmed by renal radionuclide scan, and vesicoureteral reflux is excluded by voiding cystourethrogram.

Autosomal recessive infantile polycystic kidneys typically present with bilateral large echogenic kidneys with a large abdominal circumference. If severe oligohydramnios develops, outcome is poor because of pulmonary hypoplasia (Fig. 11–11).

Skeletal Dysplasia

Skeletal dysplasias include a heterogeneous group of over 160 disorders. The prevalence is 2.4 per 10,000 births (88). Up to one-fourth of affected infants are stillborn, with another one-third dying by 1 week of age. The most common lethal dysplasias include thanatophoric dysplasia, osteogenesis imperfecta type II, and achondrogenesis. The most common nonlethal skeletal dysplasia is achondroplasia (89).

Prenatally, a systematic approach is needed to analyze skeletal anomalies. Long bones should be evaluated for size, shape, bowing, and symmetry. Shortening of the extremities can involve the proximal segment (rhizomelic), midsegment (mesomelic), distal segment (acromelic), or the entire limb (micromelic). Fractures

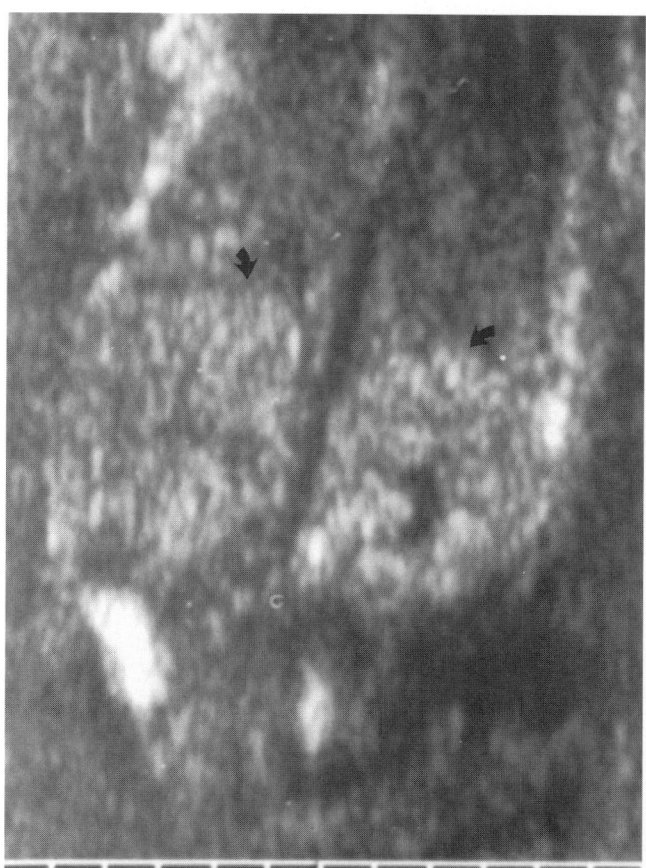

FIG. 11–11. Infantile polycystic kidney disease. Coronal image of a 24-week fetus demonstrates bilateral enlarged echogenic kidneys *(arrows)*. Severe oligohydramnios is present.

appear as bones that are irregular, angled, or bowed sonographically (Fig. 11–12). The skull should be evaluated for frontal bossing or cloverleaf deformity. Decreased skull echogenicity may be noted with osteogenesis imperfecta and hypophosphatasia. Hypertelorism, micrognathia, and abnormally shaped ears may be identified. Hands and feet should be evaluated for polydactyly, missing digits, or equinovarus deformities. The presence of hemivertebrae, scoliosis, and platyspondyly should be explored. Although short ribs may be difficult to recognize sonographically, the thoracic circumference can be measured and compared to normal values for gestational age. If gestational age is unknown, the ratio of thoracic to abdominal circumference can be used. A small thorax suggests a poor prognosis because chest restriction results in pulmonary hypoplasia and, at times, hydrops. Additional findings such as cleft lip, cardiac, and renal anomalies help narrow the differential diagnosis.

When there is a positive family history of a skeletal dysplasia, accurate prenatal diagnosis is possible. When a skeletal abnormality is noted incidentally, a precise diagnosis is more difficult. Fetal radiographs help confirm a diagnosis if fractures or joint calcifications are identified. Additional biochemical testing or karyotyping is useful. Because dysplasias may progress with time (e.g., achondroplasia and osteogenesis imperfecta), serial sonograms are useful for assessment of skeletal growth in cases at risk (90). The potential development of polyhydramnios and/or hydrops should also be noted. Differentiating intrauterine growth retardation or constitutional short stature from a true dysplasia is more difficult in the third

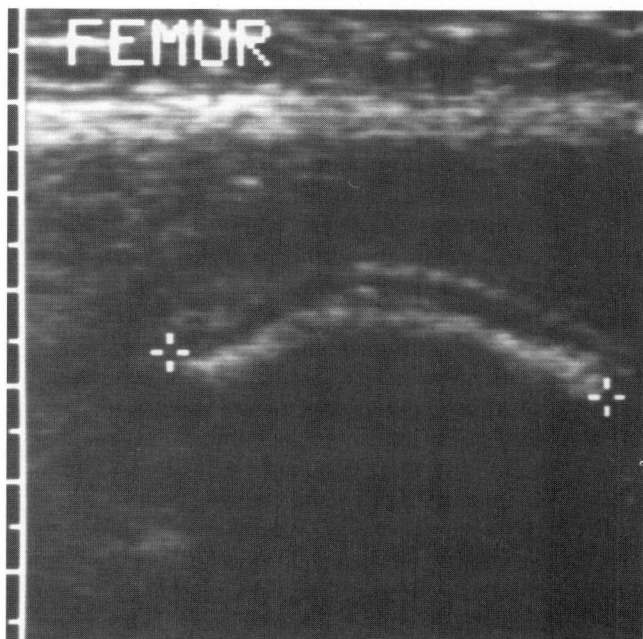

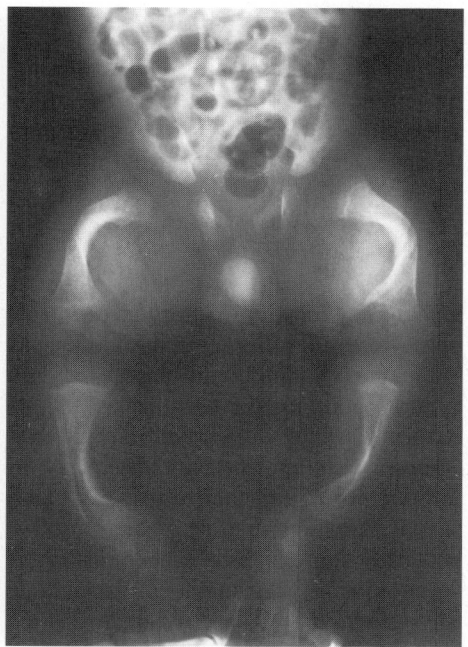

A

B

FIG. 11–12. Osteogenesis imperfecta type III. **A:** Longitudinal image of a fetal thigh at 38 weeks of gestation demonstrates a short, bowed femur *(cursors)*. **B:** Radiograph after delivery confirms the presence of short bowed femurs, tibia, and fibula bilaterally.

trimester. Assessment of fetal well-being including the biophysical profile and umbilical arterial flow patterns aids in establishing the correct diagnosis.

DETECTION OF FETAL ASPHYXIA

Fetal asphyxia is the most common cause of fetal injury or death (50% to 60%), followed by developmental anomalies (25% to 30%) (21). Fetal asphyxia is a spectrum of conditions ranging from transient episodes of hypoxemia to sustained hypoxemia with resultant metabolic acidosis. There are diverse signs of asphyxia with multiple organs potentially affected and a wide range in severity, duration, and chronicity. When asphyxia develops, the fetus redistributes cardiac output from nonvital organs (lung, kidney, skeleton) to vital organs (brain, adrenals, placenta). This protective redistribution is reflexive, resulting from hypoxemic or acidemic stimulation of aortic body chemoreceptors (29). When sustained, redistribution can be profound. Diminished amniotic fluid production develops as a result of decreased urine production. Oligohydramnios further endangers the fetus because the umbilical cord is more at risk for compression, especially during uterine contractions. Cerebral asphyxia results in alterations in biophysical activities and responses. It is unclear whether increasing degrees of hypoxemia cause progressive loss of a biophysical function or if all functions are lost simultaneously. Fetal breathing has been noted to disappear early, whereas fetal movements disappear only with more severe disease (91,92).

Identification of an asphyxiated fetus is important because emergency delivery may improve outcome. Acute fetal asphyxia is rare except in cases of cord prolapse or placental abruption. These obstetric complications can be recognized sonographically and suggest appropriate intervention (93). Unfortunately, most asphyxiated fetuses exhibit both subacute and chronic signs of asphyxia. The fetus suffering from uteroplacental insufficiency typically has intermittent hypoxemic episodes induced during episodes of uterine contraction. Between these periods, the fetus can be normally oxygenated or demonstrate minimal compensated hypoxemia. Signs of hypoxemia thus depend on the duration, progression, and frequency of hypoxemic episodes.

The biophysical signs of asphyxia may be acute, such as loss of breathing movements and heart rate reactivity, or they may be chronic, such as oligohydramnios. Biophysical responses will change during hypoxemic episodes. Experiments in fetal lambs have demonstrated a decrease in fetal breathing and gross movements during hypoxemia (94,95). Fetal muscle tone and heart rate response to movement (i.e., accelerations) also decrease during hypoxemia (96). Maternal depressant medication and fetal cerebral anomalies can alter fetal biophysical activities, so these causes should be excluded. Ultrasound

findings of chronic effects of intermittent hypoxemia include intrauterine growth retardation. Oligohydramnios should be considered a sign of fetal asphyxia unless renal abnormalities or premature rupture of membranes is identified (29).

Fetal Biophysical Profile

Monitoring fetal activity and its responses has altered the practice of perinatology (97,98). Any fetus at risk for uteroplacental insufficiency is a candidate for fetal evaluation in the third trimester. The first electronic fetal heart rate evaluation developed was the contraction stress test (CST), which relies on the fetal heart rate response to uterine contractions. The test records the fetal heart response as contractions are induced with oxytocin. If no fetal decelerations are recorded, uteroplacental function is considered normal. Disadvantages include the need to administer oxytocin intravenously and the length of the examination (average time of 90 minutes) (99).

The nonstress test (NST) evaluates fetal heart rate acceleration in response to fetal movement. As with a negative CST, a reactive NST is predictive of intrauterine survival for approximately 7 days subsequent to the test. This test has became popular because it requires relatively little time, cost, and technical skill (100). Reproducibility of NST interpretation, however, is problematic (101). Past acute asphyxial events are not excluded solely with a NST, and nonreactive patterns may exist for benign reasons.

The differentiation of the normal from the compromised fetus may be most accurate when several fetal and environmental parameters are evaluated together. Manning proposed the combined use of five ultrasound-monitored fetal variables to assess risk of asphyxia to reduce both false-positive and false-negative results. These include fetal breathing movements, gross body movements, tone, amniotic fluid volume, and heart rate reactivity (102). Each variable is evaluated according to tested criteria, and they are assigned scores of 2 when normal and 0 when abnormal (Table 11–2). Observation of each variable is continued until normal criteria are met or 30 minutes of continuous observation has been completed. The total score, termed the biophysical profile score (BPS), is an accurate method of differentiating if a fetus is normal or compromised (Table 11-3). Manning et al. reported that in a series of over 19,000 pregnancies, there was a false-normal test rate of approximately one per 1,000, with more that 97% of pregnancies tested having normal test results (103). Clinical studies from other centers have reported similar results with this method (104). In 1993, Manning et al. reported on 493 fetuses in which BPS were performed just before umbilical venous blood pH values were obtained via cordocenteses. A BPS of 0 was associated with significant fetal acidemia, whereas scores of 8 or greater were associated with a nor-

TABLE 11–2. *Biophysical profile scoring: technique and interpretation*

Biophysical variable	Normal (score 2)	Abnormal (score 0)
FBMs	At least one episode of FBM of at least 30-sec duration in a 30-min observation period	Absent FBM or no episode of ≥30 sec in 30 min
Gross body movement	At least three discrete body or limb movements in 30 min (episodes of active continuous movement are considered a single movement)	Two or fewer episodes of body or limb movements in 30 min
Fetal tone	At least one episode of active extension with return to flexion of fetal limb(s) or trunk; opening and closing of hand considered normal tone	Either slow extension with return to partial flexion or movement of limb in full extension or absent fetal movement
Reactive FHR	At least two episodes in 30 min of FHR acceleration of ≥15 bpm of at least 15-sec duration associated with fetal movement	Less than two episodes of acceleration of FHR or acceleration of <15 bpm in 30 min
Qualitative AFV	At least one pocket of AF that measures at least 2 cm in tow perpendicular planes	Either no AF pockets or a pocket <2 cm in two perpendicular planes

AF, amniotic fluid; AFV, amniotic fluid volume; bpm, beats per minute; FBM, fetal breathing movement; FHR, fetal heart rate. From ref. 34.

mal pH (105). A score of 6 was a poor predictor of abnormal outcome, but a decrease from a score of 2–4 to a score of 0 was an accurate predictor of abnormal outcome. In a similar study, for each of the four acute variables of the BPS, a substantial difference in mean umbilical venous pH was noted for the normal and abnormal results (106). Manning et al. prospectively studied the incidence of cerebral palsy in 22,336 high-risk pregnancies managed with serial BPS compared with 30,224 low-risk pregnancies that did not receive antepartum testing. Cerebral palsy diagnosed by 3 years of age was significantly associated with a low BPS. Incidence of CP was 0.8 per 1,000 when the BPS score was 10 and 250 per 1,000 when the score was 1 (107).

Because the BPS is labor intensive, abbreviated screening tests have been evaluated. When normal, the four ultrasound monitored variables appear equal to that achieved by the addition of the NST component. The NST should be performed when one or more variables are abnormal (108). Provided amniotic fluid volume is normal, a BPS of 8 to 10 by whatever combination can be considered normal. All equivocal or abnormal BPS results should be based on a complete assessment including a NST (109).

Biophysical evaluation should be performed in patients with recognized high-risk factors. It allows for accurate differentiation of the normal fetus from the compromised one, information crucial in the timing of intervention. The variables used in the fetal BPS were selected because of ease and rapidity of measurement. Additional variables such as swallowing, fine hand movement, rapid-eye-movement state, peristalsis of fetal gut, urine output, and umbilical vessel flow rates may be found to add to the more precise evaluation of the fetal condition (110).

Doppler Assessment of Blood Velocities in Umbilical and Fetal Vessels

Doppler ultrasound velocimetry can provide the clinician with important information on the hemodynamics of various vascular regions. The three main areas being studied are the umbilical artery, uteroplacental arteries,

TABLE 11–3. *Biophysical profile scoring: management protocol*

Score	Interpretation	Management
10	Normal infant, low risk for chronic asphyxia	Repeat testing at weekly intervals; repeat twice weekly in diabetics and patients over 42 weeks of gestation
8	Normal infant, low risk for chronic asphyxia	Repeat testing at weekly intervals; repeat testing twice weekly in diabetics and patients over 42 weeks of gestation; oligohydramnios is an indication for delivery
6	Suspicion of chronic asphyxia	Repeat testing in 4–6 hours; deliver if oligohydramnios present
4	Suspicion of chronic asphyxia	If past 36 weeks of gestation and favorable, deliver; if less than 36 weeks of gestation and L/S[a] <2, repeat test in 24 hrs; repeat score ≤4, deliver
0–2	Strong suspicion of chronic asphyxia	Extend testing time to 120 min; if persistent score ≤4, deliver regardless of gestational age

[a]L/S, lecithin–sphingomyelin ratio. From ref. 34.

and fetal circulation. Gestational age-related reference values have been established for maternal uterine and arcuate artery, umbilical artery, fetal descending aorta, and fetal cerebral, renal, and femoral arteries (111). Values are obtained by directing an ultrasound beam toward a vessel and recording the frequency shift (Doppler effect) in the returning echoes. The Doppler shift principle states that echoes returning from moving structures are altered in frequency, and the amount of shift is directly proportional to the velocity of the moving structure. The frequencies of echoes returning from blood moving toward the transducer are increased, whereas the frequencies of echoes returning from blood moving away from the transducer are decreased. This method may not accurately measure velocity, but it does accurately evaluate the relative resistance to flow (112). The frequency spectrum can be analyzed by comparing the systolic to diastolic flow velocities. There are several different ratios for measurement of flow impedance. These include the difference between peak systolic and diastolic flow velocity over the mean flow velocity (pulsatility index), the difference between peak systolic and diastolic flow over the peak systolic flow (resistive index), and the ratio of the peak systolic to diastolic flow (S/D ratio). All indices are independent of the angle of insonation.

A major clinical obstetric application has been in the measurement of umbilical arterial flow using the S/D ratio (Fig. 11–13). In a normal pregnancy, the placental resistance declines slowly with advancing gestational age. The umbilical artery peak systolic flow velocity

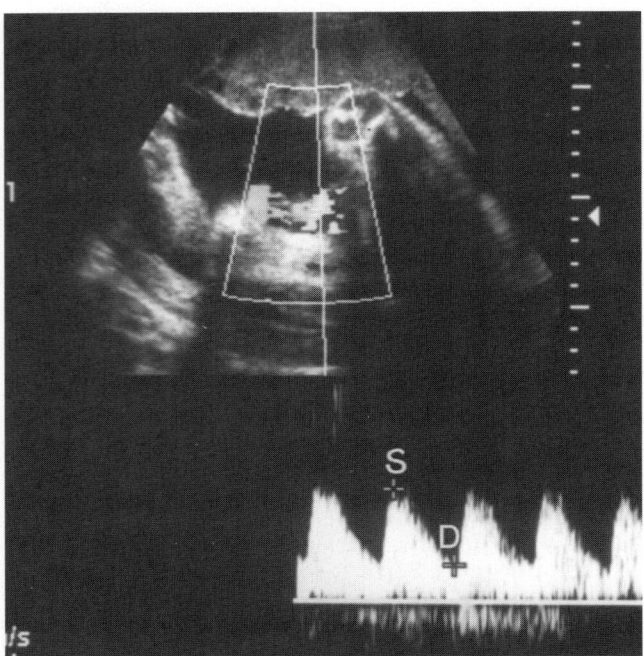

FIG. 11–13. Umbilical artery velocimetry. S, systolic velocity; D, diastolic velocity. Note S/D ratio of approximately 3.

gradually decreases while diastolic flow velocity increases. Thus, the umbilical artery S/D ratio declines with advancing gestational age and should be less than 3 after 30 weeks of gestation (113). In growth-retarded fetuses and fetuses developing intrauterine distress, the umbilical artery blood velocity waveform changes as placental vascular resistance increases. Typically, the diastolic velocity of the waveform decreases and disappears. Absent or reversed end-diastolic flow is associated with a high risk of morbidity and mortality. Several studies have compared the prediction of fetal acidosis by Doppler and cord blood gases. A statistically significant correlation has been found between an increased umbilical S/D ratio and fetal hypoxia and acidemia and is even more significant when diastolic blood flow is absent or reversed (114). In the preselected population of high-risk pregnancies, this method has a high predictive value with regard to diagnosing fetal compromise and can be used for monitoring fetal health (115). If an abnormal umbilical velocimetry is identified in an SGA fetus, fetal heart rate variability should be tested. Fetuses that remain normal after a nonstress test have a low morbidity and can be closely followed (116,117).

Absent diastolic flow velocity of the umbilical artery has been noted in up to 25% of fetuses with anomalies, typically trisomy 13 or 18 (118). Thus, if emergent delivery is not felt to be indicated, an amniocentesis may be recommended for further evaluation. Because abnormal velocimetry may indicate a chronic fetal abnormality and not acute distress, delivery should not be undertaken based on Doppler velocimetry alone (119,120). In the fetus with IUGR and equivocal umbilical blood flow studies, cordocentesis may provide additional information.

Applied as a screening test in an unselected pregnant population, umbilical velocimetry has currently not been found to be cost-effective. A significant change in indices does not develop until more than 60% of the terminal placental arteries are obliterated (121). Alfirevic and Neilson (122) performed a meta-analysis of 20 randomized controlled trials. Their findings do suggest that in a preselected population of high-risk pregnancies, Doppler velocimetry of the umbilical artery has a high predictive value with regard to diagnosing fetal compromise (122). Follow-up studies have showed an association between the abnormal intrauterine umbilical and fetal blood flow and subsequent postnatal neurodevelopmental impairment, suggesting that Doppler velocimetry can be a useful test of fetal well-being (110,122).

Measurement of flow velocity waveforms in the uterine artery has been shown to be a method for early recognition of the pregnancy at risk for preeclampsia and IUGR as well (123). Placental circulation is high-volume flow with high diastolic flow. Indices decrease as term approaches, with diastolic velocity increasing with advancing gestation. Fetal growth retardation has been reported when indices increase or notching in the waveform at end-systole develops. Flow velocity waveforms are useful to predict preeclampsia and early pathologic placental processes (120,124,125).

The fetus with an abnormal umbilical artery velocimetry will redistribute blood flow detectable as vasodilation of the main arteries of the fetus including the heart and brain (29). Measurable flow velocities of intrafetal vessels include the middle cerebral, descending aorta, and renal arteries (126,127). Although experimental, these measures provide a means of assessing the distribution of fetal blood flow and may prove useful in assessing the fetal cardiovascular adaptive responses to chronic hypoxemia. Doppler studies of the fetal circulation in intrauterine growth retardation and hypoxia have demonstrated a compensatory redistribution of arterial blood flow with increased flow to the brain and myocardium and decreased flow to the periphery. Doppler waveforms of the middle cerebral artery (MCA) can be obtained at the level of the circle of Willis. The MCA impedance decreases with advanced gestational age but remains higher than that of the umbilical artery (128). Fetal brain sparing during hypoxia is characterized by increase in diastolic and mean blood flow velocity in the MCA. If vasodilation of the MCA is lost, the fetus will begin to enter the acidotic stage. At term, evidence of fetal hemodynamic redistribution may exist in the presence of normal umbilical artery indices, so ratios such as the MCA/UA pulsatility index are currently being investigated (122,129–132).

SUMMARY

Ultrasonography has profoundly influenced the practice of perinatal medicine. The ability to distinguish the normal from abnormal pregnancy has many applications. Serious complications such as developmental anomalies, intrauterine asphyxia, and growth abnormalities may now be identified with greater frequency and accuracy as a result of advances in ultrasonography. Recognition of high-risk conditions such as placental abruption and cord prolapse as well as more chronic conditions such as intrauterine asphyxia allow for optimal preventive care. In addition, the more accurate ability to identify fetal anomalies has increased the potential for prenatal interventional care.

REFERENCES

1. Dewhurst CJ, Beasley JM, Campbell S. Assessment of fetal maturity and dysmaturity. *Obstet Gynecol* 1972;113:141.
2. Donald I. Ultrasound in obstetrics. *Br Med Bull* 1968;24:71.
3. Hellman LM, Kobayashi M, Fillisti L, et al. Growth and development of the human fetus prior to the twentieth week of gestation. *Am J Obstet Gynecol* 1969;1034:789.
4. Robinson HP, Fleming JEE. A critical evaluation of sonar crown–rump length measurement. *Br J Obstet Gynaecol* 1975;82:702.
5. Silva PD, Mahairas G, Schaper AM, et al. Early crown–rump length a good predictor of gestational age. *J Reprod Med* 1990;35:641.
6. Selbing A. Gestation age and US measurement of gestational sac, CRL and BPD during the first 15 weeks of pregnancy. *Acta Obstet Gynecol Scand* 1982;61:233.
7. Campbell S, Newman GB. Growth of the fetal biparietal diameter during normal pregnancy. *Br J Obstet Gynaecol* 1971;78:513.
8. Sabbagha RE, Hughey M. Standardization of sonar cephalometry and gestational age. *Obstet Gynecol* 1978;52:402.
9. Hadlock FP, Deter RL, Carpenter RL, et al. The effect of head shape on the accuracy of BPD I estimating fetal gestational age. *Am J Roentgenol* 1981;137:83.
10. Sabbagha RE, Turner JH, Rockette H, et al. Sonar BPD and fetal age: definition of the relationship. *Obstet Gynecol* 1974;43:7.
11. Queenan JT, O'Brien GD, Campbell S. Ultrasound measurement of fetal limb bones. *Am J Obstet Gynecol* 1980;138:297.
12. Hadlock FP, Deter RL, Harrist RB. Computer assisted analysis of fetal age using multiple fetal growth parameters. *J Clin Ultrasound* 1983;11:313.
13. Deter RL, Harrist RB, Birnholz JC, et al. Evaluation of fetal dating studies. In: Hedlock F, Deter RL, eds. *Qualitative obstetrical ultrasonography.* New York: John Wiley & Sons, 1986:31.
14. Hadlock FP, Deter RL, Harrist RB, et al. A date independent predictor of IUGR:FL/AC ratio. *Am J Roentgenol* 1983;141:979.
15. Ianniruberto A, Gibbons JM. Predicting fetal weight by ultrasonic B-scan cephalometry: an improved technique with disappointing results. *Obstet Gynecol* 1971;37:689.
16. Campbell S, Wilkin D. Ultrasound measurement of fetal abdominal circumference in the estimation of fetal weight. *Br J Obstet Gynaecol* 1975;82:689.
17. Warsof SL, Gohari P, Berkowitz RL, et al. The estimation of fetal weight by computer assisted analysis. *Am J Obstet Gynecol* 1977;128:881.
18. Shepard MJ, Richards VA, Berkowitz RL, et al. An evaluation of two equations for predicting fetal weight by ultrasound. *Am J Obstet Gynecol* 1982;142:47.
19. Lubchenco LO, Harsman C, Presser M, et al. Intrauterine growth as estimated from live born weight data at 24 to 42 weeks of gestation. *Pediatrics* 1963;32:793.
20. Deter RL, Harrist RB, Hadlock FP, et al. Longitudinal studies of fetal growth with the use of dynamic image ultrasonography. *Am J Obstet Gynecol* 1982;143:545.
21. Morrison I. Perinatal mortality. *Semin Perinatol* 1985;9:144.
22. Campbell S. Fetal growth. *Clin Obstet Gynecol* 1974;1:41.
23. Persson PH, Grennert L, Gennssar G, et al. Diagnosis of intrauterine growth retardation by serial ultrasonic cephalometry. *Acta Obstet Gynecol Scand [Suppl]* 1978;178:40.
24. O'Brien GD, Queenan JT. Ultrasound fetal femur length in relation to intrauterine growth retardation. *Am J Obstet Gynecol* 1982;144:33.
25. Tamura RK, Sabbagha RE. Percentile ranks of sonar fetal abdominal circumference measurements. *Am J Obstet Gynecol* 1980;138:475.
26. Sabbagha RE. Intrauterine growth retardation: antenatal diagnosis by ultrasound. *Obstet Gynecol* 1978;52:252.
27. Campbell S. Ultrasound measurement of the fetal head to abdomen circumference ratio in assessment of growth retardation. *Br J Obstet Gynaecol* 1977;84:165.
28. Wladimiroff JW, Bloemsma CA, Wallenburg HCS. Ultrasound assessment of fetal head and body sizes in relation to normal and retarded fetal growth. *Am J Obstet Gynecol* 1978;131:857.
29. Cohn HE, Sacks EJ, Heyman MA, et al. Cardiovascular responses to hypoxemia and acidemia in fetal lambs. *Am J Obstet Gynecol* 1974;120:817.
30. Phelan JP, Smith CV, Broussard P, et al. Amniotic fluid volume assessment with the four quadrant technique at 36-42 weeks gestation. *J Reprod Med* 1987;32:540.
31. Manning FA, Hill LM, Platt LD. Qualitative amniotic fluid volume determination by ultrasound: antepartum detection of intrauterine growth retardation. *Am J Obstet Gynecol* 1981;1139:254.
32. Marks AD, Divon MY. Longitudinal study of the amniotic fluid index in postdated pregnancy. *Obstet Gynecol* 1992;79:229.
33. Chamberlain PF, Manning FA, Morrison I, et al. Ultrasound evaluation of amniotic fluid volume: I. The significance of marginal and decreased amniotic fluid volume to perinatal outcome. *Am J Obstet Gynecol* 1984;150:245.

34. Manning FA, Morrison I, Lange IR, et al. Fetal assessment based on fetal biophysical profile scoring: experience in 12,620 referred high risk pregnancies: I. Perinatal mortality by frequency and etiology. *Am J Obstet Gynecol* 1985;151:343.

35. Petrikovsky B, Gelertner N, Oleschuk C: Fetal abdominal fat line: can macrosomia be diagnosed. *Am J Gynecol* 1996;174:428.

36. Goldstein P, Gershenson D, Hobbins JC. Fetal biparietal diameter as a predictor of mature L/S ratio. *Obstet Gynecol* 1976;438:667.

37. Strassner HT, Plat LD, Whittle M, et al. Amniotic fluid phosphatidyl-glycerol and real-time ultrasonic cephalometry. *Am J Obstet Gynecol* 1979;135:804.

38. Golde SH, Platt LD. The use of ultrasound in the diagnosis of fetal lung maturity. *Clin Obstet Gynecol* 1984;27:391.

39. Harman CR, Manning FA, Stearns E, et al. The correlation of ultrasonic placental grading and fetal pulmonic maturity in five hundred and sixty-three pregnancies. *Am J Obstet Gynecol* 1982;143:941.

40. Hubbarb AM, Adzick NS, Crombleholme TM, et al. Leftsided congenital diaphragmatic hernia: value of prenatal MR imaging in preparation for fetal surgery. *Radiology* 1997;203:636.

41. Levine D, Barnes PD, Madsen JR, Li W, Edelman RR. Fetal central nervous system anomalies: MR imaging augments sonographic diagnosis. *Radiology* 1997;204:635.

42. Siedler DE, Filly RA. Relative growth of the higher brain structures. *J Ultrasound Med* 1987;6:573.

43. Pretorius D, Davis K, Manco-Johnson M, et al. Clinical course of fetal hydrocephalus: 40 cases. *Am J Neuroradiol* 1985;6:23.

44. Drugan A, Kraus B, Canady A, et al. The natural history of prenatally diagnosed cerebral ventriculomegaly. *JAMA* 1989;261:1785.

45. Chervenak FA, Berkowitz RL, Tortora M, et al. The management of fetal hydrocephalus. *Am J Obstet Gynecol* 1985;151;933.

46. Brown IM, Bannister CM, Rimmer S, et al. The outcome for infants diagnosed prenatally as having cerebral ventriculomegaly. *J Matern Fetal* 1995;5:13.

47. Patel MD, Filly AL, Hersh DR, et al. Isolated mild fetal cerebral ventriculomegaly: Clinical course and outcome. *Radiology* 192:759,1994.

48. Benaceraff BR, Stryker J, Frigoletto FD. Abnormal US appearance of the cerebellum (banana sign). Indirect sign of spina bifida. *Radiology* 1989;171:151.

49. Van de Hof MC, Nicolaides KH, Campbell J, Campbell S. Evaluation of the lemon and banana signs in one hundred thirty fetuses with open spina bifida. *Am J Obstet Gynecol* 1990;162:322.

50. Bulas DI, Johnson D, Allen J, et al. Fetal hemangioma. Sonographic and color flow Doppler findings. *J Ultrasound Med* 1992;11;499.

51. Levitsky DB, Mack LA, Nyberg DA, et al. Fetal aqueductal stenosis diagnosed sonographically: How grave is the prognosis? *Am J Roentgenol* 1995;164:725.

52. Manning FA, Harrison MR, Rodeck C. Catheter shunts for fetal hydronephrosis and hydrocephalus: Report of the International Fetal Surgery Registry. *N Engl J Med* 1986;315:336.

53. Benson JT, Dillard RG, Burton BK. Open spina bifida: Does c-section delivery improve prognosis? *Obstet Gynecol* 1988;71:532.

54. Songster GS, Gray DL, Crane JP. Prenatal prediction of lethal pulmonary hypoplasia using US fetal chest circumference. *Obstet Gynecol* 1989;73:261.

55. Estroff JA, Parak R, Frigoletto FD, et al. The natural history of isolated fetal hydrothorax. *Ultrasound Obstet Gynecol* 1992;2:162.

56. Lein JM, Colmorgen GHC, Gehret JF, et al. Spontaneous resolution of fetal pleural effusion diagnosed during the second trimester. *J Clin Ultrasound* 1990;18:54.

57. Adzick NS, Harrison MR, Glick PL, et al. Fetal cystic adenomatoid malformation: prenatal diagnosis and natural history. *J Pediatr Surg* 1985;20:483.

58. Saltzman DH, Adzick NS, Benacerraf BR. Fetal cystic adenomatoid malformation of the lung: apparent improvement *in utero*. *Obstet Gynecol* 1988;71:1000.

59. Benya EC, Bulas DI, Selby DM, et al. Cystic sonographic appearance of extralobar pulmonary sequestration. *Pediatr Radiol* 1993;23:605.

60. Albright EB, Crane JP, Shackelford GD. Prenatal diagnosis of a bronchogenic cyst. *J Ultrasound Med* 1988;7:91.

61. Blott M, Nicolaides KH, Greenough A. Pleuroamniotic shunting for decompression of fetal pleural effusions. *Obstet Gynecol* 1988;71:798.

62. Bromley B, Parad R, Estroff JA, et al. Fetal lung masses: prenatal course and outcome. *J Ultrasound Med* 1995;14:927.

63. Songster GS, Gray DL, Crane JP. Prenatal prediction of lethal pulmonary hypoplasia using US fetal chest circumference. *Obstet Gynecol* 1989;73:261.

64. Bulas DI, Saal HM, Fonda J, et al. Cystic hygroma and CDH: early prenatal evaluation of Fryns syndrome. *Prenat Diag* 1992;12:867.

65. Adzick NS, Harrison MR, Glick PR. Diaphragmatic hernia in the fetus: Prenatal diagnosis and outcome in 94 cases. *J Pediatr Surg* 1985;20:357.

66. Wilson JM, Fauza DO, Lund DP, et al. Antenatal diagnosis of isolated CDH is not an indicator of outcome. *J Pediatr Surg* 1994;29:815.

67. Metkus AP, Filly RA, Stringer MD, et al. Sonographic predictors of survival in fetal diaphragmatic hernia. *J Pediatr Surg* 1996;31:148.

68. Harrison MR. The fetus with a diaphragmatic hernia: pathophysiology, natural history and surgical management. In Harrison MR, Bolvus MS, Filly RA, eds. *The unborn patient*, ed. 2. Philadelphia: WB Saunders, 1990:295.

69. VanderWall KJ, Skarsgard ED, Filly RA, et al. Fetendoclip: a fetal endoscopic tracheal clip procedure in a human fetus. *J Pediatr Surg* 1997;32:970.

70. Perone N. A practical guide to fetal echocardiography. *Contemp Obstet Gynecol* 1988;1:55.

71. Ott WJ. The accuracy of antenatal fetal echocardiography screening in high and low risk patients. *Am J Obstet Gynecol* 1995;172:1741.

72. Crawford DC, Chita SK, Allan LD. Prenatal detection of congenital heart disease: Factors affecting obstetric management and survival. *Am J Obstet Gynecol* 1988;159 352.

73. Hertzberg BS. Sonography of the fetal gastrointestinal tract: Anatomic variants, diagnostic pitfalls and abnormalities. *Am J Roentgenol* 1994; 162:1175.

74. McKenna KM, Goldstein RB, Stringer MD. Small or absent fetal stomach: prognostic significance. *Radiology* 1995;197:729.

75. Pretorius 1987 DH, Drose JA, Dennis MA, et al. Tracheoesophageal fistula *in utero: twenty-two cases.* J Ultrasound Med 1986;6:509.

76. Nyberg DA, Mack LA, Patten RM, et al. Fetal bowel, normal sonographic findings. *J Ultrasound Med* 1987;6:257.

77. Foster MA, Nyberg DA, Mahony BS, et al. Meconium peritonitis prenatal sonographic findings and their clinical significance. *Radiology* 1987;165:661.

78. Nyberg DA, Dubinsky TJ, Resta RG, et al. Echogenic fetal bowel during the second trimester: clinical importance. *Radiology* 1993;188:527.

79. Hertzberg BS, Bowie JD. Fetal gastrointestinal abnormalities. *Radiol Clin North Am* 1990;28:101.

80. Babcock CJ, Hedrick MH, Goldstein RB, et al. Gastroschisis: can sonography of the fetal bowel accurately predict postnatal outcome. *J Ultrasound Med* 1993;13:701.

81. Nicolaides KH, Snifders RJM, Cheng HH, et al. Fetal gastrointestinal and abdominal wall defects: associated malformation and chromosomal abnormalities. *Fetal Diagn Ther* 1992;7:102.

82. Chescheir NC, Azizkhan RG, Seeds JW, et al. Counseling and care for the pregnancy complicated by gastroschisis. *Am J Perinatol* 1991;8: 323.

83. Fitzsimmons J, Nyberg DA, Cey DR, et al. Perinatal management of gastroschisis. *Obstet Gynecol* 1988;71:910.

84. Gunn TR, Moral JD, Pease P. Antenatal diagnosis of urinary tract abnormalities by ultrasonography after 28 weeks: Incidence and outcome. *Am J Obstet Gynecol* 1995;172:479.

85. Fernbach SK, Maizels M, Conway JJ. Ultrasound grading of hydronephrosis; introduction to the system used by the Society for Fetal Urology. *Pediatr Radiol* 1993;23:478.

86. King LR, Hatcher PA. Natural history of fetal and neonatal hydronephrosis. *Pediatr Urol* 1990;35:433.

87. Hutton KE, Thomas DF, Arthur RJ, et al. Prenatally detected posterior urethral valves: Is gestational age at detection a predictor of outcome? *J Urol* 1994;152:698.

88. Camera G. Mastroizcovo P. Birth prevalence of skeletal dysplasia in the Italian multicentric monitoring system for birth defects. In Papadatos CJ, Bartsocas CCS, eds. *Skeletal dysplasias.* New York: Alan R Liss, 1982:441.

89. Clark RN. Congenital dysplasias and dwarfism. *Pediatr Rev* 1990;12:149.

90. Bulas DI, Stern HJ, Rosenbaum KN, et al. Variable prenatal appearance of osteogenesis imperfecta. *J Ultrasound Med* 1994;13:419.

91. Vintzileos AM, Rippert LSM, Sniders RJM, Nicolaides KH, et al.

Relationship of fetal biophysical profile score and blood gas values in severly growth retarded fetuses. *Am J Obstet Gynecol* 1990;163: 569.

92. Manning FA, Platt LD. Maternal hypoxemia and fetal breathing movement. *Obstet Gynecol* 1979;53:758.

93. Lange IR, Manning FA, Morrison I, et al. Cord prolapse: is antenatal diagnosis possible? *Am J Obstet Gynecol* 1985;151:1083.

94. Boddy K, Dawes GS. Fetal breathing. *Br Med Bull* 1976;31:3.

95. Natale R, Clewlow F, Dawes GS. Measurement of fetal forelimb movements in the lamb *in utero*. *Am J Obstet Gynecol* 1981;140:545.

96. Brown R, Patrick J. The non-stress test: how long is enough? *Am J Obstet Gynecol* 1981;141:646.

97. Manning FA. Dynamic ultrasound based fetal assessment: the fetal biophysical profile score. *Clinical Obstet Gynecol* 1995;3826:44.

98. William K. Amniotic fluid assessment. *Obstet Gynecol Surv* 1993;46: 795.

99. Ray M, Freeman R, Pine S, et al. Clinical experience with oxytocin challenge test. *Am J Obstet Gynecol* 1972;114:1.

100. Freeman RK. The use of oxytocin challenge test for antepartum clinical evaluation of uteroplacental respiratory function. *Am J Obstet Gynecol* 1975;121:481.

101. Hage ML. Interpretation of nonstress tests. *Am J Obstet Gynecol* 1985;153:490.

102. Manning FA, Platt LD, Sipos L. Antepartum fetal evaluation: development of a fetal biophysical profile score. *Am J Obstet Gynecol* 1980;136:787.

103. Manning FA, Morrison I, Harman CR, et al. Fetal assesment based on fetal biophysical prophile score. Experience with 19,221 referred high risk pregnancies. *Am J Obstet Gynecol* 1987;157:880.

104. Baskett TF, Gray JH, Prewett ST, et al. Antepartum fetal assessment using a fetal biophysical profile score. *Am J Obstet Gynecol* 1983; 148:630.

105. Manning FA, Snijder R, Harman CR, et al. Fetal BPS correlation with antepartum umbilical venous pH. *Am J Obstet Gynecol* 1993;169:755.

106. Vintzileos AM, Gaffney SE, Salinger LM, et al. The relationship between fetal biophysical profile and cord pH in patients undergoing C section. *Obstet Gynecol* 1987;70:196.

107. Manning FA, Harman CR, Menticoglou S. Fetal BPS and cerebral palsy at age 3 years. *Am J Obstet Gynecol* 1996;174:319.

108. Manning FA, Harman CR, Lange IR, et al. Modified fetal BPS by selective use of the NST. *Am J Obstet Gynecol* 1987;156:709.

109. Manning FA. Dynamic ultrasound based fetal assessment: the fetal biophysical profile score. *Clin Obstet Gynecol* 1995;38:26.

110. Marsal K. Rational use of Doppler ultrasound in perinatal medicine. *J Perinat Med* 1994;22:463.

111. Johnson T. Maternal perception and Doppler detection of fetal movement. *Clin Perinatol* 1994;21:765.

112. Gill RW. Measurement of blood flow by ultrasound accuracy and source of error. *Ultrasound Med Biol* 1985;11:625.

113. Giles WB, Trudinger BJ, Cook CM. Umbilical artery velocity time waveforms in pregnancy. *J Ultrasound Med* 1982;1:9.

114. Okamura K, Watanabe T, Ando J, et al. Blood gas profiles of fetuses with abnormal Doppler flow in the umbilical artery. *Am J Perinatol* 1996;13:297.

115. Weiner CP. The relationship between umbilical artery S/D ratio and umbilical blood gas measurements in specimens obtained by cordocentesis. *Am J Obstet Gynecol* 1990;162:1198.

116. Giles W. Clinical use of Doppler US in pregnancy. Information from six randomised trials. *Fetal Diagn Ther* 1993;8:247.

117. Farmakides G, Weiner Z, Mammapoulos M, et al. Doppler velocimetry. *Clin Perinatol* 1994;21:849.

118. Rochelson B, Schulman H, Farmakides G, et al. The significance of absent end diastolic velocity in umbilical artery velocity waveforms. *Am J Obstet Gynecol* 1987;156:1213.

119. Trudinger BJ, Cook CM, Giles WB, et al. Fetal umbilical artery velocity waveforms and subsequent neonatal outcome. *Br J Obstet Gynaecol* 1991;98:378.

120. Farmakides G, Weiner Z, Mammapoulos M, Nikolaides P. Doppler velocimetry. *Clin Perinatol* 1994;21:849.

121. Thompson RS, Trudinger BJ. Doppler waveform pulsatility index and resistance pressure and flow in the unbilical placental circulation. *Ultasound Med Biol* 1990;16:449.

122. Alfirevic Z, Neilson JP. The current status of Doppler sonography in obstetrics. *Curr Opin Obstet Gynecol* 1996;8:114.

123. Campbell S, Griffin DR, Pearce FMF. New Doppler ultrasound technique for assessing uteroplacental blood flow. *Lancet* 1983;1:675.

124. Fleischer A, Schumlman H, Farmakides G. Uterine artery Doppler velocimetry in pregnant women with hypertension. *Am J Obstet Gynecol* 1986;154:806.

125. Jaffe R. Multigate spectral Doppler velocimetry for fast assessment of intraplacental fetal circulation: a preliminary study *J Ultrasound Med* 1996;15:309.

126. Wladimiroff JW, Wijingaard JAGW, Degani S. Cerebral and umbilical blood flow velocity waveforms in normal and growth retarded pregnancies. *Obstet Gynecol* 1987;69:705.

127. Veille JC, Kanaan C. Duplex Doppler ultrasonographic evaluation of the fetal lamb artery in normal and abnormal fetuses. *Am J Obstet Gynecol* 1989;161:1502.

128. Dubiel M, Gudmundsson S, Gunnarson G, Marsal K. Middle cerebral artery velocimetry as a predictor of hypoxemia in fetuses with increased resistance to blood flow in the umbilical artery. *Early Hum Dev* 1997;47:177.

129. Harrington K, Carpenter RG, Nguyen M, et al. Changes observed in Doppler studies of the fetal circulation in pregnancies complicated by preeclampsia or SGA baby. *Ultrasound Obstet Gynecol* 1995;6:19.

130. Devine PA, Bracero LA, Lyskiewicz A, et al. Middle cerebral to umbilical artery Doppler ratio in post date pregnancies. *Obstet Gynecol* 1994;84:856.

131. Zimmermann P, Alback T, Koskinen J, et al. Doppler flow velocimetry of the umbilical artery, uteroplacental artery and fetal MCA in prolonged pregnancy. *US Obstet Gynecol* 1995;5:189.

132. Hecher K, Campbell S, Doyle P, et al. Assessment of fetal compromise by Doppler ultrasound investigation of the fetal circulation. *Circulation* 1995;91:129.

CHAPTER 12

Prenatal Diagnosis: Procedures and Trends

Arie Drugan, Baruch Feldman, Mark Paul Johnson, and Mark I. Evans

The introduction of techniques for culturing and karyotyping of amniotic fluid fibroblasts came in the mid-1960s (1). Invasive procedures for diagnosis of fetal genetic disorders have thus been available for more than three decades. The first diagnosis of a fetal chromosome anomaly by amniocentesis (2) was followed shortly by the diagnosis, reported by Nadler in 1968, of an enzyme deficiency in amniotic fluid cells (3). Thereafter, collaborative studies established the safety and accuracy of midtrimester amniocentesis (4,5), and this technique has become a routine part of prenatal care in high-risk patients and the gold standard against which other procedures for prenatal diagnosis have been compared.

Despite its proven efficacy, a major disdvantage of amniocentesis is the availability of results only late in the second trimester, usually after 18 weeks of gestation. The emotional and physical implications of termination of pregnancy this late in gestation are obvious. In the mid-to late 1980s, improvement in ultrasound technology and increasing expertise in ultrasound-guided procedures allowed clinicians to attempt prenatal diagnosis in the first trimester with chorionic villus sampling (CVS) and early amniocentesis. These technical developments have been backed and reinforced by increasing preference on the part of patients for first-trimester prenatal diagnosis (6). Chorionic villus sampling is usually performed between 10 and 13 weeks of gestation so that results are available by the end of the first trimester. The accuracy and safety of CVS are comparable to those of amniocentesis (7,8), and the early results allow patients privacy in reproductive decisions and an earlier and safer termination of pregnancy if they so choose. An alternative to CVS has been offered by early amniocentesis performed between 10 and 14 weeks of gestation (9). Another alternative, although still experimental, is the use of coelocentesis for prenatal diagnosis at 7 to 12 weeks of gestation. It has been recently suggested as a safe and reliable method for early prenatal diagnosis (10).

A change in the pattern of indications for prenatal diagnosis has also been observed over the years. Advanced maternal age (over 35 years) is still the most common indication for genetic counseling and prenatal diagnosis, noted in more than 70% of cases. Other standard indications include a previous affected offspring or a balanced structural rearrangement of parental chromosomes, the latter being clinically evident as recurrent pregnancy loss (Table 12–1). In recent years, increased utilization of ultrasound and biochemical maternal serum

A. Drugan: Department of Obstetrics and Gynecology, Hutzel Hospital, Wayne State University, Detroit, Michigan; and Department of Obstetrics and Gynecology, Rambam Medical Center, Haifa, Israel

B. Feldman: Division of Reproductive Genetics, Department of Obstetrics and Gynecology, Hutzel Hospital, Wayne State University, Detroit, Michigan

M. P. Johnson: Departments of Obstetrics and Gynecology, Pathology, Molecular Medicine, and Genetics, Wayne State University; and Reproductive Genetics, Department of Obstetrics and Gynecology, Hutzel Hospital/The Detroit Medical Center, Detroit, Michigan

M. I. Evans: Division of Reproductive Genetics; Center for Fetal Diagnosis and Therapy; and Human Genetics Program, Hutzel Hospital, Wayne State University, Detroit, Michigan

TABLE 12–1. *Indications for prenatal diagnosis*

Increased risk of chromosome anomalies
   Advanced maternal age
   Previous offspring with chromosome anomalies
   Parental balanced translocation or inversion
   Ultrasound diagnosis of fetal malformations or anomalies
   Abnormal biochemical screening in maternal serum
Previous offspring with neural tube defect
Parents carriers of a Mendelian genetic trait
   Molecular DNA diagnosis (i.e., CF, sickle cell anemia or Fragile X)
   Enzymatic activity in villi or amniocytes (i.e. Tay-Sachs, Refsum)
   Precursor levels in cell-free amniotic fluid (17-OH progesterone in congenital adrenal hyperplasia)

screening tests for fetal chromosome anomalies has caused more young patients, previously considered to be at low risk for fetal aneuploidy, to seek invasive prenatal testing. The combination of multiple-marker serum screening (AFP, hCG, ± UE3) and maternal age will point to the need for more detailed prenatal testing in about 65% of chromosomally abnormal conceptions. If the risk cutoff for fetal aneuploidy is taken as equal to that of a 35-year-old, some 5% of pregnant patients will test positive, and one in 50 amniocenteses performed for this indication will diagnose a chromosomally abnormal conception (11). Sonographic markers for fetal chromosome anomalies (Table 12–2) are another emerging indication for fetal karyotyping, observed in about 3% to 5% of pregnancies. The most ominous of these findings are abnormalities of the fetal neck, indicating a need for evaluation of fetal chromosomes even in association with normal biochemical serum screening in young patients (12). Moreover, the results of biochemical or ultrasound screening may be used to modulate the risk of aneuploidy in the population previously considered at risk, allowing a reduction in the number of invasive diagnostic procedures in patients of advanced maternal age (13,14). Furthermore, at-risk patients who previously would have declined amniocentesis may accept invasive prenatal diagnosis following a positive screening result (14).

The need for rapid karyotyping may arise when fetal anomalies are suspected near the legal limit for termination of affected pregnancies, that is, after an abnormal result on biochemical or ultrasound screening. In these cases, the diagnostic options are late CVS or cordocentesis and karyotyping of fetal blood lymphocytes (15). Other tests that may be performed on blood obtained by cordocentesis include hematologic, acid–base balance, and immunologic status of the fetus (16).

TABLE 12–2. *Relative risk for aneuploidy associated with isolated sonographic markers*

Sonographic marker	Prevalence	Relative risk[a]
Choroid plexus cysts	1.25%	× 9[b]
Nuchal edema or cysts	4% to 5%	
>4 mm		× 18
>5 mm		× 28
>6 mm		× 36
Lt ventricular echogenic focus	5%	× 4
Hyperechoic bowel	0.6% to 0.8%	× 14–16
Pyelectasis	2%	× 3.3–3.9
Fetal biometry		
Short CRL	7%	× 3
Short femur length	4% to 5%	× 2.7
Short humerus	4% to 5%	× 4.1
Short femur and humerus	2.4%	× 11.5

[a]Risk for trisomy 21 as calculated in relation to maternal age alone or in combination with biochemical screening.
[b]Risk specific for trisomy 18; risk for trisomy 21 is negligible.

PRENATAL DIAGNOSIS IN THE FIRST TRIMESTER

Chorionic Villus Sampling

The first attempts at first-trimester prenatal diagnosis were made in the Soviet Union and China in the early 1970s, mainly for fetal gender determination (17). It was not until 1983, however, that the laboratory techniques to obtain karyotypes from chorionic villi adequate for interpretation were developed in Milan by Simoni and Brambati (18). They were also the first to report on diagnosis of trisomy 21 by the direct method 5 hours after chorionic villus sampling was performed (19). Over the years, the quality of chromosome preparation from CVS material has improved considerably, approaching the banding quality obtained from amniocytes or blood karyotypes (20). The clinical procedure has been also refined, with the use of real-time ultrasound guidance and malleable catheters for villi aspiration. The use of variable approaches (i.e., transcervical versus transabsominal) depending on placental location has likewise improved the yield and safety of CVS (21,22).

Chorionic villus sampling can be offered to almost every patient who needs prenatal diagnosis in the first trimester. The most common indication for CVS is advanced maternal age, which accounts for 70% to 80% of cases (21). Other indications for fetal karyotyping include a previous child with chromosome anomalies or a carrier parent of a balanced translocation or inversion. Normal ranges of lysosomal enzymes in fresh and cultured villi have been also established, allowing for the diagnosis of disorders such as Tay-Sachs or the mucopolysaccharidoses (23). Chorionic villus sampling is particularly suitable for DNA molecular prenatal diagnosis of classic genetic disorders. The amount of DNA obtained from a few villi is much larger than that contained in amniocytes from 40 mL of amniotic fluid.

Technical Aspects

Chorionic villus sampling procedures, whether transcervical, transabdominal or transvaginal, are most commonly performed between 10 and 13 weeks of gestation (Fig. 12–1). After 13 weeks, the procedure is usually best done transabdominally (24,25), although the transcervical approach for late CVS using a thin biopsy forceps has also been employed successfully (26). Fetal viability and gestational age must always be confirmed before the procedure. The major determinant of approach is placental location. Fundal placentas are most commonly an indication for the transabdominal approach. However, other factors may dictate the preferable approach to CVS in specific cases. Thus, transcervical or transvaginal CVS should be avoided in patients with active vaginal or cervical infection (e.g., herpes), whereas the transabdominal approach should be avoided in cases with interposed bowel or marked uterine

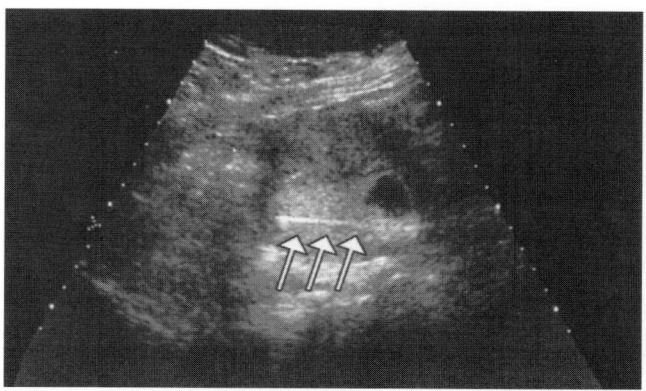

FIG. 12–1. In transcervical chorionic villus sampling (CVS), the catheter *(arrows)* is guided through the cervical canal and into the placenta.

retroversion (24). After CVS, fetal heart activity should be verified, and Rh immunoprophylaxis (anti-D IgG) should be administered to Rh-negative patients.

Some American and European centers prefer to use the transabdominal approach for CVS (27,28). In our experience, however, transabdominal sample size usually has been lower than that obtained transcervically (29). Transabdominal CVS is usually the procedure of choice for cases with anterior fundal placentas, whereas transcervical CVS should generally be performed when the placenta is posterior and low-lying. In general, tailoring the type of procedure to placental location is expected to reduce complication rates after CVS (21,30).

Transvaginal, transmural CVS should be reserved to a very limited number of cases in which the placenta is posterior, the uterus is retroverted and retroflexed, and the cervical canal points toward the mother's abdomen. In these cases, the procedure can be performed transvaginally with a needle guided by transabdominal or transvaginal ultrasound (31,32).

Safety

The complications of CVS must be judged from the perspective of the natural pregnancy loss rate in the first trimester. The likelihood of spontaneous abortion following documentation of a viable fetus at 8 to 11 weeks has been calculated by Simpson to be about 3% to 5% (33). It increases significantly with maternal age. Both the Canadian and the American collaborative studies documented an excess loss rate of 0.6 to 0.8% in the CVS group. It is not significantly different from the loss rate in the amniocentesis group (6,7). Fundal placental location, three catheter insertions, and obtaining small amounts of villi have been significantly associated with pregnancy loss after CVS. These factors may reflect technical difficulty during the procedure (24).

Concerns about the safety of CVS have been raised by Firth and Burton (34–36). In two small series, these authors claimed a 1% risk of limb reduction defects (LRDs) following CVS and reported an inverse correlation between gestational age and risk of anomalies. In contrast, evaluation of over 200,000 cases from experienced centers, worldwide, reveals that the incidence of LRDs or any other defects is identical to that of the background population and that the Firth and Burton studies had serious flaws (37). Furthermore, closer assessment has shown that several cases with LRDs reported after CVS had unaccounted familial factors (38). There may be an increased risk with CVS procedures done at 6 to 7 weeks of gestation as opposed to the reccommended time of 10 to 12 weeks of gestation, or by inexperienced personnel, but available data suggest that CVS is otherwise safe and effective.

Fetomaternal Transfusion

Another potential concern for CVS is the possibility of fetomaternal transfusion. Transiently rising maternal serum alpha-fetoprotein (AFP) levels following CVS have been reported (39). The increase is in corrolation with sample size but not with CVS technique, whether transabdominal or transcervical (40). The calculated mean volume of transfused fetal blood was 5.4 mL. Others have reported that the volume of fetomaternal transfusion following CVS could reach 21% of fetoplacental blood volume (41). Rh isoimmunization should be, thus, considered a relative contraindication to CVS. However, in practice, fetomaternal transfusion is not a significant problem.

Chromosomal Analysis

Two types of cells are observed in chorionic villi. The outer layer consists of cytotrophoblasts, which divide spontaneously, and is used for direct evaluation of metaphases. The inner mesenchymal core is used to initiate long-term cultures and is usually considered more representative of fetal karyotype. Overall, cytogenetic results are obtained by either direct analysis, long-term culture, or both in 99.6% of cases in which villi are obtained (20). Results of direct analysis are equivocal in 1% to 2% of cases, but questions raised are usually resolved by long-term CVS or amniotic cell cultures (24). In most cases, an abnormal direct result that proves to be normal on long-term culture will not be confirmed in karyotypes obtained from amniocytes or fetal lymphocytes. More rarely, a normal direct result is followed by an abnormal result in long-term culture, with the abnormality being confirmed in fetal tissue in one-half of those cases (20). Maternal cell contamination has been observed in 1.9% of long-term cultures but did not contribute to diagnostic error in any case (24).

Chromosomal mosaicism in CVS material affects about 1.2% to 2.5% of cases (average 1.3%). It is more common in direct preparations than in long-term culture, which is why direct preparations are no longer used alone for diagnosis (41). Mosaicism is restricted to extraembryonic tissue in 70% to 80% of cases. Follow-up of the cases with confined placental mosaicism (CPM) documented a significantly elevated fetal loss rate (7.5% to 16.7%), mostly in the second and third trimesters, suggesting that such placental mosaicism is not entirely benign (42,43). Intrauterine growth retardation (IUGR) also appears to be more common in this situation (44). Mosaic trisomy 3 is the most common type of mosaicism observed in placental cells (41). However, an adverse impact on pregnancy outcome seems to be most frequent in association with trisomies of chromosomes 13, 16, and 22 (45).

The diagnosis of mosaicism in CVS presents difficulties in genetic counseling because it implies uncertainty with respect to fetal genotype and phenotype. The accuracy of the diagnosis by CVS may be increased by using both a direct preparation and long-term culture. When further evaluation is needed, level II ultrasonographic screening for anomalies and amniocentesis are indicated for follow-up. The use of amniocentesis in these cases may allow earlier clarification of fetal karyotype without a significant increase in procedure-related fetal loss rate (43). In our experience, however, the frequency of mosaicism in amniotic fluid cultures is not significantly different from that observed in CVS (0.35% versus 0.56%, respectively) (46). Cordocentesis may also be employed in such cases to verify mosaicism in fetal blood (47). However, even if fetal blood karyotype is normal, there is still a small chance that mosaicism is confined to specific fetal tissues, as observed in some cases with trisomy 20 mosaicism. The finding of CPM may also represent an indication to seek cases of uniparental disomy. The conception starts out trisomic, but one copy of the three is lost in the embryo but not in the extraembryonic tissue, the placenta (48).

Early Amniocentesis

Early amniocentesis refers to aspiration of amniotic fluid for analysis less than 15 weeks from the last menstrual period. Obstetricians are familiar with the technique of amniocentesis, and an incorrect assumption followed that early amniocentesis would exhibit the same safety and accuracy as the midtrimester procedure (41,49). With improved ultrasound technology and increasing experience with ultrasound-guided needle manipulations, early amniocentesis appeared to be an attractive alternative to CVS performed in the first trimester. The procedure is relatively simple. Under continuous ultrasound guidance and utilizing aseptic technique, a 22-gauge needle is inserted into a pocket of amniotic fluid, and about 1 mL of fluid per week of gestation is aspirated into a 20-mL syringe (Fig. 12–2). Because the membranes are not yet adhered to the uterine wall, tenting of membranes ahead of the needle is relatively common in early amniocentesis. In our experience,

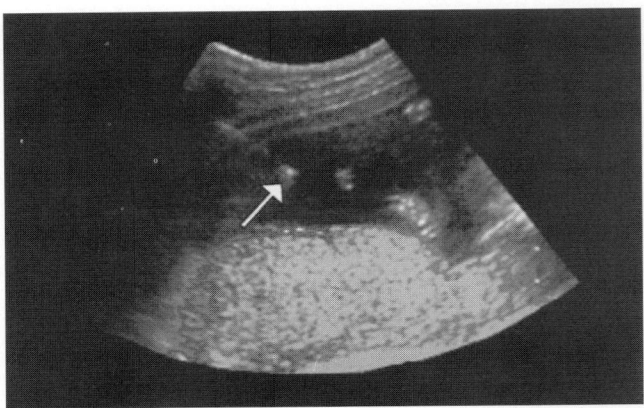

FIG. 12–2. In early amniocentesis, the needle *(arrow)* is inserted through the uterine wall and into the amniotic cavity.

aspiration of fluid is hampered by tenting of membranes in about 5% of early procedures. Rotating the needle or the use of a stylet longer than the needle allows the procedure to succeed in most cases (9,50).

Complications of early amniocentesis include bleeding, uterine cramping, leakage of fluid, and infection, as sometimes observed after amniocentesis performed at later gestational ages. Women who had a genetic amniocentesis at 11 to 14 weeks of gestation are significantly more prone to have postprocedure amniotic fluid leakage (2.9% versus 0.2%), vaginal bleeding (1.9% versus 0.2%), and fetal loss (2.2% versus 0.2%) than women undergoing amniocentesis at 16 to 19 weeks (51). The total unintentional loss rate following early amniocentesis is reported in the literature to be between 1.4% and 4.2% (Table 12–3). However, not all of these losses could be related causally to the early procedure (49–57). There seems to be a trend in all series toward increased loss rates after amniocentesis performed at 11 or 12 weeks of gestation (49). However, there are many caveats to be considered. Recently, Wilson et al., in the Canadian early versus midtrimester amniocentesis trial showed that there is an increased risk of clubfoot with procedures done before 12 weeks (58). Sundberg and associates also found an association between amniocentesis and talipes equinovarus (59). The risk is now estimated to be approximately

TABLE 12–3. *Rate of pregnancy loss following early amniocentesis*

Author	Loss rate
Penso and Frigoletto (49)	3.8%
Hanson et al. (52)	2.3%
Stripparo et al. (53)	3.1%
Nevin et al. (54)	1.4%
Elejalde et al. (57)	1.6%
Brumfield et al. (51)	2.2%
Dunn and Godmilow (55)	4.2%
Johnson et al. (56)	2.4%

1%. These findings suggest that early amniocentesis should not be done before 12 weeks, and therefore, early amniocentesis and CVS are not equivalent, as CVS can be done safely by 10 weeks. Furthermore, even a 14-week amniocentesis is not comparable to a 10-week CVS. The principal determinant of total fetal loss after any procedure is the gestational age. Our experience shows procedure-related losses of amniocentesis and CVS at comparable gestational ages to be nearly identical.

In comparison with CVS, early amniocentesis has a lower rate of pseudomosaicism and maternal cell contamination. A concern has been raised, however, about culture failure after early amniocentesis. In our experience, culture failure rate is one in 700 in midtrimester samples, about 1% following early procedures, and nearly 5% if amniocentesis is performed before 12 weeks (29,60). This rate is somewhat lower than the 1.6% rate of culture failure reported by Stripparo and colleagues (53) but higher than 0.32% reported by Elejalde and associates (57). Failure of culture of amniocytes has been reported more commonly in association with fetal chromosome abnormalities (61). Furthermore, the mean culture time may also be somewhat longer after early amniocentesis as compared to midtrimester procedures (62).

Early amniocentesis may also permit the diagnosis of fetal structural anomalies through analysis of amniotic fluid AFP and acetylcholinesterase (AChE). Alpha-fetoprotein peaks in amniotic fluid at 12 to 13 weeks of gestation and then declines gradually, in correlation with fetal serum AFP (63,64). Elevated amniotic fluid AFP levels have been observed with fetal neural tube defects (NTD) or omphalocele even in these early samples (65). Low amniotic fluid AFP values were found in some conceptions diagnosed as aneuploid, but these data are still in question. Even more challenging is the interpretation of amniotic fluid AChE results. Acetylcholinesterase is usually analyzed by gel electrophoresis as a bimodal result, either positive or negative. In early amniotic fluid samples, a faint, inconclusive band is frequently observed. In contrast to positive AChE result in midtrimester amniotic fluid samples, this observation seems to be associated with fetal anomalies in only a minority of cases (66). Thus, it appears that in early amniotic fluid samples, a negative AChE result may be reliable in the setting of elevated amniotic fluid AFP, but the interpretation of a positive result may necessitate quantitative evaluation of band density (67). A normal sonogram in this situation is reassuring in regard to fetal neural tube or abdominal wall defects, but other adverse outcomes have been reported in these pregnancies as well (68).

Chorionic Villus Sampling versus Early Amniocentesis

Most procedures for prenatal diagnosis are performed for relatively soft indications (e.g., advanced maternal age, a previous child with chromosome anomalies, parental translocation or inversion). Prenatal diagnosis in the first trimester enables us to reassure most patients with normal results 6 to 9 weeks earlier than would be possible with midtrimester amniocentesis. Although still at risk for miscarriage, patients undergoing CVS for prenatal diagnosis show a sharp drop in anxiety levels immediately after receiving results, whereas patients undergoing amniocentesis remain anxious longer (69). In the few unfortunate cases that are diagnosed as abnormal, the mother can have a less traumatic and less risky first, rather than second, trimester termination of pregnancy (70).

Which of the two procedures available for prenatal diagnosis is preferable in the first trimester? Only a few prospective, randomized studies compare CVS and amniocentesis in the first trimester (59,71,72). Byrne and associates suggest that the two techniques can be comparable in terms of accuracy and successful results (71). Nicolaides reported that the two procedures, CVS and early amniocentesis, are similar in providing a sample for evaluation (99.3% and 100%, respectively) and in giving a nonmosaic cytogenetic result (97.5% and 97.9%, respectively) (72). Spontaneous pregnancy loss following CVS was, however, significantly lower than after early amniocentesis (2.1% versus 4.9%, respectively). Furthermore, in light of the Canadian data, amniocentesis should generally not be performed before 12 weeks (58), so that these procedures are no longer comparable, and there is a definite advantage to CVS. Concerns have also been raised on fetal lung development and function following removal of amniotic fluid so early in gestation (73–75). Thus, our opinion is that CVS is the procedure of choice for karyotyping as well as for DNA molecular analysis before 12 weeks of gestation. Early amniocentesis may be preferable in certain biochemical disorders and in situations in which CVS may not truly represent fetal tissue. One example of the latter situation is a twin pregnancy with fused placentas, in which discrimination of one fetal karyotype from the other might be impossible with CVS but could be achieved with early amniocentesis (Fig. 12–2).

PRENATAL DIAGNOSIS IN THE SECOND AND THIRD TRIMESTERS

Midtrimester Amniocentesis

Midtrimester amniocentesis is the traditional, most commonly performed procedure for prenatal diagnosis. It also is considered the gold standard with which other procedures for prenatal diagnosis are compared. Indications for genetic amniocentesis include increased risk for chromosome anomalies or for structural anomalies that may be associated with elevated AFP (Table 12–1). In addition, some metabolic genetic disorders may be diagnosed by measurement of precursor levels in cell-free fluid or enzyme activity in cultured amniocytes (76).

For cytogenetic studies, amniocytes are removed from amniotic fluid by centrifugation and cultured in flasks or on cover glasses to grow in monolayers. Dividing cells are arrested in metaphase, when chromosomes are maximally condensed, using agents such as colcimide that prevent spindle formation. The cells are then harvested, placed in hypotonic saline, which causes intracellular swelling and better spreading of the chromosomes during slide preparation. After fixation, the chromosomes are stained by giemsa or quinacrine to allow microscopic analysis. The use of triple gas incubators, specific growth media that enhance cellular proliferation, and *in situ* culture on cover glass have considerably shortened the sampling-to-harvesting interval. The results are available within 2 weeks in most laboratories. Additional improvement is obtained by computerized cytoanalyzers that expedite recognition of metaphase spreads and avoid the need for photography and darkroom processing.

Technical Aspects

Amniocentesis should be performed by an obstetrician trained and experienced in the procedure. We believe genetic counseling should be a prerequisite to amniocentesis (77). Pedigree information obtained during the counseling session will allow the clinician to ascertain genetic risks more accurately and to maximize the benefits of genetic evaluation of patients seemingly at high risk for genetic disease other than the indication for referral (e.g., advanced maternal age or abnormal serum screening). A detailed ultrasound examination is performed to evaluate gestational age, placental location, and amount of amniotic fluid and to exclude fetal anomalies. After sterile preparation of the skin, a draped sterile ultrasound transducer is used to locate a suitable pocket of fluid. Under continuous ultrasound guidance, a 20- to 22-gauge, 3.5-inch-long, spinal needle is inserted in a single smooth motion into the pocket of fluid. When the needle, which is visualized on ultrasound as a bright spot, is placed satisfactorily into the pocket of amniotic fluid, the stylet is removed, and a 5-mL syringe is used to aspirate the first 1 to 2 mL of fluid, which is then discarded. This is done to minimize the risk of contamination with maternal cells collected in the path of the needle. Twenty to thirty milliliters of amniotic fluid is then gently aspirated, transferred into sterile tubes, and transported at room temperature to the laboratory for processing (78).

In Rh-negative patients, the risk of Rh isoimmunization is probably increased by transplacental passage of the needle (79). The risk of Rh isosensitization following amniocentesis in Rh-negative women with Rh-positive fetuses has been estimated to increase by 1% above the background risk of Rh isoimmunization during pregnancy for these patients (80). Thus, the patient's blood type and antibody status should be known before amniocentesis, and unsensitized Rh-negative women should receive Rh immunoprophylaxis after the procedure.

Safety and Complications

Amniocentesis is a very safe procedure when performed by trained personnel. The procedure-related pregnancy loss rate in experienced hands is 0.3% to 0.5% over and above the spontaneous loss rate at 16 weeks of gestation, which is estimated to be 2% to 3% (76). Pregnancy loss rates seem to be associated with the number of failed needle insertions at the same session and with vaginal bleeding after amniocentesis. Gestational age at the time of amniocentesis, volume of fluid removed, and repeat amniocentesis at a different session after a failed attempt do not seem to correlate with increased risk of pregnancy loss (81). In experienced hands, transplacental amniocentesis does not appear to increase the rate of fetal loss (82). Leakage of amniotic fluid through the cervix is a relatively frequent complication, affecting approximately 1% to 2% of patients following amniocentesis, but it is usually of minor long-term consequence. In most cases, it resolves with bed rest for 48 to 72 hours (83). Even patients with complete absence of fluid after amniocentesis may reaccumulate amniotic fluid and go on to have normal outcome (84). On the other hand, prolonged amniotic fluid leakage, although rare, may lead to severe oligohydramnios, which can result in fetal pressure deformities (i.e., arthrogryposis) and in pulmonary hypoplasia (85). Thus, as long as there is no evidence of infection, expectant management (for at least several days) seems prudent. The risk of severe amnionitis endangering maternal health appears to be very low, about 0.1% (76). Likewise, fetal injury by the needle should be very rare during ultrasound-guided amniocentesis. Long-term follow-up of outcomes after midtrimester amniocentesis was reported by several authers. The findings indicate that there does not appear to be a compromise of child development, behavior, growth, or health (86–88).

Cytogenetic analysis of amniotic fluid cells reflects fetal status accurately in over 99% of cases; however, mosaicism may sometimes cause confusion in the interpretation of the results. In our experience, the frequency of results needing further investigation is similar in cultures from amniocentesis and CVS (46). Differentiation between cytogenetic abnormalities that truly reflect fetal chromosome aberrations and those that are the result of laboratory artifacts may be difficult. One or more hypermodal cells limited to one colony or culture flask are identified in 2% to 3% of all amniocyte cultures and usually will be associated with a normal phenotype (89). True fetal mosaicism should be considered when hypermodal cells are identified in different culture flasks or in separate colonies in the same flask. The frequency of hypermodal cells in one or more colonies from the same flask is 0.7%, and hypermodal cells with the same abnormality originating from multiple culture flasks are observed in 0.2% of amniotic cultures (90,91). Even in the latter, however, the abnormality in culture may not represent true fetal mosaicism, as observed by Gosden and colleagues (47). Fetal blood sampling for karyotyping should help to avoid termination of pregnancy of some normal fetuses in these cases.

Late Chorionic Villus Sampling

The techniques of transabdominal CVS to obtain fetal karyotype from analysis of chorionic villi in the first trimester have been applied successfully in the second and third trimesters. Nicolaides and associates first reported six successful human placental biopsies at 14 to 37 weeks of gestation and suggested that CVS should not be confined to the first trimester (92). Chieri and Aldini performed midtrimester transabdominal placental biopsies and amniocenteses in 220 patients, 210 of whom were indicated for advanced maternal age (93). A sample of villi adequate for analysis (>2 mg) was obtained in 90.9% of cases. The success rate was 94% with an anterior or fundal placenta and 83.8% with a posterior placental location. In the latter situation, the approach to the placenta was transamniotic. Cytogenetic results were obtained in 95% of samples. No discrepancy was found between cytogenetic results obtained in villi and amniotic fluid, and therefore, when fetal anomalies were detected by CVS, they were acted on without waiting for amniocyte culture confirmation (67). Several other studies documented a sampling and diagnostic success of 98% to 99%, with a very low rate (0.3% to 1.8%) of procedure-related pregnancy loss (94–96).

The collaborative results of 2,058 late CVS procedures performed at 24 centers were reported by Holzgreve and colleagues (15). A fetal karyotype was obtained in 96% of procedures. The frequency of abnormal chromosome results was 21% when fetal anomalies were observed on ultrasound and 6.2% in patients with normal ultrasound findings. The pregnancy loss rate, excluding terminations, was 10.3% in the group with abnormal ultrasound findings and 2.3% in the normal ultrasound group. Holzgreve and associates further presented their own data on 301 CVS procedures in the second and third trimesters, 225 (74.7%) of which were performed for abnormal ultrasound scans (97). Karyotyping was successful in 99% of cases. The rate of chromosome anomalies was 20% in the group with abnormal ultrasound and increased to 38% when the ultrasound findings included abnormalities of amniotic fluid volume.

It was apparent from these studies that despite the decrease in mitotic index with placental aging, direct results could be obtained with even small amounts of placental tissue. The quality of karyotypes obtained from analysis of second- and third-trimester samples was similar to that obtained in the first trimester (94). Moreover, the risk of maternal cell contamination in late CVS samples actually may be lower than that observed in the first trimester as a result of less direct contact between villi and decidua at later gestational age (98). Thus, placental biopsies in the second and third trimesters are technically feasible procedures for prenatal diagnosis, with results apparently as accurate as those of amniocentesis and probably associated with a smaller risk of pregnancy loss than percutaneous umbilical blood sampling. The major advantage of late CVS is the possibility of obtaining rapid results in situations where such information is needed for decisions regarding pregnancy termination or fetal therapy. Such situations would include the ultrasound diagnosis of fetal anomalies late in the second trimester, close to the legal limit in gestational age after which termination of pregnancy is no longer an option. Late CVS also offers a distinct advantage over cordocentesis in cases complicated by oligohydramnios. In the third trimester, knowledge of the fetal karyotype in pregnancies complicated by severe IUGR or fetal anomalies may influence the mode of delivery, the management of intrapartum fetal distress, which is a common phenomenon in fetuses with chromosome anomalies, or the decision for surgical intervention within the first few hours after birth.

Cordocentesis

Freda and Adamson originally attempted to access the vascular system of the fetus for treatment of Rh isoimmunization by hysterotomy and fetal exposure (99). This method soon was abandoned because of the unacceptably high risk for the mother and fetus. Subsequently, the development of fiberoptics allowed the introduction of fetoscopy to visualize and sample vessels on the chorionic plate or the umbilical cord (100,101). Although the risk of maternal compromise with this method was relatively small, the high rate of pregnancy loss associated with fetoscopy (i.e., up to 11.3%) was considered a major disadvantage (102).

Introduced by Daffos and associates in 1983 (103), percutaneous ultrasound-guided umbilical blood sampling rapidly gained wide acceptance. In experienced hands, the risk of fetal loss is relatively small, between 1% to 2.3% (104,105), although numbers as high as 5.4% have also been reported (106). Other complications, usually associated with excessive needle manipulations, include hematoma of the umbilical cord and placental abruption, chorioamnionitis (0.6%), and preterm delivery (9%) (106). Fetal exsanguination from the puncture site is a relatively rare complication but has been reported infrequently (107). Maternal complications are negligible, although one case of life-threatening amnionitis has been reported (108). It appears that the risks are higher when the mother is obese, the placenta is posterior, or when the sampling is performed relatively early in gestation (i.e., before 19 weeks) (104).

Indications for cordocentesis are detailed in Table 12–4. Parental counseling before cordocentesis should include the risk of that pregnancy being affected by the conditions considered and the yield of information obtained through fetal blood sampling in such a situations. The risk and potential complications of the procedure itself also should be discussed. A detailed ultrasound examination should be performed before cordocentesis for evaluation of gestational age, placental location, and the diagnosis of fetal anomalies. Fetal blood can be obtained by puncture of the fetal heart, the intrahepatic part of the umbilical vein, or by puncture of an umbilical vessel close to its placental insertion, the latter being by far the most common site for cordocentesis. When the placenta is anterior or lateral, the needle is introduced transplacentally into the umbilical cord. In cases with a posterior placenta, the needle is introduced transamniotically, and the cord is punctured close to its placental insertion. Different guidance techniques (i.e., fixed needle guides versus freehand), needles of lengths varying from 8 to 15 cm with gauges varying from 20 to 27, and differing patient preparation protocols are used by various centers. Nicolaides and colleagues advocate an outpatient setting in the ultrasound department without need for maternal fasting, sedation, tocolytics, antibiotics, or fetal paralysis for the procedure (109).

Molecular diagnoses are available now for many of the mutations resulting in thalassemia, sickle-cell disease, and hemophilia A and B, enabling diagnosis in the first trimester by CVS, so that blood sampling need be performed only in noninformative cases or with ambiguous results. Cordocentesis is, however, necessary for the diagnosis and management of von Willebrand disease and of congenital alloimmune thrombocytopenia (110). In alloimmune thrombocytopenia, cordocentesis allows the determination of fetal platelet phenotype and count. A low fetal platelet count in this situation can be treated by weekly infusion of platelets until delivery (111,112).

In Rh isoimmunization, fetal blood sampling is performed for immediate confirmation of fetal antigenic status, obviating the need for further intervention in the Rh-negative fetus. If the fetus is Rh-positive, cordocentesis enables a more accurate assessment of fetal anemia and an immediate rise in fetal erythrocyte count on correction by intravascular transfusion. From case-control studies, it appears that intravascular correction of fetal anemia is more efficient and less risky to the mother and fetus than the intraperitoneal approach at all gestational ages or levels of disease severity (113,114). Moreover, in cases with cardiac decompensation in which the fetus may be compromised by the volume overload needed to correct the severe anemia, better results were obtained by intravascular exchange transfusion (115). It should be noted, however, that cordocentesis may enhance maternal sensitization more than amniocentesis does, especially if blood sampling is performed by a transplacental approach (116). Rh immunoprophylaxis should be offered to all Rh-negative, nonsensitized patients with an Rh-positive fetus undergoing cordocentesis.

Because IgM is too large to cross the placenta, the diagnosis of fetal infection is usually based on the demonstration of agent-specific IgM antibodies in fetal blood. Fetal blood sampling should be scheduled to allow enough time from initial exposure for IgM to appear after immunocompetence develops in the fetus. For first-trimester exposures, the best time for cordocentesis is probably after 22 weeks of gestation. In specific cases, *in utero* treatment also is available. Thus, after toxoplasmosis infection in the mother and demonstration of IgM specific for toxoplasmosis in fetal blood, antibiotic treatment with spiramycin significantly reduces the risk of congenital toxoplasmosis as well as the risk of late sequelae (117). Cordocentesis has been used for repeated blood transfusions *in utero* to hydropic fetuses with hemolytic anemia caused by parvovirus B19 infection (118).

Cordocentesis has been used for the evaluation of the small-for-dates fetus. Severe, early-onset IUGR is commonly associated with fetal chromosome anomalies. Cordocentesis allows rapid fetal karyotyping within 48 to 72 hours. Other abnormalities observed in blood samples from IUGR fetuses with normal chromosomes include hypoxemia, hypercapnia, lactic acidemia, leukopenia, thrombocytopenia, and disturbed carbohydrate, lipid, and protein metabolism. Several studies have compared the prediction of fetal acidosis by Doppler or biophysical profile with cord blood gases. Weiner demonstrated a sta-

TABLE 12–4. *Indications for cordocentesis*

Prenatal diagnosis of inherited blood disorders
    Hemoglobinopathies (e.g., homozygous thalassemia, sickle-cell disease)
    Coagulopathies (e.g., hemophilia A and B, von Willebrand disease)
Prenatal diagnosis of metabolic disorders
Fetal infections
    Toxoplasmosis: specific IgM or DNA hybridization
    Rubella: specific IgM
    Cytomegalovirus: specific IgM and blood cultures
    Varicella zoster virus: specific IgM
    Human parvovirus (B19): viral DNA
    Human immunodeficiency virus: specific IgM
Rapid fetal karyotyping
    Late booking or failed amniocentesis
    Suspected fetal mosaicism on amniocentesis
    Abnormal maternal serum screening
    Ultrasound diagnosis of fetal malformations
Evaluation of the small-for-gestational-age fetus
    Acid–base status
    Oxygenation
Assessment and treatment of fetal anemia
Diagnosis and treatment of fetal thrombocytopenia

Adapted from ref. 104.

tistically significant correlation between an increased umbilical systolic-to-diastolic ratio (>3.5) and fetal hypoxia and acidemia in cord blood (119). This relationship was even more significant with absent or reversed diastolic flow. In another study, the biophysical profile significantly correlated with changes in cord pH and, to some extent, with the degree of fetal acidemia (120). In cases of severe IUGR with equivocal biophysical score and umbilical blood flow studies, the availability of fetal PO_2 and pH may provide additional and crucial information in the balance between the risks of premature delivery versus growing in a hostile intrauterine environment.

REFERENCES

1. Steel MW, Breg WR. Chromosome analysis of human amniotic fluid cells. *Lancet* 1966;1:383.
2. Jacobson JB, Barter RH. Intrauterine diagnosis and management of genetic defects. *Am J Obstet Gynecol* 1967;99:795.
3. Nadler HL. Antenatal detection of hereditary disorders. *Pediatrics* 1968;42:912.
4. Medical Research Council. *Diagnosis of genetic disease by amniocentesis during second trimester of pregnancy.* Ottawa: Medical Research Council, 1977.
5. National Institute of Child Health and Human Development Amniocentesis Registry, 1978. *The safety and accuracy of midtrimester amniocentesis. DHEW Publication No. (NIH) 78-190.* Washington, DC: United States Department of Health, Education and Welfare, 1978.
6. Evans MI, Drugan A, Koppitch FC, et al. Genetic diagnosis in the first trimester: the norm for the 90's. *Am J Obstet Gynecol* 1989;160:1332.
7. Canadian Collaborative CVS–Amniocentesis Clinical Trial Group. Multicenter randomized clinical trial of chorionic villus sampling and amniocentesis. *Lancet* 1989;1:1.
8. Rhoads GG, Jackson LG, Schlesselman SE, et al. The safety and efficacy of chorionic villus sampling for early prenatal diagnosis of cytogenetic abnormalities. *N Engl J Med* 1989;320:609.
9. Hanson FW, Happ RL, Tennant FR, et al. Ultrasonography-guided early amniocentesis in singleton pregnancies. *Am J Obstet Gynecol* 1990;162:1376.
10. Findlay I, Atkinson G, Chambers M, et al. Rapid genetic diagnosis at 7–9 weeks gestation: diagnosis of sex, single gene defects and DNA fingerprints from coelomic samples. *Hum Reprod* 1996;11:2548.
11. Drugan A, Reichler A, Bronshtein M, et al. Abnormal biochemical serum screening versus second trimester ultrasound-detected minor anomalies as predictors of aneuploidy in low risk patients. *Fetal Diagn Ther* 1996;11(5):301.
12. Zimmer EZ, Drugan A, Ofir C, et al. Ultrasound anomalies of the fetal neck: Implications for the risk of aneuploidy and structural anomalies. *Prenat Diagn* 1997;17:1055.
13. Haddow JE, Palomaki GE, Knight GJ, et al. Reducing the need for amniocentesis in women 35 years of age or older with serum markers for screening. *N Engl J Med* 1994;330:1114.
14. Beekhuis JR, De Wolf BT, Mantingh A, Heringa MP. The influence of serum screening on the amniocentesis rate in women of advanced maternal age. *Prenat Diagn* 1994;14:199.
15. Holzgreve W, Miny P, Schloo R, et al. "Late CVS" international registry: compilation of data from 24 centers. *Prenat Diagn* 1990;10:159.
16. Hoskins IA. Cordocentesis in isoimmunization and fetal physiologic measurement, infection and karyotyping. *Curr Opin Obstet Gynecol* 1991;3:266.
17. Kazy Z, Rozovsky IS, Balchaten VA. Chorion biopsy in early pregnancy: a method of early prenatal diagnosis for inherited disorders. *Prenat Diagn* 1982;2:39.
18. Simoni G, Brambati B, Danesino C, et al. Efficient direct chromosome analyses and enzyme determinations from chorionic villi samples in the first trimester of pregnancy. *Hum Genet* 1983;63:349.
19. Brambati B, Simoni G. Letter to the editor. *Lancet* 1989;1:583.
20. Ledbetter DH, Martin AO, Verlinsky Y, et al. Cytogenetic results of chorionic villus sampling: high success rate and diagnostic accuracy in the United States Collaborative Study. *Am J Obstet Gynecol* 1990; 162:495.
21. Copeland KL, Carpenter RJ, Penolio KR, et al. Integration of the transabdominal technique into an ongoing chorionic villus sampling program. *Am J Obstet Gynecol* 1989;161:1289.
22. Jahoda MGJ, Pijpers I, Reuss A, et al. Transabdominal villus sampling in early second trimester: a safe sampling method for women of advanced age. *Prenat Diagn* 1990;10:307.
23. Evans MI, Moore C, Kolodny F, et al. Lysosomal enzymes in chorionic villi, cultured amniocytes, and cultured skin fibroblasts. *Clin Chim Acta* 1986;157:109.
24. Simpson JL. Chorionic villus sampling. *Semin Perinatol* 1990;14:446.
25. Podobnick M, Ciglar S, Singer Z, et al. Transabdominal chorionic villus sampling in the second and third trimesters of high risk pregnancies. *Prenat Diagn* 1997;17:125.
26. Borrell A, Costa D, Delgado RD, et al. Transcervical chorionic villus sampling beyond 12 weeks of gestation. *Ultrasound Obstet Gynecol* 1996;7:416.
27. Brambati B, Oldrini A, Lanzani A. Transabdominal villus sampling: a free hand ultrasound guided technique. *Am J Obstet Gynecol* 1987; 157:134.
28. Smidt-Jensen S, Hahnemann N. Transabdominal fine needle biopsy from chorionic villi in the first trimester. *Prenat Diagn* 1984;4:163.
29. Evans MI, Quigg MH, Koppitch FC, et al. First trimester prenatal diagnosis. In: Evans MI, Fletcher JC, Dixler AO, et al, eds. *Fetal diagnosis and therapy: science, ethics and the law.* Philadelphia: JB Lippincott, 1989:17.
30. Brambati B, Lanzani A, Tului L. Transabdominal and transcervical chorionic villus sampling: efficiency and risk evaluation of 2411 cases. *Am J Med Genet* 1990;35:160.
31. Ghirardini G, Popp WL, Camurri L, et al. Vaginosonographic guided chorionic villi needle biopsy. *Eur J Obstet Gynecol Reprod Biol* 1986; 23:315.
32. Sidransky E, Black SH, Soenksen DM, et al. Transvaginal chorionic villus sampling. *Prenat Diagn* 1990;10:583.
33. Simpson JL. Incidence and timing of pregnancy losses: relevance to evaluating safety of early prenatal diagnosis. *Am J Med Genet* 1990; 35:165.
34. Firth HV, Boyd PA, Chamberlain P, et al. Severe limb abnormalities after chorionic villus sampling at 56–66 days' gestation. *Lancet* 1991; 337:762.
35. Burton BK, Schulz CJ, Burd LI. Limb anomalies associated with chorionic villus sampling. *Obstet Gynecol* 1992;79:726.
36. Firth H, Boyd PA, Chamberlain P, MacKenzie IZ, Huson SM. Limb defects and chorionic villus sampling [letter; comment]. *Lancet* 1996; 347:1406.
37. Kuliev A, Jackson L, Froster U, et al. Chorionic villus sampling safety. Report of World Health Organization/EURO meeting. *Am J Obstet Gynecol* 1996;174:807.
38. Schloo R, Miny P, Holzgreve W, Horst J, Lenz W. Distal limb deficiency following chorionic villus sampling? *Am J Med Genet* 1992; 42:404.
39. Blakemore KJ, Baumgarten A, Schonfeld Dimaio M, et al. Rise in maternal serum alpha-fetoprotein concentration after chorionic villus sampling and the possibility of isoimmunization. *Am J Obstet Gynecol* 1986;155:986.
40. Shulman LP, Meyers CM, Simpson JL, et al. Fetomaternal transfusion depends on amount of chorionic villi aspirated but not on method of chorionic villus sampling. *Am J Obstet Gynecol* 1990;162:1185.
41. McGowan KD, Blakemore KJ. Amniocentesis and chorionic villus sampling. *Curr Opin Obstet Gynecol* 1991;3:221.
42. Johnson A, Wapner RJ, Davis GH, et al. Mosaicism in chorionic villus sampling: an association with poor perinatal outcome. *Obstet Gynecol* 1990;75:573.
43. Sundberg K, Lundsteen C, Philip J. Early filtration amniocentesis for further investigation of mosaicism diagnosed by chorionic villus sampling. *Prenat Diagn* 1996;16:1121.
44. Kalousek DK, Dill FJ. Chromosomal mosaicism confined to the placenta in human conceptions. *Science* 1983;221:665.
45. Leschot NJ, Schuring Blum GH, Van Prooijen-Knegt AC, et al. The outcome of pregnancies with confined placental chromosome mosaicism in cytotrophoblast cells. *Prenat Diagn* 1996;16:705.
46. Wright DJ, Brindley BA, Koppitch FC, et al. Interpretation of chori-

onic villus sampling laboratory results is just as reliable as amniocentesis. *Obstet Gynecol* 1989;74:739.

47. Gosden C, Rodeck CH, Nicolaides KH. Fetal blood sampling in the investigation of chromosome mosaicism in amniotic fluid cell culture. *Lancet* 1988;1:613.

48. Ledbetter DH, Engel E. Uniparental disomy in humans: development of an imprinting map and its implications for prenatal diagnosis. *Hum Mol Genet* 1995;4:1757.

49. Penso CA, Frigoletto FD. Early amniocentesis. *Semin Perinatol* 1990; 14:465.

50. Dombrowsky MP, Isada NB, Johnson MP, Berry SM. Modified stylet technique for tenting of amniotic membranes. *Obstet Gynecol* 1996; 87:455.

51. Brumfield CG, Lin S, Conner W, et al. Pregnancy outcome following genetic amniocentesis at 11–14 versus 16–19 weeks gestation. *Obstet Gynecol* 1996;88:114.

52. Hanson FW, Zorn EM, Tennant FR, et al. Amniocentesis before 15 weeks gestation: outcome, risks and technical problems. *Am J Obstet Gynecol* 1987;156:1524.

53. Stripparo I, Buscaglia M, Longatti L, et al. Genetic amniocentesis: 505 cases performed before the sixteenth week of gestation. *Prenat Diagn* 1990;10:359.

54. Nevin J, Nevin NC, Dornan JC, et al. Early amniocentesis; experience of 222 consecutive patients from 1987–1988. *Prenat Diagn* 1990;10: 79.

55. Dunn LK, Godmilow L. A comparison of loss rates for first trimester chorionic villus sampling, early amniocentesis and midtrimester amniocentesis in a population of women of advanced maternal age [abstract]. *Am J Hum Genet* 1990;47(Suppl):A273.

56. Johnson JM, Wilson RD, Winsor EJ, et al. The early amniocentesis study: a randomized clinical trial of early amniocentesis versus midtrimester amniocentesis. *Fetal Diagn Ther* 1996;11:85.

57. Elejalde BR, de Elejalde MM, Acuna JM, et al. Prospective study of amniocentesis performed between weeks 9 and 16 of gestation: its feasibility, risks, complications and use in early genetic amniocentesis. *Am J Med Genet* 1990;35:188.

58. The Canadian Early and Mid-trimester Amniocentesis Trial (CEMAT) Group. Randomised trial to assess safety and fetal outcome of early and midtrimester amniocentesis. *Lancet* 1998;351:242.

59. Sundberg K, Bang J, Smidt-Jensen S, et al. Randomised study of risk of fetal loss related to early amniocentesis versus chorionic villus sampling. *Lancet* 1997;350:697.

60. Rooney DE, MacLachlan N, Smith J, et al. Early amniocentesis: a cytogenetic evaluation. *Br Med J* 1989;299:25.

61. Reid R, Sepuvelda W, Kyle PM, Davies G. Amniotic fluid culture failure: clinical significance and association with aneuploidy. *Obstet Gynecol* 1996;87:588.

62. Diaz Vega M, De La Cueva P, Leal C, Aisa F. Early amniocentesis at 10–12 weeks gestation. *Prenat Diagn* 1996;16:307.

63. Drugan A, Syner FN, Greb A, et al. Amniotic fluid alpha-fetoprotein and acetylcholinesterase in early genetic amniocentesis. *Obstet Gynecol* 1988;72:33.

64. Crandall BF, Hanson FW, Tennant F, et al. Alpha-fetoprotein levels in amniotic fluid between 11 and 15 weeks. *Am J Obstet Gynecol* 1989;160:1204.

65. Crandall BF, Chua C. Detecting neural tube defects by amniocentesis between 11 and 15 weeks gestation. *Prenat Diagn* 1995;15:339.

66. Drugan A, Syner FN, Belsky RL, et al. Amniotic fluid acetylcholinesterase: implications of an inconclusive result. *Am J Obstet Gynecol* 1988;159:469.

67. Burton BK, Nelson LH, Pettenati MJ. False positive acetylcholinesterase with early amniocentesis. *Obstet Gynecol* 1989;74:607.

68. Brown CL, Colden KA, Hume RF, et al. Faint and positive amniotic fluid acetylcholinesterase with a normal sonogram. *Am J Obstet Gynecol* 1996;175:1000.

69. Robinson GE, Garner DM, Olmsted MP, et al. Anxiety reduction after chorionic villus sampling and genetic amniocentesis. *Am J Obstet Gynecol* 1988;159:953.

70. Gosden CM. First trimester fetal karyotyping: CVS or early amniocentesis? [editorial]. *Ultrasound Obstet Gynecol* 1991;1:233.

71. Byrne D, Marks K, Azar G, et al. Randomized study of early amniocentesis versus chorionic villus sampling: a technical and cytogenetic comparison of 650 patients. *Ultrasound Obstet Gynecol* 1991;1:235.

72. Nicolaides KH, Brizot ML, Patel F, Snijders R. Comparison of chori-

onic villus sampling and early amniocentesis for karyotyping in 1492 singleton pregnancies. *Fetal Diagn Ther* 1996;11:9.

73. Yuksel B, Greenough A, Naik S, et al. Perinatal lung function and invasive antenatal procedures. *Thorax* 1997;52:181.

74. Calhoun BC, Brehm W, Bombard AT. Early genetic amniocentesis and its relationship to respiratory difficulties in paediatric patients: a report of findings in patients and matched controls 3–5 years postprocedure. *Prenat Diagn* 1994;14(3):209.

75. Thompson PJ, Greenough A, Nicolaides KH. Lung function in infancy following first trimester amniocentesis or chorion villus sampling. *Fetal Diagn Ther* 1993;8(2):79.

76. Drugan A, Johnson MP, Evans MI. Amniocentesis. In: Evans MI, ed. *Reproductive risks and prenatal diagnosis.* Norwalk, CT: Appleton & Lange, 1992:191.

77. Cohn GM, Gould M, Miller RC, et al. The importance of genetic counseling before amniocentesis. *J Perinatol* 1996;16:352.

78. Hanson FW, Tennant FR, Zorn EM, et al. Analysis of 2136 genetic amniocenteses: experience of a single physician. *Am J Obstet Gynecol* 1985;152:435.

79. Golbus MS, Stephens JD, Cann HM, et al. Rh isoimmunization following genetic amniocentesis. *Prenat Diagn* 1982;2:149.

80. Murray JC, Karp LE, Williamson RA, et al. Rh isoimmunization as related to amniocentesis. *Am J Hum Genet* 1983;16:527.

81. NICHD National Registry for Amniocentesis Study Group. Midtrimester amniocentesis for prenatal diagnosis: safety and accuracy. *JAMA* 1976;236:1471.

82. Bombard AT, Power JF, Carter S, et al. Procedure related fetal losses in transplacental versus nontransplacental genetic amniocentesis. *Am J Obstet Gynecol* 1995;172:868.

83. Crane JP, Rohland BM. Clinical significance of amniotic fluid leakage after genetic amniocentesis. *Prenat Diagn* 1986;6:25.

84. Nimrod C, Varela-Gittings F, Machin G, et al. The effect of very prolonged membrane rupture on fetal development. *Am J Obstet Gynecol* 1984;148:540.

85. Gold R, Goyert G, Schwartz DB, et al. Conservative management of midtrimester post amniocentesis fluid leakage. *Obstet Gynecol* 1989; 74:745.

86. Finegan JA, Quarrington BJ, Hughes HE, et al. Child outcome following mid-trimester amniocentesis: development, behaviour, and physical status at age 4 years. *Br J Obstet Gynaecol* 1990;97(1):32.

87. Baird PA, Yee IM, Sadovnick AD. Population-based study of longterm outcomes after amniocentesis. *Lancet* 1994;344:1134.

88. Finegan JA, Sitarenios G, Bolan PL, Sarabura AD. Children whose mothers had second trimester amniocentesis: follow up at school age. *Br J Obstet Gynaecol* 1996;103(3):214.

89. Simpson JL. Amniocentesis: what it can tell you and what it can't. *Contemp Obstet Gynecol* 1988;31:33.

90. Hsu LYF, Kaffe S, Perlis ET. Trisomy 20 mosaicism in prenatal diagnosis: a review and update. *Prenat Diagn* 1987;7:581.

91. Worton RG, Stern RA. A Canadian collaborative study on mosaicism in amniotic fluid cell cultures. *Prenat Diagn* 1984;4:131.

92. Nicolaides KH, Soothill PH, Rodeck CH, et al. Prenatal diagnosis: why confine chorionic villus (placental) biopsy to the first trimester? *Lancet* 1986;1:543.

93. Chieri PR, Aldini AJR. Feasibility of placental biopsy in the second trimester for fetal diagnosis. *Am J Obstet Gynecol* 1989;160:581.

94. Smidt-Jensen S, Lundsteen C, Lind AM, et al. Transabdominal chorionic villus sampling in the second and third trimester of pregnancy: chromosome quality, reporting time and feto-maternal bleeding. *Prenat Diagn* 1993;13:957.

95. Ko TM, Tseng LH, Hwa HL, et al. Prenatal diagnosis by transabdominal chorionic villus sampling in the second and third trimesters. *Arch Gynecol Obstet* 1995;256:193.

96. Podobnik M, Ciglar S, Singer Z, et al. Transabdominal chorionic villus sampling in the secomd and third trimesters of high risk pregnancies. *Prenat Diagn* 1997;17:125.

97. Ganshirt-Ahlert D, Pohlschmidt M, Gal A, et al. Transabdominal placental biopsy in the second and third trimester of pregnancy: what is the risk of maternal contamination in DNA diagnosis? *Obstet Gynecol* 1990;75:320.

98. Holzgreve W, Miny P, Gerlach B, et al. Benefits of placental biopsies for rapid karyotyping in the second and third trimesters (late chorionic villus sampling) in high risk pregnancies. *Am J Obstet Gynecol* 1990; 162:1188.

99. Freda VJ, Adamson KJ. Exchange transfusion *in utero*. *Am J Obstet Gynecol* 1964;89:817.

100. Hobbins JC, Mahoney MJ. *In utero* diagnosis of hemoglobinopathies: technique for obtaining fetal blood. *N Engl J Med* 1974;290:1065.

101. Rodeck CH, Cambell S. Umbilical cord insertion as source of pure fetal blood for prenatal diagnosis. *Lancet* 1979;1:1244.

102. Ward RHT, Modell B, Fairweather DVI. Obstetric outcome and problems of midtrimester fetal blood sampling for antenatal diagnosis. *Br J Obstet Gynaecol* 1981;88:1073.

103. Daffos F, Cappella-Pavlovsky M, Forestier F. Fetal blood sampling via the umbilical cord using a needle guided by ultrasound: report of 66 cases. *Prenat Diagn* 1983;3:271.

104. Nicolaides KH, Sniders RJM. Cordocentesis. In: Evans MI, ed. *Reproductive risks and prenatal diagnosis.* Norwalk, CT: Appleton & Lange, 1992:201.

105. Buscaglia M, Ghisoni L, Bellotti M, et al. Percutaneous umbilical blood sampling: indication changes and procedure loss rates in a nine years experience. *Fetal Diagn Ther* 1996;11:106.

106. Bernaschek G, Yildiz A, Kolankaya A, et al. Complications of cordocentesis in high risk pregnancies: effects on fetal loss and premature deliveries. *Prenat Diagn* 1995;15:995.

107. Seligman SP, Young BK. Tachycardia as the sole fetal heart rate abnormality after funipuncture. *Obstet Gynecol* 1996;87:833.

108. Wilkins I, Mezrow G, Lynch L, et al. Amnionitis and life threatening respiratory distress after percutaneous umbilical blood sampling. *Am J Obstet Gynecol* 1989;160:427.

109. Nicolaides KH, Soothill PW, Rodeck CH, et al. Ultrasound guided sampling of umbilical cord and placental blood to access fetal well being. *Lancet* 1986;1:1065.

110. Bussel JB, Berkowitz RL, McFarland JG, et al. Antenatal treatment of neonatal thrombocytopenia. *N Engl J Med* 1988;319:1374.

111. Nicolini U, Rodeck CH, Kochenour NK, et al. *In utero* platelet transfusion for allo-immune thrombocytopenia. *Lancet* 1988;2:506.

112. Murphy MF, Pullon HWH, Metcalfe P, et al. Management of fetal allo-immune thrombocytopenia by weekly *in utero* platelet transfusions. *Vox Sang* 1990;58:45.

113. Keckstein G, Stoz F, Tschurtz S, et al. Intrauterine treatment of severe fetal erythroblastosis: intrauterine transfusion with ultrasonic guidance. *J Perinat Med* 1989;17:341.

114. Harman CR, Bowman JM, Manning FA, et al. Intrauterine transfusion: intraperitoneal versus intravascular approach: a case control comparison. *Am J Obstet Gynecol* 1990;162:1053.

115. Poissonier MH, Brossard Y, Demedeiros N, et al. Two hundred intrauterine exchange transfusions in severe blood incompatibilities. *Am J Obstet Gynecol* 1989;161:709.

116. Weiner CP, Grant S, Hudson J, et al. Effect of diagnostic and therapeutic cordocentesis on maternal serum alpha-fetoprotein concentration. *Am J Obstet Gynecol* 1989;161:706.

117. Daffos F, Forestier F, Capella-Pavlovsky M, et al. Prenatal management of 746 pregnancies at risk for congenital toxoplasmosis. *N Engl J Med* 1988;318:271.

118. Peters MT, Nicolaides KH. Cordocentesis for the diagnosis and treatment of human fetal parvovirus infection. *Obstet Gynecol* 1990;75:501.

119. Weiner CP. The relationship between the umbilical artery systolic/diastolic ratio and umbilical blood gas measurements in specimens obtained by cordocentesis. *Am J Obstet Gynecol* 1990;162:1198.

120. Ribbert LSM, Sniders RJM, Nicolaides KH, et al. Relationship of fetal biophysical profile and blood gas values at cordocentesis in severely growth retarded fetuses. *Am J Obstet Gynecol* 1990;163:569.

CHAPTER 13

Fetal Therapy

Mark I. Evans, Alan W. Flake, Mark Paul Johnson,
Wolfgang Holzgreve, and Michael R. Harrison

For nearly three decades, prenatal diagnostic techniques have been developed to detect fetal structural and functional abnormalities (1). At the same time, the legal right to consider abortion was recognized in the United States. Couples thus had the option of pregnancy termination when legally permissible. However, in limited instances it has become possible to correct selected abnormalities. In general, structural abnormalities are best approached surgically, whereas metabolic abnormalities have generally been treated pharmacologically or now genetically. Fetal therapeutic approaches have traditionally been divided into three main categories: surgical, medical, and genetic, and this chapter follows that pattern.

SURGICAL THERAPY

Over the past few years a number of advances have been made in surgical therapies. The surgical approaches have been further subdivided into those that are percutaneous, endoscopic, and open.

Percutaneous

The classic example of percutaneous therapy has been the evaluation of obstructive uropathies, seen in one of every 5,000 to 8,000 men. The natural history of obstruction may lead to hydronephrosis, renal dysplasia, and

M. I. Evans: Division of Reproductive Genetics; Center for Fetal Diagnosis and Therapy; and Human Genetics Program, Hutzel Hospital/Wayne State University, Detroit, Michigan

A. W. Flake: Department of Pediatric Surgery, Children's Hospital of Philadelphia, Philadelphia, Pennsylvania

M. P. Johnson: Departments of Obstetrics/Gynecology, Pathology, Molecular Medicine, and Genetics, Wayne State University; and Reproductive Genetics, Department of Obstetrics and Gynecology, Hutzel Hospital/The Detroit Medical Center, Detroit, Michigan

W. Holzgreve: University of Basel, Basel, Switzerland

M. R. Harrison: Department of Pediatric Surgery, University of California, San Francisco, San Francisco, California

eventually death (2). Prenatally diagnosed cases of posterior urethral valves generally have a 30% to 50% mortality. Death is most often secondary to pulmonary hypoplasia. Most of these babies die a pulmonary death because they don't live long enough to die a renal death.

The sonographic diagnosis of fetal lower urinary tract obstruction (LUTO) is suggested by a dilated and thickened bladder, hydroureters, hydronephrosis, and oligohydramnios (Fig. 13–1). In a male fetus, these findings are highly suggestive of posterior urethral valves. However, sonographicaly, urethral stricture or atresia, urethral agenesis, ureteral reflux, persistent cloaca, and megalourethra can present similarly. Thus, precise diagnosis can usually be made only after birth (3).

Patient management is complex. Major congenital anomalies are sought by detailed ultrasonography. Renal cystic dysplasia and the volume of amniotic fluid have prognostic value. We developed the concept of serial vesicocenteses to determine the functional status of the fetal kidneys by the concentrations of Na, Ca, β_2-microglobulin, and total protein in fetal urine as well as its osmolality (4,5) (Fig. 13–2). A single vesicocentesis can not adequately predict the renal reserve because two consecutive samples may be on different sides of the normal cut-off level.

The diversion of fetal urine into the amniotic cavity by ultrasound-guided vesicoamniotic shunts serves a dual purpose; it prevents the renal damage that may result from obstruction, and it allows normal pulmonary development. Decompression of the obstruction results in resolution of the urinary obstruction and improved pulmonary status at birth. Our experiences with over 100 patients evaluated for obstruction reveals that we can, with reasonable certainty, divide patients into those who appear to have a favorable prognosis and those who do not. Untreated, poor prognosis patients all die. Nevertheless, of those treated, a few may survive but as renal cripples. Good prognosis cases did better treated than not.

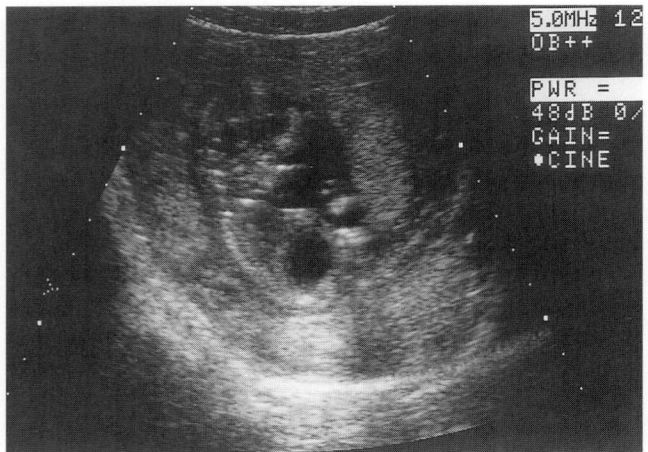

FIG. 13–1. Ultrasound of obstructive uropathy in a 13-week fetus. The enlarged bladder fills the abdomen because of urethral obstruction.

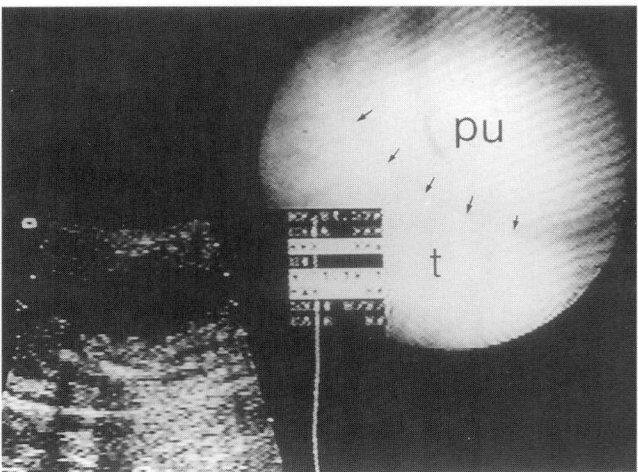

FIG. 13–3. *In utero* cystoscopic view of fetal bladder. T, trigone; PU, posterior urethra. Note markedly dilated bladder neck on ultrasound.

Treatment of fetuses with LUTO using urinary diversion procedures has significant limitations. First, they are palliative measures that defer the final treatment of the obstruction until the birth of the child. Second, vesicoamniotic shunts may become obstructed or displaced in up to 25% of cases, requiring additional interventions to replace the shunt, with their attendant complications. Fetal vesicostomy or ureterostomy via open fetal surgery have been proposed to overcome the problems associated with the percutaneously placed shunts, but they have not gained support because such procedures would be significantly more invasive.

We next introduced the concept of performing percutaneous fetal cystoscopy to evaluate fetuses affected with LUTO (6,7) (Fig. 13–3). This procedure uses the same techniques and skills as fetal vesicocentesis. A thin endoscope is passed through the lumen of the needle or trocar to observe the fetal bladder at the time of the vesicocentesis. Diagnostic fetal cystoscopy can be performed with evaluation of the musculature of the detrusor and trigone regions, the ureters, and the proximal urethra for evidence of long-standing obstruction and reflux. The endoscope is then removed, and the bladder is drained of urine to be used for evaluation of underlying renal function.

We hypothesize that percutaneous fetal cystoscopy may allow a more precise prenatal diagnosis and prognosis in fetuses with lower urinary tract obstruction. Since this procedure can be performed at the time of diagnostic vesicocentesis, it should not pose additional risks to the standard assessment of fetal renal function. In addition, those fetuses truly identified as having posterior valves may fare better if the obstruction can be eliminated in utero, avoiding the complications of vesico-amniotic shunts or the morbidity of open fetal surgery.

Other Shunt Approaches

The original disorder for which shunting was attempted was obstructive hydrocephalus. Attempts in the late 1970s and early 1980s were nearly uniformly dismal. However, in retrospect, most operated patients were, in fact, poor candidates. Many had multisystem disorders, including aneuploidy and hopeless congenital anomalies such as holoprosencephaly.

Brain shunts have been abandoned since the early 1980s, but now, with a better understanding of the poor natural history of the anomaly (8) and better, more accurate diagnostic techniques, there may be limited applications for prenatal neurologic shunting, which might once again become a possibility.

The other major percutaneous approach has been for fetal thoracic abnormalities. Shunting has been successfully performed in cases of macrocystic adenomatous malformations, presumed chylothorax, and hydrops. There is less experience with chest shunting than blad-

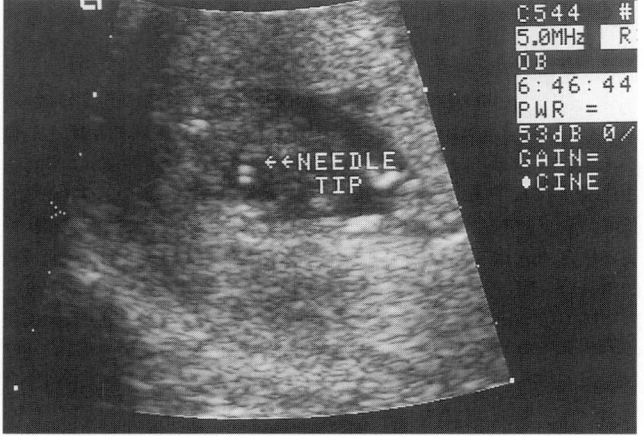

FIG. 13–2. Needle tip in bladder, draining urine from fetus of Fig. 13–1.

ders, and there is a smaller margin for error and greater risk for disaster if the shunt hits the mediastinal structures. Nevertheless, in appropriately chosen situations, drainage of a fluid-filled space, such as an isolated pleural effusion that acts as a space-occupying lesion, has allowed compensatory lung growth and improved outcomes (9).

Endoscopic Approaches

Endoscopic fetal surgery is likewise being developed for the treatment of umbilical cord ligation in acardiac twins, for laser ablation in twin-to-twin transfusion, and developments are occurring in its use for early fetal blood sampling and as an adjunct to *in utero* fetal muscle biopsy.

The next several years will be very exciting, particularly as new modifications to these techniques make the procedures safer, more reliable, quicker, and therefore more commonplace. It is likely that many applications of open fetal surgery will in fact be modified to be done endoscopically as experience continues.

Open Surgical Approaches

Open fetal surgery has been selectively performed for over a decade, primarily at the University of California, San Francisco, with recent expansion to a few other sites. Its application has been limited by appropriate concern for maternal risk, rigorous selection criteria, and somewhat frustrating results. During this time there has been constant innovation, motivated by clinical necessity, to improve the feasibility and safety of open fetal surgery for the fetus and the mother. Today, operative techniques for opening and closing the uterus, monitoring the fetus intraoperatively, maintaining fetal homeostasis, and treating a variety of anomalies have been developed and are relatively standardized (10).

Open fetal surgery is performed through a maternal hysterotomy. It is preferentially performed in the lower uterine segment. It must provide optimal exposure of a specific fetal part or region, avoid the placenta, and provide hemostasis with absolute control of the fetal membranes. The consequences of a poorly placed or technically inadequate hysterotomy include technical failure of the fetal procedure, intra- or postoperative fetal demise, postoperative amniotic fluid leak, and chorioamnionitis with associated preterm labor.

The timing of a fetal operation depends on the anomaly being treated and the pathophysiology of the specific fetus (11,12). In general, small size and tissue integrity become significantly limiting factors at less than 18 weeks of gestation. After 30 weeks of gestation, it is usually more reasonable to deliver the fetus and treat the abnormality *ex utero*. In addition, there is less time for fetal intervention to achieve the desired effect (i.e., lung growth) with late operations. There is also the unproven impression that the later a fetal operation is performed, the more reactive the uterus, and the higher the likelihood of preterm labor. For these reasons, open fetal procedures have been performed between 18 and 30 weeks gestation. Another important consideration is the magnitude of the operation and associated fetal stress. Minor, rapidly performed procedures that can be accomplished through a small hysterotomy are much less likely than prolonged, major fetal operations to induce fetal or uteroplacental physiologic derangement with secondary preterm labor and/or fetal demise.

Fetal Monitoring and Homeostasis

Reliable intraoperative monitoring has been very difficult to achieve. The confined space and small amount of exposed fetal tissue area in combination with the poor tissue integrity of the fetus make sutured electrodes less than satisfactory. Pulse oximetry has been successfully utilized, but the inherent problems and limitations of this technology are amplified in the fetus. Small size, minimal pulse pressure, moisture, and ambient light all hinder pulse oximetry, and mostly when it is critical under conditions of fetal hypotension or instability. Recently, radiotelemetry systems have been developed in cooperation with NASA that allow fetal heart rate, temperature, intraamniotic pressure, and, potentially, parameters such as pH and tissue oxygenation to be monitored (13). A small radiotelemeter is sutured to the fetal skin and sends a continuous signal to an outside antenna. This can be left in place postoperatively for monitoring and is more sensitive for detection of uterine contraction than standard tocodynanometry. Despite progress, the use of intraoperative and postoperative ultrasound remains the most reliable method of assessing fetal status, providing information on fetal heart rate, volume status, and contractility.

Fetal homeostasis is maintained by protection of uteroplacental blood flow by continued uterine relaxation and careful monitoring and control of maternal volume status and blood pressure. Care is taken to avoid umbilical cord compression, which may occur at the margins of the hysterotomy or if inadequate amniotic fluid surrounds the fetus. Every attempt is made to maintain intraamniotic volume by exteriorization of only the necessary part of the fetus and by continuous high-volume perfusion of the amniotic space with warm Ringer's lactate solution. Loss of uterine volume initiates uterine contraction.

Congenital Diaphragmatic Hernia

Congenital diaphragmatic hernia (CDH) has been the prototype for open fetal surgery. The fetal approach to CDH has undergone complete reevaluation since the first attempted CDH repair in 1986 and the first success in 1990 (14,15). Definitive repair of CDH by reduction of viscera from the chest, diaphragmatic patch placement, and abdominal silo construction (to reduce intraabdominal pressure) has proven to be a technical tour de force with unacceptable mortality, particularly when the liver has herniated into the chest. A scoring system based on the lung-to-heart ratio in the chest cavity was developed. The lower the ratio, the higher the neonatal mortality rate. Patients can thus be divided into those who are too good to need surgery, appropriate candidates, and those who, if left untreated, have a very high mortality. We have therefore abandoned definitive repair as an option for CDH and switched to *in utero* tracheal occlusion (Fig. 13–4). Tracheal occlusion induces lung growth through accumulation of pulmonary secretions, which reduces the herniated viscera from the chest and alleviates lung hypoplasia. The tracheal occlusion procedure is relatively simple and consists of exposure of the fetal neck in hyperextension, dissection of the trachea circumferentially, with care taken to avoid the recurrent laryngeal nerves, and placement of occlusive hemoclips. The fetus is then put back into the uterus. The uterine incision is then closed, with careful attention paid to hemostasis. Collaborative data on the procedure suggest that this technique is the most appropriate procedure for operative intervention in CDH. As both surgical skills and neonatal treatments improve, there is a need for continual evaluation of the relative merits of each approach and of which is better under different circumstances. It remains to be seen whether tracheal occlusion will improve on the results of conventional treatment of CDH (16).

Congenital Cystic Adenomatoid Malformation

Congenital cystic adenomatoid malformation (CCAM) is a space-occupying congenital cystic lesion of the lung that may grow and induce hydrops by causing a mediastinal shift and compromise of venous return to the heart. Fetuses with CCAM who develop hydrops have a

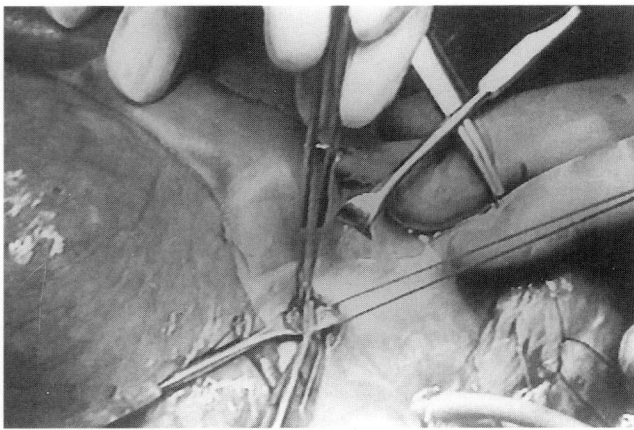

FIG. 13–4. Isolation of fetal trachea for placement of hemoclips to occlude the trachea.

mortality approaching 100%. Fetal resection of CCAM reverses hydrops and has improved survival dramatically (17). The fetal operation is performed by exposure of the arm and chest wall on the side of the lesion through the maternal hysterotomy. A large thoracotomy is performed through midthorax of the fetus, and the lobe containing the CCAM is exteriorized. The attachments of the lobe to adjacent lung tissue are bluntly divided, and the lobar hilum is divided by application of a TIA stapler or a bulk ligature. The thoracotomy is quickly closed. Although this is a major operative procedure, operative time is short compared to repair of CDH, and blood loss and fetal stress are relatively minimal.

Sacrococcygeal Teratoma

Fetal sacrococcygeal teratoma (SCT) is a tumor arising from the presacral space that may grow to massive proportions and in some fetuses induce high-output failure from tumor vascular steal. The combination of fetal SCT and high-output physiology with associated placentomegaly or hydrops uniformly results in fetal demise. The pathophysiologic rationale for fetal surgery is to ligate the vascular steal and reverse the high-output physiology. The fetal operation is performed by exteriorization of the fetal buttocks with attached tumor (18). Every attempt is made to keep the head, torso, and lower extremities of the fetus in the uterus. Because the tumor can be larger than the fetus, significant loss of uterine volume occurs, and the uterus may contract. Once exteriorized, the anus is identified, and the fetal skin is incised posterior to the anorectal sphincter complex to avoid injury to the continence mechanism. A tourniquet is then applied to the base of the tumor and brought down gradually as the tumor is finger fractured down to its vascular pedicle. The vascular pedicle is then ligated with suture ligatures or stapled, depending on the width of the pedicle. The entire fetal procedure can be performed in less than 15 minutes with minimal blood loss. Because of the increase in afterload following ligation of the low-resistance tumor circuit, the fetal hemodynamic status must be monitored closely during and in the period immediately following the ligation, by ultrasound.

Closing the Uterus

The obvious difference between fetal surgery and a cesarean section is that the fetus must be returned to the uterus and remain in the uterus for several weeks for the procedure to succeed. The primary criteria of an adequate closure are strength, healing, and avoidance of amniotic fluid leak. The closure is initiated by placement of large interrupted full-thickness monofilament retention sutures the length of the wound. This allows elevation of the wound edges during closure to minimize hemorrhage. The staple lines are excised to freshen the edges and allow apposition of muscle tissue. A fine running monofiliment is then placed to approximate the membranes. A small catheter is left in the amniotic space to reconstitute amniotic fluid and instill antibiotics before the closure is completed. A second running layer of larger monofiliment absorbable suture is placed through the myometrium to achieve broad muscular approximation. Finally, the retention sutures are tied to relieve tension on the wound and provide strength. Fibrin glue has sometimes been used as an additional sealant but has not been proven to be necessary. Before the last stitch is tied, under ultrasound guidance, the amniotic fluid volume is reconstituted with warm lactated Ringer's solution, antibiotics are instilled, and the catheter is removed.

The EXIT Procedure

The EXIT procedure is a modified fetal delivery and may be applied to deliver fetuses after fetal surgical procedures such as tracheal ligation or for fetuses with difficult airway problems such as massive cervical teratomas or cystic hygromas. The most important component of the EXIT procedure is maintenance of uteroplacental perfusion until the fetal airway is secured and ventilation is established. In direct contrast to cesarean section, where uterine contraction for hemostasis is encouraged, uterine relaxation is maintained by active tocolysis. The fetal manipulations are then performed with maternal support via the placenta. With this approach, clips can be removed, bronchoscopy performed, and stable airway access established in otherwise very difficult circumstances (Fig. 13–5).

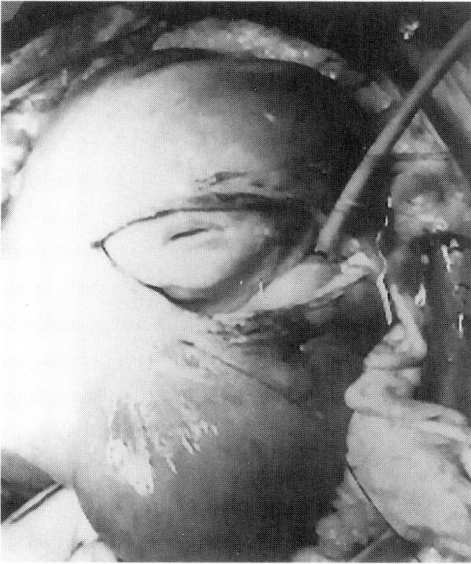

FIG. 13–5. The EXIT procedure. Fetus about to be delivered. Repair of tracheal clips and insertion of bronchial tube will occur before fetus is detached from placenta.

MEDICAL THERAPY

Congenital Adrenal Hyperplasia

Congenital adrenal hyperplasia offers the first example of an inborn error of metabolism inherited by the fetus to be treated *in utero* with prevention of malformation as the primary goal. Prenatal diagnosis has been possible since the early 1980s by using the accumulation of 17-hydroxyprogesterone in the amniotic fluid as a marker. The diagnosis later was usually performed by linkage analysis because the CAH gene was known to lie witihn the HLA region of chromosome 6. More recently the gene has been located, and diagnosis is now done directly using molecular probes. Molecular heterogeneity is the rule, and most individuals with congenital adrenal hyperplasia are compound heterozygotes at the molecular level. The primary defect is inability to transport cholesterol across the mitochondrial membrane. The clinical phenotype does show a correlation with the molecular genotypic abnormality (19) (Fig. 13–6). Chorionic villus sampling and molecular markers for the diagnosis of congenital adrenal hyperplasia now make it possible to assign disease status and gender sooner, allowing maternal steroid therapy to be avoided with male or unaffected female fetuses.

The clinical spectrum of disease associated with congenital adrenal hyperplasia ranges from a critically ill salt-wasting variety to mild virilization precociously in male or ambiguously in female fetuses. Prominent clitoromegaly with labial fusion can resemble the male genitalia so much as to cause misclassification of the newborn sex identity. This can be life-threatening if the salt-wasting variety of adrenal insufficiency is present. Virilization of the female fetus may already have occurred during weeks 9 to 16 of gestation. Therefore, prenatal *in utero* therapy aimed at the prevention of the virilization must be begun before the determination of gender or disease status (20–23). The general approach has been aimed at pharmacologically suppressing the fetal adrenal by giving the mother dexamethasone (20).

The 21-hydroxylase enzyme defect most commonly present in CAH impairs the metabolism of cholesterol to cortisol, creating excessive 17-hydroxyprogesterone. Alternate-pathway metabolism of this precursor shifts to androstenedione and other androgens (Fig. 13–7). Consequently, genetically female fetuses are exposed to high levels of androgens and can become masculinized. The abnormal differentiation can vary from mild clitoral hypertrophy to complete formation of a phallus and apparent scrotum. In the first attempt to prevent this birth defect, Evans and colleagues (21) administered dexamethasone, a fluorinated steroid, to an at-risk mother beginning in the tenth week of gestation. Maternal estriol and cortisol values indicated rapid and sustained fetal and maternal adrenal gland suppression. Forrest and David (21,23), using the same protocol of 0.25 mg of dexam-

Postpubertal virilization ⟶ Infertility	Labial fusion ⟶ Salt Loosing
Non Classical	Classical

FIG. 13–6. Spectrum of phenotypic and genotype variation in congenital adrenal hyperplasia (CAH).

ethasone four times a day but beginning at 9 weeks, reported attempts to prevent masculinization of the external genitalia in hundreds of pregnancies at risk for the severe form of 21-hydroxylase deficiency congenital adrenal hyperplasia. Recent data from hundreds of cases of CAH show that the masculinization can be either completely or mostly prevented. The data still need further analysis, but the therapy appears safe.

Because of a few reported cases of masculinization following the 9-week initiation protocol, we now begin steroid suppressive therapy at 7 weeks and continue therapy until delivery or confirmation of an unaffected fetus because of the recognized risks associated with maternal dexamethasone therapy (Fig. 13–8).

The fundamental principles addressed in these attempts to prevent masculinization of the female fetus with congenital adrenal hyperplasia are logically extended to other medical fetal therapies. The concepts of a thorough informed consent procedure, thorough documentation of progress, and high-risk obstetric management have generally been followed by investigators in these fields.

Methylmalonic Acidemia

Methylmalonic acidemia is related to a functional vitamin B_{12} deficiency. Coenzymatically active vitamin B_{12} is required for the conversion of methylmalonylcoenzyme A to succinylcoenzyme A (Fig. 13–9). Genetically determined etiologies for methylmalonic acidemia include defects in methylmalonylcoenzyme A mutase or in the metabolism of vitamin B_{12} to the conenzymatically active form, adenosylcobalamin, by the converting enzyme. Some patients respond to large-dose B_{12} therapy, which can enhance the amount of the active holoenzyme (mutase apoenzyme plus adenosylcobalamin). There are at least five complementation groups in this enzymatic classification.

Ampola and colleagues (24) were the first to attempt prenatal diagnosis and treatment of a B_{12}-responsive variant of methylmalonic acidemia. Maternal serum B_{12} level rose sixfold above normal, and the maternal urinary excretion of methylmalonic acid progressively decreased to slightly above normal by delivery. Amniotic fluid methyl-

Androgen Production in 21-Hydroxylase Deficiency (Congenital Adrenal Hyperplasia)

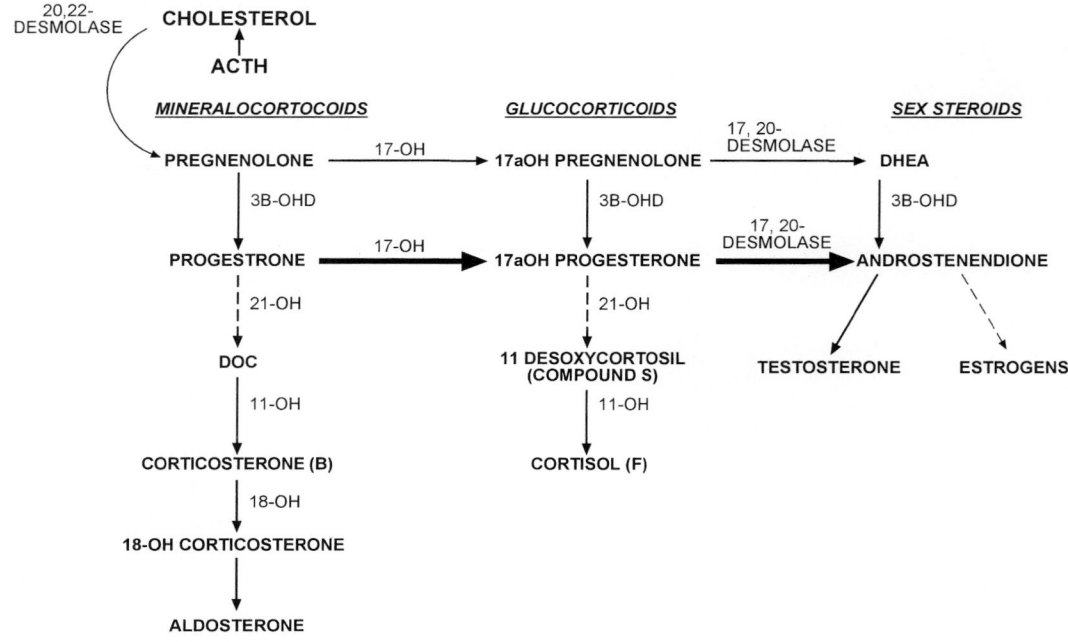

FIG. 13–7. Metabolic pathway showing diversion of pathway from elevated 17-OHP to androgens.

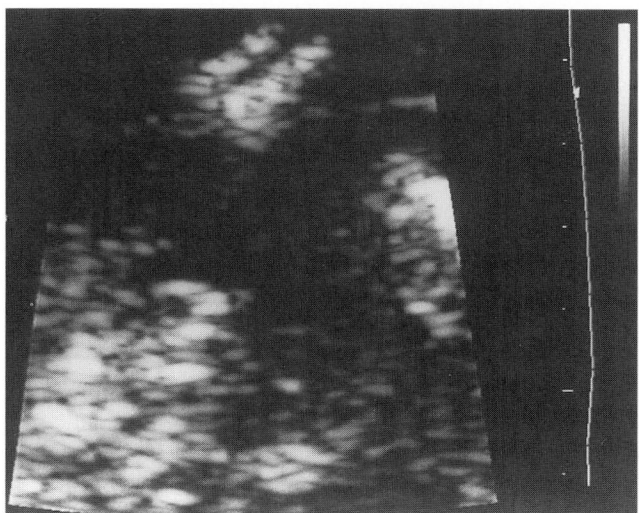

FIG. 13–8. Prenatal ultrasound of labial enlargement in first trimester in congenital adrenal hyperplasia (CAH).

malonic acid levels were three to four times the normal mean level despite prenatal treatment. Postnatally, the diagnosis of methylmalonic acidemia was confirmed. The newborn suffered no acute neonatal complications and had an extremely high serum level of vitamin B_{12}. Evans and colleagues followed a dose–response vitamin B_{12} regimen in the treatment of methylmalonic acidemia and showed a need for an increasingly higher dose as the pregnancy progressed (25). In order to maintain plasma and urinary methylmalonic acid within the normal range, vitamin B_{12} doses needed to be increased sevenfold from the first to the second trimester. In these cases, the prenatal therapy cer-

tainly improved the fetal biochemistry and secondarily the maternal biochemistry. Whether there was any significant clinical benefit to this fetus cannot be sufficiently ascertained. Nyhan (26) has suggested that an increased frequency of minor anomalies may be associated with untreated fetal methylmalonic acidemia. Thus, very early or perhaps even prophylactic treatment with vitamin B_{12} may be indicated even before prenatal diagnosis of B_{12}-responsive methylmalonic acidemia for the at-risk fetus to achieve optimal therapy. It seems likely that reduction of the fetal burden of methylmalonic acidemia should have developmental benefit and could reduce the neonatal risk. However, this remains speculative.

Multiple Carboxylase Deficiency

Biotin-responsive multiple carboxylase deficiency is an inborn error of metabolism in which the mitochondrial biotin-dependent enzymes pyruvate carboxylase, propionylcoenzyme A carboxylase, and α-methylcrotonyl-coenzyme A carboxylase have diminished activity. Affected patients present as newborns or in early childhood with dermatitis, severe metabolic acidosis, and a characteristic pattern of organic acid excretion in their urine (27). Metabolism in patients and in cells cultured *in vitro* can be restored toward normal levels by biotin supplementation. Such therapy has been utilized for fetuses affected with this severe disorder of metabolism.

Published experience provides compelling evidence that biotin administration effectively prevents neonatal complications in certain patients with biotin-responsive multiple carboxylase deficiency. No toxicity has been observed. Further experience with vitamin-responsive

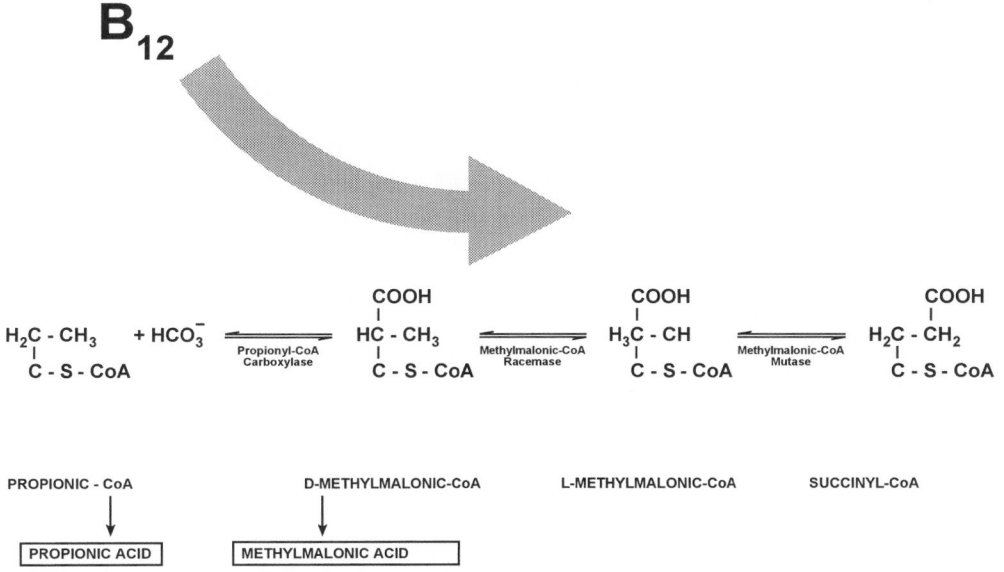

FIG. 13–9. Conversion of methylmalonic CoA to succinyl CoA is aided by excess vitamin B_{12}.

disorders will be useful in the determination of the optimal mode and dose interval for fetal therapy.

Smith–Lemli–Optiz Syndrome

Smith–Lemli–Optiz syndrome (SLOS) was first reported in 1964 (28). The reported incidence is approximately one in 20,000, established from patients who have been clinically diagnosed. The true incidence may be different now that a biochemical test is available to confirm the diagnosis. In 1993, an inborn error of cholesterol biosynthesis in a patient with SLOS was confirmed to be a deficiency of the enzyme 7-dehydrocholesterol reductase in a liver specimen (29–31).

Characteristic features of SLOS include facial phenotype, growth and mental retardation, and anomalies of the heart, kidneys, central nervous system, and limbs. Cleft palate, postaxial polydactyly, 2–3 syndactyly of the toes, and cataracts are often seen in affected patients. The 2–3 syndactyly of the toes is very specific for this disorder and is seen in over 90% of affected patients. The facial phenotype is absolutely characteristic of the syndrome. Affected patients typically present with a narrow forehead, ptosis, anteverted nares, low-set ears, and micrognathia.

The ambiguous genitalia seen in SLOS are the opposite of CAH. Patients with SLOS are deficient in cholesterol and therefore are also most likely have low levels of steroid hormones, which are necessary for masculinization of male genitalia.

The biochemical defect in SLOS is a deficiency of the enzyme 7-dehydrocholesterol reductase, which is responsible for the conversion of 7-DHC to cholesterol in the last step of cholesterol biosynthesis. Deficiency of this enzyme results in the characteristic biochemical pattern of low cholesterol and elevated 7-DHC and 8-dehydrocholesterol (8-DHC), its isomer, seen in affected patients. This pattern of decreased cholesterol and elevated 7-DHC and 8-DHC can be seen in multiple compartments from affected patients, including plasma, red cells, tissues (including brain and cataracts), fibroblasts, amniotic fluid, and chorionic villus. The diagnosis can even be made retrospectively in fixed tissue in paraffin blocks.

Prenatal diagnosis of SLOS has now been available for the last 2 years. There are approximately 11 reports in the literature since 1994 (32–42). Prenatal diagnosis is possible by either amniocentesis (13+ weeks on) or chorionic villus sampling (10 to 12 weeks).

Following identification of the cholesterol metabolic defect in a child with SLOS whose cholesterol level was 8 mg/dl (normal >100 mg/dL), a treatment protocol was tried providing exogenous cholesterol to affected patients. This form of therapy has now been provided to many patients with SLOS for the past 4 years in many centers in the United States and internationally (43–45). The goal is to raise cholesterol levels as well as decrease the levels of the precursors, 7-DHC and 8-DHC.

Fetal therapy strategies include providing cholesterol to the mother or to the fetus. The former is not possible because cholesterol does not cross the placenta well in the third trimester. Also, cholesterol is available only in a crystalline form that cannot be given intravenously or intramuscularly. It also cannot be placed in the amniotic fluid because it would precipitate, so this option is not feasible. However, cholesterol can be given to the fetus in the form of LDL-cholesterol by giving fresh frozen plasma. The group at Tufts has attempted treatment in two patients. In both cases therapy was started late in pregnancy, and the results, therefore, are inconclusive. Therefore, a major relevant principle is that in order for fetal therapy to be successful, the earlier the diagnosis, the better.

Neural Tube Defects

Animal studies suggest that neural tube defects (NTDs) can arise from a variety of vitamin or mineral deficiencies. There are historic data in humans suggesting increased NTD frequencies in subjects with poor dietary histories or with intestinal bypasses. Biochemical evidence of suboptimal nutrition is present in some women bearing infants with NTDs. In 1980, Smithells et al. suggested that vitamin supplementation containing 0.36 mg folate can reduce the frequency of NTD recurrence by sevenfold in women with one or more prior affected children. For almost a decade, there was a great deal of controversy regarding the benefit of folate supplementation for the prevention of NTDs. Finally, in 1991, a randomized double-blind trial designed by the MRC Vitamin Study Research Group demonstrated that preconceptual folate reduced the risk of recurrence in high-risk patients. Subsequently, it was shown that preparations containing folate and other vitamins also reduce the occurrence of first-time NTDs. In response to these findings, guidelines were issued calling for consumption of 4.0 mg/day folic acid by women with a prior child affected with a NTD, for at least 1 month before conception through the first 3 months of pregnancy. In addition, 0.4 mg/day folic acid is recommended to all women planning a pregnancy, to be taken preconceptually. The data on NTD recurrence prevention are now very well established, and the folate regimen has become routine for high-risk cases. The question of primary prevention is more difficult to prove because of the enormity of the size of the study that would be needed to have sufficient power. However, the majority of experts in the field believe that the primary incidence could be cut by perhaps half. As of January, 1998, the United States Food and Drug Administration has mandated that breads and grains be supplemented with folic acid. It is one of the largest public health experiments ever performed. The hope is that a 30% to 50% reduction of NTDs will be seen.

Future Developments

Vitamin therapy has been utilized in the two vitamin-responsive genetic errors of metabolism discussed above. A significant number of other vitamin-responsive defects are known. The *in utero* treatment approach would seem to be a possibility for these conditions, especially those with neonatal manifestations. We speculate that in addition to these disorders, there may be genetic defects for which prenatal vitamin E administration may be justifiable. Postnatally, vitamin E administration prevents abnormalities of leukocyte function and improves shortened red cell survival in glutathione synthetase deficiency. Because grossly lowered intracellular glutathione levels in this mutant state seem to predispose to oxidant-mediated cellular damage, it might be desirable to consider prenatal antioxidant therapy with vitamin E. Most patients with glutathione synthetase deficiency have neurologic impairment, which can be progressive. Future studies may confirm this speculation.

In abetalipoproteinemia, which is associated with very low serum vitamin E levels, progressive and fatal neurologic impairment develops. It is now known that high-dose vitamin E supplementation can slow or prevent these neurologic changes. Prenatal treatment might therefore be justifiable on an experimental basis. However, at present it is not known when this damage begins and, therefore, when *in utero* treatment should be intiated.

GENETIC THERAPIES

Genetic approaches to fetal therapy using preimplantation injection of DNA into the male pronucleus of an IVF fertilized embryo have been successful in ewes but are not likely to be used in the near future in humans. This subject has been reviewed extensively elsewhere and is not repeated here (54).

An alternative approach has been the use of hematopoietic stem cell therapy, which has recently, at long last, been shown to be unequivocally successful in the prenatal treatment of X-linked severe combined immunodeficiency disorder (SCIDS).

Hematopoietic stem cell (HPSC) therapy for the treatment of congenital disease has tremendous theoretical appeal. The replacement of defective cells with normal cells during specific periods of organ development and cellular ontogeny may have significant advantages over postnatal transplantation. Regulatory events during fetal development may favor the normal incorporation of transplanted cells and their proliferation. Early in gestation, immunologic barriers that are prohibitive to postnatal cellular therapy may not exist. Finally, successful prenatal cellular therapy could prevent prenatal and completely preempt postnatal complications of the disease. Several opportunities for prenatal cellular therapy exist that need to be explored experimentally and, when appropriate, clinically. Cells that may be transplanted to treat specific target diseases include hematopoietic stem cells (HSCs), CNS "stem cells," hepatocytes, myoblasts or fibroblasts, and vascular endothelial cells. The rationale for transplantation may be replacement of a defective cell lineage with normal cells, as in the treatment of immunodeficiency diseases by prenatal hematopoietic stem cell transplantation, or the replacement of a deficient enzyme or factor by normal or genetically engineered cells, as in the treatment of inborn errors of metabolism by CNS "stem cells," or hemophilia by hepatocytes. In addition, prenatal tolerance induction in preparation for postnatal cellular or organ transplantation may be a useful approach.

Prenatal Hematopoietic Stem Cell Transplantation

The engraftment and clonal proliferation of a relatively small number of normal HSCs can sustain normal hematopoiesis for a lifetime. This observation provides the compelling rationale for bone marrow transplantation (BMT) and is now supported by thousands of long-term survivors of BMT who otherwise would have succumbed to lethal hematologic disease. Realization of the full potential of BMT, however, continues to be limited by a critical shortage of immunologically compatible donor cells, the inability to control the recipient or donor immune response, and the requirement for recipient myeloablation to achieve engraftment. The price of human leukocyte antigen (HLA) mismatch remains high: the greater the mismatch, the higher the incidence of graft failure, graft-versus-host disease (GVHD), and delayed immunologic reconstitution. Current methods of myeloablation have high morbidity and mortality. In combination, these problems remain prohibitive for most patients who might benefit from BMT. A theoretically attractive alternative that potentially can address many of the limitations of BMT is *in utero* transplantation of HSC. This approach is potentially applicable to any congenital hematopoietic disease that can be diagnosed prenatally and can be cured or improved by engraftment of normal HSCs.

Rationale for *in Utero* Transplantation

The rationale for *in utero* transplantation is to take advantage of the window of opportunity created by normal ontogeny. There is a period, before population of the bone marrow and before thymic processing of self-antigen, when the fetus theoretically should be receptive to engraftment of foreign HSC without rejection and without the need for myeloablation. In the human fetus, the ideal window would appear to be before 14 weeks of gestation, before release of differentiated T lymphocytes into the circulation, and while the bone marrow is just beginning to develop sites for hematopoiesis. It certainly may extend beyond that in immunodeficiency states, particularly when T-cell development is abnormal. During this time, presentation of foreign antigen by thymic dendritic cells theoretically should result in clonal deletion of reactive T-cells during the negative selection phase of thymic processing. Recent advances in prenatal diagnosis have made possible the diagnosis of a large number of congenital diseases during the first trimester. Technical advances in fetal intervention make transplantation feasible by 10 to 12 weeks of gestation. The ontologic window of opportunity falls well within these diagnostic and technical constraints, making application of this approach a realistic possibility.

Because of the unique fetal environment, prenatal HSC transplantation could theoretically avoid many of the current limitations of postnatal BMT. There would be no requirement for HLA matching, which greatly expands the donor pool. Transplanted cells would not be rejected, and space would be available in the bone marrow, eliminating the need for toxic immunosuppressive and myeloablative drugs. The mother's uterus is the ultimate sterile isolation chamber, eliminating the high risk and costly 2 to 4 months of isolation required after postnatal BMT and before immunologic reconstitution. Finally, prenatal transplantation would preempt the clinical manifestations of the disease, avoiding the recurrent infections, multiple transfusions, growth retardation, and other complications that cause immeasurable suffering for the patient and often compromise postnatal treatment.

Source of Donor Cells

The source of donor cells may be critical to the success of engraftment. The most obvious advantage of the use of fetal cells is the minimal number of mature T cells in fetal liver-derived populations before 14 weeks of gestation. This alleviates any concern about GVHD and avoids the necessity of T-cell depletion, which detrimentally influences engraftment.

Although there may be important homing, proliferative, and developmental advantages to the use of fetal cells, there are practical and ethical advantages to the use of cord blood or postnatal HSC sources. There are legitimate ethical concerns regarding the use of fetal tissue for transplantation that must be addressed. In addition, fetal tissue obtained by the usual methods has a high degree of microbial contamination (11). The transplantation of transmissible viral, fungal, or bacterial disease could have disastrous consequences for the recipient fetus or mother. Finally, although the fetal liver is a rich source of HSC, small size limits total cell yield, and currently the specific donor cells are not renewable. In contrast, the use of adult-derived cells would allow a renewable, relatively infection-free, ethically acceptable source of donor cells. One appealing strategy would be tolerance induction by the *in utero* transplantation of highly purified adult bone marrow HSC from a living related donor, followed by a single or multiple postnatal "booster" injections.

Diseases Amenable to Prenatal Treatment

Generally speaking, any disease that can be diagnosed early in gestation, that is improved by BMT, and for which postnatal treatment is not entirely satisfactory is a target disease (Table 13–1). Some diseases are far more likely to benefit from prenatal transplantation than others, however. The list can be divided into three general categories: hemoglobinopathies, immunodeficiency disorders, and inborn errors of metabolism. Each of the diseases has unique considerations for treatment, and in fact, each disease may respond differently. Of particular relevance to the prenatal approach, in which experimental levels of engraftment have been relatively low, is the observation that in many of the target diseases, engrafted normal cells would be predicted to have a significant survival advantage over diseased cells. This would have the clinical effect of amplification of the level of engraftment in the peripheral circulation. In addition, even with minimal levels of engraftment, specific tolerance for donor antigen should be induced, allowing additional cells from the same donor to be given to the tolerant recipient after birth.

Hemoglobinopathies

The sickle cell anemia and thalassemia syndromes make up the largest patient groups potentially treatable by prenatal stem cell transplantation. Both groups can be diagnosed within the first trimester. Both have been cured by postnatal BMT, but BMT is not recommended routinely because of its prohibitive morbidity and mortality and the relative success of modern medical management. In both diseases the success of BMT is indirectly related to the morbidity of the disease; that is, the younger the patient, the fewer transfusions received, and the less organ compromise from iron overload, the better the results. With both diseases the primary questions relevant to prenatal transplantation are: (a) What levels of normal peripheral cell expression are necessary to alleviate clin-

TABLE 13–1. *Selected genetic disorders potentially treatable by* in utero *stem cell therapy*

Hemoglobinopathies
  Sickle cell anemia
  α- and β-Thalassemia major
  Hemophilia
Immunodeficiency diseases
  Severe combined immunodeficiency syndrome (SCID)
  Chronic granulomatous disease
  Agammaglobulinemia
  Chediak–Higashi syndrome
  Wiskott–Aldrich syndrome
Inborn errors of metabolism
  Mucopolysaccharidoses
  Krabbe disease
  Adrenal leukodystrophy
  Metachromatic leukodystrophy
  Niemann-Pick
  Gaucher disease
Neuromuscular disorders
  Duchenne muscular dystrophy
  Becker muscular dystrophy

ical disease? and (b) Can adequate levels of donor cell engraftment be achieved by *in utero* HSC transplantation? At present only indirect evidence exists to answer these questions.

In sickle cell disease (SCD) the pathophysiology is directly related to the concentration of HbS within red cells, which results in marked rheologic abnormality, including hyperviscosity, cellular adherence, and sickling, with a result of vasoocclusion and tissue ischemia. In examining the *in vitro* relationships between hematocrit (HCT) and viscosity using mixtures of sickle and normal red blood cells (RBCs), Schmalzer observed that the primary determinant of viscosity is the sickle HCT (fraction of RBCs that contain HbS). Adverse effects of HCT on viscosity were seen at a sickle HCT level in the low 20s. Oxygen delivery, as gauged by the maximal point on the HCT-versus-viscosity curve, was markedly improved by exchanging normal for sickle RBCs (even when the total HCT was held constant). The clinical correlate of this *in vitro* information is chronic exchange transfusion therapy, which is indicated after cerebrovascular accidents in SCD. Maintaining the percentage of HbS below 30% reduces the risk of recurrent stroke from between 60% and 90% to less than 10%. The maximal HbS that effectively prevents stroke is unknown, but a transfusion regimen maintaining an HbS of 50% was found to be effective in preventing recurrent stroke in a small study group of SCD.

The clinical manifestations of thalassemia are secondary to hypoxia related to severe anemia and ineffective erythropoiesis. It is now standard therapy to transfuse patients with thalassemia major chronically from an early age, which suppresses endogenous erythropoiesis and maintains oxygen delivery. When instituted at an early age, this effectively prevents the bone marrow expansion and secondary bony changes as well as the hemodynamic and cardiac manifestations of the disease. The necessary normal hemoglobin (Hb) level required is controversial, but good results have been achieved with maintenance of Hb at 9 g/dL.

Although these levels of normal Hb are higher than have been achieved experimentally (30% donor Hb is maximal), there would be a significant survival advantage of normal cells in both diseases. In SCD, erythrocytes have a circulating half-life of 10 to 20 days (normal half-life 120 days) before destruction. In thalassemia, most cells (80%) never leave the bone marrow and also have shortened survival in the periphery. Therefore, engraftment of even a few normal stem cells could result in significantly amplified levels of peripheral donor cell expression.

Immunodeficiency Diseases

These represent an extremely heterogeneous group of diseases, which differ in their likelihood of cure by achievement of hematopoietic chimerism. Once again,

the most likely to benefit from even low levels of donor cell engraftment are those diseases in which a survival benefit exists for normal cells. The best example of this situation is severe combined immunodeficiency syndrome (SCID). Several different molecular causes of SCID have been identified, with approximately two-thirds of cases being of X-linked recessive inheritance (X-SCID). The genetic basis of X-SCID has been defined recently (55) as a mutation of the gene encoding the common −y chain (−yc), which is a common component of several members of the cytokine receptor superfamily, including those for interleukin-2 (IL-2), IL-4, IL-7, IL-9, IL-15, and possibly IL-13. Children affected with X-SCID therefore have simultaneous inactivation of multiple cytokine systems, resulting in a block in thymic T-cell development and diminished T-cell response. B cells, although present in normal or even increased numbers, are dysfunctional, either secondary to the lack of helper T-cell function or because of an intrinsic defect in B-cell maturation. Another form of SCID is secondary to adenosine deaminase (ADA) deficiency. Clinical experience with HLA-matched sibling bone marrow or fetal liver or thymus transplantation generally has been successful without myeloablative therapy, which suggests that the lymphoid progeny of relatively few engrafted normal HSC have a selective growth advantage *in vivo* over genetically defective cells (56). The competitive advantage of nonaffected cells in X-SCID is best supported by the discovery of skewed X-inactivation in female carriers (57). Only T cells containing the normal X chromosome are present in the circulation. Evidence that ADA production confers a survival advantage derives from the early experience with gene therapy for ADA deficiency SCID. ADA-gene-corrected autologous T cells have persisted for prolonged periods despite discontinuation of the T-cell infusions. Transfer of ADA-gene-corrected cells versus uncorrected cells from the same SCID patient into an immunodeficient BNX mouse results in survival of the corrected cells and death of the uncorrected cells, confirming a survival advantage for ADA-producing cells even when there is normal ADA production in the surrounding environment. Unfortunately, other diseases such as chronic granulomatous disease would not be expected to provide a competitive advantage for donor cells. Nevertheless, in all these conditions, even a partial reconstitution of the defective cell or component would ameliorate at least partially the clinical manifestations of the disease and should result in donor-specific tolerance. If higher levels of engraftment are needed, further HSC transplants from the same donor could be performed after birth without fear of rejection.

We have successfully treated a fetus with X-linked SCIDS in a family where a previously afflicted child died at 7 months of age. Diagnosis by CVS in the second pregnancy showed another affected male fetus. For this couple abortion was not an option. After lengthy informed consent, paternal bone marrow was harvested, T cells depleted, and injected intraperitoneally into the fetus beginning about 16 weeks of gestation (Fig. 13–10). Subsequent injections were performed at 17 and 18 weeks. The baby presently shows a split chimerism with all of his T cells being his father's and most of his B cells being his. He has achieved normal milestones and immune progress through 2 years of age (58). Other cases have recently been tried using higher T-cell concentrations that have ended in fetal demise (59). Many details still remain to be worked out.

Inborn Errors of Metabolism

An even more heterogeneous group of diseases, inborn errors of metabolism, are caused by a deficiency of a specific lysosomal hydrolase, which results in the accumulation of substrates such as mucopolysaccharide, glycogen, or sphingolipid. Depending on the specific enzyme abnormality and the compounds that accumulate, specific patterns of tissue damage and organ failure occur. These include CNS deterioration, growth failure, dysostosis multiplex and joint disability, hepatosplenomegaly, myocardial or cardiac disease, upper airway obstruction, pulmonary infiltration, corneal clouding, and hearing loss. The potential efficacy of prenatal HSC transplantation for the treatment of these diseases must be considered on an individual disease basis. The purpose of BMT in these diseases is to provide HSC-derived mononuclear cells that can repopulate various organs in the body, including the liver (Kupffer cells), skin (Langerhans cells), lung (alveolar macrophages), spleen (macrophages), lymph nodes, tonsils, and the brain (microglia). Patients who have been corrected by postnatal BMT, such as Gaucher disease or Maroteaux–Lamy syndrome (minimal CNS involvement), are certainly reasonable candidates for prenatal treatment. In many cases postnatal BMT has corrected the peripheral manifestations of the disease and

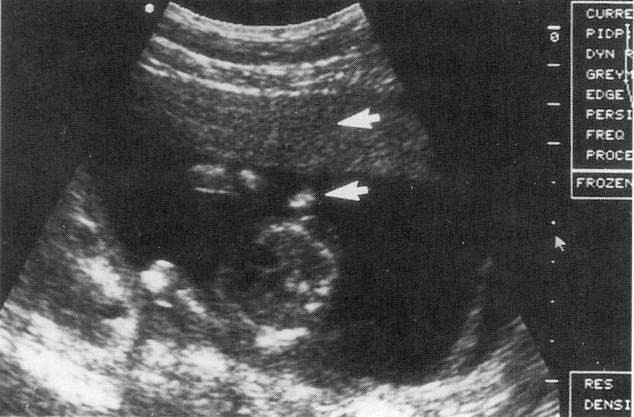

FIG. 13–10. Intraperitoneal injection of hematopoietic stem cells with *arrows* showing fluid accumulation in the peritoneum.

has arrested the neurologic deterioration but has not reversed neurologic injury that is present in such disorders as metachromatic leukodystrophy and Hurler disease. In these cases the neurologic injury may begin well before birth. Postnatal maturation of the blood–brain barrier restricts access to the CNS of transplanted cells or the deficient enzyme. These considerations suggest that prenatal treatment may be necessary for a cure. The primary question is whether donor HSC-derived microglial elements would populate the CNS, providing the necessary metabolic correction within the blood–brain barrier. In the authors' opinion, these represent the least likely group of diseases to benefit from *in utero* HSC transplantation. Experience to date with HPSC has shown it to be effective for immunodeficiencies but not yet for other disorders. It is likely to be true that there will need to be disease-specific approaches. It will take dozens to hundreds of cases to work out optimal regimens.

CONCLUSION

Although still not available for all disorders, there are an increasing number of congenital and genetic abnormalities for which *in utero* treatment is possible and, in some cases, now routine. Advances in surgical, medical, and genetic therapies have progressed at different paces for different disorders, but there is great hope and enthusiasm that progress will continue to expand the number of disorders for which therapy can be effective.

REFERENCES

1. Evans MI, ed. *Reproductive risks and prenatal diagnosis.* Norwalk, CT: Appleton & Lange, 1992.
2. Evans MI, Sacks AL, Johnson MP, Robichaux AG III, May M, Moghissi KS. Sequential invasive assessment of fetal renal function, and the *in utero* treatment of fetal obstructive uropathies. *Obstet Gynecol* 1991;77(4):545–550.
3. Freedman AL, Bukowski TP, Smith CA, Evans MI, Johnson MP, Gonzalez R. Fetal therapy for obstructive uropathy: Specific outcomes diagnosis. *J Urol* 1996;156:720–724.
4. Johnson MP, Bukowski TP, Reitlerman C, Isada NB, Pryde PG, Evans MI. *In utero* surgical treatment of fetal obstructive uropathy: a new comprehensive approach to identify appropriate candidates for vesicoamniotic shunt therapy. *Am J Obstet Gynecol* 1994;170:1770–1779.
5. Johnson MP, Flake AW, Quintero RA, Evans MI. Shunt procedures. In Evans MI, Johnson MP, Moghissi KS, eds. *Invasive outpatient procedures in reproductive medicine.* New York: Raven Press, 1997.
6. Quintero RA, Hume RF, Smith C, et al. Percutaneous fetal cystoscopy and endoscopic fulguration of posterior urethral valves. *Am J Obstet Gynecol* 1995;172:206–209.
7. Quintero RA, Johnson MP, Romero R, et al. *In utero* percutaneous cystoscopy in the management of fetal lower obstructive uropathy. *Lancet* 1995;346:537–540.
8. Drugan A, Krause B, Canady A, Zador IE, Sacks AJ, Evans MI. The natural history of prenatally diagnosed ventriculomegaly. *JAMA* 1989; 261:1785–1788.
9. James D, Smoleniec J, Weiner CP. Fetal hydrops. In James DK, Steer PJ, Weiner CP, Gonik B, eds. *High risk pregnancy: Management options.* London: WB Saunders, 1994:803–812.
10. Harrison M, ed. *The unborn patient.* Philadelphia: WB Saunders, 1991.
11. Jennings RW, Adzick NS, Harrison MR. Fetal surgery. In *Reproductive risks and prenatal diagnosis.* Norwalk, CT: Appleton & Lange, 1992: 311–320.

12. Harrison MR, Adzick NS. Fetal surgical techniques. *Semin Pediatr Surg* 1993;2:136–142.

13. Jennings RW, Adzick NS, Longaker MT, Lorenz HP, Harrison MR. Radiotelemetric fetal monitoring during and after open fetal operation. *Surg Gynecol Obstet* 1993;176:59–64.

14. Harrison MR, Longaker MT, Adzick NS, et al. Successful repair *in utero* of a fetal diaphragmatic hernia after removal of herniated viscera from the left thorax. *N Engl J Med* 1990;322:1582–1584.

15. Harrison MR, Adzick NS, Flake AW, et al. Corection of congenital diaphragmatic hernia *in utero:* VI. Hard-learned lessons. *J Pediatr Surg* 1993;28:1141–1148.

16. Hedrick MH, Estes JM, Sullivan KM, et al. Plug the lung until it grows (PLUG): A new method to treat congenital diaphragmatic hernia in utero. *J Pediatr Surg* 1994;29:612–617.

17. Adzick NS, Harrison MR, Flake AW, Howell LJ, Golbus MS, Filly RA. Fetal surgery for cystic adenomatoid malformation of the lung. *J Pediatr Surg* 1993;28:806–812.

18. Flake AW. Fetal sacrococcygeal teratoma. *Eur J Med* 1993;2:113–120.

19. Miller WL. Genetics, diagnosis and management of 21-hydroxylase deficiency. *J Clin Endocrinol Metab* 1994;78:241–246.

20. Evans MI, Chrousos GP, Mann DL, et al. Pharmacologic suppression of the fetal adrenal gland *in utero:* attempted prevention of abnormal, external genital masculinization in suspected congenital adrenal hyperplasia. *JAMA* 1985;253:1015.

21. David M, Forrest M. Prenatal treatment of congenital adrenal hyperplasia resulting from 21-hydroxylase deficiency. *J Pediatr* 1984;105:799–803.

22. Pang S, Pollack MS, Marshall RN, Immken LD. Prenatal treatment of congenital adrenal hyperplasia due to 21-hydroxylase deficiency. *N Engl J Med* 1990;322:111–115.

23. Forrest MG, David M. Prevention of sexual ambiguity in children with 21-hydroxylase deficiency by treatment *in utero. Pediatrie* 1992;47:351–357.

24. Ampola MG, Mahoney MJ, Nakamura E. Prenatal therpay of a patient with vitamin B responsive methylmalonic acidemia. *N Engl J Med* 1975;293:313.

25. Evans MI, Duquette DA, Rinaldo P, et al. Modulation of B_{12} dosage and response in fetal treatment of methylmalonic aciduria (MMA); titration of treatment dose to serum and urine MMA. *Fetal Diagn Ther* 1997;12:21–23.

26. Nyhan WL. Prenatal treatment of methylmalonic aciduria. *N Engl J Med* 1975;293:353.

27. Scriver C, Beaudet A, Valle D, eds. *The metabolic basis of inherited disease,* 7th ed. New York: McGraw-Hill, 1994.

28. Smith DW, Lemli L, Opitz JM. A newly recognized syndrome of multiple congenital anomalies. *J Pediatr* 1964;64:210–217.

29. Irons M, Elias ER, Salen G, Tint GS, Batta AK. Defective cholesterol biosynthesis in Smith–Lemli–Opitz syndrome. *Lancet* 1993;341:1414.

30. Tint GS, Irons M, Elias E, et al. Defective cholesterol biosynthesis associated with the Smith–Lemli–Opitz syndrome. *N Engl J Med* 1994;330:107–113.

31. Shefer S, Salen G, Batta AK, et al. Markedly inhibited 7-dehydrocholesterol-reductase activity in liver microsomes from Smith–Lemli–Opitz homozygotes. *J Clin Invest* 1995;96:1779–1785.

32. Gelman-Kohan Z, Nisani R, Chemke J, Appelman Z, Rappaport S, Hegesh E. Prenatal detection of recurrent SLOS type 2. *Am J Hum Genet* 1990;47:A57.

33. Hobbins JC, Jones OW, Gottesfeld MD, Persutte W. Transvaginal ultrasonography and transabdominal embryoscopy in the first-trimester diagnosis of Smith–Lemli–Opitz syndrome, type II. *Am J Obstet Gynecol* 1994;171:546–549.

34. Johnson JA, Aughton DJ, Comstock CH, von Oeyen PT, Higgins JV, Schulz R. Prenatal diagnosis of Smith–Lemli–Opitz syndrome, Type II. *Am J Med Genet* 1994;49:240–243.

35. Abuelo DN, Tint GS, Kelley R, Batta AK, Shefer S, Salen G. Prenatal detection of the cholesterol biosynthetic defect in the Smith–Lemli–Opitz syndrome by the analysis of amniotic fluid sterols. *Am J Med Genet* 1995;56:281–285.

36. Dallaire L, Mitchell G, Giguere R, Lefebvre F, Melancon B, Lambert M. Prenatal diagnosis of Smith–Lemli–Opitz syndrome is possible by measurement of 7-dehydrocholesterol in amniotic fluid. *Prenat Diagn* 1995;15:855–858.

37. Hyett JA, Clayton PT, Moscoso G, Nicolaides KH. Increased first trimester nuchal translucency as a prenatal manifestation of Smith–Lemli–Opitz syndrome. *Am J Med Genet* 1995;58:374–376.

38. Kelley RI. Diagnosis of Smith–Lemli–Opitz syndrome by gas chromatography/mass spectrometry of 7-dehydrocholesterol in plasma, amniotic fluid and cultured skin fibroblasts. *Clin Chim Acta* 1995;236:45–58.

39. McGaughran JM, Clayton PT, Mills KA, Rimmer S, Moore L, Donnai D. Prenatal diagnosis of Smith–Lemli–Opitz syndrome. *Am J Med Genet* 1995;56:269–271.

40. Rossiter JP, Hofman KJ, Kelley RI. Smith–Lemli–Opitz syndrome: Prenatal diagnosis by quantification of cholesterol precursors in amniotic fluid. *Am J Med Genet* 1995;56:272–275.

41. Mills K, Mandel H, Montemagno R, Soothill P, Gershoni-Baruch R, Clayton PT. First trimester prenatal diagnosis of Smith–Lemli–Opitz syndrome (7-dehydrocholesterol reductase deficiency). *Pediatr Res* 1996;39:816–819.

42. Sharp P, Haan E, Fletcher JM, Khong TY, Carey WF. First trimester diagnosis of Smith–Lemli–Opitz syndrome. *Prenat Diagn* 1997;17(4):355–361.

43. Irons M, Elias E, Tint GS, et al. Abnormal cholesterol metabolism in the Smith–Lemli–Opitz syndrome: Report of clinical and biochemical findings in 4 patients and treatment in 1 patient. *Am J Med Genet* 1994;50:347–352.

44. Irons M, Elias ER, Abuelo D, Bull MJ, Greene CL, Johnson VP, et al. Treatment of Smith–Lemli–Opitz syndrome: Results of a multicenter trial. *Am J Med Genet* 1997;68:311–314.

45. Elias ER, Irons MB, Hurley AD, Tint GS, Salen G. Clinical effects of cholesterol supplementation in six patients with the Smith–Lemli–Opitz syndrome (SLOS). *Am J Med Genet* 1997;68:305–310.

46. Smithells RW, Sheppard S, Schorah CJ, et al. Possible prevention of neural tube defects by preconceptual vitamin supplementation. *Lancet* 1980;1:399–340.

47. Smithells RW, Nevin NC, Seller MJ, et al. Further experience of vitamin supplementation for prevention of neural tube defect recurrences. *Lancet* 1983;1:1027.

48. Younis JS, Granat M. Insufficient transplacental digoxin transfer in severe hydrops fetalis. *Am J Obstet Gynecol* 1987;157:1268.

49. Mills JL, Rhoads GG, Simpson JL, et al. The absence of a relation between the periconceptional use of vitamins and neural-tube defects. *N Engl J Med* 1989;321:430.

50. Mulinare J, Cordero JF, Erickson JD, Berry RJ. Periconceptional use of multivitamins and the occurrence of neural tube defects. *JAMA* 1988;260:3141.

51. Schulman JD. Treatment of the embryo and the fetus in the first trimester: current status and future prospects. *Am J Med Genet* 1990;35:197.

52. MRC Vitamin Study Research Group. Prevention of neural tube defects: results of the MRC vitamin study. *Lancet* 1991;338:132–137.

53. Czeizel AE, Dudas I. Prevention of the first occurrence of neural-tube defects by preconceptional vitamin supplementation. *N Engl J Med* 1992;327:1832–1835.

54. Yaron Y, Kramer R, Johnson MP, Evans MI. Gene therapy: Is the future here yet? *Obstet Gynecol Clin North Am* 1997;24:179–199.

55. Noguchi M, Yi H, Rosenblatt HM, et al. Interleukin-2 receptor gamma chain mutation results in X-linked severe combined immunodeficiency in humans. *Cell* 1993;73:147–157.

56. Buckley RH, Schiff SE, Schiff RI, et al. Haploidentical bone marrow stem cell transplantation in human severe combined immunodeficiency (review). *Semin Hematol* 1993;30:92–104.

57. Puck JM, Stewart CC, NLssbaum RL. Maximum-likelihood analysis of human T-cell X chromosome inactivation patterns: Normal women versus carriers of X-linked severe combined immunodeficiency. *Am J Hum Genet* 1992;50:742–748.

58. Flake AW, Puck JM, Almieda-Porada G, et al. Successful *in utero* correction of X-linked recessive severe combined immunodeficiency (X-SCID): Fetal intraperitoneal transplantation of CD34 enriched paternal bone marrow cells (EPPBMC). *N Engl J Med* 1996;335(24):1806–1810.

59. Blakemore K, Bambach B, Moser H, et al. Engraftment following *in utero* bone marrow transplantation for globoid cell leukodystrophy. *Am J Obstet Gynecol* 1996;174:312.

CHAPTER 14

The Impact of Maternal Illness on the Neonate

Helain J. Landy

Progress in obstetric and neonatal care has directly contributed to improvements in neonatal outcome. The infant mortality rate, an established indicator of a nation's health status and well-being, has declined dramatically in the United States over the past 40 years (1). The latest figures from 1995, reflecting both neonatal and postneonatal mortality rates, indicate the lowest rate yet recorded: 7.5 infant deaths per 1,000 liveborn infants, a 6% reduction from the previous year (2). These encouraging data largely reflect neonatal and pediatric advances in combination with regionalization of perinatal services and delivery of high-risk mothers in tertiary centers (3).

The mother's well-being during pregnancy has direct relevance for the newborn. Potential complications such as preterm delivery, growth disturbances [intrauterine growth restriction (IUGR) or macrosomia], congenital malformations, or chronic maternal illness may be important factors. The focus of this chapter will be to discuss the impact of maternal illness on fetal development and well-being.

PRETERM DELIVERY

Preterm delivery is responsible for the majority of neonatal deaths and a major proportion of perinatal morbidity with the exception of lethal congenital anomalies (4,5). Encouraging data reveal increasingly effective care for pregnant women and neonates. This translates into a better prognosis for preterm infants, in part attributed to surfactant use, with overall survival rates surpassing 80% (6,7). Infant mortality rates from prematurity and low birth weight have declined an impressive 5% annually since 1988 (1).

H. J. Landy: Division of Maternal–Fetal Medicine, Department of Obstetrics and Gynecology, Georgetown University Medical Center, Washington, D.C.

In contrast, the preterm delivery rate in the United States has not changed since the 1950s despite intense research efforts and technological advances; compared to other industrialized nations, the United States ranks poorly (1). A number of confounding variables may explain these facts. These include a racial disparity regarding persistently higher mortality statistics for black infants, a lack of agreement in the diagnosis of preterm labor, an overlap in the characteristics of actual and threatened preterm labor, controversies over the effectiveness of available screening techniques and therapies for preterm labor, and varying dosages and administration of tocolytic medications (1).

Preterm Labor and Premature Rupture of Membranes

A significant proportion of preterm deliveries result from preterm labor and premature rupture of the membranes (PROM). Approximately 70% of preterm births may be associated with clinical evidence of ruptured membranes or underlying maternal, obstetric, or fetal conditions (Table 14–1) (8–10).

Predisposing factors for preterm labor remain largely unknown, although epidemiologic studies consistently report an association with lower socioeconomic status, nonwhite race, low prepregnancy weight, and maternal age at the extremes (either 18 years or younger or 40 years or older) (11,12). Lack of prenatal care is strongly associated with higher rates of preterm delivery, low birth weight, and maternal and infant mortality (13). A previous history of preterm birth or one or more spontaneous second-trimester abortions places an ensuing gestation at additional risk for premature delivery from preterm labor or PROM (14–18). Prostaglandins, thought to be important mediators in the onset of labor at term, may have a role in preterm labor; in the absence of intrauterine infection, however, the data are not convincing (19).

TABLE 14–1. *Underlying conditions associated with preterm birth*

Maternal conditions	Fetal conditions
Anatomic conditions	Fetal growth restriction
Uterine malformations	Multiple gestation
Unicornuate or bicornuate uterus	Fetal anomaly
Myomas	Fetal death
Cervical incompetence	
Placenta previa or abruption	
Ruptured membranes	
Medical conditions	
Systemic medical or obstetric illness	
Trauma	
Exogenous substance use	
Tobacco	
Cocaine	
Maternal *in utero* exposure to diethylstilbestrol (DES)	
Infection (subclinical or clinical)	
Urogenital tract	
Amniotic cavity	
Systemic	

Although PROM occurs in only 2% to 4% of pregnancies before term (20), it is associated with 15% to 40% of preterm deliveries (14) and represents the foremost predisposing factor for admissions to neonatal intensive care units (12). The underlying etiology remains unclear; however, evidence suggests that inflammatory weakening of the membranes is involved (21–23). Some clinical characteristics seen with PROM are also common to cases with preterm labor (e.g., poor socioeconomic status, young maternal age, and tobacco use) (14). Vaginal bleeding has been found to be an independent risk factor for PROM (14).

Recent studies confirm the increasingly important role of cervicovaginal inflammation and infection in both preterm labor and PROM (21,24–27). Bacterial vaginosis, a relatively common condition in which the normally predominant lactobacilli are overgrown by anaerobes and other peroxide-producing bacteria, is strongly associated with premature birth, preterm labor, and PROM (24,28–32) in addition to delivery of low birth weight preterm infants (33).

In most patients, spontaneous labor begins after the membranes rupture. The latent period, defined as the time between membrane rupture and onset of contractions, is shorter in patients close to term. In preterm patients, over half will be in labor within 24 hours of ruptured membranes, and more than 85% within 1 week (34,35). Premature rupture of membranes remote from viability is associated with significant rates of maternal and fetal morbidity and low rates of neonatal survival (35–38). The oligohydramnios syndrome, a tetrad of fetal complications involving pulmonary hypoplasia, orthopedic deformities, Potter's facies, and IUGR, may be seen with prolonged PROM (36).

Pharmacologic tocolysis, employed to try to prevent progression of preterm labor, is implemented most often before 34 weeks of gestation. These various agents, administered orally, subcutaneously, or parenterally, can have potentially serious maternal and/or fetal side effects (Table 14–2). In spite of the widespread use and evaluation of tocolytic agents, data have not demonstrated benefits in medical costs or improvements in neonatal sur-

TABLE 14–2. *Potential complications of various tocolytic agents*

Agent	Side effects
Magnesium sulfate	*Maternal:* Decreased respiratory drive, cardiovascular function, renal function; contraindicated in myasthenia gravis *Fetal:* Alterations in fetal heart rate patterns
Betamimetic agents (e.g., ritodrine, terbutaline)	*Maternal:* Pulmonary edema; myocardial ischemia or infarction (rare); hypotension; hyperglycemia; hypokalemia. *Fetal:* Alterations in fetal heart rate patterns
Prostaglandin synthetase inhibitors (e.g., indomethacin)	*Maternal:* Gastrointestinal bleeding *Fetal:* Constriction of ductus arteriosus; reversible, dose-dependent oligohydramnios from decreased fetal urinary output; pulmonary hypertension seen with prolonged use (rare)
Calcium-channel blockers (e.g., nifedipine)	Well tolerated

vival or other long-term outcome parameters (11). The major benefit of tocolysis lies in its ability to provide short-term pregnancy prolongation in order that corticosteroids can be administered (11). Corticosteroids, which are given to patients between 24 and 34 weeks of gestation at risk for preterm delivery, were initially utilized to induce fetal pulmonary maturity (39). Optimal benefit can be seen within 24 hours and through 7 days after administration. Data have demonstrated additional neonatal benefits such as reductions in rates of mortality and intraventricular hemorrhage and of respiratory distress syndrome, even with treatment of less than 24 hours' duration and in gestations earlier than 30 to 32 weeks with ruptured membranes (40).

Antibiotic therapy, particularly aimed at treating bacterial vaginosis and other genital tract organisms, has been associated with lower rates of preterm delivery, preterm labor, and PROM in some studies (26,41–42a), though not in others (43,44). Few reports, however, have demonstrated improvements in neonatal morbidity with routine antibiotic administration (45,46).

Screening for Preterm Delivery

Because a woman's past obstetric history may be important for subsequent pregnancies, several risk-scoring systems have been developed. The most widely applied system was devised by Papiernik and modified by Creasy (47). Application of these systems to various populations in the United States, however, has been disappointing (48). Moreover, applicability to nulliparas has not been accepted. A 1996 study of almost 3,000 gravidas that attempted to develop a risk assessment system for predicting spontaneous preterm delivery using clinical information at 23 to 24 weeks of gestation was similarly disappointing (18).

Other screening tools have been proposed to help identify the pregnancy at risk for preterm delivery. These include cervical examination, home uterine activity monitoring, screening for genital tract colonization and/or infection, and, recently, vaginal secretions containing fetal fibronectin.

Cervical Examination

The utility of routine cervical examination in otherwise uncomplicated pregnancies is controversial. Although asymptomatic cervical dilation may be the first sign of impending preterm delivery, implying cervical incompetence or undiagnosed preterm labor, it also may represent a normal anatomic variant (49,50). In 1994, a randomized, multinational trial evaluated digital cervical examination in over 5,000 patients. This study could show no statistically significant differences in preterm delivery, low birth weight, or PROM when 2,803 women who had cervical examinations at each prenatal visit were compared with 2,799 patients in whom cervical examination was avoided (51).

Recently, the dimension of sonographic cervical examination has been added in attempts at predicting preterm delivery and/or cervical incompetence. Several studies have demonstrated the superiority of sonographic evaluation of the cervix to digital assessment of cervical dilation, length, and effacement (52–56). Predictive sonographic findings for increased risks of preterm delivery include cervical shortening (generally described as less than 3 cm), funneling or ballooning of membranes at the level of the internal os, and cervical dilation (52,55,57). In conjunction with transvaginal sonography, adjunctive tools that may aid in the diagnosis of asymptomatic cervical incompetence include application of transfundal pressure (58,59) or maternal postural changes (60).

Home Uterine Activity Monitoring

The working premise behind home uterine activity monitoring (HUAM) is that uterine contractions increase in frequency in the 24 hours before the development of preterm labor (61). The use of HUAM involves tocodynamometric recording of uterine contractions combined with interpretation and daily telephone contact by health care providers to try to detect early preterm labor. Oral tocolytic agents often are used in conjunction with HUAM. Although many studies have been carried out evaluating its efficacy, data are conflicting, and the quality of supportive evidence is limited by study designs (62–64). Its use in clinical practice is widespread in spite of the lack of endorsement by the U.S. Preventive Services Task Force (63) and the American College of Obstetricians and Gynecologists (62).

Genital Tract Screening

Routine screening for various infections (e.g., syphilis, hepatitis B, and rubella) is recommended early in pregnancy. Additional testing for other sexually transmitted disorders, however, is left to the discretion of the practitioner based on the patient's history and physical examination (65).

Infections with *Neisseria gonorrhoeae, Trichomonas vaginalis, Chlamydia trachomatis,* and group B streptococci as well as urinary tract infections, asymptomatic bacteriuria, and bacterial vaginosis have been associated with premature delivery (24a,26,66). In light of the earlier discussion on the role of cervicovaginal inflammation and infection in preterm labor and PROM, guidelines that include more widespread screening of pregnant women may be warranted. More aggressive screening and treatment for these conditions during gestation as well as in women contemplating pregnancy has been recommended by some investigators (25,26). Recently adopted guidelines recommend routine late pregnancy screening for group B *Streptococcus* colonization and antibiotic treatment for carriers in labor; this strategy reflects attempts to prevent early-onset disease in newborns, however, rather than impact on rates of prematurity (67).

Fetal Fibronectin

Fetal fibronectin, a protein produced by the fetal membranes, probably functions to bind the placenta and membranes to the decidua. Disruption of this normal interface, as with preterm labor or PROM, allows leakage of fibronectin into cervicovaginal secretions. In normal pregnancy it is rarely present after 20 weeks of gestation, and it has been found to be of value in predicting preterm delivery (68). Positive tests for fetal fibronectin also are seen more commonly in women with bacterial vaginosis (68,68a). A recent study from the Maternal–Fetal Medicine Units Network has demonstrated that a positive vaginal or cervical fibronectin test predicts subsequent fetal fibronectin positivity as well as subsequent spontaneous preterm delivery (69).

A commercial enzyme immunoassay kit to detect fetal fibronectin became available in 1995 to determine a woman's risk of preterm labor in the setting of intact membranes, cervical dilation less than 3 cm, and gestational age between 24 weeks, 0 days, and 34 weeks, 6 days. Its use as a routine screening test for the general obstetric population, however, has not been endorsed by The American College of Obstetricians and Gynecologists Committee on Obstetric Practice; requirement for further study is cited (70).

MATERNAL NUTRITION

Recognition of the importance of proper nutrition during pregnancy has varied over the years. Earlier in this century, restrictions in maternal diet were implemented to lessen fetal growth in order to facilitate vaginal delivery or to decrease the rates of preeclampsia (71). Fetal growth, which is determined by complex interactions of environmental, genetic, and physiologic factors, is influenced by both maternal prepregnancy body mass index and pregnancy weight gain: low birth weight and IUGR are seen with underweight mothers or those with poor weight gain, and macrosomia is common in infants born to overweight women or those with excessive weight gain (71–73). Current weight gain recommendations for singleton pregnancies are 25 to 35 lb for women of normal weight, 28 to 40 lb for underweight, and 15 to 25 lb for overweight gravidas; in twin gestations, weight gain ideally should be 35 to 45 lb (74). Several recent epidemiologic studies show an association of fetal neural tube defects and other malformations with maternal obesity (75–78).

Although it is common for multivitamins to be prescribed to pregnant women in the United States, a balanced diet with appropriate weight gain should supply the required vitamins and make supplementation unnecessary. In certain conditions, however, specific recommendations are warranted. For instance, vitamin B_{12} and zinc are indicated for strict vegetarians; additional folic acid is suggested for women taking anticonvulsant medications, carrying multiple gestations, or with hemoglobinopathies. To prevent anemia, iron supplementation in the latter trimesters is recommended (79). In contrast, excessive vitamin A, in daily doses of at least 25,000 to 50,000 IU, has been found to be teratogenic, producing malformations similar to those seen with maternal exposure to 13-*cis*-retinoic acid (Accutane) (80).

High-dose folic acid supplementation (4 mg/day) has been shown to reduce the risk of a subsequent neural tube defect in women with a prior affected infant (81), and such doses beginning 1 month before conception and continuing through the first 3 months of pregnancy have been advocated (82). Further studies led to the additional statement from the Centers for Disease Control that all women of child-bearing age in the United States who are capable of becoming pregnant should consume 0.4 mg of folic acid daily (83). Beginning January, 1998, the U.S. Food and Drug Administration ordered folic acid fortification of bread, flour, and other grain foods to help prevent these birth defects (84).

MATERNAL ILLNESSES

Hypertension

Hypertension complicates almost 10% of pregnancies and constitutes a major cause of maternal and perinatal morbidity and mortality (85). Several subdivisions exist, although the classification and terminology are confusing. A simple but overlapping classification containing four categories was recommended by the American College of Obstetricians and Gynecologists in 1972: (a) chronic hypertension, (b) preeclampsia, (c) chronic hypertension with superimposed preeclampsia, and (d) transient hypertension. In clinical practice, however, only two distinct conditions are commonly recognized: chronic hypertension and pregnancy-induced hypertension (PIH) (86).

Chronic hypertension is defined as systolic blood pressure at least 140 mm Hg and diastolic blood pressure at least 90 mm Hg obtained on several different occasions (87). Perinatal mortality is increased as maternal blood pressure rises (88); it has been theorized, therefore, that antepartum treatment may be beneficial. Potential fetal complications associated with chronic hypertension include IUGR and fetal death. Several different antihypertensive agents are used during pregnancy. α-Methyldopa is frequently utilized, being a safe, effective agent that has been studied extensively. Newer antihypertensive drugs that are safe in pregnancy include β-blockers, labetalol (a combination α- and β-blocker), and calcium-channel blockers such as nifedipine. The use of diuretics, which was more common before the development of these newer agents, is discouraged because of the accompanying plasma volume reduction (89). Angiotensin-converting enzyme (ACE) inhibitors, commonly used in young nonpregnant adults, are both teratogenic and fetotoxic if administered during gestation. Skull defects (hypoplastic calvaria and encephalocele) and *in utero* renal failure leading to oligohydramnios, pulmonary hypoplasia, long-standing neonatal anuria, and fetal or neonatal death have been reported (90–92). Antihypertensive medication is changed to another agent once pregnancy is confirmed in women using an ACE inhibitor.

Pregnancy-induced hypertension is a disorder that commonly involves several different organ systems and may present with more clinical signs than just high blood pressure. Preeclampsia is defined as hypertension in association with proteinuria, representing renal involvement, and usually occurs after 20 weeks of gestation. Eclampsia involves the development of seizures and/or coma, which represents central nervous system involvement, in a preeclamptic patient. The triad of hypertension, proteinuria, and edema defining preeclampsia, though described classically, is nonspecific; these clinical signs may represent other conditions (85). Severe preeclampsia can be defined by the end-organ criteria listed in Table 14–3 (86,93). Thrombocytopenia with the platelet count below 100,000/μL is the most consistent finding in patients with PIH (94). The syndrome of hemolysis, elevated liver enzymes, and low platelets, which is known by the acronym HELLP, is a variant of severe preeclampsia. The HELLP syndrome occurs with a frequency of 2% to 12% (95) and may have a variety of clinical presentations (96,97). Well-recognized risk factors for the development of PIH are outlined in Table 14–4 (85,86).

TABLE 14–3. *Clinical manifestations of severe pregnancy-induced hypertension*[a]

Systolic blood pressure ≥160 mm Hg or diastolic blood pressure ≥110 mg Hg
Proteinuria >5 g/24 hr
Elevated serum creatinine
Oliguria <500 ml/24 hr
Pulmonary edema
Grand mal seizure (eclampsia)
Microangiopathic hemolysis
Thrombocytopenia
Hepatocellular dysfunction (elevated alanine and/or aspartate aminotransferase)
Intrauterine growth restriction or oligohydramnios
Other symptoms suggestive of end-organ involvement (e.g., headache, visual disturbance, epigastric or right upper quadrant pain)

[a]Modified from refs. 86 and 93.

TABLE 14–4. *Risk factors associated with the development of pregnancy-induced hypertension (PIH)*[a]

Nulliparity
Age over 40 years
African-American race
Positive family history of PIH
Prior history of PIH
Chronic hypertension
Chronic renal disease
Antiphospholipid syndrome
Diabetes mellitus
Multiple gestation
Gestational trophoblastic disease
Fetal hydrops
Angiotensinogen gene T235

[a]Modified from refs. 85 and 86.

The precise pathophysiologic factors involved in PIH have been difficult to elucidate. What is known, however, is that vasospasm appears to be responsible for many of the serious clinical manifestations (e.g., hypertension and diminished renal function). Earlier classic investigations demonstrated supportive evidence: failure of the blunted pressor response to angiotensin II present in normal pregnancy that is not seen in PIH (98) and a progressive sensitivity to the pressor effects of infused angiotensin that can be demonstrated after 18 weeks in patients destined to develop PIH (99). Other factors may involve an imbalance in the production of prostacyclin, a potent vasodilator, relative to levels of thromboxane, a vasoconstrictor, and alterations in the synthesis of nitric oxide and/or endothelin-1 (86).

Some fetal effects of PIH reflect vasospasm with regard to placental perfusion: a decrease in uteroplacental perfusion may result in abruption, IUGR, or oligohydramnios. Placental abruption, which occurs in fewer than 2% of patients with chronic hypertension (100), has been found to occur significantly more frequently (9.5%) in those with superimposed PIH (101). Neonatal thrombocytopenia is another fetal complication, noted in more infants of hypertensive than normotensive mothers (9.2% compared to 2.2%) (102).

Prematurity also contributes to the increased rates of perinatal morbidity and mortality associated with PIH. Conservative management may be attempted for women with severe PIH remote from term; however, delivery, which remains the only definitive treatment, ultimately may be required (103,104). In cases managed conservatively, patients are hospitalized at bed rest with frequent clinical and laboratory assessments. Magnesium sulfate, an agent long recognized for its anticonvulsant effects, is often administered. Although phenytoin sulfate may be used, magnesium sulfate is the preferred drug (105–107). Blood pressure control is achieved with the use of agents such as labetalol, hydralazine, or nifedipine. A protocol of high-dose corticosteroid administration has been shown to stabilize both clinical and laboratory parameters in patients with HELLP syndrome before term (108). Delay of delivery in gestations less than 34 weeks for corticosteroid administration to enhance fetal pulmonary maturation is recommended only if both mother and fetus are stable (86).

Over the years, various attempts have been made to prevent preeclampsia. A beneficial effect of low-dose aspirin (60 mg to 80 mg daily) in high-risk groups has been demonstrated (101,109–111). Its use has not been recommended in unselected, normotensive gravidas, however (86). Some studies have shown less PIH with calcium supplementation (112,113), although data are conflicting (114). Recent evaluation of the uteroplacental circulation via transvaginal Doppler sonography 12 to 16 weeks into gestation suggests an association with abnormal waveforms and increased risks of developing preeclampsia later in gestation (115,116). More study is needed in this area.

Diabetes Mellitus

Diabetes mellitus is the most common medical illness complicating pregnancy, affecting nearly 4% of pregnancies (117,118). The disease is classified based on requirement for insulin therapy into type 1 (insulin-dependent) or type 2 (non-insulin-dependent) diabetes. The White classification system for diabetes in pregnancy, developed in 1949, was based on age of onset and duration of disease as well as disease progression with respect to vascular complications (120). With continued improvements in glucose control, assessment of fetal well-being, and neonatal management, the White classification is no longer as helpful in the management of the pregnant diabetic (117). Rather, the distinction can be made between diabetes that preexisted a woman's pregnancy (pregestational diabetes) and diabetes first recognized during pregnancy (gestational diabetes).

Fetuses of diabetic mothers may have growth disturbances at both ends of the spectrum: IUGR and macrosomia. IUGR, fetal growth less than or equal to the tenth percentile for gestational age, is not an infrequent finding in pregnancies of women with vascular complications of pregestational diabetes. In diabetic pregnancies, IUGR often results from uteroplacental insufficiency, usually secondary to maternal hypertension, although fetuses with congenital anomalies also may exhibit signs of IUGR. Maternal hyperglycemia may play a role in decreased uteroplacental perfusion (121).

Infants of mothers with both pregestational and gestational diabetes are at risk for macrosomia, which refers to excessive fetal growth. Macrosomia has been defined variably as birth weight above 4,000 g, weight above the 90th percentile for gestational age, or an *in utero* estimated fetal weight of more than 4,500 g (122). In the diabetic population, macrosomia may occur in 2% to 33% of pregnancies (123–126), the wide disparity partly a result of differing definitions. The antenatal diagnosis of macrosomia is not uniformly accurate (124,127).

Macrosomia is accompanied by additional risks of prolonged labor, birth trauma from shoulder dystocia, and instrumented or cesarean deliveries (128–132). Brachial plexus palsy, often a result of shoulder dystocia, is the most serious and most frequent birth injury occurring in macrosomic infants. Shoulder dystocia occurs two to six times more frequently in deliveries of diabetic mothers than in the nondiabetic population (128,133,134). Demonstrable brachial plexus injury will be present in 15% to 30% of those macrosomic infants who experience shoulder dystocia (135–137), although the majority of cases resolve within 1 year. Permanent injury resulting from shoulder dystocia in a macrosomic infant is estimated as 0.24% to 1.8% (122).

Polyhydramnios, defined as excessive amniotic fluid, is not an unusual finding in diabetic pregnancies. Although the definition varied in the past, standardization based on a four-quadrant sonographic assessment of the amniotic fluid index (AFI) currently defines polyhydramnios as an AFI greater than the 95th percentile for gestational age (138). In diabetic pregnancies, the etiology is not clear, although fetal malformations or poor glucose control may be related. When polyhydramnios complicates maternal diabetes, higher rates of perinatal morbidity and mortality are reported (139).

Pregestational Diabetes Mellitus

Twelve percent of diabetic pregnancies are complicated by pregestational diabetes mellitus (118). Pregnancies of pregestational diabetics are at significant risk for both spontaneous abortion and fetal anomalies (140–143), the latter representing the major cause of perinatal mortality in this group of patients (144–146). The frequency of congenital anomalies among infants of diabetic mothers occurs two to three times the rate in the nondiabetic population (147). These malformations, which occur before 7 weeks of gestation, commonly include open neural tube defects, congenital heart defects, and the caudal regression syndrome (147,148).

Hyperglycemia is responsible for the increased risks of both fetal malformations and spontaneous abortion seen in diabetics (140–143,149). Poor glycemic control, combined with derangements in amino acid and lipid concentrations, is believed to underlie the development of fetal malformations (141,149), a concept known as fuel-mediated teratogenesis (150). Similarly, hypertrophic cardiomyopathy, which can cause cardiomegaly and congestive heart failure, may result from elevated maternal glucose levels throughout pregnancy (151,152). A patient's degree of hyperglycemia can be assessed by the level of glycosylated hemoglobin (hemoglobin A_{1c}), a retrospective marker of glucose control (149). Several studies have demonstrated that intensive glycemic control in the periods before conception and organogenesis can lower the frequency of congenital anomalies in infants of diabetic mothers (153–155).

In the past, a major source of perinatal mortality among diabetic pregnancies was fetal demise, often unexplained and sudden. Among well-controlled diabetics, stillbirth is an uncommon event. With diabetic ketoacidosis, however, perinatal mortality rates may be as high as 50% to 90% (156). Recent evidence employing fetal blood sampling has confirmed that these previously designated unexplained stillbirths result from hyperglycemia, metabolic disturbances, polycythemia, and acidemia (157,158). In the 1960s at the Joslin Clinic, efforts to prevent fetal demise resulted in the strategy of scheduled preterm deliveries. Even though reductions in the number of stillbirths occurred, neonatal deaths from respiratory distress syndrome were prevalent, predominantly as a result of errors in estimates of gestational age (159). Data from the 1980s suggested a delay in fetal pulmonary maturation in diabetic pregnancies (160–162a); however, recent studies have disproved this assumption, especially with good glucose control (163–166). Other complications seen in women with pregestational diabetes mellitus, especially those with end-organ dysfunction from long-standing vascular disease, include preterm delivery and PIH (117).

In the immediate neonatal period, infants of diabetic mothers are at higher risks for a number of metabolic irregularities. Hypoglycemia may occur from a rapid decline in neonatal glucose levels after delivery. This results from a combination of removal of the continued placental source of glucose and fetal islet cell hyperplasia from chronic maternal hyperglycemia. Close maternal glucose control during labor with continuous insulin and glucose infusions can lessen the development of neonatal hypoglycemia (167). Other neonatal metabolic derangements include hypercalcemia, polycythemia, and hyperbilirubinemia (158,168–170).

Gestational Diabetes Mellitus

Gestational diabetes mellitus (GDM) is diagnosed by at least two abnormal values on a 3-hour 100-g oral glucose tolerance test subsequent to an elevated 1-hour 50-g glucose challenge test (171). It occurs in fewer than 4% of pregnancies but comprises the majority of cases of diabetes in pregnancy (118). Recent estimates suggest rising prevalence rates as a result of increased detection following the 1980s recommendations for universal screening (118,172). In women with GDM, the risk of developing diabetes mellitus 20 years later is approximately 50% (173).

For most patients with GDM, glucose levels may be controlled with dietary therapy alone; insulin is administered when glucose levels exceed standard recommendations (fasting plasma glucose below 105 mg/dL or 2-hour postprandial value below 120 mg/dL) (171). As already mentioned, infants of mothers with GDM are at risk for macrosomia, operative and cesarean deliveries, birth trauma, fetal death, and neonatal hyperglycemia and/or hyperbilirubinemia (117).

Fetal Assessment

A number of tools are utilized to assess fetal well-being in diabetic pregnancies. Obstetric ultrasonography can be of value in determining early fetal viability as well as screening for various anomalies. Fetal echocardiography is employed in the midtrimester to evaluate fetal cardiac structure. In the third trimester, sonography can assess fetal growth and aid in the diagnosis of macrosomia, polyhydramnios, or septal hypertrophy. An ongoing sense of fetal well-being can be obtained through maternal perception of fetal movement counts. Serial fetal biophysical testing (e.g., nonstress tests and biophysical profiles) is usually implemented by 32 weeks in most insulin-dependent diabetics; pregnancies with well-controlled gestational diabetes, being at low risk for fetal demise, may not require testing except in the presence of other obstetric factors (159).

Autoimmune Disorders

A number of disorders that involve circulating autoantibodies and/or deposition of immune complexes may have direct effects on pregnancy. These include the rheumatologic or connective tissue diseases and conditions associated with circulating antiphospholipid antibodies.

Rheumatologic Disorders

Rheumatologic disorders are chronic inflammatory diseases usually affecting the connective tissues and joints. The most common disorders occurring in young women include systemic lupus erythematosus, rheumatoid arthritis, scleroderma, and Sjögren's syndrome.

Systemic Lupus Erythematosus

Systemic lupus erythematosus (SLE) is the most common connective tissue disorder seen among reproductive-age women. Its various clinical presentations include polyarthritis, skin manifestations, Raynaud's phenomenon, and nephritis; laboratory abnormalities such as anemia, leukopenia, thrombocytopenia, and the presence of autoantibodies are common. The disease is characterized by remissions and exacerbations. Patients with SLE have a high prevalence of fetal wastage: spontaneous abortion, IUGR, preterm delivery, stillbirth, and perinatal death (174–179). Two recent studies have shown that the increase in pregnancy complications results from early losses (179) and a high rate of preterm and term PROM (180). Fetal survival is higher when the disease is in remission (174,181–184). Other predictors of fetal wastage include active nephritis, hypertension, and circulating antiphospholipid antibodies (e.g., lupus anticoagulant or anticardiolipin antibodies) (174,181,182,184–188).

In spite of older data that supported the opinion of disease exacerbation during pregnancy, most authorities now agree that pregnancy has no effect on disease progression in SLE (187,189–191). Treatment with corticosteroids is standard (175–177,188). Salicylates and other nonsteroidal antiinflammatory agents (e.g., paracetamol) are commonly used, although high doses are discouraged (192–194). Azathioprine, an immunosuppressive that has been used predominantly in renal transplant patients (191,195–197), and antimalarial agents are used widely in SLE patients and considered to be safe during pregnancy (176,198,199,200,201). In some cases, plasmapharesis has been performed (202,203).

Infants of mothers with SLE are at risk for the neonatal lupus syndrome. This consists of abnormalities in the heart and skin or development of clinical features of SLE, occurring as a result of transplacental passage of maternal antibodies (204–205a). The most frequently seen heart abnormality is congenital complete heart block (206), occurring in fewer than 3% of infants at risk (192). The pathophysiology involves deposition of immunoglobulin, specifically circulating IgG autoantibodies directed against ribosomal nucleoprotein antigens [anti-Ro (SSA) and, to a lesser extent, anti-La (SSB) antibodies] in fetal cardiac tissue (109,205a,207). Anti-Ro (SSA) and anti-La (SSB) antibodies are detectable in 40% to 50% of SLE patients (178,206). Most cases of congenital complete heart block occur in fetuses whose mothers do not have overt clinical SLE (208); however, more than 90% of mothers with affected children have detectable anti-Ro (SSA) antibodies (206). Heart block in the absence of structural defects has been documented as early as 16 weeks of gestation (209).

The presenting finding of congenital heart block is fetal dysrhythmia; sonography may reveal a pericardial effusion or hydrops, which can result from either congestive failure or an immune mechanism (207,210,211). Maternal treatment with dexamethasone and/or plasmapheresis, used to lower circulating antibody levels and to minimize inflammatory injury, has not successfully reversed fetal heart block (212,213), though resolution of ascites has been reported with corticosteroid use (211). In one case of a hydropic 24-week fetus with heart block, *in utero* cardiac pacing was technically feasible (214); this technique may be a future option in severe cases. After birth, heart block is usually permanent; intermittent and incomplete cases, as well as unusual late presentations, have been described (215–217). For those infants that survive, cardiac pacemaking is instituted; however, mortality rates are high (12% to 28%) (215,218,219). Coexistent cardiac anomalies among infants with congenital heart block are common (220,221).

The other major organ system involved in the neonatal lupus syndrome is the skin. Cutaneous lesions are frequently widespread macular rashes, although a butterfly rash and discoid lesions are found occasionally (178). These lesions, which have a characteristic inflammatory histology (222), generally appear within the first few weeks of life and disappear spontaneously within 6 months, coexistent with the clearance of maternal autoantibodies from the neonatal circulation (178,208). Hematologic manifestations such as anemia, thrombocytopenia, glomerulonephritis, and hepatosplenomegaly are rare (206).

Rheumatoid Arthritis

Rheumatoid arthritis complicates approximately one in 1,000 to 2,000 pregnancies. Women are more commonly affected by the condition than men, and the age of onset is generally between ages 35 and 50. Rheumatoid arthritis has a familial preponderance associated with the tissue antigen HLA-DR4 (223). The disease is characterized by chronic polyarthritis and inflammatory synovitis, usually of the peripheral joints, resulting in bone and cartilage destruction and joint deformities. Other clinical manifestations include anorexia, weakness, fatigue, and vague musculoskeletal complaints. The diagnosis is made based on specific criteria outlined by the American Rheumatism Association (224).

The reason that the symptoms of rheumatoid arthritis are ameliorated during pregnancy is not known (225–227). A prevailing hypothesis involves immune complex deposition (228), although several reports have demonstrated an association between levels of α_2-pregnancy-associated globulin and disease activity (227,229). In contrast to SLE, perinatal morbidity and mortality are not increased in patients with rheumatoid arthritis.

The major therapies for rheumatoid arthritis are acetylsalicylic acid (aspirin) and nonsteroidal antiinflammatory agents; concerns for adverse fetal and/or neonatal effects (such as impaired hemostasis, premature closure of the fetal ductus arteriosus, prolonged gestation, and long labor) have been largely theoretical (161). Gold therapy, which has been shown to lower the levels of rheumatoid factor, has been used for many years; antimalarial agents are also administered (161). Although D-penicillamine has been used, some reports have shown connective tissue defects similar to Ehlers-Danlos syndrome in children with antenatal exposure (230).

Scleroderma

Scleroderma affects the skin, gastrointestinal tract (especially the esophagus), lungs, and kidneys. The typical remissions and exacerbations of the disease make it difficult to assess the effect of pregnancy. In a 1989 report on 94 cases of scleroderma in pregnancy and a review of the literature, pregnancy had either no effect on the disease or was associated with exacerbations (231). Fetal mortality may be as high as 20%, and the development of neonatal scleroderma has been described.

Sjögren's Syndrome

This rare autoimmune disorder, also known as keratoconjunctivitis sicca or sicca syndrome, involves lymphocytic infiltration of the salivary and lacrimal glands resulting in loss of saliva and tears. Sjögren's syndrome is both clinically and immunologically related to SLE. Many circulating autoantibodies are present, as well as anti-Ro (SSA) and anti-La (SSB) antibodies. Pregnancy complications of fetal loss and congenital heart block have been reported (232).

Antiphospholipid Antibodies and the Antiphospholipid Syndrome

Circulating antiphospholipid antibodies and the antiphospholipid syndrome (APS) are associated with clinical complications such as adverse pregnancy outcomes, thrombocytopenia, and thrombosis. These antibodies are directed against negatively charged phospholipids present on cell membranes, notably platelets and endothelial cells (233). The most common antiphospholipid antibodies are the lupus anticoagulant and anticardiolipin antibodies. The lupus anticoagulant was originally described as a circulating anticoagulant identified in two patients with SLE (234). It is paradoxically named, however, for the anticoagulant activity is seen *in vitro*, whereas *in vivo* it acts is as a potent thrombotic agent.

Antiphospholipid antibodies may be found in the normal population, but they are more frequently detected in patients with SLE (235,236). Diagnosis of the APS involves both clinical and laboratory parameters: the presence of the lupus anticoagulant and/or medium to high levels of IgG or IgM anticardiolipin antibodies plus one clinical parameter (thrombosis, autoimmune thrombocytopenia, or pregnancy loss) (237–239). Potential pregnancy complications include those listed in Table 14–5 (161,233,240,241). Pregnancy loss may be the only clinical marker associated with the presence of antiphospholipid antibodies, however. New evidence shows a very high rate of development of thrombotic complications after the identification of these antibodies, even in asymptomatic individuals (242).

Initial treatment of the APS involved use of low-dose aspirin (75 mg) and corticosteroids (243,243a), and successful pregnancy outcomes were reported by many investigators worldwide using similar regimens (233). Corticosteroid use may be associated with oropharyngeal candidiasis, gestational diabetes, osteoporosis, and

TABLE 14–5. *Pregnancy complications seen in association with antiphospholipid antibodies*

Fetal loss, including miscarriage and stillbirth
Intrauterine growth restriction
Placental infarction
Early-onset severe preeclampsia
Thrombosis
Unusual postpartum syndrome (e.g., cardiopulmonary disease, fever, hemolytic-uremic syndrome)

PROM (233,244–246). An alternative regimen consisting of low-dose aspirin and heparin currently is the preferred therapy (244,247,248). Potential problems associated with heparin include thrombocytopenia and heparin-induced osteoporosis, though these complications are fewer with administration of low-molecular-weight heparin (249). Intravenous immunoglobulin also has been used (250–252). In spite of aggressive treatment, however, successful pregnancy outcomes are not guaranteed.

The most striking adverse fetal outcomes associated with APS are fetal death and IUGR. Other unusual reported complications include fetal or neonatal thrombosis resulting from transplacental passage of maternal antibodies (253,254) and fetal effects of therapy.

Thyroid Disorders

Disorders of thyroid metabolism are common in women of child-bearing age. Pregnancy significantly affects thyroid physiology; normal pregnancy is characterized by hypermetabolic effects that resemble the clinical findings of hyperthyroidism. Although some thyroid function tests may be altered during pregnancy, largely by hyperestrogenemia and the resulting increase in thyroid-binding globulin, levels of free circulating hormone (T_4 and T_3) and thyroid-stimulating hormone (TSH) are unchanged. Moreover, several obstetric conditions, notably hyperemesis gravidarum or gestational trophoblastic disease, may cause abnormalities in thyroid function. These principles must be understood when making the diagnosis of thyroid disease during pregnancy.

Hyperthyroidism

Approximately one in 2,000 pregnancies will be complicated by thyrotoxicosis (255). The most frequent cause of thyrotoxicosis is Graves' disease, an autoimmune disease that affects 1% of American women and is associated with thyroid-stimulating immunoglobulins (TSI) (256,257). Another cause of hyperthyroidism is destruction-induced thyrotoxicosis, which causes glandular disruption and release of stored thyroid hormone (256). Poorly controlled or untreated hyperthyroidism in pregnancy is associated with increased rates of preeclampsia, congestive heart failure, and adverse perinatal outcomes (258). The most serious consequence of uncontrolled hyperthyroidism, thyroid storm, presents with exaggerated features of thyrotoxicosis including fever, dehydration, and heart failure (259). Usually, this rare condition is triggered by a precipitating event such as infection, trauma, or delivery (259), and treatment of the underlying condition is critical (256).

Medical treatment of hyperthyroidism involves blocking thyroid hormone production and controlling the peripheral clinical symptoms. Propylthiouracil (PTU) and methimazole, which block production of thyroid hormone, are safe in pregnancy (260). Both agents cross the placenta, but methimazole has been associated with a scalp disorder known as aplasia cutis (261). Peripheral manifestations such as tachycardia are controlled with β-blockers, notably propranolol, widely used during pregnancy. In difficult cases, thyroidectomy may be performed during pregnancy after medical control of thyrotoxicosis has been achieved. Iodides may be used for short periods in preparation for thyroidectomy or for management of thyroid storm.

Most fetal morbidity and mortality develop from uncontrolled maternal hyperthyroidism. Prolonged iodide exposure after 10 to 12 weeks of gestation may result in fetal hypothyroidism and goiter (256,257). Fetal thyrotoxicosis, which results from transplacental passage of TSI (262), has been reported in approximately 1% of infants of mothers with Graves' disease and has been associated with fetal death (256,263,264). Fetal blood sampling has been helpful in measuring fetal thyroid status (265). Infants exposed to maternal PTU may not become hyperthyroid until several days when the thyrotoxic effect of TSI remains after drug clearance has occurred (256).

Hypothyroidism

Overt hypothyroidism rarely complicates pregnancy, although uncontrolled hypothyroidism is reportedly associated with high rates of stillbirths and low-birth-weight infants (256). In many cases, hypothyroidism develops after thyroidectomy or radioiodine therapy; other causes of hypothyroidism include Hashimoto's thyroiditis, carcinoma, or insufficient thyroid replacement (257,266). Thyroid microsomal and thyroid peroxidase antibodies are common (257).

Replacement therapy with thyroxine is recommended for these patients, with TSH levels used to guide therapeutic dosages. Replacement doses of thyroxine may need to be increased during pregnancy (267,268). Pregnancies complicated by hypothyroidism may have increased risks for preeclampsia, placental abruption, anemia, postpartum hemorrhage, cardiac dysfunction, and poor perinatal outcome (266). Neonatal hypothy-

roidism needs to be excluded if maternal antenatal treatment involved radioactive iodine; however, because congenital hypothyroidism is a difficult diagnosis, screening for all infants has become routine (256,269).

Perinatal Infections

Any infection occurring during pregnancy has the potential for causing infectious or teratogenic complications in the fetus, some with devastating effects. The two important routes for fetal infection are hematogenous via the placenta and ascending via the vagina and cervix, the latter usually occurring intrapartum. The effect of an infectious agent on fetal growth and development depends on, among other things, the type of organism, the infectious load, timing in gestation, and potential organ systems affected. Many different organisms have been implicated in causing fetal infection; some of the important perinatal viral infections are listed in Table 14–6, and nonviral infections in Table 14–7.

Treatment of many perinatal infections either does not exist, as in cases with viruses, or may not prevent congenital infection, as with syphilis. Efforts to minimize the effect on the neonate, therefore, have focused primarily on prevention. Examples include cesarean delivery in cases of active maternal genital herpes infection, thereby decreasing the risk of intrapartum ascending infection, neonatal administration of the hepatitis B vaccine, or administration of prophylactic eyedrops to newborns to prevent gonococcal ophthalmia neonatorum. Attempts at preventing early-onset neonatal disease from group B *Streptococcus* have resulted in recent guidelines from the Centers for Disease Control and Prevention for universal third-trimester screening and administration of intrapartum antibiotics to carriers; these recommendations have been adopted by the American College of Obstetricians and Gynecologists (270). There is much work to be done, however, in devising strategies to prevent other perinatally transmitted illnesses such as congenital cytomegalovirus infection or human immunodeficiency virus, which may have damaging effects on a significant number of children annually.

Thromboembolic Disorders

Venous thromboembolism occurs in one of 1,000 to 2,000 pregnancies (271,272). The most constant predisposing factor for thromboembolic disease during pregnancy is venous stasis, although other factors include prolonged bed rest, operative vaginal or cesarean delivery, sepsis, hemorrhage, multiparity, and advanced maternal age (273). Recent investigations contradict older reports that demonstrated the greatest risk for development of thromboembolism to be during the third trimester and the immediate postpartum period; the older data may have been skewed by the practices of common

TABLE 14–6. *Some perinatal viral infections[a]*

Organism	Type of organism	Route of transmission	Potential severe fetal or neonatal effect(s)	Critical exposure
Cytomegalovirus	Double-stranded DNA virus	Transplacental more common than ascending	IUGR, hepatosplenomegaly, chorioretinitis, microophthalmia, cerebral calcifications, hydrocephaly, microcephaly	Timing in gestation not critical; primary infection more severe than recurrent
Rubella	RNA virus	Transplacental	Congenital heart disease, purpura, cataracts, retinopathy, IUGR, microcephaly	First trimester
Herpes simplex virus (HSV)	Double-stranded DNA virus	Ascending intrapartum	Microcephaly, mental retardation, seizures, mircoophthalmia, retinal dysplasia, meningitis, chorioretinitis (HSV-2 more important than HSV-1)	Intrapartum
Varicella–zoster	DNA herpesvirus	Transplacental	Limb hypoplasia, cutaneous scars, chorioretinitis, cortical atrophy, microcephaly; neonatal varicella if contracted peripartum	First trimester for congenital infection; neonatal varicella if contracted 5 days before or 2 days after delivery
Parvovirus B-19	Single-stranded DNA virus	Transplacental	Fetal anemia causing hydrops and/or stillbirth	First or early second trimester
Human immunodeficiency virus (HIV)	Retrovirus	Transplacental; ascending intrapartum; through breast-feeding	Neonatal acquired immunodeficiency syndrome (AIDS)	Any
Hepatitis B	DNA virus	Mostly ascending intrapartum; transplacental during acute hepatitis; through breast-feeding	Chronic hepatitis, cirrhosis	Intrapartum

[a]DNA, deoxyribonucleic acid; IUGR, intrauterine growth restriction; RNA, ribonucleic acid. Data from refs. 269a–269d.

TABLE 14–7. *Some nonviral perinatal infections[a]*

Organism (disease)	Type of organism	Route of transmission	Potential severe fetal or neonatal effect(s)	Time of critical exposure
Neisseria gonorrhoea (gonorrhea)	Gram-negative diplococcus	Ascending	Opthalmia neonatorum	Intrapartum
Group B Streptococcus	Gram-positive bacteria	Ascending	Early-onset neonatal infection: sepsis, meningitis, pneumonia	Intrapartum
Treponema pallidum (syphilis)	Spirochete	Transplacental	Hepatosplenomegaly, osteitis, hemolytic anemia, thrombocytopenia, pneumonia, hydrops, cutaneous or mucous membrane lesions, hepatitis, stillbirth	Any trimester but worse risk with first and second trimesters
Toxoplasma gondii (toxoplasmosis)	Protozoan	Transplacental	Chorioretinitis, hydrocephaly, microcephaly, stillbirth	Third trimester more important but worse effects with first trimester infection

[a]From refs. 269e–270.

operative deliveries, delaying postpartum ambulation, and suppression of lactation with oral estrogen (273,274). Newer data suggest not only equal frequencies in all trimesters but that antepartum events may occur at least as often as those postpartum (174,274–278). Some underlying medical conditions associated with higher risks of developing thromboemboli include protein C, protein S, and antithrombin III deficiencies (all autosomal dominant disorders), factor V Leiden mutation (a missense mutation in the factor V gene that is responsible for up to 95% of activated protein C resistance), hyperhomocysteinemia, and the antiphospholipid antibody syndrome (274,279–281).

The clinical diagnosis of deep vein thrombosis during gestation is imprecise. Noninvasive tests, such as impedance plethysmography or real-time Doppler sonography, which are accurate in nonpregnant patients, may be difficult to interpret during pregnancy; the data they provide as initial tests, however, may be useful (273). Venography remains the standard in diagnosing deep venous thromboembolism (282). For both pregnant and nonpregnant patients suspected of having a pulmonary embolism, the ventilation–perfusion scan is the recommended study (283).

Treatment for acute deep vein thrombosis or pulmonary embolism during pregnancy involves 5 to 10 days of intravenous heparin followed by subcutaneous heparin in doses to achieve full-dose anticoagulation for a minimum of 3 months (273,274). Antepartum prophylactic heparin therapy is indicated in patients with a previous thrombotic event (274). The preferred anticoagulant during pregnancy is heparin because it does not cross the placenta (284); the newer low-molecular-weight heparins are safe in pregnancy (249). Warfarin is avoided because of associated fetal malformations: first-trimester exposure may produce an embryopathy involving stippled epiphyses, nasal and limb hypoplasia, and hypertelorism (285,286), and second- or third-trimester exposure has been associated with central nervous system abnormalities (287). In the postpartum period, warfarin may be used in women who are breast-feeding (274).

Renal Disorders

Mild renal dysfunction typically has little, if any, effect on pregnancy outcome (288); however, adverse pregnancy events are well described in women with moderate to severe renal insufficiency (e.g., serum creatinine 1.4 mg/dL or greater) (289–291). These pregnancies are especially risky: maternal complications include anemia, vascular accidents, placental abruption, chronic hypertension, pregnancy-induced hypertension, preeclampsia, proteinuria, and worsening renal function; perinatal complications such as IUGR, stillbirth, prematurity, polyhydramnios, and midtrimester pregnancy loss are not unusual (289,291,292).

Dialysis may be utilized during pregnancies complicated by renal insufficiency. More literature is available for hemodialysis than for continuous ambulatory peritoneal dialysis (293–297). Pregnancy success rates in dialysis patients are at most 52% (294). In general, outcomes are more promising for women in whom dialysis has been initiated during pregnancy compared to patients already on dialysis before conception (293,295). Complications associated with peritoneal dialysis in pregnancy include preterm labor (293) and acute peritonitis (295,298). Hemodialysis involves intermittent and often significant fluid shifts, which may be accompanied by hypotension, electrolyte imbalances, and preterm labor (292). In one reported case, in spite of efforts to eliminate major fluid shifts and changes in arterial pressure in a patient at 32 weeks gestation, uterine artery Doppler studies showed a significant increase after hemodialysis; redistribution of flow away from the uteroplacental vascular bed during hemodialysis was postulated (292).

Pregnancy is no longer an unusual event among women of child-bearing age with functioning renal transplants, occurring in approximately one of 20 to 50 women (196,299). These pregnancies have low success rates, however: excluding elective termination, the chance of delivering a liveborn infant is at best only 19% (300), although repeated successful pregnancies have been reported (301). Hypertension before or during early pregnancy is associated with adverse perinatal events (299). Typically, pregnancy results in increased renal function, which transiently declines in late pregnancy. As many as 15% of patients with kidney disease may experience permanent renal impairment (300). High rates of preterm delivery, IUGR, hypertension and/or preeclampsia, and stillbirth are reported (196,299,300). The risk of graft rejection is not influenced by pregnancy, however (196). Cyclosporine A, a potent anti-T-cell immunosuppressive agent, has replaced older regimens of azathioprine and steroids in preventing graft rejection (302). Cyclosporine has been used successfully during pregnancy without evidence of teratogenicity (302–304).

Heart Disease

Maternal cardiac disease may be accompanied by significant maternal and perinatal morbidity and mortality. Although the etiology of cardiac disease has changed in the past 30 years, with congenital heart disease now more common than rheumatic heart disease, the underlying pathophysiology remains the same. Functional status before or early in pregnancy is an important prognostic indicator of maternal and fetal outcome. A helpful and commonly used system for assessing cardiac function is the New York Heart Association classification (Table 14–8) (305,306). Better prognoses are expected during pregnancy for women with functional classes I and II than for those with classes III or IV.

TABLE 14–8. *The New York Heart Association (NYHA) functional classification of heart disease*[a]

Class	Symptoms
Class I	Asymptomatic
Class II	Symptoms with greater than normal activity
Class III	Symptoms with normal activity
Class IV	Symptoms at rest

[a]From refs. 305 and 306.

Preconception counseling is extremely important in this group of patients. The added cardiovascular demands of pregnancy may be associated with cardiac deterioration: over 40% of women with heart disease will develop pulmonary edema for the first time during the third trimester (305,307). Maternal risks vary with the individual cardiac lesion, several specific defects being associated with especially high risks of maternal mortality (Table 14–9) (305).

Fetal risks include premature delivery, IUGR, and stillbirth, especially with maternal cyanotic heart disease (305,308). A 2% to 5% incidence of fetal cardiac anomalies has been suggested in women with congenital heart disease, although with specific lesions, the risk may be as high as 26% (305,309,310). Most of the drugs used in the treatment of cardiac disease are well tolerated and rarely associated with significant fetal problems (e.g., β-blockers, calcium-channel blockers, digitalis, and heparin) (309). Newer agents have not been well studied during pregnancy.

Cardiac surgery, if possible, should be delayed until after completion of pregnancy. If it is required, however, timing is recommended during the second trimester (309). Maternal and perinatal mortality varies with the type of procedure. In mitral valve commissurotomy, the cardiovascular procedure that has been performed the most during pregnancy, for example, maternal mortality is under 3%, and perinatal mortality is less than 10%; in contrast, with open-heart surgery, although maternal mortality is not significantly higher, fetal loss may be as high as 20% (309).

Myocardial infarction rarely occurs during pregnancy; the incidence is estimated at 0.01% (311). Cases show a preponderance during the third trimester and in multiparous women over age 33 (312), with the majority located in the anterior wall (312,313). Maternal mortality ranges from 19% to 37% (312–314). Fetal mortality is similarly high, most resulting from maternal death (312–314). Recent use of acute coronary artery angioplasty has been successful during pregnancy (315,316). Treatment with thrombolytic agents for maternal myocardial infarction has been reported during the second trimester, although the fetal risk of such therapy has not been established (317). In women with previous infarctions, subsequent successful pregnancies have been reported (318,319).

TABLE 14–9. *Some maternal congenital heart lesions in pregnancy*[a]

Cardiac lesion	Specific information
Aortic insufficiency	Well tolerated
Aortic stenosis	Valve diameter must decrease to ≤1/3 for hemodynamic significance; increased risk of angina, MI, syncope, or sudden death with severe disease because CO is fixed and may not be able to compensate; frequently associated with ischemic heart disease; most critical time is at pregnancy termination or delivery; PA catheterization may be most useful in labor
Ebstein's anomaly	Right-to-left shunt ± pulmonary HTN; association with thromboembolism, CHF, arrhythmias; 25% have Wolf-Parkinson-White syndrome and increased risk for tachyarrhythmias
Eisenmenger syndrome	Pulmonary HTN with left-to-right shunt; grave prognosis; maternal mortality 30% to 50%; high association with thromboembolism; therapeutic termination is recommended
Marfan syndrome	Autosomal dominant; aortic dissection or aortic or splenic artery aneurysm or rupture associated with worse outcomes; 50% mortality seen with aortic root diameter >40 mm
Mitral insufficiency	Well tolerated; CHF rare; pulmonary edema more likely with preeclampsia because of increase in afterload; because of increased risk of atrial enlargement and fibrillation, prophylactic digitalis recommended in severe disease
Mitral stenosis	Tachycardia may result in fall in CO and BP; fluid balance crucial; most critical time is immediately postpartum; hemodynamic monitoring is recommended
Mitral valve prolapse	Common; mostly asymptomatic; chest pain or palpitations possible; responds to beta-blockers
Tetralogy of Fallot	VSD, overriding aorta, RVH, and pulmonary stenosis; patients are cyanotic; maternal mortality 4% to 15% in uncorrected patients; corrected cases fairly good outcome
Tricuspid or pulmonic valve disease	Well tolerated

[a]BP, blood pressure; CHF, congestive heart failure; CO, cardiac output; HTN, hypertension; MI, myocardial infarction; PA, pulmonary artery; RVH, right ventricular hypertrophy; VSD, ventricular septal defect. Data from refs. 305, 306, and 309.

Women having undergone heart transplantation have had successful pregnancies (320–324). Reported cases include four patients who initially received their allograft because of peripartum cardiomyopathy from an earlier pregnancy (324). Maternal hypertension, preeclampsia, and jaundice, as well as fetal IUGR, are common (324). Immunosuppression issues are the same as those discussed for patients with renal transplants.

Cancer

Cancer develops in approximately one of 1,000 pregnancies. The most common invasive carcinoma originates in the cervix (325), affecting one of 2,200 pregnancies (326). Almost 3% of all cervical cancers are diagnosed during pregnancy (327). The second most common site for malignancy during pregnancy is the breast, with cancer estimated to occur once in every 1,360 to 3,200 pregnancies (328). Other frequently seen neoplasias include vulvar, ovarian, and colorectal carcinoma as well as leukemia, Hodgkin's disease, and melanoma. Stage for stage, comparing diagnoses in nonpregnant women, carcinoma identified during pregnancy may be more advanced. Currently, this is felt to reflect a delay in diagnosis, possibly because of the physiologic changes of pregnancy and not necessarily because the cancer is more aggressive during the pregnant state (329). It has never been substantiated that pregnancy termination alters cancer progression (329). Metastasis to the fetus or placenta has been reported in fewer than 70 cases, mostly involving the breast, cervix, leukemia, lymphoma, melanoma, and thyroid (330).

Decisions regarding the management of malignancies during pregnancy are difficult and involve risk assessment for both mother and fetus; they are compounded by the timing in gestation. In general, first-trimester treatment risks spontaneous abortion or fetal malformation, and early third-trimester therapy places the pregnancy at risk for preterm labor. Surgery can be performed at any time, although it is preferred during the second trimester. Radiation or chemotherapy exposure in the first trimester may affect organogenesis, resulting in either pregnancy loss or fetal structural defects (331–333).

During the first 3 weeks of gestation, radiation exposure of at least 250 rads (2.5 cGy) poses the greatest risk for spontaneous abortion (334). Exposure to more than 50 rads (0.5 cGy) is more commonly associated with development of severe malformations (335); however, it is unusual to see congenital anomalies in embryos exposed to 5 rads (0.05 cGy) or more (334). Some malformations associated with radiation exposure during weeks 3 to 10 include microcephaly, low birth weight, mental retardation, cataracts, retinal degeneration, and skeletal abnormalities (334,335). Radiation exposure between 11 and 20 weeks of gestation is not commonly associated with fetal

malformations (329). Pregnancy termination has been suggested when fetal exposure is greater than 10 rads (0.1 cGy) (336). In cases in which local irradiation is used to treat malignancies of the pelvis, spontaneous abortion or fetal demise usually occurs (327).

Use of cytotoxic chemotherapy is generally avoided in the first trimester, although data vary for different agents (327). Exposure beyond the first trimester has not been found to be associated with increased risks of congenital anomalies (332,333). Long-term developmental data are lacking, however. In treating patients with chemotherapeutic agents, it must be recognized that the physiologic changes of pregnancy may alter the efficacy, toxicity, and/or dosage regimens.

SUMMARY

Many maternal conditions have relevance for a developing pregnancy. Counseling pregnant women with underlying medical disorders must encompass the effects of the illness on the pregnancy, the effects of the pregnancy on the condition, as well as potential complications of therapeutic interventions and the risks of possible premature delivery. Statistics that indicate reductions in neonatal mortality rates are encouraging; however, there is much yet to be learned in perinatology in order to impact on the unacceptably high rates of premature deliveries and to improve the health of women before and during pregnancy.

REFERENCES

1. Singh GK, Yu SM. Infant mortality in the United States: trends, differentials, and projections, 1950 through 2010. *Am J Public Health* 1995;85:957–964.
2. Guyer B, Strobino DM, Ventura SJ, MacDorman M, Martin JA. Annual summary of vital statistics—1995. *Pediatrics* 1996;98: 1007–1019.
3. McCormick MC, Shapiro S, Starfield BH. The regionalization of perinatal services: summary of the evaluation of a national demonstration program. *JAMA* 1985;253:799–804.
4. McCormick MC. The contribution of low birth weight to infant mortality and childhood morbidity. *N Engl J Med* 1985;312:82–90.
5. Wilcox A, Skjærven R, Buekens P, Kiely J. Birth weight and perinatal mortality. A comparison of the United States and Norway. *JAMA* 1995;273:709–711.
6. McCormick MC, Wise PH. Infant mortality. *Curr Opin Pediatr* 1993; 5:552–557.
7. Tamura RK, Sabbagha RE, Davis CL, et al. Antenatal estimates of gestational age and fetal weight as predictors of perinatal mortality in very preterm fetuses. *J Matern Fetal Invest* 1992;1:261–265.
8. Amon E, Anderson GD, Sibai BM, Mabie WC. Factors responsible for a preterm delivery of the immature newborn infant (less than or equal to 1000 gm). *Am J Obstet Gynecol* 1987;156:1143–1148.
9. Arias F, Tomich P. Etiology and outcome of low birth weight and preterm infants. *Obstet Gynecol* 1982;60:277–281.
10. Meis PJ, Ernest JM, Moore ML. Causes of low birth weight births in public and private patients. *Am J Obstet Gynecol* 1987;156:1165–1168.
11. American College of Obstetricians and Gynecologists. *Preterm labor. ACOG technical bulletin 206.* Washington, DC: ACOG, 1995.
12. Kaltreider DF, Kohl S. Epidemiology of preterm delivery. *Clin Obstet Gynecol* 1980;23:17–31.
13. Centers for Disease Control. State-specific trends among women who

did not receive prenatal care—United States 1980–1992. *MMWR* 1994;43:939–942.

14. Harger JH, Hsing AW, Tuomala RE, et al. Risk factors for preterm premature rupture of fetal membranes: A multicenter case-control study. *Am J Obstet Gynecol* 1990;163:130–137.

15. Hoffman HJ, Bakketeig LS. Risk factors associated with the occurrence of preterm birth. *Clin Obstet Gynecol* 1984;27:539–552.

16. Keirse MJNC, Rush RW, Anderson ABM, Turnbull AC. Risk of preterm delivery in patients with a previous pre-term delivery and/or abortion. *Br J Obstet Gynaecol* 1978;85:81–85.

17. Kristensen J, Langhoff-Roos J, Kristensen FB. Implications of idiopathic preterm delivery for previous and subsequent pregnancies. *Obstet Gynecol* 1995;86:800–804.

18. Mercer BM, Goldenberg RL, Das A, et al. The preterm prediction study: a clinical risk assessment system. *Am J Obstet Gynecol* 1996; 174:1885–1895.

19. Romero R, Brody DT, Oyarzun E, Mazor M, Wu YK, Hobbins JC, Durum SK. Infection and labor. III. Interleukin-1: a signal for the onset of parturition. *Am J Obstet Gynecol* 1989;160:1117–1123.

20. Romero R, Ghidini A, Bahado-Singh R. Premature rupture of the membranes. In Reece EA, Hobbins JC, Mahoney MJ, Petrie RH, eds. *Medicine of the fetus and mother*. Philadelphia: JB Lippincott, 1992: 1430.

21. McGregor JA, French JI, Lawellin DW, Franco-Buff A, Smith C, Todd JK. Bacterial protease-induced reduction of chorioamniotic membrane strength and elasticity. *Obstet Gynecol* 1987;69:167–174.

22. Minkoff H. Prematurity: infection as an etiologic factor. *Obstet Gynecol* 1983;62:137–144.

23. Schoonmaker JN, Lawellin DW, Lunt B, McGregor JA. Bacteria and inflammatory cells reduce chorioamniotic membrane integrity and tensile strength. *Obstet Gynecol* 1989;74:590–596.

24. Gibbs RS, Romero R, Hillier SL, Eschenbach DA, Sweet RL. A review of premature birth and subclinical infection. *Am J Obstet Gynecol* 1992;166:1515–1528.

24a. Gravett MG, Nelson HP, DeRouen T, Critchlow C, Eschenbach DA, Holmes KK. Independent association of bacterial vaginosis and Chlamydia trachomatis infection with adverse pregnancy outcome. *JAMA* 1986;256:1899–1903.

25. McGregor JA, French JI. Bacterial vaginosis and preterm birth. *N Engl J Med* 1996;334:1337–1338.

26. McGregor JA, French JI, Parker R, et al. Prevention of premature birth by screening and treatment for common genital tract infections: results of a prospective controlled evaluation. *Am J Obstet Gynecol* 1995;173:157–167.

27. McGregor JA, Schoonmaker JN, Lunt BD, Lawellin DW. Antibiotic inhibition of bacterially induced fetal membrane weaking. *Obstet Gynecol* 1990;76:124–128.

28. Gravett MG, Hummel D, Eschenbach DA, Holmes KK. Preterm labor associated with subclinical amniotic fluid infection and with bacterial vaginosis. *Obstet Gynecol* 1986;67:229–237.

29. Kurki T, Sivonen A, Renkonen O-V, Savia E, Ylikorkala O. Bacterial vaginosis in early pregnancy and pregnancy outcome. *Obstet Gynecol* 1992;80:173–177.

30. Martius J, Krohn MA, Hillier SL, Stamm WE, Holmes KK, Eschenbach DA. Relationship of vaginal *Lactobacillus* species, cervical *Chlamydia trachomatis,* and bacterial vaginosis to preterm birth. *Obstet Gynecol* 1988;71:89–95.

31. McGregor JA, French JI, Richter R, et al. Antenatal microbiologic and maternal risk factors associated with prematurity. *Am J Obstet Gynecol* 1990;163:1465–1473.

32. Meis PJ, Goldenberg RL, Mercer B, et al. The preterm prediction study: significance of vaginal infections. National Institutes of Child Health and Human Development Maternal–Fetal Medicine Units Network. *Am J Obstet Gynecol* 1995;173:1231–1235.

33. Hillier SL, Nugent RP, Eschenbach DA, et al. Association between bacterial vaginosis and preterm delivery of a low-birth-weight infant. *N Engl J Med* 1995;333:1737–1742.

34. Hauth JC, Gilstrap LC 3d, Hankins GD, Connor KD. Term maternal and neonatal complications of acute chorioamnionitis. *Obstet Gynecol* 1985;66:59–62.

35. Wilson JC, Levy DL, Wilds PL. Premature rupture of membranes prior to term: consequences of nonintervention. *Obstet Gynecol* 1982;60:601–606.

36. Beydoun SM, Yasin SY. Premature rupture of the membranes before

28 weeks: conservative management. *Am J Obstet Gynecol* 1986;155: 471–479.

37. Moretti M, Sibai BM. Maternal and perinatal outcome of expectant management of premature rupture of membranes in the midtrimester. *Am J Obstet Gynecol* 1988;159:390–396.

38. Taylor J, Garite TJ. Premature rupture of membranes before fetal viability. *Obstet Gynecol* 1984;64:615–620.

39. National Institutes of Health Consensus Development Conference. *Effect of corticosteroids for fetal maturation on perinatal outcomes.* Bethesda, MD: National Institutes of Health Consensus Development Conference Statement, 1994:1–18.

40. Gardner MO, Papile L-A, Wright LL. Antenatal corticosteroids in pregnancies complicated by preterm premature rupture of membranes. *Obstet Gynecol* 1997;90:851–853.

41. Hauth JC, Goldenberg RL, Andrews WW, DuBard MB, Copper RL. Reduced incidence of preterm delivery with metronidazole and erythromycin in women with bacterial vaginosis. *N Engl J Med* 1995;333: 1732–1736.

42. Morales WJ, Schorr S, Albritton J. Effect of metronidazole in patients with preterm birth in preceding pregnancy and bacterial vaginosis: a placebo-controlled, double-blind study. *Am J Obstet Gynecol* 1994; 171:345–349.

42a. McGregor JA, French JI, Reller LB, Todd JK, Makowski EL. Adjunctive erythromycin treatment for idiopathic preterm labor: results of a randomized, double-blinded, placebo-controlled trial. *Am J Obstet Gynecol* 1986;154:98–103.

43. Klebanoff MA, Regan JA, Rao V, et al. Outcome of the Vaginal Infections and Prematurity Study: results of a clinical trial of erythromycin among pregnant women colonized with group B streptococci. *Am J Obstet Gynecol* 1995;172:1540–1545.

44. Romero R, Sibai B, Caritis S, et al. Antibiotic treatment of preterm labor with intact membranes: a multicenter, randomized, double-blinded, placebo-controlled trial. *Am J Obstet Gynecol* 1993;169: 764–774.

45. Egarter C, Leitich H, Karas H, et al. Antibiotic treatment in preterm PROM and neonatal morbidity: a metaanalysis. *Am J Obstet Gynecol* 1996;174:589–597.

46. Morales WJ, Angel JL, O'Brien WF, Knuppel RA, Finazzo M. A randomized study of antibiotic therapy in idiopathic preterm labor. *Obstet Gynecol* 1988;72:829–833.

47. Creasy RK, Gummer BA, Liggins GC. System for predicting spontaneous preterm birth. *Obstet Gynecol* 1980;55:692–695.

48. Main DM, Richardson DK, Hadley CB, Gabbe SG. Controlled trial of a Preterm Labor Detection program: efficacy and costs. *Obstet Gynecol* 1989;74:873–877.

49. Amon E. Premature Labor. In Reece EA, Hobbins JC, Mahoney MJ, Petrie RH, eds. *Medicine of the fetus and mother*. Philadelphia: JB Lippincott, 1992:1404.

50. Papiernik E, Bouyer J, Collin D. Precocious cervical ripening and preterm labor. *Obstet Gynecol* 1986;67:238–242.

51. Buekens P, Alexander S, Boutsen M, Blondel B, Kaminski M, Reid M. Randomised controlled trial of routine cervical examinations in pregnancy. European Community Collaborative Study Group on Prenatal Screening. *Lancet* 1994;344:841–844.

52. Gomez R, Galasso M, Romero R, et al. Ultrasonographic examination of the uterine cervix is better than cervical digital examination as a predictor of the likelihood of premature delivery in patients with preterm labor and intact membranes. *Am J Obstet Gynecol* 1994;171:956–964.

53. Iams JD, Goldenberg RL, Meis PJ, et al. The length of the cervix and the risk of spontaneous premature delivery. National Institute of Child Health and Human Development Maternal–Fetal Medicine Units Network. *N Engl J Med* 1996;334:567–572.

54. Iams JD, Paraskos J, Landon MB, Teteris JN, Johnson FF. *Obstet Gynecol* 1994;84:40–46.

55. Okitsu O, Mimura T, Nakayama T, Aono T. Early prediction of preterm delivery by transvaginal ultrasonography. *Ultrasound Obstet Gynecol* 1992;2:402–409.

56. Timor-Tritsch IE, Boozarjomehri F, Masakowski Y, Monteagudo A, Chao CR. Can a "snapshot" sagittal view of the cervix by transvaginal ultrasonography predict active preterm labor? *Am J Obstet Gynecol* 1996;174:990–995.

57. Quinn MJ. Vaginal ultrasound and cervical cerclage: A prospective study. *Ultrasound Obstet Gynecol* 1992;2:410–416.

58. Guzman ER, Pisatowski DM, Vintzileos AM, Benito CW, Hanley

ML, Ananth CV. A comparison of ultrasonographically detected cervical changes in response to transfundal pressure, coughing, and standing in predicting cervical incompetence. *Am J Obstet Gynecol* 1997;177:660–665.

59. Guzman ER, Rosenberg JC, Houlihan C, Ivan J, Waldron R, Knuppel R. A new method using vaginal ultrasound and transfundal pressure to evaluate the asymptomatic incompetent cervix. *Obstet Gynecol* 1994;83:248–252.

60. Wong G, Levine D, Ludmir J. Maternal postural challenge as a functional test for cervical incompetence. *J Ultrasound Med* 1997;16: 169–175.

61. Katz M, Newman RB, Gill PJ. Assessment of uterine activity in ambulatory patients at high risk of preterm labor and delivery. *Am J Obstet Gynecol* 1986;154:44–47.

62. American College of Obstetricians and Gynecologists. *Home uterine activity monitoring. ACOG Committee Opinion 172.* Washington, DC: ACOG, 1996.

63. US Preventive Services Task Force. Home uterine activity monitoring for preterm labor. Policy statement. *JAMA* 1993;270:369–370.

64. US Preventive Services Task Force. Home uterine activity monitoring for preterm labor. Review article. *JAMA* 1993;270:371–376.

65. *Guidelines for Perinatal Care,* 4th ed. Elk Grove Village, IL: American Academy of Pediatrics; and Washington, DC: American College of Obstetricians and Gynecologists, 1997:75–76.

66. Regan JA, Klebanoff MA, Nugent RP, et al. Colonization with group B streptococci in pregnancy and adverse outcome. VIP Study Group. *Am J Obstet Gynecol* 1996;174:1354–1360.

67. Centers for Disease Control. Prevention of perinatal group B streptococcal disease: A public health perspective. *MMWR* 1996;45:1–24.

68. Goldenberg RL, Mercer BM, Meis PJ, Copper RL, Das A, McNellis D. The preterm prediction study: fetal fibronectin testing and spontaneous preterm birth. National Institute of Child Health and Human Development Maternal–Fetal Medicine Units Network. *Obstet Gynecol* 1996;87:643–648.

68a. Goldenberg RL, Thom E, Moawad AH, Johnson F, Roberts J, Caritis SN. The preterm prediction study: Fetal fibronectin, bacterial vaginosis, and peripartum infection. National Institute of Child Health and Human Development Maternal–Fetal Medicine Units Network. *Obstet Gynecol* 1996;87:656–660.

69. Goldenberg RL, Mercer BM, Iams JD, et al. The preterm prediction study: patterns of cervicovaginal fetal fibronectin as predictors of spontaneous preterm delivery. National Institute of Child Health and Human Development Maternal–Fetal Medicine Units Network. *Am J Obstet Gynecol* 1997;177:8–12.

70. American College of Obstetricians and Gynecologists. *Fetal fibronectin preterm labor risk test. ACOG Committee Opinion 187.* Washington, DC: ACOG, 1997.

71. Abrams B. Maternal nutrition. In Creasy RK, Resnik R, eds. *Maternal–fetal medicine,* 3rd ed. Philadelphia: WB Saunders, 1994: 162–170.

72. American College of Obstetricians and Gynecologists. *Nutrition during pregnancy. ACOG Technical Bulletin 179.* Washington, DC: ACOG, 1993.

73. Johnson JWC, Longmate JA, Frentzen B. Excessive maternal weight and pregnancy outcome. *Am J Obstet Gynecol* 1992;167:353–372.

74. Institute of Medicine, Food and Nutrition Board, Committee on Nutritional Status During Pregnancy and Lactation, Subcommittee on Dietary Intake and Nutrient Supplements During Pregnancy and Subcommittee on Nutritional Status and Weight Gain During Pregnancy. *Nutrition during pregnancy. Part I. Weight gain.* Washington, DC: National Academy Press, 1990.

75. Shaw GM, Velie EM, Schagger D. Risk of neural tube defect-affected pregnancies among obese women. *JAMA* 1996;275:1093–1096.

76. Watkins ML, Scanlon KS, Mulinare J, Khoury MJ. Is maternal obesity a risk factor for anencephaly and spina bifida? *Epidemiology* 1996;7:507–512.

77. Waller DK, Mills JL, Simpson JL, Cunningham GC, Conley MR, Lassman MR, Rhoads GG. Are obese women at higher risk for producing malformed offspring? *Am J Obstet Gynecol* 1994;170:541–548.

78. Werler MM, Louik C, Shapiro S, Mitchell AA. Prepregnant weight in relation to risk of neural tube defects. *JAMA* 1996;275:1127–1128.

79. Institute of Medicine, Food and Nutrition Board, Committee on Nutritional Status During Pregnancy and Lactation, Subcommittee on Dietary Intake and Nutrient Supplements During Pregnancy and Subcommittee on Nutritional Status and Weight Gain During Pregnancy. *Nutrition during pregnancy. Part II. Nutrient supplements.* Washington, DC: National Academy Press, 1990.

80. American College of Obstetricians and Gynecologists. *Vitamin A supplementation during pregnancy. ACOG Committee Opinion 112.* Washington, DC: ACOG, 1992.

81. Medical Research Council Vitamin Study Research Group. Prevention of neural tube defects: results of the Medical Research Council vitamin study. *Lancet* 1991;338:131–137.

82. Centers for Disease Control. Use of folic acid for prevention of spina bifida and other neural tube defects—1983–1991. *MMWR* 1991;40: 513–516.

83. Centers for Disease Control. Recommendations for the use of folic acid to reduce the number of cases of spina bifida and other neural tube defects. *MMMR* 1992;41:1–7.

84. Survey alert. Fortified pasta coming. *Obstet Gynecol Surv* 1997;52: 191.

85. National High Blood Pressure Education Program Working Group. Report on high blood pressure in pregnancy. *Am J Obstet Gynecol* 1990;163:1691–1712.

86. American College of Obstetricians and Gynecologists. *Hypertension in pregnancy. ACOG Technical Bulletin 219.* Washington, DC: ACOG, 1995.

87. National Institutes of Health. National Heart, Lung, and Blood Institute. *The Fifth Report of the Joint National Committee Report on the Detection, Evaluation, and Treatment of High Blood Pressure. NIH Publication No. 93-1088.* Bethesda, MD: NIH, 1994.

88. Tervila L, Goecke C, Timonen S. Estimation of gestosis of pregnancy (EPH–gestosis). *Acta Obstet Gynecol Scand* 1973;52:235–243.

89. Gant NF, Madden JD, Siiteri PK, MacDonald PC. The metabolic clearance rate of dehydroisoandrosterone sulfate. IV. Acute effects of induced hypertension, hypotension, and naturesis in normal and hypertensive pregnancies. *Am J Obstet Gynecol* 1976;124:143–148.

90. Barr M, Cohen MM. ACE inhibitor fetopathy and hypocalvaria: the kidney–skull connection. *Teratology* 1991;44:485–495.

91. Hanssens M, Keirse MJ, Vankelecom F, Van Assche FA. Fetal and neonatal effects of treatment with angiotensin-converting enzyme inhibitors in pregnancy. *Obstet Gynecol* 1991;78:128–135.

92. Piper JM, Ray WA, Rosa FW. Pregnancy outcome following exposure to angiotensin–converting enzyme inhibitors. *Obstet Gynecol* 1992; 80:429–432.

93. Davey D, MacGillivray I. The classification and definition of hypertensive disorders in pregnancy. *Am J Obstet Gynecol* 1988;158: 892–898.

94. Leduc L, Wheeler JM, Kirshon B, Mitchell P, Cotton DB. Coagulation profile in severe preeclampsia. *Obstet Gynecol* 1992;79:14–18.

95. Sibai BM, Taslimi MM, El-Nazer A, Amon E, Mabie WC, Ryan G. Maternal–perinatal outcome associated with the syndrome of hemolysis, elevated liver enzymes, and low platelets in severe preeclampsia–eclampsia. *Am J Obstet Gynecol* 1986;155:501–509.

96. Martin JN Jr, Blake PG, Perry KG Jr, McCaul JF, Hess LW, Martin RW. The natural history of HELLP syndrome: patterns of disease progression and regression. *Am J Obstet Gynecol* 1991;164:1500–1513.

97. Weinstein L. Syndrome of hemolysis, elevated liver enzymes, and low platelet count. A severe consequence of hypertension in pregnancy. *Am J Obstet Gynecol* 1986;142:159–167.

98. Talledo OE, Chesley LC, Zuspan FP. Renin–angiotensin in normal and toxemic pregnancies. III. Differential sensitivity to angiotensin II and norepinephrine in toxemia of pregnancy. *Am J Obstet Gynecol* 1968;100:218–222.

99. Gant NF, Daley GL, Chand S, Whalley PJ, MacDonald PC. A study of angiotensin II pressor response throughout primigravid pregnancy. *J Clin Invest* 1973;52:2682–2689.

100. Sibai BM. Diagnosis and management of chronic hypertension in pregnancy. *Obstet Gynecol* 1991;78:451–461.

101. Sibai BM, Abdella TN, Anderson GD. Pregnancy outcome in 211 patients with mild chronic hypertension. *Obstet Gynecol* 1983;61: 571–576.

102. Burrows RF, Andrew M. Neonatal thrombocytopenia in the hypertensive disorders of pregnancy. *Obstet Gynecol* 1990;76:234–238.

103. Schiff E, Friedman SA, Sibai BM. Conservative management of severe preeclampsia remote from term. *Obstet Gynecol* 1994;84:626–630.

104. Sibai BM, Mercer BM, Schiff E, Friedman SA. Aggressive versus expectant management of severe preeclampsia at 28 to 32 weeks ges-

tation: a randomized controlled trial. *Am J Obstet Gynecol* 1994;171: 818–822.

105. Appleton MP, Kuehl TJ, Raebel MA, Adams HR, Knight AB, Gold WR. Magnesium sulfate versus phenytoin for seizure prophylaxis in pregnancy-induced hypertension. *Am J Obstet Gynecol* 1991;165: 907–913.

106. The Eclampsia Trial Collaborative Group. Which anticonvulsant for women with eclampsia? Evidence from the Collaborative Eclampsia Trial. *Lancet* 1995;345:1455–1463.

107. Lucas MJ, Leveno KJ, Cunningham FG. A comparison of magnesium sulfate with phenytoin for the prevention of eclampsia. *N Engl J Med* 1995;333:201–205.

108. Magann EF, Bass D, Chauhan SP, Sullivan DL, Martin RW, Martin JN. Antepartum corticosteroids: disease stabilization in patients with the syndrome of hemolysis, elevated liver enzymes, and low platelets (HELLP). *Am J Obstet Gynecol* 1994;171:1148–1153.

109. CLASP (Collaborative Low–Dose Aspirin Study in Pregnancy) Collaborative Group. CLASP: A randomised trial of low-dose aspirin for the prevention and treatment of pre-eclampsia among 9364 pregnant women. *Lancet* 1994;343:619–629.

110. Hauth JC, Goldenberg RL, Parker CR, et al. Low-dose aspirin therapy to prevent preeclampsia. *Am J Obstet Gynecol* 1993;168: 1083–1093.

111. Imperiale TF, Petrulis AS. A meta-analysis of low-dose aspirin for the prevention of pregnancy-induced hypertensive disease. *JAMA* 1991; 266:260–264.

112. Belizán JM, Villar J, Gonzalez L, Campodonico L, Bergel E. Calcium supplementation to prevent hypertensive disorders of pregnancy. *N Engl J Med* 1991;325:1399–1405.

113. Lopez-Jaramillo P, Delgado F, Jacome P, Teran E, Ruano C, Rivera J. Calcium supplementation and the risk of preeclampsia in Ecuadorian pregnant teenagers. *Obstet Gynecol* 1997;90:162–167.

114. Levine RJ, Hauth JC, Curet LB, et al. Trial of calcium to prevent preeclampsia. *N Engl J Med* 1997;337:69–76.

115. Harrington K, Carpenter RG, Goldfrad C, Campbell S. Transvaginal Doppler ultrasound of the uteroplacental circulation in the early prediction of pre-eclampsia and intrauterine growth retardation. *Br J Obstet Gynaecol* 1997;104:674–681.

116. Harrington K, Goldfrad C, Carpenter RG, Campbell S. Transvaginal uterine and umbilical artery Doppler examination of 12–16 weeks and the subsequent development of pre-eclampsia and intrauterine growth retardation. *Ultrasound Obstet Gynecol* 1997;9:94–100.

117. American College of Obstetricians and Gynecologists. *Diabetes and pregnancy. ACOG Technical Bulletin 200.* Washington, DC: ACOG, 1994.

118. Engelgau MM, Herman WH, Smith PJ, German RR, Aubert RE. The epidemiology of diabetes and pregnancy in the U.S., 1988. *Diabetes Care* 1995;18:1029–1033.

119. Deleted in proof.

120. White P. Pregnancy complicating diabetes. *Am J Med* 7:609–616.

121. Nylund L, Lubell NO, Lewander R, Persson B, Sarby B. Uteroplacental blood flow in diabetic pregnancy: measurements with indium 113m and a computer-linked gamma camera. *Am J Obstet Gynecol* 1982;144:298–302.

122. American College of Obstetricians and Gynecologists. *Fetal macrosomia. ACOG Technical Bulletin 159.* Washington, DC: ACOG, 1991.

123. Bruzzi P, Green SB, Byar DP, Brinton LA, Schairer C. Estimating the population attributable risk for multiple risk factors using case-control data. *Am J Epidemiol* 1985;122:904–914.

124. Elliott JP, Garite TJ, Freeman RK, McQuown DS, Patel JM. Ultrasonic prediction of fetal macrosomia in diabetic pregnancies. *Obstet Gynecol* 1982;60:159–162.

125. Gabbe SG, Mestman JH, Freeman RK, Anderson GV, Lowensohn RI. Management and outcome of class A diabetes mellitus. *Am J Obstet Gynecol* 1977;127:465–469.

126. Kek LP, Ng CS, Chng KP, et al. Extremes of foetal birthweight for gestation in infants of diabetic mothers. *Ann Acad Med Singapore* 1985;14:303–306.

127. Tamura RK, Dooley SL. The role of ultrasonography in the management of diabetic pregnancy. *Clin Obstet Gynecol* 1991;34:526–534.

128. Acker DB, Sachs BP, Friedman EA. Risk factors for shoulder dystocia. *Obstet Gynecol* 1985;66:762–768.

129. Gross TL, Sokol RJ, Williams T, Thompson K. Shoulder dystocia: a fetal–physician risk. *Am J Obstet Gynecol* 1987;156:1408–1418.

130. Keller JD, Lopez-Zeno JA, Dooley SL, Socol ML. Shoulder dystocia and birth trauma in gestational diabetes: a five-year experience. *Am J Obstet Gynecol* 1991;165:928–930.

131. Meshari AA, DeSilva S, Rahman I. Fetal macrosomia—maternal risks and fetal outcome. *Int J Gynecol Obstet* 1990;32:215–222.

132. Sacks DA. Fetal macrosomia and gestational diabetes: What's the problem? *Obstet Gynecol* 1993;81:775–781.

133. Bahar AM. Risk factors and fetal outcome in cases of shoulder dystocia compared with normal deliveries of a similar birthweight. *Br J Obstet Gynaecol* 1996;103:868–872.

134. Langer O, Berkus MD, Huff RW, Samueloff A. Shoulder dystocia: Should the fetus weighing greater than or equal to 4000 grams be delivered by cesarean section? *Am J Obstet Gynecol* 1991;165:831–837.

135. Gordon M, Rich H, Deutschberger J, Green M. The immediate and long-term outcome of obstetric birth trauma. I. Brachial plexus paralysis. *Am J Obstet Gynecol* 1973;117:51–56.

136. Hardy AE. Birth injuries of the brachial plexus: incidence and prognosis. *J Bone Joint Surg [Br]* 1981;63-B:98–101.

137. Tan KL. Brachial palsy. *J Obstet Gynaecol Br Commonw* 1973;80: 60–62.

138. Moore TK, Cayle JE. The amniotic fluid index in normal pregnancy. *Am J Obstet Gynecol* 1990;162:1168–1173.

139. Desmedt EJ, Henry OA, Beischer NA. Polyhydramnios and associated maternal and fetal complications in singleton pregnancies. *Br J Obstet Gynaecol* 1990;97:1115–1122.

140. Dicker D, Feldberg D, Samuel N, Yeshaya A, Karp M, Goldman JA. Spontaneous abortion in patients with insulin-dependent diabetes mellitus: the effect of preconceptional diabetic control. *Am J Obstet Gynecol* 1988;158:1161–1164.

141. Miller E, Hare JW, Cloherty JP, et al. Elevated maternal hemoglobin A_{1c} in early pregnancy and major congenital anomalies in infants of diabetic mothers. *N Engl J Med* 1981;304:1331–1334.

142. Miodovnik M, Mimouni F, Siddiqi TA, Khoury J, Berk MA. Spontaneous abortions in repeat diabetic pregnancies: a relationship with glycemic control. *Obstet Gynecol* 1990;75:75–78.

143. Miodovnik M, Mimouni F, Siddiqi TA, Tsang RC. Periconceptional metabolic status and risk for spontaneous abortion in insulin-dependent diabetic pregnancies. *Am J Perinatol* 1988;4:368–373.

144. Cousins L. Congenital anomalies among infants of diabetic mothers. Etiology, prevention, diagnosis. *Am J Obstet Gynecol* 1983;147: 333–338.

145. Gabbe SG. Congenital malformations in infants of diabetic mothers. *Obstet Gynecol Surv* 1977;32:125–132.

146. Kitzmiller JL, Cloherty JP, Younger MD, et al. Diabetic pregnancy and perinatal morbidity. *Am J Obstet Gynecol* 1978;131:560–580.

147. Mills JL. Malformations in infants of diabetic mothers. *Teratology* 1982;25:385–394.

148. Mills J, Baker L, Goldman AS. Malformations in infants of diabetic mothers occur before the seventh gestational week. Implications for treatment. *Diabetes* 1979;28:292–293.

149. Leslie RDG, Pyke DA, John PN, White JM. Hemoglobin A_1 in diabetic pregnancy. *Lancet* 1978;2:958–959.

150. Freinkel N. Banting Lecture 1980. Of pregnancy and progeny. *Diabetes* 1980;29:1023–1025.

151. Reller MD, Kaplan S. Hypertrophic cardiomyopathy in infants of diabetic mothers: an update. *Am J Perinatol* 1988;5:353–358.

152. Veille J-C, Sivakoff M, Hanson R, Fanaroff AA. Interventricular septal thickness in fetuses of diabetic mothers. *Obstet Gynecol* 1992;79: 51–54.

153. Kitzmiller JL, Gavin LA, Gin GD, Jovanovic-Peterson L, Main EK, Zigrang WD. Preconception care of diabetes. Glycemic control prevents congenital anomalies. *JAMA* 1991;265:731–736.

154. Lucas MJ, Leveno KJ, Williams ML, Raskin P, Whalley PJ. Early pregnancy glycosylated hemoglobin, severity of diabetes, and fetal malformations. *Am J Obstet Gynecol* 1989;161:426–431.

155. Pregnancy outcomes in the Diabetes Control and Complications Trial. *Am J Obstet Gynecol* 1996;174:1343–1353.

156. Coustan DR. Perinatal mortality and morbidity. In Reece EA, Coustan DR, eds. *Diabetes mellitus in pregnancy,* 2nd ed. New York: Churchill Livingstone, 1995:361–367.

157. Richey SD, Sandstad JS, Leveno KJ. Observations concerning unexplained fetal demise in pregnancy complicated by diabetes mellitus. *J Matern Fetal Med* 1995;4:169–172.

158. Salvesan DR, Brudenell MJ, Nicolaides KH. Fetal polycythemia and

thrombocytopenia in pregnancies complicated by maternal diabetes mellitus. *Am J Obstet Gynecol* 1992;166:1287–1293.

159. Landon MB, Gabbe SG. Fetal surveillance and timing of delivery in pregnancy complicated by diabetes mellitus. *Obstet Gynecol Clin North Am* 1996;23:109–123.

160. Bourbon JR, Farrell PM. Fetal lung development in the diabetic pregnancy. *Pediatr Res* 1985;19:253–267.

161. Cunningham FG. Connective–tissue disorders complicating pregnancy. In Cunningham FG, MacDonald PC, Gant NF, eds. *Williams obstetrics,* 18th ed, Suppl. Norwalk, CT: Appleton & Lange, 1993: 1–15.

162. Ojomo EO, Coustan DR. Absence of evidence of pulmonary maturity at amniocentesis in term infants of diabetic mothers. *Am J Obstet Gynecol* 1990;163:954–957.

162a. Cruz AC, Buhi WC, Birk SA, Spellacy WN. Respiratory distress syndrome with mature lecithin/sphingomyelin ratios: diabetes mellitus and low Apgar scores. *Am J Obstet Gynecol* 1976;126:78–82.

163. Curet LB, Olson RW, Schneider JM, Zachman RD. Effect of diabetes mellitus on amniotic fluid lecithin/sphingomyelin ratio and respiratory distress syndrome. *Am J Obstet Gynecol* 1979;135:10–13.

164. Fadel HE, Saad SA, Davis H, Nelson GH. Fetal lung maturity in diabetic pregnancies: relation among amniotic fluid insulin, prolactin, and lecithin. *Am J Obstet Gynecol* 1988;159:457–463.

165. Kjos SL, Walther FJ, Montoro M, Paul RH, Diaz F, Stabler M. Prevalence and etiology of respiratory distress in infants of diabetic mothers: predictive value of fetal lung maturation tests. *Am J Obstet Gynecol* 1990;163:898–903.

166. Parker CR Jr, Hauth JC, Hankins GD, et al. Endocrine maturation and lung function in premature neonates of women with diabetes. *Am J Obstet Gynecol* 1989;160:657–662.

167. Jovanovic L, Peterson CM. Management of the pregnant, insulin–dependent diabetic woman. *Diabetes Care* 1980;3:63–68.

168. DeMarini S, Mimouni F, Tsang RC, Khoury J, Hertzberg V. Impact of metabolic control of diabetes during pregnancy on neonatal hypocalcemia: a randomized study. *Obstet Gynecol* 1994;83:918–922.

169. Peevy KJ, Landaw SA, Gross SJ. Hyperbilirubinemia in infants of diabetic mothers. *Pediatrics* 1980;66:417–419.

170. Widness JA, Cowett RM, Coustan DR, Carpenter MW, Oh W. Neonatal morbidities in infants of mothers with glucose intolerance in pregnancy. *Diabetes* 1985;34(Suppl 2):61–65.

171. Metzger BE and the Organizing Committee. Summary and recommendations of the Third International Workshop-Conference on Gestational Diabetes Mellitus. *Diabetes* 1991;40(Suppl 2):197–201.

172. Proceedings of the Second International Workshop-Conference on Gestational Diabetes Mellitus. *Diabetes* 1985;34(Suppl 2):1–130.

173. O'Sullivan JB. Body weight and subsequent diabetes mellitus. *JAMA* 1982;248:949–952.

174. Gimovsky ML, Montoro M, Paul RH. Pregnancy outcome in women with systemic lupus erythematosus. *Obstet Gynecol* 1984;63:686–692.

175. Le Huong D, Wechsler B, Vauthier-Brouzes D, et al. Outcome of planned pregnancies in systemic lupus erythematosus: a prospective study on 62 pregnancies. *Br J Rheumatol* 1997;36:772–777.

176. Lima F, Buchanan NM, Khamashta MA, Kerslake S, Hughes GR. Obstetric outcome in systemic lupus erythematosus. *Semin Arthritis Rheum* 1995;25:184–192.

177. Mintz G, Niz J, Gutierrez G, Garcia-Alonso A, Karchmer S. Prospective study of pregnancy in systemic lupus erythematosus. Results of a multidisciplinary approach. *J Rheumatol* 1986;13:732–739.

178. Out HJ, Derksen RH, Christiaens GC. Systemic lupus erythematosus and pregnancy. *Obstet Gynecol Surv* 1989;44:585–591.

179. Petri M, Allbritton J. Fetal outcome of lupus pregnancy: a retrospective case-control study of the Hopkins Lupus Cohort. *J Rheumatol* 1993;20:650–656.

180. Johnson MJ, Petri M, Witter FR, Repke JT. Evaluation of preterm delivery in a systemic lupus erythematosus pregnancy clinic. *Obstet Gynecol* 1995;86:396–399.

181. Houser MT, Fish AJ, Tagatz GE, Williams PP, Michael AF. Pregnancy and systemic lupus erythematosus. *Am J Obstet Gynecol* 1980;138:409–413.

182. Imbasciati E, Surian M, Bottino S, et al. Lupus nephropathy and pregnancy. A study of 26 pregnancies in patients with systemic lupus erythematosus and nephritis. *Nephron* 1984;36:46–51.

183. Tozman EC, Urowitz MB, Gladman DD. Systemic lupus erythematosus and pregnancy. *J Rheumatol* 1980;7:624–632.

184. Varner MW, Meehan RT, Syrop CH, Strottmann MP, Goplerud CP. Pregnancy in patients with systemic lupus erythematosus. *Am J Obstet Gynecol* 1983;145:1025–1040.

185. Derksen RH, Kater L. Lupus anticoagulant: revival of an old phenomenon. *Clin Exp Rheumatol* 1985;3:349–357.

186. Font J, Lopez-Soto A, Cervera R, et al. Antibodies to thromboplastin in systemic lupus erythematosus: isotype distribution and clinical significance in a series of 92 patients. *Thromb Res* 1997;86:37–48.

187. Lockshin MD, Qamar T, Levy RA, Druzin ML. Pregnancy in systemic lupus erythematosus. *Clin Exp Rheumatol* 1989;7(Suppl 3):S195–S197.

188. Ogasawara M, Aoki K, Hayashi Y. A prospective study on pregnancy risk of antiphospholipid antibodies in association with systemic lupus erythematosus. *J Reprod Immunol* 1995;28:159–164.

189. Lockshin MD. Pregnancy does not cause systemic lupus erythematosus to worsen. *Arthritis Rheum* 1989;32:665–670.

190. Lockshin MD, Reinitz E, Druzin ML, Murrman M, Estes D. Lupus pregnancy. Case-control prospective study demonstrating absence of lupus exacerbation during or after pregnancy. *Am J Med* 1984;77:893–898.

191. Meehan RT, Dorsey JK. Pregnancy among patients with systemic lupus erythematosus receiving immunosuppressive therapy. *J Rheumatol* 1987;14:252–258.

192. Lockshin MD. Pregnancy associated with systemic lupus erythematosus. *Semin Perinatol* 1990;14:130–138.

193. Stuart MJ, Gross SJ, Elrad H, Graeber JE. Effects of acetylsalicylic-acid ingestion on maternal and neonatal hemostasis. *N Engl J Med* 1982;307:909–912.

194. Turner G, Collins E. Fetal effects of regular salicylate ingestion in pregnancy. *Lancet* 1975;2:338–339.

195. Alstead EM, Ritchie JK, Lennard-Jones JE, Farthing MJ, Clark ML. Safety of azathioprine in pregnancy in inflammatory bowel disease. *Gastroenterology* 1990;99:443–446.

196. Davison JM. Dialysis, transplantation, and pregnancy. *Am J Kidney Dis* 1991;17:127–134.

197. Pilarski LM, Yacyshyn BR, Lazarovits AI. Analysis of peripheral blood lymphocyte populations and immune function from children exposed to cyclosporine or to azathioprine *in utero. Transplantation* 1994;57:133–144.

198. Khamashta MA, Buchanan NM, Hughes GR. The use of hydroxychloroquine in lupus pregnancy: the British experience. *Lupus* 1996;5(Suppl 1):S65–S66.

199. Parke A, West B. Hydroxychloroquine in pregnant patients with systemic lupus erythematosus. *J Rheumatol* 1996;23:1715–1718.

200. Parke AL, Rothfield NF. Antimalarial drugs in pregnancy—the North American experience. *Lupus* 1996;5(Suppl 1):S67–S69.

201. Phillips-Howard PA, Wood D. The safety of antimalarial drugs in pregnancy. *Drug Saf* 1996;14:131–145.

202. Shumak KH, Rock GA. Therapeutic plasma exchange. *N Engl J Med* 1984;310:762–771.

203. Wei N, Klippel JH, Huston DP, et al. Randomised trial of plasma exchange in mild systemic lupus erythematosus. *Lancet* 1983;1:17–22.

204. Hardy JD, Solomon S, Banwell GS, Beach R, Wright V, Howard FM. Congenital complete heart block in the newborn associated with maternal systemic lupus erythematosus and other connective tissue disease. *Arch Dis Child* 1979;54:7–13.

205. Lockshin MD, Gibofsky A, Peebles CL, Gigli I, Fotino M, Hurwitz S. Neonatal lupus erythematosus with heart block: family study of a patient with anti-SS-A and SS-B antibodies. *Arthritis Rheum* 1983;26:210–213.

205a. Buyon JB, Winchester R. Congenital complete heart block. A human model of passively acquired autoimmune injury. *Arthritis Rheum* 1990;33:609–614.

206. Watson RM, Lane AT, Barnett NK, Bias WB, Arnett FC, Provost TT. Neonatal lupus erythematosus. A clinical, serological and immunogenetic study with review of the literature. *Medicine* 1984;63:362–378.

207. Olah KS, Gee H. Fetal heart block associated with maternal anti-Ro (SSA) antibody—current management. A review. *Br J Obstet Gynaecol* 1991;98:751–755.

208. Reichlin M, Friday K, Harley JB. Complete congenital heart block followed by anti-Ro-SS-A in adult life. Studies of an informative family. *Am J Med* 1988;84:339–344.

209. Buyon JP, Waltuck J, Kleinman C, Copel J. *In utero* identification and therapy of congenital heart block. *Lupus* 1995;4:116–121.

210. Richards DS, Wagman AJ, Cabaniss ML. Ascites not due to congestive heart failure in a fetus with lupus-induced heart block. *Obstet Gynecol* 1990;76:957–959.

211. Watson WJ, Katz VL. Steroid therapy for hydrops associated with antibody-mediated congenital heart block. *Am J Obstet Gynecol* 1991;165:553–554.

212. Buyon JP, Swersky SH, Fox HE, Bierman FZ, Winchester RJ. Intrauterine therapy for presumptive fetal myocarditis with acquired heart block due to systemic lupus erythematosus. Experience in a mother with a predominance of SS-B (La) antibodies. *Arthritis Rheum* 1987;30:44–49.

213. Herreman G, Galezewski N. Maternal connective tissue disease and congenital heart block. *N Engl J Med* 1985;312:1329.

214. Walkinshaw SA, Welch CR, McCormack J, Walsh K. *In utero* pacing for fetal congenital heart block. *Fetal Diagn Ther* 1994;9:183–185.

215. Esscher E, Scott JS. Congenital heart block and maternal systemic lupus erythematosus. *Br Med J* 1979;1:1235–1238.

216. McCarron DP, Hellmann DB, Traill TA, Watson RM. Neonatal lupus erythematosus syndrome: late detection of isolated heart block. *J Rheumatol* 1993;103:1212–1214.

217. Reed BR, Lee LA, Harmon C, et al. Autoantibodies to SS-A/Ro in infants with congenital heart block. *J Pediatr* 1983;103:889–891.

218. McCune AB, Weston WL, Lee LA. Maternal and fetal outcome in neonatal lupus erythematosus. *Ann Intern Med* 1987;106:518–523.

219. Rider LG, Buyon JP, Rutledge J, Sherry DD. Treatment of neonatal lupus: case report and review of the literature. *J Rheumatol* 1993;20:1208–1211.

220. Davison MB, Radford DJ. Fetal and neonatal congenital complete heart block. *Med J Aust* 1989;150:192–198.

221. McCue CM, Mantakas ME, Tingelstad JB, Ruddy S. Congenital heart block in newborns of mothers with connective tissue disease. *Circulation* 1977;56:82–90.

222. Provost TT, Watson R, Gammon WR, Radowsky M, Harley JB, Reichlin M. The neonatal lupus syndrome associated with U1RNP (nRNP) antibodies. *N Engl J Med* 1987;316:1135–1138.

223. Lipsky PE. Rheumatoid arthritis. In Wilson JD, Braunwald E, Isselbacher KJ, et al, eds. *Harrison's principles of internal medicine,* 12th ed. New York: McGraw-Hill, 1991:1437–1442.

224. Arnett FC, Edworthy SM, Bloch DA, et al. The American Rheumatism Association 1987 revised criteria for the classification of rheumatoid arthritis. *Arthritis Rheum* 1988;31:315–324.

225. Ostensen M, Husby G. A prospective clinical study of the effect of pregnancy on rheumatoid arthritis and ankylosing spondylitis. *Arthritis Rheum* 1983;26:1155–1159.

226. Thurnau GR. Rheumatoid arthritis. *Clin Obstet Gynecol* 1983;26:558–578.

227. Unger A, Kay A, Griffin AJ, Panayi GS. Disease activity and pregnancy associated alpha 2-glycoprotein in rheumatoid arthritis. *Br Med J* 1983;286:750–752.

228. Paget SA, Gibofsky A. Immunopathogenesis of rheumatoid arthritis. *Am J Med* 1979;67:961–970.

229. Ostensen M, von Schoultz B, Husby G. Comparison between serum alpha 2-pregnancy-associated globulin and activity of rheumatoid arthritis and ankylosing spondylitis during pregnancy. *Scand J Rheumatol* 1983;12:315–318.

230. Buchanan WW, Needs CJ, Brooks PM. Rheumatic diseases: The arthopathies. In Gleicher N, ed. *Principles and practice of medical therapy in pregnancy,* 2nd ed. Norwalk: Appleton & Lange, 1992:428–434.

231. Maymon R, Fejgin M. Scleroderma in pregnancy. *Obstet Gynecol Surv* 1989;44:530–534.

232. Julkunen H, Kaaja R, Kurki P, Palosuo T, Friman C. Fetal outcome in women with primary Sjögren's syndrome. A retrospective case-control study. *Clin Exp Rheumatol* 1995;13:65–71.

233. Branch DW. Antiphospholipid syndrome: Laboratory concerns, fetal loss, and pregnancy management. *Semin Perinatol* 1991;15:230–237.

234. Conley CL, Hartmann RD. A hemorrhagic disorder caused by circulating anticoagulant in patients with disseminated lupus erythematosis. *J Clin Invest* 1952;31:621–622.

235. Love PE, Santoro SA. Antiphospholipid antibodies: anticardiolipin and the lupus anticoagulant in systemic lupus erythematosus (SLE)

and in non-SLE disorders. Prevalence and clinical significance. *Ann Intern Med* 1990;112:682–698.

236. Ninomiya C, Taniguchi O, Kato T, Hirano T, Hashimoto H, Hirose S. Distribution and clinical significance of lupus anticoagulant and anticardiolipin antibody in 349 patients with systemic lupus erythematosus. *Intern Med* 1992;31:194–199.

237. Harris EN. Syndrome of the black swan. *Br J Rheumatol* 1987;26:324–326.

238. Hughes GRV, Harris EN, Gharavi AE. The anticardiolipin syndrome. *J Rheumatol* 1986;13:486–489.

239. Lockshin MD. Antiphospholipid antibody. Babies, blood clots, biology. *JAMA* 1997;277:1549–1551.

240. Kniaz D, Eisenberg GM, Elrad H, Johnson CA, Valaitis J, Bregman H. Postpartum hemolytic uremic syndrome associated with antiphospholipid antibodies. A case report and review of the literature. *Am J Nephrol* 1992;12:126–133.

241. Kochenour NK, Branch DW, Rote NS, Scott JR. A new postpartum syndrome associated with antiphospholipid antibodies. *Obstet Gynecol* 1987;69:460–468.

242. Silver RM, Draper ML, Scott JR, Lyon JL, Reading J, Branch DW. Clinical consequences of antiphospholipid antibodies: an historic cohort study. *Obstet Gynecol* 1994;83;372–377.

243. Lubbe WF, Butler WS, Palmer SJ, Liggins GC. Fetal survival after prednisone suppression of maternal lupus–anticoagulant. *Lancet* 1983;1:1361–1363.

243a. Lubbe WF, Liggins GC. Lupus anticoagulant and pregnancy. *Am J Obstet Gynecol* 1985;153:322–327.

244. Cowchock FS, Reece EA, Balaban D, Branch DW, Plouffe L. Repeated fetal losses associated with antiphospholipid antibodies: a collaborative randomized trial comparing prednisone with low-dose heparin treatment. *Am J Obstet Gynecol* 1992;166:1318–1323.

245. Landy HJ, Isada NB, McGinnis J, Ratner R, Grossman JH 3d. The effect of chronic steroid therapy on glucose tolerance in pregnancy. *Am J Obstet Gynecol* 1988;159:612–615.

246. Landy HJ, Kessler C, Kelly WK, Weingold AB. Obstetric performance in patients with the lupus anticoagulant and/or anticardiolipin antibodies. *Am J Perinatol* 1992;9:146–151.

247. Kutteh WH. Antiphospholipid antibody-associated recurrent pregnancy loss: treatment with heparin and low-dose aspirin is superior to low-dose aspirin alone. *Am J Obstet Gynecol* 1996;174:1584–1589.

248. Rosove MH, Tabsh K, Wasserstrum N, Howard P, Hahn BH, Kalunian KC. Heparin therapy for pregnant women with lupus anticoagulant or anticardiolipin antibodies. *Obstet Gynecol* 1990;75:630–634.

249. Fejgin MD, Lourwood DL. Low molecular weight heparins and their use in obstetrics and gynecology. *Obstet Gynecol Surv* 1994;49:424–431.

250. Kaaja R, Julkunen H, Ämmälä P, Palosuo T, Kurki P. Intravenous immunoglobulin treatment of pregnant patients with recurrent pregnancy losses associated with antiphospholipid antibodies. *Acta Obstet Gynecol Scand* 1993;72:63–66.

251. Scott JR, Branch DW, Kochenour NK, Ward K. Intravenous immunoglobulin treatment of pregnant patients with recurrent pregnancy loss caused by antiphospholipid antibodies and Rh immunization. *Am J Obstet Gynecol* 1988;159:1055–1056.

252. Spinnato JA, Clark AL, Pierangeli SS, Harris EN. Intravenous immunoglobulin therapy for the antiphospholipid syndrome in pregnancy. *Am J Obstet Gynecol* 1995;172:690–694.

253. Sheridan-Pereira M, Porreco RP, Hays T, Burke MS. Neonatal aortic thrombosis associated with the lupus anticoagulant. *Obstet Gynecol* 1988;71:1016–1018.

254. Silver RK, MacGregor SN, Pasternak JF, Neely SE. Fetal stroke associated with elevated maternal anticardiolipin antibodies. *Obstet Gynecol* 1992;80:497–499.

255. Mestman JH, Goodwin TM, Montoro MM. Thyroid disorders of pregnancy. *Endocrinol Metab Clin North Am* 1995;24:41–71.

256. American College of Obstetricians and Gynecologists. *Thyroid disease in pregnancy. ACOG Technical Bulletin 181.* Washington, DC: ACOG, 1993.

257. Mazzaferri EL. Evaluation and management of common thyroid disorders in women. *Am J Obstet Gynecol* 1997;176:507–514.

258. Davis LE, Lucas MJ, Hankins GD, Roark ML, Cunningham FG. Thyrotoxicosis complicating pregnancy. *Am J Obstet Gynecol* 1989;160:63–70.

259. Roth RN, McAuliffe MJ. Hyperthyroidism and thyroid storm. *Emerg Med Clin North Am* 1989;7:873–883.

260. Wing DA, Millar LK, Koonings PP, Montoro MN, Mestman JH. A comparison of propylthiouracil versus methimazole in the treatment of hyperthyroidism in pregnancy. *Am J Obstet Gynecol* 1994;170: 90–95.

261. Milham S Jr. Scalp defects in infants of mothers treated for hyperthyroidism with methimazole or carbimazole during pregnancy. *Teratology* 1985;32:321.

262. Matsuura N, Konishi J, Fujieda K, et al. TSH-receptor antibodies in mothers with Graves' disease and outcome in their offspring. *Lancet* 1988;1:14–17.

263. Houck JA, Davis RE, Sharma HM. Thyroid-stimulating immunoglobulin as a cause of recurrent intrauterine fetal death. *Obstet Gynecol* 1988;71:1018–1019.

264. Page DV, Brady K, Mitchell J, Pehrson J, Wade G. The pathology of intrauterine thyrotoxicosis: two case reports. *Obstet Gynecol* 1988; 72:479–481.

265. Wenstrom KD, Weiner CP, Williamson RA, Grant SS. Prenatal diagnosis of fetal hyperthyroidism using funipuncture. *Obstet Gynecol* 1990;76:513–517.

266. Davis LE, Leveno KJ, Cunningham FG. Hypothyroidism complicating pregnancy. *Obstet Gynecol* 1988;72:108–112.

267. Mandel SJ, Larsen PR, Seely EW, Brent GQ. Increased need for thyroxine during pregnancy in women with primary hypothyroidism. *N Engl J Med* 1990;323:91–96.

268. Toft AD. Drug therapy: Thyroxine therapy. *N Engl J Med* 1994;154: 785–787.

269. American Academy of Pediatrics, American Thyroid Association. Newborn screening for congenital hypothyroidism: recommended guidelines. *Pediatrics* 1987;80:745–749.

269a. American College of Obstetricians and Gynecologists. *Hepatitis in pregnancy. ACOG Technical Bulletin 174.* Washington, DC: ACOG, 1992.

269b. American College of Obstetricians and Gynecologists. *Human immunodeficiency virus infections in pregnancy. ACOG Educational Bulletin 232.* Washington, DC: ACOG, 1997.

269c. American College of Obstetricians and Gynecologists. *Perinatal herpes simplex virus infections. ACOG Technical Bulletin 122.* Washington, DC: ACOG, 1988.

269d. American College of Obstetricians and Gynecologists. *Perinatal viral and parasitic infections. ACOG Technical Bulletin 177.* Washington, DC: ACOG, 1993.

269e. Ray JG. Lues-lues: Maternal and fetal considerations of syphilis. *Obstet Gynecol Surv* 1995;50:845–850.

269f. Ricci JM, Fojaco RM, O'Sullivan MJ. Congenital syphilis: the University of Miami/Jackson Memorial Medical Center experience, 1986–88. *Obstet Gynecol* 1989;74:687–693.

269g. Walker CK, Sweet RL. HIV and other sexually transmitted diseases in pregnancy. In: Reece EA, Hobbins JC, Mahoney MJ, Petrie RH, eds. *Medicine of the fetus and mother.* Philadelphia: JB Lippincott, 1992:1193–1219.

270. American College of Obstetricians and Gynecologists. *Prevention of early-onset group B streptococcal disease in newborns. ACOG Committee Opinion 173.* Washington, DC: ACOG, 1996.

271. Franks AL, Atrash HK, Lawson HW, Colberg KS. Obstetrical pulmonary embolism mortality, United States, 1970–85. *Am J Public Health* 1990;80:720–722.

272. Rochat RW, Koonin LM, Atrash HK, Jewett JF. Maternal mortality in the United States: report from the Maternal Mortality Collaborative. *Obstet Gynecol* 1988;72:91–97.

273. Toglia MR, Weg JG. Venous thromboembolism during pregnancy. *N Engl J Med* 1996;335:108–114.

274. Barbour LA, Pickard J. Controversies in thromboembolic disease during pregnancy: a critical review. *Obstet Gynecol* 1995;86:621–633.

274a. Ginsburg JS, Brill-Edwards P, Burrows RF, et al. Venous thrombosis during pregnancy: leg and trimester of presentation. *Thromb Haemostas* 1992;67:519–520.

275. Aaro LA, Juergens JL. Thrombophlebitis associated with pregnancy. *Am J Obstet Gynecol* 1971;109:1128–1133.

276. Bergqvist A, Bergqvist D, Hallböök T. Deep vein thrombosis during pregnancy: A prospective study. *Acta Obstet Gynecol Scand* 1983;62: 443–448.

277. Hellgren M, Nygards EB. Long-term therapy with subcutaneous heparin during pregnancy. *Gynecol Obstet Invest* 1982;13:76–89.

278. Tengborn L, Bergqvist D, Mätzsch T, Bergqvist A, Hedner U. Recurrent thromboembolism in pregnancy and puerperium. Is there a need for thromboprophylaxis? *Am J Obstet Gynecol* 1989;160:90–94.

279. den Heijer M, Koster T, Blom HJ, et al. Hyperhomocysteinemia as a risk factor for deep-vein thrombosis. *N Engl J Med* 1996;334:759–762.

280. Dizon-Townson DS, Nelson LM, Jang H, Varner MW, Ward K. The incidence of factor V Leiden mutation in an obstetric population and its relationship to deep vein thrombosis. *Am J Obstet Gynecol* 1997; 176:883–886.

281. Rouse DJ, Goldenberg RL, Wenstrom KD. Antenatal screening for factor V Leiden mutation: A critical appraisal. *Obstet Gynecol* 1997; 90:848–851.

282. Weinmann EE, Salzman EW. Deep-vein thrombosis. *N Engl J Med* 1994;331:1630–1641.

283. The PIOPED Investigators. Value of the ventilation/perfusion scan in acute pulmonary embolism: Results of the Prospective Investigation of Pulmonary Embolism Diagnosis (PIOPED). *JAMA* 1990;263: 2753–2759.

284. Ginsberg JS, Hirsh J. Use of antithrombotic agents during pregnancy. *Chest* 1995;108(Suppl 4):305S–311S.

285. Hall JG, Pauli RM, Wilson KM. Maternal and fetal sequelae of anticoagulation during pregnancy. *Am J Med* 1980;68:122–140.

286. Wong V, Cheng CH, Chan KC. Fetal and neonatal outcome of exposure to anticoagulants during pregnancy. *Am J Med Genet* 1993;45:17–21.

287. Stevenson RE, Burton OM, Ferlauto GJ, Taylor HA. Hazards of oral anticoagulants during pregnancy. *JAMA* 1980;243:1549–1551.

288. Katz AI, Lindheimer MD. Does pregnancy aggravate primary glomerular disease? *Am J Kidney Dis* 1985;6:261–265.

289. Cunningham FG, Cox SM, Harstad TW, Mason RA, Pritchard JA. Chronic renal disease and pregnancy outcome. *Am J Obstet Gynecol* 1990;163:453–459.

290. Hou SH, Grossman SD, Madias NE. Pregnancy in women with renal disease and moderate renal insufficiency. *Am J Med* 1985;78:185–194.

291. Jones DC, Hayslett JP. Outcome of pregnancy in women with moderate or severe renal insufficiency. *N Engl J Med* 1996;335:226–232.

292. Krakow D, Castro LC, Schwieger J. Effect of hemodialysis on uterine and umbilical artery Doppler flow velocity waveforms. *Am J Obstet Gynecol* 1994;170:1386–1388.

293. Elliott JP, O'Keeffe DF, Schon DA, Cherem LB. Dialysis in pregnancy: a critical review. *Obstet Gynecol Surv* 1992;46:319–324.

294. Hou SH. Pregnancy in women on haemodialysis and peritoneal dialysis. *Ballieres Clin Obstet Gynaecol* 1994;8:481–500.

295. Jakobi P, Ohel G, Szylman P, Levit A, Lewin M, Paldi E. Continuous ambulatory peritoneal dialysis as the primary approach in the management of severe renal insufficiency in pregnancy. *Obstet Gynecol* 1992;79:808–810.

296. Nageotte MP, Grundy HO. Pregnancy outcome in women requiring chronic hemodialysis. *Obstet Gynecol* 1988;72:456–459.

297. Yasin SY, Beydoun SN. Hemodialysis in pregnancy. *Obstet Gynecol Surv* 1988;43:655–668.

298. Tison A, Lozowy C, Benjamin A, Usher R, Prichard S. Successful pregnancy complicated by peritonitis in a 35-year old CAPD patient. *Perit Dial Int* 1996;16(Suppl 1):S489–S491.

299. Sturgiss SN, Davison JM. Perinatal outcome in renal allograft recipients: prognostic significance of hypertension and renal function before and during pregnancy. *Obstet Gynecol* 1991;78:573–577.

300. Davison JM. Renal transplantation and pregnancy. *Am J Kidney Dis* 1987;9:374–380.

301. Ehrich JH, Loirat C, Davison JM, et al. Repeated successful pregnancies after kidney transplantation in 102 women (Report by the EDTA Registry). *Nephrol Dial Transplant* 1996;11:1314–1317.

302. Burrows DA, O'Neil TJ, Sorrells TL. Successful twin pregnancy after renal transplant maintained on cyclosporine A immunosuppression. *Obstet Gynecol* 1988;72:459–461.

303. Gaughan WJ, Moritz MJ, Radomski JS, Burke JF Jr, Armenti VT. National Transplantation Pregnancy Registry: report on outcomes in cyclosporine-treated female kidney transplant recipients with an interval from transplant to pregnancy of greater than five years. *Am J Kidney Dis* 1996;28:266–269.

304. Olshan AF, Mattison DR, Zwanenburg TS. International Commission for Protection Against Environmental Mutagens and Carcinogens. Cyclosporine A: review of genotoxicity and potential for adverse human reproductive and developmental effects. Report of a Working Group on the genotoxicity of cyclosporine A, August 18, 1993. *Mutat Res* 1994;317:163–173.

305. American College of Obstetricians and Gynecologists. *Cardiac disease in pregnancy. ACOG Technical Bulletin 168.* Washington, DC: ACOG, 1992.

306. Criteria Committee of the New York Heart Association. *Nomenclature and criteria for diagnosis of diseases of the heart and great vessels,* 8th ed. Boston: Little Brown, 1979.

307. Szekely P, Turner R, Snaith L. Pregnancy and the changing pattern of rheumatic heart disease. *Br Heart J* 1973;35:1293–1303.

308. Patton DE, Lee W, Cotton DB, et al. Cyanotic maternal heart disease in pregnancy. *Obstet Gynecol Surv* 1990;45:594–600.

309. McAnulty JH, Morton MJ, Ueland K. The heart and pregnancy. *Curr Probl Cardiol* 1988;9:589–660.

310. Whittemore R, Hobbins JC, Engle MA. Pregnancy and its outcome in women with and without surgical treatment of congenital heart disease. *Am J Cardiol* 1982;50:641–651.

311. Sheikh AU, Harper MA. Myocardial infarction during pregnancy: management and outcome of two pregnancies. *Am J Obstet Gynecol* 1993;169:2779–2784.

312. Roth A, Elkayam U. Acute myocardial infarction associated with pregnancy. *Ann Intern Med* 1996;125:751–762.

313. Badui E, Enciso R. Acute myocardial infarction during pregnancy and puerperium: a review. *Angiology* 1996;47:739–756.

314. Hankins GDV, Wendel GD Jr, Leveno KJ, Stoneham J. Myocardial infarction during pregnancy: a review. *Obstet Gynecol* 1985;65:139–146.

315. Ascarelli MH, Grider AR, Hsu HW. Acute myocardial infarction during pregnancy managed with immediate percutaneous transluminal coronary angioplasty. *Obstet Gynecol* 1996;88:655–657.

316. Eikman FM. Acute coronary artery angioplasty during pregnancy. *Cathet Cardiovasc Diagn* 1996;38:369–372.

317. Schumacher B, Belfort MA, Card RJ. Successful treatment of acute myocardial infarction during pregnancy with tissue plasminogen activator. *Am J Obstet Gynecol* 1997;176:716–719.

318. Dufour P, Berard J, Vinatier D, et al. Pregnancy after myocardial infarction and a coronary artery bypass graft. *Arch Gynecol Obstet* 1997;259:209–213.

319. Frenkel Y, Barkai G, Reisin L, Rath S, Mashiach S, Battler A. Pregnancy after myocardial infarction: Are we playing safe? *Obstet Gynecol* 1991;77:822–825.

320. Baxi LV, Rho RB. Pregnancy after cardiac transplantation. *Am J Obstet Gynecol* 1993;169:33–34.

321. Key TC, Resnik R, Dittrich HC, Reisner LS. Successful pregnancy after cardiac transplantation. *Am J Obstet Gynecol* 1989;160:367–371.

322. Kirk EP. Organ transplantation and pregnancy: a case report and review. *Am J Obstet Gynecol* 1991;164:1629–1634.

323. Löwenstein BR, Vain NW, Perrone SV, Wright DR, Boullón FJ, Favaloro RG. Successful pregnancy and vaginal delivery after heart transplantation. *Am J Obstet Gynecol* 1988;158:589–590.

324. Scott JR, Wagoner LE, Olsen SL, Taylor DO, Renlund DG. Pregnancy in heart transplant recipients: management and outcome. *Obstet Gynecol* 1993;82:324–327.

325. Antonelli NM, Dotters DJ, Katz VL, Kuller JA. Cancer in pregnancy: A review of the literature. Part I. *Obstet Gynecol Surv* 1996;125–134.

326. Hacker NF, Berek JS, Lagasse LD, Charles EH, Savage EW, Moore JG. Carcinoma of the cervix associated with pregnancy. *Obstet Gynecol* 1982;59:735–746.

327. Berman ML, DiSaia PJ. Pelvic malignancies, gestational trophoblastic neoplasia, and nonpelvic malignancies. In Creasy RK, Resnik R, eds. *Maternal–fetal medicine,* 3rd ed. Philadelphia: WB Saunders, 1994:1112–1134.

328. Donegan WL. Breast cancer and pregnancy. *Obstet Gynecol* 1977;50:244–252.

329. Schwartz PE. Cancer in pregnancy. In Reece EA, Hobbins JC, Mahoney MJ, Petrie RH, eds. *Medicine of the fetus and mother.* Philadelphia: JB Lippincott, 1992:1257–1281.

330. Dildy GA 3d, Moise KJ Jr, Carpenter RJ Jr, Klima T. Maternal malignancy metastatic to the products of conception: a review. *Obstet Gynecol Surv* 1989;44:535–540.

331. Brill AB, Forgotson EH. Radiation and congenital malformations. *Am J Obstet Gynecol* 1964;90:1149–1168.

332. Nicholson HD. Cytotoxic drugs in pregnancy. Review of reported cases. *J Obstet Gynaecol Br Commonw* 1968;75:307–312.

333. Sweet DL, Kinzie J. Consequences of radiotherapy and antineoplastic therapy for the fetus. *J Reprod Med* 1976;17:241–246.

334. Debakan A. Abnormalities in children exposed to x-irradiation during various stages of gestation: Tentative timetable of radiation injury to the human fetus. Part I. *J Nucl Med* 1968;9:471–477.

335. Brent RC. The effect of embryonic and fetal exposure to x-ray, microwaves, and ultrasound: counseling the pregnant and non-pregnant patient about these risks. *Semin Oncol* 1989;16:347–368.

336. Orr JW Jr, Shingleton HM. Cancer in pregnancy. *Curr Prob Cancer* 1983;8:1–50.

CHAPTER 15

The Effects of Maternal Drugs on the Developing Fetus

David A. Beckman and Robert L. Brent

Every conception has a risk of abortion, premature delivery, stillbirth, or serious congenital anomaly (Tables 15–1 and 15–2). Furthermore, it is axiomatic that drugs administered or taken by a pregnant woman present the mother and fetus with both risks and benefits. The controversies in this field are primarily related to the nature and magnitude of the risks from these drugs.

Abortion and birth defects have some common etiologies, but in many instances the causes of these two adverse reproductive outcomes are divergent. Most human teratogens affect the embryo during a relatively narrow period of early embryonic development (18 to 40 days for major malformations excluding genital malformations and cleft palate, which have longer periods of sensitivity). However, there are a few teratogens and many fetotoxic agents that have deleterious effects during the second and even the third trimester.

In this chapter, we evaluate the data concerning the potential risks of selected prescribed and self-administered drugs in human pregnancy. The evaluations were made after a review of the available clinical, epidemiologic, and experimental data and an analysis based on reproducibility, consistency, and biological plausibility. Only key references or reviews are cited, which will guide the reader to additional relevant literature.

CHARACTERIZATION OF ADVERSE REPRODUCTIVE OUTCOMES

Spontaneous Abortion

The definition of spontaneous abortion is based on the stage of embryonic development when viability was not possible outside the uterus. This stage is presently considered to be 20 weeks or less of gestation and a fetal weight of less than 500 g, although these criteria are not universally accepted.

The frequency of spontaneous abortion varies with the stage of gestation (Table 15–2): more than 80% of abortions occur in the first trimester, and there is a steady decline in the risk of abortion as pregnancy progresses. Therefore, it is essential that epidemiologic studies investigating the cause of abortion compare control and "exposed" populations with the same mean stage and range of abortion. Two pregnant populations with a 2-week difference in mean stage of pregnancy will have a different background incidence of abortion. Abortion in human populations includes the following causes (Table 15–3):

Chromosomal Abnormalities

The earlier a spontaneous abortion occurs, the higher the proportion of chromosomal abnormalities in the abortus (1,2). Approximately 53% of spontaneous abortions in the first trimester are caused by chromosomal abnormalities, 36% in the second trimester, and only 5% in the third trimester. Over 95% of abortuses with chromosomal abnormalities represent autosomal trisomy, double trisomy, monosomy, triploidy, or tetraploidy (3,4). Most chromosomal abnormalities are not the cause of repetitive abortion, although in about 4% of couples with two or more spontaneous abortions, a normal-appearing parent could be a carrier for a balanced translocation or may

D. A. Beckman: Division of Developmental Biology, Department of Pediatrics, Thomas Jefferson University; and Nemours Research Programs, Alfred I. duPont Hospital for Children, Wilmington, Delaware

R. L. Brent: Department of Pediatrics, Jefferson Medical College, Philadelphia, Pennsylvania; and Division of Research, duPont Hospital for Children, Wilmington, Delaware

TABLE 15–1. *Frequency of reproductive risks in the human[a]*

Reproductive risk	Frequency
Immunologically and clinically diagnosed spontaneous abortions per 10^6 conceptions	350,000
Clinically recognized spontaneous abortions per 10^6 pregnancies	150,000
Genetic diseases per 10^6 births	110,000
Multifactorial or polygenic (genetic–environmental interactions)	90,000
Dominantly inherited disease	10,000
Autosomal and sex-linked genetic disease	1,200
Cytogenetic (chromosomal abnormalities)	5,000
New mutations	3,000
Major congenital malformations per 10^6 births	30,000
Prematurity per 10^6 births	40,000
Fetal growth retardation per 10^6 births	30,000
Stillbirths per 10^6 pregnancies (>20 wk)	20,900

[a]Modified from ref. 38.

be a mosaic with abnormal karyotypes in the germ cell line. Environmental exposures during pregnancy cannot account for any of these abortions because most aneuploidies result from meiotic nondisjunction during gametogenesis before conception.

TABLE 15–2. *Estimated outcome of 100 pregnancies versus time from conception*

Time from conception	Percent survival to term[a]	Last time for induction of selected malformation[b]
Preimplantation		
0–6 days	25	
Postimplantation		
7–13 days	55	
14–20 days	73	
3–5 wk	79.5	22–23 days: cyclopia, sirenomelia, microtia 26 days: anencephaly 28 days: meningomyelocele 34 days: transposition of great vessels
6–9 wk	90	36 days: cleft lip, 6 wk: diaphragmatic hernia, rectal atresia, ventricular septal defect, syndactyly 9 wk: cleft palate
10–13 wk	92	10 wk: omphalocele
14–17 wk	96.26	12 wk: hypospadias
18–21 wk	97.56	
22–25 wk	98.39	
26–29 wk	98.69	
30–33 wk	98.98	
34–37 wk	99.26	
38 wk +	99.32	38 wk +: CNS cell depletion

[a]Data from ref. 283.
[b]Data from ref. 237.

TABLE 15–3. *Etiology of spontaneous abortion in the human*

Chromosomal abnormalities
  Chromosomal abnormalities from either the maternal or paternal gonadocytes account for 50% to 70% of abortions
Abortions with normal chromosomes (euploidy)
  Genetic abnormalities: dominant mutations (lethal), polygenic genetic abnormalities, recessive disease from either the maternal, paternal, or both parents' gonadocytes
  Severe maternal disease states: diabetes, hypothyroidism, hepatitis, collagen diseases, untreated hyperthyroidism, severe malnutrition
  Corpus luteum or placental progesterone deficiency (luteal phase deficiency)
  Maternal infection that results in fetal infection: *Treponema pallidum, Plasmodium falciparum, Toxoplasma gondii,* herpes simplex virus, parvovirus B19, or cytomegalovirus
  Antiphospholipid antibodies: lupus anticoagulant, anticardiolipin antibodies
  Maternal–fetal histocompatibility
  Overmature gametes
  Mechanical or physical problems: uterine abnormalities, multiple pregnancies, very rarely trauma
  Cervical incompetence
  Abnormal placentation: hypoplastic trophoblast, circumvallate implantation
  Embryos and fetuses with severe malformation or growth retardation

Abortions with Normal Chromosomes (Euploidy)

Hertig (1) and many other investigators reported the occurrence of malformed or blighted embryos as a cause of abortion. These embryonic losses may occur later in the first trimester and have been shown to have normal karyotypes (3). The etiologies of these abortions are manifold and include the following.

Genetic Abnormalities

Dominant mutations (lethals), polygenic genetic abnormalities, and recessive disease may rarely account for repetitive abortion, but in most instances they will occur sporadically. A review of gene knockouts and mutations in mice suggests that embryonic death resulted from disturbances in basic cellular functions, vascular circulation, hematopoiesis, or the nutritional supply from the mother rather than from alterations affecting embryonic organ systems (5).

Maternal Diabetes

Type I (insulin-dependent) diabetes mellitus with poor metabolic control increases the risk of abortion and stillbirths, but there is no increased risk with good metabolic control.

Maternal Hyper- and Hypothyroidism

Abnormal thyroid function is rare in patients with recurrent abortion.

Corpus Luteum or Placental Progesterone Deficiency (Luteal Phase Deficiency)

It is controversial whether low hormone levels after implantation result from impending abortion or are the cause of the abortion.

Maternal Infection

Infections of the genital tract could be responsible for abortion, but it is not easy to document causality. The data suggesting that infection with *Chlamydia trachomatis, Borrelia burgdorferi, Mycoplasma hominis, Listeria monocytogenes,* or *Ureaplasma urealyticum* results in abortion are not conclusive. In contrast, maternal disease resulting in fetal infection with *Treponema pallidum, Plasmodium falciparum, Toxoplasma gondii,* herpes simplex virus, parvovirus B19, or cytomegalovirus has the potential to cause stillbirth or spontaneous abortion.

Severe, Debilitating Maternal Diseases

Hepatitis, collagen diseases, untreated hyperthyroidism, Wilson's disease, or severe malnutrition can lead to abortion.

Antiphospholipid Antibodies

Lupus anticoagulant and anticardiolipin antibodies predispose women to recurrent abortion in both first and second trimesters through vascular disruption or thrombosis in the placenta.

Maternal–Fetal Histocompatibility

It is suggested that embryonic loss increases if the mother and fetus are more histocompatible at the HLA locus, which may lead to failure to develop maternal blocking antibodies against paternal antigens.

Overmature Gametes

Either the ovum or sperm could age because insemination occurred a few days before ovulation or ovulation occurred before insemination. The magnitude of this risk factor as a cause of spontaneous abortion is not known, and some investigators are skeptical that this phenomenon is clinically significant.

Mechanical or Physical Problems Related to Uterine Abnormalities, Multiple Pregnancies, or Trauma

A hostile intrauterine environment can result from submucosal or intramural myomas, adhesions (Asherman's syndrome), multiple embryos, or abnormalities of the uterus (bifid uterus, infantile uterus). Uterine trauma from a direct blow or penetrating injury may rarely be responsible for an abortion, and if this type of injury occurs, it would be more likely to result in a stillbirth at midgestation or later.

Cervical Incompetence

Cervical incompetence is more likely to result in second-trimester than first-trimester abortions.

Abnormal Placentation

Hypoplastic trophoblast and circumvallate implantation increase the risk of fetal loss.

Some Environmental Teratogens and Reproductive Toxins

Severe malformations or growth retardation increase the risk of fetal loss.

Congenital Malformations

The etiology of congenital malformations can be divided into three categories: unknown, genetic, and environmental (Table 15–4). The etiology of 65% to 75%

TABLE 15–4. *Etiology of human congenital malformations observed during the first year of life[a]*

Suspected cause	Percent of total
Unknown	65–75
Polygenic	
Multifactorial (gene–environment interactions)	
Spontaneous errors of development	
Synergistic interactions of teratogens	
Genetic	15–25
Autosomal and sex-linked inherited genetic disease	
Cytogenetic (chromosomal abnormalities)	
New mutations	
Environmental	10
Maternal conditions: alcoholism, diabetes, endocrinopathies, phenylketonuria, smoking and nicotine, starvation, and nutritional deficits	4
Infectious agents: rubella, toxoplasmosis, syphilis, herpes simplex, cytomegalovirus, varicella–zoster, Venezuelan equine encephalitis, or parvovirus B19	3
Mechanical problems (deformations): Amniotic band constrictions, umbilical cord constraint, or disparity in uterine size and uterine contents	1–2
Chemicals, drugs, high-dose ionizing radiation, hyperthermia	<1

[a]Modified from refs. 38, 43, and 206.

of human malformations is unknown. A significant proportion of congenital malformations of unknown etiology are likely to have an important genetic component. Malformations with an increased recurrent risk, such as cleft lip and palate, anencephaly, spina bifida, certain types of congenital heart disease, pyloric stenosis, hypospadias, inguinal hernia, talipes equinovarus, and congenital dislocation of the hip, fit in the category of multifactorial disease as well as in the category of polygenic inherited disease (6). The multifactorial/threshold hypothesis postulates the modulation of a continuum of genetic characteristics by intrinsic and extrinsic (environmental) factors (6). Although the modulating factors are not known, they probably include placental blood flow, placental transport, site of implantation, maternal disease states, maternal malnutrition, infections, drugs, chemicals, and spontaneous errors of development.

Spontaneous errors of development may account for some of the malformations that occur without apparent abnormalities of the genome or environmental influence. We postulate that there is some probability for error during embryonic development just because embryonic development is such a complicated process. It is estimated that 75% of all conceptions are lost before term, 50% within the first 3 weeks of development (1,2) (Table 15–2). The World Health Organization (7) estimated that 15% of all clinically recognizable pregnancies end in a spontaneous abortion, 50% to 60% of which are caused by chromosomal abnormalities (4,8) (Table 15–1). Finally, 3% to 6% of offspring are malformed, which represents the background risk for human maldevelopment. This means that, as a conservative estimate, 1,176 clinically recognized pregnancies will result in approximately 176 miscarriages, and 30 to 60 of the infants will have congenital anomalies in the remaining 1,000 live births. The true incidence of pregnancy loss is much higher because undocumented pregnancies are not included in this risk estimate.

Based on his review of the literature, Wilson (9) provided a format of theoretical teratogenic mechanisms: mutation; chromosomal aberrations; mitotic interference; altered nucleic acid synthesis and function; lack of precursors, substrates, or coenzymes for biosynthesis; altered energy sources; enzyme inhibition; osmolar imbalance or alterations in fluid pressures, viscosities, and osmotic pressures; and altered membrane characteristics. We suggest a revised list of mechanisms for teratogenesis caused by environmental teratogens and reproductive toxins (Table 15–5).

Even though an agent can produce one or more of these pathologic processes, exposure to such an agent does not guarantee that maldevelopment will occur. Furthermore, it is likely that a drug, chemical, or other agent can have more than one effect on the pregnant woman and the developing conceptus, and therefore, the nature of the drug or its biochemical or pharmacologic effects will not in themselves predict a teratogenic effect in the

TABLE 15–5. *Mechanisms of teratogenesis*

1. Cell death or mitotic delay beyond the recuperative capacity of the embryo or fetus.
2. Inhibition of cell migration, differentiation, and cell communication.
3. Interference with histogenesis by processes such as cell deletion, necrosis, calcification, or scarring.
4. Biological and pharmacologic receptor-mediated developmental effects.
5. Metabolic inhibition or nutritional deficiencies.
6. Physical constraint, vascular disruption, inflammatory lesions, or amniotic band syndrome.

human. In fact, the discovery of human teratogens has come primarily from human observations and epidemiologic studies. Animal studies and *in vitro* studies can be very helpful in determining the mechanism of teratogenesis and the pharmacokinetics related to teratogenesis (10). However, even if one understands the pathologic effects of an agent, one cannot predict the teratogenic risk of an exposure in the human without taking into consideration the developmental stage, the magnitude of the exposure, and the repairability of the embryo.

Various maternal viral, bacterial, and parasitic infections are known to cause maldevelopment in humans, including cytomegalovirus, fetal herpes virus infections (type 1 or 2), parvovirus B19 (erythema infectiosum), rubella virus, congenital syphilis *(Treponema pallidum)*. *Toxoplasmosis gondii* infection, varicella–zoster virus, and Venezuelan equine encephalitis (11). The incidence of serum antibody to human immunodeficiency virus (HIV) in pregnant women is increasing from the 1991 estimate of 1.5 per 1,000 women delivering in the United States (12); the incidence is as high as 31% in pregnant women in some African cities (13). Several studies support the conclusion that asymptomatic HIV pregnancies are not associated with an increased risk of congenital malformations, low birth weight, or abortion (15–17). It is likely that sexually transmitted diseases, opportunistic maternal infections, and symptomatic HIV pregnancies may increase the risk of low birth weight and morbidity in noninfected offspring.

The lethal or developmental effects of infectious agents are the result of mitotic inhibition, direct cytotoxicity, or necrosis. Repair processes may result in metaplasia, scarring, or calcification, which causes further damage by interfering with histogenesis. Infectious agents appear to be exceptions to some of the principles of teratogenesis because the relevence of dose and time of exposure cannot be demonstrated as readily for replicating teratogenic agents. Transplacental transmission of an infectious agent does not necessarily result in congenital malformations, growth retardation, or lethality.

Vascular disruption is a rare event associated with intrauterine death and a wide range of structural anomalies, including cerebral infarctions, certain types of visceral and urinary tract malformations, congenital limb amputations of the nonsymmetric type; and orofacial malformations such as mandibular hypoplasia, cleft palate, and Moebius syndrome, which vary too widely to constitute a recognized syndrome. Some anomalies associated with twin pregnancies can be explained by vascular disruption resulting from placental anastomoses in the shared placenta of monozygotic twins, anastomoses in a small percentage of dichorionic placentas in the case of dizygotic twins, or death of one twin resulting in emboli, intravascular coagulation, and altered fetal hemodynamics in the co-twin (18,19). Vascular disruption may also result from physical trauma such as chorionic villous sampling and exposure to some developmental toxicants such as cocaine and misoprostol. Although uterine bleeding during the first trimester may result in fetal anomalies, adverse effects associated with vascular disruption can also occur later in gestation. This topic is discussed in greater detail below with respect to specific drugs.

Adverse Effects Produced Later in Pregnancy

The fetal period is characterized by histogenesis involving cell growth, differentiation, and migration. Drugs that produce permanent cell depletion, vascular disruption, necrosis, specific tissue or organ pathology, physiologic decompensation, or severe growth retardation have the potential to cause deleterious effects throughout gestation. Sensitivity of the fetus for induction of mental retardation and microcephaly is greatest at the end of the first and the beginning of the second trimester. Other permanent neurologic effects can be induced in the second and third trimesters. Effects such as cell depletion or functional abnormalities, not readily apparent at birth, may give rise to changes in behavior or fertility that become apparent only later in life.

Two examples of drugs that present little risk to the developing embryo during organogenesis but can affect a fetus later in pregnancy are angiotensin-converting enzyme inhibitors and aspirin (discussed in more detail below).

FACTORS THAT AFFECT SUSCEPTIBILITY TO THE DELETERIOUS EFFECTS OF DRUGS

A basic tenet of environmentally produced embryo- and fetotoxicity is that teratogenic or abortagenic milieus have certain pathologic characteristics in common and follow certain basic principles. These principles determine the quantitative and qualitative aspects of developmental toxicity (Table 15–6).

Stage of Development

The induction of developmental toxicity by environmental agents usually results in a spectrum of morphologic anomalies or intrauterine death, which varies in inci-

TABLE 15–6. *Factors that influence susceptibility to developmental toxicants*

Stage of development: The developmental period at which an exposure occurs will determine which structures are most susceptible to the adverse effects of chemicals and drugs and to what extent the embryo can repair the damage.

Magnitude of the exposure: Both the severity and incidence of toxic effects increase with dose.

Threshold phenomena: The threshold dose is the dose below which the incidence of death, malformation, growth retardation, or functional deficit is not statistically greater than that of nonexposed subjects.

Pharmacokinetics and metabolism: The physiological changes in the pregnant woman and during fetal development and the bioconversion of compounds can significantly influence the developmental toxicity of drugs and chemicals by affecting absorption, body distribution, active metabolites, and excretion.

Maternal diseases: A maternal disease may increase the risk of fetal anomalies or abortion with or without exposure to a chemical or drug.

Placental transport: Most drugs and chemicals cross the placenta. The rate and extent to which a drug or chemical crosses the placenta are influenced by molecular weight, lipid solubility, polarity or degree of ionization, plasma protein binding, receptor mediation, placental blood flow, pH gradient between the maternal and fetal serum and tissues, and placental metabolism of the chemical or drug.

Genotype: The maternal and fetal genotypes may result in differences in cell sensitivity, placental transport, absorption, metabolism, receptor binding and distribution of an agent and account for some variations in toxic effects among individual subjects and species.

dence depending on the stage of exposure and the dose. The developmental period at which an exposure occurs will determine which structures are most susceptible to the deleterious effects of the drug or chemical and the extent to which the embryo can repair the damage. The period of sensitivity may be narrow or broad, depending on the environmental agent and the malformation in question. Limb defects produced by thalidomide have a narrow period of susceptibility (Table 15–7), whereas microcephaly produced by radiation has a broad period of susceptibility. Our knowledge of the susceptible stage of the embryo to various environmental influences is continually expanding and is vital to evaluating the significance of individual exposures or epidemiologic studies.

During the first period of embryonic development, from fertilization through the early postimplantation stage, the embryo is most sensitive to the embryolethal effects of drugs and chemicals. Surviving embryos have malformation rates similar to the controls not because malformations cannot be produced at this stage but because significant cell loss or chromosome abnormalities at theses stages have a high likelihood of killing the embryo. Because of the omnipotentiality of early embryo-

TABLE 15–7. *Developmental stage sensitivity to thalidomide-induced limb reduction defects in the human*[a]

Days from conception for induction of defects	Limb reduction defects
21–26	Thumb aplasia
22–23	Microtia
23–34	Hip dislocation
24–29	Amelia, upper limbs
24–33	Phocomelia, upper limbs
25–31	Preaxial aplasia, upper limbs
27–31	Amelia, lower limbs
28–33	Preaxial aplasia, lower limbs; phocomelia, lower limbs; femoral hypoplasia; girdle hypoplasia
30–36	Triphalangeal thumb

[a]Modified from ref. 228.

onic cells, surviving embryos have a much greater ability to have normal developmental potential. Wilson and Brent (20) demonstrated that the all-or-none phenomenon, or marked resistance to teratogens, disappears over a period of a few hours in the rat during early organogenesis utilizing ionizing X-irradiation as the experimental teratogen. The term *all-or-none phenomenon* has been misinterpreted by some investigators to indicate that malformations cannot be produced at this stage. On the contrary, it is likely that certain drugs, chemicals, or other insults during this stage of development can result in malformed offspring, but the nature of embryonic development at this stage will still reflect the basic characteristic of the all-or-none phenomenon, which is a propensity for embryo lethality rather than for survival of malformed embryos.

The period of organogenesis (from day 18 through about day 40 of postconception in the human) is the period of greatest sensitivity to teratogenic insults and the period when most gross anatomic malformations can be induced. Most environmentally produced major malformations occur before the 36th day of gestation in the human. The exceptions are malformations of the genitourinary system, the palate, or the brain or deformations as a result of problems of constraint, disruption, or destruction. Severe growth retardation in the whole embryo or fetus may also result in permanent deleterious effects in many organs or tissues.

Adverse effects on growth, development, and survival can be produced by drugs during the fetal period as well, as discussed above. The approximate last gestational days on which certain malformations may be induced in the human are presented in Table 15–2.

Magnitude of the Exposure

The dose–response relationship is extremely important when effects are compared among different species because doses per kilogram are, at most, rough approximations. Dose equivalence among species can be accomplished only by performing pharmacokinetic studies, metabolic studies, and dose–response investigations in the human and the species being studied. Furthermore, the response should be interpreted in a biologically sound manner. One example is that a substance given in large enough amounts to cause maternal toxicity is likely also to have deleterious effects on the embryo such as death, growth retardation, or retarded development. Another example is that because the steroid receptors that are necessary for naturally occurring and synthetic progestin action are absent from nonreproductive tissues early in development, the evidence is against the involvement of progesterone or its synthetic analogs in nongenital teratogenesis (21,22).

An especially anxiety-provoking concept is that the interaction of two or more drugs or chemicals may potentiate their developmental effects. Although this is an extremely difficult hypothesis to test in the human, it is an especially important consideration because multichemical or multitherapeutic exposures are common. Fraser (23) warns that the actual existence of a threshold phenomenon when nonteratogenic doses of two teratogens are combined could easily be misinterpreted as potentiation or synergism. Potentiation or synergism should be invoked only when exposure to two or more drugs is just below their thresholds for toxicity.

Several considerations affect the interpretation of dose–response relationships:

Active metabolites. Metabolites may be the proximate teratogen rather than the administered chemical. For example, the metabolites phosphoramide mustard and acrolein may produce the maldevelopment that follows exposure to cyclophosphamide (24).

Duration of exposure. A chronic exposure to a prescribed drug can contribute to an increased teratogenic risk, as occurs with anticonvulsant therapy; in contrast, an acute exposure to the same drug may present little or no teratogenic risk.

Fat solubility. Fat-soluble substances such as polychlorinated biphenyls (25) can produce fetal maldevelopment for an extended period after the last ingestion or exposure in a woman because they have an unusually long half-life.

Threshold Phenomena

The threshold dose is the dosage at which the incidence of death, malformation, growth retardation, or functional deficit is statistically greater than that of controls. The threshold level of exposure is usually from less than one to three orders of magnitude below the teratogenic or embryopathic dose for drugs and chemicals that kill or malform half the embryos. A teratogenic agent therefore has a no-effect dose, as compared to mutagens or carcinogens, which have a stochastic dose–response curve. The characteristics of threshold phenomena are compared to stochastic phenomena in Table 15–8. Every exogenous teratogenic agent that has been appropriately tested has exhibited threshold phenomena during organogenesis (9).

Pharmacokinetics and Metabolism

The physiologic alterations in pregnancy and the bioconversion of compounds can significantly influence the teratogenic effects of drugs and chemicals by affecting absorption, body distribution, active form(s), and excretion of the compound. Physiologic alterations in the mother during pregnancy that affect the pharmacokinetics of drugs include the following (26–28): decreased gastrointestinal motility and increased intestinal transit time, which may delay absorption of drugs from the small intestine as a result of increased stomach retention but enhance absorption of slowly absorbed drugs; decreased plasma albumin concentration, which alters the kinetics of a compound normally bound to albumin; increased plasma and extracellular fluid volumes that affect concentration-dependent transfer of compounds; renal elimination, which is generally increased but is influenced by body position during late pregnancy; inhibition of metabolic inactivation in the liver late in pregnancy; and variations in uterine blood flow, although little is known about how this affects transfer across the placenta.

The fetus also undergoes physiologic alterations that affect the pharmacokinetics of drugs (28): the amount and distribution of fat vary with development and affect the distribution of lipid-soluble drugs; the fetal circulation contains a higher concentration of unbound drug largely because the plasma fetal proteins are lower in concentration than those in the adult and may lower drug affinity; the functional development of pharmacologic receptors is likely to proceed at different rates in different tissues; and drugs excreted by the fetal kidneys may be recycled by swallowing of amniotic fluid.

The role the placenta plays in drug pharmacokinetics (25,29) involves transport (discussed in detail below); the presence of receptor sites for a number of endogenous and xenobiotic compounds (β-adrenergic, glucocorticoid, epidermal growth factor, IgG-Fc, insulin, low-density lipoproteins, opiates, somatomedin, testosterone, transcobalamin II, transferrin, folate, retinoid) (25); and the bioconversion of xenobiotics. Bioconversion has been shown to be important in the teratogenic activity of several xenobiotics. There is strong evidence that reactive metabolites of cyclophosphamide, 2-acetylaminofluorene, and nitroheterocycles (niridazole) are the proximate teratogens (30). There is also evidence in experimental animals that suggests that other chemicals undergo conversion to intermediates that have deleterious effects on embryonic development; these include phenytoin, procarbazine, rifampicin, diethylstilbestrol, some benzhydrylpiperazine antihistamines, adriamycin, testosterone, benzo(a)pyrene, methoxyethanol, caffeine, and paraquat (29,30).

The major site of bioconversion of chemicals *in vivo* is likely to be the maternal liver. Placental P_{450}-dependent monooxygenation of xenobiotics will occur at low rates unless induced by such compounds as those found in tobacco smoke (29). However, the fetus also develops functional P_{450} oxidative isozymes capable of converting proteratogens to active metabolites.

Maternal Disease

Maternal disease states such as diabetes mellitus, epilepsy, phenylketonuria, and endocrinopathies are associated with adverse effects on the fetus. In some cases, it may be difficult to determine whether it is the maternal disease itself or its treatment that plays a role in the etiology of malformations. For example, the genetic and environmental milieu that causes epilepsy may also contribute to the maldevelopment associated with exposure to diphenylhydantoin (31).

The role of maternal malnutrition is an important area for investigation because it may be a contributing factor to the teratogenic milieu. A series of investigations pro-

TABLE 15–8. *Stochastic and threshold dose–response relationships of diseases produced by environmental agents[a]*

Relationship	Pathology	Site	Diseases	Risk	Definition
Stochastic phenomena	Damage to a single cell may result in disease	DNA	Cancer, mutation	Some risk exists at all dosages; at low exposures, the risk is below the spontaneous risk	Incidence of disease increases, but severity and nature of the disease remain the same
Threshold phenomena	Multicellular injury	High variation in etiology affecting many cell and organ processes	Malformation, growth retardation, death, chemical toxicity, etc.	No increased risk below the threshold dose	Both severity and incidence of the disease increase with dose

[a]Modified from ref. 43.

vided evidence suggesting that folic acid supplementation could reduce the incidence of recurrence of neural tube defects in the human (32–35). It was later shown convincingly that periconceptional supplementation with folic acid reduces the risk of recurrence of neural tube defects in subsequent siblings of children with neural tube defects (36). Furthermore, low-dose folic acid supplementation, 0.8 mg/day, was reported to decrease the incidence of neural tube defects in a population not at increased risk for these defects (37). Although folate supplementation reduces the incidence of neural tube defects, folate supplementation will not prevent all neural tube defects. It is not known whether folic acid supplementation corrects an undefined metabolic defect or a nutritional deficiency.

Placental Transport

The exchange between the mammalian embryo and the maternal organism is controlled by the placenta, which includes the chorioplacenta, the yolk sac placenta, and the paraplacental chorion. The placenta varies in structure and function among species and for each stage of gestation. As an example, the rodent yolk sac placenta continues to function as an organ of transport for a much greater part of gestation than in the human. Thus, differences in placental function and structure may affect our ability to apply teratogenic data developed in one species directly to other species, including the human (38). As pharmacokinetic techniques and the actual measurement of metabolic products in the embryo become more sophisticated, the appropriateness of utilizing animal data to predict human effects may improve.

Historically a placental barrier was thought to exist that prevented harmful substances from reaching the embryo. It is now clear that there is no "placental barrier" per se. The fact is that most drugs and chemicals cross the placenta. It will be a rare substance that will cross the placental barrier in one species and be unable to reach the fetus in another (39). No such chemical exists except for selected proteins whose actions are species-specific.

Even before there were chemical techniques to demonstrate the presence of drugs or chemicals in the embryo, there was clear evidence that they had reached the fetus because of clinical manifestations of the drugs: anticoagulants such as warfarin can affect the clotting of fetal blood; many drugs can affect the fetal cardiac rate; changes in the fetal EEG can be demonstrated in response to many drugs that affect the central nervous system; and newborns may exhibit withdrawal symptoms from drugs taken by their mothers, either medications or substances of abuse such as alcohol or opiates.

These observations demonstrate clinically significant placental transport of drugs only in the latter portion of gestation and may not be a means of evaluating embryonic exposure during early organogenesis.

Those factors that determine the ability of a drug or chemical to cross the placenta and reach the embryo include molecular weight, lipid affinity or solubility, polarity or degree of ionization, protein binding, and receptor mediation. Compounds with low molecular weight, high lipid affinity, nonpolarity, and without protein-binding properties will cross the placenta with ease and rapidity. As an example, ethyl alcohol is a chemical that reaches the embryo rapidly and in concentrations equal to or greater than the level in the mother.

High-molecular-weight compounds such as heparin (20,000 daltons) do not readily cross the placenta, and therefore, heparin is used to replace warfarin-like compounds during pregnancy for the treatment of hypercoagulation conditions. Rose Bengal does not cross the placenta. In general, compounds with molecular weights of 1,000 or greater do not readily cross the placenta, whereas 600-dalton compounds usually do; most drugs are 250 to 400 daltons and cross the placenta (40).

In addition to the particular properties of the drug or chemical, three other conditions affect the quantitative aspect of placental transport: placental blood flow, the pH gradient between the maternal and fetal serum and tissues, and placental metabolism of the chemical or drug. The biotransformation properties of the placenta and/or maternal organism are important because a number of chemicals or drugs are not teratogenic in their original form.

The most important concept with regard to placental transport of teratogens must be reemphasized. An agent is teratogenic because it affects the embryo directly or indirectly by its ability to produce a toxic effect in the embryo or extraembryonic membranes at exposures that are attained in the human being, not because it crosses the placenta per se.

Genotype

The genetic constitution of an organism is an important factor in the susceptibility of a species to a drug or chemical. More than 30 disorders of increased sensitivity to drug toxicity or effects as a result of an inherited trait have been reported in the human (41). The effect of a drug or chemical depends on both the maternal and fetal genotypes and may result in differences in cell sensitivity, placental transport, absorption, metabolism (activation, inactivation, active metabolites), receptor binding, and distribution of an agent. This accounts for some variations in teratogenic effects among species and in individual subjects.

ESTIMATING THE DEVELOPMENTAL RISKS OF DRUGS DURING HUMAN PREGNANCY

Evaluation of Data Available for the Human

Although chemicals and drugs can be evaluated for fetotoxic potential by utilizing *in vivo* animal studies and in vitro systems, it should be recognized that these testing procedures are only one component in the process of evaluating the potential teratogenic risk of drugs and chemicals in the human. The evaluation of the teratogenicity of drugs and chemicals should include, when possible, data obtained from human epidemiologic studies, secular trend data in humans, animal developmental toxicity studies, the dose–response relationship for developmental toxicity, the relationship to the human pharmacokinetic equivalent dose in the animal studies, and considerations of biological plausibility (Table 15–9) (42,43). This method is of greatest value when utilized for the evaluation of chemicals and drugs that have been in use for some time or for evaluating new drugs that have mechanism of action, structure, pharmacology, and purpose similar to those of other, extensively studied agents. The ability to establish a causal relationship between an environmental agent and abortigenic effect is more difficult for the following reasons:

1. Abortion is a very frequent reproductive event, and therefore, the incidence can vary considerably among different populations of women. Differences in the abortion incidence between two populations in a single study may result by chance alone.
2. There are multiple causes of abortion, and most epidemiologic studies dealing with abortion make no attempt to determine the etiology of the abortions. Because most abortions are related to preconceptual or periconceptual events, it is extremely difficult to match patients in case-control studies. It would be necessary to have large increases in a particular etiologic category of environmentally induced abortion in order to demonstrate a statistically significant increase in the incidence of spontaneous abortion in an "exposed" population of pregnant women.
3. Confounding factors appear to be more significant in abortion studies than in birth defect studies (cocaine, smoking, alcohol, syphilis, narcotics, caffeine). This

further decreases the possibility that the agent being studied has a direct abortigenic effect.

4. The incidence of therapeutic abortions is difficult to estimate in most epidemiologic studies (44,45).

One of the advantages of studying multiple reproductive endpoints is that there is frequently, but not always, concordance of effects involving more than one parameter (growth, malformations, abortion, stillbirth, prematurity, etc.). Isolated abortion studies that do not study the totality of reproductive effects are at a serious disadvantage because spurious or nonetiologic results may be misinterpreted as being causally related to a drug or environmental toxicant.

Some investigators and regulatory agencies divide drugs and chemicals into developmentally toxic and nontoxic compounds. In reality, potential developmental toxicity can be evaluated only if one considers, as a minimum, the agent, the dose, the species, and the stage of gestation. Working definitions for developmental toxicity in the human are suggested in Table 15–10.

Potential human teratogens and abortifacients comprise a large group of drugs because they include all drugs and chemicals that can produce embryotoxic and fetotoxic effects in many species at some exposure. Because these exposures are not utilized or attained in the human, they represent no or minimal risks to the human embryo.

Misconceptions in Evaluating Developmental Toxicity in the Human

Misconceptions have led to confusion regarding the potential effects of even proven teratogens. Examples of erroneous concepts include: if an agent can produce one type of malformation, it can produce any malformation; an agent presents a risk at any dose, once it can be proven to be teratogenic; and an agent that is teratogenic is likely to be abortigenic.

TABLE 15–9. *Evidence for potential developmental toxicity in the human*[a]

Epidemiologic studies: Epidemiologic studies consistently demonstrate an increased incidence of pregnancy loss or of a particular spectrum of fetal effects in exposed human populations.
Secular trend data: Secular trends demonstrate a relationship between the incidence of pregnancy loss or a particular fetal effect and the changing exposures in human populations. The percentage of the population exposed must be large for this analysis.
Animal developmental toxicity studies: An animal model mimics the human developmental effect at clinically comparable exposures. Because mimicry may occur in only one animal species, if it occurs at all, it would not necessarily be observed during an initial developmental toxicology study. Developmental toxicity studies are therefore indicative of a potential hazard in general rather than the potential for a specific adverse effect on the fetus.
Dose–response relationship: Developmental toxicity in the human increases with dose, and the developmental toxicity in animals occurs at a dose that is pharmacokinetically equivalent to the human dose.
Biological plausibility: The mechanisms of developmental toxicity are understood or the results are biologically plausible.

[a]Modified from refs. 42 and 43.

TABLE 15–10. *Definitions of potential for developmental toxicity in the human[a]*

Developmental toxicant: An agent or milieu that has been demonstrated to produce permanent alterations or death in the embryo or fetus following intrauterine exposures that usually occur or are attainable in the human.

Potential for developmental toxicity: An agent or milieu that has not been demonstrated to produce permanent alterations or death in the embryo or fetus following intrauterine exposures that usually occur or are attainable in the human but that can affect the embryo or fetus if the exposure is raised substantially above the usual exposure. Most chemicals and drugs have the potential for interrupting a pregnancy or inducing developmental defects if the exposure is increased sufficiently.

Little or no potential for developmental toxicity: An agent or milieu that has been demonstrated to produce no embryo or fetotoxicity at any attainable dose in the human. In contrast, an environmental agent may be so toxic that it has no developmental toxicity in the human because it kills the mother before or at the same dose that it begins to have adverse effects on the embryo.

[a]Modified from ref. 42.

These concepts are incorrect. The data clearly indicate that proven teratogens do not have the ability to produce every birth defect. Many teratogens can be identified on the basis of the malformations that are produced. Thus, the concept of the syndrome is probably more appropriate in clinical teratology than any other area of clinical medicine. Some symptoms or signs appear in many teratogenic syndromes, such as growth retardation or mental retardation, and therefore are not very discriminating. On the other hand, rare or specific effects, such as deafness, retinitis, or a pattern of cerebral calcifications, may point to a specific teratogen. It is also true that there is substantial overlap in malformation syndromes that may not always be identifiable. Environmentally produced birth defects may be confused with genetically determined malformations. Thalidomide can serve as an example. A patient with bilateral radial aplasia and a ventricular septal defect may have the Holt Oram syndrome or the thalidomide syndrome. It may or may not be possible to make a diagnosis with absolute certainty, even if one has a history of thalidomide ingestion during pregnancy. It is possible, however, to refute the suggestion that thalidomide was responsible for congenital malformations in an individual by the nature of the limb malformation.

The specificity of some teratogens can sometimes point to the mechanism or site of action. For instance, the predominant central nervous system effects of methyl mercury are understood when one realizes the propensity for organic mercury to be stored in lipid.

Epidemiologists sometimes use poor judgment when grouping malformations. As an example, limb reduction defects are frequently studied with regard to their association with environmental teratogens, but in some studies, limb defects that are clearly related to problems of organogenesis are lumped with congenital amputations even though it is very unlikely that any agent will be responsible for both types of malformations. It is clear that epidemiologic studies could be markedly improved if there were more input from clinical teratologists in planning and performing the studies.

Case-control studies concerning spontaneous abortion may contain serious errors unless the populations being studied are similar with regard to the stage of pregnancy when abortion occurred. If not, there is the possibility that an abortion rate will differ on the basis of the selection process and not the drug or environmental agent being studied.

Unfortunately, most epidemiologic studies dealing with drug- or environmentally induced abortion do not attempt to determine the etiology of the abortion.

POTENTIAL EMBRYO- AND FETOTOXICITY OF SELECTED PRESCRIBED AND SELF-ADMINISTERED DRUGS

We evaluated the literature concerning selected drugs that cause or are suggested to cause deleterious effects during pregnancy in the human. The data included human epidemiologic studies, secular trend data in humans where appropriate, and animal developmental toxicity studies. In our analysis, we considered the dose–response relationship of teratogenicity, the relationship to the human pharmacokinetic equivalent dose in the animal studies, and biological plausibility (Table 15–9) (42,43). Table A-1 in Appendix H focuses on these drugs, listing their potential adverse effects in the human. Although these drugs account for a small percentage of all malformations and abortions, they are important because these exposures may be preventable.

Alcohol

Adverse effects in offspring from excessive alcohol consumption during pregnancy were recognized more than 200 years ago (46). It was Jones et al. (47), however, who defined the fetal alcohol syndrome in children with intrauterine growth retardation, microcephaly, mental retardation, maxillary hypoplasia, flat philtrum, thin upper lip, and reduction in the width of palpebral fissures. Cardiac abnormalities were also seen. Many of the children of alcoholic mothers had fetal alcohol syndrome, and all of the affected children evidenced developmental delay (47,48).

A period of greatest susceptibility is not clearly established, but the risk for adverse effects increases with increased consumption. Binge drinking early in pregnancy may be associated with an increased risk of alcohol-related effects (49). The risk of decreased brain growth and differentiation is greater during the second and third trimesters. Chronic daily consumption of 6 oz of alcohol constitutes a high risk, whereas the fetal alcohol syndrome is not likely when the mother consumes fewer than two drinks or no more than 1 oz of alcohol per day (50). Reduction of alcohol consumption or cessation of drinking early in pregnancy reduces the incidence and severity of alcohol-related effects (49,51–53) but may not entirely eliminate the risk of some degree of physical or behavioral impairment. The human syndrome is likely to involve the direct effects of alcohol and the indirect effects of genetic susceptibility and poor nutrition. Alcoholism can have maternally deleterious effects on intermediary metabolism and nutrition, especially if alcoholic cirrhosis is present, which can contribute to an adverse milieu for the developing embryo.

Although alcoholic mothers frequently smoke and consume other drugs, there is little doubt from the human and animal data that alcohol ingestion alone can have a disastrous effect on the developing embryo or fetus. The reported incidence of fetal alcohol syndrome varies widely in different studies but appears to be approximately 6% in offspring of women who drink heavily during pregnancy (53). Fetal alcohol syndrome may be the most commonly recognized cause of environmentally induced mental deficiency (50,54); there are at least several hundred children born each year with full fetal alcohol syndrome and probably many more with subtler fetal alcohol effects.

Aminopterin and Methotrexate

Aminopterin and methotrexate (methylaminopterin) are folic acid antagonists that inhibit dihydrofolate reductase, resulting in cell death during the S-phase of the cell cycle (55). Four aminopterin-induced therapeutic abortions resulted in malformations (hydrocephalus, cleft palate, meningomyelocele) in the abortuses (56,57). Thirteen case reports of attempted therapeutic abortions that failed included observations of growth retardation, abnormal cranial ossification, high-arched palate, and reduction in derivatives of the first branchial arch (58). Similar anomalies were reported in three offspring of women treated with methotrexate during early pregnancy (59–61).

The risk of adverse effects from aminopterin and methotrexate in the usual therapeutic range is not known precisely but appears to be moderate to high (58,62).

Androgens

Masculinization of the external genitalia of a girl was reported following *in utero* exposure to large doses of testosterone (63), methyltestosterone, and testosterone enanthate (64). The masculinization is characterized by clitoromegaly with or without fusion of the labia minora and no indication of nongenital malformations. Affected girls experience normal secondary sexual development at puberty (65).

Based on experimental animal studies, behavioral masculinization of a girl from prenatal exposure to androgens will be very rare. The available literature indicates that the effects of androgens on the fetus are dependent on the dose and the stage of development during which the exposure occured.

Angiotensin-Converting Enzyme Inhibitors

The first angiotensin-converting enzyme (ACE) inhibitor, captopril, was introduced in 1981 for the treatment of severe refractory hypertension. Since then the number of ACE inhibitors has increased, and the category now includes enalapril, lisinopril, quinapril, peridopril, fosinopril, ramipril, and cilazapril (66). Their relative effectiveness, combined with a paucity of side effects as compared to other antihypertensives, have made these drugs extremely popular for the treatment of all types of hypertension as well as congestive heart failure and diabetic nephropathy.

The ACE inhibitors are competitive inhibitors of angiotensin-converting enzyme (ACE), a carboxypeptidase that forms an integral part of the renin–angiotensin system (66). The enzyme ACE catalyzes the conversion of angiotensin I to angiotensin II, one of the most potent vasoconstrictors known. It is the same enzyme as kininase II and also catalyzes the breakdown of bradykinin. A vasodilatory peptide itself, bradykinin stimulates the release of other vasodilatory substances including prostaglandins and endothelium-derived relaxation factor (67). Both mechanisms of action contribute to the decrease in blood pressure resulting from ACE inhibition (67).

Although they are considered relatively safe for the treatment of hypertension, ACE inhibitors used during pregnancy have been associated with adverse fetal outcomes in both humans and experimental animals. The first case of adverse fetal outcome in humans was reported in 1981 (68). In that report, treatment with captopril began on the 26th week of gestation, oligohydramnios was detected 2 weeks later, and a cesarean section was performed the following week. The child was anuric and hypotensive and died on day 7. The kidneys and bladder were morphologically normal, but hemorrhagic foci were found in the renal cortex and medulla. Numerous cases of severe and often lethal adverse fetal effects associated with ACE inhibitor use during pregnancy have since been reported (69,70). The most consistent findings have been associated with a disruption of fetal renal function resulting in oligohydramnios and neonatal anuria accompanied by severe hypotension (69,70). Intrauterine growth retardation, pulmonary hypoplasia, hypocalvaria, persistent patent ductus arteriosis, and renal tubular dysgenesis have also been reported (70–72). Some of these effects may also result from the condition for which ACE inhibitors were prescribed (69). These effects have been associated with ACE inhibitor treatment only during the second and third trimesters. There are no reports of adverse fetal outcome associated with ACE inhibitor use during the first trimester (70,72). As ACE inhibitors do not appear to affect organogenesis in either human or animal studies, it is not a classical teratogen. For this reason, Pryde et al. (70) have proposed the term ACE inhibitor fetopathy to describe the characteristic syndrome that results from ACE inhibitor use during pregnancy.

The majority of adverse fetal effects associated with ACE inhibitor use during pregnancy result from the direct therapeutic action of ACE inhibitors on the fetus. The ACE inhibitors readily cross the placenta, where they inhibit fetal ACE activity (70,73). The decreased renal blood flow caused by vasodilation of renal efferent arterioles results in a loss of glomerular filtration pressure, leading to fetal anuria and oligohydramnios (73,74). This in turn may result in other adverse fetal outcomes, such as pulmonary hypoplasia. Fetal urine production and tubular function do not begin until approximately 9 to 12 weeks of gestation (73), which probably explains the lack of adverse fetal effects when ACE inhibitor treatment is discontinued in the first trimester (74). Renal dysplasia, in particular a lack of renal proximal tubule differentiation, has also been noted in some affected fetuses (71,74).

Exposure to an ACE inhibitor during pregnancy has also resulted in several cases of hypocalvaria, an ossification defect of the membranous bones of the skull that leaves the fetal brain inadequately protected (70,71). Although the pathogenesis is still unknown, inadequate perfusion of developing bone as a result of fetal hypotension combined with pressure from uterine muscles because of oligohydramnios may explain this defect (71,72). It has also been suggested that ACE inhibitors may affect ossification by acting on osteoblast-derived growth factors (71).

Despite consistent reports of adverse ACE inhibitor fetopathy, there are no controlled studies available to assess the risks associated with the use of ACE inhibitors during pregnancy. Because there is no reported incidence of adverse fetal effects from ACE inhibitor use during the first trimester of pregnancy, there is no contraindication to ACE inhibitors in women of reproductive age. If the woman becomes pregnant, therapy is then changed to an alternative antihypertensive agent that represents less risk for the fetus.

Antibiotics

The incidence of intraamniotic infection is about 1% of all pregnancies but 3% to 40% of women with ruptured membranes for 24 hours or more (75). Intraamniotic infection is associated with increased morbidity in the newborn, including pneumonia and sepsis. There is also a significant increase in perinatal mortality associated with intraamniotic infection, although, this is in part related to prematurity.

Increased neonatal mortality and morbidity, especially from group B streptococcal infection, can be largely prevented by intrapartum chemoprophylaxis. Neonatal sepsis is also significantly reduced if mothers receive intrapartum antibiotics.

Ceftriaxone Plus Doxycycline

Untreated *Neisseria gonorrhoeae* can lead to serious consequences for the infected woman. Treatment with ceftriaxone plus doxycycline has no reported adverse effects on the fetus.

Penicillin

There are no adverse fetal effects reported for any penicillins.

Erythromycin

As is the case with other sexually transmitted diseases, *Chlamydia* infection is on the increase. The infant most likely acquires chlamydial infection during parturition at an incidence of approximately 50%. Erythromycin is an effective prenatal treatment, although there may be an increased risk of cholestatic hepatitis.

Streptomycin and Kanamycin

Based on case reports, there appears to be a small increased risk of sensorineural deafness in offspring of women treated with streptomycin for tuberculosis during pregnancy (76,77). Other congenital anomalies have not been associated with *in utero* exposure to streptomycin in the human (78). Because auditory nerve damage is a toxic effect of streptomycin in the adult, and animal data show inner ear damage after high exposures *in utero* (79), it is likely that there is a small increased risk of deafness but not of malformations after *in utero* exposure to streptomycin. A related drug, kanamycin, appears to have minimal risk of causing similar adverse effects (80,81).

Tetracyclines

Tetracycline crosses the placenta but is not concentrated by the fetus. Tetracyclines complex with calcium and the organic matrix of newly forming bone without altering the crystalline structure of hydroxyapatite (82). Although tetracycline has been shown to discolor teeth without affecting the likelihood of developing caries (83,84), very high doses may depress skeletal bone growth. No congenital malformations of any other organ system have been associated with antenatal tetracycline exposures (85). Several case reports of limb reduction defects in human embryos exposed to tetracycline are not supported by epidemiologic studies or animal studies. Therapeutic doses of tetracycline are associated with no or minimally increased risk of congenital malformations, but they are likely to result in some degree of dental staining, which does not appear to have a deleterious effect on the offspring.

Cephalosporins

Cephalosporins containing N-methylthiotetrazole have been associated with testicular toxicity in experimental animals. More data are needed to determine whether this association indicates a potential fetal hazard in the human.

It appears that acute exposure to antibiotics in usual therapeutic doses poses little significant risk to the fetus, especially in comparison to the potentially devastating effects of neonatal sepsis.

Antihypertensives (Excluding ACE Inhibitors)

Clonidine

Clonidine exerts its hypotensive effect by a direct α-adrenergic agonistic action in the central nervous system. There appears to be no increased risk during pregnancy but there are few available data (36).

Hydralazine

Hydralazine is a vasodilator often used in combination with methyldopa for the treatment of preexisting hypertension in pregnancy, and its use does not appear to constitute an increased risk for the fetus. Although there is one report of fetal thrombocytopenia (86), over 120 normal pregnancies have been reported (87).

Methyldopa

Methyldopa is currently the lowest-risk antihypertensive drug available for use during pregnancy (88). Methyldopa is a centrally acting adrenergic antagonist with no reported adverse effects on the fetus or on mental and physical development.

Nifedipine

Nifedipine is a calcium channel blocker used for the treatment of preterm labor with no reported adverse fetal effects. The potential for adverse effects with its long-term use in the treatment of hypertension is unknown.

Propranolol

Propranolol is a β-blocker useful in treating preexisting hypertension during pregnancy. However, prolonged use may cause intrauterine growth retardation (89).

Aspirin

Aspirin acts principally by inhibiting prostaglandin synthesis by irreversibly acetylating and inactivating fatty acid cyclooxygenase. Low-dose aspirin (60 to 150 mg per day) is used clinically in the prevention or treatment of a variety of conditions that affect maternal and fetal health. For instance, aspirin is used for the treatment of systemic lupus erythematosus, antiphospholipid syndrome, and preeclampsia.

Of obvious concern is the potential for increased fetal and maternal bleeding associated with low-dose aspirin use near the time of delivery or higher doses used to treat preterm labor. Jankowski et al. reported a study involving 25 women threatened with premature delivery who were given 3.6 g of oral aspirin per day for 4 successive days within 10 days before delivery (90). They and others have found no adverse effects on maternal bleeding at delivery, fetal hemorrhage, or circulatory disorders.

There is some evidence that aspirin combined with dipyridamole may prevent or ameliorate intrauterine growth retardation associated with idiopathic uteroplacental insufficiency. Fetal growth was also improved with aspirin (150 mg per day) alone in fetuses with high, but not extreme, umbilical artery systolic/diastolic ratio. Third-trimester exposure to low daily doses of aspirin were not associated with adverse fetal outcome in these studies (91,92).

High fetal losses are associated with lupus anticoagulant antibodies, anticardiolipin antibodies, and systemic lupus erythematosus. Surviving fetuses experience an increased incidence of growth retardation, fetal distress, and preterm delivery. Low-dose aspirin (60 to 80 mg per day) in combination with prednisone (20 to 80 mg per day) improves pregnancy outcome and greatly reduces thrombosis (93).

Case reports suggest that 75 to 300 mg of aspirin per day in combination with dipyridamole might reduce the risk of late fetal loss in patients with arterial thromboembolism, thrombotic thrombocytopenic purpura, and idiopathic or essential thrombocythemia (93).

Although doubts concerning the safety of aspirin during pregnancy have been expressed, aspirin use during the first trimester is not associated with an increased teratogenic risk (94). Third-trimester exposure to 80 mg per day or less is not associated with an early constriction of the ductus arteriosus (95). Much larger doses of aspirin during the third trimester have been associated with an increased length of gestation, duration of labor, frequency of postmaturity and blood loss at delivery (96). These potential effects justify careful fetal surveillance.

Caffeine

Caffeine is a methylated xanthine that acts as a central nervous system stimulant. It is contained in many beverages including coffee, tea, and colas, as well as chocolate. Caffeine is also present in many over-the-counter medications, such as cold and allergy tablets, analgesics, diuretics, and stimulants. The consumption of caffeine in medicines leads to relatively minimal population intakes. In contrast, caffeine-containing foods and beverages are consumed in large quantities by most of the human populations of the world. The *per capita* consumption of caffeine from all sources is estimated to be about 200 mg/day, or about 3 to 7 mg/kg per day (97). Consumption of caffeinated beverages during pregnancy is quite common and is estimated to be approximately 144 mg per day (98).

Current evidence does not appear to implicate the usual exposure to caffeine as a human teratogen. Associations between maternal coffee drinking during pregnancy and miscarriage or poor fetal growth have been reported in epidemiologic studies (99–103). In many instances these associations are largely attributable to confounding effects of maternal cigarette smoking or other factors. Some of these studies have serious methodologic limitations (104). If maternal consumption of caffeine-containing beverages in conventional amounts during pregnancy does have an association with the rate of miscarriage or fetal growth retardation, the effect appears to be relatively small.

In other studies, no association has been found between between caffeine consumption during pregnancy and congenital defects (85,105,106). For instance, Rosenberg et al. analyzed six selected birth defects in relation to maternal ingestion of more than 8 mg/kg per day of tea, coffee, or cola (107). The defects were inguinal hernia, cleft lip/cleft palate, cardiac defects, pyloric stenosis, cleft palate (isolated), and neural tube fusion defects. None of the point estimates of relative risk was significantly greater than unity, suggesting that caffeine was not a teratogen, at least for the defects evaluated.

Interpretation of the available information pertaining to the animal and human studies regarding the teratogenicity of caffeine leads us to conclude that the usual exposure of caffeine does not represent a measurable risk in the human for any one malformation or group of malformations. There is a clear indication that the consumer must ingest a substantial amount of caffeine in order for it to have an effect on the developing embryo or fetus; total consumption of 300 mg/day may be a safe upper daily limit. Most reviewers and investigators concluded that there is a threshold below which caffeine does not exert a detrimental effect, and the usual human consumption falls in this nontoxic range. The quantity of caffeine consumed in an average cup of coffee, about 1.4 to 2.1 mg/kg (108), is believed to be below the amount that induces congenital defects in animals. Quantities of caffeine in tea and soft drinks would be even less.

Carbamazepine

Although epidemiologic and case-report studies have not yielded consistent results, exposure to carbamazepine has been associated with minor craniofacial defects, fingernail hypoplasia, developmental delay (109,110), reduced birth weight, length and head circumference (111), and neural tube defects (112). Confounding the issue is the possibility that epilepsy itself may increase the risk for malformations (113). However, an attempted suicide involving carbamazepine produced blood levels of 27 to 28 µg/ml (the therapeutic range is 8 to 12 µg/ml) during what was estimated to be 3 to 4 weeks postconception (114). The fetus was later determined to have myeloschisis, with carbamazepine the only known exogenous risk factor. This suggests that carbamazepine has the potential to produce neural tube defects at about two to three times the therapeutic level. It appears that the risk for minor defects is significant, but the risk for all teratogenic effects is not known. The risk for abortion is also unknown but appears to be small.

Cocaine

Cocaine (benzoylmethylecgonine) is one of the most commonly used illicit drugs by women of reproductive age. Reported estimates for cocaine use during pregnancy range from 3% to 17%, the highest rates occurring in inner city populations (115). Because of its widespread use during pregnancy and the growing cost of caring for cocaine-exposed neonates, there has been increasing concern over the risks associated with prenatal cocaine use for maternal and fetal health. Yet despite numerous clinical studies linking prenatal cocaine use with a variety of adverse maternal and fetal effects, methodologic limitations in these studies have made it difficult to establish a causal relationship between these alleged effects and maternal cocaine use. Not only are the timing, frequency, and dose of cocaine use hard to determine, but adverse effects related to low socioeconomic status, poor nutrition, multiple drug use, infections, and a lack of prenatal care are difficult to dissociate from effects of cocaine use alone (115). Thus, the issue of how much risk to the fetus is associated with cocaine use during pregnancy is unresolved. Nonetheless, a growing body of literature supports the concept that cocaine is a developmental toxicant. Adverse effects attributed to prenatal cocaine exposure include a higher incidence of spontaneous abortion, placental abruption, stillbirth, prematurity, low birth weight, growth retardation, decreased head circumference, intracerebral hemorrhage, congenital defects, neurobehavioral abnormalities, and a possible association with increased risk of SIDS (115,116). These effects are reduced but not eliminated in mothers receiving appropriate prenatal care. As with other developmental toxins, outcome is dependent on dose and time of use.

The majority of adverse effects associated with cocaine use during pregnancy appear to be caused by the high levels of cocaine abuse in later stages of gestation rather than in the first trimester or organogenesis (117). Moderate use of cocaine only in the first trimester does not appear to result in adverse fetal outcome and may not pose an increased risk to the fetus (118,119).

Adverse fetal outcomes associated with maternal cocaine use are thought to result primarily from the vasoconstrictive effects of cocaine on both the maternal and fetal vasculature (117). Vasoconstriction of the uterine arteries, which are normally fully dilated during pregnancy, may compromise fetal growth and development. Studies in animals have confirmed that cocaine reduces uterine artery and placental blood flow, leading to reduced oxygen and nutrient supply to the fetus (120). Fetal cardiovascular effects resulting from uterine vasoconstriction include hypertension, tachycardia, hypoxia, and an increase in cerebral blood flow (120,121). Cocaine also crosses the placenta, where it has a direct effect on the fetal vasculature flow (120). Fetal hypertension combined with increased cerebral blood flow may result in intracerebral hemorrhage or infarction, which has been reported to occur in cocaine-exposed fetuses in both human and animal studies (122–124).

Disruption of uterine and fetal vasculature may also lead to a variety of congenital anomalies that have been associated with cocaine abuse. A significant association between cocaine use and an increased incidence of genitourinary tract malformations has been found (122,124,125). Other defects reported include limb reduction defects, nonduodenal intestinal atresia, cardiac anomalies, hypospadias, prune belly syndrome from urethral obstruction, hydronephrosis, and crossed renal ectopia (121,122,124). Two cases of limb–body wall complex have also been reported (126). With the exception of genitourinary tract malformations, the sample size in these clinical studies has not been sufficient to determine a statistically significant relationship between cocaine use and these congenital anomalies (127).

Coumarin Derivatives

Nasal hypoplasia following exposure to several drugs, including warfarin, during pregnancy was reported by DiSaia (128). Kerber et al. (129) were the first to suggest warfarin as the teratogenic agent. Coumarin anticoagulants have since been associated with nasal hypoplasia,

calcific stippling of the secondary epiphysis, and central nervous system abnormalities. Warfarin embryopathy has been described, and an overview of the difficulties in relating a congenital malformation to an environmental cause has been published (130,131). There is an estimated 10% risk for affected infants following exposure during the period from the eighth through the 14th week of pregnancy, although this risk has been reported to be much lower in some series, and other factors besides dose and gestational stage seem to play a role (131). Low-dose warfarin (5 mg/day or less) throughout pregnancy did not result in any adverse effects in 20 offspring (132).

Coumarin inhibits the formation of carboxyglutamyl residues from glutamyl residues, decreasing the ability of proteins to bind calcium. The inhibition of calcium binding by proteins during embryonic/fetal development, especially during a critical period of ossification, could explain the nasal hypoplasia, stippled calcification, and skeletal abnormalities of warfarin embryopathy (131). Microscopic bleeding does not seem to be responsible for these problems early in development (130).

One case report was unique in that the time of exposure to warfarin was between 8 and 12 weeks of gestation, and the infant presented Dandy Walker malformation, eye defects, and agenesis of the corpus callosum (133). This case report is the clearest evidence for a direct effect of warfarin on the developing central nervous system rather than an effect mediated by hemorrhage, because the exposure is well defined and occurs before the appearance of vitamin K-dependent clotting factors. Further supportive evidence for a direct pathogenic role of warfarin is the report of an infant with an inherited deficiency of multiple vitamin K-dependent coagulation factors whose congenital anomalies were similar to warfarin syndrome without exposure to warfarin (134). The risk of stillbirths and spontaneous abortions is increased in pregnant women treated with warfarin, but the risk may be less if the exposure is in the latter half of pregnancy. The risk of adverse effects from hemorrhage increases later in gestation.

Cyclophosphamide

Cyclophosphamide, a widely used antineoplastic agent, is also used to treat severe rheumatoid arthritis. Cyclophosphamide is likely to be teratogenic in the human, but the magnitude of the teratogenic risk is uncertain. The reported defects include growth retardation, ectrodactyly, syndactyly, cardiovascular anomalies, and other minor anomalies (135–137). Ten normal pregnancies have been reported after cyclophosphamide exposure (138).

The mechanism of cyclophosphamide teratogenesis was reviewed by Mirkes (24): cytochrome P_{450} monooxygenases convert cyclophosphamide to 4-hydroxycyclophosphamide, which in turn breaks down to phosphoramide mustard and acrolein. Phosphoramide mustard may produce teratogenic effects by interacting with cellular DNA in an as yet undefined manner, while acrolein acts in a different manner, possibly by affecting sulfhydryl linkages in proteins (139). Tissue sensitivity to phosphoramide mustard and acrolein is thought to be related to such processes as detoxification and cellular repair.

Diethylstilbestrol

The first abnormality reported following exposure to diethylstilbestrol (DES) during the first trimester was clitoromegaly in female newborns (140). Herbst et al. (141,142) and Greenwald et al. (143) later reported an association of vaginal adenocarcinoma in female offspring following first-trimester exposures. Diethylstilbestrol is the only drug with proven transplacental carcinogenic action in the human. Almost all of the cancers occurred after 14 years of age, and only in those exposed before the 18th week of gestation. There is a 75% risk for vaginal adenosis for exposures occurring before the ninth week of pregnancy; the risk of developing adenocarcinoma is about 1:1,000 to 1:10,000 (144). Although the incidence of vaginal adenosis was related to the amount of DES administered, the incidence of vaginal carcinoma does not appear to be related to the maternal dose.

Although there does not appear to be an adverse effect on menstrual cycle functioning or on the rate of conception, the anatomic abnormalities of the uterus and cervix induced by intrauterine exposure to DES, including T-shaped uterus, transverse fibrous ridges, and uterine hypoplasia, have in some reports been associated with an increased risk of ectopic pregnancies, spontaneous abortions, and premature delivery in pregnancies of women exposed to DES *in utero* (145–148).

There have been reports that male fetuses exposed to DES *in utero* exhibited genital lesions and abnormal spermatozoa (149,150). Other studies reported no increase in the risk for the male offspring for genitourinary abnormalities or infertility (151). An association between *in utero* exposure to DES and testicular cancer in male offspring has been suggested, but the data are not conclusive (151,152). The controversial nature of the effects of DES exposure on the male fetus may be attributable to study design or, more likely, to the fact that dose levels varied greatly according to different regimens: exposure to DES during the first half of pregnancies varied from 1.5 to 150 mg per day with total doses from 135 mg to 18 g (153).

Diethylstilbestrol is a potent nonsteroidal estrogen and, as in the case of steroidal estrogens, must interact with the receptor proteins present only in estrogen-responsive tissues before exerting its effects by stimulating RNA, protein, and DNA synthesis. The carcinogenic effect of DES is most likely indirect: DES exposure results in the presence of columnar epithelium in the vagina, and this misplaced tissue may have a greater susceptibility to developing the adenocarcinoma, much as teratomas and other misplaced tissues are more susceptible to malignant degeneration.

Digoxin

Digoxin is used to correct fetal tachyarrhythmias with no substantiated adverse fetal effects (154). However, the possibility of any adverse side effects must be balanced with the fetal prognosis if the dysrhythmia persists or is likely to lead to fetal cardiac failure.

Diphenylhydantoin

Hanson and Smith (155) characterized the fetal hydantoin syndrome in infants whose mothers were treated for epilepsy with hydantoin anticonvulsants. Chronic exposure to diphenylhydantoin has been suggested to present a 5% to 10% risk for the full fetal hydantoin syndrome including ocular hypertelorism, flat nasal bridge, and distal digital hypoplasia with nail hypoplasia (31,156). Cleft lip and palate, congenital heart disease, and microcephaly have been reported, but hypoplasias of the nails and distal phalanges are possibly more common malformations in the exposed fetuses (157,158). Although the hydantoin syndrome is observed in 11% of the subjects in some studies, three times as many exhibit mental deficits (31). It should be mentioned that prospective studies demonstrate a much lower frequency of effects, and some do not demonstrate any effect; thus, the overall prospective risk may be much lower for the classically reported effects.

Factors associated with epilepsy may contribute to the etiology of these malformations (159). Based on the United States Collaborative Perinatal Project and a large Finnish registry, the incidence of malformations was 10.5% when the mother was epileptic, 8.3% when the father was epileptic and 6.4% when neither parent was affected (160).

The teratogenic action of diphenylhydantoin has been postulated to involve the cytochrome P_{450} metabolism of phenytoin to produce a reactive epoxide metabolite. The arene oxide would covalently bind to macromolecules and interfere with their function (161). Further studies have not confirmed this or other hypotheses.

Glucocorticoids

Glucocorticoids (dexamethasone, betamethasone, hydrocortisone, methylprednisone) are effective in reducing the incidence of respiratory distress syndrome in premature newborns by inducing early lung maturation as first hypothesized by Liggins (162). Endogenous glucocorticoids mediate normal pulmonary maturation. Exogeneous glucocorticoids are used to stimulate the production of surfactant. The adverse fetal effects observed in experimental animals exposed to pharmacologic doses are not seen in humans at therapeutic levels (163).

Dexamethasone is used to suppress the fetal adrenal gland in cases of congenital adrenal hyperplasia (164). 21-Hydroxylase deficiency impairs the conversion of cholesterol to cortisol and results in excess 17-hydroxyprogesterone, which in turn results in excess levels of androgens. The masculinization of female fetuses with congenital adrenal hyperplasia varies from clitoral hypertrophy to formation of a phallus. Maternal replacement doses of dexamethasone suppress both the maternal and fetal adrenal glands and prevent masculinization in most patients.

Glucocorticoids are also used in the treatment of rheumatic diseases, other acute and chronic inflammatory diseases, and organ transplantation. Glucocorticoids have not been shown to be teratogenic in humans, but chronic glucocorticoid therapy has been associated with increased risk for prematurity and intrauterine growth retardation (165–167).

Indomethacin

Oral administration of the prostaglandin synthetase inhibitor indomethacin is effective in the treatment of polyhydramnios that is either idiopathic or related to maternal diabetes mellitus. The reduction in renal prostaglandin levels achieved using indomethacin would reduce the inhibitory action of the E prostaglandins on the antidiuretic effect of arginine vasopressin and result in decreased urine production by the fetal kidneys. Oligohydramnios, constriction of the ductus arteriosus (prostaglandins are necessary to maintain the patency of the fetal ductus arteriosus), and fetal hydrops are potentially serious side effects of large doses of indomethacin later in pregnancy and warrant careful fetal surveillance (168).

Indomethacin may also be used to prevent preterm labor or intraventricular hemorrhage. Its efficacy for preventing intraventricular hemorrhage is controversial. Case reports of an increased incidence of impaired renal function, oligohydramnios, and ductus arteriosus constriction have not been confirmed in larger-scale epidemiologic studies. Indomethacin may predispose the neonate to necrotizing enterocolitis when used as a tocolytic (169,170).

Methylene Blue

Methylene blue may be used to mark the amniotic cavity during amniocentesis, but it can also be used in the treatment of methemoglobinemia. There appears to be no increased risk of congenital malformations other than intestinal (ileal) atresia or abortion from intrauterine exposure to methylene blue. The magnitude of the risk of intestinal atresia associated with exposure to methylene blue during amniocentesis is not known, but if it is causal, the risk is likely to be small.

In one study, methylene blue was injected into one amniotic cavity of 86 twin pregnancies (171); jejunal atresia occurred in one of the infants in 17 of these pregnancies. In 15 of these cases, it was possible to determine which twin was exposed to methylene blue, and in each case the twin exposed to methylene blue had jejunal atresia. Because of the generally increased incidence of congenital anomalies associated with twin pregnancies and other factors, it is not yet clear whether the association of methylene blue with intestinal atresia is causal or fortuitous.

Neonatal hemolytic anemia and jaundice have been documented in neonates exposed to methylene blue late in pregnancy (172–174). Hemolytic anemia is a complication of methylene blue therapy in children.

Misoprostol

Misoprostol is a synthetic prostaglandin E_1 methyl analog used for the prevention of gastric ulcers induced by nonsteroidal antiinflammatory drugs. It has known, but not very effective, abortifacient properties. Gonzalez et al. (175) recently reported seven newborns with vascular disruptive phenomena (limb reduction defects, Moebius syndrome) whose mothers used misoprostol early in pregnancy in an attempt to induce abortion. Although there is evidence that misoprostol is used illegally by thousands of pregnant Brazilian women as an abortifacient (176–178), controlled cohort or case-control epidemiologic studies of the fetal outcome of failed abortions are not available. Although the data available are not conclusive, the uterine bleeding produced by misoprostol and the type of malformations produced suggest a vascular disruption mechanism for misoprostol-induced teratogenesis.

If one is looking for vascular disruption, it will more likely be produced later in gestation. Therefore, classical animal teratology experiments will not detect the vascular disruptive effect of drugs or chemicals unless they are exposed beyond the period of early organogenesis (179). Furthermore, it has become clear that if an agent produces vascular disruption, it is a rare event, and therefore large populations would need to be studied before the effect could be discovered (180).

Previous case reports are also of little assistance. Collins and Mahoney (181) reported an infant with hydrocephalus and attenuated digital phalanges after exposure intravaginally to 15-methyl-$F_{2\alpha}$ prostaglandin 5 weeks after conception. Schuler et al. (182) reported that 29% of women who used misoprostol in Brazil as an abortifacient failed to abort. Seventeen children who failed to abort were observed to have no malformations. Schonhofer (183) and Fonesca et al. (184) reported five

Brazilian infants with defects of the skull and overlying scalp who were exposed to misoprostol *in utero*. These case reports indicate the low risk of misoprostol exposure and the possibility that some of the features reported may or may not be caused by misoprostol (185,186). It is too early to know the extent of the effects of misoprostol, but it is biologically plausible that they should include all of the features of vascular disruption.

Oxazolidine-2,4-diones (Trimethadione, Paramethadione)

Trimethadione and paramethadione are antiepileptic oxazolidine-2,4-diones that distribute uniformly throughout body tissues and exert their effects by means of the action of their metabolites. These drugs affect cell membrane permeability and vitamin K-dependent clotting factors, but their primary mode of action is unknown.

Zackai et al. (187), in discussing the fetal trimethadione syndrome, included the following characteristics: developmental delay, V-shaped eyebrows, low-set ears with anteriorly folded helix, high arched palate, and irregular teeth. Clinical observations of these and other associated findings, such as cardiovascular, genitourinary, and gastrointestinal anomalies, have been reviewed (187–190). The incidence of miscarriage, stillbirth, and infant death was also increased. There are wide variations in reported risk, with estimates as high as 80% for major or minor defects. Because the number of exposures is small, the actual risk could vary considerably from these figures.

D-Penicillamine

D-Penicillamine has been used in the treatment of rheumatoid arthritis and cystinuria. D-Penicillamine is a copper chelator, and copper deficiency appears to be the mechanism for teratogenicity (191). Exposure to D-penicillamine can induce a connective tissue defect including generalized cutis laxa, hyperflexibility of the joints, varicosities, and impaired wound healing (192–194). The exposure must be long enough to induce a copper deficiency sufficient to inhibit collagen synthesis and maturation. However, the condition appears to be reversible, and the risk is low, 5% or less.

Phenobarbital

In two prospective studies of patients in high-risk groups for neonatal intraventricular hemorrhage, intravenous phenobarbital administered antenatally resulted in a significant reduction in the incidence of severe cases of intraventricular hemorrhage by increasing cerebral vascular resistance (195). Phenobarbital reduces peak arterial blood pressure, thereby reducing the risk for intraventricular hemorrhage, one of the leading complications of the very-low-birth-weight preterm infant (196). Initiation of intravenous phenobarbital in the early neonatal period is probably too late to derive the potential benefits of this therapy.

Progestins

Although various progestins utilized therapeutically as progestational agents act by means of similar receptors, their potential androgenic effects can differ markedly. This point is critical to the evaluation of the virilizing effects of these compounds in the human. It has been shown, for example, that the pharmacokinetic parameters that estimate steroid bioavailability and metabolism show great variability among subjects and between steroids conveniently grouped together, such as "progestins" (197). One must assume that these differences in bioavailability and metabolism reflect differences in the biological activity of these steroids in humans.

In contrast to progesterone and 17α-hydroxyprogesterone caproate, high doses of some of the synthetic progestins have been reported to cause virilizing effects in humans. Exposure during the first trimester to large doses of 17α-ethinyltestosterone has been associated with masculinization of the external genitalia of female fetuses (198). Similar associations result from exposure to large doses of 17α-ethinyl-19-nortestosterone (norethadrone) (198) and 17α-ethinyl-17-OH-5(10)estren-3-one (Enovid-R) (199). The synthetic progestins, like progesterone, can influence only those tissues with the appropriate steroid receptors. The preparations with androgenic properties may cause abnormalities in the genital development of females offspring only if present in sufficient amounts during critical periods of development, but not in the amounts present in oral contraceptives. In 1959, Grumbach et al. (199) pointed out that labioscrotal fusion could be produced with large doses if the fetuses were exposed before the 13th week of pregnancy, whereas clitoromegaly could be produced after this period, illustrating that a specific form of maldevelopment can be induced only when the embryonic tissues are in a susceptible stage of development.

The World Health Organization (200) reported that there is a suspicion that combined oral contraceptives or progestogens may be weakly teratogenic but that the magnitude of the relative risk is small. In a large retrospective study, Heinonen et al. (201) reported a positive association between cardiovascular defects and *in utero* exposure to female sex hormones. A revaluation of some of the base data by Wiseman and Dodds-Smith (202), however, did not support the reported association. Another retrospective study conducted by Ferencz et al. (203) did not find a positive association between female sex hormone therapy and congenital heart defects. Although neither study disproved the positive association reported by Heinonen et al. (201), their findings made the association less likely.

Epidemiologic studies have reported an association between exposures to female sex hormones, oral contraceptives, or progestogens and congenital neural tube defects (204) and limb defects (205). Further studies and reevaluations have not supported either of these associations (9,21,22).

Further support for the absence of a nongenital effect of progestins comes from (a) a negative correlation between sex hormone usage during pregnancy and malformations, (b) no increased incidence in malformations following progesterone therapy to maintain pregnancy, and (c) no increased incidence in malformations following first-trimester exposure to progestogens (mostly medroxyprogesterone) administered to pregnant women who had signs of bleeding. The Food and Drug Administration has recognized that the evidence does not support an increased risk of limb reduction defects, congenital heat disease, or neural tube defects following exposure to oral contraceptives or progestins (206).

It is generally accepted that the actions of steroid hormones are mediated by specific steroid receptors (207); therefore, only those tissues with the specific receptors can be affected by steroid hormones.

Retinoids—Systemic Administration (Isotretinoin, Etretinate)

Vitamin A congeners, including retinol, retinal, all-*trans*-retinoic acid (tretinoin), and 13-*cis*-retinoic acid (isotretinoin), are all teratogenic in numerous species. Both isotretinoin (Accutane, Roche Laboratories), marketed for treating severe acne, and etretinate (Tigason, Sautier Laboratories), marketed for treating psoriasis, contained warnings by the manufacturers against exposure during pregnancy. Unfortunately, exposures have occurred. Analyses of the resulting malformations have been reviewed (208,209). Human malformations include central nervous system, cardioaortic, microtia, clefting defects, and, more controversially, limb defects. Isotretinoin has a serum half-life of 10 to 12 hours; there is no apparent risk to the fetus if maternal use is terminated before conception (210). However, an increased risk for malformations and subnormal results on standard intelligence tests has been reported for offspring of women who were treated with therapeutic doses of isotretinoin in the first 60 days after conception (211).

Etretinate exposure during the first 60 days of pregnancy is associated with a high risk of malformations. Etretinate has a very long half-life and persists in the body for months (212,213). Whether the lower concentrations of etretinate remaining in the mother's circulation over these extended periods increase the risk of malformations is not known, but if there is an increased risk, it is likely to be low.

Experimental evidence suggests that endogenous retinoic acid may act as a natural morphogen. Exogenous retinoids act either directly, resulting in cytotoxicity, or via receptor-mediated pathways to interact with DNA and alter programmed cell death (214,215). Although retinoids can influence many types of cells, Lammer (208) emphasized that neuroectodermally derived cells of the rhomboencephalon are particularly sensitive and that the resulting neural crest cell abnormality differs from that resulting in oculoauriculovertebral dysplasia or Goldenhar syndrome. The susceptibility of specific cell types to the effects of the retinoids may be determined by the intracellular concentration of cellular retinoic binding protein (208).

Retinoids—Topical Administration (Tretinoin)

There have been a number of case reports of congenital malformations occurring in the offspring of mothers who used topical tretinoin during their pregnancy. The United States Food and Drug Administration received adverse reaction reports involving approximately 17 infants who were born from mothers who used topical tretinoin during pregnancy, with a higher than expected representation of holoprosencephaly (F. Rosa, *personal communication*). Although there has not been an abundance of epidemiologic studies involving topical tretinoin, there are three reports. On the basis of Michigan Medicaid data, the incidence of birth defects in 147 pregnancies exposed to topical tretinoin was compared to the incidence of birth defects in 104,092 nonexposed; the relative risk was 0.8 in the exposed population (F. Rosa, *personal communication*). A relative risk of 0.7 for birth defects was determined in 215 pregnancies exposed to topical tretinoin as compared with 430 nonexposed mothers in data from Group Health of Puget Sound (216). De Wals et al. (217) evaluated the association between the occurrence of holoprosencephaly and topical tretinoin exposure. Among 502,189 births, there were 31 infants with holoprosencephaly. Eight patients had an abnormal karyotype, and 16 had a normal karyotype. None of the patients with a normal karyotype had been exposed to topical tretinoin during pregnancy.

Because all teratogens that have been appropriately studied have a no-effect dose, it would be paramount that topical administration of a known teratogen such as tretinoin must be absorbed and produce teratogenic concentrations in the blood. At conventional doses, the blood levels from topical administration are far below the teratogenic dose. It appears that prudent use of this topical medication presents no risk to the embryo because there would be no teratogenic exposure. The pharmacokinetics, animal studies, and human studies support this conclusion.

Rh Immune Globulin

After exposure to Rh(D)-positive red cells, usually resulting from a fetal transplacental hemorrhage that occurs to some degree in 75% of pregnancies (218), the Rh(D)-negative mother becomes Rh immunized. Rh immunization during a previous pregnancy results in brain damage of various degree or death in an Rh(D)-positive newborn in approximately 50% of cases (218). Once maternal Rh immunization has developed, it cannot be treated effectively, but it can be prevented by antenatal prophylaxis with 300 µg of RhIg at 28 weeks of gestation (218). No adverse fetal effects to immunoprophylaxis have been reported.

Smoking and Nicotine

Approximately 30% of all women of childbearing age smoke, and about 25% of all women will continue to smoke after they become pregnant (219). The evidence in humans indicates that smoking affects the fetal–placental unit directly in a dose-related manner and probably involves more than one component of smoke (220). Placental lesions and fetal growth retardation have been consistently reported in epidemiologic studies involving pregnant women who smoke cigarettes (221–223). Fetal death is 20% to 80% higher among women who smoked cigarettes while pregnant (223). However, despite suggestions that smoking during pregnancy may increase the risk of limb anomalies, there is no proven relationship between smoking and specific malformations or malformations in general (224–226). Because of the large number of pregnant women who smoke and the documented effects of smoking on the fetus, one can conclude that smoking presents a significant risk to the fetus for growth retardation and abortion.

Thalidomide

Lenz and Knapp (227) were the first to associate thalidomide exposure during pregnancy with limb reduction defects and other features of the thalidomide syndrome. Limb defects resulted from exposure limited to a 2-week period from the 22nd to the 36th days postconception: exposures from the 27th to the 30th days most often affected only the arm, whereas exposures from the 30th to the 33rd days resulted in both leg and arm abnormalities (228,229). Although there was no association with mental retardation, gross brain malformations, or cleft palate, other abnormalities included facial hemangioma, microtia, esophageal or duodenal atresia, deafness, and anomalies of the eyes, kidneys, heart, and external ears and increased incidence of miscarriages and neonatal mortality (227,228,230,231). A high proportion, about 20%, of the fetuses exposed during the critical period were affected. More recently, an increased risk for autism has been associated with exposure to thalidomide during the 20th to 24th day of gestation (232). The current use of thalidomide in Brazil for the treatment of leprosy has resulted in additional cases of embryopathy including at least 29 children born with thalidomide syndrome (233,234).

Thyroid: Iodides, Antithyroid Drugs (Thioamides)

There are several case reports of congenital goiter caused by *in utero* exposures to iodide-containing drugs (235). Maternal intake of as little as 12 mg per day may result in fetal goiter (235). Iodinated diagnostic x-ray contrast agents used for amniofetography have been reported to affect fetal thyroid function adversely (236).

Thioamides are antithyroid drugs used to treat maternal thyrotoxicosis. The thioamides block thyroid hormone synthesis by inhibiting the oxidation of iodide or iodotyrosyl. Unlike other thioamides, propylthiouracil also inhibits the peripheral deiodination of thyroxine to triiodothyronine. All thioamides are associated with a significant risk of fetal goiter and teratogenesis (237). However, in the case of propylthiouracil, the fetal goiter can be reduced with intraamniotic injections of thyroxine (238), which also prevent other abnormalities caused by inhibition of fetal thyroid function.

Tocolytics

Fetal distress can result from uterine hypertonus, umbilical cord compression, premature rupture of the fetal membranes, oligohydramnios, placental abruption, and uteroplacental insufficiency. In some cases of severe fetal hypoxemia or acidosis, prompt delivery may be recommended. However, if immediate surgery is not feasible, tocolytics may help to reduce fetal distress until delivery is possible.

In cases of hypoxemia secondary to reduced blood flow to the fetus, inhibiting uterine activity should increase the delivery of oxygen to the fetus by increasing uterine and intervillous perfusion. In addition to inhibiting uterine activity, β-adrenergic agonists both increase maternal cardiac output and dilate uterine vessels, resulting in a further increase in placental perfusion.

Ritodrine, a β2-adrenergic receptor agonist, may be administered as an intravenous bolus for acute fetal distress (239). Ritodrine's mechanism of action leads to a reduction in the intracellular calcium available for smooth muscle contraction.

Terbutaline sulfate, a nonspecific β-adrenergic agonist, is associated with a higher incidence of cardiovascular side effects than ritodine with prolonged use.

When the use of β-adrenergic agonists is contraindicated in cases of intraamniotic infection, uncontrolled maternal thyroid disease, diabetes mellitus, and cardiovascular disease, magnesium sulfate may be used as a tocolytic agent. Although its mechanism of action is unknown, it results in an uncoupling of the actin–myosin interaction in smooth muscle (240). An advantage of magnesium sulfate tocolysis is the absence of cardiovascular side effects.

The data concerning the fetal effects of tocolytic agents are restricted to case reports, but there are no reports of adverse fetal outcome resulting from exposure to therapeutic doses of terbutaline (241), ritodrine (242), or magnesium sulfate (243).

Toluene

Although occupational exposure to toluene has not been associated with congenital malformations in offspring, there are case reports of malformations resulting from the abuse of toluene. The first description of an infant with features similar to fetal alcohol syndrome born to a chronic abuser of toluene appeared in 1979 (244). This case and 22 additional cases have been described in detail (245). Thirty-nine percent of the toluene-exposed infants were born prematurely, and 9% died in the perinatal period. In the surviving infants, 52% exhibited growth deficiency, 67% were microcephalic, and 80% exhibited developmental delay. Craniofacial features similar to those in the fetal alcohol syndrome were observed in 89%. An increased incidence of prematurity, perinatal death, growth and developmental delay, and phenotypic features similar to fetal alcohol syndrome were reported in 35 pregnancies of 15 toluene abusers (246). Pearson et al. (245) suggest that the clinical and experimental data can be interpreted to imply that alcohol and toluene may have a common mechanism of facial teratogenesis. Toluene appears to have the potential for developmental toxicity in the human, but the magnitude of the risk is minimal for usual occupational exposures and has not yet been determined for toluene abusers.

Valproic Acid

Valproic acid (dipropylacetic acid) is used for the treatment of various types of epilepsy. Dalens et al. (247) were the first to report the association of valproic acid and congenital malformations in the human. Although other reports followed, Robert and colleagues (248) described the associated malformations, consisting primarily of neural tube defects, and their incidence in detail. The neural tube defect observed is usually spina bifida in the lumbar or sacral region. An increased risk appears to be correlated with higher serum levels (249,250). Other anomalies include postnatal growth retardation, microcephaly, midface hypoplasia, microagnathia, and epicanthal folds. Therapeutic dosages during pregnancy present a teratogenic risk for spina bifida of about 1% (251), but the risk for facial dysmorphology may be greater.

Valproic acid crosses the human placenta (252), but the fetal serum concentrations are not known.

Vitamins

Despite the common use of vitamin supplements in pregnant women, there have been only rare associations between excess vitamin intake and adverse effects in the human fetus. However, health fads may result in "megadoses" of vitamins with unforeseen effects.

Biotin

Biotin-responsive multiple carboxylase deficiency is an inborn error of metabolism in which there is a severe reduction in the activities of the mitochondrial biotin-dependent carboxylase enzymes. Affected individuals exhibit dermatitis, severe metabolic acidosis, and a characteristic pattern of organic acid excretion. Metabolism in these patients is restored to normal levels by biotin supplementation. Prenatal administration of 10 mg per day of oral biotin initiated during the third trimester prevented neonatal complications with no adverse fetal effects (254).

Vitamin A

Case reports have associated congenital defects in humans with massive vitamin A ingestion during pregnancy (255). Although effects similar to those produced by vitamin A congeners, namely central nervous system, cardioaortic, microtia, and clefting defects (see discussion of Retinoids above), may be predicted, no pattern of anomalies has emerged. Another 14 infants of women who ingested high doses of vitamin A (25,000 IU or more) during pregnancy had no congenital anomalies, although three additional pregnancies ended in miscarriage (256).

A review of literature concerning retinoids and birth defects entitled "Recommendations for Vitamin A Use During Pregnancy" was published by the Teratology Society (255). Although there is some controversy concerning the highest daily dose without increased risk (257), supplementation of 8,000 IU vitamin A per day should be the maximum during pregnancy, and high dosages (25,000 IU or more) are not recommended. β-Carotene as a source of vitamin A is likely to be associated with a smaller risk than an equivalent dose of vitamin A as retinol (255).

Vitamin B₁₂

Ampola et al. (258) were the first to report prenatal treatment of a vitamin-responsive inborn error of metabolism. Their report involved a fetus with a vitamin B_{12}-responsive variant of methylmalonic acidemia, a metabolic disease involving a functional deficiency in the coenzymatically active form of vitamin B_{12}. Oral cyanocobalamin, 10 mg per day, initiated at 32 weeks of gestation, resulted in only a slight increase in maternal serum B_{12} level. Oral therapy was therefore stopped at 34 weeks of gestation, and 5 mg per day of intravenous cyanocobalamin was initiated. This regimen produced a progressive increase in maternal serum B_{12} and a decrease in urinary methylmalonic acid excretion. The infant had no acute neonatal complications after delivery at 41 weeks.

Vitamin D

Excess of vitamin D has been associated with increased incidence of congenital malformations. Huge doses of vitamin D administered for rickets prophylaxis in pregnant women resulted in an increased incidence of a syndrome consisting of supravalvular aortic stenosis, elfin facies, and mental retardation in the human (259, 260). Animal studies and additional clinical reports suggest that the teratogenic risk of therapeutic doses of vitamin D is none to minimal.

DRUGS WHOSE RISK IS CONTROVERSIAL

Antituberculosis Therapy

Drugs prescribed for the treatment of tuberculosis include aminoglycosides, ethambutol, isoniazid, rifampin, and ethionamide. The ototoxic effects of streptomycin at high dose over a prolonged period (discussed above) are the only proven adverse effects of these drugs on the fetus. Other aminoglycosides have not been associated with fetal effects. Neither ethambutol nor rifampin has been associated with an increase in the incidence of growth retardation, premature birth, or malformations (76,77).

Early reports did not associate therapeutic exposures to isoniazid with an increased risk of malformations (76, 77), but there is an unconfirmed association with central nervous system dysfunction (261). There was one attempted suicide involving 50 tablets of isoniazid per day during the 12th week, which resulted in a stillbirth with arthogyryposis multiplex congenita syndrome (262). Isoniazid may have a small increased risk for adverse effects on the central nervous system, but there is no apparent increase in risk for malformations or abortions with therapeutic exposures.

Only one report associated ethionamide with an increased risk of teratogenic effects (263). However, this association is tenuous and not supported by other case reports.

The only antituberculosis drug with confirmed developmental toxicity is streptomycin, as discussed above. Although this does not eliminate the possibility of adverse effects on the fetus following exposure to the other prescribed tuberculostatic medications discussed, therapeutic exposures appear to represent a very small risk of teratogenesis and even less risk of abortion.

Benzodiazepines

The benzodiazepines, such as chlordiazepoxide (Librium), diazepam (Valium), alprazolam (Xanax), and meprobamate, are widely used as tranquilizers during pregnancy, and, therefore, it is not surprising that they have been associated with congenital malformations in some publications.

Chlordiazepoxide was associated with various anomalies after exposure during early pregnancy, but no syndrome was identified (85,264). Other studies were inconclusive or found no association (265–267). Chlordiazepoxide appears to have a minimal risk for congenital anomalies and no increased risk for abortion at therapeutic doses.

Some studies reported an association between diazepam and increased incidence of congenital malformations (267). However, a follow-up study found no associations (268). The majority of studies of fetal outcome following in utero exposure to diazepam are negative (265,269–271). Behavior alterations have been reported in infants exposed to benzodiazepines, mostly diazepam (272), but this observation must be confirmed, and the long-term developmental outcome evaluated, before it can be appropriately interpreted.

Although third-trimester exposure to diazepam can reversibly affect the fetus and neonate (273), there is minimal increased risk of congenital malformations and no demonstrated increased risk of abortions from therapeutic exposures.

Meprobamate has been weakly associated with a variety of congenital malformations (274,275). Other studies found no associations (85,266). Because of inconsistencies, the data are not sufficient to confirm or rule out a small increase risk of malformations from exposures early in pregnancy.

Benzodiazepines appear to have no or minimal increased risk of malformations at therapeutic ranges. The risk for abortion is unknown, but given the widespread use of these drugs, it is unlikely that a significant abortagenic effect would have gone unnoticed.

Lithium Carbonate

Lithium carbonate, widely used for treatment of manic–depressive disorders, was first associated with human congenital malformations in 1970 (276,277). The malformations described include heart and large vessel anomalies, Ebstein's anomaly, neural tube defects, talipes, microtia, and thyroid abnormalities. Lithium does cross the placenta (278) and appears to be a human teratogen at therapeutic dosages. More recent epidemiologic data indicate that it presents a very small risk for malformations (279,280). The results of a retrospective study suggest that lithium may also increase the risk for premature delivery (281), but, again, the magnitude of the risk is likely to be small. Transient toxic effects seen in the neonate include congenital goiter, lethargy, hypotonia, and cardiac murmur (282). Because of the value of lithium carbonate for treating manic–depressive psychosis, the risk associated with psychiatric relapse on removing the drug may be greater than the teratogenic risk. If other drugs are found for the treatment of manic–depressives that have no teratogenic potential, they could be substituted during pregnancy.

ACKNOWLEDGMENTS

The authors thank Yvonne Edney for her secretarial assistance. This work was supported in part by funds from NIH HD 29902, Harry Bock Charities, and the Nemours Foundation.

REFERENCES

1. Hertig AT. The overall problem in man. In Benirschke K, ed. *Comparative aspects of reproductive failure.* Berlin: Springer-Verlag, 1967:11–41.
2. Robert CJ, Lowe CR. Where have all the conceptions gone? *Lancet* 1975;1:498–499.
3. Kajii T, Ferrier A, Niikawa N, Takahara H, Ohama K, Avirachan S. Anatomic and chromosomal anomalies in 639 spontaneous abortions. *Hum Genet* 1980;55:87.
4. Simpson JL. Genes, chromosomes and reproductive failure. *Fertil Steril* 1980;33:107–116.
5. Copp AJ. Death before birth: Clues from gene knockouts and mutations. *Trends Genet* 1995;11:87–93.
6. Fraser FC. The multifactorial/threshold concept—uses and misuses. *Teratology* 1976;14 267–280.
7. World Health Organization. *Spontaneous and induced abortion. Technical Report Series No. 461.* Geneva: World Health Organization, 1970.
8. Boue J, Boue A, Lazar P. Retrospective and prospective epidemiological studies of 1,500 karyotyped spontaneous abortions. *Teratology* 1975;12:11–26.
9. Wilson JG. *Environment and birth defects.* New York: Academic Press, 1973.
10. Brent RL. Predicting teratogenic and reproductive risks in humans from exposure to various environmental agents using *in vitro* techniques and *in vivo* animal studies. *Cong Anom* 1988;28(Suppl): S41–S55.
11. Sever JL. Infections in pregnancy: Highlights from the collaborative perinatal project. *Teratology* 1982;25:227–237.
12. Gwinn M, Pappaioanou M, George JR, et al. Prevalence of HIV infection in childbearing women in the United States. *JAMA* 1991;265: 1704–1708.
13. Braddick MR, Kreiss JK, Embree JE, et al. Impact of maternal HIV infection on obstetrical and early neonatal outcome. *AIDS* 1990;4: 1001–1005.
14. Blanche S, Rouzioux C, Moscato MLG, et al. A prospective study of infants born to women seropositive for human immunodeficiency virus type 1. *N Engl J Med* 1989;320:1643–1648.
15. Embree JE, Braddick M, Datta P, et al. Lack of correlation of maternal human immunodeficiency virus infection with neonatal malformations. *Pediatr Infect Dis J* 1989;8:700–704.
16. European Collaborative Study. Mother-to-child transmission of HIV infection. *Lancet* 1988;ii:1039–1043.
17. Qazi QH, Sheikh TM, Fikrig S, Menikoff H. Lack of evidence for craniofacial dysmorphism in perinatal human immunodeficiency virus infection. *J Pediatrics* 1988;112:7–11.
18. Van Allen MI. Structural anomalies resulting from vascular disruption. *Pediatr Clin North Am* 1992;39:255–277.
19. Van Allen MI, Siegel-Bartelt J, Dixon J, Zuker RM, Clarke HM, Toi A. Constriction bands and limb reduction defects in two newborns with fetal ultrasound evidence for vascular disruption. *Am J Med Genet* 1992;44:598–604.
20. Wilson JG, Brent RL, Jordan HC. Differentiation as a determinant of the reaction of rat embryos to x-irradiation. *Proc Soc Exp Biol Med* 1953;82:67–70.
21. Briggs MH, Briggs M. Sex hormone exposure during pregnancy and malformations. In Briggs MH, Corbin A, eds. *Advances in steroid biochemistry and pharmacology.* London: Academic Press, 1979:51–89.
22. Wilson JG, Brent RL. Are female sex hormones teratogenic? *Am J Obstet Gynecol* 1981;114:567–580.
23. Fraser FC. Interactions and multiple causes. In Wilson JG, Fraser FC, eds. *Handbook of teratology.* New York: Plenum Press, 1977:445–463.
24. Mirkes PE. Cyclophosphamide teratogenesis: A review. *Teratogen Carcinogen Mutagen* 1985;5:75–88.
25. Miller RK. Placental transfer and function: The interface for drugs and chemicals in the conceptus. In Fabro S, Scialli AR, eds. *Drug and chemical action in pregnancy: Pharmacologic and toxicologic principles.* New York: Marcel Dekker, 1986:123–152.
26. Jackson MJ. Drug absorption. In Fabro S, Scialli AR, eds. *Drug and chemical action in pregnancy: Pharmacologic and toxicologic principles.* New York: Marcel Dekker, 1986:15–36.
27. Mattison DR. Physiologic variations in pharmacokinetics during pregnany. In Fabro S, Scialli AR, eds. *Drug and chemical action in pregnancy: Pharmacologic and toxicologic principles.* New York: Marcel Dekker, 1986:37–102.
28. Sonawane BR, Yaffe SJ. Physiologic disposition of drugs in the fetus and newborn. In Fabro S, Scialli AR, eds. *Drug and chemical action in pregnancy: Pharmacologic and toxicologic principles.* New York: Marcel Dekker, 1986:103–121.
29. Juchau MR, Rettie AE. The metabolic role of the placenta. In Fabro S, Scialli AR, eds. *Drug and chemical action in pregnancy: Pharmacologic and toxicologic principles.* New York: Marcel Dekker, 1986: 153–169.
30. Juchau MR. Bioactivation in chemical teratogenesis. *Annu Rev Pharmacol Toxicol* 1989;29:165–187.
31. Hanson JW. Teratogen Update: Fetal hydantoin effects. *Teratology* 1986;33:349–353.
32. Laurence KM, James N, Miller MH, Tennant GB, Campbell H. Double-blind randomized controlled trial of folate treatment before conception to prevent recurrence of neural tube defects. *Br Med J* 1981; 282:1509–1511.
33. Smithells RW, Seller MJ, Nevin NC, et al. Further experience of vitamin supplementation for prevention of neural tube defect recurrences. *Lancet* 1983;1:1027–1031.
34. Smithells RW, Sheppard S, Schorah CJ, et al. Apparent prevention of neural tube defects by periconceptional vitamin supplementation. *Arch Dis Child* 1981;56:911.
35. Smithells RW, Sheppard S, Wild J, Schorah CJ. Prevention of neural tube defect recurrences in Yorkshire: Final report. *Lancet* 1989;2: 498–499.
36. Medical Research Council. Prevention of neural tube defects: Results of the Medical Research Council Vitamin Study. *Lancet* 1991;338: 131–137.
37. Cziezel AE, Dudas I. Prevention of the first occurrence of neural-tube defects by periconceptional vitamin supplementation. *N Engl J Med* 1992;327:1832–1835.
38. Brent RL. Environmental factors: Miscellaneous. In Brent RL, Harris MI, eds. *Prevention of embryonic, fetal and perinatal disease. DHEW Pub. No. (NIH) 76-853.* Bethesda: DHEW, 1976:211–218.
39. Brent RL. Drugs and pregnancy: Are the insert warnings too dire? *Contemp Ob-Gyn* 1982;20:42–49.
40. Mirkin BL. Maternal and fetal distribution of drugs in pregnancy. *Clin Pharmacol Ther* 1973;14:643–647.
41. McKusick VA. *Mendalian inheritance in man: catalogs of autosomal dominant, autosomal recessive, and X-linked phenotypes, ed. 8.* Baltimore: Johns Hopkins University Press, 1988.
42. Brent RL. Method of evaluaing alleged human teratogens [editorial]. *Teratology* 1978;17:83.
43. Brent RL. Definition of a teratogen and the relationship of teratogenicity to carcinogenicity [editorial]. *Teratology* 1986;34:359–360.
44. Susser E. Spontaneous abortion and induced abortion: an adjustment for the presence of induced abortion when estimating the rate of spontaneous abortion from cross-sectional studies. *Am J Epidemiol* 1983; 117:305–308.

45. Olsen J. Calculating the risk ratios for spontaneous abortions: the problem of induced abortion. *Int J Epidemiol* 1984;13:347–350.

46. Warner RH, Rosett HL. The effects of drinking on offsrping: An historical survey of the American and British literature. *J Stud Alcohol* 1975;36:1395.

47. Jones KL, Smith DW, Streissguth AP, Myrianthopoulous NC. Outcome in offspring of chronic alcoholic women. *Lancet* 1974;1:1076–1078.

48. Streissguth AP, Grant TM, Barr HM, Brown ZA, Martin JC, Mayock DE, Ramey SL, Moore L. Cocaine and the use of alcohol and other drugs during pregnancy. *Am J Obstet Gynecol* 1991;164:1239–1243.

49. Streissguth AP, Sampson PD, Marr HM. Neurobehavioral dose–response effects of prenatal alcohol exposure in humans from infancy to adulthood. *Ann NY Acad Sci* 1989;562:145–158.

50. Streissguth AP, Landesman-Dwyer C, Martin JC, Smith DW. Teratogenic effects of alcohol in humans and laboratory animals. *Science* 1980;209:353–361.

51. Autti-Ramo I, Granstrom M-L. The effect of intrauterine alcohol exposure of various durations on early cognitive development. *Neuropediatrics* 1991;22:203–210.

52. Autti-Ramo I, Granstrom M-L. The psychomotor development during the first year of life of infants exposed to intrauterine alcohol of various durations. Fetal alcohol exposure and development. *Neuropediatrics* 1991;22:59–64.

53. Day NL, Richardson GA. Prenatal alcohol exposure: A continuum of effects. *Semin Perinatol* 1991;15:271–279.

54. Clarren SK and Smith DW. The fetal alcohol syndrome. *N Engl J Med* 1978;298:1063–1067.

55. Skipper HT, Schabel FM Jr. Quantitative and cytokinetic studies in experimental tumor models. In Holland JF, Frei E III, eds. *Cancer medicine.* Philadelphia: Lea & Febiger, 1973:629–650.

56. Goetsch C. An evaluation of amniopterin as an abortifacient. *Am J Obstet Gynecol* 1962;83:1474–1477.

57. Thiersch JB. Therapeutic abortions with a folic acid inhibitor (4-amino P.G.A.). *Am J Obstet Gynecol* 1952;63:1298–1304.

58. Warkany J. Teratogenicity of folic acid antagonists. *Cancer Bull* 1981;33:76–77.

59. Milunsky A, Graef JW, Gaynor MF. Methotrexate-induced congenital malformations with a review of the literature. *J Pediatr* 1968;72:790–795.

60. Powell HR, Ekert H. Methotrexate-induced congenital malformations. *Med J Aust* 1971;2:1076–1077.

61. Sosa Munoz JL, Perez-Santana MT, Sosa Sanchez R, Labardini JR. Acute leukemia and pregnancy. *Rev Invest Clin (Mex.)* 1983;35:55–58.

62. Aviles A, Diaz-Macqueo JC, Talavera A, Guzman T, Garcia EL. Growth and development of children of mothers treated with chemotherapy during pregnancy: Current status of 43 children. *Am J Hematol* 1991;36:243–248.

63. Grumbach MM, Conte FA. Disorders of sex differentiation. Williams RH, ed. *Textbook of endocrinology.* Philadelphia: WB Saunders, 1981:422–514.

64. Hoffman F, Overzier C, Uhde G. Zur frage der hormonalen erzengung fotaler zwittenbildugen beim menschen. *Geburtshife Frauenheilkd* 1955;15:1061–1070.

65. Reschini E, Giustina G, D'Alberton A, Candiani GB. Female pseudohermaphroditism due to maternal androgen administration: 25-year follow-up. *Lancet* 1985;1:1226.

66. Maxwell SRJ, Kendall MJ. Ace inhibition in the 1990s. *Br J Clin Pract* 1993;47:30–37.

67. Gavras I, Gavras H. Ace inhibitors: A decade of clinical experience. *Hosp Pract (Off Ed)* 1993;28:117–127.

68. Guignard JP, Burgener F, Calame A. Persistent anuria in neonate: A side effect of captopril. *Intern J Pediatr Nephrol* 1981;2:133.

69. Hanssens M, Keirse MJNC, Vankelecom F, Van Assche FA. Fetal and neonatal effects of treatment with angiotensin-converting enzyme inhibitors in pregnancy. *Obstet Gynecol* 1991;79:128–135.

70. Pryde PG, Sedman AB, Nugent CE, Barr M. Angiotensin-converting enzyme inhibitor fetopathy. *J Am Soc Nephrol* 1993;3:1575–1582.

71. Barr M Jr, Cohen MM Jr. ACE inhibitor fetopathy and hypocalvaria: The kidney–skull connection. *Teratology* 1991;44:485–495.

72. Brent RL, Beckman DA. Angiotensin-converting enzyme inhibitors, an embryopathic class of drugs with unique properties: Information for clinical teratology counselors. *Teratology* 1991;43:543.

73. Guignard JP. Effect of drugs on the immature kidney. *Adv Nephrol Neker Hosp* 1993;22:193–211.

74. Martin RA, Jones KL, Mendoza A, Barr M, Benirschke K. Effect of ACE inhibition on the fetal kidney: Decreased renal blood flow. *Teratology* 1992;46:317–321.

75. Cox SM, Williams ML, Leveno KJ. The natural history of preterm ruptured membranes: what to expect of expectant management. *Obstet Gynecol* 1988;71:558–562.

76. Snider DE, Layde PM, Johnson MW, Lyle MA. Treatment of tuberculosis during pregnancy. *Am Rev Respir Dis* 1980;122:65–79.

77. Warkany J. Antituberculosis drugs. *Teratology* 1979;20:133–138.

78. Heinonen OP, Slone D, Shapiro S. *Birth defects and drugs in pregnancy.* Littleton, MA: Publishing Sciences Group, 1977:516.

79. Nakamoto Y, Otani H, Tanaka O. Effects of aminoglycosides administered to pregnant mice on postnatal development of inner ear in their offspring. *Teratology* 1985;32:34B.

80. Jones HG. Intrauterine ototoxicity. A case report and review of literature. *J Natl Med Assoc* 1973;65:201–203.

81. Nishimura H, Tanimura T. Clinical aspects of the teratogenicity of drugs. New York: Excerpta Medica American Elsevier, 1976.

82. Cohlan SQ, Bevelander G, Tiamsic T. Growth inhibition of prematures receiving tetracycline: Clinical and laboratory investigation. *Am J Dis Child* 1963;105:453–461.

83. Baden E. Environmental pathology of the teeth. In Gorlin RJ, Goldman HM, eds. *Thomas' oral pathology,* ed. 6. St Louis: CV Mosby, 1970:189–191.

84. Brent RL, Jensh RP, Beckman DA. Medical sonography: Reproductive effects and risks. *Teratology* 1991;44:123–146.

84. Rebich T, Kumar J, Brustman B. Dental caries and tetracycline-stained dentition in an American-Indian population. *J Dent Res* 1985;64:462–464.

85. Heinonen OP, Slone D, Shapiro S. *Birth defects and drugs in pregnancy.* Littleton, MA: Publishing Sciences Group, 1977.

86. Widerlov E, Karlman I, Storsater J. Hydralazine-induced neonatal thrombocytopenia [letter]. *N Engl J Med* 1980;301:1235.

87. Bott-Kanner G, Schweitzer A, Reisner SH, Joel-Cohen SJ, Rosenfeld JB. Propranolol and hydralazine in the management of essential hypertension in pregnancy. *Br J Obstet Gynaecol* 1980;87:110–114.

89. NHBPEP. *Working Group Report on high blood pressure in pregnancy.* Bethesda, MD: Public Health Service, National Institutes of Health Publication No. 91-2039, 1991:38.

89. Witter FR, King TM, Blake DA. Adverse effects of cardiovascular drug theapy on the fetus and neonate. *Obstet Gynecol* 1981;58:100S–105S.

90. Jankowski A, Skublicki S, Wichlinski LM, Szymanski W. Clinical pharmacokinetic investigations of acetylsalicylic acid in cases of imminent premature delivery. *J Clin Hosp Pharmacy* 1985;10:361.

91. Trudinger BJ, Cook CM, Giles WB, Connelly AJ, Thompson RS. Low-dose aspirin in pregnancy. *Lancet* 1989;1:410.

92. Wallenburg HCS, Rotmans N. Prevention of recurrent idiopathic fetal growth retardation by low-dose aspirin and dipyridamole. *Am J Obstet Gynecol* 1987;157:1230.

93. Barton JR, Sibai BM. Low-dose aspirin to improve perinatal outcome. *Clin Obstet Gynecol* 1991;34:251.

94. Werler MM, Mitchell A, Shapiro S. The relation of aspirin use during the first trimester of pregnancy to congenital cardiac defects. *N Engl J Med* 1989;321:1639.

95. McParland P, Pearce JM, Chamberlain GVP. Doppler ultrasound and aspirin in recognition and prevention of pregnancy-induced hypertension. *Lancet* 1990;335:1552.

96. Lewis RB, Schulman JD. Influence of acetylsalicylic acid, an inhibitor of prostaglandin synthesis, on the duration of human gestation and labour. *Lancet* 1973;2:1159.

97. Barone JJ, Roberts H. Human consumption of caffeine. In Dews PB, ed. *Caffiene.* New York: Springer-Verlag, 1984:59–73.

98. Morris MB, Weinstein L. Caffeine and the fetus—is trouble brewing? *Am J Obstet Gynecol* 1981;140:607–610.

99. Beaulac-Baillargeon L, Desrosiers C. Caffeine–cigarette interaction on fetal growth. *Am J Obstet Gynecol* 1987;157:1236–1240.

100. Fenster L, Eskenazi B, Windham GC, Swan SH. Caffeine consumption during pregnancy and fetal growth. *Am J Public Health* 1991;81:458–461.

101. Srisuphan W, Bracken MB. Caffeine consumption during pregnancy and association with late spontaneous abortion. *Am J Obstet Gynecol* 1986;154:14–20.

102. Watkinson B, Fried PA. Maternal caffeine use before during and after pregnancy and effects upon offspring. *Neurobehav Toxicol Teratol* 1985;7(1):9–17.

103. Wilcox AJ, Weinberg CR, Baird DD. Risk factors for early pregnancy loss. *Epidemiology* 1990;1:382–385.

104. Berger A. Effects of caffeine consumption on pregnancy outcome—a review. *J Reprod Med* 1988;33:945–956.

105. Kurppa K, Holmberg PC, Kuosma E, Saxen L. Coffee consumption during pregnancy and selected congenital malformations: A nation-wide case-control study. *Am J Public Health* 1983;73:1397–1399.

106. van't Hoff W. Caffeine in pregnancy. *Lancet* 1982;1:1020.

107. Rosenberg L, Mitchell AA, Shapiro S, Slone D. Selected birth defects in relation to caffeine-containing beverages. *JAMA* 1982;247:1429–1432.

108. Felts JH. Coffee arabica. *NC Med J* 1981;42:281.

109. Jones KL, Lacro RV, Johnson KA, Adams J. Pattern of malformations in the children of women treated with carbamazepine during pregnancy. *N Engl J Med* 1989;320:1661–1666.

110. Nielsen M, Froscher W. Finger- and toenail hypoplasia after carbamazepine monotherapy in late pregnancy. *Neuropediatrics* 1985;16:167–168.

111. Bertollini R, Kallen B, Mastroiacovo P, Robert E. Anticonvulsant drugs in monotherapy: Effect on the fetus. *Eur J Epidemiol* 1987;3:164–167.

112. Rosa FW. Spina bifida in infants of women treated with carbamazepine during pregnnacy. *N Engl J Med* 1991;10:674–677.

113. Janz D. Antiepileptic drugs and pregnancy: Altered utilization patterns and teratogenesis. *Epilepsia* 1982;23:S53–S63.

114. Little BB, Santos-Ramos R, Newell JF, Maberry MC. Megadose carbamazepine during the period of neural tube closure. *Obstet Gynecol* 1993;82:705–708.

115. Slutsker L. Risk associated with cocaine use during pregnancy. *Obstet Gynecol* 1992;79:778–789.

116. Young SL, Vosper RJ, Phillips SA. Cocaine: Its effects on maternal and child health. *Pharmacotherapy* 1992;12:2–17.

117. Jones KL. Developmental pathogenesis of defects associated with prenatal cocaine exposure: Fetal vascular disruption. *Clin Perinatol* 1991;18:139–146.

118. Koren G, Graham K. Cocaine in pregnancy: Analysis of fetal risk. *Vet Hum Toxicol* 1992;34:263–264.

119. Robert E. Valproic acid and spina bifida: A preliminary report—France. *MMWR* 1982;31:515–566.

120. Woods JR, Plessinger MA. Maternal–fetal cardiovascular system: A target of cocaine. *NIDA Res Monogr* 1991;108:7–27.

121. Plessinger MA, Woods JR. Maternal, placental, and fetal pathophysiology of cocaine exposure during pregnancy. *Clin Obstet Gynecol* 1993;36:267–278.

122. Chasnoff IJ, Chisum GM, Kaplan WE. Maternal cocaine use and genitourinary tract malformations. *Teratology* 1988;37:201–204.

123. Dogra VS, Menon PA, Poblete J, Smeltzer JS. Neurosonographic imaging of small for gestational age neonates exposed and not exposed to cocaine and cytomegalovirus. *J Clin Ultrasound* 1994;22:93–102.

124. Hoyme HE, Jones KL, Dixon SD. Prenatal cocaine exposure and prenatal vascular disruption. *Pediatrics* 1990;85:743.

125. Chavez GF, Mulinare J, Cordero JF. Maternal cocaine use during early pregnancy as a risk factor for congenital urogenital anomalies. *JAMA* 1989;262:795–798.

126. Viscarello RR, Ferguson DD, Nores J, Hobbins JC. Limb-body wall complex associated with cocaine abuse: Further evidence of cocaine's teratogenicity. *Obstet Gynecol* 1992;80:523–526.

127. Lutiger BK, Graham K, Einarson TR, Koren G. Relationship between gestational cocaine use and pregnancy outcome: A meta analysis. *Teratology* 1991;44:405–414.

128. DiSaia PJ. Pregnancy and delivery of a patient with a Starr-Edwards mitral valve prosthesis: Report of a case. *Obstet Gynecol* 1966;29:469–472.

129. Kerber IJ, Warr OS, Richardson C. Pregnancy in a patient with prosthetic mitral valve. *JAMA* 1968;203:223–225.

130. Barr M, Burdi AR. Warfarin-associated embryopathy in a 17-week abortus. *Teratology* 1976;14:129–134.

131. Hall JG, Pauli RM, Wilson RM. Maternal and fetal sequelae of anticoagulation during pregnancy. *Am J Med* 1980;68:122–140.

132. Cotrufo M, deLuca TSL, Calabro R, Mastrogiovanni G, Lama D.

133. Kaplan LC. Congenital Dandy Walker malformation associated with first trimester warfarin: A case report and literature review. *Teratology* 1985;32:333–337.

134. Pauli RM, Lian JB, Mosher DF. Association of congenital deficiency of multiple vitamin K-dependent coagulation factors and the phenotype of the warfarin embryopathy: Clues to the mechanism of teratogenicity of coumarin derivatives. *Am J Hum Genet* 1987;41:566–583.

135. Greenberg LH, Tanaka KR. Congenital anomalies probably induced by cyclophosphamide. *JAMA* 1964;188:423–426.

136. Scott JR. Fetal growth retardation associated with maternal administration of immunosuppressive drugs. *Am J Obstet Gynecol* 1977;128:668–676.

137. Toledo TM, Harper RC, Moser RH. Fetal effects during cyclophosphamide and irradiation therapy. *Ann Intern Med* 1971;74:87–91.

138. Blatt J, Mulvihill JJ, Ziegler JL, Young RC, Poplack DG. Pregnancy outcome following cancer chemotherapy. *Am J Med* 1980;69:828–832.

139. Hales BF. Effects of phosphoramide mustard and acrolein, cytotoxic metabolites of cyclophosphamide, on mouse limb development *in vitro*. *Teratology* 1989;40:11–20.

140. Bongiovanni AM, DiGeorge AM, Grumbach MM. Masculinization of the female infant associated with estrogenic therapy alone during gestation: Four cases. *J Clin Endocrinol Metab* 1959;19:1004–1011.

141. Herbst AL, Kurman RJ, Scully RE, Poskanzer DC. Clear-cell adenocarcinoma of the genital tract in young females. *N Engl J Med* 1972;287:1259–1264.

142. Herbst AL, Ulfelder H, Poskanzer DC. Adenocarcinoma of the vagina: Association of maternal stilbestrol therapy with tumor appearance in young women. *N Engl J Med* 1971;284:878–881.

143. Greenwald P, Barlow JJ, Nasca PC, Burnett WS. Vaginal cancer after matrnal treatment with synthetic estrogens. *N Engl J Med* 1971;285:390–392.

144. Herbst AL, Anderson D. Clear cell adenocarcinoma of the vagina and cervix secondary to intrauterine exposure to diethylstilbestrol. *Semin Surg Oncol* 1990;6:343–346.

145. Barnes AB, Colton T, Gundersen J, Noller KL, Tilley BC, Strama T, Toensend DE, Hatab P, O'Brien PC. Fertility and outcome of pregnancy in women exposed *in utero* to diethylstilbestrol. *N Engl J Med* 1980;302:609–613.

146. Berger MJ, Goldstein, DP. Impaired reproductive performance in DES-exposed women. *Obstet Gynecol* 1980;55:25–27.

147. Herbst AL, Hubby MM, Blough RR, Azizi F. A comparison of pregnancy experience in DES-exposed and DES-unexposed daughters. *J Reprod Med* 1980;24:62–69.

148. Linn S, Lieberman E, Schoenbaum SC, Monson RR, Stubblefield PG, Ryan KJ. Adverse outcomes of pregnancy in women exposed to diethylstilbestrol *in utero*. *J Reprod Med* 1988;33:3–7.

149. Gill WB, Schumacher GFB, Bibbo M, Straus FH, Schoenberg HW. Association of diethylstilbestrol exposure *in utero* with cryptorchidism, testicular hypoplasia and semen abnormalities. *J Urol* 1979;122:36–39.

150. Shy KK, Stenchever MA, Karp LE, Berger RE, Williamson RA, Leonard J. Genital tract examinations and zona-free hamster egg penetration tests from men exposed *in utero* to diethylstilbestrol. *Fertil Steril* 1984;42:772–778.

151. Vessey MP. Epidemiological studies of the effects of diethylstilbestrol. *IARC Sci Publ* 1989;96:335–348.

152. Gershman ST, Stolley PD. A case-control study of testicular cancer using Connecticut Tumor Registry data. *Int J Epidemiol* 1988;17:738–742.

153. Herbst AL, Robboy SJ, Scully RE, Poskanzer DC. Clear-cell adenocarcinoma of the vagina and cervix in girls: Analysis of 170 registry cases. *Am J Obstet Gynecol* 1974;119:713–724.

154. Pinsky WW, Rayburn WF, Evans MI. Pharmacologic therapy for fetal arrhythmias. *Clin Obstet Gynecol* 1991;34:304–309.

155. Hanson JW, Smith DW. The fetal hydantoin syndrome. *J Pediatr* 1975;87:285–290.

156. Albengres E, Tillement JP. Phenytoin in pregnancy: A review of the reported risks. *Biol Res Pregnancy Perinatol* 1983;4:71–74.

157. Barr M, Pozanski AK, Schmickel RD. Digital hypoplasia and anticonvulsants during gestation, a teratogenic syndrome. *J Pediatr* 1974;4:254–256.

Coumarin anticoagulation during pregnancy in patients with mechanical valve prostheses. *Eur J Cardiothorac Surg* 1991;5:300–305.

158. Gaily E. Distal phalangeal hypoplasia in children with prenatal phenytoin exposure: Results of a controlled anthropometric study. *Am J Med Genet* 1990;35:574–578.

159. Keneko S. Antiepileptic drug therapy and reproductive consequences: Functional and morphological effects. *Reprod Toxicol* 1991;5:179–198.

160. Shapiro S, Slone D, Hartz SC, et al. Anticonvulsants and parental epilepsy in the development of birth defects. *Lancet* 1976;1:272–275.

161. Spielberg SP, Gordon GB, Blake DA, Mellits ED, Bross DS. Anticonvulsant toxicity *in vitro*: Possible role of arene oxides. *J Pharmacol Exp Ther* 1981;217:386–389.

162. Liggins GC, Howie RN. A controlled trial of antepartum glucocorticoid treatment for prevention of the respiratory distress syndrome in premature infants. *Pediatrics* 1972;50:515–525.

163. Collaborative Group on Antenatal Steroid Therapy. Effect of antenatal dexamethasone administration in the prevention of respiratory distress syndrome. *Am J Obstet Gynecol* 1981;141:276–287.

164. Chrousos GP, Evans MI, Loriaux DL, McCluskey J, Fletcher JC, Schulman JD. Prenatal therapy in congenital adrenal hyperplasia. Attempted prevention of abnormal external genital masculinization by pharmacologic suppression of the fetal adrenal gland *in utero*. *Ann NY Acad Sci* 1985;458:156–164.

165. Cowchuck FS, Reece EA, Balaban D, Branch DW, Plouffe L. Repeated fetal losses associated with antiphopholipid antibodies: a collaborative randomized trial comparing prednisone with low-dose heparin treatmen. *Am J Obstet Gynecol* 1992;166:1318–1323.

166. Scott JR. Fetal growth retardation associated with maternal administration of immunosuppressives. *Am J Obstet Gynecol* 1977;128:668–676.

167. Reinisch JM, Simon NG. Prenatal exposure to prednisone in humans and animals retards intrauterine growth. *Science* 1978;202:436–438.

168. Moise KJ. Indomethacin therapy in the treatment of symptomatic polyhydramnios. *Clin Obstet Gynecol* 1991;24:310.

169. Fejgin MD, Delpino ML, Bidiwala KS. Isolated small bowel perforation following intrauterine treatment with indomethacin administration. *Am J Perinatol* 1994;11:296–296.

170. Major CA, Lewis DF, Harding JA, Porto MA, Garite TJ. Tocolysis with indomethacin increases the incidence of necrotizing enerocolitis in the low-birth-weight neonate. *Am J Obstet Gynecol* 1994;170:102–106.

171. van der Pol JG, Wolf H, Boer K, et al. Jejunal atresia related to the use of methylene blue in genetic amniocentesis in twins. *Br J Obstet Gynecol* 1992;99:141–143.

172. Cowett RM, Hakanson DO, Kocon RW, Oh W. Untoward neonatal effect of intraaminotic administration of methylene blue. *Obstet Gynecol* 1976;48[Suppl]:745–755.

173. Crooks J. Haemolytic jaundice in a neonate after intra-amniotic injection of methylene blue. *Arch Dis Child* 1982;57:872–886.

174. Serota FT, Bernbaum JC, Schwartz E. The methylene blue baby. *Lancet* 1979;2:1142–1143.

175. Gonzalez CH, Vargas FR, Perez ABA, et al. Limb deficiency with or without Moebius sequence in seven Brazilian children associated with misoprostol use in the first trimester of pregnancy. *Am J Med Genet* 1993;46:59–64.

176. Coelho HLL, Misago C, Fonseca WVC, Souza DSC, Araujo JML. Selling abortifacients over the counter in pharmacies in Fortaleza, Brazil. *Lancet* 1991;338:247.

177. Costa SH, Vessey MP. Misoprostol and illegal abortion in Rio de Janeiro, Brazil. *Lancet* 1993;341:1258–1261.

178. Luna-Coelho HL, Teixeira AC, Santos AP, et al. Misoprostol and illegal abortion in Fortaleza, Brazil. *Lancet* 1993;341:1261–1263.

179. Brent RL. Relationship between uterine vascular clamping, vascular disruption, and cocaine teratogenicity [editorial]. *Teratology* 1990;41:757–760.

180. NICHD Workshop. CVS and limb reduction defects. *Teratology* 1993;48:7–13.

181. Collins FS, Mahoney MJ. Hydrocephalus and abnormal digits after failed first trimester prostaglandin abortion attempt. *J Pediatr* 1983;102:620–621.

182. Schuler LS, Ashton PW, Sanseverino MT. Teratogenicity of misoprostol. *Lancet* 1992;339:437.

183. Schonhofer PS. Brazil: Misuse of misoprostol as a abortifacient may induce malformations. *Lancet* 1991;337:1534.

184. Fonseca W, Alencar AJC, Mota FSB, Coelho HLL. Misoprostol and congential malformations. *Lancet* 1991;338:56.

185. Brent RL. Congenital malformation case reports: the editor's and reviewer's dilemma. *Am J Med Genet* 1993;47:872–874.

186. Castilla EE, Orioli IM. Teratogenicity of misoprostol: Data from the Latin-American collaborative study of congenital malformations (ECLAMC). *Am J Med Genetics* 1994;51:161–162.

187. Zackai EH, Melman WJ, Neiderer D, Hanson JW. The fetal trimetbadione syndrome. *J Pediatr* 1975;87:280–284.

188. Cohen MM. Syndromology—an updated conceptual overview. VII. Aspects of teratogenesis. *Int J Oral Maxillofac Surg* 1990;19:26–32.

189. Feldman GL, Weaver DD, Lovrien EW. The fetal trimethadione syndrome. *Am J Dis Child* 1977;131:1389–1392.

190. Smith ESO, Dafoe CS, Miller JR, Banister P. An epidemiological study of congenital reduction deformities of the limbs. *Br J Prev Soc Med* 1977;31:39–41.

191. Keen CL, Mark-Savage P, Lonnerdal B, Hurley LS. Teratogenesis and low copper status resulting from D-penicilliamine in rats. *Teratology* 1982;26:163–165.

192. Harpey JP, Jaudon MC, Clavel JP, Galli A, Darbois Y. Cutix laxa and low serum zinc after antenatal exposure to penicillamine. *Lancet* 1983;2:858.

193. Linares A, Zarranz JJ, Rodriguez-Alarcon J, Diaz-Perez JL. Reversible cutix laxa due to maternal D-penicillamine treatment. *Lancet* 1979;2:43.

194. Solomon L, Abrams G, Dinner M, Berman L. Neonatal abnormalities associated with D-pencillamine treatment during pregnancy. *N Engl J Med* 1977;296:54–55.

195. Morales WJ. Antenatal therapy to minimize neonatal intraventricular hemorrhage. *Clin Obstet Gynecol* 1991;34:328–335.

196. Morales WJ. Effect of intraventricular hemorrhage on the one-year mental and neurologic handicaps of the very low birth weight infant. *Obstet Gynecol* 1987;70:111–114.

197. Fotherby K. A new look at progestins. *Clin Obstet Gynecol* 1984;11:701–722.

198. Wilkins L. Masculinization due to orally given progestins. *JAMA* 1960;172:1028–1032.

199. Grumbach MM, Ducharine JR, Moloshok RE. On the fetal masculinizing action of certain oral progestins. *J Clin Endocrinol Metab* 1959;19:1369–1380.

200. World Health Organization. *The effect of female sex hormones on fetal development and infant health. Technical Report Series, No. 657.* Geneva: World Health Organization, 1981.

201. Heinonen OP, Sloane D, Monson RR, Hook EB, Shapiro S. Cardiovascular birth defects and antenatal exposure to female sex hormones. *N Engl J Med* 1977;296:67–70.

202. Wiseman RA, Dodds-Smith IC. Cardiovascular birth defects and antenatal exposure to female sex hormones: A reevaluation of some base data. *Teratology* 1984;30:359–370.

203. Ferencz C, Matanoski GM, Wilson PD, Rubin JD, Neill CA, Gutberlet R. Maternal hormone therapy and congenital heart disease. *Teratology* 1980;21:225–239.

204. Gal I. Risks and benefits of the use of hormonal pregnancy test tablets. *Nature* 1972;240:241–242.

205. Janerich DT, Piper JM, Glebatis DM. Oral contraceptives and congenital limb-reduction defects. *N Engl J Med* 1974;291:697–700.

206. Brent RL. The magnitude of the problem of congenital malformations. In Marois M, ed. *Prevention of physical and mental congenital defect. Part A. Basic and medical science, education and future stragegies.* New York: Alan R Liss, 1985:55–68.

207. O'Malley BW, Schrader DT. The receptors of steroid hormones. *Sci Am* 1976;234:32–43.

208. Lammer EJ, Schunior A, Hayes AM, Holmes LB. Isotretinoin dose and teratogenicity. *Lancet* 1988;2:503–504.

209. Rosa FW. Teratogen update: Penicillamine. *Teratology* 1986;33:127–131.

210. Dai WS, Hsu M, Itri LM. Safety of pregnancy after discontinuation of isotretinoin. *Arch Dermatol* 1989;125:362–365.

211. Dai WS, LaBraico JM, Stern RS. Epidemiology of isotretinoin exposure during pregnancy. *J Am Acad Dermatol* 1992;26:599–606.

212. DiGiovanna JJ, Zech LA, Ruddel ME, et al. Etretinate: Persistent serum levels of a potent teratogen. *Clin Res* 1984;32:579A.

213. Rinck G, Gollnick H, Organos CE. Duration of contraception after etretinate. *Lancet* 1989;1:845–846.

214. Alles AJ, Sulik KK. Retinoic-acid-induced limb-reduction defects:

Perturbation of zones of programmed cell death as a pathogenetic mechanism. *Teratology* 1989;40:163–171.

215. Yasuda Y, Konishi H, Kihara T, Tanimura T. Developmental anomalies induced by all-*trans*-retinoic acid in fetal mice: II. Induction of abnormal neuroepithelium. *Teratology* 1987;35:355–366.

216. Jick SS, Terris BZ, Jick H. First trimester topical tretinoin and congenital disorders. *Lancet* 1993;341:1181–1182.

217. DeWals P, Bloch D, Calabro A, et al. Association between holoprosencephaly and exposure to topical retinoids: Results of the EUROCAT survey. *Neonat Perinat Epidemiol* 1991;5:445–447.

218. Bowman JM. Antenatal suppression of Rh alloimmunization. *Clin Obstet Gynecol* 1991;34:296–303.

219. Prager K, Malin H, Speigler D, Van Natta P, Placek P. Smoking and drinking behavior before and during pregnancy of married mothers of liveborn and stillborn infants. *Public Health Rep* 1984;99:117–127.

220. Naeye RL. Effects of maternal cigarette smoking on the fetus and placenta. *Br J Obstet Gynaecol* 1979;85:732–737.

221. Chattingius S. Does age potentiate the smoking-related risk of fetal growth retardation? *Early Hum Dev* 1989;20:203–211.

222. Hjortdal JO, Hjortdal VE, Foldspang A. Tobacco smoking and fetal growth: A review. *Scand J Soc Med* 1989;45[Suppl I–II]:1–22.

223. Stillman RJ, Rosenberg MJ, Sachs BP. Smoking and reproduction. *Fertil Steril* 1986;46:545–566.

224. Erickson JD. Risk factors for birth defects: Data from the Atlanta defects case-control study. *Teratology* 1991;43:41–51.

225. Tikkanen J, Heinonen OP. Maternal exposure to chemical and physical factors during pregnancy and cardiovascular malformations in the offspring. *Teratology* 1991;43:591–600.

226. Werler MM, Pober BR, Holmes LB. Smoking and pregnancy. *Teratology* 1985;32:473–481.

227. Lenz W, Knapp K. Thalidomide embryopathy. *Arch Environ Health* 1962;5:100–105.

228. Brent RL, Holmes LB. Clinical and basic science lessons from the thalidomide tragedy: What have we learned about the causes of limb defects? *Teratology* 1988;38:241–251.

229. Lenz W. A short history of thalidomide embryopathy. *Teratology* 1988;38:203–215.

230. Kida M. *Thalidomide embryopathy in Japan.* Tokyo: Kodansha, 1987.

231. Ruffing L. Evaluation of thalidomide children. *Birth Defects* 1977;13: 287–300.

232. Rodier PM, Ingram JL, Tisdale B, Croog VJ. Linking etiologies in humans and animal models: studies of autism. *Reprod Toxicol* 1997; 11:417–422.

233. Cutler J. Thalidomide revisited. *Lancet* 1994;343:795–796.

234. Jones GRN. Thalidomide: 35 years on and still deforming. *Lancet* 1994;343:1041.

235. Carswell F, Kerr MM, Hutchinson JH. Congenital goiter and hypothyroidism produced by maternal ingestion of iodides. *Lancet* 1970;1: 1241–1243.

236. Rodesch F, Camus M, Ermans AM, Dodion J, Delange F. Adverse effect of amniofetography on fetal thyroid function. *Am J Obstet Gynecol* 1976;126:723–726.

237. Schardein JL. *Chemically induced birth defects.* New York: Marcel Dekker, 1993.

238. Clewell WP. *In utero* treatment of thyrotoxicosis. In Evans MI, Fletcher JC, Ditlen AO, Schulman JD, eds. *Fetal diagnosis and therapy: Science, ethics, and the law.* Philadelphia: JB Lippincott, 1984:124.

239. Smith CV. Reversing acute intrapartum fetal distress using tocolytic drugs. *Clin Obstet Gynecol* 1991;34:353–359.

240. Caritis SN, Darby MJ, Chan L. Pharmacologic treatment of preterm labor. *Clin Obstet Gynecol* 1988;31:635–651.

241. Egarter CH, Husslein PW, Rayburn WF. Uterine hyperstimulation after low-dose prostaglandin E$_2$ therapy: Tocolytic treatment in 181 cases. *Am J Obstet Gynecol* 1990;163:794–796.

242. Mendez-Bauer C, Shekarloo A, Cook V, Freese U. Treatment of acute intrapartum fetal distress by β2-sympathomimetics. *Am J Obstet Gynecol* 1987;156:638–642.

243. Reece EA, Chervenak FA, Romero R, Hobbins JC. Magnesium sulfate in the management of acute intrapartum fetal distress. *Am J Obstet Gynecol* 1984;148:104–106.

244. Toutant C, Lippman S. Fetal solvents syndrome. *Lancet* 1979;1:1356.

245. Pearson MA, Hoyme HE, Seaver LH, Rimsza ME. Toluene embryopathy: Delineation of the phenotype and comparison with fetal alcohol syndrome. *Pediatrics* 1994;93:211–215.

246. Arnold GL, Kirby RS, Langendoerfer S, Wilkins-Haug L. Toluene embryopathy: Clinical delineation and developmental follow-up. *Pediatrics* 1994;93:216–220.

247. Safra MJ, Oakley GP. Valium: An oral cleft teratogen? *Cleft Palate J* 1976;13:198–200.

248. Dalens B, Raynaud E-J, Gaulme J. Teratogenicity of valproic acid. *J Pediatr* 1980;97:332–333.

249. Robert E. Valproic acid as a human teratogen. *Congen Anom* 1988; 28[Suppl]:S71–S80.

250. Linhout D, Meinardi H, Meijer JWA, Nau H. Antiepileptic drugs and teratogenesis in two consecutive cohorts: changes in prescription policy paralleled by changes in pattern of malformations. *Neurology* 1992;42[Suppl 5]:94–110.

251. Omtzigt JGC, Nau H, Los FJ, Pijpers L, Lindhout D. The disposition of valproate and its metabolites in the late first trimester and early second trimester of pregnancy in maternal serum, urine, and amniotic fluid: Effect of dose, co-medication, and the presence of spina bifida. *Eur J Clin Pharmacol* 1992;43:381–388.

252. Lammer EJ, Sever LE, Oakley GP Jr. Valproic acid. *Teratology* 1987; 35:465–473.

253. Dickinson RG, Hapland RC, Lynn RK, Smith WB, Gerber N. Transmission of valproic acid across the placenta: half-lives of the drug in mother and baby. *J Pediatr* 1979;94:832–835.

254. Roth KS, Yang W, Allan L, Saunders M, Gravel RA, Dakshinamurti K. Prenatal administration of biotin: biotin responsive multiple carboxylase deficiency. *Pediatr Res* 1982;16:126–129.

255. Teratology Society. Teratology Society Position Paper: Recommendations for vitamin A use during pregnancy. *Teratology* 1987;35: 269–275.

256. Zuber C, Librizzi RJ, Vogt BL. Outcomes of pregnancies exposed to high doses of vitamin A. *Teratology* 1987;35:42A.

257. Rothman KJ, Moore LL, Singer MR, Nguyen US, Mannino S, Milunsky A. Teratogenicity of high vitamin A intake. *N Engl J Med* 1995; 333:1369–1373.

258. Ampola MG, Mahoney MJ, Nakamura E, Tanaka K. Prenatal therapy of a patient with vitamin B responsive methylmalonic acidemia. *N Engl J Med* 1975;293:313–317.

259. Friedman WF. Vitamin D and the supravalvular aortic stenosis syndrome. In Woollam DHM, ed. *Advances in teratology.* New York: Academic Press, 1968:83–96.

260. Garcia RE, Friedman WF, Kaback MM, Rowe RD. Idiopathic hypercalcemia and supravalvular stenosis: Documentation of a new syndrome. *N Engl J Med* 1964;271:117–120.

261. Monnet P, Kalb JC, Pujol M. Harmful effects of isoniazid on the fetus and infants. *Lyon Med* 1967;218:431–455.

262. Lenke RR, Turkel SB, Monsen R. Severe fatal deformities associated with ingestion of excessive isoniazid in early pregnancy. *Acta Obstet Gynecol Scand* 1985;64:281–282.

263. Potworowska M, Sianoz-Ecka E, Szufladowicz R. Treatment with ethionamide in pregnancy. *Gruzlica* 1966;34:341–347.

264. Kullander S, Kallen B. A prospective study of drugs and pregnancy. *Acta Obstet Gynecol Scand* 1976;55:25–33.

265. Czeizel A. Lack of evidence of teratogenicity of benzodiazepine drugs in Hungary. *Reprod Toxicol* 1988;1:183–188.

266. Hartz SC, Heinonen OP, Shapiro S, Siskind V, Slone D. Antenal exposure to meprobamate and chlordiazepoxide in relation to malformations, mental development, and childhood mortality. *N Engl J Med* 1975;292:726–728.

267. Rothman KJ, Fyler DC, Goldblatt A, Kreidberg MB. Exogenous hormones and other drug exposures of children with congenital heart disease. *Am J Epidemiol* 1979;109:433–439.

268. Zierler S, Rothman KJ. Congenital heart disease in relation to maternal use of Bendectin and other drugs in early pregnancy. *N Engl J Med* 1985;313:347–352.

269. Aselton P, Jick H, Milunsky A, Hunter JR, Stergachis A. First-trimester drug use and congenital disorders. *Obstet Gynecol* 1985;65: 451–455.

270. Safra MJ, Oakley GP. Association between cleft lip with or without cleft palate and prenatal exposure to diazepam. *Lancet* 1975;2:478–479.

271. Tikkanen J, Heinonen OP. Risk factors for conal malformations of the heart. *Eur J Epidemiol* 1992;8:48–57.

272. Laegreid L, Hagberg G, Lundberg A. Neurodevelopment in late infancy after prenatal exposure to benzodiazepines—A prospective study. *Neuropediatrics* 1992;23:60–67.

273. Rementeria JL, Bhatt K. Withdrawal symptoms in neonates from intrauterine exposure to diazepam. *J Pediatr* 1977;90:123–126.
274. Milkovich L, van den Berg BJ. Effects of prenatal meprobamate and chlordiazepoxide hydrochloride on human embryonic and fetal development. *N Engl J Med* 1974;291:1268–1271.
275. Saxen I. Association between oral clefts and drugs taken during pregnancy. *Int J Epidemiol* 1975;4:37–44.
276. Lewis WH, Suris OR. Treatment with lithium carbonate. Results in 35 cases. *Tex Med* 1970;66:58–63.
277. Vacaflor L, Lehmann HE, Ban TA. Side effects and teratogenicity of lithium carbonate treatment. *J Clin Pharmacol* 1970;10:387–389.
278. Rane A, Tomson G, Bjarke B. Effects of maternal lithium therapy in a newborn infant. *J Pediatr* 1974;93:296–297.
279. Cohen LS, Friedman JM, Jefferson JW, Johnson EM, Weiner ML. A reevaluation of risk of *in utero* exposure to lithium. *JAMA* 1994;271:146–150.
280. Jacobson SJ, Jones K, Johnson K, et al. Prospective multicentre study of pregnancy outcome after lithium exposure during first trimester. *Lancet* 1992;339:530–533.
281. Troyer WA, Pereira G, Lannon RA, Belik J, Yoder MC. Association of maternal lithium exposure and premature delivery. *J Perinatol* 1993;13:123–127.
282. Wilson N, Forfar JD, Godman MJ. Atrial flutter in the newborn resulting from lithium ingestion. *Arch Dis Child* 1983;58:538–539.
283. Kline J, Stein Z, Susser M, Warburton D. Environmental influences on early reproductive loss in a surrent New York City study. In Porter IM, Hook EM, eds. *Human embryonic and fetal death.* New York: Academic Press, 1980:225.
284. Friedman JM, Polifka JE, eds. *TERIS, teratogenic effects of drugs: a resource for clinicians.* Baltimore: The Johns Hopkins University Press, 1994.

CHAPTER 16

Obstetric Analgesia and Anesthesia

Mark A. Rosen

Labor and childbirth pain and techniques for its control are described in the writings of ancient civilizations from the earliest recorded times (e.g., Chinese, Babylonian, Egyptian, Persian, Hebrew, and Greek). Included are descriptions of inhaling opium, drinking alcohol, strange use of agents such as henbane and hemlock, boiled and smeared on the woman's body as a salve, and the use of bondage (Fig. 16–1). Although pain of labor has been a concern of humans from the earliest recorded times, it has been the source of considerable confusion and misconceptions. *Genesis* includes the prediction that "in sorrow, thou shalt bring forth children" (1). It was widely regarded that alleviation of labor pain may contravene the divine intent. Pope Pius XII wrote a special encyclical in 1957 about the spiritual value of childbirth pain but explained that there was no prohibition in the tradition of the Catholic Church against use of appropriate methods to alleviate labor pain.

The modern history of obstetric anesthesia began 3 months after the famous demonstration of the anesthetic properties of ether in Boston. James Simpson, a Scottish obstetrician, administered ether to a woman with a contracted pelvis to facilitate vaginal delivery in January, 1847. The first obstetric anesthetic in the United States was administered in Cambridge, Massachusetts 3 months later to Fanny Longfellow, wife of the famous poet Henry Wadsworth Longfellow. She became an outspoken enthusiast of labor analgesia. Dr. Simpson likewise became an ardent advocate of the use of obstetric analgesia and evoked significant controversy among the public as well as the medical community about its use, safety, and value.

Public controversy essentially abated, and labor analgesia gained considerable respect and acceptance when

John Snow, an English obstetrician, administered chloroform to Queen Victoria for the birth of her eighth child in 1853 and her ninth child 4 years later. He used a refinement of Simpson's technique of inhalation analgesia. Subsequently, John Snow restricted his medical practice to anesthetic administration, the first physician to do so. However, despite a growing popularity among the public, controversy continued within the medical community. Although numerous studies of obstetric anesthesia appeared in the medical literature during the later part of the 19th century and first half of the 20th century, good studies were scarce. Most studies lacked substance in defining or characterizing important issues of maternal safety or impact on the newborn.

Circumstances changed by the second half of the 20th century as a result of a number of advances that include the introduction of continuous caudal anesthesia by Hingson and Edwards (2) and later continuous epidural anesthesia; description of a simple scoring system for neonatal evaluation by obstetric anesthesiologist Virginia Apgar (3); and pioneering work by the obstetric anesthesiologists Gertie Marx (4), John Bonica, Sol Shnider (5), and others, characterizing changes in maternal physiology induced by pregnancy, efficacy and safety of obstetric analgesia, impact of techniques and medications on uterine blood flow, placental transfer of anesthetic agents, and impact of various techniques and agents on newborn well-being.

In the second half of the 20th century, impressive strides in obstetric anesthesia took place as scientific research burgeoned, scientific societies were founded, a separate subspecialty emerged with specialized training for residents and fellows, and comprehensive textbooks (6,7) and dedicated scientific journals emerged. Somewhat ironically, as the use of regional analgesia for labor became more widespread, and the science of its safe and effective use ensued, methods of so-called natural childbirth arose from direct appeals to the public by Grantly

M. A. Rosen: Department of Anesthesia and Perioperative Care and Department of Obstetrics, Gynecology and Reproductive Sciences, Moffitt–Long Hospital, University of California, San Francisco, San Francisco, California

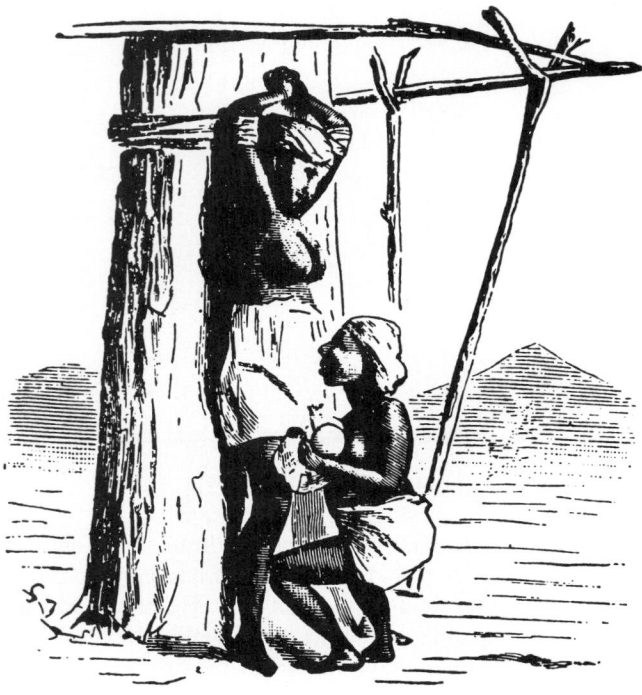

Serang Island Delivery

FIG. 16–1. Management of parturients among primitive people. Example of one form of a fixed, stressful position that may have been used to help distract the mother's attention. (Modified from Englemann CL. *Labor among primitive people, 2nd ed.* St. Louis: JH Chambers, 1883.)

Dick Read (8), a British obstetrician, and Fernand Lamaze (9), a French obstetrician.

This chapter introduces the neonatal practitioner to the scientific background and clinical techniques of modern obstetric anesthesia and discusses the consequence of these techniques on the fetus and neonate. Obstetric analgesia may benefit the parturient in painful labor, facilitate safe and painless use of forceps or vacuum devices for vaginal delivery, facilitate safe vaginal delivery of twins or a fetus in a breech presentation, and is certainly required to permit delivery by cesarean section. Although the effects of modern obstetric anesthesia on the fetus and newborn are ordinarily benign, rarely they can have an adverse impact that the neonatal practitioner should learn to recognize, comprehend, and manage.

THE PAIN OF PARTURITION

Neurotransmission

Pain is the sensation of discomfort that results from sufficient stimulation of specialized receptors in traumatized tissue. Neuronal impulses are conducted to the central nervous system (CNS) on afferent, small myelinated and unmyelinated, somatic and visceral nerves (axonal conduction), entering the spinal cord primarily through the dorsal roots that correspond to embryonic dermatomes. Painful impulses undergo complex modulation in the posterior horn of the spinal cord (primarily in the substantia gelatinosa), involving many interneurons and neurotransmitters that include enkephalins, endorphins, polypeptides such as substance P, serotonin, and many other substancess (Fig. 16–2).

From the spinal cord, pain pathways can be traced to the cerebral cortex by upward transmission of impulses primarily through the dorsal columns and the lateral-spinothalamic and anteriorspinothalamic tracts. These impulses stimulate the reticular formation and tegmental tract in the brainstem, where they evoke the typical reflex responses to pain, including tachycardia, hyperventilation, increased blood pressure, and release of catecholamines and hypothalamic hormones. The impulses then continue through the thalamus and project to the sensory cortex for localization and discrimination of pain.

Nerve fibers arise from the medulla, thalamus, and cortex with caudal projections to the dorsal horn of the spinal cord, which modulate the release of the above-mentioned neurotransmitters (descending modulation). With sufficient inhibitory descending modulation, a peripheral sensation may be perceived as a sensory modality other than "pain," for example, as "pressure," "burning," or "pruritus." Alternatively, excitatory modulation can produce disproportionate responses to other-

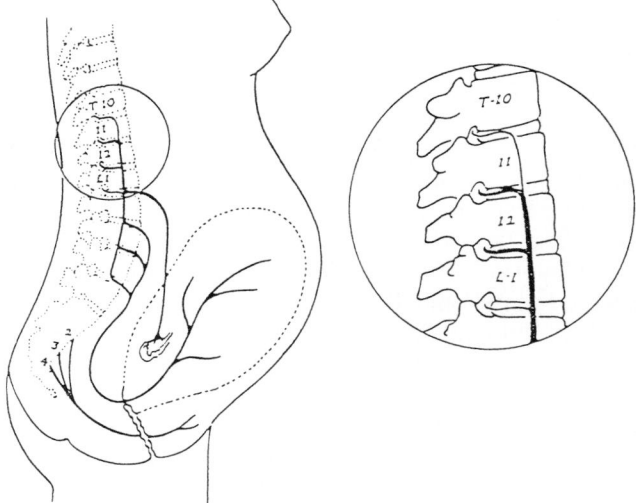

FIG. 16–2. Partuition pain pathways. Afferent pain impulses from the cervix and uterus are carried by nerves that accompany sympathetic fibers and enter the neuraxis at T-10, T-11, T-12, and L-1 spinal levels. Pain pathways from the perineum travel to S-2, S-3, and S-4 via the pudendal nerve. (Reprinted with permission from Bonica JJ. The nature of pain of parturition. *Clin Obstet Gynecol* 1975;2:511.)

wise ordinary stimuli, as occurs in hyperesthetic syndromes.

Transmission of pain impulses can be diminished by application of local anesthetics to the spinal cord or elsewhere in the CNS, which blocks axonal impulse conduction by blockade of sodium channel conductance, or by application of inhibitory neurotransmitters or their analogs (notably narcotics) or antagonists of excitatory neurotransmitters (e.g., clonidine). This is the physiologic and pharmacologic basis for analgesia induced by administration of local anesthetics, narcotics, and other agents to the CNS, particularly to the spinal cord, by spinal or epidural anesthetic techniques.

Labor and Delivery Pain

Pain during labor and delivery is caused by uterine contractions, dilation of the cervix, and distention of the perineum. Somatic and visceral afferent sensory fibers from the uterus and cervix travel with sympathetic nerve fibers to the spinal cord. These fibers pass through the paracervical tissue with the uterine artery and then through the inferior, middle, and superior hypogastric plexuses to the sympathetic chain. Nerve impulses from the uterus and cervix enter the spinal cord through the 10th, 11th, and 12th thoracic nerves (T-10 to T-12) and the first lumbar nerve (L-1). Somatic perineal pain impulses travel to the 2nd, 3rd, and 4th, sacral nerves primarily via the pudendal nerve (S-2 to S-4). Pain in the perineum, caused by distention of the vagina, perineum, and pelvic floor muscles, is associated with descent of the fetus into the pelvis during the second stage of labor, and with delivery (Fig. 16–3).

Somatic pain differs from visceral pain, with very different types of pain sensation. Somatic pain such as incisional pain or second-stage labor pain is well localized and typically described as sharp. Visceral pain such as uterine contractions in the first stage of labor is poorly localized, and usually described as dull but intense aching.

Reflex Effects

Along with the subjective sensation of pain, nerve impulses of labor pain lead to stimulation of the autonomic nervous system and create reflex cardiovascular, respiratory, endocrine, and musculoskeletal effects.

Cardiovascular

Cardiovascular sympathetic nervous system stimulation can increase cardiac output by as much as 60% during labor (10). Tachycardia, hypertension, and, rarely, arrhythmias may develop. Uterine blood vessels are particularly sensitive to sympathetic tone. Shnider and colleagues demonstrated that experimentally produced pain can reduce uterine blood flow in pregnant ewes by release of endogenous catecholamines (11). Fetuses of mothers who receive no analgesia have been found to have higher concentrations of lactate and lower pH in their blood at birth (12).

Respiratory

Hyperventilation is a common response to painful stimulation. Arterial carbon dioxide is severely reduced

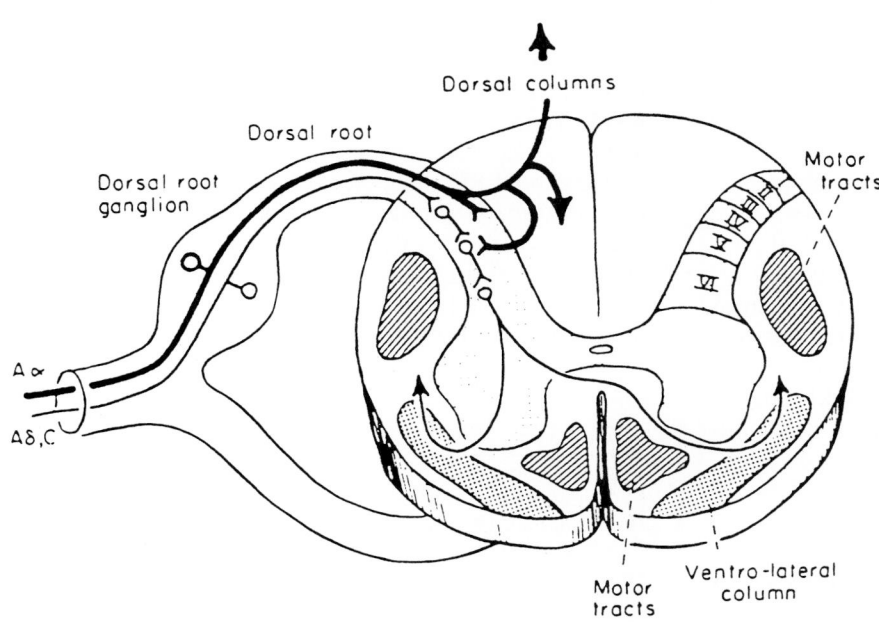

FIG. 16–3. Schematic cross section of the spinal cord. Aδ and C fibers make multiple synaptic connections in the dorsal horn. Cell bodies in lamina V send axons to the ipsilateral and contralateral ventral column to make up the spinothalamic system. (Reprinted by permission from Bonica JJ. The nature of pain of parturition. *Clin Obstet Gynecol* 1975;2:511.)

in some patients during labor. The resultant respiratory alkalosis may compromise fetal oxygenation by shifting the maternal oxyhemoglobin dissociation curve to the left (13), leading to decreased oxygen release at the placenta (14).

Endocrine

Catecholamines are released in large amounts during painful uterine contractions. Endogenous pain-controlling substances, such as endorphins and enkephalins, also are released from the placenta, fetus, and CNS during labor (15).

Musculoskeletal

Maternal skeletal muscle expulsive efforts ("bearing down") may become an uncontrollable urge as a result of labor pain. Obstetric anesthesia has been shown to control these reflexes, decreasing metabolic acidosis that results from excessive muscular efforts and halting involuntary expulsive efforts before cervical dilation is complete. Uncontrolled bearing down before the cervix is dilated can result in cervical edema, inhibiting further cervical dilation and resulting in the need for cesarean delivery.

PHYSIOLOGIC CHANGES DURING PREGNANCY WITH ANESTHETIC IMPLICATIONS

During pregnancy, labor, and delivery, women undergo fundamental changes in anatomy and physiology as a result of altered hormonal activity, biochemical changes associated with increasing metabolic demands of a growing fetus, placenta, and uterus, and mechanical displacement by an enlarging uterus. Maternal ventilation, oxygen uptake, metabolic rate, and cardiac output increase while peripheral vascular resistance significantly decreases, in part because of the low-pressure arteriovenous shunting of the uteroplacental circulation. As the uterus enlarges, the diaphragm is pushed cephalad, the heart shifts leftward, and lumbar lordosis is exaggerated. The stomach, aorta, and vena cava are compressed, and the function of the gastroesophageal sphincter is altered, contributing to reflux. Increased respiratory drive and airway edema lead to subjective symptoms of breathlessness and frequent upper respiratory infections. Cardiovascular changes result in lower extremity venous engorgement, which can cause hemorrhoids, varices, and ankle edema. Some normal physiologic changes have important implications for anesthetic administration.

Respiratory System

The neck, oropharyngeal soft tissue, and chest wall are affected by the weight gain that normally occurs during gestation. The vascularity of the respiratory tract mucosa increases, and capillaries engorge. Diaphragms elevate with cephalad pressure of the growing gravid uterus, and the chest wall diameter increases in the anteroposterior and transverse diameters. This results in the lung volume changes shown in Table 16–1.

Ventilation begins to increase significantly at about 8 weeks of gestation, most likely in response to progesterone sensitization of the respiratory center to carbon dioxide and to an increased metabolic rate. However, this increase surpasses the increase in body weight, basal metabolic rate, or oxygen consumption. Alveolar ventilation increases about 50%, primarily through increased tidal volume. Labor pain further increases ventilation. Oxygen consumption increases by about 60% in response to higher maternal metabolism and greater extraction in the uterus and placenta. The oxyhemoglobin dissociation curve shifts to the right during pregnancy, with P_{50} increasing from 26 to 30 mm Hg by term. This shift facilitates delivery of oxygen to the fetus. Airway resistance decreases 50% from the effects of progesterone on bronchial smooth muscle. Lung compliance remains unchanged, but chest wall compliance decreases.

Tracheal intubation can be difficult because of anatomic changes associated with pregnancy. These changes include weight gain with enlarged neck, breasts, and chest wall, impairing insertion of the laryngoscope, as well as airway edema, obstructing visualization of the larynx. Failed tracheal intubation is more common than in nonpregnant patients (16).

Airway manipulation requires care to prevent trauma and bleeding in the highly vascular airway mucosa, particularly the nasal airway, which is best avoided by not routinely using nasogastric tubes or nasal airways. Smaller endotracheal tubes may be required if the larynx is edematous, particularly in patients with severe preeclampsia.

Induction rate of inhalation anesthesia is increased in pregnant patients because of their decreased functional residual capacity and increased alveolar ventilation. In an analogous fashion, decreased oxygen reserve secondary to decreased FRC and increased oxygen uptake as a result of increased metabolic rate increase the risk of hypoxia and hypercarbia, which develop more rapidly during episodes of apnea, airway obstruction, or hypoventilation.

With increased alveolar ventilation, PCO_2 decreases to 30 mm Hg at term gestation; pH rises only to 7.44 since

TABLE 16–1. *Changes in pulmonary function in pregnancy*

Vital capacity (VC)	Unchanged
Expiratory reserve volume (ERV)	Decreased 20%
Residual volume (RV)	Decreased 20%
Functional residual capacity (FRC)	Decreased 20%
Inspiratory Capacity (IC)	Unchanged
Closing capacity (CC)	Unchanged

there is renal compensation to excrete HCO_3 (22 meq/L). In labor, hyperventilation during painful uterine contractions may result in hypoventilation and arterial hypoxemia between contractions.

Cardiovascular System

Hormonally induced increases in blood volume begin early in gestation and continue rapidly during the second trimester and more slowly during the remainder of gestation. Blood volume returns to normal baseline values within 2 weeks after an uncomplicated delivery.

Cardiac output increases early in gestation, most rapidly to about 35% to 45% above baseline during the second trimester, stabilizes until term gestation, when cardiac output increases substantially with labor contractions and maximally just after delivery with autotransfusion of blood from the contracting uterus. Functional flow murmurs are common in this hyperdynamic state.

Peripheral and pulmonary vascular resistance decrease significantly beginning early in gestation. Blood pressure decreases, accompanied by increased pulse pressure, as a result of the changes in peripheral vascular resistance and aortic compliance. Central venous pressures remain unchanged despite increased blood volume because the latter is accommodated by dilated pulmonary and peripheral vasculature and increased venous capacitance.

The heart shifts leftward from elevation of the left hemidiaphragm. Cardiac wall thickness and chamber volume increase. The ventricle hypertrophies and dilates, accommodating greater volume with the same preload and increasing cardiac output by increased rate, stroke volume, ejection fraction, and contractility.

Hypotension may occur in the supine position from aortocaval compression by the gravid uterus: significant aortoiliac artery compression occurs in 15% to 20% of parturients, and vena caval compression in all. Vena caval compression may contribute to lower extremity venous stasis, resulting in ankle edema and varices.

Physiologic dilutional anemia of pregnancy results from a greater increase in plasma volume than in RBC mass. Average blood loss at delivery is well tolerated because of the expanded blood volume. Average loss is 300 to 500 mL for vaginal delivery and 600 to 1,000 mL for cesarean section.

Venous compression by the gravid uterus diverts some blood returning from the lower extremities through the internal vertebral venous plexus and the azygos and epidural veins, increasing the likelihood of epidural venous puncture with epidural or spinal techniques. Full supine positioning is avoided for pregnant women during anesthetic administration in the second and third trimesters. Anesthetic techniques that interfere with increased sympathetic tone will further compromise compensatory mechanisms for vena caval compression induced by supine positioning, potentially causing profound hypotension.

Gastrointestinal System

Gastric reflux is common during gestation. The stomach is displaced cephalad and anterior, and the pylorus is displaced cephalad and posteriorly by the gravid uterus. Gastric pressure is increased by the gravid uterus and by a lithotomy position. Gastrin plasma levels increase, probably by placental production, increasing gastric acidity. Increased progesterone and estrogen levels decrease lower esophageal sphincter tone, and progesterone inhibits plasma motilin. Gut motility and gastric emptying are considerably slowed by labor or opioid administration.

Beyond midgestation, women are at increased risk for pulmonary aspiration of acidic gastric contents because of decreased competence of the lower esophageal sphincter and delayed gastric emptying with onset of labor or opioid administration. This risk of aspiration is an important consideration for the method of induction of general anesthesia and airway management by anesthesiologists.

Hepatic, Hematologic, and Renal Systems

Hepatic function remains normal despite slight elevations in hepatic enzymes. Plasma protein concentrations decrease from dilution, although circulating amounts increase. The albumin/globulin ratio decreases, with a greater decrease in albumin than serum globulin concentration. Plasma levels of fibrinogen, factor VII, VIII, X, and XII increase. Hypercoagulability with increased thrombosis can develop, partially as a result of increased coagulation factors and platelets. Plasma cholinesterase levels decrease but rarely result in clinically important prolongation of metabolism of anesthetic agents or succinylcholine. Colloid osmotic pressure decreases further at delivery.

Ureters and renal pelves dilate from the 12th week of gestation to term as a result of mechanical obstruction by blood vessels and, later, by the gravid uterus. Renal blood flow (RBF) and glomerular filtration rate (GFR) increase. Renal threshold for glucose decreases, and tubular reabsorption is inadequate for increased GFR.

With elevations in RBF and GFR, normal values of creatinine are about 50% those of nonpregnant women. Electrolyte and fluid balance remain normal because of compensatory increases in RBF and GFR in response to increased tubular reabsorption. Minor glucosuria is common from the change in renal threshold and inadequate tubular reabsorption.

Nervous System

Neural sensitivity to and diffusion of local anesthetic agents increase during pregnancy, so that lower doses of agents produce neural blockade (17–19). This change is probably related to progesterone increase. In addition, engorgement of epidural veins decreases the size of the epidural and subarachnoid spaces and results in the extended distribution of administered spinal and epidural drugs compared with nonpregnant women.

The amount of inhaled halogenated agent required to produce anesthesia decreases 25% to 40% during pregnancy, an effect probably also related to progesterone (20–22).

Uterine Blood Flow

With uterine growth, blood flow increases to about 700 mL/min, which is about 10% of cardiac output at term gestation. About 80% of the uterine blood flow perfuses the intervillous space of the placenta, and 20% the myometrium. Uterine vasculature is not autoregulated and remains essentially maximally dilated under normal conditions during pregnancy. Although uterine arteries are capable of marked vasoconstriction in response to α-adrenergic agents, their sensitivity and response are reduced in pregnancy.

Uterine blood flow (UBF) will decrease in response to decreased uterine arterial blood pressure if there is systemic hypotension from shock, general, epidural, or spinal anesthesia. It also decreases with aortocaval compression or with increased uterine venous pressure resulting from vena caval compression in supine position or uterine contractions, particularly uterine tetany, from oxytocin hyperstimulation or abruption.

ANALGESIC TECHNIQUES FOR LABOR AND VAGINAL DELIVERY

The pain of labor is highly variable and is described by many women as severe. Analgesia for labor and childbirth reduces the psychological or subjective component of pain. Factors that influence the perception of labor pain include duration of labor, use of oxytocin, parity, participation in childbirth preparation classes, fear and anxiety about childbirth, attitudes and experience of pain, and coping mechanisms. Labor analgesia may prevent reflex effects that can be deleterious for certain high-risk patients or for their fetuses, including those with severe preeclampsia, valvular heart disease, or myasthenia gravis. However, maternal request for pain relief is sufficient justification for administration of analgesics during labor. In no other circumstance would it be considered acceptable for a person to experience such severe pain when it could be safely managed under a physician's care (23).

The choice of analgesic technique resides primarily with the parturient. The medical condition of the parturient, stage of labor, condition of the fetus, and availability of qualified personnel also are factors. Many different techniques are used to alleviate labor and delivery pain. Analgesia refers to pain relief without loss of conscious-

ness; regional analgesia denotes partial sensory blockade in a specific area of the body, with or without partial motor blockade. Regional anesthesia is the loss of all sensation, motor function, and reflex activity in a specific area of the body. General anesthesia results in the loss of consciousness; goals for providing general anesthesia typically include hypnosis, amnesia, analgesia, and skeletal muscle relaxation. Of interest, agents that produce general anesthesia are not necessarily analgesic when administered in low concentrations.

Techniques for labor analgesia must be safe for mother and fetus and individualized to satisfy the analgesic requirement and desires of the parturient. They must accommodate the changing nature of labor pain and the evolving, varied course of labor and delivery whether it be spontaneous or instrumental vaginal delivery or cesarean delivery. Techniques available include nonpharmacologic techniques, administration of systemic medication, inhalation analgesia, and regional analgesia.

Nonpharmacologic Techniques: Psychological and Alternative Techniques

Psychological and alternative techniques for obstetric analgesia include hypnosis, natural childbirth as described by Dick-Read (8), the breathing techniques described by Lamaze (9) acupuncture, acupressure, the LeBoyer technique (24), transcutaneous nerve stimulation, hydrotherapy, biofeedback, and others.

Some techniques for nonmedicated labor analgesia may involve enhanced release of inhibitory neurotransmitters in the CNS, which attenuate the response to noxious stimuli, producing analgesia by descending modulation. Some of these techniques produce analgesia that is reversible with naloxone (25), implicating release of endorphins as part of their mechanism of action. Although these techniques can be effective for some pregnant women, and particularly for relatively low-intensity pain of short duration (26), they rarely provide intense analgesia for long periods. When used in conjunction with other forms of pain therapy, their effectiveness appears to be enhanced.

The breathing techniques of psychoanalgesia are designed to distract the parturient from her pain through focused exercises that minimize hyperventilation. However, some hyperventilating parturients lower their arterial carbon dioxide tensions to as low as 12 to 15 mm Hg, displacing their oxyhemoglobin dissociation curve to the left and interfering with placental oxygen exchange. Neonates of hyperventilating parturients are more acidotic than those of mothers who do not hyperventilate (27). The adverse effects of hyperventilation can be prevented with adequate obstetric analgesia. For example, fetal acid–base balance is better maintained during prolonged labor in patients who receive epidural anesthesia than in patients who receive either no analgesia or small doses of systemic narcotic drugs (28).

Psychoanalgesic techniques require a high level of personal concentration and are not entirely reliable or applicable to all deliveries. Unfortunately, some women who experience severe pain during parturition and require analgesia feel as if they have failed (29). Many women find labor more painful than anticipated (30,31). Nonetheless, the role of emotional support is important, as evidenced in observations of the positive impact of doumas providing continuous emotional support (32).

Systemic Medications

Systemic medications for labor and delivery are widely used but must be administered in limited doses because they readily cross the placenta and can depress the fetus. The use of sedative-hypnotics such as barbiturates, phenothiazine derivatives, hydroxyzine, benzodiazepines, or dissociative agents such as ketamine and scopolamine is uncommon, but the use of narcotic analgesics is more widespread. Narcotics are the most effective systemic medication for relief of pain. Excessive maternal sedation, maternal respiratory depression, loss of maternal protective airway reflexes, and the risk of neonatal depression limit the dose of narcotics safely administered for labor analgesia. The most commonly used narcotic analgesics in obstetrics are the synthetic opioids fentanyl, butorphanol, nalbuphine, and meperidine and the opiate morphine.

Sedatives and Tranquilizers

Sedatives and tranquilizers are administered to parturients to diminish the adverse motivational–affective component of labor pain. Examples of such drugs are barbiturates, phenothiazines, and benzodiazepines.

Secobarbital and pentobarbital have been used, although rarely in current practices. Because of their prolonged effects, their use is confined principally to facilitate maternal sleep in the early latent phase of labor, when delivery is unlikely before 12 to 24 hours. In some patients, barbiturates have an antianalgesic effect and may convert a minimally uncomfortable, controlled patient into a hyperventilating, confused, and unmanageable one.

Promethazine and propiomazine are phenothiazines. Hydroxyzine, although not a phenothiazine, has similar properties. These drugs are useful for relieving anxiety, modifying the response to painful stimulation, and potentiating the actions of narcotic analgesics. In addition, they are useful in controlling nausea and vomiting, which may be severe enough to produce maternal dehydration during labor. In the recommended dosages, these drugs appear to have minimal depressant effects on either mother or fetus, although they rapidly cross the placenta and may cause a decrease in beat-to-beat fetal heart rate variability (33).

Diazepam and midazolam are used as anxiolytic agents. They rapidly cross the placenta, yielding approximately equal maternal and fetal blood levels within minutes of IV administration (34). The neonate has a limited ability to excrete diazepam, so the drug and its active metabolite may persist in significant amounts for as long as a week (35). The use of benzodiazepines remains somewhat controversial, but they can reduce maternal anxiety, decrease narcotic dosage, and treat convulsions associated with local anesthetic toxicity or eclampsia. The drug may produce neonatal hypotonia, lethargy, and hypothermia when used in large maternal doses (30 mg) (36). Small doses (2.5 to 10 mg IV) produce minimal sedation and hypotonia in the neonate (37).

Dissociative Analgesia

The intramuscular or IV administration of low-dose ketamine (0.25 mg/kg) produces a state called dissociative analgesia. This state is characterized by good analgesia and amnesia, without loss of consciousness or protective airway reflexes (38). This is accompanied by a dreaming phenomenon, which may be unpleasant, but is minimized by coadministration of benzodiazepines. Used in divided doses totaling less than 1 mg/kg, ketamine can provide adequate analgesia for vaginal delivery and episiotomy repair. As the dose administered increases, airway protection is less insured. This agent is best reserved as a low-dose supplement to other techniques or for exceptional situations in which safer agents or techniques are contraindicated or where rapid control is required because mother's pain is inhibiting her cooperation in delivering a compromised fetus.

Narcotic Analgesics

The narcotic analgesics act by stimulating opiate receptors found in many locations throughout the CNS. More than one type of opiate receptor exists, each with particular drug affinities and responses (39). The majority of opiate receptors in the brain and spinal cord that produce analgesia are the μ-receptors (40). These receptors are also responsible for respiratory depression and may affect thermoregulation. κ- and δ-receptors are found primarily in the spinal cord and, when stimulated, seem to potentiate spinal analgesia (41). σ-Opiate receptors are found primarily in smooth muscle and are responsible for significant side effects of opiates such as nausea, vomiting, and urinary retention. Specificity of opiate receptors is not absolute, and most opiate or opioid agents bind to more than one receptor, but with variable affinities.

Neural transmission is altered by binding of opiate agonist agents, probably at synaptic junctions. Another class of opioid drugs binds to the receptor with high affinity but does not produce analgesia. These drugs are capable of displacing the agonist drugs from the receptor and reversing their effects and are known as narcotic antagonists (e.g., naloxone, naltrexone). A third class of agents interacts with the receptors and results in both agonist and antagonist activity. Unlike the pure antagonists, these drugs, with high receptor affinity, are capable of producing some analgesic effect (e.g., levallorphan, pentazocine, nalbuphine, and butorphanol). It is possible that receptor specificity is the explanation for the peculiar actions of the agonist–antagonist agents (42).

In general, all opioids, at equipotent doses, have similar effects on the fetus and newborn, crossing the placental barrier by passive diffusion. Although systemic opioids can alleviate labor pain, large doses are necessary to be effective, risking excessive maternal sedation, maternal respiratory depression, loss of protective airway reflexes, and newborn respiratory depression and impaired early breast-feeding and neurobehavior. In clinical use, large doses of opioids are avoided; the clinical doses used to relieve labor pain should not produce adverse effects on either mother or baby. All opioids readily cross the placental barrier and exert neonatal effects in normal doses, including decreased fetal heat rate variability. Normal doses also result in maternal side effects, including nausea, vomiting, pruritus, and decreased motility of the gastrointestinal system with delayed gastric emptying.

Intramuscular administration of opioids is technically easy but leads to uneven analgesia, the possibility of late respiratory depression, and profound neonatal effects if not properly timed (43). Intravenous administration is the most widely used technique to administer opioids in labor, with effects that are more predictable and doses more easily timed. However, achievement of a steady blood level of opiate sufficient to provide analgesia is difficult, with the parturient frequently suffering underdosage or, more rarely, overdosage. Continuous IV infusion of short-acting opiates such as alfentanil or self-administration of IV opiates may overcome this limitation. Patient-controlled analgesia (PCA) is a popular method of IV administration of these drugs because the patient usually titrates her own dose to the minimum required for analgesia, resulting in the lowest blood levels of opiates and, hence, considerably less placental transfer (44). Remifentanil, which is rapidly metabolized by nonspecific serum esterases, will possibly prove an effective opiate for continuous intravenous infusion, presuming the drug does not accumulate in the fetus.

The epidural injection of opiates alone is of limited utility for labor analgesia. Intraspinal opiates were demonstrated to produce profound analgesia in humans in 1979 (45,46). Shortly thereafter, several researchers attempted to apply this technique for the relief of labor pain. In one study, high doses (7.5 mg) of epidural morphine provided satisfactory but not excellent analgesia for 6 hours in the first stage of labor, whereas 2 or 5 mg produced barely satisfactory analgesia in fewer than onehalf of patients (47). Besides the inadequate analgesia, and the 1-hour delay in onset of relief, the side effect of pruritus was significant. When rapidly acting, lipid-soluble narcotics are administered alone into the epidural space, the analgesia achieved is equivalent to that from systemic administration (48) but inferior to that from dilute concentrations of local anesthetics and less effective for the somatic pain associated with the second stage of labor.

Subarachnoid (i.e., spinal) injections of fentanyl, meperidine, and sufentanil provide more potent analgesia than epidural or systemic administration. The effectiveness is less, and the duration shorter, than those provided by dilute solutions of local anesthetics for analgesia in the second stage (49). Reports of fetal heart rate changes after intrathecal fentanyl or sufentanil administration (50) may be related to rapid onset of analgesia and rapid decrease in circulating catecholamines, resulting in unopposed oxytocic effect on the uterus, increasing uterine tone, and decreasing uterine blood flow. This etiology is speculative by the author but supported by observed cases and case reports (51).

Systemic administration of opioids at doses safe for mother and newborn provides some analgesia but cannot substitute for the analgesia provided by regional anesthetic techniques. Systemic narcotics are recommended for administration in the smallest doses possible, minimizing any repeated dosing to avoid accumulation of drug and metabolites in the fetus. Narcotics are most useful in primiparae in early labor, as adjuncts to major regional anesthetics, and in multiparae with relatively short, predictable labors with minimal pain.

When administered into the epidural or intrathecal spaces, opioids can be useful primarily in the first stage of labor but do not provide adequate analgesia for the second stage of labor or for operative obstetric procedures. They have been most useful when coadministered into the epidural or intrathecal space with local anesthetics.

After maternal administration, the lipid-soluble, poorly ionized narcotic analgesics rapidly enter the fetal circulation, where they result in a dose-related respiratory depression. The degree of depression is a function of the dose, the timing, and the route of administration. Intramuscular administration is associated with the highest incidence of neonatal depression at 2 to 4 hours after injection. Intravenous or epidural injection produces peak neonatal depression at 30 to 60 minutes postinjection. In addition, some narcotics, most notably meperidine, have active metabolites that prolong their fetal effects far longer than the action of the parent drug.

If a neonate is suspected of narcotic-related depression, the administration of naloxone, 0.1 mg/kg IV or IM, will produce a reversal of the drug depression within 1 to 2 minutes and will last 1 to 2 hours. The indiscriminate use of naloxone in the immediate neonatal period should be discouraged, however, because neonatal cyanosis or sudden death has been reported with the use of narcotic antagonists in neonates of maternal drug abusers or in neonates whose respiratory depression was not narcotic-induced. Furthermore, neonatal depression is not likely to be caused by placental transfer of appropriate opioid doses in labor. When in doubt, the neonate should be ventilated by bag and mask as an alternative which may be safer than narcotic antagonist administration. However, when required, narcotic-induced depression can outlast the action of naloxone, so it may be necessary to repeat the dose if naloxone is used.

Inhalation Analgesia

An inhaled analgesic technique was first used by Simpson in 1847. The parturient inhaled subanesthetic concentrations of anesthetic agents. Techniques involving inhalation of low concentrations of halogenated agents such as halothane, methoxyflurane, and isoflurane are no longer used.

Some birthing centers use nitrous oxide, usually administered by a device that delivers 50% oxygen and 50% nitrous oxide, a concentration that, when used alone, is insufficient to result in unconsciousness or loss of protective airway reflexes. Appropriate equipment and fully trained personnel are essential to ensure safety by limiting the nitrous oxide concentration, avoiding administration of a hypoxic mixture, avoiding coadministration of other agents, and minimizing risk of maternal loss of protective airway reflexes.

Nitrous oxide provides a satisfactory degree of pain relief for some parturients and can be used during the first, second, or third stage of labor, alone or to supplement a regional block or local infiltration. Nitrous oxide is administered continuously or intermittently before each uterine contraction to provide pain relief, although continuous inhalation is more reliable. Use of 50% nitrous oxide in a supervised fashion is safe in that it is rapid-acting, has rapidly reversible effects, causes minimal maternal cardiovascular or respiratory depression, does not affect uterine contractility, and does not cause neonatal depression, regardless of duration of maternal nitrous oxide administration. However, 50% nitrous oxide is a weak analgesic.

Regional Analgesia

Regional analgesia, including epidural, spinal, and combined spinal–epidural techniques, has become the most widely used regional block for labor analgesia. Lumbar sympathetic blocks and paracervical blocks are rarely performed for labor analgesia, but pudendal blocks are used for delivery. Regional blocks involve administration of local anesthetic; some include coadministration

of narcotic analgesics. The future will see administration of other agents that modulate interneuronal communication (52,53).

Local Anesthetics

Many chemical compounds have nerve conduction-blocking properties, including anesthetic vapors, alcohols, barbiturates, meperidine, diphenhydramine, phenothiazines, propranolol, some antiarrhythmic agents, and biotoxins such as saxitoxin and tetrodotoxin. However, the clinically useful compounds consist of aromatic and amine moieties linked by an intermediate chain containing an ester or amide group. These agents, known as local anesthetics, reversibly block impulse conduction in sensory and motor nerves. They have chemical structures of secondary or tertiary amines, which are weak bases, and are marketed as the HCl salts to achieve aqueous solubility.

Local anesthetics produce impulse block in neural conduction by inhibition of voltage-gated sodium channels in the nerve membrane. Uncharged local anesthetic molecules are lipid soluble in free-base form and diffuse through connective tissue, nerve sheaths, and axonal membranes. Inside the axon, in the axoplasm, local anesthetic molecules are protonated to a charged cationic form, then bind receptors from the intracellular side of the nerve membrane, physically or ionically blocking sodium ion movement through sodium channels. Sodium conductance is rendered insufficient for the axonal membrane to reach its threshold potential for activation, and impulse conduction is thereby blocked.

The ester-linked local anesthetics such as procaine, chloroprocaine, and tetracaine are rapidly metabolized by plasma cholinesterase, limiting risk of maternal toxicity and placental drug transfer (54). The amide-linked local anesthetics (lidocaine, bupivacaine, ropivacaine) are slowly degraded by the liver and bind to plasma protein. Ropivacaine, the newest of these local anesthetics, is the S-enantiomer of 1-propyl-2′,6′-pipecoloxylidide, an amino amide-type local anesthetic agent with a chemical formula similar to that of bupivacaine and mepivacaine. The significant difference from the other two congener local anesthetic agents is that ropivacaine is an S-isomer rather than a racemic mixture. Vascular absorption of local anesthetics limits the safe dose that can be administered; toxic plasma concentrations produce neurologic toxicity (seizures) or cardiovascular toxicity (myocardial depression, ventricular arrhythmias). Accidental intravascular injection has resulted in maternal mortality.

Mild overdose of local anesthetic is exhibited by the neonate as a decrease in neuromuscular tone, similar to that seen with magnesium. If a direct intravascular or intrafetal injection of local anesthetics occurs, significant depression can develop, exhibited by bradycardia, ventricular arrhythmias, and severe cardiac insufficiency with acidosis.

Epidural Analgesia and Combined Spinal–Epidural Analgesia

In many centers, epidural analgesia for labor and delivery is the technique of choice. The parturient remains awake, alert, without sedative side effects; maternal catecholamine concentrations are reduced (55); hyperventilation is avoided (56); cooperation and capacity to participate actively during labor are facilitated; and excellent, predictable analgesia can be achieved, superior to the analgesia provided by all other techniques.

The technique involves insertion of a specialized needle between vertebral spinous processes in the back, through the ligamentum flavum, into the potential epidural space, but not through the dura, which forms the perimeter of the intrathecal or subarachnoid space. The placement technique is tactile, using loss of resistance with an air- or saline-filled syringe. Once the needle is properly placed, a catheter is inserted through the needle and left in place, and the needle is removed. The catheter is secured for intermittent or continuous injections. Most commonly, the needle is inserted at the lumbar epidural level (L1-2, L2-3, or L3-4), but the technique for caudal epidural anesthesia is similar.

Epidural block can be performed early in labor when the patient requests analgesia, as soon as satisfactory progress of labor is established, usually when the cervix is dilated 4 to 5 cm in nulliparae or less in multiparae. During early labor, many anesthesiologists strive for a segmental block at T-10 to L-1 to provide analgesia for the pain of uterine contractions and cervical dilation. Later, a larger volume can be administered to provide perineal analgesia. Once the catheter is placed, analgesia may be attained and continued throughout the active phase of labor and delivery, and for operative anesthesia as well as postoperative analgesia.

The mechanism by which epidural injections of local anesthetic drugs produce analgesia is to decrease both the number and frequency of afferent nerve impulses in the vicinity of the spinal cord. Local anesthetics are most effective at reducing or eliminating somatic pain. An inevitable consequence of their action is also a decrease in efferent nerve activity, leading to motor blockade. The ideal choice of a local anesthetic for labor would be one that provides safe, effective analgesia and sensory blockade while preserving motor function. Bupivacaine and ropivacaine are the local anesthetics that provide maximum sensory block with the least motor block.

Local anesthetics are typically infused continuously after incremental bolus doses to produce reliable pain relief with similar or lower blood drug concentrations than result from repetitive boluses of the same drugs (57,58). Most important, the possibility of disastrous complications of total spinal anesthesia or massive intravascular injections with cardiovascular collapse is decreased. If an epidural catheter enters an epidural vein

during continuous infusion, the analgesia merely ceases without producing neurologic or cardiovascular toxicity (59). If the catheter enters the subarachnoid space instead, the level of sensory and motor blockade increases slowly without the sudden onset of complete subarachnoid blockade that may occur with bolus techniques (60).

The choice of drug for continuous epidural infusion includes dilute solutions of lidocaine, bupivacaine, ropivacaine, or chloroprocaine (61,62). The concentration and volume of the loading dose and of the infusion are quite variable. With higher concentrations, the density of the motor blockade increases. With larger volumes, a greater dermatomal spread of analgesia is achieved. Many practitioners routinely use reduced concentrations of local anesthetics and coadminister an opioid. Dilute solutions of local anesthetics minimize the motor blockade and preserve the perception of pelvic pressure with descent of the fetus. The administration of both agents results in an additive or synergistic effect (63). Some clinicians use extremely dilute concentrations of local anesthetics combined with an opioid and allow the parturient to ambulate if there is normal neuromotor function.

One variation of the lumbar epidural technique is the combined spinal–epidural. After placement of the epidural needle, but before insertion of the epidural catheter, a long spinal needle is passed through the indwelling epidural needle to puncture the dura, and a small dose of local anesthetic or opioid or both is administered. If opioid alone is administered, and the epidural catheter is not activated, analgesia without motor blockade or sympathectomy is achieved. This allows the parturient to ambulate safely. The side effects of pruritus, nausea, and vomiting are usually not substantial with lipid-soluble opioids such as fentanyl or sufentanil, but the first-stage analgesia is limited to about 2 hours in the early active phase of labor and is rarely effective for the second phase.

If small doses of local anesthetics are administered through the spinal needle, a segmental analgesia results more rapidly than by epidural administration. The epidural placement of the catheter allows continuation of the segmental analgesia initiated by the spinal technique.

Contraindications and Complications of Regional Anesthesia

Certain conditions make regional anesthesia contraindicated, such as patient refusal, infection at the needle insertion site, coagulopathy, or hypovolemic shock.

Infrequent but occasionally life-threatening complications can result from administration of regional anesthesia. The most serious complications are from accidental intravenous or intrathecal injections. Measures to minimize complications include aspiration of the needle or catheter for presence of CSF or blood and use of test doses while observing for signs and symptoms of intrathecal or intravascular administration. Intrathecal administration is identified by the rapid onset of block, consistent with spinal but not epidural anesthesia. Intravascular injection can be identified by infusing a low dose of epinephrine, which will cause maternal tachycardia. Other techniques for test dosing have been described (64). After careful test dosing, administration of the therapeutic dose as incremental, fractionated doses are important to ensure safety.

Hypotension secondary to sympathetic blockade is the most common complication of major regional block for parturition (65). Prophylactic measures include adequate hydration, avoidance of the supine position, and displacement of the uterus off the abdominal great vessels. Treatment includes uterine displacement, IV fluids, and administration of vasopressor such as ephedrine. If treated promptly, maternal hypotension does not result in fetal depression or neonatal morbidity. Other relatively frequent complications of epidural analgesia include headache from CSF leakage after accidental dural puncture. This occurs in fewer than 1% to 2% of cases and can be conservatively treated by bed rest, palliated by theophylline or caffeine administration, or definitively treated by autologous epidural blood patch.

The most profound, immediate complications of regional anesthesia are intravenous injection of local anesthetic or an accidental high or total spinal block. High blood concentrations of local anesthetics can result in neurologic symptoms including drowsiness, lightheadedness, tinnitus, circumoral paresthesias, metallic taste in the mouth, slurred speech, blurred vision, or convulsions, unconsciousness, and cardiovascular depression or arrest. High blood concentrations result from overdosage or accidental intravascular injection. If either occurs, treatment includes immediately securing the airway, oxygen administration, with controlled ventilation if necessary, and administration of a small dose of barbiturates or benzodiazepine to terminate any convulsive activity. Aortocaval compression must be avoided, and the cardiovascular system supported with fluids and vasoactive drugs if required. Resuscitation and support of the mother will reestablish uterine blood flow and allow adequate fetal oxygenation and excretion of local anesthetic (66). Unless the mother cannot be resuscitated, delivery of the fetus should be delayed because the neonate has an extremely limited ability to excrete local anesthetics and may have prolonged convulsions (67). Measures that minimize the likelihood of accidental intravascular injection include careful aspiration before injection, test dosing, and administration of therapeutic doses in an incremental fashion.

An excessive level of neural blockade as either high or total spinal blockade may develop during initiation of a spinal, epidural, or caudal block or during an infusion, leading to blockade of the motor nerves to the respiratory muscles. Treatment includes endotracheal intubation and ventilation with oxygen. Maternal circulation must be supported by avoiding aortocaval compression and administration of additional fluids and vasopressors, if needed.

In any situation of maternal cardiac arrest with unsuccessful resuscitation, consideration must be given to urgent delivery of the fetus. When delivered within 5 minutes of maternal arrest, the chances for infant survival are maximized. Evacuation of the uterus relieves aortocaval compression, improving the chances of maternal resuscitation (68,69).

Long-term maternal neurologic injury secondary to epidural analgesia is rare. Epidural hematoma and abscess are also very rare complications. Spinal and epidural techniques are contraindicated in patients with bleeding disorders or those who are anticoagulated. Epidural techniques with resulting sympathectomy are contraindicated for septic parturients but are safe for women with chorioamnionitis.

An increase in core body temperature that results from epidural analgesia for labor is influenced by several factors, including duration, ambient temperature, and, possibly most important, the presence of shivering. During the first 5 hours of epidural analgesia, a significant rise in body temperature does not occur (70). If labor is prolonged, temperature increases at about 0.10°C/hr and may reach 38°C by 12 hours (71) in as many as 20% of parturients. The temperature rise is not associated with a change in WBC, is not associated with an infectious process, and does not require treatment. Although a temperature elevation is usually mild, it may be clinically difficult to distinguish the increase secondary to the epidural from one signaling the onset of maternal chorioamnionitis. The etiology of this epidural-induced temperature rise remains uncertain; epidural anesthesia for nonobstetric surgery or cesarean section is associated with hypothermia. Both imbalance between reduced heat loss and heat production and impairment of regulation have been postulated.

The impact of epidural analgesia on the progress of labor, length of the second stage, and requirement for instrumental vaginal delivery or for cesarean delivery has been the subject of controversy. Small randomized prospective studies have shown conflicting results, but they all suffered from flawed design (72). Women who are more likely to experience severe pain select epidural analgesia and independently are more likely to require obstetric intervention for delivery for obstetric reasons (73). The real controversy is whether a causal relationship exists between labor epidural analgesia and cesarean delivery. Retrospective population-based studies suggest that introduction of epidural analgesia or increase in its use for labor analgesia in a hospital practice does not increase the cesarean delivery rate (74–77). It is possible that some cesarean deliveries are avoided by epidural analgesia, such as delivery of the breech presenting fetus, atraumatic delivery of the preterm fetus, delivery of twins, and vaginal delivery after a previous low transverse cesarean delivery. If epidural analgesia relates to any increase in the cesarean delivery rate among nulliparous women, the increase must be extremely small in clinical settings.

Careful monitoring of the fetus and uterine tone is important during administration of regional analgesia. Fetal bradycardia from uterine hyperactivity and decreased uteroplacental perfusion is most likely due to the rapidly decreasing maternal catecholamines after administration of analgesia (78). When hypertonicity does not resolve spontaneously and promptly, nitroglycerin is effective in relaxing the uterus (79).

Spinal Analgesia

Spinal anesthesia is typically administered only immediately before delivery. A small dose of a local anesthetic dissolved in a hypertonic dextrose solution is injected into the subarachnoid space, typically with the patient in the sitting position. Injection produces immediate analgesia of the lumbosacral nerve roots and provides excellent anesthesia for episiotomy, forceps application, and delivery.

Paracervical and Lumbar Sympathetic Blocks

Paracervical block is occasionally used by obstetricians to provide pain relief in the first stage of labor. The technique involves submucosal administration of local anesthetics immediately lateral and posterior to the uterocervical junction, blocking transmission of pain impulses at the paracervical ganglion. Analgesia is not as profound as with epidural or spinal regional block, and the duration of analgesia is short (45 to 60 minutes), but complications and side effects of epidural analgesia such as hypotension, hypoventilation, and motor blockade are avoided. Convulsions may occur as a result of systemic absorption of local anesthetic. When using paracervical block, the obstetrician should closely monitor the fetus, inject just beneath the vaginal mucosa after a negative aspiration for blood, and allow a 5-minute interval between injection of the two sides. 2-chloroprocaine is often used for this block because it undergoes rapid intravascular hydrolysis and has a very short intravascular half-life, should there be accidental intravascular or fetal injection. Lidocaine is also used, but bupivacaine is contraindicated.

Paracervical block is associated with a relatively high incidence of fetal bradycardia. The etiology of this association is unclear but probably involves decreased uterine blood flow secondary to the vasoconstrictor properties of local anesthetics. Fetal bradycardia is usually limited to less than 15 minutes, and treatment is supportive, with lateral positioning and oxygen administration to the mother. Because the bradycardia is associated with increased neonatal morbidity and mortality, this block is used infrequently and should be avoided in patients with evidence of uteroplacental insufficiency or nonreassuring fetal heart rate patterns (80).

Pudendal Block

Pudendal block is performed by obstetricians using a transvaginal technique, guiding a sheathed needle to the vaginal mucosa and sacrospinous ligament just medial and posterior to the ischial spine. The technique provides analgesia for vaginal delivery or uncomplicated instrumental vaginal delivery, but the rate of failure is high, and the block that is achieved is often inadequate for forceps application, examination of the cervix and upper vagina, or manual exploration of the uterus after delivery. In many centers, this technique is reserved for occasions when epidural or spinal blocks are unavailable. Complications include vaginal lacerations, systemic local anesthetic toxicity, ischiorectal or vaginal hematoma, and fetal injection of local anesthetic.

Perineal Infiltration

Infiltration of the perineum is commonly performed by obstetricians to provide anesthesia for episiotomy and its repair. Care is taken to avoid injection into the fetal scalp and to limit the total dose. This is a common and useful technique alone or in conjunction with other regional blocks.

General Anesthesia

General anesthesia is very rarely used for vaginal delivery, but when it is, the patient's airway must be secured by placement of a cuffed endotracheal tube to prevent pulmonary aspiration of gastric contents.

ANESTHESIA FOR CESAREAN DELIVERY

Although the majority of cesarean deliveries are performed with regional anesthesia, sometimes the severity of the fetal condition requires the use of general anesthesia for its rapidity. In some conditions, regional anesthesia is contraindicated. In preparation for any cesarean delivery, women should receive a nonparticulate oral antacid to increase gastric pH; some anesthesiologists routinely coadminister an agent to accelerate gastric emptying, such as metoclopramide and an H_2-receptor antagonist such as raniditine to reduce acid production.

Epidural Anesthesia

Epidural anesthesia is an excellent choice for surgical anesthesia when an indwelling, functioning epidural catheter is already in place for labor analgesia. It is also ideal for patients with preeclampsia or cardiac disease who would not tolerate the sudden onset of a sympathectomy. The volume and concentration of local anesthetic agents used for surgical anesthesia are larger than those used for labor analgesia, but the techniques of catheter placement and test dosing are similar, as are the potential complications. Typically, the anesthesiologist attempts to provide a dense block from the T-4 level to the sacrum. This may not always alleviate the visceral pain associated with peritoneal manipulation, and adjuvant drugs may be necessary.

Spinal Anesthesia

For the patient without an epidural catheter, spinal anesthesia is the most common regional anesthetic technique used for cesarean delivery. The block is technically easier than epidural blockade, more rapid in onset, and more reliable in providing surgical anesthesia from the midthoracic level to the sacrum. The incidence of post–dural-puncture headache has decreased with the introduction of noncutting, pencil point spinal needles. Hypotension is more likely and more profound with spinal anesthesia than with epidural anesthesia because the onset of the sympathectomy is more rapid. Prehydration, avoiding aortocaval compression, and aggressive use of ephedrine result in a more favorable outcome.

Local Anesthesia

Although cesarean delivery can be performed after local anesthetic infiltration, it is not without considerable discomfort and risks the possibility of local anesthetic overdose. However, in circumstances of acute fetal distress, where a regional block is inadequate, induction of general anesthesia is considered dangerous or an anesthesiologist is unavailable, local infiltration can be helpful to deliver the baby emergently.

General Anesthesia, Intravenous Agents, Neuromuscular Blocking Agents, and Adjuvant Medications

General anesthesia is used for cesarean section typically when regional anesthesia is contraindicated or for emergencies because of its rapid, predictable action.

Before induction of general anesthesia, it is important to neutralize the stomach pH with a nonparticulate antacid, denitrogenate the lungs, ("preoxygenation") to increase the oxygen reserve, and use cricoid pressure to occlude the esophagus and decrease the likelihood of passive regurgitation and pulmonary aspiration. General anesthesia is then induced in a rapid fashion, using intravenous agents to induce unconsciousness and paralysis and to facilitate tracheal intubation. Cricoid pressure is maintained until proper placement of the cuffed endotracheal tube is confirmed.

After induction, anesthesia is maintained by administration of a combination of inhaled nitrous oxide, an inhaled potent halogenated agent, sedative-hypnotics, and narcotic analgesics. Intravenous skeletal muscle relaxants are administered to decrease muscle tone to facilitate surgery.

For some patients with morbid obesity and those with suspected abnormal or difficult airway, rapid-sequence induction of general anesthesia is contraindicated. Alternatives include awake intubation or use of regional anesthetic techniques. For the unexpected difficult airway in which intubation fails, and ventilation by mask is difficult, a predetermined protocol is crucial to ensure maternal and fetal safety, including immediate availability of emergency airway equipment, including a laryngeal mask airway and equipment to perform a cricothyroidotomy.

Induction Agents

A number of different agents are used by anesthesiologists to induce unconsciousness rapidly. Among the most commonly used are thiopental, ketamine, and, to a lesser extent, etomidate and propofol. Each agent represents a different biochemical class, and each has specific advantages and cardiovascular effects.

Sodium thiopental is a highly lipid-soluble, protein-bound barbiturate that rapidly crosses the placenta and produces a dose-related global depression in the neonate. It is the most commonly used agent for induction of general anesthesia in obstetrics. Intravenous administration of an appropriate dose renders the patient unconscious within 30 seconds of its administration but has no significant clinical impact on neonatal well-being. Although the drug undergoes hepatic oxidation to inactive, water-soluble metabolites, patients will awaken within 15 minutes of initial administration as a result of rapid redistribution of the drug from vessel-rich organs, including the brain, to muscle and fat. The neonatal depression that occurs with higher dosages of barbiturates must be treated by cardiorespiratory support until the neonate excretes the drug, a process that may take up to 2 days (81).

Ketamine is a structural analog to phencyclidine, which is more lipid-soluble and less protein-bound than thiopental. These characteristics lead to rapid brain uptake and subsequent redistribution, with awakening caused by redistribution to peripheral tissue rather than by metabolism. Ketamine is biotransformed in the liver to active metabolites, such as norketamine. In contrast to thiopental, ketamine increases arterial pressure, heart rate, and cardiac output by central stimulation of the sympathetic nervous system. Doses above those appropriate for induction of unconsciousness can increase uterine tone and decrease uterine arterial perfusion. In low doses, ketamine has profound analgesic effects but has been associated with undesirable psychotomimetic side effects such as bad dreams, which can be lessened by coadministration of benzodiazepines. This agent may be a more appropriate choice than thiopental for the parturient who is actively hemorrhaging.

Etomidate contains a carboxylated imidazole ring, which provides water solubility in acidic solutions and lipid solubility at physiologic pH. Like thiopental, it has a rapid onset of action because of its high lipid solubility, and its redistribution results in a relatively short duration of action. Although etomidate has minimal effects on the cardiovascular system, unlike thiopental and ketamine, it is painful on injection and induces extrapyramidal motor activity.

Propofol is a diisopropylphenol, available as a 1% aqueous solution in an oil-in-water emulsion containing soybean oil, glycerol, and egg lecithin. Because this preparation is preservative-free, it cannot be kept in syringes on standby for potential emergencies. For an elective cesarean section, this highly lipid-soluble drug results in a rapid onset of action similar to that of thiopental, with a very short initial distribution half-life, but with less hangover effect than thiopental. It has not been demonstrated to be superior to thiopental in maternal or neonatal outcome.

Nitrous Oxide

Nitrous oxide is a colorless, nonexplosive, nonflammable, and nearly odorless inorganic gas. Because it has relatively low solubility in blood, inhalation of nitrous oxide has both a rapid effect and a rapid elimination. Biotransformation is limited to less than 0.1%, by reductive metabolism in the gastrointestinal tract by anaerobic bacteria. Nitrous oxide inhaled at 50% is a weak analgesic, with relatively minor cardiovascular effects.

Halogenated Hydrocarbons

Halothane, enflurane, isoflurane, sevoflurane, and desflurane are all halogenated hydrocarbons that differ in chemical composition, physical properties, biotransformation, potencies, and rates of uptake and elimination. In clinical use, these volatile liquid agents are delivered by specialized vaporizers; the inhaled concentrations are carefully titrated because of their relatively profound cardiovascular effects, which differ. Uptake of these agents depends on a number of factors, including the inspired concentration, the rate of ventilation, cardiac output, solubility of the agent in blood, alveolar blood flow, and the partial pressure difference between alveolar gas and venous blood. These agents are important components of general anesthesia for cesarean section because, without them, the incidence of maternal recall of intraoperative events is unacceptably high (82,83).

Placental transfer of inhalation agents is rapid because these are nonionized, highly lipid-soluble substances of low molecular weight. The fetal concentrations of these agents depend directly on the concentration and duration of anesthetic in the mother. If excessive concentrations of anesthetic are given for inordinately long times, neonatal anesthesia, evidenced by flaccidity, cardiorespiratory depression, and decreased tone, may be anticipated (84). By itself, general anesthesia will not cause neonatal asphyxia. If neonatal depression is caused by transfer of anesthetic drugs, the infant is merely lightly anesthetized and should respond easily to simple treatment measures. Neonatal treatment should include effective ventilation to allow pulmonary excretion of the inhaled anesthetic; cardiopulmonary resuscitation is rarely necessary. Rapid improvement of the infant should follow ventilation; if not, a search for other causes of depression is indicated.

Clinicians often mistakenly ascribe the use of general anesthesia in conditions of fetal "distress" to causing the depressed or asphyxiated neonate. General anesthesia may have been employed in these cases because it is the most rapidly acting anesthetic to achieve an emergency cesarean delivery for fetal distress. The induction-to-delivery interval, by itself, is not an important determinant of neonatal asphyxia unless it includes a prolonged uterine incision-to-delivery interval, when uterine blood flow may decrease and contribute to fetal asphyxia.

Narcotic Analgesics

The narcotic analgesics have been described in a previous section. During typical general anesthesia for cesarean delivery, opioids are administered after the baby is delivered to avoid placental transfer to the neonate.

Neuromuscular Blocking Agents

Succinylcholine remains the skeletal muscle relaxant of choice for obstetric anesthesia because of its rapid onset and short duration of action. This depolarizing neuromuscular blocking agent is normally hydrolyzed in maternal blood by the enzyme pseudocholinesterase and therefore does not interfere with fetal neuromuscular activity. If the hydrolytic enzyme is present either in low concentrations (85) or in a genetically determined atypical form (86), prolonged maternal or neonatal respiratory depression secondary to muscular paralysis can occur.

Nondepolarizing neuromuscular blocking agents are titrated to the response of neuromuscular stimulation monitoring for continued neuromuscular blockade. Under normal circumstances, the poorly lipid-soluble, highly ionized, nondepolarizing neuromuscular blockers (e.g., d-tubocurarine, pancuronium, atracurium, vecuronium) do not cross the placenta in amounts significant enough to cause neonatal muscle weakness (87). This placental impermeability is only relative, however, and when large doses are given over long intervals, as in the treatment of maternal tetanus or status epilepticus, neonatal neuromuscular blockade can occur (88).

The diagnosis of neonatal depression secondary to neuromuscular blockade may be made on the basis of a maternal history of very prolonged administration of neuromuscular blockers or a history of atypical pseudocholinesterase, the present response of the mother to the drugs, and physical examination of the newborn. The paralyzed neonate will have normal cardiovascular function and, initially, good color but no spontaneous ventilatory movement, muscle flaccidity, and no reflex responses. The anesthesiologist can place a nerve stimulator on the neonate and demonstrate the classic signs of neuromuscular blockade (89). Treatment consists of respiratory support until the drug is excreted by the neonate, taking up to 48 hours. Reversal of nondepolarizing relaxants with cholinesterase inhibitors may be attempted (e.g., neostigmine, 0.06 mg/kg), but adequate respiratory support is the mainstay of treatment.

Adjuvant Medications

In addition to opioids, anesthesiologists may administer benzodiazepines, antiemetic agents, and other agents, but typically only after the baby is delivered and the cord is clamped. Rarely are these drugs administered before delivery in doses large enough that placental transfer results in a clinically important neonatal effect.

CONCLUSION

Maternal anesthetics may affect the fetus and neonate by diffusion from the maternal circulation to the fetal circulation, causing direct drug effects. These drugs are the same as those safely used for neonatal surgery and, properly managed, are not toxic to the neonate. The protein- or tissue-binding properties of anesthetic agents as well as serial dilutions and restricted doses usually protect the fetus from the effect of maternal anesthetics.

An anesthetic drug or technique may affect the fetus indirectly, producing the signs and symptoms of fetal distress and asphyxia; treatment is based on restoring placental exchange, perfusion, and gas exchange. Any technique that results in maternal hypotension or hypoxia will decrease maternal–fetal oxygen exchange and produce fetal distress. Examples of this phenomenon include overdose with narcotics or inhalation analgesia, total spinal anesthesia, or maternal aspiration of gastric contents.

Uteroplacental blood flow depends on an adequate maternal cardiac output and perfusion pressure. Anesthetic techniques that interfere with maternal cardiovascular integrity can produce fetal depression by increasing uterine arterial tone (e.g., use of drugs with primarily α-adrenergic activity), decreasing cardiac output (e.g.,

decreased venous return caused by vena cava compression by the gravid uterus; venodilation and bradycardia secondary to the sympathectomy accompanying spinal or epidural block; myocardial depression following overdose of potent inhalation anesthetic or local anesthetic drug); or by decreasing systemic blood pressure (e.g., sympathectomy from high spinal or epidural anesthesia).

An increase in uterine muscular tone can decrease uteroplacental perfusion by impeding venous outflow from the intervillous space (90). High levels of local anesthetics (e.g., after intravascular injection) or of α-adrenergic vasopressors may produce increased myometrial tone and fetal distress, particularly when combined with oxytocin stimulation.

In general, modern techniques of obstetric analgesia for labor and anesthesia for instrumental vaginal delivery or cesarean delivery are safe and effective for the mother and safe for the fetus and neonate. Administration of analgesics and anesthetics by skilled clinicians who observe appropriate precautions and understand the physiologic changes in pregnancy is necessary. Skillful labor analgesia, coupled with emotional support for the parturient, may not only reduce maternal stress but decrease intrapartum stress for the fetus as well (91,92).

ACKNOWLEDGMENT

The author gratefully acknowledges and appreciates the efforts of John Stephen Naulty, author of the predecessor to this chapter, parts of which have been incorporated into this chapter.

REFERENCES

1. *Genesis* 3:16.
2. Hingson RA, Edwards WB. Continuous caudal anesthesia: an analysis of the first ten thousand confinements thus managed with the report of the authors' first thousand cases. *JAMA* 1943;123:538–546.
3. Apgar V. A proposal for a new method of evaluation of the newborn infant. *Curr Res Anesth Analg* 1953;32:260–267.
4. Marx GF, Orkin LR. Physiological changes during pregnancy. *JAMA* 1958;19:258.
5. Shnider SM. Clinical and biochemical studies of cyclopropane analgesia in obstetrics. *Anesthesiology* 1963;24:11.
6. Bonica JJ, ed. *Obstetric analgesia and anesthesia.* Philadelphia: FA Davis, 1967.
7. Shnider S, Levinson G, eds. *Anesthesia for obstetrics, 3rd ed.* Baltimore: Williams & Wilkins, 1993.
8. Read GD. *Childbirth without fear.* New York: Harper, 1944.
9. Lamaze F. *Painless childbirth: Psychoprophylactic method* (Celestin LR, trans). London: Burke, 1956.
10. Ueland K, Hansen J. Maternal cardiovascular dynamics: II. Posture and uterine contractions. *Am J Obstet Gynecol* 1969;103:1.
11. Shnider SM, Wright RG, Levinson G, et al. Uterine blood flow and plasma norepinephrine changes during maternal stress in the pregnant ewe. *Anesthesiology* 1979;50:524.
12. Myers RE. Maternal psychologic stress and fetal asphyxia: a study in the monkey. *Am J Obstet Gynecol* 1975;122:47.
13. Motoyama EK, Rivard G, Acheson F, et al. Adverse effect of maternal hyperventilation on the fetus. *Am J Obstet Gynecol* 1975;122:47.
14. Ralston DH, Shnider SM, De Lorimer AA. Uterine blood flow and fetal acid–base changes after bicarbonate administration in the pregnant ewe. *Anesthesiology* 1974;40:348.

15. Gintzler AR. Endorphin-mediated increases in pain threshold during pregnancy. *Science* 1980;210:193.

16. Samsoon GLT, Young JRB. Difficult tracheal intubation: a retrospective study. *Anaesthesia* 1987;42:487.

17. Datta S, Lambert DH, Gregus J, et al. Differential sensitivity of mammalian nerve fibers during pregnancy. *Anesth Analg* 1983;62:1070.

18. Butterworth JF, Walker FO, Lysak SZ. Pregnancy increases median nerve susceptibility to lidocaine. *Anesthesiology* 1990;72:962.

19. Dietz FB, Jaffe RA. Pregnancy does not increase susceptibility to bupivacaine in spinal root axons. *Anesthesiology* 1997;87:610.

20. Palahniuk RJ, Shnider SM, Eger EI II. Pregnancy decreased the requirement for inhaled anesthetic agents. *Anesthesiology* 1974;41:82.

21. Gin T, Chan MTV. Decreased minimum alveolar concentration of isoflurane in pregnant humans. *Anesthesiology* 1994;81:829.

22. Datta S, Migliozzi RP, Flanagan HL, Krieger NR. Chronically administered progesterone decreases halothane requirements in rabbits. *Anesth Analg* 1989;68:4.

23. American Society of Anesthesiologists and American College of Obstetricians and Gynecologists. *Pain relief during labor.* Chicago, IL: American Society of Anesthesiologists, 1992.

24. LeBoyer F. *Birth without violence.* London: Wildwood House, 1975.

25. Bragin RE. Opioid and catecholaminergic mechanisms of different types of analgesia. *Ann NY Acad Sci* 1986;467:331.

26. Doering SG, Entwisle DR. Preparation during pregnancy and ability to cope with labor and delivery. *Am J Orthopsychiatry* 1975;45:825.

27. Saling E, Ligidas P. The effect on the fetus of maternal hyperventilation during labour. *J Obstet Gynaecol Br Commonw* 1969;76:877.

28. Zador G, Nillson BA. Low dose intermittent epidural anesthesia with lidocaine for vaginal delivery. *Acta Obstet Gynecol Scand [Suppl]* 1974;34:17.

29. Melzack R, Taenzer P, Feldman P, Kinch RA. Labour is still painful after prepared childbirth training. *Can Med Assoc J* 1981;125:357.

30. Melzack R. The myth of painless childbirth. *Pain* 1984;19:321.

31. Wahl CW. Contraindications and limitations of hypnosis in obstetric analgesia. *Am J Obstet Gynecol* 1960;16:210.

32. Kennell J, Klaus M, McGrath S, et al. Continuous emotional support during labor in a US hospital. *JAMA* 1991;265:2197.

33. Powe CE, Kiem IM, Fromhagen C, et al. Propiomazine hydrochloride in obstetrical analgesia. *JAMA* 1962;181:290.

34. Cree IE, Meyer J, Hailey DM. Diazepam in labour. *Br Med J* 1973;4:251.

35. Scher J, Hailey DM. The effects of diazepam on the fetus. *J Obstet Gynaecol Br Commonw* 1972;79:635.

36. Cohen S. Inhalation analgesia and anesthesia for vaginal delivery. In: Snider SM, Levinson G, eds. *Anesthesia and obstetrics, 3rd ed.* Baltimore: Williams & Wilkins, 1993:194.

37. McAllister CB. Placental transfer and neonatal effects of diazepam when administered to women just before delivery. *Br J Anaesth* 1980;52:423.

38. Galloon S. Ketamine for obstetric delivery. *Anesthesiology* 1976;44:522.

39. Yaksh AR. Opioid receptor systems and the endorphins: a review of their spinal organization. *J Neurosurg* 1987;67:157.

40. Yaksh TL. Spinal opiate analgesia: characteristics and principles of action. *Pain* 1981;11:293.

41. Schmauss C, Yaksh TL. *In vivo* studies on spinal opiate receptors mediating antinociception. *J Pharmacol Exp Ther* 1983;228:1.

42. Bullingham RE, McQuay HJ, Moore RA. Clinical pharmacokinetics of narcotic agonist–antagonist drugs. *Clin Pharmacokinet* 1983;8:139.

43. Shnider SM, Moya F. Effects of meperidine on the newborn infant. *Am J Obstet Gynecol* 1960;89:1009.

44. McIntosh DG, Rayburn WF. Patient-controlled analgesia in obstetrics and gynecology. *Obstet Gynecol* 1991;78:1129.

45. Wang JK, Nauss LA, Thomas JE. Pain relief by intrathecally applied morphine in man. *Anesthesiology* 1979;50:149.

46. Behar M, Magora F. Olshwang D, Davidson JT. Epidural morphine in treatment of pain. *Lancet* 1979;1:527.

47. Hughes SC, Rosen MA, Shnider SM, et al. Maternal and neonatal effects of epidural morphine for labor and delivery. *Anesth Analg* 1984;63:319.

48. Camann WR, Denney RA, Holby ED, Datta S. A comparison of intrathecal, epidural, and intravenous sufentanil for labor analgesia. *Anesthesiology* 1992;77:884.

49. Honet JE, Arkoosh VA, Norris MC, et al. Comparison among intrathecal fentanyl, meperidine, and sufentanil for labor analgesia. *Anesth Analg* 1989;69:122.

50. Cohen SE, Cherry CM, Holbrook RH, et al. Intrathecal sufentanil for labor analgesia—sensory changes, side effects, and fetal heart rate changes. *Anesth Analg* 1993;77:1155.

51. Friedlander JD, Fox HE, Cain CF, et al. Fetal bradycardia and uterine hyperactivity following subarachnoid administration of fentanyl during labor. *Reg Anesth* 1997;22:378.

52. Eisenach JC, De Kock M, Klimscha W. Alpha-adrenergic agonists for regional anesthesia. *Anesthesiology* 1996;85:655.

53. Bouaziz H, Tong C, Eisenach JC. Postoperative analgesia from intrathecal neostigmine in sheep. *Anesth Analg* 1995;80:1140.

54. O'Brien JE, Abbey V, Hinsvark O, et al. Metabolism and measurement of 2-chloroprocaine, an ester-type local anesthetic. *J Pharm Sci* 1979;68:75.

55. Shnider SM, Abboud TK, Artal R, et al. Maternal catecholamines decrease during labor after lumbar epidural anesthesia. *Am J Obstet Gynecol* 1983;147:13.

56. Levinson G, Shnider SM, DeLorimer AA, et al. Effect of maternal hyperventilation on uterine blood flow and fetal oxygenation and acid–base status. *Anesthesiology* 1974;40:340.

57. Rosenblatt R, Wright R, Denson D, et al. Continuous epidural infusions for obstetric analgesia. *Reg Anaesth* 1983;8:10.

58. Hicks JA, Jenkins JG, Newton MC, et al. Continuous epidural infusion of 0. 075% bupivacaine for pain relief in labour: a comparison with intermittent top-ups of 0.5% bupivacaine. *Anaesthesia* 1988;43:289.

59. Dathis F, Macheboeuf M, Thomas H, et al. Epidural analgesia with a bupivacaine–fentanyl mixture in obstetrics: comparison of repeated injections and continuous infusion. *Can J Anaesth* 1988;35:116.

60. Li DF, Rees GA, Rosen M. Continuous extradural infusion of 0.0625% or 0.125% bupivacaine for pain relief in primigravid labour. *Br J Anaesth* 1985;57:264.

61. Abboud TK, Afrasiabi A, Sarkis F, et al. Continuous infusion epidural analgesia in parturients receiving bupivacaine, chloroprocaine, or lidocaine: maternal, fetal, and neonatal effects. *Anesth Analg* 1984;63:421.

62. Chestnut DH, Bates JN, Choi WW. Continuous infusion epidural analgesia with lidocaine: efficacy and influence during the second stage of labor. *Obstet Gynecol* 1987;69:323.

63. Chestnut DH, Owen CL, Bates JN, et al. Continuous infusion epidural analgesia during labor: a randozmized double-blind comparison of 0.0625% bupivacaine/0.0002% fentanyl versus 0.125% bupivacaine. *Anesthesiology* 1988;68:754–759.

64. Leighton BL, Gross JB. Air: an effective indicator of intravenously located epidural catheters. *Anesthesiology* 1989;71:848.

65. Rosenblatt R, Wright R, Denson D, et al. Continuous epidural infusions for obstetric analgesia. *Reg Anaesth* 1983;8:10.

66. Morishima HO, Adamsons K. Placental clearance of mepivacaine following administration to the guinea pig fetus. *Anesthesiology* 1967;28:343.

67. Ralston DH, Shnider SM. The fetal and neonatal effects of regional anesthesia in obstetrics. *Anesthesiology* 1978;48:34.

68. Lee RV, Rodgers BD, White LM, Harvey RC. Cardiopulmonary resuscitation of pregnant women. *Am J Med* 1986;81:311.

69. American Heart Association. Special resuscitation situations. *JAMA* 1992;268:2242.

70. Mercier FJ, Benhamou D. Hyperthermia related to epidural analgesia during labor. *Int J Obstet Anesth* 1997;7:19.

71. Lieberman E, Lang JM, Frigoletto F, et al. Epidural analgesia, intrapartum fever, and neonatal sepsis evaluation. *Pediatrics* 1997;99:415.

72. Thorp JA, Hu DH, Albin RM, et al. The effect of intrapartum epidural analgesia on nulliparous labor: A randomized, controlled, prospective trial. *Am J Obstet Gynecol* 1993;169:851.

73. Wuitchik M, Bakal D, Kipshitz J. The clinical significance of pain and congitive activity in latent labor. *Obstet Gynecol* 1989;73:35.

74. Gribble RK, Meier PR. Effect of epidural analgesia on the primary cesarean rate. *Obstet Gynecol* 1995;86:783.

75. Iglesias S, Burn R, Saunders LD. Reducing the cesarean section rate in a rural community hospital. *Can Med Assoc J* 1991;145:1459.

76. Socol ML, Garcia PM, Peaceman AM, Dooley SL. Reducing cesarean births at a primarily private university hospital. *Am J Obstet Gynecol* 1993;168:1748.

77. Lagrew DC, Morgan MA. Decreasing the cesarean section rate in a private hospital: Success without mandated clinical changes. *Am J Obstet Gynecol* 1996;174:184.

78. Friedlander JD, Fox HE, Cain CF, et al. Fetal bradycardia and uterine hyperactivity following subarachnoid administration of fentanyl during labor. *Reg Anesth* 1997;22:378.

79. Segal S, Csavoy AN, Datta S. Placental tissue enhances uterine relaxation by nitroglycerin. *Anesth Analg* 1998;86:304.

80. Thiery M, Vroman S. Paracervical block analgesia during labour. *Am J Obstet Gynecol* 1972;113:988.

81. Fox FS, Smith JB, Namba Y, et al. Anesthesia for cesarean section. *Am J Obstet Gynecol* 1979;133:15.

82. Tunstall ME. The reduction of amnesic wakefulness during caesarean secton. *Anaesthesia* 1979;34:316.

83. Schultetus RR, Hill CR, Dharamay CM, et al. Wakefulness during cesarean section after anesthetic induction with ketamine, thiopental, or ketamine and thiopental combined. *Anesth Analg* 1986;65:723.

84. Moya F. Volatile inhalation agents and muscle relaxants in obstetrics. *Acta Anesthesiol Scand [Suppl]* 1966;25:368.

85. Shnider SM. Serum cholinesterase activity during pregnancy, labor and puerperium. *Anesthesiology* 1965;26:355.

86. Brada A, Haroun S, Bassili M, et al. Response of the newborn to succinylcholine injection in homozygotic atypical mothers. *Anesthesiology* 1975;43:115.

87. Kivalo I, Saaroski S. Placental transmission and foetal uptake of C-dimethyltubocurarine. *Br J Anaesth* 1972;44:557.

88. Older PO, Harris JM. Placental transfer of tubocurarine. *Br J Anaesth* 1968;40:459.

89. Ali HH, Savarese JJ. Monitoring of neuromuscular function. *Anesthesiology* 1976;45:216.

90. Vasicka A, Kretchmer H. Effect of conduction and inhalation anesthesia on uterine contractions. *Am J Obstet Gynecol* 1961;82:600.

91. Morishima HO, Pederson H, Finster M. The influence of maternal psychological stress on the fetus. *Am J Obstet Gynecol* 1978;131:286.

92. Jouppila R, Jouppila P, Hollmen A. Effect of segmental extradural analgesia on placental blood flow during normal labour. *Br J Anaesth* 1978;50:563.

PART THREE

Transition and Stabilization

CHAPTER 17

The Onset of Respiration

Nicholas M. Nelson

By the end of normal-term gestation, the fetus and its lungs are well prepared to assume responsibility for extrauterine gas exchange. The alveoli are developed by the 25th week, and, by the 35th week, the type II great alveolar pneumocyte has begun to produce adequate quantities of the surface-active material on which alveolar stability will later depend, once air breathing commences. *In utero,* the alveoli are open and stable at nearly the normal neonatal lung volume because they are "inflated" by a fetal lung liquid, probably produced by ultrafiltration of pulmonary capillary blood as well as secretion by alveolar cells (1).

The pulmonary and bronchial circulations are well developed and thoroughly admixed by multiple connections at the alveolar level. This combined circulation is characterized by high pressure and low flow because of a high degree of pulmonary vascular resistance, both passive and active. The passive resistance most likely relates to compression of pulmonary capillaries by the fetal lung liquid (2), but there is also a high degree of active vasomotor tone resulting from the hypoxic level (PO_2 of 25 mm Hg) of the pulmonary venous stream (3–6). This hypoxic increase in active pulmonary vasomotor tone is a dominant feature in the behavior of the pulmonary vasculature at all stages of development but is more active in the fetus because of a relatively much larger vascular muscle mass than that of the adult (7,8). These features are responsible for the key characteristic of the fetal circulation: pulmonary vascular resistance greatly exceeds systemic resistance (Table 17–1) and nearly 50% of the fetal cardiac output perfuses the placenta, whereas only 5% to 10% perfuses the lung (Tables 17–2 and 17–3). With the onset of inflation and ventilation of the lung at birth, these resistances will reverse, and it is the success of this reversal that principally determines the success of the cardiopulmonary adaptation to birth.

The neuromuscular controls of respiration are also laid down well before even premature birth. The fetus spends nearly 30% of its time engaged in a rapid, discoordinate form of "panting"—paradoxic motions of the chest and abdominal wall (9,10) associated with the rapid, irregular, and low-voltage electrocortical activity seen in rapid-eye-movement (REM), or "active," sleep (11,12). In the human fetus near term, as much as 600 mL of amniotic fluid per day is inhaled through such activity (13), and a lot is swallowed (14). These breathing movements can even modulate blood flow through the fetal ductus arteriosus (15). Thus, the "first breaths of life" are now, perhaps, an inaccurate label, albeit a dramatic underscoring of the events that mark the perinatal shift from placental to pulmonary gas exchange and from liquid to gaseous ventilation.

THE FIRST BREATHS

The passive phase of these events during vaginal birth is shown in Fig. 17–1, wherein the thoracic cage is compressed to pressures of 30 to 160 cm H_2O during passage through the birth canal, sometimes producing a forcible ejection of as much as 30 mL of tracheal fluid through the airways (16). The subsequent recoil of the chest wall after birth of the trunk may produce a small passive inspiration of air, perhaps accompanied by active glossopharyngeal forcing of some air into at least the proximal airways and introduction of some blood into pulmonary capillaries ("capillary erection") (17). Thus, an air–liquid interface is established within the larger airways of the lung, and with it are established the surface retractive forces that would tend to collapse the smaller airways and alveoli, were it not for the presence of a surface-active material in the alveolar lining layer.

N. M. Nelson: Department of Pediatrics, The Milton S. Hershey Medical Center, Hershey, Pennsylvania

TABLE 17–1. *Hemodynamic characteristics of the perinatal circulation*[a]

	Resistance (mm Hg × L^{-1} × kg × min)			Conductance (ml × kg^{-1} × min × mm Hg^{-1})		
	Fetal sheep	Neonatal sheep	Neonatal human	Fetal sheep	Neonatal sheep	Neonatal human
Pulmonary	530	85	140	1.9	11.8	7.1
Ductus	30	810		33.3	1.2	
Systemic	170	220	300	5.9	4.5	3.3

[a]Data from refs. 176–182.

TABLE 17–2. *Distribution of cardiac output*[a]

	Full-term fetal lamb			Human	
	Resistance (mm Hg/ml/kg/min)	Conductance (ml/kg/min/mm Hg)	F_{CO}	Fetus F_{CO}	Adult F_{CO}
Vital organs					
Brain	3.3	0.3	0.03	0.14	0.14
Heart	2.5	0.4	0.04	0.02	0.05
Lung	2	0.5	0.05	0.1	1
Placenta	0.25	4	0.4	0.33	0
Metabolic organs					
Liver	0.56	1.8	0.18		
Gut	2	0.5	0.05	0.08	0.23
Spleen	5	0.2	0.02	0.02	
Kidney	5	0.2	0.02	0.05	0.22
Adrenal				0.04	
Carcass	0.27	3.7	0.37		
Bone					0.14
Muscle					0.18
Skin					0.04

[a]Values calculated from assumed mean blood pressure of 55 mm Hg and data from refs. 183–188.

TABLE 17–3. *Organ blood flow*[a]

Tissue	Fetal sheep (ml/kg body weight/min)	Fetal human (ml/kg body weight/min)	Fetal sheep (ml/100 g tissue/min)	Fetal human (ml/100 g tissue/min)	Adult human (ml/100 g tissue/min)	
					Rest	Maximum
Vital organs						
Brain	16.5	51	132	25	50	130
Heart	22	7.3	291	165	70	400
Lung	27.5	36.3	126			
Placenta	220	120	130	11		
Metabolic organs						
Liver	99		20		50	250
Gut	27.5	29	69	101	40	200
Spleen	11	7.3	240			
Kidney	11	18.2	173	155	400	550
Adrenal		14.5		340		
Carcass	204		26		2.5	260
Bone					3	15
Muscle					3	60
Skin					10	150
Total cardiac output (both ventricles)	550	363				

[a]Data from refs. 183–187 and 189.

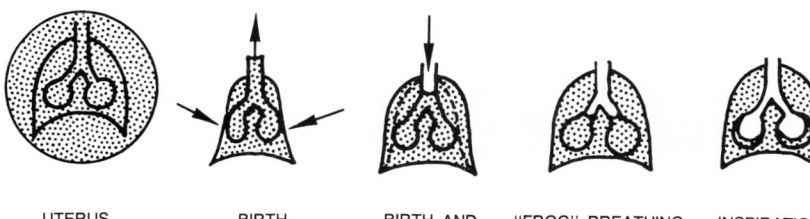

UTERUS   BIRTH CANAL   BIRTH AND RECOIL   "FROG" BREATHING CAPILLARY ERECTION   INSPIRATION

FIG. 17–1. Mechanical events of the first breaths. (From ref. 209.)

The functional life cycle of this surface-active material (18) is shown in Fig. 17–2 (19). The effective spreading and stabilization of the phospholipid (principally dipalmitoyl lecithin) monolayer has now come to be understood as the special purview of several lung-specific proteins. Of these surfactant proteins (Table 17–4), SP-A, SP-B, and SP-C are especially concerned with secretion and metamorphosis of the surface-active material from its intracellular storage sites (the lamellar bodies) to the tubular myelin of the hypophase, en route to the phospholipid interface. At that interface, an interaction of charges among the basic arginine and lysine residues of SP-B apparently helps to resist surface tension by increasing the lateral stability of the phospholipid monolayer (20). Thus, SP-B is clearly the lung-specific protein that is most critical to surfactant function (21). The critical concentration of surfactant in the lung liquid necessary to lower surface tension is about 3 mg/mL (22), but much higher concentrations appear necessary for alveolar stability in the premature infant (18). It appears that the respiratory distress syndrome may involve some sort of difficulty in the movement of phospholipid into tubular myelin, a process apparently facilitated by SP-A and SP-B (23,24).

The first opening of the alveoli (and lung) will be made easier if some fetal lung liquid is retained in at least the smaller airways of the lung before the "first" active breaths are taken (25) (Fig. 17–3). The reason for this is that inflation of the lung by air from the totally collapsed and gas-free state (dashed line) requires the exertion of considerable distending pressure across the lung—10 cm H_2O pressure is shown here, but levels up to 80 cm H_2O are not uncommon for the first full expansion—so that the spontaneous occurrence of alveolar rupture in term infants with healthy lungs becomes understandable. Note that "inflation" with liquid (solid line) requires rather less force because of the lack of an air–liquid interface. Note also that the deflation curve in air is not superimposable on its inflation curve ("hysteresis") because mobilization

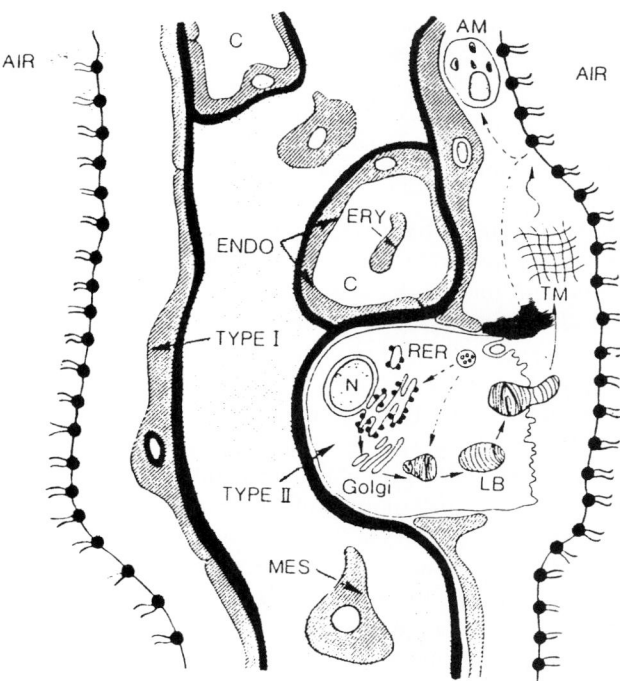

FIG. 17–2. Schematic cross-section of an alveolar wall. Surface-active material is a translation product that moves from the rough endoplasmic reticulum (RER) to storage in the lamellar bodies (LB) before being excreted into the hypophase as tubular myelin (TM), a process requiring lung-specific surfactant proteins (SP-A, SP-B, SP-C). The monolayer–air interface is indicated by the two-tailed hydrophobic ends of the phospholipid molecules, whose orientation is stabilized by SP-B. TYPE I, type I pneumocyte; TYPE II, type II pneumocyte; ENDO, endothelial cell; MES, mesenchymal cell; ERY, erythrocyte; C, capillary; N, nucleus; AM, alveolar macrophage. (From ref. 19.)

TABLE 17–4. Pulmonary surfactant proteins[a]

	SP-A	SP-B	SP-C	SP-D
Chromosome number	10	2	8	
Gene				
Length (kilobases)	5	6	3	
Content (exons)	11	11		
Translation product				
Weight (kilodaltons)	26	40	20	
Length (amino acids)	248	381	197	
Monomer				
Mass (kilodaltons)	28	9	4	43
Length (amino acids)		79	35	
Polarity	Hydro-philic	Hydro-phobic	Hydro-phobic	Hydro-philic
Function				
Feedback inhibition	+			
SAM ≥ monolayer	+	+		
Stabilize monolayer		+		

[a]Data from refs. 23 and 190.

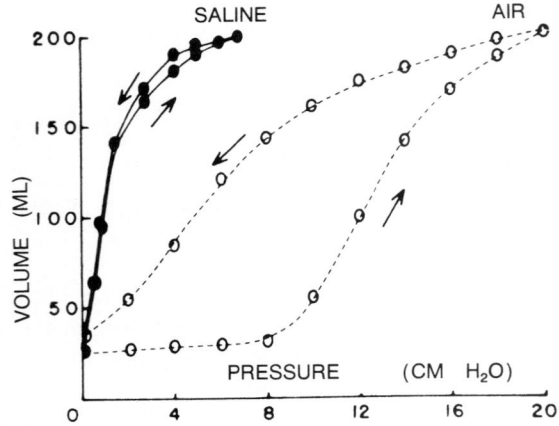

FIG. 17–3. Pressure–volume curves after air versus liquid expansion of the lung. (From ref. 210.)

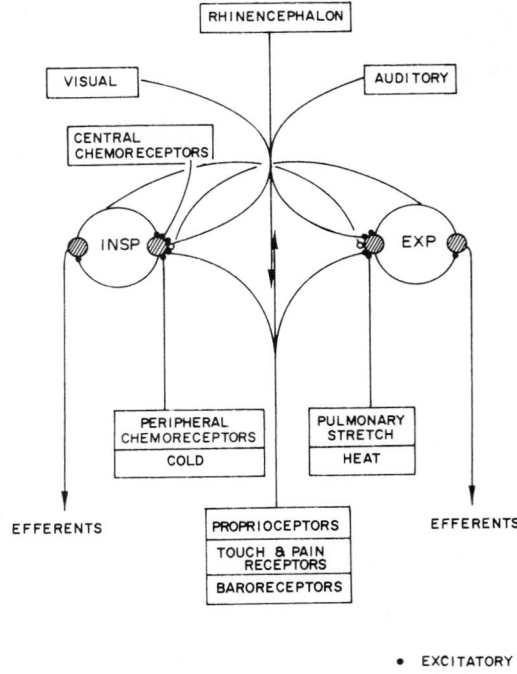

FIG. 17–4. Hypothetical functional organization of the respiratory center. EXP, expiration; INSP, inspiration. (Adapted from ref. 211.)

and orientation of alveolar surfactant molecules during deflation decrease alveolar surface tension as the alveolar surface contracts. Thus, the transpulmonary (alveolus to intrapleural space) distending pressure required to maintain lung volume at 30 mL diminishes from 10 to nearly 0 cm H_2O.

STIMULI FOR BREATHING

The precise reason or reasons for the first extrauterine inspirations will probably remain somewhat obscure because the unfamiliar stimuli to which the newborn infant is suddenly subjected are multiple: cold, light, noise, gravity, and pain, all in addition to the hypercapnea, respiratory acidosis, and hypoxia (collectively called asphyxia) that result from normal labor and its accompanying intermittent restriction of maternal placental perfusion.

The possible interplay of these stimuli around the respiratory center is shown in Fig. 17–4. The animal fetus at term has been demonstrated to be responsive to all these stimuli, although there are certain inconsistencies. Thus, the fetal carotid body (the peripheral chemoreceptor) responds to hypoxia and to hypercapnia (particularly oscillatory) (26), and neuronal traffic from these influences is regularly recordable along the carotid sinus nerve (27). Moreover, although the acidity of the fetal cerebrospinal fluid, like that of the adult, appears to be regulated at pH levels lower than those of blood, the fetal central chemoreceptor responds but poorly to the normal ventilatory drive of cerebrospinal fluid acidosis (28). Throughout all these observations has been noted the fact that the animal fetus will not breathe when warm and submerged, despite the presence of chemical stimuli for respiration, whereas when chilled and exposed, the fetus will breathe, despite the lack of chemical stimuli for respiration. The possibility thus arises of a well-tuned fetal respiratory center, quite responsive to the usual chemical

stimuli, that is repressed *in utero* but derepressed by delivery (29).

The unaroused (repressed?) fetus is apneic and appears to have its respiratory rhythm generator switched off in expiration; that is, the inspiratory neurons are inhibited, and the expiratory neurons are in tonic discharge (30). In this state, the respiratory centers appear unresponsive to chemical or sensory stimuli. This refractory state can result from vagal (pulmonary stretch afferents) (31) or superior laryngeal (laryngeal taste afferents) (32,33) discharge in states of experimental manipulation, but in the normal fetus it may more likely represent the influence of prostaglandins, particularly PGE_2 (34). In any case, states of fetal arousal (such as REM sleep) appear to be linked, possibly through the reticular formation, to a rhythmic, alternating discharge of inspiratory and expiratory neurons. The accentuation of fetal hypoxia by disruption of placental gas exchange during normal birth produces a gasping respiratory effort (35) with resultant improved cerebral oxygenation, accompanied by decreasing tonic discharge of expiratory neurons. These effects, coupled with the general sensory arousal of birth, are evidently sufficient to restore the inherent rhythmicity of discharge in the respiratory centers (36).

Figure 17–4 represents imaginary cross-connections that could explain these phenomena of possible interaction. This interactional concept portrays the inspiratory and expiratory centers as mutually inhibitory and, moreover, affected by neighboring neuronal "traffic" from both above and below (37). Thus, the general "tone" of the respiratory neurons may well be enhanced or facilitated by nonrespiratory environmental stimuli such as heat or cold, pain, change in position or pressure, noise, and light.

PULMONARY ADAPTATION

In any case, the first active breaths of air, once taken and sustained, set in motion a nearly inexorable chain of events that:

1. Converts the fetal to the adult circulation.
2. Empties the lung of liquid.
3. Establishes the neonatal lung volume and the characteristics of pulmonary function in the newborn infant.

These events are outlined in Fig. 17–5 and are analyzed separately (although they occur concurrently) in the remainder of this chapter. The upper left-hand corner of Fig. 17–5 is a reprise of the events diagrammed in Fig. 17–1. Air entry into the respiratory system establishes the lung retractive forces of surface tension (Fig. 17–3), with the consequent development of negative intrapleural and interstitial pressure, because the overlying chest wall resists collapse. These events, along with the increase in alveolar oxygen tension, are solidly established fact and are indicated as such by the solid boxes of Fig. 17–5 (less well-established events are indicated by broken-line boxes). The final and most dramatic events in the sequence are the great increases in blood and lymph flow through the lung that follow the onset of ventilation.

As lung liquid is ejected from the airways and alveoli, retractive forces become established, hydrostatic alveolar pressure on the pulmonary capillaries decreases, and these compressible vessels with tone open the "sluice gate" of the "alveolar waterfall" of blood flow through the lung (38,39). Moreover, the increasing pulmonary venous oxygen tension of the air-breathing newborn serves to decrease active vasomotor tone in the precapillary pulmonary arterioles under the influence of the endothelial relaxation factor, nitric oxide (NO) (40–42). Thus, for both reasons, intraluminal hydrostatic capillary pressure (P_c) rises as pericapillary interstitial (alveolar) pressure (P_{if}) decreases and Starling's equilibrium is perturbed, so that capillary fluid tends to transude into the interstitium (43,44), and alveolar fluid may well also be directly absorbed into the interstitial spaces at the alveolar corners (45). Starling's equilibrium is displayed as:

$$\text{Fluid transfer} = k[(P_c - \pi_{pl}) - (P_{if} - \pi_{if})]$$

where k is the filtration constant (relating to pore size), π_{pl} is plasma osmotic pressure, and π_{if} is interstitial osmotic pressure. Positive values for fluid transfer indicate transudation, and negative values indicate fluid absorption.

In the newly born lung, these events are marked by a decrease in total plasma volume, which reaches its nadir at 2 to 8 hours after birth, and by a dramatic increase in lung lymph drainage, beginning promptly on ventilation and subsiding by about 6 hours of age (46). During this

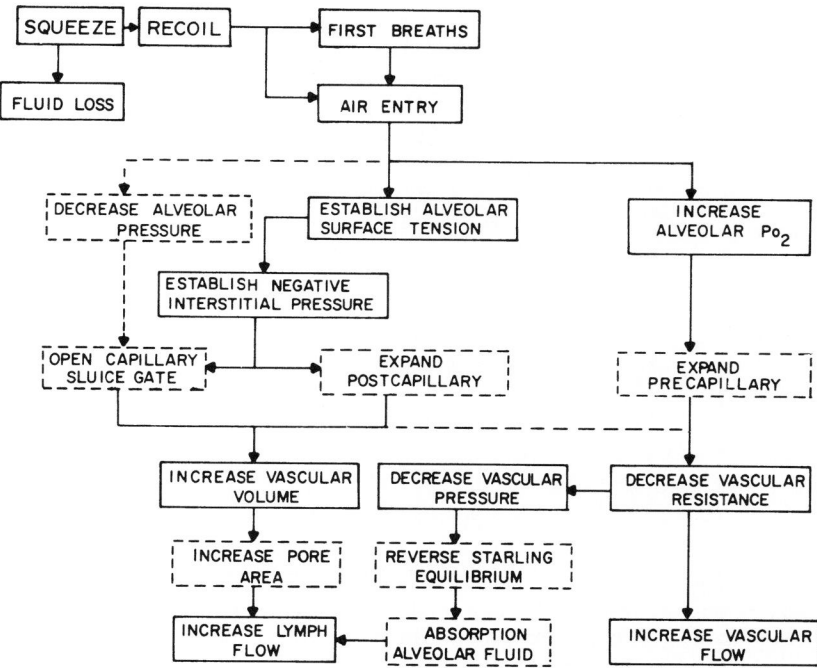

FIG. 17–5. The sequence of events following the onset of ventilation. (From ref. 209.)

early period after birth, lymphatic distension in the lung has been demonstrated both histologically (47) and radiologically (48), but the role of atrial natriuretic factor in these fluid movements is uncertain (49). It is of obvious clinical interest that infant rabbits delivered by cesarean section and immature lamb fetuses are both slow to clear their lung liquid—the former presumably denied the thoracic squeeze of vaginal birth, and the latter influenced by higher alveolar surface tensions because of lack of adequate alveolar surface-active material (50).

Infants born by cesarean section, especially where not preceded by labor, are less asphyxiated and less energized by "surges" of cortisol and catechols (51–53) than are their vaginally delivered cohorts; their lungs are wetter as well (54–57), although cesarean birth is not prerequisite to "transient tachypnea" of the newborn (clinically ascribed to slow clearance of fetal lung liquid) (58).

CIRCULATORY ADAPTATION

The magnitude of the passive and active increase in pulmonary blood flow following inflation and ventilation of the lung is shown in the experimental data of Fig. 17–6. If the lung is inflated from the fetal state and ventilated with a gas mixture that does not change the fetal composition of the blood gases (approximately pH 7.35, PCO_2 45, PO_2 25), an increase in pulmonary vascular conductance (decrease in resistance) can be achieved, as shown by the increasing flow–pressure slopes of the two right-hand curves in Fig. 17–6. This increase in conductance is most likely caused by the expansion of collapsible pulmonary capillaries (as already mentioned) as well as those vessels that are anatomically "tethered" to the pulmonary parenchyma. Then, as the blood-gas composition is changed by an increase in PO_2 and a decrease in

PCO_2 (similar to ventilation with air), further increases in vascular conductance are achieved, as shown in the left-hand pair of curves in Fig. 17–6.

The decrease in pulmonary vascular resistance thus set in motion (59,60), combined with the increase in peripheral vascular resistance that follows increasing oxygenation, the loss of the umbilical circulation, and the cold shock of birth, leads to closure of the foramen ovale within minutes of birth (Fig. 17–7). The ductus arteriosus, however, remains open for some hours, and, because systemic resistance is now higher than pulmonary resistance (the reverse of the fetal circumstance), blood flow through the ductus also reverses, now passing left to right. This is the "transitional" phase of the perinatal circulation, during which there may be reversion to the fetal pattern at any time that pulmonary vascular resistance should again rise higher than peripheral vascular resistance (61). During this phase, there is also a considerable increase in the volume load presented to the left ventricle because of the vast increase in left ventricular input (i.e., pulmonary venous return) (62). The ductus arteriosus constricts under the influence of prostaglandins interacting with rising oxygen tension in the blood coursing through it (63,64). This constriction decreases luminal blood flow, with resultant ischemia of the inner muscle wall and diminished responsiveness to prostaglandins (65). The involutional process normally begins at about 4 to 12 hours postnatally and is completed by around 24 hours of age (66).

These events are diagrammed in Fig. 17–8, along with blood flow data (in mL/kg per minute) taken from experiments in fetal sheep. In this diagram, the ventricles are shown as (electric) parallel generators with diodes

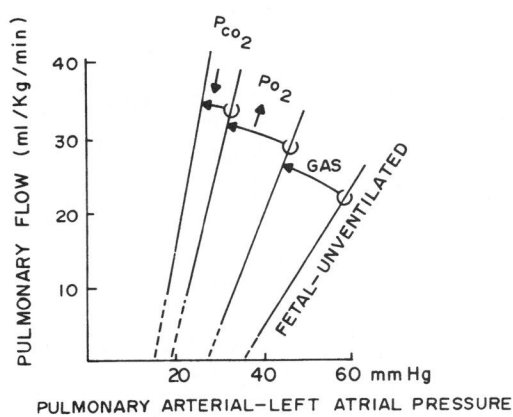

FIG. 17–6. Pulmonary vascular conductance increases with the onset of ventilation. Separate curves depict the contributions of gaseous inflation, increased PO_2 and decreased PCO_2. (Adapted from ref. 212.)

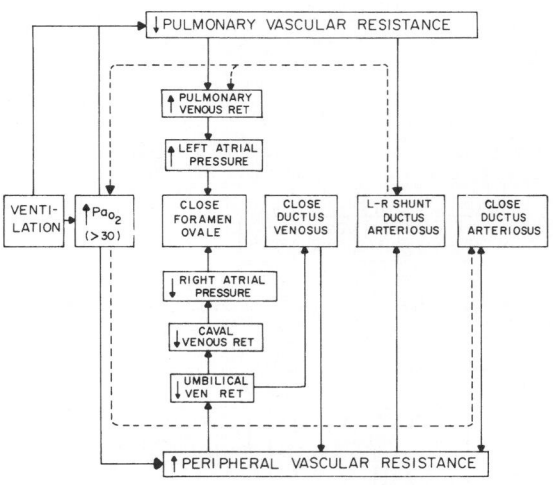

FIG. 17–7. Conversion from the perinatal to the transitional and neonatal circulations, following the onset of ventilation. L-R, left-to-right; RET, return; VEN, venous. (From ref. 209.)

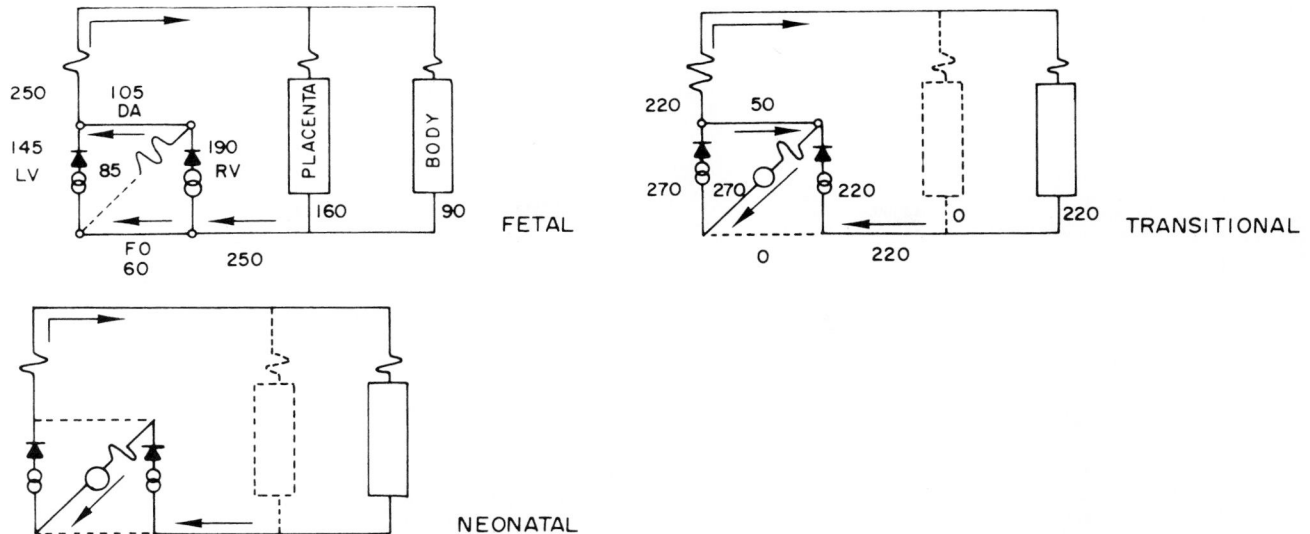

FIG. 17–8. Stages in the conversion of the perinatal circulation. Numbers refer to blood flow in mL/kg/min. LV, left ventricle; DA, ductus arteriosus; FO, foramen ovale; RV, right ventricle. (From refs. 209, 213.)

(valves) to direct the flow of blood (as a diode directs the flow of electrons). The electrical symbol for resistance indicates relative resistances in the pulmonary and systemic circuits. The large circle in the center of the pulmonary circuit represents the expanding and established alveolus. The diagrammatic sequence makes obvious the conversion of the central circulation from that of two ventricles connected in parallel circuits, where volume loads may be unequal, to a connection in series, where the right ventricular output must equal left ventricular input (and, thus, output), except for some small amount of blood stored in the "capacitance vessels" (capillaries and veins) of the pulmonary circulation.

Much of the increase in peripheral vascular resistance is a result of the cessation of the umbilical circulation. The umbilical arteries constrict vigorously under the influence of increased oxygenation and, particularly, in response to longitudinal stretch on the umbilical cord. The balance of umbilical arterial inflow to and umbilical venous outflow from the placenta, aided by the positive force of uterine contractions and the negative force of neonatal thoracic inspiration (67–69), determines the course of the transfusion of blood from the placenta to the infant, as shown in Fig. 17–9. The umbilical arteries close very rapidly, in advance of closure of the umbilical vein, resulting in an average net transfer of about 15 to 20 mL/kg of blood to the infant within 3 minutes if he or she is held below the introitus with the cord untouched.

Apart from those shown in Fig. 17–9 there are little human data to document these events, but those that are available are shown in Figs. 17–10 and 17–11. Measurements of output from both ventricles, together with appropriate pressure data, permit calculation of the resis-

tances shown in Fig. 17–10 (fetal data are taken from the sheep). The dominant events depicted include (from the top) the following:

1. The rise and subsequent fall in systemic resistance.
2. The vast decrease in pulmonary resistance.

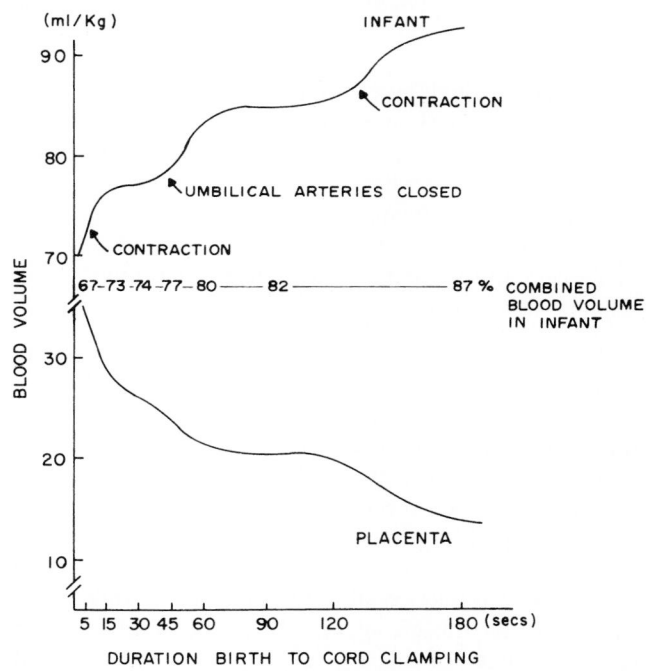

FIG. 17–9. The placental transfusion: sequence of events during the first 3 minutes of life. (From ref. 209.)

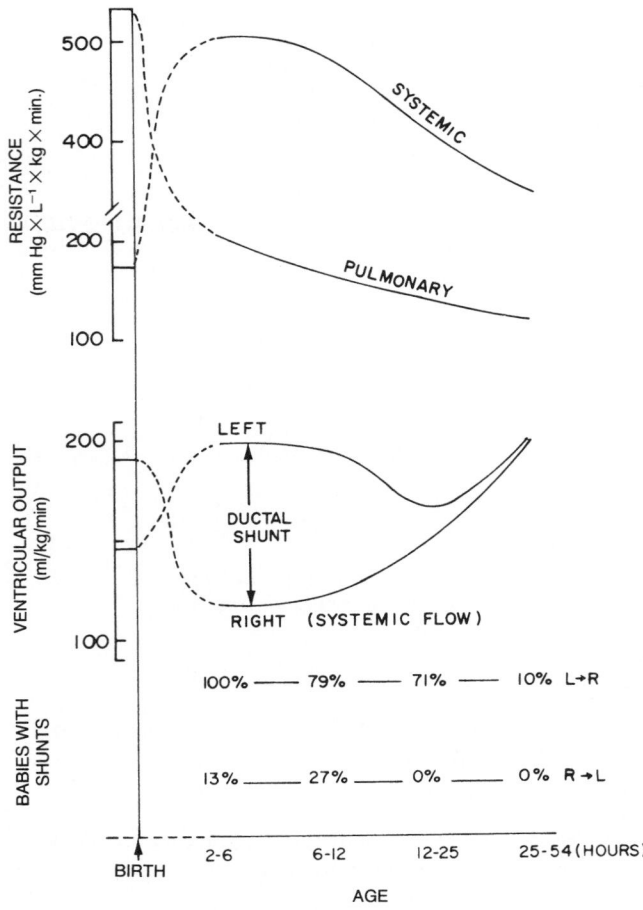

FIG. 17–10. Perinatal hemodynamics in the human showing changes in vascular resistance, ventricular output, and shunting. (From ref. 209, with data from refs. 213, 214.)

3. The large, albeit transient, increase in left ventricular volume (and pressure) work.
4. The decrease in right ventricular pressure (and, transiently, volume) work.
5. Closure of the ductus arteriosus (and equalization of ventricular volume work) between 12 to 14 hours.
6. Closure of the foramen ovale in the first minutes and hours after birth.

Human flow data (during the transitional phase of the perinatal circulation) are shown in Fig. 17–11 and document that the left ventricle is pumping nearly twice the volume load of the right ventricle (62,70,71).

However, it is pressure work that chiefly determines the behavior of the electromotive forces of the beating heart—the QRS loop remains unchanged from its rightward-dominant vector orientation over the first days of life. This is a reflection of the dominance of right-over-left ventricular muscle mass as a result of the chronic "cor pulmonale" of the fetal state. This dominance will slowly subside to the left-dominant picture of the adult over the first 3 to 6 months of life, as the ventricles

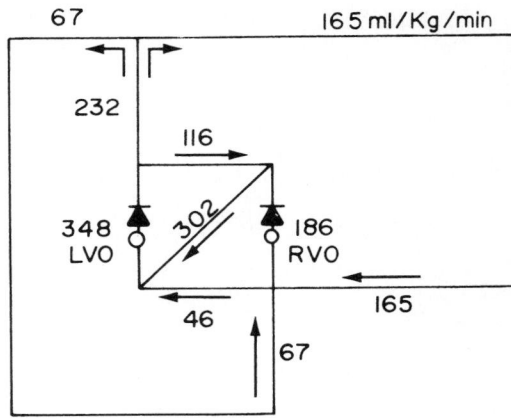

FIG. 17–11. The human perinatal (transitional) circulation is divided into cerebral blood flow **(left)** and carcass blood flow **(right).** Flow data are given in mL/kg/min. (From ref. 209, with flow data from refs. 213–216.)

become remodeled in response to decreasing right- and increasing left-ventricular pressure work. The only perinatal ECG indication of these shifting pressure/volume loads on the ventricles is the change in orientation of the T vector from leftward inferior and anterior at birth to rightward inferior and anterior at transition (about 6 hours) to leftward inferior and posterior at restitution (12 to 24 hours).

METABOLIC ADAPTATION

Many of the same stimuli that elicit the first breaths—the asphyxia of labor (by diminution of placental perfusion), the cold shock of ejection from the womb, and the subsequent independent forage for fuel (as well as oxygen), mandated by separation from the placenta—comprise the principal metabolic perturbations of birth: hypoxia, hypothermia, and hypoglycemia (72,73). These combined assaults have been likened to ejection from one's warm and friendly neighborhood pub into cold, midwinter streets, naked and without a free lunch, and each can separately elicit a surge of catechols (epinephrine, norepinephrine) from their stores in the adrenal and aortic paraganglia (Organ of Zuckerkandl) into the general circulation (Fig. 17–12) for distribution to the target tissues that will sustain the infant until his mother can reassume her responsibilities for warmth and nutrition. The immediate eightfold surge in TSH seen in Fig. 17–12 is principally the result of the cold shock of delivery (74) but may also be driven by the many ectopic (i.e., nonhypothalamic) sources of TRH (thyroid-releasing hormone) built up by the fetus (75).

Three important enzymes are activated by this surge of catechols. First, hepatic phosphorylase becomes engaged in glycogenolysis, the average infant having sufficient glycogen stores to sustain blood glucose levels during the

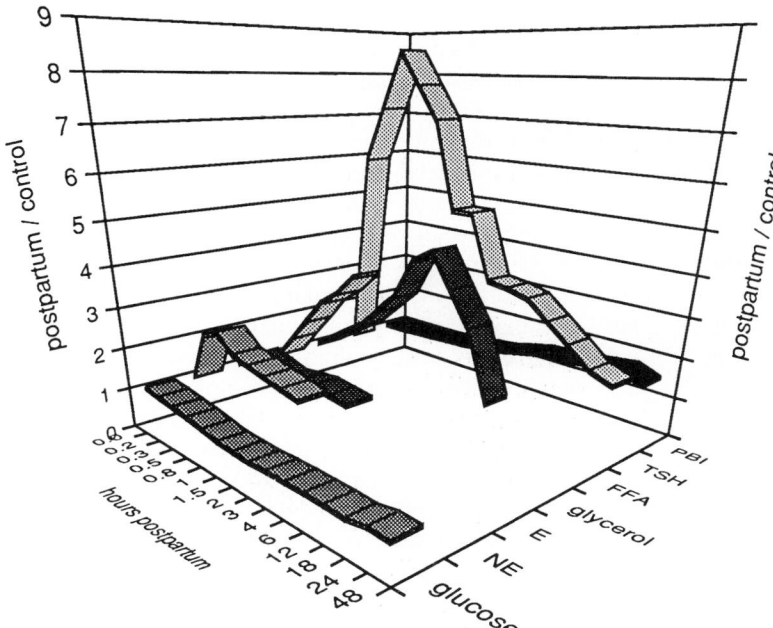

FIG. 17–12. Postnatal changes in metabolism. The value scale is the ratio of postpartum to prepartum (fetal) levels of each of these moieties. NE, norepinephrine; E, epinephrine; FFA, free fatty acids; TSH, thyroid-stimulating hormone; PBI, protein-bound iodine, which is roughly equivalent to the sum of thyroxine and triiodothyronine. (Drawn from data of refs. 53, 75–77, 217–223.)

first 12 hours of postpartum fasting. Next, lipase in adipose tissue commences hydrolyzing stored fat into glycerol and free fatty acids, which are thus made available to gluconeogenesis as a "fail-safe" source of glucose. This rapid progression from carbohydrate to adipose energy sources, during a transient period of neonatal starvation, can be monitored by the respiratory quotient (ratio of CO_2 production to O_2 consumption), which descends from 1.0 towards 0.7 until successful suckling completes the conversion from placental to peroral energy assimilation. Finally, deiodinase converts thyroxine (T_4) to triiodothyronine (T_3) with particular exuberance in brown adipose tissue. This specialized fat of the newborn serves as an "electric blanket" of nonshivering thermogenesis because its T_3 stimulates a protein, thermogenin, whose location and action are unique to brown fat; thermogenin diverts the energy of the protons within the mitochondrial respiratory chain to the production of heat rather than its usual storage as ATP (53,76,77). Thus does the stressed but sessile newborn bend the biology of "fight or flight" to his particular metabolic need.

PULMONARY MECHANICS

To return to the first few extrauterine respirations, we note in Fig. 17–13 that the first breath (I) begins with no (air) volume and no transpulmonary pressure gradient. As the chest wall (including the diaphragm) expands, the transpulmonary (distending) pressure increases until it overcomes surface tension (compare with Fig. 17–3) in the smaller airways and alveoli, usually at transpulmonary pressures below 25 cm H_2O (78). At this point, actively inspired air begins to enter and does so with

increasing ease as alveolar dimensions increase. The reason is contained in the LaPlace relationship:

$$P = 2T/R$$

This equation states that, if wall tension (T) of a spherical surface remains constant, the distending pressure (P) required to maintain equilibrium will decrease as the spherical radius (R) increases. An appropriate analogy is the increasing ease with which a child's balloon is inflated, once first expanded.

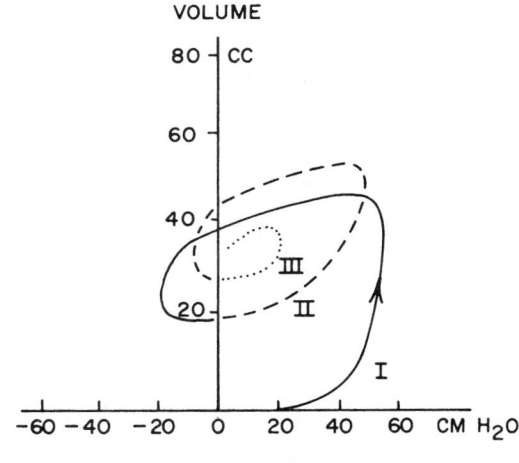

FIG. 17–13. Pressure–volume curves of the first three extrauterine breaths. (From ref. 209.)

At the maximum inspiratory level (of about 45 mL of air in this example), breath I is actively exhaled (note negative transpulmonary pressure in Fig. 17–13), but not to 0 volume. Evidently with great rapidity, the alveolar lining layer, containing surface-active material, is able to stabilize alveolar surfaces so that surface tension decreases as alveolar dimensions decrease. Thus, both T and R decrease together in the LaPlace relation, so that the transpulmonary pressure required to maintain inflation is relatively stable and of small dimensions. These dimensions are indicated in Fig. 17–14, which compares the pressure–volume characteristics of the infant lung, chest wall (and diaphragm), and total respiratory systems to those of the adult. Notable is the fact that, whereas the relaxation pressure curves for the lung alone are remarkably similar across the age span, the infant's chest wall is almost infinitely distensible (i.e., compliant) (79). This results in large part, of course, from the nonossification of the infant thorax—a matter of thoughtful convenience during the high extrinsic pressures of vaginal birth. Indeed, even some adult animals of diving species, also subjected to high extrinsic thoracic pressures, have chest walls as compliant as that of the newborn human. However, it is the opposition of the retractive forces of the somewhat expanded lung against the expansive forces of the somewhat compressed chest wall that determines the resting (end-expiratory) volume of the total respiratory system, and the higher the compliance (nonstiffness) of the chest wall, the lower will be the resting volume. Note that in Fig. 17–14, the infant's rest volume is a good deal closer to the residual, or "closing," volume of the lung than is the case for the adult. Moreover, the transpulmonary pressure at rest is also less in the infant. This tenuous situation is further detailed in Fig. 17–15, in which it is seen that some smaller airways of the infant can actually close within the range of the normal tidal volume and "trap" gas in the infant lung's periphery, so that it does not communicate with the trachea (80). Through measurement of total thoracic gas volume, in comparison to functional residual capacity, as much as 6 mL/kg of lung volume may be measured as trapped in the first 2 weeks of life (81).

Such gas trapping is the more frequently observed in the first few postnatal days (82), and intrapleural negative pressure increases to adult levels by 16 days after birth (83); these facts suggest a developmental change in respiratory system equilibrium that may be too rapid to be accounted for by ossification of the thoracic cage. It may be that this developmental change actually involves increasing tonus in the intercostal muscles (see below). This would serve to decrease the compliance of the chest wall such that the rest volume of the lung may increase to a level at which smaller airways no longer collapse during quiet breathing.

Moreover, in the first few hours and days of life, the resourceful infant tries to keep his functional residual capacity safely above his lung's rest volume by maintaining inspiratory muscle tone throughout a significant portion of passive expiration (84–86) and by laryngeal adductive "braking" of the expiration (87) through a series of passive "minigrunts" (88–92). Thus, he preserves the stability of his lung volume in a resistance (larynx)/compliance (lung and chest wall), or "RC," circuit, just as the energy of the heartbeat is stored in the elastic walls of the great vessels and then steadily discharged through the circulation under control of the peripheral vascular resistance. The basic difference is that blood flow is "direct current," whereas gas flow is "alternating current."

The larynx and pharynx must also interlock the infant's epiglottis and palate to allow simultaneous nursing and breathing by providing an "interrupt" of diaphragmatic action during a swallow (93). These airway protective mechanisms can also produce an early infantile form of breath-holding spells ("squirming Valsalva") (94) during motor activity; they are chemoreflexive in nature, gener-

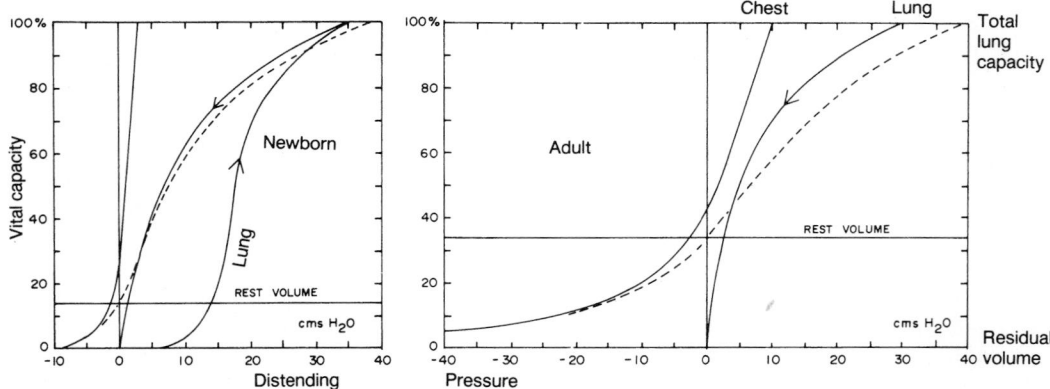

FIG. 17–14. Comparative mechanics of the infant and adult lung. (From ref. 209.)

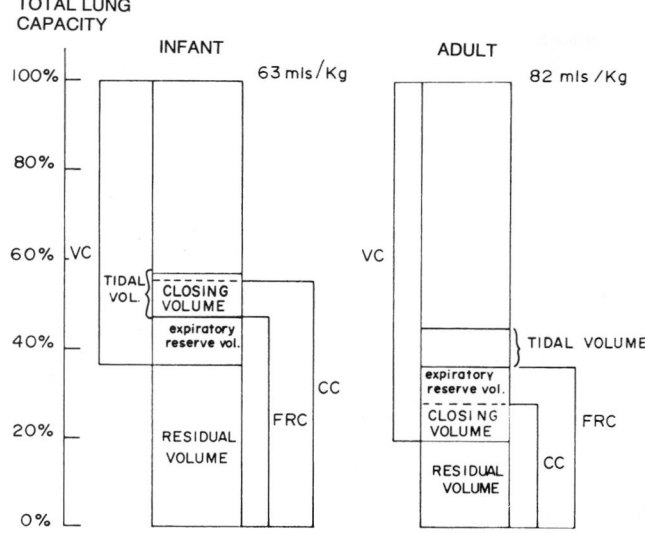

FIG. 17–15. Static lung volumes of the infant and adult. VC, vital capacity; CC, closing capacity; FRC, functional residual capacity. (From ref. 209.)

TABLE 17–5. Static lung volumes[a]

	Infant (ml/kg)	Adult (ml/kg)
TLC	63	82
IC	33	52
TGV	30–36	30
FRC	30	30
VC	30–40	66
CC	35	23
VT	6	7
ERV	7	14
CV	12	7
RV	23	16
ERV/FRC	0.23	0.47
RV/TLC	0.37	0.20
FRC/TLC	0.48	0.37
VT/FRC	0.20	0.23

CC, closing capacity; CV, closing volume; ERV, expiratory reserve volume; FRC, functional residual capacity; IC, inspiratory capacity; RV, residual volume; TGV, thoracic gas volume; TLC, total lung capacity; VC, vital capacity; VT, tidal volume.
[a]Data from refs. 170 and 191–198.

ally inhibit ventilation, and are frequently marked by bradycardia (95,96).

Despite these qualifications, the standard static lung volumes as defined by Fig. 17–16 have been measured frequently and reproducibly by many investigators of the newborn and are shown in Table 17–5. Infants delivered by elective cesarean section initially have a decreased lung gas volume, presumably because they have been denied the partial purging of fetal lung liquid provided by thoracic compression during passage through the birth canal (56,97).

The decreased lung capacities (total, inspiratory, vital), as compared to the adult in Table 17–5, may indicate an imperfect leverage exerted by a too compliant chest wall on the underlying lung. The higher residual volume and lower expiratory reserve volume of the infant may relate to gas trapped behind smaller closed airways. In any case, the first few days of life, especially in the premature, are

marked by disturbances in efficient gas exchange (requiring simultaneous and nearly equal ventilation and perfusion), which can be ameliorated by stabilization of the chest wall (98). Indeed, the prone position appears most conducive to efficient gas exchange [decreased resistance with increased compliance (99), tidal volume (100), and arterial oxygenation (101)], apparently because this position stabilizes the chest wall by "coupling" the rib cage to the abdomen (102), so as to diminish the inefficient chest distortions of paradoxic respiration.

It has become apparent that the stability of the chest wall, as well as many other integrative functions involving the respiratory system, depends on the "sleep state" of the infant (103–111). Active, or REM, sleep is the dominant state in the newborn and is one of relative arousal, characterized by intense low-voltage and fast electrocortical and reticular activity. It is associated with sucking, swallowing, increased cerebral blood flow (112), and esophageal peristalsis as well as glottic closure (113,114). Proprioceptive reflexes are generally depressed, with resultant loss of postural tone. The precise mode of this depression is incompletely understood but appears, peripherally at least, to involve an inhibition of monosynaptic muscle spindle ("γ-loop") reflexes, which sense increased local muscular loads and, in response, increase α-motoneuron discharge (103,104). Inhibition of the γ-loop reflex apparently results in loss of intercostal muscle tone during REM sleep, so that stiffness ("elastance") of the thoracic cage decreases, and diaphragmatic contraction causes inward motion of the ribs during inspiration, producing "paradoxic" respiration (Fig. 17–17). This limits the effectiveness of the diaphragm as a generator of force (115,116). Such deformation is capable of triggering the intercostal phrenic

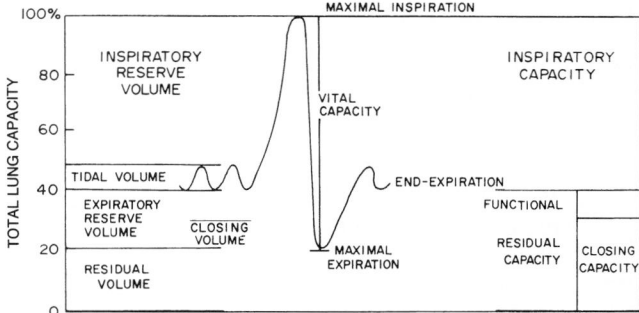

FIG. 17–16. Static lung volumes defined. A standard spirogram is shown for reference. (From ref. 209.)

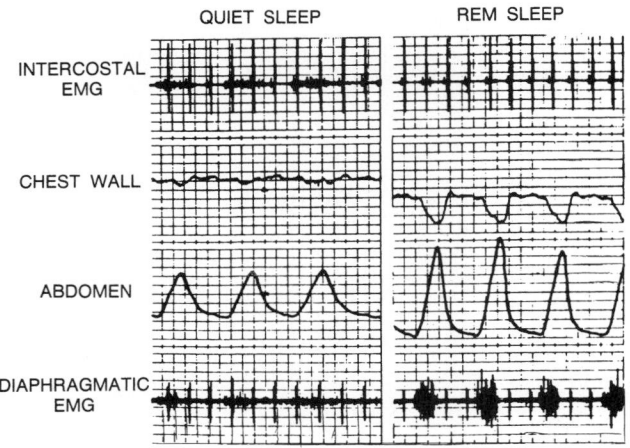

FIG. 17–17. Paradoxic respiration in rapid-eye-movement (REM) sleep. As the abdomen expands (upward deflection) and the diaphragm descends, the chest wall is drawn inward (downward deflection). Large, brief electromyographic (EMG) spikes are an electrocardiographic artifact. Note the tonic discharge of the intercostal EMG throughout inspiration in quiet sleep, compared to brief, low-voltage, phasic intercostal EMG and intense phasic diaphragmatic EMG in REM sleep. (From ref. 224.)

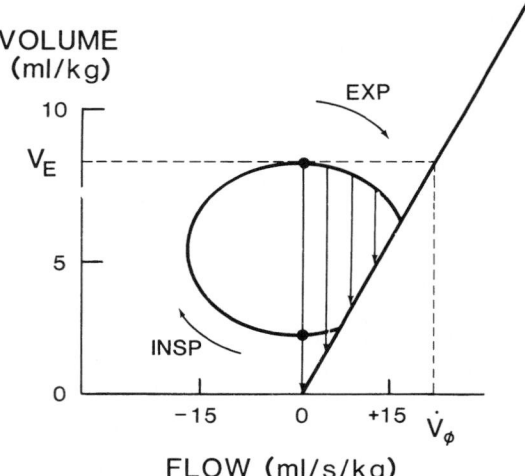

FIG. 17–18. In this low-volume loop, the slope of the linear portion of passive expiration is the time constant (resistance × compliance) of the respiratory system. The vertical distance from any point on the loop to the linear passive phase represents inspiratory muscular activity. V_E, inspiratory volume; V_ϕ, peak expiratory flow. (From refs. 85, 130.)

(inhibitory) reflex, which terminates such an inspiration early (117–119).

Thus, respiration in REM sleep is irregular and more rapid than in quiet sleep. Tidal volume is unchanged, but mean inspiratory air flow (tidal volume/inspiratory duration) is increased, as is minute volume. This is, however, a fatiguing form of respiration (120), the more so for the premature infant whose respiratory muscle fibers resist fatigue poorly (121–125). The infant is especially ill-equipped, therefore, to compensate for extra respiratory loads during REM sleep (126). The Hering-Breuer reflex, especially strong in the premature, fosters recruitment of intercostal neurons under respiratory loads, but this reflex is inhibited during REM sleep. The diminished lung volume and arterial oxygenation observed in REM sleep (127) thus become more understandable.

All these recently recognized inefficiencies of chest wall performance render suspect the traditional assessment of pleural pressure by monitoring esophageal pressure, especially in the preterm infant (128). Nearly all the data in Table 17–6 were gained from studies of esophageal pressure, so it is fortunate that a currently impeccable method (passive expiratory flow–volume plot) is now available for remeasurement of passive respiratory mechanics (Fig. 17–18) (85,129,130).

During quiet breathing, the infant's ventilatory efforts are opposed by several forces: the resistance of the lung and chest wall to stretch (elastic recoil), the resistance to movement (flow resistance) of air and tissue, and the inertial resistance offered by air and tissue at rest to any large change in their state of motion. An "equation of motion" states that the relations among these variables:

$$P = V/C + R \times F$$

where P is the muscular force (measured as transpulmonary pressure) applied to the respiratory system, V is the volume of gas in the system, C is the distensibility or compliance of the system, V/C is the force of elastic recoil, R is the flow resistance, F is air flow, and $R \times F$ is the force required to overcome the resistance to flow. (During quiet breathing the inertial resistance is negligible.)

These forces, as currently measured, are set out in Table 17–6, wherein it is apparent that the muscular force to be generated by both infant and adult are really quite comparable (about 2 cm H_2O). Nonetheless, there are certain notable differences, including the lower proportional nasal resistance of the newborn. The much higher chest wall compliance of the newborn is, again, most striking.

Now, the product of the total compliance and resistance of the system is its "time constant," an expression of how rapidly the system, once perturbed by an active inspiration, will passively return to its rest position under the force of elastic recoil operating against flow resistance. This time constant is about 0.15 to 0.20 seconds in the infant and 0.55 seconds in the adult, so that the resting respiratory rate of the infant (30 to 50 beats/min) is appropriately about twice that of the adult (20 beats/min). Further, any entity that reduces the total compliance (increases the "stiffness") of the system (e.g., fluid in the lung) must decrease the time constant and, thus, increase the resting respiratory rate.

TABLE 17–6. *Forces that oppose breathing*[a]

	Infants		Adults	
Elastic recoil (V_L/C_L)	1.5 cm H_2O		1.5 cm H_2O	
Volume (V_L)	0.1 L		2.1 L	
Compliance (C_L), total	0.0026 L/cm H_2O	0.029 L/cm H_2O/L lung volume	0.100 L/cm H_2O	0.03 L/cm H_2O/L lung volume
Chest wall	0.0236 L/cm H_2O	0.262 L/cm H_2O/L lung volume	0.200 L/cm H_2O	0.06 L/cm H_2O/L lung volume
Lung tissue	0.0050 L/cm H_2O	0.055 L/cm H_2O/L lung volume	0.200 L/cm H_2O	0.06 L/cm H_2O/L lung volume
Flow resistance ($R \times F$)	0.4 mean/1.9 max cm H_2O		0.4 mean/1.9 max cm H_2O	
Mean (pulmonary) resistance	35 cm H_2O/L/sec			
Inspiratory (total) resistance	69 cm H_2O/L/sec	100% total resistance	5.5 cm H_2O/L/sec	100% total resistance
Chest wall		26% total resistance		16% total resistance
Pulmonary	25–50 cm H_2O/L/sec		4.5 cm H_2O/L/sec	
Nose	10 cm H_2O/L/sec	21% total resistance	2.8 cm H_2O/L/sec	54% total resistance
Mouth-airway	16 cm H_2O/L/sec	34% total resistance	1.6 cm H_2O/L/sec	29% total resistance
Lung tissue	9 cm H_2O/L/sec	19% total resistance	0.1 cm H_2O/L/sec	1% total resistance
Expiratory (*i.e.*, total) resistance	97 cm H_2O/L/sec			
Chest wall				
Pulmonary	35–70 cm H_2O/L/sec			
Gas flow (mean)	0.030–0.050 L/sec			
Inspiration	0.048 L/sec			
Expiration	0.037 L/sec			

[a]Data from refs. 191, 193, 195, 197, and 199–202.

PULMONARY VENTILATION

It is this higher ventilatory rate that is chiefly responsible for the higher minute ventilation, alveolar ventilation, wasted ventilation, and oxygen consumption (normalized for body weight) of the infant, as seen in Table 17–7. Yet, when they are compared on the basis of body surface area (generally held as a better basis for metabolic comparisons), the infant and adult are, again, strikingly similar.

The chemical and neuronal drivers of neonatal respiration are becoming better defined (131), but a number of mysteries remain. It is now clear that the respiratory centers of the newborn respond normally to CO_2 and that their response becomes more powerful with increasing postconceptional age (132–134). Conceivably, this increasing respiratory response may represent, in the human, the result of a postnatal increase in excitatory respiratory neuronal synapses and consequent respiratory motor activity, as noted in other species (135).

Responses to O_2 are more complex (136), probably because they involve suprapontine centers in the brain as well as the peripheral chemoreceptors. Short-term (less than 90 seconds) responses are like those in the adult, with hyperoxia producing immediate hypoventilation (137,138), whereas hypoxia produces immediate hyperventilation (139,140), thus demonstrating the presence of functional peripheral chemoreceptors (141).

Prolonged (2 to 3 minutes) hypo- or hyperoxia, however, soon leads to reversal of both of these responses (Fig. 17–19). Postulated but unproved explanations for

TABLE 17–7. *Pulmonary ventilation*[a]

	Infant	Adult	Units
Respiratory frequency (f)	34–35	13	bpm
Tidal volume (V_T)	6–8	7	ml/kg
Alveolar volume (V_A)	3.8–5.8	4.8	ml/kg
Dead space volume (V_D)	2.0–2.2	2.2	ml/kg
Minute ventilation ($\dot{V}_E$)	200–260	90	ml/kg/min
Alveolar ventilation ($\dot{V}_A$)	100–150	60	ml/kg/min
Wasted (*i.e.*, dead space) ventilation ($\dot{V}_D$)	77–99	30	ml/kg/min
Dead space/tidal volume (V_D/V_T)	0.27–0.37	0.3	
Oxygen consumption ($\dot{V}o_2$)	6–8	3.2	ml/kg/min
Ventilation equivalent ($\dot{V}_A/\dot{V}o_2$)	16–23	19–25	
Alveolar ventilation ($\dot{V}_A$)	2.3	2.4	l/m² min

[a]Data from refs. 191, 193, 195, 201, and 203.

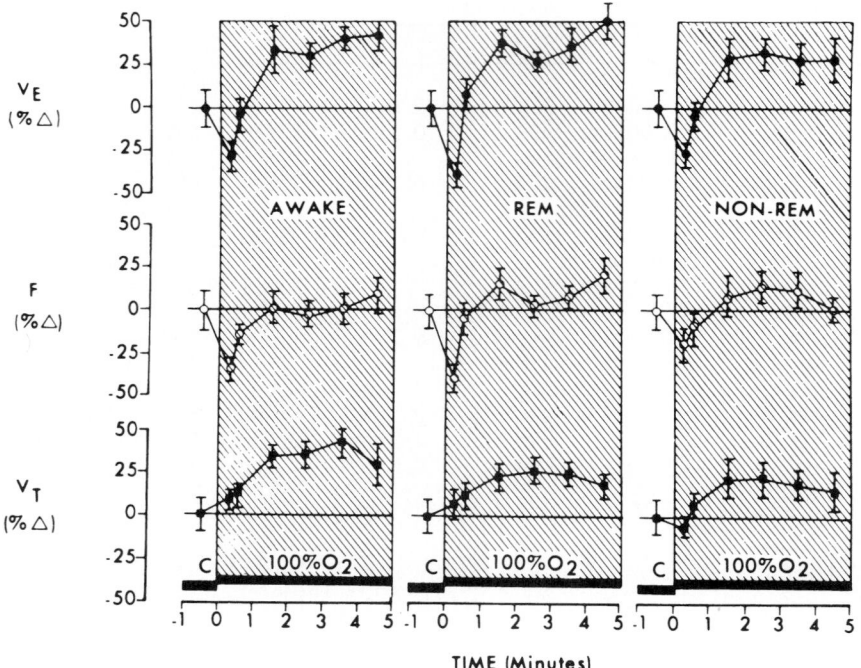

FIG. 17–19. Biphasic ventilatory responses to hyperoxia in the human newborn. The immediate ventilatory decrease in hyperoxic environments (normal adult peripheral chemoreceptor response) is not sustained. (From ref. 140.)

the biphasic hyperoxic response include cerebral vasospasm and impaired CO_2 carriage (by O_2-saturated hemoglobin), leading to local accumulation of carbonic acid and consequent direct stimulation of the respiratory centers (142). It also seems possible that the biphasic hypoxic response represents impaired facilitation by higher centers of synaptic contacts among the respiratory motor neurons (see Fig. 17–4) as the result of an imbalance between excitatory and inhibitory amino acid neurotransmitters (143). It may even prove to be the case that such a hypoxic lack of neuronal facilitation of quantitatively marginal respiratory synapses is responsible for fetal respiratory quiescence (fetal PaO_2 is about 25 mm Hg), apart from the fetal "respiration" seen to accompany the intense reticular activity of REM sleep. The interactional effects of CO_2 and O_2 breathing are, again, similar to the adult's (i.e., hypoxic enhancement of CO_2 responses, presumably caused by peripheral chemoreceptor discharge), provided the experiments are short-term (139).

It is the tidal volume that is unsustained during hypoxia (144) despite the normal increase in brain blood flow also seen in adults (145–147), possibly because of diaphragmatic fatigue. In any case, however, not having the ability to maintain ventilation during hypoxia, the newborn acclimatizes by decreasing his oxygen consumption, just as do hibernating species and those at altitude (148–150), and, if the hypoxia is chronic, by stimulated growth of the respiratory system (151).

The association of chemical drives to and neuromuscular modulation of ventilation (152) has come to be analyzed in the following equation (153):

$$\dot{V}_E = V_T/T_I \times T_I/T_{TOT}$$

where $\dot{V}_E$ is total instantaneous ventilation, and V_T is the tidal volume of each breath; T_I is the duration of a given inspiration, and T_{TOT} is the duration of the complete breath (inspiration plus expiration); V_T/T_I is the mean inspiratory gas flow per breath and serves as a representative sum of chemical stimulation (principally CO_2 and H^+) and neuronal modulation (peripheral chemoreceptor signals, rapidly adapting vagal fiber signals from "irritant" receptors in the tracheobronchial epithelium, facilitative and inhibiting influences from suprapontine centers) of the inherent rhythmicity of respiratory neuronal discharge (Fig. 17–4) (118), as well as its neuromuscular expression in gas flow. The firing of these neurons requires a critical spatial and temporal summation of input impulses such that their resting potential may be raised above the firing threshold. T_I/T_{TOT} represents the "duty cycle," which determines the duration of firing of inspiratory neurons (i.e., T_I) or of expiratory neurons ($T_E = T_{TOT} - T_I$). These controls of frequency largely rest in the pulmonary submucosal stretch receptors (slow-adapting vagal fibers) (154).

All these relations have come under intense scrutiny in the newborn through detailed and critical analysis of the Hering-Breuer reflexes (153–159). These are very well developed in the premature in quiet sleep and allow him to recruit intercostal neurons when presented with a respiratory load (e.g., airway obstruction) (160). They are not, however, active during REM sleep. With maturation, the strengths of these reflexes clearly decrease (155,157,158). It seems possible, therefore, that maturational increases in respiratory neuronal synapses ("dendritic arborization") may render the respiratory centers less susceptible to the influences of vagal stretch and irritant receptors. As higher volitional centers develop to modulate an increasingly robust group of respiratory neurons, it appears that more primeval modulation through the vagus becomes less necessary to maintain constancy of ventilation under varying respiratory loads (e.g., speech, posture).

Although earlier studies were conducted without knowledge of sleep state, there is strong evidence that hypoxia inhibits respiration in the newborn infant and that hyperoxia decreases the frequency of periodic respiration in the premature (despite its other dangers) (161,162). In animals subjected to preterminal asphyxia, the evidence suggests that suprapontine centers become hypoxically depressed, allowing activity of the respiratory neurons to be unmodulated from above and responsive, therefore, only to negative feedback from the peripheral chemoreceptors and vagal stretch receptors (163–165). In such situations, any defect in the "feedback loop" can lead to oscillatory behavior (166–168). In REM sleep, there are multiple such opportunities for disruption of feedback loops because of erratic respiratory timing. Premature infants, in addition, have in-phase oscillations of tidal volume and respiratory frequency during periodic breathing, suggesting an unstable total ventilation whereby CO_2 is either overblown or excessively retained (166–168). Periodic respiration can be induced in newborn animals with mature chemoreceptors by varying the critical ratio of $PaO_2/PaCO_2$ (169). Thus, the ancient observation that periodic respiration of the premature infant is relieved by O_2 breathing (restoring suprapontine facilitative neural influences) or CO_2 breathing (increasing pontine respiratory activity) become more understandable. Drugs such as caffeine and theophylline appear to facilitate respiration by increasing reticular activity, similar to that in REM sleep.

VENTILATION–PERFUSION IMBALANCE

Exchange of respiratory gases between the tissues and the environment is, of course, the basic purpose of respiration, both cellular and pulmonary. It is thus obvious that adequate pulmonary respiration will be to no avail if the intervening circulation cannot carry and release oxygen to the tissues. Just as this principle applies to adequate distribution of arterialized blood to tissues, so also must the distribution of venous blood flow be well matched to gaseous flow throughout the alveoli. Any inhomogeneity of the flow of gas and blood through the lungs must serve to reduce the efficiency of gas exchange. Such inhomogeneities are most frequently expressed as the ratio of ventilation to perfusion $(\dot{V}/\dot{Q})$ within given groups of alveoli. Whereas the overall $\dot{V}/\dot{Q}$ of the normal lung is nearly 1, there is a vast range of possible ratios from 0 (a "shunt") to infinity (a "dead space"). Presently available estimates for ventilation/perfusion ratios in the term newborn human at about 24 hours of age are shown in Table 17–8. It appears from this that most ventilated areas are reasonably well-perfused (i.e., little dead space or "wasted ventilation"), whereas significant perfusion is directed to atelectatic alveoli or is totally shunted around the lung. Probably little of this shunt flow passes through the foramen ovale, and rather more passes right to left across the ductus arteriosus (even after reversal of dominant flow during the transitional phase of circulatory conversion). This occurs because of phasic pressure differences across the ductus during the cardiac cycle, with the mean pressures on the pulmonary and systemic sides being essentially balanced for the first several hours (see Fig. 17–10). A presently undocumentable amount of desaturated blood may also be shunted across the lung to the left atrium by way of bronchopulmonary anastomoses.

TABLE 17–8. *Distribution of pulmonary ventilation and perfusion in the infant*

Type of alveolus	Percent total ventilation		Percent total perfusion		$\dot{V}_A/\dot{Q}_c$
Anatomically shunted	20		10		0
Atelectatic, perfused	0		15		0
Trapped gas, perfused	0		10		0
Silent (*i.e.,* atelectatic, nonperfused)	0		0		0
Low $\dot{V}_A/\dot{Q}_c$ areas	2	} 75	5	} 65	0.4
Normal $\dot{V}_A/\dot{Q}_c$ areas	68		58		1.2
High $\dot{V}_A/\dot{Q}_c$ areas	5		2		2.5
Dead space (i.e., ventilated, nonperfused)	5		0		~
Diffusion block	<1		<1		

[a]Data from refs. 193, 195, and 204–206.

TABLE 17-9. *Respiratory gas exchange and pressures of adults and infants*[a]

	Adult	Infant
Flows		
Alveolar ventilation ($\dot{V}_A$)	60 ml/kg/min	120 ml/kg/min
Pulmonary capillary flow ($\dot{Q}_C$)	75 ml/kg/min	200 ml/kg/min
Ventilation/perfusion ratio ($\dot{V}_A/\dot{Q}_C$)	0.8	0.6
Venous admixture		
Low $V_A/\dot{Q}_C$ flow/total flow ($\dot{Q}_O/\dot{Q}_T$)	0.02	0.10–0.20
Shunt flow/total flow ($\dot{Q}_S/\dot{Q}_T$)	0.05	0.05–0.15
Alveolar cases		
Oxygen (P_{AO_2})	105 mm Hg	105 mm Hg
Carbon dioxide (P_{ACO_2})	40 mm Hg	35 mm Hg
Nitrogen (P_{AN_2})	568 mm Hg	573 mm Hg
Arterial cases		
Oxygen (P_{aO_2})	95 mm Hg	80 mm Hg
Carbon dioxide (P_{aCO_2})	41 mm Hg	36 mm Hg
Nitrogen (P_{aN_2})	575 mm Hg	583 mm Hg
Gas Differences		
Oxygen (AaDO2)	10 mm Hg	24 mm Hg
Carbon dioxide (aADCO2)	1 mm Hg	1 mm Hg
Nitrogen (aADN2)	7 mm Hg	10 mm Hg

[a]Data from refs. 193, 195, 204, 205, and 207.

ALVEOLAR–ARTERIAL PRESSURE GRADIENTS

Such gas/blood flow variations are essentially responsible for the gas pressure differences established in the lung (Table 17–9), and one can estimate the approximate relative contributions of the several components to the total alveolar–arterial oxygen differences by measuring CO_2 and N_2 differences (Table 17–10). Thus, the portion of the AaDO2 attributable to high-$\dot{V}/\dot{Q}$ areas (dead space component) is reflected in the aADCO2, whereas that which is attributable to low-$\dot{V}/\dot{Q}$ areas (distribution component) is reflected in the aADN2. The summed effects of direct venoarterial shunting and perfusion of atelectatic lung can, in this manner, be separately estimated. There are certain differences between the normal term and premature infant, with the premature tending to have a higher degree of venous admixture because of increases in both true anatomic shunts and "virtual" shunts (i.e., low-$\dot{V}/\dot{Q}$ areas) (170–172). This is possibly related to alveolar instability because the magnified blood gas differences of prematures diminish if the chest is stabilized at higher lung volume (98), and they also diminish during the first 2 weeks of life.

SUMMARY

To return in brief summation to the basic focus of this chapter—the onset of respiration—we may gain from Fig. 17–20 an appreciation of just how rapidly the term newborn establishes respiration (173) and recovers from the asphyxiating influence that is normal vaginal birth.

Finer indications of the components of this achievement are shown in Fig. 17–21. The normal lung volume at rest (functional residual capacity) is essentially established by 8 to 10 minutes, although some of the dependent airways may be in intermittent collapse, as previously seen. The specific compliance (compliance normalized to lung volume) takes rather longer to achieve maximum. This most likely represents the rather slow clearance of fetal lung liquid from the parenchyma by way of the lymphatics. The airway conductance (reciprocal of resistance) increases somewhat slowly, possibly also representing clearance of fluid and "mucus" from airways and alveoli.

Figure 17–22 traces the development of respiratory gas pressure differences at the onset of respiration and indicates that, even as early as 60 minutes of age, there is insignificant wasted ventilation (i.e., minimal aADCO2).

TABLE 17–10. *Respiratory gas differences of adults and infants*[a]

	Total difference (AaDO2)	=	Diffusion component (AcDO2)	+	Dead space component (aADCO2)	+	Distribution component (aADN2)	+	Shunt component (caDO2)
Adult	10 torr	=	<l	+	1	+	7	+	2
Infant	25 torr	=	<l	+	1	+	10	+	14

[a]Data from refs. 193, 204–206, 208.

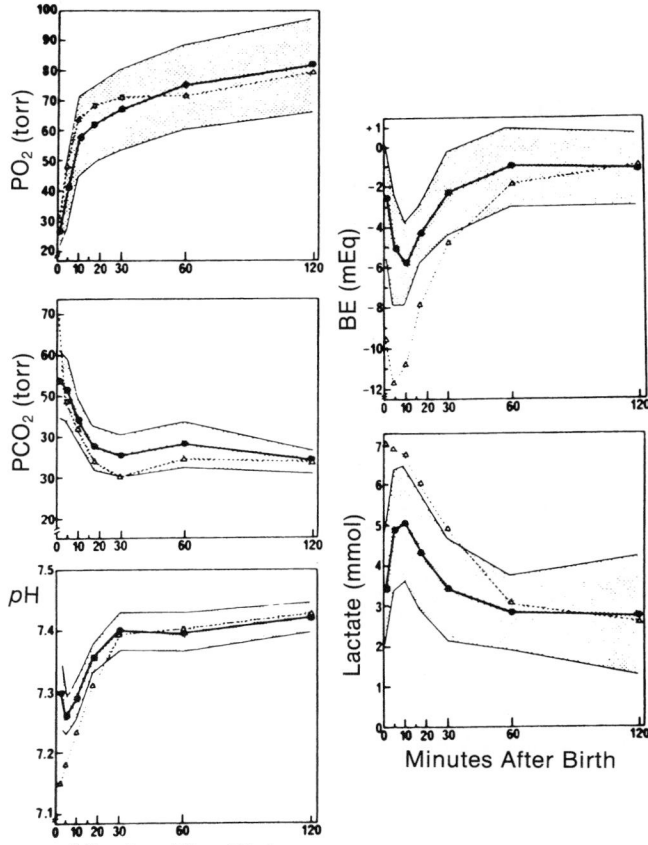

FIG. 17–20. Arterial blood gas changes in the first hours of life. *Solid circles,* mean values for normal term infants; *shaded zones,* ±1 standard deviation; *open triangles,* means for infants with fetal distress. (From ref. 198.)

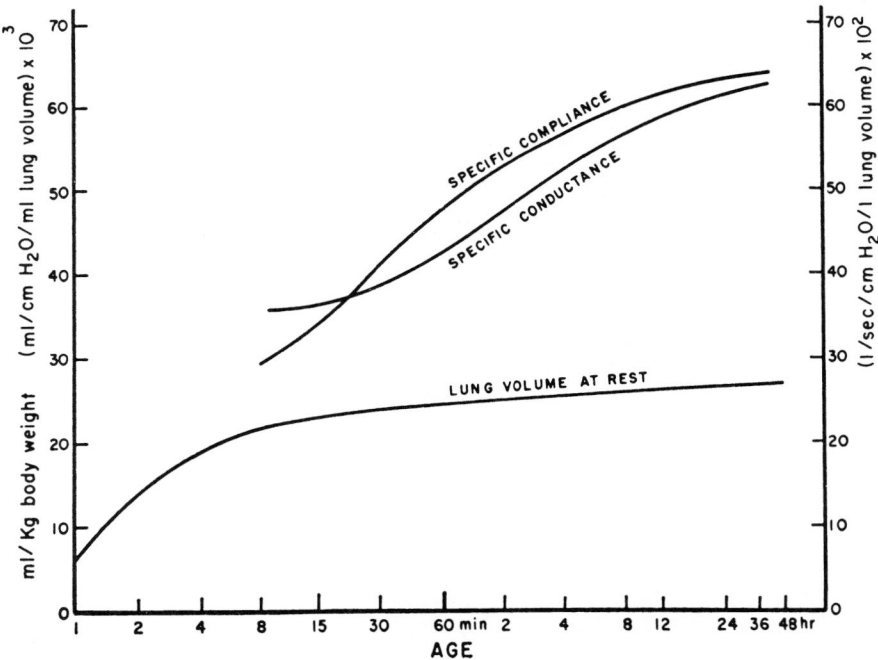

FIG. 17–21. Postnatal changes in pulmonary mechanics. (From ref. 193.)

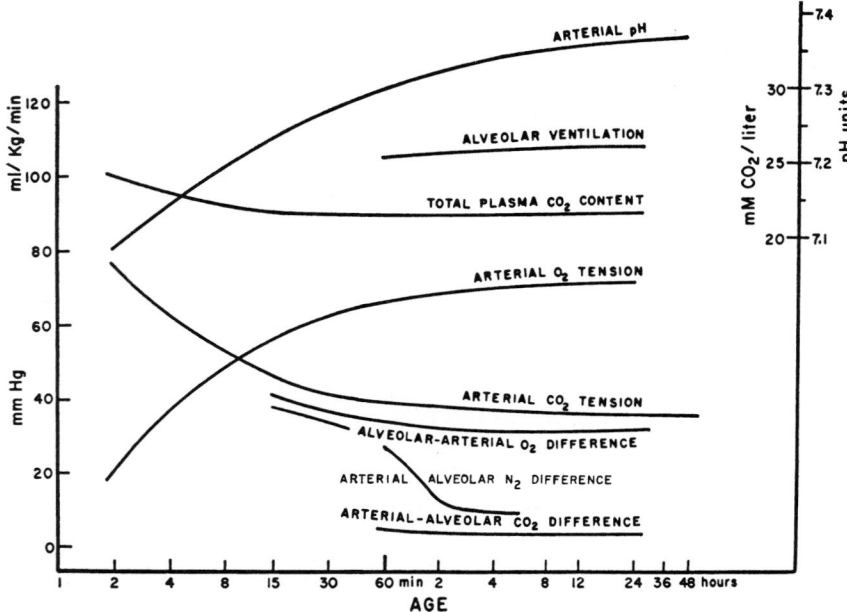

FIG. 17–22. Postnatal changes in blood gases. (From ref. 209.)

However, the large (35 mm Hg) AaDO₂ in the first 2 hours appears mainly attributable to perfusion of poorly ventilated areas of the lung (i.e., higher aADN₂) (174). Subsequently, as lung volume becomes firmly established (175) and compliance improves (fluid clears?) around 2 to 4 hours of age, low-$\dot{V}/\dot{Q}$ areas evidently become better ventilated (decreasing aADN₂). The high AaDO₂ remaining thus appears exclusively attributable to direct venoarterial shunting or to the perfusion of persistently atelectatic areas of the lung.

REFERENCES

1. Higuchi M, Murata Y, Miyake Y, Hesser J, Tyner J, et al. Effects of norepinephrine on lung fluid flow rate in the chronically catheterized fetal lamb. *Am J Obstet Gynecol* 1987;157:986–990.
2. Walker AM, Ritchie BC, Adamson TM, Maloney JE. Effect of changing lung liquid volume on the pulmonary circulation of fetal lambs. *J Appl Physiol* 1988;64(1):61–67.
3. Stenmark KR, James SL, Voelkel NF, Toews WH, Reeves JT, et al. Leukotriene C₄ and D₄ in neonates with hypoxemia and pulmonary hypertension. *N Engl J Med* 1983;309(2):77–80.
4. Cassin S, Stenmark KR, Gause G, Zapp LM, Kuck H, et al. Leukotrienes and prostaglandins in fetal lung liquid. *J Appl Physiol* 1990;68(5):2214–2222.
5. Fineman JR, Soifer SJ, Heymann MA. The role of pulmonary vascular endothelium in perinatal pulmonary circulatory regulation. *Semin Perinatol* 1991;15(1):58–62.
6. Pearce WJ, Longo LD. Developmental aspects of endothelial function. *Semin Perinatol* 1991;15(1):40–48.
7. Haworth SG, Hall SM, Chew M, Allen K. Thinning of fetal pulmonary arterial wall and postnatal remodelling: ultrastructural studies on the respiratory unit arteries of the pig. *Virchows Arch A* 1987;411:161–171.
8. Spitzer AR, Davis J, Clarke WT, Bernbaum J, Fox WW. Pulmonary hypertension and persistent fetal circulation in the newborn. *Clin Perinatol* 1988;15(2):389–413.
9. Boddy K, Mantell CD. Observations of fetal breathing movements transmitted through maternal abdominal wall. *Lancet* 1972;2:1219.
10. Patrick J, Natale R, Richardson B. Patterns of human fetal breathing activity at 34 to 35 weeks' gestational age. *Am J Obstet Gynecol* 1978;132:507–513.
11. Dawes GS, Fox HE, Laduc BM, et al. Respiratory movements and rapid-eye-movement sleep in the foetal lamb. *J Physiol* 1972;220(1):119–143.
12. Merlet C, Hoerter J, Devilleneuve C, Tchobroutsky C. Mise en evidence des mouvements respiratoires chez le foetus d'agneau *in utero* au cours du dernier mois de la gestation. *CR Acad Sci [D] (Paris)* 1970;270:2462.
13. Duenhoelter JH, Pritchard JA. Fetal respiration: quantitative measurements of amniotic fluid inspired near term by human and rhesus fetuses. *Am J Obstet Gynecol* 1976;125:306–309.
14. Wolfson VP, Laitman JT. Ultrasound investigation of fetal human upper respiratory anatomy. *Anat Rec* 1990;227:363–372.
15. van Eyck J, van der Moooren K, Wladimiroff JW. Ductus arteriosus flow velocity modulation by fetal breathing movements as a measure of fetal lung development. *Am J Obstet Gynecol* 1990;163:558–566.
16. Saunders RA, Milner AD. Pulmonary pressure/volume relationships during the last phase of delivery and the first postnatal breaths in human subjects. *J Pediatr* 1978;93:667–673.
17. Mortola JP, Fisher JT, Smith JB, et al. Onset of respiration in infants delivered by cesarean section. *J Appl Physiol* 1982;52:716–724.
18. Notter RH, Shapiro DL. Lung surfactants for replacement therapy: biochemical, biophysical, and clinical aspects. *Clin Perinatol* 1987;14(3):433–479.
19. Haagsman HP, van Golde LMG. Synthesis and assembly of lung surfactant. *Annu Rev Physiol* 1991;53:441–464.
20. Cochrane CG, Revak SD. Pulmonary surfactant protein B (SP-B): structure–function relationships. *Science* 1991;254:566–568.
21. Grossmann G, Suzuki Y, Robertson B, Kobayashi T, Berggren P, et al. Pathophysiology of neonatal lung injury induced by monoclonal antibody to surfactant protein B. *J Appl Physiol* 1997;82(6):2003–2010.
22. Kobayashi T, Shido A, Nitta K, Inui S, Ganzuka M, et al. The critical concentration of surfactant in fetal lung liquid at birth. *Respir Physiol* 1990;80:181–192.
23. Hawgood S, Shiffer K. Structures and properties of the surfactant-associated proteins. *Annu Rev Physiol* 1991;53:375–394.
24. Hawgood S, Poulain FR. Functions of the surfactant proteins: a perspective. *Pediatr Pulmonol* 1995;19(2):99–104.
25. Faridy EE. Air opening pressure in fetal lungs. *Respir Physiol* 1987;68:293–300.
26. Delacourt C, Canet E, Bureau MA. Predominant role of peripheral chemoreceptors in the termination of apnea in maturing newborn lambs. *J Appl Physiol* 1996;80(3):892–898.

27. Purves MJ, Biscoe TJ. Development of chemoreceptor activity. *Br Med Bull* 1966;22:56.
28. Hodson WA, Fenner A, Brumley G, et al. Cerebrospinal fluid and blood acid–base relationships in fetal and neonatal lambs and pregnant ewes. *Respir Physiol* 1968;4:322.
29. Rigatto H. Control of ventilation in the newborn. *Annu Rev Physiol* 1984;46:661–674.
30. Bystrzycka E, Nail BS, Purves MJ. Central and peripheral neural respiratory activity in the mature sheep foetus and newborn lamb. *Respir Physiol* 1975;25:199–215.
31. Purves MJ. Onset of respiration at birth. *Arch Dis Child* 1974;49:333–343.
32. Harned HS, Myracle J, Ferreiro J. Respiratory suppression and swallowing from introduction of fluids into the laryngeal region of the lamb. *Pediatr Res* 1978;12:1003–1009.
33. Lee JC, Stoll BJ, Downing SE. Properties of the laryngeal chemoreflex in neonatal piglets. *Am J Physiol* 1977;233:R30–R36.
34. Hollingworth SA, Jones SA, Adamson SL. Rebound increase in fetal breathing movements after 24-h prostaglandin E$_2$ infusion in fetal sheep. *J Appl Physiol* 1996;80(1):166–175.
35. St John WM. Medullary regions for neurogenesis of gasping: noeud vital or noeuds vitals? *J Appl Physiol* 1996;81(5):1865–1877.
36. Chernick V. Fetal breathing movements and the onset of breathing at birth. *Clin Perinatol* 1978;5:257–268.
37. Thomas AJ, Friedman L, MacKenzie CN, Strohl KP. Modification of conditioned apneas in rats: evidence for cortical involvement. *J Appl Physiol* 1995;78(4):1215–1218.
38. Permutt S, Riley KL. Hemodynamics of collapsible vessels with tone: The vascular waterfall. *J Appl Physiol* 1963;18:924.
39. Nelin LD, Krenz GS, Rickaby DA, Linehan JH, Dawson CA. A distensible vessel model applied to hypoxic pulmonary vasoconstriction in the neonatal pig. *J Appl Physiol* 1993;74(5):2049–2056.
40. Fike CD, Gordon JB, Kaplowitz MR. Micropipette and vascular occlusion pressures in isolated lungs of newborn lambs. *J Appl Physiol* 1993;75(4):1854–1860.
41. Domkowski PW, Cockerham JT, Crescenzo DG, Kot PA, Dyer KL, et al. Pulmonary hydraulic impedance responses to hypoxia and hypercapnia in newborn pigs. *J Appl Physiol* 1994;77(1):386–396.
42. Hislop AA, Springall DR, Buttery LD, Pollock JS, Haworth SG. Abundance of endothelial nitric oxide synthase in newborn intrapulmonary arteries. *Arch Dis Child* 1995;73(1):F17–F21.
43. Raj JU, Hazinski TA, Bland RD. Effect of hypoxia on lung lymph flow in newborn lambs with left atrial hypertension. *Am J Physiol* 1988;254:H487–H493.
44. Miserocchi G, Poskurica BH, Del Fabbro M. Pulmonary interstitial pressure in anesthetized paralyzed newborn rabbits. *J Appl Physiol* 1994;77(5):2260–2268.
45. Bland RD. Dynamics of pulmonary water before and after birth. *Acta Paediatr Scand [Suppl]* 1983;305:12–20.
46. Egan EA, Olver RE, Strang LB. Changes in non-electrolyte permeability of alveoli and the absorption of lung liquid at the start of breathing in the lamb. *J Physiol* 1975;244:161–179.
47. Aherne W, Dawkins MJR. The removal of fluid from the pulmonary airways after birth in the rabbit, and the effect on this of prematurity and prenatal hypoxia. *Biol Neonate* 1964;7:214.
48. Fletcher BD, Sachs BE, Kotas RV. Radiologic demonstration of postnatal liquid in the lungs of newborn lambs. *Pediatrics* 1970;46:252.
49. Castro R, Ervin MG, Ross MG, Sherman DJ, Leake RD, et al. Ovine fetal lung fluid response to atrial natriuretic factor. *Am J Obstet Gynecol* 1989;161:1337–1343.
50. Bland RD, Carlton DP, Scheerer RG, Cummings JJ, Chapman DL. Lung fluid balance in lambs before and after premature birth. *J Clin Invest* 1989;84:568–576.
51. Grawjer LA, Sperling MA, Sack J, et al. Possible mechanisms and significance of the neonatal surge in glucagon secretion. Studies in newborn lambs. *Pediatr Res* 1977;11:833.
52. Kaneoka T, Ozono H, Goto U, et al. Plasma noradrenalin and adrenalin concentration in feto-maternal blood. Their relation to feto-maternal endocrine levels, cardiotocographic and mechanoradiographic values, and umbilical arterial blood biochemical profiling. *J Perinat Med* 1979;7:302–310.
53. Lagercrantz H, Marcus C. Sympathoadrenal mechanisms during development. In: Polin RA, Fox WW, eds. *Fetal and neonatal physiology.* Philadelphia: WB Saunders, 1992:160–169.
54. Boon AW, Milner AD, Hopkin IE. Lung volumes and lung mechanics in babies born vaginally and by elective and emergency lower segmental cesarean section. *J Pediatr* 1981;98(5):812–815.
55. Cassady G. Effect of cesarean section on neonatal body water spaces. *N Engl J Med* 1971;285(16):887–891.
56. Milner AD, Vyas H. Lung expansion at birth. *J Pediatr* 1982;101:879–886.
57. Milner AD, Saunders RA, Hopkin IE. Effects of delivery by caesarean section on lung mechanics and lung volume in the human neonate. *Arch Dis Child* 1978;53(7):545–548.
58. Avery ME, Gatewood OB, Brumley G. Transient tachypnea of newborn. *Am J Dis Child* 1966;111:380.
59. Skinner JR, Boys RJ, Hunter S, Hey EN. Non-invasive assessment of pulmonary arterial pressure in healthy neonates. *Arch Dis Child* 1991;66:386–390.
60. Belik J, Stephens NL. Developmental differences in vascular smooth muscle mechanics in pulmonary and systemic circulations. *J Appl Physiol* 1993;74(2):682–687.
61. Musewe NN, Poppe D, Smallhorn JF, Hellman J, Whyte H, et al. Doppler echocardiographic measurement of pulmonary artery pressure from ductal Doppler velocities in the newborn. *J Am Coll Cardiol* 1990;15:446–456.
62. Stopfkuchen H. Changes of the cardiovascular system during the perinatal period. *Eur J Pediatr* 1987;146:545–549.
63. Starling MD, Elliot RB. The effects of prostaglandins, prostaglandin inhibitors and oxygen on the closure of the ductus arteriosus, pulmonary arteries and umbilical vessels *in vitro*. *Prostaglandins* 1974;8:187.
64. Sharpe GI, Larsson KS. Studies on closure of the ductus arteriosus, X. *In vitro* effects of prostaglandins. *Prostaglandins* 1975;9:703.
65. Weiss H, Cooper B, Brook M, Schlueter M, Clyman R. Factors determining reopening of the ductus arteriosus after successful clinical closure with indomethacin. *J Pediatr* 1995;127(3):466–471.
66. Milne MJ, Sung RYT, Fok TF, Crozier IG. Doppler echocardiographic assessment of shunting via the ductus arteriosus in newborn infants. *Am J Cardiol* 1989;64:102–105.
67. Creasy RK, Drost M, Green MV, Morris JA. Effect of ventilation on transfer of blood from placenta to neonate. *Am J Physiol* 1972;222:186–188.
68. Marquis L, Ackerman BD. Placental respiration in the immediate neonatal period. *Am J Obstet Gynecol* 1973;117:358–363.
69. Phillip AGS, Teng SS. Role of respiration in effecting placental transfusion at cesarean section. *Biol Neonate* 1977;31:219–224.
70. Baylen BG, Agata Y, Padbury JF, Ikegami M, Jobe AH, et al. Hemodynamic and neuroendocrine adaptations of the preterm lamb left ventricle to acutely increased afterload. *Pediatr Res* 1989;26:336–342.
71. Rein AJJT, Sanders SP, Colan SD, Oarness IA, Epstein M. Left ventricular mechanics in the normal newborn. *Circulation* 1987;76(5):1029–1036.
72. Ogata ES. Carbohydrate metabolism in the fetus and neonate and altered neonatal glucoregulation. *Pediatr Clin North Am* 1986;33(1):25–45.
73. Lagercrantz H, Slotkin TA. The "stress" of being born. *Sci Am* 1986;254(4):100–107.
74. Marchini G, Persson B, Jonsson N, Marcus C. Influence of body temperature on thyrotropic hormone release and lipolysis in the newborn infant. *Acta Paediatr* 1995;84(11):1284–1288.
75. Fisher DA, Polk DH. Fetal and neonatal thyroid physiology. In Polin RA, Fox WW, eds. *Fetal and neonatal physiology.* Philadelphia: WB Saunders, 1992:1842–1849.
76. Nedergaard J, Cannon B. Brown adipose tissue: Development and function. In Polin RA, Fox WW, eds. *Fetal and neonatal physiology.* Philadelphia: WB Saunders, 1992:314–325.
77. Power GG. Fetal Thermoregulation: animal and human. In Polin RA, Fox WW, eds. *Fetal and neonatal physiology.* Philadelphia: WB Saunders, 1992:477–483.
78. Milner AD, Saunders RA. Pressure and volume changes during the first breath of human neonates. *Arch Dis Child* 1977;52:918–924.
79. Davis GM, Coates AL, Papageorgiou A, Bureau MA. Direct measurement of static chest wall compliance in animal and human neonates. *J Appl Physiol* 1988;65(3):1093–1098.
80. Ratjen F, Zinman R, Stark AR, Leszczynski LE, Wohl MEB. Effect of changes in lung volume on respiratory system compliance in newborn infants. *J Appl Physiol* 1989;67(3):1192–1197.

81. Geubelle F, Francotte M, Beyer M, et al. Functional residual capacity and thoracic gas volume in normoxic and hyperoxic newborn infants. *Acta Paediatr Belg* 1977;30:221–225.

82. Krauss AN, Auld PAM. Pulmonary gas trapping in premature infants. *Pediatr Res* 1971;5:10.

83. Agostoni E, Mead J. Statics of the respiratory system. In: *Handbook of physiology, vol 1.* Washington, DC: American Physiological Society, 1964.

84. Colin AA, Wohl MEB, Mead J, Ratjen FA, Glass G, et al. Transition from dynamically maintained to relaxed end-expiratory volume in human infants. *J Appl Physiol* 1989;67(5):2107–2111.

85. Mortola JP, Milic-Emili J, Noworaj A, et al. Muscle pressure and flow during expiration in infants. *Am Rev Respir Dis* 1984;129:49–53.

86. Stark AR, Cohlan BA, Waggener TB, Frantz ID, Kosch PC. Regulation of end-expiratory lung volume during sleep in premature infants. *J Appl Physiol* 1987;62(3):1117–1123.

87. Diaz V, Kianicka I, Letourneau P, Praud JP. Inferior pharyngeal constrictor electromyographic activity during permeability pulmonary edema in lambs. *J Appl Physiol* 1996;81(4):1598–1604.

88. Harding R. Function of the larynx in the fetus or newborn. *Annu Rev Physiol* 1984;46:645–659.

89. Kosch PC, Davenport PW, Wozniak JA, Stark AR. Reflex control of expiratory duration in newborn infants. *J Appl Physiol* 1985;58:575–581.

90. Kosch PC, Hutchison AA, Wozniak JA, Carlo WA, Stark AR. Posterior cricoarytenoid and diaphragm activities during tidal breathing in neonates. *J Appl Physiol* 1988;64(5):1968–1978.

91. Wise PH, Krauss AN, Waldman S, Auld PAM. Flow–volume loops in newborn infants. *Crit Care Med* 1980;8:61–63.

92. Reed WR, Roberts JL, Thach BT. Factors influencing regional patency and configuration of the human infant upper airway. *J Appl Physiol* 1985;58:635–644.

93. Wilson SL, Thach BT, Brouillette RT, Abu-Osba YK. Coordination of breathing and swallowing in human infants. *J Appl Physiol* 1981;50:851–858.

94. Abu-Osba YK, Brouillette RT, Wilson SL, Thach BT. Breathing pattern and transcutaneous oxygen tension during motor activity in preterm infants. *Am Rev Respir Dis* 1982;125:382–387.

95. Mortola JP, Rezzonico R. Ventilation in kittens with chronic section of the superior laryngeal nerves. *Respir Physiol* 1989;76:369–382.

96. Wennergren G, Hertzberg T, Milerad J, Bjure J, Lagercrantz H. Hypoxia reinforces laryngeal reflex bradycardia in infants. *Acta Paediatr Scand* 1989;78:11–16.

97. Vyas H, Milner AD, Hopkin IE, Falconer AD. Role of labour in the establishment of functional residual capacity at birth. *Arch Dis Child* 1983;58(7):512–517.

98. Thibeault DW, Poblete E, Auld PAM. Alveolar–arterial O$_2$ and CO$_2$ differences and their relation to lung volume in the newborn. *Pediatrics* 1968;41:574.

99. Vanderghem A, Beardsmore C, Silverman M. Postural variations in pulmonary resistance, dynamic compliance, and esophageal pressure in neonates. *Crit Care Med* 1983;11:424–427.

100. Hutchinson AA, Ross KR, Russell G. The effect of posture on ventilation and lung mechanics in preterm and light-for-date infants. *Pediatrics* 1979;64:429–432.

101. Martin RJ, Herrell M, Rubin D, Fanaroff A. Effect of supine and prone positions on arterial oxygen tension in the preterm infant. *Pediatrics* 1979;63:528–531.

102. Fleming PJ, Muller ML, Bryan MH, Bryan AC. The effects of abdominal loading on rib cage distortion in premature infants. *Pediatrics* 1979;64:425–428.

103. Bryan MH, Knill RL, Bryan AC. Chest wall instability and its influence on respiration in the newborn infant. In Stern L, Fries-Hansen B, Kildeberg P, eds. *Intensive care in the newborn.* New York: Masson, 1976.

104. Bryan AC, Bryan MH. Control of respiration in the newborn. *Clin Perinatol* 1978;5:269–281.

105. Bolton DPG, Herman S. Ventilation and sleep state in the new-born. *J Physiol* 1974;240:67–77.

106. Finer NN, Abroms IF, Taeusch HW. Ventilation and sleep states in newborn infants. *J Pediatr* 1976;89:100–108.

107. Harding R, Johnson P, McClelland ME, et al. Laryngeal function during breathing and swallowing in foetal and newborn lambs. *J Physiol* 1977;272:14P–15P.

108. Hathorn MKS. The rate and depth of breathing in new-born infants in different sleep states. *J Physiol* 1974;243:101–113.

109. Frantz ID, Adler SM, Abroms IF, Thach BT. Respiratory response to airway occlusion in infants: sleep state and maturation. *J Appl Physiol* 1976;41:634–638.

110. Haddad GG, Lai TL, Epstein MAF, et al. Breath-to-breath variations in rate and depth of ventilation in sleeping infants. *Am J Physiol* 1982;243:R164–R169.

111. Knill R, Andrews W, Bryan AC, Bryan MH. Respiratory load compensation in infants. *J Appl Physiol* 1976;40:357–361.

112. van Eyck J, Wladimiroff JW, van den Wijngaard JAGW, Noordam MJ, Prechtl HFR. The blood flow velocity waveform in the fetal internal carotid and umbilical artery; its relation to fetal behavioural states in normal pregnancy at 37–38 weeks. *Br J Obstet Gynaecol* 1987;94:736–741.

113. Durand M, Leahy FN, MacCallum M, et al. Effect of feeding on the chemical control of breathing in the newborn infant. *Pediatr Res* 1981;15:1509–1512.

114. Read DJC, Henderson-Smart DJ. Regulation of breathing during different behavioral states. *Annu Rev Physiol* 1984;46:675–685.

115. Le Souef PN, Lopes JM, England SJ, et al. Effect of chest wall distortion on occlusion pressure and the preterm diaphragm. *J Appl Physiol* 1983;55:359–364.

116. Homma Y, Wilkes D, Bryan MH, Bryan AC. Rib cage and abdominal contributions to ventilatory response to C0$_2$ in infants. *J Appl Physiol* 1984;56:1211–1216.

117. Knill R, Bryan AC. An intercostal–phrenic inhibitory reflex in human newborn infants. *J Appl Physiol* 1976;40:352–356.

118. Hagan R, Bryan AC, Bryan MH, Gulston G. Neonatal chest wall afferents and regulation of respiration. *J Appl Physiol* 1977;42:362–367.

119. Tusiewicz K, Moldofsky H, Bryan AC, Bryan MH. Mechanics of the rib cage and diaphragm during sleep. *J Appl Physiol* 1977;43:600–602.

120. Lopes JM, Muller NL, Bryan MH, Bryan AC. Synergistic behavior of inspiratory muscles after diaphragmatic fatigue in the newborn. *J Appl Physiol* 1981;51:547–551.

121. Guslits BG, Gaston SE, Bryan MH, England SJ, Bryan AC. Diaphragmatic work of breathing in premature human infants. *J Appl Physiol* 1987;62(4):1410–1415.

122. Keens TG, Bryan AC, Levison H, Ianuzzo CD. Developmental pattern of muscle fiber types in human ventilatory muscles. *J Appl Physiol* 1978;44:909–913.

123. Le Souef PN, England SJ, Stogryn HAF, Bryan AC. Comparison of diaphragmatic fatigue in newborn and older rabbits. *J Appl Physiol* 1988;65(3):1040–1044.

124. Watchko JF, Sieck GC. Respiratory muscle fatigue resistance relates to myosin phenotype and SDH activity during development. *J Appl Physiol* 1993;75(3):1341–1347.

125. Johnson BD, Wilson LE, Zhan WZ, Watchko JF, Daood MJ, et al. Contractile properties of the developing diaphragm correlate with myosin heavy chain phenotype. *J Appl Physiol* 1994;77(1):481–487.

126. Praud J, Egreteau L, Benlabed M, Curzi-Dascalova L, Nedelcoux H, et al. Abdominal muscle activity during CO$_2$ rebreathing in sleeping neonates. *J Appl Physiol* 1991;70(3):1344–1350.

127. Henderson-Smart DJ, Read DJC. Reduced lung volume during behavioral active sleep in the newborn. *J Appl Physiol* 1979;46:1081–1085.

128. Le Souef PN, Lopes JM, England SJ, et al. Influence of chest wall distortion on esophageal pressure. *J Appl Physiol* 1983;55:353.

129. Gerhart T, Reifenberg L, Duara S, Bancalari E. Comparison of dynamic and static measurements of respiratory mechanics in infants. *J Pediatr* 1989;114:120–125.

130. Le Souef PN, England SJ, Bryan AC. Passive respiratory mechanics in newborn and children. *Am Rev Respir Dis* 1984;129:552–556.

131. Johnson SM, Smith JC, Feldman JL. Modulation of respiratory rhythm *in vitro*: role of G$_{i/o}$ protein-mediated mechanisms. *J Appl Physiol* 1996;80(6):2120–2133.

132. Frantz ID, Adler SM, Thach BT, Taeusch HW. Maturational effects on respiratory responses to carbon dioxide in premature infants. *J Appl Physiol* 1976;41:41–45.

133. Cosgrove JF, Neunburger N, Bryan MH, et al. A new method of evaluating the chemosensitivity of the respiratory center in children. *Pediatrics* 1975;56:972–980.

134. Carroll JL, Bamford OS, Fitzgerald RS. Postnatal maturation of carotid chemoreceptor responses to O$_2$ and CO$_2$ in the cat. *J Appl Physiol* 1993;75(6):2383–2391.

135. Suthers GK, Henderson-Smart DJ, Read DJC. Postnatal changes in the rate of high frequency bursts in inspiratory activity in cats and dogs. *Brain Res* 1977;132:537–540.

136. Canet E, Kianicka I, Praud JP. Postnatal maturation of peripheral chemoreceptor ventilatory response to O_2 and CO_2 in newborn lambs. *J Appl Physiol* 1996;80(6):1928–1933.

137. Reinstorff D, Fenner A. Ventilatory response to hyperoxia in premature and newborn infants during the first three days of life. *Respir Physiol* 1972;15:159–165.

138. Krauss AN, Tori CA, Brown J. Oxygen chemoreceptors in low birth weight infants. *Pediatr Res* 1973;7:569–574.

139. Albersheim S, Boychuk R, Seshia MMK. Effects of CO_2 on immediate ventilatory response to O_2 in preterm infants. *J Appl Physiol* 1976; 41:609–611.

140. Rigatto H, Kalapesi Z, Leahy FN, et al. Ventilatory response to 100% and 15% O_2 during wakefulness and sleep in preterm infants. *Early Hum Dev* 1982;7:1–10.

141. Walker DW. Peripheral and central chemoreceptors in the fetus and newborn. *Annu Rev Physiol* 1984;46:687–703.

142. Haddad GG, Mellins RB. Hypoxia and respiratory control in early life. *Annu Rev Physiol* 1984;46:629–643.

143. Lin J, Suguihara C, Huang J, Hehre D, Devia C, et al. Effect of N-methyl-D-aspartate-receptor blockade on hypoxic ventilatory response in unanesthetized piglets. *J Appl Physiol* 1996;80(5):1759–1763.

144. Rigatto H, Wiebe C, Rigatto C, Lee DS, Cates D. Ventilatory response to hypoxia in unanesthetized newborn kittens. *J Appl Physiol* 1988;64(6):2544–2551.

145. Darnall RA, Green G, Pinto L, Hart N. Effect of acute hypoxia on respiration and brain stem blood flow in the piglet. *J Appl Physiol* 1991; 70(1):251–259.

146. Longo LD, Pearce WJ. Fetal and newborn cerebral vascular responses and adaptations to hypoxia. *Semin Perinatol* 1991;15(1):49–57.

147. Suguihara C, Bancalari E, Hehre D. Brain blood flow and ventilatory response to hypoxia in sedated newborn piglets. *Pediatr Res* 1990;27: 327–331.

148. Duara S, Neto GS, Gerhardt T, Suguihara C, Bancalari E. Metabolic and respiratory effects of flow-resistive loading in preterm infants. *J Appl Physiol* 1991;70(2):895–899.

149. Downing SE, Chen V. Myocardial hibernation in the ischemic neonatal heart. *Circ Res* 1990;66:763–772.

150. Gleed RD, Mortola JP. Ventilation in newborn rats after gestation at simulated high altitude. *J Appl Physiol* 1991;70(3):1146–1151.

151. Okubo S, Mortola JP. Respiratory mechanics in adult rats hypoxic in the neonatal period. *J Appl Physiol* 1989;66(4):1772–1778.

152. Moss IR, Inman JG. Neurochemicals and respiratory control during development. *J Appl Physiol* 1989;67(1):1–13.

153. Wyszogrodski I, Thach BT, Milic-Emili J. Maturation of respiratory control in unanesthetized newborn rabbits. *J Appl Physiol* 1978;44:304–310.

154. Olinsky A, Bryan MH, Bryan AC. Influence of lung inflation on respiratory control in neonates. *J Appl Physiol* 1974;36:426–429.

155. Olinsky A, Bryan MH, Bryan AC. Response of newborn infants to added respiratory loads. *J Appl Physiol* 1974;37:190–193.

156. Taeusch HW, Carson S, Frantz ID, Milic-Emili J. Respiratory regulation after elastic loading and CO_2 rebreathing in normal term infants. *J Pediatr* 1976;88:102–111.

157. Kirkpatrick SML, Olinsky A, Bryan MH, Bryan AC. Effect of premature delivery on the maturation of the Hering-Breuer inspiratory inhibitory reflex in human infants. *J Pediatr* 1976;88:1010–1014.

158. Adler SM, Thach ET, Frantz ID. Maturational changes of effective elastance in the first 10 days of life. *J Appl Physiol* 1976;40:539–542.

159. Rabbette PS, Fletcher ME, Dezateux CA, Soriano-Brucher H, Stocks J. Hering-Breuer reflex and respiratory system compliance in the first year of life: a longitudinal study. *J Appl Physiol* 1994;76(2):650–656.

160. Moomjian AS, Schwartz JG, Wagaman MJ, et al. The effect of external expiratory resistance on lung volume and pulmonary function in the neonate. *J Pediatr* 1980;96:908–911.

161. Rigatto H, Brady JP. Periodic breathing and apnea in preterm infants: II. Hypoxia as a primary event. *Pediatrics* 1972;50:219–228.

162. Fenner A, Schalk U, Hoenicke H, et al. Periodic breathing in premature and neonatal babies: Incidence, breathing pattern, respiratory gas tensions, response to changes in the composition of ambient air. *Pediatr Res* 1973;7:174–183.

163. Guntheroth WG, Kawabori I. Hypoxic apnea and gasping. *J Clin Invest* 1975;56:1371–1377.

164. Lawson EE, Thach BT. Respiratory patterns during progressive asphyxia in newborn rabbits. *J Appl Physiol* 1977;43:468–474.

165. Webb B, Hutchison AA, Davenport PW. Vagally mediated volume-dependent modulation of inspiratory duration in the neonatal lamb. *J Appl Physiol* 1994;76(1):397–402.

166. Haddad GG, Mellins RH. The role of airway receptors in the control of respiration in infants: A review. *J Pediatr* 1977;91:281–286.

167. Waggener TB, Frantz ID, Stark AR, Kronauer RE. Oscillatory breathing patterns leading to apneic spells in infants. *J Appl Physiol* 1982;52:1288–1295.

168. Fleming PJ, Goncalves AL, Levine MR, Woollard S. The development of stability of respiration in human infants: Changes in ventilatory responses to spontaneous sighs. *J Physiol* 1984;347:1–16.

169. Canet E, Praud JP, Bureau MA. Periodic breathing induced on demand in awake newborn lamb. *J Appl Physiol* 1997;82(2):607–612.

170. Dahms BB, Krauss AN, Auld PAM. Pulmonary function in dysmature infants. *J Pediatr* 1974;84:434–437.

171. Koch G. Lung function and acid–base balance in the newborn infant. *Acta Paediatr Scand [Suppl]* 1968;181:5.

172. Parks CR, Woodrum DE, Alden ER, et al. Gas exchange in the immature lung I. Anatomical shunt in the premature infant. *J Appl Physiol* 1974;36:103–107.

173. Palme-Kilander C, Tunell R, Chiwei Y. Pulmonary gas exchange immediately after birth in spontaneously breathing infants. *Arch Dis Child* 1993;68(1 Spec No):6–10.

174. Bolton DPG. Diffusional inhomogeneity: gas mixing efficiency in the new-born lung. *J Physiol* 1979;286:447–455.

175. Sandberg K, Sjoqvist BA, Hjalmarson O, Olsson T. Analysis of alveolar ventilation in the newborn. *Arch Dis Child* 1984;59:542–547.

176. Arcilla RA, Oh W, Wallgren G. Quantitative studies of the human neonatal circulation, II. Hemodynamic findings in early and late clamping of the umbilical cord. *Acta Paediatr Scand* 1967;179:25.

177. Assali NS. Some aspects of fetal life *in utero* and the changes at birth. *Am J Obstet Gynecol* 1967;97:324.

178. McMurphy DM, Heymann MA, Rudolph AM, Melmon K. Developmental changes in constriction of the ductus arteriosus: responses to oxygen and vasoactive agents in the isolated ductus arteriosus of the fetal lamb. *Pediatr Res* 1972;6:231.

179. Wallgren G, Hanson JS, Lind J. Quantitative studies of the human neonatal circulation, III. Observations of the newborn infant's central circulatory responses to moderate hypovolemia. *Acta Paediatr Scand [Suppl]* 1967;179:45.

180. Wallgren G, Lind J. Quantitative studies of the human neonatal circulation, IV. Observations on the newborn infant's peripheral circulation and plasma expansion during moderate hypovolemia. *Acta Paediatr Scand [Suppl]* 1967;179:57.

181. Wallgren G, Hanson JS, Tabakin BS, et al. Quantitative studies of the human neonatal circulation, V. Hemodynamic findings in premature infants with and without respiratory distress. *Acta Paediatr Scand [Suppl]* 1967;179:71.

182. Drayton MR, Skidmore R. Ductus arteriosus blood flow during first 48 hours of life. *Arch Dis Child* 1987;62:1030–1034.

183. Dawes GS. *Fetal and neonatal physiology.* Chicago: Year Book, 1968.

184. Folkow B, Neil E. *Circulation.* London: Oxford University Press, 1971.

185. Harned HS. Respiration and the respiratory system. In Stave U, eds. *Physiology of the perinatal period.* New York: Appleton Century Crofts, 1970

186. Rudolph AM, Heymann MA. The circulation of the fetus *in utero:* Methods for studying distribution of blood flow, cardiac output and organ blood flow. *Circ Res* 1967;21:163.

187. Rudolph AM, Heymann MA. Circulatory changes during growth in the fetal lamb. *Circ Res* 1970;26:289.

188. Rudolph AM, Heymann MA, Teramo KAW, et al. Studies on the circulation of the previable human fetus. *Pediatr Res* 1971;5:452.

189. Reed KL, Anderson CF, Shenker L. Fetal pulmonary artery and aorta: two-dimensional Doppler echocardiography. *Obstet Gynecol* 1987;69:175–178.

190. Mendelson CR, Boggaram V. Hormonal control of the surfactant system in fetal lung. *Annu Rev Physiol* 1991;53:415–440.

191. Chu J, Clements JA, Cotton EK, et al. Neonatal pulmonary ischemia. *Pediatrics* 1967;40:709.

192. Mansell A, Bryan AC, Levison H. Airway closure in children. *J Appl Physiol* 1972;33:711.

193. Nelson NM. Neonatal pulmonary function. *Pediatr Clin North Am* 1966;13:769.

194. Phelan PD, Williams HE. Ventilatory studies in healthy infants. *Pediatr Res* 1969;3:425.

195. Polgar G, Promadhat V. *Pulmonary function testing in children: techniques and standards.* Philadelphia: WB Saunders, 1971.

196. Lacourt G, Polgar G. Development of pulmonary function in late gestation. The functional residual capacity of the lung in premature children. *Acta Paediatr Scand* 1974;63:81–88.

197. Milner AD, Saunders RA, Hopkin IE. Tidal pressure/volume and flow/volume respiratory loop patterns in human neonates. *Clin Sci Mol Med* 1978;54:257–264.

198. Tunell R, Gopher D, Persson B. The pulmonary gas exchange and blood gas changes in connection with birth. In Stetson JB, Surger PR, eds. *Neonatal intensive care.* St Louis: Warren H. Green 1976: p. 99.

199. Lacourt G, Polgar G. Interaction between nasal and pulmonary resistance in newborn infants. *J Appl Physiol* 1971;30:870.

200. Sharp JT, Druz WS, Balagot RC, et al. Total respiratory compliance in infants and children. *J Appl Physiol* 1970;29:775.

201. Davis GM, Bureau MA. Pulmonary and chest wall mechanics in the control of respiration in the newborn. *Clin Perinatol* 1987;14(3): 551–579.

202. Mortola JP. Dynamics of breathing in newborn mammals. *Physiol Rev* 1987;67(1):187–243.

203. Lees MH, Way RC, Ross BB. Ventilation and respiratory gas transfer of infants with increased pulmonary blood flow. *Pediatrics* 1967;40: 259.

204. Corbet AJS, Ross JA, Beaudry PH, Stern L. Effect of positive-pressure breathing on aADN$_2$ in hyaline membrane disease. *J Appl Physiol* 1975;38:33–38.

205. Corbet AJS, Ross JA, Beaudry PH, Stern L. Assessment of ventilation–perfusion inequality by aADN$_2$ in newborn infants. *Biol Neonate* 1979;36:10–17.

206. Krauss AN, Klain DB, Auld PAM. Carbon monoxide diffusing capacity in newborn infants. *Pediatr Res* 1976;10:771–776.

207. Avery ME, Fletcher BD. *The lung and its disorders in the newborn infant, 3rd ed.* Philadelphia: WB Saunders, 1974.

208. Nourse CH, Nelson NM. Uniformity of ventilation in the newborn infant; direct assessment of the arterial–alveolar N$_2$ difference. *Pediatrics* 1969;43:226.

209. Smith CA, Nelson NM. *Physiology of the newborn infant, 4th ed.* Springfield, IL: Charles C Thomas 1976.

210. Radford EP. *Tissue elasticity, vol 177.* Washington, DC: American Physiological Society, 1957

211. Burns BD. The central control of respiratory movements. *Br Med Bull* 1963;19:7.

212. Strang LB. The lungs at birth. *Arch Dis Child* 1965;40:575.

213. Rasmussen K. Quantitative blood flow in the fetal descending aorta and in the umbilical vein in normal pregnancies. Longitudinal and cross-sectional studies. *Scand J Clin Lab Invest* 1987;47:319–324.

214. Mandelbaum VHA, Alverson DC, Kirchgessner A, Linderkamp O. Postnatal changes in cardiac output and haemorrheology in normal neonates born at full term. *Arch Dis Child* 1991;66:391–394.

215. Burnard ED, Granang A, Gray RE. Cardiac output in the newborn infant. *Clin Sci* 1966;31:121.

216. Walther FJ, Benders MJ, Leighton JO. Early changes in the neonatal circulatory transition. *J Pediatr* 1993;123(4):625–632.

217. Padbury JF, Agata Y, Ludlow J, Ikegami M, Baylen B, Humme J. Effect of fetal adrenalectomy on catecholamine release and physiologic adaptation at birth in sheep. *J Clin Invest* 1987;80:1096.

218. Padbury JF, Polk DH, Newnham JP, Lam RW. Neonatal adaptation: Greater sympathoadrenal response in preterm than full-term fetal sheep at birth. *Am J Physiol* 1985;248:E443.

219. Broberger U, Hansson U, Lagercrantz H, Persson B. Sympathoadrenal activity and metabolic adjustment during the first 12 hours after birth in infants of diabetic mothers. *Acta Paediatr Scand* 1984;73(5):620–625.

220. Faxelius G, Lagercrantz H, Yao A. Sympathoadrenal activity and peripheral blood flow after birth: comparison in infants delivered vaginally and by cesarean section. *J Pediatr* 1984;105(1):144–148.

221. Hagnevik K, Faxelius G, Irestedt L, Lagercrantz H, Lundell B, et al. Catecholamine surge and metabolic adaptation in the newborn after vaginal delivery and caesarean section. *Acta Paediatr Scand* 1984;73(5):602–609.

222. Fisher DA, Klein AH. Thyroid development and disorders of the thyroid in the newborn. *N Engl J Med* 1981;304:702.

223. Cornblath M, Reisner SH. Blood glucose in the neonate and its clinical significance. *N Engl J Med* 1965;273:378–381.

224. Muller N, Gulston G, Cade D, Whitton J, Froese AB, et al. Diaphragmatic muscle fatigue in the newborn. *J Appl Physiol* 1979;46(4): 688–695.

CHAPTER 18

Delivery Room Management

Roderic H. Phibbs

Much of newborn intensive care is emergency medicine that requires rapid institution of appropriate diagnostic and therapeutic procedures. This is particularly true immediately after birth, when the newborn infant may have cardiac arrest and apnea. The procedures undertaken to restore life constitute resuscitation, from the Latin *resuscitate*, "to arouse again," and include those actions necessary to help an infant make the transition from dependent fetal life to independent neonatal life. Skillful resuscitation of the asphyxiated newborn infant can prevent brain damage and minimize subsequent neonatal disease. There is a high risk of asphyxia during labor, delivery, and the first minutes after birth. This is because of the arrangement of the fetal circulatory pathways and because the newborn infant must successfully inflate his or her lungs and rearrange his or her circulation immediately after birth. Failure of either to occur leads to asphyxia. A rational approach to resuscitation must be based on the physiologic changes in the circulatory and respiratory systems that occur normally as the newborn infant adapts to extrauterine life. The physiology of transition, discussed in Chapter 17, should be understood before reading this chapter.

PATHOPHYSIOLOGY OF INTRAPARTUM ASPHYXIA AND RESUSCITATION

Asphyxia occurs when the organ of gas exchange fails. When this occurs, arterial carbon dioxide partial pressure ($PaCO_2$) rises, and arterial oxygen partial pressure (PaO_2) and pH fall. Despite the low PaO_2, tissues continue to consume O_2, although at a lower rate in some organs. When the PaO_2 is very low, anaerobic metabolism occurs, producing large quantities of metabolic acids. These are buffered partly by the bicarbonate in the blood (1).

R. H. Phibbs: Department of Pediatrics, University of California, San Francisco, San Francisco, California

The human infant is particularly vulnerable to asphyxia in the perinatal period. During normal labor, transient hypoxemia occurs with uterine contractions, but the healthy fetus tolerates this well. There are five basic causes of asphyxia during labor and delivery:

1. Interruption of umbilical blood flow (e.g., cord compression)
2. Failure of gas exchange across the placenta (e.g., placental abruption)
3. Inadequate perfusion of the maternal side of the placenta (e.g., severe maternal hypotension)
4. An otherwise compromised fetus who cannot further tolerate the transient, intermittent hypoxia of normal labor (e.g., the anemic or growth-retarded fetus)
5. Failure to inflate the lungs and complete the change in ventilation and lung perfusion that must occur at birth.

The last cause may occur because of airway obstruction, excessive fluid in the lungs, or weak respiratory effort. Alternatively, it may occur as a result of fetal asphyxia from one of the first four causes, because fetal asphyxia often leads to an infant who is acidotic and apneic at birth.

The umbilical cord blood pH, partial pressure of oxygen (PO_2), partial pressure of carbon dioxide (PCO_2), and calculated base excess are standard measures of fetal asphyxia (2–4). With fetal acidosis, the pH can vary over a wide range. Consequently, it is important to remember that pH is a logarithmic function of hydrogen ion concentration. A decrease of 0.3 pH units from 7.40 to 7.10 indicates only a 40 nmol/L increase in hydrogen ion (i.e., from 40 to 80 nmol), whereas a 0.3 decrease from 7.10 to 6.80 indicates an increase of 80 nmol/L (i.e., from 80 to 160 nmol). The gradient in blood gas tensions between umbilical artery and vein gives some indication of placental perfusion at the time of birth. The slower the flow of fetal blood through the placenta, the more complete the equilibration of gas tensions between fetal and maternal blood. For example, an arterial PO_2 of 25 mm Hg with a venous PO_2 of 32 mm Hg suggests good placental blood flow. An arterial PO_2 of 12 mm Hg with a venous PO_2 of 45 mm Hg suggests very slow flow. Metabolic acidosis suggests asphyxia, although some of the increased lactic acid in the blood may be due to reduced uptake of lactate by the asphyxiated liver rather than increased lactate production from anaerobic metabolism (2,5). If asphyxia occurred just before birth, there may be lactic acid in the tissues that has not yet reached the central circulation. This will be detected only by blood gas measurements a few minutes after birth. If the fetus was asphyxiated an hour before delivery and recovered, that event will not be reflected in the umbilical cord blood gases at birth. Other indicators of asphyxia include plasma hypoxanthine, which increases because of lack of aerobic metabolism, and plasma erythropoietin, which increases in response to fetal hypoxia (5).

Asphyxia in the fetus or newborn infant is a progressive and reversible process. The speed and extent of progression are highly variable. Sudden, severe asphyxia can be lethal in less than 10 minutes. Mild asphyxia may progressively worsen over 30 minutes or more. Repeated episodes of brief, mild asphyxia may reverse spontaneously but produce a cumulative effect of progressive asphyxia. In the early stages, asphyxia usually reverses spontaneously if its cause is removed. Once asphyxia is severe, spontaneous reversal is unlikely because of the circulatory and neurologic changes that accompany it. Other sources provide a general review of these phenomena (7).

Figure 18–1 schematically represents the sequence of pathophysiologic changes that accompany asphyxia. Although there are some quantitative differences between the changes that occur in the fetus and those in the newborn infant, the scheme generally applies to both. It is useful to consider the changes in both fetus and newborn infant together, because many cases of neonatal asphyxia begin in the fetus and continue after birth. Cardiac output is maintained early in asphyxia, but its distribution changes radically. Selective regional vasoconstriction reduces blood flow to less vital organs and tissues such as gut, kidneys, muscle, and skin (8). Blood flow to the brain and myocardium increases, thereby maintaining adequate oxygen delivery despite reduced oxygen content of the arterial blood. Other organs and tissues must depend on increased oxygen extraction to maintain oxygen consumption (9,10). Pulmonary blood flow is low in the fetus. It is decreased further by hypoxia and acidosis (11). As a consequence of these adaptations, fetal oxygen consumption decreases (12).

Early in asphyxia, newborns make vigorous attempts to inflate their lungs. If successful, the lungs become adequately ventilated and perfused, but the mere presence of gasping does not ensure that this will happen. As

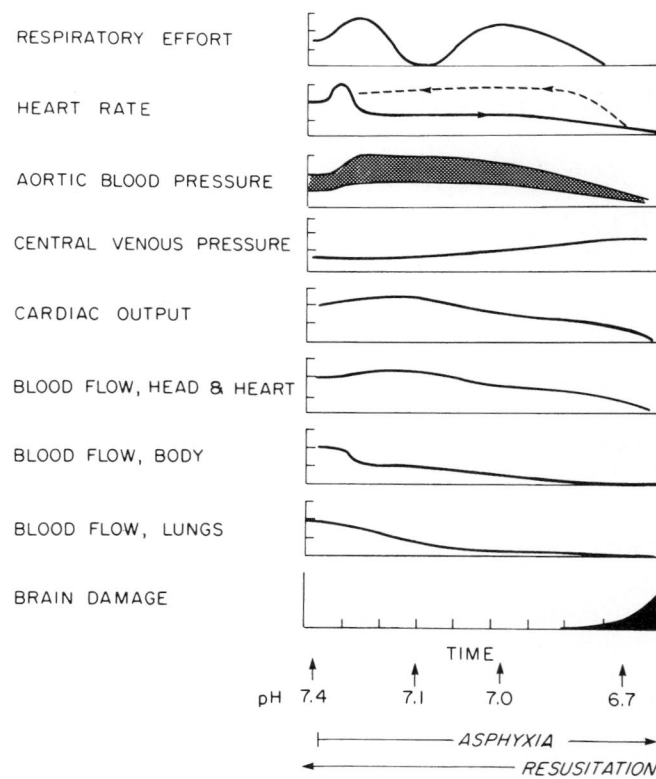

FIG. 18–1. The sequence of cardiopulmonary changes with asphyxia and resuscitation. If there is complete interruption of respiratory gas exchange, the entire process of asphyxia could occur in about 10 minutes. It could take much longer with an asphyxiating process that only partly interrupts gas exchange or one that does so completely but only for repeated brief periods. With resuscitation, the process reverses, beginning at the point to which the asphyxia has proceeded. (Adapted from ref. 7.)

asphyxia becomes more severe, the respiratory center is depressed, and the chances of an infant spontaneously establishing effective ventilation and pulmonary perfusion diminish.

If asphyxia progresses to the severe stage, oxygen delivery to the brain and heart decreases. The myocardium then uses its stored reserve of glycogen for energy. Eventually, the glycogen reserve is consumed and the myocardium is exposed simultaneously to progressively lower values of PO_2 and pH. The combined effects of hypoxia and acidosis lead to decreased myocardial function and decreased blood flow to the vital organs (13,14). Brain injury begins late during this phase (7).

This sequence of cardiovascular events is manifested by changes in heart rate and aortic and central venous pressures (see Fig. 18–1), all of which are measured easily in the newborn immediately after birth. The early bradycardia and hypertension are due to the reflexes that shunt blood away from nonvital organs. Early in asphyxia, central venous (i.e., right atrial) pressure may rise slightly, owing to pulmonary hypertension and constriction of systemic capacitance vessels. As the myocardium fails, central venous pressure rises further, aortic pressure decreases, and heart rate is reduced further.

The initial adaptations of the systemic circulation to asphyxia are mediated by reflexes (15). There also are major hormonal responses to asphyxia, including elevations in plasma corticotropin, glucocorticoids, catecholamines, arginine vasopressin, renin, and atrial natriuretic factor, and a decrease in insulin (16,17). Some of these are important in maintaining the circulatory adaptations to asphyxia. Catecholamines, which come mainly from the adrenal medulla, maintain myocardial function in the presence of asphyxia, thereby increasing survival (18,19). Arginine vasopressin helps maintain the hypertension, bradycardia, and redistribution of systemic flow (20). Increased hepatic glycogenolysis helps maintain plasma glucose concentrations (5).

The physiology of resuscitation is essentially a reversal of the pathophysiology of asphyxia. In Fig. 18–1, which illustrates both processes, asphyxia proceeds from left to right, and resuscitation from right to left. It is crucial to determine where the infant is in this sequence of pathophysiologic events when resuscitation is started. If asphyxia has proceeded to myocardial failure, resuscitation must include restoration of cardiac output as well as establishment of effective ventilation and perfusion of the lungs. Generally, myocardial failure does not occur until both pH and PaO_2 are extremely low, approximately 6.9 and 20 mm Hg, respectively. Cardiac output is reestablished through rapid correction of the severe hypoxia and acidosis. Until this is done, output must be maintained by cardiac massage. As soon as pH is raised to approximately 7.1 and PaO_2 to 50 mm Hg, the myocardium responds rapidly, heart rate rises, aortic pressures rise, and pulse pressure widens, whereas central venous pressure falls. These changes indicate that cardiac massage can be stopped. At this point, the infant usually will be hypertensive because the vasoconstriction in nonvital organs still is present. This vasoconstriction is relieved only by continued adequate oxygenation and correction of acidosis. Pressures then will fall toward normal. The vasoconstriction also is manifested by intense pallor of the skin. As the vasoconstriction is relieved, the skin becomes pink and well perfused, with rapid capillary refilling (i.e., less than 2 seconds) when blanched by pressure. As peripheral flow improves, lactic acid sequestered in these tissues enters the central circulation and a large base deficit, which may have been corrected earlier, now reappears.

If asphyxia is only moderately severe, resuscitation begins in the middle of the sequence depicted in Fig. 18–1. There is hypertension, indicating that the myocardium has not yet failed. Effective ventilation of the lungs with a high oxygen concentration may correct acidosis by lowering the PaO_2, oxygenating the blood, and adequately dilating the pulmonary vascular bed. If significant acidosis persists after alleviation of the hypercarbia, however, alkali should be given to correct the metabolic component of the acidosis, relieve pulmonary vasoconstriction, and establish good pulmonary perfusion. Generally, raising pH to 7.25 is sufficient for this purpose, but there are some important exceptions discussed later in which a higher pH is needed to dilate the pulmonary vascular bed.

When the effects of asphyxia are alleviated, spontaneous respiratory efforts return. The duration between the onset of resuscitation and reappearance of spontaneous respiratory efforts is directly proportional to the amount of brain injury that has occurred (7).

Onset of spontaneous respiratory efforts is not necessarily an indication to withdraw assisted ventilation. Often, there is residual atelectasis and the infant does not have strong, regular respiratory efforts. $PaCO_2$ may be normal, and PaO_2 may rise to a high level with assisted ventilation. But when assisted ventilation is withdrawn, effective ventilation may decrease and the whole process of asphyxia recurs. Such cases must be managed by gradual withdrawal of assisted ventilation and reduction of oxygen.

The blood volume of the asphyxiated infant may be abnormal. Intrapartum asphyxia alters the distribution of blood volume between infant and placenta at the time the cord is clamped. Asphyxia during labor usually shifts blood from the placenta to the fetus. There are certain situations, however, in which the infant's blood volume may be reduced. The most obvious of these is hemorrhage from the fetoplacental unit, which is manifested by vaginal bleeding. Three other conditions that shift blood volume from the fetus to the placenta are compression of the umbilical cord by the after-coming head in a breech delivery, in which umbilical venous flow is reduced selectively more than arterial flow; severe hypotension in the mother; and asphyxia occurring only at the end of labor (21).

Initially, it may be difficult to determine whether or not blood volume is adequate in the asphyxiated newborn. There are two reasons for this. First, many of the circulatory responses to asphyxia are similar to those associated with loss of blood volume. Either asphyxia or hypovolemia may cause bradycardia, metabolic acidosis, poor peripheral perfusion indicated by pallor and slow capillary filling, and a large difference between core and skin temperature. A low aortic pressure could be due to either the end stage of asphyxia or the shock. Only changes in central venous pressure are in the opposite direction, and even here the coexistence of the two processes can have offsetting effects. Second, the circulatory changes during asphyxia and resuscitation may determine the adequacy or inadequacy of the circulating blood volume. If an infant is moderately asphyxiated and has systemic and pulmonary vasoconstriction (see Fig. 18–1, center) and a small blood volume, aortic and central venous pressures will be nearly normal. Administration of a blood volume expander at this point would only overload the circulation. The effects of volume expansion would be even worse if the asphyxia were more severe and myocardial failure were present. Correction of asphyxia (see Fig. 18–1, left) relieves the vasoconstriction of resistance and capacitance vessels, and the small blood volume now becomes inadequate to support the circulation. Reperfusion of asphyxic and ischemic tissues also increases loss of intravascular water from these capillary beds, leading to edema and reduced plasma volume.

During recovery from asphyxia, several metabolic abnormalities appear. There may be hypoglycemia due to depletion of carbohydrate reserves during the asphyxia. Hypoglycemia must be prevented because it can cause myocardial failure in a heart recently subjected to asphyxia (22). Hyperglycemia due to excessive glucose administration similarly is dangerous during asphyxia because it worsens the acidosis by increasing lactic acid production (23). Hypocalcemia also develops, possibly as a result of increased calcitonin release during asphyxia (24), and can lead to myocardial failure.

Hyperkalemia occurs during asphyxia, when, in the process of buffering acidosis, H^+ enters the erythrocytes and K^+ is displaced from them. Although this increases plasma K^+ while the patient is asphyxiated, total body K^+ decreases as some of the K^+ is excreted by the kidney. On relief of asphyxia, the buffering processes are reversed and K^+ leaves the plasma and reenters the erythrocytes, leading to hypokalemia. An exception to this process is asphyxia that is so severe that it produces severe renal ischemia, anuria, and retention of potassium.

HIGH-RISK PREGNANCIES

Certain situations during pregnancy, labor, or delivery carry an increased risk of intrapartum asphyxia. If these high-risk deliveries are identified before birth, their progress during labor and delivery can be monitored and resuscitation can be initiated at birth. Tables 18–1 and 18–2 list some of the factors that alert the physician to a high-risk delivery. Optimal management of these cases requires good communication between obstetricians, anesthesiologists, and pediatricians. The physician responsible for care of newborn infants always should know of any patients with potential problems in the labor and delivery area.

RESUSCITATION OF THE ASPHYXIATED INFANT

If a severely asphyxiated infant is expected, a resuscitation team must be present at the birth. In almost all cases, good communication between obstetricians and pediatricians will provide timely notice of the impending delivery of an asphyxiated infant. The actual steps in the resuscitation fall into three major phases, and a typical division of duties among the team of skilled personnel is listed. One of these people should be experienced at tra-

TABLE 18–1. *Some factors that place the newborn infant at high risk for asphyxia*

Maternal conditions	Labor and delivery conditions	Fetal conditions
Diabetes mellitus	Forceps delivery other than low-elective or vacuum-extraction delivery	Premature delivery Postmature delivery
Preeclampsia, hypertension, chronic renal disease	Breech or other abnormal presentation and delivery	Acidosis determined by fetal scalp capillary blood
Anemia (i.e., hemoglobin <10 g/dL)	Cephalopelvic disproportion: shoulder dystocia, prolonged second stage	Abnormal heart rate pattern or dysrhythmia
Blood type or group alloimmunization	Cesarean section	Meconium-stained amniotic fluid
Abruptio placentae, placenta previa, or other antepartum hemorrhage	Prolapsed umbilical cord	Oligohydramnios Polyhydramnios
Narcotic, barbiturate, tranquilizer, psychedelic drug use or alcohol intoxication	Cord compression (e.g., nuchal cord, cord knot, compression by after-coming head in breech delivery)	Decreased rate of growth: uterine size or fetal size determined by ultrasonography
History of previous perinatal loss	Maternal hypotension or hemorrhage	Macrosomia
Prolonged rupture of membranes		Immaturity of pulmonary surfactant system
Lupus		Fetal malformations determined by sonography
Maternal heart disease		Hydrops fetalis
Maternal fever or other evidence of amnionitis		Low biophysical profile
Abnormal umbilical artery Doppler velocity		Multiple births; in particular, discordant, stuck, or monoamniotic

TABLE 18–2. *Fetal heart rate patterns associated with fetal and neonatal distress*

Heart rate pattern	Fetal or neonatal problems
Severe (i.e., <80 beats/min), sustained bradycardia, with loss of variability	Fetal hemorrhage, fetal asphyxia
Sustained tachycardia, uncomplicated by other abnormal patterns	Infection, often with apnea
Late decelerations with loss of variability	Asphyxia
Severe, recurrent variable decelerations, with loss of variability	Asphyxia and possible hypovolemia
Sinusoidal	Severe anemia with asphyxia

cheal intubation, ventilation of the lungs, and the general management of resuscitation, and one should be an experienced neonatal nurse. The extent of resuscitation needed can be determined only after the infant's condition is evaluated by someone with considerable clinical experience. The following list outlines the responsibilities of each member of the resuscitation team.

Member A:

1. Assess infant.
2. Manage airway and intubate the trachea, if needed.
3. Provide positive-pressure ventilation.
4. Secure endotracheal tube.

Member B:

1. Listen for heart rate and give cardiac massage, if needed.
2. Auscultate chest to be sure endotracheal tube is in proper position and gas exchange is good.
3. Catheterize umbilical vessel or vessels and maintain patency of catheters.
4. Measure intravascular pressures, assess perfusion, sample blood for pH, PO_2, and PCO_2, and draw blood cultures.
5. Administer fluids and drugs.
6. Continue assessment of infant.

Member C:

1. Blot baby dry; apply electrocardiograph (ECG) monitor leads, radiant monitor servocontrol, and transcutaneous oxygen sensor.
2. Keep timed written record of resuscitation and vital signs and calls for Apgar scores at 1 and 5 minutes and every 5 minutes thereafter until the score is 7 or greater; time and record the rate and volume of infusions such as alkali and blood volume expanders.
3. Assist member A by providing endotracheal tube suction, adjusting the fraction of oxygen inspired (FiO_2), and helping to secure endotracheal tube.
4. Help member B by providing medications and blood volume expanders in sterile syringes; B is working in a sterile field early in resuscitation.
5. Monitor baby's temperature and capillary blood glucose.

Equipment and supplies for optimal resuscitation include the following:

Resuscitation table with heat source to maintain normal body temperature

Oxygen and air sources, oxygen–air blender, and infant ventilation systems; the standard infant anesthesia bag, with tailpiece and adjustable resistance and a Norman elbow, is the most versatile system for manual ventilation[1]

Airway suction system

Infant face masks and endotracheal tubes from 2.5- to 4.0-mm internal diameter

Laryngoscope with no. 1 Miller blade for full-term infants and a no. 0 blade for preterm infants; be sure the batteries and light bulb of the laryngoscope work

Monitors

Heart rate by ECG

Transcutaneous oxygen saturation

Arterial and venous pressures with waveform displays; transducers can be connected to the catheters beforehand so that aortic pressure is displayed as soon as the umbilical artery catheter is inserted, and the venous waveform can be used to localize the catheter tip in the thoracic inferior vena cava (25)

Indirect blood pressure monitor

Catheters and catheterization tray with instruments, sterile drapes, and sterile syringes for sampling blood and flushing the lines

All emergency medicines and fluids

Tube thoracostomy tray with instruments and catheters from 10 to 14 Fr

Blood gas electrodes with a trained operator of the blood gas machines close enough to the resuscitation area so that results are available in less than 5 minutes

In selected situations (see the following), it is useful to have present in the delivery room a unit of whole blood or packed erythrocytes that were cross-matched against the mother; this blood can be kept in a cold pack and returned to the blood bank if not used.

Phase 1

Clinical Assessment of Severity of Asphyxia

The Apgar score was the first attempt at a systematic assessment of birth asphyxia (2,26). There is a loose corre-

---

[1]Self-inflating bags are less desirable because you must begin the inflation with a rapid rise in pressure in order to close the flap valve, thus preventing the desired slower, more gentle inflation.

lation between low Apgar scores and umbilical cord blood gases. However, some infants with severe acidosis have normal Apgar scores, and some with normal blood gases and pH have very low scores (27,28). Maternal anesthetics, sedatives, maternal drugs, fetal sepsis, and central nervous system pathologic conditions can lower the Apgar score; extremely premature infants often have low scores without any other evidence of asphyxia (29,30). Regardless of the cause, an Apgar score that remains low calls for action. The clinical significance of the Apgar score increases with time. Scoring should continue every 5 minutes until the score increases to 7 or above. The length of time it takes to reach a score of 7 is a rough indication of severity of asphyxia. Umbilical cord blood gases, discussed previously, are useful measures of fetal asphyxia, but this information will not be available until a few minutes after birth, and resuscitation must be started before that. Thus, their main value is in guiding subsequent management of the infant.

It is essential to maintain body temperature. When the cord is clamped, blot the infant dry with a sterile towel to reduce evaporative heat loss and place him or her under a radiant heater on the resuscitation table (31). Do not overheat the infant.

Next, clear the airway. Gently suction the oropharynx and nose. If the infant's respiration is vigorous, nothing more may be necessary. Attach ECG electrodes and pulse oximeter, and monitor the heart rate and oxygen saturations.

Initiate Ventilation

If the infant is apneic or the respiratory rate is slow and irregular, place a mask over the infant's face and ventilate with oxygen-enriched gas using intermittent positive pressure from the anesthesia bag while observing chest movements and the ventilation pressure on an aneroid manometer. Most infants can be resuscitated using 40% to 60% oxygen (32). Begin ventilation by slowly applying a pressure of 20 cm H_2O to the airway for term infants, and 30 cm H_2O to the airway for preterm infants. Maintain this inflating pressure for 1 to 2 seconds, then ventilate at a rate of 40 to 60 breaths per minute, using an inflation time of 0.3 to 0.5 seconds and enough pressure to provide a visable rise of the upper portion of the chest. Repeat the application of the initial inflating pressure pattern three to four times over the first 2 minutes. These prolonged breaths inflate regions of the lungs that were gasless and create the necessary functional residual capacity (33). Figure 18–2 illustrates this process. Avoid rapid inflation or overdistention of the lungs. If the stomach becomes inflated, pass an orogastric tube and apply suction. The very premature infant with a very small lung volume and a surfactant deficient lung presents special problems for initial ventilation that are discussed later.

In mildly asphyxiated infants, ventilation will produce a prompt increase in heart rate and the onset of regular, spontaneous respiration. If both do not occur, intubate the trachea and continue assisted ventilation. Tracheal intubation may induce severe bradycardia when the hypopharynx is stimulated, but heart rate should increase as soon as intubation is completed and assisted ventilation is begun. With severe asphyxia, the experienced resuscitator may prefer to intubate the trachea immediately. Ventilation through a properly positioned endotracheal tube is more effective than ventilation by mask and avoids distention of the stomach with gas. However, the less experienced physician who cannot intubate the trachea quickly should use mask ventilation first, then intubate the trachea later if it still is necessary. Do not continue to attempt tracheal intubation for more than about 30 seconds. If unsuccessful in that time, ventilate the infant's lungs by mask for at least 1 minute before again attempting tracheal intubation. Intubate gently to avoid trauma to the hypopharynx and vocal cords. If a stylette is used to stiffen the tracheal tube during intubation, secure the stylette so the tip of the stylette is approximately 0.5 cm back from the tip of the tube. If the stylette extends beyond the tip of the endotracheal tube, it could traumatize the airway.

As a general guideline, use a 2.5-mm diameter endotracheal tube for babies weighing 1 kg or less, 3.0 mm for 1 to 1.5 kg, 3.5 mm for 1.5 to 2.5 kg, and 4.0 mm for larger babies (see Appendices F–3 and F–4). Some bigger babies need a tube one size smaller than that recommended for their weight. In general, gas should leak from the space between the endotracheal tube and the trachea when 15 to 30 cm H_2O pressure is applied to the airway.

If the infant does not make strong respiratory efforts after initiation of assisted ventilation and the mother has received morphine or other narcotic within an hour before delivery, give naloxone hydrochloride 0.1 mg/kg intravenously or intramuscularly.

Begin Cardiac Massage

If there is no electrical activity on the ECG, no audible heartbeat, or if the heart rate remains below 50 beats/min after onset of assisted ventilation, begin cardiac massage. Give external cardiac massage by placing both hands around the infant's chest, with the fingertips over the back and the thumbs overlapping each other on the midsternum, then quickly press down firmly with both thumbs at a rate of 80 to 100 strokes per minute (34). Increase the inspired oxygen to 100% and continue cardiac massage while proceeding with other resuscitative measures until the spontaneous heart rate rises above 100 and the arterial pressure is normal. If there is no spontaneous heart rate, give epinephrine (0.1 mL/kg of 1:10,000 solution) intravenously or through the endotracheal tube. It will be absorbed rapidly from the mucosa of the airway when given into the airway (35). Most cases of presumed cardiac arrest actually are profound bradycardias that respond to effective ventilation alone or to ventilation and cardiac massage, or the latter

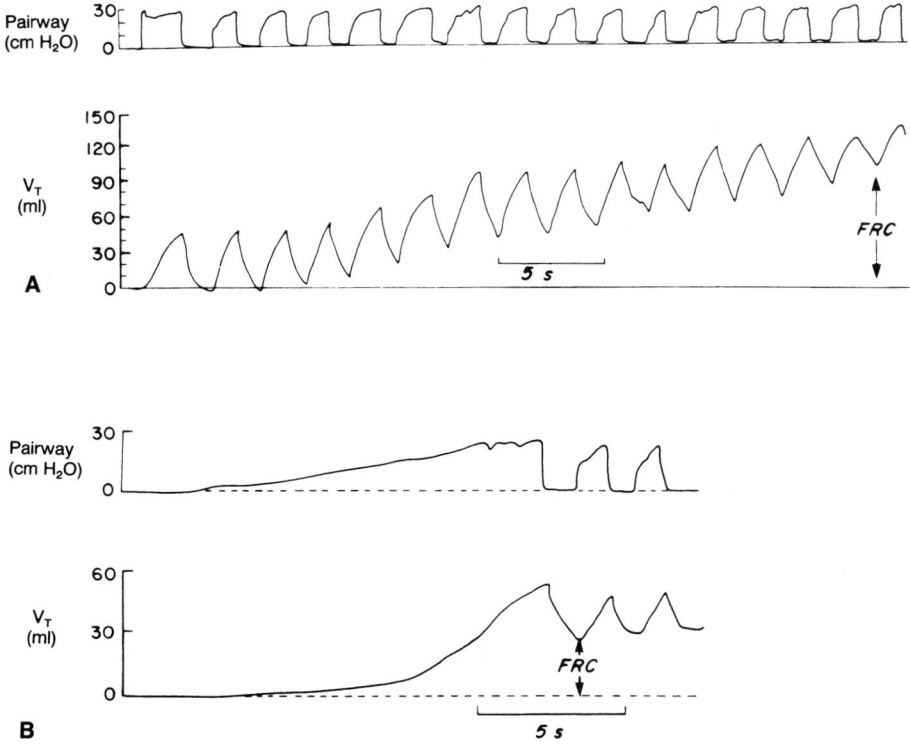

FIG. 18–2. Initial inflation of the lungs by assisted ventilation in two asphyxiated infants. **A:** An inflation pressure of 30 cm H_2O is applied repeatedly for 1 to 2 seconds. For the first several breaths, the volume entering and leaving the lungs is the same. Then the volume out is slightly less than the volume in for several breaths, and this trapped gas begins to form the functional residual capacity (FRC). **B:** The first inflation is with a pressure that is increased slowly up to 30 cm H_2O over 8 seconds and held at that pressure for 2 seconds. During exhalation, less gas leaves than what entered; therefore, some FRC has been generated with the first breath. P_{air}, pressure applied to the airway; V_T, tidal volume. (Adapted from Boon AW, Milner AD, Hopkin IE. Lung expansion, tidal exchange, and formation of the functional residual capacity during resuscitation of asphyxiated neonates. *J Pediatr* 1979;95:1031; and Vyas H, Milner AD, Hopkin IE, et al. Physiologic responses to prolonged and slow-rise inflation in the resuscitation of the asphyxiated newborn infant. *J Pediatr* 1981;99:635.)

plus epinephrine. The efficacy of massage and the return of adequate cardiac activity are judged best by monitoring aortic blood pressure. Massage can be discontinued for a few seconds to evaluate the spontaneous heart rate and blood pressure (Fig. 18–3). Infants who do not respond rapidly to these measures will require prompt correction of acidosis (see section on "Correct Severe Metabolic Acidosis," below), atropine sulfate (0.01 mg/kg), and $CaCl_2$ (0.2 mL/kg of a 10% solution). Although epinephrine is recommended primarily to start the heart, it also is quite effective in correcting bradycardia due to asphyxia.

Catheterize an Umbilical Artery and Draw a Blood Sample

Measure pH, PaO_2, and $PaCO_2$ to evaluate the efficacy of ventilation. Depending on the values obtained, adjust ventilatory rate, pressure, and inspired oxygen accordingly. Measure hematocrit, connect the catheter to a pre-calibrated pressure transducer, and measure blood pressure. Alternatively, the catheter can be connected to the transducer ahead of time and the blood pressure displayed as soon as the catheter is passed into the aorta. This also reduces the risk of accidentally injecting air bubbles through the catheter into the infant's circulation while the catheter is being connected to the transducer.

It is important to obtain a measurement of pH and PCO_2 quickly to determine that ventilation is neither inadequate nor excessive and to detect metabolic acidosis. Although a venous blood gas analysis is not as representative as an arterial one, it will suffice as an initial measurement to detect severe acidosis and to determine whether or not PCO_2 is near the normal range. Venous PCO_2 is about 6 mm Hg higher and pH about 0.06 units lower than in arterial blood (25). If there will be a delay in placing an umbilical artery catheter, a line emergently placed in the lower portion of the umbilical vein will provide access until an arterial line is in place.

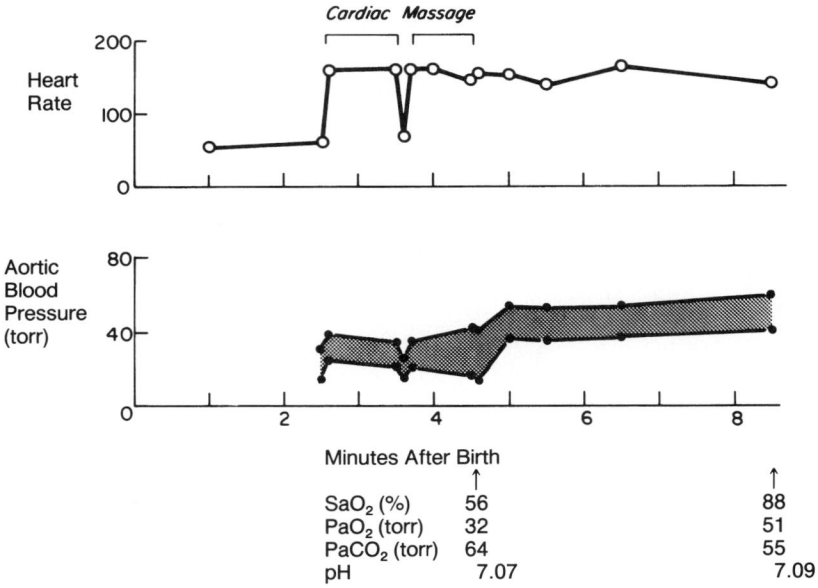

FIG. 18–3. Resuscitation and cardiac massage were performed on a 2.1-kg infant who was delivered by cesarean section due to signs of fetal asphyxia at 34 weeks of gestation. The infant was intubated and ventilated with 60% oxygen beginning 30 seconds after birth. An electrocardiogram was begun at 1 minute, and at 2.5 minutes an umbilical artery catheter connected to a pressure transducer and a recorder was passed into the descending aorta. Note persistent bradycardia despite assisted ventilation and low aortic pressure with narrow phasic pressure. Cardiac massage raised heart rate and pressure. When briefly discontinued after 1 minute, pressure and heart rate fell. After another minute of massage and assisted ventilation, good cardiac output had returned. This was manifested by a sustained higher heart rate and higher blood pressure with wider phasic pressure when massage was discontinued a second time at 5 minutes after birth. By 8.5 minutes, the infant was still acidotic, but there was adequate oxygenation and aortic pressure continued to rise. PaCO₂, arterial carbon dioxide partial pressure; PaO₂, arterial oxygen partial pressure; SaO₂, saturation of arterial blood hemoglobin with oxygen.

Correct Severe Metabolic Acidosis

If the pH is less than 7.05 due to a mixed acidosis, or the base deficit is 15 mEq/L or more, correct the metabolic component of the acidosis with an infusion of either tromethamine or $NaHCO_3$, depending on the $PaCO_2$. The immediate objectives are twofold: to reverse the myocardial failure and low cardiac output that occurs from acute metabolic, but not respiratory, acidosis (13,14,36,37); and to relieve the intense pulmonary vasoconstriction that occurs with severe acidosis, particularly in full-term infants (11,38,39). The degree of pulmonary vasoconstriction is approximately the same for metabolic and respiratory acidosis (40).

Calculate the dose of buffer from the following formula:

$$\text{mmol buffer } 0.3 \times \text{body weight (kg)} \times \text{base deficit (mEq/L).}$$

Infuse at the rate of 1 mmol/L/kg/min. $NaHCO_3$ comes as either a 1.0 or 0.5 mol/L solution. Dilute the former with sterile water, not a dextrose solution, to 0.5 or 0.3 mol/L. Tromethamine comes as a 0.3 mol/L solution that can be given without further dilution.

The ability of $NaHCO_3$ buffer to raise pH depends on the ability of the lungs to eliminate the CO_2 produced by the buffering process, as determined by the following equation:

$$H^+ + NaHCO_3 \rightleftarrows Na^+ + H_2CO_3 \rightleftarrows H_2O + CO_2$$

Do not give $NaHCO_3$ unless ventilation is adequate and $PaCO_2$ is low, normal, or declining toward normal. Continue ventilation during bicarbonate therapy to eliminate the excess CO_2 produced. CO_2 is highly diffusable, so even if ventilation is adequate, some of the CO_2 produced by buffering could enter cells and transiently increase acidosis.

Some studies suggest that there is an association between rapid infusions of large volumes of concentrated sodium bicarbonate and intracranial hemorrhage in preterm infants. The hemorrhages might be caused by transient hypernatremia from too rapid an infusion, by an acute rise in $PaCO_2$ from inadequate ventilation during the $NaHCO_3$ infusion, which would cause cerebral vasodilation, or by the asphyxia for which the drug was given. Infusion of sodium bicarbonate into the inferior vena cava at the rate of 1 mEq/kg/min, for a total dose of up to 5 mEq/kg, causes only a slight transient increase in arterial sodium concentration.

Tromethamine has the twofold advantage of reducing $PaCO_2$ and buffering metabolic acid. It is most useful for treating infants with severe mixed metabolic and respiratory acidosis and for situations of severe asphyxia with suspected extreme acidosis in which blood gas measurements are not available. Tromethamine may cause respiratory depression, so it should be used only in situations in which ventilation already is assisted. Tromethamine also may cause hypoglycemia. An earlier preparation of tromethamine was very hyperosmolar, highly alkalotic, and tended to sclerose vessels. These problems have been corrected in the 0.3 mol/L preparation, which also is adjusted to pH 8.6. Figure 18–4 illustrates correction of a severe mixed acidosis. Figure 18–5 shows how the car-diovascular effects of an infusion of alkali differ depending upon the severity of the asphyxia.

Phase II

As soon as the infant's condition is stabilized, perform a thorough examination for major anomalies, dysmorphic features, abnormalities of intrauterine growth, and evidence of infection, such as rashes and hepatospleno-megaly. It is easy to overlook a neural tube defect in a supine infant. A scaphoid abdomen and difficulty achieving adequate ventilation suggest a diaphragmatic hernia (see following). Insert an orogastric tube into the stomach and aspirate its contents. This reduces the risk of regurgitation and aspiration, which can occur despite the presence of an endotracheal tube. If the tube fails to enter the stomach, consider esophageal atresia and apply continuous suction to the tube. Suctioning of 20 mL or more of fluid from the stomach suggests obstruction of the upper gastrointestinal tract. During resuscitation, an infant often will pass urine or meconium. Note and record this, because the asphyxiated infant may not void or pass stool again for a day or longer.

Reevaluate Assisted Ventilation

Monitor for complications of assisted ventilation. The tube may be dislodged from the trachea and advance into the esophagus. Alternately, the tracheal tube may advance into the right main bronchial stem, leading to nonventilation of the entire left lung and the upper lobe of the right lung. This is the most common serious complication of tracheal intubation. Immediately after intubation, auscultate both sides of the chest to be sure the breath sounds are equal; reauscultate the chest every few minutes until the tube is removed or properly secured in position. The presence of reduced breath sounds in the left chest does not necessarily indicate partial ventilation of the left lung. In neonates, breath sounds can be transmitted from the opposite side of the chest and often can be heard over a lung that is completely collapsed. The breath sounds should be equal on both sides of the chest. If breath sounds are absent or diminished on the left side, slowly withdraw the endotracheal tube while continuing ventilation until breath sounds are equal. Some endotracheal tubes have centimeter marks on them to indicate the distance to the tracheal end of the tube. The tip of the tube generally will be in the midtrachea if the distance mark at the infant's lip is 7 cm in a 1-kg infant, 8 cm in a 2-kg infant, 9 cm in a 3-kg infant, and 10 cm in a 4-kg infant. In large preterm and full-term infants in whom a 3.0-mm or larger diameter endotracheal tube is appropriate (see section on "Initiate Ventilation" and Appendices F–3 and F–4), right main bronchial stem intubation can be avoided by using a shouldered Cole endotracheal tube. When the proper-sized tube for the baby is used, the tube tip reaches the midtracheal region when the

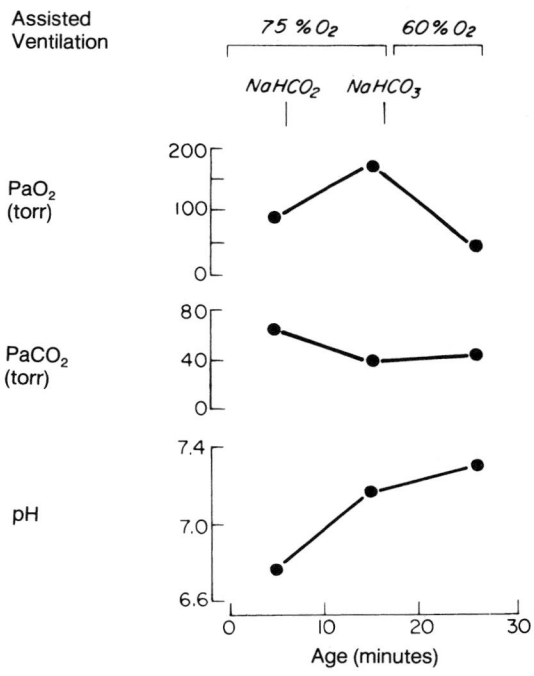

FIG. 18–4. Arterial blood gas tensions, pH, and therapy during the first 30 minutes after the birth of a 1.6-kg premature infant. There was severe mixed acidosis initially. Assisted ventilation achieved effective CO_2 elimination early in this infant, and $NaHCO_3$ could be given early to begin correcting the metabolic component of the acidosis. The base excess on the first blood specimen was beyond the limits of calculation (more than –25 mEq/L). The first infusion of $NaHCO_3$ was given between 6 and 10 minutes. When the second sample was drawn at 15 minutes, the calculated base excess was –22 mEq/L. After the second infusion of $NaHCO_3$, the base excess was –6 mEq/L, and no more alkali was given. Note that arterial carbon dioxide partial pressure $PaCO_2$ fell between the first and second measurements when $NaHCO_3$ was given. PaO_2, arterial oxygen partial pressure.

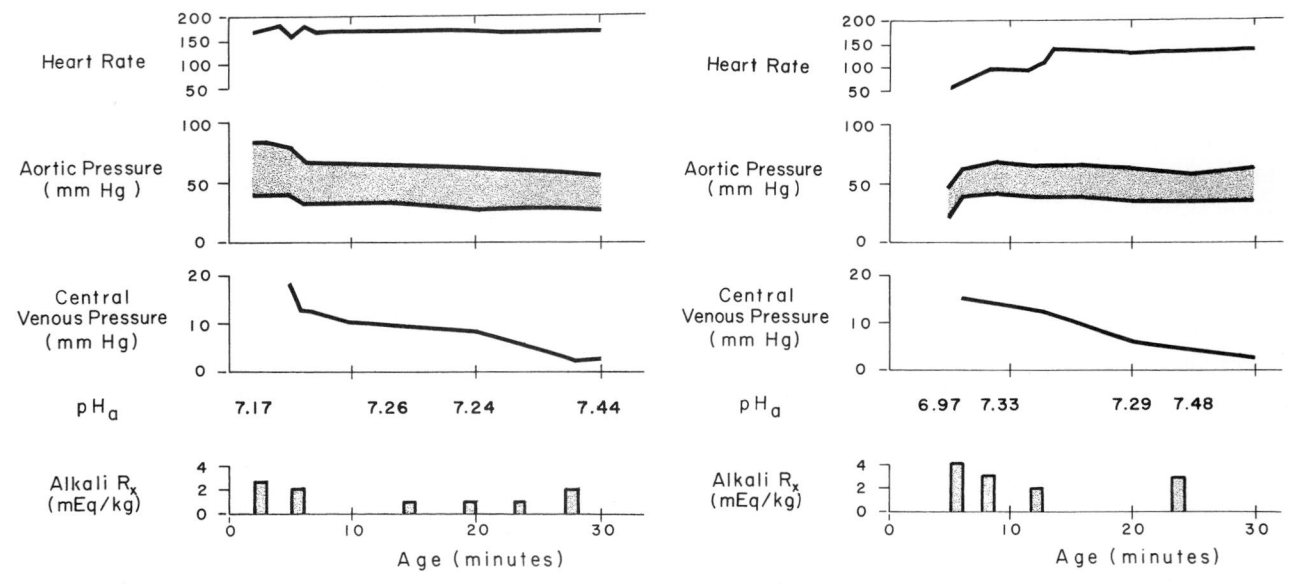

FIG. 18–5. A: Cardiovascular responses to alkali therapy in a moderately versus a severely asphyxiated infant. Age is in minutes after birth. Both infants were intubated and ventilated immediately after birth. In each case, aortic blood pressures, blood gas tensions, and pH were measured through an umbilical arterial catheter passed into the decending aorta, and central venous pressure was measured via a catheter passed through the umbilical vein into the right atrium. The 2.15 kg infant depicted in the **panel on the left** was moderately asphyxiated. The circulatory changes had progressed to a point approximately halfway through the scheme shown in Fig. 18–1. Myocardial function was fairly well preserved. The heart rate rose as soon as assisted ventilation was started and myocardial contractility was sufficient to generate systemic hypertension in the presence of peripheral vasoconstriction. However, central venous pressure was elevated, probably due a combination of pulmonary vasoconstriction and incipient myocardial failure. With correction of the metabolic acidosis, peripheral vasoconstriction was relieved, the skin color changed from pale to pink, and aortic and central venous pressures declined to normal. **B:** This 2.9 kg infant was profoundly asphyxiated, equivalent to the **far right** of the scheme shown in Fig. 18–1. Heart rate remained low after initation of ventilation, aortic pressure was low, and central venous pressure was high, indicating serious myocardial failure. As the metablic acidosis was corrected with alkali, myocardial function improved progressively, as indicated by the rising heart rate and aortic pressure and falling central venous pressure.

shoulders of the tube abut the vocal cords. The shoulders prevent the tube from advancing into the bronchus. If the tube passes easily beyond the optimal distance (i.e., it meets no resistance), one can be sure the tube is in the esophagus, not the trachea. Shouldered tubes do not work as well in smaller, preterm infants because the distal segment of the 2.5-mm diameter tube that is beyond the shoulders is long enough to reach the right main bronchial stem in the smallest infants. A shouldered tube cannot be used for long-term ventilation because it may traumatize the vocal cords, but it can be used safely for the first half-hour or hour of resuscitation. It then can be replaced with a straight tube when resuscitation is completed, should assisted ventilation still be required.

Examine the abdomen for distention. This usually is due to assisted ventilation via a face mask and can be relieved by an orogastric tube. On rare occasions, gastric distention caused by such ventilation will perforate the stomach. The resulting severe abdominal distention must be relieved by paracentesis to allow adequate ventilation.

During phase II, pulmonary function may change rapidly, leading to several complications. First, PaO_2 will rise as ventilation and perfusion become better matched and may reach high levels that are dangerous in the very premature infant. Hyperoxia is managed better initially by reducing inspired oxygen concentration *rather* than by withdrawing ventilatory assistance. Second, improved ventilation may lead to acute hypocarbia, which will reduce cerebral and myocardial blood flow (41–43). Correct hypocarbia by reducing the rate of assisted ventilation and inspiratory pressure. Figure 18–6 illustrates these changes. Third, as lung compliance increases, the ventilatory pressure that was appropriate initially will become excessive. If the excess pressure is mild, the result will be hyperventilation and hypocarbia. If it is extreme, however, there will be tamponade of the pulmonary circulation and right-to-left shunting of blood at the atrial and ductal levels and low systemic blood flow. This phenomenon is manifested by a low aortic pressure, wide fluctuations in blood pressure in phase with the pos-

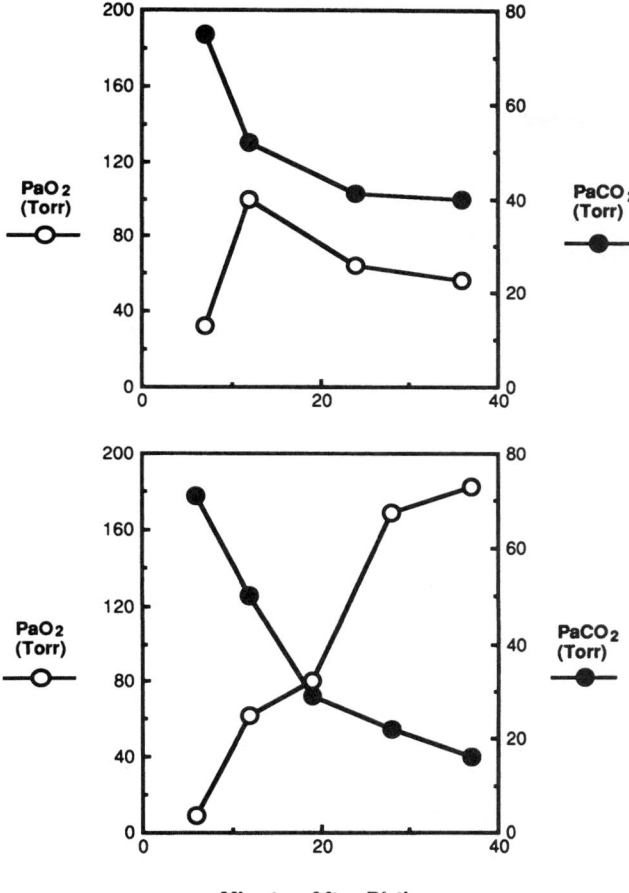

Minutes After Birth

FIG. 18–6. Changes in arterial blood gas tensions occurred during resuscitation of two very-low-birth-weight infants. Each was intubated immediately after birth, and in each the umbilical artery was catheterized before 10 minutes after birth to allow frequent measurements of blood gases. Both were hypoxic and hypercarbic at the first measurements taken 6 and 7 minutes after birth, respectively. As ventilation and oxygenation improved, ventilation pressures, rates, and inspired oxygen concentration were reduced. In the baby shown in the **upper panel,** this led to normal blood gas tensions. In the baby shown in the **lower panel,** adjustments were made too slowly, leading to hyperoxia and extreme hypocarbia. $PaCO_2$, arterial carbon dioxide partial pressure; PaO_2, arterial oxygen partial pressure.

itive-pressure ventilation, and arterial hypoxemia. This situation can be detected by briefly disconnecting the endotracheal tube from the ventilation system. Aortic pressure will rise within 5 seconds. If this occurs, restart ventilation using lower airway pressures. The hypoxia caused by the shunting of blood from right to left will decrease quickly as the lungs are ventilated with lower pressures.

Tension pneumothorax may occur during spontaneous or assisted ventilation of any infant. A tension pneumothorax of small or moderate size may restrict ventilation and cause hypoxia and hypercarbia. Pneumothorax must be suspected whenever PaO_2 decreases despite a ventilation system that is functioning properly. Sometimes the diagnosis of pneumothorax is difficult to make by physical examination. Breath sounds may be unequal bilaterally, but often they are equal. The upper portion of the affected side of the chest tends to lag behind the unaffected side during inflation of the lungs. Transillumination with a cold fiberoptic light may cause the affected side to glow brightly; however, the absence of this sign does not rule out pneumothorax, particularly in the larger infant with a thicker chest wall. The diagnosis of pneumothorax can be made best by a chest radiograph, but this often is difficult to obtain quickly in the resuscitation area. The arterial and central venous pressures may not change with small pneumothoraces. If hypoxia and hypercarbia become severe, it may he necessary to perform a diagnostic thoracentesis with a small-gauge angiocatheter and syringe before there is time to obtain a radiograph.

The situation changes when a tension pneumothorax is large. Venous return to the heart and cardiac output may fall precipitously to extremely low levels. If blood pressure, PaO_2, and $PaCO_2$ are being measured, this critical situation will be diagnosed easily because the onset of hypoxia and hypercarbia will be accompanied by severe hypotension rather than the hypertension of asphyxia (see Fig. 18–1) (44). This situation requires treatment as urgent as in cardiac arrest. One cannot wait for a confirmatory radiograph. Figure 18–7 illustrates the diagnosis and successful treatment of such a case. Satisfactory decompression of a tension pneumothorax usually requires insertion of a thoracostomy tube and continuous suction applied to the tube through an underwater suction system. Aspiration with a needle and syringe usually gives only very brief relief. While assembling equipment for decompression of the pneumothorax, however, insert a 22-gauge angiocath connected to a three-way stopcock and a 30-mL syringe. This is a convenient and relatively safe method for temporary decompression of the pneumothorax.

Evaluate Circulatory Status

The healthy newborn can compensate for loss of a large volume of blood. Asphyxia however, disrupts the newborn's ability to do so (45). Most asphyxiated infants have a normal or greater than normal blood volume; only a few have a low blood volume (21). Consequently, hypovolemic shock does not develop in most asphyxiated infants. Of the few infants in whom hypovolemic shock develops in the first hours after birth, however, almost all have had intrapartum asphyxia (46). Blood volume expansion is essential for the infant who is in hypovolemic shock, but may be harmful for the asphyxiated infant who has a normal blood volume.

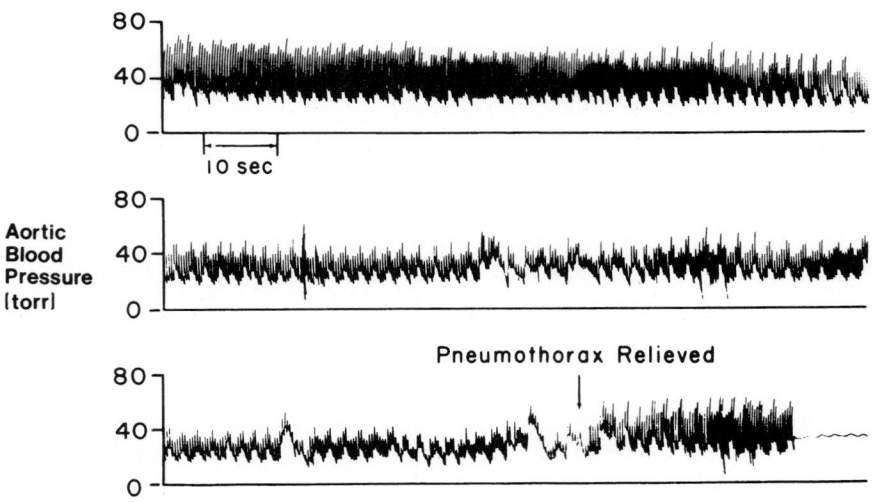

FIG. 18–7. Aortic blood pressure of a premature, 1.5-kg infant at 32 weeks' gestational age during development of a tension pneumothorax. This is a continuous tracing at 2 hours of age. Because the patient's condition was rapidly worsening, as shown by hypotension, a narrow pulse pressure, and rapidly increasing cyanosis despite assisted ventilation with 100% oxygen, thoracentesis of the right pleural cavity was done (*arrow*) before radiologic confirmation of the pneumothorax was obtained. About 50 mL of air escaped when the pleural cavity was opened. The patient's color improved, and blood pressure promptly returned to normal.

Because some circulatory changes due to asphyxia may either mimic or mask hypovolemic shock, it is impossible to identify those infants who need blood volume expansion until resuscitation has produced adequate oxygenation of arterial blood and a normal $PaCO_2$. Acute hypocarbia causes systemic hypotension (47), and severe overventilation may reduce systemic blood flow (see previous). Neither of these states requires blood volume expansion.

Signs that suggest an inadequate blood volume include the following: low aortic pressure and a narrow and abnormal aortic waveform (Figs. 18–8 and 18–9), falling hematocrit, persistent metabolic acidosis, low central venous PO_2 (i.e., less than 30 mm Hg) after correction of arterial hypoxia, cold extremities, and delayed (i.e., greater than 3 seconds) filling of capillaries in the skin after they have been blanched under pressure, provided that core temperature is normal. Tachycardia often is absent in the early stages of severe shock and may be present from too many other causes to be a useful sign (48,49).

If some findings suggest shock but the diagnosis is uncertain, it is useful to connect a second catheter to a pressure transducer, insert the catheter into the umbilical vein, and use direct pressure monitoring to locate the position of the catheter tip in the inferior vena cava or right atrium (25). Central venous pressure may be low or normal during hypovolemic shock, but it will be high with circulatory tamponade from excessive positive-pres-

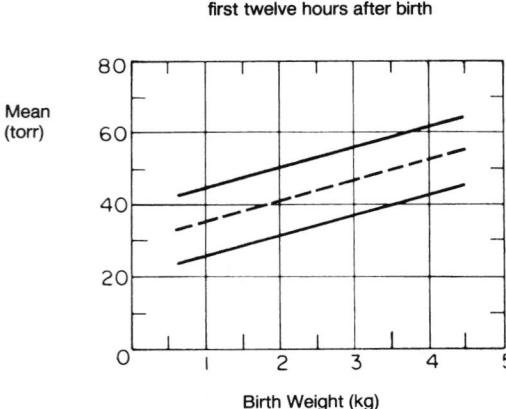

FIG. 18–8. Mean aortic blood pressure was obtained from an umbilical artery catheter. The *dashed line* is the average blood pressure at each birth weight, and the *solid lines* are the 95% confidence limits of this relationship. Blood pressure values below the lower confidence line are hypotensive. (From Versmold HT, Kitterman JA, Phibbs RH, et al. Aortic blood pressure during the first twelve hours of life in infants with birth weights 610–4220 grams. *Pediatrics* 1981;67:607.)

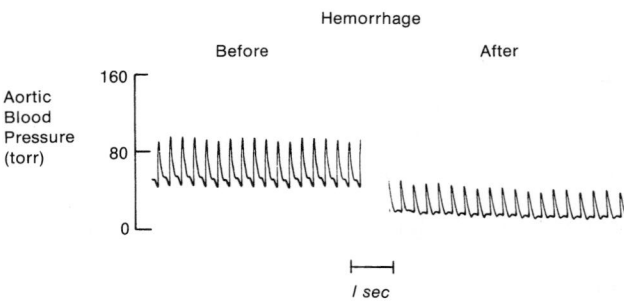

FIG. 18–9. Changes in aortic blood pressure during rapid hemorrhage in a newborn lamb. Blood pressure falls and pulse pressure (i.e., systolic minus diastolic) narrows. Note the difference in waveform before and after hemorrhage. Before the hemorrhage, pressure continues to decrease after the dicrotic notch, indicating continued systemic flow during diastole. This disappears after hemorrhage, indicating little or no systemic flow during diastole. Heart rate has not yet increased, but will do so later.

sure ventilation, tension pneumothorax, or postasphyxial myocardiopathy. The findings of low or normal central venous pressure in combination with signs of poor systemic perfusion support a trial of volume expansion. A low central venous oxygen content is a very sensitive, but nonspecific, indicator of increased oxygen extraction in the microcirculation in response to inadequate oxygen delivery from any cause. It is one of the earliest changes during hypovolemic shock (50).

Hypovolemic shock is treated best with repeated small infusions of whole blood that has been cross-matched against the mother before delivery and is available in the resuscitation area at birth (51). Group O Rh-negative blood given to newborns without cross-matching against the mother's serum occasionally has produced fatal transfusion reactions caused by incompatibility in minor blood groups and should not be used. If only packed erythrocytes are available, give equal volumes of cells and a plasma substitute, such as 5% albumin or isotonic saline. If no erythrocytes are available, use a plasma substitute for initial resuscitation, then give packed cells as soon as they are available. However, this is less effective than giving blood initially. The object of therapy is prompt restoration of adequate tissue perfusion. This must be done rapidly enough to avoid the cumulatively harmful effects of prolonged underperfusion of tissues. The latter can lead to the secondary effects of shock, including increased capillary permeability and pulmonary disease, which make therapy more difficult. Excessive speed in volume replacement also is dangerous, however. Some vascular beds, such as that of the brain, vasodilate in response to systemic hypotension. If treatment produces an abrupt rise in systemic pressure, there is no time for this vasculature to partially constrict and the higher pressure is transmitted to the capillaries, where it may cause capillary injury, edema, or hemorrhage. In most cases, shock can be treated with repeated infusions of 5 mL/kg blood given by a steady infusion over approximately 5 minutes. Observe the response to each infusion and stop therapy as soon as tissue perfusion is adequate. Usually, aortic pressure will rise after the first or first few infusions, but as these relieve systemic vasoconstriction, pressure falls again and additional volume expansion may be required, provided other signs of poor perfusion persist. Occasionally, when there has been massive hemorrhage, volume may have to be replaced more rapidly. In such a case, monitor aortic pressure continuously to avoid abrupt rises in pressures. Figure 18–10 shows the course of successful treatment during the first hour of life in an infant who lost approximately 50% of his blood volume during delivery and also suffered asphyxia. Figure 18–11 shows the course in an infant in whom hypovolemia did not become evident until assisted ventilation relieved asphyxia and unmasked hypovolemia.

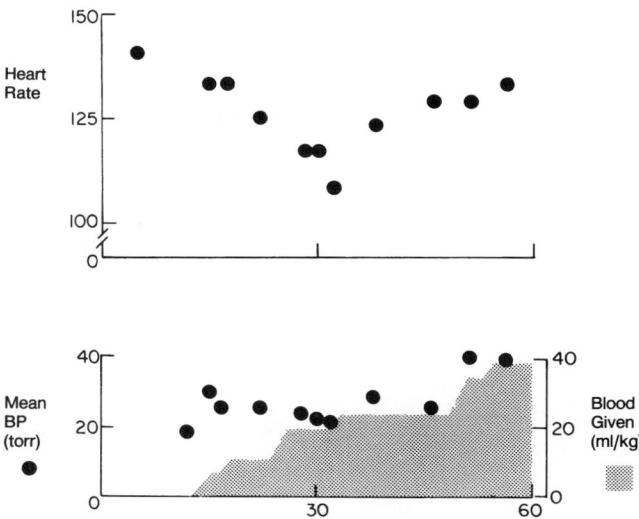

FIG. 18–10. Heart rate, aortic blood pressure, and blood volume replacement were monitored during the first hour after birth in a 2.8-kg infant who suffered massive blood loss when the anteriorly placed placenta was incised deeply at cesarean section delivery. The *shaded area* shows the cumulative volume of whole blood given expressed as mL/kg body weight. The final volume, which produced a normal aortic blood pressure and relieved signs of poor perfusion, was 40 mL/kg, approximately one-half the total blood volume for a normal newborn infant. The blood was given as a series of small transfusions guided by the changes in blood pressure. Note that the heart rate is not elevated at first, despite the extreme hypotension, and that subsequently heart rate does not change consistently in the opposite direction of blood pressure changes.

Phase III

This is the time when infants with mild asphyxia will improve quickly, whereas those who were more severely asphyxiated may begin to manifest transient failure of various organ systems secondary to asphyxia (52).

Adjust Assisted Ventilation to Changes in Pulmonary Function

Pulmonary function will improve rapidly in many infants as compliance improves with absorption of lung water. Pulmonary perfusion will increase in response to a rising pH and PO_2. On the other hand, if ischemia has caused more severe asphyxia with lung injury, there may be continued respiratory distress that is indistinguishable from early hyaline membrane disease. This will require continued ventilatory assistance. Unlike hyaline membrane disease, however, this form of respiratory failure usually begins to improve within a few hours after birth (53), whereas hyaline membrane disease due to immaturity of the surfactant system worsens over the first day after birth. When a fetus with immature lungs has suf-

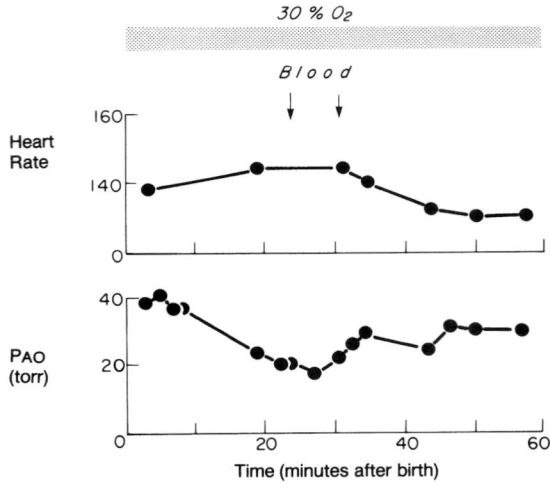

FIG. 18–11. Heart rate, aortic blood pressure (PAO), and therapy were monitored during the first hour after the birth of a 1.5-kg second twin delivered by cesarean section. There had been a large abruption of the placenta. Initially, the infant was hypoxic and acidotic, and aortic pressure was normal. As blood gas tensions normalized, aortic pressure fell and the infant continued to appear pale and poorly perfused. This probably is an example of the intense vasoconstriction of asphyxia keeping blood pressure at a normal level despite a subnormal blood volume. Relief of the asphyxia allowed sufficient vasodilation to unmask the hypovolemia.

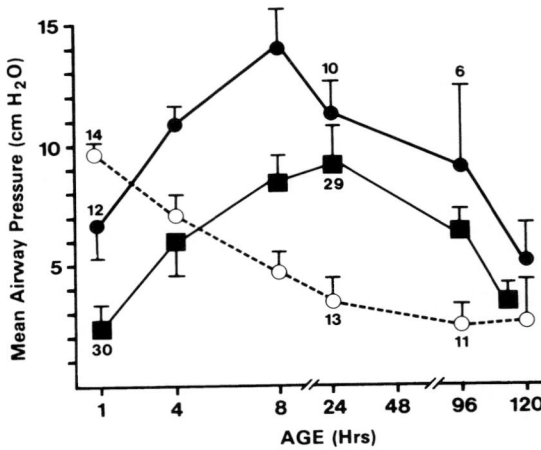

FIG. 18–12. The course of respiratory distress is characterized by changes in mean airway pressure in three groups of infants: those with severe perinatal asphyxia but no hyaline membrane disease, those with perinatal asphyxia plus hyaline membrane disease, and those with no perinatal asphyxia but hyaline membrane disease. In both groups with hyaline membrane disease, the disease worsens, as indicated by the increased mean airway pressure required over the first 24 hours. Those who also had asphyxia had more severe disease. Those with severe asphyxia but no hyaline membrane disease had a completely different course, with progressive improvement over the first 24 hours of life. ○, no respiratory distress syndrome—severe acidosis; ●, respiratory distress syndrome—severe acidosis; ■, respiratory distress syndrome—mild or no acidosis. (From ref. 54.)

fered significant intrapartum asphyxia, the ensuing hyaline membrane disease generally will be more severe (54). These divergent courses of respiratory distress are illustrated in Fig. 18–12.

Infants with early-onset hyaline membrane disease should be given exogenous surfactant as soon as the condition is apparent and the endotracheal tube is in proper position with its tip above the carina. Early treatment with surfactant is more effective than treatment that has been delayed several hours. At this early stage in the infant's course, it often is impossible to distinguish between hyaline membrane disease, postasphyxial respiratory distress, and congenital pneumonia. This is not a reason to withhold surfactant treatment, because it has no adverse effect and may be of some benefit in some infants with other pulmonary disease (55,56).

Cardiac Function

Transient myocardial failure of 1 to 2 days of duration can occur after asphyxia (22,57–59). The resulting circulatory failure is differentiated from that due to hypovolemic shock by an elevated central venous pressure. Postasphyxial myocardiopathy responds to a continuous infusion of dopamine with improved systemic perfusion and decreased central venous pressure. Start with a dose of 5 μg/kg/min and increase the dose as needed to obtain adequate systemic perfusion pressures. If possible, cor-

rect hypoxia and acidosis to improve myocardial function before starting dopamine. If pulmonary vasoconstriction and hypertension coexist with systemic hypotension due to myocardial failure, venous-to-arterial shunting of blood through the foramen ovale and ductus arteriosus often occurs. This leads to additional systemic hypoxemia and worsening metabolic acidosis. When correcting acidosis in this situation, it is important to avoid hyperventilation, because hypocarbia constricts the coronary circulation and causes systemic hypotension (42,43,47). Some infants of poorly controlled diabetic mothers have a particularly severe form of myocardiopathy. The antecedents of this myocardiopathy are asphyxia plus hypoglycemia plus hypocalcemia, and all of these must be corrected to improve myocardial performance.

Hematology

Consumption of coagulation factors may complicate severe asphyxia. This almost always is a transient process rather than continuing disseminated intravascular coagulation. Thrombocytopenia is the most consistent finding. In extreme cases, clinical bleeding occurs and requires replacement of platelets and plasma clotting factors. Other hematologic changes include a transient rise in the number of granulocytes, including immature forms, and in erythroid precursors in the peripheral blood. These can rise to very high concentrations and could be misleading when considering diagnoses such as infection and hemolytic anemia. If the changes are secondary to asphyxia, however, they will disappear in a day or less.

Glucose

When hypoxia and acidosis have been relieved, begin a continuous infusion of 10% dextrose in water at 3 mL/kg/hour to maintain a normal concentration of blood glucose. This provides 5 mg of glucose per kg per minute. Begin screening for hyperglycemia and hypoglycemia with repeated testing of capillary blood. Glucose infusions usually are not necessary until hypoxia is relieved. Hypoglycemia can be corrected by temporarily increasing the infusion rate of the 10% dextrose to 5 mL/kg/hour (8.4 mg/kg/min), which is sufficient in all but the most extreme cases of asphyxia-induced hypoglycemia. Rapid infusions of more concentrated solutions of dextrose rarely are needed to correct hypoglycemia and can be dangerous because of their hyperosmolarity and their tendency to produce serious vascular injury.

Fluid and Electrolytes

Asphyxia causes renal ischemia, which may persist after birth and resusitation (60). Many asphyxiated infants are oliguric for the first day of life and have a rising serum creatinine (52,61). Very high serum creatinine concentrations in the first days of life, however, are not due to renal failure but to tissue necrosis after severe asphyxia. When urine output increases, there is transient hematuria and oliguria. With extreme asphyxia, corticomedullary hemorrhagic necrosis occurs and the renal failure is more severe. As renal function returns, sodium, potassium, and chloride can be added to parenteral fluids. As acidosis is corrected, extracellular potassium shifts back into cells and postasphyxial infants with good renal function may become hypokalemic. The usual maintenance amounts of electrolytes may be adequate to maintain serum electrolyte concentrations, but in many cases renal losses of electrolytes are very high during this diuresis, so it will be necessary to administer higher concentrations of electrolytes. When planning sodium requirements, take into account sodium given as $NaHCO_3$ during resuscitation and the NaCl in catheter-flush solutions. Infants who are asphyxiated often become hypocalcemic by the first day after birth (24). Serum ionized calcium should be measured and supplemental calcium given as needed.

Gastrointestinal Function

During asphyxia, blood flow to the small and large bowels is reduced. Severe asphyxia may cause serious ischemic injury to these organs and gastrointestinal blood flow may remain abnormal for up to 3 days after delivery and resuscitation (60). Because of this, it may be advisable to delay enteral feedings for several days and continue intravenous fluids. Occasionally, acute necrotizing enterocolitis occurs when severely asphyxiated infants are fed in the first day or two after birth. This is particularly important in infants who also have suffered hypovolemic shock, because shock severely compromises intestinal blood flow.

Central Nervous System

Severe asphyxia can lead to hypoxic ischemic encephalopathy. Because the homeostatic responses to asphyxia tend to preserve oxygen delivery to the brain at the expense of other organs, asphyxial encephalopathy tends to occur in infants with evidence of multiorgan injury (60,61). However, there are situations in which encephalopathy appears in isolation. A significant portion of the damage to the brain is reperfusion injury, which occurs some time after recovery from asphyxia (63,64). This interval raises the potential for treatment that could prevent this portion of the injury. Several forms of therapy that might provide such neuroprotection are under investigation, but none has been shown to be effective yet (63). However, there are some lesions from these studies that are applicable to clinical care. Many studies point to hypocarbia as a contributor to neurologic injury (63,65). Closely monitoring P_aCO_2 and adjusting ventilation to avoid hypocarbia has been discussed previously. There is so much conflicting information about the benificial versus the harmful effects of hyperglycemia in the asphyxiated infant the it seems prudent to keep the blood glucose concentration in the physiologic range.

SPECIAL PROBLEMS

Meconium Aspiration

Meconium staining of amniotic fluid occurs in 10% to 15% of all deliveries (66,67). Mature fetuses pass meconium in response to various stimuli, including asphyxia. Meconium staining diminishes with decreasing gestational age and is rare before 34 weeks of gestation, whereas it is quite common in postmature fetuses (68). Infants can aspirate meconium into the airway by gasping, which may occur *in utero* in response to a variety of stimuli, including hypoxia, or by inhalation after delivery. Aspiration of meconium can cause pulmonary disease both by plugging of the airways and by producing a chemical pneumonitis. Clinical pulmonary disease is more likely if meconium staining occurs before the second stage of labor, if the meconium-stained fluid is thick with particulate matter, and if there is meconium below the vocal cords (66,69). Many infants have meconium in the hypopharynx but none below the vocal cords, and disease is unlikely to develop in them. Some have no meconium in the hypopharynx but have meconium below the cords, and these infants are at increased risk for pulmonary disease.

In some instances, asphyxia is present and requires resuscitation at birth; meconium aspiration syndrome follows immediately afterward. In other instances, infants are clinically well at birth and manifest symptoms of meconium aspiration syndrome during the first few hours after birth. Severe disease nonetheless can develop in infants with this more gradual onset of symptoms. Pulmonary air leaks are ten times as likely to develop in infants with meconium aspiration as in infants without meconium staining; the air leak often occurs during resuscitation. Pulmonary hypertension develops in some infants.

Clearing thick meconium from the airway at birth reduces the risk and severity of disease. In vertex deliveries, suctioning the oropharynx after the head has been delivered, but before delivery of the shoulders, followed by prompt tracheal intubation and suctioning of the trachea once the baby is delivered has reduced the incidence of clinical disease and reduced, but not eliminated, mortality from this disease (66,67,70,71). These prophylactic procedures should be carried out in all cases of thick or particulate meconium. Intubation and suctioning carries very little risk when done properly (72). The only reasonable exception to routine intubation and suctioning is the baby who has had the oropharynx suctioned on the perineum, has no other risk factors, and is vigorous at birth. An attempt to intubate such an infant is unlikely to be successful and may result in trauma to the upper airway or vomiting and aspiration of meconium-stained gastric contents.

Several measures should be taken to prepare for the delivery of a baby with meconium-stained amniotic fluid:

Have a second person available to help with the suctioning.

Have several endotracheal tubes available, because the first tube used may become so obstructed with thick, tenacious meconium that it cannot be reused when necessary.

Have oral suctioning ready on the resuscitation table.

Have a manually operated meconium suction device that attaches to the endotracheal tube adapter and to a source of suction that will provide a negative pressure in the range of 80 to 120 mm Hg (73), which is the amount of pressure needed to suck thick meconium through this system. The old practice of wearing a soft face mask and sucking on the endotracheal tube like a straw is unsafe and should not be used.

After delivery of the head, the obstetrician or a designated assistant should suction the oropharynx quickly while the chest is still compressed in the birth canal.

Obviously, there will be cases in which this maneuver is not possible.

After the baby is delivered, do nothing that might stimulate him or her to cry or inhale. Intubate the trachea quickly. Ideally, this should be done without first suctioning the oropharynx, which often stimulates the infant to gasp. In some cases, however, large amounts of meconium in the oropharynx obstruct the view of the vocal cords so that intubation is impossible until the oropharynx is suctioned. If there is thick meconium staining but no meconium visible in the hypopharynx, it still is appropriate to intubate the trachea and suction because there may be significant amounts of meconium below the vocal cords. As soon as the endotracheal tube is inserted into the trachea, connect it to the suction apparatus, apply suction, and withdraw the tube while maintaining the suction. In many cases, meconium will not be drawn into the suction apparatus but a plug of meconium will be drawn into the tube, lodge there, and be seen only when the tube is removed. If more than a scant amount of meconium (i.e., greater than 0.5 mL) is obtained on the first suctioning, repeat the process until no more is seen. In some instances, there may be so much meconium in the airway that it still can be recovered after suctioning the trachea five or six times. During tracheal suctioning, a second person should monitor heart rate continuously. If significant sustained bradycardia develops, discontinue suctioning and give positive-pressure ventilation with oxygen.

After clearing the airway, proceed with resuscitation as with any other infant, paying particular attention to two problems. First, have a very high index of suspicion for a tension pneumothorax, which may occur early in the resuscitation. Second, be aware that intense pulmonary vasoconstriction is more likely to occur in these infants. When it occurs, it should be treated with more aggressive correction of metabolic acidosis than is necessary in other infants.

The Extremely-Low-Birth-Weight Infant

Infants with birth weights less than 1,250 g, and particularly those less than 1,000 g, present a special set of problems. Hack and Fanaroff (74) have pointed out the value of a well-trained and experienced resuscitation team in the successful management of these infants. The smaller the infant, the weaker the muscles of respiration and the less likely he or she will be able spontaneously to achieve adequate lung inflation and create an adequate functional residual capacity, even if the surfactant system has matured. Furthermore, lung inflation stimulates surfactant release from the type II alveolar cells (75,76). This has led to the recommendation that all extremely-low-birth-weight infants should have their tracheas intubated at birth and have their lungs inflated. The findings of the only controlled trial of prophylactic intubation support this approach (77). It may be that the same result can be achieved in very vigorous babies with the application of positive end-expiratory pressure.

Initial ventilation requires special attention in the very preterm infant with a small lung volume and surfactant deficiency. Serious lung damage can be done by ventilating such lungs with very large tidal volumes for a period as short as 15 minutes (78–80). The large inflating breaths recommended earlier in this chapter for resuscitation of larger infants may not be appropriate for these infants. In experimental animals it is possible to prevent this lung injury by administering surfactant at birth (80). In clinical studies prophylactic administration of surfactant in the highest risk infants is more effective than rescue treatment of established hyaline membrane disease (81). Therefore, seriously consider prophylactic administration of surfactant to the extremely-low-birth-weight infant as soon as possible after birth unless there is evidence of a mature surfactant system. A skillful, experienced resuscitation team can give surfactant within 5 minutes after birth as a part of the initial resuscitation. However, if there is any question about the ability to do this, the initial phase of resuscitation should be completed first, then the surfactant given.

As pulmonary function improves and these smallest infants are weaned from assisted ventilation, it is important to remember that many of them cannot maintain an adequate functional residual capacity, even in the absence of lung disease, and progressive atelectasis gradually will develop unless end-expiratory distending pressure is applied to their lungs. Special attention also must be given to the inspired oxygen concentration as the infant's condition improves. The clinician's sense of time is distorted easily during a complex resuscitation and the ensuing period of recovery. What seems like minutes may be an hour or more, and failure to adjust inspired oxygen in a timely way may lead to prolonged hyperoxia.

The radiant heat required to maintain normal body temperature during resuscitation evaporates water from the infant's skin. This can produce very high insensible water losses from very premature infants. Once the endotracheal tube and catheter are in place and secured and other emergency procedures completed, cover the infant with a clear plastic wrap to reduce insensible water loss.

One of the greatest problems in a subset of extremely-low-birth-weight infants is the management of the infant at the margin of viability. This limit varies between centers and, at present, is usually in the range of gestational age from 23 to 25 weeks. It is important to have a clear understanding of the prognosis for such infants at one's own center, both for the approach to the infant at birth and for counseling the parents prior to the birth of such an infant (82,83). There is understandable reluctance to subject an infant with no chance of long-term survival to hours and perhaps days of the discomfort of intensive care. It is even worse, however, initially to withhold resuscitation from an infant thought at first to be nonvi-

able but then, because he or she continues to breathe and be vigorous, to resuscitate the infant, most likely after serious brain damage has occurred. Yu et al. (84) have pointed out that the infant's response to resuscitation is one of the determinants of viability. Figure 18–13 illustrates this concept. In these borderline cases of uncertain viability, it is better to start with vigorous resuscitation. It quickly will become evident if therapy is futile, so care can be withdrawn early.

Multiple Births

The five features of multiple births that complicate delivery room management are the following:
1. Increased incidence of preterm labor and delivery. This affects management only by increasing the number of personnel needed for resuscitation. The risk of intrapartum asphyxia is somewhat increased in the second-born of twins.
2. Increased incidence of congenital anomalies in monozygotic multiple births.
3. Increased risk of intrauterine growth retardation in one fetus in a multiple birth set because the placenta is shared unevenly. This results in the usual problems of small-for-gestational-age (SGA) infants, including intrapartum asphyxia, polycythemia, hypoglycemia, and pulmonary hemorrhage (see Chap. 26).
4. Twin-to-twin transfusion syndrome.
5. Stuck twin syndrome.

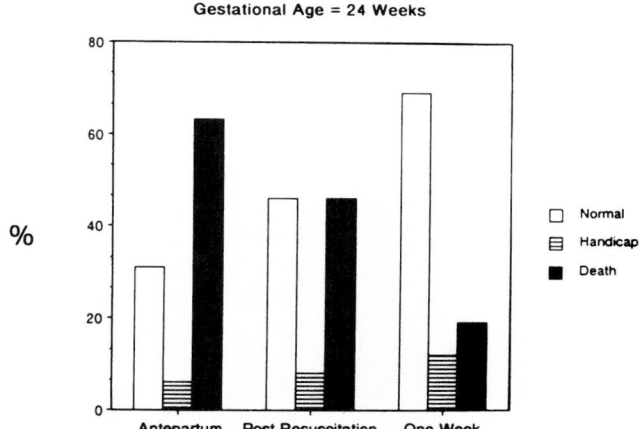

FIG. 18–13. Prognosis for infants born at an estimated 24 weeks of gestation. The prognosis is given three times: before birth, after resuscitation, and at 1 week after birth. The prognosis changes at the second and third points, because it applies only to infants who survived to those points. (From Phibbs RH. Delivery room management of the extremely low birth weight infant. In: Cowett RM, Hay WW Jr, eds. *The micropremie: the next frontier. Report of the 99th Ross Conference on Pediatric Research,* pp 13–18. Columbus, OH: Ross Laboratories, 1990. Adapted from data in ref. 84.)

The twin-to-twin transfusion syndrome, which occurs in at least 5% of multiple pregnancies, results from vascular anastomosis between the circulations of monozygotic twins, primarily with monochorionic placentas. Both the degree of transfusion from one fetus to the other and the time course are quite variable, and determine the clinical problems at birth. Bleeding may have been relatively recent, or it may have begun in the second trimester and been long-standing at the time of birth. If the transfusion is primarily in one direction, the donor twin becomes anemic and the recipient twin polycythemic. With ongoing bleeding, the recipient grows normally while the donor becomes progressively smaller for gestational age. As the process becomes more severe, polyhydramnios develops in the recipient fetus and oligohydramnios in the donor. Ultimately, either twin may become hydropic, one from volume overload and the other from anemia. In severe cases, the donor twin may die and intravascular coagulation in the dead fetus can cause emboli that pass into the recipient's circulation. When embolization occurs, it commonly involves the brain, kidneys, and gastrointestinal tract of the recipient fetus. Recent embolization of the gastrointestinal tract may cause a bowel perforation, whereas early embolization causes an atretic area of the bowel.

When twins suffering from this syndrome are delivered, management during resuscitation may be extremely complicated. Fortunately, those responsible for the resuscitation of such babies usually are forewarned of the most severe cases. Findings in the mother should lead to close ultrasonic surveillance of the fetuses and prenatal recognition of the unidirectional twin-to-twin transfusion syndrome. The polycythemic baby needs to have his or her hematocrit reduced. Management of the anemic donor is less straightforward. Recent acute blood loss requires the same management as in any other hypovolemic baby. More often, the anemia has been prolonged and severe, so the donor's circulation may be compromised and may not tolerate blood volume expansion. In this case, the proper therapy is partial exchange transfusion with packed cells to raise the hematocrit to a normal level. Both arterial and central venous pressures should be monitored beginning immediately after birth (see section on "Hydrops," below) to assess the circulatory status and make the correct adjustments in both hematocrit and intravascular volume. Have packed erythrocytes that are cross-matched against the mother available in the resuscitation area. Rapidly measure hematocrit or hemoglobin in each twin and begin the appropriate therapy.

In monochorionic twins, the vascular anastomoses may be multidirectional, so that the direction of flow is determined at least in part by the differences in circulatory resistance between the twins. Such twin-to-twin transfusions are not diagnosed so easily, nor are the hemoglobin measurements necessarily different at birth even when the blood volumes are.

The stuck twin syndrome is a poorly understood phenomenon in monochorionic twins. There is discordant growth with oligohydramnios in the SGA fetus and polyhydramnios in the appropriate-for-gestational-age fetus. The SGA fetus becomes compacted into a small volume within the uterus. Lung growth often is restricted, which leads to pulmonary hypoplasia that is lethal if severe. If mild, it requires positive-pressure ventilation at high pressures and rates. There usually are placental vascular anastomoses between the placentas, suggesting that this is a complication of the twin-to-twin transfusion syndrome. The hematocrits, however, often are nearly normal and similar in both twins. In some cases there is marked myocardial dysfunction in one or both twins, which can be detected antenatally by echocardiography. Preparations for delivery are the same as for the twin-to-twin transfusion syndrome.

Birth Injury

Severe birth injury and intrapartum asphyxia often occur together. The main problem for delivery room management of these infants is significant hemorrhage from the traumatized tissues, which complicates the resuscitation (see section on "Phase II," above). The blood loss almost always is internal and, therefore, not immediately evident. Moderate blood loss can occur in fractured limbs or into the perineum in a difficult breech delivery. Sites for major blood loss include intracranial, mediastinal, and intraabdominal (e.g., ruptured spleen, hepatic subcapsular hematoma). A subgaleal hematoma can produce a massive loss of blood volume because of the extremely large potential space. Any of these hematomas can contain several hundred milliliters of blood and are particularly dangerous because they can consume large quantities of coagulation factors and lead to generalized bleeding that perpetuates the hypovolemia. In severe cases, only early and extremely aggressive therapy can bring the situation under control. Treatment includes replacement of the lost blood volume and erythrocyte mass and, if there is depletion of clotting factors, very aggressive replacement of these factors with fresh frozen plasma, platelets, and, on occasion, cryoprecipitate.

Early detection of internal hemorrhage from birth trauma is crucial. Abdominal distention and discoloration suggest intraabdominal bleeding, which easily is confirmed by aspiration of a small amount of blood from the peritoneal cavity. Control of intraabdominal bleeding may require surgery. Intracranial hemorrhage sufficient to cause hypovolemia usually is manifested by a bulging fontanelle and can be confirmed quickly by ultrasonography. Small intracranial hemorrhages also may cause circulatory instability through their effects on the autonomic nervous system. A mediastinal hematoma does not declare itself by any physical sign, but a chest radiograph often suggests its presence when the mediastinum is widened. If suspected, it can be diagnosed quickly by an ultrasound examination of the mediastinum. Early swelling of the back of the neck from a subgaleal hematoma may be hard to recognize, but an expanding subgaleal hemorrhage pushes the ears laterally and forward. This often is the earliest sign of this condition. Subgaleal hemorrhage, too, can be confirmed by ultrasound.

Hydrops

Hydropic babies present a challenging set of problems for resuscitation. Usually, abnormal findings in the mother of a fetus with hydrops lead to an ultrasound diagnosis before delivery. Every effort should be made to establish the cause of the hydrops before delivery to help with preparations for managing the infant at birth. An ultrasound examination should be done or repeated just before delivery to assess the presence and size of pleural effusions. Assessment of fetal blood by percutaneous umbilical sampling is especially helpful for early management whenever feasible. Have whole blood or packed erythrocytes cross-matched against the mother in the resuscitation area, even if the hydrops is not due to Rh disease or other alloimmune hemolysis, because many infants with nonimmune hydrops also are anemic at birth. More personnel are needed for management of these infants than for a routine resuscitation. One member of the resuscitation team should be prepared to perform paracentesis and thoracentesis as needed. The supplies needed for partial exchange transfusion and for paracentesis, plus specimen tubes for diagnostic studies, must be on hand. Two umbilical vessel catheters should be connected to pressure transducers and a recorder with one channel calibrated for arterial pressure and the other for venous pressure. There must be equipment for measuring hematocrit or hemoglobin near the resuscitation area, and someone should have the specific assignment of obtaining blood from the umbilical cord at birth and immediately making this measurement by 5 minutes after birth.

Lung inflation and ventilation often are difficult in hydropic infants because the lungs are compressed by the diaphragm, which is elevated by ascites and by large pleural effusions. There also is low compliance due to excessive lung water. Resuscitation usually requires tracheal intubation and ventilation with oxygen at high pressures. If the abdomen is distended with ascites, perform a paracentesis in the flank region to avoid puncturing a large liver or spleen. It is necessary to remove only enough fluid so that the abdomen is soft and the diaphragms move easily with inflation. If ventilation remains difficult and there are pleural effusions, these too should be reduced to allow ventilation. Even after fluid is removed from the abdomen and chest, many of these babies continue to require high pressures to provide adequate ventilation because of excess lung water, surfactant deficiency, and, in some cases of long-standing hydrops, pulmonary hypoplasia (85).

While the baby is being ventilated and the effusions are being reduced, catheterize the umbilical artery and vein and measure blood gas tensions and pH and intravascular pressures to assess the state of the circulation. Anemia compromises tissue oxygenation, and anemic hydropic infants usually do not respond well to resuscitative measures until their hematocrit is at least 30% to 35% (86). Transfused blood is virtually 100% hemoglobin A, which transports oxygen much more efficiently after birth than hemoglobin F. How the anemia is corrected depends on the state of the circulation. Most infants with hydrops due to alloimmune disease have low or normal blood volumes (87). The blood volumes of infants with nonimmune hydrops of various causes are unpredictable. If intravascular pressures indicate that blood volume is adequate, do a partial exchange transfusion and keep blood volume constant. If there is evidence of hypovolemia, infuse more blood than is withdrawn until intravascular pressures are normal. Alternately, infuse a bolus of packed erythrocytes, as is done for the treatment of hypovolemic shock. In most cases, evidence of hypovolemia does not appear until the asphyxia is relieved (86). The most common sequence is a partial exchange transfusion that keeps blood volume constant while raising hematocrit, and then repeated small infusions of packed erythrocytes and albumin or fresh frozen plasma to support the circulation. Do not give the plasma or albumin until the anemia is corrected. Fresh frozen plasma also partially corrects the hemostatic defects that often are present (88). Most infants with alloimmune hydrops have very low concentrations of serum albumin and low plasma colloid osmotic pressures (87,89). About one-half of those with nonimmune hydrops also are hypoalbuminemic. There has been concern that giving albumin and fresh frozen plasma to these infants during resuscitation would raise plasma colloid osmotic pressure enough to draw excessive volumes of fluid into the circulation and worsen pulmonary edema. In practice, however, this rarely occurs, and if it does, it can be managed by appropriate adjustments in assisted ventilation. Pulmonary vasoconstriction, which may occur in any asphyxiated infant, is particularly common in hydropic infants (86,90). Therefore, if pulmonary perfusion has not improved after the initial steps in resuscitation, correct metabolic acidosis with alkali therapy. After resuscitation is complete, there usually is residual pulmonary disease that requires assisted ventilation. This may be transient respiratory distress, hyaline membrane disease, pulmonary hypoplasia, or some combination of these. Diuresis will improve lung function, and therapy with furosemide often is helpful.

Major Anomalies

Infants with certain congenital anomalies require special management at the time of delivery.

Diaphragmatic Hernia

The infant with a diaphragmatic hernia will have a variable degree of pulmonary hypoplasia. The degree of restricted lung growth depends upon the size and duration of the intrathoracic mass during fetal life. The unsuspected mild case will present with respiratory distress and a scaffoid abdomen. After birth, gas that enters the intestines from swallowing or from assisted ventilation by face mask will dilate the intestines in the thorax and further restrict ventilation. Infants with more severe forms of this anomaly are critically ill at birth. Fortunately, many fetuses with this anomaly are detected antenatally by ultrasound, which also can estimate the severity of the pulmonary pathology (91). The higher-risk cases should be delivered at a hospital with extracorporeal membrane oxygenation capability and with an experienced pediatric surgery team standing by at the time of delivery.

At birth, ventilation should not be attempted by face mask. The infant's trachea should be intubated immediately. A muscle relaxant should be given to prevent swallowing and gastric suction started. In addition to mechanical ventilation, immediate cardiopulmonary care includes placement of arterial and central venous catheters (usually by umbilical artery and vein) and a peripherial arterial catheter in the right radial artery. These infants often have pulmonary hypertension, and some have poor myocardial function that requires treatment with dopamine.

Abdominal Wall Defects

An infant with an omphalocele or gastroschisis has a very high evaporative water loss and heat loss from the defect. Immediate management includes establishing intravascular access and beginning liberal fluid replacement and placing the infant feet first into a plastic bag that extends up over the defect and around the upper chest. This reduces evaporative and heat losses. The mouth of the bag should not be drawn so tightly that it restricts ventilation. The infant should be placed on gastric suction and started on antibiotics.

The infant with a gastroschisis presents another life-threatening problem. Before birth the free intestines are suspended in the amniotic fluid. After birth, if the infant is supine, the free intestines will slide down to one side, which can place traction on, or kink, the mesenteric vessels. This can quickly lead to infarction of large portions of the bowel, which can be fatal. These infants should be placed on their sides and twisting of the mesentary avoided. Because of this problem, when gastroschisis is diagnosed antenatally, the infant is better managed by delivery at a center with an experienced pediatric surgery team on hand at the time of delivery.

REFERENCES

1. Torrance S, Wittnich C. The effect of varying arterial oxygen tension on neonatal acid–base balance. Pediatr Res 1992;31:112.
2. James LS, Weisbrot IM, Prince CE, et al. The acid–base status of human infants in relation to birth asphyxia and onset of respiration. J Pediatr 1958;52:379.
3. Yeomans ER, Hauth JC, Gilstrap LC, et al. Umbilical cord pH, PCO₂, and bicarbonate following uncomplicated term vaginal deliveries. Am J Obstet Gynecol 1985;151:798.
4. Goodwin TM, Belai I, Hernandez P, et al. Asphyxial complications in the term newborn with severe umbilical acidemia. Am J Obstet Gynecol 1992;167:1506.
5. Rudolph CD, Roman C, Rudolph AM. Effect of acute umbilical cord compression on hepatic carbohydrate metabolism in the fetal lamb. Pediatr Res 1989;25:228.
6. Ruth V, Fyhrquist F, Clemons G, et al. Cord plasma vasopressin, erythropoietin and hypoxanthine as indices of asphyxia at birth. Pediatr Res 1988;24:490.
7. Dawes G. Fetal and neonatal physiology. Chicago: Year Book, 1968, p 149.
8. Cohn HE, Sacks FJ, Heymann MA, et al. Cardiovascular responses to hypokalemia and acidemia in fetal lambs. Am J Obstet Gynecol 1974; 120:817.
9. Fisher DJ. Increased regional myocardial blood flows and oxygen deliveries during hypoxemia in lambs. Pediatr Res 1984;18:602.
10. Boyle DW, Host K, Zerbe GO, et al. Fetal hind limb oxygen consumption and blood flow during acute graded hypoxia. Pediatr Res 1990;28:94.
11. Rudolph AM, Yuan S. Response of the pulmonary vasculature of hypoxia and H⁺ ion concentration changes. J Clin Invest 1966;45:339.
12. Parer JT. The effect of acute maternal hypoxia on fetal oxygenation and the umbilical circulation in the sheep. Eur J Obstet Gynecol Reprod Biol 1980;10:125.
13. Fisher DJ. Acidemia reduces cardiac output and left ventricular contractility in conscious lambs. J Dev Physiol 1986;8:23.
14. Lewinsky R, Szwarc R, Benson L, Ritchie J. The effects of hypoxic acidemia on left ventricular end-systolic elastance in fetal sheep. Pediatr Res 1993;34:38.
15. Itskovitz J, LaGamma EF, Bristow J, et al. Cardiovascular responses to hypoxemia in sinoaortic-denervated fetal sheep. Pediatr Res 1991;30:381.
16. Jones CT, Roebuck MM, Walker DW, et al. The role of the adrenal medulla and peripheral sympathetic nerves in the physiological responses of the fetal sheep to hypoxia. J Dev Physiol 1988;10:17.
17. Cheung CY, Brace RA. Fetal hypoxia elevates plasma atrial natriuretic factor concentration. Am J Obstet Gynecol 1988;159:1263.
18. Fisher DJ. β-Adrenergic influence on increased myocardial oxygen consumption during hypoxemia in awake newborn lambs. Pediatr Res 1989;25:585.
19. Slotkin TA, Seidler FJ. Adrenomedullary catecholamine release in the fetus and newborn: secretory mechanisms and their role in stress and survival. J Dev Physiol 1988;10:1.
20. Perez R, Espinoza M, Riqueline R, et al. Arginine vasopressin mediates cardiovascular responses to hypoxia in fetal sheep. Am J Physiol 1989; 256:R1011.
21. Linderkamp O, Versmold HT, Messow-Zahn K, et al. The effects of intrapartum and intrauterine asphyxia on placental transfusion in premature and full-term infants. Eur J Pediatr 1978;127:91.
22. Bucciarelli RL, Nelson RM, Egen EA, et al. Transient tricuspid insufficiency of the newborn: a form of myocardial dysfunction in stressed newborn. Pediatrics 1977;59:330.
23. Longstrath WJ Jr, Kwon JM, Zelenock GB, et al. Infusion of five percent dextrose increases mortality and morbidity following six minutes of cardiac arrest in resuscitated dogs. J Clin Care 1987;2:4.
24. Venkataraman PS, Tsang RC, Chen IW, et al. Pathogenesis of early neonatal hypocalcemia: studies of serum gastrin and plasma glucagon. J Pediatr 1987;110:599.
25. Kitterman JA, Phibbs RH, Tooley WH. Catheterization of umbilical vessels in newborn infants. Pediatr Clin North Am 1970;17:895.
26. Apgar V. A proposal for a new method of evaluation of the newborn infant. Anesth Analg 1953;32:260.
27. Sykes GS, Molloy PM, Johnson P, et al. Do Apgar scores indicate asphyxia? Lancet 1982;1:494.
28. Martin M, Paes BA. Birth asphyxia: does the Apgar score have diagnostic value. Obstet Gynecol 1989;72:120.
29. Meyer BA, Dickinson JE, Chambers C, et al. The effect of fetal sepsis on umbilical cord blood gases. Am J Obstet Gynecol 1992;166:2.
30. Catlin EA, Carpenter MW, Brann BS, et al. The Apgar score revisited: influence of gestational age. J Pediatr 1986;109:865.
31. Dahn LS, James LS. Newborn temperature and calculated heat loss in the delivery room. Pediatrics 1972;49:504.

32. Ramji S, Ahuja S, Thirupuram S, et al. Resuscitation of asphyxic newborn infants with room air or 100% oxygen. *Pediatr Res* 1993;34:809.

33. Vyas H, Milner AD, Hopkin IE, et al. Physiologic responses to prolonged and slow-rise inflation in the resuscitation of the asphyxiated newborn infant. *J Pediatr* 1981;99:635.

34. Moya F, James L, Burnard L, et al. Cardiac massage in the newborn infant through the intact chest. *Am J Obstet Gynecol* 1962;84:798.

35. Lindemann R. Resuscitation of the newborn with endotracheal administration of epinephrine. *Acta Paediatr Scand* 1984;73:210.

36. Downing ES, Campbell AGN, Racamora JM, et al. Influences of hypercapnia on cardiac function in the newborn lamb. *Yale J Biol Med* 1971; 43:242.

37. Effron MB, Guarnieri T, Frederisken JW, et al. Effect of tris (hydroxymethyl) aminomethane on ischemic myocardium. *Am J Physiol* 1978;235:H167.

38. Chu J, Clements JA, Cotton E, et al. Pulmonary hypoperfusion syndrome. *Pediatrics* 1965;35:733.

39. Lewis AB, Heymann MA, Rudolph RA. Gestational changes in pulmonary vascular responses in fetal lambs in utero. *Circ Res* 1976;39:536.

40. Schreiber MD, Heymann MA, Soifer SJ. Increased arterial pH, not decreased PaCO$_2$, attenuates hypoxia-induced pulmonary vaso-constriction in newborn lambs. *Pediatr Res* 1986;20:113.

41. Patel J, Marks K, Roberts I, et al. Measurement of cerebral blood flow in newborn infants using near infrared spectroscopy with indocyanine green. *Pediatr Res* 1998;43:34.

42. Kruyswijk H, Jansen BH, Muller EJ. Hyperventilation-induced coronary artery spasm. *Am Heart J* 1986;112:613.

43. Case RB, Felix A, Wachter M, et al. Relative effect of CO$_2$ on canine coronary vascular resistance. *Circ Res* 1978;42:410.

44. Ogata ES, Kitterman JA, Gregory GA, et al. Pneumothorax in idiopathic respiratory distress syndrome (IRDS): incidence and effect on vital signs, blood gases and pH. *Pediatrics* 1976;58:177.

45. Morin F, Sola A, Brown C, et al. Hypoxia disrupts the newborn lamb's response to hemorrhage. *Pediatr Res* 1981;15:673.

46. Phibbs RH, Clements JA, Creasy RK, et al. Lung maturity, intrauterine growth, neonatal asphyxia and shock and the risk of hyaline membrane disease. *Pediatr Res* 1976;10:451.

47. Dale HH, Evans CL. Effects on the circulation of changes in carbon dioxide content of the blood. *J Physiol* 1922;56:125.

48. Sola A, Spitzer AR, Morin FC, et al. Effects of arterial carbon dioxide tension on the newborn lamb's cardiovascular responses to rapid hemorrhage. *Pediatr Res* 1983;17:70.

49. Meyers RL, Paulick RP, Rudolph CD, et al. Cardiovascular responses to acute, severe haemorrhage in fetal sheep. *J Dev Physiol* 1991;15:189.

50. Weil MH, Rackrow EC, Trevino R, et al. Difference in acid base state between venous and arterial blood during cardiopulmonary resuscitation. *N Engl J Med* 1986;315:153.

51. Paxton CL. Neonatal shock in the first postnatal day. *Am J Dis Child* 1978;132:509.

52. Martin-Ancel A, Garcia-Alix A, Cabanas F, et al. Multiple organ involvement in perinatal asphyxia. *J Pediatr* 1995;127:786.

53. Desmond MM, Kay JL, Megarity AL. The phases of transitional distress occurring in neonates in association with prolonged postnatal umbilical cord pulsations. *J Pediatr* 1959;55:131.

54. Thibeault DW, Hall TK, Sheehan MB, et al. Post-asphyxial lung disease in newborn infants with severe perinatal acidosis. *Am J Obstet Gynecol* 1984;150:393.

55. Segerer H, Stevens P, Schadow B, et al. Surfactant substitution in ventilated very low birthweight infants: factors related to response types. *Pediatr Res* 1991;30:6.

56. U.S. EXOSURF Pediatric Study Group. Effects of EXOSURF on infants with occult congenital pneumonia. *Pediatr Res* 1990;27:288A.

57. Burnard ED, James LS. Failure of the heart after undue asphyxia at birth. *Pediatrics* 1961;28:545.

58. Cabal LA, Devaskar U, Siassi B, et al. Cardiogenic shock associated with perinatal asphyxia in preterm infants. *J Pediatr* 1980;96:705.

59. Walther FJ, Siassi B, Ramadan NA, et al. Cardiac output in newborn infants with transient myocardial dysfunction. *J Pediatr* 1985;107:781.

60. Akinbi H, Hilpert P, Bhutani V. Gastrointestinal and renal blood flow velocity profile in neonates with birth asphyxia. *J Pediatr* 1994;125:625.

61. Perlman JM, Track ED. Renal injury in the asphyxiated newborn infant: relationship to neurologic outcome. *J Pediatr* 1988;113:875.

62. Crissinger KD, Granger DN. Intestinal blood flow and oxygen consumption: responses to hemorrhage in the developing piglet. *Pediatr Res* 1989;2:102.

63. Vannucci R, Perlman J. Interventions for perinatal hypoxic-ischemic encephalopathy. *Pediatrics* 1997;100:1004.

64. Fellman V, Raivio KO. Reperfusion injury as the mechanism of brain damage after perinatal asphyxia. *Pediatr Res* 1997;41:599.

65. Vannucci R, Brucklacher R, Vannucci S. Effect of carbon dioxide on cerebral metabolism during hypoxia-ischemia in the immature rat. *Pediatr Res* 1997;42:24.

66. Gregory GA, Gooding C, Phibbs RH, et al. Meconium aspiration in infants: a prospective study. *J Pediatr* 1974;85:848.

67. Wiswell TE, Tuggle JM, Turner BS. Meconium aspiration syndrome: have we made a difference? *Pediatrics* 1990;85:5.

68. Matthews TG, Warshaw JB. Relevance of the gestational age distribution of meconium passage in utero. *Pediatrics* 1979;64:1.

69. Meis PJ, Hall M, Marshall JR, et al. Meconium passage: a new classification for risk assessment during labor. *Am J Obstet Gynecol* 1978; 130:509.

70. Carson BS, Lasey BW, Bowes WA, et al. Combined obstetric and pediatric approach to prevent meconium aspiration syndrome. *Am J Obstet Gynecol* 1976;126:712.

71. Davis RO, Phillips JB, Harris BA, et al. Fatal meconium aspiration syndrome occurring despite airway management considered appropriate. *Am J Obstet Gynecol* 1985;151:731.

72. Wiswell TE, Henley MA. Intratracheal suctioning, systemic infection, and the meconium aspiration syndrome. *Pediatrics* 1992;89:2.

73. Kretlow RA. Handpowered apparatus for aspiration of meconium from the trachea. *Pediatrics* 1987;70:642.

74. Hack M, Fanaroff AA. Changes in the delivery room care of the extremely small infant (less than 750 g): effects on morbidity and outcome. *N Engl J Med* 1986;314:660.

75. Corbet A, Cregan J, Frink J. Distension-produced phospholipid secretion in postmortem in situ lungs of newborn rabbits. *Am Rev Respir Dis* 1983;128:695.

76. Massaro GD, Massaro D. Morphologic evidence that large inflations of the lung stimulate secretion of surfactant. *Annu Rev Respir Dis [Am]* 1983;127:235.

77. Drew JH. Immediate intubation at birth of the very low birth weight infant: effect on survival. *Am J Dis Child* 1982;136:207.

78. Nilsson R, Grossman G, Robertson B. Lung surfactant and the pathogenesis of neonatal bronchiolar lesions induced by artificial ventilation. *Pediatr Res* 1978;12:249.

79. Bjorklund L, Ingimarsson J, Cursiedt T, et al. Manual ventilation with a few large breaths at birth compromises the theraputic effect of subsequent surfactan replacement in immature lambs. *Pediatr Res* 1997;42:348.

80. Wada K, Jobe A, Ikegami M. Tidal volume effects on surfactant treatment responses with the initiation of ventilation in preterm lambs. *J Appl Physiol* 1997;83:1054.

81. Kendig JW, Notter RH, Cox C, et al. A comparison of surfactant as immediate prophylaxis and as rescue therapy in newborns of less than 30 weeks gestation. *N Engl J Med* 1991;324:865.

82. Kilpatrick S, Schlueter M, Piecuch R, et al. Outcome of infants born at 24–26 weeks gestation: I. Survival and cost. *Obstet Gynecol* 1997;90:803.

83. Piecuch R, Leonard C, Cooper B, et al. Outcome of infants born at 24–26 weeks gestation: II. Neurodevelopmental outcome. *Obstet Gynecol* 1997;90:809.

84. Yu VH, Lake HL, Bajuk B, et al. Prognosis for infants born at 23 to 28 weeks gestation. *Br Med J* 1986;293:1200.

85. Chamberlain D, Hislop A, Hey E, et al. Pulmonary hypoplasia in babies with severe rhesus isoimmunization: a quantitative study. *J Pathol* 1977;122:43.

86. Phibbs RH, Johnson P, Kitterman JA, et al. Cardiorespiratory status of erythroblastotic newborn infants: III. Intravascular pressures during the first hours of life. *Pediatrics* 1976;58:484.

87. Phibbs RH, Johnson P, Tooley WH. Cardiorespiratory status of erythroblastotic newborn infants: II. Blood volume hematocrit and serum albumin concentrations in relation to hydrops fetalis. *Pediatrics* 1974;53:13.

88. Hey E, Jones P. Coagulation failure in babies with rhesus isoimmunization. *Br J Haematol* 1979;42:441.

89. Baum JD, Harris D. Colloid osmotic pressure in erythroblastosis fetalis. *Br Med J* 1972;1:601.

90. Phibbs RH, Johnson P, Kitterman JA, et al. Cardiorespiratory status of erythroblastotic infants: I. Relationship of gestational age, severity of hemolytic disease and birth asphyxia to idiopathic respiratory distress syndrome and survival. *Pediatrics* 1972;49:5.

91. Albanese CT, Lopoo J, Filly R, et al. Liver position predicts outcome in fetuses with congenital diaphragmatic hernia. *Obstet Gynecol (in press)*.

CHAPTER 19

Physical Assessment and Classification

Mary Ann Fletcher

Physical assessment in neonates serves to determine anatomic normality for the first time in a new life and the state of health in a patient who is unable to describe his or her own symptoms. The improved techniques for fetal diagnosis help in predicting major malformations, but the neonatal examination carries a primary purpose of identifying physical anomalies that may be either readily apparent or subtle. A challenge is to determine which findings will be transient or are merely variations of normal and which are markers of major malformations or syndromes. Most of the clinical descriptions of specific syndromes are made of findings that become typical only after there has been sufficient growth and maturation. An example is the subtlety or absence of obvious findings in aborted fetuses or extremely premature infants with Down syndrome.

Because many of the physical signs of early disease also present as part of the normal physiologic changes occurring at birth or in the newborn period, differentiating the markers of subtle illness from transitional variations is a particular challenge in neonatal physical diagnosis. Additionally, there are unique findings that appear quite dramatic but carry little medical significance. Once the examiner has determined that findings represent a disease process, he or she then has to decide just how sick that infant is or is likely to become. To that end, there have been devised a number of acuity of illness scores that range from the very simple to complex systems that include physiologic monitoring and laboratory values (1–4). The primary advantage of such scoring systems is in forcing a systematic and quantitative assessment that can be compared among observers and over time. Because a newborn cannot tell us directly whether he or she is feeling better or worse, comparative scores assist in evaluating if therapy should be initiated and the response to treatment.

The first neonatal examination occurs immediately after birth in the assigning of Apgar scores from 0 to 10 at 5-minute intervals until the total is above 7. The scores summarize encapsulated assessments of the cardiopulmonary and neurologic systems after inspection for color, heart rate, respiratory efforts, tone, and muscle activity and assigning a value of 0, 1, or 2 for each of the five observations. Also part of this first examination is inspection for designation of gender and a cursory inspection for major anomalies. Any obvious abnormality merits more immediate evaluation, but the definitive examination in healthy infants should take place after initial transition and the first bath.

The first complete examination ordinarily occurs within the first 24 hours after birth, but if any portion of an assessment is deferred or abnormal at that time or if the infant is discharged at less than 48 hours, timely reexamination is warranted (5). During the first outpatient visit, the physician should fully reevaluate the infant, especially those systems not as easily assessed immediately after birth, e.g., the eyes, and those that undergo the greatest changes during transition, e.g., the cardiovascular and hepatobiliary systems. The areas emphasized with subsequent well-baby examinations include neuromuscular and sensory development, the heart, and the hips as well as parameters of growth including head circumference, length, and weight.

This chapter is a brief discussion of the steps for assessing the newborn infant and interpreting some of the findings. A thorough textbook on how to perform and interpret the physical examination in neonates is available (6).

M. A. Fletcher: Department of Pediatrics, The George Washington University School of Medicine and Health Sciences, Washington, D.C.; and Shady Grove Adventist Hospital, Rockville, Maryland

NEWBORN HISTORY

It is tempting to start the physical examination of neonates before reviewing the history and available laboratory information of the mother. If a newborn is critically ill, the clinician should initiate therapy for stabilization after a cursory examination and before obtaining the complete history, but too much delay can lead to missed or partial diagnoses. Historic information is just as important for neonates as for any other patient. Even if it is more practical to examine an apparently healthy newborn before obtaining the history, a complete evaluation includes all available information. A key part of the newborn's history is the mother's pregnancy history as well as her prior medical and social history. Other essential elements include general family history, the postnatal course, and information about the placental examination.

Maternal history includes the mother's age, gravidity, parity, time and type of previous fetal losses, general fertility issues, and premature births and their outcome; maternal illness before or during pregnancy; extent and location of prenatal care; results of any prenatal laboratory tests, especially those for hepatitis and sexually transmitted diseases; labor and delivery history, including duration, assessments of fetal well-being, anesthesia, and route of delivery; drug, alcohol, and tobacco use; prescription and nonprescription medication use; and her vocation.

The general family history includes current or significant past medical illnesses in other family members, including siblings; physical traits or appearance, including birth weights of other siblings; consanguinity; social information, educational levels, vocations; and ethnic or racial background. Helpful information about the newborn period of siblings includes success in breast-feeding, infections, congenital anomalies, genetic conditions, and jaundice or other concerns.

To include the postnatal course as part of the newborn history, the clinician should review events surrounding the birth and response to resuscitation, vital signs, feeding, eliminations, and behavior. If there were any complications or requirement for anything other than routine care, this information is a key part of the total neonatal history.

Placental Information

Often more overlooked than history in evaluating neonates is information about the placenta and the clues it provides about the gestational history. Several features of the placenta and cord can be readily assessed on gross examination by anyone at the time of delivery.

The placenta should be examined for size, odor, color, and the number and character of fetal membranes. In the last trimester the ratio of fresh placental weight to infant weight is normally 1:6. There should be a uniform thickness and density throughout. Depressions and adherent clots or changes in firmness on the maternal surface suggest abruption or infarction. The placenta is essentially odorless except for a slight odor of fresh blood; malodor

may indicate an infection or merely maternal ingestion of strongly spiced food.

The color of the fetal surface changes with gestational age, but pallor or plethora suggests aberrations in fetal blood volume or hemoglobin level. Elevated bilirubin in the amniotic fluid stains the placenta bright yellow. Meconium will discolor the fetal surface greenish-brown but so too can old blood. If either meconium passage or bleeding occurred more than 1 day prior to delivery, it can be difficult to differentiate the two by gross examination. If a meconium stain goes through the membranes onto the fetal surface or into the cord, the time of passage was hours before delivery. If the staining is only superficial, it was likely very recently passed.

The fetal surface should be examined for cloudiness of fetal membranes, which suggests an inflammatory reaction but not necessarily due to infection. Nodules on the amnion indicate prolonged, extreme oligohydramnios with probable fetal pulmonary hypoplasia. Their presence suggests futility if resuscitation is underway.

The umbilical cord is assessed for appearance, length and diameter, the number of vessels, and insertion site. The cord is a uniform ivory color with three fetal vessels twisting gently throughout its length. Ranging in length from 30 to 100 cm, a shorter cord suggests decreased fetal movement and a reason for fetal distress, failed descent, or avulsion. Longer cords are more likely to result in fetal entanglement or prolapse. At term, the cord diameter is an average of 1.5 cm and is relatively uniform throughout its length, without strictures. Thin cords with a paucity of Wharton jelly are more likely to undergo compression by fetal parts. Cords too thick at the fetal insertion may indicate an omphalocele or urine leakage from a patent urachus.

In multiple gestations with a single placenta, the dividing membranes should be assessed. Membranes can be teased apart and counted: four layers indicate dichorionic placentation and two layers indicate a monochorionic placenta and, therefore, monozygotic twinning. With a dichorionic placenta or completely separate placentas and same sex twins, one cannot say if they are identical or fraternal from the placental examination, but if the placenta is monochorionic, they are identical. Just as monozygotic twins can have separate placentas, dizygotic twins can have tightly fused placentas that appear to be one mass. If there are any remnants of vessels seen in translucent dividing membranes held to a light, there are four membrane layers. If there is only a transparent membrane with no choroidal remnants, it is likely to contain only amnion (see Chap. 27 for additional discussion).

GESTATIONAL AGE ASSESSMENT

For standard reporting of reproductive health statistics and as a prerequisite to determining normality, all infants should be classified by gestational age and birth weight

(5). Ultrasonography has improved the accuracy of pregnancy dating, but discrepancies in dates, physical appearance, or size require further evaluation. If there has been no prenatal care, physical assessment remains the primary clinical determinant of gestational age.

Gestational age is noted in completed weeks after the onset of the last menstrual period. For example, a fetus who is 37 weeks and 2 days is in its 38th week of gestation. A term infant is any infant whose birth occurs from the beginning of the first day of week 38 through the end of the last day of week 42 after the onset of the last menstrual period (i.e., 260 to 294 days of gestation). A preterm infant is one born before 37 completed weeks or at 36 weeks and 6 days (259 days) or less. A postterm infant is one whose birth occurs from the beginning of the first day of week 43 (i.e., after 294 days or at 42 weeks and 1 day or more). Classifying infants born at term, preterm, or postterm helps to establish the level of risk for neonatal morbidity and long-term developmental problems. The terms premature and postmature often are used clinically to connote physical or physiologic findings, not always correlating with gestational age. Postdates is an obstetric term meaning a pregnancy that has continued to any time after the expected date of confinement but is not necessarily postterm.

Assessment Techniques

Estimation of gestational age by physical examination is possible because there is a predictable pattern of physical changes that occur throughout gestation. The most popular score for gestational age assessment was originally developed in part by Saint-Anne-Dargassies (7), Amiel-Tison (8), and Dubowitz et al. (9). It was then modified by Ballard et al. (10). Compared to reliable ultrasound dates, the earlier Ballard system tended to overestimate the age of premature infants and underestimate the age of postterm infants (11). It was particularly inaccurate in very-low-birth-weight infants with a deviation of more than 2 weeks (12). Further modifications of the original system produced the New Ballard Score (NBS), which extended the range and accuracy of age assessment to within 1 week (Fig. 19–1) (13).

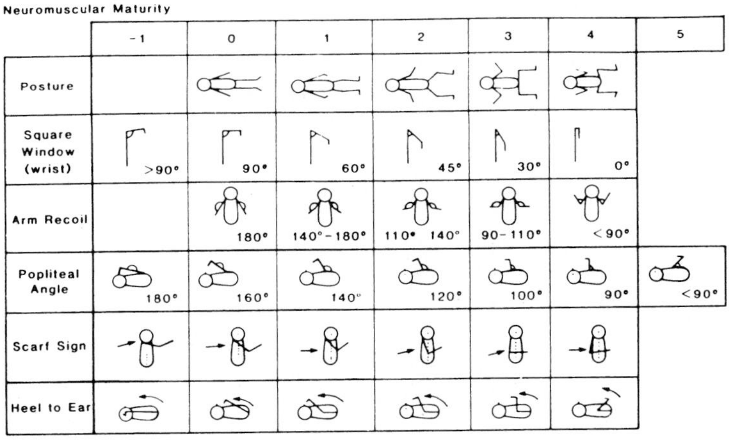

Physical Maturity

	-1	0	1	2	3	4	5
Skin	sticky friable transparent	gelatinous red, translucent	smooth pink, visible veins	superficial peeling &/or rash. few veins	cracking pale areas rare veins	parchment deep cracking no vessels	leathery cracked wrinkled
Lanugo	none	sparse	abundant	thinning	bald areas	mostly bald	
Plantar Surface	heel-toe 40-50 mm: -1 <40 mm: -2	>50mm no crease	faint red marks	anterior transverse crease only	creases ant. 2/3	creases over entire sole	
Breast	imperceptible	barely perceptible	flat areola no bud	stippled areola 1-2mm bud	raised areola 3-4mm bud	full areola 5-10mm bud	
Eye/Ear	lids fused loosely: -1 tightly: -2	lids open pinna flat stays folded	sl. curved pinna; soft; slow recoil	well-curved pinna; soft but ready recoil	formed & firm instant recoil	thick cartilage ear stiff	
Genitals male	scrotum flat, smooth	scrotum empty faint rugae	testes in upper canal rare rugae	testes descending few rugae	testes down good rugae	testes pendulous deep rugae	
Genitals female	clitoris prominent labia flat	prominent clitoris small labia minora	prominent clitoris enlarging minora	majora & minora equally prominent	majora large minora small	majora cover clitoris & minora	

Maturity Rating

score	weeks
-10	20
-5	22
0	24
5	26
10	28
15	30
20	32
25	34
30	36
35	38
40	40
45	42
50	44

FIG. 19–1. Assessment of maturity by the expanded Ballard Score. (From ref. 13.)

Accuracy in estimating gestational age requires experience and consideration of the infant's history and overall condition at the time of scoring; for example, maternal medications or drugs and the infant's fetal position or sleep state affect the neuromuscular response in a normal infant. Significant hypertonia or hypotonia is particularly powerful in affecting the neuromotor scores but would not affect the physical maturity score. Examination as soon as possible after initial stabilization or by 12 hours increases the accuracy in gestations shorter than 28 weeks (13). The use of NBS is particularly attractive for neonates who are immature and instrumented, because it does not require lifting the infant. Although described here separate from other components of the examination, the steps for assessing gestational age can be done as part of the general physical examination and provide information for the neurologic evaluation. The neurologic examination of infants during the first year continues to use a number of these assessment elements (14,15).

Neuromuscular Maturity

The resting posture, which is the posture assumed by an unrestrained, healthy infant, reflects a progressive increase in tone and flexion in a caudocephalad direction to a pattern of full flexion at term (see Fig. 19–1).

The square window is assessed by flexing the wrist and measuring the minimal angle between the palm and flexor surface of the forearm. This angle decreases with advancing gestational age. Conditions of marked intrauterine compression, such as severe oligohydramnios, increase wrist flexion. As an extremely premature newborn advances through corrected gestational age, he or she will not continue to develop as much wrist flexion after birth as the infant would have had he or she stayed *in utero*.

The scarf sign, indicative of shoulder and superior axial tone, is assessed by pulling the hand across the chest to encircle the neck as a scarf and observing the position of the elbow in relation to the midline. There is decreased range and a higher score if there is marked obesity, chest wall edema, an abnormally shortened humerus, or shoulder girdle hypertonicity. Brachial plexus injury or generalized hypotonia produces a spuriously low score.

With the infant supine and head midline, arm recoil is assessed by first flexing the elbow and holding the arm against the forearm for 2 to 5 seconds. The elbow is then fully extended and released with observation of how quickly and fully the infant resumes a flexed posture. Assessing recoil should not be done as part of testing arm traction or with forceful extension, because other responses may interfere with a normal reaction. Any pathology affecting the motor strength of the arm will decrease this score.

To determine the popliteal angle, one should first flex the hips with the thighs alongside the abdomen rather than over the front. With the hips held in flexion, the knee is then extended as far as possible to estimate the popliteal angle. If an infant was in frank breech presentation with legs extended, the popliteal angles would be greater than expected for age.

In the heel-to-ear maneuver, the legs are held together and pressed as far as possible toward the ears without lifting the pelvis from the table. The angle made by an arc from the back of the heel to the table decreases with maturity.

Physical Maturity

Skin in the most premature infants is gelatinous and almost transparent, allowing the abdominal vessels to be visible. It becomes opaque with maturity as it thickens and keratinizes, eventually shedding the lubricating vernix so it dries, cracks, and sheds.

Lanugo, which is the fine hair evenly distributed over the body, first emerges at 19 to 20 weeks but for a few weeks after initial emergence is not readily apparent. Maximally apparent at 27 to 28 weeks, lanugo sheds first from the areas of greatest contact. Lanugo is distinct from the more pigmented body hair that may be quite prominent in infants of medium to dark complexion.

Assessment of the plantar surface includes measuring the foot, because its length reliably corresponds to early gestational ages. With normal muscle activity and uterine compression, creases develop in the sole, progressing from the toes toward the heel. Inappropriate sole creasing is seen in infants with serious neuromotor deficit in the lower extremities (e.g., decreased creasing or only deep vertical creasing) or with oligohydramnios (e.g., increased creasing).

The breast develops with an increase in color, stippling of the areola, and increase in the size of the breast tissue. Although the volume of the breast somewhat depends on fetal nutrition and fat deposition, areolar development with increasing gestational age is more consistent and independent of these factors.

Ear cartilage becomes firmer with gestation if there is no continuous, extrinsic pressure and the auricular muscles have normal anatomy and activity. Unfusing of the eyelids can occur over several weeks, and a fused condition by itself is not a sign of extreme, nonviable immaturity. Opening starts by 22 weeks; complete unfusing is evident by at least 28 weeks (13). The vessels in the anterior vascular capsule of the lens mature in a predictable enough pattern in the last trimester of gestation to augment assessment of gestational age between 27 and 34 weeks, but this method has a 2-week margin of error, 1 week greater than the NBS (16). Use of the eye findings is helpful in augmenting assessment when the examination is affected by neuromotor deficits or there is a significant dating discrepancy.

Maturity of the external genitalia is one of the more reliable individual indicators of gestational age (13). Due to timed descent in the third trimester, testicular progress through the canal into the scrotum is a gestational age marker. For the scrotum to develop fully into a pendulous, ruggated, term appearance, there has to have been testicular descension at some time, even if the sac is empty at the time of birth. The appearance of term female genitalia depends on fat deposition and is abnormally immature in a poorly nourished infant. The clitoris approaches term size well before 38 weeks, so it is disproportionately large in premature females (17,18). The appearance of a pigmented vertical line, the linea nigra, above the pubis toward the umbilicus suggests a gestational age of at least 36 weeks.

Influences on Age Assessment Results

If there is a discrepancy between expected and achieved scores, factors that influence the demonstrated findings should be sought before assigning gestational age. There is no significant difference among races in the dating scores other than what can be explained by individual variation (19,20).

Resting posture reflects progressive flexion into the position assumed when a term fetus occupies virtually all available intrauterine space and is no longer in a freely floating state. To minimize the volume occupied, this flexion logically progresses in a caudal to cephalic sequence. Compression from oligohydramnios accelerates flexion; it gives an artificially advanced estimate of maturity. Conversely, poor fetal motor activity over a long period spuriously decreases estimated age. Fetuses with markedly decreased motor activity, poor swallowing, and polyhydramnios have decreased plantar and palmar horizontal creasing and inappropriately immature posturing. Any condition affecting the position or activity of the lower extremities, such as frank breech presentation with hyperextended knees or myelomeningocele with paresis, leads to an aberrantly lowered neuromotor score. Similarly, an infant who is hypotonic from illness or sedation has less flexion than normal for true gestational age.

GROWTH

Measurement Techniques

Infants weighing less than 2,500 g are low birth weight regardless of gestational age. Very low birth weight refers to a weight less than 1,500 g, and extremely low birth weight indicates an infant weighing less than 1,000 g. Classification by these weight groups helps establish the level of risk for neonatal and long-term morbidity and mortality, particularly when the weight classification is coupled with an accurate gestational age (21).

Of all measurements, crown–heel length is the most subject to variability, because it depends on achieving full extension of an infant who is more naturally in flexion.

This measurement is performed with the infant supine, the neck neutral, the leg fully extended, the ankle flexed. If there is deviation from an expected norm, the first step in evaluation would be to remeasure the infant for confirmation.

If the percentile of an accurate crown–heel length falls below those percentiles for weight and head circumference, measuring the crown–rump length establishes leg and trunk proportionality, which may be abnormal in congenital dwarfisms. When anomalies of the lower extremities make crown–heel length implausible, the crown–rump measurement may still be feasible. Crown–rump length is measured with the infant supine and the hips flexed 90 degrees. Standards for separate lengths of upper and lower limbs are available (22,23).

The head circumference is the largest dimension around the head obtained with a tape placed snugly above the ears; this is the occipital frontal circumference (OFC). Minor changes in head circumference occur during the first week after birth as scalp edema and molding resolve. The molding seen after prolonged breech positioning can lead to an OFC that is as much as 2 cm higher than it will be after molding resolves.

The OFC predictably falls on the same percentile curve as the length. If the OFC differs from length by more than one quartile, the cause should be sought, because head size in part reflects brain growth. The most frequent reason for a head percentile to exceed that of length is familial. In this situation the head circumference follows a persistently higher but consistent growth curve. In contrast, pathologic macrocephaly tends to cross to higher percentile curves as it progresses. A decreased rate of head growth, manifested by a flat curve or by dropping to a lower percentile, may indicate poor brain growth, atrophy, or premature cranial synostosis. The fetal head circumference exceeds the abdominal circumference until 32 weeks. Between 32 and 36 weeks, the two circumferences are approximately equivalent, and after 36 weeks, the abdominal circumference normally is greater.

Interpretation of Growth Parameters

Interpretation of growth parameters requires plotting the measurements on percentile charts constructed from a similar race and environmental population. If birth weight falls between the 10th and 90th percentiles for a given gestational age, the infant is appropriate for gestational age (AGA); if less than the 10th percentile, the infant is small for gestational age (SGA); and if above the 90th percentile, the infant is large for gestational age (LGA). Some literature cite the 3rd and 95th percentiles as outer limits, but for most clinical purposes, this broader range underselects for some at-risk infants, particularly in the lower sizes. Accuracy in gestational age assessment is critical in determining if a weight is appropriate. AGA infants born at term are at lowest risk for problems associated with neonatal mortality and morbidity (21).

If the three parameters of weight, length, and head circumference fall on the same curve, the infant is symmetric. The infant is asymmetric if the parameters are on different curves, usually with the weight on a curve lower than those of the head circumference or length. If an infant has either a slowing of intrauterine growth rate documented by serial fetal sonography or a presumed slowing by very low weight for length measurements, he or she is classified as having intrauterine growth retardation (IUGR). An infant can be IUGR without being SGA.

Infants who are SGA, IUGR, or LGA are at risk for perinatal and long-term problems. The problems encountered by SGA infants are discussed in Chapter 25. Several of the problems encountered by LGA infants include the following:

Iatrogenic prematurity due to overestimation of gestational age by late size estimates
Increased requirement for delivery by cesarean section
Pulmonary hypertension
Shoulder dystocia
Birth injuries
    Ecchymoses
    Local fat necrosis associated with forceps applications
    Cephalohematoma, skull fracture
    Brachial plexus injuries
    Paralysis of diaphragm
    Fracture of clavicle or humerus
Polycythemia
    Jaundice
    Hyperviscosity syndrome
    Seizures
    Renal vein thrombosis
    Increased total blood volume
Poor feeding
Hypoglycemia.

EXAMINATION

Examination Conditions

A routine neonatal examination, normally only taking 5 to 10 minutes, should be in a quiet, warm environment. The room's light should be bright enough to detect skin markings and color but not so bright as to discourage open eyes. When an infant is ill, attention to optimizing the environment and recognizing the potential effect of noxious nursery surroundings on his or her state is fundamental.

Even healthy infants do not tolerate handling in extended examinations. The sicker or more immature they are, the less they tolerate manipulation and environmental assaults. For all examinations, there must be the prevenient consideration that no harm should come by the process.

In routine care situations, having one or both parents present during an examination allows discussion about physical findings and offers the opportunity to point out behaviors that can help them better understand their infant. They can address directly any questions about history or therapy at that time as well.

General Assessment

A neonatal physical examination includes the principles of inspection, palpation, percussion, and auscultation of each body system. Inspection plays the most important role and percussion the least. Unlike examinations of adults, there is less opportunity to progress through the systems in order and more need to proceed in whatever order is practical for the infant's current state. For instance, it is important to observe the respiratory rate and pattern before touching the infant, and auscultating the heart precedes other handling if the infant is quiet. A systematic approach that includes all aspects while being efficient and nondisruptive is essential.

The specifics of neonatal examination are discussed in the following sections. Some systems that are discussed in more detail in other chapters are given less emphasis in this chapter than they would merit in an actual examination.

Inspection

Inspection begins before making any physical contact and from enough of a distance to encompass the infant as a whole. An immediate assessment of wellness can come from simply noting the state, color, respiratory effort, posture, and spontaneous activity. Even simple observations of spontaneous movement patterns can suggest future neurologic deficits or well-being (24).

State

Important indicators of infant well-being are the states or levels of arousal the infant achieves throughout the examination and throughout the day as described by the parent or nursing staff. One categorization of states listed in the following originally was defined by Prechtl and Beintema (25). Modifications have been made but are not clinically important for general assessments (26–29).

- Deep sleep
- Light sleep
- Awake, light peripheral movements
- Awake, large movements, not crying
- Awake, crying.

During examination, a healthy infant should demonstrate several levels of arousal. The most useful states for assessing an infant are those of light sleep and quiet awake, so irritating maneuvers are held until the conclusion of the assessment. What it takes to assist an infant in moving from one state to another or how well he or she does it without assistance is noteworthy. Because the deep sleep that follows a recent feeding may give an appearance of lethargy on arousal, knowing the feeding history and pattern is prerequisite to determining aptness of state.

Quieting an infant may require anything from simply stopping the handling to holding and talking to him or her. The amount of time spent in unstimulated crying is normally limited in the first 24 hours but may increase significantly each day thereafter. Excessive crying that requires more than routine consoling, particularly if there are no intervals of quiet alert states, indicates abnormal irritability but other causes include a proper response to pain or to a cold environment (30,31).

Color

Color assessment includes judging perfusion and skin color for the presence of cyanosis, jaundice, pallor, plethora, or any unusual cast and evaluating the distribution and types of pigmentation.

Respiratory Effort

The degree of respiratory effort is a primary indicator of how distressed or comfortable a newborn infant is, even if the cause of distress is not pulmonic. The physician can observe the respiratory rate, depth of excursions, use of accessory muscles with retractions or nasal flare, any emitted sounds, such as grunting or whining, and the crying pattern. Understanding the infant's pattern of respiratory effort can suggest a specific illness and direct the examination. As the severity of a condition increases, these distinctions may be lost (Table 19–1).

Posture

One of the more important clues to physical status is the resting posture assumed by an unrestrained infant. This posture reflects intrauterine positioning and general body tone, and it varies with gestational age (see Fig. 19–1). At term, the healthy infant lies with thighs partially abducted and the hips, knees, ankles, elbows, and shoulders comfortably flexed. While observing neck position, the examiner looks for symmetry between the sides and compares the upper and lower extremities. If there is lateral asymmetry and the head is turned to one side, there may be an asymmetric tonic neck reflex with the extremities on the mental side in extension and those on the occipital side in flexion. In that case, the head should be turned to the opposite side to verify that the asymmetry reverses.

If the fetal presentation is nonvertex or unknown or there is asymmetry or deformation, it is helpful to assist the infant in assuming a position reflecting his or her intrauterine attitude. The physician can fold the extremities into the fetal position by applying moderate pressure to a relaxed infant's feet while gently shaking the infant's legs and by directing the arms toward the thorax through gentle pressure on the elbows.

Spontaneous Activity

The examiner should observe what the infant does in light sleep and awake states. Does the infant stretch, move all extremities equally, open and close hands, root and start sucking when something touches his or her face, and yawn with great facial expression, or does the infant lie quietly and move only in response to stimulation?

Premature infants spend more time sleeping but should have spontaneous activity and resting postures commensurate with their gestational age (32). Because they habituate and become disorganized and stressed quickly on handling, inspection before contact in a benign environment is important.

Vital Signs

Temperature

It is unusual for neonates to develop fevers except in response to environmental temperature. If an infant's skin temperature is above 38° and remains elevated after the environment returns to normal, a rectal temperature should be obtained. Unless the temperature has been elevated for a prolonged time, the rectal temperature is less likely to be affected by environment and evaluation for

TABLE 19–1. *Patterns of neonatal respiratory effort*[a]

Condition	Pattern observed
Distal airway or lung parenchyma	Intercostal retractions, sternal retractions, flaring, tachypnea, grunt, increased work in breathing
Upper airway obstruction	Suprasternal retractions, subcostal retractions
Cardiac pattern	Tachypnea without effort, infant is quiet but not somnolent
Neurodepression	Poor effort compared with physiologic need, apnea
Metabolic acidosis of sepsis	Tachypnea, apnea, lethargy, whining, minimal retractions

[a]Early in disease process, before patterns merge with multiple system involvement.

infectious or neurologic causes is indicated (33). Infants often become hypothermic, usually in response to the environment and particularly if the infant is premature, thin, or remains quiet and does not cry vigorously. Recurrent or profound hypothermia also requires additional evaluation.

Term infants sweat, albeit poorly, in response to thermal stress. Preterm infants develop a measurable response by 2 weeks of age (34). Visible sweating at rest or on feeding in an afebrile infant is abnormal and may indicate distress, typically from cardiac disease.

Respiratory Rate and Heart Rate

The respiratory rate is obtained by looking at the upper abdomen for a full minute. As soon as an infant is touched, the respiratory rate and depth change. The normal respiratory rate is 30 to 60 inspirations per minute in a term infant, with lower rates occurring after the period of cardiopulmonary transition. When awake, some normal infants breathe shallowly and rapidly but are able to slow sufficiently to feed well. Deep sleep is characterized by a more regular breathing pattern, whereas the awake state has more bursts of rapid breathing (29,35,36).

The heart rate is 110 to 160 beats/min in healthy term infants but may vary significantly during deep sleep or active awake states. Preterm infants have resting heart rates at the higher end of the normal range. Tachycardia, with a rate persistently greater than 160, may be a sign of many conditions, including central nervous system irritability, congestive heart failure, sepsis, anemia, fever, or hyperthyroidism.

Blood Pressure

Measuring blood pressure is not a routine part of vital signs in most newborn nurseries but is used for infants requiring special care and for evaluating coarctation of the aorta. There are wide variations of normal at different gestational ages (37–39). The Committee on Fetus and Newborn of the American Academy of Pediatrics states that hypertension should be diagnosed only after three separate measurements (40).

The range of normal blood pressure in neonates depends on the method used for assessment and gestational age (see Appx. C–1: Blood pressure values). The values obtained by the blanching and flush methods are mean pressures and are lower than those registered by direct intravascular or Doppler monitoring. The flush method for obtaining mean pressure is easier in an active infant and requires only a sphygmomanometer. The Doppler methods, although providing diastolic and systolic pressures, require electronic equipment and a quieter patient. Two important elements for obtaining accurate blood pressures are a quiet infant and a properly sized cuff with a width 50% to 67% of the length of the arm.

For the flush method, the hand or foot is wrapped or squeezed firmly enough to blanch the skin (41). The cuff is inflated, the wrapping removed, and the pressure slowly lowered until there is a flush of color, at which point the pressure is read.

Facies

Assessment of facies includes looking for symmetry, size, shape, and the relations of all parts of the face and how the infant holds or uses them. A seemingly unusual facial appearance dictates analyzing the individual components to decide if the constellation represents malformation, deformation, a syndrome, or merely familial appearance.

Head and Neck

Inspection of the head includes assessment of the shape and size relative to the rest of the body and face, distribution and character of the hair, and the underlying scalp.

Head circumference was discussed previously. Even when the OFC is normal, it is important to notice if the size of the head seems appropriate for the size of the face.

The shape of the cranial vault reflects interaction of internal forces (i.e., brain anatomy, volume, intracranial pressure) against external forces (i.e., intrauterine and extrauterine molding, suture mobility). Normal intrauterine molding for a vertex presentation leads to a narrowed biparietal diameter and a maximal occipitomental dimension; after breech presentation, there may be marked accentuation of the occipitofrontal dimension with parietal flattening, an occipital shelf, and apparent frontal prominence. This normal breech shape requires differentiation from the abnormal occipital prominence found in posterior fossa masses (e.g., Dandy–Walker malformation), frontal prominence due to increased cranial volume, or the boat-shaped scaphocephaly from synostosis of the sagittal suture. Normal molding resolves within a few weeks, but other aberrations progress. Pathologic conditions that prevent normal molding of the fetal head should be suspected in infants who failed to engage in vertex and descend in labor. These conditions are all unusual but important to detect as early as possible.

Because plagiocephaly (i.e., flattening) and torticollis often coexist, occipital flattening with contralateral frontal prominence dictates determining range of motion for the neck. The infant's head should turn as far as the shoulder in both directions—farther if it is premature. Frontooccipital plagiocephaly may be manifested by a unilateral epicanthal fold or asymmetry of the ears (42). To fully assess position, the ears should be viewed *en face* and from the top of the head.

Hair and Scalp

The hair is inspected for color, texture, distribution, and directional patterns. Although hair color may change, there should be racial concordance. For example, reddish or blond hair in a dark-skinned infant may indicate albinism. Similarly, the hair color should be fairly uniform. Random patches of white hair are familial or sporadic and inconsequential, but white forelocks with other pigment defects and anomalies are associated with deafness and retardation (43). The texture of hair at birth is relatively fine. Most of the conditions associated with abnormal textures or fragility appear some time later. With immaturity, the hair is even finer and more sparse.

The hair line may vary at the frontal margin, and normal but hirsute infants have hair well down the forehead but without synophrys (i.e., grown-together eyebrows). The posterior hair line has a more consistent limitation, so that hair roots well below the neck creases, particularly at the lateral margins, suggest syndromes associated with short or webbed necks.

Although neonatal hair initially appears quite disheveled, its growth direction normally is consistent. There is usually a single, parietal hair whorl, which is to the right of center. If there are more than two or if an isolated whorl is frontal or significantly out of normal position, there may be abnormal development of the underlying brain (44). It is unusual for hair to be strongly upswept at the neck or forehead at birth. If there is extreme hair unruliness with multiple direction of growth, particularly with unusual facies, microcephaly, or SGA, there may be poor brain growth of early fetal onset (45). Unruliness is typical but not diagnostic of a number of genetic syndromes, including Cornelia de Lange and Down syndromes.

Superficial ecchymoses and abrasions of the scalp are common after vaginal deliveries, especially after extraction by forceps or vacuum. Incision sites for fetal scalp electrodes or blood sampling should be small and inconsequential, although some are deep enough to require closure. A small defect of the scalp, cutis aplasia, that appears coincidentally at a potential monitoring spot may be confused with an electrode lesion, because it sometimes appears ecchymotic or blistered.

Many telangiectatic or staining lesions appear over the scalp, neck, and face, ranging from the superficial and transient flammeus nevus or stork bite to the more intense, permanent port wine stain. These and the common skin lesions are discussed in detail in Chapter 54. The light-brown staining that sometimes develops after exposure to silver nitrate eye drops can be removed with alcohol; it disappears by 7 to 10 days.

Once an essential part of the cranial examination, transillumination of the skull is not relied on because the only abnormalities detectable involve large fluid collections. For the most part, more precise diagnostic techniques are available, but the technique should not be forgotten as a potential supplement to the physical examination. Transillumination remains an important adjunct to examining the chest, abdomen, and genitalia for fluid or air accumulations.

Palpation of the Head

Palpation detects motility and firmness of adjacent bones, size of the sutures, and bony or dermal defects. Depending on the extent and direction of molding, there is variable overlap in the sagittal, coronal, or lambdoid sutures. With craniosynostosis, the fused sutures do not move freely when alternate sides are pressed. Sutures that are overlapping but not fused feel like a mountain cliff with a drop-off from the overriding bone to the lower bone. Sutures that are fused feel more like a mountain range with an equal build-up on both sides. Isolated craniosynostosis occurs in 0.6 of 1,000 live births, with affected sutures found to be metopic in 50%, sagittal in 28%, coronal in 16.5%, and lambdoid in 5.5% (46).

Any suture, particularly the metopic, may be normally widened in the absence of increased intracranial pressure; the exception is a wide lambdoid suture, which ordinarily indicates increased pressure. Palpation of the bones adjacent to the sagittal suture may reveal a give and return similar to that felt when pressing on an aluminum can. These softer areas, indicating craniotabes, occur most often in premature infants or in term gestations if the fetal head was compressed against the maternal bony pelvis for several weeks. Physiologic craniotabes resolves within a few weeks after birth (47). Pathologic craniotabes occurs in syphilis and rickets but probably is not evident from these associations in the early neonatal period.

The fontanelles vary in size between and within race and by gestational age (48–50). Measurement of the fontanelle is not helpful as part of a routine assessment, because the normal range in size varies widely and its reproducibility is poor. There is little clinical application for measurements in otherwise normal infants, because head growth can occur despite apparently closed fontanelles; the rate of closure is independent of other growth parameters and bone age (50,51). Although aberrantly large fontanelles are seen in genetic syndromes and metabolic or endocrine diseases, they are not pathognomonic. Palpable tension in the anterior fontanelle is a late indicator of cranial hypertension; widening of the sutures, with excessive rate of head growth, occurs first.

There are several other palpable findings on the head unique to the neonatal period. The most frequent, caput succedaneum, presents at birth with pitting edema and initially is most prominent over the presenting area. It represents fluid accumulation within and under the scalp. Although a caput initially may be limited to overlying a single bone, it will shift to dependent regions and be more apparent in crossing sutures.

Cephalohematoma is less common and rarely is present immediately upon delivery. Any nonfluctuant swelling that is palpable in the delivery suite is more likely a caput. Typically, a cephalohematoma develops after delivery and expands during the first few hours as blood accumulates between the surface of a calvarial bone and its pericranial membrane (52). The cephalohematoma is rounded and discrete, with boundaries limited by suture lines. There may be pitting edema if a caput overlies a cephalohematoma, but an isolated cephalohematoma feels fluctuant. Because of periosteal reflection at the margins, there is often a false sensation of underlying bony depression. The blood contained in a cephalohematoma may take several weeks to resorb and prolongs neonatal jaundice. Unless there are neurologic indicators, radiographs to look for the occasional underlying skull fracture are not indicated.

The least frequent scalp injury is a subgaleal hematoma, which may feel crepitant, with less pitting and more discoloration than found in caput succedaneum. Because there is little anatomic restriction to accumulation of fluid under the aponeurosis, large amounts may redistribute and deplete total body volumes in massive subgaleal hemorrhage (53). Cephalohematomas and subgaleal hematomas occur most often after vacuum or difficult forceps extractions but may develop spontaneously even in cesarean or unassisted vaginal deliveries (54).

A thorough examination of the head includes auscultating for bruits over the temporal arteries and anterior fontanelle, particularly if there are conditions involving high-output cardiac failure or neuropathology.

The neck should be extended for maximal exposure to look for clefts or cysts. The isthmus of a normal thyroid is just palpable in the sternal notch on neck extension; rarely, midline enlargements represent a goiter. Other congenital neck masses include cystic hygroma, lymphangioma, and cervical teratoma (55).

Eyes

Examining the eyes of a neonate requires patience and a cooperative infant. Stimulating sucking may encourage spontaneous eye opening in dim light, but if the infant is crying inconsolably, delaying the examination is prudent. After routine eye medications are instilled, there may be enough edema of the lids that lid retractors are necessary. The neonatal eye examination is discussed in more detail in Chapter 52.

The emphasis of the neonatal eye examination is on the structure and appearance of the eye and its surroundings rather than assessment of visual acuity or extraocular muscles. Observations include determining the relative size, shape, and position of the eye in its socket and demonstrating if the infant appears to have vision by reacting to light. Because measuring is reserved for eyes that appear abnormal, one looks for symmetry and observes whether the eyes seem to fit their sockets. Both eyes should be the same size and sit neither too deeply nor too far forward. The size and shape of the socket needs to be related to the size and shape of the surrounding skull. Marked molding with depression of the forehead may make normal eyes appear to sit too far forward unless their position relative to the cheeks is considered. If the eyes are unequal, there should be a determination of which side is normal and whether one is too big or the other too small.

Chemical blepharoconjunctivitis, caused by silver nitrate, peaks on the second day of life with copious secretions and edema, but it is self-limited. Tearing or persistent eye crusting after the first 2 days calls for evaluation for glaucoma, infection, corneal abrasion, mass lesions with obstruction of the nasolacrimal duct, or absence of the puncta. The signs of congenital glaucoma that may be noticed during the neonatal examination include photophobia, excessive tearing, cloudy cornea, or eyes that appear large (56).

The pupil response to light requires a relatively dark room with only a moderately bright beam to avoid stimulating reflex eye closure. The pupil diameter decreases toward term as its response to light increases. Pupil reaction occurs consistently only after 32 weeks of gestation but may develop as early as 28 weeks of gestation. Pupils of term infants are anomalously dilated if their diameter is larger than 5.4 mm or anomalously constricted if smaller than 1.8 mm (57).

Iris color is poorly defined at birth. The iris should form a continuous circle without interruptions or unusual stretching or banding. Because of normal cloudiness in the corneas of infants at less than 28 weeks of gestation, only a cursory inspection of the iris and pupils is done, with close examination, including internal structures, deferred until general cloudiness resolves.

A thorough fundoscopic examination with mydriasis is not routine, but there should be an attempt to detect cloudiness, masses, or large hemorrhages. The fundoscopic examination is easiest when the infant is asleep and not resisting. Assessment of vision is best with an alert, quiet infant, but a startle in response to a bright light flash through closed lids even with the infant asleep indicates intact optic pathways. The corneal edema normally present the first 2 days after birth may prevent an accurate detection of a red reflex or visualization of the fundus without mydriasis. This is especially problematic in darkly pigmented eyes.

The classically described gemini red reflex (GRR) or choroidal light reflex is detected by examining both eyes simultaneously at a distance of 1 m. From a wide beam on the ophthalmoscope held at a distance, the circle of light covers much of the face. The focus is adjusted to give the brightest red glow, indicating that light is reflecting from the retina. Asymmetry in the color, brightness, position, or presence of the glow in the GRR is abnormal and warrants full ophthalmologic evaluation (58). Because GRR requires the infant to fix both eyes on a light source and is best with dilated pupils, a simple, monoccular red reflex is substituted in the newborn examination. Because this monocular reflex is not as informative as it would be if the reflex were simultaneously compared in both eyes, the GRR is assessed when bilateral fixation develops.

Ears

Each ear is examined for shape, size, position, the presence of a canal, and any extraneous tags or pits. The tympanic membranes are examined to evaluate sources of late neonatal infection. The shape of the external ear is determined in part by intrauterine forces and by the activity of extrinsic and intrinsic auricular muscles. Abnormal formation may be a sign of neuromuscular weakness or abnormalities in auricular muscles (59,60). The length of the ear roughly approximates the vertical distance from the arch of the brow to the bottom of the nose. Position of the ears depends on how complete their cephalad migration and anterior rotation are and how much molding or deformation there may be. The position at term should be similar on both sides, with at least one-quarter of the pinnae above a line extended between the medial canthi. Because a line extended between the medial and lateral canthi on one eye reflects variable slanting of the eye, it is better to use a more consistently positioned marker such as the two medial canthi.

A behavioral reaction to a standardized sound excludes only gross bilateral deficits, but it should be elicited in all neonates. Assessment of hearing by brainstem evoked potential or otoacoustic emission is specifically indicated in infants at risk for hearing deficits, particularly those with anomalies of the head and neck, a family history of childhood deafness, very low birth weight, severe asphyxia, fetal infection, meningitis, and after hyperventilation therapy and intracranial hemorrhage. Even though congenitally acquired hearing deficits may result from anomalies, infections, or other perinatal conditions, loss may not develop for months or be detectable until behavioral audiometry is feasible.

Nose

The nose is assessed for shape, size, and patency and for the presence of swelling over the nasolacrimal duct, the size of the philtrum, and definition of the nasolabial folds. It should appear appropriately sized for the face when viewed laterally and *en face.*

Nasal deformation with asymmetry of the nares and apparent deviation occurs as part of facial compression and molding. The triangular cartilage rarely may be dis-

located during delivery, causing septal deviation, which is best treated by surgical relocation during the first week. With depression of the tip of the nose, a dislocated septum appears even more angled within the nares, but a normal septum merely compresses. After release, a dislocated septum does not return to upright nor can it be readily molded into a normal shape (61).

Nasal patency is assessed by free passage of a small catheter through both nares and into the stomach. Air flow is detected by holding a strand of thread in front of each nostril and observing fluttering with breathing.

Congenital obstruction of the nasolacrimal duct, usually symptomatic in the first days or weeks of life, presents with a large tear meniscus at the lower lid, tearing without stimulation, dried mucoid residue after a nap, or a discharge during waking. A distally obstructed nasolacrimal duct is diagnosed by pressing the finger over the lacrimal sac and sliding it along the course of the duct toward the eye to express material from the puncta. Dacryocystocele is a dilation of the lacrimal drainage system due to obstruction at both ends and filling of the enclosed space. Dacryocystoceles are observed at birth as immobile, tense, sometimes blue–gray cystic swellings no more than 1 cm in length, located just below the medial canthal tendon (62,63).

Mouth and Throat

The shape of the mouth is a marker of fetal position and neuromotor activity. For the mouth to develop properly, there must be muscle activity of the tongue against an intact hard palate. If there is a large palatal defect so the tongue does not meet superior resistance, the mandible is more receded and small; if the hard palate is intact but the tongue inactive, the hard palate may have a high arch or have prominent lateral palatine ridges.

The more common oral findings have counterparts in neonatal dermatology and are benign (Table 19–2). The mouth should be observed with the infant at rest and crying. The shape and size of the mouth is best determined by looking at the mandible and how well it fits the maxilla. It should open at equal angles bilaterally. If the fetal position was with the head tilted for an extended period just before delivery, there may be mandibular deviation causing the jaw to open at an angle. This deformation resolves spontaneously, but significant oral asymmetry causes difficulty in breast-feeding on one side compared to the other. Asymmetry on crying occurs with facial nerve paresis, in which the nasolabial folds are asymmetric, or with absence of the depressor anguli oris muscle, in which the folds are symmetric (63,64). The side with the absent muscle feels thinner.

The tongue, buccal surface, palate, uvula, and back of the mouth should be visualized. The gums and hard palate are best assessed by palpating with a gloved finger for masses or submucous defects while the strengths of

TABLE 19–2. *Neonatal oral findings*

Finding	Caucasians (%)	Non-Caucasians (%)	Comments
Palatal cysts (e.g., Bohn nodules, Epstein pearls)	73–85	65–79	Yellow-white elevated cysts 1 mm in diameter; nests of epithelial cells in the midpalatal raphe at the fusion points of the soft and hard palates
Alveolar or gingival cysts	54	40	Appear similar to palatal cysts
Alveolar lymphangioma	0	4	Blue-domed, fluid-filled cysts in posterior regions; no more than one per quadrant; may cause discomfort during feeding if cysts are large
Alveolar eruption of cysts with or without teeth	<0.1	<0.1	Clear, fluid-filled cysts; mandibular central incisor; rates range from 1:2,500 in Hong Kong to 1:3,392 in Canada
Leukoedema	11	43	Filmy, white hue of mucosa, nonblanching; of no significance compared with thrush
Median alveolar notch	16	26	Reduces when teeth erupt or persists as notch between central incisors
Ankyloglossia	~2	~2	Male to female ratio of 3:1; lingual frenum prevents protrusion of tongue, extends to papillated surface of tongue, or causes fissure in tip
Commissural lip pits	1	3	Blind-ended pits at corners of mouth; autosomally dominant; associated with preauricular pits; medial pits more syndromic
Thrush			Adherent white plaques on tongue and buccal and palatal surfaces; will scrape off; caused by *Candida* sp.
Bifid uvula	<1	<1	Associated with submucous cleft palate
Ranula	<<1	<<1	Cyst of sublingual salivary gland
Epulis	<<1	<<1	Large, pedunculated cyst of incisor region

Data from refs. 80–84.

the suck and gag reflex also are assessed. If the tongue is too large, the mouth cannot be closed completely, but if the tongue protrudes because of low oral–facial tone it can be.

Skin and Lymph Nodes

The skin is assessed for general color, the presence of any extra markings or rashes, texture, turgor, edema or areas of induration, thickness of underlying fat, and maturity. Icterus progresses in a cephalocaudal pattern generally correlating with serum bilirubin in the absence of phototherapy (65). If any mark on the skin is to be considered to be a "birth mark," there is rarely an infant born without several. In view of the many variations of normal and the important signs of other diseases or syndromes that are manifested on the skin, understanding the common physical findings of the neonatal skin is fundamental. Details about dermal conditions are discussed in Chapter 54.

Lymph nodes are palpable in more than one-third of all neonates, most commonly in the inguinal region and independent of perinatal history. These nodes, from 3 to 12 mm in diameter, tend to persist (66). A benign node commonly palpable in the femoral triangle serves as a reliable landmark for finding the femoral pulse adjacent to it.

The most frequent, abnormal congenital lymphatic masses are cystic hygroma or cystic lymphangiomas, which are soft, compressible, and often poorly defined masses in almost any part of the body, but commonly in the head, neck, abdomen, and axilla. If markedly distended, the hygroma may transilluminate. Ultrasonography reveals their cystic anatomy. A discussion on the congenital abnormalities of the lymphatic system is available (67).

Chest and Abdomen

Size and Symmetry

In term neonates, the chest circumference is 1 to 2 cm less than the head circumference; it is relatively smaller with lower gestational age. The thorax is normally symmetric and wider than its anteroposterior dimension. The ribs are compliant, and their shape is easily impacted by external and internal forces. Compression from the infant's own arm or a twin's body part may lead to marked asymmetry in thoracic shape and pattern on inspiration. By encouraging the infant to assume the fetal position, the cause of a chest deformation may become apparent.

The abdomen is mildly protuberant compared with the chest. It should be softly rounded, with a diameter slightly greater above than below the umbilicus. The abdominothoracic relation is reversed in diaphragmatic defects, with herniation of abdominal contents into the thorax leaving a scaphoid abdomen. Supraumbilical fullness is increased in the presence of duodenal atresia with gastric distention or hepatomegaly, and infraumbilical fullness is increased with distention of the urinary bladder or in severe cases of IUGR with an abnormally small liver. Any significant abdominal visceral enlargement causes distention, as does forced depression of the diaphragm.

Retractions

Mild subcostal and intercostal retractions are common, even in healthy neonates because of their compliant chest walls. Suprasternal retractions, indicating proximal airway resistance, are normally less pronounced; supraclavicular retractions are never normal. In conditions notable for loss of lung volume and poor compliance, respiratory movements may become paradoxical (i.e., seesaw), with a collapse of the chest wall on inspiration as the abdominal wall expands. With air trapping and increased thoracic volume, there is an increase in the anteroposterior dimension and abdominal distention as the diaphragm is pushed down.

Because the diaphragm is the primary muscle of breathing with little contribution by accessory muscles, quiet breathing is abdominal, with only mild but equal subcostal retractions. The umbilical stump moves caudally in the midline with each contraction of the diaphragm. In the absence of abdominal abnormalities, any lateral deviation of the umbilicus with inspiration suggests a diaphragmatic paresis with the deviation toward the nonfunctioning side (68). This belly dancer sign is lost during mechanical ventilation. Albeit rare, neonatal diaphragmatic paresis occurs most often with brachial plexus injuries, and it should be considered if an arm is weak.

Auscultation of Breath Sounds

Neonatal lung sounds are relatively more tubular than vesicular because of better transmission of large airway sounds across a small chest. Changes in the pitch of the tubular sounds from one side to the other or between regions most likely represent main stem or conducting bronchial narrowing. The coarse crackle of distal airway opening is particularly common in neonates in whom there is a natural tendency in many conditions for microatelectasis. If heard at the end of inspiration, adventitial sounds represent more distal disease compared with those in beginning inspiration, which usually represent conducting airway secretions. A characteristic sound of crushing Styrofoam or walking on dry snow signals pulmonary interstitial emphysema.

Locating abnormal sounds requires listening over the extrathoracic airways, because these sounds may be transmitted well through the chest. If bowel sounds are heard, the examiner should differentiate direct transmission from herniated contents or referred abdominal sounds.

If there is stridor or wheezing, auscultation of the nose or throat may reveal a site of extrathoracic obstruction. Because there must be sufficient air flow to cause stridor or wheezing in the first place, stimulating the infant may accentuate an obstruction. If an endotracheal tube is in place and an air leak is present, a whistling sound corresponding to ventilator breaths may be evident in the periphery of the lung fields but is loudest over the upper trachea or outside the mouth.

Clavicles

The clavicles may be hypoplastic or absent as in cleidocraniodysostosis or fractured. If they are absent, the shoulders may be made almost to touch in the anterior midline. If carefully sought by radiographs or repeated examinations, clavicular fractures are found in at least 1.7% to 2.9% of term deliveries and more frequently on the right side (69). More often than not, clavicular fractures are undetected until they develop a callus and mass over the fracture site at 2 to 3 weeks of age. If a new fracture is complete, the ends may be displaced with palpation and feel crepitant as they rub against each other. An overlying hematoma may cause a visible fullness, there may be an associated brachial plexus injury or pseudoparesis, or the infant may not be willing to breast-feed on one side because of discomfort with positioning. Standing at the foot of the infant, the examiner feels each clavicle, compares ease of outlining the distinct borders of the bones, and assesses tenderness, swelling, or crepitation.

Nipples

The breasts of term infants vary in diameter from 0.5 cm to several centimeters, with clinically insignificant differences between sexes. The internipple distance varies with gestational age and body weight, but its relation to chest circumference is more constant. If the internipple distance in centimeters divided by the chest circumference is greater than 0.28, the space is more than 2 standard deviations above the mean regardless of body size (70). Larger breasts, influenced by maternal hormones, may secrete a thin, milky substance (i.e., witches' milk) for a few days or weeks. Although the degree of enlargement may not be the same in both breasts, they should never be hot, red, or notably tender. Unless there are specific signs of inflammation, enlarged breasts should be left alone.

Supernumerary nipples occur in 1.2% to 1.6% of darkly pigmented infants but are more unusual in lightly pigmented infants. These supernumerary nipples, seen in the milk line below and medial to the true breast, are rudimentary, occasionally only distinguishable because of the presence of a small pigmented mark or dimple. There is a suggested association of renal anomalies detectable on ultrasound or intravenous pyelography in

Caucasian populations that is not confirmed in black population studies (71,72).

Umbilicus

The umbilicus normally is positioned approximately halfway between the xiphoid and the pubis. A caudally placed insertion occurs in conditions of caudal regression or underdeveloped lower body segment. The neonatal appearance of the umbilicus does not indicate what the adult appearance will be, because most are relatively protuberant with redundant skin. If the umbilical cord itself is especially broad or remains fluctuant after vascular pulsations have stopped, there may be a herniation of abdominal contents into the cord. Determining the presence of two umbilical arteries is part of the first assessment at birth.

As the cord dries, it should remain odorless. The base should not appear red or indurated. After the cord falls off, the umbilicus should be examined for granuloma or continued leakage through a patent urachus.

Palpation of Abdomen

The infant tolerates palpation of the abdomen best when the organs are brought to the examining hand rather than the fingertips pushing into the abdomen and probing for the organs. Standing at the right side of the infant, with the left hand lifting the legs and raising the pelvis slightly off the mattress to relax the abdominal muscles, the examiner can keep the right hand flat and use the fingerpads rather than fingertips to palpate the abdominal organs. Palpation should start below the umbilicus on both sides and proceed toward the diaphragm. In some instances, it is helpful to palpate the abdomen with the infant in the decubitus or prone position, allowing the contents to fall toward the hand rather than being pushed away (73). Palpation of the abdomen in ill neonates increases centrally measured blood pressure by as much as 25% above baseline (74).

The liver is normally palpable 1 to 3.5 cm below the costal margin in the midclavicular line and across the midline as a left lobe that is distinguishable from the spleen felt more laterally. A left lobe larger than the right may reflect situs inversus. At term, the normal liver span, determined by percussing the upper and lower margins, is 5.9 ± 0.8 cm in the midclavicular line (75). This varies by gestational age and weight. Estimation of hepatomegaly based on lower border estimation alone is inaccurate. An effective technique to outline the margins of the liver or any solid abdominal mass is to scratch lightly across the skin surface while auscultating with the diaphragm of the stethoscope held over the mass. The pitch elevates when the stroking overlies the solid mass or liver.

The normal edge of the liver is thin and soft, and the hepatic surface is smooth. A full or firm edge commonly represents a marked increase in total blood volume, increased extramedullary hematopoiesis, chronic infection, early cirrhosis, or an infiltrative process. Hepatomegaly is a late and inconstant finding in cardiac failure. Cardiac pulsations in the liver occur in right-sided obstructive cardiac lesions, but these hepatic pulsations should be differentiated from a normally transmitted cardiac impulse or respiratory excursions. In the first 24 to 48 hours after birth, the liver often decreases markedly in size, probably reflecting redistribution of circulating blood volume.

The kidneys are palpable if the abdomen is soft, and they are moderately firm and lobulated. An enlarged ureter simulates a filled segment of large bowel, although it is less mobile.

An infant reveals abdominal tenderness by a grimace, cry, or drawing up of the legs on light palpation. True guarding is unusual. Rebound tenderness is difficult to detect, and infants with significant peritoneal disease are often too obtunded to show a reliable response. The presence of localized edema or discoloration of the abdominal wall is an important indicator of intraperitoneal disease. An unusual exception is ecchymosis caused by leaking of an umbilical vessel or urine edema from a patent urachus leaking into the subcutaneous space above the peritoneum. In either case, the dramatic findings are limited to the abdominal wall below the umbilicus.

A thin abdominal wall allows transillumination of fluid- or gas-filled masses to outline their position and size. Meconium-filled bowel loops do not transilluminate, but stomach or bowel distended with air, hydronephrotic kidneys, or a distended bladder will. A transillumination pattern that shifts with patient rotation suggests free air.

Auscultation of the abdomen includes listening for pitch and activity of bowel sounds and for bruits. Infants normally have relatively inactive bowel sounds on their first day of life or, if they are extremely premature and never fed, for several days or weeks. Even in infants with clinical ileus, bowel sounds tend to persist to some extent, but a true absence of bowel sounds is always significant. Detecting changes in the pattern of bowel sounds is more helpful than the findings of a single examination. Auscultation may reveal the presence of a bruit over the liver, indicating an arteriovenous fistula, or over the kidneys in the presence of renal artery stenosis.

Cardiovascular System

The changes that occur in the cardiovascular system during the neonatal period complicate the cardiac examination until the pulmonic and systemic pressures have reversed their fetal associations, all communications have closed, and the left ventricle becomes predominant. Each aspect of examination from inspection through auscultation plays a role, but auscultating for murmurs is not always the most helpful in determining if a newborn infant has cardiac disease. The role for most clinicians in the newborn examination is not to determine precisely what the cardiac anatomy is but to rule out cardiac disease as part of a routine newborn examination and, in a symptomatic infant, to determine if the cause is cardiac. If so, the physician must determine the urgency of the condition by asking some basic questions. Is this a cardiac disease that could be fatal if not immediately diagnosed and treated (e.g., ductal dependent lesions, cyanotic heart disease)? Is its presence aggravating or relieving other conditions (e.g., patent ductus arteriosus in the presence of lung disease or pulmonary hypertension)? Is this something that requires following the patient and potential future intervention but is not emergent and should not interfere with newborn and parental adjustment (e.g., mild pulmonic stenosis or a small septal defect)?

Murmurs persisting after the first 12 hours are likely to reflect structural abnormalities even though they may not be hemodynamically significant. Unlike the innocent murmurs of infants older than 1 month, some types of heart disease can be found on echocardiography in most cases. In one study of infants referred to the cardiology department for murmurs between 12 hours and 14 days, 84% had identifiable lesions, with ventricular septal defects (39%), pulmonic stenosis (15%), and patent ductus arteriosus (15%) most common (76). The remaining 16% had normal hearts with innocent murmurs due to tricuspid regurgitation or peripheral pulmonic stenosis. Because many murmurs are transient in the first 2 days, it requires clinical judgment as to whether or not an echocardiac evaluation is warranted if there is no option for reexamination in a timely manner. Clearly if there are other signs of cardiac disease besides a murmur, an evaluation is urgent.

Evaluation of the cardiovascular system begins in the delivery room with assessment of the Apgar scores and includes evaluation of heart rate, color, and respiratory effort. Frequently, a line of demarcation is observed, with the head, right arm, and right side of the chest pink and the rest of the infant pale or cyanotic until there is functional closure of the ductus. With vigorous crying, its disappearance indicates an appropriate drop in pulmonary vascular resistance and transductal shunting. Another reassuring milestone in cardiac transition often noticed at the first bath by nursing staff is a brief but bright red flush over the entire body and extremities. This blush, reminiscent of cooked lobster, is distinguishable from the darker, ruddy, plethoric color of polycythemia, which is accentuated in the mucous membranes and less so on the palms and soles and is more persistent. The blush is not seen in infants with cyanotic cardiac disease. Specific points to be considered in the cardiac examination are outlined in Table 19–3.

Genitourinary System

In the delivery room, one of the first documented observations of the neonate is assignment of gender. Genital abnormalities are relatively uncommon but cause significant stress to new parents, so it is important to distinguish the variations of normal from pathologic malformations (see Chap. 43). It is always urgent to start an appropriate evaluation of gender if that is in question.

The male infant should be examined by stretching the penis for an expected penile length at term of at least 2.5 cm. The presence of chordae prevents complete stretching, but a twisted median raphe is of no significance. In obese infants, the shaft may be retracted and covered by suprapubic fat, appearing to be too small unless it is stretched. The observation of the presence of erectile tissue essentially eliminates true micropenis as a consideration. The meatal opening should be located, although completely retracting the foreskin is unnecessary. Any significant glanular hypospadias generally is accompanied by incomplete foreskin and therefore is readily apparent on simple inspection. Fortunately, the newborn frequently provides opportunities to observe the origin, direction, and force of his stream on urination.

The presence of both testes deep in the scrotal sac indicates term gestation. If a testis is not felt within the sac or canal, use a lubricated finger to sweep from the anterior iliac crest along the canal while palpating the scrotum. The volume of the testes should be estimated. Table 19–4 summarizes the normal values. If the scrotum or a testis is distended but soft and nontender, transillumination may reveal a hydrocele. Deep discoloration suggests hematoma or torsion and a need for immediate surgical evaluation, but superficial scrotal cyanosis may represent benign ecchymosis after breech presentation. Hydrocele of the cord, a harbinger of inguinal hernia, is not so likely to transilluminate but is easily felt.

The female genitalia should be inspected for size and location of the labia, clitoris, meatus, vaginal opening, and the relations of the posterior fourchette to the anus (see Table 19–4).

Virtually all female newborns have redundant hymenal tissue. Hymens tend be annular (80%), with a smooth or fimbriated edge and a central or ventrally displaced opening. Tags of tissue may extend from 1 to 15 mm beyond the rim of the hymen and occur in at least 13% of female neonates. These tags disappear within a few weeks. A complete review of hymenal variations in newborns is available (77). An imperforate hymen can present with a build-up of mucoid or bloody secretions causing a mass protruding from the vagina, a hydrometroculpos, which usually resolves with spontaneous rupture or regression but can enlarge significantly and cause urinary obstruction or apparent discomfort.

Assessment for virilization in the female is difficult, because there are varying degrees of clitoral hypertrophy

TABLE 19–3. *Neonatal cardiac examination*

Findings	Key location	Points to consider
Color	Over entire surface except presenting part; inside oral mucous membranes	Peripheral cyanosis may include area around mouth but not inside mucous membranes Prominent venous-capillary plexus around mouth and eyes simulates cyanosis Acrocyanosis of extremities reverses with warming Mild cyanosis may appear as pallor or mottling Infant with PDA runoff looks washed out, particularly in the feet
Respiratory pattern	Lateral view of chest and abdomen Alae nasi	Most often have respiratory rate within normal range May be cyanotic but tachypneic without distress (e.g., retractions, labored breathing) unless there is pulmonary edema or severe acidosis
Heart rate rhythm	PMI	Resting rate 120–130 (range 100–150); higher second to the fourth weeks and in premature infants Most premature beats are transient and benign
Precordial bulge	Thorax compared side to side and to the abdomen	Thoracic asymmetry indicates bulge with AVM, tricuspid regurgitation (i.e., Ebstein), tetralogy with absent PV, intrauterine arrhythmia, or myocardopathy Most commonly, asymmetry indicates pneumothorax, diaphragmatic hernia, atelectasis, or lobar emphysema
PMI	Left parasternal area	Visible until 4–6 h of life during transition; beyond 12 h, associated with volume overload lesions (for example, AP shunt, transposition, or outflow obstruction) Normally more visible in premature infants but increases with PDA Abnormal to have PMI beyond 1–2 cm left of LSB at less than 1 wk of age Right sided indicates dextrocardia versus shift due to intrathoracic pressures Absence of increased impulse with cyanosis indicates pulmonary atresia, tetralogy, tricuspid atresia Increase with cyanosis indicates transposition Thrill: gross insufficiency of AV valve, severe pulmonary stenosis, absent pulmonary valve
Blood pressure	Right arm and leg	Pressure in lower extremities is equal to or minimally higher than pressure in upper extremities in the first week Pressures are preserved by ductal flow in the presence of severe left-sided obstructive disease Norms vary by gestational and chronologic age and method
Pulses	Right and left brachial and simultaneous femoral and right brachial	Look for equality of intensity and timing, synchronicity, slope of impulse curve, no delay in peak between preductal and postductal pulses Easily seen axillary pulses suggest runoff or wide pulse pressure
Pulse pressure	Systolic minus diastolic BP	25–30 in term; 15–25 in preterm Narrow indicates myocardial failure, vasoconstriction, vascular collapse Widened indicates AV malformation, truncus arteriosus, AP window, PDA; may not be widened until pulmonary vascular resistance has dropped
S_1	Upper LSB	Usually single and relatively accentuated; audible split indicates Ebstein anomaly or slow heat rate; decreased with CHF, prolonged AV conduction
	Lower LSB	Increased accentuation with increased flow across AV valve indicates PDA, MI, VSD, TAPVR, AVM, tetralogy
S_2	Upper LSB	Two components should be heard by 6–12 h of age Single sound indicates aortic atresia, pulmonary atresia, truncus arteriosus, transposition of great arteries Wide split indicates pulmonary stenosis, Ebstein anomaly, TAPVR, tetralogy, occasionally left-to-right atrial shunts Loud sounds indicate systemic or pulmonary hypertension
S_3 and S_4	Base or apex	S_3 indicates increased atrioventricular valve flow, PDA, CHF S_4 indicates severe myocardial disease with diminished LV compliance
Click	Lower LSB	Benign first several hours; abnormal after transition Dilation of great vessel indicates truncus arteriosus, tetralogy of Fallot, left- or right-sided ventricular outflow obstructions
Murmur	Precordium, back, under both axilla	Many serious cardiac malformations do not have their classic murmurs in early neonatal period but will have some combination of signs suggesting pathology; absence of murmur does not preclude presence of serious malformation (e.g., transposition, TAPVR) At least 60% of infants have murmurs during the first 48 h of life; PDA, peripheral pulmonary stenosis, tricuspid regurgitation Quiet is necessary to auscultate murmurs; may need to disconnect the infant from the ventilator, for a few beats Persistent murmurs first heard right after birth indicate ventricular outflow obstruction most often pulmonic stenosis
Venous pulse	Jugular vein, liver	Jugular a and v waves in sleeping infant In presence of cyanosis, pulsating liver suggests RA or RV obstruction
Abdomen	Liver (left and right)	Span greater than 5.5 cm at term; late sign of congestive heart failure; presence of left-sided or central liver suggests likely cardiac anomaly
Edema	Presacrum, eyelids, legs and feet; Chest: hydrops	Causes are more often noncardiac except when associated with abnormalities of renal blood flow (e.g., left-sided obstruction or severe hydrops associated with myocarcardiopathy such as severe anemia)

AP, aortopulmonary; AV, atrioventricular; AVM, arteriovenous malformation; BP, blood pressure; CHF, congestive heart failure; LSB, left sternal border; LA, left atrium; LV, left ventricle; MI, mitral insufficiency; PDA, patent ductus arteriosus; PMI, point of maximal impulse; PV, pulmonary valve; RA, right atrium; RV, right ventricle; S_1, first heart sound; S_2, second heart sound; S_3, third heart sound; S_4, fourth heart sound; TAPVR, total anomalous pulmonary venous return; VSD, ventricular septal defect.
From refs. 85 and 86.

TABLE 19–4. *Newborn genitalia*

	Parameter	Normal ranges	Abnormal ranges
Penis	Length	3.5 cm ± 1 cm	<2.5 cm
	Width	0.9–1.2 cm	
Testis	Volume	1–2 cm	
Anus			
Location, male	Anus to scrotum/Coccyx to scrotum	0.58 ± 0.06 cm	<0.46 cm
Location, female	Anus to fourchette/Coccyx to fourchette	0.44 ± 0.05 cm	<0.34 cm
Size	Diameter	7 mm + (1.3 × weight in kg)	
Masculinization (i.e., labioscrotal fusion)	Anus to fourchette/Anus to clitoris	<0.5 cm	>0.5 cm

From refs. 87 and 88.

and labioscrotal fusion. With clitoral size realized by 27 weeks of gestation but with little deposition of fat in the labia, there is particular confusion about clitoral hypertrophy in premature infants. Masculinization causes posterior fusion of the labioscrotal folds independent of clitoral hypertrophy. The distance of the anus from the posterior fourchette varies by gestational age and body size, but its relation relative to other genital landmarks is more constant (see Table 19–4). Measurements are made with the hips flexed and the infant relaxed so that the perineum does not bulge.

Musculoskeletal System

Examination of the spine includes observation for abnormal curving and cutaneous manifestations of underlying deformities such as sacral agenesis or spina bifida. A pilonidal sinus is suspected if the bottom of a sacral pit is not visible or there is moisture in an otherwise dry area. Long tufts of hair, an overlying hemangioma, or pigmented nevus potentially indicate a tethered cord unless well below the origin of the cauda equina. A palpable mass usually indicates a lipoma if it is covered with normal skin and moves with it. A sacrococcygeal teratoma tends to be a fixed mass just lateral to midline, and spinal dysraphism presents as a midline mass, most frequently without full skin coverage.

One assesses the extremities for symmetry, size and length, range of active and passive motion, and obvious deformity. The length of the upper extremities should allow the fingers to reach to the upper thighs on extension. The muscles are not well defined but should not feel atrophic or fibrotic.

Hand examination consists of observing its activity and appearance, including the nails, joints, and palmar creases. The creases of the fifth digit should be parallel. If there is shortening of the midphalanx, the nonparallel creases mark a radial deviation, clinodactyly. Any curve less than 10 to 15 degrees is normal. The thumb should reach just beyond the base of the index finger. Extra digits that are postaxial or on the ulnar side most often are equivalent to skin tags with no significance except in their familial occurrence, most often in families of color.

Extra digits on the preaxial or radial side are often enough associated with hematologic and cardiac abnormalities to warrant further evaluation regardless of racial background.

The neonate's hips require assessment with each visit because dislocations may not be detectable on every examination. If the femur freely dislocates, it may appear to jerk spontaneously when the infant extends or flexes his or her hip. The legs should be symmetric in length on extension and with the knees flexed as the feet rest on the bed. If they are unequal, suggesting dislocation of the shorter leg (i.e., Galeazzi sign), the next maneuver is to attempt reduction on the shorter side while stabilizing the pelvis (i.e., Ortolani maneuver). With the hip and knee flexed, the thigh is grasped with the third finger over the greater trochanter and the thumb near the lesser trochanter. The other hand stabilizes the pelvis. As the thigh is abducted, gentle pressure applied to the greater trochanter reduces the dislocated femoral head into the acetabulum with a clunking sensation. The commonly felt, benign clicks are distinct from the pathologic clunks, which often are seen as much as they are felt when the femoral head jerks into place. If the legs are of equal length or if they rest in full abduction, the first maneuver is to attempt to dislocate the head (i.e., Barlow maneuver). With the hip and knee flexed, the thigh is grasped and adducted to 15 degrees beyond midline while applying downward pressure. If the hip dislocates on the maneuver, the Ortolani maneuver should then reduce it. If the hip rides to the edge but not out of the acetabulum during the Barlow maneuver, it is subluxable. Even if dislocation is undetectable, there may be telescoping with free movement of the femur up and down, indicating some degree of instability. The Ortolani maneuver may be negative if a teratologic hip dysplasia cannot be reduced. Unless both hips are involved, discrepancy in leg length and inability to abduct fully to the affected side will be diagnostic.

Nervous System

Neurologic evaluation begins with the initial observations made on approaching the infant and continues as the infant is positioned and stimulated for the remainder of the routine physical examination. As discussed earlier, assessing gestational age includes many of the steps also used to evaluate motor tone and symmetry. Much can be learned about the neurologic state just by observing what the infant does on his or her own; little more is needed unless the observations indicate abnormality or there are particular risk factors. Subtle differences in tone or use require more specific evaluation.

Jitteriness is a frequent finding in neonates that warrants special comment. It is characterized by rhythmic tremors of equal amplitude around a fixed axis in an extremity or the jaw. It occurs more often if the infant is awake, after a startle, or after crying. Distinguishable

TABLE 19–5. *Neonatal neurologic evaluation*

Test	Technique	Normal for term	Deviant for term
Resting posture	Observe unswaddled infant without contact in quiet awake, quiet active, or light sleep states	Moderate flexion of four limbs, held off bed Equal side-to-side and upper-to-lower if head is in midline Extension of neck in face presentation or legs in breech presentation	Constant tight flexion Full extension, flaccid or forced Knees abducted to bed (i.e., frog leg) Elbows flexed with dorsum of hands on bed Tight, persistent fisting ATNR persistent ≥30 seconds Strong lateral preference
State	Deep sleep Light sleep Awake, light peripheral movements Awake, large movements, not crying Awake, crying	Moves from one to the other with appropriate stimuli Self calms Modulated cry with expression	Is difficult to move from one to the other Stays too alert or cries without physical reason Does not come to fully awake state Weak or monotonous cry
Motor activity	Observe throughout physical examination	Appropriate for state of alertness Symmetric, fairly smooth Expressive face with yawn or cry	Bicycling, swatting without stimulus Asymmetric, weak Jittery while sucking Flat facial expression
Phasic (i.e., passive) tone: resistance to movement	Measure resistance to extension (limb recoil) Scarf, heel to ear	Response appropriate for gestational age	Resists too much or too little Asymmetry
Tendon reflexes	Test patellar reflex with head midline	Patellar reflex only one reliably present at birth	Sustained clonus
Postural (i.e., active) tone: resistance to gravity			
Traction response	Pull to sitting while grasping infant's hands	Infant pulls back with flexion at elbows, knees, and ankles Head comes with body with minimal lag and falls forward when sitting is obtained	Asymmetry in pulling back No resistance Full head lag Pull to stand instead Head does not fall forward as infant goes past upright
Upright suspension	Suspend infant facing examiner with both hands in axillae	Infant supports himself then yields slowly Holds head erect, flexes hips, knees, and ankles Eyes open	Infant falls through immediately Legs extend Eyes fail to open Infant fails to relax and fall through after 1 min
Ventral suspension	Hold infant under chest and suspend in prone position	Flexes arms, extends neck, holds back straight	Hangs limply or excessively rigidly
	Galant: stroke adjacent to spine	Curves toward side of stimulus	Asymmetric incurving
	Landau: stroke caudolcephalad along spine	Extends back, lifts head and pelvis, micturates	Weak or absent response
Positive support	Hold infant to support trunk with feet touching firm, flat surface	Infant extends hips to bear his own weight and relaxes after 1 min	Infant fails to bear weight or extends too much or too long
Integrated reflexes			Unequal laterality
Moro reflex	Hold infant in supine position; support head and neck with hand; allow head to drop while still supporting it	Spreading: arms abduct, extend; hands open Hugging: arms adduct and flex; hands close	Absence of spread Asymmetry Exaggeration with disorganization in state
Tonic neck reflex	Infant in supine, neutral position; turn head to one side; repeat opposite side	Mental extension, occipital flexion primarily of arms; does not remain in position for >30 seconds	Exaggerated response and stays in position >30 seconds
Withdrawal reflex	Painful stimulus to one foot	Withdrawal of stimulated foot; variable extension of opposite leg	Absence of flexion in stimulated leg

ATNR, asymmetric tonic neck reflex.

TABLE 19–6. Assessment of cranial nerves

Cranial nerve	Assessment	Pitfalls
I	Withdrawal or grimace to strong odor (e.g., peppermint, oil of cloves)	Rarely tested clinically; rapid habituation
II	Behavioral response to light (i.e., blink, fixing, following, turning to light source); searching nystagmus	Room too bright; infant too deeply asleep; overstimulation of other senses
III, IV, VI	Ocular movement, doll's eyes, oculovestibular response, pupil size, gemini red reflex	Should not force eyes to open; ocular alignment usually poor in neonates; light for pupil response causes eye closing
VII	Facial muscle tone at rest and during crying	Poor mouth opening due to absence of depressor anguli oris muscle
V, VII, XII	Sucking strength, rooting reflex	Gestational-age dependent; infant should be hungry
VIII auditory portion	Behavioral response to horn (i.e., blink, widened eyes); quieting to voice	Room too loud; difficult to distinguish unilateral loss; rapid habituation
IX, X	Swallowing with normal gag	Irritated throat after suctioning
VII, IX	Facial expression to strong flavor	Rapid habituation
XII	Tongue fasciculation, thrust, ability to shape around nipple	Macroglossia

from clonic–tonic seizure activity because it can be stopped by stimulating sucking, it is most often a physiologic activity. If it fails to cease during sucking, it may be a sign of hypoglycemia or hypocalcemia or of irritability associated with maternal drug abuse (78,79).

The basics of the neonatal neurologic examination include assessment of state; spontaneous muscle activity for assessing amount, quality, and strength; passive and active muscle tone; and the functioning of the cranial nerves. The steps are described in Tables 19–5 and 19–6.

REFERENCES

1. Silverman WE, Andersen DH. Controlled clinical trial of effects of water mist on obstructive respiratory signs, death rate and necropsy findings among premature infants. *Pediatrics* 1956;17:1.
2. Morley CJ, Thornton AJ, Cole TJ, Hewson PH, Fowler MA. Baby Check: a scoring system to grade the severity of acute systemic illness in babies under 6 months old [see comments]. *Arch Dis Child* 1991; 66:100.
3. Gray JE, Richardson DK, McCormick MC, Workman-Daniels K, Goldmann DA. Neonatal therapeutic intervention scoring system: a therapy-based severity-of-illness index. *Pediatrics* 1992;90:561.
4. Richardson DK, Gray JE, McCormick MC, Workman K, Goldmann DA. Score for neonatal acute physiology: a physiologic severity index for neonatal intensive care. *Pediatrics* 1993;91:617.
5. AAP Committee on Fetus and Newborn and ACOG Committee on Obstetrics: Maternal and Fetal Medicine. *Guidelines for perinatal care,* 4th ed. Elk Grove Village, IL and Washington, DC: American Academy of Pediatrics and American College of Obstetricians and Gynecologists, 1997.
6. Fletcher M. *Physical diagnosis in neonatology.* Philadelphia: Lippincott–Raven Publishers, 1998.
7. Saint-Anne Dargassies S. *Neurological development in the full-term and premature neonate,* 1st ed. Amsterdam: Elsevier, 1977.
8. Amiel-Tison C. Neurological evaluation of the maturity of newborn infants. *Arch Dis Child* 1968;43:89.
9. Dubowitz LM, Dubowitz V, Goldberg C. Clinical assessment of gestational age in the newborn infant. *J Pediatr* 1970;77:1.
10. Ballard JL, Kazmaier Novak K, Driver M. A simplified score for assessment of fetal maturation of newly born infants. *J Pediatr* 1979; 95:769.
11. Alexander GR, de Caunes F, Hulsey TC, Tompkins ME, Allen M. Valid-
ity of postnatal assessments of gestational age: a comparison of the method of Ballard et al. and early ultrasonography. *Am J Obstet Gynecol* 1992;166:891.
12. Sanders M, Allen M, Alexander GR, et al. Gestational age assessment in preterm neonates weighing less than 1500 grams. *Pediatrics* 1991; 88:542.
13. Ballard JL, Khoury JC, Wedig K, Wang L, Eilers-Walsman BL, Lipp R. New Ballard Score, expanded to include extremely premature infants. *J Pediatr* 1991;119:417.
14. Ellison P. The infant neurological examination. *Adv Dev Behav Pediatr* 1990;9:75.
15. Amiel-Tison C, Grenier A. *Neurological assessment during the first year of life,* 1st ed. New York: Oxford University Press, 1986.
16. Hittner HM, Hirsch NJ, Rudolph AJ. Assessment of gestational age by examination of the anterior vascular capsule of the lens. *J Pediatr* 1977;91:455.
17. Litwin A, Aitkin I, Merlob P. Clitoral length assessment in newborn infants of 30 to 41 weeks gestational age. *Eur J Obstet Gynecol Reprod Biol* 1991;38:209.
18. Oberfield SE, Mondok A, Shahrivar F, Klein JF, Levine LS. Clitoral size in full-term infants. *Am J Perinatol* 1989;6:453.
19. Constantine NA, Kraemer HC, Kendall-Tackett KA, Bennett FC, Tyson JE, Gross RT. Use of physical and neurologic observations in assessment of gestational age in low birth weight infants. *J Pediatr* 1987;110: 921.
20. Stevens-Simon C, Cullinan J, Stinson S, McAnarney ER. Effects of race on the validity of clinical estimates of gestational age. *J Pediatr* 1989;115:1000.
21. Wilcox AJ, Russell IT. Birthweight and perinatal mortality: II. On weight-specific mortality. *Int J Epidemiol* 1983;12:319.
22. Sivan Y, Merlob P, Reisner SH. Upper limb standards in newborns. *Am J Dis Child* 1983;137:829.
23. Merlob P, Sivan Y, Reisner SH. Lower limb standard in newborns. *Am J Dis Child* 1984;138:140.
24. Prechtl H, Einspieler C, Cioni G, et al. An early marker for neurological deficits after perinatal brain lesions. *Lancet* 1997;349:1361.
25. Prechtl H, Beintema D. *The neurologic examination of the full-term newborn infant. Clinics in developmental medicine, vol. 12.* London: SIMP Heinemann, 1964.
26. Brazelton TB. *Neonatal behavioral assessment scale, 2nd ed. Clinics in developmental medicine, vol. 88.* Philadelphia: JB Lippincott Co., 1984.
27. Lester BM, Boukydis CF, McGrath M, Censullo M, Zahr L, Brazelton TB. Behavioral and psychophysiologic assessment of the preterm infant. *Clin Perinatol* 1990;17:155.
28. Thoman EB. Sleeping and waking states in infants: a functional perspective. *Neurosci Biobehav Rev* 1990;14:93.
29. Haddad GG, Jeng HJ, Lai TL, Mellins RB. Determination of sleep state in infants using respiratory variability. *Pediatr Res* 1987;21:556.

30. Poole SR. The infant with acute, unexplained excessive crying. *Pediatrics* 1991;88:450.
31. Heine RG, Jaquiery A, Lubitz L, Cameron DJ, Catto-Smith AG. Role of gastro-oesophageal reflux in infant irritability. *Arch Dis Child* 1995; 73:121.
32. Als H, Lester BM, Tronick EC, Brazelton TB. Manual for the assessment of preterm infants behavior (APIB). In: Fitzgerald HE, Lester BM, Yogman MW, eds. *Theory and research in behavioral pediatrics, vol. 1.* New York: Plenum Press, 1982:65.
33. Grover G, Berkowitz CD, Lewis RJ, Thompson M, Berry L, Seidel J. The effects of bundling on infant temperature. *Pediatrics* 1994;94:669.
34. Harpin VA, Rutter N. Sweating in preterm babies. *J Pediatr* 1982;100: 614.
35. Hathorn MK. The rate and depth of breathing in new-born infants in different sleep states. *J Physiol (Lond)* 1974;243:101.
36. Stern E, Parmelee AH, Harris MA. Sleep state periodicity in prematures and young infants. *Dev Psychobiol* 1973;6:357.
37. Hegyi T, Carbone MT, Anwar J, et al. Blood pressure ranges in premature infants. The first hours of life. *J Pediatr* 1994;124:627.
38. Park MK, Lee DH. Normative arm and calf blood pressure values in the newborn. *Pediatrics* 1989;83:240.
39. Perry EH, Bada HS, Ray JD, Korones SB, Arheart K, Magill HL. Blood pressure increases, birth weight-dependent stability boundary, and intraventricular hemorrhage [see comments]. *Pediatrics* 1990;85:727.
40. Committee on Fetus and Newborn AAoP. Routine evaluation of blood pressure, hematocrit, and glucose in newborns. *Pediatrics* 1993;92:474.
41. Goldring D, Wohltmann HJ. Flush method for blood pressure determinations in newborn infants. *J Pediatr* 1952;40:285.
42. Jones MD. Unilateral epicanthal fold: diagnostic significance. *J Pediatr* 1986;108:702.
43. Jones K, ed. *Smith's Recognizable patterns of human malformation*, 4th ed. Philadelphia: WB Saunders, 1988.
44. Smith DW, Gong BT. Scalp hair patterning as a clue to early fetal brain development. *J Pediatr* 1973;83:374.
45. Smith DW, Greely MJ. Unruly scalp hair in infancy: its nature and relevance to problems of brain morphogenesis. *Pediatrics* 1978;61(5): 783.
46. Shuper A, Merlob P, Grunebaum M, Reisner SH. The incidence of isolated craniosynostosis in the newborn infant. *Am J Dis Child* 1985; 139:85.
47. Graham JM, Smith DW. Parietal craniotabes in the neonate: its origin and significance. *J Pediatr* 1979;95:114.
48. Popich GA, Smith DW. Fontanels: range of normal size. *J Pediatr* 1972;80:749.
49. Faix RG. Fontanelle size in black and white term newborn infants. *J Pediatr* 1982;100:304.
50. Duc G, Largo RH. Anterior fontanel: size and closure in term and preterm infants. *Pediatrics* 1986;78:904.
51. Lloyd FA, Finkelstein SI. Normal head growth in infant with nonidentifiable anterior fontanel. *J Pediatr* 1975;87:490.
52. Potter EL, Craig JM. *Pathology of the fetus and the infant, vol. 1*, 3rd ed. Chicago: Year Book Medical Publishers, 1975.
53. Benaron D. Subgaleal hematoma causing hypovolemic shock during delivery after failed vacuum extraction: a case report. *J Perinatol* 1993; 13:228.
54. Govaert P, Vanhaesebrouck P, De Praeter C, Moens K, Leroy J. Vacuum extraction, bone injury and neonatal subgaleal bleeding. *Eur J Pediatr* 1992;151:532.
55. Gundry SR, Wesley JR, Klein MD, Barr M, Coran AG. Cervical teratomas in the newborn. *J Pediatr Surg* 1983;18:382.
56. Crouch ER Jr, Crouch ER. Pediatric vision screening: why? when? how? Contemp Pediatr 1991;September[Special Issue]:9.
57. Isenberg SJ. Clinical application of the pupil examination in neonates. *J Pediatr* 1991;118:650.
58. Adler R, Lappe M, Murphree AL. Pupil dilation at the first well baby examination for documenting choroidal light reflex. *J Pediatr* 1990; 118:249.
59. Smith DW, Takashima H. Ear muscles and ear form. *Birth Defects: Original Article Series* 1980;XVI:299.
60. Zerin M, Van Allen MI, Smith DW. Intrinsic auricular muscles and auricular form. *Pediatrics* 1982;69:91.
61. Silverman SH, Leibow SG. Dislocation of the triangular cartilage of the nasal septum. *J Pediatr* 1975;87:456.
62. Ogawa GSH, Gonnering RS. Congenital nasolacrimal duct obstruction. *J Pediatr* 1991;119:12.
63. Levin SE, Silverman NH, Milner S. Hypoplasia or absence of the depressor anguli oris muscle and congenital abnormalities, with special reference to the cardiofacial syndrome. *S Afr Med J* 1982;61:227.
64. Miller M, Hall JG. Familial asymmetric crying facies. Its occurrence secondary to hypoplasia of the anguli oris depressor muscles. *Am J Dis Child* 1979;133:743.
65. Kramer LI. Advancement of dermal icterus in the jaundiced newborn. *Am J Dis Child* 1969;118:454.
66. Bamji M, Stone RK, Kaul A, Usmani G, Schacter FF, Wasserman E. Palpable lymph nodes in healthy newborns and infants. *Pediatrics* 1986;78:573.
67. Hilliard RI, McKendry JBJ, Phillips MJ. Congenital abnormalities of the lymphatic system: a new clinical classification. *Pediatrics* 1990; 86:988.
68. Nichols MN. Belly dancer's sign. *Clin Pediatr* 1976;April:342.
69. Joseph PR, Rosenfeld W. Clavicular fractures in neonates. *Am J Dis Child* 1990;144:165.
70. Hassan A, Karna P, Dolanski EA. Intermamillary indices in premature infants. *Am J Perinatol* 1988;5:54.
71. Varsano IB, Lutfi J, Ben-Zion G, Mukamel MM, Grünebaum M. Urinary tract abnormalities in children with supernumerary nipples. *Pediatrics* 1984;73:102.
72. Robertson A, Sale P, Sathyanarayan. Lack of association of supernumerary nipples with renal anomalies in black infants. *J Pediatr* 1986; 109:502.
73. Senquiz AL. Use of decubitus position for finding the olive of pyloric stenosis. *Pediatrics* 1991;87:266.
74. Sinkin RA, Phillips BL, Adelman RD. Elevation in systemic blood pressure in the neonate during abdominal examination. *Pediatrics* 1985;76:970.
75. Reiff MI, Osborn LM. Clinical estimation of liver size in newborn infants. *Pediatrics* 1983;71:46.
76. Du Z-D, Roquin N, Barak M. Clinical and echocardiographic evaluation of neonates with heart murmurs. *Acta Paediatr* 1997;86:752.
77. Berenson A, Heger A, Andrews S. Appearance of the hymen in newborns. *Pediatrics* 1991;87:458.
78. Linder N, Moser AM, Asli I, Gale R, Livoff A, Tamir I. Suckling stimulation test for neonatal tremor. *Arch Dis Child* 1989;64:44.
79. Parker S, Zuckerman B, Bauchner H, Frank D, Vinci R, Cabral H. Jitteriness in full-term neonates: prevalence and correlates. *Pediatrics* 1990;85:17.
80. Jorgenson RJ, Shapiro SD, Salinas CF, Levin LS. Intraoral findings and anomalies in neonates. *Pediatrics* 1982;69:577.
81. Levin LS, Jorgenson RJ, Jarvey BA. Lymphangiomas of the alveolar ridges in neonates. *Pediatrics* 1976;58:881.
82. Fromm A. Epstein's pearls, Bohn's nodules and inclusion-cysts of the oral cavity. *J Dent Child* 1967;34:275.
83. King NM, Lee AMP. Prematurely erupted teeth in newborn infants. *J Pediatr* 1989;114:807.
84. Leung AKC. Natal teeth. *Am J Dis Child* 1986;140:249.
85. Johnson GL. Clinical examination. In: Long WA, ed. *Fetal and neonatal cardiology.* Philadelphia: WB Saunders, 1990:223.
86. Braudo M, Rowe RD. Auscultation of the heart—early neonatal period. *Am J Dis Child* 1961;101:575.
87. Flatau E, Josefsberg Z, Reisner SH, Bialik O, Laron Z. Penile size in the newborn infant. *J Pediatr* 1975;87:663.
88. Reisner SH, Sivan Y, Nitzan M, Merlob P. Determination of anterior displacement of the anus in newborn infants and children. *Pediatrics* 1984;73:216.

CHAPTER 20

Behavioral Competence

T. Berry Brazelton

It is important to assess the neonate's contribution to his or her new environment. The parents' inclination is to nurture newborns and to value their reactions to handling, voice, and vision; it is belittling to these reactions if physicians do not value them similarly. If we as physicians attend to them by changing neonatal nurseries and lying-in arrangements to value and capture the neonate's best periods of alert responsiveness, we place a stamp of approval on the parents' attention to their neonate and on the newborn as an important, interactive person from the start. As physicians, we are providing new, confused parents with a way of communicating with their infants and showing them that the neonate can lead them when they are confused.

The demands of a complex, undirected society, coupled with the lack of support of new parents in our nuclear family system, leave most parents insecure and at the mercy of tremendous internal and external pressures. They have been told that their infant's outcome will be shaped by their parenting, but there are few stable cultural values on which they can rely for guidance in setting their course as new parents.

This neonatal period offers us as professionals interested in the child and family a rare opportunity for support and guidance. An infant is not as helpless as he or she appears to be. The infant comes well equipped to signal his or her needs and gratitude, can make choices about what to accept from his parents, and can shut out what is not wanted in effective ways. The infant can be seen as a powerful force, stabilizing and influencing those around him or her.

Compared with newborns of other species, the human neonate is relatively helpless in motor capabilities and relatively precocious in sensory capabilities. This creates a motor dependence and a freedom for acquisition of the

T. B. Brazelton: Department of Pediatrics, Harvard Medical School, Cambridge; and Department of Pediatrics, Children's Hospital, Boston, Massachusetts

many patterns of sensory and affective information that are necessary for the child and adult human to master and survive in a complex world.

It is important to evaluate infants at risk as early as possible to permit the use of sophisticated preventive and therapeutic approaches when they can offer the most benefit. Premature and minimally brain-damaged infants seem to be less able to compensate in disorganized, depriving environments than well-equipped neonates, and the problems of the compromised infants with organization in development are compounded early (1). If we are to improve the outcome for these children, assessment of the risk in early infancy should mobilize preventive efforts and programs for intervention (2).

We need more sophisticated methods of assessing neonates and of predicting their role in the possible failure of the environment–infant interaction. We need to be able to assess at-risk environments, because the scarcity of resources requires the selection of target populations for our efforts at early intervention. Minimally brain-damaged babies do make remarkable compensatory recoveries in a fostering environment (3).

The behavioral responses of the neonate can be used to understand the organization of the central and autonomic nervous systems at birth. The individual differences in neonatal behaviors reflect the variations in genetic endowment and intrauterine influences. As the neonate responds to labor, delivery, and recovery in the new environment, we can begin to predict how new experiences and learning will affect him or her and how the infant will interact with the new environment.

NEONATAL BEHAVIORAL ASSESSMENT SCALE

To record and evaluate some of the integrative processes in neonatal behavior, my colleagues and I developed a behavioral evaluation scale that tests and documents the infant's changing state of consciousness and responses to various kinds of stimulation. The Neonatal Behavioral Assessment Scale (NBAS, Brazelton scale) was first published in 1973 (4). After modifications, the experiences of 20 years were summarized in an edition in 1995. Twenty centers and several hundred trained observers contributed to the revised edition. The NBAS is in use in more than 600 locations. Training centers have been established in the United States, Europe, Asia, and South America, and more than 540 published studies have appeared within the United States and in cross-cultural contexts (5,6).

Conceptual Base

The original goal for the NBAS was to record the dimensions of state—autonomic, motor, sensory-receptive, and responsive—that were integrative and interactive with each other in the normal, healthy, full-term infant. The NBAS was seen not as a set of discrete stimulus–response presentations but was considered to be an interactive assessment in which the adult participant played a major role, facilitating the performance and organizational skills of the infant. We hoped to establish the infant's capacities for and limits in contributing to the caregiving environment. We expected to gain a deeper understanding of the meaning of infant behavior as it reflected the relative contribution of these developments. We conceived of a single assessment in the neonatal period as only one brief glimpse into the continuum of the infant's adjustment to labor, delivery, and the new environment. The test was expected to reflect the infant's inborn characteristics and the behavioral responses that had been shaped by the intrauterine environment. We hoped repeated examinations would demonstrate the infant's coping capacities and capacities for using his or her inner organization to experience, integrate, and profit developmentally from the environment's stimulation. We thought that serial examinations would reflect the interaction between the infant's inborn characteristics and the shaping of them in the first few weeks (7).

As we worked with the NBAS, several issues became clear. An assessment of the newborn presents an opportunity for looking forward into the baby's future and backward into the intrauterine experience. The intrauterine influences that shape newborn behavior are becoming more commonly recognized. The newborn's behavior at birth is phenotypic and genotypic, reflecting complex behaviors that are shaped by influences *in utero* that probably act in a synergistic fashion.

Any interpretation of reactions must be made with the understanding that the neonate's reactions to all stimuli depend on his or her ongoing state of consciousness. The infant's use of state to maintain control of reactions to environmental and internal stimuli is an important capacity and reflects his or her potential for organization. State no longer need be treated as an error variable; it instead

sets a dynamic pattern to allow for the full behavioral repertoire of the infant. The NBAS tracks changes in state over the course of the examination and the lability and direction of these changes. The variability of state indicates the infant's capacities for self-organization; the child's ability to quiet himself and need for stimulation measure this adequacy.

The behavioral examination tests for neurologic adequacy with 20 reflex measures and for 28 behavioral responses to environmental stimuli, including the kind of interpersonal stimuli that mothers use in handling their infants. Best performance is accepted to overcome variability. In the examination, there is a graded series of procedures (e.g., talking, hand on belly, restraint, holding, rocking) designed to soothe or alert the infant. His or her responsiveness to animate stimuli (e.g., voice, face) and to inanimate stimuli (e.g., rattle, bell, red ball, white light, temperature change) is assessed. Estimates of vigor and attentional excitement are measured, and an assessment is made of motor activity, tone, and autonomic responsiveness as the infant changes state. In addition, criteria to include three quantitative concepts have been added: cost to the neonate of the assessment, cost to the examiner of eliciting best performance, and quality of best performance.

With this examination, given on successive days, we have been able to outline the initial period of alertness immediately after delivery, the period of depression and disorganization that follows, and the curve of recovery to optimal function after several days. The period of depression and disorganization lasts 24 to 48 hours in infants with uncomplicated deliveries and no medication effects, but it persists for 3 to 4 days in infants compromised by medications given during the delivery. The curve of recovery may be the best single early predictor of individual potential function, and it seems to correlate well with the neonate's ability on retest at 30 days (7).

Content

The revised NBAS assesses the newborn's behavioral repertoire on 28 behavioral items, each scored on a nine-point scale. The NBAS measures the coping capacities and the adaptive strategies of the infant that emerge during recovery from the stresses of labor and delivery and adjustment to the demands of the extrauterine environment. This process of adaptation can be measured by studying patterns of change, called profile or recovery curves, over repeated Brazelton-type examinations.

The following items constitute the NBAS (5,6). The numbers in parentheses refer to the optimal state for assessment, which are defined in the next section of this chapter.

Response decrement to repeated visual stimuli, such as light (1,2,3)
Response decrement to rattle (1,2,3)
Response decrement to bell (1,2,3)

Response decrement to tactile stimulation of the foot, such as a pinprick (1,2,3)

Orienting response to inanimate visual stimuli (4,5)

Orienting response to inanimate auditory stimuli (4,5)

Orienting response to inanimate visual and auditory stimuli (4,5)

Orienting response to animate visual stimuli, such as the examiner's face (4,5)

Orienting response to animate auditory stimuli, such as the examiner's voice (4,5)

Orienting response to animate visual and auditory stimuli (4,5)

Quality and duration of alert periods (4,5)

General muscle tone in resting and in response to being handled passively and actively (4,5)

Motor maturity (4,5)

Traction responses such as a pull-to-sit maneuver (4,5)

Cuddliness—responses to being cuddled by examiner (4,5)

Defensive movements—reactions to a cloth over the infant's face (3,4,5)

Consolability with intervention of examiner (6 to 4,3,2)

Peak of excitement and infant's capacity to control self (all states)

Rapidity of buildup to crying state (all states)

Irritability during the examination (all awake states)

General assessment of kind and degree of activity (alert states)

Tremulousness (all states)

Amount of startle (3,4,5,6)

Lability of skin color for measuring autonomic lability (from 1 to 6)

Lability of states during entire examination (all states)

Self-quieting activity—attempts to console self and control state (6 to 4,3,2,1)

Hand-to-mouth facility (all states)

Smiles (all states).

To be able to assess these patterns of change, at least two but preferably three or more examinations are needed for each infant. The first should be done on days 2 or 3, after the immediate stresses of labor and delivery have begun to wear off. The next examination is best performed at 7 to 14 days, and the third can be done at 1 month. Scores from the successive examinations establish a behavioral pattern of change over the first weeks of life. This pattern may be the most important measure for predicting later developmental outcome.

I believe that the behavioral items elicit important evidences of cortical control and responsiveness, even in the neonatal period. The neonate's capacity to manage and overcome the physiologic demands of this adjustment period to attend to, differentiate, and habituate to the complex stimuli of an examiner's maneuvers may be an important predictor of the baby's future central nervous system (CNS) organization. The curve of recovery of these responses during the first neonatal month is of more significance than the midbrain responses detectable in routine neurologic examinations.

Included in this examination are behavioral tests of important CNS mechanisms such as habituation or the neonate's capacity to shut out disturbing or overwhelming stimuli; choices in attention to various objects or human stimuli (i.e., a neonate shows clear preferences for female rather than male voices and for human rather than non-human visual stimuli); and control of the neonate's state to attend to information from the environment (e.g., effort to complete a hand-to-mouth cycle to attend to objects and people around him or her). All of these mechanisms are evidenced in the neonate, even in the premature infant, and are more predictive of CNS intactness than reflex responses (8).

Assessment of Behavioral States

There are predictable, directed responses from a neonate interacting socially with a nurturing adult or responding to an attractive auditory or visual stimulus. If positive rather than intrusive stimuli are used, the neonate has amazing capacities for alerting and attention and for suppressing interfering reflex responses to attend, and, with predictable behaviors, the infant responds to and interacts with his or her environment from birth (6). However, this predictability requires a knowledge of his or her ongoing state of consciousness (9). State of consciousness, or the "state" of the infant, becomes a most important matrix for interpreting neonatal behavior. The infant's reactions to all stimuli, internal and external, depend on his ongoing state of consciousness. With state used as a matrix, behavioral responses become quite predictable.

State depends on physiologic variables, such as hunger, nutrition, degree of hydration, and the timing within the wake–sleep cycle of the infant. Our criteria for state throughout this chapter are based on the descriptions by Prechtl and Beintema (9). If state is accounted for, most of the infant's reactions to negative and positive stimuli from internal and external sources are predictable. State becomes a matrix for understanding reactions. It qualifies stimulation as appropriate or inappropriate to the infant's organization. For almost any maturational level, the behavior produced by appropriate stimuli in appropriate states can demonstrate the complexity of an intact and adaptable CNS.

The matrix of state as a concept for organization in the neonate has become important since its use as a background for neurologic responses in Prechtl's assessment (9). Within the context of the optimal state of alertness, Prechtl and Dykstra (10) were able to demonstrate that the newborn could show better reflexive behavior and that the neurologic examination became a better predictive measure.

If the sleeping or awake state of the baby is accounted for, an experienced examiner can make a fairly accurate prediction of how a baby will respond to any given stimulus. For example, within a deep sleep state, a baby responds slightly to a moderately loud, brief rattle; although breathing changes and blinking may occur, the child probably stirs very little. In lighter sleep, the infant may startle, may begin to rouse, and his or her face may become alert, with his or her respiratory patterns changing markedly. In a state between sleep and awake, the infant probably startles briefly, but the startle is followed by a slower movement of the arms and legs and a writhing of the trunk, and the child will open his or her eyes to look dully for the next stimulus. In a semi-alert state, the neonate becomes more alert, begins to move about, and may even search for the rattle, with respirations becoming slower and more regular. In a wide-awake state, a newborn infant often becomes quiet, looks surprised, but remains wide awake and alert; the child shifts his or her eyes and then head to turn toward the rattle as if searching for it. Unless it is a very loud or insistent rattle, he may not stop crying to respond to the sound when in a crying state. The state of arousal is a matrix for predictable responses and is the infant's way of defending himself or herself from the world around him or her in the case of sleep states and of controlling arousal to attend to the environment in waking states. The parameters of state are relatively easy to determine by simple observation (11). The categories of behavioral states are listed with their criteria for definition.

Quiet Sleep. The infant's eyes are firmly closed and still. There is little or no motor activity, with the exception of occasional startles or rhythmic mouthing. Respiration is abdominal and relatively slow (average, 36 breaths/min), deep, and regular.

Active Sleep with Rapid Eye Movements. The infant's eyes are closed, and rapid eye movements (REMs) occur during a 10-second interval. Body activity can range from minor twitches to writhing and stretching. Respiration is irregular, costal, and generally faster than that seen in quiet sleep (average, 46 breaths/min). Facial movements may include frowns, grimaces, smiles, twitches, mouth movements, and sucking, although face movements are not seen often this category of active sleep.

Drowsy State. The infant's eyes may open and close or may be partially or fully open, but they are still and appear dazed. There may be some generalized motor activity, and respiration is fairly regular, but it is faster and more shallow than that observed in regular sleep.

Alert Inactivity. The infant's body and face are relatively quiet and inactive, and the eyes appear bright and shining.

Fussing. The characteristics of this state are the same as those for alert inactivity, but mild, agitated vocalizations are continuous, or one cry burst may occur.

Crying. The characteristics of this state are the same as those for alert inactivity, but generalized motor activity is more intense, and cry bursts are continuous.

Sleep Cycles

The length of sleep cycles (i.e., active REM and quiet sleep) changes normally with maturation of the CNS. Term infants have regular cycles of 45 to 50 minutes, but immature babies have shorter, less well-defined cycles. Newborn infants have as much active REM sleep in the first half of the deep period as in the second half. Initially, brief sleep and wake patterns coalesce as the environment presses the neonate to develop diurnal patterns of daytime wakefulness and night sleep (11,12). Appropriate feeding patterns, diet, absence of excessive parental anxiety, sufficient nurturing stimulation, and a fussing period before a long sleep have been implicated as reinforcing the CNS maturation necessary for the development of diurnal cycling of sleep and wakefulness.

Anders (13) suggests that REM sleep is regulated by brain stem mechanisms that constitute an autoregulating and stimulating system of the CNS. This state contributes to the growth and maintenance of neural tissue by cyclic excitatory activation of developing neuronal structures, which increases their differentiation. Without well-differentiated REM cycles, the neurophysiologic structures may be delayed in their development of differential responses. In immature organisms or neonates whose brain stems have been stressed by anoxia, maternal drugs, or other disorganizing factors, delays in differentiation of sleep states can be expected, and these infants may be at risk for prolonged CNS disorganization. Steinschneider (14) suggested that this kind of sleep disorganization may be a predictor for the apneic attacks found in sudden infant death syndrome.

Crying

Crying serves many purposes in the neonate, not the least of which is to shut out painful or disturbing stimuli. Hunger and pain are responded to with crying, which brings the caretaker to the infant. There is a kind of fussy crying that occurs periodically throughout the day, usually in a cyclic fashion, which seems to act as a discharger of energy and an organizer of the states that ensue (15). After a period of fussy crying, the neonate may be more alert, and he or she may sleep more deeply.

Crying seems to be an important behavior for organizing the day and for reducing disturbance within the CNS in the neonatal period. Most parents can differentiate cries of pain, hunger, and fussiness after 2 to 3 weeks and learn quickly to respond appropriately (16). The cry is of ethologic significance for eliciting appropriate care for the infant.

Studies of the cry patterns of infants with various clinical syndromes or diseases suggest that there are cry features that differentiate damaged or sick infants from healthy controls (17). The cry can be used to aid the differential diagnosis of certain diseases. Down syndrome is associated with a low-pitched, hoarse, guttural cry; a higher threshold for the production of the cry; and a longer latency from stimulation to cry onset. Infants with cri du chat syndrome and those with trisomy 13 have a fundamental frequency that is high pitched, averaging 850 Hz, in contrast to the range of 400 to 600 Hz in healthy infants.

Lester (18) found that malnourished infants had a longer cry duration, longer cry latency, higher fundamental frequency, lower amplitude of the fundamental frequency, and fewer harmonics than well-nourished infants.

SENSORY CAPACITIES

Visual Capacity

The newborn is equipped at birth with the capacity for processing complex visual information and for demonstrating ocular movements to track an object in space. Even more important to the newborn's survival is the fact that she can defend herself from visual stimuli that may otherwise force her to make excessive demands on her immature physiologic system. When a bright light is flashed into a neonate's eyes, the pupils constrict, she blinks, her eyelids and whole face contract, and she withdraws her head by arching her whole body, often setting off a complete startle as she withdraws. Her heart rate and respirations increase, and there is an evoked response registered on her visual occipital electroencephalogram (EEG).

Repeated stimulation of this nature induces diminishing responses because of the infant's capacity to shut down responses. For example, in a series of 20 bright-light stimuli presented at 1-minute intervals, we found that the infant rapidly habituated and damped out the behavioral responses (15). By the tenth stimulus, he had decreased not only his observable motor responses but also his cardiac and respiratory responses. The latency to evoked responses, as measured by EEG tracings, was increasing, and by the fifteenth stimulus, the EEG reflected the induction of a quiet, unresponsive behavioral state accompanied by trace alternans and spindles. The infant's capacity to shut out repetitious, disturbing visual stimuli protects him from having to respond to visual stimulation and frees his energy to meet physiologic demands. This capacity of the neonate has been considered a kind of neurologic habituation and is present in neonates with intact CNSs (19). The capacity to habituate to visual stimuli is decreased in immature infants (20). It is affected by medication such as barbiturates given to mothers as premedication at the time of delivery. This led Brazier (21) to postulate that the primary focus for this mechanism is in the reticular formation and midbrain. The infant finally becomes deeply asleep with tightened, flexed extremities; has little movement except jerky startles; produces no eye blinks; has deep, regular respirations; and has a rapid, regular heart rate. This state of habituation seems to signal a defensive state against the assaults of the environment.

Any newborn baby in a bright, noisy nursery is likely to be in such a habituated state. She is unlikely to be responsive to loud noises or a flashlight if they are used as test stimuli, and testing her vision or hearing would require moving her to a darker, quieter room, where complex visual responses can be captured more easily and reliably. The only justification that I can find for those who claim that newborns cannot see or do not respond with real behavioral preference to various visual stimuli is that they have tested the infants in overlighted, inappropriate settings.

Just as he is equipped with the capacity to shut out certain stimuli, the newborn demonstrates the capacity to alert to, turn his eyes and head to follow, and fix on a stimulus that appeals to him. Fantz (22) first pointed out neonatal preference for certain kinds of complex visual stimuli. He found that sharply contrasting colors, larger squares, and medium-bright objects were appealing to the neonate and brought him to a prolonged, alert state of fixation. Fantz and others found that the neonate preferred an ovoid object and one in which there were eyes and a mouth. The kind of attention and the length of fixation were reduced markedly if mothers had been medicated before delivery.

Goren et al. (23) showed that, immediately after delivery, a human neonate would fix on a drawing that resembled a human face and follow it, with eyes and head turning for 180 degrees. A scrambled face did not demand the same kind of attention, nor did the infant completely follow the distorted face with her eyes and head; the head turned to follow only one-half of the arc. My colleagues and I found that the capacity of neonates to fix on and follow a red ball was a good predictive sign of neurologic integrity (24). However, its absence is not a serious predictor, because it depends on whether the infant is in an alert state. Many conditions interfere with the neonate's capacity to come to an alert state: the CNS depression that follows delivery, hypoxia or any of the stresses of delivery, premedication given to the mother, transient effects of metabolic derangement or illness in the neonate, and normal conditions of hunger, fatigue, and an overly bright nursery. Newborns are capable of visual fixing and following during alert periods, and this may be a sensitive predictor of neurologic and visual integrity (8).

Visual acuity of the newborn is still difficult to determine. Gorman and colleagues (25) used the neonate's opticokinetic responses to a moving drum lined with stripes and found that 93 of 100 infants responded preferentially to stripes subtending a visual range of only 33.5 minutes of arc. We found that premature infants were less reliable but also could fix on and follow the same lined drum (24). Dayton and coworkers (26) found at least 20/150 vision in newborns by this same technique. Rather than being able to accommodate well, the infants have a fixed focal length of about 19 cm (27). To capture visual interest, an examiner must present a bright object at this distance.

In one long-term study, Sigman and associates (28) found that visual behavior may be one of the best predictors of an intact CNS in the neonate. They found that summary scores on the neonate's neurologic examination were significantly related to the length of first fixation on a black-and-white checkerboard as a visual stimulus. This capacity to stare at a complex object was related to an alert state, and, if infants could not be brought to such a state, the prediction was more ominous. The optimal response to visual stimulation in a neonate can be described as an initial alerting, attention that increases but that is followed by a gradual decrease in interest, and a final turning away from a monotonous presentation.

Several observers demonstrated that neonates prefer moving and somewhat complex visual patterns to stationary ones (29). If the moving object can be moved slowly parallel to the natural, lateral movements of the eyes, it is more likely to capture the baby's interest. The duration and degree of his attention may be correlated with a middle range of complexity and the similarity of the target to the ovoid shape and the structures of the human face.

Auditory Capacity

The neonate's auditory responses are specific and well organized. Assessments often are not sensitive to the complexity of the newborn's behavior. For example, the loud clackers used on the Collaborative Project of the National Institute of Neurological Diseases and Blindness for early detection of CNS defects were ineffective in loud, noisy nurseries. A large percentage of the neonates tested in the first 3 days with this routine were unresponsive; they appeared to have shut out or habituated to the ambient auditory stimuli. Another approach under these conditions would have been to use a soft rattle in a quiet setting.

In response to an interesting auditory stimulus, such as a rattle, the infant moves from a sleeping state to an alert state. His breathing becomes irregular, his face brightens, and his eyes open, and, when he is completely alert, his eyes and head turn toward the sound. In the case of a well-organized neonate, head turning is followed by a searching look on his face and scanning with his eyes to find a source for the auditory stimulus. To find out whether the neonate can respond this way, a full test of hearing should include several stimuli, animate and inanimate, with careful attention to the neonate's ongoing state of consciousness to ensure that the test breaks into his state.

Eisenberg (30) determined the differential responses to different ranges of sound that are available to the infant. In the range of human speech (i.e., 500 to 900 Hz), the neonate inhibits motor behavior. She often demonstrates cardiac deceleration as evidence of attention and orients with head turning toward the source of sound. Outside this human range, there is a less complex behavioral response. The strikingly narrow range of stimuli for positive, attending responses can be demonstrated by linking devices for recording sucking to the auditory input (31). Within this narrow human range, sucking ceases as an initial response to the stimulus and is followed by a burst–pause pattern of sucking, as if the infant is pausing to receive more of the interesting auditory input.

Various frequencies and intensities have different functional properties. High-frequency signals above 4,000 Hz are more effective in producing a response, even in crying or sleep states, but they are likely to produce distress. Signals at lower intensities (e.g., 35 to 40 dB) are effective inhibitors of distress, especially as continuous white noise (32). White noise at these levels eventually induces a sleep state, even in a crying neonate. Kearsley (33) demonstrated the importance of the rise time of the sound on the neonate's behavioral response. Sounds with prolonged onset times and low frequencies produced eye opening and cardiac deceleration followed by an attentive look, and sounds with rapid onset and high frequency produced eye closing, cardiac acceleration, increased head movements, and aversion.

There is a series of regular steps in the neonate's behavioral response to an appropriate sound. As the sound is located, the cardiac rate increases and may be accompanied by a mild startle. If the auditory stimulus is attractive to the infant, his face brightens, his heart rate decelerates, his breathing slows, and he becomes alert and searches with his eyes until the source of the sound is localized to the en face midline of the baby. This behavior, which occurs as a response to an attractive auditory stimulus (e.g., rattle, human voice), becomes a measure of the neonate's capacity to organize his central and autonomic nervous systems.

Habituation to repeated auditory stimuli becomes a further test of CNS function. If there is a damaged cortex, behavioral inhibition is not likely to occur. Bronstein and Petrova (34) found that 2-hour-old to 8-day-old infants ceased sucking on a pacifier initially, but after repeated sounds of 60 to 70 dB, they resumed sucking. Bridger (35) found that the heart rate acceleration as an initial response to an auditory stimulus ceased after several trials, and the baby essentially habituated behaviorally and autonomically to this repetitive stimulus. However, a change in frequency or a tonal change brought about an immediate increase in motor activity and a change in heart rate; this reaction represents dishabituation. Cardiac response can be used to study the infant's mental organization for repetitive, novel, and contingent responses.

Cairns and Butterfield (36) documented the differences in the neonate's responses to human or nonhuman sounds by using a sucking paradigm to detect subtle information-processing differences. They believe that monitoring for a burst–pause pattern in sucking as one changes auditory stimuli can differentiate between CNS impairments of receptive processing from the kind of peripheral impairment that is found in nerve deafness of rubella, congenital malformations, hyperbilirubinemia, and other disorders.

Olfactory Capacity

Engen and associates (37) demonstrated observable differentiated responses to odors in the neonate, concluding that the newborn is designed with a highly equipped sense of smell, ready to pick up the odors that help her adapt to her new world. For example, she acts offended by acetic acid, asafetida, and alcohol in the neonatal period but is attracted to sweet odors of milk and sugary solutions. MacFarlane (38) showed that 5-day-old neonates can reliably differentiate their own mothers' breast pads from those of other lactating mothers, although this power of discrimination was not present at 2 days of age. They turn their heads toward their own mothers' breast pads with 80% reliability after controls for laterality are imposed. The neonate perceives the odor of her mother as a learned response by the fifth day.

Taste Capacity

The newborn has fine differential responses to taste. Pratt and colleagues (39) observed different sucking responses to sugar and decreased sucking to other tastes. Johnson and Salisbury (40) reported that a newborn's taste preferences are expressed in an even more complex fashion. An infant is fed different fluids through a monitored nipple, and his sucking pattern is recorded. Saline causes such resistance that the baby is likely to aspirate. With a cow-milk formula, he will suck in a rather continuous fashion, pausing at irregular intervals. If breast milk then is fed to him by this same system, he will register his recognition of the change in taste after a short latency, and then suck in bursts with frequent pauses at regular intervals. The pauses seem to be directly related to the taste of breast milk, and his burst–pause pattern seems to indicate that he changes to a program for other stimuli (e.g., social communication) to be added to the feeding situation during the pauses.

Procedures for recording various parameters of sucking behavior have documented the fine discriminations that infants make (41). A suck apparatus connected to a polygraph has been used for recording the infant's sucking behavior under conditions in which the presentation of drops of fluid is contingent on that behavior. When sucking on a blank nipple, the infant sucks in short bursts separated by long pauses, and sucking within those bursts is quite rapid. When a sweet fluid (e.g., 15% sucrose) is delivered contingent on sucking, the infant engages in more sucks per minute, invests more sucks per burst, takes shorter rest periods, and sucks more slowly within each sucking burst. Moreover, these parameters are affected by sweetness along a continuum from 0% through 15% sucrose and by the amount of fluid received per suck (42). With increasing concentrations or increasing amounts of sucrose , infants tend to suck more slowly within bursts.

Sensitivity to Tactile Stimuli

The sensitivity of the infant to handling and to touch is apparent. A mother's first response to an upset baby is to contain him, to shut down his disturbing motor activity by touching or holding him. Fathers are more likely to tap in a playful, rhythmic fashion or to use tactile methods to excite the infant. Touch becomes a message system between the caregiver and the infant, for calming him and for exciting him to attend to cues. A patting motion of three times per second is soothing, but five to six times per second becomes an alerting stimulus (43). As with auditory stimuli, the law of initial values seems to be important. When a baby is quiet, a rapid, intrusive tactile stimulus brings him up to an alert state. When he is upset, a slow, modulated tactile stimulus seems to reduce his activity.

Swaddling is used in many cultures to replace the important constraints offered first by the uterus and then by mothers and caretakers. As a restraining influence on the overreactions of hyperactive neonates, the supportive control that is offered by a steady hand on a baby's abdomen or by holding his arms so that he cannot startle reproduces the swaddling effects of holding or wrapping. This added control of disturbing motor responses allows the neonate to attend and interact with his environment.

If an infant cannot use soothing tactile stimuli to help him adapt his state behavior, the physician must consider a diagnosis of CNS irritability. A baby with CNS irritation from a bleed or from infection demonstrates constantly increasing irritability with stimuli, especially tactile. This response should signal the examiner to investigate the infant further for evidence of CNS difficulties.

Sucking Capacity

An awake, hungry newborn exhibits active searching movements in response to tactile stimulation in the region around the mouth and even as far out on the face as the cheek and sides of the jaw and head. This is called the rooting reflex, and it is present in premature infants even before sucking itself is effective. Peiper (44) described oral pads in the cheeks and mouth, which help maintain and establish negative pressure. Sucking is facilitated by the thorax in inspiration and by fixing the jaw to maintain it between respirations. A second mechanism, expressing, is made by the tongue as it moves up against the hard palate and from the front to the back of the mouth. Swallowing and respirations must be coordinated, and the depth and rate of respiration are handled differently in nutritive and nonnutritive sucking. Peiper argues for a hierarchic control of swallowing, sucking, and breathing, in which swallowing controls sucking and sucking controls breathing. The absence of coordination between these three systems in the neonate indicates discoordination within the CNS, which may occur in damaged or very immature infants.

Gryboski (45) described a technique of monitoring three components of sucking with three transducers: a lapping mechanism at the front of the tongue, a milking action at the base of the tongue, and a suction component in the upper esophagus. The timing of the three components becomes a measure of the maturity of the CNS of a premature infant. There is a latency before they become coordinated in an effective milking mechanism; the more prolonged the latency, the more immature is the baby. The examiner can feel these three components by placing a finger in the baby's mouth. A nurse who is familiar with premature infants can tell whether they are coordinated. If there is CNS irritation, the examiner can feel the disruption of the central processes that control these mechanisms by inserting a finger into the neonate's mouth, and, when the infant is sucking, an examiner can determine for himself the presence and coordination of the three components. This is an easily available and valuable measure of the infant's stage of relative maturity and of his CNS coordination.

The infant sucks in a more or less regular pattern of bursts and pauses, with 5 to 24 sucks per burst (46). The pause between bursts has been considered a rest and recovery period, and a period during which cognitive information is being processed by the neonate. Kaye and Brazelton (47) found that the pauses were important ethologically, because they are taken by mothers as signals to stimulate the infant to return to sucking. Mothers tend to look down at, talk to, and stimulate a baby when he pauses in a sucking burst. The mother's jiggling actually prolongs the pause as the infant responds to the stimulating information given to him by his mother.

Sucking, because of the stability produced through central control early in gestation, is used by researchers to measure all sorts of behaviors in infants: sensory discrimination, conditioning, learning, orienting, and attention (31,46,48) The importance of sucking as a way of

self-regulation can be seen in a newborn as she begins to build from a quiet state to crying. Her attempts to achieve hand-to-mouth contact to keep her activity under control are fascinating. When she finally is able to insert a finger into her mouth, suck on it, and quiet herself, she seems rewarded. The sense of satisfaction and of gratification at having achieved this self-regulation are so striking that the watching adult can see that she has achieved a goal. Her face softens and alerts as she begins to concentrate on maintaining this kind of self-regulation. This is the most obvious evidence that the baby has goal-oriented behaviors that she can achieve for herself. A pacifier can achieve this same quieting in an upset baby, but a pacifier may not serve the self-regulating feedback system as richly as the baby's own maneuver.

Pairing sucking with other auditory, visual, or tactile modalities has been neglected in most neonatal nurseries. The variations and complexity of this system as it reflects CNS functions are well studied by psychologists and psychophysiologists (49). For example, Cairns and Butterfield (36) found that a neonate sucking on a nonnutritive pacifier presented a rich set of responses to human and nonhuman auditory signals. After hearing a human voice, he would increase his sucking rate as a signal to bring it on again, and he could be conditioned in 20 minutes to suck harder or to pause to produce a second vocal signal. However, with white noise or pure-tone (i.e., nonhuman) signals, he sucks less hard after the signal and learns to suck only to reduce the noise, not to repeat it or increase it.

If a human vocal sound was introduced to a neonate who was monitored by a nonnutritive pacifier, he began to produce a burst–pause pattern with prolonged pauses, as if he were waiting for the human signals to repeat themselves. Cairns and Butterfield (36) suggest that pairing nonnutritive sucking with auditory stimulation can differentiate forms of CNS difficulty by the ability of the neonate to discriminate between paired signals that differ only in this way (i.e., human vs. nonhuman). Cairn's group has been able to discriminate between the central and peripheral forms of impairment in auditory receptiveness that are the residua of rubella, hyperbilirubinemia, prematurity, and hypoxia.

Pairing two separate modalities of CNS function, such as sucking and sensory receptors, to test for fine discrimination tasks, for habituation and dishabituation to repetitive signals, and for conditioning and learning tasks suggests innovative methods for evaluating the neonate's CNS function.

ORGANIZATION OF MOTOR BEHAVIOR

One of the most neglected and illuminating sources of information about a neonate's status is gathered from simple observation of how he moves his extremities, what kind of movements he makes, and whether his movements are simple, random startles, or purposeful. One of the most exciting behaviors that can be observed in the neonatal period is demonstrated by a well-organized newborn. As he begins to rouse from sleeping and when he begins to startle and become upset, he may attempt to bring his hand up to his mouth. In this effort, he may turn his head to one side, immediately controlling one side of his body by the central monitoring effects of the tonic neck reflex. The face and arm first extend and then slow down in extension. An observer can see the infant work to bring his hand up to his mouth. The infant's body begins to relax, his face softens, and he makes real efforts to insert his clenched fist. If these efforts are successful, he maintains a quiet state of semialertness, sucking loudly on the fist. Even if he cannot insert the hand or a finger, he remains in a rewarded peaceful state, ready to listen to a sound or look at a presenting stimulus. He has demonstrated to the observer that he can achieve a complex motor act by shutting out interfering reflex startles, completing a cycle of lateralizing his motor energy by bringing his hand up to his mouth, and using this activity to maintain a quiet and alert state, receptive to information from the environment. This complex behavior embedded in the goal-oriented achievement of wanting to listen or to look is powerful evidence of optimal CNS organization in the neonate.

When this behavioral organization is not observed in a particular interval, does it mean that the neonate cannot perform well? Not necessarily. Several conditions influence her performance:

Ongoing state of arousal; if the child is too deeply asleep or too upset during an observation period, the likelihood of detecting organized behavior is reduced
Environmental conditions (e.g., too low or too high temperature, sound or light levels that reduce the child to a relative shutout state)
Ongoing chemical or humoral imbalances (e.g., mild dehydration, hypocalcemia, hypoglycemia), which render the child hypersensitive and jittery or too sleepy
State of well-being (i.e., illness, stress); relative motor disorganization may be a primary symptom of an impending illness
Degree of recovery from the stresses of labor and delivery
Perinatal stresses (e.g., hypoxia, maternal medication).

Disorganization of motor activity may become an important symptom of stress in a neonate and should be assessed carefully. Repeated examinations as she recovers over the neonatal period are essential.There are maneuvers that should be used for assessment of muscle tone and the balance of flexor and extensor muscles. The range that is possible for a given baby may be more important than any one sample of motor performance. The resting, spontaneous posture gives an idea of the preferred position. A normal full-term baby spontaneously prefers a position of flexion for both arms and legs. His extremities may extend from time to time, but he usually is found in flexed postures.

A baby who lies in full extension may be hypotonic. Hypertonicity is signaled by tightly flexed extremities with few spontaneous movements except brief, jerky startles. The examiner can determine in the first few minutes the most likely category to which the baby will be assigned. A few simple passive maneuvers of extending then flexing arms, legs, neck, and trunk confirm the degree of hypertonicity or hypotonicity. Hypertonicity is accompanied by jerky snapback of extremities or overshooting into tight flexion after the limbs are released. Hypotonicity is signaled by floppy, hyperextensive limbs, with little resistance or spontaneous movement after they are released. Organized reflex motor responses (i.e., motor stepping, placing, and prone responses; crawling movements and attempts to lift the head; traction of the neck and shoulder; girdle musculature in a pull-to-sit maneuver) confirm and elaborate the infant's motor strength and the balance between flexor and extensor groups. Jerky, clonic movements and the snapback point to an imbalance of flexor and extensor muscle groups. Smooth movements of a neonate are an indicator of good balance between these groups and reveal a well-organized CNS.

Defensive reactions to a cloth over the face or to a painful stimulus to any part of the body elicit structured motor patterns, and the baby's effectiveness in approaching and removing an obtrusive stimulus becomes a way of testing intact motor pathways and their organization. For example, covering his face with a cloth elicits a series of motor maneuvers. He first roots, then twists his head from side to side, stretches his neck backward in active arching, and finally brings each arm up to swipe at the offending cloth. Many newborns effectively push the cloth off the face. These responses (e.g., hand-to-mouth, defensive movements, other sequential motor acts) may be of equal value as elicited reflexes in assessing the upper extremities for neurologic adequacy.

LEARNING IN THE NEONATAL PERIOD

Because the neonate is equipped with remarkable capacities for responsiveness, we can improve assessments of CNS integrity at birth. Static neurologic assessments have not been particularly fruitful in predicting future function. Perhaps a model of assessment based on his capacity to use stimulation from the environment would offer us a better chance for predicting outcome.

Classic Conditioning

One of the most obvious signs of newborn learning can be seen by use of classic conditioning techniques, in which the infant is presented with a neutral stimulus (i.e., conditioning stimulus) in association with a stimulus effective in eliciting an observable response (i.e., unconditioned stimulus). Over a series of presentations in which the stimuli are paired, the neutral stimulus comes to elicit the response under investigation and demonstrates the infant's capacity to retain these associations. Denisova and Figurin (50) first demonstrated that newborns could be conditioned by being placed in the feeding position to which they had become accustomed. After only a few days, they exhibited anticipatory sucking movements.

Lipsitt and Kaye (51) used the presentation of a low-frequency, 93-dB tone in association with the insertion of a nipple in the mouths of infants 3 and 4 days of age. To a control group, the tone and nipple were presented non-contiguously. On every fifth trial, the tone was presented alone as a test for conditioning, and, after training was completed, all babies received a series of extinction trials with the test tone alone. Evidence was found for classic appetitive conditioning, although the effects of training did not manifest themselves until the extinction condition.

Papousek (52) and Siqueland and associates (53) studied the effect of contingent reinforcement of head turning to a touch at the side of the mouth. The stimulation produces the rooting reflex and head turning in 30% of preconditioning trials. After 5% dextrose solution was offered in response to successful head turning, the head turning was increased significantly by the reinforcement. Associating a tone with the positive condition enhanced head turning to a rate of 83%. If, on alternate trials, the head turns were not reinforced with dextrose solution, there was a gradual behavioral shift down to a rate of 30%. These studies demonstrated that reflexive behavior could be altered by contingent reinforcement.

Effects of Stimulation on Recovery

If these learning paradigms are capable of indicating sensory and neurologic integrity, perhaps a clinical test of the baby's future function could be based on a curve of behavioral improvement. Using the NBAS, we observed that there was a significant improvement over the first 10 days in major areas of behavior function in a low-risk group of babies (54). The infants became more alert and capable of orienting to animate and inanimate stimuli. They turned significantly more to the voice and rattle and followed the human face and a red ball with significantly more head turning and alerting. Their motor maturity, muscle tone, and integrated motor performances also improved. On behavioral items reflecting their physiologic adjustments, such as startles and tremulousness, they improved significantly. This pattern of behavioral recovery based on the items of the NBAS can serve as an important system for evaluating CNS integrity and maturity.

There is increasing evidence that sensory input that is appropriate to the state of physiologic recovery of the neonate may further his weight gain, sensory integrity, and functional outcome. Unless we pay more attention to appropriate stimulation for the infant, we may be interfering with or retarding his optimal sensory development. Pettigrew (55) found that, for kittens, specific visual input was necessary to develop the specificity of initially undifferentiated cells. Blakemore and Cooper (56) found that visual cortex neurons responded predominantly to stimuli that were equivalent to the environment in which the kittens were reared. In both cases, these effects were found only after a given level of CNS maturity had been achieved. Before that time, exposure had no effect, because it did not appropriately fit the organism's level of development.

Most of the studies on early stimulation have not been individualized to the subjects. Evidence suggests that each premature or recovering neonate must be examined for the possibility of sensory overloading (57). A premature infant responds to a soft rattle by turning his head away from the rattle and by other means of shutting it out, but a normal neonate turns toward the rattle and searches for the source of the sound (57). The finely defined thresholds for appropriate sensory stimuli, as opposed to those that must be coped with or shut out, must be taken as seriously as whether or not we offer stimulation. In the recovery phase, a high-risk baby may be too easily overwhelmed, and routine stimulation may force him into an expensive coping model, but grading the stimuli to his particular sensory needs may further his recovery and his ultimate CNS outcome.

How can we tell when the infant is being overloaded? We can tell by watching his color changes, his kind of respirations, and his state of alertness and by looking for evidence of fatigue. Using Kearsley's ideas about the relative degree of attention to a stimulus as measured against physiologic demands, we have a clearly defined areas of "appropriate" and "inappropriate" properties of stimuli that can be applied to each neonate, permitting estimation of the amount and quality of stimulation that can be offered to every at-risk neonate without undue expense (33).

The studies by Sander and associates (58) show that the infant shapes his motility and his state behavior to the environment, particularly if it is sensitive to him and his needs. Two models of regulation occurred with the neonates and caretakers they studied. The first consisted of basic regulation of endogenous biorhythmicity and was entrained by specific extrinsic cues in relation to the neonate's endogenous rhythm. Entrainment was most effective when the exogenous cue approximated the point in time at which a shift in the endogenous cycle was occurring. With the repeated establishment of contingent associations between state changes in the infant and specific configurations in caretaking events, entrainment was favored. The second model depended on the caretaker and infant achieving a regulatory balance based on mutual readiness of states, and, with this, the stage was set to facilitate initial cognitive development. As the partners appreciated a mutual regulation of states of attention, they began to learn about and from each other, and a kind of reciprocity or affective interaction ensued.

These demonstrations of behavioral and sensory responsiveness can be used to assess the neonate and enable us to enhance the parent–infant interaction by sharing this assessment with the parent. The nonverbal communication between parent and infant in the initial stages of attachment is built on the infant's behavior. As pediatricians interested in enhancing the parent–infant bond, we would do well to observe, assess, and participate in the marvelous responsive capacities of the newborn infant.

REFERENCES

1. Greenberg NH. A comparison of infant–mother interactional behavior in infants with atypical behavior and normal infants. In: Hellmuth J, ed. *Exceptional infant.* vol 2. New York: Brunner Mazel, 1971:390.
2. Brazelton TB. Touchpoints: emotional and behavioral and development. Reading: Addison-Wesley, 1993.
3. Sigman M, Parmelee AH. Longitudinal evaluation of the preterm infant. In: Field TM, ed. *Infants born at risk.* New York: Spectrum, 1979.
4. Brazelton TB. Neonatal Behavioral Assessment Scale. *Spastics international publications clinics in developmental medicine, monograph no. 50.* Philadelphia: JB Lippincott, 1973.
5. Brazelton TB. Neonatal Behavioral Assessment Scale, 3rd ed, *Spastics international medical publications clinics in developmental medicine, monograph no. 137.* Cambridge: Cambridge University Press, 1995.
6. Brazelton TB. Neonatal Behavioral Assessment Scale, 2nd ed. *Spastics international medical publications clinics in developmental medicine, monograph no. 88.* London: Blackwell Scientific Publications, 1984.
7. Brazelton TB, Nugent JK, Lester BM. Neonatal Behavioral Assessment Scale. In: Osofosky J, ed. *The handbook of infant development.* New York: John Wiley and Sons, 1987.
8. Tronick E, Brazelton TB. Clinical uses of the Brazelton Neonatal Behavioral Assessment. In: Friedlander BZ, Sterritt GM, Kirk GE, eds. *Exceptional infant, vol 3. Assessment and intervention.* New York: Brunner Mazel, 1975.
9. Prechtl H, Beintema O. *The neurological examination of the full term newborn infant.* London: William Heinemann, 1964.
10. Prechtl H, Dykstra J. Neurological diagnosis of cerebral injury in the newborn. In: Berge TS, ed. *Proceedings of symposium on prenatal care.* Groningen: Nordhoff, 1959.
11. Thoman EB. Early development of sleeping behavior in infants. In: Ellis NR, ed. *Aberrant development in infancy.* New York: John Wiley and Sons, 1975:123.
12. Michaelis R, Parmelee AH, Stern E, et al. Activity states in premature and term infants. *Dev Psychobiol* 1973;6:209.
13. Anders TF. Sleep and its disorders in infants and children: a review. *Pediatrics* 1972;50:312.
14. Steinschneider A. Nasopharyngitis and prolonged deep apnea. *Pediatrics* 1975;56:967.
15. Brazelton TB. Observations of the neonate. *J Am Acad Child Psychiatry* 1972;1:38.
16. Lester BM. The organization of crying in the neonate. *Pediatr Psychol* 1978;3:122.
17. Wasz-Hockert O, Lind J, Vuorenkoski V, et al. *The infant cry.* England: Lavenham, 1968.
18. Lester BM. Spectrum analysis of the cry sounds of well-nourished and malnourished infants. *Child Dev* 1976;47:237.
19. Ellingston RV. Cortical electrical responses to visual stimulation in the human infant. *Electroencephalogr Clin Neurophysiol* 1960;16:663.
20. Hrbek A, Mares P. Cortical evoked responses to visual stimulation in full term and premature infants. *Electroencephalogr Clin Neurophysiol* 1964;16:575.
21. Brazier MAB, ed. *The central nervous system and behavior* (translated). 2nd conf. New York: Josiah Macy Foundation, 1959.
22. Fantz RI. Visual perception from birth as shown by pattern selectivity. *Ann N Y Acad Sci* 1965;118:793.
23. Goren CC, Sarty, M, Wie PYK. Visual following and pattern discrimination by newborn infants. *Pediatrics* 1975;56:544.
24. Brazelton TB, Scholl MI, Robey JS. Visual responses in the newborn. *Pediatrics* 1966;37:284.
25. Gorman JJ, Cogan DG, Gellis SS. An apparatus for grading the visual acuity of infants on the basis of opticokinetic nystagmus. *Pediatrics* 1957;19:1088.
26. Dayton GO Jr, Jones MH, Aiu P, et al. Developmental study of coordinated eye movements in the human infant. *Arch Ophthalmol* 1964;71:856.
27. Haynes H, White BL, Held R. Visual accommodation in human infants. *Science* 1965;148:528.
28. Sigman M, Kopp CB, Parmelee AH, et al. Visual attention and neurological organization in neonates. *Child Dev* 1973;44:461.
29. Hershenson M. Visual discrimination in the human newborn. *J Comp Physiol Psychol* 1964;58:270.
30. Eisenberg RB. Auditory behavior in the human neonate: methodologic problems. *J Aud Res* 1965;5:159.
31. Lipsitt EP. Learning in the human infant. In: Stevenson HW, Rheingold HL, Hess E, eds. *Early behavior: comparative and behavioral approaches.* New York: John Wiley and Sons, 1967:225.
32. Lipton EL, Steinschnieder A, Richmond J. Auditory sensitivity in the infant: effect of intensity on cardiac and motor responsivity. *Child Dev* 1966;37:233.
33. Kearsley RB. The newborn's response to auditory stimulation: a demonstration of orienting and defensive behavior. *Child Dev* 1973;44:582.
34. Bronstein AI, Petrova EP. The auditory analyzer in young infants. In: Brackbill Y, Thompson GC, eds. *Behavior in infancy and early childhood.* New York: Free Press, 1967:163.
35. Bridger WH. Sensory habituation and discrimination in the human neonate. *Am J Psychiatry* 1961;117:991.
36. Cairns GF, Butterfield EC. Assessing infant's auditory functioning. In: Friedlander BZ, Sterritt GM, Kirk GE, eds. *Exceptional infant*, vol 2. New York: Brunner Mazel, 1975:84.
37. Engen T, Lipsitt LP, Kaye H. Olfactory responses and adaptation in the human neonate. *J Comp Physiol Psychol* 1963;56:73.
38. MacFarlane A. *Parent–infant interaction.* Oxford: Elsevier Press, 1975:103.
39. Pratt KC, Nelson AK, Sun KH. The behavior of the newborn infant. In: *Ohio State University student contributions in psychology,* vol 30. Columbus, OH: Ohio State University, 1930.
40. Johnson P, Salisbury DM. *Parent–infant interaction.* Oxford: Elsevier Press, 1975:119.
41. Lipsitt LP, Kaye H, Bosack TN. Enhancement of neonatal sucking through reinforcement. *J Exp Child Psychol* 1966;4:163.
42. Crook CK, Lipsitt LP. Neonatal nutritive sucking: effects of taste stimulation on sucking rhythm and heart rate. *Child Dev* 1976;47:518.
43. Brazelton TB, Tronick E, Adamson L, Als H, Wise S. *Parent–infant interaction.* Oxford: Elsevier Press, 1975:33.
44. Peiper A. *Cerebral function in infancy and childhood.* New York: Consultant's Bureau, 1963. Nagler B, Nagler H, translators.
45. Gryboski JD. The swallowing mechanism of the neonate: esophageal and gastric motility. *Pediatrics* 1965;35:445.
46. Kaye K. Infant sucking and its modification. In: Lipsitt LP, Spiker CC, eds. *Advances in child development and behavior*, vol 3. New York: Academic Press, 1967.
47. Kaye K, Brazelton TB. *The ethological significance of the burst–pause pattern in infant sucking.* Presented at the Society for Research in Child Development, Minneapolis, Minnesota, April 1971.
48. Haith MM, Kessen W, Collins D. Response of the human infant to level of complexity of intermittent visual movement. *J Exp Child Psychol* 1969;7:52.
49. Lipsitt LP. The study of sensory and learning processes of the newborn. *Clin Perinatol* 1977;4:163.
50. Denisova MP, Figurin NKL. Voprosu o pervykh sochetatelnykh pishchevykh refleksakh u grundykh detei. *Vopr Genet Reflek Pedol* 1929;1:81.
51. Lipsitt LP, Kaye H. Conditioned sucking in the human newborn. *Psychosom Sci* 1974;1:29.

52. Papousek H. Conditioned motor digestive reflexes in infants. II. A new experimental method for the investigation. Czekoslovakia Pediatrici 1960;15:981.

53. Siqueland ER, Lipsitt LP. Conditioned head turning in human newborns. *J Exp Child Psychol* 1966;3:356.

54. Tronick R, Wise S, Als H, et al. Regional obstetric anesthesia and newborn behavior: effect over the first 10 days of life. *Pediatrics* 1977;58:94.

55. Pettigrew JD. The effect of visual experience on the development of stimulus specificity by kitten cortical neurons. *J Physiol* 1974;237:49.

56. Blakemore C, Cooper GF. Development of the brain depends on the visual environment. *Nature* 1970;228:477.

57. Als H, Lester BM, Tronick E, Brazelton TB. Manual for the assessment of preterm infants' behavior (APIB). In: Fitzgerald HE, Lester BM, Yogman MW, eds. *Theory and research in behavioral pediatrics*, vol 1. New York: Plenum Press, 1975.

58. Sander LW, Chappell PF, Gould SB, et al. *An investigation of change in the infant-caretaker system over the first week of life.* Presented at the Annual Meeting of the Society for Research in Child Development, Denver, Colorado, 1975.

CHAPTER 21

General Care

Joan McGregor Kelly

There are aspects of general care that apply to all newborns regardless of gestational age or medical condition. This chapter deals with the general care that newborns receive during the four phases of their hospitalization: delivery, transition, hospital stay, and discharge. Infection control and general laboratory evaluation also are discussed.

DELIVERY ROOM CARE

Resuscitation

Neonatal resuscitation and the physiology of transition are discussed in Chapters 17 and 18. Practical recommendations regarding resuscitation in the delivery room can be found in the American Heart Association and American Academy of Pediatrics (AHA/AAP) Textbook of Neonatal Resuscitation.[1]

Cord Clamping and Cord Blood Collection

After delivery of the infant's head, the obstetrician must clear the infant's airway. During the 30 to 60 seconds of suctioning, usually before clamping the cord, the infant is held at the level of the introitus or abdomen to prevent a significant shift of his blood volume. Consequences of a significant shift toward the infant include polycythemia, circulatory volume overload, and hyperbilirubinemia, and these generally outweigh any potential advantage of augmenting the infant's iron reserve. Stripping the umbilical cord to enhance placental transfusion to the infant is reserved for infrequent instances of severe

J. McGregor Kelly: Division of Neonatology, Holy Cross Hospital, Silver Spring, Maryland

[1]P.O. Box 927, Elk Grove Village, IL 60009-0927.

fetal hypovolemia. As soon as possible after suctioning, the cord is clamped and cut 4 to 5 cm from the infant's abdomen (1). After the infant is dried and stabilized and if the umbilical base appears normal, an umbilical clamp is secured to the cord 1 to 2 cm distal to the abdominal wall, and any excess length is cut. If the base appears fuller than normal, which suggests an omphalocele, or if catheterization of umbilical vessels is likely, it is helpful to clamp the cord more distally. Notation should be made if fewer than three umbilical vessels exist (2).

After delivery of the placenta, blood may be collected for laboratory tests by direct needle aspiration of the fetal vessels in the cord or on the fetal placental surface. Allowing placental blood to drip from the cord directly into laboratory tubes before placental delivery may contaminate the specimen if there is not a free flow. Fetal or placental blood should not clot for at least 15 minutes after cord clamping.

Temperature Control

At delivery, the infant moves from a warm environment *in utero* into a much cooler delivery room. Although this immediate cold stress helps the infant initiate breathing, prolonged cold stress is dangerous (3). Because the neonate is particularly vulnerable to hypothermia, exquisite attention to his or her environmental support is required. The infant should be placed on a heated radiant warmer bed, dried with warm linens, and swaddled in clean ones, with a stockinet cap covering his or her head. If the parent holding the infant wishes to unwrap and inspect him or her, a radiant warmer should be placed over the parent and baby. Common potential sources of cold stress in the first few hours include cold oxygen used in resuscitation, unwarmed transport incubators, environmental drafts, and the initial weighing, bathing, and examination (see Chap. 24).

Identification and Security

Footprinting, palmprinting, or fingerprinting are the traditional methods of documenting a newborn's identity. Despite evidence that these methods are unreliable, local regulations may require them (4). Before leaving the delivery room, each infant should be identified by wrist and ankle bands that indicate the mother's name and hospital identification number and the infant's hospital number and date of birth. The mother should wear a band with identical information; the father may do so as well. Any time an infant is released to a parent, the matching bands must be verified. Parents should verify the identity of anyone asking to take their infant from their room. Because of the variety of personnel and visitors in maternity, nursery, and postpartum areas, all hospitals should follow strict security precautions to ensure the safety of each newborn.

INFECTION CONTROL

Because bacterial and viral infections can be devastating to neonates, prevention and early detection are mainstays of general care. Meticulous attention to infection control is essential, because newborns are at risk for infections acquired from their mothers, their environment, and the personnel providing their care.

Careful hand washing is the mainstay of infection control. Before entering the nursery, personnel should scrub their hands and forearms to the elbows with a sponge and an antiseptic preparation such as iodophor, chlorhexidine, or hexachlorophene. Hands should be washed and dried before and after handling each baby and after touching any object likely to be contaminated.

If there is the potential for contact with blood or body fluids, personnel should protect themselves and other patients by following universal precautions. This means simply wearing gloves for diaper changes and phlebotomy. For more invasive procedures, gown, mask, goggles, and gloves are appropriate. Contaminated linens and clothing should be disposed of properly.

Cover gowns traditionally have been used in nursery and postpartum units, but gowning decreases neither bacterial colonization of the infant's nose or umbilicus nor the incidence of sepsis (5). Gowns are valuable for protecting the caregiver's clothing and where universal precautions apply, but their routine use is unnecessary. The fact that ungowned visitors pose no greater risk to healthy newborns also has brought into question the traditional use of scrub attire in nurseries; it remains necessary for personnel who attend deliveries.

Providing each infant with his or her own clothing, diapers, and bulb syringe limits cross-contamination and essentially isolates each infant with his or her own equipment. It is common practice to wipe equipment, such as stethoscopes, with alcohol between uses on multiple infants. There is no convincing evidence that this decreases colonization or cross-contamination, but, like gowning, if the practice reminds personnel to practice careful hand washing, it is valuable. Nursery linens and infant clothing may be laundered routinely; autoclaving is unnecessary (6).

Separating infants into cohort groups by age, which allows complete cleaning of a nursery module as that cohort is discharged, is an effective means of preventing the spread of pathogens. Cohorting can be routine or instituted after an outbreak occurs.

ADMISSION PROCEDURES

After initial stabilization, bonding, and identification, the infant is transferred to an area where his or her adaptation to extrauterine life can be monitored while routine admission procedures are performed. This area may be in a specialized nursery, the routine care nursery, or the postpartum recovery room. Its staff should be attuned to the subtleties of newborn adaptation and familiar with aberrations of medical history, physical examination, or laboratory data that may necessitate immediate involvement of the infant's physician.

Transition and Initial Physical Assessment

The transition period classically refers to the first 6 to 12 hours of life, during which a healthy newborn goes through predictable patterns of alertness, vital sign changes, and gastrointestinal activity (7). Sick, stressed, or premature infants do not follow the predictable patterns. Proper interpretation of the changing physical findings in the first few hours depends on familiarity with these normal patterns.

Increasingly, the term "transition" is used interchangeably with "adaptation." Physiologic adaptation to extrauterine life occurs over the first 24 hours and is considered complete when vital signs, feeding, and gastrointestinal and renal function are normal. Infants with delayed or prolonged transitions may have persistent tachypnea, delayed hunger and feeding, or difficulty maintaining their temperature. Differentiating an otherwise healthy infant with delayed transition from an ill infant with similar symptoms sometimes is difficult. Because time alone cures one and harms the other, it is crucial to make an accurate observation.

An initial assessment of the newborn includes measurement of vital signs (e.g., heart rate, respiratory rate, temperature), body measurements (e.g., weight, length, head circumference, sometimes chest and abdominal circumference), and a complete physical examination. Assessment of vital signs, behavior, and activity continues at least every half hour until they remain stable for 2 hours. The apparently normal infant should be examined by 24 hours of age by the responsible physician (8). There is much reliance on astute nurses whose experience and judgment are invaluable in the newborn's initial care.

Vitamin K

Because of poor placental transport of vitamin K and an absence of intestinal flora to produce it, newborns have low levels of active vitamin-K–dependent clotting factors. This insufficiency may present clinically as a spontaneous bleeding diathesis, notably as gastrointestinal, skin, or intracranial hemorrhage. Hemorrhagic disease of the newborn, a potentially lethal disorder, has an incidence of 0.25% to 1.7%; breast-fed infants and infants of mothers taking anticonvulsants are at highest risk (9). Although effectively treated with vitamin K and blood products, the disease can be prevented by the administration of 0.5 to 1 mg of vitamin K, given intramuscularly within 1 hour of birth (8). Oral vitamin K is effective, although there is no consensus on optimal dosage (10). Careful documentation of vitamin K administration is important.

Eye Prophylaxis

The prevention of neonatal gonococcal ophthalmia was the original impetus for newborn eye prophylaxis. *Chlamydia*, although causing a less serious ophthalmia, is the more prevalent ocular pathogen acquired by the newborn from the maternal genital tract. Penicillinase-producing gonococci (PPGC) are becoming prevalent. Acceptable agents for eye prophylaxis are 1% silver nitrate, 0.5% erythromycin, and 1% tetracycline (11). Erythromycin and tetracycline have direct antibiotic effects; silver nitrate causes a chemical conjunctivitis, producing an inflammatory response with a secondary antibiotic effect. Each agent has limitations in its spectrum of activity. All are effective against sensitive gonococci; silver nitrate is the most effective against PPGC; no agent works particularly well against *Chlamydia* (12).

All agents are instilled into the lower conjunctival sac, and the lids are massaged to distribute the medication. Excess medication can be wiped away, but the eyes should not be flushed. To allow for uninhibited mutual gazing and parent–infant bonding in the delivery room, eye prophylaxis may be delayed until admission to the nursery, where it can be carefully administered and documented. However, it should not be delayed by more than 1 hour (11). Topical antimicrobial therapy is insufficient prophylaxis for infants of mothers with active gonococcal infections at delivery, and these infants must receive parenteral therapy as well (11).

Although evidence suggests that ocular prophylaxis is not necessary for infants delivered by cesarean section after fewer than 3 hours of ruptured membranes, the AAP recommends prophylaxis for all infants, regardless of route of delivery (13).

GENERAL LABORATORY EVALUATION

Maternal Evaluation

Several screening blood tests are recommended for all pregnant women (14):

- Hemoglobin and hematocrit levels
- Serologic test for syphilis (STS)
- Blood group, Rh type, and indirect Coombs test
- Rubella IgG
- Hepatitis B surface antigen (HBsAg)
- Alpha-fetoprotein.

In at-risk populations, screening for human immunodeficiency virus (HIV) and illicit drugs is routine, and STS in the third trimester and at delivery are recommended. The results of the tests should be available to the infant's caregivers as early diagnostic or therapeutic actions may be necessary. There should be a standard manner in which this information is transmitted to the infant's chart. Any other abnormalities or problems during the pregnancy also should be noted on the chart.

The mother with no prenatal care should have an STS, blood group and Rh, and HbsAg drawn on admission. As illicit drug use is especially prevalent in this population, screening the mother and/or infant also is necessary. Results must be available before discharge, as they will affect immediate treatment of the infant as well as follow-up arrangements. HIV testing of the mother and infant should be offered.

Neonatal Evaluation

The value of routine laboratory evaluations on all patients admitted to hospitals is a subject of debate. Previous recommendations for newborns have included blood type and direct Coombs test, STS, hemoglobin and hematocrit, glucose or rapid blood glucose screen, urinalysis, and the newborn metabolic screen. Of these, only the metabolic screen should be performed on every infant; other tests are necessary as indicated in the text that follows.

Blood Type and Coombs Test

The infants at risk for hemolytic disease due to Rh type or major blood group incompatibility are Rh-positive infants of Rh-negative mothers and type A or B infants of type O mothers. The Rh status of any infant born to an Rh-negative mother should be determined to identify candidates for maternal immunoprophylaxis; even if an Rh-positive baby is unaffected by Rh disease, RhoGAM (i.e., anti-Rh IgG) should be given to the mother postpartum to protect future Rh-positive fetuses. Blood typing all infants of type O mothers is more controversial. Infants with clinically significant hemolysis due to ABO incompatibility usually have only mild anemia; hyperbilirubinemia is the major problem. When serial observation of the infant of a type O mother is possible, infant blood type and Coombs status need be determined only if significant jaundice occurs. In populations in which close follow-up is not feasible, it is helpful to know the infant's blood type before discharge. Saving cord blood for later typing per practitioner request is more cost-effective than routinely typing all infants of type O mothers. Hospitals should have specific policies in place for keeping cord blood for an appropriate period of time and for prompt typing and communication of results when requested. Direct Coombs-negative type A or B infants have hemoglobin values, reticulocyte counts, and bilirubin levels comparable to those of type O infants. Coombs-positive infants usually have lower hemoglobin values and higher reticulocyte counts and bilirubin levels, indicating more hemolysis (15). Therefore, Coombs testing should be done on the cord blood of all type A or B infants of type O mothers. Cord or serum bilirubin levels, hemoglobin and hematocrit testing, and reticulocyte counts are optional unless therapy for hyperbilirubinemia is likely or indicated.

Glucose Screening

The incidence of hypoglycemia is decreasing as newborns are fed sooner after birth and as maternal diabetes is better controlled. Selected screening of infants who are at risk by virtue of history or size is appropriate (16). Any infant with symptoms attributable to hypoglycemia should have a glucose test. Rapid glucose screening tests are technique dependent; those tests that use reagent strips demonstrating color change may be inaccurate at high hemoglobin and hematocrit levels. Abnormal results should be confirmed by standard whole blood glucose assays.

Hemoglobin and Hematocrit Determinations

There is little justification for routine hemoglobin and hematocrit determinations on a single infant with no evidence of anemia or polycythemia by history or physical examination (17,18). Monochorionic twins, however, are at risk for twin-to-twin transfusion and its attendant complications; therefore, same-gender twins should each have blood drawn for hemoglobin and hematocrit tests (19).

Newborn Screening Programs

Programs are in place for neonatal screening for rare but potentially devastating disorders that are difficult to detect clinically, but for which there are dramatic benefits from early intervention. These disorders include phenylketonuria and congenital hypothyroidism. Most of the hospitals in the United States also screen for galac-tosemia, and some screen for other metabolic diseases and for hemoglobinopathies that are amenable to early preventive health measures (20). The techniques and the timing for sampling vary; most programs require a sample shortly after birth and 2 weeks later. Because some assays measure metabolites of ingested substrates, it is advantageous to have feedings well established; blood usually is drawn on the morning of discharge. There should be a routine procedure in place for ensuring that each screen sample is drawn, with follow-up for abnormal results.

THE HOSPITAL STAY

The practice of an infant spending long periods of time in the mother's room (i.e., rooming-in) has gained favor and forced reconsideration of practices based on fears of detriment to the infant not kept in a restricted nursery environment controlled for hygiene, attire, and visitors (21). Rooming-in has become a necessity with the shortening of postpartum hospital stay, because new mothers staying in the hospital for only 24 to 36 hours simply cannot become comfortable with infant care if contact with their infants is limited.

Although relaxation of old restrictions allows infants to be outside the nursery, attention still must be given to providing a safe environment. Particular dangers are cold-induced stress, falls, and removal of the infant from the mother's care by unauthorized persons.

When with the mother, the infant should enjoy the same level of nursing care as he or she would have within the nursery. This includes a general physical assessment and measurement of vital signs at least every 8 hours; recording of feeding volume, frequency, and behavior; recording of urine and stool output; cord and circumcision care; and any other procedures deemed necessary. The mother's assistance in all appropriate areas is desirable, because this helps ensure her competence in the care of her infant. The infant's bassinet should contain all clothing and equipment necessary for the infant's care.

Bathing and Dressing

After achieving temperature stability, the infant with an apparently normal transition can be bathed. Although vernix has lubricating and antiinfectious properties that make its presence desirable, removing it for cosmetic purposes is routine. Bathing also removes gross maternal blood, minimizing exposure of the infant and his caregivers to blood-borne viruses such as hepatitis B virus (HBV), herpes simplex virus, and HIV. In infants whose maternal history is unclear or who has a positive result for one of these viruses, injections should be delayed until after the initial bath.

Warm water alone is sufficient for bathing most infants; a mild, nonmedicated soap or chlorhexidine gluconate may be used. Hexachlorophene, which can be absorbed through intact skin and cause neurotoxicity, is not recommended for routine bathing (22). Care must be taken during bathing to minimize heat loss. After the bath, the infant is returned to the radiant warmer; when the infant's temperature is stable, he or she is dressed in a diaper, shirt, and hat; wrapped in a double blanket; and transferred to an open bassinet. After 24 hours, most infants can maintain normal temperatures without a hat or second blanket.

Before discharge, the mother should understand how to bathe her baby safely. A mild soap and shampoo can be used sparingly (23). Special baby soaps and lotions are expensive and unnecessary for infant skin care. Twice-weekly baths usually are sufficient. Overbathing dries and cracks skin; a mild hand lotion—not oil or ointment—can be applied if necessary.

Babies often are overdressed for their environments. The infant should be dressed in clothing that the parent would find comfortable, with one extra layer and a hat added in cool weather. Protection from direct and indirect sunlight is important, because infant skin burns easily.

Frequent diaper changing affords the best protection from diaper rash; creams, pastes, wipes, lotions, and powders generally are unnecessary. Warm water rinsing cleanses most soiled skin, with mild soap added as necessary. Diaper wipes are best reserved for times away from home when no sink is available. Air drying before rediapering helps keep the skin healthy. A product that adheres to the skin as a barrier to urine and stool should be applied to macerated skin; healthy skin needs nothing. Parents wishing to use powder should apply a nontalc, cornstarch type by hand; shaking the powder onto the baby may cause powder-aspiration pneumonitis (24). Neither cloth nor disposable diapers enjoy a clear advantage in maintaining infant skin health.

Umbilical Cord Care

After the first bath, the umbilical cord and surrounding skin are treated topically to decrease invasive bacterial colonization. Acceptable agents include triple dye, alcohol, bacitracin, silver sulfadiazine, and povidone–iodine (25,26). Thereafter, the cord remnant is left exposed outside the diaper to dry and mummify. The cord clamp can be removed safely after 24 hours.

Although it is unclear whether any particular subsequent treatment shortens the time of cord attachment, it is common practice to wipe the cord at least daily, usually with alcohol (26,27). The alcohol is applied underneath the dried cord to the still-moist areas. A mildly foul smell, slight oozing, a drop or two of blood, or a thin rim of erythema on the surrounding abdominal skin is normal.

Feeding

Healthy infants tolerate feeding during transition; early feeding may prevent or minimize hypoglycemia. Vigorous infants without problems may nurse in the delivery room. Formula-fed infants are offered the first feeding after stabilization in the admission nursery. Because any newborn may have an uncoordinated suck and swallow reflex or an inapparent anomaly predisposing to aspiration, the formula-fed infant should take a few sips of sterile water before the formula. If aspirated, glucose water causes as severe a chemical pneumonitis as formula, and plain water therefore is recommended (28). Subsequently, the infant can be fed room-temperature iron-fortified formula (29). Breast-fed infants need not receive sterile water before the first nursing, because aspiration of colostrum is fairly benign.

Most mothers decide long before delivery whether they will breast or formula feed their infants (30). Although breast milk is superior to formula, no mother should be subject to disapproval if she chooses to bottle feed. Because there remain many misunderstandings among first-time mothers about feeding, correcting misinformation is important.

On the first day of life, the breast-fed baby may latch onto the breast and nurse only briefly. Nursing becomes more vigorous in the second 24 hours, and by the third day, each session should last 10 to 15 minutes on each breast. Similarly, the formula-fed infant, who takes only 15 to 30 mL every 3 to 4 hours on day 1, increases to 75 to 90 mL by day 4 or 5 (31). Except when a more consistent glucose intake is required, babies should be fed on demand, when they are awake and hungry, rather than in accordance with a dictated schedule. There is no value in routinely supplementing the breast-fed infant with feedings of water, glucose water, or formula. In fact, this practice may discourage breast-feeding (32).

Parents of bottle-fed infants should know how to prepare and store formula, know how to clean bottles and nipples, and understand the range of normal feeding volumes. Breast-feeding mothers need instruction about the mechanics of nursing, techniques for awakening and encouraging a sleepy baby, pumping and storing expressed milk, formula supplementation, and nutrition during lactation. Much of this instruction should occur prenatally, when the mother is interested and energetic. It should be supplemented in the hospital by nurses, physicians, or lactation specialists who can reinforce previous learning and ensure that the mother and her infant are doing well at discharge. Videotapes can supplement reading material. Mothers should know whom to contact and when to call if breast-feeding is not going well at home. Many pediatricians schedule office visits for breast-fed babies within a few days of discharge; by this time, mother's milk supply should be adequate to stop postnatal weight loss.

Voiding and Stooling

Ninety-one percent of normal newborns void in the first 16 hours of life. Failure to do so by 24 hours should evoke concern but not panic (33). An apparently well infant is unlikely to have serious disease and can be managed expectantly (34). Similarly, 99% of term newborns pass a stool in the first 24 hours; 76% of premature infants do so, with 99% passing a stool by 48 hours (33). As feeding is established, meconium stools give way to frothy, lighter transitional stools and then to a typical, seedy, yellow–green stool. Infants may produce stool in small quantities at each feeding because of the gastrocolic reflex; less frequent stools should be more voluminous. In the breast-fed infant, scanty, infrequent stools indicate poor caloric intake (35).

Behavior

Sleeping, in approximately 4-hour cycles, occupies 20 to 22 hours of a typical newborn's day; the remainder is spent feeding and in the quiet alert state (36). Crying is minimal. Parents may be concerned that their baby is inactive, particularly in the first 2 days. Despite extended sleeping, the newborn has a sophisticated array of behavioral responses to various stimuli, and certain aspects of later behavior patterns or personalities can be predicted by responses evoked on early examinations (37). The knowledgeable caregiver can help strengthen the parent–infant bond by guiding the parents in choosing appropriate responses to their infant's behavioral cues (see Chap. 20).

Jaundice

Two-thirds of all babies appear jaundiced during the first few days of life. Although the causes of jaundice are myriad and the pathophysiology complex, most jaundiced infants are normal, and their jaundice abates without ill effects (38). Excess bilirubin resulting from hemolytic disease appears to be the only common cause of jaundice that should raise concern. The screening recommendations for Rh and ABO disease were discussed previously. The AAP has published comprehensive guidelines for the evaluation and treatment of healthy term infants with jaundice (39).

Jaundiced, breast-fed newborns have higher bilirubin levels than formula-fed infants (40). This difference disappears if infants are nursed every 2 to 3 hours, rather than every 3 to 4 hours (41). Frequent nursing has the added benefit of increasing the mother's milk supply and avoiding the problems caused by supplementation (32,41).

Risks of Perinatally Acquired Infection

Sepsis

Neonatal sepsis is a relatively rare but potentially lethal disease. Conditions that place an infant at increased risk for sepsis include the following [many of these risk factors are additive (42)]:

- Prolonged rupture of the fetal membranes
- Maternal chorioamnionitis, usually involving maternal fever, leukocytosis, uterine tenderness or irritability, purulent cervical discharge or foul-smelling amniotic fluid, or fetal tachycardia
- Maternal colonization with group B streptococci
- Prematurity
- Maternal urinary tract infection
- Perinatal asphyxia, unless clearly associated with a noninfectious cause, such as abruption
- Male gender.

Infants who manifest even subtle clinical signs of sepsis deserve full evaluation and antibiotic therapy. Otherwise healthy infants with risk factors for sepsis pose a dilemma. Most of these clinically well infants are not infected, but because neonatal sepsis can be rapidly lethal, it must be treated promptly.

The laboratory evaluation of the possibly septic infant is complicated by several unique problems: low sensitivity of blood cultures, lack of cerebrospinal fluid pleocytosis in proven meningitis, variability of leukocyte counts, and the use of intrapartum antibiotics. There are several approaches to the evaluation and treatment of at-risk, asymptomatic neonates (42,43). Although there is little agreement on the validity of specific approaches, especially when confounded by maternal antibiotics, an approach weighing risk factors and laboratory results is reasonable (Fig. 21–1) (42).

Basic science and clinical research aimed at the prevention of group B streptococcal sepsis in infants of colonized mothers has produced numerous, at times conflicting, recommendations for management. Happily, the current recommendations for maternal management (both prenatally and intrapartum) and management of at-risk newborns carry the endorsement of the professional societies for Pediatrics, Obstetrics, and Family Practice, as well as the Centers for Disease Control and Prevention (44, 45). As consensus guidelines, the approaches suggested reflect an intent to maximize prevention of neonatal group B streptococcal disease while minimizing the risks, confusion, and expense inherent in earlier approaches.

Positive Maternal Serologic Test Result for Syphilis

As the prevalence of syphilis in the general population rises, so does the incidence of congenital syphilis. Recommendations for selected screening of pregnant women or infants at risk have failed to detect all infected infants. All mother–infant pairs should be screened. Because the STS (i.e., Venereal Disease Research Laboratory [VDRL] test, rapid plasma reagin test) lacks specificity when performed on cord blood, this method of screening newborns is not recommended (46). The Centers for Disease Control (CDC) (47) recommends vigilance regarding the mother's STS:

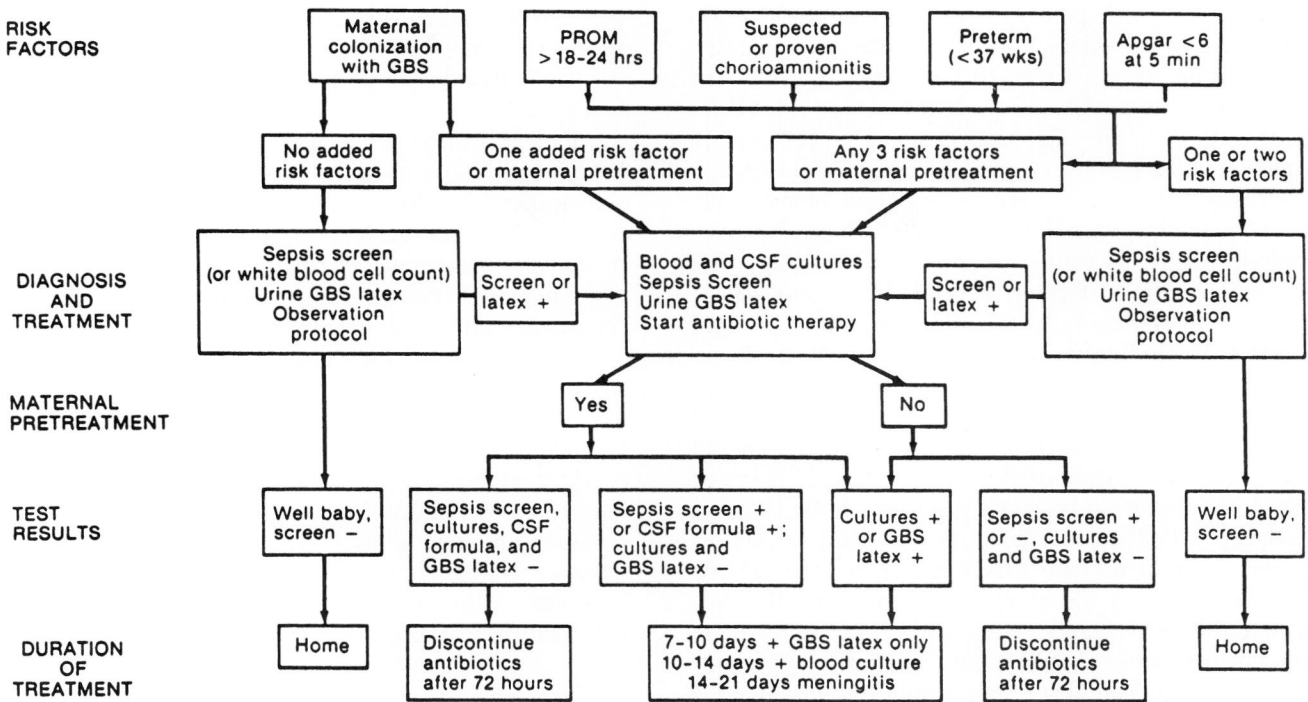

FIG. 21–1. Management of asymptomatic neonates at risk for sepsis. +, positive; –, negative; CSF, cerebrospinal fluid; PROM, prolonged rupture of membranes. (From ref. 42.)

Pregnant women should be screened early in pregnancy.... In areas of high syphilis prevalence, or in patients at high risk, screening should be repeated in the third trimester and again at delivery.... An infant should not be released from the hospital until the serologic status of its mother is known.

The CDC's recommendations for infant evaluation depend on the pediatrician's knowledge of the mother's serologies and treatment throughout pregnancy. The physician should evaluate the infant if the mother has a positive STS result confirmed by a treponemal test (e.g., the fluorescent treponemal antibody absorption test) and was untreated, had poorly documented treatment, was treated with a drug other than penicillin, was treated within 1 month of delivery, or was treated adequately but did not demonstrate at least a fourfold fall in STS titer afterward, whether due to insufficient follow-up or treatment failure (47).

Evaluation of the infant includes several measures (47):

- Complete physical examination
- STS (the same test performed on the mother so that titers can be compared)
- Lumbar puncture for analysis of cells, protein, and VDRL
- Long-bone radiographs
- Any other test clinically indicated.

Differentiating between early infection and passive transfer of maternal antibody is problematic in the infant with an otherwise negative workup, because there is no reliable assay for IgM antitreponemal antibodies. The recommendations for treatment and follow-up are necessarily conservative. Moreover, excluding the diagnosis of neurosyphilis can be so difficult that therapy must be sufficient to treat it (see Chap. 48).

Positive Maternal Test Result for Hepatitis B Surface Antigen

The HBsAg-positive mother can transmit HBV perinatally to her newborn. The spectrum of disease manifestations in the infant range from asymptomatic seroconversion to fulminant, fatal hepatitis. Perinatally infected infants are at particular risk of becoming chronic carriers, and, even if free of chronic hepatitis, they are at increased risk of developing later cirrhosis or hepatocellular carcinoma. Because immunoprophylaxis against HBV initiated at birth is 98% to 99% effective in preventing virus acquisition by the infant, identification of HBsAg-positive pregnant women is essential (48). Confining testing to high-risk women (e.g., Asian or African race, intravenous drug abuse, multiple sexual partners) misses 50% of those who are HBsAg-positive; therefore, "Prenatal HbsAg testing of all pregnant women is recommended..." (48).

Treatment of the infant whose mother is HBsAg-positive consists of immediate, thorough bathing; administration of 0.5 mL of hepatitis B immune globulin (HBIG) intramuscularly within 12 hours of birth; and the first dose of hepatitis B vaccine (0.5 mL, regardless of the product used) intramuscularly, concurrently with HBIG but at a different site. Subsequent doses of vaccine are given at 1 and 6 months of age (48). No special isolation is necessary. Although HBV is found in breast milk, breast-fed infants, even if they are not receiving immunoprophylaxis, are not at increased risk of acquiring HBV infection, and breast-feeding therefore is allowed (48).

A hepatitis B immunization series is recommended for all infants, including those of HBsAg-negative mothers. The first dose may be administered at birth, although alternate schedules are acceptable (49). If the maternal HBsAg status is unknown at delivery, the infant should receive 0.5 mL of hepatitis B vaccine within 12 hours of birth. If the mother subsequently is found to be HBsAg-positive, HBIG should be given to the infant as soon as possible and no later than 7 days of age, and the vaccine series continued. If the mother is found to be HBsAg-negative, HBIG is unnecessary, and completion of the immunization series should follow recommended schedules and dosing. Note that immunization and prophylaxis recommendations for the small (less than 2 kg) premature infant differ from those just discussed (48).

Positive Maternal Test Result for Human Immunodeficiency Virus

Vertical transmission of HIV from mother to infant occurs transplacentally and intrapartum. Treatment of infected women with zidovudine from the second trimester of pregnancy through delivery and subsequent treatment of their infants for the first 6 weeks of life has decreased the previous attack rate of 13% to 39% by approximately two-thirds (50). Maternal antibodies are transferred passively to the infant and are detectable for 15 to 18 months; therefore, HIV culture and identification of HIV proviral DNA by means of the polymerase chain reaction are the preferred diagnostic tests for the newborn. False-negative results are common within the first month of life; retesting at 4 to 6 months is recommended. All exposed infants need comprehensive follow-up.

There are documented cases of infants acquiring HIV infection through breast-feeding. The AAP recommendation states, "In the United States, where safe alternative sources of feeding are readily available and affordable, HIV-infected women should be counseled not to breast-feed their infants..." (50). No special isolation for mother or infant is necessary as long as universal precautions are followed.

Maternal Drug Use

Maternal use of cocaine should be suspected if newborn infants have congenital anomalies, particularly those that can be explained by vascular disruption; irritability, abnormal behavior, seizures, or cerebral infarction; in all cases of placental abruption; and in cases of premature labor, unless otherwise explained (51–53). Cocaine metabolites can be detected in neonatal urine after they have been cleared from maternal urine; a positive infant screen identifies drug use even if the maternal screen is negative. Cocaine-exposed infants do not go through a predictable pattern of drug withdrawal seen with opiate use. They are at risk for apnea, but there is no consensus regarding monitoring of these babies after discharge (54).

The use of other illicit drugs and of alcohol abounds, with changes to new drugs occurring as interest and availability fluctuate. Suspicious maternal or infant behavior should prompt investigation of drug use. Social services support should be available for the drug-using mother and her infant. Chapter 56 provides a general discussion of drug withdrawal syndromes in the newborn, as do other sources (55).

Mothers who use drugs are at increased risk for all sexually transmitted diseases.

The Premature or Postdate Infant

The mildly premature (35 to 37 weeks' gestation) infant may have neonatal problems such as respiratory distress syndrome, hypoglycemia, immature feeding behavior, and hyperbilirubinemia. It is not necessary to provide other than routine hospital care to those infants who appear healthy after initial stabilization. However, scrupulous monitoring for the development of early complications and meticulous follow-up after discharge are required. This would likely include additional physician visits, particularly in the first few weeks.

As the end of gestation approaches, the ability of the uteroplacental unit to nourish the fetus may deteriorate. The fetus may stop growing or lose weight. The fetus may respond to excessive hypoxia *in utero* by brisk hematopoiesis or may tolerate labor and delivery poorly, requiring nonroutine obstetric intervention or neonatal resuscitation. Postnatal sequelae can include polycythemia, hypoglycemia, meconium aspiration syndrome, and the various consequences of asphyxia, including persistent pulmonary hypertension.

Multiple Gestations

"We are faced with the undeniable fact that the human species is not designed to carry more than a single fetus *in utero* with any degree of biologic grace" (56). Twins have a mortality rate four times that of singletons, and that risk increases with increasing number of fetuses (57). Most twin pairs are somewhat growth retarded; approximately one-half are also premature. Congenital anomalies may be more common in monozygotic twins than in singletons; these twins are also at risk for twin-to-twin transfusion and its consequences(19). Parents of twins need special support; referring them to literature and support groups prenatally may help them recognize and cope better with the stresses of having two infants. Special help with breast-feeding may be necessary (58). Caregivers must remember to assess and treat twins as individuals and should encourage the family to do so as well. Parents of a sick or dying twin grieve as deeply as do parents of singletons; that the other twin is alive and well does not diminish their grief and worry (59).

Cyanotic Spell

Although the true incidence of the cyanotic or dusky spell in apparently well infants is unknown, personnel who work in well-baby nurseries see these episodes regularly. The otherwise healthy-appearing infant can have a problem as simple as spitting up or one as potentially devastating as apnea, sepsis, or intracranial hemorrhage. Sorting through the various diagnostic possibilities demands an accurate description of the event, the activities immediately before and after it, and any intervention performed. Particular attention should be paid to the cardiac, respiratory, and neurologic examination of the infant. Continuous cardiopulmonary monitoring and pulse oximetry may be necessary to help define the problem and guide the workup.

Circumcision

Removal of the foreskin was almost routine in this country before the 1970s. In 1975, the AAP (60), although recognizing the sociocultural, cosmetic, and religious reasons for circumcision, found the evidence for its postulated medical benefits (e.g., prevention of phimosis, balanitis, sexually transmitted diseases, and penile, prostatic, and cervical cancers) mostly unconvincing.

> A program of education leading to continuing good personal hygiene would offer all the advantages of routine circumcision without the attendant surgical risk.

However, there is evidence that uncircumcised males are at more risk for urinary tract infections and that lack of circumcision may enhance transmission of HIV. In 1989, the AAP (61) relaxed its stance.

> Newborn circumcision has potential medical benefits and advantages as well as disadvantages and risks. When circumcision is being considered, the benefits and risks should be explained to the parents and informed consent obtained.

There is still much debate, but no consensus, on the issue of routine neonatal circumcision.

Effective pain relief for circumcision can be provided by a dorsal penile nerve block, although this has potential risks (62,63). The simple act of sucking on a pacifier, especially if sucrose flavored, appears to lessen the infant's pain during circumcision (64). Topical anesthesia also is effective (65), and agents such as EMLA (eutectic mixture of local anesthetics) are popular, though not officially approved for use in neonates. Acetaminophen appears beneficial for pain relief after the immediate postoperative period (66).

The glans of the recently circumcised penis should be dabbed with petroleum jelly at each diaper change to prevent the friable mucosa from adhering to the diaper. A stuck glans can be atraumatically freed from the diaper by the application of warm water. The granulating tissue of the normal healing circumcision may be mistaken for pus. A swollen, oozing glans or an impaired urinary stream should prompt consultation with the physician.

An uncircumcised penis requires no special care. As the foreskin loses its adhesions to the glans, it can be retracted gently for cleansing. An excellent instructional pamphlet on care of the uncircumcised penis is offered to parents by the AAP.[2]

DISCHARGE

Car and Home Safety

Car safety should start before birth, with parental acquisition of an approved child safety seat. Because these seats often are used improperly, hospital personnel should know the principles of their use and ensure that the babies discharged from their care are protected properly. Every hospital should have resources on site or readily available in the community for families without safety seats so that they may obtain them before discharge.

Literature or videotaped material regarding home safety for infants should be available to parents. Topics addressed should include burns, falls, aspiration and strangulation, bottle propping, and control of siblings and pets.

Home Routines and Visitors

Newborns do not have routines, which, combined with the recovering mother's fatigue, makes the first few weeks at home exhausting. Moreover, newborns are particularly susceptible to infection. For these reasons, parents should be discouraged from having a houseful of visitors or taking trips out of the home that could expose the infant to the general public. All energies should be directed at new baby care and feeding until the postpartum recovery is complete and a reasonably predictable feeding schedule established.

Discharge Time and Follow-Up

Discharge from the hospital should be dictated by the well being of the mother and her infant, rather than by any other considerations. Both mother and infant should

[2]P.O. Box 927, Elk Grove Village, IL 60009-0927.

be sufficiently recovered from delivery so that continuous observation no longer is necessary. The mother should understand her postpartum care and be healthy enough to undertake it; and the parents should understand the care of their infant and how to obtain help if necessary. For the multiparous, vaginally delivered woman with a healthy, term infant and help at home, this length of time may be less than 24 hours. Obstetric, neonatal, and social considerations may preclude a rapid discharge (67).

All infants should have follow-up arrangements documented before discharge. Those who are discharged within 48 hours of delivery should be examined within 2 days (67); others should be seen no later than 2 weeks of age. As with time of discharge, time for follow-up should be individualized, with consideration given for type of feeding, infant birth weight, maternal and infant blood types, parental experience, and the hospital duration and course.

Special consideration should be given to the adolescent mother, who may need extensive care, support, and teaching both in and out of hospital. Discharge should be delayed until "…a plan to safeguard the infant is in place" (67). Especially important for the long-term benefit of the mother–infant pair are programs providing the young mother the opportunity to complete high school.

REFERENCES

1. Cunningham FG, MacDonald PC, Gant NF. *Williams' obstetrics,* 18th ed. Norwalk, CT: Appleton & Lange, 1989:307.
2. Froehlich LA, Fujikura T. Follow-up of infants with single umbilical artery. *Pediatrics* 1973;52:6.
3. Oliver TK Jr. Temperature regulation and heat production in the newborn. *Pediatr Clin North Am* 1965;12:765.
4. Thompson JE, Clark DA, Salisbury B, Cahill J. Footprinting the newborn infant: not cost effective. *J Pediatr* 1981;99:797.
5. Birenbaum HJ, Glorioso L, Rosenberger C, Arshad C, Edwards K. Gowning on a postpartum ward fails to decrease colonization in the newborn infant. *Am J Dis Child* 1990;144:1031.
6. Donowitz LG. Nosocomial infections in neonatal intensive care units. *Am J Infect Control* 1989;17:250.
7. Desmond MM, Franklin RR, Vallbona C, et al. The clinical behavior of the newly born. I: the term baby. *J Pediatr* 1963;62:307.
8. AAP Committee on Fetus and Newborn and ACOG Committee on Obstetric Practice. Postpartum and follow-up care. In: Hauth JC, Merenstein GB, eds. *Guidelines for perinatal care*, 4th ed. Elk Grove Village, IL: American Academy of Pediatrics and American College of Obstetricians and Gynecologists, 1997:155.
9. Lane PA, Hathaway WE. Vitamin K in infancy. *J Pediatr* 1985;106:351.
10. Hathaway WE, Isarangkura PB, Mahasandana C, et al. Comparison of oral and parenteral vitamin K prophylaxis for prevention of late hemorrhagic disease of the newborn. *J Pediatr* 1991;119:461.
11. Committee on Infectious Diseases, American Academy of Pediatrics. Prevention of neonatal ophthalmia. In: Peter G, Hall CB, Halsey NA, Marcy SM, Pickering LK, eds. *Report of the committee on infectious diseases*, 24th ed. Elk Grove Village, IL: American Academy of Pediatrics, 1997:601.
12. Hammerschlag MR, Cummings C, Roblin PM, Williams TH, Delke I. Efficacy of neonatal ocular prophylaxis for the prevention of chlamydial and gonococcal conjunctivitis. *N Engl J Med* 1989;320:769.
13. Isenberg SJ, Apt L, Yoshimori R, McCarty JW, Alvarez SR. Source of the conjunctival bacterial flora at birth and implications for ophthalmia neonatorum prophylaxis. *Am J Ophthalmol* 1988;106:458.
14. AAP Committee on Fetus and Newborn and ACOG Committee on Obstetric Practice. Antepartum and intrapartum care. In: Hauth JC, Merenstein GB, eds. *Guidelines for perinatal care*, 4th ed. Elk Grove Village, IL: American Academy of Pediatrics and American College of Obstetricians and Gynecologists, 1997:75.
15. Alter AA, Feldman F, Twersky J, et al. Direct antiglobulin test in ABO hemolytic disease of the newborn. *Obstet Gynecol* 1969;33:846.
16. Pagliaria AS, Karl IE, Haymond M, Kipnis DM. Hypoglycemia in infancy and childhood, part I. *J Pediatr* 1973;82:365.
17. Oski FA. The erythrocyte and its disorders. In: Nathan DG, Oski FA, eds. *Hematology of infancy and childhood*, 3rd ed. Philadelphia: WB Saunders, 1987:16.
18. Oh W. Neonatal polycythemia and hyperviscosity. *Pediatr Clin North Am* 1986;33:523.
19. McCulloch K. Neonatal problems in twins. *Clin Perinatol* 1988;15:141.
20. Coen RW, Koeffler H. *Primary care of the newborn*. Boston: Little, Brown, 1987:167.
21. Committee on Fetus and Newborn, American Academy of Pediatrics. Postpartum (neonatal) sibling visitation. *Pediatrics* 1985;76:650.
22. AAP Committee on Fetus and Newborn and ACOG Committee on Obstetric Practice. Infection control. In: Hauth JC, Merenstein GB, eds. *Guidelines for perinatal care*, 4th ed. Elk Grove Village, IL: American Academy of Pediatrics and American College of Obstetricians and Gynecologists, 1992:141.
23. Morelli JG, Weston WL. Soaps and shampoos in pediatric practice. *Pediatrics* 1987;80:634.
24. Mofenson HC, Greensher J, DiTomasso A, Okun S. Baby powder—a hazard! *Pediatrics* 1981;68:265.
25. Committee on Fetus and Newborn, American Academy of Pediatrics. Skin care of newborns. *Pediatrics* 1974;54:682.
26. Gladstone IM, Clapper L, Thorp JW, Wright DI. Randomized study of six umbilical cord care regimens. *Clin Pediatr* 1988;27:127.
27. Arad I, Eyal F, Fainmesser P. Umbilical care and cord separation. *Arch Dis Child* 1981;56:887.
28. Olson M. The benign effects on rabbits' lungs of the aspiration of water compared with 5% glucose or milk. *Pediatrics* 1970;46:538.
29. Committee on Nutrition, American Academy of Pediatrics. Iron-fortified infant formulas. *Pediatrics* 1989;84:1114.
30. Sarett HP, Bain KR, O'Leary JC. Decisions on breast-feeding or formula feeding and trends in infant-feeding practices. *Am J Dis Child* 1983;137:719.
31. Driscoll JM Jr. Routine and special care. In: Fanaroff AA, Martin RJ, eds. *Neonatal–perinatal medicine*, 4th ed. St. Louis: CV Mosby, 1987:441.
32. Lawrence RA. Breast-feeding. *Pediatr Rev* 1989;11:163.
33. Clark DA. Times of first void and first stool in 500 newborns. *Pediatrics* 1977;60:457.
34. Moore ES, Galvez MB. Delayed micturition in the newborn period. *J Pediatr* 1972;80:867.
35. Lawrence RA. Infant nutrition. *Pediatr Rev* 1983;5:133.
36. Hack M. The sensorimotor development of the preterm infant. In: Fanaroff AA, Martin RJ, eds. *Neonatal–perinatal medicine*, 4th ed. St. Louis: CV Mosby, 1987:473.
37. Brazleton TB, Parker WB, Zuckerman B. Importance of behavioral assessment of the neonate. *Curr Probl Pediatr* 1976;7:1.
38. Newman TB, Maisels MJ. Does hyperbilirubinemia damage the brain of healthy full-term infants? *Clin Perinatol* 1990;17:331.
39. Provisional Committee for Quality Improvement and Subcommittee on Hyperbilirubinemia, American Academy of Pediatrics. Practice parameter: management of hyperbilirubinemia in the healthy term newborn. *Pediatrics* 1994;94:558.
40. Schneider AP II. Breast milk jaundice in the newborn. *JAMA* 1986;255:3270.
41. Yamauchi Y, Yamanouchi I. Breast-feeding frequency during the first 24 hours after birth in full-term neonates. *Pediatrics* 1990;86:171.
42. Gerdes JS. Clinicopathologic approach to the diagnosis of neonatal sepsis. *Clin Perinatol* 1991;18:361.
43. St. Geme JW Jr, Murray DL, Carter J, et al. Perinatal infection after prolonged rupture of membranes: an analysis of risk and management. *J Pediatr* 1984;104:608.
44. Committee on Infectious Diseases, American Academy of Pediatrics. Group B streptococcal infections. In: Peter G, Hall CB, Halsey NA, Marcy SM, Pickering LK, eds. *Report of the committee on infectious diseases*, 24th ed. Elk Grove Village, IL. American Academy of Pediatrics, 1997, p 494.
45. Committee on Infectious Diseases and Committee on Fetus and Newborn, American Academy of Pediatrics. Revised guidelines for preven-

tion of early-onset group B streptococcal (GBS) infection. *Pediatrics* 1997;99:489.

46. Committee on Infectious Diseases, American Academy of Pediatrics. Syphilis. In: Peter G, Hall CB, Halsey NA, Marcy SM, Pickering LK, eds. *Report of the committee on infectious diseases.* 24th ed. Elk Grove Village, IL: American Academy of Pediatrics, 1997:504.

47. Centers for Disease Control, 1989. Sexually transmitted diseases treatment guidelines. *MMWR* 1989;38:9.

48. Committee on Infectious Diseases, American Academy of Pediatrics. Hepatitis B. In: Peter G, Hall CB, Halsey NA, Marcy SM, Pickering LK, eds. *Report of the committee on infectious diseases*, 24th ed. Elk Grove Village, IL: American Academy of Pediatrics, 1997:247.

49. Centers for Disease Control. Hepatitis B virus: a comprehensive strategy for eliminating transmission in the United States through universal childhood vaccination. *MMWR* 1991;40.

50. Committee on Infectious Diseases, American Academy of Pediatrics. HIV infection. In: Peter G, Hall CB, Halsey NA, Marcy SM, Pickering LK, eds. *Report of the committee on infectious diseases*, 24th ed. Elk Grove Village, IL: American Academy of Pediatrics, 1997;279.

51. Hoyme HE, Jones KL, Dixon SD, et al. Prenatal cocaine exposure and fetal vascular disruption. *Pediatrics* 1990;85:743.

52. Chasnoff IJ, Griffith DR, MacGregor S, Dirkes K, Burns K. Temporal patterns of cocaine use in pregnancy. *JAMA* 1989;261:1741.

53. Chasnoff IJ, Bussey ME, Savich R, Stack CM. Perinatal cerebral infarction and maternal cocaine use. *J Pediatr* 1986;108:456.

54. Bauchner H, Zuckerman B. Cocaine, sudden infant death syndrome, and home monitoring. *J Pediatr* 1990;117:904.

55. Committee on Drugs, American Academy of Pediatrics. Neonatal drug withdrawal. *Pediatrics* 1983;72:895.

56. Hendricks CH. Twinning in relation to birth weight, mortality, and congenital anomalies. *Obstet Gynecol* 1966;27:47.

57. Ghai V, Vidyasagar D. Morbidity and mortality factors in twins. *Clin Perinatol* 1988;15:123.

58. Becker PG. Counseling families with twins: birth to 3 years of age. *Pediatr Rev* 1986;8:81.

59. Wilson AL, Fenton LJ, Stevens DC, Soule DJ. The death of a newborn twin: an analysis of parental bereavement. *Pediatrics* 1982;70:587.

60. Committee on Fetus and Newborn, American Academy of Pediatrics. Report of the ad hoc task force on circumcision. *Pediatrics* 1975;56:610.

61. Task Force on Circumcision, American Academy of Pediatrics. Report of the task force on circumcision. *Pediatrics* 1989;84:388.

62. Stang HJ, Gunnar MR, Snellman L, Condon LM, Kestenbaum R. Local anesthesia for neonatal circumcision: effects on distress and cortisol response. *JAMA* 1988;259:1507.

63. Schoen EJ [letter], Stang H, Snellman L [reply]. Dorsal penile nerve block for circumcision. *JAMA* 1989;261:701.

64. Blass EM, Hoffmeyer LB. Sucrose as an analgesic for newborn infants. *Pediatrics* 1991;87:215.

65. Benini F, Johnston CC, Faucher D, Aranda JV. Topical anesthesia during circumcision in newborn infants. *JAMA* 1993;270:850.

66. Howard CR, Howard FM, Weitzman ML. Acetominophen analgesia in neonatal circumcision: the effect on pain. *Pediatrics* 1994;93:641.

67. Committee on Fetus and Newborn, American Academy of Pediatrics. Hospital stay for healthy term newborns. *Pediatrics* 1995;96:788.

CHAPTER 22

Fluid and Electrolyte Management

Edward F. Bell and William Oh

Disorders of fluid and electrolyte balance are among the most commonly encountered problems in the care of newborn infants. Careful management of fluid and electrolyte intake can enhance the outcome of most critically ill or premature infants.

The goal of fluid and electrolyte management is to replace losses of water and electrolytes so as to maintain normal balance of these essential substances during growth and recovery from disease. A subsidiary aim in the first days of life is to allow successful transition from the aquatic environment of the fetus into the arid extrauterine milieu. The principles of fluid and electrolyte management in the neonatal period are similar to those established for older children, except for some variations and specific features of body composition, insensible water loss, renal function, and the neuroendocrine control of fluid and electrolyte balance.

To manage fluid therapy of newborns appropriately, the clinician should understand the normal physiologic mechanisms that govern water and electrolyte balance and the variations in these mechanisms that can occur in sick or premature infants. The clinician should develop a systematic approach to the estimation of fluid and electrolyte requirements for correction of deficits and replacement of ongoing losses, both normal and abnormal. Finally, the results of fluid and electrolyte management must be monitored carefully so that the intakes of water and electrolytes can be adjusted as needed.

E. F. Bell: Department of Pediatrics, University of Iowa; and Divison of Neonatology, Children's Hospital of Iowa, Iowa City, Iowa

W. Oh: Department of Pediatrics, Brown University School of Medicine, Providence, Rhode Island

BODY COMPOSITION OF THE FETUS AND NEWBORN INFANT

Changes in Body Water During Growth

The total body water (TBW) is divided into two major compartments, intracellular (ICW) and extracellular (ECW). The ECW is further divided into the interstitial water and the plasma volume, which is the intravascular component of the ECW (Fig. 22–1).

In the early stages of fetal development, a large part of the body consists of water (1). It has been estimated that TBW is 94% of the body weight during the third month of fetal life. As gestation progresses, the TBW per kilogram declines. By 24 weeks, the TBW is approximately 86%, and by term it is about 78% of body weight (Fig. 22–2). There also are characteristic changes in the partition of body water between ECW and ICW during development. ECW decreases from 59% of body weight at 24 weeks of gestation to about 44% at term, and ICW increases from 27% to 34% of body weight during the same period (Table 22–1) (1–6).

After birth, TBW per kilogram of body weight continues to fall, due primarily to a contraction of the ECW (2,7–10). This mobilization of extracellular fluid is thought to be related to the concurrent improvement in renal function that occurs following birth (11–13). Various studies have shown an increase, decrease, or no change in the ICW after birth. ICW probably increases roughly in proportion to body weight in the first weeks of postnatal life (2,9,10,14). Thereafter, ICW increases faster than body weight and by 3 months exceeds ECW (see Fig. 22–2) (1,2). These postnatal changes in body water and its partition between ECW and ICW are influenced by the intake of water and electrolytes (8,15). Failure to allow the normal postnatal contraction of ECW in premature infants may increase the risk of significant patent ductus arteriosus (PDA) (16).

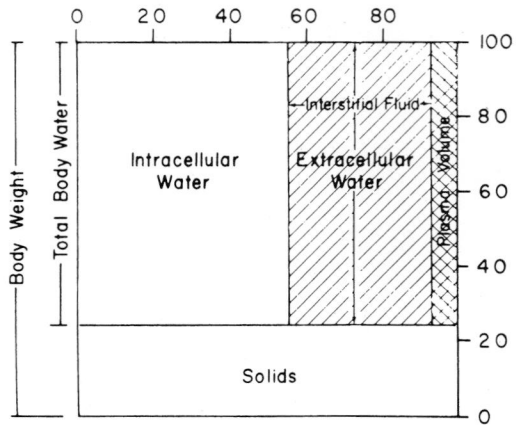

FIG. 22–1. Distribution of body water in a term newborn infant.

TABLE 22–1. *Change in body water and electrolyte composition during intrauterine and early postnatal life*

Component	Gestational age (wk)					1 to 4 wk after term birth
	24	28	32	36	40	
Total body water (%)	86	84	82	80	78	74
Extracellular water (%)	59	56	52	48	44	41
Intracellular water (%)	27	28	30	32	34	33
Sodium (mEq/kg)	99	91	85	80	77	73
Potassium (mEq/kg)	40	41	40	41	41	42
Chloride (mEq/kg)	70	67	62	56	51	48

Data from refs. 1 through 6.

Solute Distribution in Body Fluids

The major cation in the blood plasma is sodium (Fig. 22–3). Potassium, calcium, and magnesium constitute the balance of the cation fraction. The anion is primarily chloride, with protein, bicarbonate, and some undetermined anions constituting the balance of the anions. The interstitial fluid (i.e., nonplasma ECW) has a solute composition that is similar to plasma, except that its protein content is lower. The ICW contains potassium and magnesium as its primary cations, and phosphate, both organic and inorganic, is the major anion, with bicarbonate contributing a smaller fraction.

The electrolyte composition of the body fluids of the newborn infant is largely determined by gestational age. Premature infants contain more sodium and chloride per kilogram of body weight than term infants (3–5) because of their larger ECW (see Table 22–1). Total body potas-

sium content largely reflects ICW and is similar or slightly lower per kilogram of body weight in premature infants than at term (3,6). These concepts are important in the management of fluid and electrolyte therapy for newborn infants.

In the fetus, fluid and electrolyte balance depends on maternal homeostasis and placental exchange. Thus, fluid and electrolyte status at birth is influenced by the maternal fluid and electrolyte management in labor (17,18).

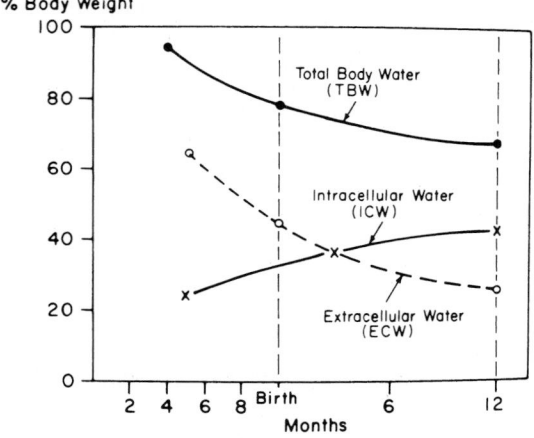

FIG. 22–2. Changes in body water during gestation and infancy. (Adapted from ref. 2, with permission.)

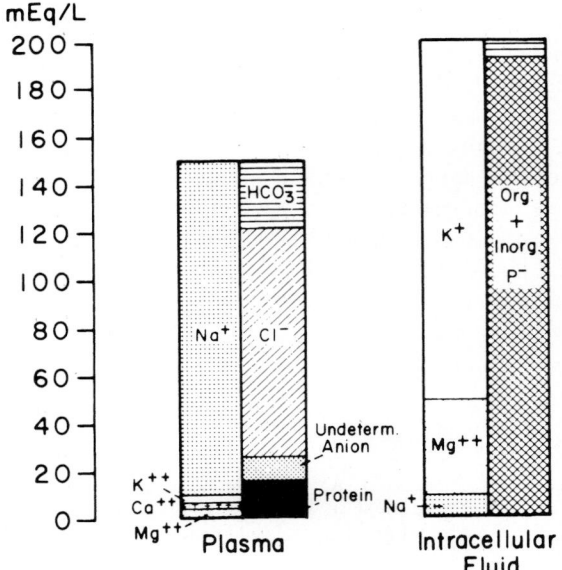

FIG. 22–3. Ion distribution in the blood plasma, which represents extracellular fluid, and in the intracellular fluid compartment.

INSENSIBLE WATER LOSS

The loss of water by evaporation from the skin and respiratory tract is known as insensible water loss (IWL). About 30% of IWL normally occurs through the respiratory tract as moisture in expired gas (19–21), with the remaining 70% lost through the skin. IWL can be expressed in reference to body surface area (m^2) or weight (kg). IWL depends more on surface area than weight, but it commonly is expressed per kilogram because weight is more easily determined than area.

Several factors are known to influence IWL in a predictable manner (Table 22–2) (22–44). When expressed per kilogram of body weight, IWL is inversely proportional to birth weight and gestation age (Figs. 22–4 and 22–5) (22,25). In other words, smaller, more immature infants have larger IWL per kilogram (Table 22–3). The same is true if IWL is expressed per square meter of body surface (26). Therefore, although the greater IWL of smaller premature infants is partly due to the increased ratio of surface area (skin and respiratory tract) to body weight, it also is thought to be related to their thinner skin, greater skin blood flow, larger body water per kilogram of body weight, and higher respiratory rate.

Factors that Increase Insensible Water Loss

Any increase in ventilation volume per minute increases the respiratory IWL, as long as the water vapor pressure is less in the inspired than in the expired gas. Increased minute ventilation may occur in infants with cardiac disease, pulmonary dysfunction, or metabolic acidosis.

Environmental temperature higher than the neutral thermal zone increases IWL in proportion to the increment in temperature (19,27,28). This effect can occur even without a rise in body temperature. In contrast, a subneutral environmental temperature is not associated with reduced IWL, although metabolic heat production is increased (28). Increased body temperature, whether caused by fever or environmental overheating, elevates IWL (19,27).

Skin breakdown or injury disrupts the barrier against cutaneous evaporation and raises IWL. Skin trauma from thermal, chemical, or mechanical injury is common among critically ill, small premature infants. Such injury may result from removal of tape and adherent monitoring devices or from prolonged skin exposure to disinfectant solutions. IWL also is increased in conjunction with the skin manifestations of essential fatty acid deficiency, a potential problem in infants receiving fat-free parenteral nutrition. Congenital skin defects, such as those seen in gastroschisis, omphalocele, and neural tube defects, are associated with increased IWL until surgically corrected.

Use of nonionizing radiant energy, in the form of either a radiant warmer or phototherapy, has been shown to increase IWL by about 50% (22,29–33). For infants in incubators with controlled air temperature, the increase in IWL with overhead phototherapy is most likely a result of increased body temperature because of the warmer incubator walls (33). For infants in incubators operated to control skin temperature, the rise in IWL with phototherapy can be explained by the lower absolute humidity resulting from the reduced air temperature that accompanies the warming of the incubator walls by the phototherapy. The impact on IWL of phototherapy delivered by fiberoptic blankets or pads is not known but is probably negligible unless the blanket produces a warmer or moister microenvironment around the infant. Studies (45,46) using separate measurements of cutaneous and respiratory water loss have not confirmed the effect of overhead phototherapy on IWL reported by earlier inves-

TABLE 22–2. *Factors affecting insensible water loss in newborn infants*

Factor	Effect on insensible water loss
Level of maturity (22,24–26)	Inversely proportional to birth weight and gestational age (Fig. 22–4)
Respiratory distress (hyperpnea)	Respiratory insensible water loss increases with rising minute ventilation when dry air is being breathed
Environmental temperature above neutral thermal zone (19,27,28)	Increased in proportion to increment in temperature
Elevated body temperature (19,27)	Increased by up to 300%
Skin breakdown or injury	Increased by uncertain magnitude
Congenital skin defect (e.g., gastroschisis, omphalocele, neural tube defect)	Increased by uncertain magnitude until surgically corrected
Radiant warmer (22,29–32,46)	Increased by about 50%
Phototherapy (22,31,33)	Increased by about 50%
Motor activity and crying (19,34,35)	Increased by up to 70%
High ambient or inspired humidity (19,21)	Reduced by 30% when ambient vapor pressure is increased by 200%
Plastic heat shield (32,36,37)	Reduced by 30% to 70%
Plastic blanket (38,39)	Reduced by 30% to 70%
Semipermeable membrane (40–42)	Reduced by 50%
Topical agents (43,44)	Reduced by 50%

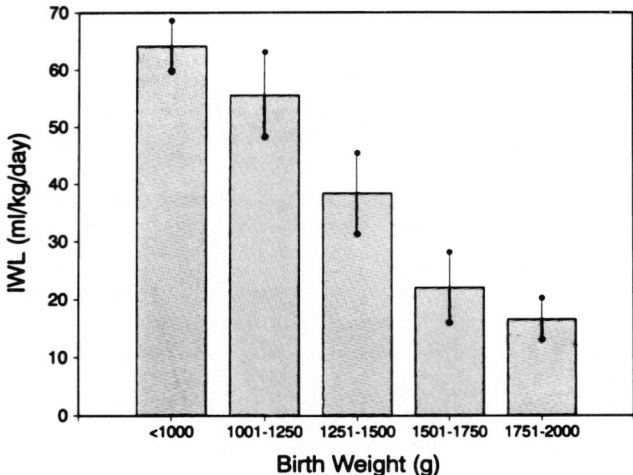

FIG. 22–4. Relation between insensible water loss (IWL) and birth weight of 5-day-old (mean) infants in incubators. (From ref. 22, as redrawn in ref. 23, with permission.)

tigators using methods based on weight loss or water balance (31,33).

If an infant's IWL is measured at the same skin temperature under a radiant warmer and in an incubator, the IWL is higher (by about 50%) under the radiant warmer. IWL is higher because absolute humidity (water vapor

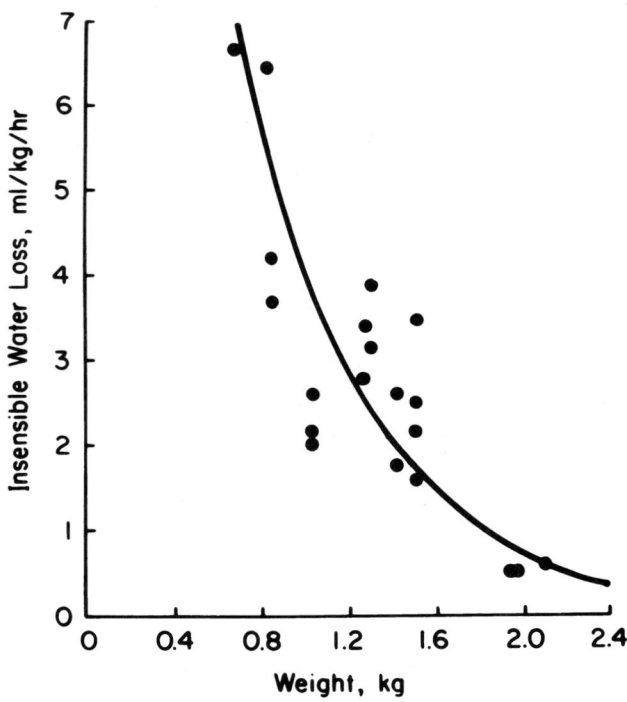

FIG. 22–5. Insensible water loss as a function of birth weight in premature infants nursed under radiant warmers. (Adapted from ref. 25.)

TABLE 22–3. *Average insensible water loss[a] of premature infants in incubators*

Age (d)	Birth weight range (kg)					
	0.50–0.75	0.75–1.00	1.00–1.25	1.25–1.50	1.50–1.75	1.75–2.00
0–7	100[a]	65	55	40	20	15
7–14	80	60	50	40	30	20

[a]Insensible water loss (mL/kg/d).
Data from refs. 22, 24, and 25.

pressure) is lower under the radiant warmer than in the incubator (32). This may be true even though relative humidity is higher under the radiant warmer (31,32), because the lower air temperature with the radiant warmer means that the saturation pressure of water vapor is considerably lower than in the incubator (Table 22–4). This finding has been confirmed using direct measurements of transepidermal water loss (47). It is now understood that the higher IWL with radiant warmers arises from the lower ambient water vapor pressure and not from higher air velocity or a direct effect of nonionizing radiation on the skin. The same phenomenon explains the effect of phototherapy on IWL of infants in incubators operated by skin temperature servocontrol. The effects on IWL of radiant warmers and phototherapy appear to be additive; the IWL with the combination is twice as large as in an incubator without phototherapy (31).

Increased motor activity and crying increase IWL by up to 70% (19,34,35). This effect may be partly due to elevated minute ventilation.

Factors that Reduce Insensible Water Loss

Increasing the humidity or water vapor pressure of inspired gas reduces respiratory IWL. The inspired humidity is raised by humidifying the air–oxygen mixture delivered to a head hood or directly to the infant's upper airway (e.g., via nasal cannula, face mask, or endotracheal tube) if respiratory support is required. Increasing ambient humidity, for example, in an incubator, reduces total IWL, but respiratory IWL is decreased more

TABLE 22–4. *Relative and absolute humidity as related to insensible water loss in incubators and under radiant warmers*

Measurement	Incubator	Radiant warmer
Air temperature (°C)	35.0	27.6
Saturation pressure (mm Hg)	42.1	27.7
Relative humidity (%)	31.4	39.0
Absolute humidity (mm Hg)	13.2	10.8
Insensible water loss (mL/kg/h)	2.37	3.40

Data from ref. 32.

than cutaneous IWL (19). A threefold increase in ambient water vapor pressure, from an average of 7 mmHg to 25 mmHg, resulted in a 30% reduction in total insensible water loss.

Plexiglas heat shields are effective in reducing the IWL of small premature infants in incubators (32,36), especially if the ends are at least partially enclosed to decrease air movement near the skin. Plexiglas heat shields are not effective for infants under radiant warmers (32,37), because Plexiglas is opaque to the infrared energy produced by the radiant heaters. Thin barriers of saran and other materials reduce IWL of infants under radiant warmers while allowing the infrared heat to reach the skin (37). These heat shields presumably reduce IWL by limiting air movement and raising water vapor pressure near the infant's body surface.

Thin plastic blankets have been found to reduce insensible water loss by 30% to 70% for infants under radiant warmers and in incubators (38,39). Semipermeable membranes (40–42) and waterproof topical agents (43,44) reduce insensible water loss from the covered areas by an average of approximately 50%.

Knowledge of these factors that influence IWL is essential for estimating the water intake required by newborn infants and for making appropriate adjustments in water intake with changes in care. The water balance of premature and critically ill infants is most highly vulnerable to influence by these variables; however, these are exactly the infants for whom precise maintenance of fluid and electrolyte balance is most important.

NEUROENDOCRINE CONTROL OF FLUID AND ELECTROLYTE BALANCE

The pituitary gland, adrenal cortex, parathyroid glands, and heart are the major organs producing hormones involved in the regulation of water and electrolyte balance in the body. The basic mechanisms by which the antidiuretic hormone, arginine vasopressin (AVP), is produced and secreted by the posterior pituitary gland appear to be intact in newborn infants (48–50), even in those who are born prematurely (51). However, it is not clear at what age precise quantitative hypothalamic control of AVP production is established. It is known that even in the first week of life, breast-fed term infants release vasopressin in response to a 10% loss of body weight (50).

Aldosterone is the most potent mineralocorticoid produced and secreted by the adrenal cortex. Its synthesis is regulated by the renin–angiotensin system, adrenocorticotrophic hormone, and the plasma concentrations of sodium and potassium. These mechanisms appear to be intact in newborn infants, even those born prematurely (52–56). Increased sodium loss in the urine of premature infants in the presence of high plasma concentrations of aldosterone and elevated urinary aldosterone excretion

suggests that the renal tubule is less responsive in premature than in term infants (54,55). Under conditions of low sodium intake, however, the high plasma aldosterone concentrations found in sick newborn infants seem to promote increased sodium reabsorption in the distal nephron (56).

Calcium concentration in the blood of newborn infants is regulated by the balance between parathyroid hormone (PTH), which is produced by the parathyroid glands, and calcitonin, which is produced in the thyroid. Serum PTH concentration is low at birth and rises slowly during the first few days, both in term and premature infants (57–59). The same pattern has been observed with serum calcitonin concentrations (58,59). Intravenous calcium infusion to large premature and term infants caused elevation of serum calcitonin and a corresponding fall in serum PTH (60). These data together indicate that the hormonal regulation of calcium metabolism is basically intact in newborn infants, even those born prematurely.

Atrial natriuretic factor (ANF) is present in the fetal heart early during development (61). In the human fetus, cardiac atrial levels of ANF increase during gestation and, by the beginning of the third trimester, exceed adult human levels; during the same period, fetal ventricular ANF levels decrease (62). Plasma ANF levels rise after birth, peaking at the time of maximal postnatal diuresis, usually 48 to 72 hours, and then returning to levels below those at birth (63–65). ANF secretion is stimulated by volume loading (66), and ANF levels correlate with atrial size (67). ANF in turn stimulates diuresis and natriuresis and seems to play an important role in the regulation of extracellular fluid volume in newborn infants (67–69). However, studies of the effects of sodium supplementation on ANF levels and sodium excretion indicate that premature infants are less responsive to ANF than are adults (68).

RENAL FUNCTION IN RELATION TO FLUID AND ELECTROLYTE THERAPY

Most aspects of renal function are incompletely developed at birth, especially in premature infants (12,70–76). Both glomerular and tubular functions increase with gestational age (12,70–72,76) at birth and with postnatal age (12,72–75). This development seems to depend most directly on postmenstrual age (gestational age plus postnatal age) and occurs at approximately the same rate, regardless of whether the infant has been born or is *in utero* (71,72,75).

In spite of the immaturity of some aspects of renal tubular function at birth, the tubules seem to respond to AVP from the first day of life, even in small premature infants (51). However, the maximal urine concentration of premature infants, typically 600 mOsm/L, is less than that of term newborn infants (800 mOsm/L) or adults

(1,200 mOsm/L) (77,78). Both term and premature infants can excrete urine with osmolarity as low as 50 mOsm/L when challenged with an acute water load (78–81). Although they can produce dilute urine, newborn infants cannot excrete a water load as rapidly as adults can (79).

The limitations in renal function in premature infants contribute to the problems of fluid and electrolyte regulation in various disease states. The glomerular and tubular functions of premature infants allow them to handle some physiologic variations in water and electrolyte load, but imbalance readily occurs when estimations of the water and electrolyte needs are misjudged, particularly in the case of extremely premature infants.

PRINCIPLES OF FLUID AND ELECTROLYTE THERAPY

As in older children, three steps should be followed in the management of infants with fluid and electrolyte disorders:

1. Estimate the deficits of fluid and electrolytes.
2. Calculate the amounts of fluid and electrolytes required for replacement of deficits, maintenance, and replacement of ongoing abnormal losses.
3. Institute a system of monitoring the response to therapy.

Estimation of Fluid and Electrolyte Deficits

Fluid Deficit

The body water deficit can be estimated on the basis of the degree of dehydration. If serial body weight measurements are available, the acute weight loss is considered to represent the water deficit. During the first week of life, however, weight loss of up to 15% occurs normally as a result of loss of ECW and tissue catabolism. Smaller infants lose a larger fraction of their weight, presumably because of their relatively larger ECW and more negative protein and energy balance. Even those small premature infants who can be enterally fed lose an average of 10% of their body weight during the first 5 days of life (82). Among infants weighing less than 1 kg who must be nourished intravenously, it is not uncommon to observe weight loss of 15% or even 20% without evidence of circulatory or renal insufficiency resulting from dehydration. The precise amount of weight loss desired during the first week of life has not been established because of a lack of reliable physiologic data. In general, smaller infants should be expected to lose larger fractions of their weight following birth. In contrast to term infants, who may lose a total of 5% to 10% of their birth weight, premature infants may lose 10% to 20% without adverse consequences. For small premature infants, a weight loss of 2% to 3% per day is a reasonable target in the first

week of life. Efforts to prevent any postnatal weight loss risk overhydration and problems with symptomatic PDA (16). Beyond the first week of life, acute weight loss should be considered to indicate nonphysiologic dehydration, and the calculated deficit of water should be replaced.

If an infant presents as an outpatient with dehydration, serial body weight data may not be available. In such cases, urine volume and concentration and physical signs can be used to estimate the degree of dehydration. Infants with 5% isotonic (i.e., serum sodium concentration 130 to 150 mEq/L) dehydration have dry mucous membranes, subnormal tear production with crying, flat or slightly sunken anterior fontanelle (when quiet in the upright position), and oliguria. Infants with 10% isotonic dehydration have dry mucous membranes, absent tears, sunken eyes and fontanelle, cool extremities, poor skin turgor, and oliguria. Infants with 15% isotonic dehydration have the aforementioned signs as well as signs of shock, such as hypotension, tachycardia, weak pulses, mottled skin, and altered sensorium. Infants with hypertonic dehydration (i.e., serum sodium concentration greater than 150 mEq/L) have less severe symptoms than infants with isotonic dehydration who have lost the same fraction of body water; the intravascular volume is preserved better with hypernatremia than with isotonic dehydration. However, infants with hypotonic dehydration (i.e., serum sodium less than 130 mEq/L) may have more severe symptoms with the same degree of dehydration.

The usual clinical signs of dehydration are more difficult to evaluate in small premature infants. Their skin and mucous membranes may appear dry because of thermal or mechanical injury, particularly in infants kept under radiant warmers. In addition, skin turgor is harder to judge because of the lack of subcutaneous fat.

Electrolyte Deficits

The nature and extent of electrolyte disturbances often can be determined by history and physical examination and by measurement of electrolyte concentrations in serum. Based on serum sodium concentration, electrolyte disturbances are divided into isotonic, hypertonic, and hypotonic abnormalities. The type of electrolyte disorder seen in a clinical situation depends on the cause of fluid and electrolyte abnormality. For example, severe acute diarrhea usually leads to isotonic dehydration. High insensible water loss, such as may occur in small premature infants under radiant warmers, may result in hypernatremic dehydration. Inadequate replacement of salt losses from diarrhea may produce hypotonic dehydration. Although it may be possible to anticipate the type of electrolyte disorder accompanying dehydration in some situations, confirmation must be made by measurement of serum electrolyte concentrations.

Calculation of Fluid and Electrolyte Requirements

After replacement of any fluid and electrolyte deficits, the requirements of newborn infants for water and electrolytes are determined by the rates of loss of these substances from the body by various routes and by the net amounts retained by body tissues during changes in body weight and composition. Knowledge of the usual rates of loss and of expected changes in body weight and composition in the first postnatal days and during subsequent growth helps to estimate water and electrolyte requirements. These estimates then are used to guide the management of fluid and electrolyte therapy.

Replacement of Fluid and Electrolyte Deficits

The deficit of fluid, or water, is calculated from the estimated degree of dehydration determined from measured body weight loss or by clinical examination. The rate and composition of initial fluid replacement depend on the severity of dehydration. As a rule, dehydration of acute onset and short duration requires more rapid correction. An exception to this rule is the case of hypertonic dehydration, in which rapid expansion of body water may cause brain swelling and convulsions.

The deficit of electrolytes is calculated on the basis of the difference between total body solute expected before dehydration and that observed in the dehydrated state (Table 22–5). It is common to replace half the water deficit over the first 8 hours and the other half over the next 16 hours. The sodium deficit is replaced over 24 hours. If the potassium deficit is large, one should replace it over a longer period (i.e., over 48 to 72 hours) to allow ascertainment of adequate renal function and to avoid the possible cardiac effects associated with rapid potassium infusion. Initiation of potassium replacement is best deferred until urine flow is established.

Maintenance Fluid and Electrolytes

Insensible water loss, urine, fecal water, and water retained in new tissues during growth are the four components that must be considered in estimating the daily maintenance water requirement. Fecal water loss is approximately 5 to 10 mL/kg/d (83). The water retained for growth is about 10 mL/kg/d, assuming a weight gain of 10 to 20 g/kg/d, 60% to 70% of which is water (3). In the first week of life, fecal water loss is small, and no water is deposited in new tissues because growth has not yet begun. In fact, water is lost from body tissues during the period of physiologic extracellular dehydration. After growth begins, replacement of fecal and growth water may require up to 20 g/kg/d, but this amount is small compared with the insensible and urine water losses, the two major routes of water loss that must be considered in estimating the water intake required to maintain the desired water balance.

A small portion of the water required to replace these normal losses is derived from the oxidation of metabolic fuels (i.e., carbohydrate, protein, and fat). This water of oxidation consists of about 0.60 mL/g of carbohydrate oxidized, 0.43 mL/g protein, and 1.07 mL/g fat (84). A newborn infant usually produces 5 to 10 mL/kg/d as water of oxidation. This amount is small enough to be neglected in most calculations but can be considered to offset the normal fecal water loss of 5 to 10 mL/kg/d.

For a term infant under basal conditions, insensible water loss is approximately 20 mL/kg/d (19). Urine volume depends on the excess of water intake over losses by other routes (i.e., IWL, feces, growth), and urine concentration is determined by the urine volume and renal solute load. The range of urinary water loss within which the infant's immature kidneys can safely excrete the total renal solute load is determined by the limits of urine concentration (volume = solute load/urine concentration) (85). A renal solute load of 15 to 30 mOsm/kg/d would require urine volume of 50 to 100 mL/kg/d to maintain an

---

TABLE 22–5. *Calculation of sodium deficit*

Type of dehydration	Serum sodium concentration (mEq/L)	Calculation of total solute deficit (mOsm/kg)[a]	Solute deficit (mOsm/kg)	Sodium deficit (mEq/kg)[b]
Isotonic (10%)	140	$(0.7 \times 280) - (0.6 \times 280)$	28	14
Hypertonic (10%)	153	$(0.7 \times 280) - (0.6 \times 306)$	12	6
Hypotonic (10%)	127	$(0.7 \times 280) - (0.6 \times 254)$	44	22

[a]Total solute deficit = $(TBW_e \times solute_e) - (TBW_o \times solute_o)$, where subscripts e and o indicate expected and observed, respectively. $TBW_e = 0.7$ L/kg; $TBW_o = 0.7 - 0.1 = 0.6$ L/kg; $solute_e = 140 \times 2 = 280$ mOsm/L, assuming total solute concentration in body water is twice the Na concentration in serum; $solute_o$ = observed serum Na × 2.

[b]Total solute deficit is assumed to be half sodium. Although the serum (and ECW) has lost this amount of sodium, only half this amount has been lost to the environment; the other half has been lost into the cells in exchange for potassium, which in turn has been lost from the body. In practice, therefore, only half the amount listed as "Na deficit" should be replaced as sodium, and the other half should be given as potassium.

average urine concentration of 300 mOsm/L. This urine concentration is near the middle of the range of urine osmolarity that can be produced by the neonatal kidneys, and it allows a margin of safety for over- or underestimation of other water requirements.

In the first days of life, a term infant receiving intravenous fluid and electrolytes would need to excrete about 15 mOsm/kg/d, assuming that endogenous solute production and tissue deposition of solute are negligible. The urine volume of 50 mL/kg/d plus the IWL of 20 mL/kg/d yield a total maintenance water requirement of 70 mL/kg/d; this assumes growth and fecal water to be small enough to be offset by the water of oxidation. If one allows for a negative water balance of 10 mL/kg/d, the true water requirement at birth is about 60 mL/kg/d. With increasing postnatal age and enteral feedings, the renal solute load and fecal water loss increase, and water is deposited in new tissues as growth begins. By the second week of life, a growing term infant needs 120 to 150 mL/kg/d.

In premature infants, the maintenance water requirement is larger because of higher IWL (22,24). Therefore, the IWL component of maintenance water should be increased with decreasing birth weight or gestation. During the first days of life, the renal solute load is less because little exogenous solute is provided. If NaCl is administered at a rate of 2 mEq/kg/d (4 mOsm/kg/d) and a solute load of 8 mOsm/kg/d resulting from tissue catabolism is assumed to be excreted (86), a urine volume of only 40 mL/kg/d is required to excrete this solute with a urine concentration of 300 mOsm/L. Thus, a small premature infant requires about 80 mL/kg/d on day 1 (60 IWL + 40 urine − 20 for negative balance). The water requirement for this same infant would be about 150 mL/kg/d in the second or third week (55 IWL + 85 urine + 10 feces + 10 growth − 10 oxidation). Very premature (less than 2 weeks of gestation) infants in the first week of life may have considerably higher IWL, raising the total water requirement to 200 or 300 mL/kg/d or even higher. The minimum water intake of premature infants is also higher than that of term infants because of the slightly lower urinary concentrating capacity (77,78). However, the aforementioned urine volumes (40 to 100 mL/kg/d) were selected to avoid taxing this limit of concentration and so are not influenced by this effect of immaturity.

The allowance for IWL should be increased by about 50% for infants under radiant warmers (22,29–32) or receiving overhead phototherapy (22,33). If both are used, the allowance for IWL should be increased by approximately 100% (31). The effect of fiberoptic phototherapy blankets or pads on IWL is not known but is probably less than that of overhead phototherapy. The IWL of infants in incubators also is increased if body or environmental temperature is too high (19,27,28). The IWL can be reduced by increasing the ambient or inspired humidity (19,21) or by using certain types of heat shields (32,36,37), plastic blankets (38,39), semipermeable membranes (40–42), or waterproof topical agents such as paraffin (43,44) (see Table 22–3).

The infant's maintenance requirements of sodium, potassium, and chloride can be estimated by adding the dermal, urinary, and fecal losses to the amounts retained in the body tissues during growth. The estimated requirements for sodium, potassium, and chloride are each between 2 and 4 mEq/kg/d (87,88). Small premature infants may require additional sodium because of increased urinary excretion (74,89–92), especially during the second and third weeks of life. The magnitude of urinary sodium excretion is inversely proportional to gestational age (70) (Fig. 22–6).

Ongoing Abnormal Losses of Fluid and Electrolytes

Ongoing abnormal losses must be replaced along with correction of established deficits and provision of maintenance fluid and electrolytes. Abnormal losses may occur with vomiting or diarrhea, ileostomy drainage, or removal by aspiration of gastrointestinal, pleural, peritoneal, or cerebrospinal fluid. The amount of extra water required can be determined by carefully measuring the volume of the losses. The additional amounts of electrolytes required can be estimated by measuring their concentrations in an aliquot of fluid (Table 22–6).

Example of Fluid and Electrolyte Calculation

Consider a 3-kg infant who presents with 10% isotonic dehydration (i.e., serum Na = 140 mEq/L). In the first 24 hours of therapy, the infant should be given 27 mEq of

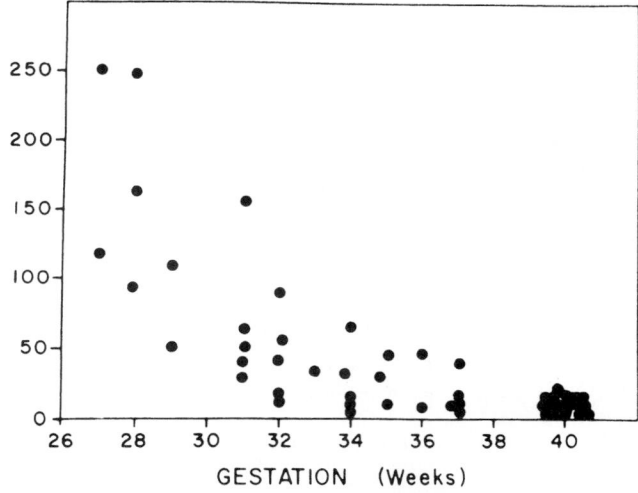

FIG. 22–6. Urinary sodium excretion in infants from 27 to 40 weeks of gestation. (Adapted from ref. 70.)

TABLE 22–6. *Electrolyte content of body fluids*

Fluid source	Sodium (mEq/L)	Potassium (mEq/L)	Chloride (mEq/L)
Stomach	20–80	5–20	100–150
Small intestine	100–140	5–15	90–120
Bile	120–140	5–15	90–120
Ileostomy	45–135	3–15	20–120
Diarrheal stool	10–90	10–80	10–110
Cerebrospinal fluid	130–150	2–5	110–130

sodium chloride in 600 mL of water as a dextrose solution (Table 22–7). If the potassium deficit is to be corrected over 72 hours, 13 mEq of potassium chloride (21/3 + 6) should be given during the first 24 hours. This fluid could then be ordered as dextrose solution with 45 mEq NaCl/L and 20 mEq KCl/L to be infused at 25 mL/h. If the infant also had significant metabolic acidosis, some or all of the sodium could be given as sodium bicarbonate or sodium acetate.

The initial glucose concentration is determined by the estimated water requirement and the desired glucose intake, which is usually 5 to 8 mg/kg/min. Smaller, more premature infants, because they require more water and may tolerate less glucose, usually are begun on fluids containing lower concentrations of glucose (e.g., 5 g/dL); larger term or near-term infants require higher glucose concentrations (e.g., 10 g/dL).

The fluid and electrolyte requirements of very small premature infants vary widely and are difficult to predict. Therefore, close monitoring of the fluid and electrolyte balance of these infants is especially important so that any imbalance can be detected as soon as possible.

Monitoring the Effectiveness of Fluid and Electrolyte Therapy

During the course of parenteral fluid therapy, detailed and organized data collection is necessary for monitoring the adequacy of fluid and electrolyte intake. Data that should be collected and recorded regularly at designated intervals include water and electrolyte intake by all routes, measurable output of water, body weight changes, serum electrolyte and creatinine concentrations, and blood urea

nitrogen concentration. In addition, clinical assessment should be made for the presence of dehydration, edema, or acute water overload. A calibrated infusion pump should be used to assure accurate administration of prescribed parenteral fluids. Accurate measurement of urine volume is difficult in small infants. It is possible to collect urine from male infants by placing the penis into a test tube that is taped to the abdomen. Urine is then aspirated from the test tube with a catheter and syringe. Urine volume also can be estimated by comparison of the weights of dry and wet diapers, provided the diaper is weighed soon enough to avoid evaporation.

Inadequate fluid may be administered if the fluid maintenance requirement is underestimated or if a preexisting deficit or ongoing loss is neglected or underestimated. Insufficient water intake leads to reduced urine volume and increased urine concentration, and if these compensatory measures are inadequate, water is mobilized from body stores to provide for obligatory insensible loss and to allow solute excretion. This results in weight loss, clinical signs of dehydration, metabolic acidosis, and hemoconcentration. As serum osmolarity rises, neurologic sequelae of hypertonicity may occur. In severe cases, untreated dehydration may lead to decreased circulating blood volume, acute renal failure, and finally to death from cardiovascular collapse.

Excessive water intake leads to increased excretion of dilute urine. If these compensatory mechanisms are overtaxed, water will be retained in the body, resulting in edema and weight gain. Rapid overhydration may produce congestive heart failure and pulmonary edema, particularly in ill infants with cardiopulmonary disorders. Even gradual daily administration of excess water (i.e.,

TABLE 22–7. *Calculation of fluid and electrolyte intake for a 3-kg infant with 10% isotonic dehydration*

	Water (mL)	Sodium (mEq)	Potassium (mEq)
Deficit	300[a]	21[b]	21[b,c]
Maintenance	300[d]	6	6
Ongoing losses	0	0	0
Total	600	27	27[c]
Total/kg	200	9	9[c]

[a]Water deficit: 0.10 × 3 kg.
[b]Electrolyte deficits calculated as in Table 22–5 (14 mEq/kg × 3 kg divided between Na and K).
[c]Potassium deficit should be replaced slowly, over 48 to 72 hours.
[d]Maintenance water requirement assumed to be 100 mL/kg/d.

volumes larger than can be readily eliminated by the kidneys) may increase the risk of heart failure from PDA in premature infants (16).

If appropriate fluid therapy is being provided, body weight should be stable or slowly increasing after the first week of life, and there should be no evidence of fluid overload or dehydration. During the first week of life, loss of as much as 15% of body weight (1% to 3% per day) is considered normal, provided urine output is adequate and there is no acidosis or evidence of dehydration. This "physiologic" weight loss is at least partly the result of a postnatal fall in the ECW volume. Efforts to prevent this weight loss are ill advised and may lead to fluid overload, edema, and significant PDA. Plotting daily weights graphically may help in detecting excessive weight loss or inappropriate weight gain.

Routine measurement of serum electrolyte concentrations is the best way to monitor the body's electrolyte status and the adequacy or excess of electrolyte intake. It is not necessary to add sodium to the parenterally administered fluid during the first 24 hours of life (93). However, adding some sodium as bicarbonate or acetate facilitates the use of permissive hypercapnia to reduce lung trauma while still maintaining acceptable arterial pH levels. In any case, It is advisable to determine the serum electrolyte concentrations soon after birth in infants who require parenteral fluids; if the mother received sodium-free fluid during labor the infant may be hyponatremic (17,18) and require immediate addition of sodium to the prescribed fluid. If not required earlier, sodium in the form of sodium chloride, sodium acetate, or sodium bicarbonate should be administered at a dose of 2 to 4 mEq/kg/d, beginning with the second day of life. The acetate and bicarbonate salts are useful in infants with metabolic acidosis from renal immaturity or other causes and to assist the kidneys in buffering the respiratory acidosis resulting from permissive hypercapnia.

During the first week of life, infants are usually in negative sodium balance as a result of the mobilization of sodium along with water from the extracellular compartment. This negative balance should be allowed as long as the serum sodium concentration remains normal. In the second and third weeks of life, small premature infants may require more sodium to replace the large amounts that are lost in the urine (74,89–92). It is important to understand that most cases of hyponatremia or hypernatremia result from excessive or inadequate intake of water.

Potassium supplementation (2 mEq/kg/d) may be started after the infant urinates unless the serum potassium concentration is elevated. In most infants, potassium should be added to the infused fluids by the second day. In very small, critically ill premature infants, however, it is often wise to wait until the serum potassium concentration falls below 4 mEq/L before administering potassium; these infants are at increased risk from hyperkalemia due to catabolism and release of potassium from cells in combination with decreased renal potassium excretion (94–97).

Hyperkalemia is the most common life-threatening electrolyte disturbance in newborn infants. If an elevated serum potassium level is reported by the laboratory, it should not be attributed to *in vitro* hemolysis without verification of the result with another blood sample obtained with good technique to minimize hemolysis. If the serum potassium concentration is higher than 6 mEq/L, only potassium-free fluids should be administered. If the serum potassium concentration is greater than 7 mEq/L, rectal administration of a potassium-binding resin (e.g., Kayexalate) should be considered. If a cardiac arrhythmia occurs in the presence of hyperkalemia, calcium, bicarbonate, and insulin with glucose should be given to force potassium into body cells. In small premature infants, hyperkalemic arrhythmias include sinus bradycardia—especially if it occurs without hypoxia—and ventricular tachycardia.

Blood urea nitrogen and serum or plasma creatinine levels (Fig. 22–7) (98) are useful for assessing renal function, although the urea nitrogen also may be elevated with dehydration.

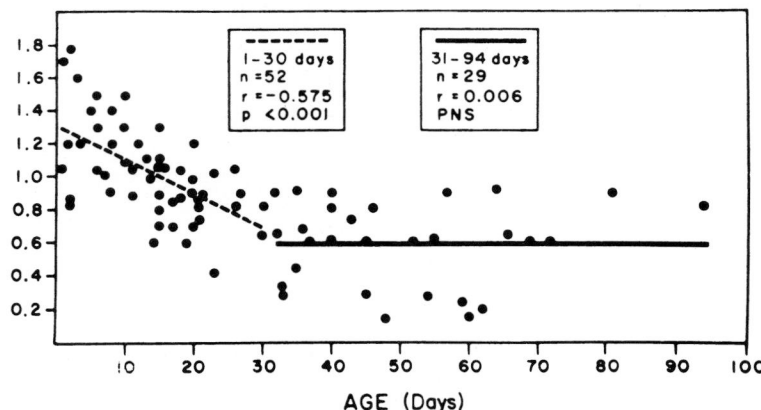

FIG. 22–7. Plasma creatinine levels of premature infants during the first 3 months of life. (From ref. 98.)

ACID–BASE BALANCE

The physiologic buffer system—primarily bicarbonate and its weak acid counterpart carbonic acid—and the renal and respiratory compensatory systems are the major mechanisms responsible for the maintenance of normal acid–base equilibrium in the body fluids. Changes in the hydrogen ion concentration in body fluids follow the Henderson–Hasselbach equation:

$$pH = 6.1 + \log ([HCO_3^-]/[H_2CO_3]),$$

in which 6.1 is the pK or dissociation constant for carbonic acid (99) and $[H_2CO_3]$ is the concentration of carbonic acid. It can be seen from this equation that any increase or decrease in the bicarbonate (HCO_3^-) concentration results in *metabolic alkalosis* or *metabolic acidosis*, respectively. Because H_2CO_3 is interchangeably linked to PCO_2 under the influence of carbonic anhydrase, any alteration in PCO_2 in body fluid also alters pH. Thus, hyperventilation, by reducing PCO_2, produces *respiratory alkalosis*, and hypoventilation, by increasing PCO_2, causes *respiratory acidosis*.

Metabolic alkalosis occurs with pyloric stenosis, because persistent vomiting results in the loss of hydrochloric acid and thus produces a relative excess of bicarbonate. Metabolic acidosis is most commonly seen as a consequence of lactic acid accumulation from anaerobic metabolism in hypoxic infants. Respiratory alkalosis may occur in an infant who is hyperventilated by a mechanical ventilator. Respiratory acidosis occurs as a result of hypercapnia in infants with respiratory distress syndrome (RDS) or other pulmonary disease.

In all types of acid–base disturbance, compensation by the lungs or kidneys occurs to restore the pH toward 7.4. Metabolic acid–base disorders are corrected by change in ventilation, and respiratory disorders are compensated for by change in renal bicarbonate excretion. If the compensation is adequate to correct the pH to normal, the acid–base disturbance is said to be compensated. For example, if an infant with RDS had a pH of 7.38, PCO_2 of 32 mm Hg, bicarbonate concentration of 18 mEq/L, and base excess of -5 mEq/L, the acid–base status would be called *compensated metabolic acidosis*. If the same infant had a pH of 7.38, PCO_2 of 50 mm Hg, bicarbonate concentration of 29 mEq/L, and base excess of +3 mEq/L, the acid–base status would be *compensated respiratory acidosis*.

FLUID AND ELECTROLYTE PROBLEMS ASSOCIATED WITH SPECIFIC CLINICAL CONDITIONS

Extreme Prematurity

Infants born at gestational ages younger than 26 weeks present special problems in fluid and electrolyte management. These infants have large insensible water losses (25,26), in some cases more than 200 mL/kg/d if the infant is nursed under a radiant warmer. The large IWL of extremely premature infants results from their meager skin barrier to evaporation and their large ratio of surface area to body weight. The average water requirement for an infant with birth weight between 500 and 750 g in the first week of life is estimated to be about 170 mL/kg/d if the infant is in an incubator with low ambient humidity and without phototherapy and perhaps 150 mL/kg/d if moderate humidity is added to the incubator; the requirement would be 210 to 220 mL/kg/d if a radiant warmer or overhead phototherapy is used and 250 to 270 mL/kg/d if both a radiant warmer and phototherapy are used (100). In the first week of life, the water requirement may be even higher in infants born after only 23 or 24 weeks of gestation. In these extremely premature infants, the cutaneous insensible water loss and consequently the total water requirement can fall rapidly near the end of the first week of life, as the stratum corneum matures and becomes less permeable to water.

Extremely premature infants, unless hyponatremic from maternal hypotonicity (17,18), should initially be started on electrolyte-free solutions of glucose (5 g/dL) in water or solutions that provide sodium in a dose of 2 to 3 mEq/kg/d as sodium acetate or sodium bicarbonate. The latter bases prevent respiratory acidosis while allowing hypercapnia with the goal of minimizing lung trauma. Administering some or all of the maintenance sodium as sodium bicarbonate or sodium acetate also serves to mitigate the metabolic acidosis present in many extremely premature infants as a result of renal immaturity and transient renal tubular acidosis. If sodium is not begun initially, it should be added by the second or third day, provided the serum sodium concentration is less than 145 mEq/L.

Hyperkalemia is a very common problem in extremely premature infants during the first week of life. This dangerous condition results from potassium release from catabolized cells in the presence of immature distal renal tubular function (94–96). Hyperkalemia is exacerbated if dehydration and oliguria occur as a result of inadequate water intake. No potassium should be given to extremely premature infants until the serum potassium concentration falls below 4 mEq/L. If the serum potassium concentration exceeds 7 mEq/L, rectal administration of a potassium-binding resin should be considered.

Respiratory Distress Syndrome and Bronchopulmonary Dysplasia

The renal function of infants with RDS is similar to that of infants of the same gestational age without respiratory distress, provided their cardiorespiratory status is not compromised (101–103). If infants with RDS become hypoxic and acidotic, however, they may have decreased glomerular filtration (inulin and creatinine clearance), renal blood flow [p-aminohippuric acid (PAH) clearance], and renal bicarbonate threshold (102–105). It has been observed that clinical improvement in infants with RDS is accompanied by an increase in urine volume that occurs on the second and third days of life (106). It is not clear whether this diuresis causes, or is caused by, the improving pulmonary function, or whether each enhances the other. These associated events may, in fact, be causally unrelated because this is the time when all infants, but especially premature infants, are in negative water balance (107,108) and undergo a contraction of the ECW.

In addition to any changes in renal function that may occur with pulmonary dysfunction resulting from severe RDS, positive-pressure ventilation also may cause water retention through effects on renal function. Continuous positive airway pressure can decrease glomerular filtration rate, sodium excretion, and free water clearance without altering renal perfusion pressure (109,110). Intermittent positive-pressure ventilation impairs water and sodium excretion by uncertain mechanisms that probably include increased aldosterone secretion (111) and increased production of antidiuretic hormone (112,113). It also is possible for impaired filtration and solute excretion to result from decreased aortic pressure and renal perfusion if excessive mean airway pressures are used during ventilatory support (114,115). Infants with RDS and other pulmonary disorders may have increased secretion of antidiuretic hormone, especially if they develop pneumothorax (49,116,117).

PDA is a problem that affects premature infants; those with RDS are more likely to develop cardiorespiratory symptoms related to PDA than those without RDS. In a randomized clinical trial, Bell and co-workers (16) compared the effects of liberal and restricted water intake on the development of significant PDA in premature infants. Infants with birth weight from 0.75 to 2.0 kg were randomly assigned to "high-volume" or "low-volume" water intake beginning on the third day of life and continuing until 30 days of age, until full enteral feedings were achieved, or until congestive heart failure or dehydration occurred. The low-volume group received only enough water to meet average estimated requirements for urinary solute excretion, fecal loss, insensible loss, and growth; the high-volume group received an excess of at least 20 mL/kg/d. The mean water intake for the 85 infants in the low-volume group was 122 mL/kg/d (standard deviation 14); for the 85 high-volume infants it was 169 mL/kg/d (standard deviation 20). The number with a typical PDA murmur (9 vs. 35) and the number with congestive heart failure due to PDA (2 vs. 11) were significantly lower in the low-volume group. Eleven of the 13 infants with hemodynamically significant PDA also had RDS, which was identified before enrollment in the study on day 3. There were more infants with dehydration in the low-volume group and more with necrotizing enterocolitis in the

high-volume group. Thus, excessive water intake during the first few weeks of life was associated with a higher risk of morbidity from PDA in premature infants, especially those with RDS.

Three other randomized clinical trials have addressed the impact of water intake on mortality and morbidity in premature infants, most of whom had RDS (118–120). A systematic review (121) of the first three studies (16,118,119) in this group found a significant reduction in the risks of PDA and necrotizing enterocolitis with restricted water intake. A more recent systematic review (122) that included all four trials (16,118–120) found, in addition, a decreased risk of death with restricted water intake when a strict intention-to-treat analysis is used. However, exclusion in one study (120) of five infants who died on the first day of life would nullify the effect of water intake on mortality (122). These analyses showed increased weight loss but no significantly increased risk of dehydration with restricted water intake (121,122).

RDS commonly is associated with a combined respiratory and metabolic acidosis resulting from hypercapnia and lactic acidemia. In severe RDS, when the acidosis is primarily respiratory, assisted ventilation should be instituted. If the acidosis is primarily metabolic, the underlying cause should be identified and corrected; if this cannot be done, sodium bicarbonate may be given to correct the acidosis. There is little evidence to support the routine use of bicarbonate in infants with RDS (121,123–125). Therefore, the current approach is to treat only significant metabolic acidosis, generally if the pH is below 7.25. When bicarbonate is used, the dose should be calculated from the following equation:

$$NaHCO_3 \text{ dose} = \text{base deficit} \times \text{body weight} \times 0.5 \text{ L/kg}.$$

The 0.5 value in the equation is the volume of distribution (i.e., bicarbonate space), which is confined mostly to the extracellular fluid compartment (see Fig. 22–3). There is some disagreement regarding the true bicarbonate space; the reported values range from 0.3 to 0.6 L/kg. The 0.5 value in the preceding equation applies to term infants; 0.6 L/kg should probably be used for premature infants because of their larger volume of ECW (1).

The calculated bicarbonate dose should be diluted to a concentration of 0.5 mEq/mL and given intravenously at a rate no faster than 1 mEq/kg/min. A slow infusion over 30 to 60 minutes is preferable, especially for premature infants, because it may reduce the risk of rapid osmolar changes in the intravascular and interstitial fluid compartments (126), which have been associated with intracranial hemorrhage in infants receiving bicarbonate infusions (127).

Infants with RDS or bronchopulmonary dysplasia often are treated with dexamethasone or other corticosteroid hormones in an attempt to ameliorate the severity of the lung disease. During dexamethasone therapy, infants may have impaired glucose tolerance, growth failure, and elevated blood urea nitrogen resulting from the catabolic effects of dexamethasone (128–130). Dexamethasone also perturbs the balance of phosphorus and potassium by increasing urinary excretion of these elements (131).

Perinatal Asphyxia

Infants with hypoxia or ischemia of the brain and kidneys during the perinatal period may suffer brain or kidney injury. Increased secretion of AVP often accompanies hypoxic encephalopathy (49,132,133). Moreover, acute renal failure may result from renal ischemia in these infants (134,135). Both conditions cause oliguria and therefore decrease the need for exogenous water. After birth asphyxia, it is advisable to restrict water intake in anticipation of possible increased AVP secretion (also known as inappropriate antidiuretic hormone secretion) or acute renal failure. During the first 24 hours of life, the water intake for asphyxiated infants should be limited to insensible water loss plus urine output minus about 20 mL/kg/d to allow for some physiologic contraction of the ECW volume. If urine production is normal by the third postnatal day, water intake can be restored to a normal level.

During the oliguric phase of acute renal failure, potassium should not be administered unless the serum potassium concentration is less than 3.5 mEq/L. With acute renal failure due to hypoxia or ischemia, the initial period of oliguria may be followed by a diuretic phase with polyuria. If urine output increases and body weight falls below the expected level (i.e., the weight before fluid retention began), the intake of water must be increased to prevent dehydration. This diuretic phase may be accompanied by large losses of sodium and other electrolytes, which must be replaced. Replacement of the urinary sodium losses is facilitated by measuring the volume and sodium concentration of a timed collection of urine.

Central Nervous System Injury

Infants with brain injury from other causes, such as intracranial hemorrhage or central nervous system infection, also may have oliguria and water retention because of inappropriately increased secretion of AVP (49,132).

Sepsis and Necrotizing Enterocolitis

Systematic reviews of randomized clinical trials of varying fluid intake in premature infants have identified overhydration as a risk factor in the pathogenesis of necrotizing enterocolitis (121,122). Infants with septicemia who also have meningitis may develop inappropriate AVP secretion, reducing their water requirement. Infants with septicemia or necrotizing enterocolitis also may develop shock from endotoxin production, from hypovolemia due to loss of intravascular water and protein to the interstitial and peritoneal spaces or to the intestinal lumen, or from frank hemorrhage resulting from thrombocytopenia, disseminated intravascular coagulopathy, or intestinal injury. In infants with shock, it is essential to replace lost water and solutes in the form of blood products or other solute-containing fluids. Even if properly treated, septic shock may cause renal injury, which would then further complicate fluid and electrolyte management.

Pyloric Stenosis

With pyloric stenosis, water, electrolytes, and hydrogen ions are lost from the stomach as a result of repeated vomiting. Infants with severe vomiting caused by pyloric stenosis have increased intracellular sodium and decreased potassium. Infants with pyloric stenosis are likely to be dehydrated and may have hypochloremic metabolic alkalosis and hypokalemia. The alkalosis may cause lethargy, hypoventilation, and, in severe cases, tetany.

Parenteral fluid therapy consists of replacing the deficits of water, potassium, and chloride. The chloride initially should be given as sodium chloride. Potassium chloride should be added after adequate urination has been established. Specific treatment of the metabolic alkalosis with acidic agents is not necessary. In most cases, cessation of vomiting from withholding of oral intake, correction of dehydration, and replacement of chloride and potassium deficits will restore the blood acid–base status to normal.

Diarrhea

The principles of parenteral fluid therapy of diarrheal dehydration in the newborn infant are similar to those applied to older infants and children. Because of their limited renal concentrating ability, newborn infants are quicker to develop severe dehydration, hypovolemia, and cardiovascular collapse. Therefore, rapid establishment of intravenous access for vascular expansion is of the utmost importance in newborn infants with moderate-to-severe dehydration from diarrhea. After stabilization, fluid and electrolyte deficits should be estimated as described earlier in this chapter. Water and electrolytes should be given to correct established deficits, meet maintenance requirements, and counteract ongoing losses.

Metabolic acidosis is a frequent finding in diarrheal dehydration. During initial volume reexpansion, preexisting acidosis may worsen as the body bicarbonate is further diluted with bicarbonate-free replacement fluids. Prerenal azotemia is common with diarrheal dehydration. It usually corrects spontaneously within several days as the infant is rehydrated.

Oral fluids and feeding should be withheld during recovery from diarrheal dehydration. Oral rehydration has been used successfully in older children with diarrhea, but there has been less experience with this technique in newborn infants (136). For this reason, oral rehydration is not recommended for newborn infants in areas where adequate personnel and supplies are available to maintain parenteral infusions. The appropriate period of fasting depends on the severity and duration of the diarrheal episode. As a rule, a more severe, protracted bout requires a longer period of fasting. How long diarrheal stools persist following the onset of fasting also helps to determine the duration of fasting. Reintroduction of oral fluids should be carried out with extreme care. Aggressive refeeding may precipitate a recurrence of diarrhea or even protracted chronic diarrhea and malabsorption with consequent growth failure.

Fluid and Electrolyte Management of Neonatal Surgical Patients

If a condition that requires surgery (e.g., pyloric stenosis) results in dehydration and electrolyte or acid–base disturbance, the infant should be restored as nearly as possible to normal fluid, electrolyte, and acid–base status before surgery. Otherwise, the risks of anesthesia and surgery might be increased by dehydration, acidosis, alkalosis, or abnormal serum potassium concentration.

During surgery, the prescribed fluid and electrolyte therapy should be continued with the same fluid composition and rate of infusion unless additional intraoperative losses require replacement. The anesthesiologist and surgeons should be apprised of the plan for parenteral fluid therapy to avoid errors resulting from lack of communication. The operative losses of fluid and blood should be recorded and replaced either during surgery or immediately thereafter.

During the initial postoperative period, some infants have reduced urine output as a result of fluid loss from the vascular compartment or increased secretion of AVP. Therefore, the fluid provided for maintenance may need to be reduced during the immediate postoperative period. However, this reduction may be offset by the extra fluid required to replace abnormal operative and postoperative losses. A system of careful monitoring of fluid and electrolyte balance is essential in the surgical patient, as in other ill newborn infants.

TECHNICAL ASPECTS OF PARENTERAL FLUID THERAPY

Blood Sampling

Sampling of capillary blood by heel puncture is a safe and commonly used technique in newborn infants. Capillary blood is adequate for determination of serum electrolyte and blood urea nitrogen concentrations because most of these values agree closely with venous samples. Serum potassium concentration is slightly higher when obtained by heel puncture, but the difference is minimized if the blood flows freely from the puncture wound so that little squeezing is required. Blood flow can be enhanced by prior warming of the foot. Because the amount of blood obtained by heel puncture is limited, the neonatal service should be supported by a laboratory in close proximity to the nurseries that is capable of performing the required analyses on blood samples of small volume. Such laboratory support is also crucial to minimize blood transfusions necessitated in part by phlebotomy blood losses (137).

Blood samples for blood gas and acid–base determination also can be obtained by heel puncture. Their reliability is enhanced by warming the skin to 44°C, which reduces the arterial–capillary differences in blood gases and pH; however, PO_2 measurements on samples obtained by heel puncture tend to underestimate true arterial PO_2, especially in the hyperoxic range. It usually is possible to combine capillary acid–base and PCO_2 values with pulse oximetry or transcutaneous oxygen tension monitoring, avoiding the need for indwelling arterial catheters. However, indwelling umbilical or radial artery catheters often are used in infants who are extremely ill and require continuous blood pressure monitoring or high levels of oxygen and ventilatory support. Because indwelling arterial catheters are associated with serious thromboembolic complications, they should be removed as soon as possible. For occasional sampling of arterial blood, direct puncture and aspiration from a peripheral artery can be used. This procedure is fairly safe in skilled hands but can cause serious complications, such as arterial obstruction or nerve injury.

Intravenous Fluid Infusion

With practice and skill, a short plastic catheter with an inner needle guide can be inserted into a peripheral vein in an extremity or the scalp. Shaving scalp hair to expose veins is distressing to many parents; the scalp should be used only if extremity sites have been exhausted and only after the procedure has been discussed with the parents. Intravenous sites must be inspected carefully on each nursing shift for evidence of infection at the insertion site or for extravasation of infusate that might injure subcutaneous tissues.

Long catheters of silicone elastomer or other materials can be inserted percutaneously so that the tip lies centrally in a large vein within the abdomen or chest. These catheters can be used for long-term intravenous access with lower risks of infection and thrombosis than occur with surgically inserted central vein catheters.

Superficial venous cutdown is seldom necessary if skilled personnel are available to insert and maintain standard intravenous catheters. Cutdowns risk local infection or septicemia and permanent venous obstruction. Moreover, catheters inserted by cutdown usually do not last as long in newborn infants as they do in older children and adults. For these reasons, superficial venous cutdown should be avoided in newborns whenever possible.

The umbilical vein is not suitable as a site for routine infusion of fluid, electrolytes, and nutrients because of the risks of infection, portal phlebitis, and liver damage. Its use should be reserved for central venous pressure monitoring and exchange transfusions. A possible exception is the use of umbilical vein catheters for fluid administration and blood sampling in extremely small premature infants in the first week of life. In such cases, a catheter with its tip in the inferior vena cava can be used for blood sampling, thereby minimizing the need for peripheral venous or capillary blood sampling, which can be traumatic to the infant's tender skin and subcutaneous tissues and disturbs his rest. If an umbilical vein catheter is used in this way, it should be removed by the end of the first week of life, when the risks of infection and thrombosis probably surpass the advantages of continued catheter use.

With any route of parenteral fluid administration to newborn infants, it is essential to use infusion pumps that can be regulated precisely and can deliver fluids at an absolutely steady rate, even when very low flow rates are used. A fluctuating infusion rate may cause erratic delivery of water, glucose and other nutrients, or drugs.

REFERENCES

1. Friis-Hansen B. Changes in body water compartments during growth. *Acta Paediatr Suppl* 1957;110:1.
2. Friis-Hansen B. Body water compartments in children: changes during growth and related changes in body composition. *Pediatrics* 1961;28:169.
3. Ziegler EE, O'Donnell AM, Nelson SE, Fomon SJ. Body composition of the reference fetus. *Growth* 1976;40:329.
4. Forbes GB, Perley A. Estimation of total body sodium by isotopic dilution. II. Studies on infants and children: an example of a constant differential growth ratio. *J Clin Invest* 1951;30:566.
5. Cheek DB. Observations on total body chloride in children. *Pediatrics* 1954;14:5.
6. Romahn A, Burmeister W. Die Körperzusammensetzung während der ersten zwei Lebensjahre: bestimmungen mit der Kalium-40-Methode. *Klin Pädiatr* 1977;189:321.
7. Cheek DB, Maddison TG, Malinek M, Coldbeck JH. Further observations on the corrected bromide space of the neonate and investigation of water and electrolyte status in infants born of diabetic mothers. *Pediatrics* 1961;28:861.
8. Kagan BM, Stanincova V, Felix NS, Hodgman J, Kalman D. Body composition of premature infants: relation to nutrition. *Am J Clin Nutr* 1972;25:1153.
9. Shaffer SG, Bradt SK, Hall RT. Postnatal changes in total body water and extracellular volume in the preterm infant with respiratory distress syndrome. *J Pediatr* 1986;109:509.
10. Bauer K, Bovermann G, Roithmaier A, Götz M, Pröiss A, Versmold HT. Body composition, nutrition, and fluid balance during the first two weeks of life in preterm neonates weighing less than 1500 grams. *J Pediatr* 1991;118:615.
11. Oh W, Oh MA, Lind J. Renal function and blood volume in newborn infant related to placental transfusion. *Acta Paediatr Scand* 1966;55:197.
12. Aperia A, Broberger O, Elinder G, Herin P, Zetterström R. Postnatal development of renal function in pre-term and full-term infants. *Acta Paediatr Scand* 1981;70:183.
13. Guignard JP. Renal function in the newborn infant. *Pediatr Clin North Am* 1982;29:777.
14. Cassady G, Milstead RR. Antipyrine space studies and cell water estimates in infants of low birth weight. *Pediatr Res* 1971;5:673.
15. Stonestreet BS, Bell EF, Warburton D, Oh W. Renal response in low-birth-weight neonates. Results of prolonged intake of two different amounts of fluid and sodium. *Am J Dis Child* 1983;137:215.
16. Bell EF, Warburton D, Stonestreet BS, Oh W. Effect of fluid administration on the development of symptomatic patent ductus arteriosus and congestive heart failure in premature infants. *N Engl J Med* 1980; 302:598.
17. Battaglia F, Prystowsky H, Smisson C, Hellegers A, Bruns P. Fetal blood studies. XIII. The effect of the administration of fluids intravenously to mothers upon the concentrations of water and electrolytes in plasma of human fetuses. *Pediatrics* 1960;25:2.
18. Tarnow-Mordi WO, Shaw JCL, Liu D, Gardner DA, Flynn FV. Iatrogenic hyponatraemia of the newborn due to maternal fluid overload: a prospective study. *Br Med J* 1981;283:639.
19. Hey EN, Katz G. Evaporative water loss in the new-born baby. *J Physiol (Lond)* 1969;200:605.
20. Sulyok E, Jéquier E, Prod'hom LS. Respiratory contribution to the thermal balance of the newborn infant under various ambient conditions. *Pediatrics* 1973;51:641.
21. Sosulski R, Polin RA, Baumgart S. Respiratory water loss and heat balance in intubated infants receiving humidified air. *J Pediatr* 1983; 103:307.
22. Wu PYK, Hodgman JE. Insensible water loss in preterm infants: changes with postnatal development and non-ionizing radiant energy. *Pediatrics* 1974;54:704.
23. Shaffer SG, Weismann DN. Fluid requirements in the preterm infant. *Clin Perinatol* 1992;19:233.
24. Okken A, Jonxis JHP, Rispens P, Zijlstra WG. Insensible water loss and metabolic rate in low birthweight newborn infants. *Pediatr Res* 1979;13:1072.
25. Costarino AT, Baumgart. Controversies in fluid and electrolyte therapy for the premature infant. *Clin Perinatol* 1988;15:863.
26. Hammarlund K, Sedin G. Transepidermal water loss in newborn infants. III. Relation to gestational age. *Acta Paediatr Scand* 1979;68:795.
27. Rutter N, Hull D. Response of term babies to a warm environment. *Arch Dis Child* 1979;54:178.
28. Bell EF, Gray JC, Weinstein MR, Oh W. The effects of thermal environment on heat balance and insensible water loss in low-birth-weight infants. *J Pediatr* 1980;96:452.
29. Williams PR, Oh W. Effects of radiant warmer on insensible water loss in newborn infants. *Am J Dis Child* 1974;128:511.
30. Jones RWA, Rochefort MJ, Baum JD. Increased insensible water loss in newborn infants nursed under radiant heaters. *Br Med J* 1976;2:1347.
31. Bell EF, Neidich GA, Cashore WJ, Oh W. Combined effect of radiant warmer and phototherapy on insensible water loss in low-birth-weight infants. *J Pediatr* 1979;94:810.
32. Bell EF, Weinstein MR, Oh W. Heat balance in premature infants: comparative effects of convectively heated incubator and radiant warmer, with and without plastic heat shield. *J Pediatr* 1980;96:460.
33. Oh W, Karecki H. Phototherapy and insensible water loss in the newborn infant. *Am J Dis Child* 1972;124:230.
34. Day R. Respiratory metabolism in infancy and in childhood. XXVII. Regulation of body temperature of premature infants. *Am J Dis Child* 1943;65:376.
35. Zweymüller E, Preining O. The insensible water loss of the newborn infant. *Acta Paediatr Scand Suppl* 1970;205:1.
36. Fanaroff AA, Wald M, Gruber HS, Klaus MH. Insensible water loss in low birth weight infants. *Pediatrics* 1972;50:236.
37. Baumgart S, Fox WW, Polin RA. Physiologic implications of two different heat shields for infants under radiant warmers. *J Pediatr* 1982; 100:787.
38. Marks KH, Friedman Z, Maisels MJ. A simple device for reducing insensible water loss in low-birth-weight infants. *Pediatrics* 1977;60:223.
39. Baumgart S. Reduction of oxygen consumption, insensible water loss, and radiant heat demand with use of a plastic blanket for low-birth-weight infants under radiant warmers. *Pediatrics* 1984;74:1022.

40. Knauth A, Gordin M, McNelis W, Baumgart S. Semipermeable polyurethane membrane as an artificial skin for the premature neonate. *Pediatrics* 1989;83:945.

41. Vernon HJ, Lane AT, Wischerath LJ, Davis JM, Menegus MA. Semipermeable dressing and transepidermal water loss in premature infants. *Pediatrics* 1990;86:357.

42. Mancini AJ, Sookdeo-Drost S, Madison KC, Smoller BR, Lane AT. Semipermeable dressings improve epidermal barrier function in premature infants. *Pediatr Res* 1994;36:306.

43. Rutter N, Hull D. Reduction of skin water loss in the newborn. I. Effect of applying topical agents. *Arch Dis Child* 1981;56:669.

44. Nopper AJ, Horii KA, Sookdeo-Drost S, Wang TH, Mancini AJ, Lane AT. Topical ointment therapy benefits premature infants. *J Pediatr* 1996;128:660.

45. Kjartansson S, Hammarlund K, Sedin G. Insensible water loss from the skin during phototherapy in term and preterm infants. *Acta Paediatr* 1992;81:764.

46. Kjartansson S, Hammarlund K, Riesenfeld T, Sedin G. Respiratory water loss and oxygen consumption in newborn infants during phototherapy. *Acta Paediatr* 1992;81:769.

47. Kjartansson S, Arsan S, Hammarlund K, Sjörs G, Sedin G. Water loss from the skin of term and preterm infants nursed under a radiant heater. *Pediatr Res* 1995;37:233.

48. Leung AKC, McArthur RG, McMillan DD, et al. Circulating antidiuretic hormone during labour and in the newborn. *Acta Paediatr Scand* 1980;69:505.

49. Wiriyathian S, Rosenfeld CR, Arant BS Jr, Porter JC, Faucher DJ, Engle WD. Urinary arginine vasopressin: pattern of excretion in the neonatal period. *Pediatr Res* 1986;20:103.

50. Marchini G, Stock S. Thirst and vasopressin secretion counteract dehydration in newborn infants. *J Pediatr* 1997;130:736.

51. Rees L, Brook CGD, Shaw JCL, Forsling ML. Hyponatraemia in the first week of life in preterm infants. Part I. Arginine vasopressin secretion. *Arch Dis Child* 1984;59:414.

52. Siegel SR, Fisher DA, Oh W. Serum aldosterone concentrations related to sodium balance in the newborn infant. *Pediatrics* 1974;53:410.

53. Dillon MJ, Rajani KB, Shah V, Ryness JM, Milner RDG. Renin and aldosterone response in human newborns to acute change in blood volume. *Arch Dis Child* 1978;53:461.

54. Aperia A, Broberger O, Herin P, Zetterström R. Sodium excretion in relation to sodium intake and aldosterone excretion in newborn preterm and full-term infants. *Acta Paediatr Scand* 1979;68:813.

55. Sulyok E, Németh M, Tényi I, et al. Postnatal development of renin-angiotensin-aldosterone system, RAAS, in relation to electrolyte balance in premature infants. *Pediatr Res* 1979;13:817.

56. Kojima T, Fukuda Y, Hirata Y, Matsuzaki S, Kobayashi Y. Effects of aldosterone and atrial natriuretic peptide on water and electrolyte homeostasis of sick neonates. *Pediatr Res* 1989;25:591.

57. David L, Anast CS. Calcium metabolism in newborn infants. The interrelationship of parathyroid function and calcium, magnesium, and phosphorus metabolism in normal, "sick," and hypocalcemic infants. *J Clin Invest* 1974;54:287.

58. David L, Salle B, Chopard P, Grafmeyer D. Studies on circulating immunoreactive calcitonin in low birth weight infants during the first 48 hours of life. *Helv Paediatr Acta* 1977;32:39.

59. Hillman LS, Rojanasathit S, Slatopolsky E, Haddad JG. Serial measurements of serum calcium, magnesium, parathyroid hormone, calcitonin, and 25-hydroxy-vitamin D in premature and term infants during the first week of life. *Pediatr Res* 1977;11:739.

60. David L, Salle BL, Putet G, Grafmeyer DC. Serum immunoreactive calcitonin in low birth weight infants. Description of early changes; effect of intravenous calcium infusion; relationships with early changes in serum calcium, phosphorus, magnesium, parathyroid hormone, and gastrin levels. *Pediatr Res* 1981;15:803.

61. Smith FG, Sata T, Varille VA, Robillard JE. Atrial natriuretic factor during fetal and postnatal life: a review. *J Dev Physiol* 1989;12:55.

62. Mercadier JJ, Zongazo MA, Wisnewsky C, et al. Atrial natriuretic factor messenger ribonucleic acid and peptide in the human heart during ontogenic development. *Biochem Biophys Res Commun* 1989;159:777.

63. Shaffer SG, Geer PG, Goetz KL. Elevated atrial natriuretic factor in neonates with respiratory distress syndrome. *J Pediatr* 1986;109:1028.

64. Liechty EA, Johnson MD, Myerberg DZ, Mullett MD. Daily sequential changes in plasma atrial natriuretic factor concentrations in mechanically ventilated low-birth-weight infants. *Biol Neonate* 1989;55:244.

65. Rozycki HJ, Baumgart S. Atrial natriuretic factor and postnatal diuresis in respiratory distress syndrome. *Arch Dis Child* 1991;66:43.

66. Robillard JE, Weiner C. Atrial natriuretic factor in the human fetus: effect of volume expansion. *J Pediatr* 1988;113:552.

67. Bierd TM, Kattwinkel J, Chevalier RL, et al. Interrelationship of atrial natriuretic peptide, atrial volume, and renal function in premature infants. *J Pediatr* 1990;116:753.

68. Tulassay T, Rascher W, Seyberth HW, Lang RE, Tóth M, Sulyok E. Role of atrial natriuretic peptide in sodium homeostasis in premature infants. *J Pediatr* 1986;109:1023.

69. Kojima T, Hirata Y, Fukuda Y, Iwase S, Kobayashi Y. Plasma atrial natriuretic peptide and spontaneous diuresis in sick neonates. *Arch Dis Child* 1987;62:667.

70. Siegel SR, Oh W. Renal function as a marker of human fetal maturation. *Acta Paediatr Scand* 1976;65:481.

71. Leake RD, Trygstad CW, Oh W. Inulin clearance in the newborn infant: relationship to gestational and postnatal age. *Pediatr Res* 1976;10:759.

72. Arant BS Jr. Development patterns of renal functional maturation compared in the human neonate. *J Pediatr* 1978;92:705.

73. Ross B, Cowett RM, Oh W. Renal functions of low birth weight infants during the first two months of life. *Pediatr Res* 1977;11:1162.

74. Sulyok E, Varga F, Györy E, Jobst K, Csaba IF. Postnatal development of renal sodium handling in premature infants. *J Pediatr* 1979;95:787.

75. Wilkins BH. Renal function in sick very low birthweight infants: 1. Glomerular filtration rate. *Arch Dis Child* 1992;67:1140.

76. Wilkins BH. Renal function in sick very low birthweight infants: 2. Urea and creatinine excretion. *Arch Dis Child* 1992;67:1146.

77. Hansen JDL, Smith CA. Effects of withholding fluid in the immediate postnatal period. *Pediatrics* 1953;12:99.

78. Calcagno PL, Rubin MI, Weintraub DH. Studies on the renal concentrating and diluting mechanisms in the premature infant. *J Clin Invest* 1954;33:91.

79. McCance RA, Naylor NJB, Widdowson EM. The response of infants to a large dose of water. *Arch Dis Child* 1954;29:104.

80. Leake RD, Zakauddin S, Trygstad CW, Fu P, Oh W. The effects of large volume intravenous fluid infusion on neonatal renal function. *J Pediatr* 1976;89:968.

81. Aperia A, Herin P, Lundin S, Melin P, Zetterström R. Regulation of renal water excretion in newborn full-term infants. *Acta Paediatr Scand* 1984;73:717.

82. Brosius KK, Ritter DA, Kenny JD. Postnatal growth curve of the infant with extremely low birth weight who was fed enterally. *Pediatrics* 1984;74:778.

83. Lemoh JN, Brooke OG. Frequency and weight of normal stools in infancy. *Arch Dis Child* 1979;54:719.

84. Williams GS, Klenk EL, Winters RW. Acute renal failure in pediatrics. In: Winters RW, ed. *The body fluids in pediatrics. Medical, surgical, and neonatal disorders of acid–base status, hydration, and oxygenation.* Boston: Little, Brown and Company, 1973:523.

85. Gamble JL, Butler AM. Measurement of the renal water requirement. *Trans Assoc Am Phys* 1944;58:157.

86. Sinclair JC, Driscoll JM Jr, Heird WC, Winters RW. Supportive management of the sick neonate. Parenteral calories, water, and electrolytes. *Pediatr Clin North Am* 1970;17:863.

87. Ziegler EE. Feeding the low birth weight infant. In: Gellis SS, Kagan BM, eds. *Current pediatric therapy 13.* Philadelphia: WB Saunders, 1990:713.

88. American Academy of Pediatrics Committee on Nutrition. Nutritional needs of preterm infants. In: Barness LA, ed. *Pediatric nutrition handbook,* 3rd ed. Elk Grove Village, IL: American Academy of Pediatrics, 1993:64.

89. Roy RN, Chance GW, Radde IC, Hill DE, Willis DM, Sheepers J. Late hyponatremia in very low birthweight infants (<1.3 kilograms). *Pediatr Res* 1976;10:526.

90. Engelke SC, Shah BL, Vasan U, Raye JR. Sodium balance in very low-birth-weight infants. *J Pediatr* 1978;93:837.

91. Rodriguez-Soriano J, Vallo A, Oliveros R, Castillo G. Renal handling of sodium in premature and full-term neonates: a study using clearance methods during water diuresis. *Pediatr Res* 1983;17:1013.

92. Al-Dahhan J, Haycock GB, Chantler C, Stimmler L. Sodium homeostasis in term and preterm neonates. I. Renal aspects. *Arch Dis Child* 1983;58:335.

93. Costarino AT Jr, Gruskay JA, Corcoran L, Polin RA, Baumgart S. Sodium restriction versus daily maintenance replacement in very low birth weight premature neonates: a randomized, blind therapeutic trial. *J Pediatr* 1992;120:99.

94. Gruskay J, Costarino AT, Polin RA, Baumgart S. Nonoliguric hyperkalemia in the premature infant weighing less than 1000 grams. *J Pediatr* 1988;113:381.

95. Shaffer SG, Kilbride HW, Hayen LK, Meade VM, Warady BA. Hyperkalemia in very low birth weight infants. *J Pediatr* 1992;121:275.

96. Sato K, Kondo T, Iwao H, Honda S, Ueda K. Internal potassium shift in premature infants: cause of nonoliguric hyperkalemia. *J Pediatr* 1995;126:109.

97. Lorenz JM, Kleinman LI, Markarian K. Potassium metabolism in extremely low birth weight infants in the first week of life. *J Pediatr* 1997;131:81.

98. Stonestreet BS, Oh W. Plasma creatinine levels in low-birth-weight infants during the first three months of life. *Pediatrics* 1978;61:788.

99. Karlowicz MG, Simmons MA, Brusilow SW, Jones MD Jr. Carbonic acid dissociation constant in critically ill newborns. *Pediatr Res* 1984;18:1287.

100. Bell EF. Nutritional support. In: Goldsmith JP, Karotkin EH, eds. *Assisted ventilation of the neonate*, 3rd ed. Philadelphia: WB Saunders, 1996:381.

101. Siegel SR, Fisher DA, Oh W. Renal function and serum aldosterone levels in infants with respiratory distress syndrome. *J Pediatr* 1973;83:854.

102. Broberger U, Aperia A. Renal function in idiopathic respiratory distress syndrome. *Acta Paediatr Scand* 1978;67:313.

103. Tulassay T, Ritvay J, Bors Z, Büky B. Alterations in creatinine clearance during respiratory distress syndrome. *Biol Neonate* 1979;35:258.

104. Torrado A, Guignard JP, Prod'hom LS, Gautier E. Hypoxaemia and renal function in newborns with respiratory distress syndrome (RDS). *Helv Paediatr Acta* 1974;29:399.

105. Guignard JP, Torrado A, Mazouni SM, Gautier E. Renal function in respiratory distress syndrome. *J Pediatr* 1976;88:845.

106. Langman CB, Engle WD, Baumgart S, Fox WW, Polin RA. The diuretic phase of respiratory distress syndrome and its relationship to oxygenation. *J Pediatr* 1981;98:462.

107. Bidiwala KS, Lorenz JM, Kleinman LI. Renal function correlates of postnatal diuresis in preterm infants. *Pediatrics* 1988;82:50.

108. Lorenz JM, Kleinman LI, Ahmed G, Markarian K. Phases of fluid and electrolyte homeostasis in the extremely low birth weight infant. *Pediatrics* 1995;96:484.

109. Fewell JE, Norton JB Jr. Continuous positive airway pressure impairs renal function in newborn goats. *Pediatr Res* 1980;14:1132.

110. Tulassay T, Machay T, Kiszel J, Varga J. Effects of continuous positive airway pressure on renal function in prematures. *Biol Neonate* 1983;43:152.

111. Cox JR, Davies-Jones GAB, Leonard PJ, Singer B. The effect of positive pressure respiration on urinary aldosterone excretion. *Clin Sci* 1963;24:1.

112. Bark H, LeRoith D, Nyska M, Glick SM. Elevations in plasma ADH levels during PEEP ventilation in the dog: mechanisms involved. *Am J Physiol* 1980;239:E474.

113. Hemmer M, Viquerat CE, Suter PM, Vallotton MB. Urinary antidiuretic hormone excretion during mechanical ventilation and weaning in man. *Anesthesiology* 1980;52:395.

114. Svenningsen NW, Andreasson B, Lindroth M. Diuresis and urine concentration during CPAP in newborn infants. *Acta Paediatr Scand* 1984;73:727.

115. Mullins RJ, Dawe EJ, Lucas CE, Ledgerwood AM, Banks SM. Mechanisms of impaired renal function with PEEP. *J Surg Res* 1984;37:189.

116. Paxson CL Jr, Stoerner JW, Denson SE, Adcock EW III, Morriss FH Jr. Syndrome of inappropriate antidiuretic hormone secretion in neonates with pneumothorax or atelectasis. *J Pediatr* 1977;91:459.

117. Stern P, LaRochelle FT Jr, Little GA. Vasopressin and pneumothorax in the neonate. *Pediatrics* 1981;68:499.

118. von Stockhausen HB, Struve M. Die Auswirkungen einer stark unterschiedlichen parenteralen Flüssigkeitszufuhr bei Früh- und Neugeborenen in den ersten drei Lebenstagen. *Klin Padiatr* 1980;192:539.

119. Lorenz JM, Kleinman, LI, Kotagal UR, Reller MD. Water balance in very low-birth-weight infants: relationship to water and sodium intake and effect on outcome. *J Pediatr* 1982;101:423.

120. Tammela OKT, Koivisto ME. Fluid restriction for preventing bronchopulmonary dysplasia? Reduced fluid intake during the first weeks of life improves the outcome of low-birth-weight infants. *Acta Paediatr* 1992;81:207.

121. Bell EF. Fluid therapy. In: Sinclair JC, Bracken MB, eds. *Effective care of the newborn infant*. New York: Oxford University Press, 1992:59.

122. Bell EF, Acarregui MJ. Restricted vs liberal water intake for preventing morbidity and mortality in preterm infants. In: Sinclair JC, Bracken MB, Soll RF, Horbar JD, eds. *Neonatal module of the Cochrane database of systematic reviews*. Available in the Cochrane Library, issue 4 [database on disk and CD-ROM]. Oxford: Update Software Ltd., 1998.

123. Sinclair JC, Engel K, Silverman WA. Early correction of hypoxemia and acidemia in infants of low birth weight: a controlled trial of oxygen breathing, rapid alkali and assisted ventilation. *Pediatrics* 1968;42:565.

124. Hobel CJ, Oh W, Hyvarinen MA, Emmanouilides GC, Erenberg A. Early versus late treatment of neonatal acidosis in low-birth-weight infants: relation to respiratory distress syndrome. *J Pediatr* 1972;81:1178.

125. Corbet AJ, Adams JM, Kenny JD, Kennedy J, Rudolph AJ. Controlled trial of bicarbonate therapy in high-risk premature newborn infants. *J Pediatr* 1977;91:771.

126. Siegel SR, Phelps DL, Leake RD, Oh W. The effects of rapid infusion of hypertonic sodium bicarbonate in infants with respiratory distress. *Pediatrics* 1973;51:651.

127. Simmons MA, Adcock EW III, Bard H, Battaglia FC. Hypernatremia and intracranial hemorrhage in neonates. *N Engl J Med* 1974;291:6.

128. Brownlee KG, Ng PC, Henderson MJ, Smith M, Green JH, Dear PRF. Catabolic effect of dexamethasone in the preterm baby. *Arch Dis Child* 1992;67:1.

129. Williams AF, Jones M. Dexamethasone increases plasma amino acid concentrations in bronchopulmonary dysplasia. *Arch Dis Child* 1992;67:5.

130. Van Goudoever JB, Wattimena JDL, Carnielli VP, Sulkers EJ, Degenhart HJ, Sauer PJJ. Effect of dexamethasone on protein metabolism in infants with bronchopulmonary dysplasia. *J Pediatr* 1994;124:112.

131. Schanler RJ, Shulman RJ, Prestridge LL. Parenteral nutrient needs of very low birth weight infants. *J Pediatr* 1994;125:961.

132. Moylan FMB, Herrin JT, Krishnamoorthy K, Todres ID, Shannon DC. Innappropriate antidiuretic hormone secretion in premature infants with cerebral injury. *Am J Dis Child* 1978;132:399.

133. Speer ME, Gorman WA, Kaplan SL, Rudolph AJ. Elevation of plasma concentrations of arginine vasopressin following perinatal asphyxia. *Acta Paediatr Scand* 1984;73:610.

134. Dauber IM, Krauss AN, Symchych PS, Auld PAM. Renal failure following perinatal anoxia. *J Pediatr* 1976;88:851.

135. Anand SK, Northway JD, Crussi FG. Acute renal failure in newborn infants. *J Pediatr* 1978;92:985.

136. Pizarro D, Posada G, Mata L, Nalin D, Mohs E. Oral rehydration of neonates with dehydrating diarrheas. *Lancet* 1979;2:1209.

137. Widness JA, Seward VJ, Kromer IJ, Burmeister LF, Bell EF, Strauss RG. Changing patterns of red blood cell transfusion in very low birth weight infants. *J Pediatr* 1996;129:680.

CHAPTER 23

Nutrition

Michael K. Georgieff

The provision of nutrition to term and preterm newborn infants remains one of the most important aspects of neonatal care. With increasing survival rates among sick newborns, the nourishment of full-term and preterm infants has assumed an increasingly greater role in the neonatal intensive care unit in the past 20 years. Great strides have been made in understanding neonatal nutritional physiology and pathophysiology in these years, allowing physicians to estimate more precisely the nutritional needs of the infants in their care. Knowledge of newborn infants' nutritional requirements, as well their neurologic, gastrointestinal, and metabolic capabilities, is a prerequisite to informed decision-making about nutritional therapy. It also is important to understand the tools available for assessment of neonatal nutritional status to judge the success or failure of nutritional therapies.

OVERVIEW

The goal of nutritional therapy in the term neonate is to ensure a successful growth transition from the fetal to the postnatal period. In the preterm infant, the goal has been to continue the process of intrauterine growth in what is now an extrauterine environment. Until lately, the goal has been to match the third trimester intrauterine rates of weight gain, linear growth, and brain growth. In successfully attaining these rates, the body composition of the preterm infant raised in an extrauterine environment nevertheless remains remarkably different than the same postconceptional aged infant who has remained *in utero* (1,2). Current efforts are aimed at understanding the metabolic processes that determine the body composition of the preterm infant.

M. K. Georgieff: Department of Pediatrics, University of Minnesota; and Department of Pediatrics, Fairview-University Medical Center, Minneapolis, Minnesota

The effect of illness on neonatal metabolism and nutritional requirements also is being recognized (3). Conditions such as bronchopulmonary dysplasia (BPD), congestive heart failure (CHF), acute respiratory distress, intrauterine growth retardation, and sepsis (and their treatments) have potential effects on neonatal energy, protein, mineral, and vitamin requirements. These conditions also may affect the digestive and absorptive capacities of the neonate.

This chapter reviews the nutritional requirements, digestive capabilities, and expected growth of term and preterm infants. It also provides an overview of various nutrient delivery systems, both enteral and parenteral. Finally, the chapter covers techniques of nutritional assessment and offers suggestions for appropriate monitoring of neonatal nutritional status.

NUTRITIONAL CAPABILITES OF THE NEWBORN INFANT

The ability to suck and swallow a meal in a coordinated fashion and then process those nutrients for utilization by the body may be one of the most complex developmental tasks facing the newborn infant (4). Success depends on a certain amount of neurologic, digestive, absorptive, and metabolic maturity. The term infant is quite mature in these respects. However, the preterm infant is progressively more immature based on the degree of prematurity.

Neurologic Maturity

The neurologically intact term infant is able to suck and swallow in a coordinated fashion within minutes of birth (5). In the preterm infant, the sucking reflex is strong at the limit of viability (23 weeks) and likely prior to that age (6). However, the ability to coordinate the suck reflex with swallowing to ensure that food is propelled into the gastrointestinal tract rather than the airway matures at approximately 34 weeks of gestation. To a great extent, this coordinated suck and swallow reflex appears to be postconceptional age mediated; that is, it does not appear that "practice" can stimulate the infant to become more mature at an earlier postconceptional age. Nevertheless, the age at which the infant matures varies widely, and some preterm infants are able to suck and swallow in a coordinated manner by 32 weeks of gestational age.

Motility in the gastrointestinal tract is dependent on neurologic maturation (7). For example, the esophagus shows a very uncoordinated pattern of peristalsis at 24 weeks of gestation, with weak peristaltic waves beginning sporadically and propagating either rostrally or caudally (8). By term, the pattern has matured into a coordinated pattern that propels food downward to the stomach (9). The lower esophageal sphincter of the very preterm infant is tenuous and provides little barrier to gastroesophageal reflux. Gastroesophageal reflux disease in the preterm infant can be associated with apnea and bradycardia, aspiration syndromes, and feeding intolerance. At term, although gastroesophageal reflux remains demonstrable in most infants, it generally is not the potentially life-threatening problem seen at earlier gestational ages.

The stomach also undergoes maturation during the third trimester. The preterm infant's stomach does not coordinately "wring" the stomach from antrum to pylorus, frequently being subject to periods of antiperistalsis, which in turn promotes gastroesophageal reflux disease (10). In addition, pyloric function is different in the preterm compared to the term infant. Gastric emptying is longer in the preterm infant, whereas stomach volume is smaller (11). The small stomach capacity frequently results in the need to feed small volumes to preterm infants on a more frequent schedule. The prolonged gastric emptying time, however, causes retention of food in the stomach and subsequent obtainment of "preaspirates" prior to the next feeding. Because the presence of preaspirates also may signify an ileus associated with more severe diseases, such as necrotizing enterocolitis (NEC), feedings often are discontinued with this sign.

The maturation of small intestinal motility has been extensively studied by Berseth (12,13) and her colleagues. They have demonstrated an orderly progression of peristaltic frequency, amplitude, and duration with increasing gestational age. The lack of a coordinated motility pattern in very preterm infants makes it more likely that they will present with signs of feeding intolerance, usually marked by abdominal distention. When compared to adults, neonates retain food in their small intestine for proportionately longer periods and in their colon for shorter periods. The newborn's ability to modulate stool water and electrolyte content is immature compared to adults.

In summary, multiple neuromaturational factors work against the preterm infant's ability to feed enterally as successfully as the term infant. These immaturities have an impact on feeding management, as will be discussed in a later section.

Digestive and Absorptive Capabilities

The newborn infant does not have the capability to digest and absorb nutrients from a complex diet. Fortunately, the term human infant has a ready source of nutrition in the form of human milk (5). Human milk is remarkably adapted to fit the digestive capacities of the term newborn and to meet the infant's nutritional needs for at least the first 6 months of life (5). Recent studies have shown the nutritional value of feeding human milk to preterm infants; however, for infants weighing less than 1,500 g, human milk needs to be fortified (14).

The functional immaturities of the gastrointestinal, hepatic, and renal systems in the newborn have an impact on the delivery of all classes of nutrients: macronutrients, minerals, trace elements, and vitamins.

Protein

Protein digestion begins in the stomach with the action of pepsin on intact protein (15). Pepsin is activated by acid hydrolysis of its precursor molecule, pepsinogen. The newborn is capable of creating an acidic stomach environment by 1 week of age (16); thus, pepsin activation is thought to be intact. Dietary protein then is acted upon by pancreatic peptidases released into the duodenum. These enzymes include trypsin, chymotrypsin, carboxypeptidases A and B, and elastase, and are amino acid selective with respect to cleavage sites, resulting in peptides of relatively small length. The peptides subsequently are cleaved once more by peptidases located in the intestinal mucosal cells, absorbed as amino acids or dipeptides, and transported to the liver. Protein digestion and absorption in adults is very efficient, with up to 95% of a protein load being fully digested. Although term and preterm infants have relatively low concentrations of chymotrypsin, the carboxypeptidases, and elastase (17), they nevertheless achieve more than 80% protein digestion.

Fat

The efficiency of fat digestion in the neonate stands in stark contrast to protein digestion. Fat is the most poorly digested macronutrient in the neonate (18). Whereas adults will absorb close to 95% of a fat meal, term infants absorb 85% to 90% and preterm infants can absorb as little as 50%, depending on the type of fat presented to them (19).

Fat digestion in the neonate begins in the stomach with the action of a lipase secreted in the mouth (lingual lipase) or by the gastric mucosa (gastric lipase) (20). The two lipases are identical, function ideally at acid pH, work primarily on medium-chain triglycerides (MCT), and do not require bile salts. Hamosh (21) has estimated that this enzyme may be responsible for up to 50% of fat digestion in the newborn. Infants fed human milk have the additional benefit of a lipase secreted into the milk by the mother (22). This lipase is found in all carnivores (but not herbivores) and functions more like pancreatic or intestinal lipases found in adults. It works primarily on long-chain triglycerides at a neutral pH, as is found in the intestine, and requires bile salts. This lipase may be responsible for the digestion of up to 20% of dietary fat (23). These two lipases are referred to as the "compensatory lipases" of the newborn and function in place of pancreatic and intestinal lipases seen in more mature humans (24).

Long-chain fatty acids are dependent on bile salts for proper micellization and uptake into the intestinal lymphatics. From there, the micelles are carried to the venous system via the thoracic duct, ultimately destined for the liver. Medium-chain fatty acids do not require micellization and can be absorbed directly into the blood stream. The bile acid, and hence bile salt, pools of the preterm newborn are low, thus restricting the fat absorption capacity of the infant. Prenatal administration of glucocorticoids to the mother can mature the fetal bile salt pool in the preterm infant less than 34 weeks of gestation to the level of the term infant (25). Without such priming, however, the preterm infant has significant impairment of fat absorption (including fat-soluble vitamins) prior to 34 weeks of gestation. Preterm infant formulas designed for infants less than 34 weeks of gestation have had their fat blend significantly modified to optimize fat absorption. They contain a higher percentage of MCT as well as higher levels of vitamins A, D, and E than formulas manufactured for term infants.

Carbohydrate

Like fats, carbohydrates can present a significant digestive challenge. The neonate has a limited ability to digest complex carbohydrates because of relatively small amounts of pancreatic amylase (26). Thus, beikost in the form of cereal rarely makes up a significant portion of the infant's diet until after 4 months of age. The term and preterm newborn readily uses glucose, which can be delivered either parenterally or enterally. Intestinal glucose uptake is seen as early as 10 weeks of gestation, long before the fetus is viable (27). However, provision of all carbohydrate calories as glucose would result in the neonatal gut being exposed to a hyperosmolar solution with a high potential for mucosal damage.

The primary carbohydrate found in mammalian milk is the disaccharide lactose. Like other disaccharides (sucrose, maltose, isomaltose), enzymatic cleavage by a disaccharidase must occur before the monosaccharides can be absorbed. In the case of lactose, glucose and galactose are produced by the action of lactase. The disaccharidases sucrase and maltase appear very early in gestation and appear to be inducible enzymes (28). In contrast, lactase begins to appear at 24 weeks of gestation and rises in concentration very slowly until term. It does not appear to be an inducible enzyme (29). The preterm infant thus is functionally somewhat lactose intolerant and will have typical symptoms of gas formation, diarrhea, and acidic stools characteristic of lactose malabsorption. Positive hydrogen breath tests have been documented in preterm infants following lactose challenges (30).

Preterm infant formulas have lower lactose contents than term formulas for this reason. Up to 60% of carbohydrate calories in preterm infant formulas are derived from linear glucose polymers, which produce a lower osmolar load than the equivalent number of individual glucose molecules. The enzyme required to digest glucose polymers (glucoamylase) is present from 24 weeks of gestation (31).

NUTRIENT REQUIREMENTS FOR TERM AND PRETERM INFANTS

Estimation of nutrient requirements is an inexact process, particularly when the goal is unclear. To date, the goal has been to achieve the same growth rates and body composition as the "reference" infant. The healthy breast-fed infant serves as the "gold standard" for the term infant; nevertheless, it is clear that breast-fed babies have different growth rates and body compositions than formula-fed infants (32). Human milk composition varies greatly among mothers, and the length of time that it remains sufficient for all the nutritional needs of the infant is not uniform. Breast-fed infants may have lower iron stores (33) and be at greater risk for vitamin D deficiency than formula-fed infants (34).

Determining the ideal growth for the infant born before term is far more problematic. Indeed, the ideal growth rate and body composition of the "healthy" preterm infant remain unknown and are likely to be different from his or her gestationally age-matched fetal counterpart. Until recently, the daily and weekly accretion rates of various nutrients in the preterm infant have been modeled on in utero accretion rates of these nutrients in gestationally age-matched fetuses. The "reference fetus" described by Widdowson and Spray (35) and again by Ziegler et al. (2) has served as the benchmark by which neonatal nutritionists judge fetal growth and body composition. Nevertheless, energy requirements are likely to be different in a 28-week-gestational-age newborn exposed to the thermal stresses of extrauterine life than in a 28-week-old fetus comfortably surrounded by amniotic fluid.

The rates of weight gain, linear growth, and head growth between the ages of 24 and 36 weeks of gestation can be calculated from the standard growth curves generated from infants born prematurely (36,37). It must be recognized that the data used to generate these plots are necessarily cross-sectional and thus need smoothing to create the resemblance of a curve. In addition, because premature birth is an abnormal event and up to 30% of very-low-birth-weight (VLBW) infants are small for dates (most likely due to the pregnancy failing over time), the reliability of newborn data to assess the growth velocity of healthy fetuses is suspect. Nevertheless, these curves are used extensively as guideposts for neonatal growth of the preterm infant. On average, these curves predict that the preterm infant should gain 10 to 15 g/kg body weight each day, grow 0.75 to 1.0 cm per week linearly, and demonstrate 0.75 cm per week of head growth. These values have been utilized to calculate the energy and protein needs of the preterm infant.

The nutrient requirements of term and preterm infants can be calculated based on fetal reference figures, balance studies, serum nutrient values, or a combination of these.

Energy Requirements

Energy requirements must take into account the amount and caloric density of the solution ingested, the route of administration (enteral vs. parenteral), the amount lost in stool or urine, and the energy requirements in the body (i.e., basal metabolic rate, cost of growth, energy cost of food processing by the body) (38). Many of these are now measurable, and reasonable estimates of energy requirements to maintain optimal growth velocities can be made for both term and preterm infants.

Energy is derived predominantly from carbohydrates and fat in the diet, which provide 4 and 9 kcal/g, respectively. The infant fed human milk receives calories predominantly from fat (39), whereas the formula-fed infant receives calories more evenly distributed between fat and carbohydrate (40). The calories derived from these sources are used first to maintain the total energy need of the infant, which consists of the basal metabolic rate, the thermic effect of feeding, and physical activity. Energy intake beyond this baseline is stored and recorded as weight gain. Protein normally is not utilized as an energy source, unless the total energy intake is less than the total energy expenditure of the infant. In those cases, certain amino acids can be deaminated and shunted into the gluconeogenic pathways to provide approximately 4 kcal/g of protein (41).

Energy requirements can be affected by numerous factors, including the route of delivery and the disease state. Energy requirements are lower when infants are fed parenterally as opposed to enterally, because no energy is excreted in the stool. Thus, the term infant who normally requires 100 kcal/kg/d enterally may be fed 90 kcal/kg/d parenterally. Diseases which increase energy needs

include CHF (42), BPD (43), acute respiratory disease (44), and overwhelming sepsis (45). Diseases that decrease energy needs include hypoxic–ischemic encephalopathy and degenerative neurologic conditions in which there is paucity of physical movement.

Term Infants

Healthy breast-fed term infants show adequate growth on as little as 85 to 100 kcal/kg body weight per day during the first 4 months of life (46). Formula-fed infants have higher energy requirements (100 to 110 kcal/kg), most likely due to a lower efficiency of digestion and absorption of fat (46). The presence of a lipase in human milk increases the digestibility of its fats.

Preterm Infants

Preterm infants have higher energy requirements than term infants because of a higher resting energy expenditure and greater stool losses due to immature absorptive capacities (47,48). Whereas the resting energy expenditure of the term infant is 45 to 50 kcal/kg/d, the preterm infant less than 34 weeks of gestation consumes 50 to 60 kcal/kg/d (47,48). Stool losses vary between 10% and 40% of intake, depending on the diet. For example, a diet in which the carbohydrate is 100% lactose and the fats are predominantly long-chain triglycerides will promote more stool losses because of the low levels of lactase and the small bile salt pools in the premature infant. Replacement of up to 50% of the lactose with glucose polymers and between 10% and 40% of the fat with MCT appears to reduce malabsorption to approximately 10% (48). The preterm infant will need an additional 50 to 60 kcal/kg/d beyond the daily energy expenditure and the loss of energy in the stool to maintain growth along the intrauterine growth curve (10 to 15 g/kg/d). Thus, barring any excess needs from diseases that increase oxygen consumption or from malabsorption, the preterm infant will gain weight adequately on approximately 120 kcal/kg/d.

Energy Sources

Carbohydrates

Newborn infants are highly dependent on a source of glucose for normal brain metabolism (49). The primary source of glucose in the term infant is lactose in human milk and cow-milk formulas. Soy-based formulas provide glucose from the metabolism of dietary sucrose or glucose polymers. Preterm infants also receive glucose, initially as dextrose in parenteral solutions, but subsequently enterally from lactose or glucose polymers. Galactose is also important to the newborn as it is needed for glycogen storage (50). The newborn infant typically utilizes between 4 and 8 mg/kg/minute of glucose (51).

This figure is commonly used as the glucose infusion rate for parenteral nutrition. Because of their low glycogen stores and poorer gluconeogenic capacities, preterm infants are more prone to hypoglycemia than term infants (52). Higher rates of glucose delivery may be required in growth-retarded infants and in infants of diabetic mothers to maintain normal glucose concentrations.

Glucose infusion rates up to 12.5 mg/kg/min commonly are used in preterm infants to promote catch-up weight gain. Beyond this rate, a cost–benefit analysis must be made. Although faster rates of weight gain can be achieved on higher glucose infusion rates (especially if the serum glucose is controlled with exogenous insulin infusion) (53), a higher metabolic rate and a shift in the respiratory quotient also will occur. Thus, a higher oxygen consumption coupled with proportionately more carbon dioxide generated by the cells may significantly affect serum carbon dioxide and ventilatory requirements. In one study, infants who received glucose and insulin remained on the respirator an average of 13 days longer than their counterparts given lower glucose infusion rates (54). Moreover, the increased "growth rates" demonstrated with high glucose infusion rates are due to fatty weight gain, without any increase in linear or brain growth (53). The overall metabolic cost of glucose infusion rates greater than 12.5 mg/kg/min must be weighed against the benefit of increased rates of nonlean weight gain.

Fats

Lipids constitute the other major energy source for neonates. Certain fatty acids, such as linoleic (omega-6 18:2) and linolenic acid (omega-3 18:3), are essential in the diet, and their absence will produce deficiency syndromes characterized by growth failure and skin rash (55). Although the full syndrome is rare, lower essential fatty acid concentrations are seen within 1 week of discontinuing lipid intake. Infants receiving parenteral nutrition or on a fat-restricted enteral diet require 0.5 mg/kg/d of an intravenous fat blend containing these fatty acids at least three times per week to prevent deficiency. The American Academy of Pediatrics (AAP) has recommended that 3% of total energy intake in infants should be in the form of linoleic acid (56).

Daily fat intake varies greatly based on the method of delivery (enteral vs. parenteral) and the dietary source (human milk vs. formula). Enterally fed term infants consume approximately 5 to 6 g/kg/d of fat, whereas parenterally fed infants rarely receive more than 4 g/kg/d, largely because of concerns about toxicity. Infants receiving human milk (especially human milk expressed by mothers who have delivered preterm) may receive up to 7 g/kg/d.

Infants fed human milk receive a unique blend of fats that has not been well replicated in infant formulas. Cow-milk fat is not well tolerated, forcing formula manufacturers to use vegetable oils as substitutes. The fatty acids found in palm, palm-olein, corn, and coconut oils are distinctly different from human milk fats. The role of omega fatty acids, such as docosahexaenoic acid (DHA) and eicosapentaenoic acid (EPA), in the infant diet has been a subject of intense research (57). These fatty acids are products of an elongation pathway from linoleic acid and are important in cell membrane structure and in myelination (58). The synthetic pathways are immature in preterm infants and for some undetermined period of time after birth in term infants (59). Sources of these fatty acids include the placenta and human milk. In contrast, cow-milk fat and vegetable oil do not contain these compounds. A number of studies are currently addressing whether these particular fatty acids are essential in the preterm and term infant (60,61). Because the preterm infant is not capable of synthesizing the compounds and would have received them *in utero,* the European Society for Pediatric Gastroenterology and Nutrition has recommended that a source of these fatty acids be added to preterm infant formula (62). Evidence of their efficacy includes studies that demonstrate better visual acuity and more mature electroretinograms (63,64). Studies of the long-term growth and developmental outcomes of infants who have been supplemented with these fatty acids are in their early stages. Any time a single component of human milk can be isolated and added to cow-milk–based infant formula, an important consideration is whether the component exerts its nutritional effect individually or in consort with other compounds (65). The potential for adverse nutrient interactions remains a concern with the addition of these fatty acids, particularly as they relate to growth. Because the long-term safety of the sources of these fats (fish oil, algae) as well as their effects on growth and neurodevelopment remain unclear, they currently have not been added to any commercially available preterm or term infant formulas in the United States.

Carnitine is another compound involved in fat metabolism in the neonate. Although carnitine deficiency is rare in the enterally fed infant because of high levels in human milk and supplementation of formulas, it remains a theoretical concern in infants receiving exclusive parenteral nutrition in which carnitine has not been supplemented (66). Carnitine supplements can be added to total parenteral nutrition (TPN), and this is recommended in infants who receive TPN for more than 3 weeks (67).

Protein Requirements

Protein requirements in humans are determined by a number of factors including protein quality and quantity, the amount of energy delivered, and the protein nutritional status of the subject (15). The latter is influenced by the degree of previous malnutrition, by the rate of catch-up growth, and potentially by inflammatory processes. The sick newborn infant is exposed to many of these influences. In addition, they have a high basal requirement for protein accretion based on *in utero* nitrogen accretion rates (2,35). Adequate energy intake is important to promote optimal protein utilization, with a nonprotein calorie-to-gram nitrogen ratio of 200:1 considered ideal. Overall protein intake in the neonate ultimately is limited to about 4 g/kg/d because of the inability of the immature kidney to excrete titratable acid, blood urea nitrogen, and ammonium ion (68).

Protein requirements, in general, and branched-chain amino acid needs, in particular, are increased in adults with physiologic instability due to septic or surgical illness (69). Recently, the possibility that similar changes might occur in sick neonates has been investigated preliminarily (44,45,70). Acute respiratory disease, sepsis, or surgical ligation of the patent ductus arteriosus does not result in increased protein requirements (44,45,70). At this time, increasing protein delivery routinely on the basis of illness or physiologic instability is not recommended.

Term Infants

The full-term breast-fed infant grows adequately and maintains normal serum and somatic (i.e., muscle) protein status on as little as 1.5 g/kg/d of protein. Although the protein content is low (1.1%), the quality of human-milk protein is excellent as the spectrum of amino acids provides a unique "match" for the amino acid needs of the newborn. The protein content is predominantly lactalbumin, as opposed to casein, which makes for smaller curds and easier digestibility. In addition, human milk is replete with nondietary nitrogen sources, including nucleotides that may enhance the immune system (71), immunoglobulins that help protect the gut epithelium (72), growth factors that stimulate intestinal growth (73), and enzymes (i.e., lipases) that aid digestion.

The term infant fed a cow-milk– or soy-based infant formula requires a greater protein delivery rate, most likely to compensate for the less than ideal protein quality. Thus, the infant on cow-milk formula typically requires 2.14 g/kg/d and the infant on soy formula up to 2.7 g/kg/d of protein (40). Cow-milk protein is predominantly casein, although a number of cow-milk–based formulas are modified to be whey predominant. The soy formulas also promote adequate growth of lean body mass. However, these formulas contain a smaller percentage of available nitrogen as essential or semiessential amino acids (74).

Protein also can be delivered to the term infant by way of protein hydrolysate formulas. These formulas are specifically designed to decrease the exposure of the infant to potentially antigenic cow or soy-milk proteins. By hydrolyzing the cow-milk–based protein such that greater than 90% of the proteins have a molecular weight of 1,250 daltons or less, allergic disease due to cow-milk allergy can be treated or potentially prophylaxed. These formulas provide approximately 2.8 g/kg/d of protein at an energy delivery of 100 kcal/kg/d.

Preterm Infants

Recommendations for protein intake in preterm infants follow many of the same parameters as in term infants. However, the needs of the preterm infant appear to be greater than the term infant. Early studies suggested that the most rapid weight gain and most efficient energy utilization was achieved with protein intakes of 3 to 5 g/kg/d (75,76). Kashyap et al. (77) refined these goals when they demonstrated that weight gain and nitrogen retention were greatest in healthy 32-week-gestational-age infants fed 3.9 g/kg/d of protein (Table 23–1). They also attempted to define the optimal energy-to-protein ratio that promoted growth, finding that approximately 30 kcal was necessary for each gram of protein delivered. In a later study by the same group, Schulze et al. (78) proposed that preterm infants tolerate 3.6 g/kg/d of protein with an energy intake of around 120 kcal/kg/d. Heird et al. (79) emphasized that increasing protein delivery requires increased energy delivery and vice versa. Their conclusions include the following:

- The low-birth-weight (LBW) infant who can take feeds soon after birth requires a protein intake of at least 2.8 g/kg/d.
- Infants who do not receive protein in the first few days of life lose at least 1% of their endogenous protein

TABLE 23–1. *Protein and energy intakes in low-birth-weight infants*

Energy intake factors	Group 1 (n = 14)	Group 2 (n = 15)	Group 3 (n = 15)
Birth weight, median (g)	1,390	1,500	1,460
Gestational age, median (wk)	32	32	32
Protein intake (g/kg/d)	2.8 ± 0.04	3.8 ± 0.04	3.9 ± 0.04
Energy (kcal/kg/d)	118 ± 1.7	119 ± 2.2	142 ± 2.4
Change in weight (g/kg/d)	16 ± 1.8	19.1 ± 3.2	21.5 ± 2.2
Head circumference at 2,200 g (cm)	33 ± 0.79	32.7 ± 0.79	32.5 ± 0.53
Energy stored (kcal/kg/d)	50 ± 3.5	49 ± 5.7	69.8 ± 4.5

From ref. 77.

stores daily. [These findings are consistent with the finding that preterm neonates were in better nutritional status if amino acids were added to dextrose solutions in the first days of life (80)].

- Infants with delayed protein intake subsequently require higher protein intakes to correct for early losses.

Finally, illnesses or medications that increase protein turnover or muscle breakdown will have an influence on protein delivery. van Goudoever et al. (81) demonstrated that the steroids used for the treatment of BPD cause negative nitrogen balance by increasing the rate of protein breakdown, but have little effect on protein synthesis.

Many preterm infants receive protein initially as part of a regimen of parenteral nutrition. Intravenous amino acid solutions have advanced to the point where they are specifically formulated for preterm infants (e.g., TrophAmine, Aminosyn-PF). These amino acid solutions are designed to normalize the plasma amino acid profile of the healthy infant, promoting levels similar to those of a 1-month-old breast-fed infant (82). Anderson et al. (80) demonstrated that dextrose solutions with amino acids given early in life promote better nutritional status than dextrose solutions without protein. Clark et al. (83) have shown that newborn preterm infants respond to parenteral nutrition with an acute increase in protein synthesis and a decrease in proteolysis. Thus, it appears that amino acid delivery in the first days of life is critical.

The recommended amount of amino acids to be delivered and the rate of advancement remain to be determined and are influenced by the infant's condition. Based on the estimates of protein loss by Heird et al. (80), it is prudent to begin amino acids on day 1; typically, there is no contraindication to beginning at 1 g/kg/d and advancing by 0.5 to 1.0 g/kg/d each day. The blood urea nitrogen and acid–base status of the infant must be followed. Studies in sick neonates suggest that 1.5 g/kg/d of amino acids on day 2 would achieve neutral nitrogen balance (44). Ultimately, the goal is to deliver between 3.0 and 3.5 g/kg/d of parenteral amino acids.

Preterm infants who begin enteral feeds in the first days after birth will be relatively protein restricted, because they typically are given human milk or dilute preterm infant formula. Although human milk from mothers delivering preterm is higher in protein (Table 23–2) compared to term human milk (84–86), the content is still relatively low and the infant will likely receive low volumes. Preterm infant formula has a high concentration of protein (3.1 to 3.6 g per 120 kcal), but it is unlikely that the infant will achieve that type of delivery in the first week (Table 23–3).

Mineral and Element Requirements

Mineral requirements in newborns are influenced by the immature status of the kidney, prematurity, and medications that affect mineral metabolism (87). In general, preterm infants require higher amounts of minerals than term infants. The daily needs of some minerals (e.g., sodium, potassium chloride) are determined by measuring serum levels, whereas others (e.g., calcium, phosphorus) are estimated from *in utero* accretion rates (2,35). A more comprehensive discussion of these needs can be found in Chapters 22 and 36 and in other sources (88). The following discussion focuses on selected minerals, comparing requirements in the preterm infant to term infants and emphasizing the effects of diseases and their treatments on mineral status.

Sodium, Potassium, and Chloride

The typical term infant requires 1 to 3 mEq/kg/d of sodium (87). Breast-fed infants have a lower sodium intake than formula-fed infants, although formula manufacturers have reduced the sodium content of cow-milk formula to levels comparable to human milk. Preterm infants have higher sodium requirements and may become hyponatremic on human milk (14,89). Baseline sodium requirements range from 2 to 4 mEq/kg/d in the preterm infant. The higher sodium requirement with lower gesta-

TABLE 23–2. *Nutrient and mineral content of preterm milk*

Element[a]	Days 3–7	Day 21	Days 29–42	Days 57–98
Protein (g/dL)	3.24 ± 0.31	1.83 ± 0.14	1.31–1.81 ± 0.12	1.8 ± 0.07
Lactose (g/dL)	5.96 ± 0.2	6.49 ± 0.21		
Fat (g/dL)	1.63 ± 0.23	3.68 ± 0.4		
Energy (kcal/dL)	51.4 ± 2.4	65.6 ± 4.3		
Sodium (mEq/dL)	2.66 ± 0.3	1.3 ± 0.18	0.76 ± 0.09	0.55 ± 0.05
Chloride (mEq/dL)	3.16 ± 0.3	1.7 ± 0.17		
Potassium (mEq/dL)	1.74 ± 0.07	1.63 ± 0.09	1.1 ± 0.1	1.1 ± 0.1
Calcium (mg/dL)	20.3–26.3 ± 1.7	20.4 ± 1.5	24.6–26.2 ± 2.2	31.5 ± 1.3
Phosphorous (mg/dL)	9.5–14.6 ± 0.7	14.9 ± 1.3	13.3 ± 0.3	
Magnesium (mg/dL)	2.8 ± .1	2.4 ± 0.1	4.9 ± 0.1	

[a]From refs. 84–86.

TABLE 23-3. Oral feeding schedule for the low-birth-weight infant

Time	Substance[a]	≤1,000 g		1,001–1,500 g		1,501–2,000 g		>2000 g	
		Amount	Frequency	Amount	Frequency	Amount	Frequency	Amount	Frequency
First feeding	Full-strength human milk or ¼-strength formula	1–2 mL/kg	1–2 h or continuous drip	2–3 mL/kg	2 h	3–4 mL/kg	2–3 h	10 mL/kg (full strength)	3 h
Subsequent feedings, 12–72 h	Formula or full-strength human milk	Increase 1 mL every other feeding to maximum of 5 mL	2 h	Increase 1 mL every other feeding to maximum of 10 mL	2 h	Increase 2 mL every other feeding to maximum of 15 mL	2–3 h	Increase 5 mL every other feeding to maximum of 20 mL	3 h
Final feeding schedule, 150 mL/kg	Full-strength formula or human milk	10–15 mL	2 h	20–28 mL	2–3 h	28–37 mL	3 h	37–50 mL, then *ad libitum*	3–4 h
Total time to full feeds			10–14 d or more for infants <750 g		7–10 d		5–7 d		3–5 d

[a]Supplemental intravenous fluids should be given to fulfill requirements of 140–160 mL/kg and caloric requirements of 90–130 cal/kg.

tional age is due predominantly to the immaturity of the proximal renal tubule in the small preterm infant. Treatment of these infants with salt-wasting diuretics (i.e., furosemide, hydrochlorothiazide) may increase the needs to 10 to 13 mEq/kg/d.

Potassium requirements in the term infant generally range between 1 and 2 mEq/kg/d. Because potassium also is reabsorbed at the proximal tubule, the preterm infant needs 2 to 4 mEq/kg/d (89). Diuretics such as furosemide, metolazone, and hydrochlorothiazide can increase requirements to 8 mEq/kg/d.

Sodium and potassium are provided in human milk and infant formulas to supply the daily need of the normal infant. However, excessive requirements from prior or ongoing losses may require supplementation. Supplements are typically in the form of chloride salts (NaCl or KCl), and the doses are based on calculations of maintenance requirements plus deficits. Infants receiving parenteral nutrition can have sodium and potassium added as chloride or as acetate, depending on the acid–base status of the infant.

Calcium, Magnesium, and Phosphorus

The term infant who has not suffered intrauterine growth retardation has bones that are well mineralized. Analysis of the reference fetus demonstrated that the average fetus accretes 80% to 90% of its calcium during the last trimester (2). If there has been no interruption of the process, the average term infant will grow well and remain well mineralized on a diet providing approximately 40 to 60 mg/kg/d of calcium and 20 to 30 mg/kg/d of phosphorus. Human milk is an excellent source for this rate of delivery. Infant formulas have higher concentrations of calcium than human milk, but there is little evidence that term infants who are formula fed are better mineralized.

LBW infants (intrauterine growth retarded or preterm) have significantly lower calcium and phosphorus contents than term, appropriate-for-dates infants. Daily calcium and phosphorus requirements in the preterm infant are estimated to be 200 and 113 mg/kg/d, respectively (90). This rate of daily accretion can only be achieved enterally. The two minerals become insoluble in typical TPN solutions when added at concentrations that would provide more than 60 mg/kg/d of calcium and 30 mg/kg/d of phosphorus (at typical fluid delivery of 150 cc/kg/d). Human milk is relatively low in calcium and phosphorus and thus must be supplemented with a fortifier to achieve adequate mineralization in the less than 1,500-g infant (91). Preterm infant formula contains enough calcium and phosphorus to deliver the daily recommended amount as well as some excess to begin to replace previously acquired deficits. This is important because most preterm infants do not tolerate full enteral feedings immediately after birth. Because parenteral nutrition results in negative calcium and phosphorus balance, preterm infants invariably will need intakes greater than the projected daily in utero requirement to avoid becoming osteopenic. Because serum calcium levels will always be maintained at the expense of the bone, following calcium levels as a way of monitoring status is not useful. Instead, indicators of bone activity (serum alkaline phosphatase) or urinary phosphorus excretion are used to monitor long-term calcium status.

As with calcium, the rates of magnesium accretion in utero are high during the third trimester. Thus, the magnesium requirement for infants born preterm are greater than those for term infants. Human milk and preterm infant formula appear to support normal magnesium levels. Magnesium delivery in parenteral nutrition is titrated based on serum magnesium levels, which should be monitored.

Iron

The majority of total body iron found in the term infant is accreted during the third trimester. The fetus maintains a constant total body iron content of 75 mg/kg during the last trimester, increasing from 35 to 40 mg at 24 weeks of gestation to 225 mg at term (92). Preterm delivery results in disruption of this process; therefore, premature infants are born with lower iron stores than term infants. Small-for-dates infants frequently are born with low iron stores, presumably because of decreased placental iron transport (93). Infants of diabetic mothers are born with low stores, presumably because much of the fetal iron is in the expanded red cell mass (94). These infants appear to be low in total body iron as well, most likely due to altered transport of iron by the diabetic placenta.

Term Infants

The appropriate-for-dates newborn infant has sufficient iron stores to last 4 to 6 months; the small-for-dates infant has closer to a 2-month supply (95). In the absence of adequate dietary iron, these stores are mobilized for hemoglobin synthesis in the rapidly expanding blood volume. An adequate source of iron (human milk or iron-fortified infant formula) generally maintains iron stores until the infant begins to obtain iron from other dietary sources in the second 6 months of life.

The major source of iron for the healthy, term infant is dietary, either through human milk or infant formula fortified with iron (96). Although human milk has a low iron content (0.3 mg/L) compared to infant formula either fortified with iron (10 to 12 mg/L) or not fortified with iron (1.15 to 4.5 mg/L), the iron is much more bioavailable due to proteins such as lactoferrin (97). Greater than 50% of the iron in human milk is absorbed, compared to only 4% to 12% of formula iron (98). The rate of iron deficiency in breast-fed infants before 6 months is relatively low, although few methodologically sound studies have been performed (99). Although iron deficiency rates of 20% to 30% have been recorded in breast-fed infants (100), it has been unclear whether the infants were exclusively breast-fed. A recent study by Innis et al. (101) showed an iron deficiency anemia rate of 15% in 8-month-old breast-fed infants. Given this, it may be wise to screen the breast-fed infant's iron status at 6 months.

The rate of iron deficiency in infants fed exclusively low-iron formula is unacceptably high, with rates between 28% and 38% (100). This compares with a rate of less than 5% in infants fed iron-fortified formula during the first 6 months of life. Indeed, the introduction of iron fortification of formulas in the early 1970s represents one of the most effective public health campaigns in this country. Nevertheless, low-iron formula continues to be available, accounting for between 9% and 30% of elective (i.e., non-Women, Infants, and Children [program]) formula sales. The reasons appear to involve the unfounded perception that iron in formula causes gastrointestinal symptoms such as colic, diarrhea, constipation, and gastroesophageal reflux. Double-blind studies have failed to support these claims (102,103). The Committee on Nutrition of the AAP supports breast-feeding for all infants, but, in lieu of that, recommends infants being fed formula receive only iron-fortified products (95). The estimated daily iron requirement for the term infant is 1 mg/kg/d.

Preterm Infants

The sick, preterm infant frequently goes into negative iron balance because of blood lost during phlebotomy. In the past, these losses were replaced by red cell transfusions, but criteria for transfusion have become more stringent because of concerns of exposure to infectious agents (104). Thus, iron supplementation of the preterm infant may need to start as early as 2 weeks of age to maintain neutral iron balance. Recombinant human erythropoietin has been used to stimulate endogenous red cell production in place of red cell transfusion and produces additional negative stress on neonatal iron balance (105). Because 3.4 mg of iron is necessary to synthesize 1 g of hemoglobin, the therapeutic use of erythropoietin significantly taxes the already low iron stores of the preterm infant. Because of these factors, the daily iron requirement for the preterm infant is 2 to 4 mg/kg/d, with the greater requirement for the more preterm infant. Infants who receive recombinant erythropoietin require at least 6 mg/kg/d of iron (106).

The issue of when to begin iron supplementation in the preterm infant has been controversial. Iron is necessary for normal growth and development of all tissues, including the brain (107). Nevertheless, iron is a very potent oxidant stress. Because preterm infants have immature antioxidant systems, there is concern that iron can exacerbate diseases that may be related etiologically to oxidation of cell membranes, including BPD and retinopathy of prematurity (ROP) (108). Definitive studies on the role of iron in these diseases on prematurity have not been performed.

Generally, human milk should be used whenever possible in preterm infants. Those who receive recombinant human erythropoietin should be supplemented earlier with iron sulfate to have an adequate erythropoietic response. It is clear that iron must be available to see a sustained erythropoietic response with recombinant erythropoietin treatment (109). Preterm infant formulas are iron fortified and should provide adequate amounts to the preterm infant.

Trace Elements

Ten trace elements are nutritionally essential for the human: zinc, copper, selenium, chromium, manganese, molybdenum, cobalt, fluoride, iodine, and iron (110). Zlotkin et al. (110) have written an excellent review of trace element requirements in newborns. Most trace elements are accreted during the last trimester. Thus, the term infant is fully replete and needs modest dietary intake of these elements (Table 23–4). Both human milk and infant formula ensure adequate intakes. The preterm infant or the term infant on prolonged TPN would rapidly go into negative balance of any of these elements if not provided with an exogenous source. While on TPN, infants receive 0.2 mL/kg body weight of neonatal trace elements (i.e., Neonate Trace-4), which supplies 0.02 mg/kg of copper, 0.3 mg/kg of zinc, 5 µg/kg of manganese, and 0.17 µg/kg of chromium. Preterm infant formulas and preterm human milk appear to supply adequate amounts of trace elements to the enterally fed premature infant (111).

TABLE 23–4. *Suggested daily intravenous intake of essential trace elements*

Element	Daily Intake
Zinc	
Premature	400 µg/kg
Full-term, <3 mo	250 µg/kg
Full-term, >3 mo	100 µg/kg
Copper[a]	20 µg/kg
Chromium[b]	0.20 µg/kg
Manganese[a]	1 µg/kg
Selenium[b]	2 µg/kg after 2 wk of parenteral nutrition
Iodine	1 µg/kg after 6 wk of parenteral nutrition; check thyroid function
Molybdenum[b]	0.25 µg/kg

[a]If evidence of liver damage appears, delete copper and manganese from total parenteral nutrition.
[b]Omit in patients with renal dysfunction.
Adapted from ref. 115.

Selenium is a potent antioxidant. Preterm infants have lower selenium stores than term infants (112), and this has been proposed as an etiology for diseases such as BPD and ROP (113). Studies linking selenium sufficiency with these diseases have not been persuasive (114), but the general consensus is that selenium status should be supported in the preterm infant (115). Selenium is not found in commercially available products and must be added separately to TPN at the rate of 2 µg/kg/d (115). Iodine is not added to TPN, but adequate amounts of iodine are absorbed through the infant's skin from iodine solutions applied topically (110). Nevertheless, a dose of 1 µg/kg/d has been recommended for infants who are on TPN for more than 6 weeks (115).

Vitamins

Vitamin requirements in newborn infants can be conceptualized most easily by considering water- and fat-soluble vitamins separately. An extensive review of all of the vitamins and their deficiencies is beyond the scope of this chapter, and the reader is referred to a source dedicated to this subject (116). This section will deal primarily with vitamins that are of particular relevance to neonates and to those with a specific risk for deficiency.

Water-soluble Vitamins

Term newborns rarely are deficient of water-soluble vitamins in the B group (116). As with all humans, neonates need a daily source of vitamin C and folate. These are provided in adequate concentrations in human milk, infant formulas, and multivitamin preparations added to parenteral nutrition. The AAP has stated that there is no need to supplement term, breast-fed infants with water-soluble vitamins unless there are extenuating circumstances during the first 6 months (5). Preterm infants also do not appear to need supplemental water-soluble vitamins once they are taking an adequate amount of formula or fortified human milk. The minimum amount of enteral feeds needed to maintain vitamin sufficiency varies among the formulas and the human milk fortifiers that are used. Infants receiving Enfamil Premature Formula or human milk fortified with Enfamil Human Milk Fortifier need no vitamin supplementation if their intake exceeds 150 mL/d. Those receiving Similac Special Care Formula or human milk fortified with Natural Care must exceed 300 mL/d to remain vitamin sufficient (117).

Fat-soluble Vitamins

Fat-soluble vitamin deficiencies also are rarely a problem for term, healthy newborns fed human milk or infant formula. Nevertheless, certain groups of infants are at risk for vitamin D deficiency (116). These include breast-fed infants whose mothers are vitamin D deficient due to their diet (vegan) or whose mothers completely protect their own skin from sunlight. Their infants also must be exposed to less than 30 minutes of sunlight per day to be at greatest risk. Most reports of rickets in breast-fed infants in these circumstances have been in far-northern climates, although in the United States the problem has been seen as far south as San Diego (118).

Virtually all infants receive vitamin K in the delivery room to prevent hemorrhagic disease of the newborn. The prevalence of this condition is very low, but the neurologic consequences are so disastrous and preventable that the current recommendation is to continue to give vitamin K at birth. Once a gut flora has been established in the first 2 postnatal days, vitamin K deficiency is exceedingly rare (119). Infants who receive broad-spectrum antibiotics, which markedly reduce the intestinal flora, however, should be supplemented with vitamin K at least twice per week (119).

Whereas infants are not wholly dependent on dietary sources for vitamin D (it can be synthesized de novo from sterol precursors by 1 week of age) and vitamin K (supplied by gut bacteria), vitamins E and A must be provided in the diet. The term infant consuming human milk or infant formula receives an adequate amount of each, assuming that there are no impediments to fat absorption, such as cystic fibrosis or short bowel syndrome. In infants with those conditions, a water-soluble A and E preparation should be utilized and serum levels monitored.

There are significant issues with fat-soluble vitamins, particularly vitamins A and E, in preterm infants less than 34 weeks of gestation because of their relatively poor digestion of fats. As with term infants, vitamin K and, most likely, vitamin D are not a major problem, although preterm infant formulas are supplemented with more vitamin D than are term formulas. Even the most premature infants are capable of synthesizing the active vitamin D metabolite by 1 week of age (120).

Vitamin A deficiency in growing mammals results in significant tissue fibrosis, particularly of the lung and liver. In 1925, Wolbach and Howe (121) noted that lambs born to vitamin A-deficient mothers had significant lung disease that, in retrospect, bears remarkable similarity to BPD (121). These animals had squamous metaplasia, loss of cilia, and loss of ciliary motility. Several investigators have noted that preterm infants have low vitamin A levels and hepatic stores (122). Moreover, preterm infants with respiratory distress syndrome who had low cord blood vitamin A concentrations are more likely to develop BPD (123). Additionally, both prenatal and postnatal steroid administration increased serum vitamin A levels in preterm infants while preventing and treating BPD, respectively (124,125). Two major studies assessed whether prophylactically administering 2,000 IU of vitamin A intramuscularly every other day from birth in infants weighing less than 1,500 g prevented BPD. Shenai et al. (126) found a significant reduction of BPD in their treated infants, from 85% to 45%, with a concomitant rise in serum vitamin A levels. The serum retinol levels of placebo-treated infants remained abnormally low (less than 20 µg/dL). In contrast, Pearson et al. (127), utilizing the same protocol, found no difference in BPD between the vitamin-A– and placebo-treated groups (46% vs. 44%) in spite of a significant rise in serum retinol concentrations in the treated group. Of note was that retinol levels remained above 20 µg/dL in the placebo group. The unifying conclusion of these two studies is that vitamin A deficiency, as seen in the control group of Shenai et al. (126), is a risk factor for BPD, but not all infants weighing less than 1,500 g are vitamin A deficient in the first month of life. Additional supplementation of infants with adequate vitamin A status does not appear to further reduce the risk of BPD according to the data of Pearson et al. (127). At this time, it appears to be prudent to check vitamin A levels in preterm infants at risk for BPD and treat those with low serum concentrations, realizing that serum concentrations are not the most reliable measure of tissue vitamin A status.

Ever since Oski et al. (128) reported on hemolytic anemia caused by vitamin E deficiency, there have been studies that assess vitamin E sufficiency in the context of oxidative stresses. Clearly, phospholipid membranes are at high risk for oxidative stresses, and, if not adequately protected by circulating antioxidants such as vitamin E, selenium, and superoxide dysmutase, they will be damaged, with subsequent cell death. Thus, it was hoped that supplementation of the preterm infant having an immature antioxidant system with vitamin E might prevent or ameliorate established BPD or ROP. Studies along those lines have been a disappointment. After initial reports that vitamin E supplementation at birth prevented BPD (129–131), subsequent studies have not been able to duplicate the effect (132). Similarly, a meta-analysis of trials of vitamin E supplementation to prevent the occurrence or progression of ROP has not shown a significant effect (133). Moreover, high vitamin E levels following supplementation appear to increase the risk of sepsis and NEC (134).

Preterm infant formulas are supplemented with vitamins E and A. For most infants fed the preterm infant formula with higher vitamin E and A concentrations, serum levels remain in the normal range. However, routine assessment of these levels in the high-risk infant weighing less than 1,500 g may be prudent, because it is likely that the deficiency state is not advantageous to the growing infant. Similarly, vitamins A and E are provided in the pediatric multivitamin preparation used in TPN.

Effect of Neonatal Illness on Nutritional Requirements

Most studies of neonatal nutritional requirements have dealt with defining the needs of the healthy growing term or preterm infant. Nevertheless, adults and older children who are ill undergo profound changes in metabolism based on the type and degree of illness (135,136). Cerra et al. (136) have investigated the independent effects of surgery, trauma, and sepsis on adult metabolism and found consistent changes in protein-energy requirements. Each increases cellular oxygen consumption and promotes more negative nitrogen balance, with sepsis having the most profound effects. Cytokines such as tumor necrosis factor (TNF-α), interleukin-6 (IL-6), and interleukin-1 (IL-1) appear to be important mediators of the response (137). The studies suggest that energy and amino acid delivery must be significantly modified in sick patients. In particular, these patients appear to require higher energy delivery and more protein to remain in neutral or positive nitrogen balance. Special amino acid solutions that are rich in branched-chain amino acids are utilized to support nitrogen balance (138).

Fewer studies have assessed these issues in preterm and term newborns. Nevertheless, some of the metabolic effects of acute lung disease, chronic lung disease, CHF, and sepsis have been studied (3). The conclusions of these studies support the concept that simply supplying the nutrients normally required by the healthy newborn will not be sufficient for infants with these illnesses.

Acute lung disease, such as hyaline membrane disease, increases the oxygen consumption of the infant in direct proportion to the degree of respiratory illness (44). Unlike adults, however, nitrogen balance appears to be unaffected by respiratory illness, with a mean protein requirement of 1.5 g/kg/d on day 2 of the disease. Severe respiratory illness is associated with a higher incidence of hypocalcemia and hypoglycemia. Thus, care must be taken to supply adequate energy in the form of dextrose to these infants. There appears to be no indication to increase protein delivery beyond what would normally be given.

BPD increases the resting energy expenditure by up to 30% (43), and infants with BPD will require energy intakes up to 150 kcal/kg/d to grow adequately. Much of the growth failure in BPD occurs in the first month, after which the rate of weight gain can be quite similar (although at a lower percentile) to infants without BPD (139). Protein requirements have not been studied extensively in infants with BPD, but those who are treated with steroids have increased muscle breakdown and a more negative nitrogen balance (81). Clearly, malnutrition plays an important role in the genesis of the disease and the rate of recovery (140). Sodium and potassium requirements are increased in infants with BPD treated with salt-wasting diuretics, occasionally requiring supplementation. Calcium balance is more tenuous due to more prolonged periods on parenteral nutrition, renal calcium wasting due to calciuric diuretics (furosemide), and bone demineralization due to corticosteroid therapy. A relationship between vitamin A deficiency and BPD has been documented (126); thus, it is important to monitor and support vitamin A status in infants with BPD.

CHF has an equally profound effect on resting energy expenditure as does BPD (141). Infants with CHF due to structural heart disease may require up to 150 kcal/kg/d on the basis of an increased metabolic rate and malabsorption due to intestinal edema. The protein requirement of infants with CHF has not been studied, although it is clear many fail to thrive and have reduced muscle mass. It is prudent to increase the protein delivery commensurate with the increase in energy delivery, maintaining a ratio of 25 to 30 kcal per gram of protein. Diuretics used to treat CHF cause the same sodium, potassium, and calcium deficiencies seen in infants with chronic lung disease. Furthermore, the use of citrated blood products to replace losses perioperatively can cause profound hypocalcemia. Persistent cyanosis places an additional nutritional stress by increasing the infant's need for iron. Because many of these infants have secondary polycythemia, there must be enough iron in the diet to support augmented erythropoiesis. Failure of a cyanotic infant to maintain an elevated hemoglobin may be due to iron deficiency, which can be screened for with a ferritin concentration and by assessing the red cell indexes for microcytosis.

The effect of sepsis on neonatal nutritional status has not been well evaluated. Infants rarely present with the overwhelming multisystem organ failure that adults routinely have with sepsis. This may be due to an incomplete cytokine response. Septic infants have increased TNF and IL-6 levels, but their levels are not nearly as high as in adults (45). Furthermore, neonatal sepsis does not result in a profoundly negative nitrogen balance. Sepsis does increase oxygen consumption, although this appears to be a nonspecific response to illness as it is seen in other nonseptic states. It appears that sepsis increases energy but not protein needs in the neonate.

NUTRIENT DELIVERY

Almost all term infants and many preterm infants more than 33 weeks of gestation will feed orally on demand immediately after birth. Breast-fed infants should be offered the breast within 30 minutes of delivery. However, ill term infants and preterm infants who are not physiologically mature or are unstable will require alternate forms of nutrient delivery. The first decision revolves around whether the infant is stable enough to be fed enterally or if parenteral nutrition is indicated. If long-term parenteral nutrition is anticipated, decisions will need to be made whether a central catheter should be placed or the nutrients should be given through a peripheral vein. If the infant is to be enterally gavage fed, the practitioner has multiple options with respect to where the gavage tube is placed, whether it remains indwelling or is replaced after each feed, and whether the feedings are by continuous drip or bolus.

Parenteral Nutrition

Indications

Parenteral nutrition is indicated in all infants in whom enteral nutrition is contraindicated or delivers less than 75% of total protein and energy requirements. Although parenteral nutrition has become a more refined nutritional tool with fewer complications over the past decade, the enteral route remains the preferred way to nourish babies. Nevertheless, many infants in neonatal intensive care units will be treated with parenteral nutrition because they are NPO [*nil per os* (nothing by mouth)] or working up slowly on enteral feedings. For all practical purposes, infants on ventilators in the acute stage of their diseases rarely are fed. It is not appropriate to simply provide these infants with a dextrose and electrolyte solution. Anderson et al. (80) demonstrated that the addition of amino acids to dextrose solutions shortly after birth improves the nutritional status of infants. Our group demonstrated that earlier initiation of parenteral nutrition was one factor associated with higher weight, length, and occipital frontal circumference percentiles at discharge and better long-term developmental outcome (141). Therefore, it is appropriate to begin parenteral nutrition for infants within 24 hours of birth, if possible. The trend in the past 5 years has been to begin feedings earlier in preterm infants to promote ongoing maturity of the intestinal tract, avoid villous atrophy due to disuse, and kindle gut hormone activity (142). Thus, infants who still require moderate respiratory support will receive "trophic" feeds, but these feedings are hypocaloric, and parenteral nutrition is indicated in these infants.

Absolute indications for parenteral nutrition include surgical lesions such as omphalocele, gastroschisis, intestinal tract atresias (e.g., tracheoesophageal atresia, duodenal atresia, ileal atresia), meconium peritonitis, diaphragmatic hernia, short bowel syndrome, and Hirschsprung's disease. Medical indications include NEC (or feeding intolerance), meconium ileus, ileus due to generalized illness, infants on extracorporeal membrane oxygen therapy, and preterm infants on slowly advancing feedings.

Routes of Delivery

The decision whether to supply parenteral nutrition centrally or peripherally requires weighing the benefits against the risks. Parenteral nutrition administered through a central line allows for greater energy delivery because solutions with dextrose concentrations greater than 12.5% can be administered. Dextrose concentrations of that magnitude and calcium infusion are poorly tolerated by peripheral veins and carry a high rate of venous sclerosis (143). Skin sloughs are likely to occur if the solution extravasates from the vein. For the same reasons, many intensive care nurseries will not allow or will limit the amount of calcium to be run through a peripheral venous line. This practice is sound, but effectively limits the amount of calcium and phosphorus that can be delivered to an infant who is already at great risk for osteopenia.

The risks of central TPN relate primarily to the risk of central venous line placement and maintenance. Umbilical venous catheters placed at birth traditionally have been used as the primary central catheter, but the incidence of venous thromboses is high (144). Clots can be detected as early as 24 hours after catheter placement. The clots are frequently infected with *Staphylococcus epidermidis,* which has become the most common pathogen isolated in the extremely-low-birth-weight (ELBW) infant after 7 days of age (145). Equally concerning is the high rate of *Candida* septicemia seen with high dextrose delivery and high serum concentrations (146).

One risk of peripheral TPN is undernutrition. The infant receiving maximal concentrations of dextrose ($D_{12.5}$%), amino acids (3.0 g/kg/d), and intravenous fat (3.5 g/kg/d) at an average fluid rate of 150 mL/kg/d will receive approximately 95 nonprotein kcal/kg/d. Although this intake meets the daily resting energy expenditure of the premature infant (65 kcal/kg/d), there are insufficient "extra" calories to sustain weight gain at 10 to 15 g/kg/d. Thus, long-term peripheral TPN will result in preterm infants slowly falling away from the growth curve. Calcium delivery also will be constrained because of either an absolute contraindication (in some nurseries) or osmolarity issues. Each day on peripheral TPN results in a larger deficit calcium balance and a higher risk of osteopenia.

Infants who are not expected to tolerate oral feedings within a week of starting parenteral nutrition should have a central line placed and be maintained on central parenteral nutrition. The choice of line also involves weighing the risks and benefits. Surgical placement of an anchored catheter (e.g., Broviac) is a riskier procedure than placement of a peripherally inserted central catheter (PICC). However, it is likely that the Broviac, placed under sterile operating room conditions, will last longer. In addition, the choice of lines (single lumen vs. double lumen, differences in gauges) is greater with surgically placed lines, and frequently blood can be drawn from one of the ports for laboratory monitoring. Conversely, the PICC lines are easily placed in the unit, can be as small as 27 gauge, and are silastic (which are less prone to clotting and infection). Their disadvantage is that they generally cannot be used for blood drawing. In our unit we try to remove all umbilical venous catheters after the infant has been stabilized following delivery room resuscitation and attempt to place a PICC line within the first 24 to 48 hours if the infant is expected to be on parenteral nutrition. Because of the low incidence of infection with these lines, we typically do not use peripheral parenteral nutrition.

Maintaining patency of the lines is important for the success of parenteral nutrition. Most centers use heparin in TPN solutions to keep central lines patent and reduce the formation of a fibrin sheath around the catheters. These fibrin sheaths are the most likely sites of infectious agents. To maintain patency, our unit utilizes the following protocol for PICC lines: for flow rates greater than 7 cc/h, no heparin is used; for flow between 2 and 7 cc/h, 0.25 U of heparin/cc is added; for flow rates less than 2 cc/h, 0.5 U of heparin/cc is added. We do not "heparin lock" our PICC lines and run them with a minimum rate of 0.5 cc/h with 1 U heparin/cc of solution. We do heparin lock surgically placed lines, administering 10 U of heparin in 1 cc of solution, given every 12 hours.

Catheter occlusions usually are treated with removal of the line because so many of the clots are infected. Nevertheless, catheter occlusions that occur without signs of sepsis (e.g., if the line was inadvertently shut off) can be treated with urokinase (5,000 U/mL). The amount of urokinase solution should approximate the internal volume of the catheter (0.2 to 0.5 mL). After instillation, the solution should be allowed to dwell in the catheter for 30 minutes. If two attempts at clearing the line fail, the catheter should be removed (147).

Nutritional Management

Parenteral nutrition should be started as soon as possible, because dextrose solutions alone cannot meet the resting energy or protein requirements of the neonate. So as not to waste TPN, which is more expensive than standard intravenous solutions, infants with rapidly changing electrolytes (and therefore electrolyte solutions) should have TPN deferred until their electrolytes are more stable.

Dextrose delivery typically should begin between 4 and 6 mg/kg/min and be advanced as tolerated. Extremely preterm infants are frequently glucose intolerant because of relative insulin hypoactivity and poor peripheral glucose utilization. Although their energy needs are higher because of their higher basal metabolic rates and higher brain to liver weight ratios, they frequently develop hyperglycemia and glycosuria. These are serious complications that must be treated immediately. Persistent glycosuria will result in a large free-water diuresis, intravascular dehydration, hypernatremia, and azotemia. Persistent hyperglycemia is a significant risk factor for fungal infection. Dextrose delivery can be slowly advanced based on how well the infant tolerates this. Typically we do not administer more than 12.5 g/kg/d because of the significant effect on the respiratory quotient. However, others have advocated rates up to 20 g/kg/d, aided by the administration of insulin to maintain normoglycemia. As stated earlier, I do not advocate this approach because the weight gain is predominantly fat rather than lean body mass and the metabolic cost of fat synthesis from glucose is high in terms of both oxygen consumption and carbon dioxide production. On the other hand, insulin is very useful in treating the hyperglycemia seen in ELBW infants in the first week of life, where glucose intolerance may necessitate decreasing dextrose delivery to unacceptably low rates (less than 4 mg/kg/min). Practices vary across the country. Table 23–5 lists the use of insulin by the group at Children's National Medical Center. The initial solution is used as the infant becomes hyperglycemic, whereas the second solution is used to wean the infant as hyperglycemia improves.

Protein in the form of amino acid solutions designed for newborns should be administered as soon as possible, usually within the first 48 hours. There are few contraindications to early protein delivery, and there is evidence that amino acid solutions improve nitrogen balance (80,45,148). At energy intakes above resting energy expenditure (65 kcal/kg/d), the main determinant of positive nitrogen balance is the nitrogen intake (149). The goal is to achieve *in utero* nitrogen accretion rates, which appears to be possible with amino acid delivery rates of 2.7 to 3.5 g/kg/d (150). Although protein requirements may be higher due to prior malnutrition, diseases that increase nitrogen turnover, or catch-up growth, it is rarely practical to give more than 3.5 g/kg/d of parenteral amino acids because of increasing blood urea nitrogen concentrations. Typically, 1 g/kg of amino acids is safe for all infants on days 1 to 2. Most infants can be advanced by 1 g/kg/d to a maximum of 3.5 g/kg/d, thus ensuring that they will be on full protein delivery by 3 to 4 days. Very unstable preterm infants and those with renal insufficiency due to indomethacin, surgery, a patent ductus arteriosus, or shock may need to be advanced more slowly. Monitoring the blood urea nitrogen allows the practitioner to decide on a daily basis whether the protein delivery can increase. A rising blood urea nitrogen is an indication that the infant is not clearing nitrogen waste and should not have the rate of amino acid infusion increased. Initially, when amino acid solutions intended

for adults were given to infants, significant complications occurred, because these solutions did not meet their metabolic needs. In the mid-1980s, improved solutions were introduced, which added the semiessential amino acids taurine, water-soluble tyrosine, and L-cysteine. Potentially toxic amino acids, such as phenylalanine and glycine, were reduced. These newer solutions promote a more normal serum amino acid profile (83), better nitrogen retention and weight gain (149,151), and lower rates of cholestasis (152). The lower rates of cholestasis may be due to the addition of taurine, which also may be important in neuronal development (153–155). Table 23–6 compares adult and pediatric amino acid solutions. There is no evidence that specialized solutions such as HepatAmine, BranchAmine, or NephrAmine are indicated in newborns. The spectrum of amino acids found in them may dangerously imbalance an infant's serum amino acid profile.

Intravenous fats provide a low-volume source of calories and shift cellular metabolism toward less carbon dioxide production, perhaps improving the respiratory load of the infant. They can be utilized within the first 3 days of life and are important in preventing essential fatty acid deficiency (156). Close monitoring of serum triglyceride levels is important during intravenous fat therapy. Intravenous fat solutions can be started at a delivery rate of 1 g/kg/d and advanced to a maximum of 4 g/kg/d. Total fat calories should be less than 60% of the diet and typically are in the 30% to 40% range. Like amino acids, intravenous fats can be advanced by 1 g/kg/d if tolerated. Because fat incorporation into cells is dependent on insulin, VLBW infants are more likely to have fat intolerance manifested by hypertriglyceridemia or, interestingly, hyperglycemia, requiring a slower rate of advancement (0.5 g/kg/d) or interruption of fat delivery. Infants with birth weights less than 1,250 g and gestational ages less than 30 weeks may need to have their fat dose held at 1 g/kg/d until their hyperbilirubinemia is resolving. This group of infants seems to be at greatest risk for intravenous lipids exacerbating hyperbilirubinemia (see Complications of Total Parenteral Nutrition). Fat emulsions are available in 10% and 20% solutions (Table 23–7) and generally are infused over no fewer than 16 hours to allow for metabolic clearing. It is important to

TABLE 23–5. *Sliding scale for insulin administration*

Factors affecting dose	Solution 1 initiating dose (25 U in 50 mL)	Solution 2 weaning dose (12.5 U in 50 mL)
Insulin concentration		
U/mL	0.5	0.25
U/0.1 mL	0.05	0.025
Blood sugar		
<150 mg/dL	0	0
150–200 mg/dL	0.1 mL/h	0.2 mL/h
200–250 mg/dL[a]	0.2 mL/h	0.4 mL/h

[a]If blood sugar is >250 mg/dL, give more insulin or decrease the glucose concentration.

TABLE 23–6. *Comparison of commonly used amino acid 10% solutions*

Solution characteristics[a]	Aminosyn 11	Freamine 111	Travasol	Aminosyn PF	TrophAmine[b]
Manufacturer	Abbott	McGraw	Clintec	Abbott	McGraw
Available solutions (%)	7, 8.5, 10	3, 6.9, 8.5, 10	5.5, 8.5, 10	7, 10	6, 10
Nitrogen (g/100 mL)	1.53	1.53	1.65	1.52	1.55
Total essential amino acids (mg/100 mL)	4,580	4,910	4,530	4,921	5,740
Total nonessential amino acids (mg/100 mL)	5,471	4,770	5,470	5,008	4,236
Total essential to total amino acid ratio (%)	45.6	50.7	45.3	49.6	52.3
Branched chain to total essential amino acid ratio (%)	47.2	46	42.2	36.6	57.5
Other components	No cysteine[c]	Cysteine[c] <20 mg/100 mL; no tyrosine, glutamic acid, or aspartic acid	No cysteine[c], glutamic acid, or aspartic acid	No cysteine[c], low tyrosine; contains taurine 70 mg/100 mL	Cysteine[c] <16 mg/100 mL; contains taurine 250 mg/100 mL
pH	5–6.5	6.5	6	5.4	5.5
mOsm/L	873	950	1000	829	875

[a]Data partially taken from the American Hospital Formulary Service and published by authority of the Board of Directors of the American Society of Hospital Pharmacists; most solutions have some electrolyte supplementation.
[b]Pediatric formulations.
[c]Cysteine may be added to all preparations.

run them separately from other solutions so as not to disturb the stability of the emulsion and to cover the solution from light to decrease breakdown. The solutions can be joined with the amino-acid–containing solution with a Y-connector near the infusion point on the infant.

Because infants initially undergo a free-water diuresis before a salt diuresis, sodium needs remain low until after day 3 of life (157). Thereafter, sodium and potassium requirements increase rapidly, and serum concentrations should be monitored at least daily while infants are on intravenous solutions. Table 23–8 lists the approximate electrolyte requirements for premature infants in the face of no extraneous losses, such as those incurred by renal failure or diuretic therapy. However, requirements may approach 10 mEq/kg/d for each if there are excessive uri-

nary losses. Chloride is the usual anion for both sodium and potassium; however, these cations also can be given as acetates, allowing for fine tuning of acid–base balance. Amino acid solutions have an inherent chloride and acetate load (e.g., TrophAmine contains 1 mEq of acetate for every gram of amino acid).

Calcium and phosphorus are the most difficult minerals to maintain balance in the preterm infant because of the large requirements for adequate mineralization, excessive losses due to calciuric diuretics and steroids, and the limited solubility of these nutrients in TPN (158). A calcium-to-phosphorus ratio of 1.7:2.0 appears to be optimal for mineralization (159). Because of solubility issues, calcium concentrations greater than 16.6 mEq/L with a concomitant phosphorus concentration of 8.3 mM

TABLE 23–7. *Available fat emulsions*

Preparation characteristics	Intralipid	Liposyn II	Liposyn III	Nutrilipid
Manufacturer	Clintec	Abbott	Abbott	McGraw
Solutions available (%)	10, 20	10, 20	10, 20	10, 20
Fat source	Soybean	Safflower	Soybean	Soybean
Fatty acids				
Linoleic (%)	50	65.8	54.5	49–60
Linoleic to linolenic ratio	5.5	15.6	6.6	8.2–6.7
Linolenic (%)	9	4.2	8.3	6–9
Oleic (%)	26	17.7	22.4	21–26
Palmitic (%)	10	8.8	10.5	9–13
Stearic (%)	3.5	3.4	4.2	3–5
Egg phosphatides (g/100 mL)	1.2	1.2	1.2	1.2
Glycerol (g/100 mL)	2.25	2.5	2.5	2.21
pH	6–8.9	6–9	6–9	6–7.9
Calories (10%–20%)/mL	1.1–2	1.1–2	1.1–2	1.1–2
mOsm/L	260	276	292	280–315

TABLE 23–8. *Daily requirements of total parenteral nutrition*

Nutrient	Requirement
Protein	2.5–3.5 g/kg
Fat emulsion	2–4 g/kg (max 3.5 g/kg in infants <2.5 kg)
Calories	90–110 kcal/kg or as needed
H_2O	125–150 mL/kg or as needed
Na	3–4 mEq/kg
K	2–3 mEq/kg
Ca	50–100 mg/kg, depending on size of infant
P	1–1.5 mM/kg
Mg	0.5–1 mEq/kg
Multivitamins (e.g., MVI Pediatric)	10 mL (40%/kg/d)

rarely are obtained. In an infant receiving 150 cc/kg/d, these values are equivalent to a calcium delivery of 50 mg/kg/d and a phosphorus delivery of 25 mg/kg/d, far less than the *in utero* accretion rate. Strategies to increase calcium retention and bone mineralization have been largely unsuccessful, but have included infusing calcium in one line and phosphorus in another and alternate infusions of higher doses of the two minerals (160,161). Monitoring of serum phosphorus and calcium levels is important. Infants are prone to hypocalcemia in the first 72 hours due to a transient hypoparathyroidism and to hypophosphatemia. Both calcium and phosphorus should be added early during TPN therapy. Calcium delivery without phosphorus delivery should be avoided because of the likelihood of hypophosphatemia. More acidic TPN solutions appear less likely to precipitate (162,163).

Infants on TPN receive 0.2 mL/kg body weight of neonatal trace elements (i.e., Neonate Trace-4), which supplies 0.02 mg/kg of copper, 0.3 mg/kg of zinc, 5 µg/kg of manganese, and 0.17 µg/kg of chromium. This supplement should be added with initiation of TPN and given daily. Selenium should be added after 2 weeks of TPN (115). Although we do not routinely measure zinc, copper, chromium, manganese, or selenium levels in infants on TPN, the practitioner should be aware that preterm infants in particular have low stores of these trace elements and that deficiencies have been described (164–166).

Water- and fat-soluble vitamins are added as a pediatric multivitamin solution (MVI Pediatric). The American Society for Parenteral and Enteral Nutrition recommends the following dosing schedule: for infants 1 to 3 kg, 3.75 mL of a 5-mL vitamin solution containing 2,300 IU of vitamin A, 400 IU of vitamin D, 7 IU of vitamin E, and 200 µg of vitamin K daily; for infants less than 1 kg, 1.5 mL of the same solution daily (167). This supplement should be added at initiation of TPN and given daily.

Complications of Total Parenteral Nutrition

Administration of parenteral nutrition remains an inexact science. Because it is not the normal mode of nutritional delivery, it is not surprising that complications occur. For the most part, complications can be divided into those associated with catheters and those related to the nutrients themselves. As discussed previously, centrally placed catheters are prone to thrombosis and infection. Thrombi can occur in the right atrium or in the veins. Of particular concern is when the superior vena cava is clotted. Superior vena cava syndrome with or without hydrocephalus can result. Occasionally, back pressure from the clot on the thoracic duct will cause a chylothorax. In addition, nonseptic complications such as skin sloughs can occur. Erosion of catheters through vessels or cardiac walls has caused pleural effusions, pericardial effusions, and endothelial damage. Improper technique of catheter insertion can result in pneumothorax or nerve injuries, whereas improper handling of fluids can result in air or fat embolisms. It is important that all personnel involved in parenteral nutrition therapy, including nurses, pharmacists, and physicians, be aware of the complications and techniques to avoid them.

Intravenous lipids have been associated with hypoxia, pulmonary hypertension, hyperbilirubinemia, and infection (168). Infants with respiratory disease have minimally lower PaO_2 values when given intravenous lipids, most likely because lipids can uncouple hypoxic vasoconstriction (169). Normally, to optimize ventilation/perfusion matching, the pulmonary vasculature supplying a poorly oxygenated alveolar area will constrict. This effect is reduced by the infusion of lipids, most likely moderated by serotonin. Similarly, higher pulmonary arterial pressures are seen in neonatal lambs infused with pharmacologic doses of lipids (6 mg/kg over 1 to 4 hours) (170). Finally, trials that have assessed whether early administration of intravenous lipids causes chronic lung disease (171,172) had mixed results. Overall, given the profound and early onset of growth failure in infants with severe lung disease, it seems prudent to start small amounts of lipids early in life.

Free fatty acids can displace bilirubin from albumin binding sites, prompting some practitioners to limit the dose of lipids to very small preterm infants. A study of infants weighing 670 to 3,360 g demonstrated adequate albumin binding of bilirubin and no effect on serum bilirubin levels (173,174). There are no reports of fat emulsions increasing the incidence of kernicterus. Theoretically, chylomicrons can be taken up by the reticuloendothelial system and interfere with fighting infection. Fat emulsions are also good media for fungi, including *Candida albicans* and *Malassezia furfur* (175). Whether these risks clinically outweigh the benefits of higher energy intake for small preterm infants has not been studied. At this time, it is likely that intravenous lipids improve the survival of infants through better growth.

Parenteral amino acids also are associated with toxicity. Excessive amino acid delivery will lead to increased serum blood urea nitrogen and ammonia levels due to the newborn infant's relatively immature renal and hepatic status. Parenteral amino acids have been associated with cholestasis, although the mechanism remains unknown (176). Infants at greatest risk are those who receive TPN for more than 3 weeks, those with intestinal disease, particularly NEC, those with sepsis, and those who remain NPO. Small amounts of trophic feeds reduce the prevalence of cholestasis, most likely by stimulating bile flow via cholecystokinin. Reduced bile flow from prolonged TPN frequently is associated with gallstones. In very rare cases, prolonged TPN with no enteral intake will lead to cirrhosis.

Aluminum toxicity is worth considering in infants who have been on TPN for more than 3 weeks. The largest contamination comes from the calcium and phosphorus salts that are added (177). The risk to the neonate is twofold. In infants with TPN, aluminum accumulates in the bones, where it is avidly taken up because of underlying osteopenia of prematurity (178). Of greater concern is the possibility that aluminum will cross the blood–brain barrier and induce an acute or chronic encephalopathy, as has been described in adult patients (179). Reduced renal capacity for excreting aluminum appears to be a necessary setting for this to occur, but it is not unusual for preterm infants to have a significant measure of renal insufficiency after treatment with indomethacin (180). Some have proposed that aluminum toxicity may be a factor in the poorer neurodevelopment of preterm infants. Because the body has no need for aluminum, manufacturers are being pressured to reduce the aluminum content of their solutions (181).

Monitoring Total Parenteral Nutrition Efficacy and Toxicity

Administering TPN is an inexact science still in the process of evolution. Matching nutrient delivery to the infant's needs presupposes knowledge of how a particular disease or its treatment affects the infant's metabolism and, therefore, the nutritional requirements. Careful monitoring of growth is indicated for any infant on TPN or partial parenteral nutrition (Table 23–9). Weight should be measured daily and length and head circumference weekly. Standards have been published for arm muscle area and arm fat area for preterm and term infants. These areas can be measured using a tape measure and skin caliper (139,182). Protein status can be assessed in two ways: somatic protein deposition (arm muscle area) and serum protein synthesis (serum albumin and prealbumin). The former provides a longitudinal view of protein accretion, whereas the latter reflects a more rapidly turned-over pool of protein. Assess-

TABLE 23–9. *Suggested monitoring for total parenteral nutrition*

Variable	First week	Later
Growth		
Weight	Daily	Daily
Length and head circumference	Weekly	Weekly
Chemistry		
Na, K, Cl, CO_2	Daily until stable	Daily
Glucose (Chemstrip bG)	Daily	Daily
Triglycerides	With each increase in IL	Twice weekly when stable
Ca (ionized Ca is most accurate)	Daily until stable	Weekly
P	Initially	Twice weekly for first week, then weekly
Albumin	Initially	Monthly
Prealbumin	Initially	Weekly (biweekly) in infants <1,000 g
Alkaline phosphatase	Initially	Weekly
Bilirubin	Initially	Every 4 wk or PRN
Mg	Initially	Weekly
Ammonia	As needed	As needed
Gamma GT	Initially	Weekly
Alanine aminotransferase	As needed	Monthly
Amino acids	As needed	As needed
Zinc		Monthly
Serum osmolarity	Initially	Weekly
Vitamin A (if infant is <1,300 g)	Weekly	Weekly while supplemented
Hematology		
Complete blood count	Initially	At least weekly
Type and screen	Initially	
Urinalysis		
Sugar	Each void	Each shift
Protein	Each void	Each shift
Specific gravity	Each void	Each shift

ment of serum concentrations of proteins with short half-lives, such as prealbumin, has been shown to reflect recent protein intake and to predict future weight gain (183). Prealbumin, also known as transthyretin, has a half-life of 1.9 days and can be measured once or twice per week to yield useful nutritional information. If the serum concentration remains stable or increases, one can expect that the infant is in reasonable nitrogen balance and will gain weight subsequently (184). A decrease of more than 10% from the previous measurement suggests relative protein-energy malnutrition and the need for a higher intake. Like most rapidly turned-over proteins, prealbumin acts as an acute phase reactant and will rise rapidly with stress, infection, and glucocorticosteroid administration (185), rendering it useless as a nutritional marker. Serum albumin, which has a half-life of 21 days, can be monitored every 2 to 4 weeks.

It is important to monitor infants on parenteral nutrition because of the toxicities associated with its administration. Table 22–9 provides guidelines for nutritional monitoring of infants on TPN. At the least, infants on TPN should have a set of electrolytes and a serum glucose checked daily. Serum glucose concentrations greater than 110 mg/dL are an indication not to increase the glucose infusion rate; concentrations greater than 150 mg/dL are an indication to reduce the rate. Serum triglyceride concentrations should be checked at least twice per week, or more frequently if the infant is showing signs of lipid intolerance. ELBW infants and infants with sepsis are especially prone to hypertriglyceridemia, even if they have tolerated intravenous fat previously. Methylxanthines and glucocorticosteroids increase the likelihood of both glucose and fat intolerance in preterm infants. A triglyceride level greater than 150 mg/dL measured with the infant off lipid infusion is an indicator of impending intolerance and lipid doses should not be increased. A triglyceride concentration greater than 200 mg/dL is considered a sign of intolerance and the lipid dose should be decreased. Because persistent hypertriglyceridemia represents a risk to the pulmonary system, daily levels should be monitored in the infant showing intolerance.

Calcium status must be monitored carefully in the first days of life, as hypocalcemia is commonly seen in ill newborns. Preterm infants, growth-retarded infants, and infants of diabetic mothers appear particularly prone to hypocalcemia. Infants receiving large amounts of citrated blood products, such as those who are postoperative, are on extracorporeal membrane oxygenation, or have disseminated intravascular coagulopathy, will require large amounts of calcium. Similarly, maintenance of normophosphatemia is important for normal metabolism. Therefore, serum calcium, phosphorus, and magnesium should be monitored daily in the first week of life, or until stable, and then weekly thereafter (see Table 23–9).

Bone mineralization is problematic for the preterm infant on long-term parenteral nutrition; therefore, close monitoring is indicated. Unfortunately, this can be quite difficult. Although osteopenia of prematurity is predominantly due to deficient intakes of calcium and phosphorus, the serum levels of these minerals will be maintained at the expense of the bones. Thus, serial measurements of calcium and phosphorus are not useful in monitoring this complication. Serum alkaline phosphatase is an indirect measure of osteopenia because its level will increase with the bone remodeling that takes place to supply the serum calcium pool. The level should be monitored weekly, particularly in preterm and growth-retarded infants. The level may be difficult to interpret, because the alkaline phosphatase will rise with cholestatic liver disease (a complication of parenteral nutrition itself) and with intestinal injury (such as NEC). Fractionating the alkaline phosphatase level into its bone and nonbone components can be done, but may take weeks depending on whether the laboratory has the capability to perform the fractionation. As with monitoring of the prealbumin concentration, the most important aspect of the alkaline phosphatase to follow is the trend. Rising alkaline phosphatase levels generally mean aggressive bone remodeling and an increased risk of osteopenia. Strategies to increase calcium and phosphorus delivery should be considered.

The incidence and severity of hepatic toxicity from parenteral nutrition has been on the decline with the introduction of more specialized neonatal amino acid solutions. The toxicity typically is cholestatic in nature, with an initial rise in serum bile acids, followed by an increase in the direct bilirubin, alkaline phosphatase. and γ-glutamyl transferase. Transaminase elevations are seen only in very severe cases. The liver toxicity was initially thought to be due to intravenous lipids (fatty liver), but now quite conclusively has been associated with amino acid solutions. Although these solutions have been refined (149), the problem persists and its cause is unknown. Total and direct bilirubin concentrations typically will be monitored in all newborns in the first week of life. Infants on prolonged TPN should have direct bilirubin measured weekly. If it is elevated, the remaining liver function tests should be assayed and followed weekly.

Trace minerals rarely are deficient in infants on TPN because of supplementation. Nevertheless, the importance of maintaining normal zinc status for growth and protein utilization (185) makes it wise to monitor the serum zinc concentration monthly, particularly if the infant is not growing adequately or has physical signs of zinc deficiency.

Vitamin status generally need not be checked in infants on TPN, with the exception of vitamins E and A. Most vitamin assays are cumbersome and are a poor reflection of total body load. The same is likely to be true for vitamins E and A. Nevertheless, the association of low serum retinol (circulating vitamin A) levels with an increased risk for BPD in the VLBW infant suggests that monitoring may be appropriate (126). An initial measurement in all infants less than 1,500 g with respiratory disease should indicate the degree of risk. Infants with levels less than 20 μg/dL should be supplemented and their levels followed weekly. The methodologies for assaying vitamin A (high-performance liquid chromatography or fluorometry) are the same as for vitamin E, and the values for both can be obtained simultaneously. As with vitamin A, it is important to keep vitamin E concentrations in the normal range, as too low a concentration has been associated with anemia (128) and perhaps ROP (129), whereas toxic levels increase the risk of sepsis and NEC (134).

Enteral Nutrition

Oral Feeding

The goal for virtually all infants prior to discharge from the hospital is full oral feedings, preferably by breast. Oral feedings come naturally to infants born at term, but can be a significant task for those born at less than 34 weeks of gestation, those with significant central nervous system disease, and those with anatomic abnormalities preventing oral feedings.

Oral feedings should be initiated within half an hour of birth by placing the infant to the mother's breast (5). Infants who are breast-fed will have a different sucking motion than those who are bottle fed. Thus, it is important that artificial nipples (and probably pacifiers) not be introduced as the infant is establishing breast-feeding (5). The oral pattern associated with breast-feeding is typically well established within 2 weeks, although a substantial number of infants who are then supplemented with bottles will demonstrate nipple confusion and may give up on breast-feeding. The healthy, breast-fed infant has no need for supplemental water, juice, or formula (5). Breast-feeding can be supported in the delivery hospital by training all of the staff to encourage mothers to breast-feed and to provide the necessary environment to promote breast-feeding. This includes allowing the mother to nurse within half an hour of delivery, having the infant room in with the mother, and having the mother learn the cues of her infant's hunger. Hospitals can contribute by not having policies about supplementing breast-fed babies and supplying charts that assess the infant's feeding and hydration status (5).

Oral feedings can be more problematic for the healthy premature infant. These infants rarely show any interest in oral feeding until approximately 32 weeks of gestation and rarely have a mature, safe feeding pattern until 34 weeks of gestation. Coordination of sucking, swallowing, and breathing is most difficult. There is little evidence that "practice" helps the gestationally immature infant to feed orally sooner. Nevertheless, Meier (186) has reported that breast-fed premature infants have longer periods of sucking with fewer obstructive apnea and desaturation spells than comparably sized bottle-fed infants. This may relate to the more metered rate of milk flow. It is important to note that preterm infants frequently are exposed to pacifiers to stimulate nonnutritive sucking, which improves gastric motility and likely increases the flow of important gastrointestinal hormones (187–189). It is unclear whether this nonnutritive sucking at an earlier postconceptional age affects the success of breast-feeding at 34 weeks of gestation.

Schanler (14) and Meier (186) have made strong cases for breast-feeding the preterm infant because of the superior performance of breast-feeding with respect to immune status and neurodevelopment, among other advantages. To successfully breast-feed the premature infant, the mother needs to be available as the infant nears 33 weeks of gestation to begin the process. Before that point, it is important that she maintain her milk supply. The intensive care nursery can help by providing a place to nurse, an electric breast pump, storage containers, and a freezer for storing the milk. An organized program with an informed leader is very useful in timing the introduction of actual breast-feeding and overseeing the progress made by the individual infant. With such a program, more than 60% of preterm infants whose mothers desire to nurse can successfully breast-feed at the time of discharge.

Preterm infants who are bottle fed also require close observation as they transition from gavage to nipple feeds. There is an energy cost to bottle feeding. Gavage feedings require between 4% and 17% less energy to process, and excessive oral feedings may tire out an infant and reduce weight gain velocity (190,191). Typically, attempts at bottling should begin around 33 weeks of gestation with one feeding per day. If the infant shows no interest or has significant obstructive apnea, it may be prudent to wait several days before attempting again. The frequency of feedings can be increased as the infant shows more aptitude. Once the infant has advanced to full oral feedings, it is important to see whether weight gain can be maintained on an *ad libitum,* on-demand schedule prior to discharge. Consistency in feeding personnel can improve the infant's performance, and in the best of all worlds, having the mother give most of the feedings is ideal.

Oral aversion is a significant problem in infants who have been NPO or on ventilators for long periods of time. Symptoms include aversive behaviors such as tongue thrusting, head turning, pooling of milk in the mouth, and occasionally breath-holding apneic spells. A barium swallowing study with fluoroscopy can help identify whether the problem is anatomic, discoordination, immaturity, or neurologic pathology. For infants with severe cases, the worst course is to force oral feedings. The involvement of an occupational or speech therapist can be invaluable in desensitizing the oral area.

Gavage Feeding

Gavage feedings are indicated for infants who can be fed enterally but not orally. For the most part, this approach is used in premature infants who are neurologically immature and the full expectation is that they will feed orally. Infants who will not be candidates for oral feeds either because of anatomic or neurologic conditions can have gastrostomy tubes placed. Gavage feedings are accomplished most frequently by placing a naso- or orogastric tube and bolusing feedings intermittently. Some practitioners prefer to place an indwelling transpyloric tube to reduce aspirates and ensure nutrient delivery. Infants can receive feeds by continuous drip as well as by bolus.

Oro- or nasogastric tube feedings can be initiated using a soft silastic 5Fr or 8Fr catheter. The tube most commonly is placed into the stomach prior to a feeding and the contents of the stomach aspirated to ensure there are no residuals from the previous feeding. The feeding is allowed to run in by gravity, although in some infants with very slow gastric emptying the feeding can be titrated in over 1 hour. The tube typically rapidly is withdrawn after the feeding, although there is some increased risk of the infant vomiting in response to this stimulus. A long-term indwelling catheter can be placed, but this type of catheter may lose flexibility over time and increase the risk of stomach perforation.

Gastric gavage feedings can be given on a schedule between every 1 and 4 hours. Typically, smaller infants do not tolerate excessive stomach distention with large-volume feedings and may exhibit respiratory compromise. They may need to be fed small amounts on a more frequent schedule. Infants less than 1,000 g can be fed on an every 1- to 2-hour bolus schedule or with continuous-drip feedings. This approach may reduce oxygen consumption and total energy expenditure, and potentially contribute to faster rates of weight gain. Infants may be fed on this schedule until they weigh 1,250 to 1,500 g, after which every-3-hour feeds are more appropriate. Nevertheless, larger infants who are not tolerating bolus feedings, those who remain on ventilators, or those with severe apnea and bradycardia may require drip feedings. Term infants who require gavage feedings may do best on an every-4-hour schedule.

Tube placement and maintenance may cause significant problems in the infant. Tubes can be malpositioned in the airway instead of the stomach. With the placement of any new tube, it is important to document its position by auscultation and by checking the pH of aspirated stomach contents. Placement of the tube can cause significant vagal stimulation, which results in apnea or bradycardia. The presence of an indwelling tube can cause apnea and bradycardia either by excessive vagal stimulation or, more commonly, by upper airway obstruction. Although nasogastric tubes are more stable, they appear to cause more problems with airway obstruction. Gastric and esophageal perforations are rare, but must be considered if there is a significant change in the infant's behavior or results of physical examination.

Gavage feedings also can be given through a transpyloric tube. The advantages of this type of feeding include ensured nutrient delivery and much less chance of gastroesophageal reflux and aspiration pneumonia. There are significant mechanical and nutritional disadvantages to this approach. The mechanical problems include difficulty in placing the tube, although this becomes easier with practice. To place the tube, the infant is turned with his or her right side down and the tube is inserted into the stomach with small amounts of injected air. As the infant remains in the right-side-down position, the tube has a reasonable chance of advancing through the pylorus into the duodenum. The tube has reached the duodenum when bile-stained fluid is returned or when the pH of the aspirated fluid changes from acidic (pH 3) to alkaline (pH 5 to 7). Infants on histamine-2 blocking agents cannot be assessed in this way. The procedure also can be done in the radiology suite under fluoroscopy with a weighted tube. The position of the tube is confirmed on x-ray film. Frequently, the tip of the tube will curl back on itself or simply move back into the stomach, and the process will need to be done again. Although rare, the most devastating complication of transpyloric feedings is intestinal perforation and peritonitis.

Transpyloric feedings pose significant nutritional risks (191–193). Bypassing the stomach decreases fat digestion and absorption, as up to 50% of fat processing takes place in the stomach by the enzymes lingual and gastric lipase. In addition, secretion of gut hormones, such as cholecystokinin and gastrin, are dependent in part on stomach distention by a meal. Potassium accretion may be impaired. Bacterial colonization of the normally sterile intestine may be a significant risk, because the normal mechanism by which the stomach acid kills bacteria has been bypassed.

Initiation of gavage feedings through any of the tubes mentioned requires careful assessment of the infant. The stable infant of birth weight more than 1,500 g typically can be fed within hours of birth, although if the infant is less than 35 weeks of gestation it is prudent to advance the strength and volume of feedings in a proscribed manner. Table 22–3 provides a sample of feeding schedules in stable infants based on birth weight. Infants with birth weights more than 1,500 g can be started on every-3-hour feedings, infants between 1,000 and 1,500 g on every-2-hour feedings, and infants less than 1,000 g on every-1-hour or continuous-drip feedings. It must be remembered that although low-volume feedings are better tolerated from a respiratory standpoint, the gastric emptying time of the preterm infant is often between 60 and 90 minutes. Therefore, it is likely that gastric aspirates will be present in an infant fed every hour or by continuous drip. In the infant fed every 2 hours or less frequently, gastric aspirates should be less than 2 cc/kg body weight. Aspirates greater than that amount may be indicative of an ileus due to feeding intolerance or impending NEC. A thorough evaluation including an abdominal examination is indicated before resuming feedings. The availability and ease of administration of parenteral nutrition make a strong argument for being conservative with feeding advancement in preterm infants.

Trophic Feeds

Slow advancement of feedings is recommended in an infant who has been ill and likely had an ileus. Infants who otherwise would remain NPO can be started with trophic feeds, which are defined as continuous-drip feedings at 1 cc or less per hour. Studies of VLBW infants begun on trophic feedings in the first week of life have shown a lower incidence of feeding intolerance and NEC, a more mature gastrointestinal tract, and a shorter duration of time to regain birth weight (194–198). Animal studies demonstrate that early feedings prevent involution of the gut villi and loss of intestinal enzymes normally seen after as few as 3 days of intravenous feedings (199). Trophic feedings can be considered more as an "oral medication" than true feedings, as little is gained nutritionally from them. Trophic feedings have not been studied in infants of birth weight less than 800 g, and it is unclear whether the benefits, if any, of early feedings in these infants outweigh the risks. Most practitioners would agree that these infants should not receive feedings while they are unstable; however, mechanical ventilation per se is not a contraindication to initiating feedings.

WHAT TO FEED NEWBORN INFANTS

What one decides to feed infants is dependent on understanding the developmental physiology of the newborn gastrointestinal tract, the requirements of the infant for normal growth and body composition, and the available mechanisms of nutrient delivery. It is not surprising that term infants will thrive on different amounts and types of foods than preterm infants, and that allowances in both groups must be made for the effect of illness on nutrient requirements.

Term Infants

Human Milk

Human milk is species-specific food for human beings (5). As such, it represents the best choice of food for the newborn infant. Substitute feedings, usually made from an animal milk base, have been available for hundreds of years and have been highly refined in this century. Nevertheless, no manufactured food can match the content of human milk for several reasons. Human milk is delivered fresh and has no "shelf life." This simple property allows live cells, growth factors, enzymes, and immune factors to remain intact and active. Formulas, which are designed to have a shelf life of 1 to 2 years (depending on the type of formulation), do not incorporate most of these factors because they would be unstable and degrade over time. The factors found in human milk are thought to be responsible for many of its immunologic and developmental advantages. Human milk is always at the correct temperature and requires no sterilization.

Approximately 60% of women in the United States elect to breast-feed their infants. This figure has remained relatively stable during the past 5 years and represents a rise from the nadir of 40% in the 1950s. It falls short of the goal of 75% set by the Healthy People 2000 initiative sponsored by the National Institutes of Health and endorsed by the AAP (5). The obstacles to improving the rate of initiation of breast-feeding include physician apathy or misinformation (200), insufficient prenatal breast-feeding education (201), and the lack of a perception of breast-feeding as culturally normal (202). By 6 months of age, only 21.6% of infants are breast-fed, even though human milk is nutritionally sufficient for infants through the first 6 months. This figure falls far short of the Healthy People 2000 goal of 50%. The decrement is due to multiple factors, but the primary ones are failure to maintain a milk supply in the first days after birth and discontinuation of breast-feeding upon the mother's return to work. The former relates to hospital and office practices, which encourage formula feeding or are, at best, ambivalent to breast-feeding. For example, early hospital discharges combined with lack of timely routine follow-up care and postpartum health visits contribute to this early loss (203,204). The late dropout relates to the fact that many mothers work and many work places are not equipped to support the mother to maintain her milk supply (205,206). The AAP recently released the report of its Breast Feeding Work Group, which reaffirms its support of breast-feeding and provides recommendations to improve the initiation and retention rates (5).

There are few absolute contraindications to breast-feeding. Infants with galactosemia should not be breast-fed (207), nor should infants whose mothers are using illegal drugs (208). Mothers with active tuberculosis and mothers in first-world countries who have human immunodeficiency virus also should not breast-feed (209,210). Mothers who are taking certain medications (e.g., amethopterin, bromocriptine, cimetidine, clemastine, cyclophosphamide, ergotamine, gold salts, methimazole, phenindione, thiouracil) should not breast-feed. Complete lists of maternal medications that contraindicate breast-feeding are available (211,212). Temporary disorders, such as maternal mastitis or engorgement, are not contraindications to breast-feeding.

Human milk is nutritionally complete for most term infants for the first 6 months of life. Its primary carbohydrate is lactose. The protein content is low (1.1%), but the amino acid spectrum is well matched for the needs of human infants, and the predominance of lactalbumin ensures a low curd tension. The fat content of human milk is high and may approach 55% of total calories. The fat blend is unique and has been difficult to imitate in formula. In particular, the presence of certain omega fatty acids (DHA and EPA) may be important for optimal retinal and neurologic development (213). Human milk is relatively low in sodium and osmolality. Not surprisingly, gastric emptying is rapid with human milk, making it ideal for infants with slow gastrointestinal motility due to illness. Human milk is relatively low in iron content but high in iron bioavailablity. The vast majority of term infants fed exclusively human milk will remain iron sufficient, although their stores at 6 months may be lower than infants fed iron-supplemented formula (101). Human milk may have a low vitamin D content, particularly in women consuming a diet low in vitamin D and having low exposure to sunshine. Their infants are at risk of rickets if they too are not exposed to sunshine or given a supplement of vitamin D.

Epidemiologic studies provide evidence for the advantages of human milk over formulas, including better immune status, fewer infections (214–217), greater psychological benefits, more rapid neurodevelopment, protection from chronic childhood diseases (218–220), protection for the mother from certain diseases (221,222), and a lower rate of allergic disease (223,224). The reader is referred to the AAP statement on breast-feeding for a more complete review of these benefits (5).

Infant Formula

Despite the advantages of human milk, many women choose formula feeding instead of breast-feeding for their infants. Infant formulas should be given for the entire first year (225). Formula manufacturers are continually attempting to improve their products, with the goal of matching human milk composition or performance. Most infant formulas are cow-milk based and are formulated at 20 cal/oz. Alternatives include soy-based formula and elemental formulas.

Carbohydrates provide approximately 40% to 45% of the calories in formula. The most commonly used cow-milk-based formulas contain lactose as the primary carbohydrate, whereas the soy formulas contain either sucrose or glucose polymers.

The protein in formula provides approximately 10% of the total calories. Cow-milk protein is casein predominant, which is reported to have a higher curd tension than whey. Formula manufacturers have increasingly processed the cow-milk protein to make the formulas whey predominant, with a whey-to-casein ratio approaching 60:40. The ratio in human milk is 70:30 (14). An additional modification is hydrolysis of the whey. Soy for-

mulas contain soy proteins, which also support normal linear growth and muscle accretion. The protein content of soy formulas is higher than cow-milk formula. Soy formulas contain phytic acid, which may bind divalent cations (Ca, Mg) in the formula. For this reason, the calcium content of soy formulas is greater than that of cow-milk formulas. Bone mineralization and linear bone growth in term infants fed soy formulas appear to be adequate.

Fat constitutes 40% to 55% of calories in infant formula and is usually a blend of vegetable oils, such as corn, coconut, soy, or palm-olein. Vegetable oils are added to cow-milk-based formulas because babies do not tolerate butterfat well. The fat blends are generally well tolerated, although infants will malabsorb up to 1 g/kg/d of ingested fat in the first 10 days of life (226). This malabsorption is lower than what is observed with whole milk (2 g/kg/d) or evaporated milk (1 to 2 g/kg/d). Recent research has focused on whether long-chain polyunsaturated fatty acids, such as DHA and EPA, are essential in the diet of newborns. Human milk contains these fatty acids, whereas cow milk does not. Newborn infants have a relatively limited ability to synthesize these fats at birth, although the rates of maturation of the enzymatic pathways (elongation and desaturation) in the postnatal period only now are being elucidated. The content of DHA in human milk decreases rapidly after 44 weeks postconception, yet infants maintain adequate DHA levels, suggesting that the synthetic process is intact near that age (227). Addition of DHA to term infant formula has yielded mixed results with respect to growth and neurodevelopment (60,61). Those studies that showed a positive effect on early retinal development or neurodevelopment failed to demonstrate long-term or permanent benefits. The safety of the sources of these oils (egg phospholipid, tuna eye-socket, algae) in infants remains under investigation.

Substantial alterations need to made to whole cow milk to create a formula that a newborn infant will tolerate and thrive on. Whole cow milk is highly osmolar, low in calcium, high in phosphorus, low in vitamins A and D, and very low in bioavailable iron. Significant adjusting of all of these nutrients, in addition to changing the protein and fat, is necessary before an infant formula is safe for newborns.

Soy formulas are indicated for infants with galactosemia or lactase deficiency, infants whose mothers choose a vegetarian diet for their family, and infants with documented immunoglobulin-E–mediated allergy to cow-milk protein (228). However, there is no evidence that soy formula prevents atopic disease. Soy formulas do not relieve colic and are not indicated for premature infants (see following).

Elemental and casein hydrolysate formulas continue to make up a larger part of the infant formula market in spite of their very high cost and poor taste. The hydrolysate formulas promote adequate growth and nitrogen retention. Their main use has been in the treatment and prevention of allergy, because 90% of the protein fragments have a molecular weight less than 1,250 daltons. These low-molecular-weight fragments are less antigenic than cow-milk protein. In spite of this, anaphylaxis to these formulas has been reported (229,230). In addition, the rate of true cow-milk protein allergy in newborns is less than 3%. Hydrolysates are not indicated for refeeding infants after gastroenteritis or for treating colic. They are more osmolar than standard cow milk or soy formulas and thus possess a potential risk to the intestinal epithelium, particularly in the preterm infant.

Preterm Infants

Human Milk

Extensive research has assessed the adequacy and desirability of human milk feedings in the preterm infant. The reader is referred to a recent review of the subject (14). This research is predicated on the argument that human milk is the ideal food for the term neonate and that the immunologic, gastrointestinal trophic, and psychological aspects are even more relevant to the preterm infant. When beginning human milk feedings in the preterm neonate, one must ask the question whether human milk is a good match for the preterm infant's nutritional requirements.

Mothers who deliver preterm produce a milk that has a higher protein, caloric density, calcium, and sodium content than milk from mothers who deliver at term (84–86). To a certain extent, these higher concentrations match the increased needs for these nutrients in preterm infants (see previous). The composition of preterm human milk changes during the first month postnatally and becomes more like term human milk thereafter. Table 22–2 demonstrates the change in content of preterm human milk in the first months of life.

Human milk provides multiple nutritional advantages for the LBW infant (14). The carbohydrate composition is predominantly lactose, but also includes oligosaccharides that are important for intestinal host defenses (231). These oligosoaccharides may play a role in protecting the human milk-fed premature infant from NEC (14).

The fat blend of preterm human milk is unique and allows up to 95% absorption of dietary fat. This is due in part to the presence of lipases in human milk but also apparently due to the fat blend. Preterm human milk also has detectable concentrations of omega-3 and omega-6 fatty acids. These fatty acids, particularly DHA, are important constituents of phospholipid membranes in the brain (232) and normally are delivered transplacentally. They are not found in cow milk, nor are they currently added to preterm infant formula in the United States. They do not appear to be readily synthesized by the preterm infant from linoleic and linolenic acid precursors and thus are considered by some to be semiessential. Studies of infants who receive a source of these fatty acids either from human milk or in preterm infant formula suggest better visual acuity (233). Studies of developmental outcome and growth, as well as safety, continue.

The protein content is predominantly whey, as opposed to the casein predominance of whole cow milk. Although preterm infant formulas are whey predominant, there are important differences in the proteins that make up the whey. The main human milk whey protein is α-lactalbumin, as opposed to β-lactalbumin in cow milk. In addition, only human milk has significant concentrations of important proteins involved in host defense, such as lactoferrin and secretory immunoglobulin A, in the whey fraction. These proteins may contribute to the observed protective effect that human milk has on the occurrence of NEC. There is evidence that these proteins act at a local (234) and systemic (235) level. Their effects may be in combination with a more benign fecal flora (236).

In spite of these advantages, the feeding of human milk to preterm infants poses several nutritional problems, particularly for the infant weighing less than 1,500 g. Preterm infants fed unsupplemented human milk have slow growth rates and higher rates of hyponatremia and osteopenia (237–241). These findings suggest that in spite of the altered content of preterm human milk, there is still not enough energy, protein, calcium, phosphorus, and sodium to sustain adequate growth and bone mineralization. There is concern that some of the energy loss occurs when fat separates from human milk (242) and adheres to delivery tubing and storage containers.

Rather than abandon human-milk feedings, the solutions to these nutritional inadequacies include preventing losses by using short tubing lengths and using a syringe and pump, maintaining the syringe upright (14).

Most importantly, human milk delivered to all infants weighing less than 1,500 g should be fortified with commercial products that increase the caloric, protein, sodium, and calcium density of the milk. Two preformulated products are currently available, a liquid and a powder. Each promotes better growth and bone mineralization than unsupplemented preterm human milk. The liquid preparation is mixed in dilutions of 1:1, 1:2, or 1:3 with human milk. Because the caloric density of human milk is presumed to be 20 kcal/oz and the undiluted fortifier contains 24 kcal/oz, it is not possible to provide a 24 kcal/oz feeding to the infant. This may be an issue in infants with BPD who require fluid restriction to 150 cc/kg/d but who require at least 120 kcal/kg/d for growth. The powdered fortifier preparation is added as one packet per 25 mL of human milk. At this concentration, the human milk can be fortified to a presumed caloric density of 24 kcal/oz and still maintain the desired base of human milk.

There is great variability in the milk expressed by mothers delivering preterm. Therefore, monitoring of nutritional status is critically important in preterm infants fed fortified human milk. In particular, growth rates, serum sodium concentrations, and bone mineralization (serum alkaline phosphatase concentration, urinary excretion of phosphorus) must be assessed with regularity in these infants. Inadequate weight gain (less than 15 g/kg/d consistently over 1 week) can be treated by giving the infant more hind milk in the diet (14). Persistent increases in serum alkaline phosphatase concentrations in spite of fortification may necessitate adding some feedings of preterm infant formula.

Care must be taken in handling human milk to protect its important nutritional and immunologic advantages. Banked human milk should not be used. Fresh human milk is best, but is often impractical, particularly if the mother lives out of town. Fresh milk can be kept refrigerated up to 24 hours, but must then be frozen. Although live cells are destroyed by deep freezing (243), proteins remain largely intact. Suboptimal freezing results in fat breakdown. Rewarming frozen human milk can be dangerous, as microwaving heats milk unevenly and can cause esophageal or gastric burns (244). It is more prudent to thaw an aliquot of milk for the entire shift or day and dispense it once it has been warmed in a water bath.

Initiating, advancing and maintaining human milk feedings in the preterm infant who cannot take oral feeds can be accomplished in many ways. Unlike preterm infant formula, human milk does not need to be diluted, as gastric aspirates are less of a problem with human milk because of better gastric emptying.

Preterm Infant Formula

The development of formulas specifically designed for the preterm infant represented an important advancement in the nutrition of these infants. Prior to the introduction of these formulas in the late 1970s through the mid-1980s, preterm infants were fed various formulations intended for infants with very different intestinal maturity, nutrient assimilation capability, and nutritional requirements. The science that went into developing preterm infant formulas carefully measured the nutrient needs of the preterm infant (described previously) and the digestive and absorptive capabilities. When these two factors were considered together, a unique formulation for preterm infants evolved. For the most part, the preterm infant formulas are designed with the physiology of the less than 34-week gestational age infant in mind. Infants at 34 weeks or more whose mothers chose not to breast-feed them should be started on term infant formulas. If they show signs of intolerance (usually diarrhea, excessive gas, abdominal distention), relative lactase insufficiency due to immature intestinal development should be suspected, and a preterm formula can be used.

Two preterm infant formulas are available in the United States, and their nutritional constituents are remarkably similar. The carbohydrate source for both is a combination of lactose and glucose polymers. The lactose content is reduced compared to term infant formulas because of the relatively lower lactase concentration found in the preterm intestine. Glucose polymers are easily digested and are low osmolar.

The protein source is cow milk that has been made whey predominant. The concentration of protein is quite high, delivering up to 3.6 g/kg/d when the formula is fed at a typical volume of 150 cc/kg/d. This high rate of delivery is designed to match the intrauterine accretion of nitrogen and follows the guidelines established by Heird et al. (79). Protein intakes at this rate maintain reasonable muscle mass accretion and support normal serum albumin and prealbumin concentrations.

The fat blend is derived from vegetable oils, as it is in term formulas. However, preterm infant formulas contain between 10% and 50% of the fat content as MCT. The necessity of MCT remains controversial. Addition of MCT was stimulated by the finding that lingual and gastric lipases are particularly effective at hydrolizing fatty acids of this length and because long-chain fatty acids require an adequate bile salt pool for absorption. As discussed previously, preterm infants have low bile salt pools, which contributes to their higher fat malabsorption rate. Excessive MCTs are not indicated, as they are poorly utilized for fat storage. They are an excellent source of energy, with the excess being excreted in the form of dicarboxylic acids (245). Preterm infant formulas currently manufactured in the United States do not contain supplemental omega-3 or omega-6 fatty acids. Their addition awaits the outcome of trials underway to determine their essentiality and safety for preterm infants.

The sodium and potassium contents of preterm infant formulas are higher than in term formulas to compensate for renal tubular immaturity. Levels of trace elements are likewise higher. The preterm infant formulas contain the most calcium and phosphorus of any formula available. The current formulations when fed at a volume of 150 cc/kg/d will provide approximately 225 mg/kg/d of calcium and 110 mg/kg/d of phosphorus. This is well in excess of intrauterine accretion rates, allowing these formulas to be utilized to provide catch-up bone mineralization for those infants who have been on prolonged parenteral nutrition or dilute formulas. In spite of this high content, most premature infants weighing less than 1,500 g have evidence of osteopenia of prematurity at the time of discharge. The bones of VLBW infants frequently are demineralized at discharge (246). Preterm infant formulas recently have been supplemented with iron in recognition of the fact that preterm infants have low iron stores and a rapid expansion of the red cell mass when catch-up growth ensues.

The preterm infant formulas are replete with water- and fat-soluble vitamins. Both formulations have higher vitamin D, E, and A concentrations compared to term formulas because of the poor fat absorption in preterm infants and the concern about the consequences of deficiency states in the infants. Studies assessing vitamin A and E levels in preterm infants fed the preterm infant formula with higher vitamin A and E concentrations demonstrated that additional supplementation with vitamins is not necessary once the infant is consuming at least 150 cc. Infants on the product with lower concentrations may need additional supplementation. In either case, serum vitamin A and E levels should be followed weekly in preterm infants of birth weighs less than 1,500 g.

Techniques for the initiation, advancement, and maintenance of preterm infant formula feedings vary widely. The formula manufacturers have recommended initiating feedings with dilute (12 kcal/oz) formula. Most infants will be on parenteral nutrition while their feedings are advanced. Although opinions vary greatly as to whether formula volume or strength should be increased first, one should keep in mind that 1 cc of fully advanced peripheral parenteral nutrition ($D_{12.5}$%, 3.0 g/kg/d of amino acids, 3.5 g/kg/d of lipids) is equivalent to approximately three-quarter-strength formula. Thus, volume-for-volume substitution of TPN with half-strength formula will dilute the caloric delivery to the infant, whereas substitution with full-strength formula will advance caloric intake.

Other Formulas

Although a large number of other formulas have been used in preterm infants, none are specifically designed to meet the nutritional needs of these infants. Any potential advantage of these formulas must be weighed against some fairly serious side effects. For example, soy formulas were used extensively in the late 1970s and early 1980s for preterm infants because they do not contain lactose and because of the concern that the preterm infant's intestine was particularly permeable to translocation of antigenic milk proteins (247). However, calcium absorption from soy formulas is very poor because the phytates in soy bind divalent cations. The incidence of osteopenia and rickets in preterm infants fed soy formulas is too high to justify recommending these products for this population (248).

Similarly, the possibility of using elemental or casein hydrolysate formulas for preterm infants has been raised. The attractiveness of these formulas stems from their more elemental nature, thus presenting less of a digestive challenge to the immature preterm intestine. Unfortunately, these formulas are a poor nutritional match for the preterm infant from a fat-soluble vitamin and mineral standpoint. The vitamin E and A contents of the hydrolysates are one-quarter to one-half that of premature infant formula. The significantly lower vitamin D levels, lower calcium levels, and poor calcium-to-phosphorus ratio (1.4:1) place the preterm infant at high risk for osteopenia of prematurity. Finally, the osmolarity of these formulas ranges from 290 to 330 mOsm/L at 20 kcal/oz, 25% higher than the preterm infant formulas, which have osmolarities of 210 to 220 mOsm/L at 20 kcal/oz and 250 to 270 mOsm/L at 24 kcal/oz. Hyperosmolarity is associated with a higher risk of NEC in preterm infants. As currently formulated, elemental or casein hydrolysate formulas are not recommended for routine use in preterm infants.

Follow-up formulas for preterm infants are available. Prior to their introduction, the preterm infant usually was switched to a formula designed for term infants prior to discharge from the hospital. This made sense from a digestive standpoint, because most intestinal capacities are similar to term by 34 weeks postconception, and preterm infants rarely leave the hospital prior to that age. Nevertheless, this practice did not take into account the large deficits in muscle stores, fat stores, and bone mineralization that occur in many of these infants, nor did they take into account the high rates of growth in preterm infants in the first year. Follow-up formulas represent a hybrid between preterm and term infant formulas. The two marketed in the United States are powders designed to be given at 22 cal/oz. At that concentration, they have a 50% higher calcium and vitamin D content than cow-milk-based formula for term infants. The carbohydrate content is a blend of lactose and glucose polymers, and the fat blend contains MCT oil similar to that in preterm infant formulas. There is less vitamin A and less sodium than in preterm infant formulas. The recommendation has been to give these formulas for the first 6 months postdischarge. An alternative approach has been to continue to feed the discharged patient premature infant formula (249). Two problems arise with this solution: the formulas are not available commercially, and the improved fat digestive capacity of the infant after 34 weeks postconception raises the possibility of excessive vitamin A absorption. Moreover, the preterm infant formulas were designed for the special physiology of the less than 1,500 g, less than 34-week gestational age infant.

NUTRITIONAL MONITORING

Any plan to nourish newborn infants should include plans for monitoring the nutritional status. For the healthy term infant, periodic plotting of the infant's weight, length, and head circumference on a standard growth curve is sufficient. The assessment of these parameters at birth provides a glimpse into the quality of fetal growth and provides a starting point for postnatal monitoring. Small-for-dates infants should be assessed for signs and symptoms of intrauterine growth retardation. Signs of intrauterine wasting include small weight for length and small mid-arm cirmcumference to head circumference ratio (250,251) and may be seen in many small-for-dates infants and some appropriate-for-dates infants. It is important to plot newborns on a population-appropriate growth curve. For example, the growth curves published by Lubchenco et al. (37) in the 1960s are widely used, but were generated from a predominantly inner-city population born at high altitude. Both factors tend to be associated with less intrauterine growth. It would not be appropriate to plot an infant of Scandinavian heritage, where birth weights are on average 11 oz higher than in the United States (252,253), born at sea level on the Lubchenco curves as it would overestimate the rate of macrosomia. The current debate is whether breast-fed infants should be plotted on their own unique curve rather than one generated from a mixed or formula-fed population.

Similarly, appropriate curves must be used to judge the growth and nutritional health of preterm infants. The recently published IHDP growth curves (Infant Health and Development Program, Ross Laboratories) have separate charts for VLBW and LBW infants and for boys and girls (254). These curves can be used for the first 2 postnatal years. The weight gain velocity of the VLBW infant is not as rapid as the LBW infant or the term infant, and little catch-up growth occurs in the first year after discharge (255). Catch-up growth has been reported to occur during late childhood (256).

The importance of monitoring protein-energy status in the hospitalized newborn cannot be overemphasized. Daily weights and weekly length and head circumference measurements should be routinely performed and charted. The effect of manipulating protein-energy delivery should be reflected with delays in the rate of weight gain. Interpretation of protein-energy status from weight measurements can be complicated by fluid retention or dehydration. Length measurements are the least reliable because of the difficulty in obtaining reproducible numbers. Assessments of energy requirements also can be made by indirect calorimetry to estimate resting energy expenditure. These measurements require special equipment and provide only a brief (usually 20 minute) glimpse into energy utilization. The daily energy expenditure is extrapolated from the short-term measurement with the potential errors introduced by the extrapolation. Stable isotope techniques, such as doubly labeled water, are the province of research institutions and are not used for clinical monitoring. Similarly, dual-energy x-ray absorptiometry has been used in research studies to assess fat and lean body mass. A more practical assessment of the infant's relative fat status can be achieved with skinfold measurements and calculation of the arm fat area (140).

Protein status can be assessed by measurements of somatic or serum proteins. Somatic protein status is best reflected in measurements of peripheral muscles, usually in the arm. The arm muscle area is calculated from the arm circumference and the skinfold thickness (257). The somatic muscle pool turns over relatively slowly, and serial measurements, like those of length, do not provide acute information with respect to recent nutritional manipulations. Serum proteins have various half-lives and, thus, give differential time information. Serum prealbumin (transthyretin) concentrations reflect recent protein intake and predict subsequent weight gain velocity (184). The half-life of the protein is 1.9 days; therefore, a weekly assessment of the serum prealbumin is useful. Serum albumin has a half-life of 10 to 21 days, can be used as a marker of chronic protein status, and can be assessed monthly if needed. It is not very responsive to recent manipulations in protein delivery. Serum transferrin concentrations, used extensively in older children and adults because of its half-life of 10 days, is not useful in premature infants for either assessing recent intake or predicting weight gain (258). It likely reflects a combination of iron and protein status and thus can be difficult to interpret. Nitrogen balance, urinary excretion of 3-methyl histidine, and stable isotope assessments using [^{15}N]glycine or [^{3}H]leucine are research tools that assess protein status.

Rapidly changing glucose, mineral, and electrolyte status is best monitored with serum levels. Infants on TPN or who are receiving diuretics should have sodium and potassium levels followed. Similarly, infants on TPN should have their serum glucose concentrations monitored. In the first days after birth, sick infants should have serum calcium, magnesium, and phosphorus levels assessed.

Chronic calcium and bone mineralization status should not be monitored solely with serum calcium and phosphorus levels, as they usually will be in the normal to low-to-normal range. The serum alkaline phosphatase concentration is an indirect measurement of bone mineralization, as it is tied closely to rapid bone turnover. An infant who is becoming osteopenic will have more rapid bone turnover and will have a higher alkaline phosphatase level. It should be expected that any growing premature infant will have relatively higher levels than a term infant, but a rapidly rising weekly alkaline phosphatase level is often indicative of active osteopenia. X-ray changes demonstrating demineralization are late findings and indicate that the bones are at least 33% demineralized. An elevated urinary excretion of phosphorus also is found during osteopenia of prematurity (259). Dual-energy x-ray absorptiometry can be used to assess bone mineralization, but is used primarily in the research setting (260).

In general, it is unnecessary to monitor trace element or vitamin status in the healthy, growing premature infant. Infants weighing less than 1,500 g who are at high risk for BPD should have a vitamin A level measured at birth and should be treated with supplemental vitamin A if the level is less than 20 µg/dL (126,127). Concomitant vitamin E measurements can be obtained. Weekly vitamin A and E levels should be followed in infants treated for deficiency.

The recent introduction of recombinant human erythropoietin has made monitoring of iron status an important consideration in the preterm infant. The iron status of the premature infant can fluctuate widely, with infants who are multiply transfused having extremely high ferritin concentrations (261). Conversely, those who receive few or no transfusions will have their meager iron stores rapidly consumed by erythropoiesis. Those treated with recombinant erythropoietin experience a decrease in their ferritin levels (105). They are likely to need iron supplementation earlier than the premature infants who were transfused. Currently, reference values for ferritin, serum iron, and transferrin concentrations in newborn infants have not been generated. Because iron has a narrow therapeutic-to-toxic ratio, better norms for assessing iron status in preterm infants are needed. At this time, it may be prudent to assay the serum ferritin concentration at 1 month of age to assess iron stores.

REFERENCES

1. Reichman B, Chessex P, Putet G, et al. Diet, fat accretion and growth in premature infants. *N Engl J Med* 1981;305:1495.
2. Ziegler EE, O'Donnell AM, Nelson SE, Fomon SJ. Body composition of the reference fetus. *Growth* 1976;40:239.
3. Wahlig TM, Georgieff MK. The effects of illness on neonatal metabolism and nutritional management. *Clin Perinatol* 1995;22:77.
4. Mathew OP. Science of bottle feeding. *J Pediatr* 1991;119:511.
5. American Academy of Pediatrics Work Group on Breastfeeding. Breastfeeding and the use of human milk. *Pediatrics* 1997;100:1035.
6. Pritchard JA. Fetal swallowing and amniotic fluid volume. *Obstet Gynecol* 1966;28:606.
7. Wood JD. Intrinsic neural control of intestinal motility. *Annu Rev Physiol* 1981;43:33.
8. Gryboski JD. The swallowing mechanisms of the neonate: I. Esophageal and gastric motility. *Pediatrics* 1965;35:445.
9. Broussard DL. Gastrointestinal motility in the neonate. *Clin Perinatol* 1995;22:37.
10. Ittmann PI, Amarnath R, Berseth CL. Maturation of antroduodenal motor activity in preterm and term infants. *Dig Dis Sci* 1992;37:14.
11. Siegel M, Lebenthal E, Krantz B. Effect of caloric density on gastric emptying in premature infants. *J Pediatr* 1984;104:118.
12. Berseth CL. Gestational evolution of small intestine motility in preterm and term intants. *J Pediatr* 1989;115:646.
13. Berseth CL. Neonatal small intestinal motility: motor responses to feeding in term and preterm infants. *J Pediatr* 1990;117:777.
14. Schanler RJ. Suitability of human milk for the low-birthweight infant. *Clin Perinatol* 1995;22:207.
15. Sunshine P. Digestion and absorption of proteins. In: Bloom RS, Sinclair JC, Warshaw JB, eds. *Selected aspects of perinatal gastroenterology.* Evansville: Mead Johnson, 1977:17.
16. Euler AR, Byrne WJ, Cousins LM, Ament ME, Walsh JH. Increased serum gastrin concentrations and gastric acid hyposecretion in the immediate newborn period. *Gastroenterology* 1977;172:1271.
17. Hadorn B, Zoppi G, Schmerling DH. Quantitative assessment of exocrine pancreatic function in infants and children. *J Pediatr* 1968;73:39.
18. Watkins JB. Mechanism of fat absorption and the development of gastrointestinal function. *Pediatr Clin North Am* 1975;22:721.
19. Balistreri WF. Anatomical and biochemical ontogeny of the gastrointestinal tract and liver. In: Tsang RC, Nichols B, eds. *Nutrition during infancy.* Philadelphia: Hanley & Belfus, Inc., 1988:33.
20. Hamosh M. Fat digestion in the newborn: role of lingual lipase and preduodenal digestion. *Pediatr Res* 1979;13:615.
21. Hamosh M. Lingual and breast milk lipases. *Adv Pediatr* 1982;29:33.
22. Jensen RG, Jensen GL. Specialty lipids for infant nutrition: I. Milks and formulas. *J Pediatr Gastroenterol Nutr* 1992;15:232.
23. Hernell O, Olvecrona T. Human milk lipases. II. Bile salt stimulated lipase. *Biochim Biophys Acta* 1974;369:234.
24. Hamosh M, Bitman J, Wood DL, Hamosh P, Mehta NR. Lipids in milk and the first steps in their digestion. *Pediatrics* 1985;75[Suppl]:146.
25. Watkins JB, Szczepanik P, Gould JB, Klein P, Lester R. Bile salt metabolism in the human premature infant. *Gastroenterology* 1975;69:706.
26. Lifschitz, CH. Carbohydrate needs in preterm and term newborn infants. In: Tsang RC, Nichols B, eds. *Nutrition during infancy.* Philadelphia: Hanley & Belfus, Inc., 1988:122.
27. Koldovsky, O. *Development of the functions of the small intestine in mammals and man.* Basel, Switzerland: S Basel and AG Karger, Publishers, 1969:168.
28. Gray GM. Carbohydrate absorption and malabsorption. In: Johnson LR, ed. *Physiology of the gastrointestinal tracts.* New York: Raven Press, 1981:1063.
29. Auricchio S, Rubino A, Murset G. Intestinal glycosidase activities in the human embryo, fetus and newborn. *Pediatrics* 1965;35:944.
30. MacLean WC Jr, Fink BB. Lactose malabsorption by premature infants: magnitude and clinical significance. *J Pediatr* 1980;97:383.
31. Lebenthal E, Lee PC. Glycoamylase and disaccharidase activities in normal subjects and in patients with mucosal injury of the small intestine. *J Pediatr* 1980;97:389.
32. Salmenpera L, Perheentupa J, Siimes MA. Exclusively breast-fed healthy infants grow slower than reference infants. *Pediatr Res* 1985;19:307.
33. Duncan B, Schifman RB, Corrigan JJ Jr, Schaefer C. Iron and the exclusively breast-fed infant from birth to six months. *J Pediatr Gastroenterol Nutr* 1985;4:421.
34. Wright AL, Holberg CJ, Taussig LM, et al. Relationship of infant feeding to recurrent wheezing at age 6 years. *Arch Pediatr Adolesc Med* 1995;149:758.
35. Widdowson EM, Spray CM. Chemical development in utero. *Arch Dis Child* 1951;26:205.
36. Babson SG, Benda GI. Growth graphs for the clinical assessment of infants of varying gestational age. *J Pediatr* 1976;89:814.
37. Lubchenco L, Hansman C, Boyd E. Intrauterine growth in length and head circumference as estimated from live births at gestational ages from 26 to 42 weeks of gestation. *Pediatrics* 1966;37:403.
38. Butte NF. Energy requirements during infancy. In: Tsang RC, Nichols B, eds. *Nutrition during infancy.* Philadelphia: Hanley & Belfus, Inc., 1988:86.
39. Hamosh M. Lipid metabolism in premature infants. *Biol Neonat* 1987;50[Suppl 1]:50.
40. Ross Pediatrics. *Composition of feedings for infants and young children. Ross ready reference.* Ross Products Division, Abbott Laboratories, Columbus Ohio, 1996.
41. Motil KJ. Protein needs for term and preterm infants. In: Tsang RC, Nichols B, eds. *Nutrition during infancy.* Philadelphia: Hanley & Belfus, Inc., 1988:100.
42. Stocker FP, Wilkoff W, Mietinen OS, et al. Oxygen consumption in infants with heart disease. *J Pediatr* 1972;80:43.
43. Weinstein MR, Oh W. Oxygen consumption in infants with bronchopulmonary dysplasia. *J Pediatr* 1981;99:958.
44. Wahlig TM, Gatto CW, Boros SJ. Metabolic response of preterm infants to variable degrees of respiratory illness. *J Pediatr* 1994;124:283.
45. Mrozek JD, Georgieff MK, Blazar BR, Mammel MC, Schwarzenberg SJ. Neonatal sepsis: effect on protein and energy metabolism. *Pediatr Res* 1997;41:237A.
46. Butte NF, Garza C, Smith EO, Nichols BL. Human milk intake and growth performance of exclusively breast-fed infants. *J Pediatr* 1983;104:187.
47. Whyte RK, Campbell D, Stanhope R, Bayley HS, Sinclair JC. Energy balance in low birth weight infants fed formula of high or low medium chain triglyceride content. *J Pediatr* 1986;108:964.
48. Sauer PJJ, Dane HF Visser HKA. Longitudinal studies on metabolic rate, heat loss, and energy cost of growth in low birth weight infants. *Pediatr Res* 1984;18:254.

49. Hay WW Jr. Fetal and neonatal glucose homeostasis and their relation to small for gestation age infants. *Semin Perinatol* 1984;8:101.

50. Kliegman RM, Morton S. Sequential intrahepatic metabolic effects of enteric galactose alimentation in newborn rats. *Pediatr Res* 1988;24:302.

51. DiGiacomo JE. Carbohydrates: metabolism and disorders. In: Hay WW Jr, ed. *Neonatal nutrition and metabolism.* St. Louis: Mosby, 1991:93.

52. Lilien LD, Pildes RS, Srinivasan G, Voora S, Yeh TF. Treatment of neonatal hypoglycemia with mini-bolus and intravenous glucose infusions. *J Pediatr* 1980;97:295.

53. Collins JW Jr, Hoppe M, Brow K, Edidin DV, Padbury J, Ogata ES. A controlled trial of insulin infusion and parenteral nutrition in extremely low birth weight infants with glucose intolerance. *J Pediatr* 1991;118:921.

54. Binder ND, Rasschko PK, Benda GI, Reynolds JW. Insulin infusion with parenteral nutrition in extremely low birth weight infants with hyperglycemia. *J Pediatr* 1989;114:273.

55. Burr GO, Burr MM. A new deficiency disease produced by rigid exclusion of fat from the diet. *J Biol Chem* 1929;82:345.

56. American Academy of Pediatrics, Committee on Nutrition. Nutritional needs of low birth weight infants. *Pediatrics* 1985;75:976.

57. Lucas A. Long-chain polyunsaturated fatty acids, infant feeding and cognitive development. In: Dobbing J, ed. *Developing brain and behaviour:* the role of lipids in infant formula. San Diego: Academic Press, 1997:3.

58. Innis SM. Essential fatty acids in growth and development. *Prog Lipid Res* 1991;30:39.

59. Innis SM. Polyunsaturated fatty acid nutrition in infants born at term. In: Dobbing J, ed. *Developing brain and behaviour:* the role of lipids in infant formula. San Diego: Academic Press, 1997:103.

60. Carson SE, Werkman SH, Tolley EA. Effect of long-chain n-3 fatty acid supplementation on visual acuity and growth of preterm infants with and without bronchopulmonary dysplasia. *Am J Clin Nutr* 1996;63:687.

61. Carlson SE, Werkman SH, Peeples JM, Cooke RJ, Tolley EA. Arachidonic acid status correlates with first year growth in preterm infants. *Proc Natl Acad Sci U S A* 1993;90:1073.

62. European Society of Paediatric Gastroenterology and Nutrition (ESP-GAN). Nutrition and feedings of preterm infants. *Acta Paediatr* Scand 1987;336[Suppl]:3.

63. Uauy RD, Birch DG, Birch EE, Tyson JE, Hoffman DR. Effect of dietary omega-3 fatty acids on retinal function of very-low-birth-weight neonates. *Pediatr Res* 1990;28:485.

64. Birch EE, Birch DG, Hoffman DR, Uauy R. Dietary essential fatty acid supply and visual acuity development. *Invest Ophtalmol Vis Sci* 1992;33:3242.

65. MacLean WC Jr, Benson JD. Theory into practice: the incorporation of new knowledge into infant formula. *Sem Perinatol* 1989;13:104.

66. Penn D, Schmidt-Sommerfeld E, Wolf H. Carnitine deficiency in premature infants receiving total parenteral nutrition. *Early Hum Dev* 1980;4:23.

67. Helms RA, Whitington PF, Mauer EC, Caterau EM, Christensen ML, Borum PR. Enhanced lipid utilization in infants receiving oral L-carnitine during long-term parenteral nutrition. *J Pediatr* 1986;109:984.

68. Lorenz JM, Kleinman LI. Otogeny of the kidney. In: Tsang RC, Nichols B, eds. *Nutrition during infancy.* Philadelphia: Hanley & Belfus, Inc., 1988:58.

69. Ziegler TR, Gatzen C, Wilmore DW. Strategies for attenuating protein-catabolic responses in the critically ill. *Annu Rev Med* 1994;45:459.

70. Keshen TH, Jaksic T, Jahoor F. Measurement of the protein metabolic response to surgical stress in extremely low birthweight neonates. *Pediatr Res* 1997;41:234A.

71. Carver JD, Pimentel B, Cox WI, Barness LA. Dietary nucleotide effects upon immune function in infants. *Pediatrics* 1991;88:359.

72. Goldman AS, Garza C, Nichold B, et al. Effect of prematurity on the immunologic system in human milk. *J Pediatr* 1982;101:901.

73. Uauy R, Stringel G, Thomas R, Quan R. Effect of dietary nucleosides on growth and maturation of the developing gut in the rat. *J Pediatr Gastroenterol Nutr* 1990;10:497.

74. Graham GG, Placko RP, Morales E, et al. Dietary protein quality in infants and children. *Am J Dis Child* 1970;120:419.

75. Davidson M, Levine SZ, Bauer CH, Dann M. Feeding studies in low-birth-weight infants. I. Relationships of dietary protein, fat, and electrolytes to rates of weight gain, clinical courses, and serum chemical concentrations. *J Pediatr* 1967;70:695.

76. Kagan BM, Stanincova V, Felix NS, et al. Body composition of premature infants: relation to nutrition. *Am J Clin Nutr* 1972;25:1153.

77. Kashyap S, Schulze KF, Forsyth MS, et al. Growth, nutrient retention, and metabolic response in low birth weight infants fed varying intakes of protein and energy. *J Pediatr* 1988;113:713.

78. Schulze KF, Stefanski M, Masterson J, et al. Energy expenditure, energy balance and composition of weight gain in low birth weight infants fed diets of different protein and energy content. *J Pediatr* 1987;110:753.

79. Heird WC, Kashyap S, Gomez MR. Protein intake and energy requirements of the Infant. *Semin Perinatol* 1991;15:438.

80. Anderson TL, Muttart C, Bieber MA, Nicholson JF, Heird WC. A controlled trial of glucose vs. glucose and amino acids in premature infants. *J Pediatr* 1979;94:947.

81. van Goudoever JB, Wattimena JDL, Carnielli VP, et al. Effect of dexamethasone on protein metabolism in infants with bronchopulmonary dysplasia. *J Pediatr* 1994;124:112.

82. Wu PYK, Edwards NB, Storm MC. Characteristics of the plasma amino acid pattern of normal term breast-fed infants. *J Pediatr* 1986;109:347.

83. Clark SC, Karn CA, Ahlrichs JA, et al. Acute changes in leucine and phenylalanine kinetics produced by parenteral nutrition in premature infants. *Pediatr Res* 1997;41:568.

84. Gross SJ, David RJ, Bauman L, Tomarelli RM. Nutritional composition of milk produced by mothers delivering preterm. *J Pediatr* 1980;96:641.

85. Schanler RJ, Oh W. Composition of breast milk obtained from mothers of premature infants as compared with breast milk obtained from donors. *J Pediatr* 1980;96:679.

86. Feeley RM, Eitenmiller RR, Jones JB, Barnhart H. Calcium, phosphorus and magnesium contents of human milk during early lactation. *J Pediatr Gastroenterol Nutr* 1983;2:262.

87. American Academy of Pediatrics. Nutritional needs of preterm infants. In: Barness LA, ed. *Pediatric nutrition handbook,* 3rd ed. Elk Grove Village, IL: American Academy of Pediatrics, 1993:69.

88. Tsang RC, ed. *Vitamin and mineral requirements in preterm infants.* New York: Marcel Dekker Inc., 1985.

89. Holliday MA. Requirements for sodium chloride and potassium and their interrelation with water requirement. In: Tsang RC, Nichols B, eds. *Nutrition during infancy.* Philadelphia: Hanley & Belfus, Inc., 1988:160.

90. Greer FR, Tsang RC. Calcium, phosphorus, magnesium and vitamin D requirements for the preterm infant. In: Tsange RC, ed. *Vitamin and mineral requirements in preterm infants.* New York: Marcel Dekker Inc., 1985:99.

91. Schanler RJ, Garza C. Improved mineral balance in very low birth weight infants fed fortified human milk. *J Pediatr* 1987;112:452.

92. Oski FA. The hematologic aspects of the maternal-fetal relationship. In: Oski FA, Naiman JL, eds. *Hematologic problems in the newborn,* 3rd ed. Philadelphia: WB Saunders, 1982:32.

93. Chockalingam UM, Murphy E, Ophoven JC, Weisdorf SA, Georgieff MK. Cord transferrin and ferritin levels in newborn infants at risk for prenatal uteroplacental insufficiency and chronic hypoxia. *J Pediatr* 1987;111:283.

94. Georgieff MK, Landon MB, Mills MM, et al. Abnormal iron distribution in infants of diabetic mothers: spectrum and maternal antecedents. *J Pediatr* 1990;117:455.

95. American Academy of Pediatrics, Committee on Nutrition. Iron supplementation. *Pediatrics* 1976;58:765.

96. Committee on Nutrition, American Academy of Pediatrics. Iron-fortified infant formulas. *Pediatrics* 1989;84:1114.

97. Siimes MA, Vuori E, Kuitunen P. Breast milk iron: a declining concentration during the course of lactation. *Acta Paediatr Scand* 1979;68:29.

98. Lonnerdal B. Iron in human milk and cow's milk-effects of binding ligands on bioavailability. In: Lonnerdal B, ed. *Iron metabolism in infants.* Boca Raton: CRC Press, 1990:87.

99. Piscane A, De Vizia B, Valiante A, et al. Iron status in breast-fed infants. *J Pediatr* 1995;127:429.

100. Pizarro F, Yip R, Dallman PR, et al. Iron status with different infant feeding regimens: relevance to screening and prevention of iron deficiency. *J Pediatr* 1991;118:687.

101. Innis SM, Nelson CM, Wadsworth LD, MacLaren IA, Lwanga D. Incidence of iron-deficiency anaemia and depleted iron stores among nine-month-old infants in Vancouver, Canada. *Can J Pub Health* 1997;88:80.

102. Oski FA. Iron-fortified formulas and gastrointestinal symptoms in infants: a controlled study. *Pediatrics* 1980;66:168.

103. Nelson SE, Ziegler EE, Copeland AM, et al. Lack of adverse reactions to iron-fortified formula. *Pediatrics* 1988;81:360.

104. Widness JA, Seward VJ, Kromer IJ, Burmeister LF, Strauss RG. Changing patterns of red blood cell transfusion in very low birth weight infants. *J Pediatr* 1996;129:680.

105. Shannon K, Keith J, Mentzer W, et al. Recombinant human erythropoietin stimulates erythropoiesis and reduces erythrocyte transfusions in very low birth weight preterm infants. *Pediatrics* 1995;95:1.

106. Ehrenkranz RA. Recombinant human erythropoietin (rHuEPO) stimulates incorporation of absorbed iron into RBCs in VLBW infants. *Pediatr Res* 1994;35:311A.

107. Abrams SA, Schanler RJ, Garza C. Bone mineralization in former very low birth weight infants fed either human milk or commercial formula. *J Pediatr* 1988;112:956.

108. Jansson LT. Iron, oxygen stress and the preterm infant. In: Lonnerdal B, ed. *Iron metabolism in infants.* Boca Raton: CRC Press, 1990:73.

109. Peters C, Georgieff ML, DeAlarcon P, et al. The effect of chronic erythropoietin administration on iron in newborn lambs. *Biol Neonate* 1996;70:218.

110. Zlotkin SH, Atkinson S, Lockitch G. Trace elements in nutrition for premature infants. *Clin Perinatol* 1995;22:223.

111. Reifen RM, Zlotkin SH. Microminerals. In: Tsang RC, Lucas A, Uauy R, et al, eds. *Nutritional needs of the preterm infant.* Baltimore: Williams & Wilkins, 1993:195.

112. Bayliss PA, Buchanan BE, Hancock RGV, et al. Tissue selenium accretion in paremature and full-term human infants and children. *Biol Trace Element Res* 1985;7:755.

113. Sinkin RA, Phelps DL. New strategies for the prevention of bronchopulmonary dysplasia. *Clin Perinatol* 1987;14:599.

114. Lipsky CL, Spear ML. Recent advances in parenteral nutrition. *Clin Perinatol* 1995;22:141.

115. Greene H, Hambridge K, Schanler R, et al. Guidelines for the use of vitamins, trace elements, calcium, magnesium, and phosphorus in infants and children receiving total parenteral nutrition: report of the Subcommittee on Pediatric Parenteral Nutrient Requirements from the Committee on Clinical Practice Issues of the American Society for Clinical Nutrition. *Am J Clin Nutr* 1988;48:1324.

116. American Academy of Pediatrics. Nutritional needs of preterm infants. In: Barness LA, ed. *Pediatric nutrition handbook,* 3rd ed. Elk Grove Village, IL: American Academy of Pediatrics, 1993:36.

117. Pereira GR. Nutritional care of the extremely premature infant. *Clin Perinatol* 1995;22:61.

118. Feldman KW, Marcuse EK, Springer DA. Nutritional rickets. *Am Fam Physician* 1990;42:1311.

119. Riedel BD, Greene HL. Vitamins. In: Hay WW Jr, ed. *Neonatal nutrition and metabolism.* St. Louis: Mosby, 1991:143.

120. Hillman L, Hoff N, Salmons SJ, Martin L, McAlister W, Haddad J. Mineral homeostasis in very premature infants: serial evaluation of serum 25 hydroxy vitamin D, serum minerals and bone mineralization. *J Pediatr* 1985;106:970.

121. Wolbach SB, Howe PR. Tissue changes following deprivation of fat-soluble vitamin A. *J Exp Med* 1925;42:753.

122. Shenai JP, Stahlman MT, Chytil F. Vitamin A delivery from parenteral alimentation solutions. *J Pediatr* 1981;99:661.

123. Shenai JP, Chytil F, Stahlman MT. Vitamin A status of neonates with bronchopulmonary dysplasia. *Pediatr Res* 1985;19:185.

124. Georgieff MK, Chockalingam UM, Sasanow SR, Gunter EW, Murphy E, Ophoven JJ. The effect of antenatal betamethasone on cord blood concentrations of retinol-binding protein, transthyretin, transferrin, retinol and vitamin E. *J Pediatr Gastroenterol Nutr* 1988;7:713.

125. Georgieff MK, Mammel MC, Mills MM, Gunter EW, Johnson DE, Thompson TR. Effect of postnatal steroid administration on serum vitamin A concentrations in newborn infants with respiratory compromise. *J Pediatr* 1989;114:301.

126. Shenai JP, Kennedy KA, Chytil F, Stahlman MT. Clinical trial of vitamin A supplementation in infants susceptible to broNchopulmonary dysplasia. *J Pediatr* 1987;111:269.

127. Pearson E, Bose C, Snidow T, et al. Trial of vitamin A supplementation in very low birth weight infants at risk for bronchopulmonary dysplasia. *J Pediatr* 1992;121:420.

128. Oski FA, Barnes LA. Vitamin E deficiency: a previously unrecognized cause of hemolytic anemia in the premature. *J Pediatr* 1967;70:211.

129. Johnson L, Schaffer D, Boggs TR. The premature infant, vitamin E deficiency and retrolental fibroplasia. *Am J Clin Nutr* 1974;27:1158.

130. Hittner HM, Godio LB, Rudolph AJ, et al. Retrolental fibroplasia: efficacy of vitamin E in a double-blind clinical study of preterm infants. *N Engl J Med* 1981;305:1365.

131. Hittner HM, Godio LB, Speer ME, et al. Retrolental fibroplasia: further clinical evidence and ultrastructural support for efficacy of vitamin E in the preterm infant. *Pediatrics* 1983;71:423.

132. Phelps DL, Rosenbaum AL, Isenberg SJ, et al. Tocopherol efficacy and safety for preventing retinopathy of prematurity: a randomized, controlled, double-masked trial. *Pediatrics* 1987;79:489.

133. Phelps DL. Retinopathy of prematurity. *Curr Prob Pediatr* 1992;22: 349.

134. Johnson L, Bowen FW, Abbasi S, et al. Relationship of prolonged pharmacologic serum levels of vitamin E to incidence of sepsis and necrotizing enterocolitis in infants with birth weights of 1500 grams or less. *Pediatrics* 1985;75:619.

135. Steinhorn DM, Green TP. Severity of illness correlates with alterations in energy metabolism in the pediatric intensive care unit. *Crit Care Med* 1991;19:1503.

136. Cerra FB, Siegel JH, Coleman B, Border JR, McMenamy RR. Septic autocannibalism: a failure of exogenous nutritional support. *Ann Surg* 1980;192:570.

137. Fleck A. Acute phase response: implications for nutrition and recovery. *Nutrition* 1988;4:109.

138. Maldonato J, Gil A, Faus MJ, et al. Differences in the serum amino acid pattern of injured and infected children promoted by two parenteral nutrition solutions. *J Parenter Enteral Nutr* 1989;13:41.

139. deRegnier R-AO, Guilbert TW, Mills MM, Georgieff MK. Growth failure and altered body composition are established by one month of age in infants with bronchopulmonary dysplasia. *J Nutr* 1996;126:168.

140. Frank L, Sosenko IRS. Undernutrition as a major contributing factor in the pathogenesis of bronchopulmonary dysplasia. *Am Rev Respir Dis* 1988;138:725.

141. Georgieff MK, Mills MM, Lindeke L, Iverson S, Johnson DE, Thompson TR. Changes in nutritional management and outcome of very-low-birth-weight infants. *Am J Dis Child* 1989;143:82.

142. Berseth CL. Minimal enteral feedings. *Clin Perinatol* 1995;22:95.

143. Roberts JR. Cutaneous and subcutaneous complications of calcium infusions. *Journal of American College of Emergency Physicians JACEP* 1977;6:16.

144. Hruszkewycz V, Holtrop PC, Batton DG, Morden RS, Gibson P, Band JD. Complications associated with central venous catheters inserted in critically ill neonates. *Infect Control Hosp Epidemiol* 1991;12:544.

145. Polin RA, St. Geme JW 3rd. Neonatal sepsis. *Adv Pediatr Infect Dis* 1992;7:25.

146. Rowen JL, Atkins JT, Levy ML, Baer SC, Baker CJ. Invasive fungal dermatitis in the less than or equal to 1000 gram neonate. *Pediatrics* 1995;95:682.

147. Duffy LF, Kerzner B, Gebus V, Dice J. Treatment of central venous catheter occlusions with hydrochloric acid. *J Pediatr* 1989;114:1002.

148. Kashyap S. Nutritional management of the extremely-low-birth-weight infant. In: Cowett RM, Hay W, eds. *The micropremie:* the next frontier. Report of the 99th Ross Conference on Pediatric Research, 1990:115.

149. Helms RA, Christensen ML, Mauer EC, et al. Comparison of a pediatric versus standard amino acid formulation in preterm neonates requiring parenteral nutrition. *J Pediatr* 1987;110:466.

150. Zlotkin SH, Bryan MH, Anderson GH. Intravenous nitrogen and energy intakes required to duplicate in utero nitrogen accretion in prematurely born human infants. *J Pediatr* 1981;99:115.

151. Helms, RA, Johnson MR, Christenson ML, et al. Evaluation of two pediatric amino acid formulations. *J Parenter Enteral Nutr* 1988; 12:4(abst).

152. Heird WC, Dell RB, Helms RA, et al. Amino acid mixture designed to maintain normal plasma amino acid patterns in infants and children requiring parenteral nutrition. *Pediatrics* 1987;80:401.

153. Hayes KC, Carey RE, Schmidt SY. Retinal degeneration associated with taurine deficiency in the cat. *Science* 1975;188:950.

154. Guertin F, Roy CC, Lepage G, et al. Effect of taurine on parenteral nutrition-associated cholestasis. *J Parenter Enteral Nutr* 1991;15:247.

155. Tyson JE, Lasky R, Flood D, et al. Randomized trial of taurine supplementation for infants <1,300 gram birth weight: effect on auditory brainstem-evoked responses. *Pediatrics* 1989;83:406.

156. White HB, Turner AC, Miller RC. Blood lipid alterations in infants receiving intravenous fat-free alimentation. *J Pediatr* 1973;83:305.

157. Costarino AT, Baumgart S. Modern fluid and electrolyte management of the critically ill premature infant. *Pediatr Clin North Am* 1986;33:153.

158. Dunham B, Marcuard S, Khazanie PG, et al. The solubility of calcium and phosphorus in neonatal parenteral nutrition solutions. *J Parenter Enteral Nutr* 1991;15:608.

159. Pelegano JF, Rowe JC, Carey DE, et al. Effect of calcium/phosphorus ratio in mineral retention in parenterally fed premature infants. *J Pediatr Gastroenterol Nutr* 1991;12:351.

160. Hoehn GJ, Carey DE, Raye JR, et al. Alternate-day infusion of calcium and phosphate in very low birth weight infants: wasting of the infused mineral. *J Pediatr Gastroenterol Nutr* 1987;6:752.

161. Kimura S, Nose O, Seino Y, et al. Effects of alternate and simultaneous administration of calcium and phosphorus on calcium metabolism in children receiving total parenteral nutrition. *J Parenter Enteral Nutr* 1986;10:513.

162. Fitzgerald KA, MacKay MW. Calcium and phosphate solubility in neonatal parenteral nutrient solutions containing Trophamine. *Am J Hosp Pharm* 1986;43:88.

163. Schmidt GL, Baumgartner TG, Fischlschweiger W, et al. Cost containment using cysteine HCl acidification to increase calcium/phosphate solubility in hyperalimentation solutions. *J Parenter Enteral Nutr* 1986;10:203.

164. Thorp JW, Boeckx RL, Robbins S, et al. A prospective study of infant zinc nutrition during intensive care. *Am J Clin Nutr* 1981;34:1056.

165. Heller RM, Kirchner SG, O'Neill JA, et al. Skeletal changes of copper deficiency in infants receiving prolonged total parenteral nutrition. *J Pediatr* 1978;92:947.

166. Lane HW, Barroso AO, Englert D, et al. Selenium status of seven chronic intravenous hyperalimentation patients. *J Parenter Enteral Nutr* 1982;6:426.

167. American Medical Association Department of Foods and Nutrition, 1975. Multivitamin preparations for parenteral use. A statement by the Nutrition Advisory Group. *J Parenter Enteral Nutr* 1979;3:258.

168. Stahl GE, Spear ML, Hamosh M. Intravenous administration of lipid emulsions to premature infants. *Clin Perinatol* 1986;13:133.

169. Hageman JR, McCullough K, Gora P, Olsen K, Pachman L, Hunt CE. Intralipid alterations in pulmonary prostaglandin metabolism and gas exchange. *Crit Care Med* 1983;11:794.

170. McKeen CR, Brigham KL, Bowers RE, Harris TR. Pulmonary vascular effects of fat emulsion infusion in unanesthetized sheep Prevention by indomethacin. *J Clin Invest* 1978;61:1291.

171. Hammerman C, Aramburo MJ. Decreased lipid intake reduces morbidity in sick premature neonates. *J Pediatr* 1988;113:1083.

172. Gilbertson N, Kovar IZ, Cox, DJ, et al. Introduction of intravenous lipid administration on the first day of life in the very low birth weight neonate. *J Pediatr* 1991;119:615.

173. Eggert LD, Rusho WJ, MacKay MW, et al. Calcium and phosphorus compatibility in parenteral nutrition solutions for neonates. *Am J Hosp Pharm* 1982;39:49.

174. Adamkin DH, Radmacher PG, Klingbeil RL. Use of intravenous lipid and hyperbilirubinemia in the first week. *J Pediatr Gastroenterol Nutr* 1992;14:135.

175. Aschner JL, Punsalang A, Maniscalco WM, Menegus MA. Percutaneous central venous catheter colonization with Malassezia furfur: incidence and clinical significance. *Pediatrics* 1987;80:535.

176. Merritt RJ. Cholestasis associated with total parenteral nutrition. *J Pediatr Gastroenterol Nutr* 1980;5:9.

177. Koo WWK, Kaplan LA, Horn J, et al. Aluminum in parenteral solutions f sources and possible alternatives. *J Parenter Enteral Nutr* 1986;10:591.

178. Koo WWK, Kaplan LA, Bendon R, et al. Response to aluminum in parenteral nutrition during infancy. *J Pediatr* 1986;109:883.

179. Alfrey AC. Aluminum. *Adv Clin Chem* 1983;23:69.

180. Sedman AB, Klein GL, Merritt RJ, et al. Evidence of aluminum loading in infants receiving intravenous therapy. *N Engl J Med* 1985;312:1337.

181. ASCN/A.S.P.E.N. Working Group on Standards for Aluminum Content of Parenteral Nutrition Solutions. Parenteral drug products containing aluminium as an ingredient or a contaminant: response to food and drug administration notice of intent and request for information. *J Parenter Enteral Nutr* 1991;15:194.

182. Sann L, Durand M, Picard J, Lasne Y, Bethenod M. Arm fat and muscle areas in infancy. *Arch Dis Child* 1988;63:256.

183. Georgieff MK, Sasanow SR, Pereira GR. Serum transthyretin levels and protein intake as predictors of weight gain velocity in premature infants. *J Pediatr Gastroenterol Nutr* 1987;6:775.

184. Georgieff MK, Sasanow SR, Mammel MC, Ophoven J, Pereira GR. Cord prealbumin values in newborn infants: effect of prenatal steroids, pulmonary maturity and size for dates. *J Pediatr* 1986;108:972.

185. Vallee BL, Galdes A. The metallobiochemistry of zinc enzymes. *Adv Enzymol* 1984;56:283.

186. Meier P. Bottle and breastfeeding effects on transcutaneous oxygen pressure and temperature in preterm infants. *Nurs Res* 1988;37:36.

187. Bernbaum JC, Pereira GR, Watkins JB, Peckham GJ. Nonnutritive sucking during gavage feeding enhances growth and maturation in premature infants. *Pediatrics* 1983;71:41.

188. Field T, Ignatoff E, Stringer S, et al. Nonnutritive sucking during tube feedings: effects on preterm neonates in an intensive care unit. *Pediatrics* 1982;70:381.

189. Widstrom AM, Marchini G, Matthieson AS, et al. Nonnutritive sucking in tube-fed preterm infants: effects on gastric motility and gastric contents of Somatostatin. *J Pediatr Gastroenterol Nutr* 1988;7:517.

190. Toce SS, Keenan WJ. Enteral feeding in very-low-birth-weight infants. *Am J Dis Child* 1987;141:436.

191. Roy RN, Pillnitz RP, Hamilton JR, Chance GW. Impaired assimilation of nasojejunal feeds in healthy low-birth-weight newborn infants. *J Pediatr* 1977;90:431.

192. Wells DH, Zachman RD. Nasojejunal feeds in low-birth-weight infants. *J Pediatr* 1975;87:276.

193. Challacombe D. Bacterial microflora in infants receiving nasojejunal tube feeding. *J Pediatr* 1974;85:113.

194. Lucas A, Bloom SR, Aynsley-Green A. Gut hormones and "minimal enteral feeding." *Acta Paediatr Scand* 1986;75:719.

195. Slagle TA, Gross SJ. Effect of early low-volume enteral substrate on subsequent feeding tolerance in the very low birth weight infants. *J Pediatr* 1988;113:526.

196. Dunn L, Hulman S, Weiner J, Kliegman R. Beneficial effects of early hypocaloric enteral feeding on neonatal gastrointestinal function: preliminary report of a randomized trial. *J Pediatr* 1988;112:622.

197. Meetze W, Valentine C, Sacks J, et al. Effects of gastrointestinal (GI) priming prior to full enteral nutrition in very low birth weight (VLBW) infants. *Pediatr Res* 1990;27:287A(abst).

198. Neu J, Valentine C, Mietze W. Scientifically-based strategies for nutrition of the high-risk low birth weight infant. *Eur J Pediatr* 1990;150:2.

199. Hughes CA, Dowling RH. Speed of onset of adaptive mucosal hypoplasia and hypofunction in the intestine of parenterally fed rats. *Clin Sci* 1980;59:317.

200. Freed GL, Clark SJ, Sorenson J, et al. National assessment of physicians' breast-feeding knowledge, attitudes, training, and experience. *JAMA* 1995;273:472.

201. World Health Organization. *Protecting, promoting and supporting breast-feeding: the special role of maternity services.* Geneva, Switzerland: World Health Organization, 1989:13.

202. Spisak S, Gross SS. Second followup report: The Surgeon General's Workshop on Breastfeeding and Human Lactation. Washington, DC: National Center for Education in Maternal and Child Health, 1991.

203. Braveman P, Egerter S, Pearl M, et al. Problems associated with early discharge of newborn infants. *Pediatrics* 1995;96:716.

204. Williams LR, Cooper MK. Nurse-managed postpartum home care. *J Obstet Gynecol Neonatal Nurs* 1993;22:25.

205. Gielen AC, Faden RR, O'Campo P, et al. Maternal employment during the early postpartum period: effects on initiation and continuation of breast-feeding. *Pediatrics* 1991;87:298.

206. Frederick IB, Auerback KG. Maternal-infant separation and breast-feeding: the return to work or school. *J Reprod Med* 1985;30:523.

207. Wilson MH. Feeding the healthy child. In: Oski FA, DeAngelis CD, Feigin RD, et al, eds. *Principles and practice of pediatrics*. Philadelphia: JB Lippincott, 1990:553.

208. Rohr FJ, Levy HL, Shih VE. Inborn errors of metabolism. In: Walker WA, Watkins JB, eds. *Nutrition in pediatrics*. Boston: Little, Brown and Company, 1983:412.

209. American Academy of Pediatrics, Committee on Drugs. The transfer of drugs and other chemicals into human milk. *Pediatrics* 1994;93:137.

210. American Academy of Pediatrics, Committee on Pediatric AIDS. Human milk, breastfeeding, and transmission of human immunodeficiency virus in the United States. *Pediatrics* 1995;96:977.

211. Centers for Disease Control and Prevention. Recommendation for assisting in the prevention of perinatal transmission of human T-lymphotropic virus type III/lymphadenopathy-associated virus and acquired immunodeficiency syndrome. *MMWR* 1985;34:721.

212. Briggs GG, Freeman RK, Yaffe SJ. *Drugs in pregnancy and lactation.* Baltimore: Williams & Wilkins, 1990.

213. Uauy-Dagach R, Mena P. Nutritional role of Omega-3 fatty acids during the perinatal period. *Clin Perinatol* 1995;22:157.

214. Kovar MG, Serdula MK, Marks JS, et al. Review of the epidemiologic evidence for an association between infant feeding and infant health. *Pediatrics* 1984;74:S615.

215. Frank AL, Taber LH, Glezen WP, et al. Breast-feeding and respiratory virus infection. *Pediatrics* 1982;70:239.

216. Saarinen UM. Prolonged breast feeding as prophylaxis for recurrent otitis media. *Acta Paediatr Scand* 1982;71:567.

217. Lucas A, Cole TJ. Breast milk and neonatal necrotising enterocolitis. *Lancet* 1990;336:1519.

218. Mayer EJ, Hamman RF, Gay EC, et al. Reduced risk of IDDM among breast-fed children. *Diabetes* 1988;37:1625.

219. Koletzko S, Sherman P, Corey M, et al. Role of infant feeding practices in development of Crohn's disease in childhood. *Br Med J* 1989;298:1617.

220. Davis MK, Savitz DA, Graubard BI. Infant feeding and childhood cancer. *Lancet* 1988;2:365.

221. Rosenblatt KA, Thomas DB. WHO collaborative study of neoplasia and steroid contraceptives. *Int J Epidemiol* 1993;22:192.

222. Newcomb PA, Storer BE, Longnecker MP, et al. Lactation and a reduced risk of premenopausal breast cancer. *N Engl J Med* 1994;330:81.

223. Saarinen UM, Kajosaari M. Breastfeeding as prophylaxis against atopic disease: prospective follow-up study until 17 years old. *Lancet* 1995;346:1065.

224. Lucas A, Brooke OG, Morley R, et al. Early diet of preterm infants and development of allergic or atopic disease: randomised prospective study. *Br Med J* 1990;300:837.

225. American Academy of Pediatrics. Formula feeding of term infants. In: Barness LA, ed. *Pediatric nutrition handbook,* 3rd ed. Elk Grove Village, IL: American Academy of Pediatrics, 1993;11.

226. Fomon SJ, Ziegler EE, Thomas LN, et al. Excretion of fat by normal full-term infants fed various milks and formulas. *Am J Clin Nutr* 1970;23:1299.

227. Henderson TR, Hamosh M, Hayman L. Serum long chain polyunsaturated fatty acids (LC-PUFA) are adequate in full term breast fed infants in spite of low milk LC-PUFA after τ3 months lactation. *Pediatr Res* 1996;39:311A.

228. American Academy of Pediatrics, Committee on Nutrition. Soy protein formulas. Recommendations for use in infant feeding. *Pediatrics* 1983;72:359.

229. Saylor JD, Bahna SL. Anaphylaxis to casein hydrolysate formula. *J Pediatr* 1991;118:71.

230. Ellis MH, Short JA, Heiner DC. Anaphylaxis after ingestion of a recently introduced hydrolyzed whey protein formula. *J Pediatr* 1991;118:71.

231. Schanler RJ. Human milk for preterm infants: nutritional and immune factors. *Semin Perinatol* 1989;13:69.

232. Uauy R, Hoffman DR. Essential fatty acid requirements for normal eye and brain development. *Semin Perinatol* 1991;15:449.

233. Carlson SE, Werkman SH, Rhodes PG, et al. Visual-acuity development in healthy preterm infants: effect of marine-oil supplementation. *Am J Clin Nutr* 1993;58:35.

234. Kleinman RE, Walker WA. The enteromammary immune system. *Dig Dis Sci* 1979;24:876.

235. Hutchens TW, Henry JF, Yip T-T, et al. Origin of intact lactoferrin and its DNA-binding fragments found in the urine of human milk-fed preterm infants. Evaluation by stable isotope enrichment. *Pediatr Res* 1991;29:243.

236. Balmer SE, Wharton BA. Diet and faecal flora in the newborn: breast milk and infant flora. *Arch Dis Child* 1989;64:1672.

237. Atkinson SA, Bryan MH, Anderson GH. Human milk feeding in premature infants: protein, fat and carbohydrate balances in the first 2 weeks of life. *J Pediatr* 1981;99:617.

238. Roy RN, Chance GW, Radde IC, et al. Late hyponatremia in very low birth weight infants (<1.3 kilograms). *Pediatr Res* 1976;10:526.

239. Schanler RJ. Calcium and phosphorus absorption and retention in preterm infants. *Exp Med* 1991;2:24.

240. Schanler RJ, Oh W. Nitrogen and mineral balance in preterm infants fed human milk or formula. *J Pediatr Gastroenterol Nutr* 1985;4:214.

241. Ziegler EE, O'Donnell AM, Nelson SE, et al. Body composition of the reference fetus. *Growth* 1976;40:329.

242. Stocks RJ, Davies DP, Allen F, et al. Loss of breast milk nutrients during tube feeding. *Arch Dis Child* 1985;60:164.

243. Bromberger P. Premature infants' nutritional needs. Part 2. Breast milk banking. *Perinatol Neonatol* 1982;10:35.

244. Pujczynski M, Rademaker D, Gatson RL. Burn injury related to improper use of microwave ovens. *Pediatrics* 1983;72:714.

245. Henderson MJ, Dear PRF. Dicarboxylic aciduria and medium chain triglyceride supplemented milk. *Arch Dis Child* 1986;61:610.

246. Koo WW, Tsang RC. Mineral requirements of low-birth-weight infants. *J Am Coll Nutr* 1991;10:474.

247. Lake AM, Walker WA. Neonatal necrotizing enterocolitis: a disease of altered host defense. *Clin Gastroenterol* 1977;6:463.

248. Hillman LS, Hoff N, Martin LA, Haddad JG. Osteopenia, hypocalcemia, and low 25-hydroxyvitamin D (25-CHD) serum concentration with use of soy formula. *Pediatr Res* 1979;13:A448(abst).

249. Cooke RJ, Griffin I, Wells J, et al. Formula feeding preterm infants after hospital discharge: 2. Effects on body composition. *Pediatr Res* 1996;39:306A.

250. Miller HC, Hassanien K. Diagnosis of impaired fetal growth in newborn infants. *Pediatrics* 1971;48:511.

251. Georgieff MK, Sasanow SR, Chockalingam UM, Pereira GR. A comparison of the mid-arm circumference/head circumference ratio and ponderal index for the evaluation of newborn infants after abnormal intrauterine growth. *Acta Paediatr Scand* 1988;77:214.

252. Bjerkedal T, Bakketeig L, Lehmann DH. Percentiles of birthweights of single live births at different gestational periods based on 125,485 births in Norway, 1967 and 1968. *Acta Paediatr Scand* 1973;62:449.

253. Sterky G. Swedish standard curves for intrauterine growth. *Pediatrics* 1970;46:7.

254. Casey PH, Kraemer HC, Berbaum J, Yogman MW, Sells JC. Growth status and growth rates of a varied sample of low birth weight, preterm infants: a longitudinal cohort from birth to three years of age. *J Pediatr* 1991;119:599.

255. Georgieff MK, Mills MM, Zempel CE, Chang P-N. Catch-up growth, muscle and fat accretion, and body proportionality of infants one year after newborn intensive care. *J Pediatr* 1989;114:288.

256. Hack M, Weissman B, Borawski-Clark E. Catch-up growth during childhood among very low-birth-weight children. *Arch Pediatr Adolesc Med* 1996;150:1122.

257. Gurney JM, Jelliffee D. Arm anthropometry in nutritional assessment: normogram for rapid calculation of muscle cicumference and cross-sectional muscle and fat areas. *Am J Clin Nutr* 1973;26:912.

258. Georgieff MK, Amarnath UM, Murphy EL, Ophoven JJ. Serum transferrin levels in the longitudinal assessment of protein energy status in preterm infants. *J Pediatr Gastroenterol Nutr* 1989;8:234.

259. Shenai JP, Jhaveri BM, Reynolds JW, et al. Nutritional balance studies in very-low-birth-weight infants: role of soy formula. *Pediatrics* 1981;67:631.

260. Koo WW. Laboratory assessment of nutritional bone disease in infants. *Clin Biochem* 1996;29:429.

261. Inder TE, Clemett RS, Austin NC, Graham P, Darlow BA. High iron status in very low birth weight infants is associated with an increased risk of retinopathy of prematurity. *J Pediatr* 1997;131:541.

CHAPTER 24

Thermal Regulation

Stephen Baumgart, Susan C. Harrsch, and Suzanne M. Touch

AN HISTORICAL PERSPECTIVE

Tarnier was an obstetrician in Paris who first applied modern concepts of incubation to human infants starting around 1830 (1,2). Tarnier's incubator, the *couveuse*, has been widely recognized as the first one designed specifically to care for premature babies. Tarnier and his student, Budin, studied premature human incubation into the next century, reporting almost doubled survival in infants born at less than 2 kg. In the United States, commercialization of the designs of Tarnier and Budin occurred, and the Rotch Incubator appeared at the Colombian Exposition in Chicago in 1893 (3–5). Thereafter, in 1933, Blackfan and Yaglou (6) provided humidity along with air warming within incubators, which improved the stability of infant temperature control. In the 1940s, Chappel in Philadelphia added air isolation techniques to incubator care to prevent neonatal septic infections recognized to occur more frequently in humid environments (7,8). In 1958, Silverman et al. (9) challenged the need for humidity in incubators and used higher air temperatures than previously reported to care for an ever smaller premature population surviving with modern techniques.

Towards Defining the Optimal, Thermal Neutral Environment

The following year, 1959, Cross and Hill from the United Kingdom described a metabolically neutral temperature for achieving the optimal environmental care of newborn animals and humans, suggesting that poor temperature maintenance resulted in increased metabolic rates of oxygen and substrate consumption (Fig. 24–1) (10–12). Physiologic responses to environmental temper-

S. Baumgart, S. C. Harrsch, and S. M. Touch: Division of Neonatology, Department of Pediatrics, Thomas Jefferson University, Jefferson Medical College, Philadelphia, Pennsylvania

ature during incubation of premature newborn infants were investigated systematically in 1962 by Kurt Bruck and co-workers (13,14) from Germany. In 1969, Sir Edmond Hey and co-workers (15–17) from the United Kingdom defined the best operational incubator temperatures for preterm babies by describing an algorithm of air and wall temperatures, taking humidification and swaddling (insulation) into account as well. The Hey and Katz nomograms for regulating incubators following preterm birth, growth, and maturation remain the benchmark standard for modern human incubation to date (Fig. 24–2).

THERMAL BALANCE AT THE BEGINNING OF LIFE

Fetal Thermal Regulation

The fetus generates heat during metabolism with cellular proliferation and differentiation, the maintenance of intra- and extracellular ion gradients, and the transport of nutrients and wastes across cell membranes. Cardiac and skeletal muscle work also generate heat *in utero* (18). Fetal ovine and human studies suggest that the rate of fetal heat production is about 33 to 47 cal/kg/min (18,19). Fetal–maternal temperature gradients in mammals and humans have demonstrated that a difference in temperature of only 0.45° to 0.50°C between the umbilical arterial and venous blood is sufficient to eliminate the majority of metabolic heat via the placental circulation (i.e., by forced convective transfer into the mother's uterine circulation) (20–22). Probably less than 10% to 20% of heat is dissipated from the fetal skin into the amniotic fluid (natural convection and conduction from the uterine wall). The mother additionally serves as a heat reservoir for the fetus, favoring the dissipation of heat as a by-product of fetal metabolism. Fatal hyperthermia may occur with an elevation of maternal temperature, or if the mother is unable to dissipate the excess heat produced during preg-

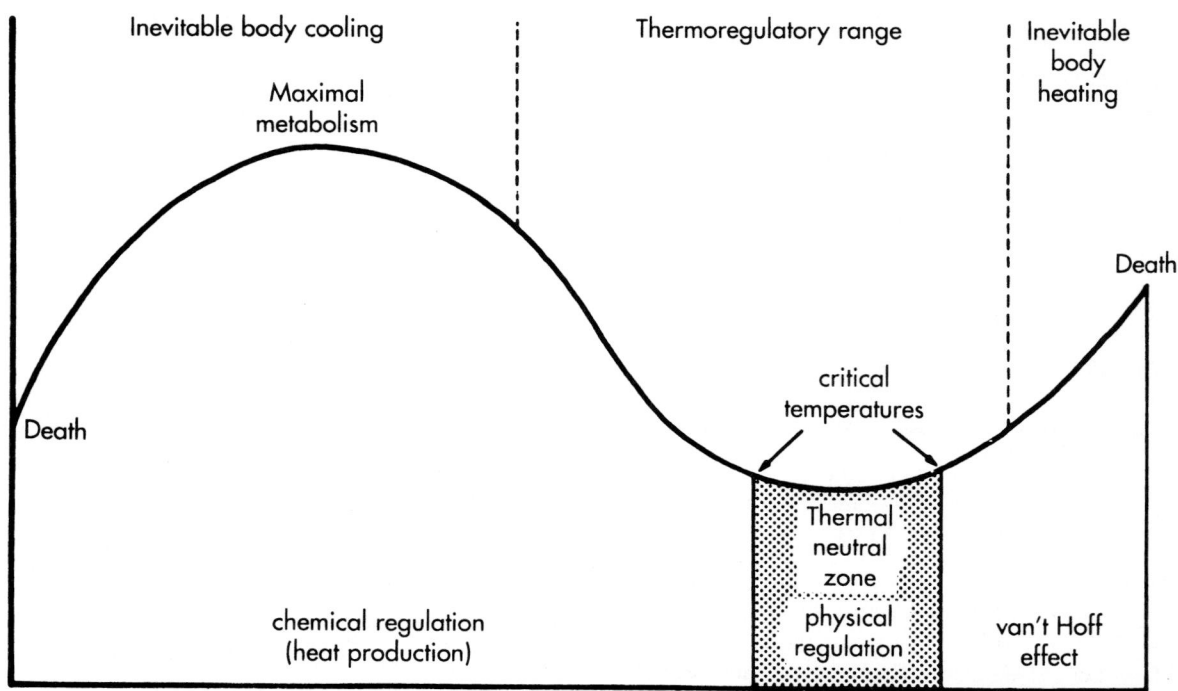

FIG. 24–1. Basic concepts for defining neonatal thermal neutral environmental temperature (horizontal axis) as the minimal observed metabolic rate (vertical axis, measured indirectly as oxygen consumption). The shaded region of this graph (the relatively narrow thermal neutral zone) is bounded by upper and lower critical temperatures for nonmetabolic or physical regulation of normal body temperature (e.g., by vasoconstriction, vasodilatation, or by changes in posture). Variation of environmental temperature outside this limited range results in a metabolic rate increase, where infant core temperature may remain normal, but at the expense of increased metabolic expenditure (e.g., cold stress). Outside the thermal regulatory range of metabolic heat production, inevitable body cooling or heating results, with eventual death at environmental extremes. (From ref. 28.)

nancy. Therefore, pregnant women are advised to avoid prolonged hot baths and exertion on hot and humid days. Maternal fever should be treated aggressively with environmental cooling and with antipyretics and antibiotics when indicated.

Transition in the Delivery Suite

At birth, a newly born infant is immediately exposed to a wet and cold environment. Without intervention, rapid cooling by convection from the neonate's skin into the cold delivery room air (at least a 10.0°C drop), and by evaporation at a tremendous rate (0.58 kcal/mL of water loss), may result in a drop of the infant's body temperature at a rate of 0.2 to 1.0°C/min. Although fetal response to cold stress is relatively insensitive prenatally (22,23), increased infant activity (crying with agitated movement characteristic of cold exposure upon birth), vasoconstriction, and nonshivering thermogenesis (shivering is not active in the human newborn) occurs the instant the baby hits the cold air, mediated by the sympathetic nervous system (24). Triggered by temperature sensation of the skin, infant metabolic rate may increase by two- to three-

fold and, thus, maintain body temperature for a period of several hours in the term subject before thermogenic reserves of glycogen and brown fat become depleted.

Physiology of Neonatal Thermal Response

Brown fat is especially thermogenic in the term newborn, with large reserves located between the scapula, in the axillae and perithymic region, and in the paraspinal and perinephric areas. Penetrated extensively by blood vessels, which give it the brown appearance and which conduct heat generated into the central circulation, these adipocytes are laden with excess triglyceride stores and numerous mitochondria. With cold stress, the sympathetic surge acts directly upon cell surface receptors, which stimulate cyclic-AMP–mediated lipoprotein lipase. Thyroid hormone also surges at birth and augments this effect (5,25,26). β-Oxidation is uncoupled in brown adipocytes, however, resulting in trigyceride breakdown and resynthesis producing heat (27).

Preterm infants with immature thermogenic response and without metabolic substrate reserves deposited over the last trimester of pregnancy fare worse. As shown in

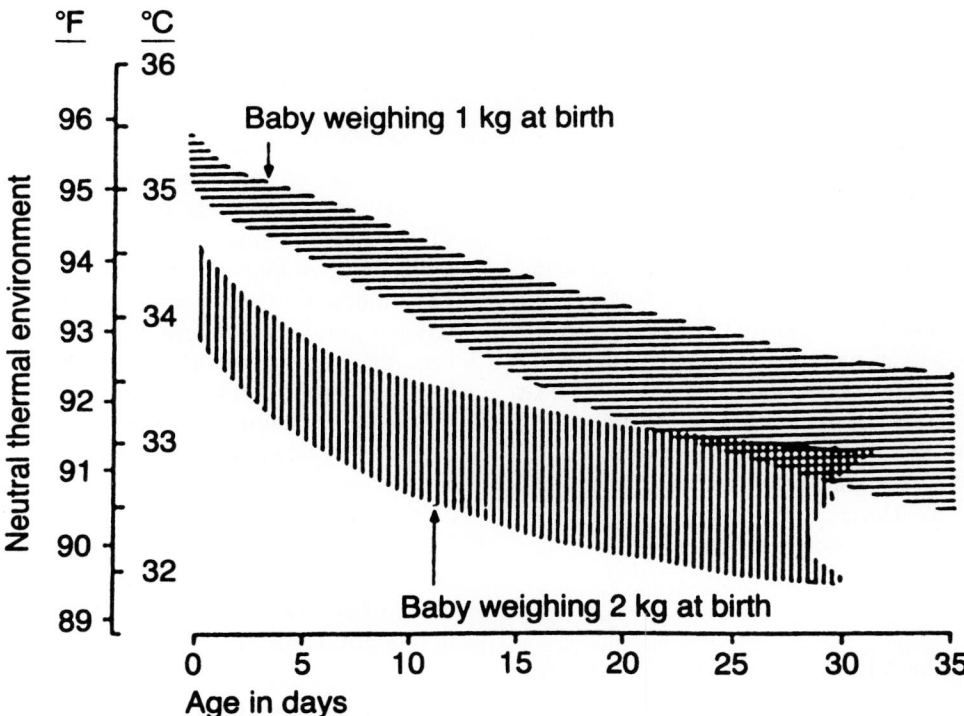

FIG. 24–2. Range of temperatures needed to provide neutral environmental conditions for babies lying naked on an insulated mattress in draft-free surroundings (at about 50% relative humidity), and when mean radiant wall temperature is the same as air temperature. The **top graph** represents a 1-kg infant at birth and the **bottom graph** a 2-kg infant. Optimum temperature probably approximates the lower limit of each neutral range as defined here. Approximately 1°C should be added to these operative temperatures to derive the appropriate neutral air temperature for a single-walled incubator when room temperature is less than 27°C (80°F), and more should be added if room temperature is very much less than this. (From ref. 15.)

Fig. 24–3, a sympathetic surge occurs at birth, with massive neurohumoral secretion of noradrenaline from paraaortic nodes and the fetal adrenal (28). Systemic and pulmonary vasoconstriction result, which may end in poor oxygen uptake and relative peripheral tissue hypoxia. Lactic acid production ensues, with demise ultimately occurring secondary to cold stress. Tarnier in the 1800s recognized this in Paris, where there was no central heating and poor home and hospital insulation.

Early Intervention

Drying infants in the delivery suite interrupts the process of evaporation, and bundling infants in cotton blankets to prevent exposure to cold air interrupts convective heat loss and provides insulation to retain the infant's metabolic heat. Placing infants at the mother's breast and cradled into her axillary fold engenders conductive heat transfer from the mother to the infant. Alternatively, and especially if early intervention is required to aid transition (e.g., suctioning or oxygen administration), the infant is dried first and then placed onto dry bedding under a radiant warmer while these procedures are performed. A con-

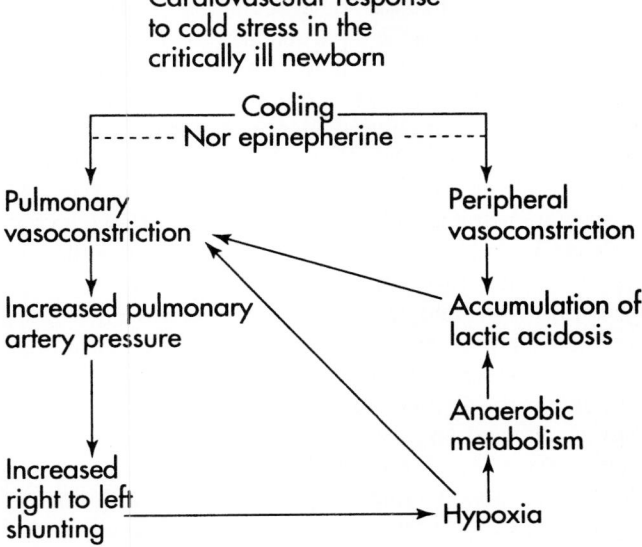

FIG. 24–3. Immediate and potentially detrimental cardiovascular response to a sympathetic surge in norepinephrine released upon birth upon exposure of the neonate's temperature-sensitive skin to a cold extrauterine environment (convection and evaporation). (From ref. 28.)

vectively warmed incubator enclosure with air temperatures ranging from 35.0° to 37.0°C and a variety of plastic swaddling heat shields have been advocated to prevent excessive cold exposure, especially during transition and hospital transport of premature infants (29–31).

Once in the nursery or in the mother's room, bundled infants may be placed into either an open bassinet or an incubator (naked or bundled) and provided close monitoring of either axillary (preferred, 36.0° to 36.5°C) or rectal (37° to 37.5°C) temperatures through the first few hours of life. Slightly premature infants (32 to 35 weeks) or small-for-gestational-age babies may appear to have normal body temperature at the expense of metabolically generated heat (9). Glass et al. (32) demonstrated that premature infants nurtured in dry, incubator environments of either 35.0°C (slightly cool) or 36.5°C in the first few days of life maintained a normal body temperature, but experienced more weight loss in the cooler environment.

Kangaroo Care

Skin-to-skin care, now termed *kangaroo care*, has been promoted for nurturing premature infants who are held naked between the mother's breasts as if in a kangaroo's pouch. The infant is in contact with the mother's warm skin and is close to the breast for unlimited feeding. Fathers also can provide thermal support in this way. Kangaroo care was first reported from Bogota, Columbia, where use of conventional incubators was limited and mortality in nonincubated preterm births high. A large randomized trial from this country recently showed infants ≤2.00 kg placed under kangaroo care shortly after birth for prolonged periods achieved transition safely and grew normally, had fewer nosocomial infections, and were discharged earlier, particularly at ≤1.80 kg (33). Significant reduction in early mortality also has been observed. During the 1980s, the kangaroo technique was promoted for nurturance of nonmechanically ventilated, growing premature infants in Scandinavian and some other European countries. Randomized clinical trials also have demonstrated enhanced mother–infant attachment, greater maternal self-esteem, prolonged and enhanced lactation, increased infant alertness, and better weight gain (34). Physiologic studies have focused on demonstrating thermal neutral metabolic response (minimal observed oxygen consumption) and temperature stability in stable growing premature babies during kangaroo care. Moreover, vital signs and oxygenation parameters were demonstrated to be more stable in preterm infants recovering from bronchopulmonary dysplasia, with absence of periodic breathing, and reduced apnea and bradycardia. Behavioral studies demonstrate more homogenous sleep patterns, less irritability later in infancy, and more direct social eye contact with caregivers (35).

In the intensive care nursery, kangaroo care may be initiated even during mechanical ventilation with uncompli-cated patients. Mothers are instructed to wear front-opening shirts, maintain careful hygiene without open sores or rashes, and avoid use of lotions, oils, or perfumes. Maximum skin surface area contact is desirable with a covering blanket to avoid outward convective and evaporative heat losses. Privacy and quiet must be provided by the nursery staff for periods of $1/2$ to 1 hour initially, and careful temperature monitoring by surface thermistor or an axillary thermometer should be performed at least every 15 minutes, along with cardiorespiratory and noninvasive oxygen monitoring where indicated. Temperature deviation more than 0.5°C of normal skin temperature (36.5° to 37.0°C) should result in termination of the session and return to incubator care. Periods up to 4 hours may be achieved. Mothers are encouraged to pump their breasts before and after sessions, because milk production is enhanced. Parents are empowered with the care of their infants, and kangaroo care integrates the family into the neonatal intensive care team. Presently, no adverse reports have been published, and the use of kangaroo care in modern intensive care settings is on the rise.

CONVECTION WARMED INCUBATORS

A modern incubator consists of an optically transparent, plastic hood (≥ 3mm thick) covering the infant, with sidewall and hand access ports. The infant lays on a bed platform, underneath which a tungsten element electronically heats the air. Air is forced over this element by a fan, circulating heated air within the hood. Temperature may be controlled thermostatically to regulate either the air or infant skin temperature (15,36).

Thermodynamics of Incubation

The physiology of mammalian (homeothermic) thermal regulation (37) may be summarized by the equation:

$$\dot{Q}_{metabolic} = \dot{Q}_{convection} + \dot{Q}_{conduction} + \dot{Q}_{evaporation} + \dot{Q}_{radiation} + \dot{Q}_{stored},$$

where $\dot{Q}$ is the *rate* of either metabolic heat production (left side of the equation), or of heat loss and heat stored (right side of the equation), generally expressed in kcal/kg/h or in W/M² (J/sec/M²). By convention, heat production and heat losses (or storage) are expressed as positive values. When a mammal is successfully maintaining normal body temperature, heat storage is zero, otherwise body temperature either increases or decreases until a new thermal equilibrium is established at another temperature. Also, when an environmental heat loss becomes a heat gain (e.g., under a radiant warmer), the gain is expressed as a negative loss.

Convection

The rate of heat transferred from an infant's skin into the incubator environment depends in part on the *insulation* provided by the dermis and the subcutaneous fascia (comprised primarily of white fat deposited late in gestation). Preterm babies have almost no fatty fascia and, therefore, are more vulnerable to heat loss through air (and skin blood flow) convection (37). Air convection is heat loss that takes place from the skin's surface into the surrounding environment and is summarized by the equation:

$$\dot{Q}_{convection} = k_1(T_{mean\ skin} - T_{air}) + k_2(T_{mean\ skin} - T_{air})V^n,$$

where two forms of skin-to-air convective heat loss occur, depending on the gradient between skin and air temperatures (ΔT), the complex geometry of surface area exposed and air thermal density k, and air movement velocity V^n (38). The first is *natural convection*, which results from the gradient of temperature between the skin surface and the surrounding air (38,39). Natural convection *cells* form as warm air rises from the skin, conveying heat and body moisture away from the surface of the baby. Air thus warmed subsequently cools and falls back toward the baby, forming the convection cell. Such cells form over the curvature of the baby's body surface area exposed. An infant in flexion leaves less surface area exposed (38). An infant extended and flaccid is able to dissipate more heat. Posture may be a valuable observation in deciding the thermal comfort or discomfort of even a preterm infant.

The second form of convection is *forced convective* air movement, usually occurring at air velocities ≥0.27 M/sec. Forced convective heat loss is roughly proportional to an exponential power (n) of the velocity (V) of air movement. Within forced convection warmed incubators, manufacturers strive to render still the air near the baby. Recent estimates of natural and forced-air convective heat loss from premature neonates nursed within incubators indicate success in this strategy, because natural convection was the only major loss observed to occur (40). Heat also is lost to a lesser degree by respiratory convection and evaporation.

An example of different incubator convection designs affecting skin-to-air heat transfer is shown in Fig. 24–4, adapted from a study of *partitional calorimetry* performed by Okken et al. (41). The left incubator partition in this figure represents a natural convection warmed incubator with no circulating fan. Air rose passively from heating elements underneath the baby's mattress to warm the interior of the incubator hood. The second partition on the right represents a more standard, fan-forced convection incubator as described previously. Nonevaporative heat loss in the passive device (non-E, the sum of convection, radiation, and conduction) was 60% compared to 47% in the forced convection warmed incubator, whereas evaporative heat loss (E) was 13% higher in the forced convective environment. These authors attributed this increased evaporative loss to disturbance by the incubator's fan of a *microenvironment* of humid air layered near the baby's skin.

Evaporation

The premature neonate loses large amounts of water (and, therefore, latent heat at 0.58 kcal/mL) through evaporation from the skin for several reasons (42–49). First and most important is the premature neonate's thin epidermis lacking keratin, which normally serves as a vapor barrier for older infants, children, and adults. Very immature skin is associated with reduced survival, and evaporative rates from infants less than 700 g may be likened to those of severe burn victims. Second, premature neonates lose excessive amounts of water and heat due to an increased body surface area/body mass ratio as demonstrated in Table 24–1 (50). The very low birth weight premature infant ≤500 g exposes six times the area of the

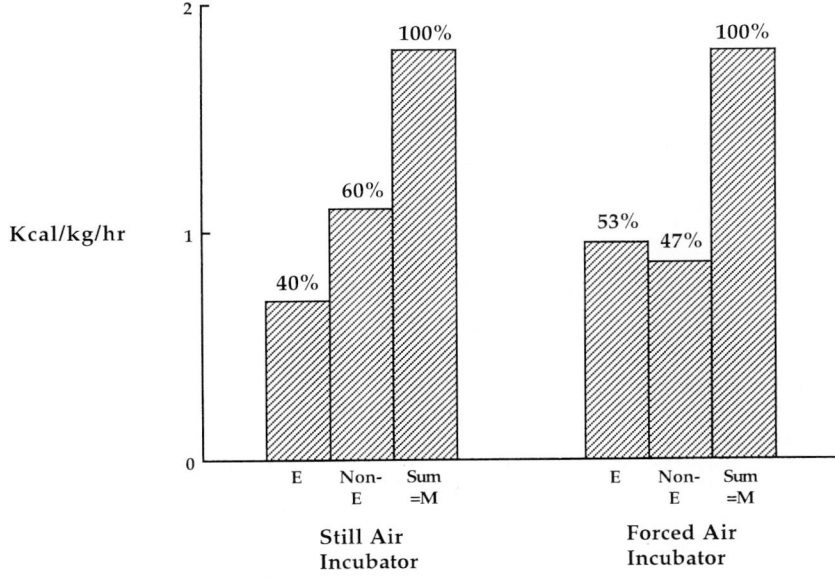

FIG. 24–4. Partitional calorimetry performed for premature infants in two different types of convection warmed incubators, natural and forced air. The rate of evaporative heat loss (E) is greater proportionally for babies nurtured in a conventional forced-air warmed environment than nonevaporative heat losses (non-E) from convection, conduction, and radiation. Heat balance is regulated by metabolic rate (M) and nonmetabolic mechanisms for thermal conservation (e.g., vasoconstriction). (Adapted from ref. 41.)

TABLE 24–1. *Calculated body surface area (BSA)/body mass ratio for adults, and for low-birth-weight (LBW) and very LBW neonates*

	Body mass (kg)	BSA (m²)	BSA/mass (cm²/kg)
Adult	70	1.73	250
LBW premature	1.5	0.13	870
LBW premature	1.0	0.10	1,000
Very LBW	0.5	0.065	1,300

Adapted from ref. 50.

adult subject per kilogram of the largely water body mass. Third, the proportion of the extracellular water mass in the very low birth weight infant, which is exposed to the external environment through the nonkeratinized epidermal layer, is significantly larger (51).

Hammerlund and Sedin (45) (Fig. 24–5) summarized the rate of transepidermal water loss in premature newborn infants, nurtured in incubators throughout the first month of life, at different gestational ages. This figure demonstrates that the newborn at 26 weeks' gestation may lose as much as 60 g of water per M²/h (more than 180 mL/kg/day or 100 kcal/kg/day). Additional amounts of water may also be lost from upper airways during respiration of nonhumidified air in incubators.

Incubator Humidification

Humidification inside modern incubators is accomplished by the evaporation of water from a reservoir located in the air path over the heating element beneath the incubator mattress (52). Earlier descriptions of humidification in incubators cited the use of nebulized mist to saturate the infant's environment (≥80% to 90% relative humidity) (53,54). These latter techniques resulted in the proliferation of pseudomonas infections and were rejected resoundingly by a number of reports (53–56). Unfortunately, abandoning all use of vapor (invisible humidification) based on infection risks encountered with particulate mists (visible humidification) has resulted in running incubator hoods completely "dry." Relative humidity levels inside dry incubators at 36° to 36.5°C may drop to less than 10% to 15%, promoting large insensible water and latent heat losses (52). In response to these concerns, the American Academy of Pediatrics presently recommends only moderate use of air humidification between 40% to 50% relative humidity in the vapor phase (i.e., gaseous), and not a particulate mist (liquid phase) (57). Put simply, if water circulating near an infant is visible, infection may be more likely.

A more recent reevaluation of incubator humidification was conducted by Harpin and Rutter (52) in 1985. Thirty-

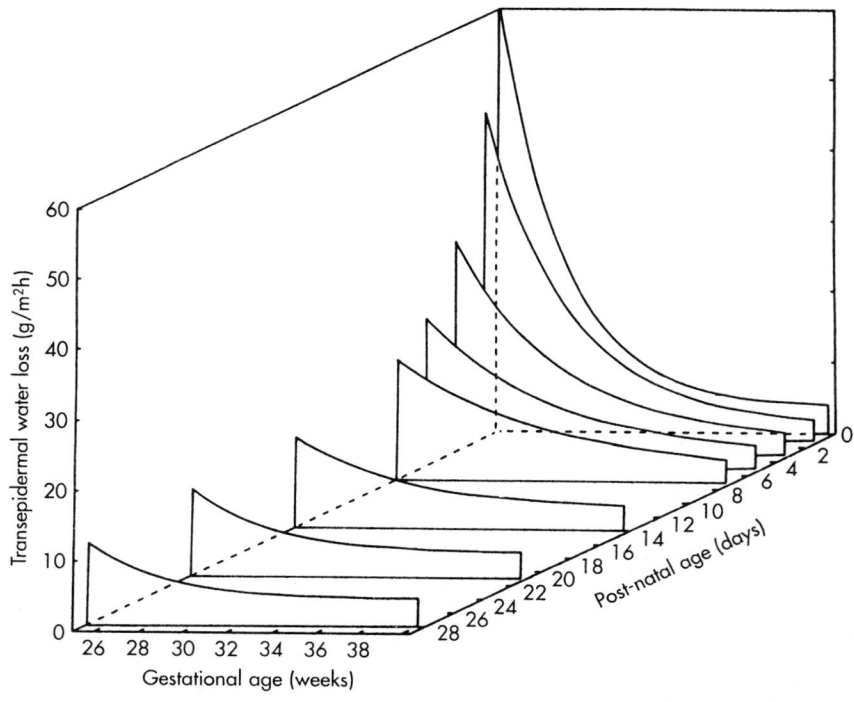

FIG. 24–5. Transepidermal water evaporation from the skin of premature neonates of gestations ranging from 25 to 40 weeks, followed longitudinally from birth over the first month of life. Dehydration is most dangerous in the most immature babies less than 28 weeks' gestation, in the first week of life before skin keratinization occurs. (From ref. 47.)

three infants less than 30 weeks of gestation and less than 2 weeks of age were nurtured in vapor-humidified incubators saturated at between 80% and 90% relative humidity. Two infants acquired pseudomonas sepsis and one died. Twenty-nine babies of similar gestation and maturity were nurtured in dry incubators: one suffered an episode of pseudomonas sepsis and died. Those who died with pseudomonas did so after the study had ended, after the first 2 weeks of life. The authors recommended that humidification be used routinely in the first 2 weeks of life to prevent evaporative losses and prevent skin desiccation. Humidification early in life may be prudent for incubation of the very-low-birth-weight infant, in whom heat and water losses are excessive and probably pathologic. Modern incubators now may be equipped with sophisticated solid-state temperature and humidity control devices to prevent condensation at higher relative humidity levels between 60% and 80%. Although verification is yet lacking, hopefully a reduced risk of infection will occur by maintaining humidity without visible condensation.

Conductive Heat Loss and Warming Mattresses

Conductive heat loss results from contact of a baby's body with the solid surface of a bed platform:

$$\dot{Q}_{conduction} = k(T_{core\ temp} - T_{mean\ skin})/D,$$

where k is contact surface area and the bed's heat conductivity constant, and (ΔT) represents the temperature gradient between the infant's body core (containing heat) and the mean skin contact surface. D is the thickness of the bed's conducting material. In general, insulating foam rubber (about 2.5-cm thickness) and double cotton blanket batting results in negligible conductive heat loss by providing insulation from the metal or plastic bed table (i.e., reducing the value of k). Recently, however, incubator manufacturers and water mattress companies have provided evidence that exogenous heat application through carefully conducted bed surfaces maintained at ≤39°C to prevent burn injury to areas of skin contact may reduce environmental heat requirements from incubators or radiant warmers for very-low-birth-weight subjects (58,59). Moreover, application of warmed mattresses during extreme environmental conditions encountered in infant transports also may prove beneficial (59,60).

Radiant Heat Loss

Radiant heat loss is the least intuitive aspect of newborn incubation. Radiant heat loss occurs as a transfer of

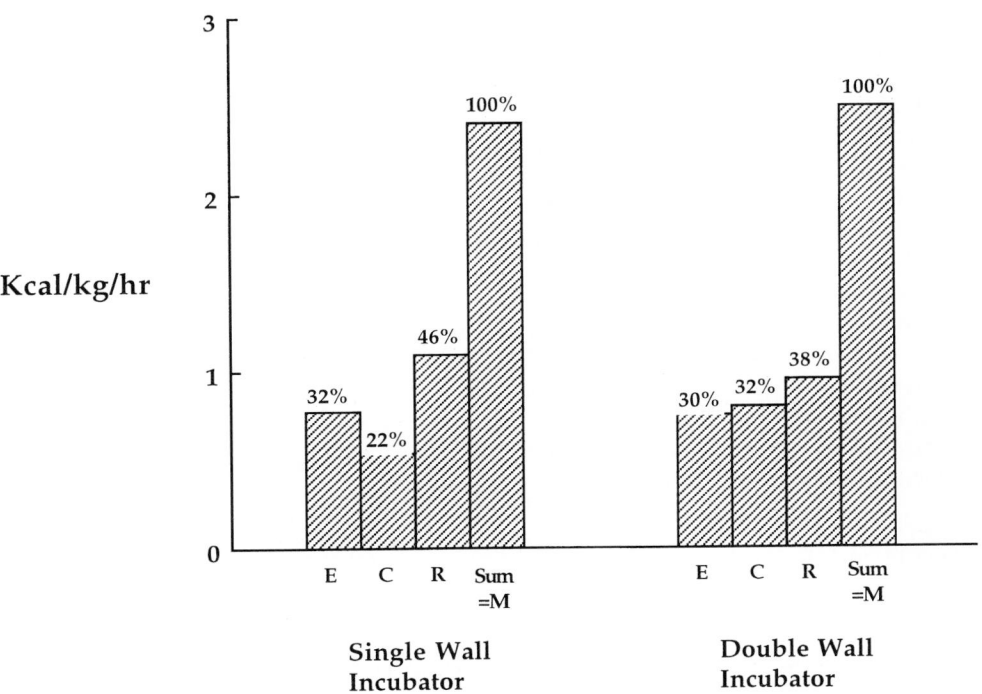

FIG. 24–6. Partitional calorimetry performed for preterm infants at steady-state, thermal neutral temperature in two forced-air, convection warmed incubators, either with only a single wall between the infant and the surrounding nursery's environmental air and wall temperatures, or with an inner wall (double-walled incubator) interposed between the infant and the incubator's outer wall. Forced air warming of both sides of the inner wall reduces radiant heat loss, resulting in lower servocontrolled incubator air temperature (higher infant convective heat loss). Evaporative loss was not altered by insertion of the double wall. (Adapted from ref. 40.)

infrared electromagnetic energy virtually instantly from one warm body to another of lesser warmth:

$$\dot{Q}_{radiation} = (\beta)(\varepsilon_1)(\varepsilon_2)(T_{mean\ skin} - T_{walls}),$$

where a radiant heat transfer constant β (Stefan–Boltzman), the physical *emissivity* of the infant's skin and the incubator's plastic walls (ε_{skin}, ε_{walls}), the absolute temperature gradient (ΔT), as well as the infant s exposed surface area and posture determine the rate of radiant heat loss within incubators (37). In a single-walled incubator, heat transfers from the infant's skin (36.5° to 37.0°C) to the mean temperature of the cooler walls of the incubator's plastic interior (about 28.0° to 36.5°C). The incubator walls then reradiate heat to the nursery walls and windows, which are even cooler (18.0 to 27.0°C). A massive heat sink is represented by the nursery walls, which may determine 60% of the operant environmental temperature perceived by the skin in room air conditions:

$$T_{operant\ environment} = 0.60\ T_{walls} - 0.40\ T_{air}.$$

Double-Walled Incubators

The importance of radiant heat transfer within incubators is demonstrated in Fig. 24–6 (40). Two incubators of different designs are compared. Partitional calorimetry for a single-walled incubator is shown on the left, whereas a double-walled incubator design is depicted on the right. The double-walled incubator constitutes a plastic chamber similar to the single-walled incubator with an additional inner wall suspended several centimeters interior to the outer wall of the incubator. Warmed air is circulated between these two incubator walls, warming both the outer and inner surfaces of the inner wall, as well as the inner surface of the outer wall of the incubator. The result is an elevated inner wall plastic temperature exposed to an infant's skin. Radiant heat loss to the inner wall of the incubator exposed to the infant's skin is significantly reduced. Convective heat loss is higher in the double-walled incubator, because a less warm air temperature is required to maintain the infant when radiant heat loss is thus conserved. Because vapor pressure was constant, evaporative heat loss was the same in both incubator devices.

Skin Surface Servocontrol Temperature

As a result of the difficulties encountered in measuring and controlling the whole environment defined by all of the parameters described previously, Silverman et al. (36) proposed that any set of environmental conditions that rendered a *normothermic* skin surface temperature would provide a thermal neutral environment. They defined a skin temperature servocontrol set point between 36.2° to 36.5°C over the anterior abdominal wall for thermostatic control of incubator air temperature warming (with or without humidification, mattress warming, or radiant

walls protection) to guarantee a minimal observed metabolic rate of oxygen consumption and, therefore, a thermal neutral environment. Proportional response, servocontolled skin temperature now has become the standard of care for regulating convection warmed incubator heating over much of the world.

Servocontrolled Incubator Homeothermy

All incubator studies demonstrating a thermal neutral environment under a variety of conditions evaluating air temperature, convection, and humidity; incubator wall temperature; and nursery temperature were performed at steady-state conditions. Infant metabolic rates often were determined in noncritical subjects at rest. Such steady-state conditions are theoretical, however, in critically ill premature neonates in thermostatically servocontrolled incuba-

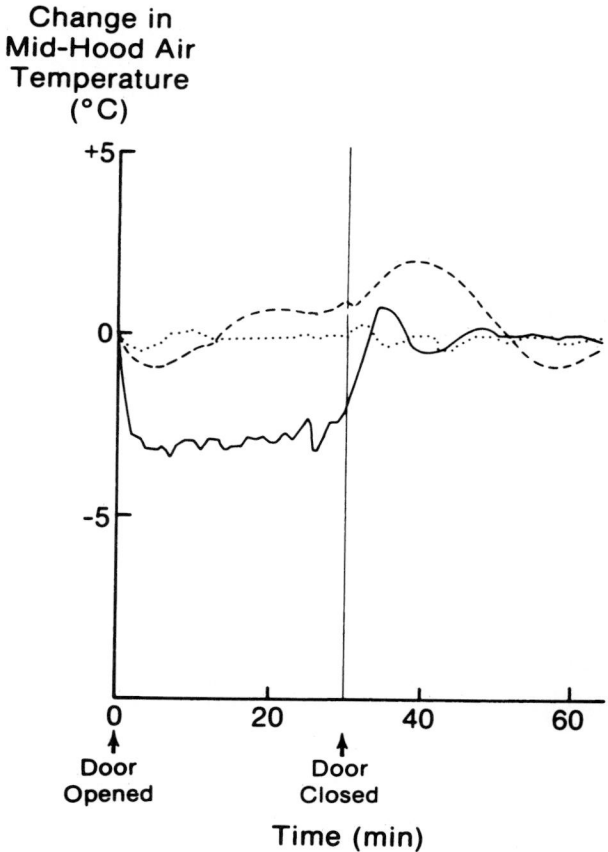

FIG. 24–7. Effect of opening and closing the incubator's front panel or hand ports on interior air temperature servocontrolled to maintain a steady state near a thermal neutral condition for premature neonates. Two different double-walled incubators commonly used are represented to demonstrate control responses to perturbation of the steady state. Overshoot and undershoot of temperature homeostasis occurs commonly, except where only the hand ports are opened. Such air temperature variations may persist more than 1 hour after returning the incubator panel to a closed position. (From ref. 61.)

tors, subjected to the many variations encountered in the modern neonatal intensive care nursery. Hand ports and doors may be opened and closed several times a day for access to nursing and minor surgical procedures, as well as radiographic, ultrasound, and echocardiographic examinations. Incubators may be invaded as often as once an hour for delivery of intensive care. Figure 24–7 demonstrates two modern double-walled incubators and their thermostatic air temperature control characteristics when the access panel or hand ports were opened and then closed (61). These incubators often demonstrated overdampening of the servocontrol system, which resulted in overshooting and undershooting air temperatures for as long as 1 hour after the door had been closed. Conceivably, such fluctuations may be experienced routinely during the entire 24-hour day of neonatal intensive care.

THE RADIANT WARMER BED

The radiant warmer bed is a variable-level, waist-high platform with a mattress surface (which may now be either heated or may incorporate an electronic scale), upon which the critically ill newborn lies without an encumbering plastic enclosure. Suspended about 80 to 90 cm above this platform is a radiant heat source with an electrically heated metal alloy wire coiled within a quartz tube. A thermostatic skin servocontrol device regulates the radiant heat, which is distributed across near and far wavelengths of the infrared spectrum (Fig. 24–8). At full power, the sum of infrared irradiance is less than 100 mW/cm^2 of surface area on the bed platform. The heat delivered in the near portion of the infrared spectrum (less than 1,000 nm) is less than 10 mW/cm^2 of surface area irradiated. These levels of radiant exposure recently have been judged as biologically safe for the developing skin and eyes in the prematurely born newborn infant when exposed briefly (62). The servocontrolled warmer generally operates at about one-half this peak power, and radiant power density delivered at bed level usually is well below the 50 to 60 mW/cm^2 felt to be potentially deleterious at longer periods of exposure. The head, foot, and sides of the radiant warmer bed platform receive less radiant power and, therefore, less warming than is delivered to the center of the bed platform. Optimally, infants are positioned in the center of this device.

Figure 24–9 demonstrates our experience with complete partitional calorimetry for critically ill premature infants nurtured under radiant warmers (63). Both radiant heat losses under a radiant warmer as well as heat gains are demonstrated. The effects of evaporation, convection, and conduction and of infant metabolic heat production are demonstrated for infants nurtured naked and supine under these devices. Heat loss comprised 64% toward convection to the surrounding cool air of the nursery's environment. The majority of convective heat loss occurred naturally, whereas a minor component was composed of forced convective air movement from doors opening and closing within the nursery, nursery personnel bustling near the bedside, as well as the cycling of heating and cooling vents supplying the nursery's ambient air control. These turbulent convective air movements contributed to evaporative heat loss, which comprised 30% of total heat loss in this figure. Thermal equilibrium is maintained under a radiant warmer by a replacement of heat losses through convection, evaporation, conduction, and radiation, by radiant heat *gain* directly from the warming element. Almost 58% of heat replacement is derived from the servocontrolled radiant warmer. Metabolic heat production M comprises 42% of the thermal balance and is overpowered by the radiant heating element.

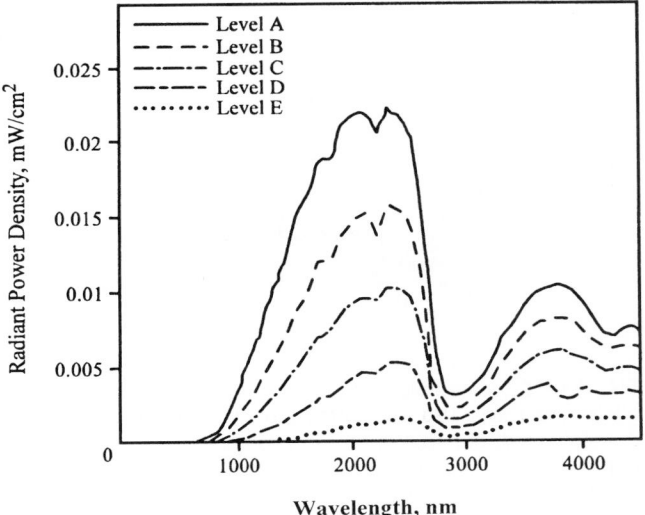

FIG. 24–8. Spectral irradiance measured at bed level with increasing power from a radiant warmer's heating element. Note two peaks of energy indicating the wire element's emission (near infrared wavelength spectrum at the **left**) and the quartz containment tube's reemission of absorbed heat from the wire (far spectrum at the **right**). The notch in the near peak probably indicates infrared adsorption by water vapor. Integrated over the entire peak emissions, levels of near and far infrared exposure are felt to be safe for the developing skin and eyes. (From ref. 62.)

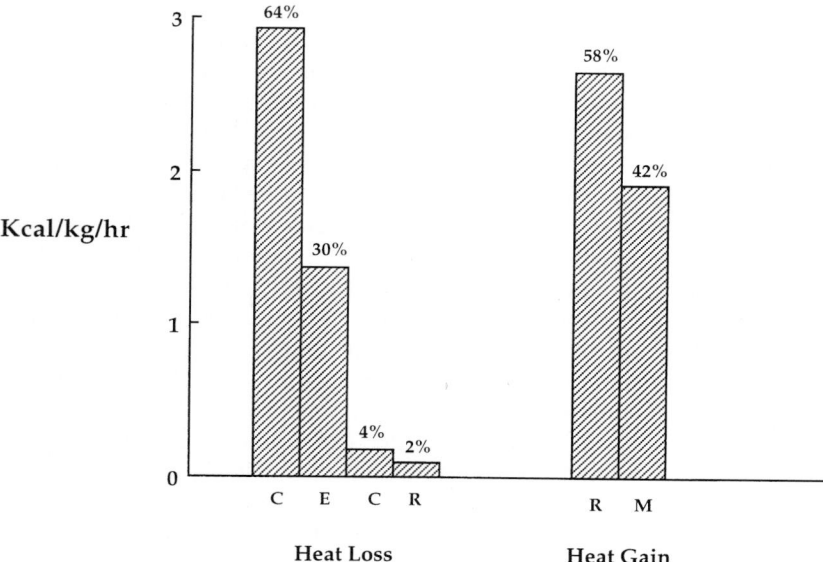

FIG. 24–9. Partitional calorimetry for infants nurtured naked under radiant warmers servocontrolled to maintain anterior abdominal wall skin temperature at 36.5°C. Shown on the **left** are convective, evaporative, conductive, and radiant heat losses (from the infant's sides), and on the **right** are radiant heat gain (facing the warmer) and heat generated by the infant's metabolism. (Adapted from ref. 63.)

Thermal Neutral Radiant Warming

Le Blanc (64) summarized a meta-analysis comparing radiant warmers to convectively heated incubators. The thermal neutral environment was defined for each warming device as the *minimal observed metabolic rate* of oxygen consumption (MOMR measured in oxygen consumption, $\dot{V}O_2$, in mL/kg/min), when skin temperature was servocontrolled between 36.0 and 36.5°C, and at steady-state conditions. Eleven of 16 infants demonstrated slightly higher rates of oxygen consumption when nursed at similar temperatures under radiant warmers ($\dot{V}O_2$ 6.84 ± 0.37 SEM vs. 7.45 ± 0.44 mL/kg/min), an increase of 8.8% in metabolic rate under radiant warmers. The assumptions involved in the calculation of MOMR are that the infant is (i) at rest and asleep, (ii) postprandial at least 2 to 3 hours, and (iii) at thermal neutral temperature conditions. Typically, premature infants demonstrate slightly higher oxygen consumptions than term infants, and small-for-gestational-age infants manifest oxygen consumptions slightly higher than premature and term infants. The minimum requirement for oxygen consumption in these studies demonstrates a metabolic rate of caloric expenditure of roughly 60 to 75 kcal/kg/day. Above this amount, 9 to 10 kcal/kg/day may be required for growth. However, intensive care conditions provided to critically ill neonates rarely approximate those of a growing premature baby at rest and at steady-state.

Figure 24–10 shows results of oxygen consumption measurements from studies conducted in our intensive care nursery in a 1.2-kg infant nurtured naked and supine under a radiant warmer while intubated endotracheally and receiving ventilatory support (65). During a 90-minute period of relatively mild cold stress (servocontrol skin temperature 35.5°C), oxygen consumption fluctuated between 5.5 and 8.5 mL/kg/min, paralleled closely

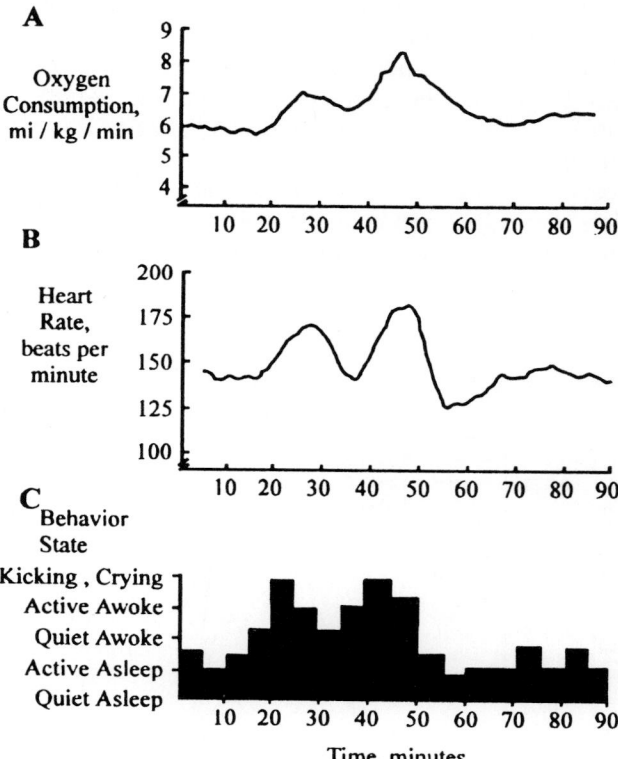

FIG. 24–10. Metabolic rate of oxygen consumption **(A)** parallels heart rate **(B)** and infant activity **(C)** with the performance of indirect calorimetry in a premature baby weighing approximately 1.0 kg. Variation with infant behavior is demonstrated in this relatively cool condition (servocontrol 35.5°C). (From ref. 65.)

by the infant's heart rate and behavior. These observations of preterm infant behavior linked to metabolism are typical, even when critically ill. Criteria for determining MOMR suggest that oxygen consumption for this subject is 5.5 mL/kg/min. However, the integrated sum of behavior over the entire study period reflects a higher rate of global metabolism. Such observations led Schulze et al. (66) speculate that a thermal neutral environment should be evaluated over periods considerably longer than 10 to 30 minutes of MOMR at steady state. Figure 24–11 shows oxygen consumption over three 90-minute periods for the same infant as shown in Fig. 24–10, at three different radiant warmer servocontrol skin temperatures— 35.5°, 36.5°, and 37.5°C (67). From these studies over longer study periods, it seems clear that infant behavior may constitute a significant part of metabolic rate determination, affecting the thermal neutral zone. Figure 24–12 shows 18 premature infants nurtured under radiant warmers demonstrating a thermal neutral environmental temperature (between 36.2° and 36.5°C servocontrolled anterior abdominal wall skin temperature), where all infant behavior was incorporated (67). Approximately 7.2 mL/kg/min VO$_2$ at the warmer's 36.5°C skin temperature set point represented optimal control under intensive care circumstances. Increasing anterior abdominal wall skin temperature above this point by 1°C resulted in no significant additional reduction in metabolic rate, and, when servocontrolled to 37.5°C, the gradient for heat loss (from the infant's core to the skin) narrowed sufficiently for a number of them to become hyperthermic (38.2° to 38.5°C). We therefore recommend avoiding skin control temperatures above 36.7° and 37.0°C for infants in the weight range studied (between 0.87 and 1.60 kg).

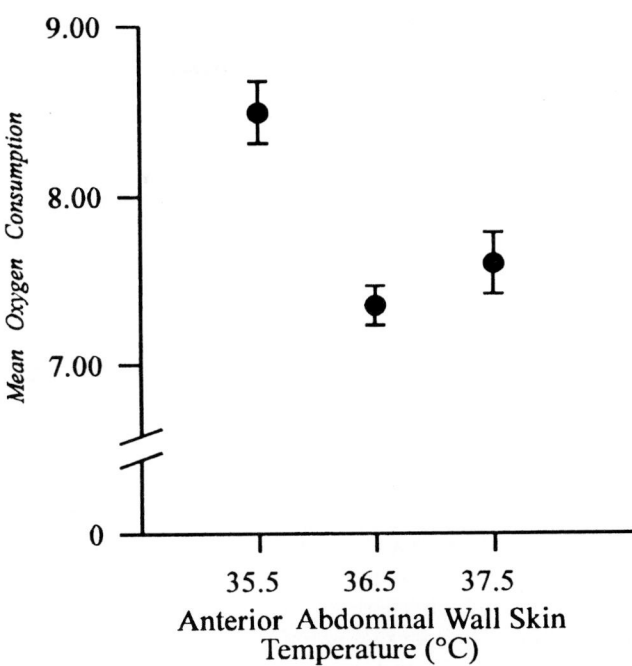

FIG. 24–12. Significantly lower oxygen consumption is demonstrated at 36.5°C compared to 35.5°C servocontrol temperature for a series of 18 infants under radiant warmers. No additional significant reduction in oxygen consumption is achieved by increasing servocontrol temperature to 37.5°C, and several infants demonstrated deep rectal hyperthermia at 37.5°C. (From ref. 67.)

HEAT SHIELDING

Rigid, Plastic Heat Shields

A 1- to 2-mm thickness of plastic used as a miniature incubator hood and placed over infants on open radiant beds has been proposed by several authors. Yeh et al. (68) reported that insensible water loss was reduced by more than 25% for infants nurtured under a plastic hood. Bell et al. (69) failed to replicate any difference in water loss using a rigid plastic body hood under radiant warmers. The configuration of the plastic hoods used in each of these studies was different, in some cases permitting free air exchange at the open ends of the hood. Moreover, the interposition of radiantly opaque plastic between infant and the radiant element may have interfered with the delivery of radiant heat to the baby's skin (70). Disruption of the servocontrol mechanism by interposition of a radiant opaque plastic heat sink between the infant and the warmer seems to be a futile strategy.

Flexible Plastic Blankets

A flexible plastic blanket made of saran seems more efficient than the body hood, particularly under a radiant warmer (Fig. 24–13) (39,71). Saran is thin, permitting

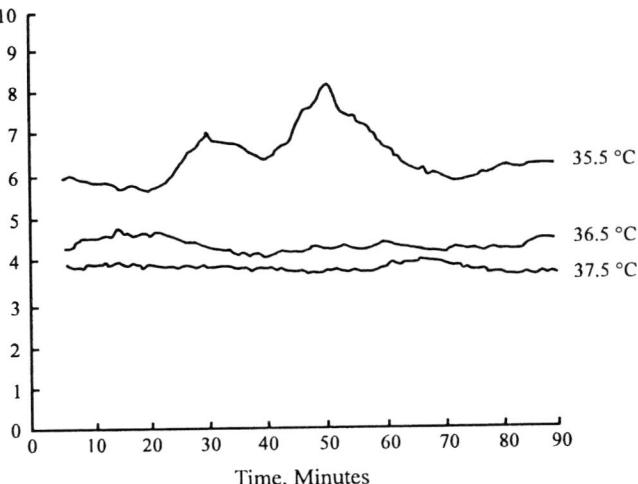

FIG. 24–11. The metabolic rates of oxygen consumption from the same infant shown in Fig. 24–10 are compared at 35.5°, 36.5°, and 37.5°C servocontrol skin temperature. Behavioral activity is attenuated, and basal metabolism is significantly reduced at warmer temperatures. (From ref. 67.)

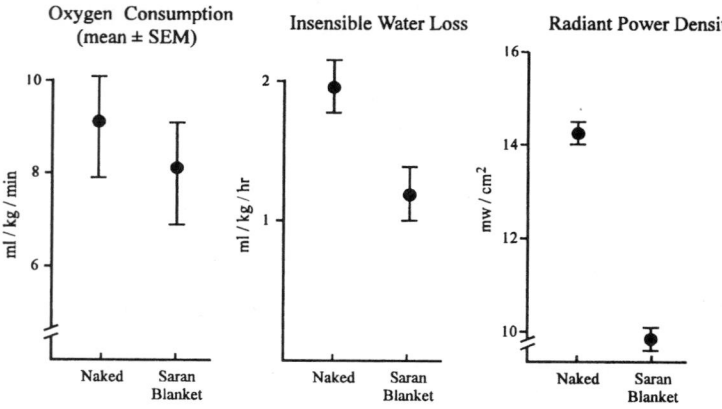

FIG. 24–13. Comparison of radiant power density delivered **(right)**, insensible water loss **(middle)**, and oxygen consumption **(left)** in preterm neonates nurtured either naked or covered by a saran plastic blanket under radiant warmers. The blanket significantly reduced all three measurements in all babies tested, suggesting better environmental maintenance under saran. (From ref. 71.)

free heat exchange without excessive evaporation (70). The flexible plastic blanket reduces the effect of forced convection, which disrupts the microenvironment of warm, humid air near the infant's skin (39). The reduction in both convective and evaporative heat losses is about 30% (71). Insensible water loss is diminished from about 2.0 to 1.2 mL/kg/hr. Oxygen consumption is reduced from 9.0 to 8.0 mL/kg/min in this study. The net effect of saran blanket heat shielding under radiant warmers renders the environment more homeothermic, with lower power required to achieve thermal equilibrium, both from the radiant warmer and the baby's rate of metabolic heat production. Adverse effects with saran plastic blankets have been cited. Although the saran plastic may stick to the immature skin causing maceration, to date, this probably remains the single most effective technique for rendering infants under radiant warmers thermal neutral.

EPIDERMAL BARRIER PROTECTION

Semiocclusive Artificial Skin

A novel strategy for thermal protection is covering the exposed surfaces of immature skin with semiocclusive polyurethane dressings, (Tegederm and Opsite) (72). In early studies using this technique, insensible water loss from days 1 to 4 of life was reduced by 30% to 50%. Upon careful removal of the artificial polyurethane dressing, skin moisture barrier development (keratinization) was consistent with development over the adjacent naked skin sites tested. A report by Porat and Brodsky (73) indicated that applying an adherent polyurethane layer over the entire torso and extremities early in very-low-birth-weight infants under 800 g improved fluid and electrolyte balance, reduced patent ductus arteriosum (PDA) and intraventricular hemorrhage (IVH), as well as improved survival. Mancini et al. (74) found a similar result and reported a decrease in bacterial growth on skin guarded by a semipermeable dressing.

Emollients and Aquaphor

Rutter and Hull (76) originally reviewed topical agents for reduction of transepidermal water loss. They found high water content creams ineffective in this regard, whereas paraffin produced a modest effect. Calculated evaporative rate was initially halved in preterm infants less than 30 weeks' gestation; however, this effect was transient, with return to a higher rate of water loss within 4 to 8 hours (75,76). Nopper et al. (77) conducted a randomized trial investigating barrier effects of a topical, petroleum-based, and preservative-free ointment (Aquaphor) applied twice daily for 2 weeks to the skin of preterm infants. Transepidermal water loss was decreased by 67% initially compared to control infants and remained at 34% below controls after 4 to 6 hours. Dermatologic scores of skin integrity were improved in treated infants, and there was a decline in bacterial colonization of axillary skin, with a significantly lower incidence of positive blood and spinal fluid cultures. The authors also suggested better temperature control and fluid balance in treated subjects. Use of Aquaphor has become popular in many nurseries, especially for very-low-birth-weight babies. Commentary by Rutter (75) on this work suggests, however, that temperature control may not be benefited in babies weighing less than 1 kg early after birth, and only high humidity incubators eliminate this problem in the smallest infants.

REFERENCES

1. Cone TE. *History of the care and feedings of the premature infant.* Boston: Little, Brown and Company, 1985.
2. Berthod P. *La couveuse et le gavage a la maternite de Paris* [Thesis]. Paris: G. Rougier, 1887.
3. Marx S. Incubation and incubators. *Am Med Surg Bull* 1896;9:311.
4. Rotch TM. Description of a new incubator. *Arch Pediatr* 1893;10:661.
5. Swanson HE. Interrelations between thyroxin and adrenalin in the regulation of oxygen consumption in the albino rat. *Endocrinology* 1956;59:217.
6. Blackfan KD, Yaglou CP. The premature infant: a study of effects of atmospheric conditions on growth and on development. *Am J Dis Child* 1933;46:1175.

7. Bolt RA. The mortalities of infancy. In: Abt I-A, ed. *Pediatrics*, vol 2, Philadelphia: WB Saunders, 1923.

8. Mauriceau F. *Traite des maladies des femmes grosses et accouchees.* Paris: Chez l'Auteur, 1669:100.

9. Silverman WA, Fertig JW, Berger AP. The influence of the thermal environment upon the survival of the newly born premature infant. *Pediatrics* 1958;22:876.

10. Cross KW, Dawes GS, Mott JC. Anoxia, oxygen consumption and cardial output in newborn lambs and adult sheep. *J Physiol* 1959;146:316.

11. Hill JR, Rahimtulla KA. Heat balance and the metabolic rate of newborn babies in relation to environmental temperature, and the effect of age and of weight on basal metabolic rate. *J Physiol* 1965;180:239.

12. Hill JR. The oxygen consumption of newborn and adult mammals: its dependence on the oxygen tension in the inspired air and on the environmental temperature. *J Physiol* 1959;149:346.

13. Bruck K, Parmelee AH, Bruck M. Neutral temperature range and range of "thermal comfort" in premature infants. *Biol Neonate* 1962;4:32.

14. Bruck K. Temperature regulation in the newborn infant. *Biol Neonate* 1961;3:65.

15. Hey EN, Katz G. The optimum thermal environment for naked babies. *Arch Dis Child* 1970;45:328.

16. Hey EN. The relation between environmental temperature and oxygen consumption in the new-born baby. *J Physiol* 1969;200:589.

17. Hey EN. Thermal neutrality. *Br Med Bull* 1975;31:69.

18. Power GG, Schroder H, Gilbert RD. Measurement of fetal heat production using differential calorimetry. *J Appl Physiol* 1984;57:917.

19. Ryser G, Jequier E. Study by direct calorimetry of thermal balance on the first day of life. *Eur J Clin Invest* 1972;2:176.

20. Morishima HO, Yeh MN, Niemann WH, et al. Temperature gradient between fetus and mother as an index for assessing intrauterine fetal condition. *Am J Obstet Gynecol* 1977;129:443.

21. Power GG, et al. Temperature responses following ventilation of the fetal sheep in utero. *J Dev Physiol* 1986;8:477.

22. Schroder H, Gilbert RD, Power GG. Computer model of fetal-maternal heat exchange in sheep. *J Appl Physiol* 1988;65:460.

23. Hodgkin DD, et al. In vivo brown fat response to hypothermia and norepinephrine in the ovine fetus. *J Dev Physiol* 1988;10:383.

24. Alexander G, Williams D. Shivering and non-shivering thermogenesis during summit metabolism in young lambs. *J Physiol (Lond)* 1968;198:251.

25. Bray GA, Goodman HM. Studies on the early effects of thyroid hormones. *Endocrinology* 1965;76:323.

26. Klein AH, Reviczky A, Padbury JF. Thyroid hormones augment catecholamine-stimulated brown adipose tissue thermogenesis in the ovine fetus. *Endocrinology* 1984;114:1065,.

27. Silva JE, Larsen PR. Adrenergic activation of triiodothyronine production in brown adipose tissue. *Nature* 1983;305:712.

28. Baumgart S. Incubation of the human newborn infants. In: Pomerance JJ, Richardson CJ, eds. *Neonatology for the clinician*. Norwalk: Appleton & Lange, 1993:139.

29. Baum JD, Scopes JW. The silver swaddler. *Lancet* 1968;1:672.

30. Besch NJ, Perlstein PH, Edwards NK, et al. The transparent baby bag. *N Engl J Med* 1971;284:121.

31. Dahm LS, James LS. Newborn temperature: heat loss in the delivery room. *Pediatrics* 1972;49:504.

32. Glass L, Silverman WA, Sinclair JC. Effect of the thermal environment on cold resistance and growth of small infants after the first week of life. *Pediatrics* 1968;41:1033.

33. Charpak N, Ruiz-Pelaez JG, de Figueroa CZ, Charpak Y. Kangaroo mother versus traditional care for newborn infants ≤2000 grams: a randomized, controlled trial. *Pediatrics* 1997;100:682.

34. Bell RP, McGrath JM. Implementing a research based kangaroo care program in the NICU. *Nurs Clin North Am* 1996;31:2.

35. Anderson GC. Current knowledge about skin-to-skin (kangaroo care) for preterm infants. *J Perinatol* 1991;11:216.

36. Silverman WA, Sinclair JC, Agate FJ Jr. The oxygen cost of minor changes in heat balance of small newborn infants. *Acta Pediatr Scand* 1966;55:294.

37. Sinclair JC. Metabolic rate and temperature control. In: Smith CA, Nelson NM, eds. *The physiology of the newborn infant*. Springfield, IL: Thomas, 1976:354.

38. Wheldon AE, Rutter N. The heat balance of small babies nursed in incubators and under radiant warmers. *Early Hum Dev* 1982;6:131.

39. Baumgart S, Engle WD, Fox WW, et al. Effect of heat shielding on convective and evaporative heat losses and on radiant heat transfer in the premature infant. *J Pediatr* 1981;99:948.

40. Bell EF, Rios GR. A double-walled incubator alters the partition of body heat loss of premature infants. *Pediatr Res* 1983;17:135.

41. Okken A, Blijham C, Franz W, et al. Effects of forced convection of heated air on insensible water loss and heat loss in preterm infants in incubators. *J Pediatr* 1982;101:108.

42. Baumgart S, Engle WD, Fox WW, et al. Radiant warmer power and body size as determinants of insensible water loss in the critically ill neonate. *Pediatr Res* 1981;15:1495.

43. Baumgart S, Langman CB, Sosulski R, et al. Fluid, electrolyte and glucose maintenance in the very low birthweight infant. *Clin Pediatr* 1982;21:199.

44. Bell EF, Neidich GA, Cashore WJ, et al. Combined effect of radiant warmer and phototherapy on insensible water loss in low-birthweight infants. *J Pediatr* 1979;94:810.

45. Hammarlund K, Sedin G. Transepidermal water loss in newborn infants. VIII. Relation to gestational age and post-natal age in appropriate and small for gestational age infants. *Acta Paediatr Scand* 1983;72:721.

46. Hey EN, Katz G. Evaporative water loss in the newborn baby. *J Physiol (Lond)* 1969;200:605.

47. Sedin G, Hammarlund K, Nilsson GE, et al. Measurements of transepidermal water loss in newborn infants. *Clin Perinatol* 1985;12:79.

48. Williams PR, OH W. Effects of radiant warmer on insensible water loss in newborn infants. *Am J Dis Child* 1974;128:511.

49. Wu PYK, Hodgman JE. Insensible water loss in preterm infants: changes with postnatal development and non-ionizing radiant energy. *Pediatrics* 1974;54:704.

50. Costarino AT, Baumgart S. Neonatal water metabolism. In: Cowett RM, ed. *Principles of perinatal–neonatal metabolism*. New York: Springer-Verlag, 1991:623.

51. Costarino AT, Baumgart S. Modern fluid and electrolyte management of the critically ill premature infant. *Pediatr Clin North Am* 1986;33:153.

52. Harpin VA, Rutter N. Humidification of incubators. *Arch Dis Child* 1985;60:219.

53. Moffet HL, Allan D, Williams T. Survival and dissemination of bacteria in nebulizers and incubators. *Am J Dis Child* 1967;114:13.

54. Moffet HL, Allan D. Colonization of infants exposed to baterially contaminated mists. *Am J Dis Child* 1967;114:21.

55. Brown DG, Baublis J. Reservoirs of pseudomonas in an intensive care unit for newborn infants: mechanism of control. *J Pediatr* 1977;90:453.

56. Hoffman MA, Finberg L. Pseudomonas infections in infants associated with high humidity environments. *J Pediatr* 1955;46:626.

57. *Guidelines for perinatal care*, 2nd ed. Elk Grove Village, IL: American Academy of Pediatrics and American College of Obstetricians and Gynecologists, 1988:278.

58. Topper WH, Stewart TP. Thermal support for the very-low-birth-weight infant: role of supplemental conductive heat. *J Pediatr* 1984;105:810.

59. Koch J. Physical properties of the thermal environment. In: Okken A, Koch J, eds. *Thermal regulation of sick and low birth weight neonates*. Berlin: Springer, 1995:103.

60. Sedin G. Physics of neonatal heat transfer, routes of heat loss and heat gain. In: Okken A, Koch J, eds. *Thermal regulation of sick and low birth weight neonates*. Berlin: Springer, 1995:21.

61. Bell EF, Rios GR. Performance characteristics of two double-walled infant incubators. *Crit Care Med* 1983;11:663.

62. Baumgart S, Knauth A, Casey FX, et al. Infrared eye injury not due to radiant warmer use in premature neonates. *Am J Dis Child* 1993;147:565.

63. Baumgart S. Radiant heat loss versus radiant heat gain in premature neonates under radiant heaters. *Biol Neonate* 1990;57:10.

64. LeBlanc MH. Relative efficacy of radiant and convective heat in incubators in producing thermoneutrality for the premature. *Pediatr Res* 1984;18:425.

65. Baumgart S. Partitioning of heat losses and gains in premature newborn infants under radiant warmers. *Pediatrics* 1985;75:89.

66. Schulze K, Kairan R, Stefanski M, et al. Spontaneous variability in minute ventilation, oxygen consumption and heart rate of low birth weight infants. *Pediatr Res* 1981.

67. Malin S, Baumgart S. Optimal thermal management for low birth weight infants nursed under high-power radiant warmers. *Pediatrics* 1987;79:47.

68. Yeh TF, Amma P, Lillian LD, et al. Reduction of insensible water loss in premature infants under the radiant warmer. *J Pediatr* 1979;94:651.

69. Bell EF, Weinstein MR, Oh W. Heat balance in premature infants: com-

parative effects of convectively heat incubator and radiant warmer, with and without plastic heat shield. *J Pediatr* 1980;96:460.

70. Baumgart S, Fox WW, Polin RA. Physiologic implications of two different heat shields for infants under radiant warmers. *J Pediatr* 1982; 100:787.

71. Baumgart S. Reduction of oxygen consumption, insensible water loss and radiant heat demand using a plastic blanket for low birthweight infants under radiant warmers. *Pediatrics* 1984;74:1022.

72. Knauth A, Gordin M, McNelis W, et al. A semipermeable polyurethane membrane as an artificial skin in premature neonates. *Pediatrics* 1989; 83:945.

73. Porat R, Brodsky N. Effect of Tegederm use on outcome of extremely low birth weight (ELBW) infants. *Pediatr Res* 1993;33:231(A).

74. Mancini AJ, Sookdeo-Drost S, Madison KC, Smoller BR, Lane AT. Semipermeable dressings improve epidermal barrier function in premature infants. *Pediatr Res* 1994;36:306.

75. Rutter N. Waterproofing our infants! [Letter] J Pediatr 1997;130:333.

76. Rutter N, Hull D. Reduction of skin water loss in the newborn. I. Effect of applying topical agents. *Arch Dis Child* 1981;56:669.

77. Nopper AJ, Horii KA, Sookdeo-Drost S, Wang TH, Mancini AJ, Lane AT. Topical ointment therapy benefits premature infants. *J Pediatr* 1996;128:660.

PART FOUR

The Low-Birth-Weight Infant

CHAPTER 25

Intrauterine Growth Restriction and the Small-for-Gestational-Age Infant

Marianne S. Anderson and William W. Hay, Jr.

INTRODUCTION

Much of the interest in infants who are small for gestational age (SGA) at birth, and much of the impetus for studying intrauterine growth restriction (IUGR) that produces SGA infants, began with the observation by pediatricians and neonatologists that newborn infants who were classified according to birth weight as small, average, or large for gestational age (SGA, AGA, and LGA, respectively) showed specific morbidities and rates of death that were unique to each of these birth weight–gestational age classifications (1). SGA infants were recognized as having more frequent problems with perinatal depression ("asphyxia"), hypothermia, hypoglycemia, polycythemia, long-term deficits in growth, neurodevelopmental handicaps, and higher rates of fetal and neonatal mortality (2) (Fig. 25–1). Although there have been tremendous improvements in perinatal diagnosis and treatment, severe IUGR and the birth of markedly SGA infants continue to be frequent problems, and the perinatal morbidity and mortality rates of IUGR fetuses and SGA infants continue to exceed those of normal fetuses and infants.

DEFINITIONS

Small for Gestational Age

SGA infants are classically defined as having a birth weight that is more than two standard deviations below the

M. S. Anderson: Neonatal-Perinatal Medicine, Department of Pediatrics, University of Colorado Health Sciences Center, Denver, Colorado

W. W. Hay, Jr.: Neonatal-Perinatal Medicine Training Program; and Neonatal Clinical Research Center, Department of Pediatrics, University of Colorado Health Sciences Center, Denver, Colorado

mean or less than the 10th percentile of a population-specific birth weight versus gestational age plot. Broader definitions include less than normal anthropometric indexes, such as length and head circumference, as well as marked differences between growth parameters, even when they are within the normal range. For example, an infant can be considered "relatively" SGA when its weight is at the 25th percentile, but its length and head circumference are at the 75th percentile. In this case, the weight/length ratio (or the Ponderal index = [weight (g)]/[length (cm)]^3) is less than normal, indicating that growth rates of adipose tissue and skeletal muscle, the principal determinants of weight, were less than normal (Fig. 25–2) (3).

Intrauterine Growth Restriction

IUGR is defined as a rate of fetal growth that is less than normal for the population and for the growth potential of a specific infant. IUGR therefore produces infants who are SGA. SGA infants can be the result of normal but slower than average rates of fetal growth, such as those constitutionally small but not abnormal infants whose parents, siblings, and more distant relatives are small (4). SGA infants also can be the result of abnormally slow fetal growth that is caused by pathophysiologic conditions or diseases. Because growth is one of the essential features of the fetus, nearly any aberration of biologic activity in the fetus can lead to growth failure. Thus, small size at birth can be either a normal outcome or one that is a result of intrinsic or extrinsic factors that limit fetal growth potential.

Birth Weight Classification of Growth

Many terms are used to describe variations in fetal growth. For example, human newborns are classified as

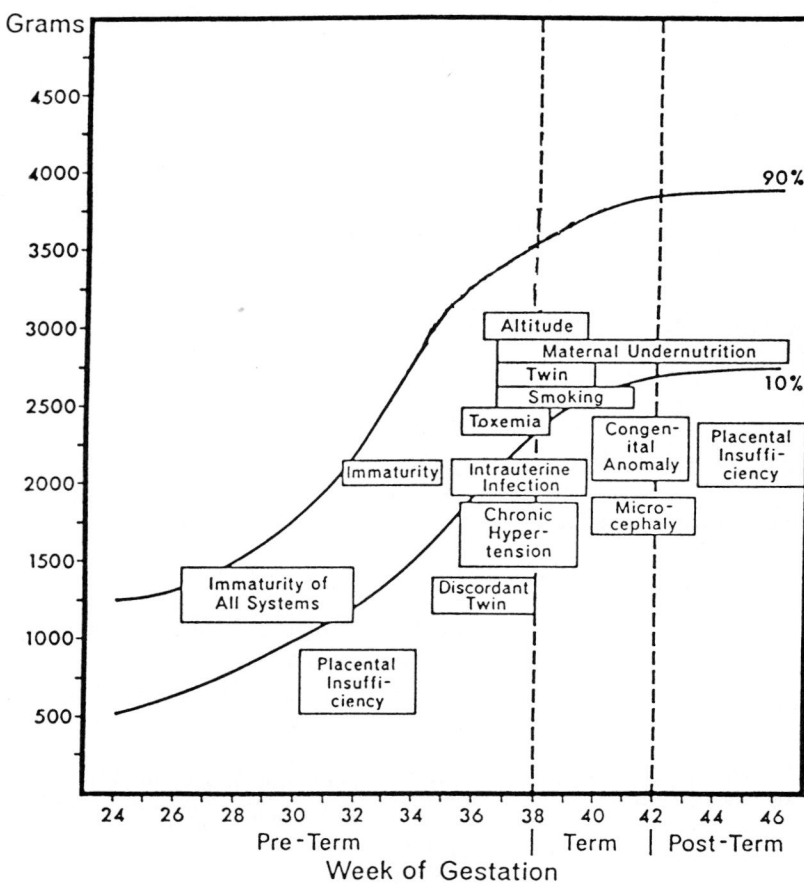

FIG. 25–1. Morbidities specific to small-for-gestational-age infants. (Adapted from Lubchenco LO. The high risk infant. In: Schaffer AJ, Markowitz M, eds. *Major problems in clinical pediatrics*, volume XIV. Philadelphia: WB Saunders, 1976:6.)

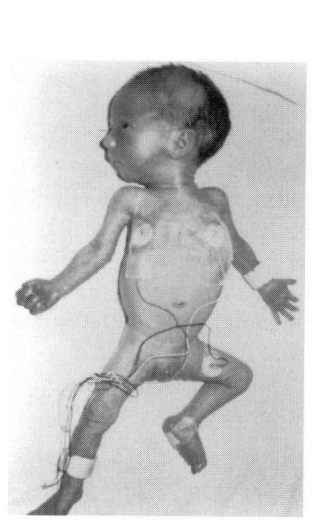

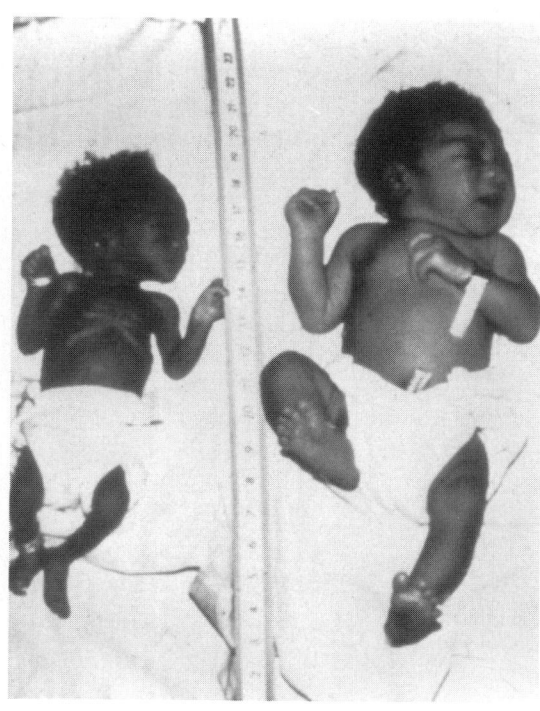

FIG. 25–2. Preterm, small-for-gestational-age infant at 34 weeks of gestation **(left)**, severely small-for-gestational-age infant at 39 weeks **(middle)**, and average-for-gestational-age infant at 40 weeks **(right)**.

Colorado Intrauterine Growth Charts

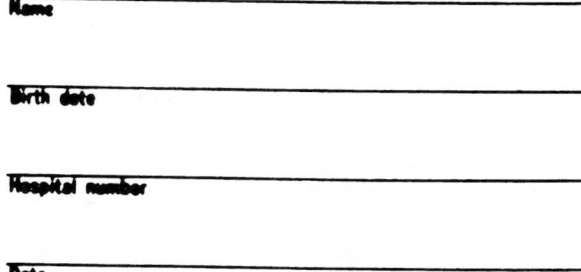

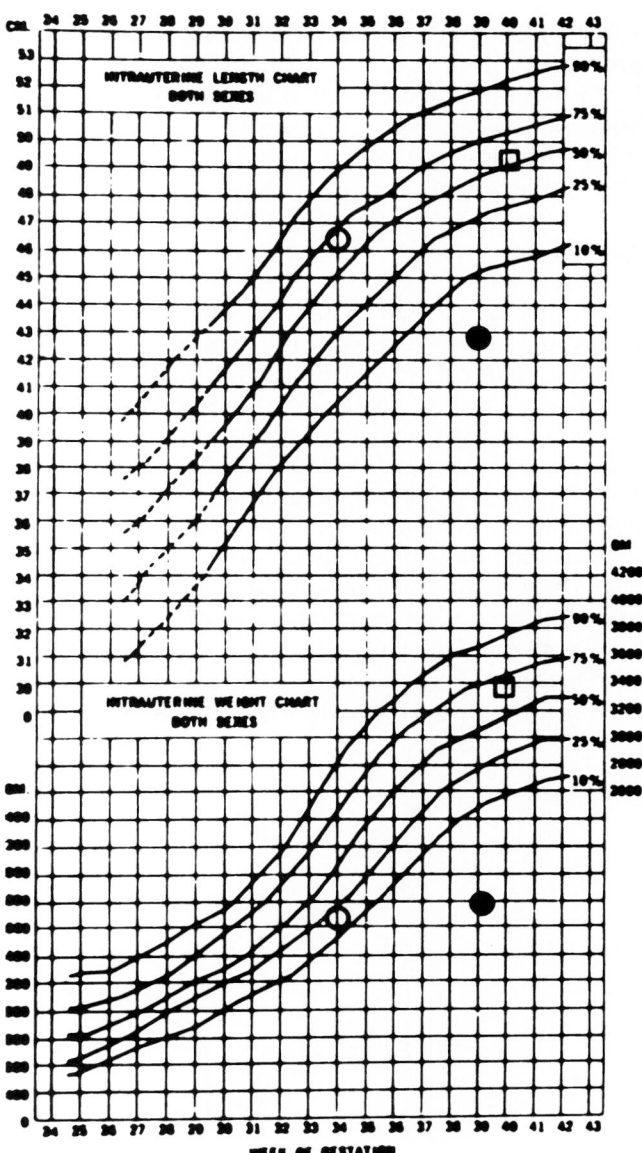

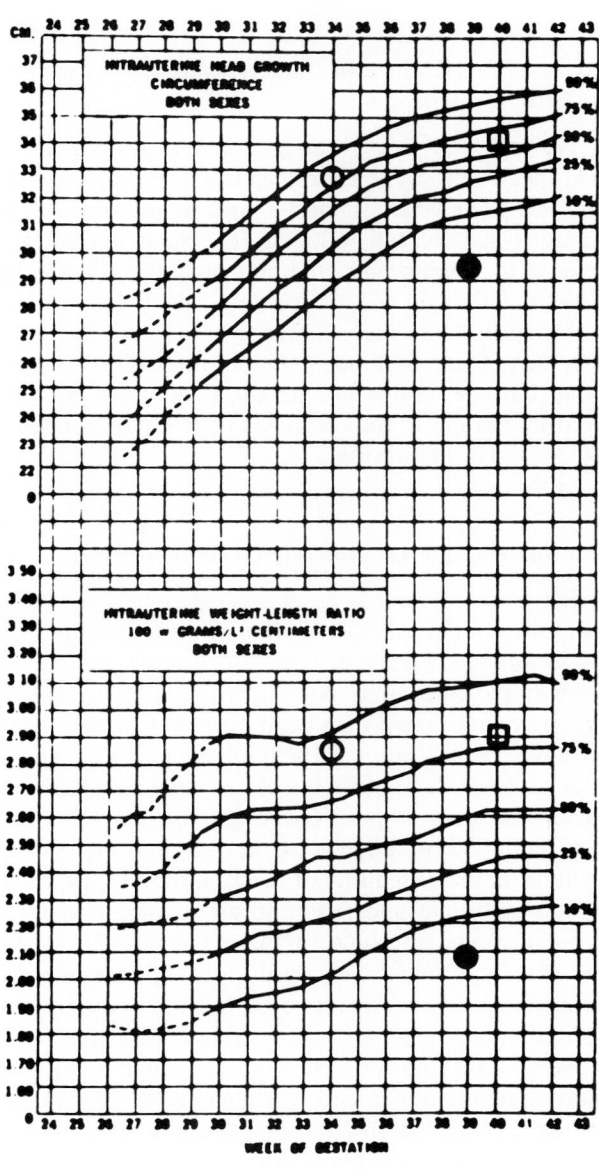

FIG. 25–3. The Colorado Intrauterine Growth Charts, including symbols that define the anthropometric measurements for the three infants shown in Fig. 25–2. (○) Preterm infant at 34 weeks of gestation, showing asymmetry of weight (15th percentile) versus length and head circumference (75th percentile) and weight-to-length ratio (85th percentile); (●) severely but symmetrically small-for-gestational-age infant at 39 weeks, showing weight, length, head circumference, and weight-to-length ratio all about equally and markedly (<10th percentile); and (□) symmetric average-for-gestational-age infant at 40 weeks, showing weight, length, head circumference, and weight-to-length ratio about the 65th to 75th percentile. (Growth charts from ref. 13.)

having normal birth weight (greater than 2,500 g), low birth weight (LBW, less than 2,500 g), very low birth weight (VLBW, less than 1,500 g), or extremely low birth weight (ELBW, less than 1,000 g). Obviously, classification by weight alone says little about fetal growth rate, as most infants with less than normal birth weights are the result of a shorter than normal gestation, i.e., they are preterm. Similarly, classifying newborns as preterm or term on the basis of birth weight is erroneous, as infants with IUGR are smaller than normal at any gestational age.

Normal Variations and the Assessment of Fetal Growth

Normal fetal growth varies almost twofold. For example, mean birth weight for neonates born in New Guinea is 2,400 g (5), whereas normal birth weights in other populations can exceed 4,000 g (6). Such variations are related to genetic and environmental factors, the latter usually reflecting local diets (e.g., the relatively obese infants of Polynesian women who eat relatively large amounts of starchy foods in their normal diet). These and other normal anthropometric variations must be considered in relation to the diagnosis of IUGR in fetuses and SGA status of newborns.

Symmetric and Asymmetric Growth Restriction

SGA infants have been classified as having symmetric or asymmetric IUGR. Symmetric IUGR implies that brain and body growth both are limited. Asymmetric growth indicates that body growth is restricted to a much greater extent than head (and thus, brain) growth. In such cases, brain growth is considered "spared." Mechanisms that allow brain growth to continue at a faster rate than adipose tissue and skeletal muscle are not completely known. Contributing factors may include an increased rate of cerebral blood flow, relative to the umbilical and systemic circulations, which has been observed in some of these infants (7). In some experimental models, cerebral glucose transporter concentrations are preserved despite fetal hypoglycemia, indicating preservation of cerebral glucose uptake capacity (8). The most severely affected infants have marked reductions in both brain and body growth. Even moderately IUGR infants have growth restrictions of both brain and body, but to varying degrees that depend on the duration and severity of the insults that inhibit growth. Asymmetric and symmetric growth restriction are best thought of, therefore, as extreme examples (Fig. 25–3). Asymmetric fetal growth differentially affects organs other than the brain. As shown in Fig. 25–4, the

heart also is larger for body weight in these infants, whereas the liver, probably representing glycogen deficit, and thymus, perhaps indicating a response to stress but also showing a potential for immunologic inadequacy, are smaller for body weight.

In general, factors intrinsic to the fetus cause symmetric growth restriction, whereas external factors cause asymmetric growth. Patterns of symmetric growth restriction develop early during fetal life, reflecting their intrinsic nature. Asymmetric patterns also can develop as early as the second trimester (9) and as much as 30% to 50% of extremely preterm neonates (less than 1,000 g) are SGA, probably reflecting pathology that produced growth restriction and led to preterm birth. Factors that limit the growth of both the fetal brain and body include chromosomal anomalies (e.g., particularly trisomy conditions), congenital infections (toxoplasmosis, rubella, cytomegalovirus), dwarf syndromes, some inborn errors of metabolism, and some drugs (10). The mechanisms by which these factors limit fetal growth are multifactorial.

Asymmetric growth restriction classically develops during the late second and third trimesters when fetal nutrients, particularly glucose and lipids, increasingly contribute to energy storage in the form of glycogen and fat (in both brown and white adipose tissue) (11). Slight reductions of energy substrate supply to the fetus limit fat and glycogen storage and the growth of skeletal muscle, but allow for continued bone and brain growth. More extreme limitations of energy substrates, for longer periods, affect both growth and energy storage. Timing is important; with decreased nutrient supply early in gestation, growth of all body organs is restricted, whereas decreased fetal nutrient supply later in gestation primarily restricts growth of glycogen content, adipose tissue, and skeletal muscle.

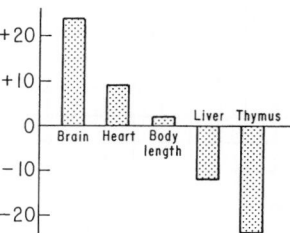

FIG. 25–4. Body length and selective organ weight percent changes from normal preterm infants of similar birth weights in necropsy series of IUGR fetuses. (After Gruenwald P. Growth patterns in the normal and deprived fetus. In: Jonxis JHP, Visser HKA, Troelstra JA, eds. *Aspects of prematurity and dysmaturity.* Springfield: Charles C. Thomas, 1968:43.)

INTERPRETATION OF FETAL GROWTH CURVES

Growth Curves Based on Neonatal Measurements

Cross-sectional growth curves have been developed from anthropometric data in populations of infants born at different gestational ages (12). Such curves have been used to demonstrate whether an infant's weight is within the normal range for a given gestational age and thus to estimate whether that infant's *in utero* growth was greater or less than normal. The normal range is defined as birth weights between the 10th and 90th percentile of the population-specific birth weight versus gestational age relationship. Fetuses and neonates who are within the 10th and 90th percentiles for weight versus gestational age are considered AGA. Those who are less than the 10th percentile are considered SGA. Those who are greater than the 90th percentile are considered LGA. Other terms for SGA infants include light for dates and small for dates.

Most growth curves usually are confined to the third trimester. Each curve is based on local populations with variable composition of maternal age, parity, socioeconomic status, race, ethnic background, body size, degree of obesity or thinness, health, pregnancy-related problems, and nutrition, as well as the number of fetuses per mother, the number of infants included in the study, and by what methods and how accurately measurements of body size and gestational age were made. Estimating gestational age, in particular, has considerable error. Such error is derived from variability in dating conception because of maternal postimplantation bleeding and irregular menses, wide variability in the development physical features of maturation in the infant, and interobserver variability in assessing an infant's developmental stage. The growth curves shown in Fig. 25–3 are those of Lubchenco and colleagues (13) in Denver, Colorado, published in 1966. They are biased to slightly lower birth weights compared with many other growth curves, especially close to term, due to the unique mix of racial and ethnic groups in the population of babies who were born at Colorado General Hospital, Denver, Colorado, at the time the data were collected. Although the higher altitude of Denver (5,280 feet or ~1,600 m) has been considered a factor in the smaller birth weights shown in these curves, the independent effect of high altitude on restricting fetal growth is not clearly demonstrable at 1 mile (1.6 km). In fact, growth curves similar to those of Lubchenco et al. have been produced at sea level among lower socioeconomic groups with a high proportion of blacks and Hispanics in the population (Fig. 25–5).

Mathematical analyses of various fetal growth curves have been used to determine growth rates over relatively short gestational periods or at discrete gestational ages (12). For example, the data used in the Lubchenco growth curves (Figs. 25–3 and 25–5) can be approximated by a simple exponential function showing fetal weight increasing at about 15 g/day/kg. This rate will vary from the smallest to the largest infants. For a given weight percentile, however, there are only differences of 1% to 2% for this exponential function among different populations and studies.

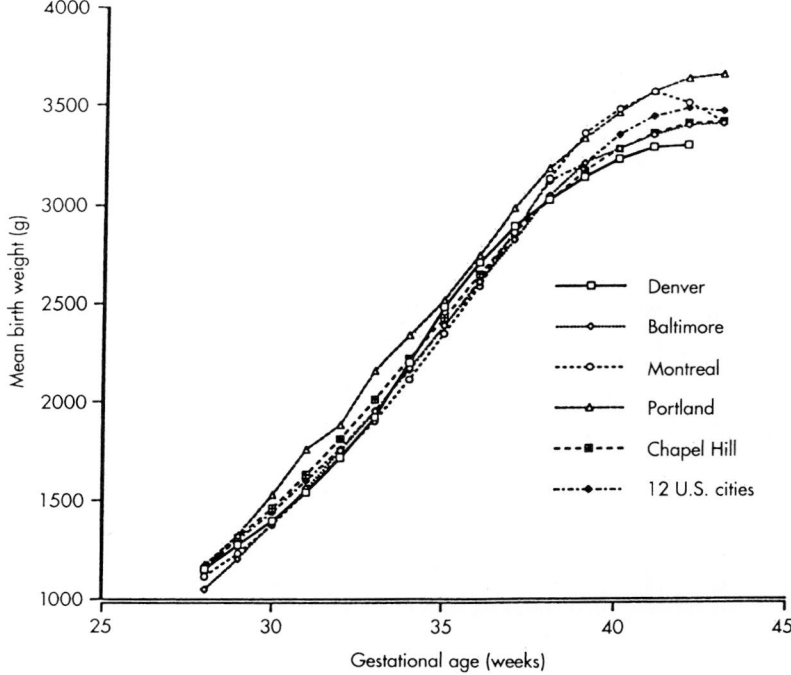

FIG. 25–5. Birth weights by gestational age from six sources. (Adapted from Naeye R, Dixon J. Distortions in fetal growth standards. *Pediatr Res* 1978;12:987.)

Growth Curves Based on Fetal Measurements

Fetal growth curves also have been developed from serial ultrasound measurements of fetuses who subsequently were born at term in healthy condition and with normal measurements, providing continuous rather than cross-sectional indexes of fetal growth. These curves can be better correlated with the expected fetal growth rate of a particular fetus than can cross-sectional, population-based growth curves. Serial ultrasound measurements of fetal growth also can more accurately determine how environmental factors, such as severe maternal illness and under

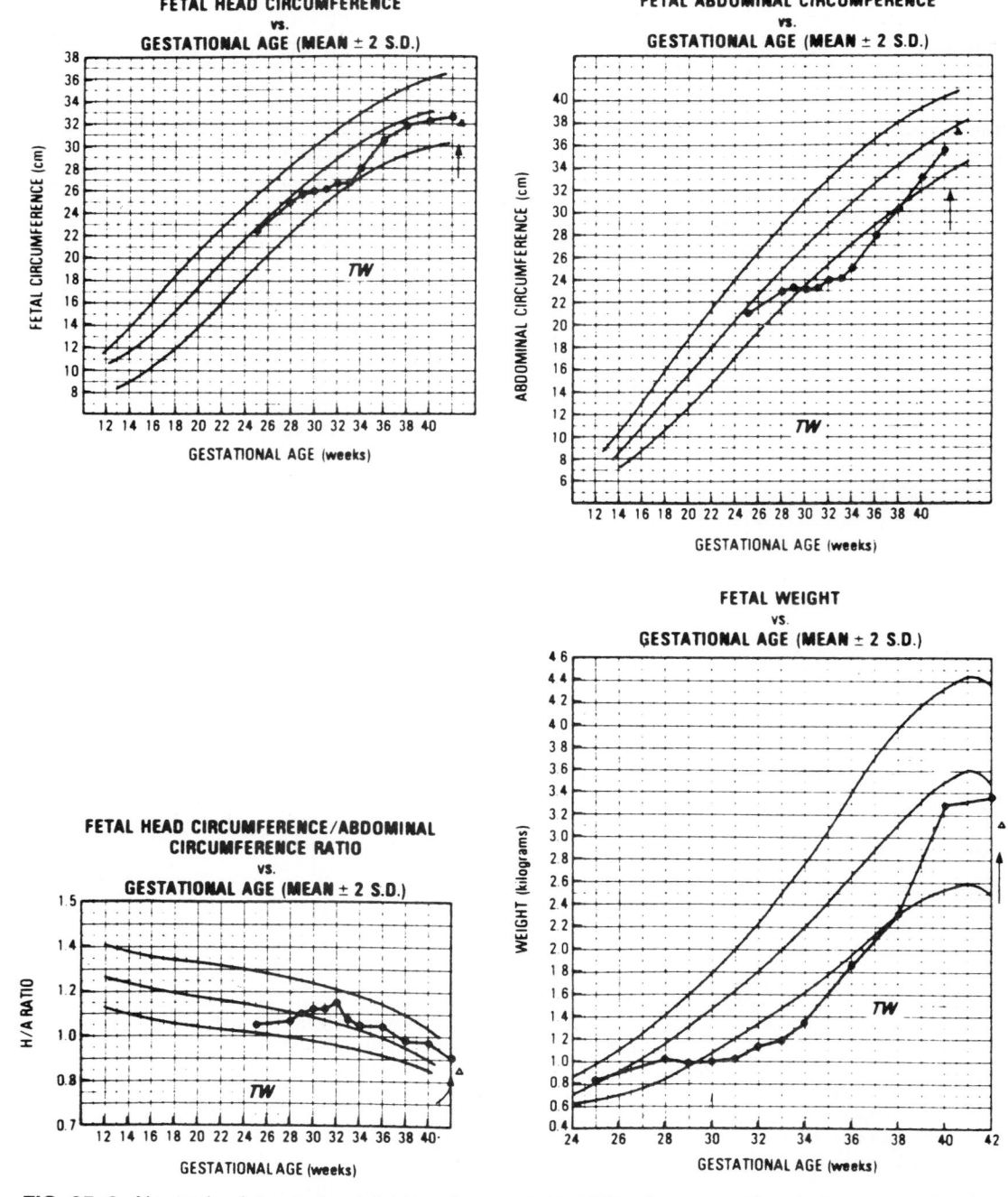

FIG. 25–6. Normative intrauterine fetal growth curves (solid lines) representing the mean ± 2 SD of a reference population of human fetuses with normal fetal growth rates according to ultrasound measurements, plus serial fetal body measurements in a mother with severe ulcerative colitis. Note that fetal growth (—•—) begins to decrease markedly in midgestation but returns to normal following the initiation of central hyperalimentation. (From Creasy RK, Resnik R. Intrauterine growth retardation. In: Creasy RK, Resnik R, eds. *Maternal-fetal medicine*, 2nd ed. Philadelphia: WB Saunders, 1989:558.)

nutrition, can inhibit fetal growth. Figure 25–6 shows an example of ultrasound data for fetal growth curves, including evidence for a particular fetus whose growth rate clearly was affected adversely by poor maternal health and beneficially by improved maternal nutrition. Further, fetal ultrasound-derived growth curves show less of the midgestational exponential increase in fetal growth rate that is typical of cross-sectional growth curves derived from neonatal measurements at different gestational ages. This observation strengthens the concept that, because preterm birth is not a normal outcome, one must be suspicious of growth parameters and growth curves derived from cross-sectional measurements of preterm infants assessed at birth. The intrauterine growth of these preterm infants probably was affected adversely by the same pathologic factors that led to their preterm birth. Thus, there probably is no ideal fetal growth curve derived from postbirth, cross-sectional measurements. Future growth curves to assess *in utero* growth of a specific newborn should be based instead on more thoroughly and accurately determined fetal growth parameters from ultrasound measurements in pregnancies with definitely known dates of conception and birth at term of normally grown and developed infants.

INTRAUTERINE GROWTH RESTRICTION AND PRETERM BIRTH

Most cases of fetal growth restriction represent only minimal growth delay and are natural, reproductively successful, although not perfect, adaptations to nutrient limitation. Most cases of IUGR, therefore, are not major causes of preterm delivery, and fetal growth rate and length of gestation usually are not related. In cases of severe IUGR, the pathophysiologic processes causing the IUGR also can lead to preterm labor and preterm delivery. Thus, IUGR frequently occurs with a variety of maternal conditions that are associated with preterm delivery (Table 25–1) (14–17).

Established maternal conditions that are associated with both IUGR and preterm delivery include very low maternal

TABLE 25–1. *Maternal conditions associated with intrauterine growth restriction and preterm delivery*

Both very young and advanced maternal age
Maternal prepregnancy short stature and thinness
Poor maternal weight gain during the latter third of
   pregnancy
Maternal illness during pregnancy
Nulliparity
Failure to obtain normal medical care during pregnancy
Lower socioeconomic status
Black race (in the United States)
Multiple gestation
Uterine and placental anomalies
Polyhydramnios
Preeclampsia
Diabetes
Intrauterine infections
Cigarette smoking, cocaine use, and other substance
   abuse

prepregnancy weight, prior preterm delivery, cigarette smoking, indirect effects of very young or advanced maternal age, and lower maternal socioeconomic status (14). Regarding race, African-American women who were born in the United States have a twofold greater incidence of both preterm birth and IUGR than do white women from the United States or African-American women who emigrated from Africa. Reasons for this are multifactorial and include nearly all of the generally associated risks and causes of IUGR and preterm delivery (15). Stretch-activated mechanisms probably induce preterm labor in cases of multiple gestation, uterine and placental space-occupying anomalies (e.g., fibroids), and polyhydramnios. Insufficient endometrial surface area for placental invasion and growth, plus abnormal placental perfusion, also combine to restrict nutrient delivery to the fetus, leading to IUGR. Poor placental growth and function limit placental supply of growth promoting hormones to the fetus, e.g., human placental lactogen (hPL), steroid hormones, and insulin-like growth factor-I (IGF-I) (18–20), and limit effective maternal–fetal nutrient exchange. In cases of polyhydramnios, IUGR often is related to the primary pathologic processes such as fetal infection, anemia, cardiac failure, and neuromuscular disorders. Intrauterine fetal infections can limit fetal growth by damaging the fetal brain and the neuroendocrine axis that support fetal growth via IGFs and insulin. Intrauterine infections also can damage the fetal heart, leading to diminished cardiac output, poor placental perfusion, and inadequate nutrient substrate uptake. Fetal infections and ascending infections of the membranes from the vagina also are associated with preterm delivery. They probably do this by enhancing the fetal supply of prostaglandins, which causes fetal and uterine production of various cytokines that are associated with or cause the onset of labor (21). Chronic placental and fetal infections also limit placental perfusion, in some cases by inhibition of nitric oxide production, which leads to uteroplacental vasoconstriction, placental insufficiency, and IUGR (22). Preeclamptic women have poor endometrial vascular support for growth of the placenta, leading to placental growth failure, fetal nutrient deficit, and IUGR (23). Fetal hypoglycemia, hypoxemia, and acidosis usually are present in such cases of poor placental development and perfusion. These factors lead to increased production of prostaglandins and the activation of labor-promoting cytokines, leading also to preterm delivery (24). Many of these cases are delivered preterm to protect the mother from eclampsia or the fetus from hypoxic–ischemic injury. Very young and very old women both produce IUGR infants who often are born prematurely. Nutritional, uterine, and vascular mechanisms may be common in these situations. Young stillgrowing adolescent girls appear less capable of mobilizing fat reserves in late pregnancy, apparently reserving them instead for their own continued development (25). Failure to mobilize such reserves can limit nutrient supply to the fetus and the rate of fetal growth (26). IUGR in cases of maternal smoking and substance abuse may be due to reduced placental blood flow, inhibition of uteroplacental vascular development, or direct fetal toxicity.

These examples illustrate that IUGR is commonly associated with conditions that also are related to preterm delivery. It is not surprising, therefore, and important to note, that IUGR is an increasingly common finding among infants born at earlier gestational ages. Whereas at term 10% of infants are classified as SGA, at less than 28 to 30 weeks gestational age, 30% to 40% of infants may be the result of IUGR (27).

FETAL GROWTH

The period of fetal growth is from the end of embryogenesis, at about the end of the first third of gestation, until term. During the embryonic period, growth occurs primarily by increased cell number (hyperplasia) (28). In the middle third of gestation, cell size also increases (hypertrophy), while the rate of cell division becomes stable. In the last third of gestation, the rate of cell division declines, while cell size continues to increase. Thus, insults that limit fetal growth in the embryonic period result in global reduction in fetal growth, whereas insults in the third part of gestation usually limit growth of fetal adipose tissue and skeletal muscle with less effect on the growth of other organs, especially the brain and heart (29).

GROWTH OF BODY COMPONENTS IN THE FETUS

Water

Fetal body water content, expressed as a fraction of body weight, decreases over gestation due to relative increases in protein and mineral accretion (Fig. 25–7) (30) and in humans because of the development of relatively large amounts of adipose tissue in the third trimester. Fetuses with marked IUGR and SGA neonates who have decreased body fat content have even lower fractional contents of body water. Extracellular water also decreases more than intracellular water as gestation advances, primarily because of increasing cell number and increasing cell size rather than the intracellular concentration of osmotic substances. Measurements of extracellular space in SGA infants usually are normal for gestational age, as adipose tissue, skeletal muscle, and mineral accretion all are decreased to about the same extent (31).

Minerals

Fetal calcium content in SGA and AGA fetuses increases exponentially with a linear increase in length, because bone density, area, and circumference increase exponentially in relation to linear growth (12). Accretion of other minerals varies more directly with body weight and according to the distribution of the minerals into extracellular (e.g., sodium) or intracellular (e.g., potassium) spaces (Table 25–2).

Nitrogen and Protein

There are very few chemical composition studies of normal human infants. Based on data from 15 studies accounting for 207 infants, nonfat dry weight and nitrogen content (predictors of protein content) show a linear relationship with fetal weight and an exponential relationship with gestational age (Fig. 25–8) (12,32). Table 25–3 shows nitrogen, protein, and selected amino acid composition and

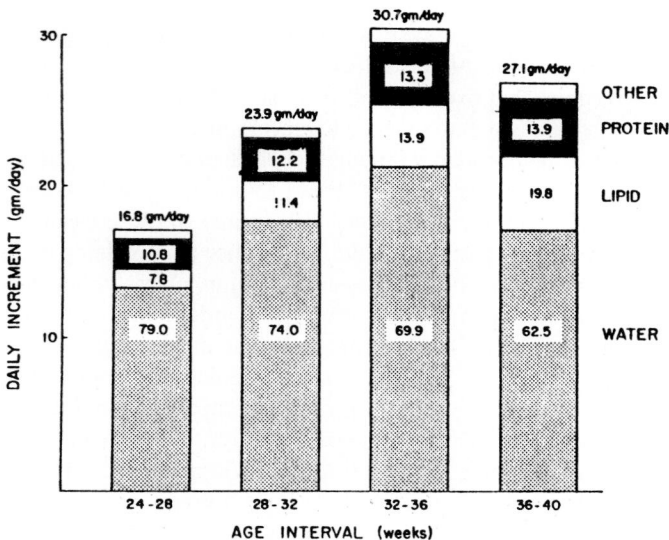

FIG. 25–7. Composition of weight gain in normal human fetuses. (From ref. 30.)

TABLE 25–2. *Chemical composition of the body of the developing fetus*

Body weight (g)	Approximate fetal age (wk)	Per kilogram whole body			Per kilogram fat-free body										
		Water (g)	Fat (g)	Water (g)	N (g)	Ca (g)	P (g)	Mg (g)	Na (mEq)	K (mEq)	Cl (mEq)	Fe (mg)	Cu (mg)	Zn (mg)
30	13	900	5	906	10	3.0	2.0	0.10	20	40	81	—	—	—
100	15	890	5	894	10	3.0	2.0	0.10	100	40	70	50	—	—
200	17	885	5	889	14	4.0	3.0	0.15	100	40	70	50	3.5	18
500	23	880	6	885	14	4.4	3.0	0.20	100	44	66	56	3.5	18
1,000	26	860	10	869	14	6.1	3.4	0.22	90	44	66	65	3.5	18
1,500	31	847	23	867	17	6.8	3.8	0.24	85	44	66	68	3.8	18
2,000	33	810	50	853	20	7.9	4.3	0.24	85	44	63	84	4.2	18
2,500	35	776	74	838	21	9.0	4.8	0.25	85	48	56	95	4.3	18
3,000	38	727	120	826	21	9.5	5.3	0.27	90	49	55	95	4.5	18
3,500	40	686	160	816	21	10.2	5.8	0.27	95	51	54	95	4.8	18

From ref. 32.

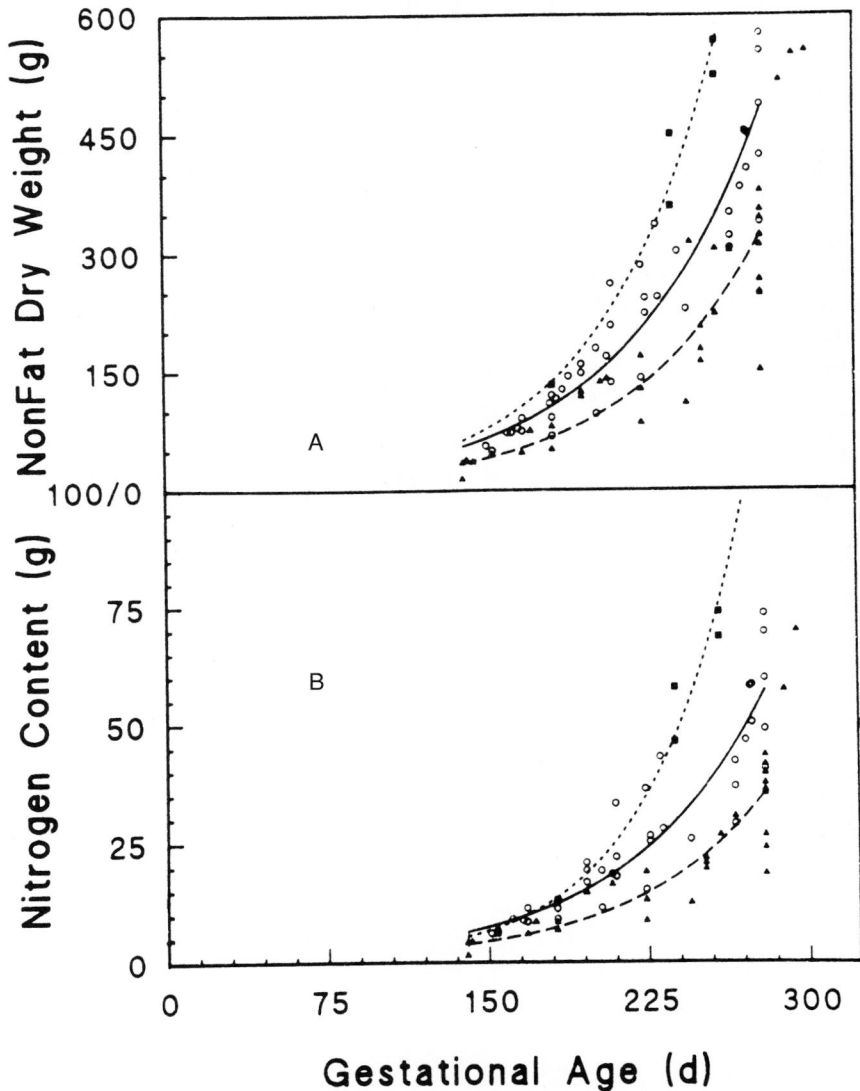

FIG. 25–8. Nonfat dry weight **(A)** and nitrogen content **(B)** versus gestational age. (■···) Large-for-gestational-age infants; (○——) average-for-gestational-age infants; (▲– –) small-for-gestational-age infants. (From ref. 12.)

TABLE 25–3. *Increments per day of nutrients in the fetal body at selected intervals during gestation*

Fetal age range (wk)	12–16	16–20	20–24	24–28	28–32	32–36	36–40
Weight range (kg)	0.02–0.1	0.1–0.3	0.3–0.75	0.75–1.35	1.35–2.0	2.0–2.7	2.7–3.4
Increments of nitrogen (N) and protein in fetal body per 24h							
Total N	29	93	243	326	386	504	714
Protein (gm) (N × 6.25)	0.18	0.58	1.52	2.04	2.41	3.15	4.46
Increments of individual amino acids in fetal body (mg/d)							
ILE	6	26	53	71	82	109	148
LEU	13	43	111	151	174	231	330
LYS	13	41	107	145	167	222	313
MET	4	11	28	39	44	59	92
PHE	7	23	61	83	95	127	184
TYR	5	17	44	59	68	91	127
THR	7	23	61	83	95	127	184
VAL	8	27	70	94	109	145	210
ARG	14	43	114	154	177	236	340
HIS	5	15	39	53	61	81	112
ALA	13	41	107	145	167	222	319
ASP	17	52	136	183	211	281	392
GLU	23	74	195	263	303	403	568
GLY	21	68	177	240	276	367	513
PRO	15	48	125	168	194	258	300
SER	8	25	66	89	102	136	191

From Widdowson EM. Chemical composition and nutritional needs of the fetus at different stages of gestation. In: Aebi H, Whitehead R, eds. *Maternal nutrition during pregnancy and lactation.* Berne: H. Huber, 1980:39–48.

accretion rates for normal human fetuses. About 80% of fetal nitrogen content is found in protein; the rest is found in urea, ammonia, and free amino acids. The data for fetal protein content and accretion in Table 25–3 thus may be high, as they are based solely on nitrogen content.

Nitrogen and Protein Accretion in Small-for-Gestational-Age Infants

Among SGA infants, nitrogen and protein contents are reduced for body weight, primarily due to deficient production of muscle mass. In fact, they often are reduced below that of fat as a fraction of body weight (33).

Glycogen

Many tissues in the fetus, including brain, liver, lung, heart, and skeletal muscle, produce glycogen over the second half of gestation (34). Liver glycogen content, which increases with gestation (Fig. 25–9), is the most important store of carbohydrate for systemic glucose needs, because only the liver contains sufficient glucose-6-phosphatase for release of glucose into the circulation. Skeletal muscle glycogen content increases during late gestation and forms a ready source of glucose for glycolysis within the myocytes. Lung glycogen content decreases in late gestation with change in cell type, leading to loss of glycogen-

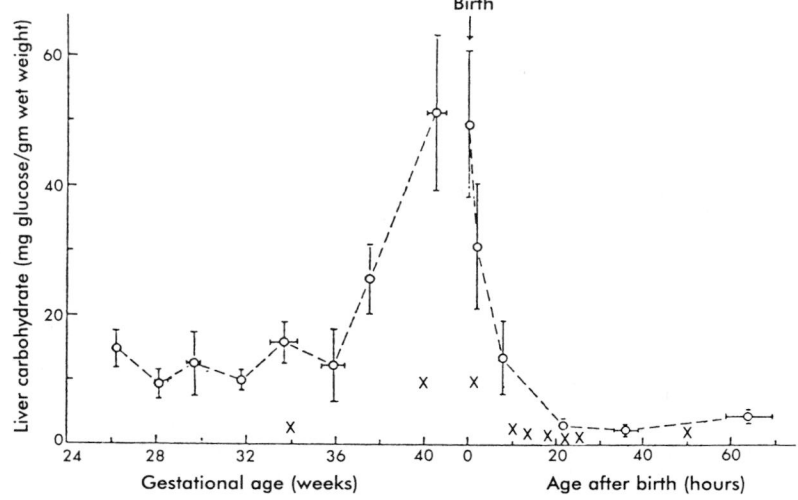

FIG. 25–9. Liver glycogen content (as carbohydrate) in normal human fetuses and newborn infants with normal birth weights for gestational age (O– –O; mean ± SEM) and infants of low birth weight for gestational age (X). (From Shelley HJ, Neligan GA. Neonatal hypoglycaemia. *Br Med Bull* 1966;22:34.)

containing alveolar epithelium, development of type II pneumocytes, and onset of surfactant production. Cardiac glycogen concentration decreases with gestation, owing to cellular hypertrophy, but cardiac glycogen appears essential for postnatal cardiac energy metabolism and contractile function. Glycogen synthesis rates are low in human fetuses, about 2 mg/d/g of liver, accounting for less than 5% of fetal glucose utilization (35). Net synthesis, degradation, and accumulation rates of fetal glycogen are controlled by the functional states of two enzymes, glycogen synthase, which promotes glycogen formation, and glycogen phosphorylase, which promotes glycogen degradation (34,36, 37). The total liver content of these two enzymes is relatively constant over gestation. Their functional states are regulated by hormone and substrate concentrations. For example, insulin acts synergistically with glucose to build hepatic glycogen stores, whereas close to term, cortisol, epinephrine, and glucagon develop the capacity to promote glycogenolysis and glucose release into the plasma.

Glycogen Deficiency in Small-for-Gestational-Age Infants

Glycogen content is markedly reduced in SGA infants, both in the liver and in the skeletal muscles (see Fig. 25–9) (34). This is due to lower fetal plasma concentrations of glucose and insulin, which are the principal regulators of glycogen synthesis. If the SGA fetus also experiences repeated episodes of hypoxemia, epinephrine secretion in response will further deplete glycogen by activating glycogen phosphorylase and increasing glycogenolysis.

Adipose Tissue

At term, fetal fat content, expressed as a fraction of fetal weight, varies markedly among species (Fig. 25–10) (37). The fat content of newborns of almost all land mammals at term is 1% to 3%, which is considerably less than the 15% to 20% fat content of human term infants. Even in those species, such as the human, that take up fat from the placenta and deposit fat in fetal tissues, the rate of fetal fatty

acid oxidation is presumed low. This condition occurs because plasma concentrations of fatty acids (and keto acid products, such as β-hydroxybutyrate and acetoacetate) are low, and because the carnitine palmitoyl transferase enzyme system is not sufficiently developed to deliver long-chain fatty acids to the respiration pathway inside the mitochondria. Fat accretion for the human fetus is shown in Fig. 25–11. Between 26 and 30 weeks of gestation, nonfat and fat components contribute equally to the carbon content of the fetal body (12,38). After that period, fat accumulation exceeds that of the nonfat components. By term, the deposition of fat accounts for more than 90% of the carbon accumulated by the fetus. The rate of fat accretion is approximately linear between 36 and 40 weeks of gestation, and, by the end of gestation, fat accretion ranges between 1.6 and 3.4 g/d/kg. At 28 weeks of gestation, it is slightly less and ranges between 1.0 and 1.8 g/d/kg.

Adipose Tissue Deficiency in Small-for-Gestational-Age Infants

By term, fat content in human fetuses with IUGR may be less than 10% of body weight (33). In these cases, the smaller placenta limits fetal fatty acid and triglyceride supply. Similarly, the smaller placenta decreases fetal glucose supply, which reduces glycerol production and triglyceride synthesis. Insulin deficiency, a result of decreased glucose and amino acid supply to the fetus, also limits fat synthesis. The insulin activation of peripheral lipoprotein lipase is thereby reduced, which normally is necessary to release fatty acids from circulating lipoproteins for adipocyte uptake and triglyceride synthesis, and to decrease the normal insulin stimulation of fatty acid synthase within adipocytes.

Calories (Total Energy Storage)

The energy value of various tissue components is shown in Table 25–4. Fat has a high energy content, 9.5 kcal/g, and a very high carbon content, approximately 78%. Thus, differences in fetal fat concentration lead to large differ-

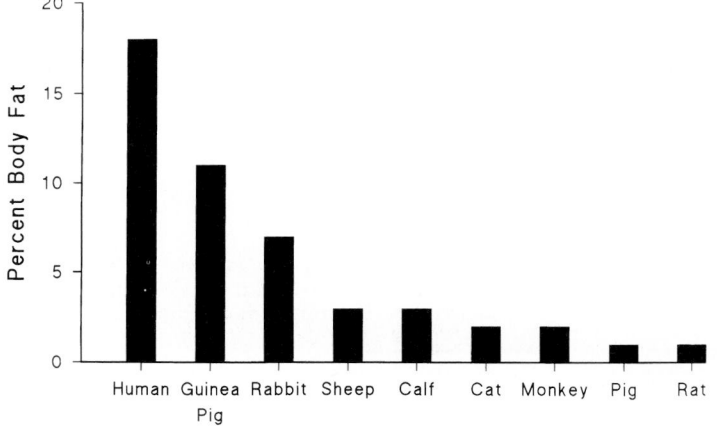

FIG. 25–10. Fetal fat content at term as a percent of fetal body weight among species. (From ref. 37.)

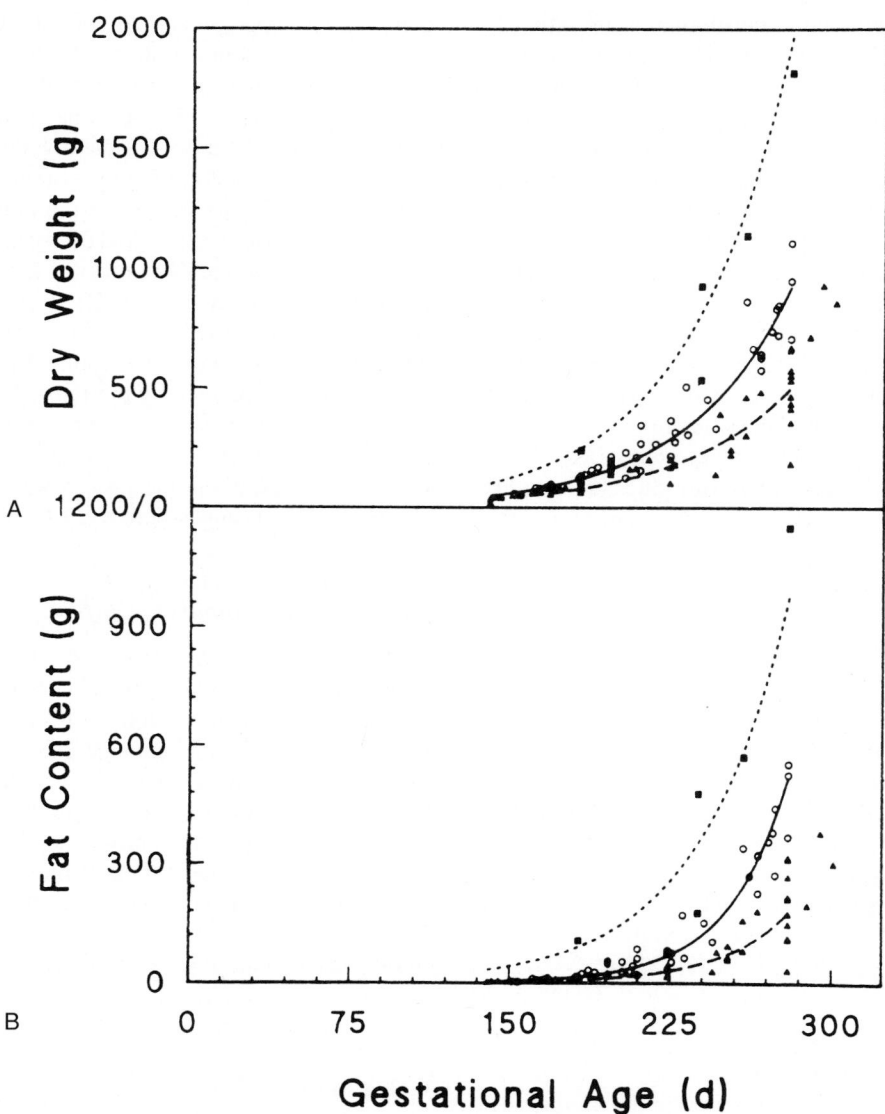

FIG. 25–11. Dry weight **(A)** and fat content **(B)** plotted against gestational age in the same newborn human infants shown in Fig. 25–7 for large-for-gestational-age (■....), average-for-gestational-age (○——), and small-for-gestational-age (▲– –) infants. (From ref. 12.)

TABLE 25–4. *Energy value of human tissue components*

Tissue component	Energy value (kcal/g)[a]
H_2O	0
Fat	9.45
Nonfat dry weight	
Pig	4.0–4.6
Lamb	4.4–4.6
Guinea pig	4.6
Carbohydrate	4.15 (3.7–4.2)
Protein	5.65
In vivo catabolism	4.35

[a]1 kcal = 4,190 J.
From ref. 46.

TABLE 25–5. *Calculation of the caloric distribution in the term human infant*[a]

	Wet weight	Fat	Nonfat wet weight	Nonfat dry weight
Weight (g)	3,450	386	3,064	511
Total calories (kcal)	5,950	3,650	2,300	2,300
Caloric concentration (kcal/g)	1.73	9.45	0.75	4.5

[a]Data from ref. 30.

ences in calculated caloric accretion rates and carbon requirements of the fetal tissues for growth. The caloric concentration of nonfat dry weight is fairly consistent at different developmental stages, indicating that the ratio of protein to nonprotein substrates in the tissues is relatively constant (Table 25–5). Thus, caloric accretion rate of any fetus can be estimated from the growth curve of the fetus and the changing fat and water concentrations (38).

Caloric Accretion Deficiency in Small-for-Gestational-Age Infants

Growth of fat and nonfat (protein plus other) tissues is metabolically linked through energy supply that is used for protein synthesis and the production of anabolic hormones (39). These promote positive protein, fat, and carbohydrate growth. Thus, restriction of nutrient supply is likely to produce growth deficits of all tissues, not just fat. Indeed, growth restriction involves limitation of muscle growth as well as fat and glycogen (33). For example, chronic selective caloric (glucose) restriction in the experimental fetal sheep model leads to increased protein breakdown as well as lower rates of fetal growth and lipid content (40). Some growth curves, such as those shown in Figs. 25–9 and 25–11 from human infants born prematurely at different times over the last third of gestation, show a bias toward thinner SGA infants with less fat relative to nonfat weight and nitrogen content (32). These infants, however, were stillborn and may have suffered extensive wasting and IUGR. Other studies have shown that human SGA infants can be markedly deficient in muscle mass, even more than for fat (33,41).

REGULATION OF FETAL GROWTH

Fetal growth is regulated by maternal, placental, and fetal factors, representing a mix of genetic mechanisms and environmental influences through which genetic growth potential is expressed and modulated.

Epidemiologic Considerations

The major maternal risk factors for IUGR that vary among populations and among individuals within populations include small maternal size (height and prepregnancy weight) and low maternal weight gain during preg-

nancy. Low maternal body mass index (the degree of thinness or fatness, defined as [weight (kg)]/[height (cm)]²) is a major predicator of IUGR. This characteristic interacts with other risk factors, such as diet, smoking, illnesses, and so forth, to affect fetal growth, especially in thin women. For example, smoking has only half the impact on fetal growth in obese versus thin women, and in black versus white women (42). Low blood pressure has a detrimental impact on fetal growth, mostly in thin women (43). Moderate obesity, therefore, protects against most growth-inhibiting risk factors except for black race and female gender. This pattern also holds for certain therapies. For example, zinc supplementation has a major impact on fetal growth in black women who have relatively low plasma zinc levels early in pregnancy, with all of the impact occurring in relatively thin women (44). Also, low-dose maternal aspirin treatment has been shown to improve fetal growth primarily in thin women (45).

Genetic Factors

Many genes contribute to fetal growth. Table 25–6 lists estimates of the quantitative contribution of fetal and parental factors to fetal growth and birth weight at term. Maternal genotype is more important than fetal genotype in the overall regulation of fetal growth. However, the paternal genotype is essential for trophoblast development, which secondarily regulates fetal growth by the provision of nutrients. More specific gene targeting studies have shown the importance of genomic imprinting on fetal growth. For example, normal fetal and placental growth in mice require that the IGF-II gene be paternal and the IGF-II receptor gene be maternal, whereas maternal disomy producing IGF-II underexpression results in fetal dwarfism (39).

Nongenetic Maternal Factors

Under usual conditions, fetal growth follows its genetic potential, unless the mother is unusually small and limits fetal growth by a variety of factors considered collectively

TABLE 25–6. *Factors determining variance in birth weight*

	Percent of total variance
Fetal	
Genotype	16
Sex	2
Total	18
Maternal	
Genotype	20
Maternal environment	24
Maternal age	1
Parity	7
Total	52
Unknown	30

Derived from Penrose LS. Proceedings of the Ninth International Congress of Genetics Part 1, 520, 1954.
From ref. 39.

as "maternal constraint." Maternal constraint represents a relatively limited uterine size, including placental implantation surface area and uterine circulation, and thus the capacity to support placental growth and nutrient supply to the fetus. A clear example of maternal constraint is the reduced rate of fetal growth of multiple fetuses in a species—human—that optimally supports only one fetus (Fig. 25–12). Obviously, small fetuses of small parents do not reflect fetal growth restriction; in fact, their rates of growth are normal for their genome and for the size of the mother. Unless maternal constraint is particularly prominent, such fetuses would not grow faster or to a larger size if more nutrients were provided, although they might grow somewhat larger if the maternal uterine endometrial surface area, and thus placental implantation and growth area, were increased. The nongenetic, maternal nature of this effect has been demonstrated by embryo transfer and cross-breeding experiments (29). For example, a small-breed embryo transplanted into a large-breed uterus will grow larger than a small-breed embryo remaining in a small-breed uterus. Furthermore, partial reduction in fetal number in a polytocous species, such as the rat, produces greater than normal birth weights in the remaining offspring. Conversely, embryo transfer of a large-breed embryo into a small-breed uterus will result in a newborn that is smaller than in its natural large-breed environment. Such evidence supports the concept that fetal growth is normally constrained, and this constraint comes from the maternal environment, i.e., the size of the uterus.

Maternal Nutrition

The single most important environmental influence that affects fetal growth is the nutrition of the fetus. Normal variations in maternal nutrition, however, have relatively little impact on fetal growth and the severity of IUGR. This is because changes in maternal nutrition, unless extreme

and prolonged, do not markedly alter maternal plasma concentrations of nutrient substrates or the rate of uterine blood flow, the principal determinants of nutrient substrate delivery and transport to the fetus by the placenta (46). Human epidemiologic data from conditions of prolonged starvation, as well as nutritional deprivation in experimental animals, indicate that severe limitations in maternal nutrition limit fetal growth only by 10% to 20%. Epidemiologic data from the Dutch during the Hunger Winter of 1944 showed an average reduction in fetal weight at term of 300 g (47), whereas birth weight at term was reduced by 500 g in women who suffered a more severe and prolonged famine in wartime Leningrad (48). Interestingly, second-generation daughters of women who suffered extreme nutritional deficit during gestation in turn tend to produce SGA infants who are 200 to 300 g less than normal at term with their first pregnancies (49). However, attempts to limit weight gain in pregnancy with a 1,200-kcal diet (50% of what is now recommended to prevent preeclampsia) increased the incidence of fetal growth restriction up to tenfold (50). Restrictions of calorie and protein intakes to less than 50% of normal for a considerable portion of gestation are needed before marked reductions in fetal growth are observed. Such severe conditions often result in fetal loss before the impact of fetal growth rate in late gestation and fetal size at birth are manifested.

Attempts to increase fetal weight gain with maternal nutritional supplements have produced mixed results. Higher caloric feeding usually increases fetal adiposity, not growth of muscle mass or gain in length or head circumference. In contrast, high protein supplements tend to produce delayed fetal growth (51). Mechanisms responsible for this phenomenon are not known.

Maternal Chronic Diseases

Chronic hypertension, pregnancy-induced hypertension, and preeclampsia, like other vascular disorders including severe and long-standing diabetes mellitus and serious autoimmune disease associated with the lupus anticoagulant, have a common effect of limiting trophoblast invasion, placental growth and development, uteroplacental blood flow, and fetal oxygen and nutrient deficiency (52). Maternal cyanotic congenital heart disease can limit fetal oxygen supply, which can limit fetal growth (53). High-altitude hypoxia also can limit fetal growth (54), but usually this is only clinically significant for nonindigenous women who move to altitudes above 10,000 feet. Severe sickle cell crises can damage uterine vasculature, leading to placental growth and transport capacities (55).

Maternal Drugs

Specific effects of drugs on fetal growth (Table 25–7) are often difficult to sort out clinically, as many women who abuse drugs do so with many drugs taken intermittently, at different doses, and at different periods of fetal vulnerability. These women also frequently suffer from

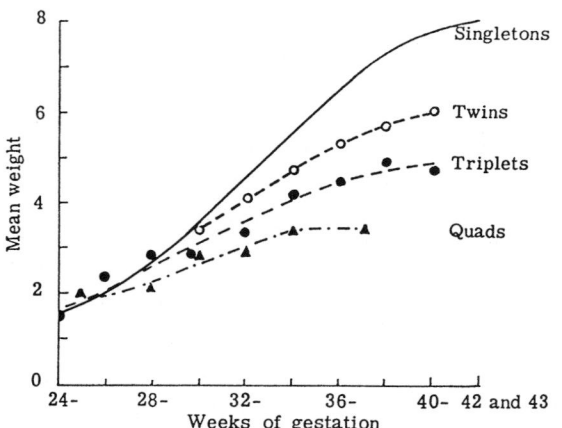

FIG. 25–12. Mean birth weight of single and multiple fetuses related to duration of gestation. (Adapted from McKeown T, Record RG. Observations on foetal growth in multiple pregnancy in man. *J Endocrinol* 1952;8:386.)

TABLE 25–7. *Drugs associated with intrauterine growth restriction*

Amphetamines
Antimetabolites (e.g., aminopterin, busulfan, methotrexate)
Bromides
Cocaine
Ethanol
Heroin and other narcotics, such as morphine and methadone
Hydantoin
Isotretinoin
Metals such as mercury and lead
Phencyclidine
Polychlorinated biphenyls (PCBs)
Propranalol
Steroids
Tobacco (carbon monoxide, nicotine, thiocyante)
Toluene
Trimethadione
Warfarin

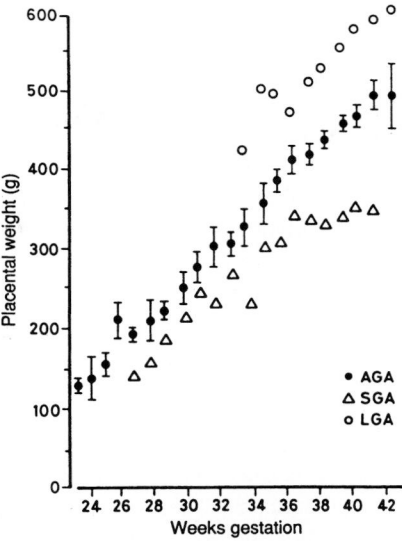

FIG. 25–13. Mean placental weights for large-for-gestational-age (○), average-for-gestational-age (●), and small-for-gestational-age (△) human infants at each gestational age. ± SEM given for AGA infants alone. (Modified from ref. 59.)

other disorders that could lead to poor fetal growth, such as poor nutrition, recurrent acute illnesses, and chronic diseases (56). Fetal growth restriction does appear to be a major part of the fetal alcohol syndrome. It is not clear when during gestation the specific effects of alcohol on fetal growth rate occur. Alcohol may exert its nonteratogenic effects by limiting placental-to-fetal amino acid transport (57). Cocaine probably exerts its primary effects on producing fetal growth restriction by causing uterine and perhaps umbilical vasoconstriction and reduced placental perfusion (58). The most consistent drug reducing fetal growth is cigarette smoking (41). Deficits of at least 300 g (about 10% of normal term weight) are not uncommon. A likely common mechanisms is the effect of nicotine, and of catecholamines released in response, to constrict the uterine and perhaps the umbilical vasculature, reducing placental perfusion. Carbon monoxide, cyanide, and other cellular toxins may limit oxygen transport to fetal tissues as well as cellular respiration.

Placenta

The size of the placenta and its directly related nutrient transport functions are the principal regulators of nutrient supply to the fetus and thus the rate of fetal growth (36). Nearly all cases of IUGR are associated with a smaller-than-normal placenta. Figure 25–13 shows a direct relationship between fetal weight and placental weight in humans, demonstrating that LGA, AGA, and SGA infants are directly associated with LGA, AGA, and SGA placentas (59). Placental growth normally precedes fetal growth, and failure of placental growth is directly associated with decreased fetal growth. Variable limitations in placental nutrient transfer capacity modulate this primary effect of placental size on fetal growth. In some cases of experimentally reduced placental size, for example, fetal weight is not reduced proportionately (60). This indicates that either the capacity of the smaller placenta to transport nutrients to the

fetus increases adaptively or the fetus develops increased capacity to grow. More characteristically, though, fetal growth fails first, or in direct relation to decreased nutrient supply. With primary fetal growth failure, placental growth can increase disproportionately, resulting in a larger than normal placental-to-fetal weight ratio for gestational age. This is characteristically seen under chronic hypoxic conditions of high altitude exposure or maternal anemia and has been seen in certain experimental situations of maternal undernutrition in early gestation (61). A variety of placental pathologic conditions are associated with IUGR (Table 25–8). In most of these cases, the placenta is simply smaller than normal. In many, there also is abnormal tro-

TABLE 25–8. *Placental growth disorders that lead to or are associated with intrauterine growth restriction*

Abnormal umbilical vascular insertions (circumvallate, velamentous)
Abruption (chronic, partial)
Avascular villi
Decidual arteritis
Fibrinosis, atheromatous changes, cytotrophoblast hyperplasia, basement membrane thickening
Infectious villitis (as with TORCH infections)
Ischemic villous necrosis and umbilical vascular thromboses
Multiple gestation (limited endometrial surface area, vascular anastomoses)
Multiple infarcts
Partial molar pregnancy
Placenta previa
Single umbilical artery
Spiral artery vasculitis, failed or limited erosion into intervillous space
Syncytial knots
Tumors, including chorioangioma and hemangiomas

phoblast development, including abnormal vascular growth in the trophoblast villi, frequently associated with limited uterine vascular perfusion of the intervillous spaces.

Placental and fetal growth both depend on an adequate supply of maternal blood to the placenta. IUGR is associated with inadequate development of the uteroplacental circulation, and radioisotope studies have demonstrated more than a twofold blood flow reduction in comparison with normal pregnancies (62). IUGR in the second half of gestation is due primarily to a failure of the normal villous vascular tree, mainly in the phase of nonbranching angiogenesis, because terminal villi are critical for oxygen and nutrient transport to the fetus (63). This angiogenesis in turn depends on cytotrophoblast invasion of the uterus and its arterioles. Cytotrophoblast invasion is actually a differentiation process whereby the cells lose the ability to proliferate and modulate their expression of state-specific antigens. These antigens include members of the integrin family of cell–extracellular matrix receptors that are required for migration and invasion of the endometrium and decidua of the uterus (64). Preeclampsia, which is associated with IUGR, is characterized by shallow cytotrophoblast invasion (65). Abnormal cytotrophoblast differentiation also occurs, evidenced by the cells' inability to switch on their integrin repertoire (66). The same observations have been made on cultured normal cytotrophoblast cells in a hypoxic environment (67). These *in vitro* results indicate that whatever leads to hypoxia of the invading cytotrophoblast cells increases cytotrophoblast proliferation over differentiation and invasion, thus setting the stage for deficient placental development that can result in deficient nutrient and growth factor supply to the fetus, producing fetal growth restriction.

At more advanced stages of placental development, placental production of growth factors and growth regulating hormones develops, leading to significant autocrine regulation of placental growth and placental regulation of fetal growth processes. Human placental lactogen is synthesized and secreted by the syncytiotrophoblast cells of the placenta (68). Fetal growth-promoting actions of placental lactogen are mediated by stimulation of IGF production in the fetus and by increasing the availability of nutrients to fetal tissues (69). Obviously, placental growth failure and/or nutrient deficit to the placenta can result in decreased placental production of growth factors that then would lead to fetal growth failure.

FETAL NUTRIENT UPTAKE AND METABOLISM AND REGULATION OF FETAL GROWTH

In general, decreased rates of fetal growth represent an "adaptation" to inadequate nutrient supply. IUGR that results from decreased nutrient supply can be interpreted, therefore, as a successful, if not perfect, adaptation to maintain fetal survival. Fetal undernutrition also appears to affect rapidly growing fetuses more than slowly growing fetuses who may have been programmed to grow more slowly for genetic or embryonic and early fetal pathologic reasons (70). Reintroduction of nutrients can return fetal growth to normal in those fetuses whose rapid growth rate was decreased by undernutrition, but too rapid an introduction of nutrients has often caused fetal pathology, including hyperlactatemia (70) and occasionally even acidosis and hypoxemia.

Glucose Uptake, Metabolism, and Regulation of Fetal Growth

Nearly all IUGR fetuses, whether studied experimentally in animal models or in women by cordocentesis (direct umbilical blood sampling), have relatively lower plasma glucose concentrations compared with normally grown fetuses (71,72). Fetal "hypoglycemia" has several consequences important to fetal adaptation and survival when maternal glucose supply is limited. First, relative fetal hypoglycemia is an important and natural compensatory mechanism that helps to maintain the maternal-to-fetal glucose concentration gradient and thus the transport of glucose across the placenta to the fetus (73). Despite this compensation, fetal hypoglycemia limits tissue glucose uptake directly by diminished mass action and indirectly by limiting fetal insulin secretion and thus the effect of insulin to promote tissue glucose uptake by skeletal muscle, heart, adipose tissue, and liver. Insulin also normally suppresses hepatic glucose production and release, and it acts as an anabolic hormone that increases net protein balance by inhibiting protein breakdown. Thus, a decrease in fetal plasma insulin concentration initially may allow fetal glucose production to take place, thereby providing glucose for both fetal and placental needs, but subsequently, combined with hypoglycemia, results in increased protein breakdown and decreased protein accretion (39,74,75).

Circulating concentrations and tissue-specific expression of growth factors such as IGF-I and IGF-II (see following) also are decreased during fetal hypoglycemia (76), which may contribute to increased fetal protein breakdown and decreased rates of fetal growth. Thus, fetal hypoglycemia in response to a decrease in maternal glucose supply acts to maintain fetal glucose supply, but it also leads to lower anabolic hormone concentrations, which limit the rate of fetal growth, thereby decreasing fetal nutrient needs.

Fetal Amino Acid Metabolism

The placenta contains a large variety of amino acid transporters, most of which use energy to actively concentrate amino acids in the trophoblast, which then diffuse into the fetal plasma, producing higher concentrations than in the maternal plasma (77). With small placentas, fetal amino acid supply is reduced, as are fetal amino acid concentrations, fetal protein synthesis, fetal protein and nitrogen balance, and, ultimately, fetal growth rate. Reduced energy supply to the placenta also reduces amino acid transport to the fetus. This is especially the case for oxygen deficit, either from primary hypoxemia or from reduced uteroplacental blood flow, and glucose deficit from chronic maternal and fetal hypoglycemia (78,79). Of course, hypoxemia and hypoglycemia could reduce fetal growth independently of reduced amino acid transport, for example, by limiting anabolic hormone and growth factor production or by decreasing energy supply, both of which are necessary to produce protein synthesis and to limit protein breakdown in fetal tissues.

The reason why amino acid and energy supplies are so important for fetal protein and nitrogen balance and for fetal growth is illustrated in Fig. 25–14. This figure shows results of experiments in fetal sheep over the second half of gestation, comparing fractional protein synthesis rates derived from tracer amino acid data and fractional body growth rates derived from carcass analysis data. The fractional rate of protein turnover per unit wet weight of fetus is several fold higher at 50% to 60% of term gestation (equivalent to about 20 to 24 weeks of human gestation). Such high rates of protein turnover require a much greater rate of amino acid supply and energy than at term, when fetal protein turnover rate is much lower. Indeed, in midgestation fetal sheep, glucose utilization rates per whole fetal weight and oxygen consumption rates per dry fetal weight are much higher in the early fetus than at term (80). These conditions result in a 50% higher rate of net protein accretion and fractional rate of fetal growth at midgestation than

at term. Clearly, amino acid and energy deficits will affect the growth rate of the fetus at earlier stages of gestation, when fetal growth normally is very rapid much more than at term, when fetal growth rate is slower.

In the normally growing fetus, net protein synthesis exceeds net protein breakdown, resulting in net protein accretion. The mechanisms underlying the reduction in protein synthesis rate over gestation appear to be intrinsic to the fetus, and not to limitation of nutrient supply by the placenta. These mechanisms include changing proportions of the organs as fractions of body mass (Table 25–9).

Fetal Endocrine and Autocrine/Paracrine-Acting Growth Factor Effects on Fetal Growth

Table 25–10 lists those hormones whose deficiency results in a reduction in fetal growth supported by experimental evidence (81). These fetal hormones promote growth (and development) *in utero* by altering both the metabolism and gene expression of fetal tissues. These hormonal actions ensure that fetal growth rate is commensurate with nutrient supply.

Insulin

Insulin has direct mitogenic effects on cellular development and thus can regulate cell number. It also enhances glucose consumption by many cells, particularly in muscle, and limits protein breakdown (75). The latter effects are associated with reduced fetal growth when insulin concentration is low. This has been produced directly by experimental surgical (82) and chemical (83) ablation of the pancreas and/or the function of the pancreatic beta cells to secrete insulin, and has been observed clinically in infants who suffer pancreatic agenesis (84). Figure 25–15 shows reduced rates of growth in fetal sheep that underwent surgical pancreatectomy and a return to normal rates of growth with insulin replacement. Much of the growth reduction with hypoinsulinemia from pancreatectomy is caused by a release of insulin's normal inhibitory role on glucose production, resulting in fetal hyperglycemia, a secondary

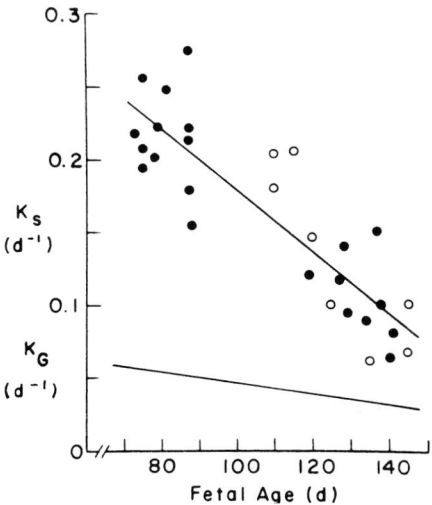

FIG. 25–14. Fractional rate of protein synthesis (K_s) over gestation in fetal sheep studied with leucine (●) and lysine (○) radioactive tracers compared with the fractional rate of growth (K_G) in the lower portion of the figure (——). (From ref. 77. Adapted from refs. 46 and 80, and from Meier PR, Peterson RG, Bonds DR, Meschia G, Battaglia FC. Rates of protein synthesis and turnover in fetal life. *Am J Physiol* 1981;240:E320.)

TABLE 25–9. *Percent contribution of organs and tissues to the body weight of human fetuses and newborn infants*

	Fetus (20–24 wk)	Full-term infant
Skeletal muscle	25	25
Skin	13	15
Skeleton	22	18
Heart	0.6	0.5
Liver	4	5
Kidneys	0.7	1
Brain	13	13

After Widdowson EM. Growth and composition of the fetus and newborn. In: Assali NS, ed. *Gestation.* New York: Academic Press, 1968:27.

TABLE 25–10. *Effects of specific endocrine deficiencies on body weight and crown–rump length, and individual tissues adversely affected by treatment in sheep fetuses delivered near term (>95% gestation)*

Endocrine deficiency	Procedure	Gestational age at onset (d)	Body weight	Crown–rump length	Tissues with specific developmental abnormalities
Insulin	Streptozotocin	70–85	↓50%	↓20%	None
	Pancreatectomy	115–120	↓30%	↓15%	None
Thyroid hormones	Thyroidectomy	80–96	↓30%	↓10%	Skeleton, skin, lungs, nervous system
		105–115	↓20%	↓10%	Skeleton, nervous system
Adrenal hormones	Adrenalectomy	110–120	↑10–15%	No change	Liver, lungs, gut, pituitary
Pituitary hormones	Hypophysectomy	70–79	↓30%	↓8%	Bones, liver, lungs, placenta
		105–110	↓20%	↓10%	Bones, liver, lungs, placenta, adrenal, gonads
		110–125	No change to ↓5%	No change	Bones, gonads, adrenal, liver
	Pituitary stalk section	108–112	↓15%	No change	Adrenals, other tissues?

From Fowden AL. Endocrine regulation of fetal growth. In: Harding R, Genkin G, Grant A, eds. Progress in perinatal physiology. *Reprod Fertil Dev* 1995;7:50.

decrease in the maternal–fetal glucose concentration gradient, and thus a decrease in glucose transport to the fetus. Without this glucose, fetal growth decreases, as has been shown by a direct decrease in glucose uptake by the fetus following the production of chronic maternal hypoglycemia (85). Fetal amino acid uptake decreases under the same circumstances. Thus, insulin deficiency, directly and indirectly, results in a decrease in fetal nutrient supply. Initially,

fetal protein breakdown results in fetal amino acid release for energy (via direct amino acid oxidation in the tricarboxylic [citric] acid cycle) and glucose production. Later on, the reduced rate of fetal growth during conditions of low insulin, glucose, and amino acid concentrations is sustained by increased protein breakdown (40); however, amino acids are used to maintain protein turnover rate and not for protein accretion, oxidation, or glucose production.

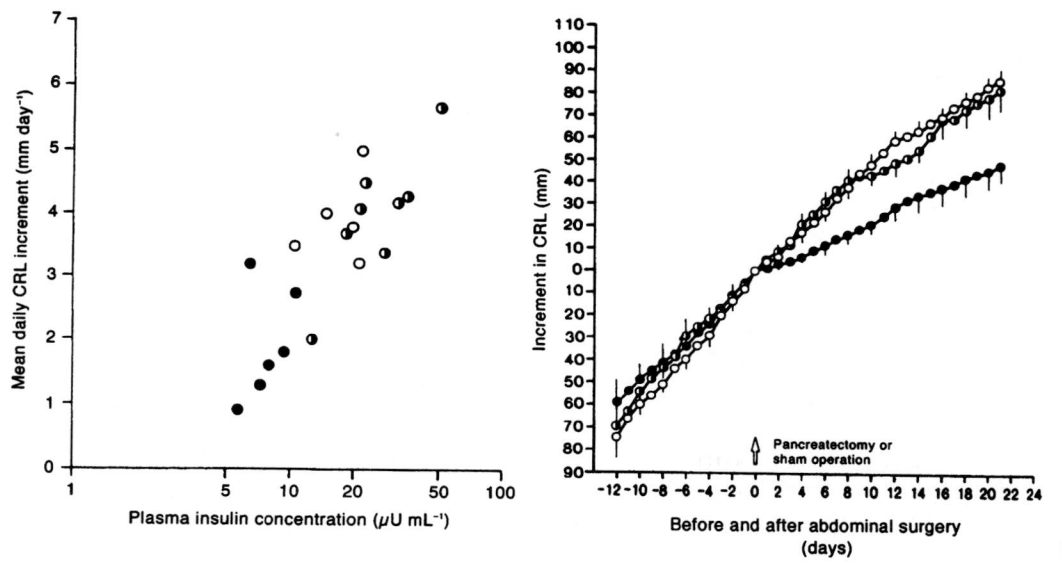

FIG. 25–15. Relationship between growth and plasma insulin concentrations in the sheep fetus. **A:** Mean daily crown–rump length (CRL) increment with respect to plasma insulin concentration in individual sheep fetuses [sham operated (○); pancreatectomized (●); pancreatectomized and given insulin treatment (◑)]. **B:** Daily increment in CRL with respect to time before and after abdominal surgery in fetuses that were sham-operated (○), pancreatectomized (●), and pancreatectomized and given insulin treatment to restore normal insulin concentrations (◑). (Data from Fowden AL. The role of insulin in prenatal growth. *J Dev Physiol* 1989;12:173. From Fowden AL. Endocrine regulation of fetal growth. In: Harding R, Genkin G, Grant A, eds. Progress in perinatal physiology. *Reprod Fertil Dev* 1995;7:50.)

Insulin-Like Growth Factor-I

IGF-I is positively regulated by glucose supply in the fetus. Infusion of IGF-I into fetal sheep decreases protein breakdown, especially when protein breakdown is increased by fasting-induced hypoglycemia. Metabolic effects of a decreased plasma concentration of IGF-I have not been studied, although, as for insulin, such effects might be difficult to separate from simultaneous changes in nutrient substrate supply and concentration. Thus, IGF-I probably can regulate metabolic processes that affect fetal protein balance and growth, but these have been difficult to measure.

Plasma IGF-I concentrations are positively related to fetal size at birth. A causative role for IGF-I has been shown by the production of transgenic models of mice that have shown that decreased expression of IGF-I results in markedly reduced rates of fetal growth. Other transgenic models with increased expression of IGF-I have been associated with increased brain growth (86,87), and this growth can be inhibited by overexpression of IGF binding protein-1 (IGFBP-1) (88). IGF-I stimulates an increase in oligodendrocytes and neuronal number, as well as neuronal outgrowth with increased dendritic arborization and axon terminal fields (89). Because IGF-I is decreased directly by reduced nutrient supply, particularly glucose, and IGFBP-1 is decreased under these circumstances, the smaller, more densely packed neuronal structure of the undernourished brain that is seen in some infants with severe IUGR may have been mediated by nutrient regulation of IGF-I and IGFBP-1 expression. Such developmental limitations might underlie the poorer neurodevelopmental outcome of severely SGA infants who have relative microcephaly.

Insulin-Like Growth Factor-II, Insulin-Like Growth Factor Binding Protein-2, Insulin-Like Growth Factor Binding Protein-3, and Vasoactive Intestinal Polypeptide

Although serum concentrations of IGF-II do not correlate with fetal size at birth in human infants, it has been shown conclusively that targeted mutation of the IGF-II gene reduces fetal size in mice (90,91). Furthermore, IGF-II is the predominant IGF expressed in the tissues of embryos and fetuses of all species. As with IGF-I and IGFBP-1, transgenic overexpression of IGF-II and IGFBP-2 shows that cellular growth is dependent on the balance between the binding protein and the IGF molecule itself. IGFBP-3 is the predominant IGF binding protein in several mammalian species including humans (92,93) and is reduced in cord blood of infants with IUGR (94). Vasoactive intestinal peptide (VIP) is another growth factor in the fetus that affects neuronal and whole body growth (95–97). Antagonists to VIP in pregnant mice produce smaller fetuses that are particularly microcephalic (98), with central nervous system neurons that show reduced mitosis and migration. These effects of VIP occur in the first half of gestation, coincident with transiently high VIP concentrations in the maternal plasma (99).

Thyroid Hormones

In all species, fetal thyroid hormone deficiency produces developmental abnormalities in certain tissues. When maternal thyroid hormones cannot compensate, as in the sheep, which does not transport maternal thyroid hormones to the fetus, fetal growth restriction develops, primarily reflecting deficient carcass growth (skin, bone, and muscle) (81). This growth restriction results from both hypoplasia (in muscle) and hypotrophy (in lung). More generally, fetal hypothyroidism decreases oxygen consumption and oxidation of glucose, thereby potentially decreasing fetal energy supply for growth. Hypothyroidism also can decrease circulating and tissue concentrations of IGF-I.

Glucocorticoids

Glucocorticoids do not have strong effects on fetal growth rate, but they are important in the maturation of many fetal enzymatic pathways (39). These include glycogen deposition, gluconeogenesis, fatty acid oxidation, induction of surfactant production and release, structural maturation of alveoli, structural maturation of the gastrointestinal tract, increased expression of digestive enzymes, increased adrenal function, switch from fetal to adult hemoglobin synthesis, and others. Many IUGR fetuses have increased cortisol concentrations that appear to result from intermittent hypoxic stress. This may account for much of the apparent increased maturation of IUGR fetuses, even when born preterm.

Growth Hormone

Growth hormone, which is the major hormonal regulator of postnatal growth, has no demonstrable effect on fetal growth (39,81).

ANTENATAL CARE OF THE INTRAUTERINE GROWTH-RESTRICTED FETUS

Diagnosis of Intrauterine Growth Restriction

Antenatal diagnosis of IUGR is difficult and often inaccurate. Despite careful attention to gestational dating by maternal history and early and serial fetal ultrasound evaluation, frequent maternal physical examinations, and repeated assessment of risks for IUGR, more than one-half of infants with IUGR may not be identified before birth (100).

Serial ultrasound evaluation of fetal growth rate and fetal body proportions and Doppler velocimetry of the uterine, placental, and fetal circulations are now the standard diagnostic approaches to determining the severity of IUGR. In particular, Doppler velocimetry has provided increasingly accurate prognostic evidence of worsening fetal condition and impending fetal death (101–106). Chronic fetal distress resulting from placental insufficiency, hypoxia, and ischemia (with or without acidosis) is associated with increased Doppler arterial waveform amplitudes that indicate increased vascular resistance and reduced systemic flow in the descending aorta and umbilical artery. Various ratios of systolic-to-diastolic flow velocity (amplitude) waveforms have been used, including the systolic-to-diastolic ratio, systolic-diastolic/systolic ratio (resistance index), and systolic-diastolic/mean ratio (pulsatility index). Ratios or indexes greater than two standard deviations from the mean are associated with IUGR, whereas reversed or absent diastolic waveforms represent severe fetal hypoxia and increased risk of fetal death. The most severely affected IUGR fetuses with the greatest risk of death demonstrate absent or reversed diastolic flow in systemic fetal arteries (104), along with increased umbilical venous pulsation and reversed flow in the abdominal vena cava. Interestingly, these same fetuses often have decreased cerebral (internal carotid artery) pulsatility index, indicating increased cerebral blood flow (105). This flow pattern has been interpreted as one way in which brain growth is spared, as body growth rate slows as a result of placental ischemia and/or placental growth failure. Doppler waveform abnormalities usually precede less specific signs of fetal distress, such as abnormal changes in fetal heart rate, spontaneously or in response to oxytocin challenge testing.

The fetus also should be examined by ultrasound for anatomic abnormalities that indicate congenital malformations, genetic syndromes, and deformations. Amniotic fluid index also is useful to identify oligohydramnios. The latter is a risk factor for congenital anomalies, severe IUGR with reduced urine production, pulmonary hypoplasia, variable decelerations from cord compression, and intrauterine fetal death in as many a 5% to 10% of affected fetuses.

Future Diagnosis and Treatment of Intrauterine Growth Restriction

Altered fetal growth rate, and pathophysiology associated with IUGR, usually develop insidiously, such that once these conditions are clinically obvious, injury has already taken place. It is important, therefore, to develop and apply diagnostic techniques to the fetus that would establish accurately and with sensitively even minimal changes in growth rate and physiologic function. Currently, Doppler ultrasound measurements of fetal cardiac output, systemic blood flow, and organ blood supply are close to achieving this goal, particularly with respect to the placental circulation (107). Other recent research trials have focused on quantifying placental transfer functions in pregnant women who are carrying a severely IUGR fetus. For example, women carrying an IUGR fetus can be given stable isotopes of nutrients normally transported across the placenta, such as glucose and selected amino acids, fol-lowed by timed cordocentesis to measure placental transfer characteristics of these substrate isotopes (108). This information can be compared with that from normal pregnancies with normal placental function and fetal growth rates.

It is also important that diagnostic techniques are developed to assess what damage is being done in the more extreme cases of IUGR. Current techniques include magnetic resonance imaging, Doppler measurements of blood flow to specific organs (107), cordocentesis (109–112), and neurologic and neuromuscular response to vibroacoustic stimulation (113). Based on such advances in fetal diagnosis, it soon may be possible to assess whether detected changes in fetal growth rate and measured fetal pathophysiology associated with IUGR are, in fact, as serious and indicative of future handicap as current postnatal follow-up studies have indicated.

Considerably more research is necessary to determine when and how damage to the fetus can be reversed or ameliorated. Some efforts have been made in animal models to improve maternal and fetal nutrition (114) and to enhance development by organ-specific hormone targeting (115). Examples of the latter include glucocorticoids that have been administered (such as betamethasone) to both the mother and the fetus to increase lung surfactant maturity (116), with additional potential benefits to the maturation of other fetal organs including the gut, heart, adrenals, and kidneys (115). Also, thyroid-releasing hormone has been administered along with corticosteroids to increase lung maturity, although currently there are mixed reports of its effectiveness (117). Continued work is necessary to assess brain development with such treatments, as well as long-term growth and development of all affected organs. More philosophically, it is important to consider whether it is wise to change normal developmental relationships among organs by using organ-specific hormone therapy; more information is needed to determine how altered patterns of organ development during fetal life are beneficial and how they may promote, or hinder, normal fetal development (118).

Antenatal Management

There are few, if any, proven treatments of IUGR. Bed rest and treatment of acute and chronic illnesses appear beneficial. Having the mother breathe supplemental oxygen improves fetal oxygenation, and in a few studies of severe IUGR fetuses with signs of chronic distress this has been associated with improved rates of fetal growth and reduced fetal aortic blood flow velocity (increased flow) (119). Trials of low-dose aspirin therapy, aimed primarily at treating preeclampsia, have not consistently improved fetal growth (120). Correction of maternal nutritional deficiencies also is useful, particularly when the mother is markedly undernourished. Maternal dietary zinc supplements have improved fetal growth when zinc deficiency was prominent. High protein intakes have not helped and, in fact, have been associated with worse IUGR and perinatal morbidity and mortality.

Fetal surveillance techniques should be instituted to determine whether the fetal condition is beginning to fail and if delivery would be more likely to result in a successful pregnancy outcome. Traditional fetal surveillance techniques have included fetal activity recordings, the oxytocin challenge test, which measures fetal heart rate changes after oxytocin-induced uterine contractions, and the nonstress test, which measures the acceleration and beat-to-beat variability of the fetal heart rate after spontaneous fetal movement. These tests, although still done, have been replaced by Doppler velocimetry and the biophysical profile, which combine analyses of fetal breathing movements, gross body movements, fetal heart rate, fetal heart rate reactivity to movement, and estimated amniotic fluid volume. The combined use of Doppler velocimetry and the biophysical profile has improved the antenatal management of IUGR (121,122). A low biophysical profile correlates with fetal hypoxia determined by absent or reversed diastolic flow in the umbilical artery and fetal blood gas and acid–base measurements obtained by cordocentesis, as well as with impending fetal demise.

Most obstetricians avoid labor when combined fetal surveillance techniques show severe fetal growth restriction and evidence of severe chronic distress (123,124), including absent or reversed diastolic flow in the fetal aorta, increased pulsations and/or reversed flow in the umbilical veins, and a low biophysical profile score. Fetuses with these conditions also usually have a nonreactive nonstress test result and a flat baseline fetal heart rate variability pattern. Such fetuses tolerate labor poorly and readily develop signs of acute distress. Saline amnioinfusion may be beneficial in the presence of oligohydramnios and an amniotic fluid index of less than 5 cm (125). Amnioinfusion to an index greater than 8 cm may decrease the incidence of meconium-stained fluid, variable decelerations in the fetal heart rate, end-stage bradycardia, and acute fetal acidosis. In all such severe cases the delivery should be coordinated with the neonatology service to provide prompt postnatal evaluation and care and to prepare for resuscitation of a depressed or asphyxiated neonate.

In the absence of repeated observations of severe or progressively worsening IUGR and signs of fetal distress, the moderately affected IUGR fetus should be left *in utero*, while providing good nutrition, perhaps bed rest, and optimal health care to the mother, and continuing fetal surveillance. Decisions to deliver these fetuses prematurely to prevent fetal death should be tempered by the difficulties of accurately diagnosing the worsening of fetal condition and successfully managing all potential neonatal problems of a preterm infant. Although lung maturity may be present, the many other problems associated with preterm delivery should add caution to a decision for early delivery, especially before 31 to 32 weeks of gestation.

CLINICAL EVALUATION AND TREATMENT OF THE SMALL-FOR-GESTATIONAL AGE INFANT

General Evaluation in the Delivery Room

SGA infants often present a variety of clinical problems immediately after birth in the delivery room. Because of their large surface area relative to body weight, SGA infants lose heat rapidly. To prevent hypothermia, they should be dried quickly and completely, placed under a radiant warmer, and protected from drafts with warmed blankets. Severely SGA infants who suffered marked oxygen and substrate deprivation *in utero* may have cardiopulmonary difficulties at birth. Closer to term they may pass meconium and present with meconium aspiration syndrome, signs of asphyxia, including hypoxemia, hypotension, mixed metabolic and respiratory acidosis, and persistent pulmonary hypertension. Immediately after birth, these infants need prompt and careful attention to their airway, breathing, and oxygen needs.

Brief Physical Examination in the Delivery Room

SGA infants have several characteristic features, even when those infants with obvious anomalies and syndromes and those born to mothers with severe illness or malnutrition are excluded (126–128). Severely SGA infants who had marked IUGR have relatively large heads for their undergrown trunks and extremities. The abdomen often appears shrunken or "scaphoid" and must be distinguished from infants with diaphragmatic hernias. The extremities appear scrawny with thin skinfolds, with evidence of decreased subcutaneous fat and skeletal muscle. The skin is loose and often rough, dry, and peeling. In term and postterm severely SGA infants, the fingernails may be long, and the hands and feet tend to look large for the size of the body. The face appears shrunken or "wizened." Cranial sutures may be widened or overriding, and the anterior fontanelle may be larger than expected, representing diminished membranous bone formation. The umbilical cord often is thinner than usual. When meconium has been passed *in utero*, the cord is yellow-green stained, as are the nails and skin.

Gestational Age Assessment of the Small-for-Gestational-Age Infant

Gestational age assessment based on physical criteria often is erroneous. Vernix caseosa frequently is reduced or absent as a result of diminished skin perfusion during periods of fetal distress or because of depressed synthesis of estriol, which normally enhances vernix production. In the absence of this protective covering, the skin is continuously exposed to amniotic fluid and will begin to desquamate. Sole creases appear more mature due to increased wrinkling from increased exposure to amniotic fluid. Breast tissue formation also depends on peripheral blood flow and estriol levels and will be reduced in SGA infants. The female external genitalia will appear less mature because of the absence of the perineal adipose tissue covering the labia. Ear cartilage also may be diminished. Specific organ maturity often continues at normal developmental rates despite diminished somatic growth in most IUGR infants. Cerebral cortical convolutions, renal glomeruli, and alveolar maturation all relate to gestational age and are not delayed with IUGR.

Neurologic Examination of the Small-for-Gestational-Age Infant

Neurologic examination for gestational age assessment may be little affected by IUGR. These infants often appear to have advanced neurologic maturity, although this observation is derived mostly from comparisons with infants of similar birth weight, not similar gestational age. Peripheral nerve conduction velocity and visual- or auditory-evoked responses correlate well with gestational age and are not impaired as a result of IUGR. These aspects of neurologic maturity are not sensitive to nutritional deprivation. Active and passive tone and posture are usually normal in SGA infants and are reliable guides to gestational age, assuming that infants with significant central nervous system and metabolic disorders are excluded.

Behavioral Observations

SGA infants demonstrate specific abnormal behaviors. They often have a "hyperalert" appearance and generally look "starved and hungry," and they often are described as being jittery and hypertonic, even without simultaneous hypoglycemia. They may be hyperexcitable, showing aberrations in tone from hypertonia to hypotonia and, in many cases, apathy. The Moro response is increased, with exaggerated extension and abduction of the arms, windmill motions, and prolongation of the tonic neck posture (129,130). When IUGR is particularly severe, SGA infants tend to show abnormal sleep cycles and a more consistent picture of diminished muscle tone, deep tendon and facial tactile reflexes, general physical activity, and excitability. These more severe changes indicate that functional central nervous system maturity is impaired, despite the presence of electrical neurologic maturity (131–133). Such severely SGA infants often appear floppy and develop exhaustion more easily after handling (134). The behavioral disorders occur even in the absence of significant central nervous system disease. The hypoexcitability indicates an adverse effect on polysynaptic reflex propagation and implies that central nervous system functional maturity does not necessarily proceed independently of the intrauterine events that result in IUGR.

Deferred Physical Examination to be Done in the Neonatal Intensive Care Unit

Careful evaluation is important as there is an increased incidence of severe malformation, chromosomal abnormality, and congenital infection among SGA infants (135,136). Dysmorphic features, "funny-looking facies," abnormal hands and feet, and the presence of palmar creases, in addition to gross anomalies, suggest congenital malformation syndromes, chromosomal defects, or teratogens. Ocular disorders, such as chorioretinitis, cataracts, glaucoma, and cloudy cornea, in addition to hepatosplenomegaly, jaundice, and a blueberry-muffin rash, suggest a congenital infection. *T*oxoplasmosis, *o*ther (syphillis, hepatitis, Zoster), *r*ubella, *c*ytomegalovirus, and *h*erpes simplex (maternal infections) (TORCH) infections resulting in IUGR are unusual in the absence of other clinical signs of chronic congenital infection; however, screening cord blood for antibodies and antigens specific to certain infections (which can be augmented by polymerase chain reaction techniques), and a urine culture for cytomegalovirus may be indicated. Radiographic examination of the long bones, looking for possible anomalies and for the quality of mineralization, may be useful. Examination of the head with ultrasonography to establish the presence of congenital anatomic abnormalities or evidence of congenital infection also may be helpful in making a diagnosis.

CLINICAL PROBLEMS OF THE SMALL-FOR-GESTATIONAL-AGE NEONATE (TABLE 25–11)

Mortality

The consequences of small size for gestational age depend on the etiology, severity, and duration of growth restriction. There continues to be much debate on this subject. Previous studies have included heterogeneous groups of infants with respect to the degree and cause of IUGR, the degree of prematurity, and the severity of clinical problems in the early neonatal period. By now, many studies have been conducted over extended periods of changing perinatal management and increasing survival rates of smaller, more preterm infants, many of whom have been classified differently at different times and among different studies as to their degree of IUGR. Some studies have indicated that the fetus responds to the "stress" of growth restriction with an acceleration of maturity, which ultimately is protective for the infant. Others have found no evidence of improved survival after perinatal stress, and SGA status has been shown to be an independent predictor of increased fetal, perinatal, and neonatal death (137). On balance, there is little evidence to support the concept of improved survival after perinatal stress in SGA infants, and the perinatal mortality rate for SGA infants with relatively severe IUGR is 5 to 20 times that of AGA infants of the same gestational age

TABLE 25–11. *Clinical problems of the small-for-gestational-age neonate*

Problem	Pathogenesis/pathophysiology	Prevention/treatment

Intrauterine death	Chronic hypoxia
	Placental insufficiency
	Growth failure
	Malformation
	Infection
	Infarction/abruption
	Preeclampsia
		Antenatal surveillance
		  Fetal growth by ultrasound
		  Biophysical profile
		  Doppler velocimetry
		Maternal treatment: ? bed rest, ?O_2
		Delivery for severe/worsening fetal distress

Asphyxia	Acute hypoxia/abruption Chronic hypoxia Placental insufficiency/preeclampsia Acidosis Glycogen depletion	Antepartum/intrapartum monitoring Adequate neonatal resuscitation

Meconium aspiration	Hypoxia	Resuscitation including tracheal
		  suctioning for definite, severe
		  aspiration

Hypothermia	Cold stress
	Hypoxia
	Hypoglycemia
	Decreased fat stores
	Decreased subcutaneous insulation
	Increased surface area
	Catecholamine depletion
		Protect against increased heat loss
		  Dry infant
		  Radiant warmer
		  Hat
		  Thermoneutral environment
		Nutritional support

Persistent pulmonary hypertension	Chronic hypoxia	Cardiovascular support Mechanical ventilation, Nitric oxide
Hypoglycemia	Decreased hepatic/muscle glycogen Decreased alternative energy sources Heat loss Hypoxia Decreased gluconeogenesis Decreased counterregulatory hormones Increased insulin sensitivity	Frequent measurement of blood glucose Early intravenous glucose support
Hyperglycemia	Low insulin secretion rate Excessive glucose delivery Increased catecholamine and glucagon effects	Glucose monitoring Glucose infusion <10 mg/min/kg Insulin administration
Polycythemia/hyperviscosity	Chronic hypoxia Maternal–fetal transfusion Increased erythropoiesis	Glucose, oxygen Partial volume exchange transfusion
Gastrointestinal perforation	Focal ischemia Hypoperistalsis	Cautious enteral feeding
Acute renal failure	Hypoxia/ischemia	Cardiovascular support
Immunodeficiency	Malnutrition Congenital infection	Early, optimal nutrition Specific antibiotic and immune therapy

(136,137). Particularly when adjusted for maternal neonatal risk factors of IUGR, including birth weight percentile, gestational age at birth, maternal height, prepregnancy weight, gestational weight gain, race, and parity, a subgroup of SGA infants is defined that has consistently and markedly higher perinatal mortality and morbidity rates than normally grown infants (138).

Intrauterine Growth Restriction/Small-for-Gestational-Age Status versus Preterm Birth, and Effects on Mortality and Morbidity

Preterm and growth-restricted infants have independent and overlapping problems. Constitutionally small infants are not likely to have increased risks of mortality or morbidity. As gestational age decreases, the problems of prematurity have a larger role in the outcome of both SGA and AGA infants. In contrast, the more mature preterm or term infant may suffer more from the impact of growth restriction. When IUGR has been severe and prolonged, these infants have a higher perinatal mortality rate than their AGA peers. Intrauterine fetal death from chronic fetal hypoxia, immediate birth asphyxia, the multisystem disorders associated with asphyxia (hypoxic–ischemic encephalopathy, persistent fetal circulation, cardiomyopathy, meconium aspiration), and lethal congenital anomalies are the main contributing factors to the high mortality rate for IUGR fetuses and neonates. Most intrauterine fetal deaths occur between 38 and 42 weeks of gestation. Improved survival depends on achieving an optimal balance between the consequences of elective preterm delivery and the risks of continued IUGR.

Asphyxia

Perinatal asphyxia is an uncommon event in SGA infants, but it does occur at increased frequency in SGA infants and can complicate the immediate neonatal course of severe IUGR infants. SGA infants frequently do not tolerate labor and vaginal delivery, and signs of fetal distress are common. In such cases, the already stressed, chronically hypoxic infant is exposed to the acute stress of diminished blood flow during uterine contractions. Cord blood lactate concentrations are often increased despite overall normal cord blood pH. Preterm SGA infants are delivered by cesarean section twice as often as preterm AGA infants (136,139). SGA infants have an increased incidence of low Apgar scores at all gestational ages (136), and these infants frequently need resuscitation.

The acute fetal hypoxia, acidosis, and cerebral depression may result in fetal death or neonatal asphyxia. Severe IUGR results in a large proportion of stillborn infants. Myocardial infarction, amniotic fluid and meconium aspiration, and cerebral edema and necrosis often are noted at autopsy in these severely IUGR stillborn infants. An inadequate resuscitation at birth adds double jeopardy to the *in utero* insults. Sequelae of perinatal asphyxia include multiple organ system dysfunction that, in the more severe cases, includes hypoxic–ischemic encephalopathy, heart failure from hypoxia–ischemia and glycogen depletion, meconium aspiration syndrome, persistent pulmonary hypertension, gastrointestinal hypoperistalsis and ischemia-induced necrosis leading to focal perforation, and acute renal tubular necrosis and renal failure. However, surfactant-deficiency respiratory distress syndrome is not increased in more mature SGA infants closer to term, despite the increased incidence of other forms of respiratory distress. Hypocalcemia may occur following asphyxia in SGA infants, although this is uncommon unless there is excessive phosphate released from damaged cells by acidosis followed by correction with sodium bicarbonate.

Neonatal Metabolism

Hypoglycemia

Hypoglycemia is extremely common in SGA infants, increasing with the severity of IUGR (Fig. 25–16) (140–148). The risk of hypoglycemia is greatest during the first 3 days of life, but fasting hypoglycemia, with or without ketonemia, can occur repeatedly up to weeks after birth. Early hypoglycemia usually is due to diminished hepatic and skeletal muscle glycogen contents (145,147). Early hypoglycemia is aggravated by diminished alternative energy substrates, including reduced concentrations of fatty acids from the scant adipose tissue and decreased concentrations of lactate from the hypo-

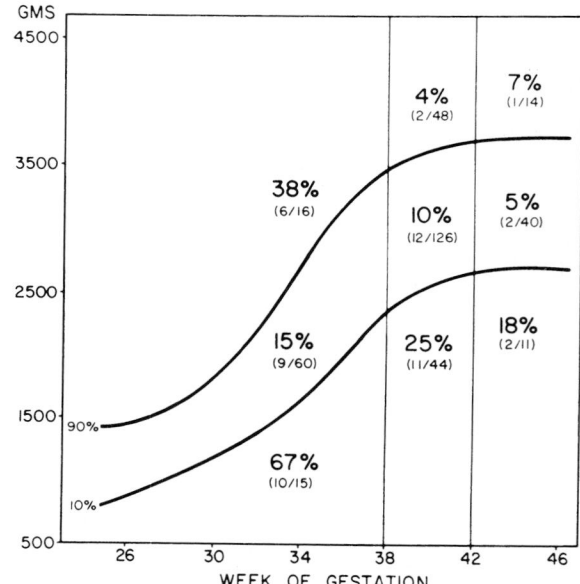

FIG. 25–16. Incidence of hypoglycemia prior to first feeding (blood glucose less than 30 mg/dL) among large-for-gestational-age, average-for-gestational-age, and small-for-gestational-age (SGA) infants, demonstrating the much greater incidence of early hypoglycemia among SGA infants at all gestational ages. (From Lubchenco LO, Bard H. Incidence of hypoglycemia in newborn infants classified by birth weight and gestational age. *Pediatrics* 1971;47:831.)

glycemia. Hyperinsulinemia, increased sensitivity to insulin, or both may contribute to a greater incidence of hypoglycemia, although there are very few, if any, accurate measures of insulin sensitivity at different times and among different conditions in SGA infants to support such assumptions (142). SGA infants also demonstrate decreased gluconeogenesis (149), and resolution of persistent hypoglycemia is coincident with improved capacity for, and rates of, gluconeogenesis.

Deficient counterregulatory hormones also contribute to the pathogenesis of hypoglycemia in SGA infants (150). Catecholamine release is deficient in these neonates during periods of hypoglycemia. Although basal glucagon levels may be elevated, exogenous administration of glucagon fails to enhance glycemia because of the decreased hepatic glycogen stores.

Fasting hypoglycemia is now less common in SGA infants as conventional nutritional treatment now involves earlier enteral and intravenous feeding as well as a more liberal use of intravenous glucose (139). All SGA infants should have early and frequent measurements of blood or plasma glucose concentrations. Blood glucose concentrations should be kept at greater than 50 mg/dL. Early enteral feeding usually can prevent hypoglycemia. In less mature infants or those who have other clinical problems, intravenous glucose should be started at 4 to 8 mg/min/kg as soon after birth as possible—preferably by 30 minutes of age. This initial infusion rate should be adjusted in response to measurements of blood glucose concentration every 30 to 60 minutes until these values are consistently greater tha 50 mg/dL. Less frequently repeated measurements should be continued until the infant is tolerating reasonably full enteral feedings. Infants with severe hypoglycemia (less than 20 mg/dL) that is persistent for more than 10 to 30 minutes, with coma and seizures, should be treated immediately with an intravenous "minibolus" of 10% dextrose in water at 200 mg/kg (2 mL/kg), followed by a glucose infusion of 10% dextrose in water at 4 to 8 mg/min/kg. Glucose concentrations should be measured at least every 30 minutes until concentrations are consistently above 45 mg/dL for blood or above 50 mg/dL plasma (or serum). Infants at greatest risk of having severe hypoglycemia are those who have been asphyxiated and those who are the thinnest according to the Ponderal index, representing those infants with the least amount of body glycogen content. Similarly, breast-fed twins who are not supplemented with a carbohydrate source are at risk, particularly the smaller twin, and they should be monitored carefully.

Hyperglycemia

Very preterm SGA infants have developmentally low insulin secretion rates and plasma insulin concentrations, which may underlie the relatively common problem of hyperglycemia in ELBW SGA infants (151). Unnecessarily high rates of glucose infusion (greater than 14 mg/min/kg) also contribute to this hyperglycemia (152). Higher concentrations of counterregulatory hormones, such as epinephrine, glucagon, and cortisol, also may contribute, although there is only limited evidence to support this commonly held assumption. In contrast, administration of insulin to even preterm SGA infants usually produces prompt decreases in glucose concentration, indicating at least normal and probably greater than normal insulin sensitivity (153).

Lipid Metabolism

SGA infants also have lower plasma free fatty acid levels than normally grown infants. Fasting blood glucose levels in SGA infants directly correlate with plasma free fatty acid and ketone body levels. In addition, once fed, SGA infants have a deficient utilization of intravenous triglycerides. After the intravenous administration of triglyceride emulsion, SGA infants have high free fatty acid and triglyceride levels, but ketone body formation is attenuated (154,155). These observations indicate that the utilization and oxidation of free fatty acids and triglycerides are diminished in SGA neonates. Free fatty acid oxidation is important because it spares peripheral tissue use of glucose, whereas the hepatic oxidation of free fatty acids may contribute the reducing equivalents and energy required for hepatic gluconeogenesis. Deficient provision or oxidation of fatty acids may be partly responsible for the development of fasting hypoglycemia in these infants.

Energy Metabolism

When nursed in a neutral thermal environment, SGA infants demonstrate the usual decline of the respiratory quotient after birth, representing a shift toward free fatty acid oxidation. During the first 12 hours after birth, basal oxygen consumption may be diminished in SGA neonates. Similar observations have been recorded *in utero* among spontaneously SGA fetal lambs, indicating a deficiency of potentially oxidizable substrates in both situations. Supporting this hypothesis is the marked increment of oxygen consumption that occurs in well-fed SGA infants (156), similar to the increase in energy production after nutritional rehabilitation of infants with marasmic kwashiorkor. The increment of oxygen consumption after fetal or infantile malnutrition represents the energy cost of growth. Partly because of enhanced caloric intake, and because metabolic rate and oxygen consumption are related more to gestational age than birth weight, SGA infants have a higher oxygen consumption rate and a higher rate of total energy expenditure (primarily due to increased resting energy expenditure) than less mature neonates (155). This also reflects an increase in cell number relative to total mass and greater heat production in response to increased heat loss. Although some nutritional balance studies of preterm SGA infants have demonstrated an increase of fecal fat and protein loss, more recent studies indicate adequate digestion of nutrients and percent nutrient retention of metabolizable nutrient intake. Thus, these infants can achieve normal, and occasionally faster, rates of growth compared with preterm AGA infants.

Those SGA infants who, because of chromosomal or infectious insults early in gestation, cannot increase their growth rate do not demonstrate increased rates of oxygen consumption after appropriate caloric intake.

Amino Acid and Protein Metabolism

SGA infants are particularly deficient in muscle mass. Improving nutrition of skeletal muscle, as well as total body protein, is a priority in these infants. There is conflicting information from a limited number of studies, however, about how well SGA infants tolerate aggressive amino acid and protein nutrition. ELBW and VLBW SGA infants have higher rates of protein loss in stools, as well as of lipids (141), with 11% to 14% lower rates of absorption. This may be partly compensated for by higher intakes, which can normalize metabolizable protein intakes. Further, although growth rate may be increased in SGA infants by increased intake of protein and nonprotein calories, specific evidence for this comes largely from preterm infants, some of whom were AGA and some SGA (157). Also, animal studies show more limited pancreatic development and intestinal size in SGA offspring (158,159), which may limit feeding tolerance, protein digestion, and the production of insulin.

Some studies have shown that amino acid turnover rates are higher in SGA LBW infants (160), but other studies show no difference (161,162). SGA infants may be more energy efficient in protein synthesis (162). This could explain faster rates of growth in SGA versus AGA infants of the same gestational age, who are fed the same diet (156,157). Thus, SGA infants possibly may tolerate higher protein intake, but the benefit of increased intake is not clear (157).

Nutritional Problems and Management

In fetal sheep that are acutely glucose deficient, amino acids are used for oxidation and for glucose production (163). With chronic glucose deficiency, protein breakdown remains increased and IUGR develops, but amino acids are not used for glucose production or oxidation more than normally (164). It is not clear if human infants born following similar patterns of IUGR and nutrient deficiency will have similar patterns of metabolism after birth, nor is it know what types and amounts of nutrients are best fed to such infants to restore normal metabolism and to reestablish normal rates of growth as quickly as possible. A rapid rate of glucose supply can lead to marked hyperglycemia, especially in the ELBW preterm SGA infant. On the other hand, amino acid intolerance is not exaggerated in SGA infants, despite some earlier evidence that amino acids are not used as readily for gluconeogenesis. If insulin and IGF-I are deficient in these infants, one would also expect lower anabolic rates until glucose and amino acid supplies and concentrations, as well as production rates of these growth factors, are restored. Similar issues may apply to lipid tolerance. Such considerations have prompted some reluctance to feed the SGA infant as aggressively as their deprived nutritional state would indicate, but large-scale, rigorous trials of different rates and amounts of nutrition to such infants have not been conducted. Such trials are needed to determine whether these infants will tolerate more aggressive feeding and whether this will result, safely, in improved nutritional rehabilitation, growth, and perhaps, neurodevelopmental outcome.

Temperature Regulation

Impaired placental function leading to ineffective heat elimination from the SGA fetus may result in a higher than normal temperature in the infant at birth (150,153). A normal increase in nonshivering thermogenesis is seen in these infants because brown fat is available (165,166). However, depletion of brown fat may occur more readily if exposure to cold is prolonged (167). *In utero* stress that depletes catecholamine stores can contribute to a failure of brown fat to produce heat. Compared with term infants, SGA infants have a narrow thermoneutral range. Heat production cannot match the rate of heat loss with continued cold stress. The rapid heat loss due to the large head-to-body ratio and increased surface area seen in all infants is

exaggerated in the SGA infant. Heat is also lost more quickly through a thin layer of subcutaneous fat insulation (165,167). Because they are gestationally more mature than their preterm peers, SGA infants do have a more generous thermoneutral range for weight and are better able to maintain the increased metabolic rate necessary to increase heat production (168). Also, SGA infants of more than 30 weeks of gestation may have increased skin maturity and less evaporative heat loss than AGA infants of comparable weight (169), indicating that thermal neutral environments should be based on gestational age and not weight alone (170). Heat production may be impaired by concurrent conditions of hypoglycemia and hypoxia seen commonly in these patients. The normal response to cold involves increased muscular activity and catecholamine (norepinephrine) release. Central nervous system depression may prevent this normal response to cold (165).

During the first few hours of life, oxygen consumption and heat production may be less than anticipated due to decreased available substrate. Fewer fatty acids are available for oxidation. Later, as nutritional support is provided, the infant may have higher than expected oxygen consumption. Brain oxygen requirements are high, and in the SGA infant brain tissue represents a large proportion of body weight. Limited availability of glucose *in utero* limits metabolic rate. After delivery, as glucose substrate is provided, the brain increases its metabolic rate and oxygen consumption. Based on brain size, increased rates of oxygen consumption are appropriate in the SGA infant (171). It is critical, therefore, that the SGA infant be resuscitated and nursed in a thermoneutral environment. The newborn should be placed immediately under a radiant warmer and dried well. A prewarmed hat will minimize excessive heat loss from the head. A flexed posture decreases exposed surface area and may slow heat dissipation.

Current and future studies of the value of selective brain cooling of infants suffering perinatal hypoxic–ischemic encephalopathy may indicate an advantage for this unique approach in SGA infants as well.

Polycythemia–Hyperviscosity Syndrome

SGA infants manifest an increased incidence of polycythemia (172). Increased red blood cell volume is likely related to chronic *in utero* hypoxia leading to increased erythropoiesis (173,174). Maternal–fetal transfusion may occur chronically with fetal hypoxia or more acutely with episodes of fetal distress. Even when not polycythemic (venous hematocrit greater than 60), SGA infants have higher than normal hematocrit (174). Approximately half of all term SGA infants have a central hematocrit above 60% and about 17% of term SGA infants have a central hematocrit above 65% in contrast to only about 5% in AGA term infants (175,176). The plasma volume of SGA infants immediately after birth averages 52 mL/kg, as opposed to 43 mL/kg in AGA infants. Once equilibrated at 12 hours of life, the plasma volume becomes equivalent in the two groups. In addition to an enhanced plasma space, the circulating red blood cell mass is expanded.

Viscosity is directly related to venous hematocrit, and increased viscosity interferes with normal tissue perfusion. Although the incidence of hyperviscosity is about 5% in the general population, it is seen much more frequently (18%) in SGA infants (175). In these cases, polycythemia is the most likely etiology of hyperviscosity. Most polycythemic infants remain asymptomatic, but SGA infants are at greater risk of symptoms and clinical consequence (176). Interestingly, male SGA infants are at highest risk. Polycythemia contributes to hypoglycemia and hypoxia. Altered viscosity interferes with neonatal hemodynamics and results in abnormal postnatal cardiopulmonary and metabolic adaptation. There is also an increased risk of necrotizing enterocolitis. In addition to correcting hypoxia and hypoglycemia in these infants, partial volume exchange transfusion should be considered to lower hematocrit and minimize the risks of polycythemia and hyperviscosity.

Immune Function and Infectious Disease Risk

Immunologic function of SGA infants may be depressed at birth and may persist into childhood, as in older infants with postnatal onset of malnutrition (177). Deficiencies have been demonstrated in lymphocyte number and function, which include decreased spontaneous mitogenesis and reduced response to phytohemagglutinin. Similarly, these infants tend to have lower immunoglobulin levels during infancy and demonstrate an attenuated antibody response to oral polio vaccine.

Miscellaneous Problems

At birth, cord prealbumin and bone mineral content are low in term SGA infants (178). Calcium and iron stores may be low due to chronic decreased placental blood flow and insufficient nutrient supply. Significant hypocalcemia can occur after stressful birth complicated by acidosis. Thrombocytopenia, neutropenia, prolonged thrombin and partial thromboplastin times, and elevated fibrin degradation products are also problems among SGA infants (179–181). Sudden infant death syndrome may be more common after IUGR. Inguinal hernias also disproportionally follow preterm IUGR.

OUTCOMES AND LONG-TERM CONSEQUENCES OF SMALL-FOR-GESTATIONAL-AGE INFANTS

Hospitalization

At term, SGA infants are admitted more frequently to the intensive care unit and have longer hospital stays than their AGA counterparts. Even among term infants well enough to avoid neonatal intensive care unit admission as newborns, the incidence of readmission to hospital during the first year is significantly increased for SGA infants. Neurologic disorders and other morbidities requiring follow-up and hospitalization are more frequent among IUGR infants, occurring 5 to 10 times more often than among AGA infants. SGA infants also are more likely to be hospitalized for serious respiratory infections, especially if the mother smoked cigarettes at the time of conception as well as at other times.

Growth and Developmental Outcome

Most studies of normal and restricted fetal growth and development support the concept that critical windows of time are present in human development during which normal growth of certain tissues (e.g., fat, muscle, bone) or organs (pancreas, brain) must occur. Insults at such times limit growth and can program persistent, even lifelong failures in growth and development (182). In rats, for example, undernutrition at a vulnerable period of brain development permanently decreases brain size, brain cell number, normal behavioral development, learning, and memory (183,184). Permanent deficits may result if growth failure occurs during these critical periods (185).

SGA infants are a heterogeneous group of babies with the potential for a variety of outcomes. Some are small from genetic or familial causes and therefore may be expected to achieve their full growth potential and have normal neurodevelopment (186). Others have specific chromosomal errors or injury from infections, which are likely to result in severe and unrecoverable failure of growth and development. Most have a less defined reason for abnormal *in utero* growth. The infant with symmetric growth restriction may have little chance for postnatal catch-up growth after an early, global disruption of growth. However, a neonate who had normal growth in early gestation, but developed growth restriction from limited nutrient availability in later gestation later, has a reasonable potential for catch-up growth and normal development.

Studies of growth-restricted infants have been plagued by methodologic problems. Many early studies included all small infants without adequate distinction between those born at different gestational ages or those with limited familial or genetic growth potential. Infants with obvious chromosomal abnormalities and evidence of congenital infection also were included. Only relatively recently have studies of outcome of IUGR and SGA infants included in the study design the recognition that the etiology of small size at birth carries great prognostic value. More recent studies of this subject also have been limited by uncontrolled confounding factors. An infant's perinatal morbidity, including inborn or outborn (requiring transport) status, presence of abnormal umbilical artery waveforms (121), as well as a variety of neonatal complications, such as asphyxia, hypoglycemia, polycythemia, and cold stress, can impact on ultimate outcome (185–187). Multiple gestation and even birth order can influence future growth potential.

Socioeconomic status and environment are among the most important, but difficult to control for, variables affecting the growth and development of SGA infants. Several studies have attempted to differentiate between the influences of biologic and environmental variables (187,188). There are strong associations between socioeconomic factors and the cognitive development and school performance of growth-restricted children.

Postnatal Physical Growth of Small-for-Gestational-Age Infants

Although measurements of weight, length (or height), and head circumference are standardized and reproducible, many authors have given more attention to one measurement over another or have been more concerned with a specific interrelationship of measurements, such as the Ponderal index (189). In general, SGA infants continue to be smaller and relatively underweight for age as they grow older, even through adolescence and early adulthood (Fig. 25–17). These infants more commonly have short stature as teenagers and young adults, indicating lifelong growth deficit.

Differences in patterns of early growth have been observed in SGA infants. Normal infants experience a period of rapid growth during the first 3 years of life. Adult size correlates with the individual growth curve after this time. Moderately affected SGA infants who had primarily a reduction in weight in the third trimester of gestation follow the same pattern of normal neonatal and infant growth, but tend to have an accelerated velocity of growth during the first 6 months (189). This catch-up growth occurs primarily from birth to 6 months of age, with some infants continuing an accelerated rate of growth for the first year. A few of these infants will achieve a normal growth percentile and thereafter have a growth rate similar to appropriately grown children (189,190). Head circumference parallels growth in length during catch-up and sustained growth periods. After the first year, no difference in the rate of growth has been noted (189,190).

Ultimate weight and height are less in SGA children when compared to their normal siblings (189,190). In one study of 4- to 6-year-old children (189), 45% of siblings were at or above the 50th percentile for weight and height, whereas only 12% of their SGA siblings achieved the 50th percentile. Interestingly, a subgroup of severely growth-restricted infants (less than 40% of expected birth weight) compared to less affected SGA peers showed no difference in weight or height at 6 months of age, adding concern for the growth outcome of even modest degrees of IUGR. Former SGA infants have been shown to have no delay in bone age, puberty, or sexual maturation at adolescence, although they were shorter, lighter, and had smaller heads. Muscle mass between the two groups was similar, but adipose tissue development was less in the SGA group (191).

Because head size correlates with brain size, volume, weight, and cellularity, head growth at the time of birth and the degree of catch-up growth thereafter are prognostic of future neurodevelopment. Deficient fetal head growth recognized by relative microcephaly at birth, whether at term or preterm, is felt to be a poor prognostic indicator, as it reflects the severity and duration of *in utero* growth failure. A lack of head sparing and small occipital-frontal circumference (OFC) is associated with poor neurologic and psychological outcome (192). Head size, if catch-up head growth has not occurred by 8 months of age, is a predictor of lower intelligence test scores at 3 years of age (193). This correlation seems to be independent of environmental or other risks. Decreased head size when compared to siblings carries significant risks of deficient mental and motor function (188).

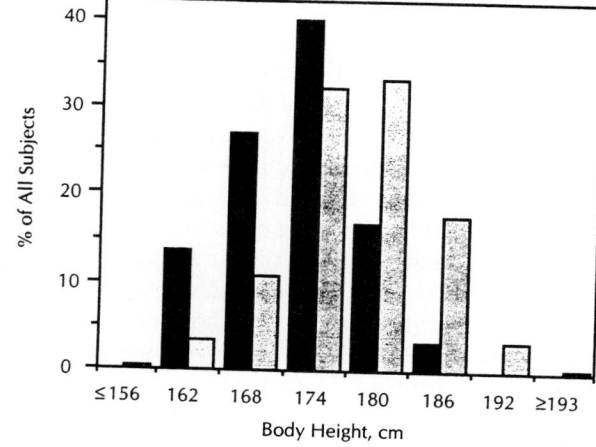
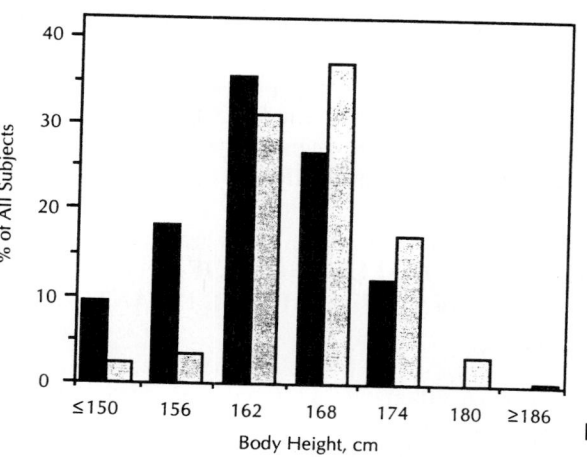

FIG. 25–17. Distribution of height at age 17 years in 30 boys **(A)** and 34 girls **(B)** born small for gestational age *(solid bars)* and their peers who were born appropriate for gestational age *(shaded bars)*. (From Paz I, Seidman DS, Danon YL, Laor A, Stevenson DK, Gale R. et al. Are children born small for gestational age at increased risk of short stature? *Am J Dis Child* 1993;147:337.)

Postnatal Neurodevelopmental Outcome of Full-Term, Small-for-Gestational-Age Infants

Neurologic disorders and other morbidities are more frequent in SGA infants as a group, occurring 5 to 10 times more often than in AGA infants. However, in full-term, mild-to-moderately SGA infants who have normal brain growth, no hypoxic–ischemic injury, and good environmental support, IUGR may have little impact on behavior or mental ability in adolescence or adulthood (185,186,192). There is no increased incidence of major handicap (189,191,193,194) and no increased risk of severe neurologic morbidity (192) in term infants born small for gestational age. Cerebral palsy is infrequent in this group (194). Routine neurologic examination is usually normal (191).

Although the absence of gross neurologic outcome in the term SGA infant is reassuring, evidence of minimal brain dysfunction among these children continues to be of concern. Many studies have revealed signs of minor brain damage, including hyperactivity, short attention span, learning problems, poor fine motor coordination, and hyperreflexia. An increased number of diffuse abnormalities are seen on electroencephalogram (194). In one study, 30% of term SGA children at 5 years of age had speech problems, which included a delayed onset of speech, immature vocabulary with persistent infantile articulation, and poor receptive and expressive abilities for age (194). In contrast, only 1.5% of the general population and about 5% of their siblings had speech difficulties.

Former term SGA infants more frequently have substandard school performance and display subtle neurologic and behavioral problems despite a normal IQ. Sensorimotor abilities are frequently affected. Overall there is no correlation between the severity of growth restriction and learning deficit, although those with poor early brain growth in infancy have more problems (193). Measures of cognition at 4 to 6 years of age correlate well with testing at adolescence. This suggests that cognitive potential is reached early, with little change later. It seems likely that environmental and socioeconomic factors play a significant role in the learning deficiencies seen in these children (188).

At adolescence, trends toward lower test scores, especially in mathematics, and an increased incidence of learning disabilities have been noted (191,194). There also is a trend toward slower alternating movements on physical examination. Most believe, however, that the cognitive and academic differences in these children are small and do not significantly affect school performance or ultimate intellectual ability.

Postnatal Neurodevelopmental Outcome in Preterm, Small-for-Gestational-Age Infants

The prognosis for preterm SGA infants is less clear and is easily confounded by other problems of preterm birth. In general, subnormal intellectual outcomes are more common among preterm SGA infants than term SGA infants. Some authors have shown that those infants suffering the dual insults of preterm birth and growth restriction are at higher risk of neurodevelopmental deficit (195,196). Among extremely preterm infants, gestational age, and not growth status, has been the most significant predictor of intellectual outcome (197). By 3 years of age, social and environmental factors play an increasing role and may impact on development in either a positive or negative way (197). Socioeconomic status is independently associated with learning disabilities in these children (187).

When compared with their appropriately grown same-weight counterparts, SGA preterm infants have a lower incidence of major developmental handicaps and cerebral palsy. Specific motor deficits are more common in AGA infants (198,199). Minor neurologic abnormalities are more frequently observed in SGA infants (198). Diffuse cerebral damage due to hypoxia and decreased intrauterine blood flow, especially to the brain, probably accounts for the differences in expression of brain damage seen in preterm AGA and SGA children (200). Restricted growth for gestational age is associated with more cognitive disability in infants who were born preterm (199,201). The need for special education is higher and becomes apparent at an earlier age in these preterm SGA infants when they reach school age (200).

Possible Adult Disorders Resulting from Intrauterine Growth Restriction

Recent epidemiologic evidence indicates that obesity, insulin resistance, diabetes, and cardiovascular disease are more common among adults who were smaller than normal at birth and very likely SGA secondary to IUGR, particularly those who had a high placental-to-fetal-weight ratio (202). A variety of animal studies support this concept, including the greater incidence of obesity, glucose intolerance, plasma lipid abnormalities, and hypertension in offspring whose mothers were fed a low-protein diet during pregnancy (203–206). These examples indicate that certain adult pathologies may be unavoidable consequences of environmentally imposed conditions, such as severe and prolonged fetal undernutrition, which lead to fetal growth restriction to ensure fetal survival. These conditions may represent an example of "programming," in which an insult, when applied at a critical or sensitive stage in development, may result in a lasting, even life-long, effect on the structure or function of the organism (183). IUGR, therefore, is increasingly seen as an adaptive physiologic process, even though it can produce adverse fetal, neonatal, and potentially adult consequences Table 25–12) (207). Mechanisms responsible for these later-life morbidities in adults, who were growth restricted *in utero*, are not yet established. There is some evidence of diminished pancreatic growth and development, which might

TABLE 25–12. *Fetal, neonatal/infancy, and adult disorders that might result from fetal programming as a consequence of fetal undernutrition at different states of gestation*

	Trimester of pregnancy		
	First	Second	Third
Consequences	Low growth trajectory	Disturbed fetal–placental relationships	Brain growth sustained, but not body
Fetal adaptation	Down regulation of fetal growth	Insulin resistance	Growth factor(s) resistance/ deficiency
Anthropometry	Symmetric	Mixed	Asymmetric
Infant growth	Reduced infant growth	Reduced infant growth	Catch-up growth possible
Adult life	Increased BP	Increased BP, NIDDM, ischemic heart disease	Increased BP, NIDDM, hypercholesterolemia, ischemic heart disease

BP, blood pressure; NIDDM, noninsulin-dependent diabetes mellitus.
From Barker D. *Mothers, babies, and diseases later in life.* London: BMJ Books, 1994.

becomes manifest in later life as pancreatic insufficiency when the adult starts and then continues eating a diet rich in simple carbohydrates and lipids. Peripheral insulin resistance may develop in the same way, and hypertension in adulthood may be the result of altered adrenal development in response to IUGR.

REFERENCES

1. Lubchenco LO, Searls DT, Brazie JV. Neonatal mortality rate: relationship to birth weight and gestational age. *J Pediatr* 1972;81:814.
2. Lubchenco LO. *The high risk infant.* Philadelphia: WB Saunders, 1976.
3. Chard T, Costeloe K, Leaf A. Evidence of growth retardation of neonates of apparently normal weight. *Eur J Obstet Gynecol Reprod Endocrinol* 1992;45:59.
4. Chard T, Yoong A, Macintosh M. The myth of fetal growth retardation at term. *Br J Obstet Gynaecol* 1993;100:1076.
5. Wark L, Malcolm LA. Growth and development of the Lumi child in the Sepik district of New Guinea. *Med J Aust* 1969;2:129.
6. Ashcroft MT, Buchanan IC, Lovell HG, Welsh B. Growth of infants and preschool children in St Christopher-Nevis-Anguilla West Indies. *Am J Clin Nutr* 1966;19:37.
7. Evans MI, Mukherjee AB, Schulman JD. Animal models of intrauterine growth retardation. *Obstet Gynecol Surv* 1983;38:183.
8. Simmons RA, Gounis AS, Bangalore SA, Ogata ES. Intrauterine growth retardation: fetal glucose transport is diminished in lung but spared in brain. *Pediatr Res* 1992;32:59.
9. Sabbagha RE. Intrauterine growth retardation. In: Sabbagha RE, ed. *Ultrasound applied to obstetrics and gynecology.* Philadelphia: JB Lippincott Co., 1987:112.
10. McGiven J, Pastor Angladi A. Regulatory and molecular aspects of mammalian amino acids transport. *Biochem J* 1993;299:321.
11. Hill RDG. Insulin as a growth factor. *Pediatr Res* 1985;19:879.
12. Sparks JW, Ross JR, Cetin I. Intrauterine growth and nutrition. In: Polin RA, Fox WW, eds. *Fetal and neonatal physiology,* 2nd ed. Philadelphia: WB Saunders, 1998:267.
13. Lubchenco LO, Hansman C, Boyd E. Intrauterine growth in length and head circumference as estimated from live births at gestational ages from 26 to 42 weeks. *Pediatrics* 1966;37:403.
14. Kramer MS. Intrauterine growth and gestational duration determinants. *Pediatrics* 1987;80:502.
15. Virgi SK, Cottington E. Risk factors associated with preterm deliveries among racial groups in a national sample of married mothers. *J Perinatol* 1991;8:347.
16. Klebanoff MA, Schulsinger C, Mednick BR, Secher NJ. Preterm and small-for-gestational-age birth across generations. *Am J Obstet Gynecol* 1997;176:521.
17. Abrams B, Newman V. Small-for-gestational-age birth: maternal predictors and comparison with risk factors of spontaneous preterm delivery in the same cohort. *Am J Obstet Gynecol* 1991;164:785.
18. Freemark M, Comer M. The role of placental lactogen in the regulation of fetal metabolism and growth. *J Pediatr Gastroenterol Nutr* 1989;8:281.
19. Lacroix MC, Devinov E, Servely JL, Puissant C, Kann G. Expression of the growth hormone gene in ovine placenta: detection and cellular localization of the protein. *Endocrinology* 1996;137:4886.
20. Gluckman PD. The endocrine regulation of fetal growth in late gestation—the role of insulin like growth factors. *J Clin Endocrinol Metab* 1995;80:1047.
21. Gibbs RS, Eschenbach DA. Use of antibiotics to prevent preterm birth. *Am J Obstet Gynecol* 1997;177:375.
22. Salas SP, Altermatt F, Campos M, Giacaman A, Rosso P. Effects of long-term nitric oxide synthesis inhibition on plasma volume expansion and fetal growth in the pregnant rat. *Hypertension* 1995;26:1019.
23. Krebs C, Macara LM, Leiser R, Bowman AW, Greer IA, Kingdom JCP. Intrauterine growth restriction with absent end-diastolic flow velocity in the umbilical artery is associated with maldevelopment of the placental terminal villous tree. *Am J Obstet Gynecol* 1996;175:1534.
24. Nicolaides KH, Economides DL, Soothill PW. Blood gases, pH, and lactate in appropriate- and small-for-gestational-age fetuses. *Am J Obstet Gynecol* 1989;161:996.
25. Scholl TO, Hediger ML, Schall JO, Chor-San K, Fischer RL. Maternal growth during pregnancy and the competition for nutrients. *Am J Clin Nutr* 1994;60:183.
26. Wallace JM, Aitken RP, Cheyne MA. Nutrient partitioning and fetal growth in rapidly growing adolescent ewes. *J Reprod Fertil* 1996; 107:183.
27. Lucas A, Gore SM, Cole TJ, et al. A multicentre trial on feeding low birthweight infants: effects of diet on early growth. *Arch Dis Child* 1984;59:722.
28. Davis JA, Dobbing J. *Scientific foundations of paediatrics.* Philadelphia: WB Saunders Co, 1974.
29. Ounsted M, Ounsted C. *On fetal growth rate. Clinics in developmental medicine no. 46.* Philadelphia: JB Lippincott Co., 1973.
30. Ziegler EE, O'Donnell AM, Nelson SE, Fomon SJ. Body composition of the reference fetus. *Growth* 1976;40:329.
31. Nimrod CA. The biology of normal and deviant fetal growth. In: Reece EA, Hobbins JC, Mahoney MJ, Petrie RH, eds. *Medicine of the fetus & mother.* Philadelphia: JB Lippincott Co., 1992:285.
32. Widdowson EM. Changes in body proportions and composition during growth. In: Davis JA, Dobbing J, eds. *Scientific foundations of paediatrics.* Philadelphia: WB Saunders, 1974:155.
33. Lapillonne A, Brailon P, Claris O, Chatelain PG, Delmas PD, Salle BL. Body composition in appropriate and in small for gestational age infants. *Acta Paediatr* 1997;86:196.
34. Shelley HJ. Glycogen reserves and their changes at birth. *Br Med Bull* 1961;17:137.
35. Philipps AF. Carbohydrate metabolism of the fetus. In: Polin RA, Fox WW, eds. *Fetal and neonatal physiology,* 2nd ed. Philadelphia: WB Saunders, 1998:560.
36. Hay WW Jr. Glucose metabolism in the fetal-placental unit. In: Cowett RM, ed. *Principles of perinatal-neonatal metabolism,* 2nd ed. New York: Springer-Verlag, 1998:337.

37. Hay WW Jr. Nutrition and development of the fetus: carbohydrate and lipid metabolism. In: Walker WA, Watkins JB, eds. *Nutrition in pediatrics*, 2nd ed. Hamilton: BC Decker Inc., 1996:364.

38. Sparks JW, Girard J, Battaglia FC. An estimate of the caloric requirements of the human fetus. *Biol Neonate* 1980;38:113.

39. Milner RDG, Gluckman PD. Regulation of intrauterine growth. In: Gluckman PD, Heymann MA, eds. *Pediatrics & perinatology:* The scientific basis, 2nd ed. London: Arnold 1993:284.

40. Carver TD, Quick AN Jr, Teng CC, Pike AW, Fennessey PV, Hay WW Jr. Leucine metabolism in chronically hypoglycemia, hypoinsulinemic growth restricted fetal sheep. *Am J Physiol* 1997;272:E107.

41. Yau K-IT, Chang M-H. Growth and body composition of preterm, small for gestational age infants at a postmenstrual age of 37–40 weeks. *Early Hum Dev* 1993;33:117.

42. Cliver SP, Goldenberg RL, Cutter GR, Hoffman HJ, Davis RO, Nelson KG. The effect of cigarette smoking on neonatal anthropometric measurements. *Obstet Gynecol* 1995;85:635.

43. Goldenberg RL, Cliver SP, Cutter GR, Davis RO, Hoffman HJ, Wen SW. Blood pressure, growth retardation, and preterm delivery. *Int J Technol Assess Health Care* 1992;8:82.

44. Goldenberg RL, Tamura T, Neggers Y, et al. The effect of zinc supplementation on pregnancy outcome. *JAMA* 1995;274:463.

45. Goldenberg RL, Hauth JC, DuBard MD, Copper RL, Cutter GR. Fetal growth in women using low-dose aspirin for the prevention of preeclampsia: effect of maternal size. *J Matern Fetal Med* 1995;4:218.

46. Battaglia FC, Meschia G. *An introduction to fetal physiology.* Orlando: Academic Press, 1986.

47. Lumey LH. Decreased birthweights in infants after maternal in utero exposure to the Dutch famine of 1944–1945. *Paediatr Perinat Epidemiol* 1992;6:240.

48. Antonov AM. Children born during the siege of Leningrad in 1942. *J Pediatr* 1947;30:250.

49. Stein Z, Susser M, Rush D. Prenatal nutrition and birth weight: experiments and quasi-experiments in the past decade. *J Reprod Med* 1978; 21:287.

50. Hickey CA, Cliver SP, Goldenberg RL, Kohatsu J, Hoffman HJ. Prenatal weight gain, term birth weight, and fetal growth retardation among high-risk multiparous black and white women. *Obstet Gynecol* 1993;81:529.

51. Rush D, Stein Z, Susser M. A randomized controlled trial of prenatal nutritional supplementation in New York City. *Pediatrics* 1980;68: 683.

52. Sibai B, Anderson GD. Pregnancy outcome of intensive therapy in severe hypertension in first trimester. *Obstet Gynecol* 1986;67:517.

53. Novy MJ, Peterson EN, Metcalfe J. Respiratory characteristics of maternal and fetal blood in cyanotic congenital heart disease. *Am J Obstet Gynecol* 1968;100:821.

54. Lichty JA, Ting RY, Bruns PD, Dyar E. Studies of babies born at high altitude. *Am J Dis Child* 1957;93:666.

55. Brown AK, Sleeper LA, Pegelow CH, Miller ST, Gill FM, Waclawisn MA. The influence of infant and maternal sickle cell disease on birth outcome and neonatal course. *Arch Pediatr Adolesc Med* 1994;148:1156.

56. Goldenberg RL, Davis RO, Nelson KG. Intrauterine growth retardation. In: Merkatz IR, Thompson JE, Mullen PD, Goldenberg RL, eds. *New perspectives on prenatal care.* New York: Elsevier, 1990:461.

57. Abel EL. Consumption of alcohol during pregnancy: a review of effects on growth and development of offspring. *Hum Biol* 1982;54:421.

58. Woods JR, Plessinger MA, Clark KE. Effect of cocaine on uterine blood flow and fetal oxygenation. *JAMA* 1986;257:957.

59. Molteni RA, Stys SJ, Battaglia FC. Relationship of fetal and placental weight in human beings: fetal/placental weight ratios at various gestational ages and birth weight distributions. *J Reprod Med* 1978; 21:327.

60. Owens JA, Falconer J, Robinson JS. Effect of restriction of placental growth on fetal and utero-placental metabolism. *J Dev Physiol* 1987;9:225.

61. Beischer NA, Sivasamboo R, Vohra S, Silpisornkosal S, Reid S. Placental hypertrophy in severe pregnancy anaemia. *J Obstet Gynaecol Br Commonwealth* 1970;77:398.

62. Nylund L, Lunell NO, Lewander R, Sarby B. Uteroplacental blood flow index in intrauterine growth retardation of fetal or maternal origin. *Br J Obstet Gynecol* 1983;90:16.

63. Macara L, Kingdom JC, Kaufman P, et al. Structural analysis of placental terminal villi from growth-restricted pregnancies with abnormal umbilical artery Doppler waveforms. *Placenta* 1996;17:37.

64. Damsky CH, Fitzgerald ML, Fisher SJ. Distribution of extracellular matrix components and adhesion receptors are intricately modulated during first trimester cytotrophoblast differentiation along the invasive pathway, in vivo. *J Clin Invest* 1992;89:210.

65. Damsky CH, Librach C, Lim K-H, et al. Integrin switching regulates normal trophoblast invasion. *Development* 1994;120:3057.

66. Zhou Y, Damsky CH, Chiu K, Roberts JM, Fisher SJ. Preeclampsia is associated with abnormal expression of adhesion molecules by invasive cytotrophoblasts. *J Clin Invest* 1993;91:950.

67. Genbacev O, Joslin RJ, Damsky CH, Polliotto BM, Fisher SJ. Hypoxia alters early gestation human cytotrophoblast differentiation/invasion in vitro and models the placental defects that occur in preeclampsia. *J Clin Invest* 1996;97:540.

68. Handwerger S. The physiology of placental lactogen in human pregnancy. *Endocr Rev* 1992;12:329.

69. Freemark M, Handwerger S. The role of placental lactogen in the regulation of fetal metabolism. *J Pediatr Gastroenterol Nutr* 1989;8:281.

70. Harding JE, Johnston BM. Nutrition and fetal growth. *Reprod Fertil Dev* 1995;7:539.

71. Thureen PJ, Trembler KA, Meschia G, Makowski EL, Wilkening RB. Placental glucose transport in heat induced fetal growth retardation. *Am J Physiol* 1992;263:R578.

72. Marconi AM, Cetin I, Davoli E, et al. An evaluation of fetal gluconeogenesis in intrauterine growth retarded pregnancies. *Metabolism* 1993;42:860.

73. Molina RD, Meschia G, Battaglia FC, Hay WW Jr. Gestational maturation of placental glucose transfer capacity in sheep. *Am J Physiol* 1991;261:R697.

74. Ross JC, Fennessey PV, Wilkening RB, Battaglia FC, Meschia G. Placental transport and fetal utilization of leucine in a model of fetal growth retardation. *Am J Physiol* 1996;270:E491.

75. Milley JR. Effects of insulin on ovine fetal leucine kinetics and protein metabolism. *J Clin Invest* 1994;93:1616.

76. Townsend SF, Briggs KK, Carver TD, Hay WW Jr, Wilkening RB. Altered fetal liver and kidney insulin-like growth factor II mRNA in the sheep after chronic maternal glucose or nutrient deprivation. *Clin Res* 1992;40:91A.

77. Hay WW Jr. Fetal requirements and placental transfer of nitrogenous compounds. In: Polin RA, Fox WW, eds. *Fetal and neonatal physiology*, 2nd ed. Philadelphia: WB Saunders, 1998:619.

78. Milley JR. Ovine fetal leucine kinetics and protein metabolism during decreased oxygen availability. *Am J Physiol* 1998;274:E618.

79. Milley JR. Ovine fetal protein metabolism during decreased glucose delivery. *Am J Physiol* 1993;265:E525.

80. Bell AW, Kennaugh JM, Battaglia FC, Makowski EL, Meschia G. Metabolic and circulatory studies of the fetal lamb at mid gestation. *Am J Physiol* 1986;250:E538.

81. Fowden A. Endocrine regulation of fetal growth. *Reprod Fertil Dev* 1995;7:469.

82. Fowden AL, Hay WW Jr. The effects of pancreatectomy on the rates of glucose utilization, oxidation and production in the sheep fetus. *Q J Exp Physiol* 1988;73:973.

83. Hay WW Jr, Meznarich HK, Fowden AL. The effects of streptozotocin on rates of glucose utilization, oxidation and production in the sheep fetus. *Metabolism* 1988;38:30.

84. Sherwood WG, Chance GW, Hill DE. A new syndrome of pancreatic agenesis. The role of insulin and glucagon in cell and cell growth. *Pediatr Res* 1974;8:360.

85. Carver TD, Anderson SM, Aldoretta PW, Esler AL, Hay WW Jr. Glucose suppression of insulin secretion in chronically hyperglycemic fetal sheep. *Pediatr Res* 1995;38:754.

86. Mathews LS, Hammer RE, Behringer RR, et al. Growth enhancement of transgenic mice expressing human insulin-like growth factor I. *Endocrinology* 1988;123:2827.

87. Behringer RR, Lewin TM, Quaife CJ, Palmiter RD, Brinster RL, D'Ercole AJ. Expression of Insulin-like growth factor I stimulates normal somatic growth in growth hormone-deficient transgenic mice. *Endocrinology* 1990;127:1033.

88. D'Ercole AJ, Dai Z, Xing Y, et al. Brain growth retardation due to the expression of human insulin like growth factor binding protein 1 (IGFBP-1) in transgenic mice: an in vivo model for the analysis of IGF function in the brain. *Dev Brain Res* 1994;82:213.

89. Ye P, Carson J, D'Ercole AJ. In vivo actions of insulin-like growth factor-I (IGF-I) on brain myelination: studies of IGF-I and IGF binding protein-1 (IGFBP-1) transgenic mice. *J Neurosci* 1995;15:7344.

90. Delhanty PJD, Han VKM. The expression of insulin-like growth factor (IGF)-binding protein-2 and IGF-II genes in the tissues of the developing ovine fetus. *Endocrinology* 1993;132:41.

91. Wood TL, Rogler L, Streck RD, et al. Targeted disruption of IGFBP-2 gene. *Growth Regul* 1993;3:3.

92. Pintar JE, Wood TL, Streck RD, Havton L, Rogler L, Hsu MS. Expression of IGF-II, the IGF-II/mannose-6-phosphate receptor and IGFBP-2 during rat embryogenesis. *Adv Exp Med Biol* 1991;293:325.

93. Wood TL, Streck RD, Pintar JE. Expression of the IGFBP-2 gene in post-implantation rat embryos. *Development* 1992;114:59.

94. Crystal RA, Giduice LC. Insulin-like growth factor binding protein (IGFBP) profiles in human fetal cord sera: ontogeny during gestation and differences in newborns with intrauterine growth retardation (IUGR) and large for gestational age (LGA) newborns. In: Spencer EM, ed. *Modern concepts of insulin-like growth factors.* New York: Elsevier, 1991:395.

95. Brenneman DE, Eiden LE. Vasoactive intestinal peptide and electrical activity influence neuronal survival. *Proc Natl Acad Sci U S A* 1986; 83:1159.

96. Hill JM, Agoston DV, Gressens P, McCune SK. Distribution of VIP mRNA and two distinct VIP binding sites in the developing brain; relation to ontogenic evens. *J Comp Neurol* 1994;342:186.

97. Gressens P, Hill JM, Gozes I, Fridkin M, Brenneman DE. Growth factor function of vasoactive intestinal peptide in whole cultured mouse embryos. *Nature* 1993;362:155.

98. Gressens P, Hill JM, Paindaveine B, Gozes I, Fridkin M, Brenneman DE. Severe microcephaly induced by blockade of vasoactive intestinal peptide function in the primitive neuroepithelium of the mouse. *J Clin Invest* 1994;94:2020.

99. Hill JM, McCune SK, Alvero RJ, et al. Maternal vasoactive intestinal peptide and the regulation of embryonic growth in the rodent. *J Clin Invest* 1996;97:202.

100. Kliegman RM. Intrauterine growth retardation. In: Fanaroff A, Martin R, eds. *Neonatal-perinatal medicine,* 6th ed. St. Louis: Mosby-Year Book, 1997:203.

101. Arduini D, Rizzo G, Romanini C. The development of abnormal heart rate patterns after absent end-diastolic velocity in umbilical artery: analysis of risk factors. *Am J Obstet Gyencol* 1993;168:43.

102. Beattie RB, Whittle MJ. Doppler and fetal growth retardation. *Arch Dis Child* 1993;69:271.

103. Hitschold T, Weiss E, Beck T. Low target birthweight or growth retardation? Umbilical Doppler flow velocity waveforms and histometric analysis of fetoplacental vascular tree. *Am J Obstet Gynecol* 1993;168:1260.

104. Karsdorp VHM, vanVugt JMG, vanGeijn HP, et al. Clinical significance of absent or reversed end-diastolic velocity waveforms in umbilical artery. *Lancet* 1994;344:1664.

105. Noordam MJ, Heydanus R, Hop WC, Hoekstra FM. Doppler colour flow imaging of fetal intracerebral arteries and umbilical artery in the small for gestational age fetus. *Br J Obstet Gynaecol* 1994;101:504.

106. Valcamonico A, Danti L, Frusca T, et al. Absent end-diastolic velocity in umbilical artery: risk of neonatal morbidity and brain damage. *Am J Obstet Gynecol* 1994;170:796.

107. Marconi AM, Ferrazzi E, Cetin I, Lanfranchi A, Pardi G, Battaglia FC. Umbilical velocimetry differentiates growth retarded fetuses at risk of acidemia. Third Congress of the International Perinatal Doppler Society, Los Angeles, California, 1990.

108. Cetin I, Marconi AM, Baggiani AM, et al. In vivo transplacental transport of 1-^{13}C-glycine and 1-^{13}C-leucine inhuman pregnancies. *Ital J Gastroenterol* 1992;24:8.

109. Marconi AM, Ferrazzi E, Cetin I, Ferrari MM, Pardi G, Battaglia FC. Lactate metabolism in normal and growth retarded human fetuses. *Pediatr Res* 1990;28:652.

110. Pardi G, Cetin I, Marconi AM, et al. Diagnostic value of blood sampling in fetuses with growth retardation. *N Engl J Med* 1993;328:692.

111. Pardi G, Cetin I, Marconi AM, et al. Venous drainage of the human uterus: respiratory gas studies in normal and fetal growth-retarded pregnancies. *Am J Obstet Gynecol* 1992;166:699.

112. Pardi G, Cetin I, Marconi AM, et al. The role of fetal blood sampling in relation to fetal heart rate and Doppler velocimetry in growth retarded fetuses. *Soc Gynecol Invest* 1993;220.

113. Richards DS. The fetal vibroacoustic stimulation test: an update. *Semin Perinatol* 1990;14:305.

114. Charlton V, Johengen M. Effects of intrauterine nutritional supplementation on fetal growth retardation. *Biol Neonate* 1985;48:125.

115. Padbury JF, Ervin MG, Polk DH. Extrapulmonary effects of antenatally administered steroids. *J Pediatr* 1996;128:167.

116. Liggins GC, Howie RN. A controlled trial of antepartum glucocorticoid treatment for the prevention of the respiratory distress syndrome in premature infants. *Pediatrics* 1972;50:515.

117. Ikegami M, Polk D, Tabor B, Lewis J, Yamada T, Jobe AH. Corticosteroid and thyrotropin-releasing hormone effects on preterm sheep lung function. *J Appl Physiol* 1991;70:2268.

118. Hay WW Jr, Catz CS, Grave GD, Yaffe SG. Workshop summary: fetal growth: its regulation and disorders. *Pediatrics* 1997;99:585.

119. Battaglia FC, Battaglia C, Artini PG, et al. Maternal hyperoxygenation in the treatment of intrauterine growth retardation. *Am J Obstet Gynecol* 1992;167:430.

120. McFarland P, Pearce JM, Chamberlain GVP. Doppler ultrasound and aspirin in recognition and prevention of pregnancy-induced hypertension. *Lancet* 1990;335:1552.

121. McDonnell M, Serra-Serra V, Gaffney G, Redman CW, Hope PL. Neonatal outcome after pregnancy complicated by abnormal velocity waveforms in the umbilical artery. *Arch Dis Child* 1994;70:F84.

122. Hobbins J. Morphometry of fetal growth. *Acta Paediatr Suppl* 1997; 423:165.

123. Gaziano EP, Knox L, Ferrera B, Brandt DG, Calvin SE, Knox GE. Is it time to reassess the risk for the growth-retarded fetus with normal Doppler velocimetry of the umbilical artery? *Am J Obstet Gynecol* 1994;170:1734.

124. Gazzolo D, Scopesi FA, Bruschettini PL, Marasini M, Espisito V, DiRenzo GC. Predictors of perinatal outcome in intrauterine growth retardation: a long-term study. *J Perinat Med* 1994;22:71.

125. Strong TH Jr, Hetzler G, Sarno AP, Paul RH. Prophylactic intrapartum amnioinfusion: a randomized clinical trial. *Am J Obstet Gynecol* 1990;162:1370.

126. Morrison J, Olsen J. Weight-specific stillbirths and associated causes of death: an analysis of 765 stillbirths. *Am J Obstet Gynecol* 1985;152:975.

127. Yogman MW, Kraemer HC, Kindon D, Tyson JE, Casey P, Gross RT. Identification of intrauterine growth retardation among low birth weight preterm infants. *J Pediatr* 1989;115:799.

128. Villar J, deOnis M, Kestler E, Bolanos F, Cerezo R, Bernedes H. The differential neonatal morbidity of the intrauterine growth retardation syndrome. *Am J Obstet Gynecol* 1990;163:151.

129. Frederickson WT, Brown JV. Gripping and moro responses: differences between small-for-gestational age and normal weight newborn. *Early Hum Dev* 1980;4:69.

130. Michaelis R, Schulte FS, Nolte R. Motor behavior of small for gestation age newborn infants. *J Pediatr* 1970;76:208.

131. Cruz Martinez A, Perez Conde MC, Ferrer MT. Motor conduction velocity and H-reflex in infancy and childhood. I: Study in newborns, twins and small-for-dates. *Electromyogr Clin Neurophysiol* 1977;17: 493.

132. Moosa A, Dubowitz V. Assessment of gestational age in newborn infants: Nerve conduction velocity vs maturity score. *Dev Med Child Neurol* 1972;14:290.

133. Schulte FJ, Michaelis R, Linke I, Nolte R. Motor nerve conduction velocity in term, preterm and small-for-dates newborn infants. *Pediatrics* 1968;42:17.

134. Als H, Tronick E, Adamson L, Brazelton TB. The behavior of the full-term but underweight newborn infant. *Dev Med Child Neurol* 1976; 18:590.

135. Chiswick ML. Intrauterine growth retardation. *BMJ* 1985;291:845.

136. Wennergren M, Wennergren G, Vilbergasson G. Obstetric characteristics and neonatal performance in a four-year small for gestational age population. *Obstet Gynecol* 1982;72:615.

137. Piper JM, Xenakis EM-J, McFarland M, Elliott BD, Berkus MD, Langer O. Do growth-retarded premature infants have different rates of perinatal morbidity and mortality than appropriately grown premature infants? *Obstet Gynecol* 1996;87:169.

138. Sciscione AC, Gorman R, Callan NA. Adjustment of birth weight standards for maternal and infant characteristics improves the prediction of outcome in the small-for-gestational-age infant. *Am J Obstet Gynecol* 1996;175:544.

139. Hawdon JM, Platt MPW. Metabolic adaptation in small for gestational age infants. *Arch Dis Child* 1993;68:262.

140. Antunes JD, Geffner ME, Lippe BM, Landaw EM. Childhood hypoglycemia: differentiating hyperinsulinemic from nonhyperinsulinemic causes. *J Pediatr* 1990;116:105.

141. Chessex P, Reichman B, Verellen G, et al. Metabolic consequences of intrauterine growth retardation in very low birthweight infants. *Pediatr Res* 1984;18:709.

142. Collins J, Leonard JV. Hyperinsulinism in asphyxiated and small for dates infants with hypoglycemia. *Lancet* 1984;2:311.

143. Frazer T, Karl IE, Hillman LS, Bier DM. Direct measurement of gluconeogenesis from [2,3¹³C₂] alanine in the human neonate. *Am J Physiol* 1981;240:615.

144. Haymond MW, Karl IE, Pagliana AS. Increased gluconeogenic substrates in the small for gestational age infant. *N Engl J Med* 1974; 291:322.

145. Kliegman RM. Alterations of fasting glucose and fat metabolism in intrauterine growth-retarded newborn dogs. *Am J Physiol* 1989; 256:E380.

146. LeDune M. Response to glucagon in small for dates hypoglycemic and nonhypoglycemic newborn infants. *Arch Dis Child* 1972;47:754.

147. Shelly HJ, Neligan GA. Neonatal hypoglycemia. *Br Med Bull* 1966; 22:34.

148. Holtrop PC. The frequency of hypoglycemia in full-term large and small of gestational age newborns. *Am J Perinatol* 1993;10:150.

149. Williams PR, Fiser RH Jr, Sperling MA, Oh W. Effects of oral alanine feeding on blood glucose, plasma glucagon, and insulin concentrations in small for gestational age infants. *N Engl J Med* 1975; 292:612.

150. Hawdon JM, Weddell A, Aynsley-Green A, Platt MPW. Hormonal and metabolic response to hypoglycemia in small for gestational age infants. *Arch Dis Child* 1993;68:269.

151. King RA, Smith RM, Dahlenberg GW. Long term postnatal development of insulin secretion in early premature neonates. *Early Hum Dev* 1986;13:285.

152. Cowett RM, Oh W, Pollak A, Schwartz R, Stonestreet BS. Glucose disposal of low birth weight infants: steady state hyperglycemia produced by constant intravenous glucose infusion. *Pediatrics* 1979;63:389.

153. Hay WW Jr. Fetal and neonatal glucose homeostasis and their relation to the small for gestational age infant. *Semin Perinatol* 1984;8: 101.

154. Bougneres PF, Castano L, Rocchiccioli F, Gia HP. Medium-chain fatty acids increase glucose production in normal and low birth weight newborns. *Am J Physiol* 1989;256:E692.

155. Sabel K, Olegard R, Mellander M, Hildingsson K. Interrelation between fatty acid oxidation and control of gluconeogenic substrates in small for gestational age (SGA) infants with hypoglycemic and with normoglycemia. *Acta Paediatr Scand* 1982;71:53.

156. Wahlig TM, Georgieff MK. The effect of illness on neonatal metabolism and nutritional management. *Clin Perinatol* 1995;22:77.

157. Hay WW Jr. Nutritional requirements of the extremel-low-birth-weight infant. In: Hay WW Jr, ed. *Neonatal nutrition and metabolism.* St. Louis: Mosby-Year Book, 1991:361.

158. De Prins FA, Van Assche FA. Intrauterine growth retardation and development of endocrine pancreas in the experimental rat. *Biol Neonate* 1981;1:16.

159. Lebenthal E, Nitzan M, Lee PC, Chrzanowski BL, Krasher J. Effect of intrauterine growth retardation on the activities of fetal intestinal enzymes in rats. *Biol Neonate* 1981;39:14.

160. Pencharz PB, Masson M, Desgranges F, Papageorgio A. Total-body protein turnover in human premature neonates: effects of birth weight, intra-uterine nutritional status and diet. *Clin Sci* 1981;61:207.

161. Cauderay M, Schutz Y, Micheli JL, Calame A, Jequier E. Energy-nitrogen balances and protein turnover in small and appropriate for gestational age low birthweight infants. *Eur J Clin Nutr* 1988;42: 125.

162. FAO/WHO/UNU. Energy and protein requirements. *World Health Organization Technical Report Series, Report of a Joint Expert Consultation.* 1985;724:1.

163. Van Veen LCP, Ten C, Hay WW Jr, Meschia G, Battaglia FC. Leucine disposal and oxidation rates in the fetal lamb. *Metabolism* 1987;36:48.

164. Carver TD, Hay WW Jr. Uteroplacental glucose metabolism and oxygen consumption after long term hypoglycemic in pregnant sheep. *Am J Physiol* 1995;269:E299.

165. Sinclair J. Heat production and thermoregulation in the small for date infant. *Pediatr Clin North Am* 1970;17:147.

166. Bhakoo ON, Scopes JW. Minimal rates of oxygen consumption in small for dates babies during the first week of life. *Arch Dis Child* 1974;49:583.

167. Aherne W, Hull D. Brown adipose tissue and heat production in the newborn infant. *J Path Bact* 1966;91:223.

168. Silverman WA, Sinclair JC, Agate FJ Jr. Oxygen cost of minor variations in heat balance of small newborn infants. *Acta Paediatr Scand* 1966;55:294.

169. Hanmerlund K, Sedis G. Transepidermal water loss in newborn infants. IV: Small for gestational age infants. *Acta Paediatr Scand* 1980;69:377.

170. Klaus MH, Fanaroff AA, eds. *Care of the high-risk neonate,* 2nd ed. Philadelphia: WB Saunders, 1979.

171. Sinclair JC, Silverman WA. Intrauterine growth in active tissue mass of the human fetus, with particular reference to the undergrown baby. *Pediatrics* 1966;38:48.

172. Hakanson DO, Oh W. Hyperviscosity in the small-for-gestational age infant. *Biol Neonate* 1980;37:109.

173. Cassady G. Body composition in intrauterine growth retardation. *Pediatr Clin North Am* 1970;17:79.

174. Snijders RJM, Abbas A, Melby O, Ireland RM, Nicolaides KH. Fetal plasma erythropoietin concentration in severe growth retardation. *Am J Obstet Gynecol* 1993;168:615.

175. Wirth FH, Goldberg KE, Lubchenco LO. Neonatal hyperviscosity. Incidence and effect of partial plasma exchange transfusion. *Pediatr Res* 1975;19:372(abst).

176. Humbert JR, Abelson H, Hathaway WE, Battaglia FC. Polycythemia in small for gestational age infants. *J Pediatr* 1969;75:812.

177. Ferguson S. Prolonged impairment of cellular immunity in children with intrauterine growth retardation. *J Pediatr* 1978;93:52.

178. Minton S, Steichen JJ, Tsang RC. Decreased bone mineral content in small for gestational age infants compared with appropriate for gestational age infants: normal serum 25-hydroxyvitamin D and decreasing parathyroid hormone. *Pediatrics* 1983;71:383.

179. Meberg A. Hermatologic syndrome of growth-retarded infants. *Am J Dis Child* 1989;143:1260.

180. Mehta P, Vasa R, Neumann L, Karpatkin M. Thrombocytopenia in the high-risk infant. *J Pediatr* 1980;97:791.

181. Perlman M, Dvilansky A. Blood coagulation status of small for dates and postmature infants. *Arch Dis Child* 1975;50:424.

182. Lucas A. Programming by early nutrition in man. In: Block GR, Whelan J, eds. *The childhood environment and adult disease (CIBA Foundation Symposium 156).* Chichester: Wiley, 1991:38.

183. Smart J. Undernutrition, learning and memory: review of experimental studies. In: Taylor TG, Jenkins NK, eds. *Proceedings of XII International Congress of Nutrition.* London: John Libbey, 1986:74.

184. Dobbing J. Nutritional growth restriction and the nervous system. In: Davison AN, Thompson RHS, eds. *The molecular bases of neuropathology.* London: Edward Arnold, 1981:221.

185. Hack M. Effects of intrauterine growth retardation on metal performance and behavior outcomes during adolescence and adulthood. *Eur J Clin Nutr* 1998;52:S65.

186. Spinillo A, Stronati M, Ometto A, Fazzi E, Lanzi G, Guaschino S. Infant neurodevelopmental outcome in pregnancies complicated by gestational hypertension and intra-uterine growth retardation. *J Perinat Med* 1993;21:195.

187. Low JA, Handley-Derry MH, Burke SO, et al. Association of intrauterine fetal growth retardation and learning deficits at age 9 to 11 years. *Am J Obstet Gynecol* 1992;167:1499.

188. Strauss RS, Dietz WH. Growth and development of term children born with low birth weight: effects of genetic and environmental factors. *J Pediatr* 1998;133:67.

189. Fitzhardinge PM, Steven EM. The small-for-date infant. I. Later growth patterns. *Pediatrics* 1972;49:671.

190. Behrman RE. Handicap in the preterm small-for-gestational age infant. *J Pediatr* 1979;94:779.

191. Westwood M, Kramer MS, Munz D, Lovett JM, Watters GV. Growth and development of full-term nonasphyxiated small-for-gestational-age newborns: follow-up through adolescence. *Pediatrics* 1983;71:376.

192. Berg AT. Indices of fetal growth retardation, perinatal hypoxia-related factors and childhood neurological morbidity. *Early Hum Dev* 1989;19:271.

193. Hack M, Breslau N, Weissman B, Aram D, Klein N, Borawski E. Effect of very low birth weight and subnormal head size on cognitive abilities at school age. *N Engl J Med* 1991;325:231.

194. Fitzharding PM, Steven EM. The small-for-date infant. II. Neurologic and intellectual sequelae. *Pediatrics* 1972;50:50.

195. Pena IC, Teberg AJ, Finello KM. The premature small-for-gestational-age infant during the first year of life: comparison by birth weight and gestational age. *J Pediatr* 1988;113:1066.

196. Allen MC. Developmental outcome and follow up of the small for gestational age infant. *Semin Perinatol* 1984;8:123.

197. Sung I, Vohr B, Oh W. Growth and neurodevelopmental outcome of very low birth weight infants with intrauterine growth retardation: Comparison with control subjects matched by birth weight and gestational age. *J Pediatr* 1993;123:618.

198. Veelken N, Stollhoff K, Claussen M. Development and perinatal risk factors of very low-birth-weight infants. Small versus appropriate for gestational age. *Neuropediatrics* 1992;23:102.

199. Hutton JL, Pharoah POD, Cooke RWI, Stevenson RC. Differential effects of preterm birth and small gestational age on cognitive and motor development. *Arch Dis Child* 1997;76:F75.

200. Kok JH, den Ouden AL, Verloove-Vanhorick SP, Brand R. Outcome of very preterm small for gestational age infants: the first nine years of life. *Br J Obstet Gynaecol* 1998;105:162.

201. McCarton CM, Wallace IF, Divon M, Vaughn HG Jr. Cognitive and neurologic development of the premature, small for gestational age infant through age 6: comparison by birth weight and gestational age. *Pediatrics* 1996;98:1167.

202. Barker DJP. Fetal and infant origins of adult disease. *BMJ* 1993;301:1111.

203. Snoeck A, Remacle C, Reusens B, Hoet JJ. Effect of a low protein diet during pregnancy on the fetal rat endocrine pancreas. *Biol Neonate* 1990;57:107.

204. Dahri S, Snoeck A, Reusesn B, Remacle C, Hoet JJ. Islet function in offspring of mothers on a low protein diet during pregnancy. *Diabetes* 1991;40:115.

205. Dahri S, Cherif H, Reusens B, Remacle C, Hoet JJ. Effect of an isolcaloric low protein diet during gestation in rat on in vitro insulin secretion by islets of the offspring. *Diabetologia* 1994;37:A80.

206. Rasschaert J, Reusens B, Dahri S, et al. Impaired activity of rat pancreatic islet mitochondrial glycerophosphate dehydrogenase in protein malnutrition. *Endocrinology* 1995;136:2631.

207. Hay WW Jr, Catz CS, Grave GD, Yaffe SJ. Workshop summary: fetal growth: its regulation and disorders. *Pediatrics* 1997;99:585.

CHAPTER 26

The Extremely-Low-Birth-Weight Infant

Apostolos Papageorgiou and Claudette L. Bardin

In the 1960s, the term low birth weight (LBW) defined all infants born with a birth weight less than 2,500 g. With improved survival of infants born weighing less than 1,500 g in the 1970s and 1980s, the term very low birth weight (VLBW) was introduced in order to express better the problems and outcomes related to infants born in this category.

In the 1990s, it became clear that a new subdivision was necessary in order to reflect the reality of the prevailing situation, namely, the large number of surviving infants born weighing less than 1,000 g. Thus, the term extremely low birth weight (ELBW) was added to identify these infants.

Indeed, few medical specialties in recent years have enjoyed the extent of progress and success that neonatology has. With regionalization of perinatal care, improved technology, and better understanding of the pathophysiology and the specific needs of ELBW infants, survival of infants born weighing less than 1,000 g has improved dramatically (1–9). Table 26–1 reflects this progress as experienced in our own perinatal center over the last 10 years. The progress is such that certain well-organized perinatal centers in North America now rarely see babies born weighing more than 1,000 g dying without lethal congenital anomalies. Our own perinatal mortality statistics at the Sir Mortimer B. Davis-Jewish General Hospital, a McGill University tertiary care referral perinatal center with 4,000 deliveries per year and a catchment area of near 12,000 deliveries,

show a neonatal mortality consistently below 1 per 1,000 live births for the last 15 years for infants weighing more than 1,000 g, including those who died from lethal congenital anomalies. The care of premature infants weighing less than 1,500 g and particularly of those weighing less than 1,000 g, occupies an important part of the daily activities of all neonatal intensive care units (NICUs) and contributes heavily to the cost of neonatal care in general (10–13).

As mortality has much decreased, concerns have been expressed as to whether morbidity has followed the same path of improvement (9,12,14–20). There is currently strong evidence that, at least for infants born weighing more thatn 750 g, the decline in morbidity is, if not completely parallel to mortality, at least significant. The question that cannot be answered clearly at this point concerns the long-term prognosis of infants born weighing less than 750 g. The data vary from country to country and from institution to institution, the numbers are still relatively small, and the survivors are still too young to draw firm long-term conclusions.

Much of what is written in this chapter is based on our own experience with the management of ELBW infants. It should be noted that this experience may be different from that in other parts of the world. It is important to appreciate that the Canadian health care system, which provides universal access to health care, emphasizes prevention and has a very successful antenatal referral policy, with the vast majority of VLBW infants being inborn. Table 26–2 indicates the number of infants weighing less than 1,500 g born in level III maternity hospitals in the province of Quebec in comparison with the number born in levels II and I.

The aim of this chapter is to present a global approach to the particular problems and to the management of the ELBW infant, referring the reader to the specific chapters for more comprehensive review of each particular problem (Table 26–3).

A. Papageorgiou: Departments of Pediatrics and Obstetrics and Gynecology, McGill University; and Departments of Pediatrics and Neonatology, SMBD-Jewish General Hospital, Montreal, Quebec, Canada

C. L. Bardin: Department of Pediatrics, McGill University; and Departments of Pediatrics and Neonatology, SMBD-Jewish General Hospital, Montreal, Quebec, Canada

TABLE 26–1. *Decline in mortality by birthweight at Jewish General Hospital, McGill University, from 1984 to 1996*

Birth weight (g)	1984–1985		1995–1996		Percent improvement
	Births	Mortality	Births	Mortality	
500–750	25	14 (56%)	34	14 (41%)	27
751–1,000	36	10 (27.7%)	56	9 (16%)	42
500–1,000	61	24 (39.3%)	90	23 (25.5%)	37

EPIDEMIOLOGY

Until recently, statistics on ELBW infants were based exclusively on birth weight analysis. Although this method offers the advantage of an objective measurement, it may not take into account the specific problems related to gestational age (21). In other words, many infants born weighing less than 1,000 g are more mature than the birth weight may indicate, hence denoting intrauterine growth restriction (IUGR) as well as prematurity. The neonatal problems and long-term prognosis can be quite different for the more mature, small-for-gestational-age infant than for the less mature, appropriate-for-gestational-age infant of the same birth weight. The distinction between appropriate-for-gestational-age and small-for-gestational-age infants born before 28 weeks of gestation became possible only in recent years, thanks to the introduction of early pregnancy ultrasonography. In Canada and particularly in the province of Quebec, systematic ultrasonography between 16 and 18 weeks of gestation has permitted not only an early detection and frequent elimination of major congenital anomalies but, at the same time, a reasonably accurate dating of all pregnancies. The possibility of being able to assign a precise gestational age to the birth weight of an infant has not only made it possible to relate a particular problem, diagnosis, and prognosis to the degree of immaturity, but also to recognize the implications of IUGR at a very early gestational age (21). In our perinatal center, in the last four years, the incidence of IUGR, defined as a birth weight beyond 2 standard deviations (SDs) below the mean for a given gestational age, has been 33% for infants born weighing less than 1,000 g. It is hoped that as gestational age dating becomes universal and more accurate, the current method of reporting perinatal statistics based on birth weight will be complemented by the gestational age, thus reflecting both the degree of maturity and the degree of appropriateness of intrauterine growth. Hence, neonatal pathology and prognosis can be based on both gestational age and birth weight.

Although mortality rates of LBW and ELBW infants are declining, the incidence of these births has not changed significantly. In the province of Quebec, the rate of live births for infants weighing 500 to 999 g remained unchanged at 0.3% between 1981 and 1993 and for those weighing 1,000 to 1,500 g was 0.4%. Similarly, the incidence of births by gestational age remains unchanged at 0.1% for less than 26 weeks, 0.2% for 26 to 28 weeks, and 0.8% for 29 to 32 weeks (22).

Factors that long have been recognized as being associated with prematurity include extremes of maternal age, socioeconomic status, low level of education, adverse social habits, maternal diseases, and gynecologic infections (23).

Significant predictors for the survival of ELBW infants include older gestational age, heavier birth weight, female gender, African-American race, singleton birth, and the absence of severe fetal growth restriction

TABLE 26–2. *Live births according to the level of hospital care in province of Québec, 1993*

Level of care	500–999 g		1,000–1,499 g	
	n = 261	%	n = 405	%
I	4	1.5	8	2.0
II	43	16.5	66	16.2
III	214	82.0	331	81.8

TABLE 26–3. *Major problems in extremely-low-birth-weight infants*

Respiratory
  Respiratory distress syndrome
  Respiratory failure
  Apnea
  Air leaks
  Chronic lung disease
Cardiovascular
  Patent ductus arteriosus
Central nervous system
  Intraventricular hemorrhage
  Periventricular leukomalacia
  Seizures
Renal
  Electrolyte imbalance
  Acid–base disturbances
  Renal failure
Ophthalmologic
  Retinopathy of prematurity
  Strabismus
  Myopia
Gastrointestinal–nutritional
  Feeding intolerance
  Necrotizing enterocolitis
  Inguinal hernias
Immunologic
  Poor defense to infection

TABLE 26–4. *Impact of birth weight on outcome in the Canadian Collaborative Study*

Gestational age	Weight (g)	Mortality
24 wk	<700	63.3%
(N = 241)	>700	37.2%
25 wk	<760	43.3%
(N = 364)	>760	35.9%

From SB Effer, *unpublished data,* 1996.

TABLE 26–5. *Impact of gestational age on survival of 533 infants aged 24 to 25 weeks in the Canadian Collaborative Study*

Gestational age (d)	No. of N.B.	Neonatal mortality (%)
168–171	125	55.2
172–176	177	47.4
177–181	171	34.5

From SB Effer et al., *unpublished data,* 1996.

(24). The importance of birth weight for the survival of infants born at 24 and 25 weeks of gestation has been demonstrated clearly in a multicenter study of Canadian tertiary care centers. In this particular study, all infants were inborn, and the gestational ages were confirmed by early ultrasonography (Table 26–4). Likewise, maturity by only a few days has been shown to add significant chances of survival, as shown in Table 26–5. Whether analysis is done by increments of 100 g or by increments of a few days gestational age, the impact of those two factors in the survival of ELBW infants is very important. Tables 26–6 and 26–7 indicate the survival rate of infants born weighing less than 1,000 g in our institution between April 1993 and March 1997, analyzed by weight and gestational age. In our experience, infants born before 27 weeks of gestation with a birth weight 2 SD below the mean are at a disadvantage compared to appropriate-for-gestational-age infants of the same gestational age in terms of acute and chronic problems, the most striking complication being the higher incidence of retinopathy of prematurity (ROP) (21).

In terms of global epidemiologic evaluation of outcomes for infants born weighing less than 1,000 g, many factors contribute to the inaccuracy of data. A number of countries, and particularly some developing ones, do not keep statistics for infants born before 28 weeks of gestation. In other countries, when death occurs rapidly in the first day of life, the death is not recorded as a neonatal death. Also, information originating from small private institutions may be inaccurate and difficult to control. National and regional data also can be affected seriously by the ratio of inborn to outborn infants. There is strong scientific evidence that the survival of ELBW infants is greater among inborns, and this in spite of the preselec-

tion of postnatally transferred infants who are generally stronger and more mature. Apart from mortality, morbidity also appears to be increased in postnatally transferred infants, as these tiny infants do not tolerate interhospital transport well. Table 26–8 indicates the survival, management, and complications of 173 infants weighing less than 1,000 g born in our center over a 4-year period (1993 to 1997), and Table 26–9 shows the incidence of complications in the 120 survivors.

PERINATAL MANAGEMENT

Prenatal

With the advent of early pregnancy ultrasonography, in the vast majority of patients presenting with premature labor, the degree of fetal maturity is fairly well established on admission to the obstetric unit. Such patients need to be taken immediately in charge by specialists in high-risk obstetrics (obstetric perinatologists), who should attempt to establish the factors predisposing to the initiation of labor and should evaluate the condition of the fetal membranes, including the presence or absence of chorioamnionitis. Also, the likelihood of controlling labor with tocolytics in order to allow adequate time for corticosteroid administration should be evaluated.

The prospective parents should receive accurate information regarding all facets of the proposed management, including the possible need for cesarean delivery, as well as information regarding the subsequent management of the newborn infant, including the potential risks related to both the degree of prematurity and the therapeutic

TABLE 26–6. *Survival rate by birth weight of 173 inborn infants weighing <1,000 g at Jewish General Hospital, McGill University from April 1993 to March 1997*

Birth weight (g)	Total births	Survivors
<500	9	3 (33%)
501–600	24	9 (38%)
601–700	30	19 (63%)
701–800	28	19 (68%)
801–900	47	37 (79%)
901–1,000	35	33 (94%)

TABLE 26–7. *Survival rate by gestational age of 173 inborn infants weighing <1,000 g at Jewish General Hospital, McGill University, from April 1993 to March 1997*

Gestational age (wk)	Total births	Survivors
<24	24	8 (33%)
24–24⁶/₇	35	9 (38%)
25–25⁶/₇	26	21 (58%)
26–26⁶/₇	34	27 (79%)
27–27⁶/₇	18	17 (94%)
28–28⁶/₇	16	14 (88%)
29–29⁶/₇	10	8 (80%)
>30	10	10 (100%)
All gestational ages	173	120 (69%)

TABLE 26–8. *Outcome of 173 inborn infants weighing <1,000 g at Jewish General Hospital, McGill University, from April 1993 to March 1997*

	No. of infants (n = 173)	%
Survived	120	69
Small for gestational age	57	33
Antenatal betamethasone		
24 h	85	49
6–23 h	43	24
Cesarean section	91	53
Oxygen	158	91
Ventilation	143	83
Respiratory distress syndrome	99	57
Surfactant for respiratory distress syndrome	57	33
Pneumothorax only	10	5.8
Pulmonary interstitial emphysema only	19	10.9
Pneumothorax + pulmonary interstitial emphysema	10	5.8
Intraventricular hemorrhage	41	24
Grades I and II	19	11
Grades III and IV	22	13
Patent ductus arteriosus	90	52
Necrotizing enterocolitis	8	5

interventions that may be necessary to keep the infant alive.

This information ideally should be provided in the presence of both the obstetric perinatologist and the neonatologist and should be based not only on general statistical information, but also on the specific institutional experience with outcomes of newborn infants of similar gestational age. In our center, the attending neonatologist provides a written consultation on all patients admitted to the obstetric high-risk unit. We meet with the family, offer an extensive review of our experience with similar cases, and answer their questions regarding risks and outcomes. The father is invited to visit the NICU and to familiarize himself with the environment and the personnel. The mother is given a book with pictures explaining each step of the baby's treatments, from the delivery room to the time of discharge.

The lowest gestational age at which resuscitation should be initiated has long been the subject of debate (25,26). Based on our experience with ELBW infants, we offer an optimistic opinion in terms of survival and potential morbidity for pregnancies of 25 weeks' gestation and over. Between 24 and 25 weeks, although we underline that the chances of survival are around 65%, we emphasize the increased risk of potential complications, such as intraventricular hemorrhage (IVH), ROP, and

TABLE 26–9. *Complications among 120 survivors <1,000 g at Jewish General Hospital, McGill University, from April 1993 to March 1997*

	No. of infants (n = 120)	%
Oxygen	106	88
28 d	82	68
36 wk	41	34
Ventilation	93	78
Respiratory distress syndrome	61	52
Intraventricular hemorrhage	19	15
Grades I and II	11	9
Grades III and IV	7	6
Patent ductus arteriosus	74	62
Closure with indomethacin	57	77
Surgery	17	23
Necrotizing enterocolitis	6	5
ROP	67	56
Stage I	19	16
Stage II	30	25
Stage III	18	15
Stage IV	0	0
Cryo-laser	7	6
Periventricular leukomalacia	6	5

chronic lung disease (CLD). For pregnancies between 23 and 24 weeks of gestation, although we emphasize the higher incidence of complications previously mentioned, we also mention the possibility of intact survival or survival with minimal handicaps. Finally, for pregnancies below 23 weeks of gestation, we make it clear to the parents that vigorous resuscitation, including intubation, will be undertaken only if the newborn has at least the degree of maturity predicted by dates and/or ultrasonography, and if, in the judgement of the neonatologist present in the delivery room, the newborn has reasonable chances of responding to resuscitation. We always make it clear to the parents that initiation of resuscitation and subsequent treatments in the NICU do not preclude discontinuation of therapy if a major complication such as severe IVH is detected in the hours or days following birth. The presence of a staff neonatologist in the delivery room is an integral part of our protocol for the management of ELBW infants.

One of the most difficult questions that parents ask, and which our obstetric colleagues continuously debate, is the safest route of delivery in the presence of either a breech presentation or evidence of fetal distress (27). In our institution, based on our own results, we advise cesarean delivery in such situations as of 25 weeks' gestation. Between 24 and 25 weeks, we feel less inclined to recommend cesarean delivery, particularly in view of the fact that many may require a classic incision. The decision to proceed with such an intervention is taken with the clear understanding by the parents of all the medical implications for both the mother and the infant. Finally, at less than 24 weeks of gestation, cesarean delivery is performed strictly for maternal indications. Our incidence of cesarean section by gestational age is indicated in Table 26–10. It is obvious that a large number of cesarean deliveries, and particularly those between 22 and 24 weeks of gestation, are performed strictly for maternal indications, i.e., severe abruption, pre-eclampsia, etc.

Another difficult management situation relates to ruptured membranes between 18 and 22 weeks of gestation, resulting in severe oligohydramnios, with the inherent risk of lung underdevelopment (28,29). Serial ultrasounds can evaluate the degree of reaccumulation of amniotic fluid and allow for a better educated decision as to whether continuation of pregnancy is advisable (30). However, in the vast majority of these cases, the outcome is very poor, and termination of pregnancy constitutes reasonable advice, particularly if rupture of membranes occurred before 20 weeks of gestation with poor reaccumulation of amniotic fluid. Amnioinfusion has been proposed and tried as a means of overcoming the problem of chest compression, so far with limited success (31).

Impending Delivery

The management of a patient with impending premature delivery should include the following: evaluation of gestational age by dates and/or early ultrasound, fetal size and position, condition of the fetal membranes, amount of amniotic fluid volume, and evidence of chorioamnionitis and other obstetric complications such as bleeding, toxemia, etc. Rectovaginal cultures for the detection of group B streptococcal colonization and initiation of therapy with penicillin also is in order (32). If cultures results return negative, penicillin can be discontinued. In all patients over 23 weeks of gestation who are not infected and for whom there is no maternal indication for immediate pregnancy termination, such as massive bleeding, and in whom the cervix is dilated less than 5 cm, we propose tocolysis with magnesium sulfate or Ritodrine and administration of betamethasone (33). Our experience over the years with the combination of tocolysis and betamethasone has been supported fully by the recent NIH Statement on Antenatal Use of Corticosteroids (34). For patients between 23 and 34 weeks' gestation, we administer two doses of 12 mg of betamethasone, 24 hours apart, and administer a "booster" dose of 12 mg weekly for those patients who continue to be at risk of delivering prematurely. Beyond 34 weeks, we use steroids only when an amniocentesis is indicated and the L/S ratio shows persistent lung immaturity. Multiple pregnancies are offered similar therapy (35). We monitor body temperature and changes in leukocyte count, keeping in mind the transient rise in leukocytosis after administration of betamethasone.

If a patient whose labor has been previously well controlled with tocolysis begins to contract actively, we discontinue tocolysis and allow labor to progress. We consider these patients as potentially infected or abrupting. If a patient has fever or demonstrates other signs of chorioamnionitis, broad-spectrum antibiotics are initiated. A number of obstetricians have started using antibiotic therapy to control premature labor or in the presence of bacterial vaginosis (36,37). This seems a reasonable approach, because between 30% and 50% of premature births are believed to be precipitated by common genital tract infections. The possibility of preventing a number of

TABLE 26–10. *Cesarean section rate in 173 infants weighing <1,000 g[a] at Jewish General Hospital, McGill University, from April 1993 to March 1997*

Gestational age (wk)	No. deliveries	No. cesarean sections
<24	24	3 (13%)
24–24$^6/_7$	35	15 (43%)
25–25$^6/_7$	26	12 (46%)
26–26$^6/_7$	34	19 (56%)
27–27$^6/_7$	18	12 (67%)
28–28$^6/_7$	16	11 (69%)
29–29$^6/_7$	10	9 (90%)
30	10	10 (100%)

[a]Where the section is otherwise indicated.

premature births with the administration of antibiotics seems an interesting proposition that needs additional study. Screening and treatment for vaginosis needs to be initiated at the first visit and repeated at 20 and 28 weeks of gestation. The most useful medications for vaginosis are erythromycin, metronidazole, and clindamycin (38).

Delivery Room Management

The successful management of ELBW infant begins in the delivery room (Table 26–11) (see also Chap. 18). A well-organized and equipped delivery room and the presence of a competent team headed by an experienced neonatologist are essential ingredients to the proper reception of these very fragile newborns. The basic principle guiding successful management should be directed toward prevention of any physiologic deviation from normality, such as hypothermia, acidosis, or hypoxia. At the same time, it is important that each intervention during the resuscitation process be adapted carefully to the size and the needs of the tiny infant. Brisk maneuvers, excessive positive pressure with bagging, or inappropriate administration of drugs and fluids can induce permanent central nervous system (CNS) or lung injuries.

It seems particularly inappropriate when high-risk mothers are referred to a tertiary care center for specialized perinatal care to have their premature newborn infants cared for in the delivery room and during the critical first hours of their lives by unsupervised in-training personnel. Major decisions, such as whether to initiate resuscitation and for how long, often have to be made in extremely short periods of time and under heavy pressure for infants at the limit of viability. This, in our view, can be done only by experienced personnel (39).

In our center, the birth of an ELBW infant is always attended by a neonatologist in addition to the pediatric house staff and a trained delivery room nurse. Appropriate equipment is used according to the American Heart Association and American Academy of Pediatrics guidelines for neonatal resuscitation, with particular emphasis on temperature control (i.e., radiant heater set at maximum temperature and prewarmed blankets).

During the initial steps of stabilization, the condition of the infant is assessed rapidly. After drying, positioning on warm blankets, and suctioning, most of the ELBW infants require immediate initiation of intermittent positive-pressure ventilation with a bag and mask. For the ELBW infants, ventilation is more effective if performed at a higher ventilatory rate than for the term infant. We use anesthesia bags and ventilate at a rate of 60 to 80 breaths per minute, adjusting the pressure to provide adequate bilateral air entry. For extremely premature infants, intubation in the delivery room may follow rapidly. Because our NICU is adjacent to the delivery room, if the infant is responding well to manual ventilation (heart rate greater than 100, pink color), he or she is transferred to the NICU for further management. Continuous ventilation and oxygenation are provided during the transfer. In hospitals with a separate resuscitation room in the delivery suite, stabilization should be provided there. Rarely in our experience will an infant require chest compressions or epinephrine. The prognosis of ELBW infants requiring these types of interventions is very guarded, particularly if their birth weight is less than 750 g. Fluid resuscitation is reserved only for those infants in whom significant blood loss has occurred and usually is performed in the NICU.

Even following optimal resuscitation, the Apgar scores of ELBW infants rarely exceed 6 or 7 in view of their decreased tone and reactivity, poor respiratory effort, and initially poor peripheral perfusion (40). The infant's heart rate is thus the best measure of the effectiveness of resuscitation efforts.

The topic of delivery room management would not be properly covered without mentioning the ethical dilemmas faced by the neonatologist, when parental and medical opinions regarding resuscitation differ, or when an ELBW infant is severely asphyxiated and requires prolonged resuscitation. It is our view that parental opinions must be respected as long as they are reasonable, and

---

TABLE 26–11. *The first 60 minutes of life*

1. Expert resuscitation in the delivery room.
2. Good thermoregulation. Dry in the delivery room and provide high humidity environment in the incubator.
3. Minimum handling and avoidance of brisk maneuvers.
4. Expert cardiorespiratory support.
   a. Intubation when indicated, avoiding excessive pressures.
   b. Continuous monitoring of oxygenation with pulse oximetry.
   c. Monitoring of blood pressure. Prudent administration of volume expenders.
   d. Catheterization of umbilical vessels when indicated.
   e. Blood gases, hemoglobin, white blood cells + differential, blood glucose
   f. Radiographic evaluation of lung pathology and position of catheters.
   g. Administration of surfactant when indicated. Rapid adjustment of ventilatory support.
5. Intravenous $D_{10}W$ and antibiotics when indicated.
6. Parental information

after full and honest discussion of the infant's chances of meaningful survival.

Admission to the Neonatal Intensive Care Unit

We believe that expert management in the delivery room and during the first hours after admission in the NICU are of paramount importance in order to prevent immediate and long-term complications in the ELBW infant. It is for this reason that all our premature deliveries are attended in the delivery room and stabilized in the NICU by a team led by a staff neonatologist, regardless of the time of day. It is well established that the majority of cerebral injuries occur around the time of delivery or in the immediate postnatal period. Acute changes in cerebral blood flow may predispose the very fragile network of periventricular vessels to rupture. Hence, it is essential to handle these very fragile infants with extreme care, avoiding unnecessary disturbances, and preventing rather than correcting physiologic deviations in acid–base balance, blood gases, blood pressure, or body temperature. Also, overly agressive ventilation in either the delivery room or the NICU may predispose to significant acute or chronic pulmonary problems, such as hyperinflation and loss of elasticity of the alveoli, pulmonary interstitial emphysema, pneumothorax, and eventually CLD. In our center, during the first hours after admission, the premature infant is placed in an open radiant warmer to allow for easier access.

The vast majority of our ELBW infants who require assisted ventilation are intubated in the NICU. Only in exceptional situations, when the infant does not respond to bag and mask ventilation, is intubation performed in the delivery room. We use the nasotracheal route, and we never use an endotracheal (ET) tube larger than 2.5 mm for infants with a birth weight less than 1,000 g. We believe that it is important to use a low-caliber ET tube in order to avoid subglottic trauma, strictures, and eventually stenosis. We have never had to perform a tracheostomy in an infant, and stridor has been very rare among our patients.

If the newborn infant is in distress, an umbilical arterial catheter is inserted, and, in infants weighing less than 750 g, we also insert an umbilical central venous line. We use the venous line to infuse fluids, thus avoiding excessive handling and disturbance to the newborn infant in the first 24 to 48 hours of life. The tip of the catheter is positioned at the junction of the inferior vena cava and the right atrium, thus avoiding the liver. This is important, particularly when infusing hypertonic solutions, such as sodium bicarbonate or calcium gluconate. The arterial line is used exclusively for blood sampling. We favor the high position of the tip of the catheter, just above the level of the diaphragm (D10). The catheter is flushed intermittently with a heparinized solution of 5% dextrose in water or 0.45% saline, depending on the levels of serum sodium or blood glucose.

Blood is analyzed for glucose, electrolytes, blood gases, hemoglobin, and leukocytes, and an intravenous with 10% dextrose is initiated at a rate varying from 85 to 100 mL/kg/d, according to the degree of immaturity and the type of incubator used (radiant heater vs. closed incubator). When almost 10% of the baby's blood volume has been removed, we replace it with packed red cells. We use a single donor, collecting the blood in small packs, which last up to 6 weeks. Donors are screened extensively for all viral illnesses. Very sick infants receive one-to-one nursing care until the condition is stabilized, at which point the ratio of nurse-to-baby becomes one-to-two.

A percutaneous central venous catheter usually is inserted between the second and third day of life for intravenous alimentation (41). As portal of entry, we use the upper extremities of the infant, and we aim for the tip of the catheter to be at the junction of the superior vena cava and the right atrium. In case of failure to properly position a central line, a venocath is introduced into one of the baby's extremities. Total parenteral nutrition (TPN) generally is started after the first 48 hours of life, when electrolytes, glucose, urea, and acid–base status are well controlled. When the mother receives intravenous fluids during her labor, a baseline electrolytic profile of the newborn shortly after birth seems to be the proper way to follow up subsequent changes. Electrolytes are repeated between 12 and 18 hours of age. During the first 72 hours, the body weight is recorded every 8 hours, and fluid intake is adjusted accordingly. The new incubators have incorporated scales, allowing recordings without excessive handling and disturbance of the newborn infant. One other major advantage of the new incubators is that they can provide a high level of humidity, thus substantially reducing the need for large volumes of fluid that, in the past, were responsible for hyperglycemia due to the delivery of an excessive glucose load.

In order to establish prognostic criteria, it is important to obtain a cranial ultrasound in the first 24 hours of life (42,43). This ultrasound needs to be repeated at least 1 week later, or as often as necessary, depending on the pathology detected on admission or if the infant's condition has deteriorated, suggesting CNS involvement. It is also important, before discharge from the hospital, to repeat the cranial ultrasound in order to evaluate the presence or absence of periventricular leukomalacia (PVL) (44). Ideally, this last ultrasound should not be done before 35 to 36 weeks of postmenstrual age.

Respiratory Support

The vast majority of infants with a birth weight less than 1,000 g will need some form of assisted ventilation in order to survive. Some controversy surrounds the timing and criteria for the initiation of assisted ventilation. Likewise, controversy also exists as to whether these tiny infants should receive prophylactic exogenous surfactant in the delivery room. We do not systematically intubate infants born weighing less than 1,000 g, and we do not administer surfactant unless the infant requires assisted ventilation and a minimum FiO_2 of 0.40. As for the choice of surfactant, the literature indicates that both the natural and the synthetic ones are effective, with probably a small edge in favor of the natural surfactants, particularly for the very premature infant (45). In our center, we favor the natural preparations.

The introduction of exogenous surfactant therapy has reduced significantly the mortality of all newborns suffering from respiratory failure secondary to respiratory distress syndrome (RDS), but its impact has been particularly important among the most premature infants (46–52). Administration of surfactant in these very tiny infants requires extra care, as rapid changes in lung compliance may not only damage the lungs by creating overinflation and overdistention, but also may predispose to acute changes in ductal circulation, which, in turn, could lead to both cerebral and/or pulmonary hemorrhage. With rapid improvement in oxygenation, persistent hyperoxia also may be detrimental to the eyes. Hence, the administration of surfactant should be performed by an experienced person, under close monitoring of ventilatory parameters and rapid reduction of peak inspiratory pressures (PIP) and oxygen concentrations. If necessary, a second dose of surfactant may be administered as soon as 6 hours after the first. However, in our experience, if the response to the second dose is not satisfactory, it is highly unlikely that the condition will improve with additional administration of surfactant. In our center, 70% of the babies improved rapidly, requiring only a single dose of surfactant.

Mechanical ventilation has improved dramatically the survival of infants weighing less than 1,000 g. In the 1970s, very few infants less than 1,000 g survived. In the early 1980s, survival of infants weighing 500 to 700 g varied from 3% to 25%, and that of infants weighing 750 to 1,000 g ranged from 30% to 70% (53). In initiating mechanical ventilation, it is imperative that minimal settings be used. Studies have shown that hyperventilation and overinflation of lungs increase the loss of surface active phospholipids (54). Also, overinflation predisposes to air leaks and particularly to pulmonary interstitial emphysema (PIE). The latter is a serious complication in the tiny infant, and it is a relatively frequent one. It is probably related to structural immaturity of the lungs, particularly to the relative lack of elastic tissue, which normally increases progressively throughout gestation (55). Also, the interstitium is larger in the more immature infant due to poor alveolization. Although drainage of a pneumothorax may lead to rapid improvement, management of PIE is far more complicated. As lung compliance is reduced, there is a need for increased PIPs to maintain adequate ventilation. This results in increased barotrauma to the small airways. Chorioamnionitis has been reported as a risk factor predisposing to PIE. In our experience, the highest incidence of PIE in tiny infants has been observed when intrauterine pneumonia complicates the RDS. In order to overcome the problems related to PIE, a number of strategies have been devised. These include acceptance of higher levels of PCO_2 and lower levels of pH, reduction of the positive end-expiratory pressure (PEEP) to between 2 and 3 cm H_2O, selective intubation of the contralateral lung, positioning the infant on the affected side, increasing the expiratory time, and systemic corticosteroid therapy. The combination of the above strategies can occasionally produce quite spectacular recovery from this condition.

A variety of ventilatory strategies have been promoted in order to maintain satisfactory ventilation and to reduce the risk of complications (56), such as high PIP–low rates, low PIP–high rates, variation in the I:E ratio, variations in the flow, permissive hypercapnia, tolerance of lower pH, and, more recently, high-frequency oscillation and even ventilation via nasal prongs. In recent years, however, the general trend is to use the lowest possible PIP to achieve acceptable ventilation and oxygenation. Of course, the question is what is considered "acceptable"? Some neonatologists will tolerate a pH as low as 7.20 and a PCO_2 as high as 65 mm Hg. Most centers also aim for PaO_2 values between 50 and 70 mm Hg. Our own approach to the ventilation of tiny infants for the last 15 years has been the following. We favor nasotracheal intubation with a 2.5-mm ET tube. Following the intubation, we hand bag the infant for 5 minutes with high rates (80 to 100 per minute) and very low pressures, while adjusting the oxygen requirements according to pulse oximetry. Subsequently, we connect the infant to the ventilator. Our PIPs rarely exceed 14 to 15 cm H_2O, and we set the PEEP at 5 cm H_2O, with initial rates of 65 to 80 per minute. We aim for PaO_2 values between 45 and 50 mm Hg, which is enough to abolish production of lactic acid and, at the same time, remains relatively close to intrauterine values. Our pulse oximeters (Ohmeda) (57) are set to alarm at a lower limit of 80% and an upper limit of 93%. We believe that this modest degree of oxygenation offers the advantage of reducing the need for high administration of oxygen concentrations, thus minimizing lung toxicity, and may help to avoid retinal damage. Our incidence of bronchopulmonary dysplasia (BPD) and ROP are shown in Table 26–9. We believe that by using the lowest possible PIP and a relatively rapid respiratory rate, we reduce overdistention and barotrauma and minimize the risk of BPD. Because, in RDS, there are compartments in the lung with relatively normal ventilation perfusion ratios and others with poor ventilation and adequate perfusion, it seems reasonable to attempt to improve ventilation of the poor ventilation perfusion (V-Q) compartment without overdistention of the normal V-Q compartment. Raising the ventilatory rate, which raises the mean airway pressure without changing the PIP, appears to accomplish this goal (58). We also have observed that with high respiratory rates, the tiny infant very rapidly stops fighting the respirator, thus making the gas exchange smoother and possibly decreasing the incidence of air leaks. These high respiratory rates also seem to be more physiologic for the very immature infant, as observed by Greenough and collaborators (59). For toilet of the airways, we use the Ballard closed suction circuit, thus avoiding disconnecting the infant from the ventilator (60). We suction sparsely, particularly during the first few days of life, when the volume of secretions is minimal.

Our ventilated babies have their umbilical vessels cannulated for blood sampling and for fluid infusion. As soon as the procedures of intubation and catheterization of the umbilical vessels are completed, we perform chest and abdominal radiography in order to assess the position of the ET tube and the umbilical catheters and, at the same time, to evaluate the severity of lung pathology. Fifteen minutes after the initiation of ventilation, we obtain an arterial blood gas and adjust the ventilatory parameters accordingly. We generally aim for a pH above 7.28 and a PCO_2 between 45 and 55 mm Hg, but when the PIPs are elevated or in the presence of PIE, we tolerate PCO_2 values up to 60 mm Hg as long as the pH is at least 7.25. When the PCO_2 is marginally higher than desirable, first we increase the respiratory rate slightly. We have rarely encountered inadvertent PEEP with rates less than 85 per minute. If the PCO_2 remains above 60 mm Hg or the pH remains below 7.25, we increase slightly the PIP. Each time we make ventilatory adjustments, we repeat the blood gases within 15 to 20 minutes, until we reach the desired values. Our ET tubes are sutured to the tape placed on the upper lip. We record the level at which sutures were placed on the ET tube, thus avoiding the need for repeated chest radiography in order to evaluate the tube position with every reintubation. Actually, we take very few radiographs, and we rely extensively on clinical assessment, blood gases, and pulse oximetry.

When the oxygen requirement exceeds 40% or the initial x-ray shows severe RDS, we immediately administer exogenous surfactant and rapidly adjust the ventilatory parameters according to the new lung compliance. In recent years, of 173 live births of infants weighing less than 1,000 g in our center, 57 infants required surfactant, representing barely 33% of the total population. However, among the 99 infants with RDS, 57 (57%) received surfactant (Table 25–8). We believe that one of the reasons for the relatively small number of infants who required surfactant therapy is our extensive use of antenatal steroids. Indeed, the mothers of 85 of the 173 infants (49%) had received the full two doses of betamethasone, and the mothers of 55 more (35%) had received one dose 6 to 23 hours before delivery.

We do not use sedation in tiny babies requiring mechanical ventilation. When this becomes necessary because an infant is very agitated or we undertake a painful procedure, we use intravenous fentanyl.

Avery et al. (61) reported in 1987 that the incidence of BPD varied between neonatal units. The unit with the lowest incidence used continuous positive airway pressure (CPAP) much more frequently than did the other units. Epidemiologic data from 36 units in the Vermont-Oxford Trial Network also indicate large differences in the incidence of BPD, from 16% to 70% for infants weighing between 501 and 1500 g (62). The incidence of BPD was lower in units allowing higher PCO_2 values. More evidence of the association of BPD and PCO_2 was provided by Kraybil et al (63). More recently, Garland et al. (64) reported the highest incidence of BPD among infants with the lowest PCO_2 before the administration of surfactant.

The concept of permissive hypercapnia for patients requiring mechanical ventilation gives priority to the prevention or limitation of severe pulmonary hyperinflation over the maintenance of normal ventilation. The principle consists of allowing the PCO_2 to rise by minimizing ventilator pressures and tidal volume (65). Potential risks of high PCO_2 values include increased cerebral perfusion, increased retinal perfusion, increased pulmonary vascular resistance, and reduction of pH. Based on epidemiologic observations, it appears that respiratory acidosis, unlike metabolic acidosis, is not associated with poor neurologic outcomes. Vannucci et al. (66) demonstrated similar findings in animal studies involving rats.

Flow rate also can affect ventilation and increase airway injury. We generally use a flow rate between 3 and 5 L/min. Only when we need very high pressures, for instance, in the presence of pulmonary hemorrhage, do we allow the flow rate to exceed 5 L/min.

Several reports in the literature have expressed concern about potential side effects of low PCO_2 values (67). Graziani et al. (68) reported that, along with other factors, a marked hypocarbia during the first 3 postnatal days was associated with increased risk of periventricular white matter injury in premature infants. The theoretical model of ischemic brain injury has been described by Wigglesworth and Pape (69). These authors hypothesize that cerebral blood flow could be decreased by several factors, including hypotension, hyperoxia, hypocarbia, and increased venous pressures. Concern also has been expressed in the literature about high-frequency ventilation, which may lead to low PCO_2 values due to effective alveolar ventilation (70,71). However, the data regarding the development of PVL among infants managed with these devices remain controversial. Most of the authors agree, however, that for hypocarbia to be dangerous for the brain, it has to reach levels below 30 mm Hg and most likely 25 mm Hg. Our policy is to avoid PCO_2 values below 40 mm Hg by first reducing PIP to around 10 to 12 mm Hg and PEEP to 3 mm Hg before reducing respiratory rates.

The time of extubation of ELBW infants is very important, because they are subsequently prone to develop severe apnea with the potential of cerebral injury. Contrary to the general trend to proceed with rapid extubation, we favor a slow weaning process (72). We maintain the infants at a very low PIP of 10 to 12 mm Hg and a PEEP of 3 mm Hg/min and rates of 15 to 25 per minute for several days while providing maximum intravenous and oral alimentation under stable conditions. When the infant is stronger and starting to gain weight, we administer caffeine and proceed directly to extubation, avoiding CPAP via the ET tube. The infant then is placed on nasal CPAP. The CPAP is discontinued when, after periodic trials, the infant can maintain good oxygenation without significant apnea, bradycardia, and desaturations.

Cardiovascular Support

By far, the major cardiovascular problem in ELBW infants is the presence of a patent ductus arteriosus (PDA). More than 50% of infants born weighing less than 1,000 g will have a PDA diagnosed during the first few days of life (73,74). The onset of clinical manifestations of the PDA is related to the timing of improvement of the infant's respiratory status, which is associated with decreasing pulmonary vascular resistance and predominantly left-to-right shunt. However, the patency of the ductus arteriosus can be documented easily in the first hours of life, with the help of echocardiography. At this early stage of life, the shunt is either right to left or bidirectional, depending on the severity of the infant's respiratory condition. In our center, the incidence of clinically significant PDA requiring therapy has been around 60% of all infants weighing less than 1,000 g. The left-to-right ductal shunting can be diagnosed as early as in the first day of life in infants with RDS who improved following surfactant therapy (75). An active precordium, with bounding pulses and visible carotid pulse, often will precede auscultation of a murmur. If left untreated, the infant may develop left-sided heart failure and pulmonary edema or hemorrhagic pulmonary edema, with significant deterioration of the respiratory status. Significant left-to-right ductal shunting may cause decreased peripheral perfusion and oxygen delivery. ELBW infants with significant PDA are at risk for IVH, necrotizing enterocolitis (NEC), renal failure, CLD, and metabolic acidosis (76). The size of the ductus arteriosus, as well as the ratio of the left atrium to aortic root, can be measured easily by echocardiography (77). We consider as significant a PDA greater than 1.5 mm and/or a ratio of left atrium to aortic root greater than 1.3.

The ductus arteriosus of the premature infant is less responsive to the vasoconstrictive effect of oxygen and is less likely to close spontaneously than that of term infants, especially in infants with RDS. The classic management of PDA first involves medical and supportive measures, i.e., fluid restriction, diuresis, distending airway pressure, and transfusion of packed red blood cells to keep the hemato-

crit above 0.4. If these measures fail to close the ductus arteriosus, pharmacologic closure is possible with a cyclooxygenase inhibitor, namely indomethacin (78–80). In ELBW infants, because closure of the ductus arteriosus is unlikely to occur spontaneously, the infant is at risk for the short- and long-term complications mentioned previously. Hence, therapy with indomethacin has become standard practice for the majority of these infants. Different protocols of treatment have been proposed. In our center, we treat most infants with 0.2 mg/kg of indomethacin every 12 hours for three doses. For infants developing clinical and/or biochemical signs of renal failure, we subsequently use 0.1 mg/kg per dose (81). A reduction in fluid intake is advisable prior to administration of indomethacin. In our experience, about 80% of the treated infants will respond with a functional closure of the ductus. However, about 30% of these may reopen, in which case, additional indomethacin is administered. If the ductus arteriosus fails to close after three courses of indomethacin, or if indomethacin cannot be administered because of significant renal dysfunction on previous treatment, then surgical ligation is necessary. In our center, 30% of infants less than 25 weeks required surgical ligation of the ductus after repeated failures of pharmacologic therapy. The more premature the infant and the greater the postnatal age at the time of treatment, the greater the failure of indomethacin (82). A group particularly resistant to indomethacin therapy are ELBW infants with severe IUGR (21). Suggested hypotheses for this high failure rate of indomethacin therapy among this group of infants include chronic hypoxia, altered levels of prostaglandin, and altered number or sensitivity of their receptors (83).

Contraindications to indomethacin therapy are renal failure, active bleeding, thrombocytopenia, and severe indirect hyperbilirubinemia. The presence of IVH does not appear to be an absolute contraindication to the use of indomethacin. Recent studies indicate that there is no progression of the severity of IVH after administration of indomethacin for PDA closure (84). Until additional data are available, it is prudent in the presence of IVH to verify the platelet count prior to the administration of indomethacin and to eliminate any bleeding diathesis.

The optimal time of administration of indomethacin is a matter of debate. Recent studies suggest that early or prophylactic use of indomethacin reduces not only the incidence of clinically significant PDA, but also may have a positive effect on the incidence of pulmonary hemorrhage, CLD, and IVH (85). At present, the trend seems to be in favor of attempting early pharmacologic closure of any ductus over 1.5 mm in those tiny infants, and this has been our approach in recent years.

Another cyclooxygenase inhibitor that seems very promising is ibuprofen (86). It has the theoretical advantage over indomethacin that it may increase the range of blood pressure over which cerebral blood flow is autoregulated, but has little effect on cerebral blood flow during normotension (87,88). In a phase I study carried out in our center, we observed a dramatic response in 12 ELBW infants treated with ibuprofen within 3 hours of birth (89). All 12 infants had their PDA permanently closed after three doses of ibuprofen. We also have observed a significant trend in the reduction of IVH and practically no side effects, particularly with regard to renal function. A large multicenter study, scheduled to start soon, may shed more light on this very promising therapy. Finally, it is our view that, in the presence of a clinically significant ductus that fails to respond to pharmacologic closure or in the presence of contraindications to the use of indomethacin, surgical ligation should not be delayed, as the presence of a continuous left-to-right shunt may contribute to ventilator and oxygen dependency with well-known consequences in terms of CLD.

With the exception of hypovolemic shock, when volume replacement is an urgent matter, we rarely use volume expanders and β-adrenergic drugs to maintain blood pressure. We pay particular attention to skin perfusion. As a rule of thumb, we aim for a mean blood pressure that is numerically slightly above the gestational age of the infant.

Fluids and Electrolytes

The management of fluids and electrolytes remains one of the most challenging aspects in the care of the ELBW infant. Knowledge of the body composition of these infants and better understanding of their renal function has helped to determine their requirements (90,91).

It is important to remember that the body of the ELBW infant is made up of 85% to 90% water, which is distributed as one-third intracellular water (ICW) and two-thirds extracellular water (ECW). Immediately following birth, glomerular filtration rate and fractional excretion of sodium (FENa) are low and urine output is minimal. This is followed by the diuretic phase, which results in a decrease in the ECW compartment. Furthermore, because of the large body surface area to body weight ratio and the underdeveloped epidermis of the ELBW infant, evaporative losses, if uncontrolled, may be of very significant magnitude, i.e., 5.7 mL/kg/h (92,93). However, the immature kidney, having a limiting concentrating ability (less than 700 mOsm), produces large amounts of diluted urine. Thus, without close control of fluid intake and the infant's environment, the infant is very vulnerable to dehydration and hypertonicity, which may predispose to IVH. One also has to be careful not to overload the infant with fluids, because this may have an impact on PDA, with possible congestive heart failure, pulmonary edema, and worsening pulmonary function (94).

For initial care of the infant under a radiant warmer, we have found it helpful to cover the head of the infant with a bonnet and to keep the body in a plastic bag with heated humidity. This significantly reduces water and heat loss. Once the infant's respiratory status has stabilized and the need for ready access to the infant is not as essential as it is during the hours following admission, the infant is transferred to an incubator, maintaining 75% to 80% humidity for the first week of life. This approach allows limitation of fluid intake to between 80 and 100 mL/kg/d for the first day of life. In addition, we monitor the infant's weight every 8 hours during the first days of life and adjust fluid intake consequently. In our experience, under these described conditions, we rarely have to exceed 180 mL/kg/d, even for infants with a birth weight less than 600 g.

Electrolyte abnormalities such as hypernatremia, hyponatremia, and hyperkalemia frequently are seen in ELBW infants. Hypernatremia is usually the result of severe insensible water loss, but can be secondary to the treatment of metabolic acidosis with large amounts of sodium bicarbonate. Hyponatremia (less than 130 mmol/L) more frequently is seen because of the high FENa during the diuretic phase. It can be present in the first day of life if the mother has received large amounts of hypotonic intravenous fluids. Hyponatremia also is seen following therapy with indomethacin without prior proper reduction of fluid intake, as well as later on when diuretics are used for the treatment of BPD.

On admission, infants receive only a 10% dextrose solution in water. We monitor blood glucose and electrolytes closely and we test all urines for glucose. We subsequently adjust the intravenous dextrose according to the blood glucose values. We start sodium supplementation only when its serum value is less than 140 mmol/L, which usually happens between the second and third days of life.

Hyperkalemia (K^+ greater than 7 mmol/L) is a severe acute problem in this ELBW group of infants, even in the absence of oliguria and potassium intake (95). A rapid rise in serum potassium can be seen during the first 24 hours of life, especially in the most immature infants. A few mechanisms have been proposed for this hyperkalemia, i.e., relative hypoaldosteronism, immaturity of the renal distal tubules, and internal potassium shift from the intracellular space to the extracellular space. Hyperkalemia is also more severe in infants with intraventricular or pulmonary hemorrhage, extensive bruising, or renal failure. It is prudent to obtain a baseline measurement of electrolytes following birth, particularly when the mother has received intravenous fluids. We routinely repeat the electrolyte measurements every 12 to 18 hours during the first few of days of life, or more frequently if indicated, especially for the smallest infants.

We treat all cases of hyperkalemia exceeding 7 mmol/L with insulin and sodium bicarbonate to allow an intracellular shift of potassium, calcium gluconate for stabilization of the myocardium, and cation exchange resin (Kayexalate) per rectum if potassium continues to rise. Potassium supplements are introduced only after the serum level has stabilized below 4.5 mmol/L.

We also monitor urine output and use the urine specific gravity and osmolality as an additional guide to assess the renal function and hydration status of the infant. Typically, the urine pH of the ELBW infant is over 7 in the first few of days of life, then decreases as the tubular reabsorption of bicarbonate increases. Microscopic hematuria consistently is seen in the urine of the ELBW infant in the first few of days after birth, regardless of the health status of the infant. Monitoring the presence of glucose in the urine can be a good indicator of the carbohydrate homeostasis of the newborn infant. Some extremely premature infants have a low glucose threshold and may be predisposed to osmotic diuresis.

Management of fluids in the ELBW infants is very much dependent on securing an intravenous line. Intravenous access may, at times, become very difficult, thus compromising fluid, electrolyte, and glucose homeostasis, thermoregulation, and physiologic stability due to the pain induced by multiple attempts to insert a venocath. The umbilical vessels usually provide an easy access route for the first days of life, subsequently, small neonatal infusion needles (IMP Group International Inc.) are inserted in the scalp or a venocath is inserted in one of the extremities. In our center, we favor the insertion of a percutaneous central venous catheter, which gives continuous venous access for as long as necessary (41). In our experience, this technique has not increased the incidence of infection when compared to peripheral catheters used for prolonged total parenteral alimentation.

The Skin of the Extremely-Low-Birth-Weight Infant

The skin of an infant born at 23 to 26 weeks of gestation is extremely immature. Maturity of the epidermis is achieved at birth only in infants born after 32 weeks of gestation (96). Prior to this time, the epidermis is underdeveloped, especially the stratum corneum, predisposing to very high transepidermal water loss, as well as the risk of trauma and percutaneous absorption of toxic agents. The skin also is permeable to gases, allowing for diffusion of oxygen and carbon dioxide. The tremendous transepidermal water loss of the ELBW infant predisposes to dehydration, electrolyte imbalance, and evaporative heat loss. Trauma to the skin may provide a portal of entry for infectious organisms. Fortunately, after birth, there is acceleration of epidermal maturation, such that, by 2 weeks of age, the skin of the premature infant almost resembles that of the term infant. Preservation of skin integrity and prevention of transepidermal water loss have been, and still are, areas of challenge in neonatology. Under a radiant warmer, water loss is extensive. Plastic shields have been used to decrease this loss, with variable success. When the infant is placed in an incubator, increasing the ambient humidity to 80% reduces total extracellular loss to a minimum. More recently, the use of the topical ointment Aquaphor was shown to reduce losses for 6 hours following application, to improve skin condition and decrease skin colonization, thus possibly reducing the risk of nosocomial infection (97). Our initial impression with Aquaphor is positive, but our experience is too limited to be able to make any recommendation.

Nutrition

Nutrition is an essential part of the care of the ELBW infant. These tiny infants are born with very low reserves of fat and carbohydrates, and they rapidly develop nutritional deficiencies in calcium, phosphorus, iron, trace minerals, and vitamins. Their endocrine and enzymatic capability is limited due to immaturity. Postnatally, they rapidly enter a catabolic state unless sufficient nutrients are given. But reversal of this catabolic state often is difficult because of limited feeding tolerance. The gastrointestinal tract is immature in terms of digestive pathways and motor function, increasing the risk of developing NEC.

Because the first goal of nutrition is to prevent catabolism, usually this will be achieved by providing a minimum of 50 kcal/kg/d. Growth will require additional caloric intake. Achieving steady growth is essential for the ELBW infant, because the growth velocity at 25 to 30 weeks' gestation is relatively higher than at term. If reasonable caloric intake cannot be provided, catch-up growth may never be achieved.

In the early days of life, satisfactory nutrition can never be achieved exclusively with milk. Parenteral nutrition provides the additional calories (98). In contrast to oral nutrition, parenteral administration of 80 to 85 kcal/kg/d can provide the necessary calories for growth. When the infant no longer is receiving intravenous nutrition, 100 to 120 kcal/kg/d are needed to maintain growth. However, these amounts of caloric intake may not be sufficient in infants suffering from CLD and other high-energy–requiring conditions (99). Appropriate growth, if one wants to mimic intrauterine growth, should be a 2% daily increase in body weight, slowing to 1% near term.

Both parenteral nutrition and oral nutrition are not without difficulties and complications in the ELBW infant. TPN requires intravenous access and, this can be associated with a variety of infections, with *Staphylococcus epidermidis* being the most common. The composition of TPN has been, and remains, an area of active research, especially with regard to the composition of essential amino acids and fatty acids. Exclusive intravenous nutrition affects the mucosal lining of the gastrointestinal tract, which is bypassed and eventually may lead to villus atrophy. TPN also requires regular metabolic monitoring for glucose, electrolytes, urea, lipids, and acid–base balance. Cholestatic jaundice is a frequent complication of TPN (100). In the vast majority of cases, this is a self-limited condition, the exact etiology of which is not completely understood, but appears to implicate both amino acids and lipids.

Enteral nutrition may consist of either breast milk or premature formulas. During fetal life, the fetus constantly swallows amniotic fluid, promoting intestinal development.

Enteral feeding, even in small amounts, has been demonstrated to stimulate trophic factors and hormonal maturation of the gastrointestinal tract, thus improving overall intestinal function and potentially improving feeding tolerance and preventing mucosal atrophy (101–103). Whether early introduction of feedings and stimulation of the gastrointestinal tract could prevent or decrease the incidence of NEC has not yet been established. Breast milk contains a lipase, which improves fat tolerance.

In our center, as soon as the infant is metabolically stable on the second or third day of life, we start TPN with 0.5 g/kg/d of amino acids, 0.5 g/kg/d of lipids, and glucose according to tolerance. Calcium, phosphorus, vitamins, and trace minerals also are added. Sodium and potassium are added according to the electrolytic profile. The intake of amino acids and lipids is increased slowly by 0.5 g/kg/d to a maximum of 3 g/kg/d. Lipids are restricted in the presence of severe indirect hyperbilirubinemia. We also adjust the amino acid intake according to urea, pH, and the degree of TPN- related cholestasis. Monitoring of urea, electrolytes, glucose, and bilirubin is performed daily for the first 4 or 5 days of life and then is reduced to twice a week. When the oral intake is half of the total caloric requirement, monitoring is performed only once a week. In our unit, during the past 4 years, the mean duration of time of TPN administration among 120 survivors born weighing less than 1,000 g was 40.9 ± 19 days (median 38.5 days, range 9 to 121 days).

In terms of enteral nutrition, we attempt to introduce minimal feedings, starting in stable infants as early as 48 hours of life. In the vast majority, we use breast milk or a premature formula (68 kcal/100 mL). It is too early to express a clear opinion on this approach, but we have not observed any obvious adverse effects. However, tolerance varies widely from one infant to the other. We encourage mothers to pump their own milk, which is used exclusively for their own babies. The progression of enteral feedings and the addition of a breast milk fortifier varies from one neonatal unit to the other. For the smallest infants, we increase the volume per feeding by 1 mL every 24 hours, up to 10 mL, and then by 1 mL every 12 hours. Generally, we add fortifier to the breast milk, thus increasing its caloric content to 81 kcal/100 mL when oral intake is between one-quarter and one-half of the total required amount. For those infants on premature formula, we also advance to a more caloric formula of 81 kcal/100 mL. Intolerance to milk feeds is not an infrequent occurrence. Tolerance of full enteral feeding, in our experience, usually is achieved between 20 and 30 days of life. In the 120 survivors mentioned previously, birth weight was regained at a mean of 14.2 ± 6.8 days (median 13 days, range 2 to 48 days). These data are comparable to that reported by Berry et al. (104).

Glucose, Calcium, and Phosphorus Homeostasis

Early hypoglycemia frequently is seen in this group of infants, because of poor glycogen reserves and the immaturity of the postnatal adaptive mechanism of endocrine as well as enzymatic control of glucose. In particular, ketogenesis and lipogenesis, which lead to the production of alternate fuels, is limited in very premature infants, making the infant more dependent on glucose (105,106). Hence, an infusion of dextrose at the rate of 5 to 7 mg/kg/min is necessary to maintain normoglycemia.

Hyperglycemia also is observed often in ELBW infants, usually secondary to high glucose infusion rates, but also because of incomplete suppression of hepatic glucose production in the presence of hyperglycemia, reflecting the immaturity of the regulatory mechanisms mentioned previously (107). Hyperglycemia poses the risk of osmotic diuresis, and thus of increased water loss, which eventually may have cerebral implications. Insulin can be used to control hyperglycemia. Although the exact mechanism of action in the extremely premature infant is not completely clear, it is thought to work by decreasing hepatic production of glucose and increasing glucose use by peripheral tissues. Hyperglycemia is a frequent and challenging complication, particularly in extremely immature infants of 23 to 24 weeks' gestation.

In our center, we monitor blood glucose within 1 hour of birth and as often as required, until stabilization. We also test all urines for glycosuria. We tolerate blood glucose values up to 8 or even 10 mmol/L, provided there is no glycosuria. If insulin infusion is used, one must remember to preflush the tubing with the infusate, because insulin adheres to plastic and, unless the binding sites are saturated prior to infusion, a very erratic infusion of insulin may occur, making the interpretation of glucose values difficult. The sudden onset of a sudden glycosuria in a previously stable infant may be an early sign of infection. Hyperglycemia also is seen frequently with initiation of dexamethasone therapy for BPD (108). Because of the slow metabolic adaptation of the ELBW infant, rapid and significant changes in glucose intake should be avoided in order to prevent episodes of hypo- or hyperglycemia, which can become difficult to control. Finally, for the treatment of acute and severe hypoglycemia, a bolus of no more than 200 mg/kg of dextrose can be administered as needed, while, at the same time, increasing the concentration of the intravenous glucose infusion.

Additional calcium is necessary in ELBW infants both in the early days of life as well as later on, when their limited calcium reserves are rapidly depleted during this period of fast growth. However, it is important to appreciate that, because of the low serum albumin of the immature infant, total serum calcium rarely exceeds 1.75 mmol/L. Measurement of ionized calcium is, of course, the ideal way to evaluate hypocalcemia. However, we found that by knowing the serum albumin level (which, incidently, is also helpful for evaluation of bilirubin binding capacity) and the total serum calcium, the management of calcium homeostasis becomes easier. Because hypocalcemia also can induce apnea, we always verify calcium levels after the first 24 hours of life. It is important to remember that metabolic acidosis can give falsely reassuring values of ionized serum calcium, which decline rapidly with the improvement of acid–base balance. Mechanisms involved in the early manifestations of hypocalcemia include parathyroid dysfunction, renal immaturity, and calcitonin stimulation. Our treatment of hypocalcemia consists of administering 500 mg/kg/d of calcium gluconate. As soon as we introduce TPN, 300 mg/kg/d of calcium gluconate is added daily to the solution, together with multivitamins. Because maternal milk has an inadequate mineral and vitamin content, we use a human milk fortifier and vitamins.

It is important to mention at this point that both the classic and hypophosphatemic forms of rickets nowadays are seen only in nutritionally neglected ELBW infants. Pediatricians also have to be reminded that the daily requirement for vitamin D in ELBW infants fed orally is not 400 IU as in term infants, but between 800 and 1000 IU.

Acid–Base Balance

No other investigation is ordered more frequently, with corrective measures taken, than measurement of acid–base balance. Both the respiratory and metabolic components need frequent adjustments. Acid–base homeostasis varies in relation to the degree of renal maturity. The renal threshold for loss of bicarbonate can be as low as 15 mEq/L. Hence, there is often a need for more buffer with sodium bicarbonate in ELBW infants. The need for supplemental sodium bicarbonate also is frequent during the introduction of amino acids in the TPN. In our center, we initiate correction of the acid–base balance as soon as the base deficit exceeds 5 mEq/L. Because TPN contains calcium, the addition of sodium bicarbonate may induce precipitation. For this reason, we have elected to administer sodium bicarbonate via slow push of 0.5 mEq/kg every 2 to 6 hours, according to the severity of the metabolic acidosis, while evaluating the progress of correction and adjusting the frequency of administration accordingly. With this approach, we do not have to discontinue intravenous alimentation, nor do we need to start a second intravenous line. The late metabolic acidosis of prematurity also is related to a combination of increased nitrogen load and low renal threshold.

Although acidosis is the main concern in the early days of life, later on, many of these tiny babies may develop a metabolic alkalosis due to the administration of diuretics, in combination with fluid restriction, as part of the management of CLD. On occasion, we have found it helpful to administer acetazolamide at a dosage of 2.5 mg/kg every 12 hours to overcome a significant metabolic alkalosis (pH more than 7.45).

Jaundice

Only on rare occasions will an infant born weighing less than 1,000 g escape the need for phototherapy. Hepatic immaturity and reduced erythrocyte lifespan, blood group incompatibilities, extensive extravasation of blood, and increased enterohepatic circulation due to poor bowel motility all contribute to the fact that ELBW infants are very prone to develop jaundice. Because the serum bilirubin binding capacity is decreased in premature infants due to the lower serum albumin, the level at which toxicity for the brain and acoustic nerves may occur is much lower than that of the more mature infant. Guidelines for the initiation of phototherapy have been proposed in the past and have undergone frequent revisions. However, some basic principles universally are accepted and govern the management of jaundice. They include the age of the baby in hours or days from birth, gestational age, presence of a hemolytic disorder, degree of bleeding in the skin or other parts of the body, and level of serum albumin. We find it helpful in our decision to initiate or discontinue phototherapy to estimate the serum binding capacity from the level of serum albumin (109). Based on this principle, we have not seen a single case of kernicterus clinically or on autopsy material. Although we do not initiate phototherapy immediately from birth, we believe that relatively early phototherapy can decrease significantly the need for exchange transfusion, which incidentally is poorly tolerated in the very immature infant. We generally initiate phototherapy when the bilirubin level has reached 80 µmol/L in the first 24 hours of life, or if we note an increment of more than 40 µmol/L/d. We consider it prudent not to allow bilirubin to exceed 250 µmol/L in stable tiny infants. When phototherapy is used, it is important to increase the fluid intake by 15% to 20% to avoid excessive insensible water loss. When the bilirubin level approaches the exchange transfusion level, it is important to avoid variations in acid–base balance, high levels of lipid infusion, hypothermia, and certain medications, which may compete with and displace bilirubin from albumin, thus precipitating kernicterus.

MAJOR MORBIDITIES OF THE EXTREMELY-LOW-BIRTH-WEIGHT INFANT

Neurologic Disorders

The neurologic examination of the newborn infant is related to gestational age and is affected greatly by any disturbance in the CNS. The ELBW infant is typically hypotonic. The primitive reflexes are absent but brain stem function (corneal, gag, oculocephalic reflexes, facial grimacing, nasal tickle) can be tested. Neuronal migration usually is completed by 24 weeks of gestation, but synaptic development and myelinization are just beginning at this age.

Intraventricular Hemorrhage

IVH is a major and unfortunately frequent complication in the ELBW infant. Its incidence is correlated with the degree of prematurity (110,111). Potential complications of IVH include hemorrhagic periventricular infarction, hydrocephalus, PVL, and seizures. The overall incidence of IVH appears to be declining in recent years (111). But as the survival rate of ELBW infants has been increasing, IVH remains a major problem. The incidence of IVH varies not only with gestational age, but also between centers. In a very large cohort of infants with a birth weight of 500 to 1,500 g from NICHD Neonatal Network, Shankaran et al. (111) observed a significant decrease in severe intracranial hemorrhage (grades III to IV) from 19% to 15% over a 3-year period, with an overall incidence of intracranial hemorrhage of 44%. In our center, in 173 infants weighing less than 1,000 g, born between April 1993 and March 1997, we observed an overall incidence of 24% (grades I and II = 11% and grades III and IV = 13%) (Table 26–8). However, among the 120 survivors, the incidence was 15% (grades I and II = 9% and grades III and IV = 6%) (Table 26–9).

The changes in the incidence of IVH could be explained by the multifactorial pathogenesis of IVH, which was well described by Volpe (112,113) in terms of intravascular, vascular, and extravascular factors, in combination with the fragility of the germinal matrix and the limited cerebral blood flow autoregulation in the ELBW group of infants.

In our center, we are particularly attentive to rapid stabilization, avoidance of hypo- and hyperoxia, as well as hypo- and hypercarbia, maintenance of normoglycemia, and control of the environment in order to prevent excessive water loss and development of hypernatremia. We attempt to maximize synchronization of the ventilator breaths to the infant's respiratory efforts and use the Ballard closed suction circuit, thus avoiding having to disconnect the infant from the ventilator. We avoid volume expanders, unless there is documented blood loss or significant hypotension, and we favor an early PDA closure. Finally, we minimize handling of the infant and provide a high humidity thermal environment. It is also important to avoid significant apnea by eliminating treatable etiologies, such as infection, hypoglycemia, and hypocalcemia, and by using methylxanthines, nasal CPAP, or mechanical ventilation, if necessary.

IVH may present acutely, leading to shock and death; it may be clinically silent; or, more commonly, it may present with cardiorespiratory instability. The timing of occurrence of IVH has been well documented. About 50% of bleeds occur during the first day of life, 25% during the second day, and 15% by the third day of life (114). It is unusual for an infant to develop IVH after 7 days of life.

Ultrasonography is the most reliable and safest technique for diagnosis of IVH. We perform a cranial ultrasound in the first 24 hours of life. If no IVH is detected, the study is repeated 1 week later, or sooner if the infant suffers from any acute event in the interim. If pathology is present, ultrasonography is repeated at intervals of 48 to 72 hours, until stabilization of the intracranial pathology has been ascertained.

The immediate management of IVH involves stabilization of the cardiovascular system, correction of any bleeding diathesis, if present, and monitoring for hyperbilirubinemia and hyperkalemia. Careful neurologic examination and serial measurements of head circumference and serial cranial ultrasounds must be performed to allow early detection of hydrocephalus. If there is rapidly progressive dilatation of the ventricles, neurosurgical intervention may be necessary for temporary or permanent drainage of the cerebrospinal fluid. We have not found repeated lumbar punctures to be helpful in dealing with this. Prognosis, morbidity, and mortality, are related to the extent of the bleed. Severe IVH with periventricular hemorrhagic ischemia usually has a mortality of more than 50% and leads to progressive ventricular dilatation in 80% of patients. The long-term neurologic sequelae are also a function of the severity of the bleed, with motor disability (spastic hemiparesis) and cognitive deficit exceeding 50% in those with severe hemorrhage (115).

Transport *in utero*, antenatal steroids, and expert delivery room stabilization are important preventive measures against IVH. In terms of pharmacologic prevention, the early administration of indomethacin or ibuprofen appears to be the most promising approach at the present time. Preliminary data indicate that Indomethacin given soon after birth significantly can reduce the incidence and particularly the severity of IVH (85).

Periventricular Leukomalacia

PVL has been reported in varying incidence from 4% to 15% and is the consequence of hypoxic-ischemic lesions, leading to necrosis of the white matter (116). Most commonly affected are the white matter near the trigone of the lateral ventricles and around the foramen of

Monro. PVL may occur in association with IVH, but also may be diagnosed independently as the only CNS lesion. Occasionally, the origin can be intrauterine. Chorioamnionitis has been reported to be associated with increased incidence of PVL (116). Postnatally acquired PVL is seen more frequently in male infants, in infants with severe RDS or infection, and in those with significant cardiovascular instability or apnea (116).

Cystic PVL among preterm infants is the single best predictor of adverse long-term neurologic outcomes (117). The frequency of cerebral palsy developing after cystic PVL has been reported to vary between 62% and 100% (118). Its central feature is a spastic paresis involving predominantly the lower extremities. However, spastic quadriplegia, visual impairment (acuity), developmental delay, or seizures in early childhood also are common observations.

The diagnosis of PVL is made by cranial ultrasonography. When the lesions have occurred *in utero*, it is possible to make the diagnosis soon after birth. However, for postnatally acquired PVL, several weeks may be necessary before the diagnosis can be secured. The characteristic evolution of PVL is the formation of multiple echolucent cysts. Because of the delayed appearance of the cystic lesions, it is important, even for those infants with normal early cranial ultrasonography, to repeat the study between 36 and 40 weeks' postmenstrual age. Consequently, the results of late neonatal cranial ultrasonography are of particular value, not only in predicting the outcome of ELBW infants with PVL, but also in planning long-term multidisciplinary follow-up.

Seizures

Despite many predisposing risk factors, seizures actually are relatively rare in the ELBW infant. Compared to full-term infants, seizures are more difficult to diagnose clinically, which probably is due to cortical underdevelopment at early gestational age. Subtle tonic and myoclonic seizures can be observed in ELBW infants, and they must be differentiated from tremors. The etiology of seizures in the ELBW infant, as for the term infant, may be related to CNS pathology, metabolic derangements (i.e., hypoglycemia, hypocalcemia, severe hyponatremia), infectious causes, and drug withdrawal.

The investigation and management of seizures is beyond the scope of this chapter. Suffice it to say that the electroencephalogram (EEG) can be difficult to interpret, because a conventional surface EEG may not detect the electrical activity of deeper structures. The treatment of seizures in ELBW infants involves correction of any metabolic abnormalities, treatment of any infection, and control of seizure activity to avoid brain injury due to alteration of cerebral energy metabolism. As in the case of the term infant, the prognosis of seizures depends on their etiology. However, the prognosis generally appears to be worse in the ELBW compared to term infants. Our order of preference for medications to control seizures is as follows: phenobarbital at a loading dose of 20 mg/kg, which, on occasion, can be increased to 30 mg/kg; phenytoin at a loading dose of 15 mg/kg; paraldehyde rectally at 0.3 mL/kg (diluted 1:1 in mineral oil); and occasionally diazepam at 0.1 to 0.2 mg/kg/dose.

Hearing Impairment

ELBW infants are at increased risk for hearing impairment because of multisystemic illnesses and the frequent use of potentially ototoxic medications, such as amino glycosides and diuretics. In 1994, the Joint Committee on Infant Hearing, in its Position Statement, recommended that all infants born weighing less than 1,500 g undergo auditory screening (119). Early diagnosis of hearing loss and the use of hearing aids as early as 6 months of age, together with speech therapy, are essential in order to reduce the disability of deafness. The most objective tests are the measure of evoked auditory brain stem responses or otoacoustic emissions (120). In our unit, we initiate screening at 3 months of corrected age, using both techniques. We have found that screening prior to this time, with current technology, may be associated with a large number of false values.

Hematologic Disorders

Anemia

Low iron stores, multiple blood tests, blood loss due to either organ hemorrhage or hemolysis, and rapid growth are some of the factors that make anemia a practically unavoidable hematologic complication for any ELBW infant. The ELBW infant usually has a hemoglobin concentration of 140 to 160 g/L at birth. Those who have suffered from IUGR may have a hemoglobin concentration as high as 200 g/L. Their blood volume is 85 to 90 mL/kg. However, these values can be affected by the extent of placental transfusion at delivery (121). We generally allow for a 10-second placental transfusion in ELBW infants not suffering from IUGR.

The need for transfusion of blood products (packed red cells, plasma, whole blood for exchange transfusion, albumin) is a source of anxiety for parents. Any measure that can decrease the frequency and severity of anemia should be implemented. These measures include limiting blood tests to those essential for appropriate management of the infant, use of microtechniques, and use of pulse oximetry and other transcutaneous devices to monitor PO_2 and PCO_2.

Although the administration of erythropoietin with iron supplementation does not eliminate completely the need for blood transfusion, it can reduce the number of transfusions (122,123). The lack of universal use of erythropoietin probably is due to the fact that it is expensive and that, at least in sick infants, it does not completely eliminate the need for blood transfusion.

To decrease the risk of infection, one unit of packed red cells from a single, properly screened donor, divided into several small bags (satellite bags), could be used for the same infant. This blood, stored in CPDA-1, is good for a period of 42 days (124). We found this approach useful and more reassuring to parents.

In our center, we also have implemented a protocol for direct blood donation from compatible parents (father or mother) who are cytomegalovirus, human immunodeficiency virus, and hepatitis B and C negative. Blood is irradiated prior to transfusion to avoid graft-versus-host disease. However, preparation of such blood requires time. The issue of blood transfusion is discussed with the family, antenatally whenever possible, or soon after admission of the infant to the NICU, and the parental decision is documented in the chart.

Our guidelines for the management of anemia with blood transfusion in ELBW infants are as follows: (i) infants born with severe anemia and/or hypovolemic shock; (ii) replacement of blood taken from an umbilical line as soon as 10% of the baby's blood volume has been lost; (iii) maintenance of hematocrit over 0.40 during the first week of life and over 0.35 during the second week; (iv) maintenance of hematocrit greater than 0.40 in infants with PDA and in those still having severe lung disease in the second week of life; (v) in infants with CLD, we maintain the hematocrit between 0.30 and 0.35; (vi) after the second week of life, the hemoglobin is allowed to decrease as long as the baby has no signs of symptomatic anemia such as poor feedings, high output cardiac failure, apnea, edema, failure to gain weight, tachycardia, and tachypnea. Finally, 4 to 6 mg/kg/d of elemental iron is commenced at 4 to 6 weeks of life and vitamin E at a dose of 25 IU is given for 2 weeks prior to the initiation of iron therapy.

When transfusion is necessary, it should be administered slowly, especially during the first weeks of life, when any acute change in blood pressure may be translated into changes in cerebral blood flow, thus predisposing to IVH, and when there is cardiorespiratory instability. We usually transfuse a volume of 10 mL/kg of packed red blood cells, which is repeated every 8 to 12 hours, according to the need. Furosemide 1 mg/kg is given with each transfusion, with the exception of blood given for replacement of blood taken from an umbilical line over a short period of time.

Hemostasis and Bleeding Diathesis

Vitamin K and Vitamin-K–dependent coagulation factors are present at low concentrations at birth (125). All our ELBW infants receive 0.5 mg of vitamin K intramuscularly immediately after delivery. Parenteral nutrition is supplemented with vitamin K (200 μg/5 mL of MVI (Pediatric Astro Pharmaceuticals).

Conditions requiring immediate administration of additional vitamin K include hemorrhagic pulmonary edema, pulmonary or gastric hemorrhage, and disseminated intravascular coagulation. The management of these conditions often will require, in addition to vitamin K, administration of fresh frozen plasma, transfusion of platelets, and treatment of the underlying condition.

Thrombocytopenia (platelets less than 100×10^9/L) commonly is observed in ELBW infants and, if severe enough, may put the infant at risk for IVH. Thrombocytopenia is frequent in infants born to preeclamptic mothers and infants with IUGR (126). Accelerated platelet destruction is seen in infants with sepsis, indwelling catheters, active bleeding, or following exchange transfusion. In practice we transfuse platelets to infants with a platelet count below 30 to 40×10^9/L. However, in case of active bleeding and a platelet count less than 60×10^9/L, transfusion of platelets should be considered.

Chronic Lung Disease

A large number of ELBW infants still require oxygen supplementation at 1 month of life, and many of them will remain oxygen dependent beyond 36 weeks of postmenstrual age. Both dates have been proposed in the literature to define CLD. It also is not rare to see a number of infants discharged on home oxygen programs. Up to 70% of infants weighing less than 1,000 g have been reported to develop CLD, and more than one-third of the survivors are discharged home on supplemental oxygen (127). Thus, for many infants, CLD seems practically unavoidable.

It is beyond the scope of this chapter to discuss the pathogenesis and pathophysiology of CLD, and we refer the reader to the Chapter 29. Hence, we will limit our discussion to a few aspects of the problem that are more specific to the ELBW infant. CLD encompasses more than the classic BPD described by Northway et al. (128) in 1969. Over the years, we have observed two distinct groups of infants developing CLD (72). The first group consists of infants with severe RDS, who require early intubation and mechanical ventilation. In our center, close to 60% of these infants receive exogenous surfactant. This is followed by a rapid decrease in oxygen requirement and need for ventilatory support. By day 3 of life, the majority of these infants are breathing room air or require a minimal amount of oxygen. However, in most of these infants, this improvement is transient, as ventilatory support needs to be increased and more oxygen supplementation becomes necessary after 7 to 10 days of life, before the final resolution of the respiratory problem. The period of deterioration usually is accompanied by the presence of increased secretions, which require frequent toilet of the airways. The second group is composed of infants who had no initial lung pathology and who required intubation for immaturity and/or apnea, but needed only minimal oxygen supplementation, if any. A number of these infants go on to develop clinical and radiologic signs of CLD. They follow the same pattern of deterioration and eventual improvement as the group with initial lung pathology. Figure 26–1 indicates the bimodal fluctuation in oxygen requirement among 120 survivors weighing less than 1,000 g in our center between 1993 and 1997.

In our population of ELBW survivors, 68% required oxygen supplementation at 28 days of age and 34% at 36 weeks' postmenstrual age (Table 26–9). The median duration of ventilation was 32 days, and the median duration of oxygen supplementation was 60 days.

Our management of the infant with CLD is based on the following principles.

Respiratory support. We accept a PCO_2 value up to 55 to 60 mm Hg, provided the pH is greater than 7.28. When the infant reaches 35 weeks of postmenstrual age, we aim for an oxygen saturation above 94% on the Ohmeda pulse oximeter in order to prevent cor pulmonale. The hematocrit generally is kept above 0.35.

Prevention of fluid overload. Early closure of the PDA, fluid restriction to 120 to 130mL/kg/d, or even less in some cases, administration of diuretics on a chronic basis, i.e., hydrochlorothiazide 1 mg/kg/dose every 12 hours and spironolactone 1 mg/kg/dose every 12 hours. Additional diuresis is obtained with furosemide, when necessary.

Nutritional support. We aim for a minimum of 120 kcal/kg/d and attempt to prevent gastroesophageal reflux and aspiration.

Control of nosocomial infections. As ET tubes become colonized, we send secretions weekly for culture and sensitivity to antibiotics. However, we do not treat the colonized infant if the condition remains stable, and we monitor the infant carefully for clinical and laboratory signs compatible with infection. We do treat, however, infants colonized with ureaplasma, mycoplasma, or chlamydia with erythromycin if the respiratory status presents an unusual progression.

Control of inflammation. Because an inflammatory response seems to be an important mechanism leading to CLD, corticosteroids have been used extensively in recent years to decrease pulmonary edema, prevent inflammation, and increase surfactant and antioxidant production. Systemic dexamethasone has been the drug of choice, and various protocols have been proposed in terms of onset and duration of treatment (129,130). We favor short courses of steroids for 14 to 21 days, usually starting between 14 and 28 days of life in infants demonstrating clinical and radiologic signs of CLD. On occasion, we have started steroids as early as the first day of life, when respiratory failure is complicated by the early appearance of interstitial emphysema. Most infants respond favorably, with rapid extubation and decrease in oxygen requirement. However, at cessation of steroid treatment, the oxygen need may increase again. Like others, we have observed with dexamethasone the well-known side effects of hypertension, flattening of the growth curve, increased risk of infection, hyperglycemia, and cardiomyopathy. When these complications occur or when O_2 requirements increase after discontinuation of therapy, we often use an intermittent administration of dexamethasone (131). This consists of giving 0.5 mg/kg/d for 3 days, followed by 7 days without therapy, and then initiation of another 3-day course of steroids. This drug regimen is repeated until stabilization and improvement of the lung condition.

Another mode of therapy that may avoid some of the side effects of systemic dexamethasone consists of administering steroids by inhalation (132). In our own study, nebulized budesonide at a dose of 500 µg twice daily did not show the same efficacy as did systemic dexamethasone. However, early administration of budes-

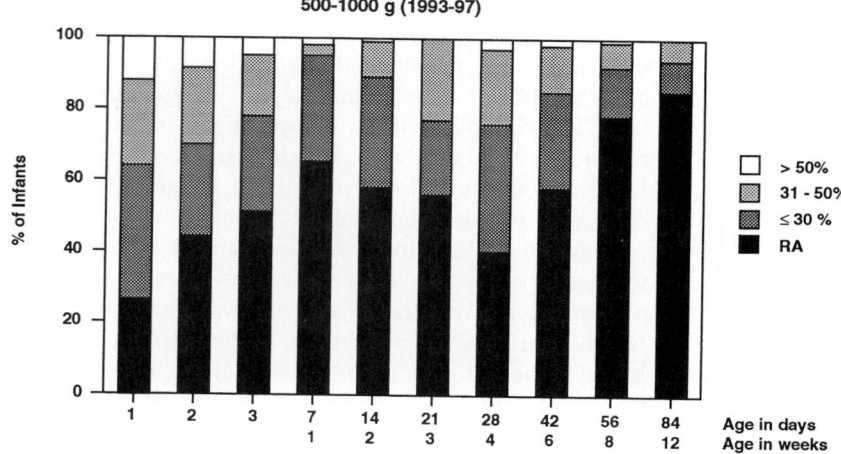

FIG. 26–1. Variation in O_2 requirement in 120 survivors. RA, room air.

onide decreased the number of infants requiring systemic administration of dexamethasone after 28 days of life (133). It remains to be determined how early and for how long one has to treat infants with systemic steroids in order to prevent or decrease the incidence of CLD. Inhaled steroids, with improved methods of pulmonary medication delivery, may be an attractive alternative in the future.

Bronchodilators. In infants with decreased air entry and wheezing, we have found that administration of nebulized salbutamol at a dose of 0.25 mL every 3 to 6 hours can be helpful (134). We often have observed that, immediately after a treatment, air entry improves and clearance of secretions becomes easier, particularly in combination with chest physiotherapy.

Home Oxygen Therapy

Despite maximum therapy, some infants remain dependent on supplemental oxygen beyond 40 weeks' postmenstrual age. Those who still require oxygen supplementation at 40 weeks, in our center, are evaluated by a pediatric pulmonologist and the parents are trained for eventual home oxygen therapy. This subgroup of infants represents 5% to 7% of our survivors born weighing less than 1,000 g.

Necrotizing Enterocolitis

Necrotizing enterocolitis (NEC) is the major gastrointestinal disorder that selectively affects the sick premature infant. Its etiology is multifactorial and includes suspected predisposing factors such as intestinal immaturity, poor intestinal motility, hypoxemia, ischemia, PDA, umbilical catheter placement, IUGR, feeding practices, exchange transfusion, and systemic infections (135).

Antenatal administration of steroids appears to accelerate intestinal maturation and provide extra protection against NEC to the prematurely born infant (136). The incidence of NEC varies widely, from center to center, between 9% and 25% for infants born weighing less than 1,000 g (137). Our incidence of NEC between 1993 and 1997 was 5% (Table 26–8). This wide variation probably reflects differences in diagnostic criteria and clinical practices. Indeed, the successful reduction in the incidence of NEC is related essentially to prevention, by avoiding all known predisposing factors and by intervening and interrupting the cascade of progression of the disease at the earliest signs, which many of us like to call "pre-NEC." These signs include increased gastric residual, mild abdominal distension, cardiovascular instability, deterioration of skin perfusion, clusters of apneic spells, and unexplained glycosuria and lipemia. In the presence of these signs and depending on their severity, it is our practice either temporarily to discontinue feedings or to decrease the volume by 50% and reevaluate the situation

in a few hours. In the presence of further abdominal distension, we do not hesitate to discontinue oral feeds and insert an orogastric catheter under continuous low suction. In the majority of cases of benign distension, the intestinal decompression reestablishes the intestinal vascular supply, and, within 2 to 4 hours, the abdomen returns to normal. In an otherwise healthy looking and active infant, we do not necessarily initiate therapy with antibiotics unless there is blood in the stools or the abdominal radiograph demonstrates, beside dilated bowel loops, signs compatible with evolving NEC, i.e., pneumatosis intestinalis. In these cases, a septic workup is performed and antibiotics are begun immediately. Our initial treatment is a combination of gentamicin and ampicillin, to which clindamycin is added in case of additional deterioration, or when the presentation is that of overwhelming NEC. With reference to the presentation of overwhelming NEC, one of the most distressing situations in neonatology is the development, in a previously healthy, stable 8- to 10-day-old premature infant in whom milk intake was progressing without complication, of fulminant abdominal distension accompanied by sepsis, profound metabolic acidosis, neutropenia, and thrombocytopenia, followed by rapid death. Fortunately, this dramatic clinical presentation is rare, as it is difficult to anticipate and to prevent.

The management of NEC, besides antibiotics and orogastric suction, requires close monitoring of vital signs, frequent abdominal radiographs, with lateral views to visualize the possible presence of free air in the peritoneal cavity, correction of metabolic abnormalities, and cardiovascular support with volume expanders and dopamine. Many infants with NEC may require assisted ventilation, as apnea frequently complicates the situation. TPN is also an integral part of the management of these infants. Persistent intractable metabolic acidosis and severe neutropenia and thrombocytopenia are ominous prognostic signs and usually reflect extensive intestinal necrosis.

For infants managed medically, the time of reintroduction of oral feeds is a critical one. We usually initiate enteric feeds after 7 to 14 days of therapy, depending on the rapidity of resolution of clinical and radiologic signs. The presence of bowel sounds, a stable condition, and a well-perfused infant without significant apnea are the basic requirements for starting oral feeds. We initially use an elemental formula and progress slowly to full enteric feeds over a period of 7 days or longer, as tolerated. For those infants on maternal milk, mother's own fresh milk is used. Post-NEC intestinal strictures are not unusual and can present several weeks after the initial episode, with milk intolerance, vomiting, and abdominal distension. Strictures are also the result of subclinical injury of the intestine and can be seen in infants in whom the diagnosis of NEC was never made before.

In summary, much still needs to be learned about NEC, its prevention, and its management. In the meantime, every neonatal unit develops its own philosophy and approach in order to reduce the risks of NEC. Our environment is no different. As we continuously learn new information, it seems that some preventive aspects deserve more attention than others. In our view, such strategies include maternal administration of steroids, use of mother's own milk, early priming of the gastrointestinal system with a very small volume of milk prior to the advancement of feedings, and, above all, careful observation of the infant's condition, with reduction or temporary discontinuation of feeds and intestinal decompression at the earliest suspicion.

Inguinal Hernias

Inguinal hernias occur frequently in ELBW infants. They can present as early as 2 weeks of age and may become extremely large. Surgical repair usually is performed prior to discharge home. Predisposing factors are weakness of the tissues and increased intraabdominal pressure, especially in the presence of CLD.

Retinopathy of Prematurity

ROP is a major threat to all ELBW infants (138) (see also Chap. 52). The etiologic factors involved in the pathogenesis of the disease are multiple and are discussed elsewhere in this book. The incidence of ROP is inversely proportional to birth weight and gestational age (139, 140). Blindness has become rare for infants born weighing more than 1,000 g, and, in our center, we have not recorded a single case in the last 20 years. But as survival has increased significantly in infants born before 26 weeks of gestation, so has the number of infants with severe ROP. Our incidence and degree of severity of ROP is shown in Table 26–9. Although the introduction of pulse oximetry and transcutaneous PO_2 and PCO_2 measurements have greatly facilitated monitoring of oxygen and ventilatory requirements in ELBW infants, they have not eliminated the problem of ROP. The frequency of ROP is so high among survivors of 23 and 24 weeks of gestation that immaturity of the retina seems to be the unsurmountable factor. And yet, a number of infants of the same gestational age escape from the severe forms of ROP. It is obvious that several aspects of retinal behavior and its pathophysiology remain poorly understood. In addition to immaturity, we have reported recently that the combination of IUGR and severe prematurity further increases the risk of severe ROP (21).

Based on current knowledge of predisposing factors and years of careful observation, we have developed a policy of keeping the PaO_2 below 50 mm Hg for all infants weighing less than 1,000 g in the first weeks of life. We set the upper limit of our Ohmeda pulse oximeter at 93% and try to avoid rapid fluctuations in PaO_2. We feel that levels around 45 mm Hg are closer to intrauterine conditions, while, at the same time, there is no pro-

duction of lactic acid. Although we favor some degree of permissive hypercapnia, we avoid longstanding values of PCO_2 over 55 mm Hg, particularly before 34 weeks of gestation. We have a low tolerance for recurrent apneic spells associated with significant desaturations. In such situations, we do not hesitate to use respiratory support [(CPAP or intermittent mandatory ventilation (IMV)] if caffeine cannot control them. Finally, our infants born weighing less than 1,000 g receive early supplementation with vitamin E.

In order to prevent severe ROP leading to blindness, a careful serial ophthalmologic examination is necessary (141). The recent joint statement of the American Academy of Pediatrics, the American Association of Pediatric Ophthalmologists, and the American Academy of Ophthalmology recommends screening of all premature infants to be performed at between 4 and 6 weeks' postnatal age or between 31 and 33 weeks' postmenstrual age. We are particularly careful not to expose our tiny infants to bright lighting because of its suspected role in the development of ROP (142).

Like others, we have observed a few cases of "rush" disease developing between 30 and 33 weeks of gestation, and even at later dates, in infants who, until then, had a benign stage I or II ROP. Initial screening in our center starts 4 weeks after birth or at 30 weeks of gestation (whichever comes first). Follow-up examinations are scheduled depending on the findings (degree of vascularization, retinal changes on the first examination) at intervals of 1 to 2 weeks. If the disease process seems to accelerate, examinations are performed twice a week. Infants with threshold and plus disease are candidates for cryotherapy or laser therapy. In our center, 6% of infants born weighing less than 1,000 g underwent cryotherapy in the past few years, with satisfactory results.

Apnea of Prematurity

Apnea of prematurity is a feature of nearly all infants with a birth weight less than 1,000 g. Its incidence and frequency decrease with advancing gestational age, but at times it may be seen up to 42 weeks of gestation (143). In the ELBW population, it is a frequent indication for mechanical ventilation, thus exposing these infants to the potential complications of ventilatory support.

Apnea usually is defined as a cessation of breathing for 20 seconds or more, or of a shorter duration if associated with cyanosis or bradycardia. Different patterns have been observed in premature infants: central apnea (absent breathing movements), obstructive apnea (breathing movements, but no airflow) or mixed apnea (central and obstructive) (144). ELBW infants are particularly prone to obstructive apnea, especially when in the supine position with the neck in the midline, because of the weakness of the muscles of the oropharynx. Apnea due to obstruction of the lower airways also has been reported, suggesting immaturity of lung mechanics. The cessation of gas exchange during a significant apneic episode is manifested by hypoxemia and/or bradycardia. Recurrent episodes of apnea may affect neurodevelopmental outcome. Although it is difficult to relate frequency and severity of apnea to outcome, one can only stress the importance of monitoring these infants by pulse oximetry. Because apneic episodes can occur in premature infants as a result a variety of underlying diseases, investigation of other pathologic causes must be undertaken before diagnosing apnea of prematurity.

Patient management will depend on the severity and frequency of apneic episodes. Methylxanthines, which stimulate the respiratory center, are the most effective pharmacologic treatment for apnea of prematurity. Methylxanthines, aside from reducing the frequency of apneic pauses, have other actions that are equally important. They increase respiratory rate, tidal volume, and minute ventilation, and they decrease diaphragmatic fatigue. They also increase the sensitivity of the chemoreceptors to carbon dioxide and improve blood pressure and cardiac output (145–147). Treatment with either aminophylline or theophylline is effective but needs to be repeated two to four times per day. In our center, we treat apnea of prematurity with caffeine, which is the metabolite of theophylline (148). We found that caffeine has fewer gastrointestinal side effects and causes less CNS irritability. It also has a much broader therapeutic index and achieves more stable plasma levels. In view of its long half-life, it needs to be given once daily. We use caffeine base at a loading dose of 10 mg/kg followed 24 hours later by a single daily dose of 2.5 mg/kg. Caffeine can be administered intravenously or orally. When given intravenously, the injection should be performed slowly, as it may otherwise be quite painful. We verify the serum level of caffeine in cases of intractable apnea or clinical signs of toxicity. Caffeine is also the drug of choice when we start weaning an infant from the mechanical ventilator. The therapeutic range of caffeine is between 23 and 104 μg/mL, and the mean half-life is 102 hours.

Another drug that has been used for the treatment of apnea is doxapram. Like methylxanthines, doxapram has been observed to improve minute ventilation and tidal volume, lower PCO_2, and increase blood pressure (149). A major disadvantage of doxapram is that it needs to be administered by continuous infusion and, overall, does not appear to offer any particular advantage over the more manageable methylxanthines. We studied the possibility of administering doxapram orally and reported on the kinetics of oral administration (150). However, in addition to a few hypertensive episodes, we also observed a rather poor oral tolerance of this drug, with excessive hypersalivation and irritability and, thus, have practically abandoned the oral route.

If we cannot control apnea in a satisfactory manner with caffeine, we rapidly initiate nasal CPAP, which, we have found, in combination with caffeine, offers very good stabilization in the vast majority of cases. Finally, if apnea persists, we do not hesitate to intubate and ventilate such an infant with low pressures and rates. In infants with persisting apnea and desaturations after 40 weeks' postmenstrual age, we perform a respirogram prior to discharging them home on either xanthines or a home monitoring program. It is important, before closing the discussion on apnea, to underline the fact that pharmacologic treatment of apnea should be considered only after proper investigation has eliminated any underlying condition requiring specific treatment, such as anemia, infection, or metabolic disorders (see also Chap. 32).

Neonatal Infections

The ELBW infant is particularly vulnerable to bacterial, viral, and fungal infections. A significant number of premature labors probably are due to infection. Chorioamnionitis is a frequent finding after a premature birth, particularly in the presence of prolonged rupture of membranes. As the clinical signs of infection often are nonspecific, the index of suspicion and the concern about the possibility of intrauterine infection should be very high in the presence of a premature birth. Hence, screening for infection should be an integral part of the evaluation of the ELBW infant. Diagnosis of neonatal infection sometimes can be difficult, as early neonatal infection often manifests with respiratory symptomatology, which is also the overwhelming pathology of prematurity. This is particularly true in the presence of group B streptococcal pneumonia, which is often indistinguishable clinically and radiologically from RDS (151). However, early appearance of recurrent apnea, poor perfusion, hypotension, and significant metabolic acidosis, often in the presence of an abnormal leukocyte count, are very strong elements in favor of infection.

In symptomatic infants, we obtain a skin surface culture, blood culture, and leukocyte count, and we initiate broad-spectrum antibiotic coverage with ampicillin and gentamicin. We do not routinely perform a lumbar puncture on admission. However, if the blood culture is positive or if there is clinical evidence of deterioration compatible with meningitis, we then perform a lumbar puncture. If the result suggests a meningitis, we adjust the duration of therapy and antibiotic dosage accordingly. If the infant's condition improves rapidly, the blood culture is negative, and the acute phase reactants are normal, we discontinue antibiotics after 3 to 5 days.

Nosocomial infections are not rare among infants whose hospitalization can be as long as 3 to 4 months. Aside from the immaturity of the immune system, predisposing factors are ventilator care, intravenous alimentation via central or peripheral lines, and exposure to extensive handling. In recent years, *Staphylococcus epidermidis* has emerged as the most common organism.

However, in ventilated infants and in those with CLD, *Pseudomonas, Klebsiella,* and *Staphylococcus aureus* are the predominant organisms found. Fungal infections are not rare and should be suspected in the presence of unexplained thrombocytopenia and clinical signs of slow deterioration.

It is our policy not to treat colonization of ET tubes with antibiotics unless there are signs of pneumonia or systemic infection. In the absence of signs of infection, the vast majority of our ventilated infants are left without antibiotic coverage under close observation, with weekly monitoring of ET colonization and sensitivity to antibiotics. This information can be used in case of clinical deterioration suggesting infection.

Concern has been expressed regarding the risk of infection in infants treated in incubators with high humidity. Our experience, using the new incubators providing high humidity, has been very positive. We do not have any evidence of an increased risk of infection.

In the past, considerable effort was placed on measures believed to protect the newborn from nosocomial infections. These efforts included the restriction of visitors, and the use of gowns, gloves, masks, and hairnets. However, no studies have shown any evidence supporting these measures (152). In our unit, despite no longer using gowns for several years, we have not observed any change in the incidence of infection. We recommend gowning only when parents handle their babies in their arms or in cases requiring strict isolation. Parental visiting is unrestricted. Moreover, we have developed a successful program of cuddling by selected volunteers for babies whose parents live far from the hospital and cannot visit very often. This is done with parental approval. On the other hand, we have implemented for everybody working in or visiting the unit a very strict program of hand washing, which appears to be the cornerstone of our relatively low incidence of nosocomial infection.

Sensory Overload and Developmental Care

During their NICU stay, preterm infants are exposed to external stimuli that are very different from those experienced by the fetus *in utero*: noise, lights, frequent disturbances, different environment (no fluid, thus alteration in body movements), and pain. In the past, pain inflicted on ELBW infants may have been a concern but mostly was ignored. In recent years, however, one has come to recognize that newborns do, indeed, experience pain (153). Ascending pain pathways are well developed by 24 weeks, but endogenous opiates and descending pathways that block incoming pain impulses are not present before 32 weeks of gestation. The physiologic and behavioral response to, as well as the long-term effect of, recurrent painful stimuli now have been studied extensively (154). Opiate and nonopiate analgesics, as well as topical local anesthetics such as EMLA®, are

being tested to determine the safest and most optimal way to manage major and minor procedures. The question of continuous pharmacologic control of pain or discomfort, other than during invasive medical interventions such as heel pricks, lumbar punctures, or drainage of pneumothoraces, requires further study, as one has to balance the long effects of discomfort versus those of the medication itself.

The sensory overload experienced by the premature newborn may affect both the cerebral pathways that normally develop only once neuronal migration is complete, as well as the usual programmed cell death. This, in turn, could lead to maladaptive developmental trajectories and influence neural maturation and organization. These concerns have led to the development and implementation in many neonatal units of individualized developmental care in order to enhance neurodevelopmental outcome (155).

Studies published thus far have shown that short-term medical outcome, as measured by duration of mechanical ventilation and oxygen supplementation, daily weight gain, tolerance to oral feedings, and length of hospitalization, is improved by individualized developmental care (155). In terms of neurodevelopmental outcome, infants who received individualized care have demonstrated improvement in behavioral organization at 2 weeks after discharge and in Bayley Mental and Psychomotor Developmental Index Scores at 9 months corrected age (155).

Our medical and nursing personnel have been, over the years, sensitized to these issues. The primary care nurse is responsible for implementing and maintaining developmental care and comfort of the infant for whom she or he is in charge by minimizing external interventions and eliminating unnecessary disturbances. Particular attention is given to the parents' needs during hospitalization. Preparation for discharge involves, aside from the NICU medical and nursing staff, the follow-up clinic nurse coordinator. Parents' group meetings, where common problems and concerns are discussed, are held on a regular basis.

FOLLOW-UP OF THE EXTREMELY-LOW-BIRTH-WEIGHT INFANT

As survival of ELBW infants has improved in the 1980s and, particularly, in the 1990s, attention has been directed toward the relatively high rate of neurodevelopmental delays and school difficulties in survivors.

Of particular concern is the study by Hack and Fanaroff (156) on school-age outcome in infants born weighing less than 750 g. The rates of mental retardation (IQ less than 70), cerebral palsy, and severe visual disabilities in this report were all far greater in infants born weighing less than 750 g compared to those born weighing between 751 and 1,499 g and to term infants. The authors concluded that infants born weighing less than

750 g were inferior in terms of cognitive ability, psychomotor skills, and academic achievements. Major ultrasonographic cerebral abnormalities were associated with mental retardation and cerebral palsy (odds ratio 5.4 and 15.2, respectively). A more recent report by the same authors indicates improvement in survival of ELBW infants but unchanged neonatal and early childhood outcomes of the survivors (157). All studies point to the importance of early cerebral abnormalities, i.e., IVH and PVL, to long-term prognosis. Allen and colleagues (6) in 1993 reported 36-month survival and morbidity rates among infants born between 22 and 25 weeks of gestation. There were no survivors at 22 weeks, whereas 15%, 56%, and 80% of infants survived at 23, 24, and 25 weeks, respectively. Only 2% of those born at 23 weeks survived without severe intracranial abnormality. For infants born at 24 and 25 weeks, the respective values of intact survival were 21% and 69%. The authors concluded that aggressive resuscitation is warranted for infants born at 25 weeks, but not for those born at 22 weeks. Whether to treat all infants born at 23 or 24 weeks of gestation presents an enormous ethical and economic dilemma that the authors could not resolve.

A regional study in Ontario, Canada, in 1993 reported the absence of any handicap at 2 years of age in 50% of surviving infants born at 23 weeks, 41% of those born at 24 weeks, and 59% of those born at 25 weeks (3). The same year, a regional study in Oxford, England, reported moderate-to-severe functional handicaps at 4 years of age in 80% of surviving infants born less than 25 weeks of gestation and 66% of those born at 25 weeks (158). In Japan, the limit of viability, as defined by the Eugenic Protection Law, was amended in 1991 from 24 completed weeks to 22 completed weeks. Nishida (159) reported that ELBW infants, treated at Tokyo Women's Medical College during the period from 1984 to 1990, had a survival rate of 84%, and that the incidence of major neurologic sequelae between 1 and 8 years of age was on the order of 17%.

All these reports, however, have to be placed in the context of ongoing advances in neonatal intensive care. Doubts about improving survival of premature infants have been revised continuously over the years with medical and technological progress. Infants with birth weights that aroused concern 15 or 20 years ago nowadays are treated routinely and successfully in our neonatal units. It is obvious that if we are to invest our energies and our budgets in the care of ELBW infants, we have to be able to demonstrate that prevention of significant cerebral, retinal, and lung damage compromising the future lives of ELBW infants is possible.

In this respect, it is important to remember that most of the studies reporting on school-age performance involve infants born in the mid or late 1980s. Certainly, much of neonatal care has evolved since that period. Some of the changes in recent years in perinatal practice that have had a particular impact on the management of ELBW infants are increased maternal transfers to tertiary care perinatal centers, more extensive use of antenatal and postnatal steroids, better ventilators and incubators, early pharmacologic closure of the PDA with indomethacin, and, finally, the use of exogenous surfactant. To all these, we also can add a better understanding of the physiology and pathophysiology of the tiny infant, and more experience on the part of physicians and nurses in handling these very fragile infants.

Our follow-up studies of infants born between 22 and 25 weeks of gestation are still in progress, and we do not yet have complete information regarding school performance. However, some interesting findings at 2 years of age are worth reporting. From April 1988 to March 1994, 108 infants born between 22 and 25 weeks of gestation were admitted to our NICU. All were inborn, and the gestational age was verified by early ultrasonography at 16 weeks of gestation and matched to the last menstrual period. The mean gestational age was 24.6 ± 0.9 weeks, and the mean birth weight was 681 ± 124 g. Six infants were born at 22 weeks, 15 at 23 weeks, 39 at 24 weeks, and 48 at 25 weeks gestation. A cranial ultrasound was performed during the first and second weeks of life to screen for IVH, and before discharge home, looking for evidence of PVL. Those infants with intracranial pathology had repeat ultrasonography, as required by their condition. Table 26–12 indicates the neonatal course of the 56 survivors. The growth parameters during the first 2 years of life are shown in Table 26–13. The number of infants with head circumference below the fifth centile increased with advanced postnatal age and is statistically significant, indicating a lack of catch-up growth.

The general IQ on Griffiths Scale is shown in Table 26–14. However, comparison between infants with a head circumference under the fifth percentile and the others did not show any difference in terms of IQ performance. This finding is particularly interesting and needs further longitudinal evaluation in view of the fact that subnormal head growth has been observed in ELBW infants by oth-

TABLE 26–12. *Neonatal course of 56 infants of gestational age 22–25 weeks at Jewish General Hospital, McGill University from 1988 to 1994*

Gestational age (wk)	24.6 ± 0.9
Birth weight (g)	681 ± 124
Intraventricular hemorrhage	7 (13%)
Grades III + IV	1 (2%)
Periventricular leukomalacia	3 (5%)
Retinopathy of prematurity	42 (75%)
Stages III + IV	18 (32%)
Cryotherapy	8 (14%)
Chronic lung disease (36 wk)	26 (36%)
Home O$_2$	5 (9%)

TABLE 26–13. *Growth parameters below the fifth percentile—change over time, 22–25 weeks gestational age at Jewish General Hospital, McGill University, from 1988 to 1994*

	3 mo	4 mo	p Value
Weight	33%	19%	NS
Head circumference	10%	33%	0.015
Length	63%	15%	<0.001

ers and has been reported to be associated with cognitive and school difficulties (160).

In terms of general health, 56% of the children required at least one rehospitalization for hernia repair, ear tubes, eye surgery, bronchiolitis-asthma, or pneumonia. The most common medical problems during the first 2 years of life were reactive airway disease in 59%, recurrent otitis media in 57%, and the need for a hearing aid in 6%. The incidence of these complications is not higher than was reported in several studies of older NICU graduates. Overall, severe impairment was diagnosed in 18% of children at age 2 years. However, contrary to previous reports, the General Developmental Index of our infants at 24 months of age was in the satisfactory range of 87 to 100, with no infant in the mentally retarded range of less than 70. This finding possibly may be explained by the very low incidence of cerebral injuries among our survivors.

From all reported studies so far, the following tentative conclusions can be made. (i) The vast majority of the survivors of ELBW infants can hope for a very meaningful life. (ii) A substantial number of ELBW infants will have significant physical and intellectual handicaps. (iii) The presence of a grade III or IV IVH, particularly in the presence of cystic PVL, is an ominous predictor for future handicaps. (iv) As survival of infants born less than 25 weeks' gestation improves, the absolute number of infants with long-term complications probably will increase, but with a concomitant increase in the number of healthy infants. (v) At present, it is safe to predict that a larger number of ELBW infants will require, in the future, multidisciplinary attention and special education. (vi) It is safe to predict that many more parents who, in the past, had no hope of taking home a healthy infant

TABLE 26–14. *General developmental index across time at Jewish General Hospital, McGill University, from 1988 to 1994*

	6 mo	12 mo	24 mo
Mean	103 ± 7	97 ± 8	96 ± 4
Median	105	97[a]	98[a]
Range	78–115	80–121	87–100

[a]p < 0.001 compared with general developmental index at 6 months.

born extremely premature can, in the future, see their hope realized more frequently.

FUTURE DIRECTIONS AND ETHICAL ISSUES

Based on available data, it is reasonable to believe that progress in the survival and quality of life of ELBW infants will continue. However, the debate regarding the lower limit of viability will continue (25,26). The barrier of 500 g already has been broken (161). Like many other centers, we have witnessed, in the last few years, the survival of infants with a birth weight less than 500 g and, more importantly, a number of them have survived with intact early development. It is our belief that society ought to support the rational care of very premature infants as much as it supports the care of older patients. It would be an untenable situation if society had to make decisions based on age and not outcomes. Hence, it is our responsibility as neonatologists to provide both short- and long-term accurate information for our patients if we want to defend our interventions with credibility. As we write these lines, there are still serious problems with the interpretation of data, and with the formulation of general guidelines that relate to variations in interventions and therapies, and to philosophical, ethical, and financial considerations in each neonatal unit, when it comes to the management of ELBW infants. It is also important to appreciate that only in recent years, thanks to early dating by ultrasonography, have gestational age-related outcomes in ELBW infants begun to be reported. Difficulties exist in the interpretation of follow-up data due to the lack of consensus on appropriate outcome measures (162). With the exception of IQ developmental tests, little standardization has been put forward.

It is also evident that not all neonatologists, or all NICUs, should undertake the treatment of ELBW infants. The management of these infants requires great expertise and ample resources. A critical mass is essential in order to maintain high medical and nursing standards. Ideally, only regional perinatal centers should be involved in the care of ELBW infants, and treatment should be undertaken only when adequate resources are available, without compromising the care of more mature infants having better chances of intact survival. Finally, the ultimate decision regarding the management and degree of intervention in the delivery room remains the responsibility of the neonatologist because, very often, there may not be time for multiple consultations and because, after all, the neonatologist is the person with the wider experience to make such decisions. However, it is also important that neonatologists involved in the care of the ELBW infant be sensitive to the wishes of the family and be objective in their presentation of information and interpretation of outcome data to the family. The neonatologist also should be prepared to advise parents when therapy has reached its limits and avoid heroic interventions when expected outcome, based on current scientific knowledge, is definitely unfavorable. In our view, as we approach the new millenium, the moving target in the management of the ELBW infant should no longer be the gestational age or the birth weight but rather the condition of the infant at birth, his or her potential to survive, the parents' desire, and our own honest evaluation of the capabilities, commitment, and resources of our own environment to provide lengthy support to the infant and to his or her family.

ACKNOWLEDGMENTS

We wish to thank our colleague, Dr. Lajos Kovacs, for critical review of the manuscript and helpful suggestions. Our thanks also to the nursing personnel of our NICU for years of competent and devoted care of the ELBW infants. Our deep appreciation to Mrs. Judi Garon for her dedication and secretarial expertise.

REFERENCES

1. Fanaroff AA, Wright LL, Stevenson DK, et al. Very low birth weight outcomes of the National Institute of Child Health and Human Development Neonatal Research Network, May 1995–December 1992. *Am J Obstet Gynecol* 1995;173:1423.
2. Tudhope D, Burns YR, Grey TA, Mohay HA, O'Callaghan MJ, Rodgets YM. Changing patterns of survival and outcomes at four years of children who weighed 500–999 grams at birth. *J Pediatr Child Health* 1995;31:451.
3. Whyte HE, Fitzhardinge PM, Shennan AT, Lennox K, Smith L, Lacy J. Extreme immaturity: outcome of 568 pregnancies of 23–26 weeks gestation. *Obstet Gynecol* 1993;82:1.
4. Papageorgiou AN, Doray JL, Ardila R, Kunos I. Reduction of mortality, morbidity and respiratory distress syndrome in infants weighing less than 1000 grams by treatment with betamethasone and ritodrine. *Pediatrics* 1989;83:493.
5. Piecuch RE, Leonard CA, Cooper BA, Sehring SA. Outcome of extremely low birth weight infants (500–999 grams) over a twelve year period. *Pediatrics* 1997;100:633.
6. Allen MC, Donohoe PK, Dusman AE. The limit of viability-neonatal outcome of infants born at 22–25 weeks gestation. *N Engl J Med* 1993;329:1597.
7. Synnes AR, Ling EWY, Whitfield MF, et al. Perinatal outcomes of a large cohort of extremely low gestational age infants (23–28 weeks gestation). *J Pediatr* 1994;125:925.
8. Ferrara TB, Hoekstra RE, Couser RJ, et al. Survival and follow-up of infants born at 23–26 weeks of gestational age (effects of surfactant therapy). *J Pediatr* 1994;124:119.
9. Kitchen WH, Doyle LW, Ford WG, et al. Changing two year outcome in infants weighing 500–999 grams at birth: a hospital study. *J Pediatr* 1991;118:938.
10. Pomerance JJ, Pomerance LJ, Gottlieb JA. Cost of caring for infants weighing 500–749 grams at birth. *Pediatr Res* 1993;4:231A.
11. McCormick MC, Bernabol JC, Eisenberg JM, Ustra SL, Finnighan E. Cost incurred by parents of very low birth weight infants after the initial neonatal hospitalization. *Pediatrics* 1991;88:533.
12. Bennett-Britton S, Fitzhardinge PM, Asby S. Is intensive care justified for infants weighing less than 801 grams at birth? *J Pediatr* 1981;99:937.
13. Bohin S, Draper ES, Field I. Impact of extremely immature infants on neonatal services. *Arch Dis Child* 1996;74:F110.
14. Saigal S, Zsatmari P, Rosenbaum P, Campbell D, King S. Cognitive abilities and school performance of extremely low birth weight infants and matched term control children at eight years: regional study. *J Pediatr* 1991;118:751.
15. Harpe M, Taylor JG, Kline N, et al. School age outcomes of children with birth weights under 750 grams. *N Engl J Med* 1994;331:753.
16. Lahayne LA, Pine TR, Jackson C, Bennet FC. Outcome of infants weighing less than 800 grams at birth: 15 years experience. *Pediatrics* 1995;96:479.
17. Saigal S, Rosenbaum P, Hattersley B, Milner AR. Decreased disability rate among 3-year old survivors weighing between 501 to 1000 gms at birth and born to residents of a geographically defined region from 1981 to 1984 compared with 1977 to 1980. *J Pediatr* 1989;114:839.
18. Halsey CR, Collin MF, Anderson CL. Extremely low birth weight children and their peers: A comparison of preschool performance. *Pediatrics* 1993;91:807.
19. Halsey CR, Collin MF, Anderson CL. Extremely low birth weight children and their peers: a comparison of school age outcomes. *Arch Pediatr Adolesc Med* 1996;150:790.
20. Zelkowitz P, Papageorgiou A, Zelazo P, Weiss MS. Behavioral adjustment of very low birth weight and normal birth weight children. *J Clin Child Psychol* 1995;24:21.
21. Bardin C, Zelkowitz P, Papageorgiou A. Comparison of outcomes of AGA and SGA infants born between 24 and 27 weeks gestation. *Pediatrics* 1997;100:1.
22. *Comité d'Enquête sur la mortalité et morbidité périnatale, Rapport pour 1992.* Collège des Médecins du Québec, 1995.
23. Vasa R, Vidyasagar D, Winegar A, Peterson P, Spellany W. Perinatal factors influencing the outcome of 501 to 1000 gram newborns. *Clin Perinatol* 1986;13:267.
24. Ott WJ. Small for gestational age fetus and neonatal outcome: reevaluation of the relationship. *Am J Perinatol* 1995;12:396.
25. American Academy of Pediatrics—Committee on Fetus and Newbor, and American College of Obstetricians and Gynecologists—Committee on Obstetric Practice. Perinatal care at the threshold of viability. *Pediatrics* 1995;96:974.
26. Fetus and Newborn Committee, Canadian Pediatric Society—Maternal Fetal Medicine Committee, Society of Obstetricians and Gynecologists of Canada. Management of the woman with threatened birth of an infant of extremely low gestational age. *CMAJ* 1994;151:547.
27. Bottoms SF, Paul RH, Iams JD, et al. Obstetric determinants of neonatal survival: influence of willingness to perform cesarean delivery on survival of extremely low birth weight infants. *Am J Obstet Gynecol* 1997;176:960.
28. Thibeault DW, Beatty EC, Hall RT, et al. Neonatal pulmonary hypoplasia with premature rupture of fetal membranes and oligohydramnios. *J Pediatr* 1985;107:273.
29. Blott M, Greenough A. Neonatal outcome after prolonged rupture of the membranes starting in the second trimester. *Arch Dis Child* 1988;63:1146.
30. Nimrod C, Davies D, Iwaniski S, et al. Ultrasound prediction of pulmonary hypoplasia. *Obstet Gynecol* 1986;68:495.
31. Vergani P, Locatelli A, Strobelt N, et al. Amnioinfusion for prevention of pulmonary hypoplasia in second-trimester rupture of membranes. *Am J Perinatol* 1997;14:325.
32. Baker CJ. Group B Streptococcal infections. *Clin Perinatol* 1997;24:59.
33. Papageorgiou A, Desgranges MF, Masson M, et al. The antenatal use of betamethasone in the prevention of RDS: a controlled double-blind study. *Pediatrics* 1979;63:83.
34. National Institutes of Health. *Effects of corticosteroids for fetal maturation on perinatal outcomes.* Bethesda, MD: National Institutes of Health, 1994;12:1.
35. Ardila J, Le Guennec JC, Papageorgiou A. Influence of antenatal betamethasone and gender cohabitation on outcome of twin pregnancies 24–34 weeks gestation. *Semin Perinatol* 1994;18:15.
36. Mercer BM, Arheart KL. Antimicrobial therapy in expectant management of preterm premature rupture of the membranes. *Lancet* 1995;346:1271.
37. Hillier SL, Nugent RR, Eschenbach DA, et al. Association between bacterial vaginosis and preterm delivery of a low birth weight infant. *N Engl J Med* 1995;333:1737.
38. John C, Hauth MD, Robert L, et al. Reduced incidence of preterm delivery with metronidazole and erythromycin in women with bacterial vaginosis. *N Engl J Med* 1995;333:1732.
39. Bhat R, Zikos-Lambropaulosi. Resuscitatory and respiratory management of infants weighing less than 1000 grams. *Clin Perinatol* 1986;13:285.
40. Hegyi T, Carbone T, Anwar M, et al. The Apgar score and its components in the preterm infant. *Pediatrics* 1998;107:77.

41. Chathas MK, Patoh JB, Fisher DE, et al. Percutaneous central venous catheterization. *Am J Dis Child* 1990;144:1246.
42. Pinto-Martin JA, Riolo S, Cnaan A, Holzman C, Susser M, Paneth N. Cranial ultrasound prediction of disabling and nondisabling cerebral palsy at age two in low birth weight population. *Pediatrics* 1995; 95:249.
43. Nwaesei CG, Papge KE, Martin DJ, et al. Periventricular infarction diagnosed by ultrasound: a post mortem correlation. *J Pediatr* 1984; 105:106.
44. Rodriguez J, Claus D, Verellen G, et al. Periventricular leukomalacia: ultrasonic and neuropathological correlations. *Dev Med Child Neurol* 1990;32:347.
45. Vermont-Oxford Neonatal Network. A multicenter, randomized trial comparing synthetic surfactant with modified bovine surfactant extract in the treatment of neonatal respiratory distress syndrome. *Pediatrics* 1996;97:1.
46. Morley CJ. Surfactant treatment for premature babies: a review of clinical trials. *Arch Dis Child* 1991;66:445.
47. Merritt TA, Hallman M, Vaucher Y, McFeeley E, Tubman TRJ. Impact of surfactant treatment in cost of neonatal intensive care. *J Perinatol* 1990;10:416.
48. Corbet A, Bucciarelli R, Zoldan S, et al. Decreased mortality rate among small premature infants treated at birth with a single dose of synthetic surfactant: a multicenter controlled trial. *J Pediatr* 1001; 118:277.
49. Kwong M, Egan E, Nutter RH, Shapiro DL. Double blind clinical trial of calf lung surfactant extract for the prevention of hyaline membrane disease in extremely premature infants. *Pediatrics* 1985;76:585.
50. Kovacs L, Bardin C, Rossignol M, Papageorgiou A. Reduction in mortality but not in chronic lung disease after surfactant therapy in infants < 1000 grams. *Pediatr Res* 1995;37:339A.
51. Ferrara TB, Hoekstra RE, Couser RJ. Effect of surfactant on outcome of infants with birth weight of 600–750 grams. *Pediatr Res* 1991; 27:243A.
52. Horbar ID, Wright EC, Oustand L, et al. Decreasing mortality associated with the introduction of surfactant therapy: an observational study of neonates weighing 601–1300 grams at birth. *Pediatrics* 1993; 92:191.
53. Brans YW, Escobedo MB, Hayashi RH, et al. Perinatal mortality in a large perinatal center: five year review of 31,000 births. *Am J Obstet Gynecol* 1984;148:284.
54. Wyszogrodski I, Kyei-Aboagye K, Taeush HW, et al. Surfactant inactivation by hyperventilation: conservation by end-expiratory pressure. *J Appl Physiol* 1975;38:461.
55. Avery ME, Fletcher BD, Williams RG. *The lung and its disorders in the newborn infants.* Philadelphia: WB Saunders, 1981.
56. Goldsmith JP, Karotkin E. *Assisted ventilation of the neonate.* Philadelphia: WB Saunders, 1996:21.
57. Thilo EH, Andersen D, Wesserstein MC, et al. Saturation by pulse oximetry: comparison of the results obtained by instruments of different brands. *J Pediatr* 1993;122:620.
58. Heicher DA, Kasting DS, Harrod JR. Prospective clinical comparison of two methods for mechanical ventilation of neonates: rapid rate and short inspiratory time versus slow rate and long inspiratory time. *J Pediatr* 1981;98:957.
59. Greenough A, Greenall F, Gamsu H. Synchronous respiration: which ventilator rates are better? *Acta Paediatr Scand* 1987;76:813.
60. Castling D, Greenough A, Giffin F. Neonatal endotracheal suction: comparison of open and closed suction techniques. *Br J Intens Care* 1995;5:218.
61. Avery ME, Tooley WH, Keller JB, et al. Is chronic lung disease in low birth weight infants preventable? A survey of eight centers. *Pediatrics* 1987;73:20.
62. Vermont-Oxford Network Database Project. Very low birth weight outcomes for 1990. *Pediatrics* 1993;91:540.
63. Kraybil EN, Runyan DK, Bose CL, Khan JH. Risk factors for chronic lung disease in infants with birth weight of 751 to 1000 grams. *J Pediatr* 1989;115:115.
64. Garland JS, Buck RK, Allred EN, Levitan A. Hypocarbia before surfactant therapy appears to increase the bronchopulmonary dysplasia risk in infants with respiratory distress syndrome. *Arch Ped Adolesc Med* 1995;149:617.
65. Feihl F, Perret C. Permissive hypercapnia. *Am J Respir Crit Care* 1994;150:1722.
66. Vannucci RC, Towfigh J, Heitjan DF, Brucklacher RM. Carbon dioxide protects the perinatal brain from hypoxic ischemic damage: an experimental study in the immature rat. *Pediatrics* 1995;95:868.
67. Fujimoto S, Togari H, Yamanuchi N, et al. Hypocarbia and cystic periventricular leukomalacia in premature infants. *Arch Dis Child* 1994;71:F107.
68. Graziani LJ,Spitzer AR, Mitchell DG, et al. Mechanical ventilation in preterm infants: neurosonographic and developmental studies. *Pediatrics* 1992;90:515.
69. Wigglesworth JS, Pape KE. An integrated model for hemorrhagic and ischaemic lesions in the newborn brain. *Early Hum Dev* 1978;2:179.
70. Wiswell TE, Graziani LS, Kornhauser MS, et al. Effects of hypocarbia on the development of cystic periventricular leukomalacia in premature infants treated with high frequency jet ventilation. *Pediatrics* 1996;98:918.
71. Goldstein RF, Lohmeyer MB, Oehler JM. Outcome of premature infants treated with high frequency ventilation: impact of disease versus technology. *Pediatr Res* 1995;37:257A.
72. Le Guennec JC, Rufai M, Papageorgiou A. Spectrum of oxygen dependency in surviving infants weighing 600 to 1000 grams: decreased incidence of severe chronic lung disease. *Am J Perinatol* 1993;10:292.
73. Clyman RI. Medical treatment of patent ductus arteriosus in premature infants. In: Long WA, ed. *Fetal and neonatal cardiology.* Philadelphia: WB Saunders, 1990:682.
74. Gonzalez A, Centura-Junca P. Incidence of patent ductus arteriosus in premature infants less than 2000 grams. *Rev Clin Pediatr* 1991;62: 354.
75. Hoekstra RE, Jackson JC, Myers T, et al. Improved neonatal survival following multiple doses of bovine surfactant in very premature neonates at risk for respiratory distress syndrome. *Pediatrics* 1991;88: 10.
76. Cotton RB, Stahlman MT, Kovar I, Catterton WZ. Medical management of small preterm infants with symptomatic patent ductus arteriosus. *J Pediatr* 1979;2:467.
77. Mellander M, Larsson LE, Ekstrom-Jobal B, Sabel KG. Prediction of symptomatic patent ductus arteriosus in preterm infants using Doppler and M-mode echocardiography. *Acta Paediatr Scand* 1987; 76:553.
78. Mahony L, Carnero V, Brett C, Heymann MA, Clyman RI. Prorphylactic indomethacin therapy for patent ductus arteriosus in very low birth weight infants. *N Engl J Med* 1982;306:506.
79. Rennie JM, Doyle J, Cooke RWI. Early adminsitration of indomethacin to preterm infants. *Arch Dis Child* 1986;61:233.
80. Fowlie PW. Prophylactic indomethacin: systematic review and meta-analysis. *Arch Dis Child* 1996;74:F81.
81. Ment LR, Oh W, Ehrenkranz KR, et al. Low-dose indomethacin and prevention of intraventricular hemorrhage: a multicenter randomized trial. *Pediatrics* 1994;93:543.
82. Robie D, Waltrip T, Garcia-Prats J, Potozay WS, Jaksic T. Is surgical ligation of a patent ductus arteriosus the preferred initial approach for the neoante with extremely low birth weight? *J Pediatr Surg* 1996;8:113.
83. Heyman MA. Prostaglandins and leukotrienes in the perinatal period. *Clin Perinatol* 1987;14:957.
84. Ment LR, Oh W, Ehrenkranz RA, et al. Low-dose indomethacin therapy and extension of intraventricular hemorrhage: a multicenter study. *J Pediatr* 1994;124:951.
85. Ment LR, Duncan CC, Ehrenkranz RA, et al. Randomized low-dose indomethacin trial for prevention of intraventricular hemorrhage in very low birth weight neonates. *J Pediatr* 1988;112:948.
86. Mitchell JA, Akarasereenout P, Thiemermann C, Flower RJ, Vane JR. Selectivity of non-steroidal anti-inflammatory drugs as inhibitors of constitutive and inducible cyclo-oxygenase. *Proc Natl Acad Sci USA* 1993;90:11693.
87. Mosca F, Bray M, Lattanzio M, Fumagelli M. Comparative evaluation of effects of indomethacin and ibuprofen on perfusion and oxygenation in preterm infants with patent ductus arteriosus. *J Pediatr* 1997;131:5.
88. Aranda JV, Varvarigou N, Beharry K, et al. Pharmacokinetics and protein binding of intravenous ibuprofen in premature newborns. *Acta Paediatr* 1997;86:289.
89. Varvarigou A, Bardin C, Beharry K, Chemtob S, Papageorgiou A, Aranda JV. Early ibuprofen administration to prevent patent ductus arteriosus in premature newborn infants. *JAMA* 1996;275:539.

90. Hellerstein S. Fluids and electrolytes: physiology. *Pediatr Rev* 1993; 14:70.

91. Guignard JP, John EG. Renal function in the tiny, premature infant. *Clin Perinatol* 1986;13:377.

92. Shaffer SG, Bradt S, Meade V, Hall RT. Extracellular fluid volume changes in very low birth weight infants during first two postnatal months. *J Pediatr* 1987;111:124.

93. Lorenz JM, Kleinman LI, Ahmed GM, Markarian K. Phases of fluid and electrolyte homeostasis in the extremely low birth weight infant. *Pediatrics* 1995;96:484.

94. Takahashi N, Hoshi J, Nishida H. Water, electrolytes and acid–base balance in extremely premature infants. *Acta Paediatr Jpn* 1994;36:250.

95. Sato K, Kondo T, Iwao H, Houda S, Neda K. Internal potassium shift in premature infants: cause of nonoliguric hyperkalemia. *J Pediatr* 1995;126:109.

96. Rutter N. The immature skin. *Eur J Pediatr* 1996;155:18.

97. Nopper AJ, Horil KA, Sookdeo-Drost S, Wang TH, Mancini AJ, Lane AT. Topical ointment therapy benefits premature infants. *J Pediatr* 1996;128:660.

98. Heird LW, Gomez MR. Parenteral nutrition in low birth weight infants. *Annu Rev Nutr* 1996;16:471.

99. Yeh TF, McClenan DA, Ayahi OA, Pildes RS. Metabolic rate and energy balance in infants with bronchopulmonary dysplasia. *J Pediatr* 1989;114:448.

100. Merritt RJ. Cholestatic jaundice with total parenteral nutrition. *J Pediatr Gastroenterol Nutr* 1980;5:9.

101. Lucas A. Gut hormones and adaptation to extrauterine nutrition. In: Nilla JP, Nullen DPR, eds. *Essentials of paediatric gastroenterology.* Edinburgh: Churchill Livingstone, 1987:302.

102. Carver JD, Barness LA. Trophic factors for the gastrointestinal tract. *Clin Perinatol* 1996;23:265.

103. Berseth CL. Effect of early feeding on maturation of the preterm infant's small intestine. *J Pediatr* 1992;120:947.

104. Berry MA, Conrod H, Usher RH. Growth of very premature infants fed intravenous hyperalimentation and calcium-supplemented formula. *Pediatrics* 1997;100:647.

105. Ogata E. Carbohydrate metabolism in the fetus and neonate and altered neonatal glucoregulation. *Pediatr Clin North Am* 1989;33:25.

106. Pildes RS, Pyatis P. Hypoglycemia and hyperglycemia in tiny infants. *Clin Perinatol* 1986;13:351.

107. Pildes RS. Neonatal hyperglycemia. *J Pediatr* 1986;5:905.

108. Ferrara TB, Couser RJ, Hoekstra RE. Side effects and long term follow-up of corticosteroid therapy in very low birth weight infants with bronchopulmonary dysplasia. *J Perinatol* 1990;10:137.

109. Odell GB, Storey GNB, Rosenberg LA. Studies in kernicterus: the staturation of serum protein bilirubin during neonatal life and its relationship to brain damage at 5 years. *J Pediatr* 1970;76:12.

110. Perlman JM, Volpe JJ. Intraventricular hemorrhage in extremely small premature infants. *Am J Dis Child* 1986;140;1122.

111. Shankaran S, Bauer CR, Bain R, Wright L, Zachary J. Prenatal and perinatal risk and protective factors for neonatal intracranial hemorrhage. *Arch Pediatr Adolesc Med* 1996;150;491.

112. Volpe JJ. Current concepts of brain injury in the premature infant. *Am J Radiol* 1989;153:243.

113. Volpe JJ. *Neurology of the newborn.* Philadelphia: WB Saunders, 1995.

114. Dolfin T, Skidmore MB, Fongk W, et al. Incidence, severity and timing of subependymal and intraventricular hemorrhages in preterm infants born in a perinatal unit as detected by serial real-time ultrasound. *Pediatrics* 1983;71:541.

115. Vohr B, Ment LR. Intraventricular hemorrhage in the preterm infant. *Early Hum Dev* 1996;44:1

116. Perlman JM, Risser R, Broyles RS. Bilateral cystic periventricular leukomalacia in premature infants: associated risk factors. *Pediatrics* 1996;97:822.

117. Levene MI. Cerebral ultrasound and neurologic impairment: telling the future. *Arch Dis Child* 1990;65:469.

118. Kuban KCK, Leviton A. Medical progress: cerebral palsy. *N Engl J Med* 1994;330:188.

119. Joint Committee on Infant Hearing 1994. Position statement. *Pediatrics* 1995;95:152.

120. Kennedy CR, Kim L, Dees DC, et al. Otoacoustic emission and auditory brain stem responses in the newborn. *Arch Dis Child* 1991; 66:1124.

121. Berry MA, Conrod H, Usher RH. Growth of very premature infants fed intraveous hyperalimentation and calcium-supplemented formula. *Pediatrics* 1997;100:647.

122. Phibbs RH. Erythropoietin therapy for the extremely premature infant. *J Perinat Med* 1995;23:127.

123. Soubasi V, Kremenopoulos G, Diamandi E, Tsantali C, Tsakiris D. In which neonates does early recombinant human erythropoietin treatment prevent anemia of prematurity? Results of a randomized controlled study. *Pediatr Res* 1993;34:675.

124. Strauss RG, Villhauer PJ, Cordle DG. A method to collect, store and issue multiple aliquots of packed red blood cells for neonatal transfusion. *Vox Sang* 1995;68:77.

125. Lane PA, Hathawy WE. Vitamin K in infancy. *J Pediatr* 1985;106:351.

126. Burrows RF, Andrew M. Neonatal thrombocytopenia in hypertensive disorders of pregnancy. *Obstet Gynecol* 1990;76:234.

127. Hudak BB, Allen MC, Hudak ML, Laughlin GM. Home oxygen therapy for chronic lung disease in extremely low birth weight infants. *Am J Dis Child* 1989;143:357.

128. Northway WH, Rosan RC, Porter DY. Pulmonary disease following respiratory therapy of hyaline membrane-bronchopulmonary dysplasia. *N Engl J Med* 1967;276:357.

129. Avery GB, Fletcher AB, Kaplan M, Brudno DS. Controlled trial of dexamethasone in respirator-dependent infants with bronchopulmonary dysplasia. *Pediatrics* 1985;75:106.

130. Cummings JJ, D Eugenio DB, Gross SJ. A controlled trial of dexamethasone in preterm infants at high risk for bronchopulmonary dysplasia. *N Engl J Med* 1989;320:105.

131. Brozanski BS, Jones JG, Gilmour CH, et al. Effect of pulse dexamethasone therapy on the incidence and severity of chronic lung disease in the very low birth weight infant. *J Pediatr* 1995;126:769.

132. Dunn MS, Magnani L, Belaiche M. Inhaled corticosteroids in severe bronchopulmonary dysplasia. *Pediatr Res* 1989;25:213A.

133. Kovacs L, Davis M, Faucher M, Papageorgiou A. Efficacy of sequential early systemic and inhaled corticosteroid therapy in the prevention of chronic lung disease of prematurity. *Acta Paediatr* 1998;87:792.

134. Kao LC, Warburton D, Platzker AC, Keens TG. Effect of isoproterenol inhalation on airway resistance in chronic bronchopulmonary dysplasia. *Pediatrics* 1984;73:509.

135. Covert RF, Neu J, Elliot MJ, et al. Factors associated with age of onset of necrotizing enterocolitis. *Am J Perinatol* 1989;6:455.

136. Bauer CR, Morrison JC, Poole WK, et al. A decreased incidence of necrotizing enterocolitis after prenatal glucocorticoid therapy. *Pediatrics* 1984;73:682.

137. Mauy RD, Fanaroff AA, Korones SB, et al. Necrotizing enterocolitis in very low birth weight infants. Biodemographic and clinical correlates. *J Pediatr* 1991;119:630.

138. Palmer EA. The continuing threat of retinopathy of prematurity. *Am J Ophthalmol* 1996;122:420.

139. Ng YK, Fielder AR, Shaw DE, Levene M. Epidemiology of retinopathy of prematurity. *Lancet* 1988;2:1235.

140. Palmer EA, Flynn JT, Hardy RJ, et al. Incidence and early course of retinopathy of prematurity. The Cryotherapy for Retinopathy of Prematurity Cooperative Group. *Ophthalmology* 1991;98:1628.

141. International Committee for the Classification of Retinopathy of Prematurity. An international classification of retinopathy of prematurity. *Pediatrics* 1984;74:127.

142. Glass P, Avery GB, Subramanian KV, Keys PM, Sostek AM, Friendly DS. Effect of bright light in the hospital nursery on the incidence of retinopathy of prematurity. *N Engl J Med* 1985;313:401.

143. Poets C, Samuels M, Southall DP. Epidemiology and pathophysiology of apnea of prematurity. *Biol Neonate* 1994;65;211.

144. Finer NN, Barrington KJ, Hayes BJ, Hugh A. Obstructive mixed and central apnea in the neonate: physiologic correlates. *J Pediatr* 1992; 121:943.

145. Davi M, Shankaran K, Simons KJ, Simons ER, Seshia MM, Rigatto H. Physiologic changes induced by theophylline in the treatment of apnea in preterm infants. *J Pediatr* 1978;92:91.

146. Gerhardt T, McCarthy J, Bancalari E. Effect of aminophylline on respiratory center activity and metabolic rate with idiopathic apnea. *Pediatrics* 1979;63:537.

147. Fesslova V, Caccano ML, Salice P, Marini A. Assessment of cardiovascular effects of theophylline in premature newborns by means of echocardiography. *Acta Paediatr Scand* 1984;73:404.

148. Aranda JV, Turmen T, Davis J, et al. Effects of caffeine on control of breathing in infantile apnea. *J Pediatr* 1983;103:975.

149. Barrington KJ, Finer N, Torok-Both C, Jamali F, Coults RT. Dose–response relationship of doxapram in the therapy for refractory idiopathic apnea of prematurity. *Pediatrics* 1987;80:22.

150. Bairam A, Gershan LA, Beharry K, Laudignon N, Papageorgiou A, Aranda JV. Gastrointestinal absorption of doxapram in newborn premature infants. *Am J Perinatol* 1991;8:110.

151. Baker CJ. Group B Sterptococcal infections. *Clin Perinatol* 1997;24:59.

152. Donowitz LG. Failure of the overgown to prevent nosocomial infection in a pediatric intensive care unit. *Pediatrics* 1986;77:35.

153. Anand KJS, Hickey PR. Pain and its effects in the human neonate and fetus. *N Engl J Med* 1987;317:1321.

154. Johnston CC, Stevens BJ. Experience in a neonatal intensive care unit affects pain response. *Pediatrics* 1996;98:925.

155. Als H, Lawhon G, Duffy FH, McAnulty C, Gibes-Grossman R, Blickman J. Individualized developmental care for the very low birth weight preterm infant-medical and neuro-functional effects. *JAMA* 1994;272:853.

156. Hack M, Fanaroff AA. Outcomes of extremely low birth weight infants between 1982 and 1988. *N Engl J Med* 1989;321:164.

157. Hack M, Friedman H, Fanaroff AA. Outcomes of extremely low birth weight infants. *Pediatrics* 1996;98:931.

158. Johnson A, Townshed P, Yudkin P, Bull D, Wilkinson AR. Functional abilities at age 4 years of children born before 29 weeks of gestation. *BMJ* 1993;306:1715.

159. Nishida H. Outcome of infants born preterm with special emphasis on extremely low birth weight infants. *Baillieres Clin Obstet Gynecol* 1993;7:611.

160. Hack M, Bresoau N, Wersman B. Effect of very low birth weight and subnormal head size on cognitive abilities at school age. *N Engl J Med* 1991;325:231.

161. Raju TNK, Hager S. The dilemma of less than 500 gram birth: epidemiologic considerations. *Am J Perinatol* 1986;3:327.

162. McCormick MC. The outcomes of very low birth weight infants: are we asking the right questions? *Pediatrics* 1997;99:869.

CHAPTER 27

Multiple Gestations

Mary E. Revenis and Lauren A. Johnson-Robbins

The products of multiple gestations comprise a disproportionate number of admissions to neonatal intensive care units and suffer greater morbidity than do singletons, but there is relatively little space devoted to their problems in most textbooks of neonatology. A review of the major problems can help the clinician to anticipate the medical needs and to prepare the parents for what lies ahead. Although some of the problems occurring in higher multiples of gestation are unique or intensified as the numbers increase, most of the issues about twins discussed in this chapter apply to all multiple gestations.

EPIDEMIOLOGY

The incidence of multiple gestation in the United States has increased dramatically during the past two decades as a result of a shift in the maternal age distribution to older ages as well as increased use of fertility enhancement therapy. The number of births from twin deliveries and higher-order multiples was 24.8 and 1.3 per 1000 live births in 1995, respectively (1). The actual rate of twin conceptions is much higher, because early fetal loss with a vanishing twin is far more common than clinically recognized (2). In 1,000 pregnancies studied early with ultrasonography, Landy et al. (2) found a twin conception rate of 3.29%, with subsequent reduction to a single fetus in 21.2% of those pregnancies.

The incidence of naturally conceived higher multiple births is mathematically described by the Hellin–Zeleny law, which states that if twins occur at a frequency of 1/N, triplets occur at a frequency of $(1/N)^2$, quadruplets at $(1/N)^3$, and so on. Because most epidemiologic studies exclude data on twins with no live-born member, they grossly underestimate the incidence of multiple gestations.

Monozygotic twinning occurs at a fairly constant rate of 3.5 per 1,000 live births, with limited variation among populations. The occurrence of monozygosity is not affected by environment, race, physical characteristics, or fertility. In contrast, rates for dizygotic twins vary greatly among populations, from 4 to 50 times per 1,000 live births. In Scotland, the overall incidence of twins is 12.4 per 1,000 live births; in Nigeria, it is 57.2 per 1,000 (3). Japan has the lowest total rate of twins, with only 4.3 per 1,000, most of which are monozygotic. Other factors that influence the incidence of dizygotic twinning include a maternally transmitted familial tendency, race, nutrition, parity, advanced maternal age, coital frequency, and seasonality. Twins are found most often in black populations and least often in Asians. Taller, heavier women bear twins at a rate 25% to 30% higher than short, undernourished women (3). Parity is an independent risk factor, with multiparous women having a greater likelihood for multiple gestations (4). Advanced maternal age predisposes to dizygotic twinning, with peak incidence at 37 years of age (4). Coital frequency has a positive affect, with a high rate of twin conceptions within the first 3 months of marriage (5). Another factor is the effect of the climatic seasons. In the Northern hemisphere, most dizygotic births are autumnal, reflecting more multiple ovulations during the winter and spring months. The seasonality of multiple births does not coincide with the peak months of singleton births (6).

High circulating levels of follicle stimulating hormone (FSH) and luteinizing hormone (LH) lead to the release of more than one ovum per menstrual cycle, making multizygotic conceptions more likely. Conception stimulants such as clomiphene citrate (Clomid, Serophene), which act by stimulating endogenous secretion of gonadotropins, raise the incidence of multiple gestations by 6.8% to 17%;

M. E. Revenis: Department of Neonatology, The George Washington University School of Medicine and Health Sciences; and Children's National Medical Center, Washington, D.C.

L. A. Johnson-Robbins: Department of Pediatrics, Albany Medical College; and Albany Medical Center, Albany, New York

exogenous gonadotropins such as Pergonal (FSH and LH) or human chorionic gonadotropins (A.P.L., Follutein, Pregnyl, Profasi HP) may increase the incidence as much as 18% to 53.5% (7). The women of the Nigerian Yoruba tribe, who have naturally elevated levels of FSH and LH, have a remarkably high rate of spontaneous, dizygotic twinning (1 in 20) (8). Martin et al. (9) examined another population and found that women with dizygotic twins have higher levels of FSH and estradiol than women bearing singletons. A phenomenon likely due to increased pituitary gonadotropin release is the twofold higher incidence of twin conceptions in the 2 months after the cessation of oral contraceptives (10). High FSH and LH levels probably account for the seasonal variation in twinning observed in many countries (11,12). The increasing use of assisted reproductive technology, such as *in vitro* fertilization, gamete intrafallopian transfer, and zygote intrafallopian transfer, during the 1980s resulted in more pregnancies complicated by multiple gestation (13,14). Currently, 33% to 40% of pregnancies resulting from assisted reproductive technology procedures are multiple gestations with the majority being dizygotic twins (13). Unexpectedly, monozygotic twinning is also more frequent in multiple gestations following assisted reproduction with an incidence of 3.2%, eight times higher than for spontaneously conceived pregnancies (15). Recently, the use of assisted reproductive technology has been seen to plateau (13,14).

ZYGOSITY

Zygosity is determined by the number of ova fertilized. Higher-order pregnancies may be monozygotic, dizygotic, or multizygotic. In 1955, Corner (16) postulated that monozygotic twins develop by splitting of the conceptus at any time from day 2 after conception through days 15 to 17. The timing of division determines whether monozygotic twins are dichorionic, monochorionic, or conjoined. Dizygotic or multizygotic gestations result if more than one ovum has undergone fertilization at the same coitus or even at different times or with different mates.

At birth, zygosity can be determined by gender differences or by direct placental examination. Other techniques have included blood typing, dermatoglyphics, and chromosome banding (17,18). The most precise technique is DNA-variant restriction fragment length polymorphisms (19). Because monozygotic twins carry significantly higher risks of morbidity and mortality prenatally and postnatally, establishing the zygosity of all multiple gestations is clinically important. More effort is going into determining zygosity prenatally using ultrasonography or genetic identification techniques.

PLACENTATION

The placenta from a twin gestation can be monochorionic or dichorionic, and, if dichorionic, it can be fused or separated, making four types of placentation possible:

1. Diamnionic, dichorionic separate,
2. Diamnionic, dichorionic fused,
3. Diamnionic, monochorionic, and
4. Monoamnionic, monochorionic.

All dizygotic twins have a diamnionic, dichorionic placenta; all monochorionic twins are monozygotic. Zygosity should be determined in the case of twins of the same gender if the placenta is not monochorionic, because these siblings may be monozygotic or dizygotic. Fusion of the placenta does not differentiate zygosity. Table 27–1 lists zygosity determination based on placental examination.

Benirschke (20) described how to determine chorionicity of a fused placenta based on examination of the dividing membranes. The amnion contains no blood vessels and is more transparent than the chorion, which contains fetal vessels and remnants of villous tissue. A monochorionic placenta is one in which the septum is composed of a thin, translucent amnion that can be easily separated and lifted from the chorionic plate. In a dichorionic placenta, the septum is thicker and more opaque. It does not separate as easily from the chorionic plate. Ultrasonography of the dividing membranes early in gestation is useful in some cases to determine the chorionicity, but it is not always technically feasible (21,22).

A monochorionic, monoamnionic placenta is formed by division of the embryonal disc at 7 to 13 days, which is after differentiation of the amnion. Only 1% to 2% of monozygotic twins are monoamnionic; the fetal mortality rate is as high as 50%, primarily due to twisting, knotting, or entanglement of the umbilical cords (23). Conjoined twins with their necessarily monoamniotic placenta result from the latest and incomplete splitting of the embryonic disc at days 13 to 15 of gestation. The monochorionic, diamnionic placenta with a dividing membrane consisting of two layers of amnion without an intervening chorion is formed at approximately 5 days of gestation. Dichorionic, diamnionic placentas are formed the earliest, within the first 3 days after conception.

TABLE 27–1. *Zygosity determination*

Clinical finding	Percentage of total deliveries	Zygosity
Different genders	35	Dizygotic
Monochorionic placenta	20	Monozygotic
Same gender and dichorionic placenta	45	8% of monozygotic and 37% of dizygotic infants[a]

[a]Further differentiation can be obtained by genotyping.
From Cameron AH. The Birmingham twin survey. *Proc R Soc Med* 1968;61:229.

ANTEPARTUM COMPLICATIONS

There are many complications of pregnancy that occur more frequently in multiple gestations. Preterm labor is the most frequent complication, occurring in 20% to 50% of multiple gestations, most likely due to uterine overdistention. Pregnancy-induced hypertension, placenta previa, antenatal and intrapartum hemorrhage, hyperemesis gravidarum, and premature rupture of membranes all occur at a higher rate (24,25). Polyhydramnios, an almost expected complication of multiple gestations, is transient in pregnancies in which there are no other complications. If persistent, the polyhydramnios suggests abnormal fetal conditions, such as twin-to-twin transfusion syndrome (TTTS) or congenital anomalies (26).

ANTENATAL MANAGEMENT

Recommendations for managing multiple gestations are controversial. The only unquestioned aspect of management is the benefit of early diagnosis, facilitating referral to an appropriate facility for high-risk infants. Antenatal management includes the following components:

- Early diagnosis,
- Nutritional intervention,
- Cervical cerclage,
- Prophylactic tocolysis,
- Steroid stimulation of fetal lung maturity,
- Therapeutic amniocentesis,
- Multifetal reduction, and
- Bed rest.

Bed rest beginning before 28 weeks commonly is advised to decrease perinatal mortality (27). The National Institutes of Health Collaborative Study showed no significant effect of antenatal betamethasone therapy in inducing fetal lung maturity in twins, but it is important to note that a relatively small number of twins were enrolled in the study (28,29). The 1994 NIH Consensus Statement on antenatal corticosteroids recommends betamethasone for all fetuses between 24 and 34 weeks of gestation including multiple gestations (30).

There are several approaches to limiting the complications seen in higher-order multiple gestation. The first is to limit the number of embryos transferred during *in vitro* fertilization to two. This results in a reduction in pre- and postnatal complications in the mother and infants without affecting the pregnancy or take-home baby rates (31,32). An alternative is the use of multifetal reduction. Reduction, most often to twins, usually is performed at 9 to 12 weeks of gestation via either the transvaginal or transabdominal route (33). Reduction of quadruplets to twins improves overall outcome, but studies on the effect of reduction of triplets to twins have had conflicting results (34,35). Several recent studies have shown an increased incidence of impaired fetal growth and a lower gestational age at delivery in infants who are the products of reduced twin gestations when compared with nonreduced twins (36,37). Selective termination is used during the second trimester in pregnancies in which one twin is discordant for a major genetic disease or anomaly (34,38).

LABOR AND DELIVERY

The total duration of labor in a twin gestation is similar to a singleton gestation, with some differences in the lengths of each stage. Friedman and Sachtelben (39) observed a shorter latent phase during twin labor but a longer active phase and second stage, probably due to dysfunctional labor in an overdistended uterus.

There are many potential complications associated with delivery of multiple gestations, including malpresentation, cord prolapse, cord entanglement, vasa previa, locked twins, and fetal distress. Locked twins occur most often if the chins interlock to prevent expulsion or extraction of the first twin. Locking occurs at a rate of 1 per 817 twin gestations, and uterine hypertonicity, monoamnionic twinning, fetal demise, and decreased amniotic fluid are all contributing factors (40).

The best method of delivery depends on the number of fetuses, the presentation of the first fetus, and the gestational age. Table 27–2 details the frequencies of each variation of presentation. If both twins are vertex, there is no evidence that cesarean section improves outcome (41). In vertex–nonvertex twin gestations longer than 32 weeks, vaginal delivery is recommended (42). Delivery of the nonvertex second twin can be by total breech extraction or external cephalic version under ultrasound guidance and epidural anesthesia (43). If the first twin is nonvertex, delivery usually is by cesarean section.

Mode of delivery of the preterm multiple gestation depends on many factors, only one of which is the fetal presentation. Historically, if premature twins present in a vertex–vertex pattern without other complications, vaginal delivery has been attempted, whereas a cesarean section is recommended for all other combinations of presentation if the gestational age is less than 34 weeks (44). When these recommendations are followed, there is no effect of mode of delivery or birth order on the incidence of intracranial hemorrhage in very-low-birth-weight (VLBW) twins (45,46). Extremely low birth weight twins (less than 1,000 g) have been shown to benefit from

TABLE 27–2. *Twin presentation*

Delivery (A–B)	Percentage of total deliveries
Vertex–vertex	42.5
Vertex–nonvertex	38.4
Nonvertex	19.1

From ref. 43.

cesarean section, regardless of their positioning, with a reduction in postnatal mortality (47).

Delayed interval delivery of multiple gestations is being reported more frequently (48–50). Management typically involves the placement of a cervical cerclage, tocolysis, and antibiotic therapy following the delivery of the first fetus to delay the delivery of the remaining fetuses as long as fetal distress is not present. The duration of pregnancy extension is highly variable, with one series achieving a mean of prolongation of 49 days (49). Delayed delivery allows for fetal maturation through either antenatal steroid administration or increasing gestational age.

MORTALITY

Multiple gestations account for 10% to 12% of perinatal deaths (51). Mortality in twins is four times higher than for singletons, with perinatal mortality rates of 15% to 31% (52,53). The increased frequencies of prematurity, preeclampsia, hydramnios, placenta previa, abruptio placentae, and cord prolapse contribute to the increased mortality. Of all intrauterine deaths in twins, 73.3% are associated with monochorionic placentation (54–56).

The frequency of single fetal demise in multiple gestation is reported as 0.5% to 6.8%, although early ultrasonography suggests a much higher rate of early loss (2,54–56). The causes of antepartum death include cord accidents, vascular anastomoses with overwhelming blood volume shifts, and velamentous insertion of the umbilical cord. Velamentous insertion, which makes the cord more vulnerable to trauma from twisting and compression, is six to nine times more common with twin gestation and increases the risks for fetal distress and for vasa previa with fetal hemorrhage (57).

After the demise of a fetal twin, the surviving fetus is at increased risk for distress, abnormal presentation, or dystocia, and the mother is at risk for toxemia, chorioamnionitis, or disseminated intravascular coagulation. In dichorionic twins, if the cause of death is intrinsic only to that fetus, complications to the surviving co-twin are rare, except from spontaneous premature labor (56). When one twin dies after at least 15 weeks of gestation in diamnionic pregnancies, a fetus papyraceous develops. The fetus loses all water content, becomes compressed, and, because of oligohydramnios, may be mistakenly identified on sonography as a stuck twin. A retained twin may be large enough to hinder labor mechanically, necessitating cesarean section (58). Before 15 weeks, the fetus is resorbed; this is called the vanishing twin phenomenon.

For most monochorionic twins, the death of one twin has little adverse effect on the surviving fetus (59). However, if vascular connections are present, the surviving twin is at risk for complications related to interfetal blood exchange, including disseminated intravascular coagulation from the release of thromboplastin by the dead twin.

After the death of one twin, partial abruptio placentae, which separates further during labor, may cause asphyxia or demise of the other twin (55). Fetal transfusion syndrome may be related to many of the antepartum deaths complicating twin pregnancy (54–56,60).

The mortality of multiple gestations higher than two is greater than for twins because of smaller fetal size and placental or cord compromise from competition for space (61). The perinatal mortality rate for triplet pregnancies is reported as 7% to 23%, and it is strongly related to gestational age at delivery (62).

TWIN-TO-TWIN TRANSFUSION SYNDROME

Interfetal blood exchange occurs almost exclusively in monochorionic twins with circulations shared through vascular anastomoses that are present in most monochorionic placentas. Only 5% to 18% of these communications are sufficiently imbalanced to produce TTTS, but the actual rate would be higher if all cases of early fetal death of one twin were identified (54,63,64). Placentas from twin pregnancies complicated by TTTS have been shown to have significantly fewer vascular anastomoses, which more commonly are deep rather than superficial in location, compared to monochorionic placentas in pregnancies not complicated by TTTS (65). Vascular anastomoses and TTTS are rare in fused dichorionic placentas of dizygotic or monozygotic twins (54,57,59,64).

Acute and chronic forms of TTTS have been described (66,67). The onset of symptoms depends on what type of vessels are in communication, with an unbalanced, arteriovenous anastomosis and unidirectional shunt leading to the earliest and most profound symptoms. If anastomoses are balanced (i.e., artery to artery, vein to vein), the onset and severity of symptoms depend on changes in perfusion pressures that may be temporary and vary throughout gestation or become problematic only after delivery or demise of one twin.

Chronic, unidirectional TTTS manifests at any time after 16 weeks and can occur when an arteriovenous anastomosis joins a high-pressure system with a low-pressure system. The donor twin becomes progressively anemic, hypovolemic, and growth retarded, with oligohydramnios, and is at risk for tissue hypoxia and acidosis from reduced perfusion (60,68). The recipient twin becomes polycythemic and hypervolemic, with polyhydramnios developing from increased urine production to relieve the circulatory volume overload. Disparities in the weight of the heart and other viscera and in the size of glomeruli and of pulmonary and systemic arterioles have been reported (60). Both twins are at risk for ischemia, thromboembolism, disseminated intravascular coagulation, and death. In the donor twin, there is hypotension and poor tissue perfusion; in the recipient, there also is poor tissue perfusion from hyperviscosity and polycythemia. Although the net transfusion is in the direction of the recipient, thrombi can exchange freely in either direction through vascular anastomoses, resulting in infarcts or the death of either twin.

Manifestations of TTTS range in severity from mild differences in blood hematocrit to the extremes of anemia and polycythemia affecting the pair (69,70). In the most severe cases, the growth-retarded donor twin may die of chronic hypoxia; the recipient develops congestive heart failure and hydrops and may die. Premature rupture of membranes, preterm labor, and delivery of compromised, premature infants are the usual sequelae. The perinatal mortality is 70% or more (71,72). Prognosis is better if symptoms, diagnosis, and delivery occur at a later gestational age or if hydrops does not develop.

In rare cases, after death of one twin with TTTS, the polyhydramnios resolves, and a healthy survivor is born at a later time. However, compromising volumes of blood may be lost from the survivor into the dead twin. Other morbidity results from the release of thrombogenic material from degenerating fetal tissues, resulting in disseminated intravascular coagulation, multiple infarcts, and tissue necrosis in the live twin (54). Possibly related to thromboembolic arterial occlusion, severe defects, such as porencephaly, multicystic encephalomalacia, renal cortical necrosis, infarcts of the spleen, cutis aplasia, small bowel atresia, colonic and appendiceal atresia with horseshoe kidney, hemifacial microsomia, and necrotic limb, have been observed in the survivor of monochorionic twins after one fetal demise (54,56,72–75). An increased incidence of these defects is not reported in dichorionic twin survivors after the death of a co-twin.

One suggested criterion for diagnosing chronic TTTS is a hemoglobin difference between twins of 5 g/dL or more. In itself, this is not sufficient to establish TTTS, because large differences in hemoglobin concentration also can occur in separate, dichorionic placentas (76). Tan et al. (65) diagnosed TTTS if a birth weight difference of 20% and a hemoglobin difference of 5 g/dL or more was found. However, a birth weight difference of more than 20% occurs with similar frequency in monochorionic and dichorionic pregnancies. The smaller twin may have polycythemia, secondary to intrauterine growth retardation (76). Fetal transfusion studies using adult cells as markers indicate significant interfetal blood exchange sufficient to cause discordant growth and amniotic fluid volumes occur far more often than differences in hemoglobin concentrations suggest (77). Because TTTS in all degrees is limited to monochorionic placentations, differentiating the type of placenta and detecting vascular anastomoses are important. Measurement of the difference in pulsatility index between fetuses by Doppler examination of umbilical arterial blood flow has been shown to be helpful in the diagnosis of TTTS even before the development of fetal hydrops (78).

Acardiac twinning (i.e., reversed arterial perfusion syndrome) is a rare but interesting variation of TTTS, occurring in 1% of monozygotic twins (79). The nonviable acardiac twin's survival depends on the existence of artery-to-artery and vein-to-vein anastomoses to the other twin (80). The structurally normal, pump twin provides the circulation for itself and for its abnormal, acardiac twin, permitting slow growth of the abnormal twin. The reversed direction of flow in the umbilical arteries of the acardiac twin, demonstrable by ultrasonography, may be responsible for preventing normal anatomic differentiation (81). Often assuming an amorphous shape, the cephalic pole is affected most severely, because it is the region most distal to the retrograde perfusion. The closer and better perfused lower part of the body is relatively spared (80). The diagnosis of acardiac twinning can be suspected prenatally by absence or marked undergrowth of the heart, head, and trunk and by increased body soft tissue (81). The acardiac twin is smaller than the pump twin, but the fetal skull and long bones may continue to grow slowly (82). Frequent complications include congestive heart failure of the pump twin developing between 22 and 30 weeks of gestation, with cardiomegaly, hepatomegaly, intrauterine growth failure, maternal hydramnios, preterm delivery, malpresentation, and fetal distress (80,83). The mortality rate of the pump twin is 50% to 55%, primarily due to prematurity (80,83).

An acute form of TTTS occurs with rapid transfer of blood through large superficial artery-to-artery or vein-to-vein anastomoses during labor and delivery, resulting in a hypovolemic donor and a hypervolemic recipient with similar birth weights (66,67). The transfusion is from the first to the second twin during the delivery of the first twin. However, if the first cord clamping is delayed, blood from the undelivered twin can be transfused into the first infant. The potential for acute volume changes during labor and delivery of monochorionic twins contributes to their vulnerability, need for resuscitation, and volume management.

Antenatal management of the TTTS previously was limited to close observation and bed rest. Acute polyhydramnios, which often complicates TTTS, is managed with serial amniocenteses of enough amniotic fluid to lessen fetal symptoms (84). In some instances, decreasing the polyhydramnios seems to stop or ameliorate the interfetal transfusion dramatically. Digoxin has been used successfully to treat cardiac failure in a recipient twin (85). Endoscopic laser coagulation of connecting vessels has been found to be effective in treating severe TTTS (86). Another approach to severe TTTS, in which the death of both twins is anticipated, is selective feticide of the donor twin with survival of the recipient twin (87).

STUCK TWIN

The stuck twin phenomenon occurs in a diamniotic pregnancy if there is a relatively acute onset of severe disparity in amniotic volumes, with one growth-retarded twin in an oligohydramniotic sac compressed against the uterine wall. If the oligohydramnios is severe enough, this twin may suffer all the complications of prolonged compression, including pulmonary hypoplasia, abnormal facies, and orthopedic deformation. The other twin is in a distended, polyhydramniotic sac, adding to compression of the smaller twin (88).

The stuck twin phenomenon occurs to some degree in as many as 35% of monochorionic diamnionic twin pregnancies, and it can develop in dichorionic pregnancies (89). In monochorionic twins, the phenomenon may be related to TTTS. Other causes, regardless of placentation, include uteroplacental dysfunction, congenital infection, discordant aneuploidy, and structural malformations. Both twins are structurally normal in 95% of cases. Disparity in volumes of amniotic fluid can occur if one twin has structural anomalies that lead to polyhydramnios (e.g., neural tube defect, upper gastrointestinal obstruction, congenital heart disease) or oligohydramnios (e.g., ruptured amnion, urinary tract anomalies, growth retardation) (90). The onset is usually between 18 and 30 weeks of gestation (89). Premature labor, possibly related to uterine distention from polyhydramnios and to preterm rupture of membranes, develops in most cases. Without intervention to reverse the fetal compression and uterine overdistention, the chance of survival of both twins is less than 20% (91).

ASPHYXIA

Despite the clinical impression that the first-born twin (twin A) does better than the second-born twin (twin B), there is no demonstrable increase in neonatal death in the second-born twin (41,53). Breech presentation is more frequent, and large placental abruptions are more common in second twins (53). Differences in the 1-minute Apgar score, umbilical venous pH, PO_2, and PCO_2 favor twin A, regardless of route of delivery, placentation, interval between twins, or presentation (92). The second-born twin has potentially greater risk for hypoxia and trauma, regardless of the route of delivery, suggesting physiologic changes after the birth of the first twin. Findings in the venous blood gases suggest compromised intervillous placental blood flow after delivery of the first twin as a major factor.

In triplet pregnancies, although preterm labor is the most frequent complication and the most important factor in perinatal morbidity and mortality, the mode of delivery is also important. If delivery is by cesarean section, triplet C has a higher 5-minute Apgar score, and triplets B and C have increased survival compared with triplets of vaginal delivery (93). If triplets are delivered by cesarean section, the three triplets have a similar acid–base status despite the finding of lower 1-minute Apgar scores for triplet C (94). The influence of birth order on acid–base status becomes significant during

vaginal births if there is a longer time *in utero* after delivery of triplet A. Triplets of more than 34 weeks of gestation and with birth weights greater than 2,000 g for each fetus tolerate vaginal delivery more successfully than smaller triplets (93).

GROWTH

Examination of fetuses between 8 and 21 weeks of gestation show similar weight-to-length ratios for singleton and twin fetuses (95). Birth weights of live-born twins up to 30 weeks of gestation are slightly smaller but similar to singletons of the same gestational age, indicating that the growth rate is similar in twins and singletons until 30 weeks of gestation (Table 27–3) (96–98). After 30 weeks, the singleton fetus has accelerated, exponential growth, and twin fetuses have a more linear rate of growth (99). Triplet growth previously was reported to decline progressively after 27 weeks of gestation (61). More recent studies indicate that growth of individual triplets and triplet sets remains linear throughout the third trimester (100).

Better growth in the third trimester for multiple gestations reflects the positive impact of more aggressive maternal nutritional and obstetric care management. In a prospective study of nutritional intervention, the incidence of preterm delivery, low birth weight (LBW), and VLBW was lowered by 30%, 25%, and 50%, respectively, compared with twin pregnancies without nutritional intervention, but the rates of intrauterine growth retardation were not affected (101).

Multiple gestations account for 17% of intrauterine growth retardation, with higher mortality rates for affected infants, particularly for the growth-retarded twin if only one is affected (51,96,102). Monochorionic twins show greater degrees of intrapair variation in birth weight than dichorionic twins, and true intrauterine growth retardation occurs more often in monochorionic twins. The individual members of twin pairs frequently are discordant for the rate of growth due to TTTS, placental insufficiency, intrauterine crowding, or an unequal impact of maternal complications that impair growth, such as preeclampsia. Ultimately, the underlying factor in most instances is a limitation of intrauterine nutrition, which may be shared unequally by the fetuses.

The incidence of discordant fetal growth as measured by biparietal diameter increases significantly as gestation

TABLE 27–3. *Birth statistics for multiple gestations*

No. of infants	Gestational age (average in wk)	Birth weight (average in g)	Reference
Twins	37.1	2,390	130
Triplets	33.0	1,720	131
Quadruplets	31.4	1,482	132

advances. It is important to differentiate discordant growth due to TTTS, in which both twins are at increased risk for morbidity and mortality often before the last trimester, from a twin gestation in which one fetus shows growth retardation, which usually becomes evident during the last trimester, and the other develops normally. With discordant growth not due to TTTS, the prognosis for the growth-retarded fetus depends on the severity of the growth failure and its cause, and the prognosis for the normally grown fetus may not be compromised. During the postnatal period, the smaller of the discordant twins has an increased incidence of hypoglycemia and is more likely to have retarded growth and development during childhood (103,104).

CONGENITAL ANOMALIES

Monozygotic twins have an increased frequency of congenital anomalies compared with dizygotic twins or singletons (75). Monozygotic twins frequently are discordant for malformations or for the severity of a given malformation. Some structural defects are related to the monozygotic twinning process, such as conjoined twins or some amorphous twins. Early embryonic malformations and malformation complexes such as sirenomelia, holoprosencephaly, and anencephaly are increased in monozygotic twins, suggesting a common cause for monozygotic twinning and early malformation complexes. Structural defects that result from the disruption of previously normal tissues are associated with the exchange of circulation in monochorionic twins with vascular connections. Those defects in which a vascular disruptive cause has been suggested include central nervous system defects (e.g., microcephaly, porencephalic cysts, hydranencephaly), gastrointestinal defects (e.g., intestinal atresia), renal cortical necrosis, hemifacial microsomia, aplasia cutis congenital, and terminal limb defects (73). Deformations due to crowding and constraint molding of the normal fetus *in utero* during late gestation are similar in type and frequency in dizygotic and monozygotic twins and include foot-positioning deformations.

Conjoined twins represent a unique structural defect of monozygotic monoamnionic twins. The nonseparated parts of the otherwise normal twins remain fused throughout the remaining period of development (105). The incidence of conjoined twins is between 1 in 80,000 to 1 in 25,000 births, and 70% to 80% of these cases are female twins (106). Approximately 40% are joined at the chest (thoracopagus), 34% at the anterior abdominal wall (xiphopagus or omphalopagus), 18% at the buttocks (pygopagus), 6% at the ischium (ischiopagus), and 2% at the head (craniopagus). With ultrasonography, the diagnosis of conjoined twins can be established as early as week 12 of gestation (107). Forty percent of conjoined twins are stillborn, and an additional 35% survive only 1 day (108). Long-term survival with or without surgical separation depends on the anatomic site of attachment and the extent of shared organs (109).

NEONATAL DISORDERS

Hyaline Membrane Disease

Twins are at increased risk of developing hyaline membrane disease due to the increase in preterm delivery (52). Both twins are usually affected by hyaline membrane disease. However, if only one twin is affected, it is usually twin B, who had a lower Apgar score at 1 minute and a higher birth weight than twin A (110). The greater risk to twin B probably is related to birth asphyxia (110). Monozygotic twins more often are born prematurely and at an earlier gestational age than dizygotic twins, and they are more prone to develop hyaline membrane disease.

Necrotizing Enterocolitis

Unique risk factors for the development of necrotizing enterocolitis have not been identified for twins or higher multiple gestations, but, as a group, they are at an increased risk due to the greater likelihood of prematurity and LBW. Comparisons of twins showed that the most significant factor in predicting the occurrence of necrotizing enterocolitis and the need for surgical intervention was a lower 1-minute Apgar score for the affected twins, predominantly twin B, compared with unaffected co-twins (111). Samm et al. (112) found that, in all their case pairs, it was twin A who had developed necrotizing enterocolitis; in no case did only twin B have necrotizing enterocolitis. In that study, the first-born infants were more stable, were fed sooner, and had feedings advanced more rapidly than the second-born twins, implicating feeding practices in the higher incidence of necrotizing enterocolitis for twin A.

Infection

One early study reported an increased rate of early-onset group B streptococcal disease in LBW twins compared to LBW singletons (113). Subsequent large population-based studies failed to show an increased risk of early-onset group B streptococcal disease in multiple gestations independent of prematurity (114,115). If just one of a pair of twins is infected or colonized with group B streptococcus *in utero*, it is most likely the twin positioned adjacent to the cervix, with the exposure due to ascending spread of group B streptococcus through the membranes. Spread of infection through the vascular connections between monochorionic twins has not been documented, although it is theoretically possible. However, spread of group B streptococcus from the amniotic fluid of an exposed twin to a co-twin may occur through intact dividing membranes (116).

The risk of neonatal listeriosis infection is increased with multiple gestations, to 2.8 and 21 times the risk for twin and triplet pregnancies, respectively, compared to singleton births (117). The risk is especially increased when maternal age is greater than 35 years. It is possible that the increased production of hormones or other inhibitors due to larger placental mass with multiple gestations versus singletons decreases immunity to listeria. Discordance of infection is 66%, with twin A at greater risk.

One study showed that multiple-birth preterm infants with bronchopulmonary dysplasia are at an increased risk of developing respiratory syncytial virus illness and pneumonia than are singletons matched for gestational age, and that if one member of a multiple gestation developed respiratory syncytial virus disease, usually the other member(s) did also. Other risk factors that contributed to this were the higher density of adults and children in the households of multiple gestations (118).

Sudden Infant Death Syndrome

Monozygotic and dizygotic twins are at some increased risk of sudden infant death syndrome (SIDS) compared with singletons, and this being especially true for LBW pairs (119). If the birth weights of the twins differs significantly, it is usually the smaller twin who dies of SIDS (119). For twins discordant for size, the risk of SIDS for the smaller of twins is greater than for LBW and premature singletons or other groups of infants at high risk for SIDS (119). It is unusual for the surviving co-twin also to die of SIDS.

POSTNEONATAL CARE AND FOLLOW-UP

In addition to the long-term impact of some of the perinatal conditions previously mentioned, twins and higher multiples continue to be at risk for medical, developmental, and social problems beyond those experienced by singletons born at similar gestational ages. A brief list of factors that should be considered in following these patients is included to assist the clinician in anticipating the problems, many of which can be lessened by preventive measures, such as the following:

- Parental stress of child-rearing (120,121),
- Child abuse and neglect (121,122),
- Intratwin favoritism (123),
- Developmental delay (e.g., performance below chronologic age, especially in language and speech) (124),
- Mental retardation (125,126),
- Cerebral palsy (125,127), and
- Growth delay (128,129).

REFERENCES

1. Guyer B, Martin JA, MacDorman MF, et al. Annual summary of vital statistics–1996. *Pediatrics* 1997;100:905.
2. Landy HJ, Weiner S, Corson SL, Batzer FR, Bolognese RJ. The "vanishing twin": ultrasonographic assessment of fetal disappearance in the first trimester. *Am J Obstet Gynecol* 1986;155:14.
3. Nylander PPS. Biosocial aspects of multiple births. *J Biosoc Sci Suppl* 1971;3:29.
4. Bulmver MG. The effect of parental age, parity and duration of marriage on the twinning rate. *Ann Hum Genet* 1959;23:454.
5. James WH. Dizygotic twinning, marital stage and status, and coital rates. *Ann Hum Biol* 1981;8:371.
6. Picard R, Fraser D, Hagay ZJ, Leiberman JR. Twinning in southern Israel. Seasonal variation and effects of ethnicity, maternal age and parity. *J Reprod Med* 1990;35:163.
7. Schenker JG, Yarkoni S, Granat M. Multiple pregnancies following induction of ovulation. *Fertil Steril* 1981;35:105.
8. Nylander PPS. Serum levels of gonadotrophins in relation to multiple pregnancy in Nigeria. *J Obstet Gynaecol Br Commonw* 1973;80:651.
9. Martin NG, Olsen ME, Theile H, et al. Pituitary-ovarian function in mothers who have had two sets of dizygotic twins. *Fertil Steril* 1984; 41:878.
10. Bracken MB. Oral contraception and twinning: an epidemiologic study. *Am J Obstet Gynecol* 1979;133:432.
11. Timonen S, Carpen E. Multiple pregnancies and photoperiodicity. *Ann Chir Gynaecol Fenn* 1968;57:135.
12. Elwood JM. Maternal and environmental factors affecting twin births in Canadian cities. *Br J Obstet Gynaecol* 1978;85:351.
13. Society for Assisted Reproductive Technology and The American Society for Reproductive Medicine. Assisted reproductive technology in the United States and Canada: 1994 results generated from the American Society for Reproductive Medicine/Society for Assisted Reproductive Technology Registry. *Fertil Steril* 1996;66:697.
14. Medical Research International and Society for Assisted Reproductive Technology, the American Fertility Society. In vitro fertilization-embryo transfer (IVF-ET) in the United States: 1990 results from the IVF-ET Registry. *Fertil Steril* 1992;57:15.
15. Wenstrom KD, Syrop CH, Hammitt DG, VanVoorhis BJ. Increased risk of monochorionic twinning associated with assisted reproduction. *Fertil Steril* 1993;60:510.
16. Corner GW. The observed embryology of human single ovum twins and other multiple births. *Am J Obstet Gynecol* 1955;70:933.
17. Robertson JG. Blood grouping in twin pregnancy. *J Obstet Gynaecol* 1969;76:154.
18. McCracken AA, Daly PA, Zolnick MR, Clark AM. Twins and Q-banded chromosome polymorphisms. *Hum Genet* 1978;45:253.
19. Hill AV, Jefreys AJ. Use of minisatellite DNA probes for determination of twin zygosity at birth. *Lancet* 1985;2:1394.
20. Benirschke K. Multiple pregnancy. In: Fox W, Polin R, eds. *Fetal and neonatal physiology.* Philadelphia: WB Saunders, 1991:97.
21. Barss VA, Benacerraf BR, Frigoletto FD. Ultrasonographic determination of chorion type in twin gestation. *Obstet Gynecol* 1985;66:779.
22. Winn HN, Gabrielli S, Reece EA, et al. Ultrasonographic criteria for the prenatal diagnosis of placental chorionicity in twin gestations. *Am J Obstet Gynecol* 1989;161:1540.
23. Timmons JD, De Alvarez RR. Monoamniotic twin pregnancy. *Am J Obstet Gynecol* 1963;86:875.
24. Newton ER. Antepartum care in multiple gestation. *Semin Perinatol* 1986;10:19.
25. Polin JI, Frangipane WL. Current concepts in management of obstetrics problems for pediatricians: II. Modern concepts in the management of multiple gestation. *Pediatr Clin North Am* 1986;33:649.
26. Hashimoto B, Callen PW, Filly RA, Laros RK. Ultrasound evaluation of polyhydramnios and twin pregnancy. *Am J Obstet Gynecol* 1986;154:1069.
27. Gilstrap LC, Hauth JC, Hankins GDV, Beck A. Twins prophylactic hospitalization and ward rest at an early gestational age. *Obstet Gynecol* 1987;69:578.
28. Loucopoulos A, Jewelewicz R. Management of multifetal pregnancies: sixteen years' experience at the Sloane Hospital for Women. *Am J Obstet Gynecol* 1982;143:902.
29. Collaborative Group on Antenatal Steroid Therapy. Effect of antenatal dexamethasone administration on the prevention of respiratory distress syndrome. *Am J Obstet Gynecol* 1981;141:276.
30. Effect of corticosteroids for fetal maturation on perinatal outcomes. *NIH Consensus Statement* 1994;12:1.
31. Roest JR, Mous HVH, van Heudsen AM, et al. A triplet pregnancy

after in vitro fertilization is a procedure-related complication that should be prevented by replacement of two embryos only. *Fertil Steril* 1997;67:290.

32. Njis M, Segal-Bertin G, Geerts L, et al. Prevention of multiple pregnancies in an in vitro fertilization program. *Fertil Steril* 1993;59:1245.

33. Evans MI, Littmann L, King M, Fletcher JC. Multiple gestation: the role of multifetal pregnancy reduction and selective termination. *Clin Perinatol* 1992;19:345.

34. Melgar CA, Rosenfeld DL, Rawlinson K, Greenberg M. Perinatal outcome after multifetal reduction to twins compared with nonreduced multiple gestations. *Obstet Gynecol* 1991;78:763.

35. Smith-Levitin M, Kowalik A, Birnholz J, et al. Selective reduction of multifetal pregnancies to twins improves outcome over nonreduced twin gestations. *Am J Obstet Gynecol* 1996;175:878.

36. Alexander JM, Hammond KR, Steinkampf MP. Multifetal reduction of high-order multiple pregnancy: comparison of obstetrical outcome with nonreduced twin gestations. *Fertil Steril* 1995;64:1201.

37. Depp T, Macones GA, Rosenn MF, et al. Multifetal pregnancy reduction: evaluation of fetal growth in the remaining twins. *Am J Obstet Gynecol* 1996;174:1233.

38. Redwine FO, Hays PM. Selective birth. *Semin Perinatol* 1986;10:73.

39. Friedman EA, Sachtelben MR. The effect of uterine overdistention on labor I. Multiple pregnancy. *Obstet Gynecol* 1964;23:164.

40. Cohen M, Kome SG, Rosenthal AH. Fetal interlocking complicating twin gestation. *Am J Obstet Gynecol* 1965;91:407.

41. McCarthy BJ, Sachs BP, Layde PM, et al. The epidemiology of neonatal death in twins. *Am J Obstet Gynecol* 1981;141:252.

42. Adam C, Allen AC, Baskett TF. Twin delivery: influence of presentation and method of delivery on the second twin. *Am J Obstet Gynecol* 1991;165:23.

43. Chervenak FA. The controversy of mode of delivery in twins: the intrapartum management of twin gestation (part II). *Semin Perinatol* 1986;10:44.

44. Cetrulo CL. The controversy of mode of delivery in twins: the intrapartum management of twin gestation (part I). *Semin Perinatol* 1986; 10:39.

45. Morales WJ, O'Brien WF, Knuppel RA, et al. The effect of mode of delivery on the risk of intraventricular hemorrhage in nondiscordant twin gestations under 1500 g. *Obstet Gynecol* 1989;73:107.

46. Pearlman SA, Batton DG. Effect of birth order on intraventricular hemorrhage in very low birth weight twins. *Obstet Gynecol* 1988;71: 358.

47. Zhang J, Bowes WA, Grey TW, McMahon MJ. Twin delivery and neonatal and infant mortality: a population-based study. *Obstet Gynecol* 1996;88:593.

48. Lavery JP, Austin RJ, Schaefer DS, Aladjem S. Asyncronous multiple birth: a report of five cases. *J Reprod Med* 1994;39;55.

49. Arias F. Delayed delivery of multifetal pregnancies with premature rupture of membranes in the second trimester. *Am J Obstet Gynecol* 1994;170:1233.

50. Ziegler WF, Welgoss J. Delayed delivery of a triplet pregnancy without surgical intervention: a case report. *Am J Perinat* 1966;13:191.

51. Manlan G, Scott KE. Contribution of twin pregnancy to perinatal mortality and fetal growth retardation: reversal growth retardation after birth. *Can Med Assoc J* 1978;118:365.

52. Ho SK, Wu PYK. Perinatal factors and neonatal morbidity in twin pregnancy. *Am J Obstet Gynecol* 1975;122:979.

53. Naeye RL, Tafari N, Judge D, Marboe CC. Twins: causes of perinatal death in 12 United States cities and one African city. *Am J Obstet Gynecol* 1978;131:267.

54. Benirschke K. Twin placenta in perinatal mortality. *N Y State J Med* 1961;61:1499.

55. Litschgi M, Stucki D. Course of twin pregnancies after fetal death in utero. *Geburtschilfe Perinatol* 1980;184:227.

56. D'Alton ME, Newton ER, Cetrulo CI. Intrauterine fetal demise in multiple gestation. *Acta Genet Med Gemellol* 1984;34:43.

57. Benirschke K. Multiple gestation: incidence, etiology and inheritance. In: Creasy RK, Resnik R, eds. *Maternal-fetal medicine.* Philadelphia: WB Saunders, 1984:511.

58. Leppert PC, Wartel L, Lowman R. Fetus papyraceus causing dystocia: inability to detect blighted twin antenatally. *Obstet Gynecol* 1979;54: 381.

59. Johnson SF, Driscoll SG. Twin placentation and its complications. *Semin Perinatol* 1986;10:9.

60. Naeye R. Human intrauterine parabiotic syndrome and its complications. *N Engl J Med* 1963;268:804.

61. McKeown T, Record RG. Observations on fetal growth in multiple pregnancy. Observations on fetal growth in multiple pregnancy in man. *J Endocrinol* 1952;8:386.

62. Egwuata VE. Triplet pregnancy: a review of 27 cases. *Int J Gynaecol Obstet* 1980;18:460.

63. Newton ER. Antepartum care in multiple gestation. *Semin Perinatol* 1986;10:19.

64. Robertson EG, Neer KJ. Placental injection studies in twin gestation. *Am J Obstet Gynecol* 1983;147:170.

65. Tan KL, Tan R, Tan SH, Tan AM. The twin transfusion syndrome. *Clin Pediatr* 1979;18:111.

66. Bajoria R, Wiglesworth J, Fisk NM. Angioarchitecture of monochorionic placentas in relation to the twin-twin transfusion syndrome. *Am J Obstet Gynecol* 1995;172:856.

67. Klebe JG, Ingomar CJ. The fetoplacental circulation during parturition illustrated by the interfetal transfusion syndrome. *Pediatrics* 1972;39:453.

68. Dudley DKL, D'Alton ME. Single fetal death in twin gestation. *Semin Perinatol* 1986;10:65.

69. Benirschke K, Driscoll SG. *The pathology of the human placenta.* New York: Springer-Verlag, 1967:87.

70. Fox H. *Pathology of the placenta.* Philadelphia: WB Saunders, 1978: 81.

71. Brennan JN, Diwan RV, Mortimer GR, Bellon EM. Fetofetal transfusion syndrome: prenatal ultrasonographic diagnosis. *Radiology* 1982; 43:535.

72. Galea P, Scott JM, Goel KM. Feto-fetal transfusion syndrome. *Arch Dis Child* 1982;57:781.

73. Hoyme HE, Higginbottom MC, Jones KL. Vascular etiology of disruptive structural defects in monozygotic twins. *Pediatrics* 1981;67:288.

74. Mannino FL, Jones KL, Benirschke D. Congenital skin defects and fetus papyraceus. *J Pediatr* 1977;91:559.

75. Schinzel AAGL, Smith DW, Miller JR. Monozygotic twinning and structural defects. *J Pediatr* 1979;95:921.

76. Danskin FH, Neilson JP. Twin-to-twin transfusion syndrome: what are appropriate diagnostic criteria? *Am J Obstet Gynecol* 1989;161:365.

77. Fisk NM, Borrell A, Hubinont C, Tannirandorn Y, Nicolini U, Rodeck CH. Fetofetal transfusion syndrome: do the neonatal criteria apply *in utero*? *Arch Dis Child* 1990;65[Suppl 7]:657.

78. Ohno Y, Ando H, Tanamura A, et al. The value of Doppler ultrasound in the diagnosis and management of twin-to-twin transfusion syndrome. *Arch Gynecol Obstet* 1994;255:37.

79. Napolitani FE, Schreiber I. The acardiac monster. A review of the world literature and presentation of 2 cases. *Am J Obstet Gynecol* 1960;80:582.

80. Van Allen MI, Smith DW, Shepard TH. Twin reversed arterial perfusion (TRAP) sequence: a study of 14 twin pregnancies with acardius. *Semin Perinatol* 1983;7:285.

81. Billah KL, Shah D, Odwin C. Ultrasonic diagnosis and management of acardius acephalus twin pregnancy. *Med Ultrasound* 1984;8:108.

82. Stiller RJ, Romero R, Pace S, Hobbins JC. Prenatal identification of twin reversed arterial perfusion syndrome in the first trimester. *Am J Obstet Gynecol* 1989;160:1194.

83. Moore TR, Gale S, Benirschke K. Perinatal outcome of forty-nine pregnancies complicated by acardiac twinning. *Am J Obstet Gynecol* 1990;163:907.

84. Radestad A, Thomasses PA. Acute polyhydramnios in twin pregnancy: a retrospective study with special reference to therapeutic amniocentesis. *Acta Obstet Gynecol Scand* 1990;69:297.

85. De Lia JE, Emery MG, Sheafor SA, Hennison TA. Twin transfusion syndrome: successful *in utero* treatment with digoxin. *Int J Gynaecol Obstet* 1985;23:197.

86. Ville Y, Hyett J, Helcher K, Nicolaides K. Preliminary experience with endoscopic laser surgery for severe twin-twin transfusion syndrome. *N Engl J Med* 1995;332:224.

87. Wittman BK, Farquaharson DG, Thomas WD, et al. The role of feticide in the management of severe twin transfusion syndrome. *Am J Obstet Gynecol* 1986;155:1023.

88. Urig MA, Clewell WH, Elliott JP. Twin-twin transfusion syndrome. *Am J Obstet Gynecol* 1990;163:1522.

89. Chescheir NC, Seeds JW. Polyhydramnios and oligohydramnios in twin gestations. *Obstet Gynecol* 1988;71:882.

90. Pretorius DH, Mahony BS. Twin gestations. In: Nyberg DA, Mahony BS, Pretorius DH, eds. *Diagnostic ultrasound of fetal anomalies.* Chicago: Year Book, 1990:592.

91. Mahony BS, Petty CN, Nyberg DA, et al. The "stuck twin" phenomenon: ultrasonographic findings, pregnancy outcome, and management with serial amniocenteses. *Am J Obstet Gynecol* 1990;163:1513.

92. Young BK, Suidan J, Antoine C, et al. Differences in twins: the importance of birth order. *Am J Obstet Gynecol* 1985;151:915.

93. Deale CJC, Cronje HS. A review of 367 triplet pregnancies. *S Afr Med J* 1984;66:92.

94. Creinin M, MacGregor S, Socol M, et al. The Northwestern University triplet study. IV. Biochemical parameters. *Am J Obstet Gynecol* 1988;159:1140.

95. Iffy L, Lavenhar MA, Jakobovits A, Kaminetzky HA. The rate of early intrauterine growth in twin gestation. *Am J Obstet Gynecol* 1983;146:970.

96. Hendricks CH. Twinning in relation to birth weight, mortality, and congenital anomalies. *Obstet Gynecol* 1966;27:47.

97. Naeye RL, Benirschke K, Hagstrom JWC, Marcus CC. Intrauterine growth of twins as estimated from live born birth-weight data. *Pediatrics* 1966;37:409.

98. Wilson RS. Twins: measures of birth size at different gestational ages. *Ann Hum Biol* 1974;1:57.

99. Arbuckle TE, Sherman GJ. An analysis of birth weight by gestational age in Canada. *Can Med Assoc J* 1989;140:157.

100. Jones JS, Newman RB, Miller MC. Cross-sectional analysis of triplet birth weight. *Am J Obstet Gynecol* 1991;164:135.

101. Dubois S, Dougherty C, Duquette MP, Hanley JA, Moutquin JM. Twin pregnancy: the impact of the Higgins Nutrition Intervention Program on maternal and neonatal outcomes. *Am J Clin Nutr* 1991;53:1397.

102. Powers WF. Twin pregnancy. Complications and treatment. *Obstet Gynecol* 1973;42:795.

103. Reisner SH, Forbes AE, Cornblath M. The smaller of twins and hypoglycemia. *Lancet* 1965;1:524.

104. Babson SG, Phillips DS. Growth and development of twins dissimilar in size at birth. *N Engl J Med* 1973;289:937.

105. Benirschke K, Temple WW, Bloor C. Conjoined twins: nosology and congenital malformations. *Birth Defects* 1978;16:179.

106. Rudolph AJ, Michaels JP, Nichols BL. Obstetric management of conjoined twins. *Birth Defects* 1967;3:28.

107. Schmidt W, Heberling D, Kubli F. Antepartum ultrasonographic diagnosis of conjoined twins in early pregnancy. *Am J Obstet Gynecol* 1981;139:961.

108. Edmonds LD, Layde PM. Conjoined twins in the United States, 1970–1977. *Teratology* 1985;25:301.

109. Filler RM. Conjoined twins and their separation. *Semin Perinatol* 1986;10:32.

110. De La Torre Verduzco R, Rosario R, Rigatto H. Hyaline membrane disease in twins. *Am J Obstet Gynecol* 1976;125:668.

111. Powell RW, Dyess DL, Luterman A, et al. Necrotizing enterocolitis in multiple-birth infants. *J Pediatr Surg* 1990;25:319.

112. Samm M, Curtis-Cohen M, Keller M, Harbhajan C. Necrotizing enterocolitis in infants of multiple gestation. *Am J Dis Child* 1986;140:937.

113. Pass MA, Khare S, Dillon HC. Twin pregnancies: incidence of group B streptococcal colonization and disease. *J Pediatr* 1980;97:635.

114. Schuchat A, Oxtoby M, Cochi S, et al. Population-based risk factors for neonatal group B streptococcal disease: results of a cohort study in metropolitan Atlanta. *J Infect* Dis 1990;162:672.

115. Schuchat A, Deaver-Robinson K, Plikaytis BD, et al. Multistate case-control study of maternal risk factors for neonatal Group B streptococcal disease. *Pediatr Infect Dis J* 1994;13:623.

116. Benirschke K. Routes and types of infection in the fetus and the newborn. *Am J Dis Child* 1960;99:714.

117. Mascola L, Ewert DP, Eller A. Listeriosis: a previously unreported medical complication in women with multiple gestations. *Am J Obstet Gynecol* 1994;170:1328.

118. Simones EAF, King SJ, Lehr MV, Groothuis JR. Preterm twins and triplets: a high-risk group for severe respiratory syncytial virus infection. *Am J Dis Child* 1993;147:303.

119. Beal S. Sudden infant death syndrome in twins. *Pediatrics* 1989;84:1038.

120. Goshen-Gottstein ER. The mothering of twins, triplets and quadruplets. *Psychiatry* 1980;43:189.

121. Tanimura M, Matsui I, Kobayashi N. Child abuse of one of a pair of twins in Japan. *Lancet* 1990;336:1298.

122. Grouthuis JR, Altemeier WA, Rubarge JP, et al. Increased child abuse in families with twins. *Pediatrics* 1982;70:769.

123. Minde K, Corter C, Goldberg S, Jeffers D. Maternal preference between premature twins up to age four. *J Am Acad Child Adolesc Psychiatry* 1990;29:367.

124. Record RG, McKeown T, Edwards JH. An investigation of the differences in measured intelligence between twins and single births. *Ann Hum Genet* 1970;34:11.

125. Durkin MV, Kaveggia EG, Pendelton E, et al. Analysis of etiologic factors in cerebral palsy with severe mental retardation. *Eur J Pediatr* 1976;123:67.

126. Kragt H, Huisjes HJ, Touwen BCL. Neurobiological morbidity in newborn twins. *Eur J Obstet Gynecol Reprod Biol* 1985;19:75.

127. Petterson B, Stanley F, Henderson D. Cerebral palsy in multiple births in Western Australia: genetic aspects. *Am J Med Genet* 1990;37:346.

128. Silva PA. The growth and development of twins compared to singletons at ages 9 and 11. *Aust Paediatr J* 1985;21:265.

129. Morley R, Cole, TJ, Powell R, Lucas A. Growth and development in premature twins. *Arch Dis Child* 1989;64:1042.

130. Newton W, Keith L, Keith D. The Northwestern University multihospital twin study: IV. Duration of gestation according to fetal sex. *Am J Obstet Gynecol* 1984;149:655.

131. Sassoon DA, Castro LC, Davis JL, Hobel CJ. Perinatal outcome in triplet versus twin gestations. *Obstet Gynecol* 1990;75:817.

132. Collins SM, Bleyl BA. Seventy-one quadruplet pregnancies: management and outcome. *Am J Obstet Gynecol* 1990;162:1384.

PART FIVE

The Newborn Infant

CHAPTER 28

Acute Respiratory Disorders

Jeffrey A. Whitsett, Gloria S. Pryhuber, Ward R. Rice, Barbara B. Warner, and Susan E. Wert

Successful adaptation to air breathing at the time of birth is the culmination of an orderly process of growth and differentiation of pulmonary cells, leading to alveolar and capillary surfaces capable of providing oxygen and eliminating carbon dioxide. Failure to achieve adequate gas exchange at birth represents a major cause of perinatal morbidity and mortality. This chapter reviews the common disorders of neonatal respiratory adaptation, including respiratory distress syndrome (RDS), pulmonary meconium aspiration syndrome (MAS), pulmonary hypertension, pneumonia, air leak, pulmonary hemorrhage, and other causes of acute respiratory dysfunction in the perinatal period. The clinical manifestations and therapy of these disorders are discussed in the context of the morphologic, biochemical, and physiologic factors critical to normal pulmonary growth, maturation, and function in the newborn.

HUMAN LUNG DEVELOPMENT

Human lung development can be divided into five distinct stages of organogenesis (1,2). The first is an early embryonic period (3 to 7 weeks of gestation) during which lung development is initiated and the major conducting airways are formed. The second is a pseudoglandular period (5 to 17 weeks of gestation) during which the bronchial tree and acinar tubules develop. The third is a canalicular period (16 to 26 weeks of gestation) during which vascularization of the surrounding mesenchyme with formation of the air–blood barrier occurs, and cytodifferentiation of bronchiolar and alveolar epithelial cells is initiated. The fourth is a saccular period (24 to 38 weeks of gestation) during which enlargement of the

peripheral air spaces occurs, resulting in the formation of primitive sac-like alveoli and thick interalveolar septa. The fifth is an alveolar period (36 weeks of gestation to 3 years of age) during which formation of thin secondary alveolar septa and remodeling of the capillary bed are initiated, giving rise to the mature alveolar organization of the adult lung (Fig. 28–1).

The human lung is a derivative of the primitive foregut and appears by 3 weeks (i.e., 22 days) of gestation as an enlargement of the caudal end of the laryngotracheal sulcus located in the median pharyngeal groove, which is an outgrowth of the ventral wall of the primitive esophagus. During the fourth week (26 to 28 days) of gestation, the respiratory primordium enlarges and subdivides into the left and right mainstem bronchi (see Fig. 28–1A,B). As the primitive lung continues to grow caudally, it expands into the mesenchyme surrounding the primitive foregut and becomes separated from the esophagus by a band of mesenchymal tissue called the tracheoesophageal septum. Between 4 and 5 weeks of gestation, the left and right primary bronchi subdivide to produce secondary, or lobar, bronchi (see Fig. 28–1C,D). Further subdivision of lobar bronchi into tertiary or segmental bronchi occurs during the sixth week of gestation, with the lung taking on a lobulated appearance as the segmental buds are formed (see Fig. 28–1E,F). The developing respiratory tract is lined by endodermally derived epithelium that forms the conducting airways and alveoli. Surrounding mesoderm is composed of mesenchymal cells that differentiate into connective tissue components such as blood vessels, fibroblasts, smooth muscle cells, and cartilage.

Preacinar blood vessels first appear at the end of week 4. Pulmonary arteries arise from the sixth pair of aortic arches and grow into the mesenchyme, where they accompany the developing airways, segmenting with each bronchial subdivision. Pulmonary veins develop as outgrowths of the atrial portion of the heart and are enveloped by mesenchyme. Intraacinar arteries and veins develop later, in parallel with alveolar formation.

J. A. Whitsett, W. R. Rice, B. B. Warner, and S. E. Wert: Department of Pulmonary Biology, Children's Hospital Medical Center, Cincinnati, Ohio

G. S. Pryhuber: Department of Pediatrics, University of Rochester, Rochester, New York

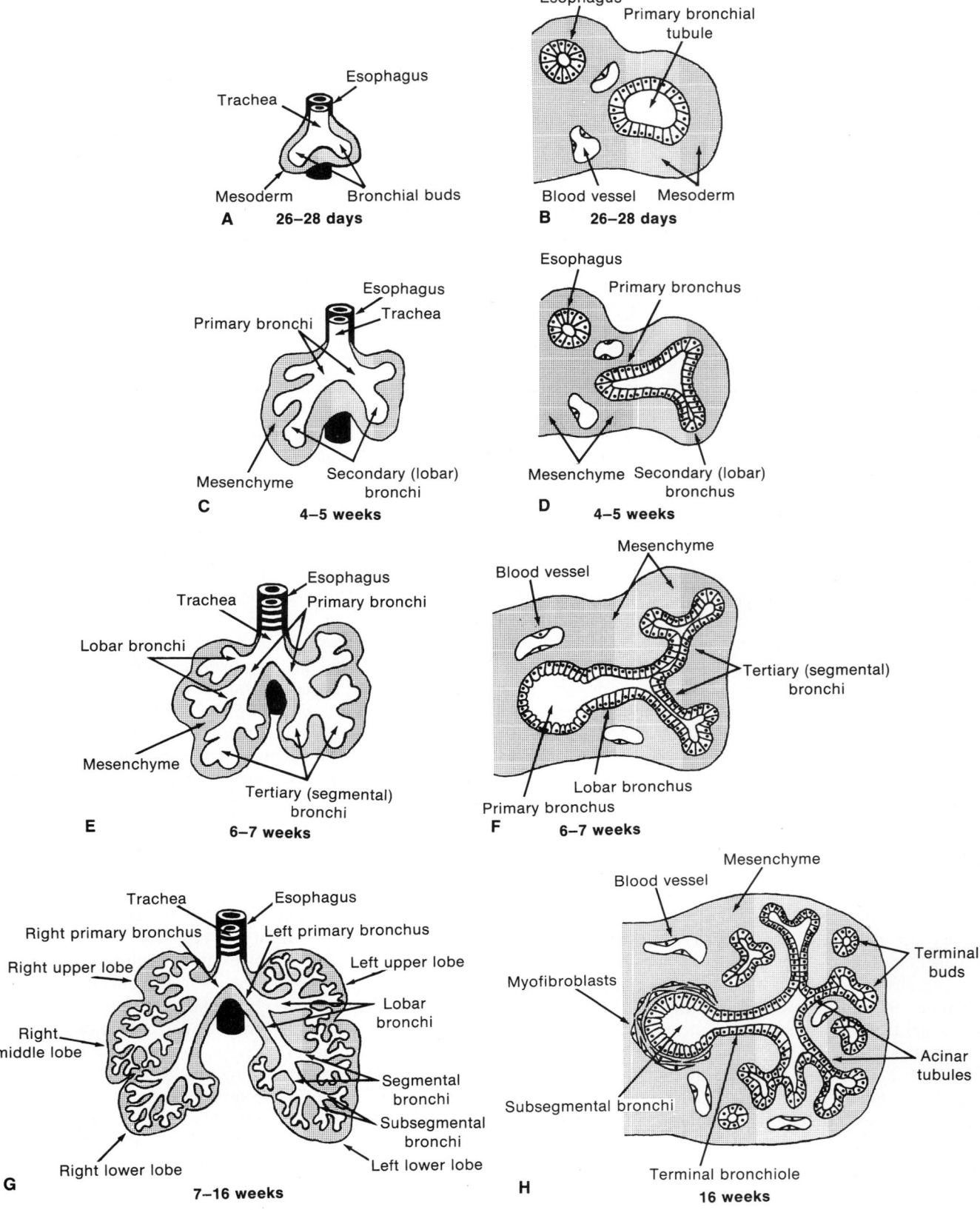

FIG. 28–1. Lung development during the embryonic **(A–F)** and pseudoglandular **(G,H)** stages of organogenesis. The overall branching pattern of the primitive lung **(left panels)** results in the development of the bronchial tree. The histologic organization of the fetal lung becomes more complex as branching morphogenesis progresses through these stages **(right panels).**

The *pseudoglandular stage* of fetal lung development extends from about 7 to 16 weeks of gestation and is marked by the formation of the bronchial portion of the lung. This occurs through a process known as branching morphogenesis, during which the segmental tubules of the developing lung undergo repetitive lateral and terminal dichotomous branching to form the primitive bronchial tree (see Fig. 28–1G,H). By week 16 of gestation, the segmental bronchi have subdivided to produce 16 to 25 generations of bronchial tubules ending in the terminal bronchioles. These bronchial tubules are lined initially by a pseudostratified columnar epithelium containing large pools of glycogen. A prominent basement membrane underlies the epithelium, and mesenchymal cells adjacent to these tubules differentiate into fibroblasts and become organized, aligning themselves in a circumferential orientation perpendicular to the long axis of the bronchial tubules. As branching progresses, pseudostratified columnar epithelium is reduced to a tall columnar epithelium, especially in distal regions of the

bronchial tree. During this period, cytodifferentiation of the airway epithelium occurs in a centrifugal direction with ciliated, nonciliated, goblet, and basal cells appearing first in the more proximal airways. Cartilage, smooth muscle cells, and mucous glands are also found in the trachea during the pseudoglandular stage of development and extend as far as the segmental bronchi.

The *canalicular stage* of lung development extends from week 16 to week 24 of gestation. By the end of week 16, the terminal bronchioles have divided into two or more respiratory bronchioles that have subdivided into small clusters of short acinar tubules and buds lined by cuboidal epithelium. These structures undergo further differentiation to become the adult respiratory unit, or pulmonary acinus, consisting of the alveolated respiratory bronchiole, alveolar ducts, and alveoli. Clusters of acinar tubules and buds continue to grow by lengthening, subdividing, and widening at the expense of the surrounding mesenchyme (Fig. 28–2A). This peripheral growth is accompanied by the formation of intraacinar

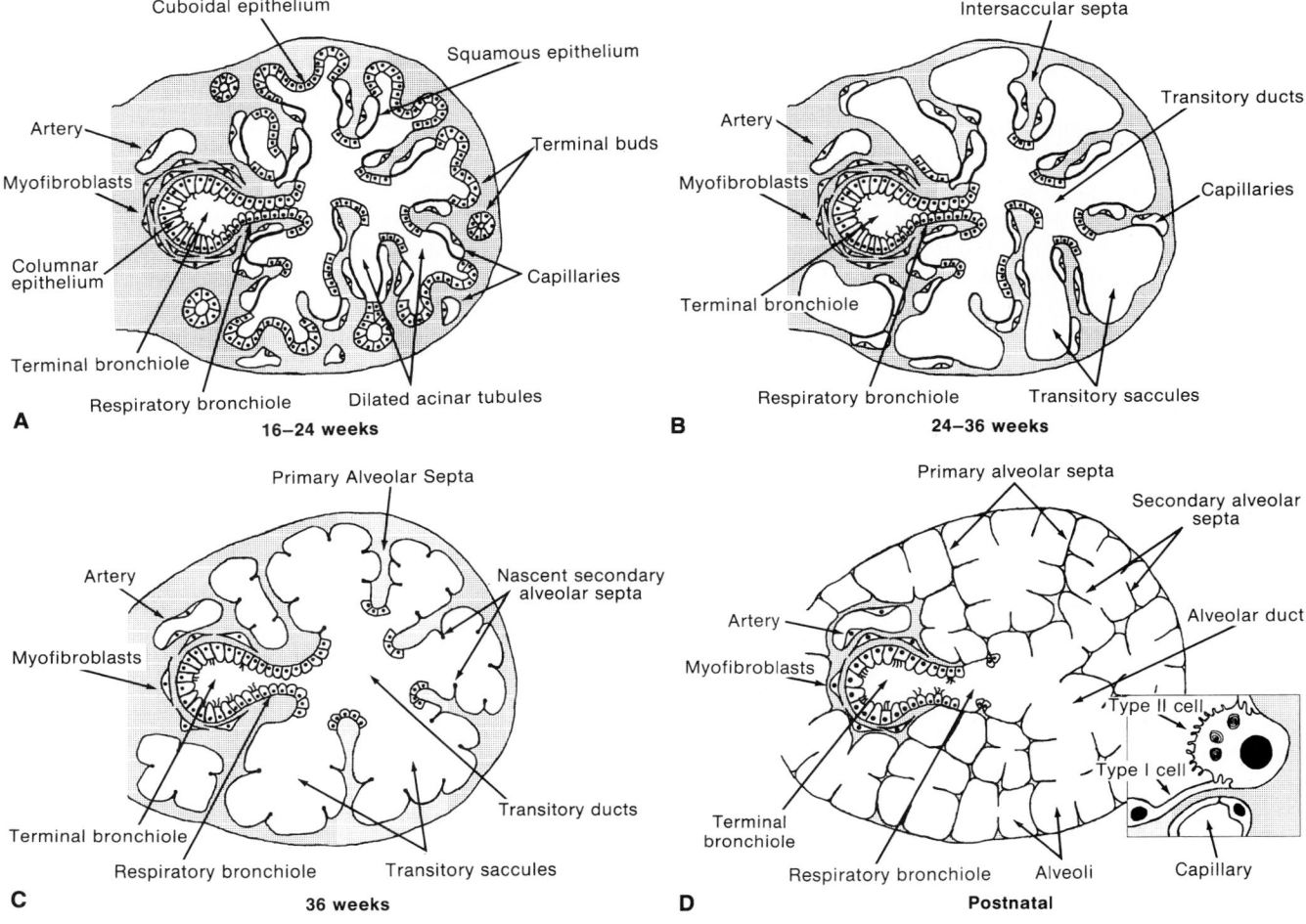

FIG. 28–2. Lung development during the canalicular **(A)**, saccular **(B)**, and alveolar stages of organogenesis **(C,D)**. Dramatic histologic changes in tissue organization occur during these periods. The adult alveolar epithelium is composed of squamous type I cells and cuboidal type II cells **(inset).**

capillaries, which align themselves around the air spaces, establishing contact with the overlying cuboidal epithelium. During this period, type II epithelial cell differentiation occurs in acinar tubules with formation of intracellular multivesicular bodies and multilamellar bodies, the storage form of pulmonary surfactant phospholipids. Type I epithelial cell differentiation occurs in conjunction with development of the air–blood barrier, wherever endothelial cells of the developing capillary system come into contact with the overlying acinar epithelial cells.

During the *saccular stage,* which extends from week 24 to week 38 of gestation, the terminal clusters of acinar tubules and buds begin to dilate and expand into thin, smooth-walled, transitory saccules and ducts that later become the true alveolar ducts and alveoli of the adult (Fig. 28–2*B*). During this period, there is a marked reduction in the amount of interstitial tissue. Intersaccular and interductal septa develop that contain a delicate network of collagen fibers and the intraacinar capillary bed. Near the end of this period, elastin is deposited in areas where future interalveolar septa will form. Increasing amounts of tubular myelin, the secretory form of pulmonary surfactant, are seen in the air spaces.

The *alveolar period,* which extends from 36 weeks of gestation to between 2 and 8 years of age, is the last stage of lung development and is marked by the formation of secondary alveolar septa partitioning the transitory ducts and saccules into true alveolar ducts and alveoli (Fig. 28–2*C,D*). This process of alveolarization greatly increases the surface area of the lung available for gas exchange. Between 20 and 70 million alveoli are formed before birth, and the postnatal formation of additional alveoli increases their number to 300 to 400 million by 2 to 8 years of age. At the beginning of this period, the secondary interalveolar septa consist of short buds or projections of connective tissue that contain a double capillary network and interstitial cells that are actively synthesizing collagen and elastic fibers. By 5 months of age, these secondary interalveolar septa have lengthened and thinned and contain only a single capillary network. This suggests that alveolar formation occurs rapidly after birth and may be complete within the first 12 to 24 months of life. Further growth of the lung occurs by expansion and further subdivision of the alveolar spaces by tertiary interalveolar septa. From birth to adulthood, the conducting airways increase in length and diameter, while airspace and capillary volume increase coordinately at the expense of interstitial volume.

DEVELOPMENTAL ANOMALIES

Each of these stages of lung development includes distinct changes in tissue organization and cellular differentiation that are important for subsequent growth and maturation of the lung. Structural and functional defects in lung development at birth can often be traced to arrested or aberrant development during one of these periods of organogenesis. Developmental anomalies of the lung occur through defective division and differentiation of the lung bud or of the left or right bronchial bud. Pulmonary agenesis, bronchial malformations, tracheoesophageal fistulas, tracheomalacia, bronchomalacia, ectopic lobes, and congenital pulmonary cysts arise during the embryonic and pseudoglandular stages of lung development. Clinical disorders related to pulmonary hypoplasia and respiratory insufficiency are associated with later periods of development. Pulmonary hypoplasia can be caused by a reduction of space within the pleural cavity, usually as a consequence of another primary developmental defect such as congenital diaphragmatic hernia, or by a reduction in the amount of amniotic fluid following premature rupture of membranes or in association with renal dysgenesis (i.e., Potter syndrome). Respiratory distress syndrome and bronchopulmonary dysplasia are associated with premature birth at a time when biochemical functions (e.g., surfactant production) and structural functions (e.g., elasticity) of the lung are still underdeveloped.

THE SURFACTANT SYSTEM

The unique physical–chemical boundary between the alveolar gases and the highly solvated molecules at the apical surface of the respiratory epithelium generates a region of high surface tension produced by the unequal distribution of molecular forces among water molecules at an air–liquid interface. Surface-active material at this interface in the alveoli provides surface-tension-lowering activity that contributes to the remarkable pressure–volume associations characteristic of the lung. This surface-active material, called surfactant, has been subject to intense study in recent decades (3–5).

Deficiency or dysfunction of pulmonary surfactant plays a critical role in the pathogenesis of respiratory diseases in the newborn period. Pulmonary surfactant exists in a variety of physical forms when isolated from the alveolar wash of the lung. These physical forms include lamellated and vesicular forms and highly organized tubular myelin. Tubular myelin is highly surface active and, although composed predominately of phospholipids, its unique structure depends on Ca^{2+} and lung surfactant proteins A (SP-A) and B (SP-B). Tubular myelin represents the major extracellular pool of surfactant from which a lipid monolayer is generated to produce an interface between the hydrated cellular surfaces and alveolar gas (Fig. 28–3). Lamellated and vesicular forms of surfactant represent nascent or catabolic forms of surfactant material; the latter is taken up by type II epithelial cells and recycled. Surfactant proteins A, B, and C (SP-C) play important roles in the organization and function of the surfactant complex regulating surfactant homeostasis. Alveolar surfactant concentrations are tightly controlled

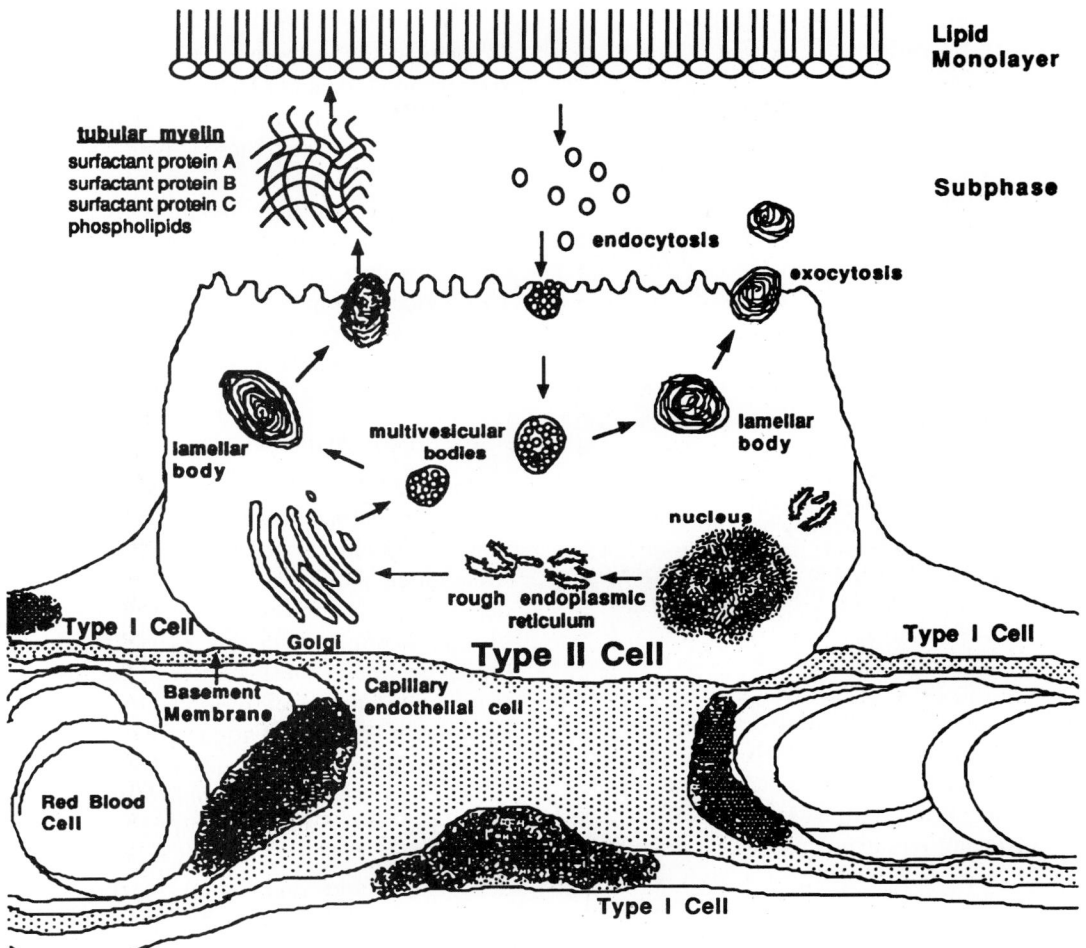

FIG. 28–3. Surfactant phospholipids are synthesized in the endoplasmic reticulum, transported through the Golgi apparatus to multivesicular bodies, and ultimately packaged in lamellar bodies before secretion. After exocytosis of the lamellar bodies, surfactant phospholipids are organized into a complex lattice called tubular myelin phospholipid that provides material for a monolayer at the air–fluid interface in the alveolus. Surfactant phospholipids and proteins are taken up by type II cells, probably transported by endosomal multivesicular bodies, and then catabolized or transported to lamellar bodies for recycling. Surfactant proteins are synthesized in polyribosomes and extensively modified in the endoplasmic reticulum, Golgi apparatus, and multivesicular bodies. Surfactant proteins are detected within lamellar bodies or in secretory vesicles closely associated with lamellar bodies before secretion into the alveolus.

by a variety of mechanisms that modulate lipid and protein synthesis, storage, secretion, and recycling.

Composition of Surfactant

Pulmonary surfactant is composed primarily of the phospholipids phosphatidylcholine and phosphatidylglycerol (Fig. 28–4). These lipid molecules are enriched in dipalmitoyl acyl groups attached to a glycerol backbone that pack tightly and generate low surface pressures (Fig. 28–5). Rapid spreading and stability of pulmonary surfactant are achieved by the interactions of surfactant proteins and phospholipids. Surfactant is synthesized and secreted by type II epithelial cells in the alveolus. Synthesis of phosphatidylcholine, surfactant proteins, and lamellar bodies, an intracellular storage form of pulmonary surfactant, increases with advancing gestation. Lamellar bodies are secreted into the lung liquid that contributes to the amniotic fluid. The measurement of amniotic fluid phosphatidylcholine, disaturated phosphatidylcholine, posphatidylglycerol, or the surfactant proteins has provided useful biochemical markers that predict lung maturation and the adequacy of lung function at birth [e.g., lecithin–sphingomyelin (L–S) ratio and phosphatidylglycerol values]. Surfactant function can be assessed by a variety of physical and physiologic tests

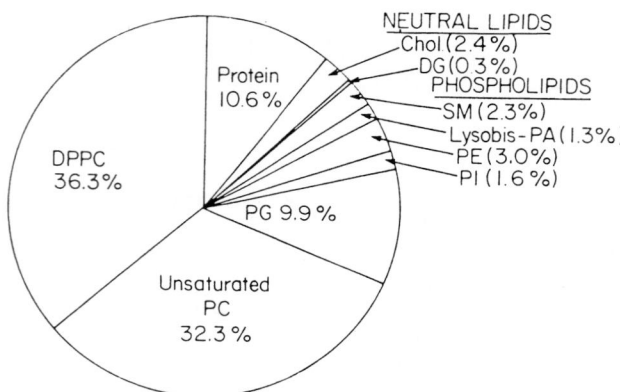

FIG. 28–4. Pulmonary surfactant components are expressed as a percentage of the total weight. Chol, cholesterol; DG, diacylglycerol; DPPC, dipalmitoylphosphatidylcholine; PA, phosphatidic acid; PC, phosphatidylcholine; PE, phosphatidylethanolamine; PG, phosphatidylglycerol; PI, phosphatidylinositol; SM, sphingomyelin. (Adapted from Possmayer F. Pulmonary surfactant. *Can J Biochem Cell Biol* 1984;62:1121.)

that measure its ability to reduce surface tension at an air–liquid interface and to spread rapidly during dynamic compression and expansion. The Wilhelmy balance, Langmuir trough, pulsating bubbleometer, and a variety of animal models have been used to assess the efficacy of surfactant and surfactant replacements.

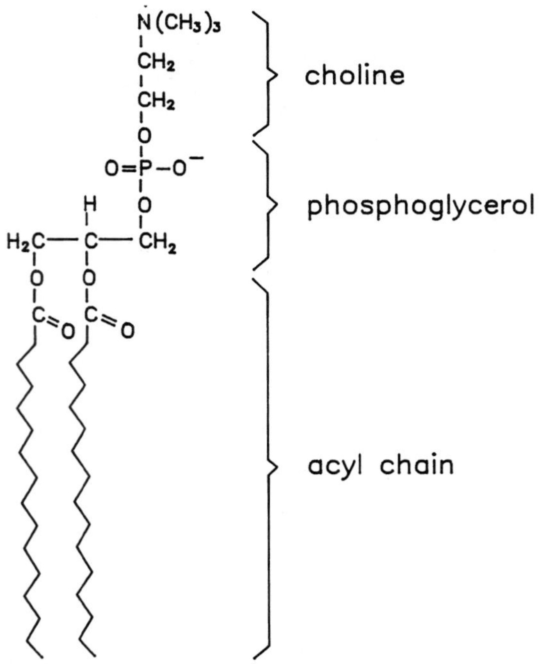

FIG. 28–5. Dipalmitoylphosphatidylcholine (DPPC) is the most abundant phospholipid in pulmonary surfactant. The acyl chains of DPPC pack tightly to form the surfactant monolayer, reducing surface tension in the alveolus.

Control of Surfactant Synthesis and Secretion

Synthesis of pulmonary surfactant is closely linked to the morphologic and biochemical differentiation of alveolar type II cells in the peripheral respiratory epithelium. Interactions between mesenchymal and epithelial cells, mediated by direct cell–cell contact or by paracrine factors, contribute to the differentiation process. Endocrine factors also modulate the differentiation of type II epithelial cells and the synthesis of surfactant components. *In vivo* and *in vitro* evidence supports the role of glucocorticoids in the modulation of morphologic differentiation and production of phospholipids and surfactant proteins by the lung.

Phospholipid Synthesis

Phosphatidylcholine is produced by type II epithelial cells using extracellular substrate and the glycogen stores that accumulate in the pre–type II cells of the fetal lung. Metabolic pathways producing phosphatidylcholine depend on the production of phosphatidic acid and a glycerophosphate backbone (see Fig. 28–5); the latter is produced as an intermediate of the glycolytic pathway (6). The synthesis of phosphatidylcholine involves the deacylation of phosphatidic acid and its reaction with cytidine diphosphocholine (CDP-choline).

Disaturated forms of phosphatidylcholine may be formed *de novo,* using disaturated acyl precursors or by remodeling (i.e., salvage pathway) of phospholipids by deacylation and reacylation reactions. Production of CDP-choline is critical to phosphatidylcholine synthesis and is achieved by phosphorylation of choline and transfer to cytidine triphosphate in a reaction dependent on choline kinase and choline phosphate cytidylyltransferase. The activities of many of the enzymes in the synthetic pathway for phosphatidylcholine increase with advancing gestation in the lung, generally increasing in the last third of gestation (6,7).

Glucocorticoid Enhancement

A variety of hormonal factors influence the rate of production of the enzymes controlling phosphatidylcholine synthesis in the developing lung (6,7). Glucocorticoids are the most clinically relevant and useful of these agents. Studies in fetal lambs and humans demonstrated that administration of glucocorticoid to the dam or mother resulted in precocious respiratory function in prematurely born offspring. The initial clinical studies of Liggins and Howie demonstrated that maternal administration of glucocorticoid decreased the incidence of respiratory distress in premature infants (8). Although the precise mechanisms by which glucocorticoids induce pulmonary maturation and lung function in premature infants have not been discerned, increased phosphatidylcholine synthesis and morphologic remodeling of the alveolar architecture, including the thinning of interstitial components of the fetal lung, are observed after glucocorticoid treatment. Glucocorticoids regulate several genes that are associated with the differentiation of the fetal lung, including the genes encoding enzymes involved in the synthesis of phosphatidylcholine and the surfactant proteins. The effects of glucocorticoid on lung cell differentiation are mediated in part by glucocorticoid receptors, which, when occupied by hormones, influence gene transcription and mRNA stability, altering the abundance of the proteins synthesized by pulmonary cells.

Other Hormonal Influences

Thyroid hormones (i.e., T_3, T_4), thyrotropin-releasing hormone (TRH), estrogens, prolactin, epidermal growth factor, β-adrenergic agents, and other agents that enhance cellular cAMP levels influence pulmonary maturation or biochemical indices of pulmonary maturation. Both T_3 and T_4 increase the synthesis of phospholipids in mammalian lung but do not readily cross the placenta.

Surfactant Secretion

Surfactant is stored within type II cells in large lipid-rich organelles called lamellar bodies. Secretion of lamellar bodies occurs by a process of exocytosis that is regulated by a number of physical and hormonal factors. Stretch, the mode of ventilation, and the labor process enhance surfactant secretion and extracellular surfactant pool sizes at birth. Catecholamines, purinoceptor agonists (e.g., adenosine triphosphate) that activate protein kinases, and Ca^{2+} ionophores enhance phospholipid secretion by type II cells in vitro (6). Surfactant protein A, hyperglycemia, and hyperinsulinemia inhibit surfactant phospholipid secretion. Newly secreted surfactant enters the extracellular space and undergoes dramatic structural reorganization to form tubular myelin, a process dependent on SP-A, Ca^{2+}, phospholipids, and SP-B. Phospholipids must move from tubular myelin to form a monolayer at the air–liquid interface.

Surfactant Recycling

The process of inflation and deflation produces spent forms of surfactant phospholipids that are taken up by type II cells and reused. Surfactant proteins A, B, and C enhance the reuptake of phospholipids in vitro. Surfactant phospholipid is reused rapidly. In the adult rabbit lung, the half-life of surfactant phospholipids is approximately 8 hours, and in newborn animals, the half-life is 3.5 days. The intracellular and extracellular pools of surfactant are generally larger in the newborn animal than in adults. A relatively small fraction of the alveolar surfactant pool is cleared by catabolism and alveolar macrophages, with most of the surfactant phospholipid recycled by type II cells. Recent studies support an important role for granulocyte/macrophage-stimulating factors and their receptors in the mediation of surfactant clearance, acting at least in part on the alveolar macrophage. Defects in GM-CSF or its receptor cause marked lipid accumulation in the postnatal lung, causing a syndrome of pulmonary alveolar proteinosis. Exogenously administered surfactant is reused efficiently by adult and newborn lungs (9). The effects of surfactant replacement therapy are therefore related to the direct surface-tension–lowering properties of surfactant introduced into the airway and to the recycling of exogenous phospholipids by type II cells.

The Role of Surfactant in Lung Disease

Quantitative and qualitative abnormalities of pulmonary surfactant contribute to the pathogenesis of lung disease in the newborn infant. In premature infants, deficiencies in surfactant production and secretion decrease intracellular and extracellular pools of surfactant, leading to alveolar surfactant insufficiency and atelectasis. Qualitative abnormalities of surfactant are also associated with many types of lung injury. Alveolar–capillary leak, hemorrhage, pulmonary edema, and alveolar cell injury fill the alveolus with proteinaceous material that inactivates surfactant. Serum and nonserum proteins, including albumin, fibrinogen, hemoglobin, and meconium, are potent inactivators of pulmonary surfactant in vivo and in vitro; SP-A, SP-B, and SP-C act synergistically to stabilize the surface properties of phospholipids in the presence of these inactivating proteins. Inhibitory factors associated with surfactant dysfunction in acute lung injury can be overcome by the administration of exogenous surfactants that contain the surfactant proteins.

Surfactant Replacement

The first successful surfactant replacement therapy in humans was reported by Fujiwara and colleagues in 1980 (10). Natural synthetic and semisynthetic surfactants have been successfully administered into the lungs of premature infants for treatment of RDS and are being tested for therapy of other lung diseases. Surfactant replacement has become standard for prevention and treatment of RDS. Animal surfactant preparations containing phospholipids, SP-B, and SP-C (e.g., Survanta, Curosurf, Infrasurf) and synthetic preparations composed primarily of phospholipids mixed with spreading agents (e.g., Exosurf) are in clinical use (4,5). The surfactant preparations containing surfactant proteins provide highly surface active material to the alveolus. Surfactant replacement also contributes to the pool size of surfactant phospholipids, providing substrate for surfactant synthesis by means of the recycling pathways.

RESPIRATORY DISTRESS SYNDROME

Respiratory distress syndrome, previously called hyaline membrane disease, is a common cause of morbidity and mortality associated with premature delivery. Respiratory distress syndrome is a developmental disorder rather than a disease process per se, and it is usually associated with premature birth. The incidence and severity of RDS generally increase with decreasing gestational age at birth and are usually worse in male infants. Infants of diabetic mothers with poor metabolic control and infants born after fetal asphyxia, maternofetal hemorrhage, or after pregnancies complicated by multiple births are at higher risk for RDS. Respiratory distress syndrome affects approximately 20,000 to 30,000 infants each year in the United States and complicates about 1% of pregnancies. Approximately 50% of the infants born between 26 and 28 weeks of gestation develop RDS, whereas fewer than 20% to 30% of premature infants at 30 to 31 weeks have the disorder.

Clinical Presentation

Infants with RDS present at birth or within several hours after birth with clinical signs of respiratory distress that include tachypnea, grunting, retractions, and cyanosis accompanied by increasing oxygen requirements. Physical findings include rales, poor air exchange, use of accessory muscles of breathing, nasal flaring, and abnormal patterns of respiration that may be complicated by apnea. Chest radiographs are characterized by atelectasis, air bronchograms, and diffuse reticular–granular infiltrates, often progressing to severe bilateral opacity characterized by the term "white-out" (Fig. 28–6). Radiographic patterns in RDS are variable and may not reflect the degree of respiratory compromise.

The infant attempts to maintain alveolar volume by prolonging and increasing expiratory pressures by breathing against a partially closed glottis, causing the grunting noise characteristic of RDS but often seen in other respiratory disorders. Increasing oxygen requirements and the need for ventilatory support often occur rapidly in the first 24 hours of life and continue for several days thereafter. The clinical course depends on the severity of RDS and the size and maturity of the infant at birth. In uncomplicated RDS, typically seen in more mature infants, recovery is rapid, and infants generally no longer require oxygen or ventilatory support after the first week of life. The most premature infants are at greatest risk for severe RDS and frequently develop complications, including central nervous system (CNS) hemorrhage, patent ductus arteriosus (PDA), air leak, and infection, which contribute to prolonged requirements for oxygen and ventilatory support.

Pathology

Pathologic findings early in the course of RDS include atelectasis, pulmonary edema, pulmonary vascular con-

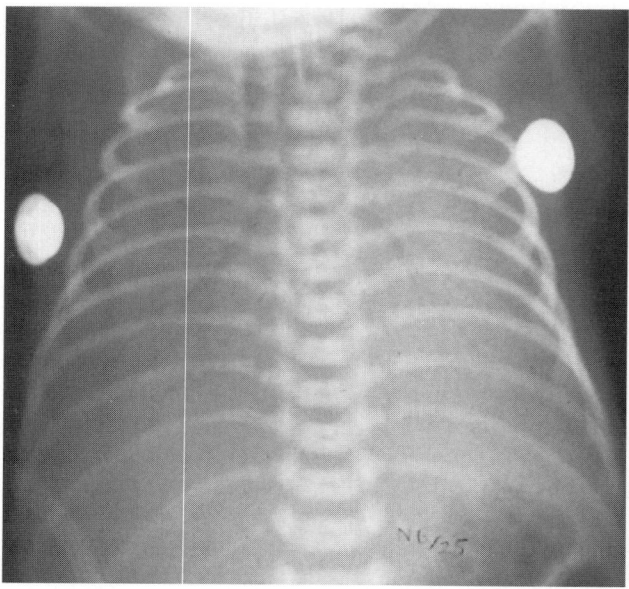

FIG. 28–6. This premature infant presented with grunting, retractions, and cyanosis after delivery. The diffuse reticular–granular opacification, air bronchograms, and decreased lung volumes in the chest x-ray film indicate respiratory distress syndrome.

gestion, pulmonary hemorrhage, and evidence of direct injury to the respiratory epithelium (Fig. 28–7). Epithelial cell injury is especially evident in the bronchiolar region of the lung. Histologic findings include the presence of hyaline membranes, the characteristic eosinophilic material derived from bronchial and bronchiolar injury to epithelial cells. Alveolar spaces are generally not inflated, and at autopsy, the lungs of infants with RDS are often airless on passive deflation. Leukocytic infiltration is not observed early in the course of RDS unless complicated by infection. Pulmonary edema, hemorrhage, and hemorrhagic edema are common pathologic features in RDS, especially if the clinical course is further complicated by PDA and congestive heart failure.

Pathophysiology

Avery and Mead first demonstrated the paucity of alveolar surfactant in the lungs of infants dying of RDS (11). Quantitative and qualitative abnormalities of the pulmonary surfactant system are critical to the pathogenesis of RDS in premature infants. Lack of pulmonary surfactant leads to progressive atelectasis, loss of functional residual capacity, alterations in ventilation–perfusion ratio, and uneven distribution of ventilation. The RDS is further complicated by the relatively weak respiratory muscles and the compliant chest wall of the premature infant, which impair alveolar ventilation. Diminished oxygenation, cyanosis, and respiratory and metabolic acidosis contribute to increased pulmonary vascular resis-

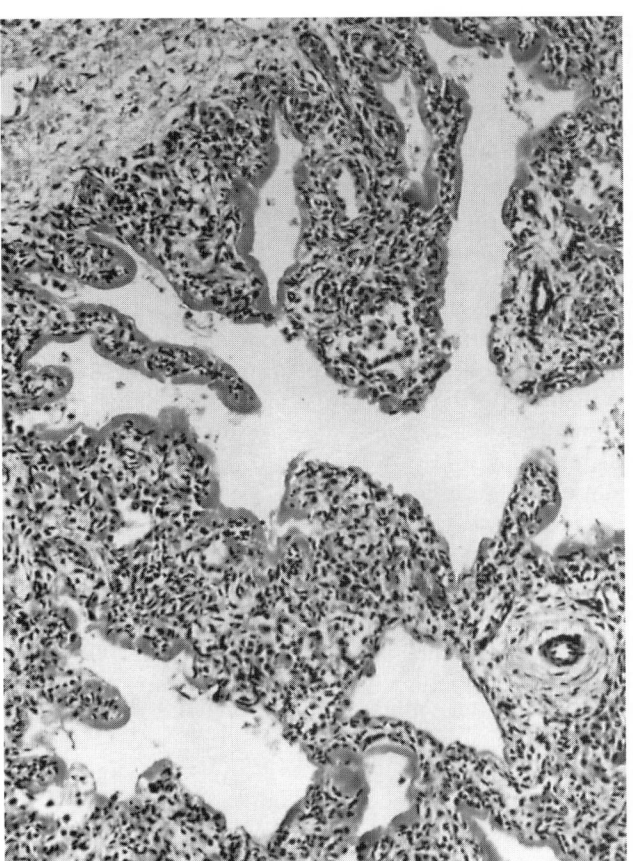

FIG. 28–7. Dilated air spaces, hyaline membranes, and extensive atelectasis are seen throughout the lung of an infant born at 28 weeks of gestation with severe respiratory distress syndrome. (Hematoxylin and eosin stain; original magnification × 250) (Courtesy of Edgar Ballard, Children's Hospital, Cincinnati, OH.)

tance (PVR). Right-to-left shunting through the ductus arteriosus, foramen ovale, and intrapulmonary ventilation–perfusion mismatch further exacerbate hypoxemia.

Prevention

Although the incidence of premature birth in the United States (approximately 7%) has not changed significantly in recent decades, the incidence of severe RDS has decreased at each gestational age as advances in maternal care and strict attention to avoidance of asphyxia and infection at birth have become standard treatment. Careful fetal monitoring, treatment of underlying maternal disorders, determination of amniotic fluid L–S or other biochemical indicators of fetal lung maturity, and administration of tocolytics and maternal glucocorticoids have decreased the incidence of RDS. Surfactant replacement further decreases its incidence and severity. Rapid restoration of blood volume after hemorrhage and correction and avoidance of anemia, acidosis, and hypothermia improve the clinical outcomes in RDS.

Positive-pressure ventilation and continuous positive airway pressure (CPAP) improve the course of severe RDS but do not prevent the disease itself.

Treatment

Postnatal therapy of RDS begins with careful assessment and resuscitation. Adequate ventilation, oxygenation, circulation, and temperature must be assured before the infant is transferred from the delivery room to the appropriate site of care. Surfactant replacement therapy may be initiated at birth in infants at risk for RDS or thereafter, as symptoms of RDS are established and the diagnosis of RDS is confirmed. Ventilatory management of neonatal respiratory disorders has been reviewed and is detailed in Chapter 30 (12).

Adequacy of ventilation and oxygenation must be established as soon as possible to avoid pulmonary vasoconstriction, further ventilation–perfusion abnormalities, and atelectasis. Positive-pressure ventilation, CPAP, and oxygen therapy may be required at any time during the course of RDS and must be readily available to the infant. Close monitoring of pH, oxygen saturation, PCO_2, and PO_2 by transcutaneous monitors and by arterial catheterization or sampling of arterialized capillary blood is critical in guiding mechanical ventilation and ambient oxygen requirements. Surfactant replacement therapy is provided through the endotracheal tube and is often used several times during the early course of RDS to maintain pulmonary function. Exogenous surfactants are given by intratracheal instillation of doses of approximately 100 mg of phospholipid per 1 kg of body weight.

Mild or moderate RDS can be managed by CPAP applied by mask, nasal cannula, nasal prongs, or endotracheal or nasopharyngeal tubes. In general, 3 to 6 cm of H_2O pressure is applied to the infant's airway. Oxygenation and effort of breathing are usually rapidly improved by CPAP. Rapid fluctuations in blood gases may occur, requiring careful monitoring of PCO_2 and PO_2. As forced inspiratory oxygen requirements decrease during recovery, airway pressure is decreased, and the infant is weaned to head hood or nasal cannula oxygen. Apnea, inadequacy of ventilation, atelectasis, mucous plugging, hyperaeration, or air leak may complicate the care of infants with RDS.

Careful attention to the mechanical details of the application of CPAP or mechanical respirators is required. Mandatory ventilation should be instituted well in advance of respiratory failure and severe respiratory acidosis to avoid severe hypoxemia and atelectasis. Ventilation is maintained through an endotracheal tube, which can be placed nasally or orally, for delivery of oxygen and positive pressure. Pressure-cycled ventilators are most frequently used in the NICU and are controlled by setting positive inspiratory pressure, rate, inspiratory–expiratory times, and positive end-expiratory pressures (PEEP).

Volume-cycled ventilators, in which fixed volumes are delivered to define the respiratory cycle, are used less frequently in the newborn. As in all respiratory therapy, critical attention to adequacy of ventilation, as assessed by PO_2, PCO_2, pH, and transcutaneous oxygen saturation, is required on an almost continual basis to adjust to the rapid changes in respiratory status occurring in these critically ill infants. Barotrauma and oxygen toxicity to the lung represent significant pulmonary complications in the therapy of RDS. Excesses in ventilation, peak or mean airway pressure, and oxygen therapy should be avoided. Because hyperoxia is associated with retrolental fibroplasia, a major cause of blindness in premature infants, arterial PO_2 must be carefully monitored, generally maintaining PO_2 between 50 to 80 mm Hg. Other forms of ventilation such as high-frequency or jet ventilators are often used in combination with exogenous surfactant for the treatment of RDS. These therapies are often considered for treatment of severely affected infants whose ventilation has not been adequately supported by conventional mandatory ventilation and surfactant therapy.

Complications

Central nervous system hemorrhage, intraventricular hemorrhage (IVH), and PDA represent significant clinical problems affecting the care of infants with RDS. Patent ductus arteriosus and subsequent congestive heart failure and pulmonary edema further compromise respiratory function, decreasing pulmonary compliance and perhaps inactivating pulmonary surfactant. Prompt diagnosis and medical or surgical treatment of PDA are indicated during the treatment of RDS. Acute CNS hemorrhage is often associated with shock, pulmonary compromise, and pulmonary hemorrhage. Fluctuations in respiratory status may contribute to IVH and can be minimized by careful attention to respiratory care and by judicious use of sedation. Intravenous fluids and administration of oral feedings must be adjusted carefully during acute and convalescent care of infants with RDS. Excessive fluid administration impairs pulmonary function and increases the risk of PDA.

MECONIUM ASPIRATION SYNDROME

Meconium-stained amniotic fluid (MSAF) occurs in approximately 12% of live births. The cause, pathophysiology, and treatment of MSAF and meconium aspiration syndrome (MAS) have been reviewed (13–15).

Meconium first appears in the fetal ileum between 10 and 16 weeks of gestation as a viscous, green liquid composed of gastrointestinal secretions, cellular debris, bile and pancreatic juice, mucus, blood, lanugo, and vernix. Meconium is approximately 72% to 80% water. The dry weight composition consists primarily of mucopolysaccharides, with less protein and lipid. Although intestinal meconium appears very early in gestation, MSAF rarely occurs before 38 weeks of gestation. Incidence of MSAF increases thereafter, and approximately 30% of newborns have MSAF after 42 weeks of gestation. The increased incidence of MSAF with advancing gestational age probably reflects the maturation of peristalsis in the fetal intestine. Motilin, an intestinal peptide that stimulates contraction of the intestinal muscle, is in lower concentrations in the intestine of premature versus postterm infants. Umbilical cord motilin concentration is higher in infants who have passed meconium than in infants with clear amniotic fluid. Intestinal parasympathetic innervation and myelination also increase throughout gestation and may play a role in the amplified passage of meconium in late gestation.

In utero passage of meconium is associated with fetal asphyxia and decreased umbilical venous blood PO_2 (Fig. 28–8). Experimentally, intestinal ischemia produces a transient period of hyperperistalsis and relaxation of anal sphincter tone, leading to the passage of meconium. Intestinal ischemia is augmented in the fetus by the diving reflex, which shunts blood preferentially to the brain and heart and away from the visceral organs during hypoxia. The gasping respiratory efforts accompanying fetal asphyxia are thought to contribute to the entry of meconium into the respiratory tract, resulting in MAS.

An association among MSAF, fetal compromise, and perinatal morbidity has been clearly demonstrated. However, most infants with MSAF do not have lower Apgar scores, more acidosis, or clinical illness than infants born with clear amniotic fluid. When normal fetal heart rate patterns are observed in cases of MSAF, the neonatal outcome is generally comparable to deliveries with clear amniotic fluid. Neonatal outcomes of deliveries complicated by MSAF associated with fetal tachycardia and decreased fetal heart rate variability are similar to those of non–meconium-stained infants with similar abnormal-

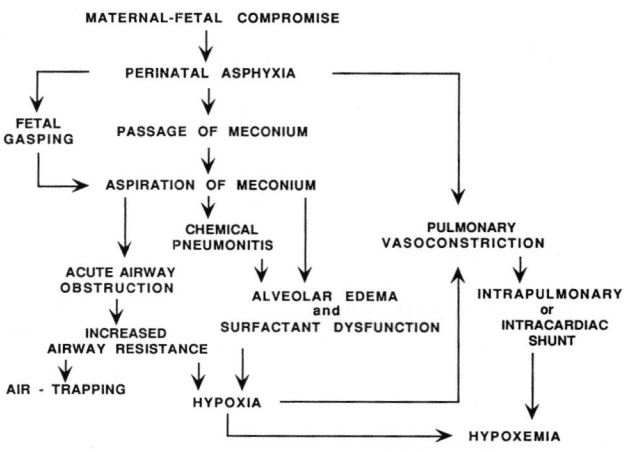

FIG. 28–8. Pathogenesis of meconium aspiration syndrome.

ities of fetal heart rate. Perinatal morbidity is increased in newborns with abnormal fetal heart rates. Meconium staining is associated with fetal compromise and demands critical evaluation of fetal well-being. However, in infants with a normal fetal heart rate pattern, MSAF generally carries a low risk for perinatal morbidity.

Clinical Presentation

Meconium found below the vocal cords defines MAS, which occurs in approximately 35% of live births with MSAF or in approximately 4% of all live births. Meconium aspiration syndrome describes a wide spectrum of respiratory disease, ranging from mild respiratory distress to severe disease and death despite mechanical ventilation. Meconium aspiration syndrome typically presents as respiratory distress, tachypnea, prolonged expiratory phase and hypoxemia soon after birth of an infant born through thick meconium or heavily stained on the nails, hair, and umbilical cord with meconium. Increased anterior–posterior dimension of the thorax or barrel chest secondary to obstructive airway disease is common in MAS. Pulmonary hypertension is also frequently observed in infants with severe MAS.

The chest radiographs of infants with MAS demonstrate coarse infiltrates, with widespread consolidation or areas of hyperaeration (Fig. 28–9). Pleural effusions are detected in approximately 30% of infants with MAS. There is an increased risk of pneumothorax or pneumo-

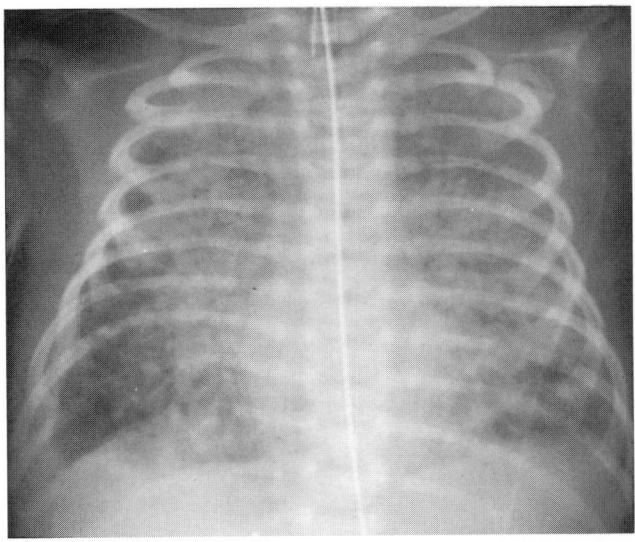

FIG. 28–9. This full-term infant was born with fetal bradycardia and thick meconium in the amniotic fluid. Cyanosis and respiratory distress were evident within minutes of delivery. The chest x-ray film demonstrates coarse, irregular infiltrates, hyperinflation (left and right diaphragms at ribs 10 to 11) and right pleural effusion indicative of meconium aspiration syndrome. Endotracheal and nasogastric tubes are in position.

mediastinum, which occur in approximately 25% of severely affected infants. Chest radiographs are abnormal in more than one-half of infants with meconium detected below the vocal cords, but fewer than 50% of the infants with abnormal radiographs have significant respiratory distress. The severity of chest radiographic abnormalities may not correlate with the severity of clinical disease.

Pathology

Postmortem examination of lungs from infants with severe MAS reveals meconium, vernix, fetal squamous cells and cellular debris in the air spaces from the airways to the alveoli. An inflammatory response with polymorphonuclear leukocytes, macrophages, and alveolar edema may be observed, but large quantities of meconium may be present without histologic signs of inflammation. Hyaline membrane formation, pulmonary hemorrhage, and necrosis of pulmonary microvasculature and parenchyma can occur. Platelet-rich microthrombi in small arterioles and increased muscularization of distal arterioles have been described in some infants dying of MAS.

Pathophysiology

The pulmonary abnormalities in MAS are related primarily to acute airway obstruction, decreased lung tissue compliance, and parenchymal lung damage (see Fig. 28–8). Instillation of meconium into adult rabbit and newborn dog tracheas causes acute mechanical obstruction of proximal and distal airways (16). A ball-valve mechanism producing partial airway obstruction contributes to air trapping, which results in increased anteroposterior chest diameter, increased expiratory lung resistance, and increased functional residual capacity. Complete obstruction of small airways may result in regional atelectasis and ventilation–perfusion inequalities. Disruption of surfactant function by serum and nonserum proteins and fatty acids contributes to atelectasis, decreased compliance, and resulting hypoxia. In more than one-half of the infants with severe MAS, pulmonary hypertension with right-to-left shunting contributes to the characteristically severe hypoxemia. Perinatal asphyxia is a critical underlying factor in the pathogenesis of MAS, increasing the risks for pulmonary hypertension and meconium aspiration.

Prevention

Before the late 1970s, it was thought that aspiration of amniotic fluid and meconium occurred during the first few breaths after delivery. Therapy was aimed at preventing MAS at the time of delivery by DeLee suctioning of the nasopharynx before delivery of the shoulders and before the first breath. The trachea was immediately intubated and suctioned to limit aspiration of meconium from the oropharynx and trachea, a procedure that remains standard in most institutions. Mortality from MAS was decreased when the trachea was suctioned immediately after birth (17). DeLee suctioning of the nasopharynx while the infant was at the perineum also decreased morbidity and mortality from MAS.

Meconium aspiration syndrome continues to occur in infants who are adequately suctioned in the delivery room. Aspiration of meconium or amniotic fluid *in utero* probably occurs in some infants with MAS, particularly in those with perinatal asphyxia. Generally, fetal lung fluid flows outward from the lungs into the amniotic sac. However, studies with radiopaque contrast and ^{51}Cr-labeled erythrocytes injected into the amniotic sac demonstrated that some amniotic fluid enters the fetal lung in the nonasphyxiated human fetus. Fetal gasping may be a critical factor in entry of meconium into the lung before birth. Gasping associated with inhalation of amniotic fluid or meconium occurs in fetal lambs, rhesus monkeys, and humans in response to fetal asphyxia induced by compression of the umbilical cord or maternal aorta. Antenatal diagnosis and treatment of fetal asphyxia is therefore critical for prevention of MAS. Clinical studies support the use of intrapartum amnioinfusion, particularly in cases of oligohydramnios, to decrease the rate of emergency cesarean section as well as to decrease morbidity related to MAS. Amnioinfusion decreases cord compression and dilutes meconium, potentially minimizing its toxicity after aspiration.

Concerns about infection risks to delivery room staff and mechanical injury to the infant related to aggressive suctioning and intubation have been raised. The use of direct tracheal suctioning for all meconium-stained infants is undergoing reevaluation (14,18). A selective approach to intubation of neonates exposed to meconium *in utero* has been proposed and is now supported by clinical studies. It is proposed that the oropharynx and nasopharynx of all meconium-exposed neonates be cleared on delivery of the head by a wall-mounted DeLee suction device. Immediate tracheal intubation and suctioning is recommended only if the infant is depressed (i.e., anticipated 1-minute Apgar score less than or equal to 7). The utilization of this type of protocol has decreased the need for emergent intubation by up to 40% without an increase in incidence or severity of meconium aspiration syndrome. Meanwhile, clearing the airway and establishing respiration and oxygenation remain basic to the resuscitation of all infants.

Treatment

Postnatal therapy for MAS begins with continuous observation and monitoring of infants at risk. Pulmonary vasoconstriction is associated with MAS, and rapid correction of hypoxemia and acidosis is critical. Chest physiotherapy and suctioning may be useful if there is airway obstruction and the infant maintains adequate oxygenation during such therapy. Studies are ongoing to determine the benefit of lung lavage with saline or with surfactant in MAS. Exogenous surfactant has been used successfully for the treatment of meconium aspiration, decreasing the need for extracorporal membrane oxygenation and air leak. Continuous monitoring of oxygenation by transcutaneous oxygen monitoring or pulse oximetry and assessment of PO_2, PCO_2, and pH by arterial catheterization should be used to guide the use of oxygen therapy and mechanical ventilation. The presence and severity of pulmonary hypertension should be evaluated. Mechanical ventilation to achieve respiratory alkalosis and infusion of sodium bicarbonate to produce a metabolic alkalosis may improve oxygenation.

Ventilatory Support

Although improvement in oxygenation was observed in patients with MAS treated with 4 to 7 cm H_2O PEEP, further studies to confirm the safety and efficacy of positive end-expiratory pressure in MAS are needed. Mechanical ventilation is required in up to 30% of infants with severe MAS and must be managed carefully. Continuous positive airway pressure or PEEP may aggravate hyperinflation associated with MAS and should be used with caution. Pneumothorax or pneumomediastinum occurs frequently during the course of MAS because of the ball-valve effect of meconium and may occur before the application of positive-pressure ventilation. Lengthening the expiratory time of the ventilatory cycle may minimize hyperinflation. Oscillation and high-frequency jet ventilation have been used in the treatment of MAS, but reports of their safety and efficacy in MAS are conflicting.

Surfactant Treatment and Other Therapeutic Considerations

Therapy of the infant with MAS includes careful observation and vigorous treatment of other sequelae of neonatal asphyxia, including temperature instability, hypoglycemia, hypocalcemia, hypotension, and decreased cardiac function. Attention needs to be given to specific therapy directed to sequelae of multiorgan hypoxemia and ischemia, including reduced renal function, reduced liver production of clotting factors, hypoalbuminemia, cerebral edema, and seizures. Recent research suggests beneficial effects of surfactant replacement therapy, inhaled nitric oxide, and high-frequency oscillatory ventilation. Meconium instilled into canine or piglet lungs or mixed with surfactant *in vitro* inactivates surfactant function, decreasing lung compliance, lung volumes, and oxygenation. Surfactant inactivation can be overcome by addition of exogenous surfactant. Several studies suggest that surfactant therapy may decrease respiratory failure associated with MAS. Findlay et al. (19) determined that surfactant replacement (6 mL/kg, Survanta) improved oxygenation and reduced the incidence of air leaks and the severity of pulmonary morbidity when begun within 6 hours after birth. Response to the first dose was moderate. However, after the second and third doses, given 6 hours apart, improvements in mean arterial-to-alveolar PO_2 ratio and in oxygenation index. Optimal dose, method, and timing of instillation of surfactant in MAS remain to be determined.

High-frequency oscillatory ventilation (HFOV) has been studied alone and in combination with inhaled nitric oxide (INO) as treatment for MAS. Kinsella et al. (20) found that the response rate of infants with MAS to HFOV plus INO was greater than the response rate to either HFOV or INO with conventional ventilation alone. Extracorporeal membrane oxygenation (ECMO) has been used successfully in treatment of severe MAS refractory to ventilatory therapy. Surfactant therapy during ECMO reduced the perfusion time required and the overall rate of complications after ECMO. Broad-spectrum antibiotics are routinely used in the therapy of MAS in infants with abnormal radiographic findings and respiratory distress, although their efficacy in MAS is unproven. Treatment of acute MAS with glucocorticoids has not been beneficial.

PERSISTENT PULMONARY HYPERTENSION OF THE NEWBORN

Gersony and colleagues (21) described hypoxemia in two infants with "persistent physiologic characteristics of the fetal circulation (PFC) in the absence of recognizable cardiac, pulmonary, hematologic, or central nervous system disease." Because the placenta is no longer present and the ductus arteriosus may or may not be patent, the term persistent pulmonary hypertension of the newborn (PPHN) is now used to describe this disorder. The pathophysiology of PPHN is related to a failure to make the transition from high pulmonary vascular resistance (PVR) and low pulmonary blood flow, characteristic of the fetus, to the relatively low PVR and high pulmonary blood flow of the postnatal infant. The clinical syndrome of PPHN has been reviewed (22–24).

Pathophysiology

The pathophysiology of PPHN can best be understood within the framework of the current knowledge of the transitional circulation. Normal transition occurs in four phases: the *in utero* phase, the immediate phase occurring in the first minutes after birth, the fast phase developing in the first 12 to 24 hours, and the final phase, which requires days or months to complete.

In Utero Circulation

The *in utero* phase (i.e., phase 1) is characterized by PVR that exceeds systemic vascular resistance, resulting in right atrial and ventricular pressures exceeding left atrial and ventricular pressures. As a result of this pressure differential, more than one-third of the oxygenated blood returning from the placenta through the inferior vena cava streams across the patent foramen ovale (PFO), is ejected from the left ventricle, and perfuses the head and neck vessels and the lower body. Venous blood returning through the superior vena cava preferentially flows into the right ventricle and main pulmonary artery. A small amount of this deoxygenated blood, comprising approximately 8% of the cardiac output and with a PO_2 less than 20 mm Hg, does perfuse the lungs, but because of elevated PVR, most is shunted across the PDA to mix with the blood in the aorta distal to the cervical and subclavian arteries. The lower body is therefore perfused with relatively less well oxygenated blood than the head and neck. Because of the large right-to-left shunt at the PFO and the PDA, blood bypasses the lungs *in utero*. Persistence of the elevated PVR after birth without the benefit of placental oxygenation results in the profound hypoxemia characteristic of PPHN. The mechanisms that maintain the fetal state of high PVR are under study. Pulmonary vasoconstriction induced by hypoxia, alterations in nitric oxide and arachidonic acid metabolism, and systemic acidosis probably contribute to physiologic abnormalities in PPHN.

Immediate Phase

The second stage of normal transition, the immediate phase, is accomplished in the first minute after birth when the fluid-filled fetal lungs are distended with air during the first breath. A rapid decrease in PVR occurs with the mechanical distention of the pulmonary vascular bed, allowing more oxygenated blood to perfuse the lungs. The entry of air into the alveoli improves the oxygenation of the pulmonary vascular bed, further decreasing PVR.

Fast Phase

The fast phase of the transitional circulation occurs for 12 to 24 hours after birth and accounts for the greatest reduction in PVR. The drop in PVR has been associated with the production of vasodilators, such as prostacyclin and endothelial-derived relaxing factor (i.e., nitric oxide). Prostacyclin is produced in the neonatal lung in response to rhythmic distension of the lungs. Pretreatment of the fetal lamb with cyclooxygenase inhibitor decreased prostacyclin production and prevented the late fall in PVR. The role of cyclooxygenase and prostacyclin in the transitional circulation may have clinical implications. Persistent pulmonary hypertension of the newborn has been observed in infants of mothers receiving aspirin or nonsteroidal antiinflammatory agents that inhibit cyclooxygenase activity. However, prostacyclin induction at birth is transient, and it does not account for pulmonary vasodilation occurring in response to increasing oxygen tension. Likewise, indomethacin did not reverse decreased PVR caused by hyperbaric oxygen. The role of pulmonary production of potent vasodilatory leukotrienes, which also occurs during the initiation of ventilation, is unclear.

The pulmonary vasodilation and increase in pulmonary blood flow occurring in response to hyperbaric oxygenation can be virtually masked by inhibitors of the endothelial-derived relaxing factor, nitric oxide. Nitric oxide (NO) is induced by oxygen, ATP, and sheer stress and is elevated in 1-day-old lamb pulmonary arteries and pulmonary veins in comparison to near-term fetuses and few-week-old lambs. Nitric oxide causes vasodilation by inducing the guanylate cyclase enzyme. The resultant increase in cGMP in turn activates a kinase that decreases intracellular calcium, allowing smooth muscle cell relaxation. The vascular effects of NO are specific and localized because of its great affinity for hemoglobin, especially deoxyhemoglobin. Thus, inhaled NO (INO) causes pulmonary vasodilation without systemic hypotension. Prostaglandin, PGI_2 in particular, and NO are believed to be the principal agents responsible for the decrease in pulmonary vascular resistance in the fast phase of transition.

Final Phase

The final phase of the neonatal pulmonary vascular transition involves remodeling of the pulmonary vascular musculature (25). In the normal fetal and term lung, fully muscularized, thick-walled preacinar arteries extend to the level of the terminal bronchioles. Intraacinar and alveolar wall arteries are not muscularized. Within days after delivery, medial wall thickness of preacinar vessels smaller than 250 μm in diameter decreases, and within months, medial wall thickness of vessels larger than 250 and smaller than 500 μm also decreases. Hypoxia at birth prevents the remodeling and regression of the smooth muscle of the preacinar bronchiolar arteries. In utero, or after birth, high-flow states and chronic hypoxia stimulate cells of the intraacinar and alveolar arteries to differentiate into smooth muscle and connective tissue, resulting in abnormally thickened and reactive arteriolar musculature. Distal extension of smooth muscle with increased numbers of adventitial fibroblasts and extracellular matrix has been described in pulmonary arteries of infants dying of severe MAS with PPHN.

Etiology

Persistent pulmonary hypertension of the newborn has a variety of causes that can be classified by the predominant abnormality involved (Table 28–1). Identification of the cause and subclass of PPHN is helpful in predicting severity and reversibility of PPHN in the neonate. Assessment of the clinical severity of PPHN helps determine the

TABLE 28–1. *Classification system for persistent pulmonary hypertension of the newborn*

Pathology	Associated diseases	Proposed mechanisms	Prognosis
Functional vasoconstriction; normal pulmonary vascular development	Acute perinatal hypoxia Acute meconium aspiration Sepsis or pneumonia (especially group B streptococci) Respiratory distress syndrome Hypoventilation CNS depression[a] Hypothermia Hypoglycemia	Response to acute hypoxia, particularly in the presence of acidemia	Good; reversible

Fixed decreased diameter; abnormal extension and hypertrophy of distal pulmonary vascular smooth muscle	Placental insufficiency
	Prolonged gestation
	In utero closure of ductus arteriosus
	  Aspirin
	  Nonsteroidal antiinflammatory agents
	Single ventricle without pulmonic stenosis
	Chronic pulmonary venous hypertension
	  TAPVR[a]
	  Obstructive left-sided heart lesions
	Idiopathic diseases
		Response to chronic hypoxia
		Excessive pulmonary blood flow in utero
		
		Elevated pulmonary venous pressure
			Poor; fixed structural lesion

Decreased cross-sectional area of the pulmonary vascular bed	Space-occupying lesions
	  Diaphragmatic hernia
	  Lung dysgenesis
	  Pleural effusions
	Congenital lung hypoplasia
	  Potter syndrome
	  Thoracic dystrophies
		Hypoplasia of alveoli and associated vessels	Poor; fixed structural lesion

Functional obstruction to pulmonary blood flow	Polycythemia Hyperfibrinogenemia	Increased blood viscosity	Good, unless chronic

[a]CNS, central nervous system; TAPVR, total anomalous pulmonary venous return.

need for referral to nurseries with ECMO and nitric oxide capability.

Clinical Presentation

Clinically, PPHN presents as labile hypoxemia that is disproportionate to the extent of pulmonary parenchymal disease. Infants with PPHN are commonly appropriate for gestational age and near term. The perinatal history frequently includes factors associated with perinatal asphyxia. Clinical symptoms include tachypnea, respiratory distress, and often rapidly progressive cyanosis, particularly in response to stimulation of the infant. The cardiovascular examination may be normal or may reveal a right ventricular heave, closely split or single loud S2, and tricuspid regurgitation suggesting that pulmonary arterial pressure is equal to or greater than systemic arterial pressure. A gradient of 10 mm Hg between right arm and lower extremity oxygen pressures suggests right-to-left shunting at the ductus arteriosus and is consistent with the diagnosis of PPHN. PPHN may occur without differential oxygen saturations if the ductus arteriosus is closed and mixing of cyanotic and oxygenated blood is occurring intrapulmonarily or at other intracardiac sites. Differential diagnosis of PPHN includes severe pulmonary parenchymal disease, such as severe MAS, RDS, pneumonia, or pulmonary hemorrhage, and congenital heart disease, such as transposition of the great arteries. Critical pulmonic stenosis, hypoplastic left ventricle, or severe coarctation should be considered in the differential diagnosis. Methods used to differentiate PPHN from pulmonary parenchymal disease or cardiac disease are outlined in Table 28–2.

The oxygenation of infants with severe pulmonary parenchymal disease without PPHN generally improves after treatment with oxygen or mechanical ventilation. Infants with PPHN often have little or no parenchymal lung disease. They are easily ventilated but remain hypoxic despite high forced inspiratory oxygen. Oxygenation will frequently improve markedly with hyperventilation and/or alkalinization of infants with PPHN. Cyanotic congenital heart disease (CCHD) is usually associated with fixed, structural mixing of venous and arterial blood. In infants with CCHD, hypoxemia is generally unresponsive to increased exogenous oxygen, mechanical ventilation, hyperventilation, or alkalinization. Diagnosis of PPHN can be complicated by the coexistence of pulmonary hypertension, parenchymal lung disease, or CCHD. Echocardiography is useful in the diagnosis of structural heart disease in this clinical setting.

Therapy

Supportive medical management includes correction of underlying abnormalities that may include polycythemia,

TABLE 28–2. *Diagnostic evaluation of severe neonatal hypoxemia*

Test	Method	Result[a]	Suggested diagnosis
Hyperoxia	Expose to 100% FiO_2 for 5–10 min	PaO_2 increases to >100 mm Hg	Pulmonary parenchymal disease
		PaO_2 increases to <20 mm Hg	Persistent pulmonary hypertension or cyanotic congenital heart disease
Hyperventilation–hyperoxia	Mechanical ventilation with 100%FiO_2 and respiratory rate 100–150 breaths/min	PaO_2 increases to >100 mm Hg without hyperventilation	Pulmonary parenchymal disease
		PaO_2 increases at a critical PCO_2, often to <25 mm Hg	Persistent pulmonary hypertension
		No increase in PaO_2 despite hyperventilation	Cyanotic congenital heart disease or severe, fixed pulmonary hypertension
Simultaneous–preductal–postductal PO_2	Compare PO_2 of right arm or shoulder to that of lower abdomen or extremities	Preductal $PO_2 \geq 15$ + postductal PO_2	Patent ductus arteriosus with right-to-left shunt
Echocardiography	M-mode	Increased RVPEP and RVET	Right ventricular systolic time interval ratio (RVSTI = RVPEP/RVET > 0.5) predicts PPHN
	Venous contrast injection	Simultaneously appears in PA and LA	Patent foramen ovale
	Two-dimensional echocardiography	Deviation of intraatrial septum to left; rule out congenital heart defect	Increased pulmonary arterial pressure
	Doppler	Failure of acceleration of systolic blood flow between large main pulmonary artery and small peripheral pulmonary artery	Suggests right-to-left PDA or intracardiac shunt

[a]LA, left atrium; PA, pulmonary artery; PDA, patent ductus arteriosus; PPHN, persistent pulmonary hypertension of the newborn; RVET, right ventricular ejection time; RVPEP, right ventricular ejection period.

hypoglycemia, hypothermia, diaphragmatic hernia, or CCHD. Metabolic acidosis and hypotension should be corrected by adequate replacement of intravascular volume and administration of sodium bicarbonate or pressors.

Specific therapy for PPHN is aimed at increasing pulmonary blood flow and decreasing right-to-left shunting. High ambient oxygen and mechanical ventilation are the pulmonary therapeutic interventions for treatment of PPHN. Ligation of the PDA is not useful, and it may be detrimental. Cardiac failure may occur after PDA ligation as the right ventricle fails in the face of high pulmonary resistance without the safety valve of the patent ductus. Shunting between the pulmonary and systemic circulations depends on the relative pressures of each system. Therefore, optimal therapy decreases pulmonary artery pressure while increasing or not changing systemic arterial pressure and cardiac output.

Infants with severe PPHN are often sensitive to activity and agitation. Transcutaneous and intravascular monitoring equipment should be used and stimulation minimized during the care of these infants. Muscle relaxants (e.g., pancuronium) and sedatives are frequently beneficial but should be used with caution. Paralysis may further compromise ventilation and may mask clinical signs of respiratory insufficiency. Sedatives should be chosen to minimize cardiovascular side effects such as systemic hypotension. Infants with PPHN, especially if asphyxiated or septic, frequently develop systemic hypotension and signs of cardiac failure. Elevated right heart pressure from increased PVR, poor venous return secondary to high intrathoracic pressures during mechanical ventilation, and previous asphyxia may contribute to myocardial dysfunction. The hematocrit should be maintained at or above 45%, and volume expanders, such as salt-poor albumin, Plasmanate, or normal saline, may be used to support the circulation. Dopamine and other pressors are commonly used for refractory hypotension but should be used with caution, as they may contribute to pulmonary vasoconstriction.

Respiratory and Metabolic Alkalosis

The often dramatic response of infants with PPHN to respiratory or metabolic alkalosis supports their use in the care of infants with severe PPHN. The degree of pulmonary parenchymal disease and risk of barotrauma may affect the clinical choice of inducing respiratory or metabolic alkalosis. It may be necessary to raise arterial pH to 7.55 or above with hyperventilation and sodium bicarbonate to reverse severe pulmonary vasoconstriction. Because of pulmonary and neurologic concerns, sustaining PCO_2 at less than 20 mm Hg is not advocated. Excessive mechanical ventilation with overdistension of the lung may increase right-to-left shunting. Pulmonary barotrauma associated with aggressive ventilation should not be underestimated. Hypocarbic alkalosis, by shifting the hemoglobin–oxygen dissociation curve, may also compromise the release of oxygen at the tissue level. Hyperoxia and hypocarbia may adversely affect cerebral blood flow. Weaning from ventilation and alkalinization must proceed with caution, because dramatic lability of PO_2 is often observed in infants with PPHN.

Nitric Oxide and High-Frequency Oscillatory Ventilation

Various vasodilators such as tolazoline and prostaglandins D_2 and E_1 have been studied for treatment of PPHN. At doses required to decrease PVR, these agents often cause undesirable systemic vasodilation and hypotension. Tolazoline has been used in therapy for PPHN but has not been shown to improve outcome.

Inhaled nitric oxide (INO) specifically dilates pulmonary vasculature. Avid binding to hemoglobin prevents INO from dilating systemic blood vessels. In addition, INO preferentially vasodilates vessels of alveoli that are patent, thus improving ventilation/perfusion (V/Q) matching. Other less specific vasodilators may increase blood flow to atelectatic alveoli, increasing V/Q mismatch. Inhaled NO combined with conventional ventilation increased oxygenation and decreased the oxygen index of approximately 30% of infants with PPHN. The likelihood of response to INO appeared inversely related to the severity of parenchymal disease (20). Approximately 25% of PPHN infants failing to respond to INO responded to INO combined with HFOV, suggesting improved response to INO if ventilation strategies are optimized to recruit atelectatic alveoli. Response to INO, especially in RDS and meconium aspiration, may be improved by cotreatment with exogenous surfactant to enhance recruitment of alveoli.

Extracorporeal Membrane Oxygenation

Extracorporeal membrane oxygenation has been useful for the treatment of severe PPHN refractory to medical management. The first newborn survivor of ECMO therapy was reported by Bartlett and colleagues in 1975 (26). In 1992, the National Registry of Neonatal ECMO reported an 87% survival rate for the 739 infants with the primary diagnosis of PPHN who were treated with ECMO (27). Most of these infants met criteria for greater than 80% risk of mortality with conventional medical management. However, criteria used to determine risk of mortality vary from institution to institution and frequently are based on retrospective chart reviews, reflecting older methods of medical management. It is impossible to determine how these infants would have done with modern conventional therapy.

Long-Term Outcome

Most infants treated for PPHN have few residual respiratory symptoms or neurologic or developmental sequelae by 1 year of age (28). Of infants with more severe parenchymal disease, qualifying for inhaled nitric oxide or ECMO, approximately 25% have persistent BPD or recurrent reactive airway disease at 1 and 2 years of age. Particularly, infants with severe MAS or congenital diaphragmatic hernia and PPHN have an increased risk for chronic pulmonary sequelae (29). Continued oxygen therapy, bronchodilators, diuretics, and enhanced nutrition may be necessary to treat residual disease and establish adequate growth. Hearing, vision, and neurologic development should be followed closely in infants treated for PPHN, especially if severely asphyxiated. Approximately 25% of infants treated with INO or ECMO for PPHN remain below 5% for weight at 1 to 2 years of age. Approximately 10% to 12% are diagnosed with severe neurodevelopmental disability. The risk of neurologic, growth, and pulmonary sequelae is greatest in infants with PPHN secondary to congenital diaphragmatic hernia (29).

PNEUMONIA

Pneumonia remains a significant cause of morbidity and mortality for preterm and term infants. The incidence of pneumonia in NICU patients exceeds 10% (30), with mortality of perinatally acquired pneumonia varying between 5% and 20% (30–32). Pneumonia may be acquired transplacentally, during the birth process, or postnatally, and it is caused by a variety of pathogens, including viruses, bacteria, and fungi (Table 28–3). Unique environmental and host factors predispose the neonate to pulmonary infections. The increased susceptibility of neonates for pneumonia may be related to immaturity of mucociliary clearance, small size of the conducting airways, and lowered host defenses. Invasive procedures, such as tracheal intubation, barotrauma, and hyperoxic damage to the respiratory tract may further impair resistance to pneumonia. The nosocomial flora of the hospital nursery, whether derived from nursery equipment or the unwashed hands of caregivers, are important vectors of pathogenic organisms.

Transplacental Viral Pneumonias

Pneumonia acquired through the transplacental route is most commonly of viral origin. Rubella, varicella-zoster, cytomegalovirus (CMV), herpes simplex virus (HSV), and human immunodeficiency virus (HIV) are acquired by this route. Transplacentally acquired pneumonitis is also associated with adenoviral, enteroviral and influenza viral infections. Viral pneumonia is usually part of a systemic illness, reflecting hematogenous spread from the mother. Severity and onset of respiratory symptoms varies from respiratory failure at delivery to chronic pneumonia evolving months after birth.

Fetal infection may result from a primary maternal infection acquired during pregnancy or from reactivation of a latent infection. *In utero* transmission of rubella occurs as a result of primary infection acquired during pregnancy. Transmission of varicella-zoster, HSV, and CMV occurs as a result of primary or recurrent maternal infection. The timing of maternal infection in relation to birth is often a critical factor in outcome. Congenital varicella typically develops when primary maternal chickenpox occurs within the 21 days preceding parturition. If maternal varicella occurs less than 5 days before birth, antepartum transfer of maternal antibody to the fetus is minimal, increasing the risk of systemic varicella infection in the neonate. Varicella pneumonia usually presents 2 to 4 days after the onset of the exanthem. Although varicella pneumonia is often self-limited, it can cause significant mortality and morbidity. Treatment with varicella-zoster immune globulin within 72 hours of birth improves clinical outcome in neonates exposed to varicella. Pneumonitis is not a common presentation in congenital CMV or herpes, but it is more common in perinatally acquired CMV and HSV. Pulmonary disease caused by transplacental transfer of the HIV virus generally presents after the neonatal period.

TABLE 28–3. *Primary pathogens of neonatal pneumonia*

Vector	Viruses[a]	Bacteria	Other agents
Transplacental	Rubella Varicella-zoster HIV CMV HSV	*L. monocytogenes* *M. tuberculosis* *T. pallidum*	
Perinatal	HSV CMV	Group B streptococci Gram-negative enteric 　(i.e., *E. coli, Klebsiella*)	*C. trachomatis* *U. urealyticum*
Postnatal	CMV HSV Community based 　(i.e., RSV, influenza, parainfluenza)	*S. aureus* *P. aeruginosa* *Flavobacterium* *S. marcescens*	*C. albicans*

[a]HIV, human immunodeficiency virus; CMV, cytomegalovirus; HSV, herpes simplex virus; RSV, respiratory syncytial virus.

Transplacental Bacterial Pneumonias

Transplacental bacterial infections are less common causes of pneumonia. *Listeria monocytogenes, Mycobacterium tuberculosis,* and *Treponema pallidum* are the most common organisms. Maternal listeriosis classically presents with a flu-like syndrome, with fever and chills occurring up to 2 weeks before delivery. Preterm labor and meconium staining of amniotic fluid, even in preterm infants, are common. Early-onset listeriosis generally presents soon after birth with respiratory distress and pneumonia. Radiographic findings are nonspecific, consisting of peribronchial or widespread infiltrates. Congenital tuberculosis occurs most commonly in infants born to women with primary infections. Respiratory symptoms in neonatal tuberculosis typically present at 2 to 4 weeks of age. Transplacental transfer of *T. palladium* occurs most commonly during primary or secondary maternal infection, usually after 20 weeks of gestation. Pneumonia alba refers to the pale, firm, and enlarged lungs seen at autopsy in congenital syphilis. Although pulmonary involvement is uncommon, the recent increase in the incidence of primary and secondary syphilis should heighten physician awareness of all manifestations of congenital syphilis.

Pneumonia Acquired in the Perinatal Period

Neonatal pneumonia is most commonly acquired during the process of labor and delivery. Infection occurs from organisms ascending from the genital tract after rupture of fetal membranes or acquired during passage of the infant through the birth canal. Respiratory symptoms are often present at delivery or have their onset in the first few days of life. Despite the abundance and heterogeneity of organisms in the genital tract, only a few commonly cause pneumonia.

In U.S. nurseries, group B *Streptococcus* (GBS) is the most frequently identified organism causing neonatal pneumonia. The second most common group of organisms to produce early-onset sepsis or pneumonia are the gram-negative enteric bacilli: *Escherichia coli, Klebsiella, Enterobacter,* and *Proteus* species. Herpes simplex and CMV are the most common viral agents causing early-onset pneumonia. Pneumonia caused by *Chlamydia trachomatis* usually begins at 2 to 8 weeks of age with upper respiratory tract symptoms, a staccato cough, and apnea. Antecedent conjunctival infection is common but not always observed. Interstitial pneumonitis and hyperinflation are associated with chlamydial pneumonia. *U. urealyticum* is a common inhabitant of the lower genital tract of women and is frequently associated with histologic evidence of chorioamnionitis. *U. urealyticum* is a cause of acute congenital pneumonia and has also been associated with chronic lung disease in infants.

Pneumonia Acquired in the Postnatal Period

Newborns exposed to respiratory equipment or humidified incubators are at risk for respiratory infection by *Pseudomonas* species, *Flavobacterium, Klebsiella,* or *Serratia marcescens.* Direct contamination by the hands of caretakers as a result of inadequate hand washing is associated with outbreaks of *Staphylococcus aureus* and gram-negative enteric organisms. Cytomegalovirus that is acquired postnatally through blood products or breast milk commonly presents as a pneumonitis. Onset of CMV disease is usually 4 to 12 weeks after exposure, presenting with tachypnea, cough, and upper respiratory symptoms.

Neonatal HSV infection is most often associated with HSV type II. However, data from the National Institute of Allergy and Infectious Disease indicate that 30% of symptomatic neonatal HSV infections were caused by HSV type I (37). Postnatal infection from HSV generally occurs from orolabial, oropharyngeal, or breast lesions. Community-based respiratory pathogens, including respiratory syncytial virus, influenza, parainfluenza, and enteroviruses, occur in the nursery. Pneumonia resulting from epidemic outbreaks of various enteroviral agents, including echovirus 22 and coxsackievirus type B, is often associated with other clinical manifestation of enteroviral disease. Risk factors for nosocomial fungal infections include very low birth weight, prolonged antibiotic therapy, intubation, central line catheter placement, intravenous alimentation, and corticosteroids. Pneumonia caused by *Candida albicans* usually presents in the context of disseminated disease. *Mycoplasma* species may also cause pneumonia in the postnatal period.

Pathologic Findings

Three common histopathologic patterns have been associated with neonatal pneumonia: hyaline membrane formation, suppurative inflammation, and interstitial pneumonitis. Hyaline membrane formation is a nonspecific response seen in lung injury associated with surfactant deficiency, pneumonia, and oxygen therapy. Damage to the alveolar epithelium results in cell necrosis and leakage of cell and serum proteins into the alveolar space. Hyaline membranes in neonatal pneumonia are often observed after GBS infection, but they are also associated with fatal pneumonia caused by *H. influenzae,* gram-negative enteric organisms, and viral agents. Bacteria are commonly seen within the hyaline membranes (Fig. 28–10). Disruption of alveolar capillary permeability and cell injury results in leakage of proteins into the alveolus that further inactivate pulmonary surfactant, leading to atelectasis. The decreased compliance, atelectasis, and hypoxemia seen in pneumonia are often indistinguishable

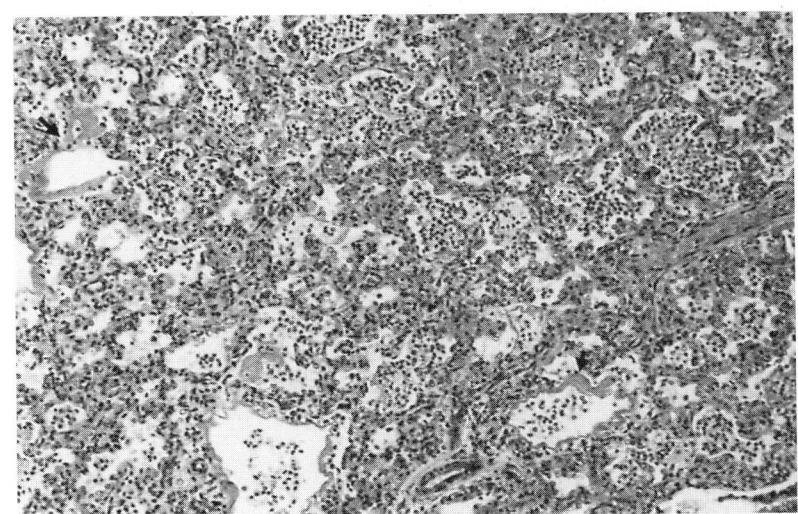

FIG. 28–10. Acute neutrophilic response with atelectasis and hyaline membranes *(arrows)* are seen in lung tissue from a full-term infant who died at 2 days of age of group B streptococcal pneumonia. (Hematoxylin and eosin stain; original magnification × 200) (Courtesy of Edgar Ballard, Children's Hospital, Cincinnati, OH.)

from findings in surfactant-deficient lungs in premature infants. The chest radiographic findings in RDS and neonatal pneumonia may be identical, although bronchopneumonia and pleural effusions are more common in GBS and other bacterial causes of neonatal pneumonia than in RDS.

Suppurative Pneumonia

Staphylococcus aureus, enteric bacilli such as *Klebsiella pneumoniae, E. coli,* and *Pseudomonas* species, and fungi can cause suppurative pneumonia. An intense inflammatory response often occurs in the lungs during these bacterial infections. Necrosis of lung parenchyma, microabscess formation, and partial obstruction of terminal bronchioles results in thin-walled, air-filled pneumatoceles. Spontaneous rupture of these structures can produce pneumothorax. Microabcesses may consolidate into larger cavities or rupture to the pleural space, causing empyema. Pneumonia may be focal or may consolidate to produce large confluent abscesses. Perfusion of consolidated lung tissue causes venous admixture and hypoxemia.

Interstitial Pneumonitis

Interstitial pneumonitis is typically caused by a virus and characterized by interstitial inflammation, edema, mononuclear infiltration, and septal hyperplasia. Alveolar spaces may remain uninvolved, but in severe cases, a serous exudate containing desquamated pneumocytes and macrophages may be associated with hyaline membrane formation. Septal wall necrosis may occur, adding a component of hemorrhage to the inflammatory exudate. Alveolar capillary block associated with the inflammation may impair respiratory function. Cytomegalovirus,

HSV, varicella-zoster, rubella, HIV, enteroviruses, and the community-based pathogens, such as respiratory syncytial, influenza and parainfluenza viruses, are commonly associated with interstitial pneumonitis.

Group B Streptococcal Pneumonia

During the 1970s, GBS pneumonia emerged as the predominant pathogen causing neonatal sepsis and pneumonia. The incidence of GBS infection in the first week of life varies from 1.3 to 3 per 1,000 live births. Despite increased awareness of the disease, GBS infection continues to be associated with mortality rates of 5% to 20% (32).

Group B streptococci are commonly found in genital and intestinal flora of 10% to 30% of pregnant women. For women with positive GBS cultures at delivery, the infant colonization rate is approximately 50%. Of colonized infants, only 0.5% to 2% develop invasive disease. Risk of infection is inversely related to birth weight. Maternal factors increasing the risk of infection include heavy colonization with GBS reflected as GBS bacteria and low levels of maternal, type-specific GBS antibodies. Obstetric factors include prolonged rupture of membranes (>18 hours), maternal intrapartum temperature at least 100.4°F, chorioamnionitis, and use of fetal monitoring devices (32).

Intrapartum chemoprophylaxis has been shown to be effective in preventing early-onset neonatal GBS disease. Efficacy of intrapartum treatment was demonstrated in high-risk pregnancies with documented prenatal GBS colonization and premature labor, rupture of membranes for more than 12 hours, or intrapartum fever. Boyer and colleagues (33) demonstrated that intrapartum intravenous ampicillin followed by treatment of the infants with intramuscular ampicillin significantly reduced early-onset GBS disease. Other studies have also shown the effectiveness of intrapartum antibiotics. A recent meta-analysis estimated a 30-fold reduction in early onset GBS with intrapartum antibiotics (34).

Early-onset GBS disease usually presents within the first week of life. Septicemia (30% to 40%), meningitis (20% to 30%), and pneumonia (30% to 40%) are the most common presentations. Regardless of the primary site of involvement, 90% of affected infants present with respiratory distress. Radiographic features of GBS infection may be indistinguishable from RDS, although pleural effusions may help differentiate GBS from RDS (Fig. 28–11). In two-thirds of affected infants, increased vascular markings or patchy infiltrates are observed on the initial chest radiographs. Respiratory distress in the absence of radiographic abnormalities may be associated with pulmonary vascular hypertension and hypoxemia. Late-onset GBS usually presents from 1 to 6 weeks after birth and is commonly associated with meningitis.

Respiratory failure in GBS pneumonia results from hyaline membrane formation, atelectasis, and pulmonary hypertension. Pulmonary hypertension is proposed to be mediated by high-molecular-weight polysaccharide exotoxin. In animals, infusion of GBS exotoxin results in an initial increase in pulmonary vascular pressures and fever, followed by a second phase characterized by granulocytopenia, granulocyte trapping in the lung, and increased pulmonary vascular permeability (35).

Isolation of GBS from cultures of blood, cerebrospinal fluid, or suppurative foci (i.e., pleural fluid) is diagnostic of GBS infection. Surface cultures of skin or mucous membranes are not be of clinical significance because of the large number of infants colonized but not infected. Urine latex agglutination tests are also not recommended as a screening tool because of the large number of false-positive and false-negative results (36). Antimicrobial therapy is usually instituted before an organism is identified and consists of a penicillin and an aminoglycoside. After the organism is identified and meningitis is excluded, therapy can continue with penicillin alone at 200,000 U/kg/day, usually for 10 to 14 days. Extensive supportive care, including oxygen, mechanical ventilation, and cardiovascular support, may also be required in treating an overwhelming infection.

Herpes Simplex Pneumonia

The incidence of neonatal HSV is increasing in the United States, affecting 1,500 to 2,200 infants per year. Classification of HSV infection is based on the site and extent of involvement; HSV may be classified as a cutaneous infection; as encephalitic, with or without cutaneous infection; and as a disseminated infection. Mortality is highest among infants with disseminated disease. The mortality rate of infants with HSV pneumonitis is approximately 79% (37). Transmission of HSV infection to the neonate is most frequently related to direct contact with virus at delivery. Most women delivering infants with symptomatic HSV disease shed virus asymptomatically at delivery, and fewer than 20% of these women reported a history of previous infection (38). Whether the maternal infection is primary or recurrent is important in the pathogenesis of neonatal HSV infection. Infants of women with serologic evidence of a recent primary infection are more likely to develop disease than infants of women with recurrent herpes. Primary infections are associated with higher titers of viral shedding and with low levels of protective antibodies, placing the neonate at higher risk. Rupture of the amniotic sac for longer than 6 hours is associated with increased risk of neonatal HSV infection, although infection after cesarean section with intact membranes has also been reported.

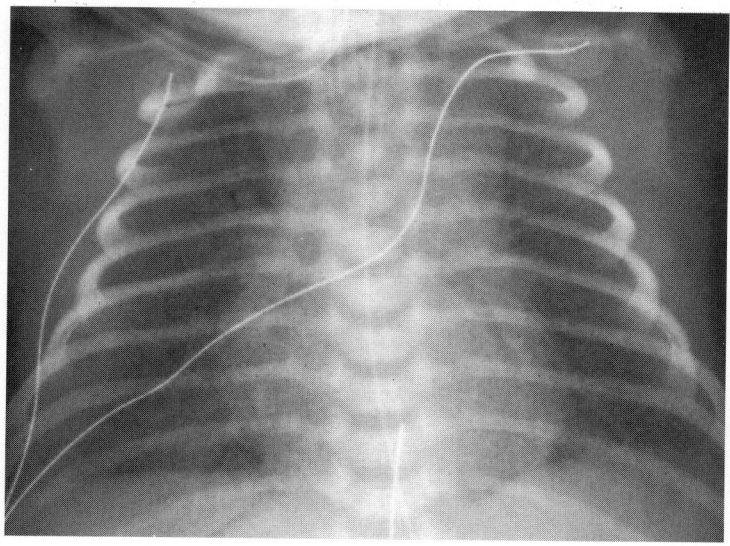

FIG. 28–11. A full-term infant of an uncomplicated pregnancy developed respiratory distress, cyanosis, and periods of apnea within 6 hours of life. The blood culture and urine latex particle agglutination assay were positive for group B streptococci. Diffuse reticulogranular pattern, air bronchograms, and right pleural effusion without significant volume loss are consistent with common radiologic features of group B streptococcal pneumonia.

Herpes simplex virus pneumonitis usually presents as part of a disseminated HSV infection. Many severely involved infants have no skin lesions. Infants typically develop signs of infection at 4 to 5 days of life. Fever, tachypnea, jaundice, and irritability, progressing to respiratory failure, shock, and disseminated intravascular coagulation are commonly seen. Diffuse interstitial pneumonitis and hemorrhagic pneumonitis are characteristic of HSV infection of the lung.

Isolation of HSV remains the definitive diagnostic method. Viral cultures should be obtained from skin lesions, cerebrospinal fluid, stool, urine, throat, nasopharynx, and conjunctiva. Hepatic dysfunction, neutropenia, bleeding diathesis, and interstitial pneumonitis are commonly associated with HSV but are not diagnostic. Serologic assays are not of clinical value, because they do not differentiate between antibodies to HSV types 1 and 2 or between maternal IgG and endogenously produced antibodies. Intranuclear inclusions and multinucleated giant cells observed in scrapings from cutaneous lesions are supportive but not diagnostic of HSV infection. Polymerase chain reaction studies on spinal fluid have recently become available and are highly sensitive and specific.

Early antiviral therapy decreases the progression from localized, cutaneous HSV infection to disseminated disease, and decreases the mortality from HSV infection. Vidarabine and acyclovir are now widely used in treatment of HSV infection in the neonate. Because of ease of administration, acyclovir is considered the treatment of choice (39).

TRANSIENT TACHYPNEA OF THE NEWBORN

Transient tachypnea of the newborn (TTN) was first described in 1966 by Avery and colleagues in a group of eight patients, seven of whom were delivered vaginally at term (38). All of the infants presented at or shortly after birth with grunting, retractions, and an increased respiratory rate. Respiratory rates of the original infants ranged from 80 to 140 breaths/min, and the symptoms persisted for 2 to 5 days. These infants could be differentiated from infants with other acute lung diseases by their clinical course and radiographic findings. Although the precise cause of TTN remains unknown, it was originally postulated that infants with TTN had reduced lung compliance because of delayed resorption of lung fluid at the time of birth. Many clinicians support the original proposal of Avery and colleagues that TTN results from distention of interstitial spaces by fluid, leading to alveolar air trapping and decreased lung compliance (40). Since the original description, others have postulated that TTN may result from mild immaturity of the surfactant system. Lack of phosphatidylglycerol in amniotic fluid samples obtained from infants with TTN supports the latter concept.

The incidence of TTN is approximately 11 per 1,000 live births. The risk factors for TTN include prematurity, maternal sedation, maternal fluid administration, maternal asthma, exposure to β-mimetic agents, and fetal asphyxia. Whether delivery by cesarean section predisposes the term infant for TTN is still debated.

Infants with TTN initially present with grunting, retractions, and increased respiratory rate. The symptoms of tachypnea may persist for several days, and most infants require less than 40% oxygen to maintain adequate systemic oxygenation. The radiographic findings in this disorder are ill defined but include increased central vascular markings, hyperaeration, evidence of interstitial and pleural fluid, prominent interlobar fissures, and cardiomegaly (Fig. 28–12). Because TTN is self-limited, no specific therapy is indicated, although adequate ventilation and oxygenation must be maintained. Because the symptoms of TTN are nonspecific and consistent with

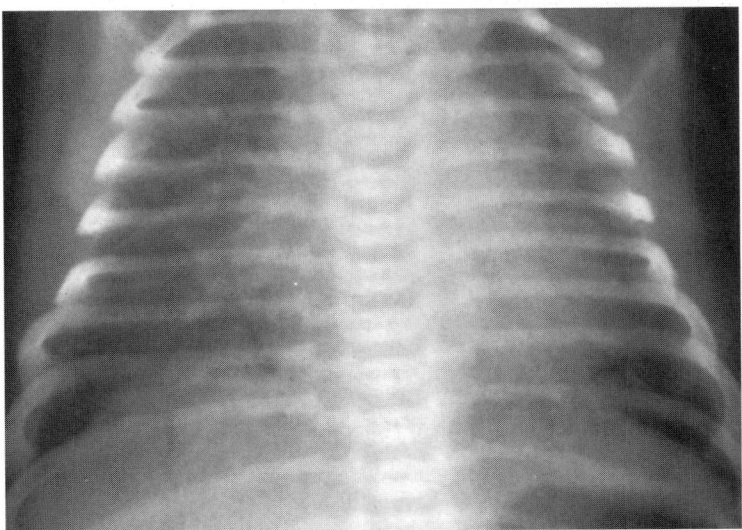

FIG. 28–12. This full-term infant was born by cesarean section and developed tachypnea and grunting that resolved 48 hours after birth. Perihilar vascular densities, streaky opacities of interstitial edema, fluid in the interlobar fissures, small pleural effusions, and cardiomegaly are observed on the radiograph. These features are indicative of transient tachypnea of the newborn.

neonatal sepsis or pneumonia, most infants with TTN are evaluated for infection and are treated with broad-spectrum antibiotics pending a definitive diagnosis.

PULMONARY HEMORRHAGE

Pulmonary hemorrhage in the newborn may vary from a focal, self-limited disorder to massive, lethal hemorrhage. The incidence of pulmonary hemorrhage in the neonatal period ranges from 0.8 to 1.2 per 1,000 live births, although the incidence was 74% of all liveborn infants in one autopsy series of 70 newborns. Asphyxia, prematurity, intrauterine growth retardation, infection, hypothermia, oxygen therapy, severe Rh hemolytic disease, and coagulopathy are associated risk factors. In some studies, surfactant therapy has been associated with an increased incidence of pulmonary hemorrhage, although this remains controversial. Although disseminated intravascular coagulation may precede pulmonary hemorrhage, most infants with pulmonary hemorrhage do not have a coagulopathy. Pulmonary hemorrhage generally presents within the first week of life, and the mortality rate after pulmonary hemorrhage is estimated to be 75% to 90%. Although most infants who develop pulmonary hemorrhage have the predisposing factors of extreme prematurity and underlying asphyxia and stress, there are a few case reports describing previously healthy, term infants with pulmonary hemorrhage associated with an inborn error of the urea cycle and elevated blood ammonia.

Clinical Findings

The observation that the hematocrit of lung effluent in pulmonary hemorrhage is lower than the hematocrit of blood supports the concept that most of these infants have hemorrhagic pulmonary edema. Neonatal pulmonary hemorrhage is therefore thought to result from shock, hypoxia, and acidosis, which lead to left ventricular failure and increased pulmonary capillary pressure with subsequent hemorrhagic pulmonary edema. Chest radiographic findings in pulmonary hemorrhage depend on whether the hemorrhage is focal or massive. Because blood or hemorrhagic edema fluid has tissue density, hemorrhagic tissue appears opacified. It is often difficult to differentiate focal hemorrhage from atelectasis or pneumonia by chest radiographs. In the case of massive pulmonary hemorrhage, the lungs can be atelectatic and opacified (i.e., whited-out). The clinical course of massive pulmonary hemorrhage usually involves rapid deterioration of ventilatory function. Affected infants develop progressive hypoxia and hypercarbia with resultant respiratory acidosis and may rapidly succumb to this disorder.

Treatment

Early detection and aggressive intervention improve the outcome of massive pulmonary hemorrhage, an oth-erwise lethal syndrome. Positive-pressure ventilation and oxygen are critical components of therapy. Blood volume and hematocrit should be vigorously restored and maintained with erythrocyte transfusions. Careful correction of hypotension, hypoxemia, and acidosis is also indicated. Coagulation abnormalities should be assessed and may be corrected with fresh-frozen plasma or appropriate clotting factors. Pressors and diuretics are indicated if congestive heart failure develops. Surfactant therapy has also been suggested as a useful adjunct in neonates with a clinically significant pulmonary hemorrhage.

AIR LEAKS

Air leaks include pneumothorax, pneumomediastinum, pneumopericardium, and pulmonary interstitial emphysema (PIE).

Pathophysiology

Pulmonary interstitial emphysema, pneumomediastinum, pneumothorax, and pneumopericardium are closely related clinical entities. Air leak begins with formation of PIE in which alveoli rupture into the perivascular and peribronchial spaces. Air may be trapped in the interstitium of the lung, leading to PIE, but it may also dissect into the mediastinum along the perivascular and peribronchial spaces, producing pneumomediastinum. Mediastinal air ruptures into the pleural space, producing pneumothorax, or into the pericardial space, producing pneumopericardium. In some instances, air can form blebs on the surface of the lung that rupture to produce pneumothorax. Rupture of the lung directly into the pleural space is thought to occur rarely.

Risk Factors

Air leaks occur in 1% to 2% of all newborn infants, but they are thought to cause symptoms in only 0.05% to 0.07%. Mechanical ventilation and CPAP are important risk factors contributing to air leak in infants with lung disease. Summarizing data from 11 studies, Madansky found that air leak occurred in 12% of infants with RDS who were not on assisted ventilation, 11% of infants on CPAP, and 26% of infants on mechanical ventilation (41). The incidence of air leak in infants admitted to the NICU is approximately 2% to 8%, but it is higher if only low-birth-weight infants are considered. As of 1986, of infants weighing 500 to 999 g at birth who developed air leak, 35% had PIE, 20% had pneumothorax, 3% had pneumomediastinum, and 2% had pneumopericardium (42). Infants developing airleak are at higher risk of death, but the risk changes with postnatal age at the time of the air leak. Aspiration syndromes, including MAS, are frequently complicated by air leak.

Radiographic Evaluation

The chest radiographs of infants with PIE have been described as demonstrating a salt-and-pepper pattern in which the radiolucent interstitial air is juxtaposed to lung parenchyma (Fig. 28–13). Radiolucent air is present in the pleural space in a pneumothorax. Because chest radiographs of neonates are usually performed in the supine position, pleural air of a pneumothorax may accumulate in the anterior chest and may be visible only on a cross-table lateral or decubitus radiograph. In a tension pneumothorax, the lung and mediastinal organs may be displaced away from the side of the pneumothorax (Fig. 28–14). The thymus may be outlined in pneumomediastinum, seen on radiographs. Pneumopericardium results in a characteristic outline of the heart by radiolucent air.

Pulmonary Interstitial Emphysema

Pulmonary interstitial emphysema occurs most frequently in smaller infants being treated by mechanical ventilation for primary lung disease. In this clinical setting, PIE is associated with a mortality rate of more than 50%. Unilateral PIE can be managed by placing the infant with the affected side down for 24 to 48 hours. Selective bronchial intubation and high-frequency or jet

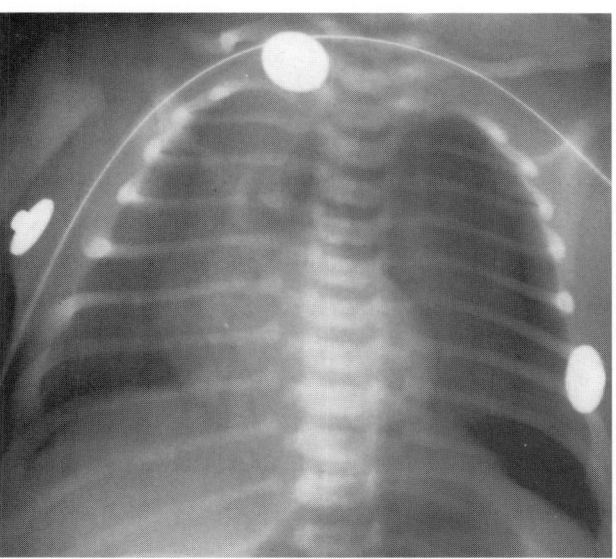

FIG. 28–14. A full-term infant born by a difficult breech delivery presented shortly after birth with crepitus in the neck area, tachypnea, grunting, and retractions. An anteroposterior chest x-ray film demonstrates bilateral pneumothorax under tension on the left. The heart and mediastinum are compressed and shifted to the right. The left pleural air herniates across the midline. The left diaphragm is depressed and inverted. Subcutaneous emphysema is seen in the soft tissues of the neck.

ventilation have been used to treat unilateral PIE along with selective lung resection. Careful attention to peak and mean inspiratory pressures may be beneficial in preventing and treating PIE. High-frequency ventilation may be helpful. Bronchopulmonary dysplasia is a frequent sequel in infants surviving PIE.

Pneumothorax, Pneumomediastinum, and Pneumopericardium

Infants with pneumothorax often present with grunting, tachypnea, cyanosis, and retractions. Accumulated air may collapse the lung or shift the mediastinum to the side opposite the air leak. A shift of the trachea or point of maximal impulse and decreased breath sounds on the affected side may be found on clinical examination. Pneumothoraces fall into two major groups: spontaneous pneumothorax in otherwise healthy, full-term infants, which most often occurs within minutes of birth, and pneumothorax in infants with significant pulmonary disease, which frequently occurs several days after birth, during therapy for pulmonary disease.

Prompt recognition of air leak is essential for effective therapy. Unexpected changes in ventilatory requirements or status and abrupt fall in blood pressure, heart rate, respiratory rate, and PO_2 may indicate an air leak. Transillumination of the thorax can be useful in the diagnosis of pneumothorax and its response to therapy. Treatment of

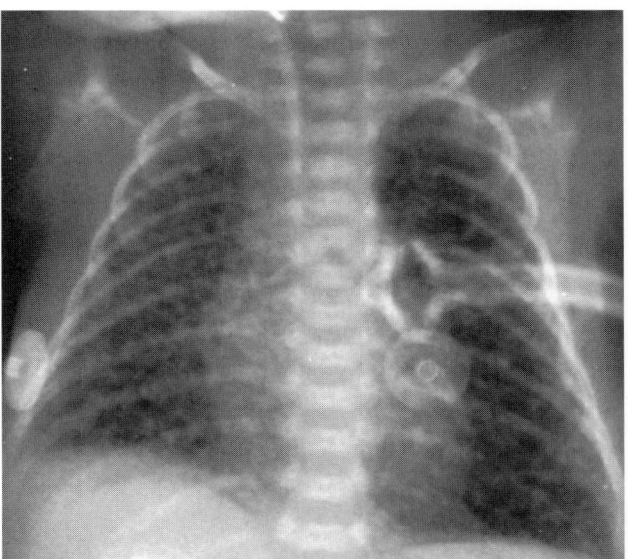

FIG. 28–13. Chest x-ray film of pulmonary interstitial emphysema (PIE). A premature infant with severe respiratory distress syndrome requiring mechanical ventilation developed worsening respiratory acidosis and hypoxia refractory to increased ventilatory support. An anteroposterior chest x-ray film demonstrates a salt-and-pepper pattern resulting from radiolucent interstitial air surrounding compressed lung tissue. A left chest tube was placed to treat pneumothorax, a common complication of pulmonary interstitial emphysema.

tension pneumothorax requires immediate surgical drainage and placement of a chest tube. For treatment of pneumothorax that does not involve tension or cardiovascular compromise, inhalation of 100% oxygen, usually for 6 to 12 hours, can be used as a nitrogen washout method in term infants. Premature infants should not be treated with hyperoxia because they are at risk for retrolental fibroplasia. Pneumomediastinum and pneumopericardium that does not unduly stress the infant can also be managed with 100% oxygen therapy. Tension pneumopericardium is life threatening, must be drained surgically, and is associated with a high incidence of morbidity and mortality.

REFERENCES

1. Burri PH. Postnatal development and growth. In Crystal RG, West JB, Barnes PJ, Cherniack NS, Weibel ER, eds. *The lung: Scientific foundations.* New York: Raven Press, 1991:677.
2. Randell SH, Young SL. Structure of alveolar epithelial cells and the surface layer during development. In Polin RA, Fox WW, eds. *Fetal and neonatal physiology.* Philadelphia: WB Saunders, 1992:962.
3. Van Golde LMG, Batenburg JJ, Robertson B. The pulmonary surfactant system: biochemical aspects and functional significance. *Physiol Rev* 1988;68:374.
4. Whitsett JA. RDS in the premature infant. In Crystal RG, West JB, Barnes PJ, Cherniack NS, Weibel ER, eds. *The lung: Scientific foundations.* New York: Raven Press, 1991:1723.
5. Shapiro DL, Notter RH. *Surfactant replacement therapy.* New York: Alan R Liss, 1989.
6. Rooney S. Regulation of surfactant associated phospholipid synthesis and secretion. In Polin RA, Fox WW, eds. *Fetal and neonatal physiology.* Philadelphia: WB Saunders, 1992:986.
7. Ballard PL. Hormonal regulation of pulmonary surfactant. *Endocrinol Rev* 1989;10:165.
8. Liggins GC, Howie RN. A controlled trial of antepartum glucocorticoid treatment for prevention of the respiratory distress syndrome in premature infants. *Pediatrics* 1972;50:515.
9. Jobe A. Phospholipid metabolism and turnover. In Polin RA, Fox WW, eds. *Fetal and neonatal physiology.* Philadelphia: WB Saunders, 1992:986.
10. Fujiwara T, Maeta H, Chida S, Morita T, Watabe Y, Abe T. Artificial surfactant therapy in hyaline membrane disease. *Lancet* 1980:55.
11. Avery ME, Mead J. Surface properties in relation to atelectasis and hyaline membrane disease. *Am J Dis Child* 1959;97:517.
12. Spitzer AR, Shaffer TH, Fox WW. Assisted ventilation: physiologic implications and application. In RA Polin, WW Fox, eds. *Fetal and neonatal physiology.* Philadelphia: WB Saunders, 1991:894.
13. Bacsik RD. Meconium aspiration syndrome. *Pediatr Clin North Am* 1977;24:463.
14. Katz VL, Barnes WA. Meconium aspiration syndrome: reflections on a murky subject. *Am J Obstet Gynecol* 1992;166:171.
15. Holtzman RB, Banzhaf WC, Silver RK, Hageman JR. Perinatal management of meconium staining of the amniotic fluid. *Clin Perinatol* 1989;16:825.
16. Tran N, Lowe C, Swieni EM, Shaffer TH. Sequential effects of acute meconium obstruction on pulmonary function. *Pediatr Res* 1980;14:34.
17. Ting P, Brady JP. Tracheal suction in meconium aspiration. *Am J Obstet Gynecol* 1975;122:767.
18. Wiswell TE, Henley MA. Intratracheal suctioning, systemic infection and the meconium aspiration syndrome. *Pediatrics* 1992;89:203.
19. Findlay RD, Taeusch W, Walther FJ. Surfactant replacement therapy for meconium aspiration syndrome. *Pediatrics* 1996;97:48.
20. Kinsella JP, Truog WE, Walsh WF, et al. Randomized multicenter trial of inhaled nitric oxide and high frequency oscillatory ventilation in severe persistent pulmonary hypertension of the newborn. *J Pediatr* 1997;131:55.
21. Gersony W, Duc G, Sinclair J. "PFC" syndrome. *Circulation* 1969;40 (Suppl III):87.
22. Clarke WR. The transitional circulation: physiology and anesthetic implications. *J Clin Anesth* 1990;2:192.
23. Hammerman C, Yousefzadeh D, Choi JH, Bui KC. Persistent pulmonary hypertension of the newborn. Managing the unmanageable? *Clin Perinatol* 1989;16:137.
24. Morin FC, Stenmark KR. Persistent pulmonary hypertension of the newborn. *Am J Respir Crit Care Med* 1995;151:2010.
25. Rabinowitz M. Structure and function of the pulmonary vascular bed: an update. *Cardiol Clin* 1989;7:227.
26. Bartlett RH, Gazzanigo AB, Huxtable RF, Schippers HC, O'Connor MJ, Jeffries MR. Extracorporeal circulation (ECMO) in neonatal respiratory failure. *J Thorac Cardiovasc Surg* 1977;74:826.
27. ECMO Life Support Organization. *ECMO registry.* Ann Arbor, MI: ECMO, 1992.
28. Ballard RA, Leonard CH. Developmental follow-up of infants with persistent pulmonary hypertension of the newborn. *Clin Perinatol* 1984;11:737.
29. Rosenberg AA, Kennaugh JM, Moreland SG, et al. Longitudinal follow up of a cohort of newborn infants treated with inhaled nitric oxide in persistent pulmonary hypertension. *J Pediatr* 1997;131:70.
30. Gaynes RP, Edwards JR, Jarvis WR, Culver DH, Tolson JS, Martor WJ, and the National Nosocomial Infection's Surveillance System. Nosocomial infections among neonates in high risk nurseries in the United States. *Pediatrics* 1996;98(3):357.
31. Zangwill KM, Schchat A, Wenger JD. Group B streptococcal disease in the United States 1990: report from a multistate active surveillance system. CDC surveillance summaries (Nov. 20). MMWR 1992;41(no. SS-6):25–32.
32. Baker CJ, Edwards MS. Group B streptococcal infections. In Remington J, Klein J. eds. *Infectious diseases of the fetus and newborn infant,* 4th ed. Philadelphia: WB Saunders, 1995:980–1054.
33. Boyer KM, Gotoff SP. Prevention of early onset neonatal group B streptococcal disease with selective intrapartum chemoprophylaxis. *N Engl J Med* 1986;314:1165.
34. Allen UD, Navas L, King SM. Effectiveness of intrapartum penicillin prophylaxis in preventing early-onset group B streptococcal infection: results of a meta-analysis. *Can Med Assoc J* 1993;149:1659.
35. Rojas J, Stahlman M. The effect of group B *Streptococcus* and other organisms on the pulmonary vasculature. *Clin Perinatol* 1984;11:591.
36. Burlington DB. *FDA safety alert: Risk of devices for direct detection of group B streptococci.* Washington, DC: FDA, 1997.
37. Whitley R, Arvin A, Prober C, et al. Predictors of morbidity and mortality among infants with herpes simplex virus infection. *N Engl J Med* 1991;324:453.
38. Whitley JR, Corey L, Arvin A, et al. Changing presentation of herpes simplex virus infection in neonates. *J Infect Dis* 1988;158:109.
39. Whitley R, Arvin A, Prober C, et al. A controlled trial comparing vidarabine with acyclovir in neonatal herpes simplex virus infection. *N Engl J Med* 1991;324:444.
40. Avery ME, Gatewood OB, Brumley G. Transient tachypnea of the newborn. *Am J Dis Child* 1966;111:380.
41. Madansky DL, Lawson EE, Chernick V, Taisusch HW. Pneumothorax and other forms of pulmonary air leak in newborns. *Am Rev Respir Dis* 1979;120:729.
42. Yu VYH, Wong PY, Bajuk B, Szymonowicz W. Pulmonary air leak in extremely low birthweight infants. *Arch Dis Child* 1986;61:239.

CHAPTER 29

Chronic Lung Disease

Jonathan M. Davis and Warren N. Rosenfeld

Bronchopulmonary dysplasia (BPD) is a chronic lung disease that develops in newborn infants treated with oxygen and positive-pressure mechanical ventilation for a primary lung disorder. The introduction of new treatment modalities (e.g., surfactant replacement therapy, high-frequency ventilation, extracorporeal membrane oxygenation) has significantly improved the outcome for many critically ill premature and term infants. As a result, more infants are surviving the newborn period and developing BPD. Approximately 7,500 new cases of BPD occur each year in the United States, and approximately 10% of these infants die in the first year of life. Bronchopulmonary dysplasia has become an extremely important complication of neonatal intensive care and the most common form of chronic lung disease in infants.

The modern history of BPD began with Northway's observations in 1967 (1). This study documented the clinical course, radiographic findings, and histopathologic lung changes in a group of infants who had received oxygen and ventilatory support for treatment of respiratory distress syndrome (RDS) and established the term bronchopulmonary dysplasia. Although Northway originally postulated that oxygen toxicity caused BPD, the exact mechanisms causing the lung injury are complex and not completely understood. Treatment with positive-pressure ventilation appears to be a critical factor in the development of BPD, although factors such as oxygen toxicity, prematurity, genetic predisposition, inflammation, and excessive fluid administration may also play important roles. Therapies for infants with BPD are directed toward improving the pathophysiologic abnormalities after they occur and include oxygen and mechanical ventilation, fluid restriction, diuretics, bronchodilators, and steroids.

J. M. Davis and W. N. Rosenfeld: Department of Pediatrics, State University of New York at Stony Brook School of Medicine, Stony Brook; Neonatology and Newborn Research; Cardiopulmonary Research Institute; and Department of Pediatrics, Winthrop-University Hospital, Mineola, New York

Many different therapies can be used in these infants, often concurrently. The optimal treatment and prevention strategies have not been established.

There has been significant debate about the exact definition of BPD, further complicated because the nature of BPD has changed with the widespread use of surfactant and other therapeutic interventions. The current form of BPD appears to be much less severe than in the past. There has been a significant decrease in the number of infants with BPD who require tracheostomy and prolonged (6 months or longer) mechanical ventilation at home or in a chronic care facility.

This chapter reviews the definition and incidence of BPD, its pathogenesis, pathophysiologic changes, treatment strategies, and long-term outcome. Newly developed approaches for the prevention of BPD in high-risk infants are presented.

DEFINITION AND INCIDENCE

In the original description of BPD, Northway defined chronic lung changes in a group of premature neonates who survived artificial ventilation for treatment of RDS (1). Northway reported 13 survivors of 32 neonates who had received mechanical ventilation. These infants had an average gestational age of 34 weeks and birth weight of 2.2 kg, distinctly different from most patients who now develop BPD.

Northway's definition of BPD included radiologic, pathologic, and clinical criteria. Bronchopulmonary dysplasia was divided into four developmental stages. The acute stages (i.e., I and II) were indistinguishable from RDS and were seen in the first 10 days of life. Stages III and IV marked the transition to the chronic stages of this disease, with the changes found in stage IV forming the basis for the definition of BPD. This stage described abnormalities that persisted beyond 1 month of age (i.e., 28 days) in patients who continued to require respiratory support (i.e., ventilation or oxygen supplementation). Chest radiographs demonstrated cyst formation and hyperexpansion alternating with areas of atelectasis.

As the care of neonates has become more sophisticated, and smaller, sicker infants have survived, the clinical and radiographic findings that define BPD have changed. Northway's original criteria depended heavily on a progression of radiographic changes, and clinical criteria were considered secondary. Further refinement was offered by Bancalari, whose criteria included ventilation for at least the first 3 days of life and respiratory symptoms (e.g., tachypnea, auscultatory rales, retractions) at 28 days of life, a need for supplemental oxygen to maintain a partial pressure (PaO$_2$) greater than 50 mm Hg and an abnormal chest radiograph at 28 days of life (2).

Many infants who eventually develop chronic lung disease do not require prolonged mechanical ventilation, nor do they have radiographs consistent with those described by Northway and Bancalari. Several studies have used less stringent criteria to define BPD such as simply the requirement for oxygen supplementation at 28 days of life (3,4). Shennan questioned the large number of normal neonates who would be included by this criterion and suggested that the need for additional oxygen at 36 weeks of postconceptual gestational age may be a more accurate predictor of ultimate pulmonary outcome (5). The definition of BPD may need to be more flexible and not restricted to a single point in time to properly define the patients who develop long-term pulmonary sequelae. This may require inclusion of patients with abnormal radiographs who require oxygen therapy for respiratory support at 28 days and those who continue to require supplemental oxygen at 36 weeks of postconceptual age.

The incidence of BPD depends on the definition used and the patient population studied. Several surfactant replacement trials have reported significantly improved survival for 750-g to 1,500-g infants with RDS after surfactant replacement therapy (6–11). This is true regardless of the type of the surfactant used (e.g., human, synthetic, surfactant-TA). The incidence of BPD, defined as oxygen dependency at 28 days with appropriate radiographic findings, was in the range of 19% to 63% for the control groups in these studies. The surfactant treatment groups had a similar incidence of BPD, in the range of 11% to 57%. It appeared from these studies that the incidence of BPD would decrease only slightly after surfactant therapy. However, the prevalence, or total number of infants with BPD, would be expected to increase because of improved survival. Fenton and associates subsequently reported that exogenous surfactant had significantly improved the survival of many low-birth-weight infants in their geographically defined population but was actually associated with a marked increase in the incidence of BPD (12). Bronchopulmonary dysplasia will continue to be an important problem for the neonatologist and pedi-

atric pulmonologist in the future. Further study of the mechanisms involved in the lung injury process and the development of possible prevention strategies are needed.

PATHOGENESIS

No single factor has been identified as the cause of BPD. Its origin is multifactorial and may depend on the nature of the injury, mechanisms of response, or the infant's inability to respond appropriately to the injury process. Northway attributed the occurrence of BPD to prolonged hyperoxia in infants with RDS (1). Since this original hypothesis, numerous other causes have been proposed.

Barotrauma/Volutrauma

With the introduction of positive-pressure ventilation for the treatment of RDS, ventilatory pressures capable of causing pathologic changes were transmitted to the lung. Although the initial phases of lung injury in BPD are the result of the primary disease process (e.g., RDS), superimposed positive-pressure mechanical ventilation appears to add to the lung injury and provoke a complex inflammatory cascade that ultimately leads to chronic lung disease. Barotrauma is the term generally used to describe the lung injury that occurs secondary to positive-pressure mechanical ventilation. Recently, some investigators have suggested that volutrauma from excessive tidal volume ventilation may be a more appropriate term to describe this lung injury process (13).

The role of barotrauma in BPD depends on several factors, including the structure of the tracheobronchial tree and the physiologic effects of surfactant deficiency. With surfactant deficiency, surface tension forces are elevated, aeration is unequal, and most terminal alveoli are largely collapsed. The pressure needed to distend these poorly compliant saccules is high is and transmitted to the terminal bronchioles and alveolar ducts. In the premature neonate, these airways are highly compliant and subject to rupture, as demonstrated by Ackerman (14). Gas then dissects into the interstitium, where it is trapped, resulting in the development of pulmonary interstitial emphysema (PIE). The occurrence of PIE increases the relative risk of developing BPD sixfold.

Whether the acute injury that leads to the development of BPD is caused by direct trauma from positive-pressure ventilation or the toxic effects of oxygen supplementation is difficult to differentiate. Nilsson and colleagues showed that even brief periods of positive-pressure ventilation can cause bronchiolar epithelial damage in the lung (15). The severity of the injury appeared to correlate well with the amount of peak pressure used. Davis and associates demonstrated that short periods of positive-pressure ventilation with relatively low inspiratory pressures were associated with compromised cell integrity in the lung, resulting in increased permeability to albumin and other proteins (16). Few other studies have been able to separate the relative contribution of barotrauma from oxygen toxicity. Davis and colleagues demonstrated that the changes of acute lung injury that precede the development of BPD were minimal in neonatal piglets subjected to positive-pressure ventilation with room air, but they were much more significant if 100% oxygen was used (17). This suggests that the damaging effects of oxygen and mechanical ventilation are additive and possibly synergistic.

Strategies to prevent barotrauma and PIE have resulted in frequent changes in methods of ventilation. Early attempts at negative-pressure ventilation successfully minimized barotrauma, but this form of ventilation was impractical and difficult to control. Recently, Samuels reported a trial of continuous negative extrathoracic pressure (CNEP) in 244 neonates with respiratory failure (18). Although fewer surviving infants treated with CNEP developed BPD, secondary analyses did show a nonsignificant increase in mortality, cranial ultrasound abnormalities, and pneumothoraces in this study group. Synchronized mechanical ventilators (SIMV) and high-frequency devices that employ rates from 120 to 1,200 cycles/min have also been developed. Bernstein and associates reported that infants (<1,000 g) receiving SIMV developed significantly less BPD than did those receiving conventional ventilation (19). A major indication for the use of high-frequency ventilators is the prevention or treatment of pulmonary barotrauma. One multicenter study failed to demonstrate that high-frequency oscillatory ventilation (HFOV) provided any advantage over conventional ventilation in the initial treatment of RDS (20). However, another smaller study did show that initial treatment with HFOV reduced the incidence of BPD (21). A randomized, controlled trial of high-frequency jet ventilation (HFJV) demonstrated that complications of pulmonary barotrauma (e.g., PIE, pneumothorax) resolved more rapidly in infants treated with HFJV than those treated with conventional ventilation (22). Another randomized trial of HFJV in infants with RDS by Keszler and colleagues found a lower incidence of BPD in infants receiving early HFJV compared to those with conventional ventilation (23). The high-frequency devices appear to be more effective in optimizing lung volume and maintaining alveolar recruitment, thus reducing lung injury and BPD. Regardless of the type of ventilation strategy used, it is imperative to avoid even brief periods of hyperventilation because hypocarbia appears to increase the risk for the development of both BPD and central nervous system abnormalities (24,25).

The major advance in the prevention of pulmonary barotrauma has been the introduction of surfactant replacement therapy. Surfactant permits more equal distribution of pressures and ventilation to all alveoli, prevents overdistention of air spaces and bronchioles, and stabilizes airways. A major benefit of surfactant therapy has been the reduction of ventilator pressures and pulmonary air leak. However, BPD continues to be a serious problem, suggesting that barotrauma is only one of many factors involved in the pathogenesis of BPD.

Oxygen and Antioxidants

Under normal conditions, a delicate balance exists between the production of free radicals and the antioxidant defenses that protect cells *in vivo*. Free radicals are molecules with extra electrons in their outer ring, and they are toxic to living tissues (Table 29–1). Oxygen has a unique molecular structure and is abundant within cells. It readily accepts free electrons generated by oxidative metabolism within the cell, producing free radicals. The balance may be disturbed by increased free-radical production under conditions of hyperoxia, reperfusion, or inflammation. Alternatively, free radicals can increase because of an inability to quench production because of inadequate antioxidant defenses. Damage caused by oxygen free radicals ranges from cell membrane destruction to the unraveling of nucleic acids.

The premature neonate may be more susceptible to free-radical damage because adequate concentrations of antioxidants may be absent at birth. Frank and associates documented the development of the antioxidant enzymes superoxide dismutase (SOD), catalase, and glutathione peroxidase in the lungs of rabbits during late gestation (Fig. 29–1) (26). The 150% increase in these enzymes during the last 15% of gestation parallels the maturation pattern of pulmonary surfactant. These developmental changes in the fetal lung allow proper ventilation by reducing surface tension and provide for the transition from the relative hypoxia of intrauterine development to the oxygen-rich extrauterine environment. Premature birth before the development of sufficient antioxidant enzymes may expose the neonate to supraphysiologic concentrations of oxygen and increase the risk for the development of BPD. Further evidence for the role of free oxygen radicals in lung injury comes from animal studies, which have shown that antioxidant supplementation

TABLE 29–1. *Free radicals*

Radical	Symbol[a]	Antioxidant
Superoxide anion	O_2^-	Superoxide dismutase, uric acid, vitamin E
Singlet oxygen	$^1O_2$	β-carotene, uric acid, vitamin E
Hydrogen peroxide	H_2O_2	Catalase, glutathione peroxidase, glutathione
Hydroxyl radical	OH•	Vitamins C and E
Peroxide radical	LOO•	Vitamins C and E
Hydroperoxyl radical	LOOH	Glutathione transferase, glutathione peroxidase

[a]L, lipid.

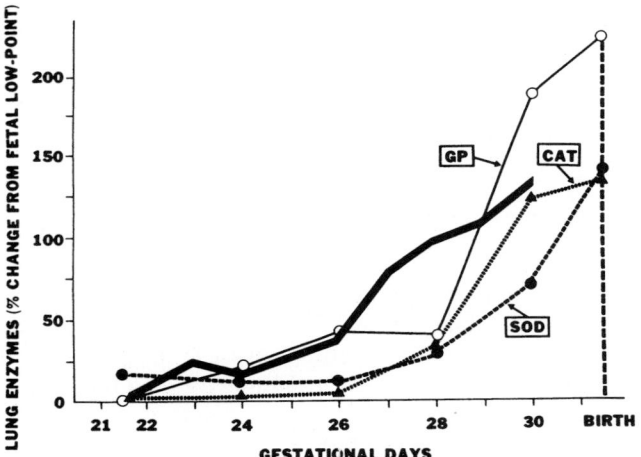

FIG. 29–1. Developmental changes in antioxidant levels and activity during gestation. The increases in superoxide dismutase (SOD), catalase (CAT), and glutathione peroxidase (GP) late in gestation are similar to those seen for pulmonary surfactant (*dark, thick line*). (From ref. 26.)

with SOD and catalase reduces cell damage, increases survival, and prevents lung injury from prolonged hyperoxia and mechanical ventilation (27–29). Genetically engineered mice overexpressing either CuZnSOD or MnSOD survive longer, whereas mice with disrupted CuZnSOD genes die more quickly in a hyperoxic environment compared to normal diploid controls (30–32). These findings confirm the role of free oxygen radicals in the development of lung injury.

Oxygen radicals have also been shown to be directly involved in the pathogenesis of BPD. Expired pentane

and ethane have been measured as indirect evidence of free-radical-induced lipid peroxidation in the first week of life and were found to be significantly elevated in neonates subsequently developing BPD (33). Similarly, plasma concentration of allantoin, an oxidation by-product of uric acid, has been shown to be significantly elevated in the first 48 hours of life in infants developing BPD compared to controls (34). Finally, Varsila and colleagues analyzed proteins in tracheal aspirates in the first week of life and found evidence of protein oxidation (carbonylation) in infants developing chronic lung disease (35). These studies all demonstrate that free oxygen radicals are intimately involved in the development of acute and chronic lung disease in newborn infants.

Inflammation

Inflammation appears to play an important role in the pathogenesis of BPD and allows many factors to be unified into a single cause of this disease. Inflammatory mediators and cellular responses are outlined in Fig. 29–2, and they have been found to be prominent in animal models of lung injury and in infants who develop BPD.

Bronchopulmonary dysplasia appears to begin as a cascade of destruction and abnormal repair that results in acute lung injury, followed by the development of chronic lung disease. The initial stimuli activating the inflammatory process in the lung may be oxygen free radicals, pulmonary barotrauma, infectious agents, or other stimuli that result in the attraction and activation of leukocytes. This leukocyte infiltration appears to occur before the development of significant pathophysiologic abnormali-

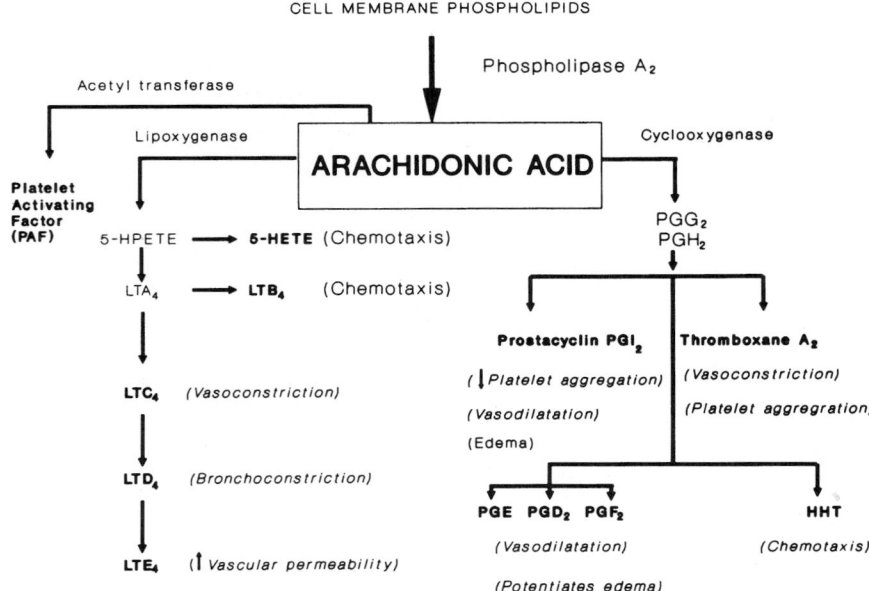

FIG. 29–2. Schematic representation of the metabolism of cell membrane lipids to arachidonic acid, which initiates the inflammatory cascade. The various metabolic pathways are shown with the agents that are produced and their function in the inflammatory process. HETE, hydroxyeicosatetraenoic acid; HHT, heptadecatrienoic acid; HPETE, hydroxyperoxyeicosatrienoic acid; LT, leukotriene; PG, prostaglandin.

ties and has been demonstrated by tagging leukocytes with indium-111 and by inspection of tracheobronchial effluent and bronchoalveolar lavage (36–38). Activated leukocytes are predominantly neutrophils and macrophages, both of which have the potential for further release of a variety of inflammatory mediators (38–40). There is also evidence suggesting that eosinophils may play a role in this inflammatory process and thus contribute to the development of BPD (41).

Among the toxic products released are the lipid products from plasma membranes that are metabolized predominantly to arachidonic acid and lysoplatelet-activating factor (see Fig. 29–2). Arachidonic acid may be catalyzed by lipoxygenase, giving rise to various cytokines and leukotrienes. Alternatively, it may be altered by cyclooxygenase to produce thromboxane, prostaglandin, or prostacyclin. These products have potent vasoactive and inflammatory properties and usually appear in elevated concentrations in tracheal aspirates within a few hours of life in infants subsequently developing BPD (40–42). These agents and the activated leukocytes that accompany them cause significant pulmonary damage, including breakdown of capillary endothelial integrity and leakage of larger molecules (e.g., albumin) into alveolar spaces. Albumin leakage and associated pulmonary edema have been postulated to be important factors in the development of BPD (43).

The release of elastase and collagenase from activated neutrophils directly destroys the elastin and collagen framework of the lung. The breakdown products of collagen (i.e., hydroxyproline) and elastin (i.e., desmosine) have been recovered in the urine of infants who develop BPD (44). The major defense against the action of elastase activity is α_1-proteinase inhibitor, which may be inactivated by oxygen radicals (45). Increased elastase activity accompanied by compromised antiproteinase function may enhance lung injury (46). This combination has been demonstrated in tracheal aspirates and serum of neonates who develop BPD (38,47,48). Therapy with exogenous antiproteases could potentially restore this delicate balance and prevent the development of BPD. This hypothesis has been tested in a pilot study in which very premature neonates requiring assisted ventilation were treated with intravenous doses of α_1-proteinase inhibitor over the first 2 weeks of life (49). There was a trend toward reductions in both the incidence of BPD and the need for continued ventilatory support with α_1-proteinase inhibitor treatment. Further studies examining the safety and efficacy of various doses are currently under way.

As the acute cycle of injury continues with further production and accumulation of inflammatory mediators, significant injury to the lung can occur during a particularly critical period of rapid growth (i.e., the six divisions from 24 to 40 weeks of gestation). It appears likely that this abnormal inflammatory process is primarily respon-sible for the acute and the chronic changes that occur in the lungs of infants with BPD.

Infection

Ureaplasma urealyticum has been recovered from cervical cultures of pregnant women and implicated as a possible cause of chorioamnionitis, prematurity, and BPD (50,51). Cassell and colleagues cultured tracheal aspirates and blood and found that BPD developed in 82% of infants (<1,000 g) colonized with *Ureaplasma,* compared with 41% of those with negative cultures (50). In contrast, other studies have found that although *Ureaplasma* was frequently detected (by culture or polymerase chain reaction) in many low-birth-weight infants, its presence was not associated with the development of BPD (52,53). Others have suggested that infection acts as a stimulus for the inflammatory response, with recruitment of leukocytes and activation of the arachidonic acid cascade, ultimately leading to BPD (54). Normal defense mechanisms against infection can be compromised in the lungs of chronically ventilated, premature infants. This makes them more susceptible to colonization and subsequent infection with a variety of infectious agents (e.g., virus, bacteria, fungi) that may affect the severity of BPD (55).

Nutrition

The nutritional status of the sick premature infant may play several roles in the development of BPD. Adequate calories and essential nutrients for growth may be lacking during a period of stress and growth; vital components for immunologic and antioxidant defenses may be inadequate; and the nutritional supplements provided may actually contribute to ongoing damage.

Premature infants have increased nutritional requirements because of increased metabolic needs and rapid growth requirements. Superimposed acute and chronic lung disease may further increase energy expenditures by 25% (i.e., increased work of breathing) in infants with limited nutritional reserves (56). If these increased energy needs are not met, the infant will develop a catabolic state, which is probably a major contributing factor in the pathogenesis of BPD. Inadequate nutrition, which could interfere with normal growth and maturation of the lung, may potentiate the deleterious effects of oxygen and barotrauma. Newborn rats with inadequate caloric intake have decreased lung weights, protein levels, and DNA content (57). These abnormalities were even greater in pups that were nutritionally deprived at birth and exposed to hyperoxia.

Antioxidant enzymes may play a vital role in the protection of the lung and the prevention of BPD. Many of these enzymes have trace elements (e.g., copper, zinc, selenium) that are an integral part of their structure. Deficiencies in these elements may compromise the premature infant's defenses and predispose the lung to further injury (58). Supplementation with these elements may provide protection to the lung and prevent hyperoxic lung injury (59). The repair of elastin and collagen is limited in animals who are undernourished, and copper and zinc may be necessary for this repair (60). Vitamin deficiency has been postulated to be important in the development of BPD. Increasing serum levels of vitamin E, a natural antioxidant that prevents peroxidation of lipid membranes, was initially thought to prevent BPD (61). However, subsequent clinical trials have been unable to demonstrate any positive effect of supraphysiologic concentrations of vitamin E in the prevention of chronic lung disease (62,63). Current nursery feeding and hyperalimentation regimens appear to provide adequate amounts of vitamin E for preterm and term infants.

Concentrations of vitamin A (i.e., retinol) may be deficient in premature neonates younger than 36 weeks of gestation (64–66). This vitamin appears to be important in maintaining cell integrity and in tissue repair. Its deficiency has been associated with changes in the ciliated epithelium of the tracheobronchial tree (67). Hustead and associates demonstrated lower serum retinol levels in cord blood and at day 21 of life in infants who developed BPD (66). Similarly, Shenai and colleagues demonstrated lower plasma retinol concentrations in the first month of life in infants who subsequently developed BPD (68). Despite adequate supplementation, some infants remain vitamin A–deficient, presumably from increased absorption of parenteral vitamin A into the tubing of the intravenous administration set or from higher nutritional requirements (69). A large, multicenter trial of vitamin A supplementation in premature infants at risk for developing BPD has recently been completed and will, we hope, determine if vitamin A deficiency is an important contributor to lung injury.

Large volumes of intravenous fluids are often administered to premature infants to provide adequate fluid requirements (from increased insensible water losses) and sufficient calories. Excessive fluid administration can be associated with the development of a patent ductus arteriosus and pulmonary edema, which can lead to an increase in oxygen and ventilator requirements and the subsequent risk of BPD (55,70). Early closure of the ductus, using indomethacin or surgical ligation, has been associated with improvements in pulmonary function, but these approaches have not affected the incidence of chronic lung disease (71).

Genetics

Numerous investigators have observed that neonates were more likely to develop BPD if there was a strong family history of atopy and asthma. Nickerson and Taussig found a positive family history of asthma in 77% of infants with RDS who subsequently developed BPD,

compared with only 33% who did not (72). Bertrand evaluated the relationship of prematurity, RDS, and need for mechanical ventilation to a family history of airway hyperactivity (73). The severity of lung disease was directly related to the degree of prematurity and the duration of oxygen exposure. However, siblings and mothers of infants with the most significant lung disease had evidence of airway reactivity, suggesting that all three factors are involved in determining long-term outcome. When histocompatibility loci (HLA) were examined, Clark and associates found that only infants with HLA-A2 developed BPD, again suggesting that other underlying factors that are poorly understood may be important in the pathogenesis of BPD (74). More recently, Hagan reported that a family history of asthma is associated with an increase in the overall severity of BPD in premature infants but does not appear to be a causative factor (75).

PATHOPHYSIOLOGIC CHANGES

Infants with BPD demonstrate abnormal findings on clinical examination, chest radiograph, pulmonary function testing, echocardiogram, and morphologic examination of the lung. The severity of BPD is directly proportional to the degree of the pathophysiologic insult and can be assessed through all of these techniques. Determining the severity of BPD is complex and has been the subject of several workshops sponsored by the National Institutes of Health and many publications. Several scoring systems have been developed to address this important issue.

Clinical Assessment

A clinical scoring system to help evaluate the severity of BPD was developed by Toce and colleagues (Table 29–2) (76). Infants with BPD are tachypneic and may have intercostal and subcostal retractions. Accessory muscles may be used to assist with respiration. Infants can be hypoxic and hypercarbic and may grow poorly despite adequate caloric intake. The Toce system attempts to standardize clinical assessment, and a severity score can be assigned to each infant at 28 days of postnatal age and at 36 weeks of postconceptual age. The clinical assessment should be adjusted if infants are receiving multiple medications for their BPD (e.g., diuretics, methylxanthines, and steroids), nasal continuous positive airway pressure, or positive-pressure mechanical ventilation.

Radiographic Abnormalities

Radiographic abnormalities characteristic of BPD were first described by Northway and associates in 1967 (1). A staging system was employed that documented the progression of the disease process through four distinct stages. The first stage was similar to uncomplicated RDS

TABLE 29–2. *Bronchopulmonary dysplasia clinical scoring system*

Variable	Score[a]			
	0 (Normal)	1 (Mild)	2 (Moderate)	3 (Severe)
Respiratory rate (average number/min)	<40	40–60	61–80	>80
Dyspnea (retractions)	0	Mild	Moderate	Severe
FiO_2 (PaO_2 50–70 mm Hg)	0.21	0.22–0.30	0.31–0.50	>0.50
$PaCO_2$ (mm Hg)	<45	46–55	56–70	>70
Growth rate (g/day)	>25	15–24	5–14	<5

[a]Score at 28 days of age or at 36 weeks of postconceptual age. Score is a mean of four measures for respiratory rate, dyspnea, and FiO_2 obtained at 6-hr intervals. Growth rate represents average daily weight gain over a 7-day period before the assignment of the score. Highest score is 15. A score of 15 is assigned if the patient is receiving mechanical ventilation. From Ref 76.

and occurred in the first few days of life. The BPD often progressed to pulmonary parenchymal opacities (stage II), a bubbly appearance (stage III), and then, finally, to an inhomogeneous appearance with marked hyperinflation, bleb formation, irregular fibrous streaks, and cardiomegaly (stage IV).

The radiographic progression of BPD is now seldom categorized by these four stages (Fig. 29–3). The radiographic classification of BPD was refined by Edwards and colleagues and then by Toce and associates to reflect the severity of the disease process (Table 29–3) (76,77). The system is based on the four most prominent radiographic findings in BPD, including lung expansion, emphysema (including bleb formation), interstitial densities, and cardiovascular abnormalities. The more severe the changes, the higher the score (maximum possible score of 10). The occurrence of hyperinflation or interstitial abnormalities on chest radiograph appears to correlate well with the development of airway obstruction later in life (78). Because the severity of BPD has continued to

change so significantly over the past 10 years, Weinstein developed a new scoring system that incorporates some of the more subtle radiographic signs that are often seen today in infants with BPD (79).

Computed tomography and magnetic resonance imaging may provide more detail of the pathologic process occurring in the lung. Computed tomography can reveal significant abnormalities that are not readily apparent on chest radiographs and can be important in determining ultimate pulmonary morbidity (Fig. 29–4) (80).

Cardiovascular Changes

The pulmonary circulation in infants with BPD can be abnormal, with endothelial cell degeneration and proliferation, medial muscle hypertrophy, peripheral extension of smooth muscle, and vascular obliteration (81). These lesions are more significant in older infants dying of severe BPD. The vascular alterations lead to increased pulmonary vascular pressures and pulmonary vascular resistance with the development of cor pulmonale. Serial electrocardiograms may reveal evidence of right ventricular hypertrophy (i.e., indirect evidence of pulmonary hypertension) (82). Echocardiograms may show elevated right ventricular systolic time intervals (RSTI) or, in more severe cases, left ventricular and septal wall thickening consistent with concentric left ventricular hypertrophy (83). Left ventricular hypertrophy may also be seen in neonates being treated with dexamethasone (84). Persistent right ventricular hypertrophy, elevated RSTI, or fixed pulmonary hypertension unresponsive to O_2 supplementation on cardiac catheterization have been associated with a poor prognosis (85).

Changes in Pulmonary Mechanics

The development of computerized pulmonary function systems has enabled more accurate measurements of pulmonary mechanics in newborn infants with BPD. In the early stages of BPD, an increase in pulmonary resistance and airway reactivity can be demonstrated (86). As the disease progresses in severity, airway obstruction can

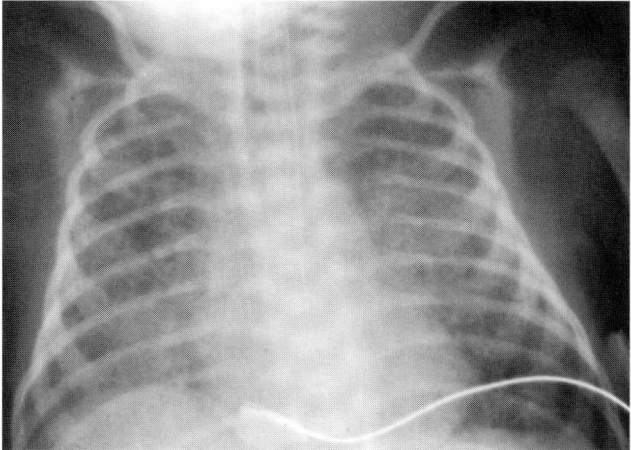

FIG. 29–3. Typical chest radiograph of a 1-month-old infant with bronchopulmonary dysplasia. The bilateral hazy appearance represents inflammatory exudate, edema, and atelectasis.

TABLE 29–3. *Roentgenographic scoring system for severity of bronchopulmonary dysplasia*

	Score[a]		
Variable	0	1	2
Cardiovascular abnormalities	None	Cardiomegaly	Gross cardiomegaly or RVH or enlarged MPA
Hyperexpansion (anterior plus posterior rib count)	≤14	14.5–16	≤16.5, or flattened hemidiaphragms
Emphysema	No focal areas	Scattered, small, abnormal lucencies	At least one large bleb or bulla
Fibrosis or interstitial abnormalities	None	Interstitial prominence; few abnormal, streaky densities	Dense fibrotic bands, many abnormal strands
Subjective	Mild	Moderate	Severe

[a]Rib counts intersecting level of the dome of the right hemidiaphragm. MPA, main pulmonary artery; RVH, right ventricular hypertrophy. From ref. 76.

become more significant, with expiratory flow limitation seen on flow–volume curves (Fig. 29–5) (87). Airway constriction can occur secondary to hypoxia and can be demonstrated with cold air provocation testing (88). The increased resistance may cause increased work of breathing and marked abnormalities in ventilation–perfusion matching. Functional residual capacity can be reduced initially because of atelectasis, but it can be elevated in later stages of BPD because of excessive air trapping and hyperinflation.

Two methods used to measure lung compliance include dynamic measurement and passive expiratory techniques after airway occlusion (89). Both methods show a reduction of lung compliance in infants with BPD. The decrease in lung compliance appears to correlate well with morphologic changes in the lung (e.g., atelectasis, edema, fibrosis). Compliance can be reduced because of increased resistance, with frequency dependence of compliance when infants are breathing rapidly (90).

The use of pulmonary function testing to follow the progression of BPD and the response of the lung to various therapeutic interventions has become widespread, but care must be used in the interpretation of results because of inherent variability in the measurement and possible error from excessive chest wall distortion (91,92).

Pathologic Changes

Detailed morphologic and biochemical analyses of lungs of infants with BPD have recently been completed by Cherukupalli and associates (93). They suggested that BPD proceeds as a continuous process through four distinct pathologic stages from acute lung injury, which is characterized by an exudative phase, to proliferative and reparative phases. If the reparative processes are successful, then BPD may resolve spontaneously. However, if lung growth and repair do not proceed normally, BPD can become significantly more severe.

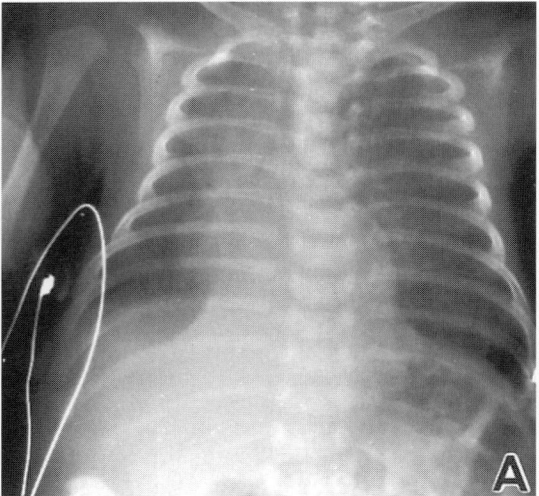
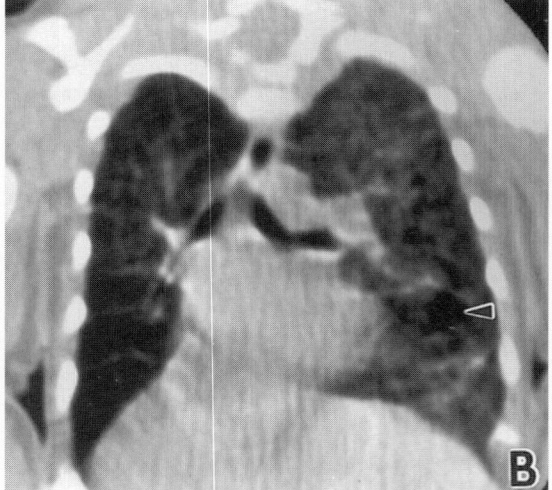

FIG. 29–4. A: Chest radiograph of a 2-month-old infant with bronchopulmonary dysplasia, showing right-sided atelectasis and a shift of the mediastinum. The lung fields have a hazy appearance. **B:** Computed tomography scan on the same infant. The major bronchi and areas of atelectasis are apparent. Fibrotic changes and a bleb are seen on the left (*arrow*).

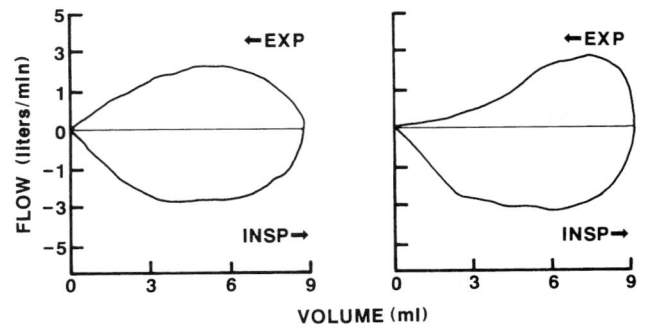

A

B

FIG. 29–5. A: Normal flow–volume loop. **B:** Expiratory flow limitation as a result of dynamic collapse of small airways during expiration. INSP, inspiration; EXP, expiration.

Airways

The large upper airways (i.e., trachea, main bronchi) of infants with BPD may reveal significant abnormalities, depending on the duration of intubation and positive-pressure ventilation. Grossly, mucosal edema or necrosis can be seen and may be focal or more diffuse (94). Necrotic areas may break down into frank ulcerations. Many of these changes are similar to those seen in necrotizing tracheobronchitis. The earliest histologic changes include patchy loss of cilia from columnar epithelial cells. These cells may become dysplastic or necrotic, resulting in breakdown of the epithelial lining. Necrotic areas may involve the mucosa alone or extend into the submucosa. Infiltration of inflammatory cells such as neutrophils and lymphocytes into these areas may be prominent. Goblet cells may become hyperplastic, resulting in increased production of mucus, which becomes mixed with dense cellular debris. Granulation tissue may develop in areas that have been damaged by the presence of the endotracheal tube or from repeated suctioning procedures. Mucosal cells may regenerate or ultimately be replaced by stratified squamous epithelium or metaplastic epithelium if the injury process continues (Fig. 29–6).

The most significant pathologic changes occurring in infants with BPD are seen in the terminal bronchioles and alveolar ducts. Hyaline membranes that appear during the acute phase of RDS become covered with a thin, dysplastic epithelial lining made up primarily of type II pneumocytes. These membranes may then become incorporated into the underlying airway. Edema, inflammation, exudate, and necrosis of epithelial cells can occur as the process continues. Necrotizing bronchiolitis may occur if the damage is particularly severe. Cellular debris, inflammatory cells, and proteinaceous exudate accumulate and obstruct many of the terminal airways; this process may actually be beneficial because it protects the distal alveoli from further damage from oxygen and mechanical ventilation. Fibroblast proliferation and activation in response to this insult may lead to peribronchial fibrosis and obliterative fibroproliferative bronchiolitis (Fig. 29–7). Smooth muscle hypertrophy may also occur, which causes narrowing of some airways and further obstruction in others.

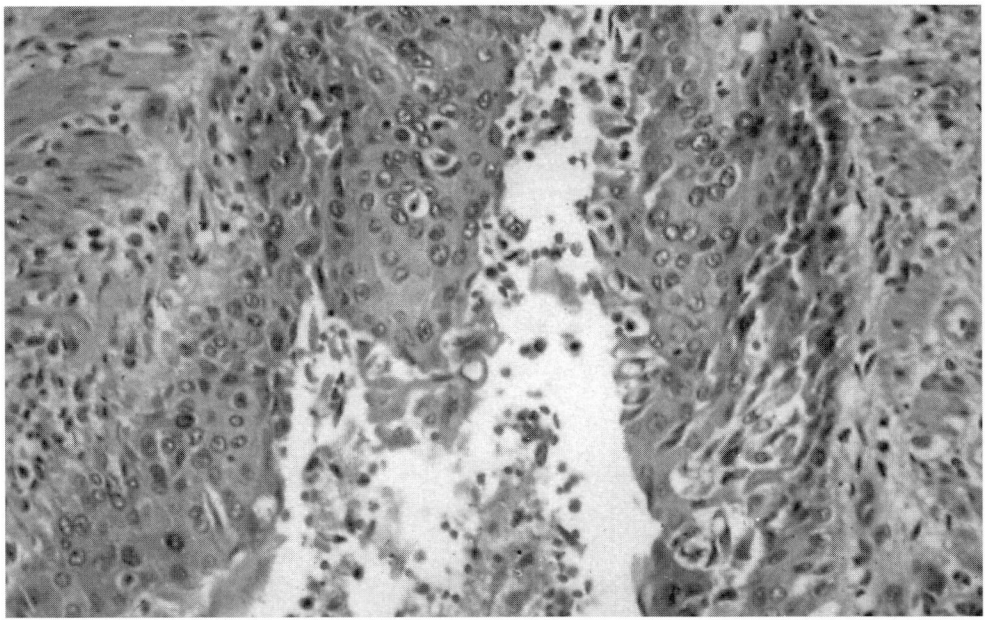

FIG. 29–6. Light micrograph from a 3-month-old infant with bronchopulmonary dysplasia shows squamous metaplasia and smooth muscle hypertrophy of a small airway. (Original magnification × 20.)

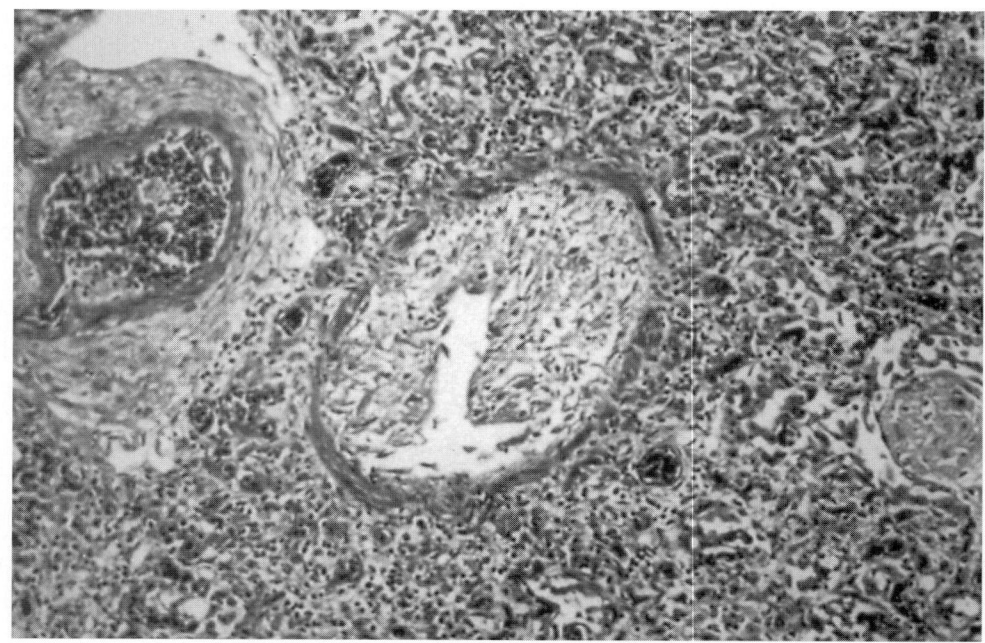

FIG. 29–7. Light micrograph from a 1-month-old infant with bronchopulmonary dysplasia shows fibrosis of a small airway. (Connective tissue stain; original magnification × 10.)

Alveoli

The earliest findings seen in the alveoli involve interstitial or alveolar edema. Focal areas of atelectasis, inflammation, exudate, and fibroblast proliferation develop later. As the disease progresses and becomes more severe, normal alveolar architecture is disrupted with areas of atelectasis becoming more widespread and alternating with areas of marked hyperinflation (Fig. 29–8). These hyperinflated areas can become emphysematous blebs. Destruction of alveoli can occur with resulting alveolar hypoplasia and a decrease in surface

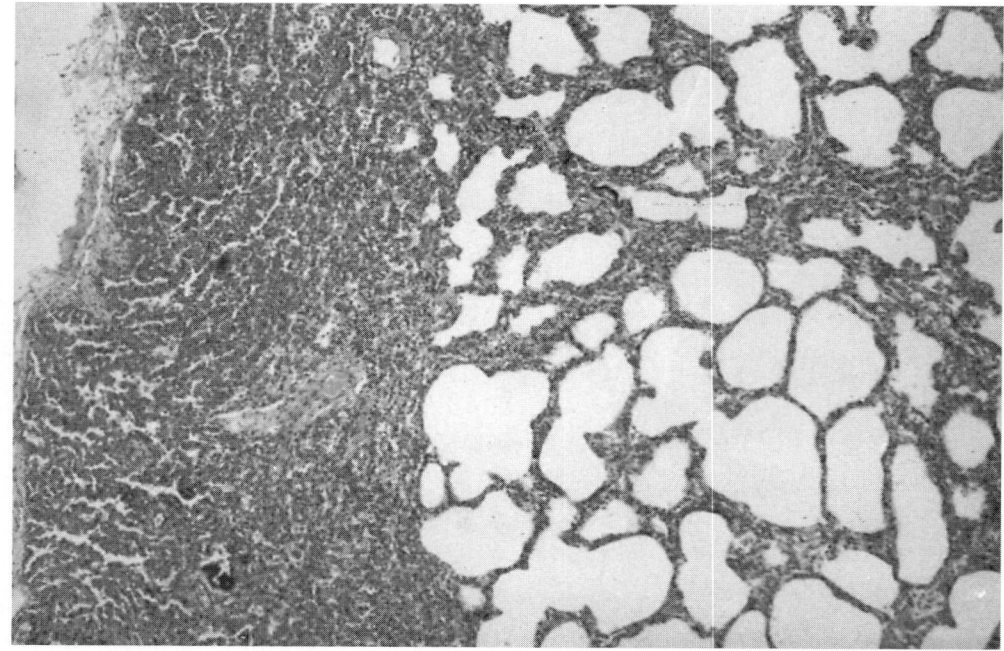

FIG. 29–8. Light micrograph from a 1-year-old infant with bronchopulmonary dysplasia shows areas of atelectasis alternating with areas of hyperinflation. (Original magnification × 4.)

area available for gas exchange. Interstitial and alveolar fibrosis can become more widespread. Capillary beds may be severely damaged, and, with medial muscle hypertrophy of pulmonary arterioles, these changes lead to marked pulmonary hypertension.

MANAGEMENT

The current approach to infants with BPD is multidisciplinary and directed toward improving the complex pathophysiologic abnormalities that have been previously described. The major treatment approaches are described in the following sections.

Mechanical Ventilation

Positive-pressure mechanical ventilation has been implicated in the pathogenesis of BPD (see Chapters 27 and 29), but the benefits from continued ventilation outweigh the risks of continued progression of chronic lung damage. Arterial blood gases should be optimally maintained with a pH of 7.25 to 7.40, PCO_2 of 45 to 60 mm Hg, and PO_2 of 55 to 70 mm Hg (95). The best method of assessing adequate oxygenation and ventilation is an arterial blood gas obtained from an indwelling arterial catheter when the infant is quiet. Intermittent arterial puncture may be accurate if obtained quickly or if local anesthesia is used, but it may not be representative if the infant is awake and agitated. Capillary blood gases should not be used to make significant therapeutic decisions because of wide variability and poor correlation with arterial blood gases (96). However, if samples are obtained properly (i.e., after adequate warming and without squeezing the heel or finger), the pH and PCO_2 may correlate with arterial values. The use of pulse oximetry and transcutaneous CO_2 measurements can assist in ventilatory management and may reflect arterial values. End-tidal CO_2 measurements may not correlate well with arterial values in infants with significant ventilation–perfusion mismatch and chronic lung disease. As mentioned previously, hypocarbia and hyperventilation may increase the risk for BPD and should be avoided (24).

Because oxygen appears to cause more significant lung damage than mechanical ventilation in animals, sufficient mean airway pressure should be used to avoid atelectasis and, if possible, maintain the fraction of inspired oxygen (FiO_2) at less than 0.5. With conventional, time-cycled ventilation, an inspiratory time of 0.4 to 0.5 seconds optimizes ventilation and improves pulmonary function (97). Inspired gas temperature should be maintained from 36.5°C to 37.5°C to ensure adequate humidity and minimize core temperature fluctuations and the progression of chronic lung disease (98).

Weaning infants with BPD from mechanical ventilation is often difficult and should be done slowly. When peak inspiratory pressures have been reduced to approximately 15 to 20 cm H_2O and FiO_2 to less than 0.4 with acceptable blood gases, the ventilator rate should be reduced slowly to allow the infant to gradually breathe more independently. This is essential because prolonged ventilation may be associated with atrophy of the muscle fibers of the diaphragm and increased diaphragmatic fatigue (99). When infants have been weaned to a ventilator rate of 10 to 20 breaths/min, infants should be extubated. With some forms of synchronized mechanical ventilation, the infant is allowed to set his/her own inspiratory time and respiratory rate. Weaning infants from this type of ventilation involves reducing the inspiratory pressure as previously described. Analysis of pulmonary mechanics before extubation does not appear to be useful in determining optimal time of extubation because multiple factors (e.g., central inspiratory drive, diaphragmatic endurance, chest wall stability) may be important (100). Infants should not be weaned to continuous endotracheal tube positive airway pressure (CPAP) because increased airway resistance and work of breathing can cause fatigue, apnea, and CO_2 retention (101). The use of methylxanthines before extubation or nasal CPAP just after extubation may facilitate successful extubation (102,103). Higgins and colleagues demonstrated that infants weighing less than 1,000 g were almost four times as likely to be successfully extubated on the first attempt when nasal CPAP was used compared with an oxyhood (76% versus 21%) (103). Chest physiotherapy and suctioning should be performed frequently to maintain a patent airway and prevent atelectasis.

Prolonged intubation and ventilation may be associated with the development of airway abnormalities (e.g., subglottic stenosis, tracheomalacia) (104). These should be considered in infants who rapidly and repeatedly fail attempts at extubation. A bronchoscopic evaluation should be performed in these infants or in any infant intubated for more than 2 to 3 months who continues to require prolonged ventilation. Surgical intervention (e.g., cricoid split, tracheostomy) should be performed as needed.

Oxygen

In infants with BPD, chronic hypoxia results in pulmonary vasoconstriction, pulmonary hypertension, and the development of cor pulmonale. This contributes significantly to the morbidity and mortality of BPD. Elevated pulmonary artery pressures and pulmonary vascular resistance have been described in infants with BPD undergoing cardiac catheterization (85,95,105). A significant reduction in pulmonary pressures were found when oxygen was administered. Oxygen is now known to act as a pulmonary vasodilator by stimulating the production of an endothelial-derived relaxing factor, which appears to be nitric oxide (NO) (106). The NO diffuses into the vascular smooth muscle and stimulates the production of cGMP, which causes vasodilation by sequestering calcium. Ideally, PO_2 should be maintained between 55 and 70 mm Hg in infants with BPD.

Pulse oximetry has become the most popular noninvasive method of neonatal oxygen monitoring. Pulse oximeters are most accurate when operating along the steep portion of the oxygen–hemoglobin dissociation curve and may be more reliable than PO_2 (107). Keeping the oxygen saturation (SO_2) between 90% to 95% should exclude values of PO_2 that are less than 45 mm Hg or greater than 100 mm Hg. Careful monitoring of oxygen status is essential because hypoxia can cause pulmonary hypertension, increased airway constriction, and growth failure. Repeated episodes of oxygen desaturation often develop in premature neonates with BPD during mechanical ventilation (108). This appears to be related to a decrease in central respiratory drive and alterations in pulmonary mechanics. Prone positioning has been shown to increase SO_2 and decrease the frequency of hypoxemic episodes (109). Hyperoxia may worsen BPD or increase the risk of retinopathy of prematurity (110). Oxygen can be administered through an endotracheal tube, hood, tent, or nasal cannula. Increased FiO_2 may be needed during periods of increased stress (e.g., during feedings). Oxygen should be withdrawn gradually and may be required for months. If oxygen-dependent infants can maintain an SO_2 of ≥92% for at least 40 minutes in room air, then it appears that they can be successfully weaned from supplemental oxygen (111). Many infants are discharged from the neonatal intensive care unit and receive oxygen at home.

The use of booster transfusions to increase oxygen-carrying capacity in infants with BPD is controversial. Traditionally, hemoglobin is maintained from 10 to 15 mg/dL in oxygen-dependent infants with BPD. Alverson and associates demonstrated significant increases in oxygen content and systemic oxygen transport and decreases in oxygen consumption and oxygen use in infants with BPD after booster blood transfusion (112). However, hemoglobin levels did not appear to correlate well with systemic oxygen transport and did not predict which infants would benefit physiologically from transfusion. The need for multiple transfusions has been significantly reduced by minimizing phlebotomy and by using human recombinant erythropoietin therapy (113).

Nutrition

Because infants with BPD have increased metabolic demands, calories must be maximized to support tissue repair and growth. Enteral feedings with fortified breast milk or with premature formulas provide the best source of calories. Feedings should be given by intermittent or continuous gavage until the infant can be fed orally. Feedings can be concentrated to increase caloric density, or glucose polymers (i.e., polycose) and medium-chain triglycerides can be added to provide optimal calories while minimizing fluid intake. Infants may require 120 to 140 calories/kg of body weight each day to gain weight (10 to 30 g/day). If fluid restriction interferes with the administration of adequate calories, a diuretic can be used to prevent fluid overload.

Intravenous nutrition should be started early to provide adequate sources of protein, fat, and carbohydrates. This may affect the ultimate outcome and severity of BPD, especially in the very-low-birth-weight infant. The early use of percutaneous Silastic central catheters has greatly enhanced the ability to provide more optimal calories to low-birth-weight infants (114). Progressive increases in intravenous protein (i.e., amino acid) concentrations should optimally provide 2.0 to 3.0 g of protein per kilogram each day. The acid–base status of the infant should be monitored because acid loads may not be well tolerated. Intravenous lipids (20% suspension) should be administered as a continuous infusion over 20 to 24 hours. Up to 3 g of lipids per kilogram each day can be safely infused if serum triglyceride levels are closely followed. However, early administration of lipids may be associated with pulmonary vascular lipid deposition, hypoxia, and more severe BPD (115,116). Intravenous glucose is a good source of calories, but excessive loads (>4 mg/kg/min) may result in increased oxygen consumption, CO_2 production, and resting energy expenditures in infants with BPD (117). Adequate calcium and phosphorus intake is necessary, especially in infants receiving furosemide, to promote bone mineralization and prevent secondary hyperparathyroidism and rickets. Vitamins and trace metals should also be supplemented. Many premature infants are deficient in vitamin A, and adequate supplementation may promote tissue regeneration and growth in the lung and decrease the incidence and severity of BPD (66). Trace metals such as copper, zinc, and selenium are essential for the structure and function of antioxidant enzymes and should be provided.

Medications

Many different types of drug therapies are used, often concurrently, to improve the clinical status of infants with BPD. The exact dosages, efficacy, mechanisms of action, pharmacokinetics, and side effects have not been well established. The following sections update and summarize a previously published extensive review (118).

Diuretics

Furosemide (Lasix) is the treatment of choice for fluid overload in infants with BPD. It acts on the ascending loop of Henle and blocks chloride transport. Furosemide increases plasma oncotic pressure and lymphatic flow and decreases interstitial edema and pulmonary vascular resistance (118,119). Several studies have demonstrated that daily or alternate-day furosemide improves clinical respiratory status and pulmonary mechanics and facilitates weaning from mechanical ventilation in infants with BPD (120,121). Side effects of furosemide are numerous and include volume depletion, contraction alkalosis, hyponatremia, hypokalemia, chloride depletion, renal calculi secondary to hypercalciuria, cholelithiasis, osteopenia, and ototoxicity (118). Supplemental potassium chloride is usually needed to prevent electrolyte depletion and alkalosis, but sodium chloride supplements should be avoided if possible. Long-term efficacy has not been determined.

The thiazides affect renal tubular excretion of electrolytes, but they are less potent than furosemide (122). Potassium and bicarbonate excretion accompany the sodium and chloride excretion produced by the thiazides. For this reason, the thiazides are usually given in conjunction with spironolactone (Aldactone), which is a competitive inhibitor of aldosterone. Spironolactone is a relatively weak diuretic that causes increased sodium, chloride, and water excretion while sparing potassium. In several randomized, controlled trials, the combination of a thiazide diuretic and spironolactone resulted in increased urine output and improvements in pulmonary mechanics in infants with moderate BPD (123,124). In contrast, Engelhardt and associates found that this combination of agents increased urine output in a manner similar to that seen with furosemide but had no effect on gas exchange or pulmonary mechanics in a similar population of infants with BPD (125). Side effects of the combination of a thiazide with spironolactone include azotemia, hyperuricemia, hyponatremia, hyperkalemia or hypokalemia, hyperglycemia, hypercalciuria, and hypomagnesemia (118,126). Long-term studies comparing furosemide with thiazide–spironolactone therapy in BPD need to be performed. Diuretic dosing is shown in Table 29–4.

Inhaled Agents

Albuterol is a specific β_2-agonist that has become the inhaled agent of choice in the treatment of reversible bronchospasm in infants with BPD. Albuterol aerosolization has been associated with acute improvements in pulmonary resistance and lung compliance secondary to bronchial smooth muscle relaxation (127). These changes in pulmonary mechanics returned to baseline by 4 hours after administration. Side effects are infrequent but can include tachycardia and hypertension. Tolerance may develop with prolonged usage, and long-term efficacy remains to be established.

Atropine is a competitive inhibitor of acetylcholine. In the lung, atropine decreases mucus secretion and transport in large airways and causes significant bronchial smooth muscle relaxation (128). Ipratropium bromide is a related muscarinic antagonist that is a much more potent bronchodilator than atropine and has significantly fewer side effects. In infants with BPD, ipratropium causes a significant improvement in pulmonary mechanics that is similar to that seen after treatment with albuterol (129). The combination of ipratropium and albuterol may be more effective than either agent alone (128,129). Because aerosolized ipratropium is so poorly absorbed, it has significantly fewer side effects than atropine. Long-term efficacy needs to be established. A selective β_2 agent should initially be used in infants with BPD; ipratropium can be added if clinical improvement is not seen. Ipratropium can be used alone if significant side effects from β agents occur.

Cromolyn inhibits the release of inflammatory mediators from mast cells (130). Limited studies have shown a reduction in inflammatory mediators from tracheobronchial aspirates of chronically ventilated infants with BPD who were treated with cromolyn, but few other clinical benefits have been definitively established (131,132). Further short- and

TABLE 29–4. *Commonly used medications for bronchopulmonary dysplasia*

Medication	Dosage[a]
Diuretics	
Furosemide	0.5–2.0 mg/kg/dose IV or PO bid (qd in infants <31 weeks postconceptual age)
Chlorthiazide	5–20 mg/kg/dose IV or PO bid
Hydrochlorthiazide	1–2 mg/kg/dose PO bid
Spironolactone	1.5 mg/kg/dose PO bid
Inhaled agents	
Albuterol	0.02–0.04 mL/kg/dose of a 0.5% solution diluted to 1–2 mL with half-normal or normal saline q4–6h
Ipratropium bromide	0.025–0.08 mg/kg diluted to 1.5–2.5 mL in half-normal or normal saline q6h; doses up to 0.176 mg may be used
Systemic agents	
Aminophylline (IV), theophylline (PO)	LD 5 mg/kg; MD 2 mg/kg/dose q8–12h; serum levels of 5–15 mg/L
Caffeine citrate	LD 20 mg/kg; MD 5 mg/kg IV or PO q24h
Dexamethasone	0.5 mg/kg/day IV or PO q12h for 3 days, decrease to 0.3 mg/kg/day for 3 days, then taper 10% to 20% every 3 days

[a]LD, loading dose; MD, maintenance dose.

long-term safety and efficacy studies need to be performed before the use of cromolyn can be recommended. Inhaled bronchodilator dosing is shown in Table 29–4.

Systemic Bronchodilators

The methylxanthines (e.g., caffeine, theophylline) are routinely used to increase respiratory drive and reduce the frequency of apnea in infants with apnea of prematurity (99). They are also used in the treatment of infants with BPD. Measurements of pulmonary mechanics in infants with BPD have shown that caffeine and theophylline can reduce pulmonary resistance and increase lung compliance, presumably through a direct bronchodilator action (133,134). These agents act as mild diuretics and improve skeletal muscle and diaphragmatic contractility. This is particularly important in chronically ventilated infants who may develop diaphragmatic atrophy and fatigue. Improved skeletal muscle contractility may stabilize the chest wall and improve functional residual capacity (135). These actions may facilitate successful weaning from mechanical ventilation. There may be a synergistic effect if theophylline and a diuretic are used concurrently (124).

The half-life of theophylline is 30 to 40 hours in newborns, and theophylline is metabolized primarily to caffeine in the liver and excreted in the urine. Adverse reactions include gastrointestinal (e.g., gastroesophageal reflux, diarrhea), central nervous system (e.g., agitation, seizures), cardiovascular (e.g., tachycardia, hypertension), and endocrine (e.g., hyperglycemia) disturbances (118). The half-life of caffeine may be as long as 100 hours. It is excreted unchanged in the urine. Side effects of caffeine are similar to those of theophylline but are rarely encountered. Caffeine is a safer drug with a wider therapeutic index and fewer side effects than theophylline and may be a more appropriate adjunct in the treatment of apnea and BPD in preterm infants. Long-term comparative studies are needed.

Two other systemic β2-agonists that act as bronchodilators and have been shown to have short-term benefits in infants with BPD include subcutaneous terbutaline and oral albuterol (136,137). However, these agents appear to offer no significant advantage to caffeine or theophylline as a primary therapy in infants with BPD. Further long-term comparative studies are needed.

Corticosteroids

Corticosteroids are synthesized by the adrenal cortex and are composed of mineralocorticoids, which affect fluid and electrolyte balance, and glucocorticoids, which affect the metabolism of many tissues and possess potent antiinflammatory properties (138). Dexamethasone is a synthetic corticosteroid that has been used in the prevention and treatment of BPD. Dexamethasone has multiple

pharmacologic effects, although the down-regulation of the inflammatory cascade is thought to be primarily responsible for the improvements in pulmonary function. Some of the effects of dexamethasone include the following:

Stabilization of cell and lysosomal membranes
Increase in serum vitamin A concentration and surfactant synthesis
Stimulation of antioxidant enzyme activity
Inhibition of leukotriene and prostaglandin synthesis
Decrease in polymorphonuclear leukocyte recruitment to the lung
Breakdown of granulocyte aggregates with improvements in pulmonary microcirculation
Reduction in pulmonary edema
Enhancement of β-adrenergic activity (139–146)

Several studies have demonstrated that early dexamethasone treatment improves pulmonary mechanics, promotes more rapid weaning from mechanical ventilation, and minimizes inflammatory changes and lung injury in infants who are at high risk for developing BPD (147–149). In contrast, other investigators have not been able to demonstrate any significant clinical benefits (150). In infants with documented BPD, dexamethasone treatment acutely reduces inflammatory markers in the tracheobronchial aspirates, improves pulmonary mechanics and clinical pulmonary status, and facilitates weaning from mechanical ventilation (151–154). A wide variety of dosing schedules have been used, although in most cases infants initially receive 0.5 mg/kg/day, which is then tapered over a variable time period. Some studies taper infants over 42 days, but others use shorter courses (7 to 10 days), pulse dosing, or lower doses, which may be just as efficacious with fewer associated side effects (147,149). It is important to note that dexamethasone administration did not significantly improve survival, duration of oxygen treatment, or total length of hospital stay in any of the studies of infants with BPD.

Dexamethasone has a relatively long half-life (i.e., 36 to 72 hours), and concurrent phenobarbital or phenytoin treatment may affect drug metabolism. If the drug is not effective after 4 to 5 days, it should be discontinued. Most studies have described frequent side effects of dexamethasone therapy including poor weight gain, hyperglycemia, hypertension, osteoporosis, gastric ulcers, adrenal suppression, cardiac abnormalities, and an increased risk of sepsis (84,118,155,156). Of greater concern is a recent report from Taiwan suggesting that although early dexamethasone improved pulmonary outcome, an increased risk of neurodevelopmental abnormalities were found at long-term follow-up (157). Unfortunately, the question of safety has not been adequately addressed through the performance of randomized controlled trials because many of the trials have had insufficient power or the control group received dexamethasone at a later point in the study. Systemic steroids should be reserved for ventilator-dependent infants with moderate to severe BPD who are resistant to more conventional treatments. Inhaled, nonabsorbable steroids such as beclomethasone may be more effective and have fewer side effects when used in the prevention and treatment of BPD (158).

Pulmonary Vasodilators

Nifedipine is a calcium channel blocker that reduces pulmonary vascular pressures in some infants with BPD. A single oral dose of 0.5 mg/kg reduces pulmonary vascular resistance and improves cardiac output in older infants with severe pulmonary artery hypertension associated with BPD (159). The effects of nifedipine appear to be greater than those observed after administration of 95% oxygen. The magnitude of the hemodynamic response appears to correlate well with plasma concentrations (160). Pharmacokinetic studies suggest that a dose of 0.5 mg/kg every 6 hours provides optimal reduction in pulmonary pressures while avoiding side effects such as systemic hypotension and decreased cardiac contractility. Nifedipine should be used cautiously because verapamil, which is a closely related agent, has caused cardiac decompensation when used in infants with supraventricular tachycardia (161). Long-term studies need to evaluate the safety and efficacy of nifedipine in infants with BPD and pulmonary hypertension.

Antibiotics

There is some evidence suggesting that infection with *Ureaplasma urealyticum* may be important in the pathogenesis and progression of BPD (50,51). Clinical trials using treatment with erythromycin as a means of reducing the incidence and severity of BPD in colonized infants have not been successful (53). Cultures of tracheal secretions should be performed intermittently to determine the types of colonizing organisms in chronically ventilated infants. If infants develop respiratory decompensation as a result of possible infection (i.e., abnormal chest radiographs and complete blood count, positive Gram stain or cultures), appropriate broad-spectrum antibiotics should be used initially, with more specific antibiotic coverage determined after the organisms are isolated. Exposure of these infants to multiple courses of broad-spectrum antibiotics may place them at higher risk for the development of invasive fungal infections.

Physical Therapy

Physical therapy may help overcome various types of motor deficits (162). Infants with RDS and BPD are at increased risk for subsequent gross motor, fine motor, or cognitive developmental delays. To optimize ventilation, these infants use neck extension and accessory muscles.

This produces abnormal posture of the neck, scapula, shoulder, and trunk. Efforts to reduce this abnormal posture and normalize tone should be provided in conjunction with a physical therapist. Infants are first positioned in a more neutral alignment. This is followed by strengthening of neck and trunk muscles, and independent movements and exploration of the environment through infant stimulation techniques are performed. A pacifier is used to facilitate and strengthen the suck reflex, especially when the infant is able to tolerate gavage feedings. When infants are fed orally, coordination of breathing, sucking, and swallowing may be difficult. Positioning the infants in natural flexion and using mandibular compression and cheek and upper palate stimulation may be helpful. Nasal oxygen is often necessary to assist the infant in feeding without tiring.

At the time of discharge, a comprehensive home therapy program is implemented. Nursing needs and home physical and occupational or speech therapy are ordered as necessary. Reevaluation at appropriate intervals is scheduled in a neonatal high-risk follow-up program, with emphasis on the possible need for a future early-intervention program. These treatment programs emphasize teaching parents specific handling, positioning, and stimulation techniques. Normalizing muscle tone and posture and stimulating desired patterns of movements are the goals of these therapies.

OUTCOME

Most neonates who develop BPD ultimately achieve normal lung function and thrive. However, this group of neonates is at higher risk of dying in the first year of life or developing significant long-term complications. During infancy, continued normal lung growth should result in slow improvement of pulmonary function and weaning from mechanical ventilation or oxygen therapy. Later in childhood, other respiratory problems (e.g., reactive airway disease) and abnormal neurologic development are additional complications that may occur and require careful follow-up.

Mortality

In Northway's original group of 32 patients, only 13 survived the first month of life (1). Nine (69%) of these survivors developed BPD, and five died within the first year of life. The remaining four infants with BPD had persistent respiratory abnormalities that resolved slowly over time. Infants with BPD in this series died primarily of pulmonary hypertension and cor pulmonale. In contrast to this 66% mortality rate, other studies have shown a marked decrease in mortality, with rates dropping to 30% to 40% (163,164). Davidson followed a group of infants weighing less than 2,500 g who were treated from 1983 to 1985 and found that infants with BPD who survived to 1 month of age had a significantly higher (30%) chance of dying in the first year of life than infants surviving without BPD (165). Causes of death included ventilatory failure (five patients), apnea (three patients), and sepsis (one patient). An increased risk of sudden infant death syndrome had been described in infants surviving with BPD, but more recent evidence suggests that infants with BPD may not be at any higher risk than other premature infants (166–168). Gibson reported that seven (47%) of 15 patients in their study who required more than 6 months of ventilation died at a mean age of 11.5 months (169). This suggested that infants chronically ventilated for treatment of moderate or severe BPD have a higher risk of dying in the first year of life. Several surfactant replacement studies have demonstrated significantly improved survival, even of infants who develop BPD. Phibbs found a 32% incidence of BPD in his surfactant treatment and control groups (170). There were no deaths from BPD in the surfactant-treated group, but three infants (25%) died in the control group. Merritt found similar rates of moderate to severe BPD in placebo and surfactant groups (9%) (7). Surfactant replacement therapy was able to significantly reduce mortality, especially from pulmonary complications. This confirms the observation that BPD is generally less severe than seen in the presurfactant era and is associated with a better outcome if it does develop.

Pulmonary Function

Although pulmonary function in most survivors with BPD improves over time with continued lung growth and permits normal activity, abnormalities detected by pulmonary function testing may remain. Follow-up studies of children with BPD have shown increased airway resistance and reactivity, decreased lung compliance, ventilation–perfusion mismatch, and blood gas abnormalities (e.g., increased PCO_2) that may continue into later years (171,172). Blayney investigated patients with BPD at 7 and 10 years of age and found that, although lung growth had occurred normally, residual volumes were increased, and forced expiratory volumes and flow rates were reduced (173). Fifty percent of these children had a history of wheezing, suggesting airway hyperactivity. Significant improvement in pulmonary function occurred from years 7 through 10, indicating that pulmonary abnormalities from BPD persist well into childhood and continue to improve slowly over time. Hakulinen found lower airway conductance and increased residual volumes in children who had BPD (174). The most significant abnormalities were found in children who had clinical respiratory symptoms, especially early in their childhood (<2 years of age).

The longest follow-up of patients was reported by Northway, who studied patients until they were 25 years of age (175). Although they appeared clinically well, patients with BPD had continued evidence of pulmonary dysfunction, including airway obstruction and hyperactivity detected on pulmonary function testing and hyperinflation seen on chest radiographs. The frequency of respiratory symptoms is increased in long-term survivors with BPD. Twenty-three percent of Northway's young adults with a history of BPD had chronic respiratory symptoms. None of the infants with BPD reported by Bader required hospitalization after their second birthdays, but 80% still had frequent wheezing or pneumonias at 10 years of age (171). Hakulinen found an increased need for hospitalization because of pulmonary problems for the first 2 years of life in his BPD survivors, but at 6 to 9 years of age, none had evidence of wheezing or respiratory distress (174). As the overall severity of BPD has decreased in recent years, so have the long-term clinical and pulmonary function sequelae. Both Jacob and Giacoia were unable to find any significant differences in pulmonary function testing of infants with BPD when compared to a matched group of premature infants without BPD (176,177). Long-term follow-up of infants developing BPD in the postsurfactant era has only recently been reported. Baraldi and colleagues demonstrated progressive improvements in pulmonary function tests over the first 2 years of life, although evidence of airway dysfunction persisted (178). It appears that abnormal pulmonary function and distress are greatest in the first 2 years of life in infants with BPD, and survival beyond that age permits children to function at normal capacity.

Cardiac Function

Cardiac failure was found by Northway to be a major cause of morbidity and mortality in infants in his original study (1). Cor pulmonale was found in 56% of his survivors, resulting in death in each case. The finding of abnormal muscularization of small pulmonary arteries (from chronic hypoxia) has been consistently identified in infants with severe BPD and may contribute to pulmonary hypertension (81). Supplementation with oxygen to alleviate pulmonary hypertension has become a mainstay of therapy, and failure to respond is a poor prognostic sign (95,105). In Northway's long-term follow-up, only one of 26 patients with BPD had evidence of right ventricular hypertrophy, suggesting that long-term survival is much improved if cor pulmonale can be prevented in infancy (175).

Infection

Increased susceptibility to infection has been found in infants with BPD. Respiratory syncytial virus (RSV) is a major pathogen that causes illness and the need for rehospitalization and mechanical ventilation in children with BPD. Infants are more susceptible to RSV infection because of impaired lung defenses secondary to damaged lung tissue (179,180). Monthly infusions of RSV-enriched immune globulin (Respigam) have recently been shown to decrease the incidence and severity of RSV infection in high-risk premature infants (181). Indications for use include significantly premature infants who are home and less than 6 months of age during RSV season (December to March), infants under 2 years of age with BPD, or any preterm infant with BPD who has received supplemental oxygen in the previous 6 months. Development of a vaccine to prevent RSV infection in high-risk populations should eventually eliminate the sequelae of RSV infection in infants with BPD. Rhinovirus, although not as common as RSV, may also be an important cause of lower respiratory tract disease in infants with BPD (182).

Growth and Neurologic Development

It is not surprising that the most critically ill and premature infants who develop BPD have an increased risk for growth failure and abnormal neurodevelopmental outcome. Infants with BPD have increased metabolic demands and caloric requirements and may grow poorly during infancy and childhood (183–185). Markestad observed that children with improving respiratory function exhibited faster catch-up growth, and those with continued respiratory problems failed to do so (186). Other studies have shown that a significant proportion of infants with BPD are consistently in the lower percentiles for height, weight, and head circumference (187). This is frequently found during the first 2 years of life, when respiratory symptoms and illness may be prominent (174).

Giacoia studied a group of preterm infants with BPD over the first 2 years of life and compared them to a group of age-matched premature infants and term controls (177). Both groups of premature infants had comparable growth rates and average mean standard scores for Wechsler IQ. However, all of the premature infants were significantly smaller than the term controls and had lower scores for performance and full-scale IQ. Vohr found no differences in full-scale IQ scores between premature infants with BPD compared to age-matched premature controls (188). Finally, Singer found no difference in intelligence between infants with BPD and age-matched premature controls at 3 years of life, but motor function was significantly impaired (189). Although the relative contribution of BPD to poor outcome remains undefined, it is associated with the sickest patients in the neonatal intensive care unit and consequently with a significant risk of poor neurodevelopmental outcome. However, perinatal factors other than BPD such as periventricular leukomalacia, intraventricular hemmorrhage, and sepsis may be more important variables in determining developmental outcome. The introduction of surfactant replacement therapy has resulted in significantly improved survival and the development of less severe BPD. It is reassuring that follow-up studies have found that the number of significant neurodevelopmental handicaps has not increased despite the survival of smaller, sicker infants who frequently develop BPD.

PREVENTION

A multidisciplinary approach to the prevention of BPD in infants is needed. The use of prenatal steroids in mothers at high risk of delivering a significantly premature infant appears to reduce the severity and incidence of BPD (190). The early use of nasal CPAP in infants with respiratory distress may eliminate the need for mechanical ventilation in some infants and facilitate successful extubation in other low-birth-weight infants (103). The use of exogenous surfactant replacement therapy in premature infants with significant RDS can reduce mortality and the severity and incidence of BPD, although the total number of survivors with BPD will increase. Exogenous surfactant may also prevent lung injury in full-term infants with pneumonia or meconium aspiration syndrome (191). Aggressive treatment of symptomatic patent ductus arteriosus may reduce the severity of BPD and should include fluid restriction, diuretics, indomethacin, or surgical closure. Ventilator pressures and inspired oxygen concentrations should be reduced as low and as soon as possible to reduce hypocarbia, volutrauma, air leak, and oxygen toxicity.

Aggressive nutritional support, initially with intravenous supplementation followed by enteral feeds when tolerated, is critical (192). Adequate nutrition helps promote normal lung growth, maturation, and repair. It also protects the lung from the damaging effects of infection, hyperoxia, and barotrauma. Supplementation with vitamin A in sufficient quantities (5,000 IU three times per week) to establish normal serum retinol concentrations has been reported, but the impact of this treatment on the incidence and severity of BPD has still not been established (193,194).

The early use of synchronized mechanical ventilation or high-frequency ventilation (HFV) in newborn infants with significant RDS may reduce the severity or incidence of BPD (19,21,23). The combined use of HFV and surfactant replacement may prevent significant lung damage in premature and term infants with significant lung disease unresponsive to surfactant replacement and conventional mechanical ventilation (195). Further conclusive evidence of the beneficial effects of both synchronized ventilation and HFV in premature infants is needed.

Extracorporeal membrane oxygenation is another technique used in the treatment of infants older than 36 weeks of gestation with severe lung disease that is unresponsive to conventional forms of therapy (196). This technique allows the lung to rest and repair itself while gas exchange is accomplished with the use of an external membrane oxygenator. The early use of ECMO before significant lung damage occurs may reduce BPD in some treated infants. Its use has been limited to term and near-term infants because of the necessity of anticoagulating treated infants. Inhaled nitric oxide (NO) is also being used clinically to treat both term and preterm infants with pulmonary hypertension secondary to severe pulmonary parenchymal disease (106). Nitric oxide has been shown to improve oxygenation and reduce the need for ECMO in many critically ill newborns. However, inhaled NO is generally administered with high concentrations of oxygen, which have been shown to cause surfactant dysfunction and synergistic pulmonary cytotoxicity in several *in vitro* and *in vivo* studies (197,198).

As described in detail previously, some studies have suggested that the early use of dexamethasone may reduce the incidence and severity of BPD, but significant concerns still exist regarding side effects and long-term outcome. The routine use of prophylactic dexamethasone can not be recommended at the present time until further long-term studies are performed to determine the optimal dose, timing, and duration of treatment to prevent BPD. The most promising method for preventing the development of BPD appears to be prophylactic supplementation of human recombinant antioxidant enzymes. This seems to be a logical strategy in preventing BPD because oxygen radicals appear to play a major role in the pathogenesis of lung injury, and premature infants are known to be relatively deficient in these enzymes at birth. Several ani-

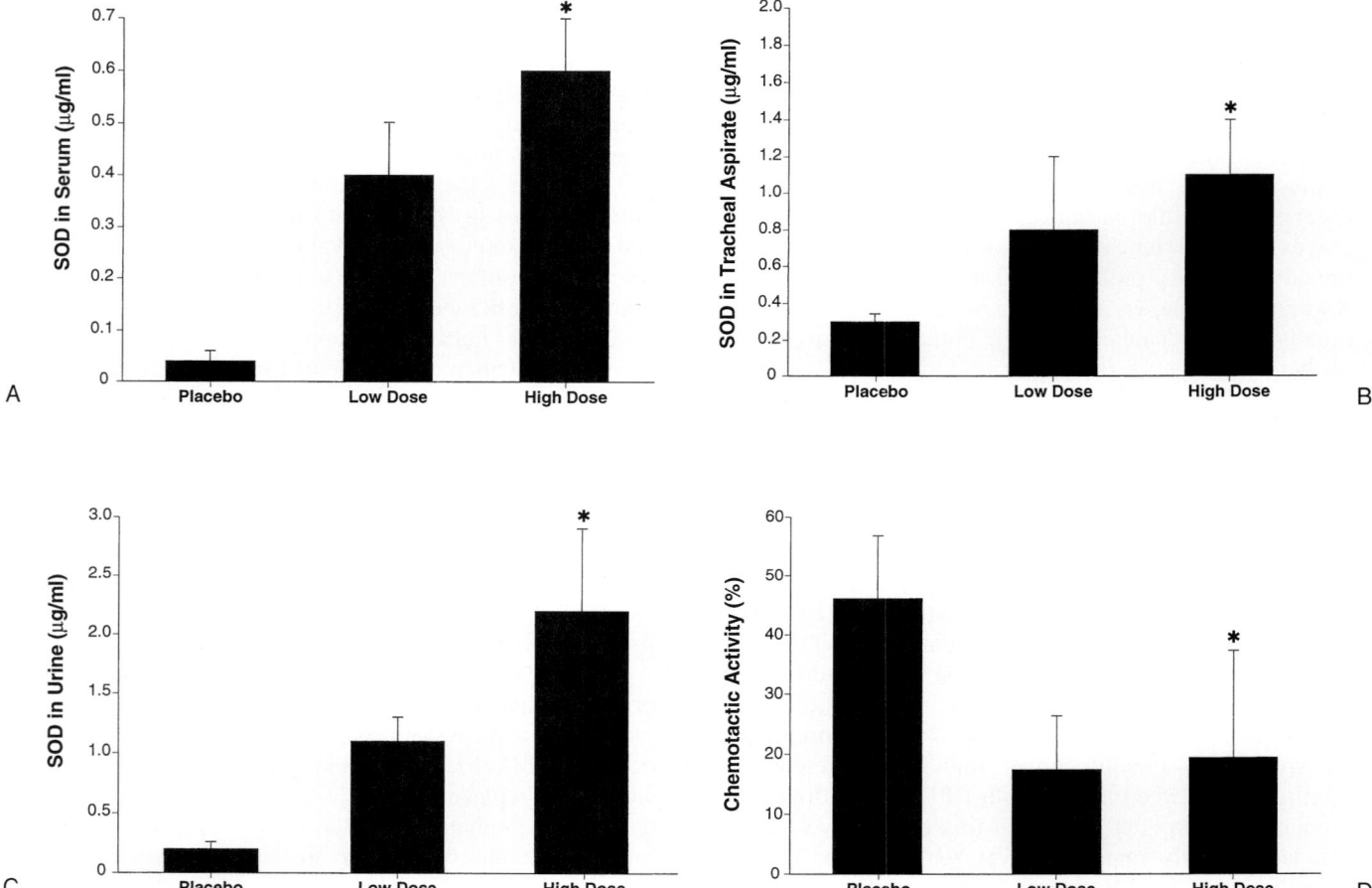

FIG. 29–9. Superoxide dismutase (SOD) concentrations in serum **(A)**, tracheal aspirates **(B)**, and urine **(C)** presented as geometric mean ± 1 SEM. No significant changes occurred in the placebo group, but both rhSOD groups were increased when first sampled on day 3 and remained elevated thereafter (*$p < 0.05$, ANOVA). Data from days 3 to 13 have been pooled and averaged. The activity of SOD correlated with its concentration. **D:** The rhSOD reduced neutrophil chemotactic activity (NCA) in tracheal aspirates. The NCA (which reflects inflammation and lung injury) in tracheal aspirates is expressed as percent of positive control (zymosan-activated serum). Baseline values were similar for all groups, but activity was significantly decreased over the 2-week dosing period in the rhSOD groups compared with the placebo. Values for each group are pooled and averaged (*$p < 0.05$). (From ref. 205.)

mal studies have shown that prolonged exposure to high oxygen concentrations can cause severe lung damage and death, and administration of antioxidants can prevent many of these complications (27–29,199–202). In a pilot study using humans, Rosenfeld and colleagues showed that subcutaneous administration of bovine SOD decreased the severity of BPD in treated infants, although total duration of respiratory support was the same for the treated and control groups (203). Human recombinant SOD has now been developed and administered prophylactically to the lung of premature infants at high risk for developing BPD (203,204). In preliminary studies in premature infants, the prophylactic use of both single and multiple intratracheal doses of human recombinant SOD appears to mitigate inflammatory changes and severe lung injury from oxygen and mechanical ventilation with no apparent associated toxicity (Fig. 29–9). In animal studies, the exogenous SOD appears to localize in both intracellular and extracellular compartments following intratracheal instillation, and significant quantities of active protein persist 48 hours after the dose is given (29,206). National collaborative trials using prophylactic SOD in premature infants at high risk for developing BPD are currently under way and may ultimately produce a therapy that can prevent or significantly ameliorate this important chronic lung disease.

REFERENCES

1. Northway WH Jr, Rosan RC, Porter DY. Pulmonary disease following respirator therapy of hyaline-membrane disease. *N Engl J Med* 1967; 276:357.
2. Bancalari E, Abdenour GE, Feller R, Gannon J. Bronchopulmonary dysplasia: clinical presentation. *J Pediatr* 1979;95:819.
3. Avery ME, Tooley WH, Keller JB, et al. Is chronic lung disease in low birth weight infants preventable? A survey of eight centers. *Pediatrics* 1987;79:26.
4. Sinkin RA, Cox C, Phelps DL. Predicting risk for bronchopulmonary dysplasia: selection criteria for clinical trials. *Pediatrics* 1990;86:728.
5. Shennan AT, Dunn MS, Ohlsson A, Lennox K, Hoskins EM. Abnormal pulmonary outcomes in premature infants: prediction from oxygen requirement in the neonatal period. *Pediatrics* 1988;82:527.
6. Hoekstra RE, Jackson JC, Myers TF, et al. Improved neonatal survival following multiple doses of bovine surfactant in very premature neonates at risk for respiratory distress syndrome. *Pediatrics* 1991;88: 10.
7. Merritt TA, Hallman M, Berry C, et al. Randomized, placebo-controlled trial of human surfactant given at birth versus rescue administration in very low birth weight infants with lung immaturity. *J Pediatr* 1991;118:581.
8. Soll RF, Hoekstra RE, Fangman JJ, et al. Multicenter trial of single-dose modified bovine surfactant extract (Survanta) for prevention of respiratory distress syndrome. *Pediatrics* 1990;85:1092.
9. Bose C, Corbet A, Bose G, et al. Improved outcome at 28 days of age for very low birth weight infants treated with a single dose of a synthetic surfactant. *J Pediatr* 1990;117:947.
10. Liechty EA, Donovan E, Purohit D, et al. Reduction of neonatal mortality after multiple doses of bovine surfactant in low birth weight neonates with respiratory distress syndrome. *Pediatrics* 1991;88:19.
11. Long W, Thompson T, Sundell H, Schumacher R, Volberg F, Guthrie R. Effects of two rescue doses of a synthetic surfactant on mortality rate and survival without bronchopulmonary dysplasia in 700- to 1350-gram infants with respiratory distress syndrome. The American Exosurf Neonatal Study Group I. *J Pediatr* 1991;118:595.
12. Fenton AC, Mason E, Clarke M, Field DJ. Chronic lung disease following neonatal ventilation. Changing incidence in a geographically defined population. *Pediatr Pulmonol* 1996;21:24.
13. Dreyfus D, Saumon G. Should the lung be rested or recruited? *Am J Respir Crit Care Med* 1994;149:1066.
14. Ackerman NB Jr, Carlson JJ, Kuechl TJ, et al. Pulmonary interstitial emphysema in the premature baboon with hyaline membrane disease. *Crit Care Med* 1984;12:512.
15. Nilsson R, Grossman G, Robertson B. Lung surfactant and the pathogenesis of neonatal bronchiolar lesions induced by artificial ventilation. *Pediatr Res* 1978;12:249.
16. Davis JM, Metlay LA, Dickerson B, Penney DP, Notter RH. Early pulmonary changes associated with high-frequency jet ventilation in newborn piglets. *Pediatr Res* 1990;27:460.
17. Davis JM, Dickerson B, Metlay L, Penney DP. Differential effects of oxygen and barotrauma on lung injury in the neonatal piglet. *Pediatr Pulmonol* 1991;10:157.
18. Samuels MP, Raine J, Wright T, et al. Continuous negative extrathoracic pressure in neonatal respiratory failure. *Pediatrics* 1996;98: 1154.
19. Bernstein G, Mannino FL, Heldt GP, et al. Randomized multicenter trial comparing synchronized and conventional intermittent mandatory ventilation in neonates. *J Pediatr* 1996;128:453.
20. HiFi Study Group. High-frequency oscillatory ventilation compared with conventional ventilation in the treatment of respiratory failure in preterm infants. *N Engl J Med* 1989;320:88.
21. Clark RH, Gerstmann DR, Null DM, deLemos RA. Prospective, randomized comparison of high-frequency oscillatory and conventional ventilation in respiratory distress syndrome. *Pediatrics* 1992;89:5.
22. Keszler M, Donn SM, Bucciarelli RL, et al. Multicenter controlled trial comparing high-frequency jet ventilation and conventional mechanical ventilation in newborn infants with pulmonary interstitial emphysema. *J Pediatr* 1991;119:85.
23. Keszler M, Modanlou HD, Brudno DS, et al. Multicenter controlled clinical trial of high-frequency jet ventilation in preterm infants with uncomplicated respiratory distress syndrome. *Pediatrics* 1997;100: 593.
24. Garland JS, Buck RK, Allred EN, Leviton A. Hypocarbia before surfactant therapy appears to increase bronchopulmonary dysplasia risk in infants with respiratory distress syndrome. *Arch Pediatr Adolesc Med* 1995;149:617.
25. Wiswell TE, Graziani LJ, Kornhauser MS, et al. Effects of hypocarbia on the development of cystic periventricular leukomalacia in premature infants treated with high-frequency jet ventilation. *Pediatrics* 1996;98:918.
26. Frank L, Groseclose EE. Preparation for birth into an O_2-rich environment: the antioxidant enzymes in the developing rabbit lung. *Pediatr Res* 1984;18:240.
27. Turrens JF, Crapo JD, Freeman BA. Protection against oxygen toxicity by intravenous injection of liposome-entrapped catalase and superoxide dismutase. *J Clin Invest* 1984;73:87.
28. Padmanabhan RV, Gudapaty R, Liener IE, Schwartz BA, Hoidal JR. Protection against pulmonary oxygen toxicity in rats by the intratracheal administration of liposome-encapsulated superoxide dismutase or catalase. *Am Rev Respir Dis* 1985;132:164.
29. Davis JM, Rosenfeld WN, Sanders RJ, Gonenne A. Prophylactic effects of recombinant human superoxide dismutase in neonatal lung injury. *J Appl Physiol* 1993;74:2234.
30. White CW, Avraham KB, Shanley PF, Groner Y. Transgenic mice with expression of elevated levels of copper-zinc superoxide dismutase in the lungs are resistant to pulmonary oxygen toxicity. *J Clin Invest* 1991;87:2162.
31. Wispe JR, Warner BB, Clark JC, et al. Human Mn-superoxide dismutase in pulmonary epithelial cells of transgenic mice confers protection from oxygen injury. *J Biol Chem* 1992;267:23937.
32. Carlsson LM, Jonsson J, Edlun T, Marklund SL. Mice lacking extracellular superoxide dismutase are more sensitive to hyperoxia. *Proc Natl Acad Sci USA* 1995;92:6264.
33. Pitkanen OM, Hallman M, Andersson SM. Correlation of free oxygen radical-induced lipid peroxidation with outcome in very low birth weight infants. *J Pediatr* 1990;116:760.
34. Ogihara T, Okamoto R, Kim HS, et al. New evidence for the involvement of oxygen radicals in triggering neonatal chronic lung disease. *Pediatr Res* 1996;39:117.

35. Varsila E, Pesonen E, Andersson S. Early protein oxidation in the neonatal lung is related to the development of chronic lung disease. *Acta Paediatr* 1995;84:1296.

36. Rinaldo JE, English D, Levine J, Stiller R, Henson J. Increased retention of radiolabeled neutrophils in early oxygen toxicity. *Am Rev Respir Dis* 1988;137:345.

37. Merritt TA, Stuard ID, Puccia J, et al. Newborn tracheal aspirate cytology: classification during respiratory distress syndrome and bronchopulmonary dysplasia. *J Pediatr* 1981;98:949.

38. Merritt TA, Cochrane CG, Holcomb K, et al. Elastase and α₁-proteinase inhibitor activity in tracheal aspirates during respiratory distress syndrome. Role of inflammation in the pathogenesis of bronchopulmonary dysplasia. *J Clin Invest* 1983;72:656.

39. Fantone JC, Feltner DE, Brieland JK, Ward PA. Phagocytic cell-derived inflammatory mediators and lung disease. *Chest* 1987;91:428.

40. Pierce MR, Bancalari E. The role of inflammation in the pathogenesis of bronchopulmonary dysplasia. *Pediatr Pulmonol* 1995;19:371.

41. Raghavender B, Smith JB. Eosinophil cationic protein in tracheal aspirates of preterm infants with bronchopulmonary dysplasia. *J Pediatr* 1997;130:944.

42. Bagchi A, Viscardi RM, Taciak V, Ensor JE, McCrea KA, Hasday JD. Increased activity of interleukin-6 but not tumor necrosis factor-α in lung lavage of premature infants is associated with the development of bronchopulmonary dysplasia. *Pediatr Res* 1994;36:244.

43. Groneck P, Gotz-Speer B, Opperman M, Eiffert H, Speer CP. Association of pulmonary inflammation and increased microvascular permeability during the development of bronchopulmonary dysplasia: a sequential analysis of inflammatory mediators in respiratory fluids of high-risk neonates. *Pediatrics* 1994;93:712.

44. Bruce MC, Wedig KE, Jentoft N, et al. Altered urinary excretion of elastin cross-links in premature infants who developed bronchopulmonary dysplasia. *Am Rev Respir Dis* 1985;131:568.

45. Ossanna PJ, Test ST, Matheson NR, Regiani S, Weiss SJ. Oxidative regulation of neutrophil elastase–alpha-1-proteinase inhibitor interactions. *J Clin Invest* 1986;77:1939.

46. Walti H, Tordet C, Gerbaut L, Saugier P, Moriette G, Relier JP. Persistent elastase/proteinase inhibitor imbalance during prolonged ventilation of infants with bronchopulmonary dysplasia: evidence for the role of nosocomial infections. *Pediatr Res* 1989;26:351.

47. Bruce MC, Boat TF, Martin RJ, Dearborn DG, Fanaroff AA. Proteinase inhibitors and inhibitor inactivation in neonatal airway secretions. *Chest* 1982;81S:44.

48. Rosenfeld W, Concepcion L, Evans H, Jhaveri R, Sahdev S, Zabaleta I. Serial trypsin inhibitory capacity and ceruloplasmin levels in prematures at risk for bronchopulmonary dysplasia. *Am Rev Respir Dis* 1986;134:1229.

49. Stiskal J, Dunn M, O'Brien K, et al. α-1 Proteinase inhibitor therapy for the prevention of bronchopulmonary dysplasia in premature infants. *Pediatr Res* 1996;39:247A.

50. Cassell GH, Waites KB, Crouse DT, et al. Association of *Ureaplasma urealyticum* infection of the lower respiratory tract with chronic lung disease and death in very-low-birth-weight infants. *Lancet* 1988;2:240.

51. Wang EEL, Ohlsson A, Kellner JD. Association of ureaplasma urealyticum colonization with chronic lung disease of prematurity: Results of a metaanlysis. *J Pediatr* 1995;127:640.

52. Da Silva O, Gregson D, Hammerberg O. Role of *Ureaplasma urealyticum* and *Chlamydia trachomatis* in development of bronchopulmonary dysplasia in very low birth weight infants. *Pediatr Infect Dis J* 1997;16:364.

53. Heggie AD, Jacobs MR, Butler VT, Baley JE, Boxerbaum B. Frequency and significance of isolation of *Ureaplasma urealyticum* and *Mycoplasma hominis* from cerebrospinal fluid and tracheal aspirate specimens from low birth weight infants. *J Pediatr* 1994;124:956.

54. Watterberg KL, Demers LM, Scott SM, Murphy S. Chorioamnionitis and early lung inflammation in infants in whom bronchopulmonary dysplasia develops. *Pediatrics* 1996;97:210.

55. Gonzalez A, Sosenko IRS, Chandar J, et al. Influence of infection on patent ductus arteriosus and chronic lung disease in premature infants weighing 1000 grams or less. *J Pediatr* 1996;128:470.

56. Weinstein MR, Oh W. Oxygen consumption in infants with bronchopulmonary dysplasia. *J Pediatr* 1981;99:958.

57. Frank L, Groseclose E. Oxygen toxicity in newborn rats: the adverse effects of undernutrition. *J Appl Physiol* 1982;53:1248.

58. Darlow BA, Inder TE, Graham PJ, et al. The relationship of selenium status to respiratory outcome in the very low birth weight infant. *Pediatrics* 1995;96:314.

59. Forman HJ, Rotman EI, Fisher AB. Roles of selenium and sulfur-containing amino acids in protection against oxygen toxicity. *Lab Invest* 1983;49:148.

60. O'Dell BL, Kilburn KH, McKenzie WN, Thurston RJ. The lung of the copper-deficient rat: a model for developmental pulmonary emphysema. *Am J Pathol* 1978;91:413.

61. Ehrenkranz RA, Bonta BW, Ablow RC, Warshaw JB. Amelioration of bronchopulmonary dysplasia after vitamin E administration: a preliminary report. *N Engl J Med* 1978;299:564.

62. Hittner HM, Godio LB, Rudolph AJ, et al. Retrolental fibroplasia: efficacy of vitamin E in a double-blind clinical study of preterm infants. *N Engl J Med* 1981;305:1365.

63. Saldanha RL, Cepeda EE, Poland RL. The effect of vitamin E prophylaxis on the incidence and severity of bronchopulmonary dysplasia. *J Pediatr* 1982;101:89.

64. Brandt RB, Mueller DG, Schroder JR, et al. Serum vitamin A in premature and term neonates. *J Pediatr* 1978;92:101.

65. Shenai JP, Rush MG, Stahlman MT, Chytil F. Plasma retinol-binding protein response to vitamin A administration in infants susceptible to bronchopulmonary dysplasia. *J Pediatr* 1990;116:607.

66. Hustead VA, Gutcher GR, Anderson SA, Zachman RD. Relationship of vitamin A (retinol) status to lung disease in the preterm infants. *J Pediatr* 1984;105:610.

67. Anzano MA, Olson JA, Lamb AJ. Morphologic alterations in the trachea and the salivary gland following the induction of rapid synchronous vitamin A deficiency in rats. *Am J Pathol* 1980;98:717.

68. Shenai JP, Chytil F, Stahlman MT. Vitamin A status of neonates with bronchopulmonary dysplasia. *Pediatr Res* 1985;19:185.

69. Hartline JV, Zachman RD. Vitamin A delivery in total parenteral nutrition solution. *Pediatrics* 1976;58:448.

70. Van Marter LJ, Leviton A, Allred EN, Pagano M, Kuban KC. Hydration during the first days of life and the risk of bronchopulmonary dysplasia in low birth weight infants. *J Pediatr* 1990;116:942.

71. Bancalari E, Sosenko I. Pathogenesis and prevention of neonatal chronic lung disease: recent developments. *Pediatr Pulmonol* 1990;8:109.

72. Nickerson BG, Taussig LM. Family history of asthma in infants with bronchopulmonary dysplasia. *Pediatrics* 1980;65:1140.

73. Bertrand JM, Riley SP, Popkin J, Coates AL. The long-term pulmonary sequelae of prematurity: the role of familial airway hyperreactivity and the respiratory distress syndrome. *N Engl J Med* 1985;312:742.

74. Clark DA, Pincus LG, Oliphant M, Hubbell C, Oates RP, Davey FR. HLA-A2 and chronic lung disease in neonates. *JAMA* 1982;248:1868.

75. Hagan R, Minutillo C, French N, Reese A, Landau L, LeSouef P. Neonatal chronic lung disease, oxygen dependency, and a family history of asthma. *Pediatr Pulmonol* 1995;20:277.

76. Toce SS, Farrell PM, Leavitt LA, Samuels DP, Edwards DK. Clinical and radiographic scoring systems for assessing bronchopulmonary dysplasia. *Am J Dis Child* 1984;138:581.

77. Edwards DK. Radiographic aspects of bronchopulmonary dysplasia. *J Pediatr* 1979;95:823.

78. Mortensson W, Andreasson B, Lindroth M, Svenningsen N, Jonson B. Potential of early chest roentgen examination in ventilator treated newborn infants to predict future lung function and disease. *Pediatr Radiol* 1989;20:41.

79. Weinstein MR, Peters ME, Sadek M, Palta M. A new radiographic scoring system for bronchopulmonary dysplasia. *Pediatr Pulmonol* 1994;18:284.

80. Oppenheim C, Mamou-Mani T, Sayegh N, de Blic J, Scheinmann P, Lallemand D. Bronchopulmonary dysplasia: value of CT in identifying pulmonary sequelae. *Am J Roentgenol* 1994;163:169.

81. Abman SH. Pulmonary hypertension in infants with bronchopulmonary dysplasia: clinical aspects. In Bancalari E, Stocker JT, eds. *Bronchopulmonary dysplasia.* Washington, DC: Hemisphere Publishing, 1988:221.

82. Harrod JR, L'Heureux P, Wagensteen OD, Hunt CE. Long-term follow-up of severe respiratory distress syndrome treated with IPPB. *J Pediatr* 1974;84:277.

83. Malnick G, Pickoff AS, Ferrer PL, et al. Normal pulmonary vascular resistance and left ventricle hypertrophy in young infants with bron-

chopulmonary dysplasia: an echocardiographic and pathologic study. *Pediatrics* 1980;66:589.

84. Bensky AS, Kothadia JM, Covitz W. Cardiac effects of dexamethasone in very low birth weight infants. *Pediatrics* 1996;97:818.

85. Berman W Jr, Yabek SM, Dillon T, Burnstein R, Corlew S. Evaluation of infants with bronchopulmonary dysplasia using cardiac catheterization. *Pediatrics* 1982;70:708.

86. Goldman SL, Gerhardt T, Sonni R, et al. Early prediction of chronic lung disease by pulmonary function testing. *J Pediatr* 1983;102:613.

87. Tepper RS, Morgan WJ, Cota K, Taussig LM. Expiratory flow limitation in infants with bronchopulmonary dysplasia. *J Pediatr* 1986; 109:1040.

88. Greenspan JS, DeGiulio PA, Bhutani VK. Airway reactivity as determined by a cold air challenge in infants with bronchopulmonary dysplasia. *J Pediatr* 1989;114:452.

89. McCann EM, Goldman SL, Brady JP. Pulmonary function testing in the sick newborn infant. *Pediatr Res* 1987;21:313.

90. Gerhardt T, Bancalari E. Lung function in bronchopulmonary dysplasia. In Bancalari E, Stocker JT, eds. *Bronchopulmonary dysplasia.* Washington, DC: Hemisphere Publishing, 1988:182.

91. Nickerson BG, Durand DJ, Kao LC. Short-term variability of pulmonary function tests in infants with bronchopulmonary dysplasia. *Pediatr Pulmonol* 1989;6:36.

92. Hanrahan JP, Tager IB, Castile RG, Segal MR, Weiss WST, Speizer FE. Pulmonary function measures in healthy infants. Variability and size correction. *Am Rev Respir Dis* 1990;141:1127.

93. Cherukupalli K, Larson JE, Rotschild A, Thurlbeck WM. Biochemical, clinical, and morphologic studies on lungs of infants with bronchopulmonary dysplasia. *Pediatr Pulmonol* 1996;22:215.

94. Stocker JT. Pathology of acute bronchopulmonary dysplasia. In Bancalari E, Stocker JT, eds. *Bronchopulmonary dysplasia.* Washington, DC: Hemisphere Publishing, 1988:237.

95. Abman SH, Wolfe RR, Accurso FJ, Koops BL, Bowman M, Wiggins JW Jr. Pulmonary vascular response to oxygen in infants with severe bronchopulmonary dysplasia. *Pediatrics* 1985;75:80.

96. Courtney SE, Weber KR, Breakie LA, et al. Capillary blood gases in the neonate. *Am J Dis Child* 1990;144:168.

97. Goldman SL, McCann EM, Lloyd BW, Yup G. Inspiratory time and pulmonary function in mechanically ventilated babies with chronic lung disease. *Pediatr Pulmonol* 1991;11:198.

98. Tarnow-Mordi WO, Reid E, Griffiths P, Wilkinson AR. Low inspired gas temperature and respiratory complications in very low birth weight infants. *J Pediatr* 1989;114:438.

99. Aranda JV, Turmen T. Methylxanthines in apnea of prematurity. *Clin Perinatol* 1979;6:87.

100. Veness-Meehan KA, Richter S, Davis JM. Pulmonary function testing prior to extubation in infants with respiratory distress syndrome. *Pediatr Pulmonol* 1990;9:2.

101. Kim EH. Successful extubation of newborn infants without preextubation trial of continuous positive airway pressure. *J Perinatol* 1989;9:72.

102. Viscardi RM, Faix RG, Nicks JJ, Grasela TH. Efficacy of theophylline for prevention of post-extubation respiratory failure in very low birth weight infants. *J Pediatr* 1985;107:469.

103. Higgins RD, Richter SE, Davis JM. Nasal continuous positive airway pressure facilitates extubation of very low birth weight neonates. *Pediatrics* 1991;88:999.

104. Miller RW, Woo P, Kelman RK, Slagle TS. Tracheobronchial abnormalities in infants with bronchopulmonary dysplasia. *J Pediatr* 1987; 111:779.

105. Goodman G, Perkin RM, Anas NG, et al. Pulmonary hypertension in infants with bronchopulmonary dysplasia. *J Pediatr* 1988;112:67.

106. Morin FC, Davis JM. Persistent pulmonary hypertension. In Spitzer AR, ed. *Intensive care of the fetus and newborn.* St Louis: CV Mosby, 1996:506.

107. Ramanathan R, Durand M, Larrazabal C. Pulse oximetry in very low birth weight infants with acute and chronic lung disease. *Pediatrics* 1987;79:612.

108. Dimaguila MA, Di Fiore JM, Martin RJ, Miller MJ. Characteristics of hypoxemic episodes in very low birth weight infants on ventilatory support. *J Pediatr* 1997;130:577.

109. McEvoy C, Mendoza ME, Bowling S, Hewlett V, Sardesai S, Durand M. Prone positioning decreases episodes of hypoxemia in extremely low birth weight infants with chronic lung disease. *J Pediatr* 1997; 130:305.

110. Higgins RD, Phelps DL. Oxygen-induced retinopathy: lack of adverse heparin effect. *Pediatr Res* 1990;27:580.

111. Simoes EAF, Rosenberg AA, King SJ, Groothius JR. Room air challenge: prediction for successful weaning of oxygen-dependent infants. *J Perinatol* 1997;17:125

112. Alverson DC, Isken VH, Cohen RS. Effect of booster transfusion on oxygen utilization in infants with bronchopulmonary dysplasia. *J Pediatr* 1988;113:722.

113. Messer J, Haddad J, Donato L, Astruc D, Matis J. Early treatment of premature infants with recombinant human erythropoietin. *Pediatrics* 1993;92:519.

114. Gilhooly J, Lindenberg J, Reynolds JW. Central venous silicone elastomer catheter placement by basilic vein cutdown in neonates. *Pediatrics* 1986;78:636.

115. Pereira GR, Fox WW, Stanley CA, Baker L, Schwartz JG. Decreased oxygenation and hyperlipemia during intravenous fat infusions in premature infants. *Pediatrics* 1980;66:26.

116. Sosenko IR, Rodriguez-Pierce M, Bancalari E. Effect of early initiation of intravenous lipid administration on the incidence and severity of chronic lung disease in premature infants. *J Pediatr* 1993;123:975.

117. Yunis KA, Oh W. Effects of intravenous glucose loading on oxygen consumption, carbon dioxide production, and resting energy expenditure in infants with bronchopulmonary dysplasia. *J Pediatr* 1989;115:127.

118. Davis JM, Sinkin RA, Aranda JV. Drug therapy for bronchopulmonary dysplasia. *Pediatr Pulmonol* 1990;8:117.

119. Bland RD, McMillan DD, Bressack MA. Decreased pulmonary transvascular fluid filtration in awake newborn lambs after intravenous furosemide. *J Clin Invest* 1978;62:601.

120. Engelhardt B, Elliott S, Hazinski TA. Short- and long-term effects of furosemide on lung function in infants with bronchopulmonary dysplasia. *J Pediatr* 1986;109:1034.

121. Rush MG, Engelhardt B, Parker RA, Hazinski TA. Double-blind, placebo-controlled trial of alternate-day furosemide therapy in infants with chronic bronchopulmonary dysplasia. *J Pediatr* 1990;117:112.

122. Weiner IM, Mudge GH. Diuretics and other agents employed in the mobilization of edema fluid. In Gilman AG, Goodman LS, Rall TW, Murad F, eds. *The pharmacological basis of therapeutics.* New York: Macmillan, 1985:887.

123. Kao LC, Durand DJ, McCrea RC, Birch M, Powers RJ, Nickerson BG. Randomized trial of long-term diuretic therapy for infants with oxygen-dependent bronchopulmonary dysplasia. *J Pediatr* 1994;124:772.

124. Kao LC, Durand DJ, Phillips BL, Nickerson BG. Oral theophylline and diuretics improve pulmonary mechanics in infants with bronchopulmonary dysplasia. *J Pediatr* 1987;111:439.

125. Engelhardt B, Blalock WA, DonLevy S, Rush M, Hazinski TA. Effect of spironolactone-hydrochlorothiazide on lung function in infants with chronic bronchopulmonary dysplasia. *J Pediatr* 1989;114:619.

126. Atkinson SA, Shah JK, McGee C, Steele BT. Mineral excretion in premature infants receiving various diuretic therapies. *J Pediatr* 1988; 113:540.

127. Wilkie RA, Bryan MH. Effect of bronchodilators on airway resistance in ventilator-dependent neonates with chronic lung disease. *J Pediatr* 1987;111:278.

128. Weiner N. Atropine, scopolamine, and related antimuscarinic drugs. In Gilman AG, Goodman LS, Rall TW, Murad F, eds. *The pharmacologic basis of therapeutics.* New York: Macmillan, 1985:130.

129. Brundage KL, Mohsini KG, Froese AB, Fisher JT. Bronchodilator response to ipratropium bromide in infants with bronchopulmonary dysplasia. *Am Rev Respir Dis* 1990;142:1137.

130. Douglas WW. Histamine and 5-hydroxytryptamine and their antagonists. In Gilman AG, Goodman LS, Rall TW, Murad F, eds. *The pharmacologic basis of therapeutics.* New York: Macmillan, 1985:605.

131. Viscardi RS, Hasday JD, Gumpper KF, Taciak V, Campbell AB. Cromolyn sodium prophylaxis inhibits proinflammatory cytokines in infants at high risk for bronchopulmonary dysplasia. *Am J Respir Crit Care Med* 1997;155:A239.

132. Watterberg KL, Murphy S, et al. Failure of cromolyn sodium to reduce the incidence of bronchopulmonary dysplasia: A pilot study. *Pediatrics* 1993;91:803.

133. Davis JM, Bhutani VK, Stefano JL, Fox WW, Spitzer AR. Changes in pulmonary mechanics following caffeine administration in infants with bronchopulmonary dysplasia. *Pediatr Pulmonol* 1989;6:49.

134. Rooklin AR, Moomjian AS, Shutack JG, Schwartz JG, Fox WW.

Theophylline therapy in bronchopulmonary dysplasia. *J Pediatr* 1979; 95:882.

135. Polgar G. Mechanical properties of the lung and chest wall. In Thibeault DW, Gregory GA, eds. *Neonatal pulmonary care.* Norwalk: Appleton-Century-Crofts, 1986:49.

136. Sosulski R, Abbasi S, Bhutani VK, Fox WW. Physiologic effects of terbutaline on pulmonary function of infants with bronchopulmonary dysplasia. *Pediatr Pulmonol* 1986;2:269.

137. Stefano JL, Bhutani VK, Fox WW. A randomized placebo-controlled study to evaluate the effects of oral albuterol on pulmonary mechanics in ventilator-dependent infants at risk of developing BPD. *Pediatr Pulmonol* 1991;10:183.

138. Haynes RC, Murad F. Adrenocorticotropic hormone; adrenocortical steroids and their synthetic analogs: inhibitors of adrenocortical steroid biosynthesis. In Gilman AG, Goodman LS, Rall TW, Murad F, eds. *The pharmacological basis of therapeutics.* New York: Macmillan, 1985:1459.

139. Wilson JW. Treatment and prevention of pulmonary cellular damage with pharmacologic doses of corticosteroid. *Surg Gynecol Obstet* 1972;134:678.

140. Georgieff MK, Mammel MC, Mills MM, Gunter EW, Johnson DE, Thompson TR. Effect of postnatal steroid administration on serum vitamin A concentrations in newborn infants with respiratory compromise. *J Pediatr* 1989;114:301.

141. DeLemos RA, Shermeta DW, Knelson JH, Kotas R, Avery ME. Acceleration of appearance of pulmonary surfactant in the fetal lamb by administration of corticosteroids. *Am Rev Respir Dis* 1970;102:459.

142. Frank L, Lewis PL, Sosenko IR. Dexamethasone stimulation of rat lung antioxidant enzyme activity in parallel with surfactant stimulation. *Pediatrics* 1985;75:569.

143. Hang SL, Levine L. Inhibition of arachadonic acid release from cells as the biochemical action of anti-inflammatory corticosteroid. *Proc Natl Acad Sci USA* 1976;73:1730.

144. Skubitz KM, Craddock PR, Hammerschmidt DE, August JT. Corticortercoids block binding of chemotactic peptic to its receptor on granulocytes and cause disaggregation of granulocyte aggregates *in vitro. J Clin Invest* 1981;68:13.

145. Kusajima K, Wax SD, Webb WR. Effects of methylprednisolone on pulmonary microcirculation. *Surg Gynecol Obstet* 1974;139:1.

146. Townley RG, Reeb R, Fitzgibbons T, Adolphson RL. The effect of corticosteroid on the beta-adrenergic receptors in bronchial smooth muscle. *J Allergy* 1970;45:118.

147. Cummings JJ, D'Eugenio DB, Gross SJ. A controlled trial of dexamethasone in preterm infants at high risk for bronchopulmonary dysplasia. *N Engl J Med* 1989;320:1505.

148. Wang JY, Yeh TF, Lin YJ, Chen WY, Lin CH. Early postnatal dexamethasone therapy may lessen lung inflammation in premature infants respiratory distress syndrome on mechanical ventilation. *Pediatr Pulmonol* 1997;23:193.

149. Brozanski BS, Jones JG, Gilmour CH, et al. Effect of pulse dexamethasone therapy on the incidence and severity of chronic lung disease in the very low birth weight infant. *J Pediatr* 1995;126:769.

150. Shinwell ES, Karplus M, Zmora E, et al. Failure of early postnatal dexamethasone to prevent chronic lung disease in infants with respiratory distress syndrome. *Arch Dis Child* 1996;74:F33.

151. Yoder MC Jr, Chua R, Tepper R. Effect of dexamethasone on pulmonary inflammation and pulmonary function of ventilator-dependent infants with bronchopulmonary dysplasia. *Am Rev Respir Dis* 1991;143:1044.

152. Gerdes JS, Harris MC, Polin RA. Effects of dexamethasone and indomethacin on elastase, α-1-proteinase inhibitor, and fibronectin in bronchoalveolar lavage fluid from neonates. *J Pediatr* 1988;113:727.

153. Avery GB, Fletcher AB, Kaplan M, Brudno DS. Controlled trial of dexamethasone in respirator dependent infants with bronchopulmonary dysplasia. *Pediatrics* 1985;75:106.

154. Harkavy KL, Scanlon JW, Chowdhry PK, Grylack LJ. Dexamethasone therapy for chronic lung disease in ventilator and oxygen dependent infants: a controlled trial. *J Pediatr* 1989;115:979.

155. Marinelli KA, Burke GS, Herson VC. Effects of dexamethasone on blood pressure in premature infants with bronchopulmonary dysplasia. *J Pediatr* 1997;130:594.

156. Rizvi ZB, Aniol HS, Myers TF, Zeller WP, Fisher SG, Anderson CL. Effects of dexamethasone on the hypothalamic-pituitary-adrenal axis in preterm infants. *J Pediatr* 1992;120:961.

157. Yeh TF, Lin YJ, Lin Ch, et al. Early dexamethasone (<12 hrs) therapy for prevention of BPD in preterm infants with RDS—a two year follow-up study. *Pediatr Res* 1997;41:188A.

158. LaForce WR, Brudno DS. Controlled trial of beclomethasone dipropionate by nebulization in oxygen and ventilator-dependent infants. *J Pediatr* 1993;122:285.

159. Brownlee JR, Beekman RH, Rosenthal A. Acute hemodynamic effects of nifedipine in infants with bronchopulmonary dysplasia and pulmonary hypertension. *Pediatr Res* 1988;24:186.

160. Johnson CE, Beekman RH, Kostyshak DA, Nguyen T, Oh DM, Amidon GL. Pharmacokinetics and pharmacodynamics of nifedipine in children with bronchopulmonary dysplasia and pulmonary hypertension. *Pediatr Res* 1991;29:500.

161. Epstein ML, Kiel EA, Victorica BE. Cardiac decompensation following verapamil therapy in infants with supraventricular tachycardia. *Pediatrics* 1985;75:737.

162. Parker A. Expert handling. *Nurs Times* 1990;86:35.

163. Northway WH Jr. Observations on bronchopulmonary dysplasia. *J Pediatr* 1979;95:815.

164. Myers MG, McGuinness GA, Lachenbruch PA, Koontz FP, Hollingshead R, Olson DB. Respiratory illness in survivors of infant respiratory distress syndrome. *Am Rev Respir Dis* 1986;133:1011.

165. Davidson S, Schrayer A, Wielunsky E, Krikler R, Lilos P, Reisner SH. Energy intake, growth and development in ventilated very-low-birth-weight infants with and without bronchopulmonary dysplasia. *Am J Dis Child* 1990;144:553.

166. Abman SH, Burchell MF, Schaffer MS, Rosenberg AA. Late sudden unexpected deaths in hospitalized infants with bronchopulmonary dysplasia. *Am J Dis Child* 1989;143:815.

167. Werthammer J, Brown ER, Neff RH, Taeusch HW Jr. Sudden infant death syndrome in infants with bronchopulmonary dysplasia. *Pediatrics* 1982;69:301.

168. Gray PH, Roger Y. Are infants with bronchopulmonary dysplasia at risk for sudden infant death syndrome? *Pediatrics* 1994;93:774.

169. Gibson RL, Jackson JC, Twiggs GA, Redding GJ, Truog WE. Bronchopulmonary dysplasia. Survival after prolonged mechanical ventilation. *Am J Dis Child* 1988;142:721.

170. Phibbs RH, Ballard RA, Clements JA, et al. Initial clinical trial of Exosurf, a protein-free synthetic surfactant, for the prophylaxis and early treatment of hyaline membrane disease. *Pediatrics* 1991;88:1.

171. Bader D, Ramos AD, Lew CD, et al. Childhood sequelae of infant lung disease: exercise and pulmonary function abnormalities after bronchopulmonary dysplasia. *J Pediatr* 1987;110:693.

172. Andreasson B, Lindroth M, Mortensson W, Svenningsen NW, Jonson B. Lung function eight years after neonatal ventilation. *Arch Dis Child* 1989;64:108.

173. Blayney M, Kerem E, Whyte H, O'Brodovich H. Bronchopulmonary dysplasia: improvement in lung function between 7 and 10 years of age. *J Pediatr* 1991;118:201.

174. Hakulinen AL, Heinonen K, Lansimies E, Kiekara O. Pulmonary function and respiratory morbidity in school-age children born prematurely and ventilated for neonatal respiratory insufficiency. *Pediatr Pulmonol* 1990;8:226.

175. Northway WH Jr, Moss RB, Carlisle KG, et al. Late pulmonary sequelae of bronchopulmonary dysplasia. *N Engl J Med* 1990;323:1793.

176. Jacob SV, Lands LC, Coates AL et al. Exercise ability in survivors of bronchopulmonary dysplasia. *Am J Respir Crit Care Med* 1997;155:1925.

177. Giacoia GP, Venkataraman PS, West-Wilson KI, Faulkner MJ. Follow-up of school-age children with bronchopulmonary dysplasia. *J Pediatr* 1997;130:400.

178. Baraldi E, Filippone M, Trevisanuto D, Zanardo V, Zacchello F. Pulmonary function until two years of life in infants with bronchopulmonary dysplasia. *Am J Respir Crit Care Med* 1997;155:149.

179. Groothuis JR, Gutierrez KM, Lauer BA. Respiratory syncytial virus infection in children with bronchopulmonary dysplasia. *Pediatrics* 1988;82:199.

180. Meert K, Heidemann S, Lieh-Lai M, Sarnaik AP. Clinical characteristics of respiratory syncytial virus infections in healthy versus previously compromised host. *Pediatr Pulmonol* 1989;7:167.

181. American Academy of Pediatrics. Respiratory syncytial virus. In Peter G, ed. *1997 red book: Report of the Committee on Infectious Diseases,* 24th ed. Elk Grove Village, IL: American Academy of Pediatrics, 1997:443.

182. Chidekel AS, Rosen CL, Bazzy AR. Rhinovirus infection associated with serious lower respiratory illness in patients with bronchopulmonary dysplasia. *Pediatr Infect Dis J* 1997;16:43.

183. Kalhan SC, Denne SC. Energy consumption in infants with bronchopulmonary dysplasia. *J Pediatr* 1990;116:662.

184. Kao LC, Durand DJ, Nickerson BG. Improving pulmonary function does not decrease oxygen consumption in infants with bronchopulmonary dysplasia. *J Pediatr* 1988;112:616.

185. Kurzner SI, Garg M, Bautista DB, et al. Growth failure in infants with bronchopulmonary dysplasia: nutrition and elevated resting metabolic expenditure. *Pediatrics* 1988;81:379.

186. Markestad T, Fitzhardinge PM. Growth and development in children recovering from bronchopulmonary dysplasia. *J Pediatr* 1981;98:597.

187. Yu VYH, Orgill AA, Lim SB, Bajuk B, Astbury J. Growth and development of very low birth weight infants recovering from bronchopulmonary dysplasia. *Arch Dis Child* 1983;58:791.

188. Vohr BR, Coll CG, Lobato D, et al. Neurodevelopmental and medical status of low-birthweight survivors of bronchopulmonary dysplasia at 10 to 12 years of age. *Dev Med Child Neurol* 1991;33:690.

189. Singer L, Yamashita T, Lilien L, Collin M, Baley J. A longitudinal study of developmental outcome of infants with bronchopulmonary dysplasia and very low birth weight. *Pediatrics* 1997;100:987.

190. Van Marter LJ, Leviton A, Kuban KC, Pagano M, Allred EN. Maternal glucocorticoid therapy and reduced risk of bronchopulmonary dysplasia. *Pediatrics* 1990;86:331.

191. Auten RL, Notter RH, Kendig JW, Davis JM, Shapiro DL. Surfactant treatment of full-term newborns with respiratory failure. *Pediatrics* 1991;87:101.

192. Frank L, Sosenko IR. Undernutrition as a major contributing factor in the pathogenesis of bronchopulmonary dysplasia. *Am Rev Respir Dis* 1988;138:725.

193. Shenai JP, Kennedy KA, Chytil F, Stahlman MT. Clinical trial of vitamin A supplementation in infants susceptible to bronchopulmonary dysplasia. *J Pediatr* 1987;111:269.

194. Kennedy KA, Stoll BJ, Ehrenkranz RA, et al. Vitamin A to prevent bronchopulmonary dysplasia in very low birth weight infants: has the dose been too low? *Early Hum Dev* 1997;49:19.

195. Davis JM, Richter SE, Kendig JW, Notter RH. High frequency jet ventilation and surfactant treatment of newborns with severe respiratory failure. *Pediatr Pulmonol* 1992;13:108.

196. O'Rourke PP, Crone RK, Vacanti JP, et al. Extracorporeal membrane oxygenation and conventional medical therapy in neonates with persistent pulmonary hypertension of the newborn: a prospective randomized study. *Pediatrics* 1989;84:957.

197. Robbins CG, Davis JM, Merritt TA, et al. Combined effects of nitric oxide and hyperoxia on surfactant function and pulmonary inflammation. *Am J Physiol* 1995;269:L545.

198. Narula P, Xu J, Kazzaz J, et al. Synergistic cytotoxicity from nitric oxide and hyperoxia in cultured alveolar epithelial cells. *Am J Physiol* 1998;274:L411.

199. de Los Santos R, Seidenfeld JJ, Anzueto A, et al. One hundred percent oxygen lung injury in adult baboons. *Am Rev Respir Dis* 1987;136:657.

200. Jacobson JM, Michael JR, Jafri MH Jr, Gurtner GH. Antioxidants and antioxidant enzymes protect against pulmonary oxygen toxicity in the rabbit. *J Appl Physiol* 1990;68:1252.

201. Tanswell AK, Freeman BA. Liposome-entrapped antioxidant enzymes prevent lethal O_2 toxicity in the newborn rat. *J Appl Physiol* 1987;63:347.

202. Walther FJ, Gidding CE, Kuipers IM, et al. Prevention of oxygen toxicity with superoxide dismutase and catalase in premature lambs. *J Free Radic Biol Med* 1986;2:289.

203. Rosenfeld W, Evans H, Concepcion L, Jhaveri R, Schaeffer H, Friedman A. Prevention of bronchopulmonary dysplasia by administration of bovine superoxide dismutase in preterm infants with respiratory distress syndrome. *J Pediatr* 1984;105:781.

204. Rosenfeld WN, Davis JM, Parton L, et al. Safety and pharmacokinetics of recombinant human superoxide dismutase administered intratracheally to premature neonates with respiratory distress syndrome. *Pediatrics* 1996;97:811.

205. Davis JM, Rosenfeld WN, Richter SE, et al. Safety and pharmacokinetics of multiple doses of recombinant human CuZn superoxide dismutase administered intratracheally to premature neonates with respiratory distress syndrome. *Pediatrics* 1997;100:24.

206. Sahgal N, Davis JM, Robbins C, et al. Localization and activity of recombinant human CuZn superoxide dismutase after intratracheal administration. *Am J Physiol* 1996;271:L230.

CHAPTER 30

Principles of Management of Respiratory Problems

W. Alan Hodson and William E. Truog

Respiratory disorders continue to be a major cause of neonatal morbidity despite a marked reduction in mortality over the past decade. The increased use of antenatal steroids and surfactant replacement therapy have decreased the incidence and severity of respiratory distress syndrome (RDS). As a greater percentage of hospitals are attempting to provide more sophisticated neonatal care, the need for specialized respiratory care increases the demand for neonatologists, nurses, respiratory therapists, and highly specialized equipment. Although the principles of management of respiratory disorders remain unchanged, the techniques of treatment have become more complex in the presence of an ever increasing and sophisticated technology. This complexity is due to the incorporation of highly technical and unique equipment and the necessary skilled personnel. The continuing and important problem of bronchopulmonary dysplasia (BPD) has had a strong influence on stimulating newer ventilatory strategies for preventing chronic lung injury as well as efforts to avoid endotracheal intubation and mechanical ventilation. Newer techniques of management have explored nonconventional means of treatment, such as high-frequency oscillatory ventilation (HFOV), liquid ventilation, and nasal pharyngeal ventilation. Knowledge of the pathophysiology of lung disorders and the maturational status of the lung is essential to the safe and efficacious application of specialized techniques of treatment.

There are standard principles of respiratory management:

- Establish airway,
- Ensure oxygenation,
- Assist ventilation,
- Assess adequacy of ventilation,
- Correct metabolic abnormalities, and
- Alleviate the cause of distress.

The goal of respiratory treatment is to provide tissue oxygenation and CO_2 removal in a safe and effective manner. Too much oxygen can be harmful. Overly aggressive lung distention can result in stretching and tearing of the lung. Respiratory and/or metabolic acidosis may constrict pulmonary blood vessels, thus affecting pulmonary blood flow. Attention to other organ system dysfunction due to hypotension (shock), hypothermia, sepsis, fluid imbalance, or metabolic derangements needs to occur in parallel with respiratory management. One of the most challenging aspects of ventilatory treatment is the dynamic way in which ventilatory status can change, due to either the treatment applied or progression of the underlying disease. This chapter reviews the rationale and principles of respiratory management and methods of continuous, accurate, and careful assessment.

OXYGEN THERAPY

Physiologic Considerations

The goal of oxygen therapy is to provide adequate tissue oxygenation without undue risk of oxygen toxicity. An arterial partial pressure of oxygen (PaO_2) of 45 mm Hg results in a saturation of fetal hemoglobin (HbF) of approximately 90%, and maintaining the PaO_2 above 50 mm Hg should be sufficient for tissue oxygen needs. Mitochondrial PO_2 is about 2 mm Hg. Unfortunately, there is no practical method for measuring tissue PO_2, and the arterial value remains the best approximation. An arbitrary ceiling of 80 mm Hg is set to minimize the risk of retinopathy of prematurity in infants weighing less

W. A. Hodson: Department of Pediatrics, University of Washington, Seattle, Washington

W. E. Truog: Department of Pediatrics, Children's Mercy Hospital, Kansas City, Missouri

than 1,500 g at birth, although retinopathy of prematurity may be unavoidable in certain extremely-low-birth-weight infants (1–3). The rationale for maintaining the PaO_2 below 100 mm Hg in larger infants is based on minimizing pulmonary oxygen toxicity. When administering oxygen, it is always useful to translate the percent of inspired oxygen to the corresponding partial pressure (PIO_2). The gap between the alveolar partial pressure of oxygen (PAO_2) and the PaO_2 indicates the magnitude of the arterial O_2 gradient across the lungs and provides an indication of the magnitude of right-to-left shunting of blood. A simplification of the alveolar air equation provides an estimate of PAO_2 (i.e., $PAO_2 = PIO_2 − PACO_2$).

Because the barometric pressure, minus water vapor pressure, is approximately 700 mm Hg, the percent of inspired oxygen multiplied by 7 equals PIO_2 in mm Hg (e.g., $21\% \approx 147$ mm Hg, $50\% \approx 350$ mm Hg). Because $PACO_2$ approximates $PaCO_2$ due to a usually insignificant arterial–alveolar CO_2 gradient ($aADCO_2$), $PaCO_2$ can be substituted for $PACO_2$, and PAO_2 can be derived. For example, if an infant is breathing 60% O_2, the measured PaO_2 is 70 mm Hg and the $PaCO_2$ is 40 mm Hg, the $PAO_2 = 420 − 40 = 380$ mm Hg, and the alveolar–arterial gradient for O_2 ($AaDO_2$) is 310 mm Hg. In an infant without lung disease or a significant right-to-left cardiac shunt, the $AaDO_2$ should not exceed 25 mm Hg while breathing ambient air. Infants with severe RDS may have an $AaDO_2$ in excess of 500 mm Hg while breathing 100% oxygen (4).

Oxygen Delivery

Each gram of HbF binds 1.37 dL of oxygen. The full-term newborn with a hemoglobin (Hb) of 17 g/dL binds and transports 23 dL of oxygen per 100 dL of blood. Less than 2% of transported O_2 is carried as oxygen dissolved in plasma. Normal tissue consumption extracts approximately four volumes percent (4 mL/100 mL) if oxygen consumption and cardiac output are normal. HbF binds oxygen with a greater affinity than adult Hb. The oxyhemoglobin saturation curve is nonlinear, and the P_{50}, the PaO_2 at which Hb is 50% saturated, increases with gestational age (Fig. 30–1). The higher the P_{50}, the greater the driving pressure for oxygen unloading. The curve gradually shifts to the right as hemoglobin A increases after birth. Several factors can adversely affect oxygen delivery, including decreased cardiac output, maldistribution of cardiac output, arterial vasoconstriction, and shifts in the O_2 dissociation curve. Oxygen unloading in the tissues is increased with a shift to the right of the O_2 dissociation curve (i.e., decreased O_2 affinity of Hb) facilitated by a local decrease in pH, increase in $PaCO_2$, and increase in temperature. A shift to the right of the O_2 dissociation curve can result from transfusion of adult red blood cells. Oxygen uptake depends on adequate alveolar ventilation ($\dot{V}_A$), an appropriate ventilation–perfusion match in the

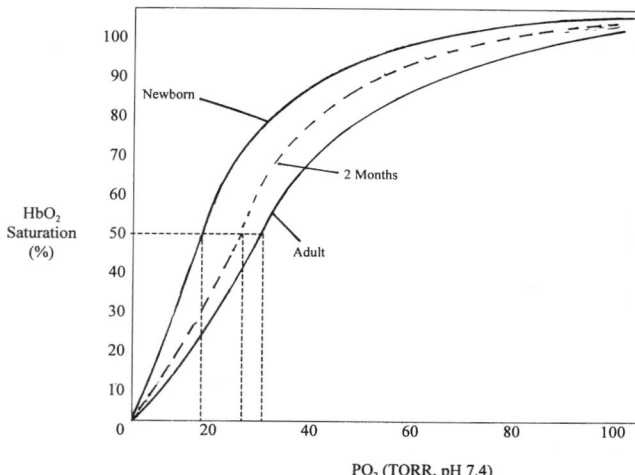

FIG. 30–1. Oxygen equilibrium curves of hemoglobin at birth, 2 months of age, and adulthood. Note the increase in P_{50} with age.

lungs, and absence of right-to-left shunting. Oxygen uptake or increased O_2 affinity of Hb (i.e., shift of curve to left) is enhanced by alkalosis, decreased temperature, decreased 2,3-diphosphoglycerate, and increased HbF.

Oxygen Administration

The concentration, humidity, and temperature of inspired oxygen should be precisely controlled. Diluting or mixing chambers can deliver only an approximate O_2 concentration, and it is necessary to have a precise analysis of the O_2 concentration being delivered to the infant's airway. An incubator is ineffective in maintaining O_2 concentrations above 30%, because opening of the portholes causes considerable dilution. Nasal prongs are the preferable route of humidified oxygen administration if there is need for chronic administration. The concentration and the rate of flow are varied, and the precise amount of oxygen delivered to the lungs by nasal prongs is difficult to determine. This is because there may be dilution of inspired air through ill-fitting prongs or through an open mouth. The impact of the concentration to be delivered should be determined by continuous monitoring of peripheral oxygen saturation and intermittently of PaO_2. The O_2–air mixture should be warmed to the same temperature as the incubator air, which should be in the range of thermal neutrality (see Chap. 24).

ASSESSMENT OF GAS EXCHANGE

Clinical Assessment

The infant with respiratory problems may present with a wide spectrum of clinical findings. The infant's response depends in large part on the degree of prematurity, lung and chest wall development, and maturation of respiratory control. The full-term infant may be able to increase the work of breathing to accomplish adequate gas exchange without treatment, including oxygen administration. The extremely premature infant will have a much weaker respiratory drive and inadequate muscular development and, thus, is less able to compensate for lung abnormalities. The classic clinical signs of respiratory distress are, therefore, still helpful in the assessment of the mature newborn infant. Nasal flaring, grunting respirations, and tachypnea are almost always present. With progression of lung disease and decreased lung compliance, chest wall retractions become more marked. With increased work of breathing, retractions progress from sternal to subcostal, to intercostal, and then to a seesaw pattern of chest and abdominal wall movement. The full-term infant may increase respiratory rate above 100 per minute, with shallow respirations. This pattern is the most efficient way to increase gas exchange, with the least costly work of breathing. Expiratory grunting represents an effort to retard or brake expiratory flow to increase end-expiratory pressure and maintain alveolar patency. It is unsafe to rely on color changes as an indication of oxygenation, as abnormalities in peripheral perfusion due to poor cardiac output, hypotension, or hypovolemia may be misleading. Similarly, infants with recurrent apnea will have intermittent deficiency in gas exchange. Auscultation assists in determining the quality of air entry in various parts of the lung as well as the presence of airway secretions or obstructions. The continuing, recurrent monitoring of clinical signs is critical to the laboratory assessment of gas exchange. Continuous oxygen saturation monitors have been a tremendous help in assisting in management decisions. However, this does not obviate the need for careful clinical observations.

The history of the pregnancy and delivery are vital to the assessment of the infant with respiratory distress. This information should include gestational age, maternal and pregnancy abnormalities, maternal medications, risks of infectious disease, mode of delivery, adaptation to birth (Apgar score), and the timing of onset of respiratory distress. Most causes of respiratory failure can be discerned from the history, clinical presentation, and chest radiograph.

Laboratory Assessment

The measurement of blood gases and pH remains a necessary part of evaluating therapy, helps to confirm clinical impressions, and verifies the values obtained by pulse oximetry, transcutaneous electrodes, and end-tidal CO_2 monitoring. Most importantly, it helps to minimize the risks of hypoxia, hyperoxia, hypocapnia, hypercapnia, and metabolic acidosis.

Blood Gases

Blood may be obtained by puncture of a peripheral artery, cannulation of a peripheral or umbilical artery, venous blood sampling, or capillary puncture. Venous and/or capillary blood values provide an approximation of arterial PCO_2 and pH but no useful information about arterial oxygenation. The PCO_2 in venous blood is approximately 6 mm Hg higher and pH 0.03 lower than in arterial blood. Peripheral arterial blood most often is sampled from the radial or posterior tibial arteries using a 23- or 25-gauge needle. Peripheral puncture is indicated when the anticipated number of samples will be small, or if arterial cannulation is unsuccessful. The painful nature of the procedure may result in altered breathing and a spurious result. The femoral artery should be avoided, as the possibility of an occlusive hematoma may seriously compromise distal circulation. There is also a risk of joint infection. After withdrawal of the needle, the site should be compressed for several minutes to prevent hematoma formation. Repeated punctures can be made at the same site. The frequency of blood gas determination is dictated by changes in clinical, radiologic, and other monitoring parameters.

Cannulation

The choice of peripheral artery or umbilical artery catheterization usually is determined by the size of the infant, the anticipated duration of the cannulation, and the need for infusions of medications and parenteral nutrition. Hypertonic solutions, including concentrated dextrose solutions, should not be given through a small peripheral arterial cannula. The major advantage of a peripheral arterial catheter is the avoidance of an umbilical cannulation and its high rate of thrombosis. A right radial arterial catheter has the unique advantage of sampling preductal PaO_2, which more accurately reflects retinal artery PO_2.

The need to insert a catheter into the umbilical artery should be based on the infant's maturation, postnatal age, and the type, severity, and expected duration of the illness. Seriously ill infants weighing less than 1,000 g at birth usually qualify. The high incidence of thrombus formation on the catheter tip, with its attendant risk of mural thrombus or emboli, must be weighed against the potential benefits to the infant. When more reliable methods of monitoring tissue oxygenation, such as near-infrared spectrometry, become available, the need for umbilical artery catheterization should be minimal.

The tip of the umbilical catheter should rest in a low or high position to avoid the risk of occlusion, thrombosis, or direct infusion into a major branching artery. The distance to various levels within the aorta is estimated from the infant's shoulder to umbilicus distance and the chart of Dunn (Fig. 30–2) (5).The high location range is between T4 (ductus arteriosus) and T11 (celiac artery), with the tip ideally resting between T7 and T10. At the lower site, the tip should be between L4 and the bifurcation of the aorta. Three studies have compared the inci-

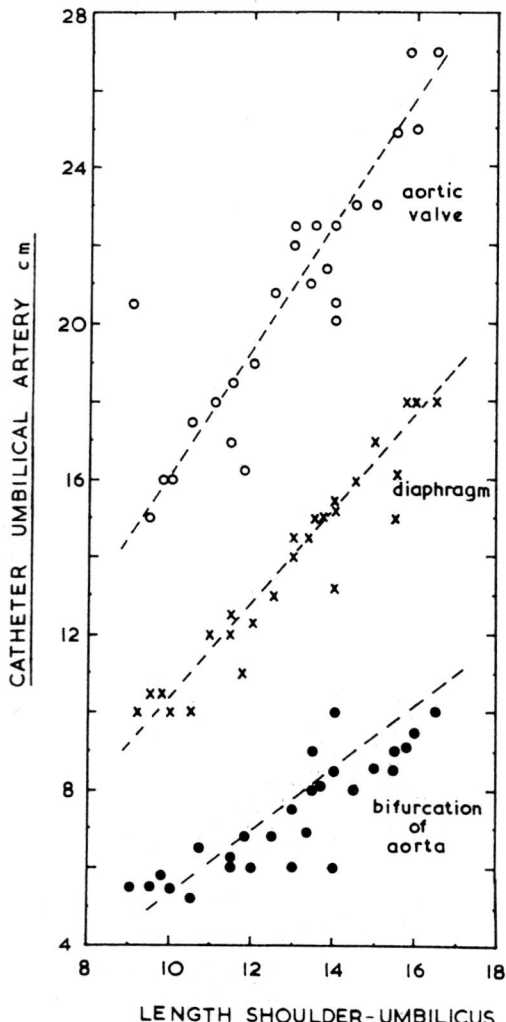

FIG. 30–2. Relation between the shoulder-to-umbilicus measurement and the length of umbilical artery catheter needed to reach the aortic bifurcation, diaphragm, and aortic valve. (From ref. 5.)

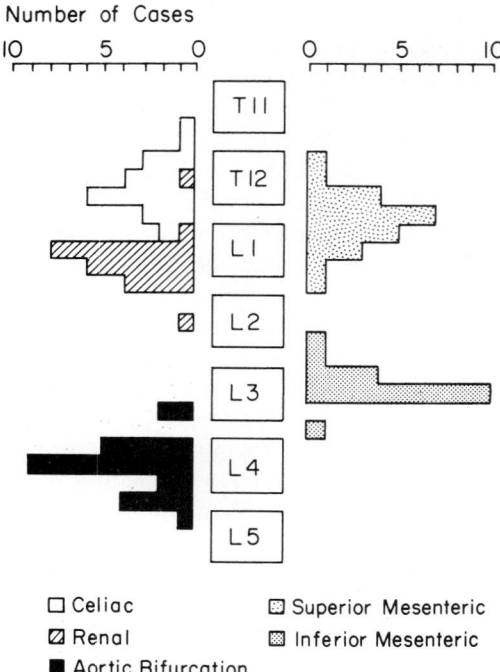

FIG. 30–3. Origins of the major arteries in relation to the vertebral bodies were determined by postmortem angiography on 27 full-term and premature infants. (Data courtesy of C. B. Graham, M.D., University of Washington, Seattle, WA.)

dence of complications of high and low catheter placement (6–8) and indicate a higher complication rate with catheters in the low position. The higher position allows greater leeway for catheter migration, although there is a greater risk of downstream embolization. A thoracoabdominal radiograph should be obtained immediately after catheter placement and before medications are infused. The vertebral landmarks and usual levels of arterial branches are depicted in Fig. 30–3.

Once the catheter is in place, there is a risk of intraluminal clotting. Therefore, a continuous infusion is required, as is flushing of the line following blood sampling. Heparinization of fluid infusions has not been shown to reduce the incidence of thrombosis. A pressure strain gauge should be connected to the catheter, with alarm limits to indicate changes in blood pressure signaling changes in blood volume or cardiac output. Dampening of the pres-

sure waveform indicates intraluminal or catheter tip narrowing or obstruction. The catheter should be removed once the infant has improved, the frequency of blood gas determinations has decreased to once or twice per day, and systemic arterial pressure monitoring no longer is essential. Occasionally the catheter may remain in place for several weeks with no evidence of complications.

The complications of umbilical artery catheterization are listed in Table 30–1. The most frequent problem is peripheral vasospasm associated with blanching or patchy cyanosis of the distal leg, foot, or toes. If this does not improve with reflex vasodilation by warming of the contralateral leg, or worsens over the next 15 to 20 minutes, the catheter should be removed. Assessment of peripheral arterial pulses by Doppler stethoscope often is helpful in deciding about catheter removal. Some thrombosis at the catheter tip is inevitable. Fortunately, the rate of complications from thrombus formation is acceptably low. Controversies exist about the risk of necrotizing enterocolitis if enteral feedings are initiated while the catheter is in place. However, the evidence for causality is poor; therefore, it is appropriate to initiate feedings gradually prior to catheter removal.

Transcutaneous PO₂ and PCO₂

Transcutaneous PO_2 monitoring should be used selectively in conjunction with pulse oximetry. Most devices

TABLE 30–1. *Complications of umbilical catheterization*

Complication	Incidence	Comment
Limb ischemia	<20%	Assess Doppler arterial and venous flow from femoral region to dorsalis pedis; if reflex and unilateral, apply warmth to contralateral extremity; if persistent (>15 min), remove catheter
Thrombosis	<90%	Assess by ultrasonographic study of aorta
Infection		Remove in presence of gram-positive blood culture if catheter was inserted
Colonization	57%	more than 24 h previously; no relation to duration of catheter
Sepsis	5%	
Blood loss	Rare	Connection to blood pressure transducer with alarm should prevent significant loss
Vascular perforation	Extremely rare	On removal, clamp for 5–10 min

contain O_2 and CO_2 electrodes. Noninvasive PO_2 measurements continue to be helpful in certain situations, particularly if transcutaneous PCO_2 also is obtained. Calibration before use and correlation with an arterial sample are necessary, but the need for subsequent blood samples should be reduced.

The PaO_2 and transcutaneous PO_2 are not identical. Differences can be due to local O_2 consumption by the skin or by the electrode itself, heating of the skin, O_2 diffusion time, and response time of the electrode (9). These differences, by acting in opposite directions, tend to cancel each other and fortuitously provide an accurate reflection of PaO_2 (10,11). Skin blood flow may be affected by vasopressor medications, hypotension, and shock (12). Use of transcutaneous PO_2 can reduce the number of blood sampling procedures, particularly during a period when rapid changes in O_2 administration or mechanical ventilatory settings are taking place. Continuous monitoring for several hours also allows assessment of changes due to position, handling, suctioning, and feeding and for comparison with SaO_2 monitoring. Second-degree burns (i.e., blistering) preclude its use for longer than 5 hours at a single site on the body. If longer use is required, the electrode site should be shifted every 3 to 4 hours and requires additional correlation with PaO_2. The short application time has made transcutaneous PO_2 monitoring less useful than oximetry for continuous assessment of oxygen over a period of many hours.

Pulse Oximetry

The now common application of pulse oximetry to the intensive care nursery has provided a safe, accurate, and noninvasive adjunct to the assessment of tissue oxygenation (13). Oxygen saturation is determined by infrared spectrometry, utilizing two electrodes and a small cuff that can be placed around a hand, foot, or toe without requiring heating or calibration. It has an extremely rapid response time. One electrode contains two diodes that emit light at two wavelengths: red at 660 nm and infrared at 940 nm. The other electrode senses the light from both of these diodes that has not been absorbed by blood or tissue. The relative concentration of hemoglobin–oxygen (HbO_2) and

deoxyhemoglobin determines the amount of transmitted light, because different forms of Hb have markedly different absorption characteristics. The ratio of the amount of light absorbed at each wavelength is used to calculate a SaO_2 value. The pulsed element of the apparatus allows the instrument to differentiate added arterial blood oxygenation and absorption from tissue, and it subtracts the amount contributed by nonpulsatile venous and arterial blood flow. With PO_2 values greater than 40 mm Hg, the saturation accurately reflects measurements of PO_2 obtained by catheter sample or by transcutaneous PO_2 (14).

A PaO_2 of 60 to 90 mm Hg results in a saturation value of 94% to 98% (see Fig. 30–1), and changes of 1% to 2% usually reflect a PaO_2 change of 6 to 12 mm Hg (13). The point of inflection at which the HbO_2 dissociation curve steepens has considerable variability and depends on proportions of hemoglobin A, HbF, PCO_2, pH, and temperature. Generally, these variables are not so critical to the interpretation of the percent SaO_2 in arterial blood as they are to PaO_2. Below 40 mm Hg, the SaO_2 falls below 90%. An alarm limit usually is set at 89%, although this lower limit may need adjustment. For example, if an infant has pulmonary hypertension, a PaO_2 below 50 mm Hg may increase pulmonary vascular resistance, and the saturation may best be maintained above 94%. If the infant is acutely ill and unstable, a correlation with PaO_2, preferably obtained by a catheter blood sample, is indicated. Poor correlation with PaO_2 exists when the SaO_2 is above a peak 98%, in which case the PaO_2 may be well above 100 mm Hg. The data of Hay et al. (13) suggest an appropriate goal is to maintain the saturation between 92% and 98% unless a specific clinical situation indicates otherwise. In very-low-birth-weight infants who require chronic oxygen administration and who are at risk for developing retinopathy of prematurity, the upper limit of saturation should be reduced to 95%. Inaccuracies may reflect improper placement, movement, or peripheral ischemia. Motion artifacts also produce invalid readings.

End-Tidal CO_2 Monitoring

The concentration of CO_2 at the mouth or nose rises to reach a plateau at the end of each breath. This plateau reflects the alveolar CO_2 concentration under normal conditions, but may be inaccurate if there is ventilation–perfusion inequality or inhomogeneity of lung disease. Recent refinements to end-tidal CO_2 detection equipment permit in-line or "mainstream" infrared monitoring just proximal to the endotracheal tube (capnography), with a continuous display of the PCO_2 waveform. There is minimal dead space of the apparatus, and sampling accuracy has improved to compensate for the low expiratory flow rates characteristic of small premature infants. End-tidal CO_2 is less reliable in extremely small premature infants. Capnography is as accurate as a capillary PCO_2 and is less precise than transcutaneous monitoring (15–17). It is helpful in the early detection of hypocapnia, which can occur following surfactant administration. It is also useful in avoiding hypercapnia with worsening respiratory failure, although its accuracy decreases as lung function declines (17,18). Arterial blood gases should be obtained when the end-tidal monitor displays readings below 28 or above 45 mm Hg.

Limiting the exposure time to hypocarbia may be important in preventing the development of cystic periventricular leukomalacia or decreasing the risk of BPD (19–21). There has been increased interest in "permissive hypercapnia," wherein modest elevations of PCO_2 to 55 to 60 mm Hg are considered acceptable. The rationale is to avoid high peak inspiratory or mean airway pressures during mechanical ventilation or to delay or avoid the initiation of mechanical ventilation (22–25). Studies of permissive hypercapnia in adults with adult respiratory distress syndrome (ARDS) have been inconclusive (26,27), and no definitive studies have clarified its role in preventing BPD. Nevertheless, continuous end-tidal CO_2 monitoring should permit rapid detection of changes in gas exchange and should facilitate weaning of ventilatory settings.

Near-Infrared Spectroscopy

Utilization of the unique light-absorbing properties of Hb and HbO_2, as used in pulsed oximetry, has led to a more sophisticated method of appraising tissue oxygenation by means of near-infrared spectroscopy. Near-infrared light penetrates the skin, bone, and various tissues and can be detected by electrodes placed on opposite sides of an infant's skull. This permits assessment of cerebral tissue O_2 and alterations in cerebral blood volume. Hb and cytochrome a and a_3 (cyt a, a_3) change their absorption characteristics according to the degree of oxygenation. The wavelength at which maximal absorption occurs is different for HbO_2, deoxygenated Hb, total Hb, and reduced and oxygenated cyt a, a_3 (28). Using photomultiplication and algorithms, the degree of oxygenation can be determined. Quantification of reduced cyt a, a_3 should provide an early indication of insufficient mitochondrial oxygen (29).

The small cranial size of the infant weighing less than 1,500 g makes cross-temple spectroscopy feasible. Preliminary studies using experimental equipment are encouraging (30,31). The light source at one temple is a fiberoptic bundle consisting of four laser diodes with different wavelengths. A second fiberoptic bundle on the opposite temple detects transmitted light of various wavelengths (30,32). The amplified signals indicate the relative amounts of HbO_2 and cyt a, a_3, providing a continuous assessment of the trends in cerebral oxygenation and blood volume (30,32,33). This important new method of assessing brain oxygenation has the potential to provide new information on changes in cerebral blood flow (34) and oxygenation resulting from infusions of drugs (e.g., vasopressors, indomethacin), changes in position, nursing procedures, paralysis, apnea and bradycardia, shock, decreased blood pressure, patent ductus arteriosus, and intrathoracic pressure variations secondary to mechanical ventilation. Further refinement of equipment and verification of its accuracy in reflecting changes in cerebral blood flow and cerebral oxygenation are needed. This method of oxygen assessment has immense potential for use in the neonatal intensive care unit (35).

CONTINUOUS POSITIVE AIRWAY PRESSURE

The application of end-expiratory pressure is intended to prevent alveoli and/or terminal airways from collapsing to airlessness. Continuous positive airway pressure (CPAP) may be applied during spontaneous breathing or as positive end-expiratory pressure (PEEP) during mechanical ventilation. This usually requires pressures between 4 to 6 cm H_2O for CPAP and 3 to 8 cm H_2O for PEEP.

The physiologic effects of CPAP/PEEP may vary depending on the underlying pulmonary pathology, although the primary goal is to prevent alveolar collapse. Observations by Harrison et al. (36) of grunting respirations in infants with respiratory distress suggested that the expiratory grunt represented laryngeal narrowing and increased resistance to expiratory flow to increase end-expiratory alveolar pressure. These observations led to the use of CPAP (24,37) and the need for PEEP once laryngeal closure was prevented by endotracheal intubation. In the surfactant-deficient state, alveoli will collapse at end-expiration unless a minimum distending pressure is maintained. CPAP of 3 to 4 cm H_2O will prevent alveolar collapse but will not recruit atelectatic alveoli. Opening pressures of 12 to 15 cm H_2O are required to inflate collapsed alveoli. The infant will need to create a high peak inspiratory pressure (PIP) in the absence of CPAP. The sheer forces from opening and closing of alveoli may contribute to alveolar epithelial damage. In addition, resultant abnormal distending forces on terminal or respiratory bronchioles will contribute to small airway injury. CPAP above physiologic levels of 3 to 4 cm H_2O

may cause overinflation of some alveoli. Therefore, Inflation and deflation may occur on the flatter portion of the pressure–volume curve and increase the work of breathing. Changes in lung mechanics and an increase in lung volume have been measured (38–40). CPAP theoretically could stimulate surfactant secretion. Maintenance of alveolar volume will reduce right-to-left shunting of blood through atelectatic alveoli, hence reducing oxygen needs. With excessive CPAP, PCO_2 may increase due to distention of airways and enlargement of the anatomic dead space. CPAP distends proximal airways with a resultant decrease in supraglottic airway resistance (41,42).

Indications

The clinical indications for CPAP are varied. Initial use was directed at infants with RDS whose oxygen requirements exceeded 60% to minimize oxygen toxicity and delay or avoid mechanical ventilation. The gestational age, birth weight, and stage and severity of respiratory disease should be factored into the decision to initiate CPAP. Full-term infants and infants greater than 33 weeks of gestation are at minimal risk of developing BPD and, therefore, the use of oxygen concentrations greater than 60% are warranted. On the other hand, if these infants have severe lung disease, e.g., meconium aspiration, hyaline membrane disease (HMD), or pulmonary hypertension, more aggressive therapy, including mechanical ventilation, usually is indicated.

It is popular to apply early nasal CPAP to infants weighing less than 1,000 g at birth who have little or no lung disease. These infants are at considerable risk for developing BPD and recurrent apneic episodes; therefore, they commonly are intubated and supported with mechanical ventilation due to their inability to sustain an adequate respiratory effort. They often develop an increasing oxygen need during the second week of life, associated with early signs of BPD and attributed, in part, to mechanical ventilation. CPAP appears to be well tolerated by such infants over a period of many days. CPAP may be beneficial in maintaining patency of extremely small terminal airways and prealveolar gas exchange units in these very immature infants. The increased enthusiasm for the use of CPAP is stimulated by the desire to minimize or prevent BPD. A comparative analysis of management protocols in eight centers in the United States indicated a similar incidence of BPD in all but one center (43). Columbia Presbyterian Hospital had a lower incidence of BPD and was unique from the other centers in its reliance on the use of early CPAP and tolerance for hypercapnia. A subsequent survey of 11 centers suggested that CPAP might have a beneficial effect on the incidence of BPD (44). Because mechanical ventilation is a major putative factor in the etiology of BPD, the use of early CPAP to avoid or minimize barotrauma has much appeal. Avoidance of endotracheal intubation should decrease the chances for tracheal injury, airway infection, abnormal mucociliary function, and overinflation from excess ventilator pressure or volume.

Brief intubation and the administration of a single dose of surfactant followed by nasal CPAP has been advocated as another method of reducing the need for mechanical ventilation in infants with moderate HMD (45). Improvement in gas exchange has been demonstrated; however, more evidence of its efficacy in reducing the incidence or severity of BPD is required.

Recurrent Apnea

CPAP helps some infants with recurrent apnea of prematurity to sustain a more regular respiratory rate. The mechanism of its action is not well understood, although an increase in functional residual capacity (FRC) may alter the Herring–Breuer reflex or stabilize the thoracic cage, minimizing chest wall distortion and possibly altering inhibitory spinal cord reflexes (46). CPAP also helps to overcome obstructive apnea (42).

Positive End-Expiratory Pressure

Some applied end-expiratory pressure is always needed during mechanical ventilation. The optimum pressure will depend on the underlying lung pathology. Usually 4 to 6 cm H_2O is adequate; however, if there has been smooth muscle hyperplasia or epithelial dysplasia of small airways, higher pressures (e.g., 8 cm H_2O) may be necessary to prevent airway closure.

Methods

Earlier methods of applying CPAP utilized an enclosed head box, face masks, and nasopharyngeal tubes. More recently, nasal prongs have been adapted to fit most infants. Continuous negative expiratory pressure, applied around the thorax, also has proven effective in improving gas exchange in infants with HMD (47,48). Continuous negative expiratory pressure requires somewhat more elaborate equipment to prevent air leak, and for this reason has not been practical. A newer device (the ALADDIN Infant Flow System, Hamilton Medical Inc., Reno, NV) appears to be well tolerated by both large and small infants. This apparatus maintains a constant flow of air by incorporating a double fluidic jet system within the apparatus. During inspiration, one jet maintains the flow to match the infant's inspiratory effort; during expiration, gas flow is reversed by a second jet to assist outflow while maintaining a constant minimum pressure. This system presumably does not add to the work of breathing and reduces the need to use high flow rates to compensate for air leak around the nasal prongs.

Complications

CPAP may have adverse effects. Overinflation can result in increased work of breathing and a decreased efficiency of gas exchange. Occasionally, pneumothorax and pneumomediastinum may result. Carbon dioxide retention may occur due to either increased dead space or ineffective ventilation of some alveoli. If the mean thoracic pressure is elevated with high levels of PEEP or CPAP, e.g., above 7 to 8 cm H_2O in the absence of lung disease, cardiac output may be decreased due to impaired venous return. The nasal prongs may cause irritation if the fit is not appropriate or the infant is active. Gastric distention may occur, making gastric feedings difficult, and often an indwelling or gastric tube is required for decompression.

Effectiveness

Does the use of CPAP decrease the need for mechanical ventilation and does it prevent or ameliorate BPD? Clinical trials have evaluated the efficacy of CPAP in infants with RDS, demonstrating an increase in PO_2, a decrease in the fraction of inspired oxygen (FiO_2), and a decrease in death rate with no significant influence on the incidence of BPD (24,37,49–53). Five trials comparing early versus late initiation of CPAP have been summarized by Bancalari and Sinclair (49). Early application resulted in a reduction in the subsequent need for mechanical ventilation. A review of available literature suggests that early nasal CPAP may be as effective as mechanical ventilation in reducing mortality rates and perhaps better in preventing BPD (54). Prophylactic CPAP has not been shown to reduce the incidence of HMD or BPD (51,55). In a Danish–Swedish multicenter study, CPAP following endotracheal administration of surfactant to infants with HMD resulted in a significant reduction in need for mechanical ventilation compared to infants not receiving surfactant (45). Other studies comparing the efficacy of conventional mechanical ventilation (CMV) to CPAP following the administration of surfactant found no differences in outcome although the number of infants studied was small (56,57).

CPAP has gained popularity as a means of facilitating weaning from mechanical ventilation. Some infants, experiencing recurrent apneic episodes, appear to benefit (58), whereas other studies have shown no benefit (59,60). Additional information is needed to confirm whether CPAP is an effective adjunct to successful extubation. The use of newer equipment, such as the ALADDIN device, may prove beneficial.

ASSISTED MECHANICAL VENTILATION

The Immature Lung

The immature lung presents a special hazard for the application of assisted ventilation. The application of positive pressure for the purpose of increasing ventilation and optimizing ventilation–perfusion ($\dot{V}_A/\dot{Q}$) matching may injure epithelial and endothelial tissues. Most alveolization occurs postnatally. In the incompletely developed lungs, structures are less elastic and more vulnerable to barotrauma. Injury to the mesenchymal and epithelial tissues that later give rise to alveolar septation and vascular formation may be irreversible. Studies in adult animals have demonstrated that otherwise healthy lungs can suffer injury, which is reflected by increased airway fluid and deterioration of gas exchange, if sufficient distending lung pressures are applied (61). The particular problems of providing assisted ventilation are illustrated in Fig. 30–4. Relative immaturity of distal bronchioles and respiratory ducts, coupled with fluid-filled and collapsed alveoli, create a set of conditions leading to overdistention of some areas and underventilation of other areas, with resultant ineffective gas exchange. This uneven ventilation, coupled with injury produced by reactive oxygen species, contributes to the common problem of chronic lung disease of prematurity. The risk of its development is proportionate to birth weight (Table 30–2).

Great strides have been made in understanding how the immature lung differs from a mature lung in phospholipid and surfactant-associated protein biosynthesis. However, there are factors other than surfactant biosynthesis that are unique to the immature lung and that increase the susceptibility to injury. These factors include, but are not limited to, incomplete development of the supportive net of collagen and elastin, incomplete development of the capillary bed in the gas exchange areas, relative softness and instability of the chest wall and its inability to maintain expiratory lung volume at an adequate FRC, and immaturity of the neural control producing sustained spontaneous respiratory effort. The metabolic function of the pulmonary endothelium is not well studied in the immature infant, but it is probably deficient in metabolizing bioactive amines and peptides.

Respiratory failure ensues when spontaneous breathing efforts fail to produce adequate ventilation. In newborn infants, this may occur because of failure of adequate output from central nervous system respiratory centers, an overly compliant chest wall that increases the work of breathing, metabolic problems due to limited energy stores, or profoundly noncompliant lungs requiring more work and depleting available energy stores. Each of these may be an indication for assisted ventilation. In most neonatal respiratory disorders, these problems occur in combination, and the diagnosis of respiratory failure cannot be ascribed to any single cause.

Establishment of an Artificial Airway

Physiologic and Anatomic Airway Peculiarities

The newborn infant has distinct anatomic and physiologic characteristics of the airways and a strong prefer-

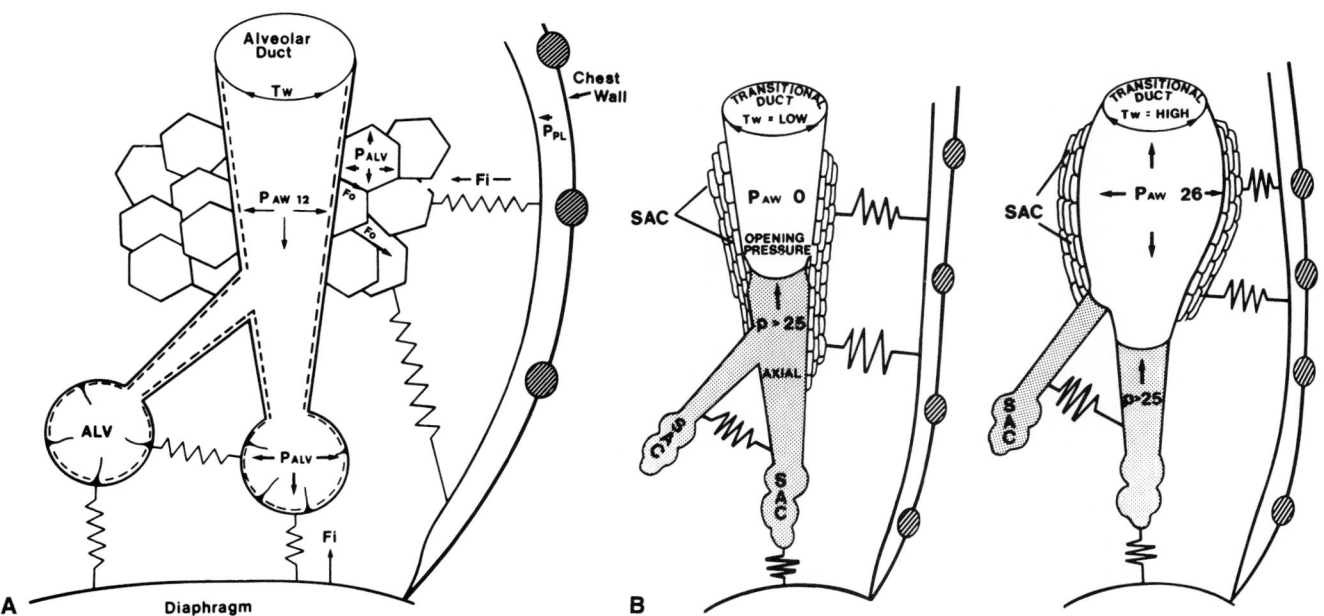

FIG. 30–4. A: A mature alveolar duct and alveoli. *Dotted line,* surfactant; P_{ALV}, alveolar pressure; P_{AW}, airway pressure; P_{PL}, pleural pressure; Fi, tissue force (stretched springs) acting inward; Fo, tissue force directed outward; Tw, wall tension or recoil pressure. **B:** The end-expiratory airway pressure (P_{aw}) equals zero in an immature distal airway **(left)**. The saccules (SAC) and airways contain fluid (*shaded area*). The axial airway is concave at the air–liquid interface due to the surface tension forces. The peripheral SACs are collapsed or fluid filled. The lax tissues are represented by relaxed springs. The inspiratory airway pressure (P_{AW}) is equal to 26 cm H2O **(right)**. The distended distal airway has a high wall tension (TW). The liquid front has been pushed peripherally, but the SACs are still not inflated. (From Thibeault DW, Lang MJ. Mechanisms and pathobiologic effects of barotrauma. In: Merritt TA, Northway WH Jr, Boynton BR, eds. *Bronchopulmonary dysplasia. Contemporary issues in fetal neonatal medicine.* Boston: Blackwell Scientific Publishers, 1988, p 82.)

ence for nasal breathing for the first few months of life (62). Nasal or nasopharyngeal obstruction due to secretions, mucosal injury, or congenital abnormalities may produce respiratory distress. Approximately one-half of the infant's airway resistance occurs in the nose, although the narrowness of the lower respiratory tract results in a total airway resistance approximately 15 times greater than that of an adult (63). Edema and inflammation can produce extremely high resistance to air flow in these narrow airways. During expiration, the airways become narrower, and resistance increases.

Endotracheal Intubation

Route

Orotracheal and nasotracheal intubation may be used for prolonged mechanical ventilation of term and premature infants. The principal advantage of the nasal route is the stabilization of the tube afforded by the close fit within the naris, but the nasal passages may limit the size of tube that can be used. Necrosis of the nasal septum or the alae nasi can occur if circulation is impaired because the tube is too large. Orotracheal intubation is more eas-

TABLE 30–2. *Mortality and development of chronic lung disease*

Birth weight (g)	Total n	% Dead	28 d alive with CLD (% survivors)	28 d alive, no CLD (% survivors)	36 Wk PCA with CLD (% alive)	36 wk PCA, no CLD (% alive)
500–750	50	46	85	15	50	50
751–1,000	46	19	70	30	27	73
1,001–1,250	49	2	46	54	15	85
1,251–1,500	52	6	10	90	8	92

Data are from combined inborn and outborn services of Truman Medical Center and Children's Mercy Hospital, Kansas City, 1995 and 1996 inclusive. Chronic lung disease (CLD) is defined as any need for supplemental oxygen therapy and/or assisted ventilation.

PCA, postconceptual age.

ily and quickly accomplished and is indicated for delivery room and emergency situations. It is the preferred route for prolonged mechanical ventilation.

The endotracheal tube should allow a small air leak between the tube and the glottis. A tube that fits too snugly within the trachea is likely to cause pressure necrosis of the mucosa. If too large a leak is allowed, it may be difficult to achieve sufficient pressure for ventilation of noncompliant lungs. A tube with a 2.5-mm inner diameter usually fits infants weighing less than 1,000 g; a 3-mm tube fits those from 1,000 to 1,500 g; a 3.5-mm tube fits those from 1,500 to 2,500 g; and a 4.0-mm tube fits larger infants.

Technique

Orotracheal intubation is a simple procedure that can be accomplished atraumatically within a few seconds. The necessary equipment consists of a straight-bladed laryngoscope, a suction catheter connected to a suction apparatus, an endotracheal tube of the appropriate size with an adapter for the bag or respirator, and an optical flexible Teflon introducer, bent to prevent its tip from protruding beyond the end of the endotracheal tube. The infant is ventilated with 100% oxygen by mask for a few breaths. A catheter to deliver oxygen can be taped to the laryngoscope blade to enhance oxygen delivery during intubation (64). The infant's neck is straightened without hyperextension by placing a small towel under the shoulders, and the head is steadied by an assistant. The laryngoscope is held in the left hand between the thumb and first two fingers. The heel of the hand is placed against the infant's left cheek to provide stability. The blade is introduced into the right side of the mouth, and the tongue is deflected to the left as the blade is advanced into the vallecula, anterior to the epiglottis. The laryngoscope is lifted rather than rotated so that the larynx is elevated and the glottis is brought into view (Fig. 30–5). The pharynx is suctioned if necessary. The endotracheal tube is introduced into the mouth to the right of the laryngoscope and gently guided into the glottis under direct vision.

Placement of the nasotracheal tube is technically more difficult and often more time consuming than orotracheal intubation. It is best, particularly in a severely compromised infant, to have an orotracheal tube in place so that the infant can be ventilated while the nasotracheal tube is being positioned. The nasotracheal tube is inserted without an introducer through the naris and gently guided along the floor of the nose. The laryngoscope is placed in the mouth to the right of the orotracheal tube, and the tip of the nasotracheal tube is seen in the posterior pharynx. A Magill forceps is held in the right hand and introduced to the right of the laryngoscope. The nasotracheal tube is grasped a few millimeters back from its tip with the forceps, and the tip of the tube is elevated until it is almost

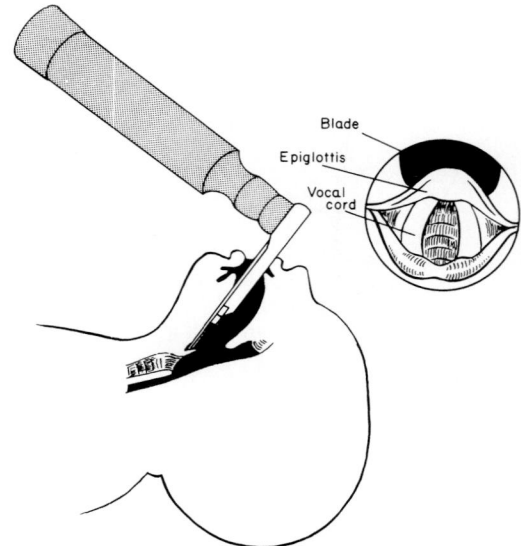

FIG. 30–5. Laryngoscopy for endotracheal intubation.

at the glottis. It is helpful to have an assistant grasp the exterior end of the nasotracheal tube to assist in advancing it. The orotracheal tube is left in place until just before insertion of the nasotracheal tube in the glottis.

Heart rate and SaO_2 should be monitored continuously during endotracheal intubation. If the heart rate falls, intubation should be deferred while the infant is ventilated with a resuscitation bag and face mask. Pretreatment with pancuronium bromide and atropine may minimize heart rate and intracranial pressure changes associated with endotracheal intubation (65,66).

Positioning

The length of the trachea from the vocal cords to the carina varies from about 3.6 cm in the smallest premature infants to 6 cm in large, term infants. Optimal positioning for the tip of an endotracheal tube is in the middle of the trachea, where it is least subject to dislodgment into the pharynx or displacement into a bronchus. The proper depth of insertion of an endotracheal tube, as determined by postmortem and radiographic measurements, is related to body weight (67). Suggested depths of insertion for either orotracheal or nasotracheal intubation are given in Table 30–3 (67,68).

Immediately after intubation, the position of the tube should be confirmed by inspection and auscultation. An adapter containing a CO_2-sensitive color detector is connected to the endotracheal tube. If there is no color change, the endotracheal tube should be withdrawn immediately. Two common errors of tube placement are intubation of the esophagus and intubation of the right main-stem bronchus. The former should be suspected if insufflation through the tube produces abdominal disten-

TABLE 30–3. *Depth of insertion of an orotracheal tube from the lips of a premature infant*

Infant weight (kg)	Depth of insertion (cm)
1.0	7
2.0	8
3.0	9
4.0	10

tion with little chest expansion and if air movement is heard better over the stomach than over the chest. Breath sounds that are louder over the right chest than the left suggest that the tube is in the right main-stem bronchus. Auscultation, although helpful, is not reliable because breath sounds are well transmitted in a small chest. A frontal chest radiograph should be obtained immediately after intubation to confirm tube placement. A lateral view can differentiate between the trachea and the esophagus, but with the CO_2 color change detector and SaO_2 monitoring, it should be obvious that an esophageal intubation has occurred and the frontal view shows the position of the tube in relation to the carina.

Care of Endotracheal Tubes

A tube in the trachea interferes with the physiologic mechanisms for clearance of respiratory secretions and may itself stimulate secretions. Meticulous care is needed to prevent accumulation and inspissation of secretions, which can obstruct the tube. Routine changing of the tube is unnecessary and subjects the infant to the repeated risk of trauma to the larynx and interruption of ventilation. However, the most common reason for sudden deterioration of an otherwise stable ventilated infant is dislodgment or blockage of the tracheal tube. The volume and quality of secretions vary with the type of pulmonary disease and with the individual patient. Suction frequency may vary from once each hour to fewer than two or three times per day.

Another important aspect of the care of artificial airways is the provision of adequate humidification. The endotracheal tube bypasses the nasal and pharyngeal mucosa, which normally warms and humidifies inspired gases. If heat and humidity are not provided from an external source, drying of the lower airway mucosa, thickened secretions, and hypothermia may result. Inspired gases should be passed through a heated nebulizer so that they are delivered to the airway already warmed to a range of 34 to 36°C, and saturated. A temperature probe to detect overheating should be positioned in the inspiratory tubing near the infant and should have an audio alarm. Inadequate humidification can contribute to airway injury (69).

Indications for Assisted Ventilation

The decision for initiation of assisted ventilation should be individualized for each baby. Factors to con-

sider include underlying disease, birth weight, gestational age, postnatal age, chest radiographic appearance, progression of clinical signs, serial arterial blood gas tension measurements, and pH measurements. The criteria indicating a need for mechanical ventilation are difficult to define, and there is lack of unanimity about a particular threshold for PaO_2, $PaCO_2$, or FiO_2. In general, the PaO_2 should be maintained at or above 50 mm Hg because of reasonable oxyhemoglobin saturation at this level, but the maximal level of inspired O_2 dictating intubation and application of assisted ventilation remains controversial. No rigid ceiling for $PaCO_2$ can be supported by morbidity or mortality data. A trend of rising $PaCO_2$ with concomitant decrease in pH and onset of apnea indicates a need for mechanical assistance. After assisted ventilation is initiated, the generally accepted goals are to maintain the PaO_2 between 45 and 70 mm Hg, $PaCO_2$ at 60 mm Hg or less, and pH at 7.25 or more while minimizing PIP and FiO_2, and optimizing mean airway pressure ($P_{AW[gas]}$) and PEEP.

Because acute lung disease is usually more severe and protracted in the more immature infant, criteria for intervention for infants weighing less than 1,000 g differ from those for larger or older infants. For example, a 750-g infant with RDS has a high probability of developing apnea, fatigue, or both, and most of these infants require assisted ventilation even if the FiO_2 need is less than 40%. A 2,500-g, 36-week-old infant with RDS has greater muscular and caloric reserve and is able to sustain rapid ventilatory rates and higher respiratory work for several days without assistance. With a normal $PaCO_2$, inspired O_2 may be increased to between 80% and 90% before intubation in some infants. The role of CPAP in the latter situation remains controversial, although it is used successfully in many centers. One factor that has changed the equation for these infants is the ability to administer surfactant to an intubated infant with RDS. Infants of gestational age 35 to 39 weeks and older than 24 hours who develop respiratory failure with RDS may benefit from surfactant treatment (70). Showing an improvement in mortality in this group with any single manipulation of assisted ventilation pattern will be difficult, because mortality rates are low using currently available techniques.

Physiologic Considerations

An understanding of the effects of mechanical ventilation on the lungs requires knowledge of the interplay among thoracic mechanics, including pulmonary compliance and airway resistance, lung volumes, respiratory control mechanisms, and alveolar gas exchange.

Lung compliance (i.e., change in lung volume per unit pressure change, in units of mL/cm H_2O) depends on the elastic properties of the tissue, which are influenced by the lung volume and abnormalities such as tissue inflammation and edema. Compliance is low if there is alveolar collapse or overdistention. Expansion from alveolar collapse requires inflation pressures of 12 to 20 cm H_2O in preterm infants with RDS. The lungs of infants with RDS have areas of collapse and overexpansion, and there is nonuniformity of compliance. Other conditions, such as pneumothorax, lobar atelectasis or consolidation, and pulmonary edema, decrease compliance. The most relevant measure of compliance, specific compliance, is calculated by normalizing compliance by end-expiratory volume. Very low or high values for FRC will reduce compliance. Changes in compliance, FRC, and gas exchange are not concordant, at least not during treatment for RDS. This has limited the value of bedside measurements of compliance, particularly without concomitant measurements in FRC. Chest wall compliance usually is high and does not present a problem to mechanical ventilation.

Airway resistance (cm H_2O/L/s) is inversely related to the fourth power of the radius during laminar air flow. Airway resistance is high in infants, increasing with low lung volumes and with obstruction of the airway. High rates of air flow increase resistance by producing turbulence in the airways.

The rate at which lung areas inflate and deflate is determined by resistance and compliance. An increase in airway resistance increases the time required for air to reach the alveoli; a decrease in compliance results in less time required to reach equilibrium. The product of resistance and compliance is the pulmonary time constant. Changes in resistance or compliance can alter the pattern or distribution of ventilation, and recognition of the variations in the time constant (e.g., short with poor compliance, prolonged with increased airway resistance) helps determine respirator settings. Unfortunately, a single time constant does not exist for all lung areas during complex pulmonary disorders. Thus, all conventional positive-pressure ventilators produce areas of overinflation and underinflation of gas exchanging areas, each contributing to suboptimal gas exchange.

Because RDS should result in a short time constant, rapid inspiratory and expiratory respirator times are permissible, and mean airway pressure should be increased to improve oxygenation. With meconium aspiration or airway edema, the time constant is slower, and sufficient time for expiration is important to avoid gas trapping, overdistention of the lungs, and possible air leak. If the expiratory time (T_E) is shorter than the time constant of the lung for expiration, overdistention results. If the overall time constant for the lung is longer than the imposed ventilator inspiratory time (T_I), inadequate ventilation could result. Unequal time constants coexisting in different parts of the lung are most likely to occur if pulmonary abnormalities are unevenly distributed, as in pneumonia, meconium aspiration, pulmonary interstitial emphysema, pneumothorax, or BPD, in which case the optimal T_I or T_E becomes difficult to determine.

It is helpful to have an understanding of lung volumes when ventilating an infant. During spontaneous breathing, the tidal volume is approximately 5 to 8 mL/kg, with approximately one-third consisting of dead space. Mechanical ventilators should permit a tidal volume in the range of 5 to 60 mL, depending on the size of the infant, with minimal apparatus dead space.

The circulatory effects of mechanically applied pressure to the alveoli are important. Normal breathing results in negative intrapleural pressure that enhances venous return and cardiac output. Positive-pressure breathing can impede venous return and may diminish cardiac output. Pressure during inspiration decreases the pulmonary capillary circulation as long as alveolar pressure exceeds capillary pressure and can affect total pulmonary blood flow and hence gas exchange.

Lung Volume Measurements During Mechanical Ventilation

Application of hot wire anemometry or pneumotachography to neonatal ventilation systems allows measurement of inspiratory and expiratory tidal volumes, minute ventilation ($\dot{V}_E$), and air leak (i.e., the difference between tidal volumes measured during inspiration and expiration) at any combination of ventilator settings. These measurements overcome a previous limitation found in time-cycled neonatal ventilators and allow a more rational selection of ventilatory settings, supplementing visual and auscultatory evidence of inadequate or excessive chest wall motion for assessing delivered tidal volume. It is possible to correlate the individual variable of tidal volume with the independently adjusted PIP, inspiratory gas flow rate, T_I, and PEEP. Knowledge of tidal volume from bedside measurements allows clinicians to determine the optimal PIP to achieve optimal tidal volume. This knowledge enables minimizing PIP, which, if excessive, otherwise may induce or exacerbate the small airway injury of BPD. However, knowledge of tidal volume and V_E does not provide knowledge of distribution of inspired ventilation and of $\dot{V}_A/\dot{Q}$ matching. Distribution of tidal volume may vary with the associated PIP; low PIP can result in tidal volume distribution only to already overinflated lung regions, resulting in worsened $\dot{V}_A/\dot{Q}$ matching, development or exacerbation of high $\dot{V}_A/\dot{Q}$ areas, and worsening of arterial CO_2 retention, despite normal or elevated $\dot{V}_E$. Despite this limitation, use of tidal volume monitoring may permit ventilation at lower PIP, possibly reducing the incidence of pneumothorax or interstitial emphysema, complications that may increase the risk of BPD (71).

General Principles of Neonatal Ventilation

Available Patterns of Assisted Ventilation

Newly developed infant respirators provide a wide range of patterns of assisted ventilation available to apply to a variety of clinical conditions. It has been 20 years since the introduction of constant-flow, time-cycled, pressure-limited, end-expiratory pressure-adjustable assisted ventilation devices. They have proven to be effective and an improvement over earlier devices to provide positive-pressure ventilation to infants. A summary of the manipulations available with this form of assisted ventilation is illustrated in Fig. 30–6.

It has been approximately 10 years since the introduction of high-frequency ventilation in neonates. However, there have been few head-to-head studies to provide evidence of superiority and safety of one pattern of ventilation over another for a specific disorder. The next several sections will discuss advantages and disadvantages of each of the two broad ventilator modes: conventional assisted ventilation, especially as modified by the various patterns of patient-triggered ventilation; and alternatively, the various patterns of high-frequency ventilation.

Appropriate ventilator settings should allow the most effective gas exchange with the least risk of lung injury. Determining appropriate settings can be difficult with the variety of adjustments available (Fig. 30–7). Excess applied airway pressure or inspired oxygen concentration should be avoided. Less certain are the safe or tolerable limits of airway pressure, including the duration of its application during a respiratory cycle. The use of a prolonged T_I, a reversed inspiratory-to-expiratory (I–E) time ratio, or an inspiratory plateau may improve oxygenation, but at a cost of local overdistention and distal airway or alveolar lining injury. There are no carefully controlled clinical studies that substantiate that reversed I–E ratios ($T_I > T_E$), limitation of PIP, or any particular pattern of ventilation can reduce the incidence of BPD. Retrospective analysis associating high airway pressure with pathologic changes in the airways at postmortem examination does not differentiate cause and effect. Already abnormal airways may have caused the use of high peak airway pressures for satisfactory gas exchange. It would seem wise to avoid the use of high airway pressures (>30 cm H_2O) unless manipulation of other variables, such as changes in PEEP, I–E ratio, and F_IO_2, fails to improve gas exchange (see Fig. 30–6).

The most common need in RDS is for an increase in PaO_2; adjustments to correct an abnormal PCO_2 are often of secondary importance. The physician decides whether to increase F_IO_2 or $P_{AW[gas]}$ by considering the prior settings and balancing the possible harmful effects of increasing $P_{AW[gas]}$ against those of increasing F_IO_2, recognizing that threshold limits are arbitrary. If the F_IO_2 is approaching 1.0, there is no choice but to increase $P_{AW[gas]}$. If PEEP is already 6 to 8 cm H_2O, the PIP or the T_I is increased. The use of PEEP helps to maintain patent small airways and prevent collapse to airlessness of those alveoli already open. Inspiratory pressures of >15 cm H_2O usually are required to open collapsed or fluid-filled acinar areas. A combination of an increase in the I–E ratio with 6 cm H_2O PEEP may be optimal during the initial phase of assisted ventilation for RDS. With subsequent opening of air spaces, the optimal T_I may need to be decreased. The use of an end-inspiratory pause or plateau should improve the distribution of inspired gas if there are regional differences in airway resistance (see Fig. 30–6). However, if the alveolar pressure exceeds capillary pressure, there will be tamponading of the pulmonary circulation and development of high $\dot{V}_A/\dot{Q}$ areas. Various effective approaches to assisted ventilation have been learned on larger babies with RDS; application of these lessons to the profoundly immature infant, now treated with surfactant, should be done with extreme caution (72).

Blood gas tensions should be measured 10 to 15 minutes after ventilatory settings are changed. If the PO_2 is below 45 mm Hg or the PCO_2 is above 65 mm Hg, adjustments may be made. Ideally, only one variable at a time should be adjusted, and the resultant changes in PO_2 and PCO_2 should be reassessed before other changes are made. A marked increase in respiratory rate could have adverse effects on the PCO_2 by increasing dead-space ventilation. A moderate degree of hypercapnia (e.g., 50 to 55 mm Hg) may be well tolerated by the infant if it is not an acute change.

Hypoxemia may persist during all combinations of ventilator settings in some conditions, and other underlying abnormalities should be suspected. The clinician should always consider the degree of air leak around the endotracheal tube when adjusting pressure and flow rates. Other management considerations are listed in Table 30–4. Reevaluation of the infant for coexisting pulmonary vascular hypertension or structural or functional heart disease is then indicated. Echocardiography may be

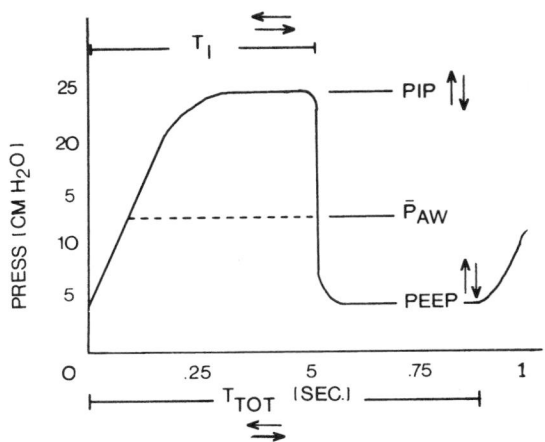

FIG. 30–6. Profile of a pressure waveform during mechanical ventilation. Bidirectional areas indicate some of the variables that can be altered to raise or lower main airway pressure. PEEP, positive end-expiratory pressure; PIP, peak inspiratory pressure; T_I, inspiratory time; T_{TOT} duration of inspiration plus expiration.

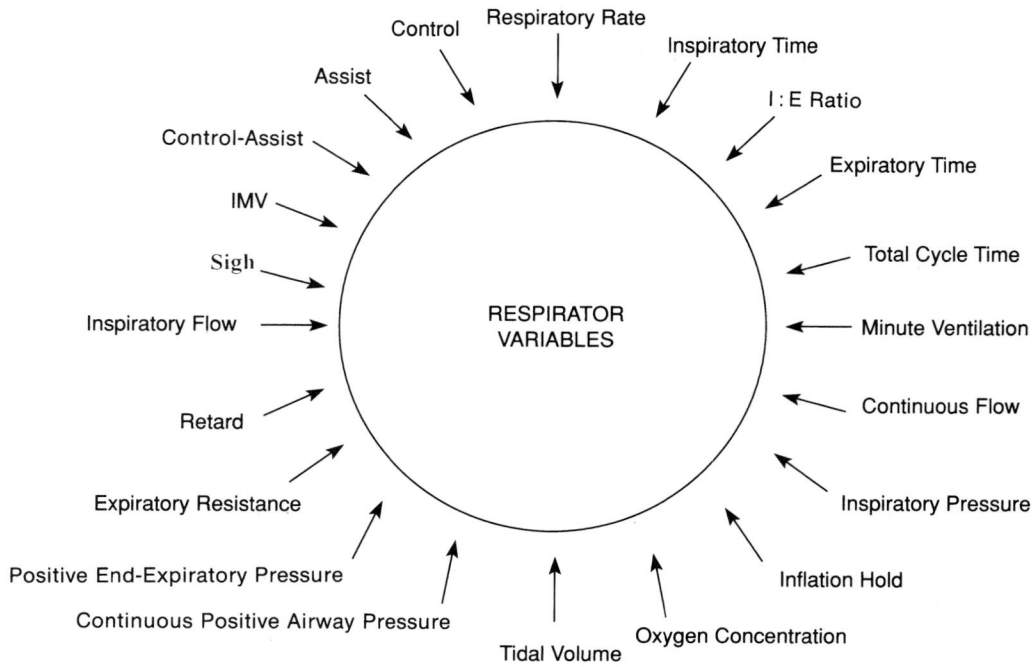

FIG. 30–7. Several respirator variables that affect the efficiency of mechanical ventilation.

a useful procedure at this point. If pulmonary hypertension is confirmed, then attempts at relieving pulmonary vasoconstriction are indicated.

If there is airway obstruction, as may occur with BPD or meconium aspiration, optimal ventilator settings may differ from those used for HMD. Because there is a relatively long time constant, the gas flow rate should not be too rapid, and there should be adequate time for expiration.

TABLE 30–4. *Management considerations*

- Utilize alternative mode of ventilation (e.g., HFV vs. IMV or SIMV versus IMV or A/C versus SIMV
- Raise the hematocrit to 45–50% with packed erythrocyte transfusions
- Reposition baby into prone position if supine or into left or right lateral positions
- Consider use of paralysis or sedation; if infant is paralyzed, discontinue its use
- Change to a larger size endotracheal tube to diminish air leak
- Consider repeated doses of exogenous surfactant beyond 24 h of age
- Administer diuretic therapy to change pulmonary fluid concentration
- Increase cardiac output and/or systemic blood pressure by administration of inotropic agents
- Reevaluate cardiac hemodynamics and degree of pulmonary hypertension with initial or repeat echocardiography
- Consider use of corticosteroids

A/C, assist/control; HFV, high-frequency ventilation; IMV, intermittent mandatory ventilation; SIMV, synchronous intermittent mandatory ventilation.

The required PIP may be below 25 cm H_2O. The use of synchronous intermittent mandatory ventilation (SIMV) or assisted control may be helpful in these circumstances.

Patient-Triggered Ventilation

The goal of patient-triggered ventilation is to maximize the efficiency of spontaneous breathing efforts while minimizing the risk of insufficient ventilation or trauma to airways (73). All patterns of patient-triggered ventilation require a rapidly responding sensor and transducer that can detect the onset of spontaneous inspiratory effort and provide the mechanical initiation of machine-assisted ventilation during the early phase of the infant's inspiration. The current methodology allows this transduction to be accomplished in as short a time as 30 to 50 ms, approximately one-tenth the duration of the inspiratory phase of a spontaneous respiratory cycle (Fig. 30–8). The means by which this signal is provided and the addition of other subtle but potentially important changes in the capabilities of a ventilator differentiate one type of conventional neonatal ventilator from another (74).

Although it is not clear that modern means of patient-triggered ventilation have achieved their optimum, these methods have already gained widespread acceptance for three reasons. These include the clinical impression that infants are more comfortable and less distressed while being ventilated with patient-triggered ventilation; there may be at least modest improvements in pulmonary gas exchange (Fig. 30–9) during patient-triggered ventilation; and there appears to be decreased need for sedation

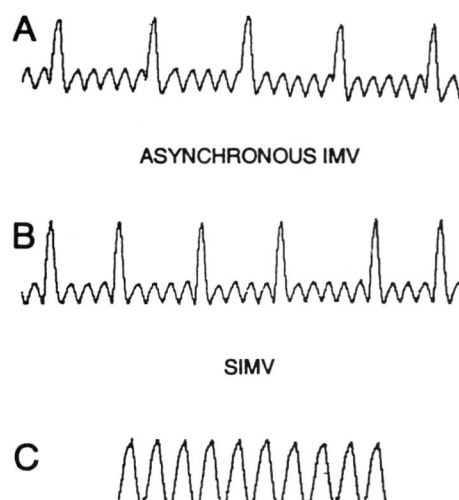

ASYNCHRONOUS IMV

SIMV

ASSIST/CONTROL

FIG. 30–10. Tidal volume tracings (inspiration = upward) demonstrating three patterns of ventilator interaction with spontaneous breathing. In this illustration, tidal volume of spontaneous breaths is less than that of ventilator breaths. **A:** Asynchronous intermittent mandatory ventilation (IMV) with ventilator breaths delivered during spontaneous expiration. During IMV, ventilator breaths occur at a constant rate, with random timing with respect to spontaneous breaths. **B:** Synchronous intermittent mandatory ventilation (SIMV) with ventilator breaths delivered early in selected spontaneous inspirations. During SIMV, ventilator breaths occur more irregularly, but the ventilator delivers the set rate synchronously with spontaneous breaths. **C:** Assist/control mode, with ventilatory breaths delivered early in all spontaneous inspirations. The assist/control mode delivers ventilatory breaths synchronously with all spontaneous breaths and may lead to increased ventilation. (From Cleary JP, Bernstein G, Mannino FL, Heldt GP. Improved oxygenation during synchronized intermittent mandatory ventilation in neonates with respiratory distress syndrome: a randomized, crossover study. *J Pediatr* 1995;126:407.)

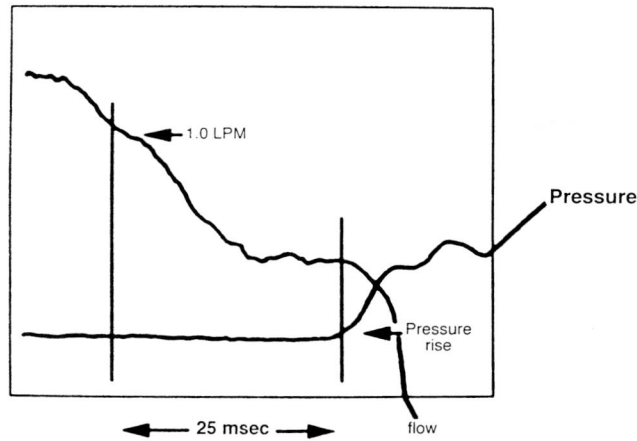

FIG. 30–8. System response time, also known as trigger delay. The flow change trigger is set at 1.0 LPM. It took 25 ms from the time this threshold was reached (*vertical line* on the **left**) until there was a measurable rise in airway pressure (*vertical line* on the **right**). (From Donn SM, Sinha SK. Controversies in patient-triggered ventilation. *Clin Perinatol* 1998; 25:49.)

and muscle relaxation. Even with patient-triggered ventilation, it is important to recognize the pitfalls that may occur when the SIMV rates are too high or when the patient is allowed to breathe in the assist/control mode (Fig. 30–10). With assist/control, hyperventilation may occur, especially if the sensor for initiation of respiration is inappropriately sensitive and triggers ventilator breaths that are not associated with patient inspiratory effort. If the goal is to avoid breaths triggered late in inspiration or

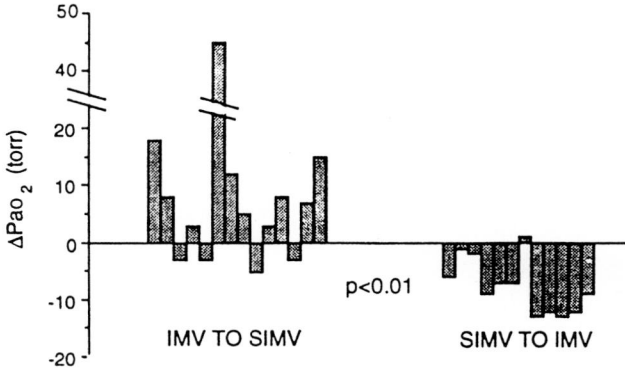

FIG. 30–9. Change in PaO₂ at each crossover. The value improved by 7.9 ± 3.4 mm Hg when crossover was from intermittent mandatory ventilation (IMV) to synchronous intermittent mandatory ventilation (SIMV), and decreased by 6.4 ± 1.4 mm Hg when crossover was from SIMV to IMV. (From Cleary JP, Bernstein G, Mannino FL, Heldt GP. Improved oxygenation during synchronized intermittent mandatory ventilation in neonates with respiratory distress syndrome: a randomized, crossover study. *J Pediatr* 1995;126:407.)

during expiration, then flow-triggering systems are less prone to auto triggering and have a shorter and more consistent response time than impedance-triggered systems (75).

A limitation of all currently available types of devices is that the individual breaths generated by the ventilator are monotonic or monophasic. Proportional assist ventilation may be one way to overcome the problem and provide even greater flexibility. With proportional assist ventilation, the relationship between patient-induced inspiratory effort and ventilator response is interactive (76). Proportional assist ventilation is a method by which, in theory, the ventilator amplifies the patient's effort throughout the inspiratory phase of the cycle. With each spontaneously generated breath, the patient can individualize the machine-initiated tidal volume and flow patterns. The method works by monitoring instantaneous flow rate and volume of gas from ventilator to patient and causing the applied pressure to change according to the equation of motion. This system may allow for both greater patient comfort and reduction of peak airway pressure required to sustain ventilation, with less likelihood of overventilation compared to assist/control modes. Preliminary use of this method in neonates has been reported and no doubt will be the subject of studies in the future.

A complex, variable-flow, assisted ventilation device (SV 300, Siemens-Elema, Solna, Sweden) also has been used successfully in the treatment of both full-term and premature infants. This ventilator provides a mode of ventilation labeled pressure-regulated, volume-controlled ventilation. Under certain circumstances, use of pressure-regulated, volume-controlled ventilation can achieve normal V_T and $\dot{V}_E$ with lower PIP than that needed by constant flow ventilators. This device also operates in SIMV modes and pressure support modes. No trials of this variable-flow ventilator compared to other conventional ventilators in the treatment of low-birth-weight infants has been reported.

Currently available neonatal ventilators are now capable of providing breath-to-breath analysis of tidal volume and hence minute ventilation. The linking of tidal volume to PIP, and to gas flow rates, duration of inspiratory time, and the PIP to PEEP difference has allowed more rational use of assisted ventilation in neonates. However, scant evidence is currently available to suggest that these sophisticated and expensive new devices have improved mortality or morbidity. Evidence for a reduction in the incidence or severity of chronic lung disorders with the use of these newer generation devices is needed to support their use.

HIGH-FREQUENCY VENTILATION

Principles of Use

A clinical definition of a high-frequency ventilator includes the following features: machine-delivered breaths at least twice that of the most rapid, spontaneously generated breathing rate in an infant and a delivered tidal volume approximately equal to or less than the spontaneously generated or conventionally delivered tidal volume. In some cases, V_T is less than the dead space. Thus, the mechanisms of gas exchange with high-frequency ventilation differ from the conventional combination of conduction and diffusion. Proposed mechanisms are outlined (Table 30–5). Various types of high-frequency ventilation are illustrated in Fig. 30–11.

Attempts have been made to differentiate high-frequency ventilators based on several ventilator-specific factors (Table 30–6) (77). The distinction among the types of high-frequency ventilators may be relevant to the

TABLE 30–5. *Means of gas exchange during high-frequency ventilation*

Facilitated or enhanced diffusion because of increased turbulence
Convective dispersion due to asymmetric velocity profiles
Direct alveolar ventilation
Axial distribution of transit times

appropriate matching of any one type of high-frequency ventilator to a particular part of the natural history of a neonatal pulmonary disorder.

Ventilation Devices and their Indications

High-Frequency Jet Ventilation

High-frequency jet ventilators are designed for the delivery of high-flow, short-duration pulses of pressurized gas directly into the upper airway through a specifically designed endotracheal tube lumen. These systems operate at rates of 150 to 600 breaths/min. Exhalation is passive. Effective tidal volumes are greater than the anatomic dead space. The ventilator is servocontrolled and operates to maintain a constant pressure at the endotracheal tube tip. The technique of high-frequency jet ventilation has been investigated to determine its efficacy in the management of very-low-birth-weight infants to reduce mortality or the development of chronic lung disease in this population (78,79).

The current status of jet ventilation as a primary mode of support for low-birth-weight infants is unclear. Keszler et al. (79) conducted a multicenter study in which 130 patients were enrolled. Half were treated with high-frequency jet ventilation and half were treated with a continuation of conventional mechanical ventilation (nonsynchronized intermittent ventilation). Virtually all the

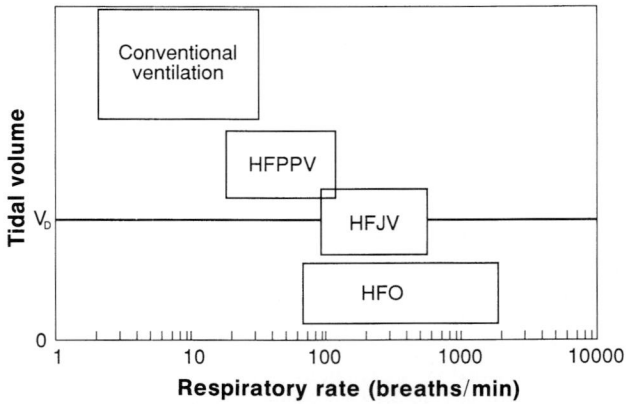

FIG. 30–11. Respiratory rate versus tidal volume. HFJV, high-frequency jet ventilation; HFO, high-frequency oscillation; HFPPV, high-frequency positive-pressure ventilation. (Adapted from ref. 77.)

TABLE 30–6. *High-frequency ventilators*

	Flow interruption	Jet ventilator	Oscillatory ventilator
Commercially available device	Infant Star (Infrasonics, San Diego, CA)	Bunnell Life Pulse (Bunnell, Salt Lake City, UT)	Sensormedics (Sensormedics, Anaheim, CA)
Indications	Failure of conventional ventilation in VLBW infants; PIE	PIE; intractable air leak; failure of conventional ventilation	Primary or rescue treatment of respiratory failure; prevention of ECMO
Variables	Rate of conventional breaths; frequency of high-frequency	Variable inspiratory "on-time" rate of 240–600 beats/min	Rate; mean airway pressure; I–E ratio
Use with conventional ventilation	Yes	Yes	No
Expiratory phase	Passive (?)	Passive	Active
Special precautions	>2 kg; no published trials	Sudden decrease in PCO_2; respiratory alkalosis	Sudden decrease in PCO_2; respiratory alkalosis

ECMO, extracorporeal membrane oxygenation; I–E ratio, inspiratory–expiratory ratio; PIE, pulmonary interstitial emphysema; VLBW, very low birth weight.

infants had been treated with exogenous surfactant. Mortality and need for ventilatory support at 28 days of life were the same in the two groups, but there was a reduction from 40% to 20% for continuing respiratory support at 36 weeks postconceptional age among infants treated with high-frequency ventilation. It is interesting to note that the 28-day BPD rate and the survival rate were comparable to that found 10 years earlier in a study comparing HFOV with conventional ventilation in infants without prior delivery of surfactant (80). These encouraging results are contrasted with another prospective randomized study in a comparable but smaller population of very-low-birth-weight infants (81). In that study with high-frequency jet ventilation, there was an increased risk of adverse outcomes, defined as large intraventricular hemorrhage, periventricular leukomalacia, or death. No difference in incidence of chronic lung disease was noted. The finding of leukomalacia had been previously associated with hypocarbia produced by treatment with high-frequency jet ventilation during the first 3 days of life (81), although no cause-and-effect relationship could be established. Earlier concerns about application of jet ventilation, which included the need to change an endotracheal tube during its initiation, as well as airway trauma and inadequate humidification, appear to have been overcome.

Problems with any large multicenter study attempting to identify an optimal means of assisted ventilation include confounding comorbidities, the changing baseline of treatment for the underlying pulmonary disorder, such as type and frequency of surfactant administration postnatally, as well as whether, and how completely, treatment with antenatal corticosteroid therapy for lung maturation was given. Using chronic lung disease as an outcome variable is difficult in any study because of the multiple confounding factors that may develop.

A hybrid device combining elements of jet and flow interruption to generate high-frequency ventilation, coupled with low-rate conventional ventilation, is available

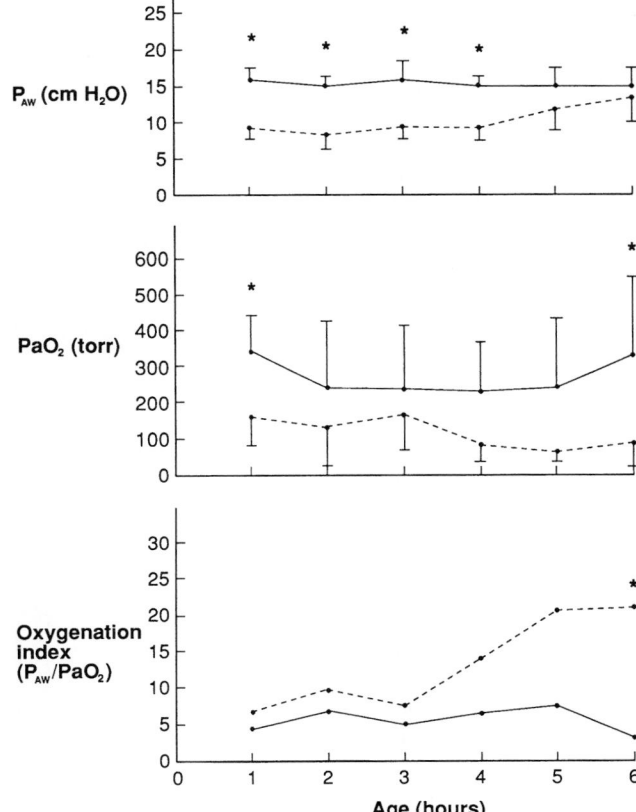

FIG. 30–12. Sequential measurements of mean airway pressure (P_{AW}) and arterial oxygen tension in 100% O_2 (mean ± SD). P_{AW} was initially higher in the high-frequency oscillatory-ventilated animals (*solid curve*), and PaO_2 was greater at the beginning and end of the study than in the conventionally mechanically ventilated (CMV) group (*broken curve*). Calculated oxygenation index was worse in the CMV group at the end of the experiment as a result of low oxygen tension despite high P_{AW}. *Asterisks* indicate statistical significance at $p < 0.05$. (Adapted from ref. 86.)

(Infrasonics, San Diego, CA). This device is operated at 10 to 15 Hz, with pauses in the high-frequency ventilator operation during the conventional breath inspiratory phase of ventilation. When operated in its mixed conventional and high-frequency mode, this device generates high-pressure, short, and nonvariable inspiratory flow with a variable shut-off phase, allowing passive lung deflation. One attractive feature is the minimal patient disturbance involved in changing from high-frequency to conventional forms of ventilation. No published study has demonstrated that this device offers any significant advantage as primary or rescue therapy compared to other types of high-frequency ventilation.

HFOV differs from the other two types by delivering smaller tidal volumes at higher rates (see Table 30–6 and Fig. 30–11) and has an active expiratory phase. The Sensormedics high-frequency ventilator (Sensormedics, Anaheim, CA) has an additional feature of operating with an independently adjustable T_I. This device has been licensed for use for primary initial treatment of assisted ventilation and for alternative therapy in intractable respiratory failure unresponsive to conventional mechanical ventilation in neonates.

Several prospective, randomized, controlled studies have been conducted using different types of HFOV (80,82–85) compared to conventional ventilation. The rationale for the postulated superiority of HFOV was that diminished distending pressures, combined with more adequate recruitment of and maintenance of lung volume, would be associated with fewer dysplastic cellular changes of the lung and less frequent or milder BPD.

Cumulatively, these studies provide evidence that HFOV can be used safely and effectively in a wide variety of newborn infants.

One question raised, but not answered, by clinical studies of HFOV is the potential benefit gained by its application at birth. Although no studies have reported use of HFOV in this situation, two studies using premature primate models of RDS demonstrated improved gas exchange if HFOV was used without any prior conventional mechanical ventilation (86,87). Jackson et al. (86) found decreased proteinaceous alveolar edema and improved gas exchange after 6 hours of HFOV applied from the first breath (Fig. 30–12). However, all animals in both treatment groups had evidence of pulmonary cellular injury. The finding of both short-term benefit and concomitant cellular damage implies that HFOV used from birth could still be associated with significant lung injury. These findings are consistent with those of Solimano et al. (88), who showed that fluid and protein leaks in preterm lambs still occurred, although HFOV was applied from the first breath after delivery.

A possible second indication for high-frequency ventilation is to preclude the need for more invasive pulmonary support with extracorporeal membrane oxygenation (ECMO). Studies enrolling patients eligible for ECMO demonstrated that approximately one-half responded favorably to HFOV and did not need ECMO (89,90). Most babies responding to high-frequency ventilation were larger infants suffering from severe RDS. Other acute pulmonary disorders, such as meconium aspiration pneumonia with severe airway obstructive

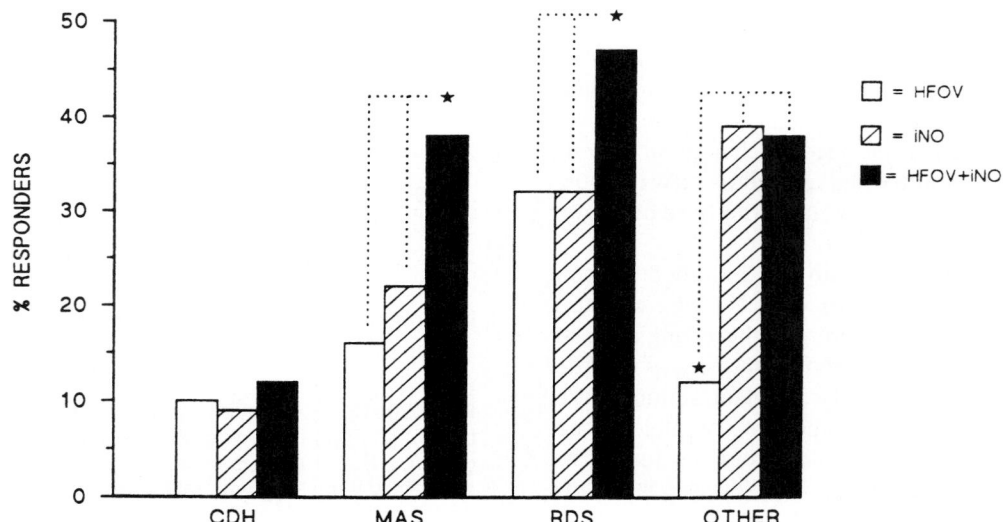

FIG. 30–13. Percentage of patients responding to high-frequency oscillatory ventilation (HFOV), inhaled nitric oxide (iNO), or combined HFOV plus iNO by disease category. More patients with RDS or MAS responded to combination therapy with HFOV plus iNO than to either treatment alone. Response to iNO during conventional ventilation was more effective than response to HFOV in patients without significant lung disease ("other" category). *Asterisk* indicates *p* < 0.05. (From ref. 91.)

changes as shown by chest radiography, may not respond as well to oscillatory ventilation. Kinsella et al. (91) recently showed that the delivery of the vasodilator gas, nitric oxide, in association with HFOV, produced an improved outcome compared to either conventional ventilation with nitric oxide or HFOV alone. There was a reduced need for ECMO, especially in near-term infants with RDS or meconium aspiration syndrome (Fig. 30–13). The synergistic effect of these two treatment modalities may help reduce dependence upon invasive ECMO support in this group of fragile term infants.

COMPLICATIONS OF ASSISTED VENTILATION

Airway-Associated Problems

Acute and chronic complications of mechanical ventilation may develop in neonates (Table 30–7). All patients with tracheal intubation demonstrate some degree of mucosal injury, usually squamous metaplasia or mucosal necrosis (92,93). In most infants, there seems to be spontaneous healing without significant sequelae. Hoarseness and stridor often occur after prolonged intubation but usually resolve in a few days. Persistent lesions may develop in some patients (94). These complications

TABLE 30–7. *Complications of mechanical ventilation*

Acute complications
  Equipment failure
    Failure of pressure in gas supply lines
    Alarm failure, with failure of staff to realize ventilation is disconnected
    Expiratory port occlusion producing inadvertent overdistention of lungs
  Endotracheal tube connection failure
    Dislodgment upward in pharynx
    Occlusion of tip of endotracheal tube
    Placement of tube tip beyond carina, providing only unilateral ventilation
    Trauma to upper airway, including tracheal perforation
  Equipment misuse
    Hypoxemia or hyperoxemia from inappropriate use of oxygen
    Arterial hypocarbia or hypercarbia from overventilation or underventilation
    Overdistention with excessive ventilatory pressure, lung rupture
  Other
    Airway blockage by excessive secretions inadequately removed by suctioning
    Trauma to airways by suctioning
    Pneumonia, produced by handling of equipment
Chronic complications
  Increased risk of chronic lung disease
  Tracheal or subglottic stenosis, or bronchomalacia
  Nasal deformities with nasotracheal tube
  Palatal deformities with endotracheal tube
  Upper airway infections (e.g., otitis media)
  Excessive prolonged dependence on mechanical ventilation (e.g., respiratory muscle impairment)

include laryngomalacia and subglottic stenosis, occasionally requiring tracheostomy. Duration of intubation, pressure from oversized tubes, inadequate humidification, and airway pressure produced by the ventilator contribute to the development of laryngotracheal lesions.

The duration of intubation is dictated by the need for continued ventilatory support. In some infants requiring assisted ventilation longer than 3 to 6 months, tracheostomy tube placement may facilitate development of normal feeding patterns and social interaction and bypass already traumatized areas of the upper airway. However, infant tracheostomy itself is associated with a significant morbidity and mortality (95). Complications can include fatal loss of airway after accidental extrusion of the tube, paratracheal soft tissue infection, severe paratracheal air leak resulting in inadequate generation of PIP, and tracheal cartilage softening, making decannulation difficult. A bedside evaluation of the airway using flexible fiberoptic endoscopy can be helpful in assessing need for additional, more invasive procedures (96).

Pulmonary Air Leak Complications

Pulmonary air leak may occur as a complication of any of the life-threatening disorders of the newborn or as a result of their treatment. The air leak may consist of pulmonary interstitial emphysema, pneumomediastinum, pneumoperitoneum, pneumopericardium, or pneumothorax. Pneumopericardium and pneumothorax usually require immediate treatment by evacuation of the free air.

Pneumothorax must be considered if there is abrupt worsening of the respiratory or circulatory status of an infant at risk. Unilateral hyperresonance, decreased breath sounds, a shift of the apical cardiac impulse, and skin mottling are useful clinical clues. High-intensity illumination may demonstrate the presence of a pneumothorax if the room can be adequately darkened (97). A definite diagnosis often can be made only by radiographic examination. The volume of the extrapulmonary air collection is not always a valid indication of tension. Interstitial emphysema, often a precursor of pneumothorax, causes the lung to remain partly expanded, even when intrapleural pressure is high (98). Bilateral pneumothorax may lead rapidly to death and must always be considered in cases of severe deterioration.

Pneumothorax in otherwise asymptomatic infants often resolves without therapy. However, marked mediastinal shift, coexisting pulmonary disease, or use of mechanical ventilation indicates a need for evacuation of the air. Aspiration with a syringe and needle may be done as an emergency procedure but is rarely adequate by itself and should be followed with tube thoracostomy.

Thoracostomy tubes should be sterile and made of nonreactive rubber or plastic. The wall thickness should be sufficient to prevent kinking, and the lumen should be large enough to prevent occlusion by exudate. The presence of at least two holes in the tube reduces the likelihood of occlusion by tissue. Polyvinylchloride feeding tubes or 8Fr (2.6-mm) to 10Fr (3.3-mm) catheters are suitable for thoracostomy use. The tube is inserted by grasping the tip with a clamp and pressing through a previously made incision through the pleura. The catheter is inserted after a skin incision has been made and can be Z-tracked over a rib for a better seal. Catheters with a trocar within the lumen often require considerable force to insert, and lung and liver puncture has been reported with their use. A novel approach to the placement of a catheter to minimize lung injury has been reported (99). A pigtail catheter is inserted over the area of suspected air leak, and the tube is inserted and rotated to form a loop within the intrapleural space.

It is not usually practical to connect a suction apparatus to the tube before it has been secured, but the pneumothorax should be aspirated with a syringe and the tube occluded with a clamp or stopcock. A single suture is placed in the skin beside the tube; this suture can be used to tie the tube securely in place. The tube may become dislodged if care is not taken at this step. Taping alone is inadequate. Pursestring sutures tend to produce larger scars without providing much additional security against tube dislodgment.

The tube is connected to continuous suction at a negative pressure of 10 to 15 cm H_2O with an underwater seal. A chest radiograph should be obtained soon after thoracostomy. If the pneumothorax has not been evacuated, the infant should be repositioned and the tube stripped or, if necessary, a second tube should be inserted.

A thoracostomy tube is left in place until air ceases to bubble from the tube and until the risk of recurrent pneumothorax is reduced (i.e., until respiratory distress has subsided or mechanical ventilation is no longer required). The tube is then clamped. If there is neither clinical nor radiographic evidence of recurrent pneumothorax, the thoracostomy tube can be removed.

Other, once common, forms of thoracic air leak, including pneumopericardium and pneumoperitoneum, are now rare.

LIQUID VENTILATION

One experimental approach to reducing the lung injury associated with gas ventilation is liquid ventilation. Lung injury may be the result of abnormal inflation patterns produced because of elevated alveolar surface tension. Liquid inflation of the lungs with saline eliminates the alveolar gas–lung liquid interface with its tendency to induce collapse and perhaps injury. However, saline is too poor a carrier of oxygen to supply the body. Liquid perfluorocarbon solutions are able to dissolve large volumes of oxygen and carbon dioxide at 1 atm. Perfluorocarbon solutions have been used as carriers for O_2 and CO_2 in moribund human infants and have been the subject of

TABLE 30–8. *Populations of infants potentially benefiting from liquid ventilation*

- Extremely-low-birth-weight infants failing to respond to surfactant therapy
- Infants with pulmonary hypoplasia secondary to congenital diaphragmatic hernia
- Term infants approaching need for extracorporeal membrane oxygenation who have failed all other conventional and experimental therapies

extensive experimental work in premature and full-term animals, including primates and lambs (100,101).

Two methods of liquid ventilation are being tested. The first is total liquid ventilation, which uses a completely perfluorocarbon-filled ventilator circuit, and a membrane oxygenator to prime the inspired liquid flow. The second is perfluorocarbon-assisted gas exchange, in which a portion of the lung volume (i.e., FRC) is filled with perfluorocarbon liquids and the lungs are ventilated with a conventional infant mechanical ventilator (102). Liquid ventilation is an attractive form of pulmonary rescue because the perfluorocarbons seem to be nontoxic and the technique, although experimental, is less invasive than ECMO. As with all forms of transpulmonary ventilation, the application of perfluorocarbon ventilation is limited by underlying anatomic conditions of immaturity in the fetal lung.

Preliminary results in very premature infants, who have failed to respond to surfactant, have been encouraging (103). There are three groups of patients who may benefit from this therapy (Table 30–8). The ultimate benefits of this treatment are unknown at the present time.

MANAGEMENT IN THE INTENSIVE CARE SETTING

Management of respiratory problems requires specialized personnel and equipment. A physician skilled in neonatal intensive care techniques should be available within the unit at all times, and other specialists should be immediately accessible for consultation.

Nurses must be carefully trained in the techniques for the intensive care of infants. Necessary skills include application of ventilatory support equipment, recognition of equipment malfunction, airway management, assessment of ventilation, and use of monitoring equipment. Nurse-to-patient ratios vary from 1:1 to 1:3, depending on the severity of the illness. Infants who are receiving assisted ventilation usually require a nursing ratio of 1:1.

Respiratory therapists are critical to the effective use of respiratory equipment. Maintenance and calibration of all oxygen administration and oxygen-measuring devices require the presence of a respiratory therapist within the hospital at all times.

Equipment needs for neonatal intensive care include wall sources of compressed air and oxygen, oxygen dilutors, heating and humidification devices, and oxygen-monitoring systems with alarms. Critically ill infants need continuous monitoring of temperature, respiratory rate, and heart rate by electrical devices with alarm systems. In the acute phase of illness, or if an umbilical or peripheral arterial catheter is in use, blood pressure monitoring and oscilloscopic electrocardiographic display must be available. Continuous electroencephalographic monitoring is possible but not in widespread use in intensive care nurseries.

The parents of severely ill infants need understanding and support. They experience feelings of anxiety, fear, guilt, and hostility. Most families are ill equipped for the unexpected emotional and financial burden imposed by the child's hospitalization. A social worker should be available exclusively to the neonatal intensive care unit to provide assistance to parents by delineating parental concerns and helping coordinate communication with the medical and nursing staff and other hospital personnel.

The physical design of the intensive care unit must facilitate the management of acute respiratory problems. Each patient area should be large enough to accommodate the necessary personnel and the enormous amount of equipment, without generating intolerable crowding. A small number of patients in each area of the nursery facilitates parental visits and alleviates the overall level of stress. The proliferation of monitors and alarms may result in monitor fatigue, with the risk that monitors are ignored (104). Although neonatology is often thought of as an acute care specialty, it more accurately is categorized as a chronic care specialty, because of the many days and weeks of specialized care that small, sick infants require. The physical design of intensive care units is catching up to that new reality.

Adequate attention paid to these ancillary features of intensive respiratory care of the newborn helps ensure the optimal outcome expected for critically ill infants.

REFERENCES

1. American Academy of Pediatrics and American College of Obstetrics and Gynecology. *Guidelines for perinatal care,* 4th ed. Elk Grove, IL: American Academy of Pediatrics, 1997:191.
2. Flynn JT, Bancalari E, Snyder ES, et al. A cohort study of transcutaneous oxygen tension and the incidence and severity of retinopathy of prematurity. *N Engl J Med* 1992;326:1050.
3. Lucey JF, Dangman B. A reexamination of the role of oxygen in retrolental fibroplasia. *J Pediatr* 1984;73:82.
4. Thibeault DW, Hobel CJ, Kwong MS. Perinatal factors influencing the arterial oxygen tension in preterm infants with RDS while breathing 100% oxygen. *J Pediatr* 1974;84:898.
5. Dunn PM. Localization of the umbilical catheter by post-mortem measurement. *Arch Dis Child* 1966;41:69.
6. Harris MS, Little GA. Umbilical artery catheters: high, low or no. *J Perinat Med* 1978;6:15.
7. Mokrohisky ST, Levine RL, Blumhagen JD, et al. Low positioning of umbilical artery catheters increases associated complications in newborn infants. *N Engl J Med* 1978;299:561.
8. Wesstrom G, Finnstrom O, Stenport G. Umbilical artery catheterization in newborns. 1. Thrombosis in relation to catheter type and position. *Acta Pediatr Scand* 1979;68:575.
9. Cassady G. Transcutaneous monitoring in the newborn infant. *J Pediatr* 1983;103:837.
10. Graham G, Kenny MA. Performance of a radiometer transcutaneous oxygen monitor. *Clin Chem* 1980;26:629.
11. The Task Force on Transcutaneous Oxygen Monitors. American Academy of Pediatrics: report of consensus meeting, December 5–6, 1986. *Pediatrics* 1989;83:122.
12. Peabody JL, Gregory GA, Willis MM. Transcutaneous oxygen tension in sick infants. *Am Rev Respir Dis* 1978;118:83.
13. Hay WW Jr, Brockway J, Eyzaquirre M. Neonatal pulse oximetry: accuracy and reliability. *Pediatrics* 1989;83:717.
14. Hay WW, Thilo E, Curlander JB. Pulse oximetry in neonatal medicine. *Clin Perinatol* 1991;18:441.
15. Epstein MF, Cohen AR, Feldman HA, Raemer DB. Estimation of $PaCO_2$ by two noninvasive methods in the critically ill newborn infants. *J Pediatr* 1985;106:282.
16. McEvedy BAB, McLeod ME, Kirpalani H, et al. End-tidal carbon dioxide measurement in critically ill neonates: a comparison of sidestream and mainstream monitors. *Can J Anaesth* 1990;37:322.
17. Rozycki HJ, Sysyn GD, Marshall MK, et al. Mainstream end-tidal carbon dioxide monitoring in the neonatal intensive care unit. *Pediatrics* 1998;101:648.
18. Sivan Y, Eldadah MK, Chea TE, Newth CJL. Estimation of arterial carbon dioxide by end-tidal and transcutaneous PCO_2 measurement in ventilated children. *Pediatr Pulmon* 1992;12:153.
19. Garland JS, Buck RK, Allred EN, Levitow A. Hypocarbia before surfactant therapy appears to increase bronchopulmonary dysplasia risk in infants with respiratory distress syndrome. *Arch Pediatr Adolesc Med* 1995;149:617.
20. Wiswell TE, Graziani LJ, Kornhauser MS, et al. Effects of hypocarbia on the development of cystic periventricular leukomalacia in premature infants treated with high frequency jet ventilation. *Pediatrics* 1996;98:918.
21. Wyatt JS, Edwards AD, Cope M, et al. Response of cerebral blood volume to changes in arterial carbon dioxide tension in preterm and term infants. *Pediatr Res* 1991;29:553.
22. Kraybill EN, Runyan DK, Bose CL, Kahn JH. Risk factors for chronic lung disease in infants with birth weights of 751–1000 grams. *J Pediatr* 1989;115:115.
23. Poets CF, Sari B. Change in intubation rates and outcome of very low birthweight infants: a population-based study. *Pediatrics* 1996;98:24.
24. Rhodes PG, Hall RT. Continuous positive airway pressure delivered by face mask in infants with the idiopathic respiratory distress syndrome: a controlled study. *Pediatrics* 1973;52:1.
25. Wung J, James LS, Kilchevsky E, James E. Management of infants with severe respiratory failure and persistence of fetal circulation, without hyperventilation. *Pediatrics* 1985;76:484.
26. Bidani A, Tzouanakis AE, Cardenas VJ Jr, et al. Permissive hypercapnia in acute respiratory failure. *JAMA* 1994;272:957.
27. Hickling KG, Joyce C. Permissive hypercapnia in ARDS and its effect on tissue oxygenation. *Acta Anesthesiol Scand Suppl* 1995;107:201.
28. Chance B. Spectrophotometry of intracellular respiratory pigments. *Science* 1954;20:272.
29. Jöbsis FF. Noninvasive, infrared monitoring of cerebral and myocardial oxygen sufficiency and circulatory parameters. Science 1977;198:1264.
30. Brazy JE. Near-infrared spectroscopy. *Clin Perinatol* 1991;18:519.
31. Wyatt JS, Cope M, Delpy DT, et al. Quantification of cerebral oxygenation and haemodynamics in sick newborn infants by near infrared spectrophotometry. *Lancet* 1986;2:1063.
32. Hampson NB, Camporesi EM, Stolp BW, et al. Cerebral oxygen availability by NIR spectroscopy during transient hypoxia in humans. *J Appl Physiol* 1990;69:907.
33. Wyatt JS, Cope M, Delpy DT, et al. Quantification of cerebral blood volume in human infants by near-infrared spectroscopy. *J Appl Physiol* 1990;68:1086.
34. Skov L, Pryds O, Greisen G. Estimating cerebral blood flow in newborn infants: comparison of near infrared spectrascopy and 133Xe clearance. *Pediatr Res* 1991;30:570.
35. Hirtz DG. Report of the National Institute of Neurological Disorders and Stroke workshop on near infrared spectroscopy. *Pediatrics* 1993;91:414.
36. Harrison VR, Heese-de V, Klein M. The significance of grunting in hyaline membrane disease. *Pediatrics* 1968;41:549.

37. Gregory GA, Kitterman JA, Phibbs RG, Tooley WH, Hamilton WK. Treatment of the idiopathic respiratory distress syndrome with continuous positive airway pressure. *N Engl J Med* 1971;284:1333.

38. Edberg KE, Sandberg K, Silberg A, et al. Lung volume, gas mixing, and mechanics of breathing in mechanically ventilated very low birth weight infants with idiopathic respiratory distress syndrome. *Pediatr Res* 1991;30:496.

39. Richardson CP, Jung AL. Effects of continuous positive airway pressure on pulmonary function and blood gases of infants with respiratory distress syndrome. *Pediatr Res* 1978;12:771.

40. Saunders RA, Milner AD, Hopkins IE. The effects of CPAP on lung mechanics and lung volumes in the neonate. *Biol Neonate* 1976;29:178.

41. Miller MJ, DiFiore JM, Strohl KP, Martin RJ. Effects of nasal CPAP on supraglottic and total pulmonary resistance in preterm infants. *J Appl Physiol* 1990;56:141.

42. Miller MJ, Waldeman AC, Martin RJ. Continuous positive airway pressure selectively reduces obstructive apnea in preterm infants. *J Pediatr* 1985;106:91.

43. Avery ME, Tooley WH, Keller JB, et al. Is chronic lung disease in low birth weight infants preventable? A survey of eight centers. *Pediatrics* 1987;79:26.

44. Horbar JD, McAuliffe TL, Alder SM et al. Variability in 28–day outcomes for very low birthweight infants: an analysis of neonatal intensive care units. *Pediatrics* 1988;82:554.

45. Verder H, Robertson B, Greisen G, et al. Surfactant therapy and nasal continuous positive airway pressure for newborns with respiratory distress syndrome. *N Engl J Med* 1994;331:1051.

46. Martin RJ, Nearman HS, Katona PG, Klaus MH. The effect of a low continuous positive pressure on the reflex control of respiration in preterm infants. *J Pediatr* 1977;90:976.

47. Fanaroff AA, Cha CC, Sosa R, Crummins RS, Klaus MH. Controlled trial of continuous negative external pressure in the treatment of severe respiratory distress syndrome. *J Pediatr* 1973;82:921.

48. Samuels MP, Raine J, Wright T, et al. Continuous negative extrathoracic pressure in neonatal respiratory failure. *Pediatrics* 1996;98:1154.

49. Bancalari E, Sinclair JC. Mechanical ventilation. In: Sinclair JC, Bracken MB, eds. *Effective care of the newborn infant.* New York: Oxford University Press, 1992;200.

50. Belenky DA, Orr RJ, Woodrum DE, Hodson WA. Is continuous transpulmonary pressure better than conventional respiratory management of hyaline membrane disease? A controlled study. *Pediatrics* 1976;58:800.

51. Han VKM, Beverley DM, Clauson C, et al. Randomized controlled trial of very early continuous distending pressure in the management of preterm infants. *Early Hum Dev* 1987;15:21.

52. Kamper J, Wulff K, Larsen C, et al. Early treatment with nasal continuous positive airway pressure in very low birth weight infants. *Acta Paediatr* 1993;82:193.

53. Roberton NRC. Does CPAP work when it really matters? *Acta Paediatr* 1993;82:193.

54. Lundstrom KE. Initial treatment of preterm infants continuous positive airway pressure or ventilation? *Eur J Pediatr* 1996;155[Suppl 2]:525.

55. Drew JH. Immediate intubation at birth of the very low birth weight infant. *Am J Dis Child* 1982;136:207.

56. Alba J, Agarwal R, Hegyi T, Hiatt IM. Efficacy of surfactant therapy in infants managed with CPAP. *Pediatr Pulmon* 1995;20:172.

57. So BH, Tamura M, Kamoshita S. Nasal continuous positive airway pressure following surfactant replacement for the treatment of neonatal respiratory distress syndrome. *Acta Paediatr Sin* 1994;35:280.

58. So BH, Tamura M, Mishima J, et al. Application of nasal continuous positive airway pressure to early extubation in very low birthweight infants. *Arch Dis Child* 1994;72:F191.

59. Annibale DJ, Halsey TC, Engstrom PC, et al. Randomized controlled trial of nasopharyngeal continuous positive airway pressure in the extubation of very low birthweight infants. *J Pediatr* 1994;124:455.

60. Tapia JL, Bancalari A, Gonzalez A, Mercado ME. Does continuous positive airway pressure (CPAP) during weaning from intermittent mandatory ventilation in very low birth weight infants have risks or benefits? A controlled trial. *Pediatr Pulmon* 1995;19:269.

61. Dreyfuss D, Saumon G. Ventilator-induced lung injury. *Am J Respir Crit Care Med* 1998;157:294.

62. Rodenstein DO, Perlmutter N, Stanescu DC. Infants are not obligatory nasal breathers. *Am Rev Respir Dis* 1985;131:343.

63. Polgar G, Kong GP. The nasal resistance of newborn infants. *J Pediatr* 1965;67:557.

64. Wung JT, Stark FI, Indyk L, et al. Oxygen supplementation during endotracheal intubation of the infant. *Pediatrics* 1977;59:1046.

65. Fanconi S, Duc G. Intratracheal suctioning in sick preterm infants: prevention of intracranial hypertension and cerebral hypoperfusion by muscle paralysis. *Pediatrics* 1987;79:538.

66. Kelly MA, Finer NN. Nasotracheal intubation in the neonate: physiologic responses and effects of atropine and pancuronium. *J Pediatr* 1984;105:303.

67. Tochen ML. Orotracheal intubation in the newborn infant: a method for determining depth of tube insertion. *J Pediatr* 1979;95:1050.

68. Kohelet D, Goldberg A, Goldberg M. Depth of endotracheal tube placement in neonates. *J Pediatr* 1982;101:157.

69. Tarnow-Mordi WO, Reid E, Griffiths P, Wilkinson AR. Low inspired gas temperature and respiratory complications in very low birth weight infants. *J Pediatr* 1989;114:438.

70. Golombek S, Truog WE. Acute effects of exogenous surfactant treatment in near term infants with RDS. *J Invest Med* 1995;43:463.

71. Hodson WA, Truog WE, Mayock DE, et al. Bronchopulmonary dysplasia: the need for epidemiologic studies. *J Pediatr* 1979;95:848.

72. Mammel MC, Bing DR. Mechanical ventilation of the newborn. Recent advances in mechanical ventilation. *Clin Chest Med* 1996;17:603.

73. Amitay M, Etches PC, Finer NN, Maidens, JM. Synchronous mechanical ventilation of the neonate with respiratory disease. *Crit Care Med* 1993;21:118.

74. Bernstein G, Cleary JP, Heldt GP, Rosas JF, Schellenberg LD, Mannino FL. Response time and reliability of three neonatal patient-triggered ventilators. *Am Rev Respir Dis* 1993;148:358.

75. Hummler HD, Gerhardt T, Gonzalez A, et al. Patient-triggered ventilation in neonates: comparison of a flow-and an impedance-triggered system. *Am J Respir Crit Care Med* 1996;154:1049.

76. Younes M, Puddy A, Roberts D, et al. Proportional assist ventilation, a new approach to ventilatory support. *Am Rev Resp Dis* 1992;145:114.

77. Slutsky AS. Nonconventional methods of ventilation. *Am Rev Respir Dis* 1988;138:175.

78. Keszler M, Donn SM, Bucciarelli RL, et al. Multi-center controlled trial comparing high frequency jet ventilation and conventional mechanical ventilation in newborn infants with pulmonary interstitial emphysema. *J Pediatr* 1991;119:85.

79. Keszler M, Madanlou HD, Brudno DS, et al. Multicenter controlled clinical trial of high-frequency jet ventilation in preterm infants with uncomplicated respiratory distress syndrome. *Pediatrics* 1997;100:593.

80. The HIFI Study Group. High-frequency oscillatory ventilation compared with conventional mechanical ventilation in the treatment of respiratory failure in preterm infants. *N Engl J Med* 1989;320:88.

81. Wiswell TE, Graziani LJ, Kornhauser MS, et al. High-frequency jet ventilation in the early management of respiratory distress syndrome is associated with a greater risk for adverse outcomes. *Pediatrics* 1996;98:1035.

82. Clark RH, Gerstmann DR, Null DM Jr, et al. Prospective randomized comparison of high-frequency oscillatory and conventional ventilation in respiratory distress syndrome. *Pediatrics* 1992;89:5.

83. Gerstmann DR, Minton SD, Stoddard RA, et al. Results of the Provo multicenter surfactant high frequency oscillatory ventilation controlled trial. *Pediatrics* 1996;98:1044.

84. HIFO Study Group. Randomized study of high frequency oscillatory ventilation in infants with severe respiratory distress syndrome. *J Pediatr* 1993;122:609.

85. Ogawa Y, Miyaska K, Kawano T, et al. A multicenter randomized trial of high frequency oscillatory ventilation as compared with conventional mechanical ventilation in preterm infants with respiratory failure. *Early Hum Dev* 1993;32:1.

86. Jackson JC, Truog WE, Standaert TA, et al. Effect of high-frequency ventilation on the development of alveolar edema in premature monkeys at risk for hyaline membrane disease. *Am Rev Respir Dis* 1991;143:865.

87. Meredith KS, de Lemos RA, Coalson JJ, et al. Role of lung injury in the pathogenesis of hyaline membrane disease in premature baboons. *J Appl Physiol* 1989;66:2150.

88. Solimano A, Bryan C, Jobe A, et al. Effects of high-frequency and conventional ventilation on the premature lamb lung. *J Appl Physiol* 1985;59:1571.

89. Carter MJM, Gerstmann DR, Clark MRH, et al. High-frequency oscillatory ventilation and extracorporeal membrane oxygenation for the treatment of acute neonatal respiratory failure. *Pediatrics* 1990;85:159.

90. Clark RH, Yoder BA, Sell MS. Prospective, randomized comparison of high-frequency oscillation and conventional ventilation in candidates for extracorporeal membrane oxygenation. *J Pediatr* 1994;124:447.

91. Kinsella JP, Truog WE, Walsh WF, et al. Randomized, multicenter trial of inhaled nitric oxide and high-frequency oscillatory ventilation in severe, persistent pulmonary hypertension of the newborn. *J Pediatr* 1997;130:55.

92. Klainer AS, Turndorf H, Wu WH. Surface alterations to endotracheal intubation. *Am J Med* 1975;58:674.

93. Rasche RF, Kuhns LR. Histopathologic changes in airway mucosa of infants after endotracheal intubation. *Pediatrics* 1972;50:632.

94. Parkin JL, Stevens MH, Jung AL. Acquired and congenital subglottic stenosis in the infant. *Ann Otol Rhinol Laryngol* 1976;85:573.

95. Filston HC, Johnson DG, Crumrire RS. Infant tracheostomy. *Am J Dis Child* 1978;132:1172.

96. Downing GJ, Kilbride HW. Evaluation of airway complications in high-risk preterm infants: application of flexible fiberoptic airway endoscopy. *Pediatrics* 1995;95:567.

97. Kuhns LR, Bednorck FJ, Wyman ML. Diagnosis of pneumothorax or pneumomediastinum in the neonate by transillumination. *Pediatrics* 1975;56:355.

98. Ogata ES, Gregory GA, Kitterman JA, et al. Pneumothorax in the respiratory distress syndrome: incidence and effect on vital signs, blood gas and pH. *Pediatrics* 1976;58:177.

99. Jung AL, Nelson J, Jenkins MB, Hodson WA. Clinical evaluation of a new chest tube used in neonates. *Clin Pediatr* 1991;2:85.

100. Greenspan JS, Wolfson MR, Rubenstein SD, Shaffer TH. Liquid ventilation of human preterm neonates. *J Pediatr* 1990;117:106.

101. Truog WE, Jackson JC. Alternative modes of ventilation in the prevention and treatment of bronchopulmonary dysplasia. *Clin Perinatol* 1992;19:621.

102. Fuhrman BP, Paczan RR, Francisis M. Perfluorocarbon associated gas exchange. *Crit Care Med* 1991;19:712.

103. Leach CL, Greenspan JS, Rubenstein SD, et al. Partial liquid ventilation with perflubron in premature infants with severe respiratory distress syndrome. *N Engl J Med* 1996;335:761.

104. Brans YW. Biomedical technology—to use or not to use. *Clin Perinatol* 1991;18:389.

CHAPTER 31

Extracorporeal Membrane Oxygenation

Billie Lou Short

In 1944, Kolff and Berk observed that blood became oxygenated as it passed through cellophane chambers of their artificial kidney membrane (1). This historic observation led to the recognition, by those involved in the fast-developing field of cardiopulmonary bypass, that blood could be oxygenated through a semipermeable membrane lung. In the bubble and disk oxygenators used during the early 1950s for open heart surgery, oxygen and blood were mixed directly. This mixing resulted in considerable damage to blood products and the potential for producing lethal fibrin emboli, making these systems unsuitable for prolonged clinical use (2). For this reason, and in light of Kolff and Berk's findings, attention was directed to the development of semipermeable membrane oxygenators that separate blood and oxygen, decreasing or eliminating the risks of the earlier oxygenators.

The first membrane lung, which used an ethylcellulose membrane, was described by Clowes in 1956 and was used successfully in open heart surgery 1 year later (3). With this report began the study of prolonged cardiopulmonary bypass and the potential application of extracorporeal membrane oxygenation (ECMO) as an artificial lung.

The 1960s witnessed intensive research on materials and techniques (2). Silicone polymers, available in thin sheets that enhanced gas transfer through membranes, began to be characterized and developed. The development of the Kolobow silicone membrane lung made the field of ECMO possible, and clinical trials, using prolonged bypass or ECMO as an artificial lung, began in the late 1960s (2,4–6).

The concept of an artificial placenta, a device capable of continuing *ex utero* the gas-exchange functions of the placenta, developed in parallel with that of an artificial lung. In 1961, Callaghan and colleagues began using animal models of respiratory distress syndrome of the newborn to test the efficacy of an extracorporeal oxygenation circuit as an artificial placenta (7). During the early 1960s, investigators, including Rashkind, White, Dorson, and Avery, used ECMO as an artificial placenta for premature infants (8–10). Although the infants died, this was an extremely important period for the development and refinement of the mechanical and surgical techniques that laid the foundation for the subsequent success of ECMO.

It was not until ECMO therapy was applied to the term infant through the pioneering work of Dr. Robert Bartlett and colleagues that its full potential as a powerful therapy for infants in severe respiratory failure was recognized. In 1976, Bartlett and his associates reported the first neonatal ECMO survivor, a term infant with severe meconium aspiration syndrome (MAS) (11). During the next 10 years, neonatal ECMO was used to treat 99 term infants with respiratory failure in three centers in the United States and produced an overall survival rate of 65%. Since 1986, ECMO therapy has developed explosively, and more than 13,000 infants have been treated in more than 90 ECMO programs, with an overall survival rate of 80% (12).

The most common use for ECMO is in the term or near-term infant with failure to oxygenate as a result of MAS, idiopathic persistent pulmonary hypertension (PPHN), congenital diaphragmatic hernia (CDH), sepsis and pneumonia, or hyaline membrane disease. Although overall survival is 80% nationally, the best results are for the MAS (94%) and PPHN (82%) groups (Table 31–1). The survival rate for the CDH population requiring ECMO has not increased over time and remains at 60% nationally, perhaps because of the heterogeneity of this group of infants, who have various degrees of pulmonary hypoplasia and pulmonary hypertension (13,14). Only 30% to 40% of the CDH population require ECMO therapy, and the remainder have

B.L. Short: Department of Neonatology, Children's National Medical Center, Washington, D.C.

TABLE 31–1. *Results of extracorporeal oxygenation[a]*

Diagnosis	Survival after therapy (%)
Meconium aspiration syndrome	94
Persistent pulmonary hypertension	82
Sepsis and pneumonia	76
Respiratory distress syndrome	84
Congenital diaphragmatic hernia	59
Total	80

[a]Data from the Extracorporeal Life Support Neonatal Registry, January 1998, 13,138 patients.

close to a 100% survival rate. Therefore, with ECMO therapy, the overall survival rate for the CDH population as a whole has increased to over 70%. Most centers are now repairing the diaphragmatic defect in the critical CDH on ECMO (13,14). The effect of this approach on survival is not known.

INDICATIONS

Among the most controversial aspects of ECMO therapy have been the clinical criteria used to determine its use (14–22). Because of the invasive nature of ECMO therapy and the potential risks associated with this therapy, the criteria are designed to select a population of infants who have an 80% or greater mortality risk with conventional therapy. Assumptions about the ability of ECMO to increase survival are valid only if the criteria are specific for each high-risk population. The ultimate test for the efficacy of ECMO, and the predictive value of ECMO criteria, is a prospective, randomized trial. Although two randomized trials have been completed, most centers have used historic controls to develop their criteria (15,16,19–21). In the prospective, randomized trial reported by O'Rourke and colleagues, a crossover design was used, which may have skewed the predictions of their criteria. In one report, however, the criteria used in O'Rourke's study, which were thought to predict a mortality over 80% based on retrospective data, predicted a mortality of only 40% when used prospectively (21). It is imperative that all centers continually evaluate their criteria, especially as less invasive therapies become available. The United Kingdom collaborative randomized trial did not involve a crossover design and therefore represents a more ideal trial for ECMO therapy (24). Of the 185 patients enrolled in the study, 93 were allocated to ECMO therapy and 92 to conventional therapy, which included high-frequency ventilation and nitric oxide therapy. Mortality was significantly different between the ECMO and conventional groups, 32% versus 59% ($p = 0.0005$). This benefit of ECMO was sustained when severe disability at 1 year of age was taken into account ($p = 0.002$). The CDH population in this study had the highest mortality rate, 82% in the ECMO group and

100% in the conventional group. Severity of illness was also a predictor, with mortality higher in the patients with an oxygen index (OI) of 60 or greater at the time of entry into the study, indicating that early transfer of these patients to an ECMO center is essential. The authors also noted that mortality was lower if the referring hospital was a teaching hospital.

The potential risks associated with ECMO therapy include those associated with ligation of the carotid artery and jugular vein, prolonged exposure to systemic heparinization, alterations in pulsatile blood flow patterns, exposure to potential toxins such as aluminum and phthalate esters (i.e., plasticizer) from the circuit, and others yet to be determined (25,26). With its long-term outcome still unknown, use of ECMO should be limited to the term or near-term infant who has a 20% or less chance of survival with conventional therapy. Although criteria developed at other centers are available, these are based on the clinical management and patient populations in those centers and may not be valid when applied to patients in other institutions (16,17,21). What is considered maximal conventional therapy (e.g., hyperventilation) in one institution may not be used in others. Differences in patient populations, such as the percentage of patients who are inborn versus outborn, may significantly alter applicability of criteria from one center to another. All ECMO centers should attempt to develop criteria based on their own management techniques and patient population.

Several important inclusion criteria for ECMO are based on known complications of the procedure. These are listed in Table 31–2.

Age and Weight Limitations

The requirement for systemic heparinization of the ECMO patient places significant limitations on the population that can be treated. Use of ECMO in the late 1960s and early 1970s in premature infants weighing less than 2,000 g or younger than 34 weeks of gestation resulted in a significant mortality rate from intracranial hemorrhage (ICH) (12,28,30). This increased risk may be a result of the combination of systemic heparinization with a more direct effect of ECMO on the brain (28,31). Concerns about an increased rate of ICH in the premature infant were corroborated by findings for infants

TABLE 31–2. *Inclusion criteria for extracorporeal membrane oxygenation*

Gestational age ≥34 weeks or birth weight ≥2000 g
No significant coagulopathy or bleeding complications
No major intracranial hemorrhage
Mechanical ventilation provided for ≤10–14 days
Reversible lung disease
No major cardiac lesion

weighing less than 2,500 g at birth who received ECMO at Children's National Medical Center in Washington, D.C. This group had a 50% incidence of ICH, representing more than 50% of the major ICHs seen in the total patient population at our center (28). Data from a review of the premature infant treated with ECMO by Hirschl and colleagues indicates that the ICH rate in the infant down to 32 weeks of gestation is lower than previously noted (32). Because of this finding, some centers are now considering treating infants in this gestational range. Although the ICH rate is lower in infants at 32 to 33 weeks of gestation than in the earlier experience with this group, the rate is still close to 50%; thus, if one is considering ECMO therapy for this population, the information given to parents should appropriately address the high risk for intracranial hemorrhage. Because of this high risk, we continue to recommend that only infants weighing more than 2,000 g at birth or older than 33 weeks of gestational age be considered candidates for ECMO. A better understanding of the pathophysiology of the intracranial bleeds seen in the ECMO population may allow us to alter the risk for this complication and thus lower the gestational age cutoff in the future (30,31).

Hematologic Limitations

The requirement for systemic heparinization places the infant with a significant coagulopathy or with bleeding complications at extreme risk. All attempts should be made to correct any coagulopathy before instituting ECMO. If the coagulopathy is severe and cannot be corrected with appropriate blood product replacement, the infant should not be considered for ECMO.

The septic infant is of particular concern because of the commonly associated coagulopathy. Although these infants are at an increased risk for bleeding complications on ECMO, correction of their coagulopathy and meticulous heparin management have resulted in successful treatment (33).

The necessity for heparinization during ECMO precludes the treatment of any infant with a major ICH. Infants with grade I intraventricular hemorrhages or small parenchymal hemorrhages can be treated if heparin management is monitored closely and activated clotting times (ACTs) are kept low (e.g., 160 to 180 seconds).

Prior Mechanical Ventilation

The limit of 10 to 14 days of assisted ventilation before ECMO therapy is imposed because of the probable development of chronic lung disease after aggressive assisted ventilation of this duration. Extracorporeal membrane oxygenation is unable to reverse this disease process within a safe period. After 3 weeks of ECMO, the risks for complications related to the ECMO procedure itself,

such as clot formation, nosocomial infections (e.g., neck wound infections), and mechanical failures (e.g., tubing ruptures), begin to increase. The maximal time that a neonatal patient can be kept on the ECMO circuit is unknown, but in view of the increasing risk of complications and usual lack of response beyond this time period, most centers limit time on the circuit to around 3 weeks. Infants with diseases, such as chronic lung disease, that do not improve in a short period should not be considered for ECMO unless there is a life-threatening underlying disease state, such as acute pulmonary hypertension, that can be rapidly reversed by ECMO.

Cardiopulmonary Disease

Candidates for ECMO must have reversible lung disease. Because of the cardiopulmonary support provided by this therapy, ECMO has allowed many infants thought to have irreversible lung disease to live. The diagnosis of irreversible lung disease has become progressively more difficult to make (13,34,35).

Significant cardiac disease must be ruled out before ECMO, but infants with severe reversible lung disease superimposed on congenital heart disease may be candidates for ECMO support before cardiac surgery.

Risk Assessment and Mortality Criteria

If the infant is failing maximal conventional therapy, ECMO should be considered. The next task is to predict which infants have a high mortality risk without ECMO.

Commonly used criteria (Table 31–3) are the alveolar–arterial oxygen gradient (AaDO$_2$), the oxygen index (OI), and arterial partial pressure of oxygen (PaO$_2$) levels less than 50 mm Hg over a specific time period (16,17,20, 21,35). The AaDO$_2$ can be calculated as follows:

$$AaDO_2 = P_B - 47 - PaCO_2 - PaO_2$$

when FiO$_2$ is 1.00, P$_B$ is the barometric pressure, and 47 is the water vapor pressure. The OI can be calculated with the following equation:

$$OI = MAP \times FiO_2 \times 100/PaO_2$$

in which MAP is the mean airway pressure.

TABLE 31–3. *Neonatal extracorporeal membrane oxygenation criteria[a]*

AaDO$_2$ 605–620 mm Hg for 4–12 hr
Oxygen index 35–60 for 0.5–6 hr
PaO$_2$ 35–50 mm Hg for 2–12 hr
pH <7.25 for 2 hr with hypotension
Acute deterioration PaO$_2$ 30–40 mm Hg

[a]Criteria used only after maximal therapy instituted; 50% of centers use more than one criterion. AaDO$_2$, alveolar–arterial oxygen gradient; PaO$_2$, arterial partial pressure of oxygen.

Deciding when to transfer an infant to an ECMO center is a difficult task. Most infants with disorders treated by ECMO improve without ECMO. Before the infant becomes too moribund for transport, the referring physician must attempt to determine which infants are at high risk for failing maximal conventional therapy. This is an enormous responsibility, which can be eased by early consultation with ECMO center personnel. Kanto and associates found that 12% of their ECMO referrals died before arrival of the transport team or during interhospital transport (37). Of these deaths, 32% occurred in infants with CDH, indicating that early referral of these patients is warranted. Data from the Children's National Medical Center show that approximately 20 infants per year (16% of ECMO referrals) died before or during transport. For the infants who died, the average peak inspiratory pressure (PIP) at the time of the referral call was 50 cm H_2O, with a PaO_2 of 28 mm Hg, compared with 45 cm H_2O and 40 mm Hg in ECMO survivors. Earlier transfer might have increased the likelihood of survival in these infants.

The typical ventilator settings and blood gas values before ECMO therapy are shown in Table 31–4. If possible, consultation for transfer should occur before these ventilator settings are reached and before the infant's PaO_2 falls below 40 mm Hg. The presence of a respiratory acidosis, as shown in Table 31–4, is associated with a significant increase in mortality and is an indication for possible early transfer.

The infant with CDH is the most difficult to manage before ECMO and should be considered for early transfer to an ECMO center. Some centers exclude infants with CDH who have not had some period with a PaO_2 more than 100 mm Hg, and other centers exclude CDH patients as candidates for ECMO because they do not have an arterial partial pressure of carbon dioxide ($PaCO_2$) less than 45 mm Hg after maximal ventilation (38–41). Most ECMO centers accept all comers because survivors have

been reported from both of the described exclusionary categories (13,14,34,35).

The studies that are performed before transfer of a patient to an ECMO center include an echocardiogram to rule out heart disease; a cranial ultrasound scan to rule out significant ICH; coagulation studies, including a partial thromboplastin time, prothrombin time, fibrinogen level, fibrin degradation products, and platelet count; calcium and electrolyte levels; leukocyte count with a differential analysis; and hemoglobin and hematocrit levels. These studies help the team at the ECMO center determine whether the patient should be considered for ECMO and, if so, assist them in anticipating difficulties.

On admission to the ECMO center, it must be determined whether the patient is an appropriate ECMO candidate. The ultrasound examination of the central nervous system (CNS) is repeated to ensure that an ICH did not occur during transport. The cardiac evaluation is repeated if there is any residual question about the possibility of cardiac disease. Doppler flow techniques are used to document the severity of pulmonary hypertension. This information can be used later if the infant does not wean from ECMO appropriately. Serum electrolyte and calcium levels, hemoglobin and hematocrit, clotting studies including fibrinogen level, fibrin degradation products, partial thromboplastin and prothrombin times, platelet count, and a baseline ACT should be obtained on admission to detect abnormalities that require correction before ECMO.

Most ECMO candidates have received muscle relaxants before admission, making the neurologic status difficult to evaluate. It is imperative to obtain a complete perinatal history, including Apgar scores, history of resuscitation and seizure activity, and a description of the neurologic status of the infant before paralysis. Infants who have sustained severe irreversible neurologic damage should not be considered for ECMO.

TABLE 31–4. *Average ventilator settings and blood gas values before extracorporeal membrane oxygenation for survivors and nonsurvivors[a]*

Ventilator and blood gas parameters[c]	Values for all patients	Values for survivors	Values for nonsurvivors
Rate (breaths/min)	97 ± 74	96 ± 74	99 ± 75
FiO_2	1.00	1.00	1.00
PIP (cm H_2O)	46 ± 11	46 ± 10	45 ± 12
PEEP (cm H_2O)	4 ± 3	4 ± 3	6 ± 3
MAP (cm H_2O)	19 ± 5	19 ± 5	19 ± 5
pH	7.39 ± 0.2	7.41 ± 0.2	7.29 ± 0.2
PCO_2 (mm Hg)	42 ± 24	39 ± 21	52 ± 32[b]
PO_2 (mm Hg)	41 ± 32	41 ± 31	38 ± 32[b]

[a]Data from the Extracorporeal Life Support Neonatal Registry, July 1990. Data displayed as mean ± SD.
[b]<0.05 survivors *versus* nonsurvivors.
[c]FiO_2, forced inspiratory oxygen; MAP, mean airway pressure; PEEP, peak end-expiratory pressure; PIP, peak inspiratory pressure.

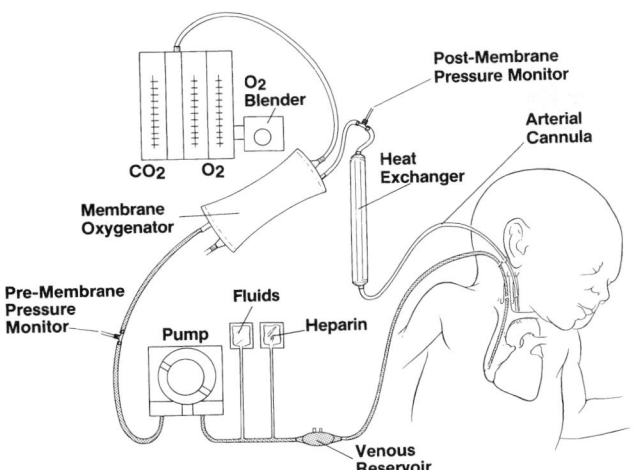

FIG. 31–1. Components of the venoarterial extracorporeal membrane oxygenation circuit. (From Short BL. Physiology of extracorporeal membrane oxygenation (ECMO). In Polin RA, Fox WW, eds. *Fetal and neonatal physiology.* Philadelphia: WB Saunders, 1992:932.)

PROCEDURE

Venoarterial Method

Venoarterial (VA) ECMO involves the use of two catheters: the venous outflow catheter in the right internal jugular vein with the tip in the right atrium and the arterial return catheter in the right carotid artery with the tip at the junction with the aortic arch. Blood is removed through the jugular catheter by means of gravity drainage into a venous reservoir (Fig. 31–1). Blood is pulled out of the reservoir by a roller occlusion pump and pushed through the membrane lung, where gas exchange occurs.

Gas transfers across the silicone membrane lung into the blood because of pressure gradients, increasing the oxygen level and removing carbon dioxide (Fig. 31–2). Blood then enters the heat exchanger, where it is warmed to body temperature and returned to the infant through the arterial catheter.

This form of bypass provides support for the lungs and cardiac support. Although most infants requiring ECMO have only a pulmonary disorder, some have cardiac dysfunction secondary to severe hypoxia and require the cardiac support that VA ECMO provides. Oxygenation is achieved by allowing the pump to support as much of the cardiac output as is needed to oxygenate the infant, usually 120 to 150 mL/kg/min in the first few days.

It is easy to support and oxygenate with VA ECMO, and it remains the gold standard for ECMO therapy. However, ligation of the carotid artery, alteration of pulsatile arterial blood flow patterns, and the possibility that particles or air in the circuit may enter the cerebral or coronary circulations remain concerns.

Venovenous Method

Venovenous (VV) techniques for ECMO have been developed because of the concerns about carotid ligation. Venovenous ECMO is currently achieved using a single double-lumen catheter placed through the internal jugular vein into the right atrium (Fig. 31–3) (42). This catheter has inflow and outflow ports that attach into the circuit. Because blood return and outflow occur in the right atrium, significant recirculation can occur, resulting in limited oxygenation with this technique (Fig. 31–4). Because the heart is the pump for VV ECMO, the use of this catheter depends on intact cardiac function (41,44–47). The advantages of this technique are the lack

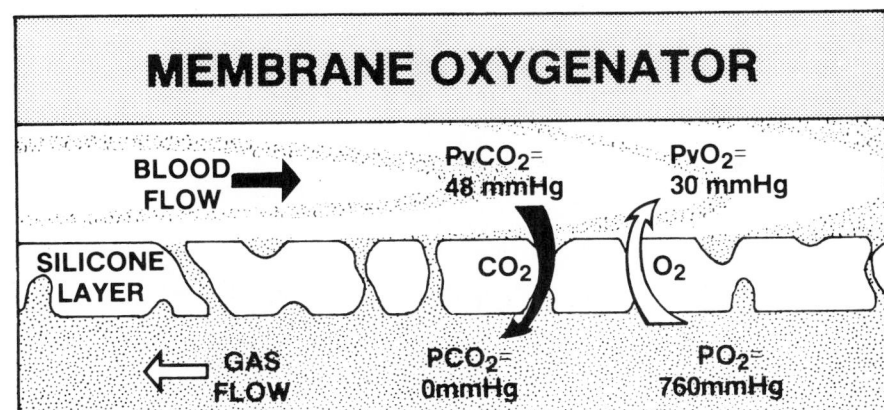

FIG. 31–2. The silicone membrane lung promotes gas transfer across a gradient for oxygen and carbon dioxide. The pore size does not allow blood products to cross. (From Short BL. Physiology of extracorporeal membrane oxygenation (ECMO). In Polin RA, Fox WW, eds. *Fetal and neonatal physiology.* Philadelphia: WB Saunders, 1992:932.)

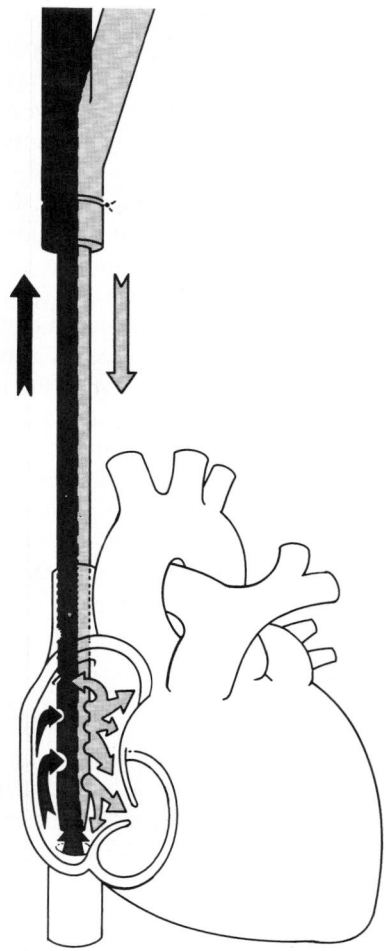

FIG. 31–3. The inflow and outflow characteristics of the venovenous catheter in the right atrium. (From Short BL, O'Brien A, Poindexter C, eds. *CNMC ECMO training manual.* Washington, DC: CNMC, 1993.)

of necessity for ligation of the carotid artery, maintenance of normal pulsatile blood flow, and the theoretical advantage that particles entering the circuit enter the lungs rather than the cerebral or coronary circulation. Disadvantages are the lack of cardiac support and limited oxygenation.

EQUIPMENT AND SYSTEMS

Most equipment currently used for ECMO therapy is modified cardiopulmonary bypass equipment designed for short-term use. To ensure safe and effective use of the ECMO equipment, the limitations of each piece of equipment must be understood and considered before it is used for long-term bypass.

There is no single ECMO machine. Each ECMO center must design an ECMO system by using equipment evaluated and designed to meet space and other specific requirements of their center. Bioengineering experts and cardiopulmonary perfusionists should be consulted in the design and evaluation of the ECMO system. The basic equipment needed for a complete system is listed in Table 31–5.

Space requirements and the possible need to transport the patient on ECMO should be taken into consideration in the design of an ECMO system (Fig. 31–5; see Fig. 31–1). The system should be on a cart or other movable base. The nondisposable equipment required includes a roller occlusion pump, a water bath to maintain normothermic bypass temperatures, a venous return monitor (VRM), gas flow meters for CO_2 and O_2 delivery into the membrane lung, an in-line venous saturation monitor, and membrane pressure monitors. Necessary disposable equipment includes the ECMO catheters (i.e., venous and arterial for VA ECMO; double-lumen venous for VV ECMO), tubing packs designed for the system, a venous reservoir, a heat exchanger, and a membrane lung.

Those involved in providing ECMO therapy must know the potential complications related to each piece of equipment, especially the thrombogenic characteristics and flow dynamics. Several of these concepts are dis-

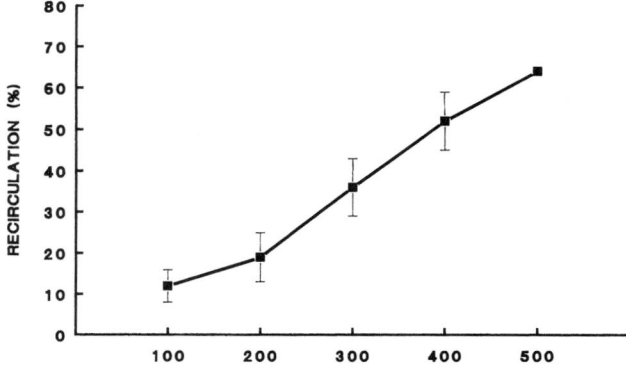

FIG. 31–4. Recirculation occurs with the use of the venovenous extracorporeal membrane oxygenation catheter. Flows greater than 400 mL/min result in greater than 50% recirculation and decrease oxygenation at this point. (Data from ref. 42.)

TABLE 31–5. *Equipment for neonatal extracorporeal membrane oxygenation*

Roller occlusion pump
Pump base
Venous return monitor
Heating unit
Coagulation timer
Membrane mounting board
Oxygen blender
Carbon dioxide or carbogen tank
O_2 and CO_2 flowmeters
In-line temperature probes
In-line oxygen saturation monitor

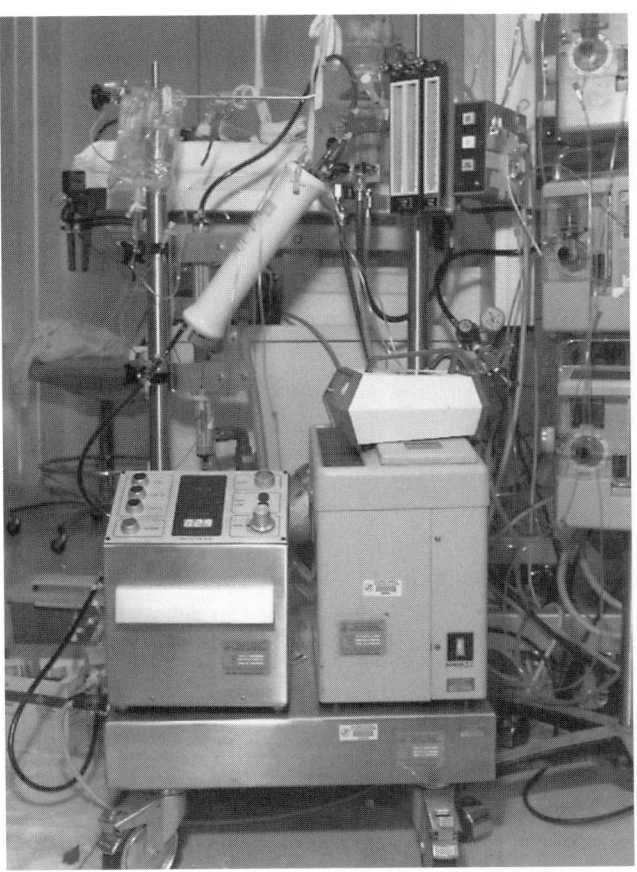

FIG. 31–5. The extracorporeal membrane oxygenation system used at the Children's National Medical Center has a modular design.

cussed in this chapter; however, additional information can be found elsewhere (43).

In VA ECMO, the venous catheter is the oxygenation catheter because the rate of blood flow through this catheter determines the percentage of the cardiac output that is supported by the ECMO pump. Oxygenation is determined by the percentage of cardiac output passing through the ECMO membrane (i.e., artificial lung) and bypassing the patient's lungs. If a small-gauge venous catheter is placed, minimal flow through the ECMO circuit occurs, and oxygenation may be compromised. Blood flow rates (Q) are directly proportional to the fourth power of the radius (r) of the tubing and inversely proportional to the length (L) of the tubing:

$$Q \propto r^4$$
$$Q \propto 1/L$$

To maximize flow into the circuit, a relatively short venous catheter with as large a lumen as possible is used.

The arterial catheter, which supplies return of flow from the circuit into the arch of the aorta, is the smallest-diameter component in the circuit and acts as the major resistance component in the circuit. A small arterial catheter may cause significant back pressure and lead to restricted blood flow, hemolysis, or eventual rupture of the circuit. Resistance to flow depends on the dimensions and geometry of the tubing and the characteristics of the fluid used. Poiseuille's Law defines this concept by the following equation:

$$R = 8\eta L/\pi r^4$$

in which $8/\pi$ is the constant of proportionality, L (cm) is the length of the tubing, η is the coefficient of viscosity (i.e., Poise = dyne $\times$ sec/cm^2), and r (cm) is the radius of the tubing. The longer the tubing and the smaller the radius, the greater is the resistance. An 8-F (2.6-mm) catheter has much greater resistance than a 10-F (3.3-mm) catheter. A short, large-lumen catheter is ideal, but the size of catheter placed is limited by the diameter of the patient's carotid artery (44).

The double-lumen catheter used in VV ECMO has a small lumen for blood return, which produces a relatively high back pressure in the circuit. Kinking of this catheter significantly increases circuit pressures and must be diligently avoided.

The VRM is an electronic device that monitors the blood flow from the patient into the ECMO circuit (see Fig. 31–1). The VRM functions as a servoregulator for the ECMO system and is designed to alarm and stop the pump if venous flow from the patient slows, ensuring that aortic blood input equals venous output. If a VRM system is not in place and venous return decreases without servoregulation, the roller pump continues to pump and causes the tubing to collapse, creating a negative pressure that pulls gas out of solution in the blood and air into the circuit at the connection points. The most common causes of loss of venous return are malplacement of the venous catheter (usually in the inferior vena cava), pneumothorax or pneumopericardium, unrecognized bleeding (e.g., ICH, hemothorax), kinking of the venous catheter, or placing an anchoring suture too tightly around the catheter during cannulation.

The only membrane lung approved for long-term ECMO use is the silicone membrane lung made by Avecor (Minneapolis, MN). The 0.8-m2 membrane is most commonly used for neonates, and can support oxygenation up to a Q of 1 L/min. Carbon dioxide transfer is so efficient with this membrane that CO_2 must be added to the gases flowing into the membrane.

PATIENT MANAGEMENT

A team approach to the management of the ECMO patient is critical. Duties of the bedside nurse, respiratory therapist, and ECMO specialist should be clearly delineated to ensure efficient and effective care (44).

Daily Medical Management

Most neonatal patients, with the exception of those with CDH, require ECMO support for 5 days. During this period, the patient who was in respiratory failure and dying before ECMO shows evidence of reversal of disease, can be slowly weaned off ECMO to minimal ventilator settings, and can usually be extubated within 24 to 48 hours after coming off the ECMO circuit. The rapidity of recovery is remarkable, given the severity of the illness suffered by these infants before ECMO. For this level of recovery to occur in such a short time, many physiologic changes must take place rapidly, making daily care of the infant a fine art. Routine care must incorporate the fact that these infants are systemically heparinized, and tasks such as suctioning of the airway should be done with caution.

As the lungs improve, less blood flow is required to pass through the artificial lung, and the ECMO blood flow can be reduced. In the first few days, a Q of 120 to 150 mL/kg/min is required to oxygenate the infant (45). With improvement of the infant's lungs, arterial blood gases improve, and the ECMO blood flow can be decreased by 10 to 20 mL/min. The venous saturation of blood in the ECMO circuit can be monitored continuously, providing a representation of a mixed venous saturation level. However, this saturation is measured in blood from the right atrium, and right atrial blood saturation does not represent true mixed venous saturation if there are intracardiac shunts. Because most infants on ECMO develop left-to-right shunts, often occurring at the level of the foramen ovale, venous saturations must be interpreted in terms of other clinical signs. The following concepts must be understood:

$$C_VO_2 = CaO_2 - \dot{V}O_2/flow$$

$$\text{Oxygen content} = Hb \times \% \text{ saturation} \times 1.36 + 0.0031 \times PO_2$$

in which C_VO_2 is venous oxygen content, CaO_2 is arterial oxygen content, $\dot{V}O_2$ is oxygen consumption, and flow is cardiac output.

For venous oxygen saturation to represent a true indication of relative arterial oxygen content, several assumptions must be made: that the cardiac output remains stable, that hemoglobin concentrations remain stable, and that the metabolic rate of the patient does not change. Any one of these factors can cause a change in the venous saturation. Therefore, the patient should be carefully evaluated before this parameter is used alone to wean the ECMO flows. Arterial blood gases are needed to determine the pH and $PaCO_2$ status of the patient and the membrane lung. If the arterial $PaCO_2$ of the membrane decreases below 35 mm Hg during VA ECMO, a decrease in respiratory rate may result because the brain detects the blood gas levels in blood from the membrane lung during VA ECMO. If the patient's respiratory rate falls, and he or she is on low bypass, the result is a deterioration in blood gas status. The problem is corrected by increasing the CO_2 coming from the membrane to stimulate the infant to breathe. A high membrane PCO_2 may indicate membrane failure and is an emergency, and a normal membrane PCO_2 with an abnormal patient PCO_2 indicates a change in the patient's clinical condition such as development of pneumothorax or secondary pneumonia.

After being stabilized on ECMO, the infant is placed on lung-rest settings on the ventilator [i.e., fraction of inspired oxygen (FiO_2) = 0.21, PIP = 15 to 18 cm H_2O; peak end-expiratory pressures (PEEP) = 5 to 6 cm H_2O; rate = 10 to 15 breaths/min]. It is typical for the lungs to appear opaque on chest radiographs during the first 1 to 3 days of ECMO (48,50). This is probably caused by the acute decrease in ventilatory settings, capillary leak, activation of complement as a result of interaction of blood products with the artificial surfaces in the circuit, and surfactant deficiency secondary to lung injury (49–52). Lotze and associates showed that surfactant replacement therapy in infants on ECMO can decrease time on ECMO for all infants except those with CDH (54). A study conducted using surfactant before ECMO revealed that a significant number of infants in the low-mortality group (OI 15 to 22) could be kept off ECMO with the use of surfactant (55). Lung compliance studies can help in predicting successful decannulation, especially in the infant who is borderline, and when a decision is being made about removing an infant from ECMO because of complications (50). A typical lung compliance curve is shown in Fig. 31–6. An old-fashioned but effective technique for assessing pulmonary improvement is to hand-ventilate the infant daily. When the chest moves easily with a peak pressure of 20 cm H_2O or less, the infant can successfully come off ECMO.

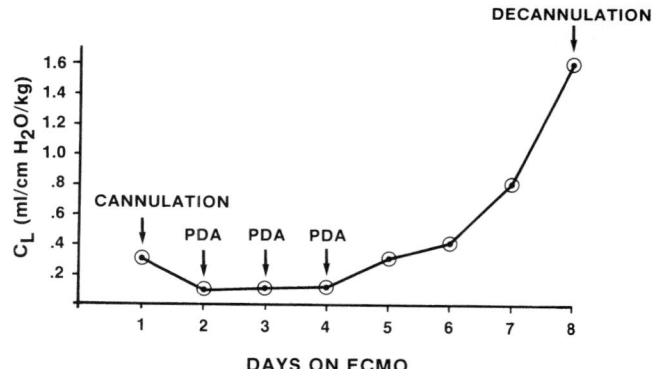

FIG. 31–6. The typical lung compliance curve for an infant with meconium aspiration syndrome on extracorporeal membrane oxygenation (ECMO). Infants in this study were successfully taken off ECMO if a lung compliance (C_L) of 0.8 mL/cm H_2O/kg was attained. (From ref. 50.)

Heparin is administered continuously into the ECMO circuit to prevent clotting (45). Heparin management will vary, depending on events before and during ECMO. Optimal heparin management can achieve the level of heparinization needed to decrease the risk for fibrin and clot formation in the circuit while minimizing the risk for bleeding complications in the patient. Because heparinization must be evaluated rapidly and at the bedside, most centers use the ACT (56). The ACT is determined in a system that uses activators, such as glass beads, to initiate the clotting cascade. The specimen is warmed to accelerate the clotting process. This test gives values of 80 to 120 seconds in a nonheparinized infant, compared with standard nonactivated bleeding time values longer than 5 minutes (57).

The primary cause of death in the ECMO population is ICH (12,58,60). The risk factors associated with the development of an ICH include significant hypoxic or ischemic cerebral insult before ECMO, sepsis with coagulopathy, or gestational age less than 37 weeks. Initial heparin management is based on pretreatment risk factors. If there is a high risk for ICH before ECMO, the ACT is maintained between 160 and 180 seconds for at least the first 24 to 48 hours. Most intracranial bleeds occur during this period. If the infant is not at risk for ICH, the ACTs are maintained between 180 and 220 seconds. The range can be narrowed, depending on the number of risk factors the infant has. The platelet count is maintained above $80,000/mm^3$ in uncomplicated cases and between 100,000 and $150,000/mm^3$ in cases complicated by bleeding (43).

Fibrin formation is related to flow rate; if there are low Qs in the circuit, the heparin dose is increased to decrease the risk for clot formation. At the beginning of an ECMO run, blood flows are high, and the ACTs can be maintained in a lower range. At the end of a run, the ACTs are increased, especially when the idling phase (i.e., 60 to 80 mL/min) is reached. When Q in the circuit is below 150 mL/min, ACTs are increased to 200 to 220 seconds. Clinical factors that affect the ACT values are renal function (heparin excretion is directly proportional to urine output), transfusion of unheparinized blood products or platelets, and a significant patent ductus arteriosus with a left-to-right shunt that may decrease renal blood flow.

Fluid requirements while on ECMO range from 80 to 120 mL/kg/day. Electrolyte requirements are significantly different from those before ECMO is started. Most infants require little sodium, usually 1 to 2 mEq/kg/day, and a large amount of potassium, usually 4 to 5 mEq/kg/day. The rationale for these requirements is unknown. Although renin levels increase on bypass, aldosterone levels decrease, and atrionatriuretic peptide levels do not change (59,60). Calcium requirements range from 20 to 40 mg/kg of elemental calcium per day.

Systemic hypertension is a common medical complication of ECMO. Hypertension (mean blood pressure > 65 mm Hg for over 3 hours) can affect as many as 70% of these patients. Hypertension usually develops shortly after cannulation and is transient, but 1% to 5% of infants require long-term antihypertensive therapy. The risk of ICH is increased by hypertension (60). Although a subject of controversy, the hypertension may be related to an increase in serum renin levels (59,61). Fluid restriction and diuretic therapy may decrease the risk for prolonged hypertension.

As pulmonary vascular resistance decreases, it is common to develop a left-to-right shunt across the patent ductus arteriosus, resulting in oxygenation difficulty (48). Most of these shunts close with fluid restriction and diuretic therapy. Few patients require surgical intervention. Indomethacin should not be used in this population, because it decreases platelet aggregation. After the shunt closes, an immediate increase in the patient's PaO_2 is observed.

Cardiac stun is an interesting complication of ECMO therapy that also occurs in patients on cardiopulmonary bypass. Cardiac stun occurs in infants with severe hypoxia or in infants in whom the tip of the arterial catheter is placed too close to the coronary arteries (61,62). This syndrome is characterized by a pulse pressure of 10 mm Hg or less on ECMO, with the patient's PaO_2 equal to or within 50 to 100 mm Hg of the pump PO_2 (e.g., a pump PO_2 of 400 mm Hg while on an FiO_2 of 1.00, with a patient PaO_2 between 300 and 350 mm Hg). The electrocardiographic pattern is normal, indicating that electrical conduction is normal, but cardiac output is markedly reduced. The pathophysiology is not understood (61,63). When data on infants with cardiac stun while on ECMO at the Children's National Medical Center were evaluated, there was a significant difference in pre-ECMO blood gases relative to infants who did not develop cardiac stun. Infants in stun were sicker before ECMO and had a higher incidence of death from ICH, indicating the marked hypoxic–ischemic insult suffered by these patients before ECMO. Treatment of cardiac stun consists of maintaining ECMO Q high enough to supply appropriate cardiac output. Afterload reduction does not improve cardiac function in this population (64). As stun resolves, the pulse pressure returns to normal, and the patient's PaO_2 no longer mirrors the pump PO_2.

Weaning from ECMO occurs slowly as the arterial blood gases and venous saturations improve. Idling flows, defined as flows at 10% of the cardiac output (i.e., 60 to 80 mL/min) are continued for 6 to 8 hours, and if blood gases are normal during this period, most infants can be successfully taken off ECMO. A lung compliance measurement of at least 0.8 mL/cm H_2O/kg indicates that the infant can successfully come off ECMO (see Fig. 31–6) (50). Typical ventilator settings for infants after completing an ECMO course are FiO_2 of 0.30 to 0.40; rate of 30 to 40 breaths/min; PIP of 18 to 20 cm H_2O; and PEEP of 5 to 6 cm H_2O.

Patient Care after Extracorporeal Membrane Oxygenation

A neuromuscular blocking agent with an intermediate half-life is used at decannulation to help the patient breathe spontaneously as soon as possible after coming off ECMO. By the end of the ECMO run, it is common for the ECMO patient to require high PaCO$_2$ levels (i.e., 45 to 55 mm Hg) to stimulate respiratory drive. These levels of PaCO$_2$ should be continued after ECMO for the first 24 to 48 hours to continue to stimulate respiratory drive. Many of these infants have been receiving narcotics such as fentanyl and may need to be weaned slowly from this therapy to avoid withdrawal symptoms. PaO$_2$ levels of 60 to 70 mm Hg are accepted, and every effort is made to wean the patient from the ventilator. In our institution, the average time to extubation post ECMO is 23 hours. The CDH patient is an exception; these patients require slower weaning to ensure that pulmonary hypertension does not recur.

Hemoglobin, hematocrit, calcium, and electrolyte measurements should be obtained 6 to 8 hours after ECMO. These can then be monitored every 24 hours or as clinically indicated. The platelet count should be followed closely (i.e., values every 8 hours for 24 hours) because rebound thrombocytopenia may occur. Intravenous sodium is increased to 2 to 3 mEq/kg/day, and potassium supplementation is decreased to 1 to 2 mEq/kg/day.

After extubation, the infant usually requires oxygen therapy for another 5 to 7 days. Most ECMO infants feed poorly and may require feeding by tube for a few days. The cause of this problem is uncertain, but it is usually transient and does not indicate long-term developmental problems.

Because not all intracranial abnormalities are detected by ultrasound, a computed tomographic or magnetic resonance scan is recommended before discharge (54). A baseline hearing screen and a neurologic assessment are also recommended before discharge. All infants should be followed in a neonatal high-risk follow-up program.

Developmental outcome is encouraging, with most centers reporting that 60% to 70% of ECMO survivors are normal at 1 to 2 years of age (65–67). Risk factors associated with poor outcome include finding a severe abnormality on neuroimaging, chronic lung disease, prematurity, and β-streptococcal sepsis (68,71). The 10% to 15% of the ECMO-treated population who are considered suspect for abnormalities at 1 to 2 years of age require close follow-up because a large percentage of these infants develop learning disabilities by 5 years of age (68).

The need for carotid artery ligation for VA ECMO has caused concern that right-sided CNS lesions may result. Schumacher and colleagues reported right-sided CNS lesions in their ECMO population, but similar findings have not been reported by others (58,59,70,71). Analysis of the first 360 patients treated at Children's National Medical Center did not reveal lateralizing hemorrhagic or nonhemorrhagic abnormalities, but there was a high incidence of posterior fossa hemorrhage, raising the concern that jugular venous ligation might increase venous back pressure and the risk of hemorrhage (58,70 72). Data published by Taylor and Walker showed that decreased sagittal sinus blood flow velocity is associated with ICH (70%) in the ECMO population (73). Whether this is cause or effect has yet to be determined. Many ECMO teams are now placing jugular bulb catheters in the right internal jugular vein to drain the venous outflow from the brain into the venous side of the circuit.

The infant with CDH may have unique long-term problems, including significant gastroesophageal reflux and chronic lung disease (74). These infants require close follow-up in a multidisciplinary clinic to prevent problems such as failure to thrive and respiratory compromise.

SUMMARY

Care of the ECMO patient requires highly trained nurses, respiratory therapists, perfusionists, and physicians. The team must continually evaluate the treatment modalities and use the information to improve techniques and to define the indications for ECMO therapy. It has been estimated that only 1,000 to 2,500 term infants require ECMO each year in the United States (75). The availability of ECMO therapy must be tailored to regional needs in an effort to maintain cost control and quality of care. In view of the developmental status of ECMO, and with possible new and less invasive therapies, such as nitric oxide, appearing on the horizon, it is clear that not every neonatal intensive care unit should develop an ECMO program (76).

REFERENCES

1. Kolff WJ, Berk HT. Artificial kidney: a dialyzer with a great area. *Acta Med Scand* 1944;17:121.
2. Kenedi RM, Courtey JM, Gaylor JDS, Gilchrsit T. *Artificial organs.* Baltimore: University Park Press, 1976:11.
3. Clowes GHA Jr, Hopkins AL, Neville WE. An artificial lung dependent upon diffusion of oxygen and carbon dioxide through plastic membranes. *J Thorac Surg* 1956;32:630.
4. Kolobow T, Stool EW, Sacko KL, Vurek GG. Acute respiratory failure, survival following ten days' support with a membrane lung. *J Thorac Cardiovasc Surg* 1975;69:947.
5. Zapol WM, Snider MT, Hil DJ, et al. Extracorporeal membrane oxygenation in severe acute respiratory failure: a randomized prospective study. *JAMA* 1979;242:2193.
6. Gille JP, Bagniewski AM. Ten years of use of extracorporeal membrane oxygenation (ECMO) in the treatment of acute respiratory insufficiency (ARI). *Trans Am Soc Artif Intern Organs* 1976;22:102.
7. Callaghan JC, delos Angeles J. Long-term extracorporeal circulation in the development of an artificial placenta for respiratory distress syndrome of the newborn. *Surg Forum* 1961;12:215.
8. Rashkind WJ, Freeman A, Klein D, Toft RW. Evolution of a disposable

plastic low volume, pumpless oxygenator as a lung substitute. *J Pediatr* 1965;66:94.

9. White JJ, Andrews HG, Risemberg H, et al. Prolonged respiratory support in newborn infants with a membrane oxygenator. *Surgery* 1971; 70:288.

10. Dorson WJ, Baker E, Cohen ML, et al. A perfusion system for infants. *Trans Am Soc Artif Intern Organs* 1969;15:155.

11. Bartlett RH, Gazzaniga AB, Jefferies MR, et al. Extracorporeal membrane oxygenation (ECMO) cardiopulmonary support in infancy. *Trans Am Soc Artif Intern Organs* 1976;22:80.

12. Stolar CJH, Snedecor SM, Bartlett RH. Extracorporeal membrane oxygenation and neonatal respiratory failure: experience from the extracorporeal life support organization. *J Pediatr Surg* 1991;26:563.

13. Breaux CW, Rouse TM, Cain WS, Georgeson KE. Improvement in survival of patients with congenital diaphragmatic hernia utilizing a strategy of delayed repair after medical and/or extracorporeal membrane oxygenation stabilization. *J Pediatr Surg* 1991;26:333.

14. Sanchez LS, O'Brien A, Anderson KD, et al. Best postductal PO_2 and PCO_2 do not predict outcome of CDH infants in extremis, stabilized with ECMO prior to surgical repair. *Pediatr Res* 1992;31:221A.

15. Bartlett RH, Roloff DW, Cornell RG, et al. Extracorporeal circulation in neonatal respiratory failure: a prospective randomized trial. *Pediatrics* 1985;76:479.

16. Beck R, Anderson KD, Pearson GD, et al. Criteria for extracorporeal membrane oxygenation in a population of infants with persistent pulmonary hypertension of the newborn. *J Pediatr Surg* 1986;21:297.

17. Cole CH, Jillson E, Kessler D. ECMO. Regional evaluation of need and applicability of selection criteria. *Am J Dis Child* 1988;142:1320.

18. Dworetz AR, Moya FR, Sabo B, et al. Survival of infants with persistent pulmonary hypertension without extracorporeal membrane oxygenation. *Pediatrics* 1989;84:1.

19. Krummel TM, Greenfield LJ, Kirkpatrick BV, et al. Alveolar–arterial oxygen gradients versus the neonatal pulmonary insufficiency index for prediction of mortality in ECMO candidates. *J Pediatr Surg* 1984;19:380.

20. Marsh TD, Wilkerson SA, Cook LN. Extracorporeal membrane oxygenation selection criteria: partial pressure of arterial oxygen versus alveolar–arterial oxygen gradient. *Pediatrics* 1988;82:162.

21. O'Rourke PP, Crone RK, Vacanti JP, et al. Extracorporeal membrane oxygenation and conventional medical therapy in neonates with persistent pulmonary hypertension of the newborn: a prospective randomized study. *Pediatrics* 1989;84:957.

22. Wung JT, James LS, Kilchevsky E, James E. Management of infants with severe respiratory failure and persistence of the fetal circulation without hyperventilation. *Pediatrics* 1985;76:488.

23. Hollenberg NK, Dzau VJ, Williams GH. Are uncontrolled clinical studies ever justified? *N Engl J Med* 1980;303:1059.

24. UK Collaborative ECMO Trial Group. UK collaborative randomised trial of neonatalextracorporeal membrane oxygenation. *Lancet* 1996;348:75.

25. Kelly AT, Short BL, Rains TC, et al. Aluminum toxicity and albumin. *Trans Am Soc Artif Intern Organs* 1989;35:674.

26. Schneider B, Schena J, Troug R, et al. Exposure to di(2-ethylhexyl)phthalate in infants receiving extracorporeal membrane oxygenation. *N Engl J Med* 1989;320:1563.

27. Cilley RE, Zwischenferger JB, Andrews AF, et al. Intracranial hemorrhage during extracorporeal membrane oxygenation in neonates. *Pediatrics* 1986;78:699.

28. Revenis ME, Glass P, Short B. Mortality and morbidity among lower birth weight (2–2.5 kg) infants treated with extracorporeal membrane oxygenation (ECMO). *J Pediatr* 1992;121:452.

29. Toomasian JM, Snedecor SM, Cornell RG, et al. National experience with extracorporeal membrane oxygenation for newborn respiratory failure. *Trans Am Soc Artif Intern Organs* 1988;34:140.

30. Short BL, Walker LK, Bendu KS, Traystman RJ. Impairment of cerebral autoregulation during extracorporeal membrane oxygenation. *Pediatr Res* 1993;33:289.

31. Short BL, Walker LK, Gleason CA, et al. Effects of extracorporeal membrane oxygenation on cerebral blood flow and cerebral oxygen metabolism in newborn sheep. *Pediatr Res* 1990;28:50.

32. Hirschl RB, Schumacher RE, Snedecor SN, et al. The efficacy of extracorporeal life support in premature and low birth weight newborns. *J Pediatr Surg* 1993;28:1336.

33. McCune S, Short BL, Miller MK, et al. Extracorporeal membrane oxygenation therapy in neonates with septic shock. *J Pediatr Surg* 1990; 25:479.

34. Newman KD, Van Meurs KP, Short BL, Anderson KD. Extracorporeal membrane oxygenation and congenital diaphragmatic hernia—should any infant be excluded? *J Pediatr Surg* 1990;25:1048.

35. Van Meurs KP, Newman KD, Anderson KD, Short BL. Effect of extracorporeal membrane oxygenation on survival of infants with congenital diaphragmatic hernia. *J Pediatr* 1990;117:954.

36. Ortiz RM, Cilley RE, Bartlett RH. Extracorporeal membrane oxygenation in pediatric respiratory failure. *Pediatr Clin North Am* 1987;34:39.

37. Boedy RF, Howell CG, Kanto WP. Hidden mortality of ECMO. *J Pediatr* 1990;117:462.

38. Langham MR, Krummel TM, Bartlett RH, et al. Mortality with extracorporeal membrane oxygenation following repair of congenital diaphragmatic hernia in 93 infants. *J Pediatr Surg* 1987;22:1150.

39. Stolar C, Dillon P, Reyes C. Selective use of extracorporeal membrane oxygenation in the management of congenital diaphragmatic hernia. *J Pediatr Surg* 1988;23:207.

40. Howell CG, Hatley RM, Boedy FR, et al. Recent experience with diaphragmatic hernia and ECMO. *Ann Surg* 1990;211:793.

41. O'Rourke PP, Lillehei CW, Crone RK, Vacanti JP. The effect of extracorporeal membrane oxygenation on the survival of neonates with high-risk congenital diaphragmatic hernia: 45 cases from a single institution. *J Pediatr Surg* 1991;26:147.

42. Anderson HL, Otsu T, Chapman RA, Bartlett RH. Venovenous extracorporeal life support in neonates using a double lumen catheter. *Trans Am Soc Artif Intern Organs* 1989;35:650.

43. Short BL. Pre-ECMO considerations for neonatal patients. In Arensman RM, Cornish D, eds. *Extracorporeal life support.* Cambridge, MA: Blackwell Scientific, 1993.

44. Van Meurs KP, Mikesell GT, Seale SR, et al. Maximum blood flow rates for arterial cannulae used in neonatal ECMO. *Trans Am Soc Artif Intern Organs* 1990;36:M679.

45. Short BL. Clinical management of the neonatal ECMO patient. In Arensman RM, Cornish D, eds. *Extracorporeal life support.* Cambridge, MA: Blackwell Scientific, 1993.

46. Knight GR, Dudell GG, Evans ML, Grimm PS. A comparison of venovenous and venoarterial extracorporeal membrane oxygenation in the treatment of neonatal respiratory failure. *Crit Care Med* 1996;24: 1678.

47. VanMeurs KP, Nguyen HT, Rhine WD, Marks MP, Fleisher FE, Benitz WE. Intracranial abnormalities and neurodevelopmental status after venovenous extracorporeal membrane oxygenation. *J Pediatr* 1994; 125:304.

48. Martin GR, Short BL. Doppler echocardiographic evaluation of cardiac performance in infants on prolonged extracorporeal membrane oxygenation. *Am J Cardiol* 1988;62:929.

49. Taylor GA, Short BL, Kreismer P. Extracorporeal membrane oxygenation: radiographic appearance of the neonatal chest. *Am J Radiol* 1986; 146:1257.

50. Lotze A, Short BL, Taylor GA. The use of lung compliance as a parameter for improvement in lung function in newborns with respiratory failure requiring extracorporeal membrane oxygenation. *Crit Care Med* 1987;15:226.

51. Keszler M, Subramanian KN, Smith YA, et al. Pulmonary management during extracorporeal membrane oxygenation. *Crit Care Med* 1989;17: 495.

52. Lotze A, Whitsett JA, Kammerman L, et al. Surfactant protein A concentrations in tracheal aspirate fluid from infants requiring extracorporeal membrane oxygenation. *J Pediatr* 1990;116:435.

53. Anderson JM, Kottke-Marchant K. Platelet interactions with biomaterials and artificial devices. In Williams DF, ed. *Blood compatibility, vol I.* Boca Raton: CRC Press, 1987:127.

54. Lotze A, Knight GR, Martin GM, et al. Improved pulmonary outcome after exogenous surfactant therapy for respiratory failure in term infants requiring extracorporeal membrane oxygenation. *J Pediatr* 1993;122(2):261.

55. Lotze A, Mitchell BR, Bulas DI, Zola EM, Shalwitz RA, Gunkel JH. Multicenter study of surfactant (beractant) use in the treatment of term infants with severe respiratory failure. Survanta in Term Infant Study Group. *J Pediatr* 1998;1321:40.

56. Hattersley P. Activated coagulation time of whole blood. *JAMA* 1966; 196:436.

57. Kay LA, ed. *Essentials of hemostasis and thrombosis,* 2nd ed. New York: Churchill-Livingstone, 1988.

58. Taylor GA, Short BL, Fitz CR. Imaging of cerebrovascular injury in

infants treated with extracorporeal membrane oxygenation. *J Pediatr* 1989;114:635.

59. Marinelli KA, Short BL, Martin GR, Goldstein D. Extracorporeal membrane oxygenation: its effect on renin, aldosterone and natriuretic peptide. *Pediatr Res* 1989;25:241A.

60. Sell LL, Cullen ML, Lerner GR, et al. Hypertension during extracorporeal membrane oxygenation: cause, effect and management. *Surgery* 1987;102:724.

61. Martin GR, Short BL, Abbott C, O'Brien AM. Cardiac stun in infants undergoing extracorporeal membrane oxygenation. *J Thorac Cardiovasc Surg* 1991;101:607.

62. Boedy RF, Goldberg AK, Howell CG, et al. Incidence of hypertension in infants on extracorporeal membrane oxygenation. *J Pediatr Surg* 1990;25:258.

63. Marban E. Myocardial stunning and hibernation. The physiology behind the colloquialisms. *Circulation* 1991;83:681.

64. Martin GR, Chauvin L, Short BL. Effects of hydralazine on cardiac performance in infants receiving extracorporeal membrane oxygenation. *J Pediatr* 1991;118:944.

65. Glass P, Miller M, Short B. Morbidity for survivors of extracorporeal membrane oxygenation: neurodevelopmental outcome at 1 year of age. *Pediatrics* 1989;83:72.

66. Schumacher RE, Palmer TW, Roloff DW, et al. Follow-up of infants treated with extracorporeal membrane oxygenation for newborn respiratory failure. *Pediatrics* 1991;87:451.

67. Towne BH, Lott IT, Hicks DA, Healey T. Long-term follow-up of infants and children treated with extracorporeal membrane oxygenation (ECMO): a preliminary report. *J Pediatr Surg* 1985;20:410.

68. Glass P, Bulas DI, Wagner AE, et al. Severity of brain injury following neonatal ECMO and outcome at age 5. *Dev Med Child Neurol* 1997;39:441–448.

69. Schumacher RE, Barks JDE, Johnston MV, et al. Right-sided brain lesions in infants following extracorporeal membrane oxygenation. *Pediatrics* 1988;82:155.

70. Bulas DI, Glass P, O'Donnell RM, Taylor GA, Short BL, Vezina GL. Neonates treated with ECMO: Predictive value of early CT and US neuroimaging findings on short-term neurodevelopmental outcome. *Radiology* 1995;195:407.

71. Bulas DI, Taylor GA, O'Donnell, Short BL, Fitz CR, Vezina G. Intracranial abnormalities in infants treated with extracorporeal membrane oxygenation: update on sonographic and CT findings. *Am J Neuroradiol* 1996;17:287.

72. Bulas DI, Taylor GA, Fitz CR, et al. Posterior fossa intracranial hemorrhage in infants treated with extracorporeal membrane oxygenation: sonographic findings. *Am J Roentgenol* 1991;156:571.

73. Taylor GA, Walker LK. Doppler US evaluation of the intracranial venous system following ligation of the right jugular vein in infants treated with extracorporeal membrane oxygenation. *Radiology* 1992;183:453.

74. Van Meurs KP, Robbins ST, Karr SS, et al. Congenital diaphragmatic hernia: long-term outcome of ECMO-treated survivors. *Pediatr Res* 1991;29:A269.

75. Southgate WM, Howell CG, Kanto WP. Need for and impact on neonatal mortality of extracorporeal membrane oxygenation in infants of greater than 2500-gram birth weight. *Pediatrics* 1990;86:71.

76. Frostell C, Fratacci MD, Wain JC, et al. Inhaled nitric oxide. A selective pulmonary vasodilator reversing hypoxic pulmonary vasoconstriction. *Circulation* 1991;83:2038.

CHAPTER 32

Sudden Infant Death Syndrome

Carl E. Hunt

Sudden infant death syndrome (SIDS) has been recognized since biblical times. SIDS is defined as the sudden death of an infant that is unexpected by history and unexplained by a thorough postmortem examination that includes a complete autopsy, investigation of the scene of death, and review of the medical history (1). An autopsy is essential in all sudden and unexpected infant deaths because the history and scene investigation do not exclude all known causes of sudden infant death, such as congenital cardiac or brain abnormalities and fatal child abuse.

SIDS is the most common cause of infant mortality in the United States after congenital anomalies and disorders relating to short gestation and low birth weight (2). SIDS is the most common cause of postneonatal infant mortality in developed countries, generally accounting for 40% to 50% of infant deaths between 1 month and 1 year of age and about 20% of all infant deaths in neonatal ICU discharges. About 3,000 infants in the United States in 1996 died of SIDS, a rate of 0.74/1,000 live births. In full-term infants, SIDS is rare before 1 month of age, the peak incidence is 2 to 4 months, and 95% of all cases have occurred by 6 months of age.

PATHOLOGY

The autopsy findings in SIDS victims have been very subtle and have yielded only supportive rather than conclusive findings to explain SIDS (1). Mild pulmonary edema and diffuse intrathoracic petechiae have been observed. Autopsy studies demonstrate structural evidence (tissue markers) of chronic asphyxia in nearly two-thirds of SIDS subjects. Infants discharged from a neonatal ICU, especially infants with a prior clinical diagnosis of bronchopulmonary dysplasia, may have residual pulmonary abnormalities at autopsy, but a diagnosis of SIDS can nevertheless be established whenever the findings are not sufficient to explain a sudden and unexpected death.

Brain-stem abnormalities in victims of SIDS include focal astrogliosis, persistent dendritic spines, and hypomyelination. The primary areas of persisting brain-stem dendritic spines are in the magnocellular nucleus of the reticular formation and dorsal and solitary nuclei of the vagal nerve. Significant increases in the number of reactive astrocytes in the medulla have also been observed in SIDS victims; these increases are not confined to areas related to respiratory neuroregulation. Substance P, a neuropeptide transmitter found in selected sensory neurons of the central nervous system, is present in increased amounts in the pons of SIDS victims. Quantitative three-dimensional anatomic studies indicate that a small subset of SIDS victims have hypoplasia of the arcuate nucleus; this region is a site of cardiorespiratory control in the ventral medulla and is integrated with other regions that regulate arousal and autonomic and chemosensory function. Recent neurotransmitter studies (3) have also identified receptor abnormalities in the arcuate nucleus; significant decreases in binding to kainate receptors and muscarinic cholinergic receptors have both been observed in some SIDS victims; there was a positive correlation between decreased densities of muscarinic cholinergic and kainate receptors. The neurotransmitter deficit in the arcuate nucleus in SIDS victims thus involves more than one receptor type relevant to CO_2 and blood pressure. Finally, tyrosine hydroxylase immunoreactivity in two brain-stem areas, vagal nuclei and area reticularis superficialis ventrolateralis, suggests that epinephrine and norepinephrine neurons are altered in SIDS victims (4).

Other postmortem observations also suggest preexisting, low-grade, chronic asphyxia. SIDS infants as a group have both prenatal and postnatal growth retardation and elevated blood cortisol levels. Elevated levels of hypox-

C. E. Hunt: Department of Pediatrics, Medical College of Ohio, Toledo, Ohio

anthine in vitreous humor have been reported in SIDS infants, suggesting a relatively long period of tissue hypoxia preceding the death. Adenosine, a precursor of hypoxanthine, is a respiratory inhibitor, and these observations thus indicate a potentially important interaction between asphyxia and hypoventilation; in response to asphyxia from any cause, the secondary acceleration of adenosine monophosphate (AMP) catabolism and adenosine accumulation will stimulate and then perpetuate hypoventilation, yielding a vicious cycle.

PHYSIOLOGIC STUDIES IN INFANTS

The most compelling hypothesis to explain SIDS is a brain-stem abnormality in cardiorespiratory control, including arousal responsiveness, and perhaps other autonomic controls such as blood pressure and sleep/wake regulation (1). The postmortem data are consistent with this hypothesis. The clinical data to support this hypothesis were initially inferred from assessments of patients with unexplained apparent life-threatening events (UALTE) or other infants at increased epidemiologic risk for SIDS (preterm infants, subsequent siblings of a previous SIDS), a few of whom later died of SIDS. These studies have identified abnormalities in respiratory pattern, chemoreceptor sensitivity, control of heart and respiratory rate or variability, cardiorespiratory interaction, and asphyxic arousal responsiveness.

Respiratory Pattern

Respiratory pattern abnormalities observed have included prolonged apnea, excess brief apneas, and periodic breathing. Dynamic respiratory patterning in infants subsequently dying of SIDS (5) has indicated restricted breath-to-breath respiratory rate variability at slow respiratory rates, caused by absence of influences that are normally present and that affect breathing.

Chemoreceptor Sensitivity

Some infants at increased risk for SIDS have diminished ventilatory responsiveness to hypercarbia and/or to hypoxia (1). Such assessments, however, are too costly and time-consuming for routine clinical use, and the extent of individual overlap between normal and at-risk infants precludes accurate identification of those infants who will later die of SIDS. Chemoreceptor sensitivity studies have generally not been performed in preterm infants and would be even less useful than in term infants if confounded by persisting lung disease and/or incomplete brain-stem maturation.

Arousal Responses

Absent arousal responsiveness renders infants incapable of responding effectively to sleep-related asphyxia, regardless of its cause. Infants at increased epidemiologic risk for SIDS (UALTE, preterm infants, and subsequent siblings of SIDS victims) who have diminished ventilatory responsiveness to hypercarbia and/or hypoxia generally have a concomitant abnormality in hypercarbic and/or hypoxic arousal responsiveness. A deficit in arousal responsiveness may be a necessary prerequisite for SIDS to occur but may be insufficient to cause SIDS in the absence of other biological and/or epidemiologic risk factor(s). Victims of SIDS may also have deficient autoresuscitation (gasping) as a complement to the asphyxic arousal response deficit. A failure of autoresuscitation in victims of SIDS would be the final and most devastating physiologic failure.

Hypoxic and hypercapnic arousal responses have been measured in some preterm infants approaching 40 weeks of postconceptional age. However, it has not been possible to establish normative values because of confounding effects of variable neurophysiologic maturation and respiratory dysfunction. In UALTE in full-term infants, however, the occurrence and severity of recurrent symptoms has correlated with arousal responsiveness.

A relationship exists between arousal and postnatal age in term infants but has not been systematically assessed in preterm infants. Most full-term infants less than 9 weeks of age arouse in response to mild hypoxia, but only 10% to 15% of normal infants older than 9 weeks of age arouse. These data thus suggest that as full-term infants mature, their ability to arouse to hypoxic stimuli diminishes as they reach the age range of greatest risk for SIDS.

Current methods for assessing arousal responsiveness in infants are cumbersome and time-consuming. Further, the overlap in individual values for healthy term controls and for infants at increased epidemiologic risk for SIDS prevents the prospective identification of infants destined to die of SIDS.

Temperature Regulation

Increased body and/or environmental temperature is associated with SIDS. There are complex interactions between temperature regulation and cardiorespiratory control. The increased sleep-related sweating that does occur in some UALTE patients may be caused by alveolar hypoventilation and secondary asphyxia, by autonomic dysfunction as part of a more generalized deficiency in brain-stem function, or may be an indication of overheating.

Cardiac Control

The ability to shorten Q-T interval as heart rate increases is impaired in some SIDS infants, suggesting that such infants may be predisposed to ventricular arrhythmias. Infants later dying of SIDS have higher heart rates in all sleep–waking states and diminished heart rate variability during wakefulness. Infants with SIDS also have significantly lower heart rate variation with respiratory frequency across all sleep–waking cycles. Even in early infancy, therefore, future SIDS victims differ in the extent to which cardiac and respiratory activity are coupled. Although heart rate variability has been studied in preterm as well as full-term infants (6), all of the variability data in SIDS victims and matched control infants have been obtained in full-term infants.

Part of the decreased heart rate variability and increased heart rate observed in infants who later die of SIDS may be associated with decreased vagal tone. This could be related to vagal neuropathy, to brain-stem damage in areas responsible for parasympathetic control of the heart, or to other factors. Furthermore, because the greatest reduction in all types of heart rate variability occurs while the infant is awake, these reductions may reflect the reduced general motility retrospectively reported in SIDS victims and also observed in infants at increased risk for SIDS.

Home cardiorespiratory monitors with memory capability have recorded some terminal events in SIDS victims. In most instances, there has been sudden and rapid progression of bradycardia, too soon to be explained by progressive desaturation from prolonged central apnea. These observations are consistent with an abnormality in autonomic control of heart rate variability or with hypoxemia secondary to obstructive apnea as the precipitating mechanism for the severe bradycardia.

EPIDEMIOLOGY

No epidemiologic differences have been of sufficient sensitivity and specificity to permit prospective identification of SIDS victims. It is not possible to determine the relative importance of each individual risk factor or to quantify the effect of combinations of risk factors. Some of these factors are likely surrogates for more fundamental risk factors, and some are probably duplicative (7).

An increased SIDS risk is associated with numerous obstetric factors, suggesting that the *in utero* environment of future SIDS victims is suboptimal. Maternal smoking during pregnancy significantly increases the risk for SIDS; infants of smoking mothers also appear to die at a younger age. The risk of death is progressively greater as daily cigarette exposure increases and as the degree of maternal anemia worsens (1,8,9). Recent data suggest that maternal smoking potentiates hyperplasia of pulmonary neuroendocrine cells, and dysfunction of these cells may contribute to the pathophysiology of SIDS (10). Both animal and clinical studies indicate decreased ventilatory and arousal responsiveness to hypoxia associated with fetal exposure to nicotine (11,12). The age-specific attenuation of hypoxic defenses following nicotine exposure focuses attention on brain catecholamine metabolism as a potential target for adverse fetal and neonatal influences (13).

Relative growth failure is evident postnatally and prenatally (1). The number of postneonatal regular care visits and immunizations are significantly less in SIDS victims than in normal infants, suggesting that postneonatal care is also suboptimal. SIDS is associated with illnesses in the last 2 weeks of life and an increased frequency of doctors' office visits in the preceding week, especially for gastrointestinal illness and/or a droopy or listless appearance. Future SIDS victims have also been observed to have repeated fatigue during feedings and profuse sweating during sleep. The fatigue is unexplained except insofar as it may be secondary to an intercurrent acute illness. The sweating may be explained by intercurrent febrile illness and/or by thermal stress related to prone sleep position or overbundling (14,15), but it could also be indicative of an autonomic deficit (see Temperature Regulation, above).

Clinical Risk Groups

Infants with an unexplained apparent life-threatening event (UALTE) are at increased risk for SIDS. There is no consensus as to the magnitude of this risk, but history of an UALTE has been reported in about 5% of SIDS victims (1). The risk of SIDS appears to be increased in infants with two or more UALTEs, but no definitive incidence rates are available. There are no data regarding the extent, if any, to which home monitoring or any other intervention might decrease the risk of SIDS in UALTE infants. Although most estimates indicate that at least 90% to 95% of all sudden, unexpected, and unexplained infant deaths are caused by SIDS, subsequent confessions or covert video recordings have confirmed that life-threatening or fatal child abuse can also be the cause of sudden and unexpected infant death (16). Filicide needs to be considered whenever the history, autopsy, and/or scene investigation yields suspicious findings.

The risks for SIDS and for infant mortality from other causes are both increased in subsequent siblings and to the same extent: 20.8 deaths/1,000 infants at risk (17). Among all second sibling deaths in families, the relative risk of dying of the same cause is 9.1 and of a dissimilar cause is 1.6. Review of multiple epidemiologic studies in subsequent siblings indicates a relative risk for repeat SIDS of about 5.2 (range of 3.6–6.0) (18). There are no data regarding the risk for SIDS in preterm infants who are siblings of a previous SIDS victim. A familial metabolic disorder should be considered in families with multiple unexplained infant deaths, especially when the history is atypical for SIDS.

Numerous studies have identified low birth weight as a risk factor for SIDS (1,7,19). A recent study of all births in 1987 in the United States analyzed risk for SIDS in relation to gestational age as well as birth weight, and in relation to postconceptional age as well as postnatal age

(20). There is an inverse relationship between risk for SIDS and birth weight/gestational age (Table 32–1). The reversal in SIDS risk below 1,000 g birth weight likely reflects increasing reluctance to diagnosis SIDS as the cause of death as the frequency and severity of (unrelated) autopsy abnormalities progressively increases. SIDS, however, should still be the correct diagnosis whenever the death was sudden, unexpected, and unexplained by the abnormalities found at autopsy. The epidemiologic characteristics of preterm infants dying of SIDS are not substantially different from those observed in full-term infants (7). However, the postnatal age of preterm infants dying of SIDS is about 5 to 7 weeks older than full-term infants, and the postconceptional age is 4 to 6 weeks younger than full-term infants (Table 32–2).

Early reports suggested a relationship between bronchopulmonary dysplasia (BPD) and risk for SIDS. A recent prospective control study (21), however, identified

TABLE 32–1. *Epidemiologic factors associated with increased risk for SIDS in preterm infants[a]*

	Adjusted odds ratio
Birth weight	
500–999 g	1.88[b]
1,000–1,499 g	3.68[b]
1,500–2,499 g	2.64[b]
>2,499 g	1.00
Gestational age	
24–28 weeks	2.32[b]
29–32 weeks	2.06[b]
33–36 weeks	1.75[b]
>36 weeks	1.00
Race	
White	1.00
Black	1.12[b]
Hispanic	0.41[b]
American Indian	1.24
Asian	0.76[b]
Gender	
Male	1.48[b]
Female	1.00
Maternal age (years)	
<18	2.56[b]
18–34	1.91[b]
>34	1.00
Marital status	
Married	1.00
Single	1.91[b]
Maternal education (years)	
<12	2.27[b]
12	1.63[b]
>13	1.00
Gravidity	
1	1.00
2–3	1.77[b]
>3	2.36[b]

[a]Based on all U.S. births in 1987 and all SIDS deaths confirmed by autopsy.
[b]Statistically significant difference from reference group.
Adapted from ref. 20.

TABLE 32–2. *Postconceptional and postnatal ages in preterm infants dying of SIDS, classified according to gestational age[a]*

Gestational	Postconceptional	Postnatal
24–28	44[b]	18[c]
29–32	45[b]	16[c]
33–36	47[b]	11
>36	50	11

[a]Adapted from ref. 20. All ages are in weeks.
[b]p < 0.05 compared to >36 weeks gestational age.
[c]p < 0.05 compared to the two older groups.

comparable incidences of UALTE in BPD and matched control preterm infants: 8.9% and 10.5%, respectively. There were no deaths from SIDS among the 78 BPD or 78 control preterm infants.

Infants with prenatal drug exposure to methadone, heroin, or cocaine also appear to have an increased risk of SIDS. This risk is estimated to be approximately five to ten times greater than in matched control infants. There are no data to indicate to what extent, if any, the presence of additional risk factors for SIDS such as prematurity are additive.

All studies of SIDS incidence have shown significantly higher rates in African-Americans than in white infants, independent of any other factors such as low birth weight, young maternal age, or high parity. The range of relative risk for African-American infants in recent years compared to white infants has been 1.7 to 5.2. Native Americans have a birth-weight-specific SIDS rate that is in the same general range as African-American infants. SIDS rates in other racial groups in the United States are comparable or better than those in white infants (Table 32–1), but assimilation into the U.S. culture may be associated with increased rates to levels comparable to those observed in African-Americans and Native Americans. Some ethnic groups in other countries also have increased SIDS rates, including Gypsy, Maori, Hawaiian, and Filipino infants.

Sleeping Position

A national "Back to Sleep" campaign was initiated in the United States in mid-1994 to advocate side or back sleeping during early infancy (22). The stimulus for this campaign was the aggregate experience from other countries of decreases of 50% or more in rates of SIDS following dramatic declines in prevalence of the prone sleep position to 10% or less (23). Prone prevalence rates in the United States progressively decreased from a high of 70% to 80% before 1992 and about 55% just before the campaign to the 18% to 30% range in 1997 (1 to 3 months, respectively). This significant decrease in prone prevalence was associated with a decrease in SIDS rates of about 35% compared to an average annual decrease before 1992 of only about 2%. Annual SIDS rates thus decreased from 1.33/1,000 live births in 1989–1991 to

1.22/1,000 in 1993 and most recently to 0.74/1,000 (provisional) in 1996 (2).

The initial back-to-sleep campaign recommendations considered side sleeping to be nearly equivalent to the supine position in reducing the risk of SIDS. More recently, however, epidemiologic data have identified both prone and side sleeping as risk factors for SIDS, with odds ratios (OR) of 13.9 and 3.5, respectively (24). The current back-to-sleep recommendations thus call for supine position for sleeping in all infants without medical contraindications, e.g., micrognathia.

Preterm infants were initially excluded from all back-to-sleep campaigns. This exclusion was based on accumulated data in preterm infants at younger postnatal ages, indicating that ventilation was optimal when sleeping was done prone, especially in the presence of lung disease (25). Epidemiologic studies, however, have now confirmed that both preterm infants and full-term infants are at greater risk for SIDS when sleeping prone or side (24); the OR for birth weights under 2,500 g were 83 and 36.6 for prone and side, respectively, and the OR for infants less than 37 weeks of gestation were 48.8 and 40.5, respectively. The current recommendation, therefore, is that supine should be the recommended sleeping position for all infants and should begin in the hospital before discharge from the neonatal ICU or nursery. Prone prevalence in the United States in 1997, among all infants, was about 18% at 1 month of age but was still about 30% in preterm infants less than 1,750 g birth weight. At 3 months, 29% of all infants and 36% of infants less than 1,750 g birth weight slept prone (research in progress).

The mechanism(s) for the epidemiologic association between decreased prone/side prevalence and decreased risk for SIDS has not been established. However, there may be an interaction between prone/side sleep position and impaired cardiorespiratory control, especially impaired ventilatory and arousal responsiveness (26). Face-down or nearly face-down sleeping does occasionally occur in prone-sleeping infants and can result in episodes of airway obstruction and asphyxia (27) in healthy full-term infants. These healthy infants all aroused before the face-down or face-nearly-down position became life-threatening, but infants with insufficient arousal responsiveness to asphyxia would be at risk for fatal asphyxia. Sleeping on a very soft surface would further increase the risk of life-threatening asphyxia in the face-down or nearly-down sleeping position. Some investigators attribute the risk of prone sleeping to thermal stress, hypothesizing that (face-down) prone sleeping causes a clinically significant degree of thermal stress. Any thermal stress could further compromise infants with deficient cardiorespiratory control. There thus may be links between epidemiologic risk factors such as soft bedding, prone sleep position, and thermal stress and links between biological risk factors such as cardiorespiratory control deficits (ventilatory and arousal abnormalities) and temperature/metabolic regulation deficits.

As prone prevalence has decreased, exposure to tobacco smoke has emerged as an even more important risk factor for SIDS (28–30). Both prenatal and postnatal smoking exposure are important; elimination just of prenatal smoking exposure could theoretically reduce the risk of SIDS an additional 30%. The effect of prenatal smoking on SIDS rates does not appear to be mediated through an effect on birth weight. Bed sharing has been a significant risk factor for SIDS in numerous studies; this association has been linked to mothers who smoke (31). Soft bedding, covers over the head, and sleeping under a comforter (duvet) have also emerged as more significant risk factors as prone prevalence has decreased (32).

PROSPECTIVE IDENTIFICATION

A major objective of SIDS research has been to develop a screening test capable of accurately identifying those infants destined to die of SIDS. To be valid and practical, such a test must have a negligible false-negative rate and an acceptable false-positive rate. The pneumogram and polysomnogram (PSG) screening studies performed prospectively in both full-term and preterm infants have focused primarily on respiratory pattern and/or cardiac abnormalities, and none has demonstrated sufficient sensitivity and specificity to be clinically useful as a screening test (1).

Prospective identification of future SIDS victims has been an even greater challenge in preterm than full-term infants because of the wider range of variability in maturational levels and in postnatal ages. It has not been possible to determine the extent to which cardiorespiratory patterns in asymptomatic preterm infants that are outside established norms for full-term infants (33) are "normal" for that postconceptional age or whether they identify a risk for clinically significant events at home and/or a risk for SIDS. Polysomnogram (PSG) recordings in preterm infants at 25 to 36 weeks of gestation, with clinical and/or hospital monitor-detected cyanosis, apnea, or bradycardia, exceeded the range established for full-term infants in 92% of instances when recorded at 36 to 44 weeks of postconceptional age. These abnormalities included apnea exceeding 20 seconds, periodic breathing for more than 15% of sleep time, bradycardia episodes below 80 beats/min, feeding hypoxia, and hypercarbia (34). Although all of these infants were discharged on a home monitor (without memory), only 16% had apparent serious events that received parental intervention, and there was no correlation between parental reports of clinically significant events and the predischarge recording. In preterm infants less than 1,500 g birth weight and having no clinical cardiorespiratory symptoms at the time of neonatal ICU discharge (35), cardiorespiratory pattern values were above the 95th percentile for healthy term infants for apnea density in 18%, for periodic breathing in 15%, and for longest apnea in 17%. These observed differences in preterm infants may be explained by a significantly lower postconceptional age in the asymptomatic infants with one or more variables above the 95th percentile (36 weeks) compared to the asymptomatic infants with all values below the 95th percentile (37.5 weeks).

The extent to which incomplete maturation in cardiorespiratory control, in preterm infants, contributes to risk for UALTE and/or for SIDS remains unresolved. It is not known whether having a cardiorespiratory pattern value outside the 95th percentile for full-term infants has any clinical significance, nor is it known whether infants with a prior history of apnea of prematurity are at greater risk for SIDS than gestational-age-matched infants without such a history. Even though 18.5% of SIDS victims are premature (7), and the risk of SIDS progressively increases as birth weight decreases, those preterm infants destined to die of SIDS cannot be accurately identified prospectively.

Symptoms related to apnea of prematurity frequently persist beyond term gestation in infants delivered at 24 to 28 weeks of gestation (36). The postconceptional age at which recurrent apnea/bradycardia episodes resolve increased with decreasing gestational age. Although the incidence of SIDS also increases with decreasing gestational age, the relationship of prolonged apnea of prematurity and/or delayed maturation of cardiorespiratory pattern to risk of SIDS remains unclarified.

New technologies utilizing event recordings now permit home memory monitoring that includes respiratory pattern, heart rate and ECG, and oxygenation (33). It is thus possible to obtain ongoing home assessments of cardiorespiratory pattern in preterm infants. Yet so far it has still not been possible to identify any specific cardiorespiratory pattern associated with increased risk for an UALTE or for SIDS.

INTERVENTION

The apnea hypothesis led to the hope that home electronic surveillance would reduce risk for SIDS. Even though respiratory pattern abnormalities may not be a critical component of the cardiorespiratory control abnormalities that appear to contribute to risk for SIDS, home monitoring could still be effective if bradycardia and/or desaturation were occurring sufficiently early so as to be amenable to intervention.

A major problem in determining the efficacy of home monitoring has been uncertainty as to the extent of monitor use or compliance. Anecdotal postmortem interviews with parents of SIDS victims dying with a monitor in the home have suggested that 50% or more of such families were not utilizing the home monitor at the time death occurred. Fewer than 10% of monitor alarms (37) are

related to physiologic events; initial parental difficulties with movement, loose leads, or other nonsignificant alarms may thus easily lead to parental frustration and noncompliance. Utilizing memory monitors to identify and minimize problems with frequent false alarms should improve family compliance. Studies can potentially be performed using memory monitors to document compliance, to identify cardiorespiratory patterns associated with true events (33), and to evaluate whether home electronic surveillance has any effective clinical role in preventing life-threatening events and SIDS.

Caffeine and theophylline have both been utilized in apnea of prematurity and UALTE. Both of these methylxanthines improve respiratory pattern and reduce the frequency and severity of clinical symptoms (1). Caffeine does decrease the auditory arousal threshold in young adults, but there are no systematic evaluations of either methylxanthine in infants with deficient arousal responsiveness or in infants identified as at increased epidemiologic risk for SIDS.

REFERENCES

1. Hunt CE. Sudden infant death syndrome. In Beckerman RC, Brouillette RT, Hunt CE, eds. *Respiratory control disorders in infants and children.* Baltimore: Williams & Wilkins, 1992:90–211.
2. Guyer B, Martin JA, MacDorman MF, Anderson RN, Strobino DM. Annual summary of vital statistics—1996. *Pediatrics* 1997;100:905–918.
3. Panigrahy A, Filiano JJ, Sleeper LA, et al. Decreased kainate receptor binding in the arcuate nucleus of the sudden infant death syndrome. *J Neuropathol Exp Neurol* 1997;56:1253–1261.
4. Obonai T, Yasuhara M, Nakamura T, Takashima S. Catecholamine neurons alteration in the brainstem of sudden infant death syndrome victims. *Pediatrics* 1998;101:285–288.
5. Schechtman VL, Lee M, Wilson AJ, Harper RM. Dynamics of respiratory patterning in normal infants and infants who subsequently died of the sudden infant death syndrome. *Pediatr Res* 1996;40:571–577.
6. Chatow U, Davidson S, Reichman BL, Akselrod S. Development and maturation of the autonomic nervous system in premature and full-term infants using spectral analysis of heart rate fluctuations. *Pediatr Res* 1995;37:294–302.
7. Hoffman HJ, Hillman LS. Epidemiology of the sudden infant death syndrome; maternal, neonatal, and postneonatal risk factors. *Clin Perinatol* 1992;19:717–738.
8. Klonoff-Cohen HS, Edelstein SL, Schneider Lefkowitz E, et al. The effect of passive smoking and tobacco exposure through breast milk on sudden infant death syndrome. *JAMA* 1995;273:795–798.
9. Schellscheidt J, Oyen N, Jorch G. Interactions between maternal smoking and other prenatal risk factors for sudden infant death syndrome (SIDS). *Acta Paediatr* 1997;86:857–863.
10. Cutz E, Perrin DG, Hackman R, Czegledy-Nagy EN. Maternal smoking and pulmonary neuroendocrine cells in sudden infant death syndrome. *Pediatrics* 1996;98:668–672.
11. Lewis KW, Bosque EM. Deficient hypoxia awakening response in infants of smoking mothers. *J Pediatr* 1995;127:691–699.
12. Milerad J, Walsh WF. Nicotine attenuates the ventilatory response to hypoxia in the developing lamb. *Pediatr Res* 1995;37:652–660.
13. Milerad J, Sundell H. Nicotine exposure and the risk for SIDS. *Acta Paediatr* 1993;82(Suppl 389):70–72.
14. Sawczenko A, Fleming PH. Thermal stress, sleeping position, and the sudden infant death syndrome. *Sleep* 1996;19(10):S267–S270.
15. Tuffnell CS, Peterson SA, Wailoo MP. Prone sleeping infants have a reduced ability to lose heat. *Early Hum Dev* 1995;43:109–116.
16. Southall DP, Plunkett MCB, Banks MW, Falkov AF, Samuels MP. Covert video records of life-threatening child abuse: Lessons for child protection. *Pediatrics* 1997;100(5):735–760.

17. Oyen N. Skjaerven R, Irgens LM. Population-based recurrence risk of sudden infant death syndrome compared with other infant and fetal deaths. *Am J Epidermiol* 1996;144:300–305.

18. Hunt CE. Sudden infant death syndrome (SIDS) in families: risk factors for recurrence. *Pediatr Res* 1999;45.

19. Black L, David RJ, Brouillette RT, Hunt CE. Effects of birth weight and ethnicity on incidence of sudden infant death syndrome. *J Pediatr* 1986;108:209–214.

20. Malloy MH, Hoffman HJ. Prematurity, sudden infant death syndrome, and age of death. *Pediatrics* 1995;96:464–471.

21. Gray PH, Rogers Y. Are infants with bronchopulmonary dysplasia at risk for sudden infant death syndrome? *Pediatrics* 1994;93:774–777.

22. Hunt CE. Prone sleeping in healthy infants and victims of sudden infant death syndrome. *J Pediatr* 1996;128(5):594–596.

23. Kattwinkel J, Brooks J, Myerberg D. Infant sleep position and SIDS in the U.S.: Joint commentary from the AAP and selected agencies of the federal government. *Pediatrics* 1994;93:820.

24. Oyen N, Markestad T, Skjaerven R, et al. Combined effects of sleeping position and prenatal risk factors in sudden infant death syndrome: The Nordic epidemiological SIDS study. *Pediatrics* 1997;100:613–621.

25. McEvoy C, Mendoza ME, Bowling S, Hewlett V, Sardesai S, Durand M. Prone positioning decreases episodes of hypoxemia in extremely low birth weight infants (1000 grams or less) with chronic lung disease. *J Pediatr* 1997;130:305–309.

26. Kahn A, Groswasser J, Sottiaux M, et al. Prone or supine body position and sleep characteristics in infants. *Pediatrics* 1993;91:1112–1115.

27. Waters KA, Gonzalez AJC, Morielli A, Brouillette RT. Face-straight-down and face-near-straight-down positions in healthy, prone-sleeping infants. *J Pediatr* 1996;128:616–625.

28. Blair PS, Fleming PJ, Bensley D, et al. Smoking and the sudden infant death syndrome: results from 1993–5 case-control study for confidential inquiry into stillbirths and deaths in infancy. *Br Med J* 1996;313: 195–198.

29. MacDorman MF, Cnattingius S, Hoffman HJ, Kramer MS, Haglund B. Sudden infant death syndrome and smoking in the United States and Sweden. *Am J Epidemiol* 1997;146:249–257.

30. Taylor JA, Sanderson M. A reexamination of the risk factors for the sudden infant death syndrome. *J Pediatr* 1995;126:887–891.

31. Mitchell EA, Tuohy PG, Brunt JM, et al. Risk factors for sudden infant death syndrome following the prevention campaign in New Zealand: A prospective study. *Pediatrics* 1997;100:835–840.

32. Fleming PJ, Blair PS, Bacon C, et al. Environment of infants during sleep and risk of the sudden infant death syndrome: results of 1993–5 case-control study for confidential inquiry into stillbirths and deaths in infancy. *Br Med J* 1996;313:191–195.

33. Hunt CE, Hufford DR, Bourguignon C, Oess MA. Home documented monitoring of cardiorespiratory pattern and O_2 saturation in healthy infants. *Pediatr Res* 1996;39:216–222.

34. Rosen CL, Glaze DG, Frost JD. Home monitor follow-up of persistent apnea and bradycardia in preterm infants. *Am J Dis Child* 1986;140: 547–550.

35. Hageman JR, Holmes D, Suchy S, Hunt CE. Respiratory pattern at hospital discharge in asymptomatic preterm infants. *Pediatr Pulmonol* 1988;4:78–83.

36. Eichenwald EC, Aina A, Stark AR. Apnea frequency persists beyond term gestation in infants delivered at 24 to 28 weeks. *Pediatrics* 1997; 100:354–359.

37. Silvestri J, Hufford DR, Durham JD, et al, and CHIME. Assessment of compliance with home cardiorespiratory monitoring in infants at risk of sudden infant death syndrome. *J Pediatr* 1995;127:384–388.

CHAPTER 33

Cardiac Disease

Michael F. Flanagan, Scott B. Yeager, and Steven N. Weindling

INCIDENCE

The incidence of congenital heart disease detectable by routine clinical examination has been most reliably estimated to be 7.5 per 1,000 live births (1). The incidence of congenital heart anomalies in neonates evident by detailed echocardigraphic examination appears to be at least three- to fourfold higher, but the difference consists mostly of tiny and clinically insignificant ventricular septal defects (2,3). Approximately 2.7 infants per 1,000 births require cardiac catheterization or cardiac surgery or die with heart disease (4). Almost one-half of these infants are first seen before the second week of life. The distributions of congenital heart anomalies in newborns seen at a primary and a tertiary pediatric cardiac center are shown in Table 33–1.

MORTALITY

Before aggressive intervention, Mitchell found that 2.3 of 1,000 live births died with cardiac problems in infancy (1). After aggressive palliation was adopted, the infant cardiac fatality rate fell to 0.8 per 1,000 births (4). Mortality has declined further since more definitive interventions have been employed in neonates and young infants. The infant cardiac fatality rate in the United States was 0.6 per 1,000 births in 1990 (5). Although the mortality in neonates with specific cardiac lesions is improved, neonatal death from congenital heart disease accounts for most neonatal deaths in referral hospitals. Prematurity and associated noncardiac anomalies influence the poten-

tial for salvaging infants with cardiac disease (Table 33–2) (4). In some situations, the mortality attributable to these problems is considerable.

SURVIVAL

With few exceptions, there is a cardiac operation or catheter intervention that can improve the quality of life or lengthen the life of a child with heart disease. Long-term survival is highly dependent on the specific diagnosis (see Table 33–2). This chapter focuses on infancy; for more information, standard texts of pediatric cardiology should be consulted (6–11). Most can expect to survive for several decades. It has been a matter of conviction among cardiologists that any improvement in survival was worth the effort, emotional drain, and cost, particularly because later progress in the field often allowed unexpected secondary interventions that provided even longer survival. The palliative shunt operations of 20 to 30 years ago unexpectedly produced candidates for later Fontan procedures. The central principle continues to be "where there is life, there is hope." The pros and cons of treating a child who has crippling extracardiac defects must be discussed with the parents in understandable language. The long-range future of patients undergoing intracardiac repair, arterial switch operations, staged multiple complex palliative operations, Fontan operations, or cardiac transplantation requires detailed discussion. Virtually all procedures have an incidence of late complications, some delayed until adulthood. The goal is not to consider the struggle to be won if the child can be coaxed to adulthood but to provide a satisfying life for many years after childhood. The possibility that brain injury or other injury may be acquired in the process of treatment should be understood (12,13). The expected physical capabilities of the patient after treatment should be delineated. After the physician is confident that the parents thoroughly understand the known facts, he or she is free

M. F. Flanagan and S. N. Weindling: Department of Pediatrics, Section of Pediatric Cardiology, Dartmouth Medical School; and Dartmouth–Hitchcock Medical Center, Lebanon, New Hampshire

S. B. Yeager: Department of Pediatrics, University of Vermont; and Division of Pediatric Cardiology, Medical Center Hospital of Vermont, Burlington, Vermont

TABLE 33–1. *Echocardiographic diagnoses in the first month of life*[a]

Diagnosis	Children's Hospital (*n* = 1,627) (%)	Dartmouth–Hitchcock (*n* = 207) (%)
Ventricular septal defect	15	33
Valvar pulmonary stenosis	5	13
Atrial septal defect secundum	5	10
Coarctation of the aorta	7	7
Cardiomyopathy	4	6
Tetralogy of Fallot	7	5
Transposition of the great arteries	17	4
Endocardial cushion defects	4	3
Hypoplastic left heart syndrome	7	2
Tricuspid atresia	2	2
Aortic stenosis	3	2
Malpositions	5	1
Total anomalous pulmonary veins	1	1
Truncus arteriosis	2	1
L-Transposition of the great arteries	1	1
Tricuspid valve diseases	5	1
Pulmonary atresia and intact interventricular septum	2	
Single ventricle	1	
Other	7	8

[a]Patients seen between 1986 and 1991. There were many infants with patent ductus arteriosus. These are not included because most were associated with respiratory distress syndrome. There were few with a diagnosis of normal heart, persistent fetal circulation, and rhythm problems. The marked difference between the two hospitals reflects the nature of their practices. The Children's Hospital in Boston includes a tertiary referral practice; and the Dartmouth–Hitchcock group has a primary referral practice.

TABLE 33–2. *Rank order of cardiac diagnoses and first-year mortality by birth weight*[a]

Birth weight > 2.5 kg (*n* = 1,552)			Birth weight < 2.5 kg (*n* = 230)		
Frequency (%)	Diagnosis	Mortality (%)	Frequency (%)	Diagnosis	Mortality (%)
17	D-TGA	9	16	VSD	5
14	VSD	2	14	PDA	9
8	PDA	8	7	MYO	6
7	HLV	50	7	COARC	38
7	TF	16	6	TF	28
6	COARC	18	6	MAL	31
5	ASD2	1	6	TRI	8
5	PS	1	5	D-TGA	17
4	MAL	28	5	ASD2	0
4	TRI	1	4	PS	0/9
4	ECD	17	3	HLV	3/8
3	MYO	6	3	ECD	2/7
2	AS	26	2	TA	2/5
2	TA	19	2	TAPVR	2/5
2	TRUNC	24	2	AS	0/5
1	PA + IVS	14	2	TRUNC	2/5
1	TAPVR	11	1	SV	1/2
1	SV	31	1	PA + IVS	1/2
1	L-TGA	0/6	1	L-TGA	0/1
6	Other	16	8	Other	28
100	Total	13	100	Total	18

[a]Data were based on 1,843 infants younger than 1 month old who were examined by echocardiography between January 1986 and January 1991. Fifty-five of those with birth weights more than 2.5 kg and six of those with birth weights less than 2.5 kg had no heart disease. There were more babies with myocardial disease and ductus arteriosus and the first-year mortality was consistently higher in the low-birth-weight group.

AS, aortic stenosis; ASD2, atrial septal defect; COARC, coarctation of the aorta; D-TGA, D-transposition of the great arteries; ECD, endocardial cushion defects; HLV, hypoplastic left heart syndrome; L-TGA, L-transposition of the great arteries; MAL, malpositions; MYO, cardiomyopathy; PDA, patent ductus arteriosus; PA + IVS, pulmonary atresia and intact interventricular septum; PS, valvar pulmonary stenosis; SV, single ventricle; TA, tricuspid atresia; TAPVR, total anomalous pulmonary veins; TF, tetralogy of Fallot; TGA, transposition of the great arteries; TRI, tricuspid valve diseases; TRUNC, truncus arteriosus; VSD, ventricular septal defect.

to express an opinion about what may be best for the child.

ETIOLOGY

Parents ask why their baby was born with a cardiac abnormality and whether it is likely to recur with a subsequent pregnancy. Until recently, the specific cause of an individual cardiac anomaly was unknown in most cases. Although fetal exposure to specific environmental, pharmacologic, biochemical, and infectious factors may increase the risk for developing a cardiac abnormality (Table 33–3) (10,14–20), these factors do not appear to explain most cases. In individual cases, it is usually difficult or impossible to identify specific extrinsic factors that may have modified the baby's genotype or genotypic expression.

Some specific cardiac anomalies are frequently associated with generalized genetic syndromes, for instance supravalvar aortic stenosis and Williams syndrome, and endocardial cushion defects with Down syndrome and heterotaxy (asplenia and polysplenia syndromes). Other cardiac anomalies are rarely associated with a noncardiac syndrome, for example, transposition of the great arteries and pulmonary atresia with intact ventricular septum (Table 33–4). Overall, approximately 8% to 13% of children with cardiac anomalies have inheritable syndromes with associated cardiovascular abnormalities (e.g., Marfan syndrome), and 13% have chromosomal syndromes associated with cardiovascular malformation (10,14,15, 19,21). The genes affected in many of these syndromes have recently been identified (Table 33–5). For instance, mutations in the genes encoding the extracellular matrix proteins fibrillin-1 and elastin are responsible, respectively, for Marfan and Williams syndrome. Recognition

TABLE 33–3. *Possible teratogens for congenital heart disease*

Vitamin deficiency
    Folate deficiency[a]
Environmental agents
    High altitude,[a] trichloroethylene, irradiation
Drugs
    Ethanol,[a] hydantoin,[a] valproic acid,[a] trimethadione,[a]
    primidone,[a] carbamazepine,[a] lithium,[a] thalidomide,[a]
    retinoic acid,[a] antineoplastic agents (?), amphetamine,
    cocaine
Metabolic factors
    Maternal diabetes,[a] maternal phenylketonuria[a]
Immune factors
    Maternal autoimmune disease with anti-Ra anti-LA
    antibodies
Infectious agents
    Rubella,[a] mumps (?), cytomegalovirus (?)

[a]It is generally accepted that these prenatal factors increase the risk for congenital heart disease.
From refs. 10, 14–18, 20, 28, 29.

TABLE 33–4. *Incidence of severe associated noncardiac anomalies among 2,220 infants with heart disease*

Diagnosis	Incidence (%)
Endocardial cushion defect	43
Patent ductus arteriosus	31
Ventricular septal defect	24
Malpositions	13
Tetralogy of Fallot	10
Coarctation of aorta	9
Pulmonary atresia with intact septum	1
D-Transposition of the great arteries	1

that a child has a syndrome associated with congenital heart disease, or vice versa, should prompt an investigation for possible associated anomalies (21,22).

Diagnostic frequency year by year, state by state, and hospital by hospital has been relatively constant, and any etiologic theory must account for this phenomenon. Increasingly, specific inherited and new genetic mutations are being recognized in many of those with isolated congenital cardiac anomalies, cardiomyopathies, and arrhythmias without generalized syndromes. Reviews of the current understanding of normal and abnormal cardiovascular embryologic development and molecular biology are available (23–26). The biology and etiology of inherited and new mutations resulting in cardiac anomalies are still being unraveled. The biochemical environment and chance events before and during fetal development may play roles in causation of new genetic mutations and in transcriptional and posttranscriptional processes (10,14–16,27). For instance, the risk for development of conotruncal anomalies is significantly reduced by periconceptual maternal intake of multivitamins and folic acid (28,29). In addition, a new adult generation of survivors with more serious cardiac anomalies is now producing children. Genetic mutations in a critical region of chromosome 22q11 involved in neural crest and cardiac development are the most common genetic mutations now recognized to result in cardiac anomaly (30), occurring in 20% to 30% of infants with isolated conotruncal malformations or interrupted aortic arch (25).

A singular abnormality results in characteristic complex cardiac malformation by altering or killing embryonic primordial cells, such as in the neural crest or endocardial cushion, before formation of cardiac structures in the conotruncus or atrioventricular valves, respectively. Animal studies have demonstrated that embryonic cervical neural crest cells migrate into the thorax and contribute to formation of the aortic arch and conotruncal outflow region of the heart. Blockage of the normal function of these embryonic neural crest cells results in aortic arch anomalies including aortic interruption; conotruncal abnormalities including tetralogy of Fallot, truncus arteriosus, and transposition; and ventricular inlet anomalies including tricuspid atresia and double-inlet single left

TABLE 33–5. *Congenital disorders associated with cardiac disease*

Disorder	Identified gene(s)	Chromosome location	% Heart disease	Cardiovascular anomalies
Autosomal dominant				
Alagille arteriohepatic dysplasia	Jagged 1	20p12	100	Multiple PA stenosis and hypoplasia, PDA, ASD, VSD
Beckwith–Wiedemann syndrome	BWS	11 pter-p15.4	15 ?	HCM, ASD, VSD, TF, PDA
de Lange syndrome	CDL	3q26.3	30	VSD, ASD, PDA, AS, EFE
CATCH 22/DiGeorge syndrome	DiGeorge chromosome region	22q11	>50	TF, interrupted Ao arch, truncus arteriosus, right Ao arch
Coffin-Siris syndrome	?	?	?	ASD, VSD, TF
Goldenhar oculoauricularvertebral	?	?	15	TF, VSD
Hereditary hemorrhagic telagiectasia Osler–Weber–Rendu	Endoglin	9q34.1	100	Pulmonary and systemic AVM, anuerysms, angiectasia
Holt–Oram heart-hand syndrome	TBX5	12q24.1	100	ASD-2, VSD or PDA in 2/3, conduc. block, HLHS, TAPVC, truncus art.
Klippel–Feil syndrome	KFSL	8q22.2	?	VSD
Marfan syndrome	Fibrillin-1	15q21.1	Up to 100%	Ao anuerysm; AR, MR, TR & prolapse
Neurofibromatosis type I	NFI	17q11.2	Rare	PS, COARC, renal artery stenosis
Noonan syndrome	NS 1	12q22-qter	?	PS/dysplasia, PDA, HCM, COARC
Rubinstein-Taybi Broad thumb-hallux syndrome	CREB binding Protein	16p13.3	35	VSD, PDA, ASD, COARC, PS Bicuspid Ao valve, complex
Saethre–Chotzen syndrome	TWIST	7p21	?	various, subalvar AS
Shprintzen velocardiofacial syndrome	DiGeorge chromosome region	22q11	80	VSD, TF, right Ao arch, aberrant right subclavian artery
Treacher Collins syndrome	TCOF1	5q32-q33.1	30	ASD, VSD, PDA
Tuberous sclerosis	TSC1	9q34	Uncommon	rhabdomyomas, rarely Ao aneuersym
Williams-Beuren syndrome	Elastin	7q11.2	50–80	Supravalvar AS, small aorta, stenoses LCA, multiple PAs, cerebral & renal arteries
Autosomal recessive				
Carpenter acrocephalopolsyndactyly	?	Unknown	33	PDA, PS, VSD, TF, TGA
Ellis van Creveld	EVC	4p16	50–60	Single atrium, primum ASD, COARC, HLHS
Mucopolysaccharidosis type 1	Iduronidase	4p16.3	>50	All types have valvular disease,
type 2	Iduronate 2-sulfat;	Xq28		Coronary disease (type 2)
type 3D	GNS	12q14		
type 6	Arylsulfatase B	5q11-q13		
Pierre Robin syndrome	?	?	?	TF, COARC, pulmonary hypertension
Smith–Lemli–Opitz syndrome 1&2	SLOS	7q32.1	20/100	VSD, PDA, ASD, TF
Trombocytopenia absent radius	unknown	Unknown	33	ASD, TF
Zellweger cerebrohepatorenal syndrome	multiple-peroxin-5,2,6,12	7q11.23		VSD, ASD, PDA
Chromosomal disorders				
Trisomy 13 Patau syndrome		13	80	PDA, VSD, ASD, COARC, AS, PS
Trisomy 18 Edwards syndrome		18	90–100	VSD, polyvalvular, ASD, PDA
Trisomy 21 Down syndrome		21	40–50	AV canal, VSD, ASD1&2, PDA, TF
XO Turner syndrome		X	>50	bicusp AV, COARC, Ao anuerysm
4p- Wolfe syndrome		4p	33	VSD, ASD, COARC
5p- Cri-du-Chat syndrome		5p	20	VSD
22+ Cat eye syndrome		22	40	TAPVC, TF
Syndromes with unknown etiology				
Asymmetric crying facies			44	VSD
CHARGE Association			65–75	TF, DORV, ASD, VSD, PDA, COARC, AV canal
VACTERL Association			10	VSD, ASD, TF
Nonrandom associations				
Cleft lip and palate			25	VSD, PDA, TGA, TF, SV
Diaphramatic hernia			25	TF
Lung agenesis			20	PDA, VSD, TF, TAPVC
Omphalocele			20	TF, ASD
Intestinal atresia			10	VSD
Renal agenesis unilateral/bilateral			17/75	VSD

Ao, aortic; AR, aortic regurgitation; AS, aortic stenosis; ASD, atrial septal defect; ASD-1, primum atrial septal defect; ASD-2, secundum atrial septal defect; AV, aortic valve; AV canal, atrioventricular canal defect; AVM, arteriovenous malformation; COARC, coarctation of the aorta; DORV, double-outlet right ventricle; EFE, endocardial fibroelastosis; HLHS, hypoplastic left heart syndrome; LCA, left coronary artery; MR, mitral regurgitation; PAs, pulmonary arteries; PDA, patent ductus arteriosus; PS, pulmonary valve stenosis; TAPVC, totally anomalous pulmonary venous connection; TF, tetralogy of Fallot; TGA, transposition of great arteries; TR, tricuspid regurgitation; truncus art., truncus arteriosus; VSD, ventricular septal defect.
From refs. 10,15,19–22,34.

ventricle (23,26). Cells in the embryonic endocardial tissue undergo a different developmental sequential process controlled by a large number of factors. Perturbation of specific steps in these embryonic cell process changes developmental sequences in characteristic ways and alters blood flow patterns affecting vascular growth downstream in characteristic ways (10,15,16,20,26,27). Because growth of specific cardiovascular structures is flow dependent, limitation of flow can cause additional hypoplasia of downstream structures (26,31,32). For example, a mildly stenotic bicommissural aortic valve may decrease blood flow through the aortic isthmus and result in coarctation.

As with gross anatomic cardiac anomalies, the specific causes of cardiac muscle diseases were unknown in most cases until recently. Many of the hypertrophic and dilated cardiomyopathies previously known as idiopathic are now known to be caused by specific gene mutations (30,33,34). Approximately half of the cases of familial isolated hypertrophic cardiomyopathy are caused by defects in sarcomeric contractile proteins, most commonly cardiac β-myosin heavy chain and troponin T_2 (30). Isolated dilated cardiomyopathy has been associated to date with a half-dozen genetic loci, and identification of more is likely (35). The nuclear and mitochondrial genetic mutations underlying a large number of metabolic disorders with cardiomyopathy have been identified (see Cardiomyopathy) (31). Specific arrhythmia syndromes are also identified as caused by specific genetic mutations. Some patients with Wolf–Parkinson–White syndrome with hypertrophic cardiomyopathy have a mutation in a gene at 7q3 (34). Prolonged QT syndrome, associated with ventricular tachycardia and sudden death, results from genetic defects in various cardiac ion channels that affect repolarization (30,36).

Certain cardiac lesions are associated with prematurity or low birth weight (see Table 33–2). Because closure of the ventricular septum may be delayed until the first months of life, it is not surprising that there is a somewhat greater incidence of ventricular septal defect among premature infants. The increased incidence of patent ductus arteriosus in prematurely born infants can be viewed as the result of birth long before the programmed time for closure of the ductus. Hypoxemia of pulmonary origin also promotes ductal patency.

FETAL CARDIOLOGY

Fetal Circulation

Extensive information about the circulatory physiology of the fetus and newborn has accumulated. The works of Barcroft (37), Dawes (38), Lind et al. (39), and Rudolph (40) should be consulted for details, but the central features are discussed here. The circulation before birth consists of parallel circuits (Fig. 33–1). Blood in the

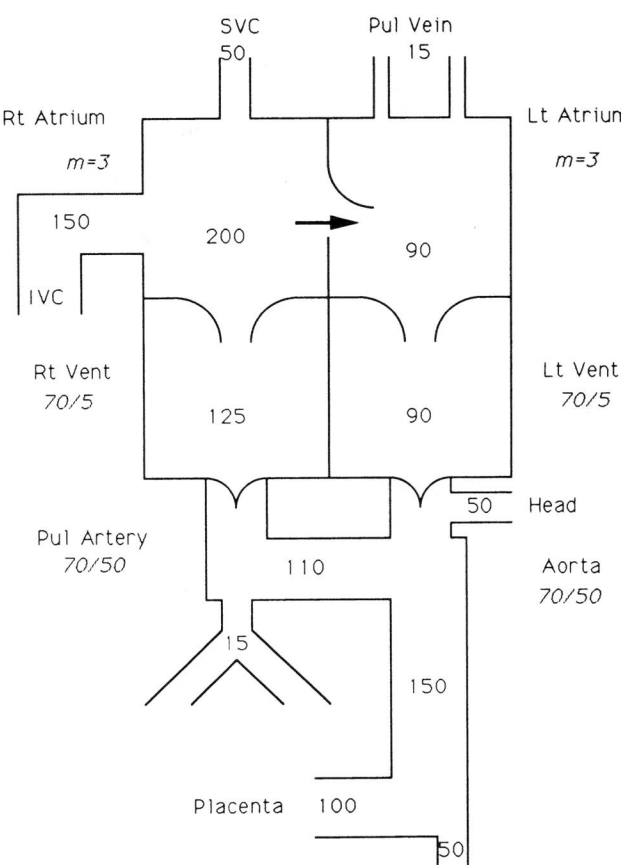

FIG. 33–1. Fetal circulation is in parallel, and the amount of blood handled by the left and right ventricles is 125 and 90 mL, respectively. Only 40 mL passes through the aortic arch to the descending aorta, and only a small fraction passes through the lungs. The numbers inside the diagram represent relative blood flow (mL); the numbers in italics are pressure measurements. (Modified from ref. 40.)

aorta may follow several routes to a capillary bed in the fetus or the placenta, back to the heart, passing through either ventricle, and out again to the aorta. The stream of newly oxygenated blood from the placenta passes through the umbilical vein, the ductus venosus, the inferior vena cava, and the right atrium. Unlike the circulation after birth, the streams of oxygenated and unoxygenated blood are not completely separated, although the more oxygenated blood from the inferior vena cava is mostly diverted through the foramen ovale into the left atrium. Consequently, blood from the left ventricle entering the ascending aorta and coronary and carotid circulations is somewhat higher in oxygen than that entering the descending aorta from the right ventricle by way of the ductus arteriosus.

Normally, the volume pumped by the right ventricle is thought to be about 62% of the combined output of both ventricles. Because both ventricles pump against the systemic resistance, the level of pressure in the two ventricles is comparable. The resistance to blood flow through the lungs is relatively great; only minimal flow through the lungs occurs *in utero,* and almost all of the right ventricular output into the pulmonary artery passes through the ductus arteriosus to the descending aorta. The parallel arrangement of the ventricles allows fetal survival despite a wide variety of cardiac lesions. With total obstruction of either ventricle, the other ventricle assumes the entire cardiac output. Reversal of the pulmonary arterial and aortic streams of blood, as occurs in transposition of the great arteries, produces no deleterious effect on the fetus. Additionally, ductal or ascending aortic flow may reverse in the presence of severe semilunar valvar stenosis or atresia. Despite this remarkable ability to adapt, grow, and survive, the fetus is affected by limitations in myocardial contractility. Prolonged, severe pressure or volume loading of the heart or primary myocardial disease may result in congestive heart failure, manifested by hydrops fetalis. The interplay between the metabolic effects of congestion in the fetus and the possible compensatory role of the placenta is not understood. Because lesions that may be expected to cause gross intrauterine difficulty are tolerated surprisingly well, the postulate that the placenta helps compensate for the metabolic abnormalities resulting from congestive heart failure is tenable.

Circulatory Adjustments at Birth

Changes in the Source of Oxygenated Blood and in the Ductus Venosus and Ductus Arteriosus

With the first breath, the resistance to pulmonary blood flow drops sharply. The oxygen content of the left heart and systemic circulation rapidly reaches levels well above that of the fetal circulation. The oxygen saturation in the ascending fetal aorta is about 65%; immediately after birth, it rises to about 93%. The ductus venosus functionally closes, establishing the portal circulation as an independent loop between two capillary beds. With removal of the low-resistance placenta, systemic resistance increases. The relative fall in the pulmonary resistance and rise in the systemic resistance result in a transitory left-to-right shunt through the ductus arteriosus. The ductus becomes functionally closed toward the end of the first day of life, becoming anatomically obliterated at about 10 days of age. Even among cyanotic newborns who are duct dependent, the ductus may inexorably close, often severing the infant's only source of pulmonary or systemic blood flow. The mechanisms causing closure of the ductus arteriosus are not completely understood but involve decreased prostaglandins and increased blood oxygen. Prostaglandin levels in the blood decrease at birth as a result of removal of their placental source of production from the circulation and increase in perfusion of the lungs, where prostaglandins are metabolized.

Foramen Ovale

Functional closure of the foramen ovale occurs soon after birth, largely as a result of increased left atrial volume and pressure secondary to the increased pulmonary venous return, the ductal left-to-right shunt, and the developing differences in diastolic pressure of the two ventricles. Anatomic closure normally is delayed for months or years. Among infants with cardiac defects, lesions with increased right atrial pressure favor indefinite patency of the foramen ovale (e.g., pulmonary stenosis), but abnormally increased left atrial pressure promotes early anatomic closure (e.g., ventricular septal defect). Before birth, the pulmonary arterioles are relatively muscular and constricted.

Pulmonary Vasculature

With the first breath, total pulmonary resistance falls rapidly because of the unkinking of the vessels with expansion of the lungs and because of the vasodilatory effect of inspired oxygen. The muscular constriction relaxes, and gradually, during the subsequent days and weeks, the muscular wall of the pulmonary arterioles thins. During the first weeks of life, the muscular arterioles retain a significant capacity for constriction. Pulmonary alveolar hypoxia normally produces an increase in pulmonary artery pressure at all ages, but in the young infant, the response is more profound and occurs more rapidly. Therefore, pulmonary hypertension equal to or greater than systemic pressure occurs commonly in neonates with severe respiratory disease.

Ventricular Work

Before birth, the two ventricles share in supplying systemic blood flow and placental flow, and after birth, the two ventricles sequentially and independently handle the entire cardiac output. At birth, the volume of blood to be pumped by the right ventricle decreases to the level of the systemic blood flow; right ventricular pressure falls as a result of the decrease in pulmonary resistance and closure of the ductus arteriosus. Although right ventricular work decreases, left ventricular work increases (Fig. 33–2). At birth, the left ventricle abruptly becomes the sole supplier of systemic blood flow, and the volume that it pumps is fractionally increased. The left-to-right shunt through the ductus arteriosus adds further volume work, and the elevated systemic resistance must be overcome. Although this is a stressful time for the left ventricle, the magnitude of these suddenly acquired burdens is not so great that detectable left ventricular difficulties are seen normally, but any impairment of myocardial function may be magnified as a consequence. Myocardial disease as a cause of symptoms is more common in the first days of life than

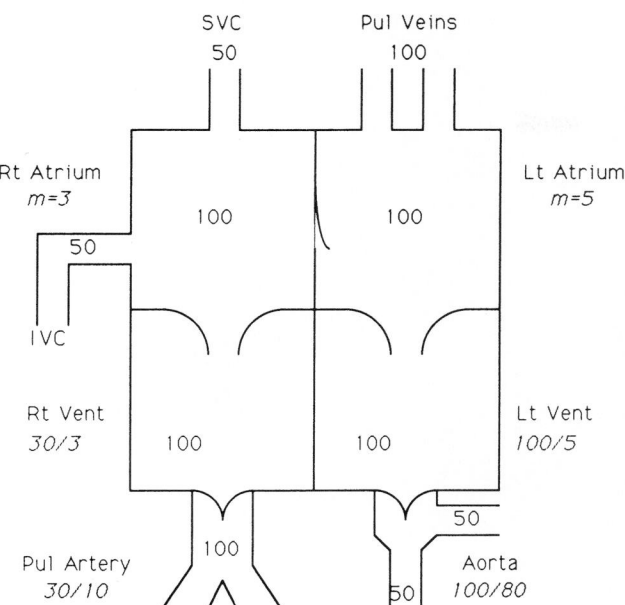

FIG. 33–2. Mature circulation is in series, and the amount of blood carried by the two ventricles is approximately the same as before birth. The lungs carry an amount equivalent to the cardiac output, as does the ascending aorta. The numbers inside the diagram represent relative blood flow (mL); the numbers in italics are pressure measurements.

at any other time during infancy; 25% of infants with myocardial disease presented in the first week of life (4).

Myocardial Function

Important changes occur in the fetus and neonate in many aspects of myocardial biochemistry and structure. These include myocyte size and number, microvascular structure, myocyte utilization of lactate and fatty acids, and antioxidant systems. Many structures and proteins involved in calcium handling within the myocyte, such as t-tubules, sarcoplasmic reticulum, Na^+–Ca^{2+} exchange, Ca^{2+}-ATPase, and phospholamban, have important developmental changes. These changes influence the effects on ventricular rhythm and function of normal development, prematurity, ischemia, cardioplegia, and various inborn errors of metabolism (41).

Fetal Echocardiography

High-resolution two-dimensional ultrasound evaluation of the fetal heart is a useful and accurate technique in the diagnosis and management of the fetus at risk for structural or functional cardiac abnormalities. Indications for prenatal echocardiography may include maternal, fetal, and genetic considerations (Table 33–6). The opti-

TABLE 33–6. *Indications for fetal echocardiography*

Suspected cardiac malformation on general ultrasound
Other malformations noted on general ultrasound
Oligo- or polyhydramnios
Fetal dysrhythmia
Suspected or known chromosomal abnormality
Family history of congenital heart disease
Family history of chromosomal abnormality
Maternal diabetes
Maternal collagen vascular disease
Rubella exposure
Evidence of hydrops fetalis
Intrauterine growth retardation
Maternal drug exposure, including:
    Lithium
    Hormones
    Anticonvulsants
    Chemotherapy
    Alcohol

mal time for performing fetal echocardiography is 18 to 24 weeks of gestation. At this age, the fetal heart is usually large enough for detailed anatomic evaluation, and the images are unimpaired by dense rib or spine calcification. There is also a relatively large volume of amniotic fluid that facilitates imaging from a variety of angles. For accurate diagnoses the examiner must be experienced in the technical aspects of fetal ultrasonography and knowledgeable in the anatomic patterns and physiologic consequences of congenital heart defects (42).

Cardiac Anatomy

Virtually all major cardiac malformations can be detected prenatally using high-resolution two-dimensional, real-time sector scanning by an experienced examiner (43). The details of systemic and pulmonary venous connections, arterial alignment, chamber size and orientation, and valve position and function can be determined (Fig. 33–3) and abnormal structures demonstrated (Figs. 33–4 and 33–5).

Cardiac Physiology

Color Doppler provides a quick and sensitive means of evaluating the function of atrioventricular and semilunar valves, the direction of flow in fetal vessels, and the presence of normal and abnormal connections (Fig. 33–5). If abnormal flow is detected, it can be evaluated further using the quantitative capabilities of pulsed or continuous-wave Doppler.

Cardiac Function

A qualitative assessment of cardiac function is obtained by visual inspection of ventricular motion dur-

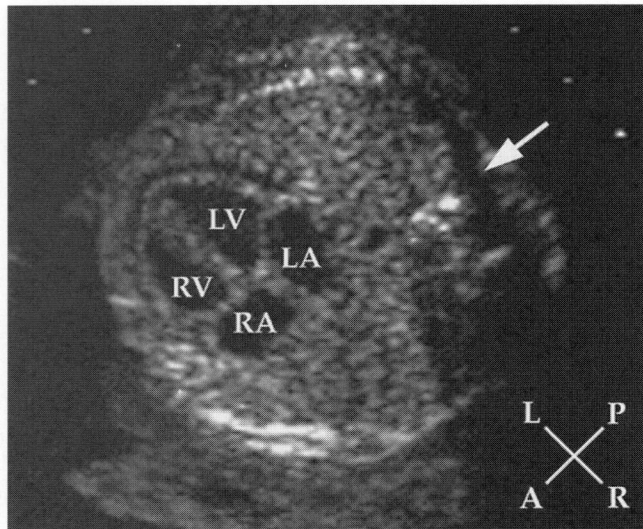

FIG. 33–3. Echocardiogram of the normal fetal heart in a four-chamber view demonstrating the position of the heart and the cardiac chambers in a cross-section of the chest. A, anterior; L, left; LA, left atrium; LV, left ventricle; P, posterior; R, right; RA, right atrium; RV, right ventricle; *arrow* denotes the spine.

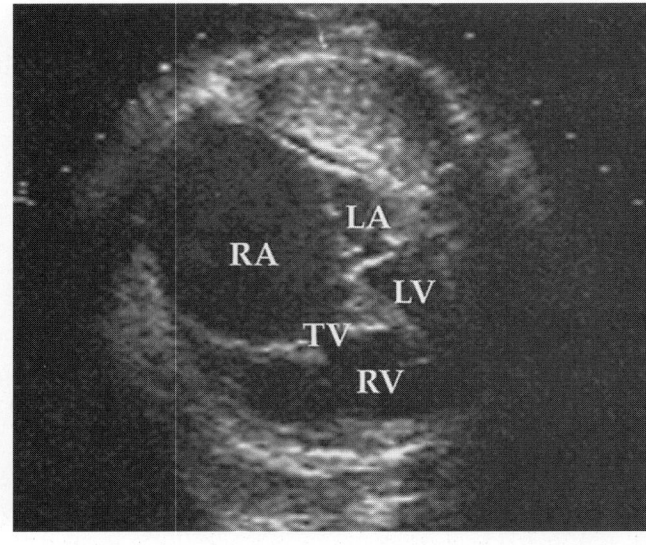

FIG. 33–4. Echocardiographic cross-sectional views of the fetal chest in an infant with Ebstein anomaly of the tricuspid valve. The right atrium (RA) is markedly dilated and fills much of the thorax. The left atrium (LA) and left ventricle (LV) are of normal size but are dwarfed by the right-sided structures. The severely regurgitant tricuspid valve has apical displacement of the septal leaflet into the right ventricle (RV).

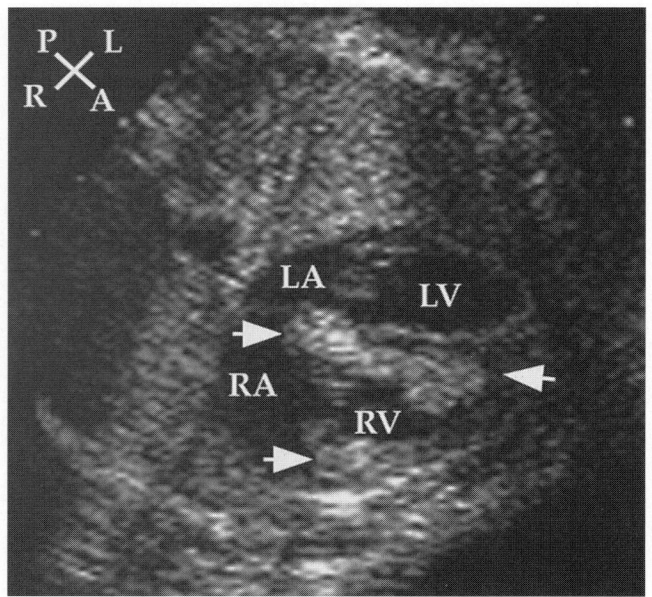

FIG. 33–5. Echocardiographic cross-sectional view of a fetus with multiple intramyocardial rhabdomyomas *(arrows)*. The infant was subsequently diagnosed with tuberous sclerosis. A, anterior; L, left; LA, left atrium; LV, left ventricle; P, posterior; R, right; RA, right atrium; RV, right ventricle.

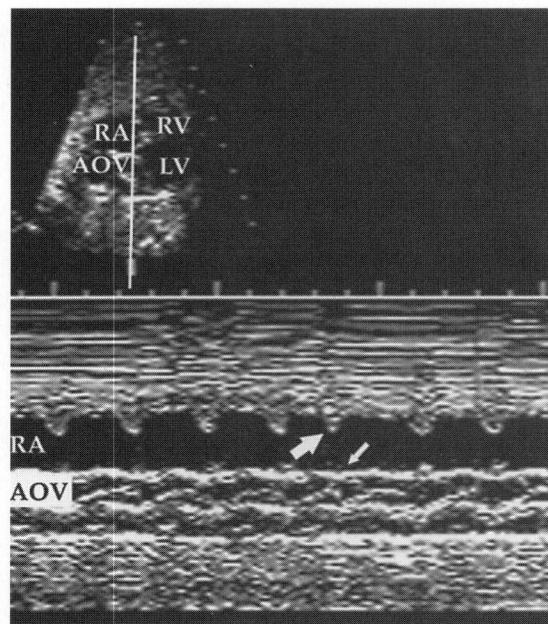

FIG. 33–6. Echocardiogram of a fetus with a premature atrial beat. The upper left image is a two-dimensional view with a cursor *(line)* through the fetal right atrium (RA) and aortic valve (AOV), demonstrating the axis of the simultaneous M-mode echocardiogram seen in the lower panel. The M-mode tracing depicts the motion of the fetal right atrial wall and aortic valve in the cursor line over a time frame of 3 seconds. A series of normal atrial wall contractions are interrupted by a premature contraction *(large arrow)* followed by opening of the aortic valve *(small arrow)*, demonstrating a premature atrial beat conducted to the ventricle. LV, left ventricle; RV, right ventricle.

ing real-time sector scanning. When more quantitative information is desired, M-mode recording can provide precise dimensions and an accurate measure of ventricular shortening (Fig. 33–6). Severe ventricular dysfunction may manifest as generalized hydrops fetalis, which is readily recognized by ultrasound as pleural and peritoneal fluid accumulation and cutaneous edema.

Arrhythmias

Tachyarrhythmias, bradyarrhythmias, and irregular cardiac rhythms are common reasons for referral for evaluation. Structural and functional abnormalities should be excluded, as described above. The mechanism of the rhythm disturbance can usually be elucidated using an M-mode tracing, which simultaneously displays the motion of an atrial wall and a semilunar valve (Fig. 33–6). By this means, the timing and sequence of atrial and ventricular activation can be deduced. The most common rhythm disturbance is isolated premature atrial contractions in a structurally normal heart or in association with an atrial septal aneurysm. Sustained tachyarrhythmia usually represents a reentrant or ectopic atrial tachycardia. These infants must be monitored closely for the development of congestive heart failure and hydrops fetalis, which would be an indication for induced delivery of the mature fetus or maternal antidysrhythmic therapy in the immature fetus. Sustained bradyarrhythmias may be secondary to heart block, nonconducted premature atrial contractions, or noncardiac sources of fetal distress. The mechanism can be inferred as described above and appropriate therapy initiated if indicated (see Arrhythmias).

PREMATURITY

The circulatory adjustments and myocardial biochemical changes at birth and in the neonatal period are modified in direct relation to the degree of prematurity. The muscular coat of the pulmonary arterioles develops late in gestation; the more premature the infant, the less muscular are the pulmonary arterioles at birth. The most notable consequence of this is that the difference between systemic and pulmonary resistance after birth is greater among premature than among normal infants. Shunting through a ductus arteriosus is often audible. Developmental biological factors in the ductus arteriosus and hypoxia, so common among premature infants, may be factors that contribute to the delay in closure of the ductus in premature infants. The propensity of the ductus to close at around 41 weeks after conception is clinically recognized. Developmental changes in myocardial structure and biochemistry may influence the function of the left ventricle in response to stress such as volume overload associated with the left-to-right shunt through a patent ductus arteriosus.

RECOGNITION OF CLINICAL FEATURES

Only a few infants are born in hospitals equipped for all eventualities. Infants with serious heart anomalies require transportation to a specially equipped and staffed cardiac center, detailed diagnostic assessment with echocardiography, and treatment, including cardiac catheterization and/or surgery. Timely clinical recognition of the likely presence of a specific cardiac anomaly, that without intervention will result in serious deterioration of the baby's condition (e.g., critical coarctation of the aorta, pulmonary valve atresia), is necessary for initiation of medical therapy to prevent and/or reverse clinical deterioration (e.g., administration of prostaglandin, inotropic agents, oxygen, and ventilation) and thereby provide the time and conditions necessary to transfer, evaluate, and treat the baby.

Initial evaluation includes assessment for cyanosis and of the infant's well-being, perfusion, pulses and blood pressure in the extremities, respiratory work and rate, precordial activity, second heart sound splitting, and murmur intensity, quality, pitch, and timing. Chest radiograph and electrocardiogram (ECG) remain cost- and time-efficient tests that aid in the initial evaluation of suspected congenital heart disease (44). Either one of these alone is rarely diagnostic. A number of lesions result in cyanosis; quite a number of lesions are also associated with loud murmurs; others are associated with little or no murmur; some cause shock (see Figs. 33–7 and 33–8). Others have chest radiographs with increased pulmonary arterial or venous markings, others have diminished pulmonary vascular markings. Most have an undistinguished electrocardio-

TABLE 33–7. *Top five diagnoses presenting at different ages*

Diagnosis	Percentage of patients
Age on admission: 0–6 days (n = 537)	
D-Transposition of great arteries	19
Hypoplastic left ventricle	14
Tetralogy of Fallot	8
Coarctation of aorta	7
Ventricular septal defect	3
Others	49
Age on admission: 7–13 days (n = 195)	
Coarctation of aorta	16
Ventricular septal defect	14
Hypoplastic left ventricle	8
D-Transposition of great arteries	7
Tetralogy of Fallot	7
Others	48
Age on admission: 14–28 days (n = 177)	
Ventricular septal defect	16
Coarctation of aorta	12
Tetralogy of Fallot	7
D-Transposition of great arteries	7
Patent ductus arteriosus	5
Others	53

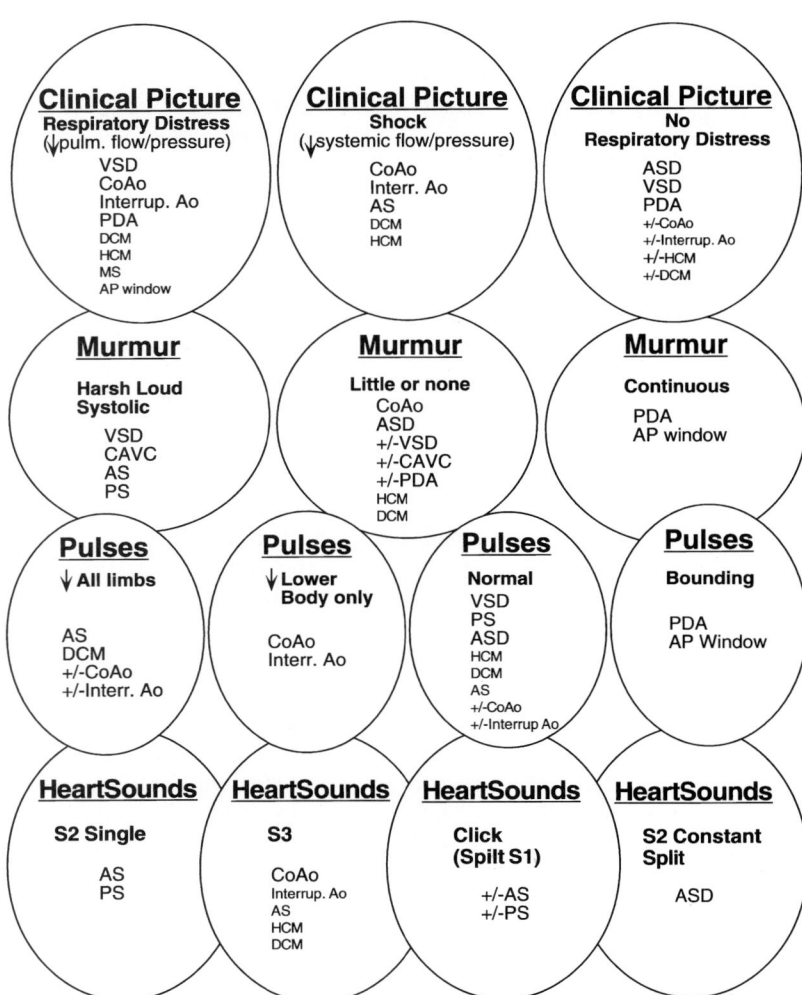

FIG. 33–7. The differential diagnosis of cardiac exam findings in acyanotic neonates. Anomalies in *larger print* are more common. +/-, sometimes; *up arrow,* increased; *down arrow,* decreased; AP window, aorticopulmonary window; AS, aortic stenosis; ASD, atrial septal defect; CAVC, complete atrioventricular canal defect; CoAo, coarctation of the aorta; DCM, dilated cardiomyopathy; HCM, hypertrophic cardiomopathy; Interrup. Ao, interrupted aortic arch; MS, mitral stenosis; PDA, patent ductus arteriosus; PS, pulmonary stenosis; VSD, ventricular septal defect.

gram at birth, while some have left axis deviation on electrocardiogram (see Figs. 33–9 and 33–10). Most cardiac anomalies vary in their characteristics at presentation. Furthermore, often it is not possible to determine with certainty if the second heart sound is split or not, or if the pulmonary vascular markings on chest radiograph are normal versus increased or normal versus decreased. Clinical analysis requires weighting of the categories of evidence as to its certainty and other possibilities. A classical diagnostic approach based on sequential analysis of data categories is limited by these types of weakness in the clinical information and is no stonger than the weakest link in the chain of information. However, interweaving of the findings provides a matrix of diagnostic information that remains intact even when one category of findings is weak. Overlapping the anomalies consistent with the clinical presentation with the anomalies consistent with the murmur findings, other physical exam findings, chest radiograph findings, and electrocardiographic findings, usually focuses the list of possible anomalies on one or two primary choices (see Fig. 33–11). The comparison of

possible anomalies suggested from history, physical examination, chest radiograph and electrocardiogram, as if with a series of Venn diagrams (see Figs. 33–7, 33–8, and 33–9), provides information that allows a careful observer to quickly determine which anomaly, or which two or three possible anomalies, is likely present. This may provide an important advantage in the timely and efficient management of potentially life threatening anomalies. For example, the combination of cyanosis, soft or no murmur, single S_2, chest radiograph with decreased pulmonary vascular markings and normal heart size, and electrocardiogram R axis of 50° suggests pulmonary atresia, which is an anomaly in which life depends upon maintaining ductal patency (see Figs. 33–8 and 33–10). Two-dimensional echocardiogram should be obtained promptly if significant cardiac disease is suspected. This technique when done by personnel trained for evaluation of congenital cardiac anomalies in neonates accurately demonstrates the anatomy, occasionally uncovering a potentially lethal lesion before symptoms. Appropriate initial management (e.g., infusion of PGE_1 in a cyanotic infant suspected to

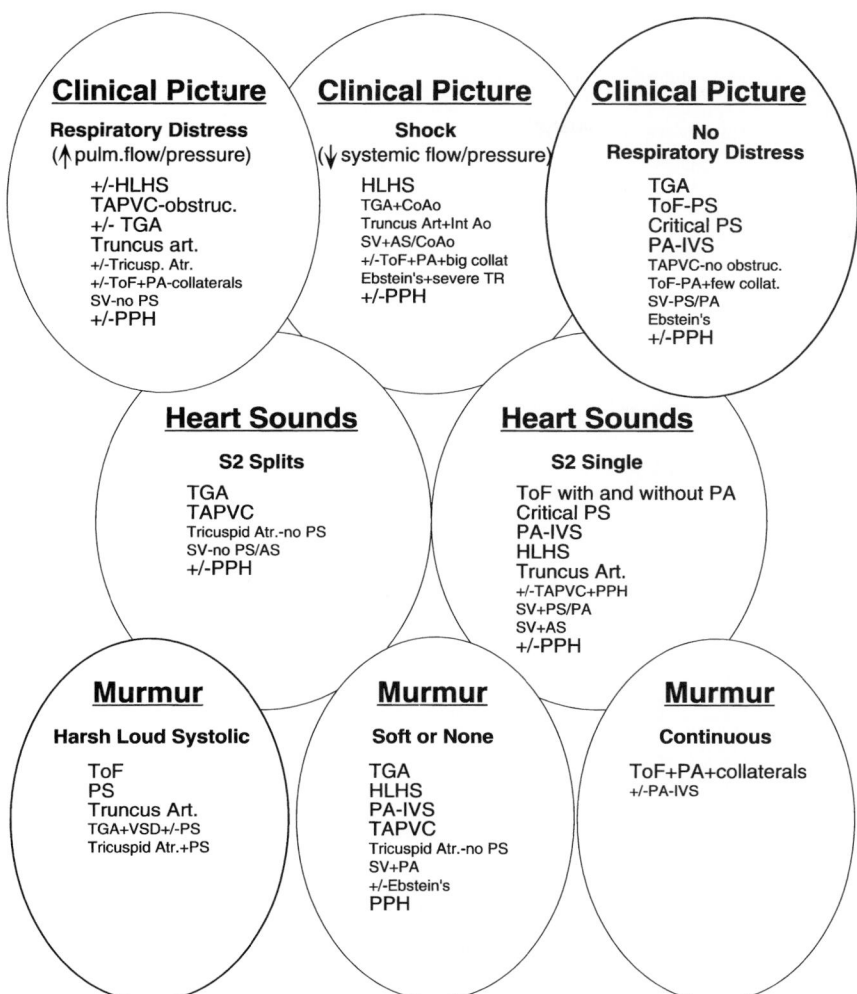

FIG. 33–8. The differential diagnosis of cardiac exam findings in cyanotic neonates. +/–, sometimes; *up arrow,* increased; *down arrow,* decreased; AS, aortic stenosis; CoAo, coarctation of aorta; collat., systemic to pulmonary artery collateral vessels; Ebstein's, Ebstein anomaly of the tricuspid valve; HLHS, hypoplastic left heart syndrome; Int Ao, interrupted aorta; PA, pulmonary atresia; PA-IVS, pulmonary atresia with intact interventricular septum; PPH, persistent pulmonary hypertension syndrome; PS, pulmonary stenosis; SV, single ventricle; TAPVC, totally anomalous pulmonary venous connection; TGA, transposition of great arteries; ToF, tetralogy of Fallot; tricuspid atr., tricuspid atresia.

have pulmonary atresia) need not await availability of echocardiography (see Management Procedures for Severe Cardiac Disease).

Age of Presentation

In New England, 35% of all those presenting with critical congenital cardiac disease in the first year of life were admitted to a treatment center within the first week of life (8). It is clinically useful to keep in mind the usual time of presentation of infants with various cardiac anomalies (Table 33–7). Although ventricular septal defect is by far the commonest congenital heart lesion discovered in neonates, transposition of the great arteries, coarctation of the aorta, and the hypoplastic left heart syndrome are the most common life-threatening anomalies presenting in the first week of life (see Table 33–2). Among those whose problem is cyanosis, transposition of the great arteries is the leading cause for admission through the third week of life; after that time, tetralogy of Fallot becomes the dominant cause of cyanosis for the

rest of childhood. Among neonatal cardiac patients admitted because of respiratory symptoms, the hypoplastic left heart syndrome is the leading cause in the first week, complex coarctation leads in the second week, and thereafter, ventricular septal defect becomes the main cause for symptomatic admission (see Table 33–6).

Physical Examination

Respiratory Symptoms

Persistent tachypnea may be the first clue to heart disease or lung disease. Cardiac abnormalities with excessive pulmonary arterial flow or pulmonary venous hypertension cause pulmonary vascular engorgement, pulmonary edema, and decreased lung compliance, often resulting in increased respiratory effort and rate. Cardiac anomalies with decreased pulmonary blood flow often have intense cyanosis that elicits a reflex "peaceful" tachypnea without respiratory distress. Grandmothers and multiparas often observe that the affected baby had

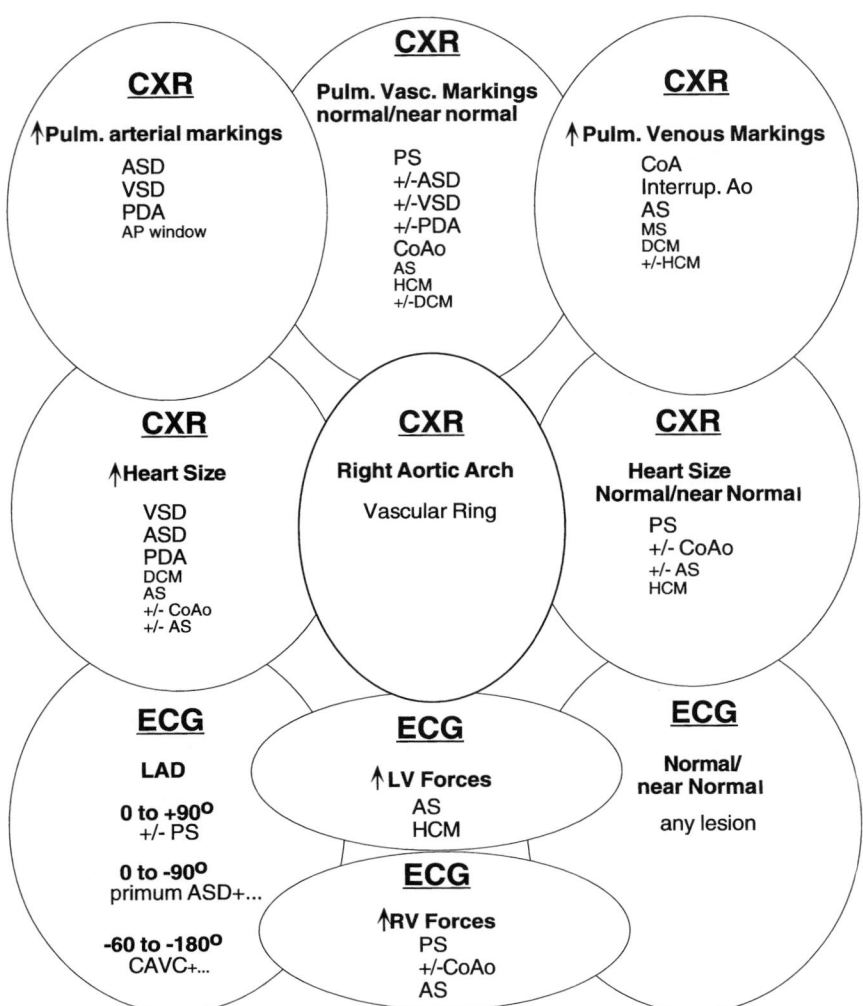

FIG. 33–9. The differential diagnosis of chest radiographic and electrocardiographic findings in acyanotic neonates. Abbreviations, see Fig. 33–7; CXR, chest X-ray; LAD; left axis deviation; LV, left ventricle; Pulm. vasc. markings, pulmonary vascular markings; RV, right ventricle.

always breathed too fast. Persistent respiratory rates of 60 per minute or greater, often with minimally labored but persistently increased depth of respiration, commonly precede other findings and may presage clinical deterioration. A chest radiograph may differentiate cardiac from pulmonary disease.

Systemic Perfusion and Pressure

Decreased systemic cardiac output is an ominous sign that requires rapid assessment and rapid appropriate management for the infant to survive. There are many potential noncardiac causes, the most common being sepsis, and important cardiac causes (see Figs. 33–7 and 33–8). Signs of diminished systemic perfusion include poorly perfused, cool, and/or mottled skin, listlessness, diminished peripheral pulse intensity, diminished systolic and pulse pressure, decreased urine output, and metabolic acidosis. Blood pressure should be measured in all four extremities in an infant who appears severely ill with these signs, particularly with coexistence of a murmur or cyanosis. Blood pressure can be quickly, noninvasively, and fairly accurately measured with an oscillometric device. It is very important to establish if the perfusion and blood pressure are diminished throughout the body or only in the postductal arterial distribution, that is, if the right arm blood pressure is similar to or higher than that in the other extremities. The latter situation is diagnostic of an aortic obstruction. The additional presence of a murmur, gallop, hepatomegaly, or cyanosis strongly suggests that a cardiac anomaly is causative.

Murmur

Hearing a murmur is the most common means of recognizing the presence of heart disease in an infant. Determining the diagnosis requires ascertaining the characteristics of the murmur. These include the history of the baby's age when the murmur was first audible and examination findings of murmur timing in systole versus dias-

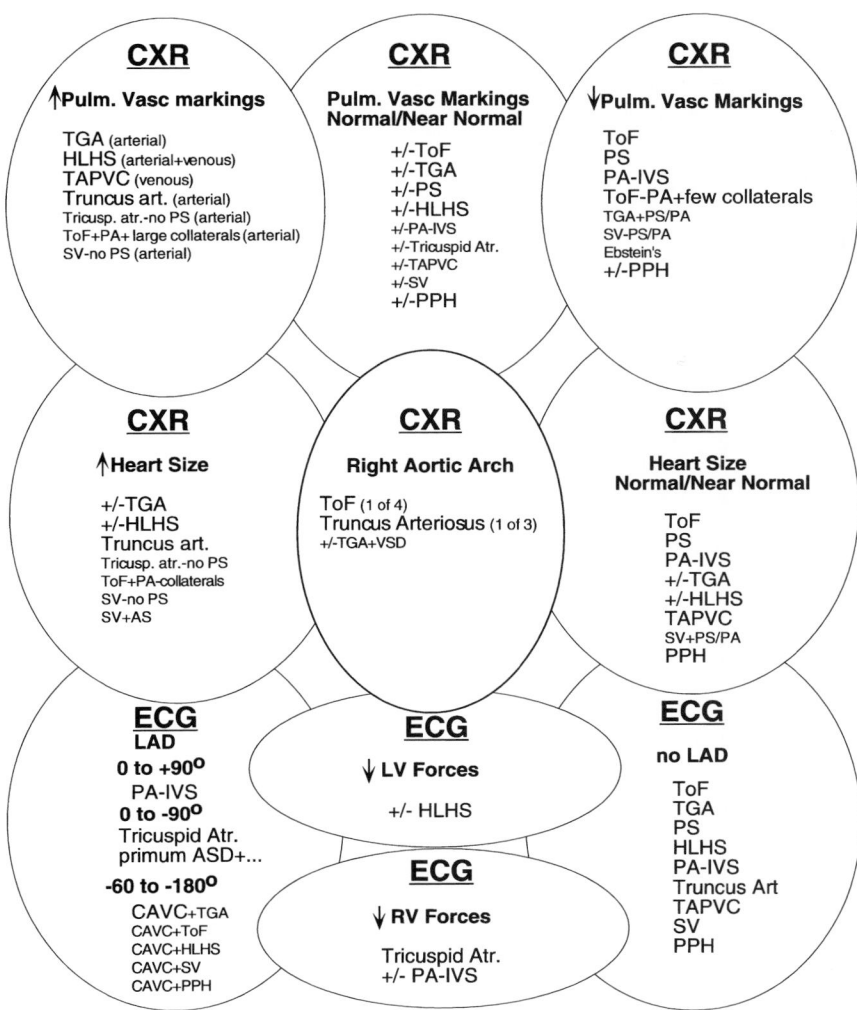

FIG. 33–10. The differential diagnosis of chest radiographic and electrocardiographic findings in cyanotic neonates. Abbreviations, see Figs. 33–8 and 33–9.

tole, loudness, pitch and the association of a thrill. The murmurs of valvar regurgitation and stenosis are audible immediately after birth, and the murmurs of septal defects are usually delayed days to weeks, or as long as several months in the case of atrial septal defects. Diastolic murmurs are rare but indicative of cardiac pathology. A prominent continuous murmur in a cyanotic neonate is also rare but is very characteristic of tetralogy of Fallot with pulmonary atresia and systemic-to-pulmonary-artery collateral vessels (the latter being the cause of the murmur). The loudness of a murmur, in combination with other findings, may suggest the likelihood of various anomalies but is often not proportional to the severity of the lesion. The absence of a murmur does not preclude serious heart disease. To the contrary, many life-threatening cardiac anomalies may be associated with little or no murmur. In a neonate with cyanosis and/or shock and suspected cardiac anomaly, the presence of little or no murmur provides a diagnostic clue (see Figs. 33–7 and 33–8). The pitch of a murmur is associated with

the pressure gradient across the abnormality causing the murmur. Tiny ventricular septal defects develop a characteristic fairly high-pitched murmur when the right ventricular pressure decreases to much less than the left ventricular pressure. Severe pulmonary or aortic stenosis can sometimes be distinguished from mild stenosis by a high-pitched harsh loud murmur and an associated thrill.

Heart Sounds

Auscultation of the heart sound splitting is the most difficult part of the cardiac examination in neonates because of the relatively rapid heart and respiratory rates in neonates. However, when abnormalities of the first and second heart sounds are strongly suspected or excluded, it provides important information. Detection of splitting of the heart sounds requires practice and a minute or so of focused attention on just that sound, using a quality stethoscope, in a quieted baby. The absence of splitting may result from a heart rate too fast

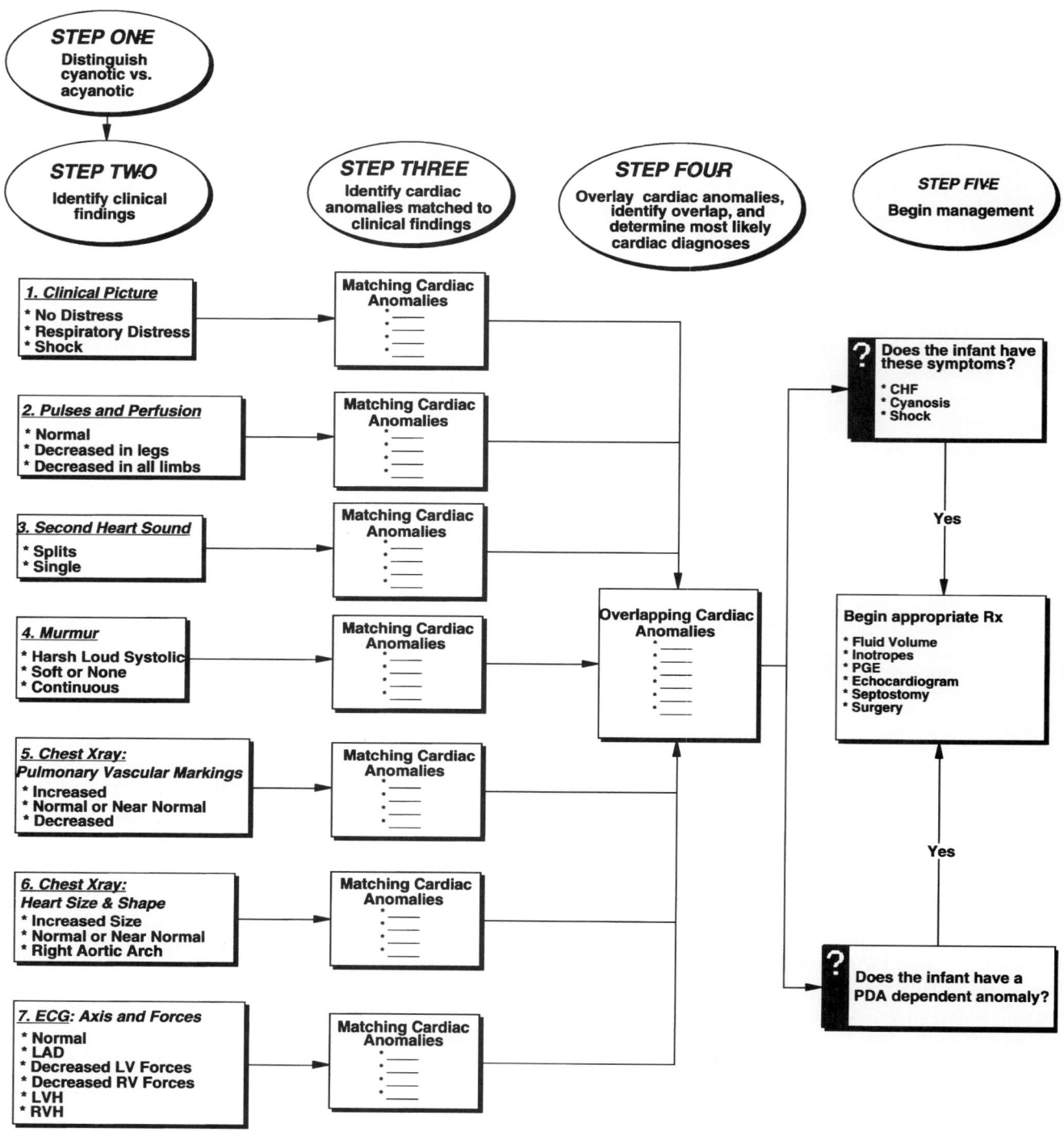

FIG. 33–11. A process for diagnosing cardiac anomalies from findings on cardiac exam, chest radiograph, and electrocardiogram. ASAP, as soon as possible; c/w, consistent with; F$_I$O$_2$, fractional percentage of inspired oxygen; PDA, patent ductus arteriosus.

to discern splitting or a truly single-component sound. A split first heart sound in a neonate suggests a click. The second heart sound emanates from closure of the aortic and pulmonary valves. Determining that the second heart sound is split (i.e., has two components) suggests that both aortic and pulmonary valves are not severely abnor-

mal; that is, it is against the presence of aortic or pulmonary valve atresia or severe stenosis. However, other serious anomalies with two semilunar valves may still be present, for example, simple transposition of the great arteries. A second heart sound that always appears single, particularly at heart rates not greater than 120 per minute, may be caused by relatively early pulmonary valve closure associated with elevation of pulmonary artery pressures comparable to aortic pressures, but it suggests that the pulmonary or aortic valve may be abnormal (as in pulmonary atresia or critical stenosis, hypoplastic left heart syndrome, truncus arteriosus). Although difficult to detect, constant splitting of the second heart sound, as opposed to the usual intermittent splitting, suggests a atrial septal defect.

Cyanosis

Much more threatening than a murmur is the presence of cyanosis. Cyanosis without pulmonary disease is almost invariably the result of a serious cardiac abnormality. Cyanosis may result from poor mixing of separate parallel circulations (e.g., transposition of the great arteries, other anomalies with transposition physiology such as Taussig–Bing-type double-outlet right ventricle); restricted pulmonary blood flow and right-to-left shunting of unoxygenated systemic venous blood to the systemic arterial circulation (e.g., tetralogy of Fallot, critical pulmonary stenosis, tricuspid atresia); or right-to-left shunting from intracardiac mixing with normal or increased pulmonary blood flow (e.g., total anomalous pulmonary venous connection without obstruction, truncus arteriosus, single ventricle without pulmonary stenosis, hypoplastic left heart syndrome). Especially in the first week of life, cyanosis may be the sole evidence of an important cardiac lesion. One-third of infants with potentially lethal congenital heart disease have cyanosis as their major symptom; another one-third have cyanosis associated with respiratory symptoms. Prompt cardiac evaluation of all cyanotic babies is mandatory because prompt infusion of prostaglandin E_1 to open the ductus arteriosus or catheter intervention to create an atrial septal defect may be necessary for survival, and most of the responsible lesions are amenable to surgery.

The clinical recognition of cyanosis is dependent on the amount of oxygen desaturation of arterial hemoglobin and therefore is influenced by the total blood hemoglobin concentration. An anemic infant may have severe arterial oxygen unsaturation without obvious cyanosis, and infants with polycythemia may appear cyanotic with normal arterial oxygen levels. Hypothermic infants may seem blue; babies viewed in fluorescent lighting may appear blue; and blue surroundings may make the estimation of cyanosis more difficult. Persistent cyanosis secondary to hypoglycemia or methemoglobinemia is rare. Cyanosis is particularly evident in the lips. Perioral or nailbed cyanosis without lip cyanosis is usually not caused by cyanotic heart disease. When cyanosis is suspected, indirect assessment of arterial oxygen saturation by the transcutaneous method can provide a rapid noninvasive check.

Acute Lung Disease and Cardiac Disease

Rapid determination of the diagnosis and initiation of appropriate management is most pressing when the infant is dyspneic and cyanotic. A chest radiograph may suggest lung disease, particularly if the findings are asymmetric. In the presence of diffuse symmetric changes possibly compatible with pulmonary edema or increased vascular markings, caution is necessary, particularly in the full-term neonate. The differential diagnosis between primary lung disease and heart disease causing pulmonary edema (e.g., total anomalous pulmonary venous connection with obstruction) can be difficult. Persistent pulmonary arterial hypertension with right-to-left shunting may coexist with lung disease and cause severe cyanosis. Although carbon dioxide retention is usually prominent among babies with primary lung disease, some severely cyanotic infants with cardiac anomalies can have marked hypercarbia. It can also be difficult to differentiate cardiac anomalies with diminished pulmonary blood flow and little murmur (e.g., pulmonary valve atresia) from persistent pulmonary arterial hypertension without other, radiographically apparent, lung parenchymal disease. Although the absence of hypercarbia suggests cardiac disease, some severely cyanotic infants with pulmonary vascular disease have normal PCO_2 values. A time-honored test has been the response of the arterial PO_2 to administration of 100% oxygen. With the exceptions noted below, the infant who responds to breathing pure oxygen with a marked rise in arterial PO_2 to 220 mm Hg or more has lung disease, and the infant who does not raise his preductal arterial PO_2 above 100 mm Hg is likely to have heart disease. Transcutaneous estimation of arterial oxygen saturation is not an accurate alternative because any arterial PO_2 greater than 70 mm Hg will result in an arterial oxygen saturation greater than 95%. Because the hyperoxia test is inconclusive when the arterial PO_2 is between 100 and 220 mm Hg, these babies should be approached as possibly having cyanotic heart disease (see Fig. 33–12). The arterial PO_2 while the baby is breathing 100% oxygen may initially be most rapidly measured from an umbilical artery catheter positioned in the descending aorta. A low arterial PO_2 measured in the descending aorta may be the result of right-to-left shunting through a ductus arteriosus with coexisting persistent pulmonary hypertension. Comparison of the PO_2 measured in blood from the right radial artery with the PO_2 measured in blood from the umbilical arterial catheter may help to differentiate persistent pulmonary hypertension from cyanotic cardiac anomaly. The former may have a high PO_2 in the right radial artery. Simultaneous mechanical hyperventilation and administration of oxygen may decrease pulmonary resistance and increase pulmonary flow, increasing the PO_2 to greater than 220 mm Hg in the descending aortic and/or right radial arterial blood, allowing differentiation of lung disease or persis-

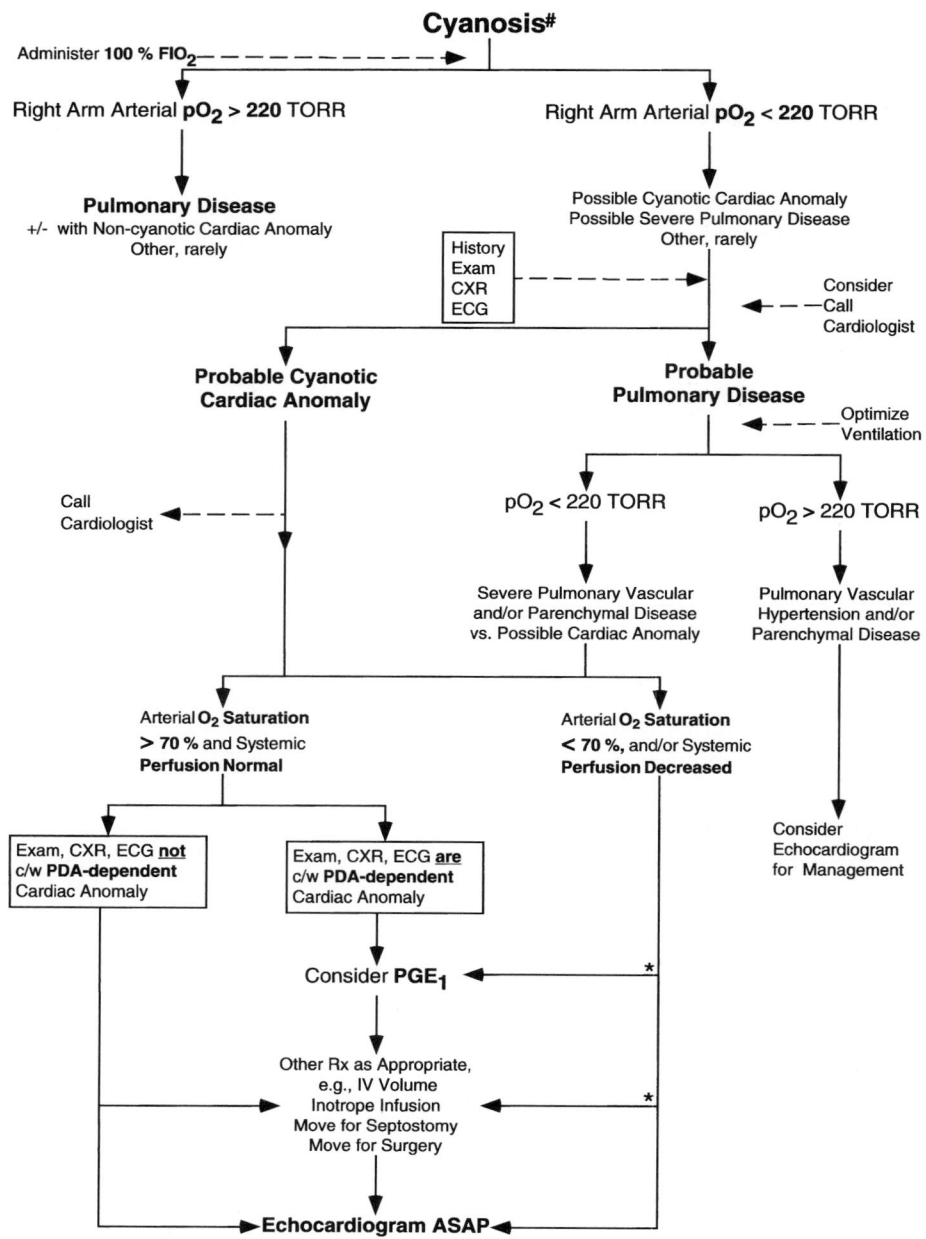

FIG. 33–12. An approach to the diagnosis and management of cyanotic infants. #, cyanosis; see text for additional details of assessment of cyanosis; +/-, possibly; *, see text concerning management of specific anomalies; ASAP, as soom as possible; c/w, consistent with; F₁O₂, fraction inspired oxygen; Rx, treatment.

tent pulmonary hypertension from cyanotic cardiac anomaly. Difficulties arise when pulmonary and cardiac pathology coexist. For example, in the baby with both lung and heart disease or those with coexistence of persistent pulmonary hypertension and predominant right-to-left shunting through the foramen ovale (see Chaps. 27 and 29) or the baby with heart disease causing pulmonary venous hypertension and pulmonary edema, results may be confusing. Arterial PO_2 often does not significantly increase in response to 100% oxygen with persistent pul-

monary hypertension and predominant right-to-left shunting through the foramen ovale. If doubt persists, the physician can make the diagnosis with two-dimensional echocardiography (see Fig. 33–12).

Noncardiac Anomalies

It is useful to know the relative frequency of the cardiac diagnostic possibilities among low-birth-weight babies (see Table 33–2) and among those who have other anomalies (see Tables 33–4 and 33–5). Among premature infants, patent ductus arteriosus, coarctation of the aorta, and ventricular septal defect occur more often. Chromosomal abnormalities and congenital syndromes are also associated with cardiac malformations (e.g., Down syndrome).

DIAGNOSTIC TOOLS

Chest Radiography

Chest radiography is rarely diagnostic of specific cardiac lesions, but it is a relatively quick and relatively inexpensive method to screen for suspected cardiac anomaly (44). Although chest radiographs may appear normal or near normal in the first day or days of life with many of the cardiac anomalies, the presence of cardiomegaly, increased pulmonary arterial or venous markings, diminished pulmonary arterial markings, or right aortic arch may provide important information as to the presence of a cardiac anomaly. In combination with other physical exam findings, chest radiographic findings may provide important information concerning the possible presence of specific cardiac anomalies that may aid in early management before an echocardiogram can be obtained. The heart size should be differentiated from the thymic shadow. Cardiomegaly is indicated by a cardiothoracic ratio greater then 0.6 in an anterior–posterior projection in the presence of an adequate inspiration. The aortic arch position can be assessed, even in the presence of a large overlying thymus, by deviation of the trachea to the opposite side. A chest radiogram may provide important information to differentiate lung disease from cardiac disease. Important associated noncardiac anomalies may be discovered by radiographic findings, for example, coexistent lung pathology, heterotaxy (asplenia syndrome, malrotation), absence of the thymus gland (DiGeorge syndrome), vertebral anomalies (VACTERL association), and abnormal sternal ossification (Down syndrome).

Electrocardiography

Electrocardiography is most valuable in neonatal cardiology in the diagnosis and management of arrhythmias. Anomalies associated with significant ventricular hypertrophy in later infancy often have findings difficult to differentiate unambiguously from normal in the neonate. Most anomalies do not have axis deviation; however, when axis deviation is present, the electrocardiogram is helpful in diagnosis and may provide a timely advantage in management (see Figs. 33–9 and 33–10).

Echocardiography

Examination of the heart by two-dimensional echocardiography with color Doppler ultrasound allows excellent analysis of the intracardiac anatomy in small infants (45). Neonates are particularly good candidates for echocardiographic imaging because they are less active and have excellent echocardiographic imaging windows. Detailed segmental examination from subxiphoid, parasternal, apical, suprasternal notch, and additional modified views as necessary delineates almost all relevant cardiac anatomy and anomalies in most neonates. The situs, ventricular relationship, great artery relationships, systemic and pulmonary venous cardiac connections, atrial and ventricular septum, valve structure, great artery anatomy and coronary origins can be accurately determined. Color Doppler visualizes the presence and direction of blood flow in patent ductus arteriosus, septal defects, systemic venous anomalies, and arteriovenous malformation. Pulsed and continuous-wave Doppler techniques enable estimation of physiologic measurements such as the pressure gradient across stenotic valves, septal defects, and patent ductus arteriosus (see Fig. 33–13). In the common case of tricuspid regurgitation, right ventricular peak systolic pressure may be estimated by Doppler measurement of the magnitude of the pressure gradient between the right ventricle and right atrium and the addition of the right atrial V-wave pressure, whether assumed or directly measured through an umbilical vein catheter (usually 3 to 10 mm Hg) (see Fig. 33–14). Right ventricular systolic pressure relative to left ventricular pressure can also be qualitatively assessed by the curvature of the interventricular septum. Contrast echocardiography with injection of agitated saline or albumin into intravenous or umbilical artery catheters can sometimes serve as a useful adjunct to color Doppler in detection of shunts.

The ventricular systolic performance, size, and wall thickness can be assessed. The shortening fraction of the left ventricular internal short-axis dimension is the most commonly used measurement to assess left ventricular systolic function. The shortening fraction measures left ventricular performance, which is a function of contractility, afterload, preload, and heart rate. Contractility can be independently assessed by measuring the relationship of end-systolic wall stress velocity to fiber shortening using directed M-mode echocardiography, indirect central pulse tracing, and phonocardiography. This technique is impaired when right ventricular hypertension results in flattening of the interventricular septal curvature in systole.

Echocardiography has limitations. Because complete examination of cardiac anatomy in neonates is labor intensive and requires expensive additional technology, the cost is generally equivalent to that of a computerized tomography or magnetic resonance scans. The evaluation has often been unsatisfactory when performed where the use of echocardiography to recognize heart disease in neonates is infrequent and echocardiographic transducers with frequencies appropriate for infants are not available. Training and performance standards for echocardio-

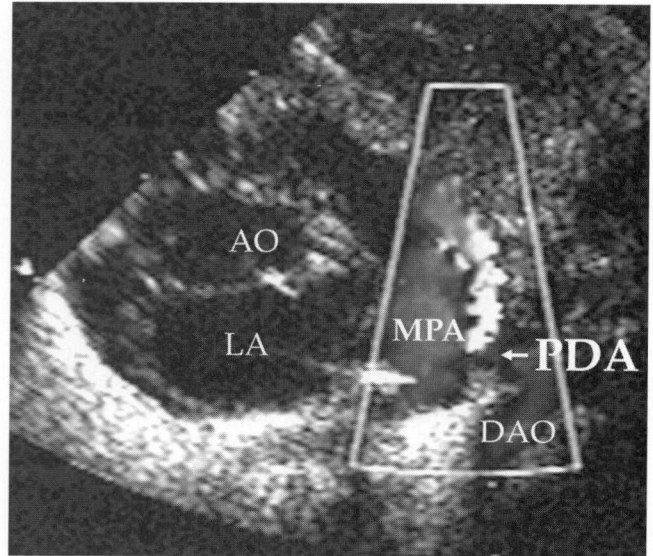

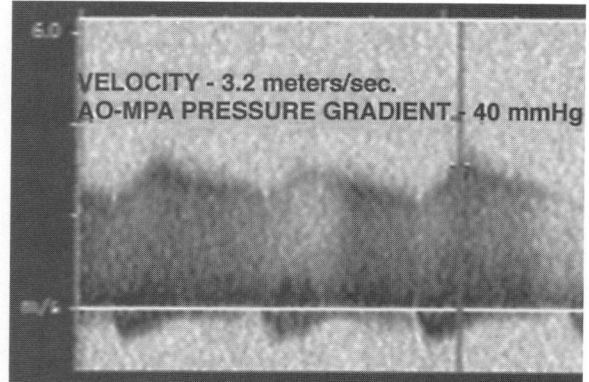

FIG. 33–13. A: Echocardiographic parasagittal parasternal view of a patent ductus arteriosus. Doppler analysis demonstrates flow away from the transducer within the pulmonary artery and aortic isthmus and, in white, a jet of flow toward the transducer through the patent ductus arteriosus into the pulmonary artery. **B:** Quantification of the velocity of the flow jet through the ductus arteriosus with a continuous-wave Doppler technique and application of the Bernoulli principle allows the aortic-to-pulmonary-artery systolic pressure gradient to be measured. The pressure gradient by this technique is 4 × (maximum instantaneous velocity)². The pulmonary artery peak systolic pressure can be estimated by the difference in the arterial systolic pressure and the pressure gradient across the ductus arteriosus. AO, aorta; DAO, descending aorta; LA, left atrium; MPA, main pulmonary artery; PDA, patent ductus arteriosus.

be best to transport the infant to the nearest center for echocardiographic examination. If personnel adequately trained in performing a complete study for congenital heart disease are available, it may be possible to send or transmit a tape of the examination for a second opinion.

Diagnostic Cardiac Catheterization and Angiography

Anatomy

Catheterization is rarely used to learn the basic anatomy of the heart. The diagnostic information necessary for most cardiac surgical procedures in neonates is now obtained noninvasively by echocardiography. Diagnostic cardiac catheterization is used to provide specific data unavailable through echocardiography that are useful in planning man-

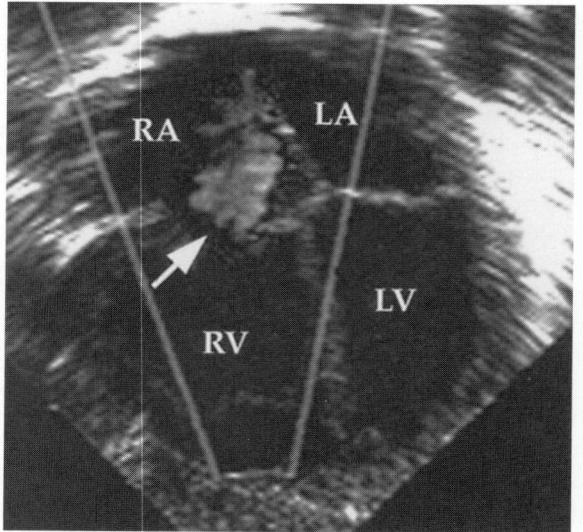

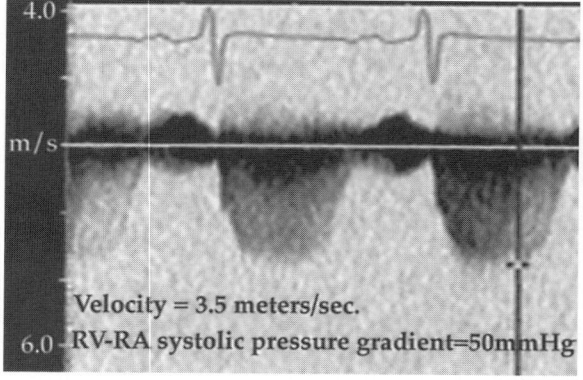

FIG. 33–14. A: Echocardiographic apical four-chamber view in systole. Doppler analysis of the right heart demonstrates tricuspid regurgitation *(arrow)*. **B:** Continuous-wave Doppler technique quantified the velocity of the regurgitant jet near the arrow in the upper panel. Application of the Bernoulli principle allows the right-ventricle-to-right-atrial peak pressure gradient to be measured and estimation of the right ventricular pressure. LA, left atrium; LV, left ventricle; RA, right atrium; RV, right ventricle.

graphic examination of congenital heart disease in fetuses and children have been disseminated (42,46). Cases of delayed transfer of babies because of erroneous diagnoses of inoperable congenital heart disease and erroneous reassurance that there is no significant lesion have been encountered. With limited experience in the diagnosis of congenital heart disease in neonates, it may

agement (47). What is the anatomy of the pulmonary arteries and systemic-to-pulmonary collaterals in the patient with tetralogy of Fallot and pulmonary atresia? Is catheter closure of the collaterals possible? What is the anatomy of the coronary arteries in the patient with pulmonary atresia and intact interventricular septum? What is the anatomy of the coronary arteries with tetralogy of Fallot or transposition where abnormality is suspected and/or echocardiographic imaging is nondiagnostic? In selected patients with cardiomyopathy, light and electron microscopic analysis of ultrastructural anatomy and biochemical analysis of myocardium obtained by biopsy may provide a diagnosis. In many situations diagnostic catheterization may be safer or more useful after initial palliative surgery, such as in hypoplastic left heart syndrome or following shunt procedures in those with complex intracardiac anomalies and pulmonary atresia.

The decision to perform a cardiac catheterization should be guided by a careful assessment of the long-term benefits in management and risk reduction versus the risk of the procedure. Before catheterization the medical condition is optimized for the anomalies present and the rapidity with which catheterization may provide critical information to further stabilize the situation. Infants with a duct-dependent anomaly are best managed with an infusion of prostaglandin E_1, begun before and continued throughout the catheterization. In the first week of life, death within 48 hours of catheterization is 15 times greater than in the fourth week of life. The risk of the catheterization procedure itself is difficult to estimate because of the high natural mortality rates associated with the lesions encountered and the association of cardiac catheterization with cardiac surgery. The potential for procedural difficulty is undeniably greater in the sick newborn (47). If only unequivocally demonstrable damage to the infant is counted, we estimate the mortality rate directly attributable to cardiac catheterization to be 1% to 2% in the neonatal period. Morbidity, such as blood loss, hypothermia, metabolic and respiratory acidosis, arrhythmia, electrolyte imbalance, hypoglycemia, thrombosis of femoral arteries, and angiographic myocardial stains, occurs during these studies and influences the outcome of subsequent cardiac surgery.

Hemodynamic Measurements

Hemodynamic data obtained by catheterization can now largely be deduced from noninvasive measurements of blood pressure, oxygen saturation, and echocardiographic Doppler measurements of pressure gradients. More direct measurement does not help neonatal surgical management of most anomalies. When catheterization is done for delineation of anatomy as outlined above, these data can be readily obtained and may help in the understanding of the clinical status and in medical management. Alternatively, information from implanted catheters may be useful for management of sick babies in the intensive care unit. Catheters in the right atrium placed through an umbilical vein, systemic vein, or transthoracically in the operating room may be used to obtain central venous pressure and blood oxygen saturation. These data can be used to infer preload and adequacy of cardiac output and, in combination with blood pressure measurements, to infer relative afterload. Catheters in the pulmonary artery, placed transthoracically at surgery or transvenously, can be used to measure left-to-right shunts and to measure pulmonary pressure to titrate pulmonary vasodilators.

The hemodynamic principals for these calculations are based on Ohm's law and the Fick principle (see Table 33–8) (47). The former, when applied to hemodynamics, is: the pressure drop across a vascular bed equals the product of the flow and resistance across it. Therefore, the resistance equals the difference of the arterial and venous pressure divided by the flow. The flow can be calculated from the Fick principal, which is based on the premise that oxygen delivery to the body equals oxygen consumption by the body. Oxygen consumption is routinely measured in

---

TABLE 33–8. *Hemodynamic calculations*

O_2 consumption = O_2 delivery
$\qquad$ = $Q \times$ (arterial O_2 content – venous O_2 content)

Blood O_2 content (mL/L) = Hgb (g/dl) $\times$ 10 (dL/L) $\times$ 1.36 (ml O_2/g Hgb) $\times$ Hgb O_2 Sat.
Average neonate O_2 consumption = 200–220 mL/min/m^2

Q_s (L/min/m^2) = O_2 consumption/Hgb $\times$ 13.6 $\times$ (arterial O_2 Sat. – venous O_2 Sat.)
Q_p (L/min/m^2) = O_2 consumption/Hgb $\times$ 13.6 $\times$ (pulm. venous O_2 Sat. – pulm. arterial O_2 Sat.)

$$Q_p/Q_s = \frac{\text{(arterial } O_2 \text{ Sat. – venous } O_2 \text{ Sat.)}}{}$$

ΔP (mmHg) = $Q \times R$ (Woods units)
R_s = Q_s/(arterial mean pressure – RA mean pressure)
R_p = Q_p/(pulm. arterial mean pressure – LA mean pressure)

Q, cardiac output or blood flow; Hgb, blood hemoglobin concentration; Sat., saturation; Q_s, systemic flow or cardiac output; Q_p, pulmonary flow; ΔP, arterial mean pressure minus arterial atrial mean pressure; pulm., pulmonary; R, vascular resistance; R_s, systemic vascular resistance; R_p, pulmonary vascular resistance.
From ref. 37.

the catheterization laboratory and, in the intensive care unit, can be assumed to be 200 to 240 mL/min/m² in neonates (48). Oxygen delivery is the product of flow and the arterial–venous oxygen content difference. Arterial and venous oxygen contents are calculated from the products of the measured blood oxygen saturations and blood hemoglobin concentration and the hemoglobin oxygen-carrying capacity (1.36 mL O²/g hemoglobin). Systemic and pulmonary flow can be calculated as in Table 33–8. In those without a hemodynamic shunt, cardiac output can be measured by the thermodilution method.

Magnetic Resonance Imaging

Magnetic resonance imaging can detect intrathoracic structures, such as peripheral pulmonary arteries, systemic-to-pulmonary collateral vessels, and the aortic arch, that often are not adequately imaged by echocardiography. Use of the available diagnostic tools in conjunction with the history and physical examination enables precise diagnosis without resorting to diagnostic cardiac catheterization in most neonates.

MANAGEMENT PROCEDURES FOR SEVERE CARDIAC DISEASE

An infant in difficulty in the first days of life because of heart disease has the potential for rapid deterioration. Too often, the baby looks as though he will survive but is near death hours later. The earlier symptoms appear, the faster deterioration can take place. By the time the infant has reached 1 or 2 months of age, concern about sudden shifts in status is less warranted.

Infants who present with severe cyanosis in the first days to weeks of life may do so because right ventricular outflow is critically obstructed and pulmonary blood flow is compromised by a closing ductus arteriosus, or because the great arteries are transposed and require a ductus arteriosus for adequate mixing of the pulmonary and systemic circulations. Babies with congestive heart failure in the first week of life often have obstructed left ventricular or aortic outflow, with descending aortic flow supplied by a closing ductus arteriosus. In these babies, survival may depend on persistent patency of the ductus arteriosus; dependency should be suspected, and prostaglandin E_1 therapy considered. If possible, echocardiography should be used to confirm a specific anatomic diagnosis, but this may not be available in many primary care facilities, and the infant's condition may not provide the time before starting treatments to transport to a facility where echocardiography is available. If a duct-dependent anomaly is suspected from physical examination, ECG, and chest radiograph (e.g., pulmonary atresia, hypoplastic left heart syndrome), or if the condition of a baby with undiagnosed cardiac anomaly is significantly worsening so that arterial oxygen saturation is <70%

(e.g., as in D-transposition of the great arteries or critical pulmonary stenosis) or there is severe congestive heart failure because of ductal closure (e.g., as in critical aortic stenosis or coarctation), prostaglandin E_1 therapy should be initiated even if echocardiography is not available (see Fig. 33–12). The usual starting dose of 0.1 µg/kg/min can frequently be reduced to 0.05 to 0.02 µg/kg/min after stabilization. The occurrence of relatively common side effects, particularly later-onset central apnea, vasodilation with hypotension, and fever should be anticipated. Endotracheal intubation should be performed prior to transport in infants receiving prostaglandins, to reduce the risk should apnea occur.

Despite prostaglandin therapy, these critically ill infants may have low cardiac output that may respond to the correction of common metabolic perturbations including hypothermia, intravascular hypovolemia, hypocalcemia, and hypoglycemia, but frequently, inotropic support is needed (Tables 33–9 and 33–10). Placement of an umbilical venous catheter may allow measurement of central venous pressure to guide fluid therapy and permit administration of concentrated infusions of dextrose, calcium, and vasoactive amines. Hyperventilation should be avoided in babies with certain lesions in which the pulmonary and systemic circulations are in parallel, such as hypoplastic left heart syndrome. Hyperventilation and oxygen administration in these babies can drop pulmonary vascular resistance to low levels, resulting in runoff into the pulmonary vasculature, systemic hypotension, and low output. After appropriate steps to correct contributing metabolic abnormalities, fluid can be given in 5- to 10-mL/kg doses until adequate response is achieved or circulatory congestion occurs. Infusion of dopamine or dobutamine (5 to 20 µg/kg/min) should be added to support pump function as needed. Higher doses or continuous infusion of epinephrine, amrinone, or isoproterenol can be considered to support refractory neonates until surgical palliation can be achieved. Digitalis preparations are much less desirable for acute inotropic support of critically ill infants who have variable renal and hepatic functions and electrolyte status.

The acyanotic cardiac infant who develops symptoms of increased respiratory work and poor feeding after 2 to 4 weeks of life often has congestive heart failure from decreasing pulmonary vascular resistance and increasing left-to-right shunt. Treatment with digoxin, diuretics, and, in refractory cases, systemic vasodilators is often indicated (see Table 33–9). Rarely, these infants have left-sided obstructive lesions or myocardial disease (e.g., anomalous left coronary artery) that requires different treatment (see below).

Therapeutic Catheterization

Infant cardiac catheterization has become a technical art demanding specific training and experience. Interven-

TABLE 33–9. *Common oral drugs for the treatment of congestive heart failure*

Genetic drug	Proprietary name	Form	Dose	Action	Toxicity
Digoxin	Lanoxin	Elixir: 50 μg = 0.05 mg/mL	Digitalizing dose: Premature, 20 μg/kg Term, 30 μg/kg Initial dose, $^1/_2$ In 6 h, $^1/_4$ In 12 h, $^1/_4$ Maintenance dose: Premature, 3–4 μg/kg/12 hr Term, 4–5 μg/kg/12 hr	Na–K ATPase inhibitor, increases contractility	Atrioventricular block (monitor ECG during loading), tachydysrhythmias, vomiting; use with caution in renal failure and myocarditis; decrease dose by one-half if used with quinidine
Furosemide	Lasix	Suspension: 10 mg/mL	1 mg/kg/12 hr PRN to 2.0 mg/kg/8 hr	Loop of Henle Cl-pump inhibition, diuretic	Hyponatremia, hypokalemia, hypochloremic alkalosis, nephrocalcinosis
Chlorothiazide	Diuril	Suspension: 10 mg/mL	10–15 mg/kg/12 hr	Blocks distal tubular Na reabsorption, diuretic	Hyponatremia, hypokalemia, hypochloremic alkalosis, hyperbilirubinemia, hyperuricemia, hyperglycemia
Spironolactone	Aldactone	Suspension: 5 mg/mL Tablet: 25 mg	1–3 mg/kg/d, $^1/_4$ tab–$^1/_2$ tab, crushed, qod–qd	Blocks tubular aldosterone receptor, diuretic	Hyperkalemia
Captopril	Capoten	Tablet: 12.5 mg, 25 mg	Term, 0.1–1.0 mg/kg/8 hr Preterm, 0.05–0.2 mg/kg/8–12 hr	Angiotensin-converting enzyme inhibition, decreases afterload	Hypotension, azotemia, proteinuria, may cause hyperkalemia when given with spironolactone or potassium; use with caution in low dose in premature neonates

TABLE 33-10. *Intravenous vasoactive drugs*

Drug	Dose (μg/kg/min)	Action	Preload	Systemic Resistance	Pulmonary Resistance	Contractility	Heart Rate	Use	Toxicity
Dopamine	2–5 5–20	D, β_1 D, β, α	+/−↓ ↓	+/−↓ ↓, ↑↑	0 ↑	↑ ↑↑	+/−↑ ↑↑	↑CO ↑BP	Tachycardia, dysrhythmias, necrosis with extravasation, ↓ renal blood flow at higher doses
Dobutamine	2–20	β_1, mild β_2, α	+/−↓	↓	↓	↑↑	↑	↑CO	Tachycardia, dysrhythmias, necrosis with extravasation
Epinephrine	0.05–1.0	α, β_1, β_2	↓, ↑	↓, ↑↑	↓, ↑	↑↑↑	↑↑↑	↑CO, ↑BP, ↑HR	Tachycardia, dysrhythmias, necrosis with extravasation, ↓ renal blood flow
Isoproteronol	0.05–2.0	β_1, β_2	↓	↓↓	↓	↑↑↑	↑↑↑	↑CO, ↑HR	Marked tachycardia, dysrhythmias, hypotension when volume depleted
Amrinone	5–10 (load: 1.0 mg/kg)	Phosphodiesterase inhibition	↓	↓↓	↓, ↑↑	↑	0	↑CO	Thrombocytopenia, dysrhythmias
Nitroprusside	0.5–5	EDRF-like action	↓↓	↓↓↓	↓	0	↑	↑CO, ↓BP	Hypotension, *V/Q* mismatch, thiocyanate toxicity
Nitroglycerin	1–5	EDRF-like action	↓↓↓	↓↓	↓	0	↑	↑CO, ↓preload	Hypotension, *V/Q* mismatch, methemoglobinemia
Phenylephrine	0.5–4.0	α	↑	↑↑↑	↑	+/−↑	+/−↓	↓TF, cyanotic spells	Cardiac output, ↓ renal blood flow

+/−, may or may not; ↓, decrease; ↑, increase; α, α-adrenergic; β, β-adrenergic; BP, blood pressure; CO, cardiac output; D, dopaminergic; EDRF, endothelial-derived relaxing factor; HR, heart rate; TF, tetralogy of Fallot; *V/Q*, pulmonary ventilation–perfusion ratio.

tions now commonly performed on neonates in the catheterization laboratory include balloon atrial septostomy by Rashkind technique for transposition of the great arteries, creation of an atrial septal defect in mitral atresia or hypoplastic left heart syndrome with restrictive atrial communication using Brockenbrough atrial puncture and balloon dilation, pulmonary and aortic valvuloplasty, pulmonary artery angioplasty, angioplasty of discrete aortic coarctation with otherwise normal caliber aortic arch, and closure of systemic-to-pulmonary arterial collateral vessels (47,49–52). To perform a therapeutic procedure and to extract vital diagnostic information with the least danger to the patient requires vigilance against a multitude of treacherous pitfalls and a finely honed sense of the clinical cost and benefit of each maneuver contemplated. The neonate undergoing study is ill, often critically ill, and may have a widely fluctuating physiologic state. Before catheterization the baby is medically stabilized as best possible as dictated by the baby's anomalies, condition, and the rapidity with which catheterization may be required to further stabilize the situation. Duct-dependent infants are managed with an infusion of prostaglandin E_1 (53,54). Careful and constant attention to maintenance of proper thermal environment, minimization of blood loss, vascular access and hemostasis, anticoagulation, metabolic status, respiratory status, and catheter manipulation optimizes the outcome.

Surgery

Heart disease in neonates is often life threatening and requires surgery. Early recognition, safe transport to a cardiac center, accurate diagnosis, and an experienced surgical team are needed for success. Anesthesiologists familiar with the problems of neonatal cardiac patients and a well-equipped intensive care unit with trained personnel contribute to successful management of these babies. The postoperative care requires fine adjustment of blood volume, body temperature, fluid and electrolyte balance, oxygenation, ventilation, and hemodynamic measurements. Close cooperation between the cardiologists, intensivists, and surgeons responsible for the care of these infants is mandatory. (See also Chap. 34.)

The timing of surgical intervention depends on the anatomic diagnosis and the likelihood of success. Only neonates who are in danger of death are candidates for immediate cardiac surgery.

In the past, there were two schools of thought concerning surgical management of infants critically ill with heart disease. The older view was that a life-saving, palliative operation should be done in infancy, followed months or years later with a reparative operation. This concept is being challenged by the conviction that single-stage repair should be used if possible. The justification for this view is the demonstrably acceptable mortality, avoidance of the double jeopardy of two cardiac opera-

tions, and increasing evidence that early repair results in improved cardiac status and neurologic function (12,55). Recent mortality data continue to support single-stage repair.

CYANOTIC LESIONS

The differential diagnosis of cyanotic heart disease includes many disorders (Table 33–11). Lesions usually associated with decreased pulmonary flow include the tetralogy of Fallot, pulmonary stenosis, tricuspid atresia, pulmonary atresia with intact ventricular septum, and Ebstein disease. Cyanotic lesions usually associated with increased pulmonary vascular markings include D-transposition of the great arteries, hypoplastic left heart syndrome, total anomalous pulmonary veins, truncus arteriosus, and single ventricle.

Anomalies with Cyanosis Caused by Separate Transposed Systemic and Pulmonary Circulations: D-Transposition of the Great Arteries

With transposition of the great arteries, the aorta arises from the right ventricle and the pulmonary artery from the left ventricle. In the most common form, D-transposition, the aorta is anterior to and to the right of the pulmonary artery rather than in its normal rightward and posterior position.

Transposition of the great arteries is one of the most common congenital heart lesions presenting in the newborn period (see Tables 33–1 and 33–2) and is a frequent cause of death among unoperated neonates with congenital heart disease. The male–female ratio is 1.8:1, and the average birth weight is greater than that for other patients with congenital heart disease, although not for the general population. Transposition is associated with other cardiac abnormalities, including ventricular septal defect, patent ductus arteriosus, pulmonary valve stenosis, hypoplastic right ventricle, and coarctation.

Pathophysiology

The systemic and pulmonary circulations are normally in series with each other, but in complete transposition, the circulations are in parallel. Systemic venous blood returns to the right atrium, enters the right ventricle, and exits through the aorta. Pulmonary venous blood, coming from the lung, enters the left atrium and the left ventricle, and then returns to the pulmonary arteries and the lungs. Without some communication between the pulmonary and systemic circulations, survival is impossible; oxygenated blood cannot be delivered to the systemic circulation, nor can systemic venous blood pick up oxygen in the lung. An atrial communication, ventricular defect, or patent ductus arteriosus, singly or in combination, may provide for mixing between the circulations (Fig. 33–15).

TABLE 33–11. *Differential diagnosis of cyanotic heart disease*

Diagnosis	Physical examination	Radiographic findings	Electrocardiographic findings
Hypoplastic left heart syndrome	Single S_2, ↑ respiratory work, ↓ pulse amplitude, ↓ perfusion, +/– SRM	↑ Pulmonary arterial markings, cardiomegaly	↓ LV force usually, develops RAE, RAD, RVH
Transposition of great arteries (IVS, VSD)[a]	Split S_2, +/– murmur, +/– ↑ respiratory work (*i.e.*, peaceful cyanosis)	↑ Pulmonary arterial markings, +/– cardiomegaly with narrow mediastinum (*i.e.*, "egg on a string")	Develops RAE, RAD, RVH
Truncus arteriosus	Split S_2, multiple clicks, soft to loud SEM, +/– DRM, ↑ respiratory work	↑ Pulmonary arterial markings, cardiomegaly	Develops RAE, RAD, BVH
Total anomalous pulmonary venous connection	Narrow S_2 split, +/– murmur, ↑ respiratory work	↑ Pulmonary venous markings, ↑ diffuse interstitial markings	Develops RAE, RAD, RVH
Tricuspid atresia			
Without PS	Split S_2, heave, SRM	↑ Pulmonary arterial markings, cardiomegaly	Left axis deviation
With PS	Single S_2, SEM	↓ Pulmonary arterial markings, +/– cardiomegaly	
Tetralogy of Fallot			
With PS	Single S_2, SEM	+/– ↓ Pulmonary arterial markings, +/– boot-shaped heart	Develops RAE, RAD, RVH
With PA	Single S_2 continuous murmur, LSB back, axillae	↑, ↓ Pulmonary arterial markings and heart size	
Pulmonary stenosis (IVS or SV)	Single S_2, click, SEM	↓ Pulmonary arterial markings	In IVS QRS axis 0°–100°, develops RAE, RAD, RVH
Pulmonary atresia (IVS or SV)	Single S_2, soft SRM	↓ Pulmonary arterial markings	In IVS QRs axis 0–80°, ↓ RV forces, +/– develops Q waves
Persistent pulmonary hypertension	Narrow split or single S_2, ↑ S_2 loudness, +/– SRM	↓ Pulmonary arterial markings, +/– parenchymal infiltrates, +/– cardiomegaly	Develops RAE, RAD, RVH

[a]Single ventricle is usually associated with transposition of the great arteries, and in the absence of PS or PA, it presents similar to transposition with ventricular septal defects.

+/–, may or may not be present; ↓, decreased; ↑, increased; BVH, biventricular hypertrophy; DRM, diastolic regurgitant murmur; IVS, intact ventricular septum; LSB, left sternal border; LV, left ventricle; PA, pulmonary atresia; PS, pulmonary stenosis; RAD, right axis deviation; RAE, right atrial enlargement; RV, right ventricle; RVH, right ventricular hypertrophy; SEM, systolic ejection murmur; SRM, systolic regurgitant murmur; SV, single ventricle; VSD, ventricular septal defect.

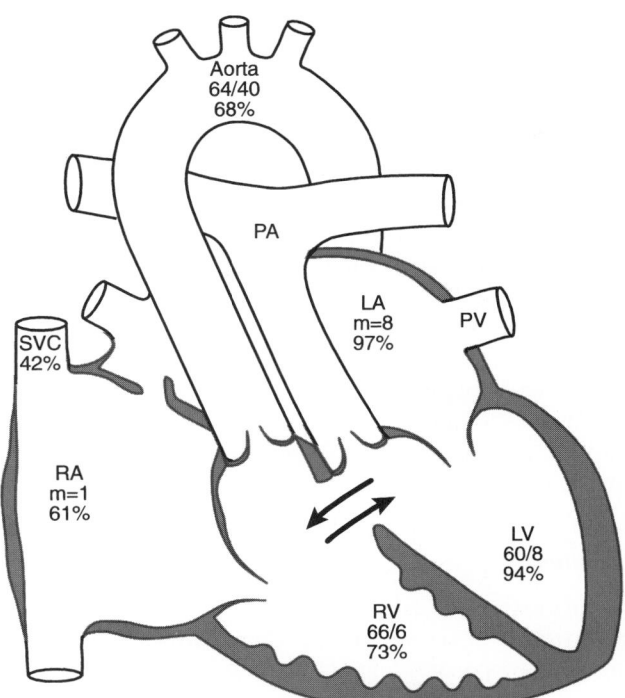

FIG. 33–15. Diagram of the anatomy and physiology of transposition of the great arteries with a single membranous ventricular septal defect in a 1-month-old baby who had mild cyanosis and controlled congestive heart failure. There is equilibration of pressure between the ventricles and elevation of left-sided diastolic pressures. After balloon septostomy, the arterial saturation rose to 75%. The numbers below the chamber name are pressure measurements (mm Hg) determined at cardiac catheterization; the percentages indicate oxygen saturation. LA, left atrium; LV, left ventricle; PA, pulmonary artery; PV, pulmonary vein; RA, right atrium; RV, right ventricle; SVC, superior vena cava. (Adapted from ref. 101.)

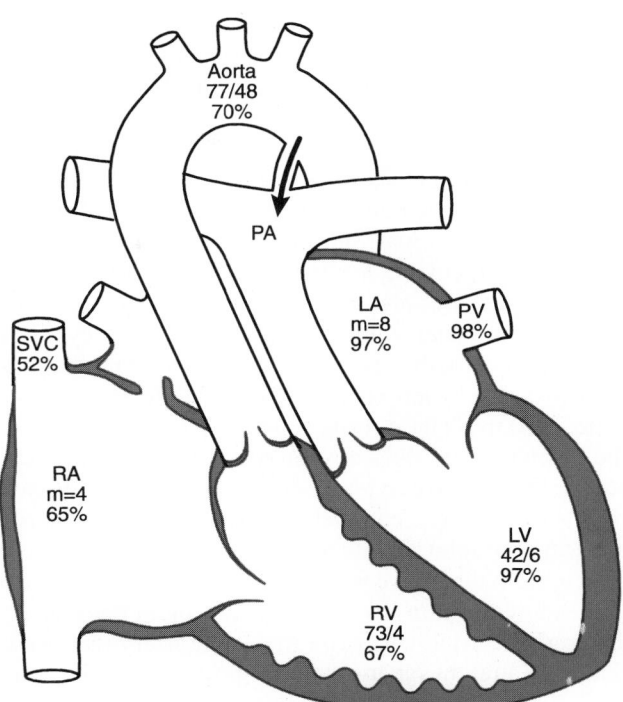

FIG. 33–16. Diagram of the anatomy and physiology of transposition with intact ventricular septum in a 1-day-old girl who was cyanotic at birth. At catheterization, she had less than systemic pressure in the left (i.e., pulmonary) ventricle. The patent ductus arteriosus shunts blood into the pulmonary circuit, and the foramen ovale shunts an equal amount out of the pulmonary circuit. If this were not the case, relative blood volume would shift to one side of the circulation in a matter of minutes. If the ductus spontaneously closed, the infant's condition would become precarious. If the ductus were dilated with prostaglandins, the infant would become pinker but might experience respiratory difficulty because of excess pulmonary flow. The numbers below the chamber name are pressure measurements (mm Hg) determined at cardiac catheterization; the percentages indicate oxygen saturation. LA, left atrium; LV, left ventricle; PA, pulmonary artery; PV, pulmonary vein; RA, right atrium; RV, right ventricle; SVC, superior vena cava. (Adapted from ref. 101.)

The foramen ovale and ductus arteriosus, both normally patent in the fetus, usually close soon after birth. Infants with transposition and intact ventricular septum become extremely cyanotic within the first few hours or days after delivery, as closure of the foramen ovale and ductus arteriosus occurs and mixing between the circulations diminishes (Fig. 33–16). The severe hypoxemia may lead to metabolic acidosis. Survival depends on prompt supportive medical care and reestablishment of patency of the ductus arteriosus and interatrial communication to improve mixing and oxygenation.

Infants born with transposition and a large ventricular septal defect are less cyanotic because the ventricular defect allows mixing. These babies may not be recognized in the newborn period but appear in subsequent weeks with congestive failure. The combination of a large pulmonary flow, pulmonary hypertension, and elevation of left atrial pressure leads to the development of congestive heart failure (see Fig. 33–15) and later pulmonary

vascular obstructive disease. Anatomic changes during the first few months of life may result in important hemodynamic changes. A large ventricular septal defect may spontaneously diminish in size or close, reducing mixing and increasing hypoxemia. Increasing pulmonary stenosis may decrease pulmonary flow and thereby increase cyanosis but improve congestive heart failure. Atrial septal defects created by balloon septostomy and those made by surgical septectomy may spontaneously diminish in size or close.

Clinical Findings

In infants with an intact ventricular septum, marked cyanosis accompanied by mild tachypnea develops soon after birth. Often the infants, though tachypneic, do not seem distressed (i.e., peaceful cyanosis). The cardiac examination, chest radiograph, and ECG may otherwise be normal. The heart sounds are normal (i.e., the second heart sound splits), and there may be no significant murmur. The ECG may show some excessive right ventricular forces. The heart and pulmonary vascularity may initially appear normal on chest radiograph, although cardiac enlargement, a narrow mediastinum, and pulmonary plethora are frequently present or develop. Because the usual clinical measures, besides cyanosis, can be unremarkable, one of the most important diagnostic tests is the hyperoxia test. Failure of the arterial PaO_2 (often <30 mm Hg in room air) to rise significantly after the inhalation of 100% oxygen for a 10-minute period is strong presumptive evidence for cyanotic heart disease, most commonly complete transposition. Subcostal echocardiography reveals the diagnosis. The great artery arising from the left ventricle has an abnormal course and then bifurcates into the right and left pulmonary artery. The right ventricle gives rise to a great artery that passes relatively straight superiorly to the posterior arching aorta (Fig. 33–17). Echocardiographic examination can also determine the patency of the foramen ovale and ductus arteriosus, the nature of associated anomalies, and the coronary anatomy relevant to the surgical arterial switch procedure.

An infant with transposition and a large ventricular septal defect usually presents with congestive failure and mild cyanosis, between 0 and 6 weeks of age. Poor weight gain, tachypnea, and excessive diaphoresis are common, and wheezing occurs in older infants. A loud systolic murmur is present maximally at the lower left sternal border, often associated with a middiastolic flow rumble. An S_3 may produce a gallop rhythm. Rales may be audible in the lungs. The ECG reveals right axis deviation and right atrial and right ventricular hypertrophy. Infrequently, if the right ventricle is hypoplastic, right ventricular forces may be absent or reduced, and left ventricular hypertrophy is present. The chest radiograph characteristically shows considerable cardiomegaly and pulmonary plethora. Echocardiography should identify the location of the ventricular septal defect and its relation to the great arteries and the atrioventricular valves and complex associated problems, including straddling or abnormal tricuspid valve, hypoplastic right ventricle, valvar or subvalvar pulmonary stenosis, coarctation of the aorta, juxtaposition of the atrial appendages, and anomalous systemic or pulmonary venous drainage.

Treatment

In those with established or suspected transposition with intact interventricular septum, prostaglandin E_1 is infused to open and maintain patency of the ductus arteriosus, to improve mixing and systemic oxygenation. Because prostaglandin E_1 may cause apnea and vasodilation, support with mechanical ventilation, volume infusion, and sometimes inotropic agents may be required. Some babies also require a widely open atrial defect for adequate oxygenation, and most do better with one. Balloon atrial septostomy usually results in considerable clinical improvement in those sick from severe cyanosis, and some require it promptly for survival (see Fig. 33–18). The anatomy of the coronary arteries and associated lesions may also be established by catheterization. The type of surgical procedure employed depends on the associated cardiac defects. "Anatomic repair" with an arterial switch operation has been demonstrated to be the procedure of choice in neonates with uncomplicated transposition (56,57). The aorta and pulmonary arteries are transected, and the distal vessels are rejoined to provide normal physiologic connections. A button of proximal aortic tissue surrounding each coronary artery origin is cut, and both coronaries with the surrounding aortic button are moved from the native transposed aorta and attached to the neoaorta. The ductus arteriosus is ligated, and the atrial septostomy is closed. Although a small number have difficulty with the coronary artery kinking, pulmonary artery compression, or anastomotic narrowing, the large majority do very well and lead essentially normal lives in childhood. Longer-term outcome is not yet known but appears promising. Midterm results are superior to the Senning and Mustard atrial baffle procedures that have frequent very serious long-term difficulties with right ventricular and tricuspid valve function and dysrhythmias (58).

Some with a ventricular septal defect but no atrial communication may require a patent ductus arteriosus

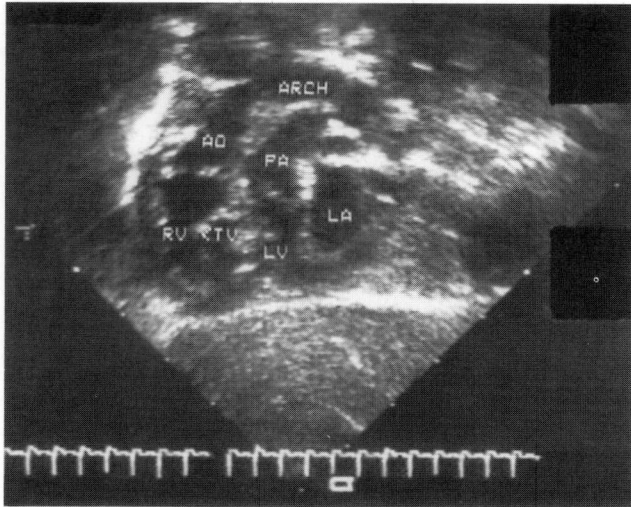

FIG. 33–17. Echocardiographic subxiphoid view of a neonate with transposition of the great arteries. (AO aorta; ARCH, aortic arch; LA, left atrium; LV, left ventricle; PA, pulmonary artery; RV, right ventricle; TV, tricuspid valve.)

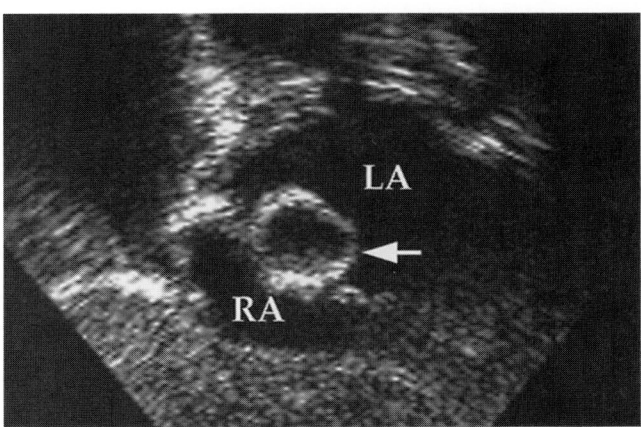

FIG. 33–18. Echocardiographic subxiphoid view demonstrating a balloon septostomy catheter with the inflated balloon *(arrow)* being pulled from the left atrium (LA) to the right atrium (RA) through the foramen ovale. This septostomy technique is used in neonates with transposition of the great arteries to create an atrial septal defect to increase intracardiac mixing of fully and incompletely oxygenated blood, thereby improving systemic oxygenation.

and balloon atrial septostomy for adequate circulatory mixing and oxygenation. Infants with transposition and isolated ventricular septal defect undergo arterial switch procedure and closure of the ventricular septal defect. The additional presence of significant pulmonary or aortic valvar or subvalvar stenosis can prohibit a straightforward arterial switch procedure. Severe pulmonary valve stenosis generally occurs with a large ventricular septal defect, and a Rastelli procedure or variation of it is done by placing a patch from the crest of the interventricular septum into the upper right ventricle to direct left ventricular blood to the transposed aorta and directing blood flow from the lower right ventricle to the pulmonary artery by interposition of a conduit (generally homograft) from a right ventriculotomy to the distal transected main pulmonary artery. The presence of native aortic valve stenosis can be dealt with by a modification of the Damus–Kaye–Stansel type in which left ventricular blood flow to the body is through anastomosis of the transected proximal main pulmonary artery to the ascending aorta, and pulmonary blood flow is through a conduit interposed between the right ventricle and distal main pulmonary artery. These procedures require revision of the surgically implanted conduits with growth and in the not infrequent occurrence of extrinsic compression. Without therapy, 95% of infants born with transpositions die within 1 year. With aggressive medical and surgical treatment, mortality is less than 10%.

Differential Diagnosis

Most infants with transposition and intact ventricular septum are readily recognized as cyanotic infants without

significant murmur and little respiratory distress. Often a split second heart sound can be distinguished on exam, and chest x-ray demonstrates cardiomegaly and increased pulmonary flow, helping to distinguish transposition from other lesions with cyanosis and little murmur, pulmonary valve atresia with intact interventricular septum, and total anomalous pulmonary venous connection. The diagnosis of transposition of the great arteries can be confused if other abnormalities, such as straddling tricuspid valve, hypoplastic right ventricle, coarctation of the aorta, or pulmonary stenosis, exist (see Table 33–11). Depending on the type and severity of the associated cardiac malformations, the clinical symptoms and findings in infants with complicated transposition of the great arteries may closely resemble those of almost any other cyanotic heart lesion.

The clinical picture in infants with transposition of the great arteries, ventricular septal defect, and pulmonary stenosis or atresia is virtually indistinguishable from that of tetralogy of Fallot or pulmonary atresia with a ventricular septal defect. If D-transposition of the great arteries is associated with a large ventricular septal defect and limited cyanosis, it is sometimes mistaken for other lesions with a large left-to-right shunt, such as a ventricular septal defect with normal aortic root or total anomalous pulmonary venous return without obstruction. The absence of cyanosis identifies the former, and echocardiography can differentiate all of these anomalies.

Anomalies with Cyanosis from Decreased Pulmonary Blood Flow

Tetralogy of Fallot

The tetralogy of Fallot is characterized by a large ventricular septal defect and infundibular pulmonary stenosis or pulmonary atresia. Both environmental factors and a number of genetic disorders are associated with tetralogy of Fallot. Many have microdeletions in a critical region of chromosome 22q11 (25,30). The primary anatomic pathologic abnormality appears to be anterior deviation of the upper part of the interventricular septum, known as the conal septum, that separates the anterior pulmonary outflow of the right ventricle from the subaortic left ventricular outflow. This results in the subaortic anterior malalignment ventricular septal defect and in the right ventricular infundibulum being hypoplastic and narrow. There is often considerable valvar pulmonary stenosis, hypoplasia of the pulmonary arteries, right ventricular hypertrophy, a relatively large ascending aorta, and a right aortic arch (25%). In infants with pulmonary atresia, pulmonary perfusion occurs by way of a patent ductus arteriosus or by systemic-to-pulmonary arterial collateral vessels. Five percent of patients have abnormal coronary distribution that may influence surgical correction. Tetralogy is one of the most common cyanotic congenital heart lesions presenting in the newborn period (see Tables 33–1 and 33–2) and is occasionally (10%) associated with severe extracardiac malformations.

Pathophysiology

Depending on the severity of right ventricular outflow obstruction, there may be intracardiac left-to-right flow or right-to-left shunt and hypoxemia. Pressures equalize between the ventricles through the large septal defect. The peripheral arterial oxygen saturation depends on the amount of systemic venous admixture and the absolute pulmonary flow (Fig. 33–19). The extent of systemic venous admixture, that is, right-to-left shunting of systemic venous blood away from the pulmonary outflow through the ventricular septal defect to the aorta, is directly related to the severity of the pulmonary stenosis and inversely related to the systemic vascular resistance. The amount of pulmonary blood flow depends on the amount of antegrade flow through the right ventricle outflow and the existence of alternative sources of flow (through a ductus arteriosus or systemic-to-pulmonary

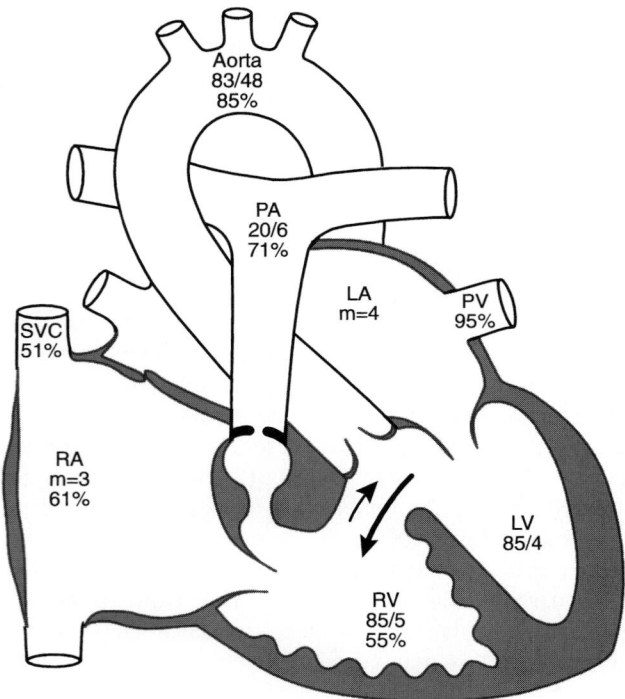

FIG. 33–19. Diagram of the cardiac anatomy and physiology in a girl with mild cyanosis and a loud murmur audible at birth. She was found to have tetralogy of Fallot and was followed without medication prior to primary reparative surgery. The numbers below the chamber name are pressure measurements (mm Hg) determined at cardiac catheterization; the percentages indicate oxygen saturation. LA, left atrium; LV, left ventricle; PA, pulmonary artery; PV, pulmonary vein; RA, right atrium; RV, right ventricle; SVC, superior vena cava. (Adapted from ref. 101.)

arterial collateral vessels). For example, in pulmonary atresia with a ventricular septal defect, the entire right heart output passes right to left through the ventricular defect, and pulmonary flow is supplied by a ductus arteriosus or collateral vessels and is usually less than normal. Cyanosis is the result. If the newborn has large aortopulmonary collateral vessels perfusing the lung, pulmonary blood flow may be large, and the infant may be barely cyanotic and some have congestive heart failure.

Tetralogy of Fallot is a progressive lesion. Clinically significant cyanosis is present at birth in 25%, by 1 year of age in 75%, and almost all have become cyanotic by 20 years of age. Infundibular hypoplasia and stenosis are progressive in both absolute and relative terms. Progression of the stenosis during the first 6 months of life is most often largely relative because of a lack of adequate infundibular expansion during rapid somatic growth and need for proportionately greater pulmonary flow (59). With time, complete atresia can occur. A patent ductus arteriosus usually closes within the first week of life, resulting in severe and often sudden hypoxemia or cyanotic spells.

Hypoxemia of rapid onset is characteristic of a "tet" spell secondary to an infundibular spasm. This may be associated with an increased adrenergic contractile state, systemic vasodilation associated with a meal, warm bath, or certain types of anesthesia, or constriction of a ductus arteriosus. Hypoxemia may result in a fall in systemic vascular resistance, metabolic acidosis, hyperpnea, and further hypoxemia. Hyperventilatory compensation for the metabolic acidosis may be ineffective because of inadequate pulmonary blood flow. The self-aggravating cycle of increasing hypoxemia and metabolic acidosis can progress to unconsciousness and convulsions.

Clinical Findings

Various degrees of cyanosis and mild tachypnea often occur soon after delivery. If hypoxemia is severe, the infant may be hypotonic, hypotensive, and bradycardic. "Tet" spells characterized by a sudden onset of irritability, hyperpnea, and increasing cyanosis may develop. Spells may end in a loss of consciousness, seizures, cerebral injury, hemiparesis, or death. The disappearance of a previously heard right ventricular outflow systolic murmur with increased cyanosis suggests a spell and constitutes an indication for immediate therapy.

There is a systolic murmur at the left sternal border, and the second heart sound is single. In a newborn with pulmonary atresia, the systolic murmur is absent; there may be a constant apical systolic ejection click and prominent continuous murmurs of a patent ductus arteriosus or aortopulmonary collaterals, audible at the base, in the axillae, and/or over the back. A patent ductus arteriosus usually does not cause a continuous murmur in the first months of life; therefore, the presence of murmurs with cyanosis and a single S_2 in a neonate strongly suggests tetralogy of Fallot with pulmonary atresia. Delay in height, weight, and skeletal maturation is common, but some infants flourish despite severe hypoxemia. Some young infants with the anatomic but acyanotic tetralogy of Fallot experience congestive heart failure, later recover from congestion, and become cyanotic. Rarely, congestive heart failure occurs in infants with pulmonary atresia and very large aortopulmonary collaterals. Although subacute bacterial endocarditis and brain abscess are common in older children with tetralogy of Fallot, these complications are extremely rare in infancy. However, spontaneous cerebrovascular accidents are common, particularly in infants with severe hypoxemia and relative anemia (<6 to 8 g/dL of oxyhemoglobin).

The chest radiograph shows a normal-sized heart, sometimes with right ventricular enlargement resulting in an upturned apex and an absent or diminished main pulmonary artery segment (i.e., boot-shaped heart), diminution of the pulmonary vasculature, and, in 25%, the aorta arching to the right. The ECG demonstrates right axis deviation, right atrial enlargement, and right ventricular hypertrophy, which at birth is often difficult to differentiate from normally prominent right ventricular forces. The echocardiographic examination shows anterior and leftward deviation of the infundibular septum, creating subpulmonary stenosis and a malalignment ventricular septal defect with a large overriding aortic root (Fig. 33–20). Additional ventricular or atrial septal defects, central pulmonary artery hypoplasia, and coronary artery anatomy can often be delineated by echocardiography but may require cardiac catheterization if these additional abnormalities are detected. Determining the possible presence of distal pulmonary artery stenosis and the anatomy of systemic-arterial-to-pulmonary-arterial collaterals may sometimes be done with magnetic resonance imaging but has generally required angiography.

Treatment

Treatment depends on the severity of the lesion. The newborn with tetralogy of Fallot and little or mild cyanosis should be carefully observed with repeated measurement of transcutaneous systemic oxygen saturation until a stable level is apparent after ductal closure. Because the right ventricular outflow obstruction is progressive, careful serial follow-up is prudent. "Tet" spells should be treated with oxygen, intramuscular or subcutaneous morphine sulfate (0.1 mg/kg), intravenous administration of saline boluses and sodium bicarbonate (approximately 1 mmol/kg), and, if needed, phenylephrine (0.1 mg/kg subcutaneously; 5 to 20 μg/kg by intravenous bolus; 0.1 to 0.5 μg/kg/min by intravenous infusion) titrated to elevate systemic vascular resistance and pressure. Prostaglandin E_1 may open a ductus arteriosus in the cyanotic newborn infant and improve pulmonary perfusion. Propranolol may be of some value in treating the infant with a reactive infundibulum. The hemoglobin concentration should be maintained high enough to permit adequate oxygen transport. The occurrence of a single "tet" spell is an indication for surgery, possibly as an emergency procedure.

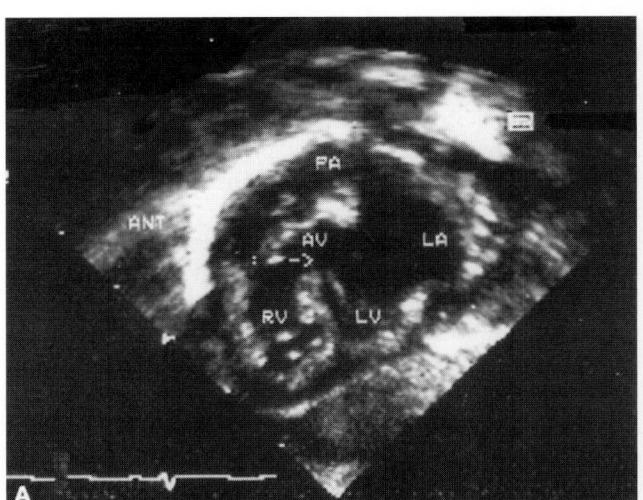 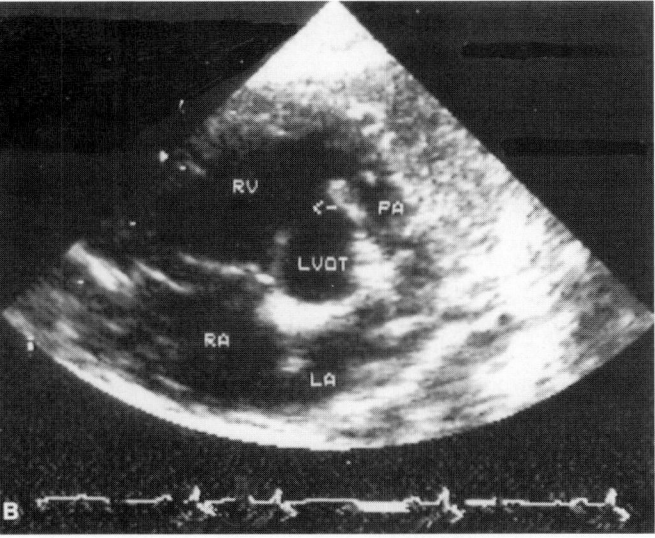

FIG. 33–20. Echocardiographic subxiphoid **(A)** and parasternal short-axis **(B)** views of an infant with tetralogy of Fallot. Anterior deviation of the conal septum (above the *arrow*) is associated with malalignment ventricular septal defect and obstruction of the right ventricular outflow above the pulmonary artery; *arrow*, ventricular septal defect and narrowed right ventricular outflow; ANT, anterior; AV, aortic valve; LA, left atrium; LV, left ventricle; LVOT, left ventricular outflow tract; PA, pulmonary artery; RA, right atrium; RV, right venticle.

In the past, critically ill infants who required surgery underwent palliative procedures, usually a shunt between the subclavian artery and branch pulmonary artery (Blalock–Taussig). The shunt was ligated during a reparative operation when the child was older. Infants with uncomplicated tetralogy of Fallot requiring surgery now undergo one-stage reparative procedures with excellent results (60). The right ventricular outflow tract is enlarged with a pericardial patch, and the ventricular septal defect is closed with a Dacron patch. There are several potential sequelae, including late dysrhythmias, but most patients with uncomplicated tetralogy of Fallot have an asymptomatic long-term course (61). Those with anomalous origin of the left anterior descending coronary from the right coronary artery and those with pulmonary atresia and hypoplastic distorted pulmonary arteries may require a palliative shunt with a more definitive repair, entailing a conduit from the right ventricle to the pulmonary artery, when the child is older.

In general, the earlier severe hypoxemia develops, the more severe is the tetralogy of Fallot, and the poorer the prognosis without surgery. The overall mortality rate without surgery is approximately 35% by 1 year of age.

Differential Diagnosis

The features of cyanosis, a harsh systolic ejection murmur, chest radiographic findings of diminished pulmonary vasculature with a normal-sized heart, and ECG evidence of right ventricular hypertrophy are characteristic of tetralogy of Fallot (see Table 33–11). The same findings with a continuous murmur suggest tetralogy of Fallot with pulmonary atresia. A few infants with tetralogy of Fallot and an underdeveloped pulmonary valve present with a characteristic to-and-fro murmur (i.e., steam engine sound) and severe respiratory distress caused by bronchial or tracheal compression by aneurysmally dilated pulmonary arteries.

Pulmonary Stenosis

Pulmonary Valve and Subvalvar Stenosis

Pulmonary valve stenosis is one of the most common intracardiac anomalies detected in the first month of life (Table 33–1). It is usually mild and not progressive. Even mild obstruction (<10 mm Hg systolic pressure gradient across the obstruction) produces a readily audible murmur. Moderate and severe pulmonary valve stenosis detected in the first week of life often progresses for a limited time over the following weeks or months. It generally presents with an isolated murmur radiating to the suprasternal notch, often but not always with an early systolic click resembling a split S_1, little or no cyanosis, and no signs of congestive heart failure. A parasternal thrill, high-pitched systolic ejection murmur, and single second heart sound indicate severe pulmonary valve stenosis. Severe valvar obstruction may produce cyanosis (Fig. 33–21) because of

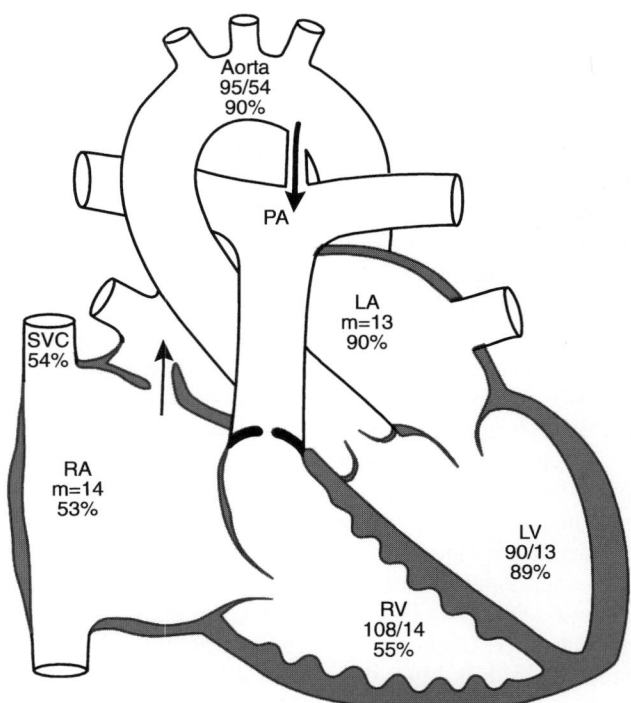

FIG. 33–21. Diagram of the cardiac anatomy and physiology in a 3-day-old baby with cyanosis from birth. There was no murmur. The pulmonary valve was nearly atretic with only a tiny orifice. A valvotomy was done, and the cyanosis resolved in 3 weeks. The numbers below the chamber name are pressure measurements (mm Hg) determined at cardiac catheterization; the percentages indicate oxygen saturation. LA, left atrium; LV, left ventricle; PA, pulmonary artery; PV, pulmonary vein; RA, right atrium; RV, right ventricle; SVC, superior vena cava. (Adapted from ref. 101.)

right-to-left shunting through a foramen ovale or rarely may present with the findings of right-sided congestive heart failure. In its most severe form, a very immobile, critically stenotic pulmonary valve requires ductal patency for adequate pulmonary blood flow and systemic arterial oxygenation. The right ventricular chamber may be small and noncompliant, resulting in some degree of right-to-left shunting though the foramen ovale, even after removal of the stenosis. Infundibular (i.e., subvalvar) obstruction as an isolated lesion is rare; its presence usually indicates an associated ventricular defect. Chest radiography demonstrates normal heart size with fairly normal contour except with occasional upturning of the apex and normal or decreased pulmonary vascular markings. At birth the electrocardiogram is usually normal, although with severe and critical stenosis there may be relative mild left axis deviation for age (R axis 60 to 90 degrees) and increased or decreased right ventricular forces (see Table 33–11). Echocardiography can determine the valve leaflet mobility, systolic pressure gradient, presence of right ventricular or infundibular hypoplasia, ductal patency, and possible associated anomalies such as atrial septal defect. Only reassurance and observation are required for the mild stenoses because progressive obstruction is rare. Because moderate obstructions in early infancy often become progressively worse with growth, the patients should be periodically examined with this in mind. The severe and critical obstructions are relieved by catheter balloon dilation (Fig. 33–22) (47,49). Recurrence is unusual. Bacterial endocarditis is rare, but the administration of antibiotics for prophylaxis before procedures that may be accompanied by bacteremia is recommended.

Pulmonary Artery Stenosis

Proximal pulmonary artery stenosis is probably the most common form of congenital heart disease discovered by hearing a murmur. The abnormality is most often acute angulation with mild narrowing of the proximal pulmonary artery branches. Minimal obstruction produces a readily audible murmur in the left upper sternal border, radiating to the clavicular regions, axillae, and back. Echocardiography can detect proximal pulmonary artery narrowing and pressure gradient and, when bilateral and severe, the presence of right ventricular hypertension. Severe peripheral pulmonary stenosis is rare and is usually associated with other problems such as tetralogy of Fallot, Williams syndrome, Alagille arteriohepatic dysplasia, and infants born of mothers with rubella. Angiography or magnetic resonance imaging is required to visualize the more distal pulmonary arteries. Pulmonary artery stenoses are usually amenable to catheter angioplasty and/or stenting.

Pulmonary Atresia with Intact Ventricular Septum

When the pulmonary valve is atretic and there is no ventricular septal defect, blood cannot pass through the right ventricle in the fetus. Without normal flow, the right ventricle cavity cannot grow normally and changes little in nature and size. It is frequently coarsely trabeculated and pea sized. There is membranous pulmonary valvar atresia and, in approximately one-third of the cases, associated infundibular hypoplasia or atresia. The tricuspid valve annulus remains proportionately small and may be stenotic or incompetent. Often, fistulous tracts connecting the right ventricular sinus to the distal coronary arteries persist, sometimes with proximal coronary artery stenosis. The right ventricle without outflow usually generates suprasystemic pressures. The high pressure probably contributes to the enlargement of fistulas that connect the right ventricle to the coronary arteries. The resultant severe coronary hypertension *in utero* may cause the coronary arteriopathy, proximal coronary artery stenoses, and myocardial fibrosis frequently seen. The pulmonary arteries are of adequate size and are perfused through a patent ductus arteriosus or, rarely, through aortopulmonary collaterals. An unrestrictive interatrial communication is essential to intrauterine survival and is present at birth. Pulmonary atresia with an intact ventricular septum is rarely associated with other cardiovascular or somatic malformations.

Pathophysiology

The major hemodynamic consequence of pulmonary atresia with intact septum is the obligatory right-to-left pas-

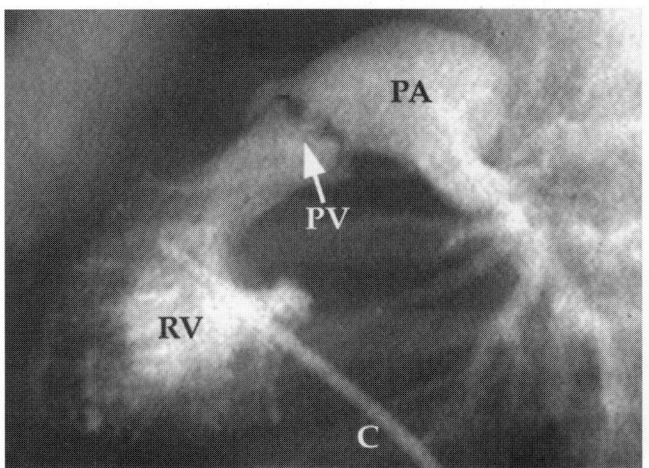

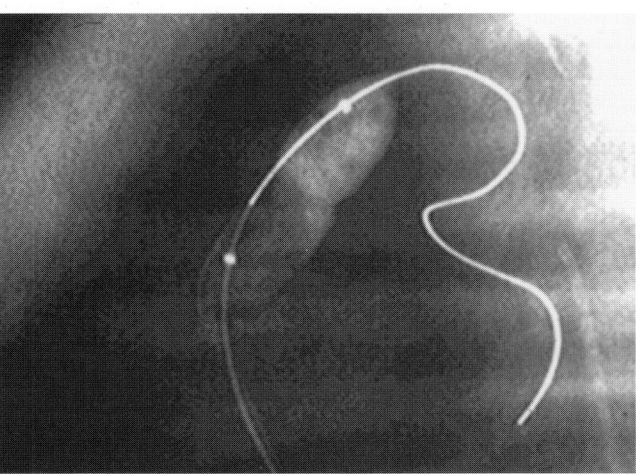

A

B

FIG. 33–22. A: Lateral view of the right ventriculogram of a neonate with mild cyanosis, loud murmur, and severe pulmonary valve stenosis. Cineangiography during injection of contrast through a catheter (C) into the right ventricle (RV) demonstrates a jet of contrast through the small orifice *(arrow)* of a thickened doming stenotic pulmonary valve (PV). There is poststenotic dilation of the main pulmonary artery. **B:** Immediately following the angiogram seen above, the pulmonary valve was crossed with a catheter, and balloon pulmonary valvuloplasty performed over a guide wire, reducing the peak-to-peak systolic pressure gradient from 82 mm Hg to 2 mm Hg.

sage of the total systemic venous return through the foramen ovale to the left atrium. A patent ductus arteriosus provides the only entrance to the pulmonary circulation. As it closes, pulmonary perfusion is greatly reduced, which results in severe hypoxemia, metabolic acidosis, and death. In those infants with fistulas from the right ventricle to the left anterior descending and/or right coronary arteries and proximal coronary artery stenosis, perfusion of the coronary arteries distal to the stenoses occurs from the high pressure right ventricle through the fistulas. Surgical establishment of continuity between the right ventricle and the pulmonary artery may result in sufficient decrease in the right ventricle pressure to cause hypoperfusion of coronary beds supplied solely by fistulas and produce myocardial infarction. The size of the infarct and its impact directly correlate with the area of distribution of the coronary vessel involved (62).

Clinical Findings

Most infants with pulmonary atresia are critically ill within the first week of life because of severe hypoxemia. With postnatal ductal constriction, severe cyanosis, hypotension, bradycardia, hypotonia, and marked acidosis occur. Signs of right-sided failure may develop but are usually absent. The precordium is quiet, and there is no thrill. S_2 is single, and there is often a pansystolic murmur of tricuspid incompetence. On the chest radiograph, the heart may appear mildly enlarged, the lung vascular markings are reduced, and the aortic arch is on the left (Fig. 33–23). The ECG usually reveals a QRS axis in the frontal plane between 0 and 80 degrees, absent or diminished right ventricular forces, and a pattern of left ventricular dominance reflecting right ventricular hypoplasia.

An echocardiogram shows normal or somewhat enlarged left-sided structures, a small tricuspid valve and right ventricle, and atresia of the pulmonary valve. If there is membranous atresia of the pulmonary valve, the membrane can move like a critically stenotic valve, and the diagnosis cannot be made with certainty without a careful Doppler flow examination. Limitations in the size of the tricuspid valve and right ventricle and the presence of tricuspid stenosis can be quantified. High-resolution two-dimensional imaging and color Doppler can detect fistulas between the right ventricle and the coronary arteries. After the presumptive clinical diagnosis is made, prostaglandin should be given to dilate and maintain patency of the ductus arteriosus and increase pulmonary blood flow. In those babies diagnosed after ductal constriction, there should be rapid improvement in oxygenation and relief of acidosis. Cardiac catheterization with selective right ventriculography and ascending aortography is done to determine the presence of fistulas and stenosis in the coronary arteries, essential for planning surgery (Fig. 33–24).

Treatment

After stabilization with prostaglandins, the treatment of choice is surgery, which is indicated as soon as feasible

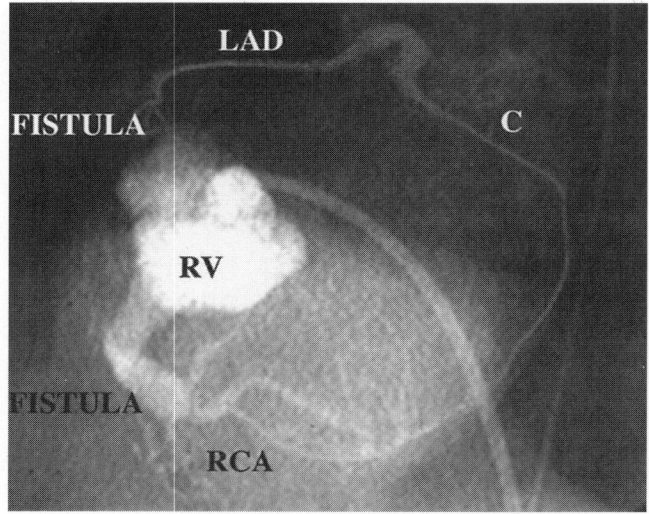

FIG. 33–24. Cineangiogram of the right ventricle (RV) in an infant who presented with severe cyanosis, no murmur, single S2, and oligemic pulmonary vascular markings on chest radiograph. Echocardiogram confirmed pulmonary valve atresia, intact interventricular septum, and a closing ductus arteriosus. The aortic origin of the right coronary artery could not be visualized, and there was evidence for coronary fistula. Prostaglandin infusion was started. Selective coronary arteriography and right ventriculography demonstrated atresia of the proximal right coronary artery. A large fistula (FISTULA, black print) from the small right ventricle perfuses the distal right coronary artery and, through collaterals, the circumflex (C). There was also fistula (FISTULA, white print) from the right ventricle to the left anterior descending (LAD). The baby successfully underwent implantation of a modified Blalock-Taussig shunt, with no attempt to connect the right ventricle to the pulmonary artery.

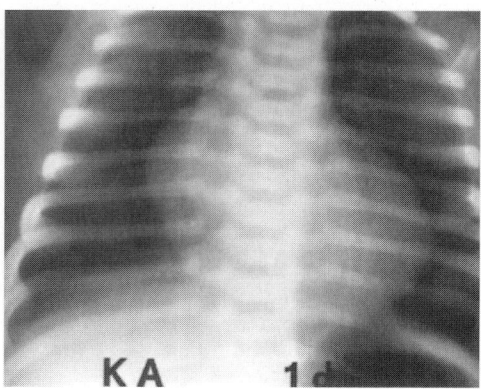

FIG. 33–23. A chest radiograph shows decreased pulmonary vascularity and mild cardiomegaly in a 1-day-old infant with pulmonary atresia and an intact ventricular septum.

after the anatomy is established by catheterization. For infants with an adequately sized right ventricle, pulmonary valvotomy or valvectomy is performed. Some infants may require placement of a patch across the right ventricular outflow tract and valve annulus for adequate relief of obstruction. Often, even when of adequate size, the right ventricle is noncompliant, resulting in persistence of marked right to left atrial shunting. In infants with severe right ventricular noncompliance or hypoplasia a systemic-to-pulmonary shunt also may be necessary for relief of hypoxemia. After a period during which the right ventricular capacity and compliance improve and the pulmonary vascular resistance decreases, these infants may no longer require shunts for maintenance of adequate pulmonary blood flow. Even infants with initially diminutive right ventricular chambers often demonstrate adequate growth of the chamber if flow through the ventricle is provided by establishing continuity between the right ventricle and pulmonary artery, and the tricuspid valve is adequate. The right ventricle cannot be decompressed in infants who have fistulas between the right ventricle and coronary arteries and stenoses involving at least two separate proximal coronary vessels, without risk of fatal infarction (62). Infants with two or more major coronary stenoses, and those with persistent severe right ventricular hypoplasia, require a staged approach with an initial neonatal shunt and a later Fontan-type cavopulmonary anastomosis or transplantation. Without therapy, the malformation is usually fatal, and with surgical treatment, more than 80% of these newborns survive to 1 year of age.

Differential Diagnosis

Pulmonary atresia with an intact septum needs to be differentiated from other cardiac causes severe cyanosis in the first week of life (see Table 33–11). The combination of peaceful cyanosis, little murmur, single S_2, chest radiograph with normal heart size and diminished pulmonary markings, and ECG with R axis of 0 to 80 degrees and diminished V_1 R wave amplitude is fairly characteristic. Critical valvar pulmonary stenosis alone, or with tetralogy of Fallot, are accompanied by a systolic ejection murmur, and right ventricular hypertrophy. Tetralogy of Fallot with pulmonary atresia has a continuous murmur and ECG with normal axis for age and prominent right ventricular forces. Transposition of the great arteries with an intact ventricular septum causes peaceful cyanosis and little murmur but is associated with a spilt S_2, chest radiograph with cardiomegaly and increased vascular markings, and ECG with normal axis for age and evidence of prominent right ventricular forces. Infants with tricuspid atresia often have a prominent murmur and have a superior frontal plane axis on the ECG. In Ebstein anomaly of the tricuspid valve, the ECG has tall wide P waves and an rsR′S′ pattern, and chest radiograph demonstrates severe cardiac enlargement

(Fig. 33–14). Echocardiography differentiates all of these.

Tricuspid Atresia

Tricuspid atresia is a relatively uncommon disease that is characterized by absence of the tricuspid valve. Except in rare cases, no valve exists, and tricuspid agenesis is therefore a more precise description of this anomaly.

Pathophysiology

The entire systemic venous return (i.e., cardiac output) enters the right atrium and exits through the foramen ovale to the left heart. The systemic and pulmonary venous streams mix in the left atrium. After passage to the left ventricle, the cardiac output passes to the aorta, and a variable amount gains access to the pulmonary artery through a ventricular septal defect, diminutive right ventricle, and a variable degree of pulmonary stenosis. Flow to the pulmonary artery is limited by the size of the ventricular defect and the amount of infundibular and valvar pulmonary stenosis. The level of cyanosis is determined by the amount of pulmonary blood flow. In early infancy, the pulmonary blood flow can be increased if needed by maintaining a patent ductus arteriosus and subsequently surgically implanting of a Blalock–Taussig shunt. Some infants have naturally balanced circulations with sufficient flow to the pulmonary arteries to allow an adequate arterial oxygen saturation of 75% to 88%, while not so much as to cause pulmonary hypertension or congestive heart failure. Occasionally, the great vessels are transposed, with the aorta arising from the right ventricle, and the systemic output may be limited by the size of the ventricular defect. A left superior vena cava is a common associated anomaly of importance to later surgery.

Clinical Findings

Babies are usually discovered to have tricuspid atresia during the first days or weeks of life because of cyanosis. Some have a harsh mixed frequency systolic murmur of left to right flow through the ventricular septal defect or ductus arteriosus, and/or a harsh high-pitched systolic ejection murmur from pulmonary stenosis. The S_2 is most often single. On chest radiographs, the heart is usually of normal size or minimally enlarged, and the pulmonary vasculature is diminished. The ECG characteristically has features distinguishing it from most other cyanotic lesions. There is a leftward superior axis similar to endocardial cushion defects (see Fig. 33–10), but usually with diminished right precordial forces. The diagnosis is readily confirmed by echocardiographic identification of a diminutive right ventricle, an absent tricuspid valve, and right-to-left flow through the foramen ovale (Fig. 33–25). The size of the ventricular septal defect and the degree of

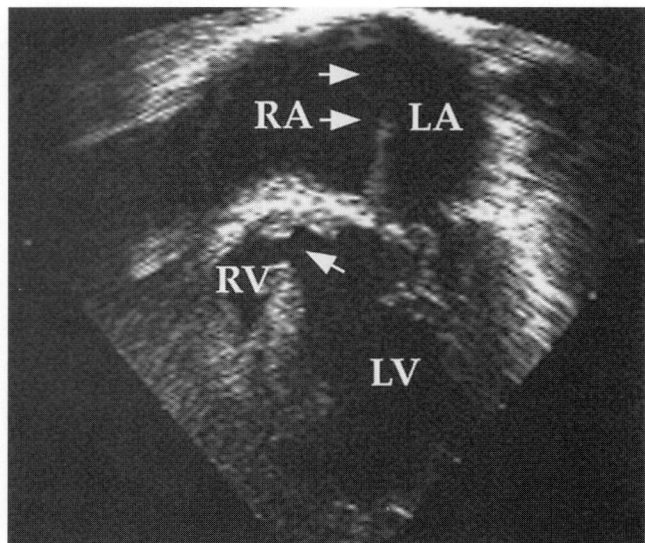

FIG. 33–25. Echocardiographic apical four-chamber view in a baby with tricuspid atresia. Systemic venous blood flows from the right atrium (RA) across a widely patent foramen ovale *(double arrows)* to the left atrium (LA) and into the left ventricle (LV). Some of the outflow of the left ventricle passes through a ventricular septal defect *(single arrow)* and hypoplastic right ventricle (RV) to the pulmonary arteries (not shown).

subvalvar and valvar pulmonary stenosis can be accurately determined.

Treatment

Infants with severe obstruction of blood flow through the ventricular septal defect and right ventricle may require infusion of prostaglandin E_1 before palliative surgery. Surgical implantation of a modified or classic Blalock–Taussig type shunt from a subclavian or innominate artery to a pulmonary artery provides the means for adequate arterial oxygenation, survival, and growth in those infants with severe intracardiac obstruction to pulmonary blood flow. After several months of age the pulmonary vascular resistance usually decreases sufficiently to permit success of bidirectional Glenn surgery connecting the upper superior vena cava carrying systemic venous blood return from the upper half of the body directly into the pulmonary artery. Variations on the Fontan operation, in which the systemic venous return from the remainder of the body is directed into the pulmonary arteries, are undertaken at or beyond the age of 1 year (63). More than 75% of infants with tricuspid atresia survive with Fontan physiology (64).

Rarely, in an infant with a large ventricular defect and no pulmonary stenosis, the pulmonary blood flow may be excessive enough to cause congestive heart failure. Anticongestive medications are usually sufficient to allow growth, although a pulmonary artery banding or other procedure may be necessary to diminish pulmonary vascular pressure and resistance.

Ebstein Anomaly of the Tricuspid Valve

Ebstein anomaly of the tricuspid valve is encountered rarely in the newborn period. The septal leaflet of the tricuspid valve is displaced downward and adheres to the ventricular septum to various degrees. The result is a dysfunctioning tricuspid valve that is regurgitant or stenotic to varying degrees. The dysfunction is compounded by the fact that the right atrium and right ventricle contract at different times, and there is an area of atrialized ventricle or ventricularized atrium, depending on the point of view. This discordant pumping of parts of each chamber contributes to the dysfunction. Those with severe prenatal tricuspid regurgitation often have massive cardiomegaly and may have pulmonary hypoplasia that is rapidly fatal after birth (Fig. 33–5). The effective right ventricular volume is reduced, and there is limited passage of blood through the right ventricle. Some right atrial blood courses through the patent foramen ovale, causing cyanosis. The severity of the defect can be described by the degree of cyanosis that, in the newborn period, can be severe because of the concomitant unresolved elevation of the pulmonary vascular resistance left over from fetal life. As the newborn's pulmonary vascular resistance regresses, the cyanosis often improves, sometimes markedly, although babies with severe regurgitation and pulmonary hypoplasia have a high mortality rate. After surviving the newborn period, the infant has a course determined by the degree of abnormality; some patients survive into late adulthood without important limitation, but others remain cyanotic and prone to supraventricular tachycardia.

Ebstein disease is recognized because of minimal or systolic low-pitched murmur of tricuspid regurgitation, multiple clicks, minimal to severe cyanosis, and cardiomegaly that may vary from minimal to some of the largest hearts encountered in the newborn period (see Fig. 33–26). The ECG has tall wide P waves and an $rsR'S'$ pattern (see Table 33–11). The diagnosis is established by echocardiography. Treatment is usually supportive. A surgical Blalock–Tauusig shunt may be required in infants who remain severely cyanotic. Treatment for supraventricular tachycardia may be needed.

Anomalies with Cyanosis as a Result of Complete Mixing of Systemic and Pulmonary Circulations

Hypoplastic Left Heart Syndrome

The hypoplastic left heart syndrome encompasses a variety of specific cardiovascular malformations producing similar hemodynamic and clinical manifestations, including aortic atresia, mitral atresia, premature closure

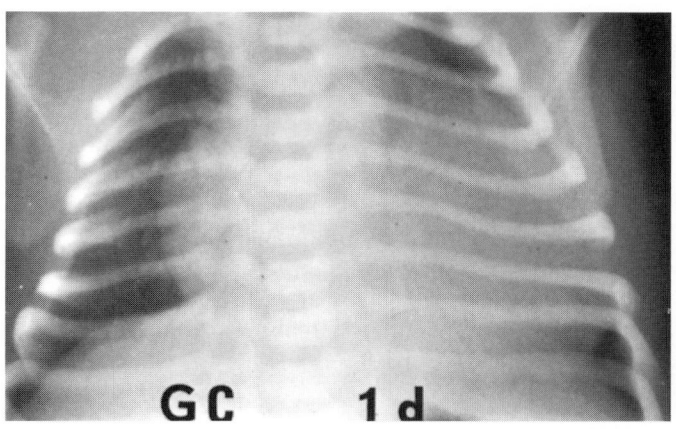

FIG. 33–26. A chest radiograph of a 1-day-old cyanotic infant with Ebstein anomaly of the tricuspid valve shows marked cardiomegaly.

of the foramen ovale, hypoplastic left ventricle with critical mitral stenosis, and aortic stenosis. Some cases of severe complex coarctation, critical aortic valve stenosis, and malaligned atrioventricular canal defects are also included in this category. The left heart chamber is usually very small, and endocardial fibroelastosis in it is common. Hypoplastic left heart syndrome occurs in 10.2% of infants with serious heart disease and is one of the most common lesions presenting in the first week of life (see Tables 33–1, 33–2, and 33–7). It is less common in very premature infants (<1.85 kg). It is usually an isolated lesion, although it has been described in association with autosomal trisomy syndromes and in infants of diabetic mothers. Familial cases occur.

Pathophysiology

Obstruction or atresia of the mitral or aortic valves limits or prevents flow through the left heart. The systemic venous return enters the right heart and is ejected into the pulmonary artery. The systemic circulation is largely or totally supplied by right-to-left flow through the ductus arteriosus. Blood traversing the lung enters the left atrium, flows through an interatrial defect or dilated foramen ovale, and returns to the right atrium to join the incoming systemic venous return. Complete mixing takes place in the right atrium, with similar oxygen saturation measured in the right ventricle, pulmonary artery, and aorta. With little or no egress through the left heart, pulmonary flow must pass left to right through an interatrial communication. Any limitation of flow through the atrial septum produces pulmonary venous hypertension.

The maintenance of adequate systemic circulation requires patency of the ductus arteriosus. In aortic atresia, the ascending aorta, brachiocephalic vessels, and coronary arteries are perfused in a retrograde fashion with blood originating from the patent ductus arteriosus. Spontaneous constriction of the ductus results in flooding of the pulmonary circulation simultaneous with low systemic blood flow, poor coronary perfusion, congestive

failure, and shock with metabolic acidosis, electrolyte imbalance, and coagulation abnormalities. Closure of the ductus stops blood flow to the body and causes immediate death.

Clinical Findings

These infants become symptomatic within the first week of life. Congestive failure and a shock-like picture may develop precipitously. The baby becomes ashen gray with poor peripheral perfusion, and all pulses are weak. Ductal constriction or flow may appear intermittent, with femoral pulses intermittently palpable. Symptoms and signs of congestive failure are associated with hypotension and, terminally, with bradycardia. S_2 is single, and a gallop may be heard. The chest radiograph shows cardiac enlargement and pulmonary plethora, and the ECG usually demonstrates right axis deviation, right atrial enlargement, right ventricular hypertrophy, and markedly diminished or absent left ventricular forces. Echocardiography demonstrates a very small or tiny left ventricle. The ascending aorta is small with retrograde flow in cases of aortic atresia, and there is frequently a discrete juxtaductal coarctation (Fig. 33–27).

Treatment

Without surgery, the mortality rate is 98% by 1 year of age. There are a few survivors with mitral atresia or hypoplasia of the left ventricle with severe aortic or mitral stenosis. Advances in cardiac surgery have encouraged several approaches to infants with this condition. Palliative surgery can be performed in the newborn period after stabilization with prostaglandin E_1, inotropic agents, volume infusion, and bicarbonate. Hyperventilation (i.e., arterial partial pressure of carbon dioxide, $PaCO_2 < 40$ mm Hg) and unnecessary supplemental oxygen administration are avoided. These measures decrease pulmonary vascular resistance and increase preferential flow of the right ventricular output into the pulmonary

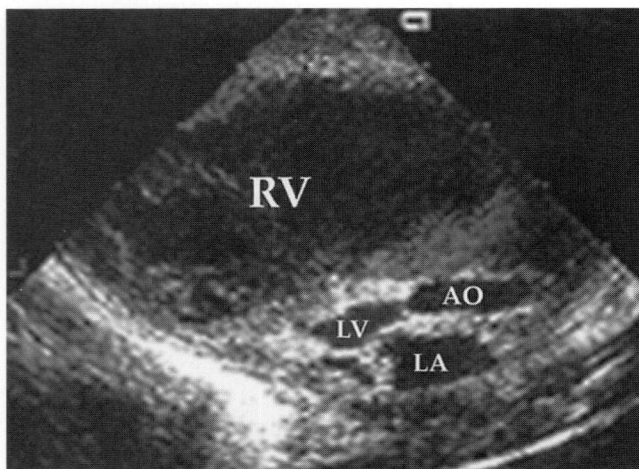

FIG. 33–27. Echocardiographic parasternal long-axis view in an infant with hypoplastic left heart syndrome. The right ventricle (RV) is near normal in size. The left atrium (LA), left ventricle (LV) and ascending aorta (AO) are tiny. Both the mitral and aortic valves are atretic.

vascular bed instead of across the ductus to the systemic vasculature, worsening the shock. Often for preoperative stabilization, mechanical hypoventilation with muscle relaxation to maintain the $PaCO_2$ 45 to 55 mm Hg, and sometimes $F_IO_2 < 0.21$ to maintain arterial O_2 saturation 70% to 75%, are required to elicit sufficient pulmonary vasoconstriction to induce adequate systemic blood flow. Surgical therapy consists of converting the circulation to single-ventricle Fontan-type physiology and/or to transplant a new heart. A Norwood first-stage procedure anastomoses an obliquely transected main pulmonary artery to the underside of the aortic arch, augments the size of the aortic arch with a patch, ligates the ductus arteriosus, supplies perfusion to the distal oversewn pulmonary artery by creation of a modified Blalock–Taussig or direct central systemic-to-pulmonary artery shunt, and leaves an atrial septectomy to allow unimpeded pulmonary venous return to the right atrium (65). The long-term outlook depends on the ability of the right ventricle to support the systemic circulation while the pulmonary circulation is supplied relatively directly with systemic venous return. Several months later, when the pulmonary resistance has dropped from relatively high neonatal values, a second-stage bidirectional Glenn procedure is done. The systemic venous return from the upper body is placed directly into the lung through a anastomosis of the upper superior vena cava to the right pulmonary artery, and the systemic-arterial-to-pulmonary-arterial shunt (with its obligate ventricular volume overload) is taken down. Finally, at a third Fontan-type procedure, systemic venous return from the lower body is also diverted directly into the pulmonary artery through a lateral tunnel within the right atrium, directing flow to a second, lower anastomosis of the lower superior vena cava to the pul-

monary artery (65). The perinatal and first-stage surgical mortality rate is between 15% and 40%, and overall during the first 5 years, it is as high as 30% to 75% (66,67). Long-range survival is undetermined.

Cardiac transplantation has been used as an alternative approach with good survival, but there are critical limitations in the timely availability of neonatal donors and limited documentation of long-range survival (68–70).

Neither reconstructive surgery leading to a Fontan procedure nor cardiac transplantation can be viewed as curative. Both methods of treatment have high fiscal and emotional costs (see Chap. 31). However, many survivors eventually do remarkably well in childhood.

Differential Diagnosis

The clinical picture of the hypoplastic left heart syndrome may be simulated by respiratory distress syndrome, interrupted aortic arch, severe complex coarctation, early neonatal myocarditis, isolated critical valvar aortic stenosis, sepsis or some inherited metabolic disorders (see Table 33–11).

Total Anomalous Pulmonary Veins

In the event of failure to connect the common pulmonary vein to the left atrium in the embryo, communications are established with available systemic venous channels that then drain the pulmonary veins. Anatomically abnormal drainage may be supracardiac (i.e., into the right or left superior vena cava), intracardiac (i.e., into the coronary sinus, right atrium), or subdiaphragmatic (i.e., through the inferior vena cava or porta hepatis). Mixed sites of drainage occur in approximately 10% of these patients. A patent foramen ovale or atrial septal defect is invariably present, permitting venous return to the left heart. Anomalous pulmonary venous return is often associated with heterotaxy.

Although isolated total anomalous venous return accounts for only 2% of newborns with serious cardiac disease (see Table 33–2), it is an important lesion because it is potentially curable and often misdiagnosed as pulmonary disease.

Pathophysiology

Infants with anomalous pulmonary venous drainage can be divided into two major categories on the basis of the hemodynamic changes produced: those with nonobstructed veins and those with obstructed veins. Nonobstructed pulmonary veins entering the systemic venous circulation or directly into the right heart result in a large left-to-right shunt, congestive heart failure, and pulmonary artery hypertension. Systemic output is maintained through right-to-left flow across an interatrial communication. Despite the obligatory right-to-left shunt through the atrium, the large pulmonary blood flow mixing with the systemic venous return at the right atrium allows a reasonable peripheral oxygen tension and produces only mild cyanosis.

If pulmonary venous return is obstructed, the circulatory effects are drastically different. The obstruction may take the form of increased resistance to flow produced by a long, common, pulmonary venous channel or localized intrinsic or extrinsic obstruction. Subdiaphragmatic anomalous pulmonary venous return is usually obstructed by constriction of the ductus venosus, obstructing flow into the inferior vena cava (Fig. 33–28). Obstruction to supracardiac pulmonary venous return may occur because of compression of the common pulmonary venous channel between the left primary bronchus and left pulmonary artery or because of narrowing at the entry of the common pulmonary vein into the right superior vena cava. Obstruction at the foramen ovale is uncommon. After birth, significant resistance to flow through the pulmonary veins becomes evident, causing pulmonary venous hypertension, pulmonary edema, marked pulmonary artery hypertension and diminished flow, and severe cyanosis. The arterial oxygen tension is low because pulmonary blood flow is markedly reduced, and the relative contribution of fully oxygenated blood to the venous return to the heart mixing in the right atrium is less than in the unobstructed form of this disorder.

Clinical Findings

Infants with total anomalous pulmonary venous return without significant obstruction usually become symptomatic after the neonatal period, when the pulmonary vascular resistance decreases and a large left-to-right shunt and congestive heart failure develop. They are mildly cyanotic with increased respiratory rate and work, often have frank congestive heart failure, and have a large heart revealed on chest radiographs.

Infants with obstructed pulmonary venous return are usually critically ill, severely cyanotic, and tachypneic within the first week of life. There are congestive heart failure and poor peripheral perfusion. In the absence of associated anomalies such as malposition with pulmonary valve or subvalvar stenosis, there is generally only a relatively soft murmur of a patent ductus arteriosus and/or tricuspid valve regurgitation. Heart size, as seen on the chest radiograph, is often normal, and there is evidence of pulmonary edema. The clinical and the radiographic pictures may resemble hyaline membrane disease or diffuse pneumonia complicated by persistent pulmonary hypertension. The ECG shows right axis deviation, right atrial hypertrophy, and right ventricular hypertrophy. The findings on two-dimensional and color Doppler echocardiography include absence of pulmonary venous connections to the left atrium, right-to-left bulging of the interatrial septum, right-to-left interatrial shunt, and pulmonary venous confluence posterior to the left atrium connecting to a systemic venous channel. The findings of severe cyanosis, little murmur, and a roentgenographic picture of a normal heart size associated with pulmonary edema are characteristic (see Fig. 33–28A and Table 33–11). Surgical success is related to the anatomy (e.g., results are poorest in the mixed variety) and to the age of onset of symptoms, as in patients with the infradiaphragmatic type. The success rate is better for infants with intracardiac drainage.

Treatment

The treatment of total anomalous pulmonary veins is surgical. Under deep hypothermic circulatory arrest, continuity or redirection of the pulmonary venous drainage into the left atrium is established. Although inotropic

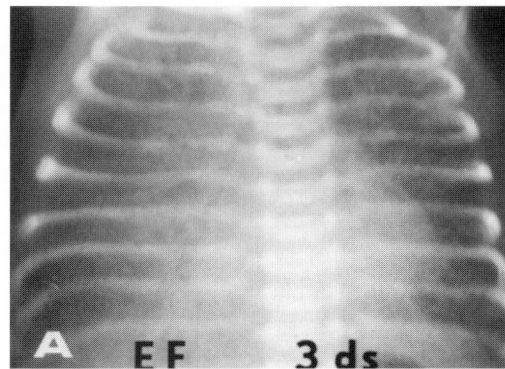 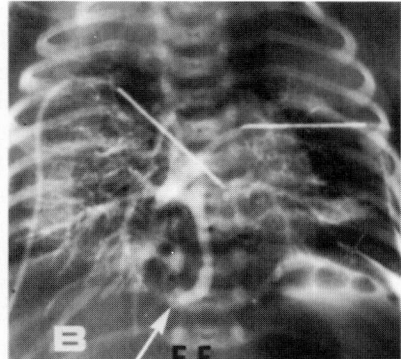

FIG. 33–28. A: A chest radiograph of a 3-day-old infant with obstructed total anomalous pulmonary venous drainage shows a ground-glass appearance of the lungs and normal heart size. A similar clinical picture may be seen in respiratory distress syndrome. **B:** Postmortem angiography shows obstruction of the common pulmonary venous channel below the diaphragm *(arrow)*.

agents, diuretics, and supportive medical treatment may help temporarily and partially with stabilization, infants with severely obstructed anomalous venous return require immediate surgical intervention. Prostaglandin E_1 therapy is not beneficial and can lead to dramatic worsening of the pulmonary edema. In most patients, surgery can be done on the basis of information from echocardiography without the delays and risks involved with cardiac catheterization. If there are associated complex congenital anomalies (e.g., heterotaxy syndrome) or intrinsic pulmonary vein stenosis is suspected, preoperative catheterization may sometimes help determine the best management. Those with unobstructed pulmonary veins and congestive heart failure with relatively normal pulmonary artery pressure may improve considerably on medical treatment, and corrective surgery may be delayed for a few weeks. Among those without additional lesions, the postoperative survivors have an excellent prognosis for a relatively normal life. A few infants develop pulmonary vein stenosis and dysrhythmias postoperatively, and close follow-up is mandatory for several years.

Differential Diagnosis

Respiratory distress syndrome and interstitial pneumonia can be clinically indistinguishable from obstructed total anomalous pulmonary venous connection. Any suggestion of an atypical course mandates echocardiography, particularly in term neonates with equally diffuse involvement of both lungs, a failed or inconclusive hyperoxia test, or any suggestion of a murmur. Two-dimensional echocardiography shows the anomalous common venous connections and obstructions. Other cardiac lesions are excluded.

Truncus Arteriosus

Failure of the conotruncus to divide into the aorta and main pulmonary artery results in the clinical problem described as truncus arteriosus. It is often associated with microdeletions in a critical region of chromosome 22q11 containing genes responsible for conotruncal development, and with related extracardiac anomalies (e.g., DiGeorge syndrome). Other factors can be responsible (28,29). The only artery arising from the heart is the common truncus arteriosus. There is one semilunar valve that may have extra valve leaflets (e.g., four or five) and is often incompetent and rarely stenotic. The pulmonary arteries arise from the left anterior aspect of the truncal root as a single main pulmonary artery, at their bifurcation, or with seperate right and left branches. Classifications in vogue are based on the level at which the pulmonary vessels take off, but they are not especially pertinent to the physiology and the clinical picture. Almost universally, there is a ventricular septal defect, usually in the subaortic septum, similar to that seen in tetralogy of Fallot. Interrupted aortic arch is an infrequent associated anomaly that should be borne in mind for timely recognition and management.

Pathophysiology

Because of the large ventricular defect and the common arterial trunk, the systemic and pulmonary venous returns are mixed, and the patient is cyanotic. The degree of cyanosis is determined by the pulmonary flow, which is a function of obstruction in the proximal pulmonary arteries. These obstructions are common, rarely severe, and located at the junction of the pulmonary artery and the trunk. If there is no obstruction, which is likely, pulmonary flow exceeds systemic output severalfold, obligating a high-output state and resulting in congestive heart failure and poor survival without surgery. Without surgery, irreversible pulmonary vascular disease is likely to develop as early as the patient's first birthday. Congestive heart failure is less of a problem if there is branch pulmonary artery stenosis, although the degree of cyanosis is greater. Proximal pulmonary artery obstructions frequently develop after surgery. When there is also interrupted aortic arch, a ductus is present, and its untreated closure results in lower body hypotension and hypoperfusion, followed by death.

Clinical Findings

Infants with truncus arteriosus resemble those with ventricular defect more than the other cyanotic defects. Except cyanosis, which may be mild, development of symptoms is delayed until the pulmonary vascular resistance has resolved enough to allow a large pulmonary flow and the features of a left-to-right shunt. Tachypnea and the other signs of congestion predominate, although cyanosis may be recognized and documented in the first days of life. There is usually a murmur that sounds like a ventricular defect, the peripheral pulses are bounding, and other signs of an aortic runoff are present. The S_2 is loud and single, and systolic clicks may be heard. On chest radiographs, the heart is enlarged, the pulmonary vasculature is engorged, and the aortic arch may be rightward (33%). The ECG inexplicably varies, showing right, left, or combined ventricular hypertrophy (see Table 33–11). If interrupted aortic arch is also present, diminished pulses, pulse pressure in the lower body, azotemia, and metabolic acidosis develop as the ductus constricts. Echocardiographic examination demonsrates the anatomy (Fig. 33–29).

Treatment

Anticongestive measures to control congestion and promote growth are rarely successful. Surgical correction is usually undertaken within the first 1 to 6 weeks of life. The

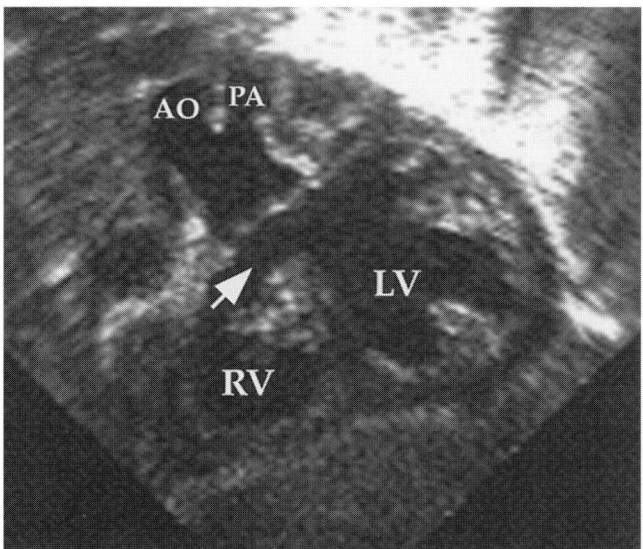

FIG. 33–29. Echocardiographic subxiphoid view in a neonate with truncus arteriosus. The right ventricle (RV) and left ventricle (LV) both pump blood through a subaortic ventricular septal defect *(arrow)* and common truncal valve into the ascending aorta (AO). The main pulmonary artery (PA) arises from the side of the ascending aorta.

later the surgery the more likely that the early postoperative course and survival will be threatened by severe elevation in pulmonary vascular resistance. Although banding of the pulmonary arteries on both sides is possible and is sometimes the only choice, it is easy to understand the difficulty of applying bands on each side equally. For this reason, and because of empirically poor results, most centers perform one-stage repair in infancy (71). This surgery consists of separating the pulmonary arteries from the trunk, establishing a conduit from the right ventricle to the pulmonary arteries, and closing the ventricular defect. Postoperative management and outcome are aided by the early use of potent pulmonary vasodilators such as nitric oxide. The long-range outcome of this type of repair involves two or three surgical revisions with larger pulmonary artery conduits to accommodate growth during childhood. Severe compression of the conduits and natural or surgery-related proximal pulmonary artery stenoses can develop and require catheter-based interventions in early childhood. The truncal semilunar valve may rarely be sufficiently incompetent to influence the outcome. However, with staged surgical intervention, the long-term survival and outcome are good (72).

Anomalies with Cyanosis with Variable and Mixed Anatomy and Physiology

Single Ventricle

There are few patients who have only one ventricle, with either two atrioventricular valves or a common atrioven-tricular valve. Most patients characterized as having a single ventricle have one dominant ventricle and a second diminutive structure that is often characterized as an outflow chamber. Because of the similarity of this syndrome to tricuspid atresia, some physicians have preferred the term univentricular heart to describe all patients with a functionally single ventricle, whether they have two atrioventricular valves, tricuspid atresia, or mitral atresia.

Seventy percent of these patients have a single left ventricle with a rudimentary anatomic right ventricular outflow chamber that is left sided (L-transposed position). The ventricular outflow chamber leads to an anterior and leftward aorta, similar to that seen in corrected transposition. Most of the remainder of patients have a single left ventricle with a rudimentary right ventricular outflow chamber that is right-sided (D-transposed position). Pulmonary stenosis coexists in 50% of these patients. In those without pulmonary stenosis, subaortic stenosis and coarctation can occur. Almost any other cardiac anomaly may be associated with single ventricle. Single right ventricles also occur, particularly with heterotaxy syndrome.

Pathophysiology

Depending on the presence or absence of pulmonary stenosis, the clinical picture may be dominated by diminished pulmonary flow and cyanosis or by excessive pulmonary flow and high-output congestive heart failure, respectively. Occasionally the pulmonary and systemic flow are balanced, and the patient is only mildly cyanotic and otherwise asymptomatic. The problems peculiar to corrected transposition, such as the tendency to develop complete heart block or develop an incompetent atrioventricular valve (usually the left), are risks. The connection between the single ventricle and the outflow chamber (i.e., ventricular defect) tends to get smaller with time in approximately 50% of patients. This has the physiologic effect of subaortic stenosis and must be considered in any management program.

Clinical Findings

The patient usually is visibly cyanotic during the neonatal period. Sometimes those with excessive pulmonary blood flow, minimal cyanosis, and congestive heart failure present later because of growth failure or tachypnea. Most have systolic murmurs from pulmonary stenosis, atrioventricular valve regurgitation, or from other associated defects. The diagnosis is made by echocardiography. Cardiac catheterization is used preoperatively in some to confirm details that may influence surgical success.

Treatment

The ultimate goal of management is to provide a cavopulmonary or atriopulmonary anastomosis (e.g.,

Fontan procedure). Rare patients who have perfectly balanced pulmonary and systemic circulations and are only mildly cyanotic and virtually asymptomatic fare well with no surgery for years. Most require a pulmonary artery band to limit pulmonary flow or a shunt procedure to increase pulmonary flow and arterial oxygenation until a Fontan procedure (i.e., direct connection of systemic venous return to the pulmonary arteries) can be performed.

Double-Outlet Right Ventricle

Double-outlet right ventricle is a rare, anatomically and physiologically heterogeneous group of anomalies. The diagnosis is applied when imaging studies demonstrate that both great arteries arise principally from the morphologic right ventricle, invariably in the presence of a ventricular septal defect. A muscular conus commonly underlies both of the great artery outflows. Although various types of double-outlet right ventricle share a common ventricular–arterial relationship, the anatomy of the ventricles, ventricular conotruncal outflows, the relationship of the great arteries, and the presence of additional anomalies are variable. Of primary importance is the relationship of the great arteries to each other and, as a consequence, to the ventricular septal defect. This determines the basic physiology and the surgical management options (73).

Pathophysiology and Clinical Findings

The most common great artery arrangement is a normal relationship, with the aortic valve posterior and rightward and the pulmonary valve leftward and anterior. The ventricular septal defect usually relates to the subaortic outflow. Many will have subvalvar and valvar pulmonary stenosis. Depending on the presence or absence of pulmonary stenosis, the physiology, clinical findings, clinical course, and therapeutic approach are, respec-

tively, like those with tetralogy of Fallot with diminished pulmonary flow or like those with an isolated large subaortic ventricular septal defect and pulmonary hyperemia and hypertension.

The second most frequent great artery relationship in double-outlet right ventricle is with the aortic valve to the right, and anterior to or alongside the pulmonary valve, and the great arteries side-by-side. The ventricular septal defect is below the pulmonary outflow. The hemodynamics, clinical findings, and course are as in transposition.

Less common types of double-outlet right ventricle include those with the aorta anterior and leftward, those with a remote uncommitted ventricular septal defect that does relate to either great artery outflow (e.g., atrioventricular inlet type defect), and those with a doubly committed ventricular septal defect that relates to both great artery outflows. Important associated anomalies in those without pulmonary stenosis, with either normally related or side-by-side great arteries, include mitral stenosis or atresia, subaortic outflow obstruction, and aortic arch hypoplasia and coarctation. Other less common associated anomalies include heterotaxy with its many related defects (see below and Table 33–12), pulmonary or aortic atresia, multiple ventricular septal defects, and superior–inferior ventricles. These associated anomalies can profoundly influence the hemodynamics, clinical course, and management. Echocardiography determines the diagnosis by showing the right ventricular–great arteries relationship and can usually determine the great artery and ventricular septal defect relationships and delineate the various associated defects. The need and timing of catheterization depend on the anatomy demonstrated by echocardiography and the therapeutic management.

Treatment

Management depends on the specific anatomic abnormalities. Medical and surgical treatment in those with

TABLE 33–12. *Common abnormalities in asplenia and polysplenia syndromes*

Asplenia	Polysplenia
Isolated levocardia or dextrocardia	Dextrocardia or levocardia
Visceral isomerism (midline liver and stomach)	Absent inferior vena cava (renal to hepatic segment)
Transposition of the great arteries	Endocardial cushion defect
Double-outlet right ventricle	Total anomalous pulmonary venous return
Total anomalous pulmonary venous return	Coronary sinus rhythm
Endocardial cushion defect	Bilateral epiarterial bronchi
Pulmonary atresia or pulmonary stenosis	
Single ventricle	
Bilateral superior vena cava	
Absent coronary sinus	
Ipsilateral inferior vena cava and abdominal aorta	
P-wave axis of atrial inversion	
Bilateral eparterial bronchi	
Bilateral trilobed lung	

normally related great arteries and no pulmonary stenosis is as with a large ventricular septal defect and in those with pulmonary stenosis as with tetralogy of Fallot. Surgical management of those with side-by-side great arteries and transposition-like physiology may be managed by intracardiac repair or arterial switch procedure. Associated anomalies may require other approaches including systemic-to-pulmonary arterial shunts, Norwood-like procedure, aortic arch repair, and later Fontan-like approach.

L-Transposition of the Great Arteries

In L-transposition of the great arteries with situs solitus, also called corrected transposition, the circulation is often physiologically corrected. The terminology refers to the position of the aorta, which is abnormally positioned, anterior and usually to the left of the pulmonary artery, as well as to the position of the ventricles. L-Transposition of the great arteries is most commonly associated with ventricular inversion as well, i.e., the ventricles undergo L-looping instead of the usual D-looping. The systemic venous blood enters the right atrium and flows into a right-sided, morphologically left, ventricle and out to the pulmonary artery. Pulmonary venous blood returns to the left atrium and by way of the tricuspid valve into the left-sided, morphologically right, ventricle to the aorta. The aorta is abnormally positioned, anterior and usually to the left of the pulmonary artery. The hemodynamic changes in patients with L-transposition of the great arteries are caused by the commonly associated cardiac abnormalities that include ventricular septal defect (50%), single ventricle (42%), and pulmonary stenosis or atresia (45%). The latter three result in cyanosis. Left atrioventricular valve regurgitation (23%), conduction disturbances, and arrhythmias, particularly supraventricular tachycardia and complete heart block, are common. This diagnosis should always be considered for a newborn with complete heart block. Medical management and surgery are directed toward correction or palliation of the associated cardiovascular malformations, such as closure of the ventricular septal defect, pulmonary valvotomy, and a cardiac pacemaker if needed.

Malpositions

The term malposition is used to describe misplacement of the heart (e.g., ectopia cordis), but it usually indicates concomitant heterotaxy (i.e., discordant sidedness) and is used to describe patients with dextrocardia with situs solitus of the abdominal organs and levocardia with abdominal situs inversus (i.e., isolated levocardia). Ambiguous location of the abdominal contents, as seen in the asplenia and polysplenia syndromes, is also described as malpositioning (Fig. 33–30). If the heart is displaced into the right chest because of pulmonary disease or

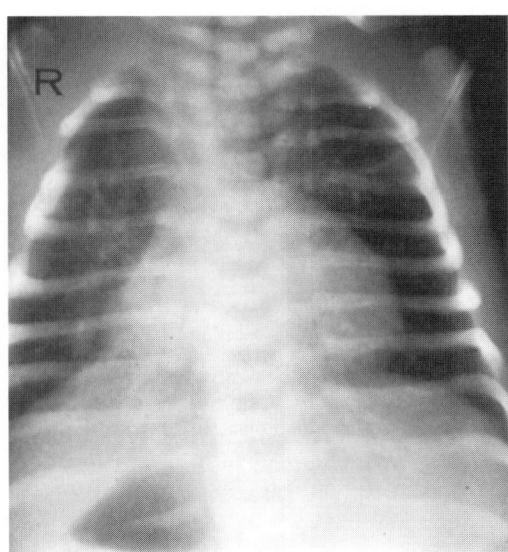

FIG. 33–30. A chest radiograph of a neonate with asplenia syndrome, tricuspid atresia, transposition of the great arteries, and a right aortic arch. The liver and stomach are on the right side.

diaphragmatic hernia or if there is total situs inversus (i.e., situs inversus universalis), there is no heterotaxy. Situs inversus universalis is rare, and the heart may be anatomically normal, unlike the more common forms of malposition.

For practical purposes, evidence of abnormal sidedness is primarily of consequence as a way to discover patients who have particularly complex combinations of congenital heart lesions. Heterotaxy may be discovered by physical examination or chest radiographs because of abnormal sidedness of the abdominal contents or because the heart is located in the right chest. After the question has been raised and regardless of the clinical appearance of the baby, it is safest to proceed with a detailed diagnostic evaluation. There is a high probability that life-threatening abnormalities exist and that the patient should be promptly turned over to a cardiac team that has the facilities and experience to handle the problem.

Table 33–12 shows the anatomic abnormalities encountered in asplenic and polysplenic patients. Incredibly, often all of these occur in combination together. For example, a baby with asplenia may have the combination of inferior vena cava crossing from one side of the midline to the other, single left or bilateral superior vena cava, dextrocardia, total and sometimes mixed pulmonary venous connections, single atrium, common atrioventricular valve, single right ventricle with double outlet, and pulmonary stenosis or atresia. The cardiologists must determine the details of anatomy and anomaly in each central systemic and pulmonary vein, cardiac chamber, valve, and great artery on a segment-by-segment basis and delineate the interconnections of the various segments of the heart.

Most patients can be palliated. On the basis of the details of the anatomy, a staged surgical management plan is devised when the patient is a neonate. The overall mortality rate tends to be higher because of the combination of lesions, particularly in those with obstruction of anomalous pulmonary veins (see Table 33–2). Those with asplenia should receive lifetime prophylactic antibiotics because of their propensity for sepsis.

ACYANOTIC LESIONS

Acyanotic diseases associated with normal pulmonary flow include those with systemic outflow obstruction such as coarctation of the aorta and aortic stenosis, mild and moderate pulmonary outflow stenosis, myocardial diseases, and arrhythmias. Acyanotic lesions usually associated with increased pulmonary blood flow include ventricular septal defect, atrial septal defect, endocardial cushion defects, patent ductus arteriosus, aortopulmonary window, and arteriovenous malformations (see Tables 33–13 and 33–14).

Acyanotic Anomalies with Systemic Outflow Obstruction

Coarctation and Interruption of the Aorta

For clinical, prognostic, and probably etiologic reasons, coarctation of the aorta is best considered in two separate categories: simple and complex. Simple coarctation is usually a discrete constriction of the aortic isthmus area, occa-

sionally associated with a patent ductus arteriosus inserting just at or below it. Complex coarctation involves tubular hypoplasia of the aortic arch, with or without discrete aortic narrowing and one or more of the following lesions: patent ductus arteriosus, ventricular septal defect, endocardial cushion defect, aortic stenosis, subaortic stenosis, mitral stenosis or regurgitation, hypoplasia of the left ventricle and ascending aorta, other cyanotic anomalies, and endocardial fibroelastosis. In its most severe form the aortic arch may be atretic and completely interrupted as in DiGeorge syndrome. In complex coarctation and interruption of the aorta, the amalgam of left-sided involvement may be secondary to reduced intrauterine flow through the left heart, with consequent underdevelopment and hypoplasia extending from the left atrium to the aortic isthmus. In simple and complex coarctation, there are great variations possible in the extent and location of the coarctation.

Coarctation occurs in 6% to 7% of newborns with heart disease (see Tables 33–1 and 33–2). It is one of the common causes of congestive failure in the neonate (see Tables 33–7 and 33–13). Among symptomatic infants, 82% have complex coarctation, and 18% have simple coarctation. It is more common in male and premature infants. Girls sometimes have Turner syndrome. Severe extracardiac anomalies, usually renal or gastrointestinal, occur in 6% to 9% of these patients (see Table 33–4).

Pathophysiology

Simple Coarctation The isthmus is normally smaller than the ascending or descending aorta in newborn

TABLE 33–13. *Findings in acyanotic 0- to 2-week-old neonates with congestive heart failure*[a]

Diagnosis	Physical examination	Radiographic findings	Electrocardiographic findings
Coarctation	↓ Leg pulses and leg BP, soft SEM in back, +/– SRM, +/– click, S_3, +/– differential cyanosis, shocklike sepsis picture	↑ Heart size, pulmonary edema	+/– RVH, develops LVH, BVH
Critical aortic stenosis	Shock, ↓ pulses and perfusion, SEM, click, S_3, single S_2	↑ Heart size, pulmonary edema	LVH, T-wave abnormalities
Patent ductus arteriosus in premature infant	Heave, ↑ pulses, ↑ pulse pressure, continuous or SRM	↑ Heart size (LV, LA), ↑ pulmonary arterial markings	Develops RVH, LVH, BVH
Cardiomyopathy	↓ Pulses, ↓ perfusion, ↓ pulse pressure, ↑ HR, SRM	Large globular heart, pulmonary edema	↓ or ↑ voltage, T-wave changes, Q waves in ALCA
Critical pulmonary stenosis	SEM, click, single S_2, most have cyanosis	Normal or ↓ pulmonary arterial markings, RAE	QRS axis 0°–90°, +/– LVH, develops RVH
Systemic arteriovenous fistula	Heave, ↑ pulses, wide pulse pressure, soft SEM or SRM, bruit, shock, +/– cyanosis	↑ Heart size, ↑ pulmonary arterial markings	Develops RVH, LVH, BVH

[a]Congestive heart failure with cyanosis may be caused by hypoplastic left heart syndrome, transposition of the great arteries, truncus arteriosus, total anomalous pulmonary venous connection, pulmonary atresia with tetralogy, tricuspid atresia, Ebstein malformation, or persistent pulmonary hypertension.

+/–, may or may not be present; ↓, decreased; ↑, increased; ALCA, anamolous left coronary artery; BVH, biventricular hypertrophy; HR, heart rate; LA, left atrium; LV, left ventricle; LVH, left ventricular hypertrophy; RAE, right atrial enlargement; RVH, right ventricular hypertrophy; S_2, second heart sound; S_3, third heart sound; SEM, systolic ejection murmur; SRM, systolic regurgitant murmur.

TABLE 33–14. *Findings in acyanotic 2- to 8-week-old neonates with congestive heart failure*[a]

Diagnosis	Physical examination	Radiographic findings	Electrocardiographic findings
Ventricular septal defect	Heave, harsh SRM, +/– S$_3$, +/– diastolic rumble, normal pulses	↑ Heart size (RV, LV, LA), ↑ pulmonary arterial markings	Develops RAE, RVH, LVH, BVH
Endocardial cushion defect	Same as ventricular septal defect, fixed split S$_2$	Same as ventricular septal defect	Left axis deviation, develops RAE, RVH, LVH, BVH
Atrial septal defect	Hyperdynamic precordium, soft SEM, fixed split S$_2$, +/– diastolic rumble	↑ Heart size (RV, normal LA and LV), ↑ pulmonary arterial markings	Develops RAD, RVH
Patent ductus arteriosus in full-term infants	Same as presentation at 0–2 weeks of age		
Cardiomyopathy	Same as presentation at 0–2 weeks of age		

[a]Murmur may be present earlier than 2 weeks of age, and congestive heart failure may occur earlier in premature infants.

+/-, may or may not be present; ↓, decreased; ↑, increased; BVH, biventricular hypertrophy; LA, left atrium; LV, left ventricle; LVH, left ventricular hypertrophy; RAD, right axis deviation; RAE, right atrial enlargement; RV, right ventricle; RVH, right ventricular hypertrophy; S$_2$, second heart sound; S$_3$, third heart sound; SRM, systolic regurgitant murmur.

infants with simple coarctation because only 10% of the combined ventricular output during fetal life passes through the isthmus into the descending aorta, whereas approximately 60% passes through the ductus arteriosus to the descending aorta. After birth, the isthmus gradually grows, but in simple coarctation, a curtain-like constricting band develops at the point of connection to the ductus arteriosus. The coarctation may become more severe in the neonatal period, as constriction of the adjacent ductal tissue occurs. During childhood, there may be progressive hypertrophy and endothelial thickening at the coarctation site, possibly engendered by high flow velocity at the narrowed point. Collateral circulation may be present at birth. In simple coarctation, the increased resistance to flow results in a pressure overload on the left ventricle. If the coarctation is not severe and there is a patent ductus arteriosus, with fall in pulmonary vascular resistance after birth, there is a reversal of flow through the ductus arteriosus from the aorta to the pulmonary artery, and a considerable left-to-right shunt may develop. If the increased pressure and volume load exceed the ability of the heart to compensate by hypertrophy or dilation, congestive failure with diminution of systemic output ensues. Left ventricular end-diastolic pressure is elevated, resulting in increased pulmonary venous pressure and development of pulmonary edema. The increased pulmonary venous pressure also produces pulmonary artery hypertension and right heart failure.

Complex Coarctation and Aortic Interruption Complex coarctation and aortic interruption are characterized by pulmonary artery hypertension with a ductus arteriosus supplying the descending aorta, usually a large intracardiac left-to-right shunt, and increased pulmonary flow. The right-sided structures are dilated and hypertrophied. There is a pressure and volume overload on both ventricles and congestive heart failure. In those with a large

ventricular septal defect and patent ductus arteriosus, the systolic pressures in the pulmonary artery, descending aorta, ascending aorta, and right ventricle are identical. Peripheral pulse pressure is normal, and the pulses are equal throughout. With ductal constriction, the femoral arterial pulsations diminish. If the aortic arch obstruction is severe or complete, perfusion to the lower one-half of the body, previously supplied by the open ductus, is reduced. Manifestations of shock, renal and mesenteric hypoperfusion, and metabolic acidosis develop. Ductus closure causes death.

Clinical Findings

Infants with isolated discrete coarctation may be asymptomatic, although some develop congestive heart failure, often after the age of 1 month. The femoral and pedal pulses are absent or diminished compared with brachial or carotid pulses. One or other brachial pulses may be decreased if the left subclavian artery on that side arises at or below the coarctation. Systolic blood pressure in the upper extremities is higher than in the lower extremities, but marked hypertension is uncommon. Pulse pressure in the lower extremities is narrow, often 10 to 15 mm Hg. S$_3$ is often prominent, and there may be an apical systolic ejection click. A systolic ejection murmur is usually heard best at the left interscapular area over the back, but it may be audible at the left upper sternal border. A continuous murmur suggests a left-to-right shunt across the ductus arteriosus. Manifestations of congestive heart failure are those of combined left and right heart failure. The chest radiograph shows cardiac enlargement and pulmonary venous congestion. The ECG usually reveals right ventricular hypertrophy in the early months and left ventricular hypertrophy only later. Echocardiographic visualization of the aortic arch usually shows the site, length, and severity of coarctation and the aortic arch branching pattern. There is characteristically a constriction from the outer posterior curvature of the aortic wall, and an anterior periductal shelf may be identified. An instantaneous systolic gradient may be derived from the velocities across the coarctation but may underestimate the severity of the lesion if cardiac output is depressed. The descending aortic flow has a characteristically diminished systolic upstroke velocity and prolonged antegrade flow.

Infants with severe isolated and complex coarctation usually present with congestive heart failure in the early neonatal period. Generally, the younger the infant, the more severe and complex are the combined malformations. Complete interruption of the aortic arch is usually associated with a ventricular septal defect and a systemic patent ductus arteriosus and is clinically indistinguishable from complicated coarctation. It is frequently seen as part of DiGeorge syndrome, which may have additional manifestations of hypocalcemia, absent thymic shadow on the initial chest radiograph, and possible impaired immune response to transfused viable nonirradiated leukocytes. Besides the findings described for simple coarctation, there is evidence of a large left-to-right shunt and pulmonary artery hypertension. Femoral pulsations may wax and wane, depending on ductal caliber. A pansystolic murmur of a septal defect or mitral regurgitation may be found. Ductal closure may result in a critically ill baby with poor perfusion, metabolic acidosis, and possibly disseminated intravascular coagulation, necrotizing enterocolitis, and renal and hepatic dysfunction. The chest radiographs show considerable cardiac enlargement, pulmonary plethora, and edema (Fig. 33–31). The ECG shows right axis deviation, right atrial hypertrophy, right ventricular hypertrophy, and often diminished left ventricular forces. Along with the aortic arch anatomy, echocardiography often reveals associated lesions, including mitral and aortic stenosis, ventricular septal defect, subaortic obstruction, and conotruncal abnormalities.

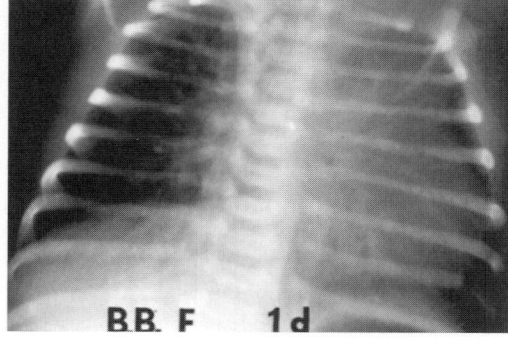

FIG. 33–31. A chest radiograph of a 1-day-old infant with complex coarctation of the aorta shows marked cardiac enlargement and pulmonary vascular engorgement.

Treatment

All neonates with congestive heart failure thought to have coarctation of the aorta should be promptly hospitalized, treated, and examined by echocardiography. Infants with complex coarctation and aortic interruption become symptomatic because of constriction of the ductus arteriosus. Prostaglandin E_1 infusion dilates the ductus, restores systemic perfusion, improves metabolic abnormalities, and supports life during the time needed to study the anatomy and arrange for surgery. Inotropic support with intravenous dopamine or adrenergic agents is often needed. In critically ill babies, there may be adverse ischemic consequences for the gastrointestinal, renal, hepatic, and coagulation systems. Echocardiography usually provides the anatomic detail needed for surgery. If needed, cardiac catheterization, digital subtraction angiography, or magnetic resonance imaging may be useful for additional delineation of the aortic arch and intracardiac anatomy.

If after initial clinical management to effect stabilization, improvement or deterioration occurs, surgery should not be unduly delayed. The surgical procedures employed depend on the severity of the lesion and include resection of the coarctation with primary anastomosis, subclavian or prosthetic patch aortoplasty, or construction of a conduit from ascending to descending aorta; division of the patent ductus arteriosus; and, if needed, intracardiac repair of additional defects such as a large ventricular septal defect. The mortality rate for infants with complicated coarctation is 85% without surgery. Surgery increases the survival rate to 85%. Regardless of the type of coarctation, the mortality is related to age of presentation and is higher for those with duct-dependent descending aortic flow. In some infants with simple and milder coarctation who respond well to medical therapy, surgery may be delayed. Those who undergo surgical coarctation repair early in infancy may develop restenosis later, which may require reoperation or catheter balloon dilation. The survivors need close medical supervision throughout childhood and may require other operations for various associated abnormalities later. The role of catheter balloon dilation of unoperated primary discrete coarctation is being investigated. It can offer palliation in the complex critically ill infant. In selected infants with an otherwise good size aortic arch, it may provide long-lasting relief (50).

Differential Diagnosis

Aortic arch obstruction should be suspected in any critically ill term baby with a septic-like shock. It should also be suspected as an associated anomaly in young babies with intracardiac anomalies such as ventricular septal defect, single ventricle, truncus arteriosus, and aortic or mitral valve disease who develop signs of poor systemic output. A thorough examination, including careful palpation of all peripheral pulses and blood pressure measurement, should lead to the correct diagnosis (see Table 33–13). Infants presenting before 1 month of age usually have severe or complex coarctation. The presence of a ductus arteriosus supplying the descending aorta may be demonstrated by the finding of a lower arterial PO$_2$ in the legs than in the arms. The hypoplastic left heart syndrome produces a similar shock-like picture or congestive failure in the first week as the ductus arteriosus closes. In these patients, there is cyanosis, the peripheral pulses are diminished throughout, and the ECG shows marked diminution in left ventricular forces.

Aortic Stenosis

Critical isolated aortic stenosis in neonates is rare. Except in circumstances of hypertrophic cardiomyopathy, the obstruction is almost always valvar. Only very severe aortic valve narrowing produces symptoms in early infancy. The symptoms are those of congestive heart failure, pulmonary edema, and sometimes peripheral vascular collapse. The baby may appear ashen and cyanotic if the pulmonary edema is severe. The cardinal features are tachypnea, a blowing systolic murmur at the upper right or middle left sternal border and an apical early systolic click resembling a split S$_1$. Chest radiographs show cardiac enlargement and pulmonary venous congestion. ECG usually has biventricular hypertrophy with T-wave changes (see Table 33–13). Echocardiographic examination demonstrates a deformed immobile aortic valve with commissural fusion. In severe aortic obstruction, transvalvar flow is diminished, and the systolic murmur and the Doppler-derived pressure gradient are of low amplitude and do not reflect the severity of the lesion. The left ventricle appears hypertrophied and may have decreased or dilated internal dimensions and poor or hyperdynamic systolic function. Some patients may have coarctation and mitral valve abnormalities.

Initial treatment of critical stenosis consists of administration of inotropic support, oxygen, and frequently prostaglandin E$_1$, to allow right ventricular support to the systemic circulation. This should be followed as soon as feasible by (Fig. 33–32) balloon valvuloplasty or surgical valvotomy (51,52). This provides effective palliation in infancy, and the majority require reintervention during childhood. Although most infants with critical aortic stenosis survive valvuloplasty or valvotomy, some have associated endocardial fibroelastosis or very small left ventricles that requires an extensive staged hypoplastic left-heart-type surgical approach for survival. The asymptomatic infant with auscultatory findings of aortic stenosis and those after valvuloplasty require continued follow-up because, over the long term, valvar aortic stenosis almost invariably progresses and recurs to some degree.

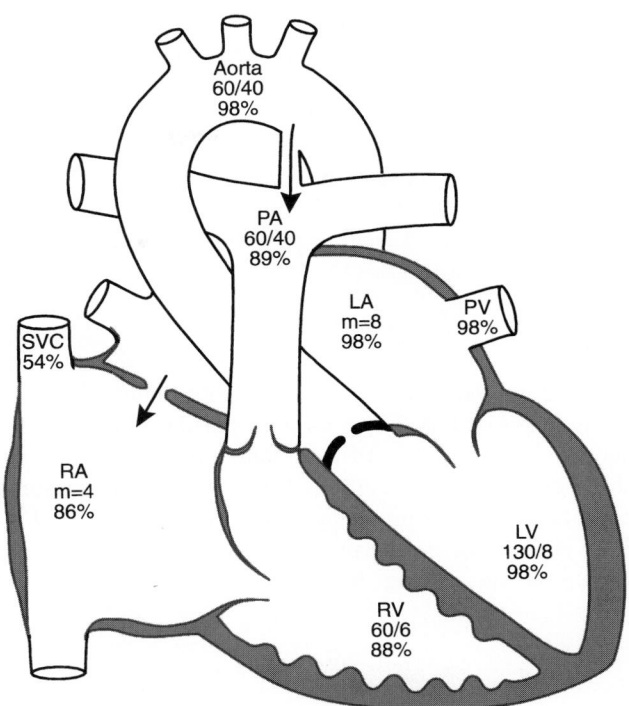

FIG. 33–32. Diagram of the cardiac anatomy and physiology in a 1-month-old infant with valvar aortic stenosis had a systolic pressure gradient of 70 mmHg across the aortic valve. The blood passing from left to right through the ductus must return again through the aortic valve, with the excess flow compounding the obstruction. The large atrial shunt, whether a true anomaly or a sprung foramen ovale, elevates left atrial pressure. The numbers below the chamber name are pressure measurements in mmHg determined at cardiac catheterization; the percentages indicate oxygen saturation data. LA, left atrium; LV, left ventricle; PA, pulmonary artery; PV, pulmonary vein; RA, right atrium; RV, right ventricle; SVC, superior vena cava. (Adapted from ref. 101.)

Acyanotic Anomalies with Left-to-Right Shunt

Ventricular Septal Defect

Ventricular septal defects may be small or large, single or multiple, and isolated or associated with other cardiovascular malformations. They are an integral part of complex congenital heart disease lesions, such as tetralogy of Fallot, truncus arteriosus, double-outlet right ventricle, and atrioventricular canal, and they have been associated with virtually every other known congenital cardiac malformation. Small, isolated self-closing muscular ventricular septal defects, frequently detectable only by echocardiography, are the most common congenital cardiac anomaly, occurring in 2% to 5% of term newborns and more frequently in infants born prematurely (see Tables 33–1 and 33–2) (2,3). Large defects occur most commonly singly in the membranous septum, less often in the low portion of the muscular septum, infrequently beneath the pulmonary valve, or posterior next to the tricuspid valve. Even though only 10% of ventricular septal defects cause symptoms, they remain the most common cause of congestive heart failure after the second week of life (see Tables 33–7 and 33–14). Extracardiac malformations occur in 24% of the patients. Recognition of a large ventricular septal defect remains paramount because without closure a large defect with pulmonary hypertension can lead to irreversible Eisenmenger-type pulmonary vascular disease by as early as the first birthday.

Pathophysiology

The common small ventricular septal defect does not produce symptoms, but a moderate or large defect in a neonate may cause significant hemodynamic alterations. If the defect is large, right and left ventricular pressures equilibrate, and pulmonary hypertension results (Fig. 33–33). The decreasing pulmonary resistance after birth allows an increasing left-to-right shunt through the

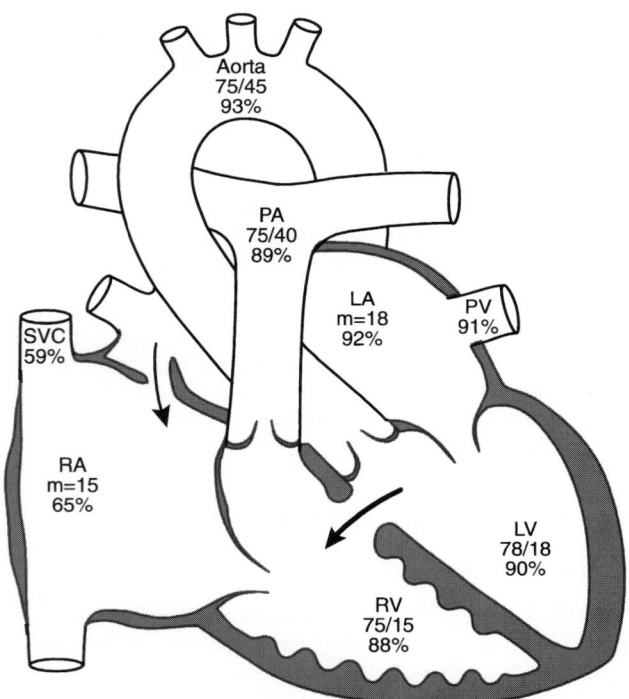

FIG. 33–33. Diagram of the anatomy and physiology with a large ventricular septal defect in a 1-month-old baby. The defect allows equilibration of pressure between the two ventricles. With pulmonary resistance much less than systemic resistance, there is a very large left-to-right shunt that caused congestive heart failure, as evidenced by the elevated atrial pressures and the reduced pulmonary venous oxygen saturation because of pulmonary edema. The numbers below the chamber name are pressure measurements in mmHg determined at cardiac catheterization; the percentages indicate oxygen saturation data. LA, left atrium; LV, left ventricle; PA, pulmonary artery; PV, pulmonary vein; RA, right atrium; RV, right ventricle; SVC, superior vena cava. (Adapted from ref. 101.)

defect. The normal regression of pulmonary resistance in the first week of life is usually delayed in these babies. Nonetheless, sufficient reduction in pulmonary resistance occurs by the second week of life to cause symptoms in many patients. Others, presumably with smaller defects or further delay in the reduction of pulmonary vascular resistance, develop symptoms as late as 3 to 4 months of age.

Symptoms are the result of congestive heart failure, not infrequently presenting with superimposed pulmonary problems such as pneumonia or atelectasis. Congestive heart failure is caused by the obligate high resting cardiac output associated with recirculation of large amounts of blood through the heart and lungs while simultaneously attempting to meet the demand for systemic flow. Cardiac pump reserve for exertions such as feeding is therefore diminished. Excessive pulmonary vascular flow and pressure decrease lung compliance, resulting in more rapid and labored, but shallower, breaths. The fixed tachypnea impairs feeding and increases caloric expenditure, resulting in diminished growth. Pulmonary congestion may not only decrease the tolerance for but increase susceptibility to recurrent respiratory infections. Mechanical pressure by enlarged structures, particularly the left pulmonary artery and atrium, may result in bronchial obstruction and pulmonary atelectasis. Because pulmonary vascular resistance is lower in premature infants at birth, the development of symptoms from a ventricular septal defect occurs earlier.

Gradual improvement and diminution in pulmonary blood flow in an infant with a moderate or large ventricular defect may occur if there is an anatomic decrease in the size of the defect. Many defects spontaneously close, and most—particularly muscular and membranous defects—become smaller with time. During childhood, but rarely in infancy, there may be progressive and irreversible development of anatomic obstructive changes in the pulmonary arterioles.

Clinical Findings

A small ventricular septal defect is characterized by an isolated readily audible harsh systolic murmur, which is localized at the lower left sternal border. Infants with large septal defects develop congestive failure in the first few months of life with symptoms of tachypnea (i.e., rate consistently >60/min), fatigue with feeding, decreased oral intake, excessive diaphoresis, and recurrent respiratory infections. Gross dyspnea is a late manifestation. Weight gain lags considerably behind height maturation. The infant often presents with a respiratory infection that may precipitate or mask underlying congestive failure. On examination, the infant is scrawny and tachypneic. The peripheral pulses are rapid and may be slightly bounding. The cardiac impulse is hyperdynamic. If pulmonary artery hypertension exists, the second heart sound may be single with an accentuated pulmonary closure. A gallop sound may be heard and is often associated with a middiastolic rumble. The systolic murmur is heard best at the lower left sternal border but is usually transmitted well to the entire precordium. There is hepatomegaly and frequently pulmonary wheezing and rales. Peripheral edema is rare.

A chest radiograph shows considerable cardiac enlargement, increased pulmonary blood flow, and sometimes pulmonary edema. The main pulmonary artery segment and left atrium are often enlarged. Atelectasis and parenchymal infiltrates are common. The ECG usually reveals left ventricular hypertrophy, and if the lesion is associated with pulmonary artery hypertension, right ventricular hypertrophy is detected. The echocardiogram can demonstrate the size, location, and number of ventricular septal defects. Associated lesions not appreciated on physical examination, including atrial septal defect, patent ductus arteriosus, coarctation of the aorta, and left and right ventricular outflow obstructions, are revealed by echocardiography. Right ventricular and pulmonary hypertension can be assessed both from the curvature of the interventricular septum and by comparison of Doppler measurement of the instantaneous systolic pressure gradient across the defect with simultaneous blood pressure. Often there is at least a trivial degree of tricuspid regurgitation to allow estimation of the right ventricular pressure from the pressure gradient between the right ventricle and right atrium. Defects with a large amount of shunt across them also show evidence of left ventricular volume overload with large left atrial and left ventricular dimensions and hyperdynamic left ventricular function. Occasionally, the infant who develops moderate congestive failure or who has evidence of borderline pulmonary artery hypertension may require cardiac catheterization to delineate the hemodynamics or determine the possible coexistence of other cardiac lesions.

Treatment

An infant with a small ventricular septal defect requires no specific treatment but should be followed. Some infants with large subaortic defects have or develop progressive pulmonary stenosis that prohibits left-to-right shunting, cardiomegaly, and congestive heart failure. These babies may develop the features of the tetralogy of Fallot. Later increasing right ventricular hypertrophy on the ECG suggests the development of pulmonary stenosis or increasing pulmonary vascular resistance and the need for careful reevaluation. In infants with congestive heart failure, administration of digitalis and diuretics may produce considerable improvement. Systemic afterload reduction with ACE inhibitors (e.g., captopril) may be beneficial in some refractory patients (see Table 33–7). If there are any pulmonary complications, antibiotics, bronchodilators, and pulmonary physiotherapy should be employed as appropriate. The use of high-caloric formulas, made by supplementation of standard formulas with additional carbohydrate (e.g., polycose) and oil (e.g., corn oil or MCT oil) up to a total of 30 kcal per ounce, is often needed for growth in babies with large defects. The total *ad libitum* oral intake should not be restricted, because growth failure and small size are a common issue in these infants.

Corrective surgery is indicated if the infant does not grow despite intensive medical therapy after a reasonable period of observation, requires repeated hospitalizations for respiratory infections, or has persistent significant pulmonary artery hypertension after 6 months of age. Primary repair in infants entails cardiopulmonary bypass, possible deep hypothermic circulatory arrest, and, in most patients, atriotomy with patch closure through the tricuspid valve. Some patients require closure through the pulmonary valve or right ventriculotomy. Small premature infants and those with multiple defects may require an initial pulmonary artery banding procedure with corrective surgery done at a later age. Of infants born with isolated, large defects requiring closure in the first year of life, as many as 10% die, usually because of associated severe extracardiac congenital anomalies, pulmonary complications, or prematurity. The long-term prognosis after transatrial surgical closure of an isolated ventricular septal defect in the first year of life is excellent, with essentially normal hemodynamics and a small risk for symptomatic dysrhythmias for most patients.

Differential Diagnosis

In the neonate, the murmur of a small ventricular septal defect is generally characteristic, but sometimes can be difficult to differentiate from that caused by a small patent ductus arteriosus or tricuspid regurgitation (see Table 33–14). Coexistence of additional malformations resulting in a large left-to-right shunt (e.g., truncus arteriosus) can be difficult to differentiate clinically from isolated large ventricular septal defects. Ascertaining their presence often requires echocardiographic examination.

Secundum and Sinus Venosus Atrial Septal Defects

Virtually all babies have a patent foramen ovale at birth. Many foramen ovale functionally close within hours of birth, but many others remain at least partly open for several months and in about 20% the foramen has some blood flow across it throughout life. This is important to the neonatologist, because umbilical vein catheters tend to follow the course of the circulation for the preceding 9 months and may pass through the foramen ovale into the left heart, providing erroneous measures of oxygen levels and allowing passage of intravenously injected materials straight to the brain, occasionally with disastrous results.

Pathophysiology and Clinical Features

An opening in the primum atrial septum around the region of the foramen ovale is a relatively common anomaly, but rarely causes symptoms or a murmur loud enough to attract attention in infants. Rarely defects occur in the atrial septum where the cavae enter, usually the superior vena cava, often with partial anomalous connection of one or more right pulmonary veins, and are clinically indistinguishable from secundum atrial septal defects. Since left ventricular compliance lessens with age, left to right shunting develops across the defect, resulting in increased flow across right heart valves (and pulmonary and tricuspid flow murmurs), persistent delayed closure of the pulmonary valve (and relatively wide fixed splitting of the second heart sound), increased right ventricular workload and increased pulmonary blood flow. Some of these defects are discovered because of concern initiated by extracardiac anomalies, and an echocardiographic examination is performed. Others are discovered during workup for failure to thrive, but most are found because a murmur of pulmonary stenosis is heard. Most small secundum defects (<5 mm diameter), many moderate-size ones (5 to 8 mm diameter) (74), and some large defects spontaneously close, or nearly close in the first several years of life. Sinus venosus defects rarely if ever close spontaneously. Because there is rarely significant congestive heart failure, treatment consists of observation and, when occasionally needed, if the defect persists, it may be closed by surgical or catheter techniques. If a large defect remains open, approximately 10% of those develop Eisenmenger-type pulmonary vascular disease later in life.

Differential Diagnosis

Rarely, a large atrial septal defect is associated with an early decrease in the pulmonary resistance and a large left-to-right shunt in the first months of life. Growth failure and congestive heart failure may raise the question of early cardiac surgery. This is a treacherous situation because any left-sided heart disease (e.g., myocardial disease) may have upset the balance of bilateral atrial outflow resistance, causing the left-to-right shunt. Surgical closure of the defect may uncover the additional problem of myocardial failure, with a disastrous outcome. The simple rule of thumb is to search diligently for associated anomalies and proceed to surgery for isolated atrial septal in early infancy with caution.

Endocardial Cushion Defects

Defects of endocardial cushion development may be partial, resulting in an ostium primum atrial septal defect; complete, resulting in additional total deficiency of the posterior inlet interventricular septum and a common atrioventricular valve (i.e., complete atrioventricular canal); or transitional with a combination of a smaller restrictive defect of the inlet interventricular septum and primum atrial septal defect, transitional atrioventricular canal defect). The atrioventricular valves, particularly the anterior mitral valve leaflet, are usually malformed, deficient, or abnormally attached to the ventricular septum. With ostium primum defect, there is usually a cleft in the mitral valve and frequently mitral regurgitation. In complete atrioventricular canal, the primitive atrioventricular valve floats like a sail over both ventricles. This malformation results in a large communication between the right and left atria and the right and left ventricles. Significant atrioventricular valve regurgitation is less common than in those with only an ostium primum defect. Occasionally, but more often in those without trisomy 21, the mitral valve has abnormal chordal attachments and is stenotic. The large atrioventricular valve is rarely primarily centered over one ventricle, and the contralateral ventricle is much smaller than normal. Endocardial cushion defects as primary lesions account for 4% of all newborns with serious heart disease (see Tables 33–1 and 33–2).

Approximately half of those with isolated complete atrioventricular canal defects have trisomy 21 (75). Forty percent of infants with Down syndrome have congenital heart disease, complete atrioventricular canals being most common. Because babies who have Down syndrome have a tendency to underventilate, causing pulmonary venous oxygen unsaturation, they may have pulmonary hypertension that, associated with a common atrioventricular canal, may limit left-to-right shunting to amounts that do not produce a murmur (Fig. 33–34). All infants with Down syndrome should be examined for congenital heart disease. When the murmur is subdued, subtle but cardinal features of cardiac anomaly are a hyperdynamic precordium and a abnormal second heart sound. An ECG will usually show leftward superior axis in those babies with Down syndrome with an atrioventricular canal defect. An echocardiogram is routinely used in the evaluation of these babies.

Pathophysiology

The hemodynamic consequence of an ostium primum atrial septal defect is volume overload, which is caused by a left-to-right shunt across the atrial septal defect or regurgitation from the left ventricle to the right atrium through the cleft mitral valve. The large volume load, particularly if aggravated by an additional overload caused by mitral regurgitation, results in congestive heart failure, which is often severe. Streaming of inferior vena cava blood across the large, low-lying defect and cleft common valve leads to mild systemic arterial oxygen unsaturation. In complete atrioventricular canal, there is an additional left-to-right shunt through a ventricular septal

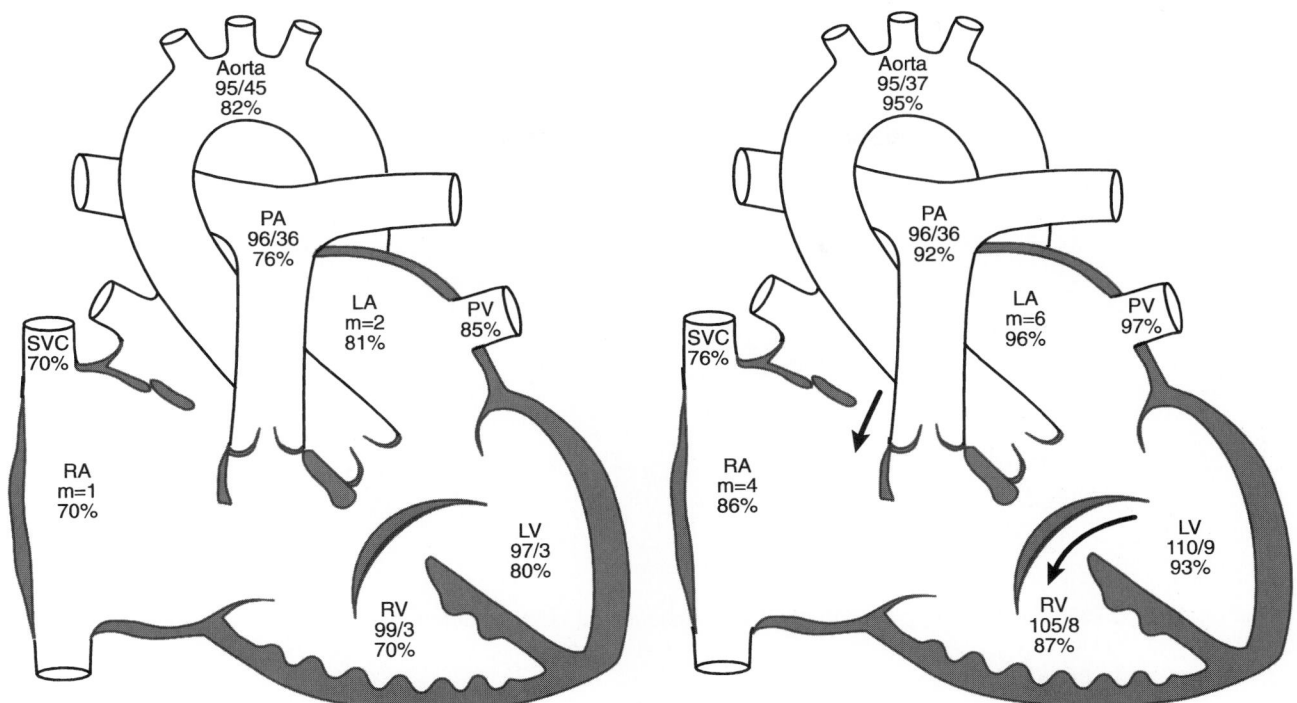

FIG. 33–34. Diagram of the anatomy and physiology of an atrioventricular canal in an asymptomatic girl with Down syndrome. There was no murmur. **A:** While she was breathing room air, the pulmonary resistance was high; there was no left-to-right shunt, and she had arterial oxygen unsaturation. **B:** When breathing oxygen, a large left-to-right shunt developed and the estimated pulmonary resistance fell sharply. The percentages indicate oxygen saturation; the numbers in italics are pressure measurements. The numbers below the chamber name are pressure measurements (mm Hg) determined at cardiac catheterization; the percentages indicate oxygen saturation data. LA, left atrium; LV, left ventricle; PA, pulmonary artery; PV, pulmonary vein; RA, right atrium; RV, right ventricle; SVC, superior vena cava. (Adapted from ref. 101.)

defect and right ventricular and pulmonary artery hypertension at a systemic level. Infants with pulmonary artery hypertension are particularly susceptible to the development of pulmonary vascular obstructive disease and its complications in later childhood.

Clinical Findings

Infants with ostium primum atrial septal defects who are symptomatic in the neonatal period usually have severe mitral regurgitation. Growth retardation may be marked, and weight lags considerably behind height maturation. Recurrent pulmonary infections are common. With complete atrioventricular canal, there is frequently mild cyanosis. The cardiac impulse is hyperdynamic, and S_1 is obscured by a loud pansystolic murmur audible at the apex or left sternal border. There is usually pulmonary hypertension, and the S_2 is accentuated. A loud S_3 and an apical middiastolic rumble are often heard. Occasionally, particularly among neonates with Down syndrome, there may be no perceptible auscultatory abnormality. The chest radiograph shows cardiac enlargement, sometimes out of proportion to the increased pulmonary vasculature, attributable to the large atria. The main pulmonary artery segment is prominent, and there is pulmonary vascular engorgement. The ECG characteristically shows a left superior QRS axis in the frontal plane, commonly 0° to −60° in primum defects and −60° to −100° in complete canal with a small Q wave in lead aVL (see Table 33–14). Significant right ventricular hypertrophy usually indicates right ventricular hypertension (Fig. 33–35).

Echocardiography demonstrates the anatomic features relevant to surgical repair, including the anatomy of the atrioventricular valve with its chordal attachments, papillary muscles, ventricular relationships, and possible regurgitation or stenosis of the atrioventricular valves (Fig. 33–36). Patients with complete atrioventricular canals may sometimes require preoperative cardiac catheterization to further delineate associated abnormalities detected by echocardiography or to evaluate pulmonary vascular resistance if there is evidence of pulmonary vascular disease. Selective left ventriculography in the case of complete atrioventricular canal shows a posterior inlet ventricular septal defect straddled by a

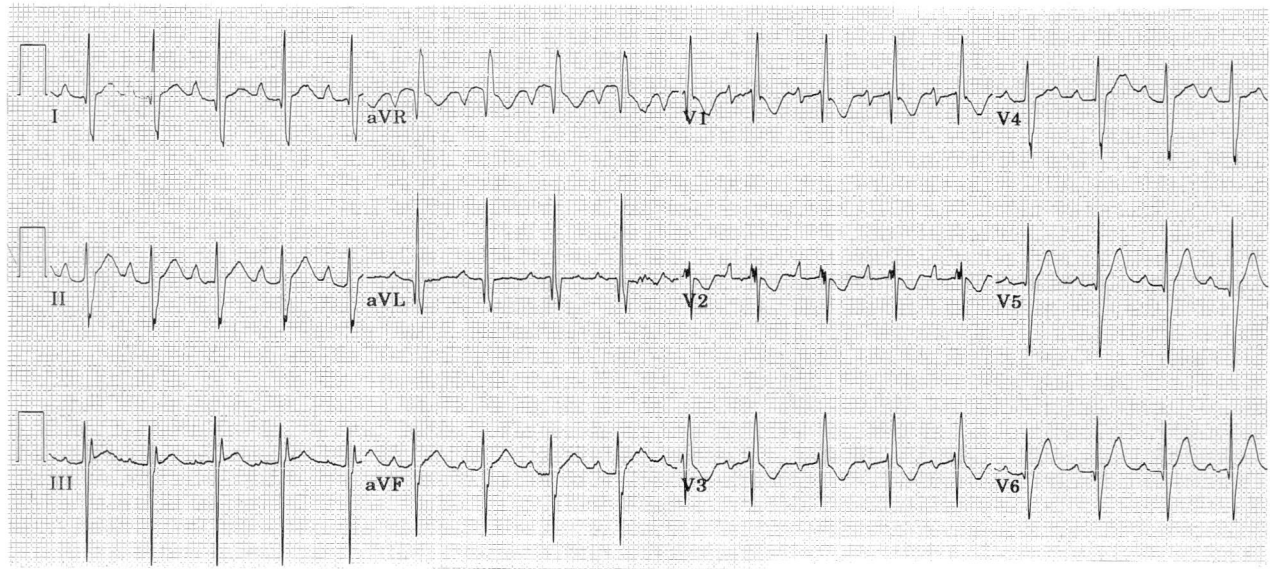

FIG. 33–35. Electrocardiogram of infant with endocardial cushion defect shows the characteristic left axis deviation.

common atrioventricular valve and diastolic anterior movement of the superior segment of the anterior mitral valve leaflet, producing an elongated and horizontal left ventricular outflow tract.

Treatment

In many patients, palliative or corrective surgery has to be performed in infancy because of refractory congestive heart failure or pulmonary hypertension. Treatment with

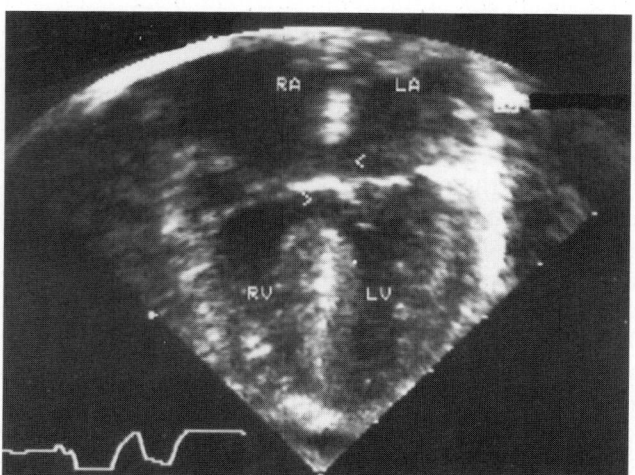

FIG. 33–36. Echocardiographic apical four-chamber view of an infant with trisomy 21 and complete atrioventricular canal defect. <, primum atrial septal defect; >, posterior inlet ventricular septal defect; LA, left atrium; LV, left ventricle; RA, right atrium; RV, right ventricle.

digitalis and diuretics may result in sufficient improvement in growth and respiratory work to delay operative repair for several months (see Table 33–9). Early caloric supplementation of formula feedings may improve growth. In some with refractory symptoms of congestive heart failure, afterload reduction may help. In infants with complete atrioventricular canals, there is pulmonary artery hypertension, and surgery is mandatory within the first year to prevent irreversible pulmonary vascular changes.

Primary complete repair is the preferred treatment. This entails cardiopulmonary bypass, atriotomy, patch closure of the atrial and ventricular septal defects, and attachment of the common valve leaflet to the patch or patches. In infants with refractory congestive heart failure weighing less than 2.5 to 3 kg or those with serious confounding noncardiac illness (e.g., duodenal atresia), pulmonary artery banding may be helpful, with complete repair accomplished later. Children with isolated uncomplicated ostium primum atrial septal defects and few symptoms can undergo complete repair without cardiac catheterization at several years of age. The long-term prognosis after surgery in infancy is excellent (76). There is often some postoperative regurgitation of the atrioventricular valve, but in most infants, this is not a significant problem. Systemic vasodilators can reduce the volume of regurgitation and may help preserve ventricular function in patients with significant postoperative mitral regurgitation. Late dysrhythmias occasionally occur. When there is severe mitral regurgitation, closure of the septal defect with valvuloplasty may result in clinical improvement, but residual mitral regurgitation may later require valve palliation or replacement. Without surgery, the prognosis is poor. Only 50% of patients with endocardial cushion defects who become symptomatic in the first month of life survive beyond 1 year of age without surgical treatment, and many of these have considerable delays in growth.

Patent Ductus Arteriosus

The ductus arteriosus, arising from the distal dorsal sixth aortic arch, is well developed by the sixth week of gestation and forms a bridge between the pulmonary artery and the dorsal aorta, inserting at the aortic isthmus. At term, it is a muscular contractile structure. In the full-term infant, functional closure occurs during the first day of life. Persistence of patency of the ductus arteriosus alone or in association with other cardiovascular lesions may produce no symptoms or severe hemodynamic changes, depending on its size.

Isolated patent ductus arteriosus, without hyaline membrane disease, is common, accounting for 4% of all newborns symptomatic with heart disease (4). It is more prevalent in female than male infants. Patent ductus arteriosus is a frequent complication of hyaline membrane disease in the premature infant, in surviving premature infants, and in infants born at high altitudes; in these patients, there is no sex difference. It is common in combination with other congenital heart lesions (e.g., coarctation of the aorta, ventricular septal defect, vascular ring). It occurs in 60% to 70% of infants born with congenital rubella.

Pathophysiology

Ductal closure occurs by constriction and then remodeling with apoptosis (77). At birth, ductal constriction is caused by multiple factors, the most important of which appear to be increased oxygen tension, the levels of circulating prostaglandins, and available ductus muscle mass. Prostaglandin E_1 is used to dilate a closing ductus in several forms of congenital heart disease in which patency of the ductus arteriosus is necessary to support pulmonary or systemic blood flow (53,54). Delayed closure frequently occurs in premature infants with respiratory distress syndrome. An inhibitor of prostaglandin synthesis (e.g., indomethacin) is used to promote closure of the ductus in this situation (78,79). The ductus arteriosus that remains patent in the term infant is abnormal and at most rarely susceptible to pharmacologic closure.

Within the first hours after birth, with a fall in pulmonary vascular resistance and a rise in systemic resistance, a left-to-right shunt may develop through the ductus arteriosus. A small right-to-left or bidirectional shunt may occur. If spontaneous closure does not occur and the ductus is small, the left-to-right shunt remains small. However, a moderate-sized patent ductus arteriosus is usually associated with a significant left-to-right shunt,

increased pulmonary blood flow, left ventricular volume overload, increased left ventricular end-diastolic volume and pressure, elevation of left atrial pressure, and the development of congestive heart failure. The run off of flow from the aorta into the ductus produces wide pulse pressure, and generates bounding peripheral pulsations. A large patent ductus arteriosus produces pulmonary artery hypertension because the pressure is transmitted directly from the aorta to the pulmonary artery through the large defect. Those with moderate and large ducts are prone to the development of pulmonary vascular obstructive disease by 1 year of age or beyond.

The premature infant may develop congestive heart failure earlier because of incomplete development of the medial musculature in the small pulmonary arterioles. The contractile function of the heart, required to handle the increased volume load, may be incompletely developed. Among those with respiratory distress syndrome, there may be an initial period of improvement as the pulmonary status improves, followed by clinical deterioration as left-to-right shunting through the ductus arteriosus increases.

Clinical Findings

Term Infants. In the neonate with a patent ductus arteriosus, as in all left-to-right shunts, the elevated but decreasing pulmonary vascular resistance determines the clinical manifestations. A continuous murmur is heard infrequently. There is usually a crescendo systolic murmur, often with clicks, sometimes detectably spilling into diastole. Often, S_2 is not clearly audible. The infant with a large patent ductus arteriosus has bounding peripheral pulses, wide pulse pressure (defined as the difference between systolic and diastolic pressure), and hyperactive cardiac impulse at the apex (see Table 33–14). There may be an apical diastolic rumble and symptoms and signs of congestive heart failure, poor weight gain, and recurrent pulmonary infections. In a full-term infant with a large patent ductus arteriosus, overt failure usually does not develop until 3 to 6 weeks of age.

The chest radiograph shows cardiac enlargement, pulmonary plethora, a prominent main pulmonary artery, and left atrial enlargement. The ECG develops left ventricular hypertrophy, occasionally left atrial hypertrophy, and in severe failure, ST-T wave changes. Echocardiography demonstrates the ductus arteriosus, its size, and the direction of the flow across the defect. Disturbed flow in the pulmonary artery, seen best with color Doppler techniques, is particularly helpful in identifying a patent ductus arteriosus. Continuous-wave Doppler allows measurement of the pressure gradient across the defect and, thereby, estimation of pulmonary pressure (Fig. 33–13). Large defects show evidence of left heart volume overload and a large left atrium and left ventricle, and right ventricular hypertension with flattening of the interventricular septum curvature. If there is associated pulmonary disease, the pulmonary resistance may be high, allowing only right-to-left shunting, which does not produce a murmur. Right-to-left ductal shunting also occurs with left heart obstructive lesions and coarctation of the aorta.

Preterm Infants. Preterm infants with a patent ductus arteriosus often have the same clinical findings as term babies. Some have a classic continuous murmur. However, many premature neonates with a large ductus arteriosus have no murmur. Most will have an increase in pulse pressure, at least intermittently. Because arterial pressure varies with age, gestational age, and illness, a rule of thumb for elevation of pulse pressure is when it exceeds half the systolic arterial pressure. Although preterm infants with a large patent ductus arteriosus may develop circulatory overload within the first week of life, some have no specific examination or radiographic signs discernible from respiratory illness. Unlike term infants, there is no substantial increased incidence of additional cardiac anomalies. However, if examination raises the likelihood of other cardiac or aortic arch anomalies, echocardiographic examination should be done before pharmacologic treatment. Echocardiographic examination of ductal diameter and length, ductal pressure gradient to estimate pulmonary artery pressure, aortic arch anatomy, and possible associated cardiovascular anomalies is indicated prior to surgical closure (Fig. 33–13).

Treatment

Term Infants. The full-term baby with a persistent patent ductus arteriosus and no evidence of cardiovascular embarrassment should be followed and catheter closure or thoracoscopic or surgical division of the ductus performed later. The choice of method and timing of closure depend on a number of factors including ductal size. Before therapeutic closure, term infants with congestive heart failure often have symptomatic improvement from treatment with digoxin and diuretics (Table 33–9).

Preterm Infants Among preterm infants with significant patent ductus arteriosus, indomethacin treatment produces closure in approximately 85% of patients. In symptomatic babies there is a corresponding resolution of findings of congestive heart failure, reduction in required respiratory support and improvement in survival (80). Its use in premature infants with a patent ductus arteriosus who do not yet manifest obvious symptoms from circulatory overload appears to improve many outcome variables including development of congestive failure symptoms, duration of ventilatory and oxygen treatment, and growth (80). Prophylactic administration of indomethacin early after birth in very premature infants decreases the incidence of patent ductus arteriosus, congestive symptoms, cerebral intraventricular hemorrhage, and possibly mortality (81–84). However, until there are data demonstrating an acceptable effect on neurologic function long term, there is uncertainty about the routine prophylactic early use of indomethacin because of the demonstrated negative effects of the drug on neonatal vasoregulation and cerebral blood flow and a theoretical increased risk for cerebral leukomalacia (83). Indomethacin can also cause deterioration of renal and platelet function, and its prophylactic use increases the incidence of oliguria and necrotizing enterocolitis (80,82). It should be avoided if there is significant renal dysfunction, thrombocytopenia, or bleeding. When available, newer prostaglandin synthesis inhibitors such as ibuprofen may have fewer side effects (85). The ductus arteriosus occasionally reopens after initially successful indomethacin treatment and may respond to a second course of treatment. Failure of indomethacin does not adversely affect subsequent surgery (86,87). Careful transfusion of packed erythrocytes in the anemic premature diminishes the left ventricular volume overload and may hasten ductal closure by increasing the arterial oxygen content. Surgical interruption of the ductus arteriosus is indicated, regardless of age or weight, in any infant with a persistent hemodynamically significant left-to-right shunt, particularly if there is pulmonary artery hypertension. Surgical mortality is low, and dramatic improvement often occurs. The procedure is performed using a left thoracotomy, or thoracoscope, in the intensive care nursery or the operating room under intravenous or inhalation general anesthesia. Catheter closure is not yet readily technically achievable in preterm small neonates.

Differential Diagnosis

The infant with congestive failure and a large left-to-right shunt caused by a ventricular septal defect may be clinically indistinguishable from the one with a large patent ductus arteriosus. Other lesions that may result in a large aortic runoff and mimic a patent ductus arteriosus include truncus arteriosus, hemitruncus (i.e., right pulmonary artery from the ascending aorta), aortopulmonary window, aneurysm of the sinus of Valsalva, and large arteriovenous malformations (see Table 33–14). In the sick neonate, clinical differentiation from other lesions is possible using echocardiography.

Aortopulmonary Window

Defects in the aortopulmonary septum are a rare anomaly resulting in a communication, usually large, between the ascending aorta and main pulmonary artery. Unlike truncus arteriosus, there are usually two normal semilunar valves, and most do not have a ventricular septal defect. In the approximately half without other cardiovascular anomalies, the physiology and clinical course are similar to truncus arteriosus with large left-to-right shunt, congestive symptoms, and pulmonary hypertension. The half with other cardiovascular anomalies most often have interrupted aortic arch and present with signs of aortic arch obstruction. Anomalous origin of the right pulmonary artery from the aortic trunk (right hemitruncus), anomalous origin of the coronary arteries from the pulmonary trunk, and other anomalies also occur with it. The diagnosis is established by echocardiography. Angiography is sometimes needed to delineate details of the anatomy needed for management. Treatment is surgical (88).

Arteriovenous Malformations

Malformation of the developing peripheral vascular system can result in abnormal connections of arteries, arterioles, and capillaries to the venous system (i.e., arteriovenous fistulae) that create a large shunt. These fistulas can involve vessels of any size and location. Large malformations presenting soon after birth with congestive heart failure occur more often in the liver and head. Capillary hemangiomas involve ongoing abnormal neovascularization. Rarely, infants with prolonged respiratory disease complicated by pneumothorax requiring multiple chest tubes may develop collateral vessels from systemic arteries in the chest wall to the pulmonary arteries. Although most infants with arteriovenous malformations have no other cardiovascular anomaly, abnormal congenital systemic-to-pulmonary vascular corrections can occur with tetralogy of Fallot with pulmonary atresia, partial anomalous pulmonary venous connection (i.e., scimitar syndrome), and bronchopulmonary sequestration.

Pathophysiology

Although most infants do not develop cardiovascular symptoms, a large systemic arteriovenous malformation can result in significant left-to-right shunt and congestive heart failure. Symptomatic babies usually have connections of relatively large arteries and veins in the cerebral or hepatic vasculature. Pulmonary arteriovenous malformations result in an intrapulmonary right-to-left shunt and cyanosis, but they do not produce congestive heart failure.

Clinical Findings

Arteriovenous fistula is one of the few cardiovascular defects that may produce severe congestive heart failure in the first day of life. Cardiovascular shock may be the predominant clinical picture. There may be a hyperdynamic precordium and pulses, flow murmur, severe congestive heart failure, and cyanosis. Bruits over the fontanelle, posterior neck, or abdomen may be audible,

and there may be an enlarged head or liver. Echocardiography can demonstrate biventricular dilation and sometimes an enlarged cava with increased flow. Arterial contrast injection demonstrates systemic arteriovenous fistulas. Systemic venous or pulmonary artery injection of contrast demonstrates pulmonary arteriovenous malformations. Ultrasonography, computed tomography, MRI, and angiography may be useful in finding and delineating the lesion.

Treatment

Malformations causing congestive heart failure usually do not spontaneously improve, except for capillary malformations that may respond to steroid or antiangiogenic drugs such as interferon. Large vessel malformations require mechanical occlusion. Surgery carries a considerable risk, and transcatheter occlusion with a variety of devices, including coils and detachable balloons, has been successful in many, usually older, patients.

VASCULAR RINGS AND SLINGS

A variety of intrathoracic vascular anomalies may encircle the trachea and esophagous and result in symptoms in the neonatal period. Depending on the degree of compression of the trachea or esophagus, several may present in infants with stridor, wheezing, cough, recurrent infections, or feeding difficulties. All of these symptoms are more commonly caused by other abnormalities, such as choanal atresia, tracheomalacia, laryngeal web, hemangioma, or gastroesophageal reflux.

Although uncommon, vascular anomalies may result in serious or life-threatening symptoms and therefore should be considered in any infant with persistent unexplained respiratory symptoms.

Right Aortic Arch with Anomalous Left Subclavian Artery

The spectrum of aortic arch anomalies is most commonly explained by the double arch model first proposed by Edwards and subsequently modified by others (89). This hypothesis explains all observed arch variants by abnormal persistence or regression of portions of a double arch present in embryologic development. The most common of the arch anomalies that has been associated with symptoms in the neonate is the right aortic arch with anomalous left subclavian artery. In this malformation, the aortic arch passes to the right of the trachea over the right mainstem bronchus, then giving rise to the left subclavian artery as the last brachiocephalic branch. A left-sided remnant of the ductus arteriosus connects the pulmonary artery with the descending aorta, resulting in a vascular ring encircling the trachea and esophagus. Symptoms, when present, are usually not severe and commonly occur beyond the newborn period. The diagnosis may be suspected on plain anteroposterior chest x-ray by leftward shifting of the trachea from the right-sided arch. Barium swallow may demonstrate a posterior, oblique indentation of the esophagous from the left subclavian artery. Echocardiography can demonstrate the position of the arch relative to the trachea as well as the branching pattern. Associated cardiac malformations, if present, can also be determined at the time of echocardiographic evaluation. Magnetic resonance imaging has proven to be a useful tool for determining vascular anatomy and be display evidence of tracheal compression.

Double Aortic Arch

Failure of the normal regression of the embryologic right arch between the right subclavian artery and the descending aorta results in a double aortic arch. The right-sided arch is the larger and more cephalad in approximately 75% of patients. The resulting vascular structure completely encircles the trachea and esophagus. Symptoms may be dramatic, even life-threatening, and usually occur within the first few months of life. The plain chest x-ray is generally nondiagnostic, but anatomy can be imaged by echocardiographic examination, magnetic resonance imaging, or angiography (Fig. 33–37). Barium swallow demonstrates bilateral indentation of the esophagus. If done, bronchoscopy will show the pulsatile compression of the trachea by the vascular ring. Surgery is indicated in symptomatic infants and consists of division of the smaller arch, usually the left. The postoperative relief of symptoms and prognosis is usually good.

Anomalous Origin of the Left Pulmonary Artery (Pulmonary Sling)

Anomalous origin of the left pulmonary artery is a rare but serious vascular defect in which the left pulmonary artery arises from the proximal right pulmonary artery and passes between the trachea and the esophagus before supplying the left lung. Respiratory symptoms are often severe, and there may be associated hypoplasia or stenosis of the trachea or right mainstem bronchus. Swallowing difficulties are uncommon. Barium esophagram demonstrates anterior compression from the aberrant vessel. Hyperinflation of the right lung as a result of selective compression of the right bronchus may be noted on plain chest x-ray. Echocardiography will generally demonstrate the key features of the anatomy, although MRI, angiography, and bronchoscopy have been recommended by some to delineate additional details (90,91). Surgery is indicated and consists of division of the left

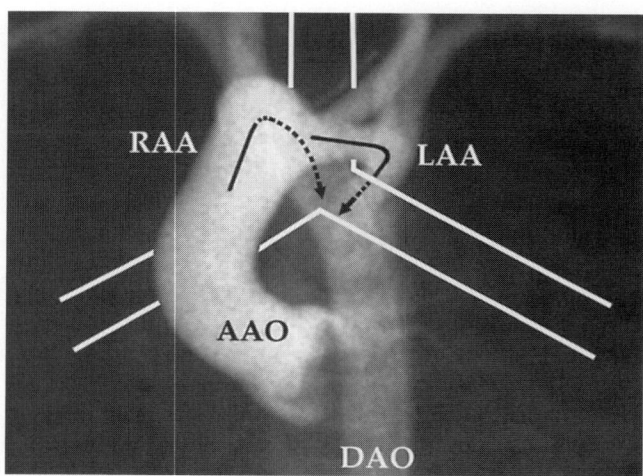

FIG. 33–37. Aortogram in the anteroposterior projection in a 2-month-old infant with a history of sudden apnea requiring resuscitation. The anatomy of a typical double aortic arch is displayed. The ascending aorta (AAO) connects to bilateral aortic arches that encircle the airways. The larger and more cephalad right aortic arch (RAA) passes over the right mainstem bronchus. The smaller, lower left aortic arch (LAA) encircles the trachea and passes over the left mainstem bronchus before rejoining the right arch to form the descending aorta (DAO). *Solid white lines* outline the trachea and mainstem bronchi. *Black arrows* show the course of the aortic arches.

pulmonary artery with reanastomosis to the main pulmonary artery in a more normal location. Outcome after surgical correction of the pulmonary artery origin has been fair, limited in part by associated lesions and by persistent pulmonary complications related to residual airway abnormalities. Residual left pulmonary artery stenosis is common after surgery.

Anomalous Origin of the Innominate Artery

Compression of the trachea by the innominate artery is a controversial source of respiratory distress in neonates and infants. It has been contended that airway compromise may result if the origin of an otherwise normal innominate artery is more distal than usual, resulting in indentation of the trachea as the vessel courses anteriorly and rightward before splitting into the right subclavian artery and right carotid artery. Bronchoscopy may reveal a pulsatile mass compressing the distal trachea. Surgical intervention to suspend the innominate from the anterior chest wall has been advocated, with reported relief of respiratory symptoms in some patients. In some series, this situation has represented a significant portion of infants undergoing surgery for airway compression (92). However, others have disputed this mechanism as a common cause of respiratory distress and suggest conservative management (93).

ACYANOTIC ANOMALIES WITH ABNORMAL CARDIAC FUNCTION OR STRUCTURE

Cardiomyopathy

Sick neonates without cardiac anatomic anomaly not infrequently develop symptoms of cardiac dysfunction and congestive heart failure as a result of myocardial dysfunction. Abnormal myocardial function or structure occurs with many abnormalities and disorders (see Tables 33–15 and 33–16). Systolic and/or diastolic dysfunction may occur as a primary event or secondary to another abnormality such as sepsis or hypothermia.

TABLE 33–15. *Dilated cardiomyopathies*

Infectious causes
  Viral (coxsackie, adenovirus, echo, CMV)
  Bacterial sepsis (endotoxemia, exotoxemia)
Myocardial ischemia
  Asphyxia
  Anomalous origin of left coronary artery
Reversible electrolyte and metabolic causes of myocardial
    dysfunction
  Hypoglycemia
  Hypocalcemia
  Hypophosphatemia
  Hypothermia
  Polycythemia
Work-overload cardiomyopathies
  Tachycardia induced (incessant SVT or VT)
  Severe pulmonary hypertension (H&D)
  Critical aortic valve stenosis (H&D)
Genetic isolated cardiomyopathy
  Dilated cardiomyopathy
    Familial dilated cardiomyopathy (1p, AD)
    Familial dilated cardiomyopathy (AD, AR)
    Familial dilated cardiomyopathy (dystrophin promoter,
      X-linked)
    Arrhythmogenic right ventricular dysplasia (AD)
    Noncompaction of the left ventricle (AD)
    Mitochondrial transfer RNA (tRNA) mutations
      T9997C tRNA Gly
      C3303T tRNA leu
  Restrictive cardiomyopathy
    Familial restrictive cardiomyopathy (AD) (R)
Neuromuscular diseases
  Duchenne muscular dystrophy (X-linked)
  Becker-type muscular dystrophy (X-linked)
  Myotubular myopathy (X-linked, also AR, AD)
  Nemaline rod myopathy (AD, AR) (H&D)
  Multicore myopathy (AR, also possible AD) (D, H, R)
  Friedreich ataxia (AD) (H&D)
  Phytanic acid oxidation disorder (Refsum disease, AR)
    (H&D)
Metabolic disorders
  Decreased Energy Production
    Disorders of mitochondrial fat oxidation
      Primary carnitine transport protein deficiency (AR)
        (H&D)
      Primary carnitine palmitoyltransferase II deficiency
        (AR) (H&D)
      Secondary carnitine deficiencies
        (many causes, e.g. methylmalonic and isovaleric
          acidemias, multiple ORT & fat acyl Co-A
          dehydrogenase deficiencies,
          Kearns-Sayre syndrome, etc.) (H&D)

Disorders of pyruvate metabolism
  Pyruvate dehydrogenase deficiency
    (Leigh necrotizing encephalopathy syndrome, AR)
    (H&D)
  Pyruvate carboxylase deficiency (Leigh syndrome,
    AR) (H&D)
Disorders of oxidative phosphorylation
  Complex I (NADH-coQ reductase) (AR, mtDNA)
  Complex III (reduced coQ-cytochrome c reductase,
    cytochrome b)
    (AR, mtDNA) (H&D)
  Complex IV (cytochrome c oxidase)
    (Leigh syndrome variants, AR, mtDNA) (H&D)
  Complex V (ATP synthetase)
    (Leigh syndrome variants, AR, mtDNA) (H&D)
  Combined respiratory chain deficiencies (H&D)
    Lethal infantile histiocytoid cardiomyopathy (AR,
      mtDNA) (WPW)
    Lethal infantile mitochondrial disease (mtDNA)
    Mitochondrial transfer RNA (tRNA) mutations
      (H&D) cardiomyopathy and myopathy
      syndromes (multiple mutations in tRNAs for
      leu, iso, gly, glu, pro) (WPW)
      MELAS syndrome (multiple tRNA leu mutations)
        (D, H, WPW)
      MERRF syndrome (multiple tRNA lys mutations)
        (D, H)
      Kearns-Sayre syndrome (multiple tRNAs leu,
        asp, cys) (HB)
    Mitochondrial DNA (mtDNA) mutations and
      deletions
      Kearns-Sayre syndrome (multiple mtDNA
        mutations, AD) (HB) others (e.g., 5 kb
        deletion, 7.4 kb deletion)
    Barth syndrome (3-methylglutaconic aciduria type
      II, X-linked) (H&D)
Infiltrative storage disorders
  Glycogen storage disease
    Type IV (Andersen disease, branching enzyme
      deficiency) (D)
  Mucopolysaccharidosis
    Type I (Hurler syndrome) (AR) (H&D)
    Type VI (Maroteaux-Lamy syndrome) (AR)
  Ganglioside degradation disorders
    G$_{M2}$ gangliosidosis (Sandhoff disease, AR) (H&D)
  Amino acid and organic acid disorders with toxic
    metabolites
    Propionic acidemia (AR)
    Ketothiolase deficiency (AR)

D, dilated cardiomyopathy; H, hypertrophic cardiomyopathy; SVT, supraventricular tachycardia; VT, ventricular tachycardia; WPW, Wolf–Parkinson–White syndrome; HB, heart block; AD, autosomal dominant; AR, autosomal recessive.
From refs. 33, 34.

TABLE 33–16. *Hypertrophic cardiomyopathy*

Hormonal causes
  Maternal diabetes mellitus
  In utero sympathomimetic exposure
  Pheochromocytoma
  Hyperthyroidism
Work overload
  Severe pulmonary hypertension
  Critical aortic valve stenosis
Genetic isolated cardiomyopathy
  Contractile protein mutation
    HCM-1 (myosin heavy chain, AD)
    HCM-2 (troponin T_2, AD)
    HCM-3 (alpha-tropomyosin, AD)
    HCM-4 (myosin binding protein C, AD)
    HCM-5 (AD)
    HCM-6 (AD) (WPW)
    HCM (AR)
  Cardiac phosphorylase kinase deficiency (AR)
  Restrictive cardiomyopathy
    Familial restrictive cardiomyopathy (AD) (R)
Genetic syndromes
  Noonan syndrome (AD)
  Cardio-facio-cutaneous syndrome (AD)
  LEOPARD syndrome (AD)
  Neurofibromatosis (AD)
  Beckwith–Wiedmann syndrome (AD)
  Cutis laxa (X-linked)
Neuromuscular diseases
  Nemaline rod myopathy (AD, AR) (D&H)
  Multicore myopathy (AR, also possible AD) (D, H, R)
  Friedreich ataxia (AD) (D&H)
  Refsum disease (D&H)
Metabolic disorders
  Decreased energy production
    Disorders of mitochondrial fat oxidation
      Primary carnitine transport protein deficiency (AR)
        (H&D)
      Primary carnitine/acylcarnitine translocase
        deficiency (AR)
      Primary carnitine palmitoyl-transferase II (AR) (D&H)
      Secondary carnitine deficiencies (H&D)
        many causes, e.g., organic acidemias, multiple ORT
          & fat acyl Co-A dehydrogenase deficiencies, etc.
      Very-long-chain acyl-CoA dehydrogenase (VLCAD)
        deficiency
      Long-chain-acyl-CoA dehydrogenase (LCAD)
        deficiency
      Long-chain 3-hydoxyacyl-CoA dehydrogenase
        (LCHAD) deficiency
    Disorders of pyruvate metabolism
      Pyruvate dehydrogenase deficiency (Leigh
        necrotizing encephalopathy syndrome, AR) (H&D)
      Pyruvate carboxylase deficiency (Leigh syndrome,
        AR) (H&D)

Disorders of oxidative phosphorylation
  Complex II (succinate-coQ reductase) (AR) (WPW)
  Complex III (reduced coQ-cytochrome c reductase,
    cytochrome b) (AR, mtDNA) (H&D)
  Complex IV (cytochrome c oxidase) (Leigh syndrome
    variants, AR, mtDNA) (H&D)
  Complex V (ATP synthetase) (Leigh syndrome variants,
    AR, mtDNA) (H&D)
  Combined respiratory chain deficiencies (D&H&WPW)
    Lethal infantile histiocytoid cardiomyopathy (AR, mtDNA)
    Lethal infantile mitochondrial disease (mtDNA)
  Mitochondrial transfer RNA (tRNA) mutations
    cardiomyopathy and myopathy syndromes
    (multiple mutations in tRNAs for leu, iso, gly, glu, pro)
    (H&D&WPW)
    MELAS syndrome (muliple tRNA leu mutations)
      (D&H&WPW)
    MERRF syndrome (multiple tRNA lys mutations) (D&H)
    Kearns-Sayre syndrome (multiple tRNAs leu, asp, cys)
      (HB)
  Mitochondrial DNA (mtDNA) mutations and deletions
    Kearns–Sayre syndrome (multiple mtDNA mutations,
      AD) (HB)
  Barth syndrome (3-methylglutaconic aciduria type II,
    X-linked) (H&D)
  Sengers cardiomyopathy with cataracts syndrome (AR)
Infiltrative storage disorders
  Glycogen storage disease
    Type II (Pompe disease, acid maltase deficiency, AR)
    Type III (Cori disease, debranching enzyme deficiency)
    Type IX (Cardiac phosphorylase kinase deficiency)
  Mucopolysaccharidosis
    Type I (Hurler syndrome, AR) (H&D)
    Type II (Hunter syndrome, X-linked)
    Type III (Sanfilippo syndrome, AR)
    Type IV (Morquio syndrome, AR)
    Type VII (Sly syndrome, AR)
  Ganglioside degradation disorders
    G_{M1} gangliosidosis (AR)
    G_{M2} gangliosidosis (Sandhoff disease, AR)
  Glycoprotein metabolic disorder
    Carbohydrate-deficient glycoprotein syndrome (AR)
  Others
    Glycosphingolipid degradation disorder (Fabry, X-linked)
    Globoside degradation disorder (Gaucher disease, AR)
    Phytanic acid oxidation disorder (Refsum disease, AR)
      (D&H)
    Tyrosinemia (AR)

D, dilated cardiomyopathy; H, hypertrophic cardiomyopathy; SVT, supraventricular tachycardia; VT, ventricular tachycardia; WPW, Wolf–Parkinson–White syndrome; HB, heart block; AD, autosomal dominant; AR, autosomal recessive.
From refs. 33, 34.

Myocardial dysfunction may be grouped by clinical and echocardiographic determination of the cardiovascular pathophysiology, without regard to etiology, as dilated, hypertrophic, and restrictive cardiomyopathy. The nature of appropriate supportive cardiac treatment depends on this cardiovascular physiologic classification. However, the outcome of supportive therapies alone is limited. Additional improvement in outcome may result from determining causation and directed treatment based on etiology.

Diagnostic evaluation should seek causation. History may provide information about family disease, possible infectious causes, maternal diabetes, and events with clear asphyxia. Physical examination may demonstrate malformations consistent with genetic syndromes, dysmorphic features and organomegaly consistent with peroxisomal or infiltrative storage disorders, encephalopathy and hypotonia consistent with various metabolic disorders and less often with neuromuscular disorders. The absence of noncardiac findings also provides diagnostic information. Although the history and exam may help point the direction, the diagnosis depends on laboratory studies. Initial evaluation should usually include blood electrolytes with measurement of total CO_2 or bicarbonate, glucose, blood urea nitrogen, creatinine, complete blood count, chest radiograph, and electrocardiogram. If infection is suspected, appropriate bacterial cultures (blood, endotracheal tube aspirate, urine, cerebrospinal fluid), viral cultures (nasophraryngeal, perirectal, cerebrospinal fluid) and serology should be obtained. Metabolic disorders can present with either dilated or hypertrophic cardiomyopathy and often clinically deteriorate with intercurrent infection. If metabolic disease is suspected, additional tests should be done, including measurement of blood ammonia, arterial blood gases, total and free carnitine, lactate, pyruvate, liver function tests, creatine kinase and urine quantitative amino acids, organic acids, and, if appropriate, mucopolysaccharides and oligosaccharides. Chromosomal analysis and skeletal x-ray analysis may be helpful if dysmorphic features are present. Ophthalmofundoscopic examination for retinal disease and cataracts may help in evaluation for disorders accompanied by these. Biopsy of skeletal muscle and/or cardiac muscle for light and electron microscopic examination, mitochondrial genomic studies and biochemical studies are often needed in the evaluation of metabolic disease (33).

Dilated Cardiomyopathies

Dilated cardiomyopathies are characterized by cardiac dilation, diminished contractility, abnormal diastolic function, and congestive heart failure. Neonates with dilated cardiomyopathy more frequently have an identifiable cause than currently achievable in older children and adults (see Table 33–15). These include identifiable infection (e.g., echo virus sepsis, Coxsackie or adenovirus myocarditis, toxoplasmosis), ischemia (e.g., anomalous origin of the left coronary artery, birth asphyxia), hemodynamic work overload (e.g., incessant tachyarrhythmia). and transiently with electrolyte or metabolic imbalance (e.g., hypothermia, polycythemia, hypoglycemia, hypocalcemia). Sometimes myocardial diseases that more commonly present in older children, such as those associated with neuromuscular disorders, have unusually early presentations in infancy. Increasingly infants are being recognized with primary biochemical disorders of energy production and metabolism that result in isolated cardiomyopathy or generalized myopathy and encephalopathy (33–35). These infants often have significant deterioration with stress, including that with birth. Caution should be used in attributing permanent or temporary cardiac dysfunction and encephalopathy entirely to "birth asphyxia" in a baby with low Apgar scores without identifiable perinatal cause for asphyxia.

Although the etiologies are diverse, in most dilated cardiomyopathies the clinical course, pathophysiology, and some molecular mechanisms are similar. Myocyte damage, from infection, cytokines, toxic metabolite, or energy deprivation from metabolic block or ischemia, results in myocardial injury. This results in a sequence of molecular and cellular changes with myocardial dysfunction, stunning, apoptosis, necrosis, and interstitial fibrosis, leading to impaired systolic contractility and diastolic compliance. Ventricular dilation, as a result of the Frank–Starling phenomenon, and tachycardia partially compensate for diminished systolic shortening fraction and support resting cardiac output but use up reserve in pump function. The impairment in diastolic compliance results in generalized edema and in pulmonary venous engorgement with tachypnea. If cardiac function worsens, resting cardiac output diminishes, and multisystem dysfunction results.

Neonatal viral myocarditis is an often fulminant disease frequently associated with hepatitis and encephalitis. The most commonly identified causes are echovirus, Coxsackie virus, particularly type B, and in some locations rubella virus. In individual cases, the cause is frequently not determined despite culturing of nasopharyngeal, tracheal, and stool swabs and serologic tests. The infection may be acquired perinatally or postnatally. Treatments including steroids, immunoglobulin, interferon, and ribavirin have been under investigation in biopsy-proven myocarditis, but supportive measures are the mainstay of treatment. Several other viruses, bacteria, mycoplasma, rickettsiae, spirochetes, and fungi rarely cause myocarditis. Myocarditis because of an autoimmune reaction may occur with maternal lupus erythematosus. Maternal IgG Ro antibodies cross the placenta, bind to the fetal myocardium, and may block conduction or cause cardiomyopathy. Steroids may be beneficial in this disease.

Anomalous origin of the left coronary artery from the pulmonary artery should be considered in all children with dilated cardiomyopathy, particularly if there is an ECG pattern of anterolateral myocardial infarction. The anomalous origin of the left coronary artery from the pulmonary artery and retrograde flow in the left anterior descending and left main coronary arteries can usually be seen on echocardiography, although angiography may be needed in some cases. Treatment is surgical and is usually successful.

Chronic supraventricular and ventricular tachycardia can lead to persistent myocardial dysfunction with the picture of cardiomyopathy. Some incessant supraventricular arrhythmias, such as ectopic atrial tachycardia and permanent junctional reciprocating tachycardia can be relatively occult, but detectable, by abnormal P waves. Effective treatment of the cardiomyopathy depends on recognition and treatment of the arrhythmia.

Treatment

General acute supportive treatment consists of correction of coexistent electrolyte, calcium, and acid–base abnormalities, providing abundant dextrose intravenously to support potentially jeopardized energy production, judiciously providing fluids to maintain cardiac output while minimizing edema, supporting the myocardial function with intravenous inotropic agents (e.g., dopamine, dobutamine, epinephrine, amrinone) (Table 33–10), and using antiarrhythmic medications as needed. (see Tables 33–17 and 33–18). In addition, antibiotics, hyperventilation, paralysis, sedation, and vasodilators may be employed. In cases with severe but presumably self-limited cardiopulmonary failure refractory to conventional therapy, venoarterial extracorporeal membrane oxygenation (ECMO) has been used with success. Although serious complications continue to exist, ECMO has become a standard treatment for critically ill neonates with self-limited cardiopulmonary failure.

Chronic supportive therapy is aimed at control of the congestive heart failure and arrhythmias (see Tables 33–9 and 33–18). Digitalization should be carried out with caution and orally if possible in infants with myocarditis,

because they may be unduly susceptible to drug-induced arrhythmias. Diuretics can help with symptoms related to pulmonary and systemic edema but do not appear to influence survival. Afterload reduction with angiotensin-converting enzyme (ACE) inhibitors can produce significant benefit in hemodynamic function, and in adults with dilated cardiomyopathy significantly improve survival. Cardiac transplantation may be considered if the course is fulminant.

Hypertrophic Cardiomyopathies

These may occur from endocrine abnormality (infant of diabetic mother, *in utero* sympathomimetic exposure) or hemodynamic work overload (e.g., pressure overload). Sometimes myocardial diseases that more commonly present in older children and adults, such as isolated hypertrophic cardiomyopathy associated with contractile gene mutations, present in infancy. Hypertrophic cardiomyopathy may occur in infants in association with genetic syndromes (e.g., Noonan syndrome) and infiltrative storage diseases (e.g., Pompe and other glycogen storage diseases, mucopolysaccharidosis). Primary metabolic disorders of energy production (disorders of fatty acid oxidation, nuclear and mitochondrial genome abnormalities in oxidative phosphorylation) cause isolated hypertrophic or dilated cardiomyopathy, or multisystem dysfunction with cardiac and skeletal myopathy and encephalopathy (see Table 33–16) (33,34). Information should be sought concerning history of maternal diabetes, exposure *in utero* to sympathomimetics and postnatally to steroid medications, family history of hypertrophic cardiomyopathy or possible metabolic disease;

TABLE 33–17. *Tachyarrhythmia diagnosis and treatment*

Type of arrhythmia	AV reciprocating tachycardia	Ectopic atrial tachycardia	Atrial flutter	Atrial fibrillation	Ventricular tachycardia
Usual QRS in arrhythmia	Unchanged	Unchanged	Unchanged	Unchanged	Abnormal
Onset and termination	Sudden	Gradual	Sudden	Sudden	Sudden or gradual
Fixed-rate tachycardia	Yes	No	V varies, A fixed	No	yes or no
A:V relationship	1:1	A > V or 1:1	A > V or 1:1	A > V	V > A or 1:1
Mechanism	Reentry	Automaticity	Reentry	Reentry	Reentry or automaticity
May respond to vagal maneuvers	Yes	Rarely	Rarely	No	Rarely
May respond to adenosine	Yes	Rarely	No	No	Rarely
May respond to esophageal pacing	Yes	No	Yes	No	No
May respond to DC countershock	Yes	No	Yes	Yes	Yes, if reentry
Antiarrhythmic agents for acute therapy	Dig, Es, Pro, Proc, Aden	Es, Flec	Dig, Pro, Flec, Sota, Aden	Dig, Pro, Flec, Sota, Aden	Lido, Proc, Es, Bret, Phen
Antiarrhythmic agents for chronic therapy	Dig, Pro, Sota, Flec, Proc, Q, oV, Amio	Pro, Flec, Sota, Amio	Dig, Proc, Q, Flec, Sota, Amio	Dig, Pro, Q, Flec, Sota, Amio	Pro, Proc, Q, Mex, Sota, Amio

A, atrial; V, ventricular; Dig, digoxin; Es, esmolol; Pro, propranolol; Proc, procainamide; Aden, adenosine; Flec, flecainide; Sota, sotalol; Lido, lidocaine; Bret, bretylium; Phen, phenytoin; Q, quinidine; oV, oral verapamil; Mex, mexiletine; Amio, amiodarone.

physical examination abnormalities of hypotonia, encephalopathy, organomegaly, dysmorphic features; and screening laboratory study abnormalities. If no abnormalities are noted, first-degree relatives should be screened with electrocardiography and echocardiography for asymptomatic hypertrophic cardiomyopathy. If physical examination or laboratory studies suggest metabolic disorder, or if echocardiographic evaluation of first degree relatives is negative or unobtainable, then additional laboratory evaluation for metabolic disorder may be helpful (33).

Infants of diabetic mothers develop a hypertrophic cardiomyopathy that is generally self-limited, although sometimes is a severe disorder. It results from the myocardial trophic response to fetal hyperinsulinemia provoked by transplacental passage of high maternal glucose loads. Clinical findings include a systolic ejection murmur, sometimes mild increase in respiratory rate and work and, rarely, evidence of frank congestive heart failure. There is an increased risk of structural heart disease in infants of diabetic mothers. Echocardiography reveals left ventricular hypertrophy that is sometimes severe, usually with involvement of the septum, and occasionally with outflow obstruction (Fig. 33–38). Treatment is supportive. Digoxin may worsen outflow obstruction and is contraindicated if the obstruction is severe.

The most common permanent hypertrophic cardiomyopathy is a genetic disorder in one of the cardiac contractile proteins, most often myosin heavy chain. In half it is inherited as an autosomal condition with variable penetrance or occurs as a new mutation. This isolated cardiac disorder is characterized by marked left ventricular hypertrophy associated with myocyte hypertrophy and disarray. There is a propensity for development of left ventricular outflow or intracavitary systolic gradients, symptoms of congestive heart failure caused by poor diastolic chamber compliance, ventricular arrhythmias, and sudden death. There can be significant progression with time, and a normal echocardiogram at birth does not exclude the possibility for phenotypic expression later in life. Because it can be subclinical and cause sudden death in older children and adults, echocardiograms and electrocardiograms should be obtained in all first-degree relatives and symptomatic relatives. Those presenting at birth appear to have the poorest prognosis. Inotropic agents and diuretics are potentially harmful and generally not used. Calcium channel blockers decrease the systolic pressure gradient, improve diastolic compliance, and may improve survival in adults. Because of hazards associated with calcium channel blockers in infants, their use in infants less than 1 year of age remains investigational. Propranolol improves symptoms but does not appear to affect the progression of hypertrophy or survival. Ventricular septal myotomy or myomectomy may improve symptoms in those refractory to medical treatment. Holter monitoring for ventricular arrhythmias should be routinely performed, and amiodarone considered in those with ventricular tachycardia or syncope. Cardiac transplantation may be required for survival in severely affected refractory patients.

Metabolic disorders of cellular energy production involving pyruvate metabolism, fatty acid oxidation, and oxidative phosphorylation may present in early infancy with clinical findings of isolated hypertrophic cardiomyopathy but are particularly likely to be present when there is associated one or more findings such as hypotonia, encephalopathy, cataracts, hypoglycemia, metabolic acidosis, elevated ketones, lactate or pyruvate. Treatment options depend on the enzyme affected.

Infiltrative disorders of the myocardium such as Pompe glycogen storage disease can present with clinical, ECG, and echocardiographic features resembling in many ways hypertrophic cardiomyopathy. Distinguishing features sometimes include skeletal muscular hypotonia, protruding tongue, short PR interval, left ventricular hypertrophy, and normal or diminished systolic function. Pompe disease is uniformly fatal.

Cardiac Tumors

Intracardiac tumors in neonates are rare. Rhabdomyoma accounts for most. Fibromas occur much less frequently, and other types occur rarely. Most babies with cardiac rhabdomyoma have tuberous sclerosis (see Table 33–5), and vice versa (94). The presence of one should prompt an investigation for the other. Cardiac rhabdomyoma may be the only manifestation of tuberous sclerosis in neonates. Neonatal cardiac rhabdomyoma are generally multiple and usually regress, often completely. Cardiac tumors 2 mm or more in diameter are readily demonstrated by echocardiography, even in the fetus. Many babies are asymptomatic, even when the tumors are large and multiple, although perivalvar masses can obstruct valve flow and development. Serious arrhythmias also sometimes occur (see Fig. 33–4).

Neonatal Tricuspid Valve Regurgitation

An abnormally functioning but anatomically normal tricuspid valve is a common finding in the newborn period. There may be right ventricular myocardial disease; perhaps asphyxial cardiomyopathy, which causes tricuspid regurgitation; or persistent pulmonary hypertension of the newborn or pulmonary hypertension resulting from pulmonary parenchymal disease. Whether there is primary myocardial dysfunction or pulmonary hypertension and secondary right ventricular dysfunction, there is secondary tricuspid regurgitation of a normal tricuspid valve. If there is right ventricular diastolic dysfunction, there may be right-to-left shunting through a patent foramen ovale. The explanation for a lower sternal murmur is documented by echocardiography and managed with

TABLE 33–18. *Neonatal antiarrhythmic drugs*

Drug (Class)	Currently commonly used	Route of metabolism/ excretion	Oral dose	IV dose	Therapeutic level	Indications	Contraindications	Toxicity
Adenosine	Yes	Red blood cells and vascular endothelium		0.075–0.10mg/kg rapid IV push, ↑ to 0.15–0.25mg/kg after 1 min if not effective		Rx-reentry SVT, DX atrial flutter		Transient AV block, ↓ HR, ↓ BP, and flushing, rare atrial fibrillation
Digoxin	Yes	Renal	Load: 20–30 μg/kg divided in 3 doses, Maintenance: 3–5 μg/kg/12 hours; ↓ w/renal hepatic dysfunction	80% of oral dose	0.8–2.2 ng/mL	SVT, atrial flutter	AV block, VT, many WPW	AV block, ↓ HR, tachyarrhythmias, vomiting, use w/caution w/renal failure, toxicity with hypocalcemia
Quinidine (IA)	Yes	Hepatic	3–15 mg/kg/6 hours; ↓ w/renal or hepatic dysfunction		2–5 μg/mL	SVT, WPW w/ propranolol, PVC, VT	Long QT, known sensitivity, IV use, conduction block, myasthenia gravis	↓ Contractility, ↑ QT, VT, conduction block, vomiting, diarrhea, rash, blood dyscrasias, ↑ HR w/atrial flutter w/o digoxin, ↑ digoxin level, need to ↓ digoxin dose by ½
Procainamide (IA)	Yes	Renal, hepatic	2.5–8 mg/kg/4 hours	7 mg/kg over 1 hour Infusion: 20–60 μg/kg/min	Procainamide[a] 4–10 μg/mL	SVT, WPW, PVC, VT	Conduction block, myasthenia gravis	Similar to quinidine, ↓ BP, lupus-like reaction, no effect on digoxin level
Disopyramide (IA)	No	Hepatic, renal	3.5–7.5 mg/kg/6 hours		2–5 μg/mL	SVT, WPW, PVC, VT	Conduction block, myasthenia gravis	Similar to quinidine, ↓ contractility, anticholinergic, hypoglycemia, no effect on digoxin level
Lidocaine (IB)	Yes	Hepatic		Bolus: 1 mg/kg/ 5–10 min Infusion: 20–50 μg/kg/min; ↓ w/ cyanosis, hepatic dysfunction	2–5 μg/mL	PVC, VT	Conduction block ↓ junctional and ventricular escape rate	CNS reactions, seizure, ↓ BP, ↓ respiratory drive
Phenytoin (IB)	No	Renal, hepatic	2–3 mg/kg/12 hours; ↓ w/hepatic dysfunction	Load: 10 mg/kg over 30–60 min Maintenance: same as oral	10–20 μg/mL	PVC, VT, digitalis intoxication	Not FDA approved for VT	CNS reactions, ↓ BP, blood dyscrasias, hepatic dysfunction, hypertrichosis, gingival hyperplasia, coarse facies, rash

Drug (Class)	FDA approved	Metabolism	Dose	Therapeutic level	Indications	Contraindications/Precautions	Side effects
Flecainide (IC)	No	Renal, hepatic	0.3–2 mg/kg/8 hours; ↓ w/renal, hepatic dysfunction	0.2–1.0 µg/mL	Refractory life-threatening SVT, PJRT, PVC, VT	Conduction block, hepatic dysfunction, myocardial dysfunction	Occasional ↑ SVT frequency w/WPW, ↑ pacing threshold and conduction block, VT, nausea, ↓ contractility
Esmolol (II)	Yes	RBC esterases	IV only. Load: 0.5 mg/kg over 1 min. Infusion: 50–100 µg/kg/min		Recurrent, sustained SVT, WPW, VT	As per propranolol	As per propranolol
Propranolol (II)	Yes	Hepatic	0.3–1.0 mg/kg/6 hours; ↓ w/chronic cyanosis, renal, hepatic dysfunction; 0.02–0.10 mg/kg over 20 min.		SVT, WPW, PVC, VT, hypertrophic cardiomyopathy, long QT	Use w/verapamil, bronchospasm, conduction block, CHF	↓ HR, conduction block, bronchospasm, ↓ BP, hypoglycemia, depression, ↓ cardiac reflexes w/anesthesia
Sotalol (II/III)	No	Renal	25–70 mg/m² BSA/8 hours		SVT, WPW & VT with structurally normal heart	Use with verapamil, bronchospasm conduction block, ? structural heart disease	As per propranolol plus ventricular arrhythmias
Amiodarone (III)	No	Hepatic	5 mg/kg/12 hours for 1 week; then 5 mg/kg/day; ↓ w/hepatic dysfunction. Load: 5 mg/kg over 15–30 min. Infusion: 10–20 µg/kg/min	1–2 mg/L	Refractory, life-threatening, SVT, VT, recurrent VF	Conduction block	Extremely long half-life, corneal deposits, thyroid and hepatic dysfunction, pulmonary fibrosis, may ↑ conduction block and digoxin and quinidine levels, need to ↓ digoxin by ½, hypotension w/IV
Bretylium (III)	No	Renal	Load: 5 mg/kg over 15 min. Infusion: 20–50 µg/kg/min.		Refractory VT, VF		Transient ↑ BP, arrhythmia, then ↓ BP
Verapamil (IV)	No	Hepatic	2–4 mg/kg/8 hours; ↓ w/hepatic, renal dysfunction, neuromuscular disease		Refractory SVT, hypertrophic cardiomyopathy some PVC, VT	IV use, conduction dysfunction, CHF, many WPW, propranolol muscular dystrophy, use w/quinidine, generally avoid in infants	↓ BP, ↓ HR, conduction block, myocardial depression, constipation, may ↑ digoxin level, need to ↓ digoxin dose ⅓ to ½

[a]To differentiate from metabolite measure by some laboratories.

Note: Continuous ECG monitoring should be done during initiation of antiarrhythmic therapy and with IV administration because of potential proarrhythmia and conduction block.

AV arteriovenous; BP, blood pressure; BSA, body surface area; CHF congestive heart failure; CNS, central nervous system; DX, diagnose; FDA, Federal Drug Administration; HR, heart rate; PJRT, permanent junctional reciprocating tachycardia; PVC, premature ventricular contractions; RX, treatment; SVT, supraventricular tachycardia; VF, ventricular fibrillation; VT, ventricular tachycardia; w/, with; WPW, Wolff–Parkinson–White syndrome.

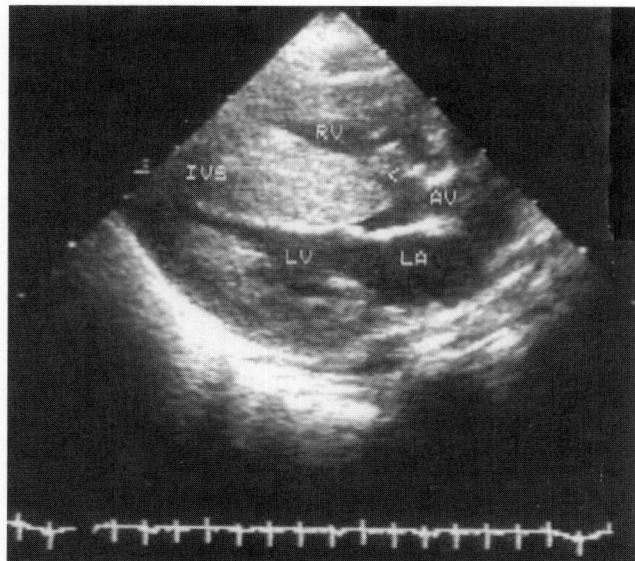

FIG. 33–38. Echocardiographic parasternal long-axis view of a diabetic mother's infant with severe hypertrophic cardiomyopathy and subaortic ventricular septal defect. <, ventricular septal defect; AV, aortic valve, IVS, interventricular septum; LA, left atrium; LV, left ventricle; RV, right ventricle.

observation, because tricuspid regurgitation of this type tends to regress as the underlying problem resolves (see Fig. 33–14).

Chronic Pulmonary Hypertension and Cor Pulmonale

Cor pulmonale is the association of right ventricular hypertrophy with pulmonary hypertension secondary to ventilatory or pulmonary disease. It frequently presents as symptoms of congestive heart failure with pulmonary disease. Patients with cor pulmonale have a structurally normal heart and must be differentiated from those with pulmonary hypertension as a consequence of intracardiac shunts or pulmonary venous obstruction. The most frequent cause in infants has been bronchopulmonary dysplasia, although its incidence has drastically declined in recent years and a large number of other causes, including airway obstruction, central hypoventilation, pulmonary hypoplasia, and diaphragmatic abnormalities, also occur.

Pathophysiology

The pulmonary artery pressure is controlled by vascular resistance that is a function of the number of small pulmonary arteries and the average luminal size. The number of vessels may be congenitally diminished by pulmonary hypoplasia or by acquired pulmonary parenchymal damage. The amount of small pulmonary artery musculature and the distance that it extends along the vessel determines the extent to which constriction may decrease average lumen caliber. The required muscle to prevent more than minimal pulmonary flow before birth is still present, although relaxed, after birth and can profoundly reconstrict with elevation of pulmonary resistance and pulmonary hypertension under the appropriate circumstances. These include alveolar hypoxia, acidemia, increased pulmonary venous pressure, and bacteremia. Polycythemia may also increase resistance. Increases in cardiac output with infection or anemia also elevate pulmonary artery pressure when pulmonary resistance is fixed. Pulmonary hypertension induces right ventricular hypertrophy and, if severe, causes right ventricular diastolic dysfunction and dilation. In addition to pulmonary hypertension, bronchopulmonary dysplasia also is frequently associated with systemic hypertension and left ventricular hypertrophy (see Chap. 28). Shifting of the interventricular septal position, elevated intraventricular pressure and biventricular hypertrophy, impair biventricular diastolic compliance and increase sensitivity to intravascular volume.

The pulmonary hypertension and cardiac sequelae seen with bronchopulmonary dysplasia generally appear to resolve when the pulmonary parenchymal disease resolves. In contrast, permanent pulmonary vascular change (i.e., Eisenmenger syndrome) occurs in patients with congenital heart disease after 1 year or more of exposure to a large left-to-right shunt with pulmonary artery hypertension.

Clinical Findings

Variable hepatomegaly and systemic venous congestion secondary to right atrial hypertension are predominant findings. Elevated left atrial pressure, especially in the presence of pulmonary parenchymal disease, may predispose to pulmonary symptoms and rales. The right ventricular impulse may be increased and the second heart sound loud and appear single. There may be a relatively soft murmur from tricuspid regurgitation, but a prominent murmur is not common and suggests possible congenital heart disease instead. Cyanosis may result from alveolar dysfunction with intrapulmonary shunting and right-to-left shunting across a patent foramen ovale. The degree of pulmonary artery hypertension and cardiac symptoms may vary with labile ventilatory or pulmonary conditions. Infants with bronchopulmonary dysplasia appear to be at increased risk for sudden death (10), similar to older patients with primary pulmonary hypertension.

Diagnostic Assessment

A variety of echocardiographic methods, some remarkably precise, some not so accurate, and most applicable to particular circumstances, can be used to assess the right ventricular pressure (see Fig. 33–14). No one technique in use is generally accepted and applicable in every patient. Sedation, often necessary for technically acceptable studies in older, active babies, may depress ventilation and should be used with caution.

Treatment

The treatment of pulmonary hypertension secondary to pulmonary or ventilatory disease is directed primarily at the underlying disorder. Judicious chronic use of oxygen as a potent pulmonary vasodilator may be useful. Bronchodilators and diuretics may be helpful for treating pulmonary parenchymal disease. Digitalis has not been found to be beneficial in most infants with congestive symptoms. With resolution of the underlying ventilatory disease, the pulmonary hypertension also resolves.

Differential Diagnosis

In patients with pulmonary hypertension, even those with lung disease, the presence of congenital heart disease should be sought. The absence of a loud murmur does not exclude a septal defect or patent ductus arteriosus in the presence of elevated pulmonary vascular resistance. Because many of the symptoms of cor pulmonale overlap those of congenital heart disease, echocardiography has been useful for excluding occult cardiovascular lesions that could lead to irreversible Eisenmenger syndrome. However, echocardiography used in cases of lung disease frequently faces the problem of poor ultrasound windows. These limitations should be realized, and the results correlated with other findings.

ARRHYTHMIAS

All forms of cardiac arrhythmias can occur in the fetus or newborn. Those most commonly encountered include sinus tachycardia and bradycardia, premature atrial depolarizations, supraventricular tachycardia, and less commonly, atrial flutter, ventricular arrhythmias, and complete heart block. Many arrhythmias are benign, occurring in otherwise normal hearts, and are of no hemodynamic consequence. Others may result in significant cardiovascular compromise, particularly if they are sustained for long periods, recur frequently, or occur in the presence of structural or functional heart disease. Thus, in evaluating patients with arrhythmias it is important to consider the hemodynamic status and whether there is evidence of structural heart disease or abnormal cardiac function. Rarely arrhythmias are the presenting sign of underlying cardiac abnormality such as cardiomyopathy or Ebstein anomaly. One should also keep in mind that arrhythmias may also result from noncardiac disease. In neonates, ventricular tachycardia, ventricular fibrillation, sinus arrest, and extreme bradycardia usually occur in association with preceding severe hypoxemia, hypotension, acidosis, electrolyte disturbance, or drug toxicity (e.g., digitalis).

Benign Arrhythmias

Sinus Bradycardia

Many infants have transient bradycardia associated with specific activities such as crying, straining or micturition. Some healthy infants persistently have a heart rate near 80 beats/min. Sustained bradycardia at less than 70 beats/min in neonates is abnormal. Noncardiac causes such as gastroesophageal reflux leading to vagal stimulation are common. Less commonly electrolyte abnormalities, hypothyroidism and exposure to medications (e.g., prenatal β-adrenergic blockers) are the cause. Bradycardia can also be produced by stimulation of the vagus nerve during procedures such as intubation and placing an nasogastric or orogastric tube. Cardiac causes, including nonconducted atrial premature beats, congenital long QT syndrome, and second- or third-degree atrioventricular block are evident on a electrocardiogram.

Sinus Tachycardia

Sinus tachycardia occurs with serious illness, fever, anemia, or pain at rates up to 230 beats/min. Tachyarrhythmias can be differentiated from sinus tachycardia by faster rates, abnormal P wave axis or PR interval, and when present by abrupt onset and termination or wide QRS complexes.

Atrial Premature Depolarizations

Premature depolarizations can originate from any conducting tissue. Atrial premature depolarizations occur in up to 30% of newborns. The diagnosis is reliably assigned when there is an identifiable, early, nonsinus P wave. However, the P wave may be "lost" in the preceding T wave. Atrial premature depolarizations may be conducted to the ventricles normally, with a bundle branch block pattern resulting in a wide QRS complex (if a bundle branch is refractory from the preceding beat), or may not be conducted to the ventricles (when very early and occurring when the AV node or proximal His bundle is refractory). When frequent, blocked atrial premature depolarizations result in ventricular bradycardia due to resetting of the sinus node with each premature atrial depolarization. In neonates with central venous catheters, frequent atrial premature depolarizations may be due to contact of the catheter with an atrial wall, and constitute an indication to withdraw the catheter from the atrium. In hemodynamically stable neonates and infants, premature atrial depolarizations generally do not warrant further evaluation. Isolated ectopic atrial depolarizations and atrial bigeminy are only rarely associated with tachycardia and usually are of no serious consequence. In most infants, these arrhythmias resolve over a few months.

Ventricular Premature Depolarizations

Premature ventricular depolarizations are early QRS complexes with a morphology different from sinus beats and without an identifiable preceding P wave. In newborns, ventricular premature depolarizations may not be much wider than normal QRS complexes. While premature ventricular depolarizations are usually benign, their identification should prompt evaluation for possible structural heart disease, electrolyte abnormalities, or the congenital long-QT syndrome. In the absence of these problems, they often resolve over a number of months. There are no data to suggest that the daily number or morphology of these complexes influences the prognosis.

Idioventricular Rhythm

An accelerated ventricular rhythm is a less common arrhythmia. There is a wide QRS rhythm, generally at a rate not more than 10% of the underlying sinus rate. This probably represents enhanced automaticity of a ventricular focus. There may be mild accelerations and decelerations of the rate. Atrioventricular dissociation is usually seen. The duration of episodes is variable. While this generally occurs in otherwise healthy infants, it has been associated with structural heart disease, electrolyte abnormalities, intracardiac tumors, intracardiac catheters, maternal heroine and cocaine use, and respiratory distress. Patients are usually asymptomatic and do not need treatment. This arrhythmia generally resolves within months (95).

Tachyarrhythmias

The heart rate alone is not enough to establish the diagnosis of a pathologic tachycardia. Infants can have a sinus tachycardia with rates up to at least 230 beats/min in response to serious illnesses, pain, fever, anemia or infusion of inotropic/chronotropic agents. Additionally, some unusual pathologic supraventricular tachycardias can have rates less than 180 beats/min. In assessing a child with a fast heart rate, one should determine if the QRS complex is narrow or wide during tachycardia, if the rate is fixed or variable, if there is a visible P wave and if so, the P wave axis. Supraventricular tachycardia typically has a narrow normal QRS complex. In general, if the QRS complex in tachycardia remains wide, the rhythm should be considered ventricular tachycardia. However, it is not uncommon for the first few beats of SVT to be wide because of aberrant conduction (right or left bundle branch block) before changing to a narrow QRS complex.

A patient with an apparently fixed high heart rate should be carefully assessed. The fixed heart rate could represent a sinus tachycardia secondary to a high-catecholamine state in an otherwise sick infant. An electrocardiogram should be obtained, and the P wave morphology clearly established. If there is no clear P wave, or the P wave does not have a sinus morphology (positive in leads I, II, and aVF; negative in lead aVR) one should strongly consider a pathologic tachycardia or structural heart disease with heterotaxy (see Table 33–17).

All neonates with documented tachyarrhythmias should have a complete cardiac evaluation, including echocardiography, to assess cardiac structure and function. It is estimated that between 8% and 25% of infants with SVT have structural heart disease, most often Ebstein malformation of the tricuspid valve, corrected transposition of the great arteries, or hypertrophic cardiomyopathy. Cardiac tumors and myocarditis rarely are predisposing causes for ventricular arrhythmias.

The clinical status of infants with tachyarrhythmias depends on the ventricular rate, duration of tachycardia, presence of underlying structural or functional heart disease, and other clinical problems. Patients may be completely asymptomatic, with the arrhythmia noted during an otherwise routine evaluation or while monitored for other reasons. The infant may not have been appearing well, with irritability, poor feeding, restlessness, or tachypnea. There may be respiratory difficulty and wheezing. With persistent tachyarrhythmias, the child may develop signs and symptoms of congestive heart failure or acidosis, becoming pale and listless. If the tachycardia persists for long enough, heart failure and a secondary dilated cardiomyopathy may develop. In the fetus with persistent or recurrent tachycardia, this is manifest as nonimmune hydrops. The time before this occurs depends on the ventricular rate, whether the tachyarrhythmia is intermittent or incessant, and the presence of structural heart disease.

Supraventricular Tachycardias

Atrioventricular Reciprocating Tachycardia and Wolff–Parkinson–White (WPW) Syndrome

The most common fetal and neonatal supraventricular tachycardias involve a reentry circuit using an accessory atrioventricular conduction pathway, atrioventricular reciprocating tachycardia (96). During supraventricular tachycardia there is conduction from the atria to ventricles over the AV node and His–Purkinje system with retrograde conduction over the accessory pathway from the ventricles to the atria. Because antegrade conduction is over the AV node and His–Purkinje system, there usually is a narrow QRS complex during tachycardia. Commonly the accessory atrioventricular conduction pathway conducts only retrograde. Therefore, during sinus rhythm all antegrade conduction is through only the AV node, and the electrocardiogram appears normal.

However, some accessory pathways conduct impulses in both directions, resulting in the WPW syndrome. During sinus rhythm the characteristic delta wave, short PR interval, and wide QRS complex result from a fusion of ventricular depolarization from conduction over the accessory pathway and normal conduction through the AV node. Because antegrade conduction during supraventricular tachycardia is usually through the AV node and His–Purkinje system, the diagnosis of WPW syndrome can not usually be made during tachycardia.

Electrocardiographically, atrioventricular reciprocating tachycardia is characterized by the abrupt onset and termination of a fairly fixed heart rate of 230 to 300 beats/min, abnormal or unidentifiable P waves that may be superimposed on the T waves, and a normal QRS morphology (see Fig. 33–39 and Table 33–17). The infant may be asymptomatic initially but then becomes irritable and fussy and refuses feeding. Congestive heart failure develops in approximately 20% after 36 hours and in 50% after 48 hours.

Persistent Junctional Reciprocating Tachycardia

One important, but unusual form of accessory pathway has slow retrograde conduction, resulting in a supraventricular tachycardia referred to as persistent junctional reciprocating tachycardia. These tachycardias are often slower than other supraventricular tachycardias, often less than 200 beats/min in newborns. This often causes an incessant or frequently recurring tachycardia that can result in a reversible dilated cardiomyopathy. Initially this arrhythmia is often well tolerated because of the slower heart rate. It can be recognized by having a fixed rapid heart rate in which there is an abnormal (nonsinus) P-wave axis.

Ectopic Atrial Tachycardia

Another potential cause of a dilated cardiomyopathy is an ectopic atrial tachycardia. This type of supraventricular tachycardia results from enhanced automaticity of a small cluster of cells in either atrium. The P-wave morphology is not normal in at least one lead. Depending on the atrial rate and possible AV block, there may be a variable A:V relationship (with more atrial than ventricular complexes). This type of SVT is characterized by a variable rate and gradual onset and termination (see Table 33–17).

Atrial Flutter and Fibrillation

Atrial flutter is less common than other types of paroxysmal supraventricular tachycardia in fetuses and neonates. It may be idiopathic or associated with the same congenital heart lesions as those producing other supraventricular tachycardias. The atrial rate may be 200 to 500 beats/min. The AV node is generally not part of the tachycardia circuit so that there need not be a 1:1 atrial:ventricular rate relationship. There is often some degree of AV node block resulting in variable conduction, frequently with a 2:1 or 3:1 atrial:venticular relationship. With a 2:1 block, the ventricular rate at the highest atrial rate would be 250 beats/min, a rate sufficient to produce congestive failure in infancy. The RR interval is constant except when the atrioventricular block changes.The rare infant without AV nodal conduction block may have a very rapid rate and shock. With higher degrees of AV nodal conduction block, a sawtoothed atrial pattern is characteristically seen, often best in leads II or V₁. In some patients the diagnosis can not be acertained from the surface electrocardiogram, especially if there is a 1:1 atrial:ventricular rate relationship. Esophageal recordings may demonstrate the atrial activity more clearly, or adenosine might be used to cause transient AV block and demonstrate the flutter waves. Adenosine, although diagnostically helpful, does not convert atrial flutter (Fig. 33–40). Overdrive atrial pacing from the esophagus or digoxin and, if necessary, cardioversion by DC countershock (initial dose 5 to 10 W-seconds) can be used to convert the rhythm to sinus. In the absence of structural heart disease, there is generally a benign course once the

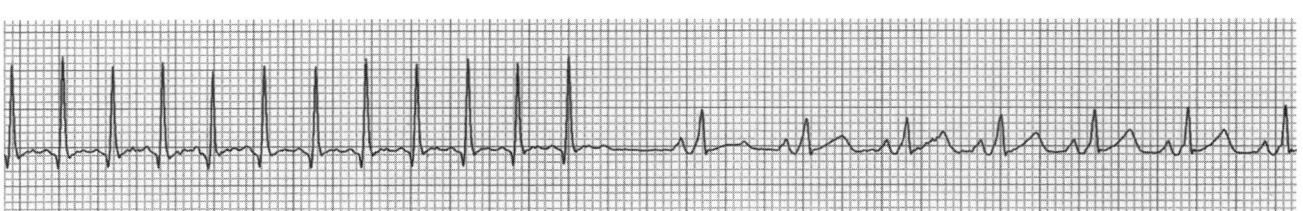

FIG. 33–39. Electrocardiogram during conversion of supraventricular tachycardia to sinus rhythm with administration of adenosine. During tachycardia at a rate of 230 beats/min, there is a normal-appearing QRS complex without a delta wave (no ventricular preexcitation), and there is no distinct P wave. After conversion to sinus rhythm, there is a short PR interval (80 milliseconds) and wide up-sloping QRS complex (90 milliseconds) representing ventricular preexcitation, indicative of the Wolff–Parkinson–White syndrome.

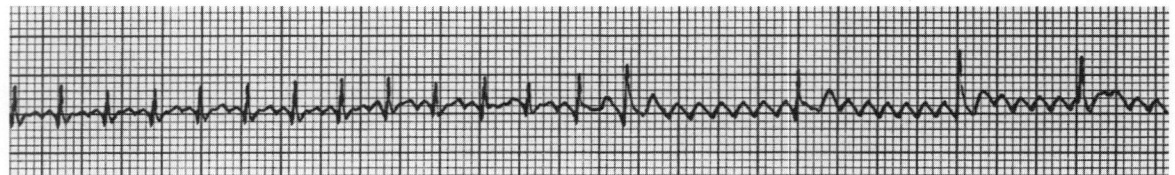

FIG. 33–40. Electrocardiogram showing the effect of adenosine on atrial flutter. Before adenosine, there is atrial flutter with 2:1 A–V conduction. The flutter waves are difficult to discern. After adenosine, there is transient slowing of AV node conduction without termination of the atrial flutter. This allows the flutter waves to be readily identified, confirming the diagnosis. The atrial rate during atrial flutter is 500 beats/minute.

arrhythmia is converted to sinus rhythm. Subsequent chronic antiarrhythmic therapy is often not necessary.

Atrial fibrillation is recognized by an irregularly irregular ventricular rhythm. It is rare in newborns and usually seen in patients with structural heart disease.

Treatments for Supraventricular Tachycardias

Treatment depends in part on the mechanism of tachycardia (see Tables 33–17 and 33–18) (96). In arrhythmias involving the AV node, such as artioventricular reciprocating tachycardias without or with the WPW syndrome, transiently slowing or blocking AV node conduction can terminate the tachycardia. Vagal maneuvers are often effective in terminating these types of supraventricular tachycardia. These include the application of ice or very cold damp cloth to the face and rectal stimulation. Ocular compression should not be used.

Rapid bolus of intravenous adenosine (0.1 mg/kg, increased to 0.2 mg/kg if needed) is the treatment of choice for most infants with supraventricular arrhythmias involving the AV node that are refractory to vagal maneuvers. Adenosine is an endogenous nucleoside with a very short half-life that can transiently block AV node conduction, interrupting these arrhythmias, resulting in abrupt conversion to sinus rhythm. It is helpful to record the patient's electrocardiogram during attempts at conversion so that one can see if there was an effect of the intervention on the arrhythmia. If there was transient termination with rapid resumption of the arrhythmia, a longer-acting agent might be necessary for control of the arrhythmia. There also might be transient evidence of WPW syndrome as the AV node conduction is briefly blocked, in the form of ventricular preexcitation from antegrade conduction down an accessory conduction pathway. Side effects appear to be rare but include initiation of atrial fibrillation.

Other antiarrhythmic agents can be used to terminate and control supraventricular tachycardia in infants, where vagal maneuvers or adenosine have resulted in only a transient termination of the arrhythmia, or for supraventricular tachycardia, which does not involve the AV node.

These might include β-blockers (i.e., esmolol or propranolol), class I antiarrhythmic agents (i.e., procainamide or flecainide), digoxin, or class III antiarrhythmic agents (i.e., sotalol or amiodarone). For ectopic atrial tachycardias, a β-blocker is often effective, and intravenous infusion of esmolol is a good first-line therapy until the arrhythmia is controlled. Intravenous verapamil has been associated with cardiovascular collapse and death in neonates and infants and should not be used in patients under 1 year of age.

If available, atrial pacing using an esophageal pacing catheter can be effective in terminating AV reciprocating tachycardias and atrial flutter. If the patient is hemodynamically unstable, DC countershock (starting with 0.5 to 1.0 Joules/kg) should be attempted for known or suspected reentry-type supraventricular tachycardias, including AV reciprocating tachycardia, atrial flutter, and atrial fibrillation.

Prophylactic antiarrhythmic therapy is prescribed for most infants with supraventricular tachycardia, as there is approximately a 20% recurrence risk of atrioventricular reciprocating tachycardias. Often the recurrance risk diminishes after a year or few years, and the medication may be discontinued (97). Athough digoxin has long been a mainstay of prophylactic antiarrhythmic therapy, its use in patients with known WPW syndrome is controversial. It still is commonly used in patients with atrioventricular reciprocating tachycardia without evident WPW syndrome. Propranolol is often used in patients with artoventricular reciprocating tachycardias, especially with WPW syndrome as well as for ectopic atrial tachycardias. For more refractory patients, combination therapy with propranolol and digoxin may be effective (96). If breakthrough occurs, switching to other agents with a greater potency and toxicity under the direction of a pediatric cardiologist may suppress recurrances. These may include drugs with a combination of actions such as sotalol or others used alone or in combination such as type IA agents (e.g., quinidine, procainamide, disopyramide), type IC agents (e.g., flecainide), oral verapamil or amiodarone, in various orders. The recommended management schemes vary between institutions and will change as more data about existing medications and new medications become available. Esophageal or intracardiac electrophysiology studies with programmed atrial stimuli can be used to determine probability of recurrence on medications or after medications have been discontinued for those with reentry supraventricular tachycardia. Rarely, radiofrequency ablation is used in infants with particularly refractory supraventricular tachycardia, often with associated ventricular dysfunction (96). Radiofrequency ablation is more safely and routinely applied in later childhood in those with persistent problematic arrhythmias.

Infants with supraventricular tachycardia may be recognized *in utero* by a rapid fetal heart rate. If the arrhythmia has been present for some time, these infants may develop hydrops. *In utero,* the administration of digoxin, flecainide, quinidine, procainamide, or sotalol to the mother, or procainamide or amiodarone directly into the umbilical vein, may be effective.

Ventricular Tachycardias

Wide complex tachyarrhythmias may represent ventricular tachycardia, SVT with aberrant conduction, atrioventricular reciprocating tachycardia in WPW syndrome with antegrade conduction over the accessory pathway and retrograde conduction over the His–Purkinje system and AV node, or any tachycardia in the presence of bundle branch or intraventricular conduction block (e.g., after cardiac surgery, hyperkalemia). In infants, the QRS complex in ventricular tachycardia may be as narrow as 0.06 to 0.11 seconds, but it is always different than in sinus rhythm (Fig. 33–41). Chronic recurrent ventricular tachycardias are rare in neonates, and are usually associated with structural or functional heart disease. When there is a polymorphic ventricular arrhythmia in the absence of apparent structural or functional heart disease, one should consider torsade de pointes associated with the long-QT syndrome. Very rarely an incessant, monomorphic ventricular tachycardia is found in infants with cardiac tumors.

The long-QT syndrome is a generally inherited abnormality of ventricular repolarization that can cause ventricular tachycardia. It can be caused by one of several mutations in proteins involved with transmembrane ionic currents (36). It can be inherited in an autosomal dominant fashion (Romano–Ward syndrome, without sensorineural hearing loss) or as an autosomal recessive condition (Jervell and Lange-Nielsen syndrome, with sensorineural hearing loss). Patients with this syndrome, including infants, generally have a prolonged corrected QT interval ($QT/RR^{1/2} > 0.46$ msec) and are at risk for torsade de pointes and sudden death. Patients identified with the long-QT syndrome are generally started on β-blockers and occasionally also require cervicothoracic sympathectomy and/or pacemakers (98). Automatic implantable defibrillators have been used in older patients with the long-QT syndrome.

Because ventricular tachycardia can be life threatening, with the potential for degeneration into ventricular fibrillation, it is safest to treat all wide complex tachycardias as ventricular tachycardia. If the patient is hemodynamically stable with a monomorphic ventricular tachycardia, antiarrhythmic therapy using lidocaine or procainamide may suppress the arrhythmia. Phenytoin can be especially useful if the arrhythmia is related to digoxin toxicity. For torsade de pointes, treatment should include magnesium sulfate, lidocaine, and possibly isoproterenol or cardiac pacing. If the patient is or becomes hemodynamically unstable, DC cardioversion should be initiated with 1 to 2 Joules/kg initially.

Complete Heart Block

In complete heart block, the ventricular rate is slower than and independent of the atrial rate. Congenital complete heart block is frequently recognized *in utero*. It is estimated to occur in 1 of 20,000 live births. In approximately 50% of infants with congenital heart block, there is an associated cardiovascular malformation (e.g., L-transposition of the great arteries, heterotaxy syndrome, endocardial cuhion defect). In the absence of structural heart disease, the heart block is usually related to mater-

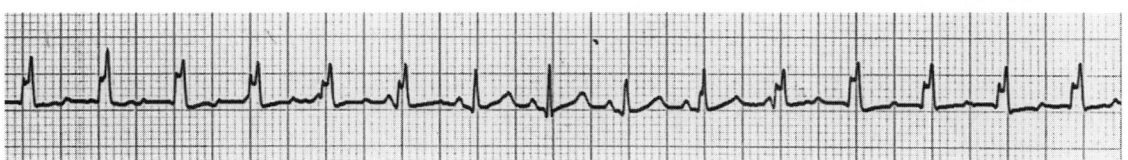

FIG. 33–41. Electrocardiogram showing ventricular tachycardia in an infant at a rate of 158 beats/min. Because of retrograde conduction block, occasional sinus beats can be conducted to the ventricles through the AV node and His–Purkinje system, resulting in a normal QRS complex. Note that the QRS complex duration of the ventricular tachycardia measures 0.08 seconds, compared a QRS duration of 0.06 seconds for the conducted sinus beats.

nal autoantibodies (anti-Ro or anti-La), which cross the placenta and interact with the developing conduction system (99). These antibodies are associated with maternal connective tissue disease, particularly lupus erythematosis and Sjögren syndrome. In newborns with heart block and no structural cardiac abnormalities, testing of their mothers for these antibodies is indicated because they may have no signs or symptoms of connective tissue disease. Occasionally newborns present with second-degree AV block and later progress to complete heart block. Therefore, those infants with persistent second-degree heart block (especially Mobitz type II) should undergo echocardiography to look for structural heart disease, and their mothers should be tested for these antibodies. Rarely myocarditis and fibrosis of the atrioventricular node or His bundle has been implicated as the cause of neonatal heart block. Complete heart block may occur as a complication of cardiac surgery, particularly in the correction of L-transposition, endocardial cushion defects, tetralogy of Fallot, and ventricular septal defects.

Most infants with isolated congenital complete heart block are asymptomatic and do not require immediate intervention. The stroke volume increases to compensate for the low ventricular rate, to maintain an adequate cardiac output. The ventricular rate may vary between 30 beats/min and 110 beats/min in infants with complete heart block. There is generally a narrow, junctional, escape rhythm. The ventricular rate tends to decrease with increasing age. Symptoms are usually related to the severity of the associated cardiovascular malformation and the degree of bradycardia. Infants without hemodynamically significant cardiac malformations tolerate bradycardia well, grow, and develop normally. Examination usually reveals cardiac enlargement from an increased left ventricular end-diastolic volume. A systolic ejection murmur and apical mid-diastolic rumble are common. Rarely, a fetus or infant with isolated complete heart block develops signs or symptoms of nonimmune hydrops or congestive heart failure. Patients with syncope or near syncope (Stokes–Adams attacks), congestive heart failure, or postsurgical block require early initiation of permanent ventricular pacing. Medical therapy with isoproterenol or with transcutaneous or transvenous cardiac pacing is helpful in the acute situation prior to surgery. The timing of pacemaker implantation in other patients is more controversial. Criteria used to select patients for permanent pacing in infants have included: awake, resting ventricular rates less than 50 beats/min; awake, resting atrial rates greater than 140 beats/min; wide QRS escape rhythms; prolonged QT intervals; frequent, complex ventricular ectopy; or ventricular tachycardia (100).

REFERENCES

1. Mitchell SC, Korones SB, Berendes HW. Congenital heart disease in 56,109 births. *Circulation* 1971;43:323.
2. Hiraishi S, Agata Y, Nowatari M, et al. Incidence and natural course of trabecular ventricular septal defect: two-dimensional echocardiography and color Doppler flow imaging study. *J Pediatr* 1992;120:409–415.
3. Roguin N, Du Z-D, Barak M, Nasser N, Hershkowitz S, Milgram E. High prevalence of muscular ventricular septal defect in neonates. *J Am Coll Cardiol* 1995;26:1545–1548.
4. Fyler DC. Report of the New England Regional Infant Cardiac Program. *Pediatrics* 1980;65(Suppl):375.
5. Gillum RF. Epidemiology of congenital heart disease in the United States. *Am Heart J* 1994;127:919–927.
6. Freedom RM, Benson LN, Smallhorn JF, eds. *Neonatal heart disease.* New York: Springer-Verlag, 1992.
7. Emmanouilides GC, Riemenschneider TA, Allen HD, Gutgesell HP. *Heart disease in infants, children and adolescents,* 5th ed. Baltimore: Williams & Wilkins, 1995.
8. Moller JH, Neal WA. *Fetal, neonatal, and infant cardiac disease.* Norwalk, CT: Appleton & Lange, 1989.
9. Garson A, Bricker JT, McNamara DG. *The science and practice of pediatric cardiology.* Philadelphia: Lea & Febiger, 1990.
10. Long WA. *Fetal and neonatal cardiology.* Philadelphia: WB Saunders, 1990.
11. Fyler DC. *Nadas' pediatric cardiology.* Philadelphia: Hanley & Belfus, 1992.
12. Newburger JW, Silbert AR, Buckley LP, Fyler DC. Cognitive function and age at repair of transposition of the great arteries in children. *N Engl J Med* 1984;310:1495.
13. Bellinger DC, Jonas RA, Rappaport LA, et al. Developmental and neurologic status of children after heart surgery with hypothermic circulatory arrest or low-flow cardiopulmonary bypass. *N Engl J Med* 1995;332(9):549–555.
14. Ferencz C, Correa-Villasenor A. Epidemiology of cardiovascular malformations: the state-of-the-art. *Cardiol Young* 1991;1:264–285.
15. Lacro RV. *Dysmorphology. Nadas' pediatric cardiology.* Philadelphia: Hanley & Belfus, 1992:37.
16. Pierpont MEM, Moller JH. *The genetics of cardiovascular disease.* Boston: Martinus Nijhoff, 1987.
17. Dawson BV, Johnson PD, Goldberg SJ, Ulreich JB. Cardiac teratogenesis of trichloroethylene and dichloroethylene in a mammalian model. *J Am Coll Cardiol* 1990;16:1304.
18. Goldberg SJ, Lebwitz MD, Graver EJ, Hicks S. An association of human congenital cardiac malformations and drinking water contaminants. *J Am Coll Cardiol* 1990;16:155.
19. Gorlin RJ, Cohen MM, Levin LS. *Syndromes of the head and neck,* 3rd ed. Oxford: Oxford University Press, 1990.
20. Smith DW, Jones KL. *Recognizable patterns of human malformation: genetic, embryologic and clinical aspects,* 3rd ed. Philadelphia: WB Saunders, 1982.
21. Greenwood RD. Cardiovascular malformations associated with extracardiac anomalies and malformation syndromes: patterns for diagnosis. *Clin Pediatr* 1984;23(3):145–151.
22. Milerad J, Larson O, Hagberg C, Ideberg M. Associated malformations in infants with cleft lip and palate: a prospective, population-based study. *Pediatrics* 1997;100:180–186.
23. Srivastava D, Thomas T, Lin Q, Kirby ML, Brown D, Olson EN. Regulation of cardiac mesodermal and neural crest development by the bHLH transcription factor, dHAND. *Nature Genet* 1997;16(2):154–160.
24. Moore KL, ed. *The developing human: Clinically oriented embryology,* 2nd ed. Philadelphia: WB Saunders, 1997.
25. Olson EN, Srivastava D. Molecular pathways controlling heart development. *Science* 1996;272:671–676.
26. Clark EB. Pathogenetic mechanisms of congenital cardiovascular malformations revisited [review]. *Semin Perinatol* 1996;20(6):465–472.
27. Kurnit DM, Layton WM, Matthysse S. Genetics, chance and morphogenesis. *Am J Human Genet* 1987;41:979.
28. Shaw GM, O'Malley CD, Wasserman CR, Tolarova MM, Lammer EJ. Maternal periconceptional use of multivitamins and reduced risk for conotruncal heart defects and limb deficiencies among offspring. *Am J Med Genet* 1995;59:536–545.
29. Botto LD, Khoury MJ, Mulinare J, Erickson JD. Periconceptional multivitamin use and the occurrence of conotruncal heart defects: results from a population-based, case-control study. *Pediatrics* 1996;98(5):911–917.

30. Maslen CL. Fundamental advances in molecular genetics: new insights and detection strategies in congenital heart disease. *ACC Edu Highlights* 1997;12(4):11–14.

31. Langille BL, Bendeck MP, Keeley FW. Adaptations of carotid arteries of young and mature rabbits to reduced carotid blood flow. *Am J Physiol* 1989;256:H931–H939.

32. Malek AM, Gibbons GH, Dzau VJ, Izumo S. Fluid shear stress differentially modulates expression of genes encoding basic fibroblast growth factor and platelet-derived growth factor B chain in vascular endothelium. *J Clin Invest* 1993;92:2013–2021.

33. Schwartz ML, Cox GF, Lin AE, et al. Clinical approach to genetic cardiomyopathy in children. *Circulation* 1996;94:2021–2038.

34. *Online Mendelian inheritance in man, OMIM (TM).* Baltimore: Center for Medical Genetics, Johns Hopkins University; Bethesda: National Center for Biotechnology Information, National Library of Medicine, 1997. World Wide Web URL: http://www.ncbi.nlm.nih.gov/omim/.

35. Grimes DA. The genetics of dilated cardiomyopathy—emerging clues to the puzzle. *N Engl J Med* 1997;337(15):1078–1079.

36. Splawski I, Timothy KW, Vincent GM, Atkinson DL, Keating MT. Molecular basis of the long-QT syndrome associated with deafness. *N Engl J Med* 1997;336(22):1562–1567.

37. Barcroft J. *Researchers of pre-natal life.* Oxford: Blackwell & Mott, 1944.

38. Dawes GS. *Foetal and neonatal physiology: a comparative study of the changes at birth.* Chicago: Year Book, 1969.

39. Lind J, Stern L, Wegelius C. *Human and foetal neonatal circulation.* Springfield, IL: Charles C Thomas, 1964.

40. Rudolph AM. *Congenital diseases of the heart.* Chicago: Year Book, 1974.

41. Gingell RL. Developmental biology of mammalian myocardium. In Freedom RM, Benson LN, Smallhorn JF, eds. *Neonatal heart disease.* London: Springer-Verlag, 1992.

42. Meyer RA, Hagler D, Huhta J, et al. Guidelines for physician training in fetal echocardiography: recommendations of the Society of Pediatric Echocardiography Committee on Physician Training. *J Am Soc Echocardiogr* 1990;3(1):1–3.

43. Yagel S, Weissman A, Rotstein Z, et al. Congenital heart defects: natural course and *in utero* development. *Circulation* 1997;96:550–555.

44. Swenson JM, Fischer DR, Miller SA, Boyle GJ, Ettedgui JA, Beerman LB. Are chest radiographs and electrocardiograms still valuable in evaluating new pediatric patients with heart murmurs or chest pain? *Pediatrics* 1997;99(1):1–3.

45. Sanders SS. Echocardiography. In *Nadas' pediatric cardiology.* Philadelphia: Hanley & Belfus, 1992:159.

46. Meyer RA, Hagler D, Huhta J, Smallhorn J, Snider R, Williams R. Guidelines for physician training in pediatric echocardiography. Recommendations of the Society of Pediatric Echocardiography Committee on Physician Training. *Am J Cardiol* 1987;60(1):164–165.

47. Lock JE, Keane JF, Mandell VS, Perry SB. Cardiac catheterization. In Fyler DC, ed. *Nadas' pediatric cardiology.* Philadelphia: Hanley & Belfus, 1992.

48. LaFarge CG, Miettinen OS. The estimation of oxygen consumption. *Cardiovasc Res* 1970;4:23.

49. Kovalchin JP, Forbes TJ, Nihill MR, Geva T. Echocardiographic determinants of clinical course in infants with critical and severe pulmonary valve stenosis. *J Am Coll Cardiol* 1997;29(5):1095–1101.

50. Kaine SF, Smith EO, Mott AR, Mullins, Geva T. Quantitative echocardiographic analysis of the aortic arch predicts outcome of balloon angioplasty of native coarctation of the aorta. *Circulation* 1996;94(5):1056–1062.

51. Zeevi B, Keane JF, Castaneda AR, Perry SB, Lock JE. Neonatal critical valvar aortic stenosis. A comparison of surgical and balloon dilation therapy. *Circulation* 1989;80(4):831–839.

52. Egito ES, Moore P, O'Sullivan J, et al. Transvascular balloon dilation for neonatal critical aortic stenosis: early and midterm results. *J Am Coll Cardiol* 1997;29(2):442–447.

53. Olley PM, Coceani F, Bodach E. E-type prostaglandins: a new emergency therapy for certain cyanotic congenital heart malformations. *Circulation* 1976;53:728.

54. Lang P, Freed MD, Rosenthal A, et al. The use of prostaglandin E$_1$ in an infant with interruption of the aortic arch. *J Pediatr* 1977;91:805.

55. Borow K, Green LH, Castaneda AR, et al. Left ventricular function after repair of tetralogy of Fallot and its relationship to age at repair. *Circulation* 1980;61:1150.

56. Jatene AD, Fontes VF, Paulista PP, et al. Anatomic correction of transposition of the great vessels. *J Thorac Cardiovasc Surg* 1976;72:364.

57. Castaneda AR, Norwood WI, Jonas RA, et al. Transposition of the great arteries and intact ventricular septum: anatomical repair in the neonate. *Ann Thorac Surg* 1984;38:438.

58. Wernovsky G, Mayer JE Jr, Jonas RA, et al. Factors influencing early and late outcome of the arterial switch operation for transposition of the great arteries. *J Thorac Cardiovasc Surg* 1995;109(2):289–301.

59. Geva T, Ayres NA, Pac FA, Pignatelli R. Quantitative morphometric analysis of progressive infundibular obstruction in tetralogy of Fallot. A prospective longitudinal echocardiographic study. *Circulation* 1995;92(4):886–892.

60. Walsh EP, Rockenmacher S, Keane JF, et al. Late results in patients with tetralogy of Fallot repaired during infancy. *Circulation* 1988;77:1062.

61. Lillehei CW, Varco RL, Cohen M, et al. The first open heart corrections of tetralogy of Fallot. A 26–31 year follow-up of 106 patients. *Ann Surg* 1986;204(4):490–502.

62. Giglia TM, Mandell VS, Connor AR, Mayer JE Jr, Lock JE. Diagnosis and management of right ventricle-dependent coronary circulation in pulmonary atresia with intact ventricular septum. *Circulation* 1992;86:1516–1528.

63. Franklin RC, Spiegelhalter DJ, Sullivan ID, et al. Tricuspid atresia presenting in infancy. Survival and suitability for the Fontan operation. *Circulation* 1993;87(2):427–439.

64. Gentles TL, Mayer JE Jr, Gauvreau K, et al. Fontan operation in five hundred consecutive patients: factors influencing early and late outcome. *J Thorac Cardiovasc Surg* 1997;114(3):376–391.

65. Norwood WI, Lang P, Hansen DD. Physiologic repair of aortic atresia—hypoplastic left heart syndrome. *N Engl J Med* 1984;308:23.

66. Forbess JM, Cook N, Roth SJ, Serraf A, Mayer JE Jr, Jonas RA. Ten-year institutional experience with palliative surgery for hypoplastic left heart syndrome. Risk factors related to stage I mortality. *Circulation* 1995;92(9 Suppl):II-262–II-266.

67. Iannettoni MD, Bove EL, Mosca RS, et al. Improving results with first-stage palliation for hypoplastic left heart syndrome. *J Thorac Cardiovasc Surg* 1994;107:934–940.

68. Razzouk AJ, Chinnock RE, Gundry SR, et al. Transplantation as a primary treatment for hypoplastic left heart syndrome: intermediate-term results. *Ann Thorac Surg* 1996;62(1):1–8.

69. Gutgesell HP, Massaro TA. Management of hypoplastic left heart syndrome in a consortium of university hospitals. *Am J Cardiol* 1995;76(11):809–811.

70. Canter C, Naftel D, Caldwell R, et al. Survival and risk factors for death after cardiac transplantation in infants. A multiinstitutional study. The Pediatric Heart Transplant Study. *Circulation* 1997;96(1):227–231.

71. Hanley FL, Heinemann MK, Jonas RA, et al. Repair of truncus arteriosus in the neonate. *J Thorac Cardiovasc Surg* 1993;105(6):1047–1056.

72. Rajasinghe HA, McElhinney DB, Reddy VM, Mora BN, Hanley FL. Long-term follow-up of truncus arteriosus repaired in infancy: a twenty-year experience. *J Thorac Cardiovasc Surg* 1997;113(5):869–878.

73. Piccoli G, Pacifico AD, Kirklin JW, Blackstone EH, Kirklin JK, Bargeron LM. Changing results and concepts in the surgical treatment of double-outlet right ventricle: analysis of 137 operations in 126 patients. *Am J Cardiol* 1983;52:549.

74. Radzik D, Davignon A, van Doesburg N, Fournier A, Marchand T, Ducharme G. Predictive factors for spontaneous closure of atrial septal defects diagnosed in the first 3 months of life [Comment]. *J Am Coll Cardiol* 1994;23(3):828–830.

75. Bharati S, Lev M. The spectrum of common atrioventricular orifice (canal). *Am Heart J* 1973;86(4):553–561.

76. Hanley FL, Fenton KN, Jonas RA, et al. Surgical repair of complete atrioventricular canal defects in infancy. Twenty-year trends. *J Thorac Cardiovasc Surg* 1993;106(3):387–394.

77. Slomp J, Gittenberger-de Groot AC, Glukhova MA, et al. Differentiation, dedifferentiation, and apoptosis of smooth muscle cells during the development of the human ductus arteriosus. *Arterioscler Thromb Vasc Biol* 1997;17(5):1003–1009.

78. Friedman WF, Hirschklau MJ, Previtz MP, et al. Pharmacologic clo-

sure of patent ductus arteriosus in the premature infant. *N Engl J Med* 1976;295:526.

79. Heymann MA, Rudolph AM, Silverman NH. Closure of the ductus arteriosus in premature infants by inhibition of prostaglandin synthesis. *N Engl J Med* 1976;295:530.

80. Nehgme RA, O'Connor TZ, Lister G, Bracken MB. Patent ductus arteriosus. In Sinclair JC, Bracken MB, eds. *Effective care of the newborn infant.* New York: Oxford University Press, 1992;281–324.

81. Ment LR, Oh W, Ehrenkranz RA, et al. Low-dose indomethacin and prevention of intraventricular hemorrhage: a multicenter randomized trial. *Pediatrics* 1994;93(4):543–550.

82. Fowlie PW. Prophylactic indomethacin: systematic review and meta-analysis. *Arch Dis Child* 1996;74:F81–F87.

83. Volpe JJ. Brain injury caused by intraventricular hemorrhage: is indomethacin the silver bullet for prevention? *Pediatrics* 1994;11:673–676.

84. Reynolds EOR. Prevention of periventricular hemorrhage. *Pediatrics* 1994;11:677–679.

85. Varvarigou A, Bardin CL, Beharry K, Chemtob S, Papageorgiou A, Aranda JV. Early ibuprofen administration to prevent patent ductus arteriosus in premature newborn infants. *JAMA* 1996;275(7):539–544.

86. Wagner HR, Ellison RC, Zierler S, et al. Surgical closure of patent ductus arteriosus in 268 preterm infants. *J Thorac Cardiovasc Surg* 1984;87:870.

87. Gersony WM, Peckham GJ, Ellison RC, et al. Effects of indomethacin in preterm infants with patent ductus arteriosus. Results of a national collaborative study. *J Pediatr* 1983;102:895.

88. Doty DB, Richardson JV, Falkovsky GE, Gordonova MI, Burakovsky VI. Aortopulmonary septal defect: hemodynamics, angiography, and operation. *Ann Thorac Surg* 1981;32:244.

89. Edwards JE. Malformations of the aortic arch system manifested as "vascular rings." *Lab Invest* 1953;2:56.

90. Yeager SB, Chin AJ, Sanders SP. Two-dimensional echocardiographic diagnosis of pulmonary artery sling in infancy. *J Am Coll Cardiol* 1986;7:625.

91. Tonkin IL, Elliot LP, Bargeron LM. Concomitant axial cineangiography and barium esophagography in the evaluation of vascular rings. *Radiology* 1980;135:69.

92. Backer CL, Ilbawi MN, Idriss FS, DeLeon SY. Vascular anomalies causing tracheoesophageal compression. *J Thorac Cardiovasc Surg* 1989;97:725.

93. Swischuk LE. Anterior tracheal indentation in infancy and early childhood: normal or abnormal? *Am J Roentgenol Rad Ther Nucl Med* 1971;112:12.

94. Nir A, Tajik AJ, Freeman WK, et al. Tuberous sclerosis and cardiac rhabdomyoma. *Am J Cardiol* 1995;76:419–421.

95. Van Hare GF, Stanger P. Ventricular tachycardia and accelerated ventricular rhythm presenting in the first month of life. *Am J Cardiol* 1991;67(1):42–45.

96. Weindling SN, Walsh EP, Saul JP. Management of supraventricular tachycardia in infants. *J Am Coll Cardiol* 1993;21:294A.

97. Perry JC, Garson A Jr. Supraventricular tachycardia due to Wolff–Parkinson–White syndrome in children: early disappearance and late recurrence. *J Am Coll Cardiol* 1990;16:1215–1220.

98. Garson A Jr, Dick M II, Fournier A, et al. The long QT syndrome in children: An international study of 287 patients. *Circulation* 1993;87:1866–1872.

99. Reed BR, Lee LA, Harmon C, et al. Autoantibodies to SS-A/Ro in infants with congenital heart block. *J Pediatr* 1983;103(6):889–891.

100. Sholler GF, Walsh EP. Congenital complete heart block in patients without anatomic cardiac defects. *Am Heart J* 1989;118:1193–1198.

101. Mullins CE, Mayer DC. *Congenital heart disease:* a diagrammatic atlas. New York: Alan R Liss, 1988.

CHAPTER 34

Preoperative and Postoperative Care of the Infant with Critical Congenital Heart Disease

Bradley S. Marino and Gil Wernovsky

PREOPERATIVE CARE: GENERAL PRINCIPLES

This section will delineate the general principles of preoperative care and is divided into the following discussions: the therapeutic and systemic implications of neonatal critical congenital heart disease, the clinical presentations of congenital heart disease in the neonate, fetal echocardiography, the evaluation of the neonate with suspected critical congenital heart disease, stabilization and transport, confirmation of the diagnosis, and evaluation of other pertinent organ systems. Whenever possible, overlap with the contents of Chapter 33 have been avoided; however, some repetition was allowed to minimize excessive cross-referencing.

The Neonate with Critical Congenital Heart Disease

Approximately one-third of all children born with congenital heart defects become critically ill during the first year of life and either die or receive surgical treatment (1). Critical congenital heart defects that are palliated or not corrected may cause progressive and irreversible secondary organ damage, principally to the heart, lungs, and central nervous system (CNS), and may interfere with normal postnatal changes, such as myocardial hyperplasia, coronary angiogenesis, and pulmonary vascular and alveolar development (2,3). In addition to these anatomic and functional sequelae, psychomotor and cognitive abnormalities may be present and limit the development of the child with palliated or uncorrected critical congen-

ital heart disease (4). Over the past decade, it has become apparent that the cumulative morbidity and mortality of palliative operations, followed by later repair, is greater than that of early corrective procedures. Primary reparative surgery in the neonate offers the opportunity to decrease the mortality caused by the primary defect and to prevent secondary damage to other organ systems (5).

Expanding the scope of reparative operations to the neonate has altered the demographic makeup of cardiac patients scheduled for surgery in the intensive care unit. Of the 2,500 annual admissions to the Cardiac Intensive Care Units of Children's Hospital of Philadelphia, Boston Children's Hospital, and C.S. Mott Children's Hospital, approximately 25% are neonates and more than 50% are less than 1 year of age (T. Kulik, M.D., and D.L. Wessel, M.D., personal communication, 1997). Optimal management requires a multidisciplinary team approach, combining the disciplines of cardiology, cardiac surgery, cardiac anesthesia, neonatology, critical care, and nursing.

Care of the critically ill neonate requires an understanding of the special structural and functional features of neonatal organ systems, the "transitional" neonatal circulation, and the secondary effects of congenital heart defects on other organ systems. The neonate responds to physiologically stressful circumstances rapidly and profoundly, with drastic changes in pH, serum lactate and glucose concentrations, and temperature (6). Neonates have diminished fat and carbohydrate reserves relative to older infants and children. They also have a higher metabolic rate and oxygen consumption, which accounts for the rapid appearance of hypoxia when these infants become apneic. Immaturity of the liver and kidney may be associated with reduced protein synthesis and glomerular filtration, such that drug metabolism is altered and hepatic synthetic function is reduced. These issues may be compounded further by the neonate's total

B. S. Marino: Division of Cardiology, The Cardiac Center, The Children's Hospital of Philadelphia, Philadelphia, Pennsylvania.

G. Wernovsky: Department of Pediatrics, University of Pennsylvania School of Medicine; and Cardiac Intensive Care Unit, The Children's Hospital of Pennsylvania, Philadelphia, Pennsylvania.

body water being greater than that of the older child and the capillary system of the neonate having the propensity to leak fluid from the intravascular space (7). This is especially prominent in the lung of the neonate, where the pulmonary vascular bed is nearly fully recruited at rest and the lymphatic recruitment required to handle increases in mean pulmonary blood flow (PBF) may be unavailable (8).

The neonate may be more likely to maintain blood pressure when a state of impending shock exists, which lures the practitioner into a false sense of security immediately prior to circulatory collapse. Systemic blood pressure is not always a reliable indicator of the adequacy of preload or satisfactory oxygen delivery. The myocardium in the neonate is less compliant than in the older child, is less tolerant of increases in afterload, and is less responsive to increases in preload (9–11). The potential for sustained or labile increases in pulmonary vascular resistance (PVR) is common in neonates, and concern over inciting pulmonary hypertensive events has deterred some from pursuing a reparative approach in neonates. Finally, the extreme stress responses to cardiopulmonary bypass (CPB) must be considered in the overall approach to the management of these patients (12,13).

These factors do not preclude intervention in the neonate, but they do dictate that effective communication among pediatric cardiologists, neonatologists, and surgeons must occur so that a management plan emerges to account for the immature physiology of the neonate. Whereas the neonate may be more physiologically labile than the older child, there is ample evidence that this age group is more resilient in the face of metabolic or ischemic stress. In fact, the neonate may be particularly capable of coping with some forms of stress. Tolerance of hypoxia in the neonate is characteristic of many species, and the "plasticity" of the neurologic system in the newborn is well described (14,15). For example, neonates with obstructive left heart lesions frequently present with profound metabolic acidosis and shock. However, effective resuscitation, without persistent organ system impairment or sequelae, is the rule rather than the exception. The elasticity and mobility of vascular structures in the neonate facilitate the technical aspects of surgery. Reparative operations in the neonate take best advantage of normal postnatal changes, allowing more normal growth and development in crucial areas such as myocardial muscle, pulmonary parenchyma, and coronary and pulmonary capillary beds. There is increasing evidence that postoperative pulmonary hypertension is more common in the infant who has been exposed to weeks or months of high pulmonary pressure and flow (16,17). This observation seems especially true in infants with truncus arteriosus, complete atrioventricular canal, and transposition of the great arteries (TGA) with ventricular septal defect (VSD). Finally, cognitive and psychomotor abnormalities associated with months of hypoxemia or

abnormal hemodynamics may be diminished or eliminated by early repair (4).

A regionalized approach to perinatal medical care, with organized transport systems and outreach education programs, has optimized the resuscitation and stabilization of newborns with congenital heart disease and has expedited the transfer of these infants to critical care units.

In critical congenital heart lesions, *the ultimate outcome depends on timely and accurate assessment of the structural anomaly, and the evaluation and resuscitation of secondary organ damage.* It is therefore critical that pediatricians, pediatric cardiologists, and neonatologists be able to rapidly evaluate and participate in the initial medical management of neonates with congenital heart disease. Because 20% of patients with severe congenital heart disease are premature neonates who weigh less than 2,500 g at birth, a multidisciplinary preoperative approach involving several subspecialty services frequently is required (18). Crucial in this process is the continued *communication* among medical, surgical, and nursing disciplines. The principles of preoperative management are listed in Table 34–1.

Clinical Presentations of Critical Congenital Heart Disease

The timing of presentation and the accompanying symptomatology depend on the nature and severity of the anatomic defect, the in utero effects (if any) of the structural lesion, and, following birth, the alterations in cardiovascular physiology secondary to the effects of the closure of the ductus arteriosus and the fall in PVR.

In the first few weeks of life, the many heterogeneous forms of heart disease present in a surprisingly limited number of ways. Signs and symptoms include (i) cyanosis, (ii) congestive heart failure or shock, (iii) asymptomatic heart murmur, and (iv) arrhythmia. Although an increasing number of neonates with congenital heart disease are diagnosed prior to delivery by fetal echocardiography (see following), the majority of neonates with congenital heart

---

TABLE 34–1. *Principles of preoperative management*

1. Initial stabilization: airway management, the establishment of vascular access, maintenance of a patent ductus arteriosus with prostaglandin E$_1$, when necessary.
2. Noninvasive delineation of the anatomic defect(s) by echocardiography.
3. Evaluation and treatment of additional organ system dysfunction, particularly of the pulmonary, renal, hepatic, and central nervous system.
4. Evaluation for additional congenital defects.
5. Genetic evaluation, if indicated.
6. Cardiac catheterization, if indicated (see text).
7. Surgical management, if indicated, when cardiac, pulmonary, renal, hepatic and central nervous system function are optimized.

anomalies are not discovered until after birth (19,20). Not infrequently, the clinician is diverted away from a diagnosis of congenital heart disease because of the report of a normal prenatal ultrasound performed for screening purposes. Conversely, the diagnosis of heart disease should not deter the clinician from performing a complete noncardiac evaluation searching for additional medical problems, such as sepsis.

Fetal Echocardiography

It is increasingly common for infants to be born with a diagnosis of probable congenital heart disease due to the increasing use of obstetric ultrasound and fetal echocardiography. The recommended timing for fetal echocardiography is 18 to 22 weeks of gestation, although reasonable images can be obtained as early as 12 to 16 weeks of gestation. Transvaginal ultrasound is being investigated for diagnostic purposes in fetuses in the first trimester. Indications for fetal echocardiography are summarized in Table 33–6 (21,22). Referral for the indications listed has resulted in the detection of significant structural and/or functional heart disease with the following approximate frequency: family history 1%, maternal diabetes 5%, fetal arrhythmia 10%, obstetrician's suspicion of congenital heart disease from screening four-chamber view 40%, other major organ system defect involving abnormal karyotype 25%, and maternal drug ingestion or abuse 1% (23).

Although the most severe forms of congenital heart anomalies can be diagnosed accurately by fetal echocardiography, some lesions, such as coarctation of the aorta, small VSDs and atrial septal defects (ASDs), total anomalous pulmonary venous return, and mild aortic or pulmonary stenosis, may be undetectable by fetal echocardiography (19,23). The main anomaly in complex congenital heart disease generally is identified by fetal echocardiography; however, complete definition of the exact anatomy of the cardiac malformation often requires postnatal echocardiography.

In utero therapy of prenatally diagnosed congenital heart disease remains limited and primarily involves redirecting delivery to a tertiary care center and drug therapy for tachyarrhythmias. Termination of pregnancy may be considered in some circumstances. Lesions that warrant delivery of the neonate with known congenital heart disease at or near a tertiary care center include:

1. Those that may require emergency surgery or catheterization (e.g., total anomalous pulmonary venous return, TGA),
2. Those that are ductal dependent for systemic blood flow (e.g., hypoplastic left heart syndrome, interrupted aortic arch (IAA), coarctation of the aorta, critical aortic stenosis),
3. Those that are ductal dependent for PBF (e.g., critical pulmonic stenosis, pulmonary atresia with intact

ventricular septum (PA/IVS), tetralogy of Fallot with pulmonary atresia (TOF/PA), tricuspid atresia, and Ebstein's anomaly).

Spontaneous delivery at term usually is preferable to elective induction, unless nonimmune hydrops fetalis is present. The full-term infant is easier to manage from a cardiorespiratory and hemodynamic standpoint and has a nutritional reserve accumulated during the third trimester that the premature neonate does not possess. The full-term neonate also is less likely to suffer from electrolyte abnormalities, respiratory distress syndrome, necrotizing enterocolitis (NEC), and intraventricular hemorrhage.

Evaluation of the Neonate with Suspected Congenital Heart Disease

The initial evaluation of the neonate with suspected congenital heart disease includes a thorough history, physical examination with four extremity blood pressures, chest radiograph, electrocardiogram, hyperoxia test, and echocardiogram, if indicated (see also Chap. 33).

Blood pressure measurement, manually or with an automated Dynamapp, should be performed on all four extremities if there is a suspicion of congenital heart disease. A systolic pressure that is more than 10 mm Hg higher in the upper body relative to the lower body is abnormal and suggests coarctation of the aorta, aortic arch hypoplasia, or IAA. It should be noted that testing for a systolic blood pressure gradient is quite specific for an arch abnormality but is not very sensitive; a systolic blood pressure gradient will not be present in the neonate with an arch abnormality in whom the ductus arteriosus is patent and nonrestrictive.

Hyperoxia Test

In all neonates with suspected critical congenital heart disease, a properly performed hyperoxia test is likely to be the most sensitive and specific tool in the initial evaluation. A hyperoxia test should be performed in neonates with resting pulse oximetry less than 95%, cyanosis, or circulatory collapse. The hyperoxia test consists of obtaining a baseline right radial (preductal) arterial blood gas when the child is breathing room air, and then repeating the measurement with the child inspiring 100% oxygen. The arterial partial pressure of oxygen (PO_2) should be measured directly via arterial puncture, although properly acquired transcutaneous oxygen monitor values for PO_2 also are acceptable. *Pulse oximetry should not be used for interpretation of the hyperoxia test,* as a neonate given 100% inspired oxygen may have an arterial PO_2 of 80 mm Hg with a pulse oximeter reading of 100% (abnormal), or an arterial PO_2 greater than 500 mm Hg with a pulse oximeter reading of 100% (normal). Measurements of PO_2 should be made at both preductal and postductal sites, as a difference in saturations is helpful diagnostically. If the preductal saturation is higher than the postductal saturation, "differential cyanosis" exists. This difference in preductal and postductal saturations is common in persistent pulmonary hypertension of the newborn, where there is desaturated blood from the pulmonary circulation entering the descending aorta through a patent ductus arteriosus (PDA). A markedly higher oxygen saturation in the upper part of the body relative to the lower part of the body is an important diagnostic clue that there may be aortic arch hypoplasia or interruption or left ventricular outflow obstruction.

There are also rare cases of "reverse differential cyanosis" in which the postductal saturation is higher than the preductal saturation. This occurs *only* in children with TGA with "reverse flow" through the PDA. If TGA is accompanied by coarctation of the aorta, interruption of the aortic arch, or suprasystemic PVR, blood flows from the pulmonary artery into the aorta through the PDA. In this circumstance the descending aorta is filled with oxygenated blood from the pulmonary system, and the lower extremities have a higher oxygen saturation than the upper extremities. Interpretation of the hyperoxia test is listed in Table 34–2 (24) and is summarized as follows: *The neonate who "fails" a hyperoxia test is very likely to have congenital heart disease with ductal-dependent systemic or PBF and should receive prostaglandin E1 until anatomic definition can be accomplished.*

When the hyperoxia test suggests that intracardiac shunting is responsible for the hypoxemia, the chest radiograph and electrocardiogram may be used to help delineate which of the cardiac structural defects is most likely until definitive echocardiography can be carried out.

Stabilization and Transport

Once a diagnosis of congenital heart disease is suspected, the infant or child must be stabilized and arrangements made to obtain a definitive anatomic diagnosis.

Initial Resuscitation

For the neonate who presents with cyanosis, congestive heart failure, or shock, simultaneous attention is devoted to the basics of advanced life support and maintenance of a PDA. A stable airway must be maintained, allowing for adequate ventilation (see following). Reliable venous access is essential; the umbilical vein should be used if patent. An arterial line assists in monitoring the blood pressure, acid–base status, and oxygenation of the patient. In the neonate this can be obtained most reliably through the umbilical artery. Volume resuscitation, inotropic support, and correction of metabolic acidosis are required to maximize cardiac output and tissue perfusion.

Blood glucose level should be checked to determine if hypoglycemia is present. In the initial evaluation of a newborn with cyanosis or circulatory collapse, a sepsis workup usually is performed, and the patient is started on appropriate antibiotics.

Airway Management and Supplemental Oxygen

In general, if respiratory distress or profound cyanosis is present, the infant should be sedated, paralyzed, intubated, and mechanically ventilated. Although intubation may be "successfully" carried out without sedation and neuromuscular blockade, there are compelling reasons to intubate with the aid of these agents in patients with con-

TABLE 34–2. *Interpretation of the hyperoxia test*

	PaO$_2$ (% saturation)		
	FiO$_2$ = 0.21	FiO$_2$ = 1.00	PaCO$_2$
Normal	70 (95)	>300 (100)	35
Pulmonary disease	50 (85)	>150 (100)	50
Neurologic disease	50 (85)	>150 (100)	50
Methemoglobinemia	70 (95)	>200 (100)	35
Cardiac disease			
Parallel circulation[a]	<40 (<75)	<50 (<85)	35
Restricted PBF[b]	<40 (<75)	<50 (<85)	35
Complete mixing without restricted PBF[c]	50–60 (85–93)	<150 (<100)	35
PPHN	Preductal	Postductal	
PFO (no right-to-left shunt)	70 (95)	<40 (<75) Variable	35–50
PFO (with right-to-left shunt)	<50 (<85)	<40 (<75) Variable	35–50

[a]D-Transposition of the great arteries with intact ventricular septum.

[b]Tricuspid atresia with pulmonary stenosis or atresia, pulmonary atresia or critical pulmonary stenosis with intact ventricular septum, or tetralogy of Fallot.

[c]Truncus arteriosus, total anomalous pulmonary venous return, single ventricle, hypoplastic left heart syndrome, tricuspid atresia without pulmonary stenosis or atresia.

PBF, pulmonary blood flow; PFO, patent foramen ovale; PPHN, persistent pulmonary hypertension of the newborn.

genital heart disease. First, the increased secretion of catecholamines with intubation may result in significant dysrhythmias in the at-risk myocardium (25). Second, vagally mediated bradycardia from hypoxemia, hypercapnia, or laryngeal stimulation may lead to asystole in these neonates with little reserve. Finally, sedation and neuromuscular blockade will dramatically reduce whole body oxygen consumption (26), raising the mixed venous oxygen saturation and improving oxygen delivery. Supplemental oxygen is a patent pulmonary vasodilator and may adversely affect neonates with increased PBF. The child with suspected congenital heart disease should receive supplemental oxygen via nasal cannula or face mask *to titrate the infant's oxygen saturation to 80% to 85%.*

Prostaglandin E₁

The neonate who "fails" a hyperoxia test, has an "equivocal" result along with other signs or symptoms of congenital heart disease, or who presents in shock within the first 3 weeks of life is highly likely to have critical congenital heart disease. These neonates are likely to have congenital lesions that depend on blood flow through a PDA for PBF, systemic blood flow, or need the PDA to promote intercirculatory mixing. The administration of prostaglandin E₁ (PGE_1) has been shown to open the ductus arteriosus and, depending on the lesion, increase PBF, systemic blood flow, or intercirculatory mixing. As the ductus becomes patent, hypoxemia is minimized and the metabolic acidosis that results from persistent hypoxemia or low systemic blood flow corrects (see also Chaps. 33 and 55) (27).

Rarely, the patient with congenital heart disease may become progressively more unstable after the institution of PGE_1 therapy. This clinical deterioration after institution of PGE_1 is an important diagnostic finding that identifies the congenital heart defect as one that has obstructed blood flow out of the pulmonary veins or left atrium. Lesions that have impaired blood flow out of the left atrium include hypoplastic left heart syndrome with restrictive patent foramen ovale, mitral atresia with restrictive patent foramen ovale, TGA with an IVS and restrictive foramen ovale, and total anomalous pulmonary venous return with obstruction. If there is clinical deterioration on PGE_1, then emergent plans for echocardiography and interventional catheterization or cardiac surgery should be made.

Adverse reactions of PGE_1, which are more common in premature and/or low-birth-weight infants, are listed in Table 34–3.

Apnea resulting from PGE_1 therapy typically occurs within the first 24 hours of administration, but *may occur at any time during administration* of the drug. For those neonates in whom transport to another facility is planned, consideration should be made for control of the airway and mechanical ventilation before transport. Factors that

TABLE 34–3. *Potential side effects of prostaglandin E1 therapy*

Potential side effects	Percent of patients
Fever	14%
Apnea	12%
Peripheral vasodilation/hypotension	10%
Bradycardia	7%
Seizures	4%
Tachycardia	3%
Edema	1%
Cardiac arrest	1%

From ref. 309.

influence the decision toward intubation are the severity of cyanosis and hemodynamic instability, gestational age of the patient, transport distance, and the skill of the transport team in emergent intubation.

PGE_1 typically causes peripheral vasodilation that manifests itself as cutaneous flushing. In many cases, peripheral vasodilation may result in hypotension. Due to this phenomenon, a separate intravenous line should be secured for volume administration in any infant receiving PGE_1, especially those who require transport. If hypotension is noted, a 10- to 20-mL/kg bolus of normal saline, lactated Ringer's solution, 5% albumin, or plasmanate generally will normalize the infant's blood pressure. It is prudent to remeasure arterial blood gas and reassess the infant's capillary refill and vital signs within 15 to 30 minutes of starting the PGE_1 infusion.

Inotropic Agents

For the neonate or infant in cardiogenic shock, continuous infusion of an inotropic agent may improve myocardial contractility and thereby enhance tissue perfusion of the vital organs and periphery. Care should be taken to replete the intravascular volume before institution of vasoactive agents (see also Chaps. 33 and 55).

Dopamine and dobutamine are recommended for the neonate with hypotension and tachycardia, as these agents have minimal chronotropic properties. A combination of low-dose dopamine, up to 5 µg/kg/min, and dobutamine, 5 to 10 µg/kg/min, may be used to minimize the potential peripheral vasoconstriction induced by high doses of dopamine while maximizing the dopaminergic effects on renal perfusion.

Isoproterenol and epinephrine are recommended for the neonate with hypotension and a normal or low heart rate, as these agents have both inotropic and chronotropic effects. *Isoproterenol* stimulates both beta-1 and beta-2 receptors. In comparison to dobutamine it has a greater chronotropic effect and a stronger vasodilatory effect via its beta-2 mechanism. Due to its strong chronotropic effect it should be started at a low dose and increased slowly to titrate effect. Chronotropic effects appear before inotropic effects in responsive hearts, and isoproterenol can produce tachyarrhythmias. The heart usually accommodates quickly to the chronotropic properties to allow the dose to be raised further for inotropic needs. *Epinephrine* has alpha-1, alpha-2, beta-1, and beta-2 effects. It is most commonly used when the previously listed inotropic infusions at high doses and in combination fail to produce the desired cardiac response.

Transport

After resuscitation and stabilization is complete, the neonate with suspected congenital heart disease often needs to be transferred to an institution that provides subspecialty care in pediatric cardiology and cardiac surgery. A successful transport involves two transitions of care for the neonate: *from the referring hospital staff to the transport team, and from the transport staff to the accepting hospital staff.* The need for accurate, detailed, and complete communication of information between the respective teams cannot be overemphasized. If possible, the pediatric cardiologist accepting the patient should be included in formulating the management plan for the neonate while the neonate is still at the referring hospital.

Reliable vascular access should be secured for the neonate receiving continuous infusions of PGE$_1$ or inotropic agents during transport. Some neonates receiving PGE$_1$ infusion will be intubated for transport. All intubated patients should have gastric decompression by nasogastric tube or orogastric tube and must not have anything by mouth or nasogastric tube (see previous for indications for sedation and neuromuscular blockade).

Acid–base status and oxygen delivery should be evaluated with arterial blood gas prior to transport. Although some patients with a structurally normal heart are transported receiving supplemental oxygen at or near 100%, this is often not the inspired oxygen concentration of choice for the neonate with congenital heart disease (see previous). This management decision for transport is particularly important for those infants with ductal-dependent systemic or PBF and complete intracardiac mixing with single ventricle physiology, and it emphasizes the need to consult with a pediatric cardiologist prior to transport to achieve optimal transport care.

In neonates, hypotension is a late finding in shock. More sensitive signs of impending decompensation include persistent tachycardia, poor tissue perfusion, and metabolic acidosis. Treatment of shock should occur prior to transport during the stabilization phase of management. Before leaving the referring hospital, the patient's most current hemodynamic status (capillary refill, heart rate, systemic blood pressure, acid–base status) should be reassessed and relayed to the receiving hospital.

Prior to transfer, the calcium and glucose status of the neonate should be evaluated. The neonatal myocardium is more dependent on calcium for inotropy than the adult myocardium, and ionized calcium levels less than 1.0 mg/dL may have a significant negative impact on neonatal myocardial contractility. If the ionized calcium is less than 1.0 mg/dL, 50 to 100 mg/kg of calcium gluconate should be given intravenously. Neonates with conotruncal anomalies are more likely to have 22q11 deletion and problems with calcium homeostasis resulting in hypocalcemia.

Confirmation of the Diagnosis

Echocardiography

Two-dimensional echocardiography, supplemented with pulsed-wave Doppler and color Doppler, has become the primary diagnostic modality for anatomic definition in pediatric cardiology (see also Chap. 33). However, the echocardiogram in the neonate is not "non-invasive"; a complete echocardiogram on a newborn suspected of having congenital heart disease may take an hour or more to perform and may not be well tolerated by a sick and/or premature neonate. Temperature instability due to exposure during this extended period may be detrimental to the newborn infant. Extension of the neck for suprasternal notch views of the aortic arch may be problematic, particularly in the neonate with respiratory distress or a tenuous airway. Subcostal imaging may result in abdominal compression and increased preload, as well as suboptimal pulmonary mechanics. Therefore, in sick neonates a medical staff person other than the individual performing the echocardiogram should observe the patient's vital signs and respiratory status.

Cardiac Catheterization

The role of pediatric cardiac catheterization has changed dramatically over the last decade. Prior to the era of Doppler echocardiography, cardiac catheterization was the primary means of defining the cardiac anatomy and assessing cardiac hemodynamics. Cardiac catheterization is presently used to:

1. Perform therapeutic interventions
2. Visualize anatomy not identified by echocardiography (e.g., distal pulmonary artery stenoses, aorticopulmonary collaterals, and coronary arteries)
3. Obtain hemodynamic information.

The usual indications for neonatal catheterization are listed in Table 34–4.

Preoperative Evaluation of Additional Organ Systems

Genetics

A careful search for other congenital anomalies is essential, as congenital heart disease is accompanied by at least one extracardiac malformation 25% of the time (28). The spectrum of associated defects in children with congenital heart disease is broad and likely reflects the complexity of the developmental process during cardiogenesis

TABLE 34–4. *Indications for neonatal catheterization*

Interventions
  Therapeutic
    Balloon atrial septostomy
    Balloon pulmonary valvotomy
    Balloon aortic valvotomy
    Balloon angioplasty of coarctation of the aorta
    Coil embolization of abnormal vascular
      communications
  Diagnostic
    Endomyocardial biopsy
Anatomic definition
  Coronary arteries
    Pulmonary atresia with intact ventricular septum
    Transposition of the great arteries
    Tetralogy of Fallot
  Aortic to pulmonary artery collateral vessels
    Tetralogy of Fallot with pulmonary atresia
  Distal pulmonary artery anatomy
Hemodynamic assessment (magnitude of shunting,
  calculation of pulmonary vascular resistance, or
  pulmonary venous gas sampling)

All the therapeutic interventions listed have alternate surgical options and their use depends on institutional experience.

(see also Chaps. 33 and 40). Children with conotruncal congenital heart lesions should have their chromosomes sent for karyotypic evaluation and fluorescent *in situ* hybridization analysis for 22q11 deletion (29).

The association of cardiovascular defects and other midline defects has been studied using the population-based registry of the Metropolitan Atlanta Congenital Defects Program (30). This group reviewed associations among neural tube defects (anencephaly, spina bifida, encephalocele), oral clefts, omphalocele, tracheoesophageal fistula, imperforate anus, conotruncal heart defects, and diaphragmatic hernia. Oral clefts, omphalocele, tracheoesophageal fistula, and imperforate anus were found to be associated with conotruncal defects more commonly than expected by chance alone. No cases of neural tube defects or diaphragmatic hernia were identified in babies with conotruncal congenital heart defects.

Central Nervous System

Imaging studies are often needed to complete the preoperative evaluation. If the child is thought to have a chromosomal anomaly, syndrome, or association that has both cardiac and CNS defects, then the brain should be imaged. Magnetic resonance imaging assists in imaging all areas of brain, including the posterior fossa and brain stem, whereas a computed tomographic scan of the head best defines cortical gray and white matter and ventricular size. If the neonate with suspected congenital heart disease is premature or may have suffered hypoxic–ischemic injury secondary to cardiac decompensation, a head ultrasound is recommended to rule out intraventricular hemorrhage prior to surgery, interventional catheterization, or placement onto an extracorporeal membrane oxygenation (ECMO) circuit. The infant or child with congenital heart disease who has seizures may need an imaging study, and/or an electroencephalogram.

Renal

Children that have ductal-dependent systemic flow are at risk of prerenal renal failure, unless arterial flow to the kidneys through the PDA can be guaranteed. If arterial flow to the kidneys is inadequate, low-dose dopamine may be started to cause dilation of the renal arterioles and the splanchnic circulation (see Chap. 42). Patency of the ductus must be reassessed if there is a suspicion of decreased systemic blood flow.

Because there is a higher incidence of urinary tract anomalies in the child with congenital heart disease, 3% to 6% of the infants with congenital heart disease compared to 1.4% of the general population, a renal ultrasound should be considered to delineate potential urinary tract malformations (31). A renal ultrasound should be strongly considered in children with midline defects, such as VACTERL (vertebral, anal, cardiac, tracheal, esophageal, renal, and limb) association, or renal dysfunction. Urinary anomalies seen with congenital heart anomalies include hydronephrosis, ureteral duplication, unilateral renal agenesis, position abnormalities, and renal dysplasia (32). Children who have both urinary tract and cardiac defects often have multiple congenital defects, and it is in this group that a complete multisystem evaluation should be undertaken.

Gastrointestinal

In neonates with ductal-dependent systemic blood flow (hypoplastic left heart syndrome, IAA, critical aortic stenosis, and coarctation of the aorta) and ductal-dependent PBF (pulmonic atresia with IVS, critical pulmonic stenosis, TOF/PA, tricuspid atresia with normally related great arteries, Ebstein's anomaly, and heterotaxy), intestinal flow may be compromised. In the great majority of lesions, intracardiac mixing results in decreased arterial PO_2. In addition, low PVR results in retrograde diastolic flow into the pulmonary vascular bed away from the splanchnic circulation ("diastolic steal"). Both of these factors decrease O_2 delivery to the intestinal mucosa. Babies with ductal-dependent systemic blood flow are at the greatest risk, as ductal constriction prior to diagnosis may severely compromise systemic blood flow, particularly to the kidneys and gastrointestinal tract. Similarly, neonates with TGA, an open ductus, and low PVR also have decreased O_2 delivery to the gastrointestinal tract (hypoxemia and "diastolic steal"). In all these cases there may be inadequate oxygen delivery to the intestine and an increased risk of NEC. The premature neonate has a much higher risk of developing NEC than the full-term neonate. Among full-term neonates it is those with critical congenital heart disease that has the highest incidence of NEC.

Full-term infants with critical congenital heart disease should be given intravenous fluid during stabilization and transport, and they usually are kept on intravenous fluid until their surgical procedure is performed. If the child's definitive procedure will not occur within the first few days of life, the newborn can be fed orally, if tolerated, or by nasogastric tube.

Because the infant with ductal-dependent systemic or pulmonary blood flow is at risk of NEC, they should be fed enterally with care, usually after the umbilical artery catheter has been removed. The advantages of enteral feeds include higher caloric intake than can be provided through a peripheral intravenous line with total parenteral nutrition, the avoidance of total parenteral nutrition cholestasis and chronic liver disease, and maintenance of a vital intestinal mucosa. The main disadvantage of giving enteral feeds to the child with critical congenital heart disease is that if there is bowel ischemia or hypoxemia, feeding the child might result in bacterial invasion into the intestinal mucosa and NEC.

Lesion-Specific Preoperative Stabilization

D-Transposition of the Great Arteries

The dominant physiologic abnormalities in the newborn with D-TGA are a deficiency of oxygen supply to the tissues and excessive right and left ventricular workload. The systemic and pulmonary circulations function in parallel rather than in series; hence, the greatest portion of the output of each ventricle is recirculated to that ventricle (Fig. 34–1A). In TGA with IVS (TGA/IVS), only a relatively small proportion of blood is exchanged by intercirculatory mixing between the two circulations and, as a result, only a small proportion of the effective circulation reaches the appropriate vascular bed (Fig. 34–1B). The systemic and pulmonary arterial oxygen saturations are thus dependent on one or more of the following anatomic paths for this exchange: *intracardiac* [patent foramen ovale, atrial septal defect (ASD), VSD] and *extracardiac* (PDA, bronchopulmonary collateral circulation).

The net volume of blood passing from the pulmonary circulation (left atrium, left ventricle, pulmonary arteries) to the systemic circulation (right atrium, right ventricle, aorta) represents the *anatomic left-to-right shunt* and is the *effective systemic blood* flow (i.e., oxygenated pulmonary venous return perfusing the systemic capillary bed). Conversely, the net volume of blood passing from the systemic circulation to the pulmonary circulation represents the *anatomic right-to-left shunt* and is the *effective PBF* (systemic venous return perfusing the pulmonary capillary bed). The effective PBF, effective systemic blood flow, net anatomic right-to-left, and net

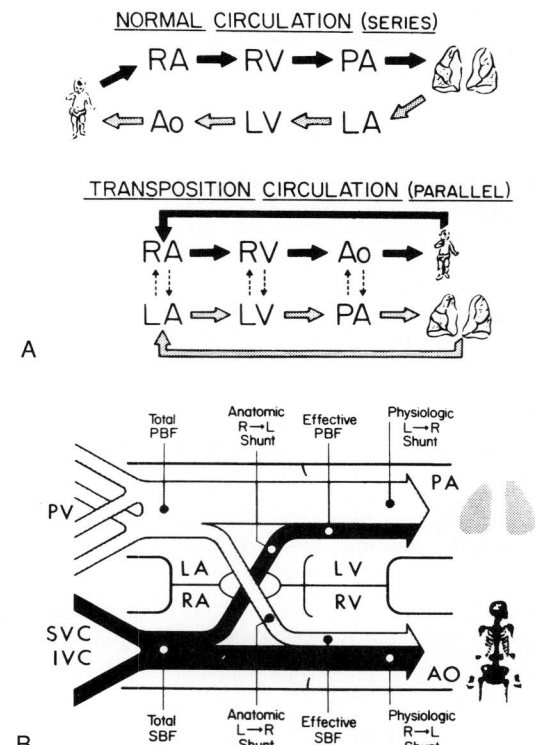

FIG. 34–1. The circulation in TGA. **A:** Systemic and pulmonary circulation pathways: in series, with normally related great arteries; in parallel, with TGA. *Solid arrows,* relatively unoxygenated blood; *stippled arrows,* oxygenated blood; *dashed arrows,* intercirculatory shunts. **B:** Circulation schema demonstrating flows and shunts in infants with TGA/IVS. Note that the anatomic left-to-right shunt constitutes the effective SBF, and the anatomic right-to-left shunt constitutes the effective PBF. AO, aorta; IVC, inferior vena cava; LA, left atrium; LV, left ventricle; L → R, left-to-right; RA, right atrium; RV, right ventricle; R → L, right-to-left; PA, pulmonary artery; PBF, pulmonary blood flow; PV, pulmonary veins; SBF, systemic blood flow; SVC, superior vena cava.

anatomic left-to-right shunts are each equal to each other. This volume is the *intercirculatory mixing,* which is the flow in TGA upon which survival depends. *The net volume exchanged between systemic and pulmonary circulations must be equal over a given short interval of time, because any major differences will result in a depletion of the blood volume of one circulation at the expense of overloading the other.*

The volumes of anatomic right-to-left and left-to-right shunted blood (i.e., "effective blood flow") that participate in functional gas exchange at the pulmonary and systemic capillary levels are relatively small in comparison to the large volumes of blood *circulating* (total systemic and pulmonary blood flow) or *recirculating* (physiologic left-to-right and right-to-left shunt flows) within each circulation. The *physiologic left-to-right shunt* represents the volume of the pulmonary venous blood recirculating through the lungs without having passed through the body, and the *physiologic right-to-left shunt* is the volume of systemic venous blood reentering the systemic circulation without having passed through the lungs.

The extent of intercirculatory mixing in TGA depends on the number, size, and position of the anatomic communications and on the total blood flow through the pulmonary circuit. In the neonate with an IVS and a closed or closing ductus arteriosus, severe hypoxemia secondary to inadequate mixing at the foramen ovale level is usually present. When the interatrial or interventricular shunting sites are of adequate size, the level of arterial oxygen saturation is influenced primarily by the pulmonary-to-systemic blood flow ratio, with a high PBF resulting in relatively high arterial oxygen saturation, as long as the ventricles can adequately maintain the high output state. If the PBF is decreased by subpulmonary or pulmonary stenosis or elevated PVR, the arterial oxygen saturation will be lowered despite adequately sized anatomic shunting sites (33–35).

The physiologic mechanisms that precisely control the equalization of interchange between the two circulations remain speculative. The shunting patterns appear to be determined by local pressure gradients that, in turn, are influenced by respiratory cycle phase, compliance of the cardiac chambers, heart rate, and the volume of blood flow and the vascular resistance in each of the circulations. With TGA/IVS, the interatrial shunt is from the right atrium to the left atrium during ventricular diastole, because left ventricular resistance to filling is less than right ventricular resistance. The shunt is from the left atrium to the right atrium in ventricular systole, because the left atrium is less distensible than the right atrium, and the net pressure in the left atrium is higher during ventricular systole. The pattern is affected by respiration, with the interatrial right-to-left (systemic-to-pulmonary) shunt increasing during inspiration when the systemic venous return increases and pulmonary venous return decreases. The effects on intercirculatory mixing from positive-pressure mechanical ventilation have not been fully studied.

Management of Profound Hypoxemia

In neonates with TGA/IVS, the combination of a very low arterial PO_2 (i.e., less than 20 mm Hg), an elevated PCO_2 (despite adequate chest motion and ventilation), and metabolic acidosis (with or without pulmonary edema on the chest radiograph) are markers for *severely decreased effective pulmonary and systemic flows* ("*poor mixing*") and requires urgent attention. The initial management of the severely hypoxemic patient with TGA includes (i) ensuring *adequate mixing* between the two parallel circuits and (ii) *maximizing the mixed venous oxygen saturation*.

Once the diagnosis of TGA is made, maintaining patency of the ductus arteriosus with PGE_1 will increase PBF and intercirculatory mixing, if PVR is lower than systemic vascular resistance *and* there is an atrial communication. *In patients who do not respond to opening the ductus arteriosus using prostaglandin with an increased arterial oxygen saturation, the foramen ovale should be emergently enlarged by balloon atrial septostomy, and ventilatory maneuvers should be utilized to decrease PVR and increase PBF.* Balloon atrial septostomy remains an elective procedure in patients with adequate oxygen delivery. Many find it helpful to perform a balloon atrial septostomy—even in the stable patient on prostaglandin—so that PGE_1 can be discontinued and surgery can take place on a more elective basis.

Despite these maneuvers, some patients remain hypoxemic despite an open ductus, an adequate sized atrial communication, and hyperventilation. In these patients, it is important to emphasize that *the majority of systemic blood flow is the recirculated systemic venous return*. In the presence of poor mixing, significant improvements in oxygen delivery can be made by increasing the mixed venous oxygen saturation, which is the major determinant of systemic arterial oxygen saturation. Maneuvers include *decreasing oxygen consumption* (muscle relaxants, sedation, mechanical ventilation) and *improving oxygen delivery* (increasing cardiac output with inotropic agents or increasing oxygen-carrying capacity by treating anemia). Coexisting causes of pulmonary venous desaturation (e.g., pneumothorax) should be identified and treated. Increasing the fraction of inspired oxygen to 100% will have little effect on the arterial PO_2, unless this serves to lower PVR and increases total PBF.

Tetralogy of Fallot

TOF results from anterior malalignment of the infundibular septum. This malalignment manifests itself as the four anatomic findings that Fallot described: anterior malalignment VSD, infundibular stenosis (subpulmonary stenosis), aortic override of the ventricular septum, and right ventricular hypertrophy. Associated anatomic abnormalities include anomalous origin of the left anterior descending coronary artery from the right coronary artery crossing the right ventricular outflow tract, dual left anterior descending supply, right aortic arch, multiple VSDs, and persistent left superior vena cava.

The preoperative physiology of TOF is mainly dependent upon the degree of subpulmonary stenosis. In patients with minimal obstruction to PBF, the physiology is similar to patients with VSD. There is little restriction of excessive blood flow into the lungs; these patients will have pulmonary overcirculation, a large pulmonary-to-systemic blood flow ratio, and symptoms of congestive heart failure. These patients have little to no right-to-left shunting and are occasionally labeled "pink tets." Alternatively, there can be severe obstruction to PBF with significant right-to-left shunting at the VSD. These patients are hypoxemic and may have oxygen saturations in the 70% to 80% range. Despite the hypoxemia, they tend to grow and develop normally. In between these two extremes are patients who are "balanced" with enough pulmonary stenosis to "protect" the pulmonary arteries from overcirculation and pulmonary hypertension. These patients may have minimal to mild hypoxemia (oxygen saturations (~90%) and are typically asymptomatic.

TOF "Spells"

The classic TOF spell includes the following symptoms: (a) agitation/irritability, (b) hyperpnea, (c) profound cyanosis, and (d) syncope. Auscultation during the spell frequently will reveal an absent murmur, due to minimal flow across the right ventricular outflow tract. If frequent or inadequately managed, these spells can, in rare cases, result in death. Initial treatment typically consists of (a) supplemental oxygen, (b) sedation (subcutaneous or intravenous morphine 0.1 mg/kg), and (c) volume expansion. Some have advocated the "knee–chest" position to increase systemic venous return and increase systemic vascular resistance. In some very irritable

infants, this positioning tends to worsen the situation, as it can be very upsetting and increase irritability. It is particularly important for physicians and nurses at the bedside to keep the situation (and patient) calm. Frequently, the most effective position for these infants is to be held by their parent across the shoulder, with their knees bent and with supplemental oxygen being given by an additional person. In the case of persistent cyanosis despite these maneuvers, agents to increase systemic afterload, such as phenylephrine (5 to 20 µg/kg/dose IV every 10 minutes), can reverse the spell in some cases. Emergency surgery or ECMO occasionally, but rarely, is indicated.

Single Ventricle Anatomies

Anatomy of Single Ventricle Complexes

Atresia of an atrioventricular or semilunar valve results in single ventricle complexes that have complete mixing of the systemic and pulmonary venous circulations. Table 34–5 lists the anatomic variants that result in single ventricle physiology. There are some children in whom there is borderline hypoplasia of an atrioventricular valve, outflow tract, or ventricle, where a separated two ventricle circula-

TABLE 34–5. *Anatomic variations in single ventricle physiology in the preoperative and postoperative states*

Anatomy	Complete intracardiac mixing	
	Preoperative	Postoperative
Variations of single left ventricle		Yes
1. Tricuspid valve atresia		Yes
a. Normally related great arteries	Yes	Yes
b. Transposed great arteries[a]	Yes	Yes
2. Double inlet left ventricle		Yes
a. Normally related great arteries	Yes	Variable[b]
b. Transposed great arteries[a]	Yes[b]	
3. Malaligned complete atrioventricular canal with hypoplastic right ventricle	Yes	
4. Pulmonary atresia with intact ventricular septum	Yes	
Variations of single right ventricle		Yes
1. Mitral valve atresia		Yes
a. Hypoplastic left heart syndrome	Yes	Yes
b. Double outlet right ventricle	Yes	Variable[b]
2. Aortic valve atresia		Yes
a. Hypoplastic left heart syndrome	Yes	Yes
b. Large ventricular septal defect and normal left ventricular size	Yes	
3. Malaligned complete atrioventricular canal with hypoplastic left ventricle	Yes	
4. Heterotaxy syndromes—most forms have pulmonary stenosis or atresia	Yes	
Two-ventricle hearts with potential single ventricle physiology		Variable[b]
1. Tetralogy of Fallot with pulmonary atresia	Yes	No
2. Truncus arteriosus	Yes[c]	No
3. Total anomalous pulmonary venous connection	Yes[c]	

[a]In tricuspid atresia or double inlet left ventricle with transposed great arteries ({S,D,D} or {S,L,L}), right ventricular hypoplasia, subaortic obstruction, arch hypoplasia, and coarctation frequently exist.

[b]Single ventricle physiology will result if a systemic-to-pulmonary artery shunt or pulmonary artery band is placed. Two ventricle repairs with normal series circulation or partial repairs with incomplete mixing are possible in certain anatomic types.

[c]Streaming may result in incomplete mixing.

Adapted from Chang AC, Hanley FL, Wernovsky G, Wessel DL, eds. *Pediatric cardiac intensive care.* Baltimore: Williams & Wilkins, 1998:272.

tion is possible. Examples of this type of lesion include Shone's syndrome, in which there are multiple left-sided obstructive lesions and unbalanced atrioventricular canal (36). Controversy exists whether patients with mild-to-moderate forms of Shone's syndrome or similar lesions should be converted to a single ventricle repair or staged toward a separated two ventricle circulation (37–39). Alternately, there are infants born with two ventricles of normal size, who have malattached or straddling atrioventricular valve or a VSD that is remote from either great vessel, which preclude a two ventricle repair. Although these infants have ventricular chambers and atrioventricular valves suitable in size for a two ventricle repair, the anatomy is such that single ventricular management must be undertaken. Examples include defects such as double-outlet right ventricle with a remote VSD; D-TGA with VSD, pulmonic stenosis, and malattached tricuspid chordae that prohibit a Rastelli repair; and D-TGA with aortic stenosis in which a Damus–Kaye–Stansel palliation must be performed.

Single Ventricle Physiology

In each of the lesions delineated previously there is essentially complete mixing of the systemic and venous returns. Mixing typically occurs at the ventricular or atrial level. A consequence of the mixing is that the ventricular output must be divided between the pulmonary and systemic arterial circuits, the two parallel circuits. In this situation, the pulmonary artery and the aortic oxygen saturations are equal, and the ventricular output is the sum of the PBF (Qp) and the systemic blood flow (Qs). The proportion of the ventricular output that goes to the pulmonary or systemic vascular bed is determined by the relative resistance to flow into the two circuits.

In almost all hearts with single ventricle physiology, one of the two outflows is obstructed. It is extremely rare to have no outflow obstruction or to have obstruction to the pulmonary *and* systemic circuits. As a result patients generally fall into two distinct categories, those with obstructed pulmonary outflow and those with obstructed systemic outflow.

Resistance to pulmonary flow is determined by:

1. The degree of subvalvar or valvar pulmonary stenosis
2. The pulmonary arteriolar resistance
3. The pulmonary venous and left atrial (LA) pressures
4. The size of the ductus arteriosus.

The LA pressure is determined by the volume of the PBF entering the left atrium and the degree of obstruction to outflow through the left atrioventricular valve and atrial septum. Resistance to systemic flow is determined by:

1. The degree of subaortic or aortic valvar stenosis, arch hypoplasia, or coarctation

2. The systemic vascular resistance
3. The size of the ductus arteriosus.

Balancing the Parallel Circulations

When managing the neonate with single ventricle anatomy, the goal is to balance the ventricular output between the systemic and pulmonary vascular beds in such a way as to provide for adequate oxygen delivery to prevent acidosis while minimizing volume load to the single ventricle. Assuming a pulmonary venous saturation of 95% to 100% and a mixed venous oxygen saturation of 55% to 60%, *an arterial oxygen saturation of 75% to 80% represents a Qp/Qs ratio of approximately 1.0.* This typically results in mild ventricular volume overload (the Qp *plus* the Qs), minimal AV valve regurgitation, and normal systemic blood flow.

The Transitional Circulation. After birth, there is a fall in PVR and a relative increase in the proportion of PBF from the combined ventricular output. As the PVR continues to fall with time, an increasing proportion of the combined ventricular output is committed to the lungs. The normal homeostatic mechanisms to improve systemic output result in an increased stroke volume and increase in heart rate.

However, the normal fall in PVR over the first few hours to days of life, in the absence of a significant obstruction to PBF, gradually results in *elevated PBF at the expense of systemic blood flow.* As the Qp/Qs ratio approaches 2.0, the single ventricle becomes progressively volume overloaded, with mildly elevated end-diastolic and atrial pressures. The neonate may show signs of respiratory distress. The greater proportion of pulmonary venous return in the mixed ventricular blood results in an elevated systemic arterial oxygen saturation (approximately 85% to 90%), and visible cyanosis may be mild or absent.

Prior to surgical intervention, a number of ventilatory and pharmacologic maneuvers may be used to "balance" the circulation (Qp/Qs ~1), resulting in adequate oxygen delivery and systemic blood flow. However, in many of these patients, ventilatory and pharmacologic management only temporizes the need for surgical intervention. Patients with unbalanced single ventricle physiology may be grouped into two physiologic extremes: (i) inadequate PBF, which results in hypoxemia, and (ii) excessive PBF, which results in congestive heart failure.

Inadequate Pulmonary Blood Flow. The newborn with single ventricle physiology and an inadequate oxygen saturation (less than 65%) may have limited PBF due to: (a) *intracardiac obstruction* (i.e., severe valvar and/or subvalvar pulmonic stenosis); (b) a *restrictive ductus arteriosus* in lesions with "duct-dependent" PBF; (c) *elevated PVR*; or (d) *obstruction to pulmonary venous outflow* causing pulmonary venous hypertension and secondary pulmonary arteriolar hypertension.

Management strategies to improve PBF in this setting should be tailored to the underlying anatomy or pathophysiology resulting in the decreased PBF. For example, patients with *intracardiac obstruction* to PBF may have maneuvers performed to increase blood pressure and systemic vascular resistance (i.e., increasing inotropic infusions), forcing more blood through the obstructed intracardiac pulmonary outflow. Interventional procedures such as pulmonary valve dilation also may be considered in this group of patients. Patients who are hypoxemic due to an *obstructive left-sided atrioventricular valve and restrictive ASD* may have transcatheter dilation of the atrial septum performed (40,41). Patients thought to be hypoxemic due to *elevated PVR* should have ventilatory maneuvers performed to decrease PVR (i.e., increased FIO_2, hyperventilation/alkalosis, nitric oxide). Most intravenous pulmonary vasodilators are nonspecific and result in unpredictable changes in pulmonary and systemic vascular resistance.

Excessive Pulmonary Blood Flow. A more common scenario in nonoperated patients with single ventricle is progressive PBF at the expense of systemic blood flow. When severe, this results in systemic hypoperfusion, metabolic acidosis, and shock. Once establishment of a PDA is confirmed, maneuvers to minimize systemic vascular resistance and maximize PVR should be employed. Hypotensive patients with a relatively high arterial oxygen saturation (greater than 90%) generally have a severe "steal" of the combined ventricular output into the pulmonary vascular circuit. In these "overcirculated" patients, excessive inotropic support (particular at alpha-doses) should be avoided and afterload reduction (i.e., sodium nitroprusside) may be especially helpful in patients with elevated systemic vascular resistance and adequate blood pressure (42).

It is important to emphasize that patients with single ventricle physiology and "high" arterial oxygen saturations actually have *decreased* oxygen delivery to the tissues. The increased oxygen content comes at the expense of reduced systemic blood flow, which results in inadequate tissue perfusion, metabolic acidosis, and low cardiac output. In addition, ventricular wall tension and oxygen consumption are increased in the dilated, volume-overloaded single ventricle, potentially contributing to myocardial dysfunction and atrioventricular valve regurgitation. A progressive metabolic acidosis, even if mild, is an extremely worrisome sign in these patients and requires urgent evaluation.

Maneuvers to increase PVR have been shown to be clinically effective in reducing excessive PBF. Supplemental inspired nitrogen (or possibly supplemental carbon dioxide) may be used to elevate PVR, by inducing alveolar hypoxia (43–45). The hematocrit should be maintained at greater than 40% to 45%, as the increased viscosity may also serve to elevate PVR. Intubation and mechanical ventilation with sedation, paralysis, and permissive hypoventilation can be used to elevate the PCO_2

to the 40 to 50 mm Hg range (46). Metabolic acidemia should be corrected with sodium bicarbonate.

It is important to emphasize that preoperative patients with marked overcirculation and systemic hypoperfusion should not undergo a lengthy period of "medical management" of their unstable physiology. If a patient requires intubation and sedation to maintain adequate systemic blood flow, the patient should undergo relatively urgent surgical management to achieve a more favorable physiology.

SURGICAL PRINCIPLES

This section will delineate general surgical principles. The discussion is divided into the timing and type of surgery, and intraoperative monitoring.

Timing and Type of Surgery

For the neonate with congenital heart disease that requires surgical intervention, the medical and surgical teams responsible must decide on the timing of the surgery and the type of surgery. In the neonate who has sustained end-organ damage secondary to hypoxemia–ischemia, medical management should continue, if possible, until there is evidence of recovery of secondary organ function, to minimize surgical morbidity and risk. In addition, the presence of sepsis should be evaluated and ruled out. Delaying surgery for a few days also allows adequate time for the family to understand the complexity of the heart defect and the proposed intervention.

The surgical procedures performed for congenital heart disease are categorized in several ways. *Operations may be open or closed, and may be palliative or corrective.* "Open" procedures are those in which the CPB machine is used, whereas "closed" procedures are those in which bypass is not used. Examples of closed procedures include repair of coarctation of the aorta, ligation of a PDA, and placement of a modified Blalock–Taussig (BT) shunt. Procedures that result in persistent intracardiac mixing are referred to as "palliative" (e.g., systemic-to-pulmonary artery shunt, pulmonary artery banding, Damus–Kaye–Stansel, stage I Norwood procedure), whereas repairs with a two ventricle circulation are referred to as "corrective."

In the past, critically ill neonates with potential two ventricle circulation were subjected to a first-stage palliative procedure, followed later by reparative surgery. These palliative operations, albeit lifesaving and low risk in many instances, may cause secondary damage to the heart, great vessels, and other organ systems. For example, systemic-to-pulmonary artery shunts impose a significant volume load on the left ventricle and possibly increase pressure and flow to the pulmonary circulation. Banding of the pulmonary artery may distort the branch pulmonary arteries or pulmonary valve, may not protect the pulmonary vasculature from high pressure or flow, and will not "grow" with the patient.

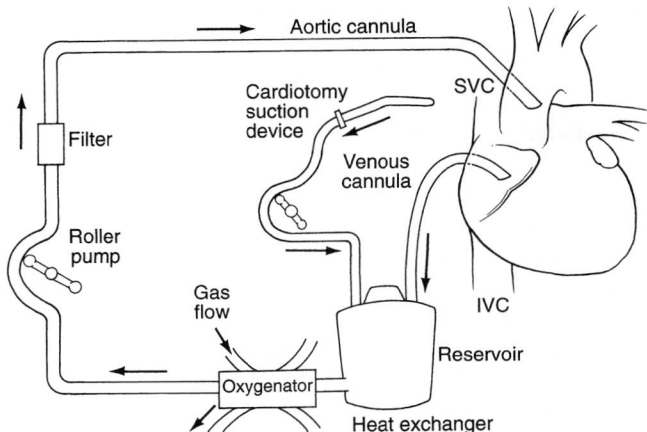

FIG. 34–2. Basic components of cardiopulmonary bypass. Venous blood is drained from the heart via a cannula in the right atrium (shown here) or, alternately, bicaval cannulation in the superior vena cava (SVC) and inferior vena cava (IVC). Blood drains by gravity to a venous reservoir and mixes with blood drained from the operative field by cardiotomy suction catheters. After passing through a heat exchanger, the blood is passed through an oxygenator, a roller pump, and a micropore filter, and back to the body via an aortic cannula. (From Mayer JE Jr. Cardiopulmonary bypass. In: Chang AC, Hanley FL, Wernovsky G, Wessel DL, eds. *Pediatric cardiac intensive care.* Baltimore: Williams & Wilkins, 1998:190, with permission.)

In patients with potential two ventricle circulation, corrective rather than palliative procedures should be performed whenever possible, even in the premature or low-birth-weight neonate. Corrective procedures on CPB may now be performed in neonates as small as 1,200 to 1,500 g, with an acceptable mortality rate, and prolonged medical therapy to achieve additional weight gain does not improve survival (47). In fact, prolonged medical therapy to achieve additional weight gain continues to expose the neonate to the risk of intensive care unit complications, and weight gain may be marginal due to the underlying congenital heart disease. Palliative procedures may be considered in the rare neonates in whom the risk of CPB is prohibitive, e.g., neonates with bleeding disorders, recent intraventricular hemorrhage, or ongoing sepsis.

Intraoperative Management

The techniques of *CPB* and myocardial preservation used in reparative and palliative open procedures are critical to provide an adequate hemodynamic result without permanent secondary organ damage. In CPB, venous blood is siphoned into the venous reservoir of the heart–lung bypass apparatus from a single cannula placed into the right atrium or two smaller catheters inserted into each vena cava. After traversing a membrane oxygenator, heat exchanger, filter, and roller pump, blood is returned to the patient in the ascending aorta via an aortic cannula.

Figure 34–2 shows the path of blood in the CPB circuit. Each component of the system is designed to minimize the priming volume required and trauma to the blood and to increase the efficiency of gas exchange and heat transfer to provide for the special needs of the neonate. Bypass is initiated by removing clamps from the venous line, which opens the siphon to the pump. Simultaneously the roller pump is started to reinfuse blood into the patient. Pump flows of 100 mL/kg/min generally are adequate to maintain tissue oxygenation. The time during which blood is continuously exchanged between the heart–lung apparatus and the patient is referred as the *total bypass time*. During this time, the patient is fully heparinized (activated clotting time greater than 500), which carries significant implications in the very-low-birth-weight neonate.

Despite notable and continuing improvements in the technical aspects of CPB, significant morbidity remains associated with its use. In addition to the anticoagulation, morbidity from CPB results from alterations in normal cardiovascular physiology and include the following: exposure of the blood to prosthetic surfaces; excessive sheer stress on blood cells, microembolization of gas bubbles and particles, hemodilution, tissue ischemia and reperfusion injury, and nonpulsatile or minimally pulsatile systemic flow. These alterations lead to the activation of neutrophils, platelets, endothelial cells, and the serum proteins that mediate blood clotting, complement fixation, and fibrinolysis (48,49). The combined effect of this activation is a generalized inflammatory response, which results in endothelial cell injury, increased capillary permeability, tissue edema, and multiple organ dysfunction in the heart, brain, lungs, and kidneys. CPB results in an increase in total body water, transient myocardial dysfunction, elevated PVR, abnormalities of gas exchange, and stress and hormonal responses leading to fluid and electrolyte disturbances. Due to the pump's priming volume being several times the neonate's blood volume, severe hemodilution occurs, which decreases oncotic pressure and increases the loss of intravascular fluid through a damaged endothelium. Dilution of clotting factors may result in severe coagulopathy after surgery, despite heparin reversal with protamine (50). Pump priming with fresh whole blood and the administration of blood components helps to prevent severe bleeding complications.

A variety of techniques have been developed to reverse tissue edema and hemodilution following CPB in children, which include ultrafiltration during CPB, postoperative peritoneal dialysis, postoperative continuous arteriovenous hemofiltration, and the use of diuretics postoperatively. In the pediatric population, ultrafiltration during CPB is restricted by the volume of the venous reservoir and provides only a limited ability to remove excess water and reverse hemodilution. A modification of standard ultrafiltration termed *modified ultrafiltration* (MUF) has been developed at the Hospital for Sick Children in London and presently is being used routinely at the Children's Hospital of Philadelphia (51,52). Unlike conventional ultrafiltration, MUF is performed in the immediate postbypass period. It removes excess water from the patient directly and provides a method of salvaging red blood cells from the circuit that may be infused during postoperative convalescence. The use of MUF after cardiac surgery in children has been demonstrated to have several beneficial effects, including improved cardiovascular hemodynamics, decreased PVR, cytokine removal and reduction in complement activation, decreased postoperative bleeding, and decreased need for blood transfusion due to hemodilution reversal (53–55).

Successful repair of complex lesions requires meticulous attention to every detail of surgical technique. A bloodless, motionless field with a nonbeating heart allows for adequate repair. This is often accomplished on bypass by clamping the ascending aorta between the root of the aorta and the aortic cannula, isolating the heart from the rest of the circulation, and instilling cardioplegia solution into the aortic root. The time during which the ascending aorta is clamped and the heart is ischemic

is referred to as the *aortic cross-clamp time. Cardioplegia* is a cold crystalloid and/or blood solution containing glucose, buffer, electrolytes, and, in particular, a high potassium concentration. With coronary cardioplegia infusion, the heart becomes flaccid, and a motionless surgical field is produced. Current techniques of myocardial protection with cardioplegia and with topical and systemic cooling allows for ischemic times greater than 2 hours to be well tolerated in most patients.

In neonatal bypass, body temperature is typically lowered to 18° to 20°C to decrease tissue oxygen consumption and to protect the heart and other organs. Body temperatures of 20°C or lower are referred to as deep *hypothermia*. Figure 34–3 shows the temperature changes during CPB. As metabolic demands decrease with hypothermia, pump flow can be temporarily reduced to as low as 25 to 50 mL/kg/min, "low flow bypass," or the pump can be turned off altogether, "circulatory arrest."

Another way to create the ideal surgical conditions is to turn the pump off once deep hypothermia levels are

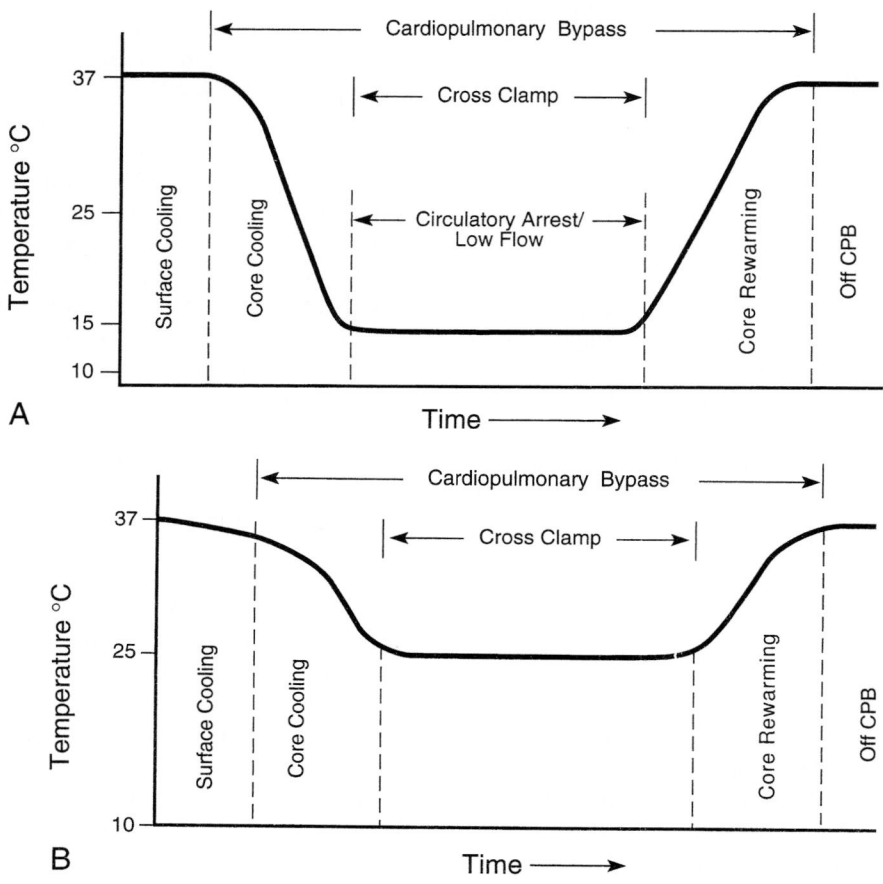

FIG. 34–3. A: Whole body temperature (y-axis) changes during cardiopulmonary bypass (CPB) using profound hypothermia. **B:** For operations not requiring profound hypothermia and circulatory arrest, cardiopulmonary bypass typically is carried out at 25° to 28°C. (From Mayer JE Jr. Cardiopulmonary bypass. In: Chang AC, Hanley FL, Wernovsky G, Wessel DL, eds. *Pediatric cardiac intensive care*. Baltimore: Williams & Wilkins, 1998:192.)

achieved throughout the body. This condition is called deep hypothermia with circulatory arrest. The time during which the pump is turned off and there is no circulation is the *circulatory arrest time*. At 18°C, circulatory arrest times less than 45 minutes are generally well tolerated, but the incidence of neurologic sequelae increases in some patients with periods greater than 60 to 75 minutes. Neurologic sequelae from deep hypothermic circulatory arrest (DHCA) are discussed later. Most surgeons use a combination of low flow and circulatory arrest to perform complex neonatal heart surgery.

POSTOPERATIVE CARE: GENERAL PRINCIPLES

Ideal postoperative care of the neonate following either reparative or palliative operations requires a thorough understanding and systematic evaluation of (a) the underlying anatomic defect, (b) the pathophysiology of the preoperative state, (c) the anesthetic regimen used during surgery, (d) the duration of CPB, aortic cross-clamp time, and circulatory arrest time, (e) the details of the operative procedure and any concerns of the surgeon regarding the potential for residual defects, and (f) data available from monitoring catheters, echocardiography, and cardiac catheterization. Optimal management of these critically ill children can best be achieved through a harmonious team approach, combining the expertise of cardiologists, neonatologists, cardiac surgeons, anesthesiologists, intensivists, nurses, and respiratory therapists.

Invasive Monitoring

Accurate measurement of systemic and pulmonary arterial pressure, ventricular filling pressures, urine output, alveolar gas exchange, cardiac output, systemic vascular resistance, and PVR allows for precise pharmacologic and ventilatory support in the perioperative period. The neonate and infant require more physiologic monitoring than the adult, because they have wider swings in physiologic variables such as heart rate, temperature, glucose metabolism, systemic vascular resistance, and PVR. Based on this principle, most patients are monitored invasively in the perioperative period. Intracardiac monitoring catheters generally are placed at the time of surgery in all patients undergoing repair of defects of any complexity greater than an isolated secundum ASD.

Continuous monitoring of the heart rate and the QRS morphology is standard practice in most intensive care units. Indwelling Foley catheters are useful for continuous, hourly assessment of urine output. The data obtained from sophisticated monitoring should not divert the physician from, or be a substitute for, less quantitative clinical measures of cardiac output such as peripheral and core temperature, urine output, capillary refill, and strength of peripheral pulses.

Intracardiac monitoring catheters have two main functions: (i) assessment of the repair for residual defects, and (ii) precise measurements of hemodynamics following surgery, allowing for rational pharmacologic manipulation of heart rate, preload, afterload, and contractility.

Following surgery, one or two right atrial (RA) catheters are placed through the RA appendage (usually through the site used for venous cannulation on CPB), and an LA catheter is placed into the right superior pulmonary vein or LA appendage. The pulmonary artery catheter is inserted through a pursestring suture in the right ventricular outflow tract. The pulmonary artery catheter may be a single lumen pressure catheter or a double lumen catheter with a thermistor for measurement of cardiac output and core temperature. Use of these catheters has been shown to have a complication rate of 1% to 2% in neonates (56–58). The most common complications noted with the use of these catheters include bleeding, entrapment, fragmentation, transient arrhythmias, and infection (56,57).

LA catheters provide indirect data on the function of the systemic ventricle and may be used for contrast (saline) injections during echocardiography to detect residual left-to-right shunts. Inspection of the pressure tracing allows assessment of the function of the systemic atrioventricular valve and may be helpful in distinguishing various arrhythmias with loss of atrioventricular synchrony.

RA catheters are used to assess the central venous pressure and for measurement of RA oxygen saturation. The RA saturation may not truly reflect the "mixed venous" saturation if the tip of the catheter is close to the renal vein flow (falsely high) or coronary sinus ostium or hepatic venous flow (falsely low). Roentgenographic confirmation of tip position is important for correct interpretation of the data. Saline contrast injections through the RA catheter during echocardiography may detect right-to-left intracardiac shunting. RA catheters may be used for vasoactive and inotropic medications and may be used for parenteral nutrition.

Pulmonary artery catheters may be used when VSDs are closed to assess residual left-to-right shunts, to determine residual right ventricular outflow tract gradients, to monitor for significant postoperative pulmonary hypertension, or when thermodilution cardiac index determinants are to be made (59–61).

The LA catheter usually is removed on the first postoperative day. The pulmonary artery catheter often also is removed at this time, although occasionally it is left indwelling in patients with significant pulmonary hypertension. RA catheters may be left in place for up to 2 weeks if necessary.

Continuous monitoring of systemic arterial pressure is routinely used. Arterial catheters allow for beat-to-beat analysis of the arterial waveform and provide insight into specific disease states, such as cardiac tamponade (narrow pulse pressure with pulsus paradoxus) or a large runoff lesion such as a BT shunt or aortic regurgitation (widened pulse pressure). Pronounced phasic variations in a patient receiving positive-pressure ventilation, coupled with low atrial pressures, are typical for significant hypovolemia. The radial artery is the most frequently used site for arterial access.

Residual Anatomic Lesions

When either the clinical course or the postoperative hemodynamic state does not conform to the expected recovery pattern, it is prudent to suspect the accuracy of the preoperative diagnosis and the adequacy of the surgical repair. The clinician should not initially assume that poor hemodynamics are due to ventricular dysfunction after CPB, although this clearly does occur. A retrospective review of 32 consecutive neonates and infants who died in the cardiac intensive care unit after cardiac surgery at Boston Children's Hospital revealed that death could be attributed to residual anatomic lesions in 12 of 18 patients who had reparative operations (62). Although low cardiac output due to myocardial ischemia does occur in neonates in the postoperative period, it can be anticipated and adequately managed.

Low Cardiac Output States

In neonates studied after the arterial switch operation, the cardiac index fell predictably by 25% from baseline values to less than 2 L/min/m^2 in 25% of the patients during the first postoperative night, whereas pulmonary and systemic vascular resistance increased (63). Factors implicated include the effects of myocardial ischemia from aortic cross-clamping, hypothermia, reperfusion injury, inadequate myocardial protection, and ventriculotomy when performed. Anticipation of this reproducible phenomenon greatly reduces the associated morbidity and potential mortality. Volume therapy to increase preload and the appropriate use of inotropic and afterload reducing agents have been shown to oppose this phenomenon (64).

Pharmacologic Support of Cardiac Output

Pharmacologic support to optimize postoperative hemodynamics can be grouped into three broad categories: (i) sympathomimetic amines, (ii) phosphodiesterase inhibitors, and (iii) vasodilators (see also Chaps. 33 and 55).

Sympathomimetic Amines

Sympathomimetic amines, either endogenous (dopamine or epinephrine) or synthetic (isoproterenol or dobutamine), have been the mainstay of therapy to improve cardiac output (see section on Stabilization and Transport).

Phosphodiesterase Inhibitors

Phosphodiesterase inhibitors such as amrinone and milrinone are bipyridine compounds that increase inotropy, cause venous and arteriolar vasodilation, and increase relaxation during diastole (65,66). Milrinone, a 2-methyl, 5-carbonitrile cogener of amrinone, is 15 times more potent than its parent compound (67,68). Phosphodiesterase inhibitors selectively inhibit cyclic nucleotide phosphodiesterase, thus increasing levels of cAMP in myocytes and smooth muscle cells.

Although clinical experience with amrinone suggests that a continuous infusion of 5 to 15 μg/kg/min after a bolus of 3.0 to 4.5 mg/kg is effective (69,70), Katz et al. (71) reported that amrinone had no inotropic effect in fetal and neonatal preparations of rat myocardial cells and avian, cat, and rabbit papillary muscles. Other studies have shown negative inotropic effects in newborn canine muscle and in neonatal piglet hearts (72,73). When administered by continuous infusion after cardiac surgery, amrinone has been shown to significantly increase cardiac index and decrease systemic vascular resistance without a significant increase in heart rate (69,74,75). Amrinone may be of particular benefit to children after CPB, who are normotensive with a low cardiac output and have elevated left ventricular afterload and coexisting pulmonary hypertension (76). Finally, amrinone has been shown to significantly increase cardiac index in children after Fontan operation (77).

Significant hypotension may be associated with intravenous administration of amrinone, particularly if the infusion is preceded by a bolus dose. This undesired effect can be precluded by administration of volume and maintenance of adequate preload (66,70). Thrombocytopenia often is seen in adults on long-term oral therapy and occasionally is seen in pediatric patients receiving infusions greater than 7 to 10 days (78).

Clinical uses for milrinone are the same for amrinone (79). Administration of milrinone in neonates with low cardiac output after cardiac surgery was demonstrated to lower filling pressures and systemic and pulmonary atrial pressures and resistance, while increasing cardiac index without increasing myocardial oxygen consumption (65). Unlike amrinone, milrinone has not been shown to have a negative inotropic effect on neonatal myocardium (79). A comparison between milrinone and dobutamine suggested that milrinone was superior in lowering systemic vascular resistance for any given increase in dP/dt (80), whereas comparison between milrinone and nitroprusside showed that milrinone was superior in increasing the peak positive rate of pressure development (dP/dt) and the stroke work of the left ventricle (81).

In contrast to amrinone, milrinone does not appear to cause thrombocytopenia as a side effect (82).

Vasodilators

Pure arterial and venous vasodilators can be used either alone or in combination with other cardiovascular drugs to improve cardiac output by reducing ventricular preload and afterload. In general, vasodilators are useful adjunctive therapy for (a) myocardial dysfunction secondary to dilated cardiomyopathy, coronary insufficiency, or cardiac surgery; (b) systemic or pulmonary hypertension; and (c) valvular regurgitation leading to volume overload. The vasodilators most commonly used in the cardiac intensive care setting include nitroglycerine, sodium nitroprusside, hydralazine, calcium channel blockers, and orally available angiotensin-converting enzyme (ACE) inhibitors. Nitroglycerine and sodium nitroprusside are the most commonly used vasodilators in the intensive care setting and are discussed here.

Nitroglycerine is a potent venous vasodilator, but it is also an effective vasodilator of the systemic and pulmonary arteries. In the vascular endothelium, nitroglycerine is converted to nitric oxide (NO). NO activates guanylate cyclase, which increases intracellular cyclic GMP, a potent relaxant of vascular smooth muscle. Intravenous nitroglycerine lowers the myocardial oxygen consumption by reducing the preload and afterload, and it lowers RA and LA pressures, left ventricular end-diastolic pressure and volume, and systemic and pulmonary arterial pressures. Nitroglycerine also has an important additional effect on the coronary vasculature, with dilation of both epicardial and collateral coronary arteries (83). When infused intravenously in children, nitroglycerine augments the cardiac output by significantly reducing systemic vascular resistance in those with myocardial dysfunction and low cardiac output after CPB (84,85). Intravenous nitroglycerine is also an effective pharmacologic agent in the treatment of systemic and/or pulmonary hypertension (84). The effective use of nitroglycerine in adults with coronary ischemia is well documented. Some centers have started using nitroglycerine in children after procedures that required manipulation of the coronary circulation, including the arterial switch operation for TGA and the Ross procedure for aortic valve disease.

Sodium nitroprusside is a nonreceptor stimulant of guanylate cyclase and increases intracellular cyclic GMP in a manner similar to nitroglycerine; it acts as a nitric oxide donor. Its clinical effect is a significant reduction in preload and afterload due to dilation of both venous and arteriolar beds. Sodium nitroprusside produces a greater reduction in systemic and pulmonary arteriolar pressures than does nitroglycerine, and it usually is used in combination with an inotropic agent. This strategy has been demonstrated to increase cardiac output and decrease systemic vascular resistance (86). There also appears to be an age-dependent response and sensitivity to nitroprusside (87).

By lowering systemic vascular resistance, sodium nitroprusside improves cardiac output of children with myocardial dysfunction secondary to postoperative heart failure, pulmonary hypertension, dilated cardiomyopathy, or mitral/aortic valve regurgitation (88). Sodium nitroprusside is most commonly used after surgery on the aortic arch, aortic root, and aortic valve to minimize hypertension, which may result in bleeding at sites of anastomosis (89). Sodium nitroprusside also has been shown to decrease diastolic dysfunction in the left ventricle after coarctation repair (90).

Thiocyanate toxicity can occur quickly if renal insufficiency occurs. Signs and symptoms of toxicity include tissue hypoxia, seizures, muscle spasms, emesis, and bone marrow suppression. Cyanide toxicity can be monitored by following: the mixed venous oxygen PO_2, which is increased in cyanide toxicity; pH, which is depressed due to metabolic acidosis; and plasma cyanide and thiocyanate levels in those infants receiving continuous infusion (91). Although toxicity can be treated with sodium thiosulfate, it is not likely to occur in children with normal hepatic and renal function (92). Finally, sodium nitroprusside, like other vasodilators, can attenuate the normal hypoxic pulmonary vasoconstriction and lead to significant intrapulmonary right-to-left shunting and hypoxemia.

Epicardial Pacing

Temporary epicardial pacing wires typically are placed on the anterior surface of the right ventricle and, increasingly, on the right atrium as well. Atrial wires may be used to increase heart rate (in the presence of sinus node dysfunction) while still allowing the ventricles to contract via the atrioventricular node and the normal His–Purkinje system. The atrial wires may be used for rapid atrial pacing, or "overdrive pacing," which is very effective in converting many types of supraventricular tachycardia to normal sinus rhythm at the bedside without the need for synchronized direct current cardioversion. In addition to the therapeutic uses, epicardial atrial wires may be used to record both unipolar and bipolar atrial electrograms for diagnostic purposes (93,94). Epicardial ventricular wires are useful in cases of atrioventricular nodal disease (e.g., complete heart block), although cardiac output may not be as effective when the ventricles contract dyssynchronously (i.e., with the right ventricle contracting prior to the left ventricle rather than through the His–Purkinje system) (95,96), and without atrioventricular synchrony (97–99). Dual chamber pacing is particularly useful in cases of complete heart block (97,98). In patients at risk of complete heart block, the temporary wires should be checked for threshold and sensitivity after arrival in the intensive care unit, and a temporary pacemaker should always be at the bedside.

Ventilatory Management

Ventilation and respiratory mechanics exert strong influences on the hemodynamics of children with congenital heart disease, especially after palliative or reparative operation (100). The uncertainties of gas exchange during spontaneous breathing in the immediate postoperative period can be minimized by using mechanical ventilation, end-expiratory pressure, and manipulation of PCO_2 and pH to optimize cardiovascular function (101,102).

Reduction in functional residual capacity decreases lung compliance and pulmonary venous oxygenation, resulting in increased work of breathing, which may substantially increase oxygen consumption (103). The most common noncardiac causes of respiratory compromise are listed in Table 34–6. Noncardiac causes of respiratory failure can be broadly grouped into CNS disorders, neuromuscular disorders, isolated neuropathies, airway abnormalities proximal to the alveoli, alveolar disease, extrinsic compression of the lungs, and chest wall abnormalities. These derangements of the respiratory system may result in impaired gas exchange, poor lung compliance, and/or ventilation/perfusion mismatch.

The most common isolated neuropathy is phrenic nerve injury resulting in hemidiaphragmatic paresis or

TABLE 34–6. *Noncardiac causes of respiratory failure after cardiothoracic surgery*

Central nervous system
  1. General anesthesia
  2. Administration of analgesics or sedative/hypnotics
  3. Hypoxic–ischemic encephalopathy
  4. Apnea of prematurity
Neuromuscular
  1. Residual neuromuscular blockade
  2. Respiratory muscle weakness—from disuse and/or malnutrition
Isolated neuropathies
  1. Hemidiaphragmatic paresis or paralysis—phrenic nerve injury (see Table 34–7)
  2. Vocal Cord Paralysis—recurrent laryngeal nerve injury
Airway abnormalities proximal to the alveoli
  1. Tracheostomy or endotracheal tube obstruction
  2. Postextubation subglottic edema
  3. Laryngotracheomalacia
  4. Left mainstem bronchomalacia—from long-standing left atrial or left pulmonary artery enlargement
  5. Congenital or acquired tracheal stenosis
Alveolar disease
  1. Acute lung injury from cardiopulmonary bypass
  2. Increased lung fluid—from left-to-right shunt lesions
  3. Atelectasis
  4. Pneumonia
  5. Pulmonary hemorrhage
  6. Pulmonary hypoplasia
Extrinsic lung compression
  1. Pleural effusion (transudate vs. exudate)
  2. Pneumothorax, hemothorax, chylothorax
Chest wall
  1. Midsternal, thoracotomy, or clamshell chest incisions

Adapted from Newth CJL, Hammer J. Pulmonary issues. In: Chang AC, Hanley FL, Wernovsky G, Wessel DL, eds. *Pediatric cardiac intensive care.* Baltimore: Williams & Wilkins, 1998:352.

TABLE 34–7. *Procedures associated with phrenic nerve injury*

Arch reconstruction
  1. Norwood palliation
  2. Interrupted aortic arch repair
  3. Coarctation repair
Hilar dissection
  1. Arterial switch operation
  2. Tetralogy of fallot
    a. TOF/APV repair: pulmonary artery plication
    b. TOF/PA: unifocalization
  3. Truncus arteriosus repair
  4. PDA ligation
Systemic-to-pulmonary artery shunt

PDA, patent ductus arteriosus; TOF/APV, tetralogy of Fallot with absent pulmonary valve; TOF/PA, tetralogy of Fallot with pulmonary atresia.

paralysis. Mechanisms of injury include nerve transection, nerve stretch, electrocautery heat trauma, and cold injury from topical cardiac hypothermia. Procedures associated with phrenic injury are listed in Table 34–7. The postoperative incidence of phrenic nerve injury has been estimated as high as 10% in children less than 2 years of age (104).

Mechanical positive-pressure ventilation minimizes postoperative pulmonary insufficiency and substantially reduces the work of breathing. Although early postoperative extubation can be accomplished successfully for some closed procedures and for children with less complex congenital heart disease repaired while on CPB, the advantages of postoperative positive-pressure ventilation have been increasingly apparent for neonates with complex congenital heart disease.

Caution must be used in suctioning the airway in infants in the immediate postoperative period. Suctioning the airway increases the levels of catecholamines and increases pulmonary and systemic vascular resistance in the neonate, which can have serious adverse effects on hemodynamics (105). Increased airway pressure, diminished motion of the chest wall, visible blood or large amounts of blood tinged or normal appearing secretions in the artificial airway are clear indications to suction the airway.

Mechanical ventilation is continued until (a) hemostasis is complete; (b) sinus rhythm or pacemaker-protected heart rate is normal for age; (c) adequate cardiac output is established; (d) the arterial waveform suggests adequate stroke volume; (e) normothermia has been achieved; (f) there is no evidence of copious secretions; and (g) the mental status is adequate to protect the airway.

If a neonate fails to tolerate postoperative weaning from mechanical ventilation, a search for residual hemodynamic causes should be initiated. Intraoperatively placed monitoring catheters and echocardiography serve to identify residual structural abnormalities remaining after surgery or those that have arisen as a result of the palliative or reparative procedure. If these modalities still do not reveal the cause of the respiratory insufficiency, cardiac catheterization should be considered.

Pain Control and Sedation

Stress responses to pain and other postoperative noxious stimuli are profound in even the youngest neonates, regardless of conceptual age (see Chap. 57) (6,106,107). These observations have led to many centers extending the anesthetic period through the first postoperative night, using high-dose continuous infusions of fentanyl at 4 to 10 µg/kg/h (following intraoperative anesthetic doses of 50 µg/kg) in neonates with unstable hemodynamics or pulmonary arterial hypertension (108). In our institution, the hemodynamically stable neonate generally receives 2 to 4 µg/kg/h during the first postoperative night. The fentanyl is then weaned off over the next 24 to 48 hours to minimize any depression of the neonate's respiratory drive after extubation. Those infants who have a protracted postoperative course may receive narcotics for a more extended period.

Fluid, Electrolyte, and Nutritional Management

Neonates may accumulate significant amounts (up to 1 L) of total body water while on CPB (63), which may result in significant edema of the chest wall, lungs, and myocardium, causing decreased total lung compliance and higher cardiac filling pressures. To minimize the detrimental cardiorespiratory effects of increased extravascular water, diuretics typically are used after the first postoperative night. Diuretic-induced electrolyte imbalances commonly occur. Several days of diuretic therapy with furosemide may result in hypokalemia, hypocalcemia, or metabolic acidosis. Long-term administration has been associated with nephrocalcinosis, especially in neonates. Intravenous administration of potassium chloride requires precise nursing protocols because of the arrhythmogenic potential of rapid administration.

Enteral nutrition is generally begun 2 to 3 days after cardiac surgery unless preoperative bowel ischemia is suspected. NEC is not uncommon in the neonate with congenital heart disease who had bowel ischemia in the preoperative period (109,110). Risk factors include left-sided obstructive lesions with mesenteric hypoperfusion following ductus arteriosus constriction, umbilical or femoral arterial catheterization, angiography, hypoxemia, and lesions with wide pulse pressures (e.g., systemic-to-pulmonary shunts, PDA, and severe aortic regurgitation). Lesions with a wide pulse pressure produce retrograde flow in the mesenteric vessels in diastole.

Ideally, caloric intake should reach 100 to 130 kcal/kg/d in infants who weigh less than 10 kg until they are weaned from mechanical ventilation. Although the enteral route is preferred, in our institution, parenteral nutrition is begun in all neonates after CPB, as adequate enteral caloric intake may take many days to achieve. Balancing carbohydrate administration with lipids is important, not only for caloric reasons, but also because it permits a respiratory quotient that avoids exclusive carbohydrate metabolism and the associated carbon dioxide production.

Infection Control

Mediastinitis occurs in up to 2% of patients undergoing cardiac surgery (111). Risk factors may include early reexploration for bleeding or reoperation (112). Mediastinitis is characterized by persistent fever, purulent drainage from the sternotomy wound, instability of the sternum, and leukocytosis. *Staphylococcus aureus* is the most common infecting organism (113). Delayed diagnosis of mediastinitis may lead to a mortality rate as high as 25% (114,115). Treatment involves surgical debridement and irrigation along with an aggressive course of parenteral antibiotics. If osteomyelitis of the sternum is present, a 42-day course of antibiotics is necessary.

In general, a longer duration of indwelling catheters is related to a higher risk of infection.

Central Nervous System Sequelae of Cardiac Surgery

Advances in the field of neonatal cardiac surgery have resulted in adverse neurologic sequelae in some children who survived complex cardiac repair. Although early corrective surgery has reduced some risk factors for CNS injury, such as chronic cyanosis, polycythemia, and right-to-left shunts, surgical techniques such as CPB and DHCA are associated with some risk of neurologic injury. In addition the decreased mortality rate of previously lethal congenital heart disease (e.g., hypoplastic left heart syndrome) has allowed surviving infants to manifest the neurologic sequelae of neonatal circulatory disturbances. During hypothermic CPB, there are multiple perfusion variables that might influence the risk of brain injury. These include, but are probably not limited to:

1. Total duration of CPB and the duration and rate of core cooling (116,117),
2. pH management during core cooling (118–120),
3. Duration of circulatory arrest (121–123),
4. Type of oxygenator (124–126),
5. Presence of arterial filtration (127), and
6. Depth of hypothermia (128–130).

Undoubtedly, there is interaction among these various elements, and CNS injury following CPB is most likely multifactorial. There is extensive literature on the CNS effects of CPB in adult patients. However, extrapolation of the adult experience to neonates with congenital heart disease must be made cautiously, as the degree of hypothermia used in adults is usually only mild to moderate, and circulatory arrest is only rarely used.

DHCA has been increasingly used in centers with expertise in neonatal and infant cardiac surgery. The major surgical advantage of this technique is the absence of perfusion cannulae and blood from the operative field. The use of DHCA assumes that there is a "safe" duration that is inversely related to body temperature. The organ with the shortest "safe" period is the brain. Evidence of transient cerebral injury during DHCA comes from numerous laboratory investigations (131–133). Experimental studies in animals on brain structure and function after use of DHCA have suggested that, at a core temperature of 15° to 20°C, a 30-minute total arrest time is safe with respect to CNS damage (134,135). A recent randomized study has suggested that a period of DHCA greater than 45 minutes was associated with a significantly greater incidence of perioperative neurologic abnormalities (136). Long-term follow-up of this cohort of patients is currently under way.

Clinical studies have primarily emphasized the incidence of seizures, choreoathetosis, and long-term developmental abnormalities. Seizures are the most frequently observed neurologic consequence of cardiac surgery using DHCA, with a reported incidence of 4% to 25% (137,138). Both focal and generalized seizures have been described, usually occurring during postoperative days 1 to 4. Although the long-term prognosis after hypoxic–ischemic seizures in the normothermic neonate may be guarded, the long-term significance of seizures occurring after hypothermic CPB with DHCA presently is being examined; long-term seizure disorders are rare.

POSTOPERATIVE LESION-SPECIFIC CARE

In addition to the general principles of postoperative care outlined previously, each specific lesion has its own special set of postoperative concerns that must be addressed to ensure successful postoperative management.

Single Ventricle Complexes

General Principles of Newborn Surgical Management

Children with single ventricle complexes will, in most cases, undergo a variation of the Fontan operation as their ultimate surgical palliation. Risk factors for poor outcome after the modified Fontan operation include (a) ventricular hypertrophy (139), (b) elevated PVR or pulmonary arterial pressure (140–142), (c) pulmonary artery distortion (143,144), (d) atrioventricular valve regurgitation (145,146), and (e) ventricular dysfunction (147). The management strategies for surgical and medical management of newborns with single ventricle anatomy must minimize these potential risk factors over the long term, even if it means that a more complex neonatal palliation must be performed. All newborn procedures for surgical palliation of the single ventricle are performed to achieve the following:

Unobstructed systemic blood flow (to minimize ventricular hypertrophy),
Limited PBF (to minimize ventricular volume load and the risk of ventricular dysfunction, atrioventricular valve regurgitation, and pulmonary arterial hypertension,
Nondistorted pulmonary arteries, and
Unrestrictive pulmonary venous return (to minimize the risk of LA hypertension, pulmonary venous hypertension, and secondary pulmonary arterial hypertension.

Surgical palliation for the single ventricle in the newborn may include placement of a systemic-to-pulmonary artery shunt, pulmonary artery banding, pulmonary artery to aortic anastomosis (Damus–Kaye–Stansel), and stage I Norwood procedures.

Palliative Procedures

Systemic-to-Pulmonary Artery Shunt

The modified BT shunt is the palliative procedure most commonly used to secure PBF in the neonate with single ventricle lesions with restrictive PBF. Depending on the size of the patient and the preexisting pulmonary arteriolar resistance, a 3.0- to 4.0-mm Gore-Tex tube is placed from the brachiocephalic vessels, usually the subclavian or innominate artery, to the pulmonary artery. Similarly, placement of a central shunt involves inserting a Gore-Tex tube between the ascending aorta and the pulmonary artery. The central shunt generally is used when there is an aberrant subclavian artery and, therefore, no innominate artery from which to place the modified BT shunt. In the past, the Waterston and Potts shunts were used to provide PBF, but they fell out of favor because they were associated with a high risk of pulmonary arterial hypertension and/or distortion of the pulmonary arteries. Figure 34–4 illustrates the classic BT, modified BT, Central, Waterston, and Potts shunts.

Pulmonary Artery Banding

In children with no restriction to systemic blood flow and little to no restriction to PBF, a pulmonary artery band may be placed to limit PBF and pulmonary arterial pressure. The pulmonary artery band is placed without CPB. Surgical staff must minimize distortion of the branch pulmonary arteries, which, as described previously, increases the risk of poor outcome of the subsequent Fontan completion procedure (148,149). By decreasing PBF there is acute reduction in the volume load on the ventricle and an immediate decrease in cavity dimension and an increase in wall thickness (150). These changes may result in acute development of subaortic stenosis, especially if systemic output is dependent upon a relatively small VSD. Figure 34–5 illustrates placement of a pulmonary artery band.

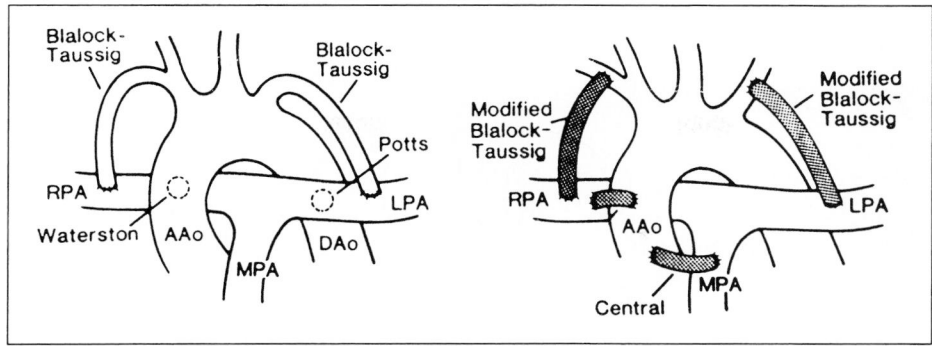

FIG. 34–4. Schematic diagram of systemic-to-pulmonary artery shunts.

Pulmonary Artery to Aortic Anastomosis (Damus–Kaye–Stansel)

The Damus–Kaye–Stansel palliation is used for children with single ventricle with subaortic stenosis with or without distal arch obstruction to allow both great arteries and semilunar valves to provide unobstructed systemic blood flow (151–154). The most common lesions for which the Damus–Kaye–Stansel operation is utilized is single left ventricle with TGA (tricuspid atresia with TGA, TGA double inlet left ventricle) and double outlet right ventricle with subaortic obstruction and a remote or doubly committed VSD where it is impossible to baffle the left ventricular outflow to great vessel without significant intracardiac obstruction. The palliation involves amalgamation of the semilunar roots, main pulmonary

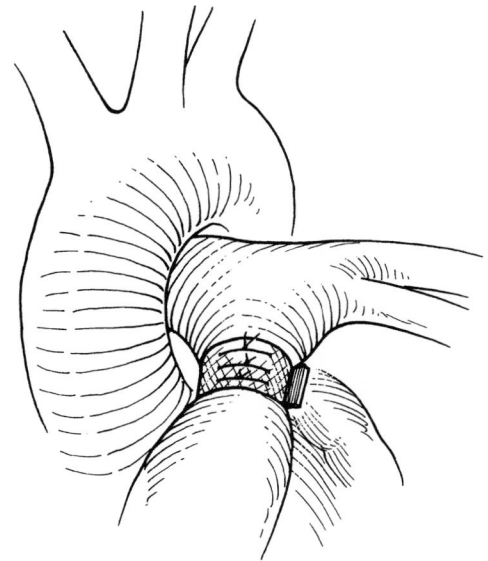

FIG. 34–5. Illustration of pulmonary artery band placement. (From Wernovsky G, Bove EL. Single ventricle lesions. In: Chang AC, Hanley FL, Wernovsky G, Wessel DL, eds. *Pediatric cardiac intensive care.* Baltimore: Williams & Wilkins, 1998:275.)

artery, and aorta to provide unobstructed systemic blood flow, and a BT shunt is placed to provide for PBF. Distal arch augmentation is necessary if distal arch hypoplasia is present, and an atrial septectomy is usually performed as well. The neoaortic (native pulmonary) valve frequently has trivial to mild insufficiency following the pulmonary artery to aortic anastomosis, but this is rarely hemodynamically significant (153,155).

Stage I Norwood

The stage I palliation, first successfully described by Norwood et al. (156) for hypoplastic left heart syndrome, is used for children with functional single ventricle and aortic atresia or severe aortic hypoplasia with subaortic obstruction (157–159). The procedure involves amalgamation of the pulmonary artery and aorta to provide unobstructed systemic blood flow, augmentation of the aortic arch, an atrial septectomy, and placement of a modified BT shunt to provide PBF. A homograft patch usually is used to augment the transverse and distal arch, and the distal main pulmonary artery is typically closed with homograft patch. Figure 34–6 shows stage I palliation.

Immediate Postoperative Management of Palliative Procedures

The physiology of the parallel circulation was described previously. Although postoperative management is similar, management strategies also must take into account the effects on myocardial function and the PVR from the procedure itself. Following the Damus–Kaye–Stansel and Norwood procedures, PVR may be transiently elevated or labile. In addition, the effects of myocardial ischemia from aortic cross-clamping may lead to globally depressed myocardial function in the first 12 to 24 hours after surgery (160).

Postoperative evaluation should assess all aspects of the specific procedure that were utilized. The patient with *low systemic cardiac output*, *excessive cyanosis* (oxygen saturation less than 65%), or relatively *high oxygen satu-*

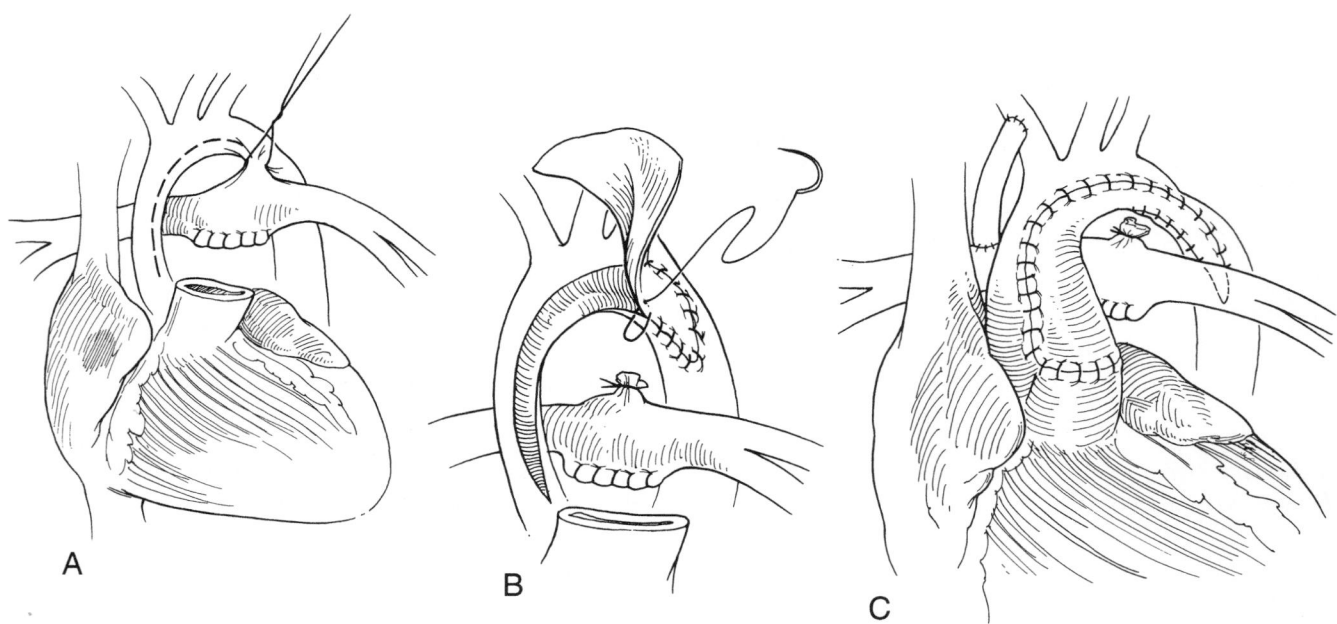

FIG. 34–6. Illustration of stage I reconstruction for hypoplastic left heart syndrome, the purpose of which is to establish unobstructed outflow to the systemic circulation and to balance the systemic and pulmonary circulations. The reconstruction involves the following. **A:** Ligating and dividing the ductus arteriosus and detaching the central and branch pulmonary arteries from the main pulmonary artery. **B:** The hypoplastic aortic arch is opened from the descending aorta retrograde to the level of the aortic valve and augmented with a patch of homograft material. **C:** The augmented arch is connected to the cardiac end of the main pulmonary artery stump. To complete the palliation, an atrial septectomy is performed to ensure unobstructed pulmonary venous outflow, and pulmonary blood flow is supplied by a right-sided modified Blalock-Taussig shunt. (From Wernovsky G, Bove EL. Single ventricle lesions. In: Chang AC, Hanley FL, Wernovsky G, Wessel DL, eds. *Pediatric cardiac intensive care.* Baltimore: Williams & Wilkins, 1998:276.)

rations (greater than 85% to 88%) must have the repair and postoperative physiology carefully evaluated.

Low Cardiac Output

Low cardiac output syndrome may occur in the first 24 to 48 hours after stage I or Damus–Kaye–Stansel palliation. Signs include tachycardia, hypotension, oliguria, and metabolic acidosis. Assessment of the arterial–venous saturation difference (A-VDO$_2$) by intermittent measurement of the mixed venous oxygen saturation (in the superior vena cava) has been shown to be a sensitive predictor of low systemic blood flow and inadequate oxygen delivery (161,162). An A-VDO$_2$ greater than 40% to 50% suggests low cardiac output and inadequate tissue delivery of oxygen. Low systemic cardiac output may be due to (a) decreased total cardiac output as a result of poor ventricular performance, (b) adequate pump performance with maldistribution of flow (increased Qp/Qs), and (c) adequate pump performance with atrioventricular valve regurgitation, which may result in maldistribution of flow from a large regurgitant fraction. A combination of these factors typically is present.

The combination of echocardiography, to evaluate ventricular and atrioventricular valve function, and measurement of the A-VDO$_2$ difference, to estimate systemic blood flow and Qp/Qs ratio, is important in establishing the cause of low cardiac output and rationally directing therapy.

Globally depressed ventricular function generally is treated by increasing inotropic support, whereas low cardiac output with adequate pump function and a high Qp/Qs ratio may improve by increasing PVR and lowering SVR. The infant with atrioventricular valve regurgitation and low cardiac output may benefit from afterload reduction, which will minimize the regurgitant fraction and improve the maldistribution of flow from the single ventricle.

Cyanosis

In the single ventricle patient after palliative procedure, differential diagnosis of cyanosis includes pulmonary venous desaturation, systemic venous desaturation, and decreased PBF. Pulmonary venous desaturation may result from pneumothorax, pleural effusion, pulmonary edema, or pneumonia. Systemic venous desaturation is seen with anemia, high oxygen consumption states, and low systemic output. Decreased PBF may occur when there is elevated PVR, pulmonary venous hypertension, a restrictive ASD, pulmonary artery distortion resulting in pulmonary artery obstruction, and an inadequate systemic-to-pulmonary artery shunt.

Elevated Oxygen Saturations

The child with parallel circulation who has a saturation greater than or equal to 90% has low PVR and PBF far in excess of systemic blood flow. This hemodynamic situation may result in inadequate systemic perfusion, renal hypoperfusion, and an inability to wean the child from mechanical ventilation. In patients with left-sided obstructive lesions who were palliated with either the Norwood or the Damus–Kaye–Stansel procedure, arch obstruction must be ruled out, as distal obstruction may force more blood through the shunt and increase Qp at the expense of Qs.

Separating the Circulation–Cavopulmonary Connections (Bidirectional Glenn, Hemi-Fontan) and the Modified Fontan Operation

General Principles

Although cavopulmonary connections improve cyanosis and minimize ventricular work, elevated PVR in the neonate precludes their use until approximately 4 months of age. Subsequent palliation for neonates with a single ventricle will be discussed only briefly.

The eventual goal of surgical palliation for single ventricle lesions is to separate the systemic and pulmonary circuits, resulting in normal or near-normal oxygen saturation. Cavopulmonary or atriopulmonary connections are utilized to divert systemic venous return directly into the pulmonary vascular bed, which provides for more effective PBF and reduces the volume load on the single ventricle. Following these procedures, the single ventricle only ejects blood to the systemic circuit with PBF derived by passive flow into the pulmonary vascular bed (at the expense of higher central venous pressure). The cavopulmonary connections utilized to stage the single ventricle patient to the modified Fontan include the bidirectional Glenn and the hemi-Fontan.

Staging to Fontan presently is performed because of the high incidence of pleural effusions and low-output myocardial failure that occurred when patients were taken directly from a single ventricle circulation to the Fontan. As described earlier in this section, the risk factors for poor outcome after the modified Fontan operation include ventricular hypertrophy, elevated PVR or pulmonary arterial pressure, pulmonary artery distortion, atrioventricular valve regurgitation, and ventricular dysfunction.

Bidirectional Glenn/Hemi-Fontan. Interim palliation with a bidirectional Glenn shunt has been increasingly utilized in the past decade, typically in infancy (4 to 9 months of age) (163–165). Usually utilizing CPB, the superior vena cava is divided with the cardiac end oversewn. The cephalic end is anastomosed end to side to the ipsilateral pulmonary artery, with pulmonary artery augmentation as indicated.

Alternately, a hemi-Fontan may be performed, in which a temporary dam is placed in the orifice of the superior vena cava separating the superior vena cava from the atrium and an anastomosis is created superior to the dam between the atrial appendage and the ipsilateral pulmonary artery (166).

Fontan Operation. The multiple technical modifications of the Fontan operation (167) in the past 2 decades [including conduits, atriopulmonary connections, intermediate cavopulmonary connections, extracardiac conduits (168,169), and the recent use of adjustable atrial defects (166) or fixed fenestrations in the intraatrial baffle (170)], combined with improved patient selection and postoperative management, have reduced the operative mortality to less than 10% in many centers, with acceptable perioperative and mid-term morbidity (141,142,171, 172). The long-term outcomes, however, continue to be in question (173). Because of the significant improvement in early mortality, attention has now been directed to decreasing the morbidity of the Fontan operation and improving the potential for long-term durability of the Fontan circulation.

Additional Lesions with Duct-Dependent Systemic Blood Flow: "Left-sided" Lesions

Critical Aortic Stenosis

Anatomic abnormalities of the aortic valve may range from a bicuspid aortic valve with little stenosis or regurgitation, to a unicommissural, myxomatous severely obstructive valve with severe left ventricular outflow tract obstruction. In the most severe cases, there is severe dysfunction of the left ventricle, endocardial fibroelastosis, and mitral and/or left ventricular hypoplasia (174).

Critical aortic stenosis may be defined as severe valvar aortic stenosis with duct-dependent systemic blood flow. In critical aortic stenosis, *in utero* obstruction results in progressive left ventricular concentric hypertrophy and eventual myocardial failure, with an elevation in end-diastolic pressure and secondary pulmonary edema. Following birth, the left ventricle may be inadequate to provide the entire systemic cardiac output. End-organ ischemia may result from decreased perfusion and lead to renal failure, NEC, and/or intracerebral hemorrhage. It is difficult to accurately define the severity of obstruction across the aortic valve by Doppler in the presence of right-to-left shunting at the ductus arteriosus and/or depressed left ventricular function.

Depending on the constellation of associated anomalies and the severity of left ventricular dysfunction, treatment for aortic stenosis may include balloon or surgical valvotomy, stage I palliation, Damus–Kaye–Stansel palliation, a neonatal Ross or Ross–Konno procedure, or cardiac transplantation (175–178).

Due to *in utero* obstruction, severe left ventricular dysfunction and/or mitral regurgitation may be present at birth. Inotropic support may be necessary. The neonate with critical aortic stenosis and a virtually intact atrial septum may remain profoundly cyanotic despite PGE_1. In these cases, atrial septostomy may be necessary to decompress the left atrium and allow pulmonary venous egress to the systemic circulation.

Coarctation of the Aorta

Coarctation of the aorta is defined as a constriction of the thoracic aorta distal to the left subclavian artery. Coarctation of the aorta typically results in narrowing of the upper thoracic aorta caused by posterior infolding or indentation opposite the insertion of the ductus arteriosus. In neonates, coarctation of the aorta is commonly associated with hypoplasia of the aortic arch and VSD (179). Rarely it also may be associated with truncus arteriosus, double outlet right ventricle, and single ventricle complexes. Coarctation of the aorta also is associated with Turner syndrome. Coarctation of the aorta also may be part of a developmental complex of left-sided obstructive lesions termed "Shone's complex," which includes parachute mitral valve, supravalvar mitral ring, subaortic stenosis, and coarctation of the aorta (36).

Coarctation of the aorta that presents in neonates and infants results in acute onset obstruction to systemic blood flow, leading to left ventricular pressure overload and failure, LA hypertension, and pulmonary edema. In neonates with coarctation of the aorta, the clinical presentation is determined by the period over which coarctation occurs, the severity of coarctation narrowing, the patency of the ductus arteriosus, and the presence of associated intracardiac lesions (e.g., VSD). A PDA allows for passage of blood from the right ventricle to the aorta, thus preserving systemic flow when coarctation of the aorta is present. If coarctation of the aorta is severe, closing of the ductus arteriosus generally results in cardiovascular collapse and shock. Similarly, the presence of a VSD protects the left ventricle from acute increases of afterload by allowing the left ventricle to eject through the VSD into the pulmonary circulation. The clinical presentation of coarctation of the aorta in the neonate varies from profound shock, metabolic acidosis, and end-organ ischemia to slowly progressive congestive heart failure.

In the critically ill neonate with coarctation of the aorta, organ systems typically involved include the central nervous (intracranial hemorrhage), renal (acute renal failure), and gastrointestinal (NEC) systems. A palpable pulse difference between the upper and lower extremities may not be present when the ductus arteriosus is open, when there is a coexistent VSD, or when the ventricular function is poor. Preoperative management includes infusion of PGE_1 to attempt to reopen the ductus arteriosus and augment systemic flow, as well as correction of metabolic acidosis to improve myocardial performance, and assessment and treatment of end-organ ischemia. Institution of PGE_1 has been shown to improve survival in neonates with coarctation of the aorta (180).

The neonate with coarctation of the aorta that is gradually progressive may be relatively asymptomatic and present with feeding intolerance, mild tachypnea, and a palpable pulse difference between the upper and lower extremities.

FIG. 34–7. The techniques that may be used to repair coarctation of the aorta include end-to-end anastomosis, end-to-side anastomosis, subclavian flap aortoplasty, and patch aortoplasty. Repair of coarctation of the aorta is accomplished through a posterolateral thoracotomy incision. Cardiopulmonary bypass is not necessary in the vast majority of cases. **A:** The end-to-end repair technique is shown. The sites of transection of the aorta are shown by the *broken lines*. The proximal aortic cross-clamp is shown in position on the aortic isthmus. The ductus arteriosus or ligamentum arteriosum is ligated and divided. An end-to-end anastomosis of the descending aorta and aortic isthmus is performed using a running suture technique. **B:** The end-to-side repair technique is shown. The *dotted lines* represent the points of incision. This technique is used when arch hypoplasia is present, typically in the newborn. The ductus arteriosus is divided and ligated, and the hypoplastic aortic isthmus is divided and ligated. The coarctation and all ductal tissue are resected from the descending aorta. The proximal side-biting clamp is placed opposite the origins of the left carotid and innominate arteries and a longitudinal incision is made under the surface of the aortic arch between the left carotid and the innominate arteries. The descending aorta then is mobilized and anastomosed end-to-side to the ascending aorta, leaving the hypoplastic distal arch as an end vessel to the left carotid and left subclavian arteries. **C:** The subclavian flap aortoplasty is shown. The *dotted lines* represent the surgical incisions. The subclavian artery is ligated distally as it exits from the thorax. The proximal stump of the subclavian artery then is opened longitudinally onto the aorta beyond the isthmus and aortic coarctation. The flap created by the opened subclavian artery is turned down onto the aorta to augment the hypoplastic area. The ductus arteriosus is ligated and divided. This is a commonly performed procedure in the neonatal period, especially when proximal arch hypoplasia is not severe. **D:** Patch aortoplasty is shown. The *dotted line* indicates the line of incision. Following aortic incision, a synthetic patch or pericardial patch is used to augment the hypoplastic area and coarctation site. The ductus arteriosus in this illustration is ligated. It should be noted that this procedure can be performed expeditiously with minimal dissection, and the ductus arteriosus can remain patent. These features occasionally make patch aortoplasty the procedure of choice; however, it is currently only rarely used as a primary procedure. (From Chang AC, Starnes VA. Coarctation of the aorta. In: Chang AC, Hanley FL, Wernovsky G, Wessel DL, eds. *Pediatric cardiac intensive care.* Baltimore: Williams & Wilkins, 1998:252.)

Treatment options include percutaneous balloon angioplasty and surgical repair. During balloon dilation, there is physical disruption of the intimal and media layers of the aorta. Due to the nontrivial incidence of aortic aneurysm formation and recoarctation with balloon angioplasty, most large centers generally manage native coarctation of the aorta with surgery (181,182). Surgical options include resection and end-to-end anastomosis, end-to-side anastomosis, subclavian flap angioplasty, and patch aortoplasty (183–185). Figure 34–7 depicts the sur-

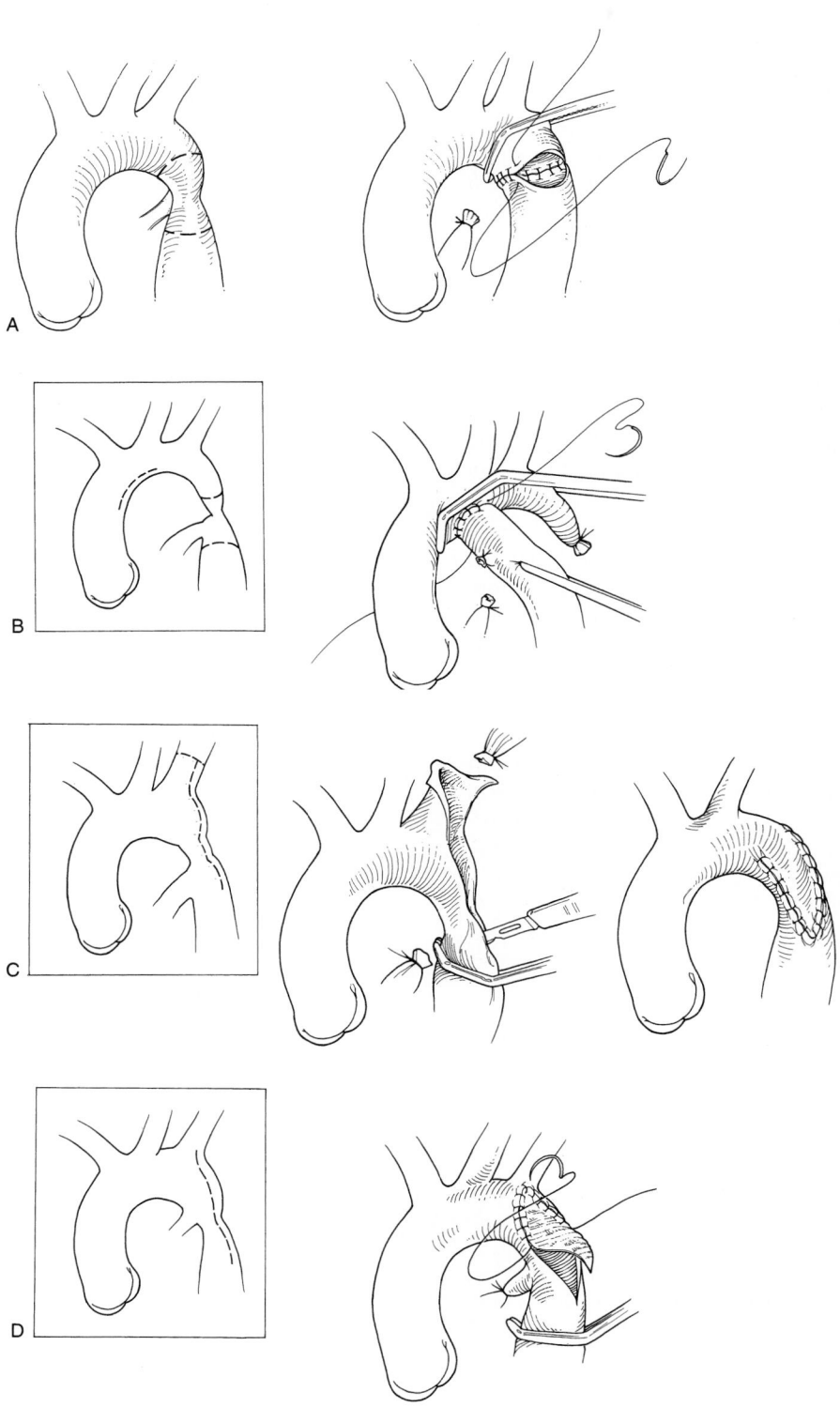

gical options to correct coarctation of the aorta. In general, neonates who present with cardiovascular collapse are repaired after resuscitation and end-organ function has been optimized in the neonatal period. When to repair the asymptomatic neonate or infant with gradually progressive coarctation has been more controversial. At the Children's Hospital of Philadelphia, these neonates usually are repaired after the first month of life to minimize the risk of "recoarctation."

Postoperative evaluation should include assessment for "residual coarctation," low cardiac output, spinal cord ischemia, and injury to structures near the aortic arch.

"Residual coarctation," defined as a systolic gradient greater than 20 mm Hg after surgical repair, is not uncommon in neonates and infants. It may be due to inadequate repair of the coarctation, inadequate repair of a hypoplastic aortic arch, or ductal remodeling. If ventricular dysfunction is present, a residual gradient across the aortic arch may not be apparent, as low cardiac output will minimize any potential gradient across the arch. If "residual coarctation" is noted and the neonate is hemodynamically and clinically stable, balloon dilation 2 months after coarctation repair is recommended. The procedure should be delayed for at least 2 months to allow for proper wound healing of the surgically altered aorta, to minimize the risk of aortic dissection during balloon dilation. If the neonate fails to wean from mechanical ventilation after surgical revision of the coarctation, echocardiography may assist in determining the presence of residual coarctation or persistent left ventricular dysfunction. "Recoarctation" is defined as a systolic gradient across a surgically repaired aortic arch after healing and remodeling of the aorta has occurred, when there was no "residual coarctation" noted after the procedure. In general, the younger the child is at the time of coarctation repair, the higher the risk of "recoarctation" (186). "Recoarctation" may be due to inadequate growth of the repaired aortic arch. "Recoarctation" also may be remedied by balloon angioplasty of the narrowed aorta.

Preoperative low cardiac output may persist in the postoperative period (187). If low cardiac output is present, "residual coarctation" and other undiagnosed cardiac lesions must be ruled out if the child does not improve. Low cardiac output is due to left ventricular dysfunction and may be treated with milrinone, which increases contractility and decreases afterload, or with an ACE inhibitor and digoxin when oral medications can be tolerated. Although most cases of postoperative myocardial dysfunction are reversible, some long-term studies have shown persistent myocardial dysfunction (188).

Spinal cord ischemia is a catastrophic complication that occurs in less than 1% of patients after coarctation repair, but it is rare in neonates and infants. This complication is not clearly correlated with aortic cross-clamp time. It may be secondary to minimal collateral circulation to the anterior spinal artery or to intrinsic anatomic abnormalities of the anterior spinal artery (189).

Complications due to injury to structures near the aortic arch include palsy or paralysis of the phrenic or recurrent laryngeal nerve, which may lead to hemidiaphragmatic paralysis and stridor, respectively (190), and disruption of the thoracic duct, which may result in chylothorax (191).

Interrupted Aortic Arch

IAA may be subdivided into three types. Figure 34–8 depicts the three types of IAA. IAA type A is often associated with TGA. IAA type B, the most common form of IAA, usually occurs with posterior malalignment of the conal septum, which results in a malalignment VSD and subaortic stenosis. IAA type C is extremely rare. IAA may be associated with truncus arteriosus, aorticopulmonary (AP) window, double outlet right ventricle, and single ventricle complexes.

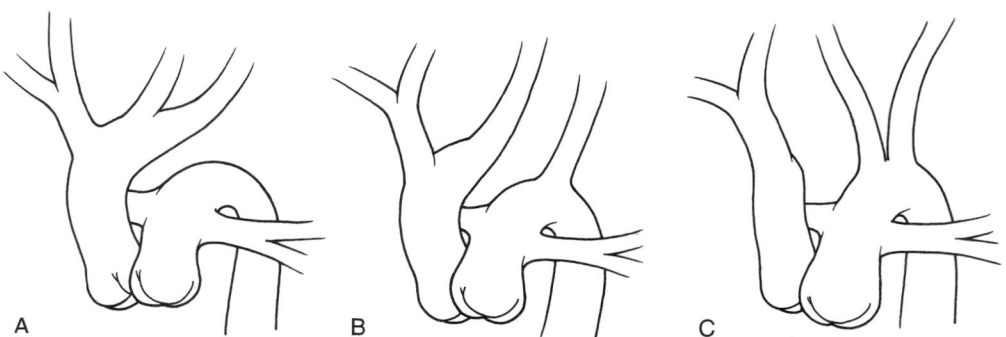

FIG. 34–8. The three types of interrupted aortic arch. **A:** In IAA type A, aortic discontinuity is distal to the left subclavian artery. **B:** In IAA type B, interruption occurs between the left subclavian artery and the left carotid artery. **C:** In IAA type C, the aorta is interrupted between the right innominate artery and the left carotid artery. (From Chang AC, Starnes VA. Interrupted aortic arch. In: Chang AC, Hanley FL, Wernovsky G, Wessel DL, eds. *Pediatric cardiac intensive care.* Baltimore: Williams & Wilkins, 1998:244.)

The clinical presentation and preoperative management is similar to coarctation of the aorta. PGE₁ is used to maintain patency of the ductus arteriosus, which provides systemic blood flow to the lower half of the body when aortic interruption is present.

In most cases, arch reconstruction can be accomplished by end-to-end anastomosis with or without patch augmentation, and VSD closure (192). In cases of severe subaortic obstruction, a Norwood-like reconstruction may be necessary to provide unobstructed systemic blood flow (193).

Postoperative evaluation and assessment of IAA is similar to that of coarctation of the aorta. Monitoring consists of an arterial line for blood pressure monitoring, central venous pressure catheter, and LA line. Specific postoperative problems include pulmonary hypertension, residual arch obstruction, residual VSD, and hyperinflation of the left lung due to compression of the left mainstem bronchus by the reconstructed aortic arch.

Lesions with Duct-Dependent Pulmonary Blood Flow: "Right-sided" Lesions

Critical Pulmonic Stenosis

Critical pulmonic stenosis may be defined as severe valvar pulmonic stenosis with duct-dependent PBF. In critical pulmonic stenosis, *in utero* obstruction results in progressive right ventricular concentric hypertrophy and elevation in right ventricular end-diastolic pressure. Following birth, the right ventricle may be inadequate to provide the entire pulmonary cardiac output. Isolated pulmonic valve stenosis, on the other hand, typically coexists with a normal-sized, hypertrophied right ventricle, a normal tricuspid valve, and normal distal pulmonary arteries. Balloon angioplasty in the cardiac catheterization laboratory is the initial procedure of choice. In some patients with a dysplastic pulmonary valve, surgical valvotomy may be necessary. Following either procedure, a small right-to-left shunt may persist at the atrial level until right ventricular hypertrophy regresses and diastolic compliance improves. Balloon valvuloplasty of the stenotic pulmonary valve is discussed in greater detail in the section on Interventional Catheterization in the Neonate.

Pulmonary Atresia with Intact Ventricular Septum

In PA/IVS, there is plate-like or membranous atresia of the valve with an IVS and variable hypoplasia of the right ventricle and tricuspid valve. The main pulmonary artery generally is present and of normal size, and PBF is supplied by a PDA. The tricuspid valve may be stenotic and/or regurgitant. The only egress of blood from the right ventricle is from tricuspid regurgitation or from coronary cameral (chamber) fistulae from the right ventricle to the coronary. A high incidence of coronary cameral fistulae is seen in children with PA/IVS, especially those that have a small hypertensive right ventricle and a small tricuspid valve annulus (194). These coronary fistulae from the right ventricle to the coronary arteries may provide the majority of coronary blood flow. A right ventricular-dependent coronary circulation (RVDCC) exists when some of the myocardium is perfused only from the high-pressure right ventricle rather than antegrade from the aorta. The presence of an RVDCC has an important impact on possible surgical management strategies (195–197).

Given that the physiology of PA/IVS is one of functional single left ventricle with duct-dependent PBF, preoperative management consists of balancing the pulmonary and systemic circulations. Preoperative cardiac catheterization is typically performed to evaluate for RVDCC. The combination of aortic root and right ventricular angiography generally are sufficient to describe the coronary artery branching pattern and distribution.

If (i) the distribution of the coronary arteries from the aorta are without discrete stenoses, (ii) there are no areas of the myocardium that are solely perfused by the right ventricle, and (iii) there is a nearly normal-sized right ventricle, tricuspid valve, and infundibulum, a staged approach to a "two ventricle" repair may be performed. The initial neonatal palliation consists of right ventricular outflow patch reconstruction to decompress the right ventricle and a modified BT shunt to ensure adequate PBF. Despite adequate relief of the right ventricular outflow tract obstruction (RVOTO), a persistent right-to-left shunt usually persists at the atrial level. This may result from tricuspid stenosis, tricuspid annular hypoplasia, and/or a diminutive and noncompliant right ventricle. If the RVOTO is appropriately relieved and the tricuspid valve and right ventricle are of "adequate" size, right ventricular hypertrophy should regress and right ventricular compliance should improve gradually over 2 to 3 months. As right ventricular compliance increases, the right ventricular contribution to PBF will increase. The BT shunt may eventually be ligated surgically or may be coil embolized in the catheterization laboratory. The final phase to repair is closure of the ASD.

In some patients, despite adequate relief of the RVOTO, the right ventricle and/or tricuspid valve may be hypoplastic, which limits the amount of PBF that can transit the right ventricle. In these patients, a "one-and-a-half" ventricle repair can be performed, with ASD closure combined with a bidirectional Glenn shunt. By this approach, the right ventricle only needs to eject the systemic venous return from the inferior vena cava (198).

Rarely, a neonate will have PA/IVS with a large compliant right ventricle and an adequate tricuspid valve without any significant fistulae, and may achieve a full repair in the neonatal period with reconstruction of the right ventricular outflow tract only.

In cases of RVDCC, decompression of the right ventricle via a valvotomy of transannular patch results in lowering of right ventricular pressure and hypoperfusion to areas of myocardium, which may result in infarction and ventricular dysfunction. As a result, these patients are staged to a single ventricle repair or undergo cardiac transplantation (196,197). Similarly, neonates without an RVDCC but who have a right ventricle or tricuspid valve that will not allow for a two ventricle repair are staged to a single ventricle repair. For these neonates, a palliative BT shunt (and PDA ligation) is performed to ensure PBF, and a cavopulmonary anastomosis and Fontan are created later. Late results for the single ventricle management pathway in patients with PA/IVS with and without RVDCC have been acceptable (199,200).

Tetralogy of Fallot

The anatomy and physiology of TOF and the treatment of hypercyanotic spells was discussed in the section on Lesion-specific Preoperative Stabilization.

Controversy still exists regarding the surgical management of symptomatic and asymptomatic infants with TOF. In asymptomatic children, recommendations for the timing of elective repair have varied from the neonatal period to 1 year of age. For symptomatic patients (neonates who are progressively cyanotic or have had a hypercyanotic spell), a staged repair (placement of a BT shunt followed by complete repair later) or early correction has been advocated. Because of the incidence of pulmonary artery stenosis at the BT shunt insertion site, as well as the fact that the infant with a two-staged repair continues to have an abnormal physiology until complete repair is undertaken, many institutions now favor complete repair at 2 to 6 months in nearly all asymptomatic patients with uncomplicated TOF. The hypercyanotic spell is seen as an indication for surgery at any age.

In general, repair of TOF involves a transventricular incision in the infundibulum that may be extended through the pulmonary annulus if there is hypoplasia of the pulmonary annulus. Through the infundibulotomy, the VSD is closed and a transannular patch is placed if the pulmonary annulus is incised. The transannular patch results in pulmonary regurgitation, which can have significant hemodynamic consequences in neonates and infants with elevated distal pulmonary artery resistance and a hypertrophied and noncompliant right ventricle (201). To minimize right ventricular dysfunction in the neonate or small infant, many centers advocate creating or leaving a small ASD to function as a popoff for high right-sided venous pressures. The ASD allows for improved cardiac output at the expense of mild cyanosis in the early postoperative period (202). Figure 34–9 illustrates the transventricular repair used to correct TOF.

If pulmonary valve annulus hypoplasia is not significant, transatrial or transpulmonary repair of the anterior malalignment VSD and subpulmonic stenosis can be undertaken. In these approaches, a transannular patch may not be necessary.

Right heart dysfunction results from a combination of right ventricular incision and pulmonary regurgitation. Diminished cardiac output also may be due to residual VSD and/or RVOTO. The child with right ventricular dysfunction typically has signs of low systemic output and signs of elevated central venous pressure, such as hepatomegaly and pleural effusions. The time course for recovery is typically 3 to 5 days. Therapy for right ventricular dysfunction includes inotropic support, diuresis, afterload reduction, and ventilatory maneuvers to minimize PVR. Those children with transient, postoperative right-sided heart failure are those who benefit the most from an atrial level communication. Children with right heart failure who do not have an atrial communication may have one created by balloon atrial septostomy in the cardiac catheterization laboratory.

Tetralogy of Fallot with Pulmonary Atresia

TOF/PA also has been referred to as PA with VSD. TOF/PA, a more extreme expression of TOF, is an extremely heterogeneous defect due to the variability of pulmonary artery architecture. When evaluating the pulmonary arteries, three subgroups of TOF/PA emerge:

1. Confluent "true" pulmonary arteries, normal to slightly small in caliber, perfused by the PDA,
2. Small mediastinal pulmonary arteries and multiple aorticopulmonary collateral arteries (MAPCAs) with multiple segments of lung receiving "dual supply," and
3. Absent or extremely diminutive "true" pulmonary arteries, less than 2 mm, with MAPCAs.

In neonates with confluent "true" pulmonary arteries, PGE₁ will ensure PBF until either a palliative aorticopulmonary shunt or complete repair can be performed (203). When complete repair is performed, a valved homograft may be placed in the right ventricular outflow tract, and the VSD is closed through the ventriculotomy that is used to attach the proximal end of the conduit. Left pulmonary artery stenosis at the ductal insertion site is common in this type of TOF/PA. In the complete repair, the conduit can be placed in such a way to "plasty" the left pulmonary artery.

The therapeutic approach to the other two subgroups, in which MAPCAs are a prominent feature, involves establishing forward flow into the "true" pulmonary arteries in the mediastinum, followed by angiography to determine the segments of the lungs that are supplied by the "true" pulmonary arteries, MAPCAs alone, or both. Surgical options to establish flow into the "true" pulmonary arteries include an aorticopulmonary shunt, a direct connection of the back of the aorta to the diminutive central pulmonary arteries, or a right ventricle to pulmonary artery conduit. Segments supplied by MAPCAs may need to be "unifocalized" into the true pulmonary arteries (204,205), whereas segments that have proximal stenoses and are supplied by the "true" pulmonary arteries may require balloon

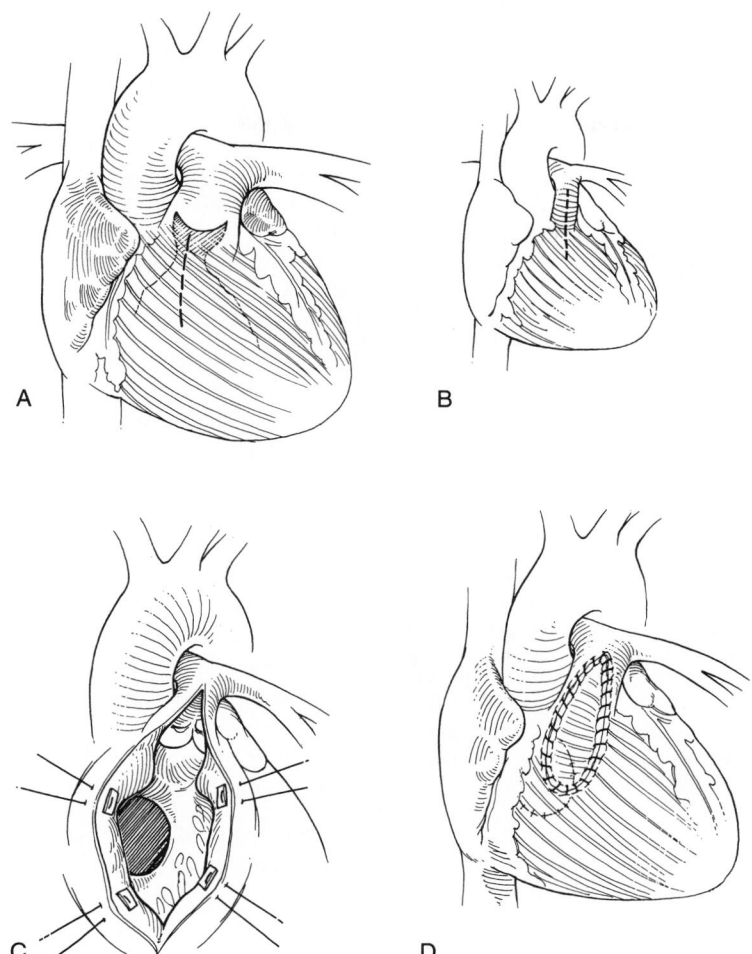

FIG. 34–9. Transventricular repair of tetralogy of Fallot. **A:** The position of the subvalvar infundibular incision is shown by the *dotted lines*. This incision is used when the pulmonary annulus is adequate and a transannular patch is not necessary. **B:** When the pulmonary valve annulus is inadequate, a transannular incision is utilized; its position is shown by the *dotted lines*. **C:** A transannular incision is shown with the edges of the infundibular muscle retracted laterally. The hypoplastic pulmonary valve is revealed along with the malalignment ventricular septal defect. The repair proceeds by resecting the hypertrophied septal and parietal bands of the infundibulum to relieve the infundibular stenosis. The ventricular septal defect is patched, taking care not to injure the overriding aorta beneath the superior aspect of the defect. **D:** A transannular patch is placed to augment the right ventricular outflow tract at the levels of the infundibulum, valve annulus, and main pulmonary artery. When a transannular patch is used, postoperative pulmonary insufficiency is almost a certainty. Some surgeons prefer to add a monocusp to the transannular patch to reduce the amount of pulmonary insufficiency in the postoperative period. (From Spray TL, Wernovsky G. Tetralogy of Fallot. In: Chang AC, Hanley FL, Wernovsky G, Wessel DL, eds. *Pediatric cardiac intensive care.* Baltimore: Williams & Wilkins, 1998:260.)

angioplasty (206). Once the cross-sectional area of the pulmonary vascular bed can tolerate normal cardiac output through the "true" pulmonary arteries without pulmonary hypertension, the VSD may be closed with acceptable postoperative right ventricular pressure (207).

Tetralogy of Fallot with Absent Pulmonary Valve

TOF with absent pulmonary valve (TOF/APV) is a variant of TOF in which there is dysgenesis of the pul-monary valve, annular stenosis, and severe pulmonary insufficiency. Massive enlargement of the branch pulmonary arteries is common due to *in utero* pulsatile pulmonary flow.

Tracheobronchomalacia typically is present due to compression from the massive branch pulmonary arteries. The external cardiac anatomy of TOF/APV is shown in Fig. 34–10.

Patients with TOF/APV may be divided clinically into two groups: neonates with severe cardiorespiratory dis-

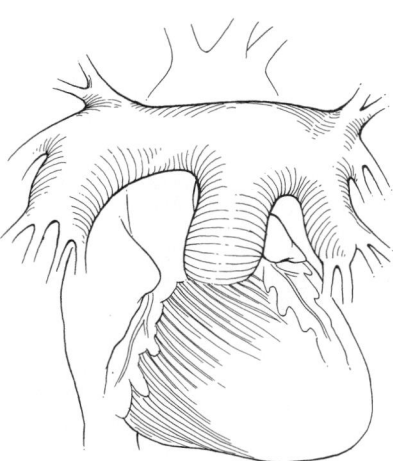

FIG. 34–10. External cardiac anatomy of tetralogy of Fallot with absent pulmonary valve. Note the massively dilated main and central, right, and left pulmonary arteries. The aneurysmal changes in the pulmonary arteries may extend into the secondary pulmonary artery branches or even into the distal pulmonary vascular bed. Tracheobronchial obstruction secondary to the massive pulmonary arteries commonly accompanies this lesion. The intracardiac anatomy is similar to that of simple tetralogy of Fallot. (From Spray TL, Wernovsky G. Tetralogy of Fallot. In: Chang AC, Hanley FL, Wernovsky G, Wessel DL, eds. *Pediatric cardiac intensive care.* Baltimore: Williams & Wilkins, 1998:263.)

tress, and older children who survived the neonatal period and exhibit physiology more typical for TOF. Neonates with TOF/APV typically present soon after birth with severe respiratory distress, cyanosis, and hyperinflation due to tracheobronchial compression. Hypoxemia results from both right-to-left shunting at the VSD and pulmonary venous desaturation from ventilation perfusion mismatch. Tracheal intubation and mechanical ventilation with high positive end-expiratory pressure may help to stent open "floppy" airways and improve gas exchange. Placing the child in the prone position may be helpful in relieving tracheal compression (208). ECMO may be required to establish stable hemodynamics and gas exchange prior to repair. Repair of this defect includes anterior and posterior plication of the pulmonary arteries, VSD closure, and placement of a monocusp or valved homograft in the right ventricular outflow tract to minimize pulmonary insufficiency (209—211). Figure 34–11 depicts pulmonary artery plication for TOF/APV. Despite adequate repair, symptomatic neonates may continue to have airway problems into childhood. The clinical spectrum varies from mild bronchospastic disease to ventilatory compromise that requires tracheostomy and chronic mechanical ventilation.

Tetralogy of Fallot with Complete Atrioventricular Canal

Independent of each other, repair of TOF and complete atrioventricular canal can be performed with low mortal-

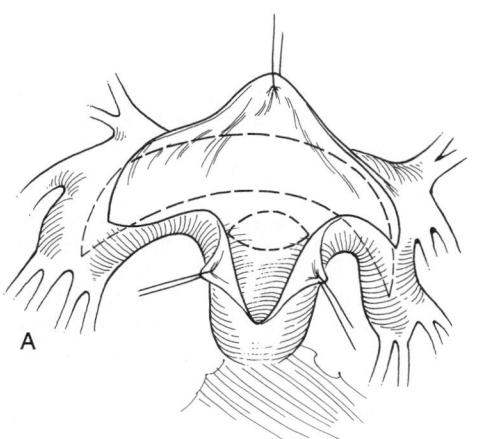
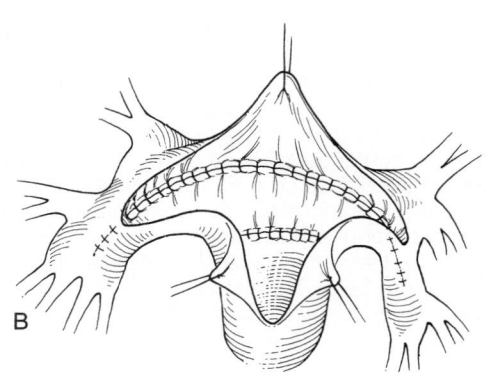

FIG. 34–11. Repair of tetralogy of Fallot with absent pulmonary valve. **A:** The aneurysmal pulmonary arteries are plicated by longitudinal anterior and posterior incisions in the enlarged pulmonary arterial segments. Redundant longitudinal strips of pulmonary artery tissues are removed, and the longitudinal incisions are closed with running suture techniques. **B:** The posterior pulmonary artery plication has been completed. Free pulmonary insufficiency will result if the absent pulmonary valve itself is not addressed. In older infants and children with this syndrome who are stable and asymptomatic at the time of repair, pulmonary insufficiency may be reasonably tolerated. However, in young infants who are unstable with both cardiac and pulmonary involvement, the best results have been achieved by using a monocusp or by placing a valved homograft in the pulmonary position. In all cases, the repair is completed by closing the typical anterior malalignment ventricular septal defect. (From Spray TL, Wernovsky G. Tetralogy of Fallot. In: Chang AC, Hanley FL, Wernovsky G, Wessel DL, eds. *Pediatric cardiac intensive care.* Baltimore: Williams & Wilkins, 1998:264.)

ity, but, in combination, the two lesions pose surgical and postoperative management problems that result in a significantly higher rate of morbidity and mortality (212, 213). Because the tricuspid valve may be regurgitant after complete atrioventricular canal repair, the combination of tricuspid regurgitation and pulmonary regurgitation from a transannular patch may result in severe right ventricular dysfunction and varying degrees of right ventricular failure in the postoperative period. In children with significant annular hypoplasia of the pulmonary valve, placement of a valved conduit should be considered to minimize the degree of pulmonary insufficiency. As in isolated TOF, leaving an atrial communication to augment cardiac output at the expense of cyanosis is particularly helpful in neonates or infants with this combined anomaly, who typically have moderate-to-severe right ventricular dysfunction postoperatively. Residual defects, such as RVOTO, atrioventricular valve regurgitation, and residual VSDs, as well as conduction disturbances, must be assessed for and treated expeditiously in these patients in the postoperative period, as it will take little provocation for the borderline right ventricle to fail.

Ebstein's Anomaly

Ebstein's anomaly results from maldevelopment of the tricuspid valve. The septal and posterior leaflets of the tricuspid valve are displaced downward, whereas the anterior leaflet is not displaced but is redundant or "sail-like." Finally, the chordae tendineae and the papillary muscles of the tricuspid valve also may be abnormal. The "atrialized" right ventricle is the proximal inlet portion of the right ventricle that is above the inferiorly displaced tricuspid valve, and the "functional" right ventricle is the remaining right ventricle that lies below the tricuspid valve. The abnormal tricuspid valve is usually regurgitant but also may be stenotic or even imperforate. Ebstein's anomaly is associated with ASD, pulmonary atresia or stenosis, PDA, and corrected TGA. In addition, there is an increased incidence of Wolff–Parkinson–White syndrome in patients with Ebstein's anomaly.

Severe tricuspid regurgitation results in a dilated right atrium with right-to-left shunting at the atrial level and decreased PBF, as well as poor left ventricular filling due to compression of the left ventricle by the dilated right ventricle. There may be massive cardiomegaly and secondary pulmonary hypoplasia or hydrops fetalis (214).

Ebstein's anomaly has a clinical spectrum that varies from hydrops fetalis to severe cyanosis and circulatory collapse in the neonate, to mild cyanosis in the child, and minimal or no symptoms in the adult (215). Cyanosis is the most common presenting symptom in infancy. Cyanosis without any other symptomatology may be managed conservatively, as the hypoxemia may resolve as PVR falls and antegrade PBF increases. Neonates with severe tricuspid regurgitation may present within the first few hours of life with cyanosis, metabolic acidosis, and circulatory collapse. Due to progressive atrial enlargement or preexisting bypass tracts, supraventricular tachydysrhythmias may be the presenting symptom. The mortality rate is at least 20% when a child with Ebstein's anomaly presents in the neonatal period (216). The child with Ebstein's anomaly who survives the neonatal period has a median age of survival of 13 years (217). Supraventricular tachydysrhythmias are a significant cause of mortality in older patients (217). The older child, adolescent, or adult with Ebstein's anomaly usually suffers from both right-sided heart failure, from tricuspid regurgitation, and left ventricular dysfunction due to right-to-left bowing of the interventricular septum from the dilated right ventricle. Compression of the left ventricular cavity decreases preload into the left ventricle and results in inefficient left ventricular ejection of blood (218).

Preoperative management of the hypoxemic neonate with Ebstein's anomaly may include institution of mechanical ventilation, initiation of PGE_1 infusion, maneuvers to lower PVR, correction of metabolic acidosis, and judicious use of inotropic agents. PGE_1 may be needed to maintain patency of the ductus arteriosus and provide PBF.

The results of surgical intervention in the symptomatic neonate with Ebstein's anomaly have been disappointing. Surgical options include (a) tricuspid valve reconstruction, (b) systemic artery to pulmonary artery shunt, (c) plication of the redundant RA tissue, atrial septectomy, insertion of an aorticopulmonary shunt, and patch closure of the tricuspid valve (219), or (d) orthotopic heart transplantation (220).

In the older child with noncritical Ebstein's anomaly, the surgeon may attempt tricuspid reconstruction or replacement (221,222) or may stage the child to a modified Fontan (223).

Specific postoperative problems include low cardiac output, pulmonary insufficiency, residual tricuspid regurgitation, and postoperative dysrhythmias. Lung hypoplasia is underappreciated in Ebstein's anomaly, and all attempts should be made to ventilate the child at his/her functional residual capacity (224). Overdistention of the airways will only increase PVR and further diminish PBF. Hypoventilation will result in respiratory acidosis superimposed on a possible metabolic acidosis, which will also increase PVR. Postoperative dysrhythmias are common after surgery for Ebstein's anomaly. Reentrant supraventricular tachycardia is not uncommon, especially if Wolff–Parkinson–White syndrome is present. Ventricular tachycardia and ventricular fibrillation have led to mortality in the postoperative period (225). The incidence of complete heart block appears higher with tricuspid valve replacement than with tricuspid valve annuloplasty.

Tricuspid Atresia

Tricuspid atresia may occur with normally or transposed great arteries. In both subtypes single ventricle physiology is present. In tricuspid atresia with transposed great arteries, right ventricular hypoplasia, subaortic obstruction, aortic arch hypoplasia, and coarctation of the aorta frequently exist; systemic blood flow is generally ductal dependent. In tricuspid atresia with normally placed great arteries, there is a right ventricle and pulmonary artery hypoplasia with restrictive communication between the normally developed left ventricle and the vestigial right ventricle. Management of tricuspid atresia involves single ventricle palliation, and eventually the modified Fontan.

Left-to-Right Shunt Lesions

Patent Ductus Arteriosus

The incidence of PDA is higher in preterm neonates. Approximately 20% of neonates weighing less than 1,750 g have a PDA (226). In the preterm infant, treatment for PDA includes medical management of left ventricular failure, indomethacin or ibuprofen therapy (227,228), and/or surgical ligation. If indomethacin or ibuprofen therapy fails to close the PDA, surgical ligation can be performed with minimal morbidity and mortality (229). Despite the risk of recanalization, ligation rather than division of the ductus arteriosus is recommended because the tissues in premature infant are very friable. Surgical closure before 10 days of age reduces the duration of ventilatory support and hospital stay, and lowers morbidity (230). In the premature neonate, surgery sometimes is performed in the neonatal intensive care unit to avoid the risks associated with transport to the operating room.

In the *term infant*, therapy for PDA includes medical management of left ventricular volume load followed by surgical ligation, transcatheter device occlusion, coil embolization, or video-assisted thoracoscopic surgery technique (231,232). Indomethacin is ineffective in term infants and therefore should not be used.

Postoperative management after PDA ligation is usually uneventful, and, in the absence of intraoperative complications, intensive care monitoring is not routine. Mediastinal complications include phrenic or recurrent laryngeal nerve injury (233), as well as pneumothorax, hemothorax, and chylothorax. Smaller neonates are at higher risk of these complications.

Aorticopulmonary Window

AP window results from failure of the aorticopulmonary septum to form. The communication between the aorta and pulmonary artery can be quite variable in size and location. The defect may be proximal, midway between the semilunar valves and the pulmonary bifurcation, or may be distal, resulting in aortic origin of the right pulmonary artery. Rarely, the right coronary artery can arise anomalously from either the AP window or from the pulmonary artery. The defect may be associated with VSD, coarctation of the aorta, or IAA.

Left-to-right shunting leads to increased PBF, and LA and left ventricular volume overload. Neonates with AP window usually present in the first month of life after PVR falls and PBF increases, resulting in congestive heart failure.

Surgical closure of an AP window involves a transaortic approach using a midline sternotomy incision in to the AP window with CPB. This approach provides optimal exposure of the defect and allows for correction of associated defects. Most centers now use the "sandwich" patch closure technique to repair the defect (234). The prognosis for children with AP window is excellent if surgical correction is performed early in life, before irreversible pulmonary vascular changes develop.

Postoperative evaluation involves assessment for residual shunt, postoperative pulmonary hypertension, and myocardial ischemia if anomalous origin of the right coronary artery is an associated defect.

Atrial Septal Defects

ASDs may be subdivided into the following types: secundum ASD, ostium primum ASD, and sinus venosus ASD. Figure 34–12 depicts the three types of ASD. Left-to-right shunting at the atrial level results in RA and right ventricular volume overload, and increased PBF. The degree of left-to-right shunting depends not only on the size of the defect but also on the relative compliance of the ventricles during diastole.

Infants and children are usually asymptomatic despite increased PBF and right ventricular volume overload. Although congestive heart failure may occur in the second or third decade of life because of chronic right ventricular volume overload, up to 5% of children with ASD will have symptoms of congestive heart failure within the first year of life (235). Pulmonary hypertension is rare in childhood, but it can occur in up to 13% of unoperated patients younger than 10 years of age with ASD (236,237).

Spontaneous closure of small secundum-type ASDs is likely to occur in the majority of cases in the first year of life. Ostium primum and sinus venosus ASDs do not close spontaneously and must be addressed surgically. The symptomatic child with an ASD has the defect closed as soon as possible. The timing of ASD repair in the asymptomatic infant or child is more controversial. In general, the defect should be repaired when circulatory arrest is not needed and when the likelihood of needing a blood transfusion is low. After 6 months of age, both of these criteria are generally met.

Postoperative problems after secundum ASD repair are extremely uncommon. Transient atrial arrhythmias or sinus node dysfunction may occur in 5% of children (238, 239).

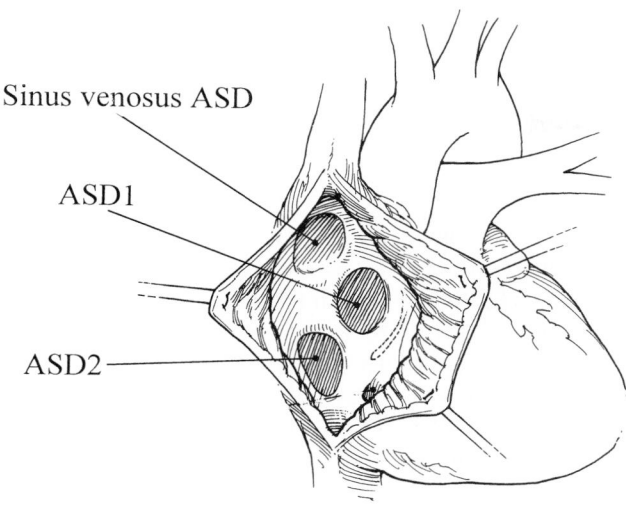

FIG. 34–12. Illustration of the atrial septum showing the three types of atrial septal defects. The ostium primum defect (ASD1) results from an endocardial cushion defect. The ostium secundum atrial septal defect (ASD2) is the most common atrial septal defect and is the only true atrial septal defect. The secundum atrial septal defect is centrally located in the region of the fossa ovalis and results from a deficiency in septum primum. The sinus venosus atrial septal defect is not a true defect in the atrial septum, but rather a defect where the atrial septum merges with the vena cavae. Sinus venosus defects are commonly associated with partial anomalous pulmonary venous return. (From Chang AC, Jacobs J. Atrial septal defect. In: Chang AC, Hanley FL, Wernovsky G, Wessel DL, eds. *Pediatric cardiac intensive care.* Baltimore: Williams & Wilkins, 1998:208.)

Children with primum ASDs typically have a cleft mitral valve, which may or may not require mitral valvuloplasty (240). Postoperative mitral valve function may be assessed by auscultation, inspection of the LA waveform, and echocardiography, if necessary. If significant

mitral valve reconstruction has been performed, systemic hypertension should be avoided, because acute increases in left ventricular pressure, due to increases in systemic vascular resistance, may result in dehiscence of the valvuloplasty sutures.

Sinus venosus ASDs may require more extensive atrial patching, as anomalous pulmonary venous connection frequently is present. If the Warden technique is used, in which the superior vena cava is transected and anastomosed to the RA appendage, postoperative evaluation should include ruling out superior vena cava and right pulmonary vein obstruction. Sinus node dysfunction is not uncommon and temporary atrial pacing may be necessary.

Ventricular Septal Defects

VSDs may be divided into the following types: muscular, conoventricular, malalignment, inlet, and conoseptal hypoplasia. Figure 34–13 illustrates the different types of VSDs, with the exception of the malalignment-type VSD. The conoventricular type, also known as membranous, perimembranous, infracristal, and subaortic, is the most common type of VSD; its defining characteristic is that the defect occurs adjacent to the membranous septum. The muscular type can be located anywhere in the muscular septum; its defining characteristic is that the entire rim of the defect is muscular. The malalignment type is a large defect created by "malalignment" between the infundibular septum and the trabecular muscular septum. The malalignment may result in anterior displacement of the infundibular septum, as in TOF, or in posterior displacement, as in IAA with subaortic stenosis. The inlet type, also known as the atrioventricular canal type, is located posteriorly near the tricuspid valve septal leaflet papillary muscle and borders the tricuspid valve annulus. The conoseptal hypoplasia VSD, also known as supracristal, subpulmonary, infundibular, or outlet, is located above the

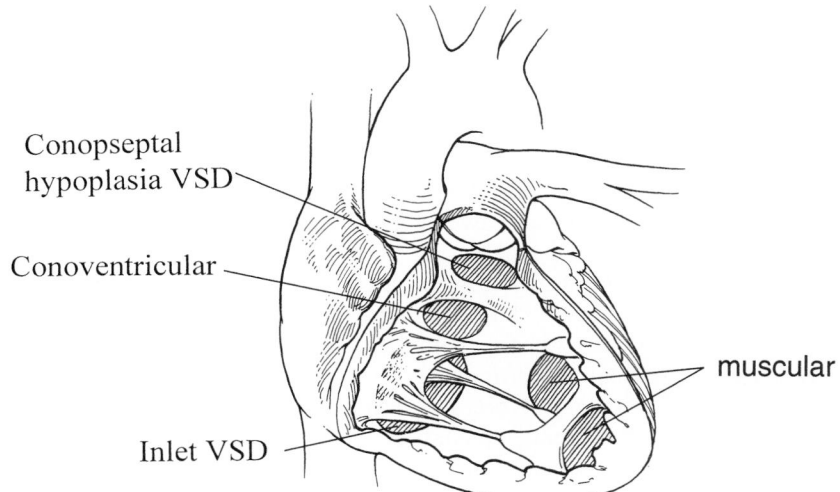

FIG. 34–13. Illustration of the ventricular septum viewed from the right ventricle showing the different types of ventricular septal defects. (From Chang AC, Jacobs J. Ventricular septal defect. In: Chang AC, Hanley FL, Wernovsky G, Wessel DL, eds *Pediatric cardiac intensive care.* Baltimore: Williams & Wilkins, 1998:213.)

crista supraventricularis within the outlet septum near the semilunar valves. The conoseptal hypoplasia defect, found more commonly in the Asian population, is associated with aortic insufficiency due to prolapse of one of the aortic cusps (most commonly right or noncoronary) into the defect. It is thought that the prolapse occurs because the VSD decreases aortic valve annular support.

Left-to-right shunting at the ventricular level results in LA and left ventricular volume overload, and increased PBF. The degree of left-to-right shunting depends not only on the size of the defect but also on the relative resistances in the pulmonary and systemic circulations. If the VSD is restrictive (significantly smaller than the aortic root diameter), the degree of shunting is determined by the size of the defect. If the VSD is unrestrictive (no pressure gradient from left to right ventricle), then the degree of left-to-right shunting is determined by the relative resistances in the pulmonary and systemic vascular beds. As PVR falls in the first weeks of life, left-to-right shunting increases and symptoms develop.

Spontaneous closure can occur in up to 50% of muscular and conoventricular defects (241). Malalignment, inlet, and conoseptal hypoplasia VSDs rarely close spontaneously. If the VSD does not close, the clinical spectrum varies from profound congestive heart failure and failure to thrive, to the asymptomatic child who takes subacute bacterial endocarditis prophylaxis when indicated.

The symptomatic child with congestive heart failure and failure to thrive is repaired at presentation. Malalignment, inlet, and conoseptal hypoplasia VSDs are electively repaired during infancy, because these defects will not close spontaneously. If the child is asymptomatic, well compensated on medical therapy, has no pulmonary hypertension, and has a conoventricular or muscular VSD that may close spontaneously, repair may be delayed. If aortic insufficiency develops in a patient with VSD, surgical closure is recommended to minimize the progression of valve insufficiency.

Conoventricular, muscular, and inlet VSDs are repaired via right atriotomy, whereas the conoseptal hypoplasia VSD is repaired via pulmonary arteriotomy. Malalignment VSD is repaired through either right atriotomy or right ventriculotomy.

Postoperative evaluation involves assessment for residual or previously undiagnosed left-to-right shunts, aortic insufficiency, and examination of the myocardial conduction system. The presence of an undiagnosed or residual shunt may be determined by auscultation, invasive monitoring, echocardiography, and/or catheterization, if indicated. If a significant VSD is present, the patient will be tachycardic, will have elevated pulmonary artery and LA pressures, an oxygen step-up from the superior vena cava or right atrium to the pulmonary artery of greater than 10%, and cardiomegaly and increased pulmonary vascular markings on chest radiograph (242). Aortic regurgitation, more common with conoseptal hypoplasia-type

VSDs, should be ruled out by auscultation, palpation of the peripheral pulses, inspection of the pulse pressure, and echocardiography, if indicated.

Continuous bedside electrocardiographic monitoring and the 12-lead electrocardiogram (ECG) are used to assess for abnormalities in the myocardial conduction system. The approach to close VSDs is most often through the RA appendage or the right ventricle, and the VSD patch is often sewn near the right bundle branch. As a result, right bundle branch block is the most common electrophysiologic complication of VSD closure. Complete heart block may occur in up to 2% to 5% of patients after VSD closure. It is most common after malalignment or conoventricular VSD repair and least common after muscular or conoseptal hypoplasia VSD repair (243). Atrioventricular synchronous temporary pacing is used to treat postoperative heart block. It is prudent to wait 10 to 14 days before implanting a permanent pacemaker, as some cases of postoperative heart block will be transient.

Common Atrioventricular Canal Defect

The endocardial cushions form the atrioventricular valves and the septum of the atrioventricular canal. The normal atrioventricular canal septum fuses with the lower portion of the atrial septum and the upper portion of the ventricular septum, thereby dividing the canal into two atria and two ventricles. When the endocardial cushions fail to join, a common atrioventricular canal results. The three discrete defects found in common atrioventricular canal include an ostium primum ASD, an inlet VSD, and a common malformed atrioventricular valve.

The common atrioventricular canal may be subdivided into three subtypes depending on how caudad or cephalad the atrioventricular valve is placed in the atrioventricular canal. The "incomplete" atrioventricular canal defect results when the atrioventricular valve is placed inferiorly so that the atrioventricular valve leaflets lay on the muscular portion of the ventricular septum. This results in a large primum ASD, a cleft mitral valve, and no VSD. In the "transitional" atrioventricular canal defect, the atrioventricular valve is placed inferiorly in the atrioventricular canal, but not upon the muscular portion of the ventricular septum, resulting in a moderate-sized primum ASD and a small restrictive VSD. The "complete" atrioventricular canal defect, which occurs when the atrioventricular valve is placed in the middle of the atrioventricular canal, results in a moderate-sized primum ASD and a large unrestrictive inlet VSD. A "gooseneck" deformity of the left ventricular outflow tract is commonly present with the complete atrioventricular canal defect. Finally, ventricular hypoplasia may result if the atrioventricular valve is not "centered" over the two ventricles. This is called an unbalanced atrioventricular canal. If significant right or left ventricular hypoplasia is present, a two ventricle repair may not be possible (37).

Signs and symptoms depend on the magnitude of the left-to-right shunt and the amount of atrioventricular valve regurgitation. The symptomatic patient should be repaired in early infancy, whereas the asymptomatic child without pulmonary hypertension (ASD physiology) may undergo elective repair within the first few years of life. Infants with a large VSD component should be repaired by 6 months to decrease the risk of pulmonary arterial hypertension and pulmonary vascular obstructive disease.

Postoperative evaluation involves assessment for (a) residual shunt by auscultation, invasive monitoring, echocardiography, and/or catheterization, if necessary; (b) postoperative pulmonary hypertension by invasive monitoring; (c) evidence of mitral regurgitation by auscultation and invasive monitoring (inspection of the LA waveform and pulmonary arterial pressure); (d) conduction abnormalities by postoperative 12-lead ECG and continuous bedside electrocardiographic monitoring; and (e) subaortic obstruction, by auscultation and echocardiography, if necessary (244,245).

The incidence of postoperative pulmonary hypertension is high and correlated with older age at operation. These episodes correlate closely to postoperative mortality (246). It is important to rule out anatomic causes of elevated pulmonary arterial pressure that mimic pulmonary hypertension, such as severe mitral regurgitation or stenosis and residual VSD with left-to-right shunting. There is also evidence that postoperative PVR is higher in children with Down syndrome than in those without it (247).

If low cardiac output is present, severe mitral regurgitation or large residual VSD must be ruled out. The incidence of reoperation for residual mitral regurgitation is approximately 5% to 10% and is a risk for death during the postoperative period. Because severe mitral regurgitation can lead to annular dilatation and worsening mitral regurgitation, aggressive afterload reduction is mandatory. Aggressive volume resuscitation should be avoided, because it may initiate a vicious cycle of annular dilation, increasing mitral regurgitation, low cardiac output, and hypotension. If the patient is hemodynamically unstable, reoperation should occur without delay.

Etiologies for elevated LA pressure include mitral valve regurgitation, mitral stenosis (especially with single papillary muscle), left ventricular outflow tract obstruction, and left ventricular dysfunction (248,249).

Transient sinus node dysfunction occurs with surprisingly high frequency, especially in children with trisomy 21 (250). Atrial pacing may improve cardiac output if sinoatrial node dysfunction is present. Atrioventricular sequential pacing is necessary if complete heart block is present and is preferable to ventricular pacing alone, as mitral regurgitation may worsen with only ventricular pacing. Junctional ectopic tachycardia is a common transient finding seen in the postoperative period.

Truncus Arteriosus

Truncus arteriosus is defined as a single arterial vessel that originates from the heart, overrides the ventricular septum, and, in order, supplies (i) the coronary circulation, (ii) the pulmonary arterial circulation, and (iii) the systemic circulation. Types I to III are characterized by increasing separation of the right and left pulmonary arteries from the truncus. Type IV is not a true subtype of truncus arteriosus. It is more accurately described as PA with MAPCAs. The VSD is a combination of malalignment and conoseptal hypoplasia types. Although the truncal valve may have three leaflets, the number of leaflets may varies from 2 to 6. The valve is often dysmorphic, and there may be truncal stenosis or regurgitation. Figure 34–14 illustrates the external anatomy of type I truncus arteriosus. In 10% to 15% of cases, the aortic arch is hypoplastic or interrupted. Coronary abnormalities are present in nearly 50% of cases. Clinically important variations include (a) high origin of the left coronary artery, which is vulnerable to surgical injury when the pulmonary arteries are explanted; and (b) anterior descending coronary artery that crosses the right ventricular outflow tract, which is vulnerable to surgical injury during right ventricle to pulmonary artery conduit placement. Truncus arteriosus also may be associated with a right-sided aortic arch, ASD, or arch interruption.

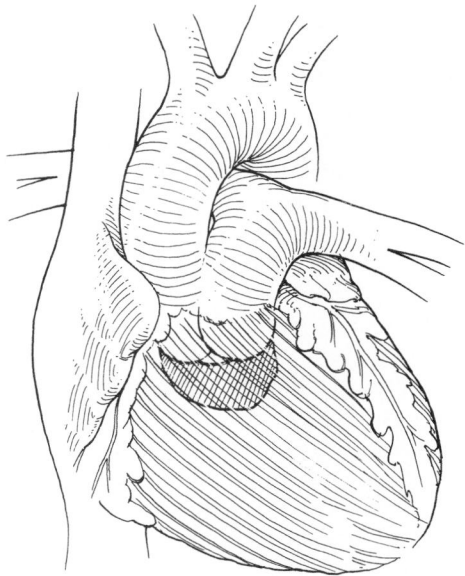

FIG. 34–14. External anatomy of type I truncus arteriosus. The ascending aorta and main pulmonary artery arise from the common trunk. Note the large truncal valve, which overrides the ventricular septum. The ventricular septal defect is a combination of malalignment and conoseptal hypoplasia types; it is generally large and unrestrictive. (From Chang AC, Reddy M. Truncus arteriosus. In: Chang AC, Hanley FL, Wernovsky G, Wessel DL, eds. *Pediatric cardiac intensive care.* Baltimore: Williams & Wilkins, 1998:229.)

The initial physiology is that of a single ventricle with complete mixing at the ventricular and arterial level, with the PBF determined by PVR and the presence of stenosis at the origin of the pulmonary artery trunk (type I) or pulmonary arteries (types II and III). Both right and left ventricles have pressure and volume overload, which can be increased further by the presence of truncal valve stenosis and/or insufficiency. In the absence of pulmonary artery stenosis, the normal fall in PVR results in significant left-to-right shunting, pulmonary overcirculation, and symptoms of congestive heart failure and failure to thrive within the first few weeks of life.

If left untreated, truncus arteriosus has a mortality rate of 90% by 1 year of age. This is due to the rapid development of pulmonary overcirculation, pulmonary hypertension, and pulmonary vascular obstructive disease that has been noted as early as 3 months of life. It has been reported that older age at repair increases the incidence of pulmonary hypertensive crises postoperatively (251). Based on this data, most centers repair infants with truncus arteriosus during the neonatal period (252). Most centers place a valved conduit from the right ventricle to the pulmonary arteries, to minimize pulmonic insufficiency and right ventricular dysfunction. An atrial level communication may be left open to preserve cardiac output if there is right ventricular dysfunction in the postoperative period. Figure 34–15 depicts the repair of truncus arteriosus.

Postoperative care after truncus arteriosus is challenging due to pulmonary hypertension and right ventricular dysfunction. Postoperative evaluation includes assessment for (a) pulmonary hypertension by invasive monitoring; (b) residual left-to-right shunt as described previously; (c) neoaortic (truncal) valve insufficiency by auscultation, palpation of the peripheral pulses, inspection of the pulse pressure, and echocardiography, if indicated; and (d) conduction abnormalities by continuous bedside electrocardiographic monitoring and 12-lead ECG.

Children older than 3 months of age are more likely to have pulmonary hypertension "crises" in the postoperative period than those repaired during the neonatal period (251,253). These paroxysmal episodes may be life threatening. In children at risk of pulmonary hypertension, pulmonary artery catheters are recommended. Hyperventilation is used to minimize PVR in the early postoperative period. If there is evidence of pulmonary hypertension, it is helpful to extend the anesthetic period with continuous neuromuscular blockade and high-dose fentanyl infusion through the first 48 hours after surgery. If pulmonary hypertension is not responsive to conventional measures, nitric oxide administration is recommended. In refractory cases, ECMO may be life saving (254).

Residual VSD following truncus arteriosus repair results in persistent left ventricular volume overload and pulmonary overcirculation. Clinical signs include tachycardia, elevated atrial and pulmonary arterial pressures, oliguria, and metabolic acidosis. Hemodynamic instabil-

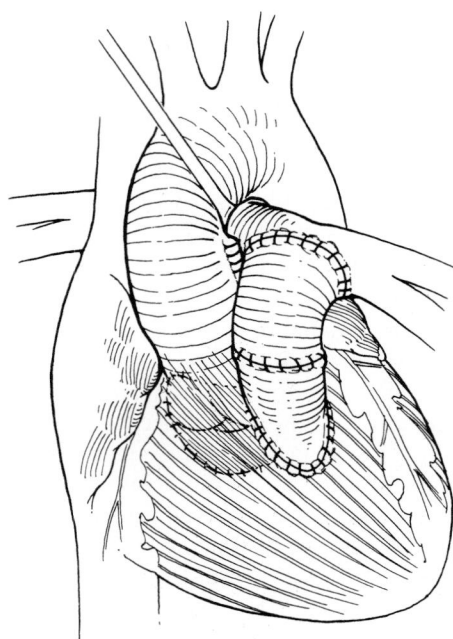

FIG. 34–15. Repair of truncus arteriosus. The procedure utilizes cardiopulmonary bypass with moderate or deep hypothermia and cardioplegic arrest. In the repair, the pulmonary arteries are removed from the trunk and the site on the trunk is oversewn with a running suture. The ventricular septal defect is closed, allowing the left ventricle to eject through the truncal valve to the aorta. A valved conduit is placed from the right ventricle to the distal main pulmonary artery. (From Chang AC, Reddy M. Truncus arteriosus. In: Chang AC, Hanley FL, Wernovsky G, Wessel DL, eds. *Pediatric cardiac intensive care.* Baltimore: Williams & Wilkins, 1998:231.)

ity from a previously unidentified VSD or a residual VSD may require catheterization and reoperation.

The presence of poor peripheral perfusion, low mixed venous saturation, metabolic acidosis, and oliguria suggest low cardiac output. Intravascular volume should be assessed, as a central venous pressure of 12 to 15 mm Hg in the immediate postoperative period is often needed to ensure adequate preload to a noncompliant dysfunctional right ventricle. Echocardiography is used to assess myocardial function and to rule out significant residual VSD, right ventricular outflow obstruction, and truncal valve insufficiency.

Right ventricular dysfunction typically is present in the postoperative period and usually is manifested by elevated RA pressure and right-to-left shunting of blood across the patent foramen ovale. The degree of shunting determines the level of systemic arterial desaturation. Right ventricular dysfunction is treated with minimization of peak ventilatory pressures, inotropic support, and afterload reduction.

Afterload reduction should be used judiciously if truncal valve stenosis is present. Truncal valve regurgitation, which can be exacerbated by slow heart rates, is treated with afterload reduction. In severe cases, truncal valve replacement sometimes is needed.

Because the repair of truncus arteriosus utilizes a right ventriculotomy, complete right bundle branch block is common. Commonly seen malignant dysrhythmias include junctional ectopic tachycardia, atrial tachycardias, and atrioventricular block. Complete heart block occurs in 3% to 5% of patients. After truncus arteriosus repair, isolated ventricular ectopy can be found, especially when hypokalemia, hypocalcemia, and/or hypomagnesemia is present.

Mixing Lesions in the Neonate

Transposition of the Great Arteries

TGA is defined as the aorta arising from the anatomic right ventricle and the pulmonary artery arising from the anatomic left ventricle. The most common form of transposition occurs when the ventricles are normally positioned and the aorta is malposed anteriorly and rightward above the right ventricle, aligned with the right ventricle via the infundibulum (D-transposition, D-TGA). Anomalies associated with TGA include VSD (40%), coronary branching anomalies (33%), coarctation of the aorta/IAA (10%), and left ventricular outflow tract obstruction (5% to 10%). Transposition physiology and preoperative care were described previously.

The distribution of VSD types is as follows: conoventricular (33%), malalignment type (30%), muscular (27%), inlet type (5%), and conoseptal hypoplasia (5%) (255). Of particular surgical importance are the malalignment-type VSDs. Anterior (rightward) malalignment of the infundibular septum is associated with varying degrees of overriding of the pulmonary annulus onto the right ventricle and subaortic stenosis, aortic arch hypoplasia, coarctation of the aorta, or, in some extreme cases, IAA (256,257). Conversely, posterior (leftward) malalignment is associated with varying degrees of subpulmonary stenosis, pulmonary annulus hypoplasia, or, in extreme cases, pulmonary valve atresia (258). Obstruction to PBF is present in 25% of all patients with TGA, in 20% of children with TGA/IVS (only 5% have hemodynamically significant obstruction to PBF), and in 30% of all children with TGA/VSD. Gradients measured preoperatively across the left ventricular outflow tract by echocardiography or during cardiac catheterization may overestimate the degree of anatomic obstruction due to greatly increased PBF in children with TGA, especially with VSD (259).

Children with D-TGA without RVOTO or left ventricular outflow tract obstruction undergo an arterial switch operation. Patients with D-TGA with significant RVOTO may require a Damus–Kaye–Stansel palliative repair, whereas children with D-TGA with left ventricular outflow tract obstruction can have either a Rastelli operation or a REV (reparation a l'etage ventriculaire) repair. In the arterial switch operation, the aorta and pulmonary artery are transected above their respective semilunar valves and switched with careful reimplantation of the coronary arteries. The arterial switch operation is illustrated in Fig. 34–16. In the Rastelli operation, the proximal main pulmonary artery is divided and oversewn, the left ventricular output is directed to the aorta by placement of an intraventricular patch-tunnel technique, and the right ventricle is connected to the main pulmonary artery by a valved extracardiac conduit. The VSD must be of adequate size to permit unobstructed outflow from the left ventricle, and enlargement of the defect by anterior excision of septal muscle may be necessary (260). The new REV procedure by Lecompte (261) involves performing a high, anterior right ventricular incision and a radical excision of the outlet septum, establishing a short and direct intraventricular tunnel from the left ventricle to the aorta, closure of the pulmonary artery orifice, and reimplantation of the transected pulmonary artery directly onto the right ventricular outflow cavity without a prosthetic conduit.

Postoperative evaluation after the arterial switch operation should include assessment of (a) left ventricular function by indexes of systemic cardiac output, LA pressure, and echocardiography, if indicated; (b) postoperative 12-lead ECG and continuous bedside electrocardiography looking for evidence of myocardial ischemia; (c) great vessel anastomoses by auscultation and echocardiography, if indicated; (d) function of the neoaortic valve by auscultation, inspection of the pulse pressure, and echocardiography, if indicated; and (e) residual shunting in those patients with coexisting VSD (262).

Left ventricular dysfunction may be due to myocardial ischemia due to coronary insufficiency or acute dysfunction due to an "unprepared" left ventricle. Arrhythmias, especially upon weaning from CPB, are frequently a marker of coronary insufficiency and should be promptly investigated and treated. Serial 12-lead ECGs are valuable in following ischemic changes.

The left ventricle frequently is poorly compliant following the arterial switch, and acute increases in preload may be followed by significant increases in LA pressure, pulmonary edema, and a fall in cardiac output. Volume infusions should be given slowly, and afterload reduction is helpful in the immediate postoperative period. Acute left ventricular failure due to an "unprepared" left ventricle is uncommon in the first few weeks of life (263), but can occur in older infants (264). Mechanical support may be needed in these patients. Hemodynamically significant great vessel anastomosis obstruction or neoaortic regurgitation are extremely uncommon early postoperative problems (262).

Total Anomalous Pulmonary Venous Connection

Total anomalous pulmonary venous connection (TAPVC) is a congenital defect in which all the pul-

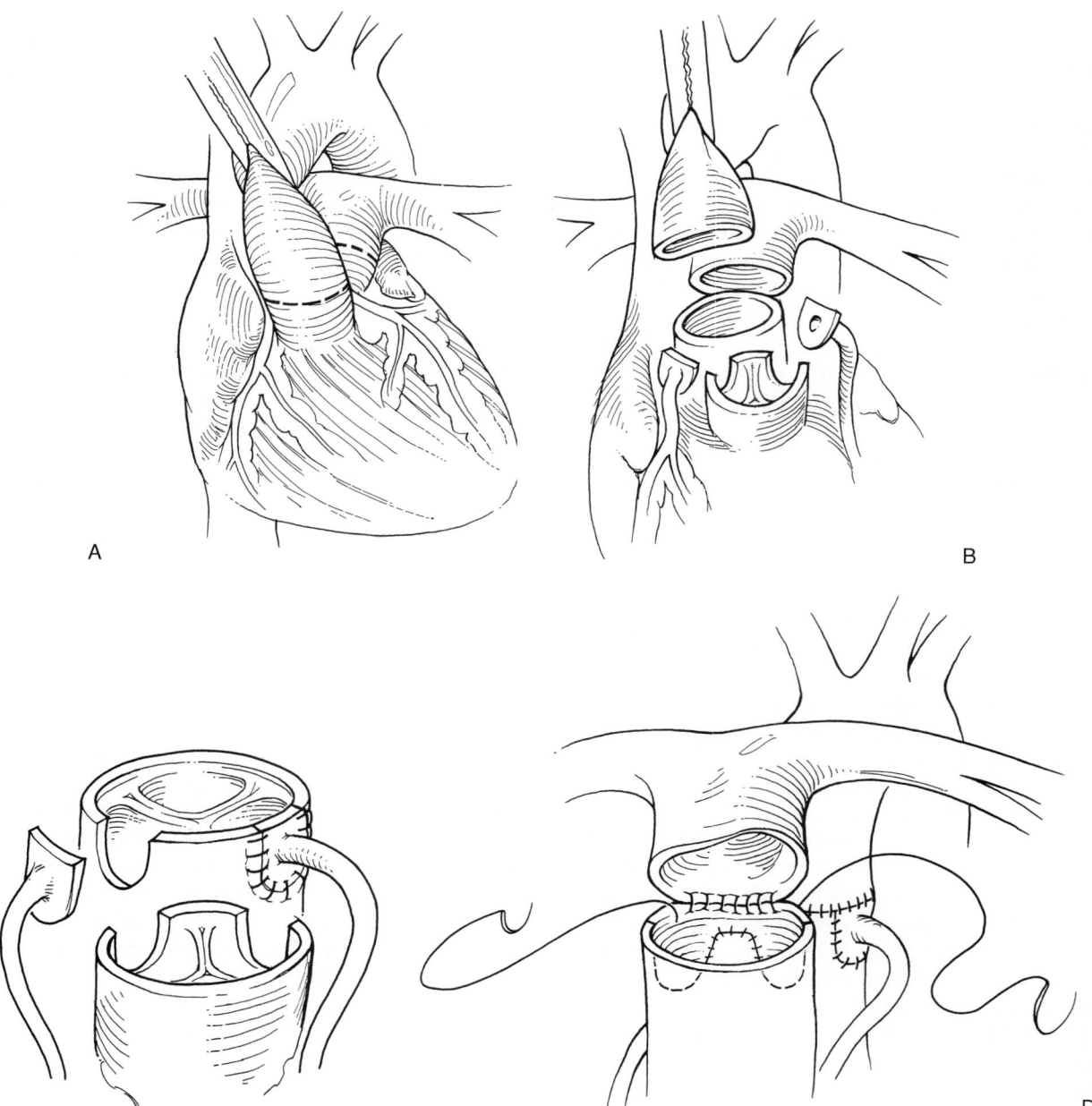

FIG. 34–16. The arterial switch operation for D-transposition of the great arteries. **A:** The external anatomy of transposition of the great arteries is shown, with the anterior and rightward aorta arising from the right ventricle and the posterior and leftward pulmonary artery arising from the left ventricle. The *dotted lines* show the sites of transection for the two great arteries. **B:** The aorta and pulmonary arteries are transected and the coronary ostia are removed from the native aortic root. **C:** The coronary buttons are transferred to the neoaortic root. **D:** The coronary transfer is completed and the neoaortic root is anastomosed to the ascending aorta. The coronary explantation sites on the neopulmonic root are repaired with a patch, and the pulmonary artery is moved anteriorly and anastomosed to the distal main pulmonary artery as described by Lecompte. (From Wernovsky G, Jonas RA. Transposition of the great arteries. In: Chang AC, Hanley FL, Wernovsky G, Wessel DL, eds. *Pediatric cardiac intensive care.* Baltimore: Williams & Wilkins, 1998:295.)

monary veins drain anomalously into a systemic venous structure rather than the left atrium. The pulmonary veins come together at a confluence behind the left atrium and then drain via the anomalous vein to the systemic venous circulation. There are four types: supracardiac, cardiac, infracardiac, and mixed type. In the *supracardiac* type, the pulmonary vein confluence drains via a vertical vein into the innominate vein or the superior vena cava. In the *cardiac* type, the pulmonary venous confluence drains into the coronary sinus or directly into the right atrium. In the *infracardiac* type, the venous confluence drains downward into the portal system of the liver; the blood then traverses the ductus venosus to get to the inferior vena cava. In *mixed drainage* patterns, the four pulmonary veins anomalously drain into more than one venous structure (e.g., the right pulmonary veins drain into the right atrium whereas the left pulmonary veins drain into a vertical vein). Anomalous pulmonary venous connection also is associated with heterotaxy syndrome.

In obstructed TAPVC with obstruction to pulmonary venous egress (typically infracardiac), pulmonary venous hypertension is noted with resultant pulmonary edema, pulmonary hypertension, and hypoxemia. In unobstructed TAPVC, pulmonary venous return is to the systemic venous circulation where blood from systemic and venous circulations mix. RA and right ventricular dilation is present, and systemic cardiac output is maintained by right-to-left shunting at the atrial level.

Obstruction to pulmonary venous return in the supracardiac type may occur if the vertical vein is compressed between the pulmonary artery and the mainstem bronchus. Although the cardiac type is rarely obstructive, obstruction may occur when there is narrowing of the venous confluence as it enters the coronary sinus. The infracardiac type, the most commonly obstructed, may be occluded at the diaphragm, the ductus venosus, or from the resistance in the liver parenchyma.

Neonates with TAPVC with obstruction present shortly after birth with severe respiratory distress, hypoxemia, and elevated pulmonary artery resistance due to severe pulmonary venous obstruction. Repair usually is performed on an emergent basis (265). In unobstructed TAPVC, the child presents later in infancy with congestive heart failure. Pulmonary hypertension can occur late in undiagnosed TAPVC without obstruction.

In supracardiac and infracardiac types of TAPVC, the pulmonary venous confluence is opened, anastomosed to the left atrium, and the anomalous vertical vein is ligated. In the infracardiac type to the coronary sinus, the coronary sinus is unroofed via a right atriotomy and a patch is placed over the foramen ovale and the coronary sinus ostium to allow both pulmonary venous blood flow and coronary sinus blood flow to drain into the left atrium.

Postoperative care after repair of TAPVC is challenging due to preoperative respiratory insufficiency and pulmonary arterial hypertension. Postoperative evaluation includes assessment for (a) respiratory insufficiency, (b) pulmonary hypertension, (c) low cardiac output, and (d) conduction abnormalities by continuous electrocardiography and 12-lead ECG.

In the neonate with obstructed TAPVC, severe respiratory compromise results from fulminant pulmonary edema prior to surgery and therefore is exacerbated by CPB. Therapy includes neuromuscular blockade and sedation to maximize ventilatory efficiency and positive end-expiratory pressure to improve alveolar oxygenation. In the most severe cases, ECMO may be necessary to support oxygen delivery.

As a result of medial hypertrophy of the pulmonary arterioles, pulmonary hypertension can occur in up to 50% of children with TAPVC; neonates are especially susceptible (265). Persistent pulmonary hypertension in the immediate postoperative period is a significant risk factor for death (266). Monitoring with a pulmonary arterial line has been helpful in lowering postoperative mortality (267). Paroxysmal severe pulmonary hypertensive "crises" have been minimized by the use of neuromuscular blockade and high-dose narcotic infusions through the first 24 to 48 hours postoperatively, and early diagnosis and repair prior to the development of significantly suprasystemic PVR (265). If pulmonary arterial pressures are elevated, residual pulmonary venous obstruction must be ruled out, either with echocardiography or cardiac catheterization, prior to maneuvers to treat the pulmonary hypertension. Nitric oxide and ECMO may be necessary to treat difficult to treat pulmonary hypertension (268).

In the preoperative period, dilated right-sided structures decrease the size of the left atrium and left ventricle and have an adverse effect on compliance of the left ventricle. As a result, low cardiac output in the postoperative period may result from a relatively noncompliant left ventricle, which has a depressed stoke volume per beat (269). Postoperative therapy consists of maintenance of optimal heart rate with either atrioventricular sequential pacing or isoproterenol, as cardiac output in this lesion may be more heart rate dependent than in other lesions. Filling pressures in the left ventricle should be maintained at 15 mm Hg, due to the poor compliance of the left ventricle. Underfilling of the left ventricle may be exacerbated by pulmonary hypertension and right heart dilatation. Overaggressive volume replacement should be avoided, because this may lead to rapid LA pressure elevation, which can lead to pulmonary hypertension and decreased PBF.

Common neonatal operations and their early postoperative sequelae are reviewed in Table 34–8.

Cardiac Transplantation in the Neonate

This section will delineate the indications for orthotopic transplantation in the neonate, postoperative management, and outcomes. Discussions on recipient selection, pretransplant management, the technical aspects of

TABLE 34–8. *Common neonatal operations and their early postoperative sequelae*

Lesion	Surgical repair (eponym) Corrective procedures	Early postoperative sequelae Common	Early postoperative sequelae Rare
COA	1. Subclavian flap repair (Waldhausen) or 2. Resection with end-to-end or end-to-side anastomosis or 3. Patch augmentation	1. Systemic hypertension 2. Absent left arm pulse (if subclavian flap repair)	1. Ileus 2. Hemidiaphragm paresis 3. Vocal cord paresis 4. Chylothorax 5. Residual obstruction
TOF	1. Patch closure of VSD via ventriculotomy or right atriotomy 2. Enlargement of RVOT with infundibular patch 3. ± Pulmonary valvotomy 4. ± Transannular RV to PA patch 5. ± RV to PA conduit	1. Pulmonary regurgitation (if transannular patch, valvotomy, or nonvalved conduit) 2. Transient RV dysfunction 3. Right-to-left shunt via PFO, which usually resolves 2 to 4 days postoperatively as RV function improves	1. Residual left-to-right shunt at VSD patch 2. Residual RVOT obstruction 3. Junctional ectopic tachycardia 4. Complete heart block
PDA	1. Ligation (± division) of patent ductus using open thoracotomy and direct visualization or video-assisted thoracoscopic visualization		1. Hemidiaphragm paresis 2. Vocal cord paresis 3. Chylothorax 4. Interruption of LPA or descending aorta
VSD	1. Repair via transatrial/transventricular or pulmonary arteriotomy approach	1. Small residual VSD 2. Right bundle branch block	1. Complete heart block 2. Junctional ectopic tachycardia 3. Large residual VSD 4. Pulmonary hypertension
CAVC	1. "Single patch" technique or 2. "Double patch" technique	1. Small residual VSD 2. Mild mitral regurgitation 3. Right bundle branch block 4. Sinoatrial node dysfunction	1. Complete heart block 2. Junctional ectopic tachycardia 3. Large residual VSD 4. Pulmonary hypertension 5. Severe mitral regurgitation 6. Subaortic stenosis
Truncus arteriosus	1. Closure of VSD; baffling LV to truncus (neoaorta) 2. Removal of PAs from truncus 3. Conduit placement from RV to PAs	1. Reactive pulmonary hypertension 2. Transient RV dysfunction with right-to-left shunt via PFO 3. Hypocalcemia (DiGeorge syndrome)	1. Truncal valve stenosis or regurgitation 2. Residual VSD 3. Complete heart block
TGA	Arterial switch operation (Jatene) 1. Division and reanastomosis of artery and aorta to anatomically correct ventricle 2. Translocation of coronary arteries 3. Closure of septal defects if present	1. Transient decrease in cardiac output 6 to 12 h after surgery	1. Coronary ostial stenosis or occlusion pulmonary (sudden death) 2. Hemidiaphragm paresis 3. Chylothorax
TAPVC	1. Reanastomosis of pulmonary venous confluence to posterior aspect of left atrium 2. Division of connecting vein	1. Pulmonary hypertension 2. Transient low cardiac output	1. Residual pulmonary venous obstruction
HLHS[a]	Stage I (Norwood) 1. Connection of MPA to aorta with reconstruction of aortic arch 2. Systemic-to-pulmonary shunt 3. Atrial septectomy	1. Low systemic cardiac output due to excessive pulmonary blood flow 2. Ventricular dysfunction 3. Tricuspid regurgitation	1. Aortic arch obstruction 2. Restrictive atrial septal defect
Complex lesions with decreased PBF[a]	1. Systemic-to-pulmonary shunt (Blalock–Taussig shunt)	1. Excessive pulmonary blood flow and mild congestive heart failure	1. Hemidiaphragm paresis 2. Vocal cord paralysis 3. Chylothorax
Complex lesions with excessive PBF[a]	1. Pulmonary artery band (prosthetic or silastic constriction of MPA)		1. PA distortion 2. Aneurysm of MPA

[a]In patients with a single ventricle, the goal is to separate pulmonary and systemic venous return, creating cavopulmonary anastomoses to route systemic venous return directly to the pulmonary arteries (bidirectional Glenn shunt, hemi-Fontan, modified Fontan operation).

CAVC, common atrioventricular canal; TGA, transposition of the great arteries; LV, left ventricle; PA, pulmonary artery; RV, right ventricle; TOF, tetralogy of Fallot; VSD, ventricular septal defect; RVOT, right ventricular outflow tract; PFO, patent foramen ovale; COA, coarctation of the aorta; PDA, patent ductus arteriosus; LPA, left pulmonary artery; TAPVC, total anomalous pulmonary venous connection; HLHS, hypoplastic left heart syndrome; MPA, main pulmonary artery; PBF, pulmonary blood flow.

Adapted from Wernovsky G, Erickson LC, Wessel DL. Cardiac emergencies. In: May HL, ed. *Emergency medicine.* Boston: Little, Brown and Company, 1992, pp 1922–1923.

the operation, and rejection surveillance and immunoregulation are beyond the scope of this chapter; the reader is referred to reviews on the topics (270,271).

Indications

Cardiac transplantation has emerged as an effective therapy for some infants with complex congenital heart disease and cardiomyopathy (272). The first successful newborn human-to-human heart transplant was accomplished at Loma Linda University Medical Center in 1985 (273). Over the last decade, increasing numbers of neonates and infants are undergoing cardiac transplantation (274,275). Presently, *primary transplantation* is performed most commonly for congenital heart disease that is lethal or is associated with a very poor prognosis and severe dilated cardiomyopathy. The most common congenital lesions treated with primary transplantation are hypoplastic left heart syndrome, unbalanced atrioventricular canal with atrioventricular valve regurgitation, and pulmonic atresia with IVS with RVDCC. The cardiac heart defects and acquired cardiac diseases for which orthotopic heart transplantation in infancy is an option are listed in Table 34–9.

Secondary transplantation generally is used when patients who have undergone reparative or palliative procedures develop ventricular dysfunction or if the child's hemodynamics preclude further procedures (e.g., the hemi-Fontan with high pulmonary arterial pressures that is unlikely to survive a lateral tunnel fenestrated Fontan completion) (276,277). ECMO has been used as a bridge to both primary and secondary orthotopic heart transplantation (278,279).

Absolute or relative contraindications to cardiac transplantation may include:

1. Recent or recurrent malignancy,
2. Serious active or recurrent infection (e.g., human immunodeficiency virus, hepatitis B),
3. Significant systemic disease (e.g., diabetes mellitus, systemic lupus erythematosus),
4. Chromosomal, metabolic, or genetic abnormality with poor long-term prognosis,
5. Other significant organ system disease (liver, kidneys, CNS),
6. Psychosocial instability, and
7. Elevated PVR.

Elevated PVR may lead to failure of the unprepared donor right ventricle, leading to a low output state. Several studies have demonstrated a significantly increased risk of mortality in children that have an indexed PVR greater than 6.0 Woods units (wU) (280). Pulmonary vasoreactivity, rather than the PVR measurement at baseline, has been shown to be more predictive of successful transplantation (281,282). If the indexed PVR is greater than 6.0 wU and unreactive to pulmonary vasodilators, most centers will not consider the patient for heart transplant alone and will list the child instead for heart–lung transplantation.

Postoperative Management

The same principles of postoperative care used with infants undergoing conventional open heart surgery apply to infants following heart transplantation. All patients are monitored aggressively in an intensive care unit. Inotropic agents (e.g., dopamine, isoproterenol, dobutamine, milrinone) are utilized frequently to maintain adequate systemic perfusion. When severe myocardial dysfunction is present, external mechanical cardiac support (right or left ventricular assist device, ECMO) may be necessary. Temporary atrial and ventricular pacing wires are used for management of postoperative arrhythmias.

Recipients of oversized donor hearts present a unique challenge. Maintaining a high heart rate with isoproterenol or atrial pacing is recommended to lower right ventricular end-diastolic volume and minimize heart size. Closure of the sternum may compress the graft and compromise its function; delayed closure of the sternotomy may be accomplished after edema is resolved.

Postoperative systemic hypertension is common after transplantation, due to immunosuppression with methylprednisolone sodium succinate (Solu-Medrol) and cyclosporine. It is aggressively controlled by the administration of sodium nitroprusside. Chronic hypertension, which generally results from FK506 and prednisone, is treated with calcium channel blockers and ACE inhibitors.

Pulmonary hypertension can be a significant postoperative problem complicating heart transplantation. It usually results from preexisting pulmonary vascular disease caused by long-standing congenital heart disease and/or cardiomyopathy, or due to issues related to CPB (discussed earlier). Severe pulmonary hypertensive

---

TABLE 34–9. *Congenital and acquired cardiac diseases for which primary orthotopic heart transplantation in infancy is an option*

Hypoplastic left heart syndrome
Severe variants of Shone's complex
Other single ventricle complexes
Critical aortic stenosis with severe endocardial
  fibroelastosis
Cardiac neoplasms with myocardial dysfunction
Severe intrauterine atrioventricular valve insufficiency with
  ventricular dysfunction
Truncus arteriosus with severe truncal valve dysplasia
Ebstein's anomaly
Cardiomyopathy
Anomalous left coronary artery with irreversible myocardial
  dysfunction

Adapted from ref. 273.

crises can be life threatening. Treatment includes hyper-oxygenation, hyperventilation, sedation, and the administration of pulmonary vasodilators such as sodium nitroprusside and inhaled nitric oxide. In some cases of pulmonary hypertension, inotropic support is needed to improve right ventricular function until the PVR decreases or the donor right ventricle adapts to the elevated afterload.

Due to diastolic dysfunction in the postoperative period, passive filling is impaired. As a result, cardiac output is quite dependent on heart rate and atrioventricular synchrony. Sinus node dysfunction of the implanted donor heart is not uncommon, and it is often necessary to use intravenous isoproterenol and, in some cases, atrial pacing to maintain adequate cardiac output. Return of normal sinus node function can take several days to weeks, and, in the rare case, normal sinus node function does not return and a permanent pacemaker is needed. Both supraventricular and ventricular arrhythmias may occur after heart transplantation, and they should be treated appropriately (283).

The most common neurologic complication following transplantation in infants is focal or generalized seizure activity. High levels of cyclosporine may be neurotoxic and may lower the seizure threshold. Other possible etiologies of postoperative seizures in the transplanted neonate include CPB and the use of DHCA, air or particulate embolization, metabolic derangement, high-output encephalopathy with or without hypertension, poor nutritional state associated with pretransplant chronic cerebral hypoperfusion, and hypoxia. Seizure episodes may be detected within the first 2 to 3 days after transplantation in 10% to 15% of infants (284). Seizure activity usually is transient and easily controlled with phenobarbital.

Due to a combination of cyclosporine therapy and/or ventricular dysfunction, many infants experience a transient period of oliguria after transplantation, which typically is self-limited and easily treated with inotropic agents and adequate preload. Those neonates with compromised renal function preoperatively may develop anuria and generalized edema that, in some cases, may require peritoneal dialysis (285).

Due to immunosuppression, marginal nutritional status, and breach of the normal protective barriers by surgery, transplant patients are especially vulnerable to infections (both nosocomial and opportunistic) in the immediate postoperative period. Infection is one of the most common causes of postoperative mortality following transplant (286). Intravenous antibiotics are started perioperatively until all intravascular catheters are removed. Infants with heterotaxy syndromes are maintained on prophylactic antibiotics indefinitely. Acyclovir is given prophylactically for a period of 3 months after transplantation to minimize the risk of herpes infection. Ganciclovir is started after transplantation to minimize

the risk of cytomegalovirus (CMV) infection, and trimethoprim-sulfamethoxazole (Bactrim) or dapsone is given prophylactically to decrease the possibility of *Pneumocystis carinii* pneumonia in the immunocompromised host.

Histamine-2 antagonists are used in the immediate postoperative period to diminish the risk of steroid-induced gastritis and/or ulceration. Postoperative nutrition must be maximized in the transplant patient for the following reasons: (a) thoracic surgical patients have tremendous caloric needs, which are increased by the malnourished preoperative state in many patients; (b) high-dose corticosteroid therapy increases the catabolic state, impairing wound healing; and (c) poor nutrition further increases the risk of infection. Enteral feedings are preferred over intravenous hyperalimentation to provide caloric intake because they have a lower incidence of systemic complications.

Outcome

Results vary, depending on the experience of the center performing the transplantation and the availability of donor organs. Early results of neonatal cardiac transplantation reported a 60% 1-year survival rate after transplantation (287). The 1-year survival rate for transplantation has improved to 90% with increasing experience and improved surgical technique (288). It is important to note that these survival rates are for those infants who survived to receive an organ. The Loma Linda University experience includes 154 orthotopic cardiac allotransplantation procedures performed on 153 infants. Early postoperative mortality in the neonate may result from primary graft failure, acute rejection, pulmonary hypertension, pneumonia, perforated duodenal ulcer, abdominal aortic thrombosis, and reperfusion pulmonary hemorrhage. All late mortality occurred within the first 14 months and resulted from chronic rejection, acute rejection, sepsis, bacterial endocarditis, and hemorrhagic shock. Late complications requiring surgical intervention include residual or recurrent coarctation, graft failure requiring retransplantation, arrhythmias requiring pacemaker placement, paralysis of the hemidiaphragm requiring plication, and wound infection necessitating sternal debridement. Recoarctation, the most common late complication, was managed successfully with percutaneous balloon angioplasty or surgical repair. Late complications requiring medical therapy include chronic renal insufficiency, hypertension, cerebrovascular accident, and feeding difficulties.

The long-term outlook for pediatric orthotopic transplantation is unclear. The 5-year actuarial survival at Loma Linda University is 75%. Graft growth and function have been essentially normal in survivors (289). Accelerated coronary artery occlusive disease has been documented at autopsy only among infants who died of unremitting rejection. Most of these children died in the first postoperative year. Systemic hypertension requiring medical therapy is uncommon beyond the first year after transplantation. Infants in whom hypertension may be a problem are those with aortic coarctation, markedly oversized grafts, excessively high cyclosporine levels, or severe chronic renal failure.

All the infants in the Loma Linda University cohort tolerated the usual childhood infections while on immunosuppressive therapy. A routine immunization schedule was maintained using toxoids and killed vaccines for diphtheria, pertussis, tetanus, and inactivated polio vaccine. Live vaccines, such as oral polio vaccine, mumps, measles, and rubella, are not utilized. *Haemophilus influenza* B vaccine was administered at 18 months and pneumococcal vaccine at 24 months. Respiratory syncytial virus occurs seasonally and may, on rare occasions, as with all viral infections, precipitate acute rejection. Forty percent of the infant survivors became CMV seropositive, but only 16.5% developed symptomatic CMV infection requiring ganciclovir and/or immunoglobulin therapy. Common CMV infections include hepatitis and retinitis.

Limitations

Heart transplantation in infants is a recent development that, like any other new modality of therapy, needs further investigation to determine its short- and long-term usefulness in the treatment of the neonate with critical congenital heart disease. The concept of managing complex congenital heart disease with this therapy is relatively new and controversial, and it is presently being evaluated by the pediatric cardiology and pediatric cardiothoracic communities.

The single most important issue that confronts the use of pediatric heart transplantation as a treatment method for certain forms of complex congenital heart disease is the limited donor organ supply. In centers where neonates with hypoplastic left heart syndrome are not staged to a modified Fontan but are instead transplanted, it is estimated that up to 40% of neonates with this complex defect do not survive to transplant or become too ill to undergo transplantation while waiting for an organ (290). Alternately, patients who undergo staged palliation at large centers have a 1-year survival equal to that of the transplanted patient (291). When the infants who died while waiting for transplant are factored into the analysis, the 1-year outcome of children being staged is similar to that of those who are placed on a transplant list. In addition, use of limited donor organs for hypoplastic left heart syndrome (or other lesions with another surgical alternative) further limits the availability of donor organs for other critical lesions with no other surgical option.

Other problems, such as the unwanted side effects of chronic immunosuppression and the lack of sensitive surveillance techniques for graft rejection, make posttransplantation follow-up problematic. Given the present allo-cation of neonatal organs, it is unlikely that pediatric heart transplantation will become the panacea that some in the pediatric medical community believe it to be.

INTERVENTIONAL CATHETERIZATION IN THE NEONATE

The indications for neonatal cardiac catheterization are outlined in Table 34–4. This section will focus on patient preparation and transport to the cardiac catheterization laboratory, special considerations when performing catheterization on a neonate, and therapeutic interventional catheterization procedures in the neonate.

Patient Preparation and Transport to the Cardiac Catheterization Laboratory

Cardiac catheterization can be performed with relatively low risk in even the most unstable of neonates. However, this is possible only if the procedure is well planned and expeditiously executed. Timely and effective communication between the catheterization physicians, surgeons, nurses, and anesthesia staff is essential.

All patients should have a baseline ECG and chest radiograph obtained prior to catheterization. Blood should be available for interventional cases. The choice of access sites used at catheterization may be critical. If indwelling catheters are to be exchanged for the procedure, additional intravenous access should be obtained and infusions should be switched before leaving the intensive care unit. Any additional studies that might be necessary during catheterization (e.g., transesophageal echocardiography, bronchoscopy, or special drug studies) should be coordinated ahead of time. Management of the critically ill patient in the catheterization laboratory is little different than in the operating room. An appropriately trained physician not involved in performing the procedure should be responsible for medical management of the patient from the time the patient leaves the intensive care unit until the patient returns and is stabilized. This individual may be a cardiologist, anesthesiologist, neonatologist, or critical care physician depending on the patient needs, institutional expertise, and staffing. To provide safe transport to the catheterization laboratory, monitors should be used and adequate personnel should be present to manage the airway, move associated apparatus, and monitor the patient. In some instances, for example, a child on ECMO, transporting the patient may be the riskiest part of the procedure and requires careful planning.

Cardiac Catheterization in the Neonate

Umbilical arterial and venous sites may be used for catheter access in neonates. Before leaving the intensive care unit, it is helpful to have umbilical lines available for catheter exchange. It is important to note that infusions given in these catheters will be interrupted during the catheterization. Alternative intravenous sources of glucose and fluid must be secured, and adequate access for inotropic support and PGE_1 must be maintained. Most newborns, particularly those receiving PGE_1 infusions, should be intubated and mechanically ventilated for catheterization. Prevention of hypothermia during catheterization may be challenging, particularly in the premature infant. Patients should be maintained on warming blankets with their heads covered and the room temperature appropriately adjusted. Radiant warming also may be required in some instances. Communication between the anesthesiologist/intensivist and the cardiologist performing the procedure must be ongoing, as changes made in ventilatory or hemodynamic support may have a profound impact on the catheterization data, and hemodynamic alterations that result from the procedure (e.g., arrhythmia, blood loss) must be dealt with in an expeditious manner.

When a newborn returns to the intensive care unit after catheterization, it is essential that the intensive care team receive a comprehensive report outlining the hemodynamic findings and any complications that may have occurred. A chest radiograph should be obtained to confirm position of invasive lines and catheters, and an ECG should be obtained after complex interventions. Repeatedly instrumenting the umbilical vessels increases the risk of infection and thrombotic complications. Therefore, patients catheterized through umbilical vessels should be closely monitored for evidence of infection, dampening of wave form, and clinical evidence of clot formation or embolism.

Therapeutic Cardiac Catheterization

Transcatheter interventions are playing an increasingly important role in the perioperative care of patients undergoing surgery for complex congenital heart defects (292, 293). Therapeutic interventions performed in the neonate include balloon atrial septostomy, balloon pulmonary valvuloplasty, balloon aortic valvuloplasty, and balloon angioplasty of coarctation of the aorta.

Septostomy Procedures

The first therapeutic catheter procedure performed for congenital heart disease, balloon atrial septostomy, remains an important modality for newborns with TGA and a restrictive ASD and (less commonly) other complex lesions. Although little has changed in the method since the technique was first described, the septostomy is now often performed under echocardiographic guidance at the bedside (294). The balloon catheter is placed across the foramen ovale, inflated, and rapidly pulled across the atrial septum, thus enlarging the atrial communication. The procedure may be performed in the catheterization laboratory when vascular access is difficult or when additional diagnostic information is needed. Other techniques for transcatheter creation of interatrial communications include blade atrial septostomy and balloon dilation of the atrial septum. These are often used as part of palliative treatment in children with left- or right-sided obstructive lesions and, in some instances, in older children with severe pulmonary hypertension to improve systemic blood flow (295,296).

Valvuloplasty

Balloon valvuloplasty is performed routinely for aortic and pulmonary stenosis in all pediatric age groups. In 1982, valvar pulmonic stenosis became the first lesion treated by balloon valvuloplasty (297), and since then it has been shown that balloon dilation of valvar pulmonic stenosis in infants and children is technically straightforward, low risk, and usually curative (298). Dilation of aortic stenosis, although generally successful, is a riskier procedure, with the potential for significant blood loss, femoral artery injury, and development of aortic insufficiency (299,300). Newborns undergoing valvuloplasty generally require intensive care after their procedure.

Critical Pulmonic Stenosis

In critical pulmonic stenosis, right ventricular outflow obstruction results in decreased PBF. PGE_1 infusion allows left ventricular output to support PBF via the PDA. An umbilical arterial catheter is used for monitoring purposes, whereas diagnostic catheterization and valvuloplasty generally are performed via the femoral vein. Included in the diagnostic evaluation is measurement of right ventricular pressure and angiography to evaluate right ventricular size, tricuspid valve size and function, and pulmonary valve annulus dimension. Rarely, patients with critical pulmonic stenosis may have associated coronary fistulae from the right ventricle.

After diagnostic evaluation, the stenotic valve is crossed and a small guidewire advanced either into a distal branch pulmonary artery or preferably through the ductus arteriosus into the descending aorta. Often the valve is predilated with a small balloon to allow passage of the larger definitive valvuloplasty balloon, which usually has a diameter 120% to 140% the annulus size. The results of dilation are measured by pull-back from the pulmonary artery to the right ventricle. Right ventricular pressure typically remains transiently elevated due to the presence of the PDA and dynamic infundibular stenosis, which occurs commonly after balloon dilation.

After completion of valvuloplasty, PGE_1 infusion is typically discontinued while the patient is observed in the intensive care unit. Right-to-left shunting at the atrial level persists for a variable time period due to the poor compliance of the hypertrophied right ventricle. As the ductus closes, patients often become progressively hypoxemic. Severe hypoxemia (PO_2 less than 25 mm Hg) after pulmonary valvuloplasty is rare and should prompt evaluation for the presence of persistent right ventricular inflow or outflow obstruction (e.g., tricuspid stenosis, inadequate relief of RVOTO, or hypoplasia of the right ventricle). In general, if RVOTO persists after balloon valvuloplasty, successful surgical management will require placement of a right ventricular outflow patch. Where anatomic obstructions are absent, reinstitution of PGE_1 for several days may allow time for sufficient remodeling of the right ventricle to permit adequate antegrade flow. In cases where inadequate right ventricular volume or poor compliance persists, a modified BT shunt may be performed to provide a stable source of pulmonary blood while right ventricular remodeling occurs (301).

Critical Aortic Stenosis

In critical aortic stenosis, left ventricular outflow obstruction prevents adequate cardiac output to the systemic circulation. PGE_1 infusion allows right ventricular output to support systemic blood flow via the PDA. The precatheterization echocardiogram is used to determine whether the left-sided anatomy is suitable for biventricular circulation and to measure the aortic annulus so an appropriately sized balloon may be chosen (302).

Catheterization laboratory management of the newborn with critical aortic stenosis entails meticulous observation, as these infants frequently are hemodynamically unstable. Rapid identification of hypovolemia, acidosis, and/or malignant arrhythmias is critical. A full diagnostic study typically is performed, including left ventriculography to estimate ventricular size, function, and aortic valve annulus size. Newborns with critical aortic stenosis have markedly diminished left ventricular shortening and forward flow; measurement of left ventricular pressure generally reveals a surprisingly low (20 to 50 mm Hg) gradient across the aortic valve. When no systolic gradient is found between the left ventricle and the aorta, it is likely that left ventricular dysfunction is irreversible or left ventricular inflow is severely restricted. Such patients should be considered candidates for Norwood palliation. In this instance, preoperative catheter creation of an ASD may be necessary. An ASD also may need to be created in patients with severe left ventricular dysfunction, little antegrade flow, and a virtually intact atrial septum.

Balloon valvuloplasty may be performed via either an antegrade approach (femoral or umbilical vein) or a retrograde arterial catheter. In general, a balloon catheter that is 75% to 90% of the annulus size is used for dilation to minimize damage to the aortic annulus and postvalvuloplasty aortic regurgitation. Retrograde dilation from the femoral artery is better tolerated by the ill newborn but risks arterial injury, and although the antegrade approach preserves arterial integrity, it generally results in more

hemodynamic instability and risks mitral valve injury. A transcarotid approach has been advocated by some for dilation of newborn aortic stenosis (303). Due to the possibility of carotid artery injury, most interventional cardiologists prefer to use this approach only in very premature infants.

After valve dilation, net ductal flow typically becomes left to right, and it may result in a "steal" from the systemic circulation. This can be confirmed by Doppler evaluation and is reflected by an increase in postductal arterial oxygen saturation. When this change has been documented, PGE_1 infusion should be discontinued, as the ductal shunt will only contribute to congestive heart failure and decrease systemic blood flow. Intravenous inotropic therapy is continued after dilation and weaned off slowly as ventricular function improves. Afterload reduction may be appropriate, particularly in cases where dilation has resulted in significant aortic insufficiency. As intravenous infusions are weaned, therapy with orally administered agents (e.g., digoxin, ACE inhibitor) should be considered.

Pedal perfusion must be assessed frequently in patients after transfemoral arterial catheterization (see section on Iliofemoral Arterial Injury).

Angioplasty

Balloon angioplasty, balloon dilation of a stenotic vascular structure, is utilized in coarctation of the aorta and branch pulmonary artery stenosis. Balloon dilation of branch pulmonary artery stenosis, which is rarely performed in neonates, is not discussed here; the reader is referred to other texts (292,293).

Coarctation of the Aorta

Both native and postoperative obstructions of the aorta have been treated by balloon angioplasty. Balloon dilation is the primary treatment for patients with *postoperative* arch obstructions (e.g., following repair of coarctation of the aorta, IAA, and Norwood palliation for hypoplastic left heart syndrome). The success rate in these groups of patients is approximately 80% (304).

Dilation usually is performed via a retrograde transfemoral arterial approach, although an antegrade transvenous approach may be applied in smaller patients or in those with single ventricle heart disease in whom the systemic venous connections still allow passage of a catheter through the ventricle to the distal arch. Patients undergoing this procedure usually do not routinely require an intensive care unit, unless there is hemodynamic instability, concern of aortic arch aneurysm formation, or peripheral vessel damage after the procedure. The most common reported complication after retrograde aortic arch dilation is femoral artery injury (305).

Dilation for *native* coarctation remains controversial. Although significant initial gradient reduction has been reported in most patients, failure rates vary from 0% to 12%, aneurysms have been reported in 4% to 15% of cases, and restenosis has occurred in 30% to 50% of patients during short-term follow-up (306). In addition, small residual arch gradients are more common after balloon dilation than after surgery.

Iliofemoral Arterial Injury

Arterial injury is more common after left heart dilations performed via the femoral artery, because angioplasty balloons have a relatively large exit profile and therefore require a large arterial sheath. The spectrum of injury varies from intimal injury with secondary arterial spasm and thrombus formation to major arterial disruption. All patients with evidence of decreased limb perfusion must be assessed carefully and continuously to determine the extent of vascular injury. Patients with occlusion of the *femoral artery* typically have a slightly cooler leg, with diminished pedal pulses and delayed capillary refill. Pedal pulses usually are present by Doppler. Limb viability rarely is compromised, because collateral flow via branches of the internal iliac artery is present. Such patients should receive intravenous heparin infusions with appropriate laboratory and clinical monitoring. Systemic thrombolytic therapy may be instituted after 24 hours if pulses and perfusion have not normalized. Although several agents may be used, the largest experience is with urokinase: an initial bolus of 4,400 U/kg is given, followed by 4,400 U/kg/h for 24 hours (307). Such therapy can be used safely even in neonates; however, there is a risk of intracranial hemorrhage, particularly in newborns who have sustained significant injury from shock or are premature (308).

Patients with occlusion of the *common iliac artery* typically will have a cold, pale, pulseless leg. Loss of limb has been reported in this group of children. Surgical management should be considered immediately to permit expeditious diagnostic evaluation and therapy.

REFERENCES

1. Fyler DC, Rothman KJ, Parisi-Buckley L, Cohn HE, Hellebrand WE, Castaneda AR. The determinants of five year survival of infants with critical congenital heart disease. *Cardiovasc Clin* 1981;11:393.
2. Rabinovitch M, Herrera-Deleon V, Castaneda AR, Reid LM. Growth and development of the pulmonary vascular bed in patients with tetralogy of Fallot, with or without pulmonary atresia. *Circulation* 1981;64:1234.
3. Flanagan MF, Fujii AM, Colan SD, Flanagan RG, Lock JE. Myocardial angiogenesis and coronary perfusion in left ventricular pressure-overload hypertrophy in the young lamb. Evidence for inhibition with chronic protamine administration. *Circ Res* 1991;68:1458.
4. Newburger JW, Silbert AR, Buckley LP, Fyler DC. Cognitive function and age at repair of transposition of the great arteries in children. *N Engl J Med* 1984;310:1495.
5. Castaneda AR, Mayer JE Jr, Jonas RA, Lock JE, Wessel DL, Hickey PR. The neonate with critical congenital heart disease: repair—a surgical challenge. *J Thorac Cardiovasc Surg* 1989;98:869.
6. Anand KJS, Sippell WG, Aynsley-Green A. Randomized trials of fentanyl anesthesia in pre-term babies undergoing surgery: effects on the stress response. *Lancet* 1987;1:62.
7. Mills, AN, Haworth SG. Greater permeability of the neonatal lung: postnatal changes in surface charge and biochemistry of porcine pulmonary capillary endothelium. *J Thorac Cardiovasc Surg* 1991;101:909.
8. Feltes TF, Hansen TN. Effects of an aorticopulmonary shunt on lung fluid balance in the young lamb. *Pediatr Res* 1989;26:94.
9. Reller MD, Morton MJ, Giraud GD. Severe right ventricular pressure loading in fetal sheep augments global myocardial blood flow to submaximal levels. *Circulation* 1992;86:581.
10. Romero TE, Friedman WF. Limited left ventricular response to volume overload in the neonatal period: a comparative study with the adult animal. *Pediatr Res* 1979;13:910.
11. Thornburg KL, Morton MJ. Filling and arterial pressure as determinants of RV stroke volume in the sheep fetus. *Am J Physiol* 1983;244:H656.
12. Anand KJS, Phil D, Hansen DD, Hickey PR. Hormonal metabolic stress response in neonates undergoing cardiac surgery. *Anesthesiology* 1990;73:661.
13. Anand KJS, Hickey PR. Halothane-morphine compared with high-dose sufentanil for anesthesia and postoperative analgesia in neonatal cardiac surgery. *N Engl J Med* 1992;326:1.
14. Fisher DJ, Heymann MA, Rudolph AM. Fetal myocardial oxygen and carbohydrate consumption during acutely induced hypoxemia. *Am J Physiol* 1982;242:H657.
15. Lenn NJ. Plasticity and responses of the immature nervous system to injury. *Semin Perinatol* 1987;11:117.
16. Clapp S, Perry BL, Farooki ZQ, et al. Down's syndrome, complete atrioventricular canal, and pulmonary vascular obstructive disease. *J Thorac Cardiovasc Surg* 1990;100:115.
17. Hanley FL, Heinemann MK, Jonas RA, et al. Repair of truncus arteriosus in the neonate. *J Thorac Cardiovasc Surg* 1993;105:1047.
18. Fyler DC. Report of the New England Regional Infant Cardiac Program. *Pediatrics* 1980;65[Suppl]:377.
19. Benacerraf BR, Sanders SP. Fetal echocardiography. *Radiol Clin North Am* 1990;28:131.
20. Flanagan MF, Fyler DC. Cardiac disease. In: Avery GB, Fletcher MA, MacDonald MG, eds. *Neonatology: pathophysiology and management of the newborn*. Philadelphia: JB Lippincott Co., 1994:524.
21. Friedman AH, Copel JA, Kleinman CS. Fetal echocardiography and fetal cardiology: indications, diagnosis, and management. *Semin Perinatol* 1993;17:76.
22. Emmanouilides GC, Allen HA, Riemenschneider TA, Gutgesell HS. *Moss and Adams' heart disease in infants, children, adolescents, including the fetus and the young adult*, 5th ed. Baltimore: Williams & Wilkins, 1995:555.
23. Allan LD, Sharland GK, Milburn A, et al. Prospective diagnosis of 1,006 consecutive cases of congenital heart disease in the fetus. *J Am Coll Cardiol* 1994;23:1452.
24. Barone, MA. *The Harriet Lane handbook*, 14th ed. St. Louis: Mosby-Year Book, 1996:155.
25. Daily WJ, Smith PC. Mechanical ventilation of the newborn infant. *Curr Probl Pediatr* 1971;1:1.
26. Fixler DE, Carrell T, Browne R, Willis K, Miller WW. Oxygen consumption in infants and children during cardiac catheterization under different sedation regimens. *Circulation* 1974;50:788.
27. Heymann MA. Pharmacologic use of prostaglandin E1 in infants with congenital heart disease. *Am Heart J* 1981;101:837.
28. Fyler DC. *Nadas' pediatric cardiology*. Philadelphia: Hanley & Belfus, 1992:37.
29. Emmanouilides GC, Allen HA, Riemenschneider TA, Gutgesell HS. Associated abnormalities in children with congenital heart disease. In: Emmanouilides GC, Allen HA, Riemenschneider TA, Gutgesell HS, eds. *Moss and Adams' heart disease in infants, children, adolescents, including the fetus and the young adult*, 5th ed. Baltimore: Williams & Wilkins, 1995:619.
30. Khoury MJ, Cordero JF, Mulinare J, Opitz JM. Selected midline defect associations: a population study. *Pediatrics* 1989;84:266.
31. Murugasu B, Yip WCL, Tay JSH, Kit-Yee C, Hui-Kim Y, Hock-Boon W. Sonographic screening for renal tract anomalies associated with congenital anomalies of the urinary system. *J Clin Ultrasound* 1990;18:79.
32. Greenwood RD, Rosenthal A, Parisi L, Fyler DC, Nadas AS. Extrac-

ardiac abnormalities in infants with congenital heart disease. *Pediatrics* 1975;55:485.

33. Aziz KU, Paul MH, Idriss FS, Wilson AD, Muster AJ. Clinical manifestations of dynamic left ventricular outflow tract stenosis in infants with d-transposition of the great arteries with intact ventricular septum. *Am J Cardiol* 1979;44:290.

34. Mair DD, Ritter DG. Factors influencing intercirculatory mixing in patients with complete transposition of the great arteries. *Am J Cardiol* 1972;30:653.

35. Mair DD, Ritter DG. Factors influencing systemic arterial oxygen saturation in complete transposition of the great arteries. *Am J Cardiol* 1973;31:742.

36. Shone JD, Sellers RD, Anderson RC, Adams P, Lillehei CW, Edwards JE. The developmental complex of "parachute mitral valve," supravalvar ring of the left atrium, subaortic stenosis, and coarctation of the aorta. *Am J Cardiol* 1963;11:714.

37. Cohen MS, Jacobs ML, WeinbergPM, Rychik J. Morphometric analysis of unbalanced common atrioventricular canal using two-dimensional echocardiography. *J Am Coll Cardiol* 1996;28:1017.

38. Bolling SF, Iannettoni MD, Dick M, Rosenthal A, Bove EL. Shone's anomaly: operative results and late outcome. *Ann Thorac Surg* 1990; 49:887.

39. Delius R, Rademecker M, deLeval M, Ellito M, Stark J. Is a high-risk biventricular repair always preferable to conversion to a single ventricle repair? *J Thorac Cardiovasc Surg* 1996;112:1561.

40. Grady RM, Canter CE, Bridges ND. Transcatheter ASD creation in infants with left heart obstruction. *J Am Coll Cardiol* 1994;27:484A (abst).

41. Perry SB, Lang P, Keane JF, et al. Creation and maintenance of adequate interatrial communication in left atrioventricular valve atresia or stenosis. *Am J Cardiol* 1986;58:622.

42. Riordan CJ, Randsbaek F, Storey JH, et al. Inotropes in the hypoplastic left heart syndrome: effects in an animal model. *Ann Thorac Surg* 1996;62:83.

43. Jobes DR, Nicolson SC, Steven JM, et al. Carbon dioxide prevents pulmonary overcirculation in hypoplastic heart syndrome. *Ann Thorac Surg* 1992;54:150.

44. Reddy VM, Liddicoat JR, Fineman JR, et al. Fetal model of single ventricle physiology: hemodynamic effects of oxygen, nitric oxide, carbon dioxide, and hypoxia in the early postnatal period. *J Thorac Cardiovasc Surg* 1996;112:437.

45. Riordan CJ, Randsbaek F, Storey JH, et al. Effects of oxygen, positive end-expiratory pressure, and carbon dioxide on oxygen delivery in an animal model in the univentricular heart. *J Thorac Cardiovasc Surg* 1996;112:644.

46. Chang AC, Zucker HA, Hickey PR, et al. Pulmonary vascular resistance in infants after cardiac surgery: role of carbon dioxide and hydrogen ion. *Crit Care Med* 1995;23:568.

47. Chang AC, Hanley FL, Lock JE, Castaneda AR, Wessel DL. Management and outcome of low birth weight neonates with congenital heart disease. *J Pediatr* 1994;124:461.

48. Kirklin JK, Westaby S, Blackstone EH, Kirklin JW, Chenoweth DE, Pacifico AD. Complement and damaging effects of cardiopulmonary bypass. *J Thorac Cardiovasc Surg* 1989;98:1100.

49. Ridley PD, Ratcliffe JM, Alberti KGMM, Elliot MJ. The metabolic consequences of a washed cardiopulmonary bypass pump-priming fluid in children undergoing cardiac operations. *J Thorac Cardiovasc Surg* 1990;100:528.

50. Kern FH, Morana NJ, Sears BS, Hickey PR. Coagulation defects in neonates during cardiopulmonary bypass. *Ann Thorac Surg* 1992;54: 541.

51. Elliot MJ. Ultrafiltration and modified ultrafiltration in pediatric open-heart operations. *Ann Thorac Surg* 1993;56:1518.

52. Darling EM, Shearer IR, Nanry K, et al. Modified ultrafiltration in pediatric cardiopulmonary bypass. *J Extracorpor Tech* 1994;26:205.

53. Davies MJ, Khan N, Gaynor JW, Elliot MJ. Modified ultrafiltration improves left ventricular systolic function after cardiopulmonary bypass. *J Thorac Cardiovasc Surg* 1998;115:361.

54. Wang MJ, Chiu IS, Hsu CM, et al. Efficacy of ultrafiltration in removing inflammatory mediators during pediatric cardiac operations. *Ann Thorac Surg* 1996;61:651.

55. Koutlas TC, Gaynor JW, Nicolson SC, Stevens JM, Wernovsky G, Spray TL. Modified ultrafiltration reduces postoperative morbidity after cardiopulmonary connection. *Ann Thorac Surg* 1997;64:37.

56. Moynihan PJ, Wernovsky G, Hickey PA, Castaneda AR. Complication rates of transthoracic intracardiac lines removed by critical care nurses. *Circulation* 1992;86[Suppl 1]:702A(abst).

57. Gold JP, Jonas RA, Lang P, Elixson M, Mayer JE Jr, Castaneda AR. Transthoracic intracardiac monitoring lines in pediatric surgical patients: a ten-year experience. *Ann Thorac Surg* 1986;42:185.

58. Hickey PR, Hansen DD, Anderson C. Cardiovascular monitoring for the pediatric patient: what's appropriate? *Anesthesiol Clin North Am* 1988;6:825.

59. Lang P, Chipman CW, Siden H, Williams RG, Norwood WI, Castaneda AR. Early assessment of hemodynamic status after repair of tetralogy of Fallot: a comparison of 24 hour (ICU) and 1 year postoperative data in 98 patients. *Am J Cardiol* 1982;50:795.

60. Vincent RN, Lang P, Chipman CW, Castaneda AR. Assessment of hemodynamic status in the intensive care unit immediately after closure of ventricular septal defect. *Am J Cardiol* 1985;55:526.

61. Chang AC, Kulik TJ, Hickey PR, Wessel DL. Real-time measurement of oxygen consumption in ventilated neonates and infants: validation using thermodilution. *Crit Care Med* 1993;2:1369.

62. Wessel DL. Perioperative care: management of the infant and neonate with congenital heart disease. In: Castaneda A, Jonas R, Mayer J, Hanley F, eds. *Cardiac surgery in the neonate and infant.* Philadelphia: WB Saunders, 1994:67.

63. Wernovsky G, Wypig D, Jonas RA, et al. Postoperative course and hemodynamics profile after the arterial switch operation in neonates and infants: a comparison of low-flow cardiopulmonary bypass and circulatory arrest. *Circulation* 1995;92:2226.

64. Wessel DL, Triedman JK, Wernovsky G. Pulmonary and systemic hemodynamic effects of amrinone in neonates folowing cardiopulmonary bypass. *Circulation* 1989;80:488.

65. Olson EM, Kem D, Smith TW. Mechanism of the positive inotropic effect of milrinone in cultured embryonic chick ventricular cells. *J Mol Cell Cardiol* 1987;19:95.

66. Meisheri K, Palmer R, van Bresman C. The effects of amrinone on contractility, calcium uptake, and cAMP in smooth muscle. *Eur J Pharmacol* 1980:61:159.

67. Rettig GF, Schieffer HJ. Acute effects of intravenous milrinone in heart failure. *Eur Heart J* 1989;10:39.

68. Borow KM, Come PC, Neuman A. Physiologic assessment of the inotropic, vasodilatory, and afterload reducing effects of milrinone in subjects without cardiac disease. *Am J Cardiol* 1985;55:1204.

69. Lawless S, Burckkart G, Diven W. Amrinone pharmacokinetics in neonates and infants. *J Clin Pharmacol* 1988;28:283.

70. Lang P, Wessel DL, Wernovsky G, Jonas RA, Mayer JE Jr, Castaneda AR. Hemodynamic effects of amrinone in infants after cardiac surgery. In: Crupi G, Parenzan L, Anderson RH, eds. *Perspectives in pediatric cardiology. Volume 2:* pediatric cardiac surgery, part 2. Mount Kisco, NY: Futura Publishing Co., 1989:292.

71. Katz AM, McCall D, Messineo FC, Pappano A, Dobbs W. Comments on "cardiotonic activity of amrinone-win 40680[5-amino-3-4"-bypyridin-6(IH)-one]." *Circ Res* 1980;46:887.

72. Binah O, Banilo P, Rosen MR. Developmental changes in the effects of amrinone on cardiac contraction. *Am J Cardiol* 1982;49:993.

73. Ross-Ascuitto N, Ascuitto R, Chen V, Downing SE. Negative inotropic effects of amrinone in the neonatal piglet heart. *Circ Res* 1987;61:847.

74. Jaccard C, Berner M, Oberhansli I. Dose response curve of amrinone immediately after cardiac surgery in children. *Pediatr Cardiol* 1987;8: 220A.

75. Skippen P, Taylor R, Bohn D. Amrinone in infants and children after cardiac surgery. *Crit Care Med* 1990;18:268S.

76. Chang AC, Atz AM, Wernovsky G, Burke RP, Wessel DL. Milrinone: systemic and pulmonary hemodynamic effects in neonates and infants after cardiac surgery. *Crit Care Med* 1995;23:1907.

77. Sorensen GK, Ramamoorthy C, Lynn AM, French J, Stevenson JG. Hemodynamic effects of amrinone in children after Fontan surgery. *Anesth Analg* 1996;82:241.

78. Ross MP, Allen-Webb EM, Pappas JB, McGough EC. Amrinone associated thrombocytopenia: pharmacokinetic analysis. *Clin Pharmacol Ther* 1993;53:661.

79. Ross-Ascuitto NT, Ascuitto RJ, Ramage D. Positive inotropic, vasodilatory, and chronotropic effects of milrinone on the postischemic neonatal pig heart. *Am J Cardiol* 1989;64:414.

80. Colucci WS, Wright RF, Jaski BE. Milrinone and dobutamine in

severe heart failure: differing hemodynamic effects and individual patient responses. *Circulation* 1986;73:175.

81. Jaski BE, Fifer MA, Wright RF. Positive inotropic and vasodilator actions of milrinone in patients with severe congestive heart failure: dose-response relationships and comparison to nitroprusside. *J Clin Invest* 1985;75:643.

82. Simonton C, Chatterjee K, Cody R. Milrinone in congestive heart failure: acute and chronic hemodynamic and clinical evaluation. *J Am Coll Cardiol* 1985;6:453.

83. Sinaiko AR. Treatment of hypertension in children. *Pediatr Nephrol* 1994;8:603.

84. Lopez-Herce J, Albajara L, Cagigas P, Garcia S, Ruza F. Treatment of hypertensive crisis in children with nifedipine. *Intens Care Med* 1988; 14:519.

85. Johnson CE, Beekman RH, Kostyshak DA, Nguyen T, Oh DM, Amidon GL. Pharmacokinetics and pharmacodynamics of nifedipine in children with bronchopulmonary dysplasia and pulmonary hypertension. *Pediatr Res* 1991;29:500.

86. Benzig GR, Helmsworth JA, Screiber JT, Kaplan S. Nitroprusside and epinephrine for treatment of low cardiac output in children after open heart surgery. *Ann Thorac Surg* 1979;27:523.

87. Balaraman V, Kullama LK, Robillard JE, Hashiro GM, Nakamura KT. Developmental changes in sodium nitroprusside and atrial natriuretic factor mediated relaxation in the guinea pig aorta. *Pediatr Res* 1990; 27:392.

88. Houde C, Bohn DJ, Freedom RM, Rabinovitch M. Profile of pediatric patients with pulmonary hypertension judged by responsiveness to vasodilators. *Br Heart J* 1993;70:461.

89. Will RJ, Walker OM, Traugott RC, Treasure RL. Sodium nitroprusside and propranolol therapy for management of post coarctectomy hypertension. *J Thorac Cardiovasc Surg* 1978;75:722.

90. Krogmann ON, Rammos S, Jakob M, Corin WJ, Hess OM, Bourgeois M. Left ventriuclar diastolic dysfunction late after coarctation repair in childhood: influence of left ventricular hypertrophy. *J Am Coll Cardiol* 1993;21:1454.

91. Linakis JG, Lacouture PG, Woolf A. Monitoring cyanide and thiocyanate concentrations during infusion of sodium nitroprusside in children. *Pediatr Cardiol* 1991;12:214.

92. Kunathai S, Sholler GF, Celermajer M, Ohalloran M, Cartmill TB, Nunn GR. Nitroprusside in children after cardiopulmonary bypass: a study of thiocyanate toxicity. *Pediatr Cardiol* 1989;10:121.

93. Humes RA, Porter CJ, Puga FJ, Schaff HV, Danielson GK. Utility of temporary atrial epicardial electrodes in postoperative pediatric cardiac patients. *Mayo Clin Proc* 1989;64:516.

94. Yabek SM, Aki BF, Berman W Jr, Neal JF, Dillon T. Use of atrial epicardial electrodes to diagnose and treat postoperative arrhythmias in children. *Am J Cardiol* 1980;46:285.

95. Park RC, Little WC, O'Rourke RA. Effect of alteration of left ventricular activation sequence on the left ventricular end-systolic pressure-volume relationship in closed-chest dogs. *Circ Res* 1985;57:706.

96. Guyton RA, Andrews MJ, Hickey PR, Michaelis LL, Morrow AG. The contribution of atrial contraction to right heart function before and after right ventriculotomy: experimental and clinical observations. *J Thorac Cardiovasc Surg* 1976;71:1.

97. Leinbach RC, Chamberlain DA, Kastor JA, Harthorne JW, Sanders CA. A comparison of the hemodynamic effects of ventricular and sequential A-V pacing in patients with heart block. *Am Heart J* 1969;78:502.

98. Rediker DE, Eagle KA, Homma S, Gillam LD, Harthorne JW. Clinical and hemodynamic comparison of VVI versus DDD pacing in patients with DDD pacemakers. *Am J Cardiol* 1988;61:323.

99. Mukharji J, Rehr RB, Hastillo A, et al. Comparison of atrial contribution to cardiac hemodynamics in patients with normal and severely compromised cardiac function. *Clin Cardiol* 1990;13:639.

100. Jenkins J, Lynn A, Edmonds J, Barker G. Effects of mechanical ventilation on cardiopulmonary function in children after open-heart surgery. *Crit Care Med* 1985;13:77.

101. Gall SA, Olsen CO, Reves JG, et al. Beneficial effects of endotracheal extubation on ventricular performance. *J Thorac Cardiovasc Surg* 1988;95:819.

102. Shapiro BA, Vender JS, Peruzzi WT. Airway pressure therapy for cardiac surgical patients: state of the art and clinical controversies. *J Cardiothorac Vasc Anesth* 1992;6:735.

103. Howlett G. Lung mechanics in normal infants and infants with congenital heart disease. *Arch Dis Child* 1972;47:707.

104. Molk Q, Ross-Russell R, Mulvey D, et al. Phrenic nerve injury in infants and children undergoing cardiac surgery. *Br Heart J* 1991;65: 287.

105. Segar JL, Merrill DC, Chapleau MW, Robillard JE. Hemodynamic changes during endotracheal suctioning are mediated by increased autonomic activity. *Pediatr Res* 1993;33:649.

106. Anand KJS, Brown MJ, Bloom SR. Studies on the hormonal regulation of fuel metabolism in the human newborn infant undergoing anesthesia and surgery. *Horm Res* 1985;22:115.

107. Anand KJS, Hickey PR. Pain and its effects in the human neonate and fetus. *N Engl J Med* 1987;317:1321.

108. Hickey PR, Hansen DD. Fentanyl and sufentanil-oxygen-pancuronium anesthesia for cardiac surgery in infants. *Anesth Analg* 1984;63: 117.

109. Kleinman PK, Winchester P, Brill PW. Necrotizing enterocolitis after open heart surgery employing hypothermia and cardiopulmonary bypass. *Am J Roentgenol* 1976;127:757.

110. Kliegman RM, Fanaroff AA. Necrotizing enterocolitis. *N Engl J Med* 1984;310:1093.

111. Demmy TL, Park SB, Liebler GA. Recent experience with major sternal wound complications. *Ann Thorac Surg* 1990;49:458.

112. Ottino G, DePaulis R, Pansini S, et al. Major sternal wound infection after open heart surgery: a multivariate analysis of risk factors in 2579 consecutive operative procedures. *Ann Thorac Surg* 1987;44:173.

113. Bor DH, Rose RM, Modlin JE. Mediastinitis after cardiovascular surgery. *Rev Infect Dis* 1983;5:885.

114. Culliford AR, Cunningham JW, Zeaff RN. Sternal and costochondral infections following open heart surgery. *J Thorac Cardiovasc Surg* 1976;72:714.

115. Engelman RM, Williams CD, Gouge TH. Mediastinitis following open heart surgery. *Am J Surg* 1973;107:772.

116. Slogoff ST, Girgis KZ, Keats AS. Etiologic factors in neuro-psychiatric complications associated with cardiopulmonary bypass. *Anesth Analg* 1982;61:903.

117. Bellinger DC, Wernovsky G, Rappaport LA, et al. Cognitive development of children following early repair of transposition of the great arteries using deep hypothermic circulatory arrest. *Pediatrics* 1991; 87:701.

118. Watanabe T, Miura M, Inui K, et al. Blood and brain tissue gaseous strategy for profoundly hypothermic total circulatory arrest. *J Thorac Cardiovasc Surg* 1991;102:497.

119. Willford DC, Moores WY, Ji S, Zhung TC, Palencia A, Daily PO. Importance of acid-base strategy in reducing myocardial and whole body oxygen consumption during perfusion hypothermia. *J Thorac Cardiovasc Surg* 1990;100:699.

120. Jonas RA, Bellinger DC, Rappaport LA, et al. Relation of pH strategy and developmental outcome after hypothermic circulatory arrest. *J Thorac Cardiovasc Surg* 1993;106:362.

121. Settergren G, Ohqvist G, Lundberg S, Henze A, Bjork VO, Persson B. Cerebral blood flow and cerebral metabolism in children following cardiac surgery with deep hypothermia and circulatory arrest: clinical course and follow-up of psychomotor development. *Scand J Thorac Cardiovasc Surg* 1982;16:209.

122. Wells FC, Coghill S, Caplan HL, Lincoln C. Duration of circulatory arrest does influence the psychological development of children after cardiac operation in early life. *J Thorac Cardiovasc Surg* 1983; 86:823.

123. Fisk GC, Wright JS, Hicks RG, et al. The influence of duration of circulatory arrest at 20°C on cerebral changes. *Anaesth Intens Care* 1976;4:126.

124. Blauth CI, Smith PL, Arnold JV, Jagoe JR, Wootton R, Taylor KM. Influence of oxygenator type on the prevalence and extent of microembolic retinal ischemia during cardiopulmonary bypass. *J Thorac Cardiovasc Surg* 1990;99:61.

125. Fish KJ. Microembolization: etiology and prevention. In: Hiberman M, ed. *Brain injury and protection during heart surgery.* Boston: Martinus Nijhoff, 1988:67.

126. Nussmeier MA, McDermott JP. Macroembolization: prevention and outcome modification. In: Hiberman M, ed. *Brain injury and protection during heart surgery.* Boston: Martinus Nijhoff, 1988:85.

127. Padayachee TS, Parsons S, Theobold R, Gosling RG, Deverall PB. The effect of arterial filtration on reduction of gaseous microemboli in the middle cerebral artery during cardiopulmonary bypass. *Ann Thorac Surg* 1988;45:647.

128. Kern FH, Jonas RA, Mayer JE Jr, Hanley FL, Castaneda AR, Hickey PR. Temperature monitoring during CPB in infants: does it predict efficient brain cooling? *Ann Thorac Surg* 1992;54:749.

129. Coselli JS, Crawford ES, Beall AC, Mizrahi EM, Hess KR, Patel VM. Determination of brain temperatures for safe circulatory arrest during cardiovascular operation. *Ann Thorac Surg* 1988;45:638.

130. Busto R, Dietrich WD, Globus MY-T, Valdes I, Scheinberg P, Ginsberg MD. Small differences in intra-ischemic brain temperature critically determine the extent of ischemic neuronal injury. *J Cereb Blood Flow Metab* 1987;7:729.

131. Greeley WJ, Kern FH, Ungerleider RM, et al. The effect of hypothermic cardiopulmonary bypass and total circulatory arrest on cerebral metabolism in neonates, infants, and children. *J Thorac Cardiovasc Surg* 1991;101:783.

132. Greeley WJ, Ungerleider RM, Smith LR, Reves JG. The effects of deep hypothermic cardiopulmonary bypass and total circulatory arrest on cerebral blood flow in infants and children. *J Thorac Cardiovasc Surg* 1989;97:737.

133. Mault JR, Ohtake S, Klingensmith ME, Heinle JS, Greeley WJ, Ungerleider RM. Cerebral metabolism and circulatory arrest: effects of duration and strategies for protection. *Ann Thorac Surg* 1993;55:57.

134. Fisk GC, Wright JS, Hicks RG, et al. The influence of duration of circulatory arrest at 20°C on cerebral changes. *Anaesth Intens Care* 1976;4:126.

135. Treasure T, Naftel DC, Conger KA, Garcia JH, Kirklin JW, Blackstone EH. The effect of hypothermic circulatory arrest time on cerebral function, morphology, and biochemistry. *J Thorac Cardiovasc Surg* 1983;86:761.

136. Newburger JW, Jonas RA, Wernovsky G. A comparison of the perioperative neurologic effects of hypothermic circulatory arrest versus low-flow cardiopulmonary bypass in infant heart surgery. *N Engl J Med* 1993;329:1057.

137. Hicks RG, Poole JL. Electroencephalographic changes with hypothermia and cardiopulmonary bypass in children. *J Thorac Cardiovasc Surg* 1992;81:781.

138. Nussmeier NA, Arlund C, Slogoff ST. Neuropsychiatric complications after cardiopulmonary bypass: cerebral protection by a barbiturate. *Anesthesiology* 1986;64:165.

139. Cohen AJ, Cleveland DC, Dyck J, et al. Results of the Fontan procedure for patients with univentricular heart. *Ann Thorac Surg* 1991;52:1266.

140. Kaulitz R, Ziemer G, Luhmer I, Kallfelz H. Modified Fontan operation in functionally univentricular hearts: preoperative risk factors and intermediate results. *J Thorac Cardiovasc Surg* 1996;112:658.

141. Knott-Craig C, Danielson G, Schaff H, Puga F, Weaver A, Driscoll D. The modified Fontan operation: an analysis of risk factors for early postoperative death or takedown in 702 consecutive patients from one institution. *J Thorac Cardiovasc Surg* 1995;109:1237.

142. Gentles TL, Mayer JE Jr, Gavreau K, et al. Fontan operation in 500 consecutive patients: factors influencing early and late outcome. *J Thorac Cardiovasc Surg* 1997;114:376.

143. Mayer JE Jr, Bridges ND, Lock JE, Hanley FL, Jonas RA, Castaneda AR. Factors associated with marked reduction in mortality for Fontan operations in patients with single ventricle. *J Thorac Cardiovasc Surg* 1992;103:444.

144. Senzaki H, Isoda T, Ishizawa A, Hishi T. Reconsideration of criteria for the Fontan operation. Influence of pulmonary artery size on postoperative hemodynamics of the Fontan operation. *Circulation* 1994;89:1196.

145. Bartmus DA, Driscoll DJ, Offord KP, et al. The modified Fontan operation for children less than 4 years old. *J Am Coll Cardiol* 1990;15:429.

146. Imai Y, Takanashi Y, Hoshino S, Terada M, Aoki M, Ohta J. Modified Fontan procedure in ninety-nine cases of atrioventricular valve regurgitation. *J Thorac Cardiovasc Surg* 1997;113:262.

147. Mayer JE Jr. Risk factors for modified Fontan operations. In: Jacobs ML, Norwood WI, eds. *Pediatric cardiac surgery*. Boston: Butterworth-Heinemann, 1992:70.

148. Jenkins KJ, Hanley FL, Colan SD, Mayer JE Jr, Castaneda AR, Wernovsky G. Function of the anatomic pulmonary valve in the systemic circulation *Circulation* 1991;84[Suppl III]:173.

149. Malcic I, Sauer U, Stern H, et al. The influence of pulmonary artery banding on outcome after the Fontan operation. *J Thorac Cardiovasc Surg* 1992;104:743.

150. Rychik J, Jacobs ML, Norwood WI. Acute changes in left ventricular geometry after volume reduction operation. *Ann Thorac Surg* 1995;60:1267.

151. Lui RC, Williams WG, Trusler GA, et al. Experience with the Damus-Kaye-Stansel procedure for children with Taussig-Bing hearts or univentricular hearts with subaortic stenosis. *Circulation* 1993;88[Part II]:170.

152. Karl TR, Watterson KG, Sano S, Mee RBB. Operations for subaortic stenosis in the univentricular heart. *Ann Thorac Surg* 1991;52:420.

153. Rychik J, Murdison KA, Chin AJ, Norwood WI. Surgical management of severe aortic outflow obstruction in lesions other than the hypoplastic left heart syndrome. Use of a pulmonary artery to aorta anastomosis. *J Am Coll Cardiol* 1991;18:809.

154. Gates R, Laks H, Elami A, et al. Damus-Stansel-Kaye procedure: current indications and results. *Ann Thorac Surg* 1993;56:111.

155. Van Son JAM, Reddy VM, Haas GS, Hanley FL. Modified surgical techniques for relief of aortic obstruction in hearts with rudimentary right ventricle and restrictive bulboventricular foramen. *J Thorac Cardiovasc Surg* 1995;110:909.

156. Norwood WI, Lang P, Hansen DD. Physiologic repair of aortic atresia with hypoplastic left heart syndrome. *N Engl J Med* 1983;308:23.

157. Jacobs M, Rychik J, Murphy J, Nicholson S, Steven J, Norwood W. Results of Norwood's operation of lesions other than hypoplastic heart syndrome. *J Thorac Cardiovasc Surg* 1995;110:1555.

158. Forbess J, Cook N, Roth S, Serraf A, Mayer J, Jonas R. Ten-year institutional experience with palliative surgery for hypoplastic left heart syndrome: risk factors related to stage I mortality. *Circulation* 1995;92:II-262.

159. Bove E, Lloyd T. Staged reconstruction for hypoplastic heart syndrome: contemporary results. *Ann Surg* 1996;224:387.

160. Wernovsky G, Wypij D, Jonas RA, et al. Postoperative course and hemodynamic profile after the arterial switch operation in neonates and infants: a comparison of low-flow cardiopulmonary bypass and circulatory arrest. *Circulation* 1995;92:2226.

161. Riordan CJ, Randsbaek F, Storey JH, Montgomery WD, Santamore WP, Austin EH. Balancing pulmonary and systemic arterial flows in parallel circulations: the value of monitoring systemic venous oxygen saturations. *Cardiol Young* 1997;7:74.

162. Rossi AF, Sommer RJ, Lotvin A, et al. Usefulness of intermittent monitoring of mixed venous oxygen saturation after stage I palliation for hypoplastic left heart syndrome. *Am J Cardiol* 1994;73:1118.

163. Chang AC, Hanley FL, Wernovsky G, et al. Early bidirectional cavopulmonary shunt in young infants: postoperative course and early results. *Circulation* 1993;88:149.

164. Bradley SM, Mosca RS, Hennein HA, Crowley DC, Kulik TJ, Bove EL. Bidirectional superior cavopulmonary connection in young infants. *Circulation* 1996;94:II-5.

165. McElhinney DB, Reddy VM, Moore P, Hanley FL. Bidirectional cavopulmonary shunt in patients with anomalies of systemic and pulmonary drainage. *Ann Thorac Surg* 1997;63:1676.

166. Laks H, Ardehali A, Grant PW, et al. Modifications of the Fontan procedure: superior vena cava to left pulmonary artery connection and inferior vena cava to right pulmonary artery connection with adjustable atrial septal defect. *Circulation* 1995;91:2943.

167. Fontan F, Baudet E. Surgical repair of tricuspid atresia. *Thorax* 1971;26:240.

168. Laschinger JC, Redmond JM, Cameron DE, et al. Intermediate results of the extracardiac Fontan procedure. *Ann Thorac Surg* 1996;62:1261.

169. Marcelletti C, Corno A, Giannico S, et al. Inferior vena cava-pulmonary artery extracardiac conduit: a new form of right heart bypass. *J Thorac Cardiovasc Surg* 1990;100:228.

170. Bridges ND, Lock JE, Castaneda AR. Baffle fenestration with subsequent transcatheter closure: modification of the Fontan operation for patient at increased risk. *Circulation* 1990;82:1681.

171. Jacobs ML, Norwood WI. Fontan operation: influence of modifications on morbidity and mortality. *Ann Thorac Surg* 1994;58:945.

172. Gentles TL, Gauvreau K, Mayer JE Jr, et al. Functional outcome after the Fontan operation: factors influencing late morbidity. *J Thorac Cardiovasc Surg* 1997;114:392.

173. Fontan F, Kirklin JW, Fernandez G, et al. Outcome after a perfect Fontan operation. *Circulation* 1990;81:1520.

174. Sharland GR, Chita SK, Fagg NLK, et al. Left ventricular dysfunction in the fetus: relation to aortic valve anomalies and endocardial fibroelastosis. *Br Heart J* 1991;66:419.

175. Rychik J, Murdison KA, Chin AJ, et al. Surgical management of severe aortic outflow obstruction in lesions other than the hypoplastic left heart syndrome: use of the pulmonary artery to aortic anastomosis. *J Am Coll Cardiol* 1991;18:809.

176. Bissett GS III, Meyer RA, Hirschfeld SS, et al. Aortic valve replacement in childhood: evaluation of left ventricular function by electrocardiography, echocardiography, and graded exercise testing. *Am J Cardiol* 1983;52:568.

177. Gerosa G, McKay R, Davies J, et al. Comparison of the aortic homograft and the pulmonary autograft for aortic valve root replacement in children. *J Thorac Cardiovasc Surg* 1991;102:51.

178. Van Son JA, Falk V, Mohr FW, et al. Ross-Konno operation with resection of endocardial fibroelastosis for critical aortic stenosis with borderline sized left ventricle in neonates. *Ann Thorac Surg* 1997;63:112.

179. Pellegrino A, Deverall PB, Anderson RH, et al. Aortic coarctation in the first three months of life: an anatomopathological study with respect to treatment. *J Thorac Cardiovasc Surg* 1985;89:121.

180. Leoni F, Huhta JC, Douglas J, et al. Effect of prostaglandin on early surgical mortality in obstructive lesions of the systemic circulation. *Br Heart J* 1984;52:654.

181. DeLezo JS, Fernandez R, Sancho M, et al. Percutaneous transluminal angioplasty for isthmus coarctation in infancy. *Am J Cardiol* 1984;54:1147.

182. Brandt B, Marvin WJ, Rose EF, et al. Surgical treatment of coarctation of the aorta after balloon angioplasty. *J Thorac Cardiovasc Surg* 1987;94:715.

183. Cobanoglu A, Teply TF, Grunkemeier GL, et al. Coarctation of the aorta in patients younger than 3 months. *J Thorac Cardiovasc Surg* 1985;89:128.

184. Campbell DB, Waldhausen JA, Pierce WS, et al. Should elective repair of coarctation of the aorta be done in infancy? *J Thorac Cardiovasc Surg* 1984;88:929.

185. Clarkson PM, Brandt PWT, Barratt-Boyes BG, et al. Prosthetic repair of coarctation of the aorta with particular reference to Dacron onlay patch grafts and late aneurysm formation. *Am J Cardiol* 1985;56:342.

186. Bergdahl L, Bjork VO, Jonasson R. Surgical correction of coarctation of the aorta: influence of age on later results. *J Thorac Cardiovasc Surg* 1983;85:532.

187. Graham TP, Atwood GF, Boerth RC, et al. Right and left heart size and function in infants with symptomatic coarctation. *Circulation* 1977;56:641.

188. Sigurdardottir LY, Helgason H. Echocardiographic evaluation of systolic and diastolic function in postoperative coarctation patients. *Pediatr Cardiol* 1997;18:96.

189. Brewer LA, Fosburg RG, Mulder GA, et al. Spinal cord complications following surgery for coarctation of the aorta: a study of 66 cases. *J Thorac Cardiovasc Surg* 1972;64:368.

190. Trinquet F, Vouhe PR, Vernant F, et al. Coarctation of the aorta in infants: which operation? *Ann Thorac Surg* 1988;45:186.

191. Park JK, Dell RB, Ellis K, Gersony WM. Surgical management of the infant with coarctation of the aorta and ventricular septal defect. *J Am Coll Cardiol* 1992;20:176.

192. Sell JE, Jonas RA, Mayer JE, et al. The results of a surgical program for interrupted aortic arch. *J Thorac Cardiovasc Surg* 1988;96:864.

193. Rychik J, Murdison KA, Chin AJ, et al. Surgical management of severe aortic outflow obstruction in lesions other than hypoplastic left heart syndrome: use of pulmonary artery to aorta anastomosis. *J Am Coll Cardiol* 1991;18:809.

194. Hanley FL, Sade RM, Blackstone EH, et al. Outcomes in neonatal pulmonary atresia with intact ventricular septum—a multiinstitutional study. *J Thorac Cardiovasc Surg* 1993;105:406.

195. Giglia TM, Mandell VS, Connor AR, et al. Diagnosis and management of right ventricular dependent coronary circulation in pulmonic atresia with intact ventricular septum. *Circulation* 1992;86:1516.

196. Dyamenahalli U, Hanna BD, Sharratt GP. Pulmonary atresia with intact ventricular septum: management of the coronary arterial anomalies. *Cardiol Young* 1997;7:80.

197. Akiba T, Becker AE. Disease of the left ventricle in pulmonary atresia with intact ventricular septum. *J Thorac Cardiovasc Surg* 1994;108:1.

198. Miyaji K, Shimada M, Sekiguchi A, et al. Pulmonary atresia with intact ventricular septum: long-term results of "one and a half ventricular repair." *Ann Thorac Surg* 1995;60:1762.

199. Hawkins JA, Thorne JK, Boucek MM, et al. Early and late results in pulmonary atresia and intact ventricular septum. *J Thorac Cardiovasc Surg* 1990;100:492.

200. Mair DD, Julsrud PR, Puga FJ, et al. The Fontan procedure for pulmonary atresia with intact ventricular septum: operative and late results. *J Am Coll Cardiol* 1997;29:1359.

201. Cullen S, Shore D, Redington A. Characterization of right ventricular diastolic performance after complete repair of tetralogy of Fallot: restrictive physiology predicts slow postoperative recovery. *Circulation* 1995;91:1782.

202. Pass RH, Mayer JE Jr, Jonas RA, et al. Course in the intensive care unit after right ventriculotomy and neonatal repair of congenital heart disease. *J Am Coll Cardiol* 1997;29:107A(abst).

203. Hennein H, Mosca R, Urcelay G, et al. Intermediate results after complete repair of teralogy of Fallot in neonates. *J Thorac Cardiovasc Surg* 1995;109:332.

204. Puga FJ, Leoni FE, Julsrud PR, et al. Complete repair of pulmonary atresia, ventricular septal defect, and severe peripheral arborization abnormalities of the central pulmonary arteries. *J Thorac Cardiovasc Surg* 1989;98:1018.

205. Reddy VM, Liddicoat JR, Hanley FL. Midline one-stage complete unifocalization and repair of pulmonary atresia with ventricular septal defect and major aortopulmonary collaterals. *J Thorac Cardiovasc Surg* 1995;109:832.

206. Rome JJ, Mayer JE, Castaneda AR, Lock JE. Teralogy of Fallot with pulmonic atresia. Rehabilitation of diminutive pulmonary arteries. *Circulation* 1993;88[Part 1]:1691.

207. Shimazaki Y, Lio M, Nakano S, et al. Pulmonary artery morphology and hemodynamics in pulmonic valve atresia with ventricular septal defect before and after repair. *Am J Cardiol* 1991;67:744.

208. Heinemann MK, Hanley FL. Preoperative management of neonatal tetralogy of Fallot with absent pulmonary valve syndrome. *Ann Thorac Surg* 1993;55:172.

209. Snir E, de Leval M, Elliot M, et al. Current surgical technique to repair Fallot's tetralogy with absent pulmonary valve syndrome. *Ann Thorac Surg* 1991;51:979.

210. Watterson K, Malm T, Karl T, Mee R. Absent pulmonary valve syndrome: operation in infants with airway obstruction. *Ann Thorac Surg* 1992;54:1116.

211. Kron IL, Johnson AM, Carpenter MA, et al. Treatment of absent pulmonary valve syndrome with homograft. *Ann Thorac Surg* 1988;46:579.

212. Ilbawi M, Cua C, Deleon S, et al. Repair of complete atrioventricular septal defect and with tetralogy of Fallot. *Ann Thorac Surg* 1990;50:407.

213. Vargas FJ, Coto EO, Mayer JE, et al. Complete atrioventricular canal and tetralogy of Fallot: surgical considerations. *Ann Thorac Surg* 1986;42:258.

214. Lang D, Obenhoffer R, Cook A, et al. Pathologic spectrum of malformations of the tricuspid valve in prenatal and neonatal life. *J Am Coll Cardiol* 1991;17:1161.

215. Celermajer DS, Bull C, Till JA, et al. Ebstein's anomaly: presentation and outcome from fetus to adult. *J Am Coll Cardiol* 1994;23:170.

216. Celermajer DS, Cullen S, Sullivan ID, et al. Outcome in neonates with Ebstein's anomaly. *J Am Coll Cardiol* 1992;19:1041.

217. Kumar AJ, Fyler DC, Mettinen OS, et al. Ebstein's anomaly: clinical profile and natural history. *Am J Cardiol* 1971;28:84.

218. Saxena A, Fong LV, Tristam M, et al. Left ventricular function in patients >20 years of age with Ebstein's anomaly of the tricuspid valve. *Am J Cardiol* 1982;49:1223.

219. Starnes VA, Pitlick PT, Berstein D, et al. Ebstein's anomaly appearing in the neonate. *J Thorac Cardiovasc Surg* 1991;101:1082.

220. Cabanero J, de Buruaga JS, Gomez JA, et al. Heart transplant in Ebstein's anomaly with endocardial fibroelastosis. *Am Heart J* 1992;124:532.

221. Carpentier A, Chauvaud S, Mace L. A new reconstruction operation for Ebstein's anomaly of the tricuspid valve. *J Thorac Cardiovasc Surg* 1988;96:92.

222. Danielson GK, Maloney JD, Devloo RAE. Surgical repair of Ebstein's anomaly. *Mayo Clin Proc* 1979;54:185.

223. Marcelletti C, Duren DR, Schuilenburg RM, et al. Fontan's operation for Ebstein's anomaly. *J Thorac Cardiovasc Surg* 1980;79:63.

224. Satomi G, Momoi N, Kikuchi N, et al. Prenatal diagnosis and outcome of Ebstein's anomaly and tricuspid valve dysplasia in relation to lung hypoplasia. *Echocardiography* 1994;11:215.

225. Danielson GK, Furster V. Surgical repair of Ebstein's anomaly. *Ann Surg* 1982;196:499.

226. Gersony WM, Peckham GJ, Ellison RC, et al. Effects of indomethacin in premature infants with patent ductus arteriosus: results of a national collaborative study. *J Pediatr* 1983;102:895.

227. Heymann MA, Rudolph AM, Silverman NH. Closure of the ductus arteriosus in premature infants by inhibition of prostaglandin synthesis. *N Engl J Med* 1976;295:530.

228. Van Overmeire B, Follens T, Hartmann S, et al. Treatment of patent ductus arteriosus with ibuprofen. *Arch Dis Child Fetal Neonatal Ed* 1997;76:F179.

229. Wagner HR, Ellison RC, Zierler S, et al. Surgical closure of patent ductus arteriosus in 268 preterm infants. *J Thorac Cardiovasc Surg* 1984;87:870.

230. Cotton RB, Stahlman MT, Berder HW, Graham TP, Catterton WZ, Kover I. Randomized trial of early closure of symptomatic patent ductus arteriosus in small preterm infants. *J Pediatr* 1978;93:647.

231. La borde F, Noirhomme P, Karam J, et al. A new video-assisted thoracoscopic surgical technique for interruption of patent ductus arteriosus in infants and children. *J Thorac Cardiovasc Surg* 1993;105:278.

232. Burke RP, Wernovsky GW, van der Velde M, et al. Video assisted thoracoscopic surgery for congenital heart disease. *J Thorac Cardiovasc Surg* 1995;109:499.

233. Burke RP, Wernovsky GW, van der Velde M, et al. Video assisted thoracoscopic surgery for congenital heart disease. *J Thorac Cardiovasc Surg* 1995;109:499.

234. Ravikumar E, Wright CM, Hawker RE, et al. The surgical management of aorticopulmonary window using the anterior sandwich patch closure technique. *J Thorac Cardiovasc Surg* 1988;29:629.

235. Hunt CE, Lucas RV. Symptomatic atrial septal defect in infancy. *Circulation* 1973;47:1042.

236. Haworth SG. Pulmonary vascular disease in secundum atrial septal defect in childhood. *Am J Cardiol* 1982;51:265.

237. Cherian G, Uthaman CB, Durairaj M, et al. Pulmonary hypertension in isolated secundum atrial septal defect: high frequency in young patients. *Am Heart J* 1983;105:952.

238. Murphy JG, Gersh BJ, McGoon MD, et al. Long term outcome after surgical repair of isolated atrial septal defect. *N Engl J Med* 1990; 323:1645.

239. Bink-Boelkens MthE, Meuzelaar KJ, Eygelaar A. Arrhythmias after repair of secundum atrial septal defect: the influence of surgical modification. *Am Heart J* 1988;11:373.

240. Lipshultz SE, Sanders SP, Mayer JE Jr, Colan SD, Lock JE. Are routine preoperative cardiac catheterization and angiography necessary before repair of ostium primum atrial septal defect? *J Am Coll Cardiol* 1988;11:373.

241. Moe DG, Guntheroth WG. Spontaneous closure of uncomplicated ventricular septal defect. *Am J Cardiol* 1987;60:674.

242. Vincent RN, Lang P, Dhipman CW, et al. Assessment of hemodynamic status in the intensive care unit immediately after closure of ventricular septal defects. *Am J Cardiol* 1985;55:526.

243. Blake RS, Chung EE, Wesley H, et al. Conduction defects, ventricular arrhythmias, and late death after surgical closure of ventricular septal defects. *Br Heart J* 1982;47:305.

244. Reeder GS, Danielson GK, Seward JB, et al. Fixed subaortic stenosis in atrioventricular canal defect: a Doppler echocardiographic study. *J Am Coll Cardiol* 1992;20:386.

245. Castaneda AR, Mayer JE Jr, Jonas RA. Repair of complete atrioventricular canal in infancy. *World J Surg* 1985;9:590.

246. Pozzi M, Remig J, Fimmers R, et al. Atrioventricular septal defect: analysis of short and mid-term results. *J Thorac Cardiovasc Surg* 1991;101:138.

247. Morris CD, Magilke D, Reller M. Down's syndrome affects results of surgical correction of complete atrioventricular canal. *Pediatr Cardiol* 1992;13:80.

248. Tandon R, Moller JH, Edwards JE. Single papillary muscle of the left ventricle associated with persistent common atrioventricular canal: variant of parachute mitral valve. *Pediatr Cardiol* 1986;7:111.

249. Chang CI, Becker AE. Surgical anatomy of left ventricular outflow obstruction in complete atrioventricular septal defect: a concept for operative repair. *J Thorac Cardiovasc Surg* 1987;94:897.

250. Portman MA, Beder SD, Ankeney JL, et al. A 20-year review of ostium primum defect repair in children. *Am Heart J* 1985;110: 1054.

251. Bando K, Turretine MW, Sharp T, et al. Pulmonary hypertension after operations for congenital heart disease: analysis of risk factors and management. *J Thorac Cardiovasc Surg* 1996;112:1600.

252. Bove EL, Lupinetti FM, Pridjian AK, et al. Results of a policy of primary repair of truncus arteriosus in the neonate. *J Thorac Cardiovasc Surg* 1993;105:1057.

253. Hanley FL, Heinemann MK, Jonas RA, et al. Repair of truncus arteriosus in the neonate. *J Thorac Cardiovasc Surg* 1993;105:1047.

254. Pearson GA, Sosnowski A, Chan KC, et al. Salvage of post-operative pulmonary hypertension crisis using ECMO via cervical cannulation in a case of truncus arteriosus. *Eur J Cardiovasc Surg* 1993; 7:390.

255. Kirklin JW, Barratt-Boyes BG. Complete transposition of the great arteries. In: Kirklin JW, Barratt-Boyes BG, eds. *Cardiac surgery*. New York: Churchill Livingstone, 1993:1383.

256. Moene RJ, Oppenheimer-Dekker A, Bartelings MM. Anatomic obstruction of the right ventricular outflow tract in transposition of the great arteries. *Am J Cardiol* 1983;51:1701.

257. Moene RJ, Ottenkamp J, Oppenheimer-Dekker A, et al. Transposition of the great arteries and narrowing of the aortic arch. *Br Heart J* 1985;53:58.

258. Kurosawa H, Van Mierop LHS. Surgical anatomy of the infundibular septum in transposition of the great arteries with ventricular septal defect. *J Thorac Cardiovasc Surg* 1986;91:123.

259. Wernovsky G, Jonas RA, Colan SD, et al. Results of the arterial switch operation in patients with transposition of the great arteries and abnormalities of the mitral valve or left ventricular outflow tract. *J Am Coll Cardiol* 1990;16:1446.

260. Rastelli GC, McGoon DC, Wallace RB. Anatomic correction of transposition of the great arteries with ventricular septal defect and subpulmonary stenosis. *J Thorac Cardiovasc Surg* 1969;58:545.

261. Lecompte Y. The REV (reparation a l'etage ventriculaire) procedure: technique and clinical results. *Cardiol Young* 1991;1:63.

262. Wernovsky G, Hougen TJ, Walsh EP, et al. Midterm results after the arterial switch operation for transposition of the great areteries with intact ventricular septum: clinical, hemodynamic, echocardiographic, and electrophysiologic data. *Circulation* 1988;78:132.

263. Davis AM, Wilkinson JL, Karl TR, Mee RBB. Transposition of the great arteries with intact ventricular septum. *J Thorac Cardiovasc Surg* 1993;106:111.

264. Mee RBB, Harada Y. Retraining of the left ventricle with a left ventricular assist device (Bio-Medicus) after the arterial switch operation [Letter]. *J Thorac Cardiovasc Surg* 1991;101:171.

265. Sano S, Brawn WJ, Mee RBB. Total anomalous pulmonary venous drainage. *J Thorac Cardiovasc Surg* 1989;97:886.

266. Lincoln CR, Rigby ML, Mercanti C, et al. Surgical risk factors in total anomalous pulmonary venous connection. *Am J Cardiol* 1988; 61:608.

267. Serraf A, Bruniaux J, Lacour-Gayet F, et al. Obstructed total pulmonary venous return: toward neutralization of a major risk factor. *J Thorac Cardiovasc Surg* 1991;101:601.

268. Lin SC, Teng RJ, Wang JK. Management of severe pulmonary hypertension in an infant with obstructed total anomalous pulmonary venous return using magnesium sulfate. *Int J Cardiol* 1996; 56:131.

269. Parr GV, Kirklin JW, Pacifico AD, et al. Cardiac performance in infancy after repair of total anomalous pulmonary venous connection. *Ann Thorac Surg* 1974;17:561.

270. Wong PC, Starnes VA. Pediatric heart and lung transplantation. In: Chang AC, Hanley FL, Wernovsky G, Wessel DL, eds. *Pediatric cardiac intensive care*. Baltimore: Williams & Wilkins, 1998:327.

271. Fricker FJ, Armitage JM. Heart and heart-lung transplantation in children and adolescents. In: Emmanouilides GC, Allen HA, Riemenschneider TA, Gutgesell HS, eds. *Moss and Adams' heart disease in infants, children, adolescents, including the fetus and the young adult*, 5th ed. Baltimore: Williams & Wilkins, 1995:495.

272. Bailey LL, Assaad AN, Trimm RF, et al. Orthotopic transplantation during early infancy as therapy for incurable congenital heart disease. *Ann Surg* 1988;208:279.

273. Razzouk AJ, Bailey LL. Infant heart transplantation. In: Emmanouilides GC, Allen HA, Riemenschneider TA, Gutgesell HS, eds. *Moss and Adams' heart disease in infants, children, adolescents, including the fetus and the young adult*, 5th ed. Baltimore: Williams & Wilkins, 1995:510.

274. Bailey LL, Gundry SR, Razzouk AJ, et al. Bless the babies: one hundred fifteen late survivors of heart transplantation during the first year of life. *J Thorac Cardiovasc Surg* 1993;105:805.

275. Starnes VA, Oyer PE, Bernstein D, et al. Heart, heart-lung and lung transplantation in the first year of life. *Ann Thorac Surg* 1992;53:306.

276. Bove EL. Transplantation after first-stage reconstruction for hypoplastic left heart syndrome. *Ann Thorac Surg* 1991;52:701.

277. Starnes VA, Griffin ML, Pitlick PT, et al. Current approach to hypoplastic left heart syndrome: palliation, transplantation, or both? *J Thorac Cardiovasc Surg* 1992;104:189.

278. Del Nido PJ, Armitage JM, Fricker FJ, et al. Extracorporeal membrane oxygenation support as a bridge to pediatric heart transplantation. *Circulation* 1994;90:II-66.

279. Galantowicz ME, Stolar CJ. Extracorporeal membrane oxygenation for perioperative support in pediatric heart transplantation. *J Thorac Cardiovasc Surg* 1991;102:148.

280. Addonizio LJ, Gersony WM, Robbins RC, et al. Elevated pulmonary vascular resistance and cardiac transplantation. *Circulation* 1987;76:V52.

281. Gajarski RJ, Towbin JA, Bricker T, et al. Intermediate follow-up of pediatric transplantation recipients with elevated pulmonary vascular resistance index. *J Am Coll Cardiol* 1994;23:1682.

282. Zales VR, Pahl E, Backer C, et al. Pharmacologic reduction of pulmonary vascular resistance pre-transplant predicts outcome following pediatric cardiac transplantation. *J Heart Lung Transplant* 1993;12:S93(abst).

283. Scott CD, Dark JH, McComb JM. Arrhythmias after cardiac transplantation. *Am J Cardiol* 1992;70:1061.

284. Razzouk AJ, Bailey LL. Infant heart transplantation. In: Emmanouilides GC, Allen HA, Riemenschneider TA, Gutgesell HS, eds. *Moss and Adams' heart disease in infants, children, adolescents, including the fetus and the young adult*, 5th ed. Baltimore: Williams & Wilkins, 1995:514.

285. Vricella L, Alonso de Begona J, Gundry SR, et al. Aggressive peritoneal dialysis for treatment of renal failure after neonatal cardiac transplant. *J Heart Lung Transplant* 1992;11:320.

286. Schowengerdt KO, Naftel DC, Seib PM, et al. Infection after pediatric heart transplantation: results of a multi-institutional study. *J Heart Lung Transplant* 1997;16:1207.

287. Backer CL, Zales VR, Harrison HL, et al. Intermediate term results of infant orthotopic cardiac transplantation from two centers. *J Thorac Cardiovasc Surg* 1991;101:826.

288. Bailey L, Gundry S, Razzark A, Wang N. Pediatric heart transplantation: issues relating to outcome and results. *J Heart Lung Transplant* 1991;11[Suppl]:267.

289. Kanakriyeh MS, Mullins CE, Cordoba M, Bailey LL. Ventricular volume and function in infant orthotopic transplantation. *J Thorac Cardiovasc Surg* 1985;89:242.

290. Wong PC, Starnes VA. Pediatric heart and lung transplantation. In: Chang AC, Hanley FL, Wernovsky G, Wessel DL, eds. *Pediatric cardiac intensive care*. Baltimore: Williams & Wilkins, 1998:329.

291. Jacobs ML, Blackstone EH, Bailey LL. Intermediate survival in neonates with aortic atresia: a multi-institutional study. *J Thorac Cardiovasc Surg* 1998;116:417.

292. Rome JJ, Lock JE. Interventional catheterization in pediatric and congenital heart disease. In: Stark J, De Leval M, eds. *Surgery for congenital heart defects*, 2nd ed. Philadelphia: WB Saunders, 1993:95.

293. Rome JJ. The role of catheter-directed therapies in the treatment of congenital heart disease. *Annu Rev Med* 1995;46:159.

294. Ashfaq M, Houston AB, Gnanpragasam JP, et al. Balloon atrial septostomy under echocardiographic control: six years' experience and evaluation of the practicability of cannulation via the umbilical vein. *Br Heart J* 1992;67:205.

295. Kerstein D, Levy PS, Hsu DT, et al. Blade balloon atrial septostomy in patients with severe primary pulmonary hypertension. *Circulation* 1995;91:2028.

296. Nihill MR, O'Laughlin MP, Mullins CE. Effects of atrial septostomy in patients with terminal cor pulmonale due to pulmonary vascular disease. *Cathet Cardiovasc Diagn* 1991;24:166.

297. Kan JS, White RJJ, Mitchell SE, et al. Percutaneous balloon valvulplasty: a new method for treating congenital pulmonary valve stenosis. *N Engl J Med* 1982;307:540.

298. Stanger P, Cassidy SC, Girod DA, et al. Balloon pulmonary valvuloplasty: results of the valvuloplasty and angioplasty of congenital anomalies registry. *Am J Cardiol* 1990;65:775.

299. Sholler GF, Keane JF, Perry SB, et al. Balloon dilation of congenital aortic valve stenosis: results and influence of technical and morphological features on outcome. *Circulation* 1988;78:351.

300. O'Connor BK, Beekman RH, Rocchini AP, et al. Intermediate-term effectiveness of balloon valvuloplasty for congenital aortic stenosis. *Circulation* 1991;84:732.

301. Hanley FL, Sade RM, Freedom RM, et al. Outcomes in critically ill neonates with pulmonary stenosis and intact ventricular septum: a multi-institutional study. *J Am Coll Cardiol* 1993;22:183.

302. Rhodes LA, Colan SD, Perry SB, et al. Predictors of survival in neonates with critical aortic stenosis. *Circulation* 1991;84:2325.

303. Asante-Korang A, Fischer DR, Sigfusson G, et al. Carotid approach for balloon valvotomy for critical aortic stenosis in early infancy: medium-term outcome. Circulation 1995;92:I-310(abst).

304. Hijazi Z, Fahey JT, Kleinman CS, et al. Balloon angioplasty for recurrent coarctation of the aorta. *Circulation* 1991;84:1150.

305. Hellebrand WE, Allen HD, Golinko RJ, et al. Balloon angioplasty for aortic recoarctation: results of valvuloplasty and angioplasty of congenital anomalies registry. *Am J Cardiol* 1990;65:793.

306. Shaddy RE, Boueck MM, Sturtevant JE, et al. Comparison of angioplasty and surgery for unoperated coarctation of the aorta. *Circulation* 1993;87:793.

307. Wessel DL, Keane JF, Fellows KE, et al. Fibrinolytic therapy for femoral arterial thrombosis after cardiac catheterization in infants and children. *Am J Cardiol* 1986;58:347.

308. Dillon PW, Fox PS, Berg CJ, et al. Recombinant tissue plasminogen activator for neonatal and pediatric vascular thrombolytic therapy. *J Pediatr Surg* 1993;28:1264.

309. *Physicians Desk Reference*, 50th ed. Montvale, NJ: Medical Economics Co. 1996:2636.

310. McDonald-McGinn DM, LaRossa D, Goldmuntz E, et al. The 22q11.2 deletion: screening, diagnostic workup, and outcome of results; report on 181 patients. *Genet Testing* 1997;1:99.

CHAPTER 35

Carbohydrate Homeostasis

Edward S. Ogata

Glucose homeostasis results from the net balance between systemic organ requirements and the production and regulation of glucose. The neonate's ability to maintain glucose homeostasis is less than optimal because it is in a metabolic transition period. The abrupt switch from intrauterine life, in which glucose and metabolic fuels are provided in a well-regulated manner, to a situation where it is an intermittent meal eater necessitates regulation of exogenous glucose and production of endogenous glucose. As the capability to perform these functions continues to develop in the neonate, clinical disorders that can afflict the neonate may perturb this balance, resulting in hypoglycemia or hyperglycemia. In addition, antecedent intrauterine events can alter the development of glucoregulatory capabilities in the fetus, resulting in altered neonatal glucose homeostasis. Diabetes in pregnancy is the *sine qua non* of changes in maternal metabolism that affect fetal development and alter neonatal glucoregulation.

To understand the processes responsible for glucose homeostasis in the normal neonate, an understanding of the development of glucoregulatory capabilities in the fetus is necessary. This chapter reviews this information and its relation to the clinical disorders associated with altered neonatal glucose homeostasis. Information on the perinatal aspects of diabetes in pregnancy also is presented.

MATERNAL METABOLISM DURING PREGNANCY

Although the metabolic alterations that develop in the pregnant woman throughout gestation favor the growth and development of the fetus, the first half of gestation also is a critical period for maternal anabolism. The increased calories ingested by the woman during early gestation not only sustain fetal growth but facilitate maternal fat deposition. This is important preparation for the second half of gestation, a period of exponential fetal growth during which these maternal stores are mobilized to meet fetal needs. The storage of maternal energy stores is facilitated by the increased secretion of insulin that occurs in women with normal carbohydrate metabolism (1–5).

From roughly midgestation onward, a number of antiinsulin factors develop in the mother to cause pregnancy to become a diabetogenic-like state. Human placental lactogen, progesterone, and estrogen, which directly antagonize maternal insulin, become increasingly available. In addition, insulin-degrading enzyme systems develop in the placenta that further deplete maternal insulin. These alterations guarantee metabolic fuel availability to the fetus during the postprandial state; the delay in clearance of glucose and other metabolic fuels from the maternal circulation as a result of the blunting of insulin's effect allows a longer period for uptake by the uteroplacental circulation (6–8). Preexisting maternal diabetes potentiates the effects of the antiinsulin factors, causing an excessive provision of glucose and other metabolic fuels to the fetus. This is the basic perturbation responsible for the problems of the infant of the diabetic mother (Fig. 35–1) (1,9).

Metabolic fuel availability is guaranteed to the fetus even during brief maternal fasting. After an overnight fast, pregnant women have significantly lower plasma glucose concentrations than fasted nongravid women (10,11); however, glucose production in the mother is significantly increased (12,13). This increased production ensures the provision of glucose to the fetus.

Prolonged maternal fasting does alter fuel provision to the fetus. As the fast progresses, maternal ketogenesis progressively increases (11,14). The human fetal brain at early gestation can use ketones (Fig. 35–2) (15). How-

E. S. Ogata: Department of Pediatrics, Northwestern University Medical School; and Children's Memorial Hospital, Chicago, Illinois

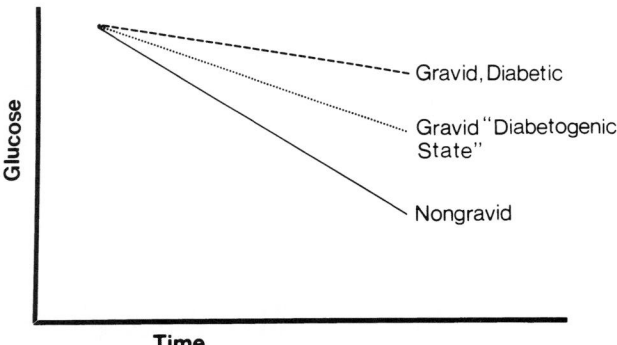

FIG. 35–1. Plasma glucose changes after glucose challenge in nongravid, gravid, and gravid diabetic women. Compared to the nongravid woman, the pregnant woman with normal carbohydrate metabolism demonstrates delayed glucose clearance from midgestation onward as a result of antiinsulin factors that develop during pregnancy. The delay in glucose clearance from the maternal circulation assures glucose provision to the fetus, particularly during the postprandial period. The blunting of maternal glucose clearance is exaggerated by the counterinsulin factors in the woman with diabetes mellitus. The decreased clearance of glucose and other metabolic fuels stimulates fetal insulin production and is responsible for many of the problems of the infant of the diabetic mother.

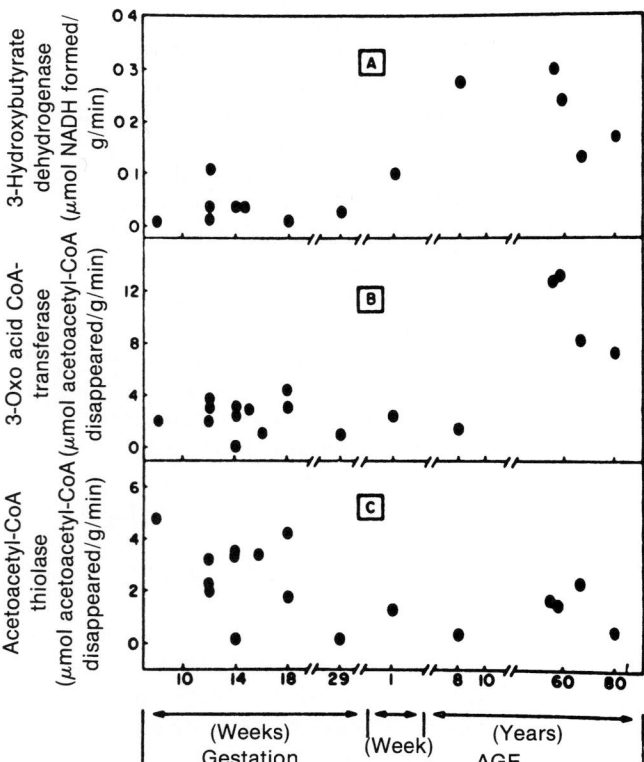

FIG. 35–2. Enzymatic activity of the three key enzymes necessary for the oxidation of ketones (i.e., [A5]β-hydroxybutyrate and acetoacetate). The activities of these enzymes are present in substantial quantities in the human fetal brain during early gestation. (From ref. 15.)

ever, this ability to use an alternative fuel may be harmful rather than beneficial to the fetus. Offspring of mothers who were ketotic during pregnancy appear to have an increased incidence of cognitive and psychomotor delay at 3 and 5 years of age (16). Whether ketone use by the fetal brain was responsible for this is unknown. Equally unclear is the duration and degree of ketone exposure necessary to cause damage. Because of this uncertainty, maternal fasting, even forgoing breakfast, should be avoided during pregnancy.

DEVELOPMENT OF GLUCOSE-PRODUCING AND GLUCOREGULATORY CAPABILITIES IN THE FETUS

To understand the problems of neonatal glucose homeostasis, the development of glucose production and regulatory capabilities in the fetus must be understood.

Glycogen

The third trimester of the human pregnancy is the first period in gestation during which some of the energy and substrate available to the fetus can be channeled from meeting needs for ongoing growth and development to energy storage. As the third trimester progresses, fat deposition and hepatic glycogen storage increase (17). The human fetus can synthesize and mobilize glycogen and respond to the signals that regulate these processes as early as the ninth week of gestation (18). Minute quantities of hepatic glycogen are detectable in early gestation; however, the great bulk of hepatic glycogen accumulates during the third trimester (18,19).

Several types of infants are at risk for neonatal hypoglycemia as a result of limited hepatic glycogen stores. Infants delivered prematurely have an abbreviated or no third trimester and thus have limited glycogen stores. Fetuses who are growth-retarded [i.e., small for gestational age (SGA)] on the basis of limited metabolic fuel availability and diminished gaseous exchange (i.e., uteroplacental insufficiency) will use these fuels for growth and not have glucose remaining for glycogen synthesis. Perinatal stress causes neonatal hypoglycemia in part because of catecholamine-stimulated mobilization of hepatic glycogen stores. This can occur at birth or during the antepartum period. In the latter situation, fetuses might recover from stress and be delivered without difficulty. As newborns, such infants have depleted glycogen stores and are at risk for hypoglycemia.

Gluconeogenesis

For many years, it was believed that maternally derived glucose was the sole metabolic fuel for the fetus and that the fetus could not produce glucose. As indicated, the fetus can use other fuels such as the ketones and can under special circumstances mobilize hepatic glycogen.

The fetus also can carry out gluconeogenesis to a limited degree, although it is likely that under normal circumstances it does not need to call on this function. Data from human abortus material have demonstrated that the four key gluconeogenic enzymes are demonstrable in fetal liver by 2 to 3 months of gestation (20,21). The activities of these enzymes are believed to increase throughout gestation and the neonatal period. Thus, all newborns including the very premature probably have some degree of gluconeogenic capability.

Endocrine Regulation

Insulin and glucagon, important hormones for regulating glucose, can be measured in fetal plasma as early as 12 weeks of gestation (22). Although plasma concentrations of these hormones are low, the relative content of these hormones in the fetal pancreas is quite high (23,24). These high concentrations may result from the limited ability of the fetal islets to secrete these hormones. Studies in premature and term infants in the newborn period indicate that their capacity to secrete these hormones in response to a glucose challenge is limited; this suggests that the fetus also has limited secretory capability (Fig. 35–3) (24–26). Of note, amino acids have a greater effect than glucose in stimulating insulin and limiting glucagon secretion (27,28).

Insulin may be more important for enhancing growth than for regulating metabolic fuels during fetal life. Insulin stimulates the growth of specific tissues (e.g., adipose, hepatic, connective, skeletal, cardiac muscle) (29,30). Excessive insulin secretion during fetal life resulting from such conditions as maternal diabetes causes the disproportionate growth of insulin-sensitive tissues, resulting in macrosomia (1,9,31,32). A lack of insulin, as in infants with transient neonatal diabetes mellitus, always is accompanied by fetal growth retardation.

Glucagon or a critical glucagon–insulin ratio is important for inducing gluconeogenic enzymes. Glucagon stimulates the induction of gluconeogenic enzymes *in vitro* and *in vivo* (33,34). Fetal plasma glucagon concentrations increase progressively during fetal life, and this is associated with a concomitant increase in gluconeogenic enzyme activity. At birth, plasma glucagon concentrations surge, coinciding with the rapid postnatal increase in gluconeogenic activity (35). Insulin may modulate glucagon's effect because it can inhibit gluconeogenic enzyme induction (34). Thus, a balance between these two hormones controls gluconeogenic enzyme induction during perinatal life.

Adrenergic mechanisms can stimulate hepatic glycogenolysis during fetal life, much as in the adult. As labor progresses, fetal sympathoadrenal activity increases, resulting in a considerable increase in circulating catecholamine levels (36,37). Cord clamping triggers an increase in glucagon secretion (38). As plasma glucose concentrations plummet with cord clamping, insulin secretion slowly decreases. These adjustments, particularly the remarkable increase in catecholamine secretion, stimulate glycogenolysis and gluconeogenesis in the neonate (Fig. 35–4).

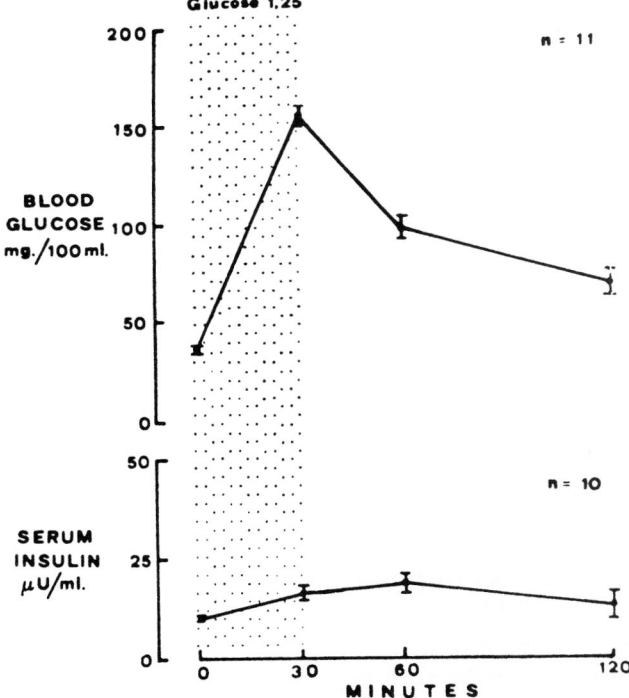

FIG. 35–3. Insulin secretion after glucose challenge in premature infants. Whereas normal adults secrete insulin briskly in response to glucagon, premature infants in the neonatal period secrete insulin only sluggishly. (From ref. 27.)

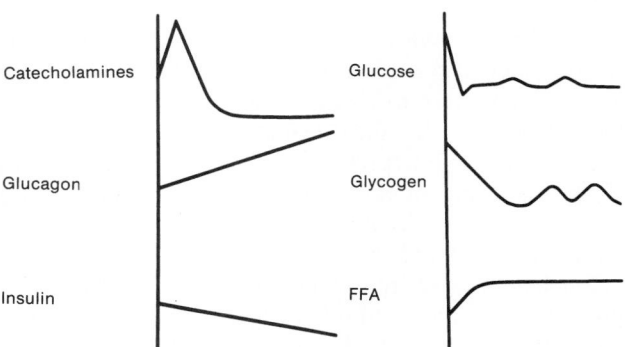

FIG. 35–4. Levels of hormone and metabolic fuels change after birth. At birth, the counterregulatory hormones (i.e., catecholamines and glucagon) increase greatly, whereas insulin secretion decreases. Neonatal plasma glucose concentrations plummet as a result of cord clamping. The changes in counterregulatory hormones and insulin favor mobilization of glucose and fat and stimulate gluconeogenesis. These changes assure adequate neonatal glucose production. FAA, free fatty acids. (From ref. 51.)

Islet cell function remains unresponsive for several weeks of neonatal life in term infants. Newborn infants increase insulin and limit glucagon secretion sluggishly in response to glucose challenge. Limited data indicate that these responses become adult-like between 1 and 2 weeks of life (39). This adaptation is critically important because the neonate, unlike the fetus, must regulate glucose production and storage through feeding and fasting cycles. Little is known about the premature infant's ability to regulate glucose in the neonatal period. The ability to modulate insulin and glucagon secretion probably develops as the neonatal period progresses.

GLUCOSE TRANSPORTERS

Glucose transporters (Glut) are a family of structurally similar proteins encoded by a family of genes and expressed in a tissue-specific manner in most mammalian tissues (40). Several isoforms have been described in the human fetus and placenta. As Gluts facilitate transfer of glucose from the maternal to fetal circulation and also uptake of glucose by most fetal and neonatal tissues, they are critically important for growth and development.

Glut 1 is the dominant isoform in most fetal tissues and the placenta (41,42). Insulin, the insulin-like growth factors, and other hormones and peptides regulate its activity and expression. The Gluts are developmentally regulated. Data from animal studies suggest that other isoforms (Glut 2 in liver, Glut 4 in muscle) appear in the neonatal period (43).

NEONATAL GLUCOSE REQUIREMENTS

The clinician makes a leap of faith in using the chemical or paper strip determination of plasma or blood glucose concentration to judge the adequacy of tissue glucose provision in the neonate. A normal plasma concentration is interpreted to mean that glucose supply to the brain and other organs is adequate for ongoing metabolic needs. To appreciate glucose requirements, glucose kinetics must be understood.

Glucose turnover represents the rate of production of glucose by the liver and other organs and the simultaneous use or uptake of glucose by the brain and other organs. Turnover is usually expressed as milligrams of glucose per kilogram of body weight per minute. Although stable isotope technology has allowed quantification of glucose turnover in neonates, this methodology cannot be directly applied for clinical purposes. Thus, the clinician must rely on the measurements of glucose concentrations, which are static, as representative of the dynamic rate of glucose production and use in a neonate. In general, plasma glucose concentrations roughly correlate with glucose turnover. Diminished plasma glucose concentrations suggest that glucose production is limited or that glucose use is increased (i.e., need is outstripping production). Elevated plasma glucose concentrations suggest either that production is excessive or, more likely, that organ uptake and use are diminished. These are the dynamic physiologic conditions that define hypoglycemia and hyperglycemia.

In the neonate, glucose production correlates directly with brain and body mass, confirming the critical role of glucose as a metabolic fuel (44–47). This holds even in the most immature of premature infants (48). Glucose turnover for newborn infants, when related to body mass, significantly exceeds that of adults (Fig. 35–5). Premature infants have even greater turnover values than term neonates. This in part reflects the ratio of brain to body mass, which is greatest in premature infants and least in adults. These relations emphasize the importance of glucose as the primary fuel for the brain (Fig. 35–6).

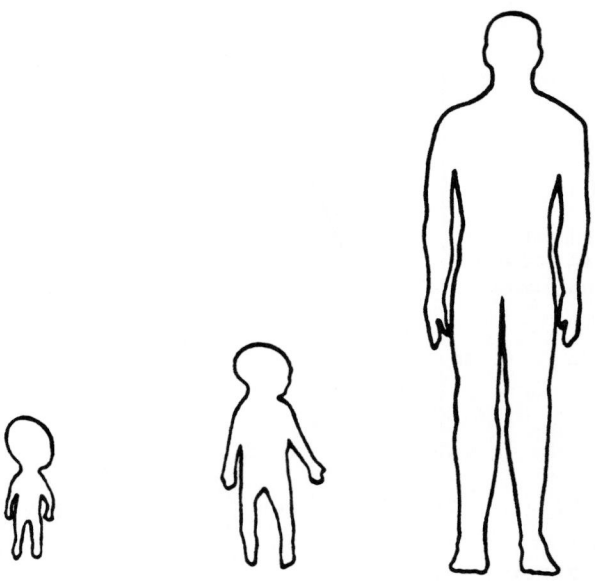

Premature Neonate Full-Term Neonate Adult
5–6 mg/kg/min   3–5 mg/kg/min   2–3 mg/kg/min

FIG. 35–5. Glucose turnover in premature and term neonates and the adult. When related to body weight, glucose turnover is greatest in the premature infant and least in the adult. The increased turnover in neonates results in part from their relatively increased brain-to-body mass ratio. (From ref. 51.)

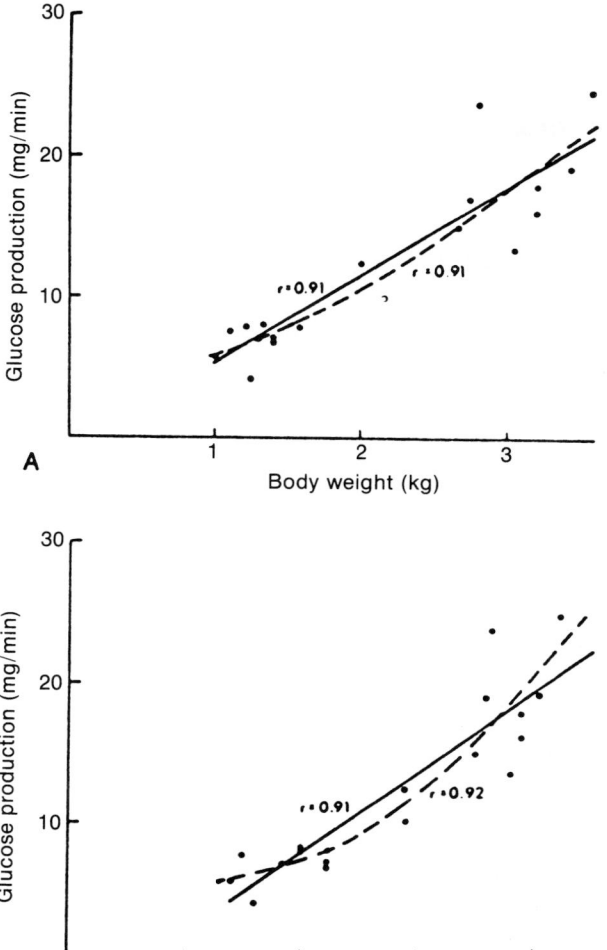

FIG. 35–6. Linear and curvilinear regression analyses indicate strong relations between glucose turnover and body mass **(A)**, and between glucose turnover and brain mass **(B)**, in newborn human infants. (From ref. 45.)

NEONATAL HYPOGLYCEMIA

A variety of blood and plasma glucose concentration values based on screening of neonates or clinical experience have been recommended as values defining hypoglycemia (49). All of these are somewhat arbitrary because they cannot be correlated directly with glucose use rate or severity of symptoms. Because plasma or blood glucose concentrations only roughly reflect glucose turnover, a plasma glucose concentration less than 40 mg/dL should be used to define hypoglycemia. When glucose turnover is sufficient to meet the needs of the organism, concentrations usually exceed this value. It also is important to note that values somewhat less than 40 mg/dL still can be associated with adequate glucose provision.

The chemical definition of hypoglycemia must take into account the methodology of glucose determinations. Glucose concentration in whole blood is approximately 10% to 15% lower than that in plasma. Delay in determination after blood sampling may result in glucose oxidation by erythrocytes, causing falsely low values. Although the use of paper strip methods to estimate glucose concentrations quickly is acceptable, their results should be corroborated by true chemical determinations.

The clinical manifestations of inadequate glucose provision to the neonatal brain range from no symptoms to lethargy or mild tremors to frank convulsions (Table 35–1). The degree of glucose limitation necessary to cause brain damage is unknown. The lack of clearly defined data on this problem and the prevailing opinion concerning the potentially damaging effects of hypoglycemia mandate that infants at risk be monitored and that asymptomatic and symptomatic infants be appropriately treated.

All conditions associated with the development of hypoglycemia in the neonate result from one or a combination of two basic mechanisms: inadequate production or excessive tissue use. Inadequate glucose production results from a lack of glycogen stores, an inability to synthesize glucose, or both (Fig. 35–7). Excessive tissue use results from increased insulin secretion. Table 35–2 categorizes infants at risk for hypoglycemia in relation to these basic mechanisms.

Inadequate Glucose Production as a Result of Limited Glycogen Stores

Premature Infants

As indicated, the third trimester of pregnancy is an important period for hepatic glycogen deposition. An infant delivered prematurely without having had the benefit of part of or the entire third trimester will have limited hepatic glycogen stores. The greater the degree of prematurity, the less glycogen will be present. Small-for-gestational-age premature infants are at extremely high risk for development of hypoglycemia because available nutrients during intrauterine life are channeled toward growth, with little set aside for glycogen storage. For this reason, SGA premature infants have extremely limited glycogen stores (50–52).

TABLE 35–1. *Symptoms of hypoglycemia*

Jitteriness
Tremors
Apnea
Cyanosis
Limpness/lethargy
Seizures

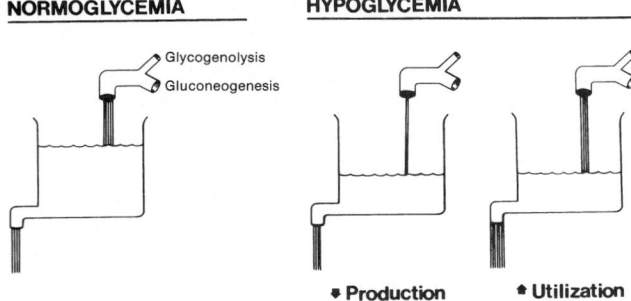

NORMOGLYCEMIA   **HYPOGLYCEMIA**

Glycogenolysis
Gluconeogenesis

↓ Production   ↑ Utilization

FIG. 35–7. The rates of glucose production and utilization are represented by the faucet and drain of the sink. The level in the sink is equivalent to plasma or blood glucose concentrations. If production from glycogenolysis and gluconeogenesis is adequate, and use is not excessive, normoglycemia exists, and the plasma or blood glucose concentration (i.e., the level in the sink) is normal. Hypoglycemia develops if production is inadequate to meet body needs or if use outstrips production. This results in decreased glucose concentrations (i.e., diminished level in sink). (From ref. 51.)

Infants Who Have Suffered Perinatal Stress

Infants who are stressed *in utero* are at increased risk for development of hypoglycemia as neonates. Hypoxia, acidosis, and alterations in fetal blood pressure and flow can stimulate catecholamine secretion *in utero,* which in turn will mobilize hepatic glycogen stores. In addition, hypoxia increases the rate of anaerobic glycolysis, thereby accelerating glucose use. These events deplete fetal glycogen stores and place the infant at risk for hypoglycemia after delivery.

TABLE 35–2. *Infants at risk for hypoglycemia*[a]

Diminished production
  Limited glycogen
    SGA
    Prematurity
    Birth stress
    Glycogen storage disorders
  Limited gluconeogenesis
    SGA
    Inborn errors
Increased utilization
  Hyperinsulinism
    IDM
    Beckwith–Wiedemann syndrome
    Nesidioblastosis or pancreatic adenoma
    Erythroblastosis fetalis
    Exchange transfusion, chlorpropamide, benzothiazides,
      β-sympathomimetics, malpositioned UA catheter
Unknown
  LGA infants who are not IDM
  Sepsis
  Polycythemia or hyperviscosity syndrome
  Congenital hypopituitarism

[a]IDM, infant of diabetic mother; LGA, large for gestational age; SGA, small for gestational age; UA, umbilical artery.

Glycogen Storage Disease

Intrinsic defects in glycogen synthesis, storage, or breakdown result in complex metabolic problems (see Chap. 39). Several types of glycogen storage disease (i.e., Ia, I, VI, 0) have hypoglycemia as one of many associated complications (49,53).

Inadequate Production as a Result of Limited Gluconeogenesis

Small-for-Gestational-Age Infants

Full-term and premature SGA neonates are at great risk for development of hypoglycemia as a result of inadequate hepatic glycogen stores. With treatment, this usually is short-lived. Approximately 1% of SGA infants in whom hypoglycemia develops have a prolonged course requiring intravenous therapy for days. A delay in the induction of gluconeogenic capability probably is responsible for this prolonged hypoglycemia. These SGA neonates have elevated plasma concentrations of gluconeogenic precursors, suggesting an inability to convert exogenous gluconeogenic precursors such as alanine to glucose (54,55).

In animal models of intrauterine growth retardation, the induction of one gluconeogenic enzyme, phosphoenolpyruvate carboxykinase, is delayed (56,57). This occurs despite appropriate increases in glucagon and decreases in insulin; these relations should favor enzyme induction. Why some SGA infants fail to induce gluconeogenic capability is unclear. Corticosteroid therapy often was used in the past to treat prolonged hypoglycemia. The success of this practice probably resulted in part from the ability of corticosteroids to induce hepatic gluconeogenic enzymes.

Many SGA infants have heightened metabolic requirements during the neonatal period. The mechanisms for this are not understood, but they may represent an attempt to compensate for the preceding intrauterine deprivation (58). This may explain the increased glucose requirements demonstrated by some hypoglycemic SGA infants.

Congenital Absence of Gluconeogenic Capability

Unlike SGA infants in whom gluconeogenic capability eventually develops, a few infants have been reported who have permanent congenital lack of gluconeogenic enzymes (59). A single infant who was unable to secrete glucagon also has been reported (60).

Excessive Tissue Use or Hyperinsulinism

A variety of disorders are associated with fetal and neonatal hyperinsulinism. In some disorders, the mechanisms for heightened β-cell function are well understood, whereas in others, the pathogenesis is unclear. In the former category are infants of diabetic mothers (IDM) and infants with altered pancreatic islets caused by conditions such as nesidioblastosis and pancreatic adenoma. Those for whom an etiology is not clear include infants with erythroblastosis and Beckwith–Wiedemann syndrome. The finding of a hypoglycemic infant who is macrosomic and requires high rates of glucose infusion (10 to 20 mg/kg body weight per minute) suggests a hyperinsulinemic state.

Infants of Diabetic Mothers

Infants of diabetic mothers are at great risk for development of hypoglycemia as a result of the carryover of the fetal hyperinsulinemic state into neonatal life. They have elevated plasma insulin concentrations and release insulin briskly in response to glucose challenge. The problems of the IDM are presented in the following sections.

Nesidioblastosis and Islet Cell Adenoma

These conditions are probably caused by several different accidents of development that result in persistent insulin secretion during fetal and neonatal life. In fact, persistent hyperinsulinemic hypoglycemia of infancy is a term often used to describe these disorders. Classically, in nesidioblastosis, pancreatic ductular cells are found in acinar tissue. Islet cell adenomas occur less frequently than nesidioblastosis (61–63). Clinically, these disorders cannot be distinguished because exuberant insulin secretion begins *in utero* and remains sustained during later fetal and neonatal life.

Nesidioblastosis or islet cell adenoma should be considered whenever a macrosomic infant has hypoglycemia with elevated plasma insulin concentrations over several days. Rebound hypoglycemia in response to excessive glucose administration is another characteristic. Increased insulin–glucose ratios and glucose requirements exceeding 10 mg/kg/min support the possibility of either nesidioblastosis or islet cell adenoma.

A number of mechanisms are probably responsible for persistent hyperinsulinemia. Somatostatin deficiency during fetal life may allow for uncontrolled insulin secretion (64). In a familial form of this disorder, a mutation of the sulfonurea receptor has been demonstrated (65); this defect leads to persistent unregulated activation of insulin-secreting mechanisms (66).

Surgical excision of a portion of the pancreas can provide definitive diagnosis and therapy. However, over the long term this may result in the development of diabetes mellitus in the patient. Both somatostatin and diazoxide have been used successfully to limit insulin secretion for as long as several months and may produce remission.

Unexplained Neonatal Hyperinsulinemia and Hypoglycemia

Infants with Beckwith–Wiedemann syndrome, erythroblastosis fetalis, and those whose mothers have taken chlorpropamide or benzothiazides are at risk for development of hypoglycemia as a result of hyperinsulinism. In 1964, Beckwith and colleagues and Wiedemann independently reported the exophthalmos–macroglossia–gigantism syndrome. Such infants frequently have omphalocele, muscular macroglossia, macrosomia, and neonatal hypoglycemia. The hypoglycemia and macrosomia are caused by hyperinsulinism resulting from β-cell hypertrophy (67,68). Some of the morbidity and mortality originally associated with this syndrome was related to unrecognized hypoglycemia. Thus, early recognition and prevention of hypoglycemia is mandatory. The gene responsible for many of the features of this syndrome is 11p15.5. Because the insulin and insulin-like growth factor genes are closely localized, combined gene dosage imbalance probably also contributes to the development of hyperinsulinism and hypoglycemia (69,70).

Infants with erythroblastosis fetalis caused by Rh incompatibility were reported in the past to be at risk for hypoglycemia from hyperinsulinism secondary to β-cell hyperplasia (71). The mechanisms responsible for islet cell hyperplasia are unknown, although it was proposed that elevated plasma glutathione concentrations might stimulate the fetal β cell to increase insulin secretion (72). The advent of direct intravascular transfusion of Rh-affected fetuses may reduce the risk of hypoglycemia. Severely affected Rh fetuses that receive serial intravascular transfusions by the percutaneous umbilical technique are normoinsulinemic despite originally having elevated glutathione concentrations. Hypoglycemia does not develop in them as neonates (73).

It is important to note that infants undergoing exchange transfusion are at risk for development of hypoglycemia because of stimulation of insulin secretion by glucose in stored erythrocytes (74). Checking for hypoglycemia during and after an exchange transfusion is therefore important.

Maternal use of chlorpropamide and benzothiazide can directly increase insulin secretion in the neonate (75,76). β-Sympathomimetic agents used to stop premature labor have been reported to cause neonatal hypoglycemia (77). These drugs stimulate glycogen breakdown and gluconeogenesis in the mother and fetus (78). Both the increased availability of maternal glucose and the β-sympathomimetic agent that crosses the placenta stimulate fetal insulin secretion, resulting in neonatal hyperinsulinism and hypoglycemia. For these reasons, infants whose mothers received tocolytic therapy shortly before delivery should be monitored for hypoglycemia.

Some debate exists as to whether glucose administered to the mother during labor and delivery stimulates fetal β-cell secretion and causes neonatal hyperinsulinism and hypoglycemia. Acute maternal glucose loading may stimulate fetal insulin secretion and increase the risk of neonatal hypoglycemia (79). If glucose infusion is well controlled, the likelihood of this is minimized. Control of maternal glucose administration is particularly important in situations where the fetus is suspected of having heightened β-cell sensitivity (e.g., maternal diabetes, Rh incompatibility) because under these circumstances even moderate excursions of glucose may stimulate fetal insulin secretion.

Malposition of the tip of an umbilical artery catheter at a level between the tenth thoracic and the second lumbar vertebrae may result in glucose-stimulated hyperinsulinism. Several infants have been reported in whom hypoglycemia was relieved only when the tip of the umbilical artery catheter was repositioned. It has been proposed that glucose from the malpositioned catheter flows into the celiac axis, thereby stimulating insulin secretion (80). Animal studies have confirmed this possibility (81), which should be considered in unexplained cases of hypoglycemia.

Large-for-gestational-age (LGA) infants whose mothers do not have diabetes mellitus are at risk for transient hypoglycemia. This is particularly true of LGA infants of obese women (82). The mechanisms responsible for hypoglycemia are unknown, although limited data suggest that hyperinsulinism is not a major factor.

Sepsis in a neonate often is heralded by hypoglycemia or hyperglycemia. The mechanisms for this are not understood. Several studies have indicated rapid glucose disposal rates after intravenous challenge in septic term neonates. Although this suggests a hyperinsulinemic state, insulin secretion in these neonates was normal (83,84). The hyperglycemia and hypoglycemia that often precede the other signs of sepsis in premature infants may be catecholamine mediated.

Hypoglycemia is a well-acknowledged complication of the neonatal polycythemia–hyperviscosity syndrome (85). Although polycythemia is more likely to occur in SGA and LGA infants who are at risk for hypoglycemia for other reasons, hypoglycemia occurs at an increased rate in polycythemic appropriately grown infants. Animal studies have documented diminished cerebral glucose uptake with polycythemia; however, the mechanisms responsible for decreasing glucose provision are unknown (86). The increased erythrocyte mass is not sufficient to reduce glucose availability. The diminished plasma volume resulting from polycythemia may limit glucose provision. These possibilities remain to be confirmed.

Congenital hypopituitarism is a rare disorder in the neonate resulting from a spectrum of developmental accidents (87,88). Congenital absence of the anterior pituitary is the common cause of this disorder, although holoprosencephaly and optic disk dysplasia also have been associated. Affected male neonates have microphallus, whereas girls have normal external genitalia (89). Neonatal hypoglycemia often develops and can be severe. The endocrine alterations resulting from congenital hypopituitarism are complex, and the mechanisms by which they cause hypoglycemia are not understood. Congenital syphilis has been reported to cause hypopituitarism and this syndrome (90). Growth hormone is important in this regard because it can reverse hypoglycemia. Because hypoglycemia can develop later in the postnatal period, infants should have growth hormone therapy initiated for the long term.

Infants who have suffered hypothermia are at increased risk for development of hypoglycemia (91). This may result from increased availability of catecholamines (92), which would deplete glycogen reserves. Tissue use of glucose also might be increased under these conditions.

Other unusual clinical conditions reported in association with hypoglycemia include salicylate administration (93), congenital adrenal hyperplasia (94), and trisomy 13 mosaicism (95). The mechanisms for these phenomena are not known.

Hypoglycemia has been noted to sometimes occur in infants who suffer poor calorie intake for prolonged periods as a consequence of inadequate maternal breast milk production. The mechanisms for this are not known but probably involve glycogen depletion and diminished release of gluconeogenic precursers by striated muscle. Severe hepatic damage, most likely as a result of impaired substrate transport and gluconeogenic capability, can also cause hypoglycemia. Disruption of intravenous glucose administration or rapid reduction in the rate of a glucose infusion can be associated with rebound hypoglycemia as a result of sluggish beta-cell responsiveness; insulin secretion may not decrease with appropriate rapidity and in response to cessation of exogenous glucose.

NEONATAL HYPERGLYCEMIA

Hyperglycemia occurs primarily in three major groups of infants: those who are very premature, those who have neonatal diabetes mellitus, and those who are septic. Altered glucoregulation in response to sepsis was discussed in the preceding section (see Unexplained Neonatal Hyperinsulinemia and Hypoglycemia).

The Very Premature Infant

Advances in perinatal care have improved the survival rate of the very premature infant. With this, the problem of glucose intolerance has greatly increased because the risk of hyperglycemia is at least 18 times greater in infants weighing under 1,000 g than in those weighing over 2,000 g. Depending on the definition, age at screening, and type of intravenous solution administered, the incidence of hyperglycemia in very premature infants has been reported to range from 20% to 86% (96,97). In general, the smaller and more premature an infant, the greater the likelihood that he or she will not tolerate exogenous glucose at maintenance rates (4–6 mg/kg/min). It is not uncommon to administer glucose at 1 to 2 mg/kg/min or less and still observe plasma glucose concentrations exceeding 200 mg/dL.

Several basic mechanisms probably are responsible for glucose intolerance in very premature infants. Many probably do not secrete glucoregulatory hormones appropriately. In addition, end organ response to these hormones may be blunted. Thus, endogenous glucose production may continue while tissue glucose uptake is limited despite intravenous glucose therapy. Limited data indicate that the premature infant will only slowly increase insulin secretion in response to glucose challenge (98–102). The amount secreted may not be sufficient to regulate glucose. Such infants may (101) or may not (103) decrease glucagon in response to glucose. In addition, very premature infants can be resistant to insulin (104). This resistance is accentuated by catecholamines, which often are quite elevated. These factors contribute to the limited ability of the premature infant to reduce glucose production in the same manner as the adult, when exogenous glucose is provided (Fig. 35–8).

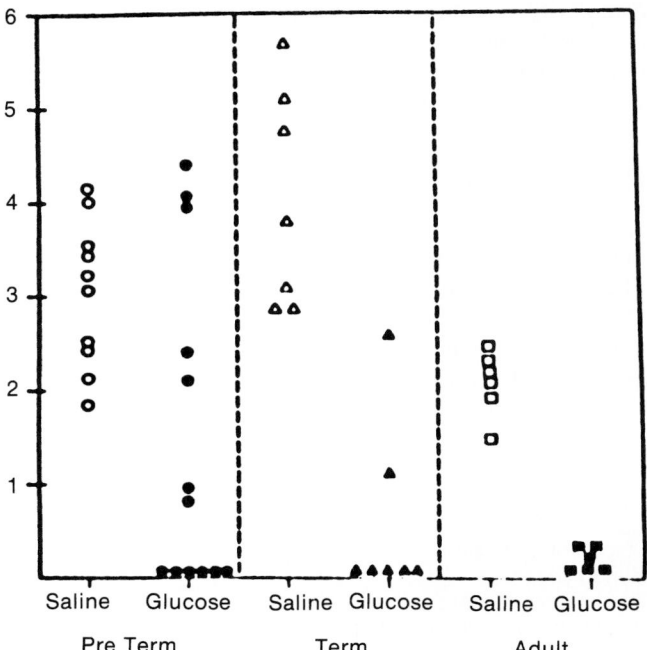

(mg·kg⁻¹min⁻¹)

FIG. 35–8. Hepatic glucose production rates (GPR) in human premature neonates, full-term neonates, and adults during either saline *(open symbols)* or glucose *(closed symbols)* infusion. With glucose infusion, adults and full-term infants but not preterm infants reduce endogenous glucose production. Many preterm infants are apparently unable to regulate glucose production; this contributes to the development of hyperglycemia in these infants. (From ref. 98.)

Neonatal Diabetes Mellitus

This is a rare disorder characterized by hypoinsulinism, progressive wasting, polyuria, and glycosuria during the neonatal period. Such infants usually are not ketotic. Of note, they are always SGA (105,106). The intrauterine growth retardation results from limited fetal insulin secretion and exemplifies the importance of insulin as a fetal growth-stimulating hormone. This disorder may be heterogeneous with respect to etiology. Synthesis of an abnormal, poorly functioning insulin molecule or receptor deficiencies are other possible causes. Neonatal diabetes mellitus usually is transient; the early acute period calls for standard diabetic therapy (i.e., monitoring caloric intake and administering exogenous insulin).

DIAGNOSIS AND TREATMENT

Hypoglycemia

All infants at risk for development of hypoglycemia should undergo frequent plasma glucose determinations. The commercially available paper strip indicators are widely used. Because their accuracy is fair, it is desirable to confirm values close to hypoglycemia or hyperglycemia with laboratory chemical determinations. Infants at risk for hypoglycemia should be checked frequently during the first 4 hours of life and then at 4-hour intervals until the risk period has passed. If an infant is feeding, blood sampling should be done before feeding. For IDMs and SGA infants, the screening should continue for at least 24 hours.

Infants who have borderline asymptomatic hypoglycemia, who do not have respiratory distress syndrome (RDS) or other serious disorders, and who are capable of enteral feedings may receive either 5% dextrose solution or formula as their initial treatment. In general, this approach can be used for infants at term who are LGA or SGA. However, because this mode of therapy is not always successful, plasma or blood glucose concentrations must be checked shortly after feeding.

Intravenous administration of glucose in a quantity sufficient to meet tissue requirements is the treatment of choice for hypoglycemia. The administration of 10% or 15% dextrose solution at 5 to 10 mL/kg body weight, followed by a continuous infusion at 5 to 6 mg/kg body weight/minute of glucose, will increase plasma glucose concentrations to 40 mg/dL or greater and acutely meet tissue requirements. The maintenance rates may require adjustment depending on the etiology of hypoglycemia.

Glucagon and epinephrine increase glucose production. Because both mobilize hepatic glycogen stores, their efficacy in treating hypoglycemia is variable, particularly in infants with limited hepatic stores. The numerous cardiovascular effects of epinephrine also limit its usefulness in infants.

Infants who are hypoglycemic for prolonged periods as a result of an inability to produce glucose can be treated with corticosteroids (hydrocortisone 5 mg/kg/day every 12 hours; prednisone 2 mg/kg/day orally). Steroids exert some of their effects by inducing gluconeogenic enzyme activity.

Hyperglycemia

Hyperglycemia in low-birth-weight infants traditionally has been treated by reducing the rate of administration of exogenous glucose. This is something of a clinical paradox because such a reduction can theoretically limit glucose availability to the brain. Attempts in the past to provide exogenous insulin as a means to regulate glucose met with variable success, primarily because of technical difficulties in providing insulin (104,107,108). New insulin delivery systems designed for children and adults provide the means to deliver minute amounts of insulin under controlled conditions. These systems have finely tuned programmable pumps and tubing that does not bind insulin (109). Application of this technology has met with preliminary success (110). Individualized continuous insulin infusion to infants at 26 weeks of gestation weighing 700 to 800 g enhanced glucose infusion and parenteral energy intake. Weight gain was significantly greater over 7 to 21 days compared with infants managed conventionally (Fig. 35–9). If further studies confirm these observations and clarify the potential metabolic consequences of this therapy, this method may prove beneficial in treating hyperglycemia in low-birth-weight infants.

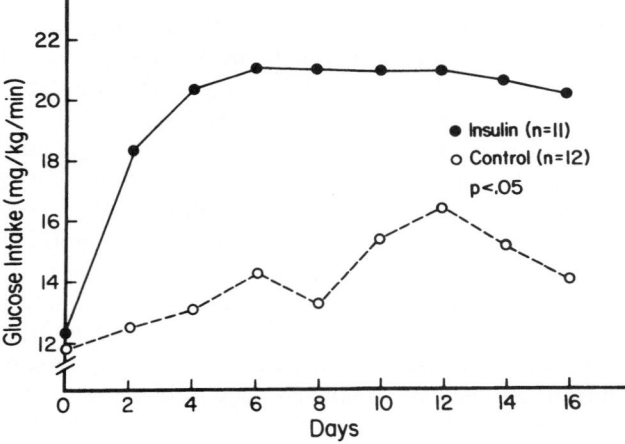

FIG. 35–9. Mean glucose infusion rates per day in insulin-treated *(solid line)* and control *(dashed line)* very-low-birth-weight infants. The controlled administration of insulin significantly increased glucose infusion from day 2 to 16. (From ref. 10.)

CONSEQUENCES

Hypoglycemia

The clinical manifestations of inadequate glucose provision to the brain range from no symptoms to mild tremors to seizures. The issue of potential long-term sequelae of hypoglycemia remains unclear. This issue is complicated by the fact that hypoglycemia often occurs in infants who have coexisting conditions that also can cause brain damage. The observations suggesting that asymptomatic hypoglycemia poses less of a risk compared to symptomatic hypoglycemia are limited, as are the observations that associate prolonged hypoglycemia with a greater risk of brain damage than brief hypoglycemia. Limited data suggest that seizures associated with hypoglycemia worsen prognosis (111–120). Because of the uncertainty in this area, all hypoglycemic infants, symptomatic or not, should be appropriately treated.

Hyperglycemia

Hyperglycemia has been associated with an increased incidence of mortality, intracranial hemorrhage, and developmental delay in very premature infants. Whether hyperglycemia causes these problems or is merely associated with their development is unclear. Increased serum osmolarity resulting from hyperglycemia might disrupt cell–serum balance and cause cell injury (96). In addition, hyperglycemia can alter cell glucose transport, which may perturb cell metabolic functions.

INFANTS OF DIABETIC MOTHERS

Table 35–3 lists the frequently occurring problems of the IDM categorized according to proposed mechanisms. The fetal and neonatal hyperinsulinism central to many of these problems results from exaggerated provision of maternal metabolic fuels to the fetus, resulting in pancreatic β-cell hypertrophy, hyperplasia, and hyperfunction (1,9). The alterations in maternal metabolism resulting

TABLE 35–3. *Problems of the infant of a diabetic mother*

Macrosomia or birth stress
Hypoglycemia
Respiratory distress syndrome
Intrauterine growth retardation
Hypocalcemia
Hyperbilirubinemia
Polycythemia or hyperviscosity
Cardiomyopathy
Congenital anomalies
Hyperinsulinism
Altered metabolic fuels, uteroplacental insufficiency
Decreased parathormone
Increased erythrocyte destruction, bruising

from diabetes mellitus that are responsible for these and other effects on the fetus have been reviewed.

Altered Fetal Growth

Macrosomia, a clinical term suggesting excessive weight for gestational age, is a well-known characteristic of IDMs (Fig. 35–10). Macrosomia in the IDM results primarily from increased adiposity because IDMs have both adipocyte hyperplasia and adipocyte hypertrophy (121). Infants of diabetic mothers also have excess non-fatty tissue. The liver and heart often are enlarged, and skeletal muscle increased. Much of this excess tissue is located in the shoulders and intrascapular area. Because IDMs have normal brain growth, this results in a disproportionality between head and shoulder size and greatly increases the risk of shoulder dystocia (Fig. 35–11). This birth complication occurs far more frequently in macrosomic IDMs than in large infants of mothers who do not have diabetes. Macrosomia is responsible for the great risk of birth trauma, meconium aspiration syndrome, persistent pulmonary hypertension, and the high incidence of cesarean section delivery in IDMs.

Because insulin has both mitogenic and anabolic effects in the fetus, the fetal hyperinsulinemic state is central to the development of macrosomia. The augmented production of insulin by the fetus stimulates the growth of insulin-sensitive tissues (e.g., adipose, muscle, connective) to cause macrosomia. Hepatic glycogen storage is exaggerated. The effect of insulin probably is mediated to some extent through stimulation of insulin-like growth factors (122). It is not surprising that head growth is normal in IDMs during intrauterine life because insulin does not stimulate brain growth to any great extent.

The excess fat in IDMs develops during the third trimester; IDMs delivered before 30 weeks of gestation rarely are LGA. Serial fetal ultrasound measurements confirm that the fetal IDM does not exceed normal growth limits until 28 to 30 weeks of gestation (31).

Despite improved maternal therapy, 20% to 30% of insulin-dependent diabetic women continue to bear macrosomic infants (123). Women with gestational diabetes, the mildest form of carbohydrate intolerance, have as great an incidence of macrosomia as women with pre-existing diabetes.

Intrauterine growth retardation is another well-known complication of diabetes in pregnancy. The development of growth retardation has been attributed to maternal vascular disease, causing uteroplacental insufficiency. More recent data suggest that growth retardation may result from alterations in maternal metabolic fuel availability during early gestation (124).

Hypoglycemia

Approximately 25% to 50% of all IDMs who manifest hypoglycemia will do so within the first 24 hours of life. Hypoglycemia is particularly likely to occur in macrosomic IDMs because hyperinsulinism is responsible for both fetal overgrowth and hypoglycemia (Fig. 35–12) (125). Several studies also suggest that these IDMs may fail to release glucagon or catecholamines in response to hypoglycemia (126). These hormonal alterations result in both increased glucose clearance and diminished glucose production.

Hypocalcemia and Hypomagnesemia

Hypocalcemia develops in 10% to 20% of IDMs during the neonatal period. This usually occurs in association with hyperphosphatemia and occasionally with hypomagnesemia. Parathormone concentrations are significantly lower in IDMs than in infants of normal mothers during the first 4 days of life (Fig. 35–13). This may be a result of hypomagnesemia, which limits parathormone secretion even in the presence of hypocalcemia. Maternal hypomagnesemia, which may occur from increased renal loss secondary to diabetes, is believed responsible for

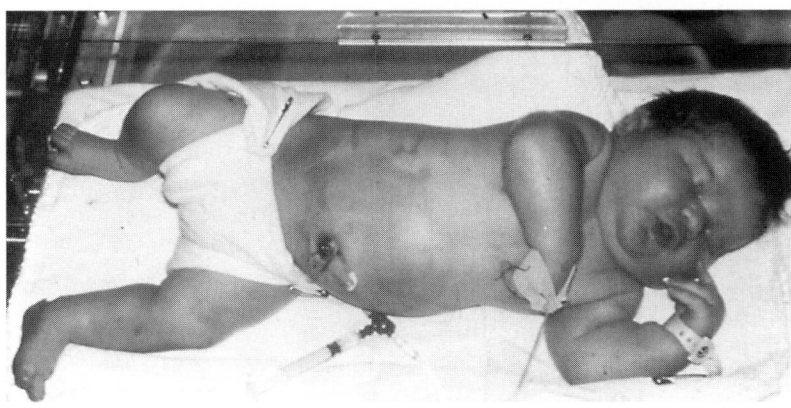

FIG. 35–10. A macrosomic infant of a diabetic mother (IDM) has head circumference and length that are at the 90th percentile; the IDM's body weight greatly exceeds the 90th percentile. The IDM has considerable fat deposition in the shoulder and intrascapular area.

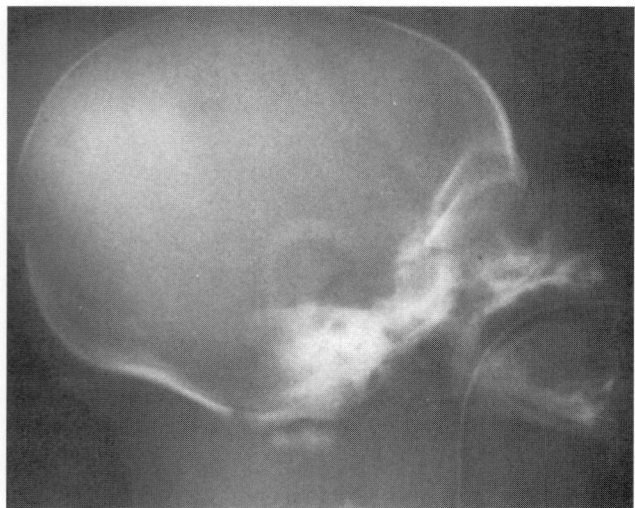

FIG. 35–11. Lateral skull and neck radiograph of an infant of a diabetic mother after a difficult vaginal delivery. Infants of diabetic mothers are at extreme risk for shoulder dystocia, which can result in severe complications, such as separation of the C1–C2 cervical spine.

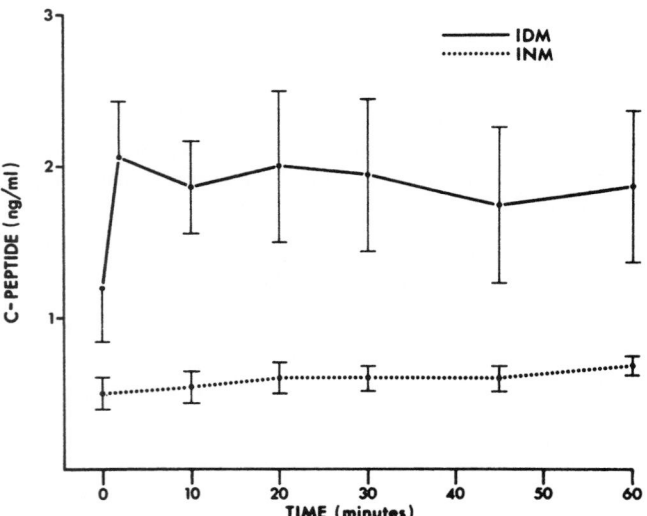

FIG. 35–12. β-Cell response to intravenous glucose challenge in infants of diabetic mothers (IDMs) and infants of mothers with normal carbohydrate metabolism (INM). C-peptide is cleared from the proinsulin molecule when the β cell is stimulated to secrete insulin. The measurement of C-peptide represents insulin on an equimolar basis and is a more accurate measure of β-cell secretion than insulin in IDMs. Infants of diabetic mothers exuberantly secrete insulin in response to glucose challenge. This adult-like response differs greatly from the normally expected sluggish insulin response of the INM. The significantly increased insulin concentration in IDMs before glucose challenge (i.e., 0 minutes) indicates that basal insulin secretion also is elevated. The increased β-cell function in IDMs is responsible for their high incidence of hypoglycemia.

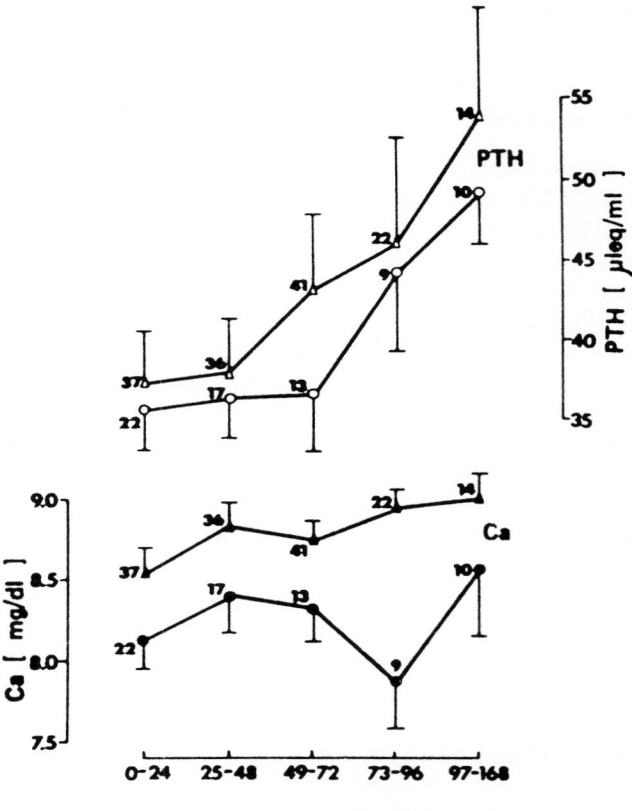

POSTNATAL AGE IN HOURS

FIG. 35–13. Parathormone (PTH) and calcium concentration in infants of diabetic mothers *(circles)* and full-term control *(triangles)* infants. Infants of diabetic mothers have lower plasma calcium and PTH concentrations during the first 6 days of life. (From ref. 127.)

fetal and neonatal hypomagnesemia (127,128). Birth asphyxia, which frequently occurs in IDMs, also causes hypocalcemia.

Hyperbilirubinemia

Indirect hyperbilirubinemia develops in 20% to 25% of IDMs. Their carbon monoxide production is increased as a result of increased hemoglobin breakdown and bilirubin production (129). The increased rate of erythrocyte breakdown in IDMs is probably linked to altered erythrocyte membrane composition resulting from changes in maternal fuel availability. Polycythemia frequently occurs in IDMs, and the normal breakdown of this increased erythrocyte mass also causes hyperbilirubinemia. Macrosomic IDMs often are bruised at birth; the resultant resorption of blood also contributes to hyperbilirubinemia.

Hyperviscosity

Infants of diabetic mothers have a 10% to 20% risk of being polycythemic and developing the neonatal hyperviscosity syndrome. Several factors are responsible for this. The hematocrit of umbilical cord blood at birth tends to be elevated, probably as a result of increased erythropoiesis (130).

The increased incidence of renal vein thrombosis reported in IDMs may be related to hyperviscosity, although this disorder does occur in IDMs with normal hematocrits.

Unexpected Fetal Death

In the past, a high incidence of unexpected fetal death occurred in late gestation. Improvement in metabolic control of maternal diabetes throughout pregnancy and new methods to assess fetal status have decreased the incidence of this tragic complication. The mechanisms of unexpected fetal death are not completely understood. In the fetal sheep, sustained hyperglycemia is associated with increased insulin secretion, elevated fetal oxygen consumption, acidosis, and death (131). This could explain the association between poor maternal metabolic control and the increased risk of fetal death.

Respiratory Distress Syndrome

Infants of diabetic mothers are at increased risk of developing RDS. In the past, IDMs have been at a fourfold to sixfold greater risk for RDS than infants of normal mothers (132). This incidence has been reduced substantially by the recent emphasis on tight control of maternal metabolism. The increased risk of RDS in poorly regulated diabetic women is due in great part to fetal hyperinsulinism. Insulin adversely affects fetal lung maturation by inhibiting the development of enzymes necessary for the synthesis of the phospholipid components of surfactant (133). Standard methods to assess fetal lung maturity antenatally may not be applicable to a diabetic pregnancy. The measurement of phosphotidyl-glycerol has greatly improved this capability.

Cardiomyopathy

Infants of diabetic mothers are at increased risk for various cardiomyopathies (134). Many have thickening of the interventricular septum and the left or right ventricular wall. The increased cardiac muscle mass results from the fetal hyperinsulinemic state. Most of these infants are asymptomatic, and the thickening is detected by electrocardiogram or echocardiogram. In a small fraction of infants, outflow obstruction severe enough to cause left ventricular failure may occur. These abnormalities generally regress over 3 to 6 months, and the condition appears to have no permanent effect on the myocardium. Those infants with congestive heart failure who survive the initial period with medical management also improve spontaneously.

Occasionally, IDMs have severe congestive heart failure at birth. Frequently, these infants have suffered intrapartum asphyxia and are hypoglycemic and hypocalcemic. Such infants generally respond to assisted ventilation and correction of their metabolic abnormalities and usually recover completely. It is unclear whether heart failure results from the combined effects of hypoglycemia, hypocalcemia, and asphyxia on an inherently normal myocardium, or whether the myocardium is abnormal and therefore more susceptible to failure.

Congenital Abnormalities

Major congenital malformations occur two to four times more frequently in IDMs than in infants born to nondiabetic women. Although many abnormalities occur in IDMs, ventricular septal defects, transposition of the great arteries, and the spinal agenesis–caudal regression syndrome occur with particular frequency (Fig. 35–14). Neural tube defects, gastrointestinal atresia, and urinary tract malformations also are relatively common. A transient anomaly unique to the IDM is known as the neonatal small left colon, microcolon, or lazy colon syndrome. This condition presents as gastrointestinal obstruction,

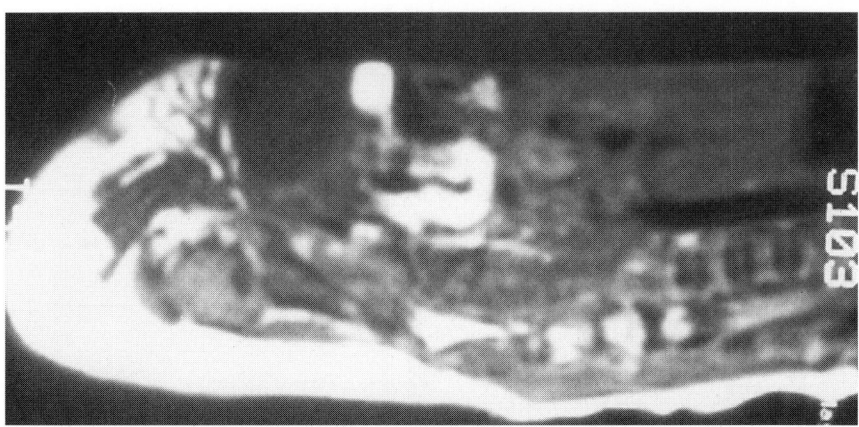

FIG. 35–14. Magnetic resonance image of an infant of a diabetic mother. The infant has spinal agenesis–caudal regression syndrome. The spinal cord is interrupted, and hip–femur relationships are malformed.

and barium contrast studies suggest congenital aganglionic megacolon. Unlike infants with Hirschsprung disease, these infants have normal innervation of the bowel and ultimately have normal bowel function.

Poor control of maternal diabetes during the first trimester, a critical period of organogenesis, has been proposed as the mechanism for the increased incidence of malformations (135,136). Infants of diabetic mothers with abnormalities have normal karyotypes (137). *In vitro* studies using embryos of laboratory animals have demonstrated that altering metabolic fuels can produce profound malformations (138). Clinical studies, however, have not confirmed a relation between birth defects and alterations in maternal metabolic variables (139).

Postnatal Problems

Infants of diabetic mothers are at increased risk for development of obesity in later life, compared to infants of mothers with normal carbohydrate metabolism (140). Studies suggest that *in utero* hyperinsulinism may be responsible for this postnatal phenomenon. Infants of diabetic mothers who become obese during childhood have the severest hyperinsulinism *in utero* (141).

Whether maternal diabetes adversely affects the long-term cognitive development of the offspring remains unanswered. In the past, the increased incidence of birth trauma and neonatal disorders probably contributed to an increased risk of poor outcome. Studies suggest that altered maternal metabolic fuel availability also may have an effect. An inverse correlation has been reported between childhood IQ and degree of abnormality of second- and third-trimester maternal lipid metabolism (142). This is consistent with the potential detrimental effect of ketones on fetal brain development.

A yet unanswered question is whether IDMs develop diabetes mellitus during postnatal life. Children and adults who were IDMs have an increased incidence of diabetes mellitus. Limited data suggest that offspring of fathers with insulin-dependent diabetes have a fivefold greater risk for development of diabetes mellitus than offspring of insulin-dependent diabetic mothers (143). Although diabetes is in part a genetic disorder, it has not been possible to delineate precisely the mode of inheritance in IDMs. It is possible that the altered metabolic state of the diabetic pregnancy may modulate this genetic predisposition. Non-insulin-dependent diabetes mellitus occurs by age 20 years in 45.5% of IDMs of insulin-dependent diabetic mothers but in only 8.6% and 1.4% of prediabetic and nondiabetic mothers, respectively (144). The mechanisms by which alterations in maternal glucose and other metabolic fuels alter fetal β-cell function are unknown.

REFERENCES

1. Freinkel N. Banting lecture 1980: of pregnancy and progeny. *Diabetes* 1980;29:1023.
2. Hytten ET, Leitch I. *The physiology of human pregnancy,* 2nd ed. Oxford: Blackwell Scientific Publications, 1971.
3. Kalkhoff R, Schalch DS, Walker JG, et al. Diabetogenic factors associated with pregnancy. *Trans Assoc Am Physicians* 1974;77:270.
4. Lind T, Billewicz WZ, Brown G. A serial study of changes occurring in the oral glucose tolerance test during pregnancy. *J Obstet Gynaecol Br Commonw* 1973;80:1033.
5. Spellacy WN, Goetz FC. Plasma insulin in normal late pregnancy. *N Engl J Med* 1963;268:988.
6. Grumbach MM, Kaplan SL, Sciarra JJ, et al. Chorionic growth hormone prolactin (CGP) secretion, disposition, biologic activity in man, and postulated function as the "growth hormone" of the second half of pregnancy. *Ann NY Acad Sci* 1968;148:501.
7. Johansson EDB. Plasma levels of progesterone in pregnancy measured by a rapid competitive binding technique. *Acta Endocrinol* 1969;61:607.
8. Kalkhoff RJ, Kissebah AH, Kim HJ. Carbohydrate and lipid metabolism during normal pregnancy: relationship to gestational hormone action. *Semin Perinatol* 1978;2:291.
9. Pedersen J. *The pregnant diabetic and her newborn,* 2nd ed. Baltimore: Williams & Wilkins, 1977.
10. Bleicher SJ, O'Sullivan JB, Freinkel N. Carbohydrate metabolism in pregnancy: V. The interrelations of glucose, insulin and free fatty acids in late pregnancy and post partum. *N Engl J Med* 1964;271:866.
11. Felig P, Lynch V. Starvation in human pregnancy: hypoglycemia, hypoinsulinemia, and hyperketonemia. *Science* 1970;170:990.
12. Kalhan SC, D'Angelo LJ, Savin SM, et al. Glucose production in pregnant women at term gestation: sources of glucose for human fetus. *J Clin Invest* 1979;63:388.
13. Ogata ES, Metzger BE, Freinkel N. Carbohydrate metabolism in pregnancy: XVI. Longitudinal estimates of the effects of pregnancy on D-(6-^{3}H) glucose and D-(6-^{14}C) glucose turnovers during fasting in the rat. *Metabolism* 1981;30:487.
14. Scow RO, Chernick SS, Brinley MS. Hyperlipemia and ketosis in the pregnant rat. *Am J Physiol* 1964;206:796.
15. Patel MS, Johnson CA, Rajan R, et al. The metabolism of ketone bodies in developing human brain: development of ketone-body-utilizing enzymes and ketone bodies as precursors for lipid synthesis. *J Neurochem* 1975;25:905.
16. Churchill JA, Berendes HW, Nemore J. Neuropsychological deficits in children of diabetic mothers. *Am J Obstet Gynecol* 1969;105:257.
17. Shelley HJ. Glycogen reserves and their changes at birth and in anoxia. *Br Med Bull* 1961;17:137.
18. Schwartz AL, Rall TW. Hormonal regulation of incorporation of alanine-U-^{14}C into glucose in human fetal liver explants: effect of dibutyryl cyclic AMP, glucagon, insulin, and triamcinolone. *Diabetes* 1975;24:650.
19. Schwartz AL, Rall TW. Hormonal regulation of glycogen metabolism in human fetal liver. *Diabetes* 1975;24:1113.
20. Greengard O. Enzymatic differentiation of human liver: comparison with the rat model. *Pediatr Res* 1977;11:669.
21. Raiha HN, Lindros KO. Development of some enzymes involved in gluconeogenesis in human liver. *Ann Med Exp Biol Fenn* 1964;47:146.
22. Kaplan SL, Grumbach MM, Shepard TH. The ontogenesis of human fetal hormones: I. Growth hormone and insulin. *J Clin Invest* 1972;51:3080.
23. Assan R, Buillet J. Pancreatic glucagon and glucagon-like material in tissues and plasma from human fetuses 6 to 26 weeks old. In Jonxis JH, ed. *Metabolic processes in the fetus and newborn infant.* Baltimore: Williams & Wilkins, 1971:210.
24. Schaeffer LD, Wilder ML, Williams RH. Secretion and content of insulin and glucagon in human fetal pancreas slices *in vitro. Proc Soc Exp Biol Med* 1973;143:314.
25. Grasso S, Distefano G, Messina A, et al. Effect of glucose priming on insulin response in the premature infant. *Diabetes* 1975;24:291.
26. Milner RDG. The development of insulin secretion in man. In Jonxis JH, ed. *Metabolic processes in the fetus and newborn infant, nutrition symposium.* Baltimore: Williams & Wilkins, 1971:310.
27. Grasso S, Messina A, Distefano G, et al. Insulin secretion in the premature infant: response to glucose and amino acids. *Diabetes* 1973;22:349.
28. Wise JK, Lyall SS, Hendler R, et al. Evidence of stimulation of glucagon secretion by alanine in the human fetus at term. *J Clin Endocrinol Metab* 1973;37:345.
29. Hill DE. Effect of insulin on fetal growth. *Semin Perinatol* 1978;2:319.

30. Susa JB, McCormick KL, Widness JA, et al. Chronic hyperinsulinemia in the fetal rhesus monkey: effects on fetal growth and composition. *Diabetes* 1979;28:1058.

31. Ogata ES, Sabbagha R, Metzger BE, et al. Serial ultrasonography to assess evolving fetal macrosomia. *JAMA* 1980;243:2405.

32. Pedersen J. Weight and length at birth of infants of diabetic mothers. *Acta Endocrinol* 1954;16:330.

33. Girard JF, Caquet D, Bal D. Control of rat liver phosphorylase and phosphoenolpyruvate carboxykinase activities by insulin and glucagon during the perinatal period. *Enzyme* 1973;15:272.

34. Girard JR, Ferre A, Kervran A, et al. Role of the insulin/glucagon ratio in the changes of hepatic metabolism during development of the rat. In Foa PP, Bajaj JS, Foa NL, eds. *Glucagon: its role in physiology and clinical medicine.* New York: Springer-Verlag, 1977:563.

35. Sperling MA, DeLamater PV, Phelps D, et al. Spontaneous and amino acid stimulated glucagon secretion in the immediate postnatal period: relation to glucose and insulin. *J Clin Invest* 1974;53:1159.

36. Padbury J, Agata Y, Ludlow J, et al. Effect of fetal adrenalectomy on catecholamine release and physiologic adaptation at birth in sheep. *J Clin Invest* 1987;80:1096.

37. Agata Y, Padbury JF, Ludlow JK, et al. The effect of chemical sympathectomy on catecholamine release at birth. *Pediatr Res* 1986;20:1338.

38. Grajwer LA, Sperling MA, Sack J, et al. Possible mechanisms and significance of the neonatal surge in glucagon secretion: studies in newborn lambs. *Pediatr Res* 1977;11:833.

39. Molsted-Pedersen L. Aspects of carbohydrate metabolism in newborn infants of diabetic mothers: II. Neonatal changes in K values. *Acta Endocrinol* 1972;69:189.

40. Bell GI, Kayano T, Buse JB, et al. Molecular biology of mammalian glucose transporters. *Diabetes Care* 1990;13:198.

41. Devaskar S, Mueckler M. The mammalian glucose transporters. *Pediatr Res* 1992;31:1.

42. Takata K, Kasahara T, Kasahara M, Ezaki D, Hirano H. Localization of erythrocyte/Hep G2 type glucose transport (Glut 1) in human placental villi. *Cell Tiss Res* 1992;267:407.

43. Simmons RA, Flozak A, Ogata ES. The effect of insulin and insulin-like growth factor I on glucose transport in normal and small for gestational age fetal rats. *Endocrinology* 1993;133:1361.

44. Bier DM, Arnold KJ, Sherman WR, et al. *In vivo* measurement of glucose and alanine metabolism with stable isotopic tracers. *Diabetes* 1977;26:1005.

45. Bier DM, Leake RD, Haymond MW, et al. Measurement of "true" glucose production rates in infancy and childhood with 6,6-dideuteroglucose. *Diabetes* 1977;26:1016.

46. Kalhan SC, Bier DM, Savin SM, et al. Estimation of glucose turnover and ^{13}C recycling in the human newborn by simultaneous [1-^{13}C]glucose and [6,6-^{2}H$_2$]glucose tracers. *J Clin Endocrinol Metab* 1980;50:456.

47. Kalhan SC, Savin SM, Adam PAJ. Measurement of glucose turnover in the human newborn with glucose-1-^{13}C. *J Clin Endocrinol Metab* 1976;43:704.

48. Sunebag A, Ewald U, Larsson A, Gustafsson J. Glucose production rate in extremely immature neonates (< 28 weeks) studied by use of deuterated glucose. *Pediatr Res* 1993;33:97.

49. Cornblath M, Schwartz R. *Disorders of carbohydrate metabolism in infancy,* 3rd ed. Boston: Blackwell Scientific Publications, 1991.

50. Pagliara AS, Karl IE, Haymond M, et al. Hypoglycemia in infancy and childhood: Parts I and II. *J Pediatr* 1973;82:365,558.

51. Ogata ES. Carbohydrate metabolism in the fetus and neonate and altered neonatal glucoregulation. *Pediatr Clin North Am* 1986;33:25.

52. Lubchenco LO, Bard H. Incidence of hypoglycemia in newborn infants classified by birth weight and gestational age. *Pediatrics* 1971;47:831.

53. Greene HL. Glycogen storage disease. *Semin Liver Dis* 1982;8:291.

54. Haymond MW, Karl IE, Pagliara AS. Increased gluconeogenic substrates in the small-for-gestational-age infant. *N Engl J Med* 1974;291:322.

55. Mestyan J, Soltesz G, Schultz K, Horvath M. Hyperaminoacidemia due to the accumulation of gluconeogenic amino acid precursors in hypoglycemic small-for-gestational age infants. *J Pediatr* 1975;87:409.

56. Bussey ME, Finley S, LaBarbera A, et al. Hypoglycemia in the newborn growth-retarded rat: delayed phosphoenolpyruvate carboxykinase induction despite increased glucagon availability. *Pediatr Res* 1985;19:363.

57. Pollak A, Susa JB, Stonestreet BS, et al. Phosphoenolpyruvate carboxykinase in experimental intrauterine growth retardation in rats. *Pediatr Res* 1979;13:175.

58. Sinclair JC, Silverman WA. Intrauterine growth in active tissue mass

59. of the human fetus, with particular reference to the undergrown baby. *Pediatrics* 1966;38:48.

59. Vidnes J, Sovik O. Gluconeogenesis in infancy and childhood: II. Studies on the glucose production from alanine in three cases of persistent neonatal hypoglycaemia. *Acta Paediatr Scand* 1976;65:297.

60. Vidnes J, Oyasaetor S. Glucagon deficiency causing severe neonatal hypoglycemia in a patient with normal insulin secretion. *Pediatr Res* 1977;11:943.

61. Garces LY, Drash A, Kenny FM. Islet cell tumor in the neonate. *Pediatrics* 1968;41:789.

62. Heitz PU, Kloppel G, Hacki WH, et al. Nesidioblastosis: the pathologic basis of persistent hyperinsulinemic hypoglycemia in infants. *Diabetes* 1977;26:632.

63. Salinas ED, Mangurten HH, Roberts SS, et al. Functioning islet cell adenoma in the newborn. *Pediatrics* 1968;41:646.

64. Otonkoski T, Andersson S, Simell O. Somatostatin regulation of β-cell function in the normal human fetuses and neonates with persistent hyperinsulinemic hypoglycemia. *J Clin Endocrinol Metab* 1993;76:184.

65. Dunne M, Kane C, Shepherd R, et al. Familial persistent hyperinsulinemic hypoglycemia of infancy and mutations in the sulfonurea receptor. *N Engl J Med* 1997;336:703.

66. Leibowitz G, Glaser B, Higazi A, Salameh M, Cerasi E, Landeau H. Hyperinsulinemic hypoglycemia of infancy (nesidioblastosis) in clinical remission: High incidence of diabetes mellitus and persistent β-cell dysfunction at long-term follow up. *J Clin Endocrinol Metab* 1995;80:386.

67. Beckwith JB. Macroglossia, omphalocele, adrenal cytomegaly, gigantism, and hyperplastic visceromegaly. *Birth Defects* 1967;5:188.

68. Wiedemann HR. E.M.G. syndrome and carbohydrate metabolism. *Lancet* 1968;2:104.

69. Normal AM. Recurrent Wiedmann-Beckwith syndrome with inversion of chromosome (II) (p11.2p15.5). *Am J Med Genet* 1992;42:638.

70. Weksburg R. Disruption of insulin-like growth factor 2 imprinting in Beckwith-Wiedemann syndrome. *Nature Genet* 1993;5:143.

71. Barrett CT, Oliver TK. Hypoglycemia and hyperinsulinism in infants with erythroblastosis fetalis. *N Engl J Med* 1968;278:1260.

72. Steinke J, Gries FA, Driscoll SG. *In vitro* studies of insulin inactivation with reference to erythroblastosis fetalis. *Blood* 1967;30:359.

73. Socol ML, Dooley SL, Ney JA, et al. Absence of hyperinsulinemia in isoimmunized fetuses treated with intravascular transfusion. *Am J Obstet Gynecol* 1991;165:1737.

74. Milner RDG, Chouksey SK, Assan R. Metabolic and hormonal effects of glucagon infusion in erythroblastotic infants. *Arch Dis Child* 1973;48:885.

75. Senior B, Slone D, Shapiro S, et al. Benzothiadiazides and neonatal hypoglycaemia. *Lancet* 1976;2:377.

76. Zucker P, Simon G. Prolonged symptomatic neonatal hypoglycemia associated with maternal chlorpropamide therapy. *Pediatrics* 1968;42:824.

77. Brazy JE, Pupkin MJ. Effects of maternal isoxsuprine administration on preterm infants. *J Pediatr* 1979;94:444.

78. Ogata ES. Isoxsuprine infusion in the rat: alterations in maternal, fetal and neonatal glucose homeostasis. *J Perinat Med* 1981;9:293.

79. Kenepp NB, Shelley WC, Gabbe SG, et al. Fetal and neonatal hazards of maternal hydration with 5% dextrose before caesarean section. *Lancet* 1982;1:1150.

80. Nagel JW, Sims S, Aplin CE, et al. Refractory hypoglycemia associated with a malpositioned umbilical artery catheter. *Pediatrics* 1979;64:315.

81. Cowett RM, Tenenbaum DG, Fatoba O, et al. The effects of arterial glucose infusion above the celiac axis in the neonatal lamb. *Biol Neonate* 1985;47:179.

82. Kliegman R, Gross T, Morton S, et al. Intrauterine growth and postnatal fasting metabolism in infants of obese mothers. *J Pediatr* 1984;104:601.

83. Leake RD, Fiser RH, Oh W. Rapid glucose disappearance in infants with infection. *Clin Pediatr* 1981;20:397.

84. Yeung CY, Lee VWY, Yeung CM. Glucose disappearance rate in neonatal infection. *J Pediatr* 1973;82:486.

85. Wiswell TE, Cornish JD, Northam RS. Neonatal polycythemia: frequency of clinical manifestations and other associated findings. *Pediatrics* 1986;78:26.

86. Rosenkrantz TS, Philipps AF, Skrzypczak PS, et al. Cerebral metabolism in the newborn lamb with polycythemia. *Pediatr Res* 1988;23:329.

87. Lovinger RD, Kaplan SL, Grumbach MM. Congenital hypopitu-

itarism associated with neonatal hypoglycemia and microphallus: four cases secondary to hypothalamic hormone deficiencies. *J Pediatr* 1975;87:1171.

88. Johnson JD, Hansen RC, Albritton WL, et al. Hypoplasia of the anterior pituitary and neonatal hypoglycemia. *J Pediatr* 1973;82:634.

89. Kauschansky A, Genel M, Walker Smith GJ. Congenital hypopituitarism in female infants. *Am J Dis Child* 1979;133:165.

90. Daaboul J, Kartchner W, Jones K. Neonatal hypoglycemia caused by hypopituitarism in infants with congenital syphilis. *J Pediatr* 1993;123:983.

91. Bower BD, Jones LF, Weeks MM. Cold injury in the newborn. *Br Med J* 1972;1:303.

92. Schiff D, Stern L, Leduc J. Chemical thermogenesis in newborn infants: catecholamine excretion and the plasma non-esterified fatty acid response to cold exposure. *Pediatrics* 1966;37:577.

93. Pickering D. Neonatal hypoglycemia due to salicylate poisoning. *Proc R Soc Med* 1968;61:1256.

94. Gemelli M, De Luca F, Barberio G. Hypoglycaemia and congenital adrenal hyperplasia. *Acta Paediatr Scand* 1979;68:285.

95. Smith VS, Giacoia GP. Hyperinsulinaemic hypoglycaemia in an infant with mosaic trisomy 13. *J Med Genet* 1985;22:228.

96. Pildes RS. Neonatal hyperglycemia. *J Pediatr* 1986;109:905.

97. Dweck HS, Cassady G. Glucose intolerance in infants of very low birth weight: I. Incidence of hyperglycemia in infants of birth weights 1,100 grams or less. *Pediatrics* 1974;53:189.

98. Cowett RM, Oh W, Schwartz R. Persistent glucose production during glucose infusion in the neonate. *J Clin Invest* 1983;71:467.

99. Hertz DG, Karn CA, Liu YM, Liechty EA, Denne SC. Intravenous glucose suppresses glucose production but not proteolysis in extremely premature newborns. *J Clin Invest* 1993;92:1752.

100. Lilien LD, Rosenfield RL, Baccaro MM, et al. Hyperglycemia in stressed small premature infants. *J Pediatr* 1979;94:454.

101. Massi-Benedetti F, Falorni A, Luyckx A, et al. Inhibition of glucagon secretion in the human newborn by simultaneous administration of glucose and insulin. *Horm Metab Res* 1974;6:392.

102. Zarif M, Pildes RS, Vidyasagar D. Insulin and growth-hormone responses in neonatal hyperglycemia. *Diabetes* 1976;25:428.

103. Grasso S, Fallucca F, Mazzone D, et al. Inhibition of glucagon secretion in the human newborn by glucose infusion. *Diabetes* 1983;32:489.

104. Goldman SL, Hirata T. Attenuated response to insulin in very low birthweight infants. *Pediatr Res* 1980;14:50.

105. Gentz JCH, Cornblath M. Transient diabetes of the newborn. *Adv Pediatr* 1969;16:345.

106. Hutchinson JH, Keay AJ, Kerr MM. Congenital temporary diabetes mellitus. *Br Med J* 1962;2:436.

107. Vaucher YE, Walson PD, Morrow G. Continuous insulin infusion in hyperglycemic, very low birth weight infants. *J Pediatr Gastroenterol Nutr* 1982;1:211.

108. Binder ND, Raschko PK, Benda GI, et al. Insulin infusion with parenteral nutrition in extremely low birth weight infants with hyperglycemia. *J Pediatr* 1989;114:273.

109. Ostertag SG, Jovanovic L, Lewis B, et al. Insulin pump therapy in the very low birth weight infant. *Pediatrics* 1986;78:625.

110. Collins JW, Hoppe M, Brown K, et al. A controlled trial of insulin infusion and parenteral nutrition in extremely low birth weight infants with glucose intolerance. *J Pediatr* 1991;118:921.

111. Creery RDG. Hypoglycaemia in the newborn: diagnosis, treatment, and prognosis. *Dev Med Child Neurol* 1966;8:746.

112. Haworth JC. Neonatal hypoglycemia: how much does it damage the brain? *Pediatrics* 1974;54:3.

113. Haworth JC, McRae KN. Neonatal hypoglycemia: a six-year experience. *Lancet* 1967;87(2):41.

114. Haworth JC, Vidyasagar D. Hypoglycemia in the newborn. *Clin Obstet Gynecol* 1971;14:821.

115. Koivisto M, Blanco-Sequeiros M, Krause U. Neonatal symptomatic and asymptomatic hypoglycaemia: a follow-up study of 151 children. *Dev Med Child Neurol* 1972;14:603.

116. Pildes RS, Cornblath M, Warren I, et al. A prospective controlled study of neonatal hypoglycemia. *Pediatrics* 1974;54:5.

117. Pildes R, Forbes AE, O'Connor SM, et al. The incidence of neonatal hypoglycemia: a completed survey. *J Pediatr* 1967;70:76.

118. Raivio KO. Neonatal hypoglycemia: II. A clinical study of 44 idiopathic cases with special reference to corticosteroid treatment. *Acta Paediatr Scand* 1968;57:540.

119. Griffiths AD, Bryant GM. Assessment of effects of neonatal hypoglycaemia. *Arch Dis Child* 1971;46:819.

120. Lucas A, Morley R, Cole TJ. Adverse neurodevelopmental outcome of moderate neonatal hypoglycaemia. *Br Med J* 1988;297:1304.

121. Fee BA, Weil WB. Body composition of infants of diabetic mothers by direct analysis. *Ann NY Acad Sci* 1963;110:869.

122. Roth S, Abernathy MP, Lee WH, et al. Insulin-like growth factors I and II peptide and messenger RNA levels in macrosomic infants of diabetic pregnancies. *J Soc Gynecol Invest* 1996;3:78.

123. Ogata ES, Freinkel N, Metzger BE, et al. Perinatal islet function in gestational diabetes: assessment by cord plasma C-peptide and amniotic fluid insulin. *Diabetes Care* 1980;3:425.

124. Eriksson UJ, Lewis NJ, Freinkel N. Growth retardation during early organogenesis in embryos of experimentally diabetic rats. *Diabetes* 1984;35:281–284.

125. Sosenko IR, Kitzmiller JL, Loo SW, et al. The infant of the diabetic mother: correlation of increased cord C-peptide levels with macrosomia and hypoglycemia. *N Engl J Med* 1979;301:859.

126. Stern L, Ramos A, Leduc J. Urinary catecholamine excretion in infants of diabetic mothers. *Pediatrics* 1968;42:598.

127. Schedewie HK, Odell WD, Fisher DA, et al. Parathormone and perinatal calcium homeostasis. *Pediatr Res* 1979;13:1.

128. Noguchi A, Eren M, Tsang RC. Parathyroid hormone in hypocalcemic and normocalcemic infants of diabetic mothers. *J Pediatr* 1980;97:112.

129. Stevenson DK, Bartoletti AL, Ostrander CR, et al. Pulmonary excretion of carbon monoxide in the human infant as an index of bilirubin production: II. Infants of diabetic mothers. *J Pediatr* 1979;94:956.

130. Widness JA, Susa JB, Garcia JF, et al. Increased erythropoiesis and elevated erythropoietin in infants born to diabetic mothers and in hyperinsulinemic rhesus fetuses. *J Clin Invest* 1981;67:637.

131. Philipps AF, Dubin JW, Matty PJ, et al. Arterial hypoxemia and hyperinsulinemia in the chronically hyperglycemic fetal lamb. *Pediatr Res* 1982;16:653.

132. Robert MF, Neff RK, Hubbell JP, et al. Association between maternal diabetes and the respiratory distress syndrome in the newborn. *N Engl J Med* 1976;294:357.

133. Bourbon JR, Farrell PM. Fetal lung development in the diabetic pregnancy. *Pediatr Res* 1985;19:253.

134. Gutgesell HP, Speer ME, Rosenberg HS. Characterization of the cardiomyopathy in infants of diabetic mothers. *Circulation* 1980;61:441.

135. Miller E, Hare JW, Cloherty JP, et al. Elevated maternal hemoglobin A_{1C} in early pregnancy and major congenital anomalies in infants of diabetic mothers. *N Engl J Med* 1981;304:1331.

136. Fuhrmann K, Reiher H, Semmler K, et al. Prevention of congenital malformations in infants of insulin-dependent diabetic mothers. *Diabetes Care* 1983;6:219.

137. Simpson JL, Elias S, Martin AO, et al. Diabetes in pregnancy, Northwestern University Series (1977–1981): I. Prospective study of anomalies in offspring of mothers with diabetes mellitus. *Am J Obstet Gynecol* 1983;146:263.

138. Freinkel N, Lewis NJ, Akazawa S, et al. The honeybee syndrome: implications of the teratogenicity of mannose in rat embryo culture. *N Engl J Med* 1984;310:223.

139. Mills JL, Knopp RH, Simpson JL, et al. Lack of relation of increased malformation rates in infants of diabetic mothers to glycemic control during organogenesis. *N Engl J Med* 1988;318:671.

140. Vohr BR, Lipsitt LP, Oh W. Somatic growth of children of diabetic mothers with reference to birth size. *J Pediatr* 1980;97:196.

141. Metzger BE, Silverman BL, Freinkel N, et al. Amniotic fluid insulin concentration as a predictor of obesity. *Arch Dis Child* 1990;65:1050.

142. Rizzo T, Metzger BE, Burns WJ, et al. Correlations between antepartum maternal metabolism and child intelligence. *N Engl J Med* 1991;325:911.

143. Warram JH, Krolewski AS, Gottlieb MS, et al. Differences in risk of insulin-dependent diabetes in offspring of diabetic mothers and diabetic fathers. *N Engl J Med* 1984;311:149.

144. Pettitt DJ, Aleck KA, Baird R, et al. Congenital susceptibility to NIDDM: role of intrauterine environment. *Diabetes* 1988;37:622.

CHAPTER 36

Calcium and Magnesium Homeostasis

Winston W. K. Koo and Reginald C. Tsang

Calcium is the most abundant mineral in the body and, together with phosphorus, forms the major inorganic constituent of bone. Magnesium is the fourth most abundant mineral and is the second most common intracellular electrolyte in the body. After birth, 99% of total body Ca is in bone. The tissue distribution of Mg varies according to the extent of bone mineralization and the rate of soft tissue growth. Near the end of the third trimester, however, about 60% of the body's Mg is in bone, 20% is in muscle, and most of the remainder is found in the intracellular space of other tissues. Although the major portions of Ca and Mg are found in the skeleton, both are essential to the function of soft tissues (1–4). It generally is agreed that about 80% of Ca and Mg accrue in the fetus between 25 weeks of gestation and term. During this period, the estimated daily accretion per kilogram fetal body weight is 2.3 to 2.98 mmol (92 to 119 mg) Ca and 0.1 to 0.14 mmol (2.51 to 3.44 mg) Mg. The peak accretion rates occur at 36 to 38 weeks of gestation. In newborn term infants, the total body Ca and Mg contents average approximately 28 g and 0.7 g, respectively (4–8).

Serum or plasma is readily available for measurement of Ca and Mg, but the fraction of each in the circulation is less than 1% of its total body content. Disturbances in serum concentrations of Ca and Mg may be associated with disturbances of physiologic function. Chronic and severely lowered serum concentrations of these minerals also may reflect the presence of a deficiency state.

Serum Ca occurs in three forms: approximately 40% is bound, predominantly to albumin; approximately 10% is chelated and complexed to small molecules such as bicar-

bonate, phosphate, or citrate; and approximately 50% is ionized. Complexed and ionized Ca are ultrafilterable.

Total Ca concentrations (tCa) in cord sera increase with increasing gestational age. Serum tCa may be as high as 3 mmol/L (1 mmol/L = 4 mg/dL) in cord blood of infants born at term, and they are significantly higher than paired maternal values at delivery. Serum tCa reaches a nadir during the first 2 days after birth; thereafter, concentrations increase and stabilize at a level generally above 2 mmol/L. In infants exclusively fed human milk, the mean serum tCa increases from 2.3 to 2.7 mmol/L over the first 6 months postnatally. Serum tCa concentrations in infants and children generally remain slightly higher than adult values (9). Normally, serum tCa in children and adults remains stable, with a diurnal range of less than 0.13 mmol/L.

Serum ionized calcium concentration (iCa) is the best indicator of physiologic blood Ca activity. Measurement of serum iCa is firmly established in clinical medicine, and the availability of highly reliable iCa analyzers allows simple, rapid, and direct determination of iCa in whole blood, plasma, and serum by ion-selective electrodes. Some differences exist in the reported values for circulating iCa as a result of differences in the design of the reference electrode, formulation of calibrating solutions, and the lack of a reference system for iCa (10,11). Cord serum iCa increases with increasing gestational age and is higher than values in paired maternal sera. With the use of newer ion-selective electrodes, serum iCa averages 1.25 mmol/L with a 95% confidence limit of 1.1 to 1.4 mmol/L (4.5 to 5.6 mg/dL) (12). Serum iCa concentrations in infants and children generally remain slightly higher than those in adults. Clinical situations may affect the measured iCa concentration. For example, the use of heparin may decrease iCa, and iCa is inversely related to blood pH. The effect of the latter may be minimized by the immediate analysis of the serum samples for iCa. Freezing serum samples in 5% CO_2-containing tubes may

W. W. K. Koo: Department of Pediatrics, Wayne State University; and Department of Pediatrics, Hutzel Hospital, Detroit, Michigan

R. C. Tsang: Division of Neonatology, Department of Pediatrics, University of Cincinnati Medical Center, Cincinnati, Ohio

minimize the impact of pH variations if measurement of iCa is delayed for 1 week.

The concentration of iCa is critical to many important biological functions, and there is finely tuned regulation of the extracellular iCa concentration and maintenance of an extremely large Ca concentration gradient across the cellular plasma membrane. The Ca messenger system is a nearly universal means by which extracellular messengers regulate cell function (1,2). Many cellular enzyme cascades are activated by a transient increase in intracellular iCa concentrations. In the cell, distribution of Ca is not uniform. The cytosolic compartment contains 50 to 150 nmol of Ca per liter of water; a larger intramitochondrial Ca pool contains 500 to 10,000 nmol of Ca per liter cell water. In contrast, the concentration of iCa in extracellular fluid is 1 million nmol/L (1 mmol/L). There are at least two adenosine triphosphate-dependent mechanisms involved in the maintenance of the Ca concentration gradient across the plasma membrane. The measurement of intracellular Ca can be affected by some *in vitro* conditions (13) and is not freely available.

Approximately 30% of serum Mg is in the protein-bound form, with the remainder in the ultrafilterable portion. Seventy to 80% of ultrafilterable Mg is in ionic form, the remainder being complexed to anions, particularly phosphate, citrate, and oxalate. Cord serum total Mg (tMg) is higher than paired maternal values and remains slightly higher in infants and young children compared to adults: 0.92 ± 0.13 mmol/L (2.2 ± 0.3 mg/dL, mean ± 2 SD) in children compared to approximately 0.88 ± 0.13 mmol/L (2.1 ± 0.3 mg/dL) in adults (14). Ion-selective electrodes are being used in the measurement of ionized Mg (iMg), which averages 62% to 70% of the tMg concentration in the cord and postnatal sera. The cord serum iMg is also higher than that in maternal serum (15,16).

The cellular Mg content of most tissues is 6 to 9 mmol/kg wet weight, and most of this Mg is localized in membrane structures (e.g., microsomes, mitochondria, plasma membranes). The much smaller pool of free Mg in the cell is maintained at about 1 mmol/L and is in an exchanging equilibrium with the membrane-bound Mg. This unbound intracellular Mg has a critical role in cellular physiology and catalyzes enzymatic processes concerned with the transfer, storage, and use of energy (3,4). Intracellular Mg usually remains stable despite wide fluctuations in serum Mg. In Mg-deficient states, however, the intracellular content of Mg can be low despite normal serum concentrations (3,4). There are a number of experimental methods available to determine the intracellular Mg concentrations (17,18). The knowledge of Mg status is critical to the regulation of Ca homeostasis. For example, hypocalcemic states may not be correctable if there is simultaneous unrecognized hypomagnesemia. Thus, appropriate attention should be paid to the early diagnosis and treatment of Mg imbalance. However, the assessment of Mg status is difficult because measurements of

tissue and intracellular Mg are not freely available (19). Nevertheless, maintenance of normal circulating Mg concentrations is a prerequisite to normal Mg homeostasis.

PHYSIOLOGIC CONTROL

Calcium Homeostasis

Calcium continuously enters the extracellular fluid from gut and bone, but Ca concentration in the extracellular fluid is maintained relatively constant by the effects of interdependent hormonal mechanisms that regulate the influx and efflux of Ca among extracellular fluid, kidney, gut, and bone. Parathyroid hormone (PTH) and 1,25-dihydroxyvitamin D [1,25(OH)$_2$D] are the hormones that primarily regulate the extracellular fluid Ca concentration through their effects on kidney, gut, and bone. Other systemic and local factors also are important in influencing Ca flux, particularly under pathologic conditions such as humoral hypercalcemia of malignancy (HHM), and their role in Ca homeostasis under physiologic conditions is being studied (see Hormonal Control).

The kidney is a major regulator of extracellular fluid Ca concentration, primarily by modulation of Ca excretion (see Chap. 42). Altered renal regulation of Ca excretion is primarily responsible for the development of some hypercalcemic states, including familial hypocalciuric hypercalcemia (FHH); it may also occur during chronic thiazide diuretic therapy. The renal capacity for acute regulation of extracellular fluid Ca concentration, however, may be overwhelmed when net Ca input into the extracellular fluid from the gut or bone exceeds the kidney's capacity for Ca excretion (20–22). The latter situation is exemplified best by hypercalcemia of malignancy. Conversely, in hypocalcemic states, the kidney cannot reduce Ca excretion sufficiently to prevent the occurrence of hypocalcemia.

The gut is important in chronic control of extracellular fluid Ca, primarily through regulation of dietary Ca absorption and the presence of hormonal stimulatory factors, including 1,25(OH)$_2$D (23,24). Gut hyperabsorption of Ca may be associated with hypercalciuria and nephrocalcinosis, but there is no major effect on the development of hypercalcemia.

There is exchange of Ca between bone fluid and extracellular fluid across the bone lining cells that is strongly related to systemic and local factors controlling bone formation and resorption (25). In growing infants, there is a net influx of extracellular fluid Ca to bone for mineralization and skeletal growth (26).

Magnesium Homeostasis

Extracellular fluid Mg is primarily controlled by the kidney and gastrointestinal tract and appears closely linked to Ca, potassium, and sodium metabolism. Magnesium is essential for the function of the parathyroid glands, metabolism of vitamin D metabolites, and adequate sensitivity of target tissues to PTH and active vitamin D metabolites. Bone metabolism is impaired under positive as well as negative Mg balance. In contrast, the control of Mg homeostasis by calciotropic hormones under physiologic conditions appears to be limited (3,4,27,28).

The kidney is the main regulator of serum concentrations and total body content of Mg. Renal excretion of Mg normally increases in proportion to the load presented to the kidney. Renal Mg excretory capacity can be overwhelmed, however, especially in developmentally less mature kidneys, as in the human infant, and in the presence of a relatively high Mg load such as that occurs *in utero* from maternal Mg loading (29,30) or postnatally in infants receiving parenteral nutrition therapy (31–33). There is renal Mg conservation, and PTH stimulates reabsorption of Mg at the renal tubule (28,34), but renal conservation of Mg is insufficient to prevent hypomagnesemia in the presence of very low intake (31,32,35) or excessive losses (e.g., from the gastrointestinal tract) (31,32,36). Other factors, including sodium and Ca loading and loop diuretics, also increase Mg loss in the urine (20,21,24,34,37).

Gastrointestinal absorption of Mg occurs in the small intestine, predominantly in the jejunum and ileum. Magnesium absorption occurs primarily by intercellular diffusion and solvent drag mechanisms, but decreased fractional absorption with larger intakes also is consistent with a facilitated diffusion or saturable component (38). Intestinal Mg absorption also may be stimulated by hormonal stimulatory factors including PTH (28). There is very little endogenous secretion of Mg into the gut, but gastrointestinal secretions contain large amounts of Mg, and increased secretory losses from gastrointestinal fistulas frequently result in Mg deficiency and hypomagnesemia (35,36).

There is limited information on the exchange of Mg between bone and extracellular fluid, but with altered Mg status, particularly in hypomagnesemic patients, there is decreased Mg–Ca exchange at the bone surface and decreased release of bone Ca (39,40), probably independent of decreased serum PTH concentrations. In contrast, PTH increases release of Mg from bone (28,41).

HORMONAL CONTROL

Parathyroid Hormone

The classic hormones important to mineral homeostasis are PTH, calcitonin (CT), and 1,25(OH)$_2$D. Parathyroid hormone is synthesized in the chief cells of parathyroid gland. It is an 84-amino-acid polypeptide with a relative molecular mass (M_r) of 9,500. In humans, the PTH gene, along with the genes for insulin, β-globulin, and CT, is located on chromosome 11p15, and restriction

site polymorphisms near the PTH gene have been detected (41,42). The initial translational product of the mRNA is a 115-amino-acid prepro-PTH. Prepro-PTH then undergoes proteolytic cleavage to remove the aminoterminal signal sequence, on translocation across the membrane of the endoplasmic reticulum, to form pro-PTH. The prohormone-specific region is cleaved further during subsequent intracellular processing to generate the 84-amino-acid secreted form of the intact hormone.

The PTH is stored in secretory granules and colocated and secreted with chromogranin A, a protein that may act in autocrine- or paracrine-regulated release of PTH. After release into the circulation, the intact PTH molecule has a serum half-life of 5 to 8 minutes and undergoes a series of cleavages by endopeptidases in the hepatic Kupffer cells. The amino-terminal fragments contain the biologically active fractions, with the 1–34 fragment having the most calcemic activity. The midregion and carboxyl-terminal fragments are biologically inert, although the latter may have some *in vitro* biological activity. The inactive fragments are cleared from the blood virtually exclusively by glomerular filtration. Normally, there are greater amounts of middle and carboxyl fragments than of the intact hormone in the circulation because of metabolic breakdown of the short-lived, intact hormone, coupled with glandular secretion of inactive fragments. Intact PTH and amino-terminal fragments constitute about 10% of PTH immunoreactivity in the peripheral circulation. Intact PTH, as measured by immunoradiometric assay (IRMA), is the most sensitive index of parathyroid gland secretory function (41,43–45). Consistency in the PTH assay methodology and serial measurements are critical to the interpretation of PTH measurements.

Parathyroid hormone concentrations in cord blood frequently are low and do not correlate with PTH concentrations in maternal sera (46,47), although by cytochemical assay, it appears that bioactive PTH may be present at a higher level than immunoactive PTH in cord sera (47,48). This may be related to the higher concentrations of parathyroid hormone-related protein (PTHrP) in the cord sera since PTH-like bioactivity was tightly correlated with levels of PTHrP in the pig (49) and the sheep (50). Serum PTH concentrations increase postnatally coincident with the fall in serum Ca in both term and preterm infants (46,47,51–53). Serum PTH concentrations are similar for children and adults but increase in the elderly (54–56). Serum concentrations of intact PTH as measured by IRMA showed no change during normal pregnancy (46,57). In adults, serum intact PTH is present in picomolar concentrations. It has a significant circadian periodicity (58–60), spontaneous episodic pulsatility with distinct peak property (59) and a significant temporal coupling with serum iCa and phosphorus concentrations (59,60) and prolactin secretion (58).

In physiologic terms, PTH is the most important regulator of extracellular Ca concentration, primarily through its effect on classic PTH target tissues, bone and kidney. It increases serum Ca concentration through mobilization of Ca from bone, probably synergistically with $1,25(OH)_2D$; increases renal distal tubular reabsorption of Ca but decreases proximal tubular reabsorption of sodium, Ca, phosphate, and bicarbonate; increases intestinal Ca absorption secondary to stimulating $1,25(OH)_2D$ production and probably also has a direct effect on intestinal Ca absorption (9,61,62). In contrast to its classic action on Ca mobilization from bone, the amino terminal fragments of PTH and PTHrP, and small pulses of PTH have an anabolic effect on bone independent of its resorptive action (63–65). Other tissues such as skin fibroblasts, cardiac cells, and vascular smooth muscle also have PTH-sensitive adenylate cyclase, but the physiologic importance of PTH in these nonclassic target tissues is not well defined (66).

Parathyroid hormone effects on end-organ systems appear to be mediated through its binding to specific receptors. The PTH (and PTHrP) receptor belongs to a superfamily of G-protein-linked cell membrane receptors (including those for CT, growth hormone-releasing hormone, glucagon, secretin, and others) with extended extracellular, ligand-binding amino-terminal and intracellular G protein–associated carboxyl-terminal domains and seven transmembrane domains (67). The gene for the PTH/PTHrP receptor is located on chromosome 3p21.1-p24.2. It contains 17 exons and encodes a mature glycoprotein of 593 amino acids (68). Signal transduction mediated by G proteins (69,70) includes both stimulatory and inhibitory responses, and functional response results from activation of secondary messengers such as cyclic adenosine monophosphate (cAMP), inositol phosphate, and cytosolic Ca.

Transcription of the PTH gene is enhanced by a decrease in extracellular ionized Ca concentration, glucocorticoid, estrogen, and progestin and inhibited by an increase in extracellular and intracellular ionized Ca, $1,25(OH)_2D$, CT, and 9-cis-retinoic acid (41,71). Secretion of PTH appears to be feedback regulated by Ca, Mg, and $1,25(OH)_2D$ (71–73) and is stimulated by β-adrenergic agonists, dopamine, and prostaglandin E_2. Hyperphosphatemia stimulates PTH secretion, probably by lowering the serum Ca concentration. A decrease in serum Mg concentration also can stimulate PTH secretion (74,75), although chronic hypomagnesemia inhibits secretion of PTH (72,75) and possibly increases target tissue resistance to PTH (39). The latter may be related to inactivity of adenylate cyclase, a Mg-requiring enzyme. The expression of PTH receptors can be downregulated. The latter plays an important role in the skeletal resistance to the calcemic effect of PTH in chronic renal failure (76).

Extracellular Ca, in turn, is the most potent regulator of PTH secretion and is mediated by the Ca-sensing receptor (CaR), which detects minute perturbations in the extracellular ionized Ca concentration and responds with alterations in cellular function that normalize iCa. The human receptor has been cloned and sequenced; the human CaR gene is located on chromosome 3q13.3-q21 and encodes a cell-surface protein of 1,078 amino acids. It contains at least seven exons of which six encode the large (~600 amino acid) amino-terminal extracellular domain and/or its upstream untranslated regions, while a single exon codes for the remainder of the receptor consisting of a seven-member membrane-spanning domain and a cytoplasmic carboxy-terminal intracellular domain. It is a member of a superfamily of G protein–coupled receptors and activates phospholipases C, A_2, and D (74,77–79).

The CaR gene is developmentally upregulated (80), and CaR transcripts are present in numerous tissues including chief cells of the parathyroid glands, kidneys (in particular the thick ascending limb), brain and nerve terminals, and also the intestine, lung, and skin (79). A variety of missense, nonsense, deletion, and insertion mutations have been identified in the CaR gene, resulting in altered receptor activity and clinical disease (78,79,81–84). It appears that the CaR probably maintains Ca homeostasis by modulating PTH (feedback inhibition) (81,82) and $1,25(OH)_2D$ production (direct inhibition and via its effect on PTH) (71,85) and regulates (decreases) the Na–K–2Cl cotransporter-dependent paracellular Ca and Mg transport, i.e., increasing renal excretion of divalent cations. The CaR also may affect renal water regulation by inhibition of vasopressin-abated water flow (79,85,86). Extracellular Ca exerts numerous other actions on parathyroid function, including modulation of the intracellular degradation of PTH, cellular respiration, membrane voltage, the hexose monophosphate shunt, etc. The role of CaR in mediating these effects is not well defined (2). Maintenance of Ca homeostasis through other organs also may be possible with the presence of CaR in the intestinal cells and probable modulation of CT secretion from intracellular calcium (79,85,87,88).

Calcitonin

Calcitonin monomer is a 32-amino-acid peptide with a M_r of 3,400. Its precursors are prepro-CT and pro-CT. The larger prohormones include peptides linked to the amino and carboxy terminals of the CT sequence (i.e., flanking peptides). Calcitonin and equimolar amounts of non-CT secretory peptides, corresponding to these flanking peptides, are generated during precursor processing. In addition, alternate processing of the initial gene transcript results in the production of another distinct RNA encoding precursor of CT gene-related peptide (CGRP). The latter is a 37-amino-acid peptide sequence (M_r 4,000). Seventy-five amino-terminal residues of each preprohormone for CT and CGRP are predicted to be identical. Pro-CT is a 116-amino-acid peptide, whereas the pro-CGRP is a 103-amino-acid peptide. Bioactivity of human calcitonin (hCT) is present in the full 32-amino-acid structure or its smaller fragments, such as hCT_{8-32} and hCT_{9-32}; the ring structure of CT enhances, but is not essential for, hormone action (9,89,90).

The CT gene is located on chromosome 11p15.2 (near the gene for PTH) and contains six exons and five introns, with exon 4 coding for CT in the thyroid C cell and exon 5 coding for CGRP in the central nervous system. Calcitonin gene transcription is positively regulated by cAMP, phorbol esters, and glucocorticoid hormones and negatively regulated by $1,25(OH)_2D$ (90–93). Secretion of CT is stimulated by an increase in serum Ca and Mg concentrations and by gastrin, glucagon, and cholecystokinin, along with several other structural analogs of these hormones (e.g., pentagastrin, prostaglandin E_2), and by norepinephrine. Hypocalcemia, propranolol and other adrenergic antagonists, somatostatin, and chromogranin A may inhibit the secretion of CT (9,92–94). Calcitonin may activate the 1-hydroxylase system independent of PTH and increase $1,25(OH)_2D$ production (95), whereas $1,25(OH)_2D$ decreases CT gene expression in adult rats but is ineffective in 13-day-old suckling rats (91). The latter observation may be related to fewer $1,25(OH)_2D$ receptors in C cells of immature rats.

Developmentally, CT-containing cells and parathyroid gland cells are thought to derive from the same tissue source as the neural crest. Calcitonin is secreted primarily from the thyroid C cells and also from many extrathyroidal tissues, including tissues from embryonic neural crest origin. Calcitonin gene-related peptide is found predominantly in nerve fibers in the central and peripheral nervous system, blood vessels, thyroid and parathyroid glands, liver, spleen, heart, lung, and possibly bone marrow. Both CT and CGRP are present in the fetus.

Circulating immunoreactive CT and CGRP are a heterogeneous mixture of different molecular forms and are recognized as long as the antigenic epitopes recognized by the antiserum are expressed. Sample preparation with initial extraction, gel chromatography, and high-performance liquid chromatography separation can improve the sensitivity and specificity of the radioimmunoassays. Two-site immunometric assays may allow further refinement in sensitivity and specificity in the measurement of these hormones (9,96,97).

In human adults, serum CT and CGRP concentrations are found in the picomolar range. Diurnal variability has been reported for serum CGRP but not for serum CT (98–100). Serum CT concentrations are high at birth compared to paired maternal CT concentrations. Serum CT concentrations further increase during the first few days after birth and may reach levels fivefold to tenfold higher than adult CT concentrations. Serum CT concentrations decrease progressively during infancy; however, in preterm infants, the mean serum CT concentrations may remain twice the adult value up to several months postnatally (9,51,52,54,101).

Calcitonin is a potent inhibitor of bone resorption and increases renal Ca excretion. There are distinct but overlapping effects of CT and CGRP. For example, CT has a potent hypocalcemic effect and inhibits bone resorption. Calcitonin decreases renal tubular reabsorption of Ca, Mg, phosphorus, and sodium and increases free water clearance in humans. In physiologic concentration, CT probably does not influence intestinal absorption of Ca and phosphorus. The net effect of CT is a lowering of serum Ca and phosphorus concentrations (9,94). Thus, the bioactivity of CT frequently is opposite that of PTH; CT probably modulates the effect of PTH on organs. Calcitonin gene-related peptide primarily affects catecholamine release, vascular tone and blood pressure, and cardiac contractility, and the influence of CGRP on Ca and phosphorus homeostasis is minor compared to that of CT. However, amylin, a pancreatic islet-derived or synthetic 37-amino-acid peptide, is a member of the CGRP family with a potent hypocalcemic effect despite sharing only 15% of its amino acid sequence with human CT. The hypocalcemic effect of amylin is thought to be mediated by the CT receptors on osteoclasts, and it is 100-fold more potent than CGRP (102). Both CT and CGRP inhibit gastric acid secretion and food intake. Calcitonin and amylin are used in the therapeutic management of hypercalcemia and pathologic states with increased bone resorption. Calcitonin also is useful as a tumor marker in the management of medullary carcinoma of the thyroid.

Calcitonin function is mediated by binding to receptors linked to G proteins and activation of adenylate cyclase and protein kinase (92,103,104). The CT receptor gene is located on chromosome 7q21.2 and encodes a 490-amino-acid, seven transmembrane G protein-linked receptor related to the superfamily of receptors that includes the PTH/PTHrP receptors. Two isoforms of human calcitonin receptor arise by alternative splicing of an exon of 48 nucleotides that encodes a 16-amino-acid insertion within the first intracellular loop. The isoform with the insertion (hCTR-1) activates only adenylate cyclase, whereas the other isofrom (hCTR-2) activates both adenylate cyclase and phospholipase C.

The kidney appears to be the dominant organ in the metabolism of human CT. A small percentage of the metabolic clearance rate of CT in humans may be accounted for by enzymatic degradation in blood. Depending on the animal species, other sites such as liver, intestine, and bone may be involved in the metabolism of CT.

Vitamin D

Dietary vitamin D (1 μg = 40 IU) is derived from plants as ergosterol (i.e., vitamin D_2) and from animals as cholecalciferol (i.e., vitamin D_3). In animals, vitamin D_3

can be synthesized endogenously in the skin after exposure to the ultraviolet B spectrum (i.e., 280 to 300 nm) of sunlight.

In mammals, vitamins D_2 and D_3 appear to metabolize along the same pathway, and there is little functional difference between their metabolites. Vitamin D (M_r 384) undergoes several major metabolic conversion steps and under *in vivo* conditions produces at least 30 vitamin D metabolites, with and without putative functions. In the liver, vitamin D is hydroxylated at carbon 25 to 25-hydroxyvitamin D (25-OHD). The vitamin D-25 hydroylase activity is found predominantly in the P_{450} CYP-27 protein on the inner surface of the mitochondrial membrane. This protein also catalyzes 27-hydroxylation of cholesterol derivatives. The CYP-27 gene is located on chromosome 2q33 and encodes a polypeptide of 531 amino acids processed to a mature protein of 498 amino acids with a molecular mass of 56.9 kD (105,106). Quantitatively, 25-OHD (1 nmol/L = 0.4 ng/mL) is the most abundant vitamin D metabolite in the circulation and is a useful index of vitamin D reserve. It is bound to vitamin D binding protein in the circulation and transported to the kidney, where it is hydroxylated further to $1,25(OH)_2D$ and 24R,25-dihydroxyvitamin D. This occurs predominantly in the mitochondria of proximal tubules.

The $1,25(OH)_2D$ is the most active vitamin D metabolite and is critical to the maintenance of mineral homeostasis, in particular the prevention of hypocalcemia, rickets, and osteomalacia (107,108). It also induces the 24-hydroxylase gene to produce 24-hydroxylated metabolites with novel hormonal activity with respect to chondrocyte differentiation and bone mineralization. The genes for 25-OHD-1α-hydroxylase and 25-OHD-24R-hydroxylase have been localized to chromosome 12q14 and 20q13.3, respectively (109–111).

Regulation of vitamin D 25-hydroxylase activity is limited. At high concentrations of vitamin D, the mitochondrial enzyme will form significant quantities of 25-OHD. The *in vivo* administration of $1,25(OH)_2D$ appears to decrease the plasma concentration of 25-OHD (112). Calcium deficiency appears to increase the metabolic clearance of 25-OHD (113).

In contrast, the production of $1,25(OH)_2D$ is tightly regulated. Parathyroid hormone, PTHrP, lower circulating concentrations of Ca, phosphorus, and $1,25(OH)_2D$, cAMP, protein kinase and insulin-like growth factor-I increase, whereas Ca, phosphorus, $1,25(OH)_2D$, and metabolites of phosphatidylinositol bisphosphate decrease the activity of the 25-OHD-1α-hydroxylase enzyme and circulating $1,25(OH)_2D$ concentrations (112–115). Conversion of $1,25(OH)_2D$ or the preceding 25-OHD metabolite to 24-hydroxylated form in response to $1,25(OH)_2D$ induction of the 24-hydroxylase gene is important in the regulation of the circulating concentration of $1,25(OH)_2D$ and catabolism of the vitamin D molecule (109,110). Other factors, such as pregnancy, steroids, prolactin, growth hormone, CT, and possibly thyroid hormone, also may increase circulating $1,25(OH)_2D$. Magnesium is a cofactor of the 1α-hydroxylase enzyme. Magnesium deficiency and hypomagnesemia in humans are associated with low serum $1,25(OH)_2D$ concentrations (75,116,117) and lower serum $1,25(OH)_2D$ response to low-Ca diet (116) but do not appear to limit $1,25(OH)_2D$ production in animals (118). In contrast to the rapid increase in PTH secretion and serum PTH concentrations, measurable alteration in serum $1,25(OH)_2D$ concentrations usually occurs only hours after exposure to an appropriate stimulus. Extrarenal production of $1,25(OH)_2D$ takes place in macrophages, particularly in granulomatous disease states. Its production is not tightly regulated, is stimulated by γ-interferon, but is not responsive to changes in dietary calcium intake (115). The physiologic role of extrarenally derived $1,25(OH)_2D$ is unclear.

Like other steroid hormones, $1,25(OH)_2D$ exerts its action through modulation of the cellular genome by binding to specific nuclear receptors (vitamin D receptor, VDR), a 424-amino-acid phosphoprotein. The VDR gene contains nine exons and is located on chromosome 12q13–14 near the site of the gene for 25 OHD-1α-hydroxylase (111,119). VDR is a member of the steroid hormone receptor superfamily that also includes the retinoic acid receptors. It has several functional domains including a zinc finger-mediated N-terminal DNA-binding domain, a C-terminal hormone-binding domain, and a hinge region important for nuclear localization. The $1,25(OH)_2D$–VDR action is modulated by a number of processes including vitamin D-responsive elements (VDREs), which are located in the 5′ upstream untranslated regulatory region of the genes stimulated or suppressed by $1,25(OH)_2D$, and by 9-*cis*-retinoic acid (109,110). Vitamin D receptors are upregulated by $1,25(OH)_2D$ at both the mRNA and protein levels. They also are increased during growth, gestation, and lactation but show an age-dependent decrease in mature animals and humans (120), supporting the notion that vitamin D receptors may be up- or downregulated, depending on Ca needs. Calcium homeostasis and bone mineralization are maintained by $1,25(OH)_2D$ through its effect on a number of target tissues, primarily by increasing vitamin D-dependent Ca absorption through the gut and renal tubules as a result of increased transcription of mRNA for Ca-binding protein and other products. Additionally, $1,25(OH)_2D$ acts on receptors of osteoblasts (enhances differentiation and inhibits proliferation) and osteocytes to promote bone formation, which in turn promotes bone resorption activities and releases bone Ca, thereby further increasing circulating Ca concentrations. Vitamin D metabolites also are important in the maintenance of phosphorus homeostasis by increasing intestinal absorption and renal reabsorption of phosphate (107–110,121).

The VDR is present in numerous cell types, and $1,25(OH)_2D$–VDR action clearly transcends bone and calcium/phosphate homeostasis. Its actions extend into cell growth and differentiation and immune, neural, and endocrine function (109,110). The multifunction of $1,25(OH)_2D$–VDR action is well demonstrated by the defect in the gene coding human VDR that results in familial target tissue insensitivity to $1,25(OH)_2D_3$, known as hereditary hypocalcemic vitamin D-resistant rickets (HVDRR). It is an autosomal recessive disorder typically with clinical features that mimic classical nutritional rickets and progressive alopecia, supporting the likely role of VDR in normal hair growth cycle in skin (122,123). In homozygous VDR knockout mice, the use of a "rescue diet" enriched with lactose, calcium, and phosphate results in normalization of circulating mineral and PTH concentrations with significant improvement in bone mineralization but not the skin or hair abnormality (124). This finding is consistent with reports that calcium therapy improves bone abnormalities in HVDRR patients (125) and supports the critical primary physiologic role of $1,25(OH)_2D$–VDR in skin and hair development independent of bone mineral homeostasis.

A rapid-onset [i.e., within minutes after exposure to $1,25(OH)_2D$], non–genome-mediated action of $1,25(OH)_2D$ on intestinal Ca transport, probably mediated through a $1,25(OH)_2D$-binding membrane receptor that "opens" voltage-gated Ca ion channels, also has been demonstrated. The physiologic role of this nongenomic action remains to be determined (61,126).

Quantification of vitamin D and its metabolites has been achieved by several different methods. The more routine approaches include high-performance liquid chromatography with detection by ultraviolet absorbance or binding assays. Immunoassays based on antibodies raised to vitamin D metabolite conjugates also are available. Values from different laboratories cannot be compared without making direct comparison of their assay procedures. Interlaboratory coefficients of variation for the measurement of 25-OHD, $24,25(OH)_2D$, and $1,25(OH)_2D$ may range between 35% and 52% (127). Furthermore, differences between vitamins D_2 and D_3 in their affinity to the vitamin D binding protein and receptors and different chromatographic behavior on various preparative chromatographic systems demand that great care be taken with assay techniques when dealing with patients who have significant vitamin D_2 intake. To ensure reliable results, appropriate vitamin D standards must be used for standard curve generation in performing competitive protein binding assays of these compounds.

Maternofetal transfer of vitamin D and its metabolites varies, depending on the species. In humans, the cord serum vitamin D concentration is very low and may be undetectable, probably because of poor maternofetal crossover; the 25-OHD concentration is directly correlated with, but is lower than, maternal values, consistent with placental crossover of this metabolite; $1,25(OH)_2D$ concentrations also are lower than maternal values, but

there is no agreement on the maternofetal relationship of this and other dihydroxylated vitamin D metabolites. *In vivo,* some placental crossover may occur after maternal exposure to pharmacologic doses of vitamin D or $1,25(OH)_2D$. Seasonal and racial variations in serum 25-OHD_3 concentrations occur, presumably from variations in endogenous production. Serum 25-OHD is lower in winter and in African-Americans; serum $1,25(OH)_2D$ is higher in African-American mothers. These differences may be reflected in cord serum values. It appears that the human fetus receives the bulk of its vitamin D already metabolized to 25-OHD (9,128).

Neonates, even very-low-birth-weight infants, appear to have adequate capacity to absorb and metabolize vitamin D. In infants receiving standard supplementary vitamin D intake, circulating 25-OHD and $1,25(OH)_2D$ concentrations may be increased to levels comparable to, and sometimes exceeding, adult values. Circulating 25-OHD and $1,25(OH)_2D$ concentrations in infants also appear to be dependent on Ca and phosphorus intake (9,32,33,128).

Parathyroid hormone and $1,25(OH)_2D$, and possibly CT, appear to maintain a stable serum Ca concentration by intermodulation of their physiologic effects on each other. Parathyroid hormone serves as the major component of rapid response to hypocalcemia, whereas $1,25(OH)_2D$, with its major effect on elevating intestinal absorption of Ca, is responsible for a slower but more sustained contribution to the maintenance of normocalcemia. Calcitonin, on the other hand, appears to function in the opposite role to PTH but with the capacity to stimulate the production of $1,25(OH)_2D$, which in theory may serve an additional regulatory role in the maintenance of Ca homeostasis. Magnesium functions primarily as a cofactor in the production of these hormones under normal circumstances, but with the exception of the Mg–PTH interaction, the interaction between Mg and these hormones during physiologic circumstances remains ill defined.

NONCLASSIC CONTROL OF CALCIUM AND MAGNESIUM HOMEOSTASIS

There is increasing evidence that maintenance of mineral homeostasis is a complex process involving more than the classic calciotropic hormones: PTH, CT, $1,25(OH)_2D$. Some factors exert their effect systemically (e.g., catecholamines, prostaglandins, growth hormone, estrogen, progesterone, cortisol, insulin-like growth factor-I, and somatostatin) by modulating the secretion or function of one or more of the calciotropic hormones or independently affecting bone resorption and/or bone formation, which in turn may affect Ca homeostasis (129–135). Local factors (e.g., transforming growth factor-β_1, lymphotoxin, tumor necrosis factor-α, and interleukins 1 and 6) in a paracrine (i.e., cell-to-cell) or autocrine (i.e., cell-to-own cell) fashion also may be important in influencing Ca flux (135–142), particularly under pathologic conditions. Interaction between systemic and local factors can occur (137,143), and some factors such as PTHrP may act both systemically and locally (144,145).

Parathyroid hormone and PTHrP genes appear to be members of the same gene family. Parathyroid hormone-related protein cDNA encodes a 177-amino-acid protein consisting of a 36-amino-acid precursor segment and a 141-amino-acid mature peptide. The mature PTHrP contains several structural or functional domains. The 1 to 13 region of PTHrP is 70% homologous with the corresponding region of PTH. Both PTH and PTHrP appear to bind to the same G-protein-linked receptor. Synthetic and recombinant PTHrPs can mimic the effects of PTH on the classic PTH target organs, involving activation of adenylate cyclase and other second messenger systems (67,144,145).

Parathyroid hormone-related protein gene expression is found in an extensive variety of normal endocrine and nonendocrine tissues. PTHrP biological activity and immunoreactivity have been found in many tissues by as early as 7 weeks of gestation, including the human fetus, placenta, lactating breasts, and mammalian milk (144–147). Circulating immunoreactive PTHrP concentrations are low or undetectable in normal subjects and increase during pregnancy. In the cord sera, concentrations of PTHrP are ten- to 15-fold higher than that of PTH (148,149) and are significantly higher than simultaneous maternal PTHrP at term (148,150). The amino-terminal fragment $PTHrP_{1-74}$ appears to be specific for HHM, whereas the carboxy-terminal fragment $PTHrP_{109-138}$ is elevated in the serum of patients with HHM or renal failure. The levels of PTHrP in these patients are similar to the concentration of PTH (i.e., 10^{-12} to 10^{-11} mol/L). The concentration of PTHrP in milk is 100-fold higher (144,147).

PTHrP, also known as PTH-like peptide, PTH-like protein, or human humoral hypercalcemic factor, is thought to be the humoral mediator that is secreted by tumors in the syndrome of HHM. Physiologically, PTHrP is an important paracrine regulator of several tissue-specific functions. Its roles in smooth muscle relaxation, placental calcium transport, lactation, and fetal bone development are becoming firmly established and it is likely to be important in the control of cellular growth and differentiation (62,144,145).

DISTURBANCES IN SERUM CALCIUM AND MAGNESIUM CONCENTRATIONS

Hypocalcemia

Neonatal hypocalcemia may be defined as a serum total Ca concentration below 2 mmol/L (1 mmol/L = 4 mg/dL) in term infants and 1.75 mmol/L in preterm

infants with iCa below 0.75 to 1.1 mmol/L (3.0 to 4.4 mg/dL), depending on the particular ion-selective electrode used. These definitions are made from a clinical viewpoint because serum Ca concentrations are maintained within narrow ranges under normal circumstances and the potential risk for disturbances of physiologic function increases as the serum Ca concentration further decreases. Changes in physiologic function (e.g., changes in cardiac contractility, blood pressure, and heart rate) may or may not be demonstrated in infants who have hypocalcemia or are undergoing Ca therapy (151–153). Children with ionized hypocalcemia, however, are reported to have a higher mortality rate in a pediatric intensive care setting (154).

Clinically, there are two peaks in the occurrence of neonatal hypocalcemia (Table 36–1). An early form typically occurs during the first few days of life, with the lowest concentrations of serum Ca being reached at 24 to 48 hours of age; late neonatal hypocalcemia occurs toward the end of the first week of life and generally presents as neonatal tetany. In some infants, the nadir of the serum Ca concentration may occur at less than 12 hours or not until some weeks after birth.

The pathophysiologic mechanisms of hypocalcemia are varied and frequently interrelated but not fully defined (Table 36–2). Several factors may contribute to the development of hypocalcemia: for example, limited milk and Ca intake, in addition to transient limited increase in the serum PTH concentration, elevated serum CT concentration, and possibly end organ resistance to $1,25(OH)_2D$. A common basis may exist for the development of hypocalcemia in a number of clinical situations: for example, a predisposing factor to early neonatal

TABLE 36–1. *Neonatal hypocalcemia*[a]

Early occurrence
  Prematurity
  Birth asphyxia
  Maternal insulin-dependent diabetes
  Maternal hyperparathyroidism
  Hypoparathyroidism[b,c]
  Activating calcium-sensing receptor mutation†
  In utero exposure to anticonvulsants (?)
  Phototherapy (?)
Late occurrence
  Intake of high-phosphate milks or cereals
  Phosphate enema
  Intestinal calcium malabsorption
  Hypoparathyroidism[b,c]
  Activating calcium-sensing receptor mutation[c]
  Hypomagnesemia
Decreased ionized calcium
  Exchange transfusions with citrated blood
  Intravenous lipid infusion (i.e. increased free fatty acid)
  Alkalosis
  In utero exposure to narcotics (?)

[a]Hypocalcemia may be [b]severe and prolonged and/or [c]present in later life.

TABLE 36–2. *Pathophysiology of neonatal hypocalcemia*

Agent	Problem	Clinical association
Calcium	Decreased intake or absorption	Prematurity; malabsorption syndrome
Ionized calcium	Increased Ca complex	Chelating agent (e.g., citrated blood for exchange transfusion, long-chain free fatty acid)
Magnesium	Decreased tissue store or absorption	Maternal hypomagnesemia; infant of insulin-dependent diabetic mother; specific Mg malabsorption (rare)
Phosphorus	Increased	Endogenous and exogenous (e.g., dietary, enema) phosphate loading
pH	Increased	Respiratory or metabolic alkalosis (e.g., shifts Ca from ionized to protein-bound fraction)
Parathyroid hormone	Decreased synthesis or secretion	Maternal hyperparathyroidism; hypoparathyroidism; DiGeorge association; hypomagnesemia
Parathyroid hormone	Decreased responsiveness	Hypomagnesemia; pseudohypoparathyroidism
Activating calcium-sensing receptor	Increased responsiveness	Autosomal dominant or sporadic hypocalcemia with hypercalciuria
Calcitonin	Increased	Infant of insulin-dependent diabetic mother, birth asphyxia, prematurity
1,25-Dihydroxyvitamin D	Decreased responsiveness	Prematurity

hypocalcemia can be inadequate Ca intake when the placental supply of Ca to the neonate is abruptly discontinued at delivery. Postnatally, even if there is maximum intestinal absorption, Ca retention with milk feeding probably is only 15 mg/kg body weight on the first day of life, rising to 45 mg/kg on the third day of life; these amounts are significantly lower than *in utero* Ca accretion rates. Some aspects of pathophysiology of hypocalcemia remain ill defined: for example, despite the hypocalcemic effects of CT, the serum CT concentrations continued to increase in neonates of normal and diabetic pregnancies irrespective of the rate of fall in serum calcium (52); and in very-low-birth-weight infants, spontaneous hypocalcemia provoked a rise in PTH but no change in CT, and a calcium infusion to treat hypocalcemia reduced the PTH but did not affect the CT concentrations (51).

Early neonatal hypocalcemia occurs most frequently in preterm infants. The frequency of hypocalcemia varies inversely with birth weight and gestational age (9,155,156). Over 50% of preterm very-low-birth-weight neonates may have hypocalcemia. Hypocalcemia also occurs in infants who have suffered birth asphyxia (157,158) and in infants of mothers with insulin-dependent diabetes (159). Infants with intrauterine growth retardation may have hypocalcemia if they are also preterm or have experienced birth asphyxia; otherwise, there is apparently no increased incidence of hypocalcemia related to growth retardation per se (156,160). The use of phototherapy and maternal anticonvulsants is reported to be associated with neonatal hypocalcemia (9).

Late neonatal hypocalcemia usually occurs toward the end of the first week of life and is less frequent than early neonatal hypocalcemia. Apart from phosphate imbalance from cow-milk–derived formulas or from early neonatal introduction of cereals, other clinical circumstances potentially associated with hypocalcemia may include intestinal malabsorption, hypomagnesemia, and hypoparathyroidism (9,24). In theory, the risk of neonatal hypocalcemia may be greater if there is preexisting maternal vitamin D deficiency.

More severe and prolonged neonatal hypocalcemia may occur with parathyroid suppression from maternal hyperparathyroidism (161) or fetal parathyroid hypoplasia or agenesis (162–165). In the former instance, the diagnosis of maternal hyperparathyroidism is often made because of the infant's condition. In the latter situations, hypocalcemia may be permanent and require continuing therapy. Hypoparathyroidism may be present in a heterogeneous group of disorders (9) and may occur sporadically or with differing Mendelian modes of inheritance, including autosomal dominant and recessive and X-linked inheritance patterns. The autosomal dominant form is associated with a point mutation in the signal peptide-encoding region of the prepro-PTH gene. The autosomal recessive form is associated with a mutation in the donor splice site leading to transcriptional loss of the second axon and prevention of translation. The X-linked recessive form is associated with embryonic dysgenesis of parathyroid glands (9,162–165).

Hypocalcemia (in varying degree of severity) from transient congenital hypoparathyroidism (TCHP) may occur in association with DiGeorge and velocardiofacial/Shprintzen syndromes. Both syndromes may represent different degrees of the same disorder with partial or complete absence of derivatives of the third and fourth pharyngeal pouches, and possibly the fifth pouch, and are often associated with defective development of the third, fourth, and sixth aortic arches (see Chap. 40). Other clinical manifestations may include some combination of congenital heart disease, primarily involving the aortic arch, decreased T-cell number or function, and possibly thyroid C-cell deficiency (9,165,166). Deletion of 22q.11 has been reported in these patients (167,168), and DiGeorge association may be inherited in an autosomal dominant fashion (169). There is increasing evidence that neonates previously diagnosed with TCHP may have recurrence of their hypoparathyroidism in later childhood (170–172).

Molecular genetic studies have demonstrated that hypocalcemia can occur in association with defects in the regulation or response to PTH, and the majority of families with autosomal forms of hypoparathyroidism probably do not have mutations of the parathyroid gene. Activating CaR mutations with reduction in EC50 (concentration of extracellular Ca required to elicit half of the maximal increase in intracellular inositol phosphate) manifested as autosomal dominant or sporadic cases of hypocalcemia with hypercalciuria have been reported (83,84). Clinical diagnosis with confirmed hypocalcemia is often delayed beyond the neonatal period, although hypocalcemia theoretically was present in the newborn period (83).

Various mutations in the α-subunit of the stimulating G protein ($G_{s\alpha}$) are responsible for the manifestations of pseudohypoparathyroidism type Ia or Albright's hereditary osteodystrophy. The gene GNAS1 is located on chromosome 20q13.2 and encodes 13 exons that are alternatively spliced to yield four $G_{s\alpha}$ proteins. The inactivating mutations of the gene result in an impaired adenylate cyclase second messenger system, leading to resistance to multiple hormones (including PTH, vasopressin, and thyrotropin) that activate $G_{s\alpha}$. Clinical manifestations include short stature, round face, brachymetacarpals and brachymetatarsals, dental dysplasia, subcutaneous calcifications, and abnormalities in taste, smell, hearing, and vision. Biochemical abnormalities include hypocalcemia, hyperphosphatemia, increased circulating PTH, and insensitivity to the administration of exogenous PTH (unaltered urinary calcium, phosphorus, and cAMP) in the absence of compromised renal function. However, the complete biochemical picture is usually not evident until 2 to 3 years after birth (173–175).

Decreases in serum iCa can occur without decreases in serum tCa. Agents that complex Ca in the blood would be expected to decrease ionized Ca (9). Such agents include citrate, which is used as an anticoagulant for blood storage. During exchange blood transfusion, iCa can be decreased to 0.5 mmol/L in spite of administration of conventional amounts of Ca (i.e., 0.5 to 1 mL of 10% Ca gluconate for each 100 mL of blood exchanged) during the transfusion. Increased levels of long-chain free fatty acids also can complex Ca *in vitro* and reduce ionized Ca. Alkalosis can result in shifts of Ca from the ionized state to the protein-bound fraction. Because alkalosis per se increases neuromuscular hyperirritability, the combination of decreased serum iCa and alkalosis may precipitate clinical tetany in an infant with borderline serum Ca status. Furthermore, *in vitro* studies have demonstrated that bicarbonate (176) as well as phosphate (177) salts may

directly bind to iCa. For reasons that are unclear, infants born to narcotic-using mothers have been reported to have a lower serum iCa if they manifest withdrawal symptoms (178).

Diagnosis

The clinical manifestation of neonatal hypocalcemia in infants may be confused easily with other neonatal disorders (e.g., hypoglycemia, sepsis, meningitis, anoxia, intracranial bleeding, narcotic withdrawal). The neonate with hypocalcemia also may be asymptomatic; the less mature the infant, the more subtle and varied are the clinical manifestations. Significant clinical signs are tremulousness, apnea, cyanosis, and seizures; infants also may be lethargic, feed poorly, vomit, and have abdominal distension. Frank convulsions are seen more commonly with late neonatal hypocalcemia. The degree of irritability of the infants does not appear to correlate with serum Ca values. The classic signs of peripheral hyperexcitability of motor nerves—carpopedal spasm (spasm of the wrists and ankles) and laryngospasm (spasm of the vocal cords)—are uncommon in newborn infants. Therefore, suspicion of hypocalcemia should be confirmed by measurement of serum tCa and iCa.

Diagnostic workup for hypocalcemia includes a history, physical examination, and relevant investigations (Table 36–3). At physiologic concentrations of hydrogen and potassium ion, tetany may develop in older infants at an iCa less than 0.8 mmol/L (3.2 mg/dL) and will almost always be manifested, with the possible exception of preterm infants, at an iCa less than 0.6 mmol/L (2.4

TABLE 36–3. *Diagnostic workup for hypocalcemia*

History
  Familial
  Pregnancy (i.e., maternal illness such as diabetes mellitus and hyperparathyroidism; intrapartum events; infant's gestational age)
  Dietary intake of infant
Physical examination
  Jitteriness, apnea, cyanosis
  Seizures
  Associated features (e.g., infant of a diabetic mother, prematurity, birth asphyxia, congenital heart defect)
Investigations
  Serum total and ionized Ca, Mg, P, glucose
  Vitamin D metabolites
  Parathyroid hormone
  Calcitonin
  Acid–base balance
  Electrocardiogram (Q–Tc > 0.4 sec or Q–oTc > 0.2 sec)
  Chest x-ray (e.g., thymic shadow, aortic arch position)
  Urine Ca, Mg, P, creatinine, drug screen
  Others (e.g., malabsorption workup, lymphocyte count, T-cell numbers and function, maternal and family screening, molecular genetic studies)

mg/dL). If serum albumin concentrations are normal, the corresponding serum tCa concentrations usually are less than 1.8 mmol/L (7.2 mg/dL). In the preterm infant, serum iCa may not decrease to the same extent as total Ca, presumably in part because of the lower serum albumin concentrations or acidosis that is found frequently in these infants. The standard nomogram relating serum tCa and total protein to ionized Ca has not been predictive of neonatal serum iCa. The measurement of electrocardiographic QT intervals, corrected for heart rate, also is of little value for prediction of neonatal hypocalcemia. Urine Ca, Mg, phosphorus, and creatinine are useful in the differential diagnosis. Molecular genetic studies may be needed to confirm a specific diagnosis.

Assays of calciotropic hormones and 25-OHD may be useful in the diagnosis of uncommon causes of neonatal hypocalcemia, such as primary hypoparathyroidism, malabsorption, and disorders of vitamin D metabolism. Other investigations listed in the tables may be important in the differential diagnosis and understanding of the pathophysiology for hypocalcemia.

Confirmation of hypocalcemia as the cause of clinical symptomatology is the reversibility of clinical signs when serum tCa or iCa has been increased to the normal range.

Therapy

Any neonate with seizures should have blood drawn for diagnostic tests before therapy. Intravenous administration of Ca salts is the most effective and most rapid means of elevating serum Ca concentrations. Seizures suspected to be caused by hypocalcemia should be treated with intravenous 10% Ca gluconate (1 mL/kg) administered over 10 minutes with constant monitoring of the heart rate. Gradual or abrupt decrease in heart rate during the infusion is an indication to slow or stop the infusion.

There is little information on comparative efficacy of Ca preparations in the treatment of neonatal hypocalcemia. In neonates, 10% Ca gluconate [0.45 mmol (18 mg) elemental Ca/kg] can effectively increase serum iCa, heart rate, and blood pressure (151–153). In children, small equimolar doses [0.07 mmol (2.8 mg) elemental Ca/kg] of 10% Ca chloride compared to 10% Ca gluconate may result in higher mean arterial blood pressure with a slightly greater mean increase (0.06 mmol/L) in the measured serum iCa (174). Thus, 10% Ca chloride (0.1 to 0.3 mL/kg) also may be used with the same precautions as above. Prolonged use of Ca chloride in high doses may be associated with acidosis and probably should be avoided. Subsequent Ca therapy will depend on symptomatic response to initial dose and repeated measurement of serum tCa and iCa concentrations.

After the resolution of the seizures, intravenous Ca solution may be continued at a dose of 1.87 mmol (75 mg) elemental Ca/kg per day until the serum Ca concentrations have remained consistently in the normal range. Thereafter, the intravenous Ca solution can be reduced in stepwise fashion (i.e., 50% for 24 hours, 25% for another 24 hours) and then discontinued.

With intravenous calcium therapy, bolus infusion may be associated with a transient slight decrease in blood pH and serum phosphorus (180) and with hypercalcemia (181). Continuous infusion probably is more efficacious than intermittent therapy because renal loss of Ca may be greater with the latter method (182). Intravenous Ca therapy may be complicated by acute hypercalcemia; extravasation of Ca solution leads to skin sloughs, tissue necrosis, and calcification. If umbilical venous catheters are used, the tips should not be intracardiac because of possible accidental administration of Ca directly into the heart. Arterial infusion of Ca in high concentrations potentially is fraught with many dangers and should be avoided if possible. Anecdotal cases of massive sloughing of soft tissue in the area perfused by the peripheral artery receiving the infusion have been reported, and inadvertent administration into a mesenteric artery theoretically can lead to necrosis of intestinal tissues. However, parenteral nutrition solutions containing standard mineral (including calcium) content can be safely infused through appropriately positioned umbilical venous or arterial cathers. Direct admixture of Ca preparation with bicarbonate or phosphate solution will result in precipitation and must be avoided.

Oral Ca therapy in the same dosage [1.87 mmol (75 mg) elemental Ca/kg per day in four to six divided doses] may be used for maintenance therapy. All Ca preparations are hypertonic, and there is a theoretical potential for precipitating necrotizing enterocolitis in infants at risk for this condition. Oral Ca preparations with a syrup base containing a high sucrose content may constitute a significant carbohydrate and osmolar load for very small infants and may be associated with an increase in frequency of bowel movements. Calcium syrup is concentrated; for example, Ca glubionate and Ca gluceptate have 2.88 and 2.25 mmol (115 and 90 mg) elemental Ca per 5 mL, respectively, if the infant is under fluid restriction. Alternatively, an intravenous preparation can be used orally if the fluid volume is tolerated.

The duration of supplemental Ca therapy varies with the course of hypocalcemia. Commonly, as little as 2 to 3 days of therapy is required, as illustrated by the treatment of early neonatal hypocalcemia. The requirement for Ca therapy may be prolonged, however, as in the case of hypocalcemia caused by malabsorption or hypoparathyroidism. The serum Ca concentrations should be measured daily during the first few days of treatment and for 1 or 2 days after discontinuation, until serum tCa and iCa concentrations are stabilized. Persistently low serum Ca concentrations should prompt further investigations even in the absence of suspicious history or physical features associated with pathologic causes of hypocalcemia. A poor response to Ca therapy often may result from concurrent Mg deficiency (see Hypomagnesemia).

Vitamin D metabolites and exogenous PTH have been used in the treatment of neonatal hypocalcemia (9). They offer no practical advantage in the treatment of acute hypocalcemia. For infants, the dose of vitamin D metabolite, $1,25(OH)_2D$, needed to maintain normocalcemia is usually higher than that employed for adults: 0.5 to 1 μg/day orally and 0.1 to 4 μg/kg per day intramuscularly or intravenously (155,183). Vigorous vitamin D treatment in patients with activating CaR mutation may be associated with worsened hypercalciuria, renal stones, nephrocalcinosis, and/or renal insufficiency, even while the patients are normocalcemic (83).

Successful management of neonatal hypocalcemia also depends on the resolution, if possible, of the primary cause of hypocalcemia. For example, in phosphate-induced hypocalcemia, high-phosphate formulas and solids should be discontinued, and human milk or a low-phosphate formula should be substituted. Use of aluminum hydroxide gel to bind intestinal phosphate should be avoided because of potential risk for aluminum toxicity (184).

Neonatal hypocalcemia may resolve spontaneously. Thus, it is possible that asymptomatic neonatal hypocalcemia may not require treatment. Because of the major physiologic importance of Ca in all cellular systems, however, hypocalcemia probably should be corrected, as it potentially can alter important cellular functions where calcium serves either as a first or second messenger in cellular activity. Treatment of asymptomatic hypocalcemia can be instituted with oral or intravenous Ca salts, using the regimen described earlier.

Pharmacologic prevention of neonatal hypocalcemia has focused primarily on the prophylactic use of Ca salts or vitamin D metabolites. In newborn infants, Ca supplementation results in sustained lowering of serum intact PTH concentrations compared to unsupplemented controls (53). Theoretically, Ca supplementation may decrease the metabolic stress from hypocalcemia and minimize the potential for depletion of tissue Ca stores. An oral dose of 1.8 to 2.0 mmol/kg per day (72 to 80 mg/kg per day) has been used successfully in low-birth-weight infants. Continuous infusion of 0.025 to 0.038 mmol (1.0 to 1.5 mg) elemental Ca/kg per hour may be needed in some infants and appears to be well tolerated in clinical practice. Vitamin D metabolites have been used in attempts to prevent neonatal hypocalcemia, with variable degrees of success. In small preterm infants, serum Ca was normalized only at pharmacologic doses of $1,25(OH)_2D$ (155). Early feeding and provision of Ca to the gut may be important in enhancing the ability of vitamin D metabolites to prevent neonatal hypocalcemia.

The most effective prevention of neonatal hypocalcemia includes prevention of prematurity and birth asphyxia, judicious use of bicarbonate therapy and mechanical ventilation, for example, during intentional induction of alkalosis in the treatment of persistent pulmonary hypertension (185). The practice of early milk feeding and, if necessary, oral or parenteral supplement of Ca salts also are useful measures. Maintenance of normal maternal vitamin D status with exogenous vitamin D supplement, if needed, may in theory be helpful in maintaining normal fetal vitamin D status and may secondarily prevent late hypocalcemia in some neonates (9). Regular follow-up monitoring of serum Ca concentration and appropriate monitoring of underlying disease (e.g., PTH concentrations) are necessary because there are no definitive measures to determine whether an infant has a "transient" hypoparathyroidism that may last for several years (170) or is at risk for "recurrence" of hypoparathyroidism and hypocalcemia, which has been reported to recur as late as adolescence (171). Maternal and family screening for calcium disorders is indicated in the absence of specific diagnosis for the neonatal hypocalcemia.

Hypercalcemia

Hypercalcemia is present when serum tCa is more than 2.75 mmol/L (11 mg/dL) or when iCa is more than 1.4 mmol/L (5.6 mg/dL). In pathologic hypercalcemia, elevation of serum iCa usually occurs simultaneously with elevation of tCa; however, elevated tCa may occur without elevation of iCa. Elevation of protein available to bind Ca (e.g., prolonged application of tourniquet before venipuncture, transudation of plasma water into tissues, in adult patients with multiple myeloma, and possibly adrenal insufficiency) may result in elevation of serum tCa. A change in serum albumin of 1 g/dL generally results in a parallel change in tCa of about 0.2 mmol/L. Conversely, reduced albumin binding of Ca may result in normal serum tCa in the presence of elevated ionized Ca.

Hypercalcemia in infants is rare. It frequently is iatrogenic and may be discovered serendipitously on a routine panel of chemistry tests. Its onset may be at birth or delayed for weeks or months. The most common clinical cause of hypercalcemia in infants (Table 36–4) is a relative deficiency in the phosphate supply and hypophosphatemia during inappropriate parenteral nutrition or enteral human milk feeding in preterm infants. Phosphate deficiency or hypophosphatemia stimulates 1α-hydroxylase and enhances synthesis of $1,25(OH)_2D$. The latter then acts through VDR to increase renal phosphate conservation by inducing phosphate-translocating proteins such as the renal sodium–phosphate cotransporter-2 (NPT2) in the kidney (186,187) and suppresses PTH synthesis (71). In contrast, hypophosphatemia associated with tumor-induced osteomalacia and X-linked hypophosphatemia (XLH) may not elicit an increase in $1,25(OH)_2D$ production and phosphate conservation. This is probably a result of an increase in phosphatonin, an uncharacterized phosphaturic hormone that is postu-

TABLE 36–4. *Neonatal hypercalcemia*

Phosphate deficiency
   Parental nutrition
   Very-low-birth-weight infants fed human milk or, less
      commonly, standard formula
Vitamin D
   Excessive maternal vitamin D intake
   Subcutaneous fat necrosis (?)
Prostaglandin-related disorder
   Bartter syndrome variant
Parathyroid
   Congenital parathyroid hyperplasia
   Maternal hypoparathyroidism
   Maternal and neonatal renal tubular acidosis
Calcium-sensing receptor defect
   Familial hypocalciuric hypercalcemia
   Neonatal severe hyperparathyroidism
Uncertain pathophysiologic mechanism
   Extracorporeal membrane oxygenation therapy
   Idiopathic infantile hypercalcemia (Williams syndrome)
   Severe infantile hypophosphatasia
   Blue diaper syndrome
   Congenital hypothyroidism
   Congenital mesoblastic nephroma
Other causes of chronic maternal hypercalcemia
   Thyrotoxicosis
   Chronic thiazide diuretic
   Chronic lithium therapy
   Vitamin A intoxication

lated to inhibit both NPT2 and 1α-hydroxylase to cause severe phosphate wasting. In XLH, the defective gene responsible for the increase in phosphatonin, phosphate wasting, and inappropriately low circulating levels of $1,25(OH)_2D$ has been identified as PEX (phosphate-regulating gene with homologies to endopeptidases located on the X chromosome) (188). Increased Ca absorbed in the presence of increased $1,25(OH)_2D$ cannot be deposited in bone in the absence of phosphate and contributes to hypercalcemia.

Neonatal hyperparathyroidism frequently results in marked hypercalcemia. It may be congenital and inherited as an autosomal-dominant or autosomal-recessive trait, or it may be secondary to maternal hypoparathyroidism (189). In affected infants, the serum Ca may be markedly elevated (>3.7 mmol/L), whereas serum phosphorus is frequently low (<1.2 mmol/L). The serum alkaline phosphatase activity may be normal or increased. Unexplained anemia or splenomegaly may be present. Radiographic skeletal demineralization, subperiosteal resorption, and pathologic fractures are frequently present. Renal calcinosis is also common. The characteristic pathologic finding in the parathyroid glands is clear-cell hyperplasia. Neonatal hyperparathyroidism also may occur in the presence of maternal or neonatal renal tubular acidosis and with FHH (78,81,82,190,191).

Neonatal hypercalcemia associated with a number of conditions can be explained by CaR mutations. The severity of hypercalcemia is related to the extent of CaR mutation. Most patients with FHH who exhibit mild hypercalcemia are heterozygous for the mutated CaR. More severe hypercalcemia with serum tCa of 3 to 3.3 mmol/L (12 to 13 mg/dL) has been attributed to coexpression of the normal and mutated CaR, with the latter having a functional equivalent of a "dominant negative" effect (81,82). Humans homozygous for inactivating CaR mutations have the most marked hypercalcemia associated with neonatal severe hyperparathyroidism; the disorder can be lethal within the first few weeks of life (78). Familial hypercalciuric hypercalcemia has been reported in patients from 2 hours to 82 years of age and is usually diagnosed in infants as part of a screening procedure after diagnosis of a family member with hypercalcemia or familial multiple endocrine neoplasia. It is inherited as an autosomal dominant trait with a high degree of penetrance (192). There usually is significant hypophosphatemia and a modest increase in serum Mg concentration, and functional parathyroid glands are needed for full expression (78,192–194). Neonatal hyperparathyroidism associated with FHH that resolves spontaneously over several months has been reported (195).

A number of other pathologic conditions associated with PTH or vitamin D may increase bone turnover, intestinal Ca absorption, and renal Ca absorption and may result in hypercalcemia. Chronic excessive exposure to vitamin D or its metabolites secondary to the treatment of maternal hypocalcemic disorders or by self-medication may result in hypercalcemia of the mother and the neonate. A Bartter syndrome variant associated with polyhydramnios, prematurity, nephrocalcinosis, and increased prostaglandin E_2 excretion may be associated with hypercalcemia in infants. Some affected subjects are reported to have increased serum $1,25(OH)_2D$ concentrations (196,197). Neonates with extensive subcutaneous fat necrosis may develop hypercalcemia. There is often a history of perinatal asphyxia, and hypercalcemia usually occurs at the end of the first week after birth and after a period of low or normal serum Ca concentrations (198). Increased prostaglandin E activity, increased release of Ca from fat and tissues, and unregulated production of $1,25(OH)_2D$ from macrophages infiltrating fat necrotic lesions have been postulated to be responsible for the hypercalcemia in these conditions (115,198,199).

Other causes of neonatal hypercalcemia in which no specific defect of vitamin D or PTH physiology has been demonstrated are listed in Table 36–4. Hypercalcemia has been reported in up to 3% of infants receiving extracorporeal membrane oxygenation therapy (200), presumably in part related to the varying amounts of Ca solutions added to the priming circuit for the ECMO system. Idiopathic infantile hypercalcemia, often considered part of Williams syndrome, is associated with varying manifestations including hypercalcemia, mental retardation, elfin facies, and supravalvular aortic stenosis. There also may be prenatal and postnatal growth failure. The presence of hypercalcemia in infants with Williams syndrome is variable, and serum Ca may be normal, but the presence of nephrocalcinosis and soft tissue calcifications in some of these infants suggests that hypercalcemia may have occurred previously. An exaggerated response to pharmacologic doses of vitamin D_2 and a blunted CT response to Ca loading may contribute to the pathogenesis of hypercalcemia of idiopathic infantile hypercalcemia. Several genetic defects in idiopathic infantile hypercalcemia, including hemizygosity at the elastin gene on the long arm of chromosome 7, have been reported (201,202). No mutation of the CT/CGRP gene has been detected (203,204). However, the cellular mechanism that led to the phenotypic expression remains unknown.

Severe infantile hypophosphatasia is associated with hypercalcemia. It is a rare autosomal recessive disorder associated with decreased synthesis of tissue nonspecific alkaline phosphatase from a deletion or point mutation in its gene located on chromosome 1. These patients have severe bone demineralization, low serum alkaline phosphatase, and elevated urinary pyrophosphate and phosphoethanolamine. The condition may be lethal *in utero* or shortly after birth because of inadequate bony support of the thorax and skull, although milder phenotypes are compatible with survival to adulthood (205).

Blue diaper syndrome is a rare familial disorder with malabsorption of tryptophan. The blue discoloration of the urine results from the hydrolysis and oxidation of urinary indican, an end product of intestinal degradation of unabsorbed tryptophan and hepatic metabolism of its intermediate metabolites. Hypercalcemia and nephrocalcinosis usually do not manifest until some months after birth (206).

Hypercalcemia may develop before and during thyroxine therapy of infants with congenital agoitrous hypothyroidism (207). In theory, deficient CT response to Ca loading or an increased degradation of CT may be responsible for the hypercalcemia (96,207). Congenital mesoblastic nephroma (208,209) may be associated with hypercalcemia in infants. It is thought that causes of chronic maternal hypercalcemia, including maternal thyrotoxicosis, chronic thiazide diuretic, lithium therapy, and vitamin A intoxication, also may affect newborn infants (9,210).

Diagnosis

Neonates with hypercalcemia may be asymptomatic, and the diagnosis made on routine screening, because of known predisposing factors, or in the presence of serious symptomatology requiring urgent treatment (154). Symptoms and signs frequently are nonspecific and include lethargy, irritability, polyuria, vomiting, constipation, dehydration, and failure to thrive. Hypertension, nephrocalcinosis, and band keratopathy of the limbus of the eye may be present in severely affected infants. Anatomic anomalies (e.g., elfin facies, evidence of congenital heart disease) may be present on physical examination. A maternal dietary and drug history or a history of polyhydramnios during pregnancy should be determined, as should a family history for evidence of disturbed Ca metabolism. Laboratory investigations are listed in Table 36–5.

Therapy

Therapy of neonatal hypercalcemia includes management of specific underlying causes (e.g., excessive vita-

---

TABLE 36–5. *Diagnostic workup for hypercalcemia*[a]

History
    Familial or maternal Ca or P disease
    Difficult labor, ECMO and pre-ECMO therapy
    Chronic excessive maternal or neonatal intake of vitamins D or A
    Chronic maternal medications (e.g., thiazide, lithium)
Physical examination
    Poor growth parameters
    Lethargy, dehydration
    Seizures, hypertension, band keratopathy (rare)
    Associated features (e.g., elfin facies, congenital heart disease, mental retardation, subcutaneous fat necrosis)
Investigation
    Serum total Ca, ionized Ca, Mg, P, alkaline phosphatase, total protein, PTH, 25-OHD
    Urine Ca, P, cAMP, creatinine
    Chest x-ray
    X-ray hands
    Renal function, abdominal ultrasound, ophthalmologic evaluation, ECG (i.e., shortened QT interval) for effect of hypercalcemia
    Maternal Ca and P and other tests including molecular genetic studies, as appropriate
    Family screening depends on primary diagnosis

[a]Abbreviations: ECMO, extracorporeal membrane oxygenation therapy; cAMP, cyclic adenosine monophosphate; ECG, electrocardiogram; 25-OHD, 25-hydroxyvitamin D; PTH, parathyroid hormone.

min D intake). Often, nonspecific therapy is the mainstay of therapy. Treatment for chronic conditions includes restriction of dietary intake of vitamin D and Ca and minimizing exposure to sunlight to decrease endogenous vitamin D production. A low-Ca, low-vitamin D_3, low-iron infant formula is available for the management of hypercalcemia in infants (Calcilo XD, Ross Laboratories, Columbus, OH). This formula contains only trace amounts of Ca (<10 mg/100 kcal) and no vitamin D. Long-term use of this formula alone will lead to calcium depletion.

For short-term treatment of acute hypercalcemic episodes, expansion of the extracellular fluid compartment with 10 to 20 mL/kg of 0.9% sodium chloride intravenously, followed by an intravenous injection of a potent loop diuretic such as 2 mg/kg of furosemide, may be effective. Care should be taken to avoid fluid and electrolyte imbalance with careful monitoring of fluid balance and serum Ca, Mg, sodium, potassium, and osmolality at 6- to 8-hour intervals. Furosemide therapy may be repeated at 4- to 6-hour intervals. Prolonged diuresis also requires replacement of Mg losses. In patients with low serum phosphorus concentrations, phosphate supplements of 0.5 to 1.0 mmol/kg of elemental phosphorus per day in divided doses may normalize the serum phosphorus concentration and lower serum Ca concentrations; excessive amounts of phosphate may result in diarrhea and hypocalcemia and a theoretical possibility of metastatic calcification.

Minimal information is available on the use of hormonal and other drug therapy for neonatal hypercalcemia. Short-term treatment with salmon CT (4 to 8 IU/kg every 12 hours, subcutaneously or intramuscularly), prednisone (0.5 to 1 mg/kg per day), or a combination may be useful. Recombinant hCT, bisphosphonates, and amylin also may be useful (102,211). Onset of action of these therapies is slow, and the hypocalcemic effect of CT may not occur. Rarely, parathyroidectomy may be necessary, although it is not always effective (212). Indomethacin, a prostaglandin synthetase inhibitor, appears to be the specific agent of choice for Bartter syndrome variant. In some instances, neonatal hypercalcemia may resolve spontaneously. The need for treatment should be reassessed at regular intervals. Family screening for hypercalcemia should be done unless a specific nonfamilial cause for hypercalcemia is established in the index case.

Hypomagnesemia

Hypomagnesemia is present when serum tMg is less than 0.06 mmol/L (1.5 mg/dL). There are no data on the level of iMg during hypomagnesemia. Tissue Mg deficiency, however, may be present despite normal serum Mg concentrations (Table 36–6) (3,4,19).

TABLE 36–6. *Neonatal hypomagnesemia*

Decreased magnesium intake
  Maternal magnesium deficiency
  Small-for-gestational-age infants
  Maternal insulin-dependent diabetes
  Specific intestinal magnesium malabsorption (isolated, familial)
  Extensive small intestine resection
Magnesium loss
  Exchange transfusion with citrated blood
  Intestinal fistula or diarrhea
  Hepatobiliary disorders
  Decreased renal tubular reabsorption
    Primary: hypokalemic alkalosis, hypomagnesemia with hypercalciuria or hypocalciuria
    Secondary: extracellular fluid compartment expansion, osmotic diuresis
  Drugs (e.g., loop diuretic, aminoglycoside)
Other causes
  Increased phosphate intake
  Maternal hyperparathyroidism

Magnesium depletion in pregnant rats results in fetal mortality, malformations, hypomagnesemia, decreased skeletal Mg content, hemolytic anemia, hypoproteinemia, and edema (213,214). Prolonged dietary Mg deprivation in human adults leads to personality change, tremor, muscle fasciculations, spontaneous carpopedal spasm, and generalized spasticity as well as hypomagnesemia, hypocalcemia, and hypokalemia (35). Clinical manifestations in human congenital hypomagnesemia (i.e., fetal Mg depletion) (215) and neonatal hypomagnesemia are less well described, especially since clinical signs overlap with the often concomitant hypocalcemia.

Postnatally, hypomagnesemia is usually associated with decreased circulating PTH concentrations, decreased production of active vitamin D metabolites, in particular $1,25(OH)_2D$, and resistance to PTH and $1,25(OH)_2D$. It occurs more frequently in infants with intrauterine growth retardation (IUGR) than in appropriate-for-gestational-age infants. Hypomagnesemia in IUGR occurs particularly in young, primiparous mothers, especially those who have toxemia of pregnancy (216,217). The severity and prevalence of hypomagnesemia in infants of insulin-dependent diabetic mothers are directly related to the severity of maternal diabetes, which is thought to reflect the severity of maternal Mg deficiency. Hypomagnesemia in infants of diabetic mothers is associated with neonatal hypocalcemia and decreased parathyroid function (159,217). Magnesium infusion in infants results in greater increases in serum Ca and PTH in those with initially low serum Mg concentrations (218), and, in children with insulin-dependent diabetes, results in greater serum Ca and PTH responses than occur in normal control subjects (117).

Specific intestinal malabsorption apparently predominates in boys (216,219,220), and hypocalcemia has occurred in all reported instances. Intestinal resection, particularly of the jejunum and ileum, the major sites of Mg absorption, increases intestinal loss through ileostomy or fecal fistulas, and rapid intestinal transit time may lead to Mg deficiency (36,216,221).

In the newborn period, exchange blood transfusions using citrate as anticoagulant result in complexing of citrate with Mg, which leads to hypomagnesemia, especially after multiple exchanges (181,222).

Magnesium content in bile, gastric fluid, and pancreatic secretion varies from 0.2 to 5.0 mmol/L (0.5 to 12 mg/dL). Diarrheal Mg content may be as high as 7.1 mmol/L (17 mg/dL). Because the typical deficit required to produce symptomatic hypomagnesemia is approximately 0.5 to 1.0 mmol (12 to 24 mg) per kilogram of body weight, fluid losses from diarrhea or a chronic intestinal fistula may be associated with significant Mg loss (36).

Infants with congenital biliary atresia and neonatal hepatitis may have low serum Mg concentrations (223). This is thought to be partly related to increased aldosterone-related renal Mg losses.

Congenital primary defects in renal tubular reabsorption of Mg may occur (224) and usually are associated with hypokalemic alkalosis with and without hypocalcemia. These defects may be classified further into a hypercalciuric group consistent with the classic Bartter syndrome, which usually presents in infancy with failure to thrive and episodes of dehydration. A variant syndrome with hypocalciuria is thought to present later with short stature, substantially lower serum Mg, and more episodes of tetany (225,226). Secondary defects in renal tubular reabsorption of Mg may result from extracellular fluid expansion caused by excessive glucose, sodium, or fluid intake or from osmotic diuresis. Loop diuretics such as furosemide and high doses of aminoglycosides such as gentamicin may cause magnesuria (227).

Increased phosphate intake may lead to decreased Mg absorption, and infants on high-phosphate milk preparations have lowered serum Mg concentrations. Further elevation of serum phosphate concentrations decreases serum Mg, possibly through the transfer of Mg from extracellular to intracellular sites. In infants with uremia, serum Mg concentrations may be decreased, possibly in relation to higher blood phosphate concentrations (228). Patients with renal failure, however, become hypermagnesemic at a Mg load that does not affect people with normal renal function (229).

Negative Mg balances may occur with hyperparathyroidism (230). Maternal hyperparathyroidism has been associated with neonatal hypomagnesemia (231). In theory, negative maternal Mg balance in this situation may account for neonatal hypomagnesemia. Alternatively, neonatal hypoparathyroidism in this situation may lead to hypomagnesemia from reduced bone-to-blood flux because PTH has a presumptive action on mobilization of bone Mg.

Symptoms and signs of hypomagnesemia, which often coexists with hypocalcemia, may be indistinguishable (4,232). Serum Mg concentrations should be measured in infants at risk for hypomagnesemia and in any infant with hypocalcemia who is resistant to the usual therapy. When hypomagnesemia coexists with hypocalcemia, a trial infusion of 6 mg elemental Mg/kg over 1 hour with pre- and postinfusion measurement of total and ionized Ca and PTH may be helpful in the diagnosis of the primary defect. An increase in serum PTH after Mg infusion is indicative of hypoparathyroidism secondary to Mg deficiency, whereas no change or a decrease in serum PTH supports the diagnosis of hypocalcemia unrelated to Mg deficiency.

Critical assessment of Mg deficiency is difficult because more than 99% of total body Mg is found in intracellular fluids or is complexed in the skeleton. It has been proposed that high Mg retention after a Mg load may reflect Mg deficiency (233). Infants generally retain large amounts of infused Mg, however, and there are large variations in response; the clinical utility of this test thus appears limited in infancy.

The treatment of choice for acute hypomagnesemic seizures is 50% Mg sulfate ($MgSO_4 \cdot 7H_2O$), 0.05 to 0.1 mL/kg (0.1 to 0.2 mmol/kg or 2.5 to 5.0 mg/kg elemental Mg) given intramuscularly or by slow intravenous infusion over 15 to 20 minutes. Repeat doses may be required every 8 to 12 hours. Possible complications of intravenous infusion include systemic hypotension and prolongation or even blockade of sinoauricular or atrioventricular conduction.

Concomitantly, oral Mg supplements can be started if oral fluids are tolerated. Fifty percent Mg sulfate can be given at a dose of 0.2 mL/kg per day. In specific Mg malabsorption, daily oral doses of 1 mL/kg per day may be required. Daily serum Mg concentrations should be measured until values are stable, to evaluate efficacy and safety (20,216). Oral Mg salts are not well absorbed, and large doses may cause diarrhea. The maintenance Mg supplement should be diluted fivefold to sixfold to allow for more frequent administration, maximizing gut absorption and minimizing side effects. Some oral preparations of Mg (e.g., Mg L-lactate dihydrate), especially those in a sustained-release form, may have greater bioavailability than other sources of Mg (e.g., Mg oxide, hydroxide, citrate). Practical experience with the use of Mg salts other than Mg sulfate in infancy is extremely limited, however.

Potassium and zinc deficiency frequently coexists with Mg-deficient states, especially when there are abnormal gastrointestinal losses or malabsorption. Appropriate replacement therapy is needed. Treatment of underlying disorders (e.g., closure of gastrointestinal fistula) should be pursued actively.

Hypermagnesemia

Hypermagnesemia is present when serum Mg is more than 1.04 mmol/L (>2.5 mg/dL). One report of cord sera with elevated serum tMg concentrations from maternal Mg therapy shows that the fraction of iMg decreases to an average of about 60% of tMg values (16), but there are insufficient data to define hypermagnesemia based on the measurement of serum iMg alone. Hypermagnesemia may result from a combination of excessive Mg load and a relatively low capacity for renal excretion of Mg. Neonatal hypermagnesemia most commonly occurs after maternal Mg sulfate administration for preeclampsia. In mothers given Mg sulfate, serum Mg concentrations have been reported from 1.1 to 5.8 mmol/L (2.6 to 14.0 mg/dL), with umbilical cord serum Mg concentrations from 0.83 to 4.8 mmol/L (2.0 to 11.5 mg/dL) (27,28). Concomitant maternal hypocalcemia also may occur secondary to decreased serum PTH concentrations (73). Variations in parenteral Mg intake resulting from high Mg content or high rate of infusion of parenteral nutrition fluids may result in hypermagnesemia, particularly in critically ill neonates (31–33). The use of Mg-containing antacids or enemas can cause hypermagnesemia (216,234). Prematurity and perinatal asphyxia may aggravate hypermagnesemia, presumably because of decreased renal Mg excretion (Table 36–7) (235).

In adults with hypermagnesemia, hypotension and urinary retention occur at serum Mg concentrations of 1.67 to 2.5 mmol/L (4.0 to 6.0 mg/dL); central nervous system depression, hyporeflexia, and electrocardiographic abnormalities (i.e., increased atrioventricular and ventricular conduction time) at 2.5 to 5.0 mmol/L (6.0 to 12.0 mg/dL); and respiratory depression, coma, and cardiac arrest above 5.0 mmol/L (12.0 mg/dL) (37,229). In newborn infants, a delay in passage of meconium (i.e., meconium plug syndrome) has been thought to be related to neonatal hypermagnesemia (236). In pregnant and newborn rats and dogs, however, hypermagnesemia does not have an effect on intestinal motility or the consistency of meconium (237). Most neonates with hypermagnesemia, particularly preterm infants, are asymptomatic, even at serum Mg concentrations of more than 1.25 mmol/L (3 mg/dL) (32,33,235). Clinical signs of neuromuscular depression with floppiness and lethargy may be the most frequent manifestations of neonatal hypermagnesemia. Clinical signs may not correlate with serum Mg concentrations, although there does appear to be a correlation with the duration of maternal Mg sulfate therapy (30), possibly representing tissue Mg content. With judicious use of Mg sulfate in the mother, however, signs of Mg intoxication should be rare in the infant (29).

Serum Ca concentrations may be normal, decreased, or increased in hypermagnesemic neonates (235). Hypermagnesemia may suppress PTH and 1,25(OH)$_2$D production and may result in lower serum Ca concentrations (73,235). Rickets has been reported when maternal Mg therapy is prolonged (e.g., in tocolysis to prevent preterm delivery) (238). It is speculated that excess Mg interferes with normal mineralization of fetal bone. Hypermagnesemia, however, might in theory displace bound Ca and lead to elevation of serum Ca concentration (239).

Calcium is a direct antagonist of Mg, and intravenous Ca given in the same dosage as for treatment of hypocalcemia may be useful for acute therapy. Loop diuretics (e.g., furosemide) with adequate fluid intake may hasten Mg excretion (4,20,34,37,227). Exchange blood transfusion with citrated blood is an effective treatment for severely depressed hypermagnesemic infants. Citrated donor blood is particularly useful because the complexing action of citrate will expedite removal of Mg from the infant. Peritoneal dialysis and hemodialysis may be considered in refractory patients. Supportive measures such as cardiorespiratory assistance and adequate hydration may be needed.

SKELETAL MANIFESTATIONS OF DISTURBED MINERAL HOMEOSTASIS

The most frequent cause of skeletal abnormalities in infancy is nutritional deficiency (Table 36–8). True fetal or congenital rickets is rare. It may result from severe maternal nutritional osteomalacia associated with Ca and

TABLE 36–7. *Neonatal hypermagnesemia*

Prematurity
Asphyxia
Maternal MgSO$_4$ administration
Neonatal Mg therapy
  Parenteral nutrition
  Antacid
  Enema

TABLE 36–8. *Risk factors for the development of osteopenia and rickets in infants*

In utero
  Severe maternal nutritional osteomalacia (i.e., Ca and vitamin D deficiency)
  Maternal hypoparathyroidism and hyperparathyroidism
  Prolonged maternal magnesium or phosphate treatment
Postnatal
  Nutritional
    Prolonged exclusive human milk feeding
    Macrobiotic diet
    Soy formula or human milk for small preterm infants
    Prolonged total parenteral nutrition with low Ca and low P
    Chronic loop diuretic therapy given to preterm infants
    Aluminum contamination (?)
  Inherited defects
    Renal tubular disorder
    Vitamin D or parathyroid hormone metabolism disorders

vitamin D deficiency (240,241), maternal hypoparathyroidism (242) or hyperparathyroidism (161), or prolonged maternal treatment with Mg sulfate (238) or phosphate-containing enemas (243).

In the Western world, rickets and osteopenia presenting during infancy occur most frequently in small preterm infants and may occur in more than 30% of extremely-low-birth-weight (<1 kg) infants (8,244). The rate of occurrence depends on the nutrient intake and is associated most frequently with prolonged intake of soy formula, human milk, and low-Ca and low-phosphorus parenteral nutrition. In infants born at term, prolonged exclusive human milk feeding with limited exposure to sunshine, macrobiotic diet, and prolonged total parenteral nutrition are factors that contribute to the development of osteopenia and rickets (241,245,246). The common underlying causes in preterm infants appear to be mineral deficiency, particularly Ca and phosphorus, whereas in term infants there may be a relative lack of Ca intake in addition to vitamin D deficiency. Isolated nutritional deficiency of copper and ascorbic acid has been reported in preterm infants with clinical and radiographic manifestations similar to rickets (8). Chronic diuretic therapy, commonly used in infants with bronchopulmonary dysplasia, and contamination of nutrients with toxins such as aluminum are added risk factors (184,246). The extent, however, to which specific risk factors are responsible for the development of osteopenia and rickets is difficult to define in individual critically ill infants receiving multiple therapies and suboptimal nutritional support.

Acquired and heritable forms of rickets that develop despite adequate availability of vitamin D usually are associated with renal tubular disorders and metabolic defects in vitamin D and PTH metabolism. These causes of rickets are rare, and their skeletal manifestations usually do not present before late infancy (161,247–249).

Most cases of rickets and osteopenia are diagnosed incidentally during the investigation of complications such as fractures or conditions unrelated to the skeleton. The presence of osteopenia and rickets is confirmed by classic radiographic features such as generalized bone demineralization and widening, cupping, and fraying of the distal metaphyses. Classic features of rickets such as severe skeletal deformities, including kyphoscoliosis and bowing of the legs, may not be present if the diagnosis is made early in infancy, before significant growth and weight-bearing have occurred. This is particularly true for the preterm infant whose skeletal problem typically is diagnosed between 2 and 6 months postnatally. Serial biochemical changes, including persistently low serum inorganic phosphate, elevated serum alkaline phosphatase activity more than 5 times the normal adult upper limit, and elevated serum bone turnover markers, may be helpful in the diagnosis. Measurement of serum 25-OHD as an indicator of vitamin D status also may be helpful. The use of photon absorptiometry allows a more accurate quantification of the degree of bone mineralization, and serial measurements of bone mineral content may be useful to monitor the progress of bone mineralization during long-term follow-up (8,250,251).

Osteopenia, rickets, and fractures in preterm infants appear to have become less frequent since the widespread use of high-Ca and high-phosphorus formulas designed specifically for preterm infants. The ingestion of the recommended daily amount of Ca and phosphorus should be adequate for otherwise healthy term infants (24,252). A total daily intake of 400 IU vitamin D appears adequate to maintain normal vitamin D status in both preterm and term infants (253–255). Human milk is likely to be low in a number of nutrients including protein, sodium, calcium, phosphorus, and possibly other nutrients for the needs of the very small preterm infant (256,257). Thus, small preterm infants receiving mother's milk require supplementation with commercially available powder or liquid fortifier containing a variety of nutrients. The use of Ca and phosphorus supplementation alone is probably inappropriate and impractical in this circumstance (250,256).

The infant's mineral intake is monitored by maintaining a normal serum Ca, phosphorus, and alkaline phosphatase while avoiding hypercalciuria [<0.15 mmol (6 mg) Ca/kg per day]. Measurement of bone turnover markers, vitamin D metabolites such as 25-OHD and $1,25(OH)_2D$, and measurement of bone mineralization with standard skeletal radiographs or photon absorptiometry are needed if pathologic bone mineralization is suspected. Recent reports of total body bone mineral content (TBBMC) based on dual-energy absorptiometry (DXA) technique in newborn (258) and postnatal (259) infants provide an added means to measure the bone mineral status in the developing skeleton.

Rickets and fractures from nutritional deficiencies respond well to adequate nutrient intake. Short-term follow-up of these infants shows no major residual physical deformity. Skeletal maturation as assessed by ossification centers of the wrists for preterm infants is similar to term infants at 1 year of age (244). However, preliminary data on TBBMC indicated that there is a relative delay in bone mineralization in preterm infants compared to weight-matched controls (260), and long-term linear growth in the extremely low-birth-weight infants may remain delayed (261), indicating that bone mineral status in the smallest preterm infants still may be suboptimal despite the relatively uncommon occurrence of radiographic rickets and fractures on follow-up. Specific therapies are required for inherited renal tubular disorders and for disorders of vitamin D and PTH metabolism and usually include phosphate and $1,25(OH)_2D$ supplementation.

REFERENCES

1. Brown E, Vassilev P, Hebert S. Calcium as an extracellular messenger. *Cell* 1995;83:679.

2. Brown EM. Homeostatic mechanisms regulating extracellular and intracellular calcium metabolism. In Bilezikian JP, Levine MA, Marcus R, eds. *The Parathyroids.* New York: Raven Press, 1994:15.

3. Gunther T. Biochemistry and pathobiochemistry of magnesium. *Artery* 1981;9:167.

4. Reinhart RA. Magnesium metabolism: a review with special reference to the relationship between intracellular content and serum levels. *Arch Intern Med* 1988;148:2415.

5. Widdowson EM, McCance RA. The metabolism of calcium, phosphorus, magnesium and strontium. *Pediatr Clin North Am* 1965;12:595.

6. Ziegler EE, O'Donnell AM, Nelson SE, et al. Body composition of the reference fetus. *Growth* 1976;40:320.

7. Ellis KJ, Shypailo RJ, Schanler RJ. Body composition of infants: human cadaver studies. *Basic Life Sci* 1993;60:147.

8. Koo WWK, Steichen JJ. Osteopenia and rickets of prematurity. In Polin R, Fox W, eds. *Fetal and neonatal physiology,* 2nd ed. Philadelphia, WB Saunders, 1998:2335.

9. Bainbridge RR, Koo WWK, Tsang RC. Neonatal calcium and phosphorus disorders. In Lifshitz F, ed. *Pediatric endocrinology: A clinical guide,* 3rd ed. New York: Marcel Dekker, 1996:473.

10. Bowers GN, Brassard C, Sena SF. Measurement of ionized calcium in serum with ion-selective electrodes: a mature technology that can meet the daily service needs. *Clin Chem* 1986;32:1437.

11. D'Orazio P, Bowers GN Jr. Design and preliminary performance characteristics of a newly proposed reference cell for ionized calcium in serum. *Clin Chem* 1992;38:1332.

12. Loughead JL, Mimouni F, Tsang RC. Serum ionized calcium concentrations in normal neonates. *Am J Dis Child* 1988;142:516.

13. Ganz MB, Rasmussen J, Bollag WB, et al. Effect of buffer systems and pH$_i$ on the measurement of [Ca^{2+}]$_i$ with fura 2. *FASEB J* 1990;4:1638.

14. Lowenstein FW, Stanton MF. Serum magnesium levels by age, sex and two racial groups in the United States, First National Health and Nutrition Examination Survey (NHANES I), 1971–1974. *J Am Coll Nutr* 1986;5:399.

15. Handwerker SM, Altura BT, Jones KY, Altura BM. Maternal–fetal transfer of ionized serum magnesium during the stress of labor and delivery: a human study. *J Am Coll Nutr* 1995;14:376

16. Koo B, Sauser K, Hammami M, Koo W. Neonatal magnesium homeostasis with and without maternal magnesium treatment. *Clin Chem* 1996;42:S309.

17. Ryzen E, Servis KL, DeRusso P, et al. Determination of intracellular free magnesium by nuclear magnetic resonance in human magnesium deficiency. *J Am Coll Nutr* 1989;8:580.

18. Elin RJ, Hosseini JM, Banks SM, et al. Precision of cellular magnesium assays. *Clin Chem* 1990;36:821.

19. Elin RJ. Assessment of magnesium status. *Clin Chem* 1987;33:1965.

20. Koo WWK, Tsang RC. Calcium and magnesium metabolism. In Werner M, ed. *CRC handbook of clinical chemistry,* vol 4. Orlando, FL: CRC Press, 1989:51.

21. Kurokawa K. The kidney and calcium homeostasis. *Kidney Int* 1994;44:S97.

22. Mundy GR. *Calcium homeostasis: hypercalcemia and hypocalcemia,* 2nd ed. Cory, NC: Martin Dunitz, 1990:17.

23. Bronner F. Current concepts of calcium absorption: an overview. *J Nutr* 1992;122:641.

24. Koo WWK, Tsang RC. Building better bones: calcium, magnesium, phosphorus, and vitamin D. In Tsang RC, Zlotkin SH, Nichols BL, Hansen JW, eds. *Nutrition during infancy: principles and practice,* 2nd ed. Cincinnati: Digital Educational Publishing, 1997:175.

25. Canalis E. Systemic and local factors and the maintenance of bone quality. *Calcif Tiss Int* 1993;53:S90.

26. Abrams SA, Yergey AL, Schanler RJ, et al. Hypercalciuria in premature infants receiving high mineral-containing diets. *J Pediatr Gastroenterol Nutr* 1994;18:20.

27. Whang R, Whang DD. Update: mechanisms by which magnesium modulates intracellular potassium. *J Am Coll Nutr* 1990;9:84.

28. Zofkova I, Kancheva RL. The relationship between magnesium and calciotropic hormones. *Magnesium Res* 1995;8:77.

29. Stone SR, Pritchard JA. Effect of maternally administered magnesium sulfate on the neonate. *Obstet Gynecol* 1970;35:574.

30. Lipsitz PJ. The clinical and biochemical effects of excess magnesium in the newborn. *Pediatrics* 1971;47:501.

31. Koo WWK, Fong T, Gupta JM. Parenteral nutrition in infants. *Aust Paediatr J* 1980;16:169.

32. Koo WWK, Tsang RC, Steichen JJ, et al. Parenteral nutrition for infants: effect of high versus low calcium and phosphorus content. *J Pediatr Gastroenterol Nutr* 1987;6:96.

33. Koo WWK, Tsang RC, Succop P, et al. Mineral vitamin D and high calcium and phosphorus needs of preterm infants receiving parenteral nutrition. *J Pediatr Gastroenterol Nutr* 1989;8:225.

34. Dirks JH. The kidney and magnesium regulation. *Kidney Int* 1983;23:771.

35. Shils ME. Experimental human magnesium depletion. *Medicine* 1969;48:61.

36. Thoren L. Magnesium deficiency in gastrointestinal fluid loss. *Acta Chir Scand* 1963;306(Suppl):1.

37. Mordes JP, Wacker WEC. Excess magnesium. *Pharmacol Rev* 1978;29:273.

38. Hardwick LL, Jones MR, Brautbar, et al. Magnesium absorption: mechanisms and the influence of vitamin D, calcium, and phosphate. *J Nutr* 1991;121:13.

39. MacManus J, Heaton FW, Lucus PW. A decreased response to parathyroid hormone in magnesium deficiency. *J Endocrinol* 1971;49:253.

40. Graber ML, Schulman G. Hypomagnesemic hypocalcemia independent of parathyroid hormone. *Ann Intern Med* 1986;104:804.

41. Kronenberg HM, Bringhurst FR, Segre GV, et al. Parathyroid hormone biosynthesis and metabolism. In Belezikian JP, Levine MA, Marcus R, eds. *The parathyroids.* New York: Raven Press, 1994:125.

42. Meyers DA, Beaty TH, Maestri NE, et al. Multipoint mapping studies of six loci on chromosome 11. *Hum Hered* 1987;37:94.

43. Solal M-EC, Sebert J-L, Boudailliez B, et al. Comparison of intact, midregion, and carboxy terminal assays of parathyroid hormone for the diagnosis of bone disease in hemodialyzed patients. *J Clin Endocrinol Metab* 1991;73:516.

44. Cosman F, Shen V, Herrington B, et al. Response of the parathyroid gland to infusion of human parathyroid hormone-(1–34) [PTH-(1–34)]: demonstration of suppression of endogenous secretion using immunoradiometric intact PTH-(1–84) assay. *J Clin Endocrinol Metab* 1991;73:1345.

45. Nussbaum SR, Potts JT Jr. Immunoassays for parathyroid hormone 1-84 in the diagnosis of hyperparathyroidism. *J Bone Miner Res* 1991;6:S43.

46. Saggese G, Baroncelli GI, Bertelloni S, et al. Intact parathyroid hormone levels during pregnancy, in healthy term neonates and in hypocalcemic preterm infants. *Acta Paediatr Scand* 1991;80:36.

47. Rubin LP, Posillico JT, Anast CS, Brown EM. Circulating levels of biologically active and immunoreactive intact parathyroid hormone in human newborns. *Pediatr Res* 1991;29:201.

48. Allgrove J, Adami S, Maning RM, O'Riordan JL. Cytochemical bioassay of parathyroid hormone in maternal and cord blood. *Arch Dis Child* 1985;60:110.

49. Abbas SK, Ratcliff WA, Moniz C, et al. The role of parathyroid hormone-related protein in calcium homeostasis in the fetal pig. *Exp Physiol* 1994;79:527.

50. MacIsaac RJ, Caple JW, Danks JA, et al. Ontogeny of parathyroid hormone-related protein in the ovine parathyroid gland. *Endocrinology* 1991;129:757.

51. Venkataraman PS, Blick KE, Fry HD, Rao RK. Postnatal changes in calcium-regulating hormones in very-low-birth-weight infants. Effect of early neonatal hypocalcemia and intravenous calcium infusion on serum parathyroid hormone and calcitonin homeostasis. *Am J Dis Child* 1985;139:913.

52. Mimouni F, Loughead J, Tsang R, Khoury J. Postnatal surge in serum calcitonin concentrations: no contribution to neonatal hypocalcemia in infants of diabetic mothers. *Pediatr Res* 1990;28:493.

53. Dilena BA, White GH. The responses of plasma ionised calcium and intact parathyrin to calcium supplementation in preterm infants. *Acta Paediatr Scand* 1991;80:1098.

54. Specker BL, Lichtenstein P, Mimouni F, et al. Calcium-regulating hormones and minerals from birth to 18 months of age: a cross-sectional study: II. Effects of sex, race, age, season, and diet on serum minerals, parathyroid hormone, and calcitonin. *Pediatrics* 1986;77:891.

55. Fujisawa Y, Kida K, Matsudea H. Role of change in vitamin D metabolism with age in calcium and phosphorus metabolism in normal human subjects. *J Clin Endocrinol Metab* 1984;59:719.

56. Insogna KL, Lewis AM, Lipinski BA, et al. Effect of age on serum immunoreactive parathyrold hormone and its biological effects. *J Clin Endocrinol Metab* 1984;53:1072.

57. Davis OK, Hawkins DS, Rubin LP, et al. Serum parathyroid hormone (PTH) in pregnant women determined by an immunoradiometric assay for intact PTH. *J Clin Endocrinol Metab* 1988;67:850.

58. Logue FC, Fraser WD, O'Reilly DSTJ, et al. The circadian rhythm of intact parathyroid hormone-(1–84): temporal correlation with prolactin secretion in normal men. *J Clin Endocrinol Metab* 1990;71:1556.

59. Kitamura N, Shigeno C, Shiomi K, et al. Episodic fluctuation in serum intact parathyroid hormone concentration in men. *J Clin Endocrinol Metab* 1990;70:252.

60. Calvo MS, Eastell R, Offord KP, et al. Circadian variation in ionized calcium and intact parathyroid hormone: evidence of sex differences in calcium homeostasis. *J Clin Endocrinol Metab* 1991;72:69.

61. Nemere I, Norman AW. Parathyroid hormone stimulates calcium transport in perfused duodena of normal chicks: comparison with the rapid effect of 1,25-dihydroxyvitamin D_3. *Endocrinology* 1986;199:1406.

62. Mallette LE. Parathyroid hormone and parathyroid hormone-related protein as polyhormones. In Belezikian JP, Levine MA, Marcus R, eds. The parathyroids. New York: Raven Press, 1994:171.

63. Tam CS, Heersche JNM, Murray TM, Parsons JA. Parathyroid hormones stimulates the bone apposition rate independently of its resorptive action: differential effects of intermittent and continuous administration. *Endocrinology* 1982;110:506.

64. Whitfield JF, Morley P. Small bone-building fragments of parathyroid hormone: new therapeutic agents for osteoporosis. *Trends Pharmacol Sci* 1995;16:382.

65. Stewart AF. PTHrP (1–36) as a skeletal anabolic agent for the treatment of osteoporosis. *Bone* 1996;19:303.

66. Gupta A, Martin KJ, Miyauchi A, et al. Regulation of cytosolic calcium by parathyroid hormone and oscillations of cytosolic calcium in fibroblasts from normal and pseudohypoparathyroid patients. *Endocrinology* 1991;128:2825.

67. Abou-Samra A-B, Juppner H, Kong XF, et al. Structure, function, and expression of the receptor for parathyroid hormone and parathyroid hormone-related peptide. *Adv Nephrol* 1994;23:247.

68. Gelbert L, Schipani EA, Juppner H, et al. Chromosomal localization of the parathyroid hormone/parathyroid hormone-related protein receptor gene to human chromosome 3p2.1.1-p24.2. *J Clin Endocrinol Metab* 1994;79:1046.

69. Birnbaumer L. Transduction of receptor signal into modulation of effector activity by G proteins: the first 20 years or so. *FASEB J* 1990;4:3068.

70. Brown EM. A cellular logic for G protein-coupled ion channel pathways. *FASEB J* 1991;5:2175.

71. DeMay MB, Kiernan MS, DeLuca HF, et al. Sequences in the human parathyroid hormone gene that bind the 1,25-dihydroxyvitamin D_3 receptor and mediate transcriptional repression in response to 1,25-dihydroxyvitamin D_3. *Proc Natl Acad Sci USA* 1992;89:8097.

72. Brown EM, Chen CJ. Calcium, magnesium and the control of PTH secretion. *J Bone Miner Res* 1989;5:249.

73. Cholst IN, Steinberg SF, Tropper PJ, et al. The influence of hypermagnesemia on serum calcium and parathyroid hormone levels in human subjects. *N Engl J Med* 1984;310:1221.

74. Toffaletti J, Cooper DL, Lobaugh B. The response of parathyroid hormone to specific changes in either ionized calcium, ionized magnesium, or protein-bound calcium in humans. *Metabolism* 1991;40:814.

75. Fatemi S, Ryzen E, Flores J, et al. Effect of experimental human magnesium depletion on parathyroid hormone secretion and 1,25-dihydroxyvitamin D metabolism. *J Clin Endocrinol Metab* 1991;73:1067.

76. Drueke TB. Abnormal skeletal response to parathyroid hormone and the expression of its receptor in chronic uremia. *Pediatr Nephrol* 1996;10:348.

77. Garrett JE, Capuano IV, Hammerland LG, et al. Molecular cloning and functional expression of human parathyroid hormone calcium receptor cDNAs. *J Biol Chem* 1995;270:12919.

78. Pearce SH, Trump D, Wooding C, et al. Calcium-sensing receptor mutations in familial benign hypercalcaemia and neonatal hyperparathyroidism. *J Clin Invest* 1995;96:2683.

79. Brown EM, Hebert SC. Calcium-receptor-regulated parathyroid and renal function. *Bone* 1997;20:303.

80. Chattopadhyay N, Baum M, Bai M, et al. Ontogeny of the extracellular calcium-sensing receptor in rat kidney. *Am J Physiol* 1996;271:F736.

81. Bai M, Quinn S, Trivedi S, et al. Expression and characterization of inactivating and activating mutations of the human Ca^{2+}-sensing receptor. *J Biol Chem* 1996;271:19537.

82. Bai M, Pearce SH, Kifor O, et al. *In vivo* and *in vitro* characterization of neonatal hyperparathyroidism resulting from a *de novo*, heterozygous mutation in the Ca^{2+}-sensing receptor gene: normal maternal calcium homeostasis as a cause of secondary hyperparathyroidism in familial benign hypocalciuric hypercalcemia. *J Clin Invest* 1997;99:88.

83. Pearce HS, Williamson C, Kifor O, et al. A familial syndrome of hypocalcemia with hypercalciuria due to mutations in the calcium sensing receptor. *N Engl J Med* 1996;335:1115.

84. Baron J, Winer KK, Yanovski JA, et al. Mutations in the Ca^{2+}-sensing receptor gene cause autosomal dominant and sporadic hypoparathyroidism. *Hum Mol Genet* 1996;5:601.

85. Hebert SC, Brown EM, Harris HW. Role of the Ca(2+)-sensing receptor in divalent mineral ion homeostasis. *J Exp Biol* 1997;200:295.

86. Brown E, Hebert S. A cloned Ca^{2+}-sensing receptor: A mediator of direct effects of extracellular Ca^{2+} on renal function? *J Am Soc Nephrol* 1995;6:1530.

87. Eskert R, Scherubl H, Petzelt C, et al. Rhythmic oscillations of cytosolic calcium in rat C-cells. *Mol Cell Endocrinol* 1989;64:67.

88. Hurwitz S. Homeostatic control of plasma calcium concentration. *Crit Rev Biochem Mol Biol* 1996;31:41.

89. Birnbaum RS, Mahoney W, Roos BA. Purification and amino acid sequence of a non-calcitonin secretory peptide derived from preprocalcitonin. *J Biol Chem* 1983;258:5463.

90. Fischer JA, Born W. Novel peptides from the calcitonin gene: expression, receptors and biological function. *Peptides* 1985;6(Suppl 3):265.

91. Besnard P, el M'Selmi A, Jousset U, et al. Effects of 1,25-dihydroxycholecalciferol and calcium on calcitonin mRNA levels in suckling rats. *Mol Cell Endocrinol* 1991;79:45.

92. MacIntyre I. The calcitonin peptide family: relationship and mode of action. *J Bone Miner Res* 1992;16:160.

93. Naveh-Many T, Raue F, Grauer A, et al. Regulation of calcitonin gene expression by hypocalcemia, hypercalcemia, and vitamin D in the rat. *J Bone Miner Res* 1992;7:1233.

94. Austin LA, Heath H III. Calcitonin, physiology and pathophysiology. *N Engl J Med* 1981;304:269.

95. Wongsurawat N, Armbrecht HJ. Calcitonin stimulates 1,25-dihydroxyvitamin D production in diabetic rat kidney. *Metabolism* 1991;40:22.

96. Zamboni G, Avanzini S, Giavarina D, et al. Monomeric calcitonin secretion in infants with congenital hypothyroidism. *Acta Paediatr Scand* 1989;78:885.

97. Zaidi M, Seth R, Girgis SI, et al. Development and performance of a highly sensitive and specific two-site immunometric assay of calcitonin gene-related peptide. *Clin Chem* 1990;36:1288.

98. Robinson MF, Body JJ, Offord KP, et al. Variation of plasma immunoreactive parathyroid hormone and calcitonin in normal and hyperparathyroid man during daylight hours. *J Clin Endocrinol Metab* 1982;55:538.

99. Trasforini G, Margutti A, Portaluppi F, et al. Circadian profile of plasma calcitonin gene-related peptide in healthy man. *J Clin Endocrinol Metab* 1991;73:945.

100. De Los Santos ET, Mazzaferri EL. Calcitonin gene-related peptide: 24-hour profile and responses to volume contraction and expansion in normal men. *J Clin Endocrinol Metab* 1991;72:1031.

101. Samaan NA, Anderson GD, Adam-Mayne ME. Immunoreactive calcitonin in the mother, neonate, child and adult. *Am J Obstet Gynecol* 1975;121:622.

102. Wimalawansa SJ, Gunasekera RD, Datta HK. Hypocalcemic actions of amylin amide in humans. *J Bone Miner Res* 1992;7:1113.

103. Nussenzveig DR, Matthew S, Gershengorn MC. Alternative splicing of a 48-nucleotide exon generates two isoforms of the human calcitonin receptor. *Endocrinology* 1995;136:2047.

104. Mbalaviele G, Jullienne A, de Vernejoul MC. Human umbilical cord blood monocytes express calcitonin receptors in culture in the presence of 1,25 dihydroxyvitamin D. *J Clin Endocrinol Metab* 1991;72:356.

105. Guo YD, Strugnell S, Back DW, et al. Transfected liver cytochrome P-450 hydroxylates vitamin D analogs at different side-chain positions. *Proc Natl Acad Sci USA* 1993;90:8668.

106. Okuda KI. Liver mitochondrial P450 involved in cholesterol catabolism and vitamin D activation. *J Lipid Res* 1994;35:361.

107. Reichel H, Koeffler HP, Norman AW. The role of the vitamin D endocrine system in health and disease. *N Engl J Med* 1989;320:980.

108. DeLuca HF, Krisinger J, Darwish H. The vitamin D system: 1990. *Kidney Int* 1990;38(Suppl 29):S2.

109. Haussler MR, Haussler CA, Jurutka PW, et al. The vitamin D hormone and its nuclear receptor: molecular actions and disease states. *J Endocrinol* 1997;154:S57.

110. Haussler MR, Whitfield GK, Haussler CA, et al. The nuclear vitamin D receptor: biological and molecular regulatory properties revealed. *J Bone Miner Res* 1998;13:325.

111. Labuda M, Fujiwara TM, Ross MV, et al. Two hereditary defects related to vitamin D metabolism map to the same region of human chromosome 12q13–14. *J Bone Miner Res* 1992;7:1447.

112. Bell NH, Shaw S, Turner RT. Evidence that 1,25-dihydroxyvitamin D_3 inhibits the hepatic production of 25-hydroxyvitamin D in man. *J Clin Invest* 1984;74:1540.

113. Clements MR, Johnson L, Fraser DR. A new mechanism for induced vitamin D deficiency in calcium deprivation. *Nature* 1987;325:62.

114. Nesbitt T, Drezner MK. Insulin-like growth factor-I regulation of renal 25-hydroxyvitamin D-1-hydroxylase activity. *Endocrinology* 1993;132:133.

115. Bell NH. Renal and nonrenal 25-hydroxyvitamin D-1α-hydroxylases and their clinical significance. *J Bone Miner Res* 1998;13:350.

116. Rude RK, Adams JS, Ryzen E, et al. Low serum concentrations of 1,25-dihydroxyvitamin D in human magnesium deficiency. *J Clin Endocrinol Metab* 1985;61:933.

117. Saggese G, Federico G, Bertelloni S, et al. Hypomagnesemia and the parathyroid hormone-vitamin D endocrine system in children with insulin-dependent diabetes mellitus: effects of magnesium administration. *J Pediatr* 1991;118:220.

118. Weaver VM, Welsh J. 1,25-Dihydroxycholecalciferol and the genesis of hypocalcaemia in magnesium-deficient chicks. *Magnesium Res* 1990;3:171.

119. Miyamoto KI, Kesterson RA, Yamamoto H, et al. Structural organization of the human vitamin D receptor chromosomal gene and its promoter. *Mol Endocrinol* 1997;11:1165

120. Ebeling PR, Sandgren ME, DiMagno EP, et al. Evidence of an age-related decrease in intestinal responsiveness to vitamin D: relationship between serum 1,25-dihydroxyvitamin D_3 and intestinal vitamin D receptor concentrations in normal women. *J Clin Endocrinol Metab* 1992;75:176.

121. Suda T, Shinki T, Takahashi N. The role of vitamin D in bone and intestinal cell differentiation. *Annu Rev Nutr* 1990;10:195.

122. Whitfield GK, Selznick SH, Haussler CA, et al. Vitamin D receptors from patients with resistance to 1,25-dihydroxyvitamin D_3: Point mutations confer reduced transactivation in response to ligand and impaired interaction with the retinoid × receptor heterodimeric partner. *Mol Endocrinol* 1996;10:1617.

123. Malloy P, Eccleshall T, Gross C, et al. Hereditary vitamin D resistant rickets caused by a novel mutation in the vitamin D receptor that results in decreased affinity for hormone and cellular hyporesponsiveness. *J Clin Invest* 1997;99:297.

124. Li Y, Pirro A, Amling M, et al. Vitamin D receptor knock-out mice develop hypocalcemia, hyperparathyroidism, rickets, osteomalacia and alopecia. *J Bone Miner Res* 1997;12(Suppl 1):S123.

125. al-Aqeel A, Ozand P, Sobki S, et al. The combined use of intravenous and oral calcium for the treatment of vitamin D dependent rickets type II (VDDRH). *Clin Endocrinol* 1993;39:229.

126. Bouillon R, Okamura WH, Norman AW. Structure–function relationships in the vitamin D endocrine system. *Endocr Rev* 1995;16:200.

127. Jongen MJM, Van Ginkel FC, van der Vijgh WJF, et al. An international comparison of vitamin D metabolite measurements. *Clin Chem* 1984;30:399.

128. Specker BL, Greer F, Tsang RC. Vitamin D. In Tsang RC, Nichols BL, eds. *Nutrition during infancy.* Philadelphia: Hanley & Belfus, 1988: 264.

129. Bilezikian JP. Estrogen and postmenopausal osteoporosis: was Albright right after all? *J Bone Miner Res* 1998;13:774.

130. Klaus G, Jux C, Leiber K, et al. Interaction between insulin-like growth factor I, growth hormone, parathyroid hormone, 1 alpha, 25-dihydroxyvitamin D_3 and steroids on epiphyseal chondrocytes. *Acta Paediatr* 1996;Suppl 417:69.

131. Saggese G, Baroncelli GI, Federico G, Bertelloni S. Effects of growth hormone on phosphocalcium homeostasis and bone metabolism. *Horm Res* 1995;44(Suppl 3):55.

132. Bachrach LK, Marcus R, Ott SM, et al. Bone mineral, histomorphometry, and body composition in adults with growth hormone receptor deficiency. *J Bone Miner Res* 1998;13:415.

133. Hayden JM, Mohan S, Baylink DJ. The insulin-like growth factor system and the coupling of formation to resorption. *Bone* 1995;17(Suppl 2):93S.

134. Hofstetter W, Wetterwald A, Cecchini MG, et al. Detection of transcripts and binding sites for colony-stimulating factor-1 during bone development. *Bone* 1995;17:145.

135. Pfeilschifter J, Laukhuf F, Muller-Beckmann B, et al. Parathyroid hormone increases the concentration of insulin-like growth factor-1 and transforming growth factor beta 1 in rat bone. *J Clin Invest* 1995;96:767.

136. Moxham JP, Kibblewhite DJ, Dvorak M, et al. TGF-beta 1 forms functionally normal bone in a segmental sheep tibial diaphyseal defect. *J Otolaryngol* 1996;25:388.

137. Mundy GR, Boyce B, Hughes D, et al. The effects of cytokines and growth factors on osteoblastic cells. *Bone* 1995;17:71S.

138. Uy HL, Mundy GR, Boyce BF, et al. Tumor necrosis factor enhances parathyroid hormone-related protein-induced hypercalcemia and bone resorption without inhibiting bone formation *in vivo*. *Cancer Res* 1997;57:3194.

139. Ellies LG, Heersche JN, Prusanski W, et al. The role of phospholipase A_2 in interleukin-1 alpha-mediated inhibition of mineralizatin of the osteoid formed by fetal rat calvaria cells *in vitro*. *J Dent Res* 1993;72:18.

140. Moe SM, Hack BK, Cummings SA, Sprague SM. Role of IL-1 beta and prostaglandins in beta 2-microglobulin-induced bone mineral dissolution. *Kidney Int* 1995;47:587.

141. Grey A, Mitnick MA, Shapses S, et al. Circulating levels of interleukin-6 and tumor necrosis factor-alpha are elevated in primary hyperparathyroidism and correlate with markers of bone resorption—a clinical research center study. *J Clin Endocrinol Metab* 1996;81:3450.

142. Kimble RB, Vannice JL, Bloedow DC, et al. Interleukin-1 receptor antagonist decreases bone loss and bone resorption in ovariectomized rats. *J Clin Invest* 1994;93:1959.

143. Kimble RB. Alcohol, cytokines, and estrogen in the control of bone modeling. *Alcohol Clin Exp Res* 1997;21:385.

144. Moseley JM, Gillespie MT. Parathyroid hormone-related protein. *Crit Rev Clin Lab Sci* 1995;32:299.

145. Martin TJ, Moseley JM, Williams ED. Parathyroid hormone-related protein: hormone and cytokine. *J Endocrinol* 1997;154:S23.

146. Moseley JM, Hayman JA, Danks JA, et al. Immunohistochemical detection of parathyroid hormone-related protein in human fetal epithelia. *J Clin Endocrinol Metab* 1991;73:478.

147. Law F, Moate PJ, Leaver DD, et al. Parathyroid hormone-related protein in milk and its correlation with bovine milk calcium. *J Endocrinol* 1991;128:21.

148. Thiebaud D, Janisch S, Koelbl H, et al. Direct evidence of a parathyroid related protein gradient between the mother and the newborn in humans. *Bone Miner* 1993;23:213.

149. Dvir R, Golander A, Jaccard N, et al. Amniotic fluid and plasma levels of parathyroid hormone-related protein and hormonal modulation of its secretion by amniotic fluid cells. *Eur J Endocrinol* 1995;133:277.

150. Seki K, Wada S, Nagata N, Nagata I. Parathyroid hormone-related protein during pregnancy and the perinatal period. *Gynecol Obstet Invest* 1994;37:83.

151. Salsbury DJ, Brown DR. Effect of parenteral calcium treatment on blood pressure and heart rate in neonatal hypocalcemia. *Pediatrics* 1982;69:605.

152. Mirro R, Brown DR. Parenteral calcium treatment shortens the left ventricular systolic time intervals of hypocalcemic neonates. *Pediatr Res* 1984;18:71.

153. Venkataraman PS, Wilson DA, Sheldon RE, et al. Effect of hypocalcemia on cardiac function in very-low-birth-weight preterm neonates: studies of blood ionized calcium, echocardiography and cardiac effect of intravenous calcium therapy. *Pediatrics* 1985;76:543.

154. Broner CW, Stidham GL, Westenkirchner DF, et al. Hypermagnesemia and hypocalcemia as predictors of high mortality in critically ill pediatric patients. *Crit Care Med* 1990;18:921.

155. Koo WWK, Tsang RC, Poser JW, et al. Elevated serum calcium and osteocalcin levels from calcitriol in preterm infants. A prospective randomized study. *Am J Dis Child* 1986;140:1152.

156. Nelson NA, Finnstrom O, Larsson L. Plasma ionized calcium, phosphate and magnesium in preterm and small for gestational age infants. *Acta Paediatr Scand* 1989;78:351.

157. Tsang RC, Chen I, Hayes W, et al. Neonatal hypocalcemia in infants with birth asphyxia. *J Pediatr* 1974;84:428.

158. Tsang RC, Steichen JJ, Chan GM. Neonatal hypocalcemia. Mechanism of occurrence and management. *Crit Care Med* 1977;5:56.

159. Mimouni F, Tsang, RC, Hertzberg VS, et al. Polycythemia, hypomagnesemia and hypocalcemia in infants of diabetic mothers. *Am J Dis Child* 1986;140:798.

160. Namgung R, Tsang R, Specker B, et al. Reduced serum osteocalcin and 1,25-dihydroxyvitamin D concentrations and low bone mineral content in small for gestational age infants: evidence of decreased bone formation rates. *J Pediatr* 1993;122:269.

161. Hanukoglu A, Chalen S, Kowardski AA. Late onset hypocalcemia, rickets and hypoparathyroidism in an infant of a mother with hyperparathyroidism. *J Pediatr* 1988;112:751.

162. Arnold A, Horst SA, Gardella TJ, et al. Mutation of the signal peptide-encoding region of the preproparathyroid hormone gene in familial isolated hypoparathyroidism. *J Clin Invest* 1990;86:1084.

163. Bilous RW, Murty G, Parkinson DB, et al. Autosomal dominant familial hypoparathyroidism, sensorineural deafness, and renal dysplasia. *N Engl J Med* 1992;327:1069.

164. Parkinson DB, Shaw NJ, Himsworth RL, et al. Parathyroid hormone gene analysis in autosomal hypoparathyroidism using an intragenic tetranucleotide (AAAT) in polymorphism. *Hum Genet* 1993;91:281.

165. Root AW. Recent advances in the genetics of disorders of calcium homeostasis. *Adv Pediatr* 1996;43:77.

166. Burke BA, Johnson D, Gilbert EF, et al. Thyrocalcitonin-containing cells in the DiGeorge anomaly. *Hum Pathol* 1987;18:355.

167. Carey AH, Kelly D, Halford S, et al. Molecular genetic study of the frequency of monosomy 22q11 in DiGeorge syndrome. *Am J Hum Genet* 1992;51:964.

168. Driscoll D, Salvin J, Sellinger B, et al. Prevalence of 22q11 microdeletions in DiGeorge and velocardiofacial syndromes: implications for genetic counselling and prenatal diagnosis. *J Med Genet* 1993;30:813.

169. Keppen LD, Fasules JW, Burks AW, et al. Confirmation of autosomal dominant transmission of the DiGeorge malformation complex. *J Pediatr* 1988;113:506.

170. Bainbridge R, Mughal Z, Mimouni F, et al. Transient congenital hypoparathyroidism: how transient is it? *J Pediatr* 1988;111:866.

171. Kooh SW, Binet A. Partial hypoparathyroidism: a variant of transient congenital hypoparathyroidism. *Am J Dis Child* 1991;145:877.

172. Paul E, Fleishman A, Greig F, Saenger P. Transient congenital hypoparathyroidism: resolution and recurrence. *Pediatr Res* 1994;35:206A.

173. Tsang RC, Venkataraman P, Ho M, et al. The development of pseudohypoparathyroidism: involvement of progressively increasing serum parathyroid hormone concentrations, increased 1,25-dihydroxyvitamin D concentrations, and "migratory" subcutaneous calcifications. *Am J Dis Child* 1984;138:654.

174. Spiegel AM, Weinsteing LS. Pseudohypoparathyroidism. In Scriver CR, Beaudet AL, Sly WS, et al, eds. *The metabolic and molecular bases of inherited disease,* 7th ed. New York: McGraw-Hill, 1995: 3073.

175. Ringel MD, Schwindinger WF, Levine MA. Clinical implications of genetic defects in G proteins: The molecular basis of McCune Albright syndrome and Albright hereditary osteodystrophy. *Medicine* 1996;75:171.

176. Hughes WS, Aurbach GD, Sharp ME, Marx SJ. The effect of the bicarbonate anion on serum ionized calcium concentration *in vitro. J Lab Clin Med* 1984;103:93.

177. Lehmann M, Mimouni F. Serum phosphate concentration. Effect on serum ionized calcium concentration *in vitro. Am J Dis Child* 1989; 143:1340.

178. Oleske JM. Experience with 118 infants born to narcotic-using mothers: does a lower serum ionized calcium level contribute to the symptoms of withdrawal? *Clin Pediatr* 1977;16:418.

179. Broner CW, Stidham GL, Westenkirchner DF, et al. A prospective, randomized, double-blind comparison of calcium chloride and calcium gluconate therapies for hypocalcemia in critically ill children. *J Pediatr* 1990;117:986.

180. Venkataraman PS, Sanchez GJ, Parker MK, et al. Effect of intravenous calcium infusions on serum chemistries in neonates. *J Pediatr Gastroenterol Nutr* 1991;13:134.

181. Dincsoy MY, Tsang RC, Laskarzewski P, et al. The role of postnatal age and magnesium on parathyroid hormone responses during "exchange" blood transfusion in the newborn period. *J Pediatr* 1982; 100:277.

182. Brown DR, Salsburey DJ. Short term biochemical effects of parenteral calcium treatment of early onset neonatal hypocalcemia. *J Pediatr* 1982;100:777.

183. Chan GM, Tsang RC, Chen IW, et al. The effect of 1,25(OH)$_2$ vitamin D$_3$ supplementation in premature infants. *J Pediatr* 1978;93:91.

184. Koo WWK, Kaplan LA. Aluminum and bone disorders: with specific reference to aluminum contamination of infant nutrients. *J Am Coll Nutr* 1988;7:199.

185. The neonatal inhaled nitric oxide study group. Inhaled nitric oxide in full-term and nearly full-term infants with hypoxic respiratory failure. *N Engl J Med* 1997;336:597.

186. Tenenhouse HS. Cellular and molecular mechanisms of renal phosphate transport. *J Bone Miner Res* 1997;12:159.

187. Taketani Y, Miyamoto K, Tanaka K, et al. Gene structure and functional analysis of the human Na$^+$/phosphate co-transporter. *Biochem J* 1997;324:927.

188. Francis F, Hennig S, Korn B, et al. A gene (PEX) with homologies to endopeptidases is mutated in patients with X-linked hypophosphatemic rickets. *Nature Genet* 1995;11:130.

189. Loughead J, Mughal F, Mimouni F, et al. Spectrum and natural history of congenital hyperpapathyroidism secondary to maternal hypocalcemia. *Am J Perinatol* 1990;7:350.

190. Igarashi T, Sekine Y, Kawato H, et al. Transient neonatal distal renal tubular acidosis with secondary hyperparathyroidism. *Pediatr Nephrol* 1992;6:267.

191. Savani R, Mimouni F, Tsang R. Maternal and neonatal hyperparathyroidism as a consequence of maternal renal tubular acidosis. *Pediatrics* 1993;91:661.

192. Auwerx J, Brunzell J, Bouillon R, et al. Familial hypocalciuric hypercalcaemia-familial benign hypercalcaemia: a review. *Postgrad Med J* 1987;63:835.

193. Firek AF, Carter WB, Heath H III. Cyclic adenosine 3′,5′-monophosphate responses to parathyroid hormone, prostaglandin E$_2$, and isoproterenol in dermal fibroblasts from patients with familial benign hypercalcemia. *J Clin Endocrinol Metab* 1991;73:203.

194. Firek AF, Kao PC, Heath H III. Plasma intact parathyroid hormone (PTH) and PTH-related peptide in familial benign hypercalcemia: greater responsiveness to endogenous PTH than in primary hyperparathyroidism. *J Clin Endocrinol Metab* 1991;72:541.

195. Wilkinson H, James J. Self limiting neonatal primary hyperparathyroidism associated with familial hypocalciuric hypercalcemia. *Arch Dis Child* 1993;69:319.

196. Seyberth HW, Rascher W, Schweer H, et al. Congenital hypokalemia with hypercalciuria in preterm infants: a hyperprostaglandinuric tubular syndrome different from Bartter syndrome. *J Pediatr* 1985;107: 694.

197. de Rovetto CR, Welch TR, Huo G, et al. Hypercalciuria with Bartter syndrome: evidence for an abnormality of vitamin D metabolism. *J Pediatr* 1989;115:397.

198. Hicks M, Levy M, Alexander J, et al. Subcutaneous fat necrosis of the newborn and hypercalcemia: case report and review of the literature. *Pediatr Dermatol* 1993;10:271.

199. Finne PH, Sanderud J, Asksnes L, et al. Hypercalcemia with increased and unregulated 1,25-dihydroxyvitamin D production in a neonate with subcutaneous fat necrosis. *J Pediatr* 1988;112:792.

200. Zwischenberger JB, Bartlett RH, eds. ECMO: extracorporeal cardiopulmonary support in critical care. Ann Arbor, MI: Extracorporeal Life Support Organization, 1996.

201. Telvi L, Pinard J, Ion R, et al. *De novo* t(X;21) (q28;q11) in a girl with phenotypic features of Williams-Beuren syndrome. *J Med Genet* 1992;29:747.

202. Nickerson E, Greenberg F, Keating MT, et al. Deletions of the elastin gene at 7q11.23 occur in 90% of patients with Williams syndrome. *Am J Hum Genet* 1995;56:1156.

203. Russo AF, Chamany K, Klemish SW, et al. Characterization of the calcitonin/CGRP gene in Williams syndrome. *Am J Med Genet* 1991; 39:28.

204. Pastores GM, Michels VV, Schaid DJ, et al. Exclusion of calcitonin/x-CGRP gene defect in a family with autosomal dominant supravalvular aortic stenosis. *J Med Genet* 1992;29:56.

205. Whyte MP. Hypophosphatasia and the role of alkaline phosphatase in skeletal mineralization. *Endocr Rev* 1994;15:439.

206. Drummond KN, Michael AF, Ulstrom RA, et al. The blue diaper syndrome: familial hypercalcemia with nephrocalcinosis and indicanuria. *Am J Med* 1964;37:928.

207. Tau C, Garabedian M, Farriaux JP, et al. Hypercalcemia in infants with congenital hypothyroidism and its relation to vitamin D and thyroid hormones. *J Pediatr* 1986;109:808.

208. Rousseau-Merck MF, Nogues C, Roth A, et al. Hypercalcemic infantile renal tumors: morphological, clinical, and biological heterogeneity. *Pediatr Pathol* 1985;3:155.

209. Ferraro EM, Klein SA, Fakhry J, et al. Hypercalcemia in association with mesoblastic nephroma: report of a case and review of the literature. *Pediatr Radiol* 1986;16:516.

210. Larkins RG. Lithium and hypercalcemia. *Aust NZ J Med* 1991;21:675.

211. Wisneski LA. Salmon calcitonin in the acute management of hypercalcemia. *Calcif Tissue Int* 1990;Suppl 46:26.

212. Ross AJ, Cooper A, Attie MF, et al. Primary hyperparathyroidism in infancy. *J Pediatr Surg* 1986;21:493.

213. Dancis J, Springer D, Cohlan SQ. Fetal homeostasis in maternal malnutrition: II. Magnesium deprivation. *Pediatr Res* 1971;5:131.

214. Cosens G, Diamond I, Theriault LL, et al. Magnesium deficiency anemia in the rat fetus. *Pediatr Res* 1977;11:758.

215. Davis JA, Harvey DR, Yu JS. Neonatal fits associated with hypomagnesemia. *Arch Dis Child* 1965;40:286.

216. Tsang RC. Neonatal magnesium disturbances: a review. *Am J Dis Child* 1972;124:282.

217. Mimouni F, Tsang RC. Perinatal magnesium metabolism: personal data and challenges for the 1990s. *Magnesium Res* 1991;4:109.

218. Shaul PW, Mimouni F, Tsang RC, et al. The role of magnesium in neonatal calcium homeostasis: effects of magnesium infusion on calciotropic hormones and calcium. *Pediatr Res* 1987;22:319.

219. Paunier L, Radde IC, Kooh SW, et al. Primary hypomagnesemia with secondary hypocalcemia in an infant. *Pediatrics* 1968;41:385.

220. Stromme JH, Nesbakken R, Normann T, et al. Familial hypomagnesemia. *Acta Paediatr Scand* 1969;58:433.

221. Opie LH, Hunt BG, Finley JM. Massive small bowel section with malabsorption and negative magnesium balance. *Gastroenterology* 1964;47:415.

222. Bajpai PC, Sugden D, Stern L, et al. Serum ionic magnesium in exchange transfusion. *J Pediatr* 1967;70:193.

223. Kobayashi A, Shiraki K. Serum magnesium level in infants and children with hepatic diseases. *Arch Dis Child* 1967;42:615.

224. Evans RA, Carter JN, George CRP, et al. The congenital "magnesium-losing kidney." *Q J Med* 1981;50:39.

225. Gitelman HJ. Hypokalemia, hypomagnesemia, and alkalosis: a rose is a rose—or is it? *J Pediatr* 1992;120:79.

226. Bettinelli A, Bianchetti MG, Girardin E, et al. Use of calcium excretion values to distinguish two forms of primary renal tubular hypokalemic alkalosis: Bartter and Gitelman syndromes. *J Pediatr* 1992;120:38.

227. Agus ZS, Wasserstein A, Goldfarb S. Disorders of calcium and magnesium homeostasis. *Am J Med* 1982;72:473.

228. Ghazali S, Hallett RJ, Barratt TM. Hypomagnesemia in uremic infants. *J Pediatr* 1972;81:747.

229. Randall RE, Cohen MD, Spray CC, et al. Hypermagnesemia in renal failure: etiology and toxic manifestations. *Ann Intern Med* 1964;61:73.

230. Hulter HN, Peterson JC. Renal and systemic magnesium metabolism during chronic continuous PTH infusion in normal subjects. *Metabolism* 1984;33:662.

231. Monteleone JA, Lee JB, Tashjian AH, et al. Transient neonatal hypocalcemia, hypomagnesemia and high serum parathyroid hormone with maternal hyperparathyroidism. *Ann Intern Med* 1975;82:670.

232. Levine BS, Coburn JW. Magnesium, the mimic/antagonist of calcium. *N Engl J Med* 1984;310:1253.

233. Byrne PA, Caddell JL. The magnesium load test: II. Correlation of clinical and laboratory data in neonates. *Clin Pediatr* 1975;14:460.

234. Brand JM. Hypermagnesemia and intestinal perforation following antacid administration in a premature infant. *Pediatrics* 1990;85:121.

235. Donovan EF, Tsang RC, Steichen JJ, et al. Neonatal hypermagnesemia: effect on parathyroid hormone and calcium homeostasis. *J Pediatr* 1980;96:305.

236. Sokal MM, Koenigsberger MR, Rose JS, et al. Neonatal hypermagnesemia and the meconium plug syndrome. *N Engl J Med* 1972;286:823.

237. Cooney DR, Rosevear W, Grosfeld JL. Maternal and postnatal hypermagnesemia and the meconium plug syndrome. *J Pediatr Surg* 1976;11:167.

238. Lamm CI, Norton KI, Murphy RJC, et al. Congenital rickets associated with magnesium sulfate infusion for tocolysis. *J Pediatr* 1988;113:1078.

239. Liu C-L, Mimouni F, Ho M, et al. *In vitro* effects of magnesium on ionized calcium concentration in serum. *Am J Dis Child* 1988;142:837.

240. Russell JGB, Hill LF. True fetal rickets. *Br J Radiol* 1974;47:732.

241. Zhou H. Rickets in China. In Glorieux FH, ed. *Rickets.* New York: Raven Press, 1991:253.

242. Gradus D, Le Roith D, Karplus M, et al. Congenital hyperparathyroidism and rickets: secondary to maternal hypoparathyroidism and vitamin D deficiency. *Isr J Med Sci* 1981;17:705.

243. Rimensberger P, Schubiger G, Willi U. Congenital rickets following repeated administration of phosphate enemas in pregnancy: a case report. *Eur J Pediatr* 1992;151:54.

244. Koo WWK, Sherman R, Succop P, et al. Fractures and rickets in very low birth weight infants: conservative management and outcome. *J Pediatr Orthop* 1989;9:326.

245. Dagnelie PC, Vergote F, van Staveren WA, et al. High prevalence of rickets in infants on macrobiotic diets. *Am J Clin Nutr* 1990;51:202.

246. Koo WWK. Parenteral nutrition-related bone disease. *J Parent Ent Nutr* 1992;16:386.

247. Schutt-Aine JC, Young MA, Pescovitz OH, et al. Hypoparathyroidism: a possible cause of rickets. *J Pediatr* 1985;106:255.

248. Glorieux FH. Rickets, the continuing challenge. *N Engl J Med* 1991;325:1875.

249. Econs MJ, Drezner MK. Bone disease resulting from inherited disorders of renal tubule transport and vitamin D metabolism. In Coe FL, Favus MJ, eds. *Bone and mineral metabolism.* New York: Raven Press, 1992:935.

250. Koo WWK, Tsang RC. Calcium, magnesium, phosphorus, and vitamin D. In Tsang RC, Lucas A, Uauy R, Zlotkin S, eds. *Nutritional needs of the preterm infant: Scientific practice and practical guidelines.* New York: Williams & Wilkins, 1993:135.

251. Koo WWK. Laboratory assessment of nutritional metabolic bone disease in infants. *Clin Biochem* 1996;29:429–438.

252. National Research Council. *Recommended dietary allowances,* 11th ed. Washington, DC: National Academy Press, 1998.

253. Koo WWK, Sherman R, Succop P, et al. Sequential serum vitamin D metabolites in very low birth weight infants with and without fractures and rickets. *J Pediatr* 1989;114:1017.

254. Greer FR, Marshall S. Bone mineral content, serum vitamin D metabolite concentrations, and ultraviolet B light exposure in infants fed human milk with and without vitamin D_2 supplements. *J Pediatr* 1989;114:204.

255. Specker BL, Ho ML, Oestreich A, et al. Prospective study of vitamin D supplementation and rickets in China. *J Pediatr* 1992;120:733.

256. Koo WWK, McLaughlin K, Saba M. Nutrition support for the preterm infant. In *The ASPEN nutrition support practice manual.* Washington, DC: American Society for Parenteral and Enteral Nutrition, 1998;26:1.

257. Koo WWK, Raju NV, Tan-Laxa MA. Infant nutrition. *Hong Kong J Pediatr (in press).*

258. Koo WWK, Walters J, Bush AJ, et al. Dual energy x-ray absorptiometry studies of bone mineral status in newborn infants. *J Bone Miner Res* 1996;11:997.

259. Koo WWK, Bush AJ, Walters J, Carlson SE. Postnatal development of bone mineral status during infancy. *J Am Coll Nutr* 1998;17:65.

260. Koo W, Walters J, Hammami M. Bone mineral status of preterm infants during late infancy. *J Bone Miner Res* 1996;11(Suppl 1):S462.

261. Hack M, Taylor HG, Klein N, et al. School-age outcomes in children with birth weights under 750 g. *N Engl J Med* 1994;331:753.

CHAPTER 37

Gastrointestinal Disease

Jon A. Vanderhoof, Terence L. Zach, and Thomas E. Adrian

Although most pediatric gastroenterologists are uncomfortable with primary care of the sick premature infant, they often are valuable consultants to the neonatologist. In evaluating a complex gastrointestinal or hepatobiliary problem, a gastroenterologist often uses an organ system-specific developmental pathophysiologic approach. In looking at a problem from a somewhat different perspective than the neonatologist, the opinion of the consultant may augment the analysis of the primary physician. It remains the responsibility of the neonatologist to put the consultant's view into perspective as it relates to the other complex problems of the sick infant.

The gastroenterologist also may offer his or her skills in invasive procedures to aid in the diagnosis of gastrointestinal and liver disease. Upper and lower gastrointestinal endoscopy, liver biopsy, rectal suction biopsy, esophageal, antroduodenal, and anorectal motility studies, and even endoscopic retrograde cholangiopancreatography can be performed in term infants and, depending on the skill and training of the gastroenterologist, in premature infants as well.

In some institutions, gastroenterologists with special expertise in nutrition provide assistance in nutritional support of parenteral nutrition-dependent or malnourished infants. Their role becomes especially important in infants with gastrointestinal or liver disease who may require long-term follow-up, such as the infant with progressive liver disease, or home parenteral nutrition, such as the infant with short bowel syndrome.

J. A. Vanderhoof: University of Nebraska Medical Center/ Creighton University, Omaha, Nebraska

T. L. Zach: Department of Pediatrics, Creighton University, Omaha, Nebraska

T. E. Adrian: Department of Biomedical Sciences, Creighton University School of Medicine, Omaha, Nebraska

DEVELOPMENT OF THE GASTROINTESTINAL TRACT

Subsequent to the development of the individual organs of the gastrointestinal tract, specialized features of the system begin to become apparent, mostly in the second and third trimesters (1). At approximately 14 weeks of gestation, differentiation of the pancreatic endocrine and exocrine tissues begins, and crypts and villi begin to form in the small intestine. A few weeks later, the colon, initially populated with villi similar to those in the small intestine, begins to develop its more characteristic surface, with gradual loss of villi. As these morphologic changes occur, numerous functional processes begin, some of which mature early *in utero*, some only at birth, and some during the first year of life.

Carbohydrate Absorption

The functional maturation of the digestive process is complex (2). There are marked differences in maturation of the digestive and absorptive processes of different nutrients (Table 37–1). In the neonate, most dietary carbohydrate is presented in the form of lactose, the predominant carbohydrate in virtually all mammalian milk. Lactose and other disaccharides are digested by enzymes located on the brush border membrane in mature enterocytes, those located on the distal and midportions of the small intestinal villi. Component monosaccharides are released after hydrolysis by disaccharidases. Lactase hydrolyzes lactose to glucose and galactose, and both subsequently are transported by active carrier-mediated transport. Other disaccharidases include maltase, which hydrolyzes maltose to two glucose units, glucoamylase, which hydrolyzes glucose oligosaccharides to glucose monomers, and sucrase, which hydrolyzes sucrose to fructose and glucose. Sucrase is actually a double enzyme, the other part of the molecule being isomaltase, which hydrolyzes α-1-6 bonds of α-limit dextrins. Disac-

TABLE 37–1. *Digestive and absorptive function in infants relative to adults*

Process	Premature infant	Full-term infant	Adult
Salivary enzymes	Normal	Normal	Normal
Gastric acid production	↓	↓ to normal	Normal
Bile acid secretion	↓↓	↓	↓
Pancreatic enzyme production	↓↓	↓	Normal
Lactase production	↓	Normal	Normal
Sucrase and isomaltase production	Normal	Normal	Normal

charidase activities are highest in the proximal and mid-jejunum and decrease distally.

Lactase activity develops later in gestation than the other disaccharidases. Lactase activity is low until the final weeks of gestation. Although other disaccharidase levels can be detected somewhat earlier in gestation and reach nearly adult levels between 26 and 34 weeks of gestational age, lactase levels are only 30% of full-term levels by that point in gestation. Because of the delayed maturation of lactase, specialized infant formulas for preterm infants have been designed, with a significant percentage of carbohydrate presented as sucrose or glucose polymers rather than lactose. The predominant enzyme for digestion of starches and glucose polymers is pancreatic amylase, which is nearly absent during the first 4 to 6 months of life and gradually matures during the latter half of the first year. An alternative pathway therefore must exist for the digestion of these glucose polymers (3,4).

Salivary glands produce an amylase that may be important in the digestion of complex carbohydrates in the newborn. This enzyme is detectable at 20 weeks of gestation and is present in significant quantities in premature infants. As with pancreatic amylase, however, the ability of the newborn to secrete salivary amylase is substantially reduced and matures throughout the first year of life. Salivary amylase is inactivated by gastric acid, but probably retains some activity in the stomach of premature infants. Glucoamylase is a brush border enzyme capable of digesting glucose units from the nonreducing ends of starch and dextrin. Glucoamylase is present in neonates and infants at 50% to 100% of adult levels.

Finally, it is probable that some malabsorbed carbohydrate is digested in the colon through the colon salvage pathway. Colonic anaerobic bacteria are capable of metabolizing carbohydrates to produce short-chain fatty acids that then are absorbed through the colonic mucosa. Considering the relative pancreatic insufficiency and lactase deficiency in the newborn infant, the colon salvage pathway may be an important mechanism by which infants absorb carbohydrates.

Fat Absorption

Fat absorption is a complex process, primarily because fat is insoluble in the aqueous environment of the small intestinal lumen (5). Solubilization, therefore, is an important part of the fat assimilation process. The first phase of fat absorption is that of enzymatic digestion or lipolysis. Because most dietary fat is present in the form of triglycerides, otherwise known as triasylglycerols, these first must be hydrolyzed by pancreatic lipase.

Phospholipids are hydrolyzed concurrently by pancreatic phospholipase. Colipase, a cofactor secreted by the pancreas, also is required, facilitating the action of lipase by binding to bile salt–lipid surfaces and improving the interaction of lipase with triglyceride. The efficiency of this process is augmented by the release of cholecystokinin (CCK) from the duodenal epithelium, which occurs in response to the presence of lipid and protein in the duodenum. CCK stimulates pancreatic secretion, gallbladder contraction, and simultaneous relaxation of the sphincter of Oddi, to mix large quantities of bile acids and digestive juices with lipids. Pancreatic lipase levels are reduced in preterm infants and intrauterine growth-retarded infants, significantly impairing lipolysis (6). Lingual lipase, secreted from the salivary glands, may facilitate lipolysis in the premature infant and partially compensate for the infant's relative pancreatic insufficiency (7). Nonetheless, fat absorption is significantly impaired in newborn infants and, to a greater extent, in premature infants, due at least in part to pancreatic insufficiency.

Closely linked with the process of enzymatic digestion of fats is micellar solubilization by bile acids (8). Bile acid molecules are complex structures with both hydrophobic and hydrophilic ends. Bile acids interface with lipids to render them water soluble by positioning the hydrophobic portion in close proximity to the lipid globules while allowing the hydrophilic portion to remain free to interact with the aqueous environment. Lipids then become enclosed in disc-shaped water-soluble micelles that contain fatty acids, monoglycerides, phospholipids, cholesterol, and fat-soluble vitamins.

Solubilization is particularly important because of the presence of the intestine's unstirred water layer. This stagnant layer of water overlies the microvillus membrane of the intestinal epithelial cells and is the primary barrier to lipid transport. The actual thickness of the unstirred water layer is complex and difficult to measure, but the layer is significantly reduced by the constant agitation of the fluid in the gastrointestinal tract due to gut motility and villus contraction. Because of the convolutions in the small intestine caused by the presence of villi and microvilli, the total surface area available to interface between the intestinal surface and the unstirred layer is much greater than the interface between the unstirred water layer and the aqueous intraluminal environment. Penetration through the unstirred layer by the disc-shaped micelles is the rate-limiting step for lipid absorption. Disease processes that increase the unstirred layer thickness will markedly inhibit fat absorption in much the same manner as disease states that render the supply of bile acids inadequate for micellar solubilization. Bile acids commonly are deficient in cholestatic liver diseases, such as neonatal hepatitis or biliary atresia, and in rare cases of congenital bile acid deficiency. Bile acids are deconjugated rapidly and reabsorbed in the presence of small intestinal bacterial overgrowth. Bile acid deficiency therefore may occur in patients with disorders that cause intestinal stasis and bacterial overgrowth, such as short bowel syndrome. In disorders of mucosal injury, the unstirred layer thickness may be increased, making penetration of the fat-containing micelles difficult and further exacerbating fat malabsorption.

Bile acids are extremely important in the fat absorption process. In the absence of bile acids, only about one-third of dietary triglycerides, a very small percentage of fatty acids, and virtually no cholesterol or fat-soluble vitamins are absorbed. Medium-chain triglycerides may be better absorbed because of their enhanced water solubility, which allows penetration of the unstirred water layer without micellar solubilization. In both preterm and term infants, bile acid synthesis is limited and the bile salt pool size is low (9). Moreover, preterm infants may have an ineffective bile salt transport process in the distal ileum, resulting in impaired enterohepatic circulation of bile salts (10). Consequently, the bile acid concentration may be less than adequate for the formation of micelles and solubilization of fat. Thus, penetration of the unstirred layer is less efficient in the term infant and further impaired in the preterm infant compared to adults.

After lipids are enclosed in the bile acid micelle and reach the lipid bilayer membrane of the small intestinal mucosal cell, absorption into the cell occurs by passive diffusion. Because of the convolutions of the gastrointestinal tract, a large surface area exists for lipid assimilation. In the absence of disease, this process progresses in the term and preterm infant relatively uninhibited. In disorders in which the absorptive surface area is reduced or damaged, however, such as short bowel syndrome or any form of diffuse enterocolitis, fat, carbohydrate, and, to a limited degree, protein are malabsorbed.

Within the enterocyte, monoglycerides and esterified fatty acids are immediately resynthesized to triglycerides. These triglycerides, along with apoproteins, phospholipids, free cholesterol, some diglycerides, and esterified cholesterol, are stabilized within chylomicrons. The outer structure of the chylomicron then fuses with the basolateral membrane and is extruded into the lamina propria, where it is carried by the lacteals and lymphatic channels and deposited into the blood stream.

Protein Absorption

The assimilation of protein begins in the stomach through the action of hydrochloric acid and pepsin. The maturational aspects of this process have been the subject of substantial study and some controversy. Conflicting data exist as to the status of acid secretion in the newborn infant. Newborn infants appear to be capable of secreting acid, although the process is somewhat immature (11). In premature infants, it is probable that the process is impaired to a greater extent (12). Pepsinogen, the proenzyme for pepsin, which facilitates protein digestion in the stomach, is secreted in preterm infants, but in much lower concentrations than in term infants (13).

The gastric aspects of protein digestion are relatively inconsequential, compared to the much more complete process in the small intestine. Enterokinase, produced in the duodenal mucosa, activates the pancreatic proteolytic enzyme trypsinogen, converting it to trypsin, which then activates essentially all of the other enzymes involved in protein digestion. Enterokinase levels have been demonstrated in human fetuses as early as 21 weeks of gestation (14). Enterokinase secretion is diminished during fetal development, however, and is only 10% of adult levels in the term newborn. In addition, pancreatic and duodenal proteolytic enzymes are present in preterm and term infants in lower concentrations than in older children and in adults. These enzymes initiate hydrolysis of proteins, and the hydrolysis process is completed by brush border and cytosolic peptidases. Protein is absorbed in the form of amino acids and dipeptides through active transport processes that appear to be well developed by 28 weeks of gestational age. Despite the relative immaturity of multiple phases of the protein assimilation process, both preterm and term infants are quite capable of absorbing adequate quantities of dietary protein. In small infants, the protein malabsorption resulting from mucosal injury is probably far less consequential than the malabsorption of the other major macronutrients.

Micronutrient Absorption

Absorption of micronutrients matures at varying rates in infancy. Water is absorbed passively in response to sodium and other electrolytes, as it is in older children and adults (15). Experimental evidence suggests that the intestinal epithelium may be more secretory during early infancy, and the increased susceptibility of infants to diarrheal disorders probably is at least partially related to this process.

Mineral absorption depends on the form in which the mineral is presented to the infant. Iron, for example, is absorbed extremely well from breast milk. Even the preterm infant is capable of absorbing nearly 50% of the iron in breast milk, whereas only a small percentage of iron is absorbed from cow-milk formulas, necessitating iron supplementation. Calcium and phosphorous also are well absorbed from breast milk (16,17). Magnesium, copper, and, to a lesser extent, zinc are well absorbed by both term and preterm infants (18). In general, minerals are absorbed somewhat better from breast milk than from cow milk. Most vitamins appear to be absorbed adequately in both term and preterm infants, although fat-soluble vitamin deficiency is common in disorders affecting fat absorption, especially disorders causing bile acid deficiency.

Gut Motility

Although nutrient assimilation is heavily dependent on the development of digestive and absorptive function, actual feeding depends greatly on the maturation of gut motility (19–21). Neuroblasts migrate in a cranial-to-caudal direction between weeks 5 and 12 of gestation. There is gradual maturation of gut motility throughout the fetal period and the first several years of postnatal life. In the fetus, normal propulsive motility in the gut probably does not appear until approximately 30 weeks of age. Interdigestive phenomena, known as migrating motor complexes, can be demonstrated by approximately 33 weeks of gestation. Motor activity in the neonatal gut differs significantly from that in adults, in that the propagation rate of the migrating motor complex is substantially slower in neonates, and the complex is not abolished by feeding as in older children.

Sucking and swallowing reflexes begin early during fetal development, but the maturation of the process is not completed until after birth. The fetus is able to swallow amniotic fluid as early as 11 to 12 weeks of gestation. Actual sucking probably does not occur until approximately 18 to 24 weeks. This type of sucking is termed nonnutritive sucking, differentiating it from the more effective nutritive sucking mechanism that develops by 34 to 35 weeks of gestation. The onset of nutritive sucking closely parallels a rapid increase in growth of the fetal stomach (22) and the acquisition of mature patterns of gastric antral and small intestinal motility.

By the time a term infant is born, sucking movements are followed in an orderly progression by swallowing, esophageal peristalsis, relaxation of the lower esophageal sphincter, and relaxation of the gastric fundus. The first stage of swallowing is an involuntary reflex in both the term and preterm infant.

Some data suggest that nonnutritive sucking may play an important role in weight gain in preterm infants. The mechanism of this effect may be related to maturational changes in the infant gastrointestinal tract, and sucking may facilitate gastric emptying and other gastrointestinal functions, primarily through stimulation of secretion of gastrointestinal regulatory peptides.

Maturation of gastrointestinal motility may have important implications for a number of conditions. Gastroesophageal reflux is common in both term and preterm infants, and probably relates to diminished lower esophageal sphincter function or inappropriate relaxation of the lower esophageal sphincter, often in association with delayed gastric emptying. The maturation of both lower esophageal sphincter function and gastric emptying has been studied extensively, with somewhat equivocal results. Depending on the technique used to measure sphincter function, the lower esophageal sphincter tone has been shown to be either low or normal in both preterm and term infants (23). Hypertonic carbohydrate solutions appear to delay gastric emptying in infants, much as they do in adults.

GASTROINTESTINAL HORMONES AND ENTERIC NEUROPEPTIDES

Gastrointestinal peptide hormones appear to play an important role in the structural and functional development of the gut, as well as in the control of alimentary functions. The function of a vast endocrine system is integrated with that of the enteric nervous system, which itself uses other regulatory peptides as local messengers.

Endocrine cells producing gastrin, somatostatin, motilin, and glucose-dependent insulinotrophic peptide (GIP) are detectable in the fetus at 8 weeks of gestation, with gastrin- and somatostatin-producing cells being most numerous (24). By 14 weeks, all of the endocrine cell types are present in the intestinal mucosa, although the anatomic distribution is more widespread than that seen in the adult (24). By the end of the second trimester, the distribution of gut endocrine cells resembles that of the adult (24). Peptidergic nerves are first demonstrable in the myenteric plexus at about 12 weeks of gestation, correlating with the known developmental pattern of enteric nerve plexuses (24). These enteric nerves then migrate through to the submucous plexus. By the third trimester, all of the regulatory peptide systems are well developed (25). At birth, the molecular forms of the gastrointestinal regulatory peptides and their distribution in the gut are similar to those of the adult (25).

Surges of gut hormones appear to be responsible for the marked growth and functional change that occur in the alimentary tract in early neonatal life. Substantial changes in gastrointestinal hormone secretion are seen during this period, triggered by the switch from intravenous to enteral feeding (26).

Gastrin is an important regulator of gastric secretion and is trophic to the gastric mucosa. At birth, cord blood levels of gastrin are already four to five times higher than those in the adult, and prefeed basal levels remain elevated for several weeks (27,28). Furthermore, gastrin levels increase in response to the first milk feed (29). After 3 to 4 weeks of life, basal gastrin levels decline, a change accompanied by development of marked elevation of levels following feeding (27,30). Gastric acid is detectable in the stomach at birth and reaches a peak in the first day or two of life (28,31). Thereafter, acid output decreases for a period of about 1 month in spite of the hypergastrinemia and rapid growth of the stomach. It has been suggested that the lack of responsiveness to gastrin could be due to a lack of receptors in the oxyntic gland mucosa. Perhaps a more likely explanation, however, is that secretion is suppressed by an inhibitor, such as peptide YY (PYY) or neurotensin, thus enabling gastrin to stimulate growth of the gastric mucosa without hyperstimulation of acid secretion (32,33).

Basal levels of the duodenal hormone, secretin, are higher at birth than in adults, and, during the first 3 weeks of life, a more marked postprandial response develops than is seen in the adult (34). Because secretin is considered to be a major factor in triggering the neutralization of acid chyme entering the duodenum, the increase in circulating secretin levels may be of considerable importance in mucosal protection during this period. It is notable that the postnatal surge of secretin, unlike that of the other alimentary hormones, occurs even in the absence of feeding, indicating the importance of this mucosal cytoprotective function (30).

CCK, released from the upper small intestine, stimulates pancreatic enzyme secretion and contracts the gallbladder. In addition, CCK has marked trophic effects on the pancreas and appears to be responsible for regeneration after resection or acute pancreatitis (35). The observed postnatal surge of plasma CCK concentrations therefore may be of importance in stimulating growth of this organ (36).

Also released from the small intestine, motilin is a hormonal peptide with powerful motor functions. These motor functions include acceleration of gastric emptying and stimulation of the interdigestive myoelectric complexes during the interprandial period. Motilin concentrations are low in cord blood, but preprandial basal concentrations show a massive postnatal surge that peaks at around 2 weeks of postnatal life (30). This peak is enhanced, but delayed, in preterm neonates. It is likely that this increase in circulating motilin concentrations is responsible for the known increase in motor activity of the gut that occurs during the neonatal period. Interdigestive motor complexes appear normal at birth in the term infant, but interdigestive cycles are incomplete in preterm neonates (37). Premature babies exhibit abnormal motor activity, with periods of motor quiescence and nonpropagating contractions. Thus, motor activity is more immature in preterm infants than in term infants (37). The relationship between maturation of the migrating motor

complexes and the late postnatal surge of motilin in preterm neonates is not clear.

The jejunal hormone, GIP, is thought to be largely responsible for the postprandial increase in circulating insulin levels (38). Basal GIP concentrations are low at birth and increase gradually throughout the first month of life, together with the development of a marked postfeeding GIP response similar to that seen in the adult after ingestion of a mixed meal (30,39). The development of the GIP response to feeding in neonates is mirrored by the postprandial insulin response, which increases through the first month of life to maintain glucose homeostasis (39).

Neurotensin is an ileal peptide that has inhibitory effects on gastric secretion and motility. Plasma neurotensin concentrations are higher in the neonate than in the adult, and an enhanced postprandial response develops in the first month of life (40). Both reduction of gastric secretion and slowing of the rate of gastric emptying will decrease the rate at which acid chyme enters the duodenum and, therefore, will result in a more steady absorption of nutrients from the gut. Thus, neurotensin may be important in the adaptation of the neonate to enteral nutrition.

PYY is an important hormone from the distal intestine that inhibits gastric emptying and slows small bowel transit (41). PYY also inhibits gastric and small bowel secretion, leading to an increase in net absorption (32). Concentrations of PYY are elevated in cord blood and rise postnatally to a peak within the first 2 weeks postpartum (33). At their peak, plasma PYY concentrations are about 50 times higher than fasting levels in normal adults (33). There is evidence to suggest that gastric emptying and intestinal transit are rapid during the first week of life, both in term and preterm infants. The triggering mechanism for the changes that then take place is unknown, but it is likely that factors such as PYY play a role (41). In addition, the very potent inhibitory effect of PYY on gastric secretion may account for the prevention of hypersecretion of acid during the early neonatal period, in spite of the marked hypergastrinemia (32).

Enteroglucagon is one of three biologically active peptides produced by posttranslational processing of the glucagon gene product in the small and large intestine. Glucagon-like peptides I and II (GLP-I and GLP-II) are the two other peptides secreted in parallel with enteroglucagon, which can serve as a marker for production of all three. GLP-I has incretin effects and physiologically enhances insulin secretion in response to ingested nutrients in the same manner as GIP. GLP-II, on the other hand, is a trophic peptide that increases growth of the small intestinal mucosa (42,43). Plasma enteroglucagon concentrations show a very marked postnatal surge, which peaks within the first week and is associated with the development of a marked postprandial response (27,30). Because an increased rate of small intestinal growth occurs in the early neonatal period, it is likely that GLP-II is important in neonatal alimentary maturation. The resulting mucosal growth increases the absorptive area for the uptake of nutrients from the gut lumen.

Temporally, the postnatal surges of gut hormones parallel the changes in gastrointestinal function that accompany the introduction of enteral feeding in the infant. It is therefore of considerable interest that these surges are not seen in infants who have never received enteral feeding (30,44). Concentrations of all gut hormones, with the exception of secretin, remain low in infants receiving only parenteral nutrition (30,44).

Precise mechanisms control the secretion of each gut hormone, and the amount of a particular peptide liberated by a meal is adequate to stimulate the appropriate digestive response (45). For example, a meal rich in long-chain triglycerides will evoke a large CCK response, not seen with medium-chain fats (46). The high circulating levels of CCK in turn stimulate pancreatic enzyme secretion and, by gallbladder contraction, release of the bile salts necessary for digestion of the long-chain fat. Medium-chain triglycerides, on the other hand, are rapidly hydrolyzed by lingual and gastric lipases; they are water soluble, do not require micelle formation, and are absorbed rapidly. Thus, bile salts and pancreatic enzymes are not required for digestion of medium-chain triglycerides, and a large CCK response is not seen when they are ingested (46). The gut endocrine system, with its sparse distribution of overlapping cell types, is designed to produce an integrated digestive response to the discontinuous stimulation of ingested food (45). Because the type of food presented can influence the integrated hormonal response, it is apparent that differences in nutrition in early neonatal life may result in changes in the growth and functional development of the neonatal alimentary tract.

Although the fetus makes little demand on its gastrointestinal tract, the situation changes dramatically at birth, when demand for nutrients necessitates the rapid maturation of the alimentary tract. This development of the gastrointestinal tract is characterized by the integrated maturation of its many functions. The observation, however, that premature infants make a satisfactory transition from intravenous nutrition through the placenta to extrauterine enteral feeding suggests that external influences can exert a substantial influence. The massive postnatal surges in circulating levels of hormones, which have trophic as well as secretory and motor functions, is compelling circumstantial evidence of a profound gut endocrine influence on alimentary development (30). This is supported further by the observation that these hormonal surges are not seen in sick infants who are on parenteral nutrition and have not been fed orally (44). It is likely that failure of secretion of trophic gut hormones is responsible for the hypoplastic gut and pancreas that accompany parenteral nutrition. Appropriate enteral stimuli or hormone replacement eventually may alleviate this problem.

ABNORMALITIES OF THE GASTROINTESTINAL TRACT

To avoid repetition, an attempt has been made to confine the abnormalities described in this section to those that might require consultation by a pediatric gastroenterologist. Some overlap with general surgery has been allowed, however, to avoid extensive cross-referencing (see Chap. 44).

Abdominal Wall Defects

Major defects of the abdominal wall, omphalocele and gastroschisis, occur in approximately 1 of 6,000 live births (47–49). In either case, a portion of the infant's gastrointestinal tract remains outside the abdominal cavity at birth. Omphalocele is a failure of the extraembryonic intestine to reenter the abdominal cavity through the umbilicus, a developmental anomaly that occurs between weeks 10 and 12 of gestational age. The defect includes the umbilicus, and the viscera typically are covered with a peritoneal sac. Occasionally, the sac may rupture, making the disorder difficult to distinguish clinically from gastroschisis. Gastroschisis is an actual defect in the abdominal wall that occurs lateral to the umbilicus. The infant with gastroschisis has a normal umbilical cord not involved in the defect. The defect usually occurs to the right of the umbilical cord. Both omphalocele and gastroschisis may occur in the presence of other intestinal anomalies. Malrotation is present in association with omphalocele. Although intestinal atresias more commonly are found in gastroschisis, atresias may be associated with either anomaly. Abdominal wall defects frequently are diagnosed prenatally by fetal ultrasound (50). The preferred route of delivery remains controversial and may depend on the size of the defect (51). Vaginal delivery may be acceptable for small defects, and cesarean section may be preferred in cases with large defects (52).

Gastroschisis or omphalocele requires immediate pediatric surgical consultation. Fluid losses and hypothermia are of primary immediate concern, especially in the case of gastroschisis because no membrane covers the bowel. Large fluid and heat losses are common, and intravenous fluid replacement should be initiated immediately. The defect should be wrapped, using warm, sterile, moist saline gauze or a sterile transparent plastic bag. Care must be taken to prevent twisting and infarction of the bowel. A nasogastric tube should be inserted to minimize intestinal distention.

Postoperative management includes sedation and mechanical ventilation for at least 48 to 72 hours because of increased intraabdominal pressure. Careful monitoring of fluids and electrolytes is essential. High fluid intake is required (53). During the postoperative period, gut motility is slow to return, especially in the case of gastroschisis. Patients with gastroschisis may demonstrate sluggish motility for up to 8 months, and a protracted course of parenteral nutrition commonly is required. Delayed onset of necrotizing enterocolitis (NEC) is not uncommon and should be suspected if bloody stools are observed.

Disorders of the Esophagus

Gastroesophageal Reflux

Gastroesophageal reflux is the most common esophageal disorder in the neonatal period (54). Gastric contents normally are retained within the stomach through the action of the lower esophageal sphincter, a zone of high pressure in the distal esophagus that remains tonically contracted except during deglutition (55). The anatomy of the stomach and esophagus, and their relationship to the diaphragm and related structures, may play a secondary role in retaining gastric contents within the stomach. Although considerable controversy exists, there is evidence to suggest that the lower esophageal sphincter may be fully functional in the normal full-term infant. Some evidence suggests that sphincter pressure may be decreased, either continuously or intermittently, in infants with gastroesophageal reflux, facilitating reflux of gastric contents into the esophagus. There is considerable controversy over the incidence of reflux in the premature infant. Reflux appears relatively more common, but some data suggest that the lower esophageal sphincter may be competent. Delayed gastric emptying and other motility problems also may play a role in reflux in premature infants.

In adults and older children, chronic esophagitis due to reflux of acid into the distal esophagus is the major concern with gastroesophageal reflux. During the neonatal period, however, esophagitis rarely occurs. Reflux typically presents with continual regurgitation and spitting up or vomiting of small quantities of formula after eating, but also may present with apnea and bradycardia. Recurrent aspiration during reflux episodes may result in pneumonitis or exacerbation of preexisting neonatal pulmonary disease. If enough formula is regurgitated, the infant may fail to thrive. In neonates, reflux also may be associated with delayed gastric emptying. Delayed gastric antral distention occurs in some very premature infants in the early postnatal period (56). Such delays in antral distention could contribute to gastroesophageal reflux and feeding intolerance commonly seen in premature infants less than 32 weeks' gestation. As in older children, reflux is encountered more frequently in infants with neurologic abnormalities.

Gastroesophageal reflux may exist as a primary disorder due to lower esophageal sphincter incompetence or intermittent relaxation, or it may be a manifestation of another disorder. First of all, it must be realized that gastroesophageal reflux may occur physiologically in all infants, although not with the frequency and severity of pathologic reflux. Any disorder that limits gastric emptying or causes a partial proximal small intestinal obstruction, such as annular pancreas or pyloric stenosis, will result in some gastroesophageal reflux. Small bowel disorders, including milk protein enterocolitis or infectious enteritis, will cause vomiting and regurgitation—in essence, gastroesophageal reflux. Finally, a variety of systemic disorders, including certain inborn errors of metabolism, chronic infection, chronic renal disease, and increased intracranial pressure, may result in chronic emesis similar to gastroesophageal reflux. Drugs, such as xanthines, which may be given because of apnea or lung disease, decrease lower esophageal sphincter pressure and may exacerbate or even cause reflux.

Several diagnostic studies are available to diagnose gastroesophageal reflux in infants; however, these studies as a rule do not separate primary from secondary causes. For example, an infant with milk protein enterocolitis or pyloric stenosis will have a postive test result for gastroesophageal reflux by any of the available studies. The most widely available test for reflux is an upper gastrointestinal series, which is preferable to a barium swallow, because the latter only examines esophageal motility. The stomach must be filled with barium to assess the patient accurately for reflux. Unfortunately, assessing a child for gastroesophageal reflux radiographically lacks sensitivity because of the short time interval during which the child is observed, and it lacks specificity because of the likelihood of physiologic reflux occurring during performance of an upper gastrointestinal series. Therefore, the primary role of an upper gastrointestinal series is to exclude gastric outlet lesions such as pyloric stenosis, or proximal small bowel partial obstructions such as duodenal webs or annular pancreas.

Twenty-four-hour pH monitoring is the most widely accepted means of assessing gastroesophageal reflux (57). The pH probe is placed approximately 2 cm proximal to the lower esophageal sphincter, and distal esophageal pH is recorded over a 24-hour period. The infant must be bolus-fed during the study, to ensure adequate gastric distention to simulate the physiologic state. Considerable controversy exists over appropriate feeding for children during 24-hour pH monitoring. The inconsistency of acid secretion in small infants makes the procedure much less reliable during the neonatal period, and, consequently, simultaneous measurement of intragastric pH often is helpful in determining the validity of the study.

A ^{99}Tc scintiscan may be used to screen for gastroesophageal reflux, although this technique is not considered as reliable as 24-hour pH monitoring. The technique is useful, however, for measuring gastric emptying delay, which may coexist with gastroesophageal reflux in a number of infants. Endoscopy with biopsy is a useful technique for detecting reflux in older infants; however, endoscopic biopsies are less useful during the neonatal period because pathologic reflux has not had sufficient time to cause esophageal mucosal injury. In older children, the presence of intraepithelial eosinophils suggests reflux, but this sign cannot be relied on in neonates, and biopsy specimens frequently are normal.

Treatment of gastroesophageal reflux is based on the severity of symptoms. If the child is thriving well and the major complaint is frequent regurgitation and spitting, the infant may be placed prone on an incline at approximately 30 degrees with the head higher than the feet. It has been demonstrated that children positioned in this manner will reflux less frequently. Although it may take several weeks for symptoms to resolve, the risk of esophagitis is lessened and reflux tends to resolve more quickly. If the volume of reflux is severe and the infant is chronically irritable, has evidence of esophagitis, or is failing to thrive, then inhibition of gastric acid secretion with agents such as antacids or H_2-receptor antagonists may be necessary. Cimetidine and ranitidine are available in liquid preparations, and they both work well. Data suggest that aluminum antacids may elevate serum aluminum levels in small infants (58). Hydrogen pump antagonists such as omeprazole are even more potent suppressors of acid secretory activity than H_2-receptor antagonists. Relatively little experience with these agents is available in neonates. The medication is supplied in encapsulated time-released beads and administered on a daily basis. Appropriate dosing for neonates has not been evaluated critically. Bethanechol, a parasympathomimetic agent, has been demonstrated to increase lower esophageal sphincter resting tone and improve weight gain in infants with failure to thrive secondary to gastroesophageal reflux (59). Unfortunately, bethanechol may have associated central nervous system side effects, such as irritability and sleeplessness. Metoclopramide also has been used to treat gastroesophageal reflux in infants. The effectiveness of metoclopramide is controversial, and it probably is most helpful when delayed gastric emptying coexists with reflux. Cisapride is another gastroprokinetic agent that acts by releasing acetylcholine from the myenteric plexus in the gut. Cisapride has been shown to be effective in the treatment of gastroesphageal reflux (60). Some clinicians thicken infants' formula with cereal. Although this may reduce spitting, it usually does not reduce reflux or its complications and results in nutrient imbalance in the infant's carefully formulated diet.

Gastroesophageal reflux may be treated successfully with surgical fundoplication in approximately 95% of cases. The most common surgical procedures include the Nissen fundoplication, in which the stomach is wrapped and sutured 360 degrees around the distal esophagus, and the Thal fundoplication, which consists of a 270-degree wrap. Complications, including gaseous distention of the stomach and dumping syndrome, may be less common with the Thal procedure. Many surgeons now perform fundoplications laparoscopically. Indications for an operation for gastroesophageal reflux include recurrent aspiration pneumonia, failure to thrive secondary to severe vomiting unresponsive to in-hospital medical management, or apparent life-threatening apnea events associated with gastroesophageal reflux (62).

Differential diagnosis of the typical neonate with chronic recurrent vomiting includes, in addition to gastroesophageal reflux, two major categories of disease. The first is upper gastrointestinal anomalies, including pyloric stenosis. Virtually all of these can be eliminated by upper gastrointestinal contrast studies; pyloric stenosis can be excluded adequately by ultrasonography in the hands of an experienced pediatric ultrasonographer. The second major diagnostic category is formula protein intolerance. Infants with formula protein intolerance commonly vomit, especially those with significant small bowel mucosal disease. Such infants often are irritable and usually have loose, Hematest-positive (Ames, Elkhart, IN) stools. Proctoscopic examinations of the rectum usually demonstrate colitis. This disorder is discussed in detail later in this chapter.

Esophageal Anomalies

The other major category of esophageal disease that presents in the neonatal period is tracheoesophageal fistula or esophageal atresia (63). These anomalies occur in approximately 1 in 4,000 live births. In addition to a prenatal history of polyhydramnios, increased salivation with coughing, choking, and cyanosis shortly after birth should raise the suspicion of tracheoesophageal fistula–esophageal atresia. The most common variety is that of atresia with the distal esophageal pouch connected to the trachea through a fistula. Such infants frequently have a stomach distended with air and respiratory symptoms due to tracheal aspiration of refluxed gastric acid. Immediate pediatric surgical consultation is required (see Chap. 44).

After surgery, gastroesophageal reflux is a virtual certainty. Patients with tracheoesophageal fistula or esophageal atresia have incompetent lower esophageal sphincter function as well as aperistaltic contractions in the midesophagus. Although swallowing usually proceeds without much difficulty, gastroesophageal reflux with chronic esophagitis and occasionally stricture formation are frequent long-term complications. Subsequent esophageal dilatations and fundoplication may be necessary.

Disorders of the Stomach and Duodenum

Congenital Anomalies

Congenital anomalies of the upper gastrointestinal tract frequently present with vomiting. The most common is pyloric stenosis, which occurs in approximately 1 in every 500 live births (64,65). The disease is most common in Caucasian males. A positive family history often is present. Pyloric stenosis usually presents with nonbilious projectile vomiting during the third to fourth week of life. The disorder often is insidious in onset. After emesis, infants are hungry and will attempt to eat to compensate for malnutrition. It is now clear that pyloric stenosis is caused by the selective inadequate development of inhibitory neurons in the myenteric plexus of the pyloric region that utilize vasoactive intestinal polypeptide and nitric oxide as neurotransmitters to relax the sphincter. Eventually, nutrition deteriorates and infants become dehydrated and alkalotic secondary to chronic vomiting of the acidic gastric contents. Unconjugated hyperbilirubinemia is present in a small percentage. Patients with pyloric stenosis have normal or firm stools, in contrast to infants with formula protein intolerance, who usually have loose stools with evidence of malabsorption, inflammation, or both. Serum electrolytes reveal potassium and chloride deficiency and metabolic alkalosis. Physical examination demonstrates visible peristalsis in the epigastric region. Careful palpation of the abdomen while feeding may reveal a pyloric olive. The olive can be felt best when the stomach is empty, particularly just after vomiting. Diagnosis usually is confirmed by an upper gastrointestinal series or ultrasonography, or both in the case of ambiguity, before proceeding with surgical intervention (66).

Before operative correction of the pyloric stenosis, infants should be rehydrated intravenously and the electrolyte imbalance and alkalosis corrected. Surgical correction consists of longitudinal incision of the hypertrophied muscle (i.e., pyloromyotomy). After the operation is completed, the patient usually can be fed within 6 to 12 hours. Pyloric stenosis has been noted to recur in rare cases. Nonoperative medical management of pyloric stenosis, consisting of anticholinergic drugs and small frequent feedings, occasionally may be helpful. This therapy, sometimes used in Europe, is rarely used in North America because of the excellent results of surgical intervention.

Other rare gastric anomalies also may present in the neonatal period. Various forms of gastric atresia or hypoplasia have been described, most of which present with vomiting at or shortly after birth. Congenital microgastria may occur in association with a variety of other anomalies, including limb abnormalities, asplenia, megaesophagus, situs inversus, midgut malrotation, and cardiac anomalies. After major reconstructive surgery of the stomach, prognosis may be quite good.

Acid Peptic Disease

Acid peptic disease may be seen in newborn infants (67–69). Ulcers in children occur most commonly in the neonatal period or during the second decade of life. In newborn infants, ulcers, whether gastric or duodenal, usually present with hematemesis. Occasionally, blood loss may be substantial, manifested by symptoms of hypovolemia and shock. Differential diagnosis of hematemesis in the newborn includes swallowed maternal blood, or blood ingested from a cracked nipple through breast-feeding. Detection of swallowed maternal blood can be determined by assaying for adult hemoglobin in the gastric contents with the Apt test.

Diagnosis of peptic ulcer disease in the neonate requires endoscopy. Radiographic studies rarely are useful because the lesions are quite superficial and difficult to image radiographically. Endoscopy can be performed easily in a newborn infant by a skilled pediatric endoscopist using appropriate equipment. The smallest pediatric upper gastrointestinal endoscopes can be used safely in term infants under conscious sedation. The minimum size of the infant in whom endoscopy can be performed safely varies with the skill of the endoscopist, but endoscopy often also can be performed safely in larger premature babies. A bronchoscope can be used in smaller infants, although the examination usually is unsatisfactory. Although ulcerations may be identified anywhere in the stomach and the duodenum, multiple superficial gastric lesions are most common in newborn infants. Ulcers may be primary, or they may be secondary, as in the case of drugs known to irritate the upper gastrointestinal tract, such as steroids or theophylline. Treatment with antacids, or preferably H_1-receptor antagonists such as cimetidine or ranitidine, for a period of 2 to 6 weeks results in complete healing of the lesion. Secondary ulcers may be treated in a similar fashion. In this instance, continuation of the offending agent requires careful assessment of the risk-to-benefit ratio, because lesions will heal more rapidly if the agents are discontinued.

Spontaneous gastric perforation is a rare occurrence in the newborn. It occurs most commonly during the first 5 days of life, especially in infants subjected to severe stress or hypoxia (70). The constellation of symptoms typically includes a sudden deterioration in clinical status between the second and fifth day of life, characterized by refusal to eat, vomiting, abdominal distention, and respiratory distress. Free intraperitoneal air and fluid are demonstrable on plain radiographs of the abdomen. Immediate surgical consultation should be sought.

Disorders of the Small Intestine

Congenital Anomalies

Of the various small intestinal disorders that present in the neonatal period, congenital anomalies that produce obstruction are likely to present earliest. Patients present with bilious vomiting, abdominal distention, and occasionally obstipation. Bilious vomiting indicates obstruction distal to the ampulla of Vater. Bilious vomiting associated with the passage of blood through the rectum suggests vascular compromise of the small intestine, necessitating immediate surgical intervention.

Malrotation or nonrotation of the gut is an anatomic defect produced by incomplete rotation and fixation of the embryonic intestine after return from its extraabdominal location at about week 10 of gestation (71). During development, the intestine rotates 270 degrees around the axis of the superior mesenteric artery to place the cecum in the right lower quadrant. When the cecum fails to rotate completely, the mesenteric attachment of the small intestine is limited to that supporting the superior mesenteric artery and vein. This permits the bowel to twist on itself and produces a midgut volvulus. In the malrotated colon, adhesive bands, otherwise known as Ladd bands, stretch anteriorly from the right peritoneal gutter over the duodenum, where they can produce obstruction. Rotational anomalies may be associated with other intestinal anomalies, usually duodenal stenosis or atresia or other small intestinal atresias. Cardiac, esophageal, urinary, and anal anomalies also may be present. Rotational abnormalities should be considered in the differential diagnosis of a high intestinal obstruction identified radiographically. Unfortunately, the diagnosis often is missed by plain abdominal radiographs because air may be present in several loops of bowel distal to the obstruction. Rotational abnormalities are identified more easily with an upper gastrointestinal series, or barium enema. The radiographic hallmark of malrotation is the identification of the cecum in the upper abdomen or to the left of the midline. Symptomatic rotational abnormalities require urgent surgical exploration, because a volvulus may result in loss of the entire midgut within hours of presentation due to vascular occlusion. Intestinal dysmotility is common following operative repair of a malrotation with or without an associated volvulus (72).

Jejunal or ileal atresias range from membranous obstructions to complete atresia. Atresias can be single or multiple (73,74). An apple peel or Christmas tree deformity of the superior mesenteric artery results in an extensive jejunal atresia followed by multiple ileal atresias that are vascularly supplied by a branch of the ileocolic artery. Unlike duodenal atresia, relatively few anomalies are associated with ileal atresia. Cystic fibrosis, however, is present in approximately 20% of infants with jejunoileal atresia.

Small intestinal atresias in the neonatal period present with bilious vomiting. The degree of abdominal distention varies with the site of the atresia. If the atresia is distal, vomiting may be delayed for up to 24 hours after birth. Depending on the location of the atresia, varying numbers of dilated loops of bowel with air–fluid levels may be present on abdominal radiographs. Because it is difficult to differentiate small intestine from colon on plain abdominal radiographs in newborns, a contrast enema should be performed to exclude colonic lesions and obstructions. Contrast enemas also are helpful in excluding disorders such as meconium plug syndrome or associated rotational abnormalities.

Meconium Ileus

Meconium ileus occurs almost exclusively in patients with cystic fibrosis. It is caused by abnormally viscid mucus glycoprotein in meconium (75). Approximately 10% to 20% of patients with cystic fibrosis have meconium ileus as the first sign of their disease. Pathologically, the lumen of the distal small intestine is obstructed by an accumulation of abnormal meconium. Infants present with bilious vomiting and abdominal distention during the first 2 days of life. A palpable sausage-like mass may be present, and rectal examination may identify hard, dry, gray-tan meconium. Abdominal radiographs demonstrate some evidence of complete obstruction, but the radiologic hallmark is the soap-bubble appearance of trapped air within the tenacious meconium in the distal small bowel. A water-soluble contrast enema occasionally is therapeutic in disrupting the meconium obstruction. Care should be taken to avoid dehydration, because contrast substances are hypertonic and can result in massive pooling of fluid within the bowel lumen. Surgical intervention is required if the contrast enema is unsuccessful.

Other disorders related to meconium may be seen in the neonatal period. Meconium peritonitis may occur when intrauterine bowel perforation, secondary to obstruction, has resulted in leakage of sterile meconium into the peritoneal cavity. Common causes include atresia, volvulus, stenosis, cystic fibrosis, meconium ileus, and Hirschsprung's disease. Small flecks of intraabdominal calcification may be identified radiographically. Ascites occasionally occurs, but may resolve spontaneously unless secondary infection develops. In severe cases, meconium peritonitis can result in adhesions that require surgical intervention.

Necrotizing Enterocolitis

The most serious gastrointestinal disorder occurring in neonates is NEC (76,77). Because NEC appears predominantly in sick, low-birth-weight infants, the incidence has increased in recent years as the mortality rate for the very-low-birth-weight infant has decreased. It has been estimated that 90% of cases occur in premature infants and that NEC may develop in 1% to 10% of infants hospitalized in neonatal intensive care units (78). Significant intercenter differences in the prevalence of NEC have been reported (73). The mortality rates vary from 10% to 50%. The age of onset of NEC is related to birth weight and gestational age. Smaller, more immature infants (less than 28 weeks of gestation) tend to have NEC at an older age than larger, more mature (greater than 31 weeks of age) infants (79). Thus, the more premature the infant, the longer the duration of risk.

The etiology of NEC is not fully known (80). Multiple factors appear to be involved, including hypoxia, acidosis, and hypotension, which may lead to ischemic damage of the mucosal barrier of the small intestine (81). Secondary bacterial invasion of the mucosa may be involved in the pathogenesis of pneumatosis intestinalis. Moreover, NEC has been observed to occur in epidemics in neonatal intensive care units, further supporting the role of microbial agents in pathogenesis. A number of conditions may predispose the larger infant to development of NEC, including cyanotic congenital heart disease, obstructive lesions of the systemic cardiac outflow (e.g., hypoplastic left heart, coarctation of the aorta), polycythemia, umbilical catheters, exchange transfusions, perinatal asphyxia, maternal preeclampsia, and maternal use of cocaine. Infants with patent ductus arteriosus also seem to be at greater risk. In this case, oxygenated blood is shunted from the intestine. All of these factors suggest that mucosal injury and ischemia are important in the development of NEC. The role of inflammatory mediators, such as tumor necrosis factor-α and platelet-activating factor, and oxygen free radicals also have received attention (82,83).

Rapid onset of enteral feeding may be a risk factor for NEC, because of changes in enteric blood flow and oxygen requirements during feeding (84,85). NEC occasionally is reported in infants who have never been enterally fed. Several factors related to enteral feeding have been studied, and a number of theories have been proposed on how enteral feedings might precipitate NEC. Hyperosmolar formulas have been implicated in the production of NEC, but these formulas differed from standard formulas in other ways as well. In addition, most hyperosmolar formulas have been reformulated to minimize this risk. Formula feedings seem to predispose to NEC more than breast-feeding, suggesting that breast milk factors, including growth factors, antibodies, and cellular immune factors, might be protective. It also is likely that formula within the gastrointestinal tract may provide a substrate for bacterial proliferation. The role of bacterial invasion in this disease has been well recognized, but is likely to be a secondary event after compromise of the intestinal mucosal barrier.

The shunting of blood away from the intestine in a fashion similar to the diving reflex in aquatic mammals has been postulated as a potential mechanism for producing the initial gut ischemia. This reflex might occur in response to a hypoxic episode and has been studied extensively in animal models.

The association of NEC with prematurity implicates immaturity of the intestinal mucosal barrier. A number of factors that affect the mucosal barrier are immature in premature infants, including acid output, intestinal motility, and enzyme production. Immaturity of the microvillus membrane itself, as well as differences in the mucus secreted by the small intestine, may play a significant role. The mucosal immune system is immature, and less secretory IgA is produced. Some interest has arisen in the possible role of oral immunoglobulin administration for prophylaxis against NEC (86).

The reported gastrointestinal hormone abnormalities in NEC patients are difficult to interpret because of the spectrum of ages at which the disease develops, the randomness of blood sample timing, and the variation in quantity of enteral feedings. Concentrations of GIP, neurotensin, and enteroglucagon in infants with NEC are lower than those normally fed infants of comparable age, but gastrin, motilin, and pancreatic polypeptide (PP) levels appear to be normal (87).

Clinical presentations vary widely. Abdominal distention usually is one of the earliest and most consistent clinical signs. Other symptoms include bloody stools, apnea, bradycardia, lethargy, shock, and retention of gastric contents due to poor gastric emptying. Thrombocytopenia, neutropenia, and metabolic acidosis may develop during bowel ischemia. Not every patient has every sign, however, and clinical presentation may vary markedly. Diagnosis is confirmed by radiographic demonstration of pneumatosis intestinalis or portal hepatic venous air. Nonspecific radiographic findings include thickening of the bowel wall, dilated loops of bowel, and ascites. The presence of reducing substances in the stool, due to carbohydrate malabsorption, may be an early finding in NEC, as may increased α_1-antitrypsin levels, which indicate protein-losing enteropathy.

Suspicion of NEC dictates that all enteral feedings should be discontinued. An orogastric tube is placed routinely to relieve distention of the alimentary tract. Intravenous access must be secured to provide fluid, electrolytes, and nutrition, because the patient will not be fed enterally for an extended period of time. Intravenous antibiotics are administered to provide coverage for enteric organisms. Inclusion of specific antianaerobic agents does not appear to be helpful (88). The duration of oral intake restriction depends on the clinical status. Patients who merely have poor feeding with increased residuals, and the presence of minimal radiographic findings, may be fed within 48 to 72 hours. In the presence of pneumatosis intestinalis and marked abdominal distention, 2 weeks of parenteral nutrition may be required before judicious gradual reintroduction of enteral feedings is considered.

Throughout the course of the disease, frequent radiographic evaluation of the abdomen for evidence of intestinal perforation is required. Apnea, bradycardia, abdominal wall discoloration or edema, or a sudden increase in intraabdominal girth should give rise to the suspicion of bowel perforation. Frequent laboratory evaluations include a complete blood count and platelet count to look for thrombocytopenia and neutropenia, both of which suggest deterioration. In infants with severe inflammation of the small intestine, large volumes of fluid and electrolytes or blood products may be required to maintain perfusion and blood pressure. This is especially true in infants in whom severe metabolic acidosis develops secondary to poor perfusion. Ventilatory support usually is necessary. Exploratory laparotomy with resection of dead bowel has been the traditional surgical approach to patients with evidence of perforation or gangrenous bowel. Peritoneal drainage prior to laparotomy may be of benefit in extremely-low-birth-weight infants or hemodynamically unstable patients (89).

Infants who require surgical intervention are at risk for postoperative complications and complications associated with total parenteral nutrition (TPN). The most common complications after surgery for NEC are sepsis, intestinal strictures, short bowel syndrome, and wound infections (90). Intraabdominal abscesses are relatively rare. In a number of infants, the mucosal inflammatory process may progress to transmural necrosis that may, if it does not lead to perforation, result in fibroblast proliferation, granulation tissue, and stricture formation. Some clinicians routinely study the gastrointestinal tract radiographically after NEC has been treated medically. It is not uncommon to find asymptomatic ileal stenosis or colonic stenosis in such patients. If symptoms of partial obstruction, such as abdominal distention, failure to thrive, or poor feeding develop in infants who have recovered from a bout of NEC, contrast studies are indicated; however, it should be noted that ileal stenosis may not be detected by these studies.

Localized Intestinal Perforation

Localized intestinal perforation recently has been recognized as a clinical entity distinct from NEC (91). Localized intestinal perforations are similar to NEC in that they occur almost exclusively in premature infants. In contrast, patients with localized intestinal perforations are less likely to have symptoms of a severe illness, such as metabolic acidosis or leukopenia, than patients with NEC (91). Patients with localized intestinal perforations are more likely to survive to discharge than patients with NEC.

The etiology of localized intestinal perforation is not known. Interruption of regional blood flow to the bowel has been hypothesized. Patients with localized perforation are more likely to have received higher dosages of indomethacin or had an umbilical artery catheter in place shortly before the perforation than patients with NEC (91).

Short Bowel Syndrome

Short bowel syndrome is defined as a malabsorptive state that occurs after bowel resection. Infants with short bowel syndrome fall into two categories: those with congenital anomalies (e.g., gastroschisis, apple peel anomaly

of the superior mesenteric artery, intestinal atresia) and anatomically normal patients who undergo bowel resection for NEC. The latter group tends to have fewer complications and a better prognosis, when equal lengths of residual small intestine remain.

After massive resection of the small intestine, the remaining small bowel undergoes an adaptation process characterized by epithelial hyperplasia (92). Within 1 to 2 days after resection, enterocytes begin replicating in the crypts. Gradual morphologic changes occur in the small intestine, including a marked lengthening of villi that results in increased mucosal surface area. This is followed by an increase in absorptive capacity that eventually enables many to survive without parenteral nutrition. The adaptation process is gradual, however, and may require weeks to years.

The major gut hormone changes seen after ileal resection are marked increases in plasma levels of PYY, enteroglucagon, and motilin (92,93). Increases of enteroglucagon (which reflect parallel changes in the trophic hormone GLP-II, and of PYY) which inhibits gastric acid secretion, small intestinal secretion, and delays gastric emptying and intestinal transit, are appropriate responses in this condition. Preservation, or even enhancement, of the PYY response would be valuable in diminishing the rapid transit and diarrhea associated with this condition. Studies in experimental animals have revealed that improvements in transit and fluid absorption are temporally related to the increase in PYY response that occurs after bowel resection (94,95).

Hypergastrinemia also accompanies intestinal resection and is responsible for the increased gastric secretion seen postoperatively. The increase of gastrin levels is triggered by the reduction in small intestinal inhibitory factors and usually subsides after a few weeks, when intestinal adaptation has taken place. Mucosal hyperplasia does not occur in the absence of enteral nutrition. In fact, mucosal atrophy may result if the patient is nourished only parenterally (96). Enteral nutrition stimulates intestinal adaptation by several mechanisms (97). Highly unsaturated long-chain fats stimulate intestinal adaptation to a greater extent than protein or carbohydrate; the mechanism by which this occurs is poorly understood. Nonetheless, careful attention to the provision of adequate enteral nutrition is important.

Management of the short bowel syndrome is a multistage process (98). During the early postoperative period, use of parenteral nutrition and careful attention to fluid and electrolyte abnormalities are essential. High-volume ostomy losses must be replaced with a solution of comparable electrolyte content to obviate the need for frequent changes in electrolyte concentration in parenteral nutrition solutions.

The presence of an ostomy may create additional problems. These vary somewhat, depending on whether the ostomy is in the ileum, from which the volume output is likely to be much greater, or in the colon, in which case stool consistency may vary markedly based on whether the ostomy was placed proximally or distally. If available, the services of an enterostomal therapist, with special training in rehabilitation of infants and children with ostomies, will assist the parents in understanding the implications of the ostomy. The ostomy should be placed away from sites such as the iliac crest, costal margin, or umbilicus, so that ostomy appliances will fit easily.

Most ostomy devices consist of an adhesive, nonallergenic wafer device with a flange that allows the transparent drainage pouch to be secured to it over the stoma. The pouch can be removed easily for draining by snapping it off the wafer, or it can be emptied through a drainage port at the bottom of the bag. When leakage occurs beneath the wafer, the device should be removed, and careful skin care around the ostomy is necessary. The skin should be washed gently with a soft cloth moistened with mild soap and tepid water. The skin should be dried thoroughly after cleansing. Many protective ointments and powders are available to apply around the stoma area to prevent skin breakdown. If skin irritation is present, tincture of benzoin or steroid preparations available in spray form may be used. The pouches often are reusable and may be washed with mild soap and water and soaked in a deodorant solution to control odor problems. Appropriate teaching will prevent many of the other problems encountered by ostomy patients, such as skin excoriation, minor stoma bleeding, stoma prolapse, and odor. Additional ostomy problems include prolapse and stenosis. The latter should be suspected in the presence of abdominal distention and vomiting. In either situation, the surgeon should be notified.

When enteral feeds are started, a slow continuous infusion of a dilute elemental formula generally works best. Formulations such as Alimentum (Ross Laboratories, Columbus, OH) or Pregestimil (Mead Johnson Laboratories, Evansville, IN), which contain significant quantities of long-chain fats, are ideal. These lactose-free preparations with hydrolyzed protein are absorbed rapidly, yet provide adequate stimulation of intestinal adaptation. Stool losses must be monitored carefully. A marked increase in fluid losses or significant evidence of carbohydrate malabsorption manifested by a low stool pH or positive stool-reducing substances are contraindications for further increasing the enteral infusion. Enteral infusions are increased as tolerated, and parenteral nutrition is decreased in a gradual isocaloric fashion. Patients then can be weaned to intermittent parenteral nutrition and prepared for home parenteral nutrition therapy (99). Intermittent parenteral nutrition allows provision of parenteral nutrients at night, primarily for the convenience of caregivers. Parenteral nutrition initially is discontinued only for short periods of time, usually 4 to 6 hours, each day. In small infants, this usually is delayed until the patient can tolerate approximately 20% of calorie intake

enterally to avoid hypoglycemia when he or she is not receiving parenteral nutrition. The duration of parenteral nutrition can be decreased gradually until all parenteral nutrition infuses over 10 to 12 hours at night. It is wise to taper the parenteral nutrition rates up and down when placing a patient on or off of parenteral nutrition, to prevent fluctuation in serum glucose levels.

Home parenteral nutrition has markedly reduced the cost of long-term management of short bowel syndrome patients and has decreased family stresses and nosocomial infections (100). It has become a standard therapy in patients with short bowel syndrome, and prolonged hospitalizations rarely are necessary. To minimize complications, careful training of home nursing personnel is essential, and coordination of activity between physician and nursing staff must be tightly controlled.

Continuous enteral infusions are used in patients with short bowel syndrome for several reasons. The percentage of calories absorbed from the continuous infusion is greater than that possible with bolus feedings, because transport carrier proteins are continually saturated. Continuous infusion provides constant stimulation of mucosal adaptation and reduces the need for parenteral calories, decreasing the risk of parenteral nutrition liver disease. Children should be fed small quantities of formula orally, so as to learn to suck and swallow. Eventually, solids can be fed around the nasogastric tube. These manipulations often will speed the transition from continuous enteral to oral feeding later in the course of therapy.

Numerous chronic complications arise in the treatment of short bowel syndrome, including bacterial overgrowth, nutritional deficiency states, watery diarrhea, parenteral nutrition liver disease, and catheter-related problems. Bacterial overgrowth is defined as increased bacterial content in the small intestine (101). Complications from bacterial overgrowth include increased malabsorption, D-lactic acidosis, and colitis-like or ileitis-like syndrome. Normal small bowel bacterial counts vary from 10^3/mL proximally to much greater numbers in the ileum. Normal antegrade peristalsis and gastric and mucosal immune factors prevent excess bacterial proliferation. In short bowel syndrome, because of disruption of normal anatomy and motility, overgrowth is likely and bacterial counts usually exceed 10^5/mL. Bacterial overgrowth should be suspected whenever motility is slowed, the bowel is dilated, or the ileocecal valve is absent. Organisms typically include facultative bacteria and anaerobes. Bacteria deconjugate bile salts, causing them to be reabsorbed, depleting the bile salt pool, impairing micelle solubilization, and resulting in steatorrhea and malabsorption of fat-soluble vitamins. More important, bacterial overgrowth causes mucosal inflammation, exacerbating malabsorption of all nutrients. Protein-losing enteropathy and loss of immunoglobulins may occur. Bacteria may compete with the host for nutrients, such as vitamin B_{12}.

Screening for bacterial overgrowth can be done with a fasting breath hydrogen or glucose breath hydrogen test, or by detecting the presence of indican in the urine. Measurement of breath hydrogen is a simple test in infants and children, although collection of samples in the neonate requires special care. A fasting breath hydrogen level greater than 42 ppm is seen only in small bowel bacterial overgrowth (102). A breath hydrogen level greater than 20 ppm after the administration of 2 g/kg of oral glucose, with measurement at 15-minute intervals after ingestion, suggests bacterial overgrowth. Measurement of indican in the urine is a simple screening test for bacterial overgrowth, because bacteria convert dietary tryptophan to indican. Unfortunately, indicanuria may occur in other conditions, and the technique lacks sensitivity (103). Bacterial overgrowth can be diagnosed definitively by culture of aspirates from the small intestine. Small intestinal biopsies demonstrating inflammatory changes suggest bacterial overgrowth.

Accumulation of D-lactate in the blood stream results in neurologic symptoms varying from frank disorientation to coma (104). Bacterial overgrowth may cause colitis-like or ileitis-like syndrome with large ulcerations characteristic of Crohn's disease, but without granulomas (105). Broad-spectrum oral antibiotics (e.g., metronidazole, TMP-SMZ, gentamicin) and antiinflammatory agents often are beneficial. Broad-spectrum antimicrobial coverage should be directed at the organisms present, usually anaerobes. Antimotility agents may improve nutrient contact with the mucosa by lengthening transit time, but tend to exacerbate bacterial overgrowth and should be used with caution. Recently, use of probiotic bacteria has been proposed for the treatment of certain patients with small bowel bacterial overgrowth (105a).

Secretory diarrhea may be a problem in some children with short bowel syndrome. This may be related to hypergastrinemia, which often occurs after resection. Because the tight junctions in the ileum are less permeable than the jejunum, the ileum plays a major role in fluid and electrolyte conservation, and ileal resections are more likely to result in major fluid and electrolyte losses than jejunal resections. Because most infants with NEC have ileal disease, this is a major problem in neonates after bowel resection. Ileal resection also results in malabsorption of bile acids, because the ileum is the primary site for bile acid reabsorption. Malabsorption of bile acids into the colon may cause fluid secretion and watery diarrhea, which may respond to a bile acid-binding resin such as cholestyramine. Unfortunately, cholestyramine may further deplete the bile acid pool, exacerbating steatorrhea.

Nutritional deficiency states may occur after parenteral nutrition is discontinued, including deficiencies of fat-soluble vitamins A, D, and E, and the minerals iron, zinc, calcium, and magnesium.

Parenteral nutrition hepatobiliary tract disease is the major complication that may result in death in infants with short bowel syndrome (100). The mechanism by which the liver injury occurs is unknown. In most instances, enteral administration of a significant percentage of calories, usually between 20% and 30% of total requirements, reduces the risk of parenteral nutrition liver disease.

Cholelithiasis develops in approximately 20% of infants receiving parenteral nutrition for short bowel syndrome because of malabsorption of bile acids, altered bilirubin metabolism, and gallbladder stasis. Cholangitis may occur in the presence of partial obstruction. Early cholecystectomy should be considered if patients are symptomatic with elevated direct bilirubin and liver enzymes.

Catheter-related infections and thrombosis are common in infants requiring long-term parenteral nutrition (106). In our experience, catheter-related infections rarely are due to intestinal bacterial overgrowth and most commonly are related to catheter care technique. Diligent parental instruction in catheter care and in the signs and symptoms of sepsis is extremely important.

During later stages of therapy, additional surgery may be indicated (107). One of the first questions usually concerns whether to close a stoma that was formed at the time of initial surgery. If the colon remains, and especially if ileum exists as well, reconnecting an ostomy may substantially conserve fluid and electrolytes, but also may result in perianal disease. In infants with dilated segments of proximal bowel, resecting a tight anastomosis or tapering the bowel to improve flow of luminal contents often reduces bacterial overgrowth. A number of procedures have been designed to slow transit time, including reverse segments of bowel, one-way valves, or colon interposition, but none is considered reliably effective, and all may increase bacterial overgrowth.

A procedure to increase the length of the bowel has been devised that involves transecting the bowel longitudinally, preserving the blood supply to both sides of the bowel, and creating a segment about twice the length and one-half of the diameter. This allows reducing the diameter of the bowel without any loss of mucosal surface area. Because it does not actually increase the mucosal surface area, it is indicated primarily to reduce bacterial overgrowth without losing absorptive surface in infants with dilated bowel. Our experience has been quite rewarding with this procedure, with 12 of 14 recent patients demonstrating significant improvement and several becoming independent of parenteral nutrition after surgery (108). It should not, however, be performed in neonates, because it is successful only after significant bowel dilation has occurred.

Intestinal transplantation has now become a reality. Well over 100 patients now have been transplanted at a number of centers in the United States and Europe (109). Patients with short bowel syndrome with evidence of parenteral nutrition-induced liver dysfunction should be referred early for intestinal transplantation. Recent evidence suggests that isolated intestinal transplantation prior to the development of irreversible parenteral nutrition-induced liver disease may be an attractive alternative to the combined liver/bowel transplantation, which has traditionally been utilized for such patients. Long-term survival 2 to 3 years following intestinal transplantation has been in the range of 50% to 70%.

It is possible for infants to survive without transplantation or permanent parenteral nutrition with surprisingly short segments of bowel (110,111). As a general rule, patients with greater than 25 cm of normal bowel at the time of neonatal resection who have an ileocecal valve, or with greater than normal 40 cm of normal bowel at the time of neonatal resection who have no ileocecal valve, have a reasonable chance of eventually becoming independent of parenteral nutrition. The ileocecal valve appears to play a major role in determining the long-term prognosis, primarily because of its ability to exclude colonic bacteria from entering the small bowel and perhaps also because of its ability to delay transit through the small intestine.

Mucosal Injury Disorders

Because of the limited small intestinal reserve in small infants, small intestinal disease perhaps is most catastrophic in infancy. In small intestinal injury, all nutrients are malabsorbed. Most symptoms, however, are related to carbohydrate malabsorption because of the osmotic diarrhea produced when these malabsorbed molecules are broken down further by intestinal bacteria into smaller and smaller osmotically active particles. The osmotic gradient overrides the ability of the ileum and colon to reabsorb fluid effectively, and watery diarrhea ensues.

Measurement of stool pH and reducing substances is an ideal means to screen for small bowel mucosal disease in infancy. When carbohydrates are malabsorbed and broken down into organic acids by colonic bacteria, the stool pH drops below 5.5. Stool pH can be measured easily with litmus paper, simply by inserting the paper into the stool. Measurement of reducing substances in stool can be done by placing five drops of stool and ten drops of water into a test tube and dropping in a Clinitest (Ames) tablet. Positive reducing substances in stool confirms the presence of carbohydrate malabsorption. Patients receiving formulas that are predominantly sucrose are less likely to demonstrate positive reducing substances in their stools because sucrose is a nonreducing carbohydrate.

Infectious Diarrhea

During the neonatal period, infectious diseases of the small intestine are relatively uncommon. A number of viruses may cause diarrhea in small infants, including rotavirus, enteric adenoviruses, and enteroviruses. Viral gastroenteritis usually presents with watery stools, with evidence of carbohydrate malabsorption. The predominant mucosa injury in viral gastroenteritis is in the proximal jejunum, where carbohydrates are absorbed. In contrast, bacterial pathogens generally produce more distal injury that involves the colon and results in Hematest-positive stools that contain leukocytes (Table 37–2). Bacterial causes of diarrhea include *Salmonella* sp, *Shigella* sp, invasive *Escherichia coli*, and *Campylobacter jejuni*. *Clostridium difficile* infection predominantly involves the large intestine and, in severe cases, produces pseudomembranous colitis. Infection with *C. difficile* usually follows a course of broad-spectrum antibiotics. Severe watery or bloody diarrhea and colonic perforation may occur. Diagnosis is difficult in neonates, because a very high percentage of small infants carry *C. difficile* without evidence of disease.

Human Immunodeficiency Virus-Associated Disease

Human immunodeficiency virus (HIV) in infants results in a variety of gastrointestinal problems. Failure to thrive is common. Chronic diarrhea and generalized lymphadenopathy often are present. Other common presentations include asymptomatic hepatosplenomegaly, which may occur in conjunction with severe interstitial pneumonia and hypergammaglobulinemia.

Chronic diarrhea in infants with acquired immunodeficiency syndrome (AIDS) presents a very difficult management problem. Diarrhea may result from opportunistic infections, tumors, including Kaposi's sarcoma and lymphoma, and direct HIV infection of the gut. Opportunistic organisms include viral agents (e.g., cytomegalovirus, rotavirus, herpes simplex, coxsackievirus, adenovirus), bacterial pathogens (e.g., *Salmonella* sp, *Campylobacter*-like organisms, *Listeria* sp, *Mycobacterium avium-intracellulare*, *Plesiomonas shigelloides*), fungal pathogens (e.g., *Candida* sp, *Aspergillus* sp), and parasitic pathogens (e.g., cryptosporidium, *Strongyloides* sp, *Giardia* sp, amoebas, *Isospora belli*). A broad spectrum of endoscopic and histologic findings is possible because of the diverse nature of the disease. Extensive viral and bacterial cultures and examinations for ova and parasites are warranted in infants and children with AIDS.

Treatment consists of therapy directed at any specific infectious pathogen identified, coupled with use of parenteral and enteral nutrition. As in almost all chronic

TABLE 37–2. *Screening stool studies in infectious diarrhea*

	Bacterial	Viral
Clinitest	−	±
pH	≥5.5	≤5.5
Hematest	+++	−
Leukocytes	+++	−

−, negative; ±, negative or positive, +++, strongly positive.

enteropathies, primary attention should be given to continuous enteral infusion with an elemental diet or protein hydrolysate formula. If malabsorption develops in the patient, as indicated by stools testing positive for reducing substances or manifesting a pH below 5.5, supplemental parenteral nutrition is needed to provide the remainder of caloric and other nutritional needs. The presence of a significant secretory component of the diarrhea may make treatment difficult, complicate the use of continuous enteral infusion, and require careful attention to intake and output of fluid and electrolytes to maintain biochemical homeostasis.

Hormonal Changes in Diarrhea

Infective diarrhea in infants is associated with a massive increase in circulating concentrations of motilin, enteroglucagon, and PYY (112,113). These abnormalities resolve once the patients are better. The gut endocrine system in infants, however, responds in a manner different from that of adults. In infants with diarrhea, plasma motilin concentrations exceed those that are known to accelerate gastric emptying and increase small bowel motility (113). Motilin is therefore likely to be involved in the motor abnormalities associated with this condition. A hormonally triggered increase in transit rate may constitute a defense mechanisms to rid the bowel of pathogens and secreted toxins. The extremely high enteroglucagon levels in neonatal infective diarrhea appear to be related to the extent of mucosal injury and its repair (114). Measurement of selected gut hormones may give information on the extent of mucosal damage or the presence of ongoing pathologic change.

Formula Protein Intolerance

One of the most common causes of chronic diarrhea in small infants is formula protein-induced enterocolitis (115,116). Small bowel involvement (i.e., enteritis), colon involvement (i.e., colitis), or concomitant small bowel and colon involvement are possible with this disorder. Protein-induced mucosal injury has been reported with cow-milk protein, soy protein, breast milk, and even beef protein. We recently have observed a number of infants who have been intolerant of protein hydrolysate formulas, but responded well to a new amino acid-based infant formula, Neocate (117).

Infants typically present before 3 months of age with bright red blood in the stool, which may be normal or loose in consistency depending on the extent of inflammation. Sigmoidoscopic examination may reveal gross friability or may appear normal until the mucosa is wiped with a cotton swab, at which time the mucosa readily bleeds. Rectal biopsy confirms inflammation, with the combination of polymorphonuclear leukocytes and eosinophils in the lamina propria. Stools may test positive for occult blood and may contain leukocytes. If the inflammation extends into the small intestine, carbohydrate malabsorption may occur, infants will have watery diarrhea, and stools will be acidic (pH less than 5.5) and test positive for reducing substances. Small intestinal biopsy will demonstrate varying degrees of mucosal injury, with shortening and blunting of the villi, inflammatory infiltrates, and an increase in mitotic activity in the crypts. Disaccharidase levels in the mucosal biopsies often are reduced.

Other symptoms that may occur as a result of formula protein-induced enterocolitis are vomiting and irritability. Infants with formula protein intolerance commonly vomit, especially those with small intestinal disease. It often is difficult to differentiate this disorder from gastroesophageal reflux, because both groups may present with irritability; however, babies with formula protein sensitivity commonly have loose stools and abnormal sigmoidoscopic examinations. This is an important distinction because the treatment is vastly different. Irritability, not dissimilar from infantile colic, may occur in infants with formula protein intolerance. In infantile colic, the irritability classically occurs at a specific time of the day and responds symptomatically to repetitive stimuli. Infants with irritability secondary to formula protein intolerance usually are inconsolably irritable, often feed poorly, have loose stools, spit up, and have abnormal sigmoidoscopic examinations or other evidence of small intestinal or colonic inflammation. A careful history and physical examination and appropriate laboratory studies can be quite specific in differentiating the two disorders.

Infants who manifest signs and symptoms of formula protein intolerance should be placed on a protein hydrolysate formula such as Nutramigen, Pregestimil, or Alimentum, because a high percentage also will be intolerant of soy formula. A small percentage of infants who do not respond to these formulas may improve on an amino acid formulation such as Neocate.

Most infants with formula protein intolerance will outgrow their sensitivity by 1 year of age. Powell (118) has described a specific challenge procedure to confirm the diagnosis of cow-milk protein intolerance. Patients should not have received the suspected antigen for at least 2 weeks before testing and should be asymptomatic. A standard dose (100 mL of cow milk or soy formula) is administered and the child is monitored carefully for reaction. Stool specimens are analyzed for occult blood, leukocytes, and reducing sugars, and a leukocyte count is obtained 6 to 8 hours later. The test result is considered positive if diarrhea develops within 24 hours, leukocytes or blood appear in stools, or the leukocyte count rises by more than 4,000 cells/mL over baseline. Approximately 20% of the infants have a delayed reaction. If the child originally had evidence of severe milk protein sensitivity, it is wise to hospitalize the infant, start with small volumes (5 to 10 mL) of formula, and gradually increase the volume to avoid severe mucosal injury, anaphylaxis, and shock. Skin testing rarely is useful in children with formula protein intolerance who have predominantly gastrointestinal symptoms.

Intractable Diarrhea of Infancy

A state of persistent diarrhea and malabsorption despite the institution of a protein hydrolysate formula and in the absence of infectious pathogens is referred to as intractable or protracted diarrhea of infancy (119). These patients demonstrate a variety of histologic abnormalities on small intestinal biopsy, including blunting or flattening of the villi, increased mononuclear cells with occasional polymorphonuclear infiltrates, cuboidalization of the surface epithelium, and a mild-to-moderate increase in mitotic activity in the crypts. Histologic lesions vary substantially, however, and correlate poorly with ultimate prognosis (120). Such infants have chronic weight loss and progressive malnutrition unless appropriate therapy is instituted. Initial therapy involves slow institution of a continuous enteral infusion of a diluted elemental formula such as Pregestimil or Alimentum (121). The rate is rapidly advanced to approximately 150 mL/kg/d or more, provided the child is not on supplemental parenteral nutrition. The concentration of the formula then is advanced sequentially over 3 to 4 days, until the patient is tolerating full caloric requirements and gaining weight. During this time, stool pH and reducing substances are monitored, and evidence of carbohydrate malabsorption suggests failure of enteral feedings. If this occurs, a period of parenteral nutrition is indicated, usually through a central venous catheter, with gradual reintroduction of enteral feedings by continuous infusion. In treating such infants, it is important to avoid using formulas that contain intact milk or soy protein, because the likelihood of protein sensitivity in such infants is high and further mucosal injury may result. Lengthy periods of parenteral or continuous enteral infusion may be necessary, but the ultimate prognosis is good.

In addition to intractable (i.e., protracted) diarrhea associated with formula protein intolerance, other rare syndromes have been reported to result in mucosal injury and chronic diarrhea. One is congenital microvillus atrophy or microvillus inclusion disease, a disorder with hypoplastic atrophy of the villi and shortening or depletion of microvilli (122). This disorder requires electron microscopic diagnosis and has a very poor prognosis. A similar disorder has been recognized electron microscopically and has been associated with "tufting" of the microvilli, hence, the term "tufting enteropathy" (123). A number of patients also have been described with an intractable diarrhea-like syndrome in association with a mild immune defect, stiff unmanageable hair, and peculiar facies (124). All of these conditions are quite rare.

Severe protracted diarrhea also may be associated with autoimmune enteropathy; however, this disorder usually presents outside the immediate neonatal period (125). Mucosal lesions are severe and the prognosis is poor. Infants with this disorder often have multiorgan autoantibodies, including gut epithelium, and frequently have pancreatic involvement with hyperglycemia or hypoglycemia.

Disorders of the Colon

Congenital Anomalies

There is substantial overlap in small bowel and colonic disease in neonates. Many of the congenital anomalies involve both the small and large intestines, and certain mucosal injury disorders, including formula protein enterocolitis and NEC, can involve both the small intestine and colon. There are some disorders that primarily affect the colon. Most are congenital and involve anatomic obstructions, such as atresias, or dysmotility, such as Hirschsprung's disease.

Anatomic Lesions

Colonic stenosis or atresia is a rare event, often associated with other skeletal anomalies. Colonic duplication also is a rare entity, which may present with delayed symptoms of obstruction. Duplications usually are cystic, gradually enlarging masses, located posterior to the rectum, which may be confused with tumors (126).

Motility Disorders

More frequent are the disorders that present with delayed passage of meconium secondary to dysmotility. Meconium plug syndrome is one such entity, in which inspissated meconium in the distal colon results in obstruction and dilatation proximally. Delayed passage of meconium is the presenting symptom, and barium enema examination reveals a large plug of meconium that often is evacuated after the barium enema. Normal feeding and stooling usually follows removal of the obstruction, but 20% to 30% of patients with meconium plug syndrome have Hirschsprung's disease. If symptoms recur after removal of the meconium plug, rectal suction biopsy is indicated.

Delayed passage of meconium also may occur with the neonatal small left colon syndrome. Radiographic examination of these infants demonstrates normal-to-dilated proximal colon with constricted or smaller distal colon, with the constricted area usually beginning around the splenic flexure. The line of demarcation is much more abrupt than is seen in neonatal Hirschsprung's disease. The disorder is more common in infants of diabetic mothers, as well as infants of mothers with hyperthyroidism. It usually resolves spontaneously, although placement of a colostomy may be necessary until normal motility returns. Colonic motility eventually will return, usually within 2 to 12 weeks, and the colostomy may be closed at that time.

Hirschsprung's disease, or congenital aganglionic megacolon, occurs in approximately 1 in 5,000 live births, more commonly in males than in females (127). The risk of recurrence in families is reported to be as high as 10%, higher in infants with total aganglionosis. The frequency is ten times higher in infants with trisomy 21. The disease is caused by a congenital absence of the ganglion cells in both the submucous and myenteric plexuses. Ganglion cells regulate normal colonic peristaltic activity. The absence of ganglion cells results in an inability of the bowel to undergo coordinated relaxation. Impaired migration of neural crest cells into the distal colon is thought to be the mechanism through which Hirschsprung's disease develops, although there is some controversy about this. The disorder almost always involves the distal rectum, but the extent varies substantially. There also is controversy as to whether or not skip areas can occur. A few such cases have been reported, but they appear to be extremely rare. In most instances, involvement does not extend proximal to the sigmoid colon. In very rare instances, the involvement may extend beyond the colon into the small intestine. The further the lesion extends, the more difficult the medical management becomes.

Most cases of Hirschsprung's disease are not diagnosed in the neonatal period. When they are, the most common clinical presentation is delayed passage of meconium, with passage of the first stool beyond 24 hours of age. This presentation probably is common but often overlooked. Infants also may appear irritable, with poor feeding and failure to thrive, which, unfortunately, is the typical presentation of a wide variety of small bowel and colonic disorders.

Some infants with Hirschsprung's disease may present with a life-threatening complication—acute enterocolitis (128). Toxic megacolon is common. Although enterocolitis may occur in the newborn period, it more commonly presents at 2 to 3 months of age. Mortality remains around 50%. The disorder presents with sudden or gradual onset of diarrhea, followed by bloody stools and eventually the clinical appearance of sepsis. The clinical overlap between infectious enterocolitis or formula protein-induced enterocolitis is such that Hirschsprung's enterocolitis also must be considered in the differential diagnosis of these more common entities. Patients who present with bloody diarrhea in infancy and have negative stool cultures, and who do not respond quickly to protein hydrolysate formula, need to have a rectal biopsy performed. If Hirschsprung's disease is suspected, surgical consultation should be obtained immediately, and attempts should be made to decompress the colon with a rectal tube or rectal irrigation. A decompressing colostomy should be placed as soon as feasible.

Diagnosis of Hirschsprung's disease usually rests with rectal suction biopsy. A small biopsy tube is inserted into the rectum and a small piece of tissue is removed from a point 2 cm proximal to the mucocutaneous junction. If the biopsy is obtained higher, patients with low-segment Hirschsprung's disease may be missed. If the biopsy is taken more distally, it will be obtained in the hypoganglionic zone, an area in which ganglion cells are normally sparse, resulting in a false-positive biopsy for Hirschsprung's disease. The biopsy must be deep enough to contain sufficient submucosa to identify ganglion cells. Superficial biopsies are inadequate to diagnose Hirschsprung's disease. Because ganglion cells are sparse, the biopsy must be serially sectioned, and 60 to 80 sections of tissue examined. Ganglion cells in newborns are somewhat immature and difficult to identify. Thus, a rectal suction biopsy is a reliable diagnostic tool, provided the biopsy is obtained from an appropriate location and depth and an experienced gastroenterologist or pathologist interprets the biopsy. If results are equivocal, a full-thickness biopsy may be performed to establish the diagnosis.

Diagnosis also can be made by inflating a balloon in the distal rectum and measuring relaxation of the internal anal sphincter, a process impaired in Hirschsprung's disease. Although this technique is performed less commonly, those who are skillful in its use believe it is as reliable as rectal biopsy. In contrast, barium enema examination in the newborn is highly unreliable in the diagnosis of Hirschsprung's disease because the transition zone has yet to develop. Therefore, proximal colonic dilation usually is not apparent in the neonate, and the clinician must look for irregular contractions in the rectosigmoid as the primary hallmark of Hirschsprung's disease.

Treatment begins with placement of a decompressing colostomy proximal to the transition zone between ganglionic and aganglionic bowel. Definitive surgery usually is done at 8 to 12 months of age. A number of different operations have been devised in which the aganglionic bowel is removed and the ganglionic bowel attached into the distal rectum. Surgical treatment generally is successful in restoring long-term fecal continence (129).

Patients with total colonic Hirschsprung's disease present major difficulties in postoperative fluid and electrolyte balance. Infants frequently require prolonged courses of parenteral nutrition. Parents should be warned about the protracted nature of the disease, and infants should be observed closely for fluid, electrolyte, and nutritional problems.

Several other intestinal motility disorders present in the neonatal period. Transient hypomotility occurs in some premature infants and is characterized by markedly delayed gastric emptying and absent or diminished small bowel motility. In most instances, these abnormalities gradually resolve with time; support with parenteral nutrition coupled with intermittent attempts at feeding is all that is indicated. Alterations in calcium and magnesium metabolism such as parathyroid dysfunction or hypothyroidism can cause diminished motility, and these disorders should be excluded in infants with apparent motility disorders. Occasionally, infants with chronic idiopathic intestinal pseudoobstruction syndrome can present during infancy. This term applies to a number of neuropathic and myopathic disorders that result in chronic progressive gastrointestinal hypomotility. A variety of histologic lesions have been described, and the prognosis for improvement is poor. Occasionally, the disorder also may involve the urinary tract, with associated megacystis and megaureter (130).

Pancreatic Disorders

Cystic Fibrosis

Disorders of the pancreas uncommonly present during the neonatal period. The most common is cystic fibrosis, which occurs in approximately 1 in 1,600 Caucasian live births (131). This autosomal recessive disorder usually presents later in childhood with failure to thrive or chronic pulmonary disease, but may present with meconium ileus in the neonatal period. After the obstruction has been relieved, therapy consists of compensating for the pancreatic insufficiency through use of elemental formulas such as Pregestimil or Alimentum, which contain hydrolyzed protein as their protein source and medium-chain triglycerides as part of their lipid component. Medium-chain triglycerides do not require digestion by pancreatic enzymes for absorption and, consequently, may facilitate nutrient assimilation in infants with pancreatic insufficiency. Despite the use of elemental formulas, replacement pancreatic enzyme therapy from birth is necessary to aid the digestion of endogenously secreted proteins.

In children with pancreatic insufficiency due to cystic fibrosis, the release of the pancreatic hormone PP is almost totally abolished. Fasting PP levels are low and the normal response to milk feeding is absent (132). Plasma insulin and GIP responses are reduced significantly in cystic fibrosis patients compared to control subjects, even though the early glucose rise is greater in the former group (132). Reduced GIP secretion in response to feeding may exacerbate the glucose intolerance that accompanies pancreatic destruction. Although plasma enteroglucagon concentrations are elevated in cystic fibrosis, levels of other hormones such as gastrin, secretin, motilin, and glucagon are quite normal (132).

The second most common cause of pancreatic insufficiency in infancy is Shwachman syndrome, a disorder characterized by pancreatic insufficiency and bone marrow dysfunction with cyclic neutropenia (133). This rare disorder should be considered in infants with steatorrhea and neutropenia. Extremely rare isolated defects in pancreatic enzyme secretion, including trypsinogen and lipase, also have been reported.

Liver Disease

Development

The liver is a complex organ serving multiple metabolic functions. From a digestive standpoint, its primary function is that of an exocrine organ producing bile for the emulsification of fats. Postnatally, the liver receives its blood from two separate sources, approximately 25% from the hepatic artery and 75% from the portal vein. The portal vein drains the splanchnic bed and allows the liver the opportunity to regulate and metabolize substances absorbed by the intestine and hormones produced in the gastrointestinal tract.

Bile is composed primarily of water. The concentration of solids in the bile are increased threefold by the gallbladder. The fetal liver is capable of synthesizing bile acids from cholesterol slowly, and the rate of synthesis increases progressively throughout gestation. The major bile salt in newborns is taurocholate. Conjugation of bile salts with glycine in preference to taurine gradually increases, and, by adulthood, most bile salts are conjugated with glycine. The bile acid pool is very small in the preterm infant, but gradually increases in the newborn and matures throughout infancy. This relatively small bile acid pool results in reduced bile salt secretion and, in addition to the relative pancreatic insufficiency, plays a role in the less efficient absorption of fat in the newborn infant. Bile acids are reabsorbed in the ileum through an active transport mechanism. There is some passive transport of bile acids in the jejunum and colon as well. In the fetus, taurocholate is absorbed passively and active ileal transport appears after birth.

Cholestatic Liver Disease

Most liver diseases in the neonatal period present with cholestasis, or conjugated hyperbilirubinemia (134,135). Although elevation of the amino transferase (i.e., transaminase) enzymes is considered the hallmark of hepatocellular injury in older children and adults, neonates may have significant hepatocellular injury even in the presence of normal amino transferase levels. There are many causes of prolonged conjugated hyperbilirubinemia in the neonatal period. These can be subdivided into general categories, including the following: infectious disorders; toxic insults such as parenteral nutrition and sepsis; metabolic disorders; anatomic disorders, including congenital hepatic fibrosis and choledochal cyst; and idiopathic infantile cholangiopathies, including primarily biliary atresia and neonatal hepatitis (136).

Neonatal Hepatitis and Biliary Atresia

After extensive evaluation of the infant with cholestasis, a diagnosis of either extrahepatic biliary atresia or idiopathic neonatal hepatitis is made in 70% to 80% of cases (137,138). Current thinking suggests that neonatal hepatitis and biliary atresia form a continuum of a pathophysiologic process directed at various levels of the hepatobiliary tract. Inflammation in the bile duct epithelium may result in sclerosis and obliteration of the bile ducts and manifest itself as extrahepatic biliary atresia. Primary hepatocellular inflammation is more likely to result in neonatal hepatitis. Reovirus type III has been found in a number of infants with both idiopathic neonatal hepatitis and biliary atresia. This virus has been implicated as a causative agent in both disorders, although there is evidence that raises questions about this hypothesis (139,140).

Idiopathic neonatal hepatitis is slightly more common than biliary atresia. Both sporadic and familial varieties exist. Neonatal hepatitis, unlike biliary atresia, is more common in low-birth-weight infants. Jaundice develops during the first week of life in most cases. A wide variety of clinical presentations may occur, from severe failure to thrive or fulminant hepatic failure to asymptomatic jaundice. Acholic stools are uncommon, but may occur if cholestasis is severe. Physical examination reveals a firm, enlarged liver and occasionally splenomegaly. The presence of other signs of congenital infection may point toward a more specific diagnosis. Liver biopsy may be helpful in making the diagnosis, but the histologic findings are relatively nonspecific. In most cases, neonatal hepatitis can be differentiated successfully from biliary atresia by percutaneous liver biopsy. Clinical management is directed toward nutritional support and medical management of clinical complications such as ascites or pruritus. The prognosis is variable, with one-half of the cases resolving with little or no sequelae. Life-threatening chronic liver disease may necessitate liver transplantation.

Extrahepatic biliary atresia accounts for about one-third of cases of neonatal cholestasis. Familial cases are uncommon, as are cases in premature infants. Patients typically present with jaundice during the first or second week of life. Acholic stools are more common than in neonatal hepatitis. The liver is firm and enlarged, and splenomegaly may be present, as in neonatal hepatitis. Infants often appear clinically well, although progressive liver injury results in nutritional deficiencies, failure to thrive, and ascites.

Differentiation between neonatal hepatitis and biliary atresia has been the subject of controversy over the years. Serum amino transferase (i.e., transaminase) levels are notoriously unreliable indicators of neonatal liver disease and may be normal even in some patients with neonatal hepatitis. Extremely elevated γ-glutamyltransferase levels are suggestive of the marked bile ductular proliferation found in biliary atresia (141). Liver biopsy demonstrates inflammatory obliteration of the extrahepatic biliary tree, with bile stasis and bile ductular proliferation in the liver. Histologic features may overlap with neonatal hepatitis, particularly early in the course of the disease, making it difficult to differentiate. Histologic transition from neonatal hepatitis to biliary atresia has been reported and may be a relatively common phenomenon. The duodenal intubation and aspiration test is a simple, rapid, inexpensive method to check for patency of the extrahepatic biliary tree. Collection of 12 2-hour aliquots of duodenal drainage from a feeding tube placed in the duodenum over a 24-hour period suggests biliary atresia if no yellow fluid is present. Aspiration of bile-stained fluid from the duodenum suggests patency of the extrahepatic biliary tract. This test is sensitive and specific for the evaluation of infantile cholestasis (142). The test has reliability comparable to, or better than, radionuclide imaging with scans, which may give abnormal results in neonatal hepatitis during periods of severe cholestasis. Reliability of the radionuclide studies may be improved by measurement of duodenal fluid counts collected by a simple string test, in which infants swallow a string that absorbs fluid from the small intestine that later can be analyzed (143). The combination of liver biopsy and imaging study or duodenal drainage usually is used to determine whether the patient is more likely to have biliary atresia or neonatal hepatitis. If bile drainage cannot be confirmed or the typical histologic picture of neonatal hepatitis is not apparent on liver biopsy, then surgical exploration and intraoperative cholangiography usually is performed to establish a final diagnosis.

If the patient has biliary atresia, a hepatoportoenterostomy with Roux-en-Y enteroanastomosis (i.e., Kasai procedure) is performed to attempt bile drainage. The Kasai procedure rarely alters the long-term outcome of biliary atresia (144), but may delay the necessity of liver transplantation. Some advocate not performing a Kasai procedure. Most, however, believe that performing the procedure does not worsen the prognosis at transplant and may allow the child to live longer so that a more suitable liver donor may be located before transplantation. For those infants with progressive liver disease after the Kasai procedure, every attempt must be made to optimize their condition before transplantation. Deficiencient absorption must be corrected by vitamin supplementation (i.e., A, D, E, and K) require supplementation. Salt and protein restriction may become necessary, as liver failure progresses.

Hepatic transplantation is the definitive treatment for biliary atresia and results in long-term survival in 70% to 85% of infants.

Other Causes of Cholestasis

Rare causes of cholestasis must be excluded before confirming the diagnosis of neonatal hepatitis or biliary

TABLE 37-3. *Steps in evaluating neonatal cholestasis*

1. Determine that hyperbilirubinemia is predominantly direct
2. Exclude metabolic and infectious causes of cholestasis
3. Perform ultrasound to exclude anatomic lesions
4. Obtain percutaneous liver biopsy and hepatobiliary scan or duodenal drainage study
5. Explore whether studies suggest biliary atresia and perform Kasai procedure if indicated

atresia (Table 37–3) (136). Infectious diseases such as cytomegalovirus, hepatitis B, HIV, rubella, herpes, toxoplasmosis, and syphilis should be excluded by standard serologic or culture techniques. Metabolic disorders to be considered include tyrosinemia, galactosemia, and hereditary fructose intolerance. Obtaining urine for reducing substances to exclude galactosemia and hereditary fructose intolerance, and succinyl acetone to exclude tyrosinemia should be done immediately. Anatomic disorders such as choledochal cysts can be diagnosed by ultrasonography. Other causes such as TPN cholestasis or sepsis should be considered, based on the clinical presentation.

Occasionally, liver biopsy will demonstrate a marked reduction in the number of intrahepatic bile ducts, revealing a disorder known as paucity of the intrahepatic bile ducts or intrahepatic biliary hypoplasia. Some of these patients fall into the category of Alagille syndrome, also known as syndromatic paucity or arteriohepatic dysplasia (145). These patients exhibit unusual facial characteristics, ocular abnormalities including posterior embryotoxon (i.e., prominent Schwalbe line), pulmonic stenosis, and vertebral arch defects, including anterior vertebral arch fusion with butterfly vertebrae. Careful cardiac examination, examination of the eyes by an ophthalmologist, and radiographic examination of the lumbosacral spine should be obtained in patients with suspected Alagille syndrome who have a paucity of intralobular bile ducts. Prognosis for long-term survival in syndromatic patients is relatively good.

There are patients with nonsyndromic paucity who have liver biopsy findings similar to those with Alagille syndrome. In general, these patients have a much poorer prognosis than those with syndromatic paucity. Life-threatening cirrhosis develops in many, and these patients may require hepatic transplantation. As in biliary atresia, liver transplantation has markedly changed the prognosis for these patients.

A number of infectious disorders, both viral and bacterial, may present during the neonatal period, and a specific diagnosis should be sought in such instances. Hepatitis B typically is found in infants whose mothers were infected during the third trimester. As many as 60% to 90% of infants born to hepatitis B surface antigen-positive mothers may be infected. Transmission from mother to infant most commonly occurs at the time of delivery.

Mothers who are hepatitis B antigen-positive are at extremely high risk to transmit hepatitis B virus to their infants. In addition, mothers who are chronic carriers of hepatitis B surface antigen also may infect their infants. Most hepatitis B in infancy is asymptomatic. Abnormal liver tests develop at approximately 6 to 8 weeks of age and may persist for up to 1 year. Nearly 50% of these children remain hepatitis B surface antigen-positive and are at risk for developing hepatocellular carcinoma. Such children should be screened annually with alpha-fetoprotein levels for evidence of liver cancer, unless their hepatitis B surface antigen determinations revert to negative. Maternal screening for hepatitis B surface antigen is essential to prevent perinatal transmission of hepatitis B. Neonates born to mothers who are hepatitis B antigen-positive should receive hepatitis B hyperimmune globulin, 0.5 mL intramuscularly at the time of birth, and hepatitis B vaccine within 12 hours of birth. Booster immunizations with hepatitis B vaccine are recommended at 1 and 6 months of age (146).

Several other viruses may produce hepatitis during the neonatal period. Hepatitis A may develop in infants of mothers with active icteric hepatitis A at the time of delivery. Hepatitis C commonly is transmitted through blood contact and produces a clinical spectrum similar to hepatitis B. Serologic tests and viral RNA assays are available to detect hepatitis C. Both hepatitis B and C run substantial risks for chronic liver disease. Recent experience has been gained with the use of alpha-interferon in the treatment of chronic hepatitis B and C, and with lamivudine in hepatitis B. Preliminary results look promising, but more experience is needed. Other viruses, such as Epstein–Barr virus, cytomegalovirus, HIV, rubella, herpes simplex, coxsackievirus, and adenoviruses may cause a wide spectrum of neonatal liver disease (147). In most instances, infection with these viruses results in spontaneous resolution without chronic injury.

Bacteria also may produce neonatal liver injury, because invasion of the liver may occur. Specific hepatic infection may result from certain bacterial diseases such as syphilis and listeriosis, as well as the parasitic disorder toxoplasmosis.

A number of metabolic diseases may present with neonatal cholestasis. The most common is α_1-antitrypsin deficiency. α_1-Antitrypsin is the major protease inhibitor in the hepatocyte. Deficiency of α_1-antitrypsin occurs in a number of inheritable phenotypes. These Pi or protease inhibitor phenotypes can be determined. Type ZZ produces the most complete deficiency state and most cases of liver disease. It is estimated that 10% to 20% of type ZZ patients develop liver disease (148). Isolated cases of type MZ and MS also have been reported with liver injury (149). The ZZ phenotype is inherited through an autosomal recessive mechanism and occurs in 1 in 2,000 live births. Patients can be identified by the measurement of a very low α_1-antitrypsin level in the blood. Diagnosis is confirmed by the determination of the ZZ phenotype, plus the classic histologic findings of periodic-acid–Schiff-positive, diastase-resistant granules on liver biopsy.

Liver disease may develop in patients with cystic fibrosis, although very few of these present during the neonatal period. Measurement of sweat chloride and specific mutational analysis to exclude cystic fibrosis should be part of the evaluation of neonatal liver disease.

Three metabolic diseases present with rather fulminant neonatal liver disease. These include galactosemia, hereditary fructose intolerance, and tyrosinemia. These disorders should be expected when coagulation abnormalities appear inappropriately severe relative to the apparent degree of liver disease. Patients with galactosemia have positive urinary reducing substances if they are being fed lactose at the time of screening. Patients with hereditary fructose intolerance also may test positive. Patients with tyrosinemia can be screened by measuring succinyl acetone content in the urine. Plasma and urine amino acids will demonstrate marked elevations of tyrosine, although this may be a nonspecific finding in any infant with neonatal liver disease. Patients with galactosemia respond to a galactose-free diet, and liver injury usually resolves spontaneously. Neonatal sepsis is a frequent occurrence in these infants, and precautions should be taken. Patients with tyrosinemia commonly undergo progressive liver and renal dysfunction and are candidates for emergent liver transplantation once the diagnosis is made.

Several lipid storage diseases produce neonatal liver disease. Niemann–Pick disease, Wolman disease, cholesterol-ester storage disease, and Gaucher disease are included in this group. Most present with an insidious onset later in life.

A number of disorders exist in which peroxisomal dysfunction occurs. The most common is Zellweger syndrome, the cerebrohepatorenal syndrome. These patients present with cholestasis, hepatomegaly, hypotonia, and dysmorphic features, and may be diagnosed by demonstration of very-long-chain fatty acids in the serum.

Defects in the urea cycle may present with hyperammonemia during the first 2 days of life. A sepsis-like picture with vomiting, lethargy, seizures, and coma suggests this diagnosis. The most common form is ornithine transcarbamylase deficiency. Serum ammonia levels are very high, provided the infant is being fed protein. Diagnosis depends on plasma and urinary amino acid levels, and liver biopsy must be assayed for specific enzymes (see Chap. 39). Protein intake should be restricted and liver transplantation should be considered. Transient hyperammonemia of the newborn also has been reported with spontaneous resolution and no long-term neurologic sequelae. Permanent resolution of the hyperammonemia usually occurs by 2 weeks of age.

Another cause of acute liver failure in the neonate is neonatal hemochromatosis or neonatal iron storage disease (150,151). This rare, apparently inherited disorder of iron storage and metabolism may present with acute and rather fulminant liver failure characterized by severe cholestasis and coagulopathy. A variety of histologic findings have been observed in the livers of these patients, but they consistently have increased iron deposition in the liver as well as in other organs. Salivary gland biopsy may be used to establish the diagnosis. The disorder is rapidly progressive and often fatal unless transplantation can be performed early. Recently, antioxidant cocktails have been advocated for such patients, and some success has been reported (152).

Cholestasis may occur in any patient on chronic parenteral nutrition, but it is far more common in sick premature infants who receive parenteral nutrition for long periods of time (153,154). The mechanism by which the liver injury occurs is unknown and perhaps multifactorial (155). Several risk factors have been identified, however, including recurrent infections, prematurity, and lack of enteral feeding. Certain components of parenteral solutions have been implicated in causing liver injury. Excessive caloric administration may play a role. Certain amino acids may be more hepatotoxic, although many of these data are derived from animal studies. Higher doses of protein may result in a more rapid rise in bilirubin, but does not appear to alter ultimate risk of development of liver disease. Available intravenous lipid preparations do not appear to cause cholestasis and may, in fact, be beneficial in this regard.

The reason premature infants are more susceptible to liver disease while on parenteral nutrition probably is related to developmental immaturity of several hepatobiliary processes. These infants have reduced and altered bile acid synthesis, decreased bile acid pool size, and, therefore, decreased intraluminal bile acids. Gallbladder function also is impaired. Bile acid reabsorption from the small bowel is underdeveloped. The premature liver also is less capable of detoxifying potentially toxic secondary bile acids.

Lack of enteral feeding definitely predisposes to parenteral nutrition cholestasis. Gastrointestinal hormones that stimulate bile flow depend on enteral feeding for their release. Reduced gut motility in the unused bowel may contribute to bacterial proliferation and the resultant production of toxic secondary bile acids. Infection, especially gastrointestinal, and gastrointestinal surgery may potentiate the liver injury through related mechanisms. Limited amounts of enteral feeding, as tolerated, may be very beneficial in preventing liver injury in the parenteral nutrition-dependent infant.

Diagnosis of parenteral nutrition liver disease depends on exclusion of other causes of cholestasis in the parenteral nutrition-dependent patient. Separation of this disorder from other causes of cholestasis is difficult using standard laboratory tests. Histologic study is nonspecific, but may be helpful in making the diagnosis (156). The disease often is reversible once parenteral nutrition is discontinued. It occasionally may progress to cirrhosis, and hepatocellular carcinoma has been reported.

Treatment is accomplished best by discontinuing parenteral nutrition. If this cannot be accomplished, the following steps should be taken:

1. Reevaluate solutions to ensure they are appropriately formulated and balanced.
2. Use low-dose enteral feedings as tolerated to stimulate bile flow and gut motility.
3. Cycle the parenteral nutrition so that it is given over only part of the day.
4. Use amino acid solutions specially formulated for infants.

Other potential therapies, yet unproven, include choleretics such as phenobarbital or ursodeoxycholic acid, hormone stimulation of bile flow, and bowel prokinetic agents. Success with combined intestinal-liver transplants suggests that this procedure may play an important role in infants with end-stage parenteral nutrition liver disease (157).

REFERENCES

1. Lebenthal E, Keung YK. Alternative pathways of digestion and absorption in the newborn. In: Lebenthal E, ed. *Textbook of gastroenterology and nutrition in infancy*, 2nd ed. New York: Raven Press, 1989:3.
2. Lebenthal E, Tucker N. Carbohydrate digestion: development in early infancy. *Clin Perinatol* 1986;13:37.
3. Cicco R, Holzman I, Brown D, et al. Glucose polymer intolerance in premature infants. *Pediatrics* 1981;67:498.
4. Lebenthal E, Lee PC. Alternate pathways of digestion and absorption in early infancy. *J Pediatr Gastroenterol Nutr* 1984;3:1.
5. Watkins JB. Lipid digestion and absorption. *Pediatrics* 1985;75 [Suppl]:151.
6. Boehm G, Bierbach U, Seuger H, et al. Activities of lipase and trypsin in duodenal juice of infants small for gestational age. *J Pediatr Gastroenterol Nutr* 1991;12:324.
7. Jensen RG, Clark RM, de Jong FA, et al. The lipolytic triad: human lingual, breast milk and pancreatic lipases: physiological implications of their characteristics in digestion of dietary fats. *J Pediatr Gastroenterol Nutr* 1982;1:243.
8. Watkins JB, Ingall D, Szczepanik P, et al. Bile salt metabolism in the newborn. *N Engl J Med* 1973;288:431.
9. Balistreri WF, Heubi JE, Suchy FJ. Immaturity of the enterohepatic circulation in early life: factors predisposing to "physiologic" malabsorption and cholestasis. *J Pediatr Gastroenterol Nutr* 1983;2:346.
10. Acra SA, Ghishan FK. Active bile salt transport in the ileum: characteristics and ontogeny. *J Pediatr Gastroenterol Nutr* 1990;10:421.
11. Euler AR, Byrne WJ, Meis PJ, et al. Basal and pentagastrin stimulated acid secretion in human newborn infants. *Pediatr Res* 1979;13:36.
12. Hyman PE, Clarke DD, Everett SL, et al. Gastric acid secretory function in preterm infants. *J Pediatr* 1985;106:467.
13. Agunod M, Yamaguchi N, Lopez R, et al. Correlative study of hydrochloric acid, pepsin and intrinsic factor secretion in newborns and infants. *Am J Digest Dis* 1969;14:400.
14. Antonowicz I, Lebenthal E. Developmental pattern of small intestinal enterokinase and disaccharidase activities in the human fetus. *Gastroenterology* 1977;723:1299.
15. Younoszai MK, Sapario RS, Laughlin M, et al. Maturation of jejunum and ileum in rats: water and electrolyte transport during in vivo perfusion of hypertonic solutions. *J Clin Invest* 1978;62:271.
16. Southgate DAT, Widdowson EM, Smits BJ, et al. Absorption and excretion of calcium and fat by young infants. *Lancet* 1969;1:487.
17. Senterre J, Putet G, Salle B, et al. Effects of vitamin D and phospho-rus supplementation on calcium retention in preterm infants fed banked human milk. *J Pediatr* 1983;103:305.
18. Voyer M, Davakis M, Antener I, et al. Zinc balances in preterm infants. *Biol Neonate* 1982;42:87.
19. Tomomasa R, Hyman PE, Itoh K, et al. Gastroduodenal motility in neonates: response to human milk compared with cow's milk formula. *Pediatrics* 1987;80:434.
20. Berseth CL. Gestational evolution of small intestine motility in preterm infants. *J Pediatr* 1989;115:646.
21. Worniak ER, Fenton TR, Milla PJ. The development of fasting small intestine motility in human neonates. In: Roman C, ed. *Gastrointestinal motility.* London: Lancaster Press, 1983:265.
22. Nagata S, Koyanagi T, Horimoto N, et al. Chronological development of the fetal stomach assessed using real-time ultrasound. *Early Hum Dev* 1990;22:15.
23. Vanderhoof JA, Rappoport PJ, Paxson CL Jr. Manometric diagnosis of lower esophageal sphincter incompetence in infants: use of a small, single-lumen perfused catheter. *Pediatrics* 1978;62:805.
24. Buchan AMJ, Bryant MG, Polak JM, et al. Development of regulatory peptides in the human fetal intestine. In: Bloom SR, Polak JM, eds. *Gut hormones.* New York: Churchill-Livingston, 1981:119.
25. Bryant MG, Buchan AMJ, Gregor M, et al. Development of intestinal regulatory peptides in the human fetus. *Gastroenterology* 1982;83:47.
26. Lucas A, Bloom SR, Aynsley-Green A. Development of gut hormone responses to feeding in neonates. *Arch Dis Child* 1980;55:678.
27. Lucas A, Adrian TE, Christofides ND, et al. Plasma motilin, gastrin and enteroglucagon and feeding in the human newborn. *Arch Dis Child* 1980;55:673.
28. Euler AP, Byrne WJ, Cousins LM, et al. Increased serum gastrin concentrations and gastric hyposecretion in the immediate newborn period. *Gastroenterology* 1977;72:1271.
29. Aynsley-Green A, Lucas A, Bloom SR. The effects of feeds of differing composition on entero-insular hormone secretion in the first hours of life in human neonates. *Acta Paediatr Scand* 1979;68:265.
30. Lucas A, Bloom SR, Aynsley-Green A. Postnatal surges in plasma gut hormones in term and preterm infants. *Biol Neonate* 1982;41:63.
31. Miller BA. Observations on the gastric acidity during the first month of life. *Arch Dis Child* 1941;16:22.
32. Adrian TE, Savage AJ, Sagor GR, et al. Effect of peptide YY on gastric, pancreatic and biliary function in humans. *Gastroenterology* 1985;89:494.
33. Adrian TE, Smith HA, Calvert SA, et al. Elevated plasma peptide YY in human neonates and infants. *Pediatr Res* 1986;20:1225.
34. Lucas A, Adrian TE, Bloom SR, et al. Plasma secretin in neonates. *Acta Paediatr Scand* 1980;69:205.
35. Johnson LR. Regulation of gastrointestinal growth. In: Johnson LR, ed. *Physiology of the gastrointestinal tract*, 2nd ed. New York: Raven Press, 1987:301.
36. Calvert SA, Soltesz G, Jenkins PA, et al. Feeding premature infants with human milk or preterm milk formula: effects on postnatal growth, intermediary metabolism and regulatory peptides. *Biol Neonate* 1985;47:189.
37. Berseth CL. Gestational evolution of small intestine motility in preterm and term infants. *J Pediatr* 1989;115:646.
38. Sarson DL, Wood SM, Holder D, et al. The effect of glucose-dependent insulinotropic polypeptide infused at physiological concentrations on the release of insulin in man. *Diabetologia* 1982;22:33.
39. Lucas A, Sarson DL, Bloom SR, et al. Developmental aspects of gastric inhibitory polypeptide (GIP) and its possible role in the enteroinsular axis in neonates. *Acta Paediatr Scand* 1980;69:321.
40. Lucas A, Aynsley-Green A, Blackburn AN, et al. Plasma neurotensin in term and preterm neonates. *Acta Paediatr Scand* 1981;17:201.
41. Savage AP, Adrian TE, Carolan G, et al. Effects of peptide YY (PYY) on mouth to cecum transit time and on the rate of gastric emptying in healthy volunteers. *Gut* 1987;70:166.
42. Drucker DJ, Ehrlich P, Asa SL, Brubaker PL. Induction of epithelial proliferation by glucagon-like peptide 2. *Proc Natl Acad Sci USA* 1996;92:7911.
43. Chance WT, Foley-Nelson T, Thomas I, Balasubramaniam A. Prevention of parenteral nutrition-induced hypoplasia by coinfusion of glucagon-like peptide-2. *Am J Physiol* 1997;273:G559.
44. Lucas A, Bloom SR, Aynsley-Green A. Metabolic and endocrine consequences of depriving preterm infants of enteral nutrition. *Acta Paediatr Scand* 1983;72:245.

45. Adrian TE, Bloom SR. Effect of food on the hormones of the gastrointestinal tract. In: Hunter JO, Jones V, eds. *Food and the gut.* Philadelphia: Bailliére Tindall, 1985:13.

46. Isaacs PET, Ladas S, Forgacs IC, et al. A comparison of the effects of ingested medium- and long-chain triglyceride on gallbladder volume and the release of cholecystokinin and other gut peptides. *Dig Dis Sci* 1987;32:481.

47. Martin LW, Torres AM. Omphalocele and gastroschisis. *Surg Clin North Am* 1985;65:1235.

48. Meller JL, Reyes HM, Loeff DS. Gastroschisis and omphalocele. *Clin Perinatol* 1989;16:113.

49. Yazbeck S, Ndoye M, Khan AH. Omphalocele: a 25 year experience. *J Pediatr Surg* 1986;21:761.

50. Dykes EH. Prenatal diagnosis and management of abdominal wall defects. *Semin Pediatr Surg* 1996;5:90.

51. Quirk JG, Forney J, Collins HB, et al. Outcomes of newborns with gastroschisis: the effects of mode of delivery, site of delivery, and interval from birth to surgery. *Am J Obstet Gynecol* 1996;174:1134.

52. Lenke RR, Hatch EI Jr. Fetal gastroschisis: a preliminary report advocating the use of cesarean section. *Obstet Gynecol* 1986;67:395.

53. Langer JC. Gastroschisis and omphalocele. *Semin Pediatr Surg* 1996;5:124.

54. Herbst JJ. Gastroesophageal reflux in infants. *J Pediatr Gastroenterol Nutr* 1985;4:163.

55. Werlin SL, Dodds WJ, Hogan WJ, et al. Mechanisms of gastroesophageal reflux in children. *J Pediatr* 1980;97:244

56. Carlos MA, Babyn PS, Marcon MA, Moore AD. Changes in gastric emptying in early postnatal life. *J Pediatr* 1997;130:931.

57. Sondheimer JM. Continuous monitoring of distal esophageal pH: a diagnostic test for gastroesophageal reflux in infants. *J Pediatr* 1980;93:804.

58. Tsou VM, Young RM, Hart MH, et al. Elevated plasma aluminum levels in normal infants using antacids containing aluminum. *Pediatrics* 1991;87:148.

59. Strickland AD, Chang JHT. Results of treatment of gastroesophageal reflux with bethanechol. *J Pediatr* 1983;103:311.

60. Scott RB, Ferreire C, Smith L, et al. Cisapride in pediatric gastroesophageal reflux. *J Pediatr Gastroenterol Nutr* 1997;25:499.

61. Deleted in proof.

62. Jolley SG, Halpern LM, Tunell WP, et al. The risk of sudden infant death from gastroesophageal reflux. *J Pediatr Surg* 1991;26:691.

63. Raffensperger JG. Esophageal atresia and tracheoesophageal stenosis. In: Raffensperger JG, ed. *Swenson's pediatric surgery,* 5th ed. Norwalk, CT: Appleton and Lange, 1990:697.

64. Benson CD, Lloyd JR. Infantile pyloric stenosis: a review of 1120 cases. *Am J Surg* 1964;107:429.

65. Dodge JA. Genetics of hypertrophic pyloric stenosis. *Clin Gastroenterol* 1973;2:523.

66. Hernanz-Schulman M, Sells LL, Ambrosino MM, et al. Hypertrophic pyloric stenosis in the infant without a palpable olive: accuracy of sonographic diagnosis. *Radiology* 1994;193:771.

67. Nord KS. Peptic ulcer disease in the pediatric population. *Pediatr Clin North Am* 1988;35:117.

68. Drumm B, Rhoads JM, Stringer DA, et al. Peptic ulcer disease in children: clinical findings, and clinical course. *Pediatrics* 1988;82:410.

69. Murphy MS, Eastham EJ. Peptic ulcer disease in childhood: long-term prognosis. *J Pediatr Gastroenterol Nutr* 1987;6:721.

70. Bell JJ. Perforation of the gastrointestinal tract and peritonitis in the neonate. *Surg Gynecol Obstet* 1985;160:20.

71. Smith EI. Malrotation of the intestine. In: Welch KJ, Randolph JG, Ravitch MM, et al, eds. *Pediatric surgery,* 4th ed. Chicago: Year Book, 1986:882.

72. Feitz R, Vos A. Malrotation: the postoperative period. *J Pediatr Surg* 1997;32:1322.

73. Grosfeld JL. Jejunoileal atresia and stenosis. In: Welch KJ, Randolph JG, Ravitch MM, et al, eds. *Pediatric surgery,* 4th ed. Chicago: Year Book, 1986:838.

74. Martin LW, Zerella JT. Jejunoileal atresia: a proposed classification. *J Pediatr Surg* 1967;11:399.

75. Holgersen LO, Stanly-Brown EG. Idiopathic post-operative intussusception in infants and childhood. *Am Surg* 1978;44:305.

76. Brown EG, Sweet AY. Neonatal necrotizing enterocolitis. *Pediatr Clin North Am* 1982;29:1149.

77. Kliegman RM, Fanaroff AA. Necrotizing enterocolitis. *N Engl J Med* 1984;310:1093.

78. Hack M, Horbar JK, Malloy MH, et al. Very low birth weight outcomes of the National Institute of Child Health and Human Development Neonatal Network. *Pediatrics* 1991;87:587.

79. Uauy RD, Fanaroff AA, Korones SB, et al. Necrotizing enterocolitis in very low birth weight infants: biodemographic and clinical correlates. *J Pediatr* 1991;119:630.

80. Kliegman RM, Walsh M. Neonatal necrotizing enterocolitis: pathogenesis, classification and spectrum of illness. *Curr Probl Pediatr* 1987;17:213.

81. Ballance WA, Dahms BB, Shenker N, et al. Pathology of neonatal necrotizing enterocolitis: a ten-year experience. *J Pediatr* 1990;117 [Suppl 1, Pt 2]:S6.

82. Kliegman RM. Neonatal necrotizing enterocolitis: bridging the basic science with clinical disease. *J Pediatr* 1990;117:833.

83. Caplan MS, Sun X-M, Hsueh W, et al. Role of platelet activating factor and tumor necrosis factor-alpha in neonatal necrotizing enterocolitis. *J Pediatr* 1990;116:960.

84. Anderson DM, Kliegman RM. The relationship of neonatal alimentation practices to the occurrence of endemic necrotizing enterocolitis. *Am J Perinatol* 1991;8:62.

85. Covert RF, Neu J, Elliott MJ, et al. Factors associated with age of onset of necrotizing enterocolitis. *Am J Perinatol* 1989;6:455.

86. Eibl MM, Wolf HM, Furnkranz H, et al. Prophylaxis of necrotizing enterocolitis by oral IgA-IgG: review of a clinical study in low birth weight infants and discussion of the pathogenic role of infection. *J Clin Immunol* 1990;10[Suppl 6]:72S.

87. Aynsley-Green A, Lucas A, Lawson GR, et al. Gut hormones and regulatory peptides in relation to enteral feeding, gastroenteritis, and necrotizing enterocolitis in infancy. *Arch Dis Child* 1990;117 [Suppl]:24.

88. Faix RG, Polley TZ, Grasela TH. A randomized controlled trial of parenteral clindamycin in neonatal necrotizing enterocolitis. *Pediatrics* 1988;112:271.

89. Morga LJ, Shochat SJ, Hartman GE. Peritoneal drainage as primary management of perforated NEC in the very low birth weight infant. *J Pediatr Surg* 1994;29:310.

90. Horwitz JR, Lally KP, Chen HW, et al. Complications after surgical intervention for necrotizing enterocolitis: a multicenter review. *J Pediatr Surg* 1995;30:994.

91. Buchheit JP, Stewart DL. Clinical comparison of localized intestinal perforation and necrotizing enterocolitis in neonates. *Pediatrics* 1994;93:32.

92. Dowling RH, Booth CC. Structural and functional changes following small intestinal resection in the rat. *Clin Sci* 1967;32:139.

93. Adrian TE, Savage AP, Fuessl HS, et al. Release of peptide YY (PYY) after resection of small bowel, colon or pancreas in man. *Surgery* 1987;101:715.

94. Besterman HS, Adrian TE, Mallinson CN, et al. Gut hormone release after intestinal resection. *Gut* 1982;23:854.

95. Armstrong DN, Ballantyne GH, Adrian TE, et al. Adaptive increase in peptide YY and enteroglucagon after proctocolectomy and pelvic ileal reservoir reconstruction. *Dis Colon Rectum* 1991;34:119.

96. Wilmore DW, Dudrick SJ, Daly JM, et al. The role of nutrition in the adaptation of the small intestine after massive resection. *Surg Gynecol Obstet* 1971;132:673.

97. Vanderhoof JA. Short bowel syndrome. In: Lebenthal EB, ed. *Gastroenterology and nutrition in early infancy,* 2nd ed. New York: Raven Press, 1990:793.

98. Vanderhoof JA. Short bowel syndrome. In: Kassirer JP, ed. *Current therapy in internal medicine,* 3rd ed. Philadelphia: BC Decker, 1991:550.

99. Vanderhoof JA. Clinical management of the short bowel syndrome. In: Balistreri WF, Vanderhoof JA, eds. *Pediatric gastroenterology and nutrition.* London: Chapman and Hall, 1990:24.

100. Goulet OJ, Revillon Y, Jan D, et al. Neonatal short bowel syndrome. *J Pediatr* 1991;119[Suppl 1, Pt 1]:18.

101. Gracey M. The contaminated small bowel syndrome: pathogenesis, diagnosis and treatment. *Am J Clin Nutr* 1979;32:234.

102. Perman JA, Modler S, Barr RG, et al. Fasting breath hydrogen concentration: normal values and clinical adaptation. *Gastroenterology* 1984;87:1358.

103. Aarbakke J, Schjonsby H. Value of urinary simple phenol and indican determinations of the stagnant loop syndrome. *Scand J Gastroenterol* 1976;2:409.

104. Hudson M, Packnee R, Mowat NA. D-lactic acidosis in short bowel syndrome: an examination of possible mechanisms. *Q J Med* 1990;74:157.

105. Taylor SF, Sondheimer JM, Sokol RJ, et al. Noninfectious colitis associated with short gut syndrome in infants. *J Pediatr* 1991;119:24.

105a.Young RJ, Vanderhoof JA. Probiotic therapy in children with short bowel syndrome and bacterial overgrowth. *Gastroenerology* 1997;112:A916.

106. Caniano DA, Starr J, Ginn-Pease ME. Extensive short-bowel syndrome in neonates: outcome in the 1980s. *Surgery* 1989;105:119.

107. Thompson JS. Recent advances in the surgical treatment of the short-bowel syndrome. *Surg Ann* 1990;22:107.

108. Thompson J, Pinch L, Murray N, et al. Experience with intestinal lengthening procedures. *J Pediatr Surg* 1991;26:721.

109. Vanderhoof JA. Short bowel syndrome in children and small intestinal transplantation. *Pediatr Clin North Am* 1996;43:533.

110. Cooper A, Floyd TS, Ross AJ, et al. Morbidity and mortality of short bowel syndrome acquired in infancy: an update. *J Pediatr Surg* 1984;19:711.

111. Dorney SFA, Ament ME, Berquist WE, et al. Improved survival in very short small bowel of infancy with use of long-term parenteral nutrition. *J Pediatr* 1985;106:521.

112. Adrian TE, Savage AP, Bacarese-Hamilton AJ, et al. Peptide YY abnormalities in gastrointestinal disease. *Gastroenterology* 1986;90:379.

113. Besterman HS, Christofides ND, Welsby PD, et al. Gut hormones in acute diarrhea. *Gut* 1983;24:665.

114. Lawson GR, Nelson R, Laker MF, et al. Gut regulatory peptides and intestinal permeability in acute infantile gastroenteritis. *Arch Dis Child* 1992;67:272.

115. Walker-Smith J, Harrison M, Kilby A, et al. Cow's milk-sensitive enteropathy. *Arch Dis Child* 1978;53:375.

116. Walker-Smith J. Cow's milk protein intolerance: transient food intolerance of infancy. *Arch Dis Child* 1975;50:347.

117. Vanderhoof JA, Murray ND, Kaufman SS, et al. Intolerance to protein hydrolysate infant formulas, an under-recognized cause of gastrointestinal symptoms in infants. *J Pediatr* 1997;131:741.

118. Powell GK. Milk- and soy-induced enterocolitis of infancy. *J Pediatr* 1978;93:553.

119. Avery GB, Villavicencio O, Lilly JR, et al. Intractable diarrhea in early infancy. *Pediatrics* 1968;41:712.

120. Goldgar CM, Vanderhoof JA. Lack of correlation of small bowel biopsy and clinical course of patients with intractable diarrhea of infancy. *Gastroenterology* 1986;90:527.

121. Orenstein SR. Enteral versus parenteral therapy for intractable diarrhea of infancy: a prospective, randomized trial. *J Pediatr* 1986;109:277.

122. Schmitz J, Ginies JL, Arnaud-Battandier F, et al. Congenital microvillous atrophy, a rare cause of neonatal intractable diarrhoea. *Pediatr Res* 1982;16:1014.

123. Patey N, Scoazec JY, Cuenod-Jabri B, et al. Distribution of cell adhesion molecules in infants with intestinal epithelial dysplasia (tufting enteropathy). *Gastroenterology* 1997;113:833.

124. Girault D, Goulet O, L-Ldeist F, et al. Intractable infant diarrhea associated with phenotypic abnormalities and immunodeficiency. *J Pediatr* 1994;125:36.

125. Unsworth J, Hutchins P, Mitchell J, et al. Flat small intestinal mucosa and autoantibodies against the gut epithelium. *J Pediatr Gastroenterol Nutr* 1982;1:503.

126. Holcomb GW III, Gheissari A, O'Neill JA Jr, et al. Surgical management of alimentary tract duplications. *Ann Surg* 1989;209:167.

127. Martin LW, Torres Am. Hirschsprung's disease. *Surg Clin North Am* 1985;65:1171.

128. Bill AJ, Chapman ND. The enterocolitis of Hirschsprung's disease: its natural history and treatment. *Am J Surg* 1962;103:70.

129. Heikkinen M, Rintala R, Luukkonen P. Long-term anal sphincter performance after surgery for Hirschsprung's disease. *J Pediatr Surg* 1997;32:1443.

130. Granata C, Puri P. Megacystis-microcolon-intestinal hypoperistalsis syndrome. *J Pediatr Gastroenterol Nutr* 1997;25:12.

131. Durie PR, Forstner GG. Pathophysiology of the exocrine pancreas in cystic fibrosis. *J R Soc Med* 1989;18[Suppl 16]:2.

132. Adrian TE, McKiernan J, Johnstone DI, et al. Hormonal abnormalities of the pancreas and gut in cystic fibrosis. *Gastroenterology* 1980;79:460.

133. Aggett PJ, Cavanagh NPC, Matthew DJ, et al. Schwachman's syndrome. *Arch Dis Child* 1980;55:331.

134. Alagille D. Management of chronic cholestasis in childhood. *Semin Liver Dis* 1985;5:254.

135. Balistreri WF. Neonatal cholestasis. In: Lebenthal E, ed. *Textbook of gastroenterology and nutrition in infancy.* New York: Raven Press, 1981:1081.

136. Sokol RJ. Medical management of neonatal cholestasis. In: Balistreri WF, Stocker JT, eds. *Pediatric hepatology.* New York: Hemisphere Publishing, 1990:41.

137. Balistreri WF. Neonatal cholestasis: medical progress. *J Pediatr* 1985;106:171.

138. Balistreri WF. Neonatal cholestasis: lessons from the past, issues for the future. *Semin Liver Dis* 1987;7:61.

139. Morecki R, Glaser JH, Cho S, et al. Biliary atresia and reovirus type 3 infection. *N Engl J Med* 1982;307:481.

140. Morecki R, Glaser J. Reovirus 3 and neonatal biliary disease: discussion of divergent results. *Hepatology* 1989;10:515.

141. Maggiore G, Bernard O, Hadchouel M, et al. Diagnostic value of serum gamma-glutamyl transpeptidase activity in liver diseases in children. *J Pediatr Gastroenterol Nutr* 1991;12:21.

142. Faweya AG, Akinyinka OO, Sodeinde O. Duodenal intubation and aspiration test: utility in the differential diagnosis of infantile cholestasis. *J Pediatr Gastroenterol Nutr* 1991;13:290.

143. Rosenthal P, Miller JH, Sinatra FR. Hepatobiliary scintigraphy and the string test in the evaluation of neonatal cholestasis. *J Pediatr Gastroenterol Nutr* 1989;8:296.

144. Raffensperger JG. A long-term follow-up of three patients with biliary atresia. *J Pediatr Surg* 1991;26:176.

145. Alagille D, Odievre M, Gautier M, et al. Syndromic paucity of interlobular bile ducts (Alagille syndrome or arteriohepatic dysplasia): review of 80 cases. *J Pediatr* 1987;110:195.

146. Tajiri H, Nose O, Shimizu K, et al. Prevention of neonatal HBV infection with the combination of HBIG and HBV vaccine and its long-term efficacy in infants born to HBeAg positive HBV carrier mothers. *Acta Paediatr Jpn* 1989;31:663.

147. Hart MH, Kaufman SS, Vanderhoof JA, et al. Neonatal hepatitis and extrahepatic biliary atresia associated with cytomegalovirus infection in twins. *Am J Dis Child* 1991;145:302.

148. Povey S. Genetics of alpha-1-antitrypsin deficiency in relation to neonatal liver disease. *Mol Biol Med* 1990;7:161.

149. Pittschieler K. Liver disease and heterozygous alpha-1-antitrypsin deficiency. *Acta Paediatr Scand* 1991;80:323.

150. Egawa H, Berquist W, Garcia-Kennedy R, et al. Rapid development of hepatocellular siderosis after liver transplantation for neonatal hemochromatosis. *Transplantation* 1996;62):1511.

151. Barnard JA, Manci E. Idiopathic neonatal iron-storage disease. *Gastroenerology* 1991;101:1420.

152. Witzleben CL, Uri A. Perinatal hemochromatosis: entity or end result? *Hum Pathol* 1989;20:335.

153. Bell RL, Ferry GD, Smith EO, et al. Total parenteral nutrition-related cholestasis in infants. *J Parenter Enteral Nutr* 1986;10:356.

154. Merritt RJ. Cholestasis associated with total parenteral nutrition. *J Pediatr Gastroenterol Nutr* 1986;5:9.

155. Balistreri WF, Novak DA, Farrell MK. Bile acid metabolism, total parenteral nutrition, and cholestasis. In: Lebenthal E, ed. *Total parenteral nutrition:* indications, *utilization, complications and pathophysiological considerations.* New York: Raven Press, 1986:319.

156. Cohen C, Olsen MM. Pediatric total parenteral nutrition, liver histopathology. *Arch Pathol Lab Med* 1981;105:152.

157. Vanderhoof JA, Langnas AN, Pinch LW, et al. Short bowel syndrome: a review. *J Pediatr Gastroenterol Nutr* 1992;14:359.

CHAPTER 38

Jaundice

M. Jeffrey Maisels

Jaundice is the most common and one of the most vexing problems that can occur in the newborn. Although most jaundiced infants are otherwise perfectly healthy, they make us anxious because bilirubin is potentially toxic to the central nervous system and, if the serum bilirubin level is very high, kernicterus (bilirubin encephalopathy) can occur.

Jaundice occurs when the liver cannot clear a sufficient amount of bilirubin from the plasma. When the problem is excessive bilirubin formation or limited uptake and conjugation, unconjugated (i.e., indirect-reacting) bilirubin appears in the blood. When bilirubin glucuronide excretion is impaired (i.e., cholestasis), conjugated monoglucuronide and diglucuronide (i.e., direct-reacting) bilirubin accumulate in plasma and, because of their solubility, also appear in the urine. There is also a fourth bilirubin fraction (unconjugated, monoglucuronide, and diglucuronide are the first three) known as δ-bilirubin. This is formed nonenzymatically from conjugated bilirubin and reacts directly with the diazo reagent (1).

In most jaundiced neonates, only unconjugated bilirubin is found in the blood, and the accumulated bilirubin is distributed by the circulation throughout the body and produces clinical jaundice. It generally is assumed that, to cross intact cell membrane barriers, the bilirubin must be free, or dissociated, from its albumin binding.

FORMATION, STRUCTURE, AND PROPERTIES OF BILIRUBIN

Bilirubin is the end product of the catabolism of iron protoporphyrin or heme, of which the major source is circulating hemoglobin. The formation of bilirubin from hemoglobin involves removal of the iron and protein moieties, followed by an oxidative process catalyzed by the enzyme microsomal heme oxygenase, in which the α-

M. J. Maisels: Wayne State University School of Medicine, University of Michigan Medical Center; and Department of Pediatrics, William Beaumont Hospital, Royal Oak, Michigan

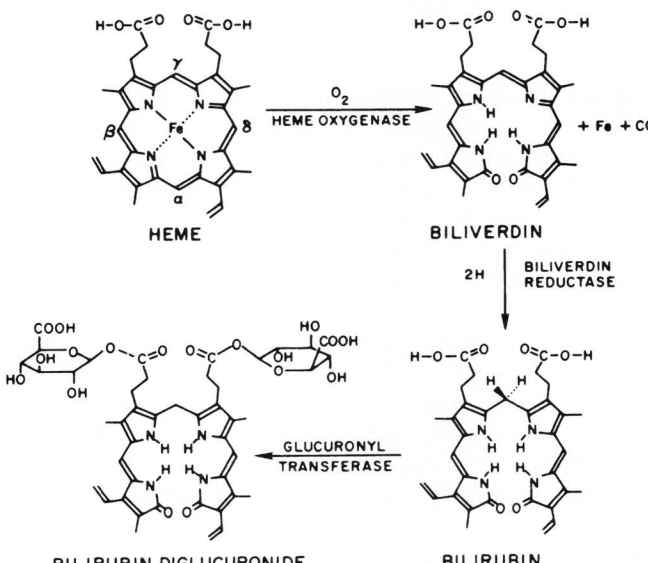

FIG. 38–1. Biosynthesis of bilirubin. (From Lightner DA, McDonagh AF. Molecular mechanisms of phototherapy of neonatal jaundice. *Accounts Chem Res* 1984;17:417.)

methane bridge of the heme porphyrin ring is opened and carbon monoxide and biliverdin are formed (Fig. 38–1).

A linear representation of bilirubin is shown in Fig. 38–2. Although conventionally illustrated as in Figs. 38–1 and 38–2, it is likely that the prevalent structure of bilirubin in plasma has the ridge–tile conformation shown in Fig. 38–3, because it is consistent with the bio-

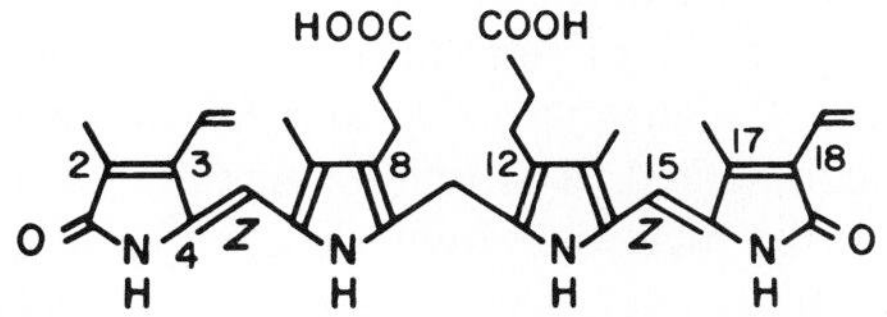

FIG. 38–2. The chemical structure of bilirubin. (From ref. 2.)

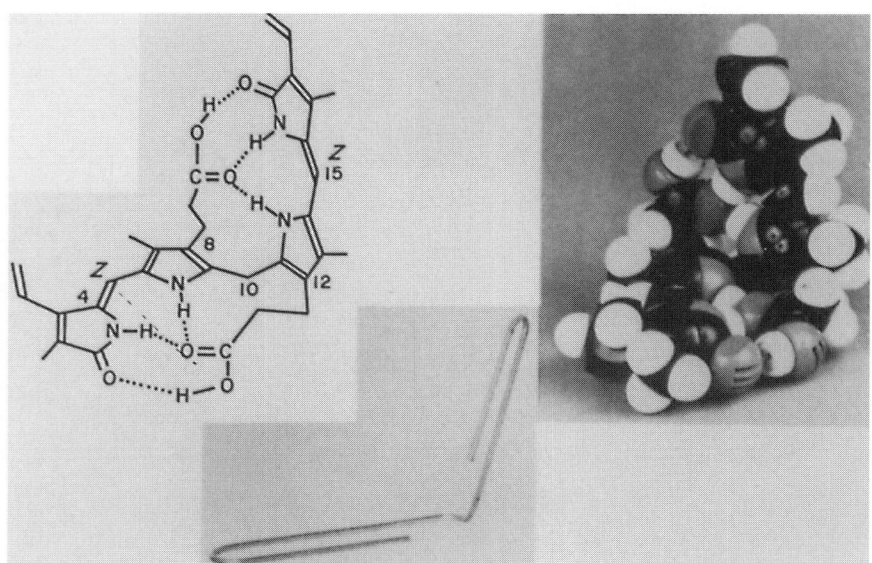

FIG. 38–3. Preferred conformation of bilirubin. Chemical structure **(left)**; bent paper clip analogy **(middle)**; space-filling molecular model **(right)**. Each representation is asymmetric and has a non-superimposable mirror image, like a D- or L-amino acid. Only one of the two possible mirror-image forms is shown in each representation. (From ref. 2.)

logical properties of bilirubin. In this conformation, the bilirubin molecule is stabilized by the presence of intramolecular hydrogen bonds, and the hydrophilic polar COOH and NH groups are not available for the attachment of water. The hydrophobic hydrocarbon groups are on the perimeter, rendering the molecule insoluble in water but soluble in nonpolar solvents, such as chloroform (2). Under these circumstances, bilirubin behaves like other lipophilic substances (e.g., dioxin, polychlorinated biphenyls)—it is difficult to excrete but crosses biological membranes, such as the placenta, blood–brain barrier, and hepatocyte plasma membrane, easily (2,3). The addition of methanol or ethanol interferes with hydrogen bonding and results in an immediate diazo reaction—the basis for measurement of indirect bilirubin by the van den Bergh reaction.

FETAL BILIRUBIN METABOLISM

Bilirubin can be detected in normal amniotic fluid after about 12 weeks of gestation, but it disappears by 36 to 37 weeks. The ability of human fetal liver to remove bilirubin from the circulation and to conjugate it is severely limited. Between 17 and 30 weeks of gestation, uridine diphosphoglucuronosyl transferase (UDPGT) activity in fetal liver is only 0.1% of adult values, but it increases tenfold to 1% of adult values between 30 and 40 weeks. After birth, activity increases exponentially, reaching adult levels by 6 to 14 weeks (Fig. 38–4). This increase is independent of gestation (4,5).

The major route of fetal bilirubin excretion is across the placenta. Because virtually all the fetal plasma bilirubin is unconjugated, it is readily transferred across the placenta to the maternal circulation, where it is excreted by the maternal liver. Thus, the newborn rarely is born jaundiced, except in the presence of severe hemolytic dis-

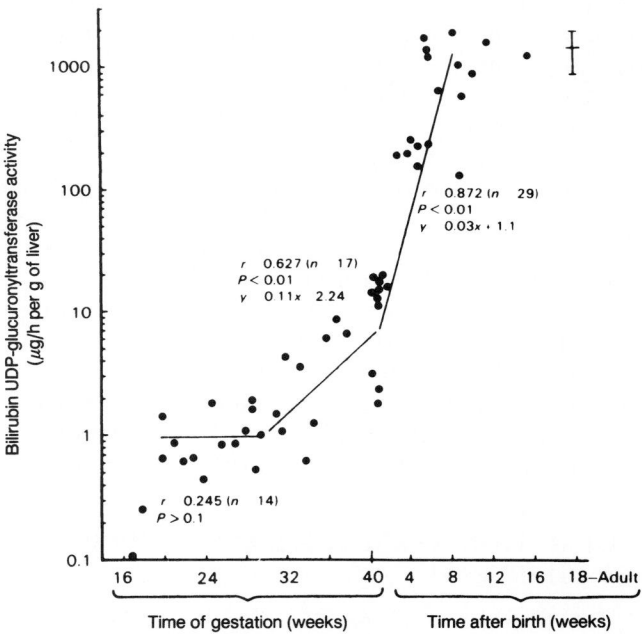

FIG. 38–4. Developmental pattern of human hepatic uridine diphosphoglucuronosyl transferase (UDPGT) activity. Samples were obtained from the livers of fetuses after elective abortions, at autopsy from premature and full-term newborns who survived less than 7 days, and from liver biopsies of infants, children, and adults undergoing laparotomy. Each point represents the activity of the liver homogenate of a single patient, but results for patients older than 18 weeks of age are shown as a mean ± SD. (From ref. 5.)

ease, when there may be accumulation of unconjugated bilirubin in the fetus. Conjugated bilirubin is not transferred across the placenta, and it also may accumulate in the fetal plasma and other tissues.

Maternal Hyperbilirubinemia and Its Effect on the Fetus

Obstetricians and pediatricians occasionally are confronted with a pregnant mother who has hyperbilirubinemia as a result of hemolytic anemia or liver disease. Reported cases in the literature provide evidence for transfer of unconjugated bilirubin from the mother to her fetus, but no clear guidelines for management (6–8).

It is possible that prolonged exposure of the fetus to a modest degree of unconjugated hyperbilirubinemia *in utero* could lead to neurologic damage (8).

NEONATAL BILIRUBIN METABOLISM

Bilirubin Production

The normal destruction of circulating erythrocytes accounts for about 75% of the daily bilirubin production in the newborn. Senescent erythrocytes are removed and destroyed in the reticuloendothelial system, where the hemoglobin is catabolized and converted to bilirubin. One gram of hemoglobin yields 35 mg of bilirubin.

A significant contribution (25% or more) to the daily production of bilirubin in the neonate comes from sources other than effete erythrocytes (Fig. 38–5). This bilirubin consists of two major components:

1. A nonerythropoietic component resulting from the turnover of nonhemoglobin heme protein and free heme, primarily in the liver.
2. An erythropoietic component arising primarily from ineffective erythropoiesis and the destruction of immature erythrocyte precursors, either in the bone marrow or soon after release into the circulation.

Transport and Hepatic Uptake of Bilirubin

Once bilirubin leaves the reticuloendothelial system, it is transported in the plasma and bound reversibly to albumin at a high-affinity primary binding site with a binding affinity of 10^7 to 10^8 M^{-1} (9). At pH 7.4, the solubility of bilirubin is very low (about 4 nm/L (0.24 mg/dL).

The parenchymal cells of the liver have a selective and highly efficient capacity for removing unconjugated bilirubin from the plasma. When the bilirubin–albumin complex reaches the plasma membrane of the hepatocyte, a proportion of the bilirubin, but not the albumin, is transferred across the cell membrane into the hepatocyte,

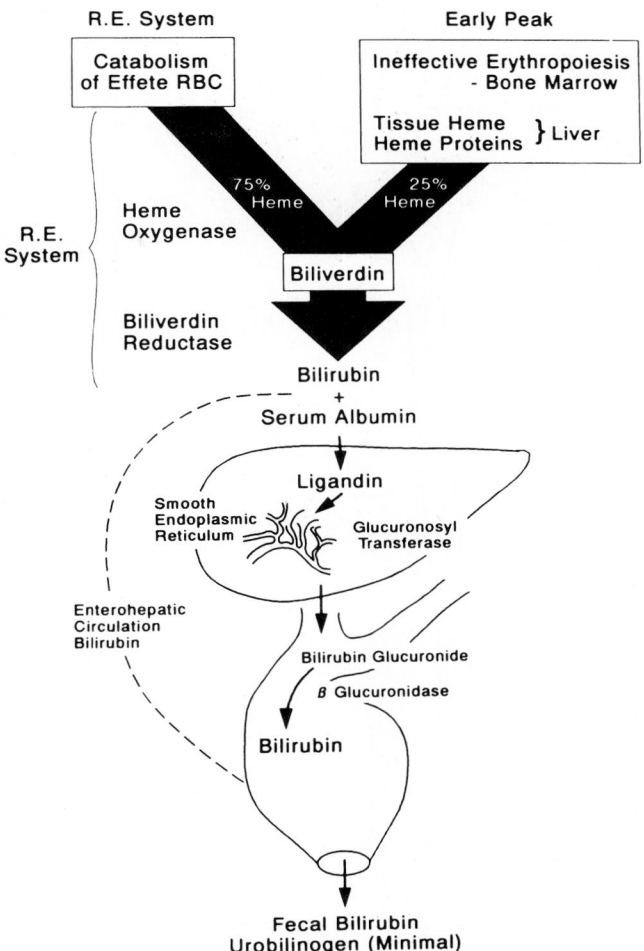

FIG. 38–5. Neonatal bile pigment metabolism. RBC, erythrocyte; R.E., reticuloendothelial.

where it is bound to ligandin and possibly other cytosolic-binding proteins (Fig. 38–6) (10).

Conjugation and Excretion of Bilirubin

Because of its hydrogen-bonded conformation (see section on Formation, Structure, and Properties of Bilirubin), unconjugated (i.e., indirect-reacting) bilirubin is nonpolar and insoluble in aqueous solutions at pH 7.4 and must be converted to its water-soluble conjugate (i.e., direct-reacting bilirubin) before it can be excreted (see Fig. 38–6). This is achieved when bilirubin is combined enzymatically with a sugar, glucuronic acid, producing bilirubin monoglucuronide and diglucuronide pigments that are more water soluble and sufficiently polar to be excreted into the bile or filtered through the kidney.

A single form of UDPGT (UDPGT1) accounts for almost all of the bilirubin glucuronidation in the human liver (11). This enzyme arises from the UDPGT1 gene

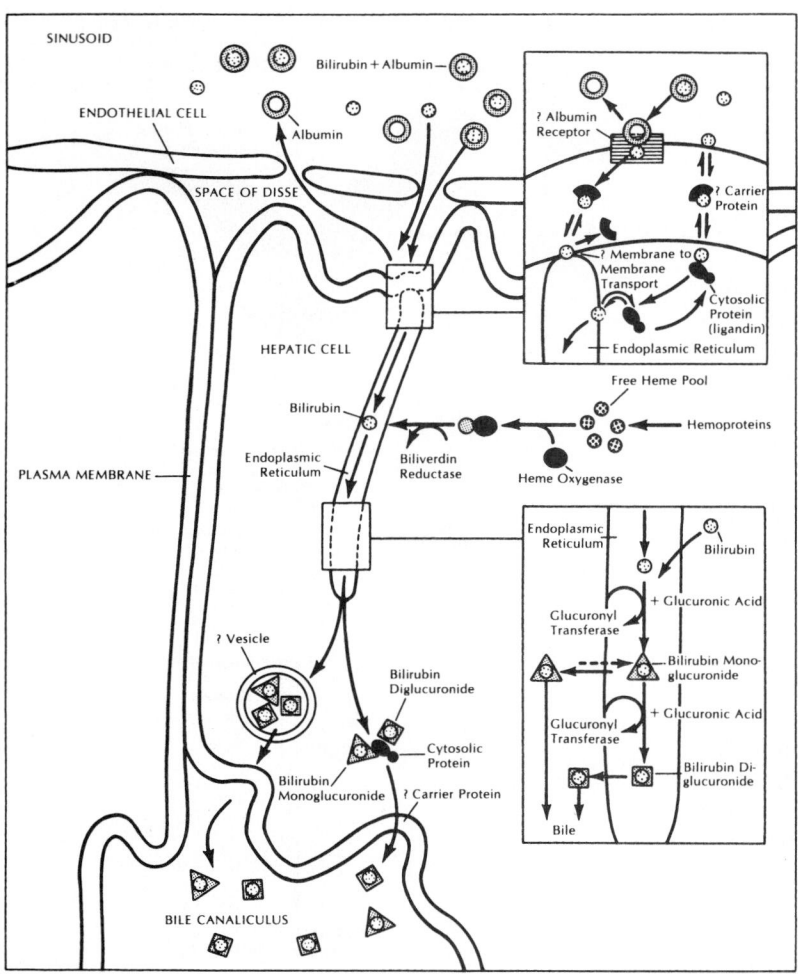

FIG. 38–6. Bilirubin transport and conjugation in the hepatocyte. Two mechanisms have been proposed for uptake of bilirubin from the extracellular environment: by means of an albumin receptor or directly. In either case, carrier protein may be involved in transmembrane passage **(upper box)**. Transport into the endoplasmic reticulum is facilitated by complexing to ligandin, but direct membrane-to-membrane transfer also may occur. Cytosolic bilirubin is in equilibrium with endoplasmic reticulum bilirubin. The hypothesis of conjugation of insoluble bilirubin to polar glucuronides **(lower box)**. Conjugated bilirubin may enter the bile canaliculi by either vesicular transport or carrier-mediated transport. (From Gollan JL, Knapp AB. Bilirubin metabolism and congenital jaundice. *Hosp Pract* 1985;February:87.)

complex whose transcription unit UDPGT1A1 encodes the UDPGT that conjugates bilirubin (12). In addition to the A1 exon, the UDPGT1 gene locus contains 12 variable exons (A2–A13) that encode other UDPGT isoforms and an exon 2–5 cluster that is common to all (i.e., constant domain) UDPGT isoforms. Bilirubin UDPGT belongs to a family of UDPGT isoenzymes that metabolize endogenous compounds and various food chemicals in most tissues. The nomenclature "glucuronosyl" is preferred to "glucuronyl," because the enzyme that glucuronidates bilirubin catalyzes the transfer of a glucuronosyl group (13).

The presence of elevated bilirubin concentrations *in utero* will prematurely induce bilirubin UDPGT activity, which suggests that bilirubin plays an important role in the initiation of its own conjugation after birth (14).

Transfer of Bilirubin into Bile and Intestinal Transport

After conjugation, bilirubin is excreted rapidly into the bile canaliculi by the liver cell, a process that requires metabolic work for the active transport of bilirubin across a large concentration gradient (see Fig. 38–6) (10). Interference with this process probably is responsible for the hyperbilirubinemia associated with hepatocellular disorders such as hepatitis.

Once in the small intestine, conjugated bilirubin is not reabsorbed. In the healthy adult, it is largely reduced by the action of colonic bacteria to a series of colorless tetrapyrroles, collectively known as urobilinogen, and an insignificant amount is hydrolyzed to unconjugated bilirubin and reabsorbed by way of the enterohepatic circulation. In the newborn, however, this enterohepatic circulation of bilirubin is significant and important (see section on Physiologic Jaundice). In conditions involving high plasma bilirubin levels and poor hepatic excretion, there is a gradient for unconjugated bilirubin from the plasma to the intestinal lumen, and significant amounts of unconjugated bilirubin may be cleared by diffusion across the intestinal wall. Figure 38–5 summarizes bile pigment metabolism in the newborn.

A recent review of the chemistry and metabolism of bilirubin can be found elsewhere (15).

PHYSIOLOGIC MECHANISMS OF NEONATAL JAUNDICE

Increased Bilirubin Load on the Liver Cell

Bilirubin Production

Measurements of carbon monoxide, which is produced in equimolar quantities with bilirubin, show that the normal newborn produces an average of 8 to 10 mg/kg (137 to 171 μmol/L) of bilirubin per day (16,17). This is more than twice the rate of normal daily bilirubin production in the adult and is explained by the fact that the neonate has a higher circulating erythrocyte volume, a shorter mean erythrocyte lifespan, and a larger early-labeled bilirubin peak. Bilirubin production decreases with increasing postnatal age but is still about twice the adult rate by age 2 weeks (16).

Enterohepatic Circulation

The newborn reabsorbs much larger quantities of unconjugated bilirubin, by way of the enterohepatic circulation, than does the adult. Infants have fewer bacteria in the small and large bowel and greater activity of the deconjugating enzyme β-glucuronidase (18). As a result, conjugated bilirubin, which is not reabsorbed, is not converted to urobilinogen but is hydrolyzed to unconjugated bilirubin, which is reabsorbed, thus increasing the bilirubin load on an already stressed liver. Studies in newborn humans and monkeys suggest that the enterohepatic circulation of bilirubin is a significant contributor to physiologic jaundice (19,20).

Decreased Clearance of Bilirubin from the Plasma

Uptake

Ligandin, the predominant bilirubin-binding protein in the human liver cell, is deficient in the liver of newborn monkeys. It reaches adult levels by 5 days of age, coinciding with a fall in bilirubin levels, and administration of phenobarbital increases the concentration of ligandin (21). Although this suggests that impaired uptake may contribute to the pathogenesis of physiologic jaundice, uptake does not appear to be rate limiting (22).

Conjugation

Deficient UDPGT activity, with resultant impairment of bilirubin conjugation, has long been considered a major cause of physiologic jaundice. In human infants, the early postnatal increase in serum bilirubin appears to play an important role in the initiation of bilirubin conjugation (14). In the first 10 days of life, UDPGT activity in full-term and premature neonates usually is less than 0.1% of adult values (see Fig. 38–4) (4,5). Thereafter, UDPGT activity increases at an exponential rate, reaching adult values by 6 to 14 weeks of age (5). The postnatal increase in UDPGT activity is independent of the infant's gestation.

Excretion

The absence of an elevated serum level of conjugated bilirubin in physiologic jaundice suggests that, under normal circumstances, the neonatal liver cell is capable of excreting the bilirubin that it has just conjugated. Nevertheless, the ability of the newborn liver to excrete conjugated bilirubin and other anions (e.g., drugs, hormones) is more limited than that of the older child or adult and may become rate limiting when the bilirubin load is significantly increased. Thus, when intrauterine hyperbilirubinemia occurs, usually as a result of isoimmunization, it is not uncommon to find an elevated serum level of conjugated bilirubin (14).

EPIDEMIOLOGY OF NEONATAL JAUNDICE

There is a wide range of factors that affect neonatal bilirubin levels (Table 38–1). Some of these factors have been identified only in large epidemiologic studies and their clinical relevance is questionable, but there are some (designated by footnotes in Table 38–1) that have been shown repeatedly to have an important influence on total serum bilirubin (TSB) levels.

Genetic, Ethnic, and Familial Influences

East Asian and Native American infants have mean maximal TSB concentrations that are significantly higher than those of Caucasian infants (23–25,26–28). Increased bilirubin production appears to be one factor contributing to the hyperbilirubinemia in these infants (28). Black infants in the United States and Great Britain have lower TSB levels than Caucasian infants (24,25,29). Neonatal jaundice runs in families (30,31). In a study of 3,301 infants, Khoury et al. (3) found that if a previous sibling had a TSB level higher than 12 mg/dL (205 μmol/L) or higher than 15 mg/dL (257 μmol/L), the risk of similar TSB levels in subsequent siblings was 3.1 and 12.5 times greater, respectively, than in siblings of infants who did not have that degree of jaundice.

Maternal Factors

Smoking

Some studies suggest that infants of mothers who smoke during pregnancy have lower serum bilirubin levels than infants of nonsmokers (24,32), but others have not found this (33,34). These data are confounded by the fact that women who smoke are much less likely to breast-feed, and the likelihood of breast-feeding is inversely related to the number of cigarettes smoked per day (35).

TABLE 38–1. *Epidemiology of neonatal jaundice*

| Associated factors | Effect on neonatal serum bilirubin levels | | |
	Increase	Decrease	No effect
Race	East Asian[a] Native American Greek	African American[a]	
Genetic or familial	Previous sibling with jaundice[a]		
Maternal	Primipara (?) Older mothers Diabetes[a] Hypertension Oral contraceptive use at time of conception First-trimester bleeding Decreased plasma zinc level	Smoking	
Drugs administered to mother	Oxytocin[a] Diazepam Epidural anesthesia Promethazine	Phenobarbital Meperidine Reserpine Aspirin Chloral hydrate Heroin Phenytoin Antipyrine Alcohol	Beta-adrenergic agents
Labor and delivery	Premature rupture of membranes Forceps delivery Vacuum extraction Breech delivery		Fetal distress Low Apgar scores
Infant	Low birth weight Decreasing gestation[a] Male gender[a] Delayed cord clamping Elevated cord blood bilirubin level Delayed meconium passage Breast-feeding[a] Caloric deprivation[a] Larger weight loss after birth[a] Low serum zinc and magnesium		
Drugs administered to infant	Chloral hydrate Pancuronium		
Other	Altitude Short hospital stay after birth[a]		

[a]Most common clinically important factors.

Diabetes

Macrosomic infants of insulin-dependent diabetic mothers are more likely to become jaundiced than control infants (36). This most likely is the result of an increase in bilirubin production, which is directly related to the degree of macrosomia in these infants (37). These infants have high erythropoietin levels and evidence of increased erythropoiesis, so that ineffective erythropoiesis and polycythemia probably are responsible for the increased bilirubin production (38,39). In addition, diabetic mothers have three times more β-glucuronidase in their breast milk than nondiabetic mothers (39). This enzyme enhances the enterohepatic reabsorption of bilirubin (see section on Breast-Feeding and Jaundice, below).

Events during Labor and Delivery

Induction and Augmentation of Labor by Oxytocin

Multiple studies and several controlled trials have shown an association between the use of oxytocin to induce or augment labor and an increased incidence of neonatal hyperbilirubinemia, although the mechanism for this is unclear (40,41).

Anesthesia and Analgesia

Epidural anesthesia, specifically, bupivacaine, has been associated with neonatal jaundice in several studies (34, 42,43).

Other Drugs

Tocolytics did not affect neonatal carboxyhemoglobin levels or the need for phototherapy (44,45).

The administration of narcotic agents, barbiturates, aspirin, chloral hydrate, reserpine, and phenytoin sodium to mothers was associated with lower TSB concentrations in their infants, whereas the use of diazepam increased TSB levels by less than 1 mg/dL (46). Antipyrine administered to the mother before delivery decreased TSB levels. and infants of heroin-addicted mothers have lower TSB levels (47). Phenobarbital, if given in sufficient doses to the mother, significantly lowers TSB levels during the first week (40,48).

Delivery Mode

Vaginally delivered term newborns had higher TSB levels than those delivered by cesarean section (49), although this was not found in a controlled trial involving low-birth-weight infants (50). When compared with forceps delivery, the use of vacuum extraction did not increase the number of babies who required phototherapy, although more clinical jaundice was seen with vacuum extraction (51,52).

Placental Transfusion and Hyperviscosity

Although a high hematocrit often is considered a risk factor for neonatal jaundice, controlled trials of an intervention for infants with symptomatic hyperviscosity using partial exchange transfusions showed no differences in the incidence of hyperbilirubinemia in the treated and control groups (53–55). In one study, infants were held 30 cm below the introitus after delivery. If cord clamping was delayed, the mean TSB level at age 72 hours was 7.7 mg/dL (132 µmol/L) compared with 3.2 mg/dL (55 µmol/L) in the early-clamped group (56).

Cord Blood Bilirubin Levels

More than 50 years ago, Davidson et al. (57) found an association between bilirubin levels in cord blood and later neonatal bilirubin concentrations. This observation has been confirmed in infants with and without hemolytic disease (58–60).

Neonatal Factors

Birth Weight and Gestation

Low birth weight and decreasing gestational age are strongly correlated with an increased risk of hyperbilirubinemia (24,34,43,61,62). Infants who are only slightly premature (less than 38 weeks) are at significantly greater risk of hyperbilirubinemia than full-term infants (34, 61,63). Compared with those at 40 weeks, infants of 36 to 38 weeks of gestation were seven to eight times, and those

less than 36 weeks were 13 times, more likely to be readmitted to the hospital with severe hyperbilirubinemia (61).

Gender

As a group, male infants consistently have higher bilirubin levels than females (34,43,61,64).

Caloric Intake and Weight Loss

Decreased caloric intake is associated with an increase in serum bilirubin in animals and humans (65). A significant association exists between hyperbilirubinemia and weight loss in the first few days after birth (34,43,61,64). The primary mechanism responsible for this appears to be an increase in the enterohepatic circulation of bilirubin (65,66).

Type of Diet

Infants fed a casein-hydrolysate formula had significantly lower TSB levels from days 10 through 18 than those fed standard casein or whey-predominant formulas (67). The cumulative stool output of the infants fed the casein-hydrolysate was lower than that of the infants fed the other formulas, suggesting that factors other than stool output and its effect on the enterohepatic circulation must explain these observations.

Breast-Feeding and Jaundice

Multiple studies over the last 25 years have found a strong association between breast-feeding and an increased incidence of neonatal hyperbilirubinemia. Although occasional studies have not found this (68), a pooled analysis of 12 studies in more than 8,000 newborns showed that breast-fed infants were three times more likely to develop TSB levels of 12 mg/dL (205 µmol) or higher and six times more likely to develop levels of 15 mg/dL (257 µmol) or higher than formula-fed infants (69). Ninety percent or more of infants readmitted to hospital in the first 2 weeks of life because of severe hyperbilirubinemia are fully or partially breast-fed (61, 63,70,71).

Jaundice associated with breast-feeding in the first 2 to 4 days of age has been called "the breast-feeding jaundice syndrome" or "breast-feeding associated jaundice" and that which appears later (at 4 to 7 days of age) has been called the "breast milk jaundice syndrome" (72). There is considerable overlap between these two entities, and evidence to support two distinct syndromes is meager. In addition to having higher TSB levels in the first 3 to 5 days (Fig. 38–7) (73), as a group, breast-fed infants have TSB levels that are higher than formula-fed infants for at least 3 to 6 weeks (67,74,75). These are the same infants who have high bilirubin levels in the first week of life,

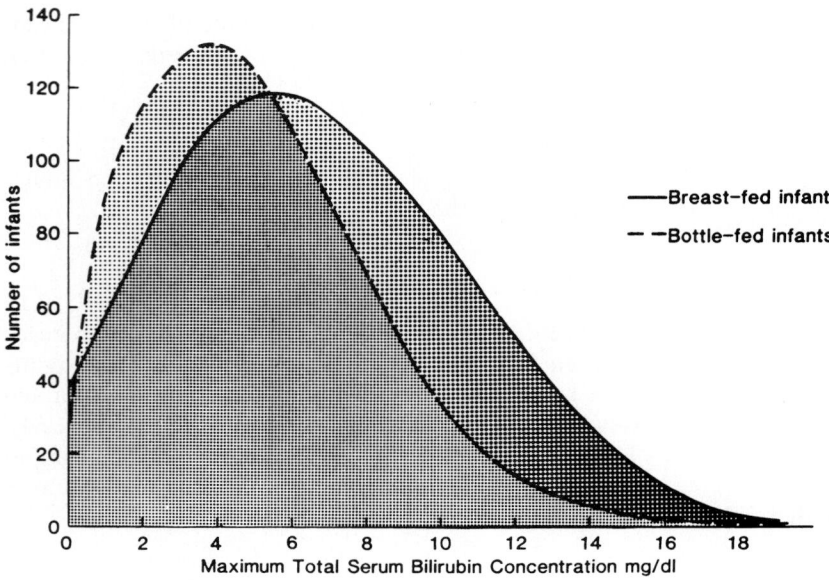

FIG. 38–7. Distribution of maximum serum bilirubin concentrations in Caucasian infants who weigh more than 2,500 g. (From ref. 73.)

and it is hard to believe that those who are still jaundiced at age 2 to 3 weeks represent a distinct group.

Prolonged indirect hyperbilirubinemia (beyond 2 to 3 weeks) occurs in 20% to 30% of all breast-feeding infants and, in some infants, may persist for up to 3 months (76). Factors that play a role in the pathophysiology of jaundice associated with breast-feeding have recently been reviewed in detail (18,72). Most studies suggest that the primary contributors to breast-feeding jaundice are a decreased caloric intake and an increase in the enterohepatic circulation of bilirubin. Some have suggested an additional role for inhibitory substances in breast milk, but the data regarding their contribution are conflicting (18,72).

Pathogenesis of Jaundice Associated with Breast-Feeding

Intestinal Reabsorption of Bilirubin. Intestinal reabsorption of bilirubin (the enterohepatic circulation) appears to be the most important mechanism responsible for the jaundice associated with breast feeding. Breast-fed infants produce lower-weight individual stools, their cumulative stool output is lower (67), and their stools contain less bilirubin than those of formula-fed infants (18,77). An increase in stool excretion in the first 21 days is associated with lower TSB levels and supports the importance of the enterohepatic circulation during this period (67). In the first 3 weeks, infants fed human milk pass significantly less stool than those fed casein-predominant formulas (67). Those infants fed casein-hydrolysate formulas pass less stool, cumulatively, than those given whey- or casein-predominant formulas (67).

Urobilinogen Formation. In adults, bilirubin in the gut is reduced rapidly by the action of colonic bacteria to urobilinogen. At birth, the fetal gut is sterile, and, although there is an increase in the bacterial content of the gut after delivery, the neonatal intestinal flora do not convert conjugated bilirubin to urobilin. This leaves bilirubin in the bowel and allows it to be deconjugated and thus available for reabsorption. Formula-fed infants excrete urobilin in their stools earlier than breast-fed infants, perhaps due to the effect of formula feeding on the intestinal flora (78). Thus, the effect of breast milk on intestinal flora, by slowing the formation of urobilin, further enhances the possibility of intestinal reabsorption of bilirubin.

Beta-Glucuronidase. Beta-glucuronidase is an enzyme that cleaves the ester linkage of bilirubin glucuronide, producing unconjugated bilirubin, which can then be reabsorbed through the gut. Significant concentrations of β-glucuronidase are found in the neonatal intestine, and its activity is higher in human milk than in infant formulas.

Gourley and Arend (79) found a positive relation between TSB levels and breast milk β-glucuronidase activity in the first 3 to 4 days after birth, but others have not been able to confirm these findings (76,80).

Meconium Passage

Because the enterohepatic circulation of bilirubin is an important contributor to neonatal hyperbilirubinemia, increasing the rate of bilirubin evacuation from the bowel should decrease the incidence of neonatal jaundice. Two randomized studies have shown that the early passage of meconium (stimulated by a rectal thermometer or a suppository) reduced peak TSB levels by about 1 mg/dL (17 μmol) when compared with control groups (81,82).

Phenolic Detergents

The use of phenolic detergents to disinfect incubators and other nursery surfaces was associated with an epidemic of neonatal hyperbilirubinemia in two hospitals (83,84). These detergents should not be used in the nursery.

Altitude

Infants born 3,100 m above sea level are four times more likely to have a bilirubin level above 12 mg/dL (205 μmol/L) than those born at sea level (85). Both short- and long-term exposure to high altitudes increases TSB levels in adults. The possible mechanisms for these observations include an increase in bilirubin load due to high hematocrits and impaired conjugation and excretion of bilirubin (86–88).

Drugs Administered to the Infant

The use of pancuronium and chloral hydrate in the neonate have been associated with an increased risk of hyperbilirubinemia (89–91). Chloral hydrate is metabolized to trichloroacetic acid and the toxic trichloroethanol, both of which accumulate in the tissues of compromised infants. The administration of chloral hydrate is associated with both indirect and direct hyperbilirubinemia (90).

Free-Radical Production

Bilirubin appears to have an important physiologic function as an antioxidant and may play a role in the prevention of oxidative membrane damage *in vivo* (see section on Physiologic Role of Bilirubin) (92). Infants with circulatory failure, sepsis, aspiration syndromes, and asphyxia—conditions believed to enhance free-radical production—had a significantly lower daily rise in mean TSB levels than control infants (93). These finding are consistent with the hypothesis that bilirubin is a free-radical scavenger and is consumed as an antioxidant. The role of bilirubin as an antioxidant is discussed later.

JAUNDICE IN THE HEALTHY NEWBORN

Normal Serum Bilirubin Levels and the Natural History of Neonatal Jaundice

Mean bilirubin levels in cord blood range from 1.4 to 1.9 mg/dL (24 to 32 μmol/L) (57,94,95), and elevated cord bilirubin levels are associated with an increased risk of hyperbilirubinemia (57,59,94,95).

Despite numerous studies, it has been difficult, if not impossible, to agree on what represents a "normal bilirubin level" in the term and near-term infant. The main reason for this is that TSB levels vary considerably, depending on the racial composition of the population, the

incidence of breast-feeding, and other genetic and epidemiologic factors (Fig. 38–8). An additional important factor is the large variation found in the laboratory measurements of serum bilirubin, a problem that has been recognized for 4 decades and shows no signs of resolution (see section on Laboratory Measurements of Bilirubin) (96,97).

Reference to Figure 38–8 gives some idea of the range of mean bilirubin values found in different populations and the natural history of neonatal jaundice. Figure 38–8 also illustrates that the studies of breast-fed populations that are restricted to hospitalized infants (unless the length of stay after birth is 5 to 7 days) are misleading, because they will miss the peak TSB levels in large portions of the population. On the other hand, since the advent of phototherapy about 30 years ago, it has been almost impossible to obtain a true picture of the natural history of neonatal jaundice. This is because some infants with higher TSB levels receive phototherapy in the first 72 to 96 hours so that what we see is a "damped" picture of neonatal hyperbilirubinemia. Recognizing these limitations, however, some recent studies have helped to clarify the picture.

An important change in the population in the United States has been a doubling in the incidence of breast-

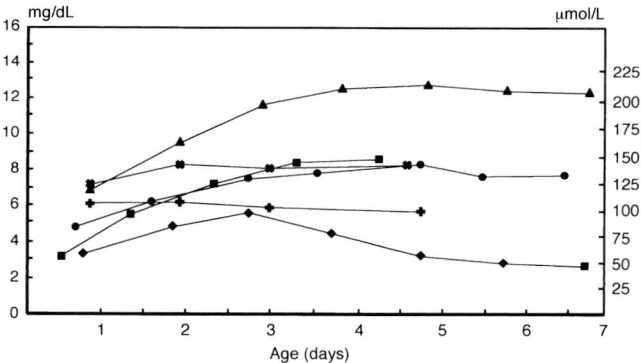

FIG. 38–8. Mean total daily bilirubin concentrations in normal full term and near-term infants. ▲, Fifty healthy Japanese newborn infants, 37 to 42 weeks of gestation, all breast-fed. Excludes Rh and ABO incompatibility. (Data from Yamauchi Y, Yamanouchi I. Transcutaneous bilirubinometry in normal Japanese infants. *Acta Paediatr Jpn* 1989;31:65.) ×, One hundred seventy-six term breast-fed Canadian infants. Excludes Rh hemolytic disease, but includes nine ABO incompatible infants with positive Coombs tests. Seventeen infants received phototherapy. +, One hundred sixty-four Canadian term formula-fed infants, seven ABO incompatible with positive Coombs tests, and three received phototherapy. (Data from ref. 94.) ■, One thousand eighty-seven term Israeli infants, 78% fully or partially breast-fed. (Data from D. Seidman, *personal communication*, 1998). •, Fifty-six Nigerian term AGA infants. Excludes ABO or Rh incompatibility and G6PD deficiency. Infants were "largely breast-fed." (Data from ref. 102.) (◆), Twenty-nine full-term American infants, all formula-fed, about 50% African-American and 50% Caucasian. (Data from ref. 19.)

feeding, from 30% in the 1960s to 60% or more today (98). In some hospitals, 85% or more of mothers are nursing their infants on discharge from the hospital. Data from the National Collaborative Perinatal Project (CPP) conducted from 1955 to 1961 (when 30% or fewer mothers breast-fed their infants) and more recent studies (73) found that about 95% of all infants had a TSB concentration that did not exceed 12.9 mg/dL (215 μmol/L), and this (95th percentile) became the accepted upper limit of "physiologic jaundice" (29).

More recent data suggest that these values no longer define normal TSB levels in the newborn population (62,99–101). We now see more jaundiced babies, and the TSB levels found in the normal population are significantly higher than previously reported. Three recent studies provide consistent information regarding the upper limits of TSB levels found in the normal population. In a study of 2,840 infants, all of whom had at least one TSB level measured after discharge from hospital, the 95th percentile was a level of 17.5 mg/dL (300 μmol/L) (100). This population was 43% white, 41% black, and 4% Asian; 59% of infants were fully or partially breast-fed. In 11 Kaiser Permanente Northern California Hospitals, the 95th percentile was a TSB level of 17.4 mg/dL (298 μmol/L) (62). In an ongoing multicenter study of infants 36 weeks or older in nurseries in the United States, Hong Kong, Japan, and Israel, 2 standard deviations above the mean for the peak TSB levels at 96 ± 6.5 hours was 17 mg/dL (291 μmol/L), and the 95th percentile was 15.5 mg/dL (265 μmol/L) (101). The consistency of these data suggests that we can now accept that the upper limit of "normal" in diverse populations is a TSB level of about 17 to 18 mg/dL (291 to 308 μmol/L). This implies that a 6-day-old breast-fed infant whose TSB level is 15 to 16 mg/dL (291 μmol/L) does not require any laboratory investigation to find out *why* the infant is jaundiced, although follow-up is necessary to ensure that the bilirubin levels do not become excessive (100). Data from studies of predominantly breast-fed infants suggest that the normal mean peak TSB level is approximately 8 to 9 mg/dL (137 to 154 μmol/L) (43,94,101–103). In the Natus multicenter study, the mean TSB level at 96 ± 6.5 hours was 9.3 mg/dL (101).

In the Japanese population and in other populations of predominantly breast-fed infants, it is clear that the TSB levels are substantially higher, reach their peak later, and remain elevated for much longer than in formula-fed infants. No significant decline in TSB is seen in any of these populations until after the fifth day (see Fig. 38–8).

Figure 38–9 shows "idealized" smoothed curves based on the data from a number of studies that provide a guide to the expected course of bilirubin levels in a primarily breast-fed (60% to 70%) western population (43,57,62, 64,94,100,101,103). Recognizing all of the limitations to these data already discussed, Fig. 38–9 should be useful

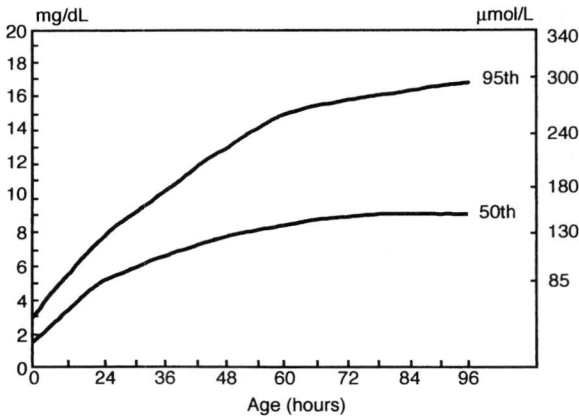

FIG. 38–9. Smoothed curves from studies in diverse populations illustrating the expected velocity of total serum bilirubin (TSB) levels and approximate values for the 50th and 95th percentiles. Data for cord blood values come from the studies of Davidson et al. (57) and Saigal et al. (94), values in the first 12 hours are from Frishberg et al. (64), and subsequent values from Bhutani et al. (100), Seidman (103), Natus Medical Inc. (101), and Wood et al. (43). Data for the 95th percentile are primarily obtained from the data of Bhutani et al. (100), but also from the studies of Newman et al. (62) and Natus Medical Inc. (101). These data represent values that might be expected in a western, predominantly breast-fed (60% to 70%) population. In view of the significant variations in different populations (see Fig. 38–8) as well as the variations found in laboratory measurement (97), the values provided should be used only as rough guidelines. Nevertheless, this graph can be useful in plotting the course of neonatal jaundice, because it will demonstrate when the velocity of the TSB increase deviates significantly from the curves shown. *Note that the values must be plotted according to the infant's age in hours, not days.* Infants who have values that exceed the 95th percentile deserve an evaluation to determine a potential cause for the jaundice, and they require careful surveillance and follow-up to prevent the development of extreme hyperbilirubinemia. Infants who have none of the epidemiologic risk factors for hyperbilirubinemia (see Table 38–9) but have TSB values that approach the upper percentiles also should receive closer scrutiny. On the other hand, those whose values fall well below the 50th percentile probably require minimal surveillance and follow-up for jaundice (100).

for plotting the course of jaundice in an infant and using the velocity of the increase in TSB to make decisions about evaluation, follow-up, and potential intervention.

Physiologic Jaundice

Because at some point during the first week of life almost every newborn has a TSB level that exceeds 1 mg/dL (17 μmol/L, the upper limit of normal for an adult), and about two-thirds or more will appear clinically jaundiced, this type of transient hyperbilirubinemia has been called "physiologic jaundice." This jaundice results from the interaction of a number of factors (Table 38–2). The term physiologic jaundice generally is applied to

TABLE 38–2. *Possible mechanisms involved in physiologic jaundice*

Increased bilirubin load on liver cell
  Increased erythrocyte volume
  Decreased erythrocyte survival
  Increased early-labeled bilirubin
  Increased enterohepatic circulation of bilirubin
Defective hepatic uptake of bilirubin from plasma
  Decreased ligandin
  Binding of Y and Z proteins by other anions
  Decreased relative hepatic uptake deficiency, phase II
Defective bilirubin conjugation
  Decreased uridine diphosphoglucuronosyl transferase activity
  Increased uridine diphosphoglucose dehydrogenase activity
Defective bilirubin excretion
  Excretion impaired but not rate limiting

newborns whose TSB level falls within the normal range. As discussed previously, however, because of the significant differences in TSB levels in different populations, it can be difficult to define what is normal or abnormal, physiologic or nonphysiologic. Second, defining the term "normal" is, in itself, a difficult task, and the definition of the term normal varies depending on whether one chooses a diagnostic, risk factor, or therapeutic definition of the term (104). A *diagnostic* definition of normal implies that if a result falls outside of a defined range, then there is a known probability of a specific disease being present. For neonatal hyperbilirubinemia, this definition does not work very well. We know that in infants who are readmitted to hospital with TSB levels of 18 to 20 mg/dL (308 to 340 µmol/L), the likelihood of finding a specific etiology is very small (less than 5%) (61,71). Hour-specific TSB levels, however, can be very informative. A TSB level of 10 mg/dL (171 µmol/L) at age 12 hours almost certainly is due to a hemolytic process, even if the precise cause of the increased bilirubin production is not yet known.

Normal also can be defined using the *risk factor approach*, which is based on the relationship of bilirubin levels in the newborn to the development of subsequent cognitive and neurologic abnormalities. Unfortunately, we have been unable, so far, to associate a specific risk of damage with a particular bilirubin level. Perhaps the most useful definition of normal levels or "physiologic" hyperbilirubinemia is the *therapeutic* definition. Here the normal range defines a bilirubin level beyond which a specific therapy will *likely do more good than harm.* Although the ranges are only approximate, the recommendations contained in the American Academy of Pediatrics (AAP) guidelines for the use of phototherapy in term newborns are examples of the application of this principle (see section on Treatment) (105). For example, the AAP recommends using phototherapy in any infant whose TSB level reaches 15 mg/dL (257 µmol/L)

between 25 and 48 hours of life. Although a level of 15 mg/dL (257 µmol/L) poses no imminent threat to the infant's well-being, *at that age* it is well above the 95th percentile (see Fig. 38–9) (100), is most likely due to an increase in bilirubin production, and, if untreated, might increase to a level that is dangerous to the infant. The suggested intervention, phototherapy, is safe and effective and, under these circumstances, is much more likely to do good than harm. Thus, with the exception of an early or rapidly rising bilirubin level that suggests hemolysis, the *diagnostic* definition of normal for indirect hyperbilirubinemia (or so-called physiologic jaundice) is of very limited value. The *risk factor* definition may have some utility, and the *therapeutic* definition is probably the most useful.

In premature newborns, the term physiologic jaundice is of little value. If untreated, low-birth-weight infants have exaggerated and prolonged hyperbilirubinemia. Although this may be considered "physiologic" because it occurs in all preterm infants, in very-low-birth-weight infants, TSB levels well within the "physiologic range" are considered potentially hazardous and are treated with phototherapy. Thus, the natural history of hyperbilirubinemia in the very-low-birth-weight infant is never observed, and defining certain bilirubin levels as "physiologic" in this population is misleading and potentially dangerous. Using a diagnostic definition of normal, a TSB level of 10 mg/dL (171 µmol/L) on day 4 in a 750-g neonate would be considered completely "physiologic," and no investigation need be done to identify a cause for this jaundice. Nevertheless, almost all neonatologists would *treat* this infant with phototherapy, implying that this value exceeds the therapeutic definition of normal and that treatment is much more likely to do good than harm. In neonatal intensive care units (NICUs) today, the term "physiologic" jaundice has no meaning and no utility and should be abandoned.

Jaundice may result from an increased load of bilirubin on the liver cell, including that contributed by the enterohepatic circulation, and a decrease in the ability of the liver to clear the bilirubin from the plasma as a result of defective uptake, conjugation, or excretion, singly or in any combination (see Table 38–2).

THE APPROACH TO A JAUNDICED INFANT

In October 1994 the Provisional Committee for Quality Improvement and Sub-Committee on Hyperbilirubinemia of the American Academy of Pediatrics published a "practice parameter" and developed an algorithm dealing with the evaluation and treatment of hyperbilirubinemia in the healthy term newborn (Fig. 38–10) (105). Additional guidelines for evaluation and follow-up of jaundiced newborns can be found in Tables 38–3 and 38–4 and Fig. 38–11.

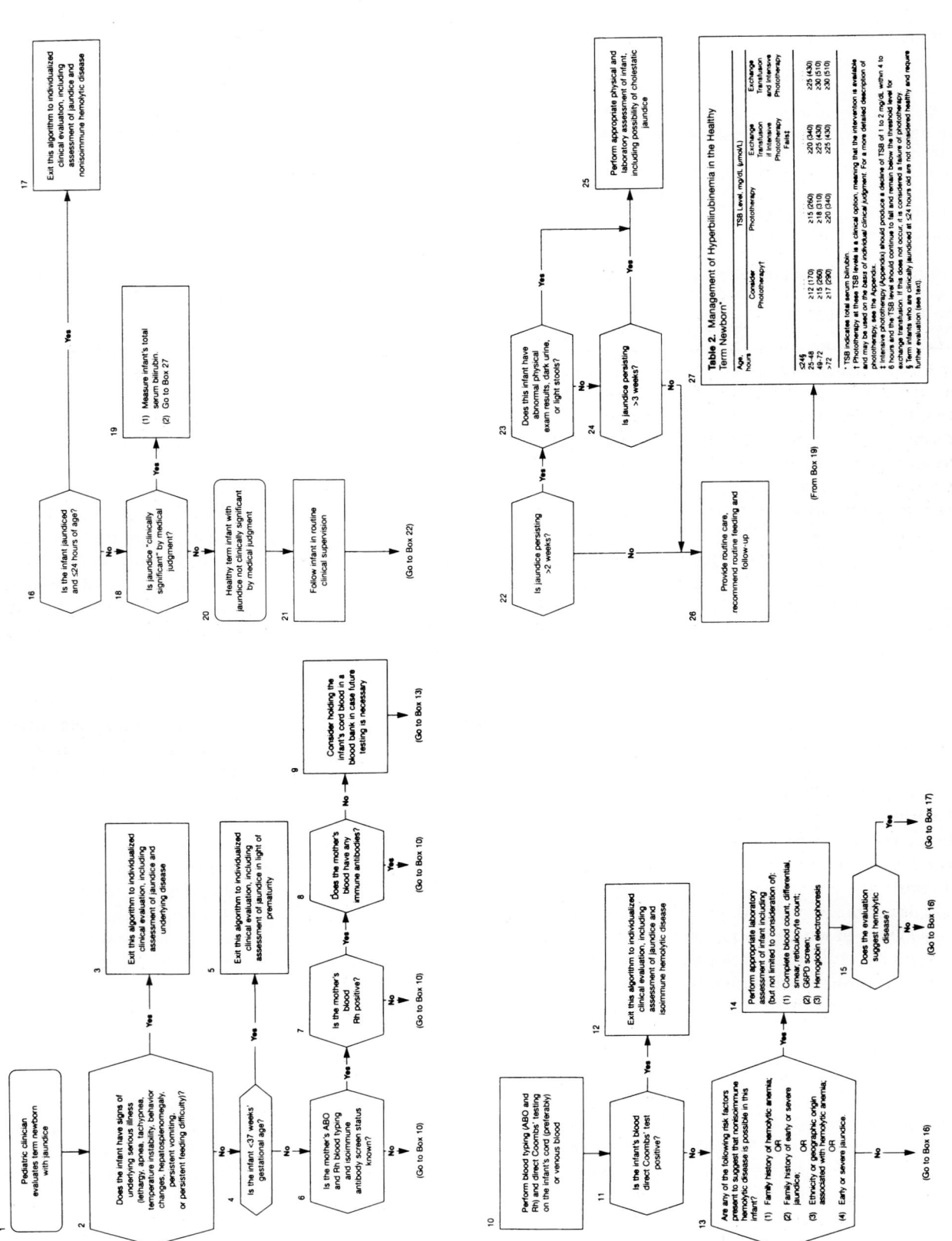

FIG. 38–10. Algorithm. Management in the healthy term infant.

TABLE 38–3. *Guidelines for initial evaluation and follow-up of jaundice in apparently healthy term and near term infants*[a]

Clinical observation	Initial actions	Other evaluations	Follow-up
Onset of jaundice in first 24 h[b]	Clinical evaluation[c] Measure TSB and TcB[d]	Blood group (ABO, Rh) Direct Coombs Test CBC, smear for red cell morphology, reticulocyte count[f]	Repeat TSB in 4–24 h[e]
Onset of jaundice 24–72 h	Clinical evaluation Assess cephalocaudal distribution[g] TcB	TSB if indicated by TcB or clinical evaluation	Clinical evaluation and/or TcB or TSB within 24–72 h and repeat as necessary

[a]These guidelines apply to the evaluation and follow-up of the majority of jaundiced newborns who are cared for in well-baby nurseries and are ≥35 wks of gestation. They cannot take into account all possible situations. The term "apparently healthy" refers to an infant who has no clinical signs suggesting the possibility of other diseases such as respiratory distress, poor feeding, lethargy, temperature instability, etc.

[b]Twenty-four hours is a long time in the life of a newborn infant. Jaundice at age 4 h is essentially always due to a hemolytic process, whereas jaundice at age 23 h may be normal.

[c]Clinical evaluation refers to a review of the obstetric history, events of labor and delivery, and physical examination of the newborn, which should include an evaluation for cephalhematomas, bruising, and hepatosplenomegaly.

[d]In some nurseries, a TcB measurement (using the Minolta/Air Shields Jaundice Meter) is used as a screening device and a decision to measure the TSB is based on the TcB level. If a TSB is done, the simultaneous measurement of a TcB allows subsequent TcB measurements to be used to follow the baby and to determine the necessity for additional bilirubin measurements. Recently developed TcB devices could largely replace TSB measurements.

[e]The frequency of obtaining repeated TSB measurements depends on the initial TSB level and the age at which it occurred. A TSB of 5 mg/dL at age 4 h must be repeated within 4 h, whereas the same level at 23 h could be repeated in 12–24 h.

[f]These investigations lack sensitivity and specificity, but may be helpful in confirming the diagnosis of ABO hemolytic disease or other rarer courses of hemolysis.

[g]Jaundice is first seen in the face. As the TSB increases, jaundice appears in the trunk, abdomen, and extremities.

TSB, total serum bilirubin; TcB, transcutaneous bilirubin.

TABLE 38–4. *Additional laboratory evaluation of the jaundiced term and near-term infant*

Indications	Maneuvers
Suspicion of hemolytic disease or anemia (e.g., pallor, early jaundice or TSB > 8 mg/dL [137 μmol/L] by 24 h or >13 mg/dL [222 μmol/L] by 48 h of life)	Blood type, group, and Coombs test, if not obtained with cord blood Complete blood count and smear Reticulocyte count
Either or both parents (or grandparents) of East Asian, Mediterranean, or Nigerian descent with TSB >15/dL (257 μmol/L). Any infant with late-onset jaundice or TSB ≥18 mg/dL (308 μmol/L)	Measure glucose-6-phosphate dehydrogenase
Jaundice beyond 3 wk of age	Direct bilirubin level, urine dipstick for bilirubin, inspect stools for color Check results of newborn thyroid screen, and evaluate infant for signs or symptoms of hypothyroidism
Infant ill	Direct bilirubin level, check urine for reducing substances, check results of newborn screen for galactosemia and other inborn errors, and evaluate for sepsis

TSB, total serum bilirubin concentration.

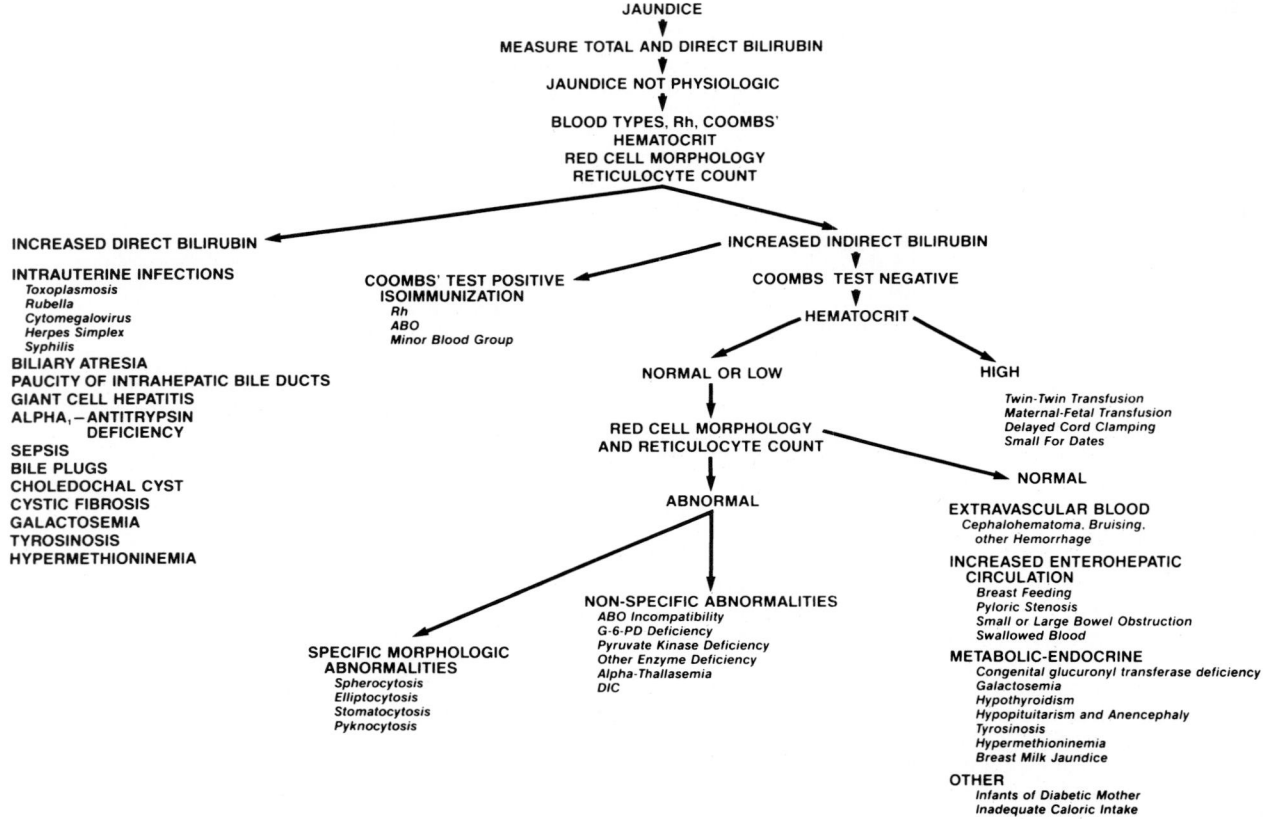

FIG. 38–11. Diagnostic approach to neonatal jaundice.

Clinical Evaluation

Identifying Clinically Significant Jaundice

The AAP algorithm (see Fig. 38–10) begins with the evaluation of a "term newborn with jaundice" and subsequently recommends measurement of the infant's TSB level if the jaundice appears to be "clinically significant" by medical judgment. The problem with this recommendation is that the ability of clinicians to diagnose "clinically significant" jaundice varies widely (57,106–108). Some studies suggest that the ability of physicians and nurses to estimate serum bilirubin levels clinically is no better than guesswork (108), whereas others have shown that newborns whose TSB levels exceed 12 mg/dL (205 μmol/L) will, at least, always be identified as "jaundiced" (57,106). Noninvasive (transcutaneous) devices for estimating serum bilirubin provide substantially greater accuracy than visual assessment (see section on Noninvasive Measurements of Bilirubin).

The Cephalocaudal Progression of Jaundice

In newborns, jaundice is detected by blanching the skin with digital pressure, thus revealing the underlying color of the skin and subcutaneous tissue. This dermal icterus is seen first in the face and then progresses in a cordad man-

ner to the trunk and extremities so that, for a given bilirubin level, the skin of the face will appear more yellow than that of the foot. First observed more than 100 years ago and confirmed by several investigators using visual observation as well as transcutaneous bilirubinometry, the cephalocaudal progression of dermal icterus is a useful clinical tool but probably is unreliable once the bilirubin level exceeds 12 mg/dL (205 μmol/L) (106,107,109–114).

Knudsen suggests that the cephalocaudal color difference in newborns is best explained by conformational change in the bilirubin–albumin complex (113). Following its formation, bilirubin is bound tightly to albumin, and the initial binding process is extremely rapid (within 10 ms). This is followed by a train of slow, relaxing changes in the conformation of the bilirubin–albumin complex commencing within 1 to 30 seconds, final conformation being reached 8 minutes after the initial binding (115). This time course suggests that, initially, there is a lower bilirubin-binding affinity to albumin (until the final stage of conformation has occurred) and thus less effective bilirubin–albumin binding in the blood immediately after it has left the reticuloendothelial system. The affinity increases after the blood reaches the distal portions of the body and the conformational changes in the bilirubin–albumin complex are completed. Knudsen suggests that some of the yellow color of the skin is the result of precipitated bilirubin acid and, in the presence of reduced bilirubin-binding affinity to albumin, there is an increased precipitation of bilirubin acid and thus an increase in the yellow color of the skin (113). This is more likely to occur in the proximal parts of the body because of the conformational changes in the young bilirubin–albumin complexes. Consistent with this hypothesis, Knudsen (113) found that there was a significant and linear correlation among the cephalocaudal color difference, the plasma bilirubin concentration, and the square of the hydrogen ion concentration. The cephalocaudal color difference was inversely related to the reserve albumin concentration, thus suggesting that the conformational change in the young bilirubin–albumin complex enhances the precipitation of bilirubin acid in the skin of the proximal parts of the body. If this is the mechanism, then objective measurement of the yellow color of the skin using transcutaneous bilirubinometry could be a better predictor of potential bilirubin encephalopathy than a serum bilirubin measurement.

Noninvasive Measurements of Bilirubin

The Ingram Icterometer (Cascade Healthcare Products, Salem, OR) is a piece of transparent plastic on which are painted five transverse strips of graded yellow hue. The instrument is pressed against the nose, the yellow color of the blanched skin is matched with the appropriate yellow stripe, and a jaundice score is assessed. This device is simple and inexpensive, and it is remarkable that, as a screening tool, it performs as effectively as the sophisticated (and much more expensive) Minolta Air Shields Jaundice Meter (116,117). The Minolta Air Shields Jaundice Meter is a hand-held rechargeable instrument. When pressure is applied to the photoprobe, a strobe light is generated by a xenon tube and passes through a fiberoptic element, penetrating the blanched skin and entering the subcutaneous tissue. The reflected light returns through a second fiberoptic bundle to the spectrophotometric module, where the intensity of the yellow color, corrected for hemoglobin, is measured and displayed as arbitrary units—the transcutaneous bilirubin index (TcB) index.

Schumacher et al. (116) and Schumacher (117) reviewed the accuracy and utility of these instruments. Readings with the Minolta Air Shields Jaundice Meter are highly reproducible and related in a linear fashion to the TSB concentration. Although these measurements are affected by the infant's race, gestational age, and birth weight (which limits the use of the jaundice meter in heterogeneous populations), when used in selected groups, the jaundice meter has performed well as a screening device (116–118). At William Beaumont Hospital, the routine use of a Minolta Air Shields Jaundice Meter in our nursery produced a 36% reduction in the number of serum bilirubin measurements obtained and, in a hospital delivering 5,000 infants annually, is estimated to save approximately $1,600 per year (118).

Because of the difficulty in using this instrument in heterogeneous populations and because it has been necessary to relate the TcB measurements to the laboratory measurements in individual hospitals, this instrument has not found widespread acceptance in the United States.

Newer devices could overcome many of these disadvantages. The Colormate III (Chromatics Color Sciences International, Inc., New York, NY) is also a hand-held colorimeter with a xenon flash tube and light sensors that are connected to a portable computer (107). The instrument measures over a band of wavelengths from 400 to 700 nm, with specific filters used to assess the reflectance of light for specific wavelengths. The algorithm incorporated into the device has been designed to examine the luminosity of the skin and incorporate the underlying color of normal skin and can account for that in the baseline evaluation. Thus, changes in the yellow component of the spectrum are observed separately and are used as a bilirubin estimate. In a study of 900 infants who had laboratory bilirubin determinations, there was a very good correlation between transcutaneous bilirubin and TSB concentrations ($r = 0.956$) (107). These measurements were made in a mixed population of white, African-American, Hispanic, and Asian infants. The study also included 53 infants weighing less than 2,000 g and 11 weighing less than 1,500 g. In addition, the instrument was tested on 61 infants who required phototherapy.

The results show that, in most circumstances, transcutaneous measurements with this type of instrument could well replace serum bilirubin determinations. This particular device has a sophisticated computer algorithm that assesses underlying skin color and permits evaluation of the yellow color regardless of the underlying skin pigmentation or degree of erythema. The accuracy of the device is improved by measurement of the underlying skin color before the onset of visual jaundice. The ability of this instrument to reflect serum bilirubin levels, even in infants undergoing phototherapy, is remarkable and suggests that it is measuring yellow color below the superficial layers of the skin and epidermis. If these results can be confirmed, the use of this and other recently developed transcutaneous instruments could prove of enormous benefit to infants and health care workers by obviating the need for serum bilirubin determinations in most circumstances. Finally, because the major concern regarding bilirubin toxicity is the amount of bilirubin in the tissue rather than the blood, the use of transcutaneous bilirubinometry ultimately may prove to be a better predictor of the potential for brain damage than serum bilirubin concentrations (114).

Laboratory Evaluation—Seeking a Cause for the Jaundice

Tables 38–3 and 38–4 and Figs. 38–10 and 38–11 provide an approach to the clinical and laboratory evaluation of the jaundiced newborn. For many years, standard texts have recommended a battery of tests for any infant whose TSB level exceeds 12 to 13 mg/dL (205 to 222 μmol) at any time, because of a belief that such levels represent potentially "pathologic" jaundice. But, as mentioned previously, not only are there significant differences in TSB levels in different populations, but recent data show that the upper limit of normal in diverse, largely breast-fed populations is a bilirubin level of about 17 to 18 mg/dL (290 to 308 μmol). Furthermore, the usual laboratory tests used (hematocrit, complete blood count, reticulocyte count, smear) are neither specific nor sensitive and rarely identify a cause for the hyperbilirubinemia (25,73). Even in infants who are readmitted to hospital in the first 2 weeks of life with clearly abnormal bilirubin levels of 18 to 20 mg/dL (308 to 340 μmol) or higher, these investigations usually are unrewarding (61,71). As can be seen in Table 38–5, in about 95% of term or near-term very jaundiced newborns, no pathologic cause of jaundice can be identified. Perhaps the ability to measure end-tidal carbon monoxide concentrations in these infants will identify some who are producing large quantities of bilirubin even though they have no obvious cause for hemolysis (119).

It makes no sense to attempt to interpret bilirubin levels without considering the infant's precise age in hours (see Fig. 38–9) (100,120) and the major epidemiologic factors that affect TSB levels (see Table 38–1 and section on An Approach to Preventing Kernicterus). Figure 38–8 illustrates the natural history of neonatal jaundice in different populations. In a mixed race population in which 60% to 70% of infants are breast-fed, the 95th percentiles for TSB levels are approximately 8 mg/dL (137 μmol/L) at 24 hours, 10 mg/dL (171 μmol/L) at 36 hours, 12 mg/dL (20 μmol/L) at 48 hours, 16 mg/dL (274 μmol/L) at 72 hours, and 17 to 18 mg/dL (291-308 μmol/L) by the fifth day (see Fig. 38–9) (100,101). Infants whose TSB levels exceed the 95th percentile, or in whom the rate of rise appears to be crossing percentiles (see Fig. 38–9), deserve evaluation and careful follow-up. Nevertheless,

TABLE 38–5. *Discharge diagnosis in 306 infants admitted with severe hyperbilirubinemia*[a]

Diagnosis	Number	Percentage
Hyperbilirubinemia of unknown cause or breast-milk jaundice	290	94.8
Cephalhematoma or bruising	3	1.0
ABO hemolytic disease[b]	11	3.6
Anti-E hemolytic disease	1	0.3
Galactosemia	1	0.3
Sepsis	0	

[a]Infants were readmitted after discharge as newborns. Mean age at admission was 5 days (range, 2–17 days), and mean bilirubin level was 18.5 ± 2.8 mg/dL (range, 12.7–29.1 mg/dL).

[b]Mother was type O, infant was type A or B, direct Coombs test was positive.

From ref. 71.

in most cases it is unlikely that a precise cause for the aberrant trend will be found.

Screening for Isoimmunization

All pregnant women should be tested for ABO and Rh (D) typing and a serum screen performed for unusual isoimmune antibodies (121). If such prenatal testing has not been performed, then a direct Coombs test, a blood type, and an Rh (D) type on the infant's (cord) blood should be done, and this should always be done if the mother is Rh negative. In addition to identification of potentially Rh-sensitized infants, this testing is obligatory because it identifies Rh-negative mothers who require anti-D γ-globulin to prevent Rh (D) sensitization.

The Diagnosis of ABO Hemolytic Disease

It is difficult to be confident about a diagnosis of ABO hemolytic disease. About 45% of Americans of western European descent have type O blood, and a similar percentage are type A. Types B and AB make up the balance. The equivalent percentages for African-Americans are 50% type O, 29% type A, 17% type B, and 4% AB (122). As a result, OA incompatibility, is by far the most common form of ABO incompatibility encountered in the United States. ABO incompatibility tends to run in families. One study found an 88% risk of recurrence of ABO hemolytic disease of the newborn in infants at risk of the disease who were born to parents whose first born child was similarly affected (123).

Ozolek et al. (124) prospectively analyzed cord blood samples of 4,996 consecutive live born infants for their blood type, hematocrit, and results of the direct antiglobulin test (DAT or Coombs test) and the indirect Coombs test. The direct Coombs test detects antibodies attached to the red cell, whereas the indirect Coombs test detects immunoglobulin G antibody in the serum. These investigators also identified the number of infants whose TSB levels was ≥12.8 mg/dL (224 μmol/L). Only 0.29% of infants (type A, B, or AB) who were incompatible with their type A or B mothers had a positive DAT result, whereas 32% of type A or B infants born to type O mothers had positive DATs. A positive DAT was the best predictor of an elevated bilirubin level, but only 20% of infants with a positive DAT developed TSB levels of ≥12.8 mg/dL (224 μmol/L). This large prospective study confirms what has been found in other smaller studies: although about one-third of group A or B infants born to group O mothers have anti-A or anti-B antibodies attached to their red cells, only 1 in 5 of those with a positive DAT have a *modest* degree of hyperbilirubinemia.

Thus, although ABO-incompatible DAT-positive infants are about twice as likely as their compatible peers to have moderate hyperbilirubinemia, severe jaundice in these infants is very uncommon (124–129). *ABO hemolytic disease is a relatively rare cause of severe hyperbilirubinemia* (see Table 38–5). Although there is certainly a wide spectrum of hemolysis in ABO hemolytic disease, this diagnosis generally should not be made unless there is a positive DAT *and* clinical jaundice within the first 12 to 24 hours. Reticulocytosis and the presence of microspherocytes on the smear help to confirm the diagnosis. Although the epidemiologic data suggest otherwise, most experienced clinicians have seen the occasional infant in whom all of the criteria for the diagnosis of ABO hemolytic disease were present yet the direct Coombs test was negative. Presumably such cases can occur, and they reflect the technical vicissitudes of Coombs testing in the laboratory.

In these days of cost containment, a question that is commonly asked is: should a blood type and direct Coombs test be performed on the cord blood of all infants of group O mothers? A recent survey suggested that 58% of hospital blood banks in the United States were routinely performing Coombs tests and blood typing on newborn cord bloods. About 36% of hospitals tested all cord bloods routinely, and 35% tested those of type O or Rh-negative mothers even though the data suggest that such routine screening is not warranted (124,130). Furthermore, even when such testing is done, there is evidence that it is often ignored by the responsible pediatrician (130,131). Thus, we do not recommend routine cord blood screening for infants of group O mothers, but we do recommend appropriate newborn follow-up (see later) so that significantly jaundiced infants are not missed.

Infants with Severe Jaundice

In those infants with severe jaundice (TSB levels greater than 18 mg/dL [308 μmol/L]), it is worth looking for ABO immunization and other causes of hemolysis (Table 38–6). If ABO or some other type of hemolytic disease is strongly suspected, these infants generally require more aggressive therapy than those with nonhemolytic jaundice. In the absence of hemolysis and any abnormal historical or physical findings, jaundice *by itself* is almost never a sign of serious illness and, although some reports have suggested that unexplained indirect hyperbilirubinemia may be the only manifestation of sepsis in otherwise healthy-appearing newborns, this is certainly a rare occurrence (132–134). Of 306 newborns admitted to our pediatric ward within 21 days of birth because of severe indirect hyperbilirubinemia (peak TSB levels 18.5 ± 2.8 mg/dL, range 12.7 to 29.1 [316 ± 4.8 μmol/L, range 217 to 498]), no cases of sepsis were identified (upper 95% confidence limits for the risk of sepsis = 1%) (see Table 38–5) (71). However, infants who exhibit some of the signs or symptoms listed in Table 38–7 deserve careful evaluation, as do those who have direct hyperbilirubinemia or something in their history, physical examination, or laboratory investigation that is out of the ordinary.

No jaundice should be dismissed as physiologic without at least a review of the maternal and infant history,

TABLE 38–6. *Causes of a pathologic indirect hyperbilirubinemia in newborn infants*

Increased production or bilirubin load on the liver
  Hemolytic Disease
    Immune
      Rh, ABO, and other blood group incompatibilities
    Heritable
      Red cell membrane defects
        Hereditary spherocytosis, elliptocytosis, stomatocytosis, pyknocytosis
      Red cell enzyme deficiencies
        Glucose-6-phosphate dehydrogenase deficiency[a] pyruvate kinase deficiency, and other erythrocyte enzyme deficiencies
      Hemoglobinopathies
        Alpha thalassemia, beta-γ-thalassemia
  Other causes of increased production
    Sepsis[a,b]
    Extravasation of blood; hematoma; pulmonary, cerebral, or occult hemorrhage
    Polycythemia
    Macrosomic infants of diabetic mothers
Increased enterohepatic circulation of bilirubin
  Breast-milk jaundice
  Pyloric stenosis[a]
  Small or large bowel obstruction or ileus
Decreased Clearance
  Prematurity
  Glucose-6-phosphate dehydrogenase deficiency
Inborn errors of metabolism
  Crigler–Najjar syndrome, types I and II, and Gilbert's syndrome
  Galactosemia[b]
  Tyrosinemia[b]
  Hypermethioninemia[b]
Metabolic
  Hypothyroidism
  Hypopituitarism[b]

[a]Decreased clearance also part of pathogenesis.
[b]Elevation of direct-reading bilirubin also occurs.

examination of the infant, and, if necessary, pursuit of further laboratory investigations. On occasion, jaundice may be one sign of serious illness, and the presence of any of the associated signs listed in Table 38–7 demands evaluation and treatment as indicted. The problem is that jaundice is common, most of the diseases the laboratory tests aim to identify are rare, and the tests themselves are neither sensitive nor specific.

TABLE 38–7. *Danger signs in jaundiced infants*

Family history of significant hemolytic disease
Onset of jaundice in first 24 h of life
Onset of jaundice after day 3 of life
Vomiting
Lethargy
Poor feeding
Fever
High-pitched cry
Dark urine
Light stools

Measuring Direct Bilirubin Concentrations

In many nurseries, routine determinations of direct bilirubin levels are obtained whenever the total bilirubin level exceeds a predetermined level. Measurements of direct bilirubin, however, are notoriously inaccurate and, when used as a screening test in the newborn nursery, direct bilirubin measurements provide a low yield and are nonspecific if the intent is to rule out treatable causes of cholestasis, such as biliary atresia or galactosemia (135, 136). Biliary atresia occurs in 10 of every 100,000 births and galactosemia in about 2 in 100,000 births. In contrast, 15,000 of 100,000 infants have significant jaundice, of whom at least 750 (5%) have a direct bilirubin level above the 95th percentile. Fortunately, galactosemia can be identified by a routine metabolic screen performed in the nursery, and biliary atresia should be diagnosed by selective testing of infants with prolonged jaundice (more than 2 weeks), light stools, or dark urine.

Every infant who is jaundiced beyond 3 weeks of age must have a measurement of direct bilirubin performed. If the level is elevated, the urine should be tested for bile and the stool color evaluated (121). This approach is essential for the early identification of infants with biliary atresia. If these infants are to benefit from the operation of portoenterostomy, surgery should be performed before 60 days of age (137). If an elevated direct bilirubin measurement is obtained while the infant is in the nursery, it must be repeated; if it remains elevated, the infant must be investigated for possible causes of cholestatic jaundice (see Fig. 38–11).

PATHOLOGIC CAUSES OF JAUNDICE

Indirect Hyperbilirubinemia

The causes of pathologic indirect hyperbilirubinemia in the neonate are listed in Table 38–6.

Increased Bilirubin Load

Hemolytic Disease

Hemolytic causes of hyperbilirubinemia are discussed fully in Chapter 45. The combination of antepartum and postpartum prophylaxis with Rh immunoglobulin has dramatically reduced the incidence of erythroblastosis fetalis, and the contribution of ABO hemolytic disease to neonatal jaundice was discussed in the section on Laboratory Evaluation. Other hemolytic processes to be considered include spherocytosis and other morphologic abnormalities of the erythrocyte, in addition to the erythrocyte enzyme deficiencies (Table 38–6). Although previous reports suggested an association between sickle cell disease and jaundice in the newborn, a matched, case-control study of 68 neonates with sickle cell disease found no increase in bilirubin levels in patients with sickle cell disease compared with controls (138).

Glucose-6-Phospate Dehydrogenase Deficiency. This problem affects hundreds of millions of people around the world, but most pediatricians in the United States do not think about this enzyme deficiency as a likely cause for significant hyperbilirubinemia (139). Although common in African-American neonates, most of these newborns do not develop severe hyperbilirubinemia and kernicterus is rare (140,141). In some other countries such as Nigeria and Greece, severe hyperbilirubinemia related to glucose-6-phophate dehydrogenase (G6PD) deficiency is much more common (142,143).

The pathogenesis of hyperbilirubinemia associated with G6PD deficiency only recently was elucidated. In a series of elegant studies, Kaplan and Hammerman (139) and Kaplan et al. (144,145) showed that, although infants with G6PD deficiency have an increased rate of red cell breakdown and bilirubin production, in those who develop significant hyperbilirubinemia, *the major problem appears to be abnormal bilirubin elimination.* Furthermore, these investigators showed that neonates who are G6PD deficient and have Gilbert's syndrome (as determined by DNA analysis) have a much higher incidence of hyperbilirubinemia than controls, whereas neither those with the Mediterranean type of G6PD deficiency alone nor those with only the variant UDPGT1 promoter (for Gilbert's syndrome) develop significant jaundice (145). On the other hand, when both genetic abnormalities were present, the incidence of hyperbilirubinemia (TSB ≥15 mg/dL) was significantly increased (145).

The risk of kernicterus in G6PD-deficient infants with TSB levels above 20 mg/dL (342 μmol/L) appears to be comparable to that associated with Rh disease. Thus, in the presence of G6PD deficiency, more aggressive treatment of these infants probably is indicated (143,146,147).

Extravascular Blood

Cephalhematomas, intracranial or pulmonary hemorrhage, or any occult bleeding may lead to an elevated serum bilirubin level from breakdown of the extravascular erythrocytes (148—150). In two reports, severe hyperbilirubinemia followed delayed absorption of intraperitoneal blood in infants who received fetal transfusions before birth (148—150). In both reported cases, despite multiple exchange transfusions, hyperbilirubinemia was not controlled until peritoneal lavage was performed.

In the very-low-birth-weight infant, the presence of periventricular-intraventricular hemorrhage (PIVH) has been associated with an increase in serum bilirubin levels in some studies (151,152) but not in others (153). Amato and colleagues (153) studied 88 infants with birth weights less than 1,500 g. Phototherapy was initiated only when serum bilirubin levels exceeded 12 mg/dL (205 μmol/L). The incidence of serum bilirubin levels greater than 12 mg/dL was 39% in the PIVH group and

46.8% in the infants without PIVH. There was no difference in the duration of phototherapy in the two groups.

Polycythemia

The catabolism of 1 g of hemoglobin produces 35 mg of bilirubin, and it is often assumed that a high hematocrit is a risk factor for neonatal jaundice, because an increase in the erythrocyte mass should increase the bilirubin load presented to the liver. Nevertheless, mean bilirubin levels and the incidence of hyperbilirubinemia were similar in polycythemic infants randomly assigned to receive either partial exchange transfusions or symptomatic treatment (see section on Epidemiology of Neonatal Jaundice) (53–55).

Increased Enterohepatic Circulation

(See sections on Physiologic Mechanisms of Neonatal Jaundice, Epidemiology of Neonatal Jaundice, and Breast-Milk Jaundice for the contribution of the enterohepatic circulation to neonatal jaundice.) Intestinal obstruction or a delay in bowel transit time increases the enterohepatic circulation by allowing more time for bilirubin deconjugation and reabsorption. Jaundice is common in infants with small bowel obstruction and occurs in infants with pyloric stenosis (154,155). Correction of the obstruction produces a prompt decline in bilirubin levels.

Infants of Diabetic Mothers

Only macrosomic infants of mothers with insulin-dependent diabetes are at increased risk of hyperbilirubinemia. This is the result of increased bilirubin production (see section on Epidemiology of Neonatal Jaundice: Maternal Factors).

Decreased Bilirubin Clearance

Inherited Unconjugated Hyperbilirubinemia–Inborn Errors of Bilirubin Uridine Diphosphoglucuronosyl Transferase Activity

Because a single form of bilirubin UDPGT (UDPGT1) accounts for almost all of the bilirubin glucuronidation activity in the human liver, inherited defects of a single enzyme will cause jaundice. Three degrees of inherited UDPGT deficiency are recognized:

Crigler–Najjar Syndrome Type I. Crigler–Najjar syndrome type I (CN-1) is inherited as an autosomal recessive gene, although there is marked genetic heterogenicity (156). Infants with this condition have virtually complete absence of bilirubin UDPGT activity, develop severe jaundice in the first 2 to 3 days of life, and often require exchange transfusion in the first week. Subsequently, intensive home phototherapy controls bilirubin levels to some extent, but as these children get older,

increasing skin thickness and pigmentation and a decrease in the surface area to body mass ratio render phototherapy less effective. A "tanning bed" phototherapy configuration is necessary to obtain adequate irradiance and surface area exposure (see section on Phototherapy). Brain damage can occur at any time, including adulthood, and plasmapheresis is used to reduce bilirubin concentrations during acute exacerbations of hyperbilirubinemia (157,158). One 16-year-old boy with CN-1 had 72 plasma exchanges over a period of 28 months before undergoing orthotopic liver transplantation (159). Liver transplantation is currently the only available definitive therapy, and serum bilirubin concentrations decline dramatically within hours of the procedure (160).

An exciting new intervention that could obviate the need for inevitable liver transplantation in patients with CN-1 is the use of human hepatocyte transplantation (161,162). Because hepatic architecture and function, except for bilirubin UDPGT activity, are normal in CN-1, transplantation of isolated liver cells is an attractive option. Fox et al. (161) infused hepatocytes (obtained from a donor liver) into the portal vein of a 10-year-old girl with CN-1. The child, who had previously required 10 to 12 hours of daily phototherapy to maintain serum bilirubin levels of 24 to 27 mg/dL (400 to 460 μmol/L), showed a decrease in serum bilirubin level to 10.6 to 14 mg/dL (180 to 240 μmol/L) and required less phototherapy to maintain those bilirubin levels. Hepatic bilirubin UDPGT activity increased from a barely detectable 0.4% to 5.5% of mean normal enzyme activity, and more than 30% of the patient's bile pigments were now bilirubin glucuronides. The ultimate treatment of the Crigler–Najjar syndrome, however, lies in the development of effective gene therapy.

The administration of tin-protoporphyrin to a 2-month-old infant with the Crigler–Najjar syndrome reduced the need for phototherapy (163). Administration of oral calcium phosphate significantly reduced serum bilirubin levels in patients with CN-1 who were receiving phototherapy (164). These two interventions may be useful adjuvants to phototherapy in the management of CN-1 (163,164).

The diagnosis of Crigler–Najjar syndrome is made using high-performance liquid chromatography analysis of serum and duodenal bile and by evaluating the response to phenobarbital (165). In CN-1 disease, phenobarbital has little or no effect on TSB concentrations, whereas in children with type II disease, TSB levels usually decrease by 30% or more during phenobarbital treatment. There is now a world registry for the CN-1 syndrome that is a unique source of information about this rare disease (166).

Suresh and Lucey (167) conducted a questionnaire survey of 42 patients ranging in age from 2 months to 21 years who had CN-1. Home phototherapy for 10 to 16 hours, principally at night, was the mainstay of postneonatal therapy. Additional therapies included oral agar, antioxidants, bilirubin oxidase, clofibrate, and cholestarimine, and liver transplantation was performed in 15 children. All patients grew normally; in 77% the neurodevelopmental status was normal. Those in school were doing well despite having had TSB levels of 15 to 29 mg/dL (257 to 496 µmol/L) for many years. Although it often is stated that sensorineural hearing loss is the most common form of bilirubin toxicity to the central nervous system, not one of 36 children evaluated had a sensorineural hearing loss, suggesting that bilirubin may not be as ototoxic as commonly believed. In these children it is important to avoid exacerbations of hyperbilirubinemia and to manage intercurrent infections promptly. Albumin infusions and plasmapheresis are effective in dealing with acute exacerbations of jaundice (165,167).

Crigler–Najjar Disease Type II. Infants with this disease (also known as Arias syndrome) generally manifest with less severe jaundice, although severe hyperbilirubinemia can occur, and kernicterus has been reported in some infants. Both infants and adults with Crigler–Najjar syndrome type II respond readily to phenobarbital therapy, with a sharp decline in serum bilirubin levels within 7 to 10 days. This response can be used to differentiate between the two syndromes (165). The pattern of inheritance for Crigler–Najjar type II disease is autosomal recessive (168).

Gilbert's Syndrome. People with Gilbert's syndrome have a mild, benign chronic unconjugated hyperbilirubinemia and no evidence of liver disease or overt hemolysis. This syndrome is common, affecting about 6% of the population, and both autosomal dominant as well as recessive patterns of inheritance have been suggested. Typically, the indirect hyperbilirubinemia is not recognized until after puberty and manifests itself during fasting or intercurrent illness.

Recently, the genetic basis for this disorder has been clarified (169). A variant promoter for the gene encoding UDPGT1 contains a two base-pair addition (TA) in the TATAA element that gives rise to seven (A[TA]$_7$TAA) rather than the more usual six (A[TA]$_6$TAA) repeats in affected subjects. This polymorphism accounts for their reduced UDPGT activity (169). Subjects with Gilbert's syndrome are homozygous for the variant promoter, providing a unique genetic marker for this disorder. The expanded A[TA]$_7$TAA promoter motif is expressed in the heterozygous form in 40% of the population (169).

Although most commonly diagnosed in young adulthood, it recently has been recognized that Gilbert's syndrome may play a role in the pathogenesis of neonatal jaundice (170). Bancroft et al. (170) have shown that newborn infants who are homozygous for the A(TA)$_7$TAA polymorphism in the promoter region of UDPGT1 have a greater increase in bilirubin levels in the first 2 days of life than do heterozygotes or A(TA)$_6$TAA homozygotes. Roy-

Chowdhury and co-workers (171) have made similar observations. In addition, as discussed previously, the combination of the Gilbert's genotype and G6PD deficiency markedly increases a newborn's risk of hyperbilirubinemia (145). We do not know if Gilbert's syndrome plays any role in the pathogenesis of extreme hyperbilirubinemia (TSB levels greater than 30 mg/dL [513 µmol/L]), but the fact that poor feeding and weight loss (a state resembling fasting) as well as very low direct bilirubin fractions are seen in some of these infants suggests that this is a possibility worthy of investigation (172).

Other Inborn Errors of Metabolism

Galactosemia. Galactosemia is a rare disease (worldwide incidence, about 1 in 50,000 infants), and jaundice may be one of the presenting features; but infants with significant hyperbilirubinemia due to galactosemia almost all have some other manifestations of the disease (e.g., vomiting, excessive weight loss, hepatomegaly, splenomegaly). Hyperbilirubinemia during the first week of life is almost exclusively unconjugated, and the conjugated fraction tends to rise during the second week, probably reflecting liver damage. The presence of a positive family history, hepatomegaly, lethargy, poor feeding, or other signs of illness merit additional diagnostic evaluation, including testing the urine for reducing substances using Clinitest.

Tyrosinemia and Hypermethioninemia. The relation between these inborn errors of metabolism and jaundice is primarily due to the presence of neonatal liver disease, which initially may manifest as indirect hyperbilirubinemia but which generally is accompanied by some evidence of cholestasis (i.e., direct hyperbilirubinemia).

Hypothyroidism. Prolonged indirect hyperbilirubinemia is one of the clinical features of congenital hypothyroidism, a condition that must be ruled out in any infant who has indirect hyperbilirubinemia beyond 2 to 3 weeks of age. Although widespread availability of screening programs for congenital hypothyroidism should allow early identification of this problem as a possible cause of jaundice, screening programs do not detect every infant, and errors are more likely to occur with early discharge of infants in whom the T4 level may still be spuriously elevated. A single case of cholestasis associated with hypothyroidism has been described in a 54-year-old woman (173).

The pathogenesis of hyperbilirubinemia associated with hypothyroidism is not clear, and administration of triiodothyronine to full-term and preterm infants does not lower peak serum bilirubin levels (174,175).

Drugs

The use of pancuronium and chloral hydrate is associated with higher bilirubin levels in sick preterm infants,

and chloral hydrate is associated with an increased risk of direct hyperbilirubinemia (see section on Epidemiology of Neonatal Jaundice) (89–91).

Breast-Milk Jaundice

See section on Breast-Feeding and Jaundice, above.

Prolonged Indirect Hyperbilirubinemia

Prolonged indirect hyprgyperbilirubinemia is defined as indirect bilirubinemia persisting beyond 2 weeks of age in the full-term infant. The causes are listed in Table 38–8.

Mixed Forms of Jaundice

Sepsis

Jaundice is one sign of bacterial sepsis. Some reports suggest that unexplained hyperbilirubinemia may be the only manifestation of sepsis in otherwise healthy-appearing newborns (132–134).

Should newborns with unexplained hyperbilirubinemia be subjected to lumbar puncture and blood and urine cultures even if they appear otherwise well? No case of sepsis was diagnosed in 306 newborns admitted to a pediatric ward within 21 days of birth with indirect hyperbilirubinemia (peak TSB level 18.5 ± 2.8 mg/dL, range 12.7 to 29.1 [316 ± 48 μmol/L, range 217 to 498]) (see Table 38–5) (71). If indirect hyperbilirubinemia is ever the *only* manifestation of bacteremia or incipient sepsis, it must be a rare occurrence. Furthermore, the finding of a positive blood or urine culture in a newborn with indirect hyperbilirubinemia does not prove that the infection is the cause of the jaundice. On the other hand, infants who appear sick, who have late-onset jaundice after icterus has resolved, or have direct hyperbilirubinemia, or something else in the history, physical examination, or laboratory investigations that is out of the ordinary, should be evaluated carefully for possible sepsis.

Hypopituitarism

Prolonged jaundice has been described in infants with congenital hypopituitarism (176,177). Most had evidence of significant cholestatic jaundice; however, in one infant, the hyperbilirubinemia was predominantly indirect. The pathogenesis of hyperbilirubinemia in this condition remains to be elucidated.

TABLE 38–8. *Causes of prolonged indirect hyperbilirubinemia*

Breast-milk jaundice	Pyloric stenosis
Hemolytic disease	Crigler–Najjar syndrome
Hypothyroidism	Extravascular blood

Other Causes

Congenital syphilis, the TORCH group of chronic intrauterine infections (i.e., toxoplasmosis, rubella, cytomegalovirus, herpes simplex), and coxsackievirus B infection are the other important causes of mixed jaundice. The clinical features and diagnoses of these conditions are described in Chapter 47.

CHANGING APPROACHES TO THE EVALUATION OF THE JAUNDICED NEWBORN

In the last few years, three factors have emerged that have colored our approach to the evaluation and management of neonatal jaundice. The first is a series of case reports suggesting the possible reemergence of kernicterus from a status of near extinction to one that is of concern to pediatricians (140,141,172,178–180). The second is the decreasing hospital stay for newborn infants, and the third is an increase in the incidence of neonatal jaundice.

A Possible Resurgence of Kernicterus

There is some anecdotal evidence that we are now seeing more kernicterus than was seen 2 or 3 decades ago (140,141,172,178–180). However, it is difficult to be confident about this perception, because there has been no uniform surveillance for the reporting of kernicterus over the last 3 to 4 decades, no agreed upon case definition for kernicterus, and, most important, no denominators for the case reports listed. In many of the reported cases, however, short hospital stays following delivery have played an important role, and an additional contributing factor could be the previously held belief that hyperbilirubinemia, no matter how extreme, is harmless if it occurs in an otherwise healthy breast-fed infant (140,178). Reports of kernicterus in such infants indicate that this is not the case (172).

Early Discharge and the Risk of Jaundice

In addition to the global trend toward a shorter hospital stay for newborns, early discharge itself seems to be associated with an increased risk of significant hyperbilirubinemia and even kernicterus (61,63,99,140,178). Recognizing (among other problems) the risk of unrecognized jaundice in infants discharged early, the AAP has recommended that those discharged before 48 hours should be seen within 2 to 3 days of discharge (105,181). However, two studies have shown that infants discharged between 48 and 72 hours are at as great a risk of readmission with significant jaundice as those discharged before 48 hours and, therefore, require similar follow-up (61,63).

It is not clear why babies discharged early should be at greater risk of developing significant hyperbilirubinemia.

The vast majority of these infants are breast-fed, and it is possible that mothers who have longer postpartum stays, are more rested, and have more time to receive advice and counsel regarding breast-feeding are able to nurse their babies more effectively. More frequent and effective lactation, as well as improved caloric intake, decreases the likelihood of hyperbilirubinemia (182,183). Early discharge also may have a negative effect on the ability of mothers to assimilate and process the information that they receive regarding lactation and infant care (184). As a result, they may nurse the infants less effectively.

Shorter hospital stays also have necessitated a readjustment in our thinking with regard to the meaning of specific bilirubin levels. To date, this has proven to be a difficult adjustment for pediatricians who have become accustomed to using a specific bilirubin level (irrespective of the baby's age) as an indication for reassurance or concern. The data of Bhutani et al. (100) graphically illustrate this point. Clinicians commonly refer to jaundice occurring on "day 2 or day 3," but reference to the data of Bhutani et al. and Fig. 38–9 indicates just how misleading this thought process can be. A TSB level of 8 mg/dL at 24.1 hours is above the 95th percentile and calls for evaluation and close follow-up, whereas the same level at 47.9 hours is below the 50th percentile and probably requires no further concern— yet both of these values occur on "day 2" (100). One point bears emphasis: *If newborns are discharged at less than 36 hours, their bilirubin levels (with very rare exceptions) can only be going in one direction, and that is up.* The recognition that jaundice is now primarily an outpatient problem will allow us to develop a consistent approach to the monitoring and surveillance of these infants and, if possible, to prevent the development of extreme hyperbilirubinemia.

More Jaundiced Newborns

There is good evidence that the incidence of neonatal jaundice is increasing. In the days of the major Collaborative Perinatal Project (CPP, 1959–1966), only 5% of infants had bilirubin levels ≥ 13 mg/dL (222 μmol/L) and less than 1% had a peak TSB level of ≥ 20 mg/dL (342 μmol/L) (29). However, in three recent studies, the 95th percentile for a population of term and near-term infants ranged from 15.5 to 18 mg/dL (62,100,101). In a study of 11 Kaiser Permanente Northern California hospitals, 2% of infants had peak TSB levels ≥ 20 mg/dL (62). Factors that may be responsible for this increase in jaundice include an increase in the number of infants breast-fed on discharge from the hospital (30% in the 1960s, 60% in 1997) and shorter hospital stays (61,62,98,99).

An Approach to Preventing Kernicterus

Although kernicterus is very rare, it is a devastating condition that is not extinct. Most of the cases reported in the last decade did not occur in infants who have ABO or Rh hemolytic disease, but in infants with G6PD deficiency, very sick newborns with low bilirubin levels, and in apparently healthy term and near-term newborns with extremely high bilirubin levels, usually well above 30 mg/dL (513 μmol/L) (140,172,178,179,185). If we can prevent extreme hyperbilirubinemia we should be able to prevent almost all cases of kernicterus, but jaundice is very common and extreme hyperbilirubinemia (30 mg/dL [513 μmol/L] or higher) is rare, occurring in only 1 in 10,000 infants (62). To ensure that we do not miss these rare infants, we need to follow and measure serum bilirubin levels in many and treat some infants with phototherapy who will never develop severe hyperbilirubinemia. There are a number of approaches that might help us to identify infants who are (or are not) at risk of developing extreme hyperbilirubinemia.

Key Epidemiologic Factors

Factors associated with an increased risk of hyperbilirubinemia were discussed in the section on Epidemiology of Neonatal Jaundice. These factors are listed in Table 38–1. The ten factors that are most commonly associated with an increased risk of nonhemolytic jaundice are listed in Table 38–9. However, because these risk factors are common and the risk of severe hyperbilirubinemia is small, they have been of limited use as predictors of infants at risk of kernicterus. Nevertheless, when some of the key factors listed in Table 38–9 are present, and certainly when several are present together, the risk of severe hyperbilirubinemia increases significantly. Some factors, such as breast-feeding, seem to play a particularly important role in the reported cases of extreme hyperbilirubinemia and kernicterus. It is remarkable that almost every recently described case of kernicterus occurred in a breast-fed infant, even when the infant had underlying G6PD deficiency (140,172,178,179). Most cases occurred in infants less than 40 weeks of gestation (172,178).

Decreasing Gestation

Decreasing gestation has been identified repeatedly as a very important contributor to hyperbilirubinemia

TABLE 38–9. *Common obstetric and neonatal factors that significantly increase the risk of nonhemolytic hyperbilirubinemia*

Previous jaundiced sibling	Male sex
East Asian descent	Breast-feeding
Oxytocin use in labor	Caloric deprivation and larger weight loss
Macrosomic infant of diabetic mother	Glucose-6-phosphate dehydrogenase deficiency
Decreasing gestation	Short hospital stay

(24,34,43,61,63). We found that infants 36 weeks or less of gestation are 13 times more likely than those 40 weeks of gestation to be readmitted for severe jaundice, and those between 36 weeks 1 day and 38 weeks of gestation are 7 times more likely to be readmitted (61). Infants of 35 to 38 weeks of gestation, although cared for in well-baby nurseries, are much more likely to nurse ineffectively, receive fewer calories, and have a greater weight loss than their truly term counterparts. When combined with less effective hepatic clearance, because of prematurity, it is not surprising that they become more jaundiced.

Universal Newborn Bilirubin Screening

We know that infants who are clinically jaundiced in the first few days are much more likely to develop significant hyperbilirubinemia later on (61,63). Bhutani et al. (100) measured serum bilirubin concentrations in 13,003 infants prior to their discharge from the hospital. In 2,840, additional bilirubin levels were measured at least once in the 5 to 6 days following discharge. Infants with ABO incompatibility and positive Coombs tests were excluded, as were Rh-sensitized infants. The investigators plotted bilirubin levels against the infant's age in hours and created percentiles that defined a high risk (above 95th percentile), a low risk (values less than 40th percentile), and an intermediate risk (40th to 95th percentile zone) (100). Using this nomogram, these investigators also followed 3,048 Coombs-negative term and near-term newborns and 224 Coombs-positive infants with ABO incompatibility. Of Coombs-negative infants whose TSB levels fell in the high-risk zone, 39.5% subsequently required phototherapy compared with 65.2% of the Coombs-positive infants. No baby, whether Coombs negative or positive, required phototherapy if the TSB level fell in the low-risk zone (125).

These data suggest that obtaining a TSB level on every baby prior to discharge can be a very useful way of predicting the risk (or absence of risk) of subsequent significant hyperbilirubinemia. If confirmed in other studies, these results suggest that there is a group of infants who, at least as far as hyperbilirubinemia is concerned, may not require an early follow-up (information that would be very useful in situations where early follow-up is difficult or impossible). Predischarge TSB levels also will alert pediatricians to those infants who, because their TSB levels fall in the high-risk zone, require much more careful surveillance and follow-up until there is clinical or laboratory evidence supporting a declining bilirubin level (see Fig. 38–9).

Measuring Bilirubin Production

When heme is catabolized, carbon monoxide (CO) is produced in equimolar quantities with bilirubin, and measurement of blood carboxyhemoglobin (COHb) concentration, CO production, or CO excretion provides a measurement of bilirubin production (17,119). The recent development of a simple noninvasive method for measuring end-tidal CO, corrected for ambient CO (ETCO$_C$), provides a technique for quantifying hemolysis (119). Measurements of ETCO$_c$ prior to discharge might identify those infants with high or low rates of bilirubin production and could provide additional help in predicting the likelihood (or lack thereof) of severe hyperbilirubinemia.

Surveillance and Follow-Up

If every baby, irrespective of risk factors for jaundice, was seen within 1 to 3 days of discharge, significantly jaundiced infants would be identified, a bilirubin level measured, and intervention (where necessary) instituted. Thus, in a perfect world, most risk assessment for hyperbilirubinemia (including bilirubin determinations) prior to discharge would be superfluous. In the real world, not only is it difficult to provide this type of follow-up for every baby but, so far, pediatricians in the United States are not convinced of its necessity (131). Although the AAP has recommended this type of early follow-up only for babies discharged before 48 hours, two studies have shown that infants discharged between 48 and 72 hours are at as great a risk of readmission with significant jaundice as those discharged before 48 hours (61,63). Thus, we recommend that any infant discharged at less than 72 hours should be seen by a health care professional within 2 to 3 days of discharge. A suggested approach to the management and follow-up of these infants is shown in Tables 38–3 and 38–4.

BILIRUBIN TOXICITY

Pathology of Kernicterus

In 1875, Orth (186) observed bilirubin pigment at autopsy in the brains of infants who were severely jaundiced. Schmorl (187) subsequently described two forms of "brain icterus," the first "characterized by a diffuse yellow coloration of the entire brain substance," and a second form in which "the jaundiced coloration appears to be completely circumscribed and...limited to the so-called `kern' or nuclear region of the brain." Full-term infants who died of kernicterus demonstrate bilirubin staining in a characteristic distribution (Table 38–10), although a variety of patterns have been described, grossly and microscopically (188). Kernicteric premature infants and Gunn rats with inherited glucuronosyl transferase deficiency display a similar topography of neuronal damage (see Table 38–10) (189). Those regions most commonly affected are the basal ganglia, particularly the subthalamic nucleus and the globus pallidus; the hippocampus; the geniculate bodies; various brainstem

TABLE 38–10. *Comparative neuropathology of kernicterus*

Topography of lesions	Full-term infants, hyper-bilirubinemia	Homozygous Gunn rats	Premature infants, low bilirubin levels
Globus pallidus	+	+	+
Subthalamus	+	+	+
Hypothalamus	+	–	–
Horn of Ammon	+	+	+
Reticular zone of the substantia nigra	+	+	+
Cranial nerve nuclei	+	+	+
Reticular formation	+		+
Central pontine nuclei			
Interstitial nucleus			
Locus ceruleus	–	+	+
Lateral cuneate nucleus of the medulla	+	+	+
Cerebellum			
Dentate nuclei	+	–	+
Nuclei of roof of fourth ventricle	+	+	+
Purkinje cells	–	+	+
Spinal cord	+	+	+

+, yellow pigment present; –, yellow pigment absent.
From ref. 189.

nuclei, including the inferior colliculus, oculomotor, vestibular, cochlear, and inferior olivary nuclei; and the cerebellum, especially the dentate nucleus and the vermis (189,190).

Neuronal necrosis is the dominant histopathologic feature after 7 to 10 days of postnatal life. For the most part, its distribution corresponds with the distribution of bilirubin staining, although there are some exceptions to this rule. For example, intense staining develops in the olivary and dentate nuclei, but there is little neuronal necrosis in these regions. The important areas of neuronal injury (as opposed to staining) include the basal ganglia, brainstem oculomotor nuclei, and brainstem auditory pathways, especially (cochlear) nuclei (190). The involvement of these regions explains some of the clinical sequelae of bilirubin encephalopathy (see section on Clinical Features of Bilirubin Encephalopathy).

Originally a pathologic diagnosis and later a well-defined acute and chronic neurologic syndrome, kernicterus or bilirubin encephalopathy appears to be a less well-circumscribed entity that includes nuclear bilirubin staining of very-low-birth-weight infants who died of other causes and, possibly, a subtle chronic encephalopathy in which extrapyramidal motor disturbances and sensorineural hearing deficit are not the predominant features.

Most, but not all, full-term infants seen today with the pathologic changes described will manifest the clinical symptomatology of this disorder, including very high serum bilirubin levels (commonly higher thatn 30 mg/dL [513 μmol/L]). Exceptions have been described. Perlman et al. (185) recently reported kernicterus at autopsy in two very sick near-term infants with maximum TSB levels of 5.2 and 14.4 mg/dL (89 to 246 μmol/L) (185).

Yellow staining of the brain also has been observed in premature infants who manifested none of the clinical signs of kernicterus during life and in whom TSB levels remained low (191,192). Turkel and colleagues (193) identified 32 infants with kernicterus at autopsy and compared them with 32 control infants of similar gestational ages without kernicterus. In the kernicteric infants, although the gross pattern of staining followed that of classic kernicterus, the typical histologic changes characteristic of kernicterus were found in only three patients. These authors suggest that the bilirubin staining they observed probably was not the same clinicopathologic entity as the kernicterus of posticteric encephalopathy. Instead of the neuronal degeneration typically seen, they found spongy change and gliosis, which both imply nonspecific damage to the brain. This suggests that prior diffuse injury may predispose the brain to bilirubin deposition at relatively low levels of serum bilirubin.

Ahdab-Barmada and Moossy (189) found kernicterus in 97 autopsies of neonates (95 younger than 36 weeks of gestation). The neuropathology in these infants was strikingly similar to that of classic kernicterus in the full-term neonate and in the Gunn rat. In the National Institute of Child Health and Human Development (NICHHD) cooperative phototherapy study, four low-birth-weight infants had autopsy-proven kernicterus (194). The neuropathologic findings in these infants were those of classic kernicterus. As can be seen from Table 38–11, the neuropathology of kernicterus is different from that of hypoxic ischemic encephalopathy. Even though hypoxic ischemic insults may predispose the brain to bilirubin deposition in some low-birth-weight infants, in others the typical histologic features of kernicterus will be found.

TABLE 38–11. *Comparative neuropathology of kernicterus and anoxic–ischemic encephalopathy in the premature neonate*

Topography of lesions[a]	Kernicterus	Anoxic–ischemic encephalopathy
Cerebral cortex	Absent	Present
Periventricular white matter	Absent	Present
Corpus striatum	Globus pallidus	Putamen and caudate nuclei
Thalamus	Subthalamus	Anterior and lateral nuclei
Horn of Ammon	Resistant sector (H2–3)	Sommer sector (H₁)
Midbrain	Interstitial nucleus	Inferior colliculi
	Nuclei of nerve III[b]	Nuclei of nerve III[b]
	Reticular portion of substantia nigra	Compact portion of substantia nigra
Pons	Locus ceruleus	Basal pontine nuclei
	Nuclei of nerves VI, VII	Superior olivary complex
	Reticular formation[b]	Reticular formation[b]
Medulla	Vestibular and cochlear nuclei	Inferior olivary nuclei
		Superior olivary nuclei
Cerebellum	Purkinje cells[b]	Purkinje cells[b]
	Nuclei of roof of fourth ventricle	Granular cells

[a]Only topographic areas considered helpful for differential diagnosis were selected in this table.
[b]Whenever neuronal damage was involved in the same structure in kernicterus and anoxic–ischemic encephalopathy, the cytopathology was different.
From ref. 189.

Autopsies on jaundiced infants reveal bilirubin staining of the aorta, pleural fluid, and ascitic fluid, or a generalized yellow cast throughout the viscera. The staining usually is not considered a sign of tissue damage unless other cytologic changes are found (188). Bilirubin staining also can be found in necrotic tissue anywhere in the body and has been described in the gastrointestinal tract, kidney, adrenals, and gonads. In infants with hemolytic disease, bile plugs commonly are found in the canaliculi between the hepatocytes, especially in the periportal areas. The kidneys may show bilirubin-stained tubular casts, bilirubin crystals in the small vessels or in edematous interstitium, and renal tubular necrosis. The bilirubin infarcts (i.e., patches of yellow staining in the renal medulla) are probably the result of focal areas of acute tubular necrosis that have been stained by bilirubin (188).

In infants dying of hyaline membrane disease, the lungs often appear grossly yellow or orange, and there is microscopic staining by bilirubin of the pulmonary hyaline membranes (i.e., yellow hyaline membrane disease) (195,196). Hyaline membranes are formed from necrotic cellular debris and transudation of plasma proteins from the capillaries after damage to the alveolar epithelium. It appears likely that the transudate also contains bilirubin, which is deposited in the membranes with albumin and other plasma molecules.

Pathophysiology of Bilirubin Toxicity

Bilirubin Chemistry and Neurotoxicity

As discussed in the section on Formation, Structure, and Properties of Bilirubin, the bilirubin molecule, in its usual conformation, is stabilized by the presence of intramolecular hydrogen bonds that saturate the hydrophilic groups of the molecule, leaving no affinities for the attachment of water and rendering it nearly insoluble in water at pH 7.4. In an alkaline medium, the hydrogen bonds are opened to form a divalent anion that has several hydrophilic groups, resulting in a molecule with much greater solubility. Because of its pronounced tendency for aggregation, bilirubin 9α (ZZ) acid is almost certainly the neurotoxic form of bilirubin (9). The pH of plasma profoundly affects the solubility of bilirubin and its binding to tissue sites, with the solubility decreasing as pH falls. Thus, when the concentration of bilirubin acid exceeds its solubility, bilirubin may gradually aggregate and come out of solution (9). Bilirubin crystals have been found in the brain cells of infants dying of kernicterus, and bilirubin in concentrations of 2 mg/dL (34 μmol/L) has been extracted from kernicteric brains (197). It is likely that even higher concentrations of pigment exist in the presence of kernicterus and may occur when aggregates of precipitated bilirubin acid are deposited in the cells of the brain (198,199). Wennberg (200) offered a different model for the development of bilirubin encephalopathy. He suggested that bilirubin monoanion and membranes form reversible complexes and that this mechanism is responsible for the development of bilirubin encephalopathy.

Cellular Toxicity of Bilirubin

Bilirubin appears to be a cell poison, but exactly how it exerts its toxic effect is not known. Cashore (201) reviewed the evidence for bilirubin toxicity to the neuron and summarized several histologic and biophysical findings from different clinical and experimental studies. These studies show a range of effects of bilirubin, including binding to cell membranes, decreased sodium–potassium exchange, increased water accumulation, axonal swelling, lowering of membrane potentials and decreased action potential, decreased activity of the auditory brainstem response, decreased phosphorylation of protein kinase and synapsone 1, decreased tyrosine uptake and dopamine synthesis, decreased methionine and thymidine uptake, and decreased mitochondrial viability (201). Bilirubin decreases the rate of tyrosine uptake and dopamine synthesis in dopaminergic striatal synaptosomes (202,203). These effects can be reversed by albumin. No single mechanism of bilirubin intoxication has been demonstrated in all cells, and specific studies of metabolism and toxicity have not been performed on basal ganglia cells, the cells commonly involved in kernicterus.

Studies using ^{31}P nuclear magnetic resonance *in vitro* and *in vivo* have demonstrated bilirubin-induced changes in energy metabolism (204,205).

The inhibition of protein phosphorylation is probably an important mechanism in bilirubin toxicity, and lysine binding may have an important role in the mediation of this toxicity (206).

It is not known why bilirubin is deposited preferentially in the basal ganglia, but it is possible that it may first attach to nerve terminals, thus lowering membrane potentials and decreasing nerve conduction, and, after further exposure, may penetrate nerve terminals or axons with retrograde uptake of bilirubin in the cell body. Cashore (201) offers a hypothetical format for the progression of bilirubin toxicity from the initial, possibly benign stage of bilirubin accumulation at the cell surface to ultimate neuronal damage and permanent sequelae (Table 38–12).

Albumin Binding and the Concept of Free Bilirubin

Bilirubin (B) is transported in the plasma as a dianion bound reversibly to serum albumin (A):

$$B^{2-} + A \leftrightarrow AB^{2-}.$$

Binding of bilirubin to the high-affinity site of albumin can be expressed as follows:

$$K = \frac{AB^{2-}}{(B^{2-})(A)}.$$

The association constant (K), derived from the equilibrium concentrations of bound (AB^{2-}) and free (B^{2-}) bilirubin, is about 10^7 to 10^8 moles. Because of this high binding affinity, equilibrium concentrations of unbound ("free") bilirubin in plasma are very low (9). Albumin has a primary binding site with the capacity for binding up to 1 molecule of bilirubin per molecule of albumin and one or more binding sites with much lower affinities. When the bilirubin–albumin ratio exceeds 1, the concentration of free or unbound bilirubin increases, but binding at the lower-affinity sites continues up to a molar bilirubin–albumin ratio of 3:1. It has been widely accepted that bilirubin toxicity occurs when free bilirubin enters the brain and binds to cell membranes (207). The presence of albumin mitigates the *in vivo* and *in vitro* toxic effects of bilirubin (207,208). Drugs, such as sulfisoxazole, that decrease albumin binding of bilirubin also increase the risk of kernicterus (29,210). These observations are consistent with the hypothesis that free bilirubin is able to move across the blood–brain barrier, bind to tissues, and damage the cells of the central nervous system. They do not exclude the possibility that, under certain circumstances, albumin-bound bilirubin may do the same.

The studies of Wennberg and Hance (208) suggest that if albumin-bound bilirubin gains access to the brain in the absence of a disrupted blood–brain barrier, it is unlikely that toxic effects will occur. Disruption of the blood–brain barrier, on the other hand, permits leakage of the albumin-bilirubin complex into the interstitium of the brain. Under these circumstances, the brain cells are exposed to the same free bilirubin concentration that exists in the serum, and the bilirubin equilibrates with binding sites on albumin and cellular membranes. If the

TABLE 38–12. *Hypothetical model of pathophysiology of bilirubin toxicity*

Site of bilirubin uptake	Effect on neurons	Duration of effect
Aggregation of bilirubin at nerve terminals ↓	Lowers membrane potentials; decreases auditory brainstem conduction ↓	Usually reversible
Bilirubin binds to cell components ↓	Impairs substrate transport, neurotransmitter synthesis, and mitochondrial functions ↓	Prevented or reversed by equimolar albumin
Retrograde uptake of bilirubin by neuronal body ↓	Dysfunction and death of neurons in acute clinical syndrome ↓	Irreversible
Pyknosis and gliosis of neurons— bilirubin staining of affected areas	Long-term clinical sequelae	Irreversible

From ref. 201.

free bilirubin concentration is sufficiently high and the reservoirs are sufficiently large, the amount of bilirubin bound to membranes might impair neuronal function.

Measurement of Free Bilirubin

Several techniques have been developed for measuring free or loosely bound bilirubin and the binding capacity and affinity of bilirubin for albumin. Acute changes in free bilirubin concentrations, however, probably are transient because there is rapid equilibration and redistribution of bilirubin between the plasma (i.e., albumin) and the tissues. Even under experimental conditions that lead to a significant increase in brain bilirubin content, the differences in free bilirubin concentrations in the serum between control and study animals is small (211).

There is a vast literature dealing with bilirubin-binding tests, but no test is currently in general use in clinical decision-making, although a relatively simple semi-automated application of the peroxidase oxidation test is in use in Japan (212). Because one molecule of albumin is capable of binding one molecule of bilirubin tightly at the primary binding site, a bilirubin–albumin molar ratio of 1 represents about 8.5 mg of bilirubin per gram of albumin. Thus, a full-term infant with a serum albumin concentration of 3 to 3.5 g/dL should be able to bind about 25 to 28 mg/dL of bilirubin (428 to 79 μmol/L). The albumin-binding capacity of sick, low-birth-weight infants is less than that of full-term infants, and their serum albumin levels often are lower. Stevenson and Wennberg (213) suggest using a factor of seven times the albumin level to predict the binding capacity of bilirubin in a healthy full-term infant and a multiple of five to six times the albumin concentration in sick, low-birth-weight infants.

Factors Affecting the Binding of Bilirubin to Serum Albumin

This subject has been reviewed in great detail (9). A few of the factors are discussed here.

Fatty Acids. Free fatty acids in plasma may compete with bilirubin for its binding to albumin, but significant interference with bilirubin binding probably does not occur until molar ratios of free fatty acids to albumin (F–A) exceed 4:1 (9).

The infusion of 1 g/kg of intralipid over a 15-hour period in infants of fewer than 30 weeks of gestation produced an F–A ratio of less than 3 and minimal increases in unbound bilirubin concentrations (214). With doses of 2 to 3 g/kg, however, higher ratios were found. Intravenous fat, given as a continuous infusion of 2 g/kg/d for 7 days to infants of 32 weeks or less of gestation (mean birth weight 1,200 g) produced F-A ratios of only 0.1 to 1.8 (215).

pH. The binding of bilirubin to albumin is unaffected by changes in the serum pH (216,217). Nevertheless, the correction of neonatal acidosis in 11 sick newborns appeared to decrease the serum free bilirubin concentration as measured by a peroxidase technique (218). The role of pH, on the other hand, may be pivotal in determining the binding of bilirubin to cells and, therefore, its deposition in the central nervous system (200,219).

Drugs. The effect of numerous drugs on bilirubin–albumin binding has been tested *in vitro* using different methods. The measured effect varies with the method used; some systems require much greater concentrations of the drug than others to demonstrate an increase in unbound bilirubin. Robertson and colleagues (220) reviewed the bilirubin displacing effect of drugs used in neonatology. They arbitrarily chose to consider an increase in the free bilirubin concentration of 5% as potentially dangerous, and they consider a drug to be a potential displacer if it occupies 5% or more of the available albumin. Knowledge of the usual peak serum bilirubin concentrations and the percentage of albumin-bound drug also can be used to calculate the concentration of bound drug. If the bound drug concentration is less than 15 μmol/L, it is unlikely that this drug will cause significant displacement of bilirubin (220).

Robertson and colleagues (220) calculated a maximal displacement factor, δ, from the K_D value, using the following equation:

$$\delta = K_D d + 1,$$

where d is the concentration of free drug in the patient's plasma, and K_D is the displacement constant, which represents the competitive effect of the drug with bilirubin for albumin binding. If K_D is 0, then $\delta = 1$, and the drug does not displace bilirubin. If $\delta = 1.2$, there has been a 20% increase of free bilirubin concentration after drug administration. Although an arbitrary value of 1.2 has been suggested as the upper permissible limit for bilirubin displacement, it is recommended that, as much as possible, drugs with the lowest δ values be selected. Appendix H–4 lists the effects of drugs used in neonatology on bilirubin–albumin binding. The free drug concentration is calculated from the serum concentration and the percentage of bound drug as taken from existing data in the literature.

Robertson et al. (221) also evaluated the effect of drug combinations on bilirubin–albumin binding. This is important because drug combinations are commonly administered to sick neonates, and the data show that the bilirubin-displacing effect of these combinations cannot be predicted from each drug's effect. For example, the administration of aminophylline with vancomycin increased the displacing effect when compared with either drug alone, but the overall effect was still minimal. In the absence of published data, drugs should be selected in which therapeutic concentrations are much lower than the usual concentration of albumin (about 2.8 mg/dL in a very-low-birth-weight newborn infant). Drugs should be selected that are not bound to albumin. Simultaneous treatment with several drugs should be limited as much as possible (221).

Other Competing Anions. It is possible that certain unidentified anions interfere with the albumin binding of bilirubin. Evidence for this is suggested by the failure of exchange transfusion to alter significantly the albumin binding of infants' serum, even though the exchange transfusion removes bilirubin, replaces much of the infant's serum albumin with bilirubin-free albumin, and lowers the free bilirubin level (222). Anions that interfere with albumin binding may not be removed by exchange transfusion.

Clinical Status of the Infant. A relation may exist between bilirubin-binding capacity and the clinical condition and gestational age of the infant. In some studies, very premature infants were able to bind less bilirubin per mole of albumin than were more mature infants (223, 224). However, no relation was found between bilirubin-binding ability and gestational age in other studies (225, 226).

Hyperbilirubinemia and Brain Bilirubin Levels

Under normal circumstances, there is a constant influx and efflux of bilirubin in and out of the brain. However, under experimental conditions, regardless of how much bilirubin is infused, it is difficult to get it to stay in the brain of healthy animals or to produce electrical central nervous system changes (227,228). Gross staining of the brain and electrophysiologic changes, however, occur readily in asphyxiated animals and in those subjected to perturbations of the blood–brain barrier or of bilirubin–albumin binding (227,230–235).

Genetic factors may be involved in determining the susceptibility of patients to bilirubin-induced neurotoxicity. For example, in different strains of Gunn rats exposed to similar bilirubin and albumin concentrations, there were significant differences in susceptibility to kernicterus and mortality, suggesting that genetic or other factors may be important in determining individual susceptibility to bilirubin toxicity (236).

Blood–Brain Barrier

A blood–brain barrier exists that limits the entry of certain substances into the central nervous system. This barrier, at the cerebral blood vessels, is due to a continuous lining of endothelial cells connected by tight junctions that restrict intercellular diffusion. The blood–brain barrier normally excludes most water-soluble substances and proteins but is permeable to lipid-soluble substances that are not protein bound. Large molecules, such as albumin, are excluded from the brain but may enter when the brain is made permeable by the infusion of a hypertonic solution (208,230,235).

Opening of the blood–brain barrier allows albumin-bound bilirubin to bathe the neurons, but whether or not free bilirubin binds to albumin or to cellular membranes may be determined by the binding of bilirubin to albumin (208). At some point, sufficient tissue binding occurs to impair neuronal function. This can be documented by changes in the electroencephalogram (208). It is likely that disruption of the blood–brain barrier and the level of free bilirubin are important in the pathogenesis of bilirubin toxicity.

Lipid Solubility

Lipid-soluble substances that are not protein bound and gases, such as carbon dioxide and oxygen, cross the blood–brain barrier easily, by simple diffusion, whereas water-soluble substances, proteins, and polar compounds (i.e., ions) do not.

Factors Affecting Blood–Brain Barrier Permeability

Anoxia, hypercarbia, and hyperosmolality open the blood–brain barrier and increase the deposition of bilirubin and albumin in the brain, producing neurophysiologic and biochemical changes as well as changes in brain physiology and energy metabolism (219,237). Thus, opening of the blood–brain barrier is likely to be one important mechanism in the pathogenesis of kernicterus, although other mechanisms undoubtedly exist. For example, during hypercarbia, the increased bilirubin that is deposited in the brain is predominantly in the unbound form, although some is also albumin bound (211,233). The regional deposition of bilirubin in the brain of piglets occurs in areas where hypercarbia produces the greatest increase in regional blood flow (233). Respiratory acidosis increases bilirubin deposition in the brain but metabolic acidosis does not (232,233).

Effect of Maturity on Blood–Brain Barrier Permeability. Is the blood-brain barrier of the neonate more permeable to bilirubin and albumin than in older children or adults? The immature brain demonstrates greater passive permeability between the blood and central nervous system for lipid-insoluble molecules (238). Studies in newborn piglets have shown that the blood–brain barrier is more permeable to bilirubin in 2-day-old than in 2-week-old piglets, whereas the permeability to albumin does not change (239). Others have found that albumin transfer into the brain of newborn Gunn rats decreases with age (240).

Mechanisms by which Bilirubin Enters the Brain

Bratlid (219) has provided a schematic presentation of possible mechanisms of bilirubin entry into the brain, its binding to neuronal cell membranes, and the potential clinical signs that may follow (Fig. 38–12). Under normal

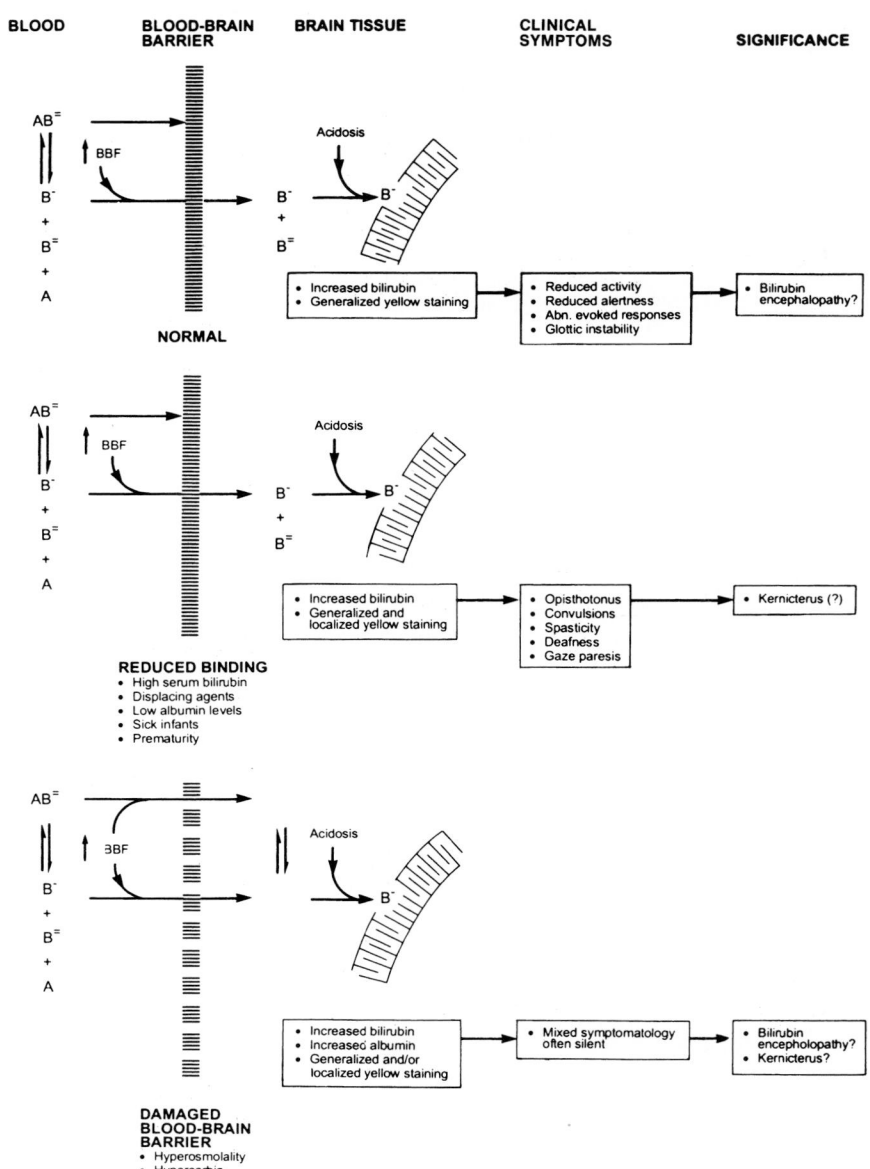

FIG. 38–12. Possible mechanisms for bilirubin entry into the brain and binding to neuronal cell membranes. The different factors affecting this process are indicated. A, albumin; AB-, albumin–bilirubin complex; B-, bilirubin monoanion; B2-, bilirubin dianion; BBF, brain–blood flow. (From ref. 219.)

circumstances, bilirubin enters the brain. Clinical confirmation of this fact is provided by the observation that modest elevations of serum bilirubin can produce clinical and electrophysiologic alterations in healthy full-term infants. Such infants demonstrate changes in behavior, characteristics of the cry, and changes in the brainstem auditory evoked response (BAER). These changes reverse as the bilirubin level decreases (241).

The second mechanism for bilirubin entry into the brain occurs when there is a marked increase in the serum level of unbound bilirubin. In the unbound state, bilirubin readily enters the brain and has the potential to produce kernicterus. Finally, bilirubin bound to albumin can enter the brain through a disrupted blood–brain bar-

rier. Even in the presence of a damaged blood–brain barrier, however, on a molar basis, more bilirubin than albumin is deposited in the brain (211,230-232). In all these situations, acidosis increases deposition of bilirubin in brain cells.

Oxidation of Bilirubin in the Brain

Mitochondria in the brain and other tissues contain a highly specific bilirubin oxidase that converts bilirubin to biliverdin and other nontoxic products (242,243). Local breakdown of bilirubin also may have a role in determining the distribution and detoxification of bilirubin in the brain (242,243).

CLINICAL FEATURES OF BILIRUBIN ENCEPHALOPATHY

Acute Bilirubin Encephalopathy or Kernicterus

In classic kernicterus, markedly jaundiced infants progress through three fairly distinct clinical phases (244–246). In the first few days, the infant becomes lethargic and hypotonic, and sucks poorly. Later in the first week, the second phase evolves. The infant becomes hypertonic and frequently develops a fever and a high-pitched cry (246). The hypertonia involves the extensor muscle groups, and most infants exhibit backward arching of the neck (i.e., retrocollis) and trunk (i.e., opisthotonus). The fever may be due to diencephalic involvement. In the third phase, usually after 1 week, hypertonia subsides and is replaced by hypotonia. Infants who manifest hypertonia during the second phase invariably develop the clinical features of chronic bilirubin encephalopathy (244,245). Van Praagh (245) found that those who were consistently neurologically normal during the first week of life never developed the features of chronic encephalopathy, but other investigators found later evidence of brain damage in some infants in whom no, or equivocal, manifestations of kernicterus were apparent in the newborn (244,247,248).

Chronic Bilirubin Encephalopathy

Temporal Evolution

There is a typical temporal evolution of chronic bilirubin encephalopathy after neonatal erythroblastosis fetalis (249). In the first year, infants typically feed poorly, develop a high-pitched cry, and are hypotonic but have increased deep tendon reflexes, a persistent tonic neck reflex, and motor delay. There is a delay in acquisition of motor skills, although most infants walk alone by 5 years of age. The other typical features of chronic bilirubin encephalopathy usually are not apparent before 1 year of age and often not for several years (246). These children generally are hypotonic at rest for the first 6 or 7 years. By the time they reach their teens, hypertonia has replaced hypotonia (250).

Clinical Features

The classic sequelae of posticteric encephalopathy constitute a tetrad consisting of extrapyramidal disturbances, auditory abnormalities, gaze palsies, and dental dysplasia (250).

Extrapyramidal Disturbances

Athetosis (i.e., involuntary, sinuous, writhing movements) may develop as early as 18 months but may be delayed as late as 8 or 9 years (249). If sufficiently severe, athetosis may prevent useful limb function. These movements are described as "uncontrollable, purposeless, involuntary and incoordinate. They may be rapid and jerky (choreiform), slow and worm-like (orthodox athetosis) or so slowed by hypertonicity that the patient may assume momentarily fixed attitudes with stiffness of the extremities (dystonia)" (250). Occasionally, extrapyramidal rigidity may predominate, rather than involuntary motion. In the opinion of Perlstein (250), "the absence of athetosis or of other forms of extrapyramidal dyskinesia, makes the diagnosis of post-icteric encephalopathy dubious, if not untenable." Severely affected children also may have dysarthria, facial grimacing, drooling, and difficulty chewing and swallowing.

Auditory Abnormalities

Some degree of hearing loss is often found in children with chronic bilirubin encephalopathy. Pathologic studies and studies of BAER indicate that injury to the brainstem, specifically the cochlear nuclei, is the principal cause of hearing loss, although occasional studies suggest possible involvement of the peripheral auditory system as well (189,212,251,252). It is noteworthy that in some frequently quoted studies, virtually all of the infants who developed severe hearing loss had received prophylactic streptomycin (an ototoxic antibiotic) prior to exchange transfusion (247,253).

Hearing loss is generally most severe in the high frequencies, and an association between moderate hyperbilirubinemia and subsequent sensorineural hearing loss has been described in low-birth-weight infants (see section on Clinical Sequelae of Hyperbilirubinemia).

Gaze Abnormalities

Limitation of upward gaze and other gaze abnormalities occur, and that full vertical eye movements during the doll's-eye maneuver are attained in most affected children suggests that the lesion is above the level of the oculomotor nuclei (190). Some patients have paralytic gaze palsies. Supranuclear palsies can be explained by bilirubin deposition and neuronal injury in the rostral midbrain, and nuclear palsies can be explained by damage to the oculomotor nuclei (189).

Dental Dysplasia

About 75% of children with posticteric encephalopathy have some degree of dental enamel hypoplasia. A smaller percentage have green discoloration of the teeth (250).

Magnetic Resonance Imaging

The diagnosis of kernicterus can now be confirmed by magnetic resonance imaging (179,254,255). The most characteristic image is a bilateral, symmetric, high-intensity signal in the globus pallidus seen on both T1- and T2-weighted images (Fig. 38–13). High signal intensity also

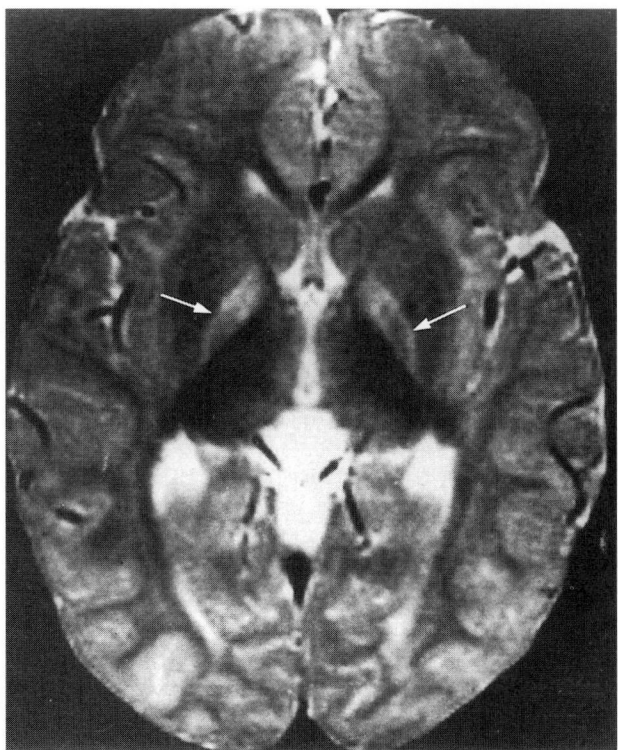

FIG. 38–13. Magnetic resonance imaging scan of a 21-month-old male infant who had erythroblastosis fetalis and presented with extreme hyperbilirubinemia and clinical signs of kernicterus at age 54 hours. Note the symmetric, abnormally high-intensity signal from the area of the globus pallidus on both sides *(arrows)*. (From ref. 255.)

has been seen in the hippocampus and the thalamus (179). We do not know how early these changes will occur and whether or not they are seen in every case. They have been seen in an 8-day-old infant as well as a 12-year-old child with a history of severe neonatal jaundice (179,254).

CLINICAL SEQUELAE OF HYPERBILIRUBINEMIA

Hsia and colleagues (256) and Mollison and Cutbush (257) first established the link between bilirubin levels and brain damage in the early 1950s, when they demonstrated that the risk of kernicterus in infants with Rh hemolytic disease increased dramatically with rising bilirubin levels and that exchange transfusion could markedly reduce the risk. Subsequent studies suggested that, in untreated infants with hemolytic disease, the incidence of kernicterus was much higher than the incidence in markedly jaundiced infants without hemolytic disease (258,259). For many years, there has been considerable disagreement about how jaundice in infants without hemolytic disease should be treated (178,259–263). Some

investigators described clinical and pathologic kernicterus in premature infants who did not have hemolytic disease and whose TSB levels were well below 20 mg/dL (342 µmol/L) (264). In some small, sick infants, yellow staining of the brain was seen at autopsy, with TSB levels less than 10 mg/dL (171 µmol/L) (264). In addition, the finding that gross bilirubin staining of the brain can occur in the absence of the typical microscopic neuronal damage described with kernicterus called into question the meaning of yellow staining of the brain in some very-low-birth-weight infants (193). Unlike the classic form of fatal kernicterus, these very-low-birth-weight infants, although they may have had kernicterus, died of other causes.

Starting in 1967 and continuing into the late 1970s, reports from the CPP, a study of 53,000 pregnant women and their offspring linked moderate elevations of neonatal serum bilirubin to lower developmental scores, lower IQ scores, and increased risk of neurologic abnormalities (265). These findings occurred at levels of bilirubin previously presumed to be safe and suggested that acute bilirubin encephalopathy or classic kernicterus was only the most obvious and extreme manifestation of a spectrum of bilirubin toxicity. At the other end of the spectrum might lie more subtle forms of neurotoxicity that occurred at much lower bilirubin levels and in the absence of any obvious abnormal clinical findings in the neonatal period.

Rh Hemolytic Diseases of the Newborn

In the only controlled clinical trial conducted on the treatment of hemolytic disease of the newborn, Mollison and Walker (266) demonstrated beyond reasonable doubt that exchange transfusion in these infants improved their chance of survival and decreased the risk of fatal kernicterus. The results of these studies, combined with subsequent uncontrolled observations, established exchange transfusion as the standard treatment for preventing kernicterus in infants with erythroblastosis fetalis and showed that kernicterus was unlikely to occur if TSB levels were kept below 20 mg/dL (342 µmol/L), an observation that has been amply confirmed by subsequent experience with the treatment of hemolytic disease (256,257).

As a complication of hemolytic disease, clinical kernicterus has largely disappeared in the western world and, because Rh disease is largely preventable, there is no reason to consider any change in this approach. It is interesting to recall, however, that these studies were performed on infants born in the late 1940s and early 1950s. These infants were commonly asphyxiated and seriously ill, and many were delivered prematurely to prevent stillbirth. Streptomycin was frequently administered to those who received exchange transfusions.

Hsia et al. (256) reported that the incidence of kernicterus in their infants was 8% for those with TSB levels of 19 to 24 mg/dL (325 to 410 µmol/L), 33% for TSB levels of 25 to 29 mg/dL (428 to 496 μmol/L), and 73% for those with bilirubin levels higher than 30 mg/dL (513 μmol/L). Later experience with Rh hemolytic disease was far more encouraging. Johnston et al. (247) studied 129 infants born between 1957 and 1958, all of whom had *indirect* serum bilirubin levels higher than 20 mg/dl (342 μmol/L). Ninety-two infants with Rh hemolytic disease were followed to age 5 to 6 years and evaluated with detailed phychometric, neurologic, and audiologic evaluations. One of 92 infants had a minimal sensorineural hearing loss (and a normal IQ) and one infant had mild athetosis, moderate sensorineural hearing loss, and a normal IQ. Thus, the risk of bilirubin encephalopathy in infants with Rh disease born from 1957 to 1958 with indirect bilirubin levels higher than 20 mg/dL (342 μmol/L) was 2 of 92 or approximately 2% (247).

In a recent study of full-term Turkish infants, those who had Coombs-positive ABO incompatibility or Rh immunization had an increase in risk of neurologic abnormalities and lower IQ scores when their indirect bilirubin levels exceeded 20 mg/dL (342 μmol/L). The median value for this population was 22.0 mg/dL (372 μmol/L) and the range 20 to 48 mg/dL (342 to 820 μmol/L). In contrast, bilirubin levels in excess of 20 mg/dL (342 (mol/L) in infants without hemolytic disease did not have these effects (267). These data appear to reinforce the belief that hemolysis is an important risk factor in bilirubin-dependant brain damage. The risk of neurologic abnormalities also was associated with the duration of indirect hyperbilirubinemia higher than 20 mg/dL (342 μmol/L). In those exposed to these bilirubin levels for less than 6 hours, the incidence of neurologic abnormalities was 2.3%. This increased to 18.7% if the exposure lasted 6 to 11 hours and to 26% with 12 or more hours of exposure (267). These data support earlier observations suggesting that the duration of hyperbilirubinemia is related to the risk of long-term neurodevelopmental outcome (268). It is difficult to define the risk of abnormal outcomes in infants with hemolysis due to causes such as red cell membrane defects and G6PD deficiency, although the risk of bilirubin encephalopathy in G6PD deficiency appears to be similar to that of Rh hemolytic disease (142).

Full-Term and Near-Term Infants without Hemolysis

There are few issues in neonatal medicine that have consistently generated such controversy as the relationship between hyperbilirubinemia and adverse developmental outcome in nonhemolyzing newborns and the indications for treating these infants. These issues have been addressed in multiple studies and the reader is referred to recent extensive reviews for details of the individual studies (258,259,265,269–271). When carefully analyzed, the data tend to demonstrate that, in otherwise healthy neonates without hemolytic disease, TSB levels

that do not exceed approximately 25 mg/dL (428 μmol/L) do not place these infants at risk of adverse neurodevelopmental consequences. Specifically, there has been no convincing demonstration of any adverse effect of such serum bilirubin levels on IQs, definite neurologic abnormalities, or sensorineural hearing loss.

No studies have looked specifically at infants 35 to 37 weeks of gestation, although the data from the very large CPP include in the study population all infants with birth weights ≥2,500 g (258,259,265). Presumably some of these infants were in the 34- to 37-week gestational age category. There are insufficient follow-up data on infants who had TSB levels of 25 to 30 mg/dL (292 to 513 μmol/L) to draw firm conclusions about this group. Nevertheless, a 21-month follow-up of 26 Coombs-negative, healthy term infants with TSB levels of 26.2 to 46.3 mg/dL (446 to 788 μmol/L) revealed no neurodevelopmental abnormalities and no hearing loss (272).

When they combined both abnormal and suspicious neurologic examination results, Newman and Klebanoff (265), in their analysis of the CPP, did demonstrate a significant increase in abnormalities associated with increasing bilirubin levels. The "suspicious" abnormalities included nonspecific gait abnormalities, awkwardness, an equivocal Babinski reflex, abnormal cremestaric refex, abnormal abdominal reflex, failure of stereognosis, questionable hypotonia, and gaze abnormalities. The most frequent abnormal findings were awkwardness and abnormal cremestaric reflexes. When the abnormal and suspiciously abnormal children were combined, the risk of abnormalities increased from 14.9% for those whose TSB levels were less than 10.0 mg/dL (171 μmol/L) to 22.4% for those whose TSB levels exceeded 20 mg/dL (340 μmol/L). Because 41,324 infants were enrolled in this study, these differences were statistically highly significant, but this finding should be kept in perspective. Even if the relationship between these findings is causal, we have no evidence that the use of a bilirubin-lowering intervention, such as phototherapy, at these low bilirubin levels would affect the outcome. Finally, as Newman and Klebanoff (265) point out, even if bilirubin levels had been prevented from exceeding 10 mg/dL (171 μmol/L) in every infant, the expected rate of abnormal or suspicious neurologic examination results would only decline from 15.13% to 14.85%.

Less reassuring information is provided by a study of a group of Israeli army draftees (n = 1,948) in which their preinduction psychological and physical examinations at age 17 years were matched with their newborn bilirubin levels. Seidman et al. (273) found an association between the risk of an IQ below 85 and a TSB level higher than 20 mg/dL (342 μmol/L) in full-term boys (but not with girls) with a negative Coombs test ($p = 0.01$). On the other hand, no association was found between bilirubin levels and mean IQ score, the risk of physical or neurologic abnormality, or hearing loss. In a more recent analysis of a similar population, however, Seidman and colleagues (274) showed a statistically significant association between increasing serum bilirubin levels and an *increase* in IQ scores!

Extreme Hyperbilirubinemia and Kernicterus

In contrast to the previous studies are the recent reports of classic kernicterus occurring in apparently healthy term and near-term newborns who did not have hemolytic disease, but who developed extreme hyperbilirubinemia (greater than 30 mg/dL [513 μmol/L]) (172,178). Every one of these infants was breast-fed, many had excessive weight loss (as a result of poor caloric intake or dehydration), and almost none were ≥40 weeks gestation. Of 21 infants reported by Brown and Johnson (178), all but one had short hospital stays and 8 were less than 37 complete weeks of gestation. These reports emphasize the importance of careful observation and surveillance of infants who are less than 38 weeks of gestation and, in particular, those who have short hospital stays. As discussed previously, short hospital stays are associated with a greater risk of readmission with severe hyperbilirubinemia, and infants with gestations below 38 weeks are at significantly greater risk of severe jaundice. Today, infants 34 to 37 weeks of gestation frequently are cared for in normal newborn nurseries, so it is often forgotten that such infants are not full term. These infants are much more likely to have difficulty nursing, poor caloric intake, and a greater weight loss than their truly term counterparts. When combined with less effective hepatic clearance, because of their prematurity, it is not surprising that they become more jaundiced.

Bilirubin-Binding Capacity and Developmental Outcome

Because bilirubin that is "free" or loosely bound to albumin is more likely to cross the blood–brain barrier (see section on Blood–Brain Barrier), the prediction of severe or mild bilirubin encephalopathy might be improved by measurement of unbound bilirubin or the reserve albumin binding capacity. A reduced albumin-binding capacity has been associated with abnormal developmental outcome in some studies (268,275) but not in others (276), although such associations have been found with abnormalities in the auditory brainstem responses (212,277,278). Currently there are no bilirubin-binding tests in routine clinical use in the United States, although a semiautomated peroxidase method has been used in Japan (212,278). Nevertheless, there are no long-term studies of the developmental outcome of infants in whom binding measurements have been obtained with this technique.

Duration of Hyperbilirubinemia

A relationship has been described between neurologic and psychometric abnormalities and the duration of exposure to TSB levels higher than 15 mg/dL (267,268, 275). Many of the infants in these studies were either premature or had hemolytic disease. In the large NICHHD collaborative phototherapy trial, a 6-year follow-up of 224 control infants who did not receive phototherapy and who had birth weights lower than 2,000 g showed no association between IQ and duration of exposure to bilirubin (279).

An 18-year follow-up of 55 boys with a history of neonatal hyperbilirubinemia (greater than 15 mg/dL [257 μmol/L]) was performed in Norway at the time of military draft physical examinations (280). Compared with the total cohort of Norwegian conscripts, there were no significant differences revealed on physical examination or tests of vision, hearing, or IQ. However, seven boys who had a history of positive Coombs tests and bilirubin in excess of 15 mg/dL (257 μmol/L) for more than 5 days had significantly lower IQ scores than the national average.

Hearing Loss and Audiometric Evoked Responses

The BAER test is an accurate and noninvasive means of assessing the functional status of the auditory nerve and the brainstem auditory pathway. The BAER tracing of a normal full-term infant is shown in Fig. 38–14. The three positive waveforms labeled in the figure are those most easily identified in the neonate. The latency for wave I represents the peripheral conduction time. Latency of waves III and V and the interpeak latency of waves I to III, III to V, and I to V all represent measurements of central conduction time. The interpeak latency I to V is referred to as the brainstem conduction time.

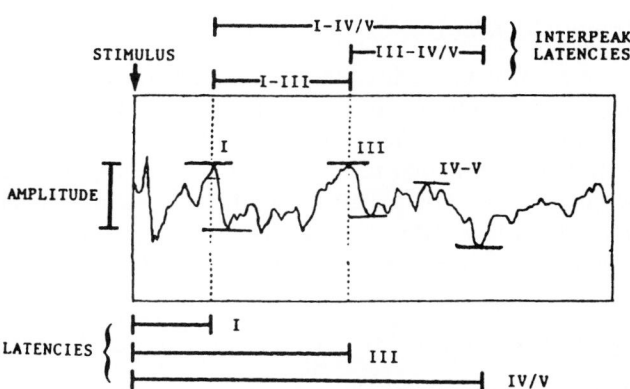

FIG. 38–14. A typical tracing of brainstem auditory evoked response has various components. Wave I reflects the response of the peripheral auditory nerve; wave III reflects the superior olive; waves IV to V reflect the inferior colliculus with peak and trough shown. Wave I peak to waves IV to V trough (i.e., interpeak latency) reflects brainstem conduction time. (From ref. 241.)

Reports also include amplitudes of the waveforms. These may decrease or be lost in response to various insults.

Several studies have documented a relationship between TSB levels and the BAER, and the acute changes seen in the BAER can be reversed by lowering the TSB level with phototherapy or exchange transfusion (241). Abnormalities of the BAER are more closely related to unbound bilirubin levels than to TSB level, but there are no studies relating abnormalities in the BAER to long-term outcome (212,278).

Despite evidence for acute bilirubin toxicity on the auditory pathway in full-term and preterm infants, there is virtually no evidence for a risk of hearing loss related to hyperbilirubinemia in full-term infants who do not have hemolytic disease (167,265,273,279). In a study of almost 17,000 children who received complete hearing evaluations at 8 years of age, the incidence of sensorineural hearing loss in those who had TSB levels 20 mg/dL or higher (342 µmol/L) was 2.2%, identical to those whose TSB levels were less than 20 mg/dL (342 µmol/L) (265). In the NICHHD phototherapy study, the incidence of sensorineural hearing loss in children followed to age 6 years was identical in the phototherapy and control groups (1.8% vs. 1.9%) (276).

Remarkably, in a follow-up of 36 children with the Crigler–Najjar syndrome, none had evidence of sensorineural hearing loss (167). Nevertheless, deficits in central hearing, speech, and language can occur in the absence of pure-tone hearing loss (270).

Cry Analysis

An abnormal cry is a sign of neurologic distress and has been associated with acute bilirubin encephalopathy (190). Modest degrees of hyperbilirubinemia also affect the infant's cry (241).

Infant Behavior

Investigators have used the Brazelton Neonatal Behavioral Assessment Scale to evaluate the effect of hyperbilirubinemia on infant behavior. Most studies show some effect, although several are confounded by the use of phototherapy (241). Jaundiced infants score lower than controls in habituation, orientation, motor performance, regulation of state, and autonomic stability (241).

Premature Infants

It is generally believed that premature infants are at greater risk of developing kernicterus or bilirubin encephalopathy than are full-term newborns exposed to similar bilirubin levels. The evidence for this, although suggestive, is not entirely convincing.

Watchko and Oski (264) have provided a detailed historical review of kernicterus in prematurity from the 1950s to the present. Reports during the years 1950 to 1965 suggested that kernicterus or the clinical sequelae of hyperbilirubinemia were unlikely to develop if exchange transfusions were used to maintain TSB levels below 18 to 22 mg/dL (308 to 376 µmol/L) (264). However, most of the infants in these studies were larger (1,250 to 2,500 g) and more mature (28 to 36 weeks of gestation) than the extremely low-birth-weight infants currently seen in NICUs.

Low-Bilirubin Kernicterus

Between 1958 and 1972, a group of studies reported the occurrence of kernicterus at TSB levels well below 20 mg/dL (342 µmol/L) (264). In general, these infants were significantly more premature and of much lower birth weight than those previously observed with kernicterus. Some were exposed to sulfisoxazole, which previously was shown in a controlled trial to be a powerful displacer of bilirubin from its binding to albumin (210). As a result of these findings, exchange transfusion in preterm infants was recommended at TSB levels of less than 20 mg/dL (342 µmol/L). Publication of data from the CPP that suggested an association between impaired psychomotor performance and TSB levels higher than 10 to 14 mg/dL (171 to 239 µmol/L) in low-birth-weight infants provided additional support for these recommendations (281,282).

In the NICHHD cooperative phototherapy study (1974 to 1976), infants were randomly assigned to a control group that received no phototherapy or to a group that received phototherapy at predetermined TSB levels. The criteria for exchange transfusion for all infants mandated exchange transfusions at low levels of serum bilirubin (10 mg/dL [171 µmol/L] in high-risk newborns with birth weights less than 1,250 g) (283). Kernicterus was found in 4 of 76 autopsied infants whose birth weights ranged from 760 to 1,270 g. Their peak TSB levels ranged from 6.5 to 14.2 mg/dL (111 to 243 µmol/L). All were asphyxiated or had hyaline membrane disease, and all had some degree of PIVH. Two had periventricular leukomalacia (PVL) (194).

Surviving infants in the study were followed and evaluated at 6 years of age with the Wechsler Verbal and Performance IQ test. No differences were found between the control and phototherapy groups in the incidence of definite and suspect cerebral palsy, clumsy or abnormal movements, hypotonia, or an IQ lower than 70. There were no differences between the two groups in growth, speech, hearing loss, or evidence of hyperactivity (279).

Scheidt and colleagues (276) also published a 6-year follow-up of 224 control children with birth weights lower than 2,000 g. None of these infants received phototherapy, but bilirubin levels were maintained below specified levels by the use of exchange transfusion. No relation was found between serum bilirubin levels and the incidence of cerebral palsy, nor was there any association between maximal bilirubin level and IQ. IQ was not associated with mean bilirubin level, time and duration of exposure to bilirubin, or measures of bilirubin–albumin binding (276).

Low-Birth-Weight Infants in the 1980s and 1990s

Two studies reviewed the risk factors previously suggested to predict the development of kernicterus. They were unable to identify any risk factor or group of factors that was associated with the development of kernicterus in the premature neonate, including birth weight less than 1,500 g, hypothermia, asphyxia, acidosis, hypoalbuminemia, sepsis, meningitis, drug therapy, and serum bilirubin levels (284,285).

It is likely that there are some risk factors for the development of kernicterus that are unknown. An excellent example of this possibility was the report from one NICU of an abrupt decrease in kernicterus at autopsy in premature infants. The incidence of kernicterus fell from 31% to 0% when the practice of flushing intravenous catheters with bacteriostatic saline that contained benzyl alcohol was stopped (286). In an earlier study from the same NICU, the incidence of kernicterus diagnosed postmortem among neonates of 25 to 32 weeks of gestation was a remarkably high 25% (189). Benzyl alcohol is an agent that increases membrane fluidity and may facilitate the passage of bilirubin into the brain (200). At the same institution, Watchko and Claasen (287) found only three cases of kernicterus in 72 autopsies performed from 1984 through 1991 on newborns of less than 34 weeks of gestation who lived at least 48 hours. This sustained decrease in the incidence of kernicterus confirms the experience in most nurseries that kernicterus in premature newborns has disappeared almost completely from the NICU. In Watchko and Claasen's population of 69 newborns who did not have kernicterus, the peak TSB level ranged from 6.3 to 20.6 mg/dL (108 to 352 μmol/L), and 56% had peak TSB values higher than those suggested for exchange transfusion by the NICHHD phototherapy study guidelines (287).

Thus, kernicterus in this population is an uncommon event, even when serum bilirubin levels are allowed to rise above those previously thought to place the premature infant at risk.

Several recent studies have failed to document an association between maximal TSB levels and developmental outcomes in very-low-birth-weight infants (288–291). van de Bor and colleagues (292) found a relation between maximal TSB concentrations in the neonatal period and cerebral palsy (not of the type characteristically found with kernicterus) at a corrected age of 2 years. No relation was found between maximal TSB concentrations and

hearing defects. However, in a follow-up of the same population at 5 years, no significant difference was found in mean maximal TSB concentrations between children with and without handicaps (288). The investigators did find, however, that children who had suffered a grade I intracranial hemorrhage were at significantly greater risk of handicap. This effect was not seen in the more severe hemorrhages, but the number of infants with severe hemorrhages was small.

Although these data are reassuring, few of the infants in the reported studies had markedly elevated bilirubin levels (288–291). Some studies have suggested an association between hyperbilirubinemia and cystic PVL in low-birth-weight infants (293–295), but others have not found this (291). Despite the associations described (all from multiple significance testing with the resultant possibility of spurious conclusions), it is unlikely that hyperbilirubinemia is causally related to cystic PVL. PVL is primarily an ischemic lesion, most likely caused by hypoperfusion of the periventricular white matter. Bilirubin normally is not deposited in the periventricular region and primarily is toxic to neurons and not the glial elements that predominate in the periventrcicular white matter.

There is little doubt that kernicterus is currently a very rare event in premature infants hospitalized in NICUs. This may be the result of overall improvements in care or of the fairly aggressive use of phototherapy. Certainly phototherapy, if used appropriately (see section on Phototherapy) is capable of controlling the bilirubin levels in almost all low-birth-weight infants, with the possible exception of the occasional infant with severe erythroblastosis fetalis or marked bruising. Thus, today exchange transfusions are rare events in most NICUs.

Hyperbilirubinemia and Pulmonary Hemorrhage

Studies from the late 1940s and early 1950s suggested an association between pulmonary hemorrhage and kernicterus (296,297). All of the infants described died of severe erythroblastosis fetalis. We know that these infants were profoundly anemic, had marked hypoalbuminemia, thrombocytopenia, and disturbances of coagulation, and occasionally were hydropic. It is not surprising that some of these infants developed hemorrhagic pulmonary edema. In an autopsy series of low-birth-weight infants with kernicterus, pulmonary hemorrhage was not found more frequently in the kernicteric infants when compared with those who did not have kernicterus (210). In animal studies, the infusion of bilirubin led to circulatory collapse and anoxia and an increased incidence of hemorrhage, including pulmonary hemorrhages (228). On the other hand, kernicteric Gunn rats showed a significantly lower prevalence of pulmonary hemorrhage when compared with nonkernicteric animals, although the kernicteric group had significantly higher bilirubin levels (298).

LABORATORY MEASUREMENTS OF BILIRUBIN

This subject was reviewed in detail by Sykes and Epstein (299) and most recently by Doumas and Eckfeldt (300). A summary of the available clinical laboratory methods is provided in Table 38–13. Although this is one of the most commonly performed laboratory measurements in the newborn and despite many advances in clinical chemistry, the measurement of serum bilirubin concentration remains remarkably inaccurate. Repeated surveys over the last 3 decades have disclosed a high level of interlaboratory variation in the measurements of both total and direct serum bilirubin concentrations in neonatal sera. In a recent study, a sample with a known TSB concentration of 14.8 mg/dL (243 µmol/L) was analyzed in 14 different university hospital laboratories. The mean (±SD) measured TSB was 15.2 ± 2.5 mg/dL (coefficient of variation 16.4%) and the range 12.1 to 18.5 mg/dL (207 to 316 µmol/L) (97). This remarkably wide range of values in skilled hands suggests that considerable caution is necessary before generalizing bilirubin levels from one institution to the wider universe of newborns. Within-laboratory variation generally is considered to be lower, but in the study of Vreman et al. (97), over time, the coeffecient of variation for repeated measurements of the same sample was as high as 17.2% in one laboratory (97).

These remarkably high variations between laboratories might explain the frequent observation in clinical practice where an infant is admitted for treatment of hyperbilirubinemia because of a high serum bilirubin level in an outside laboratory. When repeated in the hospital laboratory, the bilirubin level may be 5 or 6 mg/dL (85 to 103 µmol/L) lower. Of course, there is no way of knowing which of these two values is correct. A 16.4% coefficient of variation between laboratories means that if the true serum bilirubin value is 20 mg/dL (342 µmol/L), the 95% confidence limits of a repeat measurement at another laboratory could fall anywhere between 14.4 and 26.6 mg/dL (246 to 455 µmol/L). These observations are quite worrying and, because follow-up, surveillance, and intervention in jaundiced infants are based on serum bilirubin values, spurious underestimation of the serum bilirubin concentration might lead to withholding of necessary therapy, and overestimation will produce unnecessary clinical intervention.

TABLE 38–13. *Summary of clinical laboratory methods for analysis of total bilirubin and its fractions in serum*

Method	Bilirubin fractions available	Results obtained by	Examples of instrument type	Comments
Diazo	Total Direct Indirect	Measurement Measurement Calculation	Multiple automated instruments	Most commonly used method: well accepted for quantification of total bilirubin. Direct bilirubin assay dependent on reaction conditions, especially pH, and often underestimates conjugated bilirubin, which leads to inaccuracies in indirect bilirubin. With appropriate reference ranges, methods in most cases remain clinically acceptable.
Direct spectrophotometry	Total	Measurement	Bilirubinometer Paramax (Baxter) ACA (DuPont)	Only use during first 14–21 d of life as carotenes, etc., increase with age and cause interference. Often called "neonatal bilirubin."
Reflectance spectrophotometry	Total Conjugated Unconjugated Delta (δ) Neonatal	Measurement Measurement Measurement Calculation Calculation	Kodak Ektachem Series	DT-60 performs only total bilirubin. Generally, good correlation between fractions (by Ektachem) and HPLC results.
HPLC	Unconjugated (α) Monoconjugated (β) Diconjugated (γ) Delta (δ)	 Measurement	 HPLC	Not available as routine laboratory method, but considered good reference for bilirubin fractions.
Bilirubin oxidase	Total	Measurement	Dri-stat assay (Beckman) available on many automated instruments	Not commonly used; direct assay not available from Beckman. Correlates well with Ektachem. Probably measures δ-bilirubin.

HPLC, high-pressure liquid chromotography.
From ref. 299.

Similar concerns exist with regard to measurements of direct-reacting or conjugated bilirubin where laboratory measurements are considered, at best, "only an approximation to the true value" (301). In a recent study, measurements of direct-reacting bilirubin using the Dupont ACA or Coulter Dacos analyzer produced direct-reacting bilirubin levels in a population of full-term newborns at one hospital that were twice as high as those measured in a similar population at another institution, where a Kodak Ektachem 700 method was used (135). The Ektachem method measures *conjugated bilirubin*, whereas the other methods measure *direct-reacting bilirubin*. Although used synonymously, direct reacting is not the same as conjugated bilirubin. Direct-reacting bilirubin refers to the bilirubin that reacts directly with diazotized sulfanilic acid (i.e., without the addition of an accelerating agent), whereas conjugated bilirubin refers to bilirubin that has been made water soluble by binding with glucuronic acid in the liver.

Site of Blood Sampling

Data regarding the differences in TSB levels when measured in capillary or venous samples are conflicting (302,303). It is useful to recall, however, that virtually all of the data on TSB levels published in the literature were obtained from capillary samples; therefore, for the purposes of clinical decision-making, capillary blood samples remain the gold standard.

Sampling Technique

Because of the well-known effects of light on bilirubin, laboratory manuals recommend that blood samples be protected from light until the serum is analyzed. Using serum samples with bilirubin levels of 16.0, 11.8, and 7.9 mg/dL (273, 202, and 135 μmol/L), Sykes and colleagues

(304) found that, under the usual laboratory conditions, there was no measurable effect of ambient light on serum bilirubin levels for at least 8 hours.

TREATMENT

Mechanisms and Principles

Hyperbilirubinemia can be treated by exchange transfusion, which removes bilirubin mechanically; phototherapy, which converts bilirubin to products that can bypass the liver's conjugating system and be excreted in the bile or in the urine without further metabolism; and pharmacologic agents that interfere with heme degradation and bilirubin production, accelerate the normal metabolic pathways for bilirubin clearance, or inhibit the enterohepatic circulation of bilirubin. Phototherapy is the most common treatment in use for hyperbilirubinemia; exchange transfusions generally are reserved for phototherapy failures. The bilirubin level at which intervention is necessary is still a contentious issue.

The background to treatment decisions for hyperbilirubinemia has been provided (see section on Bilirubin Toxicity). The basic principles underlying the recommendations given in Tables 38–14 and 38–15 (see also Table 38–17) are as follows:

Healthy full-term infants without hemolytic disease are at a low risk of bilirubin toxicity unless their hyperbilirubinemia is extreme (generally ≥30 mg/dL [513 μmol/L]).

Because of the tremendous changes in obstetric and neonatal care in the past 40 years, the existing data on the use of exchange transfusion in hemolytic disease may not be applicable to infants in the 1990s.

Evidence for treatment efficacy is lacking for many infants.

Treatment is not free of risk.

TABLE 38–14. *Management of hyperbilirubinemia in the healthy term and near-term newborn*

	TSB level [mg/dL (μmol/L)]			
Age (h)	Consider phototherapy[a]	Phototherapy	Exchange transfusion if intensive phototherapy fails[b]	Exchange transfusion and intensive phototherapy
≤24[c]	—	—	—	—
25–48	≥12 (205)	≥15 (260)	≥20 (340)	≥25 (430)
49–72	≥15 (260)	≥18 (310)	≥25 (430)	≥30 (510)
>72	≥17 (290)	≥20 (340)	≥25 (430)	≥30 (510)

[a]Phototherapy at these TSB levels is a clinical option, meaning that the intervention is available and may be used on the basis of individual clinical judgment.

[b]Intensive phototherapy should produce a decline of TSB of 1 to 2 mg/dL within 4–6 h, and the TSB level should continue to fall and remain below the threshold level for exchange transfusion. If this does not occur, it is considered a failure of phototherapy.

[c]Term infants who are clinically jaundiced at ≤24 h old are not considered healthy and require further evaluation.

TSB, total serum bilirubin.
Adapted from ref. 105.

TABLE 38–15. *Approaches to the prevention and treatment of jaundice associated with breast-feeding*

Prevention
1. Encourage frequent nursing (i.e., at least eight times per day)
2. Do not supplement with water or dextrose water

Treatment options
1. Observe
2. Discontinue nursing, substitute formula
3. Alternate feedings of breast milk and formula
4. Discontinue nursing, administer phototherapy
5. Continue nursing, administer phototherapy

There is a problem with the first principle listed. Except in the most obvious circumstances (i.e., major blood group incompatibility with a rapidly rising bilirubin level), it is difficult, and sometimes impossible, to rule out an underlying hemolytic process. Standard diagnostic tests for hemolysis, such as the reticulocyte count, hematocrit, or examination of the peripheral smear, are neither sensitive nor specific. Nevertheless, today, the overwhelming majority of full-term and near-term infants with significant elevations of their serum bilirubin do not have hemolytic disease (61,70,71,305). The possibility of G6PD deficiency must be considered in areas where this condition is prevalent and in certain ethnic groups (see Chap. 45). These infants usually are not anemic and cannot be distinguished from the normal population by measurements of hematocrit or reticulocyte count (139,306).

Risks

When used properly, phototherapy is a very effective and safe method of lowering the serum bilirubin concentration. Its use has drastically decreased the need for exchange transfusion and has contributed to the virtual disappearance of kernicterus in the low-birth-weight infant.

On the other hand, in full-term and near-term newborns, phototherapy can lead to separation of the mother and infant, increase parental concern, decrease the likelihood of successful breast-feeding, and adversely affect the mother–infant relationship (307). At a time when pediatricians are trying to promote breast-feeding in the face of considerable odds (e.g., early discharge from hospital, the rapid return of mothers to the work force, commercial marketing of formulas), attention should be given to an intervention that has a negative impact on the nursing mother.

The risk of exchange transfusion includes risks from the transfused blood and from the procedure. Blood bank screening procedures have reduced the risk of human immunodeficiency virus infection and hepatitis significantly, but this risk is never zero. In experienced hands, the risk of the procedure is about 2 to 3 deaths per 1,000 procedures overall (308–310); however, this risk can be much higher in sick, low-birth-weight infants (287,311). Experience with exchange transfusion is decreasing, and with new types of phototherapy and other interventions in immune hemolytic disease, it is likely to decrease even further (312–316). It is now common for a resident to complete a 3-year pediatric training program without ever having performed an exchange transfusion. Under the circumstances, the mortality and morbidity for this procedure is likely to increase in the years ahead.

Full-Term and Near-Term Newborns

Most infants who are treated for neonatal jaundice have no identifiable pathology and no evidence of hemolytic disease (41,61,70,71). About 90% are fully or partially breast-fed (71). Guidelines for the treatment of full-term and near-term infants are given in Table 38–14. These guidelines were originally developed by the AAP for newborns of ≥37 weeks of gestation, but there are many infants at 34 to 36 weeks of gestation who are cared for in well-baby nurseries and managed no differently from those of 37 weeks of gestation. Some clinicians may prefer to use slightly lower TSB levels for intervention with phototherapy and/or exchange transfusions for infants who are 35 to 36 weeks of gestation. This is a matter of individual judgment.

No formal review of the compliance with, or efficacy of, the AAP guidelines has been carried out, but there is little doubt that if all significantly jaundiced infants were identified and these guidelines followed, essentially no cases of kernicterus would occur. One of the key differences between the AAP's practice parameter and previous guidelines is that the practice parameter contemplates exchange transfusion *only when intensive phototherapy fails* (see section on Phototherapy), unless the first TSB obtained is in excess of 30 mg/dL (513 µmol/L). Even in the face of such extreme hyperbilirubinemia, by the time blood has been obtained and typed and cross-matched for an exchange transfusion, intensive phototherapy might have reduced the TSB by as much as 10 mg/dL (171 µmol/L), in which case a decision might be made to withhold the exchange transfusion (317). In virtually every case of kernicterus reported over the last decade, the TSB level has far exceeded those at which the AAP guidelines call for intervention (140,141,172,178,179,184). Dr. William Robertson (318), who chaired the subcommittee responsible for producing the AAP's practice parameter, recently reflected on these guidelines and writes:

> How does the 1994 practice parameter on management of hyperbilirubinemia in the healthy term newborn appear through the retrospectoscope in 1998? Naturally, I am biased, but it looks good, given its purpose of providing guidance, *not certainty.* A guideline is similar to the white lines on both sides of the highway; we all try to stay between those white lines, except when unusual circumstances such as a flat tire make us pull off the road and outside the lines to attend to the crisis.

One criticism of the AAP practice parameter is that, although it is intended to provide guidelines for intervention in healthy infants, the bilirubin levels chosen for phototherapy suggest that the infants may not, in fact, be healthy. This is particularly so for bilirubin levels in the early portion of the time periods 25 to 48 hours and 49 to 72 hours. For example, the guidelines recommend phototherapy when the bilirubin level is ≥15 mg/dL (260 µmol/L) in a 25- to 48-hour-old infant (see Table 38–14), But a TSB of 15 mg/dL (260 µmol/L) at 26 hours is far above the 95th percentile and is even greater than the 95th percentile for a 48-hour-old infant (see Fig. 38–9) (100). The same can be said for a TSB of 18 mg/dL (310 µmol/L) at 49 to 72 hours and 20 mg/dL (340 µmol/L) at greater than 72 hours. Thus, although these treatment levels are quite appropriate, by definition, infants who qualify for treatment may not be healthy and may have an underlying component of increased bilirubin production or inadequate bilirubin clearance, or both. Such infants merit investigation for the cause of their hyperbilirubinemia.

Breast-Fed Infants

Of infants who develop bilirubin levels high enough to require phototherapy and who do not have evidence of isoimmunization or other obvious hemolytic disease, 80% to 90% are fully or partially breast-fed (41,71). Table 38–15 suggests an approach to the prevention and treatment of jaundice associated with breast-feeding. Observational studies show that increasing the frequency of breast-feeding during the first few days after birth decreases TSB levels (182,183,319). We performed a controlled trial in which mothers were randomly assigned to a frequent or demand breast-feeding schedule. We found no significant difference between the TSB levels measured in the two groups at an average age of 55 hours (320). Given the natural history of jaundice in breast-fed infants, however, it is certain that maximum bilirubin levels had not yet been achieved in these infants. On the other hand, the observational data of Yamauchi and Yamanouchi (183) show a very strong inverse and linear relationship between the frequency of nursing in the first 24 hours and the probability of hyperbilirubinemia on day 6.

In many hospitals it is a common practice to provide supplemental feedings of water or dextrose water to breast-fed infants in the mistaken belief that this will lower their TSB levels. On the contrary, this practice consistently *increases* TSB levels and should be abandoned (321,322). Furthermore, Kuhr and Paneth (323) found that an increase in dextrose water intake in the first 3 days of life was significantly related to a decrease in breast-milk intake on the fourth day (323).

When the TSB in a breast-fed infant reaches a level at which intervention is being considered, a number of options exist (see Table 38–15). Two randomized controlled trials evaluated some of these interventions. When TSB levels reached 15 mg/dL (257 µmol/L), Amato et al. (324) compared the effect of interrupting breast-feeding versus phototherapy. There was no difference between the groups in the amount of time needed to reduce the bilirubin to less than 12 mg/dL (205 µmol/L). In a controlled clinical trial, Martinez and colleagues (325) compared the effect of four different interventions on hyperbilirubinemia in 125 full-term breast-fed infants (Table 38–16). When the serum bilirubin level reached 17 mg/dL (291 µmol/L), the infants were assigned at random to one of the four interventions. The results are shown in Table 38–16. Although discontinuing breast-feeding and using phototherapy was the most effective strategy, in neither the study of Amato et al. nor Martinez et al. was intensive phototherapy used (326). Although it seems reasonable to offer the mother a choice of the interventions listed in Table 38–15, we believe that any interruption of nursing is undesirable and, unless very severe hyperbilirubinemia is present (TSB levels in excess of 25 mg/dL [428 µmol/L]),

TABLE 38–16. *Effect of interventions for jaundice in breast-fed infants[a]*

	Group			
	1	2	3	4
	Continue breast-feeding	Discontinue breast-feeding, substitute formula	Discontinue breast-feeding, substitute formula, use phototherapy[b]	Continue breast-feeding, use phototherapy
No.	25	26	38	36
Serum bilirubin ≥20 mg/dL (342 µmol/L)	6 (24%)	5 (19%)	1 (3%)[c]	5 (14%)

[a]When the serum bilirubin reached 17 mg/dL (291 µmol/L), infants were randomly assigned to one of four interventions.
[b]Standard, not intensive, phototherapy.
[c]Significantly different versus group 1 (*p* = 0.013) and group 2 (*p* = 0.036).
From ref. 325.

it is our practice to recommend that breast-feeding be continued while the infant is treated with intensive phototherapy (see section on Phototherapy) (326).

Low-Birth-Weight Infants

Table 38–17 provides suggested guidelines for the management of hyperbilirubinemia in low-birth-weight infants. Over the last decade, there has been a remarkable decrease in the incidence of kernicterus found by autopsy in infants who died in NICUs. Some of this may be due to the liberal use of phototherapy. Certainly, phototherapy has dramatically decreased the necessity for exchange transfusion, which, in low-birth-weight infants, is now almost exclusively carried out in the occasional infant with severe Rh hemolytic disease or extensive bruising. In a cohort of 833 infants with birth weights between 500 and 1,500 g born in North Carolina between 1985 and 1989, only two infants (0.24%) underwent exchange transfusion (290). As discussed previously, the validity of previously used criteria for exchange transfusion in the low-birth-weight population has been questioned and, with the introduction of more effective means of administering phototherapy to low-birth-weight infants, much of the debate regarding exchange transfusion in this population has become moot (287). Furthermore, exchange transfusion at low bilirubin levels is very inefficient and is less effective than phototherapy in achieving prolonged reduction of bilirubin levels in infants with nonhemolytic jaundice (327).

As shown in Table 38–17, phototherapy generally is used according to a sliding scale—the lower the birth weight, the lower the TSB level at which phototherapy is instituted. Although this practice is followed widely, there is little evidence to support it. In view of the known antioxidant properties of bilirubin, it is possible that maintaining very low TSB levels by the aggressive use of phototherapy might have other, less desirable consequences (289).

Bilirubin is a powerful antioxidant and thus may exert a protective effect against oxidant injury (92). One such injury is retinopathy of prematurity, and several studies have evaluated the relationship between TSB levels in very-low-birth-weight infants and the development of retinopathy of prematurity (289,328–332). Yeo et al. (289) found a significant association between visual loss due to retinopathy of prematurity and peak serum bilirubin concentrations less than 160 μmol/L (9.4 mg/dL), although others have not found this (328–332). Such observations do raise concerns about the aggressive use of phototherapy in extremely low-birth-weight infants, particularly those at 23 to 26 weeks of gestation who are most susceptible to the development of retinopathy of prematurity. A controlled clinical trial is necessary to settle this important question.

Special Circumstances

For term, near-term, and very-low-birth-weight infants, special circumstances may exist that require a more aggressive approach to treatment than provided in Tables 38–14 and 38–17. Table 38–18 lists some of the conditions that may modify intervention for hyperbilirubinemia.

Elevated Direct-Reacting or Conjugated Bilirubin Levels

There are no helpful data and, as a result, little guidance on how we should deal with the occasional infant who has a high TSB as well as a significant elevation of direct-reacting bilirubin. Because direct-reacting bilirubin is not toxic to the central nervous system, some authors have suggested guidelines for exchange transfusion based on the level of indirect serum bilirubin level only. More recently, however, most guidelines have either ignored the subject or have referred to TSB levels as the criteria for treatment.

TABLE 38–17. *Approaches to the use of phototherapy and exchange transfusion in low-birth-weight infants[a]*

Birth weight (g)	Total bilirubin level [mg/dL (μmol/L)[b]]	
	Phototherapy[c]	Exchange transfusion[d]
<1,500	5–8 (85–140)	13–16 (220–275)
1,500–1,999	8–12 (140–200)	16–18 (275–300)
2,000–2,499	11–14 (190–240)	18–20 (300–340)

[a]Note that these guidelines reflect ranges used in neonatal intensive care units. They cannot take into account all possible situations. In some units, prophylactic phototherapy is used for all infants who weigh <1,500 g. Higher intervention levels may be used for small-for-gestational-age infants, based on gestational age rather than birth weight.

[b]Consider initiating therapy at the these levels. Range allows discretion based on clinical conditions or other circumstances (see Table 38–18).

[c]Used at these levels and in therapeutic doses, phototherapy should, with few exceptions, eliminate the need for exchange transfusion.

[d]Levels for exchange transfusion assume that bilirubin continues to rise or remains at these levels despite intensive phototherapy (see section on Phototherapy).

TABLE 38–18. *Conditions that may modify intervention for hyperbilirubinemia*

Immediate exchange transfusion
  Clinical signs of bilirubin encephalopathy

Earlier or prophylactic phototherapy due to increased procedural risk of morbidity and mortality or technical difficulty in performing exchange transfusion
  Serious complication with previous exchange transfusions
  Serious cardiovascular, coagulation, or other disease
  Potential graft-versus-host reaction (e.g., acquired or inherited immunodeficiencies, mother exposed to immunosuppressive agents)
  Inability to use umbilical vessels (e.g., abdominal surgery, omphalocele)

Earlier phototherapy or exchange transfusion due to possible increased risk of bilirubin toxicity
  Serum bilirubin rising more than 1 mg/dL (17 µmol/L) per hour
  Serum albumin <2.5 mg/dL
  Reduced bilirubin-binding capacity, if measured
  Persistent, severe, metabolic or respiratory acidosis[a]
  Persistent, severe hypercapnia[a]
  Persistent, severe hypoxemia[a]
  Sepsis
  Very sick low-birth-weight infants

[a]Attempt to correct blood gas abnormality.

Kernicterus has been well described in infants who have elevated TSB levels but in whom the indirect-reacting bilirubin was well below 20 mg/dL (342 µmol/L) (255,333). One infant had the bronze baby syndrome, and another was a 54-hour-old male infant with erythroblastosis fetalis whose TSB level was 45.2 mg/dL (773 µmol/L), of which 31.6 mg/dL (540 µmol/L) was direct reacting. Thus, the total indirect bilirubin in this infant was only 13.6 mg/dL (255). We have seen the records of other similar cases. Kernicterus in these infants may be the result of competitive displacement (by direct-reacting bilirubin) of unconjugated bilirubin from its binding site to albumin or perhaps an elevation in delta bilirubin, preventing adequate binding of unconjugated bilirubin.

Ebbesen (334) found that infants with elevated direct bilirubin levels of 6.4 to 9.9 mg/dL (109 to 169 µmol/L) and the bronze baby syndrome had a decrease in reserve albumin binding capacity. On the other hand, some infants with extremely high, but predominantly direct-reacting, serum bilirubin levels have come to no harm. A common recommendation is that the direct bilirubin concentration should not be subtracted from the total bilirubin level unless it exceeds 50% of the TSB concentration. This course of action would not have prevented kernicterus in the infant described by Grobler and Mercer (255).

Hemolytic Disease

As discussed previously, infants with hemolytic disease appear to be at a greater risk of developing bilirubin encephalopathy than are nonhemolyzing infants with similar TSB levels. The reasons for this are not clear. In the early studies of Rh disease, almost all infants were delivered prematurely (to prevent stillbirth); many were asphyxiated and severely ill. It is unlikely that the risk of kernicterus in infants with Rh disease, treated in today's intensive care environment and with similar TSB levels, would be nearly as great. Although it has been suggested that infants with hemolytic disease may have a decrease in their bilirubin-binding capacity, when measured, this has not been found to be the case (335). Similarly, we have no obvious explanation for the increased risk of bilirubin encephalopathy in infants with G6PD deficiency.

In almost all cases of Rh hemolytic disease, phototherapy should be used quite early, as soon as there is evidence of a rapidly rising TSB level. In ABO hemolytic disease, on the other hand, an early rising TSB frequently levels off and declines spontaneously, and phototherapy often is unnecessary (127). Nevertheless, a reasonable rule of thumb for ABO hemolytic disease is to institute phototherapy at TSB levels 1 to 2 mg/dL (17 to 34 µmol/L) below those given in Tables 38–14 and 38–17. If, despite intensive phototherapy, serum bilirubin levels approach 18 to 20 mg/dL (308-342 µmol/L) in any infant with hemolytic disease, exchange transfusion should be considered.

Intravenous immunoglobulin (IVIG) has been used successfully in Rh and ABO hemolytic disease (313). In controlled trials, it has been shown to reduce the need for exchange transfusions (314,316). The use of tin and zinc-mesoporphyrin has decreased TSB levels in infants with Coombs-positive ABO incompatibility and G6PD deficiency (see section on Pharmacologic Treatment) (336, 337).

Early studies of the natural history of Rh and ABO hemolytic disease provided fairly accurate predications of whether or not the serum bilirubin concentration would reach 20 mg/dL (342 µmol/L). As a result, rules of thumb were developed for exchange transfusion based on cord blood TSB levels and on TSB levels at different ages. The use of intensive phototherapy and IVIG has rendered these guidelines largely irrelevant. If, despite intensive phototherapy and the use of IVIG, the serum bilirubin level continues to rise, or if it rapidly approaches 18 to 20 mg/dL (308 to 242 µmol/L), then an exchange transfusion is indicated.

Repeat Exchange Transfusions

In general, the criteria for repeat exchange transfusions are similar to those used for the initial exchange.

Hydrops Fetalis

The pathogenesis of hydrops fetalis, with its attendant edema and serous effusions, is not clear. It commonly occurs when the fetal hemoglobin drops below 6 to 7 g/dL. The rapid production of severe anemia in fetal sheep produced hydrops associated with an increased central venous pressure and placental edema, whereas the same degree of anemia produced over a longer period did not result in hydrops, placental edema, or an increased central venous pressure (338). In Rh isoimmunization, fetal edema may result from the extensive erythropoiesis that takes place in the fetal liver. This can disrupt the portal circulation and impair albumin synthesis (339,340). Fetuses with severe hydrops also have elevated concentrations of atrial natriuretic factor (341). Hypoxia produces myocardial dysfunction with increased umbilical venous pressure that leads to the release of atrial natriuretic factor (342). Severely affected infants die of progressive cardiorespiratory failure, in which asphyxia and hyaline membrane disease play a major role.

In one hydropic fetus with erythroblastosis fetalis, pulsed-Doppler studies of left and right ventricular outputs were obtained over time. Despite severe anemia, cardiac outputs were normal and remained normal after *in utero* percutaneous intravascular transfusions, which reversed the hydrops. These measurements of normal cardiac output *in utero* suggest that high-output failure due to anemia is not the mechanism for hydrops in these infants and supports the hypothesis that portal hypertension and disruption of normal liver function from extramedullary hematopoiesis is the primary mechanism for the development of hydrops in isoimmune hemolytic disease of the fetus (343).

Hydropic infants generally suffer significant hypoxia *in utero*. Women who are to deliver such infants should be managed exclusively in perinatal centers capable of the full range of obstetric and neonatal intensive care. Hydropic infants and those who are severely anemic (hematocrit less than 35%) and asphyxiated require immediate treatment. Exchange transfusion of about 50 mL/kg of packed cells soon after birth raises the hematocrit to about 40%. Phlebotomy should not be routinely performed on these infants because they usually are normovolemic and may be hypovolemic (343–345). No manipulations of blood volume should be performed without appropriate measurements of central venous and arterial blood pressures. For accurate monitoring of central venous pressure, however, the umbilical venous catheter must enter the inferior vena cava by way of the ductus venosus. If the catheter is in a portal vein or the umbilical vein, the pressures so measured are meaningless and preclude interpretation of the infant's circulatory status. In addition, before making therapeutic decisions based on measurements of central venous pressure, the physician must also correct acidosis, hypercarbia, hypoxia, and anemia. Serum glucose levels should be monitored carefully, because hypoglycemia is common.

Exchange Transfusion

Edwards et al. (346) reviewed the basic indications for, and contraindications to, performing exchange transfusions. They also provide a detailed description of the necessary equipment, technique, and known complications of this procedure. A few issues will be discussed here. The prevention of Rh hemolytic disease with Rh immune globulin and the more effective use of phototherapy has led to a dramatic decline in the number of exchange transfusions performed. As discussed previously, it is quite possible for a pediatric resident to complete a 3-year training program without ever having performed an exchange transfusion. As fewer and fewer of these procedures are done, it is quite likely that the risks of complications will increase. The overall mortality has been reported to be about 0.3 per 100 procedures, and significant morbidity (apnea, bradycardia, cyanosis, vasospasm, respiratory arrest, pulmonary edema, cardiac arrest) occurs in 1 to 5 per 100 procedures. In term and near-term infants who are relatively well, the risk of death is low (308,310,311). Jackson (311) reported a 15-year experience (1980 to 1995) of exchange transfusion in 106 infants. Eighty-one were healthy, and there were no deaths in these infants, although one child developed severe necrotizing enterocolitis requiring surgery. There were 25 sick infants, 3 (12%) of whom had serious complications from the exchange transfusion and 2 (8%) died. There were three additional deaths that were considered "possibly due" to the exchange transfusion. Thus, the total number of deaths in sick infants, possibly due to the exchange, was 5 of 25 (20%). Although the risk is very low, exchange transfusion nevertheless carries the usual risk of any blood product. The risk estimates (risk per tested unit) for transfusion transmitted viruses in the United States for the period from 1991 to 1993 were as follows: human immunodeficiency virus 1:493,000; human T-cell lymphotropic virus 1:641,000; hepatitis C virus 1:103,000; and hepatitis B virus 1:63,000 (347).

Bilirubin Dynamics during Exchange Transfusion

During exchange transfusion, bilirubin from the extravascular space is drawn into the plasma, and partial equilibration between extravascular and plasma bilirubin occurs almost instantaneously (348). Thus, by the end of the exchange, in which only 13% of the circulating erythrocytes remain, the serum bilirubin is still 45% of the preexchange level. Immediately after the exchange, further equilibration takes place, which is completed within 30 minutes and produces the early rebound of plasma bilirubin to 60% of the preexchange level (348).

Phototherapy

The most comprehensive reference source for phototherapy is the 1993 monograph by Jährig et al. (349), to which the reader is referred for more detailed information and additional references.

TABLE 38–19. *Factors that determine the dose of phototherapy*

Spectrum of light emitted
Irradiance of light source
Design of phototherapy unit
Surface area of infant exposed to the light
Distance of infant from light source

Terminology

It helps to understand how phototherapy works if we consider that light is an infusion of discrete photons of energy that correspond to the individual molecules of a drug in a conventional medication. Absorption of these photons by bilirubin molecules in the skin leads to the therapeutic effect in much the same way as binding of drug molecules to a receptor has a desired effect. There are five major factors that influence the dose and, therefore, the efficacy of phototherapy. These factors are listed in Table 38–19. Table 38–20 defines the radiometric quantities used in assessing the dose.

Light Spectrum

The spectrum of light delivered by the phototherapy unit is determined by the type of light source and any filters used. Because of the optical properties of bilirubin and skin, the most effective lights are those with wavelengths that are predominantly in the blue-green spectrum (350).

There is a common misconception that ultraviolet (UV) light is used for phototherapy. None of the light systems described emit any significant amount of UV radiation, and the small amount of UV light that is emitted by fluorescent tubes is in longer wavelengths than those that cause erythema. In any case, almost all UV light produced is absorbed by the glass wall of the fluorescent tube and by the plexiglass cover of the phototherapy unit.

Irradiance

There is a direct relationship between the efficacy of phototherapy and the irradiance used (Fig. 38–15) (351).

Irradiance is directly related to the distance between the light and the infant (Fig. 38–16) (326). The irradiance in a specific wavelength band is called the spectral irradiance and is expressed as $\mu W/cm^2/nm$ (see Table 38–20). Commercial radiometers measure the irradiance in a predetermined band and display the results as a spectral irradiance ($\mu W/cm^2/nm$). To do this they divide the irradiance by the width of the wavelength band. Thus, under a particular light, a radiometer might measure an irradiance of 400 $\mu W/cm^2$ in the 400- to 480-nm band (width of 80 nm) and provide a readout of the spectral irradiance of $400/80 = 5$ $\mu W/cm^2/nm$. A different radiometer (under the same light) measuring in the 425- to 475-nm band (a width of 50 nm) would display a spectral irradiance of 400/50 or 8 $\mu W/cm^2/nm$. This makes it difficult to compare published data on spectral irradiance measurements, because different radiometers and different phototherapy systems have been used.

The Relationship between Irradiance and the Distance between the Infant and the Light Source

Figure 38–16 shows that the light intensity (measured as spectral irradiance) is inversely related to the distance from the source.

The relationship between intensity and distance is almost (but not quite) linear, indicating that these data do not obey the law of inverse squares, which states that the light intensity will decrease with the square of the distance (326).

Spectral Power

This is the product of the skin surface irradiance and the spectral irradiance across this surface area. Because irradiance and the surface area of the infant exposed to phototherapy are key elements in determining the efficacy of phototherapy, the use of spectral power is the only meaningful way to compare the dose of phototherapy received by infants under the different phototherapy systems (326). Calculations of spectral power show why a much more effective dose of phototherapy is delivered to the infant by using the appropriate fluorescent tubes than can be delivered using a fiberoptic phototherapy system (326).

TABLE 38–20. *Radiometric quantities used*

Quantity	Dimensions	Usual units of measure
Irradiance (radiant power incident on a surface per unit area of the surface)	W/m^2	W/cm^2
Spectral irradiance (irradiance in a certain wavelength band)	W/m^2 per nm (or W/m^2)	$\mu W/cm^2$ per nm
Spectral power (average spectral irradiance across a surface area)	W/m	mW/nm

From ref. 326.

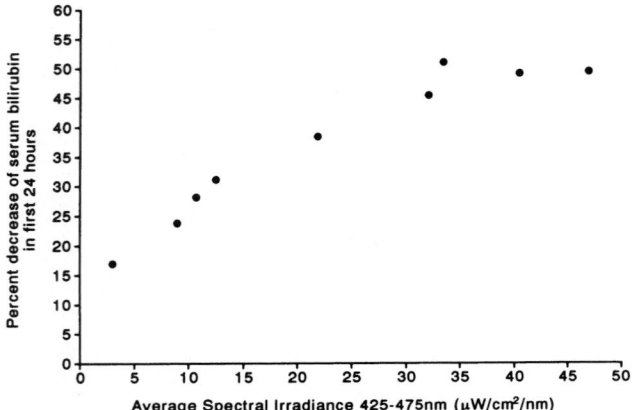

FIG. 38–15. Relationship between average spectral irradiance and decrease in serum bilirubin concentration. Full-term infants with nonhemolytic hyperbilirubinemia were exposed to special blue light (Phillips TL 52/20W) of different intensities. Spectral irradiance was measured as the average of readings at the head, trunk, and knees. Drawn from the data of Tan (351). (From ref. 326.)

Mechanism of Action

Phototherapy detoxifies bilirubin by converting it to photoproducts that are less lipophilic than bilirubin and can bypass the liver's conjugating system and be excreted without further metabolism (2). It is not known exactly where the process of phototherapy takes place, but it probably does not take place in the skin cells. It is more

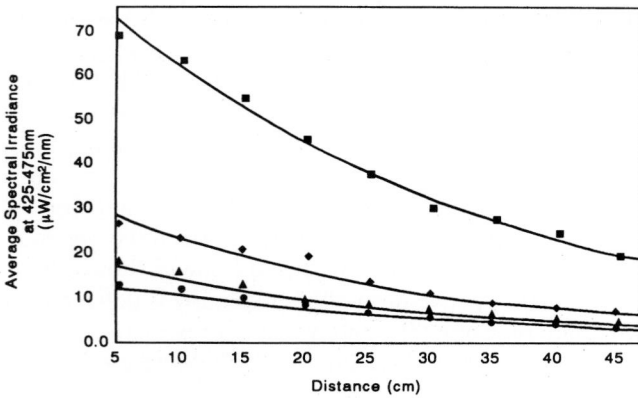

FIG. 38–16. Effect of light source and distance from the light source to the infant on average spectral irradiance. Measurements were made across the 425- to 475-nm band using a commercial radiometer (Olympic Bilimeter Mark II). The phototherapy unit was fitted with eight 24-inch fluorescent tubes. (■) Special blue, General Electric 20-W F20T12/BB tube; (♦) blue, General Electric 20-w F20T12/B blue tube; (▲) daylight blue, four General Electric 20-W F20T12/B blue tubes and four Sylvania 20-W F20T12/D daylight tubes; (•) daylight, Sylvania 20-W F20T12/D daylight tubes. Curves were plotted using linear curve fitting (True Epistat; Epistat Services, Richardson, TX). The best fit is described by the equation $y = Ae^{BX}$. (From ref. 326.)

likely that it works on bilirubin bound to albumin in the superficial capillaries or in the interstitial space (352).

Bilirubin Photochemistry

When bilirubin absorbs light, photochemical reactions occur. Although many such reactions have been observed *in vitro*, only three have been shown to occur *in vivo* during phototherapy.

Configurational (Z→ E) Isomerization

Isomers are substances that have the same molecular formula but different physicochemical properties. There are four possible configurational isomers of bilirubin (Fig. 38–17). In infants receiving phototherapy, the stable 4Z,15Z isomer is converted predominately to the 4Z,15E isomer (Figs. 38–17 and 38–18) (2). The formation of 4Z,15E bilirubin is spontaneously reversible in the dark and occurs rapidly in bile. Thus, the 4Z,15E bilirubin formed in the skin and excreted by the liver is readily converted back to ordinary unconjugated bilirubin. The conversion of the 4Z,15Z isomer to the 4Z,15E isomer is also reversible by light (2).

When infants are exposed to phototherapy, photoisomerization occurs almost instantaneously, but the clearance of the light-generated 4Z,15E isomer is very slow ($T^{1}/_{2} \sim 15$ hours). Thus, although configurational isomerization is extremely rapid and accounts for the bulk of the photochemical outcomes, it probably plays only a minor role in lowering the serum bilirubin concentration because "although it is formed fastest, it has nowhere to go" (353).

Structural Isomerization

In this reaction (Fig. 38–19), intramolecular cyclization of bilirubin (an irreversible process) occurs in the presence of light to form a substance known as lumirubin that can be excreted in bile (without the need for conjugation) and in urine (but at a much lower rate than in bile)

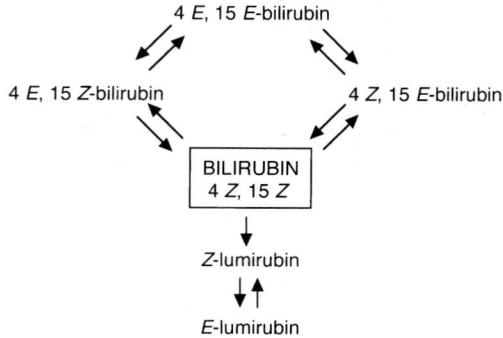

FIG. 38–17. Configurational and structural isomers of 4Z, 15Z bilirubin in infants undergoing phototherapy.

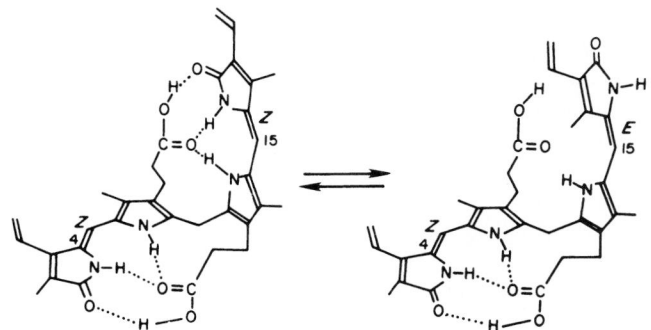

FIG. 38–18. Z-E carbon–carbon double-bond configurational isomerization of bilirubin in humans. (From ref. 2.)

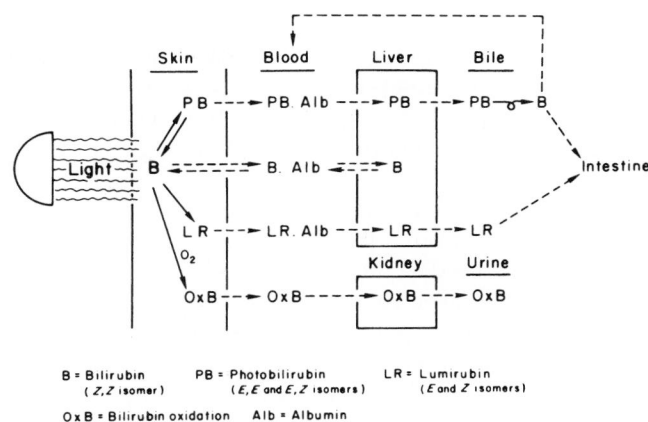

FIG. 38–20. General mechanisms of phototherapy for neonatal jaundice. Chemical reactions *(solid arrows)* and transport processes *(broken arrows)* are indicated. Pigments may be bound to proteins in compartments other than blood. Some excretion of photoisomers, particularly lumirubin, in urine also occurs. (From ref. 2.)

(353). During phototherapy, the serum concentration of lumirubin is about 2% to 6% of the TSB, which is much lower than the concentration of the configurational isomers that form about 20% of the total bilirubin. However, because lumirubin is cleared from the serum much more rapidly than the 4Z,15E isomer, it is likely that lumirubin formation is mainly responsible for the phototherapy-induced decline in serum bilirubin in the human infant (353). It is quite possible, however, that the contribution of the other isomers, 4E,15Z and 4E,15E bilirubin, also is important (354).

Photooxidation

Bilirubin can be photooxidized to water-soluble, colorless products that can be excreted in the urine. This is a slow process, however, and is probably only a minor contributor to the elimination of bilirubin during phototherapy.

Figure 38–20 summarizes the general mechanisms of phototherapy in neonatal jaundice.

Clinical Use and Efficacy

There are more than 50 published controlled trials of the clinical use of phototherapy (see Maisels [40] for a description and analysis of these studies), confirming that phototherapy is effective in preventing and treating

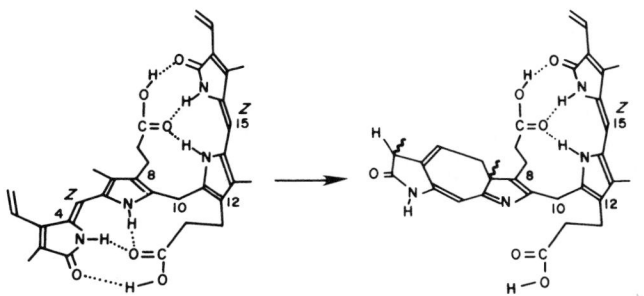

FIG. 38–19. Intramolecular cyclization of bilirubin in the presence of light to form lumirubin. (From ref. 2.)

hyperbilirubinemia and dramatically reduces the need for exchange transfusion (40).

Dose–Response Relationship

As described previously, there is a clear relationship between the dose of phototherapy and the measured decrement in the serum bilirubin level (see Fig. 38–15) (351). The factors that determine the dose are shown in Table 38–19. The other important factor is the initial bilirubin level, the rate of decline being proportional to the initial bilirubin concentration (355).

Types of Light

Fluorescent Tubes. Although daylight or cool white fluorescent tubes can provide adequate phototherapy where the objective is to control a slowly rising serum bilirubin level in a preterm or term infant, they are much less effective than "special blue" tubes (see Fig. 38–16). Special blue fluorescent tubes provide much more irradiance in the blue spectrum than other commercially available tubes and are the most effective light source currently available in the United States for phototherapy (see Fig. 38–16) (326,353). They are labeled F20-T12/BB (General Electric, Westinghouse) or TL52/20W (Phillips). Note that these are different from regular blue tubes (labeled F20-T12/B) (353). Because these tubes generally are used to treat healthy full-term infants readmitted to the hospital because of severe hyperbilirubinemia, the fact that these tubes give the infants a bluish tinge (and thus may obscure cyanosis) should be of little concern. When used in the NICU, monitoring by pulse oxymetry will be reassuring.

Halogen Lamps. These lamps have the advantage of being more compact than fluorescent systems but, unlike fluorescent lamps, *they cannot be brought close to the infant (to increase the irradiance) without incurring the risk of a burn.* In addition, the surface area covered by most halogen lamps is relatively small, and the spectral power will be less than that produced by a bank of fluorescent lights.

Fiberoptic Systems. These systems consist of a light that is delivered from a tungsten-halogen bulb through a fiberoptic cable and emitted from the sides and ends of the fibers inside a plastic pad (326,356). These systems have the advantage of not requiring eye patches. They are less bulky than conventional phototherapy equipment and provide a convenient way to deliver double phototherapy when it is necessary to expose more of the infant's surface area (see following). They also are useful for home phototherapy. Their major disadvantage is that they have very low spectral power because of their small surface area. This is the result of the inverse relationship between surface area and irradiance. For a given light source, enlarging the pad means that the light must be distributed over a greater area, thus reducing the irradiance (when compared to a small pad and the same light source). To achieve high levels of spectral irradiance, manufacturers must compromise by reducing the size of the pad, which exposes a relatively small surface area of the infant to the light (356).

Light-Emitting Diodes. A new method of delivering high-intensity, narrow-band light has been described recently (312,357). The use of high-intensity gallium nitride light-emitting diodes (LEDs) permits high irradiance in the spectrum of choice (blue, blue-green, etc.), with minimal heat generation. The device is low weight, low voltage, low power, and portable and could be an effective means of providing intensive phototherapy in the hospital or at home. To date, only limited clinical trials have been performed (357).

Full-Term and Near-Term Infants—Using Phototherapy Effectively

Phototherapy initially was used in low-birth-weight and full-term infants primarily to prevent slowly rising serum bilirubin levels from reaching levels that might require an exchange transfusion. Today, phototherapy most often is used in full term and near-term infants who have left the hospital and are readmitted on days 4 to 7 for treatment of serum bilirubin levels of ≥20 mg/dL (342 μmol/L). These infants need a therapeutic dose of phototherapy (sometimes termed intensive phototherapy) to get the bilirubin level down as soon as possible (317, 326). As discussed previously, the light spectrum, the irradiance, and the infant's exposed surface area are the key elements in determining the bilirubin response to phototherapy. Thus, to provide the most effective phototherapy for these full-term and near-term infants, we use special blue fluorescent tubes and bring them as close to the infant as possible. To do this, a full-term infant

should be in a bassinet, not an incubator, because the top of the incubator prevents the light from being brought sufficiently close to the infant. In a bassinet it is possible to bring the fluorescent lights within about 10 cm of the infant and to produce a spectral irradiance of more than 50 μW/cm²/nm (see Fig. 38–16). This does not overheat naked full-term infants. Note, however, that *halogen phototherapy lamps cannot be positioned closer to the infant than recommended by the manufacturers without incurring the risk of a burn.*

To increase the surface area of the infant exposed, fiberoptic pads should be placed below the infant. This type of "double phototherapy" is approximately twice as effective as single phototherapy in low-birth-weight infants and almost 50% better in full-term infants (358,359). Another way of increasing the surface area of the infant exposed to light is to place a reflecting material (a white sheet or aluminum foil) within or around the bassinet or incubator so that light is reflected onto the infant's skin. Different systems of surrounding the infant with fluorescent lights have been described (317,360, 361). Using such a system, Hansen (317) has reported declines in serum bilirubins of 10 to 11 mg/dL (170 to 185 μmol/L) within 2 hours. On occasion, we have used two or even three fiberoptic pads to cover almost the entire lower surface of the infant. Although data from Tan (351) suggest that there is a saturation point beyond which an increase in the irradiance produces no added efficacy, we do not know that a saturation point exists. Given that the conversion of bilirubin to excretable photoproducts is partly irreversible and follows first-order kinetics, there may not be a saturation point. Certainly with existing equipment there is no such thing as an overdose of phototherapy.

Preterm Infants

Conventional phototherapy with daylight or cool white fluorescent lights, halogen lamps, or fiberoptic pads have all been effective in decreasing TSB levels and the number of exchange transfusions performed in low-birth-weight infants. For those with severe bruising or hemolytic disease, however, intensive phototherapy (as described previously) should be used.

Intermittent versus Continuous Phototherapy

Clinical studies comparing intermittent with continuous phototherapy have produced conflicting results (349). In practice, on–off cycles complicate nursing care and probably are more trouble than they are worth. There is no doubt, however, that in the majority of circumstances phototherapy does not *need* to be continuous. It can and certainly should be interrupted during feeding or brief parental visits. On the other hand, when bilirubin levels are very high, intensive phototherapy should be administered continuously until a satisfactory decline in the bilirubin level has occurred.

Hydration and Feeding

Breast-fed infants who are readmitted to the hospital with high bilirubin levels commonly have excess weight loss due to a combination of mild dehydration and poor caloric intake. In these infants it makes sense to provide supplemental calories and fluids using a milk-based formula, because formulas inhibit the enterohepatic circulation of bilirubin and help to lower the bilirubin level. Because lumirubin is excreted in the urine, maintaining adequate hydration and good urine output also helps to improve the efficacy of phototherapy. Routine supplementation (with dextrose water) of all infants receiving phototherapy is not indicted.

Biological Effects and Complications

Even though phototherapy has been used in millions of infants for more than 30 years, reports of significant toxicity are exceptionally rare.

Skin

Bilirubin is a photosensitizer and, in some circumstances, could act as a photodynamic agent in the presence of light and produce damage. Severe blistering and photosensitivity during phototherapy for jaundice have been described in infants with congenital erythropoietic porphyria (362). The presence of congenital porphyria is a contraindication to the use of phototherapy. Two recent reports document the development of bullous eruptions in infants with hemolytic disease and transient porphyrinemia who received phototherapy (363,364). All of the infants had significant cholestasis (elevated direct-reacting bilirubin levels), and plasma proto- and coproporphyrin levels were elevated in the two infants in whom they were measured.

Significant accumulation of coproporphyrins has been well described in infants with the *bronze baby syndrome*, which occurs exclusively in phototherapy-exposed infants who also have cholestasis (365). An animal model of the bronze baby syndrome has been produced by ligating the common bile duct in adult Wistar rats and subjecting them to phototherapy (366).

Children with the CN-1 syndrome receiving phototherapy for 2 to 3 years often develop pigmented lesions and tanning as well as skin atrophy (367).

Eye Damage

Because light can be toxic to the retina, the eyes of infants receiving phototherapy should be protected with appropriate eye patches (368).

Other Complications

The products of photodecomposition have no direct neurotoxic effects. Although phototherapy can produce DNA strand breaks in cell cultures, there is no evidence that this occurs in humans. A relationship has been described between the use of phototherapy and the risk of patent ductus arteriosis in very-low-birth-weight infants (369,370). The possible mechanisms for this effect are not clear, but may be related to a mechanism similar to nitric oxide-induced vasorelaxation (370).

Pharmacologic Treatment

Pharmacologic agents used in the management of hyperbilirubinemia can accelerate the normal metabolic pathways for bilirubin clearance, inhibit the enterohepatic circulation of bilirubin, and interfere with bilirubin formation by either blocking the degradation of heme or inhibiting hemolysis.

Acceleration of Normal Metabolic Pathways for Bilirubin Clearance

Phenobarbital

Phenobarbital is a potent inducer of microsomal enzymes that increases bilirubin conjugation and excretion and increases bile flow. When given in sufficient doses to the mother, the infant, or both, phenobartital is effective in lowering serum bilirubin levels in the first week of life (48). However, concerns about long-term toxicity when given to pregnant women militates against its use for this purpose (371,372).

Decreasing Bilirubin Production by Inhibiting Heme Oxygenase

As illustrated in Fig. 38–1, the enzyme microsomal heme oxygenase is necessary for the conversion of heme to biliverdin, one of the first steps in the formation of bilirubin from hemoglobin. Certain synthetic metalloporphyrins are powerful competitive inhibitors of heme oxygenase and, therefore, suppress the formation of bilirubin. The inhibition of heme degradation to bilirubin does not result in the accumulation of heme, which is excreted in the bile in quantities that compensate for the decreased excretion of bilirubin (48).

In a series of controlled clinical trials, Valaes, Kappas and colleagues demonstrated that Sn-mesoporphyrin (SnMP) is a potent inhibitor of heme oxygenase and is highly effective in reducing maximum bilirubin levels and the requirements for phototherapy in preterm neonates (373). They also showed that SnMP in a dose of 6 μmol/kg was more effective than special blue light phototherapy in the treatment of term and near-term neonates with established hyperbilirubinemia. None of the neonates who received SnMP required phototherapy (374,375). SnMP was equally effective in controlling hyperbilirubinemia in infants with G6PD deficiency (337). The only side effect seen so far has been a transient, nondose-dependent erythema that disappeared without sequalae in infants who received phototherapy after SnMP administration (373). Sn-protoporphyrin and SnMP have both been used in the treatment of the Crigler–Najjar syndrome and have achieved a temporary reduction in serum bilirubin levels (163,376).

The idea of using these inhibitors of bilirubin production is very attractive. It requires no apparatus, infants do not need to be blindfolded, and there is no separation of mother from infant. To date, however, only 384 newborns have received SnMP (or Sn-protoporphyrin) in contolled trials. SnMP could be given prophylactically to every baby in the delivery room, but this is unlikely because it would expose some 4 million newborns in the United States to SnMP each year. If SnMP were used instead of phototherapy to treat established jaundice, at least 200,000 infants would receive SnMP annually, and it is possible that twice this number would receive the drug. With these numbers, the possibility of an unanticipated adverse event or complication surely would increase. Whether this form of treatment will become a substitute for (or even replace) phototherapy remains an open question. Certainly in developing countries or parts of the world where phototherapy is expensive and perhaps inaccessible and where conditions such as G6PD deficiency account for a substantial number of infants with extreme hyperbilirubinemia and kernicterus, the benefits of SnMP are more easily defined and surely outweigh the risks.

Decreasing Bilirubin Production by Inhibiting Hemolysis

The success of high-dose intravenous immunoglobulin (IVIG) therapy in children with isoimmune thrombocytopenia suggested that a similar approach might be useful in the treatment of isoimmune hemolytic disease. Controlled trials have confirmed that the administration of IVIG to infants with Rh hemolytic disease will significantly reduce the need for exchange transfusion (314–316). It also is likely that IVIG will help to mitigate the course of severe ABO hemolytic disease (377).

The doses used have ranged from 500 mg/kg given over 2 hours soon after birth to 800 mg/kg given daily for 3 days. Anti-D-coated erythrocytes are removed from the circulation through antibody-dependent lysis by cells of the reticuloendothelial system. The mechanism of action of IVIG is unknown, but it is possible that it might alter the course of Rh hemolytic disease by blocking Fc receptors, thus inhibiting hemolysis. The risks of IVIG therapy are certainly lower than those of exchange transfusion.

PHYSIOLOGIC ROLE OF BILIRUBIN

Despite its potential toxicity, bilirubin may have an important and positive physiologic role (92). Bilirubin is a powerful antioxidant *in vitro* (92). There is a positive relationship between serum bilirubin levels and antioxidant activity in term and preterm infants (378–380). There also is some suggestion of a physiologic role for bilirubin as an antioxidant in the human neonate (93,380,381). Because of the possibility that oxidative injury may play a role in the development of retinopathy of prematurity, investigators have evaluated the relationship between bilirubin levels and retinopathy of prematurity, but the results of these studies are conflicting (289,328–332,382).

REFERENCES

1. Weiss JS, Gautam A, Lauff JJ, et al. The clinical importance of protein-bound fraction of serum bilirubin in patients with hyperbilirubinemia. *N Engl J Med* 1983;309:147.
2. McDonagh AF, Lightner DA. "Like a shrivelled blood orange"—bilirubin, jaundice and phototherapy. *Pediatrics* 1985;75:443.
3. Ives NK, Gardner RM. Blood-brain barrier permeability to bilirubin in the rat: studies using intracarotid bolus injection and *in-situ* brain perfusion techniques. *Pediatr Res* 1990;27:436.
4. Onishi S, Kawade N, Itoh S, et al. Postnatal development of uridine diphosphate glucuronyl transferase activity towards bilirubin and o-aminophenol in human liver. *Biochem J* 1979;194:705.
5. Kawade N, Onishi S. The prenatal and postnatal development of UDP-glucuronyl transferase activity toward bilirubin and the effect of premature birth on this activity in the human liver. *Biochem J* 1981;196:257.
6. Dubey AP, Garg A, Bhatia BD. Fetal exposure to maternal hyperbilirubinemia. *Ind Pediatr* 1983;20:527.
7. Smith JF, Baker JM. Crigler-Najjar disease in pregnancy. *Obstet Gynecol* 1994;84:670.
8. Taylor WG, Walkinshaw SA, Farquharson RG, Fisken RA, Gilmore IT. Pregnancy in Crigler-Najjar syndrome. Case report. *Br J Obstet Gynaecol* 1991;98:1290.
9. Brodersen R. Binding of bilirubin to albumin. *CRC Crit Rev Clin Lab Sci* 1980;11:305.
10. Crawford JM, Hauser SC, Gollan JL. Formation, hepatic metabolism, and transport of bile pigments: a status report. *Semin Liver Dis* 1988;8:105.
11. Bosma PJ, Seppen J, Goldhoorn B, et al. Bilirubin UDP-glucuronosyl transferase 1 is the only relevant bilirubin glucuronodating isoform in man. *J Biol Chem* 1994;269:17960.
12. Clarke DJ, Moghrabi N, Monaghan G, et al. Genetic defects of the UDP-glucoronosyltransferase-1 (UGT1) gene that cause familial nonhaemolytic unconjugated hyperbilirubinemias. *Clin Chim Acta* 1997;266:63.
13. Bock KW, Burchell B, Dutton GJ, et al. UDP-glucuronosyl transferase activities. Guidelines for consistent interim terminology and assay conditions. *Biochem Pharmacol* 1983;32:953.
14. Rosenthal P, Blanckaert N, Cabra PM, Thaler MM. Formation of bilirubin conjugates in human newborns. *Pediatr Res* 1986;20:947.
15. Tiribelli C, Ostrow JD. New concepts in bilirubin and jaundice: report of the third international bilirubin workshop, April 6–8, 1995, Trieste, Italy. *Hepatology* 1996;24:1296.
16. Bartoletti AL, Stevenson DK, Ostrander CR, et al. Pulmonary excretion of carbon monoxide in the human infant as an index of bilirubin production. I. Effects of gestational age and postnatal age and some common neonatal abnormalities. *J Pediatr* 1979;94:952.
17. Maisels MJ, Pathak A, Nelson NM, et al. Endogenous production of carbon monoxide in normal and erythroblastotic newborn infants. *J Clin Invest* 1971;50:1.
18. Gourley GR. Pathophysiology of breast milk jaundice. In: Polin RA, Fox WW, eds. *Fetal and neonatal physiology,* 2nd ed. Philadelphia: WB Saunders, 1998:1499.

19. Gartner LM, Lee K-S, Vaisman S, et al. Development of bilirubin transport and metabolism in the newborn rhesus monkey. *J Pediatr* 1977;90:513.

20. Poland RL, Odell GB. Physiologic jaundice: the enterohepatic circulation of bilirubin. *N Engl J Med* 1971;284:1.

21. Wolkoff AW, Goresky CA, Sellin J, et al. Role of ligandin in transfer of bilirubin from plasma into liver. *Am J Physiol* 1979;236:E638.

22. Gartner LM, Lee K-S. Bilirubin binding, free fatty acids and a new concept for the pathogenesis of kernicterus. *Birth Defects* 1976;12:264.

23. Horiguchi T, Bauer C. Ethnic differences in neonatal jaundice: comparison of Japanese and Caucasian newborn infants. *Am J Obstet Gynecol* 1975;121:71.

24. Linn S, Schoenbaum SC, Monson RR, et al. Epidemiology of neonatal hyperbilirubinemia. *Pediatrics* 1985;75:770.

25. Newman TB, Easterling MJ, Goldman ES, Stevenson DK. Laboratory evaluation of jaundiced newborns: frequency, cost and yield. *Am J Dis Child* 1990;144:364.

26. Munroe M, Shah CP, Badgley R, Bain HW. Birthweight, length, head circumference and bilirubin level in Indian newborns in the Sioux Lookout Zone, Northwestern Ontario. *Can Med Assoc J* 1984;131:453.

27. Saland J, McNamara H, Cohen MI. Navajo jaundice: a variant of neonatal hyperbilirubinemia associated with breast feeding. *J Pediatr* 1974;85:271.

28. Johnson JD, Angelus P, Aldrich M, Skipper BJ. Exagerated jaundice in Navajo neonates: the role of bilirubin production. *Am J Dis Child* 1986;140:889.

29. Hardy JB, Drage JS, Jackson EC. *The first year of life: the Collaborative Perinatal Project of the National Institutes of Neurological and Communicative Disorders and Stroke.* Baltimore, MD: Johns Hopkins University Press, 1979.

30. Khoury MJ, Calle EE, Goesoef RM. Recurrence risk of neonatal hyperbilirubinemia in siblings. *Am J Dis Child* 1988;142:1065.

31. Nielsen H, Haase P, Blaabjerg J, Stryhn H, Hilden J. Risk factors and sib correlation in physiological neonatal jaundice. *Acta Pediatr Scand* 1977;76:504.

32. Diwan VK, Vaughan TL, Yang CY. Maternal smoking in relation to the incidence of early neonatal jaundice. *Gynecol Obstet Invest* 1989;27:22.

33. Knudsen A. Maternal smoking and the bilirubin concentration in the first three days of life. *Eur J Obstet Gynecol Reprod Biol* 1991;40:123.

34. Gale R, Seidman DS, Dollberg S, Stevenson DK. Epidemiology of neonatal jaundice in the Jerusulem population. *J Pediatr Gastroenterol Nutr* 1990;10:82.

35. Jones JB. The smoking disease. *Br Med J* 1971;1:228.

36. Jährig D, Jährig KS, Striets S, et al. Neonatal jaundice in infants of diabetic mothers. *Acta Paediatr Scand* 1989;360:101.

37. Stevenson DK, Ostrander CR, Cohen RS, et al. Pulmonary excretion of carbon monoxide in the human infant as an index of bilirubin production. II. Evidence for the possible effect of maternal prenatal glucose metabolism on postnatal bilirubin production in a mixed population of infants. *Eur J Pediatr* 1981;137:255

38. Widness JA, Susa JB, Garcia JF, et al. Increased erythropoiesis and elevated erythropoietin in infants born to diabetic mothers and in hyperinsulinemic rhesus fetuses. *J Clin Invest* 1981;67:637.

39. Berk MA, Mimouni F, Miodovnik M, Hertzberg V, Valuck J. Macrosomia in infants of insulin-dependent diabetic mothers. *Pediatrics* 1989;83:1029.

40. Maisels MJ. Neonatal jaundice. In: Sinclair JC, Bracken MB, eds. *Effective care of the newborn infant.* Oxford: Oxford University Press, 1992:507.

41. Maisels MJ, Gifford KL, Antle CE, et al. Jaundice in the healthy newborn infant: a new approach to an old problem. *Pediatrics* 1988;81:505.

42. Friedman L, Lewis PJ, Clifton P, Bulpitt CJ. Factors influencing the incidence of neonatal jaundice. *Br Med J* 1978;1:1235.

43. Wood B, Culley P, Roginski C, Powell J, Waterhouse J. Factors affecting neonatal jaundice. *Arch Dis Child* 1979;54:111.

44. Ferguson JE, II, Schutz TE, Stevenson DK. Neonatal bilirubin production after preterm labor tocolysis with nifedipine. *Dev Pharmacol Ther* 1989;12:113.

45. Caritis SN, Toig G, Heddinger LA, Ashmead G. A double-blind study comparing ritodrine and terbutaline in the treatment of preterm labor. *Am J Obstet Gynecol* 1984;150:7.

46. Drew JH, Kitchen WH. The effect of maternally administered drugs on bilirubin concentrations in the newborn infant. *J Pediatr* 1976;89:657.

47. Nathenson G, Cohen MI, Litt IF, McNamara H. The effect of maternal heroin addition on neonatal jaundice. *J Pediatr* 1972;81:899.

48. Valaes T, Harvey-Wilkes K. Pharmacologic approaches to the prevention and treatment of neonatal hyperbilirubinemia. *Clin Perinatol* 1990;17:245.

49. Yamauchi Y, Yamanouchi I. Difference in TcB readings between full term newborn infants born vaginally and by cesarean section. *Acta Paediatr Scand* 1989;79:824.

50. Wallace RL, Schifrin BS, Paul RH. The delivery route for very-low-birth-weight infants. A preliminary report of a randomized, prospective study. *J Reprod Med* 1984;29:736.

51. Dell DL, Sightler SE, Plauche WC. Soft cup vacuum extraction: a comparison of outlet delivery. *Obstet Gynecol* 1985;66:624.

52. Vacca A, Grant A, Wyatt G, Chalmers I. Portsmouth operative delivery trial: a comparison of vacuum extraction and forceps delivery. *Br J Obstet Gynaecol* 1983;90:1107.

53. Black VD, Lubchenco LO, Luckey DW, et al. Developmental and neurologic sequelae in the neonatal hyperviscosity syndrome. *Pediatrics* 1982;69:426.

54. Black VD, Lubchenco LO, Koops BL, Poland RL, Powell DP. Neonatal hyperviscosity: randomized study of effect of partial plasma exchange transfusion on long-term outcome. *Pediatrics* 1985;75:1048.

55. Goldberg K, Wirth FH, Hathaway WE, et al. Neonatal hyperviscosity II. Effect of partial plasma exchange transfusion. *Pediatrics* 1982;69:419.

56. Saigal S, O'Neill A, Surainder Y, Chua LB, Usher R. Placental transfusion and hyperbilirubinemia in the premature. *Pediatrics* 1972;49:406.

57. Davidson LT, Merritt KK, Weech AA. Hyperbilirubinemia in the newborn. *Am J Dis Child* 1941;61:958.

58. Knudsen A, Lebech M. Maternal bilirubin, cord bilirubin and placental function at delivery in the development of jaundice in mature newborns. *Acta Obstet Gynecol Scand* 1989;68:719.

59. Rosenfeld J. Umbilical cord bilirubin levels as a predictor of subsequent hyperbilirubinemia. *J Fam Pract* 1986;23:556.

60. Risemberg HM, Mazzi E, MacDonald MG, et al. Correlation of cord bilirubin levels with hyperbilirubinemia in ABO incompatibility. *Arch Dis Child* 1977;52:219.

61. Maisels MJ, Kring EA. Length of stay, jaundice and hospital readmission. *Pediatrics* 1998;101:995.

62. Newman TB, Escobar GJ, Branch PT, et al. Incidence of extreme hyperbilirubinemia in a large HMO. *Amb Child Health* 1997;3:203(abst).

63. Soskolne EL, Schumacher R, Fyock C, et al. The effect of early discharge and other factors on readmission rates of newborns. *Arch Pediatr Adolesc Med* 1996;150:373.

64. Frishberg Y, Zelicovic I, Merlob P, Reisner SH. Hyperbilirubinemia and influencing factors in term infants. *Isr J Med Sci* 1989;25:28.

65. Fevery J. Fasting hyperbilirubinemia: unraveling the mechanism involved. *Gastroenterology* 1997;113:1707.

66. Gärtner U, Goeser T, Wolkoff AW. Effect of fasting on the uptake of bilirubin and sulfobromophthalein by the isolated perfused rat liver. *Gastroenterology* 1997;113:1707.

67. Gourley GR, Kreamer B, Arend R. The effect of diet on feces and jaundice during the first three weeks of life. *Gastroenterology* 1992;103:660.

68. Rubatelli FF. Unconjugated and conjugated bilirubin pigments during perinatal development. IV. The influence of breast-feeding on neonatal hyperbilirubinemia. *Biol Neonate* 1993;64:104.

69. Schneider AP. Breast milk jaundice in the newborn. A real entity. *JAMA* 1986;255:3270.

70. Seidman DS, Stevenson DK, Ergaz Z, Gale R. Hospital readmission due to neonatal hyperbilirubinemia. *Pediatrics* 1995;96:727.

71. Maisels MJ, Kring E. Risk of sepsis in newborns with severe hyperbilirubinemia. *Pediatrics* 1992;90:741.

72. Auerbach KG, Gartner LM. Breast feeding and human milk: their association with jaundice in the neonate. *Clin Perinatol* 1987;14:89.

73. Maisels MJ, Gifford K, Antle CE, et al. Normal serum bilirubin levels in the newborn and the effect of breast feeding. *Pediatrics* 1986;78:837.

74. Kivlahan C, James EJP. The natural history of neonatal jaundice. *Pediatrics* 1984;74:364.
75. Maisels MJ, D'Archangelo MR. Breast feeding and jaundice in the first six weeks of life. *Pediatr Res* 1983;17:324A(abst).
76. Alonso EM, Whitington PF, Whitington SH, Rivard WA, Given G. Enterohepatic circulation of non-conjugated bilirubin in rats fed with human milk. *J Pediatr* 1991;118:425.
77. De Carvalho M, Robertson S, Klaus M. Fecal bilirubin excretion and serum bilirubin concentration in breast-fed and bottle-fed infants. *J Pediatr* 1985;107:786.
78. Yoshioka H. Development and differences of intestinal flora in the neonatal period in breast-fed and bottle-fed infants. *Pediatrics* 1983;72:317.
79. Gourley GR, Arend RA. Beta-glucuronidase and hyperbilirubinemia in breast-fed and formula-fed babies. *Lancet* 1986;1:644.
80. Wilson DC, Afrasiabi M, Reid MM. Breast-milk beta-glucuronidase and exaggerated jaundice in the early neonatal period. *Biol Neonate* 1992;61:232.
81. Cottrell BH, Anderson GC. Rectal or axillary temperature measurement: effect on plasma bilirubin and intestinal transit of meconium. *J Pediatr Gastroenterol Nutr* 1984;3:734.
82. Weisman LE, Merenstein GB, Digirol M, Collins J, Frank G, Hudgins C. The effect of early meconium evacuation on early-onset hyperbilirubinemia. *Am J Dis Child* 1983;137:666.
83. Daum F, Cohen MI, McNamara H. Experimental toxicologic studies on a phenol detergent associated with neonatal hyperbilirubinemia. *J Pediatr* 1976;89:853.
84. Wysowski DK, Flynt JW, Goldfield M, et al. Epidemic neonatal hyperbilirubinemia and use of a phenolic disinfectant detergent. *Pediatrics* 1978;61:165.
85. Moore LG, Newberry MA, Freeby GM, Crnic LS. Increased incidence of neonatal hyperbilirubinemia at 3,100 m in Colorado. *Am J Dis Child* 1984;138:157.
86. Atland PD, Parker MG. Bilirubinemia and intravascular hemolysis during acclimatization to high altitude. *Int J Biometeorol* 1977;21:165.
87. Berendsohn S. Hepatic function at high altitudes. *Arch Intern Med* 1962;109:256.
88. Barron ESG. Bilirubinemia. *Medicine* 1931;10:114.
89. Freeman J, Lesko S, Mitchell AA, Epstein MF, Shapiro S. Hyperbilirubinemia following exposure to pancuronium bromide in newborns. *Dev Pharmacol Ther* 1990;14:209.
90. Lambert GH, Muraskas J, Anderson CL, Myers TF. Direct hyperbilirubinemia associated with chloral hydrate administration in the newborn. *Pediatrics* 1990;86:277.
91. Reimche LD, Sankaran K, Hindmarsh KW, Kasian GF, Gorecki DKJ, Tan L. Chloral hydrate sedation in neonates and infants—clinical and pharmacologic considerations. *Dev Pharmacol Ther* 1989;12:57.
92. McDonagh AF. Is bilirubin good for you? *Clin Perinatol* 1990;17:359.
93. Benaron DA, Bowen FW. Variation of initial serum bilirubin rise in newborn infants with type of illness. *Lancet* 1991;338:78.
94. Saigal S, Lunyk O, Bennett KJ, Patterson MC. Serum bilirubin levels in breast- and formula-fed infants in the first 5 days of life. *Can Med Assoc J* 1982;127:985.
95. Knudsen A. Prediction of the development of neonatal jaundice by increased umbilical cord blood bilirubin. *Acta Pediatr Scand* 1989;78:217.
96. Mather A. Reliability of bilirubin determinations in icterus of the newborn infant. *Pediatrics* 1960;26:350.
97. Vreman HJ, Verter J, Oh W, et al. Interlaboratory variability of bilirubin measurements. *Clin Chem* 1996;42:869.
98. Ryan AS. The resurgence of breastfeeding in the United States. *Pediatrics* 1997;99:E12.
99. Lee K-S, Perlman M, Ballantyne M. Association between duration of neonatal hospital stay and readmission rate. *J Pediatr* 1995;127:758.
100. Bhutani VK, Johnson L, Sivieri EM. Predictive ability of a predischarge hour-specific serum bilirubin for subsequent significant hyperbilirubinemia in healthy-term and near-term newborns. *Pediatrics* 1999;103:6.
101. Natus Medical Inc., San Carlos, CA. Diagnosis of increased bilirubin production and prediction of hyperbilirubinemia > 95th percentile in near term and term infants. *Personal communication.* 1998.
102. Okolo AA, Omene JA, Scott-Emaukpor AB. Physiologic jaundice in the Nigerian neonate. *Biol Neonate* 1988;53:132.
103. Seidman, D. *Personal communication.* 1998.
104. Sackett BL, Haynes RB, Tugwell P. *Clinical epidemiology. A basic science for clinical medicine.* Boston: Little, Brown and Company, 1985.
105. American Academy of Pediatrics. Provisional Committee for Quality Improvement and Subcommittee on Hyperbilirubinemia. Practice parameter: management of hyperbilirubinemia in the healthy term newborn. *Pediatrics* 1994;94:558.
106. Madlon-Kay DJ. Recognition of the presence and severity of newborn jaundice by parents, nurses, physicians, and icterometer. *Pediatrics* 1997;100. http://www.pediatrics.org/cgi/contentest/fall/100/3/e3/.
107. Tayaba R, Gribetz D, Gribetz I, Holzman IR. Noninvasive estimation of serum bilirubin. *Pediatrics* 1998;102. http://www.pediatrics.org/cgi/content/fall/3/e28/.
108. Moyer VA, Ahn C, Sneed S. Accuracy of clinical judgment in neonatal jaundice. Program and abstracts. Ambulatory Pediatric Association, 38th Annual Meeting, New Orleans, Louisiana, 1998.
109. Ebbesen F. The relationship between the cephalo-pedal progress of clinical icterus and the serum bilirubin concentration in newborn infants without blood type sensitization. *Acta Obstet Gynaecol Scand* 1975;54:329.
110. Kramer LI. Advancement of dermal icterus in the jaundiced newborn. *Am J Dis Child* 1969;118:454.
111. Hegyi T, Hiatt M, Gertner I, et al. Transcutaneous bilirubinometry: the cephalocaudal progression of dermal icterus. *Am J Dis Child* 1981;135:547.
112. Knudsen A. The cephalocaudal progression of jaundice in newborns in relation to the transfer of bilirubin from plasma to skin. *Early Hum Dev* 1990;22:23.
113. Knudsen A. The influence of the reserve albumin concentration and pH on the cephalocaudal progression of jaundice in newborns. *Early Hum Dev* 1991;25:37.
114. Knudsen A, Broderson R. Skin colour and bilirubin in neonates. *Arch Dis Child* 1989;64:605.
115. Jacobsen J, Brodersen R. Albumin-bilirubin binding mechanism: kynetic and spectroscopic studies of binding of albumin and zanthobilirubic acid to human serum albumin. *J Biol Chem* 1983;10:6319.
116. Schumacher RE, Thornbery J, Gutcher GR. Transcutaneous bilirubinometry: a comparison of old and new methods. *Pediatrics* 1985;76:10.
117. Schumacher RE. Non-invasive measurements of bilirubin in the newborn. *Clin Perinatol* 1990;17:417.
118. Maisels MJ, Kring E. Trancutaneous bilirubinometry decreases the need for serum bilirubin measurements and saves money. *Pediatrics* 1997;99:599.
119. Stevenson DK, Vreman HJ. Carbon monoxide production in neonates. *Pediatrics* 1997;100:252.
120. Maisels MJ, Newman TB. Jaundice in full term and near-term babies who leave the hospital within 36 hours. The pediatrician's nemesis. *Clin Perinatol* 1998;25:295.
121. American Academy of Pediatrics, College of Obstetrics and Gynecology. *Guidelines for perinatal care,* 4th ed. Elk Grove Village, IL: American Academy of Pediatrics, 1997.
122. Giblet ER. Blood groups and blood transfusion. In: Braunwald E, Isselbacher KJ, Petersdordf RG, Wilson JD, Martin JB, Fauci AS, editors. *Harrison's principles of internal medicine,* 11th ed. New York: McGraw-Hill, 1987:1483.
123. Katz MA, Kanto WP, Korotkin JH. Recurrence rate of ABO hemolytic disease of the newborn. *Obstet Gynecol* 1982;59:611.
124. Ozolek J, Watchko J, Mimouni F. Prevalence and lack of clinical significance of blood group incompatibility in mothers with blood type A or B. *J Pediatr* 1994;125:87.
125. Bhutani VK, Johnson LH, Sivieri EM, Spitz DM. Neonatal bilirubin nomogram: a tool to facilitate practical application of AAP guidelines for management of hyperbilirubinemia in healthy term newborns. *Pediatr Res* 1998;43:167A.
126. Kanto WP, Marino B, Godwin AS, Bunyapen C. ABO hemolytic disease: a comparative study of clinical severity and delayed anemia. *Am J Dis Child* 1978;62:365.
127. Osborn LM, Lenarsky C, Oakes RC, Reiff MI. Phototherapy in full-term infants with hemolytic disease secondary to ABO incompatibility. *Pediatrics* 1984;74:3.
128. Quinn MW, Weindling AM, Davidson DC. Does ABO incompatibility matter? *Arch Dis Child* 1988;63:1258.
129. Serrao PA, Modanlou HD. Significance of anti-A and anti-B iso-

hemagglutinins in cord blood of ABO incompatible newborn infants: correlation with hyperbilirubinemia. *J Perinatol* 1989;9:154.

130. Leistikow EA, Collin MF, Savastano GD, et al. Wasted health care dollars. Routine cord blood type and Coombs' testing. *Arch Pediatr Adolesc Med* 1995;149:1147.

131. Maisels MJ, Kring EA. Early discharge from the newborn nursery: effect on scheduling of follow-up visits by pediatricians. *Pediatrics* 1997;100:72.

132. Chavalitdhamrong P-O, Escobedo MB, Barton LL, et al. Hyperbilirubinemia and bacterial infection in the newborn. *Arch Dis Child* 1975; 50:652.

133. Linder N, Yatsiv I, Tsur M, et al. Unexplained neonatal jaundice as an early diagnostic sign of septicemia in the newborn. *J Perinatol* 1988; 8:325.

134. Rooney JC, Hill DJ, Danks DM. Jaundice associated with bacterial infection in the newborn. *Am J Dis Child* 1971;122:39.

135. Newman TB, Hope S, Stevenson D. Direct bilirubin measurements in jaundiced term newborns: a re-evaluation. *Am J Dis Child* 1991;145: 1305.

136. Schreiner RL, Glick MR. Interlaboratory bilirubin variability. *Pediatrics* 1982;69:277.

137. Davenport M, Kerkar N, Mieli-Vergani G, et al. Biliary atresia: The King's College Hospital experience (1974–1995). *J Pediatr Surg* 1997;32:479.

138. Bainbridge R, Khoury J, Mimounie F. Jaundice in neonatal sickle cell disease: a case controlled study. *Am J Dis Child* 1988;148:569.

139. Kaplan M, Hammerman C. Severe neonatal hyperbilirubinemia: a potential complication of glucose-6-phosphate dehydrogenase deficiency. *Clin Perinatol* 1998;25:575.

140. MacDonald M. Hidden risks: early discharge and bilirubin toxicity due to glucose-6-phosphate dehydrogenase deficiency. *Pediatrics* 1995; 96:734.

141. Washington EC, Ector W, Abboud M, et al. Hemolytic jaundice due to G6PD deficiency causing kernicterus in a female newborn. *South Med* 1995;88:776.

142. Valaes T. Severe neonatal jaundice associated with glucose-6-phosphate dehydrogenase deficiency: pathogenesis and global epidemiology. *Acta Pediatr Suppl* 1994;394:58.

143. Slusher TM, Vreman HJ, McLaren D, et al. Glucose-6-phosphate dehydrogenase deficiency and carboxy hemoglobin concentrations associated with bilirubin related morbidity and death in Nigerian infants. *J Pediatr* 1995;126:102.

144. Kaplan M, Rubatelli FF, Hammerman C, et al. Conjugated bilirubin in neonates with glucose-6-phosphate dehydrogenase deficiency. *J Pediatr* 1996;128:695.

145. Kaplan M, Renbaum P, Levi-Lahad E, Hammerman C, Lahad A, Beutler E. Gilbert syndrome and glucose-phosphate dehydrogenase deficiency: a dose-dependent genetic interaction crucial to neonatal hyperbilirubinemia. *Proc Natl Acad Sci U S A* 1997;94:12128.

146. Brown WR, Boon WH. Hyperbilirubinemia and kernicterus in glucose-6-phosphate dehydrogenase deficient infants in Singapore. *Pediatrics* 1968;41:1055.

147. Gibbs WN, Gray R, Lowry M. G6PD deficiency and neonatal jaundice in Jamaica. *Br J Hematol* 1979;43:263.

148. Rajagopalan I, Katz BZ. Hyperbilirubinemia secondary to hemolysis of intrauterine intraperitoneal blood transfusion. *Clin Pediatr* 1984; 23:511.

149. Rose J, Berdon WE, Sullivan T, Baker DH. Prolonged jaundice as presenting sign of massive adrenal hemorrhage in newborn. *Radiology* 1971;98:263.

150. Wright K, Tarr PI, Hickman RO, Guthrie RD. Hyperbilirubinemia secondary to delayed absorption of intraperitoneal blood following intrauterine transfusion. *J Pediatr* 1982;100:302.

151. Epstein MF, Leviton A, Quban KCK, et al. Bilirubin interventricular hemorrhage and phenobarbital in very low birth weight babies. *Pediatrics* 1988;82:350.

152. Pasnick M, Lucey JF. Serum bilirubin in preterm infants following intracranial hemorrhage. *Pediatr Res* 1983;17:329A.

153. Amato M, Fouchere JC, von Muralt G. Relationship between peri-interventricular hemorrhage and neonatal hyperbilirubinemia in very low birth weight infants. *Am J Perinatol* 1987;4:275.

154. Bleicher MA, Reiner MA, Rapaport SA, Track NS. Extraordinary hyperbilirubinemia in a neonate with idiopathic hypertrophic pyloric stenosis. *J Pediatr Surg* 1979;14:527.

155. Wooley MM, Felsher BF, Asch MJ, et al. Jaundice, hypertrophic pyloric stenosis, and glucuronyl transferase. *J Pediatr Surg* 1974;9:359.

156. Labrune P, Myara A, Hadchouel M, et al. Genetic heterogeneity of Crigler-Najjar syndrome type I: a study of 14 cases. *Hum Genet* 1994; 94:693.

157. Blumenschein SD, Kallen RJ, Storey Petal. Familial non-hemolytic jaundice with late onset of neurological damage. *Pediatrics* 1968;42:786.

158. Chalasani N, Roy-Chowdhury N, Roy-Chowdury J, Boyer T. Kernicterus in an adult who is heterozygous for Crigler-Najjar syndrome and homozygous for Gilbert-type genetic defect. *Gastroenterology* 1997;112:2099.

159. Ahmad P, Pratt A, Land VJ, et al. Multiple plasma exchanges successfully maintained a young adult patient with Crigler-Najjar syndrome type I. *J Clin Apheresis* 1989;5:17.

160. Shevell MI, Bernard B, Adelson JW, et al. Crigler-Najjar syndrome type I: treatment by home phototherapy followed by orthotopic hepatic transplantation. *J Pediatr* 1987;110:429.

161. Fox IJ, Roy-Chowdhury J, Kaufman SS, et al. Treatment of the Crigler-Najjar syndrome type I with hepatocyte transplantation. *N Engl J Med* 1998;338:1422.

162. Chowdhury JR, Chowdhury NR, Strom SC, Kaufman SS, Horslen S, Fox IJ. Human hepatocyte transplantation: gene therapy and more? *Pediatrics* 1998;102:647.

163. Rubaletlli FF, Guerrini P, Reddi E, Jori G. Tin-protoporphyrin in the management of children with Crigler-Najjar disease. *Pediatrics* 1989; 84:728.

164. Van der Veere CN, Jansen PLM, Sinaasappel M, et al. Oral calcium phosphate: a new therapy for Crigler-Najjar disease? *Gastroenterology* 1997;112:455.

165. Rubaltelli FF, Novello A, Zancan L, et al. Serum and bile bilirubin pigments in the differential diagnosis of Crigler-Najjar disease. *Pediatrics* 1994;94:553.

166. Van der Veere CN, Sinaasappel M, McDonagh AF, et al. Current therapy for Crigler-Najjar syndrome type I: report of a world registry. *Hepatology* 1996;24:311.

167. Suresh G, Lucey JF. Lack of deafness in Crigler-Najjar syndrome type I: a patient survey. *Pediatrics* 1997;100:1.

168. Jansen PLM, Mulder GJ, Burchell B, Bock KW. New developments in glucuronidation research: report of a work shop on "glucuronidation, its role in health and disease." *Hepatology* 1992;15:532.

169. Bosma PJ, Roy-Chowdhury J, Bakker C, et al. The genetic basis of the reduced expression of bilirubin UDP-glucuronosyl transferase 1 in Gilbert's syndrome. *N Engl J Med* 1995;333:1171.

170. Bancroft JD, Kreamer B, Gourley GR. Gilbert's syndrome accelerates development of neonatal jaundice. *J Pediatr* 1998;132:656.

171. Roy-Chowdhury N, Deocharan B, Bejjanki HR, et al. The present of a Gilbert-type promotor abnormality increases the level of neonatal hyperbilirubinemia. *Hepatology* 1997;26:370A.

172. Maisels MJ, Newman TB. Kernicterus in otherwise healthy, breast-fed term newborns. *Pediatrics* 1995;96:730.

173. Ariza CR, Frati AC, Sierra I. Hypothyroidism-associated cholestasis. *JAMA* 1984;252:2392.

174. Lees MH, Ruthven CRJ. The effects of triiodothyronine on neonatal hyperbilirubinemia. *Lancet* 1959;2:371.

175. Shrand H, Ruthven CRJ. Effect of triiodothyronine on serum bilirubin level in neonatal development of the premature infant. *Lancet* 1960;2: 1274.

176. Copeland KC, Franks RC, Ramamurthy R. Neonatal hyperbilirubinemia and hypoglycemia and congenital hypopituitarism. *Clin Pediatr* 1981;20:523.

177. Lanes R, Bancheette V, Edwin C, et al. Congenital hypopituitarism and conjugated hyperbilirubinemia. *Am J Dis Child* 1978;132:926.

178. Brown AK, Johnson L. Loss of concern about jaundice and the reemergence of kernicterus in full term infants in the era of managed care. In: Fanaraoff AA, Klaus MH, eds. *Yearbook of Neonatal-Perinatal Medicine.* St. Louis, MO: Mosby, 1996;XVII.

179. Penn AA, Enzman DR, Hahn JS, et al. Kernicterus in a full term infant. *Pediatrics* 1994;93:1003.

180. Sola A, Kitterman JA. Changes in clinical practice and bilirubin encephalopathy in "healthy term newborns." *Pediatr Res* 1995;37: 145A.

181. American Academy of Pediatrics, Committee on the Fetus and Newborn. Hospital stay for healthy term newborns. *Pediatrics* 1995;96: 788.

182. De Carvalho M, Klaus MH, Merkatz RB. Frequency of breastfeeding and serum bilirubin concentration. *Am J Dis Child* 1982;136:737.

183. Yamauchi Y, Yamanouchi I. Breast-feeding frequency during the first 24 hours after birth in full-term neonates. *Pediatrics* 1990;86:171.

184. Eidelman AL, Hoffman MW, Kaitz M. Cognitive deficits in women after childbirth. *Obstet Gynecol* 1993;81:764.

185. Perlman JM, Rogers B, Burns D. Kernicterus findings at autopsy in 2 sick near-term infants. *Pediatrics* 1997;99:612.

186. Orth J. Ueber das vorkommen von bilirubinkrystallen bei neugebornen kindern. *Virchows Arch [A]* 1875;63:447.

187. Schmorl G. Zur kenntnis des ikterus neonatorum, Insbesondere der dabei auftretenden gehirnveranderungen. *Verh Dtsch Ges Pathol* 1904;15:109.

188. Turkel SB. Autopsy findings associated with neonatal hyperbilirubinemia. *Clin Perinatol* 1990;17:381.

189. Ahdab-Barmada M, Moossy J. The neuropathology of kernicterus in the premature neonate: diagnostic problems. *J Neuropathol Exp Neurol* 1984;43:45.

190. Volpe JJ. *Neurology of the newborn,* 3rd ed. Philadelphia: WB Saunders, 1995.

191. Cashore WJ, Oh W. Unbound bilirubin and kernicterus in low birthweight infants. *Pediatrics* 1982;69:481.

192. Gartner LM, Snyder RN, Chabon RSetal. Kernicterus: high incidence in premature infants with low serum bilirubin concentration. *Pediatrics* 1970;45:906.

193. Turkel SB, Miller CA, Guttenberg ME, et al. A clinical pathologic reappraisal of kernicterus. *Pediatrics* 1982;69:267.

194. Lipsitz PJ, Gartner LM, Bryla DA. Neonatal and infant mortality in relation to phototherapy. Pediatrics 1985;75[Suppl]:422.

195. Doshi N, Klinsky B, Fujikura TEA. Pulmonary yellow hyaline membranes in neonates. *Hum Pathol* 1980;11:520.

196. Valdes-Dapena MA, Nissim JE, Arey JB, et al. Yellow pulmonary hyaline membranes. *J Pediatr* 1976;89:128.

197. Claireaux A. Icterus of the brain in the newborn. *Lancet* 1953;2:1226.

198. Brodersen R, Robertson A. Chemistry of bilirubin and its interaction with albumin. In: Levine RL, Maisels MJ, eds. *Hyperbilirubinemia in the newborn:* report of the 85th Ross Conference on Pediatric Research. Columbus, OH: Ross Laboratories, 1983:91.

199. Brodersen R, Stern L. Deposition of bilirubin acid in the central nervous system: a hypothesis for the development of kernicterus. *Acta Paediatr Scand* 1990;79:12.

200. Wennberg RP. Cellular basis of bilirubin toxicity. *N Y State J Med* 1991;91:493.

201. Cashore WJ. The neurotoxicity of bilirubin. *Clin Perinatol* 1990;17:437.

202. Cashore WJ, Kilgress NV. Inhibition of synaptosomal tyrosine uptake by bilirubin. *Pediatr Res* 1989;25:209A.

203. Cashore WJ, Kilgress NV, Chung CE. Effects of bilirubin and albumin on dopamine synthesis in striatal synaptosomes. *Pediatr Res* 1989;25:210A.

204. Ives NK, Cox DWG, Gardner RM, et al. The effects of bilirubin on brain energy metabolism during normoxia and hypoxia: an in-vitro study using 31P nuclear magnetic resonance spectroscopy. *Pediatr Res* 1988;23:569.

205. Ives NK, Bolas NM, Gardner RM. The effects of bilirubin on brain energy metabolism during hyperosmolar opening of the blood brain barrier: in-vivo study using 31P nuclear magnetic resonance spectroscopy. *Pediatr Res* 1989;26:356.

206. Hansen TWR, Mathiesen SBW, Walaas SI. Polylysine, but not polyglutamine or polyarginine, blocks the inhibitory effect of bilirubin on phosphorolation of phospholemman by the catalytic subunit of cAMP-dependent kinase. *Pediatr Res* 1995;37:210A.

207. Wennberg RP, Ahlfors CE, Rasmussen LF. The pathochemistry of kernicterus. *Early Hum Dev* 1979;31:353.

208. Wennberg RP, Hance AJ. Experimental encephalopathy: importance of total bilirubin, protein binding and blood brain barrier. *Pediatr Res* 1986;20:789.

209. Harris RC, Lucey JF, MacLean JR. Kernicterus in premature infants associated with low concentrations of bilirubin in the plasma. *Pediatrics* 1958;21:875.

210. Silverman WA, Andersen DH, Blanc WA, et al. A difference in mortality rate and incidence of kernicterus among premature infants allotted to two prophylactic antibacterial regimens. *Pediatrics* 1956;18:614.

211. Hansen ØyasÆter S, Stiris T, et al. Effects of sulfisoxazole, hypercarbia, and hyperosmolality on entry of bilirubin and albumin into brain regions in young rats. *Biol Neonate* 1989;56:22.

212. Nakamura H, Takada S, Shimabuku R, et al. Auditory and brainstem responses in newborn infants with hyperbilirubinemia. *Pediatrics* 1985;75:703 .

213. Stevenson DK, Wennberg RP. Predictors of a new therapy for jaundice. *West J Med* 1990;153:648.

214. Spear ML, Stahl GE, Paul MH, et al. The effect of 15-hour fat infusions of varying dosage on bilirubin binding to albumin. *JPEN* 1985;9:144.

215. Nizar L, Vyhmeister N, Ross R, et al. A jaundiced look at intravenous fat administration and the risk factor for kernicterus. *Clin Res* 1990;38:197A.

216. Levine RL. Fluorescence quenching studies of the binding of bilirubin to albumin. *Clin Chem* 1972;23:2292.

217. Nelson P, Jacobsen J, Wennberg RP. Effect of pH on the interaction of bilirubin with albumin and tissue culture cells. *Pediatr Res* 1974;8:963.

218. Kozuki K, Oh W, Widness J, Cashore W. Increase in bilirubin binding to albumin with correction of neonatal acidosis. *Acta Paediatr Scand* 1979;68:213.

219. Bratlid D. How bilirubin gets into the brain. *Clin Perinatol* 1990;17:449.

220. Robertson A, Carp W, Broderson R. Bilirubin displacing effect of drugs used in neonatology. *Acta Paediatr Scand* 1991;80:1119.

221. Robertson A, Carp W, Broderson R. Effect of drug combinations on bilirubin-albumin binding. *Dev Pharmacol Ther* 1991;17:95.

222. Valaes T, Hyte M. Effect of exchange transfusion on bilirubin binding. *Pediatrics* 1977;59:881.

223. Cashore WJ, Horwich A, Karotkin EH, et al. Influence of gestational age and clinical status on bilirubin-binding capacity in newborn infants. *Am J Dis Child* 1977;131:898.

224. Cashore WJ, Oh W, Brodersen R. Reserve albumin and bilirubin toxicity index in infant serum. *Acta Paediatr Scand* 1983;72:415.

225. Ritter DA, Kenny JD, Norton HJ, et al. A prospective study of free bilirubin and other high-risk factors in the development of kernicterus in premature infants. *Pediatrics* 1982;69:260.

226. Robertson A, Sharp C, Karp W. The relationship of gestational age to reserve albumin concentration for binding of bilirubin. *J Perinatol* 1988;8:17.

227. Jirka JH, Duckrow B, Kendig JW, Maisels MJ. Effect of bilirubin on brainstem auditory evoked potentials in the asphyxiated rat. *Pediatr Res* 1985;19:556.

228. Rozdilsky B, Olszewski J. Experimental study of the toxicity of bilirubin in newborn animals. *J Neuropathol Exp Neurol* 1961;20:193.

229. Lucey JF, Hibbard E, Behrman RE, et al. Kernicterus in asphyxiated newborn rhesus monkeys. *Exp Neurol* 1964;9:43.

230. Bratlid D, Cashore WJ, Oh W. Effect of serum hyperosmolality on opening of blood brain barrier for bilirubin in rat brain. *Pediatrics* 1983;71:909.

231. Bratlid D, Jori G. Mechanism of bilirubin entry into the brain in an animal model. In: Rubaltelli FF, ed. *Neonatal jaundice:* new trends in phototherapy. New York: Plenum Press, 1984:23.

232. Bratlid D, Cashore WJ, Oh W. Effects of acidosis on bilirubin deposition in rat brain. *Pediatrics* 1984;73:431.

233. Burgess GH, Oh W, Bratlid D, et al. The effects of brain blood flow on brain bilirubin deposition in newborn piglets. *Pediatr Res* 1985;19:691.

234. Burgess GH, Stonestreet BS, Cashore WJ, Oh W. Brain bilirubin deposition and brain blood flow during acute urea-induced hyperosmolality in newborn piglets. *Pediatr Res* 1985;19:537.

235. Levine RL, Fredericks WR, Rapoport SI. Entry of bilirubin into the brain due to opening of the blood brain barrier. *Pediatrics* 1982;69:255.

236. Stobie PE, Hansen CT, Hailey JR, et al. A difference in mortality between two strains of jaundiced rats. *Pediatrics* 1991;87:5918.

237. Cashore WJ. Bilirubin metabolism and toxicity in the newborn. In: Polin RA, Fox WW, eds. *Fetal and neonatal physiology,* 2nd ed. Philadelphia: WB Saunders, 1998:1493.

238. Saunders NR, Mollgard K. Development of the blood-brain barrier. *J Dev Physiol* 1984;6:45.

239. Lee C, Oh W. Permeability of the blood-brain barrier for 125I-albumin-bound bilirubin in newborn piglets. *Pediatr Res* 1989;25:452.

240. Ohsugi M, Sato H, Yamamura H. Transfer of bilirubin covalently bound to 125I-albumin from blood to brain in the Gunn rate newborn. *Biol Neonate* 1992;62:47.

241. Vohr BR. New approaches to assessing the risks of hyperbilirubinemia. *Clin Perinatol* 1990;17:293.

242. Hansen TWR, Allen JW. Bilirubin-oxidizing activity in rat brain. *Biol Neonate* 1996;70:289.

243. Hansen TWR, Allen JW. Oxidation of bilirubin by brain mitochondrial membranes-dependence on cell type and postnatal age. *Biochem Mol Med* 1997;60:155.

244. Gerrard J. Kernicterus. *Brain* 1952;75:526.

245. Van Praagh R. Diagnosis of kernicterus in the neonatal period. *Pediatrics* 1961;28:870.

246. Connolly AM, Volpe JJ. Clinical features of bilirubin encephalopathy. *Clin Perinatol* 1990;17:371.

247. Johnston WH, Angara V, Baumal R, et al. Erythroblastosis fetalis and hyperbilirubinemia. A five-year follow-up with neurological, physiological and audiological evaluation. *Pediatrics* 1967;39:88.

248. Jones MH, Sands R, Hyman CB, et al. Longitudinal study of incidence of central nervous system damage following erythroblastosis fetalis. *Pediatrics* 1954;14:346.

249. Byers RK, Paine RS, Crothers V. Extrapyramidal cerebral palsy with hearing loss following erythroblastosis. *Pediatrics* 1955;15:248.

250. Perlstein MA. The late clinical syndrome of post-icteric encephalopathy. *Pediatr Clin North Am* 1960;7:665.

251. Chin KC, Taylor MJ, Perlman M. Improvement in auditory and visually evoked potentials in jaundiced preterm infants after exchange transfusion. *Arch Dis Child* 1985;60:714.

252. Pearlman M, Fainmesser P, Sohmer H, et al. Auditory nerve-brainstem evoked responses in hyperbilirubinemic neonates. *Pediatrics* 1983;72:658.

253. Hyman CB, Keaster J, Hanson V, et al. CNS abnormalities after neonatal hemolytic disease or hyperbilirubinemia. *Am J Dis Child* 1969;117:395.

254. Martich-Kriss V, Kollias SS, Ball WS. MR findings in kernicterus. *AJNR* 1995;16:819.

255. Grobler JM, Mercer MJ. Kernicterus associated with elevated predominately direct-reacting bilirubin. *S Afr Med J* 1997;87:146.

256. Hsia DYY, Allen FH, Gellis SS, Diamond LK. Erythroblastosis fetalis. VIII. Studies of serum bilirubin in relation to kernicterus. *N Engl J Med* 1952;247:668.

257. Mollison PL, Cutbush M. Haemolytic disease of the newborn. In: Gairdner D, ed. *Recent advances in pediatrics.* New York: P. Blakiston & Son, 1954:110.

258. Newman TB, Maisels MJ. Does hyperbilirubinemia damage the brain of healthy full-term infants? *Clin Perinatol* 1990;17:331.

259. Newman TB, Maisels MJ. Evaluation of jaundice in the term newborn: a kinder, gentler approach. *Pediatrics* 1992;89:809.

260. Merenstein GB. "New" bilirubin recommendations questioned. *Pediatrics* 1992;89:822.

261. Cashore WJ. Hyperbilirubinemia: should we adopt a new standard of care? *Pediatrics* 1992;89:824.

262. Gartner LM. Management of jaundice in the well baby. *Pediatrics* 1992;89:826.

263. Johnson L. Yet another expert opinion on bilirubin toxicity! *Pediatrics* 1992;89:829.

264. Watchko JF, Oski FA. Kernicterus in preterm newborns: past, present and future. *Pediatrics* 1992;90:707.

265. Newman TB, Klebanoff MA. Neonatal hyperbilirubinemia and long-term outcome: another look at the collaborative perinatal project. *Pediatrics* 1993;92:651.

266. Mollison PL, Walker W. Controlled trials of the treatment of haemolytic disease of the newborn. *Lancet* 1952;1:429.

267. Ozmert E, Erdem G, Topcu M. Long-term follow-up of indirect hyperbilirubinemia in full-term Turkish infants. *Acta Paediatr* 1996;85:1440.

268. Johnson L, Boggs TR, Schaffer R, Simopoulous AP. Bilirubin-dependent brain damage: incidence and indications for treatment. In: Odell GB, ed. *Phototherapy in the newborn:* an Overview. Washington, DC: National Academy of Sciences, 1974:122.

269. Watchko JF, Oski FA. Bilirubin 20 mg/dl = vigintiphobia. *Pediatrics* 1983;71:660.

270. Johnson L. Hyperbilirubinemia in the term infant: when to worry, when to treat. *N Y State J Med* 1991;91:483.

271. Johnson L, Bhutani VK. Guidelines for management of the jaundiced term and near-term infant. *Clin Perinatol* 1998;25:555.

272. Raghubir KV, Fox GF, Inwood S, Kelly EN. Follow up of term neonates with extremely high unconjugated bilirubin. *Pediatr Res* 1996;39:276A.

273. Seidman DS, Paz I, Stevenson DK, Laor A, Danon YL, Gale R. Neonatal hyperbilirubinema and physical and cognitive performance at age 17 years. *Pediatrics* 1991;88:828.

274. Seidman DS, Laor A, Paz I, Gale R, Isacsohn M, Stevenson DK. Neonatal hyperbilirubinemia in healthy term infants and cognitive outcome in late adolescence. *Pediatr Res* 1998;43:194A.

275. Odell GB, Storey GNB, Rosenberg LA. Studies in kernicterus: III. The saturation of serum proteins with bilirubin during neonatal life and its relationship to brain damage at five years. *J Pediatr* 1970;76:12.

276. Scheidt PC, Graubard BI, Nelson KB, et al. Intelligence at six years in relation to neonatal bilirubin level: follow-up of the National Institute of Child Health and Human Development Clinical Trial of Phototherapy. *Pediatrics* 1991;87:797.

277. Nwaesei CG, Van Aerde J, Boyden M, Perlman M. Changes in auditory brainstem responses in hyperbilirubinemic infants before and after exchange transfusion. *Pediatrics* 1984;74:800.

278. Funato M, Tamai H, Shimada S, Nakamura H. Vigintiphobia, unbound bilirubin, and auditory brainstem responses. *Pediatrics* 1994;93:50.

279. Scheidt PC, Bryla DA, Nelson KB, Hirtz DG, Hoffman HJ. Phototherapy for neonatal hyperbilirubinemia: Six year follow-up of the NICHD clinical trial. *Pediatrics* 1990;85:455.

280. Nilsen ST, Finne PH, Bergsjo P, Stamnes O. Males with neonatal hyperbilirubinemia examined at 18 years of age. *Acta Paediatr Scand* 1984;73:176.

281. Naeye RL. Amniotic fluid infections, neonatal hyperbilirubinemia, and psychomotor impairment. *Pediatrics* 1978;62:497.

282. Scheidt PC, Mellits ED, Hardy JB, Drage JS, Boggs TR. Toxicity to bilirubin in neonates. Infant development during first year in relation to maximum neonatal serum bilirubin concentration. *J Pediatr* 1977;91:292.

283. Brown AK, Kim MH, Wu PYK, et al. Efficacy of phototherapy in prevention and management of neonatal hyperbilirubinemia. *Pediatrics* 1985;75[Suppl]:393.

284. Kim MH, Yoon JJ, Sher J, Brown AK. Lack of predictive indices in kernicterus. A comparison of clinical and pathologic factors in infants with or without kernicterus. *Pediatrics* 1980;66:852.

285. Turkel SB, Guttenberg ME, Moynes DR, Hodgman JE. Lack of identifiable risk factors for kernicterus. *Pediatrics* 1980;66:502.

286. Jardine DS, Rogers K. Relationship of benzyl alcohol to kernicterus, intraventricular hemorrhage, and mortality in preterm infants. *Pediatrics* 1989;83:153.

287. Watchko J, Claasen D. Kernicterus in premature infants: current prevalence and relationship to NICHD phototherapy study exchange criteria. *Pediatrics* 1994;93:996.

288. van de Bor M, Ens-Dokkum M, Schreuder AM, et al. Hyperbilirubinemia in low birthweight infants and outcome at 5 years of age. *Pediatrics* 1992;89:359.

289. Yeo KL, Perlman M, Hao YMP. Outcomes of extremely premature infants related to their peak serum bilirubin concentrations and exposure to phototherapy. *Pediatrics* 1998;102:1426.

290. O'Shea TM, Dillard RG, Klinepeter KD, et al. Serum bilirubin levels, intracranial hemorrhage, and the risk of developmental problems in very low birth weight infants. *Pediatrics* 1992;90:888.

291. Graziani LJ, Mitchell DG, Kornhauser M, et al. Neurodevelopment of preterm infants: neonatal neurosonographic and serum bilirubin studies. *Pediatrics* 1992;89:229.

292. van de Bor M, van Zeben-van der Aa TM, Verloove-Vanhorick SP, et al. Hyperbilirubinemia in very preterm infants and neurodevelopmental outcome at two years of age: results of a national collaborative survey. *Pediatrics* 1989;83:915.

293. Ikonen RS, Kuusinen EJ, Janas MO, Koivikko MJ, Sorto AE. Possible etiologic factors in extensive periventricular leucomalacia of preterm infants. *Acta Paeditr Scand* 1988;77:489.

294. Trounce J, Shaw DE, Levine MI, Rutter N. Clinical risk factors and periventricular leucomalacia. *Arch Dis Child* 1988;63:17.

295. Ikonen RS, Koivkko MJ, Laippala, Kuusinen EJ. Hyperbilirubinemia, hypocarbia and periventricular leukomalacia in preterm infants: relationship to cerebral palsy. *Acta Paediatr* 1992;81:802.

296. Ahvenainen EK, Call JD. Pulmonary hemorrhage in infants. A descriptive study. *Am J Pathol* 1952;28:1.

297. Zuelzer WW, Mudgett RT. Kernicterus: etiologic study based on an analysis of 55 cases. *Pediatrics* 1950;6:452.

298. Johnson L, Sarmiento F, Blanc WA, Day R. Kernicterus in rats with an inherited deficiency of glucouronyl transferase. *Am J Dis Child* 1960;97:591.

299. Sykes E, Epstein E. Laboratory measurement of bilirubin. *Clin Perinatol* 1990;17:397.

300. Doumas BT, Eckfeldt JH. Errors in measurement of total bilirubin: A perennial problem. *Clin Chem* 1996;42:845.

301. Watkinson LR, St John A, Penberthy LA. Investigation into paediatric bilirubin analyses in Australia and New Zealand. *J Clin Pathol* 1982; 35:52.

302. Leslie GI, Philips JB, Cassady G. Capillary and venous bilirubin values: are they really different? *Pediatrics* 1963;32:416.

303. Eidelman AI, Schimmel, Algur N, et al. Capillary and venous bilirubin values: they are different—and how! *Am J Dis Child* 1989;143: 642.

304. Sykes E, Maisels MJ, Kusack S. The effect of ambient light on serum bilirubin levels. *Pediatr Res* 1971;29:326A.

305. Maisels MJ, Gifford K. Neonatal jaundice in full-term infants: role of breastfeeding and other causes. *Am J Dis Child* 1983;137:561.

306. Kaplan M, Abramov A. Neonatal hyperbilirubinemia associated with glucose-6-phosphate dehydrogenase deficiency in Sephardic-Jewish infants: incidence, severity and the effect of phototherapy. *Pediatrics* 1992;90:401.

307. Kemper K, Forsyth B, McCarthy P. Jaundice, terminating breast-feeding, and the vulnerable child. *Pediatrics* 1989;84:773.

308. Ellis MI, Hey EN, Walker W. Neonatal death in babies with rhesus isoimmunization. *Q J Med* 1979;48:211.

309. Hovi L, Siimes MA. Exchange transfusion with fresh heparinized blood is a safe procedure: experiences from 1069 newborns. *Acta Paediatr Scand* 1985;74:360.

310. Keenan WJ, Novak KK, Sutherland JM, et al. Morbidity and mortality associated with exchange transfusion. Pediatrics 1985;75[Suppl]: 417.

311. Jackson JC. Adverse events associated with exchange transfusion in healthy and ill newborns. *Pediatrics* 1997;99:5. http://www.pediatrics.org/cgi/content/fall/99/5/e7.

312. Vreman HJ, Wong RJ, Stevenson DK. Light-emitting diodes: a novel light source for phototherapy. *Pediatr Res* 1998;44:804.

313. Sato K, Hara Y, Kondo T, Iwao H, Honda S, Ueda K. High-dose intravenous gammaglobulin therapy for neonatal immune haemolytic jaundice due to blood group incompatibility. *Acta Paediatr Scand* 1991; 80:163.

314. Dagoglu T, Ovali F, Samanci N, et al. High-dose intravenous immunoglobulin therapy for haemolytic disease. *J Int Med Res* 1995; 23:264.

315. Voto LS, Sexer H, Ferreiro G, et al. Neonatal adminstration of high-dose intravenous immunoglobulin and rhesus hemolytic disease. *J Perinat Med* 1995;23:443.

316. Rubo J, Albrecht K, Lasch P, et al. High-dose intravenous immune globulin therapy for hyperbilirubinemia caused by Rh hemolytic disease. *J Pediatr* 1992;121:93.

317. Hansen TW. Acute management of extreme neonatal jaundice—the potential benefits of intensified phototherapy and interruption of enterohepatic bilirubin circulation. *Acta Paediatr* 1997;86:843.

318. Robertson WO. Personal reflections on the AAP practice parameter on management of hyperbilirubinemia in the healthy term newborn. *Pediatr Rev* 1998;19:75.

319. Varimo P, Simili S, Wendt L, Kolvisto M. Frequency of breast feeding and hyperbilirubinemia. *Clin Pediatr* 1986;25:112.

320. Maisels MJ, Vain N, Acquavita AM, et al. The effect of breast-feeding frequency on serum bilirubin levels—a randomized controlled trial. *Am J Obstet Gynecol* 1994;170:880.

321. De Carvalho M, Holl M, Harvey D. Effects of water supplementation on physiological jaundice in breast fed babies. *Arch Dis Child* 1981;56:568.

322. Nicoll A, Ginsburg R, Tripp JH. Supplementary feeding and jaundice in newborns. *Acta Pediatr Scand* 1982;71:759 .

323. Kuhr M, Paneth N. Feeding practices and early neonatal jaundice. *J Pediatr Gastroenterol Nutr* 1982;1:485.

324. Amato M, Howald H, von Muralt G. Interruption of breast-feeding vs.

325. Martinez JC, Maisels MJ, Otheguy L, et al. Hyperbilirubinemia in the breast-fed newborn: a controlled trial of four interventions. *Pediatrics* 1993;91:470.

326. Maisels MJ. Why use homeopathic doses of phototherapy? *Pediatrics* 1996;98:283.

327. Tan KL. Comparison of the effectiveness of phototherapy and exchange transfusion in the management of nonhemolytic neonatal hyperbilirubinemia. *J Pediatr* 1975;87:609.

328. Heyman E, Ohisson A, Girschek P. Retinopathy of prematurity and bilirubin [Letter]. *N Engl J Med* 1989;320:256.

329. Boynton BR, Boynton CA. Retinopathy of prematurity and bilirubin [Letter]. *N Engl J Med* 1989;321:193.

330. Fauchére JC, Meier-Gibbons FE, Koerner F, Bossi E. Retinopathy of prematurity and bilirubin—no clinical evidence for a beneficial role of bilirubin as a physiological antioxidant. *Eur J Pediatr* 1994;153: 358.

331. Gaton DD, Gold J, Axer-Siegel R, Wielunsky E, Naor N, Nissenkorn I. Evaluation of bilirubin as possible protective factor in the prevention of retinopathy of prematurity. *Br J Ophthalmol* 1991;75:532.

332. DeJonge MH, Khuntia A, Maisels MJ, Bandagi A. Bilirubin (BR) and severe retinopathy of prematurity (ROP) in 23-26 week estimated gestational age (EGA) infants. *Pediatr Res* 1998;43:171A.

333. Clark CF, Torii S, Hamamoto Y, Kaito H. The "bronze baby" syndrome: postmortem data. *J Pediatr* 1976;88:461.

334. Ebbesen F. Low reserve albumin for binding of bilirubin in neonates with deficiency of bilirubin excretion and bronze baby syndrome. *Acta Paediatr Scand* 1982;71:415.

335. Catterton Z, Carp W, Bunyaten C, et al. Bilirubin binding capacity in ABO hemolytic disease of the newborn. *Clin Res* 1979;27:817A.

336. Kappas A, Drummond GS, Manola T, et al. Sn-protoporphyrin use in the management of hyperbilirubinemia in term newborns with direct Coombs'-positive ABO incompatibility. *Pediatrics* 1988;81:485.

337. Valaes T, Drummond GS, Kappas A. Control of hyperbilirubinemia in glucose-6-phosphate dehydrogenase-deficient newborns using an inhibitor of bilirubin production, Sn-mesoporphyrin. *Pediatrics* 1998; 101:5. http://www.pediatrics.org/cgi/content/fall/101/5/e1.

338. Blair DK, Vander Straten MC, Gest AL. Hydrops fetalis in sheep from rapid induction of anemia. *Pediatr Res* 1994;35:560.

339. Nicolaides K, Warensky J, Rodeck C. The relationship of fetal plasma protein concentration and hemoglobin level to the development of hydrops in Rhesus isoimmunization. *Am J Obstet Gynecol* 1985;152: 341.

340. Grannum P, Kopel J, Moya F, et al. The reversal of hydrops fetalis by intravascular intrauterine transfusion in severe isoimmune fetal anemia. *Am J Obstet Gynecol* 1988;158:914.

341. Moya FR, Granham PAT, Riddick L, et al. Atrial natriuretic factor in hydrops fetalis caused by Rh isoimmunization. *Arch Dis Child* 1990; 65:683.

342. Weiner C. Non-hematologic effects of intravascular transfusion on the human fetus. *Semin Perinatol* 1989;13:338.

343. Barss VA, Doubilet PM, St. John-Sutton M, Cartier MD, Frigoletto FD. Cardiac output in the fetus with erythroblastosis fetalis: assessment using pulsed Doppler. *Obstet Gynecol* 1987;70:444.

344. Phibbs RH, Johnson P, Tooley WH. Cardiorespiratory status of erythroblastotic newborn infants. II. Blood volume, hematocrit, and serum albumin concentration in relation to hydrops fetalis. *Pediatrics* 1974;53:13.

345. Nicolaides K, Clewell W, Rodeck C. Measurement of human fetoplacental blood volume in erythroblastosis fetalis. *Obstet Gynecol* 1988; 157:50.

346. Edwards MC, Fletcher MA. Exchange transfusions. In: Fletcher MA, MacDonald MG (eds). *Atlas of procedures in neonatology,* 2nd ed. Philadelphia: JB Lippincott, 1993:363.

347. Schreiber GB, Busch MP, Kleinman SH, Korelitz JJ. The risk of transfusion-transmitted viral infections. *N Engl J Med* 1996;334:1685.

348. Valaes T. Bilirubin distribution and dynamics of bilirubin removal by exchange transfusion. Acta Paediatr Scand Suppl 1963;52:149.

349. Jährig K, Jährig D, Meisel P, eds. *Phototherapy:* treating neonatal jaundice with visible light. München: Quintessenz Verlags-GmbH, 1998.

350. Agati G, Fusi F, Donzelli GP, Pratesi R. Quantum yield and skin fil-

tering effects on the formation rate of lumirubin. *J Photochem Photobiol B* 1993;18:197.

351. Tan KL. The pattern of bilirubin response to phototherapy for neonatal hyperbilirubinemia. *Pediatr Res* 1982;16:670.

352. Christensen T, Kinn G. Bilirubin bound to cells does not form photoisomers. *Acta Paediatr* 1993;82:22.

353. Ennever JF. Blue light, green light, white light, more light: treatment of neonatal jaundice. *Clin Perinatol* 1990;17:467.

354. McDonagh AF, Maisels MJ. Photoisomerization of bilirubin in Crigler-Najjar patients. In: Kappas A, Lucey J, eds. *Treatment of Crigler-Najjar syndrome. Conference proceedings.* New York: Rockefeller University, 1996.

355. Jährig K, Jährig D, Meisel P. Dependence of the efficiency of phototherapy on plasma bilirubin concentration. *Acta Paediatr Scand* 1982;71:293.

356. ECRI. Fiberoptic phototherapy systems. *Health Devices* 1995;24:134.

357. Seidman DS, Moise J, Ergaz Z, et al. A new blue light emitting phototherapy device vs conventional phototherapy: a prospective randomized controlled application in term newborns. *Pediatr Res* 1998;43:193A.

358. Holtrop PC, Ruedisueli K, Maisels MJ. Double versus single phototherapy in low birth weight newborns. *Pediatrics* 1992;90:674.

359. Tan KL. Efficacy of bidirectional fiberoptic phototherapy for neonatal hyperbilirbinemia. *Pediatrics* 1997;99:5.

360. Tan KL, Lim GC, Boey KW. Efficacy of "high-intensity" blue-light and "standard" daylight phototherapy for non-haemolytic hyperbilirubinemia. *Acta Paediatr* 1992;81:870.

361. Garg AK, Prasad RS, Hifzi IA. A controlled trial of high-intensity double-surface phototherapy on a fluid bed versus conventional phototherapy in neonatal jaundice. *Pediatrics* 1995;95:914.

362. Tonz O, Vogt J, Filippini L, Simmler F, Wachsmuth ED, Winterhalter KH. Severe light dermatosis following phototherapy in a newborn infant with congenital erythropoietic urophyria. *Helv Paediatr Acta* 1975;30:47.

363. Mallon E, Wojnarowska F, Hope P, Elder G. Neonatal bullous eruption as a result of transient porphyrinemia in a premature infant with hemolytic disease of the newborn. *J Am Acad Dermatol* 1995;33:333.

364. Paller AS, Eramo LR, Farrell EE, Millard DD, Honig PJ, Cunningham BB. Purpuric phototherapy-induced eruption in transfused neonates: relation to transient porphyrinemia. *Pediatrics* 1997;100:360.

365. Rubaltelli FF, Jori G, Reddi E. Bronze baby syndrome: a new porphyrin-related disorder. *Pediatr Res* 1983;17:327.

366. Jori G, Reddi E, Rubaltelli FF. Bronze baby syndrome: an animal model. *Pediatr Res* 1990;27:22.

367. Kappas A, Lucey J. *Treatment of Crigler-Najjar syndrome. Conference proceedings.* New York: Rockefeller University, 1996.

368. Messner KH, Maisels MJ, Leure-DuPree AE. Phototoxicity to the newborn primate retina. *Invest Ophthalmol Vis Sci* 1978;17:178.

369. Rosenfeld W, Sadhev S, Brunot V, Jhavri R, Zabaleta I, Evans HE. Phototherapy effect on the incidence of patent ductus arteriosus in premature infants: prevention with chest shielding. *Pediatrics* 1986;78:10.

370. Barefield ES, Dwyer MD, Cassady G. Association of patent ductus arteriosus and phototherapy in infants weighing less than 1000 grams. *J Perinatol* 1993;13:376.

371. Yaffe SJ, Dorn LD. Effects of prenatal treatment with phenobarbital. *Dev Pharmacol Ther* 1990;15:215.

372. Reinisch JM, Sander SA, Mortensen EL, et al. In utero exposure to phenobarbital and intelligence deficits in adult men. *JAMA* 1995;274:1518.

373. Valaes T, Petmezaki S, Henschke C, et al. Control of jaundice in preterm newborns by an inhibitor of bilirubin production: studies with tin-mesoporphyrin. *Pediatrics* 1994;93:1.

374. Kappas A, Drummond G, Henschke C, et al. Direct comparison of Sn-mesoporphyrin, an inhibitor of bilirubin production, and phototherapy in controlling hyperbilirubinemia in term and near-term newborns. *Pediatrics* 1995;95:468.

375. Martinez JC, Garcia HO, Othegui L, et al. Control of severe hyperbilirubinemia in full-term newborns with the inhibitor of bilirubin production Sn-mesoporphyrin (Sn-MP). *Pediatrics* 1999;103:1.

376. Galbraith RA, Drummond GS, Kappas A. Suppression of bilirubin production in the Crigler-Najjar type I syndrome: studies with the heme oxygenase inhibitor tin-mesoporphyrin. *Pediatrics* 1992;89:175.

377. Hammerman C, Kaplan M, Vreman HJ, Stevenson DK. Intravenous immune globulin in neonatal ABO isoimmunization: factors associated with clinical efficacy. *Biol Neonate* 1996;70:69.

378. Hammerman C, Goldstein R, Eiran M, Kaplan M, Eidelman AI, Garnter LM. Antioxidant potential of bilirubin in the premature infant. *Pediatr Res* 1997;41:152A.

379. Belanger S, Lavoie JC, Chessex P. Influence of bilirubin on the antioxidant capacity of plasma in newborn infants. *Biol Neonate* 1997;71:233.

380. Gopinathan V, Miller NJ, Milner AD, Rice-Evans CA. Bilirubin and ascorbate antioxidant activity in neonatal plasma. *FEBS Lett* 1994;349:197.

381. Hegyi T, Goldie E, Hiatt M. The protective role of bilirubin in oxygen radical disease of the preterm infant. *J Perinatol* 1989;14:300.

382. Saugstad OD. Mechanisms of tissue injury by oxygen radicals: implicates for neonatal disease. *Acta Paediatr* 1996;85:1.

CHAPTER 39

Inherited Metabolic Disorders

Barbara K. Burton

Major advances in the recognition and treatment of inborn errors of metabolism have made it more essential than ever that the neonatologist be familiar with the clinical presentation of these disorders. Many of the diseases in this group are associated with symptoms in the neonatal period, and many affected infants find their way into neonatal intensive care units. The likelihood of establishing a diagnosis often is directly related to the level of awareness of the neonatologist responsible for the infant's care. Although many of the individual inborn errors of metabolism occur infrequently, collectively, they are not rare. With current diagnostic methods and mass screening programs operating in several states, many of these disorders have been found to be significantly more common than previously believed. There is no doubt that a significant number of children with these disorders are undiagnosed. Every geneticist has had the experience of diagnosing an inborn error of metabolism in a child and discovering that the parents have had one or more other children who died in early infancy of vague or undetermined causes. In such cases, it is reasonable to assume that the other children were similarly affected but undiagnosed. Autopsy findings in such cases are often nonspecific and unrevealing unless special biochemical studies are done. Infection often is suspected as the cause of death, and sepsis is a common accompaniment of inherited metabolic disorders.

The significance of the precise diagnosis of metabolic disease cannot be overemphasized. Increasingly, these disorders are lending themselves to successful medical management. If treatment means the prevention of significant mental retardation or death, even when the numbers are small, the diagnosis is clearly worth pursuing. However, the success of most treatment regimens depends on the earliest possible institution of therapy, stressing the importance of early clinical diagnosis. Even when no effective therapy exists or an infant cannot be salvaged, diagnosis is critical for purposes of genetic counseling.

Inborn errors of metabolism are all genetically transmitted, typically in an autosomal recessive or X-linked recessive fashion, and there is usually a substantial risk of recurrence. Prenatal diagnosis is available for many conditions in this group. Awareness of the diagnosis before birth of an at-risk infant can lead to earlier therapy and an improved prognosis.

This chapter defines the constellation of findings in the newborn that should alert the clinician to the possibility of inherited metabolic disease. The discussion is confined to the disorders for which manifestations are observed in the first few months of life and does not include the many disorders (e.g., most lysosomal storage diseases) that typically present in later infancy or childhood. The laboratory tools used to evaluate infants suspected of having inherited metabolic disease are discussed. Treatment of important groups of metabolic disorders are addressed, focusing on the stabilization and acute management of patients with these conditions.

A list of the major inborn errors of metabolism that have been described clinically in early infancy is shown in Table 39–1. This table cannot be considered complete because it includes only the disorders for which manifestations in the first few months of life have been documented in the literature. It is likely that disorders typically occurring later in childhood occasionally may present as early as the first month of life. New disorders causing neonatal disease undoubtedly will continue to be described. A single literature reference is listed for each disorder in the table, and detailed information about most of the disorders listed can be found in recent editions of reference textbooks (1,2).

B. K. Burton: Division of Genetics and Metabolism, Department of Pediatrics, University of Illinois College of Medicine; and Center for Medical and Reproductive Genetics, Michael Reese Hospital, Chicago, Illinois

TABLE 39–1. *Inborn errors of metabolism that present in early infancy*

Disorder	Reference
Disorders of Carbohydrate Metabolism	
Galactosemia (i.e., galactose-1-phosphate uridyl transferase deficiency)	38
Hereditary fructose intolerance (i.e., fructose-1-phosphate aldolase deficiency)	39
Fructose-1,6-diphosphatase deficiency	40
Glycogen storage disease type I (i.e., von Gierke disease, glucose-6-phosphatase deficiency)	41
Glycogen storage disease type II (i.e., Pompe disease, alpha-glucosidase deficiency)	42
Glycogen storage disease type III (i.e., limit dextrinosis, debrancher deficiency)	41
Glycogen storage disease type IV (i.e., amylopectinosis, brancher deficiency)	43
Disorders of Amino Acid Metabolism	
Maple syrup urine disease	44
Homocystinuria	45
Nonketotic hyperglycinemia	46
Phenylketonuria	47
Hereditary tyrosinemia	48
Hyperornithinemia–hyperammonemia–homocitrullinuria syndrome	49
Lysinuric protein intolerance	50
Methylene tetrahydrofolate reductase deficiency	51
Pyridoxine dependency with seizures (i.e., presumed glutamic acid decarboxylase deficiency)	52
Organic Acidemias	
Methylmalonic acidemia	53
Methylmalonic acidemia with homocystinuria	54
Propionic acidemia	55
Isovaleric acidemia	56
3-Methyl crotonyl CoA carboxylase deficiency	57
Holocarboxylase synthetase deficiency (i.e., early-onset multiple carboxylase deficiency)	58
Biotinidase deficiency (i.e., late-onset multiple carboxylase deficiency)	59
Glutaric acidemia type I	60
Glutaric acidemia type II (i.e., multiple acyl CoA dehydrogenase deficiency, severe)	61
Ethylmalonic-adipic aciduria (i.e., later-onset glutaric acidemia type II, multiple acyl CoA dehydrogenase deficiencies, mild)	62
3-Hydroxy-3-methylglutaric acidemia	63
2-Methylacetoacetyl-CoA thiolase deficiency	64
Mevalonic aciduria	65
Pyroglutamic aciduria	66
3-Hydroxyisobutyric aciduria	67
3-Methylglutaconic aciduria	68
Urea Cycle Disorders	
Carbamyl phosphate synthetase deficiency	69
Ornithine transcarbamylase deficiency	69
Citrullinemia	69
Argininosuccinic aciduria	69
Arginase deficiency	70
N-Acetylglutamate synthetase deficiency	71
Fatty Acid Oxidation Defects	
Short-chain acyl CoA dehydrogenase deficiency	72
Medium-chain acyl CoA dehydrogenase deficiency	73
Very-long-chain acyl CoA dehydrogenase deficiency	74
Long-chain 3-hydroxyacyl-CoA dehydrogenase deficiency	75
Carnitine-acylcarnitine translocase deficiency	76
Carnitine transporter deficiency (i.e., primary systemic carnitine deficiency)	77
Carnitine palmitoyl transferase II deficiency	78
Lactic Acidemias	
Pyruvate dehydrogenase deficiency	32
Pyruvate carboxylase deficiency	79
Phosphoenolpyruvate carboxykinase deficiency	80
NADH-CoQ reductase (i.e., complex I) deficiency	81
Cytochrome oxidase (i.e., complex IV) deficiency	82
Transport Disorders	
Cystic fibrosis	83
Infantile free sialic acid storage disease	84
Hartnup disease	85
Lysosomal Storage Disorders	
GM$_1$ gangliosidosis type I (i.e., generalized gangliosidosis, beta-galactosidase deficiency)	86

TABLE 39–1. *Continued*

Disorder	Reference
Gaucher disease type II (i.e., glucocerebrosidase deficiency)	87
Niemann–Pick disease types A and B (i.e., sphingomyelinase deficiency)	88
Niemann–Pick disease type C	89
Mannosidosis (i.e., alpha-mannosidase deficiency)	90
Fucosidosis (i.e., alpha-fucosidase deficiency)	91
Farber disease (i.e., acid ceramidase deficiency)	92
Wolman disease (i.e., acid lipase deficiency)	93
Krabbe disease (i.e., galactocerebrosidase deficiency)	94
Mucopolysaccharidosis type VI (i.e., Maroteaux–Lamy syndrome, arylsulfatase B deficiency)	95
Mucopolysaccharidosis type VII (i.e., beta-glucuronidase deficiency)	96
Mucolipidosis type II (i.e., I-cell disease)	97
Mucolipidosis type IV	98
Multiple sulfatase deficiency	99
Sialidosis type II (i.e., neuraminidase deficiency)	100
Peroxisomal Disorders	
Zellweger syndrome	101
Neonatal adrenoleukodystrophy	101
Hyperpipecolic acidemia	101
Rhizomelic chondrodysplasia punctata	101
Disorders of Metal Metabolism	
Menke kinky hair disease	102
Molybdenum cofactor deficiency	103
Sulfite oxidase deficiency	104
Neonatal hemochromatosis	105
Other Disorders	
Congenital adrenal hyperplasia	106
Carbohydrate deficient glycoprotein syndrome	107
Hereditary orotic aciduria	108
Hypophosphatasia	109
Crigler–Najjar syndrome	110
Alpha₁–antitrypsin deficiency	111
Canavan disease (i.e., aspartoacylase deficiency)	112
Steroid sulfatase deficiency	113
Senger syndrome	114
Smith–Lemli–Opitz syndrome	33
Lowe syndrome	115

CLINICAL MANIFESTATIONS OF INBORN ERRORS OF METABOLISM

Acute Metabolic Encephalopathy

Several groups of inherited metabolic disorders, most notably the organic acidemias, urea cycle defects, and certain disorders of amino acid metabolism, typically present with acute life-threatening symptoms in the neonatal period. Because they are associated with protein intolerance, symptoms usually begin after feedings have been instituted. Affected infants are typically full term and usually appear normal at birth. The interval between the first protein feeding and clinical symptoms ranges from hours to weeks. The initial findings are usually those of lethargy and poor feeding, as seen in almost any sick infant. Although sepsis is often the first consideration in infants who present in this way, these symptoms in a full-term infant with no specific risk factors strongly suggest a metabolic disorder. Infants with inborn errors of metabolism rather quickly may become debilitated and septic; therefore, it is important that the presence of sep-

sis not exclude consideration of other possibilities. The lethargy associated with these conditions is an early symptom of a metabolic encephalopathy that may progress to coma. Other signs of central nervous system (CNS) dysfunction, such as seizures and abnormal muscle tone, may exist. Evidence of cerebral edema may be observed, and intracranial hemorrhage occasionally occurs (3).

An infant with an inborn error of metabolism who presents more abruptly or in whom the lethargy and poor feeding go unnoticed may first come to attention because of apnea or respiratory distress. The apnea is typically central in origin and a symptom of the metabolic encephalopathy, but tachypnea may be a symptom of an underlying metabolic acidosis, as occurs in the organic acidemias. Infants with urea cycle defects and evolving hyperammonemic coma initially exhibit central hyperventilation, which leads to respiratory alkalosis.

Vomiting is a striking feature of many of the inborn errors of metabolism associated with protein intolerance, although it is somewhat less common in the newborn than in the older infant. If persistent vomiting occurs in the neonatal period, it usually signals significant underlying disease. Inborn errors of metabolism should always be considered in the differential diagnosis. It is common for an infant to be diagnosed as having a metabolic disorder after having undergone surgery for suspected pyloric stenosis (4). Formula intolerance frequently is suspected, and many affected infants have numerous formula changes before a diagnosis finally is established.

The basic laboratory studies that should be obtained for an infant who has acute life-threatening symptoms consistent with an inborn error of metabolism are listed in Table 39–2.

Hyperammonemia

Among the most important laboratory findings associated with inborn errors of metabolism presenting with an acute encephalopathy is hyperammonemia. A plasma ammonia level should be obtained for any infant with unexplained vomiting, lethargy, or other evidence of an encephalopathy. Significant hyperammonemia is observed in a limited number of conditions. Inborn errors of metabolism, including urea cycle defects and many of the organic acidemias, are at the top of the list. Also in the differential diagnosis is a condition referred to as transient hyperammonemia of the newborn (THAN) (5). Ammonia levels in these conditions frequently exceed 1,000 μmol/L. The finding of marked hyperammonemia provides an important clue to diagnosis and indicates the need for urgent treatment to reduce the ammonia level. The degree of neurologic impairment and developmental delay subsequently observed in infants with urea cycle defects depends on the duration of the neonatal hyperammonemic coma (6).

A flow chart for the differentiation of conditions producing significant hyperammonemia in the newborn is shown in Figure 39–1. The timing of the onset of symptoms may provide an important clue. Infants with urea cycle defects typically do not become symptomatic until after 24 hours of age. Patients with some of the organic

acidemias, such as glutaric acidemia type II, or with pyruvate carboxylase deficiency may exhibit symptomatic hyperammonemia during the first 24 hours. Symptoms in the first 24 hours are characteristic of THAN, a condition that is poorly understood but apparently not genetically determined. The typical patient with this disorder is a large premature infant (mean gestational age of 36 weeks) who has symptomatic pulmonary disease, often from birth, and severe hyperammonemia. Survivors do not have recurrent episodes of hyperammonemia and may or may not exhibit neurologic sequelae, depending on the extent of the neonatal insult. There are some affected infants who survive with normal intelligence despite extraordinarily high ammonia levels (5).

Infants who develop severe hyperammonemia after 24 hours of age usually have a urea cycle defect or an organic acidemia; infants with organic acidemias typically exhibit a metabolic acidosis and ketonuria as well. Urine organic acids should always be obtained, regardless of whether or not acidosis is present. Metabolic acidosis is not a feature of the urea cycle defects. Plasma amino acid analysis is helpful in the differentiation of the specific defects in this group. Characteristic amino acid abnormalities provide a definitive diagnosis of citrullinemia and argininosuccinic aciduria. Although no diagnostic amino acid elevations are observed in carbamyl phosphate synthetase deficiency or ornithine transcarbamylase deficiency, a low or undetectable level of plasma citrulline is observed in both of these conditions. This finding is helpful in differentiating these two conditions from THAN, in which the plasma citrulline level is normal. However, plasma citrulline is not accurately measured in all laboratories performing amino acid analysis, probably because it is important in few other clinical settings. In clinical situations in which this is a critical diagnostic test, samples should be sent to laboratories with expertise in the differentiation of urea cycle defects. Carbamyl phosphate synthetase deficiency and ornithine transcarbamylase deficiency may be differentiated by measuring urine orotic acid, which is low in the former and elevated in the latter. The pattern of inheritance of the two may also help to differentiate them; ornithine transcarbamylase deficiency, an X-linked disorder, rarely produces severe hyperammonemia in a female infant, whereas carbamyl phosphate synthetase deficiency, an autosomal recessive disorder, occurs with equal frequency in the two genders.

Although the clinical and laboratory evaluation outlined should lead to a specific tentative diagnosis for virtually all patients, liver biopsy may be indicated for enzymatic confirmation of the diagnoses of carbamyl phosphate synthetase and ornithine transcarbamylase deficiencies, because these diagnoses dictate rigid lifelong therapy or consideration of hepatic transplantation. Acute treatment should be based on the presumptive diagnosis, with biopsy considered only after the infant is stabilized.

TABLE 39–2. *Laboratory studies for an infant suspected of having an inborn error of metabolism*

Complete blood count with differential
Urinalysis
Blood gases
Electrolytes
Blood glucose
Plasma ammonia
Urine reducing substances
Urine ketones if acidosis or hypoglycemia is present
Urine ferric chloride test
Plasma and urine amino acids, quantitative
Urine organic acids
Plasma lactate

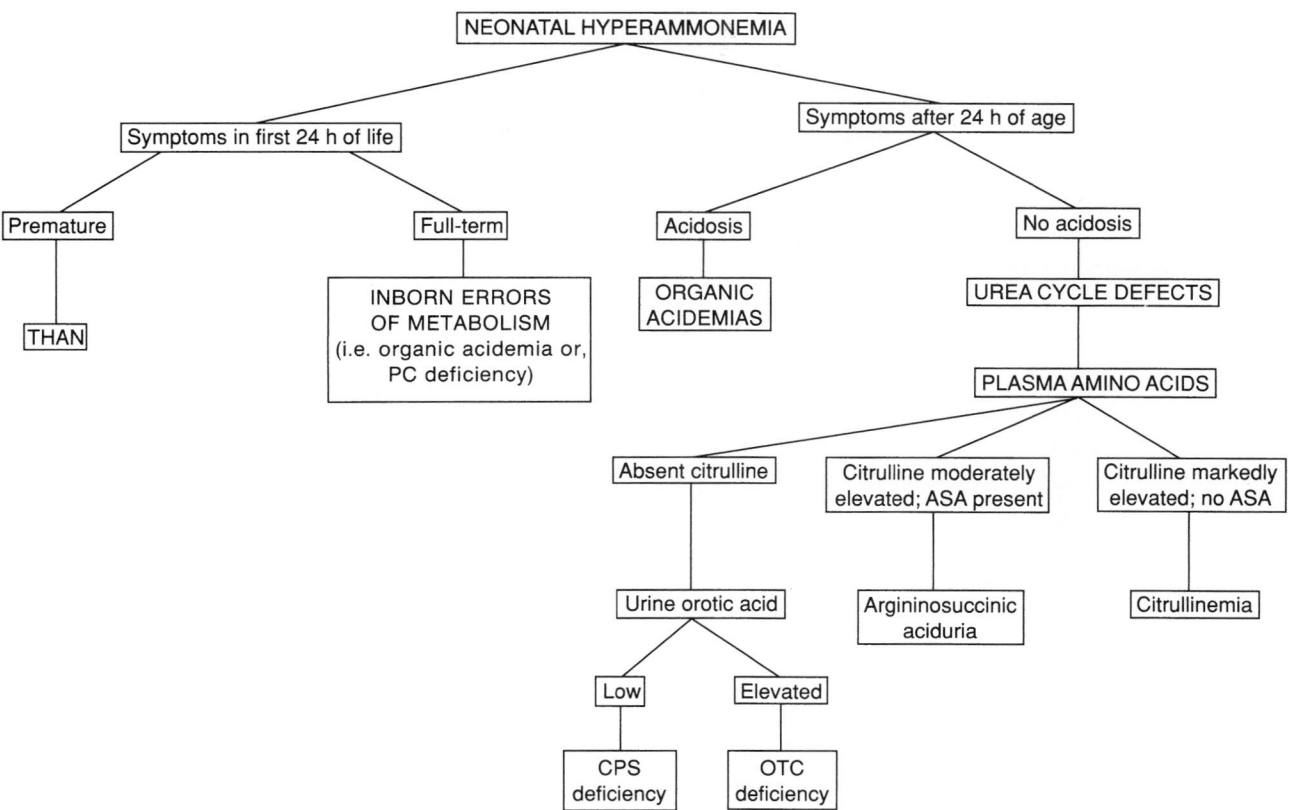

FIG. 39–1. Differentiating between conditions that produce severe neonatal hyperammonemia. ASA, argininosuccinic acid; CPS, carbamyl phosphate synthetase; OTC, ornithine transcarbamylase; PC, pyruvate carboxylase; THAN, transient hyperammonemia of the newborn.

Less significant elevations of plasma ammonia than those associated with inborn errors of metabolism and THAN can be observed in a variety of other conditions associated with liver dysfunction, including sepsis, generalized herpes simplex infection, and perinatal asphyxia. Liver function studies should be obtained in evaluating the significance of moderate elevations of plasma ammonia. However, even in cases of severe hepatic necrosis, it is rare for ammonia levels to exceed 500 μmol/L or 900 g/100 mL (7). Mild transient hyperammonemia with ammonia levels as high as twice normal is relatively common in the newborn, especially in the premature infant, and is usually asymptomatic. It appears to be of no clinical significance, and there are no long-term neurologic sequelae (8).

Metabolic Acidosis

The second important laboratory feature of many of the inborn errors of metabolism during acute episodes of illness is metabolic acidosis with an increased anion gap, readily demonstrable by measurement of arterial blood gases or serum electrolytes and bicarbonate. A flow chart for the evaluation of infants with this finding is shown in

Figure 39–2. An increased anion gap (greater than 16) is observed in many inborn errors of metabolism and in most other conditions producing metabolic acidosis in the neonate. The differential diagnosis of metabolic acidosis with a normal anion gap essentially is limited to two conditions, diarrhea and renal tubular acidosis. Among the inborn errors, the largest group typically associated with overwhelming metabolic acidosis in infancy is the group of organic acidemias, including methylmalonic acidemia, propionic acidemia, and isovaleric acidemia. The list of disorders in this group has expanded dramatically as new disorders have been defined through the use of organic acid analysis.

In addition to specific organic acid intermediates, plasma lactate often is elevated in organic acidemias as a result of secondary interference with coenzyme A (CoA) metabolism. Neutropenia and thrombocytopenia commonly are observed and further underscore the clinical similarity of these disorders to neonatal sepsis. Hyperammonemia, sometimes as dramatic as that associated with urea cycle defects, is seen commonly but not uniformly in critically ill neonates with organic acidemias.

The metabolic acidosis associated with organic acidemias and certain other inborn errors of metabolism

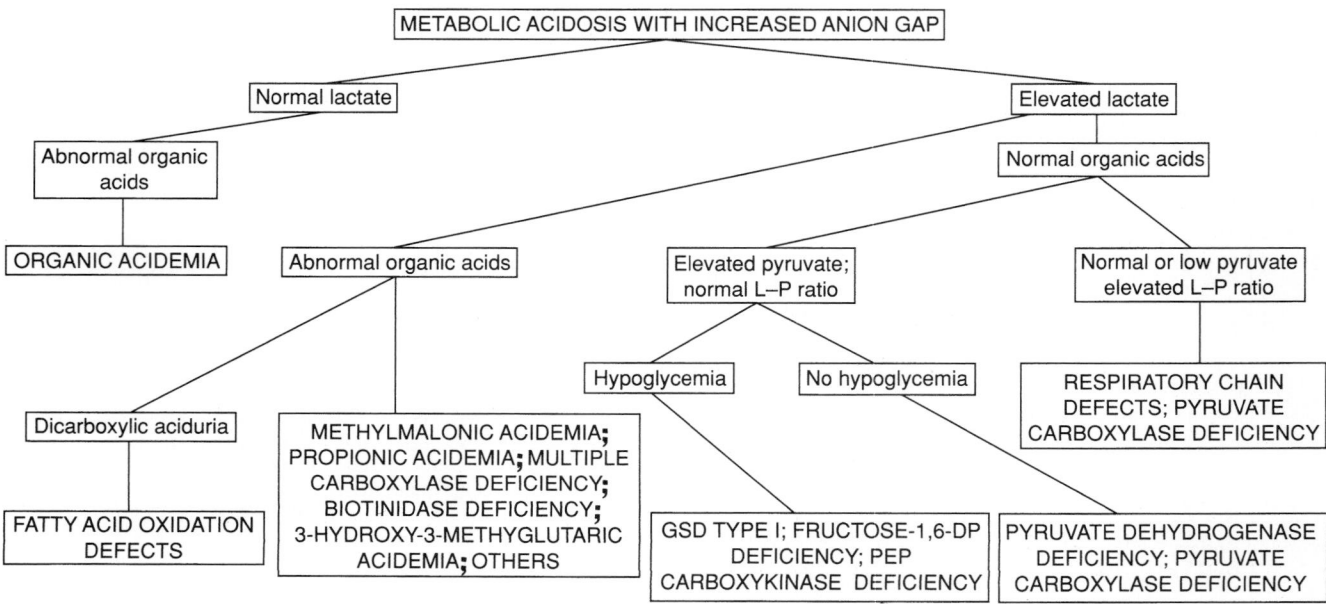

FIG. 39–2. Evaluating metabolic acidosis in the young infant. fructose-1,6-DP, fructose-1,6-diphosphatase; GSD, glycogen storage disease; L/P, lactate/pyruvate.

may have significant adverse impact on many different organ systems, which may lead to the erroneous diagnosis of a wide variety of seemingly unrelated disorders. I had the experience of caring for an infant with isovaleric acidemia who presented at 10 days of age with respiratory distress, severe metabolic acidosis, a dilated heart, and poor cardiac output. The infant was suspected of having the hypoplastic left heart syndrome or other severe congenital heart disease. Cardiac catheterization was performed, even though members of the nursing staff had observed that the infant had a strong unpleasant odor, reminiscent of sweaty feet. Personnel in the catheterization laboratory also noticed that the blood had a strong peculiar odor, but it was not until 18 hours later, long after significant heart disease had been ruled out, that the diagnosis of metabolic disease was first considered. Despite attempts at therapy with dialysis and other measures, the child succumbed to the disease. In this case, the metabolic acidosis led to poor function of the myocardium and not the reverse.

Another child subsequently found to have methylmalonic acidemia was admitted through the emergency room with severe metabolic acidosis and a tight, distended abdomen with evidence of multiple air–fluid levels on x-ray films. The history revealed that the child had fed poorly since birth and had repeated episodes of vomiting despite several formula changes. Intestinal obstruction was suspected, and the child was taken to the operating room, where most of the small intestine was found to be infarcted, presumably secondary to the acidosis and poor tissue perfusion. No anatomic abnormalities were found. Postoperatively, metabolic disease was considered,

and the diagnosis of a vitamin B$_{12}$-responsive form of methylmalonic acidemia was made. The infant died of complications of the disease even though the early diagnosis and treatment of this disorder, before the terminal episode, should have been associated with a good prognosis.

Defects in pyruvate metabolism or in the respiratory chain may lead to primary lactic acidosis presenting as severe metabolic acidosis in infancy (9,10). Unlike most of the other conditions presenting acutely in the newborn, the clinical features of these disorders are unrelated to protein intake. Disorders in this group should be considered in patients with lactic acidosis who have normal urine organic acids. Differentiation of the various disorders in this group can be facilitated by measuring plasma pyruvate and calculating the lactate/pyruvate ratio. A normal ratio (less than 25) suggests a defect in pyruvate dehydrogenase (PDH) or in gluconeogenesis, and an elevated ratio (greater than 25) suggests pyruvate carboxylase deficiency, a respiratory chain defect, or a mitochondrial myopathy.

Not all infants with life-threatening metabolic disease have metabolic acidosis or hyperammonemia. For example, patients with nonketotic hyperglycinemia typically present in the neonatal period with evidence of severe and progressive CNS dysfunction, but do not exhibit metabolic acidosis or hyperammonemia (11). Even patients with galactosemia rarely may present with symptoms of acute CNS toxicity, which may progress to cerebral edema, when galactose-1-phosphate levels rise precipitously. Therefore, a series of laboratory studies designed to screen for inborn errors of metabolism should be obtained for any infant with clinical findings suggesting an inborn error of metabolism, even if metabolic acidosis and hyperammonemia are not present. These studies are listed in Table 39–2. Most are self-explanatory. Although not available in many hospital laboratories, amino acid and organic acid analysis can be obtained in any part of the country through reference laboratories or through referral of samples to medical center genetics units. It is important to insist that any reference laboratory used for this purpose provide prompt test results and reference ranges and provide interpretation of abnormal results.

Urine testing for reducing substances should be performed using Benedict reagent (Clinitest tablets, Miles, Elkhart, IN). If the result is positive, the urine should be tested for glucose by dipstick. A nonglucose reducing substance in the urine is probably galactose, but there are other possibilities (Table 39–3). The urine ferric chloride test is a simple and rapid test that can lead to the early recognition of maple syrup urine disease, before results of amino acid analysis are available. In addition to the branched chain ketoacids, there are several other substances and disorders that produce a color change with ferric chloride. These are shown in Table 39–4. These tests are simple and straightforward and can be performed at the bedside. Reagents should be available in any hospital chemistry laboratory.

Several disorders associated with an acute metabolic encephalopathy in the neonate deserve special mention because they typically are not associated with hyperammonemia or metabolic acidosis. One of these is nonketotic hyperglycinemia, a condition that typically results in severe and progressive CNS dysfunction, including obtundation, seizures, and altered muscle tone. Routine laboratory studies all yield normal findings. The first diagnostic clue is usually the finding of elevated glycine on plasma amino acid analysis. The diagnosis is confirmed by measurement of cerebrospinal fluid (CSF) glycine and demonstration of an elevated CSF to plasma glycine ratio. Although therapy of infants with nonketotic hyperglycinemia has been attempted with dietary protein restriction, sodium benzoate, and a variety of other drugs, the results have been disappointing. Most infants with

this disorder die or exhibit significant neurologic impairment.

A second disorder that produces a progressive encephalopathy with no clues on routine laboratory studies is molybdenum cofactor deficiency. The neurologic findings in the affected infant are virtually indistinguishable from those associated with hypoxic-ischemic encephalopathy. Surviving infants exhibit similar neurologic sequelae including cerebral palsy, mental retardation, and seizures. The diagnosis may be suggested by the finding of hypouricemia or, beyond the neonatal period, by ectopia lentis noted on ophthalmologic examination. If it is suspected, urine should be screened for the presence of sulfites, a finding attributable to a deficiency of the enzyme sulfite oxidase, which accompanies the disorder.

The inborn errors of metabolism most likely to be associated with an acute encephalopathy in the newborn are summarized in Table 39–5. The typical laboratory findings in each condition or group of conditions also are listed.

Emergency Treatment of the Infant with an Acute Metabolic Encephalopathy

When an inborn error of metabolism, such as an organic acidemia or urea cycle defect, is suspected in a critically ill infant, immediate treatment should be initiated even if a definitive diagnosis may not yet be established. Within 48 to 72 hours, the results of amino acid and organic acid analyses should be available, allowing diagnostic confirmation in most cases. Appropriate and aggressive treatment before the confirmation of a diagnosis may be life saving and may avert or reduce the neurologic sequelae of some of these disorders. The immediate treatment of infants with disorders in this group has two primary goals. The first is the removal of accumulated metabolites, such as organic acid intermediates or ammonia. At the first suspicion of a disorder associated with protein intolerance, protein intake in the form of breast milk, infant formula, or hyperalimentation should be discontinued immediately. In critically ill infants with hyperammonemia, arrangements should be made for hemodialysis. Although peritoneal dialysis, continuous arteriovenous hemoperfusion, and exchange transfusion all have been used in the past to lower plasma ammonia levels, all are substantially less effective than hemodialysis (12). In infants who are comatose, ventilator dependent, or exhibit evidence of cerebral edema, dialysis should be instituted immediately without waiting to see if there is a response to dietary manipulation, medication, or other less aggressive therapy. Maximal supportive care should be provided simultaneously. In patients suspected of having a urea cycle defect because of significant hyperammonemia without acidosis, an infusion of 6 cc/kg of 10% arginine HCl (0.6 g/kg) can be given intravenously over 90 minutes. In patients with cit-

TABLE 39–3. *Disorders associated with nonglucose reducing substances in urine*

Disorder	Compound
Galactosemia	Galactose
Hereditary fructose intolerance	Fructose
Hereditary tyrosinemia	p-Hydroxy-phenylpyruvic acid
Galactokinase deficiency	Galactose
Essential fructosuria	Fructose
Pentosuria	Xylulose
Severe liver disease with secondary galactose intolerance	Galactose

TABLE 39–4. *Disorders associated with a positive ferric chloride reaction*

Disorder	Urine	
	Major compound	Color
Phenylketonuria	Phenylpyruvic acid	Green
Hereditary tyrosinemia	p-Hydroxy-phenylpyruvic acid	Green, fading rapidly
Maple syrup urine disease	Branched-chain ketoacids	Gray-green
Histidinemia	Imidazolepyruvic acid	Blue-green
Alkaptonuria	Homogentisic acid	Dark brown
Diabetic ketoacidosis	Acetoacetic acid	Cherry red
Pheochromocytoma	Catecholamines	Blue-green
Drug intoxication	Salicylates	Purple
	Phenothiazines	Purple
	p-Amino-salicylic acid	Red-brown
	Lysol	Green
Conjugated hyperbilirubinemia	Bilirubin	Green

rullinemia and argininosuccinic aciduria, this often results in a precipitous drop in the plasma ammonia level. An intravenous arginine preparation is commercially available and should be readily accessible from any hospital pharmacy.

If an organic acidemia is suspected, vitamin B_{12} (1 mg) should be given intramuscularly in case the patient has a vitamin B_{12}-responsive form of methylmalonic acidemia. Biotin (10 mg) should be given orally or by nasogastric tube, because some patients with multiple carboxylase deficiency are biotin responsive. If acidosis exists, intravenous bicarbonate should be administered liberally. Calculations of bicarbonate requirements appropriate for the treatment of other conditions rarely are adequate in these disorders because of ongoing production of organic acids or lactate. The acid–base status should be monitored frequently, with therapy adjusted accordingly.

After removing toxic metabolites, the second major goal of therapy in infants with inborn errors of metabolism should be to prevent catabolism. Ten percent glucose should be liberally administered intravenously, because it is important to provide as many calories as possible. Intravenous lipids can be given to infants with urea cycle defects and other disorders in which dietary fat plays no role. Protein should not be withheld indefinitely. If clinical improvement is observed and a final diagnosis has not been established, some amino acid intake should be provided after 2 to 3 days of complete protein restriction. Essential amino acids or total protein can be provided orally or intravenously at an initial dose of 0.5 g protein/kg body weight/24 hours. This should be increased incrementally to 1.0 g/kg/24 hours and held at that level until the diagnostic evaluation is complete and plans can be made for definitive long-term therapy. Therapy should be planned in conjunction with a geneticist or specialist in metabolic disease. Until then, supplemental calories and nutrients can be provided orally using protein-free diet powder (Product 80056, Mead Johnson, or Prophree, Ross Laboratories).

The chronic therapy of urea cycle defects and most of the organic acidemias involves restriction of dietary protein. Depending on the specific diagnosis, this may be accomplished by simple restriction of total protein intake in breast milk or standard infant formula or by use of special formulas designed for individual inborn errors of metabolism. Formulas have been developed for many of the more common metabolic disorders and are commercially available. These specialized formulas typically are

TABLE 39–5. *Major inborn errors of metabolism presenting in the neonate as an acute encephalopathy*

Disorders	Characteristic laboratory findings
1. Organic acidemias (includes MMA, PA, IVA, MCD, and many less common conditions)	Metabolic acidosis with increased anion gap; elevated plasma and urine ketones; variably elevated plasma ammonia and lactate; abnormal urine organic acids
2. Urea cycle defects	Variable respiratory alkalosis, no metabolic acidosis; markedly elevated plasma ammonia; elevated orotic acid in OTCD; abnormal plasma amino acids
3. Maple syrup urine disease	Metabolic acidosis with increased anion gap; elevated plasma and urine ketones; positive ferric chloride test; abnormal plasma amino acids
4. Nonketotic hyperglycinemia	No acid–base or electrolyte abnormalities; normal ammonia; abnormal plasma amino acids
5. Molybdenum cofactor deficiency	No acid–base or electrolyte abnormalities; normal ammonia; normal amino and organic acids; low serum uric acid; elevated sulfites in urine

IVA, isovaleric acidemia; MCD, multiple carboxylase deficiency; MMA, methylmalonic acidemia; OTCD, ornithine transcarbamylase deficiency; PA, propionic acidemia.

deficient in one or several specific amino acids. Dietary treatment alone may be effective in management of some patients with organic acidemias and in several disorders of amino acid metabolism, such as maple syrup urine disease.

In several of the vitamin-responsive disorders, such as methylmalonic acidemia, multiple carboxylase deficiency, and homocystinuria, dietary protein restriction may be combined with specific cofactor therapy. In the organic acidemias and certain other disorders, L-carnitine, usually beginning with a dose of 100 mg/kg/d, may be given. Acyl-CoAs accumulating in these disorders combine with carnitine to produce acylcarnitines that are water soluble and excreted in the urine. Without treatment, many patients with these disorders develop a secondary carnitine deficiency. Treatment with exogenous carnitine prevents the development of symptoms of carnitine deficiency and provides a measure of protection against recurrent episodes of metabolic decompensation by providing an augmented mechanism for excretion of accumulated metabolites.

Patients with urea cycle defects require supplementation with oral arginine or, in some cases, citrulline, which is converted to arginine in the body. In normal persons, adequate amounts of arginine are synthesized via the urea cycle. Patients with a defect in urea synthesis have deficient arginine production and must depend on dietary supplementation. In the case of carbamyl phosphate synthetase and ornithine transcarbamylase deficiencies, the most severe of the urea cycle defects, drug therapy also is required. These disorders were formerly almost uniformly lethal in the neonatal period. The development of novel drugs that provide an alternate pathway for waste nitrogen excretion has allowed survival of many affected infants (13). Sodium benzoate and sodium phenylacetate were the agents originally used, but these have been replaced largely for oral use by sodium phenylbutyrate.

Despite rigorous therapy and intensive surveillance, patients with urea cycle defects remain at risk for intercurrent episodes of hyperammonemia, which may result in death or neurologic sequelae. The risk appears to be greatest for patients with carbamyl phosphate synthetase and ornithine transcarbamylase deficiency. Liver transplantation should be considered seriously for patients with these disorders, if they can be stabilized.

Hypoglycemia

Hypoglycemia and its associated symptoms occasionally may be seen in infants with disorders of protein intolerance, but it more commonly is seen in disorders of carbohydrate metabolism or of fatty acid oxidation. Among the best known inborn errors of metabolism associated with hypoglycemia are the glycogen storage diseases, of which types I (i.e., von Gierke disease or glucose-6-phosphatase deficiency) and III (i.e., limit dextrinosis or

debrancher deficiency) are the most likely to be associated with manifestations in the neonatal period. The hypoglycemia in these disorders is related to the inability of the liver to release glucose from glycogen, and it is most profound during periods of fasting. Hypoglycemia, hepatomegaly, and lactic acidosis are prominent features of these disorders. Hypoglycemia is not a feature of glycogen storage disease type II (i.e., Pompe disease), because cytoplasmic glycogen metabolism and release are normal in this disorder, in which glycogen accumulates within lysosomes as a result of the deficiency of the lysosomal enzyme α-1,4-glucosidase. The clinical manifestations of this disorder include macroglossia, hypotonia, cardiomegaly with congestive heart failure, and hepatomegaly. Cardiomegaly is the most striking and may be apparent in the neonatal period. Congestive heart failure is the cause of death in most cases.

A disorder that presents clinically with findings virtually indistinguishable from the hepatic glycogen storage diseases types I and III is fructose-1,6-diphosphatase deficiency, a disorder of gluconeogenesis. Several other disorders of gluconeogenesis have been described. The basic immediate treatment of all of these disorders is frequent feedings and glucose administration. The definitive diagnosis is made by liver biopsy and assay of appropriate hepatic enzymes. In some cases, enzymatic assays can be performed using lymphocytes or cultured skin fibroblasts.

A number of inherited defects in fatty acid oxidation have been identified in infants presenting with hypoglycemia. Although many of the disorders in this group typically present after 2 months of age, neonatal manifestations may be observed. These disorders are important because of their apparent frequency and because of the variability of the initial presentation. Affected infants have an impaired capacity to use stored fat for fuel during periods of fasting and readily deplete their glycogen stores. Despite the development of hypoglycemia, acetyl CoA production is diminished, and ketone production is impaired. The hypoglycemia occurring in these conditions typically is characterized as nonketotic, although small amounts of ketones may be produced. Hypoglycemia may occur as an isolated finding or may be accompanied by many of the other biochemical derangements typically associated with Reye's syndrome, such as hyperammonemia, metabolic acidosis, and elevated transaminases. Hepatomegaly may or may not be present. Any infant presenting with findings suggesting Reye's syndrome should be evaluated for fatty acid oxidation defects. As the incidence of true Reye's syndrome has decreased, most children presenting at any age with this constellation of findings have an inherited metabolic disorder.

The most common of the fatty acid oxidation defects is medium-chain acyl-CoA dehydrogenase deficiency, which is estimated to occur in 1 of 15,000 births, an incidence similar to that observed for phenylketonuria (PKU)

(14,15). It is among the most common inborn errors of metabolism. In addition to presenting as nonketotic hypoglycemia or a Reye's-like syndrome, it may present as sudden death or an acute life-threatening event. Many infants diagnosed as having medium-chain acyl-CoA dehydrogenase deficiency have a history of a sibling who died of sudden infant death syndrome (16). Fat accumulation in the liver or muscle of any infant who dies unexpectedly should strongly suggest the possibility of this or a related disorder of fatty acid oxidation. Very-long-chain fatty acyl-CoA dehydrogenase deficiency is associated with similar clinical findings, although there may be evidence of a significant cardiomyopathy. Infants with this defect may present with cardiac arrhythmias or unexplained cardiac arrest. Defects in the carnitine cycle or in carnitine uptake also may lead to a profound defect in fatty acid oxidation and result in sudden neonatal death.

The accumulation of fatty acyl-CoAs in patients with fatty acid oxidation defects leads to a secondary carnitine deficiency, probably as a result of excretion of excess acylcarnitines in the urine (17,18). Urine organic acid analysis and measurement of serum carnitine and analysis of the plasma acylcarnitine profile are the most helpful laboratory studies in the initial screening for defects in fatty acid oxidation. These studies are sufficient to establish the diagnosis of medium-chain acyl-CoA dehydrogenase deficiency, which is associated with the presence of a characteristic metabolite, octanoylcarnitine, on the acylcarnitine profile. Enzymatic assays may be necessary for the definitive diagnosis of some of the fatty acid oxidation defects. As is true for the defects in carbohydrate metabolism leading to hypoglycemia, treatment of the fatty acid oxidation defects involves avoidance of fasting and provision of adequate glucose. Restriction of dietary fat intake and supplemental L-carnitine therapy at a dose of 50 to 100 mg/kg/d is recommended. With appropriate therapy, patients with medium-chain acyl-CoA dehydrogenase deficiency appear to have an excellent prognosis. The prognosis for the other fatty acid oxidation defects is more variable.

Jaundice and Liver Dysfunction

Jaundice or other evidence of liver dysfunction may be the presenting finding in a number of inherited metabolic disorders in the neonatal period. These are listed in Table 39–6, along with the laboratory studies useful in diagnosis. For most of the inborn errors of metabolism associated with jaundice, the elevated serum bilirubin is of the direct-reacting type. This generalization does not include those inborn errors of erythrocyte metabolism, such as glucose-6-phosphate dehydrogenase deficiency or pyruvate kinase deficiency, which occasionally are responsible for hemolytic disease in the newborn. The best-known metabolic disease associated with jaundice is galactosemia, in which the deficiency of the enzyme galactose-1-phosphate uridyl transferase results in an accumulation of galactose-1-phosphate and other metabolites, such as galactitol, which are thought to have a direct toxic effect on the liver and on other organs. Jaundice and liver dysfunction in this disorder are progressive and usually appear at the end of the first or during the second week of life, with vomiting, diarrhea, poor weight gain, and eventual cataract formation if the infant is receiving breast milk or a galactose-containing formula. Hypoglycemia may be observed. The disease may present initially with indirect hyperbilirubinemia resulting from hemolysis secondary to high levels of galactose-1-phosphate in erythrocytes. Alternatively, the effects of acute galactose toxicity on the brain rarely may cause the CNS symptoms to predominate and, in some cases, *Escherichia coli* sepsis is the presenting problem.

If galactosemia is suspected, the urine should be tested simultaneously with Benedict reagent and with a glucose oxidase method. The glucose oxidase method is specific for glucose, and Benedict reagent can detect any reducing substance. A negative dipstick for glucose with a positive Benedict reaction means that a nonglucose reducing substance is present. With appropriate clinical findings, this is most likely to be galactose. Paper or thin-layer chromatography can be used to identify positively the reducing substance. If a child with galactosemia has been on intravenous fluids and recently has not been receiving galactose in the diet, galactose may not be present in the urine.

If the diagnosis of galactosemia is suspected, whether or not reducing substances are found in the urine, galactose-containing feedings should be discontinued immediately and replaced by soy formula or other lactose-free

TABLE 39–6. *Inborn errors of metabolism associated with neonatal liver disease and laboratory studies useful in diagnosis*

Disorder	Laboratory studies
Galactosemia	Urine reducing substances; red blood cell galactose-1-phosphate uridyl transferase
Hereditary tyrosinemia	Plasma quantitative amino acids; urine succinylacetone
Alpha₁-antitrypsin deficiency	Quantitative serum alpha₁-antitrypsin; protease inhibitor (Pi) typing
Neonatal hemochromatosis	Serum ferritin; liver biopsy
Zellweger syndrome	Plasma very-long-chain fatty acids
Niemann–Pick disease type C	Skin biopsy for fibroblast culture; studies of cholesterol esterification and accumulation
Glycogen storage disease type IV (brancher deficiency)	Liver biopsy for histology and biochemical analysis or skin biopsy with assay of branching enzyme in cultured fibroblasts

formula, pending the results of appropriate enzyme assays on erythrocytes to confirm the diagnosis. Untreated galactosemics, if they survive the neonatal period, have persistent liver disease, cataracts, and severe mental retardation. Many affected infants die of *E. coli* sepsis in the neonatal period, and the early onset of sepsis may alter the presentation of the disorder (19).

Treatment of the disorder by maintenance of strict dietary restriction of galactose, if started early, results in complete reversal of liver disease and enables many affected individuals to develop normal or near-normal intelligence. Unfortunately, there continues to be an increased incidence of mental retardation even among treated patients. In addition, there are some late sequelae of the disorder that appear to be unaffected by current therapy. These include premature ovarian failure in females and a late-onset neurologic syndrome involving ataxia and tremors in both genders (20,21). Many states have newborn screening programs for galactosemia, but clinical manifestations of the disorder often appear before the results of screening studies are available; therefore, it is critical that physicians remain alert to this possibility.

Another inborn error of metabolism that occasionally presents in the newborn period with jaundice, hepatomegaly, and the presence of reducing substances in the urine is hereditary fructose intolerance, which is characterized by episodes of profound hypoglycemia, vomiting, and metabolic acidosis. This disorder is seen uncommonly in the neonate, because most newborns are not exposed immediately to a fructose-containing diet unless they have been given a soy formula with sucrose as the carbohydrate source. In the uncommon event that an infant who has been receiving fructose should present with these findings, this diagnosis should be considered. Analysis of the urine reveals the presence of a nonglucose reducing substance that can be demonstrated by chromatography to be fructose. Treatment involves elimination of fructose from the diet and results in complete resolution of all clinical signs and symptoms. Confirmation of the diagnosis is by assay of the deficient enzyme fructose-1-phosphate aldolase in liver tissue, but this rarely is necessary.

α_1-Antitrypsin deficiency, a puzzling disorder that is among the most common of all inherited metabolic diseases, also may present with neonatal jaundice (22). The clinical manifestations of this disorder may be identical to those of traditional neonatal or giant cell hepatitis, and a determination of serum α_1-antitrypsin should be a part of the initial evaluation of all children presenting with this syndrome. Infants with deficient levels of α_1-antitrypsin on quantitative analysis should have protease inhibitor typing performed to confirm the diagnosis. There is no specific treatment for the liver disease associated with α_1-antitrypsin deficiency, but approximately one-half of all affected infants eventually exhibit com-

plete resolution of the liver dysfunction. Others may progress to end-stage disease and require liver transplantation. A history of chronic pulmonary disease in adult family members may be obtained.

Hereditary tyrosinemia is another disorder that presents with liver disease in early infancy. The biochemical hallmarks of this disorder include marked elevations of plasma tyrosine and methionine and generalized aminoaciduria with a disproportionate increase in the excretion of tyrosine. However, these findings are relatively nonspecific and may be observed as a secondary phenomenon in other forms of liver disease. Hereditary tyrosinemia once was among the most difficult of inborn errors of metabolism to diagnose clinically. The finding of succinylacetone in the urine of patients with this disease has led to a helpful diagnostic test for the disorder (23). It also has become possible to establish the diagnosis definitively by demonstrating a deficiency of the enzyme fumarylacetoacetate fumarylhydrolase in lymphocytes and cultured skin fibroblasts of affected individuals (24).

Neonatal hemochromatosis, a recently described and poorly understood disorder, may be the most common cause of congenital cirrhosis. Its fulminating course distinguishes it from many of the other metabolic disorders associated with neonatal liver disease. In addition to being associated with severe liver failure from birth, the disorder is characterized by distinctive hepatic morphology and hepatic and extrahepatic parenchymal iron deposition. Serum ferritin and iron typically are elevated, whereas total transferrin is low, but these findings are not diagnostic. The definitive diagnosis is established by liver biopsy or autopsy. If liver biopsy is contraindicated because of a secondary coagulopathy, biopsy of the salivary glands is a useful alternative. Most affected infants succumb to the disorder during the early weeks of life. The only clearly effective mode of therapy is liver transplantation; intensive chelation therapy may be attempted but largely has been unsuccessful. At present, it is not clear whether iron storage is the primary defect or is secondary to fetal liver disease that may be causally heterogeneous. There are familial recurrences, so at least some cases appear to have a genetic basis, although the mode of inheritance is not well established.

Less common metabolic causes of neonatal liver dysfunction include Niemann–Pick disease type C and glycogen storage disease type IV. Infants with Niemann–Pick disease type C exhibit cholestatic jaundice, which typically resolves by several months of age. They then are clinically normal for a period of months to years before developing findings of a degenerative neurologic disorder. Infants with glycogen storage disease type IV accumulate an abnormal form of glycogen in the liver as a result of a deficiency of the glycogen branching enzyme. This leads to progressive cirrhosis and generalized hepatic dysfunction. Hypoglycemia is not a prominent feature, as it is in some other forms of glycogen storage disease.

Zellweger syndrome, formerly referred to as the cerebrohepatorenal syndrome, is another cause of neonatal jaundice and hepatic dysfunction, but it usually is recognizable clinically because of the associated hypotonia and dysmorphic features. It is the prototype of the peroxisome assembly disorders and is associated with generalized peroxisomal dysfunction.

In contrast to disorders in which there is an elevation of the direct-reacting bilirubin, a persistent elevation of indirect bilirubin beyond the limits of physiologic jaundice, without evidence of hemolysis, suggests the diagnosis of the Crigler–Najjar syndrome. The hyperbilirubinemia in this disorder is related to a partial or complete deficiency of glucuronyl transferase, the liver enzyme responsible for the normal conjugation of bilirubin to bilirubin diglucuronide. There is no effective long-term therapy for all patients with this disorder, but the standard modalities of phototherapy and exchange transfusion may prevent the development of kernicterus in the neonatal period (25,26). Hepatic transplantation has been performed successfully in patients with this disorder. Patients with a partial deficiency of the enzyme may respond to phenobarbital therapy (26).

Findings Suggestive of a Storage Disease

Many of the well-known lipid storage diseases typically do not present in the neonatal period. Among those that occasionally may be associated with hepatosplenomegaly in the neonatal period are GM_1-gangliosidosis type I, Gaucher disease, Niemann–Pick disease, and Wolman disease. The glycogen storage diseases that are associated with hepatomegaly in the newborn have previously been discussed in reference to hypoglycemia. Infants with the most common mucopolysaccharidoses, such as the Hurler and Hunter syndromes, uncommonly exhibit clinical abnormalities in the first month of life. Newborns with the typical features of these syndromes, such as coarse facial features, hepatosplenomegaly, skeletal abnormalities, and hernias, are more likely to have GM_1-gangliosidosis or a mucolipidosis, such as I-cell disease. Beta-glucuronidase deficiency, also classified as mucopolysaccharidosis type VII, may present in the neonatal period with features virtually indistinguishable clinically from those seen later in the Hurler and Hunter syndromes. An infantile form of sialidosis (i.e., neuraminidase deficiency) typically is associated with findings at birth. The clinical manifestations of several of these conditions may be so severe *in utero* that fetal hydrops develops.

If one of these disorders is suspected, urine screening tests for mucopolysaccharides and oligosaccharides should be performed. These can be helpful diagnostically, but negative results do not rule out the possibility of a storage disorder. False-positive mucopolysaccharide spot tests are not uncommonly observed in neonates. The definitive diagnosis of most disorders of lipid or mucopolysaccharide metabolism is made by appropriate biochemical studies on leukocytes or cultured skin fibroblasts.

Abnormal Odor

Abnormal body or urinary odor, more commonly observed by nurses or mothers rather than physicians, is an important but often overlooked clue to the diagnosis of several of the inborn errors of metabolism and may be the most specific clinical finding in these patients. It is best described for PKU, for which the urine was found to have a peculiar musty odor years before the biochemical basis of the disease was understood. In the acutely ill neonate with an abnormal odor, isovaleric acidemia, glutaric acidemia type II, and maple syrup urine disease are the most likely entities to be encountered. In maple syrup urine disease, the urine has a distinctive sweet odor, said to be reminiscent of maple syrup or burnt sugar. The odor associated with isovaleric acidemia and glutaric acidemia type II is pungent and unpleasant and similar to that of sweaty feet.

Dysmorphic Features

There formerly appeared to be a clear distinction between inborn errors of metabolism and dysmorphic syndromes, both of which may be inherited in a similar fashion. Infants with inherited metabolic disease were thought to be phenotypically normal at birth, with no evidence of major or minor structural anomalies. It is becoming increasingly apparent that inherited metabolic disorders may be associated with consistent patterns of birth defects, suggesting that metabolic derangements *in utero* may disrupt the normal process of fetal development.

This phenomenon is illustrated clearly by the group of disorders associated with multiple defects in peroxisomal enzymes, including those involved in fatty acid oxidation and plasmalogen synthesis (27,28). These include Zellweger syndrome (i.e., cerebrohepatorenal syndrome), neonatal adrenoleukodystrophy, and several variant conditions, all of which are associated with congenital hypotonia and dysmorphic features, such as epicanthal folds, Brushfield spots, large fontanelles, simian creases, and renal cysts. Patients with glutaric acidemia type II, one of the organic acidemias, have a characteristic phenotype, including a high forehead, hypertelorism, low-set ears, abdominal wall defects, palpably enlarged kidneys, hypospadias, and rocker bottom feet (29,30). An energy-deficient mechanism (i.e., fuel-mediated teratogenesis), similar to that postulated for maternal diabetes mellitus, has been suggested to explain these findings. Several of the other organic acidemias, such as mevalonic aciduria, and 3-hydroxyisobutyric aciduria, as well PDH, have been associated with multiple dysmorphic features.

Some infants with PDH deficiency have dysmorphic facial features resembling those observed in the fetal alcohol syndrome (FAS) (31). The specific findings observed include a narrow forehead with frontal bossing, a broad nasal bridge, short nose with anteverted nostrils, and a long philtrum. The resemblance to FAS has been explained by suggesting that there is a common mechanism in the two disorders, involving a deficiency of PDH activity. It has been postulated that, in FAS, acetaldehyde from the maternal circulation inhibits fetal PDH, which leads to malformations.

The Smith–Lemli–Opitz syndrome is an autosomal recessive disorder associated with a wide range of malformations, including dysmorphic facies, cleft palate, congenital heart disease, hypospadias, polydactyly, and 2–3 syndactyly of the feet. Recent observations have revealed that this disorder is an inborn error of cholesterol biosynthesis. Affected infants have decreased levels of plasma cholesterol accompanied by markedly elevated levels of the cholesterol precursor 7-dehydrocholesterol (32).

Isolated malformations may be even more commonly associated with inherited metabolic disorders than are specific malformation patterns. Patients with nonketotic hyperglycinemia frequently have agenesis of the corpus callosum and may have gyral malformations related to defects in neuronal migration as well (33). Patients with PDH deficiency also may exhibit agenesis of the corpus callosum (34). It is not uncommon for patients with almost any of the inborn errors of metabolism to exhibit one or more dysmorphic features or anomalies that are nonspecific. The observation of dysmorphic features in an infant in no way should preclude consideration of an inherited metabolic disorder. In selected circumstances, it may heighten the clinical suspicion.

Abnormal Eye Findings

Abnormal eye findings typically are associated with many of the inborn errors of metabolism, although they are not always found at the time of initial presentation. Cataracts classically are associated with galactosemia and other disorders of galactose metabolism, but also are observed in disorders such as Zellweger syndrome and Lowe syndrome. Dislocated lenses, seen in homocystinuria, molybdenum cofactor deficiency, and sulfite oxidase deficiency, may be found as early as the first month of life and are an important clue to diagnosis. Retinal degenerative changes are typical of the peroxisomal disorders, including Zellweger syndrome and neonatal adrenoleukodystrophy, and are observed in several other conditions. Other abnormalities that may be associated with inborn errors of metabolism include corneal clouding and congenital glaucoma. A careful eye examination, preferably by an ophthalmologist, should be performed whenever an inherited metabolic disorder is suspected. A summary of some of the inherited metabolic disorders associated with specific ocular abnormalities is shown in Table 39–7.

Samples to Obtain from a Dying Child with a Suspected Inborn Error of Metabolism

If death appears imminent in a child suspected of having an inborn error of metabolism, it is important to

TABLE 39–7. *Eye abnormalities associated with inborn errors of metabolism*

Eye finding	Associated disorders
Cataracts	Galactosemia
	Homocystinuria
	Lowe syndrome
	Zellweger syndrome
	Rhizomelic chondrodysplasia punctata
	Senger syndrome
	Hypophosphatasia
Ectopia lentis	Homocystinuria
	Molybdenum cofactor deficiency
	Sulfite oxidase deficiency
Cherry red spot	Niemann–Pick disease types A and B
	Gaucher disease type II
	GM$_2$ gangliosidosis (Tay–Sachs; Sandhoff)
	Sialidosis type II
	Farber disease
Corneal clouding	Mucopolysaccharidoses
	Mucolipidoses
	Lowe syndrome
	Homocystinuria
Pigmentary retinopathy	Zellweger syndrome
	Neonatal adrenoleukodystrophy
	Long-chain 3-hydroxyacyl-CoA dehydrogenase deficiency

obtain the appropriate samples for postmortem analysis. This is critical for resolution of the cause of death and is essential for subsequent genetic counseling and prenatal diagnosis. The following samples should be collected and stored: urine, frozen; plasma, separated from whole blood and frozen; and a small snip of skin obtained using sterile technique and stored at room temperature or 37°C in tissue culture medium, if available, or sterile saline. The latter sample can be obtained by slipping a 25-gauge needle under the skin, lifting the skin, and snipping a 2- to 3-mm ellipse with a sterile scissors, which can be found in a suture removal tray. The skin should be cleansed with alcohol. If an autopsy is performed, a sample of unfixed liver tissue should be obtained as soon as possible after death and frozen at -20°C for subsequent biochemical studies. Additional tissue should be preserved for electron microscopy. If consent for autopsy is denied, consent for a postmortem needle biopsy of the liver should be requested. The liver tissue should be frozen in total or in part if histologic studies appear to be indicated. As soon as possible after death, the case should be reviewed with a metabolic specialist and plans made for the transport of samples to the appropriate laboratory.

NEWBORN SCREENING FOR INHERITED METABOLIC DISORDERS

All 50 states and the District of Columbia in the United States and many other countries have newborn screening programs in place for genetic disorders. In the United States, there are significant state-to-state differences in the disorders that are included, the methods of screening, and follow-up.

The only two disorders for which screening is routine in all 50 states and the District of Columbia are PKU and hypothyroidism. Because neonates with PKU usually are asymptomatic, neonatologists rarely encounter this condition, except in the context of following abnormal screening test results. Because phenylalanine levels are normal in the cord blood of infants with this condition and rise only after milk feedings have been initiated, newborn screening samples should be obtained after 24 hours of age. In the case of infants discharged before 24 hours, most states recommend that a sample be obtained at discharge and subsequently repeated. In the case of sick infants who are not being fed, the initial newborn screening sample should not be withheld indefinitely but should be submitted at the recommended time (often 7 days), because screening for some other disorders, such as hypothyroidism, is not affected by the feeding history. For PKU screening, however, another specimen should be submitted after feedings are instituted. If the phenylalanine level is elevated on the first sample, a repeat specimen may be requested. If it is elevated again, referral for definitive diagnosis should be made immediately. This includes quantitative plasma amino acids and analysis of urinary pterins to rule out disorders of biopterin metabolism, which result in hyperphenylalaninemia. Newborn screening and early dietary treatment of PKU have altered completely the natural history of this disorder, which once accounted for 1% of all institutionalized mentally retarded persons. Children whose disorder is maintained under strict dietary control now can be expected to exhibit normal growth and intellectual development.

Several other inherited metabolic disorders are included in the newborn screening programs of selected states. The specific disorders and the number of states engaged in newborn screening for each are as follows: galactosemia 37; maple syrup urine disease 20; homocystinuria 19; biotinidase deficiency 12; hereditary tyrosinemia 7; congenital adrenal hyperplasia 5; and cystic fibrosis 3. A likely candidate for the future may be medium-chain acyl-CoA dehydrogenase deficiency. Although there is no simple screening test for the abnormal metabolites in this disorder, a single DNA mutation has been identified that accounts for approximately 90% of the defective genes (14). It may be possible to implement newborn screening by direct DNA analysis, and several pilot screening programs have been conducted to test this approach. This disorder appears to be an excellent candidate for newborn screening, because it is estimated to be among the most common of the inborn errors of metabolism, with an incidence of approximately 1 in 15,000, and is associated with an excellent prognosis if recognized and treated.

Neonatologists should attempt to be actively involved in the evaluation of disorders considered for inclusion in newborn screening programs. Several criteria should be met before screening is considered on other than a research basis. The disorder should be sufficiently common to justify screening. A relatively simple, accurate, and inexpensive screening test should be available. Treatment for the disorder should be available, and there should be some demonstrable benefit to starting treatment before clinical symptoms appear and the diagnosis is made on clinical grounds. It is on the basis of the last criterion that newborn screening for cystic fibrosis often has been criticized. Newborn screening for purposes of genetic counseling alone, when there is no clear benefit to the affected infant, generally is not viewed as appropriate. It is a inefficient method of identifying couples at risk of having a child with a recessively inherited disorder, because it identifies such couples only after the birth of an affected child. Carrier testing in the child-bearing age group is a far more appropriate approach to the identification of at-risk couples.

MATERNAL METABOLIC DISORDERS

With advances in therapy for inborn errors of metabolism, it is now common for patients with many of these disorders to reach adult life with normal or near-normal intelligence and the desire to have families of their own. This has led to serious concerns about the potential adverse effects of maternal metabolic derangements on fetal growth and development. The real potential for adverse consequences is illustrated by the experience that has accumulated with maternal PKU. In the past, patients with PKU were severely retarded and did not reproduce. This changed completely with the initiation of newborn screening programs and early dietary management. Dietary therapy was once maintained until 5 to 6 years of age and then discontinued. Treatment now is continued indefinitely in most cases, because it has been demonstrated that some patients exhibit neurologic deterioration and loss of IQ points after discontinuation of the diet. Nonetheless, most patients with PKU who are now adults have been off the diet for years and have high phenylalanine levels. After women with PKU began reproducing, it became clear that the maternal metabolic environment in this condition had extremely harmful effects on fetal development. A spectrum of findings referred to as "maternal PKU syndrome" is observed in a large percentage of exposed infants, most of whom do not themselves have PKU (35,36). More than 90% of exposed infants exhibit mental retardation, and microcephaly occurs in 72%, growth retardation in 40%, and congenital heart disease in 12%. Altered facial features, similar to those observed in FAS, may be observed. Mothers with benign hyperphenylalaninemia, a condition that is associated with lower phenylalanine levels than classical PKU and does not require treatment, may be at increased risk for fetal abnormalities.

There is some suggestion that dietary treatment of pregnant women before conception and throughout pregnancy, with careful control of phenylalanine levels, may reduce the risk (37). This is a difficult goal to achieve, because the phenylalanine-restricted diet is an onerous one to patients who have ever been on a normal diet, and some adult patients, despite early therapy, may have borderline intellectual functioning. A national collaborative study is in progress to address many of the issues related to the identification and treatment of maternal PKU. There has been no evidence for an increased risk of birth defects or any other problems in infants born to fathers with PKU.

Pregnancies have been reported in mothers with a variety of other inherited metabolic disorders, including several forms of glycogen storage disease, propionic acidemia, isovaleric acidemia, homocystinuria, hereditary orotic aciduria, and several others, with no adverse outcomes clearly attributable to the maternal disorder. The collaborative experience with many disorders, however, is limited to single cases or small numbers of patients. It is probable that other maternal metabolic disorders will be identified that adversely affect fetal development.

REFERENCES

1. Scriver CR, Beaudet AL, Sly WS, Valle D, eds. *The metabolic and molecular bases of inherited disease*, 7th ed. New York: McGraw-Hill, 1995.
2. Emery AEH, Rimoin DL, eds. *Principles and practice of medical genetics*, 3rd ed. New York: Churchill Livingstone, 1996.
3. Fischer AQ, Challa VR, Burton BK, McLean WT. Cerebellar hemorrhage complicating isovaleric acidemia: a case report. *Neurology* 1981;31:746.
4. Nyhan WL. Patterns of clinical expression and genetic variation in the inborn errors of metabolism. In: Nyhan WL, ed. *Heritable disorders of amino acid metabolism*. New York: John Wiley and Sons, 1974;3.
5. Ballard RA, Vinocur B, Reynolds JW, et al. Transient hyperammonemia of the preterm infant. *N Engl J Med* 1978;299:920.
6. Msall M, Batshaw ML, Suss R, et al. Neurologic outcome in children with inborn errors of urea synthesis. *N Engl J Med* 1984;310:1500.
7. Goldberg RN, Cabal LA, Sinatra FR, et al. Hyperammonemia associated with perinatal asphyxia. *Pediatrics* 1979;64:336.
8. Batshaw ML, Wachtel RC, Cohen L, et al. Neurologic outcome in premature infants with transient asymptomatic hyperammonemia. *J Pediatr* 1986;108:27.
9. Robinson BH, Taylor J, Sherwood WG. The genetic heterogeneity of lactic acidosis: occurrence of recognizable inborn errors of metabolism in a pediatric population with lactic acidosis. *Pediatr Res* 1980;14:956.
10. Robinson BH, Glerum DM, Chow W, et al. The use of skin fibroblast cultures in the detection of respiratory chain defects in patients with lactic acidemia. *Pediatr Res* 1990;28:549.
11. Carson NAJ. Non-ketotic hyperglycinemia—a review of 70 patients. *J Inherit Metab Dis* 1982;2[Suppl 5]:126.
12. Wiegand C, Thompson T, Bock GH, et al. The management of life-threatening hyperammonemia: a comparison of several therapeutic modalities. *J Pediatr* 1980;96:142.
13. Batshaw ML, Brusilow SW, Waber L, et al. Treatment of inborn errors of urea synthesis: activation of alternative pathways of waste nitrogen synthesis and excretion. *N Engl J Med* 1982;306:1387.
14. Matsubara Y, Narisawa K, Tada K, et al. Prevalence of K329E mutation in medium-chain acyl-CoA dehydrogenase gene determined from Guthrie cards. *Lancet* 1991;1:552.
15. Ziadeh R. Medium chain acyl-CoA dehydrogenase deficiency in Pennsylvania: neonatal screening shows high incidence and unexpected mutation frequencies. *Pediatr Res* 1995;37:675.
16. Duran M, Hofkamp M, Rhead WJ, et al. Sudden death and "healthy" affected family members with medium-chain acyl coenzyme A dehydrogenase deficiency. *Pediatrics* 1986;78:1052.
17. Stanley CA, Hale DE, Coates PM, et al. Medium chain acyl-CoA dehydrogenase deficiency in children with non-ketotic hypoglycemia and low carnitine levels. *Pediatr Res* 1983;17:877.
18. Engel AG, Rebouche CJ. Carnitine metabolism and inborn errors. *J Inherit Metab Dis* 1984;1[Suppl 7]:38.
19. Levy HL, Sepe SJ, Shih VE, et al. Sepsis due to Escherichia coli in neonates with galactosemia. *N Engl J Med* 1977;297:823.
20. Kaufman FR, Kogut MD, Donnell GN, et al. Hypergonadotropic hypogonadism in female patients with galactosemia. *N Engl J Med* 1981;304:994.
21. Friedman JH, Levy HL, Boustany RM. Late onset of distinct neurologic syndromes in galactosemic siblings. *Neurology* 1989;39:741.
22. Cutz E, Cox DW. Alpha₁-antitrypsin deficiency: the spectrum of pathology and pathophysiology. *Perspect Pediatr Pathol* 1979;5:1.
23. Lindbland B, Lindstedt S, Stein G. On the enzymic defects in hereditary tyrosinemia. *Proc Natl Acad Sci USA* 1977;74:4641.
24. Kvittingen EA, Halvorsen S, Jellum E. Deficient acetoacetate fumarylhydrolase activity in lymphocytes and fibroblasts from patients with hereditary tyrosinemia. *Pediatr Res* 1983;14:541.
25. Karon M, Imach D, Schwartz A. Phototherapy in congenital non-obstructive non-hemolytic jaundice. *N Engl J Med* 1970;282:377.
26. Garodischer R, Levy G, Krasner J, Yaffe SJ. Congenital non-obstructive non-hemolytic jaundice: effect of phototherapy. *N Engl J Med* 1970;282:375.
27. Schutgens RBH, Heymans HSA, Wanders RJA, et al. Peroxisomal disorders: a newly recognized group of genetic diseases. *Eur J Pediatr* 1986;144:430.
28. Wilson GN, Holmes RD, Hajra AK. Peroxisomal disorders: clinical commentary and future prospects. *Am J Med Genet* 1988;30:771.

29. Sweetman L, Nyhan WL, Trauner DA, et al. Glutaric acidemia type II. *J Pediatr* 1980;96:1020.

30. Chalmers RA, Tracy BM, King GS, et al. The prenatal diagnosis of glutaric acidemia type II using quantitative gas chromatography–mass spectroscopy. *J Inherit Metab Dis* 1980;3:67.

31. Robinson BH, McMillan H, Petrova-Benedict R, Sherwood WG. Variable clinical presentation in patients with deficiency of pyruvate dehydrogenase complex. A review of 30 cases with a defect in the E component of the complex. *J Pediatr* 1987;111:525.

32. Opitz JM, de la Cruz F. Cholesterol metabolism in the RSH/Smith–Lemli–Opitz syndrome: summary of an NICHD conference. *Am J Med Genet* 1994;50:326.

33. Dobyns WB. Agenesis of the corpus callosum and gyral malformations are frequent manifestations of nonketotic hyperglycinemia. *Neurology* 1989;39:817.

34. Wick H, Schweizer KK, Baumgartner R. Thiamine dependency in a patient with congenital lactic acidemia due to pyruvate dehydrogenase deficiency. *Agents Actions* 1977;7:405.

35. Lenke RR, Levy HL. Maternal phenylketonuria and hyperphenylalaninemia. An international survey of untreated and treated pregnancies. *N Engl J Med* 1980;303:1202.

36. Levy HL, Waisbren SE. Effects of untreated maternal phenylketonuria and hyperphenylalaninemia on the fetus. *N Engl J Med* 1983;309:1269.

37. Rohr FJ, Doherty LB, Waisbren SE, et al. New England Maternal PKU project. Prospective study of untreated and treated pregnancies and their outcomes. *J Pediatr* 1987;11:391.

38. Fishler K, Koch R, Donnell GN, Wenz E. Developmental aspects of galactosemia from infancy to childhood. *Clin Pediatr* 1980;19:38.

39. Baerlocher K, Gitzelmann R, Steinmann B, Gitzelmann-Cumarasamy N. Hereditary fructose intolerance in early childhood: a major diagnostic challenge. Survey of 20 symptomatic cases. *Helv Paediatr Acta* 1978;33:465.

40. Pagliara AS, Karl IE, Keating JP, et al. Hepatic fructose-1,6-diphosphatase deficiency. A cause of lactic acidosis and hypoglycemia in infancy. *J Clin Invest* 1972;51:2115.

41. Moses SW, Gutman A. Inborn errors of glycogen metabolism. *Adv Pediatr* 1972;19:95.

42. Huijing F, van Creveld S, Losekoot G. Diagnosis of generalized glycogen storage disease (Pompe's disease). *J Pediatr* 1963;63:984.

43. Levin B, Burgess EA, Mortimer PE. Glycogen storage disease type IV: amylopectinosis. *Arch Dis Child* 1968;43:548.

44. Clow CL, Reade TM, Scriver CR. Outcome of early and long-term management of classical maple syrup urine disease. *Pediatrics* 1981;68:856.

45. Mudd SH, Skovby F, Levy HL, et al. The natural history of homocystinuria due to cystathionine beta-synthase deficiency. *Am J Hum Genet* 1985;37:1

46. Baumgartner R, Ando T, Nyhan WL. Nonketotic hyperglycinemia. *J Pediatr* 1969;75:1022.

47. Smith I, Wolff OH. Natural history of phenyketonuria and influence of early treatment. *Lancet* 1974;2:540.

48. Kvittingen EA. Hereditary tyrosinemia type I—an overview. *Scand J Clin Lab Invest* 1986;46:27.

49. Fell V, Pollitt RJ, Sampson GA, Wright T. Ornithinemia, hyperammonemia and homocitrullinuria. A disease associated with mental retardation and possibly caused by defective mitochondrial transport. *Am J Dis Child* 1974;127:752.

50. Simell O, Perheentupa J, Rapola J, Visakorpi JK, Eskelin L-E. Lysinuric protein intolerance. *Am J Med* 1975;59:229.

51. Allen RJ, Wong PWK, Rothenberg SP, et al. Progressive neonatal leukoencephalomyopathy due to absent methylene-tetrahydrofolate reductase, responsive to treatment. *Ann Neurol* 1980;8:211.

52. Scriver CR, Whelan DT. Glutamic acid decarboxylase (GAD) in mammalian tissue outside the central nervous system, and its possible relevance to hereditary B_6 dependency with seizures. *Ann N Y Acad Sci* 1969;166:83.

53. Matsui SM, Mahoney MJ, Rosenberg LE. The natural history of the inherited methylmalonic acidemias. *N Engl J Med* 1983;308:857.

54. Mitchell GA, Watkins D, Melancon SB, et al. Clinical heterogeneity in cobalamin C variant of combined homocystinuria and methylmalonic aciduria. *J Pediatr* 1986;108:410.

55. Wolf B, Hsia YE, Sweetman L, et al. Propionic acidemia: a clinical update. *J Pediatr* 1981;99:835.

56. Newman CGH, Wilson BDR, Callaghan P, Young L. Neonatal death associated with isovaleric acidemia. *Lancet* 1967;2:439.

57. Finnie MDA, Cottrall K, Seakins JWT, Snedden W. Massive excretion of 2-oxoglutaric acid and 3-hydroxyisovaleric acid in a patient with a deficiency of 3-methylcrotonyl-CoA carboxylase. *Clin Chim Acta* 1976;73:513.

58. Burri BJ, Sweetman L, Nyhan WL. Heterogeneity of holocarboxylase synthetase in patients with biotin-responsive multiple carboxylase deficiency. *Am J Hum Genet* 1985;37:426.

59. Wolf B, Heard GS, Weissbecker KA, et al. Biotinidase deficiency: initial clinical features and rapid diagnosis. *Ann Neurol* 1985;18:614.

60. Leibel RL, Shih VE, Goodman SI, et al. Glutaric acidemia: a metabolic disorder causing progressive choreoathetosis. *Neurology* 1980;30:1163.

61. Goodman SI, Stene DO, McCabe ERB, et al. Glutaric acidemia type II: clinical, biochemical and morphologic considerations. *J Pediatr* 1982;100:946.

62. Mantagos S, Genel M, Tanaka K. Ethylmalonic-adipic aciduria: in vivo and in vitro studies indicating deficiency of activities of multiple acyl-CoA dehydrogenases. *J Clin Invest* 1979;64:1580.

63. Wysocki SJ, Hahnel R. 3-Hydroxy-3-methylglutaryl-CoA lyase deficiency: a review. *J Inherit Metab Dis* 1986;9:225.

64. Robinson BH, Sherwood WG, Taylor J, et al. Acetoacetyl CoA thiolase deficiency: a cause of severe ketoacidosis in infancy simulating salicylism. *J Pediatr* 1979;95:228.

65. Hoffmann G, Gibson KM, Brandt IK, et al. Mevalonic aciduria—an inborn error of cholesterol and nonsterol isoprene biosynthesis. *N Engl J Med* 1986;314:1610.

66. Hagenfeldt L, Larsson A, Zetterstrom R. Pyroglutamic aciduria. Studies of an infant with chronic metabolic acidosis. *Acta Paediatr Scand* 1974;63:1.

67. Fang-Jong D, Nyhan WL, Wolff J, et al. 3-Hydroxyisobutyric aciduria: an inborn error of valine metabolism. *Pediatr Res* 1991;30:322.

68. Kelley RI, Cheatham JP, Clark BJ, et al. X-linked dilated cardiomyopathy with neutropenia, growth retardation, and 3-methylglutaconic aciduria. *J Pediatr* 1991;119:738.

69. Hudak ML, Jones MD Jr, Brusilow SW. Differentiation of transient hyperammonemia of the newborn and urea cycle enzyme defects by clinical presentation. *J Pediatr* 1985;107:712.

70. Cederbaum SD, Shaw KNF, Valente M. Hyperargininemia. *J Pediatr* 1977;90:569.

71. Bachmann C, Krahenbiihl S, Colombo JP, et al. *N*-acetylglutamate synthetase deficiency: a disorder of ammonia detoxification. *N Engl J Med* 1981;304:543.

72. Amendt BA, Greene C, Sweetman L, et al. Short chain acyl-CoA dehydrogenase deficiency: clinical and biochemical studies in two patients. *J Clin Invest* 1987;79:1303.

73. Stanley CA. New genetic defects in mitochondrial fatty acid oxidation and carnitine deficiency. *Adv Pediatr* 1987;34:59.

74. Strauss AW. Molecular basis of human mitochondrial very-long-chain acyl-CoA dehydrogenase deficiency causing cardiomyopathy and sudden death in childhood. *Proc Natl Acad Sci USA* 1995;92:10496.

75. Sewell AC. Long chain 3-hydroxyacyl-CoA dehydrogenase deficiency: a severe fatty acid oxidation disorder. *Eur J Pediatr* 1994;153:745.

76. Chalmers RA, Stanley CA, English N, Wigglesworth JS. Mitochondrial carnitine-acylcarnitine translocase deficiency presenting as sudden neonatal death. *J Pediatr* 1997;131:220.

77. Rinaldo P, Stanley CA, Hsu BYL, Sanchez LA, Stern HJ. Sudden neonatal death in carnitine transporter deficiency. *J Pediatr* 1997;131:304.

78. Hug G, Bove KE, Soukup S. Lethal neonatal multiorgan deficiency of carnitine palmitoyl-transferase II. *N Engl J Med* 1991;325:1862.

79. Robinson BH, Oei J, Sherwood WG, et al. The molecular basis for the two different clinical presentations of classical pyruvate carboxylase deficiency. *Am J Hum Genet* 1984;36:283.

80. Clayton PT, Hyland K, Brand M, Leonard JV. Mitochondrial phosphoenolypyruvate carboxykinase deficiency. *Eur J Pediatr* 1986;145:46.

81. Robinson BH, DeMeirlier L, Glerum M, et al. Clinical presentation of patients with mitochondrial respiratory chain defects in NADH-coenzyme Q reductase and cytochrome oxidase: clues to the pathogenesis of Leigh disease. *J Pediatr* 1987;110:216.

82. Dimauro S, Mendell JR, Sahenk Z, et al. Fatal infantile mitochondrial

myopathy and renal dysfunction due to cytochrome-C oxidase deficiency. *Neurology* 1980;30:795.

83. The Cystic Fibrosis Genotype-Phenotype Consortium. Correlation between genotype and phenotype in patients with cystic fibrosis. *N Engl J Med* 1993;329:1308.

84. Stevenson RE, Lubinsky M, Taylor HA, et al. Sialic acid storage disease with sialuria: clinical and biochemical features in the severe infantile type. *Pediatrics* 1983;72:441.

85. Scriver CR, Mahon B, Levy HL, et al. The Hartnup phenotype: mendelian transport disorder, multifactorial disease. *Am J Hum Genet* 1987;40:401.

86. O'Brien JS, Stern MB, Landing BH, et al. Generalized gangliosidosis. *Am J Dis Child* 1965;109:338.

87. Barranger JA, Murray GJ, Ginns EI. Genetic heterogeneity of Gaucher's disease. In: Barranger JA, Brady RO, eds. *Molecular basis of lysosomal storage disorders.* New York: Academic, 1984:311.

88. Besley GT, Elleder M. Enzyme activities and phospholipid storage patterns in brain and spleen samples from Niemann–Pick disease variants: a comparison of neuropathic and non-neuropathic forms. *J Inherit Metab Dis* 1986;9:59.

89. Funk JK, Filling-Katz MR, Sokol J, et al. Clinical spectrum of Niemann-Pick disease type C. *Neurology* 1989;39:1040.

90. Autio S, Louhimo T, Helenius M. The clinical course of mannosidosis. *Ann Clin Res* 1982;14:93.

91. Dawson G, Spranger JW. Fucosidosis: a glycosphingolipidosis. *N Engl J Med* 1971;285:122.

92. Antonarakis SE, Valle D, Moser HW, et al. Phenotypic variability in siblings with Farber disease. *J Pediatr* 1984;104:409.

93. Young LW, Sty JR, Babbitt JP. Wolman's disease. *Am J Dis Child* 1979;133:959.

94. Clarke JTR, Ozere RL, Krause VW. Early infantile variant of Krabbe globoid cell leukodystrophy with lung involvement. *Arch Dis Child* 1981;8:640.

95. Spranger JW, Koch F, Mekusick VA, et al. Mucopolysaccharidosis VI (Maroteaux–Lamy's disease). *Helv Paediatr Acta* 1970;25:337.

96. Nelson A, Peterson L, Frampton B, Sly WS. Mucopolysaccharidosis VII (beta-glucuronidase deficiency) presenting as nonimmune hydrops fetalis. *J Pediatr* 1982;101:574.

97. Leroy JG, Spranger JW, Feingold M, Dopitz JM. I-cell disease: a clinical picture. *J Pediatr* 1971;79:360.

98. Amir N, Zlotogora J, Bach G. Mucolipidosis type IV: clinical spectrum and natural history. *Pediatrics* 1987;79:953.

99. Burk RD, Valle D, Thomas GH, et al. Early manifestations of multiple sulfatase deficiency. *J Pediatr* 1984;104:574.

100. Aylsworth AS, Thomas GH, Hood JL, et al. A severe infantile sialidosis: clinical, biochemical and microscopic features. *J Pediatr* 1980;96:662.

101. Wilson GN, Holmes RD, Hajra AK. Peroxisomal disorders: clinical commentary and future prospects. *Am J Med Genet* 1988;30:771.

102. Danks DM, Campbell PE, Stevens BJ, et al. Menkes kinky hair syndrome: an inherited defect in copper absorption with widespread effects. *Pediatrics* 1972;50:188.

103. Duran M, deBree PK, deKlerk JBC, et al. Molybdenum-cofactor deficiency: clinical presentation and laboratory diagnosis. *Int Pediatr* 1996;11:334.

104. Mudd SH, Irreverre F, Laster L. Sulfite oxidase deficiency in man: demonstration of the enzymatic defect. *Science* 1967;156:1599.

105. Verlos A, Temple IK, Hubert A-F, et al. Recurrence of neonatal haemochromatosis in half sibs born of unaffected mothers. *J Med Genet* 1996;33:444.

106. White PC, New MI, Dupont B. Congenital adrenal hyperplasia. *N Engl J Med* 1987;316:1519.

107. Jacken J, Stibler H, Hagberg B. The carbohydrate-deficient glycoprotein syndrome: a new inherited multisystemic disease with severe central nervous system involvement. Acta Paediatr Scand Suppl 1991;375:1.

108. McClard RW, Black MJ, Jones ME, et al. Neonatal diagnosis of orotic aciduria: an experience with one family. *J Pediatr* 1983;102:85.

109. Kozlowski K, Sutcliffe J, Barylak A, et al. Hypophosphatasia: review of 24 cases. *Pediatr Radiol* 1976;5:103.

110. Berk PD, Jones EA, Howe RB, Berlin NI. Disorders of bilirubin metabolism. In: Bondy, PK, Rosenberg LE, eds. *Metabolic control and disease,* 8th ed. Philadelphia: WB Saunders, 1980:1009.

111. Sveger T. Liver disease in alpha₁-antitrypsin deficiency detected by screening of 200,000 infants. *N Engl J Med* 1976;294:1316.

112. Matalon R, Michals K, Sebesta D, et al. Aspartoacylase deficiency and *N*-acetylaspartic aciduria in patients with Canavan disease. *Am J Med Genet* 1988;29:463.

113. Shapiro LJ, Buxman MM, Weiss R, et al. Enzymatic basis of typical X-linked ichthyosis. *Lancet* 1978;2:756.

114. Cruysberg JRM, Sengers RCA, Pinckers A, et al. Features of a syndrome with congenital cataracts and hypertrophic cardiomyopathy. *Am J Ophthalmol* 1986;102:740.

115. Charnas LR, Bernardini I, Rader D, et al. Laboratory findings in the oculocerebrorenal syndrome of Lowe with special reference to growth and renal function. *N Engl J Med* 1991;324:1318.

CHAPTER 40

Congenital Anomalies

Scott D. McLean[1]

In a busy nursery, caring for a newborn with a congenital malformation is nearly a daily activity. This chapter will review some common birth defects and malformation syndromes, many of which have significant morbidity and mortality. The consultative services of a clinical geneticist or dysmorphologist often are quite helpful, but this resource may not be immediately available, and the role must be assumed, at least temporarily, by the attending pediatrician or neonatologist. Naturally, such a task brings many challenges—cognitive, managerial, and emotional—for which the practitioner often feels unprepared and overwhelmed. A logical approach and a good fund of knowledge are invaluable; a multigenerational perspective also proves quite useful, even essential. Uncovering the subtle or obvious genetic clues hidden in a pedigree or in the physiognomy of parents and siblings, even aunts, uncles, and grandparents, will materially influence diagnostic and therapeutic activity. The entire realm of newborn pathology is always daunting for parents, so a visible departure from the norm multiplies their fear, concern, worry, and guilt. This highly charged emotional milieu easily can overwhelm parents and becomes very stressful for nurses and physicians as well. The physician-leaders of the health care team should prepare themselves by becoming well informed regarding the nature and natural history of congenital malformations, in order to optimize care for the infant and to project confidence and control in an intrinsically unsettling situation.

A congenital anomaly is any alteration, present at birth, of normal anatomic structure. It may be major or minor, isolated or part of a larger constellation of defects, of clear or uncertain cause. Several genetic and environmental etiologies are well delineated (Table 40–1), but the term congenital implies no particular causation. The fundamental cause of nearly half of all birth defects is unknown (1).

Individual birth defects are rare; consequently, some practitioners are tempted to dismiss them as flukes of nature that warrant sympathy but not significant attention or investigation. In aggregate, however, birth defects are surprisingly common and ubiquitous among all cultures, ethnic groups, and socioeconomic strata. Numerous epidemiologic studies place the incidence of major malformations in newborns at 2% to 3% (2,3). An equal percentage are estimated to harbor occult anomalies that eventually are detected by midchildhood, giving a cumulative incidence of major birth defects of 5% to 6%: about one of every 20 newborn children. Assuming a birth rate of almost 4 million per year (4), one may anticipate that, in the United States alone, an infant with a congenital anomaly is born every 2 minutes 15 seconds. Although their mortality has been declining since 1979, birth defects remain the leading cause of death in infancy and the second leading cause of death in children between the ages of 1 and 4 years (4). These figures bluntly indicate that congenital anomalies constitute more than a trivial burden on the public health. The Centers for Disease Control and various state health agencies have developed a number of birth defects registries to track these phenomena. Central to these initiatives is the commitment of individual practitioners to diagnose and report all congenital defects accurately and reliably.

In developed countries, the economic impact of caring for children with birth defects is considerable. In 1978, one center reported that approximately one in four pediatric inpatients had a disorder with a significant genetic component (5). Because comprehensive and cost-effective outpatient management for medically fragile children is a challenging and often elusive goal for most systems of modern health care, it would seem reasonable to posit that the socioeconomic burden associated with congenital anomalies will continue unabated for the foreseeable

S. D. McLean: Medical Genetics, Department of Pediatrics, Wilford Hall Medical Center, Lackland Air Force Base, Texas

[1]The opinions and assertions herein contained are those of the author and do not necessarily represent those of the Department of the Army or the Department of Defense.

TABLE 40–1. *Causes of malformations in newborns*

	Percent
Genetic causes	
Chromosome abnormalities	10.1
Single mutant genes	3.1
Familial	14.5
Multifactorial inheritance	23.0
Teratogens	3.2
Uterine factors	2.5
Twinning	0.4
Unknown cause	43.2

Modified from ref. 1.

future. In Maryland in 1995, 2,200 individuals, 90% of whom were children, with 30 rare diseases, representing less than 2% of the Medicaid population, generated $100 million in Medicaid payments (6).

DEFINITIONS AND CLASSIFICATIONS

The terminology for various birth defects and malformation syndromes can be a source of confusion for both the novice and veteran clinician alike. Categories of anomalies may seem arbitrary and capricious, but a developmental or embryologic perspective often will cast light upon the rationale behind a particular designation. The term "birth defect," although considered by some authorities to be antiquated, enjoys wide usage and conveys immediate meaning for parents. "Congenital anomaly" is fundamentally equivalent, *indicating an abnormality of anatomic structure present at birth.* It may be

further refined in terms of *severity* ("major" and "minor"), *pathogenesis* ("malformation," "deformation," "disruption," "dysplasia"), or *pattern* ("isolated," "syndromic"). These terms are defined in Table 40–2.

The great majority of congenital anomalies occur in isolation, as a single phenomenon, and are postulated to arise because of a primary, intrinsic malformation of a fetal structure that occurs at 10 weeks of gestation or earlier. Usually, the family history is bereft of similarly affected individuals, but these defects tend to recur occasionally, on the order of 3% to 5% for each subsequent pregnancy for the parents of an affected child. Classic mendelian genetics does not adequately explain this situation, but another model, multifactoral inheritance, has proven quite useful. A constellation of factors, including multiple genes inherited from each parent, as well as poorly defined environmental influences, seems to allow a developing fetal structure to cross a threshold of "liability," beyond which morphogenesis proceeds abnormally (7). This type of multifactorial heritability accounts for most isolated major malformations.

Figure 40–1 illustrates the proportionate incidence of etiologic categories for minor and major anomalies. Multiple major anomalies suggest that the underlying cause is a sequence, developmental field defect, association, or syndrome, which in turn may be caused by a chromosomal anomaly, a single-gene mutation, a teratogen, or unknown factors. Minor anomalies deserve special attention because, in terms of diagnostic significance, they are the equals of the major malformations (8), often providing the linchpin of clinical recognition of a rare syn-

TABLE 40–2. *Terminology*

Major Anomaly	An anatomic abnormality severe enough to reduce normal life expectancy or compromise normal function, e.g., neural tube defect, cleft lip.
Minor Anomaly	A structural alteration that either requires no treatment or can be corrected in a straightforward manner, with no permanent consequences, and present in less than 4% of the normal population, e.g., preauricular skin tag, small ventricular septal defect.
Minor Variant	A physical feature, often familial, that is present in only a small proportion (1% to 5%) of normal individuals, e.g., simian crease of the palm, epicanthal folds.
Malformation	A morphologic defect of an organ, part of an organ, or region due to an *intrinsically abnormal developmental process;* e.g., microphthalmia, ectrodactyly
Deformation	An abnormal form, shape, or position of a part of the body caused by *unusual mechanical forces on normal tissue,* e.g., club feet, plagiocephaly.
Disruption	A morphologic defect due to extrinsic interference with a normal developmental process resulting in *breakdown of normal tissue,* e.g., amniotic band sequence, fetal alcohol syndrome.
Sequence	Several anomalies that occur due to a cascade of events, caused by a single initiating event or anomaly, e.g., Potter sequence, Pierre Robin sequence.
Developmental Field Defect	A set of morphologic defects that share a common or contiguous region during embryogenesis, e.g., hemifacial microsomia
Association	A nonrandom set of anomalies in which the specific components occur together more frequently than would be expected by chance and for which cause is not established, e.g., VATER association, CHARGE association.
Syndrome	A recognizable pattern of anomalies that "run together" e.g., Down syndrome, Smith–Lemli–Opitz syndrome

CHARGE, *c*oloboma, *h*eart disease, *a*tresia choanae, *r*etarded growth and development and/or CNS anomalies, *g*enital hypoplasia, and *e*ar anomalies or deafness; VATER, *v*ertebral defects, imperforate *a*nus, *t*racheo*e*sophageal fistula, and radial and *r*enal dysplasia.

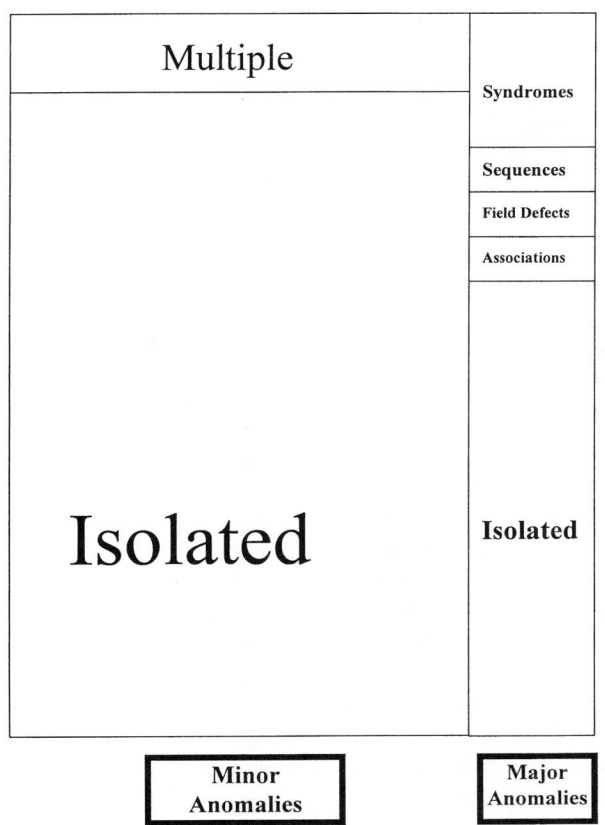

FIG. 40–1. Proportionate incidence of etiologic categories for minor and major anomalies. (Adapted from ref. 18.)

An integrated approach to management of a newborn with congenital anomalies (10) encompasses three parallel and simultaneous lines of activity, as outlined in Fig. 40–2. Urgent interventions for the infant are undertaken immediately. From the outset, the family is provided with support in the form of information, preliminary interpretation, and acknowledgment of their distress and concern. The third simultaneous activity is data collection—history, physical, laboratory studies and imaging, and preliminary definition of the nature of the problem. All efforts should be made to verify information and to amass a complete database.

History

Prenatal information, beginning with conception, must be specifically sought from both the mother and her obstetric records. The nature and timing of maternal illnesses, including febrile episodes, can suggest a direct infectious disruption, such as rubella or cytomegalovirus. Maternal trauma and use of alcohol, drugs, medications, or tobacco—degree, timing, and duration—should be documented. Quickening, the date at which there is maternal sensation of fetal movement, as well as the subsequent vigor and frequency of fetal activity, reflects central nervous system integrity and peripheral muscular function. Prenatal ultrasonography, especially if per-

drome. A single minor anomaly is present in 13% of neonates, but more than one is decidedly less common—two minor anomalies occur in only 1%, and three minor anomalies in just 0.05% (9). As the numbers of minor anomalies increase, the search for occult major anomalies and the consideration that a syndromic diagnosis is possible should increase proportionately.

MANAGEMENT STRATEGY

The basic approach to managing an infant with one or more congenital anomalies is much the same as the management of any other clinical scenario. Effective clinical management is organized around an understanding of the natural history of the condition at hand; consequently, an accurate diagnosis is invaluable. History taking begins with conception and includes a detailed family tree. Physical features must be scrutinized, measured, and documented with precision, and confirmatory studies must be carefully chosen and interpreted. Common pitfalls include incomplete ascertainment of all relevant information, impetuous diagnosis and prognostication, and failure to communicate with parents in a straightforward and compassionate manner.

Simultaneous Activities:

Gather Data	Therapeutic Intervention	Psychosocial Support
History	**Resuscitation**	family
prenatal		staff
perinatal	**Urgent procedures**	**Within 24 hours**
family		meet with family
Physical examination	**Formulate overall plan**	define anomalies
detailed		discuss
multisystem	**Define long-term issues**	investigation
measurements		intervention
family members	**Preventive measures**	**At regular intervals**
Ancillary studies	Genetic counseling	review diagnosis
photographs		reformulate plans
radiographs	**Reevaluate** plans and	continue support
cytogenetics	therapies regularly	
DNA analysis		
Define problem(s)		
categorize process		
diagnosis		

FIG. 40–2. Integrated approach to management. (Modified from ref. 5.)

formed serially and with careful attention to detail, may yield critical information regarding the amount of amniotic fluid and malformations of the kidneys, brain, heart, and gastrointestinal system. Review of the obstetric record or the ultrasound study, as well as a discussion with the attending obstetrician or perinatologist, can save valuable time and effort. Maternal serum and amniotic fluid alpha-fetoprotein levels and prenatal chromosomal studies should be verified and documented in the infant's medical record. Late trimester problems with fetal position, such as transverse or breech lie, potentially indicate neuromuscular or structural abnormalities of the fetus. These infants not uncommonly also have a history of perinatal distress and poor transition to extrauterine life. Finally, it often is useful to inquire about any prenatal event or factors that the parents suspect, even remotely, may have caused their infant's problems. Concerns about witnessing a solar or lunar eclipse, for example, are best made explicit, if only for the purpose of assuaging guilt.

Family History

A systematic and detailed inquiry into the age, health, development, and congenital anomalies of all members of the immediate family comprises the core of an adequate family history. All second-degree relatives, such as grandparents, aunts, uncles, nieces, and nephews, should be considered, and more distant relatives may contribute valuable data. A three-generation pedigree provides a concise picture of patterns of inheritance. One must specifically clarify the biologic parentage for each individual. Spontaneous abortions, miscarriages, stillbirths, and infant deaths clearly are germane, but this information typically is omitted by parents unless the interviewer specifically inquires. Consanguinity also should be directly but tactfully questioned. A "quick pedigree" is an oxymoron; routinely the entire process requires patience and time, as much as an hour for some extensive kindreds. With this in mind, the interviewer will be sympathetic, on the day of delivery, to parents who are understandably terrified, exhausted, and disoriented. After rest, time, and a chance to speak with relatives, they may be more prepared to help refine and expand on their complete family history.

Physical Examination

It is axiomatic that a proper newborn physical examination is detailed and complete. The careful observer, especially one who repeats the examination several times, will recognize departures from the norm. Several points are worth keeping in mind when examining infants with a malformation or a generalized dysmorphic appearance.

- *Be alert.* There is a heightened chance that additional, initially unsuspected anomalies are present. Although a malformation may be minor in severity, it might represent the most important, critical clue to the diagnosis.

- *Collect "clues" systematically,* by closely examining each topographical segment of the body and by scrutinizing progressively more detailed regions. For example, on initial observation it may be noted that the fingers are disproportionately short; a closer examination may reveal that the fourth and fifth fingers are stiff and rigidly extended, with faint flexion creases, especially at the distal interphalangeal joints, that the nails are short and narrow, and almost absent on the fifth finger. The placenta may be examined with the obstetrician or pathologist in order to seek evidence of cryptic twinning, umbilical cord anomalies, or amniotic bands.
- *Document the examination with great care,* using appropriate morphologic terms and sufficient detail, and strongly consider supplementing written findings with clinical photographs.
- *Measure* those features that are obviously or potentially abnormal in size, shape, position, or symmetry. Normal standards are available for virtually any anatomic structure, encompassing all ages from preterm infant to adulthood (11,12). Hall (8) admonishes, *"Never make a clinical judgment on a measurable parameter without measuring it."*
- *Examine both parents,* if possible, seeking any signs of similar anomalies. Dominant conditions frequently manifest a subtle but distinctive phenotype in adults.

Adjunctive Investigations

Imaging studies and consultations with pediatric subspecialists will be dictated by the emerging clinical picture. For example, a newborn with Down syndrome, even when a cardiac murmur is absent, merits the attention of a pediatric cardiologist, because significant structural defects of the heart are present in 50%, but may be missed on clinical examination. A newborn girl with puffy hands and feet, a webbed neck, and coarctation of the aorta also should receive a renal ultrasound, because kidney malformations commonly are associated with Turner syndrome. When the diagnosis is unclear and several malformations are present, occult anomalies of the central nervous system, heart, kidneys, vertebrae, and eyes are reasonable to pursue, especially when the known birth defects are multiple and severe. Skeletal films, to include hands, feet, long bones, pelvis, vertebrae, chest, and cranium, are helpful when length is less then the 5th percentile for gestational age or when the limbs are disproportionately short. These studies often require interpretation by a pediatric radiologist skilled in this area.

Chromosomal Analysis

Forty-six chromosomes are present in most normal human cells. Formation of ova and sperm, however, is a surprisingly error-prone process: nearly two-thirds of all fertilizations result in aneuploidy or abnormal chromosomal number or structure, with subsequent reproductive loss. Some of this prenatal loss occurs late enough to be recognized as a miscarriage or spontaneous abortion, but most wastage is occult. Ninety-eight percent of these chromosomal defects are lethal (13).

An abnormal karyotype occurs in 1 of 170 liveborn infants. Among chromosomally abnormal neonates, one-third have an extra sex chromosome with mild or no phenotypic manifestations in the newborn period, one-fourth have trisomy of an autosome, such as trisomy 21 or trisomy 18, and 40% have a variation of chromosomal structure, such as a deleted or duplicated segment, or a translocation, most (79%) of which are balanced and generally do not cause birth defects. Approximately 10% of infants who die in the perinatal period secondary to multiple congenital malformations have abnormal cytogenetic studies (13).

Which infants deserve chromosomal studies? Truly isolated malformations very infrequently are caused by a cytogenetic defect. On the other hand, neonates with multiple major malformations or a recognized syndrome, as well as stillborn infants, with or without malformations, should have cytogenetic testing. Between these extremes lies a sizable "gray area." Factors in favor of chromosomal testing include intrauterine growth retardation, an abnormal neurologic exam, a major malformation accompanied by several minor malformations, and a history of multiple pregnancy losses for the mother or in close relatives.

Peripheral blood lymphocytes are the tissue of choice for most cytogenetic analysis, but many other tissues can be used, including skin fibroblasts, bone marrow, placenta, and pericardium, usually harvested postmortem. Two to three milliliters of venous or arterial blood, collected in a sodium heparin (green top) tube, generally are sufficient. This should be kept at room temperature or refrigerated, never frozen, in transit. The cells usually will remain viable for 1 or 2 days, but the shortest possible transit time increases the chances for useful results. If the sample is shipped, overnight couriers are required. The lymphocytes are separated, incubated in the presence of a mitogen to stimulate cell division, which is then abruptly halted with colchicine, and the cell membranes are disrupted gently while being placed on a glass slide. After enzymatic preparation and staining, the "spread" of chromosomes is analyzed in approximately 20 cells. Generally, 550 or more bands are visible with Giemsa staining of 46 chromosomes at metaphase. Several cells are photographed and arranged in standard groupings, a karyotype. Turnaround time for cytogenetic analysis is typically 72 hours, although some laboratories are able to provide results in slightly less time. Because of the high percentage of dividing cells in bone marrow, karyotypes from this tissue may be obtained in a matter of hours, although the quality of the banding frequently is inadequate for high-resolution analysis of small or subtle abnormalities. To achieve the latter, a special request for pro-metaphase analysis should accompany a peripheral blood sample.

In the past several years, an increasing number of syndromic conditions have been found to be caused by tiny chromosomal deletions that are not visible by routine karyotyping, even at pro-metaphase levels of detail. Molecular probes that will hybridize at these loci with great specificity have been developed. These DNA probes are complexed with a fluorescent marker and become powerful tools for detecting submicroscopic chromosomal deletions. This technique, termed fluorescent *in situ* hybridization (FISH), has been adapted for whole, entire chromosomes, is available in different fluorescent spectra, and effectively can identify the nature of many chromosomal anomalies, such as translocations. A metaphase spread can, in essence, be painted with several single-locus or whole-chromosome FISH probes simultaneously, providing a highly specific, and colorful, picture of genomic structure.

Metabolic Studies

As a general rule, inborn errors of metabolism do not result in dysmorphism or congenital malformations, with several important exceptions. Several mendelian disorders of peroxisomes, subcelluar organelles involved in lipid metabolism, result in distinctive phenotypes. Zellweger syndrome, also known as cerebrohepatorenal syndrome, and rhizomelic chondrodysplasia punctata exemplify this class of disease. Screening for peroxisomal conditions is accomplished by searching for high levels of very-long-chain fatty acids in serum. Smith–Lemli–Opitz syndrome, another multiple congenital anomaly syndrome, recently has been discovered to be caused by defective synthesis of cholesterol. High levels of the precursor, 7-dehydrocholesterol, are diagnostic. Other malformation syndromes no doubt will be found to be caused by biochemical anomalies.

Synthesis and Analysis of Data

Every clinician develops a unique, individual strategy of diagnosis. Acquiring a deep and broad fund of knowledge is arguably fundamental and, oftentimes, sufficient in itself. Unfortunately, the sheer numbers of conditions and syndromes impose some limits on the "brute force" approach; the *London Dysmorphology Database,* for instance, contains more than 2,750 multiple congenital anomaly syndromes (14).

Precise diagnosis is neither possible nor necessary in the immediate newborn period for many neonates with a multiple congenital anomaly syndrome. More than half of all individuals with congenital anomalies never receive a firm diagnosis, even after the most definitive of workups, and remain an "unknown." Categorization of an anomaly as a malformation, disruption, or deformation, however, is a feasible and useful first step. These terms have been defined and discussed previously. An isolated major anomaly in the absence of any similarly affected relative would suggest a multifactoral etiology. If there are multiple malformations, one of the following strategies may be useful:

- Instant recognition, or *gestalt* diagnosis, which depends on the clinician's previous experience and strength of visual memory. Certain caveats apply, however: many disorders have a considerable range of phenotypic variation, and other conditions, or phenocopies, may mimic the one that has instantly come to mind.
- Perusal of an atlas or illustrated text, such as *Smith's Recognizable Patterns of Human Malformation,* to match a photograph with the patient. This simple strategy often yields excellent results.
- Pattern analysis, in which all phenotypic and clinical "problems" are enumerated, grouped, combined, recombined, and weighed in order to discern developmental relationships, sequences, and influences. Major organ systems or classes of disease (e.g., skeletal dysplasias) then become entry points for further comparison, matching the patient's pattern against published descriptions while attempting to take into account phenotypic variability.
- Focusing the initial investigation on the anomaly that is most distinctive, rare, or unusual. Clinodactyly of the fifth finger is very common, but a coloboma of the iris is fairly unusual. A variety of texts or electronic databases then can be consulted and a relatively short list of diagnostic possibilities generated.

Once a preliminary analysis has generated a differential diagnosis, all reasonable efforts are made to test each competing hypothesis. Often, a clinical finding can corroborate a possibility. For instance, a lateral radiograph of the knee may allow confirmation of chondrodysplasia punctata by demonstrating the typical stippled, punctate mineralization of the epiphyses. Although many diagnoses are purely clinical, molecular tools are becoming extremely helpful. An electronic literature search or querying an internet resource, such as *Online Mendelian Inheritance in Man,* can help determine whether a novel approach using direct DNA sequence analysis, FISH, or linkage analysis has been developed for the disease in question.

More often than not, the diagnostician will achieve only the generic exclusive diagnosis, etiology unclear. When this is the case, there is a temptation to "force" a diagnosis, analogous to hammering a somewhat square peg into a slightly round hole. This may not be in the best interests of the patient so that, in these situations, there is honor in admitting ignorance. Certain characteristics of many syndromic conditions, such as the so-called "elfin" facies of Williams syndrome, are not apparent in the new-born period. The most useful diagnostic decision may be to wait and start afresh at a later time, recollecting data, recombining features into new patterns, and researching the literature.

Other Management Issues

Communication with the parents of a child with congenital anomalies will require a compassionate, timely, and honest presentation of the facts. Prematurity and sepsis, however, are sometimes more comprehensible than malformations, especially if those anomalies are multiple or bizarre. One's choice of terminology is important but often challenging. Many parents find it quite helpful for the principal caregiver to examine the infant in their presence, pointing out the features that seem to be unusual, as well as delineating those that are normal. Parents naturally feel responsible for the birth defect, which they might interpret as a reflection of their own shortcomings, real or imagined. Guilt is as common for the parents of a malformed child as pride is for the parents of a normal newborn. Although it is not always possible to convince parents to set aside unreasonable guilt, they can at least be reassured that they had no control over the events causing the abnormality and that they have permission to not feel guilty.

Expect the full spectrum of grief from both parents. They have experienced the loss of a much-anticipated "normal" child. Shock, denial, bargaining, and acceptance will all occur, even when their child does not have a lethal condition. The physicians and nursing personnel involved in the care of the malformed infant work as a team to keep track of this process and be alert for dysfunctional grief. Social work services, clergy, and support groups are important adjuncts. The National Organization for Rare Disorders, the Alliance of Genetic Support Groups, and specific support groups can provide up-to-date information and lay contacts for interested parents.

If the malformed infant dies and there is any question regarding the precise diagnosis, a full, unrestricted autopsy can prove extremely useful. Visceral, central nervous system, and skeletal anomalies frequently come to light at postmortem examination. Clinical photography and cytogenetic analysis of fibroblasts obtained from sterile skin biopsy, fascia, or pericardium also may yield important insights. Tissue, cells in culture, and extracted DNA can be stored in a long-term repository and later reanalyzed in light of new research or collaboration.

Families often are reluctant to grant permission for an autopsy. In many instances, however, this procedure has profound implications for the parents' reproductive options and even those of distant relatives. Cultural and social beliefs and practices must, of course, be carefully respected regarding the care of the child's body after death. Nevertheless, an autopsy can be recast in the light of a final gift of the child to his family, perhaps even to the world, if in fact a diagnosis is thereby established or medical science advanced.

SELECTED EXAMPLES

Teratogenic Conditions

A teratogen, from the Greek root *teras,* meaning monster or marvel, is any environmental factor that causes a structural or functional abnormality in the developing fetus or embryo. These environmental agents include infections, medications, drugs, chemicals, and maternal metabolites, such as phenylalanine (Table 40–3). By their very nature, teratogens induce a disruption or sequence of disruptions of inherently normal tissue. Extensive compendia of these agents have been studied in humans and laboratory animals, and several excellent resources are available for the clinician. In addition, regional teratogen hot lines can be accessed by both professionals and patients.

Ethanol is the most common human teratogen. As many as 1 of 300 newborns will manifest the prenatal effects of exposure, ranging from cerebral palsy to learning disability. Up to one-fifth of mental retardation (usually mild) is attributable to fetal alcohol syndrome (FAS). Unfortunately, the dysmorphisms of FAS are overlooked routinely in the newborn nursery. Numerous structural anomalies have been reported; common and salient features are listed in Table 40–4.

Multifactoral Disorders

The multifactoral model of inheritance, as discussed previously, was developed to explain how certain common, isolated malformations arise. It assumes that multi-

TABLE 40–3. *Selected teratogens and their effects*

Teratogen	Anomalies	Comments
Phenytoin (Dilantin)	Growth deficiency Wide anterior fontanelle Hypertelorism Cleft lip and palate Hypoplastic distal phalanges Small nails	Similar facial features seen with exposure to carbamazepine, valproate, mysoline, phenobarbital. Full spectrum in 10%, milder effects in one-third.
Warfarin (Coumadin)	Nasal hypoplasia Stippled epiphyses Short fingers Seizures	Critical period between 6 and 9 week's gestation. One-third of exposed fetuses are affected.
Retinoic acid (Accutane)	Microtia or anotia Hypertelorism Micrognathia Conotruncal cardiac defects Hydrocephalus Microcephaly Cortical, cerebellar dysplasia	If exposed more than 15 days after conception, one-third have embryopathy.
Rubella	Growth deficiency Microcephaly Deafness Cataracts Microphthalmia Chorioretinitis Cardiac septal defects Patent ductus arteriosus Peripheral pulmonic stenosis	Fifty-percent chance of effects if exposed in first trimester, but risk extends into second trimester. May have late, persistent infectious sequelae, e.g., diabetes mellitus.
Varicella	Mental deficiency Seizures Cortical atrophy/microcephaly Growth deficiency Limb hypoplasia/club foot Cutaneous scars	One to two percent with effects when exposed between 8 and 20 weeks' gestation; wide spectrum of severity.
Maternal phenyketonuria	Mental retardation (73% to 92%) Hypertonia Low birth weight (52%) Microcephaly (73%) Cardiac defects (15%) Spontaneous abortion (30%)	Even when "on diet," phenylalanine levels may rise above 4 to 10 mg/dL, the apparent threshold for fetal effects. Percentages cited here are for levels >16 mg/dL. Normal is <2.

TABLE 40–4. *Structural anomalies in fetal alcohol syndrome*

Growth deficiency of prenatal onset
Mental retardation
Microcephaly
Short palpebral fissures
Maxillary hypoplasia
Cervical vertebral malformations (10%–20%)
Short nose
Smooth philtrum
Thin upper lip
Ventricular septal defect, atrial septal defect
Small distal phalanges
Small fifth fingernails

ple genes and environmental factors govern the extent to which a particular structure may develop abnormally. The susceptibility, or genetic *liability,* of a malformation in a population is described in terms of a continuous distribution in which there is a point, or *threshold,* above which, in an all-or-none fashion, a structural defect will occur. Using this model, one can predict that, within a particular extended family, there may be an overall enrichment for susceptibility genes or environmental factors and, consequently, some clustering of a particular congenital anomaly, such as pyloric stenosis. This recurrence risk for nearly all multifactoral conditions can be predicted via mathematical formulas (approximately the square root of the incidence in a population) to be between 2% and 5%. That is, for each and every subsequent pregnancy for the parents of an affected child, the risk will be 1 in 20 to 1 in 50. The same probability applies to other first-degree relatives, such as siblings.

These theoretical risks prove to be quite similar to empirical data. Table 40–5 lists some common multifactoral disorders and their recurrence risks. Other predictions of the model also are borne out: when a second child is affected, the risk for a third occurrence is on the order of 10% to 15%; the more severe the malformation, the higher the recurrence risk; and if a sex predisposition is observed, as for males and pyloric stenosis, then the recurrence risk is higher when the affected child is of the lesser affected sex, e.g., a girl with pyloric stenosis.

TABLE 40–5. *Multifactoral disorders*

Disorder	Empiric recurrence risk
Cleft lip with or without cleft palate	4%–5%
Cleft palate	2%–6%
Ventricular septal defect	3%–4%
Pyloric stenosis	3%
Hirschsprung anomaly	3%–5%
Clubfoot	2%–8%
Congenital hip dysplasia	3%–4%
Neural tube defects	3%–5%
Atrial septal defect (secundum)	2%–3%

Important examples of multifactoral disorders are the neural tube defects (NTDs). From a morphogenetic point of view, NTDs, including anencephaly and spina bifida at various vertebral levels, generally are considered equivalent manifestations of failed neural tube folding before 28 days' gestational age. Many syndromic and teratogenic (ethanol, valproic acid) causes are well delineated; however, most NTDs are isolated, multifactoral phenomena with recurrence risks of the usual order of magnitude (3% to 5%). One must keep in mind, of course, that recurrences in a family may embrace the entire spectrum of neural tube folding errors, from meningocoele to anencephaly, rather than duplicate the NTD present in the proband. The risk of NTD is decreased with adequate maternal intake of folic acid; 0.4 mg/d for all women of childbearing age and, for women who have previously borne an affected child, 4.0 mg/d, beginning 1 month prior to conception through at least the third month of gestation.

Chromosomal Abnormalities

Since 1956, when the normal diploid number of human chromosomes was established as 46 (15), an astounding variety of cytogenetic aberrations have been observed. These include triploidy (69 chromosomes per cell), trisomies, monosomies, reciprocal and robertsonian translocations, insertions, deletions, duplications, isochromosomes, ring chromosmes, and inversions. Some aneuploidies, such as trisomy 16, the most common trisomy in humans, are uniformly lethal in the prenatal period. Other departures from the norm have no phenotypic consequences, such as many balanced translocatons, and others result in remarkably few structural or functional anomalies in the newborn period, such as 47,XXY, Klinefelter syndrome. Multiple congenital anomalies that involve several developmental fields often are caused by chromosomal aneuploidy, and clinicians with a high index of suspicion not uncommonly are rewarded with a precise diagnosis. Several of the more common chromosomal abnormalities observed in liveborn infants are described below.

Trisomy 21

Down Syndrome is the most common chromosomal aberration recognized at birth, with an incidence of about 1 per 700 live births. Only one of four conceptions that result in trisomy 21 is viable (16). The phenotype is quite variable, but distinctive facies (Fig. 40–3) and mental retardation are always present. It generally is believed that, because the gestalt recognition of Down syndrome usually is uncomplicated, diagnosis is more straightforward than for other chromosomal anomalies. However, of the children referred to a clinical geneticist because of suspected Down syndrome, only 72% to 87% actually

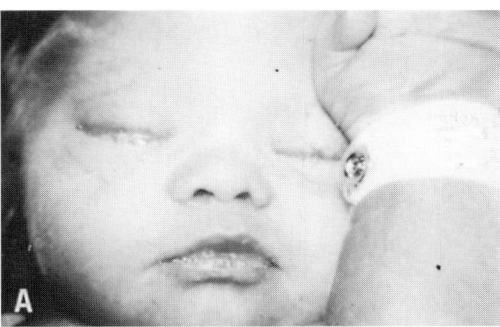

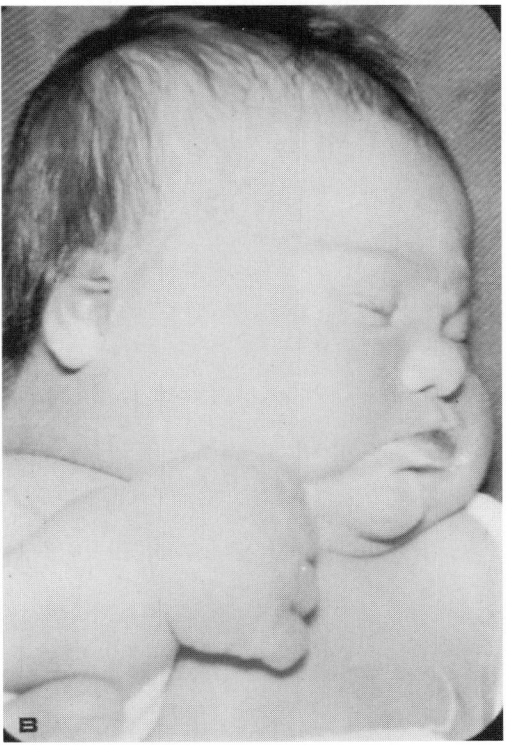

FIG. 40–3. **A**: Trisomy 21. **B**: Down syndrome.

TABLE 40–6. *Major anomalies at birth in Down syndrome*

Cardiac: all types		40%
Atrioventricular canal	16%–20%	
Ventricular septal defect	16%	
Patent ductus arteriosus	3%–5%	
Atrial septal defect	4%–10%	
Gastrointestinal: all types		10%–18%
Duodenal stenosis/atresia	3%–5%	
Imperforate anus	2%	
Other	6%	
Hematologic: leukemoid reaction		Common
Hypothyroidism (congenital)		1%

From refs. 17a–17c.

this chromosome. Table 40–8 demonstrates the well-recognized relationship between Down syndrome and advancing maternal age; 90% of trisomy 21 is due to nondisjunction at maternal meiosis (16). Translocation of chromosome 21 to another acrocentric chromosome occurs in 1 of 30 Down syndrome infants. These possibilities must be assayed via karyotyping, in order to provide accurate genetic counseling. Any chromosomal pattern other than trisomy 21 mandates analysis of parental karyotypes. For example, if an isochromosome 21 is present in the infant, parental chromosomal analysis may disclose that a parent carries the same isochromosome. Recurrence risk for that parent is then 100%. Straightforward trisomy 21 in the infant is not associated with chromosomal abnormalities of either parent and their testing is unnecessary. Recurrence risks are then 1% plus the age-related maternal risk.

have had trisomy 21 (17). As with most dysmorphologic diagnoses, never are all or even most of the "typical" findings present in any one child. Table 40–6 lists the major anomalies that have been observed in children with Down syndrome. Cardiac anomalies, atrioventricular canal in particular, may not be apparent on clinical examination. An echocardiogram is recommended for all newborns with suspected or confirmed Down syndrome, ideally prior to discharge, certainly by 1 month of age. Table 40–7 lists those minor anomalies of Down syndrome that the practitioner is likely to observe and weigh in working toward a clinical diagnosis.

For 95% of newborns with Down syndrome, nondisjunction during either maternal or paternal meiosis results in the formation of a gamete with two copies of chromosome 21, although many other mechanisms of abnormal gametogenesis can give rise to an extra copy of

TABLE 40–7. *Minor anomalies in Down syndrome*

Microbrachycephaly	75%
Upslanting palpebral fissures[a]	80%
Epicanthal folds	59%
Speckling of iris (Brushfield spots)[b]	56%
Flat facial profile[a]	90%
Low nasal bridge	68%
Small ears[b]	100%
Mildly dysplastic ears[a]	50%
Short neck	61%
Excess skin at nape of neck[a,b]	80%
Protruding tongue	47%
Narrow palate	76%
Open mouth	58%
Short hands and fingers	
Clinodactyly (curving) of the fifth finger[a]	60%
Simian crease[a]	45%
Wide gap between the first and second toes[b]	68%
Poor Moro reflex[a]	85%
Hyperflexibility of joints[a]	80%
Hypotonia[a]	80%

[a]Among the ten cardinal features set forth by Bryan Hall (32).

[b]Cited by Rex and Preus (17) as having superior discriminative efficacy and power.

From refs. 17a, 17b, 17d.

TABLE 40–8. *Incidence of Down syndrome as a function of maternal age*

Maternal age (yr)	Incidence
20	1:1667
25	1:1250
30	1:952
35	1:385
36	1:295
37	1:227
38	1:175
39	1:137
40	1:106
41	1:82
42	1:64
43	1:50
44	1:38
45	1:30
46	1:23
47	1:18
48	1:14
49	1:11

From D'Alton ME, DeCherney AH. Prenatal diagnosis. *N Engl J Med* 1993;328:114.

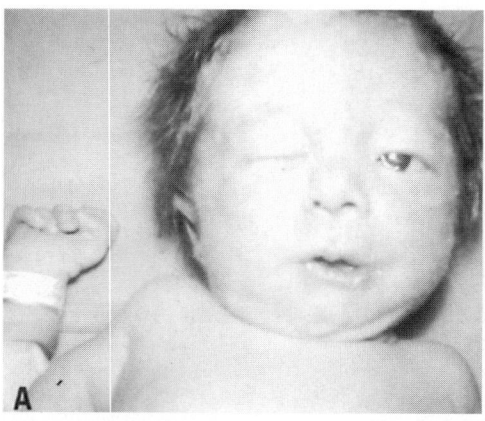

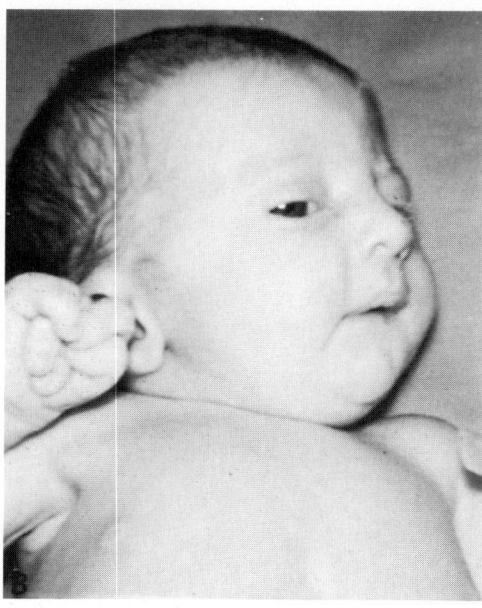

FIG. 40–4. A,B: Trisomy 18.

Trisomy 18

Described by Edwards et al (20) in 1960, trisomy 18 affects 1 of 5,000 newborns. Girls outnumber boys at a 4:1 ratio, and a maternal age effect is well established: *de novo* nondisjunction during meiosis accounts for 90%. One-tenth represent mosaicism, and various translocations and isochromosomal anomalies occasionally are seen. Life expectancy is markedly reduced, with 90% mortality in the first year and frequent demise in the neonatal period. The congenital anomalies in trisomy 18 neonates usually are multiple, severe, and associated with considerable morbidity. Severe psychomotor retardation always is present. Figure 40–4 demonstrates typical facial features.

Considerable overlap with trisomy 13 syndrome results in frequent diagnostic uncertainty in the newborn period, pending cytogenetic analysis. Table 40–9 lists some features that are common to both conditions, and Table 40–10 includes those findings that are more common to trisomy 18. Careful communication with the cytogenetic laboratory will ensure that chromosomal data are available as soon as possible, a helpful adjunct for decision-making when the clinical management options include expectant care and minimal intervention. In selected instances, there may be some benefit from rapid analysis via FISH probes for chromosome 13 and 18 markers. Bear in mind, however, that, on occasion, these modalities may not detect trisomic states that involve translocations or partial duplication and that full chromosomal analysis is superior and definitive. These results usually are available 48 to 72 hours after the laboratory receives the specimen.

TABLE 40–9. *Anomalies common to both trisomy 13 and trisomy 18*

Growth deficiency
Severe developmental retardation
Microcephaly
Ear anomalies
Microphthalmia
Highly arched palate
Micrognathia
Excessive neck skin
Congenital heart defects, various
   Ventricular septal defect, patent ductus arteriosus
Umbilical hernia
Renal anomalies
   Cystic kidneys
Cryptorchidism
Overlapping, flexed fingers
Prominent heels

TABLE 40–10. *Findings more common to trisomy 18*

Prominent occiput
Narrow palpebral fissures
Small mouth
Short sternum
Widely spaced nipples
Cardiac: polyvalvular disease
Prominent clitoris
Hypoplastic labia
Hip dislocation
Clubfoot
Hypoplastic nails
Syndactyly between toes 2 and 3
Hammertoes
Seizures

TABLE 40–11. *Findings more common to trisomy 13*

Scalp defects
Holoprosencephaly
Sloping forehead
Capillary hemangiomas
Ocular hypotelorism
Iris coloboma
Prominent nasal bridge
Cleft lip
Cleft palate
Short neck
Hypoplastic nipples
Cardiac: dextrocardia
Polydactyly (postaxial)
Apnea

Trisomy 13

This is the third most common autosomal trisomy recognized at birth, affecting 1 of 12,000 newborns, and initially was delineated in 1960 by Patau et al (21). Three-fourths are straightforward trisomy 13; a maternal age effect is apparent. Twenty percent are caused by translocations, mostly robertsonian, in which the long arm of the acrocentric chromosome 13 becomes attached via the centromere to another acrocentric chromosome, commonly chromosome 14. A small percentage of these translocations are familial, so parental karyotyping is essential for adequate recurrence risk counseling. Mosaicism is seen in 5%. Mean life expectancy is 130 days; 14% survive to 1 year of age. As with trisomy 18, cognitive and motor development is profoundly affected. Table 40–11 lists some of the anomalies that tend to be encountered more commonly in trisomy 13. Figure 40–5 shows typical facies.

The Support Organization for Trisomy 18, 13, and Related Disorders[2] is a grass-roots, lay group that serves as an excellent resource for parents, professionals, and other interested parties regarding trisomies 13 and 18 in particular.

Segmental Aneuploidies

Deletions, duplications, and translocations of segments of chromosomes theoretically are possible in an unlimited variety. Unequal or nonhomologous crossing over during meiosis may be a common theme, but certain chromosomal segments are involved with enough frequency to suggest that these loci are especially susceptible to rearrangement through an as-yet-undefined process. Deletions and duplications often have broadly predictable phenotypes. The deleted or duplicated segment may be interstitial, involving the midsection of one of the arms of a chromosome, or terminal. Because each band of a chromosome contains hundreds to thousands of genes, even the smallest of deletions is not trivial. As a general rule, the larger the deletion or duplication, the more severe the somatic and functional effects. For example, terminal or interstitial deletions of the short arm of chromosome 5, which occur in 1 of 50,000 births, result in a distinctive phenotype, cri-du-chat syndrome, which takes its name from the high-pitched cry of affected infants. Facial features include microcephaly, round

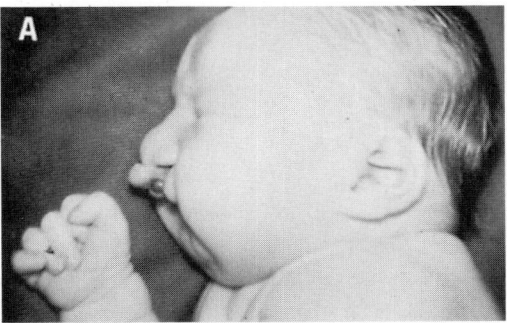

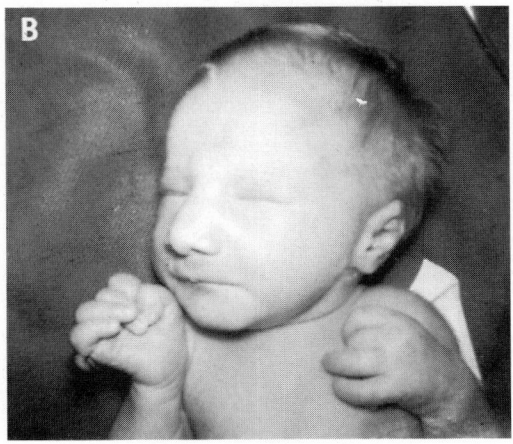

FIG. 40–5. A,B: Trisomy 13.

[2]S.O.F.T., 2982S Union St., Rochester, NY 14624; (716) 594-4621; http://www.trisomy.org.

facies, hypertelorism, broad nasal bridge, epicanthal folds, posteriorly rotated malformed ears, preauricular skin tags, and small chin (Fig. 40–6). Various other malformations may be present, including cleft lip with or without cleft palate, heart defects, and megacolon. Hypotonia and mental retardation are typical. The severity of cri-du-chat syndrome can be correlated roughly with the extent of the deletion: at a minimum, band 5p14-15 is missing—these individuals may have few major anomalies and mild retardation, but usually have some facial features and an unusual cry. Other common segmental aneuploidies are summarized in Table 40–12.

Chromosomal rearrangements are often *de novo,* spontaneous events that have occurred in a single egg or sperm, with no parental age effect, and therefore are unlikely to recur. Some, however, are the consequence of parental translocations, balanced and benign for that parent, or inversions of a chromosomal segment that spans the centromere (pericentric). Because 70% of the human genome consists of noncoding DNA, these molecular breaks and rejoinings, when no gain or loss of material is involved, usually have neutral consequences. If the break falls within a gene, some phenotypic effects may ensue. Careful analysis of translocations has, in fact, provided the critical link for mapping and cloning several important genes. During formation of eggs or sperm at meiosis, however, these rearrangements may yield gametes that have significant deletions, duplications, or more complex anomalies, with serious consequences for the offspring. Unbalanced translocations, in which there is both a duplicated chromosomal segment and a deletion, produce phenotypes that are unique, because they are a mixture of a partial monosomy syndrome and a partial trisomy. Not uncommonly, an unbalanced translocation is the consequence of a balanced translocation in a parent. Chromosomal studies on both mother and father then are critical for providing adequate recurrence risk counseling.

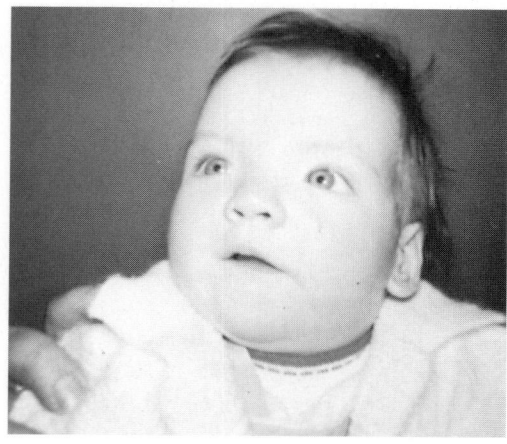

FIG. 40–6. Cri-du-chat syndrome (5p-).

TABLE 40–12. *Selected chromosomal anomaly syndromes*

Karyotype	Features
4p-	Poor growth, microcephaly, prominent glabella, hypertelorism, downturned corners of mouth, micrognathia, cleft lip/palate, cryptorchidism, heart defects, profound developmental retardation. May involve only a small region, to include 4p16, requiring high-resolution banding or FISH for confirmation. Also known as the Wolf–Hirschhorn syndrome.
Dup 9p	Poor growth, macrocephaly, hypertelorism, downslanting palpebral fissures, prominent nose, downturned corners of mouth, cupped ears, short fingers and toes, developmental retardation.
Del 11p13	Mental deficiency, poor growth and microcephaly, aniridia, cataracts, blindness, cryptorchidism, hypospadias, Wilms tumor (50%). The interstitial deletion encompasses a tumor-suppressor gene and provides the *de facto* "first hit" in tumorigenesis.
13q-	Growth deficiency, mental deficiency, microcephaly, prominent nasal bridge, hypertelorism, microphthalmia, colobomata, bilateral retinoblastoma, micrognathia, anomalous auricles, hypoplastic thumbs, congenital heart disease, genitourinary anomalies. Band q14 is the locus of the RB gene, a tumor-suppressor gene implicated in retinoblastoma.
18p-	Mild growth deficiency and microcephaly, psychomotor retardation, ptosis, epicanthal folds, hypertelorism, wide mouth, protruding ears, small hands and feet, pectus excavatum.
18q-	Short-stature hypotonia, variable mental deficiency, conductive deafness, auricular anomalies, long hands, tapering digits, cardiac defects.
Dup 22q	Highly variable, also known as cat-eye syndrome, after the bilateral inferotemporal colobomata of the irides, which also may involve the choroid and retina. Mild developmental delays, normal growth, slight hypertelorism, downslanting palpebral fissures, preauricular tags or pits, cardiac defects, anal atresia, renal agenesis. Forty-seven chromosomes are present: the "extra" chromosome is composed of one or two chromosome 22 fragments, joined by their acrocentric short arms, creating trisomy or tetrasomy 22 q. FISH provides confirmation of the nature of the small "marker" chromosome. Parental karyotypes are necessary because a mildly affected parent also may have the marker.

FISH, fluorescent *in situ* hybridization.

Abnormalities of the Sex Chromosomes

With the exception of Turner syndrome, sex chromosome aneuploidies tend to be phenotypically bland in newborn children. Klinefelter syndrome, 47,XXY, is associated with a few, occasional congenital anomalies, such as cryptorchidism and hypospadias. Variants with more than one Y or more than two X chromosomes tend to have greater mental deficiency and more minor anomalies.

Turner syndrome is caused by complete or partial absence of one X chromosome and occurs in 1 of 2,500 newborn girls. One half have a 45,X karyotype; a large number of other X chromosome anomalies, ranging from various isochromosome X patterns to simple deletions, ring chromosomes, and mosaics, account for the remainder. Almost all conceptuses with Turner syndrome are spontaneously aborted but, of those that are live born, only one-third are recognized in the newborn period. Clinical findings may include prominent ears, low posterior hairline, webbed neck, broad chest with widely spaced nipples, and puffiness of the dorsa of the hands and feet (Fig. 40–7). Although short stature is common in older girls, mean birth length is 47 cm, just within two standard deviations of the population mean. Ovarian dysgenesis (greater than 90%), renal anomalies (40% to 60%, horseshoe kidney in particular), and cardiac malformations (10% to 20%, especially coarctation of the aorta) will require directed investigations once this diagnosis is suspected (22).

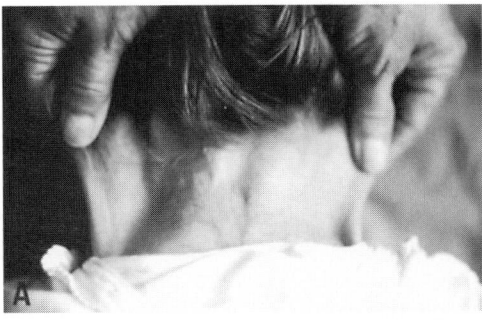
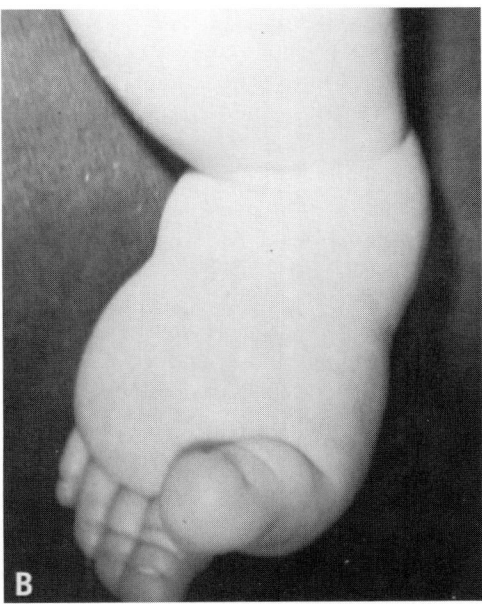

FIG. 40–7. A,B: Turner syndrome.

Microdeletion Syndromes

The difference between the deletion of a single nucleotide and deletion of an entire chromosome is primarily one of degree. It is not surprising, then, to find that many dysmorphologic syndromes are caused by monosomy or haploinsufficiency to an intermediate degree—very small chromosomal deletions, usually submicroscopic and undetectable by standard cytogenetic techniques, yet occasionally detectable by high-resolution banding. These microdeletions amount to a loss of several contiguous genes, with recognizable but variable phenotypic consequences. In some instances, microdeletions may be transmitted from parent to child as an autosomal dominant trait, but most occur *de novo,* with unaffected parents, as a consequence of imprecise alignment of homologous chromosomes and unequal crossing over during meiosis. For most microdeletion syndromes, a molecular probe for the minimal critical region of deleted DNA has been developed and can be hybridized to a fluorescent marker, enabling rapid analysis via FISH. Table 40–13 lists several microdeletion syndromes, their loci, and general features.

Single Gene Disorders

Achondroplasia

The most common skeletal dysplasia recognized at birth, achondroplasia is an autosomal dominant condition characterized by short limbs, frontal bossing, a large head, midface hypoplasia, and distinctive radiographic findings. In the newborn period, a thoracolumbar gibbus, or sharp kyphotic angulation of the vertebrae, may be present, followed in early childhood by lumbar lordosis. There is distinctive midface hypoplasia, a low nasal root, and relative prognathism (Fig. 40–8), which become more pronounced in childhood. The limb shortening is of the rhizomelic type, involving the humeri and femurs more than the distal extremities. There may be limitation of elbow extension, yet other joints may be relatively hyperextensible. The fingers often display a trident pattern, with a splay or gap between the third and fourth digits. Mild hypotonia is common. The enlarged head circumference is associated with mild ventriculomegaly in some cases, and in older children and adults a narrow foramen magnum has, on occasion, caused symptomatic cervicomedullary compression. Cognitive development is normal.

TABLE 40–13. *Microdeletion syndromes*

Syndrome	Locus	Features
Wolf–Hirschhorn syndrome	4p16	Hypotonia, microcephaly, hypertelorism, prominent glabella, severe mental deficiency.
Cri du chat	5p16	Low birth weight, cat-like cry, microcephaly, downslanting palpebral fissures.
Grieg cephalopolysyndactyly	7p13	Polydactyly, syndactyly, frontal bossing.
Williams syndrome	7q11.23	Supravalvular aortic stenosis, hyperacussis, stellate irides, prominent lips, mild mental retardation.
Larger–Giedion syndrome	8q24	Multiple exostoses, bulbous nose, protruding ears, loose skin (infancy).
WAGR	11q13	Wilms tumor, aniridia, genital anomalies, growth retardation.
Retinoblastoma	13q14.11	Retinoblastoma plus growth deficiency, microcephaly, prominent nasal bridge, hypoplastic thumbs, cardiac defects.
Prader–Willi syndrome	15q12	Paternal deletion in 70%, maternal 15q disomy in 30%. Hypotonia, hypogonadism, mental retardation, poor growth in infancy, hyperphagia and morbid obesity in childhood.
Angelman syndrome	15q12	Maternal deletion in 60%, paternal disomy in 5%. Severe mental retardation, seizures, ataxic gait microcephaly, paroxysms of laughter.
ATR-16	16p13.3	Alpha thalassemia, mild mental retardation.
Rubinstein–Taybi syndrome	16p13.3	CBP gene deletion in 25%, growth deficiency, mental retardation, small mouth, beaked nose, broad thumbs and toes.
Miller–Dieker syndrome	17p13	Lissencephaly, high forehead with vertical furrowing while crying.
Smith–Magenis syndrome	17p11.2	Brachycephaly, broad nasal bridge, short philtrum, prominent jaw, broad hands.
Alagile syndrome	20p11.23	Deep-set eyes, broad forehead, chronic cholestasis, vertebral defects, peripheral pulmonary artery stenosis.
DiGeorge sequence	22q11.2	Aortic arch anomalies, parathyroid and thymic deficiency leading to hypocalcemia and diminished cellular immunity.
Velo-cardio-facial syndrome	22q11.2	Cleft palate, prominent nose with narrow alar base, conotruncal cardiac defects, tapering fingers

Through positional cloning, achondroplasia has been localized to chromosome 4p16.3 (23) and the fibroblast growth factor receptor-3 gene (FGFR3) at that locus implicated in pathogenesis. Remarkably, heterozygosity for a single point mutation at nucleotide 1138, which converts a glycine residue to arginine, is responsible for all cases (24). Homozygosity for this FGFR3 mutation, as occurs in one-fourth of the conceptions when both parents have achondroplasia, results in a lethal, severely abnormal phenotype quite similar to another skeletal dysplasia, thanatophoric (Greek for "death seeking") dysplasia. Interestingly, thanatophoric dysplasia also is caused by mutations of FGFR3 involving other nucleotides (25).

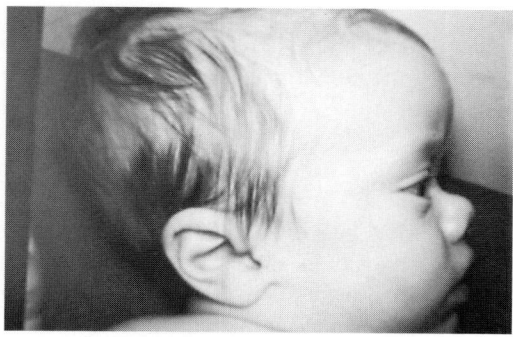

FIG. 40–8. Achondroplasia.

Smith–Lemli–Opitz Syndrome

As mentioned previously in this chapter, Smith–Lemli–Opitz syndrome is a multiple congenital anomaly syndrome recently found to be the consequence of a metabolic error, namely a deficiency of 7-dehydrocholesterol reductase (26). Like many other enzymatic deficiencies, this condition is inherited in an autosomal recessive fashion. The reductase, which maps to chromosome 7q32.1, is responsible for the last step in cholesterol synthesis. Consequently, serum cholesterol tends to be low (although in 10% it falls within normal limits) and the immediate precursor, 7-dehydrocholesterol, is markedly elevated. A variable spectrum of anomalies may be seen, including microcephaly, various central nervous system structural defects, hypotonia, growth deficiency, and distinctive facies with a high, square forehead, ptosis, a short nose, anteverted nares, and micrognathia (Fig. 40–9). Peripheral and central neural myelinization is reduced. About three-fourths of males have genital anomalies—cryptorchidism, ambiguous genitalia, even complete sex reversal. Syndactyly between the second and third toes is nearly universally present. More severely affected individuals may have visceral defects, such as renal cysts or agenesis, cardiac anomalies, pancreatic hyperplasia, hepatic dysfunction, cataracts, severe growth retardation, postaxial polydactyly, and may die in the neonatal period. Recurrence risk is 25%.

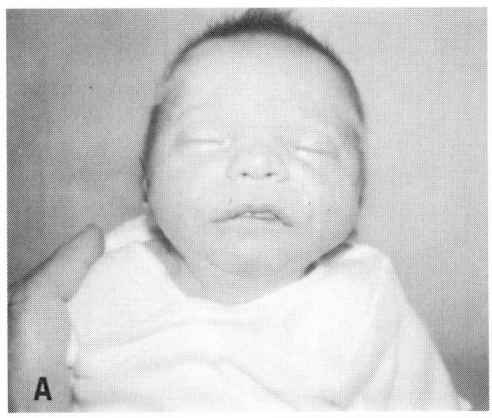

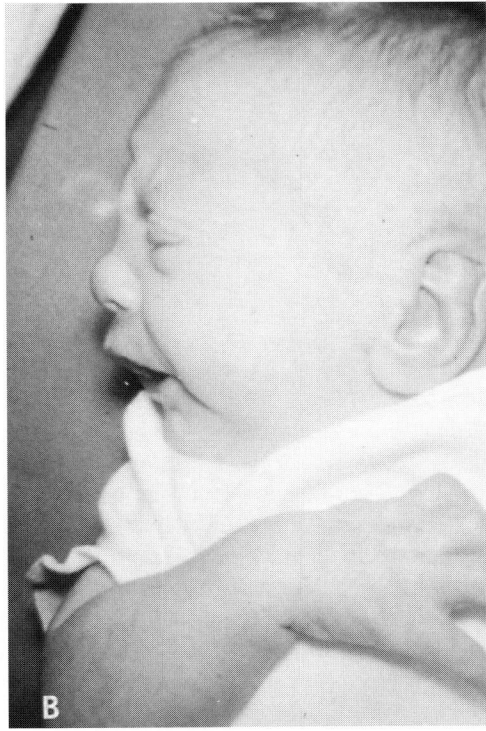

FIG. 40–9. A,B: Smith–Lemli–Opitz syndrome.

Chondrodysplasia Punctata, Rhizomelic Type

Rhizomelic chondrodysplasia punctata is an inborn error of peroxisome metabolism, inherited as an autosomal recessive trait, which is manifest as a distinctive skeletal dysplasia. Birth length is reduced and the proximal limbs ("rhizome" = root) are particularly affected. In addition, there is microcephaly, full cheeks, a depressed nasal bridge, cataracts, ichthyosis, coronal clefts of the vertebral bodies, and congenital heart disease (Fig. 40–10). Punctate calcific stippling of the epiphyses is readily demonstrable via lateral radiographs of the knee. Severe psychomotor retardation is the rule, and death usually occurs in the first year of life. Very-long-chain fatty acids and phytanic acid are increased in serum, and plasmalogen biosynthesis is deficient. Peroxisomes are found to be absent or markedly abnormal by electron microscopic studies of hepatocytes.

Treacher Collins–Franceschetti Syndrome

Also known as mandibulofacial dysostosis, this autosomal dominant condition was first described in the mid-1800s and fully delineated decades later by those after whom it is named. Clinical features vary widely within and between families, but may include a narrow face with downslanting palpebral fissures, zygomatic underdevelopment, a small chin, and an extension of scalp hair onto the cheek (Fig. 40–11). The lower eyelids are notched at the outer third; medial to this coloboma, the eyelashes are sparse or absent. The ears often are crumpled and small. One-third lack the external auditory canal and/or manifest conductive hearing loss because of ossicular defects. Ear tags and preauricular fistulae are common. In one-third there is overt palatal clefting, and an equal number have occult, submucous clefts. Intelligence is usually normal. In the early 1990s, several investigators localized the gene to chromosome 5q32-33.2 using linkage analysis and FISH. In 1996, the gene, designated TCOF1, was positionally cloned (27). The gene product, named "treacle" (British for "molasses," derived from the Middle English term for an antidote for poison), is predicted to be truncated in most TCOF1 patients due to the introduction of a premature termination codon via various deletions, insertions, and splicing alterations.

Apert Syndrome

This autosomal dominant craniosynostosis syndrome is readily recognized by the combination of an unusual head shape and characteristic limb anomalies. The premature fusion of cranial sutures is irregular but typically involves the coronal sutures, leading to brachycephaly with a full forehead and flat occiput, flat midface, shallow orbits, and downslanting palpebral fissures. There is syndactyly of the fingers and toes, both cutaneous and osseous, as well as broad thumbs (Fig. 40–12). Other anomalies may involve the cardiac, gastrointestinal, central nervous, and genitourinary systems. Most cases are sporadic. Mutations of the fibroblast growth factor receptor-2 gene at chromosome 10q25-26 have been implicated; other mutations in this gene cause several other dominant craniosynostosis syndromes, such as Crouzon syndrome and Pfeiffer syndrome (28).

Malformation Sequences

These patterns of anomalies represent the denouement of precise cascades of fetal events that, in many cases, are in turn initiated by a primary event, often a mechanical or vascular disruption of a specific developmental field. A

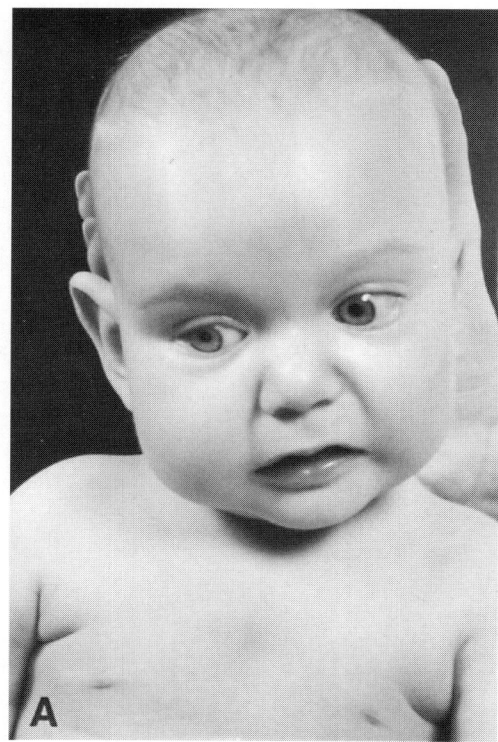

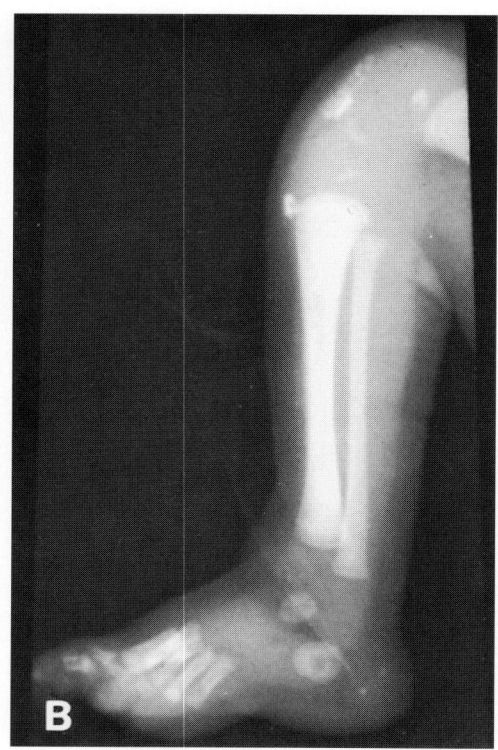

FIG. 40–10. A,B: Rhizomelic chondrodysplasia punctata.

malformation sequence may stand alone as a recognizable entity or may be a component of a larger picture, associated with a chromosomal defect, microdeletion, or single-gene disorder. The Pierre Robin sequence, for example, is recognized as a cleft of the posterior palate, often in the shape of a "U," in a child with a markedly retruded, small mandible. At 5 to 9 weeks' gestation, a malpositioned jaw allows the tongue to interfere with the medial apposition of the posterior palatal shelves as they migrate toward the midline, thereby mechanically prohibiting their fusion. The newborn not uncommonly experiences significant airway obstruction and will require very close observation and occasional surgical intervention. Robin sequence may be isolated or may occur as an element of a multitude of

FIG. 40–11. Treacher Collins–Franceschetti syndrome.

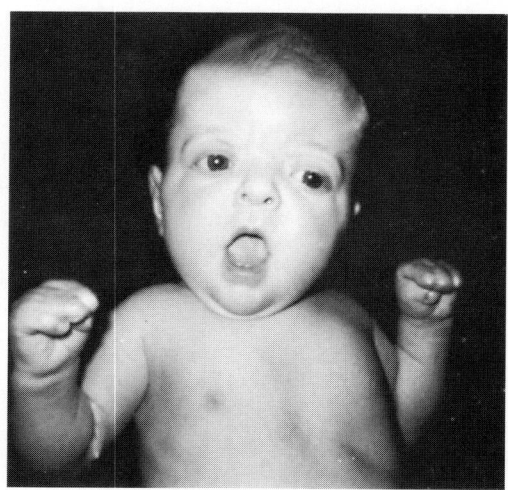

FIG. 40–12. Apert syndrome.

syndromes, such as trisomy 18, velo-cardio-facial syndrome, Beckwith–Wiedemann syndrome, Miller–Dieker syndrome, FAS, and many others.

Other Mechanisms

Recent developments in molecular biology have elucidated a number of mechanisms that lie beyond the classic paradigms of genetic disease. Anticipation, uniparental disomy, and imprinting are three such phenomena that deserve mention, although it should be kept in mind that many of the resulting disorders do not feature congenital anomalies. *Anticipation* refers to the progressive increase in severity of an inherited condition over successive generations in a pedigree. This phenomenon is exemplified by myotonic dystrophy and fragile X syndrome; in both, a marked expansion in the number of tandemly repeated trinucleotides is correlated with predictably more dysfunctional phenotypes. *Uniparental disomy* involves the inheritance of both copies of a particular chromosome or chromosome segment from only one parent and has been observed in cystic fibrosis, Russell–Silver syndrome, Prader–Willi syndrome, and Angelman syndrome, among others. *Imprinting* refers to how a gene may function differently, depending on whether it is inherited from the mother or the father.

Beckwith–Wiedemann syndrome (BWS) occurs in 1 of 17,000 live births. It features somatic overgrowth, macroglossia, omphalocoele, visceromegaly, and dysplasia of the renal medulla. Transitory, symptomatic hypoglycemia is present in 30%, and a number of neoplasms, including Wilms tumor, adrenal cortical carcinoma, and hepatoblastoma, are common, especially in individuals with hemihypertrophy, which affects about 13% of patients. Glabellar nevus flammeus, linear grooves of the ear lobes, and posterior helical ear pits are valuable diagnostic signs (Fig. 40–13). About 85% of cases are spo-

radic, and a number of these individuals have a small, interstitial duplication of chromosome 11 involving band p15.5; invariably the duplicated region is paternal in origin. Other individuals, who do not have duplicated segments, derive both 11p15.5 regions from their father. They have the normal number of chromosomes—that is, they are disomic for this region—but have inherited both segments from only one parent, i.e., uniparental disomy. These data also suggest that BWS is caused by a dosage effect related to a gene or genes that are differentially expressed in maternally and paternally derived alleles, i.e., imprinting. Several studies recently have implicated the p57 gene (KIP2) in BWS (29), but the complexities of this condition continue to be investigated.

Disorders of Unknown Etiology

Cornelia de Lange Syndrome

This rare, sporadic condition of unknown etiology often is recognizable based on the facial gestalt: the eye-

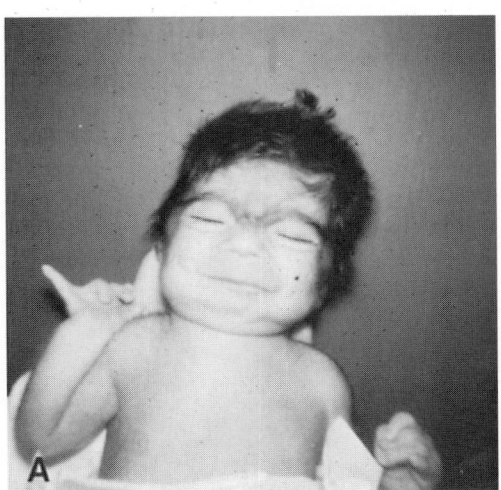

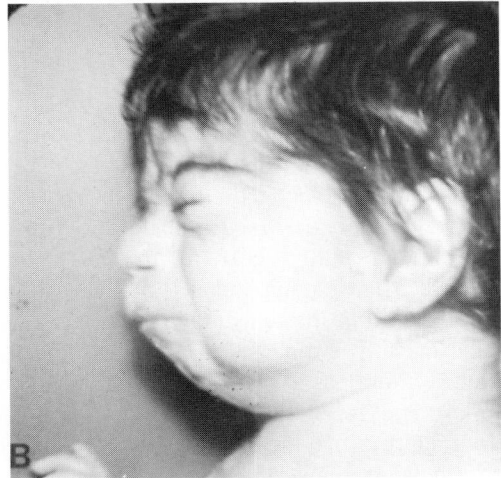

FIG. 40–14. A,B: Cornelia de Lange syndrome.

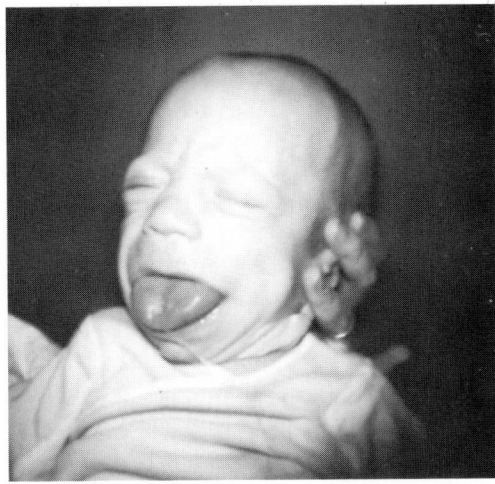

FIG. 40–13. Beckwith–Wiedemann syndrome.

brows are crescent shaped, neatly defined, and often meet in the midline (synophrys); the anterior hairline is low; the nose is short and the nostrils upturned; and the lips are thin with downturned corners, likened to that of a carp (Fig. 40–14). Microcephaly and mental retardation are common but not invariable. Growth is deficient prenatally and postnatally. About one-fourth have upper limb anomalies, which can range from proximally placed thumbs to severe reduction defects. Empiric recurrence risk is estimated to be 2% to 5%. Duplication of the long arm of chromosome 3 causes a very similar malformation pattern (phenocopy) and must be excluded.

GENETIC COUNSELING

In general terms, genetic counseling has been practiced throughout the millennia as a form of interpretation and, welcome or not, advice giving for individuals, couples, or families for whom a congenital anomaly has personal significance. As a portent, omen, or prophecy, the malformation of a newborn has been inferred to be the visitation of a god, of celestial forces, of bad seed or bad morals, sure to bring ruin to the bearer of bad fruit. Even as we shake our heads at such a legacy, one would be wise to recall that, a century ago, an eugenic approach to genetic counseling was the norm and not the exception. Genetic counseling now is a process of communicating with an individual or couple about what exactly has caused a genetic problem, how they might understand it, and what options they have for the future. Informally, many clinicians perform these activities as an integral component of fundamental caregiving. Formally, however, genetic counseling is a complex and comprehensive activity that has blossomed as a discipline in its own right. It is learned didactically and practically via postgraduate, degree-conferring programs in medical genetics and genetic counseling, with board certification (and recertification) incumbent on thoroughly documented case workups, close supervision by experienced preceptors, and successful performance on rigorous, standardized examinations.

The goals of genetic counseling have evolved over the past several decades. The provision of advice regarding reproductive choice and behavior, with an eye toward reducing the amount of genetic disease in future generations, has been superseded by other aims. The genetic counselor fundamentally seeks to provide information with clarity, sensitivity, and support to enable the person seeking information, the consultand, to understand well and decide capably. Emphasis is placed on the psychological and cultural aspects of this interactive process, and support and follow-up are key elements. Genetic counseling requires that the diagnosis be established with as much precision as possible, that an accurate and full pedigree be obtained, and that up-to-date information regarding the diagnosis be researched. Recurrence risk calculations may be simple and straightforward, or they may require more sophisticated analysis, often involving the use of Bayes theorem. This theorem, created more than 200 years ago, allows the laws of probability to be applied to a specific clinical scenario and quantifies the risk of recurrence by iincorporating multiple observations into a complex formula (30). These data, the natural history of the disorder in question, management options, and the full spectrum of reproductive options are discussed in detail with the consultand, often with explicit attention to the significance these have for that individual, the psychological and practical burden perceived in the context of the social structure, finances, and personal experience. Principles of genetic counseling also include a commitment to strive for a nondirective approach, truth telling, avoidance of paternalism, respect for autonomy and dignity, and anticipation of ongoing psychological needs and issues. A concerted effort is made to identify and facilitate outside sources of information and support, such as from clergy, genetic support groups, and social services.

Difficult Decisions

Some infants are born with anomalies that are irreparable and incompatible with life. For these newborns, the decision to limit intervention, although deeply saddening, is clear. Bilateral renal agenesis and anencephaly are salient examples—no amount of intervention will help; solace and support are the only options. Other newborns, whose malformations are profound, but who may respond to heroic therapy, demand greater courage on the part of parents and clinicians—courage to analyze carefully in the face of chaos, in the context of a health care system whose bias is to act, simply because action is possible, and without much time in which to reach a decision. These decisions often are aided materially by genetic or dysmorphologic analysis or consultation.

The critical data, to be sought rapidly in this scenario, is a precise diagnosis, for with diagnosis comes knowledge of natural history, worst case and best case, which may portend a high likelihood of good neurologic outcome, as in the case of VATER association, or a more grim future, as in trisomy 13 or trisomy 18. The dignity of the child compels the caregiver to have as clear a vision of the future as possible, to deal with decisions such as whether or not to intubate, transplant an organ, etc. The infant with thanatophoric dysplasia may well live, with extraordinary care, to several years of age, as has been reported in two children, and one in ten infants with trisomy 18 lives to the first birthday, albeit with significant psychomotor retardation. However, these facts are a starting point for an individualized analysis, shared between family and physician, and not the foundation of policy to either routinely offer maximal intervention or insist that care be denied.

In the United States, economic arguments typically are reserved for the macrocosmic debate over whether treatment has value for infants with a limited lifespan and limited cognitive potential. Some parents and professionals would point out accurately that these are value judgments, susceptible to the failings of the "slippery slope"—where can one draw an acceptable line regarding which children are "worth it"? Not long ago, individuals with Down syndrome were managed expectantly, cardiac surgery was rarely considered an option, and home life and normal socialization discouraged. Many families now perceive a similar paradigm of disfavor within medical institutions toward their infants with trisomy 13 or trisomy 18 and are aggressively seeking out those practitioners who will perform major surgery. When confronted with the argument that their children are profoundly and permanently disabled, these same families counter that they find richness and reward in their child, which they feel is reciprocated, and that this judgment regarding "quality of life" is theirs, and theirs alone, to make.

The clinician in the midst of these challenges may do worse than to fall back on basic principles—complete ascertainment of facts, diagnostic precision, and solid understanding of the natural history. One cannot underestimate the power of careful and frequent communication with the family, with the dual aims of appreciating the family's points of view and of presenting, with clarity, the medical point of view.

ADDENDA

The Internet

Particularly in the field of clinical genetics, information access can be both critical and problematic. On the one hand, many of the classic papers that delineate syndromes remain superb resources and guideposts to diagnosis and natural history. On the other hand, the spectrum of variability for many conditions is continually being expanded through focused study and improved analysis. In addition, as a direct consequence of the Human Genome Project and related research, tremendous strides are taken on a nearly daily basis regarding the molecular underpinnings of many clinical conditions. In the past several years, it has become clear that many compendia of genetic disease become obsolete by the time their ink is dry. Consequently, the internet has emerged as an important resource for both the research community and those medical practitioners who bridge the gap between basic or applied research and the bedside. Several internet sites are especially useful for those who need current data about a particular genetic entity not only for scientific information, such as whether the gene has been identified recently and whether a diagnostic test has been developed, but also for support materials, such as information sheets for parents and where to find a support group. As always, one should bear in mind that the internet is public domain; personal, institutional, and patient information are subject to the same common-sense, legal, and ethical standards regarding privacy as apply elsewhere. The following is a selected list of resources that may be helpful entry points into the wealth of information on the internet:

- Gibbs S, Sullivan-Fowler M, Rowe NW. *Mosby's medical surfari*. St. Louis: Mosby-Year Book, Inc., 1996. Subtitled "A guide to exploring the internet and discovering top health care choices," this printed text may be helpful for those not yet wired and who want an introduction in a comfortable context.
- *Information for Genetic Professionals*, University of Kansas Medical Center (http://www.kumc.edu/GEC/prof/geneprof.htm). This is one of the original online clearing houses of practical genetic information. More than 1,500 internet links to other genetic web sites are available via this home page (D. Collins, *personal communication*).
- *Online Mendelian Inheritance in Man* (OMIM), National Center for Biotechnology Information-Johns Hopkins University (http://www3.ncbi.nlm.nih.gov/Omim/). Originally published in print form as the opus of Dr. Victor McKusick, this catalogue of mendelian genetics reigns as one of the most definitive and current sources of information, with search capabilities and links to MEDLINE, graphics, and clinical photographs, as well as access to DNA sequence data.
- *Directory of National Genetic Voluntary Organizations*, The Alliance of Genetic Support Groups (1-800-336-4363; http://www.medhelp.org/agsg/agsgsup.htm). For current information on support groups and information understandable by patients and their families, this site is the definitive resource.

REFERENCES

1. Nelson K, Holmes LB. Malformations due to presumed spontaneous mutations in newborn infants. *N Engl J Med* 1989;320:19.
2. Chung CS, Myrianthopoulos NC. Congenital anomalies: mortality and morbidity, burden and classification. *Am J Med Genet* 1987;27:505.
3. Van Regemorter N, Dodion J, Druart C. Congenital malformations in 10,000 consecutive births in a university hospital: need for genetic counseling and prenatal diagnosis. *J Pediatr* 1984;104:386.
4. Guyer B, Martin JA, MacDorman MF, Anderson RN, Strobino DM. Annual summary of vital statistics 1996. *Pediatrics* 1997;100:905.
5. Hall JG, Powers EK, McIlvaine RT, Ean VH. The frequency and familial burden of genetic disease in a paediatric hospital. *Am J Med Genet* 1978;1:416.
6. Panny S. *Strategies for integrating genetics into managed care.* Texas Genetics Network (TEXGENE) Annual Conference, Austin, Texas, June 14, 1996.
7. Bishop DT. Multifactoral inheritance. In: Emery AEH, Rimoin DL,

eds. *Principles and practice of medical genetics*, 2nd ed, vol 1. Edinburgh: Churchill Livingstone, 1990:165.

8. Hall BD. The state of the art of dysmorphology. *Am J Dis Child* 1993; 147:1184.

9. Stevenson RE, Hall JG. Terminology. In: Stevenson RE, Hall JG, Goodman RM, eds. *Human malformations and related anomalies*, vol 1. New York: Oxford University Press, 1993:21.

10. Hall JG. An approach to malformation syndromes. In: Berg K, ed. *Medical genetics: past, present, future.* New York: Alan R. Liss, 1985:275.

11. Hall JG, Froster-Iskenius UG, Allanson JE. *Handbook of normal physical measurements.* Oxford: Oxford University Press, 1989.

12. Saul RA, Stevenson RE, Rogers RC, Skinner SA, Prouty LA, Flannery DB. Growth references from conception to adulthood. *Proceedings of the Greenwood Genetic Center*, 1988[Suppl 1].

13. Opitz JM. Study of the malformed fetus and infant. *Pediatr Rev* 1981;3:57.

14. Winter RM, Baraitser M. *London dysmorphology database.* Oxford: Oxford University Press, 1996.

15. Tjio JH, Levan A. The chromosome number of man. *Hereditas* 1956; 42:1.

16. Hook EB. Chromosome abnormalities: prevalence, risks, and recurrence. In:Brock DH, Rodeck CH, Ferguson-Smith MA, eds. *Prenatal diagnosis and screening.* Edinburgh: Churchill Livingstone, 1992:351.

17. Rex AP, Preus M. A diagnostic index for Down syndrome. *J Pediatr* 1982;100:903.

17a. Gorlin RJ, Cohen MM Jr, Levin LS, eds. *Syndromes of the Head and Neck,* 3rd ed. New York: Oxford University Press, 1990:33–40.

17b. Jones KL. *Smith's Recognizable Patterns of Human Malformation,* 5th ed. Philadelphia: WB Saunders Company, 1997:8–13.

17c. Tolmie JL. Down Syndrome and other autosomal trisomies. In: Emery AEH, Rimoin DL, eds. *Principles and Practice of Medical Genetics,* 2nd ed., vol. 1. Edinburgh: Churchill Livingstone, 1990:925–945.

17d. Epstein CH. Down Syndrome. In: Scriver CR, Beaudet AL, Sly WS, Valle D, eds. *The Metabolic Basis of Inherited Disease,* 6th ed. New York: McGraw-Hill, 1989:291–326.

18. Aase J. Dysmorphologic diagnosis for the pediatric practitioner. *Pediatr Clin North Am* 1992;39:135.

19. Hall JG. When a child is born with congenital anomalies. *Contemp Pediatr* 1988;August:78.

20. Edwards JH, Harnden DG, Cameron AH. A new trisomic syndrome. *Lancet* 1960;1:787.

21. Patau K, Smith DW, Therman E, et al. Multiple congenital anomalies caused by an extra autosome. *Lancet* 1960;1:790.

22. Robinson A, de la Chapelle A. Sex chromosome abnormalities. In: Emery AEH, Rimoin DL, eds. *Principles and practice of medical genetics*, 2nd ed, vol 1. Edinburgh: Churchill Livingstone, 1990:973.

23. Francomano CA, Ortiz de Luna RI, Hefferon TW. Localization of the achondroplasia gene to the distal 2.5 Mb of human chromosome 4p. *Hum Mol Genet* 1994;3:787.

24. Shiang R, Thompson LM, Zhu Y-Z, et al. Mutations in the transmembrane domain of FGFR3 cause the most common form of dwarfism, achondroplasia. *Cell* 1994;78:335.

25. Tavormina P, Shiang R, Thompson L, et al. Thanatophoric dysplasia (types I and II) caused by distinct mutations in fibroblast growth factor 3. *Nat Genet* 1995;9:321.

26. Opitz JM, de La Cruz F. Cholesterol metabolism in the RSH/Smith-Lemli-Opitz syndrome: summary of an NICHD Conference. *Am J Med Genet* 1994;50:326.

27. The Treacher Collins Syndrome Collaborative Group. Positional cloning of a gene involved in the pathogenesis of Treacher Collins syndrome. *Nat Genet* 1996;12:130.

28. Wilkie AOM, Slaney SF, Oldridge M, et al. Apert syndrome results from localized mutations of FGFR2 and is allelic with Crouzon syndrome. *Nat Genet* 1995;9:165.

29. Hatada I, Ohashi H, Fukushima Y, et al. An imprinted gene p57 (KIP2) is mutated in Beckwith-Wiedemann syndrome. *Nat Genet* 1996;14:171.

30. Young ID. Risk estimation in genetic counseling. In: Rimoin DL, Connor JM, Pyeritz RE, eds. *Principles and practice of medical genetics,* 3rd ed, vol 1. Edinburgh: Churchill Livingstone, 1996:521.

CHAPTER 41

Endocrine Disorders of the Newborn

Thomas Moshang, Jr. and Paul S. Thornton

Almost from the moment of conception, endocrine physiologic processes are actively involved in the growth and development of the human fetus. Disturbances of the interplay of these complex hormonal processes can cause somatic or biochemical alterations in the fetus and newborn infant. Therefore, the clinical disorders of endocrine function in the newborn are reflections of altered physiologic function, in either the fetus or the mother, during intrauterine life. Moreover, the disturbances of endocrine physiologic function can occur during different stages of fetal development, resulting in different clinical situations. Knowledge about the physiologic fetomaternal hormonal processes and the ontogeny of the fetal endocrine glands makes the clinical disorders of endocrine function in the newborn more readily understandable.

DISORDERS OF SEXUAL DIFFERENTIATION

Normal Sexual Differentiation

A schematic representation of the controls of sexual development is depicted in Fig. 41–1. The gonadal anlagen are recognized as genital ridges by the fifth or sixth week of gestation. These primitive gonads are bipotential, consisting of cortical (i.e., ovarian) and medullary (i.e., testicular) components. The genital ridge is composed of three cell types: (i) germ cells destined to become prespermatagonia in the male or oocytes in the female, (ii) supporting cells destined to become Sertoli cells (male) or follicular cells (female), and (iii) the steroid cells destined to become Leydig cells (male) or theca cells (female). Although the determination of gender is made

at conception based upon chromosomes and the associated genes, the critical step in gender differentiation may be based upon whether the supporting cell differentiates as a Sertoli cell as opposed to a follicular cell.

In 1959, Ford et al. (1) determined that the Y chromosome was necessary for male development, which was further localized to the short arm of the Y chromosome in 1966 (2). In 1986, Page et al. (3) postulated that a gene coding for a zinc finger protein in region one (Yp1A2) on the short arm of the Y chromosome was the testicular-determining factor). More recently, however, Sinclair et al. (4) localized a gene in the Yp1A1 region of the short arm of the Y chromosome that is present in all 46XY males, all 46XX males, and not found in any 46XY females. This gene is referred to as the SRY gene (the sex-determining region of the Y chromosome) (4). However, this complex story certainly is not complete, because the SRY gene has not been found in most 46XX true hermaphrodites in whom testicular tissue is present. Furthermore, infants with camptomelic dysplasia show a female predominance, with 75% of the XY genotype infants having a female phenotype (5). These patients have mutations in the SOX-9 gene (SRY-related HMG Box genes). The SOX-9 gene is very highly conserved throughout nature. It is proposed that SRY is a transcription factor that turns on the expression of SOX-9, which in turn causes differentiation of the supporting cells of the gonadal ridge into Sertoli cells (6). The Sertoli cells stimulate production of testosterone and mullerian-inhibiting substance (MIS) by the Leydig cells. These hormones respectively cause development of the wolfian structures and regression of the mullerian structures, resulting in the male phenotype. A third gene, DAX-1, appears to be antagonistic to SRY by inhibiting SOX-9 expression (7). DAX-1 is expressed in males and females. However, in males, SRY has a dominant effect over DAX-1, resulting in expression of SOX-9 in males. The current concept is that the SRY gene is the primary testicular-

T. Moshang, Jr.: Department of Pediatrics, University of Pennsylvania; and Department of Pediatrics, Children's Hospital of Philadelphia, Philadelphia, Pennyslvania

P. S. Thornton: National Metabolic Unit, The Children's Hospital, Dublin, Ireland

NORMAL SEXUAL DIFFERENTIATION

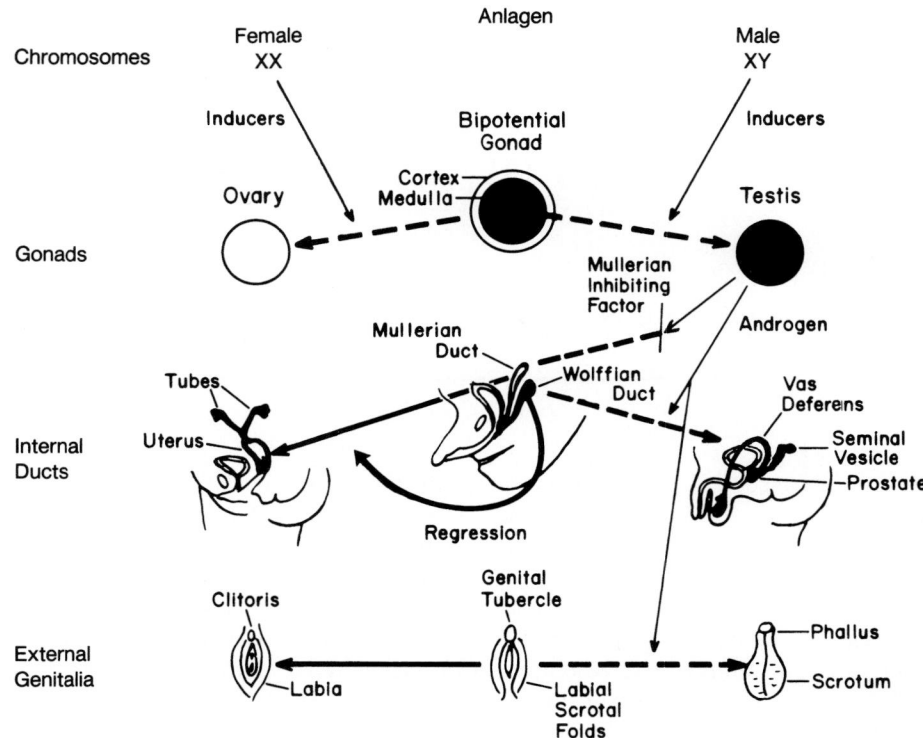

FIG. 41–1. Various inducers (*thin arrows*) are necessary for differentiation of the gonads and masculine development (*dashed arrows*). In the absence of these inducers, the differentiation is female (*thick arrows*).

determining factor, but more than one factor downstream of the SRY gene is involved in testicular determination.

The differentiated gonads play a critical role in directing the differentiation of the internal genital ducts, as well as the external genitalia. In the presence of the SRY gene or SOX-9, the primary sex cords develop into testes and the supporting cells become Sertoli cells. The development of testes and regression of mullerian structures is complete by 6 to 7 weeks of gestation. The Leydig cells in the seminiferous tubules secrete MIS, a 140-kilodalton glycoprotein, by 7 weeks. MIS causes degeneration of the mullerian duct with resultant absence of the uterus, fallopian tubes, and proximal two-thirds of the vagina. Leydig cells in the testes, stimulated by human chorionic gonadotropin (hCG), secrete testosterone, which locally stimulates the wolffian ducts to proliferate into the vas deferens, seminal vesicle, and epididymis. Testosterone is converted locally, by 5α-reductase, to dihydrotestosterone (DHT), which causes fusion of the urogenital slit and genital tubercle and development of the scrotum and penis. Male genital development is completed by 12 weeks of gestation. In the second trimester, abdominal descent of the testes is stimulated by MIS. Further descent of the testes into the scrotum and penile growth

in the second and third trimesters of gestation is in response to increasing testosterone production. This increase in testosterone production is stimulated by pituitary gonadotropins.

In the absence of the SRY gene or SOX-9, and in the presence of two XX chromosomes, the primary sex cords become follicles and the ovaries are formed by 10 weeks of gestation. In Turner syndrome, where there is a deficiency of the second X chromosomes, ovarian formation is limited. The fetal ovaries, in the absence of androgens and MIS, do not descend. The mullerian ducts persist, with resultant formation of the uterus, fallopian tubes, and vagina. There is no stimulus to the wolffian duct. The development of female external genitalia does not depend on hormone action or the presence of functioning gonads.

Sexual Ambiguity and Gonadal Disorders

The first thought in most parents of a newborn infant is the gender of the child. Even when many parents today are aware of the probable gender of a child because of prenatal ultrasonography or amniocentesis, the declaration of gender at birth is necessary. In those situations when gender is unclear or discordant from prenatal chromosomal findings, the situation is truly a medical emergency. It is important for attending physicians at the birth of such infants to be extremely cautious but simultaneouly reassuring to parents that the gender of such a child will be discerned in a short period of time.

Disorders of Chromosomal Sex

The normal complement of sex chromosomes directs the bipotential gonad to differentiate into either ovary or testicle. Many varieties of sex chromosome aberrations have been reported (see Chap. 40). Some of these are lethal to the fetus (e.g., YO), and some probably cause very few somatic or biochemical abnormalities in terms of sexual differentiation (e.g., XXX). It is clear that aberrations of sex chromosomes influence gonadal differentiation. In contrast to the autosomal chromosomes, extra genetic material from the X chromosome can be tolerated with minor untoward effects. This is because, both in normal 46XX females and in patients with an extra X chromosome (e.g., 47XXX), the second and subsequent X chromosomes are inactivated and do not contribute to the pool of genetic information. Studies of natural chromosomal disorders indicate that at least two X chromosomes are required for complete ovarian development. Although more than two X chromosomes do not interfere with gonadal differentiation, a percentage of the reported patients with X polyploidy have manifested early menopause (8). It generally is true that a Y chromosome is necessary for testicular development; however, case reports of true hermaphrodites and normal male phenotypes with only XX chromosomes are well documented (9,10). The etiology of the 46XX true hermaphrodite is still not fully understood, because the SRY gene has not been found in most 46XX true hermaphrodites.

The classic sex chromosome aberrations occur relatively frequently as determined by newborn screening. In the New Haven Study, XXY occurred once in 545 males, XYY occurred once in 728 males, XXX occurred once in 727 females, and only one case of 45 XO occurred in 2,181 female newborns (11). The diagnosis of Turner syndrome, however, is made with greater frequency than the other sex chromosome aberrations because of the associated somatic abnormalities. Various combinations and deletions of sex chromosomal material have been reported, which cause a range of abnormalities of gonadal and sexual differentiation. Common sex chromosome abnormalities other than Turner syndrome (e.g., XXX, XXY, XYY) do not present with problems during the neonatal period.

Turner Syndrome

The classic chromosomal abnormality is total loss of an X chromosome. Other chromosomal abnormalities have been reported, such as mosaicism of cells with an XO cell line with normal 46XX cells, 46XY, or deletion of part of an X chromosome (e.g., 46X isochromosome X). Chromosomal analysis of girls with Turner syndrome suggests that over 50% are 45XO, 17% are isochromosome mosaic 46X,i(Xq), 8% are 45XO/46XX, and all of the other mosaics comprise the remainder (12). It is known that concepta that are 45XO often abort before week 28 of gestation (13), and that 1 in 15 spontaneous abortions are 45XO.

The loss of some of the genetic information in the X chromosomes results in varying degrees of the somatic abnormalities of Turner syndrome. The presence of a 46XX cell line in mosaicism does not modify the short stature or somatic abnormalities to a great degree, but does seem to influence gonadal development. In the study by Goldberg et al. (14), spontaneous female sexual development occurred in 3 of 25 patients with mosaic karyotypes but in none of the XO group.

The Turner phenotype in the newborn is secondary to the lymphangiectasia and lymphedema. The webbed neck, in the newborn, is most often seen as redundant folds about the posterior neck. The lymphedema involves the dorsa of the hands and feet. A host of associated somatic defects have been described in this syndrome, most of which become more readily identifiable with age and growth of the child (15). The most common defects include triangular facies with low-set ears, high-arched palate, low hairline, shield-like chest with widespread and hypoplastic areolae, and cubitus valgus. Coarctation of the aorta is a common cardiovascular abnormality; however, the more benign condition of bicuspid aortic valves is more common. Skin manifestations include hemangiomas, cutis laxa, pigmented nevi, dysplastic nails, and tendency to keloid formation. Skeletal abnormalities such as "beaking" of the medial tibial condyle, drumstick-shaped distal phalanges, and vertebral anomalies have been described (16). Short metacarpals, resulting in the knuckle sign, may be detected clinically or radiologically. Palmar simian creases, distal axial triradius, and increased number of digital ulnar whorls are documented as dermatoglyphic abnormalities. The most consistent characteristics, short stature and sexual infantilism, are seen in the older child.

There is no specific therapy for this syndrome in the newborn period unless the developmental anomalies, such as coarctation of the aorta, create a clinical problem. These children have a high incidence of recurrent otitis media, chronic lymphocytic thyroiditis, and idiopathic hypertension. There is an increased incidence of mental retardation, but many Turner syndrome children are intellectually normal or even bright. Estrogen/progesterone therapy at the appropriate age is indicated for the treatment of sexual infantilism.

One of the major psychological problems for girls with Turner syndrome is short stature. Recombinant growth hormone does increase final height and is now approved for treatment of the short stature of Turner syndrome (17). The combination of early use of growth hormone (before 5 years of age) and low-dose estrogen replacement at an appropriate age is thought to give the best outcome in terms of height and pyschosexual development.

The question of fertility in later life might arise even in the newborn period. Studies have indicated that women with Turner syndrome can achieve pregnancy, with successful outcome, using *in vitro* fertilization of donor oocytes and hormonal therapy, at a rate similar to couples with infertility for other reasons (18).

In Turner syndrome with XO/XY or XX/XY mosaicism or variations, the gonadal elements frequently will contain testicular components. Various external genitalia phenotypes have been documented in this mosaic variant of Turner syndrome, including normal female, normal male, intersex female with clitoromegaly, and male with hypospadias and unilateral cryptorchidism. The most frequent phenotype of the mosaic Turner syndrome combined with a Y chromosome, however, is normal male with descended testes. Previously, due to selection bias, it was believed that the most common phenotype was female, although occasionally with clitoromegaly (19). It is now clear due to prenatal amniotic chromosomal studies that the majority of these children are phenotypically male.

In this type of mosaicism, the presence of both medullary and cortical elements in gonadal remnants is referred to as mixed gonadal dysgenesis. In mixed gonadal dysgenesis, in the presence of a Y chromosome, the likelihood of malignant degeneration of the gonadal tissues is markedly increased in the intraabdominal gonads. In those children with a female phenotype, early gonadectomy is recommended because any gonadal hormone function is more likely to be androgenic (20).

Disorders of Gonadal Sex

A number of conditions have been documented in which there is gonadal failure of one degree or another. The etiologies of these disorders may include sex chromosome aberrations, but in many reported conditions no chromosome aberrations have been noted. Certainly, various teratogens, including radiation, viruses, and drugs, might cause *in utero* gonaditis and damage to the developing gonad. The degree and timing of the damage to the developing testis will cause varying levels of failure of development of the internal ducts and external genitalia.

Pure Gonadal Dysgenesis

Complete dysgenesis of the genital ridges results in normal phenotypic females. Affected girls tend to be tall and eunuchoid and have primary amenorrhea and sexual infantilism. The chromosomal karyotype may be either 46XX or 46XY. In the 46XX females, the condition can be inherited in an autosomal recessive manner and is associated with sensory neural deafness (21). In the 46XY females, the condition also is inherited in an autosomal recessive fashion but also may be transmitted as an X-linked mutation (22). Teratogenic factors also may cause gonadal dysgenesis. A high incidence of neoplasia has been reported in pure gonadal dysgenesis. Most infants with 46XY gonadal dysgenesis will be detected in the neonatal period only if chromosome studies are done for other reasons, such as amniotic studies, because the infants are phenotypically normal females.

Partial Gonadal Dysgenesis

Teratogenic factors that damage the testis at later stages of fetal development cause varying clinical situations. Destruction of the testis from between weeks 9 and 12 of gestation will not prevent involution of the mullerian structures, because MIS will have been secreted, but will result in failure of fusion and development of the external genitalia, which is dependent on testosterone production by the testes. Thus, the external genitalia will be phenotypically female but there will be no gonads, uterus, or fallopian tubes. If the testes disappear late in the second trimester (i.e., vanishing testes syndrome), the infant will have congenital anorchia with otherwise normal male external and internal genitalia. Lesser damage occurring between these times in gestation may cause micropenis or cryptorchidism.

True Hermaphroditism

In true hermaphroditism, both ovarian and testicular elements are present. Findings may consist of an ovary on one side and a testis on the contralateral side, an ovary or a testis and a contralateral ovotestis, or two ovotestes. Therefore, this terminology also includes those patients with mixed gonadal dysgenesis associated with sex chromosome aberrations (e.g., 45XO/46XY). In true hermaphrodite patients without chromosome aberrations, two-thirds have a 46XX karyotype, and one-third have a 46XY karyotype. It is interesting to note that of the true hermaphrodite patients with 46XX karyotype, very few have the SRY gene, yet 50% express the H-Y antigen. This contrasts with the 46XX males, of whom 90% carry the SRY gene. It has been suggested that the 46XX true hermaphrodite has an autosomal or X-linked mutation of a gene downstream of the SRY gene that plays a role in gonadal differentiation.

The development and differentiation of the internal duct structures and external genitalia in the true hermaphrodite depend on the degree of functioning testicular tissue. The sex differentiation of the gonaduct corresponds to the gonad on the same side, because it is apparent that MIS acts locally. Most true hermaphrodites have ambiguous external genitalia.

Disorders of Phenotypic Sex

Disorders of phenotypic sex result when the anatomic development of the external genitalia does not correspond to the chromosomal or gonadal sex. This condition is called pseudohermaphroditism and may either be a genotypic male with inadequate virilization or a virilized genotypic female. These conditions usually occur in the presence of normal gonads and sex chromosomes. Such derangements may be secondary to teratogens causing defective embryogenesis, genetic defects causing abnormal and inappropriate hormonal changes, or receptor abnormalities.

The external genitalia may be truly ambiguous—that is, the sex of the infant cannot be ascertained by physical examination. Alternatively, the phenotype may be completely normal but inappropriate for the genotype and detected only because the genotype was known for other reasons.

Female Pseudohermaphroditism

Masculinization of the female fetus is caused by androgens, either produced by the fetus or transferred across the placenta from the mother. Exposure to androgens prior to week 12 of gestation results in fusion of the urogenital sinus and genital folds. Labial scrotal fusion may occur at the same time. With exposure to androgens after week 12 of gestation, however, only clitoral enlargement may occur. Clitoral enlargement also may occur with postnatal androgen exposure.

Congenital Adrenal Hyperplasia This condition is the most common cause of virilization in the female. The more common inherited enzymatic deficiencies of adrenal biosynthesis (i.e., 21-hydroxylase, 11-hydroxylase, and 3β-hydroxysteroid dehydrogenase defects) all cause virilization of the female. The gonaducts remain normal, with persistence and development of the mullerian ducts. This is as expected, because these patients are true females without testes and, therefore, do not have MIS to suppress mullerian duct development. The excess adrenal androgens, however, cause fusion of the labia, fusion of the urogenital sinus with the genital fold, and clitoral enlargement. In the 21-hydroxylase and 3β-hydroxysteroid dehydrogenase forms of congenital adrenal hyperplasia, the virilization often is associated with salt-losing adrenal crisis presenting in the first week of life. The various enzymatic defects of this disorder and the methods of diagnosis and treatment are discussed more fully in the section on adrenal disorders.

Drug-Induced Female Pseudohermaphroditism A number of female newborns have been virilized by progestational agents or androgens used during the first trimester of pregnancy (23). The incidence of drug-induced female pseudohermaphroditism has decreased because, with recognition of this iatrogenic cause of virilization of the fetus, there has been a decreased use of the incriminated drugs. Such drugs were used most commonly during the first trimester of gestation, for prevention of spontaneous abortion or maintenance of pregnancy in patients with habitual abortion. When these drugs are used during the first trimester of gestation, the anatomic changes are similar to those found in congenital adrenal hyperplasia. There will be fusion of the labioscrotal folds with formation of a urogenital sinus and clitoromegaly. Rarely, virilization can be so extreme as to cause complete external masculinization. When used after the first trimester, these drugs will cause only clitoral enlargement, without fusion of the labioscrotal folds. The bone age often is advanced at birth. Unlike congenital adrenal hyperplasia, however, there is neither progressive virilization nor progressive acceleration of growth, bone age, or sexual development postnatally. The androgens are not elevated. These children will feminize normally at puberty and are capable of bearing children. The only therapy necessary is surgical correction of the labioscrotal fusion and clitoromegaly, when these findings are present.

Virilizing Disorders in the Mother The virilization of a female fetus as the result of an androgen-producing tumor of the mother is a relatively rare condition. These tumors almost always are caused by an ovarian lesion, although in one report the lesion was a benign adrenal adenoma (24). The reported tumors have included arrhenoblastomas, Krukenberg tumors, luteomas, a lipoid tumor of the ovary, and a stromal cell tumor. Haymond and Weldon (25) reviewed the reported cases and noted that maternal virilization has been characterized by clitoromegaly, acne, deepening of the voice, decreased lactation, hirsutism, and elevated excretion of urinary 17-ketosteroids. The offspring tend to have a low birth weight as well as virilization. The degree of virilization of the fetus is variable.

Idiopathic Female Pseudohermaphroditism There are two forms of idiopathic female pseudohermaphroditism. There is a small group of genotypically normal females in whom virilization of the external genitalia is seen in association with congenital anomalies of the gastrointestinal and urinary tracts. The reported anomalies include imperforate anus, renal agenesis, urinary tract obstructions, urethrovaginal fistulas, and defective formation of the mullerian ducts. The masculinization of these infants cannot be explained on the basis of androgens and is thought to be caused by nonhormonal factors. There is another group of female pseudohermaphrodites in whom there are no associated anomalies and no history of maternal exposure to androgens. It is possible that, in this last form, there is an as yet unknown disturbance of steroid metabolism in either the mother or the placenta.

Male Pseudohermaphroditism

Incomplete masculinization of the male fetus may be secondary to an enzymatic deficiency of testosterone synthesis, unresponsiveness to testosterone action (i.e., androgen-resistance syndromes), or teratogenic damage to either the gonad or the genital anlagen (see section on Disorders of Gonadal Sex).

Congenital Adrenal Hyperplasia This disorder can cause incomplete masculinization of the male fetus when the enzyme deficient in the adrenal also is deficient in the testes and is necessary for testosterone synthesis. Deficiency of the 3β-hydroxysteroid dehydrogenase enzyme causes a block early in the biosynthetic pathway of cortisol and aldosterone synthesis, resulting in a severe salt-losing syndrome (26). The inability to form testosterone indicates that the genetic defect affects both testicular and adrenal steroid biosynthesis (27). This results in a variable degree of ambiguity of the external genitalia, because the high levels of dehydroepiandrosterone have mild androgenic effects, ranging from mild coronal hypospadias to severe perineoscrotal hypospadias and micropenis. The testes are usually in the scrotum. Other, and more rare, defects of adrenal steroid biosynthesis affecting testicular synthesis of testosterone include genetic mutations for 17α-hydroxylase, 17-ketosteroid reductase, and 17,20-lyase enzymes as well as deficiency of the steroidogenic acute regulatory protein. In the latter two disorders, there may be a normal female phenotype due to the complete absence of any androgens, and absence of both mullerian and wolffian structures. The full details of these disorders, including diagnosis and treatment, are outlined in the section on adrenal hyperplasia.

Syndromes of Androgen Insensitivity This is a group of disorders characterized by normal regression of the mullerian duct structures and normal synthesis of testosterone. The androgen insensitivity syndrome occurs when there is either a defect in the conversion of testosterone to DHT caused by deficiency of 5α-reductase, or abnormalities of the androgen receptor or postandrogen receptor.

In the 5α-reductase deficiency, the testis produces both MIS and testosterone. Thus, there is regression of mullerian structures and normal development of the wolffian structures; however, because external genitalia fuse and develop secondary to the local action of DHT, which is absent in this syndrome, these patients may have a blind vaginal pouch, a small phallic structure with chordee and a hooded prepuce, and severe hypospadias. At puberty, these patients will masculinize under the influence of testosterone and develop pubic hair, penile enlargement, and descent of the testes. The diagnosis is suspected by demonstrating that the patients have 46XY chromosomes and an elevated testosterone-to-DHT ratio, both basally (ratio greater than 35) and following hCG stimulation (ratio increases to greater than 74). The diagnosis is confirmed by finding reduced 5α-reductase activity in fibroblasts from genital skin.

Complete androgen insensitivity syndrome previously was referred to as the testicular feminization syndrome. Affected patients are XY male pseudohermaphrodites with normal female external genitalia, absent wolffian and mullerian structures, but with testes that may be located in the abdomen, inguinal canal, or in inguinal hernias. There is a blind vaginal pouch, due to loss of the uterus and upper third of the vagina. Unlike patients with 5α-reductase deficiency, they do not virilize at puberty, and breasts do develop secondary to the peripheral conversion of the high levels of testosterone to estradiol. There is normal estrogenization of the labia minora and the vagina. Most affected patients have very little pubic hair, and approximately one-third have total absence of sexual hair. In all other respects, including height, habitus, voice, and breast development, these individuals are completely feminine. They frequently marry and have normal sexual relations. Some patients with complete androgen insensitivity syndrome have difficulty during intercourse because of the short vaginal length and will require corrective surgery. There are many patients who report difficulties in adjusting to the diagnosis, including the lifelong problem of infertility, which cannot be corrected due to the absence of a uterus. When the diagnosis is made during childhood, it usually is because of prenatal amniotic chromosome studies or discovery of testicular masses or testicular tissue during a herniorrhaphy. Because of the lack of formation of a uterus, these patients also frequently will come to attention because of primary amenorrhea. These patients may be either androgen receptor-negative or androgen receptor-positive. Molecular studies have demonstrated mutations in the androgen receptor gene, accounting for the variations in receptor binding of androgens (28). Testosterone levels are in the male range after puberty. This syndrome is inherited as an X-linked disorder.

There are incomplete forms of androgen insensitivity, including Reifenstein syndrome, where qualitatively abnormal or reduced binding to the androgen receptor results in defective virilization of the fetus and subsequent feminization at puberty. These abnormalities were previously referred to as partial testicular feminization syndromes. They present with either phenotypic female genitalia and 46XY chromosomes or variable degrees of sexual ambiguity.

Phenotype Inconsistent with Chromosomal Sex

Chorionic villus sampling or amniocentesis is being performed more routinely for a variety of reasons. Chromosomal sex generally is determined during such procedures. A problem ensues at birth when the phenotype, with completely normal external genitalia, is inconsistent with the chromosomal sex determined during amniocentesis or chorionic villus sampling. One possible explanation is that there was an error in the initial karyotyping. There are, however, a number of conditions that present at birth with normal external genitalia that are discordant with chromosomal sex. Table 41–1 lists these conditions.

TABLE 41–1. *Etiology of normal phenotype inappropriate for the genotype*

Disorder	Genotype	Phenotype	Etiology
Pure gonadal dysgenesis	XY	Female	AR, XLR
46XX Males	XX	Male	SRY translocation
46XY Females	XY	Female	SRY deletion
Congenital lipoid hyperplasia	XY	Female	CAH
17,20-Lyase deficiency	XY	Female	CAH
17-Hydroxylase deficiency	XY	Female	CAH
Androgen resistance syndrome	XY	Female	XLR/AD

AD, autosomal dominant; AR, autosomal recessive; CAH, congenital adrenal hyperplasia; SRY, testicular determining gene; XLR, X-linked recessive; XLR/AD, may be either X-linked recessive or autosomal dominant.

These children always should be raised according to the phenotypic sex.

Hypospadias and Cryptorchidism

Twenty-five percent of infants born with undescended testes and hypospadias have a disorder of intersex. This incidence of intersex increases with severity of the hypospadias and bilateral undescended testes. The incidence of isolated hypospadias is 8 in 1,000 newborn males, and most cases have no associated endocrine abnormality. However, severe hypospadius combined with cryptorchidism must be evaluated for congenital adrenal hyperplasia and other causes of sexual ambiguity.

Micropenis

Isolated micropenis generally is not considered as ambiguous genitalia, but identification of its cause should be carried out with urgency. The evaluation of micropenis is dealt with in the section on hypopituitarism.

Evaluation of Sexual Ambiguity

The evaluation of a newborn with ambiguous genitalia should be treated as an emergency, for several reasons. First, life-threatening illness can occur in several of the types of congenital adrenal hyperplasia. Second, the uncertainty of a child's gender, if handled poorly, can cause parents to have long-term psychological concerns, which may in turn affect the child's own perception of body image.

Parents should be informed immediately that, although gender cannot be determined at that moment by physical examination, a definitive gender will be determined within several days. This allows enough time (generally 72 hours) for most experienced cytogenetic laboratories to provide sex chromosome determination. The parents should be reassured that appropriate gender will be established in their child. It is our general philosophy not to discuss the pending studies in detail because there are occasions for gender assignment that are not consistent with either chromosomal or gonadal sex. As in any diagnostic problem, the approach to the child with ambiguous genitalia should begin with a thorough history, a careful physical examination, and then laboratory and radiologic testing. Table 41–2 outlines the different causes of sexual ambiguity.

The history may provide some clues. It is important to ask about drug ingestion during the pregnancy, particularly in the first trimester, and to inquire about the possibility of any recent androgenic changes in the mother that might suggest the cause for female pseudohermaphroditism. A history of infection or exposure to teratogens in the first trimester might suggest partial gonadal dysgenesis. The family history of a previous sibling who died in the first 10 days of life, or siblings who are overvirilized

TABLE 41–2. *Etiology of ambiguous genitalia*

Virilization of females
  Congenital adrenal hyperplasia
    21-Hydroxylase deficiency
    11-Hydroxylase deficiency
    3β-Hydroxysteroid dehydrogenase deficiency
  Chromosomal aberrations
    XO/XY
    XX/XY
    Variants
  Maternal virilization
    Drug-induced
    Excess androgen production by mother
  True hermaphroditism
  Idiopathic
    Isolated
    Associated with midline congenital anomalies
Inadequate masculinization of males
  Congenital adrenal hyperplasia
    3β-Hydroxysteroid dehydrogenase deficiency
  Partial androgen resistance syndromes
    5α-Reductase deficiency
    Partial androgen receptor defects
  Testicular dysgenesis
  True hermaphroditism
  Idiopathic
    Isolated
    Associated with midline congenital anomalies

TABLE 41–3. *Studies to evaluate ambiguous genitalia*

Immediate studies
  Chromosomal analysis
    Bone marrow
    Blood
  Pelvic ultrasonography
  Serum
    17-Hydroxyprogesterone
    17-OH pregnenolone
    Testosterone
    11-Deoxycortisol
    Dihydrotestosterone
Later studies
  Vaginogram
  Exploratory laparotomy and gonadal biopsy
  Radiologic studies, intravenous pyelography, barium enema
  Skin biopsy to evaluate testosterone metabolism

or had precocious puberty, might suggest the possibility of congenital adrenal hyperplasia.

Physical examination is important, but on no account should a diagnosis be made purely on the grounds of physical examination. The presence or absence of palpable gonads is very important and can direct appropriate laboratory and radiologic investigations. The measurement of the length and diameter of the penis is valuable both for prognostic information and as a baseline if treatment is given in an attempt to enlarge the penis. Severe micropenis or agenesis, despite the presence of testes or a normal 46XY karyotype, may necessitate a gender reassignment to female gender. The urethral opening should be identified and the existence or absence of a vagina should be determined. The degree of fusion of the labia

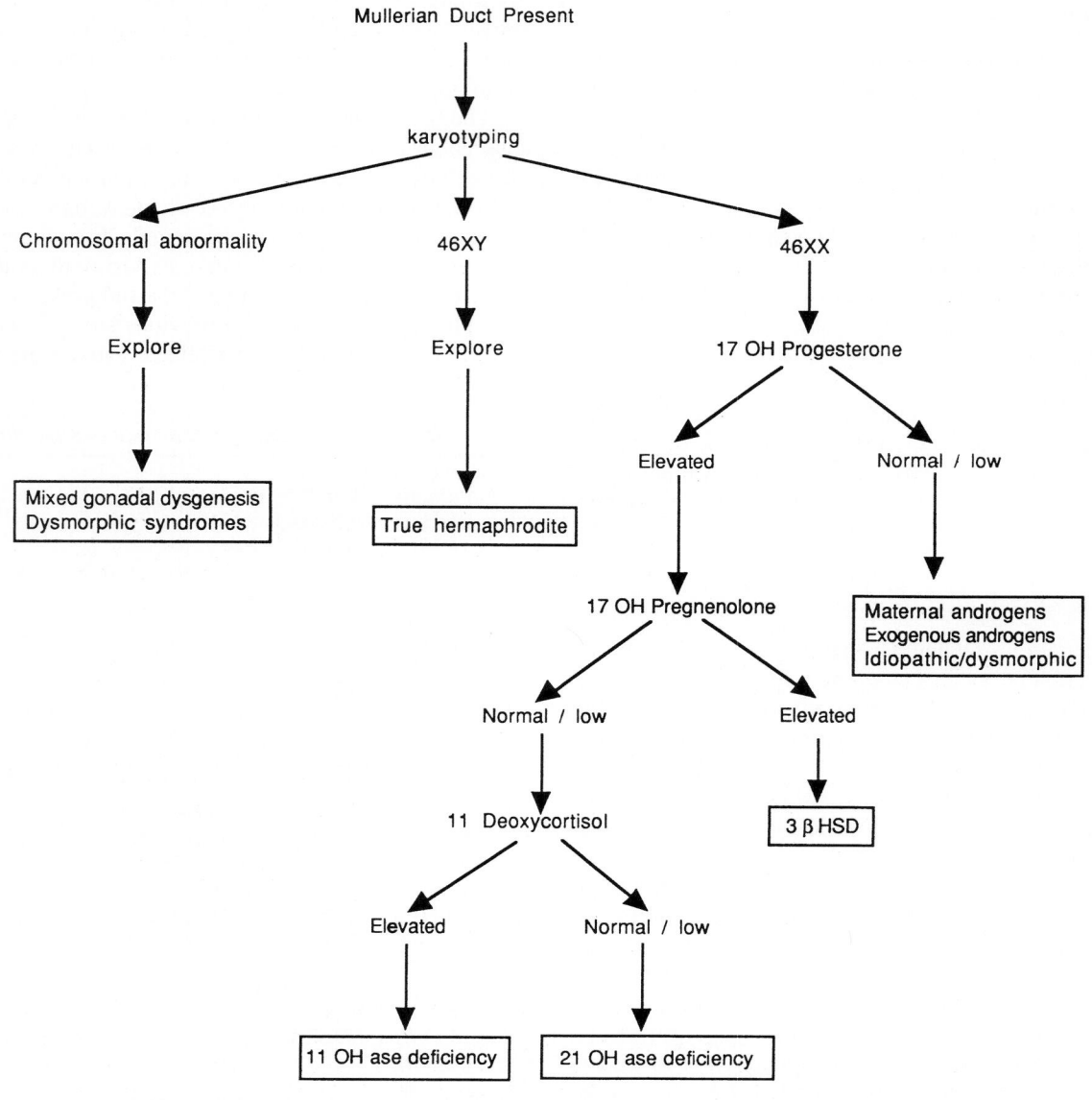

FIG. 41–2. An algorithm for evaluating sexual ambiguity in infants with mullerian structures.

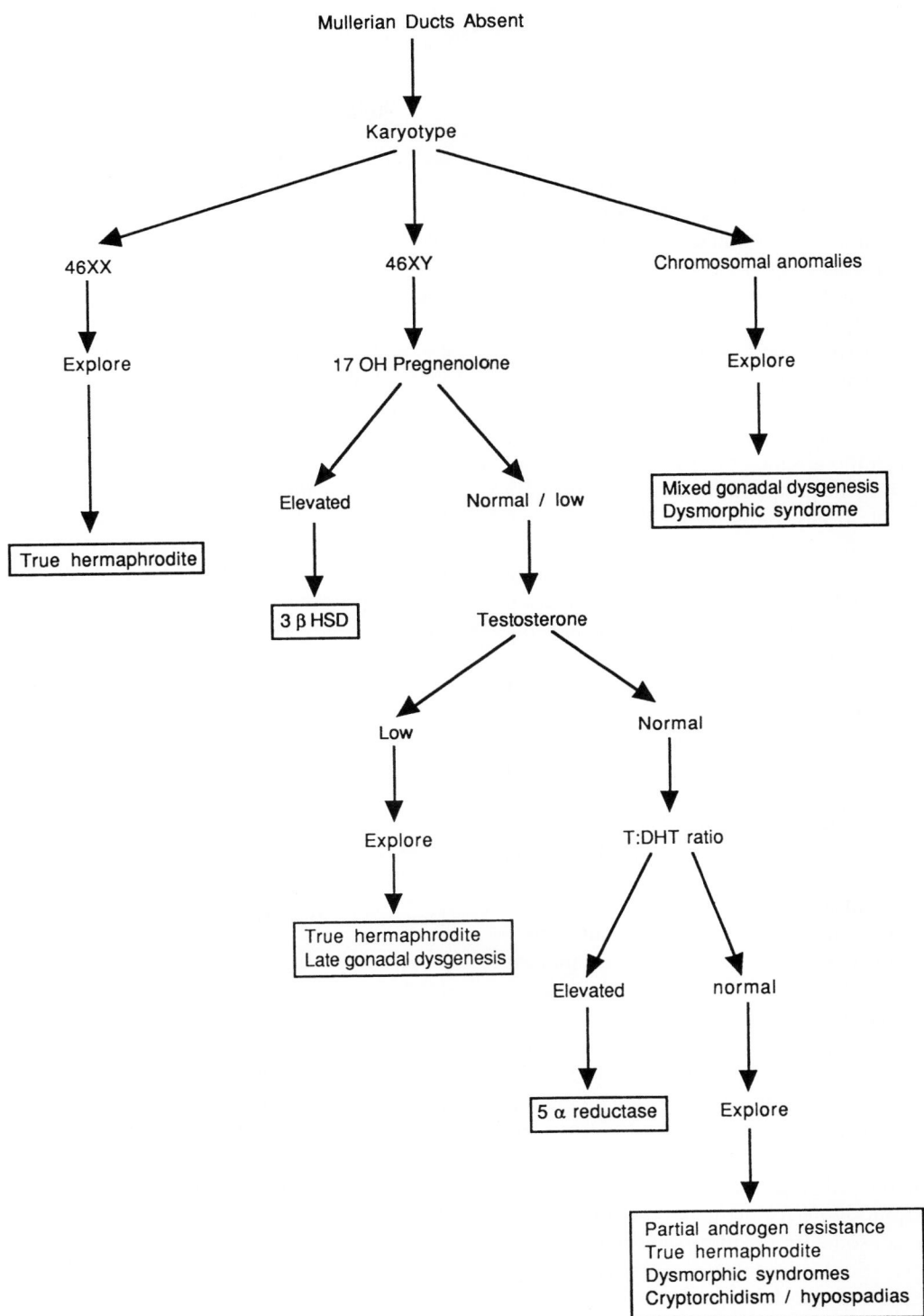

FIG. 41–3. An algorithm for evaluating sexual ambiguity in infants without mullerian structures.

should be assessed. Finally, the presence of any abnormalities involving the urinary tract or anal region and any of the other organ systems should be evaluated.

Certain tests should be obtained as soon as it is apparent that there is sexual ambiguity, to determine the appropriate gender of the infant (Table 41–3). Other tests may be required at a later time to make an accurate diagnosis. It should be stressed, however, that gender determination does not require that all studies leading to a final diagnosis be completed (e.g., the exact type of congenital adrenal hyperplasia may be important for genetic counseling and future prenatal diagnosis, but not for gender assignment).

Some laboratories can use bone marrow for chromosomal estimation and have a karyotype result available in 6 hours; however, this should be used as an adjunct to standard chromosomal analysis because bone marrow karyotyping may miss mosaicism. The determination of whether the infant is a virilized female or an inadequately virilized male is dependent upon the chromosomal studies. The karyotype, however, should not be used per se as the major factor in gender determination because gonadal function and future sexual function are more important.

Pelvic ultrasound should be undertaken by an experienced radiologist as soon as possible, to determine the presence or absence of uterus and gonads. The presence of a uterus indicates the absence of any functioning testicular tissue early on in gestation, and almost certainly indicates that the child, no matter what the karyotype, should be raised as a female. Conversely, the absence of mullerian structures implies the presence of functioning testicular tissue at 7 to 9 weeks of gestation and secretion of MIS. Their absence also almost certainly indicates the presence of the SRY gene and probably an XY karyotype. This finding alone should not determine a male gender assignment. Karyotype, phallic size, degree of hypospadias, and the continued presence of testicular tissue, as suggested by testosterone concentrations, are all part of the equation in gender determination. Ultrasonography may identify gonads previously nonpalpable and may even define them as either ovarian or testicular tissue, depending on the echogenic pattern (29). Measurement of MIS may be helpful in the determination of the presence of testesticular tissue (30). The results of chromosomal analysis, ultrasound, and steroid determinations should be available within 48 to 72 hours. Gender assignment should be made by this time.

To evaluate further the possible cause of sexual ambiguity, secondary studies may be necessary. The algorithms in Figs. 41–2 and 41–3, which are based on the initial ultrasound findings, delineate the steps that may be necessary to make a definitive diagnosis. These algorithms do not include those patients with a normal phenotype that is inappropriate for the genotype. In cases of androgen resistance, some time will be required to evaluate the skin biopsy. Surgical exploration frequently will be required in cases of true hermaphroditism; this also may be done at a later time. It should be stressed that the final pathophysiologic diagnosis is not necessary for gender assignment.

When the baby has been fully evaluated, including consultations from an endocrinologist, a urologist, and possibly a psychiatrist, there must be a consensus of agreement as to the appropriate gender, with future heterosexual function and fertility as major determining factors, before discussion with the parents. The attending physician should then discuss the condition fully with the parents, including expectations for future sexual function and fertility and whether any hormonal medications or surgery will be needed.

Gender assignment for most infants with ambiguous genitalia is not difficult, because chromosomal sex and gonadal sex will correlate with the internal structures. The external genitalia will, in general, require minor to moderate surgery to improve function and cosmetic appearance. In some cases, hormonal therapy may be required later on in life, but not during the neonatal period. Rarely, as in cases of incomplete androgen resistance syndromes or in true hermaphroditism or mixed gonadal dysgenesis, gender assignment contrary to chromosomal or gonadal sex must be considered. In this case, careful consideration must be given to the likelihood of adequate normal sexual function as an adult. If it is thought that the penis will be very small and nonfunctional as an adult (less than 4 cm), it often is more considerate to raise the child as a female. However, equal emphasis and effort must be directed at vaginal depth to ensure properly functioning female genitalia. Intersex patients need care by centers where psychosocial help is available as well as a full complement of experienced specialists knowledgeable in gender assignment. There are a number of anecdotal reports of genotypic males raised as females who are considerably dissatisfied with their gender of raising (31).

DISORDERS OF THE ENDOCRINE HYPOTHALAMUS AND PITUITARY

Development of the Hypothalamic–Pituitary Axis

The hypothalamus and pituitary glands regulate the fetal endocrine system after week 12 of gestation. In general terms, the hypothalamus regulates the anterior pituitary by secreting stimulatory hormones and inhibiting hormones. The stimulatory hormones identified include growth hormone-releasing hormone, thyrotropin-releasing hormone (TRH), corticotropin-releasing hormone (CRH), and gonadotropin-releasing hormone (GnRH). Somatostatin inhibits pituitary growth hormone release and prolactin inhibitory factor inhibits prolactin release. In response to these hypothalamic controlling hormones, the anterior pituitary secretes growth hormone, thyroid-stimulating hormone (TSH), adrenocorticotropic hormone (ACTH), prolactin, luteinizing hormone, and follicle-stimulating hormone. The posterior pituitary secretes vasopressin and oxytocin.

The pituitary gland is formed of two distinct parts. The anterior pituitary, or adenohypophysis, arises embryonically from an invagination of the oral ectodermal cavity called the Rathke pouch. This diverticulum arises at 3 weeks of gestation, and by 5 weeks has migrated to its final position and separates completely from the oral cavity. At approximately the same time in gestation, the posterior pituitary, or neurohypophysis, is formed from an invagination of the floor of the diencephalon. This invagination grows downward and joins up with the Rathke pouch, to form the posterior portion of the pituitary gland. Neural fibers migrate from the hypothalamus down to the posterior pituitary to form the neurohypophyseal tract. The hypothalamus itself arises by proliferation of neuroblasts in the intermediate zone of the diencephalic wall. The supraoptic and periventricular nuclei of the hypothalamus are formed. By 12 weeks of gestation, both the hypothalamus and pituitary gland are functioning.

Most disorders of the hypothalamic–pituitary axis in the newborn period, except for the syndrome of inappropriate secretion of antidiuretic hormone (SIADH), are those of insufficiency. In the newborn, most hypothalamic and pituitary problems are related to malformations, trauma, infection, or genetically inherited disorders, unlike in older children and adults, in whom tumors may both secrete hormones and disrupt hormone function. Causes of disorders of the hypothalamic–pituitary axis in the newborn child are outlined in Table 41–4.

Disorders of the Anterior Pituitary

Disorders of anterior pituitary function often are difficult to detect in the newborn; however, there is a series of characteristic findings that may occur. The predominant symptoms of anterior pituitary insufficiency are hypoglycemia, micropenis, and, occasionally, cholestatic jaundice. The hypoglycemia may be quite severe and comparable to that seen in infants with congenital hyperinsulinism. The infants may even have a brisk glycemic response to glucagon causing further confusion (32). The cholestatic jaundice starts as unconjugated and

TABLE 41–4. *Etiology of disorders of the hypothalamic–pituitary axis*

Malformations
  Cleft lip and palate
  Optic nerve atrophy
  Septooptic dysplasia
  Transphenoidal encephalocele
  Holoprosencephaly
  Anencephaly
Trauma associated with breech delivery
Congenital infection
  Rubella
  Toxoplasmosis
Tumor
  Hypothalamic hamartoblastoma (i.e., Pallister Hall
    syndrome)
  Rathke pouch cyst
  Craniopharyngioma
Isolated or combined familial or idiopathic pituitary hormone
    deficiency
Autosomal recessive or X-linked recessive familial
    panhypopituitarism

becomes predominantly conjugated and often will resolve only after hormone replacement. There may be combined deficiency of multiple hormones of the anterior pituitary or isolated deficiency of a single hormone. The molecular basis of multiple hormone deficiency is established for a number of genetic defects. Transcription factors that are now recognized include Pit-1, Prop-1, P-OTX, Rpx, and P-Lim. Evidence for the role of these transcription factors comes from mouse work with the identification of Pit-1 as the cause of the Snell dwarf mouse (33), Prop-1 as the cause of the Ames dwarf mouse (34), and the generation of P-Lim knockout mice (35). In humans, P-Lim is associated with deficiencies of all anterior pituitary hormones except ACTH, in conjunction with retinal colobomas. On the other hand, Pit-1 defects result in pituitary gland hypoplasia and deficiencies of GH, TSH, and prolactin. Prop-1 (Prophet of Pit-1) is essential for the expression of Pit-1; therefore, defects in Prop-1 expression result in an identical clinical picture. P-OTX and Rpx play an important role in anterior pituitary development. However, there are no known examples of defects resulting from deficiencies of these factors in mice or humans.

Growth Hormone Deficiency

Deficiency of growth hormone does not present as intrauterine growth retardation. Intrauterine growth is determined by maternal factors, including nutritional status, placental function, and gestational infection or drugs. During early postnatal life, thyroid hormone, insulin, and nutrition are more important growth determinants than growth hormone. The effect of growth hormone deficiency on linear growth often is not discerned until 6 to 9 months of age. Growth hormone deficiency in the neonate may present as hypoglycemia, micropenis, or both. A family history of short stature is pertinent because familial autosomal dominant inheritance of growth hormone deficiency is well recognized.

Gonadotropin Deficiency

Micropenis most often is secondary to gonadotropin deficiency, which can occur as either isolated hypogonadotropic hypogonadism or combined multiple pituitary hormone deficiency. Micropenis is defined as penile size less than 2.5-cm stretched length. In female infants, there are no clinical signs of hypogonadotropic hypogonadism at birth.

Adrenocorticotropic Hormone Deficiency

Adrenocorticotropic hormone deficiency rarely presents as adrenal crisis; it is more likely to result only in cortisol insufficiency and to present as hypoglycemia or hyponatremia without hyperkalemia. Occasionally, cholestatic jaundice (i.e., conjugated hyperbilirubinemia) is associated with ACTH deficiency in the newborn. Newborn patients with prolonged direct hyperbilirubinemia should be evaluated for pituitary insufficiency (36). Isolated ACTH deficiency is extremely rare, but defects in the CRH gene is reported (37). The combination of both growth hormone and ACTH deficiency may cause hypoglycemia of such severity that it is difficult to differentiate from congenital hyperinsulinism.

Thyroid-Stimulating Hormone Deficiency

TSH deficiency results in secondary hypothyroidism in the newborn. This generally is not detected clinically, and more often is detected by the newborn screening tests as a low thyroxine (T_4) level but a normal TSH level. This finding may be misinterpreted as the euthyroid sick syndrome (see section on Disorders of the Thyroid) in a stressed neonate. Furthermore, secondary hypothyroidism may be missed in those countries using only TSH determinations for thyroid screening. Isolated TSH deficiency, like ACTH deficiency, is extremely rare, and TSH deficiency usually is seen only in panhypopituitarism. Thus, in an infant with any of the abnormalities outlined in Table 41–4, the routine newborn screening procedures should not be relied on to detect secondary hypothyroidism.

Diagnosis

The diagnosis of hypothalamic and pituitary deficiency may be made by stimulation tests, as well as by determination of random hormone levels. Growth hormone levels are tonically elevated in the first few days of life, and, as a screening test, a random growth hormone level greater than 10 ng/mL suggests adequate growth hormone function. A random low growth hormone level requires provocative growth hormone testing to confirm growth hormone deficiency. Provocative growth hormone testing in normal newborn infants often results in growth hormone levels of 25 ng/mL or higher, whereas growth hormone deficient infants will not respond to provocative testing. ACTH deficiency and adrenal insufficiency are unlikely if a random cortisol level is greater than 20 µg/dL, because newborns normally have very low cortisol levels, without diurnal variation. In general, ACTH stimulation testing is necessary to test the hypothalamic–pituitary–adrenal axis. GnRH will stimulate pituitary secretion of luteinizing hormone and follicle-stimulating hormone during the first few months of life but, subsequently, normal children will not respond to GnRH. Therefore, to assess gonadotropin function, GnRH testing should be performed in the first 2 to 3 months of life.

In those infants suspected of anterior pituitary deficiency, ultrasonography through the open fontanelle may discern malformations of the brain, including the defects seen in septooptic dysplasia. To evaluate further the possibility of septooptic dysplasia in suspected infants, ophthalmologic examination also should be performed. In those infants in whom malformation is strongly suspected, magnetic resonance imaging or computed tomography scanning may be useful in delineating the abnormality.

Treatment

Anterior pituitary deficiency often is not detected clinically during the neonatal period because the hypoglycemia may be very modest, micropenis—obviously not a clinical feature in hypopituitary females—is marginal, and jaundice is not severe. Treatment considerations, therefore, are based on the severity of symptoms. The child who is severely hypoglycemic will require growth hormone and glucocorticoid replacement. The dose of these hormones for replacement therapy can be relatively modest. Recombinant growth hormone is injected subcutaneously, at a dose of 0.04 mg/kg daily. Data indicate that the production rate of cortisol is less than previously believed, and, based on this information, replacement of glucocorticoid insufficiency requires 8 to 10 mg/m^2 of oral hydrocortisone per day (38). If the newborn is ill, it is recommended that initially the child be treated with at least three times the replacement dose. In male infants with micropenis, a short trial of hCG, testosterone, or both, is recommended to stimulate the penis to grow. Not only will this improve penile size, but such treatment provides an opportunity to evaluate testicular response to hCG and penile response to testosterone. If undescended testes are associated with micropenis, the administration of 5,000 IU/m^2 of HCG with measurement of testosterone at baseline and after 2 and 4 days will assist in the determination of the presence and function of the testes, as well as determination of MIS levels. Testosterone can be administered by injecting testosterone enanthate, 25 mg intramuscularly every month, for a total of three injections. Penile response to this treatment can be assessed at the end of 3 months. Some authors have recommended a prolonged course of hCG, which will test both testicular response and penile growth in response to endogenous testosterone production.

Disorders of the Posterior Pituitary

There are two hormones secreted from the posterior pituitary, vasopressin or antidiuretic hormone (ADH) and oxytocin. Oxytocin has no known function in the neonate. ADH is manufactured in the supraoptic and periventricular nuclei of the hypothalamus. It is bound to neurophysin and is transported by axonal transport along the neurons of the neurohypophyseal tract to the posterior pituitary, where it is stored and released as necessary. ADH can be found in the fetus after 12 weeks of gestation; ADH secretion is stimulated by hyperosmolar states and volume depletion. ADH release is inhibited predominantly by volume overload. It acts on the collecting tubules of the kidney by increasing the permeability to water and urea. There are two main disorders of ADH secretion, diabetes insipidus (DI) and SIADH.

Diabetes Insipidus

DI in the newborn may be due to central ADH insufficiency or renal unresponsiveness to ADH (nephrogenic DI). This section will deal only with central DI.

DI in the neonate may present with failure to thrive, irritability, fever, vomiting, and hypernatremia. There may be a history of polyhydramnios in the mother. Polyuria is difficult to detect in newborn infants because normal newborn infants will void up to 20 times a day (39). DI should be suspected, however, in symptomatic, cachectic-appearing, hypernatremic infants. Sustained urine output greater than 60% of fluid input is unusual, and single-void volumes of greater than 6 mL/kg suggest DI. The diagnosis is confirmed by demonstrating inappropriately dilute urine in the presence of a hyperosmolar serum, and by demonstrating an appropriate concentration of the urine after administration of vasopressin. Unresponsiveness to vasopressin indicates renal problems rather than central DI. Water deprivation tests should not be done in newborn infants, because acute dehydration and hypernatremia may cause permanent brain damage.

A list of causes of central DI is given in Table 41–5. Secondary DI is more common than primary DI in the neonatal period. DI should be strongly suspected in infants with the listed malformations.

Treatment

Treatment of DI requires strict management of fluid balance. These infants require enormous quantities of free water; it is not unusual to provide several times usual maintenance quantities of water as 5% glucose intravenously, while providing nutrition and electrolytes by the oral route. Desmopressin is a long-acting analog of vasopressin and can be given intranasally or sublingually. Intranasal administration is the best and most consistent route of administration; however, sublingual administration can be helpful in patients with cleft lip and palate. The dose and dose interval must be carefully evaluated, by trial and error, in each child individually. Dosing should start at 1 to 2 μg once or twice daily. Rarely would more than 5 μg be required. Rapid shifts in the serum sodium caused by excessive fluid input or urine output should be avoided. An alternative approach that avoids the possibility of water overload is to use a diluted formula. This treatment is based on the principle that hunger rather than thirst is the driving force behind fluid intake in the neonate. Thus, providing the total daily caloric intake as one-third strength formula will usually result in good fluid balance. It does require two- to three-hourly feeding even during the night. In emergency treatment of severe dehydration, intravenous aqueous vasopressin (Pitressin) infusion, rather than desmopressin, is recommended. The short half-life of Pitressin allows precise control of fluid balance. Rapid shifts in the serum sodium, caused by excessive fluid input or urine output, should be avoided.

Syndrome of Inappropriate Antidiuretic Hormone Secretion

It is clearly documented that ADH levels are elevated in the premature infant (40). Increased ADH secretion occurs for many reasons in sick premature infants, and these are outlined in Table 41–6. A common mechanism for the elevated ADH levels in many of the pathologic cases is intravascular volume depletion. Intravascular volume depletion is detected by stretch receptors in the left atrium. Thus, the elevated ADH levels are appropriate for the volume status, but inappropriate for the osmolar status.

TABLE 41–5. *Etiology of central diabetes insipidus*

Primary
  Familial
    X-linked recessive
    Autosomal dominant
  Idiopathic
Secondary
  Malformation sequences
    Optic atrophy
    Septooptic dysplasia
    Holoprosencephaly
  Birth trauma
  Periventricular hemorrhage
  Infection
    Meningitis
    Encephalitis

TABLE 41–6. *Causes of elevated levels of antidiuretic hormone in the newborn*

Birth asphyxia
Acute deterioration of hyaline membrane disease and
  bronchopulmonary dysplasia
Respiratory syncytial virus infection
Pneumothorax
Pulmonary interstitial emphysema
Artificial ventilation
Acute blood loss
Periventricular hemorrhage
Surgery
Pain
Syndrome of inappropriate ADH secretion

ADH, antidiuretic hormone.

SIADH, by definition, occurs when there is hyponatremia associated with a urine osmolarity that is less than maximally diluted and with continued sodium loss in the urine (i.e., urine sodium greater than 20 to 30 mEq/L). These circumstances are present in the absence of volume depletion, renal failure, or adrenal insufficiency. True SIADH is uncommon in neonates (41), and this condition should be differentiated from appropriately elevated ADH levels. It is vitally important to control water and sodium intake and prevent hyponatremia in SIADH, but equally important to treat the volume depletion states causing appropriate ADH secretion.

Hyponatremia occurs commonly in newborn premature infants who have a higher fractional excretion of sodium than term infants. The most common nonphysiologic cause of hyponatremia is renal sodium wasting due to diuretics. The differential diagnosis of hyponatremia in the newborn also must include prerenal failure, renal failure, adrenal insufficiency, and SIADH. Unlike volume depletion states, SIADH is treated by fluid restriction. If volume depletion is evident, combined with polyuria, urinary sodium loss, and hyponatremia, cerebral salt wasting should be suspected.

DISORDERS OF THE ADRENAL GLAND

Development and Function of the Adrenal Gland

The adrenal gland is two separate glands, the adrenal cortex and the adrenal medulla. The fetal adrenal cortex is of mesodermal origin, whereas the chromaffin cells of the adrenal medulla are of neuroectodermal origin. The classes of hormones secreted by these two glands differ and are independent of each other. Inasmuch as diseases of the adrenal medulla during the neonatal period are extremely rare, this section will focus on the adrenal cortex.

The anlage of the adrenal cortex arises as two large masses on either side of the aorta, at about the level of the first thoracic nerve. Immediately adjacent are the medullary cells that have migrated from the neural crest. Fetal adrenal cortical cells can be identified by 4 weeks of gestation. By 7 weeks of gestation, the medullary cells begin to migrate to the interior of the adrenal cortex. The original adrenal cortical cells make up the fetal zone of the adrenal cortex. There is a second downgrowth of coelomic epithelium that envelops the original cortical cells and remains as an outer shell. The fetal adrenal gland is large during gestation, but involutes during the last half of pregnancy and especially after birth. The adult adrenal cortex slowly develops from the outer shell, with involution of the fetal zone. The fetal zone is active in steroid metabolism, and the rapid involution after birth suggests a role in the maintenance of pregnancy.

The trophic hormonal control of the fetal adrenal is not clear. In anencephalic fetuses, the fetal adrenal appears to be normal during the first 12 weeks of gestation, with subsequent involution of the gland. In patients with enzymatic defects of cortisol biosynthesis, however, the excessive androgen production in association with hyperplasia of the adrenal glands during the first 12 weeks of gestation suggests that ACTH must play some role during that time.

The adrenal cortex secretes three main groups of steroid hormones, glucocorticoids, mineralocorticoids, and androgens. The glucocorticoids, of which cortisol (hydrocortisone) is the most important, exert their major physiologic effects on carbohydrate, protein, and fat metabolism. The mineralocorticoids, desoxycorticosterone and aldosterone, maintain salt and water balance by promoting sodium retention in exchange for hydrogen and potassium in the distal convoluted tubules of the kidney. The adrenal androgens, dehydroepiandrosterone (DHEA), δ4-androstenedione, and 11β-hydroxyandrostenedione, are protein anabolic and responsible for the development of sexual hair in girls at puberty. Adrenal androgens are secreted during the neonatal period. The slightly higher levels of adrenal androgens during the neonatal period may be secondary to the relative deficiency of 3β-hydroxysteroid dehydrogenase in the fetal zone of the fetal adrenal cortex, which is reflected in the higher concentrations of δ5 steroids (e.g., DHEA, 17-OH pregnenolone) noted especially in premature infants.

The production of adrenocortical steroids is controlled by a hypothalamic–pituitary–adrenal homeostatic mechanism. Hypothalamic CRH provokes release of pituitary ACTH. The hypothalamic CRH center is sensitive both to tissue levels of cortisol and to stress. ACTH, in turn, stimulates adrenocortical steroid biosynthesis, mainly cortisol. Increased levels of cortisol inhibit the production of ACTH, probably acting at the level of the hypothalamus.

The regulation of aldosterone, however, is influenced by many factors. The main regulatory homeostatic mechanism controlling aldosterone secretion is the renin–angiotensin system. Acute changes in pressure receptors control the release of renin from the juxtaglomerular cells of the kidney. Increased levels of circulating renin, in turn, increase angiotensin II. Angiotensin II acts on the zona glomerulosa of the adrenal cortex to increase aldosterone secretion and directly to cause vascular contractility. Increased pressure within the arterial receptors, secondary to the contracted vessels and the increased blood volume produced by elevated aldosterone, operates a negative-feedback inhibition of the renin–angiotensin system.

Other mechanisms are involved in a secondary fashion in the control of aldosterone secretion. A low sodium or high potassium intake will increase aldosterone excretion. ACTH also will cause a transient, albeit unsustained, increase in aldosterone excretion (42), and aldosterone secretion will be diminished in the absence of ACTH (43). Finally, cortisol itself may have a permissive role in aldosterone action at the tissue level.

Adrenal Insufficiency

The disorders of the adrenal cortex during the neonatal period consist almost entirely of those conditions that cause adrenal insufficiency. The inborn errors of steroid biosynthesis (i.e., congenital adrenal hyperplasia) can cause excessive production of various steroids, but Cushing syndrome or cortisol excess rarely occurs during the neonatal period. Cushing syndrome may occur secondary to exposure to exogenous steroids such as dexamethasone. Adrenal cortical tumors resulting in Cushing syndrome can present very early in life (within several months of age) but not in the neonate. Cushing disease has not been described in the very young infant. Adrenal insufficiency can result from lack of trophic hormone stimulation, ACTH receptor abnormalities, damage to fetal adrenal gland, inherited degenerative disorders, or inborn errors of steroid biosynthesis.

Adrenocorticotropic Hormone Insufficiency

There have been a number of neonatal deaths, after shock and peripheral vascular collapse associated with severe hyponatremia and hyperkalemia, in which the adrenal glands were noted to be hypoplastic at autopsy. Some of these cases of failure of development of the adrenal cortex after involution of the fetal zone have been reported in infants with anencephaly and in patients with partial or total pituitary aplasia. The probable basis of the developmental failure in these cases is the lack of ACTH. The possibility, however, that the lack of another central nervous system factor also might be involved in these cases is suggested in the patients with congenital hypopituitarism. In the latter group of patients, the adrenal insufficiency produces decreased cortisol production, but mineralocorticoid function remains normal. Such patients tend to have hypoglycemia, poor feeding, and failure to thrive. These patients can, in general, maintain water and electrolyte balance and can respond to sodium deprivation with increase in aldosterone excretion; however, hyponatremia with normokalemia has been noted in hypopituitarism and isolated glucocorticoid insufficiency. The limitation of the developmental failure to the zona fasciculata and reticularis, in ACTH deficiency, can be explained by the fact that the trophic hormone for zona glomerulosa function is not ACTH but angiotensin II.

ACTH Unresponsiveness

Migeon et al. (44) postulated that the dichotomy of control of the various zones of the adrenal cortex may be the explanation for a familial syndrome of isolated glucocorticoid deficiency. This syndrome was reported initially by Shepard et al. (45) in 1959. It presents in early childhood with hyperpigmentation, hypoglycemia, failure to thrive, and poor feeding. These patients have cortisol insufficiency and cannot increase 17-hydroxysteroid excretion in response to ACTH stimulation. These patients can, however, respond to sodium deprivation with increased aldosterone excretion and decreased sodium excretion. Migeon et al. (44), based on in vitro experiments, suggested that this syndrome is the result of an inherited defect in the ACTH receptor system. This syndrome has since been referred to as the syndrome of ACTH unresponsiveness. A family with this syndrome has been reported, however, in whom the pathogenesis of the disorder appears to be more compatible with a degenerative process (see section on Familial Isolated Glucocorticoid Insufficiency) (46). It is probable that this familial syndrome is caused by a variety of defects, including ACTH unresponsiveness.

Damage

Adrenal insufficiency can occur during the newborn period as a result of damage to the relatively large and hyperemic adrenal glands. Trauma in association with a difficult delivery, particularly breech delivery, hemorrhagic diseases, or infectious processes can damage the adrenal glands. Minor hemorrhage or unilateral damage may not cause adrenal insufficiency and may present subsequently as calcification of the adrenal glands detected on an abdominal radiograph obtained for other purposes. All patients with shock symptoms in association with hyponatremia should be suspect for adrenal insufficiency. The highly sensitive ACTH determinations, using monoclonal antibodies and immunoradiometric assays, can detect elevated levels of plasma ACTH, diagnostic of primary adrenal insufficiency.

Degenerative Disorders

The most common cause of chronic adrenal insufficiency is idiopathic atrophy, or degeneration of the adrenal glands. Chronic adrenal insufficiency (i.e., Addison disease), however, is extremely uncommon in childhood and unheard of during the newborn period, if the cases of congenital hypoplasia of the adrenal glands are excluded. It is possible that some of the cases of congenital hypoplasia of the adrenals are caused by a degenerative process, especially when the central nervous system, including the pituitary gland, is intact.

Familial Isolated Glucocorticoid Insufficiency

This disorder can occur during the neonatal period. Affected infants present during the neonatal period with shock, hyperpigmentation, and hypoglycemia. Some of the families with this syndrome probably have a defect in ACTH responsiveness; however, there are a substantial number of case histories with a clinical course suggestive of an inherited degenerative process.

A family was studied, of which five siblings had hyperpigmentation, hypoglycemia, convulsions, and deficient glucocorticoid production (46). Mineralocorticoid function was normal. Of these five children, two were studied during early infancy, and glucocorticoid function initially was normal. The development of deficient glucocorticoid production at a later age in these two patients suggests an inherited degenerative process of the adrenal glands as the pathogenetic basis for this syndrome in this family.

Congenital Adrenal Hyperplasia

This is a genetic disorder involving deficiency of one of several enzymatic systems required for normal steroid biosynthesis. The various clinical manifestations of this syndrome can be correlated with the different defects of cortisol synthesis. The biochemical basis of this syndrome

has been extensively reviewed (47). The principal biochemical reactions in the conversion of cholesterol into active adrenocortical steroids require a series of hydroxylations (Fig. 41–4). These hydroxylations actually are mediated by cytochrome P450 oxidases. The initiation of steroidogenesis requires that the steroidogenic acute regulatory (STAR) protein form contact sites between the outer and inner membranes of mitochondria, allowing cholesterol to enter into the mitochondria. The side chain cleavage of cholesterol is then mediated by P450scc. The most common disorder is lack of 21-hydroxylation. Hydroxylation of both progesterone and 17-hydroxyprogesterone is mediated by a single enzyme, P450c21. A single enzyme, P450c11, mediates 11β-hydroxylase, 18-hydroxylase, and aldehyde synthase activities. Similarly, a single enzyme, P450c17, mediates 17α-hydroxylase and 17,20-lyase activities. There are probably several 3β-hydroxysteroid dehydrogenase enzymes, which are not P450 enzymes. The gene for one of these enzymes, located on chromosome 1, has been cloned and has been identified to be responsible for the disease, 3β-hydroxysteroid dehydrogenase deficiency (48).

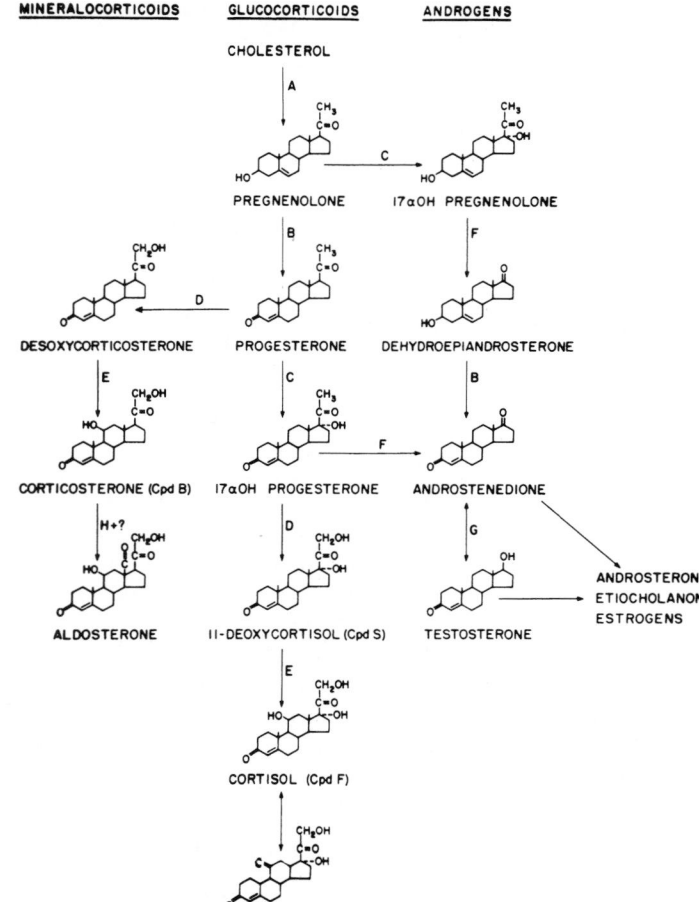

FIG. 41–4. The biosynthetic pathway of adrenal steroid. The classic enzyme terminology is represented by the alphabetical letters with the appropriate cytochrome P450 oxidases in parentheses. A, 20,22-desmolase (P450scc); B, 3β-hydroxysteroid dehydrogenase; C, 17α-hydroxylase (P450c17); D, 21-hydroxylase (P450c21); E, 11-hydroxylase (P450c11); F, 17,20-lyase ({P450c17); G, 17-keto reductase; H+, 18-hydroxylase + 18-oxidase (P450c11).

The three synthetic pathways produce mineralocorticoids, glucocorticoids, and androgens. Both steroidogenesis and adrenocortical growth are stimulated by the trophic influence of ACTH. Deficient cortisol synthesis secondary to an enzymatic deficiency causes increased ACTH production. Increased ACTH production, in turn, causes a compensatory hypertrophy of the adrenal cortex, and in this manner the block in the biosynthetic pathway may be partially overcome. This increased production of ACTH, however, also leads to an increased production and accumulation of precursor steroids. The clinical findings and the steroidal patterns of the individual defects are summarized in Table 41–7.

Virilization

Virilization of the female is secondary to the elevation of adrenal androgens caused by those enzymatic defects subsequent to 17-hydroxylation. In most cases, there is some fusion of the labioscrotal folds with clitoral enlargement, which may be bound down by chordee. Occasionally, virilization may be so severe that a phallic urethra develops. Virilization of the male generally is not noted during the neonatal period, and, in the nonsalt-losing forms of this disorder, the male often will be undetected until age 5 or 6 years. At this time, he may be noted to be large for his age and muscular, demonstrating secondary sexual changes. The classic virilizing form of congenital adrenal hyperplasia is the result of a deficiency of the cytochrome P450c21 (i.e., 21-hydroxylase deficiency). This defect also is the most common, accounting for almost 90% of recognized cases. As discussed later, elevation of 17-hydroxyprogesterone is not diagnostic of 21-hydroxylase deficiency. A mistaken diagnosis of 21-hydroxylase deficiency can result in errors in genetic counseling and prenatal treatment.

Incomplete Masculinization

Failure of complete masculine development occurs in those forms of adrenal hypoplasia in which synthesis of testosterone is blocked. The incomplete masculinization in the male, which is under fetal testicular control, suggests that the enzymatic deficiency in these defects occurs in both the adrenal gland and the testis. The lack of 3β-hydroxysteroid dehydrogenase activity occurring in both the adrenal gland and the testis has been demonstrated (26). In the 3β-hydroxysteroid dehydrogenase defect, the block results in secretion of steroids that consist almost entirely of compounds with δ5-3β-hydroxy configuration. The lack of the enzyme in the fetal testis causes incomplete masculinization in the male by interfering with testosterone synthesis (27). The marked elevation of δ5-3β-hydroxyadrenal androgens, especially DHEA, however, accounts for the virilization of the female infant. The elevation of serum 17-hydroxypregnenolone is diagnostic of 3β-hydroxysteroid dehydrogenase deficiency. In 3β-hydroxysteroid dehydrogenase deficiency, however, 17-hydroxyprogesterone concentrations also are markedly elevated (49). Therefore, the finding of elevations of 17-hydroxyprogesterone requires further studies to delineate the exact enzymatic defect. The reported cases of genetic males with both congenital lipoid hyperplasia and the 17α-hydroxylase defect support the hypothesis that the adrenal and testicular enzymatic mechanisms for testosterone biosynthesis share common genetic controls.

Hypertension

Hypertension has been associated with enzymatic blocks resulting in excessive secretion of mineralocorticoids. A defect of cytochrome P450c11 (i.e., 11-hydroxy-

TABLE 41–7. *Clinical and biochemical findings of the common variants of congenital adrenal hyperplasia*

| Enzyme deficiency (classic) | Phenotype | | Other clinical manifestations | Predominant steroids |
	46XX	46XY		
Congenital lipoid hyperplasia	Female	Female	Salt-wasting crisis	Low level—all steroids No response to ACTH
3β-Hydroxysteroid dehydrogenase deficiency	Virilized	Hypospadias	Salt-wasting crisis	Dehydroepiandrosterone 17-OH pregnenolone Increased Δ5-Δ4 ratio of steroids
21-Hydroxylase deficiency	Virilized	Male	Pseudoprecocious puberty in male Late virilization in female Salt-wasting crisis	17-OH progesterone Androstenedione Testosterone
11α-Hydroxylase deficiency	Virilized	Male	Pseudoprecocious puberty in male Hypertension	11-Deoxycortisol 11-Deoxycorticosterone Androstenedione Low renin
17α-Hydroxylase deficiency	Female	Female	Sexual infantilism Hypertension	Corticosterone 11-Deoxycorticosterone (Low renin)

ACTH, adrenocorticotrophic hormone.

lase deficiency) causes an accumulation of desoxycorticosterone, a potent mineralocorticoid, as well as 11-deoxycortisol (50). The 17α-hydroxylase defect (i.e., P450c17) blocks 17-hydroxylation of progesterone, interfering with cortisol and androgen biosynthesis, and the mineralocorticoid excess results in hypertension (51). Hypertension in these forms of congenital adrenal hyperplasia, however, is an inconstant feature. Whether the hypertension is related to the duration of excessive secretion of mineralocorticoid, the degree of the defect (i.e., variations of the genetic mutation), or variations in sodium intake is not clear. It is not known whether hypertension occurs during the newborn period in infants with these forms of the congenital adrenal hyperplasia syndrome.

Salt Loss

The salt-losing form of the 21-hydroxylase defect, and the 3β-hydroxysteroid dehydrogenase defect block steroid synthesis early in the biosynthetic pathway, result in mineralocorticoid insufficiency and severe sodium loss. The electrolytes initially are normal, but, within 1 week of life, serum sodium concentration will slowly decrease with a concomitant increase in serum potassium concentration. These infants may manifest acute adrenal crisis with shock, peripheral collapse, and dehydration by 10 to 14 days of age.

The underlying metabolic defects for two varieties of the 21-hydroxylase enzyme defect are now understood. Eberlein and Bongiovanni (52) postulated that both varieties are the result of the same hydroxylase deficiency. In the salt-loser patient, there is almost complete 21-hydroxylase deficiency, whereas in the compensated patient there is sufficient 21-hydroxylase to permit aldosterone synthesis. It is clear that a single gene mediates the hydroxylation of both progesterone and 17-hydroxyprogesterone, and it is likely that variations in the mutation of the P450c21 gene account for the heterogeneity of 21-hydroxylase deficiency disorders, including the nonclassic late-onset variant.

A few instances of aldosterone deficiency caused by a specific defect of 18-dehydrogenase, the last enzymatic transaction toward aldosterone, have been described (53,54). There is salt and water loss, without the other clinical consequences of congenital adrenal hyperplasia. These disorders probably are secondary to point mutations of the P450c11 enzyme that mediates these activities.

Congenital Lipoid Hyperplasia

Previously, this disorder was thought to be due to a deficiency of the enzyme, 20,22 desmolase (P450scc), which is necessary for conversion of cholesterol to pregnenolone. This disorder is now known to be due to both an inborn error of steroidogenesis, a genetic defect of the STAR protein necessary for acute steroidogenesis, and cellular damage of the mitochondrion necessary for steroidogenesis due to accumulation of cholesterol esters. The recent description of the genetic mutations (55) explain the variations in timing of presentation with adrenal crisis. The phenotype includes normal external female genitalia, neonatal hyponatremia, hyperkalemia, and dehydration. However, the age at presentation varies from the newborn period to several months of age and later. No steroids are detected in this disorder and the adrenal glands are markedly enlarged, filled with cholesterol esters.

Prenatal Diagnosis and Treatment of Congenital Adrenal Hyperplasia

It is possible, using molecular and genetic techniques, to diagnosis 21-hydroxylase deficiency in the fetus prenatally. It should be stressed, however, that these techniques should be considered experimental, and such diagnosis and treatment should be performed in major medical centers well versed in performing them. It is equally important to stress that only 21-hydroxylase deficiency can be diagnosed prenatally with any degree of confidence. A proband diagnosed to have 21-hydroxylase deficiency on the basis of elevated 17-hydroxyprogesterone levels, without confirmation by measurement of other steroids, can lead to a mistaken diagnosis (49).

Once the diagnosis of 21-hydroxylase deficiency has been established in a propositus, genetic evaluation of the mutation for P450c21 should be done in the propositus and the parents. The parents should be tested with ACTH, to confirm biochemically that they are genetic heterozygotes for 21-hydroxylase deficiency. The management of the pregnancy, the techniques used for diagnosis, the treatment of the female fetus with 21-hydroxylase deficiency, and the problems with these techniques have been reviewed (56,57). In brief, the mother is started on dexamethasone early in the first trimester and, subsequently, chorionic villus sampling or amniocentesis is performed to determine the sex and genetic studies. DNA is extracted from cultured tissue and analyzed using appropriate cDNA probes. If molecular and genetic techniques confirm the diagnosis and the fetus is female, dexamethasone treatment is continued to term.

Diagnosis of Adrenal Insufficiency

It is difficult to make the diagnosis of acute adrenal insufficiency in the newborn. There must be a high index of suspicion in any acutely ill infant with shock, peripheral collapse, and a rapid and weak pulse, and in any infant with poor feeding, failure to thrive, intermittent pyrexia, or even hypoglycemia and convulsions. A subtle sign of congenital adrenal hypoplasia is hyperpigmentation, especially in the extensor creases and genitalia; however, this sign is recognized most often after the diagnosis has been made. Decreased serum sodium and chloride and increased serum potassium levels are suggestive of mineralocorticoid deficiency. Isolated hyponatremia does not exclude glucocorticoid insufficiency and should be viewed as a possible sign of adrenal insufficiency. Certainly, ambiguous external genitalia at birth always should suggest the possibility of congenital adrenal hyperplasia.

The serum cortisol levels are low in all newborns, and especially in premature infants. There is no diurnal variation of cortisol levels; therefore, cortisol determinations without stimulation testing are not useful. In clinical situations highly suggestive of adrenal insufficiency, it is recommended that a rapid, 1-hour ACTH stimulation test be performed and that pharmacologic doses of glucocorticoids be administered, along with fluid and mineral resuscitation, after testing. Plasma concentrations of ACTH are elevated in those infants with primary adrenal insufficiency, including congenital adrenal hyperplasia. A plasma sample for ACTH determination should be obtained before ACTH testing.

Delineation of the specific enzyme defect in congenital adrenal hyperplasia can be determined by measuring serum concentrations of the various steroidal precursors to cortisol synthesis (see Table 41–7). The serum concentration of 17-hydroxyprogesterone is elevated in the affected newborn and may serve as a screening device using a filter paper technique (58). Normal newborn levels are less than 100 ng/dL (59) and may increase to levels as high as 200 ng/dL in the male infant at 1 to 2 months of age. Stressed newborns may have higher levels. This is especially true in the preterm sick newborn, in whom 17-hydroxyprogesterone values can be above 600 ng/dL. However, the 17-hydroxyprogesterone levels in stressed infants are significantly less than the values noted in patients with 21-hydroxylase deficiency. Serum levels of 17-hydroxyprogesterone are normally elevated in cord blood, with values ranging between 900 and 5,000 ng/dL. The serum levels rapidly decrease by the second or third day of life, and values above 1,000 ng/dL are suspect. Affected infants with 21-hydroxylase deficiency often have serum levels markedly above 2,000 ng/dL. It is important to recognize that elevated serum concentrations of 17-hydroxyprogesterone are not diagnostic of the 21-hydroxylase defect. Serum levels of 17-hydroxyprogesterone can be mildly elevated in the 11-hydroxylase defect and can be markedly elevated in the 3β-hydroxysteroid dehydrogenase defect secondary to peripheral conversion of 17-hydroxypregnenolone to 17-hydroxyprogesterone (49). Serum levels of 17-hydroxypregnenolone are especially elevated in the premature infant, and levels up to 2,000 ng/dL are normal (60).

Treatment of Adrenal Insufficiency

The immediate need of the critically ill infant in adrenal crisis is for cortisol. If possible, cortisol should be withheld until the diagnosis can be established, either by ACTH testing or by obtaining serum and plasma assay for determination of the appropriate steroids and ACTH. However, if a newborn infant is in shock and *in extremis*, the use of glucocorticoids as a lifesaving measure is justified, whatever the diagnosis. In the usual situation, salt and water alone will relieve the clinical crisis. Intravenous isotonic saline in 5% glucose water should be infused at a rate of 100 to 120 mL/kg during the first 24 hours. If the infant is in severe shock, the use of plasma or 5% albumin, 10 to 20 mL/kg, as well as cortisol, is often necessary. Hydrocortisone hemisuccinate or phosphate, 1.5 to 2 mg/kg, should be given intravenously immediately. Constant infusion of hydrocortisone hemisuccinate or phosphate ($30 mg/m^2/d$) should be continued. Hydrocortisone hemisuccinate, 2 mg/kg, can be given intramuscularly if intravenous access is a problem. The infant with severe shock may at times require a vasopressor. In severe adrenal cortical insufficiency, vasopressor drugs may be without effect until after the administration of hydrocortisone.

Hydrocortisone or cortisone acetate, 10 to 12 $mg/m^2/d$, is the mainstay for long-term treatment of patients with adrenal insufficiency. Cortisone acetate also can be given intramuscularly every 3 days for long-term replacement therapy, but this regimen seldom is necessary. During severe stress, such as pernicious vomiting or surgery, cortisone acetate ($30 mg/m^2$) should be given parenterally on a daily basis.

Often a mineralocorticoid is a necessary adjunct for the chronic treatment of adrenal insufficiency. The dose of the oral mineralocorticoid, 9α-fludrocortisone (Florinef) is 0.05 to 0.1 mg/d, which is sufficient for most forms of adrenal insufficiency. In the salt-losing forms of congenital adrenal hyperplasia, occasionally higher doses of fludrocortisone are necessary. It has been recognized that even the compensated (i.e., nonsalt-losing) form of the 21-hydroxylase defect may be treated better when a small amount of mineralocorticoid is added to the therapeutic regimen.

Iatrogenic Adrenal Insufficiency

It often is necessary during the neonatal period to use pharmacologic doses of glucocorticoids for adjunctive treatment of a number of diseases, such as bronchopulmonary dysplasia. There are no good studies, especially in newborn infants, as to the dose and duration of glucocorticoid therapy that will result in adrenal insufficiency. It is probable, however, that high-dose glucocorticoid therapy for a very brief duration (less than 1 week) will not cause adrenal insufficiency, but treatment longer than 30 days may result in at least transient adrenal insufficiency. Therefore, after a very short course of pharmacologic glucocorticoid therapy, tapering glucocorticoids in decrements is not necessary in terms of adrenal function.

The clinical course of the primary condition, however, may worsen with rapid discontinuation of glucocorticoids. After prolonged glucocorticoid therapy, the dose of glucocorticoids can be decreased by one-half every several days until a physiologic replacement dose (10 mg of hydrocortisone/m^2/d orally) is achieved. The dose can then be lowered more gradually, by 20% increments every 4 or 5 days.

It is likely that adrenal function will be suppressed for some time after prolonged pharmacologic glucocorticoid therapy. Again, there are no studies correlating dose, duration of pharmacologic treatment, and time needed for recovery of adrenal function after high-dose glucocorticoid therapy. There are anecdotal reports of adrenal crisis occurring during stress 6 months and longer after discontinuation of pharmacologic glucocorticoid therapy. It is possible to evaluate periodically the adrenal response to exogenous ACTH to determine when iatrogenic adrenal insufficiency has resolved. Alternatively, the empiric use of pharmacologic doses of glucocorticoids during situations of stress, for at least 1 year after discontinuation of prolonged high-dose glucocorticoid therapy, is not inappropriate. A minimal dose of glucocorticoid to be used during stress situations is 30 mg of hydrocortisone/m^2/d, orally.

DISORDERS OF THE THYROID

Development and Function of the Thyroid

The fetal thyroid begins as a thickening of epithelium at the base of the tongue. The thyroid anlage subsequently migrates down the trachea, leaving the thyroglossal duct as an embryonic remnant. During its caudal migration, the thyroid anlage assumes a more bilobate shape. Thy-

roid function is apparent by 12 weeks of gestation, with the ability to accumulate and concentrate iodide present. Organification of iodine, with synthesis of T$_4$ and triiodothyronine (T$_3$), occurs by 14 weeks of gestation. The fetal hypothalamic–pituitary feedback mechanisms are operative by the latter part of gestation, and the fetal thyroid is responsive to TSH. There is no placental transfer of maternal or fetal TSH, although thyroid-stimulating immunoglobulins (TSI) will cross the placenta. Free T$_4$ and, more so, T$_3$ are capable of crossing the placenta in either direction (61,62). The gradient in transfer of thyroid hormones, except in the hypothyroid fetus, is fetus to mother.

The biosynthesis of thyroid hormones is illustrated in Fig. 41–5. Circulating plasma iodide is concentrated by the thyroid gland. The concentrated iodide is then oxidized by a thyroid peroxidase and bound to tyrosine to form monoiodotyrosine (MIT) and diiodotyrosine (DIT). The iodotyrosines are held in peptide linkage to thyroglobulin. These iodotyrosines are then coupled to form T$_3$ and T$_4$, still linked to thyroglobulin. The thyroid hormones are cleaved from thyroglobulin by thyroid proteases, and T$_3$ and T$_4$ are secreted into the circulatory system. Intrathyroidal iodotyrosines and iodothyronines are deiodinated by dehalogenase enzymes and remain within the intrathyroidal iodide pool to be reused. The thyroid gland secretes both T$_3$ and T$_4$; however, a large percentage of the circulating T$_3$ is secondary to deiodination of T$_4$ by the peripheral tissues (63). The iodide released from the peripheral metabolism of iodothyronines enters the circulatory system to be reconcentrated by the thyroid gland or excreted by the kidneys. The iodothyronines are transported in the plasma by proteins. Thyroxine-binding globulin (TBG), an α-globulin, is the major carrier of T$_4$, but TBG also will bind T$_3$ to a lesser extent. Thyroxine

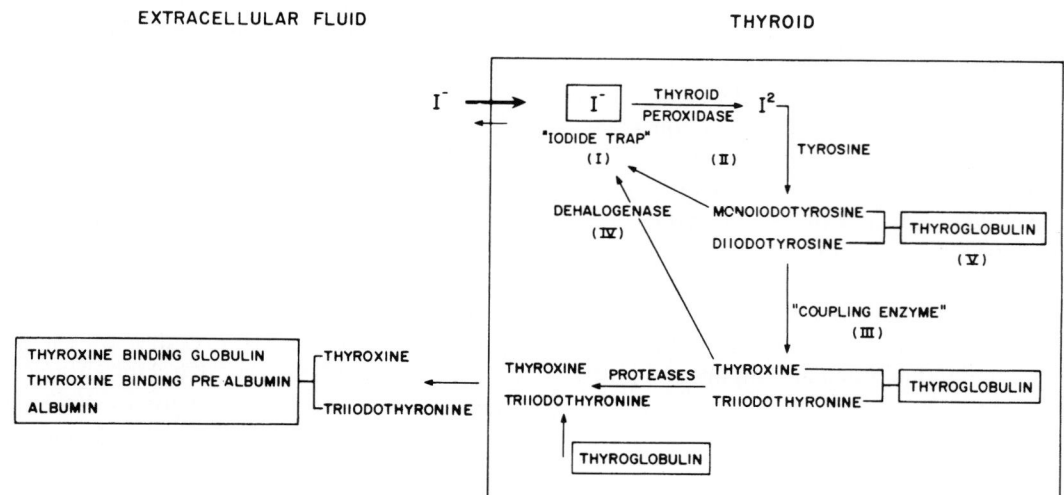

FIG. 41–5. Thyroid hormone synthesis. The roman numerals represent described enzymatic defects of thyroxine synthesis.

also is bound by T_4-binding prealbumin and by albumin. At the cellular level, free T_3 and T_4 are active. Disorders, either genetic or acquired, that quantitatively change the concentration of TBG will alter the level of total T_4 in serum without altering biological thyroid status.

The secretion of the thyroid hormones is under hypothalamic–pituitary control. The hypothalamus secretes a tripeptide, TRH, which stimulates release of TSH from the pituitary (64,65). TSH, in turn, stimulates the production of thyroid hormones. Every step of thyroid hormone biosynthesis and release, from iodide accumulation to proteolysis of thyroglobulin, is under TSH stimulation. The thyroid hormones, in turn, exercise negative feedback control of TSH response to TRH at the pituitary level.

Thyroid Function Tests

Thyroid function tests in the newborn are elevated compared to values obtained for older children. This is secondary to the surge of TSH that occurs in the immediate postnatal period. The total T_4 ranges from 7.3 to 22.9 µg/dL during the first month of life, with mean values greater than 10 µg/dL (Tables 41–8 and 41–9). The thyroid function tests remain elevated compared to the values found in older children, for the first several months of life. The TBG levels are elevated, secondary to maternal estrogen effect, causing the increased T_4 levels. Thyroid function tests normally are lower in premature and sick newborns than in healthy term newborn infants (Table 41–10). This also is an effect of TBG levels, which are decreased in the premature infant.

Congenital Hypothyroidism

The causes of congenital hypothyroidism are many and include disorganized embryogenesis, genetic disorders, including errors of T_4 biosynthesis, and environmental factors. It is useful to classify congenital hypothyroidism into the following subgroups:

- Agenesis of the thyroid gland (athyrotic cretinism) or dysgenesis of the thyroid gland (thyroid hypoplasia, thyroid ectopia),
- Endemic goitrous hypothyroidism,
- Inborn errors of T_4 synthesis (familial goitrous cretinism),
- Drug-induced hypothyroidism,
- End-organ unresponsiveness to thyroid hormone,
- Thyroid unresponsiveness to thyrotropin,
- Secondary hypothyroidism (pituitary hypothyroidism), and
- Tertiary hypothyroidism (hypothalamic hypothyroidism).

Agenesis or Dysgenesis of the Thyroid Gland

Disordered embryogenesis of the thyroid gland is the most frequent cause of congenital hypothyroidism in the United States. Although congenital endemic goitrous hypothyroidism may have been more prevalent throughout the world at one time, the frequency of this disorder has declined with the introduction of iodine into endemic areas.

Little is known of the causes of defective fetal thyroid development. There may be genetic factors. Athyrotic congenital hypothyroidism has been documented in siblings (66,67) and in identical twins (68). Nonetheless, athyrosis generally is a sporadic disorder. Thyroid antibodies have been detected with increased incidence among mothers of children with hypothyroidism (69). Most mothers with thyroid antibodies have normal children, however, and, conversely, most mothers who deliver children with congenital hypothyroidism do not have thyroid antibodies. Thyroid hypoplasia has been reported in children with congenital toxoplasmosis, but *in utero* infectious disorders have not been implicated commonly as a cause of thyroid dysgenesis.

Endemic Goitrous Hypothyroidism

Although endemic goiter is one of the widespread nutritional diseases in the world, the introduction of iodine into various foods, including infant formulas, has markedly decreased the incidence of endemic goitrous hypothyroidism. The dietary requirements for iodine vary, but 40 to 100 µg/d is sufficient for most children. In areas with endemic goiters, it is probable that factors

TABLE 41–8. *Range of mean values for thyroid and thyroid-stimulating hormones during the neonatal period in full-term infants*

	T_4 (µg/dL)	T_3 (ng/dL)	TBG (mg/dL)	TSH (µU/mL)
Cord blood	10.9 (7–13)	48 (12–90)	5.4 (1.2–9.6)	9.5 (2.4–20)
2 h of age	22.1	217		86
24–72 h of age	17.2 (12.4–21.9)	125 (89–256)	5.4	7.3 (<2.5–16.3)
2 wk of age	12.9 (8.2–16.6)	250	5 (1–9)	
6 wk of age	10.3 (7.9–14.4)	163 (114–189)	4.8 (2–7.6)	2.5 (<2.5–6.3)

T_3, triiodothyronine; T_4, thyroxine; TBG, thyroxine-binding globulin; TSH, thyroid-stimulating hormone.

TABLE 41–9. *The upper limit of normal for measurements of thyroid-stimulating hormone in the first 5 days of life*

Age at collection (d)	Standard TSH cutoff		Age-adjusted TSH cutoff	
	No. of infants	TSH value (mU/L)	No. of infants	TSH value (mU/L)
0–1	19	>20	8	>30
2	54	>20	26	>25
3	136	>20	45	>25
4	30	>20	30	>20
5	34	>20	34	>20
Total	273		143	

Retrospective study of 37,927 infants with definite abnormal results during a 6-month period (1988–1989).
TSH, thyroid-stimulating hormone.
From Allen DB, Sieger JE, Litsheim T, Duck SC. Age-adjusted thyrotropin criteria for neonatal screening of hypothyroidism. *J Pediatr* 1990;117:310.

other than iodine (e.g., enzymatic defects, other genetic factors, and other dietary factors such as goitrogens), contribute to goiter formation. The contributory factors are suggested by the evidence that females are more commonly afflicted than males, many of the population within the endemic area may not be afflicted, and the incidence of endemic cretinism varies in different areas. In the Alps, deaf-mutism is a common finding in association with endemic cretinism, suggesting possibly an associated enzymatic defect of organification of iodide. When cretinism occurs in conjunction with an endemic goiter, the signs and symptoms are similar to the dysgenetic form of cretinism, except for the presence of a goiter and an elevated radioactive iodine uptake.

Inborn Errors of Thyroxine Synthesis

The inherited disorders of T_4 synthesis involve deficiencies in one or more of the enzymes necessary for hormonogenesis or release of thyroid hormones, resulting in hypothyroidism. A compensatory increase in TSH production produces hyperplasia and enlargement of the thyroid gland, creating the clinical picture of familial goitrous cretinism. These defects of T_4 biosynthesis have been reviewed by Dumont et al. (70).

TABLE 41–10. *Mean values for thyroid and thyroid-stimulating hormones in cord blood of full-term and premature infants*

	T_4 (μg/dL)	T_3 (ng/dL)	TSH (μU/mL)
Term	10.9	48	9.5
35 wk of gestation	9.5	29	12.7
32 wk of gestation	7.6	15	

T_3, triiodothyronine; T_4, thyroxine; TSH, thyroid-stimulating hormone.

Iodide Trap Defect

The thyroid gland has the ability to concentrate iodide, so that the intrathyroidal iodide concentration may be 40-fold greater than the serum concentration. In this rare inherited defect of T_4 synthesis, this ability is lost. As would be anticipated, the 24-hour radioactive iodine uptake is negligible. Thyroid scans do not demonstrate the presence of thyroid tissue, although there may be some uptake, but the gland is detected by ultrasonography. Several other organs, including the salivary glands, share the ability to concentrate iodide, and this defect can be distinguished from athyrosis because the salivary iodide concentration also is low and there usually is a goiter. The serum T_4 is low in this defect, but the TSH is elevated. In a manner of speaking, this defect represents iodine deficiency, and high dosages of iodide can overcome this defect to some degree.

Organification or Peroxidase Defect

A defect in the organification of iodide is one of the more frequent defects of T_4 synthesis. In this defect, the thyroid has an increased uptake of iodide but is unable to oxidize it and cannot combine it with tyrosine. This leads to the accumulation of free iodide in the gland, and the administration of anions such as perchlorate or thiocyanate will cause a discharge or release of the unbound iodide. Iodine that is bound to tyrosine or thyronines cannot be discharged. These findings have led to a simple test for the organification defect. The patient is given a tracer amount of radioactive iodine, and the radioactivity over the thyroid gland is noted. In a patient with the organification defect, the radioactive iodine is rapidly concentrated into the gland. When the radioactivity over the gland has leveled off, a dose of potassium perchlorate or thiocyanate given orally (0.5 to 1 g) will displace the unorganified iodine, causing a rapid discharge of the radioactive iodine from the thyroid gland. The measurement of T_4 usually is low or low normal, but the TSH is elevated.

A variant of this form of familial goiter secondary to a defect in organification is associated with deaf-mutism (or Pendred syndrome). The clinical pattern differs slightly from the full organification defect, in that patients with the Pendred syndrome often have only small goiters and the perchlorate discharge is not as complete. The hearing loss in this variant is neurosensory. Intelligence usually is normal.

Coupling Defect

The failure of coupling of MIT and DIT into T_4 and T_3 is a cause of goitrous hypothyroidism. The coupling of the iodotyrosines into the final product of the thyroid hormones is a complex intermediate step involving many processes, and the block should not be thought of as a defined enzymatic deficiency. The inability of the thyroid gland to couple MIT and DIT into T_4 and T_3 leads to the accumulation of large amounts of MIT and DIT in the gland, with the small amounts of T_4 and T_3 synthesized being immediately released into the circulation. Thus, when extracts of the thyroid gland are subjected to chromatographic analysis after radioactive iodine labeling, large amounts of MIT and DIT are detected with only trace quantities of T_4 and T_3. The TSH is elevated. The radioactive iodine uptake by the thyroid gland is rapid and high. Definitive diagnosis requires thyroid biopsy and chromatographic analysis of the iodotyrosines and iodothyronines.

Dehalogenase Defect

The deiodination of the iodotyrosines and iodothyronines occurs in the thyroid as well as in the liver, kidneys, and other organs. The inherited inability of the thyroid to deiodinate MIT and DIT causes leakage of these precursors from the gland and depletion of iodide stores. This loss of iodide causes decreased hormone synthesis, resulting in compensatory TSH release, thyroid hyperplasia, and increased synthesis of MIT, DIT, and the iodothyronines. The goitrous hypothyroidism in this defect is not caused by a biosynthetic block but, in a sense, by iodine deficiency. Radioactive iodine is rapidly accumulated and turned over. Large amounts of iodine can permit adequate hormone synthesis. The T_4 is low or low normal, and the TSH is elevated. Because this defect is extrathyroidal as well as intrathyroidal, administered radioactive MIT and DIT appear unchanged in the urine.

Abnormal Thyroglobulin

Thyroglobulin is synthesized exclusively within the thyroid. The iodination of the tyrosyl residues with the thyroglobulin complex leads to the formation of MIT and DIT, and coupling of these iodinated tyrosyl residues leads to formation of T_4 and T_3. The defects of thyroglobulin formation incorporates a group of disorders. Errors of thyroglobulin synthesis, as well as decreased synthesis, are possible. Deficient protease activity for thyroglobulin degradation also has been postulated to result in deficiency of thyroid hormone release.

These disorders are characterized by abnormal iodoproteins in the thyroid and the serum. These peptides sometimes have been described as albumin-like, and have been identified by Savoie et al. (71,72) as the iodoalbumin thyroalbumin, in which the major iodinated compounds appear to be monoiodohistadines and diiodohistadines. These investigators concluded that the abnormality of thyroglobulin causes iodination of inappropriate proteins, mainly albumin, with a subsequent low yield of T_4. A compensatory increase in TSH secretion causes thyroid hyperplasia and a rapid turnover of T_4 or albumin. Proteolysis of the iodohistadinethyroalbumin results in a high secretion of iodohistadine, which can be detected in the urine.

Drug-Induced Neonatal Goiter

Many drugs have been demonstrated to be goitrogenic. In the newborn infant, the most commonly implicated drugs are iodides and thiourea derivatives used for treatment of maternal thyrotoxicosis. The use of these drugs not only has caused goiter in the newborn but also has been associated with scattered reports of hypothyroidism (73). Although the correlation between the dose of the drug and the occurrence of goiter is poor, prolonged administration of thiourea drugs to the mother increases the risk of fetal goiter. Herbst and Selenkow (74) suggest lowering the dose of thiourea drugs during the last trimester and concurrent use of thyroid hormone, in the treatment of a thyrotoxic pregnant woman. In the infants of hyperthyroid mothers, it is necessary to distinguish the drug-induced goiter from the long-acting TSI-induced goiter. A low T_4 suggests that the goiter is secondary to the drug, whereas a high T_4 is more compatible with a TSI-induced goiter and possible neonatal hyperthyroidism. Treatment usually is not necessary for the infant with a drug-induced goiter unless the goiter is asphyxiating or, more rarely, the infant is hypothyroid. Thyroid hormone will cause the goiter to subside.

Concerns have been raised as to the appropriate use of antithyroid agents in the lactating mother. It has generally been accepted that propylthiouracil is safe in lactating mothers (75). Because of adverse drug reactions some lactating mothers may need to be discontinued from propylthiouracil treatment. There have been studies of the safety of carbimazol and methimazole as alternative treatment for lactating hyperthyoid mothers. Both reports showed that, although the drugs are passed into the milk, the dosage the infant receives is minimal and appears to be safe (76,77). Nonetheless, thyroid function should be monitored in the infant.

Unresponsiveness to Thyroid Hormones

Refetoff et al. (78) reported a family with deaf-mutism, stippled epiphyses, delayed bone age, goiter, and an elevated serum T_4. The children clinically appeared to be euthyroid. The serum thyroid hormone-binding proteins and hormone biosynthesis were normal. This family represents tissue unresponsiveness to thyroid hormone. It is clear that there are several expressions of this syndrome. Refetoff's patients probably represent a variant that is totally resistant to thyroid hormones and, despite elevated T_4 levels, is basically hypothyroid. There are patients with isolated central resistance to thyroid hormone who are mildly hyperthyroid or euthyroid in infancy and childhood (79).

Unresponsiveness to Thyroid-Stimulating Hormone

Stanbury et al. (80) reported a severely retarded 8-year-old boy with a normal thyroid gland, a low protein-bound iodine (PBI), normal radioactive iodine uptake, and high endogenous levels of biologically active TSH. Exogenous TSH neither stimulated the thyroid gland *in vivo* nor increased glucose metabolism by thyroid slices *in vitro*. TSH unresponsiveness of the thyroid gland was postulated by these investigators as an explanation for this clinical syndrome.

Secondary and Tertiary Hypothyroidism

These conditions are due to failure of secretion of TSH and TRH from the pituitary and hypothalamus, respectively. Newborn infants with these disorders may be missed in some of the newborn screening programs because detection is directed toward primary hypothyroidism, which is associated with both low T_4 and elevated TSH levels. All patients with the midline abnormalities outlined in Table 41–4 should be suspected of possible secondary or tertiary hypothyroidism. Therefore, they should have more complete thyroid studies (including a free T_4 determined by dialysis, ultrasensitive TSH, and TRH testing) because of the risk that they might be missed by the newborn screening test.

Symptoms

Symptoms of agenesis of the thyroid gland are detectable by 6 weeks of age; however, a number of infants will have clinical manifestations at birth or during the immediate neonatal period. The signs during the early neonatal period are subtle and include prolonged neonatal jaundice, poor suck, poor feeding, lethargy (i.e., the quiet baby), respiratory difficulties, bradycardia, consti-

pation, and intermittent cyanosis. Later, the more classic symptoms of cretinism appear. The progressive myxedema causes coarsening of the facies, with puffy eyelids, flattened nasal bridge, and enlarged tongue. The cry is hoarse secondary to myxedema of the larynx and epiglottis. The infant is extremely lethargic and hypotonic. Constipation, poor feeding, poor weight gain, dry hair, umbilical hernia, and pallor become more notable with time.

There is considerable evidence for the essential role of the thyroid hormones in the growth and development of the central nervous system (81). The final outcome of mental development in children with congenital hypothyroidism depends on the severity, time of onset, and duration of thyroid insufficiency. By the time the symptoms are clinically evident, it is likely that brain injury has occurred.

Infants with ectopic or residual thyroid tissue or inborn errors of T_4 synthesis often will produce enough thyroid hormone to delay the onset of clinical symptoms. Although the signs and symptoms are similar to those for the athyrotic cretin, the prognosis for mental function is greatly improved.

Diagnosis

The incidence of congenital hypothyroidism has been estimated to be 1 in 4,000 births. In view of the desirability of early diagnosis and treatment, screening of newborn infants, using filter paper spots, as for phenylketonuria testing, is standard in the United States. Some 34% of low T_4 values detected by this method are not the result of true hypothyroidism, but represent diminished levels of TBG. If the initial T_4 is in the lowest 10% of the samples being tested, a repeat T_4 and a TSH are determined on the same sample. If the repeat T_4 is still low (less than 6 µg/dL) or the TSH is elevated, confirmatory tests are requested. A serum sample should be obtained and studied in detail. A low T_4 and a normal TSH may represent secondary or tertiary hypothyroidism or TBG deficiency. Low T_4 levels also are found normally in premature infants and severely ill newborn infants and are not necessarily indicative of hypothyroidism (see section on Euthyroid Sick Syndrome). If the T_4 is greater than 7 µg/dL, it is regarded as normal in premature or sick infants (82). Note the need to avoid using specimens obtained in the early hours after birth because of the normal surge of TSH (see Tables 41–8 and 41–9).

The diagnosis should be confirmed by serum T_4 and TSH levels, as well as some determination of T_4 binding (e.g., T_3 resin uptake). In those cases suggestive of deficient thyroid hormone binding, a direct measurement of TBG should be determined. TBG deficiency is an X-linked disorder and occurs in 1 in 2,000 screening studies of boys. The initial confirmatory serologic studies should not include TBG measurements, because the test is more expensive than a T_3 resin uptake and will miss binding abnormalities involving other proteins. Radiographic skeletal age is often useful, because one-half of full-term infants with congenital hypothyroidism will not have the osseous centers normally present at birth. It is important to perform a thyroid scan on all patients with congenital hypothyroidism to identify those patients with inborn errors of T_4 synthesis so that appropriate genetic counseling may be given.

The incidence figures for various forms of congenital hypothyroidism, as determined by the newborn screening studies, are listed in Table 41–11. It is probable that the hypothalamic–hypopituitary forms of hypothyroidism have been underestimated by the newborn screening studies, because many of the TSH-deficient patients have normal serum T_4 concentrations at birth. Also, the syndromes of T_4 resistance and thyroid resistance to TSH can be missed by the newborn screening method. Probably the most common cause of undetected congenital hypothyroidism is omitting the screening study. This is more likely to occur in intensive care situations, because of the magnitude of other ongoing problems. The problems with newborn screening for congenital hypothyroidism have been reviewed (83).

Treatment and Prognosis

The dose of thyroid hormone prescribed should be sufficient to achieve high euthyroid levels of serum T_4 within 2 weeks of starting therapy. This usually is achieved with a starting dose of L-thyroxine, during the newborn period, of 10 μg/kg/d. A dose of 37.5 μg/d is a convenient starting dose for most full-term infants, as the smallest tablet size is 25 μg. Once treated, the serum T_4 returns to normal before the serum TSH. It is recommended that, to avoid overdosing with L-thyroxine during the first 4 weeks, the serum concentration of T_4 should be used as the laboratory guide for adequate treatment. After 4 to 6 weeks of therapy, however, the TSH level is the best monitor of treatment, and if the TSH remains elevated, the dose of L-thyroxine should be increased.

The prognosis for mental development has been correlated with time of onset of therapy. Klein et al. (84) studied 31 patients. In nine patients treated before the age of 3 months, the mean IQ was significantly greater than that of the children treated after 3 months of age. The prognosis for mental development in children with congenital hypothyroidism who have treatment started within 1 month of life is good. There is some evidence that there may be an increase in learning disabilities even in those infants treated within 1 month of age (85). Another survey, however, indicated no differences in IQ testing or other psychometric parameters studied when children with congenital hypothyroidism treated within 1 month of age were compared to matched normal controls (86). In the latter study, the only factor that correlated with poor IQ levels was inadequate treatment.

Recently, controversy has arisen over the issue of transient hypothyroxinemia in preterm infants and neurologic outcome. It is suggested by a retrospective analysis of thyoid levels in premature infants that severe transient hypothyroxinemia during the immediate neonatal period is an important cause of problems in neurologic and mental development detected at 2 years of age (87). None of the infants were subsequently diagnosed as having permanent hypothyroidism. Despite adjusting for many variables, it is still not clear whether those children with the impaired neurologic and mental outcome had lower thyroxine levels causing the worse outcome or because these children were sicker, which resulted in the worse outcome and lower thyroxine levels. Perhaps the answer lies in a paper by van Wassenaer et al. (88), which showed that thyroid replacement in a randomized double-blind, placebo-controlled study of 200 infants less than 30 weeks of gestation did not improve developmental outcome. No firm recommendations may be made at this time and further studies are awaited.

Euthyroid Sick Syndrome

The euthyroid sick syndrome is a reflection of adaptive physiologic processes that occur during acute and chronic illness. Thyroid hormones increase basal metabolism, cardiac output, and oxygen consumption. Reduced production of thyroid hormones, especially T_3, which reduces oxygen consumption and basal metabolic rate, is beneficial for certain illnesses (e.g., catabolic or hypoxic conditions). In animal studies, hypophysectomized rats survive longer during oxygen deprivation than intact animals. The euthyroid sick syndrome has been noted in both premature and full-term sick newborn infants.

The euthyroid sick syndrome is characterized by a low normal T_4 concentration, an extraordinarily low T_3 concentration, and a normal TSH level. The latter two findings distinguish the euthyroid sick syndrome from primary and secondary hypothyroidism. T_3 levels generally are in the low normal range in both primary and secondary hypothyroidism, with TSH levels markedly elevated in primary hypothyroidism. In those cases difficult to distinguish from secondary hypothyroidism, administration of TRH to a patient with the euthyroid sick syn-

TABLE 41–11. *Incidence of various forms of congenital hypothyroidism*

Disorder	Incidence
Congenital thyroid agenesis or dysgenesis	1:4000
Inborn errors of thyroxine synthesis	1:30,000
Hypothalamic–hypopituitary hypothyroidism	1:66,000[a]

[a]Hypothalamic–hypopituitary hypothyroidism incidence is based on newborn screening studies.

drome results in a normal rise and prompt decline of TSH. After TRH administration, patients with hypothalamic hypothyroidism will demonstrate a marked and prolonged increase in TSH and patients with pituitary hypothyroidism will demonstrate no increase in TSH. Unlike older infants and children, reverse T_3 is not useful in the diagnosis of euthyroid sick syndrome, because it is elevated normally in the newborn infant. Euthyroid sick syndrome does not require any treatment other than correction of the primary disease.

Congenital Thyrotoxicosis

Thyrotoxicosis in the neonatal period is relatively uncommon. Affected infants almost always are born of mothers who have either active Graves' disease or who have a history of previous Graves' disease. Neonatal thyrotoxicosis may also present in infants born to mothers with Hashimoto thyroiditis. Fewer than 5% of infants born to mothers with Graves' disease will have thyrotoxicosis in the newborn period. It is thought that the etiologic factor for neonatal thyrotoxicosis is the placental transfer of maternal thyroid-stimulating immunoglobulins. Thyroid-stimulating immunoglobulins have been demonstrated in more than 90% of studied cases (89).

Neonatal thyrotoxicosis is manifested by poor weight gain or excessive weight loss, goiter, irritability, tachycardia, flushing, and exophthalmos. A number of these infants tend to be small for gestational age. In an infant of a thyrotoxic mother, a high normal T_4 should be viewed with suspicion and the child followed closely. A low or suppressed TSH is further suggestive of neonatal thyrotoxicosis. Onset of symptoms usually occurs within the first week of life, but may be delayed until the second week. Arrhythmias, such as paroxysmal atrial tachycardia (90), cardiac failure, and death may occur if thyrotoxicity is especially severe. The prognosis is good because the thyrotoxic state is transient. Most cases will have resolved by 9 months of age. In several reported cases, there has been a rapid advance in skeletal maturation, with advanced bone age and premature closure of the cranial sutures (91,92).

Major therapeutic concerns in neonatal thyrotoxicosis are tracheal obstruction secondary to goitrous encroachment and cardiac failure. Subtotal thyroidectomy is rarely required to relieve tracheal obstruction. In nonneonatal thyrotoxicosis, iodide usually is reserved for preoperative management of thyrotoxicosis, because the duration of its therapeutic effects is limited. However, because neonatal thyrotoxicosis is a self-limiting disorder, iodide (one drop every 8 hours of saturated solution of potassium iodide), along with a β-adrenergic blocking agent such as propranolol hydrochloride, is used to control the thyrotoxicosis. Iodide has the advantage of interfering not only with T_4 synthesis but also with release of thyroid hormones. In the most severe cases, digitalis, sedation, or glucocorticoids may be necessary to prevent cardiovascular collapse.

REFERENCES

1. Ford CE, Jones KW, Polani PE, et al. A sex-chromosome anomaly in a case of gonadal dysgenesis. *Lancet* 1959;1:711.
2. Jacobs PA, Ross A. Structural abnormalities of the Y chromosome in man. *Nature* 1966;210:352.
3. Page DC, Mosher R, Simpson EM, et al. The sex-determining region of the human Y chromosome encodes a finger protein. *Cell* 1987;51:1091.
4. Sinclair AH, Berta P, Palmer MS, et al. A gene from the human sex determining region encodes a protein with homology to a conserved DNS binding motif. *Nature* 1990;346:240.
5. Kwoc C, Weller PA, Guioli S, et al. Mutations in SOX9, the gene responsible for campomelic dysplasia and autosomal sex reversal. *Am J Hum Genet* 1995;57:1028.
6. Swain A, Lovell-Badge R. A molecular approach to sex determination in mammals. *Acta Paediatr Suppl* 1997;423:46.
7. Muscatelli F, Strom TM, Walker AP, et al. Mutations in the DAX-1 gene give rise to both X-linked adrenal hypoplasia congenita and hypogonadotropic hypogonadism. *Nature* 1994;372:672.
8. Johnston AW, Ferguson-Smith MA, Handmaker SD Jr, et al. The triple-X syndrome: clinical, pathological and chromosomal studies in three mentally retarded cases. *Br Med J* 1961;2:1047.
9. Anderson M, Page DC, de la Chapelle A. Chromosome Y-specific DNA is transferred to the short arm of X chromosome in human XX males. *Science* 1986;233;786.
10. Winters SJ, Wachtel SS, White BJ, et al. H-Y antigen mosaicism in the gonad of a 46XX true hermaphrodite. *N Engl J Med* 1979;300:745.
11. Lus HA, Rudd FH. Chromosomal abnormalities in the human population: estimation of rates based on New Haven Newborn Study. *Science* 1970;169:496.
12. Lippe BM. Primary ovarian failure. In: Kaplan SA, ed. *Clinical pediatric endocrinology.* Philadelphia: WB Saunders, 1990;325.
13. Carr DH, Gedeon M. Population cytogenetics in human abortuses. In: Hook EB, Porter IH, eds. *Population cytogenetics.* New York: Academic Press, 1977;1.
14. Goldberg MD, Scully AL, Solomon IL, et al. Gonadal dysgenesis in phenotypic female subjects. *Am J Med* 1968;45:529.
15. Haddad HM, Wilkins L. Congenital anomalies associated with gonadal aplasia. *Pediatrics* 1959;23:885.
16. Preger L, Steinbach HL, Moskowitz P. Roentgenographic abnormalities in phenotypic females with gonadal dysgenesis. *AJR* 1968;104:899.
17. Rosenfeld RG, Hintz RL, Johanson AJ, et al. Three year results of a randomized prospective trial of methinyl human growth hormone and oxandrolone in Turner syndrome. *J Pediatr* 1988;113:393.
18. Serhal PF, Craft IL. Oocyte donation in 61 patients. *Lancet* 1989;1:1185.
19. Morishima A, Grumbach M. The interrelationship of sex chromosome constitution and phenotype in the syndrome of gonadal dysgenesis and its variants. *Ann NY Acad Sci* 1968;155:695.
20. Moshang T, Vallet HL, Cintron C, et al. Gonadal function in XO/XY or XX/XY Turner's syndrome. *J Pediatr* 1972;80:460.
21. Pallister PD, Opitz JM. The Perrault syndrome: autosomal recessive ovarian dysgenesis with facultative, non-sex-limited sensorineural deafness. *Am J Med Genet* 1979;4:239.
22. Sternberg WH, Barclay DL, Kloepfer HW. Familial XY gonadal dysgenesis. *N Engl J Med* 1968;278:695.
23. Grumbach MM, Ducharme J, Moloshok RE. On the fetal masculinizing action of certain oral progestins. *J Clin Endocrinol* Metab 1959;19:1369.
24. Murset G, Zachman M, Prader A, et al. Male external genitalia of a girl caused by virilizing adrenal tumor in the mother. *Acta Endocrinol* 1970;65:627.
25. Haymond MW, Weldon VV. Female pseudohermaphroditism secondary to a maternal virilizing tumor. *J Pediatr* 1973;82:682.
26. Bongiovanni AM. Adrenogenital syndrome with deficiency of 3β-hydroxysteroid dehydrogenase. *J Clin Invest* 1962;41:2086.
27. Bongiovanni AM, Eberlein WR, Goldman AS, et al. Disorders of adrenal steroid biogenesis. *Recent Prog Horm Res* 1967;23:375.
28. Griffen JE, Wilson JD. Syndromes of androgen resistance. *Hosp Pract* 1987;22:159.

29. Eberenz W, Rosenberg HK, Moshang T, et al. True hermaphroditism: sonographic determination of ovotestes. *Radiology* 1991;179:429.

30. Lee MM, Donahoe PK, Silverman BL, et al. Measurements of serum mullerian inhibiting substance in the evaluation of children with non-palpable gonads. *N Engl J Med* 1997;336:1480.

31. Diamond M, Sigmundson HK. Sex reassignment at birth. Long term review and clinical implications. *Arch Pediatr Adolesc Med* 1997;151:298.

32. Stanley CA. Hyperinsulinism in infants and children. *Pediatr Clin North Am* 1997;44:363.

33. Pfaffle R, Kim C, Otten, et al. Pit-1: clinical aspects. *Horm Res* 1996;45[Suppl]:25.

34. Sornson MW, Wu W, Dasen JS, et al. Pituitary lineage determination by the Prophet of Pit-1 homeodomain factor defective in Ames mouse. *Nature* 1996;384:327.

35. Bach I, Rhodes SJ, Pearse RV II, et al. P-Lim, a LIM homeodomain factor is expressed during pituitary organ and cell committment and synergizes with Pit-1. *Proc Natl Acad Sci USA* 1995;92:2720.

36. Fitzgerald JF. Cholestatic disorders of infancy. *Pediatr Clin North Am* 1989;35:357.

37. Kyllo J, Collins MM, Vetter KL, et al. Linkage of congenital isolated adrenocorticotropic hormone deficiency to corticotropin releasing hormone locus using sequence repeat polymorphisms. *Am J Med Genet* 1996;62:262.

38. Linder BL, Esteban NV, Yergey AL, et al. Cortisol production rate in childhood and adolescence. *J Pediatr* 1990;117:892.

39. Goellner MH, Ziegler EE, Fomon SI. Urination during the first three years of life. *Nephron* 1981;28:174.

40. Rees L, Brook CGD, Shaw JCL, et al. Hyponatremia in the first week of life in preterm infants: parts I and II. *Arch Dis Child* 1984;59:414.

41. Judd BA, Haycock GB, Dalton N, et al. Hyponatremia in premature babies and following surgery in older children. *Acta Paediatr Scand* 1987;76:385.

42. Newton MA, Laragh JH. Effect of corticotropin on aldosterone excretion and plasma renin in normal subjects, in essential hypertension and in primary aldosteronism. *J Clin Endocrinol Metab* 1968;28:1006.

43. David JO, Yankopoulos NA, Lieberman F, et al. Role of the anterior pituitary in the control of aldosterone secretion in experimental secondary hyperaldosteronism. *J Clin Invest* 1960;39:765.

44. Migeon CJ, Kenny EM, Kowarski A, et al. The syndrome of congenital adrenocortical unresponsiveness to ACTH. *Pediatr Res* 1968;2:501.

45. Shepard TH, Landing BH, Mason DG. Familial Addison's disease. *Am J Dis Child* 1959;97:154.

46. Moshang T Jr, Rosenfield RL, Bongiovanni AM, et al. Familial glucocorticoid insufficiency. *J Pediatr* 1973;82:821.

47. Miller WL, Levine LS. Molecular and clinical advances in congenital adrenal hyperplasia. *J Pediatr* 1987;111:1.

48. Simard J, Rheaume E, Sanchez R, et al. Molecular basis of congenital adrenal hyperplasia due to 3β-hydroxysteroid dehydrogenase deficiency. *Mol Endocrinol* 1993;7:716.

49. Cara J, Moshang T, Bongiovanni AM. Elevated 17 hydroxyprogesterone and testosterone in a newborn male with 3β-hydroxysteroid dehydrogenase deficiency. *N Engl J Med* 1985;313:618.

50. Eberlein WR, Bongiovanni AM. Plasma and urinary corticosteroids in hypertensive form of congenital adrenal hyperplasia. *J Biol Chem* 1956;223:85.

51. Goldsmith O, Solomon DH, Horton R. Hypogonadism and mineralocorticoid excess: the 17-hydroxylase deficiency syndrome. *N Engl J Med* 1967;277:673.

52. Eberlein WR, Bongiovanni AM. Defective steroidal biogenesis in congenital adrenal hyperplasia. *Pediatrics* 1958;21:661.

53. Ulick S, Gautier E, Vetterik K, et al. An aldosterone biosynthetic defect in a salt-losing disorder. *J Clin Endocrinol Metab* 1964;24:669.

54. Visser HK, Cost WS. A new hereditary defect in the biosynthesis of aldosterone: urinary C 21-corticosteroid pattern in three related patients with a salt-losing syndrome, suggesting an 18-oxidation defect. *Acta Endocrinol* 1964;47:589.

55. Bose HS, Sugawara K, Strauss JF III, et al. The pathophysiology and genetics of congenital lipoid hyperplasia. *N Engl J Med* 1996;335:1870.

56. Pang S, Pollack MS, Marshall RN, et al. Prenatal treatment of congenital adrenal hyperplasia due to 21-hydroxylase deficiency. *N Engl J Med* 1990;322:111.

57. Speiser PW, Laforgia N, Kato K, et al. First trimester prenatal treatment and molecular genetic diagnosis of congenital adrenal hyperplasia (21-hydroxylase deficiency). *J Clin Endocrinol Metab* 1990;70:838.

58. Pang S, Hotchkiss J, Drash AL, et al. Microfilter paper method for 17-hydroxyprogesterone RIA: screen for congenital adrenal hyperplasia. *J Clin Endocrinol Metab* 1977;45:1003.

59. Weiner D, Smith J, Dahlem S, et al. Serum adrenal steroid levels in full term infants. *J Pediatr* 1987;110:122.

60. Lee MM, Rajagopalen L, Berg GJ, et al. Serum adrenal steroid concentrations in premature infants. *J Clin Endocrinol Metab* 1989;69:1133.

61. Fisher DA, Hobel CJ, Garza R, et al. Thyroid function in the preterm fetus. *Pediatrics* 1970;46:208.

62. Dussault J, Row VV, Lickrish G, et al. Studies of serum triiodothyronine concentration in maternal and cord blood: transfer of triiodothyronine across the human placenta. *J Clin Endocrinol Metab* 1969;29:595.

63. Pittman CS, Chambers JB Jr, Read VH. The extrathyroidal conversion rate of thyroxine to triiodothyronine in normal man. *J Clin Invest* 1971;50:1187.

64. Burgus R, Dunn TF, Desiderio DM, et al. Characterization of ovine hypothalamic hypophysiotropic TSH-releasing factor. *Nature* 1970;226:321.

65. Nair RMG, Barret JF, Bowers CX, et al. Structure of porcine thyrotropin releasing hormone. *Biochemistry* 1970;9:1103.

66. Lowrey GH, Aster RH, Carr EA, et al. Early diagnostic criteria of congenital hypothyroidism. *Am J Dis Child* 1958;96:131.

67. Childs B, Gardner LI. Etiologic factors in sporadic cretinism. *Ann Hum Genet* 1954;19:90.

68. Greig WR, Henderson AS, Boyle JA, et al. Thyroid dysgenesis in two pairs of monozygotic twins and in a mother and child. *J Clin Endocrinol Metab* 1966;26:1309.

69. Blizzard RM, Chandler RW, Landing BH, et al. Maternal autoimmunization to thyroid as a probable cause of athyrotic cretinism. *N Engl J Med* 1960;262:327.

70. Dumont JE, Vassart G, Refetoff S. Thyroid disorders. In: Scriver CR, Beaudet AC, Sly WS, et al, eds. *The metabolic basis of inherited disease*, 6th ed. New York: McGraw-Hill, 1989:1843.

71. Savoie JC, Thompoulos P, Savoie F. Studies on mono and di-iodohistidine: I. The identification of histidines from thyroidal iodoproteins and their peripheral metabolism in the normal man and rat. *J Clin Invest* 1973;52:106.

72. Savoie JC, Massin JP, Savoie F. Studies on mono and di-iodohistidine: II. Congenital goitrous hypothyroidism with thyroglobulin defect and iodohistidine-rich iodoalbumin production. *J Clin Invest* 1973;52:116.

73. Burrow GN. Neonatal goiter after maternal propylthiouracil therapy. *J Clin Endocrinol Metab* 1965;5:403.

74. Herbst AL, Selenkow JA. Hyperthyroidism during pregnancy. *N Engl J Med* 1965;273:627.

75. Kampmann JP, Johansen K, Hansen JM, Helweg J. Propylthiouracil in human milk: revision of a dogma. *Lancet* 1980;1:736

76. Lamberg BA, Ikonen E, Osterlund K, et al. Antithyroid treatment of maternal hyperthyroidism during lactation. *Clin Endocrinol* 1984;21:81.

77. Azizi F. Effect of methimazole treatment of maternal thyrotoxicosis on thyroid function in breastfeeding infants. *J Pediatr* 1996;128:855.

78. Refetoff S, DeWind LT, DeGroot LJ. Familial syndrome combining deaf-mutism, stippled epiphyses, goiter, and abnormally high PBI: possible target organ refractoriness to thyroid hormone. *J Clin Endocrinol Metab* 1967;27:279.

79. Bode HH, Danon M, Weintraub BD, et al. Partial target organ resistance to thyroid hormone. *J Clin Invest* 1973;52:776.

80. Stanbury JB, Rocmans P, Butler UK, et al. Congenital hypothyroidism with impaired thyroid response to thyrotropin. *N Engl J Med* 1968;279:1132.

81. French FS, Van Wyk JJ. Fetal hypothyroidism: I. Effects of thyroxine on neural development. II. Fetal versus maternal contributions to fetal thyroxine requirements. III. Clinical implications. *J Pediatr* 1964;64:589.

82. Committee on Genetics, American Academy of Pediatrics. Screening for congenital deficiency of thyroid hormone. *Pediatrics* 1977;60:389.

83. Willi SM, Moshang T Jr. Diagnostic dilemmas: results of screening tests for congenital hypothyroidism. *Pediatr Clin North Am* 1991;38;555.

84. Klein AH, Meltzer S, Kenny FM. Improved prognosis in congenital hypothyroidism treated before age 3 months. *J Pediatr* 1972;81:912.

85. Glorieux J, Dussault J, Letarte J, et al. Preliminary results on the mental development of hypothyroid infants detected by the Quebec screening program. *J Pediatr* 1983;102:19.

86. New England Congenital Hypothyroidism Collaborative. Characteristics of infantile hypothyroidism discovered on neonatal screening. *J Pediatr* 1984;102:539.

87. Reuss ML, Paneth N, Pinto-Martin JA, et al. The relation of transient hypothyroxinemia in preterm infants to neurologic development at two years of age. *N Engl J Med* 1996;334;821.

88. van Wassenaer AG, Kok JH, de Vijlder JJ, et al. Effects of thyroxine supplementation on neurologic development in infants born at less than 30 weeks' gestation. *N Engl J Med* 1997;336:21.

89. Foley TP Jr, White C, New A. Juvenile Graves' disease: usefulness and limitations of thyrotropin receptor antibody determinations. *J Pediatr* 1989;110:378.

90. Riopel DA, Mullins CE. Congenital thyrotoxicosis with paroxysmal atrial tachycardia. *Pediatrics* 1972;50:140.

91. Farrehi C. Accelerated maturity in fetal thyrotoxicosis. *Clin Pediatr* 1968;7:134.

92. Hollingsworth DR, Mabry CC, Eckard JM. Hereditary aspects of Grave's disease in infancy and childhood. *J Pediatr* 1972;81:446.

CHAPTER 42

Renal Disease

Luc P. Brion, Lisa M. Satlin, and Chester M. Edelmann, Jr.

DEVELOPMENTAL PHYSIOLOGY

The kidneys play a central role in the physiologic transition from fetal to postnatal life. Whereas homeostasis *in utero* is maintained largely by the placenta, adaptation to the extrauterine environment requires that the kidneys assume responsibility for regulating water and solute balance. Although the neonatal kidney traditionally has been characterized as dysfunctional, closer analysis indicates that the kidney functions at a level that is appropriate to the growing infant's physiologic needs, except in very-low-birth-weight (VLBW) infants.

Embryology

Embryologic development of the definitive mammalian kidney, the metanephros, is preceded by the transient appearance of two primitive kidneys: the rudimentary pronephros, which appears at 3 weeks and disappears by 5 weeks of fetal life, and the mesonephros, which appears at 5 weeks and degenerates by 12 weeks (1). The ureteric bud, an offshoot of the mesonephric duct, ultimately forms the ureter, pelvis, calyces, and collecting ducts of the metanephros. Importantly, the ureteric bud induces formation of nephrons within the metanephric blastema. The nephroblastic cells of the blastema, on contact with the ureteric bud, differentiate into the glomerulus, proximal convoluted tubule, loop of Henle, and distal convoluted tubule of the metanephric kidney, which first appears at 5 weeks and begins to produce urine by 10 weeks of gestation (2).

Nephronogenesis proceeds in a centrifugal pattern. Thus, the first nephrons to develop are those residing in the juxtamedullary region, whereas the youngest are located in the superficial cortex, in the nephrogenic zone. In the 22-week-old human fetus, all glomeruli present belong to juxtamedullary nephrons. At a conceptional age of 40 to 42 weeks, the juxtamedullary glomeruli are about twice the size of the outer cortical glomeruli. By 1 year of age, the juxtamedullary glomeruli are only about 20% larger than cortical glomeruli, similar to the relationship observed in the adult.

The full complement of approximately 1 million nephrons per kidney in the human is achieved at a body weight of about 2,300 g or 36 weeks' gestational age (GA) (3). When birth occurs before 36 weeks' conceptional age, nephron formation continues until a full complement is achieved. Once complete, nephronogenesis never is resumed, even after extensive loss of renal tissue. Thus, the full-term infant is born with as many nephrons as he or she will have for the duration of life.

Physiologic, biochemical, and enzymatic maturation of newly formed nephrons may lag behind anatomic maturation by weeks or months. Thus, the immature kidney is characterized by structural and functional heterogeneity arising from the concurrent presence of nephrons in diverse stages of differentiation.

Renal Physiology

Urine produced by the metanephric kidneys of 10- to 16-week-old fetuses contributes to the formation of amniotic fluid (2,3). Although renal function is not necessary for long-term regulation of fetal water and electrolyte homeostasis, a process assumed by the placenta, evidence indicates its importance in normal growth (4), lung development (5), and protection from acute changes in fetal

L. P. Brion: Department of Pediatrics, Albert Einstein College of Medicine and Jack D. Weiler Hospital of the Montefiore Medical Center, Bronx, New York

L. M. Satlin: Division of Pediatric Nephrology, Department of Pediatrics, Mount Sinai School of Medicine, New York, New York

C. M. Edelmann, Jr.: Department of Pediatrics, Albert Einstein College of Medicine, Bronx, New York

vascular volume (6). The hourly rate of urine production in normal fetuses is about 5 mL at 20 weeks, 10 mL at 30 weeks, increasing to up to 50 mL at 40 weeks (2,7).

Renal Blood Flow

Renal blood flow (RBF) in the human fetus, measured by Doppler ultrasonography, increases from 20 mL/min at 25 weeks of gestation to more than 60 mL/min at 40 weeks (8). The effective renal plasma flow (ERPF) has traditionally been calculated from the renal clearance of the organic acid para-aminohippurate (PAH), corrected for the fraction of PAH extracted by the kidney (9); the value for ERPF divided by (100 − hematocrit [%])/100 provides an estimate of RBF. The ERPF increases from 20 mL/min/1.73 m^2 at 30 weeks of GA to 45 mL/min/1.73 m^2 by 35 weeks and 83 mL/min/1.73 m^2 at term (9). During the first 3 months of postnatal life, ERPF increases rapidly to 300 mL/min/1.73 m^2; by 24 months of age, ERPF averages 650 mL/min/1.73 m^2, similar to adult values (9).

Because the renal extraction ratio for PAH varies with age, calculated values of ERPF must be interpreted with caution in the fetus and neonate. Indeed, the rate of extraction of PAH in the full-term newborn at 1 week of age is only about 60%, reaching 90%, the adult value, by 5 months (10). PAH clearance averages 148 mL/min/1.73 m^2 in full-term infants at 2 weeks of life, increasing to 200 mL/min/1.73 m^2 by 2 to 3 months (11). PAH clearance, corrected for body surface area (BSA), reaches adult levels sometime between 1 and 2 years of age (9). The incomplete PAH extraction early in life appears to arise from the relatively greater blood flow to juxtamedullary nephrons and efferent arteriovenous shunting in cortical nephrons (see following), thereby allowing blood to bypass PAH-transporting segments of the nephron. In addition, the organic acid secretory pathways in the proximal tubule are immature early in development (12). Thus, RBF and renal plasma flow (RPF) will be underestimated by PAH clearance alone in neonates, particularly in premature infants, in the absence of determination of the PAH extraction ratio.

The rate of RBF is determined by the cardiac output and the ratio of renal to systemic vascular resistance. Developmental changes in both hemodynamic determinants contribute to the postnatal increase in RBF.

The two kidneys of the adult, which comprise 0.5% of the total body mass, receive approximately 20% to 25% of the total cardiac output, corresponding to a RBF of 4 mL/min/g kidney weight. In contrast, the previable fetus receives only about 5% of the cardiac output, and the 1-week-old term infant receives about 9% (13).

Although it has been proposed that imposition of functional demand at birth causes a dramatic increase in RBF, experimental evidence suggests that clamping of the umbilical cord does not, in itself, result in an immediate increase in RBF (14). Indeed, RBF has been shown to increase progressively to 6% of cardiac output by the end of the first week, reaching 15% to 18% by the end of the first month of life (15). Because additional increases in the percentage of cardiac output received by the kidneys occur in parallel with increases in renal mass, the rate of RBF per unit kidney weight thereafter remains relatively constant.

The intrarenal distribution of RBF in the newborn differs from that reported in the adult, reflecting the relative size and number of glomeruli present in the different regions of the kidney at that stage of development. The newborn kidney has a greater percentage of blood flow to the inner cortical and medullary areas compared to the adult (Fig. 42–1) (16,17). Maturation is accompanied by a redistribution of blood flow toward the superficial cortex, so that the ratio of inner cortical to outer cortical blood flow becomes progressively less than in the fetus (15,16–18). At maturity, about 93% of RBF goes to the cortex, which constitutes about 75% of the renal mass, whereas only 7% is distributed to the renal medulla and perirenal fat.

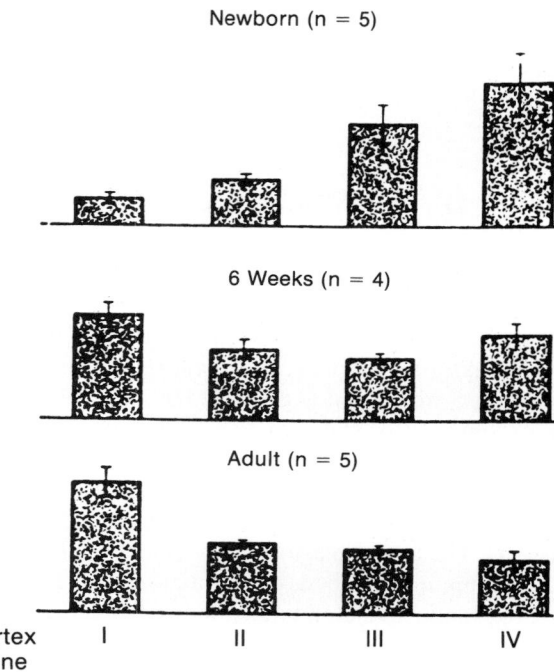

FIG. 42–1. Postnatal changes in the intrarenal distribution of blood flow. Relative rates of blood flow per glomerulus in the four cortical zones of the canine kidney. Zone I represents the most superficial region, and zone IV represents the deepest. The total height of the bars in each age group is equal. At birth, the blood flow to the superficial cortex was lowest, with most blood flow perfusing the deep cortex. By 6 weeks of age, this pattern was reversed. Maturation is accompanied by an increase in blood flow to the outer cortex, due primarily to a decrease in renal vascular resistance. (From ref. 17, with permission.)

The primary factor responsible for the maturational increase in RBF and change in intrarenal distribution is a decrease in renal vascular resistance (19), with the rise in cardiac output and mean arterial blood pressure (MAP) accounting only partially for postnatal changes in renal hemodynamics (19,20). Indeed, the intrarenal vascular resistance, localized both at the afferent and efferent arterioles (21), is much higher in the newborn than in the adult (19,22). The maturational decrease in vascular resistance in the kidney is of greater magnitude than in other organs. Note that the decrease in renal vascular resistance occurs at a time when the systemic vascular resistance increases approximately sixfold.

A major contribution to the evolution of the kidney from a high-resistance, low-flow organ, with most of the blood supplying the inner cortex, into a low-resistance, high-flow organ, with most of the blood supplying the outer cortex, is provided by anatomic changes in the renal vasculature (21). Because RBF can be acutely increased during the neonatal period by volume expansion (23,24), anatomic immaturity cannot be solely responsible for the low perfusion rate of the newborn kidney; a functional constraint also must exist.

Several vasoactive substances suggested to have a role in the regulation of RBF include the renin–angiotensin system, the kallikrein–kinin system, prostaglandins (PG), vasopressin, and atrial natriuretic peptides. The renal nerves and adrenergic nervous system also may play important roles in regulating renal vascular resistance in the neonate. These factors are considered in subsequent sections.

Anatomic Maturation of Vascular Structures

Experimental evidence indicates that the postnatal increase in RBF may be due, in part, to glomerulogenesis or structural changes in the vascular bed, or both. Although development and formation of new glomeruli may continue after birth in premature infants of less than 34 to 36 weeks of conceptional age, the increase in RBF continues long after nephronogenesis is complete (25,26), suggesting that other factors are involved.

The intrarenal vascular system distal to the afferent arteriole in the neonate differs from that in the adult. Variability in the complexity of the glomerular capillary network exists early in postnatal life, with some glomeruli in the nephrogenic zone possessing only a single capillary loop (27). Inner cortical glomeruli at this age generally have a smaller number of capillaries than the adult, although they appear similar in overall structure.

Efferent arterioles in the outer cortex of the neonatal kidney join the venous system by way of venous channels or sinusoids (28). Few of the efferent arterioles descend into the medulla to divide to form the vasa recta and peritubular capillaries. Thus, the renal vasculature of the neonatal kidney is characterized by fewer vessels and by efferent arterioles that connect directly to the venous system, thereby bypassing the proximal tubules (21).

Renin–Angiotensin System

The renin–angiotensin system is very active in the fetus and newborn. The fetus produces renin as early as 17 weeks of GA (29). Plasma renin activity (PRA) is inversely related to GA, decreasing from 60 ng/mL/h at 30 weeks to about 10 to 20 ng/mL/h at term (30). PRA in the newborn may be 20-fold greater than in the adult (31). It increases gradually to a maximum by 3 to 6 days, then falls by 3 to 6 weeks to a level that still exceeds normal adult levels (31).

The localization of renin within the kidney changes with development. Whereas the majority of renin-containing cells are located in the juxtamedullary apparatus in both the newborn and adult, renin is also present in the interlobular arteries and glomeruli in the fetus (32).

The high levels of PRA in the neonate may be due to increased secretion, decreased clearance, or a smaller volume of distribution (33). PRA increases as expected in response to changes in position from recumbent to upright, volume depletion (e.g., hemorrhage, administration of furosemide), and hypoxia (24,33–38). Activity levels decrease after volume expansion with isotonic saline and administration of substances such as the β-adrenergic antagonist propranolol, the PG synthetase inhibitor (PGSI) indomethacin, or vasopressin (33,39–41). The administration of saralasin, a competitive antagonist of angiotensin II (AII), results in an increase in PRA, indicating a functional short-loop feedback mechanism in the newborn (42).

The high levels of PRA in the neonate are associated, in general, with levels of AII and aldosterone (43) that exceed those in the adult. Despite this, in contrast to the adult, systemic blood pressure is low and systemic vascular resistance is very low. Circulating levels of plasma AII decrease during postnatal life in parallel with PRA (44).

Although the renin–angiotensin system does not appear to play a major role in the control of basal blood flow in the fetus and newborn, the system may be important under conditions of stress. An acute reduction in blood volume or onset of hypoxia in the fetus or neonate results in significant increases in renin and AII levels (7,45,46). AII constricts the efferent arteriole more than the afferent arteriole, thereby maintaining glomerular capillary pressure. The action of AII on the fetal and neonatal renal vasculature may be offset by vasodilatory PGs (see later).

Kinins

Bradykinins are potent vasodilator peptides generated from the protein precursor kininogen by the proteolytic enzyme kallikrein. The kinins are inactivated by two kininases, kininase I, which is a carboxypeptidase, and kininase II, which is a peptidyl dipeptide hydrolase and is also known as angiotensin-converting enzyme (ACE). Thus, inhibition of ACE by drugs such as captopril not only decreases AII production but also prevents breakdown of kinins.

Premature infants have undetectable levels of urinary kinins (47); urinary excretion of kallikreins and kinins is lower in newborns than older children (48). The role of these substances in modulating the function of the immature kidney remains unclear.

Prostaglandins

Complex interactions between PGs and the renin–angiotensin and kinin systems have been described, making it difficult to identify the specific effects of PGs on regulation of blood pressure, RBF, and electrolyte and water homeostasis.

Prostaglandins E_2, D_2, and I_2 (PGE_2, PGD_2, PGI_2) have been shown to reduce renal vascular resistance and increase RBF (49,50); prostaglandin $F_{2\alpha}$ ($PGF_{2\alpha}$) and thromboxane A_2 (TXA_2) contribute to vasoconstrictor tone (49,51). The urinary excretion of PGs, including PGE_2, $PGF_{2\alpha}$, and metabolites of PGI_2 and TXA_2, is high in the fetus (52,53), presumably reflecting a high rate of renal synthesis. Urinary excretion of PGE_2 and prostacyclin metabolites in the premature infant is five times that noted at term and 20 times that measured in older children (54). Although rates of excretion decrease after birth, urinary PG excretion remains significantly higher in neonates, especially premature infants, than in children or adults (55,56).

Evidence suggests that PGs produced by the fetal kidney are involved in the regulation of RBF (57). Inhibition of PG synthesis by maternal administration of nonsteroidal antiinflammatory drugs such as indomethacin results in reduction in RBF in the fetus (57,58). In contrast, administration of indomethacin to the unstressed adult causes little change in RBF.

Urinary excretion of PGs decreases in parallel with changes in PRA; however, it remains unclear whether the effects on RBF are mediated by PGs or through their effects on the renin–angiotensin system. Thus, in the newborn, as in the adult, PGs probably play little or no role in control of RBF in the normal subject at rest. PGs may, however, attenuate renal vasoconstriction in pathologic conditions.

Renal Nerves and the Adrenergic System

Circulating catecholamine levels, particularly norepinephrine, are very high just before and immediately after birth (59). The abrupt decrease in catecholamine release postnatally is not associated with any change in renal vascular resistance. It has been suggested that the high vascular resistance of the maturing kidney is due to a high sensitivity of the neonatal renal vasculature to circulating catecholamines, acting directly on α-adrenergic receptors or indirectly on β-adrenergic receptors by means of renin–angiotensin release (60).

In general, the renal vascular bed of the newborn seems to be more sensitive, but less reactive, than that of the adult in response to renal nerve stimulation. The sensitivity of the newborn renal vasculature to the effects of the adrenergic nervous system may be related, in part, to differences in adrenergic receptor density compared to the adult. Innervation of the developing kidney is incomplete at birth (61), and most of the adrenergic receptors in the fetal and neonatal kidney are α-type (62). α-Adrenergic–mediated vasoconstrictor effects are enhanced, whereas β-adrenergic and dopaminergic vasodilatory responses are decreased in the newborn compared to those in the adult (63–65). The gradual appearance of β-adrenergic receptors in the developing kidney may account for some vasodilation of the renal circulation (66).

Dopamine and Dopamine Receptors

Exogenous administration of dopamine, which results in an increase in RBF in the adult, has no effect in the young animal unless there also is an increase in systemic blood pressure and cardiac output (67–69). Renal cortical dopamine-1 receptor density does not appear to change with age, whereas that of dopamine-2 receptors decreases (70).

Arginine Vasopressin

The plasma concentration of arginine vasopressin (AVP) in neonates increases abruptly after birth and is highest in infants whose mothers labored before vaginal delivery (71). Although AVP has the potential to contribute to the increased renal vascular resistance characteristic of the neonate through its action on vascular and glomerular V_1 receptors, its role in regulating basal renal hemodynamics remains to be defined. Infusion of synthetic AVP does not alter RBF and renal vascular resistance in fetal sheep (41); however, AVP may play a role in certain stress-induced reductions in renal hemodynamics. For example, during hemorrhage, but not during hypoxemia, the marked decrease in RBF and increase in renal vascular resistance have been correlated closely with the rise in plasma AVP (7,45,72).

Atrial Natriuretic Factor

Atrial natriuretic peptides and messenger ribonucleic acids (mRNA) are present in both atria and ventricles of the fetus in several species, and circulating levels of these peptides are significantly elevated compared to those of the adult (73–75), due in part to decreased renal clearance. Although the plasma levels of atrial natriuretic factor (ANF) fall to adult levels within the first few weeks of life (75), ANF release appears to respond to various stimuli that are associated with volume overload.

The role of ANF in volume and sodium homeostasis early in life remains uncertain. Infusion of ANF into the renal artery of sheep results in renal vasodilation and an increase in RBF in fetal and newborn animals (76); systemic infusion causes a decline in MAP and thereby reduces RBF (77).

Autoregulation of Renal Blood Flow

Autoregulation in the mature kidney allows for constancy of RBF as renal perfusion pressure varies over a wide range, from about 80 to 150 torr. Although systemic blood pressure in the fetus (i.e., 40–60 torr) and neonate (see Clinical Evaluation) is less than the lower limit of autoregulatory range defined for adults, experimental evidence suggests that the fetus and newborn are able to autoregulate RBF efficiently at their prevailing low arterial pressure (78–80). The autoregulatory response probably is mediated in part by a myogenic response of the renal afferent arteriole (81), which dilates in response to a decrease in renal perfusion pressure, as well as by hormonal factors.

Glomerular Filtration

Initiation of glomerular filtration in the human fetus occurs between weeks 9 and 12 of GA (82,83). It has been suggested that the functional demand placed on the neonatal kidney by cessation of placental function at birth stimulates glomerular filtration rate (GFR) to increase. However, accurate estimates of GFR, assessed by inulin clearance (C_{in}) or true creatinine methodology, indicate a good correlation with GA, a relationship that obtains whether the fetus remains *in utero* or is born prematurely (84–87). Specifically, GFR averages approximately 8 to 10 mL/min/1.73 m^2 at 28 weeks of GA and increases only slightly before 34 weeks conceptional age, although body size and kidney weight increase appreciably during this time. After about 34 weeks conceptional age, at which time GFR averages 25 mL/min/1.73 m^2 regardless of postnatal age, GFR increases rapidly, often by threefold to fivefold within 1 week (84,86,88), coincident with completion of nephronogenesis (Fig. 42–2). Thus, an infant born prematurely at 28 weeks of GA shows little increase in GFR until the infant is about 6 weeks old (i.e., until a conceptional age of 34 weeks is attained). The GFR of neonates who are small for GA is similar to that of infants whose body weight is appropriate for the same GA.

Changes in GFR immediately after birth are variable. In the human, however, the general pattern is one of an

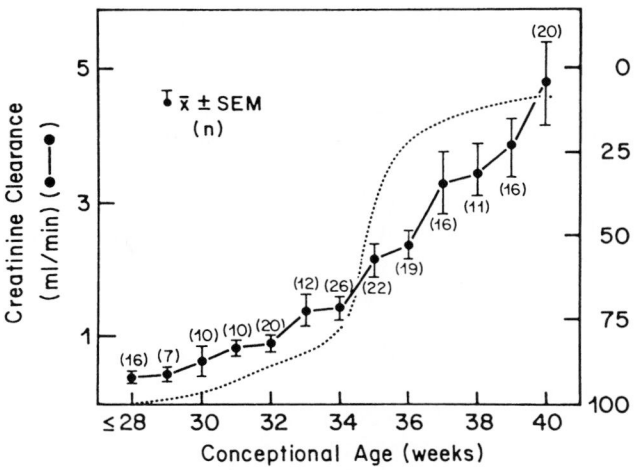

FIG. 42–2. Changes in glomerular filtration rate (mL/mi), estimated by creatinine clearance, and nephrogenic activity in the kidney cortex (%) are plotted as a function of postconceptional age in the human infant. There is a temporal relationship between the accelerated rate of increase in glomerular filtration rate and completion of nephrogenesis after 34 weeks of gestation. (From Arant BS. Neonatal adjustments to extrauterine life. In: Edelmann CM Jr, ed. *Pediatric kidney disease.* Boston: Little, Brown and Company, 1992:1021.)

increase in GFR in the first 2 hours, followed by a decrease to lower values at 4 hours (89). During the first 4 months of life, GFR increases rapidly relative to body size, kidney weight, and BSA (8). Thereafter, a slower rise is noted until adult values, determined on the basis of BSA, are reached by 2 years of age (8,90,91). The postnatal increase in GFR in premature infants may lag behind that observed in full-term newborns; at 9 months of age, the GFR of VLBW infants was approximately 70% of that measured in full-term infants of identical age (92). Overall, the increase in absolute GFR (in milliliters per minute) observed during development in a number of species is about 25-fold.

Total kidney GFR (TKGFR) is determined by the number of functional nephrons and the rate of filtration per nephron. Increases in either one or both of these can account for the postnatal increase in GFR.

Analysis of the similar developmental pattern of change in GFR for several mammalian species indicates that an accelerated rate of increase in GFR is observed around the time nephronogenesis is complete. Thus, those species that complete nephronogenesis *in utero*, including the full-term human neonate (2), sheep (15), and guinea pig (93), show a rapid increase in GFR after birth (84,93). In contrast, premature infants continue to produce new nephrons after birth (2,94); GFR increases rapidly only after nephronogenesis has been completed (95).

Glomeruli are formed in the nephrogenic zone of the kidney, that area of the renal cortex directly under the renal capsule. With maturation, these glomeruli migrate to deeper zones of the renal cortex. At birth, the more mature glomeruli in the juxtamedullary cortex, which are nearly as large as glomeruli in the adult kidney, have higher filtration rates than the most recently formed glomeruli in the superficial cortex, some of which may not begin filtration for some time. Thus, GFR, similar to RBF, matures centrifugally. As nephrons enlarge and forces that regulate filtration permit, GFR increases, with most of the surge due to enhanced perfusion of superficial nephrons (15,20,25,93,96), related temporally to the increase in total RBF and its centrifugal redistribution within the renal cortex.

The addition of newly functioning nephrons is insufficient, however, to account for the large increases in GFR observed during maturation. A substantial rise in rate of filtration per nephron also must occur. Measurements of single-nephron GFR (SNGFR) and TKGFR by micropuncture techniques in superficial nephrons of the guinea pig show little increase in SNGFR in the first 2 weeks of life, followed by a surge thereafter that continues until the SNGFR of the adult, about 20 nL/min, is reached by 4 to 5 weeks (93). During this time period, TKGFR increases at a constant rate. These data indicate that the increase in TKGFR arises initially from an increase in SNGFR of deep nephrons; superficial nephrons appear to contribute to TKGFR later.

The process of urine formation starts with ultrafiltration of plasma through the glomerular capillary membrane. The rate of filtration depends on filtration characteristics of the membrane and on the net ultrafiltration pressure, represented by the difference between hydrostatic pressure (i.e., glomerular capillary hydraulic pressure minus the Bowman space pressure) and colloid osmotic pressure within the capillary loop. The capillary hydrostatic pressure promotes filtration, whereas the colloid osmotic pressure of the blood and the hydrostatic pressure in the Bowman space oppose it.

The postnatal increase in GFR may result from changes in all of these variables, including surface area available for filtration, permeability of the filtering membrane, and effective filtration pressure. The variables that must be considered in describing changes in GFR are described by the following formula:

$$SNGFR = P_{uf} \times k \times S,$$

where P_{uf} is the net ultrafiltration pressure, k is the hydraulic conductivity of the glomerular capillary per unit surface area (i.e., index of membrane permeability), and S is the surface area for filtration.

Net Ultrafiltration Pressure

The low systemic blood pressure in the immediate postnatal period, substantially less than in the adult in many mammalian species, suggests that glomerular capillary pressure might be low as well. In fact, measurements of glomerular capillary pressure performed in newborn guinea pigs indicate an increase from 18 to 38 torr between days 1 and 30 of life. During this same period, MAP increases from 40 to 60 torr (21). Concomitantly, plasma oncotic pressure rises, as does proximal tubular pressure, an index of the pressure in the Bowman space. The net effect of these changes is a 2.5-fold increase in net ultrafiltration pressure between birth and 50 days of life, an increase accounting for only about 10% of the 25-fold increase in GFR observed with maturation (21).

K_f

K_f, the product of the total surface area available for filtration (S) and the hydraulic conductivity of the capillary (k), provides an index of the net permeability property of the glomerular capillary. An increase in K_f appears to be necessary for the increases in glomerular plasma flow and SNGFR observed during the later stages of maturation.

Measurements of hydraulic conductivity, or water permeability per unit surface area, have not been performed during development. Analysis of the clearance of macromolecules in dogs suggests that changes in the permeability characteristics of the glomerular capillary membrane play only a small role in the increase in GFR with development (97).

Glomerular capillary surface area increases during development by an average of fourfold in the juxtamedullary glomeruli and by tenfold in the superficial glomeruli, providing a combined increase in capillary surface area of approximately eightfold during the first 6 weeks of life (98–100), indicating that the maturational increase in GFR is caused primarily by an increase in glomerular surface area.

Many of the vasoactive substances known to affect RBF also influence GFR. Cortisone and growth hormone have been reported to increase GFR concomitant with an increase in RBF (101,102). AII, a powerful vasoconstrictor of both afferent and efferent arterioles, present in high circulating levels in the infant, is known to reduce RBF and constrict the glomerular mesangium, thereby reducing the surface area available for filtration (103); thus, it may determine glomerular blood flow and hydrostatic pressure within glomerular capillaries. A role for PGs in regulation of GFR has been suggested by the observation that administration of PGSI to newborn babies results in a transient decrease of GFR (104,105).

Autoregulation of Glomerular Filtration Rate

In the adult, RBF and GFR are maintained over a wide range of MAPs (i.e., 60–150 torr). This autoregulation is accomplished primarily by changes in renal vascular resistance at the level of the afferent and efferent arterioles. As MAP falls, efferent arteriolar resistance increases, resulting in maintenance of glomerular capillary pressure and preservation of filtration rate. If MAP falls below a critical lower value, however, renal perfusion pressure and GFR decrease and prerenal azotemia ensues. On the other hand, as MAP increases, afferent arteriolar resistance increases to limit a rise in glomerular hydrostatic pressure and thus protect the glomeruli from the effects of systemic hypertension. Experimental evidence indicates that the full-term newborn also can autoregulate, albeit at a lower range of MAP (78,106). The autoregulatory range, however, has not been established.

Filtration Fraction

The normal balance between GFR and RBF is calculated as the filtration fraction (GFR/RPF) and averages 0.2 in the adult kidney. Evidence indicates that the developmental increase in filtration fraction appears to be determined mainly by changes in GFR. RBF increases in a linear fashion that parallels renal growth, whereas GFR increases in a nonlinear pattern until nephronogenesis is complete.

Tubuloglomerular Feedback

Maturational relationships between tubular flow and GFR (i.e., tubuloglomerular feedback) also occur with growth; this mechanism is thought to contribute to the autoregulatory maintenance of RBF and GFR. A stimulus (e.g., tubular flow rate, ion concentration) at the macula densa is transmitted to the vascular structures of the nephron that control GFR. The feedback system aims at maintaining a constant rate of water and salt delivery to distal segments of the nephron in which reabsorption is regulated to maintain fluid balance. The tubuloglomerular feedback mechanism (i.e., change of SNGFR induced by a given change in tubular flow rate) is maximally sensitive in a range that corresponds to the values of SNGFR and tubular flow rate under normal conditions. As GFR increases with maturation, the maximal response and flow range of maximum sensitivity also increase, so that the relative sensitivity of the tubuloglomerular feedback mechanism is unaltered during growth (107,108).

Tubular Function

Sodium, bicarbonate, phosphate, amino acids, and glucose are reabsorbed primarily by the proximal tubule. Although most filtered potassium also is reabsorbed proximally, net urinary potassium secretion occurs in the distal tubule, primarily in the cortical collecting duct. Tubular secretion of organic acids occurs in the proximal tubule. Hydrogen ion transport occurs in both the proximal and distal tubules.

Sodium

Term infants are in a state of positive sodium balance, a requisite for growth, particularly of bone. Although the sodium intake per unit of BSA is generally smaller in the newborn than in the adult, the magnitude of this positive balance remains relatively constant within a wide range of sodium intakes (109,110). The tendency of the neonatal kidney to retain sodium may become problematic under conditions of salt loading. Exogenous administration of a sodium load to an adult is followed by immediate expansion of the extracellular fluid (ECF) space. This signals the kidney to decrease tubular sodium reabsorption, resulting in increased excretion of sodium and a relatively rapid return of the ECF space to the baseline condition. Full-term newborn infants given a sodium load in excess of 12 mEq/kg/d experience a rise in serum sodium levels, abnormal increase in weight, and generalized edema (111). The limited capacity of the neonatal kidney to excrete a sodium load compared to its mature counterpart appears to be due more to factors related to tubular sodium reabsorption than to the low GFR (112).

The fractional excretion of sodium (FENa), which may be as high as 20% during fetal life, decreases progressively during gestation (113—115), so that the FENa in the full-term newborn generally averages about 0.2% (115,116). After the first few hours of postnatal life, the FENa and urinary sodium excretion decline rapidly, possibly secondary to contraction of the ECF volume (113). Premature infants of less than 30 weeks of GA continue to show elevated values of FENa, similar to those observed in the fetus, which may exceed 5% during the first few days of life (115,117). In these infants, excessive urinary sodium losses exceeding dietary sodium intake (e.g., breast milk, low-salt formula) often create a state of negative sodium balance and loss of body weight during the first 2 weeks of life (i.e., hyponatremia of prematurity). It has been estimated that these infants require at least 2 mEq/kg/d of supplemental sodium to maintain a normal sodium concentration and remain in positive balance (118,119). Conditions that may augment the FENa include hypoxia, respiratory distress, hyperbilirubinemia, acute tubular necrosis (ATN), administration of theophylline or diuretics, polycythemia, and increased fluid and salt intake (54,120–122).

Studies in several mammalian species demonstrate parallel and proportionate increases in GFR and the reabsorptive capacity of the proximal tubule after birth, consistent with maintenance of glomerulotubular balance during postnatal development. Thus, the fractional reabsorption of sodium in the proximal tubule remains constant at about 70% in euvolemic animals (25,92). Functional glomerulotubular imbalance may exist in the premature infant whereby the reabsorptive capacity of the proximal tubule lags behind the capacity for glomerular filtration (123,124).

The observation that the fractional reabsorption of sodium in the proximal tubule of the full-term newborn is similar to that observed in the adult indicates that the sodium retention characteristic of the full-term infant must arise from enhanced reabsorption in more distal segments of the nephron (125). The avidity of the distal nephron for sodium reabsorption, which increases with GA (124), may be related to the high levels of aldosterone prevailing early in postnatal life (34). Clearance studies in premature infants (43,126), however, and investigations in neonatal laboratory animals (127,128) reveal a relative insensitivity of the immature kidney to aldosterone. Sulyok et al. (43) showed that infants born between 30 and 32 weeks of GA and studied at 1 week of age, while receiving 1.5 to 2.0 mEq/kg/d of sodium, generally were in negative sodium balance with high urinary sodium excretion rates. PRA was directly related to urinary sodium loss but was inversely related to plasma aldosterone concentration and sodium balance. There was a positive correlation between plasma aldosterone concentration and sodium balance, however, suggesting that premature infants can augment their PRA in response to salt wasting, but that their adrenals initially fail to respond adequately to this stimulation. The relative hypoaldosteronism results in an inability to conserve sodium, manifested clinically by weight loss and hyponatremia.

The sodium wasting characteristic of the premature infant may also be due to a paucity of sodium-selective channels in the luminal membrane of the distal nephron (129), that segment responsible in the adult for the final renal reabsorption of urinary sodium. Paradoxically, preterm infants of 34 to 36 weeks of GA excrete a sodium load more efficiently than do term newborns, but not as efficiently as adults (86,117,126). In these subjects with decreased proximal reabsorption under basal conditions, the further depression in proximal reabsorption during saline loading increases distal delivery even further, presumably exceeding the reabsorptive capacity of this segment.

In addition to the renin–angiotensin–aldosterone system, sodium excretion during maturation is regulated by circulating catecholamines, renal sympathetic innervation, ANF, and glucocorticoids. Studies in newborns indicate a relatively poor natriuretic response to ANF compared to their adult counterparts (73,130,131). Renal PGE_2 and PGI_2 are natriuretic in the adult. Thus, administration of indomethacin to the adult reduces sodium excretion; in contrast, however, this inhibitor causes a natriuresis when administered to fetal sheep, despite a decrease in fetal RBF (57). Administration of cortisol to fetal sheep is associated with depression of proximal sodium reabsorption (101,132).

Potassium

Potassium is transported actively across the placenta from mother to fetus (133). Indeed, fetal potassium is maintained at levels exceeding 5 mEq/L even in the face of maternal potassium deficiency (133,134).

Unlike adults who are in zero balance, growing infants maintain a state of positive potassium balance (43,135). The relative conservation of potassium early in life generally is associated with higher plasma potassium values than in the adult (124,135—137); plasma potassium levels average 5.2 mEq/L from birth to age 4 months, decreasing to 4.2 mEq/L by 3 years of age (137). The renal clearance of potassium in the infant is less than in the older child, even when corrected for GFR (137). Children and adults ingesting a regular diet containing sodium in excess of potassium excrete urine with a sodium-to-potassium ratio greater than 1, as expected. Although the sodium-to-potassium ratio of breast milk and commercial infant formulas averages 0.5, the urinary sodium-to-potassium ratio of the newborn also is greater than 1, consistent with significant potassium retention.

Infants, like adults, can excrete potassium at a rate that exceeds its glomerular filtration when given a potassium load, indicating the capacity for net tubular secretion (138); however, the rate of potassium excretion per unit body weight in response to exogenous potassium loading is less in newborn than older animals (139). Clearance studies in saline-expanded dogs also provide indirect evidence for a diminished secretory and enhanced reabsorptive capacity of the immature distal nephron to potassium (140).

Filtered potassium is reabsorbed almost entirely in proximal segments of the nephron, urinary potassium being derived predominantly from distal potassium secretion. Therefore, potassium balance, at least in the adult, is maintained by renal secretion rather than reabsorption. Approximately 50% of the filtered load of potassium is reabsorbed along the proximal tubule in both newborns and adults (136). Up to 40% of the filtered load of potassium reaches the superficial distal tubule of the newborn, in contrast to about 10% in mature animals, providing evidence for functional immaturity of the loop of Henle (136,141).

Potassium secretion in the cortical collecting duct, that segment responsible for urinary potassium secretion in the adult, is low early in life and cannot be stimulated by high urinary flow rates (142). Although Na–K–ATPase activity in the neonatal collecting duct segments has been reported to be only 50% of that measured in the mature nephron (143), cell potassium content is similar in neonatal and mature collecting ducts (144), consistent with a low membrane permeability of this segment to potassium. Electrophysiologic analysis has confirmed the absence of functional potassium secretory channels in the luminal membrane of the neonatal cortical collecting duct (145); these unique channels appear only after the second week of postnatal life, coincident with the appearance of potassium secretion in this segment (145). Plasma aldosterone concentrations in the fetus and newborn are high compared to that in the adult; yet, clearance studies demonstrate a relative insensitivity of the potassium secretory process to this hormone early in life (146).

Acid–Base

The acid–base status of the fetus is maintained by placental function and maternal mechanisms. The fetal kidney in the second one-half of pregnancy, however, is able to acidify the urine (147,148). Immediately after birth, the acid–base state of the full-term newborn is characterized by a metabolic acidosis (149). Recovery occurs within 24 hours in the full-term infant, an increase accomplished in large measure through pulmonary excretion of CO_2 (150).

The normal range for serum bicarbonate is lower for preterm infants (16 to 20 mmol/L) and full-term infants (19 to 21 mEq/L) than for children and adults (24 to 28 mmol/L), presumably due to a low renal tubular bicarbonate threshold (151—154). The low threshold may arise from a relatively expanded ECF compartment in the neonate or a low fractional reabsorption of bicarbonate in the proximal tubule (151,155,156). The transcription, translation, and activation of selective proximal tubular transport proteins responsible for bicarbonate absorption may be stimulated early in postnatal life by a perinatal surge in glucocorticoid levels (157). Experimental evidence suggests that renal tubular carbonic anhydrase activity, already present in the human fetal kidney in late gestation (158), does not limit the capacity of the neonatal kidney for bicarbonate reabsorption.

Term newborns generally are able to excrete a maximal acid load within the first 2 months of life (159). Premature infants born at 34 to 36 weeks of GA and studied 1 to 3 weeks after birth exhibit rates of excretion of net acid, titratable acid, and ammonium that are about 50% lower than term babies of similar postnatal age; net acid excretion increases to levels observed in term newborns only after 3 weeks of age (159,160). In response to acid loading with ammonium chloride, urinary pH of premature infants rarely decreases below 5.9 until the second month of life (161). In contrast, by the end of the second postnatal week, urine pH values of 5.0 or lower, comparable to those in the adult, are consistently observed in term infants (153,162).

The capacity of the neonatal kidney for renal acidification is blunted, due in part to a limited excretion of urinary buffers, including phosphate and ammonium ions. The rates of ammonia synthesis and excretion are low in the neonate (163) and, in response to acid loading, do not increase to mature values until 2 months of age (153,154,164). Phosphate loading, administration of cow milk that is rich in protein and phosphate instead of breast milk, or high-protein feeding enhances the ability of the newborn to excrete titratable acids and ammonia (162). Before feeding, newborns excrete 10% to 25% of H^+ as titratable acid. In 1-week-old babies fed cow milk, net acid excretion per kilogram body weight is high, and 60% of urinary acid is in the form of titratable acid (165). In contrast, 1-week-old breast-fed babies, who ingest a milk low in phosphate and protein, excrete 60% less net acid than cow-milk–fed infants, and only 20% of this is titratable acid (165).

The final site of urinary acidification is the renal collecting duct. Functional immaturity of this segment and the acid–base transporting intercalated cells therein may further limit the ability of the neonate to eliminate an acid load (166,167). Postnatal differentiation of intercalated cells has been shown to include an increase in density of proton pumps (168) and base-extruding anion exchangers (169).

Up to 10% of preterm infants develop a partially compensated hyperchloremic metabolic acidosis during weeks 1 to 3 of life (i.e., late metabolic acidosis) (154), despite an otherwise healthy appearance. Typically, spontaneous remission occurs in the subsequent 2 weeks. These infants are characterized further by an apparent delay in postnatal weight gain despite ample dietary intake, suggesting a high rate of endogenous acid formation in infants whose dietary intake exceeds their anabolic capacity (170). Although infants provided supplemental sodium bicarbonate to maintain acid–base homeostasis showed greater increases in length than controls, there were no differences in weight gain between the two groups (152,171). Because supplementation with sodium results in an increase in serum bicarbonate, it has been suggested that the late metabolic acidosis and low bicarbonate threshold results in part from large urinary sodium losses.

Calcium

Urinary excretion of calcium varies inversely with GA in the first week of life and varies directly with urine flow and sodium excretion (see Chap. 36) (172). High rates of calcium excretion may contribute in part to early neonatal hypocalcemia, which occurs in the first 24 to 48 hours of life (173). The urinary calcium-to-creatinine ratio in full-term infants ranges from 0.05 to 1.2 during the first week of life, but may exceed 2 in premature neonates (172,174). In children more than 1 year of age, the ratio is approximately 0.2, and in adults, the ratio is less than 0.11 (175). Urinary calcium excretion from 1 to 15 years of age averages 2.4 mg/kg/d, with an upper limit of 4 mg/kg/d (175).

The high fractional excretion of calcium in preterm infants may be related to maturational changes in the tubular handling of calcium. Approximately 50% of filtered calcium is reabsorbed along the superficial proximal tubule in mature rats, yet only 1% of filtered calcium is excreted (136). Thus, in the adult, almost one-half of the filtered calcium is reabsorbed at a site beyond the proximal tubule or in deep nephrons (136). The fractional reabsorption of calcium in the loop of Henle, like that for sodium, potassium, and chloride, is low in the neonate (136). Furosemide, methylxanthines, and dexamethasone, drugs frequently administered to premature infants with pulmonary disease, increase urinary calcium excretion, thus increasing the risk for nephrocalcinosis and nephrolithiasis (176—178).

The roles of parathyroid hormone (PTH) and calcitonin in the regulation of renal calcium excretion in the neonatal period are unclear. In mature animals and in adults, PTH decreases the urinary excretion of calcium (179), whereas calcitonin at high doses increases calciuria (180). PTH–responsive adenylate cyclase has been found in renal cortical homogenates from preterm rabbits (181) and in the thick ascending loop of Henle in 2-day-old puppies (182). It has been suggested that neonatal hypocalcemia may be due to end-organ unresponsiveness to PTH. In premature and full-term newborns, however, the administration of exogenous PTH increases urinary excretion of cyclic adenosine monophosphate (cAMP) (183,184), results in a calcemic response, but affects calciuria and phosphaturia only minimally (185). Recent evidence suggests that the postnatal increase in tubular responsiveness to PTH may be related to increasing levels of expression of the recently cloned extracellular calcium-sensing receptor in the developing kidney (186).

Magnesium

Ninety-seven percent of the filtered magnesium is reabsorbed by the mature nephron, largely in the thick ascending limb of the loop of Henle (187). Micropuncture analysis of magnesium transport in developing rats showed efficient renal tubular reabsorption of magnesium in this segment early in life; the fractional reabsorption of magnesium in the loop of Henle had already reached mature values of about 60% in the youngest animals (136). Postnatal maturation is associated with a decrease in the fractional reabsorption of magnesium in the proximal tubule (136). The avid retention of magnesium by the immature kidney likely contributes to the inverse relationship noted between plasma magnesium and somatic maturity in early postnatal life (188).

Phosphate

In contrast to most other transport processes, the capacity of the immature kidney to reabsorb phosphate is greater than in the adult (see Chap. 36) (189,190). The tubular reabsorption of phosphate increases from 85% of the filtered load at 28 weeks of GA to 99% at term and decreases thereafter to about 85% between 3 and 20 months of age. An increase in phosphate load, provided by a change in formula from breast milk to cow milk, results in doubling in the renal clearance of phosphate and a decrease in fractional reabsorption from 95% to 80% (191).

Clearance studies performed in infants and children suggest that phosphate retention in the young is due in large part to the low GFR (190,191). Studies in experimental animals, however, demonstrate enhanced tubular reabsorption early in life (192,193). Younger subjects have a higher maximal net reabsorption (Tm) of phosphate per unit glomerular filtrate (Tm/GFR) than adults (193–195). Micropuncture analysis of newborn and adult guinea pigs confirm a higher fractional reabsorption of phosphate in the newborn proximal tubule (75%) compared to the adult (65%); distal phosphate reabsorption also is higher in younger than older animals (196).

The high intrinsic rate of sodium phosphate cotransport observed in neonatal proximal tubules has been attributed to an abundance of sodium-phosphate transporter proteins in the luminal membrane (197), a high membrane fluidity of the immature nephron (198), a low intracellular phosphate concentration (199), and the hormonal milieu prevailing in the perinatal period (197,198). Glucocorticoids, hormones circulating in high concentrations early in postnatal life, inhibit and growth hormone stimulates proximal tubular phosphate transport (198,200). The high reabsorptive capacity of the immature kidney for phosphate persists after parathyroidectomy (193,195). Serum levels of PTH are low immediately after birth, increasing substantially thereafter to levels in infancy exceeding those observed in later childhood (201,202). Exogenous administration of PTH to humans or experimental animals results in a blunted phosphaturic effect in immature kidneys (181,192). By the end of the first week of life, however, full-term infants exhibit a prompt phosphaturic response and an increase in urinary cAMP excretion after PTH administration.

Glucose

Premature infants of less than 34 weeks of GA have a higher urinary glucose concentration, higher fractional excretion of glucose, and lower maximal reabsorption of glucose than full-term infants and older children (84). However, the maximal reabsorption of glucose factored by GFR, the fractional reabsorption of glucose, is similar in newborn infants and adults (84). Similar observations have been made in experimental animals (95,203). These results provide additional evidence for preservation of glomerulotubular balance, at least in term infants. The lower renal threshold for glucose in newborns compared to their adult counterparts is believed to reflect a greater degree of nephron heterogeneity early rather than later in life (95).

Studies in the rat and guinea pig indicate that the neonatal proximal tubule possesses both high- and low-affinity sodium-coupled glucose transporters mediating reabsorption of filtered glucose in the kidney; interestingly, only the low-affinity high-capacity system is present in adults (204–206). It is not clear when the high-affinity system disappears during maturation, but its presence early in life may enable the anatomically immature kidney to reabsorb sugar more efficiently from the glomerular filtrate.

Organic Acids

Organic acids, including PAH (see Renal Blood Flow) and endogenously produced uric acid, are eliminated by filtration and proximal tubular secretion. Organic acids are transported from the peritubular circulation across the basolateral surface of the proximal tubule to the tubular fluid. The renal clearance of organic acids is low in the neonate, even when corrected for body size, and increases gradually with age (14,207,208). As discussed previously, the limitation in tubular excretion of weak acids may be due in part to the preponderance of blood flow to the juxtamedullary region, bypassing tubular secretory sites. Additional variables that may account for the limited clearance of organic acids include the low GFR, limited energy for transport, and restricted expression of organic anion transporter proteins (209).

Amino Acids

The renal reabsorption of many amino acids, including threonine, serine, proline, glycine, and alanine, is lower in newborn animals and humans than in adults, often resulting in aminoaciduria (210,211). This does not appear to be a generalized defect in amino acid reabsorption because other filtered amino acids (e.g., methionine, isoleucine, leucine, tyrosine) are reabsorbed more completely. Specific transport systems for acidic, basic, and neutral amino acids have been identified in the luminal membrane of proximal tubules in newborn kidneys (212–215). The transient limitation in net transtubular reabsorption of amino acids characteristic of the neonate may arise from intrinsic differences in activity and transport capacity of discrete transport systems, and/or a lower rate of amino acid efflux out of the cell into the peritubular circulation in the neonate compared to the adult, a mechanism that also would account for the high intracellular concentrations of amino acids observed early in life (212).

Urinary Concentration

In mammals, fetal urine is hypotonic with respect to fetal plasma. Yet, the fetal kidney is able to concentrate urine, evidenced by the observation that maternal water deprivation (216) or infusion of AVP into the fetus (217) reduces the fetal urine flow rate and free water clearance.

Urine voided at or shortly after birth generally is hypotonic with respect to plasma (89,218). Maximal urinary concentrating ability in the neonate has been shown to be less than that of children and adults. After fluid deprivation for 12 to 24 hours, the maximal urine osmolality achieved in both premature infants and full-term newborns averages about 500 mOsm/kg (219–222), a value roughly 60% that observed in older children and adults. A few 1- to 2-month-old infants may be able to achieve a urine osmolality as high as 1,000 mOsm/kg, a maximal value generally not seen before 12 months of age (220,222).

The limited ability of infant kidneys to concentrate urine may be related to several factors, including low GFR (see Glomerular Filtration), inability to maintain a corticomedullary osmotic gradient, and diminished responsiveness of the distal nephron to antidiuretic hormone (ADH).

Medullary Gradient. The capacity to concentrate the urine has been directly related to elongation of the loops of Henle and their penetration into the medulla (223). The inner medulla and renal papillae are poorly developed in the immature kidney. In the rat, the 1.6-fold increase in length of the renal medulla correlates well with the 1.5-fold increase in urine osmolality observed between 10 and 20 days of age (223). Associated with this anatomic maturation is the build-up of a high interstitial solute concentration gradient in the medulla. Generation of the corticopapillary osmotic gradient reflects the postnatal maturation of several processes involved in urinary concentration: sodium reabsorption and urea sequestration by the thick ascending limb of the loop of Henle and functional activation of aldose reductase, an enzyme necessary for generation of intracellular osmolytes, important for maintenance of cell function in the concentrated milieu (224–226). These structural and functional limitations of the countercurrent multiplication and exchange systems prevent build-up and maintenance of a medullary gradient in the immature kidney.

Antidiuretic Hormone. The limited ability of the immature kidney to concentrate urine is not due to an inability of the fetus or neonate to synthesize and secrete ADH. Circulating levels of ADH are elevated in preterm and term infants and decrease rapidly in term infants within 24 hours of birth (227,228). Studies in fetal and newborn animals (45,229,230), as well as in human infants (228,231), indicate a qualitatively appropriate response to osmolar or volume stimuli known to affect ADH release. Furthermore, exogenous administration of AVP or 1-des-amino-8-d-AVP (DDAVP) to healthy 1- to 3-week-old newborns leads to a response, albeit of shorter duration and reduced magnitude than that observed at 4 to 6 weeks (232). Thus, the limited concentrating ability of the fetus and newborn also has been attributed to a blunted sensitivity of the immature nephron to ADH, proposed to be due to a paucity of AVP receptors (233), inefficient coupling between AVP receptor binding and cAMP generation (182,234,235), and/or absence of AVP-regulated water channels (236).

The effect of ADH on water transport in the medullary collecting duct is minimal in the neonate. Although expression of the gene encoding the AVP V_2 receptor is detected early in gestation (237), the developmental appearance of the protein has not been rigorously characterized. Cumulative evidence suggests that the AVP intracellular signaling pathway is the immature collecting duct is disrupted at several steps both proximal and distal to cAMP generation (234,235). Recent studies demonstrate that the expression of the renal AVP-regulated water channel, aquaporin-2, is developmentally regulated with low levels observed in the immediate postnatal period; the postnatal increase in abundance of transcript/protein correlates well with the development of urine concentrating ability (236).

Although infants excrete more PGE_2 per unit BSA than do older children (see Prostaglandins), inhibition of PG synthesis in fetal lambs has no effect on urinary concentrating ability (57). Studies at the level of the single collecting duct also indicate that inhibition of endogenous PG production by indomethacin does not substantially increase AVP-stimulated water permeability. In sum, these data suggest that PGs contribute little to the postnatal maturation of renal concentrating ability.

Thus, the limited ability of the neonatal kidney to concentrate the urine is due to structural and functional constraints that together prevent generation of the requisite corticopapillary osmotic gradient.

Urinary Dilution

Premature infants (less than 35 weeks of GA) studied under conditions of maximal water diuresis decrease urine osmolality to 70 mOsm/kg, whereas infants more than 35 weeks of GA are able to reduce urine osmolality to 50 mOsm/kg (124). This is associated with a significantly greater osmolar clearance in the premature infants, indicating that they cannot dilute their urine as well as term infants or adults. Although there is greater proximal sodium rejection in preterm than term infants, the high avidity of the distal nephron for sodium reabsorption allows the neonate, especially the preterm infant, to generate a free water clearance greater than that in adults (112,125,140). Despite the greater capacity for free water clearance, the ability of the neonate to excrete a hypotonic load is limited, presumably due to the low GFR.

CLINICAL EVALUATION OF RENAL FUNCTION AND DISEASE

Early diagnosis of a renal anomaly may help to prevent complications, including those related to the kidney itself

(e.g., progressive loss of renal function due to systemic hypertension, obstructive or reflux uropathy, or infection) and those related to other organs (e.g., cerebral hemorrhage, seizures or congestive heart failure [CHF] secondary to hypertension, ventricular arrhythmia secondary to hyperkalemia, urosepsis). In this section, we review clinical and laboratory features that should raise suspicion of a renal problem and present an approach to establish the correct diagnosis.

Incidence of Renal and Urinary Tract Malformations

Studies using neonatal abdominal palpation as the screening method have shown an incidence of renal and urinary tract malformations of 0.2% to 0.6% (238–240), whereas neonatal autopsy series have had an incidence of 7% to 9% (Table 42–1) (241,242). Series using routine prenatal ultrasound (US) have detected anomalies in 0.1% to 1.4% of fetuses (243–247), of which several cases of mild pyelectasis were diagnosed as normal on postnatal US. Prospective studies using routine US screening in cohorts of neonates or older infants (with or without prenatal US) found an incidence of 1% to 2% (248–252). We found a similar incidence (1.3%) using a perinatal approach that combined family history, prenatal US, physical examination, and case-oriented neonatal imaging (251). In one large series, the male-to-female ratio for hydronephrosis was 2.4:1, compared to 1.4:1 for parenchymal anomalies (253).

History

Family History

Positive family history should be sought for hereditary disease, including renal cystic disease, tubular disorders, and nephrotic syndrome. There is a 9% incidence of asymptomatic renal malformations—most often unilateral renal agenesis—in the first-degree relatives of infants with agenesis or dysgenesis of both kidneys or agenesis of one kidney and dysgenesis of the other (254). A study using US has confirmed that, in some families, bilateral agenesis or dysplasia is inherited as an autosomal dominant trait (renal adysplasia) (255). The clinician should keep in mind that some autosomal dominant diseases have variable penetrance or time of presentation (e.g., adult-type polycystic disease) and that new mutations may occur. In addition, the history for prior fetal loss should be carefully reviewed, with autopsy review if possible.

Teratology

The risk of renal or urinary tract malformations is increased by maternal diabetes and by certain medications or drugs, including alcohol, trimethadione, thalido-

TABLE 42–1. *Incidence of renal and urinary tract malformations in infancy*

Author	No. of subjects	Selection criteria	Method of screening	Most common anomalies (final diagnosis)	No. of subjects with anomalies (% of total)
Sherwood 1956	12,160	Consecutive NN	Palpation confirmation by IVU	Ectopia (7), horseshoe/fused kidneys (5), obstruction (6), Wilms (1)	22 (0.2%)
Museles 1971	12,150	Consecutive NN	Palpation confirmation by IVU	Ectopia (7), horseshoe (4), agenesis (3)	22 (0.2%)
Brion 1984	1,200	Consecutive NN	Prenatal US (2/3), physical examination, US screening for various indications	Hypoplasia/agenesis (4), obstructive uropathy (8), reflux (1)	15 (1.3%)
Helin 1986	11,986	Consecutive pregnancies	Prenatal US	Hydronephrosis (9), VUR (3), mild dilatation (10), cystic disease (3)	33 (0.3%)
Steinhart 1988	437	Healthy infants	US	VUR (3), obstructive uropathy (3)	6 (1.4%)
Gillerot 1988	900	NN autopsies	Autopsy	Dysplasia/agenesis (30), polycystic kidneys (18), obstructive uropathy (11), cloacal exstrophy (4)	63 (7%)
Scott 1991	1,061	NN in well-baby nursery	Postnatal US, followed by appropriate workup	Duplex kidney (1), solitary kidney (2), hydronephrosis	11 (1.0%)
Scott 1993	242,628	Northern Region Fetal Abnormality Survey	Population survey including both prenatal US and postnatal US	Hydronephrosis (97), VUR (16), renal agenesis (33), MKD (15), dysplasia (6), PKD (11), duplex kidney (15), megaureter (10), urethral valves	451 (2%)
Jelen 1993	1,021	Consecutive neonates	Postnatal US	Hydronephrosis (6), MKD (2), duplication (4), agenesis (2)	20 (2%)
Fugelseth 1994	22,310	Consecutive pregnancies	Prenatal US at 17 and 32 wk	Hydronephrosis (24), MKD (10)	47 (0.2%)
Gunn 1995	3,856	Consecutive pregnancies	Prenatal US after 28 wk, confirmed by postnatal US at 6 d to 6 wk	Transient pylectasis (216), obstructive uropathy (23), VUR (14), MKD (8), urethral valves (3)	54 (1.4%)
Kim 1996	5,442	Consecutive pregnancies	Prenatal US confirmed by US	Hydronephrosis (37), MKD (5), PKD (2), renal agenesis (2), ectopic kidney (1), hypoplastic kidney (1)	48 (0.9%)

IVU, intravenous urography; MKD, multicystic kidney dysplasia; NN, newborn infants; PKD, polycystic kidney disease; US, ultrasonography; VUR, vesicoureteral reflux.

mide, and cocaine (see Appendix I–1). Maternal diabetes, at least in the absence of tight diabetic control initiated before conception, is associated with urogenital malformations, with an incidence of 2.6%, compared to an incidence of 1.2% in controls (256), as well as with neonatal renal venous thrombosis. The risk for renal or urinary tract malformations is high when an infant of a diabetic mother has either a caudal regression syndrome or a femoral hypoplasia–unusual facies syndrome (see Appendix I–1). Fetal alcohol syndrome is associated with unilateral renal agenesis, renal hypoplasia, ureteral duplication, and hydronephrosis (257). A meta-analysis showed that maternal cocaine abuse is associated with an odds ratio of genitourinary malformations of 5.0 (95% confidence interval 1.1 to 23.6); the odds ratio was 6.1 (95% confidence interval 1.2 to 31.3) in studies comparing cocaine–polydrug users to polydrug users without cocaine (258).

Pregnancy

The diagnosis of a urologic problem may be obtained by US performed as a routine examination or as a part of the workup for another anomaly. A high maternal serum or amniotic alpha-fetoprotein (AFP) concentration is associated with several anomalies, including bladder exstrophy or myelodysplasia (which are associated with urinary tract malformations, see Appendix I–1), and with congenital nephrotic syndrome of the Finnish type (CNF). Increased maternal serum AFP concentration is associated with pyelectasis and thick-walled bladder (259). Oligohydramnios may result from amniotic sac rupture or leakage or from fetal oligoanuria. The latter can result from bilateral congenital renal disease, bilateral or lower urinary tract obstruction, or acquired fetal renal disease, e.g., due to maternal administration of indomethacin or ACE inhibitors (260–262) or severe pregnancy-induced hypertension. Among many causes, polyhydramnios may be the first clue to the diagnosis of a nephrogenic defect of urinary concentration, whereas fetal hydrops may be the first sign of congenital nephrotic syndrome.

Dysmorphism

Renal and Urinary Tract Anomalies Associated with Multiple Congenital Anomalies

Any dysmorphic feature (e.g., abnormal ears) should lead the clinician to look for other anomalies and structural defects. Appendix I–1 lists the major signs of multiple congenital anomalies associated with renal and urinary tract anomalies (see Chaps. 40 and 43). The most typical sequence related to kidney disease is the oligohydramnios sequence (i.e., Potter syndrome). This sequence can be due either to prolonged leakage of amniotic fluid

or to intrauterine oligoanuria secondary to bilateral renal agenesis, lower urinary tract obstruction, polycystic kidneys, or renal hypoplasia–dysplasia–aplasia–dysgenesis. Fetal deformation caused by severe oligohydramnios includes Potter facies, characterized by a redundant skin, flat nose, low-set ears, bilateral skinfolds arising at the inner canthus and receding chin; wrinkled skin; and malposition of the hands and feet (263). Lung hypoplasia results from fetal compression due to the oligohydramnios (264) and, in some cases, massive abdominal distention. Even a short duration (1 week) of oligohydramnios can induce hypoplasia of the lung during the pseudoglandular period (12 to 16 weeks of GA) and the canalicular period (17 to 28 weeks of GA) (263–266).

Associations of Renal and Urinary Tract Anomalies with Single Signs

Upper urinary tract anomalies may be associated with several isolated anomalies (e.g., abnormal vertebrae, anorectal malformations) (see Appendix I–2); however, some of these associations are controversial (267–269). Ultrasonographic screening of 112 infants with isolated single umbilical artery (UA) showed an incidence of urinary tract malformations of 7% (268). The presence of specific index signs should raise the suspicion of a known multiple congenital anomaly; the presence of vertebral or anorectal anomalies can suggest a possible VATER syndrome (i.e., vertebral defects, anal atresia, tracheoesophageal fistula with esophageal atresia, and radial and renal defects). The risk of finding renal or urinary tract anomalies increases with the number of additional system anomalies and, in the case of hypospadias, with its severity (267). Some signs may be an indication for performance of US only in some families (e.g., preauricular pits) (269). Thus, it appears justified to obtain a US but not an intravenous urogram in newborn infants who are suspected clinically of having a recognized multiple congenital anomaly, as well as in those with several anomalies. In the absence of rigorous large-scale studies, decisions must be made on an individual basis.

Physical Examination

Vital Signs and General Examination

Shock and asphyxia can lead to prerenal or intrinsic renal failure. Tachycardia, peripheral vasoconstriction, hypotension, or narrowing of the pulse pressure suggests hypovolemia or low-output cardiac failure, which places the infant at risk for prerenal failure. Tachyarrhythmia, premature ventricular contractions, or abnormal QRS complexes on cardiac monitoring may be the first sign of hyperkalemia, which may be due to, or related to, renal immaturity or renal failure. Seizures or coma may be due to hypertension or complications of renal failure.

Measurement and Evolution of Blood Pressure in the Neonatal Period

Although a direct technique is the gold standard for measuring blood pressure, artifacts may result from the presence of air bubbles or blood clots or from using a low resonant frequency system (270). Indirect methods, i.e., computerized oscillometric and Doppler techniques, provide accurate assessment of the systolic and mean blood pressure, unless the patient is in shock (271). Accurate indirect measurements of diastolic blood pressure may be obtained by some oscillometric devices (272). Care should be taken to use an adequate cuff size, i.e., a 0.4 to 0.6 ratio between the width of the inflatable part (i.e., bladder) of the cuff and the arm circumference for the Doppler technique (273), or a 0.45 to 0.70 ratio between cuff width and arm circumference for the oscillometric technique (271). The length of the bladder should be 80% of the arm circumference (274). Coarctation of the aorta should be suspected if the systolic blood pressure in the upper limbs is more than 10 torr higher than that in the thigh or 15 torr higher than in the calf (275,276).

There is a wide variability in blood pressure among infants and among reported studies (see Appendices C–1a through C–1d) (277–279). Although blood pressure during the first hours of life is correlated with GA and weight (278), this correlation is significant only in premature infants with low Apgar scores, whose blood pressure tends to be lower than in healthy infants (279) (see Hypertension). Blood pressure increases with the awake state (see Appendix C–1d), knee–chest position, crying, pain, and during physical examination and procedures (280,281). In some infants, blood pressure follows a circadian pattern (282). Arterial blood pressure in normal infants increases by approximately 1 torr per day during the first week of life and then by 1 torr per week until 5 to 6 weeks of life (see Appendices C–1a through C–1d). The upper limit of normal systolic blood pressure in infancy is 113 torr (283). Tracking (i.e., a trend for the same individual) of blood pressure already starts during the first months of life (284).

Chest

A small chest suggests hypoplastic lungs, which can be associated with renal and urinary tract malformations. Polythelia (supernumary nipples) raises the suspicion of urinary tract anomalies. CHF, patent ductus arteriosus (PDA), and severe respiratory distress all can cause prerenal failure.

Abdomen

The physical examination of a newborn infant should include bimanual palpation of the abdomen for the presence of a normal kidney in each flank (238,239,251). The examination is easiest in the delivery room, before the bowel is filled with gas; later on, it is facilitated by relaxation of the abdominal wall musculature obtained, for instance, by eliciting the sucking reflex. Several characteristics of the kidneys should be evaluated, including their location (normally in the flank; an ectopic kidney may be located in the pelvis), size (the normal size for a 3.3 ± 0.5 [mean ± SD] kg infant is 4.2 to 4.3 ± 0.5 cm) (285), and long axis (normally cephalocaudal). A horseshoe kidney may be suspected if the lower pole is closer to the midline than the upper pole. The consistency normally is firm, as opposed to a cyst or a hydronephrotic kidney, which may be depressible. The surface normally is smooth, as opposed to large cysts in multicystic or autosomal dominant polycystic kidneys. Abdominal masses most often are of renal or urologic origin (286) and may be due to a polycystic or multicystic kidney, renal vein thrombosis, renal tumor, congenital hydronephrosis, or acquired hydronephrosis (e.g., fungus ball, papillary necrosis). A suprapubic mass suggests bladder distention. In some patients, one or both kidneys cannot be palpated. This may be due to a less than optimal examination (e.g., absence of patient relaxation, bowel distention), unilateral renal agenesis, renal malposition (in which case the kidney may be felt at another place in the abdomen), or renal hypoplasia or aplasia. Some abnormalities of the abdominal wall, such as bladder exstrophy, cloacal exstrophy, and prune-belly syndrome, are associated with renal anomalies. The umbilical cord should be examined for the number of UAs. Anorectal anomalies or ambiguous genitalia, including severe hypospadias (267), should raise the suspicion of renal or urologic malformations. Percussion of the abdomen may disclose ascites or a large bladder. In the absence of hydrops fetalis, neonatal ascites commonly is due to the rupture of an obstructed urinary tract (7 of 27 patients [26%]) (287). Sphincter dysfunction may suggest an occult spinal dysraphism.

Limbs

Motor and sensory dysfunction of the lower limbs suggests an occult spinal dysraphism. Several limb anomalies are part of syndromes or sequences associated with renal or urinary tract malformations, such as skeletal dysplasia, caudal regression syndrome, radial aplasia, femoral hypoplasia, rocker bottom feet, compression deformation, polydactyly, syndactyly, and hemihypertrophy.

Hydration

Serial measurements of net body weight (i.e., without equipment such as arm boards) should be compared to the normal postnatal weight evolution (288). Signs of dehydration include weight loss, dry skin and mucosae, sunken fontanelle, sometimes with signs of hypovolemia. In newborn infants, generalized edema usually starts around the eyes, at the perineum, and on the lateral sides of the trunk. Because edema fluid and third-space fluid do not participate in the effective ECF volume, hydration status should be based on a complete history and physical examination, as well as assessment of urine output and serum and urine biochemical analysis (see Chap. 22). Edema may be a sign of renal failure or nephrotic syndrome, among other causes.

Clinical Observations

Time of the First Postnatal Voiding

With early feeding, 97% of all infants void within 24 hours after birth (including in the delivery room) (Table 42–2) (289–292). Urine produced *in utero* normally is very dilute, with an average osmolality less than 200 mOsm/kg. Higher osmolality *in utero* may result from obstructive urinary tract disease caused by poor tubular reabsorption of sodium, from administration of oxytocin or indomethacin to the mother, or from acute or subacute intrauterine asphyxia. In contrast, urine produced after birth usually is isotonic or hypertonic, probably as a result of increased release of oxytocin and ADH.

Urine Output

In full-term infants, urine output after the first day of life increases progressively, in parallel with daily intake. In LBW and VLBW infants, three phases occur in the early postnatal period: an oliguric phase, during which the urine output is always lower than the intake; a polyuric phase starting between 24 and 72 hours of age, during which the output is always greater than the intake; and an adaptive phase, during which the kidney adjusts to the rate of fluid intake (293,294). A diuretic phase is observed in most infants, regardless of respiratory status or environment. The diuretic phase is associated with a high excretion of sodium and chloride, and, in much smaller amounts, potassium and bicarbonate (295). The diagnosis and treatment of oligoanuria and polyuria are discussed elsewhere in this chapter (see Acute Renal Failure; Tubular Dysfunction).

Characteristics of Urination

The baby should be observed for dribbling or persistence of a large bladder after urination, suggesting either posterior urethral valves or neurogenic bladder. Urination through an abnormal location suggests hypospadias or ambiguous genitalia, or both. Additional discussion can be found in Chapter 43.

Urinalysis

Urinalysis at the bedside includes the dipstick, which can help diagnose proteinuria, excretion of hemoprotein (hematuria, hemoglobinuria or myoglobinuria), glucosuria, and leukocyturia, and the measurement of urine specific gravity (SG) by refractometry. The amount of physiologic proteinuria in neonates changes with GA and postnatal age (Table 42–3). The differential diagnosis of pink urine and of hemoprotein is discussed later in this chapter (see Differential Diagnosis of Hematuria). Glucosuria usually is absent until the glycemia is greater than 150 mg/dL, although mild glucosuria is common in VLBW infants even when glycemia is normal. Urine SG is inversely proportional to urine output. In neonates, the relationship between SG and osmolarity differs from that in older subjects (296), and dipsticks do not provide a reliable assessment of urine osmolarity (297).

Laboratory Evaluation

Measurement of Glomerular Filtration Rate Using Exogenous Substances

To be an adequate marker for GFR, a substance must not be metabolized, must be completely filtered through the glomerulus, must not be secreted by the tubule, and must be eliminated from the body only by the kidney, unless GFR is determined by a classic clearance method

TABLE 42–2. *Time of first postnatal voiding*

| | Criteria | No. | Cumulative % of infants passing first urine within | | | | |
			Delivery room	≤20 h	≤24 h	≤30 h	≤48 h
Pynnönen 1972[a]	Boys	155	16%	94%		97%	
	Girls	164	4%	92%		99%	
Clark 1977	Full-term	395	13%		100%		
	Premature	80	21%		100%		
	Postterm	25	12%		100%		
Chih 1991	>2,500 g	920	19%		96%		100%
	<2,500 g	80	20%		96%		100%
Wang 1994	<1,500 g	111	3%		97%		100%
Total		1819	15%		97%		

[a]Physical examination did not show any overt abnormalities, significant for this study.

TABLE 42–3. *Proteinuria during the first days of life*

Gestational age (wk)	No. of infants	Mean and range (mg/m²/h)
≤28	5	0.86 (0.2–1.33)
30	12	2.08 (0–9.4)
32	15	2.32 (0–5.22)
34	15	2.48 (0–13.07)
36	17	1.27 (0–4.60)
40	26	1.29 (0–6.14)

From ref. 84.

(298). Adequate markers include inulin, polyfructosan, and radionuclides such as ^{99m}Tc-diethylenetriaminepentacetic acid (DTPA). Renal clearance can be measured by classic clearance techniques with collection of samples of blood and urine, by the rate of constant infusion that is associated with a steady-state plasma concentration, or by a noncompartmental analysis or a double-slope analysis of the plasma concentration after a single injection (299–301). The duration of infusion (for constant infusion technique) and the sampling time (for single injection technique) need to be as long as 24 to 72 hours in preterm infants (300).

Assessment of Glomerular Filtration Rate Using Creatinine Clearance or Plasma Creatinine Concentration

In the clinical setting, GFR often is estimated by creatinine clearance (C_{cr}) or by comparing P_{cr} to normal values for GA and postnatal age (Fig. 42–3) (302–304). Limitations of C_{cr} as an assessment of GFR have been attributed to inaccurate determination of P_{cr}, effect of maternal creatinine load on creatinine concentration, tubular secretion of creatinine, and difficulty in obtaining complete urine collections in newborn infants, especially in girls. Measuring P_{cr} is difficult, especially at levels below 1 mg/dL; the clinician should know the accuracy and the precision of the technique used in the laboratory, as well as possible sources of interference (305,306). Cord blood creatinine concentration is almost equivalent to the maternal level. In normal full-term infants, P_{cr} decreases exponentially during the first few days of life, with a half-life of 2.1 days (307); the rate of this decrease is a better indicator than the absolute value of P_{cr} when the mother is in renal failure. The correlation between P_{cr} and C_{in} on the second day of life in LBW infants signifies that, within 36 hours of life, the P_{cr} no longer simply reflects maternal GFR (308). In normal LBW infants, P_{cr} remains relatively high for weeks because GFR, although increasing progressively, remains lower than in full-term infants (302,308,309). Although in children C_{cr} tends to overestimate GFR at low values of C_{in} (304), the agreement between C_{cr} and C_{in} in LBW infants suggests that creatinine secretion is minimal in immature tubules (308).

Urine can be collected either from diapers, taking care to limit evaporation and to correct for losses by weighing diapers serially; by applying an adhesive plastic collection bag on the perineum; by using a modified metabolic bed; or by catheterizing the bladder if hourly urine output

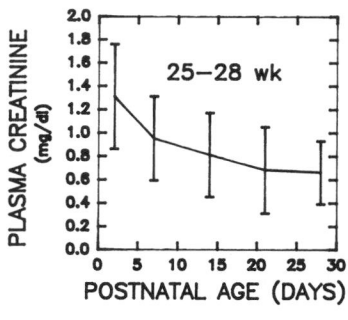

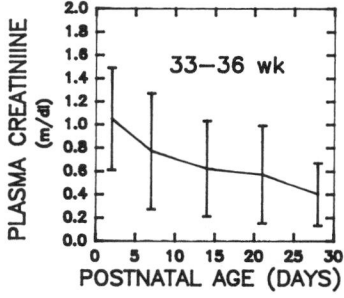

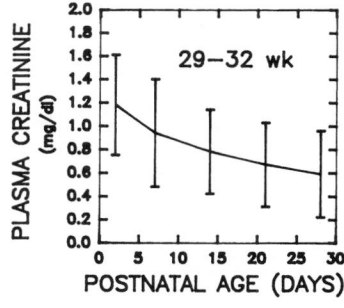

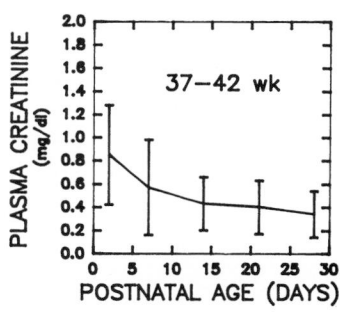

FIG. 42–3. The normal values of plasma creatinine concentration (mean ± 2 SD) during the first month of life are shown at four gestational age ranges. Infants were excluded from this study if they had congenital heart disease, heart failure with patent ductus arteriosus, indomethacin therapy within 48 hours, postasphyxic oligoanuria, renal anomalies, or muscle disease. These values were obtained using a kinetic Jaffé technique with a Beckman Creatinine Analyzer 2. This method reportedly had no interference with bilirubin up to 400 μmol/L (23 mg/dL); the addition of 0.1 mmol/L of pyruvate produced a rise of 5 μmol/L (0.06 mg/dL) in the creatinine value. (Adapted from ref. 303, using a conversion factor of 1 IU = 0.0113 mg/100 mL.)

measurement or bladder decompression is necessary. GFR may be expressed in mL/min; mL/min/1.73 m² of BSA; mL/min/kg of weight; or mL/min/kg of lean body mass; which of these units is most appropriate for infants is controversial (310).

If measured reliably, P_{cr} is correlated with the half-life of medications eliminated by the kidney (311–313). Nevertheless, the relationship between GFR and P_{cr} is hyperbolic, so that a fall in GFR of 50% may not be detectable by a change in P_{cr}.

The relationship between P_{cr} and GFR includes urinary creatinine excretion:

$$GFR \sim C_{cr} = U_{cr} \times V /P_{cr},$$

where C_{cr} is creatinine clearance (mL/min), V is urinary volume (mL/min), U_{cr} is the urinary creatinine concentration (mg/dL), and P_{cr} is plasma creatinine concentration (mg/dL). Daily production of creatinine depends on the rate of biotransformation of creatinine in striated muscle and on the amount of muscle (314). For the same GFR, P_{cr} increases with creatinine production and thus with muscle mass; for the same P_{cr}, GFR increases with muscle mass (314). To take this into account, Schwartz et al. developed a formula designed to estimate GFR corrected for BSA in steady-state individuals with normal body composition for age (and thus normal hydration) and stable renal function:

$$GFR = kL/P_{cr},$$

where GFR is glomerular filtration rate (mL/min/1.73 m²), the constant k is the rate of urinary creatinine excretion per unit of body size for a group of similar body habitus (mg/100 min/cm/1.73 m²), L is body length (cm), and P_{cr} is plasma creatinine concentration (mg/dL). Using a modified Technicon Autoanalyzer to measure P_{cr} (302), the average value of k was 0.45 in appropriate-for-GA full-term infants, 0.33 in LBW infants, 0.33 in small-for-GA full-term infants, and 0.31 in large-for-GA full-term infants (309,314,315), reflecting the low muscle mass in the latter three groups. During the first week of life in LBW infants, the formula kL/P_{cr} gave values similar to those obtained by C_{in} (309). However, because k has a large coefficient of variation (30% to 35%), kL/P_{cr} gives only an approximation of GFR.

Thus, the clinician usually can use P_{cr} for routine estimation of GFR in most newborn infants, except immediately after birth or during sudden changes in GFR; the latter are reflected by sequential measurements of P_{cr}. Formal measurements of C_{cr} or GFR are recommended for patients with renal impairment.

Beta₂-Microglobulin

This low-molecular-weight (LMW) protein is freely filtered by the glomerulus and reabsorbed and catabolized by the tubule; in contrast with creatinine, it does not cross the placenta. Its serum concentration in normal fetuses is independent of GA. Preliminary data suggest that serum beta₂-microglobulin concentration in fetuses suspected of urinary tract malformation may help predict their postnatal GFR (316,317).

Blood Urea Nitrogen

A high value of blood urea nitrogen (BUN) can result from catabolism, dehydration, high protein load (e.g., oral, intravenous, gastrointestinal bleeding), or renal failure. A low value of BUN can result from ECF expansion or decreased production of urea. The latter may be observed in association with anabolism, low protein intake, urea cycle disorder, liver failure, or liver immaturity (318).

Uric Acid

Serum concentration of uric acid is higher in cord blood than in maternal blood. Renal handling of uric acid along the nephron includes glomerular filtration, tubular reabsorption, tubular secretion, and further reabsorption distal to the secretory site. Fractional excretion of uric acid during the first 24 hours decreases from about 70% at 29 to 31 weeks of GA to 39% ± 14% (mean ± SD) at 38 to 40 weeks of GA (319) and decreases with postconceptional age, to reach less than 20% at 1 year of age and less than 10% in adults. This results from progressive tubular maturation (320). Urinary uric acid concentration is lowest on day 7 in full-term infants; its concentration in premature infants is highest on day 1 and remains significantly higher than in full-term babies during the first month of life (321). A high urinary uric acid to creatinine ratio is a marker of perinatal asphyxia (322).

Plasma Renin Activity

The most common indication for the measurement of PRA is the evaluation of hypertension. Normal levels of PRA are higher in the newborn infant than in older children or adults. This is discussed further in the section on Hypertension.

Genetic, Biochemical, and Molecular Diagnosis

The number of tests available for the diagnosis of congenital disorders is rapidly increasing (see Chaps. 9,12,39, and 40). Classic chromosome analysis can be enhanced by high-resolution methods. Biochemical diagnosis is possible either by measuring enzyme activity or a chemical in a biologic fluid (e.g., high AFP concentration in maternal serum or amniotic fluid suggesting a diagnosis of congenital nephrotic syndrome in a high-risk family) or in cultured cells obtained from chorionic villi, amniotic cells, or fibroblasts (e.g, for diagnosing cystinosis).

In many disorders, the gene has been mapped to a specific chromosomal locus and is genetically linked to DNA markers. Genetic diagnosis is then possible on amniotic fluid, chorionic villous, or blood samples, if one or more specific alleles are informative (i.e., characteristic for the disease) in a given family or in a given population (e.g., in CNF, see later in this chapter). Depending on the gene of interest, such alleles may be recognized by using restriction fragment length polymorphism (RFLP), variable number of tandem repeats (VNTR), or polymerase chain reaction (PCR) using allele-specific primers (ASO). In addition, if the gene responsible for a particular disease has been cloned and sequenced, the specific mutation in an affected individual or family can be determined by PCR, followed by sequence analysis or single-stranded conformational polymorphism (SSCP). Molecular diagnosis may be complicated by the fact that a similar phenotype may result from mutations of one of two or more genes; this is the case for autosomal dominant polycystic kidney disease (ADPKD) (chromosomes 16, 4, and 2) (323–327) and for nephrogenic diabetes insipidus (NDI) (see section on Nephrogenic Diabetes Insipidus).

Urinary Acidification

Immaturity of renal tubular acidification results in a significantly lower value of serum bicarbonate concentration in VLBW infants than in full-term infants. In parallel, the serum base deficit is often between -5 and -10 mEq/L in VLBW infants, compared with 0 to -5 mEq/L in full-term infants, and the anion gap, obtained by the difference between sodium concentration and the sum of chloride and bicarbonate concentrations, is normally 15 to 22 mEq/L in premature infants, compared to 12 ± 2 mEq/L (less than 15 mEq/L) in full-term infants. In newborn infants, metabolic acidosis often is secondary to asphyxia, hypoxia, shock, or sepsis. If metabolic acidosis is persistent, a defect in tubular acidification, among other diagnoses, should be suspected, whether urine pH is low or high; measurement of urine-to-blood carbon dioxide tension gradient is indicated to rule out distal tubular acidosis (328) (see Tubular Function).

Microscopic Examination of Urine

The shape of erythrocytes in freshly voided urine should be observed under the microscope. The presence of deformed cells suggests hematuria of glomerular origin, whereas undeformed cells predominate in either massive hematuria or lower urinary tract disease. Leukocyturia is common in normal infants during the first few days of life (329); yet, leukocyturia may be lacking in a newborn infant with a positive urine culture, in contrast to older children. The presence of bacteria on a gram stain may be a better predictor of urinary tract infection

(UTI). The presence of erythrocyte casts in the urine suggests the diagnosis of glomerulopathy, whereas leukocyte casts can be observed during UTI.

Urine Electrolytes and Osmolality

The measurement of urinary and blood osmolality, urea, creatinine, and electrolytes is indicated for the differential diagnosis of polyuria and for the early diagnosis of oligoanuria.

Proteinuria

Maturation is associated with a decrease in the daily rate of proteinuria (see Table 42–3) and with qualitative changes, which can be analyzed by two-dimensional gel electrophoresis (330). The first voided urine in 22- to 28-week-old infants contains many serum proteins and peptides, whereas urine in full-term infants contains much less polypeptides. Urinary excretion of lysosomal and brush border enzymuria and that of LMW proteins follow specific developmental patterns (331). LMW proteins (i.e., beta$_2$-microglobulin, myoglobin, and retinol-binding globulin) are filtered through the glomerulus and reabsorbed and catabolized by the tubule. Because the tubular reabsorption of beta$_2$-microglobulin increases with maturation, its fractional excretion decreases until 2 years of age (332). The urinary concentration of LMW proteins is a sensitive indicator of tubular renal damage due to asphyxia or medications (see Acute Renal Failure). Another identified protein is called the Tamm–Horsfall glycoprotein, which is derived from the tubule.

Imaging of the Kidney and the Urinary Tract

Ultrasonography and Doppler Flow Analysis

Ultrasonography is performed to screen for renal and urologic malformations or as one of the first steps in the workup of renal failure, oligoanuria, hypertension, UTI, or hematuria (333). Indications for the performance of neonatal US are shown in Table 42–4. In a series using similar indications, 71 of 1,500 newborns had neonatal US performed, and 15 (21%) were found to have a congenital renal or urinary tract malformation (250). The size of the kidneys should be compared to normal for size, GA, and gender (285). The examiner should assess not only the kidneys but also the adrenal glands, aorta, renal arteries, renal veins, inferior vena cava, ureters, and bladder. The differential diagnosis of US anomalies is presented in Table 42–5 (334–338).

Blood flow through renal vessels can be assessed by Doppler US, which is indicated for the evaluation of hematuria, hypertension, and acute renal failure (ARF), especially in a patient with UA catheterization. Pulsed-Doppler flow analysis (i.e., duplex scanning) allows the

TABLE 42–4. *Indications for ultrasonography to rule out renal–urinary tract malformations and/or acquired renal disease in newborn infants*

History[a]
  Family history
    First-degree relative with Potter's syndrome (bilateral renal agenesis/dysgenesis), autosomal dominant polycystic kidney disease
    Sibling with autosomal recessive polycystic kidney disease
    Abnormal prenatal ultrasonography (kidney, bladder, ascites)
    Oligohydramnios, unless normal postnatal renal function and oligohydramnios attributed to
    Prolonged rupture of the membranes
    Postdate delivery, subacute fetal distress
  Physical examination or evidence for other congenital anomaly[a,b]
    Syndrome, sequence or field defect described in Appendix I–1[b]
    Any part of a possible VATER syndrome (vertebral anomalies, anorectal anomalies, tracheoesophageal fistula)
    Preauricular pits, if family history
    Supernumerary nipples
    Congenital diaphragmatic hernia with additional anomalies
    Lung hypoplasia, symptomatic spontaneous pneumothorax
    Abnormal abdominal examination
      Abnormal kidney palpation
      Abdominal mass
      Bruit[c]
    Ascites
    Single umbilical artery
    Second- or third-degree hypospadias
    Ambiguous genitalia
  Evidence for renal disease
    Renal failure, oligoanuria[c]
    Systemic hypertension[c]
    Urinary tract infection
    Hematuria[c]
    Significant proteinuria
    Nephrotic syndrome

[a]The best timing of ultrasonography remains to be determined. A negative test immediately after birth does not rule out hydronephrosis and/or vesicoureteral reflux. A repeat test should be obtained within a few weeks (or earlier of clinically indicated).

[b]The frequency of urinary tract anomalies in many of these entities has not been determined. Because a cost–benefit analysis has not been performed, the indication for neonatal ultrasonographic screening should be decided on an individual basis. The frequency of fetal urinary tract anomalies in association with maternal diabetes or cocaine use is probably too low to justify neonatal ultrasonography in asymptomatic infants.

[c]These patients also should have Doppler ultrasonography.

Modified from ref. 251.

TABLE 42–5. *Renal ultrasonographic patterns in newborn infants*

Normal appearance
  Prerenal failure
  Renal artery thrombosis
  Congenital renal disease, e.g., renal tubular acidosis
  Renal cystic disease (in which cysts develop late)
  Developing hydronephrosis or vesicoureteral reflux
Increased cortical echogenicity
  With increased corticomedullary differentiation in large kidneys
    Beckwith–Wiedemann syndrome
  With normal corticomedullary differentiation
    Prerenal failure
    Renal ischemia
    Mild renal dysplasia
    Congenital nephrotic syndrome, Finnish type
  With loss of corticomedullary differentiation in normal to small kidneys[a]
    Severe renal dysplasia
    Pyelonephritis, including renal candidiasis (often heterogeneous)
    Renal tubular dysgenesis/glomerular dysgenesis[b]
  With loss of corticomedullary differentiation in large kidneys[a]
    Renal vein thrombosis
      Edema results in decreased echoes
      Hemorrhage results in increased echoes
    Corticomedullary necrosis[c]
    Autosomal recessive polycystic kidney disease
    Renal glomerular dysgenesis/tubular dysgenesis
    Transient nephromegaly (benign)
    Contrast nephropathy
    Lymphangioma
    Mesoblastic nephroma[d]
Cysts(s)[e]
  See Appendix I–3
Increased medullary echogenicity
  Nephrocalcinosis
  Medullary cystic disease
  Tamm–Horsfall proteinuria, acute tubular necrosis
  Medullary sponge kidney
Intrapyelic echogenicity
  Renal candidiasis ("fungus ball")
  Lithiasis
Hydronephrosis

This list does not include findings shown by Doppler ultrasonography.

[a]Diffuse or heterogenous hyperechogenicity of cortex or whole kidney.

[b]Renal size may be enlarged.

[c]Renal size may be normal or enlarged.

[d]Solid mass causing distortion of intrarenal collecting system, with occasional cystic areas corresponding to necrosis or hemorrhage.

[e]Absence of cysts visualized by ultrasonography does not rule out a renal cystic disease in a newborn infant. Some entities result in development of cysts later in life, whereas others (e.g., autosomal recessive polycystic kidney disease) result in hyperechogenicity.

Modified from ref. 334.

measurement of blood flow velocity, which gives an assessment of RBF, and calculation of the ratio of end-diastolic minimum velocity to systolic peak velocity (i.e., diastolic-to-systolic ratio), which gives an assessment of renal artery vascular resistance (339–341).

Voiding Cystourethrogram

Vesicoureteral reflux (VUR) and bladder obstruction should be ruled out in patients with hydronephrosis, trabeculated bladder, bladder distention, or myelomeningocele (342). It has been suggested that in patients with UTI, the voiding cystourethrogram (VCUG) be delayed, because VUR that is present during the UTI may disappear within 4 to 6 weeks. However, it may be important to know that VUR does occur in the presence of UTI. Sterile technique is imperative to prevent iatrogenic infection; the role of prophylactic antibiotic therapy has not been evaluated.

Renal Radionuclide Scan

The most commonly used radionuclides in the study of newborn infants include ^{99m}Tc, which is preferred because it is a pure γ-ray emitter and has a half-life of only 6 hours, and ^{123}I, which also emits x-rays and has a half-life of 13 hours. ^{131}I should be avoided in infants because of its long half-life. ^{99m}Tc-DTPA is eliminated mostly by glomerular filtration and very little by tubular secretion. Analysis of the radioactivity due to this compound can be used for assessing renal perfusion (if measurements are taken immediately after the injection), renal mass (if measurements are taken within 1 to 3 minutes after the injection), and GFR (if using a double-compartment analysis of radioactivity in sequential blood measurements or convolution analysis after a single injection), as well as for visualizing the urinary tract (343). In contrast, ^{99m}Tc-dimercaptosuccinic acid (DMSA) binds to the tubules and is only minimally excreted into the urine; it is preferred for the analysis of renal morphology and differential function. Typical indications for radionuclide studies include renovascular hypertension, lack of visualization of a kidney by US, preoperative evaluation of the severity of urinary tract obstruction, and evaluation of differential renal function. In normal newborn infants, however, routinely measuring GFR using radionuclides is not ethically justifiable, even though the amount of radioactivity is minimal. Therefore, normal values for age are not available. Chapter 43 provides details on anatomic diagnoses.

Intravenous Urography

In newborn infants, intravenous urography largely has been replaced by US, because of the improved resolution of the new generations of US probes, increased recogni-

tion of the nephrotoxicity of standard radiopaque products, and the poor contrast obtained, which is due to the low GFR during the first weeks of life. If needed, a low-osmolality contrast material is preferred (see Nephrotoxicity). Optimally, the procedure is delayed a few weeks, at which time improved renal function usually results in better visualization.

Percutaneous Antegrade Pyelography

This technique may be diagnostic in some cases of cystic disease or urinary tract obstruction (344).

Angiogram

The frequency of this procedure, mostly used during cardiac catheterization, has decreased dramatically since the development of two-dimensional echocardiography. The anatomy of the kidneys always should be examined during cardiac catheterization. Angiography may be indicated in case of an abdominal tumor, renovascular hypertension, or an aortic thrombus.

Computed Tomography and Magnetic Resonance Imaging

Computed tomography (CT) and magnetic resonance imaging (MRI) are indicated in case of an abdominal tumor. In addition, MRI appears to be more sensitive than US in detecting a tethered cord in a patient with bladder distention and lack of VUR or urethral stenosis on VCUG.

Renal Pathology

Renal biopsy is indicated in nephrotic syndrome and may be indicated in polycystic kidney disease, hematuria, or persistent severe renal failure of unclear origin. Major contraindications to renal biopsy include bleeding diathesis, anticoagulant therapy, moderate or severe hypertension, solitary kidney, and intrarenal tumor (345). The technique involves visualization of the kidney using US, radioisotope, or radiopaque contrast. The most common complication is macroscopic hematuria, which occurs in 5% to 7% of biopsies.

ACUTE RENAL FAILURE AND OLIGOANURIA

ARF, usually defined as an acute deterioration in the ability of the kidneys to maintain the homeostasis of body fluids (346), is associated with an acute decrease in the rate of glomerular filtration, as opposed to isolated acute tubular dysfunction. Because the placenta fulfills that role *in utero*, congenital malformations associated with limitation of renal function will not lead to renal failure until birth.

Incidence

The incidence of intrinsic oliguric ARF in newborn infants admitted to the neonatal intensive care unit (NICU) ranges between 1% and 6% in retrospective studies, and between 6% and 8% in prospective studies (347–349). In a prospective study on 314 NICU admissions, Norman and Assadi (349) found 72 infants (23%) with azotemia (i.e., BUN ≥20 mg/dL) and urine output ≤25 mL/kg/d for at least 24 hours. In that series, the incidence of prerenal failure was 17%, whereas that of intrinsic renal failure was 6%. Stapleton et al. (348) found an incidence of oliguric renal failure (i.e., urine output less than 1 mL/kg/h unresponsive to fluid challenge, accompanied by a P_{cr} greater than 1.5 mg/dL) of 8% in NICU patients.

Diagnosis

Intrauterine oligoanuria can be suspected when oligohydramnios develops in the absence of amniotic fluid leakage or rupture of the amniotic membranes; it can be due to a congenital urinary tract anomaly (e.g., urinary tract obstruction, renal agenesis, dysgenesis), to toxins (e.g., ACE inhibitors, indomethacin) (262,350,351), or to intrauterine asphyxia. If urine output alone is used to assess renal function, ARF often will be both overlooked and overdiagnosed. Indeed, normal urine output is found in approximately one-third of neonates with ARF (347,352), and anuria may occur as a result of the syndrome of inappropriate ADH secretion (SIADHS), in the absence of ARF. Renal function should be evaluated for possible ARF in infants who have been subjected to perinatal asphyxia, shock, hypoxemia, or various nephrotoxins (Fig. 42–4). Clinical signs of ARF include syndromes or signs suggestive of renal or urogenital malformations, oligoanuria, polyuria, hematuria, proteinuria, fluid overload, dehydration, cardiac arrhythmia, and systemic hypertension. Other signs include decreased activity, seizures, anemia, vomiting, and anorexia. Sometimes ARF is suspected on the basis of electrolyte abnormalities or elevated plasma levels of medications (e.g., aminoglycosides).

ARF is characterized by decreased GFR and renal tubular function compared to normal values for either postconceptional age or GA and postnatal age. Although the diagnosis of ARF is strongly suggested by a P_{cr} that is above the upper limit of normal, during the first days of life such an elevation also may result from abnormal maternal renal function. Thus, measuring GFR or following P_{cr} over time is required to diagnose ARF in a newborn infant during the first few days of life. Because renal tubular function changes with maturation, it is important to use criteria appropriate for age; indexes developed for more mature subjects are not indicative of intrinsic renal failure in VLBW infants.

Etiology

A wide variety of malformations and prenatal, perinatal, and postnatal events may cause neonatal renal failure (Table 42–6) (348–359). The most common type of acute intrinsic renal failure is ATN, which is discussed in the next section.

Pathophysiology of Acute Tubular Necrosis

The evolution of ATN is characterized by three successive phases: initiation, maintenance, and recovery. Although ATN may be precipitated by a single event, its development is multifactorial and involves vascular (i.e., hemodynamic), nephronal, and cellular (i.e., metabolic) factors (346).

Vasoconstriction of the afferent arterioles plays a major role in the initiation phase of ATN (360–362). Increased renal vascular resistance results from changes in the relative concentrations of vasoconstrictive agents such as PRA, adenosine, thromboxane (TX), endothelin, and platelet activating factor, and vasodilator agents such as natriuretic peptides, nitric oxide (NO), PGs, and prostacyclin. The increase in PRA, which results from the stimulation of the juxtaglomerular apparatus by the high solute content of damaged tubules, helps maintain glomerular filtration by vasoconstricting the efferent arteriole. ACE inhibitors, in contrast with other types of vasodilators, aggravate the renal insult (see section on Nephrotoxicity).

During the maintenance phase of ATN, the main factors are nephronal and cellular. A decrease in GFR and in tubular flow may result from obstruction of the tubule by cellular debris (363) and from backleak of fluid and solutes secondary to loss of integrity of the proximal tubule (346,363). In addition, glomerular membrane permeability may decrease during ARF. Cellular factors include cessation of oxidative phosphorylation, which results in depletion of adenosine triphosphate (ATP); disruption of major cellular functions, e.g., Na^+/K^+-ATPase, and cell swelling; formation of free radicals, lipid alterations, and membrane damage; calcium influx; and activation of several genes and mediators (346). The interaction between interstitial inflammatory cells and adhesion molecules play a major role in the severity of tubular ischemic lesions (364).

The production of local growth factors decreases during the early phase of ATN; the tubular epithelium only regenerates during the recovery phase. GFR initially increases in parallel with a decrease in intratubular pressure and casts; GFR then increases in parallel with PRF and urine output (349). Unless enough fluid is provided to compensate for the large amounts of urine lost during the polyuric phase, hypovolemia may develop and slow the recovery or even cause a secondary deterioration of renal function. Randomized trials are needed to determine the best specific therapy to reduce the severity of

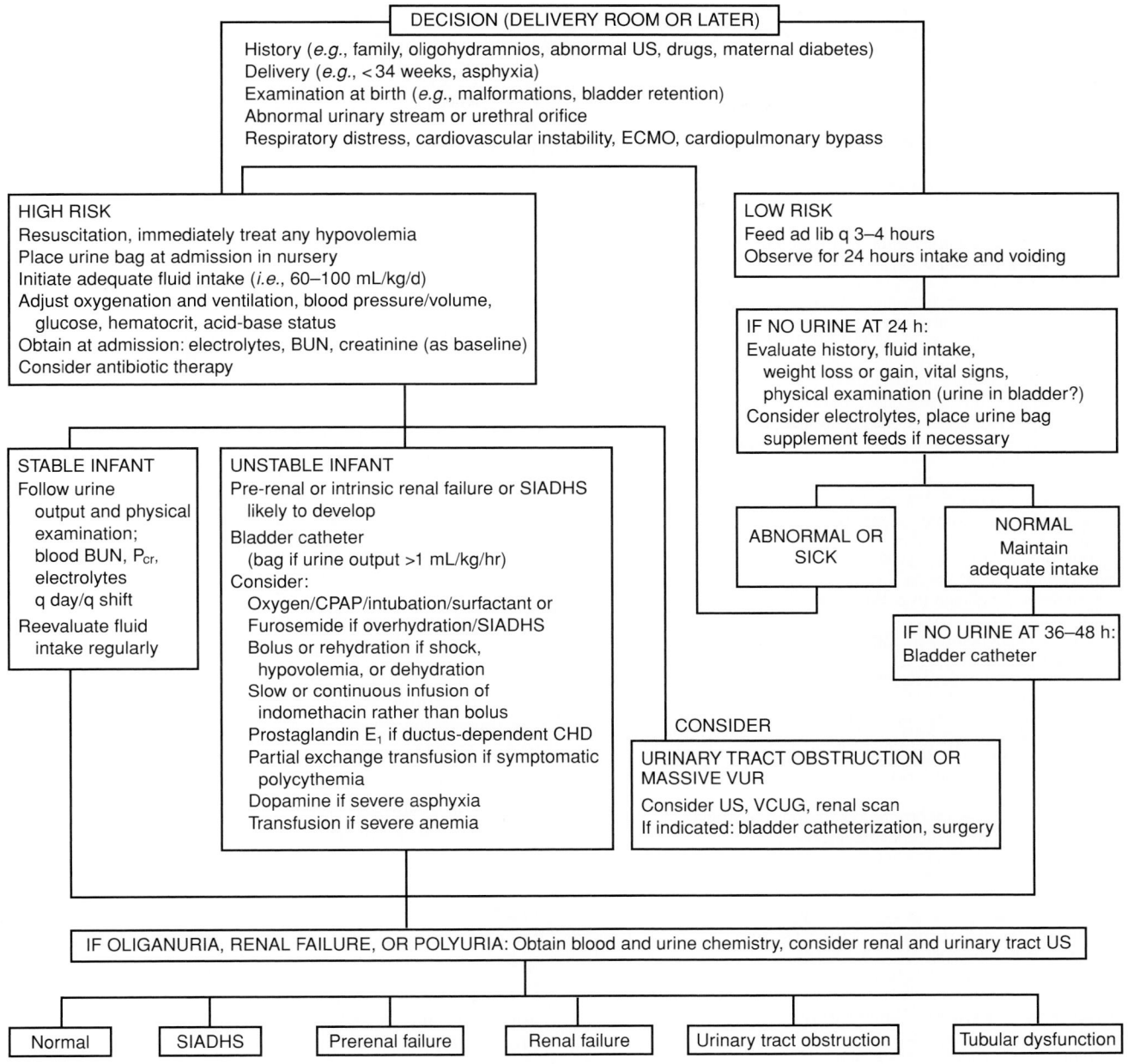

FIG. 42–4. Proposed approach for monitoring urinary output and preventing prerenal failure. ad lib, *ad libitum*; BUN, blood urea nitrogen; CHD, congenital heart disease; CPAP, continuous positive airway pressure; P$_{cr}$, plasma creatinine concentration; PDA, patent ductus arteriosus; q, every; SIADHS, syndrome of inappropriate antidiuretic hormone secretion; US, ultrasonography; VCUG, voiding cysto-urethrogram.

ARF (e.g., vasodilators or drugs targeting the inflammatory reaction) and to improve its recovery (e.g., growth factors) with the least side effects (365).

Prevention of Prerenal Failure and Early Diagnosis of Acute Renal Failure

The first step is to identify infants at high risk for renal failure or oligoanuria immediately after birth or after pre-disposing events (see Fig. 42–4). In these infants, urine collection should be initiated right away, and vital signs, electrolytes, and renal function should be followed serially. If urinary tract anomalies are suspected, a complete urologic workup should be considered (see Chap. 43). Decompression of the urinary tract by bladder catheterization or surgical intervention, or both, may be indicated. In VLBW infants, PDA, low blood pressure, and mechanical ventilation are associated with lower GFR and higher

TABLE 42–6. *Etiologic classification of acute neonatal renal failure*

Parenchymal malformation[a]
  Renal agenesis
  Renal hypoplasia
    Simple hypoplasia
    Oligonephronic hypoplasia
  Renal dysplasia
    Multicystic
    Hypoplastic
    Aplastic
    Associated with urinary tract obstruction or
      vesicoureteral reflux
  Nephron dysgenesis
    Tubular dysgenesis: congenital hypernephronic
      nephromegaly with tubular dysgenesis = congenital
      tubular dysgenesis = isolated congenital renal tubular
      immaturity
    Glomerular dysgenesis:
      Idiopathic
      Secondary to maternal administration of
        indomethacin or angiotensin-converting enzyme
        inhibitors
  Polycystic kidney disease
    Adult type (autosomal dominant)
    Infant type (autosomal recessive)
    Other
Acquired renal dysfunction or lesion[b]
  Asphyxia/hypoxia/ischemia
    Functional (may lead to prerenal or intrinsic renal
      failure)
      Systemic hypotension, shock, hypovolemia, severe
        dehydration
      Renal artery vasoconstriction, e.g., nephrotoxins,
        endotoxin, endothelin
      Reverse diastolic blood flow (preeclampsia, patent
        ductus arteriosus)
      Prenatal/perinatal/postnatal asphyxia
      Respiratory distress, hypoxemia
      Sepsis
      Heart failure, extracorporeal membrane oxygenation,
        cardiopulmonary bypass surgery
      Hyperviscosity, polycythemia
      Severe anemia
    Vascular
      Arterial/arteriolar thrombosis/embolism/stenosis
      Cortical/medullary necrosis, renal infarction
      Venous thrombosis
  Urinary tract obstruction (see Table 42–7)
  Urinary tract infection
  Disseminated intravascular coagulation
  Drugs
    Antibiotics (aminoglycosides, amphotericin, acyclovir)
    Indomethacin
    Tolazoline
    α-Adrenergic agents
    Angiotensin-converting enzyme inhibitors
    Radiocontrast agents
    Cyclosporine
  Toxins
    Hemoglobinuria
    Myoglobinuria
    Hyperoxaluria
    Benzyl alcohol
    Polysorbate
    Ethylene glycol
    Uric acid nephropathy
  Glomerular disease
    Membranous glomerulonephritis (IgG-mediated)
    Congenital syphilis
    Diffuse mesangial sclerosis

[a]May not cause acute renal failure until after the neonatal period.
[b]May occur *in utero*.

FENa (366). Oliguric renal failure develops in 22% of patients on venoarterial extracorporeal membrane oxygenation (ECMO) and may develop in patients on venovenous ECMO in the absence of changes in cardiac output, blood pressure, or hypoalbuminemia; the exact pathophysiology of the renal dysfunction remains to be elucidated (367,368).

Renal Blood Flow

Decreased RBF may result from multiple mechanisms such as reverse diastolic flow, hypotension, heart failure, and vasoconstriction (Table 42–6). In mothers with preeclampsia, absent or retrograde diastolic blood flow in the fetal aorta and UA predicts several perinatal complications, including renal failure (369).

RBF velocity remains low for at least 1 week in VLBW infants with intrauterine growth retardation (370). Prevention of prerenal failure includes correction of any abnormality in and maintenance of adequate oxygenation, ventilation, blood pressure, cardiac output, hydration (see Chap. 22), blood glucose, and hematocrit, as well as prevention and early treatment of sepsis. Preliminary data suggest that indomethacin-mediated renal vasoconstriction and ARF may be reduced by using prior volume expansion and by using a low dose and a slow infusion of indomethacin (371). The effect of furosemide on indomethacin-mediated nephrotoxicity is controversial (372,373).

In hypotensive premature infants (29 to 34 weeks of GA) with respiratory distress syndrome, the infusion of dopamine at a rate of 0.5 to 2 µg/kg/min resulted in a transient elevation in blood pressure compared to controls, followed by increases in urine output, creatinine clearance, and natriuresis (374–375). In another series, the administration of low-dose dopamine to premature infants with respiratory distress syndrome increased blood pressure and natriuresis, but the increase in GFR and urine output did not reach significance (376). Low-dose dopamine may stimulate PRA in the absence of any change in blood pressure (377). Dopamine may decrease indomethacin-mediated oliguria (378).

Urine Output

In asymptomatic low-risk full-term infants receiving routine care, low or even absent urine output (detected by checking the number of wet diapers) during the first 24 hours of life is a normal event, assuming adequate fluid intake. If spontaneous urination is not observed within an additional 12 hours (i.e., at 36 hours of life), the baby should be reexamined for possible urine retention in the bladder, and the bladder should be catheterized.

In contrast, in premature infants and in patients with significant history, symptoms, or physical examination, urine output should be measured from birth. A urine dipstick test, done on a sample obtained noninvasively, may provide the first evidence for hematuria or myoglobinuria (379). If there is no urine by 24 hours of life or if subsequent output is less than 1 mL/kg/h, the bladder should be catheterized (see Fig. 42–4); suprapubic pressure (i.e., Credé maneuver) is not the preferred method, because of the risk for VUR, and rarely for bladder or renal rupture (380). Patients at high risk for renal failure (e.g., shock, ECMO, or major surgery) should have their bladder catheterized to measure the hourly urine output. If little or no urine is obtained, oligoanuria is suspected (see Oligoanuria).

If polyuria develops, possible diagnoses include hypervolemia, tubular dysfunction, diabetes insipidus, glucose overload, polyuric phase of ATN, and polyuric phase of postrenal failure (e.g., after decompression of the bladder by catheterization).

Perinatal Asphyxia

The risk for and severity of ARF increases with the severity of asphyxia (381–383). Early diagnosis of ARF secondary to perinatal asphyxia is suggested by the finding of increased tubular (LMW) proteinuria immediately after birth (384–386). Asphyxiated infants with a urine output less than 1 mL/kg/h for 36 hours usually have a high urinary concentration of beta$_2$-microglobulin as well as clinical signs of hypoxic–ischemic encephalopathy. A dipstick may help detect hematuria, myoglobinuria, and proteinuria. Oligoanuria in these infants may result from prerenal (i.e., functional) failure mediated in part by endothelin (387), intrinsic renal failure (e.g., ATN), or SIADHS. One prospective randomized study showed that infusion of dopamine at low dose (2 to 5 μg/kg/min) in severely asphyxiated newborn infants increased systolic blood pressure and urine output and decreased the incidence of abnormal P_{cr} (388).

General Approach in Oligoanuria

The diagnosis of oligoanuria (i.e., urinary output less than 0.5 to 1.0 mL/kg/h) should be confirmed by reviewing the chart and demonstrating the absence of urine by bladder catheterization, using a 3.5Fr or 5Fr lubricated feeding tube, which then is left in place and connected to a sterile system for continued monitoring of the hourly urine output. Delayed micturition has been described in association with transient bladder distention attributed to severe perinatal asphyxia (389). Bladder puncture should be avoided because of the high likelihood of causing trauma.

Once oligoanuria is confirmed, the history should be reviewed for severe asphyxia, respiratory failure, hypotension, shock, and renal toxins. Intake and output over the last few days should be reviewed. The physical examination should seek evidence of weight loss, dehydration, malformations, respiratory failure, CHF, shock, hypotension, and central nervous system disease. General care should be optimized, including measures to support ventilation, oxygenation, cardiac output, functional circulatory volume, and extracellular volume.

Urine and Blood Analysis

The differential diagnosis of oligoanuria includes not only renal failure but also SIADHS and decreased urine production secondary to the administration of ADH or its analogs (Table 42–7). The differentiation between prerenal and true renal ARF is presented in Table 42–8.

Urine should be examined promptly for protein, cellular elements and crystals, electrolytes, creatinine, and SG or osmolality. A blood sample should be obtained for hematocrit, electrolytes, creatinine, BUN, and glucose; other tests (e.g., serum concentration of xanthine or uric acid, oxaluria) may be indicated based on history or initial results. Plasma osmolality can be either measured or calculated from the following formula:

$$\text{Posm (mOsm/kg)} \; 2 \times \text{Na (mEq/L)} + \text{glucose (mg/dL)}/18 + \text{BUN (mg/dL)}/2.8.$$

Use of this formula is not recommended for infants with a birth weight less than 1,000 g, in whom it may substantially underestimate true osmolality (390).

TABLE 42–7. *Differential diagnosis of oligoanuria*

Renal failure
  Prerenal (see Table 42–6)
  Intrinsic (see Table 42–6)
  Postrenal
    Bladder retention
      Urethral valves
      Meningomyelocele, tethered cord
      Massive vesicoureteral reflux
    Bilateral ureteral obstruction
      Ureteropelvic junction obstruction
      Ureterovesical junction obstruction, ureterocele
      Lithiasis
      Fungus ball
    Extrinsic compression
    Uroascites (i.e., ruptured urinary tract)
      Secondary to urinary tract obstruction
      Bladder perforation (umbilical artery catheterization or direct bladder trauma)
Syndrome of inappropriate secretion of antidiuretic hormone
Exogenous administration (to the mother or the newborn infant) of
  Antidiuretic hormone, desmopressin
  Oxytocin
  Indomethacin
Acute bladder distension without renal failure
  Curarization
  Neurogenic bladder
  Hematoma of the anterior wall of the bladder (traumatic suprapubic aspiration)

TABLE 42–8. *Differential diagnosis: prerenal vs. intrinsic oliguric renal failure*[a]

	Prerenal	Intrinsic
FeNa	≤2.5%	>3%
UNa	≤20	>50
Uosm	≥350	≤300
U/P osm[b]	≥1.2	0.8–1.2
U_{SG}	>1,012	<1,014
Urine retinol binding protein[c]	<20 mg/mmol creatinine	>27 mg/mmol creatinine
Urine myoglobin[c]	<0.5 mg/mmol creatinine	>1.5 mg/mmol creatinine
Ultrasonography[d]	Normal	May be abnormal[d]
BUN/Pcr	>30	<20
Response to challenge[e]	UO >2 mL/kg/h	No ↑ UO

[a]FENa and UNa are high (falsely suggesting an intrinsic renal failure) after diuretic administration, volume expansion, urinary excretion of nonabsorbable solutes (glycosuria, mannitol, glycerol, bicarbonate [in metabolic alkalosis]), adrenal insufficiency, or gestational age <28 wk. FENa increases transiently in normal full-term infants immediately after birth and in premature infants during the diuretic phase. FENa is also high in case of prolonged urinary tract obstruction and in chronic renal failure. Conversely, FENa and UNa are low (falsely suggesting prerenal failure) in acute renal failure due to severe vasoconstriction (e.g., indomethacin, radiocontrast nephropathy, sepsis, early phase of myoglobinuria), in acute urinary tract obstruction, and in some cases of nonoliguric ATN.

[b]Although plasma osmolality can be estimated using the formula:
Posm: 2 × PNa (mEq/L) + gl (mg/dL)/18 + BUN (mg/dL)/2.8
the measured value of Posm is preferable, especially in critically ill patients, because of large differences in the case of sick cell syndrome (leaking cellular membranes), and in infants with a birth weight <1,000 g (Giacoia 1992).

[c]Transient tubular dysfunction secondary to neonatal asphyxia is characterized by moderate proteinuria with normal or mildly decreased GFR and normal or mildly increased FeNa. Very high urine levels of myoglobin or retinol binding protein may, in some cases, precede the increase in FeNa of intrinsic renal failure (Kojima 1985).

[d]The ultrasonography in "intrinsic" renal failure may show increased echogenicity of the pyramids, which probably corresponds to precipitation of Tamm–Horsfall protein, signs of renal vein thrombosis, renal artery thrombosis, adrenal hemorrhage, hydronephrosis, cystic kidney disease, renal dysplasia/hypoplasia, or other pathology (see Table 42–5).

[e]The challenge corresponds to the administration of 20 mL/kg of crystalloid (more should be given if there is evidence of hypovolemia) and/or 1 mg/kg of furosemide. Normalization of the urine output after such a challenge may correspond to a prerenal failure or to the polyuric phase following an oliguric renal failure. See text for additional comments.

BUN/Pcr, ratio of blood urea nitrogen to plasma creatinine concentration; FeNa, fractional excretion of sodium; GFR, glomerular filtration rate; gl, glycemia; PNa, plasma sodium concentration; UNa, urinary sodium concentration; UO, urine output; Uosm, urine osmolality; U/P osm, ratio of urine to plasma osmolality, U_{SG}, urine specific gravity.

While waiting for the results of these tests and ordering a renal US, and in some instances a renal scan, an initial therapeutic decision often can be made. This is especially important in patients in whom no urine can be obtained for analysis. Prerenal failure is a reasonable presumptive diagnosis in the presence of respiratory failure, CHF, dehydration, or shock, if osmolality or SG is high in the absence of casts in the urine. Rapid correction of the problem may be the only therapeutic intervention needed. The SIADHS can be suspected on the basis of severe neurologic dysfunction, pneumothorax, or pleural effusion, with weight gain, oligoanuria, and high urinary SG.

The urine obtained initially (i.e., before any diuretic or fluid challenge) should be sent for urinalysis and urine chemistry for the assessment of tubular function. Various indices and tests have been proposed to differentiate ATN from prerenal or functional failure, by the presence of tubular dysfunction in ATN (391,392). Fractional excre-

tion of sodium is the preferred index; it is obtained from the following formula:

$$\text{FENa (\%)} = 100 \times U_{Na}/U_{cr} \times P_{cr}/P_{Na}$$

where U_{Na} is the urinary concentration of sodium (mEq/L), U_{cr} is the urinary concentration of creatinine (mg/dL), P_{Na} is the plasma sodium concentration (mEq/L), and P_{cr} is the plasma creatinine concentration (mg/dL). The FENa is the ratio of the sodium clearance to the creatinine clearance, expressed as a percent. A FENa greater than 3% suggests a diagnosis of intrinsic failure and a value less than 2.5% a prerenal failure; however, several exceptions exist (Table 42–8).

Asphyxiated newborn infants may manifest transient tubular dysfunction associated with a normal or mildly decreased GFR and a normal or decreased urine output. Their tubular dysfunction is characterized by a positive dipstick test for blood, moderate tubular proteinuria (i.e.,

LMW proteins and N-acetyl-β-d-glucosaminidase [NAG]), and a FENa that is either normal or mildly increased (384,385,393–395). In contrast, ATN is associated with marked proteinuria, markedly decreased GFR, and often oligoanuria. Urinary concentration of myoglobin and retinol-binding protein, but not NAG, can be used to differentiate between normal transient tubular dysfunction and ATN (384,385). Renal and bladder US may establish a diagnosis of urinary tract obstruction, uroascites, or renal cystic disease (see Appendix I–3), suggest renal vein or artery thrombosis, adrenal hemorrhage, or show abnormal cortical, medullary, or pyelocalicial echogenicity (see Table 42–5) (334–338, 396–398). One common finding is increased echogenicity of the pyramids (396,397), which may correspond to the precipitation of Tamm–Horsfall protein in patients with ATN.

The diagnosis of SIADHS is suggested by a plasma osmolality less than 280 mOsm/kg, a ratio of urinary to plasma osmolality that is greater than 1, high urine SG, and an inappropriate increase in weight. The strict criteria used for the diagnosis of SIADHS in adults rarely are met in newborn infants. In most instances, inappropriate levels of ADH are found in patients with abnormal renal function, because asphyxia is a common cause of both problems. The treatment of SIADHS usually includes fluid restriction with a normal sodium intake; hypertonic glucose may be necessary to treat severe hypoglycemia secondary to drastic fluid restriction, and furosemide (with careful replacement of the sodium lost in the urine) may be needed in patients with severe CHF secondary to fluid overload. Hypertonic saline is indicated to raise natremia to 125 mEq/L in patients developing central nervous system signs (e.g., seizures, coma) associated with severe hyponatremia.

Challenge Test

A challenge test is indicated only if the etiology of the renal failure is not evident from the assessment of risk factors, clinical signs, US, and urine indexes (see Table 42–8). This can be a fluid challenge (20 mL/kg of crystalloid solution, e.g., isotonic saline) or a diuretic challenge (usually furosemide 1 mg/kg intravenously). Although patients who fail to respond to furosemide may respond to bumetanide (5 μg/kg/dose intravenously), a more potent loop diuretic, this medication has not been evaluated prospectively in acute neonatal oligoanuria. Whereas mannitol (1 g/kg) has been used for this purpose (399), its administration has resulted in ARF in adult patients (400) and may enhance the risk for intraventricular hemorrhage in VLBW infants through an acute increase in serum osmolality.

A diuretic challenge test should be done first in patients thought to be hypervolemic or in heart failure, whereas a fluid challenge should be done first in those thought to be hypovolemic. If no satisfactory response, defined by a normal urine output, is obtained after the first challenge test, the other test should be considered. Although normalization of the urine output is most commonly observed in prerenal failure, it also may be coincidental with the beginning of the polyuric phase of an intrinsic renal failure, or with the transformation of an oliguric into a nonoliguric renal failure (401). The correct diagnosis may be suggested by renal US and by the rapidity of GFR recovery, rather than by the FENa, which is increased by the challenge itself. In any of these situations, the prognosis usually is good. In contrast, if anuria persists despite optimization of general care and double-challenge test, the diagnosis of intrinsic renal failure is likely, severe fluid restriction is indicated, and the prognosis is guarded. Nonrandomized studies in adult patients with oliguria and azotemia suggest that the administration of low-dose dopamine may result in improvement of urine output and creatinine clearance in some patients, even though they may be refractory to furosemide (402,403). A prospective study is required to evaluate the possible role of dopamine in the early management of diuretic-resistant oliguria in newborn infants.

Nonoliguric Renal Failure

Nonoliguric renal failure is characterized by a sudden decrease in GFR and tubular function in the absence of oligoanuria. Thirty to fifty percent of neonates with ARF are nonoliguric (347,404). The ARF observed in one-third of patients who receive cardiopulmonary bypass surgery typically is nonoliguric (353). Renal failure without oliguria may be overlooked in the absence of routine measurement of blood chemistries and urinalysis (347,348). It may be confused initially with the polyuric phase of an intrinsic or postrenal renal failure, especially after an undiagnosed oligoanuric episode, or with prerenal failure that has been treated by the administration of fluids or low-dose dopamine for shock or hypovolemia (401). Although the prognosis of nonoliguric renal failure usually is better than oliguric renal failure (352), it can be complicated by symptomatic hyperkalemia (405).

Treatment of Acute Renal Failure

In our experience, prevention of ARF and its complications avoids the need for renal replacement therapy (e.g., dialysis, hemo[dia]filtration) in most patients. Some researchers, however, argue that early institution of replacement therapy may result in improved mortality and morbidity.

Supportive Treatment and Prevention of Complications

Supportive treatment of infants with ARF should be aimed at comprehensive homeostasis of all vital systems.

Some patients may need major respiratory and cardiovascular support (406), and all such patients require adequate fluid and electrolyte balance and adjustment of the dosage of medications that are eliminated by the kidney (347,407,408). Early diagnosis and treatment may help prevent many complications of ARF, such as water or medication intoxication and hyperkalemia. The prognosis of ARF depends not only on the severity and the duration of the renal injury, but also, and perhaps mainly, on the overall status of the patient.

Fluid and Electrolytes

Water and Sodium. In the presence of oligoanuria refractory to the initial fluid and diuretic challenge, fluid restriction is indicated. Fluid intake is limited to ongoing sensible losses (i.e., gastrointestinal losses, urinary output, third-space losses, drainage), plus 25 mL/kg/24 hours in a full-term infant, and 50 to 100 mL/kg/24 hours in a LBW or VLBW infant to replace insensible water loss. Neither sodium nor potassium should be administered routinely during this phase. On the other hand, high doses of calcium may be required to treat hypocalcemia or for the electrocardiographic consequences of hyperkalemia. If fluid restriction is not initiated early in the course of ARF, fluid overload will result, with potential CHF, pulmonary edema, and pulmonary hemorrhage. If massive fluid overload leads to severe CHF, hemo(dia)filtration may be indicated.

Hyperkalemia. Patients with ARF often develop hyperkalemia, i.e., a potassium concentration greater than 6.5 mEq/L (409,410). Factitious hyperkalemia can result from hemolysis or clot formation during sampling (i.e., release of potassium from erythrocytes or platelets) or from interference with the measurement of potassium concentration by benzalkonium released from a heparin-coated umbilical catheter (411). If hyperkalemia is associated with hyponatremia, hypoglycemia, and hypotension, a diagnosis of adrenal insufficiency should be considered (see Chap. 41). This most often results either from congenital adrenal hyperplasia or from bilateral adrenal hemorrhage; the latter may be suspected on the basis of anemia with thrombocytopenia, jaundice, and bilateral abdominal masses, and confirmed by US.

The treatment of hyperkalemia includes discontinuing all potassium intake; discontinuing any medication that could cause hyperkalemia (e.g., indomethacin, ACE inhibitors, potassium-sparing diuretics); and correcting hypovolemia using isotonic saline to promote tubular secretion of potassium. Simultaneous administration of several forms of therapy (Table 42–9) often is required for treatment of life-threatening hyperkalemia (404,409, 412–419).

If electrocardiographic changes are associated with hyperkalemia, administration of calcium chloride or calcium gluconate is indicated; this will rapidly, but only transiently, decrease myocardial cell excitability, but will not decrease potassium concentration (see Table 42–9) (413). Thus, the administration of calcium should be followed immediately by at least one method to decrease the potassium concentration.

Cellular uptake of potassium can be induced by an infusion of sodium bicarbonate or the combination of glucose and insulin. Because their mechanisms are different, more than one method may be used; none has been shown to be superior to the others. If glucose and insulin are infused, the initial ratio for VLBW infants (500 to 1,000 g) should be approximately 2.2 g/U (414); the ratio should be adjusted (range 1 to 3 g/U) according to the evolution of the glycemia. Salbutamol infusion also is effective in treating hyperkalemia (415). Its action is mediated by an induction of Na^+/K^+-ATPase through cAMP, enhancing the movement of potassium into cells. This is independent of the action of insulin or aldosterone.

Although cation-exchange resins offer the potential advantage of removing potassium from the body rather than increasing cellular uptake, the effect of the resin is much slower than that of glucose and insulin (417). Repetitive use of sodium polystyrene sulfonate may cause sodium overload; this complication can be avoided by using a resin with calcium instead of sodium. Sorbitol should be administered concomitantly to prevent fecal impaction. Oral administration of cation-exchange resins is not recommended (418), whereas repetitive rectal administration may cause local bleeding.

If these techniques fail to correct hyperkalemia, exchange transfusion with washed, packed erythrocytes reconstituted with plasma or albumin is extremely efficient in normalizing potassium concentration for as long as 12 hours (419). It is the treatment of choice in patients in whom renal replacement therapy is contraindicated by peritonitis or cardiovascular instability. Renal replacement therapy, especially hemo(dia)filtration, is the procedure of choice for infants with severe oliguric ARF and for those on ECMO (420).

Acid–Base and Mineral Disturbances. Metabolic acidosis develops rapidly in most infants with ARF. It may require the administration of large doses of sodium bicarbonate, which may aggravate fluid overload.

Hypocalcemia develops rapidly in almost all patients with ARF. It may result from hyperphosphatemia and increased deposition of calcium in injured tissues, especially in rhabdomyolysis; skeletal resistance to PTH, which results from decreased hydroxylation of vitamin D (421); and, in aminoglycoside-induced ARF, parathyroid dysfunction secondary to hypomagnesemia, which is due to increased tubular loss (422). Hypercalcemia may occur as a late complication of rhabdomyolysis, as a result of reabsorption of calcium deposited in necrotic tissues. Hyperphosphatemia is due to tissue damage (e.g., severe asphyxia, shock, rhabdomyolysis) and decreased urine

TABLE 42–9. *Treatment of hyperkalemia in renal failure*

Medication	Dose (iv unless otherwise specified)	Mechanism	Onset of action	Duration
Calcium chloride	0.25–0.5 mEq/kg over 5–10 min	Modifies myocardial excitability	1–3 min	30–60 min
Calcium gluconate	0.5–1 mEq/kg over 5–10 min			
Sodium bicarbonate	1 mEq/kg over 10–30 min	Intracellular uptake of K	5–10 min	2 h
Glucose	0.5 g/kg/h	Intracellular uptake of K	30 min	4–6 h
+Insulin	1 U/2.2 g glucose (1–3)[a]			
Salbutamol (albuterol)	4–5 µg/kg over 15–20 min[c]	Intracellular uptake of K	30–40 min	>120 min
Cation exchange resin (Na/Ca polystyrene sulfonate)	1 g/kg intrarectally q 6 h[b]	Exchange of K for Na or Ca	1–2 h	6 h
Exchange transfusion	2/3 washed RBCs reconstituted with 5% albumin	Uptake of K by RBCs	Minutes[d]	>12 h
Peritoneal dialysis	Use a dialysate with low K concentration	Dialysis	Minutes[d]	No limit
Hemo(dia)filtration		Filtration (and dialysis)	Minutes[d]	Days

[a]The preparation of an insulin drip requires saturating the plastic tubing with the insulin solution before infusing to the patient. The average ratio of glucose to insulin associated with maintenance of normal glycemia in very-low-birth-weight infants is 2.2 ± 0.6 g/U (mean ± SD) (Lui).

[b]Oral administration of polystyrene resin should be avoided in very-low-birth-weight infants and those with poor peristalsis (risk for concretions) (Ohlson). Substantial load of calcium or sodium may result from the respective resin. The effect on potassium concentration is slower than glucose insulin combination.

[c]The iv preparation is not available in the United States. Salbutamol is also efficient by aerosol, but no experience is available in newborn infants.

[d]These techniques are both rapid and extremely effective in correcting potassium levels. The time to set them up may be the limiting factor; other techniques may be used to stabilize the infant initially.
Modified from ref 413.

excretion (421). In addition, ARF usually causes hypermagnesemia, which may result from decreased excretion and from shift from the intracellular space (423). The polyuric phase of ATN is associated with increased urinary excretion of phosphate and magnesium. Hypocalcemia should be prevented or treated with early intravenous administration of calcium gluconate or chloride. During the oliguric phase, no intake of magnesium (e.g., antacids) or phosphate should be provided, to limit both hypermagnesemia and hyperphosphatemia.

Polyuric Phase. The oliguric phase of ARF is followed by a polyuric phase. During this phase, serial measurements of urine electrolytes and hourly monitoring of the urine output are imperative to adequately replace urinary losses and prevent dehydration, hyponatremia, and hypokalemia. In some cases, bicarbonate, phosphate, and magnesium need to be given to replace urinary losses. When GFR approaches normal levels, fluid intake should be decreased gradually and carefully, while following weight, serum chemistries, and urine output. Replacing the urine output volume for volume for an indefinite duration would cause an adaptive persistence of the polyuria. However, some patients may not recover a normal urinary concentrating ability despite normalization of GFR; these patients still need high fluid intake (424).

Nutrition

If fluid restriction is required, glucose intake often is minimal and severe hypoglycemia may develop, unless a hypertonic solution of glucose is infused through a central venous catheter. If refractory hypoglycemia occurs because of low glucose intake, steroids or a continuous infusion of glucagon can be given. If this is unsuccessful, hemofiltration should be initiated. This technique will allow increased fluid and glucose intake while rapidly correcting the hypervolemia.

Adequate nutrition should be provided to assure anabolism, thereby reducing renal load (425). Breast milk or low-protein formula should be initiated as soon as possible; if the infant cannot be fed, total parenteral nutrition (TPN) should be initiated. If the ARF is severe, the usual amino acid solution should be replaced by essential L-amino acids supplemented with L-histidine (Levamin Essential; Leiras, Turku, Finland), initially given at a dose of 0.5 to 1 g/kg/d.

Hematologic Disturbances

Anemia associated with ARF may result from several factors, including decreased erythropoietin production, abnormal or ineffective erythropoiesis, impaired iron use, and shortened erythrocyte survival. Transfusion of packed erythrocytes may be necessary. Bleeding tendency may result from abnormal platelet function and, in some patients (e.g., those with renal venous thrombosis), from thrombocytopenia.

Adjustment of Medication Dosage

The interval of administration of medications with renal elimination (e.g., antibiotics, paralyzing agents, tolazoline, theophylline, antiepileptic drugs, and digoxin) should be adjusted to actual renal function (spontaneous or renal replacement therapy) to avoid toxic levels. The latter might, in turn, increase the severity of the renal failure (see Nephrotoxicity). Although there are insufficient data to calculate adjustment of dosage in newborn infants, predictions can be made from the relationship between P_{cr} and the half-life of serum concentration of a particular drug (311–313). Additional adjustments can be made by monitoring drug levels. When possible, medications with minimal or no renal toxicity should be chosen.

Renal Replacement Therapy

Renal replacement therapy is indicated only if aggressive symptomatic treatment fails to manage life-threatening complications due to massive fluid overload, hyperkalemia, or hypertension (426). Modalities include peritoneal dialysis, hemodialysis, hemofiltration, and hemodiafiltration (427–437).

Peritoneal dialysis is contraindicated in patients with respiratory failure and should be used with caution in those with peritonitis (428). In patients with liver failure, the dialysis solution should contain bicarbonate (instead of lactate) (429). The other techniques require either heparinization, which is contraindicated in premature infants because of the risk of intraventricular hemorrhage, or prostacyclin (431). Hemo(dia)filtration is the technique of choice for the treatment of massive fluid overload. Availability of large-bore intravascular catheters in a patient on ECMO makes this technique particularly easy to initiate. Hemo(dia)filtration is done by arteriovenous route, or, if MAP is too low or if arterial access is impossible, by venovenous route with pump assistance (432). Renal transplantation should be considered after the neonatal period (see Chronic Renal Failure).

Before renal replacement therapy is initiated, serious consideration should be given to the possibility that the patient may have either a dysmorphic syndrome with a very poor future quality of life, or severe irreversible multiorgan failure. Immediate survival depends mostly on nonrenal problems, whereas ultimate prognosis also depends on the severity of bilateral renal parenchymal disease (436,437).

Prognosis

The short-term prognosis for neonatal ARF depends on the general condition of the infant and the status of all major organs and systems. A team approach to management is crucial and should include a neonatologist, nephrologist, urologist, geneticist, and radiologist.

Acquired Renal Failure

In one series, the mortality rate in patients with oliguric ARF due to acquired conditions (i.e., asphyxia and sepsis) was 60% and even higher in those with congenital heart disease (348). A similar mortality rate (61%) was observed in a series of infants requiring peritoneal dialysis in the first 60 days of life (427). For newborn infants in whom ARF develops while on ECMO, the prognosis is grim. In contrast, the prognosis for nonoliguric renal failure or for prerenal failure is excellent, unless major arrhythmia secondary to hyperkalemia develops or multiorgan failure develops. Long-term abnormalities in GFR and in tubular function are common in acquired as well as congenital causes of ARF. In one series, limited urinary concentrating ability tested using DDAVP was observed at 1 to 36 months of age in 11% of patients who had a neonatal $P_{cr} \geq 1.5$ mg/dL (424). Fanconi syndrome has been reported as a sequela of renovascular accident in the neonatal period (438).

Congenital Urinary Tract Malformations

Immediate mortality of infants with congenital urinary tract malformations depends primarily on the severity of respiratory failure associated with lung hypoplasia and pulmonary hypertension (439). Infants with severe pulmonary hypoplasia, often associated with typical Potter syndrome, die within the first postnatal hours or days; the treatment of moderate lung hypoplasia and pulmonary hypertension (406) is discussed in Chapter 28. The presence of bilateral renal parenchymal disease is the major factor predicting poor renal function in cases with congenital renal or urinary tract malformations. Patients with prenatal diagnosis of bilateral urinary tract obstruction should have a comprehensive assessment, including family history, ultrasonography, karyotype, AFP, specific biochemical or genetic tests as indicated, and urine biochemical analysis (Table 42–10) (440–442). If prenatal assessment demonstrates severe urinary tract obstruction with oligohydramnios in a fetus without a lethal disease and without evidence for renal dysfunction suggestive of bilateral renal dysplasia (316,317,440), intervention may be indicated to alleviate oligohydramnios and thus limit or prevent lung hypoplasia. Depending on GA, one may then consider either intrauterine decompression of the urinary tract or elective premature delivery after steroid administration to the mother. Serial determinations of urine indicators appear more reliable to predict long-term renal function than single measurements (440–442). Chronic renal failure (CRF) may develop despite early surgical intervention for urinary tract obstruction or reflux (443).

Special Considerations

Structural anomalies of the kidneys and urinary tract are discussed in Chapter 43.

Tubular Dysgenesis

Several cases of perinatal ARF have been described in association with immature nephrons, predominantly with either glomerular lesions or tubular lesions. Oligohydramnios developed in most patients during the second trimester. These infants died *in utero* or soon after birth.

Autosomal Congenital Tubular Dysgenesis

Congenital tubular dysgenesis (i.e., congenital oligomeganephronic nephromegaly with tubular dysgenesis, congenital renal tubular immaturity) has been described in 1% of 500 consecutive perinatal autopsies (444). This autosomal recessive syndrome is characterized by short and undifferentiated tubules and lack of identifiable proximal tubules by lectin staining, contrasting with the presence of numerous glomeruli (445–449). Renal US shows normal or increased cortical echogenicity, decreased corticomedullary differentiation, and variable renal size (336,445). Oligohydramnios develops during the second trimester, usually after 20 weeks of gestation, and results in Potter sequence and perinatal death. Some cases have been described in association with twin-to-twin transfusion or polymalformations.

Other Types of Tubular Dysgenesis

The administration of ACE inhibitors during pregnancy can result in oligohydramnios, lung hypoplasia, neonatal renal failure with oligoanuria for 3 to 9 days, hypotension, hypoplasia of the calvaria, and, in many cases, perinatal death (260,261,351). Pathologic examination may show tubular dysgenesis with abundant presence of renin in glomeruli and preglomerular arterioles, suggesting up regulation of the renin–angiotensin system (450). Similar lesions may occur in one kidney, with renal artery stenosis secondary to arteritis or medial arterial calcinosis (451).

Prenatal administration of PGSIs (e.g., indomethacin) has been associated with perinatal death, bleeding diathesis, ileal perforation, premature ductal closure, fetal oligoanuria, oligohydramnios, and transient or prolonged neonatal renal failure (requiring chronic dialysis) with hematuria and casts (335,336,452). Pathology may show immature tubules and glomeruli, massive cortical necrosis, or ischemic changes in the cortex associated with cystic dilation of the superficial nephrons and increased intrarenal renin (262).

Renal Artery Thrombosis

The clinical presentation of renal artery thrombosis is a variable combination of hyperreninemic systemic hypertension, hematuria, severe oligoanuric ARF (if the lesion is bilateral), and loss of femoral pulses and of

TABLE 42–10. *Assessment of the fetus with bilateral renal mass*

Procedure	Significance and interpretation
Family history	Autosomal dominant polycystic kidney disease, autosomal recessive polycystic kidney disease, hereditary renal dysplasia
Comprehensive ultrasonography	Dysmorphic syndrome (e.g., skeletal dysplasia)
	Lung hypoplasia (secondary to abdominal mass, oligohydramnios, or both)
	Abnormality of central nervous system, spinal cord, heart, gastrointestinal tract, limbs
	Tumor (obstructing urinary flow)
	Hydrops, ascites
	Oligohydramnios, polyhydramnios
	Cortical cysts or abnormal echogenicity suggest renal dysplasia; however, hydronephrosis may be difficult to differentiate from cystic dysplasia
	Large trabeculated bladder in a male suggests a diagnosis of posterior urethral valves
DNA analysis	Fetal karyotype to rule out trisomy 13, 18, 9
	Molecular genetics (for specific diagnoses)
Alpha-fetoprotein	If abnormal for gestational age:
	Low: consider diagnosis of trisomy
	High: consider myelomeningocele
Assessment of renal function	
	Abnormal fetal urine composition (especially progressive worsening on serial analysis) predicts poor long-term renal function and thus is a contraindication to fetal intervention
	Sodium >95th percentile for gestational age (100 mEq/L at 20 wk)
	Chloride >90 mEq/L
	Osmolality >210 mOsm/kg
	Calcium >2 mmol/L (8 mg/dL)
	Phosphate >2 mmol/L
	Beta 2-microglobulin >4 mg/L
	Protein >20 mg/dL
	Urine output <2 mL/h
	Abnormal amino acid concentration for gestational age
	High fetal serum level of $beta_2$-microglobulin: >4.9 mg/L (95% confidence interval at 18–39wk) or >5.6 mg/L

blood flow to the lower extremities. Renal artery thrombosis is often but not always (453) associated with a history of UA catheterization (454–457). The incidence of thrombi in infants with a UA catheter in place ranges between 24% and 95% (458,459). These thrombi may become symptomatic when massive or when embolism occurs.

Renal US may be normal or show increased cortical echogenicity or nephromegaly. Real-time US may show a blood clot in the aorta or a renal artery, and Doppler flow studies may show decreased renal arterial flow. Isotopic renogram may show absence of RBF or a localized defect. If the UA catheter is still in place, angiography may be performed, preferably using a low-osmolality radiocontrast agent (see Nephrotoxicity).

ARF associated with bilateral renal artery thrombosis may require prolonged replacement therapy (e.g., peritoneal dialysis) (455). The indications for surgical treatment are not clear (455,460,461). Thrombolysis and, if it fails, thrombectomy should be considered for patients with refractory hypertension and those with massive aortic thrombus resulting in major complications (e.g., compromised limb perfusion or anuria) (455,460,461). The other patients usually can be treated with antihypertensive agents and symptomatic management of the compli-

cations of ARF; heparinization may help limit further extension of the thrombus. The therapeutic decision should take into account the risk of disseminated bleeding and intraventricular hemorrhage, especially in premature infants.

Although renal artery thrombosis often results in localized or diffuse renal hypotrophy, renal function often improves to a level that is close to normal, and hypertension resolves in most patients within a few months (462,463). Fanconi syndrome may occur in rare patients (463).

Renal Venous Thrombosis

Neonatal renal venous thrombosis is an uncommon condition. It may be associated with polycythemia; severe perinatal asphyxia; severe dehydration, sometimes with shock; maternal diabetes; angiography for congenital cyanotic heart disease; and adrenal hemorrhage (464,465). Suboptimal fibrinolysis in stressed newborn infants may be an important factor (466). Renal venous thrombosis presents clinically as the association of a unilateral or bilateral palpable flank mass with hematuria, proteinuria, and, in some cases, oligoanuria. Ultrasonography and Doppler studies show whether the thrombosis extends to the inferior vena cava. Ultrasonography of the kidney shows a typical image, characterized by enlargement of the kidney, loss of definition of the corticomedullary junction, abnormal focal or generalized increase in echo amplitude of the renal parenchyma, and decrease in the size and echo amplitude of the central echo complex (465). The acute complications of renal venous thrombosis include ARF, systemic hypertension, and disseminated intravascular coagulation. The lesion ultimately may result in renal atrophy (467,468).

Conservative and supportive therapy are indicated. The indications for surgery are not clear. In the presence of consumption coagulopathy, administration of heparin may be considered, although unproven. In cases associated with bilateral renal venous thrombosis or inferior vena cava thrombosis, similar results have been reported using either thrombectomy or thrombolysis (469,470).

Cortical Necrosis and Medullary Necrosis

Renal cortical or medullary necrosis is the most severe type of ARF. The most common causes of renal necrosis include severe asphyxia and shock (471,472). Idiopathic arterial calcification is a rare cause of renal infarction (473). The symptomatology is not specific and includes oligoanuric ARF, proteinuria, and hematuria that is often grossly apparent. The kidneys often are enlarged; renal US shows homogeneously hyperechoic kidneys, with loss of sharp corticomedullary definition (337). The renal scan shows either very poor renal function or nonvisualization of the kidneys. Calcifications may become visible both on the US and the abdominal radiography. The treatment is similar to that described previously for ATN. The prognosis of bilateral global cortical necrosis is dismal; the diagnosis has been made most often at autopsy. Patients with focal or unilateral necrosis may recover, but often have chronic hypertension and CRF. Infants with medullary necrosis typically have persistent limitations in urinary concentrating ability.

Postrenal Failure

Postrenal failure may result from urinary tract anomalies, extrinsic compression of the urinary tract, fungal infection (fungus ball) or, rarely, urolithiasis (474) (see Hypercalciuria, Nephrocalcinosis, and Nephrolithiasis, and Chap. 43). The medical treatment of postrenal failure is similar to that of intrinsic renal failure. Decompression of the urinary tract (see Chap. 43) often results in an increase in GFR as well as a polyuric phase that usually is transient. During the polyuric phase, severe dehydration, hyponatremia, and hyperkalemia may develop despite adequate increase of serum aldosterone levels (475). Sequential adjustment of fluid and electrolyte intake to these losses may help prevent or limit such complications. When GFR comes to baseline within 1 week

after surgery, fluid intake should be reduced slowly and carefully, taking into account the fact that limited urine-concentrating ability is expected in association with dysplastic kidneys. The evolution of renal function depends on the degree of renal dysplasia, which is very common in congenital urinary tract obstruction, and the frequency of UTI, which is related to VUR, urinary stasis, and the presence of an indwelling catheter.

NEPHROTOXICITY: DRUGS AND TOXINS

Several drugs that cross the placenta (see Chap. 15) can damage the fetal kidney, including aminoglycosides, heavy metals, alcohol (476), and organic solvents (Table 42–11) (477). Chapters 15 and 55 provide a discussion of the relevant pharmacokinetics. Nephrotoxicity may result from renal ischemia or direct cytotoxicity, or both. Direct cytotoxicity is related to the concentration of drug or metabolite in renal tubular cells, which depends on the concentration of free drug in the plasma, GFR, and tubular transport.

Nephrotoxicity may present as oligoanuria, ARF, drug toxicity caused by decreased clearance of a medication with renal excretion, hypotension, hematuria, proteinuria, renal tubular acidosis (RTA), nephrocalcinosis or nephrolithiasis, polyuria, abnormal plasma electrolyte concentrations, or cardiac arrhythmia (see Table 42–11). Because most NICU patients are exposed to multiple drugs as well to episodes of hypoxemia and ischemia, it often is very difficult to determine whether a particular drug is the major renal offender.

Prevention of nephrotoxicity includes avoiding teratogens during pregnancy, adjusting the daily dose of medications excreted by the kidney according to measured or predicted GFR and to serum drug levels, avoiding known toxins (355,478,479), and avoiding, if possible, nephrotoxic drugs, especially synergistic combinations.

Specific Considerations

Aminoglycosides

Aminoglycosides cause renal vasoconstriction mediated by TXB_2 (480) and direct cellular toxicity, especially in the proximal tubule, which absorbs the drug and stores it in lysosomes. Eventually, tubular necrosis, tubular atrophy, intratubular myeloid bodies, and interstitial nephritis may develop (481,482).

Aminoglycoside nephrotoxicity often presents as isolated proteinuria, reversible polyuric ARF with a high FENa, or transient tubular dysfunction (483,484). Laboratory findings may include proteinuria, decreased GFR, decreased urine-concentrating ability, glucosuria, increased urinary excretion of sodium, potassium, calcium, and magnesium, alterations in tubular transport of organic acids, and, rarely, a Fanconi syndrome (423,

TABLE 42–11. *Nephrotoxic effects of various drugs and toxins*

Substance	Renal side effects
Drugs	
Aminoglycosides	Proteinuria, increased urinary excretion of Na, K, Mg, and glucose, Fanconi syndrome, myelin figures, decreased concentrating ability, decreased RBF, polyuric ARF, ATN, interstitial nephritis
Methicillin	Interstitial nephritis
Amphotericin B	Hyperkaliuria, hyposthenuria, NDI, hypernatriuria, ATN, oliguria, RTA, nephrocalcinosis
Acyclovir	Crystalluria, obstructive nephropathy
Indomethacin	Decreased RBF, ATN, oligoanuria, hyponatremia, hyperkalemia, nephron dysgenesis, and oligohydramnios (*in utero*)
Tolazoline	Hypotension and hypoxemia resulting in decreased GFR, ATN, oliguria, hematuria
α-Adrenergic agents	Decreased RBF, ATN
ACE inhibitors	Hypotension, decreased RBF, ATN, nephron dysgenesis (*in utero*)
Radiocontrast agents	Decreased RBF, oliguric ATN, Tamm–Horsfall proteinuria, nephromegaly with US similar to ARPKD, increased urinary excretion of uric acid
Cyclosporine	Renal vasoconstriction, decreased RBF and GFR, interstitial nephritis
Loop diuretics	Nephrocalcinosis, nephrolithiasis
Ifosfamide	Fanconi syndrome
Toxins	
Hemoglobin	ATN
Myoglobin	ATN
Oxalate	Nephrocalcinosis, nephrolithiasis, oxalosis with ARF
Benzyl alcohol	Cardiovascular collapse, ATN
Polysorbate (in iv tocopherol)	ATN
Uric acid	Crystalluria, ATN
Organic solvents (toluene)	Fanconi syndrome, aminoaciduria, hyperchloremic acidosis
Alcohol (fetal alcohol syndrome)	Distal RTA
Ethylene glycol (in paracetamol)	ARF, metabolic acidosis

ACE, angiotensin-converting enzyme; ARF, acute renal failure; ARPKD, autosomal recessive polycystic kidney disease; ATN, acute tubular necrosis; GFR, glomerular filtration rate; NDI, nephrogenic diabetes insipidus; RBF, renal blood flow; RTA, renal tubular acidosis.

483–487). The most sensitive indicator of nephrotoxicity is the detection of proteinuria (initially brush border enzymes, e.g., trehalase, and LMW proteins; after 1 week of therapy, cytoplasmic and lysosomal enzymes, e.g., NAG) (488–490) or phospholipiduria (491).

Gentamicin, kanamycin, and tobramycin are more nephrotoxic than amikacin or netilmicin (482,488). Studies in infants and children, in contrast with those in adults, have failed to show an additive toxicity of vancomycin and aminoglycosides (492–494). The daily dose of aminoglycosides should be adjusted according to P_{cr} and to serum drug levels. P_{cr}, serum electrolytes, urinalysis, and urine output should be followed serially in high-risk patients; sodium and potassium intake should be adjusted to urine losses. In patients with severe nephrotoxicity and in those with renal failure, a less toxic antibiotic should be used.

Indomethacin

Indomethacin is excreted into the urine through the organic secretory pathway of the proximal tubule, which explains higher levels in more immature patients (495). Indomethacin administration was found to transiently decrease RBF in premature infants with symptomatic PDA (340). Some patients develop transient renal dysfunction, associated with a fall of PRA from the high levels that are attributed to renal hypoperfusion before closure of the PDA, and a transient rise in the plasma level of AVP (496). During prolonged administration of indomethacin (i.e., up to 1 week), hormonal levels normalize, and renal function tends to improve (496,497). Indomethacin causes NAG enzymuria and increases the proximal tubular reabsorption of solutes (e.g, Na^+), the corticomedullary gradient, and the hydroosmotic effect of ADH. The latter two changes result in an increased ratio of urine to plasma osmolality and decreased free water clearance, leading to water retention and dilutional hyponatremia (498–500). Indomethacin administration may also cause oliguric ARF and decreased renal K^+ excretion, resulting in hyperkalemia. The latter may result from hyporeninemic hypoaldosteronism, decreased Na^+ delivery to the distal tubule, or ARF. Maternal administration of indomethacin may induce nephron dysgenesis (see Acute Renal Failure) (262,335), oligohydramnios, and neonatal renal failure (498).

Indomethacin is contraindicated if P_{cr} is elevated (i.e., P_{cr} greater than 1.8 mg/dL) and in the presence of oligoanuria or hyperkalemia. The incidence of nephrotoxicity is increased by the combination of indomethacin with other nephrotoxins. Preliminary data suggest that prior volume expansion may reduce indomethacin-induced nephrotoxicity and that simultaneous administration of dopamine or furosemide may reduce the incidence of oliguria even in the absence of an improvement in GFR (371,373,378). During a course of indomethacin, P_{cr}, serum electrolyte concentrations, and urine output should be monitored. The interval of drug administration should be adjusted according to P_{cr} or GFR, and fluid intake should be adjusted according to urine output. If oligoanuria develops, a challenge dose of furosemide should be given; fluid restriction should be initiated if oligoanuria persists.

Tolazoline

In newborn infants, tolazoline is a nonspecific vasodilator (i.e., acting on both the pulmonary and the systemic vasculature, presumably as an α-antagonist). Tolazoline is excreted into the urine by glomerular filtration and by tubular secretion (501). Renal complications, including oliguria, transient oliguric ARF, and hematuria, are common in neonates in whom tolazoline induces systemic hypotension (502).

Amphotericin B

Amphotericin B causes nephrotoxicity by renal vasoconstriction (503) and by its affinity to sterols, which are important components of membranes. Functional tubular alterations include an increase in urinary pH, in fractional excretion of Na^+, K^+, and phosphate, and in NAG enzymuria (504). Prolonged administration results in glomerular lesions, interstitial edema, focal tubular atrophy, and nephrocalcinosis (505).

In newborn infants, amphotericin often results in increased P_{cr} and BUN, and transient hypokalemia (506); the latter can be prevented by increasing potassium intake. Acute signs of nephrotoxicity may include decreased RBF and GFR, azotemia, oligoanuria, increased urinary excretion of Na^+, K^+, phosphate, and bicarbonate, and hyposthenuria. Later complications may include NDI, distal RTA, and nephrocalcinosis (505,507). The incidence and prognosis of renal damage depend on the total dose of amphotericin administered (505). Nephrotoxicity may be limited by using a slow infusion (508), adjusting the daily dose to GFR and to minimum inhibitory and fungicidal concentrations (509), and avoiding hypercholesterolemia (510). If oligoanuric ARF develops, amphotericin should be withheld temporarily and restarted later, either at a lower dose or preferentially using a liposomal formulation at a similar or higher dose (511). Liposomal amphotericin has limited toxicity and is well tolerated in neonates (512).

Acyclovir

Acyclovir administration may result in an increase in urine beta$_2$-microglobulin and an obstructive nephropathy mediated by crystalluria that may lead to ARF (514). The risk of nephropathy can be minimized by adjusting the interval of administration for GA and renal function, by using a slow infusion, and by providing sufficient fluid intake to maintain adequate urinary output (514,515). If acyclovir is considered in a patient who also needs fluid restriction, the urine should be checked regularly for crystalluria and increased P_{cr}. If renal dysfunction is observed, the dose of acyclovir should be withheld or decreased, and fluid intake increased temporarily.

Radiocontrast Agents

Radiocontrast agents may cause ischemia, direct toxicity, and tubular obstruction by Tamm–Horsfall protein (516) or by uric acid crystals resulting from increased uricosuria (517). Histopathologic features include vacuolization of proximal tubular cells, mild dilation of proximal tubules, areas of luminal inspissation by waxy debris, and interstitial edema (518). Although there is no study comparing low- and high-osmolality products in infants, only the latter cause a decrease in GFR in immature rabbits (519).

The signs of radiocontrast nephrotoxicity may include poor visualization or a prolonged nephrogram, proteinuria with casts, and oliguric ARF (516). One premature infant, who had no visualization after injection of an iodinated product, had a transient oligoanuric ARF with an SG of 1.020, low FENa, and nephromegaly (518); US suggested the diagnosis of ARPKD.

Intravenous urography is best avoided in the neonatal period, especially during the first days of life. In newborn infants who need angiography or CT with contrast, a low-osmolality agent is preferred. Adequate hydration should be provided before the procedure.

Angiotensin-Converting Enzyme Inhibitors

Administration of ACE inhibitors during pregnancy has been associated with tubular dysgenesis, oliguric ARF, hypotension, hypoplasia of the calvaria, and perinatal death, and is therefore contraindicated (see Acute Renal Failure) (260,261,351). Neonates born in ARF after maternal ACE inhibition have a high mortality rate using conservative management; peritoneal dialysis may be considered to treat the ARF and to remove the ACE inhibitor (351). Postnatal ACE inhibition may cause profound hypotension, decreased RBF, and oliguric ARF (520,521), especially in association with hypovolemia. These hypotensive events respond to massive volume expansion but not to inotropes. ACE inhibition also enhances the renal toxicity of aminoglycosides (480).

Cyclosporine A

Cyclosporine induces reversible renal vasoconstriction (522) and interstitial fibrosis. Its nephrotoxicity is enhanced by high serum levels of the drug, ischemia, concomitant administration of nephrotoxic drugs, and low GFR (523), and is reduced by using a continuous, rather than a 4-hour, infusion (523). Cyclosporine nephrotoxicity develops in two-thirds of patients treated after liver transplantation (524). It may present as a variable combination of systemic hypertension, high P_{cr} and BUN, hyperkalemia, hypomagnesemia, metabolic acidosis, NAG enzymuria, and proteinuria, or, rarely, as ARF (524,525). Cyclosporine-induced nephrotoxicity often is easily controlled medically; other immunosuppressive drugs should be considered if severe nephrotoxicity has developed.

Myoglobinuria–Hemoglobinuria

Rhabdomyolysis causes major shifts between intra- and extracellular electrolytes, shock, severe renal vasoconstriction, hyperuricemia, thrombi in the glomerular capillary tufts due to disseminated intravascular coagulation, intratubular hemoprotein casts, formation of free radicals, and peroxidation of lipids (526,527). In adults with crush syndrome (526,528), forced alkaline diuresis, with mannitol for patients with oligoanuria, prevents hypovolemia and intratubular hemoprotein casts. However, a similar approach cannot be recommended for neonates, because it may increase the risk for brain edema, intraventricular hemorrhage, pulmonary edema, and PDA. The low incidence of neonatal rhabdomyolysis (379,529,530) may result from the low myoglobin content of immature muscle, especially in premature infants (531). Myoglobinuria should be suspected in severely asphyxiated full-term infants with a strongly positive reaction for heme in the absence of microscopic hematuria (379).

CHRONIC RENAL FAILURE

The definition of chronic renal insufficiency is a reduction in GFR to a level between 25% and 50% of normal, whereas that of CRF is a reduction in GFR to less than 25% of normal for at least 3 months (532). End-stage renal disease (ESRD) is the stage at which the patient requires chronic dialysis or renal transplantation for survival.

Incidence

The incidence of ESRD is three to eight cases per one million children (age range 0 to 16 years) (532–534). Only 6% of children with ESRD are under 3 years of age (532). In 1989, of the 754 children (age range 0 to 18 years) who received 761 renal transplants in the United States, less than 7% were under 2 years of age, and less than 2% were under 1 year of age (535).

Etiology

Most reports of CRF in children combine patients who developed CRF as neonates with those in whom CRF developed as a result of a later insult to the kidney (Table 42–12) (536). Many patients in CRF under 24 months of age have aplastic–hypoplastic–dysplastic kidneys or obstructive uropathy (535–537). Typically, the course in infants is characterized by slow, progressive deterioration of renal function.

Diagnosis

History, physical examination, US, measurement of GFR using a radionuclide for the estimation of the functional level of each kidney, urinalysis, and urine culture should be obtained initially. In patients with hydronephrosis, meningomyelocele, or UTI, a VCUG is indicated and a furosemide radionuclide scan should be considered. In certain patients, intravenous urography, percutaneous antegrade pyelography, or a renal biopsy may be indicated (see Clinical Evaluation of Renal Function and Disease).

The signs and symptoms suggestive of CRF are nonspecific, especially in infants, and include growth failure, anorexia, vomiting, pallor, edema, seizures, dehydration, heart failure, hypertension, polyuria, fever, hematuria, proteinuria, and pyuria. In children, symptoms such as lassitude, fatigue, headache, and nausea can be present. The diagnosis of CRF is confirmed by a persistently low GFR corrected for postconceptional age.

Pathophysiology and Treatment

The patient should have periodic physical examinations, including measurement of blood pressure, regular monitoring of growth rate and GFR, and serial measurements of plasma or serum creatinine concentration,

TABLE 42–12. *Etiology of chronic renal failure in 75 patients ≤2 yr of age*

Diagnosis	No. of patients	Percentage
Hypoplasia	24	32
Obstructive uropathy	15	20
Oxalosis	8	11
Congenital nephrotic syndrome	6	8
Hemolytic uremic syndrome[a]	4	5
Cortical necrosis	3	4
Infantile polycystic kidney disease	3	4
Glomerulonephritis[a]	3	4
Steroid-resistant nephrotic syndrome	2	3
Birth hypoxia with renal failure	2	3
Jeune's syndrome	1	1
Drash syndrome	1	1
Anatomic problems	1	1
Unknown	2	3

Note that "infancy" here is defined as <2 yr of age.
[a]These diagnoses are virtually not seen during the neonatal period.
From ref. 536.

acid–base status, serum electrolytes, mineral metabolism, hemoglobin, and hematocrit. Urinalysis, including dipstick, urinary electrolytes, pH, and calcium, should be done serially, and UTI should be excluded on a regular basis. The goal of the treatment is to optimize growth rate and homeostasis, while limiting the rate of progression of the renal disease toward ESRD (532,538–540). The daily dose of medications excreted by the kidney needs to be modified, based on the level of renal function or their removal by means of dialysis (see section on Acute Renal Failure). Growth failure associated with CRF may result from multiple factors, including acidosis, reduced caloric intake, anemia, hypertension, renal osteodystrophy, aluminum intoxication, abnormalities of growth hormone and somatomedins, recurrent episodes of fluid and electrolyte disturbances, recurrent infections, and administration of steroids (541–544).

Nutrition

Infants with chronic renal insufficiency should have the same amount of protein intake as the recommended dietary allowance (RDA) for normal infants (545–547). Breast milk, SMA (Wyeth Ayerst, Radnor, PA), and Similac PM 60/40 (Ross, Columbus, OH) provide adequate high-quality protein and minerals with limited phosphate and sodium content. The formula often needs to be supplemented with carbohydrates and with medium-chain triglycerides to reach 120% to 180% of the caloric RDA. Continuous nocturnal feeding through a nasogastric tube or a gastrostomy tube, and, in a few patients, TPN, may be required (546).

As the degree of renal failure increases (i.e., GFR less than 25% of normal), protein intake should be decreased to maintain a BUN below 100 mg/dL, using milk with high-quality proteins (i.e., at least 35% essential amino acids), such as breast milk, SMA, Similac PM 60/40, or Special Formula S-29 (Wyeth Ayerst). Patients with severe renal failure may require either special diets poor in total protein and supplemented with essential amino acids or their corresponding keto acids, or TPN with essential amino acids (e.g., Nephramine; American McGaw, Santa Ana, CA) (547).

Maintenance of Adequate Fluid and Electrolyte and Acid–Base Balance

Most patients with chronic renal insufficiency are able to maintain normal serum levels of sodium, potassium, and bicarbonate; however, they have limited ability to concentrate urine. Therefore, additional water may be required to compensate for polyuria. The requirements in electrolytes and base should be assessed for every patient from the measurement of serum and urinary electrolytes. For instance, hydronephrosis is often associated with distal tubular acidosis, hyperkalemia, and excessive free water diuresis (548). Acute episodes of fluid or electrolyte imbalance, characterized by hyponatremia, hyperkalemia, azotemia, hypocalcemia or hypercalcemia, metabolic acidosis, and hyperphosphatemia can be precipitated by diarrhea, UTI, sepsis, or increased catabolism associated with poor nutritional intake. Peritoneal dialysis may be required to rapidly correct the imbalance.

Cardiovascular System

Rigorous control of hypertension is important to avoid the complications of hypertension and its known effect of accelerating progression of renal failure. A discussion is presented elsewhere in the chapter (see Hypertension).

Mineral Metabolism and Renal Osteodystrophy

Chronic loss of renal function is associated with a decreased 1-α-hydroxylation of vitamin D and an increased secretion of PTH (543). Initially, the latter is an appropriate response to low serum ionized calcium, but in CRF the set point for the inhibition of PTH secretion by extracellular calcium is raised, which corresponds to secondary hyperparathyroidism. When GFR decreases further, the serum concentration of $1,25(OH)_2D_3$ decreases (549). If phosphate intake is limited, renal 1-α-hydroxylase is stimulated, resulting in a decrease in PTH (Table 42–13). However, when GFR is less than 25% of normal, hyperphosphatemia develops. The radiographic signs of renal osteodystrophy may include rickets-like lesions (i.e., radiolucent bands), signs of osteitis fibrosa related to increased PTH secretion (i.e., subperiosteal resorption zones and metaphyseal changes), and slipped epiphyses (550). Prevention and treatment of renal osteodystrophy include the administration of vitamin D analogs and calcium carbonate, limitation of phosphate intake, and removal of all sources of aluminum (Table 42–14) (544,551,552). Calcium carbonate not only provides calcium, but also is an efficient phosphate-binding agent.

Although aluminum is no longer used in dialysis fluids or phosphate-binding agents (553), its presence in some parenteral solutions, in combination with a low GFR (e.g., in normal premature infants or in patients with CRF) may lead to neurotoxicity and osteodystrophy (554–556). Aluminum intoxication is suggested by hypercalcemia, a normal alkaline phosphatase level, normal PTH levels, and solid metaphyseal bands (543). Severe intoxication is associated with bone pain, proximal myopathy, fractures, and encephalopathy (557). If aluminum intoxication is confirmed by a serum level greater than 100 µg/L (558), by an intravenous desferrioxamine test, or by bone biopsy, parenteral administration of desferrioxamine is indicated (559).

Hematologic Disturbance

CRF is associated with a normochromic, normocytic, hypoproliferative anemia, resulting from many factors,

TABLE 42–13. *Disturbances in mineral metabolism associated with chronic loss of renal function in children*

Stage	Ionized calcium	Phosphate	1,25(OH)$_2$D$_3$	iPTH	Alkaline phosphatase
Early (GFR 70–80%)	Low	Low (when fasting); Normal (during day time)	Normal (inadequate for low Ca)	High	Normal–high
Moderate (GFR <50%)					
Normal P intake	Low	Normal	Low	High	High
Restricted P intake	Normal (low)	Low	Normal	Normal	
Advance (GFR <25%)	Low	High	Low	High	High
Aluminum intoxication	High (while on vitamin D); normal	Normal/high	Normal	Normal (high)	Normal (high)

Pathophysiology in patients with moderate loss of renal function

Normal phosphate intake
  Loss of renal function   ⟶   Increased set point of inhibition of PTH ⟶

                                                        ⎤ Increased iPTH
  Low 1α-hydroxylase   ⟶   Decreased calcitriol   ⟶   Decreased ionized Ca ⟶⎦
Effect of reduction in phosphate intake
  Decreased phosphate diet   ⟶   Normalized calcitriol   ⟶   Improved ionized Ca   ⟶   Normalized iPTH

1,25(OH)$_2$D$_3$, serum concentration of 1,25 dihydroxy-vitamin D$_3$ or calcitrol; iPTH, serum level of immunoreactive parathyroid hormone; GFR, glomerular filtration rate (expressed in % of normal); Ca, calcium; P, phosphate.

including low erythropoietin (Epo) levels, shortened erythrocyte survival, iron and folate deficiency, and aluminum intoxication. Steady-state levels of Epo are low relative to the degree of anemia, because reduced synthesis of Epo by endothelial cells of the peritubular capillary in the renal cortex and outer medulla is not compensated by extrarenal sites (560–562). Two-thirds of patients respond to the administration of 50 U/kg of Epo two to three times a week (563). Epo administration increases hematocrit, improves symptomatology, and prevents iron overload from multiple blood transfusions. Side effects include hypertension, thromboocclusion of vascular access, and, rarely, seizures and elevated liver enzymes. Patients with ESRD and a hematocrit below 30% should receive Epo (see Table 42–14), with iron supplementation at a dose that may need adjustments according to ferritin levels (564–566).

Growth Hormone

CRF is associated with high baseline levels of growth hormone with alterations of the peaks, normal total serum concentration of insulin-like growth factor (IGF)-1, and controversial changes in IGF-binding proteins (567–571). Thus, growth failure in CRF could result either from a decrease in free IGF-1 or from hormonal resistance. The administration of recombinant human growth hormone accelerates growth in growth-retarded children with ESRD (569–573), without accelerating bone maturity or the decline in renal function, and increases final adult length; however, recombinant human growth hormone has been associated with slipped femoral epiphysis and benign intracranial hypertension (573).

Surgical Treatment

Surgical treatment of urinary tract obstruction and of severe VUR has an important role but may not prevent progressive loss of renal function (574). Bilateral nephrectomy is commonly performed in patients with CNF and allows preparation of the infant for renal transplantation.

TABLE 42–14. *Initial doses and side effects of medications commonly used in chronic renal failure*

Medication	Initial dose	Mineral metabolism and growth	Kidney	Other
Vitamin D		Hypercalcemia	Renal failure (metastatic calcifications)	Metastatic calcifications
1,25(OH)$_2$D$_3$	20–60 ng/kg/d			
DHT	15–40 μg/kg/d			
1 α-OHD$_3$	1–2 μg/kg/d			
CaCO$_3$	10–20 mg/kg/d of elemental Ca	Hypercalcemia	Hypercalciuria	
Erythropoietin	25–50 U/kg three times a week		Hypertension	Seizures (hypertension)

TABLE 42-15. *Prognosis of various congenital diseases at risk for end-stage renal disease*

Diagnosis	Transplant offered	n	Percentage survival neonatal period (causes of death)	Percentage survival at 1 yr	Percentage of those surviving neonatal period who develop ESRD (age)	Long-term survival	Reference
Posterior urethral valves	Yes	50	98% (UTI + sepsis)	98%	8%	96% at 2–12 yr (6.8)	Connor 1990 (593)
Prune-belly syndrome	No	50	72% (respiratory renal failure)	68%	6%	68% at ? yr (≤35)	Burbige 1987 (595)
	Yes	32	72% (respiratory failure)	66%	48%	63% at ? yr	Reinberg 1991 (594)
	Yes	7	57% (CHF, stillborn, bronchopneumonia)	57%	50% (13–14 yr)	57% at 3–14 yr	Reinberg 1991 (594)
ARPKD	No	46[a]	NA	79% (from birth)	23% (1 mo–>10 yr)	46% at 15 yr (actuarial)	Kaplan 1989 (596)
	Yes	17 (sample)		88% (from 1 mo)	41% (8 mo–16 yr)	88% at 6.1 ± 4.3 yr	Cole 1987 (597)
	Yes	52[b]	87% (respiratory failure)	86% (from 1 mo) 77% (from birth)	18% (1–43 yr)	67% at 15 yr (actuarial)	Roy 1997 (598)
Nephrotic syndrome	No	14	100%	NA	100%	0% at 4 yr	Mahan 1984 (599)
	Yes	27	100%	NA	100% (8–90 mo)	75% until transplant; recipients: 82% at 2 yr after transplant	Mahan 1984 (599)
	Yes	46	NA	NA	89% [nephrectomy]	93%	Holmberg 1996 (600)

[a]This series involved 23 neonatal PKD, 23 infantile PKD, and 7 patients diagnosed after 1 yr of age. Seven patients were lost to follow-up.
[b]This series includes some of the patients reported in Kaplan (1989). Five patients were lost to follow-up.

ARPKD, autosomal recessive polycystic kidney disease; CHF, congestive heart failure; ESRD, end-stage renal disease; NA, not available; UTI, urinary tract infection.

Infection

Infants with CRF are at risk for infections because of urinary stasis, malnutrition, peritoneal dialysis, and immunosuppression at the time of transplantation. Chemoprophylaxis for UTI is indicated in infants at increased risk because of VUR, ADPKD, or urinary tract obstruction, and at the time of invasive procedures. The incidence of peritonitis in children receiving continuous ambulatory peritoneal dialysis (CAPD) or continuous cyclic peritoneal dialysis (CCPD) is one episode every 5 to 12 months (575,576). The most common agents include *Staphylococcus* sp, gram-negative organisms, and *Candida* sp (575).

Central Nervous System

CRF-related polyneuropathy and encephalopathy can result from aluminum intoxication, hypertension, and electrolyte imbalance. Aluminum-related encephalopathy is characterized by regression of developmental milestones, ataxia, seizures, myoclonus, dementia, and loss of bulbar function (557,577,578). Nowadays, most acute central nervous system complications related to CRF are limited by removal of all sources of aluminum intake, careful monitoring of renal function and of blood pressure, and early initiation of dialysis. Nevertheless, one often observes some motor and mental delay, as well as electroencephalographic abnormalities (579,580). Successful transplantation may be associated with a significant improvement in mental performance and in an acceleration in head growth (580).

Dialysis

The rate of transfer of solutes across the peritoneum is high in young patients (581). Early initiation of CAPD, in association with nasogastric feeding to augment caloric intake, appears to be the treatment of choice for treatment of ESRD in infants (582). Usually, four to five exchanges are performed per day, using a Silastic Tenckhoff catheter (539). The side effects of CAPD are the burden to the family, the risk of peritonitis, anorexia, and chronic loss of protein, amino acids, calcium, and phosphate. For CCPD, five to eight 2-hour exchanges are performed automatically at night (583). The North American Pediatric Renal Transplant Cooperative Study (NAPRTCS) has reported an annual mortality of 14% and a 24-month mortality probability of 0.21 in infants on peritoneal dialysis (540).

Transplantation

Renal transplantation may improve growth and development compared to long-term dialysis (580,584,585). The success of renal transplantation has increased in par-

allel with improvements in preoperative condition, graft survival after multiple preoperative transfusions (586), quality of antigen matching, made possible by the availability of large multicenter organizations and by the increased use of grafts from living related donors, duration of cold storage of the graft, anesthetic and postoperative therapy (587), and immunosuppression (587–591). The complications of renal transplantation include postoperative renal failure, fluid and electrolyte disturbances, hypertension, hypotension, infection, and the side effects of the medications. Difficult problems include the early detection of rejection and the differentiation of renal failure due to cyclosporine from rejection or other complications of the transplant.

Undertaking renal transplantation before or after the age of 1 year remains a controversial issue. The NAPRTCS data show that graft survival for cadaveric transplants improves when the recipient age is greater than 24 months, whereas the prognosis for living donor transplants improves after the age of 12 months and a weight of approximately 8 kg (537,590). The mortality rate of cadaveric transplant recipients younger than 2 years of age is 14%, compared to 4.7% to 8% in older groups (591). In contrast, a few centers have reported excellent results using cadaveric transplants during the second year of life, and living related donor kidneys in recipients with a weight of 5 to 7 kg or a length of 65 cm (584,585,592). Preemptive transplants (i.e., before initiating dialysis) are now offered routinely.

Prognosis

The prognosis for infants with CRF has improved considerably over the last two decades (Table 42–15) (593–600). This may have resulted not only from changes in treatment but also from a change in the patient population associated with an earlier diagnosis. For obstructive urinary tract disease and for prune-belly syndrome, the presence of associated renal dysplasia–hypoplasia is the main prognostic factor (593–595). Isolated posterior urethral valves are associated with a low mortality rate and a low risk of ESRD (593). Neonates diagnosed with ARPKD but without lung hypoplasia may develop ESRD, hypertension, and portal hypertension (596–597). Only limited data are available on ADPKD. Of five infants who survived the neonatal period and were followed until the age of 3.5 ± 3.4 years (mean ± SD), ESRD developed in only one (597). CNF, which used to be a fatal disease, now has a much better prognosis, using bilateral nephrectomy followed by renal transplantation (599,600).

HYPERTENSION

Systemic hypertension is defined as a blood pressure that persistently exceeds the mean + 2 SD for normal subjects of similar GA, size, and postnatal age (see Appendices C–1a through C–1d). Hypertension is very likely to occur if the blood pressure consistently exceeds 90/60 torr in a full-term infant or 80/50 torr in a premature infant (601), and is likely in an infant after the neonatal period if systolic blood pressure is higher than 113 torr (283).

Incidence

The reported incidence of neonatal hypertension ranges between 0.2% and 43% (602–604). This variability may result, in part, from the criteria for sample selection, the methods used for measuring blood pressure, and the normative values used. Neonatal hypertension is relatively common in patients with a history of UA catheterization (3%) (605) and those with bronchopulmonary dysplasia (BPD) (as much as 43%) (603). In one series, it also was associated with PDA and intraventricular hemorrhage (604).

Etiology and Pathophysiology

An etiology (see Appendices C–1e and C–1f) can be determined in only approximately one-third of hypertensive newborn infants (606,607). The most common mechanisms of neonatal hypertension include iatrogenic disease, renovascular hypertension, and renal disease (606).

Hypertension may develop after discharge from the nursery (608). Maternal hypertension, intrauterine growth retardation, and low ponderal index at birth, but not the type of diet, are associated with the development of hypertension in childhood and adulthood (609–612). Low ponderal index and small head circumference are associated with syndrome X (noninsulin-dependent diabetes mellitus, hypertension, and hyperlipidemia) (613). Low birth-weight is associated with a reduction in the number of nephrons, thereby predisposing to hypertension (614).

Clinical Features

Mild-to-moderate hypertension may be asymptomatic (615–617). The symptoms associated with hypertension are nonspecific (Table 42–16) and may be due to the underlying disease, the hypertension itself, or its complications (e.g., neurologic, cardiovascular) (618,619). The infant's chart should be reviewed carefully for the administration of excessive fluids or medications causative of hypertension. Infants with a UA catheter may have had transient episodes of blood pressure elevation associated with an increase in P_{cr} and hematuria, all suggestive of renal artery thromboembolism. Pertinent points of the physical examination are listed in Table 42–16.

Investigation

The first step is to determine whether the infant is indeed hypertensive, or if the blood pressure rises only during periods of agitation, pain, crying, feeding, or performance of procedures. All hypertensive neonates should have a urinalysis and routine blood chemistry tests (see Appendix C–1f). If hypertension appears to be iatrogenic or secondary to drug withdrawal, specific therapy can be tried before additional investigations are performed.

A thorough workup should be initiated in every patient with persistent or severe hypertension (see Appendix C–1f), to rule out cardiovascular complications, to reach a specific diagnosis (see Appendix C–1e), and to assess for possible complications. Ambiguous genitalia in a hypertensive infant should raise the suspicion of congenital adrenal hyperplasia. The association of a maternal history of Graves' disease and neonatal systolic hypertension and tachycardia with or without a goiter suggests the diagnosis of neonatal hyperthyroidism. The association of metabolic alkalosis and hypertension can be observed in congenital adrenal hyperplasia, primary hyperaldosteronism,

TABLE 42–16. *Signs and symptoms associated with neonatal hypertension*

System	History/observation	Physical examination
Growth	Failure to thrive	Weight and length may be small for age
Vital signs	Tachypnea, fever	Tachypnea, tachycardia, fever
Respiratory	Apnea, cyanosis, tachypnea	Apnea, central cyanosis, tachypnea, rales
Cardiovascular	Sweating	Hyperdynamic precordium, heart murmur, congestive heart failure, tachyarrhythmia, mottling, peripheral cyanosis and poor perfusion, abdominal bruit, increased pulse, differential pulse (upper vs. lower extremities: coarctation of the aorta), ischemia of the lower extremities with absent pulse (probable aortic thrombus)
Fluids/renal	Edema, hematuria, weight loss, polyuria	Edema, abdominal mass
Gastrointestinal/liver	Anorexia, abdomen distension	Hepatomegaly
Neurologic	Irritability/lethargy/seizures	Irritability, tremors, seizures, lethargy, coma, bulging fontanelle increased/decreased/asymmetric tone, facial palsy, abnormal reflexes, abnormal optic fundus
Genitalia		Hypogonadism (congenital adrenal hyperplasia)

Note that some of these findings are directly related to hypertension, whereas other signs are related to the primary cause.

or rarely in unilateral renovascular hypertension (620). The association of metabolic acidosis, hyperkalemia, and hypertension suggests the diagnosis of Gordon syndrome (see section on Renal Causes of Hypertension).

If no cause is evident, or if a renal or renovascular etiology is suspected, the workup usually will include US of the kidneys, adrenals, aorta, and bladder, with a flow study (i.e., Doppler US with duplex scan) of the aorta and the renal arteries, as well as a renal scan and PRA (621). Intravenous urography, angiography, MRI, or CT may be indicated in specific patients. If there is any suspicion of hydronephrosis or reflux, urine obtained by suprapubic aspiration or bladder catheterization should be sent for bacterial and fungal culture. Of 17 patients with fungal uropathy, hypertension was one of the presenting signs in seven (622).

If PRA is elevated compared to age-appropriate normal values for the same laboratory, a perfusion renal scan should be obtained in addition to the renal US and Doppler, because the scan is more sensitive for the detection of small defects. Renal microemboli from a UA catheter, however, can elude detection by any of these means. High PRA may be secondary to the administration of diuretics or adrenergic medications or to severe respiratory disease, and mild elevations of PRA may be seen in normal infants. Conversely, one normal value of PRA does not exclude hyperreninemic hypertension (601).

Hypertension can affect the cardiovascular system, the kidneys, the retina, and the brain (623). Hypertension may result in high serum BUN and creatinine, proteinuria, hematuria, and increased natriuresis (624). The latter may become very severe and lead to dehydration. If myocardial dysfunction, cardiomegaly, or heart failure develops, the blood pressure should be reduced rapidly. Reversible retinal changes are common in hypertensive neonates (623). Malignant hypertension may result in central nervous system dysfunction and intracranial bleeding.

Treatment

The treatment of chronic or subacute hypertension usually is aimed at a rapid decrease of blood pressure to a level that is not less than approximately three-fourths of the initial value, followed by progressive normalization. A rapid decrease of blood pressure to a normal level might place the infant at risk for both cerebral ischemia and renal failure (521), secondary to compromised central nervous system and RBF, respectively. In many patients, etiologic treatment should be tried before antihypertensive medications (see Specific Considerations). In patients with sodium or volume overload, sodium restriction with or without diuretics may control mild hypertension (see Diuretics). Many newborn infants in whom hypertension develops already are receiving diuretics, however, and more intensive diuretic therapy may cause dehydration and a further increase in PRA.

Various modalities of treatment for neonatal hypertension have been recommended. The first-line antihypertensive medication may be hydralazine, α-methyldopa, or a β-blocker (preferably metoprolol). Hydralazine is used frequently in combination with a diuretic or a β-blocker, or both, to limit the side effects of hydralazine, i.e., fluid retention and tachycardia, and to increase its efficacy. Preliminary data suggest that nicardipine, an intravenous calcium channel blocker that acts as a vasodilator with limited effects on the inotropic and dromotropic functions of the myocardium, is effective and well tolerated in premature infants (625). Isradipine, an oral calcium channel blocker, has been used successfully in hypertensive children including neonates (626).

Malignant hypertension should be corrected immediately and vigorously to prevent central nervous system hemorrhage. The best treatment is probably the combination of sodium and fluid restriction, a loop diuretic, and a potent short-term vasodilator. The effect of diazoxide, an arteriolar vasodilator (627), is difficult to predict. Titration of the rate of infusion of sodium nitroprusside, an arteriolar and venous vasodilator (628), achieves rapid and excellent control of the blood pressure; however, prolonged administration produces cyanide and thiocyanate, which cause metabolic acidosis and reduce tissue oxygen extraction (628). Labetolol yields a gradual improvement in blood pressure (617); it is effective even in patients with renal failure (629). ACE inhibitors (e.g., enalapril, captopril) are extremely potent and have been used successfully in some newborn infants (630,631). However, they are long-acting and may cause, at any time during therapy, profound hypotensive episodes, which can be complicated by renal failure, central nervous system dysfunction, or even cerebral infarction (521). The rate of infusion of nicardipine can be titrated to achieve rapid and excellent control of blood pressure without side effects (632); however, only limited data are available in neonates (625).

Specific Considerations

Iatrogenic Hypertension

Direct or indirect iatrogenic causes of neonatal hypertension are listed in Appendix C–1e. If the infant is hypervolemic secondary to excessive administration of sodium or fluids, intake should be restricted and a diuretic—usually furosemide—administered. It is imperative to eliminate hidden sources of sodium, such as isotonic saline used to flush an arterial line and sodium-containing medications (e.g., antibiotics). If fluid restriction is not possible and severe hypertension with CHF is present, hemofiltration should be strongly considered.

If hypertension is induced by a medication, one may consider withholding it, decreasing the dose, or using an infusion instead of repeated injections. Hypertension induced by pancuronium probably is mediated by release of catecholamines (633–635); blood pressure may normalize after replacing pancuronium with vecuronium.

Many infants with BPD develop hypertension (603,608). UA catheterization and the administration of corticosteroids are contributing factors in some infants, but the etiology in many remains unknown. Because hypertension often develops after discharge from the NICU, frequent monitoring of blood pressure during follow-up is important (607,608). Hypertension in these infants tends to resolve progressively (636). As much as 30% of infants receiving dexamethasone for BPD manifest hypertension (637). If severe hypertension develops, the risk of intraventricular hemorrhage, CHF, and renal failure may outweigh the possible beneficial effects of steroids on the lung disease.

Hypertension develops in 11% to 92% of neonates receiving ECMO (638–640). Although in some patients hypertension due to fluid retention responds well to diuretic administration, in others its pathophysiology remains unclear.

Hypertension may develop after surgery. Of four patients who developed hypertension after surgical repair of an abdominal wall defect, three had edema of the lower extremities and normal PRA, and one had evidence for ureteropelvic obstruction and high PRA (641). The duration of hypertension in these patients ranged from 12 days to 6 months. Hypertension appearing after primary closure for bladder exstrophy may be related to traction for skeletal immobilization (642).

Renovascular Hypertension

Hyperreninemia is present in most infants with renovascular hypertension. The most common cause of neonatal renovascular hypertension is aortic or renal thromboembolism related to UA catheterization (605). Hypertension develops in approximately 3% of infants with UA catheterization (605). Hypertension may develop either while the catheter is in place or long after its removal (643) and may be associated with a history of renal failure or hematuria. Associated signs may include hematuria, ARF in patients with bilateral involvement, and loss of femoral pulses and blood flow to the lower extremities in patients with extensive aortic thrombosis. Although the treatment remains controversial, a selective approach seems justified (see Acute Renal Failure). A thrombus that compromises only renal perfusion usually can be treated using antihypertensive agents; heparinization should be considered. If hypertension cannot be controlled by medical therapy, or if massive aortic thrombosis results in other major complications, thrombolysis

should be considered, using urokinase, streptokinase, or thromboplastin antecedent (460,461,605). If severe hypertension persists despite antihypertensive treatment and thrombolysis, thrombectomy or nephrectomy should be considered. Although hypertension resolves within a few months in most patients, refractory hypertension may develop in rare patients, and nephrectomy ultimately may be necessary.

Congenital vascular anomalies responsible for neonatal renovascular hypertension include stenosis or hypoplasia of the renal artery (644,645) and segmental intimal hyperplasia (646). All these conditions may involve the aorta as well as the renal arteries. Unilateral renovascular stenosis may cause a reversible syndrome characterized by hypokalemic alkalosis, salt-losing syndrome, and hyperechogenicity of the contralateral kidney (620). If medical treatment controls the hypertension, it can be continued until surgical correction at a later age; some infants with unilateral renal artery disease may need unilateral nephrectomy (645,647).

Hypertension may rarely result from two types of infiltration of the arterial wall. Idiopathic arterial calcification of infancy is characterized by calcium deposits in all layers of the arteries, including the aorta and the coronary arteries, as well as in the heart valves (473,648–650). Some of these deposits may be visible on a plain radiogram. Most cases have been diagnosed at autopsy. Hypertension typically fails to respond to standard antihypertensive medication and to nephrectomy; biphosphonate, calcium antagonists, or PGE_1 may be successful (650,651). Galactosialidosis may result in intimal infiltration by sialyloligosaccharides and hyperreninemic hypertension (652).

Other causes of renovascular hypertension include neonatal renal arterial embolism in the absence of UA catheterization (453), intramural hematoma of the renal artery (653), renal vein thrombosis (467), and external compression of the renal artery by hydronephrosis (654), adrenal hemorrhage (655), or urinoma (656). Hyperreninemic hypertension associated with renal tumors can be either primary (i.e., renin within the tumor itself) or secondary (i.e., increased renin in hypertrophied juxtaglomerular cells adjacent to residual glomeruli entrapped in the tumor) (657,658).

The choice of antihypertensive medications is controversial. Whereas ACE inhibitors are considered the drugs of choice for adults and children with renovascular hypertension and some centers have had good success in neonates as well, many neonatologists have serious concerns about the potential major side effects (521). Other medications, such as a β-blocker or, in the case of a hypertensive crisis, a potent vasodilator, should be tried first. The advantage of a β-blocker such as propranolol is that it reduces the secretion of renin and the release of norepinephrine. Because of the side effects of propranolol (e.g., bronchoconstriction, hypoglycemia), one may consider using either labetolol or a more specific β_1-blocker, metoprolol.

Renal Causes of Hypertension

Hypertension is a common complication of renal anomalies and diseases such as polycystic kidney disease (PKD) (597), renal dysplasia (659), tumors, of which mesoblastic nephroma is the most common in newborn infants (660,661), hydronephrosis (662), and interstitial nephritis (606). Hypertension may develop in patients with ATN as a result of fluid and sodium overload. Surgical correction of hydronephrosis, VUR, or renal compression (see Chap. 43) usually results in cure of the hypertension, unless there is postoperative edema with postrenal failure or renal dysplasia (663). If hydronephrosis is present, antibiotic therapy should be initiated, pending results of the culture. The presence of yeast in the urine should lead to initiation of systemic amphotericin therapy. If hydronephrosis is secondary to a fungus ball, surgical relief of the obstruction should be followed by local irrigation with amphotericin. Hypertension due to PKD or cystic dysplasia sometimes is severe. If medical therapy fails, nephrectomy may have to be performed.

Gordon syndrome, the association of hypertension with hyperkalemia and metabolic acidosis, may rarely be diagnosed during the neonatal period in patients with a family history (664). Although the exact mechanism of this syndrome is unclear, hyperactivity of the Na–KCl cotransporter of the loop of Henle has been postulated. This syndrome responds to the administration of thiazides.

Liddle's syndrome, or pseudoaldosteronism, is a rare autosomal dominant syndrome, which results from an increase in the reabsorption of Na in the distal renal tubule due to constitutive activation of the amiloride-sensitive epithelial sodium channel or *ENaC*. Activation of *ENaC* may result from mutations of any of its three subunits, α, β, and γ, mapped, respectively, to chromosomes 12p, 16p, and 16p (665–667). This syndrome, rarely observed in infancy, presents as an association of hypertension, polyuria, polydipsia, failure to thrive, hypokalemic metabolic alkalosis, and minimal PRA and aldosterone secretion. This condition must be differentiated from 11β-hydroxysteroid dehydrogenase deficiency (see Chap. 41). Some patients with Liddle's syndrome have hypercalciuria and develop nephrocalcinosis. The treatment, i.e., the administration of KCl and an aldosterone-independent K-sparing diuretic, results in normalization of the electrolyte and acid–base balance and the blood pressure.

Coarctation of the Aorta

Coarctation of the aorta (see Chaps. 33 and 34) produces hypertension limited to the upper extremities or to the right arm, with hypotension and decreased pulse volume in lower extremities and normal PRA.

Neurologic Hypertension

Neurologic causes of hypertension include intracranial hypertension, drug withdrawal, seizures, and familial dysautonomia. Seizures are common complications of severe hypertension; in turn, blood pressure may increase transiently during seizure episodes (668). Narcotic withdrawal should be treated as described in Chapter 56. Appropriate pain relief should be given before and after surgical procedures (see Chap. 57). A discussion of treatment of intracranial hypertension is presented elsewhere (see Chaps. 49 and 50).

Endocrine Hypertension

Several adrenal disturbances can induce hypertension directly; they should be differentiated from Liddle's syndrome. Hyperthyroidism is associated with systolic hypertension and sustained tachycardia and, sometimes, with episodes of supraventricular tachycardia (669). Neural crest tumors are uncommon in newborn infants (670).

Prognosis

The use of routine monitoring should allow early detection of most infants with hypertension, before the development of neurologic complication. The prognosis of neonatal hypertension depends on etiology, timing of the diagnosis, presence of complications, and response to therapy. Patients in whom hypertension is diagnosed on the basis of either neurologic, cardiovascular, or renal decompensation have a high mortality rate. The mortality rate of patients with idiopathic calcification of the arteries or with massive aortic thrombosis remains high despite aggressive therapy. The long-term prognosis for newborn infants with thromboembolism of the renal artery or the aorta is good, often with progressive resolution of the hypertension within a year and only mild-to-moderate decrease in renal function (460,462). Most hypertensive neonates with PKD or dysplastic kidney eventually will require nephrectomy. Hypertension in patients with BPD tends to resolve after 6 months of age (636).

DIURETICS

This section reviews the major characteristics of the various types of diuretics, classified according to their major site of action along the nephron, from proximal to distal (Table 42–17) (671).

TABLE 42–17. *Effects of various types of diuretics of urinary output*

Type of diuretic	Site of major action	Elimination	FeNa (%)	Volume	Urine characteristics						
					CH₂O	K⁺	Ca²⁺	Mg²⁺	H₂PO₄⁻	Cl⁻	HCO₃⁻
CA inhibitors	PCT	Secretion	3–6	+	+	+++	0,+	0,+	++	0	+++
Osmotic	Loop	Filtration	>10	+++	+	+	+	+	++	+	+
Loop	TAl > PCT[a]	Secretion	15–30	+++	+,−[b]	++	+++	++	++	+++	+,[c]
Thiazides	DCT > PCT	Secretion	5–10	++	0	++	−,+[d]	++	++	+++	+,−[c]
Metolazone	DCT > PCT	Secretion	4–7	+++	0,−	0	−	+	+	+++	0
Spironolactone	CD	metabolization	2–3	+	—	−	++	+	+	+	0
Other K⁻ Sparing	CD > DCT[e]	Variable[f]	2–3	+	0	—	−	−	+	+	+

Most of these studies were performed in adults,

+, increase; 0, no change; −, decrease.

CA, carbonic anhydrase; CD, connecting tubule and collecting duct; CH₂O, free water clearance; DCT, distal convoluted tubule; FeNa, fractional excretion of sodium; loop, thin Henle's loop; PCT, proximal convoluted tubule; TAL, thick ascending loop of Henle.

[a]Ethacrynic acid at usual doses does not have any significant effect on proximal tubule reabsorption. Note that ethacrynic acid is not recommended because of its ototoxicity.

[b]Decreased CH₂O during water loading and increased CH₂O during dehydration.

[c]Despite decreased reabsorption of bicarbonate related to the inhibition of carbonic anhydrase, the acute result is a "contraction" alkalosis. Chronic administration results in increased urine acidification in the distal part of the nephron (see text).

[d]Thiazides may be associated with hypercalciuria after salt loading.

[e]Amiloride causes mild metabolic acidosis by decreasing Na⁺/H⁺ exchange, especially in the DCT.

[f]Amiloride is not metabolized and acts on the luminal side. Triamterene is hydroxylated in the liver. Modified from ref. 67.

Types of Diuretics

Carbonic Anhydrase Inhibitors

Carbonic anhydrase inhibitors, e.g., acetazolamide, reduce bicarbonate and water reabsorption in the proximal tubule. The diuretic action of acetazolamide is limited by metabolic acidosis, which results from carbonic anhydrase inhibition. The combination of acetazolamide and furosemide (672) may be indicated in some VLBW infants with posthemorrhagic hydrocephalus (see Chap. 49). The dose of acetazolamide should be increased gradually, while titrating the amounts of supplementary sodium, potassium, and base that are needed.

Osmotic Diuretics

Although mannitol has been used in newborn infants, its risk-to-benefit ratio has not been assessed (399,673). It is contraindicated in premature infants because of the risk of inducing an intraventricular hemorrhage. The efficacy of mannitol in the treatment of cerebral edema in newborn infants is controversial; no benefit was observed in a randomized study (see Chap. 49) (674,675).

Loop Diuretics

Loop diuretics—diuretics with a main site of action in the loop of Henle—have multiple actions that can affect blood pressure and fluid and electrolyte balance. First, they increase RBF and redistribute renal cortical and pulmonary blood flow. The vasodilator action, observed before any diuretic effect, is responsible for the rapid improvement of blood gas exchange and pulmonary compliance in patients with pulmonary edema (e.g., in CHF and in BPD) (676). Second, loop diuretics are secreted into the renal tubular lumen, where they reach their site of action. They inhibit chloride reabsorption at the cortical thick ascending loop of Henle, by blocking the Na^+–K^+–$2Cl^-$ cotransporter (677). The increased CH_2O induced by loop diuretics may be useful for the treatment of fluid retention and hyponatremia (678). Loop diuretics also decrease the lumen-positive transepithelial potential in the thick ascending loop of Henle, thereby decreasing passive reabsorption of calcium. A less important effect is a decrease in proximal tubular fluid reabsorption, which results in part from weak inhibition of carbonic anhydrase activity. Third, loop diuretics stimulate renin secretion and PG synthesis (679). Increased PG synthesis may be an important mediator of the effects of these diuretics; indomethacin prevents or limits all the effects of furosemide (680).

Indications for loop diuretics include oligoanuria and fluid retention with hyponatremia (e.g., SIADHS, CHF, nephrotic syndrome, liver failure). In newborn infants, the effect of intravenous furosemide starts within 1 hour and lasts for approximately 6 hours (see Chap. 55). In infants with a postconceptional age of fewer than 31 weeks, the secretory clearance of furosemide is very low, suggesting that the amount of diuretic reaching the site of action is entirely dependent on GFR. Bumetanide is much more potent than furosemide on a weight basis (677); pharmacologic data are becoming available in neonates (681).

Benzothiazides or Thiazides

The benzothiazides are secreted into the tubule to reach their site of action. Their primary action is an inhibition of the Na–Cl cotransporter located at the early distal convoluted tubule. A second effect is the inhibition of proximal reabsorption of chloride, which may be mediated in part through the inhibition of carbonic anhydrase activity. Finally, thiazides decrease NaCl and fluid reabsorption at the inner medullary collecting duct. Because thiazides do not impair the urine concentrating mechanism, dilutional hyponatremia may develop if water intake is not limited. Thiazides may decrease calciuria by enhancing reabsorption of calcium at the level of the proximal convoluted tubule in response to ECF contraction, as well as at the level of the distal convoluted tubule. Thiazide administration may result in a positive calcium balance and a prolonged increase in total and ionized serum calcium concentration, except after salt loading or during sodium replacement (682,683).

Thiazides generally are ineffective in patients with renal failure. Long-term administration of a thiazide and a potassium-sparing diuretic improves lung mechanics and fractional oxygen requirement in VLBW infants with BPD (684,685). In addition, because of their hypocalciuric effect, they are indicated for the prevention and the treatment of nephrocalcinosis in patients with hypercalciuria (see Hypercalciuria). Finally, they are used for the treatment of NDI in association with a PGSI (see Tubular Dysfunction).

Quinazoline

Like the thiazides, metolazone, a quinazoline, is an inhibitor of the reabsorption of sodium and chloride at the diluting segment, but its action is more complete and more prolonged; it also decreases calciuria. In contrast to thiazides, metolazone causes little or no increase in urinary potassium excretion, and it does not affect carbonic anhydrase. It also has an antihypertensive action. Metolazone is efficient even in patients with CRF, if higher dosage is used (686). It has been used successfully in adults and children with edema refractory to furosemide and thiazides (687), as well as in VLBW infants with BPD in whom tolerance to furosemide develops (688).

Potassium-Sparing Diuretics

Potassium-sparing diuretics inhibit sodium reabsorption by the principal cells of the connecting tubule and the cortical collecting duct and thereby decrease potassium secretion. Spironolactone—a steroid analog—and its metabolites compete with aldosterone for binding to intracellular receptor proteins. Amiloride and triamterene block an electrogenic Na^+ channel on the luminal membrane of the collecting duct, thereby reducing K^+ secretion. In addition, amiloride decreases Na^+ reabsorption and completely blocks K^+ secretion at the distal convoluted tubule, causing a mild metabolic acidosis by decreasing $Na^+–H^+$ exchange in this segment. Spironolactone increases calciuria, whereas amiloride and triamterene decrease it.

In neonates, potassium-sparing diuretics are used most often in addition to a thiazide. They are especially useful in situations associated with primary hyperaldosteronism (see Chap. 41) or secondary hyperaldosteronism secondary to CHF, nephrotic syndrome, liver failure, or administration of a thiazide or of a loop diuretic (689). They also may be used for the treatment of Bartter syndrome and, in association with a PGSI, for the treatment of NDI (see Tubular Dysfunction) (690). Triamterene or amiloride is indicated to treat Liddle's syndrome.

Strategy in Using Diuretics

The choice of diuretic depends on the acuity of hypertension or fluid overload, the adequacy of renal function, and the expected side effects. For emergencies (e.g., cardiovascular or respiratory failure as a result of fluid overload), loop diuretics are the best choice because of their rapidity of action and their potency. In most patients, fluid restriction should be initiated along with diuretic therapy. Hyponatremia is a common complication of thiazides initiated without fluid restriction, because they do not impair urinary concentrating ability. Mild hyponatremia (130 to 135 mEq/L) does not justify additional sodium intake; the latter would initiate the vicious cycle of diuretic–low serum sodium concentration–increased sodium intake–more hypertension or lung edema–more diuretic. However, potassium and chloride depletion should be prevented.

Both hypokalemia and hypochloremic metabolic alkalosis may occur during thiazide or loop diuretic administration, unless the patient has renal failure or appropriate preventive therapy is initiated (691). Acute thiazide or loop diuretic administration results in a "contraction" alkalosis because of a reduction of the ECF volume and a relatively low bicarbonate concentration in the urine (692,693). During chronic diuretic administration, metabolic alkalosis results from increased distal urine acidification, which may be due to hypokalemia, mineralocorticoid excess, and increased delivery of Na^+ to the distal convoluted tubule, where protons are secreted in exchange for Na^+. There is serious concern about the effects of metabolic alkalosis associated with diuretic therapy in patients with chronic lung disease (692). Thus,

both potassium depletion and metabolic alkalosis should be prevented by adding KCl or a potassium-sparing diuretic as soon as diuretic therapy is initiated, except in the presence of renal failure.

Resolution of peripheral edema is neither an emergency nor a priority. An effective circulatory volume and a normal blood pressure should be maintained at all times; this is especially critical during vasodilation (e.g., antihypertensive medications, general anesthesia). In a patient with low circulatory volume and abnormally low serum protein concentration (e.g., postoperative phase, third-space losses, nephrotic syndrome, hydrops fetalis) with visceral (e.g., pleural, peritoneal, pericardiac) fluid accumulation, the circulatory volume should be expanded with colloids before administration of diuretics.

Thiazides (or metolazone if CRF) have been used as first choice for chronic diuretic therapy, to minimize bone calcium loss and prevent nephrocalcinosis and nephrolithiasis. However, this calcium-sparing effect disappears after sodium load during sodium replacement, and with the addition of spironolactone. During chronic therapy, the efficacy of a single diuretic decreases progressively, because of compensatory mechanisms at other sites of the nephron (688,694). Thus, the combination of two diuretics from different groups often is required. The association of a thiazide and spironolactone is efficient in premature infants with BPD (684); intermittent doses of furosemide can be added to this regimen when necessary. In refractory patients, the association of metolazone and furosemide should be considered (688). Patients on chronic diuretics should have regular ultrasonographic screening (see Nephrocalcinosis and Nephrolithiasis).

BACTERIURIA AND URINARY TRACT INFECTIONS

In infants, bacteriuria can be diagnosed with certainty only by culturing samples obtained by invasive techniques (i.e., bladder catheterization, suprapubic aspiration). There is no consensus, however, about the magnitude of bacteriuria required to reach significance (Table 42–18). In one series, *Candida* spp were responsible for 25 of 60 (42%) hospital-acquired UTI in an NICU (695). Bacteriuria in newborn infants can be either asymptomatic or an indication of pyelonephritis, which is characterized by local and systemic inflammatory response. Similarly, candiduria can be asymptomatic, cause hydronephrosis, or be part of a disseminated infection. Lower UTI (i.e., cystitis) usually cannot be diagnosed on clinical grounds in newborn infants, except when associated with hematuria.

Frequency in Newborn Infants

The frequency of bacteriuria ranges between 0% and 2.0% in an unselected neonatal population and between

TABLE 42–18. *Methods of diagnosis of bacteriuria urinary tract infection in newborn infants*

	Suprapubic aspiration	Bladder catheterization
Contraindications	No (clinical or US) evidence for presence of urine in the bladder Abdominal distension, peritonitis, organomegaly Hemorrhagic tendency, thrombocytopenia Local skin infection	Hypospadias, phimosis, local skin infection
Complications[a]	Microscopic hematuria (common); gross hematuria, hypovolemia requiring transfusion; bladder wall hematoma, urinary tract obstruction; aspiration of bowel content; bowel perforation, peritonitis, perforation of abdominal organ; abdominal wall abscess; sepsis, death	Microscopic hematuria (common), gross hematuria (rare), urinary tract infection
Positive culture	$\geq 10^2$ or 10^5 organisms/mL[b]	$\geq 10^4$ or 10^5 organisms/mL[b]
Indeterminate	$< 10^2$ or 10^5 organisms/mL	$< 10^4$ or 10^5 organisms/mL

[a]Except for hematuria, most complications are very rare.
[b]Some authors use as definition of urinary tract infection a count $\geq 10^5$/mL of a single bacterial species (Herzog, Wiswell, Ginsburg).

0.6% and 10% in an NICU population (696–702). Risk factors include prematurity (frequency of bacteriuria is 0% to 10%) (697,699,701,702), male gender (male-to-female ratio ranges from 1:1 to 9:1 in newborn infants) (699–702), and absence of circumcision (relative risk of UTI during the first month of life is ten times as high in uncircumcised as in circumcised males) (700–702). Although the frequency of UTI in circumcised male newborn infants is similar to that in females (700), it rises for 2 weeks after ritual Jewish circumcision (703). The frequency of UTI also is increased in infants with urinary tract anomalies.

Pathophysiology

The risk of UTI depends on bacteriologic factors (see Chap. 48) and host characteristics. Periurethral cultures obtained in uncircumcised infants show higher total bacterial counts, as well as a higher prevalence of *Escherichia coli* than cultures obtained in circumcised infants (704). The normal defense against UTI includes maintenance of an adequate flow of urine, complete emptying of the bladder, and presence of an anatomic barrier (i.e., the bladder outlet). These defense mechanisms may be compromised by urinary tract obstruction, VUR (see Chap. 43), bladder dysfunction (e.g., neurogenic bladder), or manipulation (e.g., prolonged or repeated bladder catheterization) (705,706). Immune defenses in general are described in Chapter 46. In the case of pyelonephritis, endocytosis of bacteria is performed by inflammatory cells and by proximal tubular cells.

Pathology

Acute pyelonephritis commonly is associated with nephromegaly. It is characterized by the presence of polymorphonuclear leukocytes in the glomeruli, tubules, and interstitium (707). Some glomeruli are completely destroyed, whereas others are infiltrated with leukocytes and surrounded by fibrin. The tubules are necrotic, dilated, and their lumens are filled with leukocytes and bacteria. Suppuration may develop in the kidney, often with multiple abscesses at autopsy, as well as other parts of the genitourinary tract. Chronic or recurrent pyelonephritis is characterized by infiltration of inflammatory cells, loss or hyalinization of glomeruli, and atrophy of tubules, with obstruction of the lumen with colloid casts. The development of renal scars may not occur until after 1 year of life.

Clinical Presentation

The percentage of infections that are asymptomatic is high in some series (697) and low in others (699). The clinical presentation of UTI in newborn infants may include one or more of the following signs:

Growth failure and gastrointestinal symptoms. Failure to thrive, excessive weight loss, poor feeding, diarrhea, and vomiting are the most common clinical features of neonatal UTI.

Jaundice. The hyperbilirubinemia observed in newborn infants with UTI may be either direct or indirect and sometimes is associated with hemolytic anemia. It is commonly the main clinical feature at presentation and may be the only sign of UTI in some infants (708).

Temperature instability or fever (temperature $\geq 38°C$). UTI has been reported in 7.5% to 11% of febrile infants presenting to the emergency room during the first 8 to 12 weeks of life (709,710).

Irritability, lethargy.

Abnormal urination. This includes poor urinary stream, malodorous urine, and polyuria, which may lead to severe dehydration.

Signs associated with bacteremia (e.g., respiratory distress) or with focal infection (e.g., mucocutaneous candidiasis, omphalitis).

Hypertension. This may develop as a result of hydronephrosis associated with the UTI (see Complications) (711).

Laboratory Features

Urinalysis

Based on specimens obtained by bladder catheterization or suprapubic aspiration, only one-half of febrile outpatients with documented UTI during the first 3 months of life had an abnormal urinalysis, defined either by the presence of more than five leukocytes per high power field or by the presence of any bacteria (709). The positive predictive value of pyuria on samples obtained by suprapubic aspiration ranges between 71% (pyuria greater than 10 leukocytes/mm^3) (696) and 96% (pyuria $\geq$20 leukocytes/mm^3) (701). Thus, the presence of pyuria, at least on a sample obtained by suprapubic aspiration, is suggestive of UTI, whereas the absence of pyuria is insufficient to rule it out (702,712,713). Microscopic demonstration of yeast cells in urine obtained by suprapubic aspiration or bladder catheterization is very suggestive of candiduria.

Urine Culture

The incidence of UTI during the first 3 days of life is very low, making urine culture superfluous during an evaluation for sepsis at that age (714,715). If antibiotic therapy is to be started immediately because of suspicion of sepsis in an infant who is more than 3 days of age, urine should be obtained by suprapubic aspiration or by bladder catheterization. Only these latter two techniques yield valid positive cultures, as shown by the fact that they only rarely yield equivocal bacterial counts, in contrast to bag-collected samples (i.e., bacterial counts most often are either greater than 10^5/mL or less than 10^3/mL (see Table 42–18) (716). If urine culture is a screening procedure, a noninvasive technique (clean voided urine or urine collected by a bag) is adequate; this may avoid the need for invasive collection of urine in a large number of patients (697). Agents most commonly responsible for neonatal UTI include *Escherichia coli* and other gram-negative rods; *Candida* spp also are frequent in UTI acquired in the NICU (717).

Complications

Acute complications of UTI in newborn infants include bacteremia, suppuration, VUR, urolithiasis, urinary tract obstruction, sometimes associated with hypertension or ARF, severe hydromineral imbalance (718),

methemoglobinemia (719). and ARF, which may be associated with urinary tract obstruction or massive VUR.

Bacteremia develops in 29% of infants with UTI under 1 month of age and in 31% to 43% of neonates with UTI (720–722). Occasionally, UTI is also associated with meningitis. Among NICU patients with hospital-acquired UTI (VLBW infants), bacteremia was present in only 3 of 35 cases (8%), whereas candidemia was present in 13 of 25 (52%) infants with candidal UTI (717). Suppurative complications of UTI, extremely rare in newborn infants, may occur in the kidney, the perirenal area, the prostate, and other genitourinary organs (723,724).

Vesicoureteral reflux is observed commonly during the acute stage of UTI (725); it often decreases or disappears after treatment and may reappear at the time of recurrent infections (726). Intraparenchymal reflux is associated with a high risk of renal scarring (see Chap. 43). Bacterial UTI can be associated with urolithiasis or with hypertension in hydronephrotic infants (662). As much as one-third of mycotic UTIs lead to the development of fungus balls (717), which may obstruct the renal pelvis or the bladder outlet (622,711,727,728). This obstruction may lead to the development of an abdominal mass, systemic hypertension, and anuria.

Investigation

Pyelonephritis versus Bacteriuria

Pyelonephritis, which presents a high risk for renal scarring, should be differentiated from asymptomatic bacteriuria, which presents a low risk. Clinical and laboratory features suggesting the diagnosis of pyelonephritis include fever, an increase in leukocyte count with a left shift, an elevated sedimentation rate, an increase in the serum concentration of C-reactive protein, and renal tubular dysfunction (729–731). Unfortunately, none of these tests, alone or in combination, can reliably establish the diagnosis or predict the development of renal scars (729). This is best done by imaging (see Imaging).

Imaging

Imaging for UTI includes US, followed by VCUG or DMSA scan, or both (732). Ultrasonography of the entire urinary tract should be obtained immediately to detect urinary tract malformations, hyperechogenic areas suggestive of pyelonephritis (337,728), and renal pyelectasis or ballooning during voiding, both suggestive of VUR (733,734). Color Doppler cystogram may show signals from the bladder to the ureter during the course of bladder filling (735). Whereas US and color Doppler are sensitive to detect VUR, the sensitivity of US to detect pyelonephritis has not been evaluated.

The VCUG may be done immediately after documenting sterilization of the urine. Alternatively, if the US is negative, the VCUG may be delayed for approximately 1 month, i.e., after resolution of transient, low-grade, UTI-related VUR (726). Significant VUR is very unlikely, and VCUG may be avoided, if US (especially with color Doppler cystography) and DMSA scan are all normal (732–736).

Cortical defects observed on DMSA scans performed 1 month after a UTI are associated with pyelonephritis, VUR, and the development of renal scars (737–739). Because ^{99m}Tc-DMSA binds to the proximal tubules and is excreted only minimally into the urine, it yields excellent visualization of the parenchyma and detection of cortical defects (343). The presence of areas of decreased cortical uptake of DMSA is a reliable indicator of pathologic inflammatory changes of acute pyelonephritis (737). The role of VCUG and DMSA scan in extremely LBW infants with UTI has not been established (739a).

Sepsis

On diagnosing UTI, a systemic infection must be ruled out.

Renal Function

Renal glomerular and tubular function should be assessed at the time of the diagnosis and during treatment and follow-up. Especially in patients with obstructive urinary tract disease, UTI can result in transient or permanent decrease in GFR or in tubular dysfunction, characterized by RTA, pseudohypoaldosteronism, decreased urine concentrating ability, or increased NAG enzymuria (740).

Treatment

The treatment of UTI is discussed in Chapter 48. The interval of administration of the antibiotics may have to be adjusted according to their levels and to P_{cr} (311). Third-generation cephalosporins, piperacillin, and aztreonam (741) are alternatives to the ampicillin–gentamicin combination and are chosen according to local epidemiology. A repeat urine culture should be obtained during treatment and after completion of the antibiotic therapy. In the case of failure to respond to treatment, US should be repeated, antibiotic therapy may have to be adjusted, and a systemic infection or other foci should be ruled out. Low-dose antibiotic therapy may be indicated after the initial 10-day course until the VCUG or the DMSA scan is performed, at least in those patients with abnormal US (742). Long-term prophylaxis may be used in patients with high risk of recurrence (e.g., severe VUR).

Therapy for asymptomatic bacteriuria in the absence of bacteremia can be given orally after the first few days. It is possible that shorter courses for the treatment of asymptomatic bacteriuria may be adequate (742), but this has not been evaluated in newborn infants. Although most neonatologists recommend treating bacteriuria regardless of the presence or absence of symptoms (743,744), growing evidence supports simple observation of infants and children with asymptomatic bacteriuria (742,745). Additional experience in newborn infants must be obtained before withholding therapy for asymptomatic bacteriuria can be recommended.

Surgical intervention may be required for patients with severe VUR and those with urinary tract obstruction (see Chap. 43) (746–748). If a fungus ball is associated with urinary tract obstruction or does not disappear during systemic treatment, daily washings with amphotericin B through a bladder catheter or a nephrostomy tube usually are a necessary addition to systemic therapy (747,748).

Long-Term Complications and Follow-Up

In patients with pyelonephritis or urinary tract anomalies, GFR, urinary concentrating ability, and tubular acidification should be assessed serially. In addition, US may demonstrate the formation of urolithiasis (749–751). The development of renal failure, once a common complication of UTI in small children, is observed only rarely, except in patients with major urinary tract malformations and renal dysplasia.

Although the association between segmental hypoplasia of the kidney (i.e., Ask–Upmark kidney), VUR, and UTI has been known for years (752,753), the development of renal scars remains a serious potential complication (754). In patients in whom UTI develops before 1 year of age, approximately one-half of the kidneys with VUR will develop renal scars, and 70% of the kidneys that eventually develop scars have VUR (736). Several risk factors for formation of renal scars can be identified early, including UTI associated with specific strains of E. coli (733), grades III to IV VUR, especially if complicated by recurrent infections (754,755), and abnormal DMSA scan at the time of the UTI (738). In the piglet model, the DMSA scan was shown to have a sensitivity of 85% and a specificity of 97% for detection of scars caused by VUR and UTI (756). Infants at risk for chronic renal scarring need long-term follow-up by a nephrologist and a urologist, including repeat urine cultures and sequential isotopic scans, and they should be considered for prophylactic antibiotic therapy (726).

Prevention

Circumcision is associated with a 12-fold reduction in the incidence of UTI in infancy, so that the incidence of UTI in circumcised males is similar to that in females (757). However, there is an association between ritual circumcision and a transient increased risk of UTI (722,758).

Intermittent bladder catheterization with anticholinergic medication is often performed in infants with neurogenic bladder associated with myelodysplasia. This method has been shown to result in a lower frequency of long-term deterioration of the radiologic appearance of the kidney, despite a relatively high incidence (19% to 42%) of bacteriuria–UTI (759,760). It appears that prophylactic antibiotic administration may reduce the risk for UTI, but this has not been evaluated prospectively (760).

Chemoprophylaxis usually is recommended after a first UTI for infants with VUR or other urinary tract anomalies (761). The role of chemoprophylaxis in newborn infants with prenatally diagnosed urinary tract malformations has not been established. In one series of 25 infants, prenatal dilation of the urinary tract led to early diagnosis of VUR in the neonatal period (762). Chemoprophylaxis was associated with absence of infection in 17 infants, a single infection in 3, and 2 or more infections in only 5.

TUBULAR DYSFUNCTION

In this section, tubular disorders that present commonly in the neonatal period are discussed, in addition to those for which early onset of treatment during the neonatal period may modify or delay the evolution toward renal failure. The reader is referred to other sources for discussion of uncommon disorders not included here (763).

Hypercalciuria, Nephrocalcinosis, and Nephrolithiasis

Normal values of the urinary calcium-to-creatinine ratio in full-term infants are less than 0.86 mg/mg (2.42 mmol/mmol) between 5 days and 7 months (764). Nephrocalcinosis and nephrolithiasis are increasingly recognized in infants with hypercalciuria, most often in premature infants (see next section) (Table 42–19). Prenatal development of nephrocalcinosis has been detected in neonatal familial hyperparathyroidism (765). Hypercalciuria may result from increased calcium intake or ingestion, decreased tubular reabsorption (766), or increased bone calcium reabsorption or uptake. Nephrocalcinosis and nephrolithiasis also may result from the precipitation of calcium phosphate or oxalate in the absence of hypercalciuria. Finally, nephrolithiasis may result from high urinary concentrations of cystine, uric acid, xanthine, 2,8-dihydroxyadenine, or acyclovir (see Nephrotoxicity), and may occur in association with UTI and with obstructive urinary tract malformations (749–751). Nephrocalcinosis may decrease renal tubular function, whereas nephrolithiasis may cause hematuria, colic, dysuria, UTI, hydronephrosis, ARF, and CRF. The treatment of asymptomatic urolithiasis is high fluid intake and specific therapy when available; lithotripsy and surgical treatment are discussed in Chapter 43.

TABLE 42–19. *Mechanisms of nephrocalcinosis and nephrolithiasis in infancy*

Hypercalciuria
  Increased calcium intake or absorption with/without hypercalcemia
    Excessive calcium intake (PO or IV)
    Rapid calcium infusion
    Hypervitaminosis D
    Fanconi syndrome if excessive vitamin D administration
    Phosphate depletion, low phosphate intake
    X-linked hypophosphatemia (during phosphate and vitamin D administration)
  Decreased renal tubular reabsorption
    Diuretics (loop diuretics, spironolactone, thiazides if sodium intake or extracellular volume is increased)
    Osmotic diuresis
    Distal renal tubular acidosis (RTA type I)
    Arthrogryposis multiplex congenita with renal and hepatic anomalies
    Bartter's syndrome
    Hyperprostaglandinuric tubular syndrome
    Autosomal dominant hypocalcemia
    Dent's disease (hypercalciuric nephrolithiasis)[a]
  Increased bone reabsorption or decreased bone uptake
    Primary hyperparathyroidism (including neonatal familial hyperparathyroidism)
    Secondary hyperparathyroidism
    Acidosis
    Chronic corticosteroid therapy
    Hypophosphatasia
    Hyperthyroidism
  Idiopathic hypercalcemia
Other mechanisms
  Factors facilitating precipitation of calcium phosphate/oxalate
  Low urine output
  Alkaline urine
  Absence of inhibitors: citrate, inorganic phosphate, magnesium
  Oxaluria (primary or secondary)
  Other causes of nephrolithiasis
    Cystinosis
    Cystinuria
    Oxaluria (primary or secondary)
    Hyperuricemia
    Classical hereditary xanthinuria
    Adenine phosphoribosyltransferase deficiency (2,8-dihydroxyadenine lithiasis)
    Acyclovir
    Urinary tract infection
    Obstructive urinary tract malformations

[a]Youngest patient described is 1.5 yr old.

Nephrocalcinosis and Nephrolithiasis in Premature Infants

Nephrocalcinosis or nephrolithiasis, detected by ultrasonography in 25% to 60% of premature infants with a GA less than 32 weeks, is predominantly due to hypercalciuria (767–771). The latter may result from increased calcium intake or gastrointestinal absorption, decreased renal tubular calcium reabsorption, and abnormal regulation of bone mineral content (Table 42–19) (772).

Chronic use of discontinuous daily calcium infusions is associated with recurrent periods of hypercalcemia and hypercalciuria. High enteral calcium intake may be associated with hypercalciuria in the absence of hypercalcemia (773). Insufficient phosphate intake may result in hypophosphatemia, hypercalcemia, hypercalciuria, and osteopenia of prematurity (774). Increasing the phosphate intake in these patients reduces calcemia and calciuria (775). Diuretic administration is the most frequent cause for hypercalciuria in LBW infants (768,770,776). A single dose of furosemide induces a tenfold increase in calciuria (777); chronic administration is associated with a mild increase in calciuria (768) and a negative calcium balance (778), and may induce secondary hyperparathyroidism and demineralization (779). Hypercalciuria also may be induced by spironolactone (780,781) or by thiazides in patients with increased sodium intake or extracellular volume (see Diuretics) (682,683,772). Hypercalciuria associated with TPN in adults has been attributed to excessive calcium intake (782), high protein intake (783), and the acid load (784). Addition of acetate to the TPN reduced calciuria without affecting serum levels of calcium, PTH, or vitamin D (784). Acute as well as chronic acid loading induces bone calcium reabsorption and hypercalciuria. Finally, the risk for lithiasis and nephrocalcinosis increases with high saturation levels, which result from low urine output or from hyperoxaluria associated with TPN or with prematurity (785,786).

To prevent hypercalciuria, VLBW infants should receive enough phosphate and should receive neither discontinuous calcium infusions nor excessive doses of vitamin D. If chronic diuretic therapy is indicated, the drug of choice is a thiazide (or metolazone if CRF), without sodium supplementation, and renal US should be done to assess for possible nephrocalcinosis or nephrolithiasis. Patients with persistent calcifications at 1 to 2 years of age show signs of tubular dysfunction, including a decrease in tubular reabsorption of phosphate, increase in FENa, and limitation of distal renal tubular acidification (787). Thus, hypercalciuric patients with nephrolithiasis or nephrocalcinosis should receive a thiazide without sodium supplementation; if an additional diuretic is required, amiloride or triamterene may be considered in some but not all patients (788).

Primary Hyperoxaluria and Oxalosis

Primary hyperoxaluria, a rare autosomal recessive disorder associated with urolithiasis, has two types of presentation. Type I (i.e., glycolic aciduria) is due to a functional deficiency of the hepatic peroxisomal enzyme alanine:glyoxylate aminotransferase (AGT), for which pyridoxine is a cofactor (789). The AGT gene has been cloned and mapped to chromosome 2q36-37 (790–792). Mutations may lead to mistargeting of the enzyme from peroxisomes to mitochondria, intraperoxisomal AGT aggregation, absence of catalytic activity, or absence of catalytic activity and immunoreactivity (763). AGT functional deficiency results in excessive production of oxalate, glyoxylic acid, and glycolic acid. The severity of type I is related to the progressive accumulation of calcium oxalate in various tissues, a condition called oxalosis. Type II hyperoxaluria (i.e., L-glyceric aciduria) is a very rare disorder, which causes urolithiasis but not oxalosis (763).

The diagnosis of hyperoxaluria is strongly suggested by a high oxalate-to-creatinine ratio in the urine for GA age and postnatal age (793–796) in the absence of a secondary cause for oxaluria (e.g., TPN or vitamin B_6 deficiency). The diagnosis is further supported by measuring glycolic aciduria and L-glyceric aciduria (795). Definitive prenatal and postnatal diagnosis is possible by measuring AGT in a liver biopsy and by DNA analysis. Approximately 12% of patients with primary hyperoxaluria present in infancy, with anorexia, failure to thrive, vomiting, dehydration and fever; presentation in the neonatal period is rare (797–799). Renal damage in hyperoxaluria type I includes nephrocalcinosis, urolithiasis, and renal failure. In some patients with type I hyperoxaluria, early administration of high doses of pyridoxine may limit the development of oxalosis (800). In these patients, therapy includes pyridoxine, inhibitors of calcium oxalate precipitation, large fluid intake (2 $L/m^2/d$), and eventually dialysis and renal transplantation (801,802). In pyridoxine-resistant patients, the treatment of choice is either early liver transplantation or combined hepatorenal transplantation (803).

Disorders of Purine Metabolism

Two disorders of purine metabolism may lead to nephrolithiasis in infancy: classic xanthinuria and adenine phosphoribosyltransferase deficiency.

Classic Xanthinuria

Classic xanthinuria is an autosomal recessive disorder with two genotypes. Type I is an isolated defect of xanthine dehydrogenase, which has been mapped to chromosome 2p22 (804). Type II is a combined defect of xanthine dehydrogenase and aldehyde oxidase (805). This disease should be differentiated from xanthinuria associated with molybdenum cofactor deficiency or with isolated sulfite oxidase deficiency. Both disorders cause severe neonatal encephalopathy, lens dislocation, and microcephaly. In addition, xanthinuria may result from the administration of allopurinol (inhibitor of xanthine oxidase) to a patient with high uric acid production (i.e., Lesch–Nyhan syndrome or treatment of malignancy). Classic xanthinuria may present with complications of xanthine urolithiasis or with ARF; some patients eventually develop CRF, duodenal ulcers, myopathy, or arthropathy, whereas others remain asymptomatic. The association of ARF with a history of hematuria or red-brown deposits on the diaper or in the urine sediment should raise the suspicion of classic xanthinuria (806). Ultrasonography may show the lithiasis. Classic xanthinuria is diagnosed by demonstrating high levels of xanthine and hypoxanthine and low-to-undetectable levels of uric acid in plasma and urine. The treatment or xanthinuria includes high fluid intake and a diet low in purines.

Adenine Phosphorib osyltransferase Deficiency

Adenine phosphoribosyltransferase deficiency is an autosomal recessive disorder due to mutations of the adenine phosphoribosyltransferase deficiency gene, which has been cloned and mapped to chromosome 16q24 (807–809). Two types have been characterized: patients with type I (mainly Caucasians) have no enzyme activity in their erythrocyte lysates, whereas those with type II (Japanese) have some residual activity. DNA analysis (PCR and SSCP) shows that these two types correspond to different mutations (810). The defect causes an increase in urinary excretion of 2,8-dihydroxyadenine, which is very poorly soluble. The disease presents with the complications of lithiasis, which can develop even in the neonatal period. The diagnosis can be suspected by visualizing round brown crystals in the urine sediment and confirmed by measuring erythrocyte adenine phosphoribosyltransferase deficiency activity and by DNA analysis. The treatment of this disorder includes a high fluid intake, allopurinol, alkali, and a diet low in purines.

Familial Hypocalciuric Hypercalcemia

Familial hypocalciuric hypercalcemia (FHH) may correspond to three different genotypes. Type I, the most common, is an autosomal dominant disorder resulting from defect of the human Ca^{2+}-sensing receptor (CaR) gene, which has been cloned and mapped to chromosome 3q21-q24 (811–813). Type II is linked to chromosome 19p13.3, whereas the gene for the third type is not yet been mapped (814,815). Inactivating mutations of the CaR gene increase both the parathyroid calcium set-point (i.e., serum calcium concentration that results in a 50% reduction in maximum PTH release) and the set-point for renal tubular reabsorption of calcium. Analysis of several families has shown that FHH is the heterozygous, benign, form, whereas neonatal severe hyperparathyroidism is the life-threatening homozygous form (816,817). In contrast, inactivating mutations of the calcium-sensing receptor gene result in autosomal dominant hypocalcemia, which is associated with urolithiasis (see Table 42–19) (766).

The diagnosis of FHH is based on family history of hypercalcemia, a low urine calcium-to-creatinine ratio (less than 0.03 mg/mg), a low fractional excretion of calcium (less than 0.016, or 1.6%), and high magnesium and low phosphate concentrations in the serum (818–820). Hypercalcemia and hypermagnesemia result from an increase in their tubular reabsorption and in their release from bone, whereas hypophosphatemia results from a decrease in renal tubular reabsorption. In most patients with FHH, PTH levels are within normal limits for normocalcemic controls but inappropriately high for the serum Ca^{2+} concentration. The differential diagnosis includes other causes of neonatal hypercalcemia (see section on Nephrocalcinosis and Nephrolithiasis and Chap. 36), and multiple endocrine neoplasia syndromes (see Chap. 41). FHH is usually a benign disorder that fails to respond to parathyroidectomy (821). However, some patients with FHH have recurrent pancreatitis. Some neonates with FHH have transient self-limited hyperparathyroidism (822). In contrast, those with neonatal severe hyperparathyroidism have severe hypercalcemia, high serum alkaline phosphatase activity, and typical radiographic bone changes; these patients may require total parathyroidectomy followed by administration of $1,25(OH)_2D_3$ (823).

Fanconi Syndrome

Fanconi syndrome is characterized by generalized dysfunction of the proximal tubule. The cardinal signs are renal glucosuria, renal phosphaturia, and generalized aminoaciduria; other features, present inconsistently, include RTA (see Renal Tubular Acidosis), tubular proteinuria, increased urinary excretion of urate, sodium, potassium, and calcium, and decreased ability to concentrate the urine and to secrete PAH (824). In some cases, distal tubular dysfunction is present, and the disease evolves toward renal failure, with less evidence of tubular dysfunction. Because several transport systems are deficient in this syndrome, the pathophysiologic process presumably involves a global disturbance, such as an alteration of the integrity of the tubular membranes or of sulfhydryl-requiring enzymes (824).

Idiopathic cases of Fanconi syndrome most often are sporadic, although autosomal recessive, autosomal dominant, and X-linked recessive transmission have been described (825). Fanconi syndrome occurs in association with a variety of acquired and congenital disorders (Table 42–20), the most common of which is cystinosis (826). Dent's disease is an X-linked disorder due to a mutation of a putative renal chloride channel, which has been mapped to chromosome Xp11.22 (827–830). This syndrome causes LMW proteinuria, hypercalciuria, nephrocalcinosis, metabolic bone disease, and progressive renal failure. The youngest patient described with Dent's disease was 1.5 years of age. Disorders associated with late-onset renal dysfunction, such as glycogenosis type I and Wilson disease, will not be reviewed here. General discussions of galactosemia, fructose intolerance, tyrosine-

TABLE 42–20. *Causes of Fanconi syndrome in infancy*

| Idiopathic | Secondary | |
	Inherited (AR unless specified)	Acquired
Isolated	Cystinosis	Renovascular accident in neonatal period
Deal syndrome (autosomal recessive)	Fructose-1-phosphate aldolase deficiency	Interstitial nephritis
	Hepatorenal tyrosinemia type 1	Medications: valproate, aminoglycosides, ifosfamide[a]
	Galactosemia	
	Glycogenosis with Fanconi S (Fanconi–Bickel S)	Renal transplantation
	Oculocerebrorenal (Lowe) syndrome (X-linked)	Toluene, heavy metal poisoning
	Vitamin D-dependent rickets	Vitamin D deficiency rickets
	Disorders of the energy metabolism	Dysproteinemia
	Pearson's syndrome (maternofetal transmission)	Nephrotic syndrome
	Cytochrome-c oxidase deficiency	
	Pyruvate carboxylase deficiency	
	Carnitine palmitoyl transferase I deficiency	

[a]Fanconi syndrome also has been reported after administration of other medications in older patients.
S, syndrome.

mia, and vitamin-D–deficient rickets can be found in Chapters 36 and 39.

The clinical presentation of Fanconi syndrome includes polyuria, polydipsia, dehydration, and failure to thrive. Signs include acidosis, hypophosphatemia, and rickets. The diagnosis is confirmed by the demonstration of glucosuria in the presence of a normal glycemia (less than 120 to 150 mg/dL), decreased tubular reabsorption of phosphate, and generalized hyperaminoaciduria. The prognosis of Fanconi syndrome depends on the underlying disorder.

The treatment includes administration of sodium citrate or bicarbonate, and as required, water, potassium, phosphate, and carnitine (831). Once rickets has developed, careful administration of vitamin D is required; excess vitamin D may result in hypercalciuria and nephrocalcinosis. Indomethacin, a PGSI, has been given successfully to some patients (832,833). Specific dietary therapy for fructose intolerance, galactosemia, or tyrosinemia results in disappearance of the Fanconi syndrome. In many other diseases, treatment serves only to slow the deterioration of renal function.

Special Considerations

Cystinosis

The reported incidence of cystinosis ranges between 1:20,000 and 1:326,000 (763). It is an autosomal recessive lysosomal storage disease, due to a defect in the carrier-mediated transport of cystine from the lysosomes to the cytosol (834). The infantile (i.e., nephropathic) type of cystinosis is the most severe form (763,835).

At birth, patients with cystinosis appear normal except for lighter skin and hair pigmentation than in siblings. Signs of Fanconi syndrome appear by 3 to 12 months of age. In some patients, the initial presentation may suggest a diagnosis of Bartter syndrome or of NDI (835). Retinopathy may be detected within the first weeks of life

(836), whereas characteristic corneal opacities appear only after 1 year. Laboratory findings include urinary excretion of typical cystine crystals, generalized hyperaminoaciduria, mild-to-moderate glucosuria, severe phosphaturia, RTA, marked increase in urinary excretion of nonaminated organic acids, and tubular or mixed glomerular and tubular proteinuria (826). Progressive deterioration of the GFR leads to ESRD at a median age of 9.2 years (837). Prenatal diagnosis is made by direct measurement of cystine in chorionic villi samples or by measurement of cystine in cultured amniocytes or chorionic villi cells.

The treatment of cystinosis in infancy includes alkalinization and supplementation of water, potassium, carnitine (831), phosphate, and vitamin D. Indomethacin, a PGSI, may reduce urinary losses and improve growth; however, it also may transiently decrease GFR (832,833). The treatment of choice is the administration of cysteamine (i.e., β-mercaptoethylamine) hydrochloride or phosphocysteamine (which lacks the foul taste and odor of cysteamine), which helps deplete cells of cystine. This treatment improves growth and delays the progression towards renal failure (838,839), especially if initiated soon after birth (840).

Deal Syndrome

Deal et al. (841) described a new, probably autosomal recessive, syndrome, characterized by ichthyosis, jaundice, musculoskeletal deformities, diarrhea, failure to thrive, and early onset Fanconi syndrome. All six patients with this syndrome died within the first 6 months of life (841).

Glycogenosis with Fanconi Syndrome

More than 20 patients have been described with Fanconi–Bickel syndrome (i.e., glycogenosis with Fanconi syndrome), an autosomal recessive disorder characterized by impaired use of galactose and glucose and hepatorenal glycogenosis (825). In the kidney, glycogen accumulation is limited to the proximal tubule, with maximal levels in the straight part. The etiology is unknown. This syndrome should be differentiated from phosphorylase b kinase deficiency (842) or from glycogenosis type I (often due to glucose-6-phosphatase deficiency), which is associated with late onset of proximal tubular dysfunction in approximately 15% of the cases (843).

Fever, vomiting, growth failure, and rickets develop in the patients within 6 weeks to 10 months of birth, followed by hepatomegaly, protuberant abdomen, moon-shaped face, and fat deposition around the shoulder and the abdomen (825,844). Laboratory findings include glucosuria on the first day of life, galactosemia on the fourth day, and hypophosphatemia by the eighth week. The Fanconi syndrome, initially severe, tends to improve. Hepatic glycogenosis causes a tendency toward hypoglycemia, ketonuria, hypercholesterolemia, and hypertriglyceridemia, but no lactic acidosis. The diagnosis of Fanconi–Bickel syndrome is confirmed by normal enzyme activity in liver or kidney biopsy. Particular attention should be given to treating possible acute decompensations at the time of surgery or infections. Hypoglycemia can be prevented by frequent protein-enriched feedings, by uncooked cornstarch (845), and restriction of galactose intake. The treatment of the nephropathy is nonspecific.

Galactose-1-Phosphate Uridyl Transferase Deficiency

Galactosemia (see Chap. 39) is an autosomal recessive disorder that results in intracellular accumulation of galactose-1-phosphate in various tissues, including the kidney. The cDNA coding for galactose 1-phosphate uridyltransferase has been cloned and sequenced, and the gene has been mapped to chromosome 9p13 (846–848). The activity of the red blood cell enzyme is measured routinely by most neonatal screening programs. Symptoms often develop in the neonatal period, soon after initiating lactose intake (i.e., milk), and include hypoglycemia, anorexia, vomiting, diarrhea, hepatomegaly, jaundice, and hypoprothrombinemia (849). Renal dysfunction develops within 2 weeks after initiation of galactose intake; it is characterized by severe proteinuria, generalized aminoaciduria, and a significant defect in transport of phosphate, bicarbonate, and PAH (849–851). Lactose intake leads to galactosuria, which produces a positive test for reducing substances but no glucosuria. Removing lactose and galactose from the diet results in rapid resolution (849).

Hereditary Fructose Intolerance

Hereditary fructose intolerance is an autosomal recessive disorder due to deficiency in fructose-1-phosphate aldolase (liver aldolase B), which normally is present in the liver, small intestine, and renal cortex (see Chap. 39). The gene has been cloned and mapped to chromosome 9q21.3-q22.2 (852,853). In patients with fructose intolerance, ingestion of fructose results in the accumulation of fructose-1-phosphate in these tissues. Although fructose is not part of the normal diet in the neonatal period, the routine use of sucrose has been recommended for sedation during neonatal procedures (854,855). A single dose of fructose will induce immediate hypophosphatemia, generalized hyperaminoaciduria, RTA, proteinuria, and phosphaturia, and transient fructosuria or glucosuria, or both (856,857). The diagnosis of fructose intolerance is suggested by the history of fructose or sucrose intake, the presence of reducing substances in the urine, hyperaminoaciduria, and high plasma concentrations of methionine and tyrosine. However, the pattern of aminoaciduria is similar to that seen in tyrosinemia. Removal of fructose and sucrose from the diet results in normalization of tubular function within 2 weeks.

Hepatorenal Tyrosinemia

Hereditary tyrosinemia type I (i.e., hepatorenal tyrosinemia, tyrosinosis) (see Chap. 39) is an autosomal recessive disorder due to a deficiency in fumarylacetoacetate hydrolase (FAH or fumarylacetoacetase) (858). The disorder is most common in the Saguenay-Lac St.-Jean region of the province of Quebec and in Scandinavia (859). The gene coding for this enzyme has been cloned and mapped to chromosome 15q23-q25 (860–862). Renal tubular dysfunction results from the accumulation of succinylacetoacetate and succinylacetone. Prenatal diagnosis is possible by measurement of succinylacetone in amniotic fluid and of FAH activity in amniocytes or chorionic villi and by RFLP in informative families (860–862). Hepatorenal tyrosinemia can be differentiated from transient neonatal tyrosinemia by a high blood concentration of succinylacetone in the former.

Clinical presentation includes failure to thrive, a cabbage-like odor, vomiting, diarrhea, severe metabolic acidosis, hepatomegaly, jaundice, melena, ascites, edema, fever, and tubular dysfunction (863,864). Renal dysfunction includes hyperaminoaciduria, severe phosphaturia, and variable degrees of RTA, glucosuria, and proteinuria (863,864). Early presentation (less than 2 months) of tyrosinemia type I is associated with liver failure and death by the age of 1 year in most untreated patients. Removal of phenylalanine, tyrosine, and methionine from the diet normalizes tubular function but does not prevent death from liver failure, recurrent bleeding, hepatocellular carcinoma, or porphyria-like syndrome with respiratory failure (865,866). Liver transplantation has considerably changed the survival rate; these patients have normal GFR but tubular dysfunction (866). Promising results suggest that administration of 2-(2-nitro-4-trifluoromethylbenzoyl)-1,3-cyclohexanedione (NTBC) may decrease the production of succinylacetone, the incidence of crises, and the need for liver transplantation (867,868).

Oculocerebrorenal Syndrome of Lowe

Oculocerebrorenal (OCRL) syndrome of Lowe is a disorder of the inositol phosphate metabolism that causes major abnormalities in the eyes (including cataracts), the nervous system, and the kidneys (see Appendix I–1). This X-linked recessive syndrome is due to mutations of the OCRL1 gene, which has been cloned and mapped to chromosome Xq25-q26 (869–871). The OCRL1 gene product, a 105-kildalton phosphatidylinositol 4,5-bisphosphate (PtdInsP2) 5-phosphatase, is normally expressed in the Golgi apparatus (872). Lowe syndrome should be suspected in a fetus if US detects cataracts, if maternal serum AFP is higher than normal for GA, or if amniotic fluid AFP is elevated without detectable acetylcholinesterase activity (872,873). However, negative results do not exclude Lowe syndrome. Molecular diagnosis is possible prenatally using RFLP analysis and mutation analysis by PCR. Fanconi syndrome appears in infancy, includes proteinuria, generalized aminoaciduria, phosphaturia, intermittent glucosuria, RTA, and carnitine wasting, and causes rickets and failure to thrive (874). Glomerular involvement develops progressively in childhood and eventually leads to renal failure in the second to fourth decade (875,876). The treatment of the Fanconi syndrome includes alkalinization therapy (Polycitra) with carnitine supplements, supplementation of phosphate once serum alkaline phosphatase increases (suggesting bone resorption), and, in some patients, supplementation with potassium or calcium (see Chronic Renal Failure).

Disorders of Energy Metabolism

These disorders have a wide range of presentation, including multiorgan dysfunction, lactic acidosis, hematologic disturbances (e.g., pancytopenia), growth failure, liver failure, pancreatic insufficiency, myopathy, cardiopathy, nervous system and sensorial disturbances, and nephropathy (see Chap. 39). Some of the genes involved are coded by nuclear DNA, whereas other genes are coded by mitochondrial DNA, resulting in maternal inheritance (877). Renal involvement most often consists of Fanconi syndrome, although some patients develop RTA, Bartter syndrome, chronic tubulointerstitial nephritis, nephrotic syndrome, or renal failure (878). Pathology may show cytoplasmic vacuolization of tubular cells and giant mitochondria. Neonatal or infantile involvement of the kidney may occur in several disorders, including Pearson's marrow-pancreas syndrome (maternal inheritance), fatal infantile mitochondrial myopathy, cytochrome c oxidase deficiency, pyruvate carboxylase deficiency, carnitine palmitoyl transferase I deficiency, and phosphoenolpyruvate carboxykinase deficiency (877–885).

Nephrogenic Diabetes Insipidus

The differential diagnosis of polyuria in infancy includes central diabetes insipidus (see Chap. 41) and nephrogenic defects in urinary concentration. The latter defects can result from either a decreased effect of ADH on tubular permeability to water or a decreased corticomedullary osmotic gradient (Table 42–21). Several entities, congenital (886) or acquired, may result in impaired urinary concentration. Many of these disorders are discussed in other sections of this chapter and in Chapter 41; therefore, only NDI is reviewed here.

NDI is characterized by an ADH-resistant defect in urinary concentration. Congenital NDI is most often transmitted as an X-linked trait, due to mutations of the AVPR2 gene (886), coding for the basolateral vasopressin V_2 receptor in the collecting duct (887). The gene has been cloned and mapped to chromosome Xq28 by linkage analysis (888). In some families, NDI is an autosomal recessive trait, which results from mutations of the apical aquaporin-2 water channels (889).

Symptoms of congenital NDI include polyuria, dehydration, fever, constipation, and failure to thrive. Pertinent laboratory findings include a persistently low urine osmolality despite hypernatremic dehydration, without other tubular dysfunction. In the past, severe episodes of dehydration with hypertonic encephalopathy resulted in a 16% prevalence of long-term neurologic problems (890). Although a more recent series showed a 14% risk for cognitive delay and a 47% risk for attention deficit hyperactivity disorder, there was no association between test performances and hypernatremia (891).

The diagnosis of NDI is confirmed by the failure to concentrate the urine and to increase urinary cAMP in response to intranasal administration of DDAVP, in contrast to patients with central diabetes insipidus (i.e., ADH deficiency) (892). Patients with defective V_2 receptors, but not those with defective aquaporin 2, have abnormal extrarenal response of the V_2 receptors to administration of DDAVP or desmopressin (889). Aquaporin 2 cannot be detected in the urine from patients with mutations in the aquaporin-2 gene and is found at lower concentration than normal in those with mutations of the V_2 receptor (893). Diagnosis in utero can be made by linkage analysis if other family members have the disease (888). Female carriers of the X-linked trait are asymptomatic, but may have mild impairment of urine-concentrating ability.

Treatment of acute hypernatremic dehydration includes correction of the free-water deficit, i.e.:

$$\text{Water deficit} = 0.6 \times \text{body weight} \times [(Na/140) - 1],$$

where water deficit is in liters, body weight is in kg, and Na is plasma sodium concentration in mM/L.

TABLE 42–21. *Etiology of nephrogenic defect in urinary concentration*

	Decreased effect of antidiuretic hormone on tubular permeability to water	Decreased corticomedullary concentration gradient

Congenital	Nephrogenic diabetes insipidus
	Hypokalemia
	  Bartter's syndrome
	  Hyperprostaglandinuric tubular syndrome
	  Pseudohypoaldosteronism
	  Proximal renal tubular acidosis
	  Duplication of the mitochondrial genome
		Medullary cystic disease, polycystic kidney disease
		Bilateral dysplastic kidneys
		Urinary tract obstruction

Acquired	Drug: PGE_2, PGE_1, amphotericin, lithium Hypokalemia Hypercalcemia	Polyuria: water/osmotic diuresis Obstructive disease (before and after treatment) Chronic/acute renal failure Pyelonephritis Nephrocalcinosis Medullary necrosis Malnutrition

PG, prostaglandin.

Chronic therapy to reduce urine output most often includes the combination of chlorothiazide, indomethacin, and potassium supplements (894,895). Preliminary data suggest that an alternative may be the use of amiloride and hydrochlorothiazide, without potassium supplements (888).

Hypokalemic Alkalosis

The differential diagnosis of hypokalemic alkalosis in infancy is given in Table 42–22. The discussion in this section is limited to the renal causes.

TABLE 42–22. *Differential diagnosis of hypokalemic alkalosis*

Inadequate intake
  Cl⁻-deficient diet
  Insufficient K and Cl in iv
Gastrointestinal losses
  Vomiting, pyloric stenosis
  Gastric suction
  Cl⁻ diarrhea
Kidney
  Diuretics: loop diuretics, thiazides
  Hypovolemia + other cause for hypokalemia (e.g., proximal RTA, cystinosis)
  Bartter's syndrome
  Gitelman syndrome
  Hyperprostaglandinuric tubular syndrome
  Liddle's syndrome (pseudohyperaldosteronism)
  Unilateral renovascular disease (rarely)
Endocrine
  Primary hyperaldosteronism
  Cushing syndrome
  Congenital adrenal hyperplasia (with hypertension):
    11β-hydroxylase deficiency
    17α-hydroxylase deficiency
    11β-hydroxysteroid dehydrogenase deficiency
Cystic fibrosis

Bartter Syndrome

Bartter syndrome is a sporadic or autosomal recessive disorder, characterized by hypokalemic alkalosis, hypercalciuria, impaired urinary-concentrating ability, hyperaldosteronism, hyperreninemia, hyperplasia of the juxtaglomerular apparatus, and normal blood pressure (896). Most patients are homozygous for the same mutation of the bumetanide-sensitive Na–K–2Cl cotransporter (NKCC2) of the ascending loop of Henle (897,898). Normal blood pressure results from antagonism between increased PRA and sympathoadrenal activities, and increased concentrations of vasodilators (prostacyclin, PGE_2, and bradykinin). Decreased urinary diluting ability results from the defect in chloride reabsorption, whereas decreased urinary concentrating ability results from the combination of hypokalemia, increased PGE_2, and a decreased corticomedullary gradient.

Patients with Bartter syndrome typically present with failure to thrive, polyuria, polydipsia, and a tendency to dehydration. Laboratory abnormalities include hypokalemic, hypochloremic alkalosis, elevated PRA, a high serum aldosterone, creatinine, and uric acid, and in some patients a low magnesium concentration. Renal abnormalities include hyperkaliuria, hypercalciuria, high excretion of PGE_2 and 6-keto-prostaglandin-$I_{1\alpha}$, decreased fractional water clearance, decreased concentrating ability, and, in some patients, high excretion of magnesium. Most if not all patients previously described as having neonatal variant of Bartter syndrome with hypercalciuria and nephrocalcinosis (899,900) probably had another disorder (see next section, Hyperprostaglandinuric Tubular Syndrome). The treatment includes supplementation with KCl and, if necessary, $MgCl_2$. If this is insufficient, either a potassium-sparing diuretic or a PGSI is indicated. The administration of indomethacin decreases PG, bradykinin, PRA, and sympathoadrenal activity, but fails to correct the excessive urinary potassium and chloride excretion.

Hyperprostaglandinuric Tubular Syndrome

Hyperprostaglandinuric tubular syndrome also has been called calcium-losing tubulopathy, neonatal variant of Bartter syndrome, hypercalciuric Bartter syndrome, and congenital hypokalemia with hypercalciuria (899,902). The syndrome results from mutations in the renal potassium channel ROMK (KCNJ1) (903). Loss of tubular K channel function probably prevents apical membrane potassium recycling with secondary inhibition of Na-K-2Cl cotransport (904); this mechanism might explain the lack of natriuretic and diuretic response to furosemide in these patients (905). Prostaglandin E_2 hypersecretion contributes to increased bone resorption, increased renal 1-α-hydroxylase, decreased tubular reabsorption of calcium, and decreased urinary concentration ability (906–908).

Clinical features include polyhydramnios, premature labor, failure to thrive, and episodes of fever, vomiting, diarrhea, renal electrolyte and water wastage, hypermagnesiuria, and hypercalciuria with nephrocalcinosis and osteopenia (909). In contrast with Bartter syndrome, there is no increase in prostacyclin, hypokalemia may be mild or intermittent, and fractional water excretion is normal. Prolonged treatment with indomethacin results in substantial improvement of clinical and most biochemical features.

Gitelman Syndrome

Gitelman syndrome, or magnesium-losing nephropathy (i.e., primary renal tubular hypokalemic metabolic alkalosis with hypocalciuria and magnesium deficiency) (910), is an autosomal recessive disorder, which results from one of several mutations in the thiazide-sensitive NaCl cotransporter (TSC) located on chromosome 16q13 (911,912). Most patients are compound heterozygotes. This syndrome typically has late onset (childhood or adulthood), is often complicated with febrile seizures and tetanic episodes, and is not associated with polyhydramnios, prematurity, defect in urinary concentration, or hypercalciuria (900,913).

Renal Tubular Acidosis

Metabolic acidosis in newborn infants usually is normochloremic, with an increased serum anion gap. The most common cause is lactic acidosis resulting from asphyxia, ischemia, hypoxemia, or local tissue damage. Less commonly, it is due to a congenital metabolic disorder (see Chap. 39) or to renal failure.

Hyperchloremic metabolic acidosis results from bicarbonate losses through the gastrointestinal tract or the urinary tract. Increased bicarbonaturia may result from either RTA or a defect in urinary acidification attributed to a deficit in distal sodium delivery; the latter commonly is observed in association with diarrhea (914,915). In contrast to adults, the urinary anion gap is not a valid measurement in newborn infants (916).

Clinical presentation of RTA includes polyhydramnios, polyuria with episodes of dehydration, failure to thrive, vomiting, and serum biochemical disturbances. Failure to thrive appears to be a direct consequence of acidosis; correction of acidosis often results in catch-up growth, unless other complications (e.g., rickets, renal failure) have developed.

Differential Diagnosis

Four types of RTA have been described: classic distal (i.e., type I), proximal RTA (i.e., type II), hyperkalemic distal (i.e., type IV), which is the most common type of RTA, and mixed proximal and distal (i.e., type III) (Table 42–23) (917). The differential diagnosis depends on the findings of hypertension, hyponatremia and salt wasting, hyperkalemia, generalized proximal tubular dysfunction, decreased ability to acidify the urine, UTI, nephrocalcinosis, or urinary tract malformation. Further workup (e.g., measurement of urinary ammonium, titratable acid, or PCO_2; ammonium chloride, sodium sulfate, or bicarbonate loading) may be required in specific cases, in consultation with a nephrologist (916–919).

Proximal Renal Tubular Acidosis

Proximal RTA or type II may be caused by an isolated defect of one of the mechanisms involved in bicarbonate absorption in the proximal tubule or, most often, may occur in association with other signs of proximal tubular dysfunction (e.g., Fanconi syndrome). The diagnosis is suspected when the serum bicarbonate concentration is low for age and urinary pH is inadequately low in the presence of mild-to-moderate acidosis. The diagnosis is confirmed either by the presence of a Fanconi syndrome or by measuring the urinary concentration of bicarbonate at various serum levels during a bicarbonate infusion.

Treatment consists of the administration of sodium bicarbonate or citrate (initially 5 to 10 mEq/kg/d) and potassium citrate. In some patients, acidosis will persist despite administration of high doses of alkali; hydrochlorothiazide or PGSI may be beneficial. Patients with Fanconi syndrome require additional therapy (see Fanconi Syndrome).

Distal Renal Tubular Acidosis

Several criteria have been proposed for the diagnosis of defects in distal RTA (920–922), including the inability to decrease urinary pH during metabolic acidosis, limited urinary ammonium concentration, limited urinary PCO_2, and decreased difference between urinary and arterial blood PCO_2.

TABLE 42–23. *Etiology of renal tubular acidosis in infancy*

Proximal RTA (type 2)	Hyperkalemic RTA (type 4)	Distal RTA (type 1)	Mixed (Type 3)
Primary AR, AD Sporadic transient	Early childhood hyperkalemic RTA	With bicarbonate wasting in infancy and early childhood) AR with sensorineural deafness (Chevalier) AD, sporadic With cystic fibrosis	Familial hyperparathyroidism with hypercalciuria and RTA (Nishiyama) VLBW infant
Secondary Fanconi syndrome Metachromatic leukodystrophy[a] Mitochondrial diseases Hereditary nephritis Tetralogy of Fallot[a] Vitamin D deficiency Vascular accident in NN period Hereditary nephritis Carbonic anhydrase inhibition Carbonic anhydrase II deficiency with osteopetrosis (AR) Drugs and toxins: valproic acids, heavy metals	1: Primary hypoaldosteronism, adrenal insufficiency 2–3: Hyporeninemic hypoaldosteronism[b] with chronic renal disease 4: Pseudohypoaldosteronism with or without salt wasting 5: Partial unresponsiveness to aldosterone toxins Tubulointerstitial disease Urinary tract obstruction, UTI Unilateral dysplastic kidney or RVT Drugs (e.g., KCl, K-sparing diuretics, heparin, ACE inhibitors, PGSI, cyclosporine)	Hypergammaglobulinemia (i.e., maternal Sjögren syndrome) Fetal alcohol syndrome Toluene, amphotericin B, lithium Hypercalcemic hyperthyroidism Vitamin D intoxication Nephrocalcinosis Medullary sponge kidney Urinary tract obstruction Carnitine palmitoyltransferase type I deficiency (1) Carbonic anhydrase II deficiency with osteopetrosis (AR)	Carbonic anyhdrase II deficiency (with osteopetrosis) (AR) Hyperparathyroidism Nephrocalcinosis and Fanconi syndrome Renal transplantation

Renal tubular acidification also may be deficient in the case of renal failure (i.e., normochloremic metabolic acidosis) or of acute diarrhea (hypochloremic metabolic acidosis) (see text).

[a]The only patients with this type of RTA were diagnosed after 12 mo of age.

[b]Types 2 and 3, associated with hyporeninemic hypoaldosteronism, are mostly seen in adults.

ACE, angiotensin-converting enzyme; AD, autosomal dominant; AR, autosomal recessive; NN, neonatal; PGSI, prostaglandin synthetase inhibitor; RTA, renal tabular acidosis; RVT, renal venous thrombosis; UTI, urinary tract infection; VLBW, very low birth weight.

Hyperkalemic Distal Renal Tubular Acidosis

Hyperkalemic distal RTA or type IV is the most common type of distal RTA. It results from the association of defects in K^+ and H^+ secretion at the level of the collecting duct. Primary type IV RTA or early-childhood hyperkalemic RTA has been described in some infants and children who presented with failure to thrive and frequent vomiting (922a). These patients had isolated signs of distal RTA with hyperkalemia, without nephrocalcinosis, and responded well to alkali therapy. Secondary cases of type IV RTA can be divided into five groups, which include hypoaldosteronism and impaired or absent renal response to aldosterone (see Table 42–23) (918,922a). The treatment of type IV RTA includes correction of the metabolic acidosis, limitation of potassium intake, and specific therapy for each specific disorder, e.g., surgical correction of obstructive uropathy (918).

Classic Distal Renal Tubular Acidosis

In classic or type I RTA, there is no defect of potassium secretion; nephrocalcinosis and nephrolithiasis are common (923). The development of nephrocalcinosis is attributed to the association of hypercalciuria, high urine pH, and low citraturia (924). Idiopathic RTA type I in infants can be associated with bicarbonate wastage. It can be hereditary and may be associated with several other conditions (see Table 42–23). The treatment includes the administration of sodium bicarbonate or citrate and potassium citrate. Administration of citrate is important for the prevention of nephrolithiasis.

Mixed Renal Tubular Acidosis

In some disorders, both proximal and distal RTA are present; this is known as mixed RTA or type III (see Table 42–23). VLBW infants during the first days or weeks of life have a mild degree of mixed tubular acidosis, with lower normal values of serum bicarbonate concentration and higher urine pH despite metabolic acidosis (see Renal Physiology). Patients with the carbonic anhydrase II deficiency syndrome may have proximal, distal, or mixed RTA. This autosomal recessive disorder results from one of several mutations of the CA II gene, which has been cloned and mapped to chromosome 8q22 (925,926). Patients with this disorder develop metabolic acidosis, osteopetrosis, growth retardation, mental retardation, and cerebral calcifications (927).

Pseudohypoaldosteronism

Pseudohypoaldosteronism (PHA) consists of unresponsiveness of the collecting duct to mineralocorticoids. PHA type I (PHA1, OMIM 264350) is an autosomal recessive disorder characterized by severe neonatal salt wasting, hyperkalemia, and metabolic acidosis. PHA-1 results from a mutation of either one of the three subunits of the amiloride-sensitive epithelial sodium channel or ENaC (928,929). The disease locus maps to chromosome 16p12.2-13.11 in some families and to 12p13.1-pter in the other families. The clinical presentation may include polyhydramnios, polyuria, anorexia, failure to thrive, and vomiting (930). Patients often develop hypercalciuria and nephrocalcinosis (931). The differential diagnosis of hyponatremia with hyperkalemia and metabolic acidosis with normal anion gap includes adrenal insufficiency and hypoaldosteronism (see Chap. 41), and acquired partial PHA (or unresponsiveness to aldosterone) (see Table 42–23). Laboratory findings in PHA includes hyperreninemia, hyperaldosteronism, and increased urinary excretion of aldosterone and tetrahydroaldosterone; in contrast, urinary excretion of 17-hydroxy- and 17-ketosteroids should be interpreted cautiously (930,932). Prenatal diagnosis of PHA may be suggested by polyhydramnios with high concentrations of sodium and aldosterone in the amniotic fluid (930). The treatment of PHA consists of administering large amounts of sodium chloride while limiting potassium intake. Indomethacin administration may help reduce urine output, natriuresis, calciuria, and nephrocalcinosis; however, it also may decrease GFR (932).

Hyperphosphaturic Syndromes

Hyperphosphaturia results from decreased proximal tubular reabsorption. Whereas severe hyperphosphaturia may result from hyperparathyroidism or Fanconi syndrome, mild hyperphosphaturia occurs after administration of diuretics (e.g., loop diuretics, carbonic anhydrase inhibitors, thiazides) or from drugs or toxins that are toxic to the proximal tubule. Other causes of hypophosphatemia (e.g., rickets and phosphate depletion) are discussed in Chapter 36. We will review briefly the hereditary forms of hyperphosphaturia that are pertinent to infancy.

X-Linked Hypophosphatemia

X-linked hypophosphatemia, also called familial hypophosphatemic rickets or vitamin-D–resistant rickets, is the most common disease associated with hyperphosphaturia in infancy. It is due to a mutation of the PEX gene, a phosphate-regulating gene that is flanked by RFLPs. It is mapped to chromosome Xp22.1-p22.2 and has been cloned (933–935). Clinical signs, including bone deformations, usually appear after the first year of life. In neonates from affected families, hypophosphatemia and low tubular reabsorption of phosphate can already be detected during the first month of life (936). The treatment includes oral phosphate supplementation and $1(OH)D_3$ or $1,25(OH)_2D_3$. This therapy improves but does not cure the bone disease, causes nephrocalcinosis in 60% of the patients (937,938), and may cause renal failure or hyperparathyroidism. Preliminary results suggest beneficial effects of using $24,25(OH)_2D_3$ instead of $1,25(OH)_2D_3$. (939).

Hypophosphatemic Rickets with Hypercalciuria

Hypophosphatemic rickets with hypercalciuria is an autosomal recessive disorder with rickets, bone pain, muscle weakness, hypophosphatemia with hyperphosphaturia, normocalcemia with hypercalciuria, a high plasma $1,25(OH)_2$-D_3 concentration, a low PTH concentration, and elevated plasma alkaline phosphatase activity. The treatment consists of the administration of supplemental phosphate (940,941).

Autosomal Dominant Hypophosphatemic Rickets

Autosomal dominant hypophosphatemic rickets is a rare, less severe disorder, with autosomal dominant inheritance with variable penetrance (942). Patients with early presentation show phosphate wasting, rickets, and lower extremity deformities as early as 1 year of age. The corresponding gene has not been cloned. Treatment consists of administration of vitamin D, with phosphate supplementation in some patients.

Vitamin-D–Dependent Rickets Type I

Vitamin-D–dependent rickets type I (VDDRI) is an autosomal recessive disorder, also called pseudo vitamin D deficiency type I (PDDR) or hereditary selective deficiency of $1,25(OH)_2D_3$. Increased phosphaturia results from hyperparathyroidism, in turn due to a defect of 1-α-hydroxylation of vitamin D in the proximal tubule (943). The gene has been mapped to chromosome 12q4 by linkage analysis (944). Infants with this disorder present typical signs of rickets, including hypotonia, tetany, irritability, motor retardation, deformations, and growth failure. Serum levels of $1,25(OH)_2D_3$ are very low or undetectable, resulting in decreased gastrointestinal absorption of calcium. This disorder should be differentiated from other causes for deficiency in 1-α-hydroxylase (e.g., Fanconi syndrome, RTA, or X-linked hypophosphatemia). Patients with VDDRI respond to the administration of physiologic doses of 1-α-OHD$_3$ or $1,25(OH)_2D_3$ (943).

Hereditary Generalized Resistance to $1,25(OH)_2D_3$

Hereditary generalized resistance to $1,25(OH)_2D_3$ is an autosomal recessive disorder, also called vitamin-D–dependent rickets type II (VDDRII) or vitamin D dependency type II or pseudo vitamin D deficiency type II. In most patients with this disorder, lack of sensitivity of target organs to $1,25(OH)_2D_3$ (945) results from a defect of the vitamin D receptor (946). The gene has been cloned and mapped to chromosome 12q13-14, i.e., close to the gene for PDDR (946,947). Patients present with rickets and some with alopecia by 2 to 12 months of life (948). Serum levels of $1,25(OH)_2D_3$ are very high. These patients respond to extremely high doses of $1,25(OH)_2D_3$ (948).

Glucosuria

Several disorders are associated with renal glucosuria: an isolated defect, or primary glucosuria, which is a benign condition, congenital glucose-galactose malabsorption, Fanconi syndrome, and other rare entities. They all are associated with mild-to-moderate glucosuria, which does not require specific therapy (949,950).

Neonates with glucose-galactose malabsorption develop severe, watery, acidic diarrhea and dehydration. This disorder is due to one of several mutations of the intestinal Na–D-glucose cotransporter (SGLT1). The corresponding gene, mapped to chromosome 22q13.1, has been cloned; mutations can be detected prenatally by SSCP (951–953).

In VLBW infants, the incidence of glucosuria is increased because of two factors: decreased tubular reabsorption of glucose (see Renal Physiology) and instability of glycemia (954). At a mean GA of 29 weeks, glucosuria appears when glycemia exceeds 152 ± 8 mg/dL (954). Massive glucosuria is uncommon in VLBW infants; however, it may lead to osmotic diuresis and, thus, dehydration and loss of electrolytes (954,955).

Uric Acid

Hyperuricemia

Hyperuricemia may result from a decrease in urinary excretion of uric acid, from an increase in its production, or from both. Uric acid excretion decreases after administration of several drugs (e.g., diazoxide, diuretics, dopamine, ethambutol), during lactic acidosis, maternal toxemia, ECF contraction, renal failure, hypertension, and lead intoxication. Decrease in urinary excretion of uric acid may result in higher serum levels but not in renal toxicity.

Increased production of uric acid is observed after perinatal asphyxia, after fructose administration (especially in patients with fructose intolerance), in Down syndrome, neoplasia, hypoxanthine-guanine phosphoribosyltransferase deficiency (Lesch–Nyhan syndrome), superactivity of 5-phosphoribosyl-a-1-pyrophosphate synthetase, and type I glycogenosis. In the latter, hyperuricemia results both from an increased production and from decreased excretion due to lactic acidosis. Because the risk of uric acid precipitation is favored by a high urinary concentration and a low urine pH, the newborn infant is at relatively low risk for tubular obstruction by uric acid crystalluria, despite low ability of the immature renal tubule to reabsorb uric acid. The prevention of uric acid nephropathy in patients at high risk includes maintaining a high tubular flow rate by the administration of high volumes of alkaline fluids (956). Uric acid crystalluria with tubular obstruction has been described rarely in newborn infants with ARF secondary to perinatal asphyxia (957). ARF may be observed also in Lesch–Nyhan syndrome (474). Allopurinol is indicated for infants with hyperuricemia secondary to neoplasia and should be given before chemotherapy in specific patients (958).

Defects of Tubular Handling of Uric Acid

Increased urinary excretion of uric acid may result from various medications (e.g., ascorbic acid, glycine, citrate, and iodinated radiocontrast agents) and from rare defects in tubular handling of uric acid. These disorders may be suspected on the basis of family history, low serum concentration of uric acid, or crystalluria. Early diagnosis may allow specific therapy and prevention of urolithiasis, which may develop later in childhood.

Aminoacidurias

Several systems of tubular transport of aminoacids are known. For many of the defects of these transporters, a firm diagnosis can be made only after a few months of age, i.e., when the normally high excretion of amino acids in infants starts to decrease. We discuss here only those disorders of amino acid transport that may cause symptoms in infancy, i.e., Fanconi syndrome (see corresponding section in this chapter), cystinuria, and lysinuric protein intolerance (LPI).

Cystinuria

Cystinuria is an autosomal recessive disorder due to a defect of the D2H or human rBAT protein, which is responsible for renal and gastrointestinal transport of cystine, lysine, arginine, and ornithine (763,959). The corresponding gene (SLC3A1 transporter gene) has been cloned and mapped to chromosome 2p. It is flanked by RFLP markers (959–963). Three variants can be distinguished in heterozygotes. Genetic and linkage analysis suggests that type III cystinuria might involve another, yet uncharacterized, genetic locus (964,965). Urolithiasis usually develops within the first 2 decades but rarely may occur by the end of the first year of life.

Neonatal urinary screening programs have shown an average prevalence of approximately 1 in 7,000, with a range of 1:2,000 in England to 1:15,000 in the United States (966). Neonatal screening offers the possibility of monitoring children before formation of cystine stones; this is particularly important for patients at highest risk for lithiasis (type I/I homozygous cystinuria) (964). Prevention of stone formation includes hydration and alkalinization of the urine; D-penicillamine and α-mercaptopropionylglycine are effective in decreasing the rate of stone formation in patients with lithiasis (967).

Lysinuric Protein Intolerance

LPI (hyperdibasic aminoaciduria type 2, or familial protein intolerance) is an autosomal recessive disorder due to a defect of the basolateral transport of the cationic amino acids lysine, arginine, and ornithine in the renal tubule and the gastrointestinal tract (763). A candidate gene for LPI, ATRC1, encoding a cationic amino acid transporter, has been mapped to chromosome 13 (13q12-q14) (968). Half of the patients with LPI have been described in Finland, where the prevalence is 1:60,000. Most breast-fed infants are asymptomatic, although some may develop symptoms of hyperammonemia during the neonatal period. Within 1 week of weaning or increase in the protein intake, most infants affected with this disorder develop nausea, vomiting, and mild diarrhea. Patients later present with poor feeding, failure to thrive, severe hypotonia, hepatosplenomegaly, osteoporosis, and developmental delay. Some may develop interstitial pulmonary infiltration, alveolar proteinosis, or severe renal involvement, including glomerular and tubular damage, which progresses rapidly to CRF (969,970).

The diagnosis is made by showing markedly increased lysinuria in contrast to only moderate increase in ornithine and arginine. Other findings include abnormal plasma amino acid concentrations, anemia, leukopenia, thrombocytopenia, and postprandial increases in urinary orotic acid and plasma ammonia. The treatment consists of administering a low-protein diet supplemented with citrulline. Hyperammonemic episodes are treated with ornithine, arginine, or citrulline, sodium benzoate, and sodium phenylacetate.

Storage Disorders

Storage disorders that may affect the neonatal kidney include Deal syndrome and Fanconi–Bickel syndrome (see Fanconi Syndrome), and two lysosomal storage disorders, i.e., sialidosis and galactosialidosis.

Sialidosis Type II

Sialidosis is an autosomal recessive disorder due to a defect of α-neuraminidase, which normally cleaves terminal a2→3 and a2→6 sialyl linkages (763). The gene coding for this enzyme maps to chromosome 10pter-q23 (971). The deficiency results in lysosomal accumulation of sialylglycoproteins and oligosaccharides. Patients with sialidosis type II develop visceromegaly, dysostosis multiplex, and mental retardation, and may later develop cherry red spot macula and myoclonus. Patients with the congenital form develop ascites and/or hydrops fetalis and die either in the neonatal period or during infancy. Some patients develop nephrosialidosis, which is characterized by severe proteinuria and progressive nephrotic syndrome. Pathology consists of foamy enlargement of glomerular and tubular epithelial cells (972). Prenatal diagnosis is possible by demonstrating absence of neuraminidase activity in amniotic or chorionic villi cells (973).

Galactosialidosis

Galactosialidosis is an autosomal recessive disorder due to a defect of a lysosomal protein, called protective protein/cathepsin A (PPCA), which normally forms a complex with β-galactosidase and neuraminidase, thereby protecting these two enzymes from proteolysis (763). The gene coding for PPCA has been mapped to chromosome 20q13.1 and cloned (974,975). Deficiency in PPCA results in the accumulation of sialyloligosaccharides. Patients with the early infantile form of this disease develop fetal hydrops, visceromegaly, ascites, and skeletal dysplasia and die early. The renal lesion usually consists of membrane-bound vacuoles in the glomerulus and in tubular cells; in addition, endothelial vacuolization may occur, leading to hyperreninemic hypertension (652). Prenatal diagnosis may be suggested by a high concentration of sialyloligosaccharides in the amniotic fluid (a nonspecific finding) (976) and confirmed by measuring β-galactosidase and neuraminidase in cultured amniotic cells (977). In addition, cultured fibroblasts (and one patient's amniotic and chrorionic villi cells) from 12 patients with the early infantile form had almost no cathepsin A activity of the protective protein, whereas those from eight patients with later presentation of the disease had 2% to 5% residual activity (978).

CONGENITAL NEPHROTIC SYNDROME

Nephrotic syndrome is defined by the association of marked proteinuria (more tham 1 g/m^2/d) with hypoalbuminemia (less than 2.5 g/dL). A nephrotic syndrome is called congenital if it presents within the first 3 months of life. This definition is based on the natural history of the Finnish type, the most common type of nephrotic syndrome in newborn infants.

Finnish Type

The incidence of CNF is estimated to be 1.2 per 10,000 births in Finland (979). CNF should be suspected if there is a history of CNF in a sibling, hydrops fetalis or edema of the placenta (i.e., placental weight greater than 25% of birth weight), or an elevated AFP or total protein concentration in the amniotic fluid. Because the disease begins *in utero* in all patients, an increased AFP (more than 10 SD above the mean amniotic fluid concentration during the second trimester) is a reliable indicator of the disease (979).

Linkage analysis has shown that the gene responsible for CNF in Finnish families is localized on chromosome 19q13.1 (980). In Finnish families, four main CNF haplotype categories have been observed (981). Analysis of non-Finnish families suggests that most patients with CNF share the same disease locus (982).

The natural history of the disease is based on experience before the availability of renal transplantation in young patients (599,979–984). The mean GA was 36.6 ± 1.8 weeks (mean ± SD), and 42% of the infants were premature (less than 37 weeks of GA). Many infants were small for gestational age, especially those with a GA at or above 37 weeks. In some patients, the typical signs of nephrotic syndrome (i.e., edema, proteinuria, hypoalbuminemia) did not develop until the third month of life. The disease was resistant to steroids or cytotoxic medications (599). Complications included severe failure to thrive and ascites in all patients, severe bacterial infections in 85%, hypothyroidism, pyloric stenosis in 12%, and thrombotic events in 10% (599). An increase in P_{cr} or BUN was observed in 20% of the patients, but none had frank uremia. One-half of the patients died by 6 months of life, and all of them by 4 years.

The proteinuria, initially very selective (i.e., almost entirely albumin as a result of increased permeability of the glomerulus only for small proteins), increases progressively and becomes nonselective, corresponding to increased sieving coefficient and to tubular damage (984). Blood chemistry is significant for low serum albumin concentration and total thyroxine concentration (as a result of urine loss of thyroxine-binding globulin) (985), a normal or mildly elevated P_{cr}, and hyperlipidemia. Ultrasonography shows enlarged kidneys, increased echogenicity of the renal cortex, decreased differentiation between cortex and medulla, and poor visualization of the pyramids (986). Tubular dilations may be misinterpreted as other causes of cystic disease, including ARPKD (987).

The diagnosis of CNF can be confirmed by linkage analysis or by renal biopsy. The latter shows irregularities of the glomerular basement membrane and thinning of the lamina densa (988), followed by fusion of the epithelial cell foot processes, all of which are similar to the findings in minimal-change, steroid-sensitive nephrotic syndrome. On light microscopy, the mature glomeruli initially typically show only minimal abnormalities, including mild mesangial hypercellularity and an increase in mesangial matrix. Immature-appearing glomeruli show a dilated urinary space surrounding a small glomerular tuft. Progressive changes include obliteration of capillary loops and glomerular hyalinization, as well as dilated tubules from both proximal and distal origin (microcystic disease). Immune deposits become visible by electron microscopy within the mesangium only at late stages of the disease (989).

Infants with CNF require intensive management, which includes repetitive administration of albumin and diuretics for ascites, thyroxin, anticoagulation, oral and parenteral hyperalimentation, and the treatment of multiple complications (599). Chronic renal insufficiency develops between 6 and 23 months of age. As a consequence, most patients eventually receive dialysis while waiting for transplantation. Aggressive therapy, including bilateral nephrectomy (performed in one series at a mean age of 1.2 years) and peritoneal dialysis until transplantation, allows normal growth and development, a patient survival rate of 97%, and a graft survival rate of 94%, 81% and 81% at 1, 3, and 5 years after transplant (600). CNF patients have an increased tendency for posttransplantation steroid-resistant nephrosis (990). Preliminary data in two patients suggest that CNF-related proteinuria may improve with long-term administration of captopril and indomethacin (991).

Other Causes

Differential Diagnosis

The entities associated with congenital nephrotic syndrome may be differentiated by the natural history of the disease; by the presence of associated anomalies (e.g., in the Drash syndrome, see following); by maternal and neonatal serology (TORCH syndrome and lupus); by measuring AFP concentration in the amniotic fluid, which is consistently elevated only in CNF; by DNA analysis in specific families; and by renal biopsy. Nevertheless, classification of a patient into one of the major entities may not be possible (983). Specific therapy may be available for some patients (e.g., those with congenital infection).

Diffuse Mesangial Sclerosis

The second most common cause of congenital nephrotic syndrome is diffuse mesangial sclerosis, which appears to be a heterogenous group (983). The onset varies between the second trimester of gestation and 33 months of age. In contrast to CNF, CRF develops rapidly in these patients and is the major cause of death in the absence of dialysis and renal transplantation. Renal venous thrombosis is a frequent complication. In most families, diffuse mesangial sclerosis is transmitted as an autosomal recessive trait. Histologic examination of the glomeruli shows mesangial cells embedded in a periodic acid-Schiff–positive and silver-positive fibrillar network occluding the capillaries. Tubular changes are similar to

those seen in CNF, and interstitial fibrosis is more pronounced than in CNF.

Patients present with proteinuria, with or without nephrotic syndrome, sometimes hematuria, often arterial hypertension, and progressive CRF leading to ESRD within a few months to 2 years from the onset. In some infants, diffuse mesangial sclerosis is part of a Drash syndrome, which also includes ambiguous genitalia—most often male pseudohermaphroditism (i.e., 46XY karyotype)—and Wilms tumor (992). Several patients have presented with incomplete forms of Drash syndrome (i.e., only two of the three signs of the triad) (992). Diffuse mesangial sclerosis is common in Galloway–Mowat syndrome, an autosomal recessive disorder that includes microcephaly, abnormal gyral pattern, developmental delay, and nephrotic syndrome. Renal pathology in this syndrome may show diffuse mesangial sclerosis, focal segmental sclerosis, mesangial proliferation, or basement membrane and tubular anomalies (993,994). In a consanguineous family with previously affected siblings, prenatal diagnosis may be suggested by demonstration of enlarged hyperechogenic kidneys with amniotic fluid at the upper limit of normal and normal amniotic fluid concentration of AFP (995).

Congenital Infection

Nephrotic syndrome due to congenital infection is seen most commonly in congenital syphilis (996,997), in which case the lesion is characterized by epimembranous or proliferative glomerulopathy, with diffuse deposits of γ-immunoglobulin and treponemal antigen along the glomerular capillaries and subepithelial electron-dense deposits (996). The condition responds very well to the administration of penicillin. The nephrotic syndrome associated with congenital toxoplasmosis is less common (998,999). The lesion is characterized by the deposition in the glomeruli of immunoglobulins, complement, and *Toxoplasma* antigen and antibody. It may respond to administration of pyrimethamine, sulfadiazine, and steroid. Congenital nephrotic syndrome has been reported in a few patients with congenital cytomegalovirus infection (1000,1001).

Other Causes

Even though some infants with congenital nephrotic syndrome have been found to have minimal change disease on biopsy, corticosteroid and cyclophosphamide therapy has not proven useful. Some cases of congenital nephrotic syndrome are associated with dysmorphic features, such as pachygyria, microcephaly, buphthalmos, or disturbances of neuronal migration. Nephrotic syndrome may result from sialidosis type II (see Sialidosis) or from type I carbohydrate-deficient glycoprotein syndrome (1002–1005). Transient cases of congenital nephrotic syndrome have been described due to maternal transmission (1006), intoxication with mercury, or nail patella syndrome (1007). Of three infants reported to have infantile systemic lupus erythematosus and congenital nephrotic syndrome, one had steroid-responsive membranous glomerulopathy (1008,1009).

HEMATURIA AND PROTEINURIA

Differential Diagnosis of Hematuria

Pink or red urine or coloration of the diaper may result from hematuria, hemoglobinuria, myoglobinuria, uric acid, porphyria, or bile pigments. Red-brown deposits on the diaper may result from xanthinuria. The presence of blood on the diaper also may result from rectal bleeding or vaginal mucoid sanguinous discharge caused by maternal hormone withdrawal. On a dipstick test, the reagent strip based on the orthotolidine peroxidase reaction will give a positive reaction with hemoglobinuria, myoglobinuria, hematuria, or other oxidants, such as hydrogen peroxide and ascorbic acid. A dipstick can detect 5 to 20 intact erythrocytes per microliter of urine, and 0.05 to 0.3 mg of free hemoglobin per 100 mL of urine, which corresponds to 2 to 10 lysed erythrocytes per microliter. The diagnosis of hematuria requires visualization of an excessive number of erythrocytes in an uncontaminated specimen of urine.

During the first week of life, Addis counts in normal full-term newborn infants range between 0 and 630,000 erythrocytes per 12 hours (mean 90,219) (329). Erythrocytes are most abundant during the first few days of life. Although most urine samples during the first week of life contain zero to four erythrocytes per microliter, more than one-half of the samples do not contain any erythrocytes. After the first week of life, erythrocytes are sparse. The presence of erythrocyte casts always is abnormal (329,1010).

Incidence

Gross hematuria during the first month of life occurred in 35 of 132,050 admissions (0.21 of 1000) to a major tertiary center between 1950 and 1967 (1011). In a more recent series, the incidence of hematuria during the first 48 hours of life was much lower in normal full-term infants (0 of 63) than in patients admitted to the NICU (48 of 78); none of these patients, however, had abnormalities on physical examination or had proteinuria, hypertension, or abnormal values of P_{cr} or BUN (1012). Transient hematuria was found in 76% of asphyxiated newborns (1013). In another series, hematuria was estimated to occur in 62% of newborn infants with UA catheter in place and US evidence of an arterial clot, and in 25% in those without evidence for a clot (1014). Hematuria was present in one-half of infants with ARF

secondary to cardiac surgery and in two-thirds of newborn infants with irreversible ARF (1015,1016).

Etiology

Hematuria may occur in a wide variety of diseases, including bleeding diathesis and renal and postrenal disorders. PGSI-mediated hematuria may be due to platelet dysfunction, ATN, or tubular dysfunction. Congenital infections (e.g., syphilis, toxoplasmosis, cytomegalovirus) may cause thrombocytopenia or, rarely, glomerulonephritis. Common congenital causes of hematuria include hydronephrosis, PKD, tumors, and sponge kidneys. Acquired causes include asphyxia, coagulation abnormalities, infectious and vascular disorders, and nephrotoxicity.

Evaluation

The first step is to confirm the diagnosis of hematuria by the demonstration of erythrocytes in fresh urine voided spontaneously or after gentle suprapubic pressure (Fig. 42–5). Suprapubic aspiration is contraindicated, because it can cause microscopic or macroscopic hematuria. If the patient is anuric, despite treating possible conditions that might be causing prerenal failure and despite a diuretic challenge and a fluid challenge (see Acute Renal Failure), the bladder should be catheterized using a lubricated 3.5Fr to 5Fr catheter.

The history may disclose familial nephritis. Maternal history may be positive for diabetes (suggesting renal venous thrombosis, infection, thrombocytopenia, glomerulonephritis), autoimmune disease, or recent use of PGSI. The patient's history should be reviewed, especially for asphyxia, sepsis, shock, hypertension, renal failure, medications, and placement of a UA line. Pertinent points in the physical examination include hypertension, bruising, edema suggesting ARF or glomerulonephritis, an abdominal mass that may indicate hydronephrosis, cystic disease, adrenal hemorrhage, and, rarely, renal trauma and bruit (suggesting renovascular disease). In some patients, the presumptive etiology is obvious (e.g., bleeding disorder, bladder trauma, severe asphyxia, ATN, renovascular disease, glomerulonephritis, nephrotic syndrome).

The initial workup should include a microscopic examination of the urine, dipstick test, and measurement of urine output, BUN, and P_{cr} (see Fig. 42–5). Most patients should have a bladder and renal US and a urine culture. Microscopic examination of the urine may show dysmorphic erythrocytes or erythrocyte casts indicating glomerulonephritis, bacteriuria, yeast forms, or crystalluria. The latter may be the first clue to a diagnosis of urolithiasis. The dipstick may show glucosuria or proteinuria. If any of these is present, additional specific investigations should be obtained. If a glomerular disease

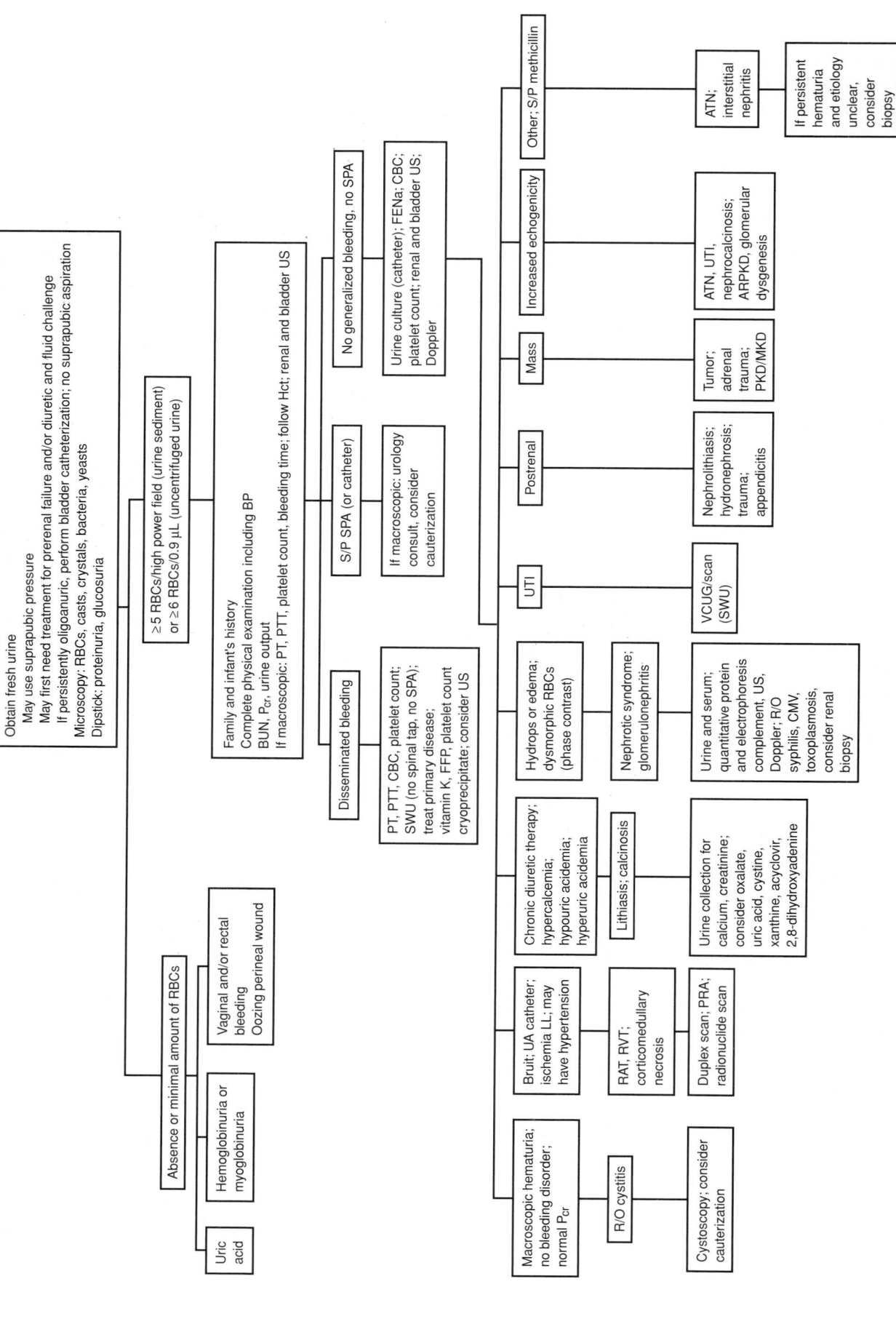

is suspected, fresh urine should be examined using phase contrast microscopy, which is the method of choice for identifying the presence of dysmorphic erythrocytes; however, this method is unreliable in determining the origin of massive hematuria.

Transient microscopic hematuria during the first 48 hours of life may be insignificant (1012), as long as the infant is asymptomatic (i.e., has no bleeding diathesis) and does not exhibit other evidence of a renal lesion (e.g., no familial renal disease; normal physical examination, blood pressure, urine output, P_{cr}, BUN and US; no erythrocyte casts in the urine).

In patients with macroscopic hematuria, the first diagnoses to exclude are bleeding disorder, trauma, and cystitis. In those patients, coagulation tests, platelet count, and bleeding time should be assessed, and a renal and bladder US should be obtained. Purpura, excessive bleeding after venipuncture, or thrombocytopenia suggests that hematuria is due to a bleeding disorder. Specific treatment for sepsis or endocarditis and the bleeding disorder should be initiated. If renal function and urine output are normal, and hematuria disappears after resolution of the bleeding diathesis, no additional renal workup is required. It should be remembered, however, that thrombocytopenia with hematuria may occur in association with renal diseases, such as renal venous thrombosis and UTI with sepsis. Macroscopic hematuria also may occur after suprapubic aspiration or catheterization of the bladder; if hematuria disappears rapidly, US is normal, and urine output, BUN, and P_{cr} remain normal, no additional investigations are required. In patients with massive hematuria in whom a bleeding disorder has been excluded, cystoscopy should be performed, unless the presumptive etiology is renal.

All other patients should have a urine culture, as well as a renal and bladder US, which may disclose an intravascular thrombus, renal venous or arterial thrombosis, cystic kidney disease, lithiasis or nephrocalcinosis, hydronephrosis, adrenal hemorrhage, or other anomalies. The association of hematuria with UA catheterization, an abdominal bruit, or blanching of the lower extremities,

---

FIG. 42–5. Differential diagnosis of hematuria. ARF, acute renal failure; ARPKD, autosomal recessive polycystic kidney disease; ATN, acute tubular necrosis; BP, blood pressure; BUN, blood urea nitrogen; CBC, complete blood count; CMV, cytomegalovirus; FeNa, fractional excretion of sodium; Hct, hematocrit; LL, lower limbs; MKD/PKD, multicystic/polycystic kidney disease; P_{cr}, plasma creatinine concentration; PRA, plasma renin activity; PT, prothrombin time; PTT, partial thromboplastin time; RAT, renal artery thrombosis; RBC, erythrocyte; R/O, rule out; RVT, renal venous thrombosis; S/P, status post; SPA, suprapubic aspiration; SWU, sepsis workup; UA, umbilical artery; UO, urine output; US, ultrasonography; UTI, urinary tract infection; VCUG, voiding cystourethrogram.

especially with hypertension, strongly suggests the diagnosis of a renovascular etiology (1014,1017). Hematuria is an unusual complication of nephrolithiasis or nephrocalcinosis during the neonatal period; it has been reported in one 10-week-old patient with familial hypercalciuria (1018).

Glomerulonephritis is a rare occurrence in newborn infants. It should be suspected if the patient has either hydrops or generalized edema with massive proteinuria or erythrocyte casts or dysmorphic erythrocytes. Although hematuria of glomerular origin is suggested by the presence of erythrocyte casts, severe proteinuria, or dysmorphic erythrocytes, it is not excluded by their absence. These patients should be assessed for possible congenital syphilis, toxoplasmosis, cytomegalovirus infection, various causes of nephrotic syndrome, familial nephritis, and immune-mediated glomerulonephritis. A decrease in the serum concentration of the third factor of complement has been described in glomerulonephritis due to congenital syphilis and in one mother–infant pair with a benign glomerulonephritis with isolated hematuria (1019). Consultation with a pediatric nephrologist should be obtained, and a renal biopsy should be considered.

For the other patients, the differential diagnosis includes a wide range of diseases; US is the most important initial investigation. Further workup depends on the clinical presentation (e.g., hypertension, ARF) or presumed etiology (e.g., ATN, cystic disease, tumor). If hematuria persists without obvious etiology, a renal biopsy should be considered.

Differential Diagnosis of Proteinuria

Proteinuria may be suggested by a strongly positive dipstick test. Significant proteinuria is diagnosed by a timed collection to quantify proteinuria. Abnormal proteinuria is defined according to normal values for age (see Table 42–3).

Incidence

Increased proteinuria occurs frequently in newborn infants admitted to the NICU; it is associated with various types of renal injury. The detection of increased tubular proteinuria is a sensitive screening test for renal damage after perinatal asphyxia (1020), as well as for tubular damage due to nephrotoxicity (see Acute Renal Failure; Nephrotoxicity).

Etiology

Proteinuria of tubular origin, the most common type, never is massive. It includes LMW proteins (i.e., less than 60,000 kilodalton), which, as in the normal situation, are freely filtered through the glomerulus. In addition, in some patients, lysosomal proteins such as NAG can be

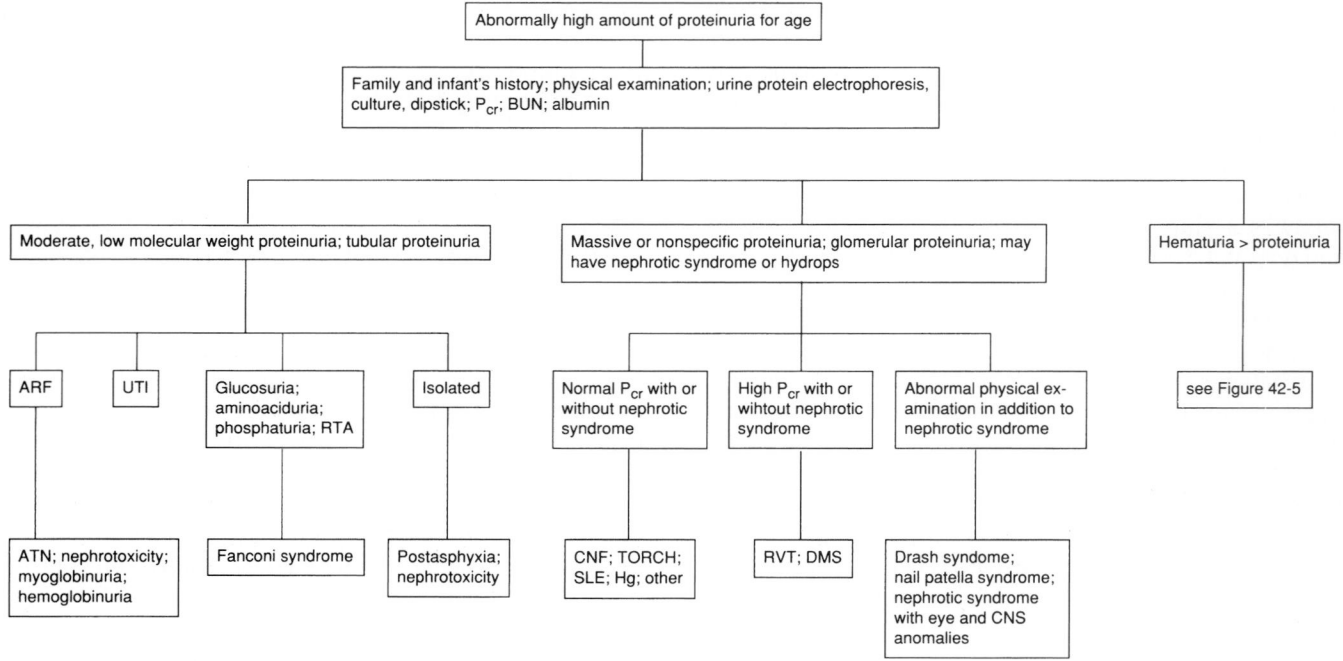

FIG. 42–6. Differential diagnosis of proteinuria. AFR, acute renal failure; ATN, acute tubular necrosis; BUN, blood urea nitrogen; CNF, congenital nephrotic syndrome (Finnish type); DMS, diffuse mesangial sclerosis; Hg, mercury intoxication; P_{cr}, plasma creatinine concentration; RTA, renal tubular acidosis; RVT, renal venous thrombosis; SLE, systemic lupus erythematosus; UTI, urinary tract infection.

found in the urine. Although tubular proteinuria can be isolated, it is associated most often with perinatal asphyxia or renal ischemia, UTI, ARF, Fanconi syndrome, or nephrotoxicity (see Acute Renal Failure; Tubular Dysfunction).

In contrast, proteinuria of glomerular origin includes proteins with higher molecular weight such as albumin. It may become massive and lead to nephrotic syndrome (see Congenital Nephrotic Syndrome, above).

Evaluation

Because proteinuria occurs frequently, an extensive workup is not indicated unless there is evidence for renal disease. Apart from history and physical examination, a major step in the differential diagnosis is the differentiation between tubular and glomerular proteinuria. This can be obtained by electrophoresis of urinary proteins or by quantitative measurement of specific LMW proteins and albumin (Fig. 42–6). In addition, there may be evidence of tubular damage (e.g., glucosuria, RTA). Discussions of specific disorders are provided elsewhere in this chapter.

REFERENCES

Developmental Physiology

1. Saxen L. *Organogenesis of the kidney.* Cambridge, MA: Harvard University Press, 1987.
2. Rabinowitz R, Peters MT, Vyas S, et al. Measurement of fetal urine production in normal pregnancy by real-time ultrasonography. *Am J Obstet Gynecol* 1989;161:1264.
3. Potter EL, Thierstein ST. Glomerular development in the kidney as an index of foetal maturity. *J Pediatr* 1943;22:695.
4. Thorburn GD. The role of the thyroid gland and kidneys in fetal growth. *Ciba Found Symp* 1974;27:185.
5. Perlman M, Levin M. Fetal pulmonary hypoplasia, anuria, and oligohydramnios: clinicopathologic observations and review of the literature. *Am J Obstet Gynecol* 1974;118:1119.
6. Gomez RA, Meernick JG, Kuehl WD, et al. Developmental aspects of the renal response to hemorrhage during fetal life. *Pediatr Res* 1984;18:40.
7. Wladimiroff JW, Campbell S. Fetal urine production rates in normal and complicated pregnancy. *Lancet* 1974;1:151.
8. Veille JC, Hanson RA, Tatum K, Kelley K. Quantitative assessment of human fetal renal blood flow. *Am J Obstet Gynecol* 1993;169:1399.
9. Rubin MI, Bruck E, Rapoport MJ. Maturation of renal function in childhood: clearance studies. *J Clin Invest* 1949;28:1144.
10. Calcagno PL, Rubin MI. Renal extraction of para-amino-hippurate in infants and children. *J Clin Invest* 1963;42:1632.
11. Barnett HL, Hare WK, McNamara H, et al. Influence of postnatal age on kidney function of premature infants. *Proc Soc Exp Biol Med* 1948;69:55.
12. Schwartz GJ, Goldsmith DI, Fine LG. p-Aminohippurate transport in the proximal straight tubule: development and substrate stimulation. *Pediatr Res* 1978;12:793.
13. Rudolph AM, Heymann MA, Teramo KAW, et al. Studies on the circulation of the previable human fetus. *Pediatr Res* 1971;5:452.
14. Aperia A, Broberger O, Herin P, et al. Renal hemodynamics in the perinatal period: a study in lambs. *Acta Physiol Scand* 1977;99:261.
15. Robillard JE, Weismann DN, Herin P. Ontogeny of single glomerular perfusion rate in fetal and newborn lambs. *Pediatr Res* 1981;15:1248.
16. Kleinman LI, Reuter JH. Maturation of glomerular blood flow distribution in the newborn dog. *J Physiol (Lond)* 1973;228:91.
17. Olbing H, Blaufox MD, Aschinberg LC, et al. Postnatal changes in

renal glomerular blood flow distribution in puppies. *J Clin Invest* 1973;52:2885.

18. Aschinburg LC, Goldsmith DI, Olbing H, et al. Neonatal changes in renal blood flow distribution in puppies. *Am J Physiol* 1975;228:1453.

19. Gruskin AB, Edelmann CM Jr, Yuan S. Maturational changes in renal blood flow in piglets. *Pediatr Res* 1970;4:7.

20. Aperia A, Broberger O, Herin P. Maturational changes in glomerular perfusion rate and glomerular filtration rate in lambs. *Pediatr Res* 1974;8:758.

21. Spitzer A, Schwartz GJ. The kidney during development. In: Windhager E, ed. *The handbook of physiology.* Bethesda, MD: American Physiology Society, 1992:475.

22. Ichikawa I, Maddox DA, Brenner BM. Maturational development of glomerular ultrafiltration in the rat. *Am J Physiol* 1979;236:F465.

23. Elinder G, Aperia A, Herin P, et al. Effect of isotonic volume expansion on glomerular filtration rate and renal hemodynamics in the developing rat kidney. *Acta Physiol Scand* 1980;108:411.

24. Drukker A, Goldsmith DI, Spitzer A, et al. The renin angiotensin system in newborn dogs: developmental patterns and response to acute saline loading. *Pediatr Res* 1980;14:304.

25. Horster M, Valtin H. Postnatal development of renal function: micropuncture and clearance studies in the dog. *J Clin Invest* 1971;50:779.

26. Jose PA, Logan AG, Slotkoff LM, et al. Intrarenal blood flow distribution in canine puppies. *Pediatr Res* 1971;5:335.

27. Vernier RL, Birch-Andersen A. Studies of the human fetal kidney: I. Development of the glomerulus. *J Pediatr* 1962;60:754.

28. Evan AP, Stoeckel JA, Loemker V, et al. Development of the intrarenal vascular system of the puppy. *Anat Rec* 1979;194:187.

29. Ljungqvist A, Wagermark J. Renal juxtaglomerular granulation in the human foetus and infant. *Acta Pathol Microbiol Scand* 1966;67:257.

30. Richer C, Hornych H, Amiel-Tison C, et al. Plasma renin activity and its postnatal development in preterm infants. *Biol Neonate* 1977;31:301.

31. Kotchen TA, Strickland AL, Rice TW, et al. A study of the renin–angiotensin system in newborn infants. *J Pediatr* 1972;80:938.

32. Graham PC, Kingdom JCP, Raweily EA, et al. Distribution of renin-containing cells in the developing human kidney: an immunohistochemical study. *Br J Obstet Gynaecol* 1992;99:76.

33. Pelayo JC, Eisner GM, Jose PA. The ontogeny of the renin–angiotensin system. *Clin Perinatol* 1981;8:347.

34. Van Acker KJ, Scharpe SL, Deprettere AJR, et al. Renin–angiotensin–aldosterone system in the healthy infant and child. *Kidney Int* 1979;16:196.

35. Smith FG, Lupu AN, Barajas L, et al. The renin–angiotensin system in the fetal lamb. *Pediatr Res* 1974;8:611.

36. Mott JC. The place of the renin angiotensin system before and after birth. *Br Med Bull* 1975;31:64.

37. Siegel SR, Fisher DA. The renin angiotensin–aldosterone system in the newborn lamb: response to furosemide. *Pediatr Res* 1977;11:837.

38. Lumberg ER, Reid GC. Effects of vaginal delivery and caesarian section on plasma renin activity and angiotensin II levels in human umbilical cord blood. *Biol Neonate* 1977;31:127.

39. John EG, Zeis PM, Samayo C. Renin–aldosterone system response to chronic salt loading and volume contraction in puppies. *Int J Pediatr Nephrol* 1981;2:9.

40. Sulyok E, Varga F, Nemeth M, et al. Furosemide-induced alterations in the electrolyte status, the function of renin angiotensin–aldosterone system and the urinary excretion of prostaglandins in newborn infants. *Pediatr Res* 1980;14:765.

41. Robillard JE, Weitzman RE. Developmental aspects of the fetal response to exogenous arginine vasopressin. *Am J Physiol* 1980;238:F407.

42. Fiselier R, Monnens L, Lameire N, et al. Effects of angiotensin II blockade in the canine puppy under different salt-intake. *Kidney Int* 1984;26:823.

43. Sulyok E, Nemeth M, Tenyi I, et al. Relationship between maturity, electrolyte balance and the function of the renin–angiotensin–aldosterone system in newborn infants. *Biol Neonate* 1979;35:60.

44. Arant BS Jr, Stephenson WH. Developmental change in systemic vascular resistance compared with prostaglandins and angiotensin II concentration in arterial plasma of conscious dogs. *Pediatr Res* 1982;16:120A.

45. Robillard JE, Weitzman RE, Fisher DA, et al. The dynamics of vasopressin release: blood volume regulation during fetal hemorrhage in the lamb fetus. *Pediatr Res* 1979;13:606.

46. Nakamura KT, Ayres NA, Gomez RA, et al. Renal responses to hypoxemia during renin–angiotensin system inhibition in fetal lambs. *Am J Physiol* 1985;249:R116.

47. Tortorolo G, Porcelli G, Cuatalo P. Urinary kallikreins in premature, small at term and normal newborns and in children. In: Pisano JJ, Austen KF, eds. *Chemistry and biology of kallikrein: kinin system in health and disease.* Washington, DC: PHEW (National Institutes of Health), 1974:76.

48. Godard C, Vallotton MB, Favre L. Urinary prostaglandins, vasopressin, and kallikrein excretion in healthy children from birth to adolescence. *J Pediatr* 1982;100:898.

49. Gerber JG, Nies AS. The hemodynamic effects of prostaglandins in the rat: evidence for important species variation in renovascular responses. *Circ Res* 1979;44:406.

50. Lifschitz MD. Prostaglandins and renal blood flow: in vivo studies. *Kidney Int* 1981;19:781.

51. Moncada S, Vane JR. Pharmacology and endogenous roles of prostaglandin endoperoxides, thromboxane A_2 and prostacyclin. *Pharmacol Rev* 1979;30:293.

52. Walker DW, Mitchell MD. Prostaglandins in urine of foetal lambs. *Nature* 1978;271:161.

53. Walker DW, Mitchell MD. Presence of thromboxane B_2 and 6-keto-prostaglandin F1-α in the urine of fetal sheep. *Prostaglandins Med* 1979;3:249.

54. Arant BS Jr. Renal disorders of the newborn infant. *Pediatr Nephrol* 1984;12:111.

55. Robillard JE, Weismann DN, Gomez RA, et al. Renal and adrenal responses to converting-enzyme inhibition in fetal and newborn life. *Am J Physiol* 1983;244:R249.

56. Benzoni D, Vincent M, Betend B, et al. Urinary excretion of prostaglandins and electrolytes in developing children. *Kidney Int* 1981;20:386.

57. Matson JR, Stokes JB, Robillard JE. Effects of inhibition of prostaglandin synthesis on fetal renal function. *Kidney Int* 1981;20:621.

58. Millard RW, Baig H, Vatner SF. Prostaglandin control of the renal circulation in response to hypoxemia in the fetal lamb in utero. *Circ Res* 1979;45:172.

59. Lagercrantz H, Bistoletti P. Catecholamine release in the newborn infant at birth. *Pediatr Res* 1973;11:889.

60. Jose PA, Slotkoff LM, Lilienfield LS, et al. Sensitivity of neonatal renal vasculature to epinephrine. *Am J Physiol* 1974;226:796.

61. McKenna OC, Angelakos ET. Adrenergic innervation of the canine kidney. *Circ Res* 1968;22:345.

62. Felder RA, Pelayo JC, Calcagno PL, et al. Alpha adrenoceptors in the developing kidney. *Pediatr Res* 1983;17:177.

63. Buckley NM, Brazeau P, Fraiser ID. Cardiovascular effects of dopamine in developing swine. *Biol Neonate* 1983;43:50.

64. Buckley NM, Brazeau P, Charney AN, et al. Cardiovascular and renal effects of isoproterenol infusions in young swine. *Biol Neonate* 1984;45:69.

65. Fildes RD, Eisner GM, Calcagno PL, et al. Renal α-adrenoceptors and sodium excretion in the dog. *Am J Physiol* 1985;248:F128.

66. Felder CC, Piccio MM, Mckelvey AM, et al. Ontogeny of renal beta-adrenoceptors in the sheep. *Pediatr Nephrol* 1990;4:635.

67. Nakamura KT, Matherne GP, Jose PA, et al. Ontogeny of renal β-adrenoceptor mediated vasodilation in sheep: comparison between endogenous catecholamines. *Pediatr Res* 1987;22:465.

68. Feltes TF, Hansen TN, Martin CG, et al. The effects of dopamine infusion on regional blood flow in newborn lambs. *Pediatr Res* 1987;21:131.

69. Driscoll DJ, Gillette PC, Lewis RM, et al. Comparative hemodynamic effects of isoproterenol, dopamine, and dobutamine in the newborn dog. *Pediatr Res* 1979;13:1006.

70. Felder RA, Nakamura KT, Robillard JE, et al. Dopamine receptors in the developing kidney. *Pediatr Nephrol* 1988;2:156.

71. Pohjavuori M, Fyhrquist F. Hemodynamic significance of vasopressin in the newborn infant. *J Pediatr* 1980;97:462.

72. Weismann DN, Robillard JE. Renal hemodynamic responses to hypoxemia during development: relationship to circulatory vasoactive substances. *Pediatr Res* 1988;23:155.

73. Chevalier RL, Gomez RA, Carey RM, et al. Renal effects of atrial

natriuretic peptide infusion in young and adult rats. *Pediatr Res* 1988;24:333.

74. Tulassay T, Rascher W, Seyberth HW, et al. Role of atrial natriuretic peptide in sodium homeostasis in premature infants. *J Pediatr* 1986; 109:1023.

75. Wei Y, Rodi CP, Day ML, et al. Developmental changes in the rat atriopeptin hormonal system. *J Clin Invest* 1987;79:1325.

76. Varille VA, Nakamura KT, McWeeny OJ, et al. Renal hemodynamic response to atrial natriuretic factor in fetal and newborn sheep. *Pediatr Res* 1989;25:291.

77. Robillard JE, Nakamura KT, Varille VA, et al. Ontogeny of the renal response to natriuretic peptide in sheep. *Am J Physiol* 1988;254: F634.

78. Chevalier RL, Kaiser DL. Autoregulation of renal blood flow in the rat: effect of growth and uninephrectomy. *Am J Physiol* 1983;244: F483.

79. Jose PA, Slotkoft LM, Montgomery S, et al. Autoregulation of renal blood flow in the puppy. *Am J Physiol* 1975;229:983.

80. Buckley NM, Brazeau P, Frasier ID. Renal blood flow autoregulation in developing swine. *Am J Physiol* 1983;245:H1.

81. Semple SJG, deWardener HE. Effect of increased venous pressure on circulatory "autoregulation" of isolated dog kidneys. *Circ Res* 1959;7:643.

82. Altschule MD. The changes in the mesonephric tubules of human embryos seven to twelve weeks old. *Anat Rec* 1930;46:81.

83. Gersh I. The correlation of structure and function in the developing mesonephros and metanephros. *Contrib Embryol* 1937;153:35.

84. Arant BS Jr. Developmental patterns of renal functional maturation compared in the human neonate. *J Pediatr* 1978;92:705.

85. Coulthard MG. Maturation of glomerular filtration in preterm and mature babies. *Early Hum Dev* 1985;11:281.

86. Aperia A, Broberger O, Elinder G, et al. Postnatal development of renal function in pre-term and full-term infants. *Acta Paediatr Scand* 1981;70:183.

87. Leake RD, Trygstad CW, Oh W. Inulin clearance in the newborn infant. Relationship to gestational and postnatal age. *Pediatr Res* 1976;10:759.

88. Oh W, Arcilla RA, Oh MA, et al. Renal and cardiovascular effects of body tilting in the newborn infant: a comparative study of infants born with early and late cord clamping. *Biol Neonate* 1966;10:76.

89. Strauss J, Daniel SS, James LS. Postnatal adjustment in renal function. *Pediatrics* 1981;68:802.

90. Barnett HL. Renal physiology in infants and children: I. Method for estimation of glomerular filtration rate. *Proc Soc Exp Biol Med* 1940;44:654.

91. Arant BS Jr. Postnatal development of renal function during the first year of life. *Pediatr Nephrol* 1987;1:308.

92. Vanpee M, Blennow M, Linne T, et al. Renal function in very low birth weight infants: normal maturity reach during early childhood. *J Pediatr* 1992;121:784.

93. Spitzer A, Brandis M. Functional and morphologic maturation of the superficial nephrons: relationship to total kidney function. *J Clin Invest* 1974;53:279.

94. MacDonald MS, Emery JL. The late intrauterine and postnatal development of human renal glomeruli. *J Anat* 1959;93:331.

95. Arant BS Jr, Edelmann CM Jr, Nash MA. The renal reabsorption of glucose in the developing canine kidney: a study of glomerulo-tubular balance. *Pediatr Res* 1974;8:638.

96. Aperia A, Herin P. Development of glomerular perfusion rate and nephron filtration rate in rats 17–60 days old. *Am J Physiol* 1975; 228:1319.

97. Goldsmith DI, Jodorkovsky RA, Sherwinter J, et al. Glomerular capillary permeability in developing canines. *Am J Physiol* 1986;251:F528.

98. John E, Goldsmith DI, Spitzer A. Quantitative changes in the canine glomerular vasculature during development: physiologic implications. *Kidney Int* 1981;20:223.

99. Fetterman GH, Sheeplock NA, Philipp FJ, et al. The growth and maturation of human glomeruli and proximal convolutions from term to adulthood: studies by microdissection. *Pediatrics* 1965;35:601.

100. Knutson DW, Chieu F, Bennett CM, et al. Estimation of relative glomerular capillary surface area in normal and hypertrophic rat kidneys. *Kidney Int* 1978;14:437.

101. Hill KJ, Lumbers ER, Elbourne I. The actions of cortisol on fetal renal function. *J Dev Physiol* 1988;10:85.

102. Corvilain J, Abramow M. Effect of growth hormone on tubular transport of phosphate in normal and parathyroidectomized dogs. *J Clin Invest* 1964;43:1608.

103. Ausiello DA, Kreisberg JI, Roy C, et al. Contraction of cultured rat glomerular cells of apparent mesangial origin after stimulation with angiotensin II and arginine vasopressin. *J Clin Invest* 1980;65:754.

104. Friedman Z, Demers LM, Marks KH, et al. Urinary excretion of prostaglandin E following the administration of furosemide and indomethacin to sick low-birth-weight infants. *J Pediatr* 1978;93: 512.

105. Cifuentes RF, Olley PM, Balfe JW, et al. Indomethacin and renal function in premature infants with persistent ductus arteriosus. *J Pediatr* 1979;95:583.

106. Aperia A, Herin P. Effect of arterial blood pressure reduction on renal hemodynamics in the developing lamb. *Acta Physiol Scand* 1976;98: 387.

107. Briggs JP, Schubert G, Schnermann J. Quantitative characterization of the tubuloglomerular feedback response: effect of growth. *Am J Physiol* 1984;247:F808.

108. Muller-Suur R, Ulfendahl HR, Persson AEG. Evidence for tubuloglomerular feedback in juxtamedullary nephrons of young rats. *Am J Physiol* 1983;244:F425.

109. Gordon HH, Levine SZ, Marples E, et al. Water exchange of premature infants: comparison of metabolic (organic) and electrolyte (inorganic) methods of measurement. *J Clin Invest* 1939;18:187.

110. McCance RA, Widdowson EM. The response of the newborn puppy to water, salt and food. *J Physiol (Lond)* 1958;141:81.

111. Aperia A, Broberger O, Thodenius K, et al. Renal response to an oral sodium load in newborn full-term infants. *Acta Paediatr Scand* 1972;61:670.

112. Aperia A, Elinder G. Distal tubular sodium reabsorption in the developing rat kidney. *Am J Physiol* 1981;240:F487.

113. Nakamura KT, Matherne GP, McWeeny OJ, et al. Renal hemodynamics and functional changes during the transition from fetal to newborn life in sheep. *Pediatr Res* 1987;21:229.

114. Robillard JE, Sessions C, Kennedey RL, et al. Interrelationship between glomerular filtration rate and renal transport of sodium and chloride during fetal life. *Am J Obstet Gynecol* 1977;128:727.

115. Siegel SR, Oh W. Renal function as a marker of human fetal maturation. *Acta Paediatr Scand* 1976;65:481.

116. Engelke SC, Shah BL, Vasan U, et al. Sodium balance in very low birth-weight infants. *J Pediatr* 1978;93:837.

117. Aperia A, Broberger O, Thodenius K, et al. Developmental study of the renal response to an oral salt load in preterm infants. *Acta Paediatr Scand* 1974;63:517.

118. Lorenz JM, Kleinman LI, Kotagal UR, et al. Water balance in very low-birth-weight infants: relationship to water and sodium intake and effect on outcome. *J Pediatr* 1982;101:423.

119. Al-Dahhan J, Haycock GB, Nichol B, et al. Sodium homeostasis in term and preterm neonates: III. The effect of salt supplementation. *Arch Dis Child* 1984;59:945.

120. Broberger U, Aperia A, Thodenius K, et al. Renal function in infants with hyperbiliremia. *Acta Paediatr Scand* 1979;68:75.

121. Aperia A, Bergqvist G, Brogerger O, et al. Renal function in newborn infants with high hematocrit values before and after isovolemic haemodilution. *Acta Paediatr Scand* 1974;63:878.

122. Harkavy KL, Scanlon JW, Jose P. The effects of theophylline on renal function in the premature newborn. *Biol Neonate* 1979;35:126.

123. Merlet-Benichou C, de Rouffignac C. Renal clearance studies in fetal and young guinea pigs: effect of salt loading. *Am J Physiol* 1977;232:F178.

124. Rodriguez-Soriano J, Vallo A, Oliveros R, et al. Renal handling of sodium in premature and full-term neonates: a study using clearance methods during water diuresis. *Pediatr Res* 1983;17:1013.

125. Kleinman LI. Renal sodium reabsorption during saline loading and distal blockade in newborn dogs. *Am J Physiol* 1975;228:1403.

126. Aperia A, Broberger O, Herin P, et al. Sodium excretion in relation to sodium intake and aldosterone excretion in newborn preterm and full term infants. *Acta Paediatr Scand* 1979;68:813.

127. Vehaskari VM. Ontogeny of cortical collecting duct sodium transport. *Am J Physiol* 1994;267:F49.

128. Stephenson G, Hammet M, Hadaway G, et al. Ontogeny of renal mineralocorticoid receptors and urinary electrolyte responses in the rat. *Am J Physiol* 1984;247:F665.

129. Satlin LM and Palmer LG. Apical Na⁺ conductance in maturing rabbit principal cell. *Am J Physiol* 1996;270:F391.

130. Brace RA, Bayer LA, Cheung CY. Fetal cardiovascular, endocrine, and fluid responses to atrial natriuretic factor infusion. *Am J Physiol* 1989;257:R580.

131. Semmekrot BA, Wiesel PH, Monnens LAH, et al. Age differences in renal response to atrial natriuretic peptide in rabbits. *Life Sci* 1990; 46:849.

132. Wintour EM, Coghlan JP, Towstoless MK. Cortisol is natriuretic in the immature ovine fetus. *J Endocrinol* 1985;106:1213.

133. Serrano CV, Talbert LM, Welt LG. Potassium deficiency in the pregnant dog. *J Clin Invest* 1964;43:27.

134. Dancis J, Springer D. Fetal homeostasis in maternal malnutrition: potassium and sodium deficiency in rats. *Pediatr Res* 1970;4:345.

135. Sulyok E. The relationship between electrolyte and acid–base balance in the premature infant during early postnatal life. *Biol Neonate* 1971;17:227.

136. Lelievre-Pegorier M, Merlet-Benichou C, Roinel N, et al. Developmental pattern of water and electrolyte transport in rat superficial nephrons. *Am J Physiol* 1983;245:F15.

137. Satlin LM. Maturation of renal potassium transport. *Pediatr Nephrol* 1991;5:260.

138. Tuvdad F, McNamara H, Barnett HL. Renal response of premature infants to administration of bicarbonate and potassium. *Pediatrics* 1954;13:4.

139. McCance RA, Widdowson EM. The response of the new-born piglet to an excess of potassium. *J Physiol* 1958;141:88.

140. Kleinman LI, Banks RO. Segmental nephron sodium and potassium reabsorption in newborn and adult dogs during saline expansion. *Proc Soc Exp Biol Med* 1983;173:231.

141. Zink H, Horster M. Maturation of diluting capacity in loop of Henle of rat superficial nephrons. *Am J Physiol* 1977;233:F519.

142. Satlin LM. Postnatal maturation of potassium transport in rabbit cortical collecting duct. *Am J Physiol* 1994;266:F57.

143. Schmidt U, Horster M. Na-K-activated ATPase: activity maturation in rabbit nephron segments dissected in vitro. *Am J Physiol* 1977; 233:F55.

144. Satlin LM, Evan AP, Gattone V III, et al. Postnatal maturation of the rabbit cortical collecting duct. *Pediatr Nephrol* 1988;2:135.

145. Satlin LM, Palmer LG. Apical K⁺ conductance in maturing rabbit principal cell. *Am J Physiol* 1997;272:F397.

146. Robillard JE, Nakamura KT, Lawton WJ. Effects of aldosterone on urinary kallikrein and sodium excretion during fetal life. *Pediatr Res* 1985;190:1048.

147. Vaughn D, Kirschbaum TH, Bersentes T, et al. Fetal and neonatal response to acid loading in the sheep. *J Appl Physiol* 1968;24:135.

148. Smith FG Jr, Schwartz A. Response of the intact lamb fetus to acidosis. *Am J Obstet Gynecol* 1970;106:52.

149. Weisbrot IM, James LS, Prince CE, et al. Acid–base homeostasis of the new-born infant during the first 24 hrs of life. *J Pediatr* 1958;52: 395.

150. Smith CA. *The physiology of the newborn infant.* Springfield, IL: CC Thomas, 1959:320.

151. Robillard JE, Sessions C, Burmeister L, et al. Influence of fetal extracellular volume contraction on renal reabsorption of bicarbonate in fetal lambs. *Pediatr Res* 1977;11:649.

152. Schwartz GJ, Haycock GB, Edelmann CM Jr, et al. Late metabolic acidosis: a reassessment of the definition. *J Pediatr* 1979;95:102.

153. Ranlov P, Siggaard-Andersen O. Late metabolic acidosis in premature infants. *Acta Paediatr Scand* 1965;54:531.

154. Edelmann CM Jr, Rodriguez-Soriano J, Boichis H, et al. Renal bicarbonate reabsorption and hydrogen ion excretion in normal infants. *J Clin Invest* 1967;46:1309.

155. Schwartz GJ, Evan AP. Development of solute transport in rabbit proximal tubule: I. HCO₃ and glucose absorption. *Am J Physiol* 1983;245:F382.

156. Moore ES, Fine BP, Satrasook SS, et al. Renal reabsorption of bicarbonate in puppies: effect of extracellular volume contraction on the renal threshold for bicarbonate. *Pediatr Res* 1972;6:859.

157. Baum M, Biemesderfer D, Gentry D, Aronson PS. Ontogeny of rabbit renal cortical NHE3 and NHE1: effect of glucocorticoids. *Am J Physiol* 1995;268:F815.

158. Lonnerholm G, Wistrand PJ. Carbonic anhydrase in the human fetal kidney. *Pediatr Res* 1983;17:390.

159. Svenningsen NW. Renal acid–base titration studies in infants with and without metabolic acidosis in the postneonatal period. *Pediatr Res* 1974;8:659.

160. Kerpel-Fronius E, Heim T, Sulyok E. The development of the renal acidifying processes and their relation to acidosis in low-birth-weight infants. *Biol Neonate* 1970;15:156.

161. Sulyok E, Heim T. Assessment of maximal urinary acidification in premature infants. *Biol Neonate* 1971;19:200.

162. Svenningsen NW, Lindquist B. Postnatal development of renal hydrogen ion excretion capacity in relation to age and protein intake. *Acta Paediatr Scand* 1974;63:721.

163. Goldstein L. Ammonia metabolism in kidneys of suckling rats. *Am J Physiol* 1971;220:213.

164. Peonides A, Levin B, Young WF. The renal excretion of hydrogen ions in infants and children. *Arch Dis Child* 1965;40:33.

165. McCance RA, Widdowson EM. Renal aspects of acid–base control in the newly born: I. Natural development. *Acta Paediatr Scand* 1960;49:409.

166. Satlin LM, Schwartz GJ. Postnatal maturation of rabbit renal collecting duct: intercalated cell function. *Am J Physiol* 1987;253:F622.

167. Mehrgut FM, Satlin LM, Schwartz GJ. Maturation of HCO₃ transport in rabbit collecting duct. *Am J Physiol* 1990;259:F801.

168. Matsumoto T, Fejes-Toth G, Schwartz J. Postnatal differentiation of rabbit collecting duct intercalated cells. *Pediatr Res* 1996;39:1.

169. Satlin LM, Matsumoto T, Schwartz GJ. Postnatal maturation of rabbit renal collecting duct. III. Peanut lectin-binding intercalated cells. *Am J Physiol* 1992;262:F199.

170. Kildeberg P, Engel K, Winters RW. Balance of net acid in growing infants: endogenous and transintestinal aspects. *Acta Paediatr Scand* 1969;58:321.

171. Radde IC, Chance GW, Bailey K. Growth and mineral metabolism in very low birth-weight infants: I. Comparison of the effects of two modes of NaHCO₃ treatment of late metabolic acidosis. *Pediatr Res* 1975;9:564.

172. Arant BS Jr. Renal handling of calcium and phosphorus in normal human neonates. *Semin Nephrol* 1983;2:94.

173. Brown DR, Steranka BH. Renal cation excretion in the hypocalcemic premature human neonate. *Pediatr Res* 1981;15:1100.

174. Karlen J, Aperia A, Zetterstrom R. Renal excretion of calcium and phosphate in preterm and term infants. *J Pediatr* 1985;106:814.

175. Ghazali S, Barratt TM. Urinary excretion of calcium and magnesium in children. *Arch Dis Child* 1974;49:97.

176. Campfield T, Braden G, Flynn-Valone P, Powell S. Effect of diuretics on urinary oxalate, calcium, and sodium excretion in very low birth weight infant. *Pediatrics* 1997;99:814.

177. Zanardo V, Dani C, Trevisanuto D, et al. Methylxanthines increase renal calcium excretion in preterm infants. *Biol Neonate* 1995;68: 169.

178. Kamitsuka MD, Williams MA, Nyberg DA, et al. Renal calcification: a complication of dexamethasone therapy in preterm infants with bronchopulmonary dysplasia. *J Perinatol* 1995;15:359.

179. Jahan I, Pitts RF. Effect of parathyroid on renal tubular reabsorption of phosphate and calcium. *Am J Physiol* 1948;155:42.

180. Ardaillou R. Kidney and calcitonin. *Nephron* 1975;15:250.

181. Linarelli LG, Bobick J, Bobick C. The effect of parathyroid hormone on rabbit renal cortex adenyl cyclase during development. *Pediatr Res* 1973;7:878.

182. Imbert-Teboul M, Chabardes D, Clique A, et al. Ontogenesis of hormone-dependent adenylate cyclase in isolated rat nephron segments. *Am J Physiol* 1984;247:F316.

183. Mallet E, Basuyau J-P, Brunelle P, et al. Neonatal parathyroid secretion and renal receptor maturation in premature infants. *Biol Neonate* 1978;33:304.

184. Linarelli LG. Nephron urinary cyclic AMP and developmental renal responsiveness to parathyroid hormone. *Pediatrics* 1972;50:14.

185. Tsang RC, Light IJ, Sutherland JM, et al. Possible pathogenetic factors in neonatal hypocalcemia of prematurity. *J Pediatr* 1973;82:423.

186. Chattopadhyay N, Baum M, Bai M, et al. Ontogeny of the extracellular calcium-sensing receptor in rat kidney. *Am J Physiol* 1996;271:F736.

187. Quamme GA, Dirks JH. Intraluminal and contraluminal magnesium on magnesium and calcium transfer in the rat nephron. *Am J Physiol* 1980;238:F187.

188. Ariceta G, Rodriguez-Soriano, Valo A. Magnesium homeostasis in premature and full-term neonates. *Pediatr Nephrol* 1995;9:423.

189. Smith FG Jr, Adams FH, Borden N, et al. Studies of renal function in the intact fetal lamb. *Am J Obstet Gynecol* 1966;96:240.

190. Brodehl J, Gellison K, Weber HP. Postnatal development of tubular phosphate reabsorption. *Clin Nephrol* 1982;17:163.

191. McCrory WW, Forman CW, McNamara H, et al. Renal excretion of inorganic phosphate in newborn infants. *J Clin Invest* 1952;31:357.

192. Johnson V, Spitzer A. Renal reabsorption of phosphate during development: whole kidney events. *Am J Physiol* 1986;251:F251.

193. Caversazio J, Bonjour JP. Fleisch H. Tubular handling of Pi in young growing and adult rats. *Am J Physiol* 1982;242:F705.

194. Senterre J, Salle B. Renal aspects of calcium and phosphorus metabolism in preterm infants. *Biol Neonate* 1988;53:220.

195. Haramati A, Mulroney SE, Webster SK. Developmental changes in the tubular capacity for phosphate reabsorption in the rat. *Am J Physiol* 1988;255:F287.

196. Kaskel FJ, Kumar AM, Feld LG, et al. Renal reabsorption of phosphate during development: tubular events. *Pediatr Nephrol* 1988;2:129.

197. Prabhu S, Levi M, Dwarakanath V, et al. Effect of glucocorticoids on neonatal rabbit renal cortical sodium-inorganic phosphate messenger RNA and protein abundance. *Pediatr Res* 1997;41,20.

198. Arar M, Levi M, Baum M. Maturational effects of glucocorticoids on neonatal brush-border membrane phosphate transport. *Pediatr Res* 1994;35,474.

199. Barac-Nieto M, Dowd TL, Gupta RK, et al. Changes in NMR-visible kidney cell phosphate with age and diet: relationship to phosphate transport. *Am J Physiol* 1991;261:F153.

200. Hammerman MR, Karl IE, Hruska KA. Regulation of canine renal vesicle Pi transport by growth hormone and parathyroid hormone. *Biochim Biophys Acta* 1980;603,322.

201. Arnaud SB, Goldsmith RS, Stickler GB, et al. Serum parathyroid hormone and blood minerals: interrelationships in normal children. *Pediatr Res* 1973;7:485.

202. David L, Anast CS. Calcium metabolism in newborn infant: the interrelationship of parathyroid function and calcium, magnesium, and phosphorus metabolism in normal sick and hypocalcemic newborns. *J Clin Invest* 1974;54:287.

203. Robillard JE, Sessions C, Kennedy RL, et al. Maturation of the glucose transport process by the fetal kidney. *Pediatr Res* 1978;12:680.

204. Roth KS, Hwang SM, Yudkoff M, et al. The ontogeny of sugar transport in kidney. *Pediatr Res* 1978;12:1127.

205. Beck JC, Lipkowitz MS, Abramson RG. Characterization of the fetal glucose transporter in rabbit kidney: comparison with the adult brush border electrogenic Na$^+$-glucose symporter. *J Clin Invest* 1988;82:379.

206. You G, Lee WS, Barros EJ, et al. Molecular characteristics of Na(+)-coupled glucose transporters in adult and embryonic rat kidney. *J Biol Chem* 1995;270:29365.

207. Horster M, Lewy JE. Filtration fraction and extraction of PAH during neonatal period in the rat. *Am J Physiol* 1970;219:1061.

208. Friis C. Postnatal development of renal function in piglets: glomerular filtration rate, clearance of PAH and PAH extraction. *Biol Neonate* 1979;35:180.

209. Lopez-Nieto CE, You G, Bush KT, et al. Molecular cloning and characterization of NKT, a gene product related to the organic cation transporter family that is almost exclusively expressed in the kidney. *J Biol Chem* 1997;272:6471.

210. Brodehl J, Gellissen K. Endogenous renal transport of free amino acid in infancy and childhood. *Pediatrics* 1968;42:395.

211. Webber WA, Cairns JA. A comparison of the amino acid concentrating ability of the kidney cortex of newborn and mature rats. *Can J Physiol Pharmacol* 1968;46:165.

212. Chesney RW, Jones D, Zelikovic I. Renal amino acid transport: cellular and molecular events from clearance studies to frog eggs. *Pediatr Nephrol* 1993;7:574.

213. Roth KS, Hwang SM, London JW, et al. Ontogeny of glycine transport in isolated rat renal tubules. *Am J Physiol* 1977;233:F241.

214. Hwang SM, Serabian MA, Roth KS, et al. l-proline transport by isolated renal tubules from newborn and adult rats. *Pediatr Res* 1983;17:42.

215. Segal S, Smith I. Delineation of separate transport systems in rat kidney cortex for l-lysine and l-cystine by developmental patterns. *Biochem Biophys Res Commun* 1969;35:771.

216. Ross MG, Sherman DJ, Ervin MG, et al. Maternal dehydration-rehydration: fetal plasma and urinary responses. *Am J Physiol* 1988;255:E674.

217. Woods LL, Cheung CY, Power GG, et al. Role of arginine vasopressin in fetal renal response to hypertonicity. *Am J Physiol* 1986;251:F156.

218. McCance RA, Widdowson EM. Renal function before birth. *Proc R Soc Lond (Biol)* 1953;141:488.

219. Hansen JDL, Smith CA. Effects of withholding fluid in the immediate postnatal period. *Pediatrics* 1953;12:99.

220. Edelmann CM Jr, Barnett HL, Troupkou V. Renal concentrating mechanisms in newborn infants: effect of dietary protein, and water content, role of urea and responsiveness to antidiuretic hormone. *J Clin Invest* 1960;39:1062.

221. Calcagno PL, Rubin MI, Weintraub DH. Studies on the renal concentrating and diluting mechanisms in the premature infant. *J Clin Invest* 1954;33:91.

222. Polacek E, Vocel J, Neugebauerova L, et al. The osmotic concentrating ability in healthy infants and children. *Arch Dis Child* 1965;40:291.

223. Trimble ME. Renal response to solute loading in infant rats: relation to anatomical development. *Am J Physiol* 1970;219:1089.

224. Horster MF, Gilg A, Lory P. Determinants of axial osmotic gradients in the differentiating counter-current system. *Am J Physiol* 1984;246:F124.

225. Edelmann CM Jr, Barnett HL, Stark H. Effect of urea on concentration of urinary nonurea solute in premature infants. *J Appl Physiol* 1966;21:1021.

226. Schwartz GJ, Zavilowitz BJ, Radice AD et al. Maturation of aldose reductase expression in the neonatal rat inner medulla. *J Clin Invest* 1992;90:1275.

227. Hadeed AJ, Leake RD, Weitzman RE, et al. Possible mechanisms of high blood levels of vasopressin during the neonatal period. *J Pediatr* 1979;94:805.

228. Rees L, Forsling ML, Brook CGD. Vasopressin concentrations in the neonatal period. *Clin Endocrinol* 1980;12:357.

229. Leake RD, Weitzman RE, Weinberg JA, et al. Control of vasopressin secretion in the new-born lamb. *Pediatr Res* 1979;13:257.

230. Weitzman RE, Fisher DA, Robillard JE, et al. Arginine vasopressin response to an osmotic stimulus in the fetal sheep. *Pediatr Res* 1978;12:35.

231. DeVane GW, Porter JC. An apparent stress-induced release of arginine vasopressin by human neonates. *J Clin Endocrinol Metab* 1980;51:1412.

232. Svenningsen NW, Aronson AS. Postnatal development of renal concentration capacity as estimated by DDAVP-test in normal and asphyxiated neonates. *Biol Neonate* 1974;25:230.

233. Rajerison RM, Butlen D, Jard S. Ontogenic development of kidney and liver vasopressin receptors. In: Spitzer A, ed. *The kidney during development:* morphology and function. New York: Masson, 1982:249.

234. Schlondorff D, Weber H, Trizna W, et al. Vasopressin responsiveness of renal adenylate cyclase in newborn rats and rabbits. *Am J Physiol* 1978;234:F16.

235. Bonilla-Felix M, John-Phillip C. Prostaglandins mediate the defect in AVP-stimulated cAMP generation in immature collecting duct. *Am J Physiol* 1994;267:F44.

236. Bonilla-Felix M, Jiang W. Aquaporin-2 in the immature rat: expression, regulation, and trafficking. *J Am Soc Nephrol* 1997;8:1502.

237. Ostrowski NL, Young WS II, Knepper MA, Lolait SJ. Expression of vasopressin Via and V2 receptor messenger ribonucleic acid in the liver and kidney embryonic, developing, and adult rats. *Endocrinology* 1993;133:1849.

Clinical Evaluation of Function and Disease

238. Museles M, Gaudry CC Jr, Bason WM. Renal anomalies in the newborn found by deep palpation. *Pediatrics* 1971;47:97.

239. Sherwood DW, Smith RC, Lemmon RH, et al. Abnormalities of the genitourinary tract discovered by palpation of the abdomen of the newborn. *Pediatrics* 1956;36:127.

240. Perlman M, Williams J. Detection of renal anomalies by abdominal palpation in newborn infants. *Br Med J* 1976;2:347.

241. Gillerot Y, Koulischer L. Major malformations of the urinary tract: anatomic and genetic aspects. *Biol Neonate* 1988;53:186.

242. Rubenstein M, Meyer R, Bernstein J. Congenital abnormalities of the urinary system: I. A postmortem survey of developmental anomalies and acquired congenital lesions in a children's hospital. *J Pediatr* 1961;58:356.

243. Helin I, Persson PH. Prenatal diagnosis of urinary tract abnormalities by ultrasound. *Pediatrics* 1986;78:879.

244. Livera LN, Brookfield DSK, Egginton JA, et al. Antenatal ultrasonography to detect fetal renal abnormalities: a prospective screening programme. *Br Med J* 1989;298:1421.

245. Gunn TR, Mora JD, Pease P. Antenatal diagnosis of urinary tract abnormalities by ultrasonography after 28 weeks' gestation: incidence and outcome. *Am J Obstet Gynecol* 1995;172:479.

246. Kim EK, Song TB. A study on fetal urinary tract anomaly: antenatal ultrasonographic diagnosis and postnatal follow-up. *J Obstet Gynaecol Res* 1996;22:569.

247. Fugelseth D, Lindemann R, Sande HA, et al. Prenatal diagnosis of urinary tract anomalies. The value of two ultrasound examinations. *Acta Obstet Gynaecol Scand* 1994;73:290.

248. Scott JES, Lee REJ, Hunter EW, et al. Ultrasound screening of newborn urinary tract. *Lancet* 1991;2:338:1571.

249. Rubecz I, Kodela I, Gasztonyi V, et al. Postnatal screening examination of renal developmental anomalies: classical diagnosis, screening of risk group and routine screening. *Orv Hetil* 1991;132:585.

250. Steinhart JM, Kuhn JP, Eisenberg B, et al. Ultrasound screening of healthy infants for urinary tract abnormalities. *Pediatrics* 1988;82:609.

251. Brion L, Rondia G, Avni FE, et al. Importance of deep abdominal palpation in the perinatal diagnosis of urologic malformations. *Biol Neonate* 1984;46:215.

252. Jelen Z. The value of ultrasonography as a screening procedure of the neonatal urinary tract: a survey of 1021 infants. *Int Urol Nephrol* 1993;25:3.

253. Scott JE, Renwick M. Urological anomalies in the Northern Region Fetal Abnormality Survey. *Arch Dis Child* 1993;68:22.

254. Roodhooft AM, Birnholz JC, Holmes LB. Familial nature of congenital absence and severe dysgenesis of both kidneys. *N Engl J Med* 1984;310:1341.

255. McPherson E, Carey J, Kramer A, et al. Dominantly inherited renal adysplasia. *Am J Med Genet* 1987;26:863.

256. Neave C. Congenital malformation in offspring of diabetics. *Perspect Pediatr Pathol* 1984;8:213.

257. Havers W, Majewski F, Olbing H, et al. Anomalies of the kidneys and genitourinary tract in alcohol embryopathy. *J Urol* 1980;124:108.

258. Lutiger B, Graham K, Einarson TR, et al. Relationship between gestational cocaine use and pregnancy outcome: a meta-analysis. *Teratology* 1991;44:405.

259. Petrikovsky BM, Nardi DA, Rodis JF, et al. Elevated maternal serum alpha-fetoprotein and mild fetal uropathy. *Obstet Gynecol* 1991;78:262.

260. Barr M Jr, Cohen MM Jr. ACE inhibitor fetopathy and hypocalvaria: the kidney–skull connection. *Teratology* 1991;44:485.

261. Cunniff C, Jones KL, Phillipson J, et al. Oligohydramnios sequence and renal tubular malformation associated with maternal enalapril use. *Am J Obstet Gynecol* 1990;162:187.

262. van der Heijden BJ, Carlus C, Narcy F, et al. Persistent anuria, neonatal death, and renal microcystic lesions after prenatal exposure to indomethacin. *Am J Obstet Gynecol* 1994;171:617.

263. Thomas IT, Smith DW. Oligohydramnios, cause of the nonrenal features of Potter's syndrome, including pulmonary hypoplasia. *J Pediatr* 1974;84:811.

264. Nimrod C, Varela-Gittings F, Machin G, et al. The effect of very prolonged membrane rupture on fetal development. *Am J Obstet Gynecol* 1984;148:540.

265. Moessinger AC, Collins MH, Blanc WA, et al. Oligohydramnios-induced lung hypoplasia: the influence of timing and duration in gestation. *Pediatr Res* 1986;20:951.

266. Thibeault DW, Beatty EC Jr, Hall RT, et al. Neonatal pulmonary hypoplasia with premature rupture of fetal membranes and oligohydramnios. *J Pediatr* 1985;107:273.

267. Khuri FJ, Hardy BE, Churchill BM. Urologic anomalies associated with hypospadias. *Urol Clin North Am* 1981;8:565.

268. Bourke WG, Clarke TA, Mathews TG, et al. Isolated single umbilical artery—the case for routine renal screening. *Arch Dis Child* 1993;68:600.

269. Lachiewicz AM, Sibley R, Michael AF. Hereditary renal disease and preauricular pits: report of a kindred. *J Pediatr* 1985;106:948.

270. Rothe CF, Kim KC. Measuring systolic arterial blood pressure: possible errors from extension tubes or disposable transducer domes. *Crit Care Med* 1980;8:683.

271. Kimble KJ, Darnall RA Jr, Yelderman M, et al. An automated oscillometric technique for estimating mean arterial pressure in critically ill newborns. *Anesthesiology* 1981;54:423.

272. Baker DM, Maisels MJ, Marks KH. Indirect BP monitoring in the newborn: evaluation of a new oscillometer and comparison of upper- and lower-limb measurements. *Am J Dis Child* 1984;138:775.

273. Lum LG, Jones MD Jr. The effect of cuff width on systolic blood pressure measurements in neonates. *J Pediatr* 1977;91:963.

274. Kirkendall WM, Feinleib M, Freis ED, et al. Recommendations for human blood pressure determination by sphygmomanometers: Subcommittee on the AHA Postgraduate Education Committee. *Circulation* 1980;62:1146A.

275. Piazza SF, Chandra M, Harper RG, et al. Upper- vs lower-limb systolic blood pressure in full-term normal newborns. *Am J Dis Child* 1985;139:797.

276. Park MK, Lee DH. Normative arm and calf blood pressure values in the newborn. *Pediatrics* 1989;83:240.

277. Tan KL. Blood pressure in very low birth weight infants in the first 70 days of life. *J Pediatr* 1988;112:266.

278. Versmold HT, Kitterman JA, Phibbs RH, et al. Aortic blood pressure during the first 12 hours of life in infants with birth weight 610 to 4,220 grams. *Pediatrics* 1981;67:607.

279. Hegyi T, Carbone MT, Anwar M, et al. Blood pressure ranges in premature infants. I. The first hours of life. *J Pediatr* 1994;124:627.

280. Spahr RC, MacDonald HM, Mueller-Heubach E. Knee–chest position and neonatal oxygenation and blood pressure. *Am J Dis Child* 1981;135:79.

281. Sinkin RA, Philips BL, Adelman RD. Elevation in systemic blood pressure in the neonate during abdominal examination. *Pediatrics* 1985;76:970.

282. Gemelli M, Manganaro R, Mami C, et al. Circadian blood pressure pattern in full-term newborn infants. *Biol Neonate* 1989;56:315.

283. de Swiet M, Fayers P, Shinebourne EA. Systolic blood pressure in a population of infants in the first year of life: the Brompton Study. *Pediatrics* 1980;65:1028.

284. Zinner SH, Lee YH, Rosner B, et al. Factors affecting blood pressures in newborn infants. *Hypertension* 1980;2[Suppl 1]:I-99.

285. Scott JES, Hunter EW, Lee REJ, et al. Ultrasound measurement of renal size in newborn infants. *Arch Dis Child* 1990;65:361.

286. Longino LA, Martin LW. Abdominal masses in the newborn infant. *Pediatrics* 1958;596.

287. Griscom NT, Colodny AH, Rosenberg HK, et al. Diagnostic aspects of neonatal ascites: report of 27 cases. *AJR* 1977;128:961.

288. Shaffer SG, Quimiro CL, Anderson JV, et al. Postnatal weight changes in low birth weight infants. *Pediatrics* 1987;79:702.

289. Clark DA. Time of first void and first stool in 500 newborns. *Pediatrics* 1977;60:457.

290. Pynnönen AL, Kouvalainen K, Jäykkä S. Time of the first urinations in male and female newborns. *Acta Paediatr Scand* 1972;61:303.

291. Chih TW, Teng RJ, Wang CS, et al. Time of the first urine and the first stool in Chinese newborns. *Acta Paediatr Sin* 1991;32:17.

292. Wang PA, Hang FY. Time of the first defaecation and urination in very low birth weight infants. *Eur J Pediatr* 1994;153:279.

293. Bidiwala KS, Lorenz JM, Kleinman LI. Renal function correlates of postnatal diuresis in preterm infants. *Pediatrics* 1988;82:50.

294. Lorenz JM, Kleinman LI, Ahmed G et al. Phases of fluid and electrolyte homeostasis in the extremely low birth weight infant. *Pediatrics* 1995;96:484.

295. Ramiro-Tolentino SB, Markarian K, Kleinman L. I. Renal bircarbonate excretion in extremely low birth weight infants. *Pediatrics* 1996;98:256.

296. Benitez OA, Benitez M, Slynen T, et al. Inaccuracy in neonatal measurement of urine concentration with a refractometer. *J Pediatr* 1986;108:613.

297. Gouyon JB, Houchan N. Assessment of urine specific gravity by reagent strip in newborn infants. *Pediatr Nephrol* 1993;7:77.

298. Coulthard MG, Ruddock V. Validation of inulin as a marker for glomerular filtration in preterm babies. *Kidney Int* 1983;23:407.
299. Summerville DA, Potter CS, Treves ST. The use of radiopharmaceuticals in the measurement of glomerular filtration rate: a review. In: Freeman LM, ed. *Nuclear medicine annual 1990.* New York: Raven Press, 1990:191.
300. Coulthard MG. Comparison of methods of measuring renal function in preterm babies using inulin. *J Pediatr* 1983;102:923.
301. Wilkins BH. Renal function in sick very low birthweight infants: 1. Glomerular filtration rate. *Arch Dis Child* 1992;67:1140.
302. Sonntag J, Prankel B, Waltz S. Serum creatinine concentration, urinary creatinine excretion and creatinine clearance during the first 9 weeks in preterm infants with a birth weight below 1500 g. *Eur J Pediatr* 1996;155:815.
303. Rudd PT, Hughes EA, Placzek MM, et al. Reference ranges for plasma creatinine during the first month of life. *Arch Dis Child* 1983; 58:212.
304. Arant BS Jr, Edelmann CM Jr, Spitzer A. The congruence of creatinine and inulin clearances in children: use of the Technicon autoanalyzer. *J Pediatr* 1972;84:559.
305. Weber JA, van Zanten AP. Interferences in current methods for measurements of creatinine. *Clin Chem* 1991;37:695.
306. Clermont MJ, Brion L, Schwartz GJ. Reliability of plasma creatinine measurement in children. *Clin Pediatr* 1986;25:569.
307. Schwartz GJ, Feld LG, Langford DJ. A simple estimate of glomerular filtration rate in full term infants during the first year of life. *J Pediatr* 1984;104:849.
308. Brion L, Fleischman AR, McCarton C, et al. A simple estimate of glomerular filtration rate in low birth weight infants during the first year of life: non invasive assessment of body composition and growth. *J Pediatr* 1986;109:698.
309. Bueva A, Guignard JP. Renal function in preterm neonates. *Pediatr Res* 1994;36:572.
310. Coulthard MG, Hey EN. Weight as the best standard for glomerular filtration in the newborn. *Arch Dis Child* 1984;59:373.
311. Brion LP, Fleischman AR, Schwartz GJ. Gentamicin interval in newborn infants determined by renal function and postconceptional age. *Pediatr Nephrol* 1991;5:675.
312. Koren G, James A, Perlman M. A simple method for the estimation of glomerular filtration rate by gentamicin pharmacokinetics during routine monitoring in the newborn. *Clin Pharmacol Ther* 1985;38: 680.
313. Kildoo CW, Lin LM, Gabriel MH, et al. Vancomycin pharmacokinetics in infants: relationship to postconceptional age and serum creatinine. *Dev Pharmacol Ther* 1990;14:77.
314. Schwartz GJ, Brion L, Spitzer A. The use of plasma creatinine concentration for estimating glomerular filtration rate in infants, children and adolescents. *Pediatr Clin North Am* 1987;34:57.
315. Schwartz GJ, Haycock G, Edelmann CM Jr, et al. A simple estimate of glomerular filtration rate in children derived from body length and plasma creatinine. *Pediatrics* 1976;58:259.
316. Tassis BMG, Trespidi L, Tirelli AS, et al. Serum β_2-microglobulin in fetuses with urinary tract anomalies. *Am J Obstet Gynecol* 1997;176: 54.
317. Berry SM, Lecolier B, Smith RS, et al. Predictive value of fetal serum β_2-microglobulin for neonatal renal function. *Lancet* 1995; 345:1277.
318. Oyanagi K, Nakamura K, Sogawa H, et al. A study of urea-synthesizing enzymes in prenatal and postnatal human liver. *Pediatr Res* 1980;14:236.
319. Stapleton FB. Renal uric acid clearance in human neonates. *J Pediatr* 1983;103:290.
320. Stapleton FB, Arant BS Jr. Ontogeny of renal uric acid excretion in the mongrel puppy. *Pediatr Res* 1981;15:1513.
321. Tsukahara H, Hiraoka M. Hori C, et al. Urinary uric acid excretion in term and premature infants. *J Paediatr Child Health* 1996;32:330.
322. Bader D, Gozal D, Weinger-Abend M. Neonatal urinary uric acid/creatinine ratio as an additional marker of perinatal asphyxia. *Eur J Pediatr* 1995;154:747.
323. Germino GG, Barton NJ, Lamb J, et al. Identification of a locus which shows no genetic recombination with the autosomal dominant polycystic kidney disease gene on chromosome 16. *Am J Hum Genet* 1990;46:925.
324. Saris JJ, Breuning MH, Dauwerse HG, et al. Rapid detection of polymorphism near gene for adult polycystic kidney disease. *Lancet* 1990;335:1102.
325. International Polycystic Kidney Disease Consortium. Polycystic kidney disease: the complete structure of the PKD1 gene and its protein. *Cell* 1995;81:289.
326. Fossdal R, Bothvarsson M, Asmundsson P, Ragnarsson J, Peters D, Breuning MH, et al. Icelandic families with autosomal dominant polycystic kidney disease: families unlinked to chromosome 16p13.3 revealed by linkage analysis. *Hum Genet* 1993;91:609.
327. Kimberling WJ, Kumar S, Gabow PA, Kenyon JB, Connolly CJ, Somlo S. Autosomal dominant polycystic kidney disease: localization of the second gene to chromosome 4q13-q23. *Genomics* 1993; 18:467.
328. Lin JY, Lin JS, Tsai CH. Use of the urine-to-blood carbon dioxide tension gradient as a measurement of impaired distal tubular hydrogen ion secretion among neonates. *J Pediatr* 1995;126:114.
329. Aas K. The cellular excretion in the urine of normal newborn infants. *Acta Paediatr* 1961;50:361.
330. Kronquist KE, Crandall BF, Tabsh KM. Characterization of fetal urinary proteins at midgestation and term. *Biol Neonate* 1984;46:267.
331. Simeoni U. Specific developmental profiles of lysosomal and brush border enzymuria in the human. *Biol Neonate* 1994;65:1.
332. Van Oort A, Monnens L, van Munster P. Beta-2-microglobulin clearance, an indicator of renal tubular maturation. *Int J Pediatr Nephrol* 1980;1:80.
333. Gordon I, Barratt TM. Imaging the kidneys and urinary tract in the neonate with acute renal failure. *Pediatr Nephrol* 1987;1:321.
334. Slovis TL. Pediatric renal anomalies and infections. *Clin Diagn Ultrasound* 1989;24:157.
335. Restaino I, Kaplan BS, Kaplan P, et al. Renal dysgenesis in a monozygotic twin: association with in utero exposure to indomethacin. *Am J Med Genet* 1991;39:252.
336. Lusiri A, Salinas-Madrigal L, Noguchi A, et al. Renal tubular dysgenesis. *AJR* 1991;157:383.
337. Shackelford GD, Kees-Folts D, Cole BR. Imaging the urinary tract. *Clin Perinatol* 1992;19:85.
338. Shultz PK, Strife JL, Strife CF, et al. Hyperechoic renal medullary pyramids in infants and children. *Radiology* 1991;181:163.
339. Glickstein J, Friedman D, Schacht R, et al. Renal artery Doppler waveforms in neonates with umbilical artery catheters. *Clin Res* 1991;39:669A.
340. Cleary GM, Higgins ST, Merton DA, et al. Developmental changes in renal artery blood flow velocity during the first three weeks of life in preterm neonates. *J Pediatr* 1996;129:251.
341. Van Bel F, Guit GL, Schipper J, et al. Indomethacin-induced changes in renal blood flow velocity waveform in premature infants investigated with color Doppler imaging. *J Pediatr* 1991;118:621.
342. Gaum LD, Wese FX, Alton DJ, et al. Radiologic investigation of the urinary tract in the neonate with myelomeningocele. *J Urol* 1982;127:510.
343. Ash JM, Antico VF, Gilday DL, et al. Special considerations in the pediatric use of radionuclides for kidney studies. *Semin Nucl Med* 1982;12:345.
344. Kullendorf CM, Salmonson EC, Laurin S. Diagnostic cyst puncture of multicystic kidney in neonates. *Acta Radiol* 1990;31:287.
345. Edelmann CM Jr, Churg J, Gerber MA, et al. Renal biopsy: indications, technique, and interpretation. In: Edelmann CM Jr, ed. *Pediatric kidney disease,* 2nd ed. Boston: Little, Brown and Company, 1992:499.

Acute Renal Failure and Oligoanuria

346. Simon EE. Review: new aspects of acute renal failure. *Am J Med Sci* 1995;310:217.
347. Chevalier RL, Campbell F, Norman A, Brenbridge AG. Prognostic factors in neonatal acute renal failure. *Pediatrics* 1984;74:265.
348. Stapleton FB, Jones DP, Green RS. Acute renal failure in neonates: incidence, etiology and outcome. *Pediatr Nephrol* 1987;1:314.
349. Norman ME, Asadi FK. A prospective study of acute renal failure in the newborn infant. *Pediatrics* 1979;63:475.
350. Hanssens M, Keirse MJNC, Vankelecom F, et al. Fetal and neonatal effects of treatment with angiotensin-converting enzyme inhibitors in pregnancy. *Obstet Gynecol* 1991;78:128.

351. Bhatt-Mehta V, Deluga KS. Fetal exposure to lisinopril: neonatal manifestations and management. *Pharmacotherapy* 1993;13:515.

352. Grylack L, Medani C, Hultzen C, et al. Non oliguric acute renal failure in the newborn: a prospective evaluation of diagnostic indexes. *Am J Dis Child* 1982;136:518.

353. Asfour B, Bruker B, Kehl HG, et al. Renal insufficiency in neonates after cardiac surgery. *Clin Nephrol* 1996;46:59.

354. McCroy WW. Congenital malformations causing renal failure in the neonatal period. *Contrib Nephrol* 1979;15:55.

355. Arrowsmith JB, Faich GA, Tomita DK, et al. Morbidity and mortality among low birth weight infants exposed to an intravenous vitamin E product, E-Ferol. *Pediatrics* 1989;83:244.

356. Tack ED, Perlman JM. Renal failure in sick hypertensive premature infants receiving captopril therapy. *J Pediatr* 1988;112:805.

357. Parchoux B, Bourgeois J, Gilly J, et al. Hypertrophic kidneys in utero and neonatal renal failure by diffuse mesangial sclerosis. *Pédiatrie* 1988;43:219.

358. Nauta J, de Heer E, Baldwin III WM, et al. Transplacental induction of membranous nephropathy in a neonate. *Pediatr Nephrol* 1990;4:111.

359. Ridgen SPA, Barratt TM, Dillon MJ, et al. Acute renal failure complicating cardiopulmonary bypass surgery. *Arch Dis Child* 1982;57:425.

360. Isenberg G, Racelis D, Oh J, et al. Prevention of ischemic renal damage with prostacyclin. *Mt Sinai J Med* 1982;49:415.

361. Schramm L, Heidbreder E, Lukes M, et al. Endotoxin-induced acute renal failure in the rat: effects of urodilatin and diltiazem on renal function. *Clin Nephrol* 1996;46:117.

362. Schramm L, Heidbreder E, Lopau K, et al. Influence of nitric oxide on renal function in toxic acute renal failure in the rat. *Miner Electrolyte Metab* 1996;22:168.

363. Myers BD, Chui F, Hilberman M, et al. Transtubular leakage of glomerular filtrate in human acute renal failure. *Am J Physiol* 1979;237:F319.

364. Kelly KJ, Williams WW Jr, Colvin RB, et al. Antibody to intercellular adhesion molecule 1 protects the kidney against ischemic injury. *PNAS* 1994;91:812.

365. Hammerman MR. New treatments for acute renal failure: growth factors and beyond. *Curr Opin Nephrol Hypertens* 1997;6:7.

366. Vanpée M, Ergander U, Herin P. Renal function in sick, very low-birth-weight infants. *Acta Paediatr* 1993;82:714.

367. Kelly RE, Phillips JD, Foglia RP. Pulmonary edema and fluid mobilization as determinants of the duration of ECMO support. *J Pediatr Surg* 1991;26:1016.

368. Roy BJ, Cornish JD, Clark RH. Venovenous extracorporeal membrane oxygenation affects renal function. *Pediatrics* 1995;95:573.

369. Yoon BH, Lee CM, Kim SW. An abnormal umbilical artery waveform: a strong and independent predictor of adverse perinatal outcome in patients with preeclampsia. *Am J Obstet Gynecol* 1994;171:713.

370. Kempley ST, Gamsu HR, Nicolaides KH. Renal artery blood flow velocity in very low birth infants with intrauterine growth retardation. *Arch Dis Child* 1993;68:588.

371. Leititis JU, Burghard R, Gordjani N, et al. Effect of a modified fluid therapy on renal function during indomethacin therapy for persistent ductus arteriosus. *Acta Paediatr Scand* 1987;76:789.

372. Yeh TF, Wilks A, Singh J, et al. Furosemide prevents the renal side effects of indomethacin in premature infants with patent ductus arteriosus. *J Pediatr* 1982;101:433.

373. Romagnoli C, Zecca E, Papacci P, et al. Furosemide does not prevent indomethacin-induced renal side effects in preterm infants. *Clin Pharmacol Ther* 1997;62:181.

374. Seri I, Tulassay T, Kiszel J, et al. Cardiovascular response to dopamine in hypotensive preterm neonates with severe hyaline membrane disease. *Eur J Pediatr* 1984;142:3.

375. Tulassay T, Seri I, Machay T, et al. Effects of dopamine on renal functions in premature neonates with respiratory distress syndrome. *Int J Pediatr Nephrol* 1983;4:19.

376. Cuevas L, Yeh TF, John EG, et al. The effect of low-dose dopamine infusion on cardiopulmonary and renal status in premature newborns with respiratory distress syndrome. *Am J Dis Child* 1991;145:799.

377. Sulyok E, Seri I, Tulassay T, et al. The effect of dopamine administration on the activity of the renin–angiotensin–aldosterone system in sick preterm infants. *Eur J Pediatr* 1985;143:191.

378. Seri I, Tulassay T, Kiszel J, Csomor S. The use of dopamine for the prevention of the renal side effects of indomethacin in premature infants with patent ductus arteriosus. *Int J Pediatr Nephrol* 1984;5:209.

379. Kasik JW, Leuschen MP, Bolam DL, et al. Rhabdomyolysis and myoglobinemia in neonates. *Pediatrics* 1985;76:255.

380. Reinberg Y, Fleming T, Gonzalez R. Renal rupture after the Credé maneuver. *J Pediatr* 1994;124:279.

381. Martín-Ancel A, García-Alix A, Cabañas FGF, et al. Multiple organ involvement in perinatal asphyxia. *J Pediatr* 1995;127:786.

382. Karlowicz MG, Adelman RD. Nonoliguric and oliguric acute renal failure in asphyxiated term neonates. *Pediatr Nephrol* 1995;9:718.

383. Elçioğlu, Sirin A, Can G, et al. Renal function disorders in newborns with perinatal asphyxia. *Geburtsh U Frauenheilk* 1995;55:160.

384. Perlman JM, Tack ED. Renal injury in the asphyxiated newborn infant: relationship to neurologic outcome. *J Pediatr* 1988;113:875.

385. Roberts DS, Haycock GB, Dalton RN, et al. Prediction of acute renal failure after birth asphyxia. *Arch Dis Child* 1990;65:1021.

386. Kojima T, Kobayashi T, Matsuzaki S, et al. Effects of perinatal asphyxia and myoglobinuria on development of acute, neonatal renal failure. *Arch Dis Child* 1985;60:908.

387. Proverbio MR, Di Pietro A, Coletta M. Studio delle modificazioni dell'emodinamica renale in corso di insufficienza renale acuta nel neonato anossico. *Pediatr Med Chir* 1996;18:33.

388. DiSessa TG, Leitner M, Ti CC, et al. The cardiovascular effects of dopamine in the severely asphyxiated neonate. *J Pediatr* 1981;99:772.

389. Ivey HH. The asphyxiated bladder as a cause of delayed micturition in the newborn. *J Urol* 1978;120:498.

390. Giacoia GP, Miranda R, West KI. Measured vs calculated plasma osmolality in infants with very low birth weights. *Am J Dis Child* 1992;146:712.

391. Ellis EN, Arnold WC. Use of urinary indexes in renal failure in the newborn. *Am J Dis Child* 1982;136:615.

392. Matthew OP, Jones AS, James E, et al. Neonatal renal failure: usefulness of diagnostic indices. *Pediatrics* 1980;65:57.

393. Tack ED, Perlman JM, Robson AM. Renal injury in sick newborn infants: a prospective evaluation using urinary β_2-microglobulin concentrations. *Pediatrics* 1988;81:432.

394. Cole JW, Portman RJ, Lim Y, et al. Urinary β_2-microglobulin in full-term newborns: evidence for proximal tubular dysfunction in infants with meconium-stained amniotic fluid. *Pediatrics* 1985;76:958.

395. Tsukahara H, Yoshimoto M, Saito M, et al. Assessment of tubular function in neonates using urinary β_2-microglobulin. *Pediatr Nephrol* 1990;4:512.

396. Chiara A, Chirico G, Comelli L, et al. Increased renal echogenicity in the neonate. *Early Hum Dev* 1990;22:29.

397. Avni EF, Spehl-Robberecht M, Lebrun D, et al. Transient acute tubular disease in the newborn: characteristic ultrasound pattern. *Ann Radiol (Paris)* 1983;26:175.

398. Dmochowski RR, Crandell SS, Corriere JN Jr. Bladder injury and uroascites from umbilical artery catheterization. *Pediatrics* 1986;77:421.

399. Gouyon JB, Guignard JP. Drugs and acute renal insufficiency in the neonate. *Biol Neonate* 1986;50:177.

400. Dorman HR, Sondheimer JH, Cadnapaphornchai P. Mannitol-induced acute renal failure. *Medicine (Baltimore)* 1990;69:153.

401. Myers BD, Moran SM. Hemodynamically mediated acute renal failure. *N Engl J Med* 1986;314:97.

402. Davis RF, Lappas DG, Kirklin JK, et al. Acute oliguria after cardiopulmonary bypass: renal functional improvement with low-dose dopamine infusion. *Crit Care Med* 1982;10:852.

403. Lindner A. Synergism of dopamine and furosemide in diuretic-resistant, oliguric acute renal failure. *Nephron* 1983;33:121.

404. Medani CR, Davitt MK, Huntington DF, et al. Acute renal failure in the newborn. *Contrib Nephrol* 1979;15:47.

405. Brion LP, Schwartz GJ, Campbell D, et al. Early hyperkalemia in very low birthweight infants in the absence of oliguria. *Arch Dis Child* 1989;64:270.

406. Gibbons MD, Horan JJ, Dejter SW. Extracorporeal membrane oxygenation: an adjunct in the management of the neonate with severe respiratory distress and congenital urinary tract anomalies. *J Urol* 1993;150:434.

407. Finn WF. Diagnosis and management of acute tubular necrosis. *Med Clin North Am* 1990;74:873.

408. Karlowicz MG, Adelman RD. Acute renal failure in the neonate. *Clin Perinatol* 1992;19:139.

409. Lackmann GM, Mader R, Tollner U. Serumkaliumspiegel bei asphyktischen und gesunden Neugeborenen in den ersten 144 Lebensstunden. *Klin Padiatr* 1991;203:399.

410. Shaffer SG, Kilbride HW, Hayen LK, Meade VM, Warady BA. Hyperkalemia in very low birth weight infants. *J Pediatr* 1992;121:275.

411. Gaylord MS, Pittman PA, Bartness J, et al. Release of benzalkonium chloride from a heparin-bonded umbilical catheter with resultant factitious hypernatremia and hyperkalemia. *Pediatrics* 1991;87:631.

412. Gruskay J, Costarino AT, Polin RA, et al. Nonoliguric hyperkalemia in the premature infant weighing less than 1000 grams. *J Pediatr* 1988;113:381.

413. Smith JD, Bia MJ, DeFronzo RA. Clinical disorders of potassium metabolism. In: Arieff AI, DeFronzo RA, eds. *Fluid, electrolyte, and acid–base disorders,* vol 1. New York: Churchill-Livingstone, 1985:413.

414. Lui K, Thungappa U, Nair A, et al. Treatment with hypertonic dextrose and insulin in severe hyperkalaemia of immature infants. *Acta Paediatr* 1992;81:213.

415. Murdoch IA, Dos Anjos R, Haycock GB. Treatment of hyperkalemia with intravenous salbutamol. *Arch Dis Child* 1991;66:527.

416. Kemper MJ, Harps E, Müller-Wiefel DE. Hyperkalemia: therapeutic options in acute and chronic renal failure. *Clin Nephrol* 1996;46:67.

417. Malone TA. Glucose and insulin versus cation-exchange resin for the treatment of hyperkalemia in very low birth weight infants. *J Pediatr* 1991;118:121.

418. Ohlsson A, Hosking M. Complications following oral administration of exchange resins in extremely low-birth-weight infants. *Eur J Pediatr* 1987;146:571.

419. Setzer ES, Ahmed F, Goldberg RN, et al. Exchange transfusion using washed red blood cells reconstituted with fresh-frozen plasma for treatment of severe hyperkalemia in the neonate. *J Pediatr* 1984;104:443.

420. Sell LS, Cullen ML, Whittlesey GC, et al. Experience with renal failure during extracorporeal membrane oxygenation: treatment with continuous hemofiltration. *J Pediatr Surg* 1987;22:600.

421. Llach F, Felsenfeld AJ, Haussler MR. The pathophysiology of altered calcium metabolism in rhabdomyolysis-induced acute renal failure: interactions of parathyroid hormone, 25-hydroxy-cholecalciferol and 1,25-dihydroxycholecalciferol. *N Engl J Med* 1981;305:117.

422. Patel V, Savage A. Symptomatic hypomagnesemia associated with gentamicin therapy. *Nephron* 1979;23:50.

423. Arieff AI, Massry SG. Effects of uremia, hemodialysis, and parathyroid hormone. *J Clin Invest* 1974;53:837.

424. Zamarella P, Zorzi C, Pavanello L, et al. The prognostic significance of acute neonatal renal failure. *Child Nephrol Urol* 1991;11:15.

425. Kekömaki M. Uremic catabolism in a neonate: reversal by parenteral nutrition. *J Pediatr Surg* 1981;16:35.

426. Coulthard MG, Vernon B. Managing acute renal failure in very low birthweight infants. *Arch Dis Child* 1995;73:F187.

427. Matthews DE, West KW, Rescorla FJ, et al. Peritoneal dialysis in the first 60 days of life. *J Pediatr Surg* 1990;25:110.

428. Mattoo TK, Ahmad GS. Peritoneal dialysis in neonates after major abdominal surgery. *Am J Nephrol* 1994;14:6.

429. Nash MA, Russo JC. Neonatal lactic acidosis and renal failure: the role of peritoneal dialysis. *J Pediatr* 1977;91:101.

430. Bishof NA, Welch TR, Strife CF, et al. Continuous hemodiafiltration in children. *Pediatrics* 1990;85:819.

431. Zobel G, Ring E, Müller W. Continuous arteriovenous hemofiltration in premature infants. *Crit Care Med* 1989;17:534.

432. Ellis EN, Pearson D, Robinson L. Pump-assisted hemofiltration in infants with acute renal failure. *Pediatr Nephrol* 1993;7:434.

433. Reeves JH, Butt WB, Sathe AS. A review of venovenous haemofiltration in seriously ill infants. *J Paediatr Child Health* 1994;30:50.

434. Ronco C, Brendolan A, Bragantini L, et al. Treatment of acute renal failure in newborns by continuous arterio-venous hemofiltration. *Kidney Int* 1986;29:908.

435. Sadowski RH, Harmon WE, Jabs K. Acute hemodialysis of infants weighing less than five kilograms. *Kidney Int* 1994;45:903.

436. Coulthard MG, Sharp J. Haemodialysis and ultrafiltration in babies weighing under 1000 g. *Arch Dis Child* 1995;73:F162.

437. Blowey DL, McFarland K, Alon U, et al. Peritoneal dialysis in the neonatal period: outcome data. *J Perinatol* 1993;13:59.

438. Stark H, Geiger R. Renal tubular dysfunction following vascular accidents of the kidney in the newborn period. *J Pediatr* 1973;83:933.

439. Callan NA, Blakemore K, Park J, et al. Fetal genitourinary tract anomalies: evaluation, operative correction, and follow-up. *Obstet Gynecol* 1990;75:67.

440. Glick PL, Harrison MR, Golbus MS, et al. Management of the fetus with congenital hydronephrosis: II. Prognostic criteria and selection for treatment. *J Pediatr Surg* 1985;20:376.

441. Elder JS, O'Grady JP, Ashmead G, et al. Evaluation of fetal renal function: unreliability of fetal urinary electrolytes. *J Urol* 1990;144 [Pt 2];144:574.

442. Muller F, Parvy P, Dommergues M, et al. Acides aminés libres de l'urine foetale et pronostic de la fonction rénale dans les uropathies obstructives bilatérales. *Ann Biol Clin* 1994;52:651.

443. Bensman A, Baudon JJ, Jablonski JP, et al. Uropathies diagnosed in the neonatal period: symptomatology and course. *Acta Paediatr Scand* 1980;69:499.

444. Genest DR, Lage JM. Absence of normal-appearing proximal tubules in the fetal and neonatal kidney: prevalence and significance. *Hum Pathol* 1991;22:147.

445. Swinford AE, Bernstein J, Toriello HV, et al. Renal tubular dysgenesis: delayed onset of oligohydramnios. *Am J Med Genet* 1989;32:127.

446. Schwartz BR, Lage JM, Pober BR, et al. Isolated congenital renal tubular immaturity in siblings. *Hum Pathol* 1986;17:1259.

447. Allanson JE, Pantzar JT, Mac Leod PM. Possible new autosomal recessive syndrome with unusual renal histopathological changes. *Am J Med Genet* 1983;16:57.

448. Voland JR, Hawkins EP, Wells TR, et al. Congenital hypernephronic nephromegaly with tubular dysgenesis: a distinctive inherited renal anomaly. *Pediatr Pathol* 1985;4:231.

449. Lorentz WB, Trillo AA. Neonatal renal failure and glomerular immaturity. *Clin Nephrol* 1983;19:154.

450. Bernstein J, Barajas L. Renal tubular dysgenesis: evidence of abnormality in the renin-angiotensin system. *J Am Soc Nephrol* 1994;5:224.

451. Landing BH, Ang SM, Herta N, Larson EF, Turner M. Labeled lectin studies of renal tubular dysgenesis and renal tubular atrophy of postnatal renal ischemia and end-stage kidney disease. *Pediatr Pathol* 1994;14:87.

452. Kaplan BS, Restaino I, Raval DS, et al. Renal failure in the neonate associated with in utero exposure to non-steroidal anti-inflammatory agents. *Pediatr Nephrol* 1994;8:700.

453. Durante D, Jones D, Spitzer R. Neonatal renal arterial embolism syndrome. *J Pediatr* 1976;89:978.

454. Malin SW, Baumgart S, Rosenberg HK, et al. Nonsurgical management of obstructive aortic thrombosis complicated by renovascular hypertension in the neonate. *J Pediatr* 1985;106:630.

455. Payne RM, Martin TC, Bower RJ, et al. Management and follow-up of arterial thrombosis in the neonatal period. *J Pediatr* 1989;114:853.

456. Kennedy LA, Drummond WH, Knight ME, et al. Successful treatment of neonatal aortic thrombosis with tissue plasminogen activator. *J Pediatr* 1990;116:798.

457. Seibert JJ, Northington FJ, Miers JF, et al. Aortic thrombosis after umbilical artery catheterization in neonates: prevalence of complications on long-term follow-up. *AJR* 1991;156:567.

458. Umbilical Artery Catheter Trial Study Group. Relationship of intraventricular hemorrhage or death with the level of umbilical artery catheter placement: a multicenter randomized clinical trial. *Pediatrics* 1992;90:881.

459. Schmidt B, Andrew M. Neonatal thrombotic disease: prevention, diagnosis and management. *J Pediatr* 1988;113:407.

460. Caplan MS, Cohn RA, Langman CB, et al. Favorable outcome of neonatal aortic thrombosis and renovascular hypertension. *J Pediatr* 1989;115:291.

461. Vailas GN, Brouillette RT, Scott JP, et al. Neonatal aortic thrombosis: recent experience. *J Pediatr* 1986;109:101.

462. Seibert JJ, Northington FJ, Miers JF, et al. Aortic thrombosis after umbilical artery catheterization in neonates: prevalence of complications on long-term follow-up. *AJR* 1991;156:567.

463. Adelman RD. Long-term follow-up of neonatal renovascular hypertension. *Pediatr Nephrol* 1987;1:35.
464. Rasoulpour M, McLean RH. Renal venous thrombosis in neonates. Initial and follow-up abnormalities. *Am J Dis Child* 1980;134:276.
465. Lam AH, Warren PS. Ultrasonographic diagnosis of neonatal renal venous thrombosis. *Ann Radiol* 1981;24:7.
466. Corrigan JJ Jr, Jeter MA. Tissue-type plasminogen activator, plasminogen activator inhibitor, and histidine-rich glycoproteins in stressed human newborns. *Pediatrics* 1992;89:43.
467. Evans DJ, Silverman M, Bowley NB. Congenital hypertension due to unilateral renal vein thrombosis. *Arch Dis Child* 1981;56:306.
468. Mocan H, Beattie TJ, Murphy AV. Renal venous thrombosis in infancy: long-term follow-up. *Pediatr Nephrol* 1991;5:45.
469. Clark AGB, Saunders A, Bewick M, et al. Neonatal inferior vena cava and renal venous thrombosis treated by thrombectomy and nephrectomy. *Arch Dis Child* 1985;60:1076.
470. Bromberg WD, Firlit CF. Fibrinolytic therapy for renal vein thrombosis in the child. *J Urol* 1990;143:86.
471. Kurnetz R, Bernstein J. Neonatal blood loss and hematuria. *J Pediatr* 1974;84:452.
472. Anand K, Northway JD, Smith JA. Neonatal renal papillary and cortical necrosis. *Am J Dis Child* 1977;131:773.
473. Van Reempts PJ, Boven KJ, Spitaels SE, et al. Idiopathic arterial calcification of infancy. *Calcif Tissue Int* 1991;48:1.
474. Jenkins EA, Hallett RJ, Hull RG. Lesch-Nyhan syndrome presenting with renal insufficiency in infancy and transient neonatal hypothyroidism. *Br J Rheumatol* 1994;33:392.
475. Terzi F, Assael BM, Claris-Appiani A, et al. Increased sodium requirement following early postnatal surgical correction of congenital uropathies in infants. *Pediatr Nephrol* 1990;4:581.

Nephrotoxicity: Drugs and Toxins

476. Assadi FK. Renal tubular dysfunction in fetal alcohol syndrome. *Pediatr Nephrol* 1990;4:48.
477. Lindemann R. Congenital renal tubular dysfunction associated with maternal sniffing of organic solvents. *Acta Paediatr Scand* 1991;80:882.
478. Brown WJ, Buist NR, Gipson HT, et al. Fatal benzyl alcohol poisoning in a neonatal intensive care unit. *Lancet* 1982;1:1250.
479. Gershanik J, Boeckler B, Enlsey H, et al. The gasping syndrome and benzyl alcohol poisoning. *N Engl J Med* 1982;307:1384.
480. Klotman PE, Boatman JE, Volpp BD, et al. Captopril enhances aminoglycoside nephrotoxicity in potassium-depleted rats. *Kidney Int* 1985;28:118.
481. Cronin RE, Bulger RE, Southern P, et al. Natural history of aminoglycoside nephrotoxicity in the dog. *J Lab Clin Med* 1980;95:463.
482. Cojocel C, Dociu N, Ceacmacudis E, et al. Nephrotoxic effects of aminoglycoside treatment on renal protein reabsorption and accumulation. *Nephron* 1984;37:113.
483. Cojocel C, Hook JB. Aminoglycoside nephrotoxicity. *Trends Pharmacol Sci* 1983;4:174.
484. Giapros VI, Andronikou S, Cholevas VI, et al. Renal function in premature infants during aminoglycoside therapy. *Pediatr Nephrol* 1995;9:163.
485. Heimann G. Renal toxicity of aminoglycosides in the neonatal period. *Pediatr Pharmacol* 1983;3:251.
486. Russo JC, Adelman RD. Gentamicin-induced Fanconi syndrome. *J Pediatr* 1980;96:151.
487. Casteels-Van Daele M, Corbeel L, Van de Casseye W, et al. Gentamicin-induced Fanconi syndrome. *J Pediatr* 1980;97:507.
488. Rajchgot P, Prober CG, Soldin S, et al. Aminoglycoside-related nephrotoxicity in the premature newborn. *Clin Pharmacol Ther* 1984;35:394.
489. Ylitalo P, Mörsky P, Parviainen MT, et al. Nephrotoxicity of tobramycin: value of examining various protein and enzyme markers. *Methods Find Exp Clin Pharmacol* 1991;13:281.
490. Sasai-Takedatsu M, Kojima T, Taketani S. Urinary trehalase activity is a useful maker of renal proximal tubular damage in newborn infants. *Nephron* 1995;70:443.
491. Ibrahim S, Langhendries JP, Bernard A. Urinary phospholipids excretion in neonates treated with amikacin. *Int J Clin Pharm Res* 1994;14:149.
492. Nahata MC. Lack of nephrotoxicity in pediatric patients receiving concurrent vancomycin and aminoglycoside therapy. *Chemotherapy* 1987;33:302.
493. Swinney VR, Rudd CC. Nephrotoxicity of vancomycin-gentamicin therapy in pediatric patients. *J Pediatr* 1987;110:497.
494. Goren MP, Baker DK Jr, Shenep JL. Vancomycin does not enhance amikacin-induced tubular nephrotoxicity in children. *Pediatr Infect Dis J* 1989;8:278.
495. Bhat R, Vidyasagar D, Vadapalli M, et al. Disposition of indomethacin in preterm infants. *J Pediatr* 1979;95:313.
496. Seyberth HW, Rascher W, Hackenthal R, et al. Effect of prolonged indomethacin therapy on renal function and selected vasoactive hormones in very-low-birth-weight infants with symptomatic patent ductus arteriosus. *J Pediatr* 1983;103:979.
497. Hammerman C, Aramburo MJ. Prolonged indomethacin therapy for the prevention of recurrences of patent ductus arteriosus. *J Pediatr* 1990;117:771.
498. vd Heijden AJ, Provoost AP, Grose W, et al. Renal functional impairment in preterm neonates related to intrauterine indomethacin exposure. *Pediatr Res* 1988;24:644.
499. John EG, Vasan U, Hastreiter AR, et al. Intravenous indomethacin and changes of renal function in premature infants with patent ductus arteriosus. *Pediatr Pharmacol* 1984;4:11.
500. Hammerman C, Zaia W, Wu HH. Severe hyponatremia with indomethacin: a more serious toxicity than previously realized? *Dev Pharmacol Ther* 1985;8:260.
501. Brodie BB, Aronow L, Axelrod J. The fate of benzazoline (Priscoline) in dog and man and a method for its estimation in biological material. *J Exp Pharmacol Ther* 1952;106:200.
502. Trompeter RS, Chantler C, Haycock GB. Tolazoline and acute renal failure in the newborn. *Lancet* 1981;1:1219.
503. Heyman SN, Clark BA, Kaiser N, et al. In-vivo and in-vitro studies on the effect of amphotericin B on endothelin release. *J Antimicrob Chemother* 1992;29:69.
504. Joly V, Dromer F, Barge J, et al. Incorporation of amphotericin B (AMB) into liposomes alters AMB-induced acute nephrotoxicity in rabbits. *J Pharmacol Exp Ther* 1989;251:311.
505. Reynolds ES, Tomkiewicz ZM, Dammin GJ. The renal lesion related to amphotericin B treatment for coccidioidomycosis. *Med Clin North Am* 1963;47:1149.
506. Baley JE, Meyers C, Kliegman RM, et al. Pharmacokinetics, outcome of treatment, and toxic effects of amphotericin B and 5-fluorocytosine in neonates. *J Pediatr* 1990;116:791.
507. Leenders AC, de Marie S. The use of lipid formulations of amphotericin B for systemic fungal infections. *Leukemia* 1996;10:1570.
508. Rubin SI, Krawiec DR, Gelberg H, et al. Nephrotoxicity of amphotericin B in dogs: a comparison of two methods of administration. *Can J Vet Res* 1989;53:23.
509. Baley JE, Kliegman RM, Fanaroff AA. Disseminated fungal infections in very-low-birth-weight infants: therapeutic toxicity. *Pediatrics* 1984;73:153.
510. Vadiei K, Lopez-Berestein G, Luke DR. Disposition and toxicity of amphotericin-B in the hyperlipidemic Zucker rat model. *Int J Obes* 1990;14:465.
511. Lopez-Berenstein G, Bodey GP, Frankel LS, et al. Treatment of hepatosplenic candidiasis with liposomal-amphotericin B. *J Clin Oncol* 1987;5:310.
512. Friedlich PS, Steinberg I, Fujitani A. Renal tolerance with the use of intralipid-amphotericin B in low-birth-weight neonates. *Am J Perinatol* 1997;14:377.
513. Deleted in proof.
514. Bianchetti MG, Roduit C, Oetliker OH. Acyclovir-induced renal failure: course and risk factors. *Pediatr Nephrol* 1991;5:238.
515. Englund JA, Fletcher CV, Balfour HH. Acyclovir therapy in neonates. *J Pediatr* 1991;119:129.
516. Berdon WE, Schwartz RH, Becker J, et al. Tamm-Horsfall proteinuria: its relationship to prolonged nephrogram in infants and children and to renal failure following intravenous urography in adults with multiple myeloma. *Radiology* 1969;92:714.
517. Sleasman JE, Stapleton FB, Tonkin II. Marked uricosuric effect of contrast media during cardiac catheterization in children. *Pediatr Res* 1986;17:219A(abst).
518. Avner ED, Ellis D, Jaffe R, et al. Neonatal radiocontrast nephropathy simulating infantile polycystic kidney disease. *J Pediatr* 1982;100:85.

519. Harvey LA, Caldicott WJH, Kuruc A. The effect of contrast media on immature renal function: comparison of agents with high and low osmolality. *Radiology* 1983;148:429.

520. Wood EG, Bunchman TE, Lynch RE. Captopril-induced reversible acute renal failure in an infant with coarctation of the aorta. *Pediatrics* 1991;88:816.

521. Perlman JM, Volpe JJ. Neurologic complications of Captopril treatment of neonatal hypertension. *Pediatrics* 1989;83:47.

522. Mehring N, Neumann KH, Rahn KH, et al. Mechanisms of cyclosporin A-induced vasoconstriction in the isolated perfused rat kidney. *Nephron* 1992;60:477.

523. McDiarmid SV. Renal function in pediatric liver transplant patients. *Kidney Int* 1996;49[Suppl 53]:77.

524. Eid A, Steffen R, Porayko MK, et al. Beyond 1 year after liver transplantation. *Mayo Clin Proc* 1989;64:446.

525. McDiarmid SV. Renal function in pediatric liver transplant patients. *Kidney Int* 1996;49[Suppl 53]:S77.

526. Ward MM. Factors predictive of acute renal failure in rhabdomyolysis. *Arch Intern Med* 1988;148:1553.

527. Martin W, Villani GM, Jothianandan D, et al. Selective blockade of endothelium-dependent and glyceryl trinitrate-induced relaxation by hemoglobin and by methylene blue in the rabbit aorta. *J Pharmacol Exp Ther* 1985;232:708.

528. Better OS, Stein JH. Early management of shock and prophylaxis of acute renal failure in traumatic rhabdomyolysis. *N Engl J Med* 1990;322:825.

529. Haftel AJ, Eichner J, Haling J, et al. Myoglobinuric renal failure in a newborn infant. *J Pediatr* 1985;93:1015.

530. Turner MC, Naumburg EG. Acute renal failure in the neonate: two fatal cases due to group B streptococci with rhabdomyolysis. *Clin Pediatr* 1987;26:189.

531. Kagen LJ, Christian CL. Immunologic measurements of myoglobin in human adult and fetal skeletal muscle. *Am J Physiol* 1966;211:656.

Chronic Renal Failure

532. Foreman JW, Chan JCM. Chronic renal failure in infants and children. *J Pediatr* 1988;113:793.

533. Potter DE, Holliday MA, Piel CF, et al. Treatment of end stage renal disease in children: a 15-year experience. *Kidney Int* 1980;18:103.

534. Pistor K, Olbing H, Schärer K. Children with chronic renal failure in the Federal Republic of Germany: I. Epidemiology, modes of treatment, survival. *Clin Nephrol* 1985;23:272.

535. Alexander SR, Arbus GS, Butt KMH, et al. The 1989 report of the North American Pediatric Renal Transplant cooperative study. *Pediatr Nephrol* 1990;4:542.

536. Najarian JS, Frey DJ, Matas AJ, et al. Renal transplantation in infants. *Ann Surg* 1990;212:353.

537. McEnery PT, Stablein DM, Arbus G, et al. Renal transplantation in children: a report of the North American Pediatric Renal Transplant Cooperative Study. *N Engl J Med* 1992;326:1727.

538. Hanna JD, Foreman JW, Chan JCM. Chronic renal insufficiency in infants and children. *Clin Pediatr* 1991;30:365.

539. Tapper D, Watkins S, Burns M, et al. Comprehensive management of renal failure in infants. *Arch Surg* 1990;125:1276.

540. Warady BA, Sullivan EK, Alexander SR. Lessons from the peritoneal dialysis patient database: a report of the North American Pediatric Renal Transplant Cooperative Study. *Kidney Int* 1996;49[Suppl 53]:S68.

541. Miller LC, Bock GH, Lum CT, et al. Transplantation of the adult kidney into the very small child: long-term outcome. *J Pediatr* 1982;100:675.

542. Rees L, Rigden SPA, Ward GM. Chronic renal failure and growth. *Arch Dis Child* 1989;64:573.

543. Mehls O, Salusky IB. Recent advances and controversies in childhood renal osteodystrophy. *Pediatr Nephrol* 1987;1:212.

544. Chesney RW, Dabbagh S, Uehling DT, et al. The importance of early treatment of renal bone disease in children. *Kidney Int* 1985;28[Suppl 17]:S75.

545. Wassner SJ, Abitbol S, Alexander S, et al. Nutritional requirements for infants with renal failure. *Am J Kidney Dis* 1986;7:300.

546. Brewer ED. Growth of small children managed with chronic peritoneal dialysis and nasogastric tube feedings: 203-month experience in 14 patients. *Adv Perit Dial* 1990;6:269.

547. Feld LG. Total parenteral nutrition in children with renal insufficiency. In: Lebenthal E, ed. *Total parenteral nutrition: indications, utilization, complications and pathophysiological considerations.* New York: Raven Press, 1986:385.

548. Chandar J, Abitbol C, Zilleruelo G, et al. Renal tubular abnormalities in infants with hydronephrosis. *J Urol* 1996;155:660.

549. Portale AA, Booth BE, Tsai HC, et al. Reduced plasma concentration of 1,25-dihydroxy-vitamin-D in children with moderate renal insufficiency. *Kidney Int* 1982;21:627.

550. Mehls O, Ritz E, Krempien B, et al. Slipped epiphyses in renal osteodystrophy. *Arch Dis Child* 1975;50:545.

551. Chesney RW, Moorthy AV, Eisman JA, et al. Increased growth after long-term oral 1-α-25-vitamin-D₃ in childhood renal osteodystrophy. *N Engl J Med* 1978;298:238.

552. Chan JCM, Kodroff MB, Landwehr DM. Effects of 1,25-dihyroxyvitamin-D₃ on renal function, mineral balance and growth in children with severe chronic renal failure. *Pediatrics* 1981;68:559.

553. Polinsky MS, Gruskin AB. Aluminum toxicity in children with chronic renal failure. *J Pediatr* 1984;105:758.

554. ASCN/ASPEN Working Group on Standards for Aluminum Content of Parenteral Nutrition Solutions. Parenteral drug products containing aluminum as an ingredient or a contaminant: response to Food and Drug Administration notice of intent and request for information. *JPEN J Parenter Enteral Nutr* 1991;15:194.

555. Bishop NJ, Morley R, Day JP, et al. Aluminum neurotoxicity in preterm infants receiving intravenous-feeding solutions. *N Engl J Med* 1997;336;1557.

556. Koo WWK, Kaplan LA, Krug-Wispe SK, et al. Response of preterm infants to aluminum in parenteral nutrition. *JPEN J Parenter Enteral Nutr* 1989;13:516.

557. Alfrey AC, LeGendre GR, Kaehny WD. The dialysis encephalopathy syndrome: possible aluminum intoxication. *N Engl J Med* 1976;294:184.

558. Alfrey AC. Aluminum intoxication. *N Engl J Med* 1984;310:1113.

559. Freundlich M, Zilleruelo G, Faugere MC, et al. Treatment of aluminum toxicity in infantile uremia with deferoxamine. *J Pediatr* 1986;109:140.

560. Chandra M, Clemons GK, McVicar MI. Relation of serum erythropoietin levels to renal excretory function: evidence for lowered set point for erythropoietin production in chronic renal failure. *J Pediatr* 1988;113:1015.

561. Lacombe C, Da Silva J-L, Bruneval P, et al. Peritubular cells are the site of erythropoietin synthesis in the murine hypoxic kidney. *J Clin Invest* 1988;81:620.

562. Beckman BS, Brookins JW, Garcia MM, et al. Measurement of erythropoietin in anephric children: a report of the Southwest Pediatric Nephrology Study Group. *Pediatr Nephrol* 1989;3:75.

563. Kitagawa T, Ito K, Komatsu Y, et al. The clinical studies of recombinant human erythropoietin (Epoetin) in children with renal anemia. *Jpn J Pediatr* 1988;41:3251.

564. Eschbach JW, Adamson JW. Guidelines for recombinant human erythropoietin therapy. *Am J Kidney Dis* 1989;14:2.

565. Stivelman JC. Resistance to recombinant human erythropoietin therapy: a real clinical entity? *Semin Nephrol* 1989;9[Suppl 2]:8.

566. Sinai-Trieman L, Salusky IB, Fine RN. Use of subcutaneous recombinant human erythropoietin in children undergoing continuous cycling peritoneal dialysis. *J Pediatr* 1989;114:550.

567. Bercu BB, Corden BJ, Schulman JD, et al. Circulating somatomedin C levels in nephropathic cystinosis. *Isr J Med Sci* 1984;20:236.

568. El-Bishti MM, Counahan R, Bloom S, et al. Hormonal and metabolic responses to intravenous glucose in children on regular hemodialysis. *Am J Clin Nutr* 1978;31:1865.

569. Tönshoff B, Mehls O, Heinrich U, et al. Growth-stimulating effects of recombinant human growth hormone in children with end-stage renal disease. *J Pediatr* 1990;116:561.

570. Rees L, Maxwell H. The hypothalamo-pituitary-growth hormone insulin-like growth factor 1 axis in children with chronic renal failure. *Kidney Int* 1996;49[Suppl 53]:S109.

571. Tönshoff B, Blum WF, Mehls O. Derangements of the somatotropic hormone axis in chronic renal failure. *Kidney Int* 1997;51[Suppl 58]:S106.

572. Fine RN, Kohaut EC, Brown D. Growth after recombinant human

growth hormone treatment in children with chronic renal failure: report of a multicenter randomized double-blind placebo-controlled study. *J Pediatr* 1994;124:374.

573. Fine RN. Recombinant human growth hormone in children with chronic renal insufficiency-Clinical update: 1995. *Kidney Int* 1996; 49[Suppl 53]:S115.

574. Warshaw BL, Edelbrock HH, Ettenger RB, et al. Progression to end-stage renal disease in children with obstructive uropathy. *J Pediatr* 1982;100:183.

575. Hogg RJ. Continuous ambulatory and continuous cycling peritoneal dialysis in children: a report of the Southwestern Pediatric Nephrology Study Group. *Kidney Int* 1985;27:558.

576. Fennell RS, Orak JK, Garin EH, et al. Continuous ambulatory peritoneal dialysis in a pediatric population. *Am J Dis Child* 1983;137: 388.

577. Baluarte HJ, Gruskin AB, Hiner LB, et al. Encephalopathy in children with chronic renal failure. *Proc Dial Transpl Forum* 1977;7:95.

578. Sedman AB, Wilkening GN, Warady BA, et al. Encephalopathy in childhood secondary to aluminum toxicity. *J Pediatr* 1984;105: 836.

579. Bock GH, Conners CK, Ruley J, et al. Disturbances of brain maturation and neurodevelopment during chronic renal failure in infancy. *J Pediatr* 1989;114:231.

580. Davis ID, Pi-Nian C, Nevins TE. Successful renal transplantation accelerates development in young uremic infants. *Pediatrics* 1990; 86:594.

581. Warady BA, Alexander SR, Hossli S, et al. Peritoneal membrane transport function in children receiving long-term dialysis. *J Am Soc Nephrol* 1996;7:2385.

582. Alexander SR. CAPD in infants less than one year of age. In: Fine RN, Gruskin AB, eds. *End stage renal disease in children.* Philadelphia: WB Saunders, 1984:149.

583. Offner G, Latta K, Hoyer PF. CAPD in children with special aspects of renal transplantation. *Contrib Nephrol* 1991;89:243.

584. So SK, Chang PN, Najarian JS, et al. Growth and development in infants after renal transplantation. *J Pediatr* 1986;110:343.

585. Najarian JS, Almond PS, Mauer M, et al. Renal transplantation in the first year of life: the treatment of choice for infants with end-stage renal disease. *J Am Soc Nephrol* 1992;2:S228.

586. Opelz G, Graver B, Terasaki PI. Induction of high kidney graft survival rate by multiple transfusions. *Lancet* 1981;1:1223.

587. Beebe DS, Belani KG, Mergens P, et al. Anesthetic management of infants receiving an adult kidney transplant. *Anesth Analg* 1991;73: 725.

588. Almond PS, Matas AJ, Gillingham K, et al. Pediatric renal transplants: results with sequential immunosuppression. *Transplantation* 1992;53:46.

589. So SK, Gillingham K, Cook M, et al. The use of cadaver kidneys for transplantation in young children. *Transplantation* 1990;50:979.

590. Stablein DM, Tejani A. Five-year patient and graft survival in North American children: a report of the North American Pediatric Renal Transplant Cooperative Study. *Kidney Int* 1993;43:S16.

591. Warady BA, Hébert D, Sullivan EK, et al. Renal transplantation, chronic dialysis, and chronic renal insufficiency in children and adolescents. The 1995 Annual Report of the North American Pediatric Renal Transplant Cooperative Study. *Pediatr Nephrol* 1997;11:49.

592. Matas AJ, Chavers BM, Nevins TE. Recipient evaluation, preparation and care in pediatric transplantation: The University of Minnesota protocols. *Kidney Int* 1996;49[Suppl 53]:S99.

593. Connor JP, Burbige KA. Long-term urinary continence and renal function in neonates with posterior urethral valves. *J Urol* 1990;144: 1209.

594. Reinberg Y, Manivel JC, Pettinato G, et al. Development of renal failure in children with the prune belly syndrome. *J Urol* 1991;145:1017.

595. Burbige KA, Amodio J, Berdon WE, et al. Prune belly syndrome: 35 years of experience. *J Urol* 1987;137:86.

596. Kaplan BS, Fay J, Shah V, et al. Autosomal recessive polycystic kidney disease. *Pediatr Nephrol* 1989;3:43.

597. Cole BR, Conley SB, Stapleton FB. Polycystic kidney disease in the first year of life. *J Pediatr* 1987;111:693.

598. Roy S, Dillon MJ, Trompeter RS. Autosomal recessive polycystic kidney disease: long-term outcome of neonatal survivors. *Pediatr Nephrol* 1997;11:302.

599. Mahan JD, Mauer SM, Sibley RK, et al. Congenital nephrotic syndrome: evolution of medical management and results of renal transplantation. *J Pediatr* 1984;105:549.

600. Holmberg C, Laine J, Ronnholm K, et al. Congenital nephrotic syndrome. *Kidney Int* 1996;49[Suppl 53]:S51.

Hypertension

601. Adelman RD. The hypertensive neonate. *Clin Perinatol* 1988;15: 567.

602. Ingelfinger J. Hypertension in the first year of life. In: Ingelfinger J, ed. *Pediatric hypertension.* Philadelphia: WB Saunders, 1982:229.

603. Abman SH, Warady BA, Lum GM, et al. Systemic hypertension in infants with bronchopulmonary dysplasia. *J Pediatr* 1984;104:928.

604. Singh HP, Hurley RM, Myers TF. Neonatal hypertension. Incidence and risk factors. *Am J Hypertens* 1992;5:51.

605. Adelman RD, Merten D, Vogel J, et al. Nonsurgical management of renovascular hypertension in the neonate. *Pediatrics* 1978;62:71.

606. Buchi KF, Siegler RL. Hypertension in the first month of life. *J Hypertens* 1986;4:525.

607. Friedman AL, Hustead VA. Hypertension in babies following discharge from a neonatal intensive care unit: a 3-year follow-up. *Pediatr Nephrol* 1987;1:30.

608. Sheftel DN, Hustead V, Friedman A. Hypertension screening in the follow-up of premature infants. *Pediatrics* 1983;71:763.

609. Law CM, de Swiet M, Osmond C, et al. Initiation of hypertension in utero and its amplification throughout life. *Br Med J* 1993; 306:24.

610. Himmelmann A, Svensson A, Hansson L, et al. Relation of maternal blood pressure during pregnancy to birth weight and blood pressure in children. The Hypertension in Pregnancy Offspring Study. *J Intern Med* 1994;235:347.

611. Barker DJ, Godfrey KM, Osmond C, et al. The relation of fetal length, ponderal index and head circumference to blood pressure and the risk of hypertension in adult life. *Paediatr Perinatal Epidemiol* 1992;6:35.

612. Lucas A, Morley R. Does early nutrition in infants born before term programme later blood pressure? *Br Med J* 1994;309:304.

613. Barker DJP, Hales CN, Fall CHD, et al. Type 2 (non-insulin-dependent) diabetes mellitus, hypertension and hyperlipidaemia (syndrome X): relation to reduced fetal growth. *Diabetologia* 1993;36:62.

614. Mackenzie HS, Brenner BM. Fewer nephrons at birth: a missing link in the etiology of essential hypertension? *Am J Kidney Dis* 1995; 26:91.

615. Guignard JP, Gouyon JB, Adelman RD. Arterial hypertension in the newborn infant. *Biol Neonate* 1989;55:77.

616. Goble MM, Rocchini AP. Neonatal hypertension: why it happens, what to do about it. *Contemp Pediatr* 1990;7:89.

617. Rasoulpour M, Marinelli KA. Systemic hypertension. *Clin Perinatol* 1992;19:121.

618. Miall-Allen VM, deVries LS, Whitelaw AGL. Mean arterial blood pressure and neonatal cerebral lesions. *Arch Dis Child* 1987;62: 1068.

619. Moore P, Fiddler GI. Facial palsy in an infant with coarctation of the aorta and hypertension. *Arch Dis Child* 1980;55:315.

620. Castelló Girona F, Yeste Fernández D, Porta Ribera R, et al. Renovascular hypertension due to unilateral renal artery stenosis with hypokalemic alkalosis, the hyponatraemic syndrome and reversible hyperechogenicity of the contralateral kidney. A study of two infants. *An Esp Pediatr* 1996;45:49.

621. Stringer DA, de Bruyn R, Dillon MJ. Comparison of aortography, renal vein renin sampling, radionuclide scans, ultrasound and IVU in the investigation of childhood renovascular hypertension. *Br J Radiol* 1984;57:111.

622. Baetz-Greenwalt B, Debaz B, Kumar ML. Bladder fungus ball: a reversible cause of neonatal obstructive uropathy. *Pediatrics* 1988; 81:826.

623. Skalina MEL, Annable WL, Kliegman RM, et al. Hypertensive retinopathy in the newborn infant. *J Pediatr* 1983;103:781.

624. Gouyon JB, Bernardini S, Semama DS. Salt depletion and dehydration in hypertensive preterm infants. *Pediatr Nephrol* 1997;11:201.

625. Gouyon JB, Geneste B, Semama DS, et al. Intravenous nicardipine in hypertensive preterm infants. *Arch Child Dis Fetal Neonatal Ed* 1997;76:F126.

626. Johnson CE, Jacobson PA, Song MH. Isradipine therapy in hypertensive pediatric patients. *Ann Pharmacother* 1997;31:704

627. McLaine PN, Drummond KN. Intravenous diazoxide for severe hypertension in childhood. *J Pediatr* 1971;79:829.

628. Benitz WE, Malachowski N, Cohen RS, et al. Use of sodium nitroprusside in neonates: efficacy and safety. *J Pediatr* 1985;106:102.

629. Bunchman TE, Lynch RE, Wood EG. Intravenously administered labetolol for treatment of hypertension in children. *J Pediatr* 1992; 120:140.

630. Wells TG, Bunchman TE, Kearns GL. Treatment of neonatal hypertension with enalaprilat. *J Pediatr* 1990;117:664.

631. O'Dea RF, Mirkin BL, Alward CT, et al. Treatment of neonatal hypertension with captopril. *J Pediatr* 1988;113:403.

632. Tobias JD, Pietsch JB, Lynch A. Nicardipine to control mean arterial pressure during extracorporeal membrane oxygenation. *Paediatr Anaesth* 1996;6:57.

633. Bancalari E, Gerhardt T, Feller R, et al. Muscle relaxation during IPPV in prematures with RDS. *Pediatr Res* 1980;14:590.

634. Greenough A, Gamsu HR, Greenall F. Investigation of the effects of paralysis by pancuronium on heart rate variability, blood pressure and fluid balance. *Acta Paediatr Scand* 1989;78:829.

635. Cabal LA, Siassi B, Artal R, et al. Cardiovascular and catecholamine changes after administration of pancuronium in distressed neonates. *Pediatrics* 1985;75:284.

636. Emery EF, Greenough A. Blood pressure levels at follow-up of infants with and without chronic lung disease. *J Perinat Med* 1993; 21:377.

637. Ferrara TB, Couser RJ, Hoekstra RE. Side effects and long-term follow-up of corticosteroid therapy in very low birthweight infants with bronchopulmonary dysplasia. *J Perinatol* 1990;10:137.

638. Sell LL, Cullen ML, Lerner GR, et al. Hypertension during extracorporeal membrane oxygenation: cause, effect, and management. *Surgery* 1987;102:724.

639. Boedy RF, Goldberg AK, Howell CG Jr, et al. Incidence of hypertension in infants on extracorporeal membrane oxygenation. *J Pediatr Surg* 1990;25:258.

640. Roy BJ, Cornish JD, Clark RH. Venovenous extracorporeal membrane oxygenation affects renal function. *Pediatrics* 1995;95:573.

641. Adelman RD, Sherman MP. Hypertension in the neonate following closure of abdominal wall defects. *J Pediatr* 1980;97:642.

642. Husmann DA, McLorie GA, Churchill BM. Hypertension following primary bladder closure for vesical exstrophy. *J Pediatr Surg* 1993; 28:239.

643. Merten DF, Vogel JM, Adelman RD, et al. Renovascular hypertension as a complication of umbilical arterial catheterization. *Radiology* 1978;126:751.

644. Angella JJ, Sommer LS, Poole C, et al. Neonatal hypertension associated with renal artery hypoplasia. *Pediatrics* 1968;41:524.

645. Wilson DI, Appleton RE, Coulthard MG, et al. Fetal and infantile hypertension caused by unilateral renal arterial disease. *Arch Dis Child* 1990;65:881.

646. Schmidt DM, Rambo ON Jr. Segmental intimal hyperplasia of the abdominal aorta and renal arteries producing hypertension in an infant. *Am J Clin Pathol* 1965;44:546.

647. Bendel-Stenzel M, Najarian JS, Sinaiko AR. Renal artery stenosis in infants: long-term medical treatment before surgery. *Pediatr Nephrol* 1996;10:147.

648. Milner LS, Heitner R, Thomson PD, et al. Hypertension as the major problem of idiopathic arterial calcification of infancy. *J Pediatr* 1984;105:934.

649. Van Dyck M, Proesmans W, Van Hollebeke E, et al. Idiopathic infantile arterial calcification with cardiac, renal and central nervous system involvement. *Eur J Pediatr* 1989;148:374.

650. Meradji M, de Villeneuve VH, Huber J, et al. Idiopathic infantile arterial calcification in siblings: radiologic diagnosis and successful treatment. *J Pediatr* 1978;92:401.

651. Ciana G, Colonna F, Forleo V, et al. Idiopathic arterial calcification of infancy: effectiveness of prostaglandin infusion for treatment of secondary hypertension refractory to conventional therapy: case report. *Pediatr Cardiol* 1997;18:67.

652. Nordborg C, Kyllerman M, Conradi N, et al. Early-infantile galactosialidosis with multiple brain infarctions: morphological, neuropathological and neurochemical findings. *Acta Neuropathol* 1997;93:24.

653. Takahashi G, Nakano H, Ueda K, et al. Neonatal renovascular hypertension: haematoma within the renal arterial wall: a case report. *Z Kinderchir* 1984;39:341.

654. Davis RS, Manning JA, Branch GL, et al. Renovascular hypertension secondary to hydronephrosis in a solitary kidney. *J Urol* 1973;110: 724.

655. Bensman A, Neuenschwander S, Lavollay B, et al. Hypertension artérielle et compression du pédicule vasculaire rénal par un hématome de la surrénale chez un nouveau-né. *Ann Pediatr (Paris)* 1982; 29:670.

656. Patel MR, Mooppan MMU, Kim H. Subcapsular urinoma: unusual form of "page kidney" in newborn. *Urology* 1984;23:585.

657. Roth A. An unusual renal tumor, associating a nephroblastoma, nephroblastomatosis, a teratoma, cystic dysplasia, hypertension and the secretion of α-foetoprotein. *J Urol (Paris)* 1984;90:7.

658. Yokomori K, Hori T, Takemura T, et al. Demonstration of both primary and secondary reninism in renal tumors in children. *J Pediatr Surg* 1988;23:403.

659. Tokunaka S, Takamura T, Osanai H, et al. Severe hypertension in an infant with unilateral hypoplastic kidney. *Urology* 1987;29:618.

660. Chan HSL, Cheng MY, Mance K, et al. Congenital mesoblastic nephroma: a clinicoradiologic study of 17 cases representing the pathologic spectrum of the disease. *J Pediatr* 1987;111:64.

661. Malone PS, Duffy PG, Ransley PG, et al. Congenital mesoblastic nephroma, renin production and hypertension. *J Pediatr Surg* 1989; 24:599.

662. Munoz AI, Baralt JF, Melendez MT. Arterial hypertension in infants with hydronephrosis: report of six cases. *Am J Dis Child* 1977; 131:38.

663. Hendren WH, Kim SH, Herrin JT, et al. Surgically correctable hypertension of renal origin in childhood. *Am J Surg* 1982;143:432.

664. Gereda JE, Bonilla-Felix M, Kalil B, et al. Neonatal presentation of Gordon syndrome. *J Pediatr* 1996;129:615.

665. Vania A, Tucciarone L, Mazzeo D, et al. Liddle's syndrome: a 14-year follow-up of the youngest diagnosed case. *Pediatr Nephrol* 1997;11:7.

666. Shimkets RA, Warnock DG, Bositis CM, et al. Liddle's syndrome: heritable human hypertension caused by mutations in the subunit of the epithelial sodium channel. *Cell* 1994;79:407.

667. Hansson JH, Nelson-Williams C, Suzuki H, et al. Hypertension caused by a truncated epithelial sodium channel subunit: genetic heterogeneity of Liddle syndrome. *Nat Genet* 1995;11:76.

668. Perlman JM, Volpe JJ. Seizures in the premature infant: effects on cerebral blood flow velocity, intracranial pressure and arterial blood pressure. *J Pediatr* 1983;102:288.

669. Schoenwetter BS, Libber SM, Jones D, et al. Hypertension in neonatal hyperthyroidism. *Am J Dis Child* 1983;137:854.

670. Kaufman BH, Telander RL, Van Heerden JA, et al. Pheochromocytoma in the pediatric age group: current status. *J Pediatr Surg* 1983; 18:879.

Diuretics

671. Chemtob S, Kaplan BS, Sherbotie JR, et al. Pharmacology of diuretics in the newborn. *Pediatr Clin North Am* 1989;36:1231.

672. Shinnar S, Gammon K, Bergman EW, et al. Management of hydrocephalus in infancy: use of acetazolamide and furosemide to avoid cerebrospinal fluid shunts. *J Pediatr* 1985;107:31.

673. Velasquez Jones L, Rivera Acosta F, Gordillo Paniagua G. Evaluation of the urinary and plasma urea ratio and osmolarity in newborn infants and malnourished children with pathological and normal renal function. *Bol Med Hosp Infant Mex* 1976;33:651.

674. Adhikari M, Moodley M, Desai PK. Mannitol in neonatal cerebral oedema. *Brain Dev* 1990;12:349.

675. Levene MI, Evans DH. Medical management of raised intracranial pressure after severe birth asphyxia. *Arch Dis Child* 1985;60:12.

676. Najak ZD, Harris EM, Lazzara A, et al. Pulmonary effects of furosemide in preterm infants with lung disease. *J Pediatr* 1983;102: 758.

677. Imai M. Effect of bumetanide and furosemide on the thick ascending limb of Henle's loop of rabbits and rats perfused in vitro. *Eur J Pharmacol* 1977;41:409.

678. Schrier RW, Lehman D, Zacherle B, et al. Effect of furosemide on free water excretion in edematous patients with hyponatremia. *Kidney Int* 1973;3:30.

679. Sulyok E, Varga F, Nèmeth F, et al. Furosemide-induced alterations in the electrolyte status, the function of renin–angiotensin–aldosterone system, and the urinary excretion of prostaglandins in newborn infants. *Pediatr Res* 1980;14:765.

680. Friedman Z, Demers LM, Marks KH, et al. Urinary excretion of prostaglandin E following the administration of furosemide and indomethacin to sick low-birth-weight infants. *J Pediatr* 1978;93:512.

681. Wells TG, Fasules JW, Taylor BJ, et al. Pharmacokinetics and pharmacodynamics of bumetanide in neonates treated with extracorporeal membrane oxygenation. *J Pediatr* 1992;121:974.

682. Brickman AS, Massry SG, Coburn JW. Changes in serum and urinary calcium during treatment with hydrochlorothiazide: studies on mechanisms. *J Clin Invest* 1972;51:945.

683. Costanzo LS, Windhager EE. Calcium and sodium transport by the distal convoluted tubule of the rat. *Am J Physiol* 1978;235:F492.

684. Albersheim SG, Solimano AJ, Sharma AK, et al. Randomized, double-blind, controlled trial of long-term diuretic therapy for bronchopulmonary dysplasia. *J Pediatr* 1989;115:615.

685. Kao LC, Durand DJ, McCrea RC, et al. Randomized trial of long-term diuretic therapy for infants with oxygen-dependent bronchopulmonary dysplasia. *J Pediatr* 1994;124:772.

686. Dargie HJ, Allison MEM, Kennedy AC, et al. High dosage metolazone in chronic renal failure. *Br Med J* 1972;4:196.

687. Arnold WC. Efficacy of metolazone and furosemide in children with furosemide resistant edema. *Pediatrics* 1984;74:872.

688. Segar JL, Robillard JE, Johnson KJ, et al. Addition of metolazone to overcome tolerance to furosemide in infants with bronchopulmonary dysplasia. *J Pediatr* 1992;120:966.

689. Bull MB, Laragh JH. Amiloride: a potassium-sparing natriuretic agent. *Circulation* 1968;37:45.

690. Knoers N, Monnens LAH. Amiloride-hydrochlorothiazide versus indomethacin-hydrochlorothiazide in the treatment of nephrogenic diabetes insipidus. *J Pediatr* 1990;117:499.

691. Perlman JM, Moore V, Siegel MJ, et al. Is chloride depletion an important contributing cause of death in infants with bronchopulmonary dysplasia? *Pediatrics* 1986;77:212.

692. Cannon PJ, Heinemann HO, Albert MS, et al. "Contraction" alkalosis after diuresis of edematous patients with ethacrynic acid. *Ann Intern Med* 1965;62:979.

693. Loon NR, Wilcox CS, Kanthanatana S, et al. Metabolic alkalosis during furosemide infusion in man: roles of volume contraction and acid excretion. *Kidney Int* 1987;31:208(abst).

694. Mirochnick MH, Miceli JJ, Kramer PA, et al. Renal response to furosemide in very low birth weight infants during chronic administration. *Dev Pharmacol Ther* 1990;15:1.

Bacteriuria and Urinary Tract Infections

695. Phillips JR, Karlowicz MG. Prevalence of Candida species in hospital-acquired urinary tract infections in a neonatal intensive care unit. *Pediatr Infect Dis J* 1997;16:190.

696. Gower PE, Husband P, Coleman JC, et al. Urinary infection in two selected neonatal populations. *Arch Dis Child* 1970;45:259.

697. Edelmann CM Jr, Ogwo JE, Fine BP, et al. The prevalence of bacteriuria in full-term and premature newborn infants. *J Pediatr* 1973;82:125.

698. Drew JH, Acton CM. Radiological findings in newborn infants with urinary infection. *Arch Dis Child* 1976;51:628.

699. Maherzi M, Guignard JP, Torrado A. Urinary tract infection in high-risk newborn infants. *Pediatrics* 1978;62:521.

700. Wiswell TE, Hachey WE. Urinary tract infections and the uncircumcised state: an update. *Clin Pediatr* 1993;32:130.

701. Olusanya O, Owa JA, Olusanya OI. The prevalence of bacteriuria among high risk neonates in Nigeria. *Acta Paediatr Scand* 1989;78:94.

702. Vilanova Juanola JM, Canos Molinos J, Rosell Arnold E, et al. Urinary tract infection in the newborn infant. *An Esp Pediatr* 1989;31:105.

703. Cohen HA, Drucker MM, Vainer S, et al. Postcircumcision urinary tract infection. *Clin Pediatr* 1992;31:322.

704. Wiswell TE, Miller GM, Gelston HM, et al. Effect of circumcision status on periurethral bacterial flora during the first year of life. *J Pediatr* 1988;113:442.

705. Fernandez Escribano A, Garcia Meseguer C, Pastor Abascal I, et al. Neonatal pelvic ectasia. *An Esp Pediatr* 1989;31:570.

706. Ehrlich O, Brem AS. A prospective comparison of urinary tract infections in patients treated with either clean intermittent catheterization or urinary diversion. *Pediatrics* 1982;70:665.

707. Neumann CG, Pryles CV. Pyelonephritis in infants and children. *Am J Dis Child* 1962;104:215.

708. Moraga Llop FA, del Alcázar Muñoz R, Casado Toda M, et al. Jaundice associated with urinary infection in the first three months of life: study of 66 cases. *An Esp Pediatr* 1980;13:5.

709. Crain EF, Gershel JC. Urinary tract infections in febrile infants younger than 8 weeks of age. *Pediatrics* 1990;86:363.

710. Krober MS, Bass JW, Powell JM, et al. Bacterial and viral pathogens causing fever in infants less than 3 months old. *Am J Dis Child* 1985;139:889.

711. Pappu LD, Purohit DM, Bradford BF, et al. Primary renal candidiasis in two preterm neonates: report of cases and review of the literature on renal candidiasis in infancy. *Am J Dis Child* 1984;138:923.

712. Newman CGH, O'Neill P, Parker A. Pyuria in infancy, and the role of suprapubic aspiration of urine in diagnosis of infection of urinary tract. *Br Med J* 1967;2:277.

713. Bonadio WA. Urine culturing technique in febrile infants. *Pediatr Emerg Care* 1987;3:75.

714. Visser VE, Hall RT. Urine culture in the evaluation of suspected neonatal sepsis. *J Pediatr* 1979;94:635.

715. DiGeronimo RJ. Lack of efficacy of the urine culture as part of the initial sepsis workup of suspected neonatal sepsis. *Pediatr Infect Dis J* 1992;11:764.

716. Nelson JD, Peters PC. Suprapubic aspiration of urine in premature and term infants. *Pediatrics* 1965;36:132.

717. Phillips JR, Karlowicz MG. Prevalence of Candida species in hospital-acquired urinary tract infections in a neonatal intensive care unit. *Pediatr Infect Dis J* 1997;16:190.

718. Vaid YN, Lebowitz RL. Urosepsis in infants with vesicoureteral reflux masquerading as the salt-losing type of congenital adrenal hyperplasia. *Pediatr Radiol* 1989;19:548.

719. Luk G, Riggs D, Luque M. Severe methemoglobinemia in a 3-week-old infant with a urinary infection. *Crit Care Med* 1991;19:1325.

720. Wiswell TE, Geschke DW. Risks from circumcision during the first month of life compared with those for uncircumcised boys. *Pediatrics* 1989;83:1011.

721. Ginsburg CM, McCracken GH, Jr. Urinary tract infections in young infants. *Pediatrics* 1982;69:409.

722. Goldman M, Barr J, Bistriztzer T. Urinary tract infection following ritual Jewish circumcision. *Isr J Med Sci* 1996;32:1098.

723. Crawford DB, Rasoulpour M, Dhawan VM, et al. Renal carbuncle in a neonate with congenital nephrotic syndrome. *J Pediatr* 1978;93:78.

724. Walker KM. Suprarenal abscess due to group B streptococcus. *J Pediatr* 1979;94:970.

725. Wang SF, Huang FY, Chiu NC, et al. Urinary tract infection in infants less than 2 months of age. *Acta Paediatr Sin* 1994;35:294.

726. Edwards D, Normand ICS, Prescod N, et al. Disappearance of vesicoureteral reflux during long-term prophylaxis of urinary tract infection in children. *Br Med J* 1977;2:285.

727. Yadin O, Ben-Ezer DG, Golan A, et al. Survival of a premature neonate with obstructive anuria due to *Candida*: the role of early sonographic diagnosis and antimycotic treatment. *Eur J Pediatr* 1988;147:653.

728. Tung KT, MacDonald LM, Smith JC. Neonatal systemic candidiasis diagnosed by ultrasound. *Acta Radiol* 1990;31:293.

729. Hellerstein S, Duggan E, Welchert E, et al. Serum C-reactive protein and the site of urinary tract infections. *J Pediatr* 1982;100:21.

730. Johnson CE, Shurin PA, Marchant CD, et al. Identification of children requiring radiologic evaluation for urinary tract infection. *Pediatr Infect Dis* 1985;4:656.

731. Pylkkänen J, Vilska J, Koskimies O. The value of level diagnosis of childhood urinary tract infection in predicting renal injury. *Acta Paediatr Scand* 1981;70:879.

732. Rickwood AMK, McKendrick T, Williams MPL, et al. Current imaging of childhood urinary tract infections: prospective survey. *Br Med J* 1992;304:663.

733. Dremsek PA, Gindl K, Voitl P, et al. Renal pyelectasis in fetuses and neonates: diagnostic value of renal pelvis diameter in pre- and postnatal sonographic screening. *AJR* 1997;168:1017.

734. Haberlik A. Detection of low-grade vesicoureteral reflux in children by color Doppler imaging mode. *Pediatr Surg Int* 1997;12:38.

735. Hiraoka M, Kasuga K, Hori C, et al. Ultrasonic indicators of ureteric reflux in the newborn. *Lancet* 1994;343:519.

736. Gleeson FV, Gordon I. Imaging in urinary tract infection. *Arch Dis Child* 1991;66:1282.

737. Rushton HG, Majd M, Chandra R, Yim D. Evaluation of ^{99m}technetium-dimercapto-succinic acid renal scans in experimental acute pyelonephritis in piglets. *J Urol* 1988;140[Pt 2]:1169.

738. Verber IG, Meller ST. Serial ^{99m}Tc dimercaptosuccinic acid (DMSA) scans after urinary infections presenting before the age of 5 years. *Arch Dis Child* 1989;64:1533.

739. Rossleigh MA, Wilson MJ, Rosenberg AR, et al. DMSA studies in infants under one year of age. *Contrib Nephrol* 1990;79:166.

739a. Eliakim A, Dolfin T, Korzets A, et al. Urinary tract infection in premature infants: the role of imaging studies and prophylactic therapy. *J Perinatol* 1997;17:305.

740. Rodríguez-Soriano J, Vallo A, Oliveros R. Transient pseudohypoaldosteronism secondary to obstructive uropathy in infancy. *J Pediatr* 1983;103:375.

741. Constantopoulos A, Thomaidou L, Loupa H, et al. Successful response of severe neonatal gram-negative infection to treatment with aztreonam. *Chemotherapy* 1989;35[Suppl 1]:101.

742. Feld LG. Urinary tract infections in childhood: definition, pathogenesis, diagnosis, and management. *Pharmacotherapy* 1991;11:326.

743. Zhanel GG, Harding GKM, Guay DRP. Asymptomatic bacteriuria: which patients should be treated? *Arch Intern Med* 1990;150:1389.

744. Leung AKC, Robson WLM. Urinary tract infection in infancy and childhood. *Adv Pediatr* 1991;38:257.

745. Wettergreen B, Hellstrom M, Stockland E, et al. Six year follow up of infants with bacteriuria on screening. *Br Med J* 1990;13:845.

746. Dore B, Irani J, Istin A, et al. Vesicorenal reflux in children under age 2: indications and results of surgery. *J Urol (Paris)* 1990;96:365.

747. Rehan VK, Davidson DC. Neonatal renal candidal bezoar. *Arch Dis Child* 1992;67:63.

748. Matsumoto AH, Dejter SW Jr, Barth KH, et al. Percutaneous nephrostomy drainage in the management of neonatal anuria secondary to renal candidiasis. *J Pediatr Surg* 1990;25:1295.

749. Rickwood AMK, Reiner I. Urinary stone formation in children with prenatally diagnosed uropathies. *Br J Urol* 1991;68:541.

750. Naoumis A, Dumas R, Belon C, et al. La lithiase urinaire de l'enfant. Enquête étiologique. *Arch Fr Pédiatr* 1989;46:347.

751. Royer P, Lévy M. La lithiase urinaire du nourrisson. *Acq Méd Récent* 1969:51.

752. Arant BS Jr, Sotelo-Avila C, Bernstein J. Segmental "hypoplasia" of the kidney (Ask-Upmark). *J Pediatr* 1979;95:931.

753. Welch TR, Nogrady MB, Outerbridge EW. Roentgenologic sequelae of neonatal septicemia and urinary tract infection. *Am J Roentgenol Radium Ther Nucl Med* 1973;118:28.

754. Holland NH, Jackson EC, Kazee M, et al. Relation of urinary tract infection and vesicoureteral reflux to scars: follow-up of thirty-eight patients. *J Pediatr* 1990;116:S65.

755. Majd M, Rushton HG, Jantausch BG, et al. Relationship among vesicoureteral reflux, P-fimbriated *Escherichia coli*, and acute pyelonephritis in children with febrile urinary tract infection. *J Pediatr* 1991;119:578.

756. Arnold AJ, Brownless SM, Carty HM, et al. Detection of renal scarring by DMSA scanning—an experimental study. *J Pediatr Surg* 1990;25:391.

757. Wiswell TE, Roscelli JD. Corroborative evidence for the decreased incidence of urinary tract infections in circumcised male infants. *Pediatrics* 1986;78:96.

758. Cohen HA, Drucker MM, Vainer S, et al. Postcircumcision urinary tract infection. *Clin Pediatr* 1992;31:322.

759. Joseph DB, Bauer SB, Colodney AH, et al. Clean, intermittent catheterization of infants with neurogenic bladder. *Pediatrics* 1989;84:74.

760. Kasabian NG, Bauer SB, Dyro FM, et al. The prophylactic value of clean intermittent catheterization and anticholinergic medication in newborns and infants with myelodysplasia at risk of developing urinary tract deterioration. *Am J Dis Child* 1992;146:840.

761. Anderson PAM, Rickwood AMK. Features of primary vesicoureteric reflux detected by prenatal sonography. *Br J Urol* 1991;67:267.

762. Gordon AC, Thomas DFM, Arthur RJ, et al. Prenatally diagnosed reflux: a follow-up study. *Br J Urol* 1990;65:407.

Tubular Dysfunction

763. Scriver CR, Beaudet AL, Sly WS, et al, eds: *The metabolic and molecular basis of inherited disease.* New York: McGraw-Hill, 1995.

764. Sargent JD, Stukel TA, Kresel J, Klein RZ. Normal values for random urinary calcium to creatinine ratios in infancy. *J Pediatr* 1993;123:393

765. Nishiyama S, Tomoeda S, Inoue F, et al. Self-limited neonatal familial hyperparathyroidism associated with hypercalciuria and renal tubular acidosis in three siblings. *J Pediatr* 1990;86:421.

766. Pearce SHS, Williamson C, Kifor O, et al. A familial syndrome of hypocalcemia with hypercalciuria due to mutations in the calcium-sensing receptor. *N Engl J Med* 1996;335:1115.

767. Hufnagle KG, Khan SN, Penn D, et al. Renal calcifications: a complication of long-term furosemide therapy in preterm infants. *Pediatrics* 1982;70:360.

768. Jacinto JS, Modanlou HD, Crade M, et al. Renal calcification incidence in very low birth weight infants. *Pediatrics* 1988;88:31.

769. Noe HN, Bryant JF, Roy S III, et al. Urolithiasis in pre-term neonates associated with furosemide therapy. *J Urol* 1984;132:93.

770. Short A, Cooke RWI. The incidence of renal calcification in preterm infants. *Arch Dis Child* 1991;66:412.

771. Woolfield N, Haslam R, Le Quesne G, et al. Ultrasound diagnosis of nephrocalcinosis in preterm infants. *Arch Dis Child* 1988;63:86.

772. Coe FL, Bushinsky DA. Pathophysiology of hypercalciuria. *Am J Physiol* 1984;16:F1.

773. Rowe JC, Goetz CA, Carey DE, et al. Achievement of in utero retention of calcium and phosphorus accompanied by high calcium excretion in very low birth weight infants fed a fortified formula. *J Pediatr* 1987;110:581.

774. Senterre J, Salle B. Renal aspects of calcium and phosphorus metabolism in preterm infants. *Biol Neonate* 1988;53:220.

775. Chessex P, Pineault M, Zebiche H, et al. Calciuria in parenterally fed preterm infants: role of phosphorus intake. *J Pediatr* 1985;107:794.

776. Ezzedeen F, Adelman RD, Ahifors CE. Renal calcification in preterm infants: pathophysiology and long-term sequelae. *J Pediatr* 1988;113:532.

777. Savage MO, Wilkinson AR, Baum JD, et al. Furosemide in respiratory distress syndrome. *Arch Dis Child* 1975;50:709.

778. Warshaw BL, Anand SK, Kerian A, et al. The effect of chronic furosemide administration on urinary calcium excretion and calcium balance in growing rats. *Pediatr Res* 1980;14:1118.

779. Venkatarman PS, Han BK, Tsang RC, et al. Secondary hyperparathyroidism and bone disease in infants receiving long term furosemide therapy. *Am J Dis Child* 1983;137:1157.

780. Atkinson SA, Shah JK, McGee C, et al. Mineral excretion in premature infants receiving various diuretic therapies. *J Pediatr* 1988:113:540.

781. Fischer AF, Parker BR, Stevenson DK. Nephrolithiasis following in utero diuretic exposure: an unusual case. *Pediatrics* 1988;81:712.

782. Adelman RD, Abern SB, Merten D, et al. Hypercalciuria with nephrolithiasis: a complication of total parenteral nutrition. *Pediatrics* 1977;59:473.

783. Bengoa JM, Sitrin MD, Wood RJ, et al. Amino acid-induced hypercalciuria in patients on total parenteral nutrition. *Am J Clin Nutr* 1983;38:264.

784. Berkelhammer CH, Wood RJ, Sitrin MD. Acetate and hypercalciuria during total parenteral nutrition. *Am J Clin Nutr* 1988;48:1482.

785. Campfield T, Braden G, Flynn-Valone P, et al. Urinary oxalate excretion in premature infants: effect of human milk versus formula feeding. *Pediatrics* 1994;94:674.

786. Hoppe B, Hesse A, Neuhaus T, et al. Urinary saturation and nephrocalcinosis in preterm infants: effect of parenteral nutrition. *Arch Dis Child* 1993;69:299.

787. Downing GJ, Egelhoff JC, Daily DK, et al. Kidney function in very low birth weight infants with furosemide-related renal calcifications at ages 1 to 2 years. *J Pediatr* 1992;120:599.

788. Leppla D, Browne R, Hill K, et al. Effect of amiloride with or without hydrochlorothiazide on urinary calcium and saturation of calcium salts. *J Clin Endocrinol Metab* 1983;57:920.

789. Watts RWE. Alanine glyoxylate aminotransferase deficiency: biochemical and molecular genetic lessons from the study of a human disease. *Adv Enzyme Regul* 1992;32:309.

790. Danpure CJ, Purdue PE, Fryer P, et al. Enzymological and mutational

analysis of a complex primary hyperoxaluria type 1 phenotype involving alanine:glyoxylate aminotransferase peroxisome-to-mitochondrion mistargeting and intraperoxisomal aggregation. *Am J Hum Genet* 1993;53:417.

791. Takada Y, Kaneko N, Esumi H, et al. Human peroxisomal L-alanine:glyoxylate aminotransferase. Evolutionary loss of a mitochondrial targeting signal by point mutation of the initiation codon. *Biochem J* 1990;268:517.

792. Danpure CJ. Molecular and clinical heterogeneity in primary hyperoxaluria type 1. *Am J Kidney Dis* 1991;17:366.

793. von Schnakenburg C, Byrd DJ, Latta K, et al. Determination of oxalate excretion in spot urines of healthy children by ion chromatography. *Eur J Clin Chem Clin Biochem* 1994;32:27.

794. Sonntag J, Schaub J. The identification of hyperoxaluria in very low-birthweight infants—which urine sampling method? *Pediatr Nephrol* 1997;11:205.

795. Morgenstern BZ, Milliner DS, Murphy ME, et al. Urinary oxalate and glycolate excretion patterns in the first year of life: a longitudinal study. *J Pediatr* 1993;123:248.

796. Reusz GS, Dobos M, Byrd D, et al. Urinary calcium and oxalate excretion in children. *Pediatr Nephrol* 1995;9:39.

797. De Zegher FE, Wolff ED, vd Heijden AJ, et al. Oxalosis in infancy. *Clin Nephrol* 1984;22:114.

798. Morris MC, Chambers TL, Evans PWG, et al. Oxalosis in infancy. *Arch Dis Child* 1982;57:224.

799. Furuta M, Torii S. Congenital oxalosis: first report of two neonatal cases. *Ann Paediatr Jpn* 1967;13:42.

800. Rose GA, Arthur LJH, Chambers TL, et al. Successful treatment of primary hyperoxaluria in a neonate. *Lancet* 1982;1:1298.

801. Leumann EP, Wegmann W, Largiadèr F. Prolonged survival after renal transplantation in primary hyperoxaluria of childhood. *Lancet* 1986;2:340.

802. Allen AR, Thompson EM, Williams G, et al. Selective renal transplantation in primary hyperoxaluria type 1. *Am J Kidney Dis* 1996;27:891.

803. Jamieson NV, on behalf of the European PH1 Transplantation Study Group. The European Primary Hyperoxaluria Type 1 Transplant Registry report on the results of combined liver/kidney transplantation for primary hyperoxaluria 1984–1994. *Nephrol Dial Transplant* 1995;10[Suppl 8]:33.

804. Rytkönen EM, Halila R, Laan M, et al. The human gene for xanthine dehydrogenase (XDH) is localized on chromosome band 2p22. *Cytogenet Cell Genet* 1995;68:61.

805. Reiter S, Simmonds HA, Zöllner N, et al. Demonstration of a combined deficiency of xanthine oxidase and aldehyde oxidase in xanthinuric patients not forming oxipurinol. *Clin Chim Acta* 1990;187:221.

806. Badertscher E, Robson WLM, Leung AKC, et al. Xanthine calculi presenting at 1 month of age. *Eur J Pediatr* 1993;152:252.

807. Fratini A, Simmers RN, Callen DF, et al. A new location for the human adenine phosphoribosyltransferase gene (APRT) distal to the haptoglobin (HP) and fra(16)(q23)(FRA16D) loci. *Cytogenet Cell Genet* 1986;43:10.

808. Broderick TP, Schaff DA, Bertino AM, et al. Comparative anatomy of the human APRT gene and enzyme: nucleotide sequence divergence and conservation of a non-random CpG dinucleotide arrangement. *Proc Natl Acad Sci USA* 1987;84:3349.

809. Hidaka Y, Tarlé SA, O Toole TE, et al. Nucleotide sequence of the human APRT gene. *Nucleic Acids Res* 1987;15:9086.

810. Kambayashi T, Nakanishi T, Suzuki K, et al. Two siblings with 2,8-dihydroxyadenine urolithiasis. *Hinyokikka Kiyo* 1994;40:1097.

811. Garrett JE, Capuano IV, Hammerland LG. Molecular cloning and functional expression of human parathyroid calcium receptor cDNAs. *J Biol Chem* 1995;270:12919.

812. Janicic N, Soliman E, Pausova Z, et al. Mapping of the calcium-sensing receptor gene (CASR) to human chromosome 3q13.3-21 by fluorescence in situ hybridization, and localization to rat chromosome 11 and mouse chromosome 16. *Mamm Genome* 1995;6:798.

813. Pollak MR, Brown EM, Chou YH, et al. Mutations in the human Ca^{2+}-sensing receptor gene cause familial hypocalciuric hypercalcemia and neonatal severe hyperparathyroidism. *Cell* 1993;75:1297.

814. Heath H III, Jackson CE, Otterud B, et al. Genetic linkage analysis in familial benign (hypocalciuric) hypercalcemia: evidence for locus heterogeneity. *Am J Hum Genet* 1993;53:193.

815. Trump D, Whyte MP, Wooding C, et al. Linkage studies in a kindred from Oklahoma, with familial benign (hypocalciuric) hypercalcaemia (FBH) and developmental elevations in serum parathyroid hormone levels, indicate a third locus for FBH. *Human Genet* 1995;96:183.

816. Pollak MR, Chou YH, Marx SJ, et al. Familial hypocalciuric hypercalcemia and neonatal severe hyperparathyroidism. Effects of mutant gene dosage on phenotype. *J Clin Invest* 1994;93:1108.

817. Marx SJ, Fraser D, Rapoport A. Familial hypocalciuric hypercalcemia. Mild expression of the gene in heterozygotes and severe expression in homozygotes. *Am J Med* 1985;78:15.

818. Law WM, Heath H. Familial benign hypercalcemia (hypocalciuric hypercalcemia). Clinical and pathogenetic studies in 21 families. *Ann Intern Med* 1985;102:511.

819. Kristiansen JH, Brøchner-Mortensen J, Pedersen KO. Renal tubular function in familial hypocalciuric hypercalcemia. *Contrib Nephrol* 1987;56:210.

820. Watanabe H, Sutton RAL. Renal calcium handling in familial hypocalciuric hypercalcemia. *Kidney Int* 1983;24:353.

821. Marx SJ, Stock JL, Attie MF, et al. Familial hypocalciuric hypercalcemia: Recognition among patients referred after unsuccessful parathyroid exploration. *Ann Intern Med* 1980;92:351.

822. Page LA, Haddow J. Self-limited neonatal hyperparathyroidism in familial hypocalciuric hypercalcemia. *J Pediatr* 1987;111:261.

823. Dezateux CA, Hyde JC, Hoey HMCV, et al. Neonatal hyperparathyroidism. *Eur J Pediatr* 1984;142:135.

824. Roth KS, Foreman JW, Segal S. The Fanconi syndrome and mechanisms of tubular transport dysfunction. *Kidney Int* 1981;20:705.

825. Manz F, Bickel H, Brodehl J, et al. Fanconi-Bickel syndrome. *Pediatr Nephrol* 1987;1:509.

826. Worthen HG, Good RA. The de Toni-Fanconi syndrome with cystinosis. *Am J Dis Child* 1958;95:653.

827. Wrong OM, Norden AG, Feest TG. Dent's disease: a familial proximal renal tubular syndrome with low-molecular-weight proteinuria, hypercalciuria, nephrocalcinosis, metabolic bone disease, progressive renal failure and a marked male predominance. *Q J Med* 1994;87:473.

828. Pook MA, Wrong O, Wooding C, et al. Dent's disease, a renal Fanconi syndrome with nephrocalcinosis and kidney stones, is associated with a microdeletion involving DXS255 and maps to Xp11.22. *Hum Mol Genet* 1993;2:2129.

829. Lloyd SE, Pearce SH, Fisher SE, et al. A common molecular basis for three inherited kidney stone diseases. *Nature* 1996;379:445.

830. Fisher SE, Black GCM, Lloyd SE. Isolation and partial characterization of a chloride channel gene which is expressed in kidney and is a candidate for Dent's disease (an X-linked hereditary nephrolithiasis). *Hum Mol Genet* 1994;3:2053.

831. Gahl WA, Bernardini IM, Dalakas MC, et al. Muscle carnitine repletion by long-term carnitine supplementation in nephropathic cystinosis. *Pediatr Res* 1993;34:115.

832. Usberti M, Pecoraro C, Federico S, et al. Mechanism of action of indomethacin in tubular defects. *Pediatrics* 1985;75:501.

833. Haycock GB, Al-Dahhan J, Mak RHK, et al. Effect of indomethacin on clinical progress and renal function in cystinosis. *Arch Dis Child* 1982;57:934.

834. Gahl WA, Tietze F, Bashan N, et al. Defective cystine exodus from isolated lysosome-rich fractions of cystinotic leucocytes. *J Biol Chem* 1982;257:9570.

835. Lemire J, Kaplan BS. The various renal manifestations of the nephropathic form of cystinosis. *Am J Nephrol* 1984;4:81.

836. Wong VG, Lietman PS, Seegmiller JE. Alterations of pigment epithelium in cystinosis. *Arch Ophthalmol* 1967;77:361.

837. Gretz N, Man F, Augustin R, et al. Survival time in cystinosis: a collaborative study. *Proc Eur Dialys Transplant Assoc* 1982;19:582.

838. Gahl WA, Reed GF, Thoene JG, et al. Cysteamine therapy for children with nephropathic cystinosis. *N Engl J Med* 1987;316:971.

839. Clark KF, Franklin PS, Reisch JS, et al. Effect of cysteamine-HCl and phosphocysteamine dosage on renal function and growth in children with nephropathic cystinosis. *Clin Res* 1992;40:113A.

840. Reznik VM, Adamson M, Adelman RD, et al. Treatment of cystinosis with cysteamine from early infancy. *J Pediatr* 1991;119:491.

841. Deal JE, Barratt M, Dillon MJ. Fanconi syndrome, ichthyosis, dysmorphism, jaundice and diarrhoea: a new syndrome. *Pediatr Nephrol* 1990;4:308.

842. Sanjad SA, Kaddoura RE, Nazer HM, et al. Fanconi's syndrome with hepatorenal glycogenosis associated with phosphorylase b kinase deficiency. *Am J Dis Child* 1993;147:957.

843. Chen YT, Scheinman JI, Park HK, et al. Amelioration of proximal renal tubular dysfunction in type I glycogen storage disease with dietary therapy. *N Engl J Med* 1990;323:590.

844. Garty R, Cooper M, Tabachnik E. The Fanconi syndrome associated with hepatic glycogenosis and abnormal metabolism of galactose. *J Pediatr* 1974;85:821.

845. Lee PJ, Van't Hoff WG, Leonard JV. Catch-up growth in Fanconi-Bickel syndrome with uncooked cornstarch. *J Inherit Metab Dis* 1995;18:153.

846. Sparkes RS, Sparkes MC, Funderburk SJ, et al. Expression of GALT in 9p chromosome alterations: assignment of *GALT* locus to 9cen→9p22. *Ann Hum Genet* 1980;43:343.

847. Reichardt JKV, Berg P. Cloning and characterization of a cDNA encoding human galactose-1-phosphate uridyl transferase. *Mol Biol Med* 1988;5:107.

848. Flach JE, Reichardt JKV, Elsas LJ II. Sequence of a cDNA encoding human galactose-1-phosphate uridyl transferase. *Mol Biol Med* 1990;7:365.

849. Komrower GM, Schwarz V, Holzel A, et al. A clinical and biochemical study of galactosemia: a possible explanation of the nature of the biochemical lesion. *Arch Dis Child* 1956;31:254.

850. Hsia DY-Y, Hsia H-H, Green S, et al. Amino-aciduria in galactosemia. *Am J Dis Child* 1954;88:458.

851. Darling S, Mortensen O. Aminoaciduria in galactosaemia. *Acta Paediatr* 1954;43:337.

852. Dreyfus JC, Schapira F, Besmond C, et al. Study of hereditary fructose intolerance by methods of molecular biology. *Ann Méd Int* 1985;136:456.

853. Lebo RV, Tolan DR, Bruce BD, et al. Spot-blot analysis of sorted chromosomes assigns a fructose intolerance disease locus to chromosome 9. *Cytometry* 1985;6:478.

854. Editorial. Pacifiers, passive behaviour, and pain. *Lancet* 1992;1:275.

855. Blass EM, Hoffmeyer LB. Sucrose as an analgesic for newborn infants. *Pediatrics* 1991;87:215.

856. Levin B, Snodgrass GJAI, Oberholzer VG, et al. Fructosaemia. *Arch Dis Child* 1968;45:826.

857. Mass RE, Smith WR, Walsh JR. The association of hereditary fructose intolerance and renal tubular acidosis. *Am J Med Sci* 1966;251:516.

858. La Du BN. The enzymatic deficiency in tyrosinemia. *Am J Dis Child* 1967;113:54.

859. Bergeron P, Laberge C, Grenier A. Hereditary tyrosinemia in the province of Québec: prevalence at birth and geographic distribution. *Clin Genet* 1974;5:157.

860. Grompe M, St.-Louis M, Demers SI, et al. A single mutation of the fumarylaceto-acetate hydrolase gene in French Canadians with hereditary tyrosinemia type I. *N Engl J Med* 1994;331:353.

861. Labelle Y, Phaneuf D, Leclerc B, et al. Characterization of the human fumarylacetoacetate hydrolase gene and identification of a missense mutation abolishing enzymatic activity. *Hum Mol Genet* 1993;2:941.

862. Demers SI, Phaneuf D, Tanguay RM. Hereditary tyrosinemia type I: strong association with haplotype 6 in French Canadians permits simple carrier detection and prenatal diagnosis. *Am J Hum Genet* 1994;55:327.

863. Halvorsen S, Pande H, Løken AC, et al. Tyrosinosis: a study of 6 cases. *Arch Dis Child* 1966;41:238.

864. Gentz J, Jagenburg R, Zetterström R. Tyrosinemia: an inborn error of tyrosine metabolism with cirrhosis of the liver and multiple renal tubular defects (de Toni-Debré-Fanconi syndrome). *J Pediatr* 1965;66:670.

865. van Spronsen FJ, Thomasse Y, Smit GPA, et al. Hereditary tyrosinemia type I: a new clinical classification with difference in prognosis on dietary treatment. *Hepatology* 1994;20:1187.

866. Laine J, Salo MK, Krogerus L, et al. The nephropathy of type I tyrosinemia after liver transplantation. *Pediatr Res* 1995;37:640.

867. Lindstedt S, Holme E, Lock EA, et al. Treatment of hereditary tyrosinaemia type I by inhibition of 4-hydroxyphenylpyruvate dioxygenase. *Lancet* 1992;340:813.

868. Kvittingen EA. Tyrosinaemia—treatment and outcome. *J Inherit Metab Dis* 1995;18:375.

869. Silver DN, Lewis RA, Nussbaum RL. Mapping the Lowe oculocere-

870. Attree O, Olivos IM, Okabe I, et al. The Lowe's oculocerebrorenal syndrome gene encodes a novel protein highly homologous to inositol polyphosphate-5-phosphatase. *Nature* 1992;358:239.

871. Nussbaum RL, Orrison BM, Jänne PA, et al. Physical mapping and genomic structure of the Lowe syndrome gene OCRL1. *Hum Genet* 1997;99:145.

872. Miller RC, Wolf EJ, Gould M, et al. Fetal oculocerebrorenal syndrome of Lowe associated with elevated maternal serum and amniotic fluid alpha-fetoprotein levels. *Obstet Gynecol* 1994;84:77.

873. Gaary EA, Rawnsley E, Marin-Padilla JM, et al. In utero detection of fetal cataracts. *J Ultrasound Med* 1993;12:234.

874. Charnas LR, Bernardini I, Rader D, et al. Clinical and laboratory findings in the oculocerebrorenal syndrome of Lowe, with special reference to growth and renal function. *N Engl J Med* 1991;324:1318.

875. Van Acker KJ, Roels H, Beelaerts W, et al. The histologic lesions of the kidney in the oculo-cerebro-renal syndrome of Lowe. *Nephron* 1967;4:193.

876. Witzleben CL, Schoen EJ, Tu WH, et al. Progressive morphologic renal changes in the oculo-cerebro-renal syndrome of Lowe. *Am J Med* 1968;44:319.

877. Rötig A, Cormier V, Blanche S, et al. Pearson's marrow-pancreas syndrome. A multisystem mitochondrial disorder in infancy. *J Clin Invest* 1990;86:1601.

878. Niaudet P, Rötig A. Renal involvement in mitochondrial cytopathies. *Pediatr Nephrol* 1996;10:368.

879. DiMauro S, Mendell JR, Sahenk Z, et al. Fatal infantile mitochondrial myopathy and renal dysfunction due to cytochrome-c-oxidase deficiency. *Neurology* 1980;30:795.

880. Ogier H, Lombes A, Scholte HR, et al. De Toni-Fanconi-Debré syndrome with Leigh syndrome revealing severe muscle cytochrome c oxidase deficiency. *J Pediatr* 1988;112:734.

881. Gruskin AB, Patel MS, Linshaw M, et al. Renal function studies and kidney pyruvate carboxylase in subacute necrotizing encephalomyopathy (Leigh's syndrome). *Pediatr Res* 1973;7:832.

882. Buist NRM. Is pyruvate carboxylase involved in the renal tubular reabsorption of bicarbonate? *J Inherit Metab Dis* 1980;3:113.

883. Falik-Borenstein ZC, Jordan SC, Saudubray JM, et al. Renal tubular acidosis in carnitine palmitoyl transferase I deficiency. *N Engl J Med* 1992;327:24.

884. Clayton PT, Hyland K, Brand M, et al. Mitochondrial phosphoenolpyruvate carboxykinase deficiency. *Eur J Pediatr* 1986;145:46.

885. Rötig A, Bessis JL, Romero N, et al. Maternally inherited duplication of the mitochondrial genome in a syndrome of proximal tubulopathy, diabetes mellitus, and cerebellar ataxia. *Am J Hum Genet* 1992;50:364.

886. Wildin RS, Antush MJ, Bennett RL, et al. Heterogenous AVPR2 gene mutations in congenital nephrogenic diabetes insipidus. *Am J Hum Genet* 1994;55:266.

887. Anderson JG, Notmann DD, Springer J. Studies in nephrogenic diabetes insipidus. *Clin Res* 1969;27:477A.

888. Knoers NV, van der Heyden H, van Oost BA, et al. Linkage of X-linked nephrogenic diabetes insipidus with DXS52, a polymorphic DNA marker. *Nephron* 1988;50:187.

889. van Lieburg AF, Knoers VVAM, Mallmann R, et al. Normal fibrinolytic responses to 1-desamino-8-D-arginine vasopressin in patients with nephrogenic diabetes insipidus caused by mutations in the aquaporin 2 gene. *Nephron* 1996;72:544.

890. Macaulay D, Watson M. Hypernatraemia in infants as a cause of brain damage. *Arch Dis Child* 1967;42:485.

891. Hoekstra JA, van Lieburg AF, Monnens LAH, et al. Cognitive and psychosocial functioning of patients with congenital nephrogenic diabetes insipidus. *Am J Med Genet* 1996;61:81.

892. Ohzeki T. Urinary adenosine 3'5'-monophosphate (cAMP): response to antidiuretic hormone in diabetes insipidus (DI): comparison between congenital nephrogenic DI type 1 and 2, and vasopressin sensitive DI. *Acta Endocrinol* 1985;108:485.

893. Deen PMT, van Aubel RA, van Lieburg AF, et al. Urinary content of aquaporin 1 and 2 in nephrogenic diabetes insipidus. *J Am Soc Nephrol* 1996;7:836.

894. Libber S, Harrison H, Spector D. Treatment of nephrogenic diabetes insipidus with prostaglandin synthesis inhibitors. *J Pediatr* 1986;108:305.

brorenal syndrome to Xq24-q26 by use of restriction fragment length polymorphisms. *J Clin Invest* 1987;79:282.

895. Rasher W, Rosendahl W, Hendrichs IA, et al. Congenital nephrogenic diabetes insipidus-vasopressin and prostaglandins in response to treatment with hydrochlorothiazide and indomethacin. *Pediatr Nephrol* 1987;1:485.

896. Bartter FC, Pronove P, Gill JR Jr, et al. Hyperplasia of the juxtaglomerular complex with hyperaldosteronism and hypokalemic alkalosis: a new syndrome. *Am J Med* 1962;33:811.

897. Simon DB. Lifton RP. The molecular basis of inherited hypokalemic alkalosis: Bartter's and Gitelman's syndromes. *Am J Physiol* 1996; 271:F961.

898. Simon DB, Karet FE, Hamdan JM, et al. Bartter's syndrome, hypokalaemic alkalosis with hypercalciuria, is caused by mutations in the Na-K-2Cl cotransporter NKCC2. *Nat Genet* 1996;13:183.

899. Moorthy MB, Cade MSJ. Bartter's syndrome: a rare cause of a severe metabolic abnormality in a pre-term neonate. *J R Army Med Corps* 1992;138:46.

900. Bettinelli A, Blanchetti MG, Girardin E, et al. Use of calcium excretion values to distinguish two forms of primary renal tubular hypokalemic alkalosis: Bartter and Gitelman syndromes. *J Pediatr* 1992;120:38.

901. Houser M, Zimmerman B, Davidman M, et al. Idiopathic hypercalciuria associated with hyperreninemia and high urinary prostaglandin E. *Kidney Int* 1984;26:176.

902. Seyberth HW, Rascher W, Schweer H, et al. Congenital hypokalemia with hypercalciuria in preterm infants: a hyperprostaglandinuric tubular syndrome different from Bartter syndrome. *J Pediatr* 1985; 107:694.

903. International Collaborative Study Group for Bartter-like Syndromes. Mutations in the gene encoding the inwardly-rectifying renal potassium channel, ROMK, cause the antenatal variant of Bartter syndrome: evidence for genetic heterogeneity. *Hum Mol Genet* 1997;6:17.

904. Derst C, Konrad M, Köckerling A, et al. Mutations in the ROMK gene in antenatal Bartter syndrome are associated with impaired K-channel function. *Biochem Biophys Res Commun* 1997;230:641.

905. Köckerling A, Reinalter SC, Seyberth HW. Impaired response to furosemide in hyperprostaglandin E syndrome: evidence for a tubular defect in the loop of Henle. *J Pediatr* 1996;129:519.

906. Roman RJ, Skelton M, Lechene C. Prostaglandin–vasopressin interactions on the renal handling of calcium and magnesium. *J Pharmacol Exp Ther* 1984;230:295.

907. Yamada M, Matsumoto T, Takahashi N, et al. Stimulatory effect of prostaglandin E_2 on $1\alpha,25$-dihydroxyvitamin D_3 synthesis in rats. *Biochemistry* 1983;216:237.

908. Raisz LG, Dietrich JW, Simmons HA, et al. Effect of prostaglandin endoperoxides and metabolites on bone resorption in vitro. *Nature* 1977;267:532.

909. Seyberth HW, Rascher W, Schweer H, et al. Congenital hypokalemia with hypercalciuria in preterm infants: a hyperprostaglandinuric tubular syndrome different from Bartter syndrome. *J Pediatr* 1985; 107:694.

910. Karolyi L, Ziegler A, Pollak M, et al. Gitelman's syndrome is genetically distinct from other forms of Bartter's syndrome. *Pediatr Nephrol* 1996;10:551.

911. Pollak MR, Delaney VB, Graham RM, et al. Gitelman's syndrome (Bartter's variant) maps to the thiazide-sensitive cotransporter gene locus on chromosome 16q13 in a large kindred. *J Am Soc Nephrol* 1996;7:2244.

912. Simon DB, Nelson-Williams C, Bia MJ, et al. Gitelman's variant of Bartter's syndrome, inherited hypokalaemic alkalosis, is caused by mutations in the thiazide-sensitive Na-Cl cotransporter. *Nat Genet* 1996;12:24.

913. Gitelman HJ. Hypokalemia, hypomagnesemia, and alkalosis: a rose is a rose—or is it? *J Pediatr* 1992;120:79.

914. Battle DC, Hizon M, Cohen E, et al. The use of the urinary anion gap in the diagnosis of hyperchloremic metabolic acidosis. *N Engl J Med* 1988;318:594.

915. Izraeli S, Rachmel A, Frishberg Y, et al. Transient renal acidification defect during acute infantile diarrhea: the role of urinary sodium. *J Pediatr* 1990;117:711.

916. Sulyok E, Guignard JP. Relationship of urinary anion gap to urinary ammonium excretion in the neonate. *Biol Neonate* 1990;57:98.

917. Carlisle EJF, Donnelly SM, Halperin ML. Renal tubular acidosis (RTA): recognize the ammonium defect and pHorget the urine pH. *Pediatr Nephrol* 1991;5:242.

918. Rodríguez-Soriano J, Vallo A, Oliveros R, et al. Transient pseudohypoaldosteronism secondary to obstructive uropathy in infancy. *J Pediatr* 1983:103:375.

919. Svenningsen NW. Renal acid-base titration studies in infants with and without metabolic acidosis in the postneonatal period. *Pediatr Res* 1974;8:659.

920. Dubose TD Jr, Pucacco LR, Green JM. Hydrogen ion secretion by the collecting duct as a determinant of the urine to PCO_2 gradient in alkaline urine. *J Clin Invest* 1982;69:145.

921. Wrong O. Distal tubular acidosis: the value of urinary pH, pCO_2 and NH_4^+ measurements. *Pediatr Nephrol* 1991;5:249.

922. Alon U, Hellerstein S, Warady BA. Oral acetazolamide in the assessment of (urine-blood) PCO_2. *Pediatr Nephrol* 1991;5:307.

922a McSherry E. Renal tubular acidosis in childhood. *Kidney Int* 1981; 20:799.

923. Brenner RJ, Spring DB, Sebastian A, et al. Incidence of radiographically evident bone disease, nephrocalcinosis, and nephrolithiasis in various types of renal tubular acidosis. *N Engl J Med* 1982;307:217.

924. Norman ME, Feldman NI, Cohn RM, et al. Urinary citrate excretion in the diagnosis of distal renal tubular acidosis. *J Pediatr* 1978;92:394.

925. Nakai H, Byers MG, Venta PJ, et al. The gene for human carbonic anhydrase II (CA 2) is located at chromosome 8q22. *Cytogenet Cell Genet* 1987;44:234.

926. Hu PY, Lim EJ, Ciccolella SP, et al. Seven novel mutations in carbonic anhydrase II deficiency syndrome identified by SSCP and direct sequencing analysis. *Hum Mutat* 1997;9:383 [corrections 576].

927. Sly WS, Hewett-Emmett D, Whyte MP, et al. Carbonic anhydrase II deficiency identified as the primary defect in the autosomal recessive syndrome of osteopetrosis with renal tubular acidosis and cerebral calcification. *Proc Natl Acad Sci USA* 1983;80:2752.

928. Chang SS, Grunder S, Hanukoglu A, et al. Mutations in subunits of the epithelial sodium channel cause salt wasting with hyperkalaemic acidosis, pseudohypoaldosteronism type 1. *Nat Genet* 1996;12:248.

929. Strautnieks SS, Thompson RJ, Gardiner RM, et al. A novel splice-site mutation in the subunit of the epithelial sodium channel gene in three pseudohypoaldosteronism type 1 families. *Nat Genet* 1996;13:248.

930. Abramson O, Zmora E, Mazor M, et al. Pseudohypoaldosteronism in a preterm infant: intrauterine presentation as hydramnios. *J Pediatr* 1992;120:129.

931. Shalev H, Ohali M, Abramson O. Nephrocalcinosis in pseudohypoaldosteronism and the effect of indomethacin therapy. *J Pediatr* 1994;125:246.

932. Wolthers BG, Kraan GP, van der Molen JC, et al. Urinary steroid profile of a newborn suffering from pseudohypoaldosteronism. *Clin Chim Acta* 1995;236:33.

933. Tennenhouse HS, Scriver CR. X-linked hypophosphatemia: a phenotype in search of a cause. *Int J Biochem* 1992;24:685.

934. The HYP Consortium. A gene (PEX) with homologies to endopeptidases is mutated in patients with X-linked hypophosphatemic rickets. *Nat Genet* 1995;11:130.

935. Rowe PSN, Goulding J, Read A, et al. Refining the genetic map for the region flanking the X-linked hypophosphatemic rickets locus (Xp22. 1-22.2). *Hum Genet* 1994;93:291.

936. Chan JCM, Alon U, Hirschman GM. Renal hypophosphatemic rickets. *J Pediatr* 1985;106:533.

937. Reusz GS, Latta K, Hoyer PF, et al. Evidence suggesting hyperoxaluria as a cause of nephrocalcinosis in phosphate-treated hypophosphataemic rickets. *Lancet* 1990;335:1240.

938. Alon U, Donaldson DI, Hellerstein S, et al. Metabolic and histologic investigation of the nature of nephrocalcinosis in children with hypophosphatemic rickets and in the Hyp mouse. *J Pediatr* 1992; 120:899.

939. Carpenter TO, Keller M, Schwartz D, et al. Dihydroxyvitamin D supplementation corrects hyperparathyroidism and improves skeletal abnormalities in X-linked hypophosphatemic rickets—a clinical research center study. *J Clin Endocrinol Metab* 1996;81:2381.

940. Tieder M, Modai D, Samuel R, et al. Hereditary hypophosphatemic rickets with hypercalciuria. *N Engl J Med* 1985;312:611.

941. Tieder M, Modai D, Shaked U, et al. "Idiopathic" hypercalciuria and hereditary hypophosphatemic rickets. Two phenotypical expressions of a common genetic defects. *N Engl J Med* 1987;316:125.

942. Econs MJ, McEnery PT. Autosomal dominant hypophosphatemic rickets/osteomalacia: clinical characterization of a novel renal phosphate-wasting disorder. *J Clin Endocrinol Metab* 1997;82:674.

943. Delvin EE, Glorieux FH, Marie PJ, et al. Vitamin D dependency: replacement therapy with calcitriol. *J Pediatr* 1981;99:26.

944. Labuda M, Morgan K, Glorieux FH. Mapping autosomal recessive vitamin D dependency type I to chromosome 12q14 by linkage analysis. *Am J Hum Genet* 1990;47:28.

945. Brooks MH, Bell NH, Love L, et al. Vitamin-D-dependent rickets type II: resistance of target organs to 1,25-dihydroxyvitamin D. *N Engl J Med* 1978;298:996.

946. Hughes MR, Malloy PJ, Kieback DG, et al. Point mutations in the human vitamin D receptor gene associated with hypocalcemic rickets. *Science* 1988;242:1702.

947. Labuda M, Fujiwara M, Ross MV, et al. Two hereditary defects related to vitamin D metabolism map to the same region of human chromosome 12q13-14. *J Bone Miner Res* 1992;7:1447.

948. Balsan S, Garabedian M, Liberman UA, et al. Rickets and alopecia with resistance to 1,25-dihydroxyvitamin D: two different clinical courses with two different cellular defects. *J Clin Endocrinol Metab* 1983;57:803.

949. Elsas LJ, Hillman RE, Patterson JH, et al. Renal and intestinal hexose transport in familial glucose–galactose malabsorption. *J Clin Invest* 1970;49:576.

950. Horowitz L, Schwarzer S. Renal glycosuria: occurrence in two siblings and a review of the literature. *J Pediatr* 1955;47:634.

951. Turk E, Martín MG, Wright EM. Structure of the human Na$^+$/glucose cotransporter gene SGLTI. *J Biol Chem* 1994;269:15204.

952. Martín MG, Turk E, Lostao MP, et al. Defects in Na$^+$/glucose cotransporter (SGLT1) trafficking and function cause glucose-galactose malabsorption. *Nat Genet* 1996;12:216.

953. Martín MG, Turk E, Kerner C, et al. Prenatal identification of a heterozygous status in two fetuses at risk for glucose-galactose malabsorption. *Prenat Diagn* 1996;16:458.

954. Stonestreet BS, Rubin L, Pollak A, et al. Renal functions of low birth weight infants with hyperglycemia and glucosuria produced by glucose infusions. *Pediatrics* 1980;66:561.

955. Wilkins BH. Renal function in sick very low birthweight infants: 4. Glucose excretion. *Arch Dis Child* 1992;67:1162.

956. Conger JD, Falk SA. Intrarenal dynamics in the pathogenesis and prevention of acute urate nephropathy. *J Clin Invest* 1977;59:786.

957. Ahmadian Y, Lewy PR. Possible urate nephropathy of the newborn infant as a cause of transient renal insufficiency. *J Pediatr* 1977;91:96.

958. Krakoff IH, Murphy ML. Hyperuricemia in neoplastic disease in children: prevention with allopurinol, a xanthine oxidase inhibitor. *Pediatrics* 1968;41:52.

959. Pras E, Raben N, Golomb E, et al. Mutations in the SLC3A1 transporter gene in cystinuria. *Am J Hum Genet* 1995;56:1297.

960. Gasparini P, Calonge MJ, Bisceglia L, et al. Molecular genetics of cystinuria: identification of four new mutations and seven polymorphisms, and evidence for genetic heterogeneity. *Am J Hum Genet* 1995;57:781.

961. Pras E, Sood R, Raben N, et al. Genomic organization of SLC3A1, a transporter gene mutated in cystinuria. *Genomics* 1996;36:163.

962. Purroy J, Bisceglia L, Calonge MJ, et al. Genomic structure and organization of the human rBAT gene (SLC3A1). *Genomics* 1996;37:249.

963. Zhang XX, Rozen R, Hediger MA, et al. Assignment of the gene for cystinuria (SLC3A1) to human chromosome 2p21 by fluorescence in situ hybridization. *Genomics* 1994;24:413.

964. Goodyer PR, Clow C, Reade T, et al. Prospective analysis and classification of patients with cystinuria identified in a newborn screening program. *J Pediatr* 1993;122:568.

965. Calonge MJ, Volpini V, Bisceglia L, et al. Genetic heterogeneity in cystinuria: the SLC3A1 gene is linked to type I but not to type III cystinuria. *Proc Natl Acad Sci USA* 1995;92:9667.

966. Levy HL. Genetic screening. In: Harris H, Hirschhorn K, eds: *Advances in human genetics.* New York: Plenum Press, 1973;4:1.

967. Chow GK, Streem SB. Medical treatment of cystinuria: results of contemporary clinical practice. *J Urol* 1996;156:1576.

968. Albritton LM, Bowcock AM, Eddy RL, et al. The human cationic amino acid transporter [*ATRC1*]: physical and genetic mapping to 13q12-q14. *Genomics* 1992;12:430.

969. DiRocco M, Garibotto G, Rossi GA, et al. Role of haematological, pulmonary and renal complications in the long-term prognosis of patients with lysinuric protein intolerance. *Eur J Pediatr* 1993;152:437.

970. Parenti G, Sebastio G, Strisciuglio P, et al. Lysinuric protein intolerance characterized by bone marrow abnormalities and severe clinical course. *J Pediatr* 1995;126:246.

971. Mueller OT, Henry WM, Haley LL, et al. Sialidosis and galactosialidosis: Chromosomal assignment of two genes associated with neuraminidase deficiency disorders. *Proc Natl Acad Sci USA* 1985;83:1817.

972. Maroteaux P, Humbel R, Strecker G, et al. Un nouveau type de sialidose avec atteinte rénale: La néphrosialidose, 1. Etude clinique, radiologique et nosologique. *Arch Fr Pédiatr* 1978;35:819.

973. Johnson WG, Thomas GH, Miranda AF, et al. Congenital sialidosis: biochemical studies: clinical spectrum in four sibs; two successful prenatal diagnoses. *Am J Hum Genet* 1980;32:43A.

974. Fukuhara Y, Takano T, Shimmoto M, et al. A new point protection of protective protein gene in two Japanese siblings with juvenile galactosialidosis. *Brain Dysfunct* 1992;5:319.

975. Galjart NJ, Gillemans N, Harris A, et al. Expression of cDNA encoding the human "protective protein" associated with lysosomal b-galactosidase and neuraminidase: homology to yeast proteases. *Cell* 1988;54:755.

976. Kleijer WJ, Hoogeveen A, Verheijen FW, et al. Prenatal diagnosis of sialidosis with combined neuraminidase and beta-galactosidase deficiency. *Clin Genet* 1979;16:60.

977. Sewell AC, Pontz BF. Prenatal diagnosis of galactosialidosis. *Prenat Diagn* 1988;8:151.

978. Kleijer WJ, Geilen GC, Janse HC, et al. Cathepsin A deficiency in galactosialidosis: studies of patients and carriers in 16 families. *Pediatr Res* 1996;39:1067.

Congenital Nephrotic Syndrome

979. Huttunen NP. Congenital nephrotic syndrome of Finnish type: study of 75 patients. *Arch Dis Child* 1976;51:344.

980. Kestilä M, Männikkö M, Holmberg C, et al. Congenital nephrotic syndrome of the Finnish type maps to the long arm of chromosome 19. *Am J Hum Genet* 1994;54:757.

981. Männikkö M, Kestilä M, Holmberg C. Fine mapping and haplotype analysis of the locus for congenital nephrotic syndrome on chromosome 19q13.1. *Am J Hum Genet* 1995;57:1377.

982. Männikkö M, Lenkkeri U, Kashtan CE, et al. Haplotype analysis of congenital nephrotic syndrome of the Finnish type in non-Finnish families. *J Am Soc Nephrol* 1996;7:2700.

983. Norio R, Rapola J. Congenital and infantile nephrotic syndromes. In: Bartsocas CS, ed. *Genetics of kidney disorders.* New York: Alan R. Liss, 1989:179.

984. Huttunen NP, Vehaskari M, Vihikari M, et al. Proteinuria in congenital nephrotic syndrome of the Finnish type. *Clin Nephrol* 1980;13:12.

985. Mattoo TK. Hypothyroidism in infants with nephrotic syndrome. *Pediatr Nephrol* 1994;8:657.

986. Lanning P, Uhari P, Koulavainen K, et al. Ultrasonic features of the congenital nephrotic syndrome of the Finnish type. *Acta Paediatr Scand* 1989;78:717.

987. Bratton VS, Ellis EN, Seibert JT. Ultrasonographic findings in congenital nephrotic syndrome. *Pediatr Nephrol* 1990;4:515.

988. Autio-Harmainen H, Rapola J. The thickness of the glomerular basement membrane in congenital nephrotic syndrome of the Finnish type. *Nephron* 1983;34:48.

989. Rapola J, Sariola H, Ekblom P. Pathology of fetal congenital nephrosis: immunohistochemical and ultrastructural studies. *Kidney Int* 1984;25:701.

990. Laine J, Jalanko H. Holthöfer H, et al. Post-transplantation nephrosis in congenital nephrotic syndrome of the Finnish type. *Kidney Int* 1993;44:867.

991. Pomeranz A, Wolach B, Bernheim J, et al. Successful treatment of Finnish congenital nephrotic syndrome with captopril and indomethacin. *J Pediatr* 1995;126:140.

992. Habib R, Loirat C, Gubler MC, et al. The nephropathy associated with male pseudohermaphroditism and Wilms' tumor (Drash syndrome): a distinctive glomerular lesion—report of 10 cases. *Clin Nephrol* 1985;24:269.

993. Garty BZ, Eisenstein B, Sandbank J, et al. Microcephaly and congenital nephrotic syndrome owing to diffuse mesangial sclerosis: an autosomal recessive syndrome. *J Med Genet* 1994;31:121.

994. Cooperstone BG, Friedman A, Kaplan BS. Galloway-Mowat syndrome of abnormal gyral patterns and glomerulopathy. *Am J Med Genet* 1993;47:250.

995. Hofstaetter C, Neumann I, Lennert T, et al. Prenatal diagnosis of diffuse mesangial glomerulosclerosis by ultrasonography: a longitudinal study of a case in an affected family. *Fetal Diagn Ther* 1996;11:126.

996. Wiggelinkhuizen J, Kaschula ROC, Uys CJ, et al. Congenital syphilis and glomerulonephritis with evidence for immune pathogenesis. *Arch Dis Child* 1973;48:375.

997. Papaioannou AC, Asrow GG, Schuckmell NH. Nephrotic syndrome in early infancy as a manifestation of congenital syphilis. *Pediatrics* 1961;27:636.

998. Shahin B, Papadopoupou ZL, Jenis EH. Congenital nephrotic syndrome associated with congenital toxoplasmosis. *J Pediatr* 1974; 85:366.

999. Couvreur J, Alison F, Coccon-Gibod L, et al. Rein et toxoplasmose. *Ann Pediatr (Paris)* 1984;31:847.

1000. Amir G, Hurvitz H, Neeman Z, et al. Neonatal cytomegalovirus infection with pancreatic cystadenoma and nephrotic syndrome. *Pediatr Pathol* 1986;6:393.

1001. Batisky D, Roy S III, Gaber LW. Congenital nephrosis and neonatal cytomegalovirus infection: a clinical association. *Pediatr Nephrol* 1993;7:741.

1002. Shapiro LR, Duncan PA, Farnsworth PB, et al. Congenital microcephaly, hiatus hernia and nephrotic syndrome: an autosomal recessive syndrome. *Birth Defects* 1976;12:275.

1003. Robain O, Deonna T. Pachygyria and congenital nephrosis disorder of migration and neuronal orientation. *Acta Neuropathol* 1983;60:137.

1004. Palm L, Hägerstrand I, Kristofferssen U, et al. Nephrogenesis and disturbances of neuronal migration in male siblings: a new hereditary disorder? *Arch Dis Child* 1986;61:545.

1005. van der Knaap MS, Wevers RA, Monnens L, et al. Congenital nephrotic syndrome: a novel phenotype of type I carbohydrate-deficient glycoprotein syndrome. *J Inherit Metab Dis* 1996;19:787.

1006. Lagrue G, Branellec A, Niaudet P, et al. Transmission of nephrotic syndrome to two neonates: spontaneous regression. *Presse Med* 1991;20:255.

1007. Similä S, Vesa L, Wasz-Höckert O. Hereditary onycho-osteodysplasis (the nail-patella syndrome) with nephrosis-like renal disease in a newborn boy. *Pediatrics* 1970;46:61.

1008. Ty A, Fine B. Membranous nephritis in infantile systemic lupus erythematosus associated with chromosomal abnormalities. *Clin Nephrol* 1979;12:137.

1009. Massengill SF, Richard GA, Donnelly WH. Infantile systemic lupus erythematosus with onset simulating congenital nephrotic syndrome. *J Pediatr* 1994;124:27.

Hematuria and Proteinuria

1010. Halvorsen S, Aas K. Observation on the urine of asphyxiated and dysmature newborn infants. *Acta Paediatr* 1962;51:417.

1011. Emmanuel B, Aronson N. Neonatal hematuria. *Am J Dis Child* 1974;208:204.

1012. Cramer A, Steele A, Wishne P, et al. Transient hematuria in premature and sick neonates. *Pediatr Res* 1981;15:692.

1013. Thullen JD, Fanaroff AA, Makker SP. Renal manifestations of perinatal asphyxia. *Pediatr Res* 1979;13:380.

1014. Seibert JJ, Taylor BJ, Williamson SL, et al. Sonographic detection of neonatal umbilical-artery thrombosis: clinical correlation. *AJR* 1987;148:965.

1015. Chesney RW, Kaplan BS, Freedom RM, et al. Acute renal failure: an important complication of cardiac surgery in infants. *J Pediatr* 1975;87:381.

1016. Pillion G, Sonsino E, Beaufils F. Insuffisance rénale aiguë du nouveau-né. *J Annu Pédiatr (Paris)* 1982;29.

1017. Willis J, Duncan C, Gottschalk S. Paraplegia due to peripheral venous air embolus in a neonate: a case report. *Pediatrics* 1981;67: 472.

1018. Kalia A, Travis LB, Brouhard BH. The association of idiopathic hypercalciuria and asymptomatic gross hematuria in children. *J Pediatr* 1981;99:716.

1019. Linshaw MA, Stapleton FB, Cuppage FE, et al. Hypocomplementemic glomerulonephritis in an infant and mother: evidence for an abnormal form of C_3. *Am J Nephrol* 1987;7:470.

1020. Miltényi M, Pohlandt F, Boka G, et al. Tubular proteinuria after perinatal hypoxia. *Acta Paediatr Scand* 1981;70:399.

CHAPTER 43

Structural Abnormalities of the Genitourinary System

George W. Kaplan and Irene M. McAleer

A discussion of neonatal pediatric urology in essence encompasses most of pediatric urology. Admittedly, there are age-specific problems that do not present in early infancy, but there are many more problems that present primarily or specifically in the neonatal months. It is these latter lesions on which this discussion will focus. The development of antenatal ultrasonography over the past two decades has had a profound effect on detection, management, and understanding of many lesions of the urinary tract. Genitourinary anomalies account for approximately 50% of all antenatally sonographically detected lesions; hydronephrosis represents about two-thirds of these genitourinary abnormalities (1). Information from ultrasonography can be further amplified with fetal bladder urine specimen measurements of electrolytes, osmolality, and beta$_2$-microglobulin. *In utero* surgical therapy now is also possible with improved fetal surgical techniques, although the benefits derived from fetal surgery are not clear (2).

To properly understand and interpret the symptoms and findings that are seen in most urologic problems, an understanding of the significant events of embryogenesis of the lesions seen is essential. Abnormalities of embryogenesis will be addressed as the resulting lesions are covered.

The ureteral bud arises from the mesonephric duct at 4 to 5 weeks of gestation, the kidney begins to form at 6 weeks, and the bladder develops during the sixth to seventh week. The wolffian duct is then incorporated into the bladder (Fig. 43–1). It is not until week 10 of gestation that urine production begins, and it is usually not until 14 to 16 weeks of gestation that the urinary tract is evident on antenatal ultrasonography (3). A number of anomalies may result from disordered embryogenesis of the ureter or kidney. Although some of the abnormalities are familial and others are related to chromosomal abnormalities, most seem to be sporadic in occurrence.

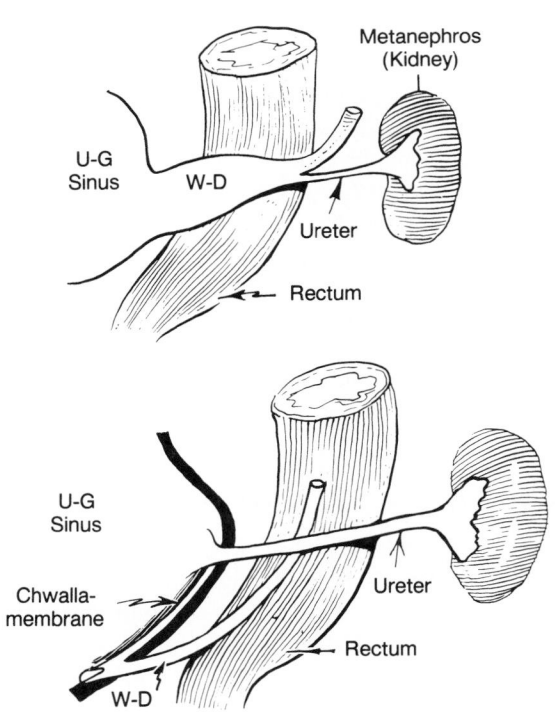

FIG. 43–1. Incorporation of the wolffian (i.e., mesonephric) duct (W-D) into the urogenital sinus (U-G). (From Kelalis PP, King LR, Belman AB, eds. *Clinical pediatric urology, vol. 1.* Philadelphia: WB Saunders, 1976:504.)

G. W. Kaplan: Department of Surgery and Pediatrics, School of Medicine, University of California, San Diego; and Division of Urology, Children's Hospital, San Diego, California

I. M. McAleer: Department of Surgery, School of Medicine, University of California, San Diego; and Division of Urology, Children's Hospital, San Diego, California

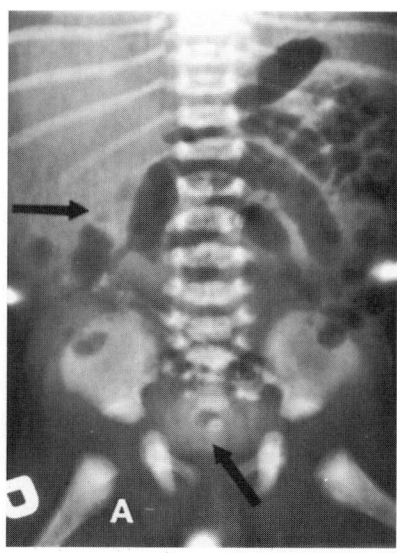 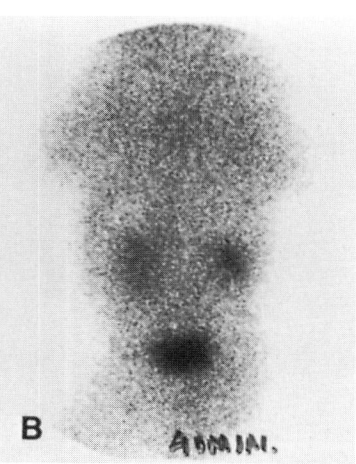

FIG. 43–2. A: An excretory urogram in a newborn infant. The right kidney barely concentrates contrast (*arrow*); there is no evidence of the left kidney. Contrast is apparent in the bladder (*arrow*). **B:** An isotope renal scan the next day demonstrates the presence and function of two kidneys. The child was normal.

IMAGING

The overall incidence of detection of fetal anomalies is currently about 1%. Urologic diagnostic imaging in the fetus, the newborn, and, to some extent, in the infant, is limited by the renal function (see Fig. 43–1). Even though renal functional parameters may be sufficient to maintain homeostasis, they may not suffice to produce the accuracy of diagnosis that would be expected from some imaging examinations when used in older children and adults.

Ultrasonography and voiding cystourethrography are not dependent on renal function and, hence, assume even greater diagnostic import than in other age groups. Improved ultrasonographic equipment, resolution, and techniques are identifying fetal anomalies with accuracy closer to imaging techniques used in children and adults. Intravenous urography and, to a lesser extent, renal scintigraphy depend on renal function to produce images and consequently may be less reliable than in the adult; newer scintigraphic agents have made evaluation of the neonatal kidneys more reproducible and reliable (Fig. 43–2).

ANOMALIES OF THE KIDNEY

With normal embryogenesis as background, the anomalies and problems that are likely to be encountered can be anticipated, because most have an embryologic basis. Some are incompatible with life, some may lead to an early demise, some are of no clinical significance, but most are potential sources of morbidity that can be minimized if the children are treated at an early age.

Renal anomalies include the cystic diseases as well as abnormalities of number, position, and rotation. If the pronephros fails to develop, the mesonephros will not develop, resulting in renal and ureteral agenesis and absence of the ipsilateral genital ducts in the male. If the mesonephric duct develops but the mesonephros does not, there will be renal agenesis but the genital ducts will be present and there might be a blind-ending ureter.

Because nephrogenesis is induced by the ureter, normal nephrogenesis depends on the ureteral bud meeting normal metanephrogenic blastema (4). Should the ureter fail to do so, a blind-ending ureter might result. If the ureter meets a degenerating portion of the metanephrogenic blastema (i.e., the cephalic or caudal end of the blastema), renal dysplasia might result (4).

Renal Agenesis

Renal agenesis can be unilateral or bilateral. Bilateral renal agenesis obviously is incompatible with extrauterine life. In cases of bilateral renal agenesis, there is no *in utero* urine production; thus, there is marked oligohydramnios and the affected fetus may exhibit the deformational changes of Potter syndrome (5). Because adequate amniotic fluid is required for normal lung development, the lungs may be hypoplastic. The incidence of bilateral renal agenesis is roughly 1 in 4,000 to 5,000 births (5). Renal agenesis sometimes may be associated with sirenomelia (5). Bilateral renal agenesis can be diagnosed antenatally by a combination of sonographic findings that include lack of identifiable renal masses, absent bladder, and severe oligohydramnios (3). For reasons that are unclear, some infants with this diagnosis have normal or near-normal levels of amniotic fluid. Renal agenesis must be considered postnatally when Potter facies are noted, when there is no urinary output within 24 to 48 hours, or when there is evidence of ventilatory failure with small lungs on chest radiograph. The postnatal diagnosis can be confirmed ultrasonographically by the absence of identifiable kidneys as well as the absence of urine in the bladder. Renal scintigraphy can prove that there are no identifiable functioning renal units. When the postnatal diagnosis of bilateral renal agenesis is made and confirmed, attempts at life support, which may have been initiated because of respiratory distress, should, in our opinion, be abandoned.

The incidence of unilateral renal agenesis is roughly 1 in 500 to 1,500 (5,6). There is a higher incidence of contralateral renal abnormality in patients with unilateral renal agenesis when compared to the general population, and many of these may be obstructive or refluxing in nature. One-third of the patients with a solitary kidney in one series required some form of surgical procedure on the solitary unit (7). Unilateral renal agenesis also is associated with congenital scoliosis as well as with vaginal and uterine agenesis (8,9). It is the most common nonskeletal anomaly seen with imperforate anus (10). Unilateral renal agenesis previously was not thought to affect longevity or health as long as the contralateral kidney was normal. Recent experimental studies have suggested that renal injury may be produced in the solitary kidney by hyperfiltration and that a reduced protein diet may be somewhat protective. Clinical studies of patients with a solitary kidney (e.g., transplant donors, trauma victims) have, at this point, failed to confirm this (11).

Renal Ectopia and Fusion

Failure of renal ascent will result in a pelvic kidney and may be associated with vaginal or vertebral anomalies (8). If the two metanephrogenic masses come into contact with each other in the pelvis, they may fuse and form a pancake or a horseshoe kidney (9). The embryogenesis of crossed ectopia, with or without fusion, is harder to explain but might result from lateral bending and rotation of the tail bud of the embryo, thereby altering the course of ascent (9).

Renal malrotation, or incomplete rotation, occurs when the kidney, as it ascends, maintains its early fetal orientation in which the renal pelvis is directed anteriorly. Malrotation is present routinely in fusion anomalies and in pelvic and crossed ectopias, and occasionally is seen in kidneys located in the renal fossa. It is of no clinical significance but does introduce difficulties in interpretation of some imaging studies; occasionally it is of surgical import in planning reconstructive procedures.

Abnormalities of renal position (i.e., ectopia) are interesting anomalies that, in themselves, are of no clinical import but may become apparent because of trauma (i.e., hematuria), a palpable mass, or associated urologic abnormality. The ectopic kidney may be located in the chest or the pelvis. Thoracic kidneys usually are associated with eventration of the diaphragm and are of no clinical significance except as a finding on a chest radiograph (12). Pelvic ectopia is the most common of the

abnormalities of position and often is associated with vesicoureteral reflux or ureteropelvic junction obstruction (13). In addition, girls with müllerian anomalies have an increased incidence of pelvic kidney compared to the general population; hence, the finding of a pelvic kidney in a girl warrants further investigation of the genital tract to uncover associated anomalies (14).

Fusion anomalies, such as horseshoe or pancake kidneys, may present in the same way that anomalies of position present. Horseshoe kidneys are found with increased frequency in girls with Turner syndrome (15). There is an increased incidence of ureteropelvic junction obstruction in horseshoe kidneys (13). Some patients with horseshoe kidneys may have increased stone formation due to relative urinary stasis with drainage from the nondependent renal pelvis. Crossed ectopia with or without fusion (i.e., one kidney is found on the opposite side of the side of ureteral bud development) is uncommon. When crossed ectopia occurs, the left kidney more commonly crosses to the right side than vice versa (16). By definition, the ipsilateral ureteral orifice is located on the anatomically appropriate side of the body (i.e., the left ureter is on the left side of the trigone and the right ureter is on the right side of the trigone). There is an increased incidence of vesicoureteral reflux and of ureteropelvic junction obstruction in crossed ectopic kidneys (13). Patients with crossed ectopia have an increased incidence of skeletal and cardiac abnormalities (10).

Supernumerary Kidney

The presence of a supernumerary (i.e., third) renal mass is a very rare anomaly, the clinical significance of which is determined by any associated pathologic condition (17). The supernumerary kidney usually is small, and more often caudal than cranial to the normally placed kidney. Many patients and some physicians confuse a supernumerary kidney with a duplication of the collecting system and commonly, but incorrectly, refer to ureteral duplication as a third kidney.

Cystic Disease

Renal cystic diseases are a group of disorders seen in pediatric urologic practice that sometimes will present in the neonatal period. Because there is no uniform system of classification, there can be difficulty in communication between disciplines. An accurate diagnosis is needed for prognosis and for genetic counseling. It is for this reason that communication must be clear. Table 43–1 is a classification scheme that has been of some clinical utility in our practice.

Autosomal recessive polycystic kidney disease, as the name implies, is an inherited disorder whose mode of transmission follows a mendelian recessive pattern. Its

TABLE 43–1. *Classification of renal cystic disease*

Polycystic Disease
    Autosomal recessive
    Autosomal dominant
Renal Cortical Cysts in Hereditary Syndromes
    Tuberous sclerosis
    von Hippel–Lindau disease
    Meckel syndrome
    Zellweger cerebrohepatorenal syndrome
    Jeune asphyxiating thoracic dysplasia
    Syndromes of multiple malformations that include cortical cysts
Renal Medullary Cysts
    Familial juvenile nephronophthisis
    Medullary cystic disease
    Renal retinal dysplasia
    Medullary sponge disease
Renal Dysplasia
    Multicystic kidney disease
    Other cystic dysplasias
    Multilocular mesoblastic nephroma
Other Cystic Diseases
    Simple cysts, single or multiple
    Unilateral segmental cystic disease

reported incidence is between 1 in 6,000 to 1 in 14,000 pregnancies. In this disorder, formerly known as infantile polycystic disease, the kidneys are very large and often occupy the entire retroperitoneum (Fig. 43–3). The cysts in this disorder are small and, in reality, are enlargements of the collecting ducts (18). The liver almost always is abnormal. At times there will be periportal hepatic fibro-

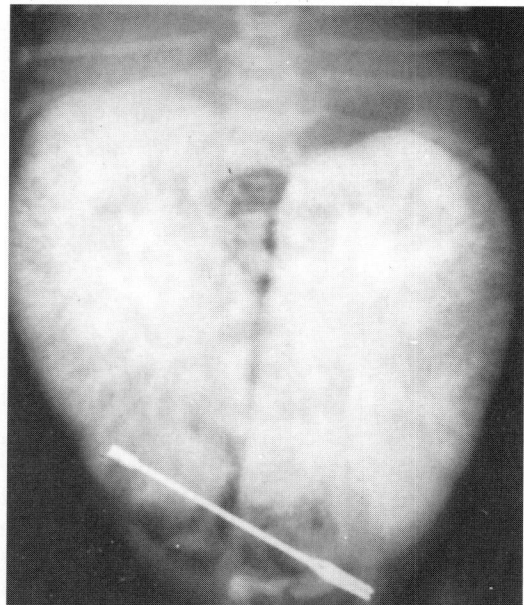

FIG. 43–3. An excretory urogram in a 2-day-old girl with infantile polycystic kidney disease shows the sunray appearance of the contrast material and the enormous renal size. (From Kelalis PP, King LR, Belman AB, eds. *Clinical pediatric urology, vol. 2.* Philadelphia: WB Saunders, 1976:686.)

sis as a significant part of this complex. Death in the neonatal period is secondary to either renal or pulmonary failure. Those who survive the neonatal period usually will exhibit decreased renal function and hypertension, but at times liver failure due to hepatic fibrosis may be the most prominent part of the clinical picture (19). Imaging studies such as antenatal or postnatal ultrasonography and intravenous urography usually are diagnostic.

Autosomal dominant polycystic kidney disease is inherited in a mendelian dominant fashion and is more common than the recessive form. However, it usually does not present until adult life, hence its former name, adult polycystic disease. These patients usually present with hypertension, hematuria, urinary tract infection, or renal failure. When this problem presents in childhood, it may do so as an abdominal mass or may be found with ultrasound as either antenatal evaluation, screening for polycystic disease, or by coincidence when ultrasound is being obtained for some other evaluation. Imaging studies will prove diagnostic, because multiple large cysts that splay and distort the collecting system will be present. Although there often are associated hepatic cysts, liver failure is not usually a clinical feature of this disorder. Microdissection studies have shown that the cysts are due to abnormal branching of the collecting tubules and cystic dilations of portions of the nephron (20). Detectable cysts may not develop in affected people until middle to late adult life, however; the disease is undetectable clinically until they appear.

Tuberous sclerosis can mimic both autosomal recessive and autosomal dominant polycystic disease in that lesions grossly similar to either form of polycystic disease can be found in the tuberous sclerosis complex (21). Microscopically, lesions characteristic of tuberous sclerosis will be seen on biopsy of the affected kidneys. Angiomyolipomas (i.e., renal hamartomas), however, are the more usual renal lesion in patients with tuberous sclerosis.

Multicystic kidney disease, with a frequency of 1 in 3,000 pregnancies (7), is the most common form of cystic disease seen in neonates. As originally defined by Spence et al. (22), this is a unilateral lesion in which the entire kidney is replaced by cysts of varying sizes. Grossly, there is no recognizable renal tissue present, but microscopically there may be dysplastic renal elements in the septa between the cysts (Fig. 43–4). Bilateral multicystic kidney disease is incompatible with life. Multicystic kidney disease is sporadic and is not inherited. Some multicystic kidneys involute, probably by absorption of the cyst fluid. This can occur antenatally or in the first few months of life. It is likely that many cases of presumed renal agenesis are multicystic kidneys that have undergone involution. Multicystic kidneys usually are detectable with antenatal ultrasonography but they occasionally present during infancy as palpable masses. Ultrasonography will demonstrate multiple, different-sized cysts in a random pattern (Fig. 43–5), and there usually is

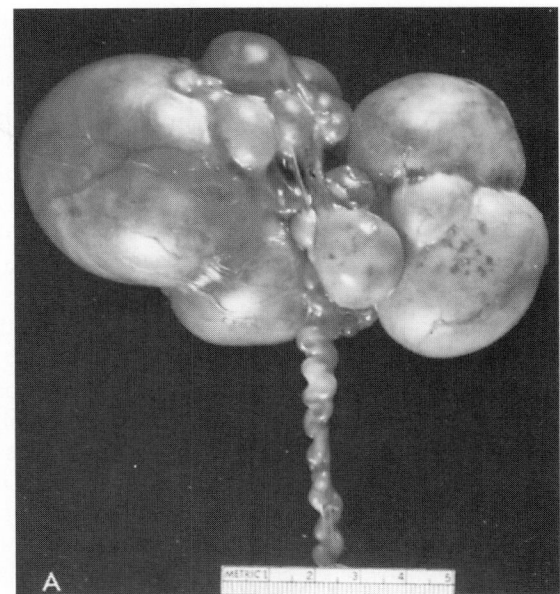

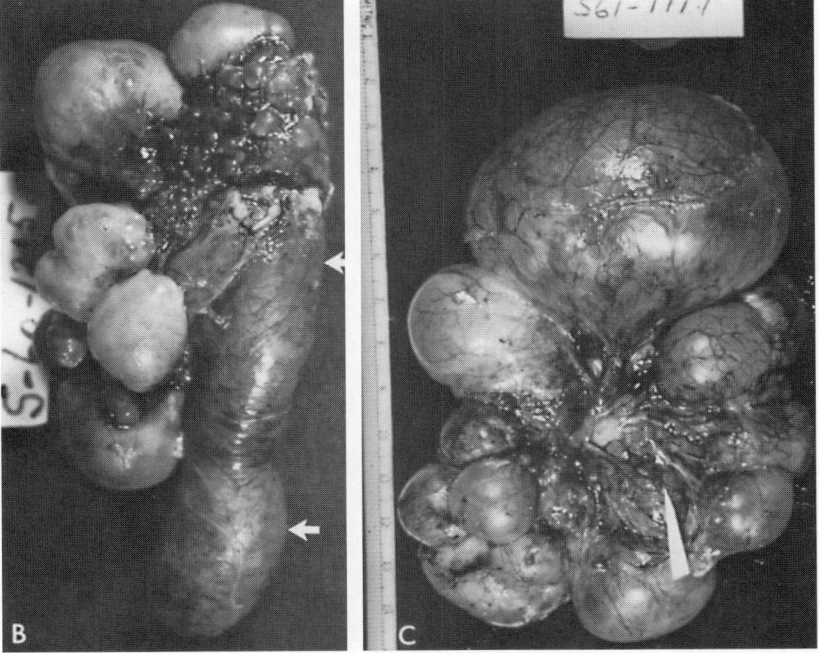

FIG. 43–4. Three examples of the variety of multicystic diseases. **A:** Multicystic kidney with a torturous atretic ureter. The cysts vary in size and appear to be held together by fibrous tissue. **B:** Multicystic kidney in a 1-month-old girl. The dilated pelvis and proximal ureter are indicated (*arrows*). **C:** Multicystic kidney in a 4-day-old girl. No ureter was found during the nephrectomy. (From Kelalis PP, King LR, Belman AB, eds. *Clinical pediatric urology, vol. 2.* Philadelphia: WB Saunders, 1976:210.)

no function noted on renal scan or intravenous urography. There is a great deal of controversy surrounding the management of these lesions; traditional therapy had been nephrectomy, but many pediatric urologists advocate observation because the incidence of sequelae such as infection, pain, hypertension, or malignancy is very low. Nephrectomy seems a reasonable alternative to lifelong

follow-up, however, and is our current recommendation if the kidney does not completely involute within 6 to 12 months. At the present time, a Multicystic Kidney Registry is collecting data on these kidneys in cases that are followed with observation. Roughly 25% of the patients with multicystic kidney disease have an obstructive lesion such as ureteropelvic junction obstruction on the

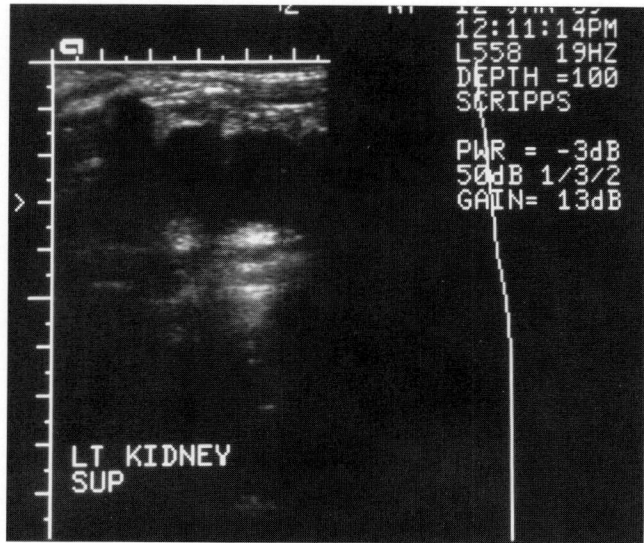

FIG. 43–5. An abdominal ultrasonographic study carried out in an infant with multicystic (i.e., cystic dysplastic) kidney.

contralateral side, and it is this fact that will determine the patient's ultimate prognosis. Since the inception of the Multicystic Kidney Registry, vesicoureteral reflux has been found to be more common than obstruction (23).

ANOMALIES OF THE URETERS AND BLADDER

Duplication and Triplication of the Ureters

Multiple ureteral buds or premature division of the ureteral bud could produce ureteral duplication or tripli-

cation (24). If there are multiple ureteral buds, one bud is likely to meet degenerating rather than normal nephrogenic tissue. This could account for the increased incidence of renal dysplasia in the upper pole of a duplicated system (4). Duplication of the urinary collecting system is one of the more common abnormalities seen in the urinary tract; its occurrence is about 0.8% (24). Duplication can be either complete or incomplete. Incomplete duplication usually is of no clinical significance, although, rarely, there can be ureteroureteral reflux between the two limbs of the partial duplication that can result in dilation of one of the moieties, usually the lower one. Complete duplication occurs once in every 500 cases (24). Complete duplication by itself is of no clinical significance, but it is associated with a higher incidence of other abnormalities in the urinary system. These abnormalities include both vesicoureteral reflux and obstruction.

Vesicoureteral reflux probably is the more common of the anomalies associated with ureteral duplication and usually occurs into the lower moiety of a duplicated system (Fig. 43–6). Duplication is seen in approximately one in five people with vesicoureteral reflux, which is much higher than its incidence in the general population (26). The grade of reflux associated with a complete duplication usually is greater than that seen with a single system. When the upper moiety of a complete duplication is abnormal, obstruction is the more common abnormality. Both obstruction and vesicoureteral reflux associated with duplications may present as either mass lesions or urosepsis; many of these are diagnosed *in utero*, with hydronephrosis seen in the upper or lower segments of the duplicated systems.

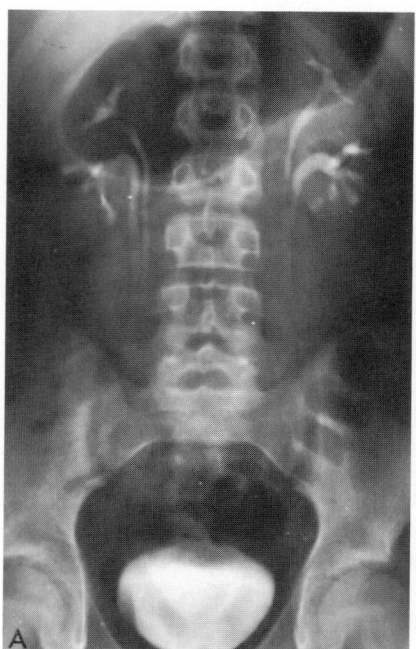
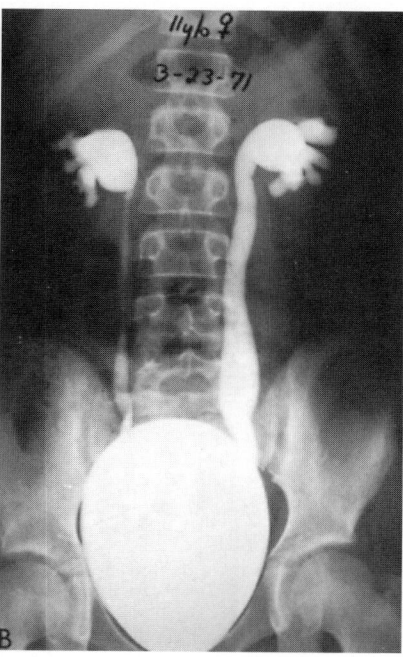

FIG. 43–6. A: An intravenous urogram in a girl with complete, bilateral duplication of the collecting system. Note the blunting of the lower calyces. **B:** A cystogram in the same child demonstrates reflux into both lower collecting systems only. (From Belman AB. The clinical significance of vesicoureteral reflux. *Pediatr Clin North Am* 1976;23:707.)

If the ureteral bud arises from a locus that is more cranial or caudal than normal, ureteral ectopia, vesicoureteral reflux, or paraureteral diverticula might be produced (27). Ectopic ureteroceles probably result from abnormalities of the ureteral bud as well as ureteral ectopia (28). Simple ureteroceles are thought to be produced by persistence of the Chwalla membrane (i.e., the membrane covering the distal end of the ureter during development) (29).

Ureteral obstructions occur primarily at the ureteropelvic and ureterovesical junctions. These obstructions usually are intrinsic in nature, and the ureter may be of normal or reduced caliber externally (30,31). Multicystic kidney disease has been said to result from ureteral obstruction early in gestation but, in our opinion, is more likely to be secondary to disordered induction of the metanephrogenic mass by a faulty ureteral bud (32).

Bladder Anomalies

Agenesis of the bladder could result if the allantoic stalk failed to develop (33). It also could occur if there was bilateral failure of ureteral migration with bilateral ureteral ectopia, because migration of the ureters is necessary for formation of the trigone, which, in turn, might be necessary for enlargement of the allantoic stalk (34). Urachal anomalies occur because of a general mesodermal failure, as in the prune-belly syndrome, or because of delayed closure of the urachus (35). Duplications of the bladder and urethra often are associated with duplications of the hindgut and lower spinal cord. Hence, it would seem that splitting of the hind end of the embryo might be responsible for this type of anomaly (36).

Posterior urethral valves probably result from abnormal insertion and persistence of the mesonephric ducts distal to the Müllerian tubercle (type I), or from persistence of the cloacal membrane (type III) (37). Type II valves probably do not exist as an obstructing lesion (see Fig. 43–17).

Ureteral Ectopia

Ureteral ectopia exists when the ureter opens in a position other than its normal location at the corner of the trigone. Ectopia may occur in ureters of single or duplex kidneys (Fig. 43–7). The most common form of ureteral ectopia is lateral ureteral ectopia in which the ureteral orifice lies within the bladder lateral to its normal position. This is the etiologic mechanism for primary vesicoureteral reflux (see Vesicoureteral Reflux). Significant medial or distal ureteral ectopia is less common than lateral ureteral ectopia and causes clinical pathologic conditions that vary depending on the location of the ureteral orifice and the gender of the patient. An abnormal proximal budding locus on the mesonephric duct allows the ureteral bud to remain in prolonged contact with the wolffian duct so that the medially ectopic ureteral orifice may open anywhere along the course of the wolffian duct (Fig. 43–8). In males, this

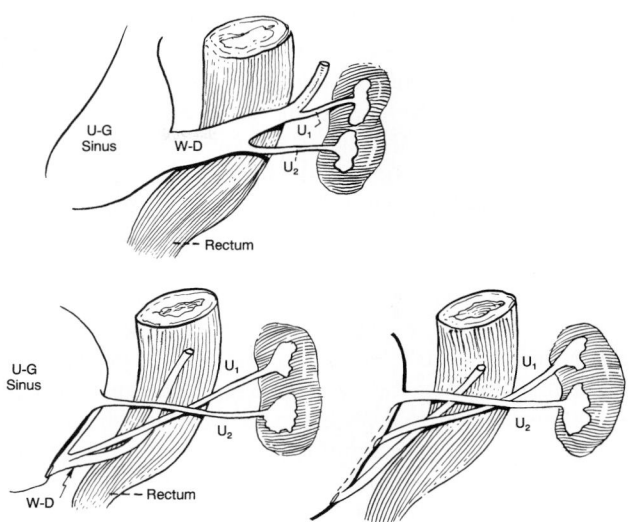

FIG. 43–7. Development of ectopic ureter. U, ureter; U-G, urogenital; W-D, wolffian duct. (From Kelalis PP, King LR, Belman AB, eds. *Clinical pediatric urology, vol. 1.* Philadelphia: WB Saunders, 1976:510.)

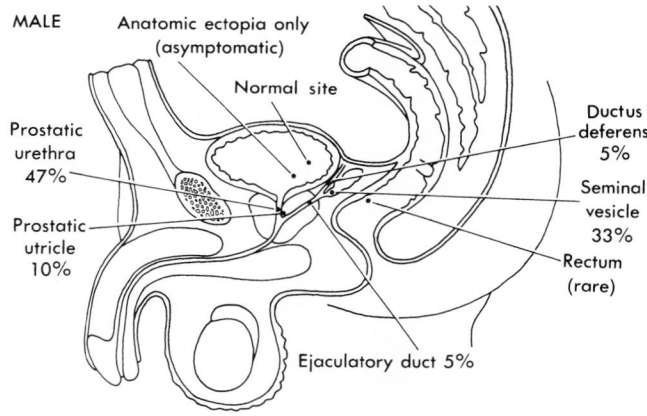

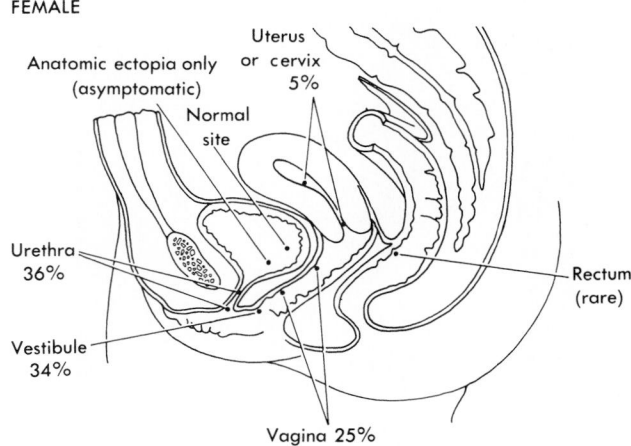

FIG. 43–8. Sites of ectopic ureteral orifices and their relative frequencies of occurrence in men and women. (From Gray SW, Skandalakis JE. *Embryology for surgeons.* Philadelphia: WB Saunders, 1972:536.)

includes the posterior urethra, seminal vesicles, vas deferens, or epididymis (38). In females, the ectopic ureter may open into the urethra, the uterus, or proximal vagina, or anywhere along the course of the Gartner duct in the anterolateral wall of the vagina. If a medially ectopic ureter opens within the confines of the bladder, no clinical abnormality occurs. If, however, the ureter opens within the confines of the bladder neck mechanism, obstruction of the involved renal unit or vesicoureteral reflux may occur.

In females, ectopic ureteral orifices that lie distal to the internal sphincter mechanism of the bladder neck can cause incontinence (39). Older girls usually present with constant dampness that is associated with an otherwise symptom-free, normal voiding pattern. Infant girls may be constantly wet or have a purulent discharge if the system is infected. Physical examination suggests the diagnosis if urine can be seen to well up in the vagina or if a spurt of urine is seen coming from the perineal ectopic ureteral orifice. Many are not diagnosed by physical findings alone. Eighty percent of these ectopic ureters arise from the upper pole segment of a total ureteral duplication, and diuretic renography with radionuclide agents frequently will better delineate the anatomy. Occasionally, intravenous urography also may suggest the diagnosis (39). Because the ectopic segment in these patients frequently functions poorly, it may not be visible on excretory urography despite the use of delayed radiographs. A high index of suspicion and an awareness of the radiographic clues to a nonvisible duplication (i.e., the drooping lily sign) often will lead to the diagnosis (Fig. 43–9). Because an ectopic

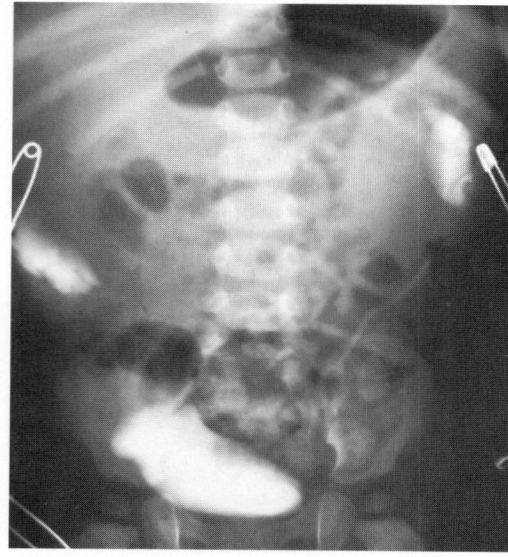

FIG. 43–9. Excretory urogram in an infant with ureteral duplication. Ectopic ureters from upper segments produced massive displacement of lower segments, leading to a misdiagnosis of abdominal mass and neuroblastoma. (From Kelalis PP, King LR, Belman AB, eds. *Clinical pediatric urology, vol. 1.* Philadelphia: WB Saunders, 1976:518.)

vaginal ureter may drain a poorly functioning and thus nonvisualizable single renal unit, congenital absence of one kidney in a girl with incontinence must not be accepted as a diagnosis without a thorough investigation that should include abdominal sonography, nuclear renal scan, and occasionally computed tomography (40).

Treatment of the ectopic ureter depends on the presence or absence of significant function in the involved renal unit. If the ureter drains an otherwise healthy system, ureteral reimplantation into the bladder will correct the problem and preserve maximal renal function. If the ureteral anomaly is associated with a duplex kidney and there is good function in both segments of the kidney, ipsilateral ureteroureterostomy is indicated. In the more usual case in which the involved renal unit functions poorly, excision of the involved segment is indicated. The distal ureteral stump is left undisturbed to avoid compromise of the normal sphincter mechanisms. The male infant with an ectopic ureter more frequently presents with a mass, urinary tract infection, or epididymitis (38). In boys, an ectopic ureter will arise more frequently from a nonduplicated kidney and can drain into the male genital tract anywhere from the prostatic urethra to the epididymis. Treatment is similar to that in females.

Ureterocele

A ureterocele is a cystic dilation of the distal submucosal or intravesical portion of a ureter. Ureteroceles account for a broad spectrum of associated or secondary pathologic conditions and constitute one of the more complex and confusing groups of anomalies of the lower urinary tract (41).

Ureteroceles in children most commonly involve the end of the upper pole ureter of a duplex kidney (i.e., ectopic ureterocele), but may less commonly involve a single-system ureter (i.e., simple ureterocele) (42). The etiology of ureteroceles is uncertain. Failure of reabsorption of the Chwalla membrane from over the ureteral orifice has been proposed as an obstructive etiology (29). It seems more likely that ureteroceles result from an intrinsic defect in the ureteral bud itself, and from faulty or delayed incorporation of the ureteral bud into the urethra and bladder base (39).

Ureteroceles associated with a single-system ureter (i.e., simple ureteroceles) tend to be intravesical and in the normal position. Intravesical ureteroceles in children often are associated with hydronephrosis of varying degrees (43).

Ureteroceles may be associated with significant derangement of the upper and lower urinary tract. Because the ureterocele most commonly associated with secondary pathology originates from the upper pole ureter of a duplex kidney, the most frequently noted associated pathologic condition is hydronephrosis and impaired function of the upper pole system and obstruction or reflux in the ipsilateral lower pole system (Fig. 43–10). Contralateral reflux or obstruction also may occur. The pathophysiology of the associated findings is understood easily when it is recognized that a ureterocele may dissect under the trigonal epithelium and cause deformity of the ipsilateral or contralateral ureterovesical junction, causing various combinations of vesicoureteral reflux or obstruction in any or all of the ureters (44). Ten percent of ureteroceles occur bilaterally (41). If the ureterocele prolapses into, or otherwise occludes, the bladder outlet, bilateral hydronephrosis and relative bladder outlet obstruction may occur. The upper pole system associated with a ureterocele frequently is minimally functional and may show evidence of dysplasia on microscopic evaluation.

Ureteroceles occur more commonly in females and usually manifest in early childhood; the ratio of occurrence in males and females is 1:6 cases (41). One-third of our patients have presented during the first year of life. Many of these are now diagnosed antenatally with ultrasound but, historically, the most common presentation was that of a febrile infant found to have a urinary tract infection. If the ureterocele prolapses into the urethra, difficult voiding or azotemia may prompt evaluation. Ureterocele is the most common cause of urinary retention in the female infant. Rarely, a ureterocele will prolapse through the external urethral meatus in a female and present as an introital mass.

In the classic situation, the diagnosis of a ureterocele should be fairly straightforward. Renal and bladder ultrasonography will reveal the upper tract dilation and the

wall of the ureterocele in the bladder (45). This can be seen antenatally. The intravenous urogram most commonly reveals an ipsilateral complete ureteral duplication and upper pole hydronephrosis coupled with the characteristic lucency of the ureterocele in the bladder. Cystography is necessary to establish the presence or absence of associated vesicoureteral reflux and to assess the integrity of the detrusor muscle backing the ureterocele. A diuretic renal scan can outline the function of the involved upper pole segment as well as any measurable obstruction of any of the segments and is helpful in determining the best surgical approach.

The choice of treatment of a ureterocele depends on several factors. The age and clinical condition of the patient, the presence or absence of significant function in the involved renoureteral unit, and the presence of reflux or obstruction in the ipsilateral or contralateral uninvolved ureters all influence the choice of therapy. In the critically ill, septic infant, transurethral or transvesical unroofing or puncture of the ureterocele may provide decompression and allow stabilization of the child until his or her clinical condition allows definitive treatment. Alternatively, placement of a temporary percutaneous nephrostomy into the involved renal unit often can be done without the need for general anesthesia. The best form of definitive treatment has been debated over the years. If an intravesical ureterocele is associated with a single kidney and minimal hydronephrosis, simple excision of the ureterocele and reimplantation of the involved ureter may suffice. Even if the system is duplex, an *en bloc* ureteral reimplantation can be performed if the ureters are not too dilated (41).

Generally, definitive management of the hydronephrotic upper tract associated with a ureterocele depends on the function of the obstructed segment. If sufficient function exists in the involved unit, pyeloureterostomy or ureteroureterostomy to the ipsilateral uninvolved unit is appropriate (41). In the most common situation, however, function usually is so poor that removal of the involved upper pole unit is necessary (41). Some centers have described definitive endoscopic treatment of the ureterocele by puncturing the ureterocele with an electrocautery probe (46). This is appropriate treatment for unstable or septic patients. Woodard found that 80% of his patients required further surgery when transurethral puncturing of ureteroceles was used as primary therapy (150). Debate centers over the management of the distal ureter and ureterocele itself. Once upper pole nephrectomy has been accomplished, the distal ureter and ureterocele may collapse, alleviating any associated pathologic condition caused by the mass effect of the ureterocele. If there is significant reflux prior to initial surgical intervention, into the ureter associated with the ureterocele (which is uncommon) or if the ureterocele tends to evert because of poor detrusor muscle backing, upper pole nephroureterectomy, excision of the involved ureter and ureterocele, and reconstruction of the bladder

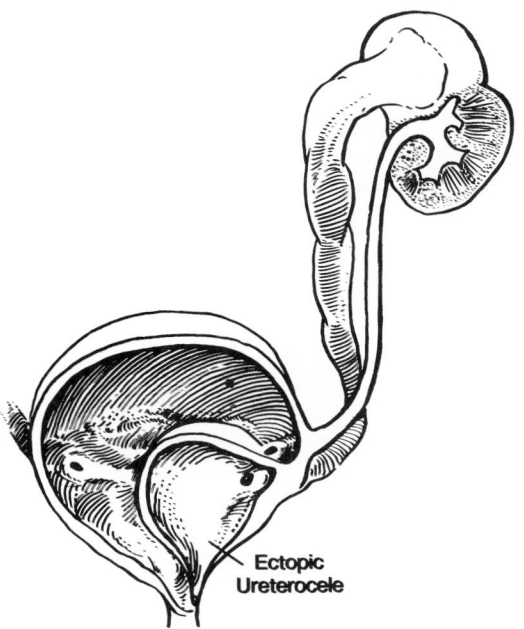

FIG. 43–10. Ectopic ureterocele. (From Malek RS, Kelalis PP, Burke EC, et al. Simple and ectopic ureterocele in infancy and childhood. *Surg Gynecol Obstet* 1972;134:611.)

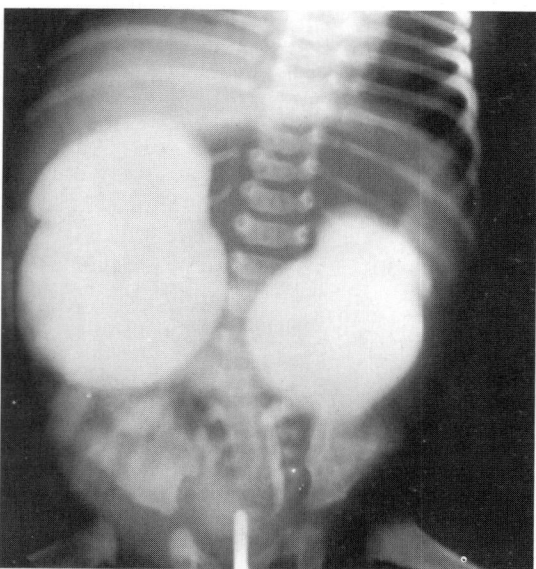

FIG. 43–11. Severe bilateral hydronephrosis secondary to ureteropelvic junction obstructions.

base is preferred. This obviates the need for a secondary, delayed surgical excision of the ureterocele because of recurrent urinary tract infections or persistent reflux (44). At times, preliminary cutaneous diversion of the involved ureter with delayed reconstruction is warranted, to allow maximal recovery of function before deciding on the need for nephrectomy versus reconstruction (41).

Ureteropelvic Junction Obstruction

Obstruction at the ureteropelvic junction probably is the most common cause of a palpable abdominal mass in the newborn and is the most common cause of antenatal hydronephrosis. This lesion usually is the result of narrowing of the ureter at the junction of the renal pelvis with the ureter. Because the renal pelvis is compliant,

there can be a great deal of renal preservation despite massive dilation of the kidney behind the obstruction (Fig. 43–11) (47).

The diagnosis of ureteropelvic junction obstruction can be made sonographically because there is a sonolucent central mass within the renal area surrounded by thin renal parenchyma (Fig. 43–12*A*). A grading system has been suggested by the Society for Fetal Urology to better standardize terminology and interpretation of renal ultrasound findings (48). The system is based on the severity of renal pelvis and calyceal dilatation as well as describing the renal parenchymal thickness (Fig. 43–13). Vesicoureteral reflux must be excluded from the differential diagnosis, and this is done by voiding cystography. The function of the obstructed kidney can be determined by radionuclide scanning (Fig. 43–12*B*). One of the advantages of radionuclide scintigraphy is that the physiologic significance of dilatation can be determined by administering furosemide (49). If the dilatation is of significance, there will be retention of the radionuclide behind the obstruction, whereas if there is no physiologic significance to the hydronephrosis, the administered diuretic will cause the radionuclide to wash out rapidly from the dilated system. It is becoming apparent that some instances of what was formerly thought to be significant hydronephrosis in the newborn are physiologically insignificant and, with time, stabilize or improve and require no treatment. In instances that are physiologically significant, repair, usually consisting of a dismembered pyeloplasty, results in improvement in drainage and renal function in most instances (47).

Ureterovesical Obstruction

Obstruction at the ureterovesical junction is not nearly so common as obstruction at the ureteropelvic junction, but it is far from rare (31). Lower ureteral obstruction may present as marked hydroureteronephrosis (i.e., a mass), but also sometimes presents as urinary infection

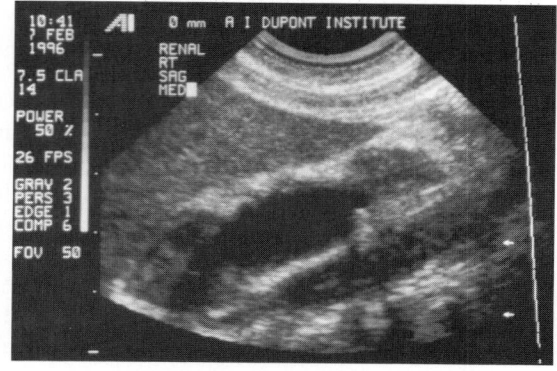

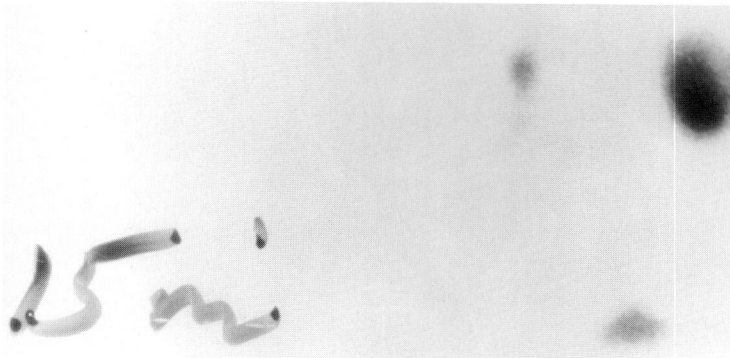

A   B

FIG. 43–12. A: An abdominal ultrasonogram in a newborn infant demonstrates a single, large echo-free region consistent with hydronephrosis. **B:** A delayed renal scan in a newborn infant with right hydronephrosis secondary to ureteropelvic junction obstruction.

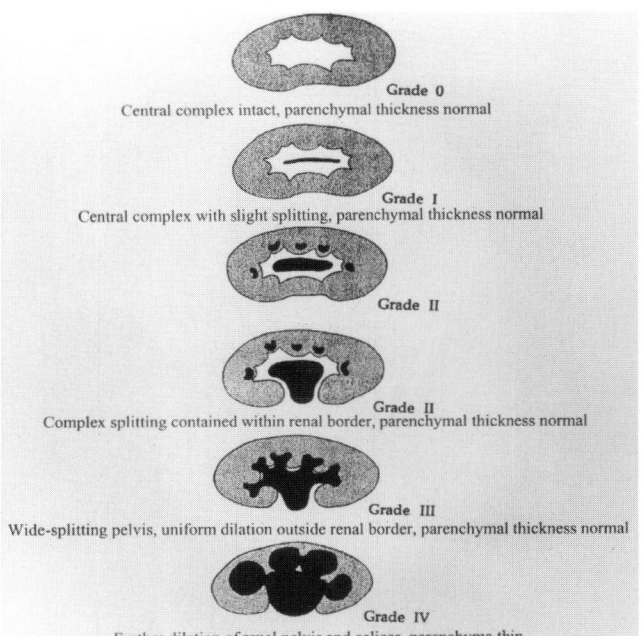

FIG. 43–13. Society for Fetal Urology grading system for ultrasonographically detected hydronephrosis. (From ref. 2, with permission. Modified by Curt Powell, M.D.)

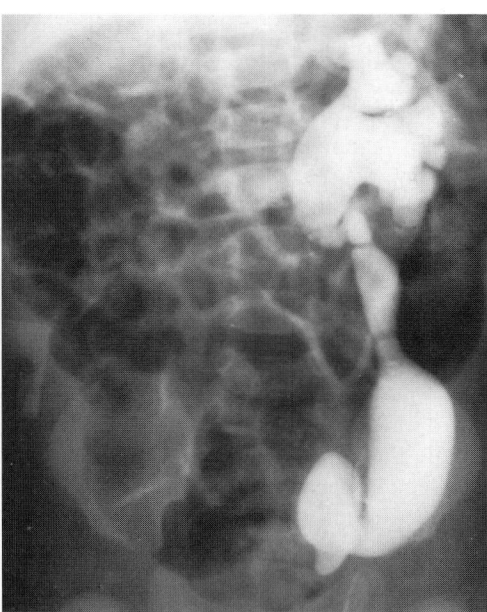

FIG. 43–14. Left ureterovesical obstruction in a 3-month-old boy who presented with unresponsive diarrhea. Urine culture was positive, and radiographic evaluation demonstrated significant pathology, as is evident in this illustration. The diarrhea resolved with treatment of the urinary infection. The ureterovesical obstruction was treated surgically. (From Kelalis PP, King LR, Belman AB, eds. *Clinical pediatric urology, vol. 1.* Philadelphia: WB Saunders, 1976:276.)

(Fig. 43–14). Just as with ureteropelvic obstruction, it has become apparent with experience that not all ureterovesical obstructions are physiologically significant; therefore, some require no treatment. Radionuclide scanning with diuretics is helpful in making the diagnosis of a physiologic obstruction (49). At times, however, an antegrade pyelogram with a pressure perfusion study is necessary to determine the significance or lack of significance of an apparent narrowing at the ureterovesical junction (50). These lesions, when identified to be obstructive, are treated by excision of the obstructing segment, tailoring or tapering of the dilated ureter, and reimplantation of the ureter into the bladder (51).

Vesicoureteral Reflux

Vesicoureteral reflux is the most common abnormality of the urinary system seen in children; it may occur in 1 of 100 births (8). The actual incidence is unknown, but there is no question that it is at least as common as cryptorchidism or hypospadias.

Vesicoureteral reflux is known to be a familial problem. When one child in a family is identified as having reflux, as many as 30% to 50% of the siblings of that child may have vesicoureteral reflux (52). For that reason, it is thought that all younger siblings of any proband identified to have reflux should be screened (53). It also has been found that transmission of reflux from a previously refluxing parent to his or her children is approximately 66% (52). The normal ureterovesical junction is a rela-

tively efficient mechanism that allows egress of urine into the lumen of the bladder, but, because of its oblique course through the ureteral wall, prevents the bladder urine from reentering the ureter (Fig. 43–15) (54). It is obvious that there is maturation of the ureterovesical junction with both time and growth, because infants have

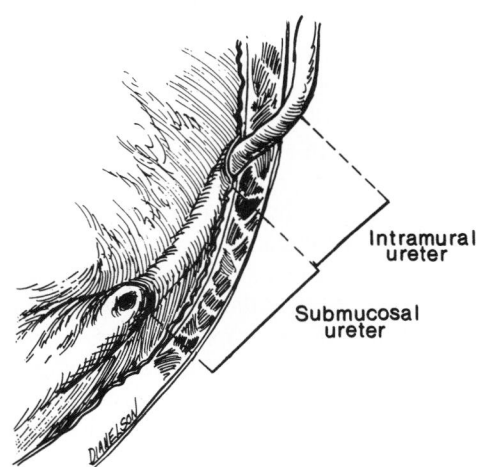

FIG. 43–15. Normal ureterovesical junction. (From Harrison JH, et al, eds. *Campbell's urology,* 4th ed. Philadelphia: WB Saunders, 1979:1597.)

a much higher incidence of vesicoureteral reflux than do older children (55).

Reflux is graded on a scale of 1 to 5 (56). The major significance of this grading system is that the higher the grade of reflux, the more likely it is that reflux will persist despite somatic growth, and the more likely that there is associated or eventual reflux nephropathy. Conversely, the lower the grade of reflux, the more likely there will be spontaneous resolution of the vesicoureteral reflux without reflux nephropathy (57).

Although the presence of hydronephrosis suggests an abnormality in the urinary tract, the radiologic confirmation of vesicoureteral reflux is accomplished by voiding cystourethrography. Generally, this should not be performed while the child is actively infected, but, in those in whom infection has been the presenting sign, once the urine is sterile and the patient afebrile, there is no need to delay investigation. Because renal scarring is produced easily in the neonate, it is especially important to establish the presence or absence of vesicoureteral reflux before discontinuing antibiotics in patients who have presented with urinary infection.

Once reflux is demonstrated, especially in the infant, the patient should be maintained on low-dose antibacterial therapy until resolution of the reflux, hopefully to prevent urinary tract infections. The choices of agents are limited in the newborn, but amoxicillin is a reasonable alternative until hepatobiliary maturation is sufficient to allow the use of sulfa or nitrofurantoin. A reasonable initial daily suppression dose would be 10 mg/kg of amoxicillin. Breakthrough infection, especially while the patient is on antibacterial suppression or due to poor parental compliance, suggests the need for surgical repair.

Exstrophy

Exstrophy of the bladder is a rare, but extremely significant, abnormality (Fig. 43–16). It affects roughly 1 child in every 25,000 live births. Exstrophy is not commonly associated with abnormalities in other organ systems, and the remainder of the urinary tract usually is normal in these children. Functional reconstruction of the exstrophic bladder, although a formidable surgical undertaking, in experienced hands sometimes can result in a continent child with a relatively normal upper urinary tract (58). The major factor affecting the success of closure in terms of continence seems to be the size of the exstrophic bladder at presentation.

The epithelium of the exstrophic bladder is grossly normal at birth, but becomes hyperplastic very shortly thereafter if the bladder is not closed. It is preferable, if possible, that the exstrophic bladder be left uncovered and kept moist using plastic wrap pending closure, assuming that closure can be accomplished in the newborn period. Gauze or petroleum gauze should not be used, as this can dry on the bladder surface and denude the urothelium.

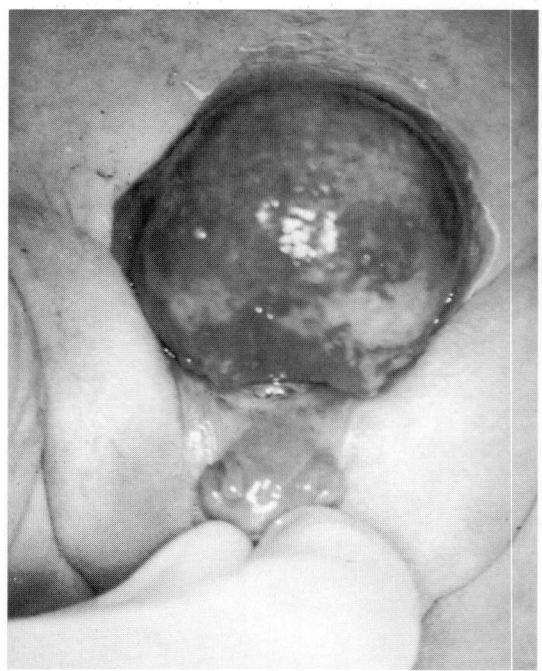

FIG. 43–16. Complete bladder exstrophy in a male child. Note that the penis is epispadiac, short, and stubby.

Functional closure of exstrophy is usually a staged procedure. In the first stage, iliac osteotomies are performed to facilitate closure. Even though osteotomy can be omitted, especially in newborns, success rates are higher when osteotomy is used (59). The exstrophic bladder is dissected free from the anterior abdominal wall, closed into a sphere, and dropped back into the pelvis. The abdominal wall then is closed over the bladder. There is no attempt at the first stage to produce urinary continence. After 2 to 3 years, a second-stage procedure is performed in an attempt to produce urinary control. Mitchell has incorporated bladder closure with epispadias repair for a one-stage bladder closure and epispadias repair with good initial results (60). In the past, ureterosigmoidostomy was used as an alternative to functional closure. In this operation, the ureters were anastomosed to the colon and the patient voided a mixture of urine and stool. There are metabolic abnormalities (e.g., hyperchloremic acidosis) associated with this form of diversion, and it has become apparent that patients who have been treated by ureterosigmoidostomy have an increased risk for development of adenocarcinoma of the colon at some time after their diversion (61). These patients should have routine surveillance colonoscopy. Similarly, the unclosed exstrophic bladder is at high risk for development of adenocarcinoma of the bladder in the second or third decade of life (62). Functional closure seems to obviate this latter risk.

Exstrophy of the cloaca is a severe anomaly, once thought incompatible with long-term survival. In this anomaly, two halves of an exstrophic bladder are separated by a midline strip of exteriorized cecum (Fig. 43–17) (63). The ileum may prolapse through the bowel plate. In addition, the child has an imperforate anus with almost no colon present distal to the exstrophic bowel plate. The small intestine is often short and there may be a malrotation anomaly. The genital tubercle is split and widely separated. Hence, it is almost impossible to produce a functional penis in boys with this anomaly (64). Genetic males with cloacal exstrophy were previously raised as females, but this practice is now questioned as some gender reassigned patients have expressed the view that they are uncomfortable with their assigned role (65). Some of these individuals are now being reassigned based on their genotypic karyotype. Each patient's ultimate gender of rearing should be carefully discussed and determined with the parents, with great thought and open discussion about these complexities. These children often have spinal dysraphism and a neurogenic bladder and bowel. For this reason, as well as the very short colon, a functional anus is almost impossible to produce, and permanent colostomy, incorporating the exstrophic bowel, is the bowel diversion of choice. Even though the colon is short, it is best to preserve as much of it as possible to improve water reabsorption. Permanent ileostomy, although used in the past, may lead to problems with dehydration and short gut syndrome. The bladder in these children can be closed and reconstructed using iliac osteotomy and then uniting the two halves of the exstrophic bladder before anterior closure. Although normal urinary control usually is not possible, dryness provided by clean intermittent catheterization is a reasonable goal.

Patent Urachus

The urachus is a tube that connects the urogenital sinus and the allantois between months 3 and 5 of intrauterine life. The urachus normally regresses first to a small-caliber, epithelialized tube and then into a sealed, obliterated cord by term or during the neonatal period. It may remain patent up to the infraumbilical area in the premature infant (66). Thirty-two percent of all bladders have tubular remnants of the urachus noted at necropsy (67). Significant urachal anomalies are rare; they occur twice as often in males as females (67).

Complete failure of obliteration results in a persistent communication between the bladder and the umbilicus that leaks urine intermittently or continuously. It is the most common urachal anomaly encountered. The etiology of this condition is unknown. It has been suggested that bladder outlet obstruction may be a contributing factor, although the chronology of embryologic events suggests that the urachal lumen obliterates before urethral tubularization. The diagnosis may be confirmed by retrograde fistulography, instillation of methylene blue into the tract or intravesically, or injection of indigo carmine intravenously. A voiding cystourethrogram occasionally will demonstrate the communication, but this study is more useful in ruling out other associated lower urinary tract anomalies such as obstruction or vesicoureteral reflux. A persistent omphalomesenteric duct must be considered in the differential diagnosis. In infants with minimal umbilical drainage that causes a small stain on the diaper, an umbilical granuloma or a patch of gastric mucosa may be at fault (68). Iatrogenic creation of a vesicoumbilical fistula, during an umbilical artery cutdown, has been reported (66). Treatment of a patent urachus consists of complete extraperitoneal excision of the urachus with an attached cuff of bladder to completely remove any urachal remnant in the bladder to prevent possible cancer development in residual tissue. Attempts should be made to preserve the umbilicus as well.

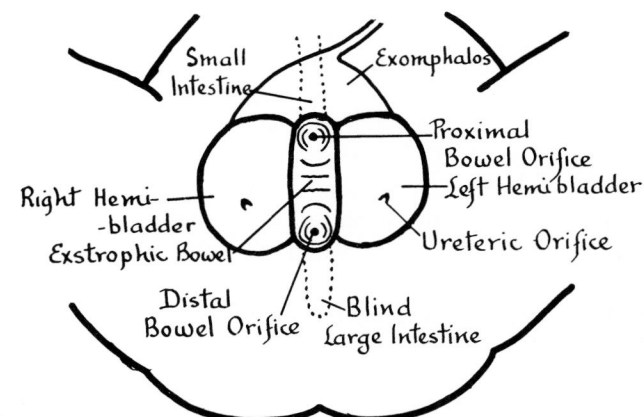
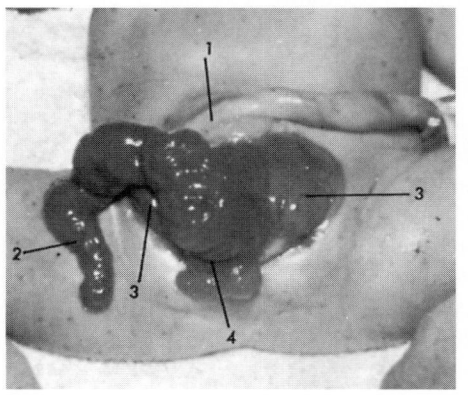

FIG. 43–17. Exstrophy of the cloaca. **A:** Diagram of the external anatomy. **B:** In a patient with exstrophy of the cloaca, the anatomic features as numbered include exomphalos (1), ileum that has prolapsed through the proximal bowel orifice (2), and the hemibladders lying on either side of the exstrophic bowel (3). Note the absence of an anus (4) and of definable external genitalia. (From ref. 63.)

Megalocystis Microcolon Intestinal Hypoperistalsis Syndrome

Megalocystis microcolon intestinal hypoperistalsis syndrome was first described in 1976 and is considered rare (69). The disorder primarily affects full-term female neonates and generally is fatal within the first year of life. Presentation includes abdominal distention, an abdominal mass (i.e., a distended bladder), and functional intestinal obstruction characterized by bilious vomiting and absent or decreased bowel sounds. The small bowel is short, dilated, and hypoactive, with an accompanying microcolon but no anatomic obstruction. There is associated incomplete bowel rotation and the abdominal musculature generally is lax.

The etiology is unknown, but the dilated bladder may be seen on antenatal ultrasound. Treatment consists of parenteral alimentation and urinary diversion by means of a cutaneous vesicostomy. Patients with Ochoa urofacial syndrome also may present with megalocystis in infancy (70).

Posterior Urethral Valves

The most common lesion obstructing the lower urinary tract in a boy is the lesion termed posterior urethral valves (Fig. 43–18). The name is a misnomer, because the valves are really a diaphragm that traverses the urethra from a point just distal to the verumontanum to the proximal limit of the membranous urethra (71). Embryologically, these occur because there is an abnormal anterior insertion and persistence of the distal extent of the wolffian duct (37). To understand the clinical picture of urethral valves, one must consider the dynamics and pathophysiologic consequences of the obstruction itself. The valves are best considered a rigid band or membrane, despite their frequently flimsy nature. The vesical neck also is a relatively rigid area. With antegrade flow of fluid, this membrane obstructs. When obstruction is present, the urethra dilates proximally and elongates. The detrusor hypertrophies in response to the extra work involved in voiding, with resultant trabeculation and sacculation. Detrusor hypertrophy also produces relative hypertrophy of the vesical neck.

The prostatic urethra becomes dilated in a fusiform manner between the two relatively rigid points, creating a subvesical chamber. If there is a primary abnormality of the ureterovesical junction or if a paraureteral saccule develops, vesicoureteral reflux may result. The presence of bilateral vesicoureteral reflux increases the possibility that renal failure will eventually occur. Hydroureteronephrosis may develop, with or without reflux. Renal parenchymal damage in the form of renal dysplasia or interstitial nephritis, with or without superimposed pyelonephritis, often is concomitant or a result of valvular obstruction. Renal dysplasia frequently is present at birth in infants with posterior

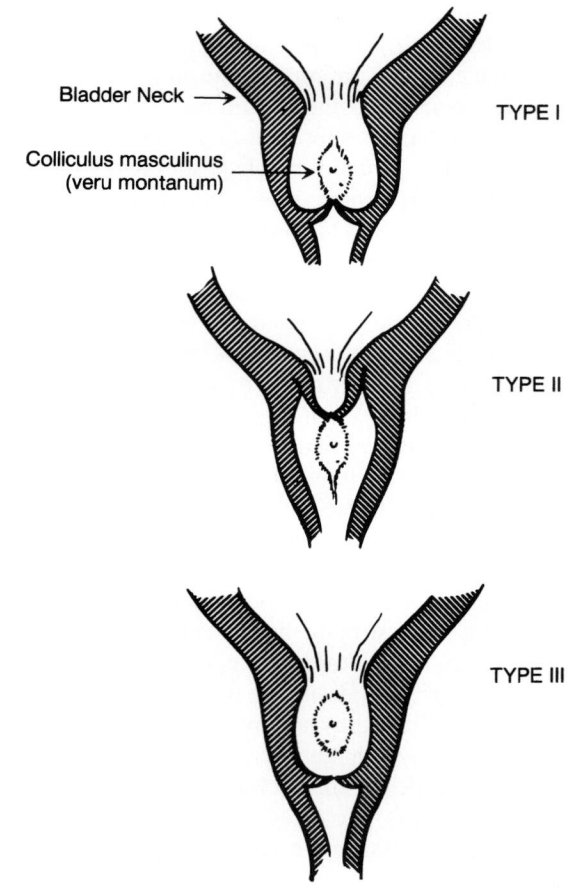

FIG. 43–18. Young classified valves into three types. The type II valve probably does not exist. (From Kelalis PP, King LR, Belman AB, eds. *Clinical pediatric urology, vol. 1.* Philadelphia: WB Saunders, 1976:306.)

urethral valves and has been found at as early as 15 weeks of gestational age in the fetus (72).

Osathanondh and Potter (73) state that dysplasia is a consequence of intrauterine urinary obstruction. In experimental animals, intrauterine urethral obstruction early in gestation usually has led to a patent urachus, without hydronephrosis or dysplasia—a situation that does not correspond to the clinical sequence in humans (74). Later in gestation, experimental intrauterine urethral obstruction results in hydronephrosis without dysplasia (75).

Clinically, dysplasia is found more often in association with severe vesicoureteral reflux (76). In addition, dysplasia often is unilateral and not bilateral, as one would expect if it resulted from intrauterine urethral obstruction. Maizels and Simpson (77), using chick embryos, showed that dysplasia results from problems associated with the renal blastema and not from obstruction of the ureter. It seems that dysplasia, when present, may represent a primary abnormality of the ureterorenal unit and may have no direct causal relationship to the presence of intrauterine urethral obstruction.

The clinical presentation of the infant with posterior urethral valves often is related to the severity of the obstruction. Virtually all of the signs and symptoms seen in the boy with posterior urethral valves are secondary to the obstructive nature of the valves, the effect of intrauterine oligohydramnios, or the presence of superimposed urinary infection or azotemia. Between 48% and 50% of boys with posterior urethral valves are diagnosed antenatally via ultrasonography (6,78).

If not detected antenatally, 25% to 50% of boys with posterior urethral valves present during the neonatal period (79). The nonrenal features of Potter syndrome may be seen in newborns with posterior urethral valves, including intrauterine growth deficiency, pulmonary hypoplasia, limb positioning defects (e.g., talipes equinovarus), and the characteristic Potter facies. All are thought to be due to a deficiency of amniotic fluid and subsequent fetal compression. The incidence of anomalies in other organ systems not directly attributable to urethral obstruction is low (80). A palpably enlarged bladder, urinary tract infection, ascites, pulmonary difficulties, such as isolated pneumothorax, failure to thrive, or gastrointestinal disturbances may lead to investigation. A strong urinary stream does not preclude the diagnosis of posterior urethral obstruction (81). Pulmonary hypoplasia will present with respiratory distress, especially with spontaneous pneumothorax or pneumomediastinum. This is an unusual but important symptom of valves in newborns. Any full-term boy with respiratory distress should be suspect for a renal problem. Hydronephrosis is present in 90% of infants with valves (81).

Boys who present with posterior urethral valves in infancy have a poorer prognosis than children who present symptomatically at an older age, especially if serum creatinine levels are higher than 0.8 or 1.0 mg% at 1 month after treatment of the valves. Presumably, this is because there is a high incidence of renal dysplasia associated with this type of presentation.

Urinary ascites is one of the rarer forms of presentation of children with posterior urethral valves (82). The presence of ascitic fluid in a newborn infant should prompt investigation of the urinary tract, because urinary ascites is responsible for one-third of all cases of neonatal ascites (83). Although the ascites rarely may be secondary to frank perforation of the urinary tract (84), most often it is due to leakage of urine through the renal fornices and transudation of fluid across the peritoneal membrane into the peritoneal cavity (85). The ascitic fluid usually has a chemical content equivalent to that of serum, because the high urea and creatinine content of urine has dialyzed passively across the peritoneal membrane and into the vascular system. These children may not have marked hydronephrosis because the urinary tract has been decompressed by leakage of urine (85). These boys often present as extremely ill infants, but occasionally may appear initially healthy except for abdominal distention.

Their prognosis with regard to renal preservation often is better than that of a child who does not present with urinary ascites, presumably because the leakage of urine from the distended system protects the upper urinary tract from the ravages of high intraluminal pressure (85). Occasionally, a localized retroperitoneal urinoma will form. The diagnosis of urinary ascites usually is made clinically and confirmed by ultrasound examination or a plain radiograph of the abdomen demonstrating bowel displaced to the central abdomen and a ground-glass appearance of the remainder of the abdomen.

Twenty-five to fifty percent of patients with posterior urethral valves have vesicoureteral reflux at presentation (6,86). In one-half of cases, the reflux is bilateral. When there is massive unilateral vesicoureteral reflux associated with posterior urethral valves, the kidney on the refluxing side often is dysplastic and does not function at presentation or subsequently. This is the so-called VURD syndrome (valves, unilateral reflux, and dysplasia). Marked hydronephrosis without vesicoureteral reflux usually carries a better prognosis for long-term renal function than does the presence of bilateral vesicoureteral reflux. In patients with posterior urethral valves, if reflux is present, it will resolve with relief of obstruction in one-third to one-half of cases (86).

Obstructive uropathy will be suggested on ultrasonography by findings such as bilateral hydronephrosis or by a distended, thick-walled bladder. Patients with posterior urethral valves often have a dilated and elongated posterior urethra that can be imaged sonographically and has been termed the keyhole urethra. Perirenal urinoma or ascites also can be detected.

The single most important study in the diagnosis of infravesical obstruction is the voiding cystourethrogram. An adequate study requires complete visualization of the urethra from the bladder neck to the meatus and oblique and lateral projections of the urethra during voiding without a catheter in the urethra, because an indwelling catheter may obscure the lesion.

Posterior urethral valves appear as a sharply defined transverse or oblique lucency, with proximal urethral elongation and distention and diminution of flow distal to the valve. The bladder neck in valve cases may be secondarily thickened and collar-like. The bladder usually is trabeculated with saccules or diverticula, especially paraurethral diverticula (Fig. 43–19). Vesicoureteral reflux often is present at diagnosis, and the refluxing ureters frequently are grossly dilated and tortuous.

Functional imaging studies of the upper urinary tracts will determine the degree of upper tract damage produced by lower tract obstruction. Historically, intravenous urography has been used routinely in upper tract imaging but may be inconclusive, especially if renal function is poor. If function is sufficient for radiographic visualization and if delayed radiographs are obtained, marked hydroureteronephrosis should be evident. Delayed filling,

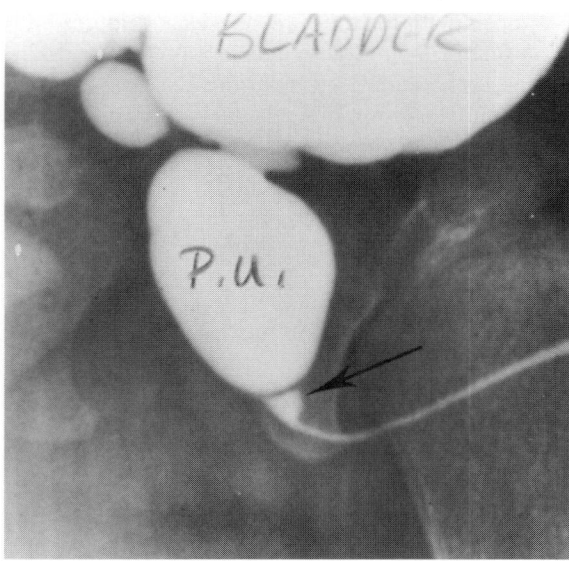

FIG. 43–19. Voiding cystourethrogram in a newborn boy with posterior urethral value (*arrow*). The prostatic urethra (PU) is dilated, and the bladder is trabeculated with multiple diverticula (*upper left*).

visualizing a poorly functioning renal unit, may be secondary to vesicoureteral reflux rather than evidence of renal function. In the newborn or azotemic infant in whom obstruction is suspected, a radionuclide renal scan usually provides more information than excretory urography. A scan allows estimation of differential renal function. Scintigraphy also is safer than excretory urography because it eliminates the need for iodinated contrast agents, which have a risk for associated morbidity.

When these infants first present, resuscitative measures may be necessary to treat associated urinary infection, replace fluid and electrolytes, and, most important, drain the urinary tract. A small intraurethral catheter (e.g., a feeding tube) often will suffice to drain the urinary tract for a few days. Once the child is stable, the valves must be either transurethrally resected primarily or the urinary tract should be drained for a prolonged period using a cutaneous vesicostomy. Many of these infants are expected in advance because of antenatal imaging, and they can be followed closely immediately after birth and may not require resuscitative measures, because the child generally is evaluated almost immediately after birth.

The long-term outlook for infants who present with posterior urethral valves is only fair, because approximately 50% of boys who present with posterior urethral valves eventually will progress to renal failure and transplantation despite treatment (87). This does not mean that a fatalistic attitude must be adopted, but, nonetheless, expectations must be realistic. If the serum creatinine is normal at 2 years of age, the prognosis for long-term normal renal function is good but not perfect (88). In a long-term follow-up of 11 to 22 years of children with urethral valves, one-third had poor renal function: 10% who survived childhood had died of renal failure; 21% had end-stage renal disease or chronic renal failure; and 46% had diurnal enuresis. Diurnal enuresis

increased the likelihood that there would be progression to renal failure (89).

Renal Tumors

Fortunately, tumors of the urinary tract are rare in infancy and those that do occur tend to exhibit a benign behavior. Variants of Wilms tumor can be seen in the neonatal period and include mesoblastic nephroma (90), nephroblastomatosis (91), and benign cystic nephroma (92). With the advent of frequent *in utero* ultrasonographic screening, many of these lesions are found as abnormally large kidneys or kidneys with a recognizable mass on ultrasound. Otherwise they usually will present in infancy as a palpable flank mass and occasionally can produce hypertension (93).

Mesoblastic nephroma is the most frequent of these tumors. This recognized variant of Wilms tumor behaves in an almost uniformly benign manner (90). Histologically, mesoblastic nephroma is composed largely of mesenchymal stroma with spindle-shaped fibrous or leiomyomatous cells. Ultrasonography will demonstrate a solid intrarenal mass. Computerized tomography will delineate better the composition of the mass and may demonstrate extension outside of the renal bed. Radionuclide scans will show the mass to be nonfunctioning tissue, and intravenous urography will reveal distortion of the calyceal architecture by the tumor. Neither of these tests is routinely obtained, however, as ultrasound and computerized tomography will demonstrate the tissue characteristics more clearly than scintigraphy or pyelography. Nephrectomy is curative, but there have been a few reports of local recurrence and rare reports of distant metastasis (90). Chemotherapy and radiation therapy are not necessary adjuncts to therapy.

Nephroblastomatosis can be diffuse or nodular (91). Diffuse nephroblastomatosis usually presents as marked enlargement of both kidneys. The kidneys are grossly enlarged and have a whitish hue. Biopsy reveals primitive metanephric epithelium resembling that seen in Wilms tumor. This lesion usually responds to chemotherapy (i.e., actinomycin D). Nodular renal blastoma consists of microscopic foci of primitive metanephric epithelium and often is an incidental autopsy finding in infants. It is thought that Wilms tumor may, in some instances, arise from foci of nodular renal blastema.

Benign cystic nephroma occasionally is classified with the cystic diseases, but more properly belongs with the renal tumors because elements of Wilms tumor may be found in the septa between the cysts (94). As with the other tumors, patients with cystic nephroma present with a palpable mass. Ultrasonography will identify the mass as multiple cysts or as complex (i.e., mixed cystic and solid). Although enucleation of the mass is a theoretical therapeutic option, nephrectomy usually is the treatment of choice. Despite the presence of Wilms tumor elements in the septa, chemotherapy is not necessary for cure.

Renal Vein Thrombosis

Another renal lesion that has a definite predilection for the neonatal period is renal vein thrombosis (95). This problem usually results from hemoconcentration secondary to dehydration and is seen in infants of diabetic mothers. It also may be seen in infants with cyanotic congenital heart disease, sickle-cell disease, or perinatal stress or sepsis. Sludging in the intrarenal venules occurs, with subsequent thrombosis. The thrombus then tends to propagate centrally. The infants present with a palpable mass, hematuria, albuminuria, and thrombocytopenia. If both kidneys are involved, the infant will become uremic. Treatment is supportive and involves correction of the underlying problems. Surgery (i.e., nephrectomy) was once thought essential to survival; however, it is recognized that nephrectomy is unnecessary and that, if collateral circulation is present, there may be renal recovery. Thrombectomy is of no help because the problem is in the peripheral rather than the central veins. Thrombolytic agents developed for clot lysis may be considered for treatment of bilateral renal vein thrombosis.

Adrenal Hemorrhage

At times, either spontaneously or in association with renal vein thrombosis, there may be hemorrhage into the adrenal gland (96). Hemorrhage also can occur following a traumatic delivery, sepsis, or asphyxia. The infant may present with icterus (from absorption of hemoglobin) and an abdominal mass. Ultrasonography will demonstrate a sonolucent or solid mass above the kidney. Over the course of a few weeks, the mass will be reabsorbed or, rarely, will form an adrenal pseudocyst (97). If the latter occurs, percutaneous drainage is the preferred mode of therapy. Otherwise, no therapy is necessary. Adrenal calcification often is seen several weeks after an adrenal hemorrhage. Adrenal hemorrhage can occur bilaterally in 10% of patients, and it occurs more commonly on the right side.

Prenatal Ultrasonography

The advent of high-resolution, real-time ultrasonography has allowed the antenatal diagnosis of many anomalies of the urinary tract. It has become apparent with time, however, that diagnostic accuracy *in utero* is not complete and that the natural history of some lesions is not as clear-cut as once thought (98). The hope that antenatal intervention might result in improvement in outcome has proven ill-founded (99). The maternal risk of morbidity with intervention has been reported to be as high as 4% to 5% (100), and there are no clear-cut examples of improvement in fetal outcome as a result of such interventions (6,101). Studies of the results of postnatal treatment after antenatal identification of lesions have, however, clearly demonstrated improved outcome (100). There seems to be no advantage to early delivery; thus, the timing of delivery in fetuses with hydronephrosis generally is determined best by obstetric factors rather than fetal concerns (102).

As stated earlier, the fetal kidneys can be identified in the early part of the second trimester of pregnancy. Dilation of the renal pelvis and calices in a nonduplex system, without identification of a dilated ureter, suggests the presence of ureteropelvic obstruction. It has become apparent that some instances of hydronephrosis resolve spontaneously and completely *in utero,* whereas others that are present at birth may stabilize or improve with time. Conversely, some seem to dilate progressively with time. Hence, not all dilations of the upper urinary tract are obstructive in nature (98). Most of those that are of significance prove to be secondary to narrowing at the ureteropelvic junction. In the hope of standardizing the descriptive terminology for the ultrasound findings with hydronephrosis, the Society for Fetal Urology has graded the severity of the hydronephrosis based on the extent of renal pelvis and calyceal dilatation and parenchymal thinning or atrophy (48).

In a duplicated system, there can be dilation of either the lower pole system or the upper pole system. Dilations of the lower pole system usually are due to ureteropelvic junction obstruction or to vesicoureteral reflux. Obstructions of the upper pole system usually are associated with hydroureter and often are accompanied by a ureterocele. Solid intrarenal lesions most commonly are mesoblastic nephromas, with neuroblastoma occurring infrequently.

Ureteral dilation can, at times, be massive and may be confused with bowel on sonography; however, following the ureter from a dilated upper system down to the bladder usually will distinguish the dilated ureter from bowel because dilated ureters often do not demonstrate peristalsis. Bilateral hydroureter, although it may be associated with bilateral ureterovesical obstruction, more commonly is due to either high-grade vesicoureteral reflux, posterior urethral valves, or the prune-belly syndrome.

In a male fetus, a thick-walled, enlarged bladder often is secondary to posterior urethral valves or the prune-belly syndrome, especially if a keyhole posterior urethra is identified. In females, an enlarged bladder may be due to the megalocystis microcolon syndrome. Ureteroceles also can be identified by sonography in the bladder. If no bladder is identified on serial ultrasonography, this suggests bilateral renal agenesis, bilateral single ureteral ectopy, or exstrophy of the bladder.

Lesions associated with hydronephrosis and normal amounts of amniotic fluid generally carry a good prognosis, whereas those associated with increased renal echogenicity and decreased amounts of amniotic fluid generally carry a poor prognosis for pulmonary maturation as well as renal function (103).

Abdominal Masses

The finding of an abdominal mass is not infrequent in the newborn nursery. An unselected series of infants in the newborn nursery revealed abdominal masses arising from the genitourinary tract in approximately 1 in every 500 admissions (104). It is quite clear from multiple reports that the urinary tract often is the source of a palpable abdominal mass in infants (105,106). In most reported series, approximately two-thirds of the infants presenting with an abdominal mass are found to have lesions in the urinary tract. In infancy, hydronephrosis and cystic kidneys are the most common lesions producing abdominal masses, whereas in older children tumors are more common (107). The obvious inference from these data is that ultrasonography, because the urinary tract is easily visualized, is the study most likely to identify the source of a palpable abdominal mass. The physical, sonographic, and urographic or renographic characteristics of the common abdominal masses of renal origin are listed in Table 43–2.

Hematuria

Hematuria in the infant can be a sign of renal vein thrombosis, acute tubular necrosis, renal calculi, urinary infection, or urinary tract obstruction (108). The presence of hematuria must be confirmed by examination of the urine, both chemically and microscopically. A positive chemical test may reflect hemoglobinuria, rather than hematuria, which implies the presence of cellular elements in the urine. Even more common than the presence of hematuria or hemoglobinuria, however, is concern about a red diaper in an infant. Two relatively common causes for red diapers are the presence of urates in the urine, which can give a pink hue to the urine, especially in the diaper, and, if cloth diapers are used, the growth of *Serratia* sp. on urine-soaked diapers left standing in the diaper pail. Obviously, these latter two situations are of no clinical consequence but must be separated from true hematuria or hemoglobinuria in diagnostic considerations.

GENITAL ABNORMALITIES

Cryptorchidism

Undescended testes are a very common finding in the newborn period, affecting perhaps as many as 1 in every 50 newborn males (109). Most testes that are undescended at birth, however, will descend during the first 6 to 9 months of life, so that the incidence of cryptorchidism at 1 year of age is approximately 0.7% to 0.8%, which is exactly the same incidence that has been found in postpubertal males (109). The newborn examination is important in determining testicular position, because the cremasteric reflex at that time is weak to absent (110). If the testis is well descended in a newborn, it is unlikely that there will be problems with true cryptorchidism later in life. Because it is thought that optimal results from treatment of cryptorchidism are produced by interventions after the possibility of testicular descent has passed (i.e., beyond 9 months of age) and before adverse effects of testicular nondescent are seen histologically (i.e., approximately 1.5 to 2 years of age), the optimal

TABLE 43–2. *Abdominal masses of renal origin*

Mass	Texture	Renal scan or excretory urogram	Ultrasonogram
Hydronephrosis	Smooth	Delayed drainage	Sonolucent
Multicystic kidney (i.e., cystic dysplasia)	Irregular	Nonfunction	Multiple large and small cysts
Polycystic kidney	Smooth (recessive); irregular or smooth (dominant)	Delayed function; distortion of collecting system	Diffuse small cysts (recessive)
			Multiple large and small cysts (dominant)
Tumor	Smooth	Distortion of collecting system	Solid
Renal vein thrombosis	Smooth	Poor function to nonfunction	Relatively normal renal architecture; enlarged kidney

time for treatment of cryptorchidism would seem to be approximately 1 year of age (111).

Penile Agenesis

Although many of the penile anomalies are common, some, such as agenesis of the penis, are rare, occurring in 1 in 10 to 30 million live births (Fig. 43–20). Penile agenesis suggests an early embryologic failure in the development of the genital tubercle. The urethra usually exits on the perineum or near the anal verge. Previously these children were raised as females, with castration and reconstruction of the external genitalia performed at an early age (112). As previously noted, current management of this and other previously sex reassigned conditions is in flux, as recent reports on long-term follow-up of these patients have called the practice of gender reassignment into question (65).

Penile Duplication

Penile duplication (i.e., true diphallia) is a rare anomaly that also may involve duplications of the urethra and bladder (Fig. 43–21) (113). Reconstruction of these anomalies involves complex decisions about functional capability of the urinary, genital, and gastrointestinal tracts, as well as appearance.

Microphallus

The boy born with an abnormally small phallus presents a true therapeutic dilemma. Most cases of microphallus are due to hypogonadism (113) and will respond to testosterone, but an occasional patient with microphallus has end-organ failure and will not respond to exogenous testosterone. It is notable that, despite the relatively common finding of microphallus in the newborn nursery, it is an extremely rare event to find an adult with a phallus so small that it is incapable of sexual function.

The normal full-term newborn phallus measures approximately 3 to 3.5 cm in stretched length; the definition of microphallus requires a phallus that is less than 2.5 cm in stretched length excluding ambigous genitalia, or the penis with hypospadias or chordee (114). To determine whether or not microphallus will respond to hormonal stimulation, 25 mg of testosterone enanthate is

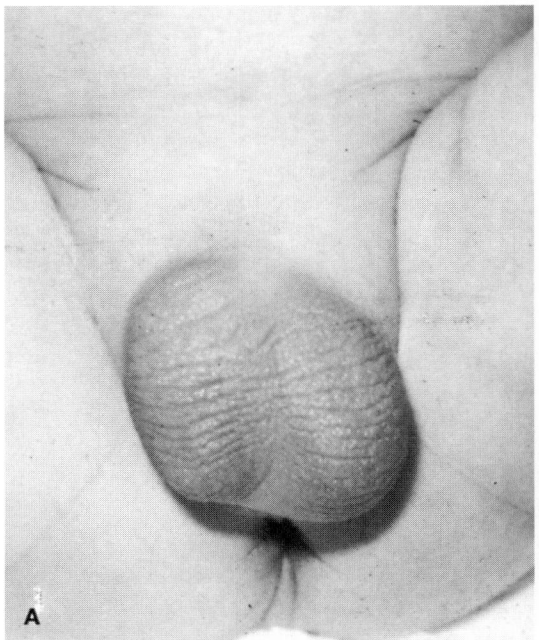
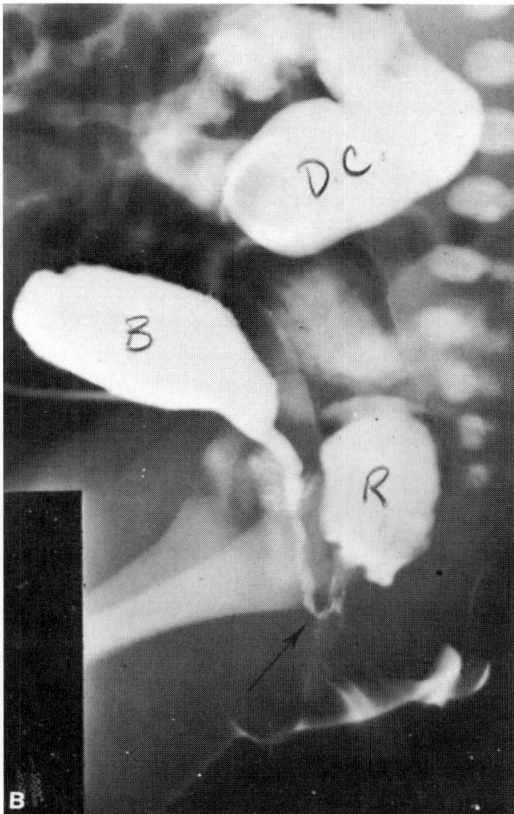

FIG. 43–20. A: Genetic boy born with complete penile agenesis. **B:** An antegrade cystourethrogram in a genetic boy with penile agenesis. The bladder is full (B), and there is communication between the urethra and rectum (*arrow*). The rectum (R) and descending colon (DC) are filled with voided contrast material.

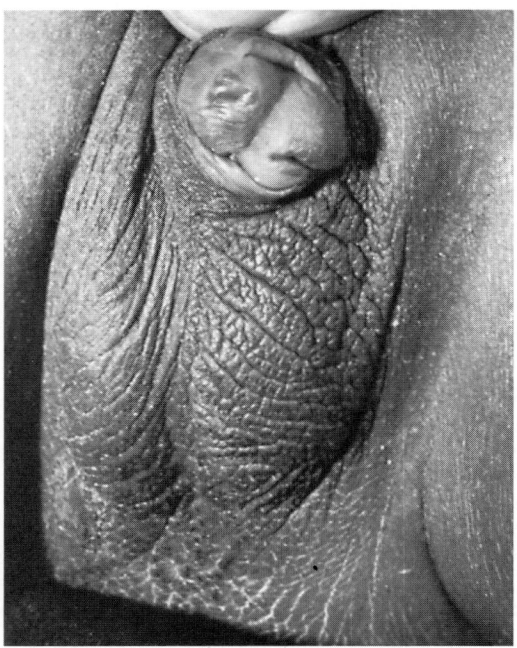

FIG. 43–21. Duplication of the glans in a 2-year-old boy. (From Kossow JH, Morales PA. Duplication of bladder and urethra and associated anomalies. Urology 1973;1:71.)

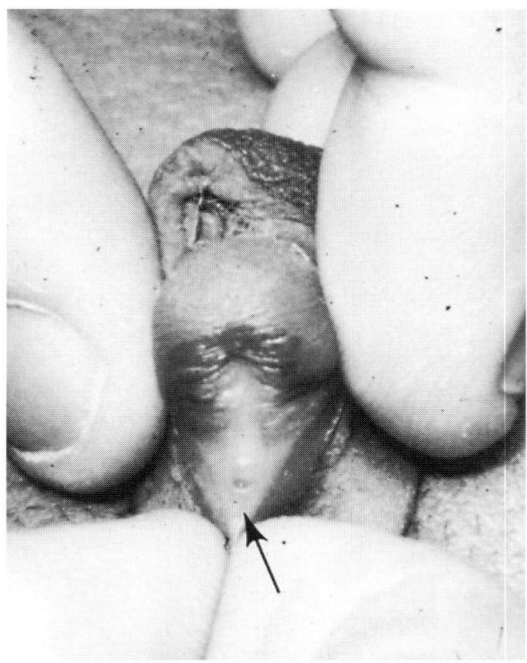

FIG. 43–22. The hypospadiac meatal position (*arrow*) is demonstrated by pulling the ventral shaft of skin away from the penis.

administered intramuscularly every 4 weeks for a total of 75 mg (see Chap. 41) (115). Some element of response usually is evident after the first dose. In most instances, after the course is completed, the child has a relatively normal phallus. If there is no response to testosterone, gender reassignment can be considered, but genotypic imprinting must be taken into consideration prior to reassignment.

Hypospadias

The term hypospadias, by definition, refers to the abnormal location of the urethral meatus somewhere ventral to the normal glanular tip (Fig. 43–22); however, the term actually encompasses a complex that includes chordee (i.e., a ventral curvature of the penis on erection) as well as an abnormality of the prepuce. Although it is traditional in some circles to categorize hypospadias by degrees (i.e., first, second, and third), it is more helpful to describe hypospadias by the location of the meatus and the presence or absence of chordee (Fig. 43–23). At times, the hypospadiac meatus is quite stenotic and can be very difficult to see, especially in the newborn.

It has become obvious that the sibling of a child with hypospadias has an increased (14%) chance of having hypospadias (116). It is thought that hypospadias is inherited as a multifactorial problem. It once was thought that there might be associated abnormalities of the upper urinary tract in children with hypospadias, but critical analysis of series of children with hypospadias who have been

uniformly investigated reveals that there is no increased incidence of upper tract abnormalities when children with hypospadias are compared to those of the general population (117).

Most forms of hypospadias can be surgically corrected and, although there is no ideal age for genital surgery, it is thought preferable to perform this surgery in the first year of life, typically after 6 months of age. The presence of the foreskin greatly facilitates the repair of these problems, and it is for this reason that circumcision should be delayed in children with hypospadias. Clinical clues that hypospadias may be present are an abnormality of the foreskin, an incomplete foreskin, and penile torsion or chordee. Whenever these abnormalities are noted, circumcision should be delayed until the surgeon who will be involved in the hypospadias repair, should it be necessary, can assess the child and determine whether the foreskin will be necessary for the repair.

Epispadias

Epispadias usually is associated with exstrophy but occasionally appears as an isolated defect (Fig. 43–24). The incidence of isolated epispadias previously reported as 1 in 100,000 live births has now been estimated as occurring in 1 in 40,000 live births (118). The repair of this lesion is moderately difficult. The more severe degrees of epispadias usually are associated with urinary incontinence and are more common than those associated

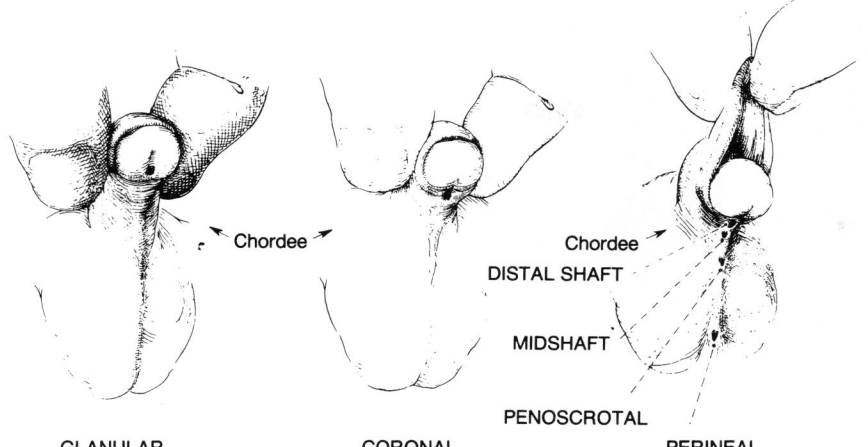

FIG. 43–23. Classification of hypospadias based on anatomic location of the urethral meatus. The associated chordee is best described in terms of its severity (mild, moderate, or severe). (From Kelalis PP, King LR, Belman AB, eds. *Clinical pediatric urology, vol. 1.* Philadelphia: WB Saunders, 1976:577.)

with continence. In incontinent cases, the bladder neck must be reconstructed. Children with epispadias tend to have a relatively short phallus and, although attempts at lengthening the phallus are somewhat helpful, this aspect of the problem sometimes defies correction.

Urethral Duplication

Urethral duplication is an uncommon anomaly that can present either as a partial or complete duplication. The

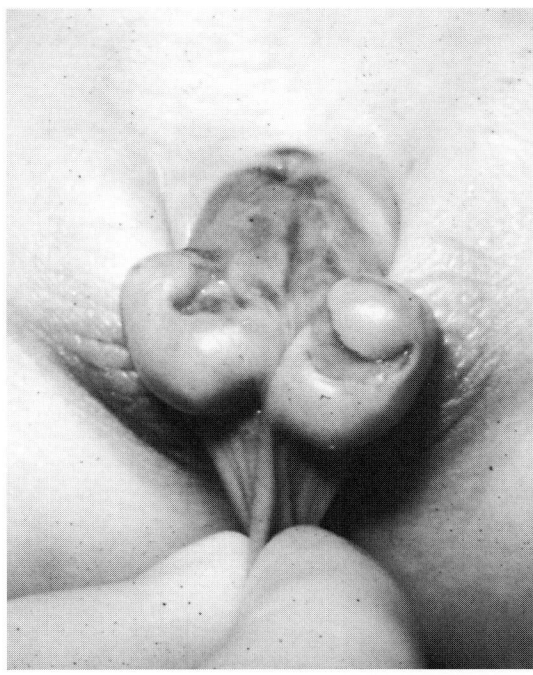

FIG. 43–24. Isolated epispadias without exstrophy. The bladder neck is intact in this child, who has good but not excellent urinary continence. Note also the incomplete duplication of glans.

more ventral urethra usually is the functional urethra, and the dorsal urethra often is stenotic and unusable (119). Repair of these anomalies must be tailored to the individual situation.

Ambiguous Genitalia

Ambiguity of the external genitalia is a quandary encountered with some regularity in the newborn nursery (see Chap. 41). These patients often pose difficult diagnostic and therapeutic challenges. It is important to establish a diagnosis rapidly. On physical examination, the presence or absence of palpable gonads is very helpful. If a gonad is palpably present, it almost certainly is a testis. Hence, bilaterally palpable gonads suggest very strongly that the patient is a genetic male. If a gonad is palpable only unilaterally, there probably is a testis on that side. There could conceivably be a normal testis, a streak gonad, or an ovary on the other side. If no testes are palpable, the patient could be an XX female, an XY male with abdominal testes or mixed gonadal dysgenesis, or a true hermaphrodite.

Chromosomal gender is established by karyotype. An XY male who is undervirilized could have Klinefelter syndrome, true hermaphroditism, 5α-reductase deficiency, hypopituitarism, 17-hydroxylase deficiency, or 3β-hydroxy steroid deficiency.

If the patient is an XX female, ambiguity could be produced by excessive maternal androgens or the adrenogenital syndrome, which is most commonly caused by a 21-hydroxylase deficiency. This latter must be considered in any phenotypically male patient with nonpalpable gonads even if the genitalia appear completely masculinized, to avoid an addisonian crisis in a patient with a salt-losing adrenogenital syndrome (Fig. 43–25).

Gender assignment (i.e., gender of rearing) should be accomplished with some dispatch to avoid excessive parental anxiety; however, assignment should not be

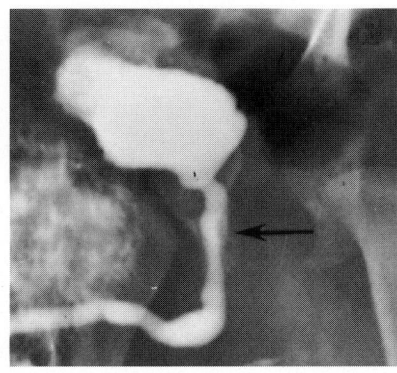
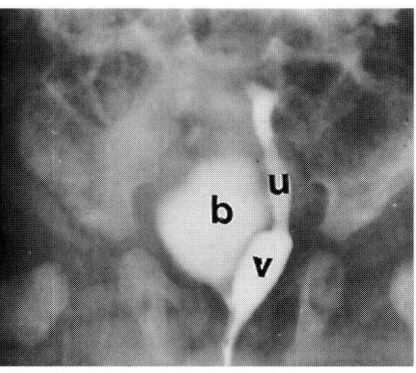

FIG. 43–25. Voiding cystourethrogram in a genetic girl who was totally masculinized by adrenal hyperplasia. **A:** Utriculus masculinus (*arrow*), as would normally be expected in a male. **B:** Retrograde vaginohistogram reveals a normal vagina (v) and uterus (u), as well as an overflow of contrast into the urinary bladder (b).

made in a cavalier manner. Anxiety produced by indecision over gender assignment is exponentially increased by changes in gender assignment. The elements that should be considered are potential fertility, capacity for sexual function, and the possibility for satisfactory reconstruction. This last factor mandates that an experienced surgeon participate in the decision regarding gender of rearing. Psychological implications are an increased concern following reports of patient dissatisfaction with gender reassignment typically expressed most strongly in adolescence and adulthood.

Development of the Prepuce and Circumcision

The prepuce forms as a roll of epithelium that fuses ventrally at the frenulum. If there is failure of urethral development, this will interfere with development of the prepuce so that abnormalities of the prepuce are very suggestive of other penile abnormalities (e.g., hypospadias, chordee, epispadias). Once the prepuce has covered the glans, its inner epithelial surface fuses with the epithelium of the glans and does not separate from it until some time in childhood (120). It is unusual for a male to have a completely retractable foreskin at birth. In the process of separation of the inner epithelial layer from the glans, cystic spaces form between the two layers and sometimes are filled with desquamated epithelial cells that form white, pearl-like beads that can be seen through the overlying skin. These areas of infantile smegma resemble sebaceous cysts and occasionally become inflamed or infected, although they more commonly drain spontaneously.

Because circumcision is so common in the United States, the natural history of preputial development has been lost, and one must depend upon observations made in countries where circumcision usually is not practiced. The foreskin in the newborn normally is not retractable. In a large series from Denmark, the foreskin was not completely retractable in most boys until puberty (121). Phimosis is defined as the inability to retract the foreskin. In early childhood, this is the normal physiologic state. Although by definition this may be phimosis, there is

every anticipation that the child will develop normally and will not have problems as a result of the temporary inability to retract the foreskin. Forcible retraction of the prepuce tends to produce tears in the preputial orifice, with resulting scarring that may lead to pathologic phimosis.

Circumcision is performed for a multitude of reasons. Medically, it is true that carcinoma of the penis, pathologic phimosis, paraphimosis, some sexually transmitted diseases, and some urinary infections in infancy may be prevented by circumcision (122). If the overall population is considered from a public health and economic basis, however, the advantages to the individual patient perhaps may be mitigated by the cost of circumcising the entire male population to prevent problems in a minority.

At times, the benefits of circumcision are offset by the complications that may arise from this surgical procedure, because complications occur after circumcision just as after any surgical procedure (123). The most common complications seen are hemorrhage and wound infection. Both of these usually prove to be easily treated, minor annoyances. Serious complications occur rarely. These include sepsis, amputation of part of the glans, loss of the entire penis, urethrocutaneous fistulas, bands of scar between the shaft and the glans (Fig. 43–26), denudation of the skin of the entire shaft of the penis, recurrent phimosis (Fig. 43–27), and urethral fistulas (Fig. 43–28) (124). At times, parents are very unhappy with the cosmetic appearance of the penis if an inadequate amount of skin has been excised, even though the functional result is good.

Testicular Torsion

Torsion of the testis in the newborn usually presents as a firm, slightly enlarged testis. There rarely is much abnormality of the overlying skin. Neonatal torsion seems to be painless and actually may be an antenatal event in as many as 72% of the cases (125,126). Twenty-eight percent of the neonatal cases develop in the postnatal period. Exploration of the testis that has undergone torsion in the newborn period probably is of extremely

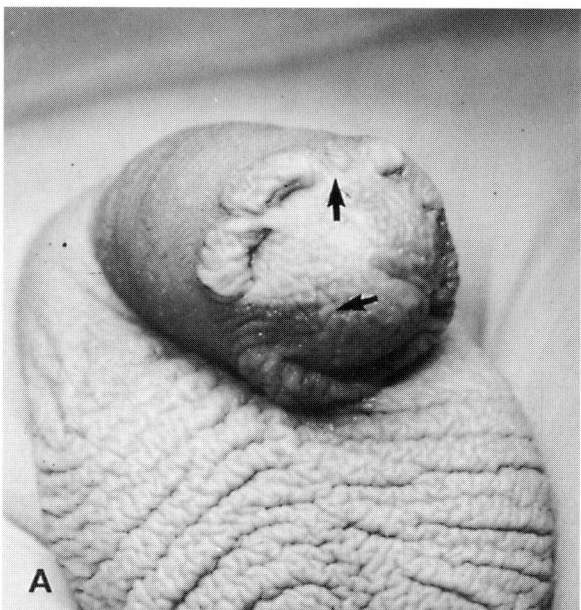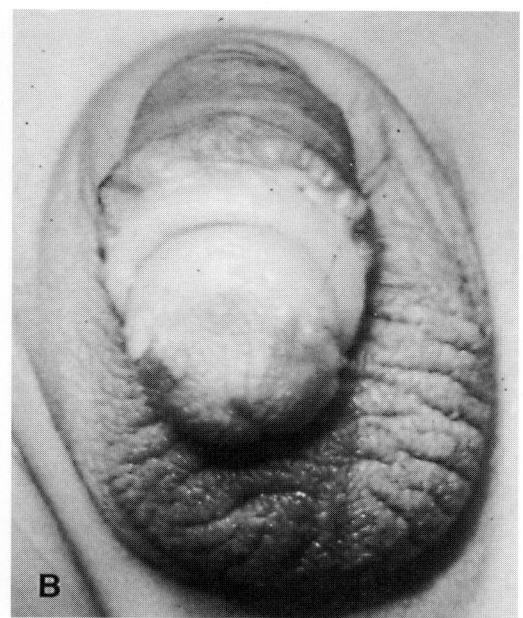

FIG. 43–26. Adhesions (*arrows*) between the distal foreskin and glans penis before **(A)** and after **(B)** surgical transection.

limited value, because it generally is too late for testicular salvage (127). Ten percent of neonatal torsions are bilateral; some are asynchronous, and some are of the intravaginal rather than the extravaginal type. Exploration for neonatal torsion is warranted if the changes are found shortly after birth and performed expeditiously (less than 6 hours from the time of change in testicular examina-

tion). In one series, using an inguinal approach, up to 20% of testes torsed acutely in the neonatal period were be salvaged (128); this may overrepresent actual salvage rates in the newborn time period. In the case of an obviously infarcted testis, contralateral exploration and testicular fixation when the infant is stable may prevent contralateral torsion (129).

Testicular Tumors

Tumors of the testis occasionally present at birth or in early infancy (130). Teratomas of the testis, occurring in 19.7% of cases registered in the Prepubertal Testicular Tumor Registry, are benign and are treated by excision (131). On some occasions, this can be excision of the tumor only, leaving the remainder of the testis *in situ*. On other occasions, because the entire testis has been destroyed, orchiectomy is necessary. A common tumor presenting in the newborn testis is one of the gonadal stromal tumors (131,132); Sertoli cell tumors are the most common of these. Although these tumors histologically may appear malignant, in infancy they invariably exhibit a benign behavior, and, for this reason, orchiectomy is curative. This is in contradistinction to gonadal stromal tumors appearing in later childhood, where malignant behavior has been documented.

Yolk sac tumors occur in infancy, with approximately 30% of recorded testis tumors in infancy. These malignant tumors are best treated by radical orchiectomy. As long as there is no evidence of metastatic disease, adjunctive chemotherapy, node dissection, or radiation therapy is thought to be unwarranted (133). Alpha-fetoprotein

FIG. 43–27. In this patient with circumcision injury, excessive removal of skin from the shaft resulted in skin regeneration over the retracted glans, obscuring the glans. The appearance is that of amputation of the glans. (From Belman AB. The penis. *Urol Clin North Am* 1978;5:17.)

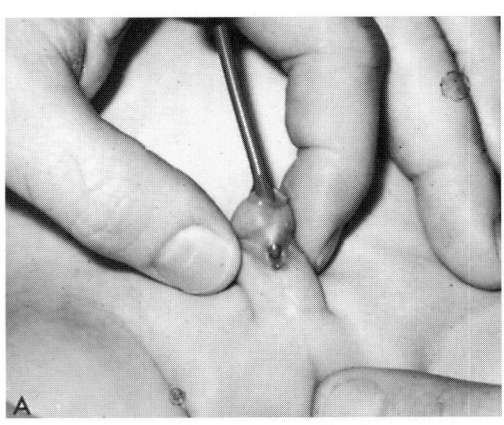
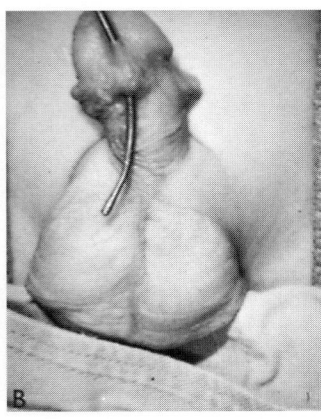

FIG. 43–28. A, B: Two examples of circumcision injuries with secondary coronal fistulas. (From Belman AB. The penis. *Urol Clin North Am* 1978;5:17.)

(AFP) levels are elevated in patients with yolk sac tumors. In infancy, AFP levels normally are elevated compared with measurements obtained in adults. Using age-adjusted AFP levels will improve the usefulness of AFP measurements as a tumor marker in infants (134).

URINARY TRACT INFECTION

Infancy is one period of life during which there is reversal in the gender incidence of bacteriuria. The overall incidence of neonatal urinary tract infections is somewhere between 1.5 to 5 cases per 1,000 live births. The male-to-female ratio is somewhere between 3:1 and 5:1 (135), whereas later in childhood and until later adult life, there is a female preponderance of patients with urinary infections. It has been documented that uncircumcised males are ten times more likely to have urinary infections than are circumcised males (136). The incidence of urinary infection in uncircumcised males approximates 1 per 100. At times, the source of the urinary infection is hematogenous rather than ascending (137).

It is imperative that there be radiographic evaluation of any newborn with culture documented bacteriuria. Vesicoureteral reflux is present in approximately one-half of those evaluated, and obstructive uropathy is not an unusual finding (138). Therefore, at a minimum, urinary tract evaluation with voiding cystourethrography and ultrasonography is indicated.

UROLOGIC ASPECTS OF MYELODYSPLASIA

Almost any child with myelodysplasia will have involvement of the urinary tract. This may be of little consequence in the newborn period, but it is essential that the patient be appropriately evaluated shortly after birth and that a surveillance program be instituted. It was thought that hydronephrosis was found at birth in roughly 10% of children with myelodysplasia, but studies have suggested that some of the hydronephrosis formerly detected actually was a result of spinal shock after closure of the neurologic

lesion and in many children resolved spontaneously (139). Although manual expression of the bladder (Credé manuever) has been used to empty the bladders of children with myelodysplasia, it is not recommended because the intravesical pressures that are produced can be quite high, which can lead to upper tract deterioration, especially in patients with associated vesicoureteral reflux (140). Intermittent catheterization can be used successfully in both male and female infants if needed, and, where these procedures are not successful or acceptable and bladder emptying is thought to be necessary, temporary cutaneous vesicostomy is a proven management modality (141). Children with myelodysplasia, if at all possible, should be managed by a multidisciplinary team that includes neurosurgeons, urologists, and orthopedic surgeons. With this approach, these children have an excellent chance of survival and development as productive citizens in modern society.

PRUNE-BELLY SYNDROME

This lesion is a spectrum of abnormalities characterized by the triad of abdominal wall deficiency, hydronephrosis, and, in males, cryptorchidism. It is the abdominal wall defect that gives the characteristic appearance leading to its name. The incidence of this lesion has been estimated to be 1 per 35,000 to 50,000 live births (6,142). Males are affected ten times more frequently than females (143). There is no clear-cut evidence that this is an inherited disorder. Theories of embryogenesis include obstructive uropathy and mesenchymal dysplasia (144).

There can be massive hydroureteronephrosis and the bladder often is very dilated. There is prostatic hypoplasia with dilation of the prostatic urethra; thus, antenatal studies may not differentiate these patients from boys with posterior urethral valves. The kidneys often are dysplastic, and it is the renal dysplasia that will determine prognosis (145). Although some affected children die in infancy, many today will survive. Reconstruction of the urinary tract, orchiopexy, and repair of the abdominal wall defect often are helpful in altering the outlook for these children (146).

UROLOGIC IMPLICATIONS OF IMPERFORATE ANUS

Because of the intimate relationships of the lower urinary and gastrointestinal tract in their respective development, it is not at all surprising that the urinary tract will be affected in a high proportion of children with imperforate anus; the higher the lesion, the greater the chance of urinary involvement (147). It is for this reason that all newborns with imperforate anus should be screened for urinary tract abnormalities with ultrasonography and a voiding cystourethrogram at the very least. There often are other associated anomalies, and the constellation has come to be known as the VACTERRL association (*v*ertebral, *a*norectal, *c*ardiac, *t*racheo*e*sophageal, *r*enal, *r*adial, and *l*imb abnormalities). When two elements are present, the other should be sought, because three elements qualify as the association. This is a nongenetic, sporadically occurring lesion.

FEMALE GENITAL ABNORMALITIES

The female reproductive system is formed by the müllerian or paramesonephric ducts. The müllerian system will differentiate into a female organ system when müllerian inhibitory substance is absent. During the sixth to eighth week of gestation, the müllerian ducts will form lateral to the wolffian ducts, cross medially, and fuse in the midline incorporating the UG sinus to form the uterovaginal canal by the tenth week of gestation. The fallopian tubes develop from the lateral ends of the müllerian ducts. The vagina develops from the fused müllerian ducts and the UG sinus. It is believed that the upper four-fifths of the vagina is müllerian derived and the lower fifth is from the UG sinus. Vaginal formation is completed by the fifth month of gestation.

The external genitalia differentiates *in utero* during the 12th to 16th weeks. Passive development of the genital tubercle into the clitoris, the urethral folds into the labia minors, and the genital swellings into the labia majors occurs in the absence of fetal androgens.

Vaginal Agenesis

Vaginal agenesis (Meyer–Rokitansky–Kuster–Hauser Syndrome) occurs when the vaginal plate does not canalize. The incidence is reported as 1 in 4,000 to 5000 live female births (148). The patients generally are 46XX females presenting with primary amenorrhea but having normal secondary female sex features. The ovaries and the external genitalia generally are normal, but the vaginal plate is not canalized and the uterus may be rudimentary. It is common to have associated genitourinary anomalies; renal anomalies are seen in 34% of the patients (149). Renal agenesis and ectopia are the most common findings. Patients also may have skeletal anomalies, particularly in the spine and ribs. Combinations of these anomalies has been termed as the MURCS association (*mü*llerian duct aplasia, *r*enal aplasia, and *c*ervicothoracic *s*omite malformations). Surgical correction is individualized based on the location and development of the uterine and vaginal remnants (149).

Hydrocolpos and Hydrometrocolpos

If the vaginal canalization is incomplete, the hymen may be imperforate or a high transverse vaginal septum may be present. The infant may then present with distention of the vagina with glanular secretions stimulated by maternal estrogens, known as hydrocolpos, or distention of the vagina and the uterus with the same secretions, known as hydrometrocolpos. With current antenatal ultrasonography, this can be found prior to delivery, but many infants still present with an abdominal mass, possible urinary obstruction, and a bulging introital mass. Ultrasound imaging may demonstrate a fluid-filled or mixed density fluid-filled pelvis mass and possibly a distended bladder with or without hydroureteronephrosis, if there is secondary urinary obstruction (Fig. 43–29).

Definitive treatment depends on the extent of vaginal canalization; this can be a simple hymenotomy or vaginoplasty or vaginal pull-through if there is a high septal defect. Occasionally, needle aspiration of the fluid and radiographic contrast injection and imaging are necessary to delineate better the length of the vaginal plate remaining.

Duplication or Fusion Anomalies

Duplication of the uterus and vagina occur if fusion of the müllerian ducts is incomplete. The child may have two uteri, one or two cervices with either a single vagina or two separate vaginas, or one or both vaginas may be

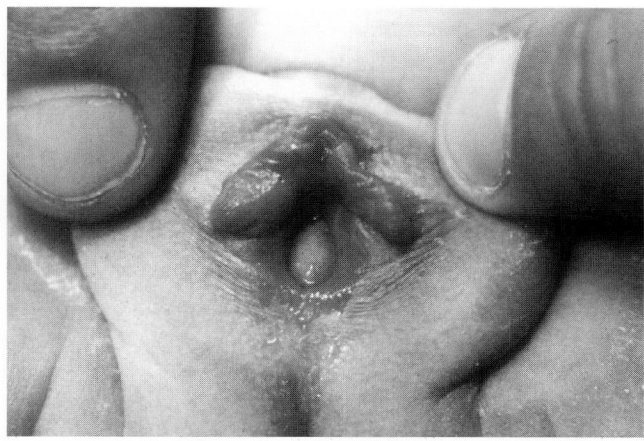

FIG. 43–29. Newborn female with imperforate hymen.

open to the perineum. These malformations can be identified early in life by ultrasonography but frequently will not present until adolescence. The typical presentation is a menstruating female having cyclic pelvic pain associated with menses and an enlarging pelvic mass. Treating vaginal duplication usually only requires incising the longitudinal vaginal septum. Successful pregnancies have been reported in some women with duplicated uteri.

Urogenital Sinus and Cloacal Abnormalities

Having a common urogenital sinus is a normal part of development in both sexes. If müllerian ductal development arrests during the first trimester, a persistent urovaginal confluence or common urogenital sinus will be found at birth. Varying locations for the junction of the vagina and urethra occur depending on the degree of vaginal differentiation. The earlier the arrest occurs, the higher the connection will be located. The anus may be located in its normal location or may be more anteriorly placed. These infants are found to have a common introital opening for urethra and vagina and a second opening for the anus. A flush genitogram will delineate the length of the common urogenital channel and the connections of the urethra and vagina. This is performed by placing a feeding tube or urethral catheter just inside the common opening and injecting contrast material in a retrograde fashion. The type of surgical reconstruction required is determined by the length of the common channel and the location of the urethral vaginal junction. This corrective surgery can be performed during the first year of life in the lower lesions and after the first year with the more proximal connections (149).

A combined urogenital sinus and anorectal malformation is termed a cloacal anomaly. By 4 to 6 weeks of gestation, the urorectal septum should divide the common allantoic–hindgut confluence. If this does not occur, a common cloaca will be present at birth. Because of the imperforate anus, these infants have abdominal distention and a single perineal opening. Delineating the anatomy is important for appropriate surgical management. This generally requires a combined approach with pediatric general surgery and urology input. These infants typically will require diverting colostomy as initial treatment. A flush genitogram can define the urethral, vaginal, and bowel junctions to better plan ultimate reconstruction with bowel pull-through, formal vaginoplasty, and urethroplasty or a simple cutback vaginoplasty. Complete reconstruction can be contemplated during infancy and may be easier near 1 year of age. Delaying reconstruction until late childhood or puberty generally is more difficult due to previous scarring from anal pull-through and the deeper, less mobile pelvis present in older girls (Fig. 43–30).

Ovarian Cysts

Ovarian cysts develop in the presence of hormonal stimulation and more commonly are seen after puberty. The fetal ovary is stimulated by fetal gonadotrophins, maternal estrogens, and placental chorionic gonadotrophin and may develop cysts during fetal development and infancy. Ovarian cysts are being found more frequently with the advent of prenatal ultrasonographic imaging. More than 250 cysts have been reported since 1975 (150). Many of these infants underwent surgical therapy with oophorectomy, cystectomy, or cyst aspiration because of the risk of ovarian torsion due to the cyst increasing the ovarian size and concerns about the occasional ovarian tumor. If discovered *in utero* by ultrasonography, the cysts can be followed until delivery. Vaginal delivery is possible in most cases, with cesarean section being reserved for very large cysts. Postnatally, small ovarian cysts (<4 cm) can be followed with serial ultrasonography, because most cysts will regress in

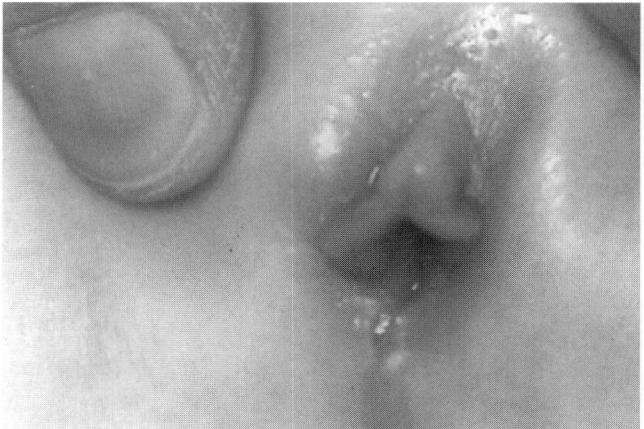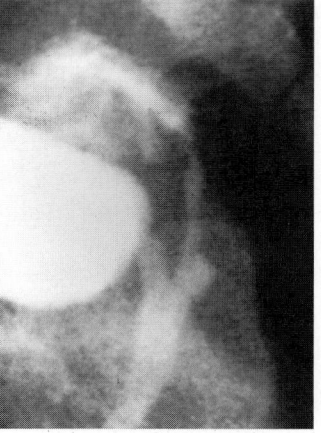

A   B

FIG. 43–30. A: Newborn female with cloacal anomaly. Note single perineal orifice. **B:** Flush genitogram demonstrating a high confluence of the bladder, vagina, and bowel into a common cloaca.

the first 3 to 4 months of life. Larger cysts can be followed for involution or can be aspirated to provide conservation of the ovary. Open surgery should be contemplated if there are complex ovarian cysts, symptomatic cysts, or cysts recur after aspiration. Every attempt should be made to conserve ovarian tissue by removing or unroofing the cyst.

Introital Masses

Introital masses generally are determined at the first examination of the infant. The differential diagnosis for introital masses in female infants include imperforate hymen, prolapsing ureterocele, and Skene's or Gartner's cysts. Prolapsing ureteroceles may extrude through the urethral meatus. Paraurethral cysts (Skene's or Gartner's) also are present in newborn girls and present with lateral displacement of the urethral meatus. These cysts involute or rupture spontaneously, so treatment usually is unnecessary.

ACKNOWLEDGMENT

We would like to thank A. Barry Belman, M.D., M.S., for his generosity in allowing the republication of illustrations from his chapter in the third edition of this book.

REFERENCES

1. Mandell J, Peters CA, Retik AB. Current concepts in the perinatal diagnosis and management of hydronephrosis. *Urol Clin North Am* 1990;17:247.
2. Baskin LS. Prenatal hydronephrosis. In: Baskin LS, Kogan BA, Duckett JW (eds). *Handbook of pediatric urology*. Philadelphia: Lippincott–Raven Publishers, 1997:11.
3. Townsend RR, Manlo-Johnson M. Prenatal diagnosis of urinary tract abnormalities with ultrasound: a review. *Scand J Urol Nephrol* 1991; 138[Suppl]:13.
4. Mackie GG, Stephens FD. Duplex kidneys: a correlation of renal dysplasia with position of the ureteral orifice. *J Urol* 1979;114:274.
5. Potter EL. *Normal and abnormal development of the kidney*. Chicago: Year Book, 1972:86.
6. Cendron M, Elder JS, Duckett JW. Perinatal urology. In: Gillenwater JY, Grayhack JT, Howards SS, Duckett JW, eds. *Adult and pediatric urology*, 3rd ed. St. Louis: Mosby-Year Book, 1996, pp 2075–2170.
7. Emanuel B, Nachman R, Aronson N, et al. Congenital solitary kidney: a review of 74 cases. *Am J Dis Child* 1974;127:17.
8. McGee MD, Lucey DT, Fried FA. A new embryologic classification for urogynecological malformations: the syndrome of mesonephric duct induced müllerian deformities. *J Urol* 1979;121:265.
9. Cook WA, Stephens FD. Fused kidneys: morphologic study and theory of embryogenesis. In: Bergsma D, Duckett JW, eds. *Urinary system malformations in children. Birth Defects:* Original Article Series. New York: March of Dimes, 1977:327.
10. Belman AB, King LR. Urinary tract abnormalities associated with imperforate anus. *J Urol* 1972;108:823.
11. Brenner B, Meyer TW, Hostetter TH. Dietary protein intake and the progressive nature of kidney disease: role of hemodynamically mediated glomerular injury in the pathogenesis of progressive glomerular sclerosis in aging, renal ablation and intrinsic renal disease. *N Engl J Med* 1983;307:652.
12. Burke EC, Wenzel JE, Utz DC. The intrathoracic kidney: report of a case. *Am J Dis Child* 1967;113:487.
13. Kelalis PP, Malek RS, Segura JW. Observations on renal ectopia and fusion in children. *J Urol* 1973;110:588.
14. Leduc B, Van Campenhout J, Simaro R. Congenital absence of the vagina: observations on 25 cases. *Am J Obstet Gynecol* 1968;100:512.
15. Elli F, Stalder G. Malformations of kidney and urinary tract in common chromosomal aberrations. *Hum Genet* 1973;18:1.
16. McDonald JH, McClellan DS. Crossed renal ectopia. *Am J Urol* 1957; 93:995.
17. N'Guessan G, Stephens FD. Supernumerary kidney. *J Urol* 1983;130: 649.
18. Osathanondh V, Potter EL. Pathogenesis of polycystic kidneys: type I due to hyperplasia of interstitial portions of collecting tubules. *Arch Pathol* 1964;77:466.
19. Blythe H, Ockenden BG. Polycystic disease of kidneys and liver presenting in childhood. *J Med Genet* 1971;8:257.
20. Osathanondh V, Potter EL. Pathogenesis of polycystic kidneys: type 3 due to multiple abnormalities of development. *Arch Pathol* 1964;77: 485.
21. Stapleton FB, Johnson DL, Kaplan GW, et al. The cystic renal lesion in tuberous sclerosis. *J Pediatr* 1980;97:574.
22. Spence HM, Baird SS, Ware EW Jr. Cystic disorders of the kidney: classification, diagnosis, treatment. *JAMA* 1957;163:1466.
23. Wacksman J, Phipps L. Report of multicystic kidney registry: preliminary findings. *J Urol* 1993;150:1870.
24. Campbell MF. Embryology and anomalies of the urogenital tract. In: Campbell MF, ed. *Clinical pediatric urology*. Philadelphia: WB Saunders, 1951:198.
25. Campbell MF. Anomalies of the ureter. In: Campbell MF, ed. *Urology*, 3rd ed. Philadelphia: WB Saunders, 1970:1487.
26. Ambrose SS, Nicholson WP. Ureteral reflux into duplicated ureters. *J Urol* 1964;92:439.
27. Stephens FD, Lenaghan D. The anatomical basis and dynamics of vesicoureteral reflux. *J Urol* 1962;87:669.
28. Stephens FD. Caecoureterocele and concepts of the embryology and aetiology of ureteroceles. *Aust N Z J Surg* 1971;40:239.
29. Chwalla R. The process of formation of cystic dications of the vesical end of the ureter and of diverticula at the ureteral ostium. *Urol Cutan Rev* 1927;31:499.
30. Johnston JH. The pathogenesis of hydronephrosis in children. *Br J Urol* 1969;41:724.
31. McLaughlin AP III, Pfister RC, Leadbetter WF, et al. Pathophysiology of primary megaureter. *J Urol* 1973;109:805.
32. Osathanondh V, Potter EL. Pathogenesis of polycystic kidneys: type 2 due to inhibition of ampullary activity. *Arch Pathol* 1964;77:459.
33. Glenn JF. Agenesis of the bladder. *JAMA* 1959;169:2016.
34. Williams DI. The development of the trigone of the bladder. *Br J Urol* 1951;23:123.
35. Bauer SB, Retik AB. Urachal and related umbilical disorders. *Urol Clin North Am* 1978;5:195.
36. Satler EJ, Mossman HW. A case of double bladder and double urethra in the female child. *J Urol* 1968;79:274.
37. Stephens FD. *Congenital malformations of the urinary tract*. New York: Praeger, 1983.
38. Das S, Amar AD. Extravesical ureteral ectopia in male patients. *J Urol* 1981;125:842.
39. Brock WA, Kaplan GW. Voiding dysfunction in children. *Curr Probl Pediatr* 1980;2:10.
40. Weiss JP, Duckett JW, Snyder HM. Single unilateral vaginal ectopic ureter: is it really a rarity? *J Urol* 1984;132:1177.
41. Brock WA, Kaplan GW. Ectopic ureteroceles in children. *J Urol* 1978;119:800.
42. Mandel J, Colodny AH, Lebowitz R, et al. Ureteroceles in infants and children. *J Urol* 1980;123:921.
43. Snyder HM, Johnston JH. Orthotopic ureteroceles in children. *J Urol* 1978;119:543.
44. Scherz HC, Kaplan GW, Packer MG, et al. Ectopic ureteroceles: surgical management with preservation of continence: review of 60 cases. *J Urol* 1989;142:538.
45. Somner TE, Crowe JE, Resnick MI. Diagnosis of ectopic ureterocele using ultrasound. *Urology* 1980;15:82.
46. Blyth B, Passerini-Glazel G, Camuffo C, et al. Endoscopic incision of ureteroceles: intravesical versus ectopic. *J Urol* 1993;149:556.
47. White JM, Kaplan GW, Brock WA. Ureteropelvic junction obstruction in children. *Am Fam Physician* 1984;29:211.
48. Maizels M, Reisman ME, Flum ES, et al. Grading nephroureteral dilatation detected in the first year of life: correlation with obstruction. *J Urol* 1992;148:609.
49. Koff SA, Thrall JH, Keyes JW Jr. Assessment of hydroureteronephrosis in children using diuretic radionuclide urographs. *J Urol* 1980;132:531.

50. Whitaker RH. Methods of assessing obstruction in the dilated ureter. *Br J Urol* 1973;45:15.

51. Johnston JH. Reconstructive surgery of megaureter in childhood. *Br J Urol* 1967;39:17.

52. Noe HN, Wyatt RJ, Peeden JN, et al. The transmission of vesicoureteral reflux from parent to child. *J Urol* 1992;148:1869.

53. Dwoskin JY. Sibling uropathology. *J Urol* 1976;115:726.

54. Paquin AJ. Ureterovesical anastomosis: the description and evaluation of a technique. *J Urol* 1954;82:573.

55. Baker R, Maxted W, Maylith J, et al. Relation of age, sex, and infection to reflux: data indicating high spontaneous cure rate in pediatric patients. *J Urol* 1966;95:27.

56. Levitt SA, Duckett J, Spitzer A, et al. Medical versus surgical treatment of primary vesicoureteral reflux: report of the International Reflux Study Committee. *Pediatrics* 1981;67:392.

57. Dwoskin JY, Perimutter AD. Vesicoureteral reflux in children: a computerized review. *J Urol* 1973;109:888.

58. Jeffs RD. Exstrophy and cloacal exstrophy. *Urol Clin North Am* 1978;5:127.

59. Scherz HC, Kaplan GW, Sutherland DH, et al. Fascia late and early apica casting as adjuncts in closure of bladder exstrophy. *J Urol* 1990;144:550.

60. Ngan JH, Grady RW, Carr MC, et al. An argument for complete one-stage anatomic repair of exstrophy in the newborn. Abstract, American Urological Association, 92nd Annual Meeting, 1997.

61. Eraklis A, Folkman J. Adenocarcinoma at the site of ureterosigmoidostomies for exstrophy of the bladder. *J Pediatr Surg* 1978;13:730.

62. McIntosh JF, Worley G Jr. Adenocarcinoma arising in exstrophy of the bladder: report of two cases and review of the literature. *J Urol* 1955;73:820.

63. Johnston JH, Penn IA. Exstrophy of the cloaca. *Br J Urol* 1966;38:302.

64. Tank ES, Lindenauer SM. Principles of management of exstrophy of the cloaca. *Am J Surg* 1970;119:95.

65. Diamond M, Sigmundson HK. Sex Reassignment at birth: long term review and clinical implications. *Arch Pediatr Adolesc Med* 1997;151:298.

66. Waffarn F, Devasker UP, Hodgman JE. Vesico-umbilical fistula: a complication of umbilical artery cutdown. *J Pediatr Surg* 1980;15:211.

67. Walden TB, Karafin L, Kendall AR. Urachal diverticulum in a 3 year old boy. *J Urol* 1979;122:554.

68. Bambirra EA, Miranda D. Gastric polyp of the umbilicus in an 8 year old boy. *Clin Pediatr* 1980;19:430.

69. Berdon WE, Baker DH, Becker JA, et al. Megacystis—microcolon intestinal hypoperistalsis syndrome: a new cause of intestinal obstruction: report of radiologic findings in five newborn girls. *AJR* 1976;126:957.

70. Ochoa B, Curlin RJ. Urofacial (Ochoa) syndrome. *Am J Med Genet* 1987;27:661.

71. Robertston WB, Hayes JA. Congenital diaphragmatic obstruction of the male posterior urethra. *Br J Urol* 1969;41:592.

72. Rattner WH, Meyer R, Bernstein J. Congenital abnormalities of the urinary system: IV. Valvular obstruction of the posterior urethra. *J Pediatr* 1963;63:94.

73. Osathanondh V, Potter EG. Pathogenesis of polycystic kidneys: type 4 due to urethral obstruction. *Arch Pathol* 1964;77:502.

74. Javadpour N, Graziano MF, Terrill R. Experimental induction of patent allantoic duct by intrauterine bladder outlet obstruction. *J Surg Res* 1974;17:341.

75. Tanagho EA. Surgically induced partial urinary obstruction in the fetal lamb: II. Urethral obstruction. *Invest Urol* 1972;10:25.

76. Johnston JH. Vesicoureteral reflux with urethral valves. *Br J Urol* 1979;51:100.

77. Maizels M, Simpson SB Jr. Primitive ducts of renal dysplasia induced by cultured ureteral buds and condensed renal mesenchyme. *Science* 1983;219:509.

78. Churchill BM, McLorie MD, Khoury AE, et al. Emergency treatment and long-term follow up of posterior urethral valves. *Urol Clin North Am* 1990;17:343.

79. Cass AS, Stephens FD. Posterior urethral valves: diagnosis and management. *J Urol* 1974;112:519.

80. Sheldon CH, Gonzales R, Bauer MS, et al. Obstructive uropathy, renal failure, and sepsis in the neonate: a surgical emergency. *Urology* 1980;16:457.

81. Egami K, Smith ED. A study of the sequelae of posterior urethral valves. *J Urol* 1982;127:84.

82. Scott TW. Urinary ascites secondary to posterior urethral valves. *J Urol* 1976;116:87.

83. Tank ES, Carey TC, Seifert NL. Management of neonatal urinary ascites. *Urology* 1980;16:270.

84. Weller MH, Miller KE. Unusual aspects of urine ascites. *Radiology* 1973;129:665.

85. Parker RM. Neonatal urinary ascites: a potentially favorable sign in bladder outlet obstruction. *Urology* 1974;3:589.

86. Johnston JH. Vesicoureteral reflux with urethral valves. *Br J Urol* 1979;51:100.

87. Johnston JH, Kulatilake AE. The sequelae of posterior urethral valves. *Br J Urol* 1971;43:743.

88. Mayor G, Genton N, Tobrado A, et al. Renal function in obstructive uropathy: long-term effect of reconstructive surgery. *Pediatrics* 1975;56:740.

89. Parkhouse HF, Barratt TM, Dillon MJ, et al. Long term outcome of boys with posterior urethral valves. *Br J Urol* 1988;62:59.

90. Howell CG, Othersen HB Jr, Kiviat NE, et al. Therapy and outcome in 51 children with mesoblastic nephroma: a report of the National Wilms' Tumor Study. *J Pediatr Surg* 1982;6:826.

91. Machin GA. Persistent renal blastema (nephroblastomatosis) as a frequent precursor of Wilms' tumor: a pathological and clinical review: 2. qSignificance of nephroblastomatosis in the genesis of Wilms' tumor. *Am J Pediatr Hematol Oncol* 1980;2:253.

92. Gonzalez-Cirraso F, Kidd JM, Hernandez RJ. Cystic nephroma: morphologic spectrum and implications. *Urology* 1982;20:88.

93. Ganguly A, Gribble J, Tune B, et al. Renin-secreting Wilms' tumor with severe hypertension: report of a case and brief review of renin-secreting tumors. *Ann Intern Med* 1973;79:835.

94. Joshi VV, Banarsee AK, Yadak K, et al. Cystic partially differentiated nephroblastoma: a clinicopathologic entity in the spectrum of infantile renal neoplasia. *Cancer* 1977;40:789.

95. Belman AB, King LR. The pathology and treatment of renal vein thrombosis in the newborn. *J Urol* 1972;107:852.

96. Khuri FJ, Alton DJ, Hardy BE, et al. Adrenal hemorrhage in neonates: report of 5 cases and review of the literature. *J Urol* 1980;124:684.

97. Levin S, Collins D, Kaplan GW, et al. Neonatal adrenal pseudocyst mimicking metastatic disease. *Ann Surg* 1974;174:186.

98. Blane CE, Koff SA, Bowerman RA, et al. Non-obstructive fetal hydronephrosis: sonographic recognition and therapeutic implications. *Radiology* 1983;147:95.

99. Elder JS, Duckett JW Jr, Snyder HM. Intervention for fetal obstructive uropathy: has it been effective? *Lancet* 1987;2:1007.

100. Murphy JL, Kaplan GW, Packer MG, et al. Prenatal diagnosis of severe urinary tract anomalies improves renal function and growth. *Child Nephrol Urol* 1988;89:290.

101. Manning FA, Harrison MR, Rodeck C, et al. Catheter shunts for fetal hydronephrosis: report of the International Fetal Surgery Registry. *N Engl J Med* 1985;315:336.

102. Montana MA, Cyr DR, Lenke RR, et al. Sonographic detection of fetal ureteral obstruction. *AJR* 1985;145:595.

103. Glick PL, Harrison MR, Golbus MS, et al. Management of the fetus with congenital hydronephrosis: II. Prognostic criteria and selection for treatment. *J Pediatr Surg* 1985;20:376.

104. Sherwood DW, Smith RC, Lemmon RH, et al. Abnormalities of the genitourinary tract discovered by palpation of the abdomen of the newborn. *Pediatrics* 1956;18:782.

105. Wedge JJ, Grosfeld JL, Smith JP. Abdominal masses in the newborn: 63 cases. *J Urol* 1971;106:770.

106. Raffensberger J, Abdusleiman A. Abdominal masses in children under one year of age. *Surgery* 1968;63:514.

107. Melicow MM, Uson AC. Palpable abdominal masses in infants and children: a report based on a review of 653 cases. *J Urol* 1959;81:705.

108. Emanuel B, Nachman R, Aronson N, et al. Congenital solitary kidney. *Am J Dis Child* 1974;127:17.

109. Scorer CG. The descent of the testicle. *Arch Dis Child* 1964;39:605.

110. Scorer CG, Farrington GH. *Congenital deformities of the testis and epididymis.* London: Butterworths, 1971.

111. Kogan JJ, Tennenbaum SY, Gill B, et al. Efficacy of orchiopexy by patient age 1 year for cryptorchidism. *J Urol* 1990;144:508.

112. Kessler WO, McLaughlin AP. Agenesis of the penis: embryology and management. *Urology* 1973;1:226.

113. Rodriguez C. Report of a case of diphallus. *J Urol* 1965;94:436.

114. Lee PA, Mazur T, Danish R, et al. Micropenis: criteria, etiologies, and classification. *Johns Hopkins Med J* 1980;146:156.

115. Burstein S, Grumbach MM, Kaplan SL. Early determination of androgen responsiveness is important in the management of microphallus. *Lancet* 1979;2:983.

116. Bauer SB, Retik AB, Colodny AH. Genetic aspects of hypospadias. *Urol Clin North Am* 1981;8:559.

117. Cerasaro TS, Brock WA, Kaplan GW. Upper urinary tract anomalies associated with congenital hypospadias: is screening necessary? *J Urol* 1986;135:537.

118. Canning DA, Koo HP, Duckett JW. Anomalies of the bladder and cloaca. In: Gillenwater JY, Grayhack JT, Howards SS, Duckett JW, eds. *Adult and pediatric urology*, 3rd ed. St. Louis: Mosby-Year Book, 1996, pp 2445–2488.

119. Williams DI, Kenawi MM. Urethral duplications in the male. *Eur Urol* 1975;1:209.

120. Gairdner D. The fate of the foreskin: a study of circumcision. *Br Med J* 1949;2:1433.

121. Oster J. Further fate of the foreskin. *Arch Dis Child* 1968;43:200.

122. Wiswell TE. Routine neonatal circumcision: a reappraisal. *Am Fam Physician* 1990;41:859.

123. MacDonald MG. Circumcision. In: Fletcher MA, MacDonald MG, eds. *Atlas of procedures in neonatology*, 2nd ed. Philadelphia: JB Lippincott, 1993:378.

124. Kaplan GW. Complications of circumcision. *Urol Clin North Am* 1983;10:543.

125. Burge DM. Neonatal testicular torsion and infarction: etiology and management. *Br J Urol* 1987;59:70.

126. Das S, Singer A. Controversies in perinatal torsion of the spermatic cord: a review, survey and recommendations. *J Urol* 1990;143:231.

127. Jerkins GR, Noe HN, Hollabauch RS, et al. Spermatic cord torsion in the neonate. *J Urol* 1983;129:121.

128. Pinto KJ, Noe HN, Jerkins GR. Management of neonatal torsion. *J Urol* 1997;158:1196.

129. Kaplan GW, Silber I. Neonatal torsion: to pex or not? In: King LR, ed. *Neonatal problems in urology*. Philadelphia: JB Lippincott, 1988:386.

130. Kaplan GW. Prepubertal testicular tumors. *World J Urol* 1984;2:238.

131. Kay R. Prepubertal testicular tumor registry. *Urol Clin North Am* 1993;20:1.

132. Kaplan GW, Chromie WJ, Kelalis PP, et al. Gonadal stromal tumors: a report of the Prepubertal Testicular Tumor Registry. *J Urol* 1986;136:300.

133. Kaplan GW, Chromie WJ, Kelalis PP, et al. Prepubertal yolk sac testicular tumors: report of the Testicular Tumor Registry. *J Urol* 1988;140:1109.

134. Wu JT, Book L, Sudar K. Serum alpha-fetoprotein (AFP) levels in normal infants. *Pediatr Res* 1981;15:50.

135. Drew JH, Acton CK. Radiologic findings in newborn infants with urinary infection. *Arch Dis Child* 1976;51:628.

136. Wiswell TE, Smith FR, Bass JW. Decreased incidence of urinary tract infections in circumcised male infants. *Pediatrics* 1985;75:401.

137. Stamey TA. *Urinary infections*. Baltimore: Williams & Wilkins, 1972.

138. Bergstrom T, Larson H, Lincoln K, et al. Studies of urinary tract infections in infancy and childhood: XII. Eighty consecutive patients with neonatal infection. *J Pediatr* 1972;80:858.

139. Chiaramonte RM, Horowitz EM, Kaplan GW, et al. Implications of hydronephrosis in the newborn with myelodysplasia. *J Urol* 1986;136:147.

140. Barbalias GA, Klauber GT, Blaivas JG. Critical evaluation of the Credé maneuver: a urodynamic study of 207 patients. *J Urol* 1983;130:720.

141. Cohen JS, Harbach LS, Kaplan GW. Cutaneous vesicostomy for temporary diversion in infants with neurogenic bladder dysfunction. *J Urol* 1978;119:120.

142. Garlinger P, Ott J. Prune belly syndrome: possible genetic implications. *Birth Defects* 1974;10:173.

143. Rabinowitz R, Schillinger JF. Prune belly syndrome in the female subject. *J Urol* 1977;118:454.

144. Silverman FM, Huang N. Congenital absence of the abdominal muscle associated with malformation of the genitourinary and alimentary tracts: report of cases and review of literature. *Am J Dis Child* 1950;80:9.

145. Williams DI, Parker RM. The role of surgery in the prune belly syndrome. In: Johnston JH, Goodwin WF, eds. *Review of pediatric urology*. Amsterdam: Excerpta Medica, 1974:315.

146. Woodard JR, Parrott TS. Reconstruction of the urinary tract in prune belly syndrome. *J Urol* 1978;119:824.

147. Fleisher MH, McLorie GA, Churchill BM, et al. The yield of investigation of the urinary tract in imperforate anus. *J Urol* 1985;133:142.

148. Hensle TW. Genital anomalies. In: Gillenwater JY, Grayhack JT, Howards SS, Duckett JW, eds. *Adult and pediatric urology*, 3rd ed. St. Louis: Mosby-Year Book, 1996, pp 2529–2548.

149. Brandt ML, Luks FI, Filiatrault D, et al. Surgical indications in antenatally diagnosed ovarian cysts. *J Pediatr Surg* 1991;26:276.

150. Smith C, Gosalbez R, Parrott TS, et al. Transurethral puncture of ectopic ureteroceles in neonates and infants. *J Urol* 1994;152:2110.

CHAPTER 44

General Surgery

Gary E. Hartman, Michael J. Boyajian, Sukgi S. Choi,
Martin R. Eichelberger, Kurt D. Newman, and David Mann Powell

Successful management of newborns with surgical conditions requires close cooperation among neonatologist, surgeon, anesthesiologist, and radiologist. The fragile nature and limited reserve of these infants are superimposed on the stress of the surgical condition and its operative correction. In addition to the physiologic concerns related to the surgical condition, special attention must be directed toward (a) temperature regulation, (b) fluid, blood, and glucose administration, and (c) monitoring of respiratory and cardiovascular performance.

Venous and arterial access for fluid administration and monitoring may be challenging. Peripheral venous access with a 22- or 24-gauge catheter provides adequate access for the most vigorous fluid resuscitation. Central venous access may be necessary in the unstable newborn or if peripheral access is unsuccessful. Umbilical artery catheterization provides vascular access and arterial monitoring and is a well-established procedure in even the smallest prematures. The umbilical catheter may be maintained in most operative procedures. Peripheral arterial access may be obtained using radial, ulnar, or posterior tibial puncture or cutdown.

G. E. Hartman, K. D. Newman, and D. M. Powell: Departments of Surgery and Pediatrics, The George Washington University School of Medicine; and Department of Pediatric Surgery, Children's National Medical Center, Washington, D.C.

M. J. Boyajian: Departments of Surgery and Pediatrics, The George Washington University School of Medicine; and Department of Plastic Surgery, Children's National Medical Center, Washington, D.C.

S. S. Choi: Departments of Otolaryngology and Pediatrics, The George Washington University School of Medicine; and Department of Otolaryngology, Children's National Medical Center, Washington, D.C.

M. R. Eichelberger: Departments of Surgery and Pediatrics, The George Washington University School of Medicine; and Emergency Trauma Services, Children's National Medical Center, Washington, D.C.

Fluid requirements are usually significantly greater than maintenance, especially in situations with intestinal obstruction, peritonitis, or gastroschisis. Before the operation there are extraordinary losses from the gastrointestinal tract or inflamed peritoneum. These losses continue in the postoperative period and are superimposed on the sodium and water retention associated with the stress response. The endocrine, metabolic, and cytokine response to operative stress, which has been well documented in adults, has been confirmed in neonates (1–3). Postoperatively, decreased urine volume may result from the surge in antidiuretic hormone, intravascular volume depletion, or both, limiting the utility of urine volume alone as a monitor of adequacy of fluid replacement. Additional assessments including skin temperature, quality of peripheral pulses, serial measurements of weight, hematocrit, and serum electrolytes and osmolality supplement urine volume as indicators of adequate volume replacement (4).

Temperature maintenance is a critical concern for all newborns, but in particular for those undergoing diagnostic studies and operative procedures in radiology and operating suites. A variety of means of temperature support may be utilized, including warming the environment, heat lamps, heating blankets, scalp and extremity wrapping, heated intravenous fluids and blood products, and heated inhaled anesthetic agents and surgical irrigating fluids. Temperature must be constantly monitored, and every effort made to minimize exposure to cold stress. Hypothermia is a potentially lethal condition, and the importance of temperature support cannot be overemphasized (5).

Anesthetic and postoperative pain management can minimize the magnitude of the stress response and accelerate the neonate's return to normal homeostasis in terms of cortisol, catecholamine, and insulin modulation (6). The expertise of all the specialists involved may be the advantage necessary to achieve survival and mandates close collaboration.

LESIONS OF THE HEAD AND NECK

Congenital abnormalities of the head and neck occur commonly in the newborn. Because of the short, fat neck of the baby, some of these lesions are not immediately apparent, and the examiner must be alert to their possibility to detect them.

Cleft Lip

Clefts of the lip or palate occur in approximately one of every 600 to 700 Caucasian newborns. The frequency is doubled in Asians and halved in African-Americans. Cleft lip occurs somewhat more often in male patients and on the left side. The defect probably results from lack of the mesodermal reinforcement of the junction of the nasomedial and lateral facial processes that normally takes place in the sixth to seventh week of gestation. Multiple genetic influences seem to be more important than environmental factors. The cleft deformity ranges from minor notching to complete separation of the entire lip and nasal floor (Fig. 44–1). The defect may involve the lip, the lip and palate, or only the palate, and it may be unilateral or bilateral. Median cleft lip is rare and is usually associated with hypotelorism, microcephaly, and early death.

Airway obstruction is not typically a consequence of isolated cleft lip or palate. Initial care focuses on feeding the infant and counseling the parents. Swallowing and airway protection should be normal, but the negative pressure of the normal suck is vented through the cleft,

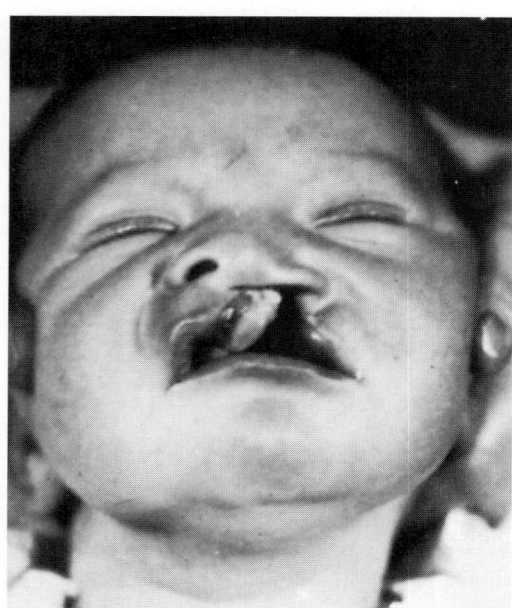

FIG. 44–1. Complete congenital cleft of the lip with associated cleft of the palate that extends forward through the alveolar ridge.

resulting in inadequate inflow. Fatigue during feeding is common and may mimic satiation. Although suckling is not altogether discouraged, a baby with a complete cleft lip or any degree of cleft palate should be expected to suffer mechanical feeding difficulty. The solution may be to rely on an enlarged nipple aperture, a compressible bottle, or a syringe feeder. With the use of a positive-pressure delivery system, the feeding schedule should be normal.

Lip closure is usually carried out at around 3 months of age. The major goals are muscle continuity, balanced lip height, the normal Cupid's-bow lip shape, a smooth and pout-free lip margin, a good nasal sill, adequate sulcus lining, and a minimal, well-placed scar. The wide, complete unilateral and the complete bilateral clefts present greater challenges. Preliminary lip adhesion for the unilateral case or presurgical orthodontics can improve anatomic associations and facilitate the definitive surgery. Residual nasal deformity is often a stubborn problem and may require secondary surgery.

Cleft Palate

The embryologic palatal shelves initially hang vertically and then rise to meet and fuse from front to back between weeks 7 and 12 of gestation. Interference with this process may result in complete, incomplete, or submucous cleft of the palate. Initial care is discussed in the section on cleft lip.

The major significance of this defect is the effect on speech. Normal modulation of speech requires reliable, dynamic palatal separation of the mouth from the nose. This requires a palate of adequate length, suppleness, and muscle power. Velopharyngeal incompetence or incomplete nasal closure results in hypernasal speech and significant communication disability.

Chronic or recurrent effusion and infection in an otherwise normal ear is common in the child with a cleft palate because eustachian tube function is compromised. This child usually needs myringotomies and ventilation tubes.

Early surgery seems to have a negative effect on facial growth, but the trend is toward closure during infancy because of the improved speech results. Most American surgeons choose 9 to 12 months of age as optimal timing for a single-stage closure.

Palatal closure is accomplished with local soft tissue. Mucoperiosteal flaps are mobilized and closed in the midline, with oral and nasal lining, effecting muscle apposition and retroposition. No bone reconstruction is involved. The goal is normal speech, and this is achieved in approximately 85% of patients. A second operation produces good results for almost all the remaining infants.

An essential concept in the treatment of these children is a multidisciplinary approach. The patient should be followed through adolescence by a team consisting of a plastic surgeon, otolaryngologist, audiologist, pedodontist, orthodontist, speech pathologist, geneticist, pediatrician, and social worker.

Pierre–Robin Sequence

The Pierre–Robin sequence is characterized by retrognathia or microgenia (i.e., small or recessed jaw or chin), glossoptosis, airway obstruction, and cleft palate. The lack of forward support of the tongue allows it to fall back and compromise the airway. The basic defect may result from intrauterine restriction of mandibular growth.

Intensive monitoring, including a home apnea monitor, is necessary for many patients. The airway can usually be maintained by conservative measures. Prone positioning allows the tongue to fall forward. An appropriately apertured board may facilitate this positioning, and a nasal airway may be useful. Early gavage feedings may obviate hazardous oral feedings. A lip–tongue adhesion may be performed in more difficult cases, but its effectiveness varies. Tracheostomy should be avoided, if possible, but it is sometimes the only safe choice. Management should be as conservative as the clinical situation permits. The airway problem is typically self-limited, resolving as the child grows.

Masses in the Neck

Masses in the neck are common in children and may be congenital, infectious, or neoplastic. Thyroglossal duct remnants, branchial apparatus anomalies, and lymphangiomas (i.e., cystic hygromas) are the most common congenital pediatric lesions in the neck.

Thyroglossal Duct Remnants

Thyroid tissue left behind in an abnormal location during normal developmental descent can result in a thyroglossal duct cyst, which presents in the midline of the neck. Infection may lead to a cutaneous salivary fistula. After appropriate therapy for infection, treatment consists of resection of the cyst, the central portion of the hyoid bone, and dissection of the tract up to its origin at the foramen cecum (Sistrunk operation) (7–9).

Branchial Cleft Anomalies

Branchial clefts with their corresponding arches and pouches are embryologic structures that give rise to many of the components of the lower face and neck. Abnormal persistence of any portion of the branchial apparatus leads to specific anomalies about the face and neck (10,11).

Preauricular Tabs and Sinuses

These lesions are not true branchial cleft remnants because they originate from an abnormal formation of the ear rather than a branchial cleft component. The preauricular sinus almost always ends blindly, and excision is indicated to prevent recurrent infection in later years.

Cervical Fistulas

Fistulas that originate from the first branchial arch present in the neck just below the ear and communicate with the external auditory canal. A fistula originating from the second branchial arch is the most common branchial cleft remnant. The fistula usually extends from the skin of the lower neck upward along the sternocleidomastoid muscle and then passes inward between the internal and external carotid arteries to attach to the posterolateral pharynx just below the tonsillar fossa (Fig. 44–2). The presenting complaint is usually related to persistent or intermittent drainage onto the neck. Complete surgical extirpation is necessary for cure. A large incision in the neck can be

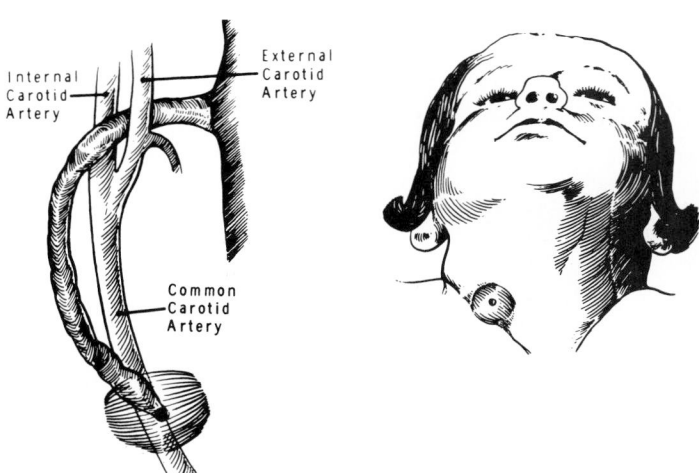

FIG. 44–2. Brachial cleft cyst, which presents low in the neck as a mass or an opening in the skin, extends upward and laterally in the neck, and passes between the branches of the carotid artery to connect with the pharynx below the tonsillar facia. (From Nardi GL, Zuidema GD. *Surgery,* 3rd ed. Boston: Little, Brown, 1972, with permission.)

avoided by the use of two or three small, neat, transverse stair-step incisions.

Branchial Cyst

Approximately 10% of persistent branchial deformities are cystic. These invariably arise low in the anterior triangle of the neck and present as smooth cysts anterior to the sternocleidomastoid muscle. Dissection with excision is curative.

Cervical Cutaneous Tabs

Occasionally, a baby presents with a cutaneous tab in the skin of the anterior aspect of the neck. A small, irregular mass of cartilage may be contained in the skin tab. The cartilage is never associated with a fistula, and removal of this small appendage is not urgent.

Cystic Hygroma

Cystic hygroma (i.e., lymphangioma) is a congenital deformity arising from abnormal development of lymphatic channels (Fig. 44–3) (12). About 80% of these watery cysts occur in the neck, and most are located posterior to the sternocleidomastoid muscle. Other sites of occurrence are the groin, the axilla, and the mediastinum. The term "hygroma" suggests the watery fluid contained in the endothelium-lined spaces. The cyst may be unilocular, but more often there are numerous cysts of various sizes that permeate the surrounding structures and distort the local anatomy. Supporting connective tissue often shows extensive lymphocytic infiltration. Except in the case of a single large cyst, no definite cleavage plane is found between hygroma and normal tissue.

The lesion is usually evident at birth. Occasionally, the mass occupies the entire submandibular region, distorting the subglottic area and compromising the airway. A supraclavicular mass may become prominent with the Valsalva maneuver. This form of cystic hygroma is usually associated with a mediastinal component. Some cystic hygromas contain nests of poorly supported vascular channels that are prone to bleeding and may produce sudden enlargement and discoloration of the lesion.

Symptoms are related entirely to the location and size of the mass. Disfigurement is often severe. Infection in the mass may lead to dangerous regional cellulitis, but after the infection subsides, the resultant intracystic fibrosis and scar may significantly reduce the size of the tumor mass. Prenatal ultrasonography has been used to diagnose cystic hygroma (13). This modality has demonstrated a hidden mortality with a high incidence of associated anomalies, including abnormal karyotypes and hydrops fetalis, when lymphangiomas are detected before 30 weeks of gestation.

Repeated aspiration of the cyst with injection of sclerosing agents is not recommended because any surgical excision that is subsequently required is rendered significantly more difficult by the sclerosing procedure. Elective surgical excision between 4 and 12 months of age is indicated for asymptomatic patients. Airway compression or recurrent infections may necessitate removal at an earlier age (14). Total excision is often impractical because of the extent of the hygroma and its proximity to vital structures. Important nerves and vascular structures must not be sacrificed in an attempt to achieve total excision of this benign lesion; multiple excisions of the residual hygroma are preferable. Postoperative wound drainage using closed-suction drains may reduce recurrence.

UPPER AIRWAY OBSTRUCTION CAUSING RESPIRATORY DISTRESS

A neonate is essentially an obligate nasal breather for the first several months of life. [Recently this belief has been challenged, and some investigators have proposed that a neonate is a preferential nasal breather (15).] Therefore, during the first few months of an infant's life,

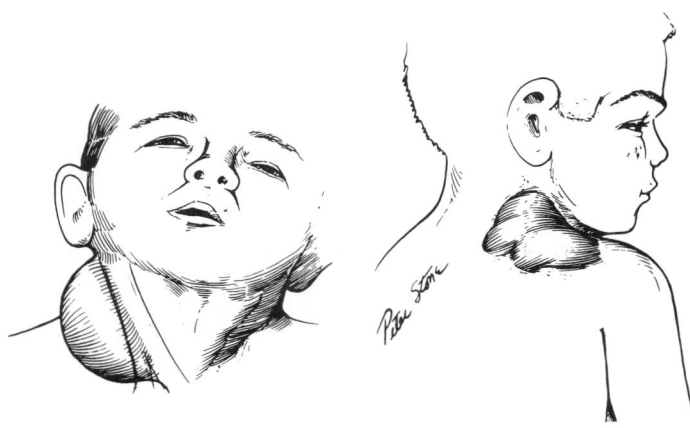

FIG. 44–3. The typical cystic hygroma occurs in the lateral neck. The mass may extend into the scapular, axillary, or thoracic compartments, or the hygroma may present separately in any of these locations. Although depicted here as a single cyst, the hygroma is often a multiloculated, ill-defined mass. (From Nardi GL, Zuidema GD. *Surgery,* 3rd ed. Boston: Little, Brown, 1972.)

any nasal condition causing obstruction can cause respiratory difficulties. Typically a neonate with nasal obstruction presents with cyclic cyanosis.

A newborn's epiglottis is softer and bulkier than that of older children and adults and is often tubular in shape. Excessive and redundant mucosa over the epiglottis and arytenoids can contribute to inspiratory stridor. The larynx in a newborn is a well-developed organ; however, it is one-third the size of an adult larynx. The subglottis of a neonate measures approximately 4.5 mm in diameter. Because of the smaller dimension, 1 mm of circumferential edema in the subglottis can reduce the cross-sectional area of a neonate's airway by more than 60% (16). The trachea and bronchi are also smaller in dimensions and are shorter than those in an adult. In addition to these anatomic differences, the airway structures in a neonate are more pliable, and its mucosa more reactive. Therefore, conditions that affect the airway such as epiglottitis and croup can have proportionately greater effect on a small infant's airway.

Evaluation of airway obstruction begins with a careful history regarding the characteristics of the stridor or other upper airway noises, voice quality, severity of airway symptoms, feeding difficulties, previous intubation history or other manipulation of the airway, other associated anomalies, and symptoms of gastroesophageal reflux or aspiration. The great majority of airway abnormalities causing obstructive symptoms can be identified from the history alone (17). History is supplemented by physical examination and other evaluation modalities. High-kilovolt anterior–posterior and lateral soft tissue film of the neck can help in evaluation of the areas from nasal cavity to subglottis. Posterior–anterior and lateral chest x-rays can help to delineate tracheal and bronchial pathology. Other studies such as computed tomography (CT) scans and magnetic resonance imaging (MRI) may be needed to evaluate airway obstruction involving the nasal cavity, nasopharynx, and trachea.

Flexible nasopharyngoscopy and laryngoscopy can be performed at the bedside with monitoring. Areas from nasal vestibule to the vocal cords can be evaluated for functional and anatomic abnormalities. Flexible bronchoscopy with sedation is often suboptimal for evaluation of the subglottic, tracheal, and bronchial airways and is inferior to rigid endoscopy. Rigid endoscopy is usually performed in the operating room under general anesthesia but with spontaneous ventilation (no paralysis). This type of anesthesia enables the surgeon to evaluate the dynamics of the airway as well as any anatomic abnormalities.

Nasal Obstruction

Nasal Pyriform Aperture Stenosis

Congenital nasal pyriform aperture stenosis (anterior nasal stenosis) is secondary to the overgrowth of the nasal

process of the maxilla (18). In this condition, the entrance into the nasal cavity known as the pyriform aperture is reduced to a slit-like opening. Because the pyriform aperture is the narrowest part of the nasal airway, even small changes in the cross-sectional area at this level can result in significant increase in nasal airway resistance and airway obstruction. Clinically, nasal obstruction causes apneic episodes and cyclic cyanosis, which is relieved by crying. Physical examination shows a bony, shelf-like projection of the posterior portion of the vestibule that almost completely obstructs the nasal cavity. The CT scan is the study of choice and helps to confirm the diagnosis as well as to define the anatomy of the nasal cavity and posterior choanae. Association of anterior nasal stenosis with midfacial dysostosis and endocrine and central nervous system abnormalities has been reported (19). Therefore, a genetic consult should be considered.

The infant is initially managed with a McGovern nipple or an oral airway with close monitoring. Gavage feeding may be necessary. If the infant is doing well, then discharge to home with an apnea monitor and a plan for close follow-up evaluations can be considered. If the infant does not tolerate an oral airway or continues to have significant nasal obstruction despite conservative management, then surgical intervention is necessary before discharge from the hospital. Sublabial approach with the use of microinstruments to remove portions of the nasal process of the maxilla is recommended (18). When the obstruction is mucosal rather than bony in nature, the diagnosis is likely to be stuffy nose syndrome, and it requires symptomatic medical treatment only.

Deviated Nasal Septum

Careful intranasal examination shows some septal deformities in as many as 70% of newborns, which may be secondary to intrauterine or birth trauma (20,21). Significant deviation of nasal septum secondary to traumatic delivery or the use of forceps is seen in approximately 1% of neonates. Physical examination shows tilted columella, deviation of the nasal septum and asymmetry of the nasal alae. Radiographic studies are not helpful. Closed reduction of the nasal septum by the use of gentle traction should be carried out during the first week of life. Careful examination of the nasal cavities to detect septal hematoma is essential. If this is present, a septal hematoma must be evacuated emergently because hematoma can lead to abscess formation and saddle nose deformity. Parents should be counseled that nasal growth disturbances can occur following trauma and that further nasal surgery may be necessary when the child is older.

Choanal Atresia

The simplest and the most widely held theory regarding pathogenesis of choanal atresia is that it results from the persistence of bucconasal membranes that normally involute during the seventh week of gestation. The incidence of choanal atresia is approximately one in 5,000 to 8,000 live births. Unilateral choanal atresia is twice as frequent as bilateral choanal atresia. Ninety percent of the atresia is bony; 10% is membranous. The female-to-male ratio is reported to be 2:1. In approximately 50% of the patients with choanal atresia, other associated anomalies are seen. The most common anomaly associated with choanal atresia is the CHARGE association (coloboma, heart disease, atresia of the choana, retarded growth and development, genitourinary anomalies, ear anomalies and/or deafness) (22). For these reasons, a genetic consultation may be indicated for patients diagnosed with choanal atresia.

In cases of unilateral atresia, unilateral mucoid nasal rhinorrhea may be seen; however, significant respiratory distress is usually absent. In bilateral choanal atresia, characteristic cyclic respiratory obstruction is seen. Nasal obstruction leads to increasing respiratory effort and distress until the child cries and the nasal obstruction is bypassed temporarily. Diagnosis is established by the inability to pass a 6-Fr suction catheter through the nostril beyond 3 to 4 cm into the nasopharynx. The atretic plate can also be visualized using a fiberoptic nasopharyngoscope. The best method of delineating the atresia is by CT scan.

A neonate with bilateral choanal atresia is initially managed with oral airway or McGovern nipple and gavage feedings. Tracheotomy is rarely needed. Choanal atresia can be addressed by transnasal, transpalatal or endoscopic approaches (23,24). Emergent surgical correction for bilateral choanal atresia is seldom required and is reserved for those infants that can not be managed conservatively. Under these circumstances, a transnasal repair can be performed with a staged definitive transpalatal repair when the child is older. In a neonate who is easily managed by conservative means alone, surgical correction can be deferred for 1 to 2 years. Restenosis requiring revision surgery is not uncommon.

Congenital Midline Nasal Masses

Encephaloceles and gliomas arise from faulty closure of the foramen caecum at the third week of fetal development (25). Gliomas are locally aggressive lesions that can cause symptoms by enlargement and pressure effects on the surrounding structures. Approximately 30% of gliomas are intranasal and thus can cause nasal obstruction and septal deviation. Fifteen percent of gliomas have a fibrous connection to the dura. Basal encephaloceles herniate through a defect in the cribriform plate and usually present as intranasal masses and cause nasal obstruction.

Congenital midline nasal masses are best evaluated by a combination of CT scan and MRI. Depending on whether there is a connection to the dura, gliomas may require a combined approach by the neurosurgery and otolaryngology services. Encephaloceles always have an intracranial connection and thus require an intracranial exploration. Early surgical intervention is advised in order to decrease the risk of meningitis and further enlargement of the mass with resulting cosmetic deformity.

Oropharyngeal Obstruction

Glossoptosis

Pierre–Robin sequence (PRS) consists of micrognathia, glossoptosis, and U-shaped cleft palate; it represents the best-known cause of glossoptosis. Pierre–Robin sequence results secondary to arrest in development of mandible at the seventh to the 11th week of gestation, which then leads to high position of tongue in the oral cavity and prevention of fusion of palatal shelves (26). It may present as an isolated anomaly or as a part of a syndrome such as Stickler's syndrome (see Chap. 40). Genetic consultation is advised.

Airway obstruction in neonates with PRS occurs because of the micrognathia, which causes posterior displacement of the tongue base. Obstruction is more severe in supine position and worsens during sleep or induction of anesthesia. Airway obstruction can be managed by positioning, placement of a nasopharyngeal airway, intubation, and tracheotomy (27). Most patients without other significant airway or neurologic deficits can be managed conservatively (28). For neonates with severe airway symptoms who do not respond to positioning or nasopharyngeal airway, a tracheotomy is required. Once it is performed, the tracheotomy tube remains in place until the cleft palate repair is completed.

Macroglossia

Macroglossia is seen in neonates with Beckwith–Wiedemann syndrome (BWS). In addition, patients with BWS may have omphalocele, adrenal cytomegaly, and visceromegaly (29). BWS occurs secondary to sporadic mutation and has a mortality rate of over 20%. The airway obstruction seen in these patients is secondary to macroglossia. Initial management consists of tracheotomy, followed by a tongue reduction procedure at a later date.

True macroglossia and relative macroglossia (a small oral cavity) can also be seen in neonates with Down syndrome; however, the size of the tongue rarely necessitates surgical intervention.

Laryngeal Obstruction

Laryngomalacia

Laryngomalacia is the most common cause of stridor in infants (30). Laryngomalacia describes the collapse of supraglottic structures on inspiration. The pathophysiology of laryngomalacia is unknown. Usually, it is a self-limited condition with mild symptoms that resolve by age 18 to 24 months.

Infants with laryngomalacia present with variable inspiratory stridor that worsens with crying, feeding, and upper respiratory infections and improves with prone position. A small number of infants have more severe symptoms of airway obstruction consisting of retraction, feeding difficulties, failure to thrive, and cyanosis. Diagnosis is confirmed by flexible laryngoscopy, which shows inward collapse of the epiglottis, aryepiglottic folds, and the mucosa over the arytenoids during inspiration. In fewer than 5% of the infants, surgery is indicated to relieve severe obstruction and prevent pulmonary and cardiac complications (31). Surgery consists of trimming the supraglottic tissue with carbon dioxide laser or by sharp dissection (32). A tracheotomy is an alternative to supraglottoplasty (epiglottoplasty).

Vocal Cord Paralysis

Vocal cord paralysis accounts for approximately 10% of all congenital laryngeal anomalies (30). Unilateral paralysis does not cause significant airway symptoms; however, the infant may have a hoarse and breathy cry. Surgical intervention is usually not required. An infant with bilateral vocal cord paralysis (BVCP) presents with normal voice and cry, but with an inspiratory stridor. Central nervous system anomalies, in particular Arnold–Chiari malformation, are often associated with BVCP (30,33). The diagnosis of BVCP is made by flexible laryngoscopy. Radiographs of the airway and chest and, if indicated, CT scan of the brain should be obtained.

In BVCP associated with Arnold–Chiari malformation, neurosurgical decompression will result in resolution of BVCP. In most infants with idiopathic BVCP, tracheotomy is required to establish an airway. During tracheotomy, the entire airway should be inspected to exclude any additional airway anomalies. Definitive vocal cord lateralizing procedures can be done at a later date, if spontaneous resolution of the paralysis does not occur (34).

Laryngeal Atresia/Web

During embryogenesis, epithelium temporarily obliterates the laryngeal lumen. This epithelial plug is then resorbed during the seventh to eighth week of gestation (35). Failure of this resorption process can result in laryngeal web, subglottic stenosis (SGS), and laryngeal atresia. Laryngeal atresia is a rare and life-threatening condition that must be recognized in the delivery room and must be followed by an emergent placement of tracheotomy tube if the infant is to survive.

The most common laryngeal web is seen at the glottic level and affects the vocal cords (36). The web may be thick, causing severe obstruction, or thin and membranous. Infants with laryngeal web present with abnormal cry, stridor, and respiratory distress. Laryngeal web can cause cyanosis or unexplained airway obstruction at birth, which requires intubation or a tracheotomy. Laryngeal web is often associated with SGS. Diagnosis is made by airway films and rigid endoscopy. Definitive treatment options to allow decannulation include dilation, endoscopic microsurgical or laser division of the web, and an open repair (36).

Posterior Laryngeal Cleft

Posterior laryngeal cleft is often associated with other congenital anomalies such as esophageal atresia, tracheoesophageal fistula, and tracheal and bronchial stenosis. Posterior laryngeal cleft is difficult to diagnose, particularly if the cleft is limited to the interarytenoid region. Posterior laryngeal cleft has been classified into four types, with type 1 being a mild interarytenoid cleft above the level of the vocal cords and type 4 representing a complete laryngotracheoesophageal cleft (37).

Presenting symptoms depend on the extent of the cleft. Airway obstruction is not a prominent feature. Rather, aspiration, choking, cyanosis, and feeding difficulties are seen commonly. Stridor and voice abnormalities can be seen but are not common. Diagnosis is made by careful inspection of the posterior glottis during endoscopy. Laryngeal cleft can be repaired endoscopically or by an external approach using laryngofissure or lateral pharyngotomy.

Subglottic Stenosis

Subglottic stenosis (SGS) is defined as narrowing of the airway at the level of the cricoid to less than 4 mm in a full-term infant and 3 mm in a premature infant. It is considered to be congenital if there has not been any previous airway manipulation. The stenosis may be cartilaginous or membranous. Many of the infants with congenital SGS may have only mild symptoms and go undiagnosed, whereas others may get intubated and thus diagnosed as having acquired SGS. Thus, the true incidence of congenital SGS is unknown. Acquired SGS is most commonly secondary to prolonged endotracheal intubation. One percent to 8% of infants who require prolonged intubation may acquire SGS (38). The injury to the subglottis is related to the duration of intubation, the size of the endotracheal tube (ETT), the degree of ETT motion, and the number of reintubations.

Infants with SGS can present with stridor, respiratory distress, and croupy barking cough. Others present with recurrent or prolonged croup and inability to be extubated after intubation, or obstructive apnea. Airway radiographs can show narrowing of the subglottic airway; however, the definitive diagnosis is made on rigid endoscopy. For infants who have severe airway obstruction and fail repeated attempts at extubation, a tracheotomy or anterior cricoid split (ACS) can be considered. An ACS can be performed only in infants without other underlying airway abnormalities that contribute to the airway obstruction and who have good pulmonary reserve (39). Any need for ventilatory support, oxygen requirement over 30%, congestive heart failure, and respiratory infection are contraindications to ACS.

Anterior cricoid split involves opening of the upper two tracheal rings, cricoid cartilage, and lower half of the thyroid cartilage in the anterior midline and presumably works by decompressing the airway. Postoperative intubation for 7 to 10 days and meticulous care to avoid ETT plugging and accidental extubation are imperative. Systemic corticosteroid is administered beginning 24 hours preextubation and continues for 72 hours postextubation. If ACS is successful, a tracheotomy can be avoided. Patients who fail ACS can undergo revision ACS or a tracheotomy followed by a formal laryngotracheal reconstruction at a later date.

Subglottic Hemangioma

Hemangiomas represent malformation of vasoformative tissue. Hemangioma in the airway usually occurs in the submucosa of the subglottic region; it increases in size over 6 to 18 months, followed by involution (40). Hemangioma may extend beyond the airway into the mediastinum. Approximately 50% of infants with airway hemangioma have cutaneous hemangioma in the head and neck region.

Infants with subglottic hemangioma present with inspiratory stridor, hoarseness, barky cough, and airway obstruction. Airway film shows soft tissue swelling in the subglottis, which is often asymmetric. Endoscopy shows a lesion that is localized to the posterior subglottis and is soft and compressible. Biopsy is usually not necessary unless diagnosis is in question, and the endoscopist should be prepared to manage possible hemorrhage into the airway. Treatment of subglottic hemangioma depends on the degree of airway obstruction and the extent of airway involved by the hemangioma. Treatment options include tracheotomy followed by expectant waiting for involution of the hemangioma, corticosteroids, and laser excision. More recently, interferon-α_{2a} administration has been introduced as a treatment for airway hemangiomas (41).

Tracheal Obstruction

Tracheal Stenosis

Tracheal stenosis may be secondary to mucosal webs of variable thickness without any gross deformity of the underlying cartilage. Stenosis of the trachea can also be caused by complete tracheal rings of variable length. The segment with complete tracheal rings lacks the posterior membranous portion of the trachea.

Symptoms of airway obstruction from tracheal stenosis depends on the diameter of the narrowed airway lumen. Neonates with tracheal stenosis can present with persistent cough, respiratory distress, expiratory stridor, and wheezing. Symptoms tend to worsen following an upper respiratory infection, and sudden and complete obstruction can occur from mucus plugging of the narrowed segment. Many patients also tend to have feeding difficulties. The diagnosis is suggested by history, airway films, and fluoroscopy; however, a definitive diagnosis is made by endoscopic evaluation. Mucosal web may respond to dilation alone. Short segments of tracheal stenosis are resected with end-to-end anastomosis (42). Long segments of stenosis require tracheoplasty using pericardial and/or cartilage grafts (43). These surgical procedures are associated with high morbidity and mortality rates.

Tracheomalacia

In tracheomalacia there is increased flaccidity of the tracheal walls, which leads to anterior–posterior collapse of the airway and obstruction (44). Primary tracheomalacia is an isolated finding that usually resolves by age 2 years. Secondary tracheomalacia is seen in neonates with tracheoesophageal fistula (TEF) or external vascular compression. In primary tracheomalacia and in secondary tracheomalacia associated with TEF, deficiency in the tracheal cartilage may cause the abnormal collapse of the trachea (44,45).

Clinical symptoms of tracheomalacia range from mild to severe. Common features of severe cases include inspiratory and/or expiratory stridor, wheezing, persistent coughing, recurrent respiratory infections, reflex apnea, and difficulty with clearing airway secretions. Reflex apnea describes a respiratory arrest that can progress to a cardiac arrest and is seen in patients with tracheobronchial compression (46). Diagnosis of tracheomalacia can be suggested by fluoroscopy, but a definitive diagnosis can only be made by endoscopic examination of the airway under spontaneous ventilation. Widened semicircular cartilages, ballooning of the posterior membranous wall, and collapse of tracheal lumen are seen. In severe cases tracheotomy is required until the condition resolves. The use of positive airway pressure through the tracheotomy tube may be necessary to maintain patency of the airway below the tracheotomy tube (47).

Vascular Compression

Innominate artery compression of the trachea can occur when there is an anomalous distal origin of the innominate artery from the aortic arch. The innominate artery crosses the trachea in a left-inferior-to-right-superior direction and causes compression of the trachea. Infants with this condition present with stridor, recurrent respiratory infections, feeding difficulties, and reflex apnea. Diagnosis is best made by endoscopy and MRI. Surgery is necessary only in infants with severe stridor or reflex apnea. Suspension of the innominate artery through thoracotomy or median sternotomy and reimplantation of the innominate artery are available surgical options (48).

Other less common vascular anomalies causing airway obstruction include double aortic arch, right aortic arch with left ligamentum arteriosum, and pulmonary artery sling. Evaluation of these conditions includes chest radiographs, MRI, and endoscopy. In symptomatic infants, the appropriate surgical procedure should be undertaken by a cardiothoracic surgeon.

THORACIC LESIONS CAUSING RESPIRATORY DISTRESS

Congenital Lobar Emphysema

Congenital lobar emphysema can be severe or life-threatening as a result of hyperexpansion of a single lobe of the lung. Air is permitted into the involved lobe but denied egress. The lobe becomes emphysematous, resulting in compression of adjacent pulmonary parenchyma and mediastinal displacement. Symptoms may appear shortly after birth and invariably develop before 4 months of age (49). The cause is unknown. An inherent, cartilaginous defect in the bronchus has been postulated, but the bronchial abnormality is not always recognizable in the resected specimen.

A chest radiograph is characteristic, showing hyperaeration of the involved lobe with mediastinal shift away from the affected side. The lobar distribution of the hyperaeration can be appreciated, and adjacent pulmonary parenchyma is compressed. The upper lobes are most frequently involved, but the condition may be seen in the middle lobe. Rarely, the lesion is bilateral (50).

Treatment is surgical, and prompt thoracotomy and lobectomy are undertaken after the diagnosis is made. An infant may remain compensated for some weeks and then deteriorate rapidly from acute hyperinflation of the involved lobe. There is no place for expectant management of congenital lobar emphysema.

An identical clinical picture may be seen in the neonate who has been ventilated for a prolonged time and develops a large pneumatocele as a result of respiratory tract barotrauma. It is often difficult for the physician to determine whether respiratory distress is caused by the pneumatocele or by generalized pulmonary parenchymal disease. Surgical excision of the pneumatocele is indicated if the lesion is enlarging and the respiratory status is worsening without another apparent cause.

Cystic Adenomatoid Malformation

Cystic adenomatoid malformation (CAM) is a pulmonary maldevelopment that presents with cystic replacement of pulmonary parenchyma. If the cysts are small (i.e., microcystic CAM) and constitute a small portion of one lung, the child may be asymptomatic. If the lesion is microcystic and replaces a large portion of the lung, the fetus may develop hydrops, and the prognosis is poor (51). If the cysts are macroscopic and the child is in respiratory distress at birth, the problem may be misdiagnosed as congenital diaphragmatic hernia. Appropriate therapy for the symptomatic neonate with CAM is thoracotomy and resection of the involved lung. Postoperative support with extracorporeal membrane oxygenation (ECMO) has been necessary for infants developing severe persistent pulmonary hypertension after CAM excision (52).

Bronchogenic Cyst

Bronchogenic cyst is another lung bud anomaly in which the normal bronchiole-to-bronchiole communication is absent or atretic, resulting in a mucus-producing cyst that may obstruct the trachea, bronchus, or esophagus. This seldom causes severe problems in the neonate, but it must be considered if a space-occupying lesion is detected on a chest x-ray film obtained for investigation of respiratory distress. Excision of the bronchogenic cyst is the preferred treatment.

Iatrogenic Airway Injury

As aggressive management of the pulmonary disease of newborns has developed, there has been a concurrent increase in injury to the airway or pulmonary parenchyma. Long-term intubation and high peak inspiratory pressure settings on the ventilator place these children at an increased risk of airway injury. It has been known since 1976 that perforation of bronchi, particularly the bronchus of the right lower lobe, can be prevented by careful measurement of suction catheters so that they do not extend more than 1 cm beyond the carina (53). The development of a bronchopulmonary fistula after chest tube evacuation of a pneumothorax can be life-threatening and may require surgical closure of the fistula, although some children have been successfully treated nonoperatively (54).

Complications of high-pressure ventilation include development of interstitial emphysema and bronchopulmonary dysplasia. The interstitial emphysema is usually self-limited, although some infants may benefit from a surgical approach to the problem (55). Surgery can be curative for granulomas within the airway of chronically intubated neonates, particularly if the lesions contribute to air trapping or stenosis. The best management for iatrogenic airway injury is prevention, and although not totally avoidable, careful attention to ventilator management and suction techniques should reduce the incidence and severity of these problems.

Diaphragmatic Hernia

Development of the diaphragm is generally complete the 12th week of gestation, by which time the bowel has returned to the abdominal cavity. Failure of the development of the posterolateral portion of the diaphragm results in persistence of the pleuroperitoneal canal or foramen of Bochdalek, which allows the viscera to occupy the chest cavity, and the abdomen is underdeveloped and scaphoid. Both lungs are hypoplastic, more so on the side of the hernia. Bronchial branching, lung weight, and lung volume are decreased. The pulmonary arteries are hypoplastic (56,57). The lesion occurs in one of every 3,000 live births, with equal frequency in male and female infants. Sporadic occurrence is the rule, but a familial pattern has been reported (58,59).

The prenatal diagnosis of congenital diaphragmatic hernia (CDH) can be made using fetal sonography as early as 15 weeks of gestation (60). Sonographic findings include herniated abdominal viscera, abnormal anatomy of the upper abdomen, and mediastinal shift away from the herniated viscera (61). The high-risk fetus is identified by a diagnosis early in gestation, a dilated stomach in the chest, low lung-to-thorax ratio, low lung-to-head ratio, and polyhydramnios. Amniocentesis with a fetal karyotype identifies chromosomal defects; trisomy 18 and 21 are most common. More than 40% of newborns with CDH have associated anomalies of the heart, brain, limbs, genitourinary system, or craniofacial region (62).

Typically, babies with congenital Bochdalek hernia present dramatically with cyanosis and severe respiratory distress immediately after birth. Because the abdominal viscera are dislocated through the defect into the chest, the abdominal contour is scaphoid. Breath sounds are diminished or absent, and because the mediastinal structures have been displaced, the heart sounds are heard in the right chest. As the bowel fills with gas, respiration and cardiac action are further compromised, hypoxia and respiratory acidosis are increased, and death is inevitable unless appropriate intervention is undertaken. Congenital diaphragmatic hernia is no longer considered a surgical emergency unless the viability of the herniated bowel is in question. In some instances, the infants remain relatively asymptomatic in the early hours and days of life, and rarely, a diaphragmatic hernia is an incidental finding in an older child. The respiratory symptoms demand an immediate x-ray film, which is diagnostic. The hernia is on the left side in 90% of these infants, and the air-filled bowel is seen occupying the left hemithorax, with resultant displacement of the mediastinum to the right (Fig. 44–4). The

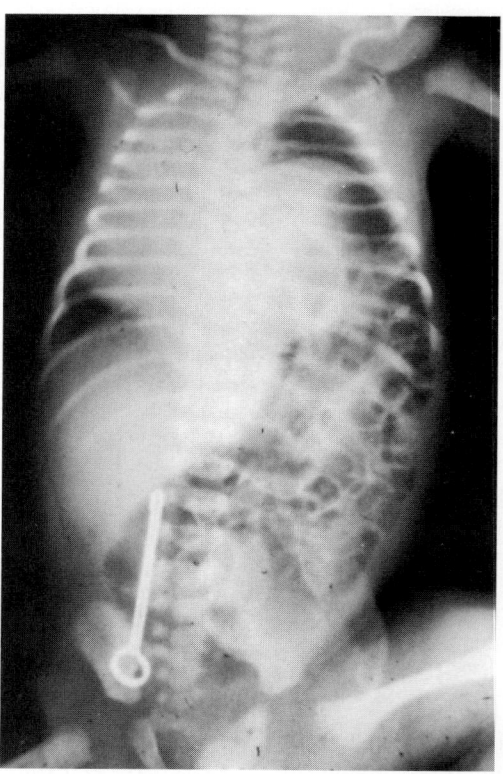

FIG. 44–4. X-ray film of left diaphragmatic hernia with loops of bowel well up into the chest. Although most diaphragmatic hernias do not have a sac, the smooth curve of the sac in this instance is visible. Notice that the heart is displaced to the border of the right chest.

abdomen is gasless. Additional x-ray films are unnecessary, and contrast studies for additional confirmation are contraindicated.

Many newborns with CDH have respiratory failure within minutes of birth, and urgent stabilization is mandatory to reverse hypoxia, hypercarbia, and metabolic acidosis. Prompt and aggressive preoperative care is essential (63,64). This generally includes mechanical ventilation with 100% oxygen, sedation with narcotics, muscle paralysis, controlled alkalosis with hyperventilation and intravenous sodium bicarbonate, and vasopressors. Permissive hypercarbia and gentle ventilation have proven effective in a number of centers. Regardless of the mode of therapy, the goal is to reverse the baby's persistent pulmonary hypertension with right-to-left shunting of oxygen-poor blood across the open foramen ovale and the ductus arteriosus.

Some infants do not improve despite aggressive therapy, and many centers use ECMO before hernia repair to stabilize these desperately ill infants (65,66). Venovenous or venoarterial bypass is used, depending on the infant's hemodynamic stability. Bypass is continued until the pulmonary hypertension is reversed and lung function is improved. Most infants respond within 7 to 10 days, but some require up to 3 weeks of support. Newborns who have not improved after this time probably have such severe pulmonary hypoplasia that further extracorporeal life support is futile.

There are no absolute respiratory criteria that exclude newborns with CDH from consideration for ECMO support (67,68). Approximately 60% of infants with CDH who are supported by ECMO are expected to survive (see Chap. 31).

The surgical findings are usually those of a posterolateral defect in the left diaphragm, with most or all of the abdominal viscera in the chest. The surgeon reduces the hernia gently by withdrawing the viscera from the chest. If a sac is present, it is delivered and excised. There may be adequate diaphragmatic tissue to accomplish direct suture repair. If a significant portion of the diaphragm is lacking, prosthetic material is used to close the defect. Before completion of the repair, a small chest tube may be placed in the left hemithorax and brought out through an intercostal space.

The temptation to expand the compressed lung at the time of initial surgery must be resisted. Aggressive attempts at expansion can result in pneumothorax on the contralateral side, which, if unrecognized, is a disastrous complication.

The abdominal viscera have been located in the thorax throughout most of the developmental period of the fetus; thus, there is insufficient room within the abdomen to accommodate the intestine without dangerously increasing the intraabdominal pressure, compressing the vena cava, and compromising respirations by elevating the diaphragm. To avoid these potential problems, the surgeon may omit anatomic closure of the abdominal wall. Skin flaps are quickly mobilized, and only the skin is closed, or the abdomen is closed by creating a silastic silo as for gastroschisis or a large omphalocele. The ventral pouch created accommodates the intraabdominal organs; diaphragmatic action and venous return are unimpeded. The ventral hernia is repaired after the infant has been weaned off the ventilator and is in stable clinical condition.

Ten percent of infants with Bochdalek hernias present with the defect on the right side. The difference in incidence on the two sides may be explained by the presence of the liver, which partially blocks the pleuroperitoneal canal and limits the amount of bowel that can herniate into the chest. Symptoms in babies with right-sided hernias may be less severe, but when a right diaphragmatic hernia of Bochdalek presents as an emergency, it is managed as described.

After CDH repair and removal from ECMO, ventilation is continued with ventilation rates and oxygen concentrations necessary to maintain adequate oxygenation. Continuous transcutaneous oxygen monitoring of upper and lower body areas is useful. To avoid relapse into pulmonary hypertension, weaning from the ventilator should

be achieved by making small incremental changes in the inspired oxygen and ventilator rate.

New modalities being investigated may offer an increased chance of survival for infants with CDH. These include surfactant replacement therapy, liquid ventilation, intratracheal pulmonary ventilation, and pulmonary lobar transplantation (69,70). Prenatal repair of the diaphragmatic hernia has been abandoned, as there was no improvement in survival or morbidity in a randomized trial. Current prenatal therapy of CDH is directed at occluding the trachea, which results in enlargement of the lungs with retained fluid. The baby is then delivered by planned cesarean section, at which time the trachea is repaired or intubated, with the baby remaining on placental support. Initial discouraging results with this technique have been improved with recent modifications; however, fetal tracheal plugging remains an experimental procedure that is being evaluated in a limited number of centers (71,72).

Babies who present after the first day of life with signs and symptoms prompting a diagnosis of diaphragmatic hernia are almost always hardier patients and have greater pulmonary reserve, and they can be expected to make a satisfactory recovery.

The anterior retrosternal hernia of Morgagni is rarely encountered in the newborn. The diagnosis is confirmed by chest radiograph in the lateral projection. The standard treatment is surgical reconstruction, beginning with an abdominal approach through a thoracoabdominal incision. The prognosis is usually favorable, and these lesions are not associated with the severe cardiopulmonary complications seen with Bochdalek hernias in the neonatal period.

Eventration of the Diaphragm

Eventration of the diaphragm may be congenital or acquired. The congenital presentation may mimic that of a congenital diaphragmatic hernia with a sac. The acquired lesion results from paralysis of the diaphragm, most commonly caused by operative trauma or birth injury (73).

Large eventrations and diaphragmatic paralysis are poorly tolerated by infants (74). Paradoxic cephalad motion of the diaphragm on inspiration produces a shift of the mobile, neonatal mediastinum that limits the function of the contralateral lung. Moderate or severe respiratory distress is evident; many newborns with eventration require ventilatory support.

Diagnosis is suggested by a marked elevation of a hemidiaphragm on a chest radiograph. Fluoroscopic examination identifies paradoxic movement of the diaphragm. Treatment is plication of the diaphragm with nonabsorbable sutures that reef up or overlap the diaphragm. The taut diaphragm results in less abnormal motion and improved ventilation.

LESIONS OF THE ESOPHAGUS

Esophageal Atresia and Associated Anomalies

The success story of the management of infants born with esophageal atresia and tracheoesophageal fistula is one of the most dramatic and satisfying that the pediatric surgeon, the neonatologist, and the pediatrician can point to. In the early 1900s, virtually all babies born with esophageal atresia and tracheoesophageal fistula died. In 1941, Haight and Towsley were the first to bring an infant with esophageal atresia and tracheoesophageal fistula successfully through the rigors of primary transthoracic reconstruction (75). This landmark accomplishment occurred before antibiotics, respiratory support, or sophisticated intravenous nutrition were available. This surgical approach formed the basis of modern operative and postoperative care of infants born with this anomaly. Fifty years after the first survivor was announced, every baby born with atresia of the esophagus who is spared coexisting fatal abnormalities and is offered appropriate care has an excellent chance of leading a normal life.

Embryologic and Genetic Considerations

The cause of esophageal atresia is unknown, but it is related to the common origin of the esophagus and trachea (76). The embryonic trachea and esophagus are first recognized as a ventral diverticulum of the foregut approximately 22 or 23 days after fertilization (77). As the diverticulum elongates, a proliferation of endodermal cells appears on the lateral walls. These cell masses become ridges of tissue that ultimately divide the foregut into tracheal and esophageal channels. The division into separate tubes is completed between 34 and 36 days after fertilization. Many embryologic studies indicate that interruption of development in the fourth fetal week allows persistence of fistulas and clefts between the esophagus and trachea and permits incomplete development of the esophagus.

There are reports of familial occurrences of esophageal atresia, which raises the possibility of a heritable genetic factor. Numerous accounts of twins and siblings with esophageal atresia have been reported (78). Conversely, certain commonly coexistent anomalies, such as the VACTERL (i.e., vertebral, anal, cardiac, tracheal, esophageal, renal, and limb anomalies) association (see Chap. 40) and other malformations, strongly suggest that the developing fetus is affected by a teratogen or defect of embryogenesis (79).

In many babies with esophageal atresia, it is the associated anomalies that alter treatment and affect survival. Congenital heart defects and chromosomal abnormalities are the most worrisome. Major anomalies that may seriously affect the infant but that are not usually fatal include imperforate anus and other congenital obstructions of the gut. Grosfeld and Ballantine found that 31 (37%) of 84 infants had cardiac anomalies; 18 (21.4%) had gastrointestinal malformations, of whom 11 (13%) had imperforate anus; and six (7%) had the VACTERL association (80). A ventricular septal defect is the most common cardiac lesion, followed in frequency by patent ductus arteriosus and tetralogy of Fallot. Piekarski and Stephens suggest that the high incidence of coexisting anomalies is a reflection of generalized damage to the mesenchymal tissue in the fourth week of gestation (81).

Esophageal Atresia with Tracheoesophageal Fistula

Esophageal atresia occurs in approximately one of 3,000 to 4,500 births. In the most common form of esophageal anomaly (86% of patients), the blind-ending upper esophageal segment usually extends into the upper portion of the thorax, and the lower portion of the esophagus is connected to the trachea at or just above the tracheal carina (Fig. 44–5) (82). This connection is 3 to 5 mm

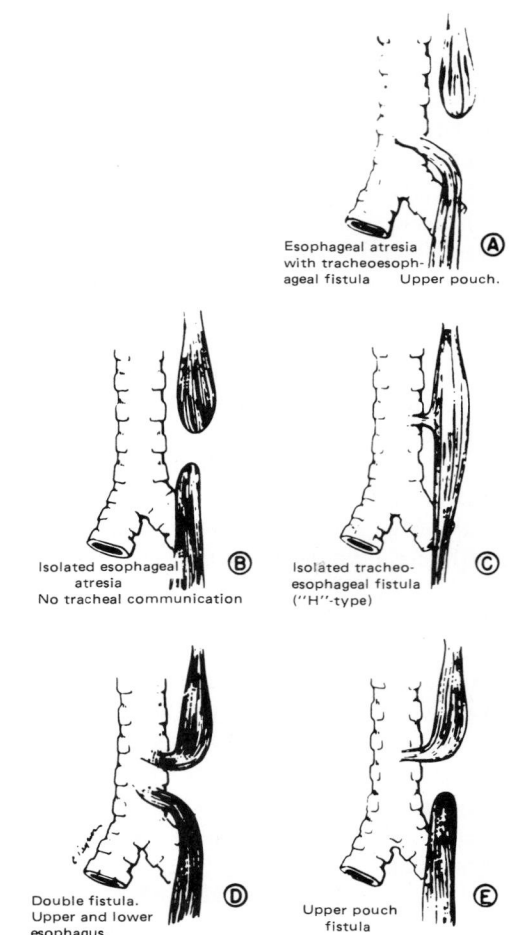

FIG. 44–5. The various forms of esophageal malformations are shown in the order of the frequency in which they occur. (From Nardi GL, Zuidema GD. *Surgery,* 3rd ed. Boston: Little, Brown, 1972.)

in diameter and easily admits inspired air or, in a retro-grade fashion, acidic gastric secretions. The earliest clinical sign of esophageal atresia is excessive oral secretions or regurgitation of saliva. The saliva pools in the blind-ending esophagus and then accumulates until it is apparent around the lips as excessive mucus. The first feeding is followed by choking, coughing, and regurgitation. Abdominal distension is a prominent feature, occurring as inspired air is transmitted through the fistula and distal esophagus into the stomach. Gastric juice may pass upward in the distal esophagus, traversing the tracheoesophageal fistula and spilling into the trachea and lungs, leading to chemical pneumonia. Pulmonary difficulties are compounded by atelectasis and diaphragmatic elevation secondary to gastric distension.

Diagnosis

The diagnosis of many infants with esophageal atresia is made prenatally. Polyhydramnios is the most frequent finding, particularly in infants with pure esophageal atresia. Those with a tracheoesophageal fistula may not develop polyhydramnios if the communication is large enough to permit swallowing of the amniotic fluid through the fistula. An additional finding on a prenatal ultrasound is failure to identify the fetal stomach, which should raise the suspicion for esophageal atresia. The prenatal diagnosis of esophageal atresia permits the search for other anatomic anomalies and possible chromosomal defects. Appropriate prenatal counseling and preparation of the family can be initiated, specifically with arrangement for postnatal correction, unless contraindicated by coexistent abnormalities.

Once the infant is born, attentive members of the nursing staff who are feeding the baby are often the first to suspect the esophageal blockage. Esophageal atresia may not be obvious on the initial newborn examination unless an attempt is made to pass a tube into the stomach. Thin, flexible feeding catheters should be avoided because they may coil up in the esophagus and give the misleading impression that they have passed into the stomach. A larger, stiffer catheter carefully advanced will meet the obstruction. Occasionally, a tube dissects into the wall of a normal esophagus, leading to a misdiagnosis of esophageal atresia, particularly in a premature infant. A contrast x-ray film rules this out and confirms the diagnosis of atresia; a lateral projection with 1 mL of dilute barium or an isoosmolar contrast agent (e.g., metrizamide) shows the length of the upper pouch, defines its precise extension into the chest, and demonstrates the rare upper pouch fistula (Fig. 44–6*A,B*). Air seen in the bowel confirms the presence of a tracheoesophageal fistula. The existence of pneumonia or atelectasis also can be demonstrated on the initial radiographs.

Evaluation of the heart and great vessels with echocardiography is important to identify potential cardiac anomalies and verify the aortic arch position. A right-sided arch may alter the surgical approach and exposure. Bronchoscopy is useful to identify the level of the fistula and to exclude upper pouch fistulas and laryngotracheoesophageal clefts.

Management

After the diagnosis is secure, the following measures should be instituted promptly:

Basic supportive measures, such as an infant warmer.
Place the infant in a 30- to 40-degree head-up position.
Give nothing orally.
Provide intravenous antibiotics for possible aspiration.
Place a sump suction catheter in the upper pouch to remove the excess secretions (Fig. 44–7).
Consult with the appropriate pediatric surgical service.

The traditional approach to the timing of surgical repair was based on the increased risk of operating on infants with low birth weight and pneumonia. However neonatal care has evolved to the point that neither low birth weight nor the presence of pneumonia is a risk factor for poor survival (83). Severe anomalies and their consequences are now the crucial determinants of survival. Therefore, at Children's National Medical Center (CNMC), each baby admitted with esophageal atresia is managed according to his or her physiologic status alone (84). If the infant is stable, immediate primary repair is undertaken. If unstable, surgery is delayed until the clinical status is stabilized, the impact of associated anomalies is determined, and the infant can be anesthetized and operated on safely.

Of historic interest, a classification developed by Waterston and colleagues in 1962 was useful in the stratification of patients for different management plans and the comparison of outcomes (85). The infants were classified as follows:

Category A: Birth weight over 2.5 kg (5.5 lb) and otherwise well
Category B: Birth weight of 1.8 to 2.5 kg and well, or higher birth weight but moderate pneumonia and other congenital anomalies
Category C: Birth weight under 1.8 kg, or higher birth weight but severe pneumonia and severe congenital anomaly.

Immediate Operative Repair

A thoracic incision provides exposure of the upper pouch and tracheoesophageal fistula. A right thoracotomy is standard unless the aortic arch is on the right, which would interfere with the dissection. A retropleural approach affords protection of the lung by maintaining its pleural envelope. If an anastomotic leak occurs, it will not communicate with the pleural cavity but can be drained posteriorly from the mediastinum with less morbidity.

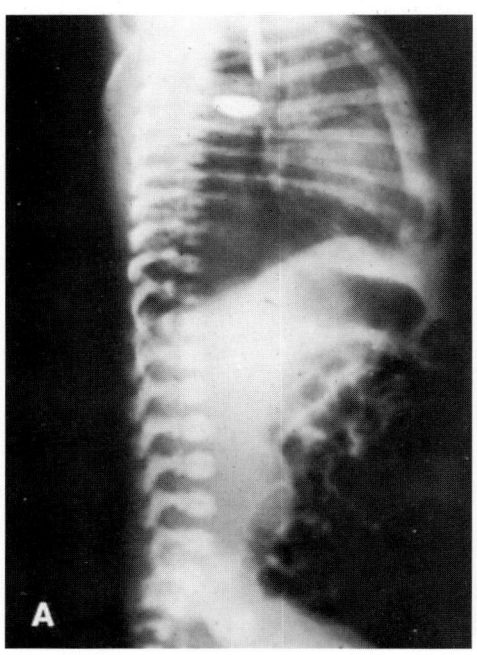
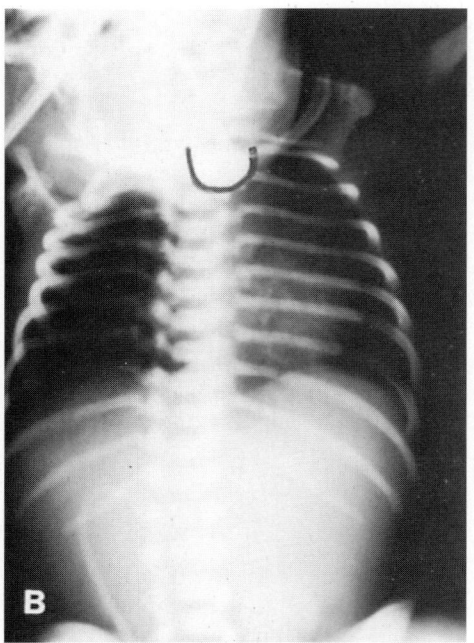
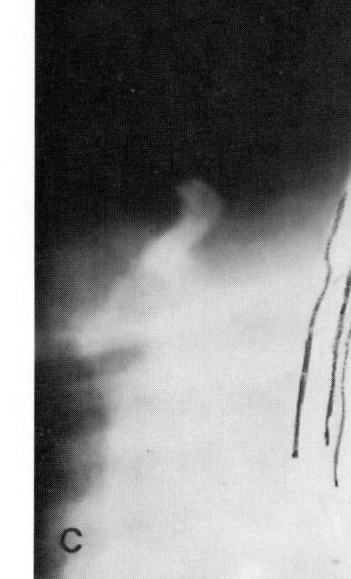

FIG. 44–6. A: Lateral radiograph of a baby with esophageal atresia and tracheoesophageal fistula reveals a small meniscus of barium in the upper pouch. Gas is present in the stomach and intestinal tract because of the fistulous connection to the trachea. In this radiograph, some air in the lower esophageal segment can be seen in the posterior mediastinum. **B:** In a radiograph of a patient with isolated esophageal atresia, the upper pouch is outlined by barium. There is no air below the diaphragm. **C:** In a barium swallow in a patient with H-type isolated tracheoesophageal fistula, a normal-sized lumen of the esophagus is seen. Dye has spilled into the trachea, outlining the upper trachea and larynx. The fistula is at the level of the clavicle.

The fistula is identified and carefully divided from the trachea. The tracheal opening is closed with several sutures, with care to avoid narrowing the tracheal lumen. Although some centers have advocated simple ligation of the fistula, this procedure is rarely performed because it is associated with an unacceptably high rate of recurrence (86).

The circumference of the lower esophageal fistula is usually small and is enlarged by trimming and spatulating its open end. The tip of the upper pouch is mobilized extensively and cut across to expose the lumen. Most sur-

geons employ a single-layer circumferential anastomosis to approximate the two ends instead of the classic two-layer Haight anastomosis (87).

Avoiding undue tension on the repair and averting compromise of the blood supply to the two ends are key factors in obtaining good results. The upper pouch is more amenable to mobilization than the distal fistula because the blood supply comes submucosally from the neck. The blood supply to the distal fistula is more easily compromised because it derives from tiny branches off the aorta. If the ends do not come together easily, there

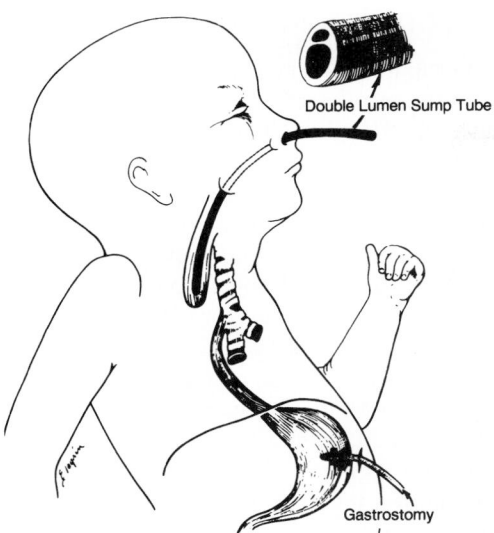

FIG. 44–7. Temporary care of a patient with esophageal atresia and tracheoesophageal fistula is performed with the patient in the upright position. A gastrostomy is in the stomach, and a double-lumen sump tube is in the upper pouch to clear secretions and saliva.

are surgical techniques available for extending the length of the upper pouch (88).

Although once routine, gastrostomy is now rarely used in stable infants. Postoperatively, infants are maintained on intravenous nutrition. Some surgeons employ a transanastomotic feeding tube so that early enteral feedings can be initiated. A chest tube is placed to drain the mediastinum and pleural space if necessary. The chest tube is connected to suction and monitored for evidence of air leak, blood loss, or saliva, which indicate an anastomotic leak. Postoperative management requires meticulous care to avoid potential disruption of the tracheal suture line, particularly if suctioning or reintubation is required. A contrast swallow is usually obtained on the fifth or sixth postoperative day. If all looks well, and there is no leak, feedings are begun and quickly advanced. Some surgeons routinely dilate the esophagus of all infants before discharge to prevent potential stricture formation.

Delayed Primary Repair and Staged Repair

If the infant is unstable, an intermediate plan allows correction of minor difficulties before repair. This plan involves delay of the surgical repair for several days. Management of these babies includes upper pouch suction with a Replogle tube, head-up position, antibiotics, and parenteral nutrition. These maneuvers provide for stabilization, improvement of pulmonary status, and diagnosis and management of certain higher-priority malformations, particularly cardiac lesions. Primary

retropleural repair, as described previously, is undertaken when the infant's condition is stable and the risk of surgery has been reduced.

Unstable infants with serious coexisting anomalies or severe prematurity have diminished chances for survival. For these infants, a gastrostomy is placed, and repair is postponed. This approach uses early retropleural fistula division without anastomosis, gastrostomy feedings, and continuous sump suction of the upper pouch. Division of the fistula is important to prevent reflux of gastric contents. In some premature infants with noncompliant lungs, division of the fistula is required to allow adequate ventilation, in essence closing off the lower-resistance pathway through the fistula and stomach. Immediate closure of the fistula may be lifesaving in these instances.

Gastrostomy and fistula division without anastomosis requires constant, intensive nursing care, but it can be safely maintained for many weeks. Coupled with the holding pattern provided by suction of the upper pouch and gastrostomy drainage, infants with esophageal atresia and tracheoesophageal fistula can be maintained indefinitely by intravenous nutrition while weight and pulmonary status are improved and other congenital anomalies are studied and corrected. Later, the definitive transthoracic operation is performed, and the esophageal anastomosis is accomplished electively.

Results

At the Children's National Medical Center in Washington, D.C., over 150 patients with a blind upper esophageal pouch and a fistula arising from the bifurcation of the trachea were treated between 1966 and 1997. Approximately 90% of these patients survived. Since 1982, the physiologic status of the infant has been the sole guide to therapy. The survival for infants who were classified as stable and had primary repair is 100%. Survival in the unstable group who had staged repair is 60%. The deaths were from associated anomalies, including congenital diaphragmatic hernia and hypoplastic left heart. As a result of this experience with high-risk infants, we concluded that a staged procedure, even one that abandons the esophagus, is preferable to primary repair for selected infants in the highest-risk group. This decision is controversial. Most pediatric surgeons eschew the staged approach, preferring primary repair in most infants with esophageal atresia and tracheoesophageal fistula.

Complications

Complications are not uncommon and require scrupulous diagnostic evaluation. Strictures, gastroesophageal reflux, poor motility, recurrent fistula, and tracheomalacia produce similar respiratory symptoms and may be difficult to differentiate.

Gastroesophageal reflux after repair of esophageal atresia has become increasingly recognized as a clinical problem because of more sensitive diagnostic tools, such as 24-hour pH monitoring. Werlin and co-workers showed that all of the 14 postoperative esophageal atresia patients they studied exhibited severe esophageal motor dysfunction. Only five of the 14 had a swallowing problem (89). In 1980, Jolley and others studied 25 young patients between 3 and 83 months after repair of esophageal atresia and tracheoesophageal fistula. Seventeen of 25 had significant gastroesophageal reflux demonstrated by prolonged pH monitoring, and 12 of these patients had significant symptoms in the form of vomiting, respiratory difficulty, or esophagitis (90). Wheatley and Coran concluded that esophageal dysmotility and gastroesophageal reflux were serious problems in combination and recommended fundoplication in selected patients (91).

Esophageal stricture is a common complication (i.e., 31% in our series) after the anastomosis of the esophagus. Stricture may present early with an inability to swallow, choking, or failure to thrive, but symptoms may develop later, particularly at the time of transition to solid foods. In most infants esophageal dilation is successful, but some require repetitive dilations as often as every 2 weeks for 1 year. Occasionally, a recalcitrant stricture requires operative resection.

Anastomotic disruption with leakage of saliva, gastric juice, and swallowed liquid into the mediastinum or thoracic space was once a dreaded complication after surgery. It is no longer universally fatal because of improvements in nutrition and antibiotics. The leak may be identified on a contrast study obtained before feeding or by an increase in the output from the chest tube or the drainage of saliva through the chest tube. If the operative repair has been accomplished with a retropleural approach and the pleura remains intact, external drainage posteriorly from the mediastinum is a relatively simple matter. If transthoracic repair is followed by esophageal disruption, the leak is best treated by extensive drainage, parenteral nutrition, and delayed surgical intervention. If the baby is deteriorating, it may be wise to abandon the esophagus and create a diverting cervical esophagostomy.

Recurrent fistulas may develop in a few infants (92). Usually, there is a history of a perioperative leak. The symptoms are often those of recurrent respiratory problems, such as bronchitis or pneumonia, related to silent aspiration. Reoperation is required to divide the fistula.

Tracheomalacia is an uncommon complication, but it is difficult to manage. It may be related to a congenital weakness of the trachea or operative injury. The spectrum of presentation ranges from complete collapse of the airway, with an inability to ventilate without positive pressure, to mild tracheal compromise. Bronchoscopy reveals the level and degree of collapse. In severe cases, operative suspension of the aorta and trachea is curative.

Esophageal Atresia without Fistula

Esophageal atresia may occur without a fistulous connection to the respiratory tract. This variant accounts for approximately 8% of esophageal malformations. As with other forms of esophageal atresia, these babies cannot swallow food or saliva. Because there is no tracheoesophageal fistula, air is absent from the gastrointestinal tract, and the abdomen is noticeably scaphoid. The radiologic findings of a blind upper pouch coupled with the absence of air below the diaphragm are pathognomonic of isolated esophageal atresia.

For many years, the standard treatment of isolated esophageal atresia included cervical esophagostomy and gastrostomy. At a later time, a feeding pathway would be created with a segment of small bowel or colon or with construction of a reversed gastric tube. This time-proven practice still has a place in the treatment of pure esophageal atresia. Since the mid-1970s, new methods for bridging the gap between the disparate esophageal segments have evolved. Howard and Myers reported a technique for elongating the blind upper pouch using daily stretching by bougie dilators, allowing the two esophageal ends to be successfully united after several months (93). Mechanical stretching of the pouches may not be necessary. Natural growth in the first months of life produces impressive elongation of the esophageal pouches. During the interval, meticulous nursing care is required to prevent aspiration of saliva and ensure adequate nutrition. In many infants, the wisest course may still be cervical esophagostomy and gastrostomy, with later esophageal replacement (94). This course is even more appropriate for the premature infant, especially if respiratory distress proves troublesome.

The decision to preserve or abandon the esophagus rests on the patient's weight, pulmonary status, presence of other serious anomalies, and general hardiness during the early diagnostic and sustaining maneuvers. Our experience has led us to treat the last 20 consecutive infants who presented with isolated atresia of the esophagus by cervical esophagostomy and gastrostomy, reconstructing the esophagus at 1 year of age using a reversed gastric tube. The latter is a tube created from the greater curve of the stomach, brought up through the chest, and anastomosed to the upper esophageal segment. Nineteen of the 20 infants survived and are growing well.

Isolated Tracheoesophageal Fistula

Isolated (i.e., H-type) tracheoesophageal fistula is a rare lesion, representing approximately 4% of esophageal anomalies. Although congenital tracheoesophageal communication without atresia may be found at any level, most of these fistulas occur in the upper portion of the trachea and the esophagus, at or above the level of the second thoracic vertebra (95). Larger fistulas and communications extending throughout the length of the trachea have been seen, defects appropriately called laryngotracheoesophageal clefts.

The infant suffering from congenital tracheoesophageal fistula usually chokes and coughs with feeding. Prompt relief may be achieved by gavage feeding. Frequently the diagnosis is not made in infancy because the symptoms can be subtle. Pneumonitis often develops in the early days of life and recurs frequently as patchy bronchopneumonia. With continued aspiration through the fistula, a constant state of bronchopneumonia supervenes, attended by all of the manifestations of chronic infection. For any child with recurrent pneumonia, a wide variety of disease entities must be considered, but the list should include H-type tracheoesophageal fistula.

A contrast esophageal swallow with a dilute or isoosmolar medium may reveal the fistula (see Fig. 44–6C). Tracheobronchoscopy is usually successful in demonstrating this anomaly, but simultaneous esophagoscopy may be required. The fistula can be exposed through a cervical collar incision in most instances. A thoracic approach is necessary in 10% to 15% of patients. Surgery produces complete cures for most patients.

LARYNGOTRACHEOESOPHAGEAL CLEFT

Although once uniformly fatal, laryngotracheoesophageal clefts can now be repaired with good results. Early diagnosis is essential to prevent repeated aspiration through the communication between the trachea and esophagus below the vocal cords. Bronchoscopy allows identification of the cleft and its severity. Defects range from those involving only the upper trachea to those extending the entire length and beyond the carina. Management involves tracheostomy and an antireflux procedure to prevent aspiration, with later repair of the defect (96).

GASTROESOPHAGEAL REFLUX

In 1947, Berenberg and Neuhauser defined a condition they called "chalasia," or abnormal relaxation of the gastroesophageal junction (97). The affected babies manifest relentless regurgitation that may present as spitting, mild vomiting, or vigorous vomiting after every feeding. The deleterious effects of gastroesophageal reflux in infants have been recognized with increasing frequency (98–100). The spectrum of symptoms caused by gastroesophageal reflux in the infant is distinctly different from that seen in the adult. In infants, the main symptoms of gastroesophageal reflux are regurgitation, significant growth retardation, aspiration pneumonia, apneic spells, stridor, and esophagitis (91,92,101,102). The abnormality is the absence of a normal valvular mechanism at the gastroesophageal junction that allows unimpeded reflux of gastric content. Associated medical conditions affect many infants. Congenital or acquired central nervous system disorders are most frequent, including severe asphyxia, cerebral palsy, chromosomal anomalies, and microcephaly.

Infants with repaired esophageal atresia and tracheoesophageal fistula may have reflux that leads to anastomotic strictures, poor weight gain, or aspiration pneumonias.

Most infants with gastroesophageal reflux have some form of vomiting from birth. In some babies, the vomiting suggests the diagnosis of pyloric stenosis. Retardation of growth and development is the second most common presenting symptom, occurring in approximately 50% of our patients. These babies rank below the tenth percentile on their growth chart or show a marked falling off of growth progression. Recurrent aspiration with pneumonia occurs in approximately one-third of infants with pernicious gastroesophageal reflux. Reflux may also be the underlying cause of severe apnea in some infants (100).

A barium swallow demonstrates reflux in about 75% of symptomatic patients. However, reflux can also be shown in many otherwise normal, healthy infants, and radiologists have understandable difficulty in defining gastroesophageal reflux that is pathologic. Gastroesophageal reflux can be documented and quantified with radionuclide material. This examination permits an accurate appraisal of the pathophysiologic effects of reflux in most patients. It has proved adaptable to infants, and when serial observations are extended over several hours, normal reflux can usually be differentiated from pathologic reflux. Gastric emptying is also measured by this scan.

Monitoring of pH at different levels of the esophagus can demonstrate gastric acid reflux. With timed studies, physicians can now chart reflux in relation to sleeping, various body positions, and during eating, documenting episodes that lead to characteristic symptoms or life-threatening incidents (103). Esophagoscopy helps physicians to document the presence of esophagitis in selected infants.

Every effort should be made to reverse the consequences of pernicious gastroesophageal reflux by conservative therapy. Medical therapy of symptomatic infants with gastroesophageal reflux consists of maintaining a semiupright posture and small frequent feedings of thickened material. Bethanechol has yielded little or no benefit, but metaclopramide, which increases the tone and amplitude of gastric contraction, relaxes the pyloric sphincter, and accelerates gastric emptying, has proved more helpful.

In rare instances, the extent of a baby's nutritional depletion or chronic pneumonitis may demand hospitalization. In infants sick enough to be hospitalized, 3 weeks is an ample period to determine whether their symptoms can be controlled by intensive medical measures. Infants less severely affected should be evaluated in an outpatient setting over 2 to 4 months. If symptoms are controlled by medical means, reflux usually disappears by 15 months, coincident with the development of upright posture. In our experience, medical therapy fails for approximately 15% of patients.

With worsening or protraction of symptoms despite adherence to conservative treatment, surgical correction is recommended if the infant fails to gain weight and grow adequately, has recurrent pneumonitis, has life-threatening apnea spells, or has esophagitis. Prompt operative correction is thought appropriate without medical trial for those patients with thoracic translocation of a significant portion of the stomach and esophageal stricture.

Surgical intervention is undertaken to place the gastroesophageal junction well below the diaphragm (i.e., lengthen the intraabdominal esophagus), recreate an acute angle of His, and create a valve-like mechanism to force the fundus of the stomach against the esophagus. The Nissen fundoplication involves wrapping the fundus of the stomach completely around the esophagogastric junction (Fig. 44–8). In the Thal procedure, the wrap is partial (i.e., 210 to 270 degrees). Postoperative problems such as dysphagia and inability to burp and vomit (i.e., gas-bloat syndrome) appear less likely with the Thal procedure (102). Gastroesophageal reflux is discussed in more detail in Chapter 37.

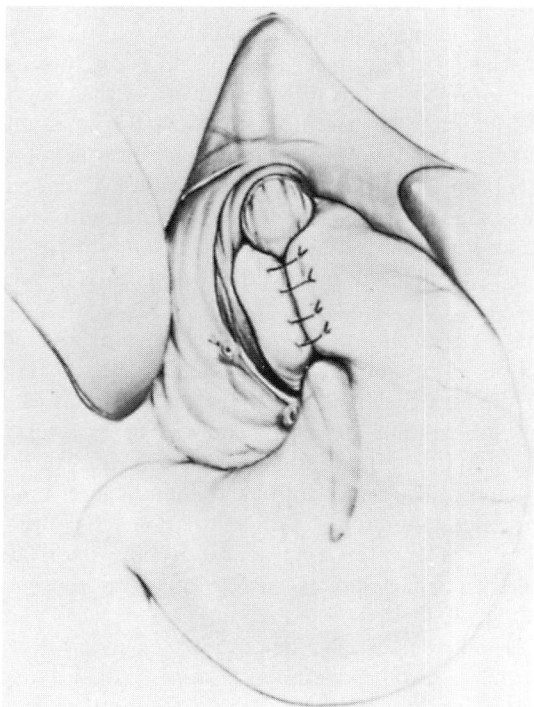

FIG. 44–8. A successful method for the surgical correction of gastroesophageal reflux employs gastric fundoplication as described by Nissen.

ABDOMINAL SURGERY

The indications for abdominal surgery are distension and bilious vomiting. To these should be added the scaphoid contour seen if there is high intestinal obstruction or the abdominal viscera are in an ectopic location, as in infants with congenital diaphragmatic hernia. Extreme degrees of abdominal distension are associated with intestinal and gastric perforation. Tenderness signifying peritoneal irritation can be elicited by careful examination. A tender, erythematous abdominal wall is a reliable sign of an intraabdominal catastrophe with resultant peritonitis and ischemic intestine. Reliance on bowel sounds can be misleading. Peristalsis can exist despite peritonitis or be absent when intestinal distension is caused by mechanical obstruction.

Pertinent radiologic studies to be obtained in all cases of suspected intraabdominal surgical lesions are the flat and upright views of the abdomen. The left lateral decubitus radiograph may be substituted for the upright radiograph if pneumoperitoneum is suspected. Intestinal obstruction can be diagnosed and the level of obstruction determined by the configuration of the air–fluid levels. Pneumoperitoneum is usually readily appreciated on abdominal x-ray films. Supine radiographs may show the football sign produced by superimposition of the falciform ligament on a large bubble of free air (Fig. 44–9). The bowel wall may be outlined by air outside and inside the bowel lumen. The left lateral decubitis radiograph may show air around the liver. Not infrequently, the findings on radiographs may be subtle and require an alert physician to make the diagnosis. Distended bowel and the absence of air–fluid levels in intestinal loops of various sizes suggest obstruction secondary to meconium ileus. Calcifications scattered within the abdomen indicate intrauterine perforation with meconium peritonitis.

Unless precluded by a deteriorating clinical condition, a contrast enema, usually of isoosmotic Gastrografin initially, requires only a short delay that is usually justified by the information obtained. The enema need not be an elaborate study in these precarious subjects.

The diagnosis of malrotation is most accurately made with a small amount of contrast placed into the stomach to confirm the position of the ligament of Treitz. Incomplete obstructions of the gastrointestinal tract, such as those caused by congenital stenosis or intraluminal web, are often the most difficult congenital lesions to diagnose and require contrast studies of the upper gastrointestinal (UGI) tract with careful attention to every centimeter of intestine on fluoroscopy.

Pneumoperitoneum: Gastric Perforation

Spontaneous perforation of a hollow viscus is most frequently seen in distressed neonates who have undergone resuscitation immediately after birth. The presence

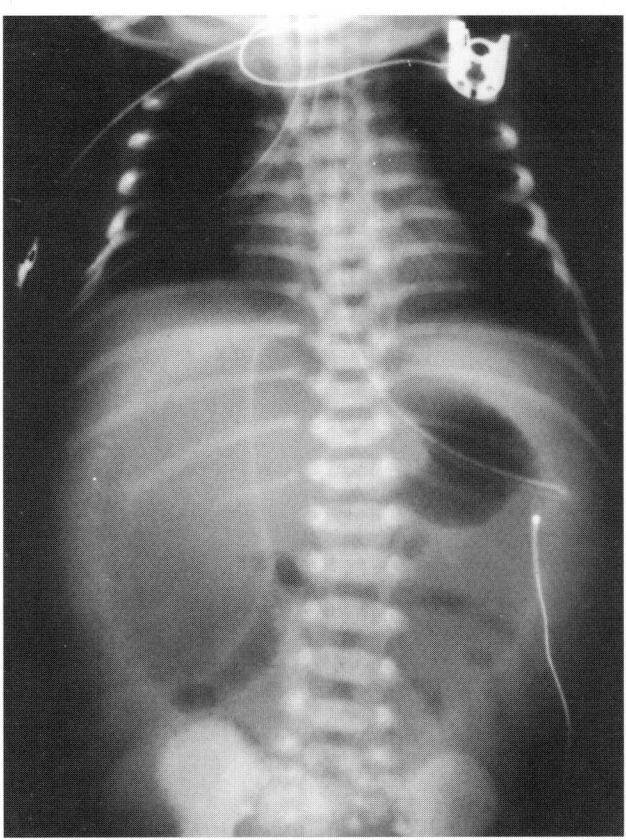

FIG. 44–9. Supine abdominal x-ray film demonstrates a massive intraperitoneal air collection. The air is seen as a large central bubble on which is superimposed a dense linear opacity produced by the falciform ligament. The falciform ligament forms the lace for the football sign.

of free air in the peritoneal cavity may be secondary to perforation anywhere in the gastrointestinal tract and is a surgical emergency. The surgeon approaching the infant with pneumoperitoneum must be prepared to investigate systematically the entire gastrointestinal tract and anticipate problems such as Hirschsprung disease, gastric perforation, necrotizing enterocolitis (NEC), or other ischemic insults to the intestine resulting in perforation (104–106).

After perforation, egress of air into the peritoneal cavity usually leads to impressive abdominal distension. Elevation of the diaphragm occurs with potential embarrassment of the infant's respiratory dynamics. A temporary but lifesaving maneuver is needle aspiration of the peritoneal cavity, which diminishes air under pressure, allowing the diaphragm to return to a more normal position. There is usually dramatic relief of abdominal distension and respiratory distress. It is not hazardous to insert a needle adapted to a 50-mL syringe through the anterior abdominal wall. The bowel is usually compressed against the posterior parietes and is not likely to be injured by this maneuver.

Surgical intervention must be prompt. When massive distension of the abdomen occurs, a gastric perforation can be anticipated. Typically, the rent occurs high on the greater curvature of the stomach. Because the perforation may be located on the posterior wall, thorough exploration of relatively inaccessible areas of the stomach must be carried out. Although it has been suggested that perforation of the stomach results from congenital deficiency of musculature in the gastric wall, this explanation is questionable. The apparent absence of musculature at the margin of the perforation probably represents retraction of the muscles of an overdistended stomach, with a ballooning of mucosa between the muscle fibers.

Repair is accomplished by primary closure in two layers after debridement of the margins of the perforation. A gastrostomy tube, inserted through a noninvolved area of the stomach, is advisable to ensure postoperative decompression. The subsequent course of the infant is usually uncomplicated if the underlying problem for which resuscitation was required is controlled. Cautious feedings can be started within a few days of surgical repair. For diagnosis and management of perforations occurring elsewhere in the gastrointestinal tract, see Meconium Peritonitis and Necrotizing Enterocolitis.

Temporary Diversion of the Intestinal Tract

Newborn intestinal emergencies often demand a temporary vent or enterostomy. Although not as desirable as an end-to-end union of the bowel, these measures may be lifesaving in fragile infants who are critically ill as the result of intestinal obstruction or peritonitis or who are threatened by serious congenital defects. An abdominal stoma in the infant does not carry the same implications as in the adult; the physician must stress this fact to allay the fears and doubts of a worried parent. Most enterostomies are temporary, and the outlook for restoration of complete intestinal continuity is good.

Gastrostomy

The stomach requires venting for two reasons. First, decompression of the gastrointestinal tract is necessary in the face of any abdominal catastrophe. Placement of the gastrostomy obviates the need for a nasogastric tube. It is more efficient and eliminates the danger of pressure necrosis of the alar cartilage of the infant's nose and the respiratory hazards that attend nasogastric tubes. Second, the gastrostomy tube provides access for feeding a depleted neonate.

Gastrostomy can be performed under local anesthesia, although it is usually done under general anesthesia. Frequently, the procedure complements a primary abdominal operation. A simple Stamm gastrostomy is preferred, and it is not difficult to remove or replace the tube as an office procedure. If the gastrostomy tube is to be maintained for a long time, it may be replaced after 1 month with a gastrostomy button, which is easier for the parents to care for at home (107).

Ileostomy

Temporary ileostomy is less desirable than primary union of the bowel, but there are clinical circumstances in which its creation as a temporary diverting procedure is prudent, including inflammatory necrosis of the distal small bowel with intraperitoneal soiling and peritonitis, ischemic insult with marginal viability of the bowel, and marked disparity in lumen size, as in intestinal atresia or meconium ileus.

A properly performed ileostomy is usually well tolerated and rarely causes skin breakdown. With appropriate supportive care, weight gain and healing proceed, and intestinal reconstruction can be carried out electively with greater safety for the infant. We recommend closure of the ileostomy when the infants weigh 2.5 to 3.0 kg to minimize fluid and electrolyte imbalances that these babies may develop (108).

In very sick infants or in babies with other underlying conditions such as meconium ileus, the double-barrel enterostomy of Mikulicz has proved valuable. The common wall that has been created is gradually crushed with a special clamp, partly reestablishing intestinal continuity. Complete closure of the bowel can be achieved without reentering the peritoneal cavity. Another effective technique of intestinal venting that permits access to the distal gastrointestinal tract is the end-to-side enteroenterostomy described by Bishop and Koop (109). This technique has particular application for lesions in the proximal gastrointestinal tract, such as jejunal and high ileal atresia.

Colostomy

The four usual indications for colostomy in the neonate are impending or actual perforation of the colon, colonic atresia with huge disparity of the bowel lumen, Hirschsprung disease, and high imperforate anus. The loop colostomy has the advantage of simplicity and speed in critically ill babies. An end-colostomy is mechanically sound, easily managed, and avoids spillage into the distal loop, which is an advantage in treating Hirschsprung disease and imperforate anus. A diaper neatly covers the colostomy during the early months of life, until definitive surgical correction of the primary problem is accomplished and the colostomy can be closed (see Chap. 37).

Rotational Abnormalities

Malrotation

In the developing embryo, the elongating intestine must undergo rotation as it returns to the celomic cavity so that it can be accommodated within the confines of the abdominal cavity. The proximal small intestine assumes the characteristic C-shaped contour, and the duodenum is fixed to the left of the midline at the ligament of Treitz. The cecum takes a counterclockwise rotation, reaching its final location in the right lower abdomen (110). Incomplete intestinal rotation with consequent inadequate fixation of the intestinal mesentery may be an asymptomatic occurrence, may give rise to subtle symptoms difficult to diagnose, or may present as a life-threatening intraabdominal catastrophe. An understanding of the mechanism by which the lesion becomes symptomatic is necessary if the physician is to recognize and prevent the devastating complications that can accompany midgut volvulus.

If rotation is abnormal, bands are formed between the ectopic cecum, located in the right upper quadrant, and the right lateral abdominal wall. As these bands course from the cecum to the abdominal wall, they traverse the duodenum and can cause intermittent, incomplete duodenal obstruction. Symptoms of partial duodenal obstruction are often baffling. The infant may experience intervals of normal feeding pattern that are interspersed with exasperating episodes of vomiting. Because the obstruction is high in the gastrointestinal tract, abdominal distension does not occur. The telltale sign of an underlying mechanical problem is bile in the vomitus. This lesion, more than any other, supports the contention that bile-stained vomitus in an infant necessitates a thorough diagnostic workup to detect a malrotation and subsequent midgut volvulus. More than 50% of babies present with symptoms before 1 week of age, but 10% remain asymptomatic until after 1 year of age (111).

The most reliable diagnostic study is a UGI series for localization of the ligament of Treitz. Surgical correction of malrotation of the colon prevents a future volvulus of the midgut and relieves the partial duodenal obstruction. The bands binding the cecum to the right abdominal wall are lysed, and the large bowel is freed and transposed to the left side of the abdomen. The duodenum is mobilized on its medial aspect, where the narrow mesentery is intimately associated with the superior mesenteric artery. As the mesentery of the small bowel is freed medially, it assumes a broad position over the posterior abdominal wall. With the mesentery splayed, the potential for torsion is eliminated. It is unnecessary to fix the intestine in its new position with sutures (112). The appendix, because it now lies on the left side of the abdomen, is usually removed or inverted. Operative correction of malrotation in this manner is known as the Ladd procedure.

Malrotation with Midgut Volvulus

If fixation of the mesentery of the small bowel has not occurred normally, the intestine is subject to torsion on the axis of the superior mesenteric artery. This mechanism of obstruction must be considered for an infant with bile-stained vomiting, especially if there is no abdominal distension. Abdominal tenderness is an ominous finding.

Roentgenographic abnormalities are often characteristic, with evidence of duodenal obstruction and scanty gas distributed through the remainder of the bowel. The air–fluid levels typical of intestinal obstruction elsewhere in the gastrointestinal tract are not usually associated with this malrotation. An airless abdomen is an ominous sign and usually indicates that infarction of the intestine has already taken place. Bloody stools imply that significant compromise to the intestinal vasculature has occurred. A UGI series shows a corkscrew-like constriction of the third portion of the duodenum.

If midgut volvulus is diagnosed or suspected as the underlying mechanism for the infant's illness, emergency surgical exploration is undertaken. If the findings are favorable and the bowel is viable, the torsion is reduced by counterclockwise rotation, and a Ladd procedure is carried out as described for the treatment of malrotation without volvulus. The prognosis is favorable as long as the viability of the intestine is not in question. However, if the diagnosis has been delayed or the volvulus has been an intrauterine event, intestinal ischemia, infarction, or both may be encountered in the distribution of the superior mesenteric artery. Initial judgments regarding the viability of the intestine are not easy; intestinal resection at the time of initial exploration is contraindicated. The ischemic intestine must be given every opportunity to recover after the torsion has been reduced. The first operation consists of untwisting the small bowel and establishing a gastrostomy.

Reexploration is undertaken 24 to 36 hours later, and areas of obvious infarction are identified. These are resected, and appropriate enterostomies are brought out to the abdominal wall; anastomosis is contraindicated. Any intestine of marginal viability is retained in hope that it will recover. Reexploration to determine recovery or further loss of small bowel is repeated after another interval of 36 to 48 hours. After the full extent of intestinal loss has been established and the margins of viable bowel exteriorized, the surgeon is faced with the management of a desperately ill infant at risk from sepsis, disseminated intravascular coagulation, and the inevitable nutritional crisis attending a short-bowel syndrome.

A central venous catheter for total parenteral alimentation is established, and nourishment is provided by this technique throughout the early postoperative weeks. After the infant has achieved positive nitrogen balance and the reestablishment of intestinal continuity is complete, there is then a difficult period of weaning from parenteral onto oral feedings. About 40 cm of residual small intestine seems to be required for successful adaptation of the intestine in full-term infants, although adaptation has been reported for children with considerably less than 40 cm of intestine (113). If the distal ileum and ileocecal valve are intact, slightly less bowel may be tolerated. Infant formulas that are fat-free and contain monosaccharides and hydrolyzed protein should be used to feed these babies because these formulas require only a minimal absorptive surface and little enzyme activity for assimilation. Gradually, the volume and concentration of these substances may be increased until all calories are taken orally. The process of weaning the infant from total intravenous to total oral alimentation may take months. This underscores the devastating complications of a midgut volvulus and indicates the need for vigilance by pediatrician and surgeon in the pursuit of the diagnosis of malrotation.

Hypertrophic Pyloric Stenosis

Pyloric stenosis occurs in approximately one of 300 to 1,000 live births. Its cause is obscure. Boys are affected about four times as frequently as girls, and the disease seems to have a predilection for the first-born child. There is a familial tendency, with a 2.5% to 20% incidence of pyloric stenosis in children of affected parents; the variation in incidence depends on the genders of the affected parent and child (114). It has been speculated that hypertrophy of the circular muscles of the pylorus results from propulsion of milk curds against the spastic pyloric canal, producing edema, additional spasm, and subsequent hypertrophy of the musculature, leading to complete obstruction. Some researchers have postulated that the muscle hypertrophy is a response to vagal stimulation. This is somewhat substantiated by the observation that infants undergoing surgery for esophageal atresia and tracheoesophageal fistula seem to have a higher incidence of pyloric stenosis, a result perhaps of vagal nerve irritation in the operative field. No infectious agent has been isolated despite the apparent seasonal incidence of the disease. The clinical onset of bile-free projectile vomiting at 2 to 8 weeks of age in a first-born boy strongly suggests the diagnosis of congenital hypertrophic pyloric stenosis. Occasionally, the onset is insidious, and these babies can present to the pediatrician as perplexing feeding problems. A typical history reveals intermittent vomiting that gradually increases in frequency and intensity over a week, until the baby vomits most ingested feedings with impressive force.

Abdominal examination is carried out with the stomach empty. If the infant has not just vomited, the physician may need to use a nasogastric tube to ensure an adequate examination. The baby can be given a pacifier for relaxation. Visible peristalsis may be observed moving across the upper abdomen. The examiner stands to the left, elevating the baby's feet with his left hand to relax the abdominal muscles and then palpates gently in the right upper quadrant. The pyloric olive is palpable to the experienced examiner in 90% of patients, and radiographic studies are usually not needed. If pyloric stenosis is suspected but the olive cannot be palpated, the diagnostic procedure of choice is abdominal ultrasonography, which is more than 90% accurate in centers experienced with this technique (115). A UGI series is usually reserved for those patients with vomiting but a normal ultrasonographic examination, in whom another cause of obstruction is suspected. Hyperbilirubinemia is seen in 8% of babies with pyloric stenosis. Almost all the bilirubin is of an indirect type and may be related to a decreased level of hepatic glycuronyl transferase (116). Jaundice clears after pyloromyotomy.

Infants with pyloric stenosis are conveniently grouped according to their clinical condition at the time they are seen by the surgeon. About one-half are well hydrated and in a satisfactory nutritional state. Serum electrolytes are normal, and the urine, although concentrated, is of adequate volume. These babies can undergo surgical correction without preoperative preparation. For the remaining infants, preparation before surgery is necessary. The typical pattern of electrolyte disturbance is that of mild or moderate metabolic alkalosis. The hypokalemia may not be reflected in the serum electrolytes, but potassium supplements must be provided before the alkalosis can be corrected. Salt-losing adrenogenital syndrome can present with symptoms identical to pyloric stenosis. However, this condition is characterized by an elevated serum potassium and metabolic acidosis.

These moderately dehydrated infants usually can be corrected within 12 hours with 5% dextrose–half-normal saline solution at a rate half to twice that of maintenance. After urine production is certain, potassium should be replaced at 2 mEq/kg for the 12-hour period of therapy.

A few infants present with severe dehydration and malnutrition and are often well below their birth weight. In this group, extensive rehydration is mandatory before surgery. The infants are profoundly alkalotic and potassium deficient. Their protein stores are depleted, urine is scanty, and they may be anemic. Intensive therapy for 2 to 3 days is required to bring these infants into metabolic balance. Fluids, electrolytes, colloid, and even blood may be necessary. Fortunately, it is rare to see such children today.

A Ramstedt–Fredet pyloromyotomy is best performed through a transverse skin incision placed in the right upper quadrant of the abdomen. This short, safe, surgical procedure accomplishes division of the hypertrophic circular muscles of the gastric outlet and reestablishes patency of the pyloric channel (Fig. 44–10). In most cases, glucose water feedings can be reinstituted 6 to 8 hours postoperatively. If the child tolerates the first feeding, slow advancement of the volume of his regular formula is encouraged. The infant commonly vomits a few times postoperatively, but this should not alter his feeding advancement. Explanation to the parents that this vomiting is common can allay their anxiety. The child is generally ready for discharge on the second or third postoperative day, when he attains adequate oral intake. Typically, the babies enjoy a growth spurt in the immediate postoperative weeks, much to the satisfaction of the parents.

Duodenal Atresia, Stenosis, and Annular Pancreas

Duodenal obstruction may be complete or partial and results from intrinsic causes or external compression (117). An intraluminal diaphragm can cause partial, inter-

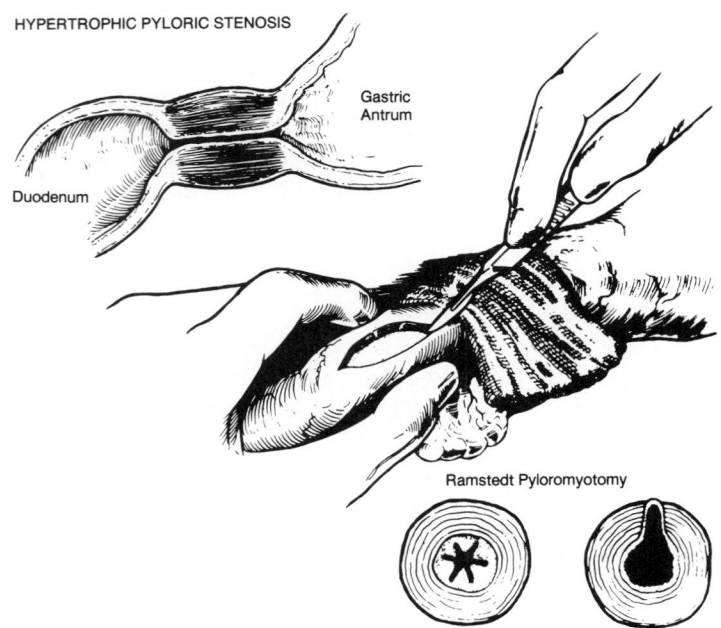

HYPERTROPHIC PYLORIC STENOSIS

Gastric Antrum

Duodenum

Ramstedt Pyloromyotomy

FIG. 44–10. A Ramstedt pyloromyotomy is made through all layers of the pylorus except the mucosa. The cross section demonstrates how the mucosa of the pylorus expands into the defect created, enlarging the cross-sectional diameter of the pyloric channel.

mittent obstruction that is difficult to recognize. Only a carefully performed UGI series outlines an intraluminal web and determines the site of obstruction. Annular pancreas, duodenal stenosis, and congenital bands are other causes of partial duodenal obstruction in which the need for early surgical intervention is more apparent.

Duodenal atresia results in complete obstruction. In instances of complete duodenal obstruction, swallowed air is prevented from passing beyond the duodenum, and the middle and lower abdomen are scaphoid. The characteristic x-ray finding is that of a double bubble of ingested air filling the stomach and blind-ending duodenum (Fig. 44–11). Duodenal atresia is often associated with trisomy 21.

Unless the underlying cause of obstruction is related to malrotation, an initial period of nasogastric drainage and resuscitation with intravenous fluids and electrolytes is appropriate before duodenal obstruction is surgically corrected. Surgical therapy is tailored to the particular lesion encountered. The intraluminal web can be resected through a transduodenal approach. It may be necessary for the surgeon to perform a gastrotomy or duodenotomy, through which a Foley catheter with the balloon minimally inflated is passed, to identify the site at which the web is attached.

Some stenotic lesions can be managed by local duodenoplasty, but obstruction from duodenal atresia requires

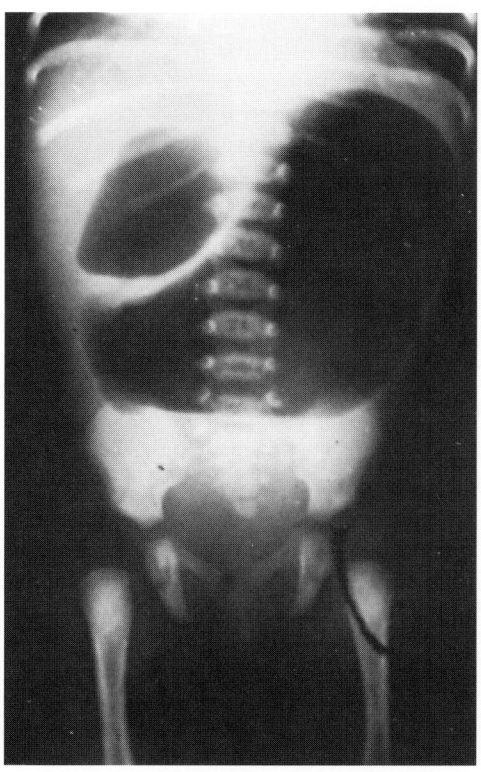

FIG. 44–11. Characteristic double bubble of congenital duodenal obstruction.

bypass for relief. Obstruction secondary to duodenal atresia or annular pancreas is best treated by creating a duodenoduodenostomy (118). A duodenojejunostomy is an alternative method to establish intestinal continuity.

Jejunoileal Atresia

Atresia of the bowel probably results from an ischemic insult to the intestine during its development (119). The atresia may be discrete, involving only a short segment of jejunum or ileum (Fig. 44–12), or it may involve the intestine over many centimeters (120). Atretic areas are sometimes multiple, and although the intervening bowel is normal, considerable length may be missing. Abdominal distension and bile-stained vomitus are the usual presenting symptoms. Radiographs show air–fluid levels distributed throughout the abdomen (Fig. 44–13). In cases of distal ileal obstruction, the contrast enema adds confirmation, showing the typical microcolon.

A short period of restoration with fluids, electrolytes, and colloid may be necessary, but this should never exceed a few hours. The method of surgical correction depends on the intraoperative findings. If the intestinal length is normal, the dilated proximal end is excised back to near-normal-caliber bowel, and an end-to-back anastomosis is performed. In the infant with a large-gap atresia, the proximal end is tapered, and anastomosis is then accomplished (121,122). The end-to-side reconstruction, described by Bishop and Koop, has proved safe and effective and has the added advantage of providing access to the gastrointestinal tract for irrigations postoperatively (109). This type of repair is particularly helpful if there is a major disparity in the size of the ends of the intestine. A Mikulicz enterostomy or simple end-enterostomy may be lifesaving in critically ill, depleted newborns with distal bowel obstruction.

Incomplete obstruction resulting from stenosis of the bowel can be puzzling and hazardous because there is a confusing clinical picture. The infants feed poorly, occasionally vomit, or become distended without pattern. These symptoms continue despite changes in the formula. The pediatrician may consider food allergies, nonspecific failure to thrive, and even a nervous mother as underlying causes. The obstruction finally becomes complete, or the bowel perforates. Surgical exploration may be needed to confirm a diagnosis of ileal stenosis, and this approach is considered even if x-ray examinations of the intestine have been normal when the clinical course of the infant suggests this diagnosis. Cure is achieved by appropriate intestinal tailoring procedures such as a Y–V plasty or longitudinal incision and transverse closure (i.e., Heineke–Mikulicz principle).

Meconium Plug Syndrome

The meconium plug syndrome is a benign form of colon obstruction in the neonate caused by a firm white

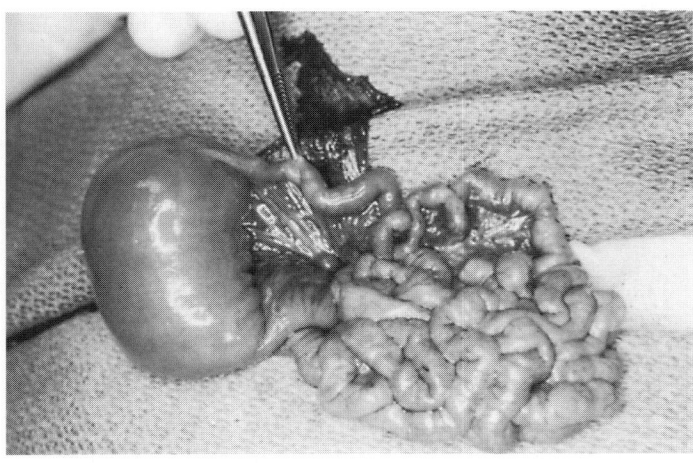

FIG. 44–12. In this patient with jejunal atresia, a dilated proximal segment and a narrow distal jejunum are evident.

plug of mucus. These babies usually present with abdominal distension. Abdominal x-ray films reveal distended loops of bowel. A barium enema shows a long radiolucency within the descending colon. The plug is passed after the barium enema or a saline rectal irrigation. Although meconium plug syndrome is found in otherwise completely normal infants, it can be difficult to differentiate from Hirschsprung disease and to rule out cystic fibrosis, so many surgeons routinely perform a rectal biopsy and obtain a sweat chloride test in infants with meconium plug syndrome.

Meconium Peritonitis

Meconium peritonitis usually follows antenatal intestinal obstruction and perforation of the bowel above the obstruction in conditions such as bowel atresia, volvulus, meconium ileus, and neonatal Hirschsprung disease. If it occurs early in gestation, the perforation may have sealed off, but the chemical peritonitis gives rise to tiny scattered foreign-body reactions that may become calcified and be visible radiographically. If the perforation occurs closer to birth, calcifications are usually not seen on radiographs, and chemical peritonitis may be followed by bacterial peritonitis. More frequently, the presenting signs are those of intestinal obstruction.

Meconium Ileus

Intestinal obstruction resulting from viscid meconium impacted in the terminal ileum is seen as the earliest manifestation of cystic fibrosis. This problem affects about 10% of the cystic fibrosis population. Infants with meconium ileus subsequently develop other complications of their underlying disease, but the later respiratory sequelae are not necessarily more severe (123).

The clinical presentation of meconium ileus is not unlike that seen with other forms of distal intestinal obstruction. Abdominal distension and bile-stained vomitus are characteristic. The upright radiograph of the abdomen is especially helpful in this form of intestinal obstruction in the newborn. The characteristic soap bubble mass in the right lower abdomen and a paucity of air–fluid levels despite the presence of many gas-filled loops of intestine is pathognomonic (Fig. 44–14). The air–fluid levels characteristic of obstruction do not develop because air is trapped by the tenacious meco-

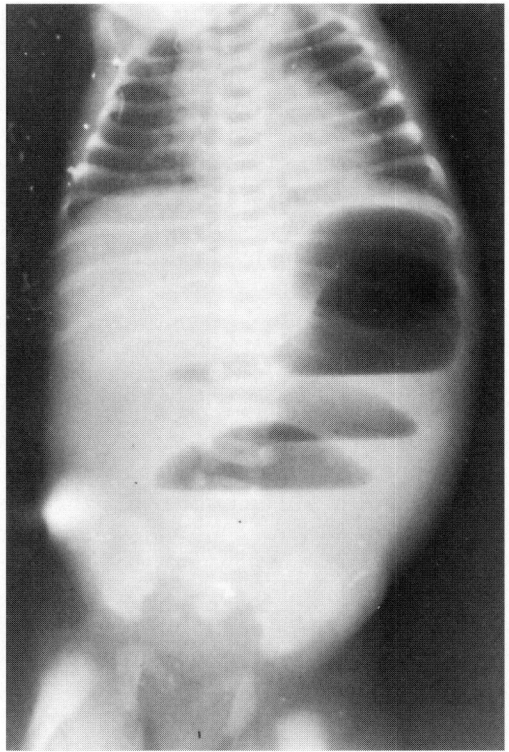

FIG. 44–13. An upright abdominal x-ray film of a patient with jejunal atresia shows gastric distension and approximately three loops of bowel with no gas beyond the obstruction.

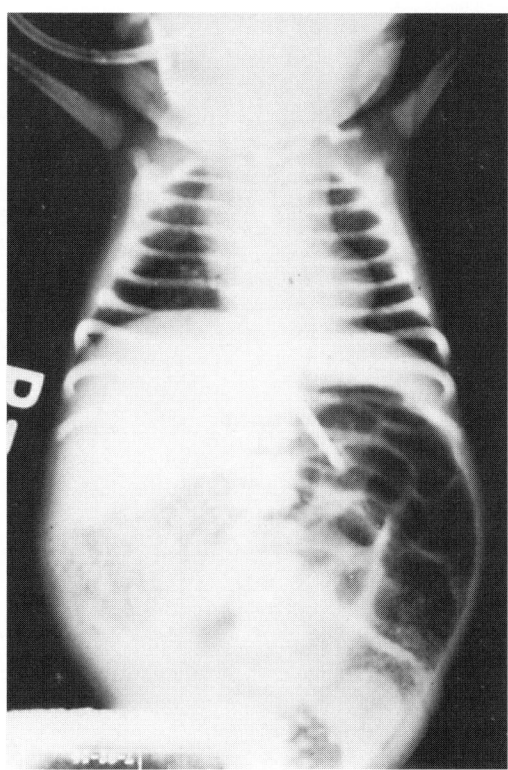

FIG. 44–14. An x-ray film of a newborn infant with meconium ileus reveals many gas-filled loops, but little fluid is seen. The right lower quadrant is filled with a large loop of intestine distended by meconium. Gas trapped in the meconium gives the typical ground-glass appearance.

nium, and a clear interface is not produced. The contrast enema shows a microcolon, unused because of the distal ileal obstruction. Concretions of meconium in the terminal ileum immediately proximal to the ileocecal valve are often seen.

Surgical intervention may be required for relief of obstruction, but enemas of Gastrografin often eliminate the obstructing mass of meconium (124). At our institution, the Gastrografin is diluted 1:4 with saline so that the complications of a hyperosmolar fluid enema are avoided. This radiopaque contrast material contains a wetting agent (i.e., Tween 80) in which the thick meconium is soluble. If the Gastrografin can be successfully advanced through the microcolon and into the obstructed distal ileum, there is reasonable expectation that meconium will be passed spontaneously with relief of obstruction (125). When the first attempt moves some meconium out, but the infant's obstruction is not completely relieved, a second enema is justified several hours later. Complete removal of the meconium may take several Gastrografin enemas over a few days. If these maneuvers fail to relieve the obstruction, or if meconium peritonitis is present, surgical exploration is the only acceptable treatment.

If surgical correction is necessary, technical problems associated with evacuating the tar-like meconium from the distended ileum and establishing intestinal continuity between the dilated proximal intestine and the distal microcolon have been solved in various ways. Irrigation through an ileostomy with dilute acetylcysteine has proved effective in some infants. A rapid and safe anastomosis involving the Bishop–Koop technique is well suited for this problem (109). A Mikulicz enterostomy has the virtue of speed while providing decompression and establishment of continuity. These techniques allow access to the distal intestine for postoperative irrigations with acetylcysteine. With use, the colon has the potential to function normally, and the vent established by the Mikulicz or Bishop–Koop procedure is closed surgically. In selected infants, resection and primary anastomosis can be performed at the first operation. In the postoperative period, the infant is subject to respiratory difficulty secondary to impacted secretions. These may require tracheal suctioning or bronchoscopy for relief. When oral feedings are instituted, exogenous pancreatic supplements are provided so that digestion and use of calories are ensured.

Duplications

An uncommon cause of intestinal obstruction in the newborn is that arising secondary to duplications of the bowel. These can exist at any level of the intestine and may cause obstruction when the lumen is compromised by the gradually expanding duplication or by the duplication acting as a focus for segmental intestinal volvulus. Because they occur on the mesenteric aspect of the bowel, duplications are intimately involved with the blood supply to the normal intestine. Small, cystic duplications are easily resected with a segment of the adjacent bowel (126). However, extensive fusiform or intramural duplications may tax the surgeon's ingenuity. In these instances, resection of the common wall, with creation of a single conduit, may enable the surgeon to preserve an extensive segment of normal intestine (127). Gastric mucosa can exist within a duplication and result in gastrointestinal hemorrhage (128). This cause of gastrointestinal bleeding is considered in the evaluation of a baby with melena.

Hirschsprung Disease

The clinical presentation of Hirschsprung disease (i.e., aganglionic megacolon) may be subtle and go unrecognized for months or years until the classic symptoms of constipation and abdominal distension are unmistakable. However, the history of constipation goes back to the early days of life in most patients with Hirschsprung disease. The consequences of aganglionosis can be life-threatening in the newborn period (129). The absence of ganglion cells modifies neuromuscular conduction and prevents proper evacuation of the bowel. Abdominal distension or debilitating enterocolitis brings the infant to the surgeon's attention.

Failure of an infant to pass meconium in the first 36 hours of life should alert the pediatrician to the possibility of Hirschsprung disease. Retention of a meconium plug requiring mechanical assistance for its evacuation is another presumptive sign that the colon may be aganglionic. A positive barium enema, even in a newborn, can be a reliable indication of Hirschsprung disease (130). The characteristic terminal narrow segment, with transition to dilated bowel in the area of the rectosigmoid, is a classic finding in older children but may not be present in neonates. Anal dilation produced by a rectal examination may confuse the findings. A normal barium enema in the neonate does not exclude the diagnosis of aganglionosis, and confirmatory evidence must be obtained by rectal biopsy.

Several techniques of biopsy have been described, but any one that provides an adequate specimen of the rectal wall can establish the diagnosis. The absence of ganglion cells in the submucosal or muscular plexus confirms the diagnosis. Experienced pathologists can interpret the more superficial biopsies, which include only the submucosal tissue. The advantage of partial-thickness biopsy is that there is less intramural scarring to complicate the definitive surgical procedure for correction of Hirschsprung disease. A suction biopsy technique is available that is readily adapted for use in infants (131). This bedside procedure provides adequate submucosal tissue for interpretation by an experienced pediatric pathologist. A histochemical technique estimating acetylcholinesterase activity has been helpful in establishing the diagnosis in some centers and has the added advantage of requiring only tiny fragments of bowel tissue (132).

The clinical presentation of Hirschsprung disease varies. Intestinal obstruction is not always typical. Enterocolitis is often the presenting complaint in a newborn, and this may be confused with NEC, seen primarily in premature infants with respiratory distress. The effects of enterocolitis associated with Hirschsprung disease can be devastating unless recognized and treated appropriately (133). Enterocolitis often presents with diarrhea and signs of collapse. Sepsis may be fatal if not promptly recognized and treated. The enterocolitis can sometimes be controlled by careful rectal lavage with quarter-normal solutions of saline. It is vital that the volume of solutions instilled be recovered during the lavage.

Whether the symptoms are those of obstruction or enterocolitis, after the infant has been resuscitated, the safest course of action is the performance of a colostomy in an area of bowel containing ganglion cells. Most babies have a transition somewhere in the rectosigmoid, and a high sigmoid colostomy usually ensures normal innervation (134). The presence of ganglion cells at the site of the colostomy should be verified by biopsy at the time of colostomy formation. In desperately ill infants, the condition may preclude a controlled laparotomy with frozen-section confirmation of the transition area. In these babies, a right transverse colostomy ensures that ganglionic bowel has been exteriorized in 98%. The few remaining infants have total colonic aganglionosis or aganglionic small bowel and present special problems in management. In these infants, barium enema is helpful, showing marked foreshortening of the entire colon. The basic surgical principle is to achieve exteriorization of the most distal normally innervated bowel.

Definitive surgical therapy is deferred until the infants are managed through the initial crisis and have achieved a weight of about 7 to 9 kg. At that time, the ganglionic intestine is transposed to the anus by one of the several pull-through techniques now available. These include the classic operation described by Swenson (135) and the modification popularized by Duhamel (136). Many centers favor the endorectal pull-through procedure of Soave (137). Several centers have advocated surgery in the newborn period with a pull-through operation and no colostomy (138). The early results are promising, but the follow-up period has been too short to allow proper scrutiny.

If the physician suspects Hirschsprung disease, the diagnosis is made early. The outlook for these infants is favorable because currently available operations have now become standardized (139). Minor constipation is the most frequent sequela of surgery. Most babies with congenital megacolon achieve excellent functional results (140).

Necrotizing Enterocolitis

Necrotizing enterocolitis is a condition predominantly seen in premature infants. It is characterized by partial- or full-thickness intestinal ischemia, usually involving the terminal ileum. The cause is unknown, but the common pathway appears to be a combination of factors that leads to intestinal ischemia (141). Studies suggest that the combination of ischemia and reperfusion injury may be a factor in the development of NEC (142). Known risk factors include prematurity, neonatal stress, formula feedings, and surgery in the newborn period. Other factors considered to increase the risk of NEC are umbilical artery catheterization, infection with certain types of bacteria, and hypoalbuminemia (143).

Although the cause is uncertain, the histopathology is well established. Initially, the disease begins as mucosal ischemia, with resultant sloughing of this layer. As the disease progresses, gas develops within the muscular layers (Fig. 44–15) and may be seen on x-ray films as pneumatosis cystoides intestinalis. If full-thickness necrosis occurs, perforation and peritonitis develop. The rapidity

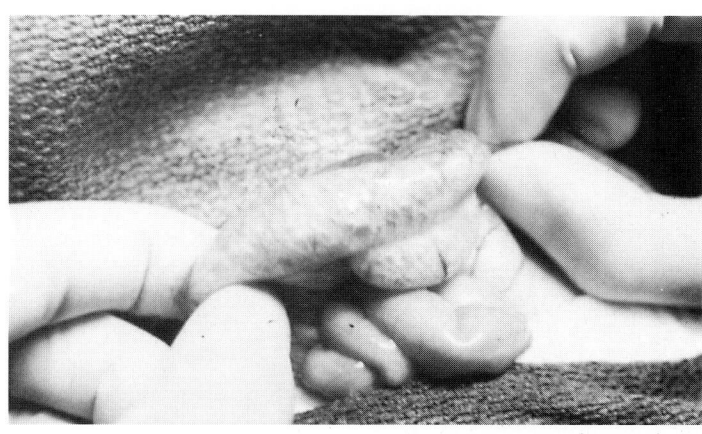

FIG. 44–15. Operative photograph of a loop of intestine affected by necrotizing enterocolitis. The gas in the seromuscular layer distorts the segment of intestine. Normal loops of uninvolved intestine also are evident.

of disease progression differs in each patient, but those who perforate usually do so within the first few days of the disease.

The diagnosis of NEC is based on clinical assessment and x-ray studies. The earliest signs are often an intolerance of feedings with vomiting. In about one-half of the patients, the vomitus is bile stained. Abdominal distension is a common early finding. Hematest-positive stools help confirm the diagnosis, but blood may be absent or a late finding. Abdominal wall erythema and a palpable abdominal mass are commonly late findings and signify more extensive disease. The use of paracentesis to choose surgical candidates has been advocated by Kosloske (144) and Ricketts (145).

Radiographic findings in early NEC may show only separated loops of distended intestine, suggesting bowel wall thickening. Pneumatosis cystoides intestinalis is pathognomonic for NEC and may be present early in the disease process. A persistent large loop of intestine seen on a series of x-ray films has been used by some as an indication for surgery, but in our experience, many children with persistent loops have been successfully treated medically.

Hepatic portal venous gas usually implies a particularly severe or extensive form of the disease, and more than 80% of children with this finding required surgery. Free intraperitoneal air is an absolute indication for surgery, although pneumoperitoneum from air dissecting down from the chest in the ventilator-dependent child must be ruled out so that an unnecessary laparotomy is not performed (dissecting air – PO_2 of air in abdomen $\approx$ FiO_2 provided to infant by the ventilator; pneumoperitoneum peritoneum – PO_2 of air in peritoneum = 21 torr).

Initial management of the child with NEC without pneumoperitoneum is standardized. The child receives nothing orally, the stomach is decompressed with a gastric sump tube, and intravenous antibiotics are begun. Antibiotics must cover gram-negative and gram-positive aerobic organisms, but anaerobic bacteria coverage is less necessary (146). Fungal infection is common after surgi-

cal treatment of NEC, and oral nystatin (Mycostatin) is recommended postoperatively (147). The best method of determining which babies require surgery consists of repeated physical examinations by the same examiner; flat and left lateral decubitus abdominal radiographs every 4 to 6 hours for detection of pneumoperitoneum; careful monitoring of the respiratory status and acid–base balance; and monitoring of the leukocyte and platelet counts for signs of sepsis.

In our experience, indications for surgery include pneumoperitoneum, persistent metabolic acidosis (i.e., pH less than 7.2), rapidly worsening pulmonary status, and unremitting neutropenia or thrombocytopenia (148). Because many of our patients with hepatoportal venous gas come to surgery, we operate on these children if they do not improve promptly on medical therapy. Our experience is similar to that of others in that mortality is higher in patients who have perforated before surgery, and it is therefore better to operate before perforation has occurred.

Surgery in these infants should be expeditious and conservative. The frankly necrotic or perforated intestine should be removed, and ileostomies formed. Although routine primary anastomosis in NEC has been advocated by some, most surgeons prefer ileostomy formation in almost all patients (149). When massive resection is necessary, the chance for the child's survival is limited, but the premature infant's intestine still has potential for growth and adaptation, and rarely is the entire intestine involved in the disease. Drainage of the peritoneum under local anesthesia in the infant weighing under 1,500 g has been advocated for perforated NEC by Ein and colleagues, although many babies managed by this method eventually require formal laparotomy (150).

If ileostomy is performed, the mucous fistula should be exteriorized close to the functioning ileostomy, and closure should be planned when the child is large enough (i.e., approximately 2 kg) and at a sufficient time after the event (i.e., at least 4 to 6 weeks) to minimize the possibility of recurrence (151). Because of a 20% incidence of stricture after medical or surgical treatment of NEC in our patients, barium enema is performed in all our surgical patients before ileostomy closure and in any medical patients with feeding difficulties. Other physicians have advocated a UGI study for all babies with medically treated NEC before feeding (152).

The children are not fed orally for at least 2 to 3 weeks after the onset of NEC, and it frequently takes more than 1 month for those patients successfully treated medically to attain adequate oral caloric intake. Hyperalimentation is mandatory in these children as soon as NEC is diagnosed, and we prefer central intravenous alimentation for most children with NEC.

The long-term success rate for treatment for NEC has been good despite long hospitalization for gastrointestinal adaptation when massive resection is necessary. The quoted survival rate for children with medically treated NEC is now more than 80%, and the survival rate for those requiring surgery is approximately 50%. At CNMC, the survival rate for NEC has steadily increased since 1980 and is 80% for the surgical and medical groups combined (148). Successful medical treatment may be followed by late-onset intestinal obstruction as a result of scarring, and an interesting long-term complication of ileocolic anastomosis in infancy is the development of anastomotic ulcers. These ulcers present as painless rectal bleeding or melena years after the NEC surgery (153). Necrotizing enterocolitis is discussed in more detail in Chapter 37.

Imperforate Anus

Imperforate anus affects male and female infants with equal frequency and occurs in approximately one of every 20,000 live births. The lesion results from a failure of differentiation of the urogenital sinus and cloaca. Associated anomalies include urogenital, cardiac, spinal cord, and esophageal malformations, especially esophageal atresia and tracheoesophageal fistula. The latter lesion occurs in 10% of patients with imperforate anus (154).

Imperforate anus can be broadly classified as high or low, depending on the relationship of the distal rectal pouch to the levator complex. High imperforate anus in either gender implies that the rectal pouch is above the sphincter muscle complex. Low imperforate anus implies that the rectum has descended past this level, with an abnormal location in the perineum. Because the levator musculature is actually funnel shaped, these associations are somewhat approximate and should be considered as guidelines. Infants with low imperforate anus can be expected to have rectal continence after repair. The sphincter muscle complex must be precisely located and preserved in infants with high imperforate anus, and a normal relationship to the rectum established surgically for continence to be achieved.

Eighty percent of girls with imperforate anus have the low type. Usually, the rectum terminates by means of a fistula anterior to the normal location of the anus on the perineum (Fig. 44–16A), on the vaginal fourchette (Fig. 44–16B), or low in the vagina. Because the termination of the colon is accessible and colostomy is not necessary, early therapy can be directed at decompression of the bowel by catheter irrigation and dilation of the fistula.

It is possible to transpose the anus from the posterior vagina or perineum to its normal position in the newborn period. This is not always necessary if the bowel is easily decompressed or the baby can stool spontaneously through the fistula. A judicious interval is appropriate to allow the baby to grow before surgery is carried out. Definitive repair usually can be accomplished by means of perineal operation because the rectum is properly related to the muscles of continence. In instances in which the fistula cannot be identified, it is usually high in the vagina and not accessible to dilation or surgical revision in the newborn period. In this 20% of female infants, a colostomy is necessary. Definitive therapy for high imperforate anus in the female infant is deferred until the baby weighs 7 to 9 kg.

In boys, the incidences of high and low imperforate anus are equal. Approximately one-half of the babies present with a fistula placed ectopically on the perineum, anterior to the normal location of the anus. The fistula can terminate as far forward as the penoscrotal junction. At birth, the opening of the fistula is not always apparent, and an interval of 12 to 24 hours may be required until the bowel fills with air or meconium reaches the most distal point in the gastrointestinal tract (Fig. 44–17A). When a spot of meconium or beads of mucus can be identified on the perineum, there is assurance that the rectal pouch is low, implying that the rectum has traversed the sphincter muscle complex, and continence is expected after repair. In babies with these findings, a perineal anoplasty in the newborn period accomplishes decompression of the bowel, and no colostomy is needed.

If no fistula is visible on the perineum, the male infant can be presumed to have a high imperforate anus. The fistula usually communicates with the posterior urethra. A colostomy is needed for decompression, and the definitive pull-through operation is generally deferred until the baby is about 1 year of age. Improved results in children with high imperforate anus are being reported with the use of the posterior sagittal anoplasty, described by Pena and DeVries, at approximately 1 year of age (155).

The value of an x-ray film with the infant in the upside-down position (i.e., Wangensteen–Rice position) is limited in the diagnosis of the level of imperforate anus (Fig. 44–17B) and is primarily of historic interest (156). Although it may help when it shows the rectal pouch at or near the perineum, it can also be misleading if the distal rectum is filled with meconium that prevents air from reaching the most distal aspect of this pouch, and com-

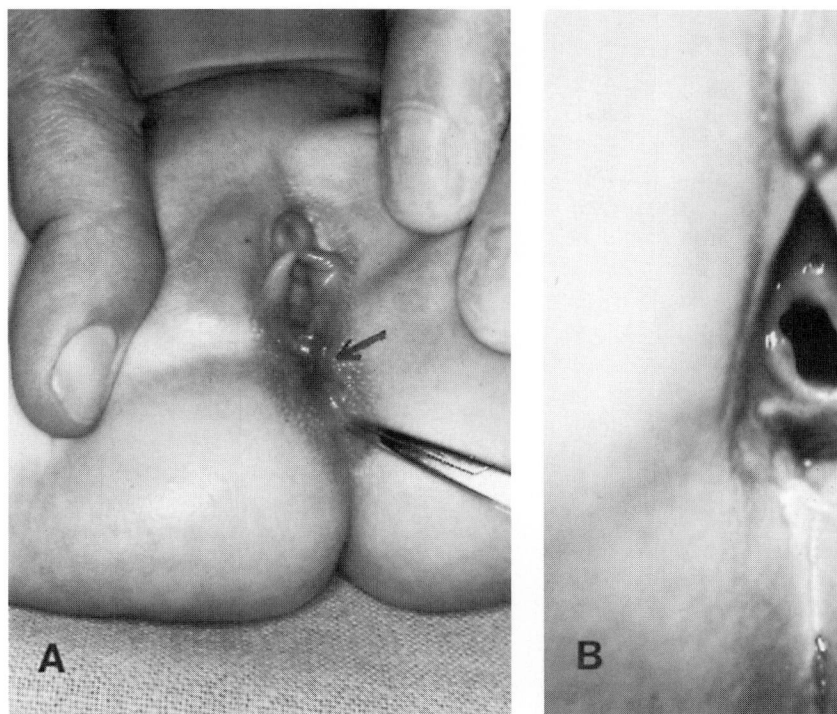

FIG. 44–16. A: Female infant with an imperforate anus. The *arrow* demonstrates the opening of the perineal fistula. The clamp is at the point where a normal anus would open. **B:** Close-up photograph of imperforate anus and an introital fistula just inside the labia minora and immediately beneath the hymenal ring. This is the most common form of fistulous opening in a female imperforate anus.

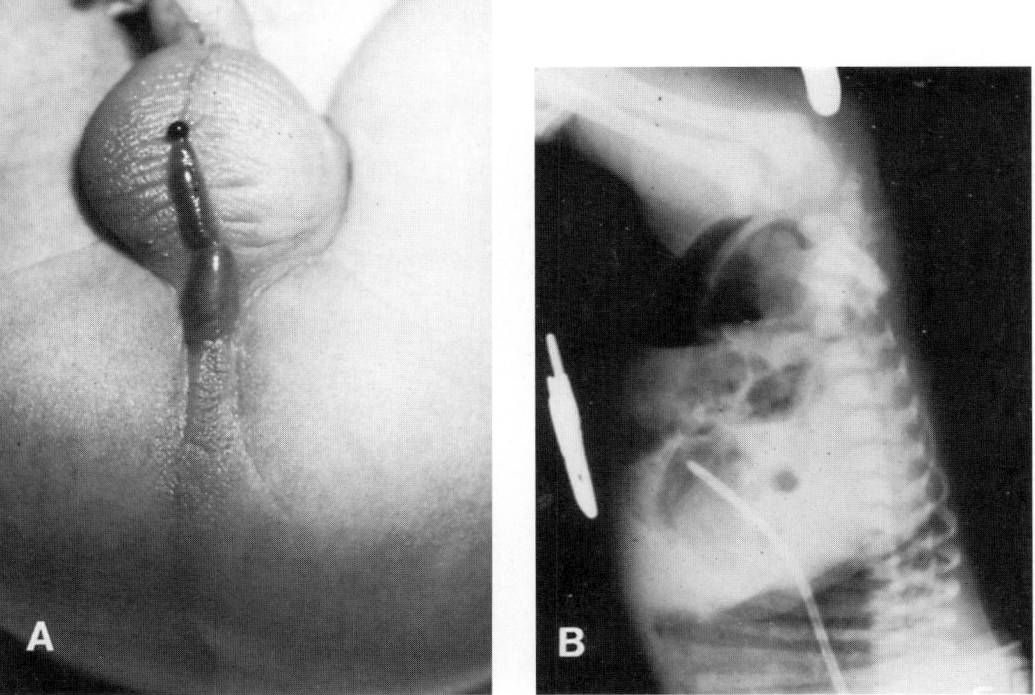

FIG. 44–17. A: Imperforate anus and partly covered perineal fistula that opens on the scrotum always occurs with a low pouch. The rectum has traversed the levator sling musculature properly. **B:** Upside-down radiographic technique of Wangensteen–Rice using a metal marker at the anus shows the distance between the rectal pouch and the anal skin. It is clearly above a line drawn between the pubis and lower border of the sacrum. There is a second gas-containing space anterior to the rectum. This indicates the presence of a rectourethral fistula with air trapped in the bladder.

plete reliance on this view for the selection of therapy is ill advised. Ultrasonography may be helpful in locating the rectal pouch.

Needle aspiration for detecting meconium in the blind perineum, with or without injection of contrast material, has been advocated by some physicians but should be performed only by the pediatric surgeon responsible for the child's care (157). If there is no fistula, and a low imperforate anus cannot be diagnosed with certainty, a colostomy is advised. Risk of a colostomy performed for a low imperforate anus is preferable to prejudicing the chances of a successful pull-through procedure by an ill-advised perineal exploration in the newborn period. With realization of the importance of the accurate transposition of the rectal pouch to the perineum, successful functional restoration has become the rule.

DISORDERS OF THE GENITALIA

Vaginal and Uterine Anomalies

Anomalies of the female reproductive tract range from simple imperforate hymen to complex forms of vaginal atresia and uterine malformations (158). These anatomic abnormalities result from errors in müllerian duct or urogenital sinus development. In the newborn, because of obstruction and accumulation of reproductive tract secretions, these conditions usually present during physical exam with either an abnormal perineum or a pelvic mass. In babies with imperforate hymen, the bulging hymen is easily identified, and hymenectomy or hymenotomy via a perineal approach provides relief of the distal vaginal obstruction. More proximal anomalies require additional ultrasonographic, radiographic, or endoscopic investigation to determine the location of the obstruction. The subsequent surgical strategy depends on the severity of the defect and may include a combined abdominal and perineal approach with complex reconstructive techniques. In children with vaginal agenesis, a neovagina is created from a segment of colon.

Ovarian Masses

The use of prenatal ultrasound has led to the increased detection of ovarian cysts in newborns (159). Formed in response to maternal hormones, presumably many of these cysts will resolve spontaneously following birth. For simple cysts, the decision regarding treatment, there-fore, lies in the increased risk of ovarian torsion. Small cysts, less than 5 cm in size, should be followed with serial ultrasound examinations. Larger cysts and all complex ovarian masses should be excised, with care taken to preserve ipsilalteral ovarian tissue.

Ambiguous Genitalia

Disruption of the orderly molecular and biochemical events in sexual differentiation lead to incomplete anatomic differentiation and clinically manifest as inter-sex abnormalities. These may be classified as true hermaphroditism (ovarian and testicular tissue present), male pseudohermaphroditism (testicular feminizaton), female pseudohermaphroditism (congenital adrenal hyperplasia), and mixed gonadal dysgenesis (160).

Optimal care of the infant born with ambiguous genitalia requires a team approach with input from parents, neonatologists, endocrinologists, and pediatric surgeons. When a newborn presents with ambiguous genitalia, the diagnostic and therapeutic goals include immediate determination of the type of abnormality based on physical examination of the gonads and cytologic analysis (Table 44–1), prompt gender assignment based on the type of abnormality and external anatomic considerations, and early medical management of congenital adrenal hyperplasia. These goals should be accomplished if possible within the first 24 hours of life. Genetically female infants should be assigned the female gender regardless of the degree of virilization. For genetically male babies, assignment depends largely on the size of the phallus because satisfactory surgical techniques do not exist to reconstruct an adequate phallus. However, follow-up studies have indicated a high incidence of emotional problems among genetic males assigned as females.

The timing or type of surgical intervention is determined by gender assignment and subsequent radiographic or endoscopic investigations. Gonads associated with gonadal dysgenesis or inconsistent with gender assignment are excised to prevent malignant degeneration and contradictory hormone secretion, respectively. Reconstructive procedures such as clitiroplasty and vaginoplasty must take into account preservation of sensation and function as well as the location and division of a urethrovaginal fistula. Infants assigned the male gender require hypospadias repair.

TABLE 44–1. *Diagnosis of intersex abnormality based on chromosome analysis and gonad physical examination*

	Symmetric gonads	Asymmetric gonads
XY	Male pseudohermaphroditism (testicular feminization)	Gonadal dysgenesis
XX	Female pseudohermaphroditism (congenital adrenal hyperplasia)	True hermaphroditism

OBSTRUCTIVE JAUNDICE

A variety of neonatal cholestatic syndromes overlap in presentation with obstructive jaundice from biliary atresia. Many conditions causing direct hyperbilirubinemia have been grouped under the term "neonatal hepatitis." To some extent, this is misleading because hepatitis implies an inflammatory process within the liver. It is preferable to separate the infants into one group with cholestatic syndromes and another group with extrahepatic obstruction, such as biliary atresia. In the former group, specific disease entities are further identified by serologic testing or metabolic screening (see Chap. 37). A common metabolic condition that causes neonatal jaundice is α_1-antitrypsin deficiency. Screening for this inherited disorder is recommended for all infants with conjugated hyperbilirubinemia. Infants with cystic fibrosis may present with obstructive jaundice that mimics biliary atresia, and infants receiving intravenous hyperalimentation for weeks or months may develop cholestatic jaundice.

Advances in hepatobiliary imaging using ^{99m}Tc scans have made it possible to differentiate cholestatic from obstructive jaundice with a high degree of accuracy, particularly after administration of phenobarbital for 5 days before the scan (161). Numerous diagnostic blood tests have been recommended, but none is completely reliable, and most represent unnecessary procrastination. The infant who has an obstructive profile on liver function tests and hepatic scan, with a negative evaluation for cystic fibrosis and α_1-antitrypsin deficiency, should be evaluated with an abdominal ultrasound to identify the gallbladder and extrahepatic biliary ducts and with a percutaneous liver biopsy. Absence of the extrahepatic duct on ultrasound and the finding of extrahepatic cholestasis on biopsy mandate surgical exploration.

An initial exploration is made through a limited right subcostal incision. If a normal gallbladder is seen, a transcholecystic cholangiogram is obtained. If the extrahepatic biliary tree appears normal, a liver biopsy is obtained, and the incision is closed.

If the gallbladder is atretic, or the liver is obviously cirrhotic, suggesting an obstructive process, the incision is enlarged so that the extrahepatic biliary system can be formally explored. Any remnant of the gallbladder or extrahepatic biliary duct through which a cholangiogram can be performed is used. In the infant with extrahepatic biliary atresia, only thread-like remnants of the biliary tree are identified. The atretic ducts are transected at their confluence, deep into the porta hepatis, and an anastomosis is created to a segment of the small intestine. This procedure is called a portoenterostomy (Kasai procedure). When the operation is performed in infants younger than 3 months of age, there is reasonable expectation that bile will drain into the intestine (162). Children who fail to drain bile after the portoenterostomy may be rescued by liver transplantation before 1 year of age, although the complication rate in these infants is higher than in older children with liver transplants (163).

Other causes of jaundice that can be relieved surgically are choledochal cysts, common duct stones, and inspissated sludge in the bile ducts. True choledochal cysts are rarely encountered in the newborn period but should be treated by cyst excision and intestinal drainage of the hepatic duct, using a technique similar to the Kasai procedure. Bile peritonitis after spontaneous rupture of the bile duct may resemble a choledochal cyst to the unwary surgeon. These babies require only drainage of the area, with anticipation that the perforation will heal spontaneously while the infant is maintained on antibiotics (164,165).

Biliary hypoplasia is a descriptive term for the radiologic finding of a diminutive extrahepatic ductal system. This may be a secondary condition resulting from intrahepatic cholestasis. Biliary hypoplasia has been associated with intrahepatic disease conditions, such as the cholestasis seen in α_1-antitrypsin deficiency (166). A cholangiogram confirms the patency of these structures and their narrow caliber. Liver biopsy invariably shows cholestasis, and there is often a paucity of intrahepatic bile ducts. Speculation that there is an inflammatory component associated with biliary hypoplasia and that it represents a phase of a dynamic process, leading perhaps to total biliary obstruction, has prompted the use of corticosteroids for treatment. In some instances of steroid therapy, the jaundice resolved, and subsequent biopsies reverted to normal.

With the increased use of abdominal ultrasonography, cholelithiasis has been diagnosed in infants with increasing frequency, particularly in infants with ileal resection or long-term intravenous hyperalimentation (167). In the asymptomatic baby, observation often is rewarded with spontaneous disappearance of the gallstones, although symptomatic cholelithiasis should be managed by cholecystectomy (168). Obstructive jaundice is discussed in more detail in Chapters 37 and 38.

HERNIA AND HYDROCELE

Inguinal hernia and hydrocele occur commonly, especially in male infants. They result from the persistence of a patent processus vaginalis, a finger-like projection of the peritoneum accompanying the testicle as it descends into the scrotum. In the female infant, the peritoneal extension accompanies the round ligament and can remain patent, becoming a potential hernia sac. A hydrocele is often associated with an inguinal hernia, or it may be an isolated finding. The fluid may be in communication with the peritoneal cavity, and the hydrocele may therefore wax and wane in size, or it may be separated and completely isolated in the scrotum, in the inguinal canal, or, in female infants, the canal of Nuck. A hydrocele presents a smooth, cylindric contour, with the superior margin generally distinct. It is not tender and is often asymptomatic. The hernia is often large enough that it is easily appreciated as a swelling in the groin or scrotum. The mass can usually be reduced back into the abdominal cavity.

The special anatomic associations of infants puts them at particular risk for incarceration of a hernia. The internal inguinal ring is narrow, and intestine finding its way into the hernia sac in the inguinal canal can become trapped and be reduced only with great difficulty. The incidence of inguinal hernia is dramatically increased in children born earlier than 36 weeks of gestation, with as many as 35% of them developing hernias.

In premature infants in our neonatal unit, we repair the hernias before discharge. If the premature infant has a hernia that freely moves in and out of the inguinal canal, has no history of incarceration, and is first seen as an outpatient, we prefer to delay elective repair until the baby is at least 46 weeks of gestation to minimize postoperative apnea (6), especially in the anemic child (169). If a troublesome hernia in a premature infant must be repaired earlier than the elective 46 weeks of gestational age, we prefer to use spinal anesthesia rather than general anesthesia to minimize the risk of postoperative apnea (6).

If there is diagnostic confusion between an incarcerated hernia and a hydrocele, a rectal examination with bimanual palpation of the internal inguinal ring delineates the structures passing through the ring into the inguinal canal. The vas deferens is a constant reference point, and the intestine adjacent to the vas and between the examining fingers confirms the diagnosis of a hernia. Surgical repair is indicated in all cases of inguinal hernia.

If incarceration of a hernia occurs, moderate bimanual pressure, applied by compressing the sac from below while providing a gentle downward counterforce with the hand above the inguinal ring, usually achieves reduction. Occasionally, these hernias reduce spontaneously after sedation is given and struggling and crying are terminated. If the hernia fails to reduce, or if there is obvious intestinal obstruction and systemic toxicity, emergency surgical reduction and repair are necessary.

An inguinal hernia in a female infant is often diagnosed by palpation of a nontender ovoid mass in the groin. The mass represents an ovary herniated into the open sac. Although the gonad can usually be reduced back into the abdomen, it often prolapses in and out until surgical repair is carried out. If the inguinal hernia is apparent unilaterally, the opposite side is routinely explored in all children younger than 1 year of age because the incidence of bilateral hernias in these children is approximately 50%.

ABNORMALITIES OF THE UMBILICUS AND ABDOMINAL WALL

Umbilical Hernia

Umbilical hernia is a common condition of the newborn, presenting as a central fascial defect beneath the umbilicus. Incarceration is a rare complication in patients with umbilical hernia, but it occurs more commonly in patients with smaller defects of the fascia, such as those seen in the neonate. Umbilical hernias are more common in African-Americans, in premature infants, and in patients with congenital deficiencies of thyroid hormone.

Most babies with umbilical hernia require no surgical treatment because the hernia disappears spontaneously up to 9 years of age. With persistence of the hernia until 4 years of age, repair is indicated. In a few patients, there is progressive enlargement of the skin of the umbilicus until a prominent proboscis is produced. Surgical repair is indicated early. A simple repair suffices for all these patients and can be accomplished through a small semilunar incision made in the curve of the umbilicus. Complicated fascial flap repairs, such as may be required in adults, are unnecessary and contraindicated in young patients. The umbilicus is never excised.

Adhesive dressings with coins and metallic or plastic objects have no place in the management of umbilical hernia because they are ineffective and merely cover the defect at the expense of irritating the surrounding skin.

Primary Infection of the Umbilicus

With the advent of prenatal care, the incidence of infection around the umbilicus (i.e., omphalitis) has been markedly reduced. Potentially serious complications can result from infections in this area. Cellulitis of the abdominal wall, with direct spread into the peritoneal cavity and resultant peritonitis of the newborn, has been recorded. The most serious consequence is ascending infection along the umbilical vein to the portal system and liver. Before antibiotics, the resultant multiple hepatic abscesses were often fatal. A more common sequela is portal vein thrombosis, which is a major cause of portal hypertension in children. In the past, this was a significant cause of esophageal varices in young patients, and although this condition now occurs less often, it must be avoided by prompt local and systemic antibiotic treatment of suspected infections in and around the umbilicus.

Umbilical Granuloma

The formation of weeping granulation tissue at the umbilicus is common in the newborn. Failure of the umbilical epithelium to grow over the severed stump of the umbilicus results in a persistent crusting mass of granulomatous tissue. Cauterization with silver nitrate is diagnostic and therapeutic. Applications of silver nitrate twice weekly for 1 month clear most umbilical granulations. With persistence of fluid at the umbilicus, a patent omphalomesenteric duct or patent urachus should be considered.

Patent Omphalomesenteric Duct

During fetal development, the omphalomesenteric duct forms a connection from the intestinal tract to the placenta. If this duct fails to involute, a tubular attachment persists between the ileum and the abdominal wall (Fig. 44–18). Liquid ileal content refluxes out of this duct.

Diagnosis of a congenital fistula at the umbilicus is made by inspection, sonography, and probing of the tract. The introduction of radiopaque material into the ostium at the umbilicus demonstrates a connection to the intestinal lumen on lateral x-ray films of the abdomen.

Treatment for patent omphalomesenteric duct is elective abdominal exploration with division and closure of the fistula at its origin in the ileum and total excision of the fistula, including its attachment to the undersurface of the umbilicus. This procedure must not be postponed because there is a potential for intestinal volvulus to occur around the post-like attachment between the umbilicus and the ileum.

In rare instances, if the patent omphalomesenteric duct opening is large, the peristaltic activity of the bowel can result in eversion of proximal intestine, as in intussusception, through the opening onto the abdominal wall. Clinically, this appears as a mucosa-covered extrusion, and the resulting mass is easily confused with a small ruptured omphalocele. Careful inspection of the neck of the defect at the border of the abdominal skin discloses the true nature of the lesion. The bowel has in effect turned inside out and prolapsed through the patent omphalome-

senteric duct. Immediate operation, with reduction and repair, is indicated.

Patent Urachus

During embryologic development, there is free communication between the urinary bladder and the abdominal wall. Persistence of this tract establishes a communication between the urinary bladder and the umbilicus through which urine may pass. Although this passage is small, the umbilicus is constantly wet. The first sign of a patent urachus may be urinary infection. In some patients, a portion of the urachus has obliterated with only a partially patent remnant or cyst remaining beneath the umbilicus. Urachal cysts may present after the newborn period as an infected infraumbilical mass caused by colonization with skin organisms from the umbilicus; sonography reveals this anatomy.

In the diagnostic workup of a newborn suspected of having a patent urachus, the cystogram in lateral projection demonstrates the abnormal tract. Another diagnostic technique is the introduction of a colored dye into the bladder through the urethral catheter. The appearance of dye on the abdominal wall confirms the connection between the umbilicus and the bladder. Extraperitoneal surgical exploration of the infraumbilical area allows complete excision of the urachal tract and closure of the bladder. Partial urachal remnants, sinus tracts, and cysts are easily excised.

Omphalocele

Developmental arrest of those somites that form the peritoneal, muscular, and ectodermal layers of the abdominal wall results in a central defect called an omphalocele. The defect is covered by a translucent membrane overlying the bowel and solid viscera and may vary in size from a small hernia of the cord that is 1 or 2 cm in diameter to a huge mass containing essentially all the abdominal viscera (Fig. 44–19). Usually, the sac remains intact, but it is occasionally ruptured during delivery.

The diagnosis of this lesion is made entirely by inspection because it is readily apparent immediately after delivery of the baby. The abdomen is wrapped carefully with well-padded, saline-soaked gauze and an outer dry layer in preparation for transport. Placement of a nasogastric tube to decompress the stomach and attention to maintenance of a normal core temperature are essential initial maneuvers. No pressure is placed on the omphalocele in an attempt to reduce it. This is hazardous to the integrity of the sac, may interfere with venous return, and may impede the infant's respiratory efforts.

Small omphaloceles are usually amenable to complete one-stage surgical repair. For larger omphaloceles (6 cm), a sheet of Silastic with interwoven Marlex can be sewn

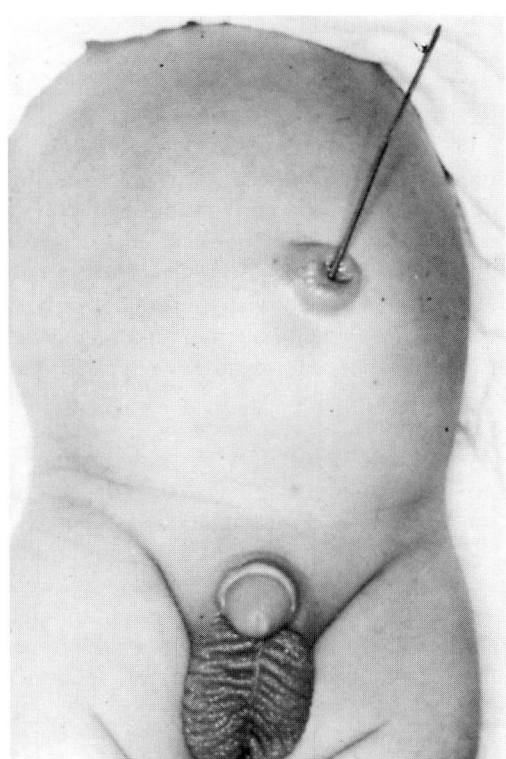

FIG. 44–18. A probe indicates that the umbilical opening which connects with the intestinal tract (i.e., patent omphalomesenteric duct).

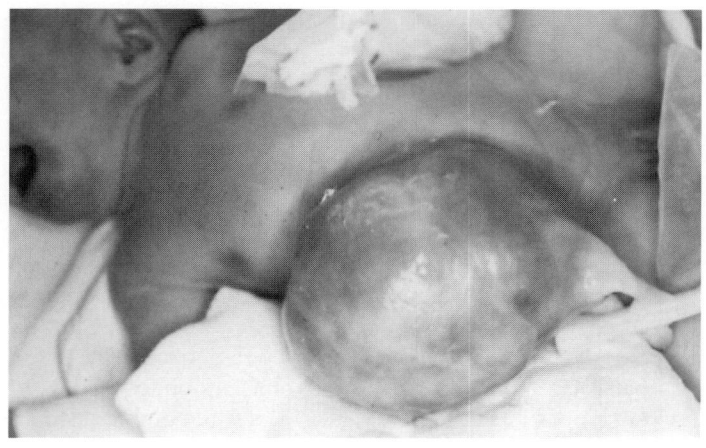

FIG. 44–19. Large omphalocele. Notice the covering of the sac and its relation to the umbilicus, which protrudes from the lower portion.

around the edge of the defect to envelop the omphalocele (170,171). Steady pressure on the prosthesis and a reduction in size over several days bring about gradual reduction of the omphalocele so that surgical closure can be accomplished. Irrigation with povidone–iodine (Betadine) solution or coverage with a layer of silver sulfadiazine (Silvadene) has been effective in reducing surface contamination throughout the time for which the prosthesis is required.

Coexisting anomalies, such as exstrophy of the cloaca or congenital heart disease, may make surgical closure inappropriate. Painting the omphalocele sac with 4% mercurochrome promotes a firm, strong crust to cover the defect. This protection serves until the natural process of epithelialization occurs. Although success with a plastic prosthesis has obviated the need for the painting method, it is still a useful treatment in rare instances; mercury toxicity is possible.

Congenital malrotation of the colon usually occurs in patients born with omphalocele. Although it is in itself not a serious defect, the anomaly can lead to midgut volvulus, and symptoms of intestinal obstruction in a baby who has previously recovered from treatment of omphalocele must be considered a dire emergency.

Gastroschisis

Originally confused as a type of omphalocele, gastroschisis is now recognized as a separate entity. It differs embryologically in that the abdominal wall has completed its development but a defect remains at the base of the umbilical stalk, through which a portion of the intestinal tract has escaped. Gastroschisis always occurs as a defect lateral to the base of the umbilicus, and the defect may represent an isolated congenital defect in the abdominal wall. An alternative theory of the embryogenesis of gastroschisis holds that closure of the celomic cavity has been completed while a portion of the intestinal tract remained trapped outside the abdomen in the base of the umbilical cord. It is postulated that this hernia of the cord then ruptures, allowing the intestine to float freely in the amnion while the umbilical arteries and vein remain attached to the baby.

The escape of the intestine into the amniotic cavity can occur at different times in fetal development. This conclusion follows the observation that in some infants the intestines are glistening and normal looking, as if they had escaped a celomic envelope just before birth. Many infants with gastroschisis, however, are born with edematous and matted intestinal loops that appear to have been exposed to the amniotic fluid for many weeks (Fig. 44–20).

Immediate treatment in the delivery room consists of wrapping the baby and the exteriorized intestine in saline-soaked gauze and dry sterile dressings. Prompt surgical repair is undertaken. In about one-half of the patients, the viscera can be returned to the abdomen and secure closure obtained. In favorable cases, peristalsis returns in a few days, and normal bowel function can be expected. If the bowel is matted and edematous, it may take many weeks before intestinal function recovers. Nutrition can be successfully supported during this interval by intravenous hyperalimentation. Previously, many of these babies died of malnutrition before intestinal function returned.

If the abdominal wall cannot be closed without undue tension, which interferes with respiration and venous return, an extraabdominal prosthetic compartment must be fashioned. As in staged omphalocele repair, Silastic-covered Marlex is well suited for this purpose because its surface is inert and does not adhere to the bowel. After the prosthesis is fastened to the fascial margins, the capacity of the plastic compartment is gradually reduced until complete surgical closure is possible, usually within 7 to 10 days. This staged maneuver, coupled with intravenous alimentation, has resulted in an increased percentage of survivors from a previously lethal anomaly (172). Intestinal atresia occurs in about 10% of patients with gastroschisis. In these babies, the clinical course is

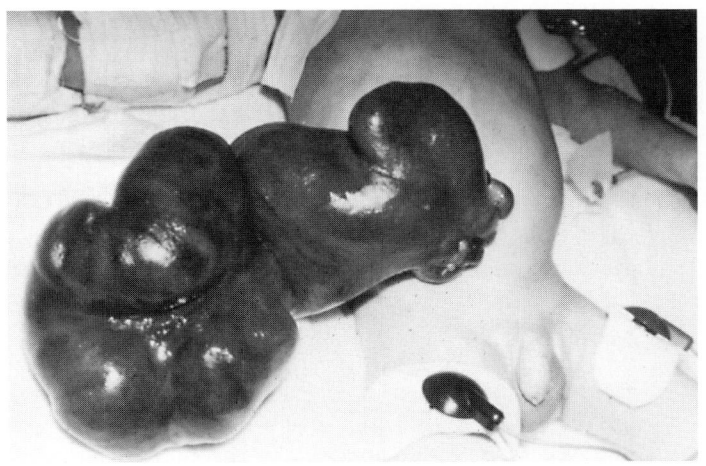

FIG. 44–20. Patient with gastroschisis. The edematous, matted bowel is the result of the intestines floating freely in the amniotic fluid. Remarkably, these distorted viscera ultimately fit back into the abdominal cavity and assume normal appearance and function.

one of early complete obstruction, which requires abdominal exploration if the lesion has been inadvertently overlooked at the time of initial repair of the gastroschisis.

Congenital Deficiency of the Abdominal Muscle

The prune-belly syndrome consists of three major anomalies:

1. Deficiency of the abdominal musculature
2. Dilation of the urinary collecting system
3. Bilateral cryptorchidism.

By definition, all patients with this syndrome are male, but a similar condition has been reported in female patients. In severely affected infants, there is marked wrinkling of the skin of the abdomen and no muscular substance beneath (Fig. 44–21). Lower abdominal musculature is most frequently and severely involved.

The bladder is characteristically large, and the ureters are dilated and tortuous. The kidneys may be hypoplastic, but usually there is enough renal parenchyma for ade-quate function from at least one side. There is an increased incidence of patent urachus, particularly if the renal function is poor.

The cause of the condition is unknown. It has been proposed that all these infants have some degree of urethral obstruction, with resultant overdistension of the bladder and abnormal pressure on the developing muscular somites (173). Others have suggested that the primary deficiency is in the abdominal musculature, allowing overdistension of the bladder with secondary changes in the urinary collecting system. It is probable that neither of these explanations is completely valid and that some more comprehensive explanation exists for the coexistence of the unusual abdominal deficiency and the distortion of the collecting system.

The treatment of these infants is conservative and nonoperative if their renal function is good (174). If the renal function is poor, urinary diversion may be necessary in the neonatal period to eliminate pressure in the collecting system. Abdominal wall reconstruction and bilateral orchiopexy can be performed between 1 and 2 years of age if the renal function is stable. Reconstruction of the

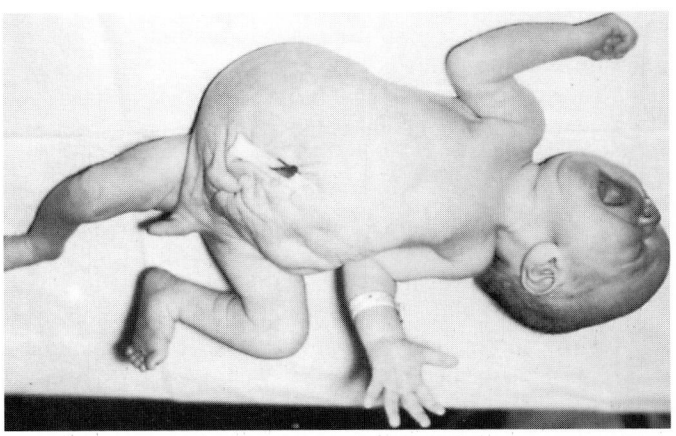

FIG. 44–21. An infant with congenital deficiency of the abdominal musculature shows the typical prune-belly appearance.

abdominal wall is best performed through a low transverse incision so that the use of normal upper abdominal musculature is maximized (175).

SACROCOCCYGEAL TERATOMA

A sacrococcygeal teratoma is an unusual tumor that is usually detected in the newborn or neonate (176). Most teratomas present as a large mass arising from the coccyx. The mass is made of mature and immature elements of different cell types. The mass may be several centimeters in diameter, or it may rival the size of the newborn infant (177). In the newborn period, the tumor is usually benign; however, when it is discovered later, the incidence of malignancy rises (178).

The diagnosis is frequently made at the time of prenatal ultrasound (179). A large solid or cystic mass is observed in the sacral region. The maternal serum alpha-fetoprotein level may be elevated. Occasionally, the blood flow through the tumor is large enough to produce heart failure and hydrops in the fetus (180). Langer and colleagues proposed using a large mass and heart failure as an indication for fetal surgery to arrest the tumor growth (181). If a sacrococcygeal teratoma is diagnosed prenatally, a multidisciplinary approach to the pregnancy and delivery is indicated (182).

The key to the management of an infant born with a sacrococcygeal teratoma is an expeditious surgical resection. The infant is stabilized, with careful attention to high-output cardiac failure. Hypothermia can be a major problem in the nursery and the operating room because of the large surface area of the mass. After a search for coexisting anomalies, and after appropriate resuscitation, the mass is resected. Complete resection is usually possible without long-term sequelae, although bowel continence can be a problem if the sphincter mechanism is disturbed by the tumor or the surgery. It is important to remove the coccyx to prevent recurrence. The tumors are rarely malignant in the newborn period, and complete surgical resection is curative.

VASCULAR ACCESS

An excellent text, *Atlas of Procedures in Neonatology,* is recommended for an in-depth review of vascular access techniques in the infant (183). The traditional method of maintaining vascular access in the neonate for blood sampling, medications, and parenteral nutrition has been to use an umbilical vessel catheter. When the umbilical vessel catheter must be maintained for an extended period of time, the risk of complications, such as emboli, thrombosis, and infections, becomes prohibitive, and the line must be removed. The use of transcutaneous pulse oximetry has reduced the need for arterial umbilical lines in neonates with pulmonary problems. When arterial access

is required, the right radial artery is a useful alternative because its preductal location accurately reflects intracerebral blood oxygenation.

Even in the smallest babies, a radial artery line can be placed by cutdown with optical magnification. Placing an arterial line percutaneously is preferable to the cutdown technique, with the aim of maintaining future arterial patency. However, multiple attempts to access the radial artery percutaneously should be discouraged to avoid damage to the artery, preventing access by cutdown. The posterior tibial artery is an alternate site for arterial lines in neonates. More proximal arterial lines in the brachial artery have been used in selected patients, although the risk of extremity ischemia is substantial with this location. Access via the femoral artery is contraindicated.

Establishing reliable venous access in the preterm infant has become one of the most common procedures done by pediatric surgeons. The placement of a catheter into the central venous circulation allows the use of more concentrated intravenous solutions and eliminates the risk of subcutaneous infiltration of solutions and resultant skin sloughs. In the past, central venous catheters were placed predominantly by a percutaneous approach; this is now restricted to larger neonates, using a Seldinger technique. In preterm infants, a Silastic catheter is placed by cutdown, with a Dacron cuff attached to the catheter placed beneath the skin to prevent catheter infection and accidental removal. A percutaneous ultrathin Silastic catheter that can be threaded from a peripheral vein to the central venous system is used with increasing frequency at the CNMC, but many children continue to require the cutdown technique.

The site of venous catheter placement depends on patient anatomy, disease, location of previous catheters, and surgeon preference. The sites of choice are the external jugular or facial vein to avoid damage to the internal jugular vein. In the infant weighing less than 1,000 g, the internal jugular vein may be the only one of adequate size, and its use unilaterally should not cause serious problems. When the line is placed in the neck, the tip of the catheter should be in the superior vena cava just cephalad to the right atrium. Silastic catheters within the atrium may cause atrial thrombus formation, atrial perforation, or dysrythmias.

If the superior vena caval system cannot be used, the saphenous vein, at its junction with the femoral vein, can usually be cannulated, even in infants weighing less than 1,000 g. If the saphenous vein is used, it is best to keep the catheter tip caudad to the renal veins (i.e., below the level of L1 to L2).

Central venous catheters in neonates are plagued with complications. Infection remains the most common complication, occurring in approximately 10% of infants. Although catheter infection can be successfully treated with intravenous antibiotics, it is better to remove the catheter, give intravenous medications and nutrition temporarily through a peripheral intravenous line, and replace the central line, if still needed, after all cultures are free of infection. Most of the organisms that contaminate central venous lines originate from the infant's skin or from careless decontamination of the connecting tubing before line changes or the administration of medication.

Central vein thrombosis is a serious problem that may lead to superior vena caval syndrome, which includes head and arm swelling and pleural effusions as a result of obstruction of the thoracic duct drainage. Babies weighing less than 1,000 g are at particularly high risk of developing thrombus (184). Management of vena caval thrombosis with thrombolytic agents, such as urokinase, may be beneficial, but the risk of systemic anticoagulation must always be considered. Some reduction in the risk of thrombosis may be achieved by the use of 1 U of heparin per 1 mL of intravenous solution.

REFERENCES

1. Anand KJ, Brown MJ, Causon RC, et al. Can the human neonate mount an endocrine and metabolic response to surgery? *J Pediatr Surg* 1985;20:41.
2. Tsang TM, Tam PK. Cytokine response of neonates to surgery. *J Pediatr Surg* 1994;29:794.
3. Kucukaydin OH, Ustdal KM. The endocrine and metabolic response to surgical stress in the neonate. *J Pediatr Surg* 1995;30:625.
4. Rowe MI, Lloyd DA, Lee M. Is the refractometer specific gravity a reliable index for pediatric fluid management? *J Pediatr Surg* 1986; 21:580.
5. Roe CF, Santulli RV, Blair CS. Heat loss in infants during general anesthesia and operations. *J Pediatr Surg* 1966;1:266.
6. Welborn LG, Rice LJ, Hannallah RS, et al. Postoperative apnea in former preterm infants: prospective comparison of spinal and general anesthesia. *Anesthesiology* 1990;72:838.
7. Gross RE, Connerly JL. Thyroglossal cysts and sinuses. *N Engl J Med* 1940;223:616.
8. Brown PM, Judd ES. Thyroglossal cysts and sinuses: results of radical (Sistrunk) operation. *Am J Surg* 1961;102:494.
9. Athow AC, Fagg NL, Drake DP. Management of thyroglossal cysts in children. *Br J Surg* 1989;76:811.
10. Gray SW, Skandalakis JE. The pharynx and its derivatives. In Gray SW, Skandalakis JE, eds. *Embryology for surgeons: the embryologic basis for the treatment of congenital defects.* Philadelphia: WB Saunders, 1972.
11. Bill AH Jr, Vadheim JL. Cysts, sinuses, and fistulas of the neck arising from the first and second branchial clefts. *Ann Surg* 1955;142:904.
12. Gray SW, Skandalakis JE. The lymphatic system. In Gray SW, Skandalakis JE, eds. *Embryology for surgeons: the embryologic basis for the treatment of congenital defects.* Philadelphia: WB Saunders, 1972.
13. Langer JC, Fitzgerald PG, Desa D, et al. Cervical cystic hygroma in the fetus: clinical spectrum and outcome. *J Pediatr Surg* 1990;25:58.
14. Grosfeld JL, Weber TR, Vane DW. One stage resection for massive cervicomediastinal hygroma. *Surgery* 1982;92:693.
15. Rodenstein DO, Perlmutter N, Stanescu DC. Infants are not obligatory nasal breathers. *Am Rev Respir Dis* 1985;131:343–347.
16. Eckenhoff JE. Some anatomic considerations of the infant larynx influencing endotracheal anesthesia. *Anesthesiology* 1951;12: 401–410.
17. Wiseman NE, Sanchez I, Powell RE. Rigid bronchoscopy in the pediatric age group: diagnostic effectiveness. *J Pediatr Surg* 1992;27: 1294–1297.
18. Brown OE, Myer CM, Manning SC. Congenital nasal aperture stenosis. *Laryngoscope* 1989;99:86–91.
19. Arlis H, Ward RF. Congenital nasal pyriform aperture stenosis. *Arch Otolaryngol Head Neck Surg* 1992;118:989–991.
20. Hinderer KH. Nasal problems in children. *Pediatr Ann* 1976;52: 499–509.
21. Kirchner JA. Traumatic nasal deformity in the newborn. *Arch Otolaryngol* 1955;62:139–142.
22. Pagon RA, Graham JM Jr, Zonana J, Young SL. Coloboma, congenital heart disease, and choanal atresia with multiple anomalies: CHARGE association. *J Pediatr* 1981;99:223–227.
23. Stankiewicz JA. The endoscopic repair of choanal atresia. *Otolaryngol Head Neck Surg* 1990;103:931–937.
24. Theogaraj SD, Hoehn JG, Hagan KF. Practical management of congenital choanal atresia. *Plast Reconstr Surg* 1983;72:634–642.
25. Hengerer AS, Yanofsky SD. Congenital malformation of the nose and paranasal sinuses. In: Bluestone CD, Stool SE, Kenna MA, eds. *Pediatric otolaryngology.* Philadelphia: WB Saunders, 1996:831–842.
26. Sadewitz VL. Robin sequence: changes in thinking leading to changes in patient care. *Cleft Palate Craniofac J* 1992;29:246–253.
27. Benjamin B, Walker P. Management of airway obstruction in the Pierre Robin sequence. *J Pediatr Otorhinolaryngol* 1991;22:29–37.
28. Tomaski SM, Zalzal GH, Saal HM. Airway obstruction in the Pierre Rob sequence. *Laryngoscope* 1995;105:111–114.
29. Gorlin RJ Cohen MM, Levin LS. Overgrowth syndromes and postnatal onset obesity syndromes. In: Corlin RJ, Pindborg JJ, Cohen MM, eds. *Syndromes of the head and neck,* 3rd ed. New York: Oxford University Press, 1990:323–352.
30. Holinger LD, Holinger PC, Holinger PH. Etiology of bilateral abductor vocal cord paralysis: a review of 389 cases. *Ann Otol Rhinol Laryngol* 1976;85:428–436.
31. Mancuso RF, Choi SS, Zalzal GH, Grundfast KM. Laryngomalacia: the search for the second lesion. *Arch Otolaryngol Head Neck Surg* 1996;122:302–306.
32. Holinger LD, Konior RJ. Surgical management of severe laryngomalacia. *Laryngoscope.* 1989;99:136–142.
33. Cohen SR, Geller KA, Birns JW, Thompson JW. Laryngeal paralysis in children: a long-term retrospective study. *Ann Otol Rhinol Laryngol* 1982;91:417–424.
34. Bower CM, Choi SS, Cotton RT. Arytenoidectomy in children. *Ann Otol Rhinol Laryngol* 1994;103:271–278.
35. Tucker JA, O'Rahilly R. Observations on the embryology of the human larynx. *Ann Otol Rhinol Laryngol* 1972;81:520–523.
36. Cohen SR. Congenital glottic webs in children: a retrospective review of 51 patients. *Ann Otol Rhinol Laryngol* 1985;14:2–16.
37. Benjamin B, Ingles A. Minor congenital laryngeal clefts: diagnosis and classification. *Ann Otol Rhinol Laryngol* 1989;98:417–420.
38. Ratner I, Whitfield J. Acquired subglottic stenosis in the very-low-birth-weight infant. *Am J Dis Child* 1983;137:40–43.
39. Cotton RT, Seid AB. Management of the extubation problem in the premature child: anterior cricoid split as an alternative to tracheotomy. *Ann Otol Rhinol Laryngol* 1980;89:508–511.
40. Sie KC, McGill T, Healy GB. Subglottic hemangioma: ten years experience with the carbon dioxide laser. *Ann Otol Rhinol Laryngol* 1994; 103:167–172.
41. Ohlms LA, Jones DT, McGill TJ, Healy GB. Interferon alpha-2a therapy for airway hemangiomas. *Ann Otol Rhinol Laryngol* 1994;103:1–8.
42. Grillo HC, Zannini P. Management of obstructive tracheal disease in children. *J Pediatr Surg* 1984;19:414–416.
43. Idriss FS, DeLeon SY, Ilbawi MN, et al. Tracheoplasty with pericardial patch for extensive tracheal stenosis in infants and children. *J Thorac Cardiovasc Surg* 1984;88:527–536.
44. Benjamin B. Tracheomalacia in infants and children. *Ann Otol Rhinol Laryngol* 1984;93:438–442.
45. Wailoo MP, Emery JL. The trachea in children with tracheo-esophageal fistula. *Histopathology* 1979;3:329–338.
46. Fearon B, Shortreed R. Tracheobronchial compression by congenital cardiovascular anomalies in children: syndrome of apnea. *Ann Otol Rhinol Laryngol* 1963;72:949–969.
47. Wiseman NE, Duncan PG, Cameron CB. Management of tracheobronchomalacia with continuous positive airway pressure. *J Pediatr Surg* 1985;20:489–493.
48. Hawkins JA, Bailey WW, Clark SM. Innominate artery compression of the trachea: treatment of reimplantation of innominate artery. *J Thorac Cardiovasc Surg* 1992;103:817–820.
49. Murray GF. Congenital lobar emphysema. *Surg Gynecol Obstet* 1967; 124:611.
50. Ekkelkamp S, Vos A. Successful surgical treatment of a newborn with bilateral congenital lobar emphysema. *J Pediatr Surg* 1987; 22:1001.
51. Adzick NS, Harrison MR, Glick PL, et al. Fetal cystic adenomatoid

malformation: prenatal diagnosis and natural history. *J Pediatr Surg* 1985;20:483.

52. Atkinson JB, Ford EG, Kitagawa H, et al. Persistent pulmonary hypertension complicating cystic adenomatoid malformation in neonates. *J Pediatr Surg* 1992;27:54.

53. Anderson KD, Chandra R. Pneumothorax secondary to perforation of sequential bronchi by suction catheters. *J Pediatr Surg* 1976;11:687.

54. Gangitano ES, Pomerance JJ, Gans SL. Successful surgical repair of iatrogenic lung perforation in a neonate. *J Pediatr Surg* 1981;16:70.

55. Zerella JT, Trump DS. Surgical management of neonatal interstitial emphysema. *J Pediatr Surg* 1987;22:34.

56. Geggel RL, Murphy JD, Langleben D. Congenital diaphragmatic hernia: arterial structural changes and persistent pulmonary hypertension after surgical repair. *J Pediatr Surg* 1985;92:805.

57. Levin DL. Morphologic analysis of the pulmonary vascular bed in congenital left-sided diaphragmatic hernia. *J Pediatr Surg* 1978;92: 805.

58. Crane JP. Familial congenital diaphragmatic hernia: prenatal diagnostic approach and analysis of twelve families. *Clin Genet* 1979;16:244.

59. Cannon C, Dildy GA, Ward R, et al. A population-based study of congenital diaphragmatic hernia in Utah: 1988–1994. *Obstet Gynecol* 1996;87:959.

60. Adzick NS, Vacanti JP, Lillehei CW. Fetal diaphragmatic hernia: ultrasound diagnosis and clinical outcome in 38 cases. *J Pediatr Surg* 1989;24:654.

61. Adzick NS, Harrison MR, Glick PL. Diaphragmatic hernia in the fetus: prenatal diagnosis and outcome in 94 cases. *J Pediatr Surg* 1985;20:357.

62. Benjamin DR, Juul S, Siebert JR. Congenital posterolateral diaphragmatic hernia: associated malformations. *J Pediatr Surg* 1988;23:899.

63. Nakayama DK, Motoyama EK, Tagge EM. Effect of preoperative stabilization on respiratory system compliance and outcome in newborn infants with congenital diaphragmatic hernia. *J Pediatr Surg* 1991; 118:793.

64. Frenckner B, Ehren H, Granholm T, et al. Improved results in patients who have congenital diaphragmatic hernia using preoperative stabilization, extracorporeal membrane oxygenation, and delayed surgery. *J Pediatr Surg* 1997;32:1185.

65. Breaux CW, Rouse TM, Cain WS, et al. Improvement in survival of patients with congenital diaphragmatic hernia utilizing a strategy of delayed repair after medical and/or extracorporeal membrane oxygenation stabilization. *J Pediatr Surg* 1991;26:333.

66. Connors RH, Tracy T, Bailey PV, et al. Congenital diaphragmatic hernia repair on ECMO. *J Pediatr Surg* 1990;25:1043.

67. Van Meurs KP, Newman KD, Anderson KD, et al. Effect of extracorporeal membrane oxygenation on survival of infants with congenital diaphragmatic hernia. *J Pediatr Surg* 1990;117:954.

68. Newman KD, Anderson KD, Van Meurs K, et al. Extracorporeal membrane oxygenation and congenital diaphragmatic hernia: should any infant be excluded? *J Pediatr Surg* 1990;25:1048.

69. Wilson JM, Thompson JR, Schnitzer JJ, et al. Intratracheal pulmonary ventilation and congenital diaphragmatic hernia: a report of two human cases. *J Pediatr Surg* 1993;28:484.

70. Crombleholme TM, Adzick NS, Hardy K, et al. Pulmonary lobar transplantation in neonatal swine: a model for treatment of congenital diaphragmatic hernia. *J Pediatr Surg* 1990;25:11.

71. Harrison MR, Langer JC, Adzick NS. Correction of congenital diaphragmatic hernia *in utero*: initial clinical experience. *J Pediatr Surg* 1990;25:47.

72. VanderWall KJ, Skarsgard ED, Filly RA, Eckert J, Harrison MR. Fetendo-clip: a fetal endoscopic tracheal clip procedure in a human fetus. *J Pediatr Surg* 1997;32:970.

73. Haller JA, Pickard LR, Tepas JJ, et al. Management of diaphragmatic paralysis in infants with special emphasis on selection of patients for operative plication. *J Pediatr Surg* 1979;14:779.

74. Langer JC, Filler RM, Coles J, et al. Plication of the diaphragm for infants and young children with phrenic nerve palsy. *J Pediatr Surg* 1988;23:749.

75. Haight C, Towsley HA. Congenital atresia of the esophagus with tracheoesophageal fistula. Extrapleural ligation of fistula and end to end anastomosis of esophageal segments. *Surg Gynecol Obstet* 1943; 76:672.

76. Tondury G. Embryology of esophageal atresia. *Z Kinderchir* 1975;17:6.

77. Skandalakis, Gray SW, Ricketts R. The esophagus. In Gray SW, Skandalakis JE, eds. *Embryology for surgeons, 65.* Baltimore: Williams and Wilkins, 1994.

78. Pfeiffer RA. Genetic and epidemiologic aspects of esophageal atresia. In Willital GH, Nihoul-Fekete C, Myers N, eds. *Management of esophageal atresia,* vol 2. Munich: Urban & Schwarzenburg, 1990.

79. Rokitansky A, Kolankayah A, Bichler B, et al: Analysis of 309 cases of esophageal atresia for associated congenital malformations. *Am J Perinatol* 1994;11:123.

80. Engum SA, Grosfeld JL, West KW, et al. Analysis of morbidity and mortality in 227 cases of esophageal atresia and/or tracheoesophageal fistula over 2 decades. *Arch Surg* 1995;130:502.

81. Piekarski DH, Stevens FD. The association and embryogenesis of tracheoesophageal and anorectal anomalies. *Prog Pediatr Surg* 1976;9: 63.

82. Holder TM, Cloud DT, Lewis JE Jr, et al. Esophageal atresia and tracheoesophageal fistula. A survey of its members by the Surgical Section of the American Academy of Pediatrics. *Pediatrics* 1961;34:542.

83. Pohlson EC, Schaller R, Tapper D. Improved survival with primary anastomosis in the low birth weight neonate with esophageal atresia and tracheoesophageal fistula. *J Pediatr Surg* 1988;23:418.

84. Randolph JG, Newman K, Anderson KD. Current results and repair of esophageal atresia with tracheoesophageal fistula using physiologic status as a guide to therapy. *Ann Surg* 1989;209:525.

85. Waterston DJ, Bonham-Carter RE, Aberdeen E. Oesophageal atresia: tracheoesophageal fistula—a study of survival in 218 infants. *Lancet* 1962;1:819.

86. Spitz L. Esophageal atresia: past, present and future. *J Pediatr Surg* 1996;31:19.

87. Manning P, Morgan RA, Coran A, et al. 50 years' experience with esophageal atresia in tracheoesophageal fistula. *Ann Surg* 1987;204: 446.

88. Livaditas A. Esophageal atresia, a method of overbridging large segmental gaps. *Z Kinderchir* 1973;13:298.

89. Werlin SC, Dodds WJ, Hogan WJ, et al. Esophageal function in esophageal atresia. *Dig Dis Sci* 1981;26:796.

90. Jolley SJ, Johnson DG, Roberts CC, et al. Patterns of gastroesophageal reflux in children following repair of esophageal atresia and distal tracheoesophageal fistula. *J Pediatr Surg* 1980;15:857.

91. Wheatley MJ, Coran AG, Wesley JR. Efficacy of the Nissen fundoplication in the management of gastroesophageal reflux following esophageal atresia repair. *J Pediatr Surg* 1993;28:53.

92. Ghandour KE, Spitz L, Brereton RJ, et al. Recurrent tracheoesophageal fistula: experience with 24 patients. *J Paediatr Child Health* 1990;26:89.

93. Howard R, Myers NA. Esophageal atresia: a technique for elongating the upper pouch. *Surgery* 1965;58:725.

94. Ein SH, Shandling B. Pure esophageal atresia: a 50 year review. *J Pediatr Surg* 1994;29:1208.

95. Schneider JM, Becker JM. The H-type tracheoesophageal fistula in infants and children. *Surgery* 1962;51:677.

96. Donahoe PK, Gee PE. Complete laryngotracheoesophageal cleft: management and repair. *J Pediatr Surg* 1984;19:143.

97. Neuhauser EBD, Berenberg W. Cardioesophageal relaxation as cause of vomiting in infants. *Radiology* 1947;48:480.

98. Randolph JG, Lilly JR, Anderson KD. Surgical treatment of gastroesophageal reflux in infants. *Ann Surg* 1974;180:479.

99. Foglia RM, Fonkalsrud EW, Ament ME, et al. Gastroesophageal fundoplication for management of chronic pulmonary disease in children. *Am J Surg* 1980;140:72.

100. Leape LL, Holder TM, Franklin JD, et al. Respiratory arrest in infants secondary to gastroesophageal reflux. *Pediatrics* 1977;50:924.

101. Nielson DW, Heldt GP, Tooley WH. Stridor and gastroesophageal reflux in infants. *Pediatrics* 1990;85:1034.

102. Randolph JG. Experience with the Nissen fundoplication for correction of gastroesophageal reflux in infants. *Ann Surg* 1983;198:579.

103. Halpern LM, Jolley SG, Tunell WP, et al. The mean duration of gastroesophageal reflux during sleep as an indicator of respiratory symptoms from gastroesophageal reflux in children. *J Pediatr Surg* 1991;26:686.

104. Holgersen LO. The etiology of spontaneous gastric perforation of the newborn: a reevaluation. *J Pediatr Surg* 1981;16:608.

105. Bell MJ. Perforation of the gastrointestinal tract and peritonitis in the neonate. *Surg Gynecol Obstet* 1985;160:20.

106. Tan CE, Krily EM, Agrawal M, et al. Neonatal gastrointestinal perforation. *J Pediatr Surg* 1989;24:888.

107. Gauderer MWL, Olsen MM, Stellato TA, et al. Feeding gastrostomy "button"—experience and recommendations. *J Pediatr Surg* 1988;23: 24.

108. Gertler JP, Seashore JH, Touloukian RJ. Early ileostomy closure in necrotizing enterocolitis. *J Pediatr Surg* 1987;22:140.

109. Bishop HC, Koop CE. Management of meconium ileus: resection, Roux-en-Y anastomosis and ileostomy irrigation with pancreatic enzymes. *Ann Surg* 1957;145:410.

110. Moore K. *The developing human,* 3rd ed. Philadelphia: WB Saunders, 1981.

111. Ford EG, Senac MO, Srikanth MS, et al. Malrotation of the intestine in children. *Ann Surg* 1992;215:172.

112. Stauffer UG, Herrmann P. Comparison of late results in patients with corrected intestinal malrotation with and without fixation of the mesentery. *J Pediatr Surg* 1980;15:9.

113. Cooper A, Floyd TF, Ross AJ, et al. Morbidity and mortality of short-bowel syndrome acquired in infancy: an update. *J Pediatr Surg* 1984; 19:711.

114. Carter CO, Evans KA. Inheritance of congenital pyloric stenosis. *J Med Genet* 1969;6:233.

115. Tunell WP, Wilson PA. Pyloric stenosis: diagnosis by real time sonography, the pyloric muscle length method. *J Pediatr Surg* 1984; 19:795.

116. Woolley MM, Feesher BF, Asch MJ, et al. Jaundice, hypertrophic pyloric stenosis and hepatic glucuronyl transferase. *J Pediatr Surg* 1974;9:359.

117. Fonkalsrud EW, deLorimier AA, Hays DM. Congenital atresia and stenosis of the duodenum—a review compiled from the members of the surgical section of the American Academy of Surgery. *Pediatrics* 1969;43:79.

118. Merrill JR, Raffensperger JG. Pediatric annular pancreas: twenty year experience. *J Pediatr Surg* 1976;11:921.

119. Louw JH, Barnard CN. Congenital intestinal atresia: observations on its origin. *Lancet* 1955;1:1065.

120. de Lorimier AA, Fonkalsrud EW, Hays DM. Congenital atresia and stenosis of the jejunum and ileum. *Surgery* 1969;65:819.

121. Thomas CG. Jejunoplasty for the correction of jejunal atresia. *Surg Gynecol Obstet* 1969;129:545.

122. Weber TR, Vane DW, Grosfeld JL. Tapering enteroplasty in infants with bowel atresia and short gut. *Arch Surg* 1982;117:684.

123. LoPresti JM, Altman RP, Kulczychi L. Meconium ileus: operative therapy and pulmonary complications in the newborn. *Clin Proc Child Hosp DC* 1972;28:221.

124. Noblett HR. Treatment of uncomplicated meconium ileus by Gastrografin enema: a preliminary report. *J Pediatr Surg* 1969;4:190.

125. Mabogunje OA, Wang CI, Mahour H. Improved survival of neonates with meconium ileus. *Arch Surg* 1982;117:37.

126. Bishop HC, Koop CE. Surgical management of duplication of the alimentary tract. *Am J Surg* 1964;107:434.

127. Wrenn EL. Tubular duplication of the small intestine. *Surgery* 1962; 52:494.

128. Leape LL. Case records of the Massachusetts General Hospital: Duplication of the ileum. *N Engl J Med* 1980;302:958.

129. Fraser GC, Berry C. Mortality of neonatal Hirschsprung's disease: with particular reference to enterocolitis. *J Pediatr Surg* 1967;2:205.

130. Taxman TL, Ulish BS, Rothstein FC. How useful is the barium enema in the diagnosis of infantile Hirschsprung's disease? *Am J Dis Child* 1986;140:881.

131. Campbell PE, Noblett HR. Experience with rectal suction biopsy in the diagnosis of Hirschsprung's disease. *J Pediatr Surg* 1969;4:410.

132. Huntley CC, Shaffner LdeS, Challa VR, et al. Histochemical diagnosis of Hirschsprung's disease. *Pediatrics* 1982;69:755.

133. Teich S, Schisgall RM, Anderson KD, et al. Ischemic enterocolitis as a complication of Hirschsprung's disease. *J Pediatr Surg* 1986;21:143.

134. Harrison MW, Dytes DM, Campbell JR, et al. Diagnosis and management of Hirschsprung's disease. *Am J Surg* 1986;152:49.

135. Swenson O, Bill AH Jr. Resection of rectum and rectosigmoid with preservation of the sphincter for benign spastic lesions producing megacolon. An experimental study. *Surgery* 1948;24:212.

136. Duhamel B. Retrorectal and transanal pullthrough procedure for the treatment of Hirschsprung's disease. *Dis Colon Rectum* 1964;7:455.

137. Soave F. Hirschsprung's disease: a new surgical technique. *Arch Dis Child* 1964;39:116.

138. Carcassonne N, Guys J, Morisson-Lacombe G, et al. Management of Hirschsprung's disease: curative surgery before 3 months of age. *J Pediatr Surg* 1989;24:1032.

139. Foster P, Cowan G, Wrenn EL, et al. 25 years' experience with Hirschsprung's disease. *J Pediatr Surg* 1990;25:531.

140. Sherman JO, Snyder ME, Weitzman JJ, et al. A 40-year multi-national retrospective study of 880 Swenson procedures. *J Pediatr Surg* 1989; 24:833.

141. Touloukian RJ, Posch JN, Spencer R. The pathogenesis of ischemic gastroenterocolitis of the neonate: selective gut mucosal ischemia in asphyxiated neonatal piglets. *J Pediatr Surg* 1972;7:194.

142. Czyrko C, Steigman C, Turley DL, et al. The role of reperfusion injury in occlusive intestinal ischemia of the neonate: malonaldehyde-derived fluorescent products and correlation of histology. *J Surg Res* 1991;51:1.

143. Atkinson SD, Tuggle DW, Tunell WP. Hypoalbuminemia may predispose infants to necrotizing enterocolitis. *J Pediatr Surg* 1989;24:674.

144. Kosloske AM, Lilly JR. Paracentesis and lavage for diagnosis of intestinal gangrene in neonatal necrotizing enterocolitis. *J Pediatr Surg* 1978;13:315.

145. Ricketts RR. The role of paracentesis in the management of infants with necrotizing enterocolitis. *Am Surg* 1986;52:61.

146. Mollitt DL, Tepas JJ, Talbert JL. The microbiology of neonatal peritonitis. *Arch Surg* 1988;123:176.

147. Smith SD, Tagge EP, Miller J, et al. The hidden mortality in surgically treated necrotizing enterocolitis: fungal sepsis. *J Pediatr Surg* 1990; 25:1030.

148. Buras R, Guzzetta P, Avery GB, et al. Acidosis and hepatic portal venous gas: indications for surgery in necrotizing enterocolitis. *Pediatrics* 1986;78:273.

149. Harberg FJ, McGill CW, Saleem MM, et al. Resection with primary anastomosis for necrotizing enterocolitis. *J Pediatr Surg* 1983;18:743.

150. Ein SH, Shandling B, Wesson D, et al. A 13-year experience with peritoneal drainage under local anesthesia for necrotizing enterocolitis perforation. *J Pediatr Surg* 1990;25:1034.

151. Musemeche CA, Kosloske AM, Ricketts RR. Enterostomy in necrotizing enterocolitis: an analysis of techniques and timing of closure. *J Pediatr Surg* 1987;22:479.

152. Radhakrishnan J, Blechman G, Shrader C, et al. Colonic strictures following successful medical management of necrotizing enterocolitis: a prospective study evaluating early gastrointestinal contrast studies. *J Pediatr Surg* 1991;26:1043.

153. Parashar K, Kyawhla S, Booth IW, et al. Ileocolic ulceration: a long term complication following ileocolic anastomosis. *J Pediatr Surg* 1988;23:226.

154. Kiesewetter WB. Rectum and anus. In Ravitch MM, Welch KJ, Benson CD, et al, eds. *Pediatric surgery,* vol 2. Chicago: Year Book, 1979: 1059.

155. Pena A, DeVries PA. Posterior sagittal anoplasty: important technical considerations and new applications. *J Pediatr Surg* 1982;17:796.

156. Wangensteen OH, Rice CO. Imperforate anus: a method of determining the surgical approach. *Ann Surg* 1930;92:77.

157. Danis RK, Graviss ER. Imperforate anus: avoiding a colostomy. *J Pediatr Surg* 1978;13:759.

158. Reynolds, M. Neonatal disorders of the external genitalia and vagina. *Semin Pediatr Surg* 1998;7:2.

159. Brandt ML, Luks FI, Filiatrault D, et al. Surgical indications in antenatally diagnosed ovarian cysts. *J Pediatr Surg* 1991;26:276.

160. Donahoe PK, Powell DM, Lee MM. Clinical management of intersex abnormalities. *Curr Probl Surg* 1991;28:519.

161. Majd M, Reba RC, Altman RP. Effect of phenobarbital on ^{99m}Tc-IDA scintigraphy in the evaluation of neonatal jaundice. *Semin Nucl Med* 1981;11:194.

162. Karrer FM, Lilly JR, Stewart BA, et al. Biliary atresia registry, 1976 to 1989. *J Pediatr Surg* 1990;25:1076.

163. Stevens LH, Emond JC, Piper JB, et al. Hepatic artery thrombosis in infants: a comparison of whole livers, reduced-size grafts, and grafts from living-related donors. *Transplantation* 1992;53:396.

164. Lilly JR, Weintraub WW, Altman RP. Spontaneous perforation of the extrahepatic bile ducts and bile peritonitis in infancy. *Surgery* 1974;75:664.

165. Megison SM, Votteler TP. Management of common bile duct obstruction associated with spontaneous perforation of the biliary tree. *Surgery* 1992;111:237.

166. Altman RP, Chandra R. Biliary hypoplasia consequent to alpha-1-antitrypsin deficiency. *Surg Forum* 1976;37:377.

167. King DR, Ginn-Pease ME, Lloyd TV, et al. Parenteral nutrition with associated cholelithiasis: another iatrogenic disease of infants and children. *J Pediatr Surg* 1987;22:593.
168. Jacir NN, Anderson KD, Eichelberger MR, et al. Cholelithiasis in infancy: resolution of gallstones in three of four infants. *J Pediatr Surg* 1986;21:567.
169. Welborn LG, Hannallah RS, Luban NLC, et al. Anemia and postoperative apnea in former preterm infants. *Anesthesiology* 1991;74:1003.
170. Schuster SR. A new method for the staged repair of large omphaloceles. *Surg Gynecol Obstet* 1967;125:837.
171. Yazbeck S, Ndoye M, Khan AH. Omphalocele: a 25-year experience. *J Pediatr Surg* 1986;21:761.
172. Caniano DA, Brokaw B, Ginn-Pease ME. An individualized approach to the management of gastroschisis. *J Pediatr Surg* 1990;25:297.
173. Moerman P, Fryns JP, Goddeeris P, et al. Pathogenesis of the prune-belly syndrome: a functional urethral obstruction caused by prostatic hypoplasia. *Pediatrics* 1984;73:470.
174. Tank ES, McCoy G. Limited surgical intervention in the prune-belly syndrome. *J Pediatr Surg* 1983;18:688.
175. Randolph J, Cavett C, Eng G. Surgical correction and rehabilitation for children with "prune-belly" syndrome. *Ann Surg* 1981;193:757.
176. Tapper D, Lack EE. Teratoma in infancy in childhood: a 54-year experience at the Children's Hospital Medical Center. *Ann Surg* 1983;198:389.
177. Altman RP, Randolph JG, Lilly, JR. Sacrococcygeal teratoma: American Academy of Pediatric Surgical Section Survey. *J Pediatr Surg* 1974;9:389.
178. Billmire DF, Grosfeld JL. Teratomas in childhood: analysis of 142 cases. *J Pediatr Surg* 1986;21:548.
179. Sepulveda WH. Prenatal sonographic diagnosis of congenital sacrococcygeal teratoma and management. *J Perinat Med* 1989;17:93.
180. Smith KG, Silverman NH, Harrison MR, et al. High output cardiac failure in fetuses with large sacrococcygeal teratoma: diagnosis by echocardiography and Doppler ultrasounds. *J Pediatr* 1989;114:1023.
181. Langer JC, Harrison MR, Schmidt KG, et al. Fetal hydrops and deaths from sacrococcygeal teratoma: rational for fetal surgery. *Am J Obstet Gynecol* 1990;163:682.
182. Nakayama DK, Killian A, Hill LM, et al. The newborn with hydrops and sacrococcygeal teratoma. *J Pediatr Surg* 1991;26:1435.
183. Fletcher MA, MacDonald MG, eds. *Atlas of procedures in neonatology,* 2nd ed. Philadelphia: JB Lippincott, 1993.
184. Mehta S, Connors AF, Danish EH, et al. Incidence of thrombosis during central venous catheterization of newborns: a prospective study. *J Pediatr Surg* 1992;27:18.

CHAPTER 45

Hematology

John J. Doyle, Barbara Schmidt, Victor Blanchette, and Alvin Zipursky

ANEMIAS

Erythroid Development

Early hematopoietic cells originate in the yolk sac. By the eighth week of gestation, more definitive fetal erythropoiesis is taking place in the liver. The liver remains the primary site of erythroid production throughout the early fetal period. By 6 months of gestation, the bone marrow becomes the principal site of erythroid cell development. Later during gestation, a switch occurs in the type of hemoglobin being formed, with adult hemoglobin (HbA) replacing fetal hemoglobin (HbF). The site of production of erythropoietin (EPO) switches from the less sensitive hepatic to the more sensitive renal site (1).

The earliest characterized erythroid precursor is the burst-forming unit (BFU-E), which gives rise to colony-forming units (CFU-E). These are identified by their growth characteristics in culture. Neonatal BFU-E and CFU-E are as sensitive as their adult counterparts to EPO stimulation (2,3). Earlier development is a function of other factors, including interleukins and burst-promoting activity. The numbers of BFU-E progressively decline along the series of fetal blood, cord blood, adult bone marrow, and adult blood. More than 40 times the number of BFU-E can be cultured from fetal blood as from adult blood (1). Measurement of the peripheral blood pool does not indicate the size of the total body pool, so it cannot be inferred that the fetus has a markedly greater erythropoietic potential than an adult does (4). It is probably at least comparable.

The major difference between fetal and adult erythropoiesis is in the response to EPO. Erythropoiesis is controlled by a feedback loop involving EPO. A decrease in erythrocyte mass is reflected by an increase in EPO, which drives erythropoiesis to increase erythrocyte mass and diminish EPO production. The expected correlation between EPO and measures of oxygen delivery (e.g., hemoglobin, mixed venous oxygen tension, and available oxygen) can be detected in premature neonates, providing evidence that the same feedback loop exists (5–7). The measured levels of EPO are much lower than those of older children and adults with corresponding degrees of anemia. Brown and colleagues presented evidence that the magnitude of the EPO response was lowest in the least mature infant (i.e., 27 to 31 weeks of gestation) (7). Forestier and associates found low EPO values in cordocentesis samples from infants between 18 and 37 weeks of gestation (8). Surprisingly, there was no correlation between gestational age and EPO level. This poor EPO response persists through the neonatal period, resulting in a reduced erythropoietic stimulus and lower hemoglobin levels in premature infants.

Normal Hemoglobin Levels

In the newborn period, the hemoglobin concentration is undergoing constant physiologic change. A clear definition of the normal hemoglobin range is important for proper evaluation and management.

Normal hemoglobin values at birth have been determined through measurement of levels in cord blood of newborn infants. In a review of normal blood values in the newborn, Oski and Naiman cite a range of 13.7 to 20.1 g/dL, with a mean of 16.8 g/dL (9). Blanchette and Zipursky obtained similar results in studies of healthy newborns, yielding cord hemoglobin values (mean ± 1 SD) of 16.9 ± 1.6 g/dL in full-term infants and 15.9 ± 2.4 g/dL in premature infants (10). Definitive values for pre-

J. J. Doyle, V. Blanchette, and A. Zipursky: Division of Hematology/Oncology, The Hospital for Sick Children; and Department of Pediatrics, University of Toronto, Toronto, Ontario, Canada

B. Schmidt: Chedoke McMaster Hospital; and Department of Pediatrics, McMaster University, Hamilton, Ontario, Canada

mature infants are known as a result of cordocentesis sampling. Data from Forestier and colleagues for 18 to 29 weeks of fetal life and our (V.B., A.Z.) own data for fetuses older than 36 weeks of gestation are given in Table 45–1 (8). Based on these data, cord hemoglobin levels less than 13.0 g/dL should be considered abnormal in term and premature (<36 weeks of gestation) neonates. In the very premature infant (<26 weeks of gestation), values as low as 12.0 g/dL may be acceptable. If anemia is confirmed, a prompt and careful search for the cause should be initiated.

One factor that can significantly influence the hemoglobin level in newborn infants is the amount of placental transfusion. At birth, blood is rapidly transferred from the placenta to the infant, with one-fourth of the placental transfusion occurring within 15 seconds of birth and one-half by the end of the first minute (11). The placental vessels contain 75 to 125 mL of blood at birth (12). Usher and associates demonstrated that the blood volume of an infant could be increased by as much as 61% by delayed cord clamping (13). In that study, the average erythrocyte mass in a group of infants with delayed cord clamping was 49 mL/kg at 72 hours of age compared with 31 mL/kg in a group in whom the cord was clamped immediately after birth. Although infants delivered after delayed cord clamping have higher hemoglobin values, it should be recognized that the placental transfusion may be markedly reduced or prevented if the infant is held above the level of the placenta at the time of delivery; in this situation, it is possible for an infant to lose blood into the placenta and be born anemic (14).

Physiologic Anemia and the Anemia of Prematurity

The hemoglobin concentration of healthy full-term and premature infants undergoes typical changes during the first weeks of life (15–18). After birth, there is a transient increase in hemoglobin concentration as plasma moves extravascularly to compensate for the placental transfusion and an increase in circulating erythrocyte volume that occurs at the time of delivery (19). Thereafter, the hemoglobin concentration gradually falls, to reach minimal levels of 11.4 ± 0.9 g/dL in term infants by 8 to 12 weeks of age and 7.0 to 10.0 g/dL in premature infants by 6 weeks of age (see Fig. 45–1) (18).

There are several reasons for the fall in hemoglobin. The first is the decline in erythrocyte production that occurs in the first few days of life and is evidenced by a fall in reticulocyte counts during that time (Fig. 45–2). Normally, reticulocyte counts may be elevated during the first 1 or 2 days of life (200 to 300×10^9/L) but then fall to low levels (50×10^9/L) through the remainder of the neonatal period. This diminution of erythropoiesis is probably related to decreased EPO production. The reduced EPO response persists until approximately 6 weeks of age, at which time erythrocyte production increases, as evidenced by a sharp rise in reticulocyte numbers in the blood and an increase in total-body hemoglobin (see Fig. 45–2). Other factors that contribute to the physiologic anemia in newborns, particularly the more profound anemia in premature infants, are the shortened survival of neonatal erythrocytes and rapid body growth (see Fig. 45–2) (20,21). Trials of folate, iron, and vitamin E have not shown any evidence of benefit in preventing the physiologic anemia of infancy (22). Optimal protein supplementation is important for maintaining good hematopoiesis (23–28).

The signs and symptoms of this early anemia in premature infants are nonspecific and reflect changes in metabolic rate or cardiorespiratory function and perfusion. Controversy exists about whether tachycardia, tachypnea, periodic breathing, and apnea are reliable indicators of anemia (29–35). Stockman and Clark demonstrated an improvement in weight gain in premature infants with poor weight gain after transfusion (36). Others have not found improved weight gain following transfusion (29,34,35). Lactate measurements and cardiac output can be shown to decrease following transfusion, but neither measurement on its own can be considered a surrogate for diagnosing anemia (34,37).

Several groups have tested blood transfusion as therapy for the anemia of prematurity. Blank et al. (38) and Meyer et al. (39) were unable to demonstrate clinical benefit in their transfused arms versus their nontransfused group other than improved hematocrit. In both studies several children were transfused for tachycardia, apnea, bradycardia, or other clinical signs interpreted as signs and symptoms of anemia. Others have shown benefit in these clinical parameters from transfusion in selected asymptomatic infants (40–42), although hemo-

TABLE 45–1. *Normal erythrocyte values during gestation*[a]

Weeks of gestation	Erythrocytes ($\times 10^{12}$/L)	Hemoglobin (g/dL)	Hematocrit (%)	Mean corpuscular volume (fL)
18–21	2.85 ± 0.36	11.7 ± 1.3	37.3 ± 4.3	131.11 ± 10.97
22–25	3.09 ± 0.34	12.2 ± 1.6	38.6 ± 3.9	125.1 ± 7.84
26–29	3.46 ± 0.41	12.9 ± 1.4	40.9 ± 4.4	118.5 ± 7.96
>36	4.7 ± 0.4	16.5 ± 1.5	51.0 ± 4.5	108 ± 5

[a]Values are given ±1 standard deviation.

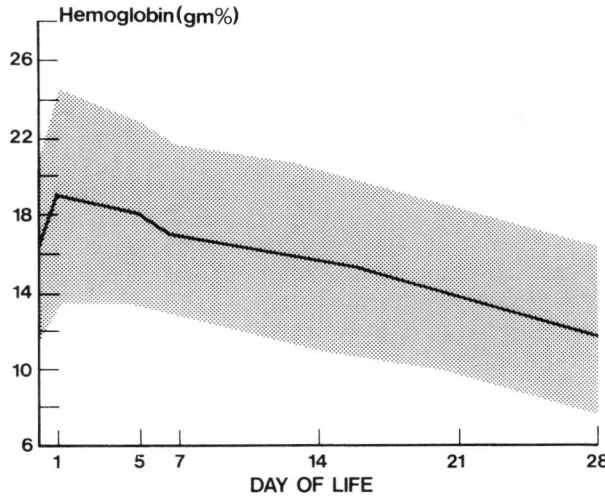

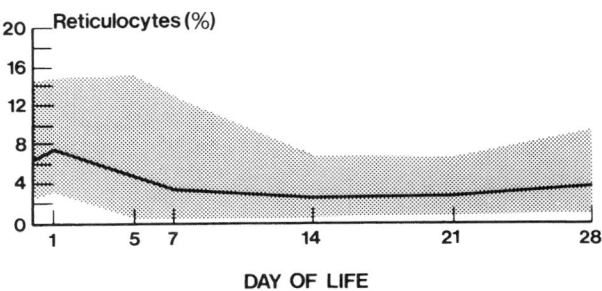

FIG. 45–1. Hemoglobin values of 178 normal premature infants ≤ 36 weeks of gestation. Data at the first point, day 0, are cord blood values. Subsequent points represent data from capillary blood samples on 1, 5, 7, 14, and 28 days of life. The dark line represents the mean value, and the shaded area includes 95% of all values.

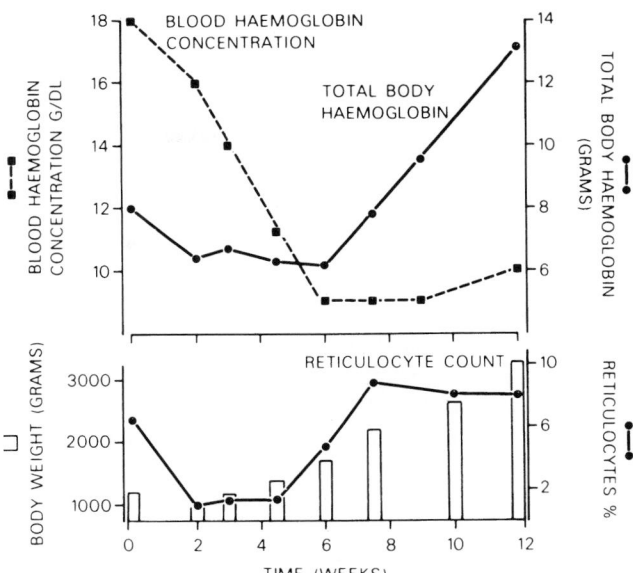

FIG. 45–2. Changes in total body hemoglobin, blood hemoglobin concentration, reticulocyte count, and body weight in a representative premature infant. The vertical bars represent the infant's body weight. During the first 6 weeks of life, the blood hemoglobin concentration and total body hemoglobin fall as a result of decreased erythrocyte production, as evidenced by the low reticulocyte count. The more rapid decline in blood hemoglobin concentration from the third to the sixth week is the result of the increasing body size and dilution of the hemoglobin mass. After 6 weeks of age, hemoglobin production increases, as evidenced by the increased reticulocyte count and the rapid increase in total body hemoglobin. The blood hemoglobin concentration during that period may rise slightly, or not at all, because the total body size increases at approximately the same rate as the total hemoglobin mass.

globin values are not necessarily the best indicator of need (40). Surveys of blood product use in neonatal units show that most transfusion practices are based on a preset hemoglobin value or what the clinician interprets as signs and symptoms of anemia (apnea, poor weight gain, etc.) (43). Similar clinical criteria have been incorporated into guidelines for the transfusion of premature infants (44). Trials of transfusion therapy at certain values have not demonstrated clear benefit and may expose these infants to infection [e.g., cytomegalovirus (CMV), hepatitis, human immunodeficiency virus (HIV)] (45). Infective and other risks from blood products can be minimized through irradiation of blood products, the use of CMV-negative product, the use of repeated dosing from a single unit (46,47), or the use of autologous transfusion by separating the plasma needed for lab tests and returning the erythrocytes to the infant (48). Trials of transfusion therapy for anemia in premature infants require a better-defined end point before they can yield a definitive result. Prevention of anemia would be a better intervention.

The desire to prevent the use of blood products coupled with the need to treat symptomatic anemia has led to trials of recombinant human erythropoietin in premature newborns. Erythropoietin has been started either early (within the first week of life) (49–55) or late (about 3 weeks of age) (23,25,56–63). In general, infants receiving the larger doses (>600 U/kg/week) at both starting points have shown improvement in reticulocyte counts and hemoglobin levels and a decrease in the number of transfusions per infant. Important to note, however, is that with early initiation of therapy there is no reduction in the number of infants transfused, and in the late group most blood exposures have already occurred before erythropoietin therapy. Alternative transfusion strategies, as indicated previously, may be equally effective in preventing multiple donor exposure and more cost-effective. Currently, the most prudent approach is for individual units to determine the availability of multiuse blood units, autologous transfusion, and the cost-benefit of erythropoietin in their population rather than using routine erythropoietin therapy (64).

Evaluation

Anemia is characterized by an abnormally low erythrocyte mass; in clinical practice, the hemoglobin concentration is assumed to reflect the circulating erythrocyte mass, and an abnormally low hemoglobin concentration defines the anemic state. After diagnosis, causes of anemia are traditionally considered under the pathophysiologic categories of decreased erythrocyte production, increased destruction (i.e., hemolysis), and blood loss. In newborn infants, this classic approach to anemia is complicated by a hemoglobin concentration that undergoes constant physiologic change during the first few weeks of life. The site of blood sampling, quantity of blood sampled for laboratory monitoring, and the effect of rapid growth can significantly influence the hemoglobin values observed in newborn infants. Failure to consider these factors may lead to errors in diagnosis and result in unnecessary investigation and therapy.

Accuracy of Capillary Hemoglobin Levels

Blanchette and Zipursky compared capillary hemoglobin values obtained by duplicate puncture of the right and left heels of 35 healthy full-term infants (65). The standard deviation of the difference in hemoglobin concentration of the duplicate samples was 0.8 g/dL; in an infant with a hemoglobin concentration of 17.0 g/dL, 95% of hemoglobin values obtained fall between 15.4 and 18.6 g/dL. It is evident that a difference as large as 1.5 g/dL of hemoglobin in consecutive laboratory reports may reflect the error inherent in the technique of capillary blood sampling in the newborn infant.

Effect of the Sampling Site on Hemoglobin Levels

In newborn infants, hemoglobin levels measured in capillary blood samples may be significantly higher than values obtained from simultaneously collected venous blood samples. Oettinger found an average difference of 3.6 g/dL between simultaneous capillary and venous hemoglobin determinations in 24 infants studied on the first day of life (66). Other investigators have reported similar differences (Fig. 45–3) (65,67,68). These differences have been found in term and premature infants, and they persist through the first 6 weeks to 3 months of life (65,69). The difference in capillary and venous hemoglobin levels is most marked in the more premature infants (69). Linderkamp and colleagues suggested that warming of the heel reverses the poor circulation and stasis in peripheral vessels that is largely responsible for capillary and venous differences (68). If the heel is prewarmed before collection of a capillary sample, the difference in capillary and venous hemoglobin values decreases significantly (65,67).

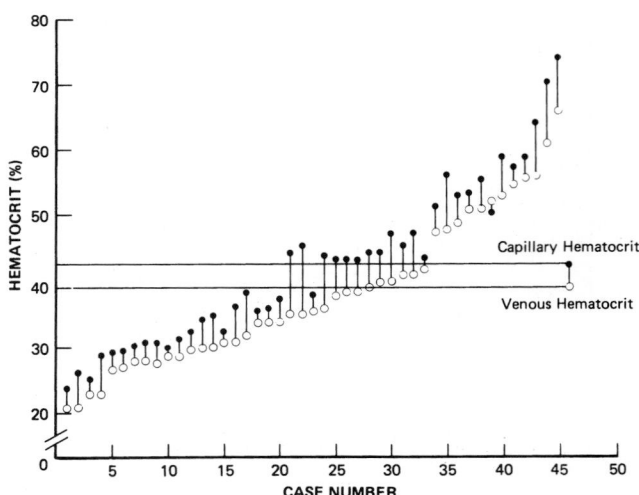

FIG. 45–3. Simultaneous capillary *(dark circles)* and venous *(open circles)* hematocrit levels in 45 premature infants studied during the first 6 weeks of life. Each vertical line represents values for 1 infant, and the horizontal solid line represents mean capillary and venous hematocrit levels for the whole group. Data are not shown for 5 infants in whom capillary and venous hematocrit levels were identical.

Correlation of Capillary Hematocrit Levels and Total Erythrocyte Mass

Erythrocyte mass is probably the best measurement of anemia. In adults, it correlates directly with hemoglobin values, which can be used as a valid means of determining anemia. In infants, the correlation between erythrocyte mass and hemoglobin values, although statistically significant, is poor (65,70). Figures 45–4 and 45–5 show the results of measurements made using a microtechnique using ^{51}Cr to measure erythrocyte mass in premature infants in the first and sixth weeks of life (65). Extremely wide variations in erythrocyte mass occur for any given hematocrit value. The capillary hematocrit is often a poor reflection of the circulating erythrocyte mass in newborn infants. This is particularly true for ill infants, in whom a poor peripheral circulation may exaggerate capillary and venous hematocrit differences, and for premature infants during periods of rapid body growth, when increases in the total circulating blood volume may influence hemoglobin levels through hemodilution (68).

Of the many techniques available for measuring erythrocyte mass, the use of chromium-labeled erythrocytes (^{51}Cr) remains the gold standard (71). This technique allows a direct measurement of erythrocyte mass and does not depend on approximations involving the use of measured plasma volumes, body weights, hematocrit values, or dilution of fetal hemoglobin after transfusion. The values shown in Fig. 45–4 agree with those obtained by other researchers (72–76). A nonradioactive technique involving the use of biotinylated erythrocytes has been

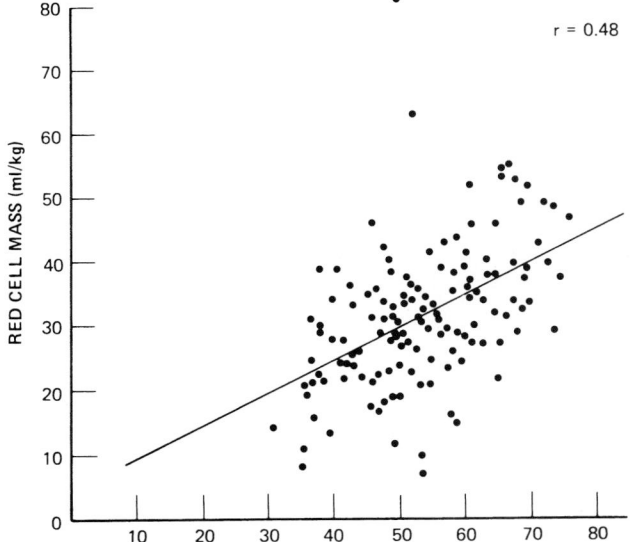

FIG. 45–4. Simultaneous capillary hematocrit and circulating erythrocyte mass levels in 135 premature infants who had birth weights less than 1500 g and were studied during the first week of life. (r, correlation coefficient.)

applied in neonates and yields values similar to those obtained with ^{51}Cr (77,78).

Effect of Growth on Hemoglobin Levels

Healthy premature infants are in a phase of rapid growth when active erythropoiesis, as evidenced by a

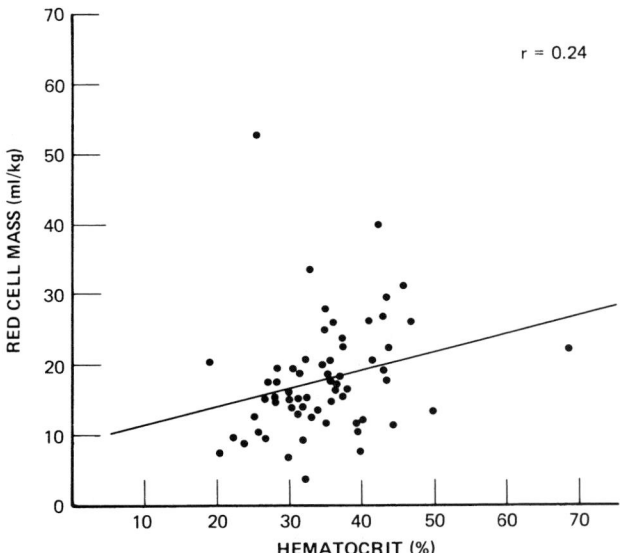

FIG. 45–5. Simultaneous capillary hematocrit and circulating erythrocyte mass levels in 63 premature infants who had birth weights less than 1500 g and were studied at 6 weeks of age. r, correlation coefficient.

mild reticulocytosis, resumes at 6 to 8 weeks of age. Associated with this rapid gain in body weight is an obligatory increase in the total circulating blood volume. The resultant hemodilution may cause a peripheral hemoglobin concentration that is static or even falls slightly. The apparent paradox of a stable or falling hemoglobin concentration despite active erythropoiesis (i.e., mild reticulocytosis and an increasing erythrocyte mass) gradually corrects, and the peripheral hemoglobin concentration increases (see Fig. 45–2). Failure to recognize the important effect of rapid body growth on the peripheral hemoglobin concentration may lead to erroneous investigation and treatment of apparent anemia (79,80).

Impact of Blood Sampling on Hemoglobin Levels

Despite the use of micromethods using small volumes of blood by most laboratories (Table 45–2), cumulative blood losses through sampling for laboratory monitoring are often surprisingly large in small infants. Blanchette and Zipursky measured an average blood loss of 22.9 mL of packed cells from 59 premature infants studied through the first 6 weeks of life (65). Forty-six percent (26 of 57) of the infants studied had cumulative losses that exceeded their circulating erythrocyte mass at birth (Fig. 45–6); in a few cases, losses were equivalent to two or three times the infants' initial circulating erythrocyte masses. Because these losses must be replaced, at least in part, by erythrocyte transfusions, some infants had the equivalent of a double- or triple-volume exchange transfusion simply as a result of blood sampling for laboratory tests. Approximately 10% of all blood loss during sampling for laboratory monitoring was hidden and represented blood on cotton swabs or in the dead space of syringes or tubing of butterfly sets used to collect blood samples (81).

There is a correlation between the volume of blood sampled and that transfused (Fig. 45–7), suggesting that much of the erythrocyte transfusion requirement of ill, premature infants is a direct consequence of blood loss for essential laboratory monitoring (65). In the study by Blanchette and Zipursky, significantly more blood was

TABLE 45–2. *Volume of whole blood required for common laboratory tests*

Test	Volume (mL)
Hemoglobin, total leukocytes, platelets	0.11
Blood gases	0.44
Electrolytes	0.21
Bilirubin	0.14
Calcium	0.14
Protein (total), albumin	0.21
PT, PTT, TCT fibrinogen[a]	0.9

[a]PT, prothrombin time; PTT, partial thromboplastin time; TCT, thrombin clotting time.

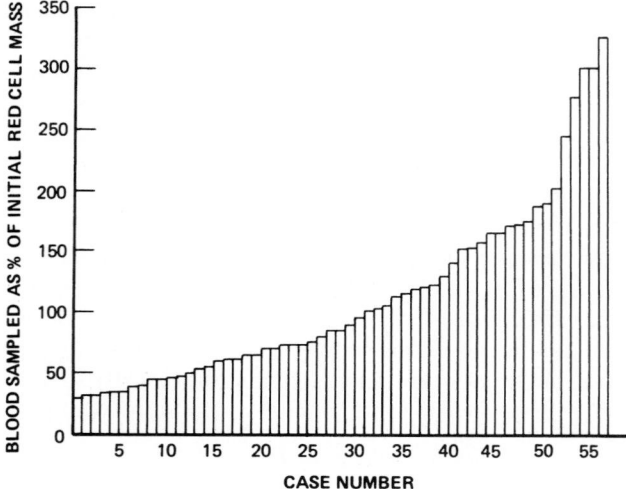

FIG. 45–6. Cumulative blood losses through sampling in premature infants, expressed as a percentage of their erythrocyte mass at birth. Infants were studied during the first 6 weeks of life, and each vertical bar represents a single infant.

sampled from infants judged to be clinically ill than from healthy premature infants (65). Iatrogenic blood loss through sampling was significant in both groups (mean ± 1 SD = 26.9 ± 9 and 14.6 ± 5 mL, respectively). These comparative volumes may not appear large, but the actual values must be compared with a total erythrocyte mass that varies between 32.3 and 45.5 mL/kg (72–76). The

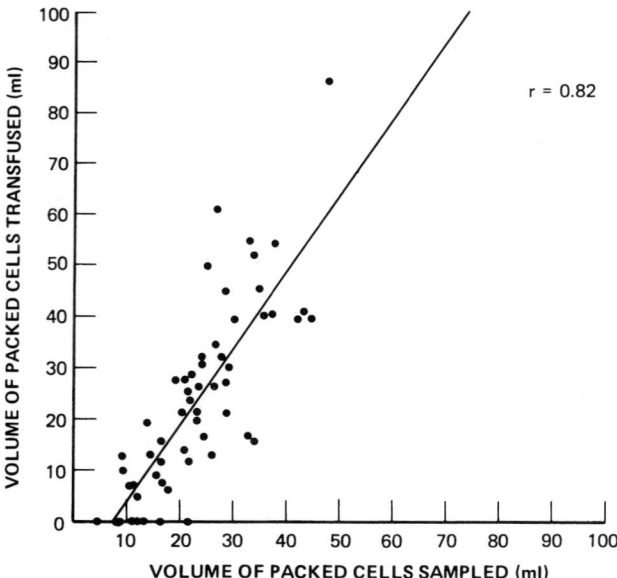

FIG. 45–7. Relation during the first 6 weeks of life between the cumulative volumes of blood sampled from and transfused into 57 premature infants who had birth weights less than 1500 g. Volumes represent milliliters of packed erythrocytes. (r, correlation coefficient.)

removal of 1 mL of blood from a 1-kg infant is equivalent to removing 70 mL of blood from an average adult, and it is therefore not surprising that repeated blood sampling, even with capillary samples, can have a profound effect on the hemoglobin concentration of small, premature infants. Ballin and colleagues have demonstrated that, if the erythrocytes that are discarded from samples drawn in which only the plasma was used were instead reinfused, the fall in hemoglobin concentration could be substantially reduced (48).

Classification

Anemia at birth or appearing during the first few weeks of life can be broadly categorized into three major groups. The anemia may be the result of blood loss, hemolysis, or underproduction of erythrocytes.

Anemia Caused by Blood Loss

Blood loss resulting in anemia may occur prenatally, at the time of delivery, or postnatally. Blood loss may be a result of occult hemorrhage before birth, obstetric accidents, internal hemorrhages, or excessive blood sampling for diagnostic studies (Table 45–3). Faxelius and colleagues associated a low erythrocyte volume with a

TABLE 45–3. *Types of hemorrhage in the neonate*

Occult hemorrhage before birth
Fetomaternal
Traumatic amniocentesis
Spontaneous
After external cephalic version
Twin-to-twin
Obstetric accidents, malformations of the placenta and cord
Nuchal cord with placental blood trapping
Rupture of a normal umbilical cord
Precipitous delivery
Entanglement
Hematoma of the cord or placenta
Rupture of an abnormal umbilical cord
Varices
Aneurysm
Rupture of anomalous vessels
Aberrant vessel
Velamentous insertion
Communicating vessels in multilobed placenta
Incision of placenta during cesarean section
Placenta previa
Abruptio placentae
Internal hemorrhage
Intracranial
Giant cephalohematoma
Subgaleal
Retroperitoneal
Laceration of the liver
Ruptured spleen
Pulmonary

maternal history of bleeding in the late third trimester, placenta previa, abruptio placentae, nonelective cesarean section, deliveries associated with cord compression, Apgar scores less than 6, an early central venous hematocrit less than 45%, and a mean arterial pressure less than 30 mm Hg (70).

Occult Hemorrhage before Birth

Occult hemorrhage before birth may be caused by bleeding of the fetus into the maternal circulation or by bleeding of one fetus into another in multiple pregnancies. In approximately 50% of all pregnancies, some fetal cells can be demonstrated in the maternal circulation (82). In about 8% of pregnancies, from 0.5 to 40.0 mL of blood is transferred from the fetus to the mother at birth, and in 1% of pregnancies, the blood loss exceeds 40 mL. Fetomaternal hemorrhages are more common after traumatic diagnostic amniocentesis or external cephalic version.

Fetomaternal Hemorrhage. The clinical manifestations of a fetomaternal hemorrhage depend on the volume of the hemorrhage and the rapidity with which it has occurred. If the hemorrhage has been prolonged or repeated during the course of the pregnancy, anemia develops slowly, giving the fetus an opportunity to develop hemodynamic compensation. These infants may manifest only pallor at birth. After acute hemorrhage just before delivery, the infant may be pale and sluggish, with gasping respirations and signs of circulatory shock.

The degree of anemia varies. Usually, the hemoglobin is less than 12.0 g/dL before the physician recognizes signs and symptoms of anemia. Hemoglobin values as low as 3.0 to 4.0 g/dL have been recorded in infants who were born alive and survived. If the hemorrhage has been acute, and particularly in hypovolemic shock, the hemoglobin value may not reflect the magnitude of the blood loss. Several hours may elapse before hemodilution occurs and the magnitude of the hemorrhage is appreciated. In general, a loss of 20% of the blood volume acutely is sufficient to produce signs of shock and is reflected in a fall in hemoglobin concentration within 3 hours of the event.

In acute and chronic hemorrhage, the erythrocytes usually appear normochromic and normocytic. Rarely in chronic hemorrhage, the cells appear hypochromic and microcytic, indicating fetal iron deficiency anemia (83).

If anemia is a direct result of a fetal-to-maternal hemorrhage, the Coombs test is negative, and the infant is not jaundiced. Infants with anemia secondary to blood loss generally have lower than average bilirubin values throughout the neonatal period as a consequence of their reduced erythrocyte mass.

The diagnosis of a fetomaternal hemorrhage great enough to result in anemia at birth can be made with certainty only by the demonstration of fetal cells in the maternal circulation. The Kleihauer technique of acid elution is the simplest and most commonly employed method for the detection of fetal cells (84). The test is based on the property of HbF to resist elution from the cell in an acid medium. The acid elution technique can be relied on with certainty for diagnosis only when other conditions capable of producing elevations in maternal HbF levels are absent. These include maternal thalassemia minor, sickle-cell anemia, hereditary persistence of HbF, and in some normal women, a pregnancy-induced rise in HbF production (85). In these conditions, the appearance of the Kleihauer test, with many cells containing variable amounts of HbF, is easily differentiated from that of a true transplacental hemorrhage, in which the fetal cells containing high concentrations of HbF are readily differentiated from the maternal cells containing no HbF.

Diagnosis of a fetomaternal hemorrhage may be missed in situations in which the mother and infant are incompatible in the ABO blood group system. In such instances, the infant's A or B cells are rapidly cleared from the maternal circulation by the maternal anti-A or anti-B and may not be seen in the Kleihauer preparation.

Twin-to-Twin Transfusion. Twin-to-twin transfusion is observed in 13% to 33% of monozygotic multiple births with monochorial placentas (86). In approximately 70% of monozygotic twin pregnancies, a monochorial placenta exists. Blood exchange between twins may produce anemia in the donor and polycythemia in the recipient. If a significant hemorrhage has occurred, the difference in hemoglobin between the twins exceeds 5.0 g/dL. There is a maximal discrepancy of 3.3 g/dL in cord blood hemoglobin concentration in dizygotic twins. The anemic twin may develop congestive heart failure and hydrops, and the plethoric twin may manifest symptoms and signs of the hyperviscosity syndrome, disseminated intravascular coagulation (DIC) and hyperbilirubinemia.

The hemorrhage may be acute or chronic. Tan and associates, on the basis of a review of 482 twin pairs in which 35 were found to have the transfusion syndrome, pointed out how the difference in weight of the twins could be used to establish the timing of the hemorrhage (86). If the weight difference exceeded 20% of the weight of the larger twin, the transfusion was chronic, and the smaller infant was invariably the donor. The anemic, smaller twin displayed reticulocytosis. If the difference in the weight of the twins did not exceed 20% of the weight of the larger twin, the larger twin was the donor in almost 50% of cases. In these presumably acute transfusions around the time of birth, significant reticulocytosis was not observed in the anemic donor.

If twin-to-twin transfusion is suspected, attempts to confirm it by placental examination should be made. The placentas of all multiple pregnancies should be routinely examined for purposes of genetic counseling. If hematologic evidence has not been obtained, and the infants have died, other findings may suggest the diagnosis, including polyhydramnios of the recipient's amniotic sac and oligohydramnios of the donor and marked differences in the size and organ weights of the twins.

With the advent of accurate ultrasound assessment of the fetus, the diagnosis of twin-to-twin transfusion *in utero* has become possible. Where severe, the donor (anemic) twin is smaller, and there is associated oligohydramnios; the recipient (polycythemic, hypervolemic) twin is larger, and there is associated polyhydramnios. Intrauterine diagnosis is therefore dependent on identification of same sex, size difference, oligohydramnios/polyhydramnios, and monochorionic placenta. When diagnosed *in utero*, twin-to-twin transfusion untreated has a high mortality rate (87). Therapy has included repeated amniocentesis to reduce the polyhydramnios (87) and laser therapy to occlude the causative arteriovenous anastomoses (88).

Obstetric Accidents and Complications

Obstetric accidents and malformations of the placenta and cord may be responsible for major blood loss at the time of delivery. These accidents may be unreported to the pediatrician and may result in diagnostic confusion about the cause of shock in the early hours of life or the presence of pallor and unexplained anemia during the second or third day of life.

The obstetric conditions that can produce neonatal hemorrhage are listed in Table 45–3. Severe and often fatal fetal hemorrhage may accompany placenta previa, abruptio placentae, or accidental incision of the placenta or umbilical cord during a cesarean section. A tight nuchal cord may cause venous obstruction leading to excessive blood trapping in the placenta and resulting in severe hypovolemia (89) and anemia (90). A prospective study of red cell mass suggested that babies born with a tight nuchal cord had a significantly lower red cell mass than controls (91).

In women with late-third-trimester bleeding, Clayton and associates were able to anticipate the birth of a possible anemic infant by examining the vaginal blood for the presence of fetal erythrocytes, employing the acid elution technique of Kleihauer (84,92).

It is good pediatric practice to obtain a hemoglobin measurement routinely at the time of delivery of all babies born of women with late-third-trimester bleeding. This determination should be repeated in 6 to 12 hours to observe the expected fall in hemoglobin resulting from the hemodilution that follows recent blood loss.

Severe bleeding as a result of an obstetric accident or complication of delivery often results in the birth of a pale, limp infant. Respirations, which usually commence spontaneously, are often irregular and gasping. They are not associated with retraction, as in conditions accompanied by primary pulmonary disease. Cyanosis is minimal, and the infant's pale color is not improved by oxygen administration. The peripheral pulses are weak or absent, and the blood pressure is reduced. The venous pressure measured after the insertion of an umbilical catheter is found to be extremely low.

Internal Hemorrhage

Anemia that appears in the first 24 to 72 hours of life and is not associated with significant jaundice is commonly caused by hemorrhage at the time of birth or by a postnatal internal hemorrhage. Traumatic deliveries may result in subdural or subarachnoid hemorrhages or cephalohematomas of sufficient magnitude to produce anemia. Subaponeurotic or subgaleal hemorrhages are relatively common after vacuum extraction and may lead to significant neonatal anemia.

Breech deliveries may be associated with hemorrhage into the adrenals, kidney, spleen, or retroperitoneal area. Rupture of the liver or subcapsular hemorrhage into the liver may occur more commonly than is clinically recognized (93–95). An infant with a ruptured liver may appear well for the first 24 to 48 hours of life and then suddenly go into shock. The abdomen may appear distended, and a mass contiguous with the liver is often palpable. Shifting dullness on abdominal percussion can often be demonstrated, and an elevation of the right hemidiaphragm may be seen on the radiograph. Splenic rupture may occur after a difficult delivery or as a result of the extreme distension of the spleen that is often seen in babies with severe erythroblastosis fetalis. The physician should always suspect a rupture of the spleen when an anemic, and often hydropic, infant with erythroblastosis is found to have a low initial venous pressure at the time of exchange transfusion. The diagnosis of intraabdominal hemorrhage is readily made with ultrasonography.

In infants with birth weights less than 1,500 g, bleeding into the cerebral ventricles, subarachnoid space, and parenchyma can also produce significant decreases in hemoglobin concentration.

Iatrogenic Anemia

Anemia appearing during the first week of life is often caused by blood removal for diagnostic studies required for the frequent monitoring of critically ill infants. Removal of more than 20% of a subject's blood volume produces anemia. In an infant of 1,500 g, this represents a blood loss of only 25 mL. If frequent blood sampling is necessary, a flow sheet should be used to record the amount removed at any given time. This simple technique often converts a diagnosis of idiopathic anemia to one of iatrogenic anemia.

Treatment

The treatment of anemia secondary to blood loss depends on the degree of anemia and the acuteness of the hemorrhage. For acute hemorrhage, the following measures must be employed:

1. If the infant is pale and limp at birth, clear the airway, administer oxygen, and intubate if necessary.
2. Obtain venous access immediately. In some circumstances, this may be through the insertion of an umbilical venous line. Blood specimens for hematologic determinations and crossmatching should be drawn. If an umbilical line is placed, it may be possible to measure a central venous pressure.
3. As soon as it is apparent that pallor is a result of hypovolemic shock or profound anemia and not a consequence of asphyxia, administer 20 mL/kg of the available solution, i.e., O Rh-negative blood, plasma, 5% albumin, or isotonic saline. Infants with acute external blood loss usually demonstrate dramatic improvement after such a procedure. Infants with massive internal hemorrhages show less evidence of response.
4. A repeat injection of 10 to 20 mL/kg of whole blood may be given after the first transfusion, particularly if whole blood was not administered initially and the venous pressure and arterial pressure have not returned to normal.

After resuscitating the infant, make efforts to determine the cause of blood loss. Examine the placenta and cord for evidence of abnormalities. Obtain a blood sample from the mother for the detection of a fetomaternal hemorrhage. The infant who is mildly anemic at birth as a consequence of chronic blood loss and who is in no distress may not require transfusion.

For anemic infants still requiring intensive supports, especially mechanical ventilation, it is probably appropriate to treat anemia with blood transfusion. The decision to transfuse must be based on the hemoglobin level and on the clinical condition of the baby. The exact guidelines are not determined. During the first 72 hours of life, an infant requiring multiple blood tests should receive transfusion after 10% of the calculated blood volume has been removed, if further blood sampling is expected.

Hemolytic Anemia

Anemia as a consequence of a hemolytic process is common in the newborn period and has multiple causes. Hemolytic anemia in the newborn period is almost always associated with elevation of the serum bilirubin value to 170 μmol/L (10 mg/dL) or greater. In general, a hemolytic process is first detected during the investigation of jaundice occurring during the first week of life.

Diagnosis of Hemolytic Disease

Detection and diagnosis of hemolytic disease in newborn infants are difficult because many of the tests used in older children and in adults are of little value during the first days of life. Hemolytic disease in adults is diagnosed if there is evidence of a rapidly falling hemoglobin concentration, increased erythrocyte production in the absence of hemorrhage, abnormal erythrocyte morphology, and increased erythrocyte destruction within the bloodstream with the release of free hemoglobin or within the reticuloendothelial system with production of bilirubin. In the newborn infant, these signs of a hemolytic process are of limited value and require additional interpretation.

Rapidly Falling Hemoglobin Concentration. The assessment of anemia in newborn infants was described previously. Hemolytic disease may be suspected if there is anemia or if hemoglobin levels fall rapidly in the absence of hemorrhage, significant removal of blood for testing, or fluid shifts.

Evidence of Increased Erythrocyte Production. In adults, an increased reticulocyte count with a stable or falling hemoglobin concentration is evidence of increased erythrocyte production and, in the absence of hemorrhage, is diagnostic of a hemolytic process. The reticulocyte count in normal newborns has a wide range, limiting its value except in severe hemolytic disease.

Erythrocyte Morphology. The shape of erythrocytes in newborns differs from that in adults. Abnormally shaped cells are frequent in newborn infants, particularly in premature infants. Quantitative assessment of the three-dimensional shape of the erythrocyte is of considerable value in the diagnosis of hemolytic disease in newborns [96] Erythrocyte morphology found in newborn infants is shown in Fig. 45–8, and the percentage of these cells found in full-term and premature infants is shown in Table 45–4.

Evidence of Erythrocyte Destruction. The catabolism of erythrocytes results in the equimolar production of bilirubin and carboxyhemoglobin [97,98]. A rapid increase in the degree of hyperbilirubinemia is a cardinal sign of erythrocyte destruction. The measurement of blood carboxyhemoglobin or in the rate of carbon monoxide excretion [99] also correlates with hemolysis [100–103].

In adults and children, intravascular hemolysis is evidenced by increased levels of hemoglobin in the plasma (i.e., hemoglobinemia), a fall in serum haptoglobin, and the appearance of hemoglobinuria and methemalbuminemia. In the normal newborn, haptoglobin levels may be zero, and plasma hemoglobin levels are above those found in adults. Gross elevations in plasma hemoglobin and hemoglobinuria are evidence of intravascular hemolysis, but the value of these tests in detecting mild hemolysis in newborn infants is limited.

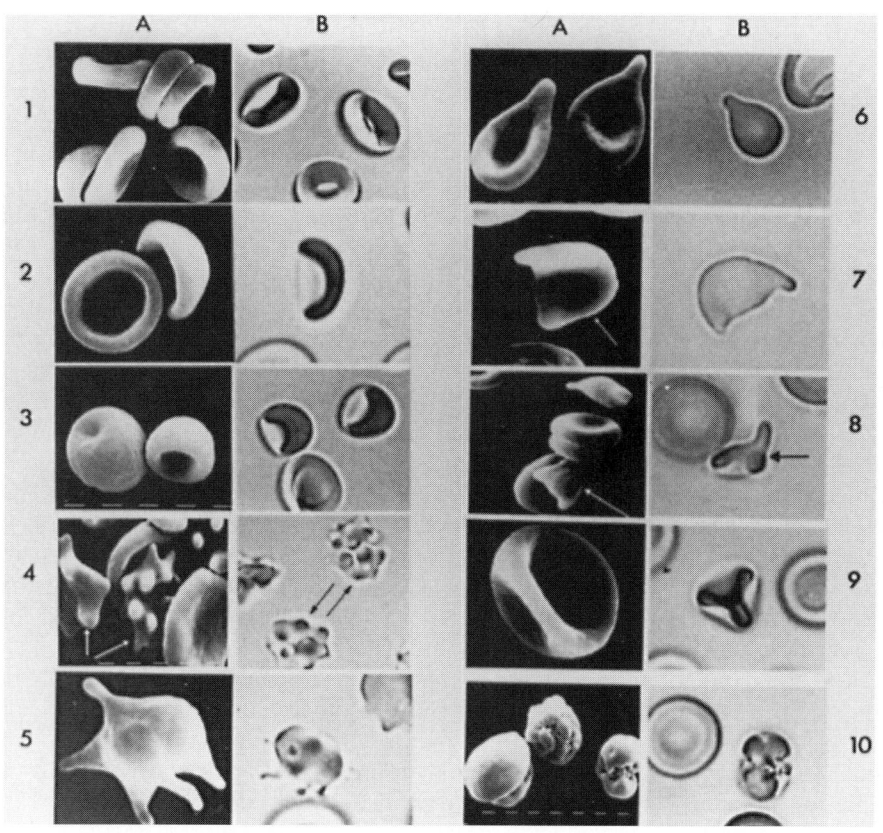

FIG. 45–8. The three-dimensional appearance of erythrocytes as seen by scanning electron microscopy **(A)** and by light microscopy **(B)** of glutaraldehyde-fixed cells. (1, discocytes; 2, bowls; 3, spherocytes; 4, echinocytes; 5, acanthocytes; 6, dacrocytes; 7, keratocytes; 8, schizocytes; 9, knizocytes; 10, immature erythrocytes.)

When erythrocytes are destroyed in the reticuloendothelial system, bilirubin is produced, with elevation of indirect bilirubin in the blood. In the newborn, there are many other causes of hyperbilirubinemia (see Chap. 38). In newborns, unlike adults, indirect hyperbilirubinemia is not a specific or helpful sign of hemolytic disease. Unusually rapid appearance of jaundice, partic-

ularly in the first 24 hours, suggests hemolytic disease. Because there are many causes of indirect hyperbilirubinemia, all newborns with abnormally high indirect bilirubin levels must be studied for evidence of hemolytic disease.

In summary, there are several signs of hemolytic disease in newborn infants:

TABLE 45–4. *Erythrocyte differential counts in adults and neonates*

	Median (5%–95%)[a]		
Erythrocytes	Adults	Full-term infants[b]	Premature infants[c]
Number studied	53	31	52
Disks	78 (42–94)	43 (18–62)	39.5 (18–57)
Bowls	18 (4–50)	40 (14–58)	29 (13–53)
Ratio of disks to bowls	2 (0–4)	2 (0–5)	3 (0–10)
Spherocytes	0 (0–0)	0 (0–1)	0 (0–3)
Echinocytes	0 (0–3)	1 (0–4)	5.5 (1–23)
Acanthocytes	0 (0–1)	1 (0–2)	0 (0–2)
Dacrocytes	0 (0–1)	1 (0–3)	1 (0–5)
Keratocytes	0 (0–1)	2 (0–5)	3 (0–7)
Schizocytes	0 (0–1)	0 (0–2)	2 (0–5)
Knizocytes	1 (0–4)	3 (0–8)	1 (0–6)
Others	1 (0–4)	3 (0–7)	4 (1–11)

[a]All values are expressed as a median plus the 5% to 95% range, because the distribution of most values was nongaussian.
[b]Of the sample, 29 were ABO compatible, 1 was AB with an A mother, and 1 was AB with a B mother.
[c]Includes ABO-compatible and ABO-incompatible infants.

1. Rapid fall in hemoglobin concentration in the absence of hemorrhage.
2. Increased erythrocyte production (i.e., reticulocytosis) with a stable or falling hemoglobin concentration.
3. Abnormal erythrocyte morphology.
4. Hemoglobinuria.
5. Jaundice during the first 24 hours of life.
6. Elevation of carboxyhemoglobin levels.

Isoimmune Hemolytic Disease

Hemolytic disease in the newborn as a consequence of isoimmunization of the mother is caused by the passage of fetal erythrocytes into the maternal circulation, where they stimulate the production of antibody. Antibodies of the IgG class return to the fetal circulation, attach to antigenic sites on the surface of the erythrocyte, and cause its rapid removal and destruction. The incidence and clinical manifestations of isoimmunization depend on the type of blood group incompatibility between the mother and fetus. This topic has been the subject of many comprehensive reviews (104–107).

Rhesus Hemolytic Disease. The incidence of Rh incompatibility in a population depends, in large part, on the prevalence of the Rh-negative antigens. The prevalence of the Rh-negative genotype ranges from approximately zero in Japanese, Chinese, and North American Indian populations to 5.5% among African-Americans and 15% among American Caucasians. Among Caucasian women, it has been estimated that in approximately 9% of all pregnancies, an Rh-negative woman carries an Rh-positive fetus. In 6% of pregnancies at risk, isoimmunization of the mother occurs if there is no immunoprophylaxis.

The severity of Rh hemolytic disease varies greatly from infant to infant. It is estimated that, without antenatal diagnosis and treatment, the perinatal mortality in this disease would be approximately 17.5%, with stillbirths accounting for about 14% of deaths (107). Although hemolytic disease tends to be more severe in a second pregnancy than in a first one in which sensitization has occurred, the severity of disease in subsequent pregnancies tends to be uniform.

Pathogenesis. The entry of fetal cells into the maternal circulation is the cause of Rh isoimmunization. As few as 0.05 to 0.1 mL of cells, particularly if transferred repeatedly, are sufficient to produce immunization. Rh immunization tends to occur more frequently in pregnancies that have been complicated by toxemia, cesarean section, or manual removal of the placenta, because transplacental hemorrhages occur with greater frequency and in greater volume under these circumstances. It is estimated that 1% of Rh-negative women develop antibodies as a consequence of these transplacental hemorrhages before the delivery of their first child. An additional 7.5% manifest evidence of sensitization within 6 months of the delivery of their first child, and another 7.5% show no evidence of immunization 6 months after delivery but develop antibodies during their next pregnancy if their fetus is Rh-positive, presumably as a consequence of a sensitization during the first pregnancy.

Destruction of fetal erythrocytes by anti-D. The transfer of antibody from the mother into the fetal circulation is responsible for the clinical manifestations of the hemolytic process. The erythrocyte, coated with an antibody of the IgG class, is removed primarily in the spleen of the fetus. The rate of destruction is proportional to the amount of antibody on the cell. At very high levels of antibody, the cell may be destroyed by intravascular hemolysis and splenic sequestration.

Before birth, the chief danger of excess erythrocyte destruction is profound anemia. After birth, the infant is primarily at risk from the toxic products of erythrocyte breakdown, such as bilirubin. *In utero*, the infant responds to the increased breakdown of cells by increasing the rate of erythrocyte production. This is reflected by an elevation of reticulocyte count and the presence of nucleated erythrocytes in the peripheral circulation. This accelerated demand for erythrocytes results in active erythropoiesis in nonmarrow sites such as the liver, spleen, and lung. A major portion of the hepatosplenomegaly observed in infants with hemolytic disease is a result of this extramedullary erythropoiesis.

In infants with severe Rh incompatibility, the liver and pancreas exhibit pathologic changes. Islet cell hyperplasia can be observed in the pancreas, and focal cellular necrosis with cholestasis may be seen in the liver.

The most severely affected infants manifest hydrops fetalis. This massive edema with pleural effusions and ascites is not strictly related to the hemoglobin level of the infant. Other factors play a role in the development of hydrops, including intrauterine hypoxia, hypoproteinemia, and a lowering of the nonprotein oncotic pressure of the plasma. Hydrops fetalis has been observed in a variety of other conditions (Table 45–5).

Clinical Manifestations. The main signs of hemolytic disease in the newborn are jaundice, pallor, and enlargement of the liver and spleen. Jaundice usually becomes evident during the first 24 hours of life, frequently within the first 4 to 5 hours of life, and becomes maximal by the third or fourth day. Jaundice and the metabolism of bilirubin are extensively discussed in Chapter 38.

The degree of anemia reflects the severity of the hemolytic process and the infant's capacity to respond to it with increased erythrocyte production. Late anemia may develop in infants with Rh isoimmunization. This is observed in two clinical settings. In one, the infant does not become sufficiently jaundiced in the initial newborn period to require exchange transfusion. This is more common since the advent of light therapy, which may control the jaundice even though the hemolytic process continues.

TABLE 45–5. *Some causes of hydrops fetalis*

Severe chronic anemia *in utero*
  Parvovirus infection
  Erythroblastosis fetalis
  Homozygous alpha-thalassemia
  Chronic fetomaternal transfusion or twin-to-twin
    transfusion
  Glucose-6-phosphate dehydrogenase deficiency (rarely)
Cardiac failure
  Severe congenital cardiomyopathy or myocarditis
  Premature closure of foramen ovale
  Large arteriovenous malformation (e.g., hemangioma)
  Intrauterine arrhythmias
Hypoproteinemia
  Renal disease
    Congenital nephrosis
    Renal vein thrombosis
  Congenital hepatitis
Intrauterine infections
  Syphilis
  Toxoplasmosis
  Cytomegalovirus
Miscellaneous
  Maternal diabetes mellitus
  Parabiotic syndrome of multiple pregnancies
  Sublethal umbilical or chorionic vein thrombosis
  Fetal neuroblastoma
  Cystic adenomatoid malformation of the lung
  Pulmonary lymphangiectasia
  Chorioangioma of the placenta (108)
  Transient leukemia of Down syndrome (109)

Continued erythrocyte destruction occurs, and the infant can develop severe or fatal anemia between 7 and 21 days of life. The other, more common situation occurs in infants who have had exchange transfusions. In these infants, a gradual fall in hemoglobin may be observed, with hemoglobin values of 5 to 6 g/dL being reached by 4 to 6 weeks of life. This results from continued destruction of residual and newly formed Rh-positive cells. Spontaneous correction can be expected by 6 to 8 weeks of age.

Petechiae and purpura may be observed in infants with severe anemia as a result of thrombocytopenia and a disturbance in the intrinsic system of coagulation. This disturbance may result from DIC or from hepatic dysfunction with consequent inability to synthesize the vitamin K-dependent factors (110,111)

Laboratory findings. Decreased hemoglobin concentration, increased reticulocyte count, and increased numbers of nucleated erythrocytes in the peripheral blood reflect the presence of the hemolytic process. Hemoglobin determinations performed on venous samples most accurately reflect the severity of the hemolytic process. Values less than 13 g/dL in the cord blood should be regarded as abnormal. The reticulocyte count is usually greater than 6% and may reach 30% to 40%. In the peripheral blood, nucleated erythrocytes may be observed in addition to some degree of polychromasia and aniso-

cytosis. Spherocytes are not found in patients with Rh hemolytic disease.

The erythrocytes of infants with Rh hemolytic disease test positive on direct Coombs testing, indicating the presence of maternal IgG on the erythrocyte surface.

Prevention. The management of Rh hemolytic disease focuses primarily on prevention of the disease by the administration of anti-Rh immunoglobulin to the mother after the delivery or abortion of an Rh-positive infant and on the prevention of the intrauterine death of the infant at risk.

The early proposals for the use of anti-Rh immunoglobulin were based on the observation that ABO incompatibility offered protection against the development of Rh sensitization, probably by allowing destruction of the fetal erythrocytes in the mother before they could stimulate Rh antibody formation. Because most major transfers of fetal erythrocytes occur at the time of delivery, efforts were undertaken to destroy such cells soon after delivery. The development of a human immunoglobulin concentrate of anti-D (RhoGAM) greatly facilitated application of this means of prevention. Prevention of Rh sensitization is now about 90% effective with the use of anti-D immune globulin at the time of delivery. Failures appear to be caused by hemorrhages that occur before term or by massive hemorrhages that occur at the time of delivery in which the amount of anti-D immunoglobulin administered is inadequate to destroy the large numbers of cells that have entered the circulation. The physician can detect massive hemorrhages at delivery by examining maternal blood for fetal erythrocytes by the Kleihauer technique. It has been estimated that approximately one in 250 deliveries involves a transplacental hemorrhage of more than 30 mL (107). In such instances, a larger dose of anti-D immunoglobulin should be given.

Immunization before delivery occurs in approximately 1% of women at risk (107). The Rh immunization can be prevented by administration of anti-D immunoglobulin at week 28 of gestation. It has been suggested that this may not be cost-effective therapy; however, this matter has been discussed in detail elsewhere, and it is the researchers' recommendation that all Rh-negative women with Rh-positive partners should be treated at week 28 of gestation with anti-D immunoglobulin to prevent Rh immunization (112).

Stillbirths are prevented by intrauterine transfusions or by the early termination of pregnancy. The pregnant woman at risk is one who is Rh (D)-negative, has an Rh (D)-positive partner, and has anti-D antibodies in her serum. All such women must be followed carefully during pregnancy (106,113).

Intrauterine diagnosis and treatment. The most accurate assessment of severity of disease in the fetus is the estimation of amniotic fluid bilirubin levels. Amniotic fluid is normally clear and colorless. It acquires a yellow pigmentation in cases of severe hemolytic disease because of the passage of bilirubin into it. The amount of bile pigment in the amniotic fluid more accurately reflects the degree of fetal involvement than does the maternal antibody titer. The concentration of bilirubin pigments, usually measured by spectrophotometry of amniotic fluid, is approximately 350 to 700 nm. Normal amniotic fluid, when plotted on a logarithmic scale, describes a straight line, but when a pigment is present, a bulge appears at approximately 450 nm. This can be measured, and the change in optical density (OD) as a function of gestational age can be employed to gauge the severity of the hemolytic process (113,114) Women who should be considered for amniocentesis are those with a history of hemolytic disease in previous infants and those whose anti-D titers are greater than 0.125 by the indirect Coombs test, remembering that titers may vary from laboratory to laboratory.

Analysis of the amniotic fluid indicates whether the infant is suffering from severe disease, and this is used as a guide to therapy, which may include continued observation with amniocentesis at 2-week intervals, premature induction after 33 weeks of gestation, or intrauterine blood transfusion.

In severe cases, in which the amniotic OD is high, it is recommended that fetal blood be sampled from the umbilical vein to determine directly the hemoglobin level in the fetal blood and the severity of the hemolytic disease.

The treatment of severe hemolytic disease *in utero* has been by intrauterine transfusions into the peritoneum of the fetus. The preferred method now is direct intrauterine transfusion through the umbilical vein. With intrauterine diagnosis (e.g., amniotic fluid or fetal blood analyses), most fetuses with severe Rh disease can be salvaged. Those who reach 33 weeks of gestation can be induced prematurely, and the survival rate is expected to be the same as for a full-term infant with Rh disease. For those with more severe disease who would not survive to 33 weeks of gestation, intrauterine transfusion beginning at 20 to 22 weeks of gestation results in salvage of as many as 87% of patients (115).

Management. Newborns with Rh hemolytic disease are at risk of death or damage, primarily from anemia or hyperbilirubinemia. As soon as the infant has been delivered and respirations have been established, the infant should be evaluated in an attempt to judge the severity of the hemolytic process. Assess pallor, organomegaly, petechiae, edema, ascites, respiratory rate, pulse, and blood pressure. Cord blood samples should be analyzed for hemoglobin concentration, reticulocyte count, nucleated erythrocyte count, blood type, direct Coombs reaction, and serum bilirubin concentration, direct-reacting and total.

In the infant with a positive-reacting Coombs test, the major initial decision is whether to perform an immediate exchange transfusion or to observe the infant's clinical status. In many instances, the outcome of previous preg-

nancies and the result of amniocentesis during the current pregnancy provide valuable information about what to anticipate in the way of severity. Except for the obviously pale or edematous child, the decision to perform an immediate exchange transfusion is based on laboratory findings.

It has been suggested that a cord hemoglobin less than 11.0 g/dL or a cord bilirubin higher than 4.5 mg/dL is an indication for immediate exchange transfusion (113). The value of immediate transfusion is that it is more efficient to remove a "potential bilirubin" (i.e., antibody-coated erythrocytes) than to allow hemolysis to occur, with distribution of bilirubin throughout the tissues, from which it is removed with greater difficulty by exchange transfusion.

For less severely affected infants, exchange transfusion is indicated if it becomes apparent that the rate of bilirubin rise is such that total indirect bilirubin will exceed 20 mg/dL (330 μmol/L) in otherwise healthy full-term infants. The physician needs to use lower maximal bilirubin levels in sick or premature infants (see Chap. 38).

ABO Hemolytic Disease. ABO hemolytic disease results from the action of maternal anti-A or anti-B antibodies on fetal erythrocytes of the corresponding blood group. Although approximately 20% of all pregnancies are associated with ABO incompatibility between the mother and fetus, the incidence of severe hemolytic disease is low. Anti-A and anti-B antibodies are found in the IgA, IgM, and IgG fractions of plasma. Only the IgG antibodies cross the placenta and are responsible for the production of disease. These naturally occurring antibodies result from continuous immune stimulation by A and B substances that exist in foods and gram-negative bacteria. It is not understood why some women develop high anti-A or anti-B titers. They may be the result of repeated, asymptomatic bacterial infections. ABO hemolytic disease tends to occur in the newborns of mothers with high levels of IgG anti-A or anti-B titers.

Fewer A or B antigenic sites are present on the erythrocytes of the newborn, which is responsible for the weakly reactive Coombs test in infants with ABO hemolytic disease. The sparse distribution of A and B sites on the erythrocytes of the newborn also explains why the erythrocyte life span in ABO hemolytic disease is only slightly shortened. Adult group A erythrocytes transfused into a baby with maternally acquired anti-A antibody are rapidly destroyed and may produce severe intravascular hemolysis.

The diagnosis of ABO hemolytic disease is often difficult and may first require the exclusion of other causes of hyperbilirubinemia. Usually, the diagnosis is suspected when hyperbilirubinemia appears in the group A or B baby of a blood group O mother. The disease is more common and more severe in black infants. Jaundice appearing in the first 24 hours (i.e., icterus praecox) is particularly characteristic of ABO hemolytic disease. Anemia may be mild or not exist. Evidence of isoimmunization is difficult to interpret because the Coombs test may be negative or only weakly positive. A positive Coombs test in ABO incompatible infants does not necessary indicate disease; it has been observed that one-third of all A or B babies of O mothers have a positive direct Coombs test (116) In approximately two-thirds of these babies, an elution test demonstrated anti-A or anti-B on the surfaces of their erythrocytes (116) The Coombs and elution tests are not specific for ABO hemolytic disease because these tests are frequently positive in infants who are not affected with disease.

The diagnosis of ABO hemolytic disease is supported by the finding of increased numbers of spherocytes; these are best detected by evaluating the three-dimensional shape of the erythrocyte (Fig. 45–9). Increased erythrocyte production is also demonstrated by an increased reticulocyte count. The diagnosis of ABO hemolytic disease is supported by the following tests and findings:

1. Indirect hyperbilirubinemia.
2. Jaundice during the first 24 hours.
3. An A or B baby of an O mother.
4. Increased numbers of spherocytes in the blood.
5. Increased erythrocyte production evidenced by reticulocytosis or an elevated carboxyhemoglobin concentration.

The levels of IgG, anti-A, or anti-B in the mothers of babies with ABO hemolytic disease are significantly higher than those in mothers whose infants do not have the disease. These tests are often not available and, unfortunately, are not high in specificity or sensitivity in the diagnosis of ABO hemolytic disease.

Treatment of this disease is directed primarily toward the prevention of hyperbilirubinemia. Phototherapy reduces the need for exchange transfusion (117): prophylactic phototherapy may be beneficial when the cord bilirubin is at least 4 mg/dl (118).

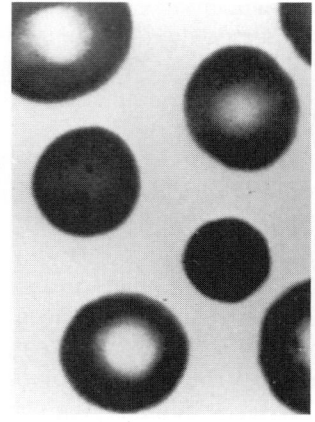 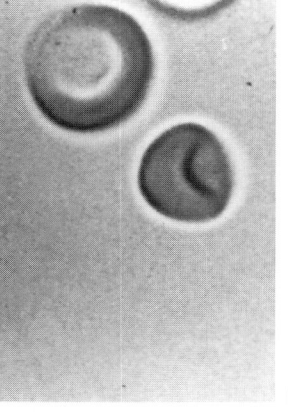

A   B

FIG. 45–9. The erythrocytes of a patient with hereditary spherocytosis, as seen on a stained blood smear **(A)** and by three-dimensional viewing **(B)** of glutaraldehyde-fixed cells.

Hemolytic Disease Resulting from Minor Blood Group Incompatibility. Hemolytic disease related to maternal erythrocyte antibodies other than anti-D, anti-A, or anti-B is relatively uncommon. In one study, minor group antibodies were found in 121 (0.08%) of 142,800 pregnant women (119). The principal antibodies found were anti-E, anti-c, and anti-Kell. Anti-Kell antibodies may cause severe hemolytic disease in newborn infants, including hydrops and neonatal death (120). In a report of 30 cases of hemolytic disease of the newborn, the following antibodies were responsible: 14 anti-c, nine anti-E, two anti-Ce, two anti-Kell, one anti-Fya, one anti-JKa, and one anti-U (121). It is recommended that all pregnant women should have their blood screened for antibodies at least once during pregnancy before week 34 of gestation.

Congenital Defects of the Erythrocyte

Inherited defects of erythrocyte metabolism, membrane function, and hemoglobin synthesis all may manifest themselves in the newborn period. Defects of erythrocyte metabolism include glucose-6-phosphate dehydrogenase (G6PD) deficiency and less common disorders such as pyruvate kinase deficiency.

Glucose-6-Phosphate Dehydrogenase Deficiency. The major function of the erythrocyte is the delivery of oxygen to the tissues. The cell is constantly exposed to oxygen, and the erythrocyte membrane and cytoplasm are subjected to oxidative damage. Oxidation causes the formation of precipitates of denatured hemoglobin (Heinz bodies), which appear to be associated with a shortened erythrocyte life span *in vivo* (Fig. 45–10). The erythrocyte has a metabolic system that can prevent oxidative damage (Fig. 45–11). Glucose-6-phosphate dehydrogenase is an enzyme in this system; if it is absent, there is a risk of oxidative damage to the erythrocyte, particularly if the cell is stressed by chemicals or drugs capable of oxidative damage (Table 45–6).

Glucose-6-phosphate dehydrogenase deficiency is a common genetic disorder affecting millions of people in the world (122). There are three major types of deficiency, all of which are inherited as a gender-linked recessive disorder. The most severe deficiency occurs rarely and is associated with a chronic hemolytic anemia. With this type of deficiency, the person has a mild or moderate anemia throughout life and may have severe hemolytic disease as a newborn. The second type affects Asians (e.g., 5.5% of Chinese) and many populations in the Middle East and Mediterranean region (e.g., 0.7% to 3% of Greeks, with the highest incidence of 53% among Kurds). These persons are healthy but are at risk of developing hemolytic anemia when exposed to oxidative drugs or chemicals (e.g., sulfa drugs, fava beans). The anemia may be of sudden onset and may be severe. In the absence of fava beans or drug exposure, hemoglobin levels are

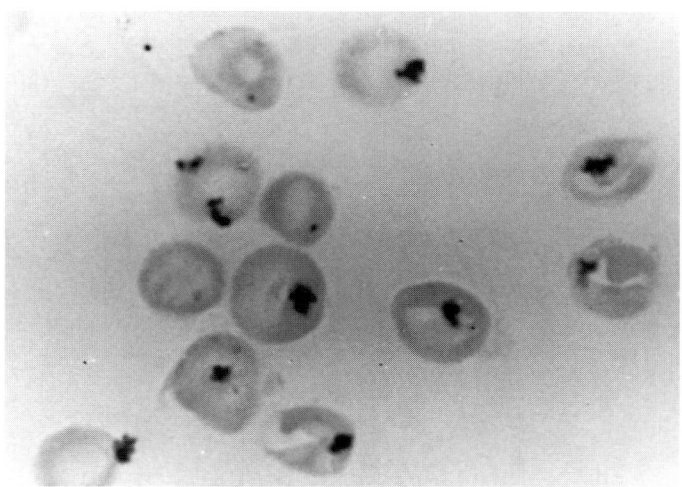

FIG. 45–10. Heinz bodies in a newborn who developed hemolytic anemia after exposure to naphthanlene in mothballs.

normal, although there is evidence that the erythrocyte life span is slightly shorter than normal.

The third type of deficiency affects blacks (e.g., 10% to 14% of African-Americans), in whom the severity of the defect usually is not as great as in those with the other two types. Anemia appears only with drug exposure, is less severe than that of the Asian–Mediterranean type, and tends to be self-limited.

Glucose-6-phosphate dehydrogenase deficiency and neonatal jaundice. Because their erythrocytes have a diminished capacity to deal with oxidative stress as a result of lower levels of glutathione peroxidase and catalase and a relative deficiency of vitamin E, newborn infants with G6PD deficiency are at greater risk of developing hemolytic anemia than are adults (see Fig. 45–10). It appears that G6PD deficiency is associated with an increased incidence of neonatal hyperbilirubinemia, especially in the more severe type affecting the Asian and

Mediterranean groups. Hyperbilirubinemia in G6PD-deficient boys has been reported in newborns in Greece, Italy, Singapore, and Thailand (123,124). Full-term African-American infants with G6PD deficiency do not develop hyperbilirubinemia more frequently than normal infants do, although the incidence in premature infants may be slightly higher (132). It has been reported from Africa, however, that black male infants with G6PD deficiency have a significantly higher incidence of hyperbilirubinemia than do controls (133). Although the hyperbilirubinemia is associated with G6PD deficiency, there is a tendency for the jaundice to occur more frequently in particular families and communities, indicating that genetic and environmental factors must influence the incidence of the disease.

In this group of patients, jaundice may be severe and may lead to kernicterus (100,101,125–127). In most cases, however, hemoglobin and reticulocyte counts are

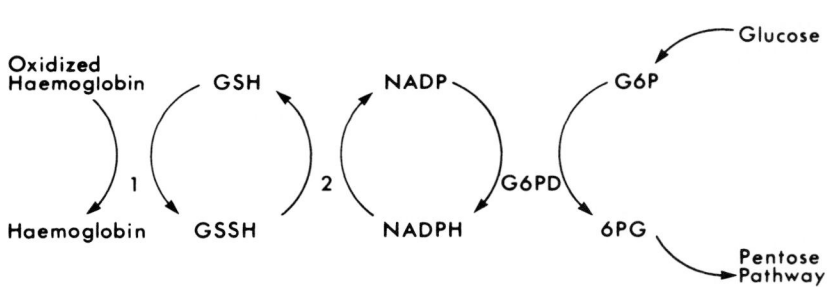

FIG. 45–11. Protection against oxidative stress in erythrocytes. The erythrocyte is constantly exposed to oxygen; as a result, there is formation of hydrogen peroxide (H_2O_2), lipid peroxides in the membrane, and oxidized products of hemoglobin such as methemoglobin and Heinz bodies. To prevent the formation of and to reduce the levels of these oxidized products, the erythrocyte has a system by which a series of enzyme steps link the metabolism of glucose through the pentose pathway to the reduction of oxidized products. (1, glutathione peroxidase; 2, glutathione reductase; G6PD, glucose-6-phosphate dehydrogenase; 6PG, 6-phosphogluconate; G6P, glucose-6-phosphate; GSH, reduced glutathione; GSSH, oxidized glutathione; NADP, nicotinamide-adenine dinucleotide phosphate; NADPH, nicotinamide-adenine dinucleotide phosphate, reduced.)

TABLE 45–6. *Drugs, chemicals, and other factors that cause glucose-6-phosphate dehydrogenase deficiency hemolytic disease*

Antimalarials
  Primaquine
  Pamaquine
  Pentaquine
Antipyretics and analgesics
  Aspirin[a]
  Acetanilid
  Acetophenetidin (phenacetin)[a]
  Acetaminophen[a]
Diabetic acidosis
  Vitamin K analogs
Infections
  Respiratory viruses
  Infectious hepatitis
  Infectious mononucleosis
  Bacterial pneumonia
Nitrofurans
  Nitrofuranto (Furadantin)
  Furazolidone (Furoxone)
  Furaltadone (Altafur)
  Nitrofurazone (Furacin)
Sulfonamides
  Sulfanilamide
  N²-Acetylsulfanilamide
  Sulfacetamide (Sulamyd)
  Sulfamethoxazole (Gantanol)
  Salicylazosulfapyridine (Azulfidine)
Sulfones
  Thiazolesulfone
Others
  Methylene blue
  Toluidine blue
  Naphthalene
  Phenylhydrazine
  Acetylphenylhydrazine
  Fava beans
  Nalidixic acid (Neggram)
  Niridazole (Ambilhar)
  Chloramphenicol

[a]Of doubtful significance.

normal, although in some affected infants the cord blood contains increased bilirubin and decreased hemoglobin levels, suggesting the presence of a mild hemolytic process *in utero*. There is no evidence of intravascular hemolysis in most of these patients. Slusher et al. (128) demonstrated elevated carboxyhemoglobin (a sensitive indicator of hemolysis) values in Nigerian children with G6PD deficiency and hyperbilirubinemia. Studies of Sephardic-Jewish neonates have yielded opposite results, with no elevation of carboxyhemoglobin values over non-jaundiced G6PD-deficient controls (129,130). The latter observation has been coupled with data suggesting deficient hepatic bilirubin conjugation in neonates with G6PD deficiency (131).

Clinical manifestations. The jaundice that occurs in these infants usually appears to be an accentuation of the physiologic jaundice of newborns with a late peak (around 5–6 days), although jaundice may appear in some during the first 24 hours of life. There is seldom evidence of a hemolytic process. Abnormal erythrocyte morphology has been documented during hemolytic episodes in adults, but this is seldom described in newborns. However, a more severe hemolytic anemia may appear, with evidence of abnormal erythrocyte morphology, Heinz bodies in the peripheral blood, and intravascular hemolysis. This may be the result of infection or exposure to drugs or chemicals (e.g., naphthalene in mothballs) (134). However, it is unusual to elicit the latter from the perinatal history.

Diagnosis. The presence of unexplained hyperbilirubinemia in an infant of a high-risk (racial intermarriage must be taken into account) population may suggest G6PD deficiency. The enzyme defect can be detected by one of many screening tests (135,136). Screening tests are based on changes in either fluorescence or color resulting from the activity of NADPH, thus indirectly measuring the activity of G6PD. Current screening tests are very effective, yielding good sensitivity and specificity, but an abnormal result should be followed up with a definitive measurement of G6PD activity based on spectrophotometric measurement of the reduction of $NADP^+$ to NADPH (137). A false normal screen result can occur in infants with significant hemolysis, which destroys the older, more G6PD-deficient red cells.

The finding of G6PD deficiency in a jaundiced infant does not in itself prove that the jaundice was caused by the enzyme defect. Other causes of jaundice must be excluded. In a study on Sephardic-Jewish neonates, neonates with both ABO incompatibility and G6PD deficiency showed no increased evidence of hemolysis when compared with neonates with only ABO incompatibility (138). Glucose-6-phosphate dehydrogenase deficiency is most severe and frequent in male infants because it is a recessive gender-linked disorder. However, female infants may be affected because they have two populations of erythrocytes, one with normal and one with low levels of G6PD, in keeping with the Lyon hypothesis. Given the high gene frequency, it is also possible for a female infant to be homozygous for the deficiency.

Treatment. Treatment is the same as that for hyperbilirubinemia described in Chapter 38. Drugs and chemicals likely to produce hemolytic anemia (see Table 45–6) should be avoided by these patients.

Other Metabolic Abnormalities of the Erythrocyte. Other abnormalities are far less common than G6PD deficiency and are unusual causes of a hemolytic process during the newborn period. Virtually all the recognized defects have been associated with jaundice and anemia during the first week of life. Of this group, erythrocyte pyruvate kinase deficiency appears to be most commonly responsible for a severe hemolytic process during the first week of life. These disorders are usually characterized by the presence of a normal osmotic fragility of unincubated blood, few or no spherocytes in the peripheral blood smear, and failure of splenectomy in later life to correct the hemolytic process. Unless the infant is a member of a high-risk group (i.e., the Amish population in the United

States), it is practical to defer diagnosis of these infants until approximately 3 months of life, after it has been established that the hemolytic process observed in the neonatal period is chronic and that the more common reasons for it have been excluded.

Abnormalities of the Erythrocyte Membrane: Hereditary Spherocytosis and Elliptocytosis. In approximately 50% of patients with hereditary spherocytosis, a history of neonatal jaundice can be obtained. Hyperbilirubinemia may require exchange transfusions. Untreated hyperbilirubinemia has resulted in kernicterus in infants with hereditary spherocytosis.

Although most patients with hereditary spherocytosis are anemic, the degree of anemia, reticulocytosis, and hyperbilirubinemia is quite variable. The hemoglobin may fall rapidly during the first several weeks of life, reaching values of 5.0 to 7.0 g/dL by 1 month of age. Neither the hematologic values observed during the immediate newborn period nor the values observed during the first several months of life are reliable indicators of the eventual severity of the disease. Hemoglobin levels of 4.0 to 7.0 g/dL during the first several months of life may subsequently stabilize in the range of 7.0 to 10.0 g/dL. Repeated transfusions are rarely needed except during the course of infections or aplastic crises. Splenectomy, if indicated, should be deferred until at least 3 or 4 years of age so that the risk of postsplenectomy infections is minimized.

Hereditary spherocytosis can be diagnosed during the newborn period. Examination of the peripheral blood reveals characteristic microspherocytes, and the osmotic fragility of erythrocytes is increased. The osmotic fragility of the erythrocytes of normal newborn infants is lower than that of adults' erythrocytes, and if an infant is suspected of having spherocytosis, the osmotic fragility should be compared with normal newborn standards. If possible, the osmotic fragility test should be deferred until the child can readily spare the necessary blood volume for the test. Family studies are extremely useful in confirming the diagnosis, although an affected parent is identified in only approximately 70% of cases.

Hereditary elliptocytosis may manifest in the newborn period as a hemolytic anemia. Only 12% to 15% of newborns with this morphologic abnormality have a shortened erythrocyte survival in later life, but many more appear to have a hemolytic anemia during the first several weeks or months of life. In the newborn period, hereditary elliptocytosis may manifest as hyperbilirubinemia and anemia associated with the presence of fragmented and deformed erythrocytes in the circulation. This is referred to as neonatal poikilocytosis. The erythrocytes of these infants are unusually susceptible to fragmentation after heating. This defect disappears within the first few months of life, and the erythrocytes assume an elliptic appearance, usually with no or minimal evidence of hemolytic disease. As in hereditary spherocytosis, demonstration of an affected parent or sibling helps to establish the diagnosis.

Most patients do not require treatment, although an exchange transfusion may be required for infants with hyperbilirubinemia. For patients with persistent hemolytic anemia, splenectomy has proved beneficial, but as in hereditary spherocytosis, it should be deferred until the patient is at least 3 or 4 years of age.

Disorders of Hemoglobin Synthesis. The predominant hemoglobin in the newborn infant is HbF ($\alpha_2\gamma_2$); therefore, it is not surprising that abnormalities in β-chain production (e.g., sickle-cell disease, β-thalassemia) do not manifest during the first month of life. Thalassemia has been diagnosed as early as the second month of life (139). Patients with sickle-cell disease are usually found to be anemic by 3 months of age, but cases of jaundice and systemic signs during the neonatal period have been reported (140).

Abnormalities in γ-chain production have been described during the first month of life, although most of these are not clinically significant. Heinz body hemolytic anemia with an unstable γ-chain abnormality has been reported (141). Cases of microcytic anemia in newborns with reduced γ-chain synthesis have been described as part of a γ-β-thalassemia syndrome (142–145).

α-Chain disorders occur frequently in the newborn period. Although there are many structural defects of the α-chain that have been reported in the newborn, these are rarely of clinical significance. α-Thalassemia manifests clinically in newborn infants and can be serious. The α-thalassemia group of diseases represents abnormalities in the synthesis of the α-chains of hemoglobin. Synthesis of these chains is determined by two pairs of α genes. A deletion of one or more of these four α genes results in one of the α-thalassemia disorders. The severity of the disease in the newborn and in the adult depends on the number of genes deleted. If one gene is lacking, the patient is hematologically normal unless he or she is a newborn, in which case there is a slight elevation of Bart hemoglobin ($\gamma4$). If two genes are absent (i.e., two missing from one chromosome or one missing from each of the two chromosomes), the patient has α-thalassemia trait, which manifests as microcytosis in the newborn (mean corpuscular volume < 95 μm^3/cell) and elevation of Bart hemoglobin. If three genes are deleted, the patient has hemoglobin H (HbH; β_4) disease, a lifelong hemolytic anemia that manifests in the newborn as jaundice and anemia. If all four genes are absent, the patient can form no α-chains and cannot form HbA or HbF. As a result, the infant is usually born dead or severely hydropic, with death occurring several hours after birth. There are now several examples of such children being maintained on transfusion therapy (170). The hemoglobin of these infants is predominantly Bart hemoglobin.

In patients with HbH disease, one parent is lacking one α gene (i.e., a silent carrier), and the other is lacking two α-genes on one chromosome (i.e., α-thalassemia trait). In the patient with homozygous α-thalassemia, each parent is lacking two genes on one chromosome. It is now thought that the α-thalassemia trait that is found in 2% to 10% of blacks is in the *trans* form in which one abnormal gene is present on each of the two chromosomes (i.e., −1α, −1α), and that the *cis* form (−−,αα) does not occur in blacks but does occur with various frequencies in populations in Southeast Asia and the Mediterranean region. This is the reason homozygous α-thalassemia and HbH disease are not found in blacks.

The incidence of α-thalassemia can be determined through measurement of levels of Bart hemoglobin in newborns. Silent carriers (i.e., −α,αα) have as much as 2% of Bart hemoglobin. Those with α-thalassemia trait (−−,αα or −α,−α) have 2% to 9% Bart hemoglobin. Those with HbH disease (−α,−−) have up to 20% of Bart hemoglobin.

Acquired Defects of the Erythrocyte

Infections and drugs can produce a hemolytic anemia in the newborn infant who has no underlying inherited defect of erythrocyte metabolism. It is frequently suggested that neonatal sepsis causes a hemolytic process. Certain infections in the newborn are associated with hyperbilirubinemia, which initially may be indirect and subsequently include direct hyperbilirubinemia. Hemolytic anemia infrequently complicates sepsis. One exception is *Clostridium welchii* sepsis, in which severe hemolytic anemia associated with microspherocytosis occurs.

Congenital syphilis, toxoplasmosis, cytomegalic inclusion disease, rubella, generalized coxsackie B infections, and *Escherichia coli* septicemia are examples of infections in which anemia and jaundice are common. Some of the nonhematologic manifestations of these diseases (e.g., rash, chorioretinitis, purpura, and hepatosplenomegaly) are useful in differentiating these disorders from isoimmunization or other primary erythrocyte abnormalities.

The erythrocytes of the newborn infant are particularly sensitive to the toxic effects of oxidant drugs. The erythrocytes of infants, particularly those of premature babies, demonstrate increased numbers of Heinz bodies, marked glutathione instability, and an increased tendency to develop methemoglobinemia when incubated with acetylphenylhydrazine or menadione. In many respects, the cells of these infants mimic the metabolic abnormalities observed in cells from patients with G6PD deficiency. Severe Heinz body hemolytic anemia (see Fig. 45–10), which occurs in infants with severe G6PD deficiency, is also seen in normal newborns who are exposed to oxidant drugs. The best and most frequent example of this is naphthalene-induced hemolytic anemia caused by exposure to mothballs. This disease is associated with a severe hemolytic anemia, hemoglobinuria, and the presence of fragmented erythrocytes and spherocytes in the circulation. If these are detected, a careful search for exposure to naphthalene or other oxidant drugs (see Table

45–6) should be carried out. This increased susceptibility to oxidative damage may be related to the low levels of antioxidants, including glutathione peroxidase, catalase, and vitamin E, in the newborn infant. Idiopathic Heinz body hemolytic anemia probably reflects a similar mechanism, resulting in hyperbilirubinemia and anemia with Heinz bodies present, but the infant has normal G6PD levels, a normal hemoglobin electrophoresis, and a negative heat test for the presence of unstable hemoglobins (146). Evaluation of the family yields no evidence of an inherited disorder, and in the affected neonate, the disorder appears to be self-limited, disappearing within the first several months of life. Vitamin C supplementation may be a factor in the etiology of idiopathic Heinz body hemolytic anemia; however, a randomized controlled trial of vitamin C in small premature newborns was unable to demonstrate hemolysis in supplemented infants (147).

Anemia Caused by Impaired Erythrocyte Production

Diamond–Blackfan Syndrome

Impaired erythrocyte production appears to be an unusual cause of anemia in the newborn. The most common cause is the Diamond–Blackfan syndrome, also known as congenital hypoplastic anemia or pure erythrocyte aplasia. In approximately one-third of infants with this abnormality, anemia exists at birth (148). The leukocyte count and platelet count are normal. Diagnosis may be established by demonstrating anemia, reticulocytopenia, and a marked decrease in the bone marrow erythroid–myeloid ratio in an otherwise healthy newborn. Erythroid–myeloid ratios range from 1:6 to more than 1:200. Low birth weight affects about 10% of these patients, about half of whom are small for gestational age. Physical anomalies are found in about 30% of patients. Anomalies apparent at birth include microcephaly, cleft palate, eye defects, web neck, and abnormalities of the thumb including triphalangeal thumbs (149). A trial of prednisone is recommended, and a response, reflected by a reticulocytosis and a rise in the hemoglobin level, often occurs within 2 weeks. After the hemoglobin has returned to normal, the medication is reduced to the lowest dose necessary to maintain hemoglobin in the acceptable range. Most patients become refractory to steroid therapy and require a lifelong transfusion program or bone marrow transplantation.

Parvovirus Infection

Hydrops fetalis is the most common manifestation of *in utero* parvovirus (HPV-B19) infection. This usually manifests during the second trimester of pregnancy and causes profound reduction of erythrocyte production, with resulting anemia and hydrops fetalis, which may be fatal. Approximately 18% of cases of nonimmune hydrops fetalis are caused by parvovirus infection (150). Locally in Toronto, eight children with parvovirus-induced nonimmune hydrops fetalis were diagnosed during the second trimester (E. Kelly and G. Ryan, *personal communication*). The four most severely affected were transfused. One died during the procedure. The hydrops resolved in the remaining seven. Six of the seven survivors were normal at 2 years of age. Thus, careful observation and transfusions are required, and because the disease is self-limited, most cases recover and are normal thereafter. Although rare, failure of red cell production has sometimes continued after birth (151). Diagnosis of parvovirus infection can be made by serologic and virologic studies of maternal blood, and infection of the fetus by viral studies of amniotic fluid or fetal blood (152).

Vitamin Deficiencies

Specific vitamin deficiencies may cause anemia in newborn infants because of decreased erythrocyte production, increased erythrocyte destruction, or a combination of these two mechanisms.

Nutritional anemia secondary to iron or folate deficiency is uncommon in neonates (153). Studies by Seip and Halvorsen indicate that stainable iron disappears from bone marrow aspirates by 12 weeks of age in premature infants and by 20 to 24 weeks in term infants, and it is only after this period that iron deficiency manifests in infants who do not receive supplemental iron (154). To prevent the development of iron deficiency, premature infants should receive supplemental iron from no later than 2 months of age. Although most premature infants have low serum folate levels by 1 to 3 months of age, they rarely manifest evidence of a megaloblastic anemia. Cases of megaloblastic anemia resulting from folate deficiency typically involve infants receiving goat's milk or phenytoin therapy and infants with chronic diarrhea or infection. Folic acid and vitamin B_{12} deficiencies are rare disorders of later infancy and have been reviewed by Shojania (155).

A syndrome thought to have been vitamin E deficiency anemia in newborn infants was first described by Hassan and colleagues in 1966 and typically occurred in premature infants (birth weight <1,500 g) at 6 weeks of age (156). Characteristic features included anemia, reticulocytosis, thrombocytosis, decreased serum vitamin E levels (<0.5 mg/dL), increased fragility of erythrocytes in the presence of dilute solutions of hydrogen peroxide, and shortened erythrocyte survival (157). Damage to the erythrocyte membrane by lipid peroxides, formed naturally during peroxidation of polyunsaturated fatty acids (PUFA) in the erythrocyte membrane, was thought to be the mechanism of the anemia; vitamin E, a biological antioxidant, inactivates lipid peroxides and protects against erythrocyte damage. The anemia may be exaggerated by increasing the PUFA content of the diet, particularly if infants are also given supplemental iron, a catalyst in the autooxidation of PUFA to free radicals and lipid peroxides (158). After the association among the PUFA content of the diet, iron supplementation, and the vitamin E requirement of premature infants was recognized, the PUFA content of infant formulas was reduced. Vitamin E deficiency as described above has become rare in premature infants, and there is no evidence that routine vitamin E supplementation is of benefit in preventing the anemia of prematurity (159).

Diagnosis

At no other time does such a variety of disorders result in anemia as in the first week of life. The need for rapid treatment often adds to the diagnostic confusion. It is because of the multiple causes and the need for prompt therapy that the fundamentals of diagnosis should be appreciated and practiced without delay. Attempts at diagnosis begin with a history if the cause is not immediately apparent. In the family history, attention should be paid to anemia in other members of the family or to unexplained episodes of jaundice, cholelithiasis, or splenectomy. A positive family history is frequently obtained in cases of infants with hereditary spherocytosis, but a history of affected siblings may be encountered in cases of patients with enzymatic defects of the erythrocyte.

In the maternal history, information should be obtained concerning both her and her husband's ethnic origins and her drug ingestion near term. Information about drugs known to initiate hemolysis in cases of G6PD deficiency should especially be sought and any history of recent exposure to mothballs containing naphthalene.

The obstetric history should provide information about vaginal bleeding during pregnancy, placenta previa, abruptio placentae, vasa previa, and cesarean section. Additional questions should be answered. Was the birth traumatic? Did the cord rupture? Was it a multiple birth?

The age at which anemia is first noticed is also of diagnostic value. Marked anemia at birth is usually the result of hemorrhage or severe isoimmunization. Anemia manifesting itself during the first 2 days of life is frequently caused by external or internal hemorrhages, but anemia appearing after the first 48 hours of life is most commonly hemolytic and is usually associated with jaundice.

One approach to the differential diagnosis of anemia in the newborn period is presented in Fig. 45–12. The physician should first decide whether the low hemoglobin level can be explained by blood loss from sampling. Cumulative losses, particularly in ill premature infants, may be extremely large, and correct interpretation of rapid changes in hemoglobin level can be made only if careful attention is paid to exact volumes of blood sampled and transfused. If the cause of anemia remains unknown, several laboratory tests may aid in diagnosis: reticulocyte count, a direct antiglobulin test (i.e., Coombs test) of the

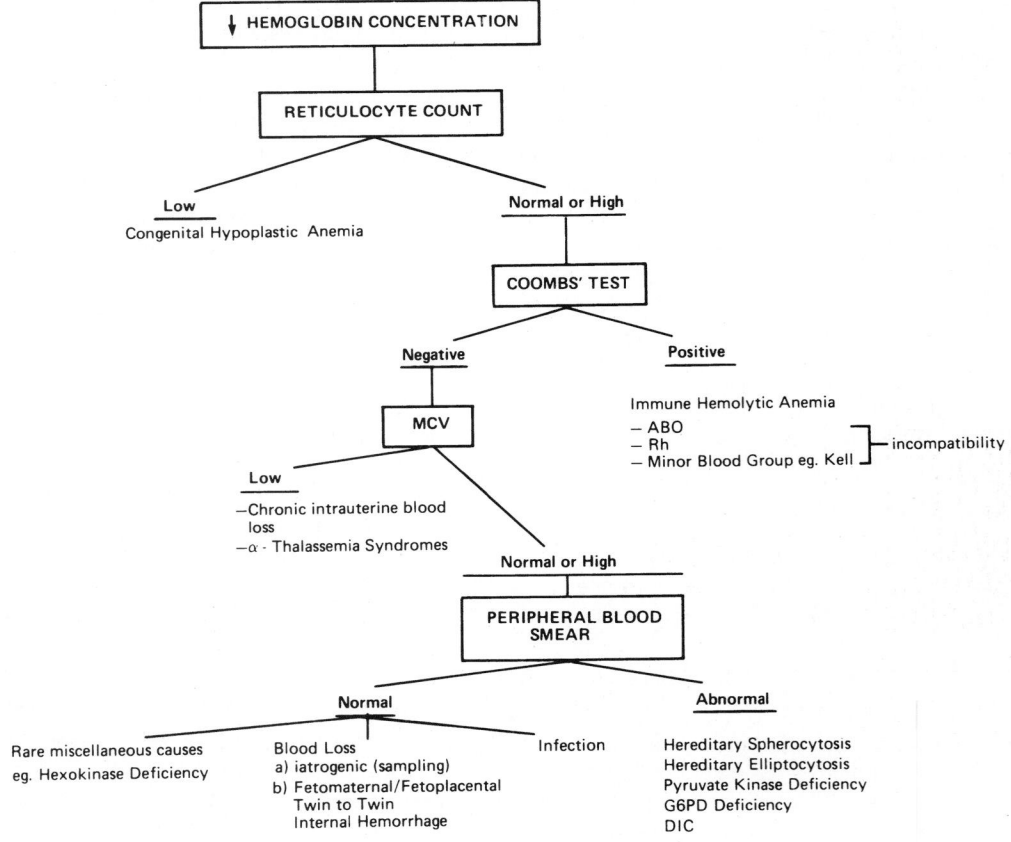

FIG. 45–12. Diagnostic approach to anemia in the newborn infant.

infant's blood, examination of a peripheral blood smear, and examination of the maternal blood smear for fetal erythrocytes. Ultrasound examination of the head or abdomen is useful to detect occult blood loss. From these studies and the history, a diagnosis often can be made, or at least the list of diagnostic possibilities can be greatly shortened.

POLYCYTHEMIA

A venous hemoglobin exceeding 22.0 g/dL or a venous hematocrit more than 65% during the first week of life should be regarded as polycythemia. Although neonatal polycythemia may be the result of fetal disorders such as twin-to-twin transfusion, placental insufficiency, and certain metabolic disorders (Table 45–7), most cases occur in otherwise normal infants. Most of these infants have been full term, appropriate for gestational age, and without asphyxia at birth. Polycythemia occurs in 1.5% to 4% of newborn infants (160–162).

The symptoms observed in the polycythemic infant appear to be primarily a consequence of hypervolemia and an increase in blood viscosity. After the central venous hematocrit reaches 60% to 65%, the increase in blood viscosity becomes much greater as a result of the

TABLE 45–7. *Neonatal polycythemia*

Possible causes by placental hypertransfusion
  Twin-to-twin transfusion
  Maternofetal transfusion
  Delayed cord clamping
    Intentional
    Unassisted home delivery
Possible associations
  Placental insufficiency
    Small-for-gestational-age infants
    Postmaturity birth
    Toxemia of pregnancy
  Placental previa
  Endocrine and metabolic disorders
    Congenital adrenal hyperplasia
    Neonatal thyrotoxicosis
    Maternal diabetes
  Miscellaneous
    Trisomies 21, 13, and 19
    Hyperplastic visceromegaly (i.e., Beckwith syndrome)
    Erythroderma icthyosiforme congenita

exponential relationship between hematocrit and viscosity (163). Plasma and erythrocyte factors also affect the viscosity of neonatal blood (164–166).

Respiratory distress, cyanosis, congestive heart failure, convulsions, priapism, jaundice, renal vein thrombosis, hypoglycemia, and hypocalcemia appear to be more common in infants with polycythemia (160). Many infants with polycythemia are asymptomatic.

In addition to supportive care, partial exchange transfusion with 5% albumin has been used for the treatment of polycythemia. Reduction of the venous hematocrit to less than 60% may improve symptoms, but it has not been shown to improve long-term neurologic outcome (167–169).

FETAL HEMOGLOBIN, NEONATAL ERYTHROCYTES, AND 2,3-DIPHOSPHOGLYCERATE

Human tissue metabolism depends critically on an adequate supply of oxygen. The oxygen transport system in humans is the erythrocyte, which contains the iron–protein conjugate hemoglobin. The erythrocyte's primary function is to bring oxygen to the tissues in adequate quantities at a partial pressure sufficient to permit its rapid diffusion from the blood. The ultimate supply of oxygen to the cell is determined by a number of factors, including the content of oxygen in the inspired air, the pulmonary and alveolar ventilation, the diffusion of oxygen from the alveolar air to the capillary bed, the cardiac output, the blood volume, the hemoglobin concentration, and the passive diffusion of oxygen from the capillaries to the cells. The initial passive diffusion of oxygen from the lungs and its final release to the tissues are largely determined by the affinity of hemoglobin for oxygen.

The oxygen–hemoglobin equilibrium curve reflects the affinity of hemoglobin for oxygen (Fig. 45–13). As blood circulates in the normal lung, arterial oxygen tension rises from 40 mm Hg and reaches approximately 110 mm Hg, sufficient to ensure at least 95% saturation of the arterial blood. The shape of the curve is such that a further increase in the oxygen tension in the lung results in only a small increase in the degree of saturation of the blood. As blood travels from the lung, the oxygen tension falls as oxygen is released to the tissues from hemoglobin. In the normal adult, when the oxygen tension has fallen to approximately 27 mm Hg, at a pH of 7.4 and a temperature of 37°C, 50% of the oxygen bound to hemoglobin has been released. The P_{50}, the whole-blood oxygen tension at 50% oxygen saturation, is 27 mm Hg. If the affinity of hemoglobin for oxygen is reduced, more oxygen is released to the tissues at a given oxygen tension. In such situations, the oxygen–hemoglobin equilibrium curve is shifted to the right of normal. It has long been recognized that increases in blood acidity, carbon dioxide content, ionic concentration, and temperature are

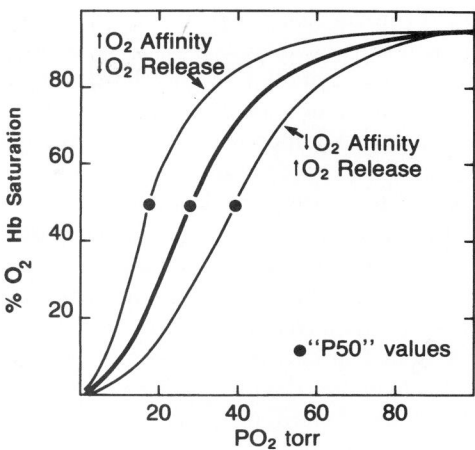

FIG. 45–13. The oxygen dissociation curve of normal adult blood. The oxygen tension at 50% oxygen saturation (P50) is approximately 27 torr. As the curve shifts to the right, the oxygen affinity of the hemoglobin decreases, and more oxygen is released at a given oxygen tension. With a shift to the left, the opposite effects are observed. A decrease in pH or an increase in temperature decreases the affinity of hemoglobin for oxygen.

capable of decreasing the affinity of hemoglobin for oxygen and shifting the curve to the right. If the affinity of hemoglobin for oxygen is increased, as occurs with alkalosis or a decrease in temperature, the equilibrium curve appears shifted to the left, and the tension must drop lower than normal before the hemoglobin releases an equivalent amount of oxygen.

The oxygen dissociation curve of the erythrocytes of newborn infants is shifted to the left, reflecting an increase in the affinity of the hemoglobin for oxygen, compared with the blood of adults (see Fig. 45–13). This shift results primarily from the fact that binding of 2,3-diphosphoglycerate to HbF is less than that to HbA (171). As a result, the unloading of oxygen in the tissues requires a greater fall of oxygen tension in the newborn than in adults. Conversely, the uptake of oxygen in the lung is enhanced in newborns. It is not clear whether this phenomenon is a benefit or handicap to newborns; presumably, its role in intrauterine life was to permit greater movement of oxygen from the mother to the fetus. There is no evidence that provision of blood containing HbA improves tissue oxygenation in the newborn.

BLEEDING DISORDERS

The hemostatic system is not completely developed at birth, and this may affect the appearance and interpretation of bleeding disorders. There is little evidence to suggest that this incomplete development places neonates at increased risk of hemorrhage, although they may be more prone to thrombosis. However, in the neonatal period, many hemorrhagic problems appear as a result of the diseases and disorders that occur at that time of life. The study of hemorrhagic disorders in the newborn period demands an understanding of the development of the hemostatic system, of congenital and acquired factors that can affect it, and appreciation of the role of disease in producing disturbances in the system.

Because of the incomplete development of the hemostatic system, interpretation of laboratory tests requires knowledge of normal values for infants of similar gestational and postnatal age, as shown in Table 45–8. The complexity of hemorrhagic disorders in the neonatal period demands that laboratory testing be as complete as possible. This requires the use of microtechnology for the assessment of the hemostatic system in the newborn. A complete assessment can be done with as little as 0.2 mL of plasma.

There are several important features of the coagulation system in the newborn (see Table 45–8). The prothrombin time of full-term and premature infants is only slightly outside the adult range of 10 to 12 seconds. The partial thromboplastin time (PTT), which is a frequently used screening test in adults, is much longer in newborn infants, particularly premature infants. Prolongation of the PTT in newborns often results from a reduction in contact factors XI and XII and may not pose a bleeding problem. Factors XI and XII are low in premature infants (a mean of 23% and 25% of adult values, respectively), rising to 30% and 38%, respectively, in full-term infants (172). Substantial prolongation of the PTT (by depression of factors XI and XII) has been observed in children with sepsis without evidence of hemorrhage, leading to the conclusion that the PTT is of little value in the sick newborn. The two-unit thrombin time is a valuable screening test because it can detect heparin contamination and fibrinogen deficiency. Bleeding disorders in newborn infants are best separated into local bleeding problems and generalized hemorrhagic diatheses.

Local Bleeding Problems

Bleeding in newborn infants can occur from the cord, into the scalp, into the gastrointestinal tract, into the abdomen (e.g., liver, adrenal glands), and into the lung. There is little evidence to suggest that the physiologically low levels of coagulation factors in the newborn play any role in the genesis of these disorders.

Intraventricular hemorrhage (IVH) is a major problem of premature infants (see Chaps. 49 and 50). There is little evidence to suggest that a hemorrhagic diathesis underlies this disorder. Therapeutic trials of infusing plasma or coagulation factor concentrates have been equivocal or unsuccessful. Although it is likely that IVH occurs as a result of local phenomena related to hypoxia, hemodynamic changes, and prematurity, it is possible that a deficiency of hemostasis may contribute to the continuation of the hemorrhage. Supportive evidence for this is found in the preliminary trials of ethamsylate, an agent that appears to affect the platelet capillary component of hemostasis and that was found in one study to prevent or diminish the severity of IVH (173).

Acquired Hemorrhagic Diathesis

Major causes of generalized acquired hemorrhagic diatheses as a result of blood coagulation factor deficiency in the newborn period are vitamin K deficiency hemorrhagic disease of the newborn, disseminated intravascular coagulation (DIC), and liver disease.

Vitamin K Deficiency

Newborn infants have a tendency to hemorrhage spontaneously in the first days of life. This has been referred to as hemorrhagic disease of the newborn. It was shown many years ago that the administration of vitamin K at birth prevented hemorrhagic disease of the newborn, the

TABLE 45–8. *Screening tests for bleeding disorders[a]*

Test	Adults	Full-term infants	Disease-free premature infants[b]
Prothrombin time (seconds)	12 ± 1	14 ± 1.3	14 ± 1.3
Partial thromboplastin time (seconds)	42 ± 4	51 ± 10	57 ± 10.5
Thrombin clotting time (2 U)	25 ± 2	23 ± 2.9	23 ± 2.4
Factor II (%)	81 ± 17[c]	50 ± 14.5	31 ± 8.6
Factor V (%)	90 ± 19	79 ± 17	70 ± 22
Factor VII–X (%)	93 ± 20	54 ± 12.2	37 ± 11
Factor VIII (%)	87 ± 27	126 ± 56	116 ± 73
Factor IX (%)	99 ± 23	35 ± 12.6	28 ± 11
Factor X (%)	89 ± 23	45 ± 12	31 ± 9.0
Antithrombin III (%)	99 ± 10	58 ± 9.6	33 ± 9.0
Fibrinogen (mg/dL)[d]	315 ± 60	215 ± 35	256 ± 20

[a]All results are expressed as means ± SD.
[b]Infants of birth weight less than 1,500 g who were free of any clinical disease.
[c]Data from Johnston M, Zipursky A. Microtechnology for the study of the blood coagulation system in newborn infants. Can J Med Technol 1980;42:133.
[d]Data from Hathaway WE, Bonnar J. *Perinatal coagulation.* New York: Grune & Stratton, 1978:56.

classic form of which occurs in the first week of life. It has become an accepted procedure to administer 1 mg of vitamin K_1 oxide intramuscularly at birth, and as a result, hemorrhagic disease in the newborn has virtually disappeared. However, there has been controversy about the question of vitamin K deficiency in newborns and the need for prophylactic treatment. Vitamin K is a cofactor necessary for the γ-carboxylation of a prothrombin precursor to active prothrombin. In the absence of vitamin K, this precursor [proteins induced by vitamin K absence (PIVKA)] can be detected in the plasma (174). Because PIVKA was found in only one-third of term infants, it has been suggested that not all infants are vitamin K–deficient, and not all need to receive prophylactic vitamin K (175), Some studies have shown that, unlike adults, normal newborns demonstrate no vitamin K in their serum, and therefore, relative to adults, they are vitamin K deficient (176). In several cases of hemorrhagic disease of the newborn, Dreyfus and colleagues observed low levels of vitamin K–dependent factors and high levels of PIVKA and a response to vitamin K (176). Current evidence suggests that many newborn infants are vitamin K deficient, even though elevated PIVKA levels are not found in all of them. Because it is not possible to select babies who are likely to bleed, it is recommended that all babies receive 1 mg of vitamin K_1 at birth.

Babies born to mothers who are on anticonvulsant medication are at particularly high risk of having vitamin K deficiency (e.g., early hemorrhagic disease of the newborn), and these mothers should receive vitamin K before delivery (177). Late hemorrhagic disease of newborns (i.e., vitamin K deficiency hemorrhagic disease) manifests at 4 to 6 weeks of age. Infants with this disease characteristically have not received vitamin K prophylaxis at birth; have been maintained on breast milk, which is low in vitamin K; and may have suffered from diarrhea or cholestatic liver disease (178). This disorder continues to be reported from areas in which routine prophylaxis is not given (179) or in which oral Vitamin K has been used as a single dose during the first days of life (180). Oral vitamin K is effective in preventing early hemorrhagic disease but is not effective in preventing late hemorrhagic disease (181–183). There have been reports that intramuscular vitamin K prophylactic therapy in newborns may increase the risk of malignant disease in childhood. Recent studies including two fully designed case-control studies have proven that this is not a risk (180). It is recommended, therefore, that vitamin K be given intramuscularly to all infants in order to prevent hemorrhagic disease of the newborn (180).

Disseminated Intravascular Coagulation

There have been many reports of disseminated intravascular coagulation (DIC) in newborn infants associated with a variety of diseases. Some reports suggest that most cases of DIC in neonates are caused by cardiovascular collapse (184). This refers to those infants who have had an episode of cardiac arrest, an Apgar score of 0 to 1, or an episode of profound hypotension.

The infant is found to have a generalized hemorrhagic diathesis with bleeding from venipuncture sites, bruising, and widespread internal hemorrhage. Blood studies reveal prolongation of screening tests (e.g., prothrombin time, PTT, thrombin time), elevated fibrin split products or D-dimers, depressed factor V levels, and hypofibrinogenemia. Platelet counts may be normal or only slightly depressed. The findings in this syndrome should be differentiated from those observed in sepsis or necrotizing enterocolitis, in which thrombocytopenia is severe, coagulation factors may be normal or slightly reduced, and bleeding is minimal (184).

Disseminated intravascular coagulation in newborns is treated first by the correction of cardiovascular collapse. If the circulation is restored to normal, the coagulopathy will correct itself spontaneously. If bleeding is a problem, replacement therapy with cryoprecipitate, 0.5 U/kg (10 mL/kg), and, if necessary, platelet concentrate should be given. After correction of the coagulopathy, patients should be monitored at 4-hour intervals with prothrombin time and fibrinogen levels. If fibrinogen falls, the DIC is continuing.

The syndrome of DIC is typically a difficult problem, complicating a serious illness in an infant. Diagnosis and treatment of the hemorrhagic diathesis are relatively straightforward. Unfortunately, the underlying disease and the ischemic damage caused by the cardiovascular collapse and the DIC result in high mortality rates (184).

Other Causes of Acquired Bleeding Disorders

Profound liver disease can produce a hemorrhagic diathesis as a result of vitamin K deficiency or a primary failure of production of coagulation factors.

Despite the use of small doses of heparin to maintain intravenous and intraarterial catheters, a hemorrhagic diathesis from heparin therapy is unusual. However, it is not uncommon in studies of newborn infants for blood samples to be contaminated with heparin. All laboratories studying blood coagulation in newborns should be able to detect heparin contamination.

Congenital Hemorrhagic Disorders in the Neonatal Period

Hemophilia A (factor VIII deficiency) and hemophilia B (factor IX deficiency) may present with bleeding symptoms in the newborn period (185). Because of gender-linked inheritance, male infants are affected. All cases of hemophilia A can be diagnosed at birth because the lower limit of the reference range for factor VIII (<50% or 0 to 0.05 U/mL) is similar to the adult value.

Although the severe (<1%) and moderate (1% to 5%) forms of hemophilia B can be confidently diagnosed in the neonatal period, children with the mild forms may require investigation in later infancy because their levels of factor IX may fall within the lower limit of the reference range for full-term and premature infants at birth (see Table 45–8) (186). The delay in confirming the diagnosis is usually of no consequence because children with mild deficiencies of factor IX are not at risk for spontaneous bleeding.

The bleeding manifestations of neonatal hemophilia include scalp hematomas, prolonged bleeding from venipuncture sites or from surgical procedures such as circumcision, and intracranial hemorrhage. Management of bleeding involves the infusion of factor VIII or IX to restore hemostasis; the replacement product of choice is a factor concentrate treated during preparation to inactivate the acquired immunodeficiency syndrome (AIDS) and hepatitis viruses (187). Factor IX concentrates should not be used in newborns other than those with known factor IX deficiency (hemophilia B) because of the risk of inducing thrombosis secondary to low antithrombin III levels.

Deficiencies of factors II, V, VII, VIII, and X and of fibrinogen are inherited in an autosomal manner. The homozygous forms of the disorders may present with bleeding in the newborn period. Delayed bleeding from the umbilical stump is characteristic of homozygous factor XIII deficiency or of a severe quantitative or qualitative abnormality of fibrinogen (188). Screening coagulation tests (e.g., prothrombin time, PTT, thrombin time) are normal in patients with factor XIII deficiency, and the diagnosis should be confirmed by specific factor assay. Treatment of the coagulation factor deficiencies involves infusion of stored plasma (except for factor V), fresh-frozen plasma, or specific factor concentrates.

Bleeding is uncommon in newborns with von Willebrand disease (189). The diagnosis of von Willebrand disease cannot be made with confidence in the newborn period because levels of von Willebrand factor are elevated at birth, masking the presence of most forms of von Willebrand disease (190).

Platelet Disorders

A platelet count less than 150×10^9/L is abnormal in term and premature infants (191). The level of platelets in the blood reflects a balance between their production and destruction. Thrombocytopenia may result from decreased production, increased destruction, or a combination of both. Examination of a well-stained smear of peripheral blood to assess platelet morphology and number and of bone marrow to assess megakaryocyte morphology and number has traditionally yielded important information concerning the mechanism of thrombocytopenia. Decreased numbers of platelets and megakaryocytes indicate a production defect, and megakaryocytic hyperplasia and the presence of megathrombocytes (i.e., young large platelets) in a peripheral blood smear are characteristic of thrombocytopenic states in which there is increased peripheral destruction of platelets. Unfortunately, these indices are not as useful in newborn infants as in older children or adults because the number of megakaryocytes in bone marrow aspirates obtained even from healthy newborn infants often appears reduced. In our (V.S., A.Z.) experience, aspirates obtained from the iliac crest are more satisfactory than those obtained from the tibia.

There are many causes of thrombocytopenia in the newborn. The most common of these disorders appear in Table 45–9 and have been reviewed elsewhere (191,192).

Neonatal Immune Thrombocytopenia

Immune thrombocytopenia occurs when antibody-sensitized platelets are prematurely destroyed in the reticuloendothelial system, particularly the spleen. Characteristic laboratory features include isolated thrombocytopenia and an increased number of immature megakaryocytes in a bone marrow aspirate. Elevated levels of platelet-bound IgG can be demonstrated in many cases.

A variety of conditions are associated with the transplacental passage of antibody, resulting in immunologic destruction of the infant's platelets. The antibody may be formed against an antigen on the platelets of the infant (isoimmune or alloimmune thrombocytopenia, in which case the mother's platelet count is normal) or an antigen present on the platelets of the mother (autoimmune thrombocytopenia, in which case both the mother and child may have thrombocytopenia), as occurs in

TABLE 45–9. *Causes of neonatal thrombocytopenia*

Decreased production of platelets
  Congenital megakaryocytic hypoplasia
    Thrombocytopenia–absent radius syndrome
    Megakaryocytic hypoplasia without anomalies
  Congenital leukemias and histiocytoses
  Inherited thrombocytopenias
    Wiskott–Aldrich syndrome
    Other X-linked or recessively transmitted
    thrombocytopenias
Increased destruction of platelets
  Immune thrombocytopenias
    Neonatal alloimmune thrombocytopenia
    Neonatal autoimmune thrombocytopenia
    Drug-induced thrombocytopenia
  Giant hemangioma syndrome
  Other states with disseminated intravascular coagulation
Both decreased production and increased destruction
    of platelets
  Infections
    Congenital, usually viral
    Acquired, usually bacterial
  Osteopetrosis

maternal immune thrombocytopenic purpura (ITP) or thrombocytopenia associated with a collagen vascular disorder such as systemic lupus erythematosus.

Neonatal Isoimmune Thrombocytopenia

In neonatal isoimmune or alloimmune thrombocytopenia, the infant possesses a platelet antigen of paternal origin that is lacking in the mother. Typically, the infant's platelets cross the placenta into the maternal circulation during pregnancy or at the time of delivery and cause immunization of the mother, with the formation of antibodies against the foreign platelet antigen. Less frequently, the cause of immunization is exposure of an antigen-negative mother to antigen-positive platelets during transfusion. During pregnancy, transplacental passage of the maternal IgG antibodies leads to sensitization of fetal platelets. Sensitized platelets are rapidly destroyed in the fetal reticuloendothelial system, particularly the spleen, and the result may be thrombocytopenia in utero and in the infant at the time of delivery. This mechanism is analogous to that causing hemolytic disease of the newborn.

The platelet-specific antigen system most often involved in cases of neonatal alloimmune thrombocytopenia is PlA1 (193,194). Other platelet-specific antigens are involved less frequently (195–201). In the largest series of cases of suspected neonatal alloimmune thrombocytopenia, 91% (120 of 132) of serologically proven cases involved PlA1 alloantibodies (197). Of the remaining 12 cases, the pathologic alloantibodies were anti-Bra-9, anti-PlA2-1, anti-Baka with HLA antibody-1, and blood group B isoagglutinins-1. Although HLA alloantibodies often develop as a result of pregnancy, they rarely are the cause of severe neonatal thrombocytopenia.

The incidence of neonatal alloimmune thrombocytopenia is estimated to be one per 5,000 live births or less (202). In fact, the incidence of platelet alloimmunization is probably higher, on the order of one in 1,000 to 2,000 pregnancies in a Caucasian population. This opinion is based on the finding of three cases of PlA1 alloimmunization in a prospective study of 5,000 pregnant women (203).

The typical infant with neonatal alloimmune thrombocytopenia is term, and thrombocytopenia is unexpected. Cutaneous manifestations of severe thrombocytopenia (e.g., bruising, petechial rash) are often the only abnormalities found on physical examination. A complete blood count shows severe isolated thrombocytopenia with a normal hemoglobin and leukocyte count.

Affected infants are at risk for serious hemorrhage, particularly into the central nervous system (CNS). In a review by Pearson and colleagues, the incidence of fatal hemorrhage was 10% to 15% (202). In some cases, CNS hemorrhage occurs in utero before delivery (204–208). Bussell and colleagues estimated that as many as 25% of CNS hemorrhage cases associated with neonatal alloimmune thrombocytopenia occur antenatally (209).

Early diagnosis and effective therapy of infants with neonatal alloimmune thrombocytopenia is important. The disorder should be suspected in all infants with severe, isolated thrombocytopenia in whom a specific cause for the thrombocytopenic state cannot be identified (e.g., sepsis, DIC, and skeletal anomalies such as absent radii) and if the maternal platelet count is normal. These infants should receive antigen-negative, compatible platelets harvested from the mother or a phenotyped blood donor. If maternal platelets are used, supernatant plasma with pathologic antibody should be removed by centrifugation or washing, and the compatible maternal platelets infused after irradiation. In clinical practice, severely thrombocytopenic infants (i.e., platelet counts $< 30 \times 10^9$/L) are often initially transfused with a unit of random donor platelets; in such cases, the platelet response is of diagnostic value (210,211). Because most persons type positively for the PlA1 and Baka antigens (98% and 88%, respectively), most random donor platelets are incompatible in cases of neonatal alloimmune thrombocytopenia because of these alloantigens, and their infusion fails to produce a satisfactory posttransfusion platelet increment. In situations in which alloimmune thrombocytopenia is clinically suspected, this pattern of response provides additional evidence for the diagnosis, and it is then most important that severely affected infants receive compatible antigen-negative platelets collected from the mother or blood donors of known antigen type. Regional blood centers serving large neonatal intensive care units should be encouraged to develop a small bank of blood donors phenotyped for common platelet antigens who are readily available for donation. In selected cases, it may be useful to harvest and store in the frozen state the platelets from mothers or antigen-negative donors for immediate use if an affected infant is anticipated (212).

Other therapeutic interventions for neonatal alloimmune thrombocytopenia include exchange transfusion to remove pathologic antibody and intravenous administration of large doses of immunoglobulin G. This latter strategy is of proven benefit in children with ITP and has been used with variable success in infants with alloimmune thrombocytopenia (213–218). However, if compatible platelets can be quickly obtained, these additional therapeutic interventions are rarely indicated. If compatible platelets cannot be obtained, or if a significant delay can be anticipated before this ideal product will be available, the therapy of choice is a trial of high-dose intravenous IgG. Current practice is to administer a total dose of 2 g/kg of body weight, given as 1 g/kg over 6 to 8 hours on each of two consecutive days. Corticosteroid therapy (e.g., prednisone) is of no proven benefit if used in the traditional dose of 1 to 2 mg/kg/day.

The risk of the disorder recurring in subsequent pregnancies is high; approximately 75% of the offspring of a sensitized PlA1-negative woman manifest thrombocytopenia. Because of the significant risk of CNS hemorrhage *in utero*, especially in cases of PlA1 alloimmunization with a history of a previously severely affected infant, most experts involved with management of these high-risk pregnancies advocate determination of the fetal platelet count by percutaneous umbilical vessel sampling (PUBS) at 18 to 20 weeks of gestation. If the fetus is determined to have severe thrombocytopenia, weekly administration of intravenous IgG to the mother is started and continued until delivery (209,219).

There is good evidence now from a randomized controlled trial that intravenous γ-globulin administered to the mother is effective in preventing CNS hemorrhage (220). It is recommended, therefore, that this be the therapy of choice but that the fetus should be followed by repeated PUBS (221). This procedure presents the danger of exsanguination, and accordingly, it should be followed by a platelet transfusion of the fetus (221). Although the benefit of *in utero* transfusion of compatible platelets has been reported, the relatively short half-life of even compatible donor platelets makes this approach impractical (219). The route of delivery is determined by the fetal platelet count obtained by PUBS or scalp vein sampling before delivery; of these two methods, PUBS is preferred because of its higher accuracy. If the fetal platelet count is less than 50×10^9/L, delivery by cesarean section is recommended. At the time of delivery, a cord blood platelet count should be obtained, and thrombocytopenia should be verified in a peripheral blood sample obtained shortly after delivery. If the infant is severely thrombocytopenic, compatible platelets should be infused immediately. These high-risk pregnancies should be managed by a team of perinatologists, neonatologists, and hematologists.

Neonatal Autoimmune Thrombocytopenia

Clinical and laboratory features of neonatal autoimmune thrombocytopenia parallel those of the alloimmune state. In both disorders, the observation of ecchymoses, a petechial rash, or both in an otherwise well infant may be the first clue to the disorder. Measurement of a maternal platelet count and examination of a peripheral blood smear obtained from the mother can help to differentiate autoimmune from alloimmune neonatal thrombocytopenia. In neonatal alloimmune thrombocytopenia, the maternal peripheral blood smear and platelet count are normal, but in the autoimmune condition (i.e., mothers with ITP), the platelet count is reduced, and the existing platelets are often large (i.e., megathrombocytes). Occasionally, the finding of unexpected thrombocytopenia in an infant may lead to the diagnosis of previously unrecognized ITP in the mother. Autoimmune thrombocytopenia may occur in infants of mothers with ITP who have normal platelet counts after splenectomy. Occasionally in mothers with ITP, increased bone marrow activity can compensate for accelerated destruction of antibody-sen-

sitized platelets. These women may have normal platelet counts, but their infants are at risk of developing acquired thrombocytopenia.

Management of infants with autoimmune neonatal thrombocytopenia differs from that of those with the alloimmune form of the disease. Compatible platelets cannot be found because platelet autoantibodies react with all donor platelets. Therapeutic options include exchange transfusion to remove passively acquired maternal autoantibodies, corticosteroids, and high-dose intravenous immunoglobulin G. In infants with significant thrombocytopenia (i.e., platelet counts $<50 \times 10^9$/L) or clinical bleeding, the authors favor administration of immunoglobulin G in a dose of 1 g/kg daily for two consecutive days. A marked increment in platelet count can be anticipated within 24 to 48 hours in 75% of patients (222,223). If this response is not observed, exchange transfusion should be considered and oral corticosteroids started (e.g., prednisone or an equivalent corticosteroid at a dose of 3 to 4 mg/kg/day initially, with rapid tapering once the platelet count increases above 50×10^9/L). Splenectomy should not be considered in newborn infants unless there is a real clinical emergency with life-threatening bleeding into the CNS and no effective alternative.

The same considerations apply to the route of delivery as have been outlined in the discussion of neonatal alloimmune thrombocytopenia. The maternal platelet count and levels of platelet-bound IgG and serum platelet antibody do not predict with certainty which infants will be thrombocytopenic (224–226). The management of the pregnant woman with chronic ITP (or ITP in remission after splenectomy) has been controversial. Recent studies indicate that the severity of the disease is much less than previously reported and that the occurrence of intracranial hemorrhage is rare (227,228). Accordingly, intrauterine diagnosis by cordocentesis is rarely indicated because it does not contribute to management and is a risk to the fetus. Although the benefit of cesarian section in these cases has not been established, it has been recommended for those fetuses who are severely thrombocytopenic (as determined by scalp sampling) (228).

Other Forms of Thrombocytopenia

A variety of other disorders may produce a reduction in platelet count. Thrombocytopenia is particularly common in ill infants admitted to neonatal intensive care units. In a prospective study of 807 consecutive infants admitted to a regional intensive care neonatal center, Castle and colleagues reported a 22% incidence of thrombocytopenia, defined as a platelet count of less than 50×10^9/L (229). In 38% of thrombocytopenic infants, the platelet count was 50 to 100×10^9/L, and in 20%, the platelet count was less than 50×10^9/L. Thrombocytopenia was associated with laboratory evidence of increased platelet destruction or DIC in

52% and 21% of patients, respectively. There was an association of thrombocytopenia with birth asphyxia. Although only 7% of the thrombocytopenic infants had positive blood cultures, sepsis is an important cause of neonatal thrombocytopenia, and a low platelet count may be an early clue to infection in this patient population (218). Inherited defects in platelet production or platelet function also manifest themselves during this period of life.

An approach to the multiple diagnostic possibilities is outlined in Fig. 45–14. In this scheme, it is as important to study the mother as it is to study the infant and to examine the placenta (i.e., for multiple hemangiomas). Points requiring specific inquiry include a history of previous bleeding in the form of purpura, bruising, or nosebleeds that might suggest a diagnosis of maternal ITP at some time in the past; ingestion of drugs that may cause thrombocytopenia in the mother and infant (e.g., quinidine, quinine); previous siblings affected with purpura, suggesting one of the immune or inherited thrombocytopenias; and skin rash or exposure to rubella in the first 8 weeks of pregnancy. Serologic evidence of congenital infections (e.g., syphilis, CMV, herpesvirus, toxoplasmosis) should be sought and recorded. An accurate maternal platelet count should be performed as soon as possible after delivery so that immune neonatal thrombocytopenia caused by maternal ITP can be differentiated from that caused by platelet isoimmunization, in which case the mother's platelet count is normal.

Physical findings of importance in differential diagnosis of the affected newborn include hepatosplenomegaly and congenital anomalies. Hepatosplenomegaly is often accompanied by jaundice and suggests an infectious process as the most likely cause of thrombocytopenia. In some cases, congenital leukemia may have to be considered. Among the congenital anomalies associated with neonatal thrombocytopenia, the commonest group recognizable at birth is that occurring in the rubella syndrome (i.e., congenital heart defects, cataracts, and microcephaly). Deformity and shortening of the forearms should suggest bilateral absence of the radii, with associated amegakaryocytic thrombocytopenia. A single large hemangioma or multiple smaller hemangiomas point to possible platelet trapping and indicate a search for bruits produced by internal hemangiomas.

A complete blood count on the infant should include hemoglobin determination, leukocyte count, platelet count, and a smear. Associated anemia may result from blood loss, concurrent hemolysis (e.g., in an infectious processes), or marrow infiltration caused by congenital leukemia. Leukocytosis of a mild degree may accompany infection or blood loss, but if this exceeds 40,000 to 50,000/μL, it may point to congenital leukemia. Bone

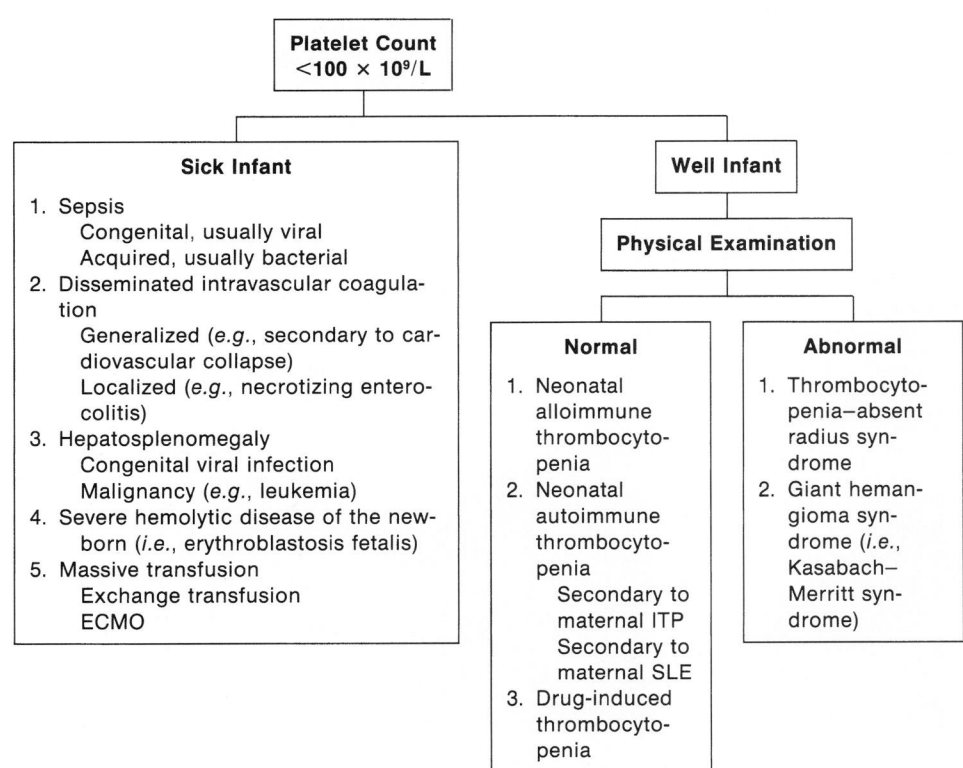

FIG. 45–14. Approach to the diagnosis of the thrombocytopenic newborn. (ECMO, extracorporeal membrane oxygenation; ITP, immune thrombocytopenic purpura; SLE, systemic lupus erythematosus.)

marrow examination should be considered if thrombocytopenia is persistent and a specific cause cannot be identified. Serologic tests for platelet antibodies and platelet antigen typing are available in reference laboratories. If isoimmune thrombocytopenia is suspected by the finding of an otherwise normal newborn with thrombocytopenia and a healthy mother with a normal platelet count, blood should be drawn from the parents soon after delivery for serologic testing. Characteristically, the maternal serum contains an antibody reactive against paternal platelets. Platelet antigen typing should be performed on both parents, if available; in cases of neonatal alloimmune thrombocytopenia, the mother will type negative and the father positive for the pathologic platelet-specific antigen. In this situation, the infant's platelet type is assumed to be identical to that of the father because it is usually not possible to obtain sufficient blood from severely thrombocytopenic newborn infants for extensive serologic testing. Results of platelet studies may not be available for some time, and therapy should not be delayed pending their results.

LEUKOCYTE DISORDERS

A diverse group of leukocyte disorders is encountered in newborn infants. Different blood cells are involved (e.g., neutrophils, lymphocytes, eosinophils), and the disorders may be quantitative or qualitative in nature. This section focuses on abnormalities that are particularly relevant to newborn infants because of the frequency with which they are encountered (e.g., neutrophil changes associated with bacterial infections) or because they are unique to this age group (e.g., congenital leukemia, neonatal alloimmune neutropenia).

Neutrophil Disorders

Normal Leukocyte Count in the Neonatal Period

Counts of segmented and band (i.e., nonsegmented, young) neutrophils of healthy full-term infants studied by us during the first 5 days of life are illustrated in Fig. 45–15 (230).

In premature infants, neutrophil counts during the first 5 days of life are similar to or slightly lower than those in full-term infants (see Fig. 45–15). In a series of 180 premature infants, mean values were found at 0, 24, and 120 hours to be 4,000, 7,500, and 3,500/mm³, respectively (Fig. 45–16) (231). Similar values have been found by others (232–234). Peak values excluding the top 2.5% were 8,000, 15,500, and 8,500/mm³, which is significantly lower than the values for full-term infants (see Fig. 45–16).

The lower limit for a normal neutrophil count in full-term and premature infants is not clearly established. In a series of 180 infants, some of the infants were found to have values of 0 without a cause (231). Xanthou (232), Coulombel (233), and Lloyd and Oto (234) reported smaller series that indicated that a neutrophil count less than 1,000/mm³ would be considered abnormal. A helpful rule of thumb is to consider a neutrophil count less than 1,000/mm³ to be abnormal in full-term and premature infants.

During the first month of life, the neutrophil count in premature infants falls slowly, so that at 30 days the mean value is approximately 2,000/mm³, with a range of 1,000 to 6,000/mm³ (232,233).

For studies by one of us (A.Z.), a cell was considered to be a segmented neutrophil if its nucleus was distinctly segmented into two or more lobes connected by a thin filament. Cells with no lobulation and those in which the

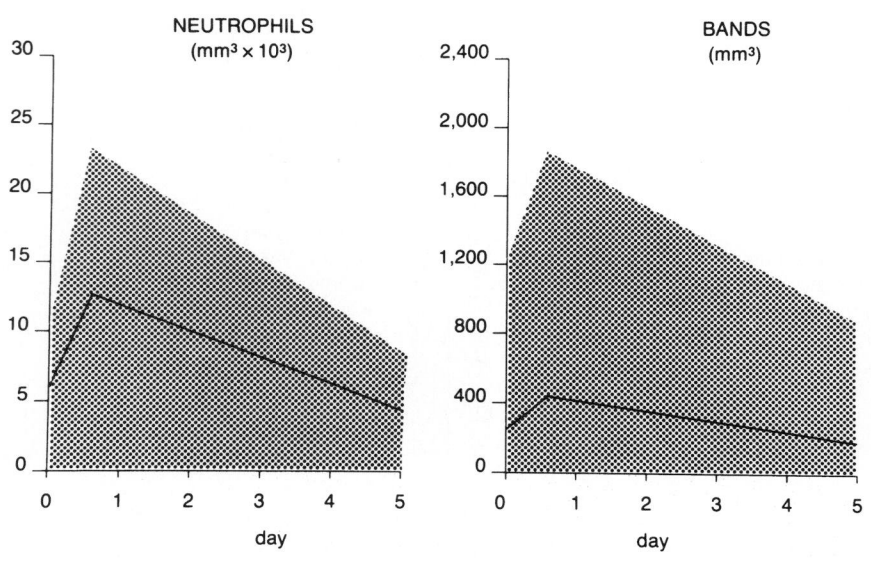

FIG. 45–15. Neutrophil and band counts of 169 normal full-term infants. Data at the first point, day 0, are cord blood values. Subsequent points represent data from capillary blood samples on 1 and 5 days of life. The heavy line represents the mean at each point. The shaded area includes 95% of the patients, excluding the top and bottom 2.5% of the group. The mean of all values on blood collected from 4 to 24 hours of age is plotted at 14 hours.

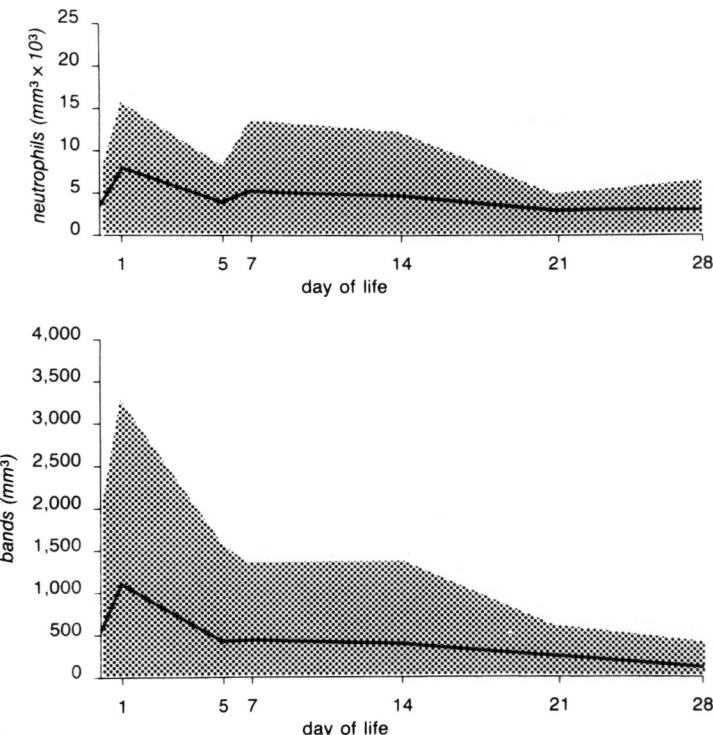

FIG. 45–16. Neutrophil and band counts of 180 premature infants. Data at the first point, day 0, are cord blood values. Subsequent points represent data from capillary blood samples on 1, 5, 7, 14, 21, and 28 days of life. The heavy line represents the mean at each point. The shaded area includes 95% of the subjects, excluding the top and bottom 2.5% of the group.

width of the narrowest segment of the nucleus was greater than one-third the width of the broadest segment were referred to as nonsegmented neutrophils or bands (Fig. 45–17). During the first 2 weeks of life for full-term and premature infants, a band–segmented neutrophil ratio greater than 0.3 was considered to be abnormal (230). Other investigators have reported reference ranges for total neutrophil and immature neutrophil counts in newborn infants throughout the first 28 days of life (235–237). Examination of a peripheral blood smear during the first few days of life characteristically reveals an excess of polymorphonuclear neutrophils. Particularly in premature infants, some immature forms (e.g., promyelocytes, myelocytes) may be seen. Sometime between the fourth and seventh days of life, the lymphocyte becomes the predominant cell and remains so until the fourth year of life.

Changes in Blood Neutrophils During Bacterial Infection

In newborn infants, clinical signs of infection may be minimal, and the speed of evolution of disease may be rapid. Changes in neutrophil number and appearance are often helpful in the diagnosis of bacterial infections in this age group.

Changes in Neutrophil Numbers

In infants with systemic bacterial infection, the total neutrophil count may be increased (i.e., neutrophilia), decreased (i.e., neutropenia), or fall within normal limits. In a study of 24 newborn infants with proven bacterial sepsis (e.g., positive bacterial cultures from the blood, cerebrospinal fluid, bladder-tap urine, or peritoneal fluid), neutropenia was observed in five, neutrophilia was seen in three, and normal neutrophil counts were observed in the remaining 16 (230). Although neutrophilia is a relatively nonspecific finding and may occur in conditions other than sepsis, the finding of neutropenia is highly significant in newborn infants and may be the first clue to bacterial infection. In the study of Manroe and colleagues, neutropenia was observed in 77% of counts associated with confirmed or suspected bacterial disease; neutrophilia was absent almost as often in infected infants (42%) as it was present (58%) (237). In addition to neutropenia, increased numbers of immature neutrophils (i.e., band forms) and an elevated band–segmented neutrophil ratio are of considerable value in the diagnosis of bacterial infection. In a study of premature infants with proven bacterial infection, 73% (11 of 15) of the infants had elevated band counts and a reversed band–segmented neutrophil ratio (231).

Changes in Neutrophil Morphology

During infection, the neutrophils of newborn infants have increased numbers of Döhle bodies (i.e., aggregates of rough endoplasmic reticulum), vacuoles, and toxic granules (231).

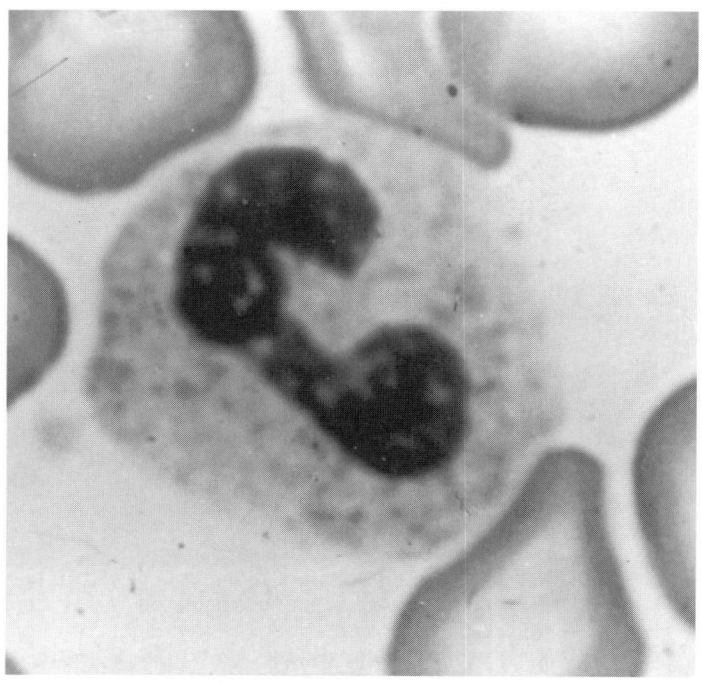

FIG. 45–17. A band neutrophil.

Neutrophil Response to Bacterial Infection

There is a characteristic pattern of neutrophil response that can assist greatly in the diagnosis of infection in newborn infants. When bacterial infection occurs, neutrophils migrate from the circulating pool to the walls of blood vessels. Massive infection may produce neutropenia by causing complement-dependent neutrophil aggregation, with disappearance from the circulation. If the demand is sufficient, neutropenia occurs. The baby's response is a release of its marrow storage pool, which consists mostly of young or band neutrophils. This is evidenced by an increase in the band–segmented neutrophil ratio and slowly thereafter by an increase in the absolute band count. The body continues to produce neutrophils, and the resulting neutrophil count is then a balance between demand and production. In the newborn infant, there is evidence that marrow reserves are relatively limited compared with those of the adult; neutrophilia may not occur, or if it does, it may be seen only late in the disease. With increased production under the stress of infection, abnormal neutrophils (i.e., those containing vacuoles, Döhle bodies, toxic granulations) are produced, providing further evidence of bacterial infection. As a myeloid response continues, it is not unusual to find in the bloodstream early myeloid precursors such as promyelocytes or even myeloblasts.

Neutrophil response to infection is also of importance in terms of understanding the susceptibility of newborns to infection. Neutrophil function, particularly chemotaxis and phagocytosis, is reduced in newborns and may con-tribute to their susceptibility to infection (238). The neutrophil storage pool is lower in newborns, accounting for the neutropenia frequently seen in association with neonatal infections and contributing to the relative inability of the newborn to fight infections (239).

There is evidence that the reduced function of the neutrophils may be secondary to relatively low levels of humoral factors (i.e., antibody, complement) in the plasma of newborns. The low neutrophil counts during infection may be reversed by administration of γ-globulin (240).

Because of the occurrence of neutropenia, the reduced marrow storage pools, and decreased neutrophil function, it has been suggested that leukocyte transfusions may be valuable in the treatment of neonatal sepsis. There have been several contradictory reports regarding the benefit of such transfusions (238). Because of the risks of leukocyte transfusions and the difficulty in obtaining leukocyte concentrates, this therapy is rarely used.

Administration of the cytokine granulocyte colony-stimulating factor (G-CSF) increases neutrophil counts in adults and children with neutropenia. There have been several reports of its use in neutropenic newborns. Administration of G-CSF resulted in an increase in neutrophil count in septic neutropenic newborns (241,242). This treatment has been reported to reduce mortality in neonates with sepsis in comparison to historic controls (242). There is, however, no prospective, controlled, randomized trial that has proven the effectiveness of G-CSF in the treatment or prevention of sepsis in neutropenic newborn infants. Nevertheless, there is evidence at the present time that supports the need for such studies and the probable effectiveness of G-CSF in the treatment of neonatal neutropenia.

Neutropenia

Causes of neutropenia include decreased production of neutrophils, increased destruction, or a combination of both mechanisms (Table 45–10).

Decreased Production of Neutrophils

Impaired granulopoiesis and neutropenia are features of a number of inherited disorders. In Kostmann syndrome and reticular dysgenesia, severe neutropenia from birth leads to early diagnosis. In the other syndromes described in this section, persistent or periodic neutropenia does not typically present a problem in the neonatal period, and these disorders are usually diagnosed later in life.

Kostmann Syndrome. Congenital neutropenia is severe in patients with Kostmann syndrome; cases are reported in which there was striking neutropenia from the first day of life (243). Bone marrow smears typically reveal normal cellularity, with a maturation arrest at the promyelocyte–myelocyte level. Serious bacterial infections occur early in life, and the disorder is usually fatal. However, infusions of the cytokine G-CSF have proven to be successful therapy for this disease (244). Inheritance is autosomal recessive in most cases.

Reticular Dysgenesia. In their original report, deVaal and Seynhaeve described premature monozygotic twins in whom recognizable leukocytes were absent from the peripheral blood (245). Both infants died of infection within the first 2 weeks of life. At autopsy, thymic tissue and lymph node tissue were absent. Smears of aspirated marrow showed normal erythroid and megakaryocytic development, with absent myeloid and lymphocytic cells.

Shwachman–Diamond Syndrome. In 1964, Shwachman and colleagues described five children with evidence of pancreatic insufficiency and neutropenia (246). Growth retardation, normal sweat electrolytes, and absence of pulmonary disease ordinarily characteristic of cystic fibrosis were other features of the disorder. Bone marrow findings include hypocellularity with maturation arrest of myeloid elements. Inheritance appears to be autosomal recessive.

Neutropenia Associated with Immunodeficiency Syndromes. Approximately one-third of boys with X-linked agammaglobulinemia are neutropenic at some time (247). Neutropenia may also be associated with deficiencies of IgG and IgA (248).

Cyclic Neutropenia. Cyclic neutropenia is a sporadic or familial disorder characterized by a regular, repetitive decrease in peripheral blood neutrophils at approximately 21-day intervals (249,250). The disorder reflects a regulatory abnormality of the stem cell pool and is rarely diagnosed in the neonatal period.

Neutropenia in Babies of Toxemic and/or Hypertensive Mothers. Neutropenia occurs frequently in infants of hypertensive or preeclamptic mothers. This appears to result from a production defect (251). In one series 48% of 301 low-birth-weight babies born to mothers with preeclampsia were found to be neutropenic, and there was a significantly higher incidence of sepsis in the neutropenic group (251). The administration of G-CSF (10 µg/kg) produced a rise in neutrophil count within 6 hours, which was sustained by daily injections of G-CSF (252).

Increased Destruction of Neutrophils

Neonatal Alloimmune Neutropenia. Neonatal alloimmune neutropenia is the neutrophil counterpart of the erythrocyte disorder of hemolytic disease of the newborn. The incidence of alloimmune neutropenia is reported to be in the range of one in 500 to one in 2,000 newborn infants (253,254). Alloimmune neutropenia occurs when a mother becomes sensitized to a foreign antigen present on the neutrophils of her infant and is then stimulated to form specific IgG antibody directed against this fetal antigen. Transplacental passage of IgG antibody into the fetal circulation results in neutropenia. Because neutropenia is the direct consequence of transplacentally acquired maternal IgG, the condition is self-limiting, and neutropenia persists for only a few weeks or months. The severity of neutropenia is influenced by the titer and subclass of the maternal IgG neutrophil antibody, the phagocytic activity of the infant's reticuloendothelial system, and the capacity of the infant's marrow to compensate for the shortened survival of antibody-sensitized neutrophils.

Investigation of infants with neonatal alloimmune neutropenia has contributed much to current knowledge of

---

TABLE 45–10. *Causes of neonatal neutropenia*

Decreased production of neutrophils
  Kostmann syndrome
  Reticular dysgenesia
  Shwachman–Diamond syndrome
  Neutropenia associated with cartilage–hair hypoplasia
  Neutropenia associated with immunodeficiency
    syndromes
  Cyclic neutropenia
Increased destruction of neutrophils
  Neonatal alloimmune neutropenia
  Neonatal autoimmune neutropenia
  Drug-induced neutropenia
Decreased production and increased destruction of
    neutrophils
  Infections
    Congenital, usually viral
    Acquired, usually bacterial
  Drug-induced neutropenia

neutrophil-specific antigens, and the antigen systems most often involved are NA1, NA2, and NB1 (255). The neutrophil-specific antigens NA1 and NA2 are located on the neutrophil Fc-γ receptor III (FcRIII), and antibodies to this neutrophil membrane glycoprotein have caused neonatal neutropenia (256,257). Although HLA antigens are present on granulocytes, and alloimmunization to these antigens is common in pregnancy, HLA antibodies are not thought to be a significant cause of neutropenia in newborn infants. It appears that maternal HLA antibodies are effectively absorbed by HLA antigens in placental tissue; the antibodies that reach the fetus are neutralized by soluble antigens or weakened by having to react with antigens on various cells distributed in the blood and other tissues. In contrast, neutrophil-specific antibodies cross the placenta without any obstacle and concentrate on the target antigen, which occurs only on the relatively small mass of mature neutrophils.

The clinical course of infants with alloimmune neutropenia is of interest. Neutropenia is usually severe. In a review of 19 affected infants reported before 1974, Lalezari found that 12 infants had total absence of circulating neutrophils for at least part of their course (255). The duration of neutropenia ranged from 2 to 17 weeks, with a mean of 7 weeks. Infections were common, and most were with *Staphylococcus aureus*. Two infants died, one with staphylococcal septicemia and the other with pneumonia and possible meningitis. Alloimmune neutropenia is not a benign disorder. Affected infants with severe neutropenia are at risk for serious bacterial infections, and therapeutic intervention may be necessary. In the past, in addition to intravenous antibiotic therapy for infants with suspected or proven infection, possible therapies include exchange transfusion to remove passively acquired maternal neutrophil antibodies, transfusion with compatible antigen-negative granulocytes harvested from the mother or known antigen-negative blood donors, corticosteroids, and high-dose intravenous IgG. However, recently G-CSF has been shown to be effective in rapidly returning the neutrophil count to normal (258). This now must be considered the preferred treatment for those children who require therapy.

There is little evidence that steroids are of value in this condition. The response to high-dose intravenous γ-globulin therapy varies (259–261). My (A.Z.) experience is limited to therapy of twins with severe neutropenia caused by maternally derived anti-NA1 antibody; both infants failed to respond to 2 g/kg of intravenous IgG. It is possible that higher doses of IgG may be required in the therapy of immune neutropenia. The use of exchange transfusion or transfusion with compatible antigen-negative neutrophils should be reserved for infected infants who have failed an adequate trial of high-dose intravenous IgG (2 to 5 g/kg administered as 1 g/kg/day for 2 to 5 days) and who are not responding to broad-spectrum intravenous antibiotic therapy.

Neonatal Autoimmune Neutropenia. Transient neutropenia in the neonatal period may reflect transfer of IgG neutrophil antibodies from mother to fetus during pregnancy. In these cases, the maternal serum contains the pathologic neutrophil antibodies, and the mother may be neutropenic and may have a history of an autoimmune disorder, such as systemic lupus erythematosus. Therapy of the affected neonate, if clinically indicated, is high-dose intravenous IgG (2 to 5 g/kg administered as 1 g/kg/day for 2 to 5 days). Such therapy produces dramatic, albeit transient, increases in absolute neutrophil counts in older children with autoimmune neutropenia (262).

Evaluation of the Infant with Neutropenia. The unexpected finding of neutropenia in a newborn infant should prompt consideration of bacterial infection. A peripheral blood smear should be carefully examined for Döhle bodies, vacuolization, and toxic granulation, and the band–segmented neutrophil ratio should be determined. In infants with some combination of neutropenia, an increased band–segmented neutrophil ratio, and morphologic features suggestive of bacterial infection, empirical broad-spectrum antibiotic therapy should be started until the results of cultures are known. If there is no clinical or laboratory evidence of infection, other causes of neutropenia must be considered; however, it is still prudent to utilize broad-spectrum antibiotic coverage until it is clear from cultures and the infant's clinical course that sepsis is not the etiology of the neutropenia. As noted above, preeclampsia and/or hypertension in the mother must be considered as a common cause of neutropenia. A maternal history, including a drug history, and a maternal neutrophil count should be obtained to exclude maternal illness (e.g., systemic lupus erythematosus) as a cause of neutropenia. The physician should obtain a careful family history, asking specifically about family members with documented neutropenia or a history of severe or unusual infections. This information may provide an important clue to the possibility of an inherited neutropenic syndrome (e.g., Kostmann syndrome). Physical examination of affected infants suggests or excludes hypersplenism and congenital viral infections as likely causes of neutropenia. In well infants with no apparent cause for the neutropenic state, neonatal alloimmune neutropenia should be considered. In such cases, a search should be made for neutrophil antibodies in a sample of maternal serum; these antibodies are typically reactive against paternal neutrophils. In some infants, a bone marrow aspirate may be necessary to exclude the possibility of an intrinsic marrow disorder such as congenital leukemia.

Congenital Leukemia and Leukemoid Reactions

Congenital leukemia is an extremely rare disorder. The predominant form of congenital leukemia is acute myeloid leukemia, commonly either monoblastic or myelomonocytic leukemia; in older children, acute leukemia is typically lymphoblastic. In all forms of congenital leukemia, the prognosis is poor. Approximately 50% of infants with congenital leukemia manifest skin nodules. The nodules are bluish and feel like fibromatous tumors deep within the skin. Other presenting features include hepatosplenomegaly, poor weight gain, fever, diarrhea, pallor, and petechiae. There are a number of disorders that can appear similar to acute leukemia in the newborn. Congenital infections such as CMV disease, toxoplasmosis, and syphilis may manifest as hepatosplenomegaly with a pronounced leukemoid response in the peripheral blood. Severe bacterial infections also may be associated with a leukemoid blood picture, and neuroblastoma may present with similar skin nodules.

Special mention should be made of the transient leukemia seen in patients with Down syndrome. Although the incidence of acute leukemia is higher in Down syndrome, there is also an unusual syndrome of transient leukemia in newborn infants in which a picture of acute megakaryoblastic leukemia appears and then, during the subsequent weeks, regresses and disappears (263).

Some cases of transient leukemia are severe, with evidence of hydrops fetalis, hepatosplenomegaly, liver disease, or congestive failure (109,264,265). Most cases of transient leukemia recover completely without antileukemic therapy. However, approximately 20% of these patients subsequently develop acute megakaryoblastic leukemia during the first 4 years of life, a disease that is fatal unless treated.

Lymphopenia

In the newborn infant, an absolute lymphocyte count consistently less than 1,500/µL is abnormal and requires evaluation. During this period, lymphopenia is most often associated with immunodeficiency disorders, including reticular dysgenesis, Swiss-type agammaglobulinemia, agammaglobulinemia associated with short-limb dwarfism, X-linked recessive agammaglobulinemia, and lymphopenia with dysgammaglobulinemia (e.g., Nezelof syndrome). Affected infants should be promptly investigated for defects of cellular and humoral immune function. If they require blood transfusions, they should be given only irradiated blood products so that graft-versus-host disease does not develop.

Eosinophilia

An elevated eosinophil count is common in premature infants. Normal values for a group of healthy premature infants studied by us are illustrated in Fig. 45–18. The upper limit of normal (95th percentile) for absolute eosinophil counts in a group of 167 full-term infants was 1,016/µL, 1,323/µL, and 1,372/µL at 0, 1, and 5 days, respectively. The corresponding mean values were 475/µL, 496/µL, and 540/µL. In a prospective study of 45 premature infants, Bhat and colleagues found the incidence of eosinophilia to be 75.5% (266). Similar results have been reported by other investigators (267–269). In Bhat's study, an absolute eosinophil count of more than 700/µL was considered to be abnormal. The frequency and severity of eosinophilia were greatest in the subgroup of infants younger than 30 weeks of gestational age. There was a significant association between the development of eosinophilia and number of blood transfusions administered, use of parenteral nutrition, and duration of intubation. The causative nature of these associations is uncertain because these features are common in ill, premature infants. Prolonged processing of antigens at the cellular level is required for the development of eosinophilia, and the investigators suggest that eosinophilia in the premature infant may be a physiologic process needed to handle foreign antigens. The fact that eosinophilia is more frequent in premature infants than in term infants may reflect immaturity of barrier mechanisms in the gastrointestinal tract, respiratory tract, or both.

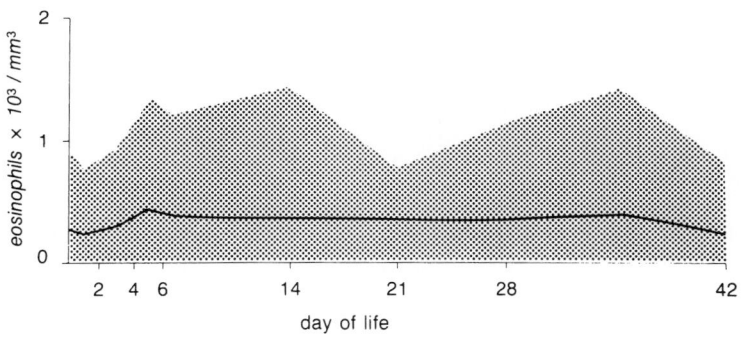

FIG. 45–18. Eosinophil counts in 142 healthy, premature infants. Data at the first point, day 0, are cord blood values. Subsequent points represent data from capillary blood samples on 1, 5, 7, 14, 28, 35, and 42 days of life. The heavy line represents the mean of each point. The shaded area includes 95% of the infants studied, excluding the top and bottom 2.5% of the group.

TRANSFUSION OF BLOOD AND BLOOD PRODUCTS

Transfusions of blood products to newborn infants are essential in many clinical situations, and guidelines for transfusion practice in this patient population have been published (270). However, guidelines simply provide a list of acceptable clinical situations in which transfusions may be given, and they should not serve as absolute indications for transfusion therapy. In all cases, the responsible physician should take into account the general condition of the infant. The decision to transfuse blood products should reflect careful consideration of the risk–benefit ratio for the individual patient.

Erythrocyte Transfusions

Transfusion of erythrocytes in newborn infants, particularly in premature newborns, is a common practice. The indications are those that hold for any other time of life: hypovolemia and anemia. Transfusion for anemia has created much controversy. Anemia is defined as a hemoglobin concentration lower than that which is normal for the given patient. This concept of normality is difficult to apply to the premature infant, who as part of his normal course may require respiratory assistance, may have apneic spells, and may have much blood sampled for laboratory tests. There is significant controversy about whether a low hemoglobin concentration is harmful to the infants or whether transfusions to maintain an arbitrary hemoglobin concentration improve their clinical condition. The following guidelines for administering a blood transfusion, although lacking definitive proof, include the caution that is necessary in view of the risks of this procedure:

Shock secondary to blood loss

Venous hemoglobin level less than 13 g/dL in neonates younger than 24 hours of age

Removal of blood for diagnostic purposes when the volume removed exceeds 10% of the infant's blood volume and significant continuing iatrogenic losses are anticipated

Hemoglobin less than 13.0 g/dL in newborn infants with severe pulmonary disease, cyanotic heart disease, or heart failure

Hemoglobin less than 8 g/dL in stable newborn infants; transfusion may be considered if the infant has symptoms (e.g., tachycardia, tachypnea, recurrent apnea, decreased vigor, poor weight gain unexplained by other causes) that can be improved by blood transfusion

The decision for transfusion should be made by the physician caring for the infant after consideration of the relative risks and benefits of the procedure. In recent years the use of blood in neonatal units has decreased, as

reviewed by Hume (271). Boulton et al. (272) compared the transfusion practices in the years 1984–1985 and 1994–1995. The percent of infants transfused decreased from 100% to 59%, and the number of transfusions per infant from 5.5 to 1.4. It is clear that the above guidelines must be tempered by considerations of risk and potential benefit.

Preparation of Blood for Transfusion and Crossmatching

There are several principles of blood transfusion and crossmatching that should be understood by those caring for neonates. First, omission of the crossmatch for initial and subsequent transfusions of neonates is recommended if the initial antibody screen does not demonstrate unexpected antibodies and the erythrocytes transfused are of an ABO and Rh type that is compatible with the baby and mother. This recommendation reflects the fact that newborn infants appear unable to form alloantibodies to erythrocyte antigens (273,274). Repeated blood sampling for pretransfusion testing only contributes to phlebotomy losses from small newborn infants. Second, the practice of using fresh-frozen plasma to adjust erythrocyte preparations to a predetermined hematocrit value for small-volume transfusions (i.e., not exchange transfusion) may lead to exposure of newborn infants to two different donors per transfusion. This practice should be discouraged (275). If necessary, isotonic saline (preferred) or albumin should be used to adjust hematocrit.

Exchange Transfusions

The authors recommend that blood for exchange transfusion be as fresh as possible and less than 5 days old. Because extracellular potassium increases rapidly during storage of erythrocyte concentrates at 4°C, it is recommended that erythrocyte units for exchange transfusion of ill premature infants be saline washed before reconstitution with fresh-frozen plasma. Manual and automated saline wash processes are effective (276). This maneuver effectively eliminates any chance of iatrogenic hyperkalemia, a complication reported in ill premature infants after exchange transfusion (277).

Efficient Use of Blood

Because newborn babies require only small volumes of blood for transfusion (approximately 10 mL/kg), there can be a great waste from a unit of blood, which usually contains 250 mL of packed erythrocytes. As a result, a number of methods of efficient use of blood have been employed; for example, a single unit may be collected into a quadruple pack. These individual bags may be used for transfusion of as many as four infants. Use may be improved by subsampling from a single erythrocyte unit through a sterile docking system, which means that one bag of blood may provide transfusion for ten or more infants. The problem with this technique is that, although it provides for efficient use of blood, the small infant who requires several transfusions during his hospital stay may receive blood from many donors, with the increasing risks associated with each donation.

The ideal system of transfusion of blood would be one that uses only one donor for each patient. Donor exposure can be kept to a minimum by designating for use by a single baby 1 unit of blood divided into a quadruple pack or aliquoting through a sterile docking system. Because red blood cells are suitable for transfusion after as long as 42 days of storage (using preservative solutions containing adenine), it is feasible to use one bag to provide most, if not all, the red cell transfusions for one baby. The use of such stored blood is not only theoretically safe (271) but was found to be as safe as using fresh blood (278).

Platelet Transfusions

A platelet count less than 150×10^9/L in a newborn infant is abnormal and requires investigation. In older children and adults, the risk of serious internal hemorrhage, particularly intracranial hemorrhage, increases significantly when the platelet count falls below 20,000/μL. Donor platelets are usually infused prophylactically when this degree of thrombocytopenia occurs. The situation in newborn infants is less clear. Particularly in ill premature infants, in whom the risk of hemorrhage into the CNS is high, factors other than the absolute platelet count may play a role. Many of these infants are on medications, such as antibiotics, that may impair platelet function. Immaturity of blood vessels in the periventricular area and changes in cerebral blood flow and pressure associated with fluid and ventilation therapy may play a role. Alternatively, intraventricular hemorrhage (IVH) may be the final result of cerebral infarction, perhaps related to asphyxia, with hemorrhage into the infarcted area. The clinical impact of significant neonatal thrombocytopenia (i.e., platelet counts $<100 \times 10^9$/L) in infants weighing less than 1,500 g at birth has been studied prospectively by Andrew and associates (279). The incidence of IVH in 97 thrombocytopenic infants was 78%, compared with 48% in nonthrombocytopenic control infants. The more severe grades of IVH (i.e., grades III or IV) were more frequent in the thrombocytopenic infants. Despite this, a trial of platelet transfusion for platelet counts less than 150×10^9/L during the first 7 days of life failed to decrease the incidence of developing or extending intraventricular hemorrhage in sick premature infants (280).

Guidelines for transfusion of platelet concentrates are outlined in Table 45–11. The standard platelet product available from blood banks is harvested from a single whole-blood donation of approximately 450 mL. After

TABLE 45–11. *Guidelines for transfusion of platelet concentrates in neonates*[a]

Premature infants (Gestational Age <37 wk)
Blood platelets $<30 \times 10^9$/L in a stable infant
Blood platelets $<50 \times 10^9$/L in a sick infant
All other infants
Blood platelet count $<20 \times 10^9$/L
Blood platelet count $<50 \times 10^9$/L with active bleeding or the need for an invasive procedure
Blood platelet count $<100 \times 10^9$/L with active bleeding plus disseminated intravascular coagulation or *other coagulation abnormalities*[b]
Bleeding with *qualitative platelet defect* and *marked prolongation* of bleeding time, regardless of the platelet count
Cardiovascular bypass surgery with unexplained *excessive bleeding,* regardless of the platelet count

[a]Adapted from ref. 270.
[b]Statements in *italics* require additional definition by a local transfusion committee.

centrifugation of this whole-blood unit, platelet-rich plasma (PRP) is separated from the erythrocyte fraction, and the PRP is further centrifuged to yield 1 unit of fresh-frozen plasma and 1 unit of random donor platelets. Each platelet concentrate contains approximately 0.7×10^{11} platelets in a volume of 50 mL; this product can be stored for as long as 5 days at 22°C. The objective of most platelet transfusions is to increase the infant's platelet count to more than 100×10^9/L. This can be achieved by the infusion of 10 mL of a standard platelet concentrate per kilogram of body weight. Generally, this volume is not excessive, providing intake of other fluids is monitored and adjusted as needed. Although methods exist to reduce the volume of platelet concentrates, additional processing should be performed with care because of possible platelet loss, clumping, and dysfunction caused by the additional handling (281). Platelets should be administered through a standard 170-μm blood filter as rapidly as the infant's overall condition permits and certainly within 2 hours. A microaggregate filter should not be used because it will trap a large number of platelets.

Granulocyte Transfusions

Although granulocyte transfusions have been beneficial in some forms of neutropenia (282), they are now rarely used in neonatal units. The reasons for this are the difficulty in obtaining their preparations and the apparent efficacy of G-CSF in rapidly elevating neutrophil counts in neutropenic infants with sepsis (241), alloimmune neutropenia (258), or other causes of neutropenia (252).

Risks

Potential complications of blood transfusion have been reviewed by Mollison (283). For newborn infants, posttransfusion hepatitis, CMV infection, HIV infection, and graft-versus-host disease are of particular concern. Because of these potential complications, it is important that physicians order blood or blood product support for newborns only in situations in which the infant will clearly benefit from such therapy.

Hepatitis

Transfusion-associated hepatitis may be caused by the hepatitis A or B viruses or more commonly by the hepatitis C virus (HCV) (284,285) Cases of HCV were previously classified as non-A, non-B hepatitis. Unfortunately, little information is available concerning HCV infection in newborn infants. In adults, the incidence of hepatitis C was previously reported to be 5% to 15% among persons who received 1 to 5 units of blood (286). More than 90% of these cases have now been confirmed to be caused by HCV infection. Approximately 50% of all patients with HCV develop chronic persistent or chronic active hepatitis. A subgroup of those with chronic hepatitis ultimately develop cirrhosis or hepatocellular carcinoma. These data are derived from studies of adults; the natural history of transfusion-acquired hepatitis in newborn infants is unknown.

Cytomegalovirus Infection

Transfusion-acquired CMV infection can occur when at-risk CMV antibody–negative infants are infused with CMV antibody–positive blood products. In the study by Yeager and colleagues, 13.5% (10 of 74) of seronegative infants who received CMV antibody–positive erythrocytes developed CMV infection (287). Infection did not occur in 90 seronegative infants who received only CMV antibody–negative blood. Two of the ten infected infants in this series died, and three others developed serious symptoms including pneumonia, hepatitis, hemolytic anemia, and thrombocytopenia. All of the fatal or other serious infections occurred in infants with a birth weight less than 1,200 g; infection was more common in infants who received 50 mL or more of blood. Similar data have been reported by Adler and colleagues, and other reports have stressed the morbidity and mortality that may be associated with transfusion-acquired CMV infection in neonates (288–290).

Based on these studies, it has been recommended that CMV antibody–negative blood products be made available to preterm infants of birth weight 1,250 g or less who are CMV antibody–negative. A study by Preiksaitis and colleagues challenges this recommendation for all neonates (291). In this prospective study of 120 seronegative infants, only one case of acquired CMV infection was observed. Because no mortality and little morbidity could be attributed to transfusion-acquired CMV, the investigators did not recommend that all neonatal units provide specialized blood components for the prevention of CMV infection. The indications for use of CMV-seronegative blood products in newborn infants have been comprehensively reviewed by Preiksaitis and associates (292). They include low-birth-weight (LBW) neonates (i.e., birth weight < 1,500 g) born to seronegative mothers in centers that have documented a high incidence of transfusion-acquired CMV infection in neonates; LBW neonates born to seronegative or seropositive mothers and who require granulocyte transfusions; and neonates receiving extracorporeal membrane oxygenation (ECMO).

The importance of breast milk as a source of CMV infection in newborn infants has also been stressed (293,294). In future studies of transfusion-acquired CMV infection in newborn infants, it will be important to control for this variable, particularly in nurseries in which pooled breast milk is used. If a decision to transfuse CMV low-risk blood products to selected LBW infants is made, and CMV-seronegative erythrocytes are not available, products that are associated with a low risk of transmitting CMV infection include frozen, deglycerolized erythrocytes; washed erythrocytes; and filtered erythrocytes (295–297).

It is now recommended that in order to avoid transfusion-induced CMV infection in newborns, they receive either blood products from CMV-negative donors or filtered blood, which in recent studies appears to be highly effective in preventing CMV infection even in immunosuppressed patients (298).

Acquired Immunodeficiency Syndrome

Since the first report of AIDS in 1981, much has been learned about the disorder (299). The causative agent of the syndrome is now known to be the HIV-1 virus. The virus can be grown in culture, and antibody to the virus can be detected with immunologic techniques, such as an enzyme-linked immunosorbent assay. Blood donations are routinely screened for evidence of antibodies to the HIV-1 virus, and the risk of HIV-1 transmission by blood products is extremely small. However, HIV-1 transmission has occurred in newborn infants, and this potentially fatal complication demands that blood or blood component therapy be restricted to situations in which therapy is clinically indicated and is likely to be of benefit to the newborn infant (300–302). The potential complication of HIV infection is a major reason to limit the number of blood donors to whom a given newborn infant is exposed.

Graft-versus-Host Disease

Graft-versus-host disease has been reported in congenitally immunodeficient infants, after blood transfusion in premature infants, after ECMO, and in apparently normal infants with Rh isoimmunization who have received intrauterine transfusions followed by exchange transfusion (303–307). Features of transfusion-associated graft-versus-host disease, usually a fatal disorder, include fever, generalized rash, diarrhea, hepatitis, and pancytopenia. Irradiation of blood products to prevent graft-versus-host disease is recommended for the following groups:

- Neonates with known or suspected congenital immunodeficiency disorders
- Neonates requiring intrauterine transfusions
- Neonates who received intrauterine transfusions and who require transfusion postnatally
- Recipients of cellular blood products from first-degree blood relatives
- Premature infants weighing less than 1,500 g at birth

Data supporting the last recommendation are not available. However, very-low-birth-weight infants (<1,500 g) may have an associated immunodeficiency, and it is reasonable to offer protection to this group of infants (308). The dose of irradiation used varies among centers, ranging from 1,500 to 5,000 cGy; a dose of 1,500 cGy is most frequently used (309).

Plasma Derivatives

Albumin

Albumin is available in 5% and 25% solutions. Although albumin infusion has been recommended as a means of drawing more bilirubin into the intravascular space before exchange transfusion, convincing data in support of such a practice is lacking.

Fresh-Frozen Plasma

Centrifugation of a single donor unit of whole blood within 6 hours of collection yields a concentrate of erythrocytes and 1 unit of fresh-frozen plasma. If stored at −30°C, the plasma product has a shelf life of 12 months and contains all coagulation factors.

Cryoprecipitate

Cryoprecipitate is prepared from fresh-frozen plasma derived from multiple donors by slow thawing at 2°C to 4°C. Each unit of cryoprecipitate contains approximately 80 units of factor VIII and 250 mg of fibrinogen in 5 to 10 mL of plasma. If stored at -30°C, the product has a shelf life of 12 months. Cryoprecipitate also contains various amounts of factor XIII.

Factor VIII and IX Concentrates

Concentrates of factor VIII and IX are commercially manufactured from large pools (2,000 to 20,000 donors) of plasma. Each concentrate lot is assayed for coagulation factor activity, and this value is stated in units on each vial. Traditionally, concentrates of factors VIII and IX have not been used in newborn infants or young children because of the increased risk of hepatitis associated with infusion of factor VIII and IX concentrates and of DIC and thrombotic complications associated with infusion of factor IX concentrates because of thrombogenic materials in such concentrates and low antithrombin III levels in newborns. Disseminated intravascular coagulation is particularly likely if liver dysfunction occurs. The introduction of high-purity virus-inactivated factor concentrates appears to have eliminated the risk of HIV-1 infection and to have significantly reduced the incidence of hepatitis, altering the previous general recommendations. However, factor IX concentrates are not recommended for use in newborns other than those with proven congenital factor IX deficiency (hemophilia B). Most North American hemophilia centers now recommend that infants with newly diagnosed severe hemophilia immediately receive hepatitis B immunization, and then they can be started on virus-inactivated factor replacement therapy, as clinically indicated for prevention or control of bleeding (187).

Hyperimmune Serum Globulin

Prevention of Hepatitis B Virus Infections

Infants of mothers who are positive for hepatitis B surface antigen (HBsAg) are frequently infected with hepatitis B virus. Infection is most likely to occur if mothers are also positive for hepatitis B e antigen. Approximately 90% of infants whose mothers are positive for both markers will become infected, and most of these infants will be permanent carriers of the hepatitis B virus. It is estimated that one in four infants who are chronic carriers after perinatal infection will later develop cirrhosis or hepatocellular carcinoma (310).

Infants receive greatest protection from a combination of active immunization with three doses of hepatitis B vaccine, together with passive immunization using hepatitis B immune globulin (HBIG). The following schedule is recommended: at birth, 0.5 mL of HBIG and 10 μg of hepatitis B vaccine (310). Both the vaccine and the immunoglobulin are given intramuscularly and can be administered at the same time if separate sites are used. At 1 and 6 months, 10 μg of hepatitis B vaccine is given. Infants should be tested for presence of anti-HBsAg at 9 months. If they are found to be negative (<10% of all cases), a repeat dose of the vaccine should be given.

Prevention of Cytomegalovirus Infections

The administration of CMV hyperimmune globulin to CMV antibody-negative patients who undergo bone marrow transplantation decreases the incidence of transfusion-acquired CMV infection. Whether a similar approach may be beneficial for the CMV antibody-negative premature infant exposed to multiple blood products is unknown.

THROMBOSIS AND EMBOLISM

The reported incidence of symptomatic thrombosis and embolism in newborn infants is approximately one case per 500 admissions to a neonatal intensive care unit (311), or one case per 20,000 births (312).

The vessels affected are numerous; they include renal, adrenal, portal, hepatic, and cerebral veins; peripheral, cerebral, pulmonary, coronary, renal, and mesenteric arteries; and the aorta, vena cava, and right atrium (313). Signs and symptoms may be fairly specific, such as a cool, pale, and pulseless limb in the case of peripheral arterial obstruction. Often, however, the clinical presentation is very nonspecific: examples include respiratory insufficiency and profound hypoxemia caused by pulmonary emboli (314) and seizures caused by arterial stroke or cerebral venous thrombosis (315–318). Occasionally, thrombosis is suspected only retrospectively when sequelae of vessel occlusion become apparent (e.g., portal hypertension as a consequence of portal vein thrombosis). Table 45–12 summarizes the major sites of thrombotic vessel obstruction and their clinical symptoms and signs in the newborn infant.

RISK FACTORS AND PATHOGENESIS

Three major factors contribute to the formation of thrombi (Virchow's triad): abnormalities of the vessel wall, disturbances of blood flow, and changes in blood coagulation.

Abnormal Vessel Wall

Intravascular Catheters

Abnormalities of the vessel wall are most frequently caused by intravascular catheters that damage the endothelium in addition to introducing a foreign surface with thrombogenic properties. Intravascular catheters have become the single most important risk factor for neonatal thrombotic disease (311). The placement of such catheters carries a potential risk of thrombosis, regardless of which vessel is used; possibly because of their widespread use, umbilical catheters have received the most attention to date.

In a retrospective review of 4,000 infants who underwent umbilical artery catheterization in the 1970s, severe symptomatic vessel obstruction was observed in approximately 1% of patients (319). Clinically silent thromboses have been detected more often at autopsy or during contrast angiography in asymptomatic infants with an umbilical artery catheter in place. Between 3% and 59% of cases have had postmortem evidence of catheter-related thrombosis (320–328). In six prospective angiographic studies, thrombosis was demonstrated in 10% to 95% of patients (329–334). Very recently, thrombi associated with a correctly placed umbilical venous catheter were documented venographically at the time of elective catheter removal in 30% (14/47) of asymptomatic infants

TABLE 45–12. *Clinical presentation of thromboembolic disease in newborn infants*

Site of vessel obstruction	Clinical signs and symptoms
Venous	
Vena cava inferior	May be associated with renal venous thrombosis; edema and cyanosis of legs
Vena cava superior	Soft-tissue edema of head, neck, and chest; chylothorax
Cerebral	Seizures
Renal	Enlarged kidney(s); hematuria
Adrenal	Often associated with adrenal hemorrhagic necrosis
Portal and hepatic	Mainly clinically silent during acute phase
Arterial	
Aorta	Congestive heart failure; systolic gradient between upper and lower limbs; decreased femoral pulses; renal failure
Peripheral	Pulselessness; fall in skin temperature; discoloration
Cerebral	Prolonged apnea; seizures
Pulmonary	Respiratory distress; pulmonary hypertension
Coronary	Congestive heart failure cardiac shock
Renal	Systemic hypertension (usually self-limiting if microemboli in end arterioles); congestive heart failure
Mesenteric	Signs of "necrotizing enterocolitis"

(335). In the same study, it was found that real-time and Doppler flow ultrasonography was not sufficiently accurate to diagnose such thrombi. Before this report, neonatal thrombosis, which was associated with central venous catheters, had been estimated to occur in approximately 14% of asymptomatic infants, based on serial echocardiography (336,337).

Abnormal Chorionic Vessels

These are present in a range of maternal disorders such as pregnancy-induced hypertension or placental infection. Abnormal chorionic vessels predispose to the development of chorionic thrombi, which can embolize into the fetal circulation, particularly into the pulmonary arteries and portal veins (338,339). Paradoxic placental emboli have also been reported as the cause of neonatal cerebral infarction (340).

Abnormal Blood Flow

Blood flow is a critical determinant of thrombus formation, site, location, and structure. Increased blood viscosity (as a consequence of polycythemia or dehydration) has been implicated in cases of neonatal thrombotic disease (311,312). Hyperviscosity caused by polycythemia is also thought to contribute to the alleged thrombotic tendency in infants with diabetic mothers (313).

Shock is another example of a severe disturbance of blood flow, predisposing to thrombosis and necrosis.

Abnormal Blood Coagulation

Epidemiologic studies in adults have confirmed several hereditary disorders and coexistent genetic defects as risk factors for thromboembolism (341). Much less is known about hereditary thrombophilia in newborn infants, although the rare; occurrences of homozygous protein C and S deficiences have been strongly linked with severe neonatal thrombotic disease (342,343). Heterozygous deficiencies of antithrombin and factor V Leiden (resistance to activated protein C) have also been associated with neonatal thrombosis and purpura fulminans in isolated case reports (344,345). Most reported cases of thrombosis in infants and children with resistance to activated protein C, however, have had additional risk factors such as leukemia, sepsis, or intravascular catheters (346).

MANAGEMENT

Clinical investigators of adult cardiovascular diseases have made considerable progress through a series of well-designed studies that enabled them to make firm recommendations on the diagnosis and treatment of thromboembolism. In contrast, the literature on neonatal thrombotic disease consists almost entirely of case reports and case series (347). Such anecdotal observations are poor guides to management, as they are uncontrolled and fraught with bias (347). Extrapolation of findings in adult patients to newborn infants may be inappropriate because the etiology, the localization of thrombi, the coagulation system, and its response to antithrombotic and fibrinolytic agents differ markedly between the two age-groups. The following recommendations are in keeping with those recently endorsed by the Scientific and Standardization Subcommittee on Neonatal Hemostasis of the International Society on Thrombosis and Haemostasis (348). Current approaches to the management of neonatal thrombosis remain to be validated in future clinical trials.

Diagnosis

Whenever thrombotic disease is suspected in the newborn (Table 45–12), every effort should be made to confirm or refute the diagnosis. Contrast angiography with the use of nonionic contrast media is the "gold standard" imaging technique for the confirmation of thrombosis before embarking on thrombolytic or surgical therapy. Other, less invasive tests such as real-time ultrasonography, Doppler flow studies, or radioisotope scans may be helpful adjunctive measures, but their precision and accuracy in neonatal thrombotic disease are still uncertain (348).

Predisposing factors should be sought and eliminated where possible. A family history of thrombotic disease should be taken. Patient and parents should be tested for hereditary deficiencies of protein C, protein S, antithrombin, as well as for the factor V Leiden mutation, and hyperhomocysteinemia.

Treatment

Organ or limb dysfunction as a result of thrombosis is the most compelling indication for active intervention. The lack of strong evidence for the benefits and safety of antithrombotic therapy in this population does not usually justify aggressive therapy for asymptomatic thrombosis or thrombosis with very minor symptoms.

Intracranial hemorrhage or hemorrhagic infarction should be ruled out by suitable imaging techniques before anticoagulant or fibrinolytic drugs are prescribed. In all infants who receive antithrombotic therapy, the platelet count should be maintained above $50 \times 10^9/L$, and the fibrinogen concentration greater than 1 g/L (348).

Heparin

At present, standard heparin is the most commonly used anticoagulant in infants with thrombotic disease

(311,312), although some investigators have begun to use low-molecular-weight heparins (349). The latter are easier to administer and monitor; the previous claim that low-molecular-weight heparins cause less bleeding than unfractionated heparin has recently been questioned (350).

Heparin has been used in newborn infants at an initial loading dose of 50 units/kg body weight by intravenous injection followed by approximately 20 units/kg per hour by continuous intravenous infusion (351). Laboratory monitoring should be performed to avoid excessive heparinization as indicated by plasma levels of heparin that are considered unsafe in adult patients.

There is, however, no validated therapeutic range for heparin therapy in newborn infants, and the optimum heparin assay for neonatal plasma has yet to be found. In adults, the activated partial thromboplastin time (aPTT) is widely used to monitor heparin therapy, but the use of the aPTT in heparinized newborn infants has been less successful because the aPTT may become unmeasurably prolonged in the presence of even low concentrations of heparin (348).

Thrombolytic Agents

The experience with thrombolytic agents (streptokinase, urokinase, tissue plasminogen activator) is limited in newborn infants (352,353). Over the years, a gradual shift seems to have occurred from streptokinase to urokinase and, more recently, to tissue plasminogen activator (353). A wide range of doses have been used; both successes and failures have been reported with all three agents (311,312,352,353). In the absence of any controlled data in this population on the superiority of one thrombolytic agent over the others, the choice of drug should be determined by familiarity and cost.

Any clinician who is contemplating thrombolytic therapy in sick neonates must weigh the risk of prolonged vessel occlusion and the uncertain drug benefits against the infant's risk of suffering from serious bleeding complications.

Surgery

The main objectives of surgical intervention in neonatal large vessel thrombosis have been, first, to remove the occluding clot and, second, to resect a nonviable product of the vessel obstruction (amputation for limb gangrene; resection of necrotic bowel). Thrombectomy may be used in selected cases, particularly if the thrombus obstructs a major artery.

Because of the devastating functional loss with all ensuing problems, amputation in peripheral arterial occlusion should be postponed as long as possible. The main aim is to prevent superimposed secondary infection. Ideally, surgical intervention should be delayed until the

necrotic parts are well demarcated. In some cases, surgery is not necessary at all because autoamputation occurs, which results in the least possible loss of tissue.

Prognosis

The vast majority of infants with thrombotic disease survive; mortality rates are highest among infants with aortic thrombosis or with central venous catheter–associated thrombosis affecting the right atrium or the superior vena cava (311). Data on long-term follow-up of neonatal thrombosis are very limited. Two of the relatively better studied sites are renal venous thrombosis and aortic thrombosis.

A total of 58 neonates with renal venous thrombosis have been followed for 0.1 to 17 years by four different investigator teams (354). Persistent hypertension was found in 28% of all children, and 21% had residual renal tubular defects (354).

The available follow-up data on survivors of aortic thrombosis suggests that blood pressure and renal function are likely to normalize during early childhood, but persistent hypertension, leg-growth discrepancies, and abnormalities in renal size and function have been described (355–358).

Prophylaxis

To reduce the risk of thromboembolic disease in the newborn, intravascular catheters should be used judiciously, and blood flow should be optimized at all times.

Heparin has been advocated as a possible means of preventing catheter-related thrombosis. There is good evidence from controlled clinical trials that the continuous infusion of low doses of heparin (<200 U/kg per day) prolongs the patency of umbilical artery catheters (357–360). Unfortunately, none of the published trials has had sufficient power to conclusively answer the question whether low doses of heparin also reduce catheter associated thrombus formation.

REFERENCES

1. Brown MS. Fetal and neonatal erythropoieisis. In Stockman JA, Pochedly C, eds. *Developmental and neonatal hematology.* New York: Raven Press, 1988:39.
2. Shannon KM, Naylor GS, Torkilson JC, et al. Circulating erythroid progenitors in the anemia of prematurity. *N Engl J Med* 1987;317:728.
3. Rhondeau SM, Christensen RD, Ross MP, et al. Responsiveness to recombinant human erythropoietin of marrow erythroid progenitors from infants with the "anemia of prematurity." *J Pediatr* 1988;112:935.
4. Christensen RD. Hematopoiesis in the fetus and neonate. *Pediatr Res* 1989;26:531.
5. Stockman JA III, Garcia JF, Oski FA. The anemia of prematurity. Factors governing the erythropoietin response. *N Engl J Med* 1977;296:647.
6. Stockman JA III, Graeber JE, Clark DA, et al. Anemia of prematurity: determinants of the erythropoietin response. *J Pediatr* 1984;105:786.
7. Brown MS, Garcia JF, Phibbs RH, et al. Decreased response of plasma

immunoreactive erythropoietin to "available oxygen" in anemia of prematurity. *J Pediatr* 1984;105:793.

8. Forestier F, Daffos F, Catherine N, et al. Developmental hematopoiesis in normal human fetal blood. *Blood* 1991;77:2360.

9. Oski FA, Naiman JL. Normal blood values in the newborn period. In Oski FA, Naiman JL, eds. Hematologic problems in the newborn, 3rd ed. Philadelphia: WB Saunders, 1982:11.

10. Blanchette VS, Zipursky A. Neonatal hematology. In Avery GB, ed. *Neonatology: Pathophysiology and management,* 3rd ed. Philadelphia: JB Lippincott, 1987:639.

11. Yao AC, Moinian M, Lind J. Distribution of blood between infant and placenta after birth. *Lancet* 1969;2:871.

12. Colozzi AE. Clamping of the umbilical cord: its effect on the placental transfusion. *N Engl J Med* 1954;250:629.

13. Usher R, Shephard M, Lind J. The blood volume of the newborn infant and placental transfusion. *Acta Paediatr* 1963;52:497.

14. Gunther M. The transfer of blood between baby and placenta in the minutes after birth. *Lancet* 1957;1:1277.

15. O'Brien RT, Pearson HA. Physiologic anemia of the newborn infant. *J Pediatr* 1971;79:132.

16. Schulman I, Smith CH, Stern GS. Studies on the anemia of prematurity. *Am J Dis Child* 1954;88:567.

17. Stockman JA III. Anemia of prematurity. *Clin Perinatol* 1977;4:239.

18. Stockman JA III, Oski FA. Physiologic anemia of infancy and the anemia of prematurity. *Clin Hematol* 1978;7:3.

19. Gairdner D, Marks J, Roscoe JD. Blood formation in infancy. Part II. Normal erythropoiesis. *Arch Dis Child* 1952;27:214.

20. Bratteby LE, Garby L, Groth T, et al. Studies on erythrokinetics in infancy. XIII. The mean life span and life span frequency function of red blood cells formed during foetal life. *Acta Pediatr Scand* 1968;57:311.

21. Pearson HA. Life-span of the fetal red blood cell. *J Pediatr* 1967;70:166.

22. Doyle JJ, Zipursky A. Neonatal blood disorders. In Sinclair JC, Bracken MB, eds. *Effective care of the newborn infant.* Oxford: Oxford University Press, 1992:425.

23. Bechensteen AG, Hågå P, Halvorsen S, et al. Erythropoietin, protein, and iron supplementation and the prevention of anaemia of prematurity. *Arch Dis Child* 1993;69:19.

24. Bechensteen AG, Halvorsen S, Hågå P, et al. Erythropoietin (Epo), protein and iron supplementation and the prevention of anaemia of prematurity: effects on serum immunoreactive Epo, growth and protein and iron metabolism. *Acta Paediatr* 1996;85:490.

25. Rønnestad A, Moe PJ, Breivik N. Enhancement of erythropoiesis by erythropoietin, bovine protein and energy fortified mother's milk during anaemia of prematurity. *Acta Paediatr* 1994;83:809.

26. Rönnholm KAR, Siimes MA. Hemoglobin concentration depends on protein intake in small preterm infants fed human milk. *Arch Dis Child* 1985;60:99.

27. Kivivuori SM, Järvenpää AL, Salmenperä L, et al. Erythropoiesis of very-low-birth-weight infants dependent on prenatal growth rate and protein status. *Acta Paediatr* 1994;83:13.

28. Brown MS, Shapiro H. Effect of protein intake on erythropoiesis during erythropoietin treatment of anemia of prematurity. *J Pediatr* 1996;128:512.

29. Lachance C, Chessex P, Fouron J-C, et al. Myocardial, erythropoietic, and metabolic adaptions to anemia of prematurity. *J Pediatr* 1994;125:278.

30. Sasidharan P, Heimler R. Transfusion-induced changes in the breathing pattern of healthy preterm anemic infants. *Pediatr Pulmonol* 1992;12:170.

31. Joshi A, Gerhardt T, Shandloff P, et al. Blood transfusion effect on the respiratory pattern of preterm infants. *Pediatrics* 1987;80:79.

32. Keyes WG, Donohue PK, Spivak JL, et al. Assessing the need for transfusion of premature infants and the role of hematocrit, clinical signs and erythropoietin level. *Pediatrics* 1989;84:412.

33. Bifano EM, Smith F, Borer J. Relationship between determinants of oxygen delivery and respiratory abnormalities in preterm infants with anemia. *J Pediatr* 1992;120:292.

34. Izraeli S, Ben-Sira L, Harell D, et al. Lactic acid as a predictor for erythrocyte transfusion in healthy preterm infants with anemia of prematurity. *J Pediatr* 1993;122:629.

35. Böhler T, Janecke A, Linderkamp O. Blood transfusion in late anemia of prematurity: effect on oxygen consumption, heart rate, and weight gain in otherwise healthy infants. *Infusionsther Transfusionsmed* 1994;21:376.

36. Stockman JA III, Clark DA. Weight gain. a response to transfusion in selected preterm infants. *Am J Dis Child* 1984;138:828.

37. Möller JC, Schwarz U, Schaible TF, et al. Do cardiac output and serum lactate levels indicate blood transfusion requirements in anemia of prematurity? *Intensive Care Med* 1996;22:472.

38. Blank JP, Sheagren TG, Vajaria J, et al. The role of RBC transfusion in the premature infant. *Am J Dis Child* 1984;138:831.

39. Meyer J, Sive A, Jacobs P. Empiric red cell transfusion in asymptomatic preterm infants. *Acta Paediatr* 1993;82:30.

40. Alverson DC, Isken VH, Cohen RS. Effect of booster blood transfusions on oxygen utilization in infants with bronchopulmonary dysplasia. *J Pediatr* 1988;113:722.

41. Ross MP, Christensen RD, Rothstein G, et al. A randomized trial to develop criteria for administering erythrocyte transfusions to anemic preterm infants 1 to 3 months of age. *J Perinatol* 1989;9:246.

42. Stute H, Greiner B, Linderkamp O. Effect of blood transfusion on cardiorespiratory abnormalities in preterm infants. *Arch Dis Child* 1995;72:F194.

43. Levy GJ, Strauss RG, Hume H, et al. National survey of neonatal transfusion practices. I. Red blood cell therapy. *Pediatrics* 1993;91:523.

44. Fetus and newborn committee Canadian Pediatric Society. Guidelines for transfusion of erythrocytes to neonates and premature infants. *Can Med Assoc J* 1992;147:1781.

45. Schreiber GB, Busch MB, Kleinman SH, et al. The risk of transfusion-transmitted viral infections. *N Engl J Med* 1996;334:1685.

46. Liu EA, Mannino FL, Lane TA. Prospective, randomized trial of the safety and efficacy of a limited donor exposure transfusion program for premature neonates. *J Pediatr* 1994;125:92.

47. Lee DA, Siagle TA, Jackson TM, et al. Reducing blood donor exposures in low birth weight infants by the use of older, unwashed packed red blood cells. *J Pediatr* 1995;126:280.

48. Ballin A, Arbel E, Kenet G, et al. Autologous umbilical cord blood transfusion. *Arch Dis Child* 1995;73:F181.

49. Obladen M, Maier R, Segerer H, et al. Efficacy and safety of recombinant human erythropoietin to prevent anaemias of prematurity. European randomized multicenter trial. *Contrib Nephrol* 1991;88:314.

50. Emmerson AJB, Coles HJ, Stern CMM, et al. Double blind trial of recombinant human erythropoietin in preterm infants. *Arch Dis Child* 1993;68:291.

51. Soubasi V, Kremenopoulos G, Diamandi E, et al. In which neonates does early recombinant human erythropoietin treatment prevent anemia of prematurity? Results of a randomized controlled study. *Pediatr Res* 1993;34:675.

52. Soubasi V, Kremenopoulos G, Diamanti E, et al. Follow-up of very low birth weight infants after erythropoietin treatment to prevent anemia of prematurity. *J Pediatr* 1995;127:291.

53. Maier RF, Obladen M, Scigalla P, et al. The effect of epoetin beta (recombinant human erythropoietin) on the need for transfusion in very-low-birth-weight infants. *N Engl J Med* 1994;330:1173.

54. Carnielli V, Montini G, Da Riol R, et al. Effect of high doses of human recombinant erythropoietin on the need for blood transfusions in preterm infants. *J Pediatr* 1992;121:98.

55. Ohls RK, Osborne KA, Christensen RD. Efficacy and cost analysis of treating very low birth weight infants with erythropoietin during their first two weeks of life: a randomized placebo-controlled trial. *J Pediatr* 1995;126:421.

56. Donato H, Rendo P, Vivas N, et al. Recombinant human erythropoietin in the treatment of anemia of prematurity: a randomized, double-blind, placebo-controlled trial comparing three different doses. *Int J Pediatr Hematol/Oncol* 1996;3:279.

57. Shannon KM, Mentzer WC, Abels RI, et al. Recombinant human erythropoietin in the anemia of prematurity. results of a placebo-controlled pilot study. *J Pediatr* 1991;118:949.

58. Chen J-Y, Wu T-S, Chanlai S-P. Recombinant human erythropoietin in the treatment of anemia of prematurity. *Am J Perinatol* 1995;12:314.

59. Shannon KM, Mentzer WC, Abels RI, et al. Enhancement of erythropoiesis by recombinant human erythropoietin in low birth weight infants: a pilot study. *J Pediatr* 1992;120:586.

60. Shannon KM, Keith JF III, Mentzer WC, et al. Recombinant human erythropoietin stimulates erythropoiesis and reduces erythrocyte

transfusions in very low birth weight preterm infants. *Pediatrics* 1995; 95:1.

61. Meyer MP, Meyer JH, Commerford A, et al. Recombinant human erythropoietin in the treatment of the anemia of prematurity: results of a double-blind, placebo-controlled study. *Pediatrics* 1994;93:918.

62. Ohls RK, Christensen RD. Recombinant erythropoietin compared with erythrocyte transfusion in the treatment of anemia of prematurity. *J Pediatr* 1991;119:781.

63. Bader D, Blondheim O, Jonas R, et al. Decreased ferritin levels, despite iron supplementation, during erythropoietin therapy in anaemia of prematurity. *Acta Paediatr* 1996;85:496.

64. Doyle JJ. The role of erythropoietin in the anemia of prematurity. *Semin Perinatol* 1997;21:20.

65. Blanchette VS, Zipursky A. Assessment of anemia in newborn infants. *Clin Perinatol* 1984;11:489.

66. Oettinger L Jr, Mills WB. Simultaneous capillary and venous hemoglobin determinations in the newborn infant. *J Pediatr* 1949;35:362.

67. Oh W, Lind J. Venous and capillary hematocrit in newborn infants and placental transfusion. *Acta Pediatr Scand* 1966;55:38.

68. Linderkamp O, Versmold HT, Strohhacker I, et al. Capillary–venous hematocrit differences in newborn infants. I. Relationship to blood volume, peripheral blood flow, and acid–base parameters. *Eur J Pediatr* 1977;127:9.

69. Rivera LM, Rudolph N. Postnatal persistence of capillary–venous differences in hematocrit and hemoglobin values in low-birth-weight and term infants. *Pediatrics* 1982;70:956.

70. Faxelius G, Raye J, Gutberlet R, et al. Red cell volume measurements and acute blood loss in high-risk newborn infants. *J Pediatr* 1977;90: 273.

71. International Committee for Standardization in Haematology. Recommended methods for measurement of red-cell and plasma volume. *J Nucl Med* 1980;21:793.

72. Mollison PL, Veall N, Cutbush M. Red cell and plasma volume in newborn infants. *Arch Dis Child* 1950;25:242.

73. Bratteby L-E. Studies on erythro-kinetics in infancy. XI. The change in circulating red cell volume during the first five months of life. *Acta Paediatr Scand* 1968;57:215.

74. Bratteby L-E. Studies on erythro-kinetics in infancy. X. Red cell volume of newborn infants in relation to gestational age. *Acta Paediatr Scand* 1968;57:132.

75. Dyer NC, Brill AB, Faxelius G, et al. Blood volume and hemorrhage timing in newborn infants with respiratory distress using the stable tracer ^{50}Cr. *Proc Am Nucl Soc* 1971;5:46.

76. Francoual C, Relier JP, Thérain F. Interet de la mesure du volume globulaire total chez le nouveau-né en detresse respiratoire. *Arch Fr Pédiatr* 1977;34:83.

77. Hudson IRB, Cavill IAJ, Cooke A, et al. Biotin labeling of red cells in the measurement of red cell volume in preterm infants. *Pediatr Res* 1990;28:199.

78. Cavill I, Trevett D, Fisher J, et al. The measurement of the total volume of red cells in man. a non-radioactive approach using biotin. *Br J Haematol* 1988;70:491.

79. Schulman I, Smith CH, Stern GS. Studies on the anemia of prematurity. *Am J Dis Child* 1954;88:567.

80. Schulman I. The anemia of prematurity. *J Pediatr* 1959;54:663.

81. Bell EF, Nahmias C, Sinclair JC, et al. The assessment of anemia in small premature infants. *Pediatr Res* 1977;11:467.

82. Zipursky A, Hull A, White FD, et al. Foetal erythrocytes in the maternal circulation. *Lancet* 1959;1:451.

83. Pai MKR, Bedritis I, Zipursky A. Massive transplacental hemorrhage. clinical manifestations in the newborn. *Can Med Assoc J* 1975;112:585.

84. Kleihauer E, Hildegard B, Betke K. Demonstration von fetalem Hamoglobin in den Erythrocyten eines Blutausstrichs. *Klin Wochenschr* 1957;35:637.

85. Pembrey ME, Weatherall DJ, Clegg JB. Maternal synthesis of hemoglobin F in pregnancy. *Lancet* 1973;1:1350.

86. Tan KL, Tan R, Tan SH, et al. The twin transfusion syndrome. Clinical observations on 35 affected pairs. *Clin Pediatr* 1979;18:111.

87. Dennis LG, Winkler CL. Twin-to-twin transfusion syndrome: aggressive therapeutic amniocentesis. *Am J Obstet Gynecol* 1997;177:342.

88. Ville Y, Van Peborgh P, Gagnon A, et al. Surgical treatment of twin-to-twin transfusion syndrome: coagulation of anastomoses with a Nd:YAG laser, under endoscopic control. Forty-four cases. *J Gynecol Obstet Biol Reprod (Paris)* 1997;26:175.

89. Vanhaesebrouck P, Vanneste K, De Praeter C, et al. Tight nuchal cord and neonatal hypovolemic shock. *Arch Dis Child* 1987;62:1276.

90. Shepherd AJ, Richardson J, Brown JP. Nuchal cord as a cause of neonatal anemia. *Am J Dis Child* 1985;139:71.

91. Cashore WJ, Usher RH. Hypovolemia resulting from a tight nuchal cord at birth. *Pediatr Res* 1975;7:399.

92. Clayton EM, Pryor JA, Wiersdma JG, et al. Fetal and maternal components in third-trimester obstetric hemorrhage. *Obstet Gynecol* 1964; 24:56.

93. Henderson JL. Hepatic hemorrhage in stillborn and newborn infants; clinical and pathologic study of 47 cases. *J Obstet Gynaecol Br Commonw* 1941;48:377.

94. Holmberg E. Rupture of liver in newborn observed at General Lying-in Hospital in Helsingfors from 1924 to 1932. *Finska Lak-Sallsk Handl* 1933;75:1067.

95. Potter EL. Fetal and neonatal deaths. a statistical analysis of 2000 autopsies. *JAMA* 1940;115:996.

96. Zipursky A, Brown E, Palko J, et al. The erythrocyte differential count in newborn infants. *Am J Pediatr Hematol Oncol* 1983;5:45.

97. Schacter BA. Heme catabolism by heme oxygenase: physiology, regulation, and mechanism of action. *Semin Hematol* 1988;25:349.

98. Rodgers PA, Vreman HJ, Dennery PA, et al. Sources of carbon monoxide (CO) in biological systems and applications of CO detection technologies. *Semin Perinatol* 1994;18:2.

99. Ostrander CR, Cohen RS, Hopper AO, et al. Paired determinations of blood carboxyhemoglobin concentration and carbon monoxide excretion rate in term and preterm infants. *J Lab Clin Med* 1982;100:745.

100. Necheles TF, Rai US, Valaes T. The role of haemolysis in neonatal hyperbilirubinemia as reflected in carboxyhaemoglobin levels. *Acta Paediatr Scand* 1976;65:361.

101. MacDonald MG. Hidden risks: early discharge and bilirubin toxicity due to glucose-6 phosphate dehydrogenase deficiency. *Pediatrics* 1995;96:734.

102. Bjure J, Fallström SP. Endogenous formation of carbon monoxide in newborn infants. I. Non-icteric and icteric infants without blood group incompatibility. *Acta Pediatr Scand* 1963;52:361.

103. Alden ER, Lynch SR, Wennberg RP. Carboxyhemoglobin determination in evaluating neonatal jaundice. *Am J Dis Child* 1974;127:214.

104. Liley AW. Diagnosis and treatment of erythroblastosis in the fetus. *Adv Pediatr* 1968;15:29.

105. Naiman JL. Current management of hemolytic disease of the newborn infant. *J Pediatr* 1972;80:1049.

106. Queenan JT. *Modern management of the Rh problem.* New York: Harper & Row, 1967.

107. Zipursky A. Erythroblastosis fetalis. In Nathan DG, Oski FA, eds. *Hematology of infancy and childhood.* Philadelphia: WB Saunders, 1974:46.

108. Cassady G, Daniel SJ. Non-immunologic hydrops fetalis associated with large hemangioendothelioma. *Pediatrics* 1968;42:828.

109. Zipursky A, Rose T, Skidmore M, et al. Hydrops fetalis and neonatal leukemia in Down syndrome. *Pediatr Hematol/Oncol* 1996;13:81.

110. Hathaway WE. Coagulation problems in the newborn infant. *Pediatr Clin North Am* 1970;17:929.

111. Chessells JM, Wigglesworth JS. Haemostatic failure in babies with rhesus isoimmunization. *Arch Dis Child* 1971;46:38.

112. Torrance GW, Zipursky A. Cost-effectiveness of antepartum prevention of Rh immunization. *Clin Perinatol* 1984;11:267.

113. Bowman JM, Friesen RF. Hemolytic disease of the newborn. In Gellis SS, Kogan BM, eds. *Current pediatric therapy,* vol 4. Philadelphia: WB Saunders, 1970:405.

114. Bowman JM, Pollack JM. Amniotic fluid spectrophotometry and early delivery in the management of erythroblastosis fetalis. *Pediatrics* 1965;35:815.

115. Zipursky A, Bowman JM. Erythroblastosis fetalis. In Nathan DG, Oski FA, eds. *Hematology of infancy and childhood.* Philadelphia: WB Saunders, 1993:4.

116. Desjardins S, Blajchman MA, Chintu C, et al. The spectrum of ABO hemolytic disease of the newborn infant. *J Pediatr* 1979;95:447.

117. Kaplan E, Herz F, Scheye E, et al. Phototherapy in ABO hemolytic disease of the newborn. *J Pediatr* 1971;79:911.

118. Risemberg HM, Mazzi E, MacDonald MG, et al. The correlation of cord bilirubin levels with hyperbilirubinemia in ABO incompatibility. *Arch Dis Child* 1977;52:219.

119. Kornstad L. New cases of irregular blood group antibodies other than anti-D in pregnancy. *Acta Obstet Gynecol Scand* 1983;62:431.

120. Pepperell RJ, Barrie JU, Fliegner JR. Significance of red cell irregular antibodies in the obstetric patient. *Med J Aust* 1977;2:453.

121. Giblett ER. Blood group antibodies causing hemolytic disease of the newborn. *Clin Obstet Gynecol* 1964;7:1044.

122. Beutler E. G6PD deficiency. *Blood* 1994;84:3613.

123. Lu TC, Wei H, Blackwell RQ. Increased incidence of severe hyperbilirubinemia among Chinese infants with G6PD deficiency. *Pediatrics* 1966;37:994.

124. Doxiadis SA, Valaes T, Karaklis A, et al. Risk of severe jaundice in glucose-6-phosphate dehydrogenase deficiency of the newborn. *Lancet* 1964;2:1210.

125. Olowe SA, Ransome-Kuti O. The risk of jaundice in glucose-6-phosphate deficient babies exposed to menthol. *Acta Paediatr Scand* 1980; 69:341.

126. Fessas P, Doxiadis S, Valaes T. Neonatal jaundice in glucose-6-phosphate dehydrogenase-deficient infants. *Br Med J* 1962;2:1359.

127. Kaplan M, Renbaum P, Levy-Lahad E, et al. Severe neonatal icterus in some glucose-6-phosphate dehydrogenase (G-6-PD)-deficient infants is explained by the combined effect of G-6PD deficiency and the UDP-Glucoronyltransferase 1 (UDPGT1) promoter polymorphism of Gilbert's syndrome. A new paradigm for multigenic disease. *Blood* 1997;90:8a.

128. Slusher TM, Vreman HJ, McLaren DW, Lewison LJ, Brown AK, Stevenson DK. Glucose-6-phosphate dehydrogenase deficiency and carboxyhemoglobin concentrations associated with bilirubin-related morbidity and death in Nigerian infants. *J Pediatr* 1995;126:102.

129. Kaplan M, Abramov A. Neonatal hyperbilirubinemia associated with glucose-6-phosphate dehydrogenase deficiency in Sephardic-Jewish neonates: incidence, severity, and the effect of phototherapy. *Pediatrics* 1992;90:401.

130. Kaplan M, Vreman HJ, Hammerman C, Leiter C, Abramov A, Stevenson DK. Contribution of haemolysis to jaundice in Sephardic Jewish glucose-6-phosphate dehydrogenase deficient neonates. *Br J Haematol* 1996;93:822.

131. Kaplan M, Rubaltelli FF, Hammerman C, et al. Conjugated bilirubin in neonates with glucose-6-phosphate dehydrogenase deficiency. *J Pediatr* 1996;128:695.

132. Eshaghpour E, Oski FA, Williams M. The relationship of glucose-6-phosphate dehydrogenase deficiency to hyperbilirubinemia in Negro premature infants. *J Pediatr* 1967;70:595.

133. Bienzle U, Effiong C, Luzatto L. Erythrocyte glucose-6-phosphate dehydrogenase deficiency (G6PD type A) and neonatal jaundice. *Acta Pediatr Scand* 1976;65:701.

134. Valaes T, Doxiadis SA, Fessas P. Acute hemolysis due to naphthalene inhalation. *J Pediatr* 1963;63:904.

135. Beutler E, Mitchell M. Special modifications of the fluorescent screening method for glucose-6-phosphate dehydrogenase deficiency. *Blood* 1968;32:816.

136. Motulsky AG, Campbell-Kraut JM. Population genetics of glucose-6-phosphate dehydrogenase deficiency of the red cell. In Blumber BS, ed. *Proceedings of the conference on genetic polymorphisms and geographic variations in disease*. New York: Grune & Stratton, 1961:159.

137. Kaplan M, Leiter C, Hammerman C, Rudensky B. Comparison of commercial screening tests for glucose-6-phosphate dehydrogenase deficiency in the neonatal period. *Clin Chem* 1997;43:1236.

138. Kaplan M, Vreman HJ, Hammerman C, Leiter C, Rudensky B, MacDonald MG, Stevenson DK. Combination of ABO blood group incompatibility and glucose-6-phosphate dehydrogenase deficiency: effect on hemolysis and neonatal hyperbilirubinemia. *Acta Paediatr* 1998;87(4):455–457.

139. Erlandson ME, Hilgartner M. Hemolytic disease in the newborn period. *J Pediatr* 1959;54:566.

140. Hegye T, Delphin ES, Bank A, et al. Sickle cell anemia in the newborn. *Pediatrics* 1977;60:213.

141. Lee-Potter JP, Deacon-Smith RA, Simpkiss MJ, et al. A new cause of hemolytic anemia in the newborn. A description of an unstable fetal hemoglobin. F Poole, $\alpha_2 G\gamma_2$ 130 tryptophan-glycine. *J Clin Pathol* 1975;28:317.

142. Piratsu M, Kan YW, Lin CC, et al. Hemolytic disease of the newborn caused by a new deletion of the entire beta-globin gene cluster. *J Clin Invest* 1989;72:602.

143. Oort M, Roos HD, Flavell RA, et al. Haemolytic disease of the newborn and chronic anemia induced by gamma-beta thalassemia in a Dutch family. *Br J Haematol* 1981;48:251.

144. Kan YW, Forget BG, Nathan DG. Gamma-beta thalassemia: a cause of hemolytic disease of the newborn. *N Engl J Med* 1972;286:129.

145. Fearon ER, Kazazian HH, Waber PG, et al. The entire beta-globin gene cluster is deleted in a form of delta-beta-gamma thalassemia. *Blood* 1983;61:1273.

146. Ballin A, Brown EJ, Zipursky A. Idiopathic Heinz body hemolytic anemia in newborn infants. *Am J Pediatr Hematol Oncol* 1989;11:3.

147. Doyle J, Vreman H, Stevenson D, et al. Does vitamin C cause hemolysis in premature newborns? Results of a multicentre, double-blind randomized, controlled trial. *J Pediatr* 1997;130:103.

148. Diamond LK, Wang WC, Alter BP. Congenital hypoplastic anemia. *Adv Pediatr* 1976;22:349.

149. Aase JM, Smith DW. Congenital anemia and triphalangeal thumbs. A new syndrome. *J Pediatr* 1969;74:471.

150. Jordan JA. Identification of human parvovirus B19 infection in idiopathic nonimmune hydrops fetalis. *Am J Obstet Gynecol* 1996;174:37.

151. Brown KE, Green SW, Antunez de Mayolo J, et al. Congenital anaemia after transplacental B19 parvovirus infection. *Lancet* 1994; 343:895.

152. Zerbini M, Musiani M, Gentilomi G, et al. Comparative evaluation of virological and serological methods in prenatal diagnosis of parvovirus B19 fetal hydrops. *J Clin Microbiol* 1996;34:603.

153. Dallman PR. Iron, vitamin E and folate in the preterm infant. *J Pediatr* 1974;85:742.

154. Seip M, Halvorsen S. Erythrocyte production and iron stores in premature infants during the first months of life. The anemia of prematurity—aetiology, pathogenesis, iron requirement. *Acta Paediatr* 1956;45:600.

155. Shojania AM. Folic acid and vitamin B12 deficiency in pregnancy and in the neonatal period. *Clin Perinatol* 1984;11:433.

156. Hassan H, Hashim SA, Van Itallie TB, et al. Syndrome in premature infants associated with low plasma vitamin E levels and high polyunsaturated fatty acid diet. *Am J Clin Nutr* 1966;19:147.

157. Oski FA, Barness LA. Vitamin E deficiency. a previously unrecognized cause of hemolytic anemia in the premature infant. *J Pediatr* 1967;70:211.

158. Williams ML, Shott R, O'Neal PL, et al. Role of dietary iron and fat on vitamin E deficiency anemia of infancy. *N Engl J Med* 1975; 292:887.

159. Zipursky A, Brown EJ, Watts J, et al. Oral vitamin E supplementation for the prevention of anemia in premature infants: a controlled trial. *Pediatrics* 1987;79:61.

160. Wiswell TE, Cornish JD, Northam RS. Neonatal polycythemia: frequency of clinical manifestations and other associated findings. *Pediatrics* 1986;78:26.

161. Stevens K, Wirth FH. Incidence of neonatal hyperviscosity at sea level. *Pediatrics* 1980;97:118.

162. Wirth FH, Goldberg KE, Lubchenco LO. Neonatal hyperviscosity. I. Incidence. *Pediatrics* 1979;63:833.

163. Shohat M, Reisner SH, Mimouni F, et al. Neonatal polycythemia. II. Definition related to time of sampling. *Pediatrics* 1984;73:11.

164. Linderkamp O, Versmold HT, Roegel KP, et al. Contributions of red cells and plasma to blood viscosity in preterm and full term infants and adults. *Pediatrics* 1984;74:45.

165. Linderkamp O, Wu PYK, Meiselman HJ. Deformability of density separated red cells in normal newborn infants and adults. *Pediatr Res* 1982;16:964.

166. Riopel L, Fouron J, Bard H. Blood viscosity during the neonatal period. the role of plasma and red blood cell type. *J Pediatr* 1982;100:449.

167. Black VD, Camp BW, Lubchenco LO, et al. Neonatal hyperviscosity is associated with lower achievement and IQ scores at school age. *Pediatr Res* 1988;23:442A.

168. Black V, Camp BW, Roberts L, et al. Neonatal hyperviscosity. outcome at school age following a randomized trial of partial plasma exchange. *J Dev Behav Pediatr* 1986;7:202.

169. Black VD, Lubchenco LO, Koops BL, et al. Neonatal hyperviscosity. randomized study of effect of partial plasma exchange transfusion on long-term outcome. *Pediatrics* 1985;75:1048.

170. Olivieri N. Fetal erythropoiesis and the diagnosis and treatment of hemoglobin disorders in the fetus and child. *Semin Perinatol* 1997;21:63.

171. Bauer C, Ludwig I, Ludwig M. Different effects of 2,3-diphosphoglycerate and adenosine triphosphate on the oxygen affinity of adult and foetal human hemoglobin. *Life Sci* 1968;7:1339.

172. Andrew M. The relevance of developmental hemostasis to hemorrhagic disorders of newborns. *Semin Perinatol* 1997;21:70.

173. Morgan MEI, Benson JWT, Cooke RWI. Ethamyslate reduces the incidence of periventricular hemorrhage in very low birth weight infants. *Lancet* 1981;2:830.

174. Bloch CA, Rothberg AD, Bradlow BA. Mother–infant prothrombin status at birth. *J Pediatr Gastroenterol Nutr* 1984;3:101.

175. Shearer MJ, Rahin S, Barkhan P, Stimmlier L. Plasma vitamin K in mothers and their newborn babies. *Lancet* 1982;2:460.

176. Dreyfus M, Lelong-Tissier MC, Lombard C, Tchernia G. Vitamin K deficiency in the newborn. *Lancet* 1979;1:1351.

177. Blayer WA, Skinner AL. Fetal neonatal hemorrhage after maternal anticonvulsant therapy. *JAMA* 1976;235:626.

178. Loughnan PM, McDougall PN. Epidemiology of late onset hemorrhagic disease. A pooled data analysis. *J Pediatr Child Health* 1993; 29:177.

179. Ekelund H. Late hemorrhagic disease in Sweden 1987–88. *Acta Paediatr Scand* 1991;80:966.

180. Zipursky A. Vitamin K at birth. *Br Med J* 1996;313:179.

181. Sann L, Leclerq BSC, Guillaumont BS, et al. Serum vitamin K, concentration after oral administration of vitamin K_1, in low birth weight infants. *J Pediatr* 1985;107:608.

182. Hathaway WE, Isarangkura PB, Mahasandana C, et al. Comparison of oral and parenteral vitamin K prophylaxis for prevention of late hemorrhage disease of the newborn. *J Pediatr* 1991;119:461.

183. von Kries R. Neonatal vitamin K. *Br Med J* 1991;303:1083.

184. Zipursky A, deSa D, Hsu E, et al. Clinical and laboratory diagnosis of hemostatic disorders in newborn infants. *Am J Pediatr Hematol Oncol* 1979;1:217.

185. Baehner RL, Straus HS. Hemophilia in the first year of life. *N Engl J Med* 1966;275:524.

186. Andrew M, Paes B, Milner R, et al. Development of the human coagulation system in the full-term infant. *Blood* 1987;70:165.

187. Brellter DB, Levine PH. Factor concentrates for treatment of hemophilia: which one to choose? *Blood* 1989;73:2067.

188. Lorand L, Losowsky MS, Miloszewski KJN. Human factor XIII fibrin stabilizing factor. *Prog Hemostas Thromb* 1980;5:245.

189. Croizat P, Revol L, Favre-Gilly J, et al. Les Hémorrhagies néo-natales dans les diethesis hemorrhagiques congénital. *Nouv Rev Fr Hematol* 1964;4:181.

190. Katz JA, Moake JL, McPherson PD, et al. Relationship between human development and disappearance of unusually large von Willebrand factor multimers from plasma. *Blood* 1989;73:1851.

191. Andrew M, Kelton J. Neonatal thrombocytopenia. *Clin Perinatol* 1984;1:359.

192. Pearson HA, McIntosh S. Neonatal thrombocytopenia. *Clin Haematol* 1978;7:111.

193. von dem Borne AE, van Leeuwen EF, von Riesz LE, et al. Neonatal alloimmune thrombocytopenia. detection and characterization of the responsible antibodies by the platelet immunofluorescence test. *Blood* 1981;57:649.

194. Mueller-Eckhardt C, Kiefel V, Grubert A, et al. 348 cases of suspected neonatal alloimmune thrombocytopenia. *Lancet* 1989;1:363.

195. von dem Borne AEGK, von Riesz E, Verheugt FWA, et al. Baka a new platelet-specific antigen involved in neonatal alloimmune thrombocytopenia. *Vox Sang* 1980;39:113.

196. Friedman JM, Aster RW. Neonatal alloimmune thrombocytopenic purpura and congenital porencephaly in two siblings associated with a "new" maternal antiplatelet antibody. *Blood* 1985;65:1412.

197. Mueller-Eckhardt C, Becker T, Weisheit M, et al. Neonatal alloimmune thrombocytopenia due to fetomaternal Zwb incompatability. *Vox Sang* 1986;50:94.

198. Shibata Y, Miyaji T, Ichikawa Y, Matsuda I. A new platelet system, Yuka/Yukb. *Vox Sang* 1986;51:334.

199. Kiefel V, Santoso S, Katzmann B, Mueller-Eckhardt C. A new platelet-specific alloantigen Bra. Report of 4 cases with neonatal alloimmune thrombocytopenia. *Vox Sang* 1988;54:101.

200. Kroll H, Kiefel V, Santoso S, Mueller-Eckhardt C. Sra, a private platelet antigen on glycoprotein IIIa associated with neonatal alloimmune thrombocytopenia. *Blood* 1990;76:2296.

201. Kaplan C, Morel-Kopp MC, Kroll H, et al. HPA-5b [Br(a)] neonatal alloimmune thrombocytopenia: clinical and immunological analysis of 39 cases. *Br J Haematol* 1991;78:425.

202. Pearson HA, Shulman NR, Marder VJ, Cone TE Jr. Isoimmune neonatal thrombocytopenic purpura; clinical and therapeutic considerations. *Blood* 1964;23:154.

203. Blanchette VS, Chen L, de Friedberg ZS, et al. Alloimmunization to the P1A1 platelet antigen: results of a prospective study. *Br J Haematol* 1990;74:209.

204. Herman JH, Jumbelic MI, Ancona RJ, Kickler TS. *In utero* cerebral hemorrhage in alloimmune thrombocytopenia. *Am J Pediatr Hematol Oncol* 1986;8:312.

205. Lester RB, Sty JR. Prenatal diagnosis of cystic CNS lesions in neonatal isoimmune thrombocytopenia. *J Ultrasound Med* 1987;6:479.

206. Burrows RF, Caco CC, Kelton JF. Neonatal alloimmune thrombocytopenia. spontaneous *in utero* intracranial hemorrhage. *Am J Hematol* 1988;28:98.

207. Manson J, Speed I, Abbott K, Crompton J. Congenital blindness, porencephaly, and neonatal thrombocytopenia: a report of four cases. *J Child Neurol* 1988;3:120.

208. de Vries LS, Connell J, Bydder GM, et al. Recurrent intracranial hemorrhages *in utero* in an infant with alloimmune thrombocytopenia. Case report. *Br J Obstet Gynaecol* 1988;95:299.

209. Bussel JB, Berkowitz RL, McFarland JG, et al. Antenatal treatment of neonatal alloimmune thrombocytopenia. *N Engl J Med* 1988;319: 1374.

210. Gill FM, Schwartz E. Platelet transfusion as a diagnostic and therapeutic aid in the newborn. *Pediatr Res* 1971;5:409.

211. McIntosh S, O'Brien RT, Schwartz AD, Pearson HA. Neonatal isoimmune purpura. response to platelet infusions. *J Pediatr* 1973;82:1020.

212. McGill M, Mayhaus C, Hoff R, Carey P. Frozen maternal platelets for neonatal thrombocytopenia. *Transfusion* 1987;27:347.

213. Massey GV, McWilliams NB, Mueller DG, et al. Intravenous immunoglobulin in treatment of neonatal isoimmune thrombocytopenia. *J Pediatr* 1987;111:133.

214. Suarez CR, Anderson C. High-dose intravenous gammaglobulin (IVG) in neonatal immune thrombocytopenia. *Am J Hematol* 1987;26: 247.

215. Beck R, Reid DM, Lazarte R. Intravenous gammaglobulin therapy for neonatal alloimmune thrombocytopenia. *Am J Perinatol* 1988;5:79.

216. Kaplan M, Abramov A, Goren A. Repeated single-dose intravenous immunoglobulin therapy for neonatal passive immune thrombocytopenia. *Isr J Med Sci* 1987;23:844.

217. Mueller-Eckhardt C, Kiefel V, Grubert A. High-dose IgG treatment for neonatal alloimmune thrombocytopenia. *Blut* 1989;59:145.

218. Pietz J, Kiefel V, Sontheimer D, et al. High-dose intravenous gammaglobulin for neonatal alloimmune thrombocytopenia in twins. *Acta Paediatr Scand* 1991;80:129.

219. Bussel J, Kaplan C, McFarland J, The Working Party on Neonatal Immune Thrombocytopenia of the Neonatal Hemostasis Subcommittee of the Scientific and Standardization Committee of the ISTH. Recommendations for the evaluation and treatment of neonatal autoimmune and alloimmune thrombocytopenia. *Thromb Haemostas* 1991; 65:631.

220. Bussel JB, Berkowitz RL, Lynch L, Lesser ML, Paidas MJ, Huang CL, McFarland JG. Antenatal management of alloimmune thrombocytopenia with intravenous gammaglobulin. a randomized trial of the addition of low-dose steroid to intravenous gamma-globulin. *Am J Obstet Gynecol* 1996;174:1414.

221. Johnson JM, Ryan G, Al-Musa A, Farkas S, Blanchette VS. Prenatal diagnosis and management of neonatal alloimmune thrombocytopenia. *Semin Perinatol* 1997:21:45.

222. Ballin A, Andrew M, Ling E, et al. High-dose intravenous gammaglobulin therapy for neonatal autoimmune thrombocytopenia. *J Pediatr* 1988;112:789.

223. Hanada T, Saito K, Nagasawa T, et al. Intravenous gammaglobulin therapy for thromboneutropenic neonates of mothers with systemic lupus erythematosus. *Eur J Hematol* 1987;38:400.

224. Kelton JG, Inwood MJ, Barr RM, et al. The prenatal prediction of thrombocytopenia in infants of mothers with clinically diagnosed immune thrombocytopenia. *Am J Obstet Gynecol* 1982;144:449.

225. Cines DB, Dusak B, Tomaski A, et al. Immune thrombocytopenic purpura and pregnancy. *N Engl J Med* 1982;306:826.

226. Kelton JG. Management of the pregnant patient with idiopathic thrombocytopenic purpura. *Ann Intern Med* 1983;99:796.

227. Karpatkin M, Porges RF, Karpatkin S. Platelet counts in infants of women with autoimmune thrombocytopenia: effects of steroid administration to the mother. *N Engl J Med* 1981;305:936.

228. Christiaens GC, Nieuwenhuis HK, von dem Borne AE, et al. Idiopathic thrombocytopenic purpura in pregnancy: a randomized trial on the effect of antenatal low dose corticosteroids on neonatal platelet count. *Br J Obstet Gynaecol* 1990;97:893.

229. Castle V, Andrew M, Kelton J, et al. Frequency and mechanism of neonatal thrombocytopenia. *J Pediatr* 1986;108:749.

230. Akenzua GI, Hui YT, Milner R, et al. Neutrophil and band counts in the diagnosis of neonatal infection. *Pediatrics* 1974;54:38.

231. Zipursky A, Palko J, Milner R, Akenzua GI. The hematology of bacterial infections in premature infants. *Pediatrics* 1976;57:839.

232. Xanthou M. Leukocyte blood picture in healthy full-term and premature babies during neonatal period. *Arch Dis Child* 1970;45:242.

233. Coulombel L, Dehan M, Tchernia G, et al. The number of polymorphonuclear leukocytes in relation to gestational age in the newborn. *Acta Paediatr Scand* 1979;68:709.

234. Lloyd BW, Oto A. Normal values from mature and immature neutrophils in very preterm babies. *Arch Dis Child* 1982;57:233.

235. Zipursky A, Jaber HM. The hematology of bacterial infection in newborn infants. *Clin Hematol* 1978;7:175.

236. Gregory J, Hey E. Blood neutrophil response to bacterial infection in the first month of life. *Arch Dis Child* 1972;47:747.

237. Manroe BL, Weinberg AG, Rosenfeld CR, Browne R. The neonatal blood count in health and disease. I. Reference values for neutrophilic cells. *J Pediatr* 1979;95:89.

238. Berger M. Complement deficiency and neutrophil dysfunction as risk factors for bacterial infection in newborns and the role of granulocyte transfusion in therapy. *Rev Infect Dis Suppl* 1990;4:S401.

239. Christensen RD, Rothstein G. Exhaustion of mature marrow neutrophils in neonates with sepsis. *J Pediatr* 1980;96:316.

240. Christensen RD, Brown MS, Hall DC, et al. Effect on neutrophil kinetics and serum opsonic capacity of intravenous administration of immune globulin to neonates with clinical signs of early-onset sepsis. *J Pediatr* 1991;118:606.

241. Gillan AR, Christensen RD, Suen Y, et al. A randomized, placebo controlled trial of recombinant human granulocyte colony-stimulating factor administration in newborn infants with presumed sepsis: significant induction of peripheral and bone marrow neutrophils. *Blood* 1994;84:1427.

242. Barak Y, Leibovitz E, Mogilner B, et al. The *in vivo* effect of recombinant human granulocyte-colony stimulating factor in neutropenic neonates with sepsis. *Eur J Pediatr* 1997;156:643.

243. Kostmann R. Infantile genetic agranulocytosis. *Acta Paediatr Scand* 1975;64:362.

244. Boxer L, Hutchinson R, Emerson S. Recombinant human granulocyte colony-stimulating factor in the treatment of patients with neutropenia. *Clin Immunol Immunopathol* 1992;62:539.

245. DeVaal OM, Seynhaeve V. Reticular dysgenesia. *Lancet* 1959;2:1123.

246. Shwachman H, Diamond LK, Oski FA, et al. The syndrome of pancreatic insufficiency and bone marrow dysfunction. *J Pediatr* 1964;65:645.

247. Buckley RH, Rowlands DT Jr. Agammaglobulinemia, neutropenia, fever and abdominal pain. *J Allergy Clin Immunol* 1973;51:308.

248. Rosen FS. The dysgammaglobulinemias and X linked thymic dysplasias. In Bergsma D, ed. *Immunologic deficiency diseases in man.* New York: National Foundation March of Dimes, 1968:67.

249. Page AR, Good RA. Studies on cyclic neutropenia. *Am J Dis Child* 1957;94:623.

250. Guerry DIV, Dale DC, Omine M, et al. Periodic hematopoiesis in human cyclic neutropenia. *J Clin Invest* 1973;52:3220.

251. Al-Mulla ZS, Christensen RD. Neutropenia in the neonate. *Clin Pediatr* 1995;22:711.

252. Makhlouf RA, Doron MW, Bose CL, Price WA, Stiles AD. Administration of granulocyte colony-stimulating factor of neutropenic low birth weight infants of mothers with pre-eclampsia. *J Pediatr* 1995;126:454.

253. Levine DH, Madyastha PR. Isoimmune neonatal neutropenia. *Am J Perinatol* 1986;3:231.

254. Minchinton RM, McGrath KM. Alloimmune neonatal neutropenia—a neglected diagnosis? *Med J Aust* 1987;147:139.

255. Lalezari P, Radel E. Neutrophil-specific antigens: immunology and clinical significance. *Semin Hematol* 1974;11:281.

256. Huizinga TW, Kuijpers RW, Kleijer M, et al. Maternal genomic neutrophil FcRIII deficiency leading to neonatal isoimmune neutropenia. *Blood* 1990;76:1927.

257. Stroncek DF, Skubitz KM, Plachta LB, et al. Alloimmune neonatal neutropenia due to an antibody to the neutrophil Fc-gamma receptor III with maternal deficiency of CD16 antigen. *Blood* 1991;77:1572.

258. Rodwell RL, Gray PH, Taylor KM, Minchinton R. Granulocyte colony stimulating factor treatment for alloimmune neonatal neutropenia. *Arch Dis Child* 1996;75:F57.

259. Hanada T, Shin R, Hosoi M, et al. Intravenous gammaglobulin in treatment of isoimmune neonatal neutropenia. *Eur J Pediatr* 1988;148:218.

260. Jarvenpa AL, Koskimies S, Rajantie J. Alloimmune granulocytopenia in three newborn infants of two families. *Acta Paediatr Scand* 1990;79:1244.

261. Cartron J, Tchernia G, Celton JL, et al. Alloimmune neonatal neutropenia. *Am J Pediatr Hematol Oncol* 1991;13:21.

262. Bussel J, Lalezari P, Fikrig S. Intravenous treatment with gammaglobulin of autoimmune neutropenia of infancy. *J Pediatr* 1988;112:298.

263. Zipursky A, Peeters M, Poon A. Megakaryoblastic leukemia and Down's syndrome. *Pediatr Hematol Oncol* 1987;4:211.

264. Miyauchi J, Ito Y, Kawaivo T, et al. Diffuse liver fibrosis accompanying transient abnormal myelopoiesis in Down's syndrome. *Blood* 1991;78:40A.

265. Ruchelli ED, Uri A, Dimmick JE, et al. Severe perinatal liver disease and Down syndrome. an apparent relationship. *Hum Pathol* 1991;22:1274.

266. Bhat AM, Scanlon JW. The pattern of eosinophilia in premature infants. *J Pediatr* 1981;98:612.

267. Gibson EL, Vaucher Y, Corrigan JJ Jr. Eosinophilia in premature infants: relationship to weight gain. *J Pediatr* 1979;95:99.

268. Lawrence R Jr, Church JA, Richards W, Lipsey AI. Eosinophilia in the hospitalized neonate. *Ann Allergy* 1980;44:349.

269. Rothberg AD, Cohn RJ, Argent AC, et al. Eosinophilia in premature neonates. Phase 2 of a biphasic granulopoietic response. *South Afr Med J* 1983;64:539.

270. Blanchette VS, Hume HA, Levy GJ, et al. Guidelines for auditing pediatric blood transfusion practices. *Am J Dis Child* 1991;145:787.

271. Hume H. Red blood cell transfusions for preterm infants; the role of evidence-based medicine. *Semin Perinatol* 1997;21:8.

272. Boulton JE, Jeffries AL, O'Brien KK, Fernandes BJ. Changing transfusion practices in the NICU. *Pediatr Res* 1996;39:197A.

273. Floss AM, Strauss RG, Goeken N, Kox L. Multiple transfusions fail to provoke antibodies against blood cell antigens in human infants. *Transfusion* 1986;26:419.

274. Ludvigsen CW Jr, Swanson JL, Thompson TR, McCullough J. The failure of neonates to form red cell alloantibodies in response to multiple transfusions. *Am J Clin Pathol* 1987;87:250.

275. Sacher RA, Strauss RG, Luban NLC, et al. Blood component therapy during the neonatal period: a national survey of red cell transfusion practice, 1985. *Transfusion* 1990;30:271.

276. Blanchette VS, Gray E, Hardie MJ, et al. Hyperkalemia after neonatal exchange transfusion: risk eliminated by washing red cell concentrates. *J Pediatr* 1984;105:321.

277. Scanlon JW, Krakaur R. Hyperkalemia following exchange transfusion. *J Pediatr* 1980;96:108.

278. Liu C, Mannino E, Lane TA. A prospective randomized trial of the safety and efficacy of a limited donor exposure transfusion program for premature infants. *J Pediatr* 1994;125:92.

279. Andrew M, Castle V, Saigal S, et al. Clinical impact of neonatal thrombocytopenia. *J Pediatr* 1987;110:457.

280. Andrew M, Vegh P, Caco C, Kirpalani H, Jefferies A, Ohlsson A, Watts J, Saigal S, Milner R, Wang E. A randomized controlled trial of platelet transfusions in thrombocytopenic premature infants. *J Pediatr* 1993;123:285.

281. Moroff G, Friedman A, Robkin-Kline L, et al. Reduction of the volume of stored platelet concentrates for use in neonatal patients. *Transfusion* 1984;24:144.

282. Christensen RD, Rothstein G, Anstall HB, et al. Granulocyte transfusions in neonates with bacterial infection, neutropenia, and depletion of mature marrow neutrophils. *Pediatrics* 1982;70:1.

283. Mollison PL. *Blood transfusion in clinical medicine,* 6th ed. London: Blackwell Scientific Publications, 1979:617.

284. Giacoia GP, Kasprisin DO. Transfusion in acquired hepatitis A. *South Med J* 1989;82:1357.

285. Azimi PH, Roberto RR, Guralnik J, et al. Transfusion in acquired hepatitis A in a premature infant with secondary nosocomial spread in an intensive care nursery. *Am J Dis Child* 1986;140:23.

286. Dienstag JL, Alter HJ. Non-A, non-B hepatitis: evolving epidemiologic and clinical perspective. *Semin Liver Dis* 1986;6:67.

287. Yeager AS, Grumet FC, Hafleigh EB, et al. Prevention of transfusion-acquired cytomegalovirus infections in newborn infants. *J Pediatr* 1981;98:281.

288. Adler SP, Chandrika T, Lawrence L, Baggett J. Cytomegalovirus infections in neonates acquired by blood transfusions. *Pediatr Infect Dis* 1983;2:114.

289. de Cates CR, Roberton NR, Walker JR. Fatal acquired cytomegalovirus infection in a neonate with maternal antibody. *J Infect* 1988;17:235.

290. Weston PJ, Farmer K, Croxson MC, Ramirez AM. Morbidity from acquired cytomegalovirus infection in a neonatal intensive care unit. *Aust Paediatr J* 1989;25:138.

291. Preiksaitis JK, Brown L, McKenzie M. Transfusion-acquired cytomegalovirus infection in neonates. A prospective study. *Transfusion* 1988;28:205.

292. Preiksaitis JK. Indications for the use of cytomegalovirus-seronegative blood products. *Trans Med Rev* 1991;5:1.

293. Rawls WE, Wong CL, Blajchman M, et al. Neonatal cytomegalovirus infections: the relative role of neonatal blood transfusion and maternal exposure. *Clin Invest Med* 1984;7:13.

294. Wu J, Tang ZY, Wu YX, Li WR. Acquired cytomegalovirus infection of breast milk in infancy. *Chin Med J* 1989;102:124.

295. Taylor BJ, Jacobs RF, Baker RL, et al. Frozen deglycerolyzed blood prevents transfusion-acquired cytomegalovirus infections in neonates. *Pediatr Infect Dis* 1986;5:188.

296. Luban NLC, Williams AE, MacDonald MG, et al. Low incidence of acquired cytomegalovirus infection in neonates transfused with washed red blood cells. *Am J Dis Child* 1987;141:416.

297. Gilbert GL, Hayes K, Hudson IL, James J. Prevention of transfusion-acquired cytomegalovirus infection in infants by blood filtration to remove leukocytes. Neonatal Cytomegalovirus Infection Study Group. *Lancet* 1989;1:1228.

298. Bowden RA, Slichter SJ, Sayers M, et al. A comparison of filtered leukocyte-reduced and cytomegalovirus (CMV) seronegative blood product for the prevention of transfusion-associated CMV infection after marrow transplant. *Blood* 1995;86:3599.

299. Shannon KM, Ammann AJ. Acquired immune deficiency syndrome in childhood. *J Pediatr* 1985;106:332.

300. Ammann AJ, Cowan MJ, Wara DW, et al. Acquired immunodeficiency in an infant. possible transfusion by means of blood products. *Lancet* 1983;1:956.

301. Shannon K, Ball E, Wasserman RL, et al. Transfusion-associated cytomegalovirus infection and acquired immune deficiency syndrome in an infant. *J Pediatr* 1983;103:859.

302. McCarthy VP, Charles DL, Unger JL. Transfusion-associated HIV infection in a neonate from a seronegative donor. *Am J Dis Child* 1987;141:1145.

303. Seemayer TA, Bolande RP. Thymic involution mimicking thymic dysplasia: a consequence of transfusion-induced graft-versus-host disease in a premature infant. *Arch Pathol Lab Med* 1980;104:141.

304. Berger RS, Dixon SL. Fulminant transfusion-associated graft-versus-host disease in a premature infant. *J Am Acad Dermatol* 1989;20:945.

305. Funkhouser AW, Vogelsang G, Zehnbauer B, et al. Graft versus host disease after blood transfusions in a premature infant. *Pediatrics* 1991;87:247.

306. Hatley RM, Reynolds M, Paller AS, et al. Graft-versus-host disease following ECMO. *J Pediatr Surg* 1991;26:317.

307. Bastian JF, Williams RA, Ornelas W, et al. Maternal isoimmunization resulting in combined immunodeficiency and fatal graft-versus-host disease in an infant. *Lancet* 1984;1:1435.

308. Luban NLC, Ness PM. Irradiation of blood products: indications and guidelines and comment. *Transfusion* 1985;25:301.

309. Leitman SF, Holland PV. Irradiation of blood products: indications and guidelines. *Transfusion* 1985;25:293.

310. Committee on Infectious Diseases. Prevention of hepatitis B virus infections. *Pediatrics* 1985;75:362.

311. Schmidt B, Andrew M. Neonatal thrombosis. Report of a prospective Canadian and international registry. *Pediatrics* 1995;96:939.

312. Nowak-Göttl U, von Kries R, Göbel U. Neonatal symptomatic thromboembolism in Germany: two year survey. *Arch Dis Child* 1997;76:F163.

313. Schmidt B, Zipursky A. Thrombotic disease in newborn infants. *Clin Perinatol* 1984;11:461.

314. Levin DL, Weinberg AG, Perken RM. Pulmonary microthrombi syndrome in newborn infants with unresponsive persistent pulmonary hypertension. *J Pediatr* 1983;102:299.

315. de Vries LS, Groenendaal F, Eken P, van Haastert IC, Rademaker KJ, Meiners LC. Infarcts in the vascular distribution of the middle cerebral artery in preterm and fullterm infants. *Neuropediatrics* 1997;28:88.

316. Estan J, Hope P. Unilateral neonatal cerebral infarction in full term infants. *Arch Dis Child* 1997;76:F88.

317. Barron TF, Gusnard DA, Zimmerman RA, Clancy RR. Cerebral venous thrombosis in neonates and children. *Pediatr Neurol* 1992;8:112–116.

318. Rivkin MJ, Anderson ML, Kaye EM. Neonatal idiopathic cerebral venous thrombosis: an unrecognized cause of transient seizures or lethargy. *Ann Neurol* 1992;32:51.

319. O'Neill JA Jr, Neblett WW III, Born ML. Management of major thromboembolic complications of umbilical artery catheters. *J Pediatr Surg* 1981;16:972.

320. Cochran WD, Davis HT, Smith CA. Advantages and complications of umbilical artery catheterization in the newborn. *Pediatrics* 1968;42:769.

321. Gupta JM, Roberton NRC, Wigglesworth JS. Umbilical artery catheterization in the newborn. *Arch Dis Child* 1968;43:382–387.

322. Larroche JC. Umbilical catheterization: its complications. *Biol Neonate* 1970;16:101.

323. Wigger JH, Bransilver BR, Blanc WA. Thrombosis due to catheterization in infants and children. *J Pediatr* 1970;76:1–11.

324. Egan EA, Eitzman DV. Umbilical vessel catheterization. *Am J Dis Child* 1971;121:213.

325. Symansky MR, Fox HA. Umbilical vessel catheterization: indications, management and evaluation of the technique. *J Pediatr* 1972;80:820.

326. Tooley WH. What is the risk of an umbilical artery catheter? *Pediatrics* 1972;50:1.

327. Marsh JL, King W, Barrett C, et al. Serious complications after umbilical artery catheterization for neonatal monitoring. *Arch Surg* 1975;110:1203.

328. Tyson JE, deSa DJ, Moore S. Thromboatheromatous complications of umbilical arterial catheterization in the newborn period. Clinicopathological study. *Arch Dis Child* 1976;51:744.

329. Neal WA, Reynolds JW, Jarvis CW, et al. Umbilical artery catheterization: demonstration of arterial thrombosis by aortography. *Pediatrics* 1972;50:6.

330. Goetzman BW, Stadalnik RC, Bogren HG, et al. Thrombotic complications of umbilical artery catheters: a clinical and radiographic study. *Pediatrics* 1975;56:374.

331. Olinsky A, Aitken FG, Isdale JM. Thrombus formation after umbilical arterial catheterization. An angiographic study. *S Afr Med J* 1975;49:1467.

332. Mokrohisky ST, Levine R, Blumhagen JD, et al. Low positioning of umbilical artery catheters increases associated complications in newborn infants. *N Engl J Med* 1978;299:561.

333. Saia OS, Rubaltelli FF, D'Elia RD, et al. Clinical and aortographic assessment of the complications of arterial catheterization. *Eur J Pediatr* 1978;128:169.

334. Wesstrom G, Finnstrom O, Stenport G. Umbilical artery catheterization in newborns. I. Thrombosis in relation to catheter type and position. *Acta Paediatr Scand* 1979;68:575.

335. Roy M, Turner-Gomes S, Gill G, Way C, Mernagh J, Schmidt B. Incidence and diagnosis of neonatal thrombosis associated with umbilical venous catheters. *Pediatr Res* 1997;41:173A.

336. Mehta S, Connors AF Jr, Danish EH, Grisoni E. Incidence of thrombosis during central venous catheterization of newborns: a prospective study. *J Pediatr Surg* 1992;27:18.

337. Tanke RB, van Megen R, Daniels O. Thrombus detection on central venous catheters in the neonatal intensive care unit. *Angiology* 1994;45:477.

338. DeSa DJ. Intimal cusions in foetal placental veins. *J Pathol* 1973;110:347.

339. Rayne SC, Kraus FT. Placental thrombi and other vascular lesions: classification, morphology, and clinical correlation. *Pathol Res Pract* 1993;189:2.

340. Scully RE, Mark EJ, McNeely WF, Ebeling SH, Phillips LD, eds. Case records of the Massachusetts General Hospital: case 15-1997. *N Engl J Med* 1997;336:1439.

341. Seligsohn U, Zivelin A. Thrombophilia as a multigenic disorder. *Thromb Haemostas* 1997;78:297.

342. Marlar RA, Montgomery RR, Broekmans AW, the Working Party on Diagnosis and Treatment of Homozygous Protein C Deficiency. Report of the Working Party on Homozygous Protein C Deficiency of the Subcommittee on Protein C and Protein S, International Committee on Thrombosis and Haemostasis. *J Pediatr* 1989;114:528.

343. Mahasandana C, Suvatte V, Marlar RA, Manco-Johnson MJ, Jacobson LJ, Hathaway WE. Neonatal purpura fulminans associated with homozygous protein S deficiency. *Lancet* 1990;335:61.

344. Jochmans K, Lissens W, Vervoort R, Peeters S, De Waele M, Liebaers I. Antithrombin-Gly 424 Arg. A novel point mutation responsible for type 1 antithrombin deficiency and neonatal thrombosis. *Blood* 1994;83:146.

345. Pipe SW, Schmaier AH, Nichols WC, Ginsburg D, Bozynski ME, Castle VP. Neonatal purpura fulminans in association with factor V R506Q mutation. *J Pediatr* 1996;128:706.

346. Nowak-Göttl U, Koch HG, Aschka I, et al. Resistance to activated protein C (APCR) in children with venous or arterial thromboembolism. *Br J Haematol* 1996;92:992.

347. Roy M, Schmidt B. Neonatal thrombosis. are we doing the right studies? *Semin Thromb Hemostas* 1995;21:313.

348. Schmidt B, Andrew M. Report of Scientific and Standardization Subcommittee on Neonatal Hemostasis. Diagnosis and treatment of neonatal thromboses. *Thromb Haemostas* 1992;67:381.

349. Massicotte P, Adams M, Marzinotto V, Brooker LA, Andrew M. Low-molecular weight heparin in pediatric patients with thrombotic disease: a dose finding study. *J Pediatr* 1996;128:313.

350. Thomas DP. Does low molecular weight heparin cause less bleeding? *Thromb Haemostas* 1997;78:1422.

351. McDonald MM, Hathaway WE. Anticoagulant therapy by continuous heparinization in newborn and older infants. *J Pediatr* 1982;101:451.

352. Corrigan JJ. Neonatal thrombosis and the thrombolytic system: pathophysiology and therapy. *Am J Pediatr Hematol Oncol* 1988;10:83–91.

353. Leaker M, Massicotte P, Brooker LA, Andrew M. Thrombolytic therapy in pediatric patients: a comprehensive review of the literature. *Thromb Haemostas* 1996;76:132.

354. Mocan H, Beattie TJ, Murphy AV. Renal venous thrombosis in infancy: long-term follow up. *Pediatr Nephrol* 1991;5:45.

355. Adelman R. Long-term follow-up of neonatal renovascular hypertension. *Pediatr Nephrol* 1987;1:35.

356. Caplan MS, Cohn RA, Langman CB, et al. Favorable outcome of neonatal aortic thrombosis and renovascular hypertension. *J Pediatr* 1989;115:291.

357. Payne RM, Martin TC, Bower RJ, et al. Management and follow-up of arterial thrombosis in the neonatal period. *J Pediatr* 1989;114:853.

358. Seibert JJ, Northington FJ, Miers JF, et al. Aortic thrombosis after umbilical artery catheterization in neonates. prevalence of complications on long-term follow-up. *Am J Roentgenol* 1991;156:567.

359. Rajani K, Goetzman BW, Wennberg RP, et al. Effect of heparinization of fluids infused through an umbilical artery catheter on catheter patency and frequency of complications. *Pediatrics* 1979;63:552.

360. David RJ, Merten DF, Anderson JC, et al. Prevention of umbilical artery catheter clots with heparinized infusates. *Dev Pharmacol Ther* 1981;2:117.

CHAPTER 46

Immunology of the Fetus and Newborn

Joseph A. Bellanti, Barbara J. Zeligs, and Yung-Hao Pung

Immunology has come a long way since 1905, when the Russian biologist Eli Metchnikoff prophetically wrote:

> Within a very short period, immunity has been placed in possession not only of a host of medical ideas of the highest importance, but also of effective means of combating a whole series of maladies of the most formidable nature in man and the domestic animals. Science is far from having said its last word, but the advances already made are amply sufficient to dispel pessimism in so far as this has been suggested by the feat of diseases and the feeling that we are powerless to struggle against them (1).

Once the branch of medicine that dealt exclusively with the study of protection of the host against microorganisms, immunology now enjoys a much broader biologic scope and is concerned with the host processes that recognize and eliminate foreignness. Immunologic responses serve three functions: defense (i.e., resistance to infection by microorganisms), homeostasis (i.e., removal of worn-out host cells), and surveillance (i.e., perception and destruction of mutant cells) (2). Although not fully developed, the cells of the immunologic system of the fetus and neonate manifest a striking capacity for response to the environment. However, the fetus and newborn appear to be particularly vulnerable to injury caused directly by immunologic mechanisms or inflicted by infectious agents that take advantage of the relatively immature and inexperienced immune system. Immaturity refers to the genetically programmed low response or lack of response of the fetal and newborn immune system. Inexperience refers to the fact that the newborn immune system has not yet had its first immunologic encounter.

J. A. Bellanti: Department of Pediatrics and Microbiology-Immunology, Georgetown University Medical Center, Washington, D.C.

B. J. Zeligs: Department of Pediatrics, Georgetown University School of Medicine; and International Center for Interdisciplinary Studies of Immunology, Washington, D.C.

Y.-H. Pung: Department of Pediatrics, Georgetown University School of Medicine, Washington D.C.

Those who care for newborns must understand these processes because they form the basis for the prevention, diagnosis, and treatment of many diseases that afflict these patients (Table 46–1).

DEVELOPMENT OF THE IMMUNE SYSTEM

Role of the Environment

The development of the immune response may be visualized as a series of adaptive cellular responses to an ever-changing and potentially hostile environment. Development can be considered at several levels: the species, the individual, or the cell (Table 46–2). From an evolutionary standpoint, the effect of a hostile macroenvironment provided the selective pressures leading to the survival of those life forms within the species that were best adapted to that environment (i.e., phylogeny). Within the developing fetus, the microenvironment in which undifferentiated progenitor cells exist (e.g., thymus, bursa of Fabricius) provides yet another type of inductive environment, permitting the full expression of immunity within the developing infant. The immunologically mature person may be considered as the best-selected form resulting from this type of development (i.e., ontogeny). The molecular environment (i.e., antigen) in which immunologically reactive cells exist provides the best-studied inductive stimulus leading to the proliferative and differentiating events commonly associated with cellular immune responses. Memory cells may be considered the best-adapted form for this environment. Fetal and neonatal development of the immunologic system is best understood in terms of the developing host responding to his environment. The cells and functions that constitute the immune system appear early in fetal life, but at least some of them are fully activated only after birth, after interaction of the neonate with his environment. Under certain circumstances (e.g., intrauterine infections), the environment of the developing fetus may be so altered

1093

TABLE 46–1. *Applications of immunology for the neonatologist*

Type	Example of immunologic procedure	Disease
Prevention	Rhogam	Hemolytic disease of the newborn
Diagnosis	Elevated IgM globulins in cord serum	Intrauterine infections
Therapy	Fresh blood transfusions	Acute sepsis of the newborn

that the immune system begins activation *in utero*. The neonatologist and others entrusted with the care of the newborn must be concerned with the deleterious effect of factors introduced to the fetus from the ever-changing and complex external environment. Threatening agents that may gain access to the fetus during prenatal development include maternal drugs, infecting organisms, and antibiotics. The obstetrician and the neonatologist, who have already made significant contributions to the understanding of teratogenic effects of these agents, must be made aware of their effects on the developing immunologic system.

The glucocorticoids, toxic agents that frequently are administered to human fetuses for prevention of respiratory stress syndrome, also act on their immune system. Glucocorticoid administration results in the inhibition of several cellular and humoral systems including cytokine production and T-cell activation, both of which are already significantly decreased in the newborn. In addition, neonatal immune cells are more sensitive to glucocorticoids than adult immune cells (3). Further, it has long been noted that sex hormones appear to play a significant role in modulation of immune function (4). It has been repeatedly observed in studies of serious bacterial infections in infants, i.e., sepsis, pneumonia, and meningitis, that a preponderance of male infants exists over females (5–8). There are variety of humoral and cellular deficiencies compared to the adult levels that may contribute to this male susceptibility, including the following: lower numbers of white blood cells and polymorphonuclear neutrophil leukocytes (PMN) in males (9); lower numbers of CD3 and CD4 cells and higher numbers of CD8 and natural killer (NK) cells in males (10); higher immunoglobulin M (IgM) levels in females (11); and greater antimicrobial antibody responses that have longer duration persist in females (12).

Development of Components

For ease of discussion, the immunologic system may be considered under two major headings. The nonspecific immune system, which functions primarily during inflammatory responses, includes the phagocytic cell system (i.e., PMNs), mononuclear phagocytes (i.e., monocytes and macrophages), and several amplification systems, including complement, coagulation, and kinin systems. The specific immune system consists of cell-mediated (i.e., T-cell) and humoral (i.e., B-cell) systems. It is important to stress that the nonspecific and specific systems are intimately interrelated and interdependent. For example, the activation of the complement system by immunoglobulins (i.e., IgM and IgG) or the production of chemotactic factors and other cytokines plays a significant role in the whole inflammatory response. The monocyte or macrophage may function in inflammatory responses and play a significant role in the processing of antigen—steps that are essential to induction of the specific immune response. The macrophage forms part of the nonspecific and specific immune systems and is important to the afferent and efferent limbs of the immune response. The cytokines are other products secreted by cells that play a role in nonspecific and specific immune mechanisms. Several abnormalities of nonspecific immunity may affect the newborn infant, including abnormalities of quantitative and qualitative factors of cellular function (e.g., neutrophils, mononuclear phagocytes) and humoral factors (e.g., specific antibody, complement, fibronectin) (13–15). The quantitative cellular abnormalities are related to size and ability to regenerate mature cells for the storage pools of phagocytic cells in the fetal liver, neonatal spleen, bone marrow, and local sites such as lung and skin. The qualitative cellular abnormalities are related to the adherence and directed migration (i.e., chemotaxis) of phagocytic cells in response to and toward a chemoattractant that is exogenous (e.g., bacterial proteins) or endogenous (e.g., cellular or plasma products), the attachment and internalization (i.e., phagocytosis) of the source of the inflammation after its precoating (i.e., opsonization) by specific plasma factors such as antibody or complement, and the inactivation (i.e., microbicidal activity) and digestion (i.e., antigen processing) of the phagocytosed material. The deficiencies in the neonatal phagocytic cell system that may predispose to infection are summarized in Table 46–3.

TABLE 46–2. *Effect of environment on the development of the immune response*

Target	Inductive environment	Process	Selected form
Species	Macroenvironment	Phylogeny	Existing life forms
Individual	Microenvironment	Ontogeny	Immunologically mature individual
Cell	Molecular environment (i.e., antigen)	Induction of immune response	Memory cells

TABLE 46–3. *Deficiencies in neonatal host defenses that predispose to infection*

Anatomic barriers
  Injuries during delivery (e.g., skin abrasions)
  Invasive procedures in the nursery (e.g., umbilical artery catheters, endotracheal tubes)
Phagocytic cells
  Small polymorphonuclear leukocyte storage pool
  Decreased polymorphonuclear leukocyte adherence
  Decreased polymorphonuclear leukocyte and monocyte chemotaxis
  Decreased polymorphonuclear leukocyte intracellular killing in stressed neonates
  Decreased phagocytosis in stressed neonates
Complement
  Decreased levels of complement
  Decreased expression of complement receptors
Cellular immunity
  Possible defects in T-cell immunoregulation
Humoral immunity
  Decreased IgA, IgM
  Decreased IgG in premature neonates
  Impaired antibody function
  Decreased levels of fibronectin
  Decreased levels of cytokine (e.g., interferon-τ, tumor necrosis factor)

INFLAMMATORY RESPONSE

After tissue injury or invasion by microorganisms, a cascade of systemic and local events is triggered. This generalized response to injury is referred to as an inflammatory response. The febrile response is believed to reflect enhanced metabolic activity and to be related to the release of endogenous pyrogens (i.e., cytokines interleukin-1 [IL-1] and tumor necrosis factor [TNF]) from the host's leukocytes, which then trigger a hypothalamic response (16). Because these pathways are not particularly well developed in the neonate, fever is not a valuable sign of infection in this age group. Similarly, leukocytosis and an increased rate of sedimentation, commonly associated with bacterial infections in the older infant and child, are not particularly useful predictive markers of inflammation in neonates. However, other parameters in the inflammatory response, such as the increase in alpha- and beta-globulins with the elevation of C-reactive protein, occur in the neonatal period and are commonly used in the diagnosis of infectious diseases in the neonate. An elevation in total neutrophil count is an inconsistent and unreliable index of neonatal sepsis; neutropenia during sepsis is more common in the neonate. If neutropenia reflects storage pool exhaustion, it is a poor prognostic sign, even with appropriate antibiotic therapy (17–19). An important event accompanying nonspecific immune responses in the newborn is activation of the coagulation system, with disseminated intravascular coagulation, as seen in bacterial sepsis. The measurement of clotting factors and fibrin split products may provide another marker for infection.

Cellular Components

Cellular responses are carried out primarily by phagocytic cells, such as PMNs, monocytes, and macrophages, and secondarily by eosinophils and lymphocytes. The storage pool size and the function of PMNs play a critical role in the inflammatory response.

Polymorphonuclear

Polymorphonuclear Leukocyte Storage Pools

Leukocytes are first produced in the liver at about 2 months of gestation. By 5 months of gestation, the bone marrow has become the primary hematopoietic center, and liver production has diminished (20). PMN storage pools are considerably smaller per kilogram of body weight in the premature and full-term newborn than in adults (21,22). Neonates are less capable of increasing their PMN numbers because the proliferative rate of their progenitor cells is already near maximum compared with adults (23).

Polymorphonuclear Leukocyte Adherence, Mobility, and Chemotaxis

The skin of the newborn is relatively deficient in expressions of nonspecific immunity. After introduction of a foreign substance into the skin, several inflammatory cells begin to adhere to the wall of vessels near the substance and move in a directed fashion toward it in response to a chemical released from the foreign material or surrounding tissue. This adherence phenomenon is now recognized to occur through the action of cell surface receptors that function as adhesion molecules (i.e., adhesins), including integrins, immunoglobulin superfamily, selectins, and other adhesion molecules that are described later. An absence of leukocyte adhesins is seen in an autosomal recessive disorder, the leukocyte adhesion defect syndrome type 1. This is associated with a defective synthesis of the integrin, CD11/CD18 (LFA-1, Mac-1, p150,95), β-chain that occurs in monocytes, macrophages, PMNs, and certain lymphocytes and is associated with impaired cell adhesion. It is clinically seen in infants with delayed separation of the umbilical cord and in recurrent bacterial and fungal life-threatening infections. In the adult inflammatory response, prominent PMN infiltration occurs during the first 4 to 12 hours, followed by a predominant mononuclear response consisting of macrophages and lymphocytes. In the newborn, the shift from a PMN response to a mononuclear cell response is slower and less intense than in the adult, reflecting maturational deficiency. In some studies, a curiously high percentage of eosinophils is observed in the 2- and 4-hour exudate of newborns older than 24 hours but not in those younger than 24 hours. Although the precise mechanisms for this eosinophilic response are unknown, it is of interest that the lesions of erythema toxicum, well known to neonatologists, consist primarily of eosinophilic leukocytes. Mobility or movement encompasses a series of cellular events that are decreased in the neonate and include cell responsiveness to chemoattractants (24–28). The latter reflects expression of cell surface receptors (particularly complement receptor [CR]3), adherence, deformability, and aggregation, all of which are necessary for normal chemotaxis (29–36). Chemotaxis does not appear to reach adult levels until 16 years of age (37). Neonatal PMNs exhibit less chemotactic activity than do adult cells because of deficiencies of intrinsic cellular factors and extrinsic humoral factors. The primary deficient humoral factors are complement components C5 (38).

Phagocytosis

Once mobilized, the phagocytic cells mount an attack on their target by a process of phagocytosis. In the adult, many foreign substances, such as damaged tissue or nonvirulent organisms, may be ingested by phagocytic cells through unenhanced processes involving cell receptors (e.g., integrins, fibronectin), nonspecific plasma, and tissue factors. More virulent organisms require opsonization by a specific antibody or complement. The newborn may have compromised cellular and humoral factors involved in phagocytosis. Of the immunoglobulins, only the IgG globulins are transmitted across the placenta. The complement factors do not cross the placenta (39). Complement and fibronectin levels are deficient in the neonate (15,40). Several investigations of phagocytosis in the neonate had conflicting results. In some studies, phagocytosis by neonatal leukocytes is abnormal when they are suspended in neonatal serum. Normal activity is restored when the same cells are resuspended in adult serum. However, under certain *in vitro* and *in vivo* conditions, neonatal PMNs are deficient in phagocytic capacity compared with the adult PMN (41). For example, if the concentration of adult serum is varied or if phagocytes are taken from sick full-term infants, phagocytic activity is deficient relative to that in normal full-term neonates. The decreased phagocytic activity may be related to the decreased expression of the complement receptor CR3 in the newborn, which is reported to reach only 60% to 70% of adult levels during stimulation (39). This receptor is important for complement-dependent adherence, surface adherence with albumin and fibronectin, and penetration of PMN into tissues (39). Decreased expression of C3 may contribute to the relatively poor adherence and chemotaxis of neonatal cells.

Microbicidal and Metabolic Activity

After particle uptake by phagocytes, there is an increase in oxygen consumption and in glucose use by the hexose monophosphate pathway, events that are collectively referred to as the "respiratory burst" (2). The formation of hydrogen peroxide, the result of increased hexose monophosphate pathway activity, is considered to be of major importance in the killing of many bacteria by the oxygen-dependent antimicrobial system. A second antimicrobial system, which is oxygen independent and granule associated, plays an important role in phagocytic cell function.

Oxygen-Dependent Systems. Phagocytic leukocytes, such as PMNs, respond to a particulate or soluble stimulus with a respiratory burst of increased oxygen consumption and the production of toxic microbicidal oxygen radicals, including superoxide (O_2^-), hydrogen peroxide (H_2O_2), and hydroxyl radicals. When the cell membrane is stimulated, NADPH oxidase (i.e., membrane-associated oxidative enzymatic system), which consists of the oxidase and nonmitochondrial flavoprotein and cytochrome components, is activated and transfers electrons to molecular oxygen, reducing it to the free-radical superoxide anion (24,42). Chronic granulomatous disease (CGD) is a genetic disorder in which the PMNs and monocytes are incapable of generating the oxidative burst necessary to produce the antimicrobial oxygen metabolites (i.e., hydrogen peroxide and related compounds). This is the result of a deficiency of one of the components of the NADPH oxidase complex (24,42). The consequent loss of the important antibacterial mechanisms of the human host defense is the basis for recurrent bacterial and fungal infections in these children. There has been marked clinical improvement in CGD patients treated with interferon-γ (IFN-γ) (24,42). The production of high-energy oxygen radicals and superoxide by the newborn's PMNs is evaluated differently by various researchers. The O_2^- generation system seems to be efficient in the normal newborn and human fetus (43,44). There is some evidence that the NADPH oxidase system in granulocytes generating O_2^- is completely developed during fetal life, but triggering mechanisms are probably deficient. The release by fetal and newborn bone marrow of many immature phagocytic cells with significantly reduced phagocytic function into the peripheral blood and the relatively rapid exhaustion of this cell reservoir may explain the defect in granulocyte function observed in stressed and infected newborns (45).

Oxygen-Independent Systems. The oxygen-independent microbicidal system is demonstrated by the ability of phagocytic cells to kill organisms in anaerobic conditions and by non-O_2-dependent microbicidal activity of the cells from patients with CGD. The active components of the O_2-independent system reside in the phagocytic cell granules. In the PMN, the primary (i.e., azurophilic) granules contain acid hydrolases, neutral proteases, lysozyme, bactericidal cationic protein, and myeloperoxidase, a critical component in the O_2-dependent system, which catalyzes the generation of toxic oxyhalide ($HOCl^-$) from H_2O_2. The specific granules contain vitamin B$_{12}$-binding protein, phospholipase-A2, collagenase, more lysozyme, and lactoferrin, which has an important role in OH$^-$ generation by the O$_2$-dependent system. The secondary granules contain stores of cell receptors for complement components (e.g., CR3) and chemoattractant. It is clear from the contents of the granules that degranulation plays a key role in both microbicidal systems and that deficiencies in granule population could result in a poor inflammatory response. This is particularly demonstrated by the role that the first granules to be released play in the amplification of the complement cascade, generation of chemoattractant C5a, release of a monocyte chemoattractant, and promotion of PMN adherence to endothelial cells (46). The granule complement is established early in cell differentiation. Primary granules appear in the promyelocyte stage and secondary granules in the myelocyte stage. Except under extreme conditions, when very immature cells are released from the bone marrow (e.g., severe neonatal sepsis), the granule content of neonatal phagocytes is similar to that of the adult. The results obtained in studies of bactericidal activity of neonatal PMNs are similar to those found in studies of phagocytosis; results obtained under apparently normal conditions differ from those obtained under stress. A deficient bactericidal activity has been shown in PMNs from neonates with a variety of clinical abnormalities, including sepsis, meconium aspiration, respiratory distress syndrome, hyperbilirubinemia, and premature rupture of the membranes (47). When subjected to the demands of adjustment to extrauterine life, relative deficiencies of the bactericidal activities of PMNs contribute significantly to the compromised host defense mechanisms of the neonate.

Monocytes and Macrophages

The other major phagocyte system involved in immunologic processes is the mononuclear phagocyte system, which consists of circulatory monocytes and tissue macrophages. Tissue macrophages comprise a wide network of phagocytic cells, including alveolar and gastrointestinal tract macrophages important for initial defense at major portals of entry and dendritic cells important in antigen processing and presentation of antigen at local sites (i.e., Langerhans cells in the skin). Liver (i.e., Kupffer cells) and spleen macrophages are vital for the systemic clearance of microorganisms, cellular debris, and immunocomplexes. Monocytes–macrophages perform a variety of functions, from microbicidal activity to secreting more than 100 molecules important in inflammatory regulation (48). These secretory products include cytokines, growth factors, eicosanoids, enzymes, enzyme inhibitors, clotting factors, complement components, plasma-binding proteins, and low-molecular-weight reactive oxygen and nitrogen products. Macrophages play a vital role in angiogenesis and wound healing. Inflammation, which is a vital part of the immune defense, is marked by the rapid movement of monocytes out of the circulation in response to several factors, including bacterial protein, complement components, fibrinopeptides, and several cytokines (e.g., transforming growth factor, platelet-derived growth factor, IL-1, TNF, IL-2). During this inflammatory response, the monocytes may be further primed by cytokines (e.g., IFN-γ], IL-2, granulocyte–macrophage colony-stimulating factor [GM-CSF]). IFN-γ activated macrophages are more bactericidal, tumoricidal, and express more major histocompatibility complex class II (MHC II) molecules on their surface. They are enabled to present antigens to lymphocytes and are primed to release cytokines (e.g., TNF-α) (48). Monocytes–macrophages can express several plasma membrane receptors, such as those for immunoglobulin (i.e., FcR) and complement components (i.e., CR1 and CR3), which enhance their function, and carbohydrate receptors (e.g., MMR on resident macrophages only). Although studies of Fc and C3b receptors on newborn monocytes reflect a level similar to those in adult cells, cord blood monocytes are less efficient in the phagocytosis of group B streptococci and intracellular killing of *Staphylococcus aureus* and group B streptococci (49). The reason for this defective intracellular killing is unknown, but the characteristic susceptibility of the newborn to group B streptococcal (GBS) infections may depend, in part, on the immunologic immaturity of the mononuclear phagocyte system. Monocytes, particularly cytokine-activated macrophages, are the first and the most important defense against many intracellular microorganisms (e.g., *Toxoplasma gondii*). Although the antibacterial activity of the newborn's monocytes is comparable to that of the adult, these cells probably have only an initial role in limiting infection. The high incidence (65%) of congenital toxoplasmosis after maternal infection during the third trimester and the significant incidence of serious tissue damage in the fetus may result from deficient activation of the fetal tissue macrophages. Decreased generation by neonatal lymphocytes of IFN-γ, which is necessary for killing of intracellular pathogens, for the increased expression of MHC II and cytokine production, and for normal inflammatory response and antigen presentation, may facilitate the survival and replication of *T. gondii* in fetal tissues (50,51). Macrophage function is deficient in the neonate (52). This may be related to decreased cytokine production. Investigation has focused on the functional capabilities of monocytes in neonates, including chemotaxis, phagocytosis, microbial killing, and antibody-dependent cellular cytotoxicity. Only chemotaxis has been shown to be primarily deficient, although the total number and the function of alveolar macrophages has been reported to be deficient in the neonatal period (37,53). This observation may partially explain the newborn's susceptibility to GBS pneumonia.

Humoral Component

Complement System

The complement system is a key component in the production of innate or natural resistance to infection in vertebrates. Deficiencies of complement components can contribute to the susceptibility of the neonatal host to infection. Despite its significant biologic role, relatively little is known about the complement system in the neonate, except that it is deficient in this period and the components do not cross the placenta from mother to fetus (39). The third component of complement, C3, can be synthesized in different tissues in the human conceptus, beginning as early as 290 days of gestation (54). The sites of synthesis for C3 appear to be the fibroblast, the lymphoid cell, and the macrophage. There is some evidence that the liver is the major producer of C3 in adults. Serum concentration of C3 in the fetus rises almost exponentially, from 1.9 mg/dL at 5.5 weeks of gestation to between 52 and 167 mg/dL at 28 to 41 weeks (54). The mean level in cord blood is ±90 mg/dL, approximately one-half the maternal levels. Studies of C3 phenotypes indicate that C3 is synthesized in utero. The concentration of complement in the newborn falls slightly after birth and recovers before the infant is 3 weeks of age. By 6 months of age, C3 reaches adult levels. Phagocytosis of bacterial products enhances production of complement components. It can be deduced that antigen stimulation after birth may play a role in the induction of complement synthesis. Complement components C3, C4, and C5 are deficient in premature and full-term infants compared with maternal and adult standards. Propp and Alper (55) found that C1q, C3, C4, and C5 in cord blood from full-term neonates were approximately 50% of the respective maternal levels. Low levels of properdin, factor B(C3PA), C1, C2, C3, and C4 also have been reported in cord blood. Levels of C1q, C2, C3, C4, C5, factor B(C3PA), properdin, and total hemolytic complement are lower in the neonatal period. Most of the biologic effects of complement, including opsonization, immune adherence, complement-dependent viral neutralization, generation of anaphylactic and chemotactic factors, and production of cell membrane lesions, require only the first five complement components. Because the fetus can synthesize each of these components in biologically active form within the first trimester of development—however, in smaller quantities than the adult—all these immunologic functions could be affected to some degree by complement levels. There is a decreased expression of CR3, the receptor for the complement component C3bi on neonatal PMNs, which is important in a variety of adhesion reactions, such as cell adherence, mobility, and phagocytosis (39).

Fibronectin and Adhesion Molecules

Fibronectin is a nonimmune opsonin that exists in an insoluble form on most cells and in a soluble form in plasma and interstitial fluid (15). Newborn infants have fibronectin levels in the plasma that are one-third to one-half those found in the adult. These levels are further reduced in premature infants and under various pathologic conditions in the newborn (e.g., sepsis, malnutrition, respiratory distress syndrome, asphyxia) (15,41,56). Fibronectin is a glycoprotein with a molecular weight of 450,000 that promotes clearance by phagocytic cells of fibrin, platelets, immune complexes, and collagenous debris. Fibronectin is also an important opsonic factor for numerous pathogenic microorganisms, including Staphylococcus aureus, Streptococcus sp, and some gram-negative bacteria. It functions as a chemoattractant for phagocytic cells alone, as for macrophages, or by increasing the response in PMNs. Fibronectin induces the expression of the complement receptors (i.e., CR1 and CR3), amplifying functions of the phagocytic cell system (39). Low levels of fibronectin may contribute to hypofunction of the neonatal phagocytic cell system, predisposing to the development of sepsis. Adhesion molecules are a group of glycoproteins on cells that mediate cell-to-cell or cell-to-matrix (e.g., fibronectin, basement membrane) attachments. These include four groups of adhesin molecules, i.e., integrins, immunoglobulin superfamily molecules, selectins, and other adhesin molecules. The attachment occurs through ligand–receptor interaction, as with ICAM-1, VCAM-1, and ELAM-1 on endothelial cells with the integrins LFA-1 (CD11a/CD18), Mac-1 (CD11b/CD18), p150,95 (CD11c/CD18), VLA-4, and slex integrin–adhesin molecules on phagocytic cell plasma membranes (48,56). This binding facilities recruitment of these cells into inflammatory sites. Activation of phagocytic cells by a variety of events, including adherence, and by cytokines such as TNF and IL-1, induces the expression of the adhesion molecules. If the cytokine production is deficient, the adhesion molecule expression also may be reduced. Deficient cytokine production may be responsible for the decreased inflammatory response seen in newborns (51).

Cytokines

There are a group of hormone-like proteins, or glycoproteins, secreted primarily by lymphocytes and macrophages and a variety of other cells, that act as mediators of systemic inflammatory and immune responses by being molecular messengers between participating cells. Some of these were previously referred to as lymphokines or monokines, based on their cellular origin, but they are all generically referred to as cytokines. A summary of the major cytokines appears in Table 46–4, listing their primary cell sources and principal functions. In the neonatal period, there are deficiencies in two very important cytokines that may be key in the age-dependent susceptibility of the infant to viral and bacterial infections. These include IFN-γ and TNF-α, both of which display reduced mRNA expression and protein production

TABLE 46–4. *Characteristics of major cytokines*

Cytokine	Molecular weight	Primary cell sources	Activity	Principal effects
IL-1 (IL-1α, IL-1β)	17,500	Macrophages, NK and B cells, Epithelial cells	Immunoaugmentation: T-cell and macrophage activation	Inflammation and hematopoiesis; fever
IL-2	15,500	T lymphocytes and LGL	T- and B-cell growth factor	Activates T and NK cells
IL-3	28,000	T lymphocytes	Hematopoietic growth factor	Promotes growth of early myeloid progenitor cells
IL-4	20,000	TH cells	T- and B-cell growth factor; promotes IgE reactions	Promotes IgE switch and mast cell growth
IL-5	50,000–60,000	TH cells	Stimulates B cells and eosinophils	Promotes IgA switch and eosinophilia
IL-6	25,000	Fibroblasts and others	Hybridoma growth factor; augments inflammation	Growth factor for B cells and polyclonal immunoglobulin production
IL-7	25,000	Stromal cells	Lymphopoietin	Generates pre-B and pre-T cells and is lymphocyte growth factor
IL-8	8,800	Macrophages and others	Chemoattracts neutrophils and T lymphocytes	Regulates lymphocyte homing and neutrophil infiltration
IL-9	30,000–40,000	Activated T lymphocytes	T-cell growth factor; stimulation of hematopoiesis	Together with IL-2 increases fetal thymocyte proliferation; stimulates erythroid precursor cell proliferation
IL-10	18,000	B and T lymphocytes (TH2) and thymocytes	Effects on T cells, B cells, and mast cells; inhibition of cytokine synthesis by TH1 cells; IL-10 shows homology with EBV proteins	Proliferation of mature and immature thymocytes in presence of IL-2 and IL-4; stimulates mast cells only when combined with IL-3 and/or IL-4; interference with antigen presentation
IL-11	23,000	Bone marrow stroma cells	Functions as cofactor in hematopoiesis; B-cell growth factor; regulator of stem cell cycle	Stimulates megakaryocyte colony-forming units; stimulates Ig synthesis in the presence of T cells
IL-12	70,000	B cells, macrophages	Activates NK cells, induces CD4 T-cell differentiation to Th1-like cells	Activates macrophages; enhancement of cell mediated cytotoxicity; induces IFN-γ secretion
IL-13	9,000–17,000	T cells	B-cell growth and inhibits macrophage inflammatory cytokine production	Stimulates B-cell growth and differentiation
IL-14	60,000	B cell of non-Hodgkin's lymphoma	B-cell growth factor (BCGF)	Stimulates rapid proliferation of non-Hodgkin's lymphoma B cell
IL-15	14,000–15,000	T cells	IL-2–like; stimulates growth of intestinal epithelium	T-cell proliferation
IL-16	56,000	CD8+ T cells, mast cells, respiratory epithelial cells, CD4+ T cells, eosinophils	Potent chemoattractant for CD4+ T cells, monocytes, and eosinophils	Chemoattractant; modulator of T-cell activation; inhibitor of HIV replication; induces functional IL-2 receptors in CD4+ T cells
IL-17	28,000–31,000	Activated CD4+ T cells	Stimulates endothelial, epithelial, and fibroblast to produce PGE$_2$ and cytokines (IL-6, IL-8, G-CFS)	Stimulates cytokine production
IL-18	18,300	Activated macrophages Kupfer cells, epidermal keratinocytes	Stimulates T-cell proliferation	Induces IFN-γ and GM-CFS in activated T cells; enhances NK cells activity
G-CSF	18,000–22,000	Monocytes and others	Myeloid growth factor	Generates neutrophils
M-CSF	18,000–26,000	Monocytes and others	Macrophage growth factor	Generates macrophages
GM-CSF	14,000–38,000	T cells and others	Monomyelocytic growth factor	Myelopoiesis
IFN γ	18,000	Leukocytes	Antiviral, antiproliferative, and immunomodulating	Stimulates NK and phagocytic cells; induces cell membrane antigens (eg, MHC)
IFN β	20,000	Fibroblasts		
IFN τ	20,000–25,000	TH lymphocytes and NK cells		
TNFα	17,000	Macrophages and others	Inflammatory, immunoenhancing, and tumoricidal	Vascular thromboses; tumor necrosis; enhances phagocytic cell function
LT=TNFβ	25,000	T lymphocytes		
TGFβ	25,000	Platelets, bone, and others	Fibroplasia and immunosuppression	Wound healing and bone remodeling

B, bursal dependent; EBV, Epstein–Barr virus; G-CSF, granulocyte–colony-stimulating factor; GM-CSF, granulocyte-macrophage–colony-stimulating factor; IL, interleukin; IFN, interferon; LGL, large granular lymphocytes; M-CSF, macrophage-colony-stimulating factor; MHC, major histocompatibility complex; NK, natural killer; T, thymus derived; TGF, transforming growth factor; TH, thymic; TNF, tumor necrosis factor.

(57,58). The primary deficiency appears to result from an immaturity in T-cell function, particularly in the production of IFN-γ in the neonate, which is reported to be 10-fold less than in the adult (51). IFN-γ has antiviral effects and is an important immune cell modulator. It increases MHC II expression as well as the cellular functions, particularly of NK cells, PMNs, and microbicidal activity of macrophages. It induces T-cell differentiation and IgG and TNF production, which augments antimicrobial activity of phagocytic cells. In the neonate, the T-cell production of TNF is 50% less than in the adult, and IFN-enhanced mononuclear phagocyte production of TNF is 7% less than adult levels. TNF plays a major role in enhancing phagocytic cell function and inducing a variety of other antimicrobial, inflammatory, and immune functions, such as the expression of adhesion molecules (i.e., integrins ICAM-1, VCAM-1, ELAM-1 on endothelial cells and phagocytic cells) alone or by inducing the production of other cytokines (58). A recent study has reported that both IL-12 mRNA expression by cord blood mononuclear cells and IL-12 production are greatly reduced compared to adult levels. IL-12 is an important cytokine in the regulation of NK and T-cell function. It is hypothesized that the impaired capacity of IL-12 production in the neonate may contribute to the decreased production of IFN-γ and NK cytotoxicity (59). Further, Zola et al. (60) have reported significantly lower expression of some of the cytokine receptors on CD4 and CD8 T lymphocytes as well as on B lymphocytes. These include the following: decreased IL-2(p55) and TNFR(p75) on CD4, CD8 T cells, and on B cells; decreased IL-2(p75) on CD4 and CD8 T cells; decreased IL-6 and IL-7 on CD4 T cells; decreased IFN-γ on CD 8T cells; and decreased IL-4 on B cells (60,61). Collectively, these deficiencies in the neonatal cytokine repertoire may, in part, contribute to the immaturity of the immune response of the newborn and may play a major role in their increased susceptibility to infections.

Antibodies

Antibodies react with antigens, and they appear to play a significant role in events mediating inflammatory responses, such as phagocytosis, chemotaxis, and the release of mediators. The extent to which the antibodies affect these functions in the fetus and newborn depends on the permeability of the placenta to a given antibody and maturation of the antibody-producing system. Silverstein and colleagues (62) studied the maturation of immunologic capability and lymphoid tissues in the normal fetal lamb *in utero* (Fig. 46–1) They established the sequence of the antibody response to different antigens. Bacteriophage OX174 given on day 37 elicited the earliest antibody response, at 41 days of gestation. This is a remarkable observation, because the fetal sheep has little organized lymphoid tissue at this stage. At approximately

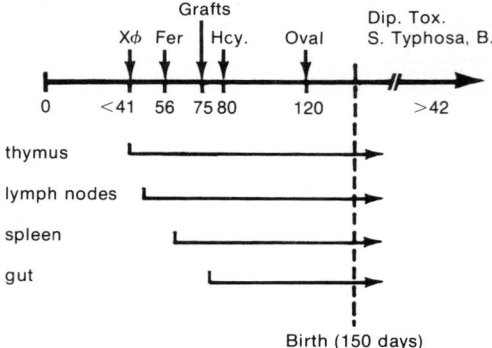

FIG. 46–1. Comparison of immunologic and lymphoid development in the fetal lamb. Numbers on the upper horizontal axis show the earliest times at which antibody responses and graft rejection could be detected. The order in which lymphocytes appear in different tissues is as follows: bacteriophage (Xφ), horse ferritin (Fer); snail hemocyanin (Hcy); hen albumin (Oval); diptheria toxoid (Dip Tox). (Adapted from Silverstein A, Prendergast R. The maturation of lymphoid tissue structure and function in ontogeny. In: Lindahl-Kiessling K, Alm G, Hanna MG Jr, eds. *Morphological and functional aspects of immunity.* New York: Plenum Press, 1971:39.)

66 days of gestation, the fetus becomes able to respond to the protein ferritin, but not until 125 days of gestation can it respond to egg albumin. Antibodies against *Salmonella typhi* or bacillus Calmette–Guérin appear only after birth. The researchers were unable to induce tolerance until the lamb reached the age at which it was able to recognize the antigen and produce antibody. It is possible to draw an analogy between this phenomenon and the poor response of human newborn infants to the polysaccharide antigens. These phenomena must be understood in the human if adequate immunization techniques are to be developed and allergic diseases are to be prevented (Table 46–5).

Opsonic Capacity

The opsonic capacity of blood refers to the enhancement of phagocytosis and includes the activities of antibodies, complement, and other proteins that are not well defined. IgM appears to have the greatest opsonic activity. Full-term and premature human newborns appear to be relatively deficient in opsonic activity toward a variety of agents. The degree of deficiency varies with different agents and probably particularly involves antibodies of the IgM type. This deficiency of antibodies may account for the susceptibility of the newborn to gram-negative infections, because IgM antibodies do not traverse the placenta. However, Miller (41) observed that addition of purified IgM to neonatal sera does not enhance opsonization of yeast particles. Complement and other heat-labile factors amplify the opsonic activity of IgM to a much greater extent than they amplify IgG opsonic activity. The deficit in opsonic activity derives from deficiencies of complement, particularly of components C3, C5, and

TABLE 46–5. *Development of the immune system in the fetus*

Gestation (wk)	Findings
4	First blood centers appear in yolk sac
5.5	Synthesis of complement is detected
7	Lymphocytes appear in peripheral blood, about 1000/mm^3
7–9	Lymphocytes appear in the thymus
11	CD2 receptors (i.e., E rosette) develop in thymus lymphocytes; B-cell maturation occurs in liver and spleen, with IgG, IgA, IgM, and IgD surface markers; serum IgM levels can be detected
12	Antigen recognition is demonstrable
13	Graft-versus-host reactivity is present
14	Phytohemagglutinin response by thymus lymphocyte occurs
17	Serum IgM levels can be detected
20	Secondary lymphoid complex is present
20–25	Lymphocytes in blood number about 10,000/mm^3
22	Complement levels detectable in serum
30	IgA level detectable in serum

Adapted from Cauchi MN. Immunological aspects of pregnancy and the newborn. In: Cauchi MN, Gilbert GL, Brown JB, eds. *The clinical pathology of pregnancy and the newborn infant.* London: Edward Arnold Publishers, 1984:325.

C3PA. In the premature infant, lowered levels of IgG may play a role in the opsonic deficiency (63). Rigorously controlled studies of the opsonic capacity of the fetus and newborn are needed so that the usefulness of potentially harmful treatments, such as fresh plasma transfusion in the septicemic neonate, can be determined. One of the important clinical sequelae of deficient antimicrobial antibody is seen in GBS infection of the newborn. The increased susceptibility of newborns to GBS infection has been correlated with deficiency of maternal antibody directed against the type-specific polysaccharides of the organism.

SPECIFIC IMMUNE MECHANISMS

The maturation of specific immune responses in the human begins *in utero* between 8 and 12 weeks of gestation. The differentiation of cells destined to perform these functions appears to arise from a population of progenitor cells, referred to as stem cells, that are located within the yolk sac, fetal liver, and bone marrow of the developing embryo (Fig. 46–2). Depending on the type of microchemical environment surrounding these cells, differentiation occurs along at least two avenues: hematopoietic and lymphopoietic.

Hematopoietic Differentiation

One type of microchemical environment leads to the proliferation and differentiation of stem cells into myeloid, erythroid, and megakaryocyte precursors. The products of these cell lines are the monocytes, granulocytes, erythrocytes, and platelets of the circulation. In the human, granulocytic cells are first observed in the liver of the fetus in the second month of gestation. Leukocyte production by the fetal liver declines at about the fifth month of gestation, when bone marrow activity increases.

Lymphopoietic Differentiation

Classically, the lymphoid system develops along two independent pathways leading to morphologically and functionally distinct populations of immune lymphocytes: the thymus-derived system of cell-mediated immunity (CMI), whose principal effector cells are the T lymphocytes, and the bursal-dependent system of antibody-mediated immunity, which is effected by the B lymphocytes. The T lymphocyte is commonly identified by the T-cell receptor–CD3 (TCR–CD3) complex or CD2 surface marker (i.e., binding site for sheep erythrocytes). The B lymphocyte is recognized primarily by its surface CD19 or CD20 markers or immunoglobulin.

T-Cell System

The basic cell type differentiates into lymphoid cells when the progenitor cells are influenced by certain microchemical environments. The first is the thymus, which leads to the differentiation of T cells (64,65). The thymus gland is derived from the epithelium of the third and fourth pharyngeal pouches at about the sixth week of fetal life. The parathyroid glands also begin their development at about this time from the same pouches. With further differentiation, a caudal migration of epithelium occurs, and, beginning in the eighth week, blood-borne stem cells enter the gland and begin lymphoid differentiation. With further development, the thymus is infiltrated with lymphocytes and is differentiated into a dense cortex containing many small lymphocytes and a less dense, central medulla with relatively more epithelial elements. Thymocyte precursors are probably derived from multipotential hematopoietic precursors in the fetal liver and later in the bone marrow (66–68). Under the influence of thymic epithelium-derived chemoattractants, pro-T cells initially localize to the thymic corticomedullary junction. These CD4-negative, CD8-negative T-cell precursors

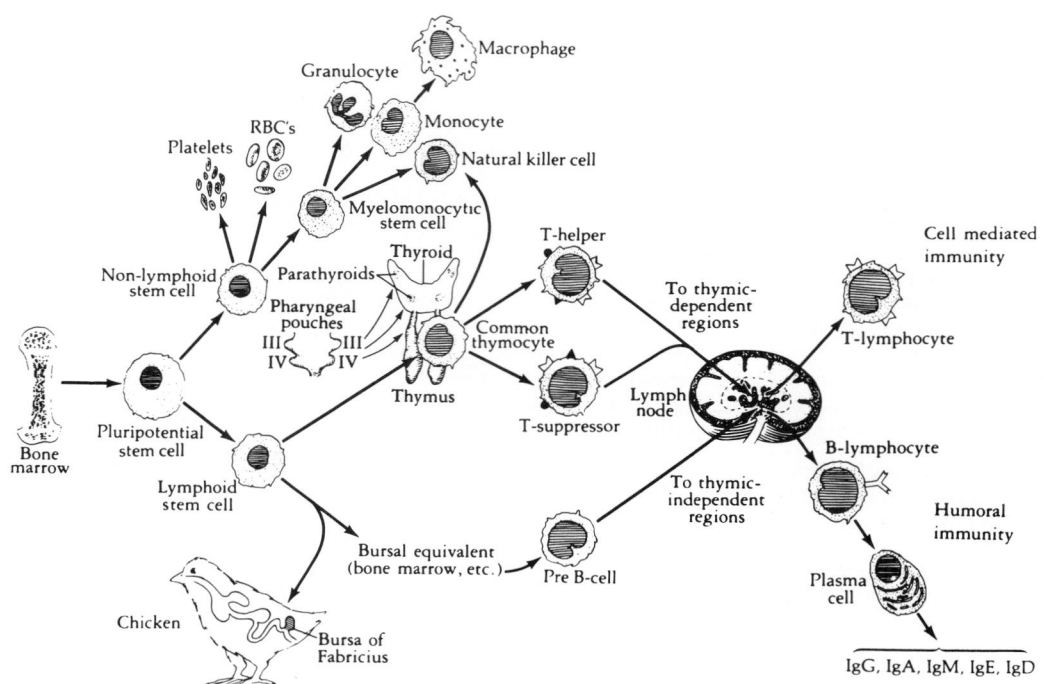

FIG. 46–2. Ontogeny of immune response, showing differentiation of progenitor cells into hematopoietic and immunocompetent cells. (From Bellanti JA. *Immunology III.* Philadelphia: WB Saunders, 1985:48.)

undergo extensive gene rearrangement, phenotypic alteration, and biochemical modification to yield the population of thymocytes that undergoes intrathymic selection. First, precursor T cells with affinity for self-MHC (i.e., usually CD4-positive and CD8-positive) are positively selected in the cortex of the thymus. Subsequently, in the medulla, they undergo negative selection, and those that recognize self-antigens are deleted. More than 95% of the thymocytes, which includes cells that have not been positively selected and those that have been negatively selected, proceed to programmed cell death, a process called apoptosis. The selected mature thymocyte, usually bearing mature TCRs with CD8 or CD4 molecules (i.e., single positive), seed the peripheral lymphoid tissue. In the developing thymus, there exists a dynamic interplay of cytokines that act in a coordinated and temporal manner to control the passage of the precursor cell through different stages of development in the thymus (Fig. 46–3). In particular, IL-1, IL-2, IL-4, and IL-7 may play central roles in precursor proliferation and differentiation (69). T-cell differentiation within the thymus appears to be regulated by several factors synthesized by the thymic epithelial cells. Several peptides have been described, and they share some properties that may result from their relative impurity (70). One of the best characterized of these thymic hormones is thymopoietin (molecular weight 5,562), which promotes prothymocyte to thymocyte differentiation, as demonstrated in the appearance of typical T-cell surface markers (71). Some synthetic polypeptide molecules that seem to have all the differentiation-induc-

ing properties of the original molecule are being evaluated. Although the characterization of hormones is preliminary, the use of thymosin has intriguing applications in clinical medicine as a replacement therapy for immunoincompetence. The clinical importance of the simultaneous embryogenesis of the parathyroid and thymus is seen in one of the immunologic deficiency disorders of infancy, the DiGeorge sequence. The DiGeorge sequence is a developmental defect in which derivatives of pharyngeal pouches III and IV do not arise, usually because of inadequate neural crest contributions. The conditions in which this occurs include exposure to teratogens, cytogenetic abnormalities, and mendelian disorders. The facies and cardiovascular defects that occur are very characteristic. Recently, DiGeorge sequence has been associated with a cluster of developmental anomalies, including velocardiofacial or Shprintzen syndrome and conotruncal atresia. These are all associated with a deletion of the long arm of the 22 chromosome (72). There is no known feature that uniformly occurs, and the diagnosis of DiGeorge sequence usually is based on two or more of the following: (1) typical facies (e.g., hypoplastic mandible, short philtrum, hypertelorism, ears low set or malformed, or both); (2) characteristic heart lesion (e.g., conotruncal malformation, usually interrupted aortic arch [IAA] type B; (3) persistent hypocalcemia with onset in the first month of life; (4) documented inability to identify the thymus at surgery or autopsy; (5) decrease in T-cell response to mitogens; and (6) decrease in T-cell number (73,74). Two rare conotrun-

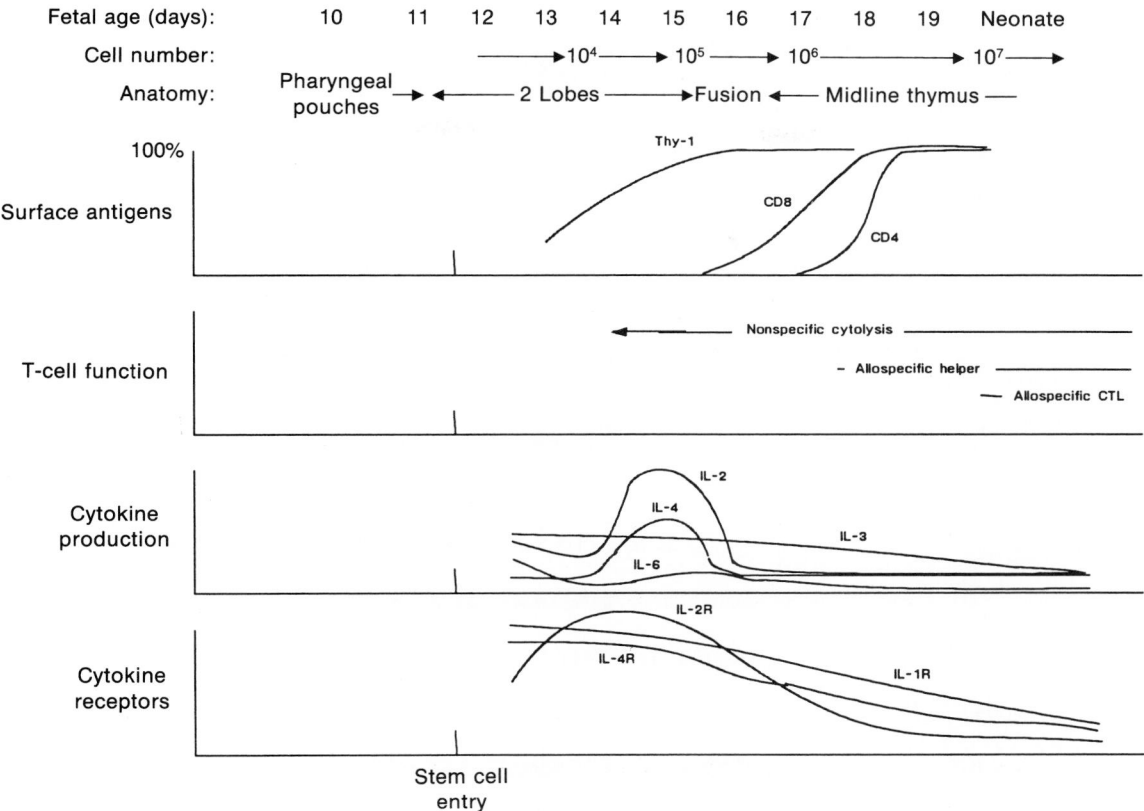

FIG. 46–3. Temporal relations among the production of cytokines, expression of cytokine receptors, and the differentiating events occurring in precursor cells in the murine fetal thymus during T-cell ontogeny. CTL, cytotoxic T lymphocytes. (Adapted from ref. 69.)

cal anomalies, type B IAA and truncus arteriosus, account for more than one-half of the cardiac lesions seen in the DiGeorge sequence. Of all patients with IAA type B, 68% had DiGeorge sequence; of all patients with truncus arteriosus, 33% had DiGeorge sequence. Failure of descent of the thymus is extremely common in DiGeorge sequence, but immunodeficiency that requires correction occurs in only approximately 25% of the patients. The term, complete DiGeorge sequence, should be reserved for patients in need of reconstitution of the immune system. The physician can identify patients requiring treatment of the thymic defect by T-cell enumeration and *in vitro* proliferation assays. Two alternatives for therapy are thymus transplantation and bone marrow transplantation from a HLA-matched sibling. After emigration of the T cells from the thymus, they circulate through the lymphatic and vascular systems as the long-lived lymphocytes (i.e., the recirculating pool), which then populate certain restricted regions of the lymph nodes, the thymic-dependent subcortical areas, and the periarteriolar regions of the spleen. Removal of the thymus in neonatal mice renders them deficient in the number of circulating T cells and leads to depletion of the thymic-dependent areas in lymphoid tissue. The long-lived nature of these lymphocytes and the degree of competence in the human

may explain in part why, after thymectomy, immediate deficits are not usually seen in the newborn period, although they may become apparent later in life. After birth, the thymus plays a continually changing role in relation to body size. It is largest compared with body size during fetal life; at birth, it weighs 10 to 15 g (2). The gland continues to increase in size, reaching a maximum of 30 to 40 g at puberty, after which involution occurs. The increased incidence of autoimmunity and malignancy with aging have been associated with senescence of thymic function.

T Cells

The stages in the life history of T cells are marked by the gradual appearance of a variety of membrane-bound glycoproteins (Fig. 46–4). Many of them have been identified using monoclonal antibodies. Immature thymocytes are characterized by expression of some surface markers acquired during intrathymic development, such as transferrin receptor (CD71), CD1, CD2, CD4, CD8, and the TCR–CD3 complex. After the T cells enter the circulation, they lose the transferrin receptor and CD1 molecule. In the peripheral blood, approximately 70% of T cells express the CD4 marker, and CD8 is found on

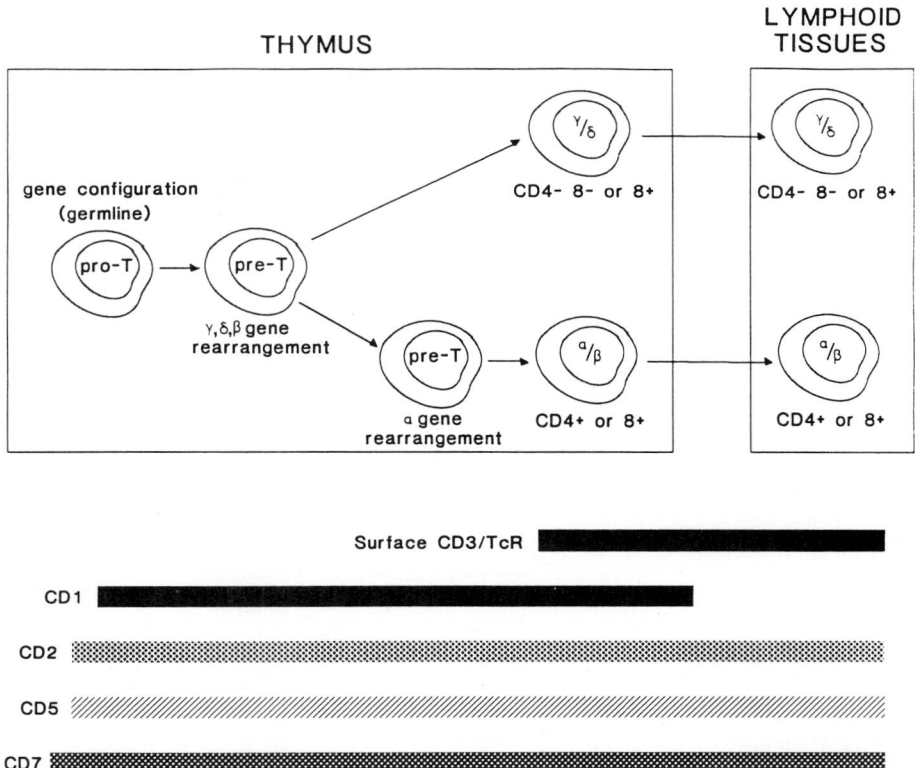

FIG. 46–4. Temporal relation among T-cell maturation, differentiation, and cell surface antigen expression.

approximately 30%. T cells that acquire helper activity characteristically express CD4, and suppressor T cells have CD8 but not CD4 on their surface. The CD4 receptor with antigen-specific TCR–CD3 complex allows the helper T cell to recognize antigens combined with antigen-presenting cell surface MHC II molecules. Helper T cells are induced to undergo blast transformation and cell division after interaction with antigen and MHC II molecules on the macrophage and other antigen-presenting cells. T-cell activation leads to the production of a variety of cytokines (e.g., IL-2, IL-3, IL-4, IL-5, IL-6, GM-CSF, IFN-γ, TNF), cell proliferation, and increased cell surface receptor expression (e.g., CD71, IL-2 receptor). Significantly decreased production of IL-4 and IFN-γ by neonatal T cells has been observed after activation (75). Recently, T helper cell populations have been further subdivided into Th1 and Th2 subsets. These subsets are identified by their different patterns of cytokine production: Th1 produces IFN-γ, IL-2, TNF-β; Th2 produces IL-4, IL-5, IL-6, IL-9, IL-10, IL-13 (76). The functions of Th1 and Th2 cells appear to correlate with their distinctive cytokine production, i.e., Th1 cells are involved in cell-mediated immune reactions and delayed-type hypersensitivity; Th2 cells are involved in antibody production and atopic disease (77). T-cell helper function in newborns is quite low, but it develops almost to adult levels by 6 months of age. T-cell–mediated suppression of immune responsiveness is somewhat higher in the infant than in the adult. The percentage of putative suppressors with the CD8 phenotype is lower in cord blood than in adult blood (78). However, in functional assays, neonatal T cells elicit increased spontaneous suppressor activity compared with adult T cells. Moreover, suppressor T cells exert a strong cytostatic effect on adult B- and T-cell proliferation, probably to prevent graft-versus-host (GVH) reaction by maternal cells transferred to the fetus. NK CD3-negative, CD56-positive cell activity is extremely low in the neonatal period, and it reaches the adult level by between 1 and 5 months of age. Although the percentage of NK cells in the peripheral mononuclear cell population is decreased in neonates, the absolute number of these cytotoxic NK cells is high in infancy and even higher from 1 month to 4 years of age compared with that in adults (79). The increased number of NK cells with adequate cytotoxic abilities present from 1 month to 4 years of age indicates the predominance of NK immunity during infancy to early childhood, in the presence of immaturity in other aspects of immunologic system. In the neonatal period, the decreased NK cell activity predisposes to increased severity of viral infections. As a general rule, T cells acquire immunocompetence (i.e., strong proliferation in mixed lymphocyte culture [MLC] and antigen binding) early during fetal life, even though their functional capacities are not always comparable to those of the adult.

Newborns, particularly premature infants, have a significantly lower rate and degree of skin sensitization to dinitrochlorobenzene, and rejection of skin allografts is slower in newborns than in normal adults. Delayed hypersensitivity can be induced in newborns during the first month of life. The newborn's inconsistency in this capacity appears to be caused more by a decreased inflammatory response and macrophage function than by depressed T-cell activity. Depressed T-cell function may be a consequence of neonatal viral infection, hyperbilirubinemia, corticosteroid therapy, or maternal medications taken late during pregnancy. Specific T-cell immunity can result from antigenic exposure *in utero* to certain antigens such as penicillin, mumps virus, *Escherichia coli*, diphtheria and tetanus toxoid, and dental plaque in the mother. There are some suggestions that specific CMI can be acquired from the ingestion of T cells contained in colostrum or breast milk or transferred through the placenta. The proliferative capabilities of immature lymphocytes are well developed early in gestation and, at the time of birth, are equal to or may exceed those of adult lymphocytes; the inflammatory response and macrophage functions, however, appear to be impaired in the newborn period.

B-Cell System

If the progenitor cells fall under the influence of a second type of microchemical environment, differentiation produces a population of lymphocytes and plasma cells concerned with humoral immunity or antibody synthesis (see Fig. 46–2). This B-cell population comes under the influence of the bursa of Fabricius in birds (80). In humans, bone marrow constitutes one of the equivalents of the bursa, but all available evidence indicates that the human fetal liver is the analog of the bursa of Fabricius in humans. The process of B-cell differentiation from a multipotent stem cell begins in fetal liver between 8 and 9 weeks of gestation, with the appearance of pre-B cells. Pre-B cells have MHC II antigens on their surface and the CD19 receptors (i.e., pan-B cell marker) shown in Figure 46–5. These cells begin to synthesize the cytoplasmic μ, the heavy chain of IgM, that later becomes the surface IgM that appears on "baby" or immature B cells. CD21, which

is the receptor for complement C3d and Epstein–Barr virus, also begins to appear on the immature B-cell surface. Although these cells continue to express surface IgM, they begin to express one of the surface immunoglobulins (i.e., IgA, IgG, IgD) shown in Figure 46–6.

Recently, a new molecular ligand has been described that governs the IgM-IgG isotype class switch referred to as the CD40 receptor (CD40-R) found on the T cells, which binds to a CD40 ligand on B cells. A deficiency of the CD40 ligand has been described in hyperimmunoglobulin M syndrome. The CD40 ligand is deficient developmentaly in the newborn and accounts for the prominent IgM responses of the fetus and newborn as described in the following (81,82). After stimulation by antigen and helper T cells through CD40/CD40 ligand, the immature cells become mature plasma cells or memory cells (83). As in T-cell development, B-cell development involves several cytokines, such as IL-3, IL-4, IL-5, IL-6, and IL-7. These cytokines influence B-cell growth and differentiation but also regulate, with CD40/CD40 ligand interaction, the immunoglobulin class switch and secretion. The cytokines that are responsible for isotype switching from IgM have been partially elucidated; IL-10 induces the switch to IgG1 or IgG3; transforming growth factor induces the switch to IgA1 or IgA2, and IL-4 associated with IL-13 induces the switch to IgE and IgG4 (84). IL-6 induces the committed B cells to become a mature immunoglobulin-secreting plasma cell. The first surface immunoglobulin expressed by a B cell is an IgM; at 13 weeks of fetal life, most B cells express IgM and IgD. In the next differentiation step, B-cell clones start to express IgG (i.e., subclasses 1, 2, 3, 4), IgA (i.e., subclasses 1, 2), or IgE. Full-term babies probably have a complete repertoire of B-cell clones, and they can theoretically synthesize each type of immunoglobulin. However, human newborns fail to respond efficiently to all antigens; for example, they are unable to mount an antibody response to polysaccharide antigens. Infants respond to protein antigens (i.e., T-dependent antigens), mainly with IgM production and a slow progression, compared with that of the adult, to IgG response. Children younger than 18 months fail to respond with an IgG2 production to *Haemophilus influenzae* type B cap-

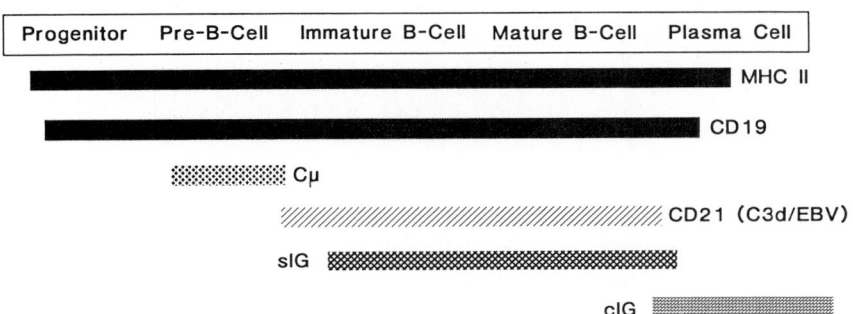

FIG. 46–5. Temporal relation among B-cell maturation, differentiation, and cell surface marker or antigen expression.

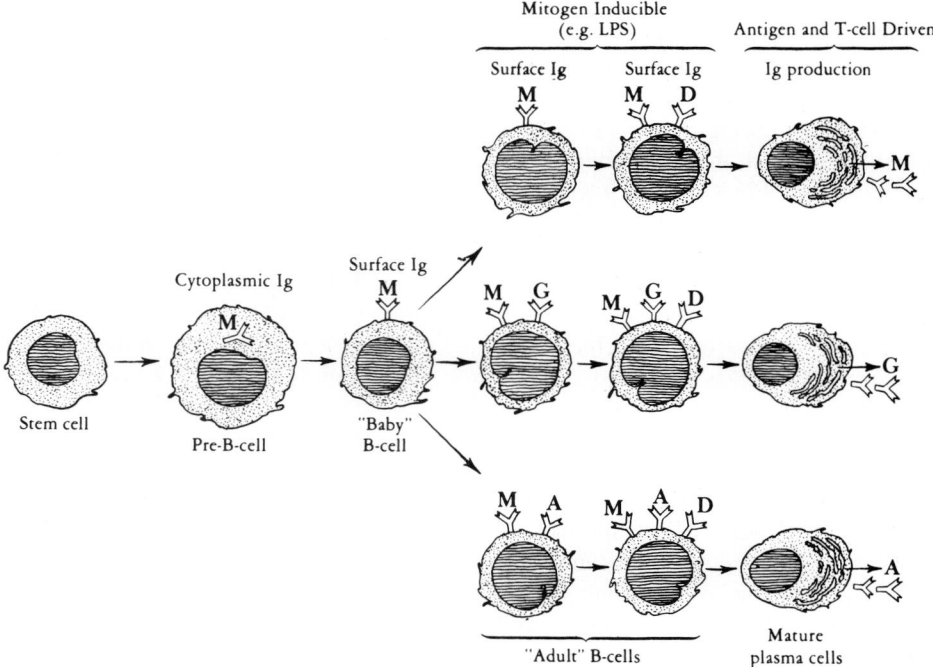

Mitogen Inducible
(e.g. LPS)

Antigen and T-cell Driven

FIG. 46–6. Mammalian B-cell differentiation model. B cells differentiate from a stem cell to a rapidly dividing pre-B cell lacking functional antibody receptors. These cells initially synthesize cytoplasmic IgM that later becomes surface IgM (i.e., baby B cells). These baby B cells can easily be made tolerant and are pivotal for further differentiation of immunoglobulin-producing cells. Although they continue to express surface IgM, they begin to express one of the surface IgG subclasses or IgA, followed later by the appearance of surface IgD. When these double or triple cells are triggered by antigen, helper T cells, or B-cell mitogens, they become mature plasma cells or memory cells (not illustrated in this figure). The antigen-dependent T-cell–driven stage requires the presence of surface IgD that is lost after antigenic stimulation. LPS, lipopolysaccharide. (Adapted from Cooper MD, Seligmann M. General Immunobiology. In: Bellanti JA, ed. *Immunology III.* Philadelphia: WB Saunders, 1985:52.)

sular antigen; this deficient synthesis of IgG2, which is the predominant subclass of antibody against *H. influenzae*, may explain the frequent appearance of *H. influenzae* infections in young children. The acquisition of adult levels of immunoglobulins is achieved by approximately 1 year of age for IgM, at 5 to 7 years for IgG, and at 10 to 14 years for IgA (85). The reasons for this defective antibody response are believed to be related in part to diminished expression of CD40 ligand (CD40L) by activated neonatal T cells as well as decreased production of cytokines (82). In addition, the expression of CD40L is a function of age: reduced at birth, increasing during the first few months, and reaching a plateau in the second decade. This is reportedly due to maturation of the CD4+ subset and has been correlated with expression of CD45RO antigen (81). Excessive suppressor T-cell activity in newborn blood, defective regulatory cytokine production, and a partial immaturity of the B cell have been suggested as limiting factors in the perinatal response (75,86,87). The relative deficiency of antibody responses of infants less than 2 years of age to polysaccharide antigens has been overcome by vaccines that utilize carrier proteins with the polysaccharide antigen, e.g., Hib vac-

cine. The fetal liver occupies the central role in B-cell development, as it probably does in T-cell development. The B cells constitute a much smaller part of the recirculating pool of lymphocytes than the T cells and populate the thymic-independent regions of the lymphoid tissue, including the germinal centers of lymph nodes. Removal of the bursa or its mammalian equivalent leads to a profound deficiency of gamma-globulin with little or no effect on CMI (88). Antibody provides a major defense against encapsulated high-grade pyogenic pathogens, including *Streptococcus pneumoniae, H. influenzae,* and *Neisseria meningitidis.* The development of immunity in the fetus and the newborn must not be considered separate from maternal influences.

MATERNAL, FETAL, AND NEONATAL INTERACTIONS

In the human, the predominant transfer of antibody occurs by passage of the IgG immunoglobulins from the maternal circulation to that of the fetus. This is accomplished by active transport of this immunoglobulin by a receptor located on one portion of the molecule. In this manner, the fetus receives a library of preformed antibody from his or her mother, reflecting most of her experiences with infectious agents. The secretory IgA immunoglobulins found in breast milk also provide local protection of the mucous membranes of the gastrointestinal tract. Although these antibodies are not absorbed, their unique structure renders them more effective in these sites and may explain the lower incidence of enteric infections seen in breast-fed infants. It has been shown that as much as 11 g of IgA may be delivered initially to the newborn infant in 24 hours, based on total output in the early colostrum. Subsequently, total IgA output appears to decrease significantly, and, between 3 and 50 days postpartum, as much as 3 g of IgA may be delivered to the breast-fed infant (89). The fate of ingested IgA has not been clearly defined. A small amount may be absorbed from the intestine and appear in the circulation within the first 24 hours of life (90). Significant numbers of granulocytes, macrophages, and B and T lymphocytes appear in breast milk (91). The B lymphocytes in human milk can produce IgA antibodies (91). Secretory antibodies in milk are directed against antigens occurring in the gastrointestinal tract: E. coli O and K antigens, *Shigella* O antigen, *Vibrio cholerae* O antigen, E. coli and V. *cholerae* enterotoxins, poliovirus, and rotavirus. There appears to be a direct relation between the extent of intestinal antigenic exposure and the level of specific secretory antibodies in milk. It is possible that, after antigenic stimulation, the lymphoid cells from the Peyer patches of the gastrointestinal tract home by way of the mesenteric lymph nodes and the blood to the mammary gland tissue and appear in the milk. As a result of this homing mechanism, human milk contains secretory IgA antibodies against many microorganisms harbored in the maternal intestine at the time of lactation (i.e., microorganisms that the baby is most likely to be exposed to after birth). Because of the same homing mechanism, human milk contains IgA antibodies to many food protein antigens (e.g., cow-milk proteins). It is possible, particularly in infants with atopic predisposition, that the frequency and magnitude of food allergy may be decreased by a prolonged period of breast-feeding (92). In the early period of life, when the infant's own secretory IgA system is maturationally deficient, breast-feeding may provide the infant with antibodies that support the local immune defense system. Decreasing the antigenic exposure or influencing the infant immune response by prolonged breast-feeding may prevent or delay the development of atopic disease. Other protective factors are present in human milk, such as lactoferrin, lactoperoxidase, *Lactobacillus bifidus* factor, complement components, and leukocytes. Necrotizing enterocolitis, a disease seen primarily in premature infants who have suffered severe perinatal stress, affects predominantly formula-fed infants. Neonatal rats subjected daily to a short period of hypoxia developed a reproducible model of the disease.

All animals died as a result of necrotizing enterocolitis if they were formula-fed, but not if breast-fed. The viable macrophages in their breast-feedings appear to have afforded the survivors protection and to have prevented the mortality seen in control animals. However, studies carried out after naturally acquired maternal cytomegalovirus infection or other viral and bacterial infections have demonstrated acquisition of neonatal infections in breast-feeding babies of infected mothers (93). Occasionally, fetal cells or other proteins may gain access to the maternal circulation and actively immunize the mother to the paternal allotypes found on these substances. This process, referred to as isoimmunization, may lead to serious disease in the infant, such as hemolytic disease of the newborn, thrombocytopenia, and leukopenia. The development of serum immunoglobulins during intrauterine life and postnatally is shown in Figure 46–7. The amount and type of gamma-globulin found in the blood of the newborn at birth is higher than those of the mother and are made up almost exclusively of the IgG immunoglobulins. There are few or no IgA and IgM globulins in cord sera because the fetus is usually protected *in utero* from antigenic stimuli. If challenged *in utero* as a consequence of immunization of the mother with *Salmonella* vaccine or infection (e.g., congenital rubella, cytomegalic inclusion disease, toxoplasmosis), the fetus responds with antibody production, mostly of the IgM variety. The exclusion of other classes of antibody is beneficial to the fetus in many cases. For example, the exclusion of the IgM isohemagglutinins, leukoagglutinins, or the IgE antibodies of allergy prevents disease that may be produced by these antibodies. However, it also prevents the passage of other maternal antibodies that would be beneficial to the newborn, such as the IgM antibodies important in bacterial defense (e.g., opsonins, agglutinins, bactericidal antibodies) against gram-negative bacteria. This may explain the increased susceptibility of the newborn to infection with gram-negative organisms such as E. coli. There is great variability in the types of antibodies that are obtained transplacentally by the fetus (Table 46–6). This reflects the quantity of antibodies in the maternal circulation and of their molecular sizes. For example, low-molecular-weight IgG antibodies (e.g., rubeola antibody), present in high concentrations in maternal serum, are readily transferred. IgG antibodies in lower concentrations (e.g., *Bordetella pertussis)* are poorly transferred, and macroglobulin antibodies (e.g., Wassermann antibody) are completely excluded. Because the IgG immunoglobulins are passively transferred, they have a finite half-life, between 20 and 30 days, and their concentration in serum falls rapidly within the first few months of life, reaching its lowest level between the second and fourth months. This period is referred to as physiologic hypogammaglobulinemia. During the course of the first few years, the levels of gamma-globulin increase because of exposure of

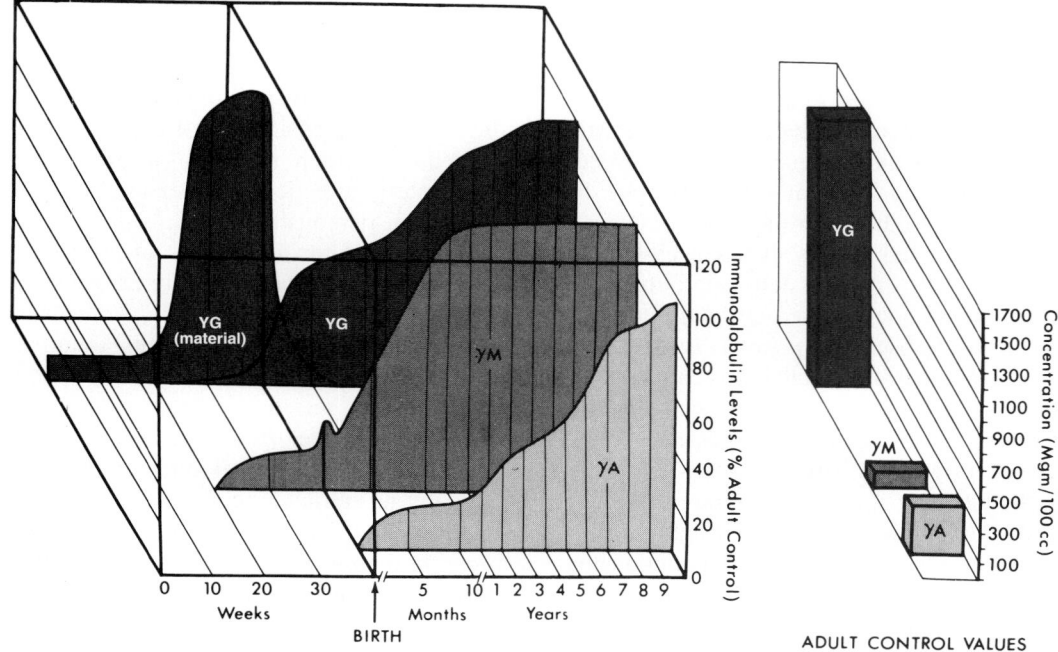

FIG. 46–7. Development of serum immunoglobulins (denoted by γ or Ig) in the human during maturation. (From Bellanti JA. General Immunobiology. *Immunology III.* Philadelphia: WB Saunders, 1985:49.)

the maturing infant to antigens in the environment. There appears to be a sequential development in the gamma-globulins at different rates. The IgM globulins attain adult levels by 1 year of age. Under physiologic conditions, little or no IgA synthesis is observed *in utero.* Plasma cells appear in the intestinal lamina propria of the neonate shortly after birth. IgA is not detectable in the serum or in the secretions during the first 2 to 3 days of life, although IgA frequently is present in the secretions after the fourth day of life. The secretory IgA concentration matures rapidly, reaching adult levels by 4 to 6 weeks of life. Serum IgA levels rise more slowly, and adult levels are observed after 10 to 14 years. This pattern of appearance of immunoglobulins recapitulates that seen in phylogeny and appears to parallel that seen after antigenic exposure during the primary immune response. In addition to providing protection to the newborn, passively acquired IgG antibodies may interfere with active antibody synthesis after immunization procedures. Several studies have confirmed that passively acquired antibody to diphtheria and pertussis may actually inhibit active antibody formation after active immunization. This occurs in the case of killed vaccines, appears to be dose related, and can be overcome by increasing the inoculum size. In the case of immunization with live virus vaccines, the effect of passively acquired antibody is to neutralize the vaccine virus, inhibiting successful immunization with parenteral live vaccines. Immunization at 2 to 3 months of age with killed vaccines (e.g., diphtheria, pertussis, tetanus) does not appear to be appreciably inhibited by this passive antibody. Live virus immunization procedures usually are delayed until the end of the first year of life because of the

TABLE 46–6. *Relation of antibody type and transplacental transfer*

Good passive transfer	Poor passive transfer	No passive transfer
Diphtheria antitoxin	*Hemophilus influenzae*	Enteric somatic (i.e., O) antibodies (*Salmonella*
Tetanus antitoxin	*Bacillus pertussis*	*sp., Shigella sp., Escherichia coli*)
Antierythrogenic toxin	Dysentery	Skin-sensitizing antibody
Antistaphylococcal antibody	Streptococcus MG	Heterophile antibody
Salmonella flagella (H) antibody		Wasserman antibody
Antistreptolysin		
All the antiviral antibodies present		
in maternal circulation (e.g.,		
rubeola, rubella, mumps, poliovirus)		
VDRL antibodies		

VDRL, veneral disease research laboratory.

TABLE 46–7. *Maternal antibodies that can produce harmful effects in the infant*

Maternal disease	Antibodies	Effect on infant
Hyperthyroidism	LATS	Transient hyperthyroidism
Idiopathic thrombocytopenia	Platelet antibodies	Transient thrombocytopenia
Isoimmunization (e.g., platelets, neutrophils, red blood cells)	Platelet, neutrophil, isohemagglutinins, Rho(D) antibodies	Transient thrombocytopenia, neutropenia, anemia
Lupus erythematosus	Autoantibodies to blood elements (e.g., LE-cell factor, Coombs test, platelets)	Transient LE-cell phenomenon, neutropenia, thrombocytopenia, congenital heart disease (i.e., AV block)
Myasthenia gravis	Cholinergic receptor antibody	Transient neonatal myasthenia gravis

Adapted from Bellanti JA, ed. *Immunology III*. Philadelphia: WB Saunders, 1985:579.
AV, arteriovenous; LATS, long-acting thyroid stimulation; LE, lupus erythematosus.

inhibitory effect of the passive antibody. Another situation in which passive acquired antibody may interfere with active antibody synthesis is the natural immunity acquired by the newborn infant from breast milk. IgA in breast milk may interfere with successful immunization with live poliovirus vaccines by neutralizing virus in the gastrointestinal tract. Poliovirus immunizations are not usually delayed, even in breast-fed infants, because active immunization follows sequential poliovirus administration according to recommended immunization schedules for infants and children. Maternal antibodies can have harmful effects, as shown in Table 46–7.

IMMUNOLOGIC CONSEQUENCES OF INTRAUTERINE INFECTIONS

The possibility of intrauterine infection should be suspected in a newborn infant if there is a known exposure of the mother to an infectious disease during pregnancy or if the infant is small for gestational age or fails to thrive. Manifestations of intrauterine infection include petechiae, hepatosplenomegaly, congenital malformation, thrombocytopenia, and unusual skin rash (see Chap. 47). An IgM concentration greater than 20 mg/dL in the cord blood or in the infant serum is considered abnormal. It should be pointed out that an elevated IgM level may be the result of leakage of maternal blood into the fetus; under these circumstances, the infant's IgA level usually exceeds the IgM level, reflecting the ratio of IgA to IgM in maternal blood. IgM concentration test repeated after 3 to 4 days disclose a significant fall in the case of maternal transfusion, but the amount of IgM actively synthesized by the newborn will have increased. Congenital infections frequently become chronic and persist for weeks or years, with signs and symptoms that are not seen in children or adults with the same infection. The agents that produce persistent infection of the human fetus exhibit a predilection for the reticuloendothelial system. Impaired function of reticuloendothelial cells may be associated with the development of immunodeficiency. In the congenital rubella syndrome, infection results from transmission of the virus

from the pregnant mother to the fetus in the first 5 months of gestation. The infection of the child continues after birth for 6 months to 3 years, despite passive antibody acquired from the mother and active antibody synthesis by the infant. After birth, the child may continue to shed virus while making antibody. A variety of abnormal antibody responses have been reported in children with congenital rubella, including increased levels of IgM with low IgG and absent IgA and low levels of IgM with low levels of IgG and absent IgA (94,95). Reports have appeared of poor antibody responses in patients with congenital rubella as determined by delayed appearance of isohemagglutinins, suboptimal vaccine responses, immune paresis with no response to tetanus or *S. typhi* vaccines, and impaired CMI as demonstrated by impaired lymphoproliferative responses to phytohemagglutinin and decreased lymphocytotoxicity (96–98). These abnormal responses have been associated with an increased frequency of infections. Many of the alterations reverted to normal responses later, when the child was no longer excreting virus (99). This could represent a form of immunologic blockade while the child is shedding virus, reversal of which may be linked to the maturity of the immunologic systems. Cytomegalovirus and herpesviruses produce infections that persist for years or throughout life, when infection is acquired *in utero*. CMI appears to be particularly important in these infections. In one study, eight infants with congenital cytomegalovirus infection and six of their mothers showed decreased specific CMI (100). The decreased CMI in the mothers may have contributed to transmission of the infection to the infant. The earlier the infection, the more devastating is the effect on the ontogeny of the immune system. If an insult occurs to the thymus in the first trimester, the normal development of T-cell function is affected; if the insult occurs in the third trimester, no resulting damage should be expected. Viral infection of the fetus may be limited by the degree of cellular immune competence, as exemplified by the infants with proven congenital infection and intact cellular responses who are no longer shedding virus at birth. The cellular competence of the fetus also may modulate the manifestations of intrauterine infection. Intrauterine syphilis, for example, presents in late pregnancy, at which time the body mounts a brisk cellular immune response to the spirochete. Infection occurring early in gestation may go unnoticed because the spirochete has neither a toxic nor a teratogenic effect on the fetus. The spirochete is teratogenic only when the immune response to the organism is activated. In contrast, rubella in very early gestation has primarily teratogenic effects (e.g., congenital defects). In later pregnancy (2 to 4 months), a primarily inflammatory effect is seen (e.g., hepatitis, iridocyclitis, meningitis). These differences may result from an intact cellular immune response characteristic of the older fetus, but, in some cases, the immune response of the child may fail to limit or clear these infections.

IMMUNOLOGIC EVALUATION

The functional significance of the two-compartment system is important in clinical medicine. It provides a useful basis on which understanding of the primary immunodeficiency disorders rests and a framework for a more logical approach to the management of maturational deficiencies in the newborn period. Selective deficiencies of the thymic-independent B system (i.e.,

agammaglobulinemias) present with recurrent bacterial infections. Selective deficiencies of the thymic-dependent tissues are associated with fungal and viral infections. Patients with combined B- and T-cell defects have the most serious of all the immunodeficiency syndromes, with profound deficiencies in cell- and antibody-mediated functions; they present with a diversity of infections. Evaluation of the immune system during the perinatal period is not an easy task. The evaluator must take into consideration the dynamic, rapidly growing, and adaptive parameters of the immune function in response to a changing internal and external environment. Table 46–8 shows some of the major classes of immunodeficiencies that can be diagnosed in the newborn period, with their time of onset and associated infections. A detailed history, with emphasis on family background and a careful physical examination, should offer a solid foundation for interpretation of clinical and research laboratory data. Table 46–9 presents some suggestions for clinical evaluation of the newborn. Table 46–10 lists some of the pertinent clinical and historic information that could be useful in the diagnosis of immunodeficiency disorders in the newborn period. Although most immunologic defects are not clinically apparent until postnatal life, it is not unlikely that, in

TABLE 46–8. *Immunodeficiency disorders that can be diagnosed in the neonatal period*

Disorder	Example	Genetics	Time of onset	Type of infection
Phagocytic disorders				
Quantitative	Neutropenia	Variable	At birth	Virulent bacteria
	Congenital asplenia	Variable	At birth or later	Gram-negative
Qualitative	Chronic granulomatous disease	X-linked, autosomal recessive	At birth	Less virulent bacteria
Disorders of antibody-forming cells	Agammaglobulinemia	Variable	>6 mo of age, earlier if infant is premature or small for dates	Virulent bacteria
T-cell immunodeficiency (i.e., cell-mediated or delayed hypersensitivity)	Congenital aplasia of thymus (i.e., DiGeorge sequence)	Variable	At birth	Fungal, viral
	Chronic mucocutaneous candidiasis	Sporadic forms, autosomal recessive		Fungal
	Pediatric acquired immunodeficiency syndrome	None	At birth or later	Bacterial, fungal, protozoal, viral, *Pneumocystis carinii*
Combined B- and T-cell immunodeficiency	Severe combined immunodeficiency	X-linked recessive, autosomal recessive, sporadic forms	6 mo	Bacterial, fungal, viral, *Pneumocystis carinii*
	Cellular immunodeficiency with abnormal immunoglobulins (i.e., Nezelof syndrome)	Variable	Variable	Bacterial, viral, fungal
Complex (i.e., multisystem) immunodeficiencies	Immunodeficiency with ataxia and telangiectasia	Autosomal recessive	>6 mo	Bacterial, viral, fungal
	Immunodeficiency with eczema and thrombocytopenia (i.e., Wiskott–Aldrich syndrome)	X-linked recessive	>6 mo	Bacterial, viral, fungal, *Pneumocystis carinii*
Disorders of early and late components of complements	Deficiency of C1, C2, C4, and later components of complement have been described	Variable	At birth	Gram-negative

TABLE 46–9. *Clinical evaluation of the immune system in neonates*

History
    Previous newborn deaths in the family; history of immune diseases
    Previous isoimmunization in mother (e.g., due to pregnancy or transfusions [Rh, ABO] or to γ-globulin
      administration)
    Previous diseases in the mother (e.g., autoimmune diseases: SLE, thyroiditis, myasthenia gravis,
      idiopathic thrombocytopenia purpura)
    History of medications in mother (e.g., quinine, guinidine, Sedormid, chlorpromazine)
    History of infections during pregnancy (e.g., rubella, cytomegalic inclusion diseases, toxoplasmosis,
      syphilis, herpes simplex, UTI, vaginal infections, TB)
Physical examination
    General appearance (i.e., assess degree of activity: if there is hyperactivity, consider hyperthyroidism,
      passive transfer of LATS; if there is hypoactivity or muscle weakness, consider myasthenia gravis
      with transfer of antibodies to muscle; if there is purpura, consider thrombocytopenia due to the
      passive transfer of antibodies to platelets)
    Skin (e.g., jaundice in first 24 h of life, petechiae are characteristic of isoimmunization such as
      erythroblastosis fetalis)
    Eyes (e.g., exophthalmos due to LATS)
    Chest (e.g., pneumonitis seen in many intrauterine infections)
    Cardiovascular (e.g., evaluate for congenital heart disease, congenital heart block in infants of mothers
      with SLE)
    Abdomen (e.g., hepatosplenomegaly seen in severe erythroblastosis fetalis, in congenital intrauterine
      infections, in GVH reactions, and in absence of spleen)
    Extremities (e.g., deformities and other birth defects)
    Neurologic (e.g., convulsions, weakness)

GVH, graft-versus-host; LATS, long-acting thyroid stimulation; SLE, systemic lupus erythematosus; TB, tuberculosis; UTI, urinary tract infection.
From Bellanti JA, ed. *Immunology III.* Philadelphia: WB Saunders, 1985:578.

certain instances, the result of immunologic deficiency may be intrauterine infection with a resultant damaged baby at birth or an aborted conceptus. Cohen and Zuelzer (101) have shown maternal blood-formed elements in fetal circulation. Theoretically, early passage of immunologically active mononuclear cells from the mother to the fetus could be responsible for GVH reaction. Although direct proof of GVH reactions in the fetus is lacking, several clinical situations suggest that such processes may occur in the newborn and fetus. Among these can be cited the report of an XX/XY chimerism in a 12-week-old abortus of a mother who had several repeated spontaneous abortions (102). A case was reported by Naiman and colleagues (103), in which, after three exchange transfusions, the infant developed jaundice, aplastic anemia, and marked histio-

TABLE 46–10. *Diagnostic clues for immunodeficiency disorders in neonates*

Findings	Comments

Hypocalcemic tetany
  Absence of thymic shadow
  Moniliasis
	DiGeorge sequence—characteristic features are *in vitro* lymphocyte stimulation with phytohemagglutinin and MLR

History of immunodeficiency in other family members	Most immunologic defects genetically determined; gender-linked most common
Agammaglobulinemia	Quantitative immunoglobulins not useful because of passive transfer of IgG; determination after 2 to 4 mo helpful in establishing diagnosis; allotypes helpful; B-cell (CD19) enumeration
Chronic granulomatous disease	NBT helpful as screening test only because there may be nonspecific elevation; tests of bactericidal function fail to reach normal values in presence of adult sera
Poor growth, splenomegaly, hepatomegaly, diffuse dermatitis, diarrhea	GVH—laboratory findings include anemia, decrease in serum complement, histiocytic infiltration of bone marrow, and erythrophagocytosis; skin biopsy shows mummified cells
Howell—Jolly bodies in peripheral smear, absence of spleen, shadow in x-ray film	Congenital absence of spleen and other associated malformations
Seborrheic dermatitis	C5 deficiency (i.e., Leiner disease)
Chronic diarrhea	Defect in phagocytosis of baker's yeast particles secondary to failure of sera to opsonize yeast

GVH, graft-versus-host; MLR, mixed lymphocyte reaction; NBT, nitroblue tetrazine.

cytosis. This infant also showed chimerism of the mononuclear cells, with one line representing donor cells.

Neonatal Immune Response to Human Immunodeficiency Virus

The immune response to human immunodeficiency virus (HIV) infection in neonates is described in greater detail in Chapter 47. The complexity of the immune response to HIV infection seen in the adult is equal or greater in the newborn. HIV has a tropism for human CD4-positive T cells and bone-marrow-derived dendritic cells, megakaryocytes, cells of monocyte–macrophage lineage, and the macrophage–microglial and endothelial cells of the central nervous system. A characteristic depletion of CD4-positive cell numbers is seen in HIV infections, after which there is a continuous but variable rate of decline of CD4 cells. In adults there is acute loss of CD4-positive T cells around the time of seroconversion and in the late symptomatic phase of disease. There are several proposed mechanisms to explain the depletion of CD4 cells, because infection of the cell is not necessarily cytopathic. One possible mechanism is that discharge of virions may be vigorous enough to disrupt the cell and cause death, depleting cell numbers. Alternatively, expression of viral antigens on the cell surface can result in CMI cytotoxicity. These losses may be compounded by the inability of the bone marrow to respond appropriately to replenish CD4 cells. Because CD4 cells play a pivotal role in many immunoregulatory functions, the loss in these cells is responsible for a reduction in their helper-inducer function and a decrease in other T-cell, B-cell, and monocyte activities, resulting in wide-ranging functional defects in cellular and humoral immunity. Immune dysregulation and nonspecific immune activation are features of HIV disease. Generalized immune activation evidenced by polyclonal hyper-gammaglobulinemia and elevated activation markers (e.g., β_2-microglobulin, neopterin) is recognized, and the levels of these activation markers are used to predict disease progression. HIV encoding a superantigen has been suggested; this may play a role in the generalized polyclonal activation and subsequent clonal deletion of T cells. One of the most perplexing clinical problems for the pediatrician and neonatologist is the diagnosis of acquired immunodeficiency syndrome in children younger than 15 months of age, because maternal IgG antibody to HIV is passively transferred across the placenta and may persist until 15 to 18 months of age in uninfected infants. Detection of HIV antibody is therefore not reliable for infants younger than 15 months of age. Moreover, viral culture and P24 antigen assays have a low sensitivity (i.e., viral culture detects approximately 50% of infected neonates). Although potentially useful, polymerase chain reaction (PCR) assay is limited by the

high false-positive results due to contamination or carry-over during testing, the complexity of the test and required laboratory facilities, and the cost. With improved quality control, PCR can identify as many as 50% of asymptomatic perinatally infected infants at birth. Viral-specific IgA antibody (i.e., HIV-IgA) immunoblot assay has a high sensitivity (99.4%) and high specificity (99.7%) for children older than 3 months of age but a much lower sensitivity in neonates. As a practical approach, identification of the infected infant relies on identification of the infected mother, followed by careful clinical and laboratory monitoring of the infant throughout the first year of life. Suggested laboratory tests include serial HIV antibody testing (i.e., ELISA and immunoblot); serial P24 antigen testing; HIV culture; immunoglobulin levels; T-cell numbers and subsets, remembering that neonates have significantly higher T-cell numbers than older children; and one or more other diagnostic techniques (e.g., PCR, HIV-IgA, immunoblot assay). The aim is to diagnose HIV infection before the onset of severe opportunistic infection, especially *Pneumocystis carinii* pneumonia.

Evaluation of the Humoral Immune System

Table 46–11 summarizes the evaluation of the humoral immune system. Pure humoral immunodeficiency syndromes are not clinically manifested in the prenatal period because of the protective effect of maternal IgG. However, very premature infants, particularly those born at less than 32 weeks of gestation, may have IgG serum levels below 400 mg/dL.

Small-for-gestational-age infants also have decreased IgG, some impairment of specific antibody responses (e.g., to attenuated polio virus), reduction in specific IgG secretory antibody responses, and an increased incidence of antibodies to food (104). Another factor to be considered is hypogammaglobulinemia in the mother, which, although rare, can lead to inadequate levels of IgG in the newborn.

Evaluation of the Cell-Mediated Immune System

Table 46–12 summarizes the evaluation of the CMI system of the newborn. Evaluation of the CMI system begins with a total and differential leukocyte count. Lymphopenia is seen in most of the CMI deficiencies, but the lymphocyte count may be normal in some patients. The number of T cells, B cells, CD4 helper cells, and CD8 suppressor cells can be ascertained by flow cytometry, using specific monoclonal antibody for individual cell markers (e.g., CD3 for T cells, CD19 or CD20 for B cells). *In vitro* lymphoblastogenic responses of T cells to specific antigens also are informative for host CMI, provided the antigens have been encountered previously (e.g., *Candida* for a baby with history of

TABLE 46–11. *Diagnostic tests for evaluation of humoral immunofunction in neonates*

Test	Comment
Practical	
Quantitative measurement of immunoglobulins	May reveal elevated IgM or IgA; does not differentiate maternal from fetally produced IgG
B-cell mitogen stimulation (e.g., pokeweed)	As with PHA (routine test), Ig synthesis determined in supernatant or cells stained with intracytoplasmic immunofluorescence techniques
IgG subclass determination	IgG3 increases in prenatal period and reaches adult levels after 3 months; IgG1, IgG2, IgG4 close to adult levels years later
Determination of total number B cells by CD19 or CD20 markers	Does not necessarily correlate with decreased Ig synthesis; helpful to elucidate level of B-cell defect
Specialized	
Specific antibody responses to *de novo* sensitization (e.g., Salmonella sp.)	O antigen induces IgM; H antigen induces IgG
Regional lymph node biopsy after immunization	Helpful for humoral and cell-mediated immunity

PHA, phytohemagglutinin.

thrush). Tests of lymphoproliferative responses should be performed with different concentrations of T-cell mitogens, such as, concanavalin A and phytohemagglutinin. Newborn lymphocytes seem to respond better than those of adults at low dosages of mitogens; at higher concentrations, they are less responsive than adult lymphocytes (105). Mixed lymphocyte culture reactions may be helpful in diagnosing CMI deficiencies. A dissociation of low phytohemagglutinin, with normal MLC, can be seen in some patients with CMI deficiency. On the basis of phylogeny and ontogeny, it can be speculated that such a defect originates at a higher level of T-cell differentiation. Lack of MLC responses suggests a defect occurring earlier in ontogenic development. Determinations of enzymes, such as adenine deaminase and nucleoside phosphorylase, may help clarify some of the cases of severe combined immunodeficiency and motivate the clinician to investigate enzyme replacement therapy or possible gene therapy. Skin testing with fungal, bacterial, and viral antigens for delayed hypersensitivity has not proved useful in the newborn. Skin testing with phytohemagglutinin (PHA) is claimed to be somewhat more sensitive (106). Contact sensitization to dinitrochlorobenzene offers advantages over intradermal testing. Dinitrochlorobenzene is positive in 90% of normal persons. Viral infections sometimes depress CMI, and some of the patients who are referred to us may show anergy because of persistent viral infections. In these cases, sound medical judgment, patience, and repeated studies are necessary. Fetal growth retardation and malnutrition also depress CMI and humoral responses for several months after birth (104). Evaluation of the nonspecific immune responses in the newborn is almost limited to testing

TABLE 46–12. *Diagnostic tests for evaluation of cell-mediated immunity in neonates*

Test	Comment
Practical	
Leukocyte and differential counts	Normal lymphocyte count does not rule out CMI deficiency; low count compatible but not diagnostic
Determination of absolute number of T cells by CD2/CD3 marker; T-cell subsets by CD4 and CD8 markers	No functional test, but correlates well with CMI status
Mitogen stimulation of lymphocytes (e.g., PHA)	Optimal, suboptimal, and overoptimal concentrations of PHA should be used
Specific antigen stimulation of lymphocytes	Previously known exposure required (e.g., *Candida*)
Specialized	
Skin testing with DNCB	Positive result practically rules out CMI deficiency
MLR	Could be positive in absence of responses to PHA
Lymph node biopsy after stimulation with *de novo* organism	To determine whether dependent areas are normal
Biopsy of thymus	To be performed in patients with obvious CMI; helps elucidate different types of CMI deficiencies that could orient new therapeutic measures
MHC I and MHC II antigen expression	Such as bare lymphocyte syndrome (i.e., MHC II deficiency)

CMI, cell-mediated immunity; DNCB, dinitrochlorobenzene; MHC, major histocompatibility complex; MLR, mixed lymphocyte reaction; PHA, phytohemagglutinin.

TABLE 46–13. *Diagnostic tests for polymorphonuclear lymphocyte function in neonates*

Test	Comment
Peripheral blood count and differential	Often of help, count important (e.g., neutropenia); morphology of cells important (e.g., Chediak–Higashi syndrome)
Rebuck skin window	May give general clue to defect of inflammatory function, particularly ability to marshal leukocytes to site of infection
Phagocytosis	Results vary with assay used; particle being phagocytized critical; assay used must distinguish humoral and cellular components of process
Chemotaxis	Decreased in cellular and humoral activity during neonatal period
Quantitative NBT	Screening test; if normal or high, does not rule out CGD
Bactericidal activity	Measured by direct killing assay; CGD can be diagnosed during neonatal period
Measurement of specific leukocyte enzymes	Not done routinely

CGD, chronic granulomatous disease; NBT, nitroblue tetrazine.

PMN function with the Rebuck skin-window technique (Table 46–13), which has not yet been standardized for the newborn. The nitroblue tetrazine test may be used as a screening test for CGD; the results should be confirmed by bactericidal assay. Lowered numbers of complement components have been described in the prenatal and cord blood. The extent to which these reflect actual functional abnormalities of complements is uncertain. Phagocytic tests should include evaluation of influences of C3 and C5. Separate evaluation of the complement effects on phagocytosis, chemotaxis, and bactericidal activities must be made. A functional deficiency of C5 activity has been described in Leiner disease. Monocyte function, although important, is not usually clinically evaluated because of a lack of adequate methods. Poplack and colleagues (107) have shown that, in humans, antibody-dependent cellular cytotoxicity activity against erythrocytes depends only on the monocyte. It is hoped that this test will prove significant in the evaluation of the monocyte in the fetus and newborn infant.

IMMUNOLOGIC THERAPY

Because newborn infants are less immunologically competent than adults and premature infants are even more susceptible to serious infections than full-term infants, several replacement therapies have been tried with variable results.

Prevention of Infection in Low-Birth-Weight Infants

There is little transport of maternal IgG to the fetus before 32 weeks of gestation, and endogenous synthesis does not begin until about 24 weeks after birth (108–111). In low-birth-weight infants, serum IgG levels by 3 months of age are only 60 to 150 mg/dL, compared with 100 to 350 mg/dL for infants born at term (108, 112–114). It is reasonable to consider intravenous immunoglobulin (IVIG) prophylaxis in premature infants. Some pilot studies indicated a lower rate of severe infec-

tion in IVIG-treated low-birth-weight infants compared with placebo-treated patients (115–118). In a randomized, double-blind, placebo-controlled trial involving 588 infants with birth weights of 500 to 1,750 g, mortality was not significantly reduced among IVIG recipients (119). However, the number of infections was significantly reduced among IVIG recipients. There was some evidence that the beneficial effect may vary by birth-weight category, and significantly more placebo patients were small for gestational age. Information about long-term results (less than 56 days) is not available from this trial. Preliminary analysis of other trials indicates no significant differences in infection rates between IVIG recipients and placebo recipients (120,121). Another multicenter, randomized, controlled trial, involving more than 2,000 neonates with birth weights between 500 and 1,500 g, has been completed (122). IVIG was initiated at less than 72 hours of age and continued every 2 weeks until hospital discharge or a weight of 1.8 kg. No significant difference was seen in the rate of nosocomial infection or in the mortality rate between control and treated groups.

The disparity in these results may be due to several variables. For instance, these studies are complicated by the fact that multiple factors contribute to the predisposition to infection in premature neonates and that different predominant pathogens occur in different nurseries. There are differences in the titers of antibodies to various pathogens, especially GBS infection, in different lots of IVIG preparations. Moreover, differences in the study design and IVIG dosage and schedule make direct comparison of the various trials difficult. At this time, IVIG cannot be recommended as standard prophylaxis for low-birth-weight infants.

Treatment of Presumed Neonatal Infection

Small trials using primarily historic controls have yielded mixed results. Questions remain concerning dose, schedule, and patient selection. Sidiropoulos and colleagues (123) treated successively admitted infants suspected of neonatal sepsis with antibiotics or antibiotics plus IVIG (0.5 to 1.0 g/d for 6 days). A reduction of mortality was found. Two of 20 infants treated with antibiotics plus IVIG died, compared with 4 of 15 infants treated with antibiotics alone (10% vs. 26%; $p = 0.16$). Among premature infants weighing less than 2,500 g, IVIG made a significant difference. Four (44%) of 9 patients who received antibiotics alone died, compared with 1 (9%) of the 11 who received antibiotics plus IVIG ($p < 0.05$). Haque and associates (124) studied 60 preterm infants of 28 to 37 weeks of gestation who were suspected of having bacterial sepsis. One-half of the group was treated with antibiotics alone and one-half was treated with antibiotics plus IgM-enriched IVIG. The doses were 190 mg/kg/d of IgG and 30 mg/kg/d of IgM for 4 days. Six (20%) of the 30 infants who received antibiotics alone died, compared with 1 (3.3%) of the 30 who received antibiotics plus IVIG, a statistically significant difference. Christensen and associates (125) used IVIG plus antibiotics in neonates with clinical signs of sepsis. They found IVIG recipients to have a more rapid correction of neutropenia, a more rapid appearance of immature neutrophils in the peripheral circulation suggesting release of neutrophils from marrow storage pools, and an increase in arterial oxygen tension compared with control infants receiving albumin. There were no deaths in either group, and no difference in mortality rates were observed. These studies suggest, but do not prove, that IVIG is a valuable form of therapy in septic premature newborns.

Group B Streptococcal Infection

GBS infection is one of the serious diseases in the newborn period. The use of IVIG in this condition has been addressed by Fischer et al. (126–128) and Santos et al. (129). Some of these preparations are opsonic for multiple strains of group B streptococci *in vitro* and protect animals against experimental GBS disease. Such passively administered IgG could ensure that premature infants who are at high risk of infection or already ill are protected by antibody to group B streptococci, even if little of it has been obtained transplacentally. However, not all GBS strains are uniformly susceptible to opsonization by antibody to group B streptococci. Lot-to-lot variation in antibody activity to group B streptococci has been observed. To ensure that an appropriate quantity of antibody is administered, screening of immunoglobulin lots for functional activity and pharmacokinetic studies in neonates are necessary. Studies by Hill and colleagues (130) indicated that administration of IVIG in neonatal rats improved the outcome of GBS pneumonia and sepsis by increasing opsonization and enhancing PMN migration. The mechanisms of these actions are unclear, but antibody may prevent neutrophil depletion by localizing bacteria to the lung where they can be phagocytized by pulmonary leukocytes and may generate inflammatory mediators, causing the release of PMNs from the marrow (130–132). Combined use of other plasma factors may provide even better protection against bacterial pathogens. Neonatal rats with GBS infection had significantly lower mortality rates if given IVIG and fibronectin than if given fibronectin alone (130). If IVIG is used, it seems reasonable to normalize the IgG level to between 700 and 1,000 mg/dL, using frequent infusions and determination of IgG levels. A dose of 100 mg/kg usually raises serum IgG by about 100 mg/dL.

Specific Antibody Replacement Therapy

Variability in IVIG preparations and lots creates several difficulties in predicting results of treatment for specific organisms. There is a potential role for directed preparations containing specific antibodies. IVIG apparently has minimal short-term side effects or complications (13,119,121,122). Nevertheless, large, multicenter studies must be completed before possible long-term problems such as hepatitis or inhibition of subsequent antibody synthesis can be identified or ruled out. That IVIG has known immunomodulating properties should be kept in mind when one is considering its use in persons without antibody deficiency (133). Passively administered antibodies are potent antigen-specific immunosuppressive agents, as illustrated by the high degree of efficacy of Rho(D) immune globulin (RhoGAM) in preventing sensitization of Rh-negative women to the Rh-D antigen on the erythrocytes of their Rh-positive fetuses. Recent studies in patients with systemic vasculitis demonstrated a 51% decrease in antineutrophil cytoplasm antibodies after high-dose therapy with IVIG, and this decrease was maintained during follow-up (134). Although there are no controlled clinical studies of the suppression of immune responses to other antigens by passively administered antibody, there is no reason to believe that antibodies to the Rh-D and neutrophil cytoplasm antigens are unique in this regard. There is evidence from animal and *in vitro* studies that IVIG can suppress antibody formation, T-cell proliferation, and NK cell activity (135–139). In addition to the masking of antigens, IVIG has many potential mechanisms for suppressing the immune response, including interaction with Fc receptors on the membranes of various cells of the immune system and the combination of antiidiotypic antibodies with antibody-producing cells or secreted antibodies (134,140). Antiidiotypic antibodies in IVIG could impair the capacity of B cells from even immune hosts to secrete antibody. Blockade of the Fc receptor by high doses of IVIG, as in the treatment of idiopathic thrombocytopenic purpura, or by the formation of immune complexes of IVIG with antigens also could impair the normal clearance of opsonized infectious agents and lead to overwhelming infection (140). There are many reasons not to administer IVIG unless there is a demonstrated broad antibody-deficiency state or other accepted clinical indications. Furthermore, studies in neonatal animals have shown that, in some situations, survival rates are reduced with high concentrations of IVIG plus antibiotic compared with antibiotic alone. The routine use of IVIG as adjuvant therapy of neonatal infections cannot be recommended at this time (141).

Summary of Recent Considerations Concerning the Use of Intravenous Immunoglobulin in Neonatal Sepsis

A review of studies of IVIG therapy up to and including 1991 by Weisman et al. (142) reports that, although IVIG is safe, the studies do not prove efficacy in treatment or prevention of neonatal bacterial infection. It suggests that pathogen-specific antibody IVIG products are required and larger and more careful trials need to be performed. In support of this, a more recent report of the safety and efficacy of monthly prophylaxis with respiratory syncytial virus immune globulin (RSV-IVIG) showed positive results. This was a randomized study of 510 children with bronchopulmonary dysplasia and/or prematurity. The children received 750 mg/kg of RSV-IVIG or placebo intravenously every 30 days. The results suggest that monthly administration was safe and well tolerated, and reduced hospitalization by 41% in children receiving RSV-IVIG treatment (143). Following this study, the use of RSV-IVIG was approved by the Food and Drug Administration for prevention of severe RSV infections in infants younger than 24 months with bronchopulmonary dysplasia or history of premature birth (144).

Active Immunization of Pregnant Women

Although the results of specific antibody replacement therapies seem promising, the availability and delay of the initiation of therapy (i.e., using it only when the condition is clinically suspected) are of concern. If pregnant women could be safely immunized at the beginning of the third trimester, producing high levels of protective antibody that then cross the placental barrier, this would probably give protection to neonates early enough to significantly decrease the incidence of the infection. GBS sepsis develops in approximately three neonates per 1,000 live births, resulting in approximately 11,000 cases annually in the United States. Mortality and morbidity from these infections continue to be substantial (145–148) Because human immunity to group B streptococci correlates with type-specific anticapsular antibodies and low levels of these antibodies predict susceptibility to invasive disease, to actively immunize women with capsular polysaccharide antigens of group B streptococci to stimulate production of type-specific, IgG antibody for transplacental protection of the fetus might be a valuable therapeutic or prophylactic approach (149–152). Baker

and associates (153) immunized 40 pregnant women, at a mean gestation of 31 weeks, with a single 50-μg dose of the type III capsular polysaccharide of group B streptococci. Twenty-five women (63%) responded to the vaccine. Of the infants born to these women, 80% continued to have protective levels of antibody (e.g., IgG-specific antibody ≥2 μg/mL) at 1 month of age, and 64% had protective levels at 3 months. Serum samples from infants with ≥2 μg/mL of antibody to type III group B streptococci uniformly promoted efficient opsonization, phagocytosis, and bacterial killing *in vitro* of type III strains. This effect may be mediated exclusively by the alternative complement pathway. Although this vaccine, with an overall response rate of 63%, is not optimally immunogenic, this study suggests that maternal immunization is feasible and can provide passive immunity against systemic infection with type III group B streptococci in most newborns. Larger trials with better vaccines are required to evaluate the safety and clinical effectiveness of this strategy.

Use of Recombinant Human Granulocyte Colony-Stimulating Factor or Granulocyte—Macrophage Colony-Stimulating Factor

Recently, several studies have investigated the use of recombinant human granulocyte colony-stimulating factor (rh G-CSF) or recombinant human granulocyte—macrophage colony-stimulating factor (rh GM-CSF) in newborn infants with presumed sepsis. This is based on the reported lower levels of these cytokines in the premature infant as well as an inability of the mononuclear cells of the neonate to produce significant amounts after stimulation (154,155). The first study consisted of 42 newborn infants 26 to 40 weeks of age with presumed bacterial sepsis within 3 days of life who were randomized to receive either placebo or varying doses of rh G-CSF, i.e., 1, 5, or 10 μg/kg every 24 hours or 5 or 10 μg/kg every 12 hours. The results showed that rh G-CSF was well tolerated and induced a significant dose-dependent increase in peripheral blood and bone marrow absolute neutrophil concentration and in C3bi expression (155). A 2-year follow-up of neonates treated with rh G-CSF showed that there were no associated long-term adverse effects (156). In a second study, 20 very-low-birth-weight neonates 72 hours old were randomized to receive either placebo or rh GM-CSF at varying doses intravenously per day. The results revealed that, in infants receiving rh GM-CSF, there was a significant increase in the circulating absolute neutrophil count as well as their C3bi receptor expression and monocyte count. In addition, there was a significant increase in bone marrow absolute neutrophil concentration (154). One important consideration for the use of G-CSF or GM-CSF in the prevention of neonatal infection is that the use of these cytokines alone only stimulates an increase in phagocytic cell numbers. This may not be sufficient, and prevention may require the use of antimicrobial specific antibody and/or complement, e.g., fresh-frozen plasma, as a source of opsonins.

Plasma Component Transfusion

Neonates have significant impairment in humoral and cellular immune factors. Augmentation of deficient humoral factors by transfusion of transfer factor, fresh-frozen plasma, antibody, or whole blood has been protective in humans or neonatal animals with infection (31, 126,129,131,157–165). Because of the extensive interaction between cellular and humoral factors, the positive effect of these therapies is thought to be produced, at least partially, by their improvement of neonatal neutrophil function. One study showed that replacement of humoral factors and PMNs is superior to replacement of humoral factors alone (84). Transfer factor is a dialyzable extract from human leukocytes with chemoattractant activity. The results of its use in patients with chemotactic defects vary. Some investigators found that transfer factor corrected the PMN chemotactic defect in patients with candidiasis and the hyper-IgE syndrome, but others found that it suppressed PMN function in several patients with the hyper-IgE syndrome (159,165). Fresh-frozen plasma contains antibody, complement, fibronectin, and other proteins that help protect against infection and have been found to be deficient in the neonate, especially the premature infant (166–168). A preliminary study suggests that fresh-frozen plasma transfusions improve PMN chemotaxis in newborn infants (158). Whether this improvement results in decreased morbidity or mortality from infection is unknown.

Neutrophil Transfusion Therapy

Bone marrow reserve for PMN in neonates is limited, and bone marrow pool exhaustion during neonatal infection is common. The most direct way to correct the impairment in neonatal PMN function and reserve is to transfuse adult PMNs into newborn infants. Several studies of transfusion of adult PMNs in human neonates with sepsis have produced mixed results (18,169–174). The first clinical trial of PMN transfusion in human neonates was carried out by Laurenti and associates (173). In this nonrandomized study, the mortality rate was 10% in the transfused group and 72% in the non-transfused group. No untoward effects of the transfusions were observed. The striking improvement in morbidity and mortality rates in the transfused group suggested that PMN transfusions could benefit septic newborns. Christensen and colleagues (18) carried out a prospective trial of adult PMN transfusion in 26 septic neutropenic neonates. Ten neonates with moderate or no depletion of their marrow PMN reserve did not receive PMN transfusion, and none died. Eight (89%) of 9 neonates with severe depletion of marrow PMN reserve who did not receive PMN transfusion died. These data indicate that septic neutropenic neonates with normal marrow PMN reserve who are given standard antibiotic and supportive care are likely to survive without PMN transfusion. In contrast, septic neutropenic neonates with severe marrow PMN depletion have a high mortality rate despite antibiotics and supportive care, and they probably can benefit from adult PMN transfusions. Two studies on the use of transfusion of PMNs from whole blood buffy coat layers failed to demonstrate a beneficial effect in septic neonates (169,174). Baley and associates (169) conducted a prospective, randomized, controlled trial of PMN transfusions for septic neonates who failed to demonstrate any improvement in survival. Several researchers recommended bone marrow examination before neonatal PMN transfusion to detect bone marrow exhaustion. Neonates with marrow exhaustion have a poor prognosis and may benefit most from PMN transfusion. Because this procedure is invasive and delays delivery of PMNs to neonates with fulminant infection, a rapid, accurate, and easily performed test to document marrow exhaustion would be useful. There are several potential problems associated with PMN transfusion. PMN sequestration in the lung, resulting in pulmonary decompensation (e.g., decreased PaO_2), occurs in adults and children (175,176). GVH disease has been reported after PMN transfusion in the immunocompromised host (177). Irradiation of leukocytes with a minimum of 3,000 cGy should be sufficient to impair lymphocyte function and prevent GVH disease without altering PMN number and function. HIV transmission from PMN transfusion is another potential concern. Although minimized with current antibody screening programs, an estimated 1 in 100,000 to 1,000,000 U of antibody-negative blood may contain transmissible virus as a result of recent HIV infection in the donor (178). Whether the risk of HIV transmission is greater with PMN transfusion than with whole blood or packed cell transfusions is unknown. Cytomegalovirus, Epstein–Barr virus, and hepatitis virus are other infectious agents that may be transmitted by PMN transfusion. Use of one of the recipient's parents, preferably the mother, as the PMN donor minimizes the risk of viral transmission. Although the results of studies of PMN transfusion in neonates appear promising, large prospective randomized trials must be carried out before it can be concluded that the potential benefits of PMN transfusion outweigh the risks. PMN transfusion cannot be recommended for routine adjunctive therapy of neonatal sepsis at this time (19,179). Polymorphonuclear leukocyte transfusion can be considered for the subgroup of septic neonates with neutrophil storage pool depletion, because this group of high-risk infants appears to be the most likely to benefit.

REFERENCES

1. Metchnikoff E. *Immunity in infective diseases.* London: Cambridge University Press, 1905.
2. Bellanti JA. *Immunology III.* Philadelphia: WB Saunders, 1985.
3. Kavelaars A, Zijlstra J, Bakker J, et al. Increased dexamethasone sensitivity of neonatal leukocytes: different mechanisms of glucocorticoid inhibition of T cell proliferation in adult and neonatal cells. *Eur J Immunol* 1995;25:1346.
4. Bellanti JA, Zeligs BJ, MacDowell AL. The maternal-neonatal interaction: role of gender and hormonal effects on the maturational deficiency in newborn phagocytic cell function. *Pediatr Res* 1997;41:745.
5. Bakwin H. The sex factor in infant mortality. *Hum Biol* 1920;1:90.
6. Ciocco A. Sex differences in morbidity and mortality. *Q Rev Biol* 1940;15:59.
7. Schlegel RJ, Bellanti JA. Increased susceptibility of males to infection. *Lancet* 1969;ii:826.
8. Washburn TC, Medearis DN, Childs B. Sex differences in susceptibility to infection. *Pediatrics* 1965;35:57.
9. Ohlsson A, Wang E, Myhr T, Willan B. The interaction of maternal smoking in pregnancy and newborn sex on total white blood cell counts (TWBC) and total neutrophil counts (TNC) in the first 24 hours (HRS) of life. *Pediatr Res* 1997;40:218A.
10. Motley D, Meyer MP, King RA, Naus GJ. Determination of lymphocyte immunophenotypic values for normal full-term cord blood. *Am J Clin Pathol* 1996;105:38.
11. Afoke AO, Eeg-Olofsson O, Hed J, Kjellman NM, Lindblom B. Seasonal variations and sex differences of circulating macrophages, immunoglobulins and lymphocytes in healthy school children. *Scand J Immunol* 1993;37:209.
12. Terres G, Morrison SL, Habicht GS. A quantitative difference in immune response between male and female mice. *Proc Soc Exp Med* 1968;127:664.
13. Baker CJ. Group B streptococcal infections in newborns. *Pediatr Rev* 1979;64:5.
14. McCracken GH, Mize SG. A controlled study of intrathecal antibiotic therapy in gram-negative enteric meningitis of infancy. *J Pediatr* 1976;89:66.
15. Polin RA. Role of fibronectin in diseases of newborn infants and children. *Rev Infect Dis* 1990;12:428.
16. Vogel SN, Nogan MM. Role of cytokines in endotoxin-mediated host responses. In: Opperheim JJ, Shevach EM, eds. *Immunophysiology. The role of cells and cytokines in immunity and inflammation.* New York: Oxford University Press, 1990:238.
17. Christensen RD, Bradley PP, Rothstein G. The leukocyte left shift in clinical and experimental neonatal sepsis. *J Pediatr* 1981;98:101.
18. Christensen RD, Rothstein G, Anstall HB, et al. Granulocyte transfusions in neonates with bacterial infection, neutropenia, and depletion of mature marrow neutrophils. *Pediatrics* 1982;70:1.
19. Krause PJ, Herson VC, Eisenfeld L, Johnson GM. Enhancement of neutrophil function for treatment of neonatal infections. *Pediatr Infect Dis J* 1989;8:362.
20. Playfair JHL, Wolfendale MR, Kay HEM. The leukocytes of peripheral blood in the human foetus. *Br J Haematol* 1963;9:336.
21. Cartwright GE, Athens JW, Wintrobe MM. The kinetics of granulopoiesis in normal man. *Blood* 1964;24:780.
22. Erdman SH, Christensen RD, Bradley PP, et al. The supply and release of storage neutrophils: a developmental study. *Biol Neonate* 1982;41:132.
23. Christensen RD, Hill HR, Rothstein G. Granulocyte stem cell (CFU$_c$) proliferation in experimental group B streptococcal sepsis. *Pediatr Res* 1983;17:278.
24. Abramson JS, Wheeler JG, Quie PG. The polymorphonuclear phagocytic system. In: Stiehm ER, ed. *Immunologic disorders in infants and Children.* Philadelphia: WB Saunders, 1989:68.
25. Anderson DC, Hughes BJ, Edwards, et al. Impaired chemotaxigenesis by type III group B streptococci in neonatal sera: relationship to diminished concentration of specific anticapsular antibody and abnormalities of serum complement. *Pediatr Res* 1983:17:496.
26. Miller ME. Phagocytic function in the neonate: selected aspects. *Pediatrics* 1979;64[Suppl]:709.
27. Mohandes AE, Touraine JL, Osman M, et al. Neutrophil chemotaxis in infants of diabetic mothers and in preterms at birth. *J Clin Lab Immunol* 1982;8:117.

28. Sacchi F, Rondini G, Mingrat G, et al. Different maturation of neutrophil chemotaxis in term and preterm newborn infants. *J Pediatr* 1982;101:273.
29. Anderson DC, Freeman KL, Heerdt J, Hughes BJ, Jack RM, Smith CW. Abnormal stimulated adherence of neonatal granulocytes: impaired induction of surface MAC-1 by chemotactic factors or secretagogue. *Blood* 1987;70:740.
30. Anderson DC, Hughes BJ, Smith CW. Abnormal mobility of neonatal polymorphonuclear leukocytes. *J Clin Invest* 1981;68:683.
31. Bruce MC, Baley JE, Medvik K, et al. Impaired surface membrane expression of C3bi but not C3b receptors on neonatal neutrophils. *Pediatr Res* 1987;21:306.
32. Krause PJ, Maderazo EG, Scroggs M. Abnormalities of neutrophil adherence in newborns. *Pediatrics* 1982;69:184.
33. Miller MH. Cell elastimetry in the study of normal and abnormal movement of human neutrophils. *Clin Immunol Immunopathol* 1979;14:502.
34. Nunoi H, Endo F, Chikazawa S, et al. Chemotactic receptor of cord blood granulocytes to the synthesized chemotactic peptide N-formylmethionyl-leucyl-phenylalanine. *Pediatr Res* 1983;17:57.
35. Olson TA, Ruymann FB, Cook BA, et al. Newborn polymorphonuclear leukocyte aggregation: a study of physical properties and ultrastructure using chemotactic peptides. *Pediatr Res* 1983;17:993.
36. Yasui K, Masuda M, Matsuooka T, et al. Abnormal membrane fluidity as a cause of impaired functional dynamics of chemoattractant receptors on neonatal polymorphonuclear leukocytes: lack of modulation of the receptors by a membrane fluidizer. *Pediatr Res* 1988;24:442.
37. Klein RB, Fischer TJ, Gard SE, et al. Decreased mononuclear and polymorphonuclear chemotaxis in human newborns, infants and young children. *Pediatrics* 1977;60:467.
38. Miller ME. Chemotactic function in the human neonate: humoral and cellular function. *Pediatr Res* 1971;5:487.
39. Berger M. Complement deficiency and neutrophil dysfunction as risk factors for bacterial infection in newborns and the role of granulocyte transfusion in therapy. *Rev Infect Dis* 1990;12[Suppl 4]:S401.
40. Roth P, Polin RA. Adherence of human newborn infants' monocytes to matrix-bound fibronectin. *J Pediatr* 1992;121:285.
41. Miller ME. Phagocytosis in the newborn infant: humoral and cellular factors. *J Pediatr* 1969;74:255.
42. Gallin JI. Interferon-γ in the management of chronic granulomatous disease. *Rev Infect Dis* 1991;13:973.
43. Ambruso DR, Altenburger KM, Johnston RB Jr. Defective oxidative metabolism in newborn neutrophils: discrepancy between superoxide anion and hydroxyl radical generation. *Pediatrics* 1979;64:722.
44. Newburger PE. Superoxide generation by human fetal granulocytes. *Pediatr Res* 1982;16:373.
45. Shigeoka AO, Charette RP, Wyman ML, Hill HR. Defective oxidative metabolic responses of neutrophils from stressed neonates. *J Pediatr* 1981;98:392.
46. Falloon J, Gallin JI. Neutrophil granules in health and disease. *J Allergy Clin Immunol* 1986:77:653.
47. Wright DG, Robichaud KJ, Pizzo PA, et al. Lethal pulmonary reactions associated with the combined use of amphotericin B and leukocyte transfusions. *N Engl J Med* 1981;304:1185.
48. Stein M, Keshav S. The versatility of macrophages. *Clin Exp Allergy* 1992;22:19.
49. Marodi L, Leijh PCJ, Van Furth R. Characteristics and functional capacities of human cord blood granulocytes and monocytes. *Pediatr Res* 1984;18:1127.
50. Wilson CB, Haas JE. Cellular defenses against *Toxoplasma gondii* in newborns. *J Clin Invest* 1984;73:1606.
51. Wilson CB, Lewis DB. Basis and implications of selectively diminished cytokine production in neonatal susceptibility to infection. *Rev Infect Dis* 1990;12[Suppl 4]:S410.
52. Blaese RM. Macrophages and the development of immunocompetence. In: Bellanti JA, Dayton DH, eds. *The phagocytic cell in host resistance.* New York: Raven Press, 1975:309.
53. Weston WL, Carson BS, Barkin RM, et al. Monocyte—macrophage function in the newborn. *Am J Dis Child* 1977;131:1291.
54. Gitlin D, Biasucci A. Development of gamma G, gamma M, beta 1c, beta 1a, C′81 esterase inhibitor, ceruloplasmin, transferrin, hemopexin, haptoglobin, fibrinogen, plasminogen, alpha-1-antitrypsin, orosomucoid, beta-lipoprotein, α2-macroglobulin and pre-albumin in the human conceptus. *J Clin Invest* 1969;48:1433.

55. Propp RP, Alper CA. C'83 synthesis in the human fetus and lack of transplacental passage. *Science* 1968;162:672.

56. Zimmerman GA, Prescott SM, McIntyre TM. Endothelial cell interactions with granulocytes: tethering and signaling molecules. *Immunol Today* 1992;13:93.

57. English K, Burchett S, English J, et al. Production of lymphotoxin and tumor necrosis factor by human neonatal mononuclear cells. *Pediatr Res* 1988;24:717.

58. Weatherstone K, Rich E. Tumor necrosis factor/cachectin and interleukin-1 secretion by cord blood monocytes from premature and term neonates. *Pediatr Res* 1989;25:342.

59. Lee SM, Suen Y, Chang L, et al. Decreased interleukin-12 (IL-12) from activated cord versus peripheral blood mononuclear cells and upregulation of interferon-γ, natural killer, and lymphokine-activated killer activity by IL-12 in cord blood mononuclear cells. *Blood* 1996; 88:945.

60. Zola H, Fusco M, Weedon H, et al. Reduced expression of the interleukin-2-receptor chain on cord blood lymphocytes: relationship to functional immaturity of the neonatal immune response. *Immunology* 1996;87:86.

61. Zola H, Fusco M, Macardle PJ, Flego L, Roberton D. Expression of cytokine receptors by human cord blood lymphocytes: comparison with adult blood lymphocytes. *Pediatr Res* 1995;38:397.

62. Silverstein A, Uhr J, Kramer K, et al. Fetal response to antigenic stimulus: II. Antibody production by the fetal lamb. *J Exp Med* 1963;117: 799.

63. Froman ML, Stiehm ER. Impaired opsonic activity but normal phagocytosis in low birth-weight infants. *N Engl J Med* 1969;281:926.

64. August CS, Berkel AJ, Driscoll B, et al. Onset of lymphocyte function in the human fetus. *Pediatr Res* 1971;5:539.

65. Stites DP, Carr MC, Fudenberg HH. Development of cellular immunity in the human fetus: dichotomy of proliferative and cytotoxic responses of lymphoid cells to phytohemagglutinin. *Proc Natl Acad Sci U S A* 1972;69:1440.

66. Boyd RL, Hugo P. Towards an integrated view of thymopoiesis. *Immunol Today* 1991;12:71.

67. Finkel TH, Kubo RT, Cambier JC. T-cell development and transmembrane signaling: changing biological responses through an unchanging receptor. *Immunol Today* 1991;12:79.

68. Nikolic-Zugic J. Phenotypic and functional stages in the intrathymic development of αβ T cells. *Immunol Today* 1991;12:65-70.

69. Carding SR, Hayday AC, Bottomly K. Cytokines in T-cell development. *Immunol Today* 1991;12:239.

70. Low TL, Goldstein AL. Thymic hormones: an Overview. *Methods Enzymol* 1985;116:213.

71. Goldstein G, Scheid M, Boyse EA, et al. Thymopoietin and bursopoietin: induction signals regulating early lymphocyte differentiation. *Cold Spring Harbor Symp Quant Biol* 1977;41:5.

72. Leana-Cox J, Pangkanon S, Eanet KR, Curtin MS, Wulfsberg EA. Familial DiGeorge/velocardiofacial syndrome with deletions of chromosome area22q11.2: report of five families with a review of the literature. *Am J Med Genet* 1996;65:309.

73. Bastian J, Law S, Vogler L, et al. Prediction of persistent immunodeficiency in the DiGeorge anomaly. *J Pediatr* 1989;115:391.

74. Hong R. The DiGeorge anomaly. *Immunodef Rev* 1991;3:1.

75. Lew DB, Yu CC, Meyer J, English BK, Kahn SJ, Wilson CB. Cellular and molecular mechanisms for reduced interleukin 4 and interferon-γ production by neonatal T cells. *J Clin Invest* 1991;87:194.

76. Romagnani S, Parronchi P, D'Elios MM, et al. An update on human Th1 and Th2 cells. *Int Arch Allergy Immunol* 1997;113:153.

77. Mosmann TR, Sad S. The expanding universe of T-cell subsets: Th1, Th2 and more. *Immunol Today* 1996;17:138.

78. Haywood AR, Loyword L, Lyslyard PM, et al. Fc receptor heterogeneity of human suppressor T cells. *J Immunol* 1978;121:1.

79. Yabuhara A, Kawai H, Komiyama A. Development of natural killer cytotoxicity during childhood: marked increases in number of natural killer cells with adequate cytotoxic abilities during infancy to early childhood. *Pediatr Res* 1990;28:316.

80. Cooper MD, Lawton AR. The mammalian "bursa equivalent": does lymphoid differential along plasma cell lines begin in the gut-associated lymphoepithelial tissues (GALT) of mammals? In: Hanne MG, ed. *Contemporary topics in immunobiology*. New York: Plenum Press, 1972:49.

81. Brugnoni D, Airo P, Graf D, et al. Ontogeny of CD40L expression by activated peripheral blood lymphocytes in humans. *Immunol Lett* 1996;49:27.

82. Nonoyama S, Penix LA, Edwards CP, et al. Diminished expression of CD40 ligand by activated neonatal T cells. *J Clin Invest* 1995;95:66.

83. Lindhout E, Koopman G, Pals ST, et al. Triple check for antigen specificity of B cells during germinal centre reactions. *Immunol Today* 1997;18:573.

84. Caligaris-Cappio F, Ferranini M. B cells and their fate in health and disease. *Immunol Today* 1996;17:206.

85. Rosen FS, Cooper MD, Wedgewood RJP. The primary immunodeficiencies. *N Engl J Med* 1984;311:235.

86. Andersson U, Bird G, Britton S. Cellular mechanisms of restricted immunoglobulin formation in the human neonate. *Eur J Immunol* 1980;10:888.

87. Gathings WE, Kubagawa H, Cooper MD. A distinctive pattern of B cell immaturity in perinatal human. *Immunol Rev* 1981;57:107.

88. Cooper MD, Lawton AR, Kincade PW. A two stage model for development of antibody producing cells. *Clin Exp Immunol* 1972;2:143.

89. Losonsky GA, Ogra PL. Development of immunocompetence in the products of lactation. In: Ogra PL, ed. *Monograph on neonatal infections: nutritional and immunologic interactions*. New York: Grune & Stratton, 1983:48.

90. Ogra SS, Weintraub D, Ogra PL. Immunologic aspects of human colostrum and milk. III. Fate and absorption of cellular and soluble components in the gastrointestinal tract of newborns. *J Immunol* 1977; 119:245.

91. Smith EV, Goldman AS. The cell of human colostrum: I. In vitro studies of morphology and functions. *Pediatr Res* 1968;2:103.

92. Hanson LA, Ahlstedt S, Carlsson B, Fallstrom SP. Secretory IgA antibodies against cow's milk proteins in human milk and their possible effect in mixed feeding. *Int Arch Allergy Appl Immunol* 1977;54:457.

93. Ogra PL, Greene HL. Human milk and breast feeding: an update on the state of the art. *Pediatr Res* 1982;16:266.

94. Alford CA Jr. Studies on antibody in congenital rubella infections. *Am J Dis Child* 1965;110:455.

95. Bellanti JA, Artenstein MS, Olson LC, et al. Congenital rubella: clinicopathologic, virologic, and immunologic studies. *Am J Dis Child* 1965;110:464.

96. Fuccillo DA, Steele RW, Henson SA, et al. Impaired cellular immunity to rubella virus in congenital rubella. *Infect Immun* 1974;9:81.

97. Michaels RH. Suspension of antibody response in congenital rubella. *J Pediatr* 1972;80:583.

98. South MA, Montgomery JR, Rowls WE. Immune deficiency in congenital rubella and other viral infections. *Birth Defects* 1975;9:234.

99. Stern LM, Forbes IJ. Dysgammaglobulinemia and temporary immune paresis in case of congenital rubella. *Aust Paediatr J* 1975;77:38.

100. Rola-Pleszczynski M, Frenkel LD, Fuccillo DA, et al. Specific impairment of cell-mediated immunity in mothers and infants with congenital infection due to cytomegalovirus. *J Infect Dis* 1977;135:386.

101. Cohen F, Zuelzer WW. Mechanism of isoimmunization. II. Transplacental passage and postnatal survival of fetal erythrocytes in heterospecific pregnancy. *Blood* 1967;30:796.

102. Taylor AI, Polani PE. XX/XY mosaicism in man. *Lancet* 1965;1:1226.

103. Naiman TL, Punnet HH, Lischner HW, et al. Possible graft-versus-host-reaction after intrauterine transfusion for Rh erythroblastosis fetalis. *N Engl J Med* 1969;281:697.

104. Chandra RH. Fetal malnutrition and postnatal immunocompetence. *Am J Dis Child* 1975;129:450.

105. Stites DP, Wybran J, Carr MC, et al. Development of cellular immunocompetence in man. In: Porter R, Knight J,eds. *Ontogeny of acquired immunity:* Ciba Foundation symposium. Amsterdam: Elsevier/North Holland, 1972:113.

106. Bonforte RJ, Topilsky M, Siltzbach LE, et al. Phytohemagglutinin skin test: a possible in vivo measure of cell-mediated immunity. *J Pediatr* 1972;81:775.

107. Poplack DG, Bonnard GD, Holiman BJ, et al. Monocyte-mediated antibody-dependent cellular cytotoxicity: a clinical test of monocyte function. *Blood* 1976;48:809.

108. Ballow M, Cates KL, Rowe JC, et al. Development of the immune system in very low birth weight (less than 1500 g) premature infants: concentrations of plasma immunoglobulins and patterns of infections. *Pediatr Res* 1986;20:899.

109. Hobbs JR, Davis JA. Serum γ-globulin levels and gestational age in premature babies. *Lancet* 1967;1:757.

110. Stiehm ER. Role of immunoglobulin therapy in neonatal infections: where we stand today. *Rev Infect Dis* 1990;12[Suppl]:S439.

111. Yoder MC, Polin RA. Immunotherapy of neonatal septicemia. *Pediatr Clin North Am* 1990;33:481.

112. Noya FJD, Rench MA, Courtney JT, et al. Pharmacokinetics of intravenous immunoglobulin in very low birth weight neonates. *Pediatr Infect Dis J* 1989;8:759.

113. Noya FJD, Rench MA, Garcia-Prats JA, et al. Disposition of an immunoglobulin intravenous preparation in very low birth weight neonates. *J Pediatr* 1988;112:278.

114. Sasidharan P. Postnatal IgG levels in very-low-birth weight infants: preliminary observations. *Clin Pediatr (Phila)* 1988;27:271.

115. Buaael JB. Intravenous gammaglobulin in the prophylaxis of late sepsis in very-low-birth weight infants: preliminary results of a randomized, double-blind, placebo-controlled trial. *Rev Infect Dis* 1990;12[Suppl]:S2457.

116. Chiricl G, Rondini G, Plebani A, et al. Intravenous gammaglobulin therapy for prophylaxis of infection in high-risk neonates. *J Pediatr* 1987;110:437.

117. Clapp DW, Kliegman RM, Baley JE, et al. Use of intravenously administered immune globulin to prevent nosocomial sepsis in low birth weight infants: report of a pilot study. *J Pediatr* 1989;115:973.

118. Haque KN, Zaidi MH, Haque SK, et al. Intravenous immunoglobulin for prevention of sepsis in preterm and low birth weight infants. *Pediatr Infect Dis* 1986;5:622.

119. Baker CJ, Melish ME, Hall RT, et al. Intravenous immune globulin for the prevention of nosocomial infection in low-birth-weight neonates. *N Engl J Med* 1992;327:213.

120. Magny J-F, Bremard-Oury C, Brault D, et al. Intravenous immunoglobulin therapy for prevention of infection in high-risk premature infants: report of a multicenter, double-blind study. *Pediatrics* 1991;88:437.

121. Stabile A, Sopo SM, Romanelli V, et al. Intravenous immunoglobulin for prophylaxis of neonatal sepsis in premature infants. *Arch Dis Child* 1988;63:441.

122. Fanaroff A, Wright E, Korones S, et al. A controlled trial of prophylactic intravenous immunoglobulin (IVIG) to reduce nosocomial infection (N.I.) in VLBW infants. *Pediatr Res* 1992;33:202A(abst).

123. Sidiropoulos D, Boehme U, Von Muralt G, et al. Immunoglobulin supplementation in prevention or treatment of neonatal sepsis. *Pediatr Infect Dis* 1986;5:S193.

124. Haque KN, Zaidi MH, Bahakim H. IgM-enriched intravenous immunoglobulin therapy in neonatal sepsis. *Am J Dis Child* 1988;142:1293.

125. Christensen RD, Brown MS, Hall DC, Lassiter HA, Hill HR. Effect on neutrophil kinetics and serum opsonic capacity of intravenous administration of immune globulin to neonates with clinical signs of early-onset sepsis. *J Pediatr* 1991;118:606.

126. Fischer GW, Hemming VG, Hunter KW, et al. Intravenous immunoglobulin in the treatment of neonatal sepsis: therapeutic strategies and laboratory studies. *Pediatr Infect Dis* 1986;5:S171.

127. Fischer GW, Hunter KW, Wilson SR. Modified human immune serum globulin for intravenous administration: in vitro opsonic activity and in vivo protection against group B. streptococcal disease in suckling rats. *Acta Paediatr Scand* 1982;71:639.

128. Fischer GW, Hunter KW, Wilson SR, Hensen SA. The role of antibody in group B streptococcal disease. In: Alving BM, Finlayson JS, eds. *Immunoglobulins:* characteristics and uses of intravenous preparations, vol 1. Washington, DC: US Government Printing Office, 1980:81.

129. Santos JI, Shigeoka AO, Rote NS, Hill HR. Protective efficacy of a modified immune serum globulin in experimental group B streptococcal infections. *J Pediatr* 1981;99:873.

130. Hill HR, Shigeoka AO, Pineus S, Christensen RD. Intravenous IgG in combination with other modalities in the treatment of neonatal infection. *Pediatr Infect Dis* 1986;5:S180.

131. Hall RT, Shigeoka AO, Hill HR. Serum opsonic activity and peripheral neutrophil counts before and after exchange transfusion in infants with early onset Group B streptococcal septicemia. *Pediatr Infect Dis* 1983;2:356.

132. Stiehm ER. Intravenous immunoglobulins in neonates and infants: an overview. *Pediatr Infect Dis* 1986;5:S217.

133. Dwyer JM. Intravenous therapy with gamma globulin. *Adv Intern Med* 1987;32:111.

134. Jayne DRW, Davies MJ, Fox CJV, Black CM, Lockwood CM. Treatment of systemic vasculitis with pooled intravenous immunoglobulin. *Lancet* 1991;337:1137.

135. Bussel J, Pahwa S, Porges A, et al. Correlation of in vitro antibody synthesis with the outcome of intravenous γ-globulin treatment of chronic idiopathic thrombocytopenic purpura. *J Clin Immunol* 1986;6:50.

136. Engelhard D, Waner JL, Kapoor N, Good RA. Effect of intravenous immune globulin on natural killer cell activity: possible association with autoimmune neutropenia and idiopathic thrombocytopenia. *J Pediatr* 1986;108:77.

137. Hashimoto F, Sakiyama Y, Matsumoto S. The suppressive effect of gammaglobulin preparations on in vitro pokeweed mitogen-induced immunoglobulin production. *Clin Exp Immunol* 1986;65:409.

138. Kawada K, Terasaki PI. Evidence of immunosuppression by high-dose gammaglobulin. *Exp Hematol* 1987;15:133.

139. Stohl W. Cellular mechanisms in the in vitro inhibition of pokeweed mitogen-induced B cell differentiation by immunoglobulin for intravenous use. *J Immunol* 1986;136:4407.

140. Bussel JB. Intravenous immunoglobulin therapy for the treatment of idiopathic thrombocytopenic purpura. *Prog Hemost Thromb* 1986;8:103.

141. NIH Consensus Conference. Intravenous immunoglobulin. *JAMA* 1990;264:3189.

142. Weisman LE, Cruess DF, Fischer GW. Standard versus hyperimmune intravenous immunoglobulin in preventing or treating neonatal bacterial infections. *Clin Perinatol* 1993;20::211.

143. The PREVENT Study Group. Reduction of respiratory syncytial virus hospitalization among premature infants and infants with bronchopulmonary dysplasia using respiratory syncytial virus immune globulin prophylaxis. *Pediatrics* 1997;99:93.

144. American Academy of Pediatrics Committee on Infectious Disease, Committee on Fetus and Newborn. Respiratory syncytial virus immune globulin intravemous: indication for use. *Pediatrics* 1997;99:645.

145. Baker CJ, Edwards MS. Group B streptococcal infections. In: Remington JS, Klein JO, eds. *Infectious diseases of the fetus and newborn infant*, 2nd ed. Philadelphia: WB Saunders, 1983:820.

146. Dillon HC Jr, Khare S, Gray BM. Group B streptococcal carriage and disease: a 6-year prospective study. *J Pediatr* 1987;110:31.

147. Institute of Medicine, National Academy of Sciences. *New vaccine development:* establishing priorities, *Vol 1. Diseases of importance in the United States.* Washington, DC: National Academy Press, 1985:424.

148. Wald ER, Bergman I, Taylor HG, et al. Long-term outcome of group B streptococcal meningitis. *Pediatrics* 1986;77:217.

149. Baker CJ, Kasper DL. Correlation of maternal antibody deficiency with susceptibility to neonatal group B streptococcal infection. *N Engl J Med* 1976;294:753.

150. Baker CJ, Kasper DL, Tager IB, et al. Quantitative determination of antibody to capsular polysaccharide in infection with type III strains of group B streptococcus. *J Clin Invest* 1977;59:810.

151. Boyer KM, Gotoff SP. Prevention of early-onset neonatal group B streptococcal disease with selective intrapartum chemoprophylaxis. *N Engl J Med* 1986;314:1665.

152. Stewardson-Kreiger PB, Albrandt K, Nevin T, et al. Perinatal immunity to group B beta-hemolytic Streptococcus type Ia. *J Infect Dis* 1977;136:619.

153. Baker CJ, Rench MA, Edwards MS, et al. Immunization of pregnant women with a polysaccharide vaccine of Group B streptococcus. *N Engl J Med* 1988;319:18:1180.

154. Cairo MS, Christensen R, Sender LS, et al. Results of a phase I/II trial of recombinant human granulocyte-macrophage colony-stimulating factor in very low birthweight neonates: significant induction of circulatory neutrophils, monocytes, platelets, and bone marrow neutrophils. *Blood* 1995;86:2509.

155. Gillan ER, Christensen RD, Suen Y, et al. A randomized, placebo-controlled trial of recombinant human granulocyte colony-stimulating factor administration in newborn infants with presumed sepsis: significant induction of peripheral and bone marrow neutrophilia. *Blood* 1994;84:1427.

156. Rosenthal J, Healey T, Ellis R, et al. A two-year follow-up of neonates with presumed sepsis treated with recombinant human granulocyte colony-stimulating factor during the first week of life. *J Pediatr* 1996;128:135.

157. Bortulussi R, Fischer GW. Opsonic and protective activity of immunoglobulin, modified immunoglobulin and serum against neonatal E. coli K1 infection. *Pediatr Res* 1986;20:175.

158. Eisenfeld L, Krause PJ, Herson VC, et al. Enhancement of neonatal polymorphonuclear leukocyte (PMN) motility with adult fresh frozen plasma (FFP). Abstract 1409. Washington, DC: The Society for Pediatric Research Meetings, 1986.

159. Friendenberg WR, Marx JJ Jr, Hensen RL, et al. Hyperimmunoglobulin E syndrome: response to transfer factor and ascorbic acid therapy. *Clin Immunol Immunopathol* 1979;12:132-142.

160. Givner LB, Edwards MS, Baker CJ. A polyclonal human IgG preparation hyperimmune for type III Group B Streptococcus: in vitro opsonophagolytic activity and efficacy in experimental models. *J Infect Dis* 1988;158:724.

161. Harper TE, Christensen RD, Rothstein G, et al. Effect of intravenous immunoglobulin G on neutrophil kinetics during experimental Group B streptococcal infection in neonatal rats. *Rev Infect Dis* 1986;8:S401.

162. Santos JI, Shigeoka AO, Hill HR. Functional leukocyte administration protection against experimental neonatal infection. *Pediatr Res* 1980;14:1408.

163. Shigeoka AD, Gobel RJ, Janatova J, et al. Neutrophil mobilization induced by complement fragments during experimental Group B streptococcal (GBS) infection. *Am J Pathol* 1988;133:623.

164. Shigeoka AO, Hall RT, Hill HR. Blood transfusion in Group B streptococcal sepsis. *Lancet* 1978;1:636.

165. Snyderman R, Altman LC, Frankel A. Defective mononuclear leukocyte chemotaxis: a previously unrecognized immune dysfunction. Studies in a patient with chronic mucocutaneous candidiasis. *Ann Intern Med* 1973;78:509.

166. Cates KL, Rowe JC, Ballow M. The premature infant as a compromised host. *Curr Prob Pediatr* 1983;13:63.

167. Gerdes JS, Yoder MC, Douglas SD, et al. Decreased plasma fibronectin in neonatal sepsis. *Pediatrics* 1983;72:877.

168. Miller ME, Stiehm ER. Immunology and resistance to infection. In: Remington JS, Klein JO, eds. *Infectious diseases of the fetus and newborn infant.* Philadelphia: WB Saunders, 1983:27.

169. Baley JE, Stork EK, Warentin PI, et al. Buffy coat transfusions in neutropenic neonates with presumed sepsis, a prospective radomized trial. *Pediatrics* 1987;80:712.

170. Cairo MS, Rucker R, Bennetts GA, et al. Improved survival of newborns receiving leukocyte tranfusions for sepsis. *Pediatrics* 1984;74:887.

171. Cairo MS, Worcester C, Rucker R, et al. Role of circulating complement and polymorphonuclear leukocyte transfusion in treatment and outcome in critically ill neonates with sepsis. *J Pediatr* 1987;110:935.

172. Laing IA, Boulton FE, Hume R. Polymorphonuclear leukocyte transfusion in neonatal septicaemia. *Arch Dis Child* 1983;58:1003.

173. Laurenti F, Ferro R, Giancarlo I, et al. Polymorphonuclear leukocyte transfusion for the treatment of sepsis in the newborn infant. *J Pediatr* 1981;98:118.

174. Wheeler JG, Chauvenet AR, Johnson CA, et al. Buffy coat transfusion in neonates with sepsis and neutrophil storage depletion. *Pediatrics* 1987;79:411.

175. Strauss RG, Connett JE, Gale RP, et al. A controlled trial of prophylactic granulocyte transusion during induction chemotherapy for acute myelogenous leukemia. *N Engl J Med* 1981;305:597.

176. Wright WC Jr, Ank BJ, Herbert J, et al. Decreased bactericidal activity of leukocytes of stressed newborn infants. *Pediatrics* 1975;56:578.

177. Rosen RC, Huestis DW, Corrigan JJ. Acute leukemia and granulocyte transfusion: fatal graft-*versus*-host reaction following tranfusion cells obtained from normal donors. *J Pediatr* 1978;93:268.

178. Friedland GH, Klein RS. Transmission of the human immunodeficiency virus. *N Engl J Med* 1987;317:1125.

179. Hill HR. Phagocyte tranfusion: ultimate therapy of neonatal disease? *J Pediatr* 1981;98:59.

CHAPTER 47

Chronic Infections

Bishara J. Freij and John L. Sever

Maternal infections acquired shortly before conception or during gestation can adversely affect pregnancy outcome indirectly through nonspecific effects of severe maternal illness (e.g., increased rates of spontaneous abortions, stillbirths, or premature births associated with measles infection during pregnancy) or directly through microbial invasion of the fetus or neonate (1). Pathogens can be transmitted from mothers to their infants through hematogenous spread across the placenta (e.g., cytomegalovirus [CMV], *Toxoplasma gondii*), ascension from an infected cervix (e.g., herpes simplex virus [HSV]), or intimate contact between a fetus and infected genital secretions during vaginal delivery (e.g., HSV, hepatitis B virus [HBV], human immunodeficiency virus type 1 [HIV-1], papillomaviruses) (2–4). Maternal coinfection by other microorganisms may enhance the risk of fetal infection by either or both pathogens (5). Iatrogenic fetal infections can occur after invasive procedures such as fetal scalp monitoring or intrauterine transfusions.

The outcome of a fetal or neonatal infection depends on the stage of pregnancy during which infection occurs, virulence of the pathogen, preexisting maternal immunity to the infecting agent, and efficacy of drug therapy for maternal or neonatal disease. Intrauterine infections may lead to resorption of the embryo, fetal demise resulting in a spontaneous abortion or stillbirth, or delivery of an infected neonate. Infected infants who are asymptomatic at birth may develop chronic problems in late infancy or early childhood (e.g., HIV-1, CMV, hepatitis C virus [HCV]) or during adulthood (e.g., rubella, HBV) (6–9).

Others suffer from severe acute neonatal disease such as pneumonia or hepatitis (e.g., HSV, syphilis), congenital malformations (e.g., CMV, rubella), intrauterine growth retardation, or prematurity (7,10,11). The number of infants born each year with these conditions is substantial (Table 47–1), and the lifetime expenditures for their medical and educational needs are considerable (12–19).

The acronym TORCH (*T. gondii*, "other," rubella virus, CMV, HSV) has long been used as a reminder that a number of pathogens can cause clinically indistinguishable illnesses in the neonate. These agents originally were grouped together because of shared clinical features (e.g., microcephaly, hepatosplenomegaly, petechiae, ocular abnormalities), their ability to cause asymptomatic infections in the mother and newborn, and their propensity for causing long-term sequelae that may be inapparent at

B. J. Freij: Division of Infectious Diseases, Department of Pediatrics, William Beaumont Hospital, Royal Oak; Department of Pediatrics, Wayne State University School of Medicine, Detroit, Michigan

J. L. Sever: Departments of Pediatrics, Obstetrics and Gynecology, Microbiology, and Immunology, The George Washington University School of Medicine, Children's National Medical Center, Washington, D.C.

TABLE 47–1. *Estimated number of infants with selected chronic congenital or perinatal infections born annually in the United States*

Infection	Number of infants	Year of estimate
Congenital cytomegalovirus (12)	40,000	1992
Hepatitis B virus (8)		
Exposed	22,113	1988
Chronic carriers[a]	6,012	1988
Congenital toxoplasmosis (13)	4,100	1995
Congenital syphilis (14)	1,049	1997
Perinatal human immunodeficiency virus type 1 (15)	516	1996
Neonatal herpes (16)	700–1,000	1995
Congenital rubella syndrome (14)[b]	5	1997

[a]If not given hepatitis B immune globulin and hepatitis B recombinant vaccine at birth.

[b]Due to the passive nature of the reporting system and to missed diagnoses of less severe cases, this figure probably only represents 20% to 30% of the actual cases (17,18).

birth (20). Because many other agents (e.g., HIV-1, *Treponema pallidum*, varicella-zoster virus [VZV], coxsackievirus, human parvovirus B19, *Mycobacterium tuberculosis*) are capable of causing similar illnesses, the diagnostic workup of infants suspected of having a TORCH infection should not be restricted to the original four agents, as is common in medical practice (21). The clinical utility of this mnemonic is limited, and its use should be minimized or abandoned altogether (22,23).

The epidemiology, clinical manifestations, diagnosis, and treatment of maternal and fetal infections caused by *T. pallidum* subsp *pallidum*, *T. gondii*, rubella virus, HIV-1, CMV, HSV, VZV, human parvovirus B19, hepatitis B, and hepatitis C are summarized in this chapter. Strategies for the prevention of maternal infection by these organisms or their vertical spread to the fetus or newborn infant are emphasized.

SYPHILIS

T. pallidum subsp *pallidum*, the causative agent of syphilis, is a motile, nonculturable, gram-negative, microaerophilic spirochete that is too slender to be observed by light microscopy. The laboratory differentiation of *T. pallidum* from the other pathogenic treponemes that cause yaws (e.g., *T. pallidum* subsp *pertenue*), endemic syphilis (e.g., *T. pallidum* subsp *endemicum*), or pinta (e.g., *T. carateum*) is difficult. Ultrastructurally, *T. pallidum* has an outer cell membrane (i.e., envelope), periplasmic flagella that arise at each end of the cell, cell wall, and a multilayer cytoplasmic membrane; a capsule-like amorphous layer coats the organism (24). Several outer membrane-associated proteins have been identified, and these are present in 100-fold lower amounts than typically is found in gram-negative bacteria. This property has been related to the chronicity of syphilitic infection (25).

Person-to-person transmission of *T. pallidum* occurs primarily through contact with infectious lesions during sexual activity. The organism enters the body through sites of minor trauma that disrupt mucosal or epithelial barriers (26). Fibronectin receptors appear to mediate the attachment of *T. pallidum* to epithelial or mucosal cells (27). Parenteral transmission of this spirochete through transfusions is rare because of routine serologic screening of blood or blood products, but intravenous drug users occasionally acquire syphilis by sharing needles contaminated with *T. pallidum*-infected blood (28). Intrauterine transmission from an infected mother to her developing fetus accounts for most congenitally infected infants; rarely, infection is acquired at birth through contact with a genital lesion (11). *In utero* transmission can occur as early as 9 to 10 weeks of gestation. The most important determinant for the risk of fetal infection is the maternal stage of syphilis. Mothers with primary, secondary, early latent, or late latent stages of syphilis have at least a 50%, 40%, or 10% risk, respectively, of delivering an infant with congenital syphilis (11). The risk of fetal infection also may be higher in more advanced stages of pregnancy (29). Concomitant maternal infection with *T. pallidum* and HIV-1 may enhance the transplacental spread of either pathogen to the fetus (11).

Natural and experimental *T. pallidum* infections elicit complex cellular and humoral immune responses. Most antitreponemal antibodies produced during the course of a syphilitic infection cross-react with antigens from nonpathogenic treponemes (i.e., culturable treponemes that are part of the normal oral, intestinal, or genital flora) and are not pathogen specific (30,31). Antibodies directed against integral membrane lipoproteins with molecular masses of 47, 44.5, 17, and 15.5 kilodaltons appear to be *T. pallidum* specific; their detection on Western immunoblot assays indicates syphilitic infection (32–34). A variety of other host immunologic defenses are activated after *T. pallidum* infection, including infiltration of inoculation sites with polymorphonuclear leukocytes that contain treponemicidal peptides (i.e., defensins), T-lymphocyte activation and proliferation with interferon-γ production, cytokine secretion, macrophage-mediated phagocytosis and intracellular killing of opsonized *T. pallidum*, and complement activation (35–38). Autoantibodies to blood cells, serum components, fibronectin, and collagen also are generated (39). Some treponemes manage to evade these clearance mechanisms during the acute phase of untreated infection, which allows them to disseminate and establish a chronic infection (37,40).

Maternal Syphilis

Epidemiology

The number of primary and secondary syphilis cases in the United States has decreased from 93,545 (66.4 per 100,000 population) in 1947 to 8,550 (3.2 per 100,000 population) in 1997 (14,41). This decline has been due largely to the introduction of penicillin and the organization of a national venereal disease control program (42). The rates are higher in urban areas and in southern states, and for nonwhites (30-fold higher rate than that of whites in 1993) (41). Cyclic national epidemics occur every 7 to 10 years. In 1996 and 1997, Baltimore, Maryland, had the highest rate for primary and secondary syphilis among United States cities, and the rate of congenital syphilis was 10-fold higher than the national rate. Adequate prenatal care and timely syphilis screening and treatment during pregnancy could have prevented about 90% of the congenital syphilis cases (43). Factors contributing to the occurrence of syphilis include cocaine use (especially crack cocaine) and exchange of drugs for sex, frequently with multiple, anonymous sex partners. Partner notification for diagnosis and treatment purposes is especially difficult under these circumstances (44,45). Other risk factors include lack of prenatal care and residence in an area with high morbidity from syphilis (43,46–48).

Pregnant women with syphilis are usually in their twenties (60% to 80%), unmarried (65% to 90%), and African-American (45% to 70%) or Hispanic (25% to 55%). They usually receive no prenatal care (45% to 65%) and are likely to be substance abusers (55% to 70%) (49–51).

Clinical Manifestations

Approximately 10 to 90 days (mean 21) after sexual contact with an infected person, a painless chancre with regional lymphadenopathy develops (i.e., primary syphilis) (26). Chancres heal within 3 to 6 weeks, even without specific therapy.

Secondary syphilis develops after hematogenous spread of T. pallidum. Its most recognizable manifestations include widely distributed rashes (e.g., macular, maculopapular, pustular, follicular) that typically involve the palms and soles, alopecia, condyloma lata (i.e., broad, flat, painless, highly infectious papules found in moist areas such as the vulva or anus), oropharyngeal lesions (e.g., mucous patches, erosions, ulcers), constitutional symptoms (e.g., low-grade fever, myalgias, sore throat, malaise, weight loss), and generalized painless lymphadenopathy. Asymptomatic central nervous system (CNS) involvement is found in 8% to 40%; headache or meningismus occurs in 1% to 2%. Hepatitis, glomerulonephritis, nephrotic syndrome, osteitis, bursitis, and arthritis are uncommon.

Secondary syphilis can resolve spontaneously without specific treatment. Untreated patients enter a latent phase of their illness, which is subdivided into an early stage, defined as 1 year of disease duration by the Centers for Disease Control and Prevention (CDC) and as 2 years by the World Health Organization, and a late stage. About 25% of patients in this phase experience relapses of secondary syphilis within 4 years, with approximately 75% of these relapses occurring during the first year (11,26).

Tertiary syphilis is a slowly progressive inflammatory process that develops after several years in about one-third of untreated patients. Manifestations include the invasion of various organs with gumma formation (i.e., late benign tertiary syphilis) or cardiovascular and CNS disease. Infection does not spread to the fetus during this stage.

The natural history of syphilis may be altered in patients coinfected with HIV-1. Support for this concept stems from several case reports describing unusual or florid symptoms and signs of disease, atypical skin rashes, and uveitis (26). Delayed healing of primary lesions and impaired immune responses to syphilis have been observed in HIV-1–infected rabbits and simian immunodeficiency virus-infected rhesus macaques (52,53).

Women with untreated gestational syphilis are at increased risk of spontaneous abortion, stillbirth, nonimmune hydrops, premature delivery, and neonatal death (29,54). Congenitally infected infants who are asymptomatic at birth subsequently develop clinical manifestations if left untreated.

Laboratory Diagnosis

Several methods currently are available for the direct detection of T. pallidum in suspicious lesions (e.g., chancre, condyloma lata, mucous patch), body fluids (e.g., nasal discharge, amniotic fluid), placentas, umbilical cords, and tissue biopsy or autopsy specimens. The organism can be visualized using dark-field microscopy, and it can be differentiated from nonpathogenic treponemes by its corkscrew appearance, characteristic 90-degree flexion centrally, and motility (26). A practical alternative to dark-field examination is the direct fluorescent antibody test for T. pallidum (DFA-TP), which uses pathogen-specific monoclonal antibodies as reagents (34). Another method involves the intratesticular or intradermal inoculation of animals with cerebrospinal fluid (CSF) or other clinical specimens (i.e., rabbit infectivity test) and examining them for evidence of a syphilitic infection over several weeks; this method is impractical for clinical purposes (34). The polymerase chain reaction (PCR) allows detection of minuscule amounts of T. pallidum deoxyribonucleic acid (DNA) in CSF, amniotic fluid, lesion exudate, serum, or biopsy specimens (34). The PCR does not distinguish between viable and dead treponemes, and the method is less sensitive than the rabbit infectivity test in detecting T. pallidum in CSF or serum.

Despite their limitations, serologic methods are the most popular and practical means of diagnosing syphilis. Two different types of antibodies are measured: nonspecific, nontreponemal reaginic (i.e., Wassermann) antibodies and specific, antitreponemal antibodies (55).

Nontreponemal tests detect immunoglobulin G (IgG) and immunoglobulin M (IgM) antibodies directed against cardiolipin-lecithin-cholesterol antigens (26). The Venereal Disease Research Laboratory (VDRL) test and the rapid plasma reagin (RPR) 18-mm-circle card test are the two most popular tests in use. These flocculation tests are inexpensive and simple to perform, making them suitable for screening purposes. Quantitative results can be obtained, and the measured titers are helpful in monitoring the response to therapy and detecting reinfections (26). These antibodies are detectable in 70% to 80% of patients with primary syphilis and in almost 100% of those with secondary syphilis. They may disappear even without specific therapy in 25% of patients with latent disease. The RPR or VDRL tests may become nonreactive within 1 or 2 years of adequate treatment of patients with primary or secondary syphilis, respectively. The length of time needed to serorevert depends on pretreatment titers (56). Some adequately treated patients remain positive for life (serofast status).

False-positive VDRL or RPR test results occur in 1% to 2% of the general population and in about 10% of intravenous drug users. Many infectious conditions (e.g., hepatitis, leptospirosis, HIV-1 infection, infectious mononucleosis, viral pneumonia, varicella, measles, bacterial endocarditis, chancroid, tuberculosis, malaria, leprosy, *Mycoplasma* pneumonia, Lyme disease) and noninfectious conditions (e.g., pregnancy, chronic liver disease, connective tissue disease, multiple blood transfusions) are associated with false-positive test results, and specific treponemal tests are required for confirmation of the diagnosis. The titers in false-positive reactions usually are low (less than 1:8) (26,34,57). Prozone (i.e., false-negative) reactions occur in 1% to 2% of patients with secondary syphilis because of the excess reaginic antibodies that prevent flocculation; diluting the serum and retesting yields high RPR or VDRL titers (58,59).

Specific treponemal tests include fluorescent treponemal antibody-absorption (FTA-ABS), *T. pallidum* immobilization, microhemagglutination assay for antibody to *T. pallidum* (MHA-TP), and the hemagglutination treponemal tests for syphilis (26,34,55). These tests are expensive and cumbersome to perform and are not suitable for screening purposes. Reactive test results are obtained in 65% (by MHA-TP) to 85% (by FTA-ABS) of women with primary syphilis, in 100% with secondary syphilis, and in 95% to 98% with later stages of disease. Because these tests remain positive indefinitely in most patients, they are not helpful in detecting reinfections. However, the FTA-ABS and MHA-TP tests have been shown to serorevert in 24% and 13%, respectively, of patients with primary or secondary syphilis within 36 months of adequate treatment (56). The specific treponemal tests are most useful in differentiating a syphilitic infection from a false-positive reaction on the VDRL or RPR tests. False-positive treponemal test reactions occur in about 1% of the general population; these are usually transient. Conditions associated with false-positive reactions include infectious mononucleosis, leprosy, leptospirosis, Lyme disease, and systemic, discoid, or drug-induced lupus erythematosus (26).

Newer serologic techniques under evaluation include enzyme immunoassays and Western blots for the detection of IgG and IgM antibodies to *T. pallidum* and antigen-capture enzyme immunoassays. These tests may help differentiate active from previously treated syphilis and aid in the accurate diagnosis of congenital infection (26,34).

Treatment

Penicillin remains the drug of first choice for the treatment of maternal syphilis and for the prevention of fetal infection (29). The drug dosage and duration of treatment vary with the stage of the disease. Early syphilis (i.e., primary, secondary, early latent) is treated with 2.4 million U of benzathine penicillin G given once intramuscularly; the cure rate with this regimen is about 95%. A second dose of benzathine penicillin G (2.4 million U given intramuscularly) may be administered 1 week after the initial dose (60). For syphilis of longer than a 1-year duration (i.e., late syphilis), 2.4 million U of benzathine penicillin G are given intramuscularly once weekly for 3 consecutive weeks. A variety of regimens are used for neurosyphilis. About 40% to 45% of treated pregnant women have Jarisch–Herxheimer reactions within a few hours of starting benzathine penicillin G therapy; reactions typically are at their peak at 6 to 12 hours and usually resolve within 24 to 36 hours. These reactions consist of fever, myalgias, headache, tachycardia, and mild hypotension. Uterine contractions, decreased fetal movements, and variable decelerations occur commonly (29,61).

Formal recommendations for syphilis therapy are the same for HIV-positive and HIV-negative patients; however, many reports have documented the failure of standard penicillin therapy in curing early syphilis in HIV-1–infected patients (26). Consequently, many experts in the field now use higher doses of penicillin for the HIV-1–positive patient (60).

The failure of maternal penicillin treatment to prevent congenital syphilis in some infants is well documented (62). Most of these failures occur when treatment is given during the last 4 weeks of pregnancy.

Antimicrobials other than penicillin probably are effective in the treatment of syphilis. Tetracyclines can be used in the penicillin-allergic patient, but their use during pregnancy is contraindicated. Erythromycin has a lower cure rate in early syphilis compared with penicillin. It is not well tolerated because of gastrointestinal adverse effects, and its transplacental transfer is unpredictable. Congenital syphilis after maternal erythromycin therapy has been observed repeatedly (63). Limited data on the use of first-generation cephalosporins (e.g., cephalothin, cephalexin), ceftriaxone, nafcillin, amoxicillin, azithromycin, and chloramphenicol suggest that they may be acceptable alternatives to penicillin in adults with early syphilis. Information on their use during pregnancy is minimal (26,60,64,65). Aminoglycosides, clindamycin, and rifampin are considered ineffective (64).

Penicillin-allergic pregnant women should be skin tested for reactions to major and minor penicillin determinants (60). If results of the skin tests are negative, penicillin can be used for the treatment of syphilis. If the result of the skin test is positive, desensitization with oral penicillin over 3 to 4 hours should be attempted and the patient subsequently treated with standard doses of the drug (66,67).

Follow-up of treated pregnant women is essential. Monthly nontreponemal serologic tests should be performed. A fourfold decline in titer should be observed within 6 months after therapy. If the decline in titer does not occur or if the titer rises, retreatment is recommended (60). Such women should be evaluated for HIV-1 infection, even if they previously had been seronegative.

Prevention

All pregnant women should be tested for syphilis on their first antenatal visit. For high-risk women, additional tests at 28 weeks of gestation and at delivery should be performed. Screening is performed with quantitative nontreponemal tests, and positive results are confirmed with treponemal tests to exclude biologic false-positive reactions. Women who test positive for syphilis should be investigated for other sexually transmitted pathogens, especially HIV-1 (60,68). In one study, 46% of women who delivered an infant with congenital syphilis in their first pregnancy delivered another infant with congenital syphilis in a subsequent pregnancy. Continued cocaine use was the single most important identifiable risk factor (69).

Congenital Syphilis

Epidemiology

The number of cases of congenital syphilis reported to the CDC increased steadily between 1980 and 1991, reflecting a true increase in the number of primary and secondary maternal syphilis cases and a change since 1989 in the surveillance case definition for congenital syphilis (70). The new surveillance case definition (Table 47–2) was implemented to provide guidelines for reporting but not for making a clinical diagnosis of congenital syphilis (71). In essence, the change involved considering stillbirths and infants born to women with untreated syphilis as presumptively infected, regardless of symptoms or results of subsequent follow-up evaluations. Because vertical transmission of *T. pallidum* does not occur in all instances, the new definition leads to the inclusion of a number of uninfected infants in the "presumptive case" category (71). The older surveillance case definition led to underestimates of the true incidence of congenital syphilis. Many infants in whom the diagnosis could not be made at birth were treated presumptively but not reported because the diagnosis could not be confirmed; others were reported inconsistently or lost to follow-up. The new case definition improved sensitivity at the expense of specificity (72,73). Compared with traditional criteria for diagnosis, the new definition results in about a fivefold increase in the reported number of congenital syphilis cases (11,74).

Most infants with congenital syphilis are African-Americans. In 1993, they accounted for 2,300 (72%) of 3,173 reported cases. The rate of congenital syphilis was 344.9 per 100,000 live births among African-Americans compared with 6.1 per 100,000 live births for non-Hispanic whites (41). Although the total number of congenital syphilis cases declined to 1,162 in 1996, the rate of congenital syphilis in Baltimore, Maryland, increased from 62 per 100,000 live births in 1993 to 282 per 100,000 live births in 1996; the rate for African-Americans increased from 113 to 564 per 100,000 live births during that period (43).

Clinical Manifestations

The pathologic and morphologic alterations of congenital syphilis are due to host immune and inflammatory responses to spirochetal fetal invasion (75–77). The most prominent histopathologic abnormalities are vasculitis with resultant necrosis and fibrosis (54). Syphilitic stillbirths usually are macerated with *T. pallidum*-rich vesiculobullous cutaneous lesions, hepatosplenomegaly, and protuberant abdomen.

TABLE 47–2. *Centers for Disease Control and Prevention surveillance case definition for congenital syphilis*

Confirmed case
    An infant in whom *Treponema pallidum* is identified by dark-field microscopy, fluorescent antibody, or other specific stains in specimens from lesions, placenta, umbilical cord, or autopsy material
Presumptive case
    Any infant whose mother had untreated or inadequately treated syphilis at delivery, regardless of findings in the infant[a]
    Any infant or child who has a reactive treponemal test for syphilis and any one of the following:
        Any evidence of congenital syphilis on physical examination
        Any evidence of congenital syphilis on long-bone radiograph
        Reactive cerebrospinal fluid Venereal Disease Research Laboratory test
        Elevated cerebrospinal fluid cell count or protein without other cause
        Quantitative nontreponemal serologic titers that are fourfold higher than the mother's when both are drawn at birth
        Reactive test for FTA-ABS-19S-IgM antibody
Syphilitic stillbirth
    Fetal death in which the mother had untreated or inadequately treated syphilis at delivery of a fetus of more than 20 weeks of gestation or of a fetus weighing more than 500 g[a]

[a]Inadequate treatment consists of any nonpenicillin therapy, or penicillin given <30 days before delivery.
From ref. 71.

Most infants with congenital syphilis are asymptomatic at birth. Infants who develop clinical manifestations during the first 2 years of life are considered to have early congenital syphilis, whereas features that appear later, usually near puberty, comprise late congenital syphilis (54).

The placenta may be larger and paler than normal. The main histopathologic abnormalities are a focal, proliferative villitis with necrosis and focal mononuclear cell infiltration; endovascular and perivascular proliferation in villous vessels, leading to vascular obliteration; and focal or diffuse villous immaturity. *T. pallidum* is demonstrable in the placenta using immunohistochemical stains; silver staining methods are difficult to perform and easy to misinterpret (78). PCR of placental tissue may confirm the diagnosis of congenital syphilis, even in some cases that do not have the histopathologic features (79). The focal placental villitis and obliterative arteritis are associated with increased resistance to placental perfusion. Antenatal measurements of uterine and umbilical systolic-to-diastolic ratios using Doppler velocity waveform analysis reveal higher mean ratios in pregnancies complicated by syphilis compared with noninfected controls (80). Necrotizing funisitis, a deep inflammatory process involving the matrix of the umbilical cord and accompanied by phlebitis and thrombosis, is common in syphilitic stillbirths and infants symptomatic at birth (81,82).

Clinical signs of congenital syphilis appear in approximately two-thirds of affected infants during the third to eighth week of life and in most by 3 months of age (54). Symptoms may be generalized and nonspecific (e.g., fever, lymphadenopathy, irritability, failure to thrive). Alternatively, the highly suggestive triad of snuffles, palmar and plantar bullae, and splenomegaly may be apparent (54). The severity of the clinical illness can vary from mild to fulminant, life-threatening disease (83–86). Premature infants are more likely to have hepatomegaly, respiratory distress, and skin lesions than similarly infected term neonates (87).

Congenitally infected infants may be small for their gestational ages (54). However, a carefully conducted study by Naeye (88) of 36 stillborn and newborn infants with congenital syphilis revealed that fetal growth was almost normal despite widespread evidence of tissue destruction. The observed growth retardation in some reports may be related to confounding factors such as maternal intravenous drug use or coinfection with other pathogens.

Hepatosplenomegaly occurs in 50% to 90% of infants with early congenital syphilis (11,54). The enlargement is caused mainly by abundant extramedullary hematopoiesis and by subacute hepatic and splenic inflammation. Jaundice, with direct and indirect hyperbilirubinemia, occurs in about one-third of infants and may be contributed to by hepatitis or hemolysis (11).

Syphilitic hepatitis is common and may worsen with penicillin therapy (84,89–91). Alkaline phosphatase elevation is a frequent biochemical abnormality (84). Transaminase and γ-glutamyltransferase concentrations may be high at presentation and increase with antimicrobial therapy to levels approaching 150 times normal (89). Fulminant syphilitic hepatitis can manifest with hypoglycemia, lactic acidosis, encephalopathy, disseminated intravascular coagulation, and shock, mimicking metabolic or other infectious causes of acute liver failure (85,92). Hepatic and splenic abnormalities may persist for as long as 1 year after treatment (54). Liver cirrhosis is uncommon (11).

Generalized lymphadenopathy is found in 20% to 50% of infants with congenital syphilis (54). The enlarged nodes are firm and nontender.

The mucocutaneous lesions of congenital syphilis are varied and occur in 30% to 60% of infants (54). The most characteristic are vesiculobullous eruptions that are most pronounced on the palms and soles. The blister fluid abounds with active spirochetes and is highly infectious (54). When a blister ruptures, it leaves behind a macerated red surface that rapidly dries and crusts. The most commonly encountered rash consists of oval, red, maculopapular lesions that are most prominent on the buttocks, back, thighs, and soles; they later change to a copper-brown color with superficial desquamation. Other lesions may be annular, circinate, petechial, or purpuric, or have a blueberry-muffin appearance (54). Mucous patches involving the nares, palate, tongue, lips, and anus can occur; these lesions become deeply fissured and hemorrhagic and subsequently result in rhagades (i.e., Parrot radial scars of late congenital syphilis) (54). Condyloma lata usually are encountered later in infancy in untreated patients. These raised, flat, moist, and wartlike lesions most commonly affect perioral (e.g., nares, angles of mouth) and perianal areas (11).

Rhinitis (i.e., snuffles) is encountered in 10% to 50% of infected infants and usually precedes the appearance of cutaneous eruptions by 1 to 2 weeks (54,84,93). The extremely contagious discharge initially is watery, but it later becomes thicker, purulent, and even hemorrhagic (54). Without treatment, the nasal cartilage ulcerates with ensuing chondritis, necrosis, and septal perforation (i.e., saddle-nose deformity of late congenital syphilis) (11). Throat involvement can produce hoarseness or aphonia (54).

Roentgenographic abnormalities are detected in 20% to more than 95% of infants with early congenital syphilis (93–98). The lower rates usually are seen in asymptomatic infants (96). Multiple, symmetric bony lesions are common. The metaphyses and diaphyses of long bones, particularly those of the lower extremities, are most commonly affected. Radiologic changes include osteochondritis, periostitis, and osteitis (11). The earliest changes occur in the metaphysis and consist of transverse, serrated radiopaque bands (i.e., Wegner sign) alternating with zones of radiolucent osteoporotic bone (54,95). Osteochondritis becomes evident radiographically 5 weeks after fetal infection (54). The metaphysis may become fragmented. Focal erosions involving the proximal medial tibia are referred to as Wimberger's sign (Fig. 47–1). Periosteal reactions may consist of a single layer of new bone formation, multiple layers (i.e., "onion peel periosteum"), or a severe lamellar form (i.e., periostitis of Pehu) (95). Periostitis is radiologically apparent after at least 16 weeks of fetal infection (54). Osteitis can give rise to a celery-stick appearance of longitudinal translucent lines that extend into the diaphysis or lead to a diffuse moth-eaten rarefaction of the shaft. Dactylitis, absence of lower extremity ossification centers, cranial nodules, and pathologic fractures or joint involvement leading to immobility of the affected limb (i.e., pseudoparalysis of Parrot) occasionally are seen (54,95, 99,100).

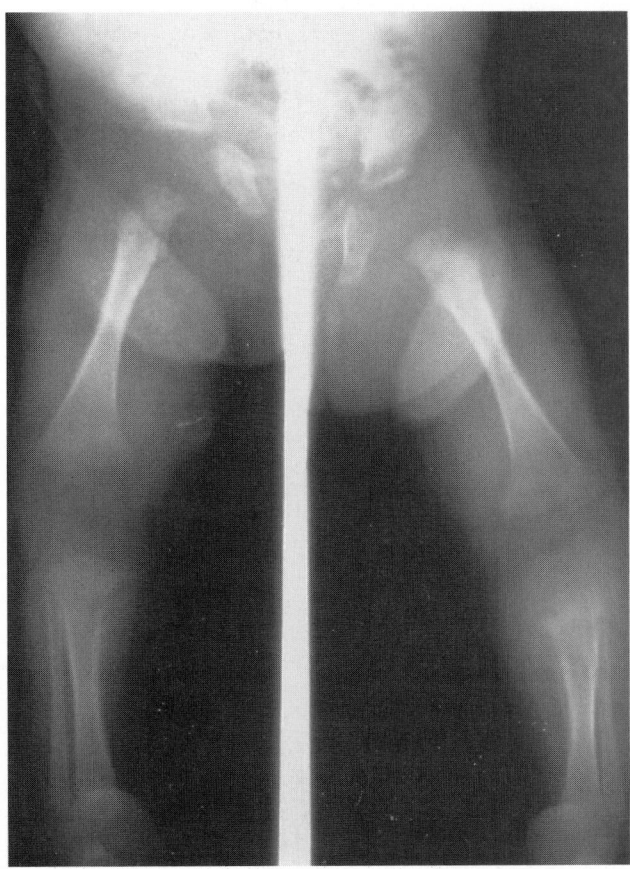

FIG. 47–1. Bone abnormalities in an infant with early congenital syphilis. Findings include bilateral, symmetric tibial periosteal new bone formation, and bilateral bony erosions involving the proximal tibial metaphysis medially (i.e., Wimberger's sign).

Hematologic abnormalities are common and include anemia, leukocytosis, leukopenia, and thrombocytopenia (93). Anemia may be due to Coombs-negative hemolysis, replacement of bone marrow by syphilitic granulation tissue, or maturation arrest in the erythroblastoid cell line (11). Thrombocytopenia is due to shortened peripheral platelet survival.

Clinically silent CNS involvement occurs in as many as 60% of infants with congenital syphilis (11). Acute syphilitic meningitis may present with neck stiffness, vomiting, bulging anterior fontanelle, and a positive Kernig's sign. CSF examination reveals a normal glucose concentration, modestly elevated protein content, and mononuclear pleocytosis (usually less than 200 cells/μL), a pattern consistent with aseptic meningitis. Chronic meningovascular syphilis develops in untreated infants and manifests in late infancy with progressive, communicating hydrocephalus, cranial nerve palsies, optic atrophy, and cerebral infarctions leading to hemiplegia or seizure disorders (54,101).

Other less common pathologic changes of early congenital syphilis involve the eyes (e.g., salt and pepper chorioretinitis, glaucoma, chancres of eyelids, uveitis), lungs (e.g., pneumonia alba, interstitial scarring, extramedullary hematopoiesis), and kidneys (e.g., nephrotic syndrome, glomerulonephritis) (54,102,103). Nonimmune hydrops is found in one-sixth of liveborn infants with congenital syphilis (50). Myocarditis, hypopituitarism, pancreatitis, diarrhea, and malabsorption also occur (54,104).

The clinical manifestations of late congenital syphilis represent residual scars after therapy of early congenital infection or persistent inflammation in untreated persons. Abnormalities of dentition are secondary to early damage incurred by developing tooth buds and can be prevented by penicillin treatment during the neonatal period or in early infancy. Unilateral or bilateral interstitial keratitis occurs in about 10% of patients and usually is diagnosed between 5 and 20 years of age. Saddle-nose deformity, high-arched palate, and poor maxillary growth are late consequences of syphilitic rhinitis. Eighth-nerve deafness occurs infrequently (3% of patients) and is due to osteochondritis of the otic capsule and resulting cochlear degeneration. Rhagades are linear scars that radiate from sites of earlier mucocutaneous lesions of the mouth, nares, and anus. Skeletal manifestations are caused by persistent or recurrent periostitis and its associated bone thickening (54,105,106).

Diagnosis

Antenatal sonography may reveal placental thickening or fetal abnormalities such as hydrops, hepatomegaly, ascites, or dilated small bowel loops (107–111). Musculoskeletal abnormalities may be visualized on rare occasions with antenatal ultrasonography (112). Spirochetes can be visualized in amniotic fluid samples using dark-field microscopy or indirect immunofluorescent staining (107,109,113). The presence of *T. pallidum* or its DNA in amniotic fluid can be demonstrated by rabbit infectivity tests or PCR techniques, respectively (114,115). With the availability of umbilical blood sampling, intrauterine infection has been confirmed as early as 24 weeks of gestation by detecting the spirochete or its DNA in fetal blood and by measuring specific IgM antibodies directed against the 47-kilodalton antigen of *T. pallidum* in fetal serum (107,110,114). By testing amniotic fluid using the rabbit infectivity test and PCR analysis, some investigators have been able to confirm intrauterine *T. pallidum* infection antenatally as early as 17 weeks of gestation (115).

At birth, the diagnosis of congenital syphilis is best established by demonstrating the spirochete or its DNA in tissues or body fluids as previously alluded to. Serologic data obtained from cord blood or neonatal sera are helpful if interpreted with their limitations in mind.

Rapid plasma reagin measurements on cord blood samples yield false-positive and false-negative results in 10% and 5% of cases, respectively (116). Serum from the infant, rather than from the umbilical cord, should be used because of lower false-positive and false-negative reactions (117). If an infant's RPR or VDRL titer is at least fourfold higher than a concomitantly obtained maternal titer, the diagnosis of congenital syphilis is likely. The RPR may be negative in infants whose mothers had acquired syphilis shortly before delivery (84). The FTA-ABS-IgM test yields false-positive and false-negative results in 35% and 10% of cases, respectively (11). This is due to interference with test performance by rheumatoid factor (i.e., fetal IgM antibodies directed against maternal IgG). This problem can be overcome by separating the IgG and IgM fractions of the serum and then testing the IgG-depleted fraction with FTA-ABS-IgM. This assay is known as FTA-ABS-19S-IgM, and it is still investigational (34). The detection of IgM antibodies against specific *T. pallidum* antigens, especially the 47-kilodalton outer membrane protein antigen, by Western immunoblot assays is diagnostically helpful (11,118,119).

In addition to serologic tests for syphilis, the complete diagnostic evaluation of an infant with congenital syphilis should include bone radiography, CSF examination, complete blood count, platelet count, liver enzyme concentrations, and HIV-1 antibody determination. However, Moyer and colleagues (98) recently demonstrated that the results of long-bone radiographs in newborns do not differentiate between active and past infection, and that the results do not alter the management of infants being evaluated for congenital syphilis.

The diagnosis of congenital neurosyphilis is difficult to ascertain. CSF abnormalities such as mononuclear pleocytosis (≥25 cells/µL), elevated protein concentra-

tion (greater than 170 mg/dL), and reactive CSF VDRL are widely used criteria (11). However, the CSF VDRL can be positive in the absence of neurosyphilis because of passive diffusion of nontreponemal IgG antibodies from serum to CSF and in infants with traumatic lumbar punctures (11). The yield of lumbar punctures in asymptomatic newborns with congenital syphilis is poor (120). A specific IgM response to the *T. pallidum* 47-kilodalton antigen has been detected in the CSF of some infants with congenial syphilis, and this may prove helpful for the diagnosis of neurosyphilis. CSF IgM reactivity can be present in infants with negative CSF VDRL test results (55). The presence of *T. pallidum* in the CSF of some infants with normal CSF cell counts, protein concentrations, and VDRL test results has been demonstrated using sensitive rabbit infectivity tests or PCR methods (11,121).

Treatment

Infants should be treated at birth if they are symptomatic, if maternal therapy was inadequate or unknown, or if follow-up cannot be ensured. Adequate maternal therapy is defined as penicillin treatment at a dose appropriate for the stage of syphilis and started at least 30 days before delivery (60).

One of two dosage regimens can be used for confirmed or presumptive congenital syphilis:

1. Aqueous crystalline penicillin G at a dose of 100,000 to 150,000 U/kg/d administered intravenously as 50,000 U/kg/dose every 12 hours during the first 7 days of life, and every 8 hours thereafter for a total of 10 days.
2. Procaine penicillin G at a dose of 50,000 U/kg/dose given intramuscularly once daily for 10 days.

If more than 1 day of therapy is missed, the entire course should be restarted (60). Benzathine penicillin G given as a single intramuscular dose of 50,000 U/kg is recommended only for infants whose evaluation (complete blood count and platelets, CSF examination, long-bone radiographs) is normal and follow-up is certain. The Jarisch–Herxheimer reaction occurs in some infants within hours of initiation of penicillin therapy.

The VDRL titers should be monitored every 2 to 3 months until they become nonreactive or the titer declines by at least fourfold. Untreated infants should have FTA-ABS tests. Passively acquired maternal antibodies usually disappear by 6 to 12 months of age in uninfected infants (122). If the VDRL titers are stable or rising or if the FTA-ABS test result remains positive beyond 15 months of age, the infant should be thoroughly reexamined and treated. The VDRL titers of adequately treated infants with congenital syphilis gradually decline, but FTA-ABS reactivities persist. Infants with CSF abnormalities should be retested at 6 months of age. If the

CSF VDRL is positive at that time, a second course of penicillin is indicated. Follow-up examinations should emphasize developmental assessment and a careful search for stigmata of congenital syphilis.

TOXOPLASMOSIS

Toxoplasmosis is a common zoonosis, afflicting approximately one in three people worldwide. Infections of immunocompetent hosts are typically asymptomatic or benign, but intrauterine infections and illnesses in immunosuppressed patients can be severe or fatal. The causative organism, *T. gondii*, is an obligate intracellular protozoan that can be encountered in the form of a tachyzoite, tissue cyst, or oocyst. In addition to humans, *T. gondii* can infect other warm-blooded animals such as cats, dogs, sheep, swine, and some birds; cats and other felines are the only known complete hosts for this parasite (13).

The life cycle of *T. gondii* usually is divided into an enteroepithelial sexual phase that occurs only in felines and an extraintestinal asexual phase that takes place in definitive (e.g., cats) and intermediate (e.g., humans) hosts (123). Susceptible cats can acquire *Toxoplasma* infection by ingesting oocysts or parasite-harboring tissues of other animals. Some of the organisms released in cat intestines invade gut epithelial cells and undergo sexual differentiation into microgametes and macrogametes; the gametocytes later fuse to produce a zygote. After a rigid wall forms around the zygote, it is excreted in feces as an oocyst. Acutely infected cats generally shed millions of oocysts in their feces daily for periods of 1 to 3 weeks. Parasites that do not undergo sexual differentiation may instead penetrate the gut wall and spread to other tissues by way of the blood and lymphatics; this extraintestinal or asexual stage can occur in humans and other susceptible animals as well.

The tachyzoite is the actively proliferating form that is encountered in organs during the acute stage of infection. Tachyzoites gain entry into the cytoplasm of host cells and multiply rapidly. Infected cells subsequently burst and release progeny parasites that go on to attack neighboring host cells, which leads to the formation of necrotic areas that are surrounded by an inflammatory cellular reaction. This process eventually is curtailed by specific cellular and humoral host immune responses. In immunodeficient persons, the acute infection can continue relentlessly and cause serious illnesses.

After the host develops specific immunity against *T. gondii*, the organism can remain in organs in a viable, clinically inapparent tissue cyst form. *T. gondii* tissue cysts most commonly are found in the brain, eyes, myocardium, and skeletal muscles, and can be detected as early as 6 to 12 days postinfection in experimentally infected animals (124). Each cyst contains a number of slowly propagating or dormant parasites. Encysted organisms can reactivate and cause serious illnesses, such as encephalitis and pneumonia, in patients who become immunodeficient later in life because of malignancy, acquired immunodeficiency syndrome (AIDS), or immunosuppressant therapy (e.g., organ transplants).

T. gondii is transmitted to humans primarily through the ingestion of oocyst-contaminated water or food or the consumption of cyst-containing raw or undercooked beef, pork, mutton, or chicken. Unwashed hands can serve as vehicles for the transport of contaminating oocysts from the soil, dust, or cat litter box material into the mouth. Transmission occasionally can occur by eating raw infected eggs, transfusion of infected blood or blood products, heart or kidney transplants from seropositive donors to seronegative recipients, or accidental self-inoculation of laboratory workers who are in contact with infected animals, needles, or glassware. Direct human-to-human transmission occurs only in the context of transplacental spread of the parasite to a developing fetus (125).

Maternal Toxoplasmosis

Epidemiology

The prevalence of anti-*Toxoplasma* antibodies among women of child-bearing age varies geographically, ranging from none to more than 90%. A seroprevalence of 39% was found in a large study of 22,845 pregnancies from diverse parts of the United States conducted between 1959 and 1966 (126). More recent surveys demonstrate the divergence of seroprevalence figures by region: Denver, Colorado, 3.3%; Palo Alto, California, 10%; Boston, Massachusetts, 14%; and Birmingham, Alabama, 30%. Seroprevalence figures for women of child-bearing age from other countries include Australia with a rate of 4%, Finland 20%, Poland 36%, Italy 40%, Ethiopia 48%, Belgium 53%, Panama 63%, France 71%, and El Salvador 75% (13,125,127–129).

The incidence of acute *T. gondii* infection during pregnancy varies by locale. Reported frequencies per 1,000 pregnancies include Alabama with 0.6, Finland with 2.4, Australia with 5, Germany with 7.5, and Belgium with 14.3 (13,128). The risk of infection is greatest for pregnant women leaving a region with a low incidence of toxoplasmosis to reside in an area where the infection is prevalent (127). Specific risk factors for acquisition of *T. gondii* infection in pregnancy may include consumption of cured pork and raw meat (including tasting raw meat while preparing food), eating unwashed raw vegetables or fruits, infrequent washing of hands or kitchen utensils after preparation of raw meat before handling another food item, and cleaning cat litter boxes (129,130).

Clinical Manifestations

Acute toxoplasmosis is asymptomatic in 80% to 90% of pregnant women. Those with clinically evident illnesses most commonly present with lymphadenopathy, primarily of the head and neck region; a single node is involved in about two-thirds of patients (131). *T. gondii* causes about 1% to 5% of infectious mononucleosis cases and should be considered a likely etiologic agent in patients with negative heterophile antibody test results (132). Complications such as hepatitis, pneumonia, myocarditis, encephalitis, and deafness are rare in immunocompetent women (125,133,134). Psychiatric complications such as psychoses with schizophreniform features, anxiety, and depression have been encountered on rare occasions (135). Fulminating illnesses are common in immunosuppressed patients (134,136).

T. gondii spreads transplacentally to involve the developing fetus in 25%, 54%, or 65% of pregnant women with untreated primary toxoplasmosis during the first, second, or third trimester, respectively (125). Proper maternal therapy reduces the overall incidence of fetal infection by more than 50%, and fewer infected infants manifest with severe congenital toxoplasmosis (137,138). These data underscore the importance of accurate and timely diagnosis of acute toxoplasmosis in pregnant women.

Diagnostic Tests

A clinical diagnosis of toxoplasmosis should be considered dubious unless supported by appropriate laboratory test results. *T. gondii* can be isolated from infected blood, CSF, aqueous humor, amniotic fluid, or homogenized tissues (e.g., placenta, brain, muscle) by inoculating these specimens into the peritoneal cavities of mice or onto tissue cultures. Tissue culture techniques are faster (≈1 week) but less sensitive than intraperitoneal inoculation methods (≤6 weeks); both methods are impractical for clinical purposes. Tachyzoites can be visualized in tissue sections or smears of body fluids, especially if labeled specific anti-*Toxoplasma* antibodies are used for staining; their presence denotes acute infection. The demonstration of tissue cysts on histopathology can be consistent with an acute or a chronic *Toxoplasma* infection (139).

Other immunologic techniques that have been used for the diagnosis of toxoplasmosis include intradermal skin tests and transformation of lymphocytes on exposure to *Toxoplasma* antigens, both of which connote chronic infection (125). *Toxoplasma* antigens can be detected in CSF, urine, serum, or amniotic fluid using enzyme-linked immunosorbent assays (ELISA) or immunoblotting methods. A positive antigen test result indicates that the infection is recent. This is particularly helpful in newborns and immunodeficient persons in whom antibody responses to infection may be absent or unpredictable (13,140). The antigen test is not available commercially. The PCR has been used successfully for the direct detection of *T. gondii* DNA in clinical samples by amplification of the *P30* or *B1* genes of the parasite; amplification

of TGR1$_E$ (a repetitive DNA sequence) and a part of the small subunit ribosomal DNA (rDNA) also have been used (141–143).

The diagnosis of toxoplasmosis most often rests on serologic confirmation. The Sabin–Feldman dye test, traditionally the reference test against which newer methods are compared, requires the use of live parasites. Positive titers are usually in the 1:256 to 1:128,000 range. Most laboratories have abandoned the dye test in favor of simpler techniques that use killed antigens, such as the indirect fluorescent antibody (IFA), ELISA, agglutination, and indirect hemagglutination (IHA) tests.

Toxoplasma-specific IgM antibodies can be measured by IFA, ELISA, or IgM immunosorbent agglutination assay (IgM-ISAGA). False-positive IgM-IFA or IgM-ELISA are encountered in sera containing rheumatoid factor; this problem is circumvented if a double-sandwich IgM-ELISA (DS-IgM-ELISA) is performed (139). Specific IgM antibodies usually become positive within 1 to 2 weeks of infection and continue to be detectable for months or years, especially when measured by very sensitive assays such as DS-IgM-ELISA or IgM-ISAGA. The detection of specific IgM antibodies should not be considered proof that an infection is acute. High specific IgM titers suggest acute infection, especially if accompanied by high specific IgG titers of about 1:1,000 or greater as measured by IFA or the Sabin–Feldman dye test. Low specific IgM titers measured by DS-IgM-ELISA or IgM-ISAGA generally are encountered in patients whose infections occurred several months earlier. IgM-IFA tests are considerably less sensitive than DS-IgM-ELISA or IgM-ISAGA and are positive in only 60% to 70% of patients with acute infections and 25% to 50% of infants with congenital toxoplasmosis. Fewer than 25% of patients are still positive by the IgM-IFA assay 9 months after an acute infection. It is important to know the type of assay used to measure specific IgM antibodies in pregnant women to interpret correctly the significance of positive and negative results (13,139). Commercially available test kits for *Toxoplasma* IgM measurements unfortunately are unreliable as the sole determinant of recent *T. gondii* infection during pregnancy, and reliance on a single test result can lead to misdiagnoses and possibly inappropriate interventions (FDA Public Health Advisory: Limitations of *Toxoplasma* IgM Commercial Test Kits, July 25, 1997).

Anti-*Toxoplasma* IgG antibodies usually appear early during an infection. IgG titers peak at about 2 months, gradually drop thereafter, but remain detectable for years. The predominant IgG antibody response is of the IgG1 subclass (144). A single high specific IgG titer is considered only suggestive of an acute infection. The strength of the binding of specific IgG to multivalent *Toxoplasma* antigens (IgG avidity) has been shown to be low in acute infections and high in chronic infections. Low IgG avidity can persist for longer than 20 weeks. IgG avidity greater than 20% indicates that the infection occurred at least 20 weeks earlier. Thus, detection of high-avidity IgG antibodies to *Toxoplasma* antigens in pregnant women during the first half of their pregnancies can provide reassurance that their infections were remote in relation to the pregnancies (145,146).

Anti-*Toxoplasma* IgA antibodies directed against the major surface protein of tachyzoites (P30) are present in more than 95% of patients with acute infections (139). These antibodies are detected at the end of the first month of infection and usually disappear within 4 to 7 months, but can last up to 12 months or occasionally longer (139,147,148). Specific IgA antibodies are found rarely in patients with chronic infections (147).

Specific serum IgE antibodies are present in about 86% of women who seroconvert during pregnancy. They appear shortly before or concomitantly with specific IgA antibodies, and they usually persist for less than 4 months (occasionally up to 8 months) (139,148).

Antibodies detected by IHA are different from those measured by the dye test, ELISA, or IFA. The titers take several weeks before becoming positive, making the test unsuitable for diagnosis of acute toxoplasmosis during pregnancy (13).

The differential agglutination test (AC/HS test) compares IgG titers obtained using acetone- or methanol-fixed (AC) tachyzoite antigens with those measured using formalin-fixed (HS) tachyzoite antigens. AC antigens detect acute phase-specific IgG antibodies. The AC-to-HS ratio is used to determine the timing of the primary infection. The test shows an acute pattern for up to 14 months (148,149).

Serologic Diagnosis of Maternal Infection

Acute infection in immunologically normal women can be diagnosed if seroconversion or a fourfold or greater rise in antibody titers occurs when serum samples are collected 3 to 6 weeks apart (125). The absence of *Toxoplasma*-specific IgM antibodies as measured by the DS-IgM-ELISA or IgM-ISAGA essentially excludes the diagnosis of acute toxoplasmosis. Elevated titers obtained by these assays are considered suggestive of the diagnosis, especially if specific IgG titers are high as well. Positive IgM-IFA results are more likely to represent recent infection. Specific antibodies detected by IgM-ISAGA or DS-IgM-ELISA usually persist at low levels for months or years after infection. High levels measured many years after the acute infection are rare (150). The detection of *Toxoplasma*-specific serum IgA or IgE antibodies indicates a recent infection; conversely, absence of these antibodies in a seropositive woman suggests that the infection is old (139,147,151).

Immunodeficient women with acute *T. gondii* frequently are unable to mount a specific IgM response, and their IgG responses may be absent or low. Use of the more sensitive antibody assays may be helpful, but direct detection of the parasite or its components (e.g., antigen, DNA) in body fluids or tissues is sometimes the only means of establishing the diagnosis of acute toxoplasmosis (125,152).

Diagnosis of Intrauterine Infection

Estimation of the duration of maternal *T. gondii* infection usually is difficult, and, consequently, assessment of the true risk to the fetus is often fraught with uncertainties. The parasite can be transmitted to the developing fetus at any stage of pregnancy and, in some cases, at or shortly before conception (13,153,154). The risk of fetal infection is estimated to be less than 1% if the initial stages of maternal infection occur before conception (154,155). This creates considerable anxiety for parents, who may choose an unwarranted end to the pregnancy or unnecessary maternal chemotherapy with potentially toxic drugs.

Prenatal diagnosis of fetal toxoplasmosis can be achieved safely and reliably. Pregnant women shown to have acquired acute *Toxoplasma* infections during the course of their pregnancies can undergo amniocentesis and ultrasound-guided cordocentesis. Parasite isolation studies, if available, include inoculation of these clinical samples into mice or onto tissue cultures. Fetal blood should be shown to be free of maternal blood contamination, using the Kleihauer–Betke stain or hemoglobin electrophoresis, before it is assayed for *Toxoplasma*-specific IgM antibodies or other nonspecific indicators of fetal infection (e.g., leukocyte and differential cell counts, platelet count, total IgM content, lactic dehydrogenase level, γ-glutamyltransferase concentration). Serial ultrasound examinations should be done at 2-week intervals to detect ventricular dilation, cerebral or hepatic calcifications, ascites, hydrops, or other fetal abnormalities (125,156).

Daffos and colleagues (157) applied this approach to prenatal diagnosis to 746 women with gestational toxoplasmosis occurring within the first 25 weeks of pregnancy. All mothers were treated with spiramycin. Fetal infection occurred in 42 pregnancies, 39 (93%) of which were successfully identified prenatally. The most sensitive test in this study proved to be parasite isolation from amniotic fluid or fetal blood (81%). Despite the use of the sensitive IgM-ISAGA assay, only 21% of infected fetuses tested positive. Serial ultrasound examinations showed abnormalities in 45% of fetuses. Among nonspecific tests, γ-glutamyltransferase or total IgM contents of fetal blood were elevated in more than one-half of the patients. Results of prenatal testing led to pregnancy terminations in 62% of cases; the diagnosis was confirmed postnatally in the remainder. No false-positive diagnoses of fetal toxoplasmosis were made in this study, although other investigators have encountered this problem (158,159).

Because maternal IgA and IgE antibodies do not cross the placenta, fetal serum IgA and IgE have been explored as possible markers for intrauterine *T. gondii* infection. Decoster and colleagues (160) were able to detect specific IgA antibodies in fetal blood as early as 23 weeks of gestation. The sensitivity of the assay was only 50%, slightly higher than that for *Toxoplasma*-specific IgM. No false-positive results were obtained. The sensitivity and specificity of *Toxoplasma*-specific fetal serum IgA measurement was 77% and 96%, respectively, in another study of 286 patients (161). *Toxoplasma*-specific IgA antibodies found in amniotic fluid are probably of maternal origin and are not useful for the diagnosis of fetal toxoplasmosis (162). Pinon and colleagues (163) were unable to detect specific anti-*Toxoplasma* IgE antibodies in fetal blood.

PCR methods have been used in prenatal diagnosis of fetal toxoplasmosis (164–169). Cazenave and colleagues (165) studied 80 women with documented acute toxoplasmosis during pregnancy. PCR analysis (using *P30* gene amplification) of the amniotic fluid was negative in 70 cases without intrauterine infection and positive for all ten with fetal toxoplasmosis. In this study, the PCR was considerably more sensitive than recovering the parasite from amniotic fluid using culture methods (40%) or detection of specific fetal IgM (40%) (165). Similarly, Grover and associates (164) amplified the *B1* gene and found the PCR method to be more sensitive than the traditional techniques used for the prenatal diagnosis of toxoplasmosis. Hohlfeld and coinvestigators (167) evaluated 339 consecutive women with gestational toxoplasmosis using PCR analysis (*B1* gene amplification) of their amniotic fluids and found that 37 of 38 infected fetuses had positive amniotic fluid test results; no false-positive results were encountered. The PCR was more sensitive than the conventional methods used for prenatal diagnosis of fetal toxoplasmosis (97.4% vs. 89.5%, respectively) (167). Other researchers found their PCR assays on amniotic fluid to have lower sensitivities than indicated by these reports (166,168). Because the PCR test for *Toxoplasma* DNA is not standardized, interlaboratory variability in test results can be encountered (170). The PCR can provide results within hours compared with tissue cultures, which require a minimum of 4 days or animal inoculation techniques, which take at least 5 weeks to complete (165). The sensitivity of PCR analysis, coupled with its rapidity, makes it promising as a diagnostic tool because it can minimize the rate of late pregnancy terminations with their relatively increased risk.

Treatment

Acute toxoplasmosis in the healthy, nonpregnant woman usually requires no specific therapy because of its benign, self-limited nature. Drugs used to treat toxoplas-mosis are active against tachyzoites, but they generally have no effect on the encysted form of the parasite.

The option of pregnancy termination should be confined to women who become infected during the first one-half of their pregnancy. Although the risk of transmission of the parasite to the fetus is at its lowest during this stage, the severity of fetal disease is usually at its greatest. Acutely infected women who elect to proceed with their pregnancies should be treated with spiramycin as soon after diagnosis as possible (149). Spiramycin is a macrolide antibiotic that is active against *T. gondii* and can cross the placenta to enter the cord blood and amniotic fluid (171). It achieves high tissue levels, especially in the placenta. The main adverse effects of spiramycin are nausea, vomiting, and diarrhea. The drug reduces the risk of intrauterine transmission of the parasite, but it does not alter fetal pathology after infection has developed. Spiramycin is only available by request from the Food and Drug Administration; the adult dose is 1 g per dose, given orally three times daily (172). It is not known whether clarithromycin or azithromycin are effective alternatives to spiramycin in preventing intrauterine *T. gondii* infection.

If prenatal diagnosis is attempted and a fetus is shown to be infected, drugs such as pyrimethamine and sulfadiazine are added. Pyrimethamine, an antimalarial drug, is a folic acid antagonist. Its half-life in adults is about 100 hours, and it achieves tissue concentrations (e.g., brain) that are higher than in serum (125). The drug causes bone marrow suppression with resultant anemia, granulocytopenia, and thrombocytopenia; severe pancytopenia occasionally occurs (173). Other side effects include a bad taste in the mouth, headache, and gastrointestinal discomfort. Pyrimethamine has been shown to be teratogenic in animals receiving massive doses of the drug early in organogenesis, and it should not be used before the fifth month of pregnancy (125). Sulfadiazine (and its hydroxylated metabolites) or the trisulfapyrimidines act synergistically with pyrimethamine against *Toxoplasma* tachyzoites; other sulfonamides show less synergy and are not used (174). These drugs are folic acid antagonists. Side effects include bone marrow suppression, rashes, crystalluria, hematuria, and reversible acute renal failure (125). One regimen used to treat pregnant women with an infected fetus incorporates 3-week courses of a combination of pyrimethamine (50 mg/d), sulfadiazine (3 g/d), and leucovorin supplements (10 mg/d), alternating with 3 weeks of spiramycin (3 g/d) (137). Leucovorin (folinic acid) is used to counteract the bone marrow suppressive effects of pyrimethamine and sulfadiazine. This treatment regimen is thought to reduce the occurrence of severe congenital infection and increase the proportion of infants born with asymptomatic toxoplasmosis. For ethical reasons, the study inferring that the drugs were efficacious did not include a control group of patients and relied on historic comparisons for its conclusions (137).

Prevention

A vaccine against *T. gondii* is not yet available. Primary prevention rests on educating susceptible pregnant women on how to avoid becoming infected with this parasite. Cats that are kept indoors and only eat dried, cooked, or canned food are unlikely to get infected and shed oocysts. Contact with cat feces should be avoided; disposable gloves should be worn when handling cat litter boxes or while gardening. Cat litter boxes should be emptied of cat feces daily and disinfected by adding boiling water to the empty box for 5 minutes. Covering children's sandboxes decreases the risk of contamination. Meat should be cooked at 66°C or higher temperatures, smoked, or cured in brine. Hands should not touch the eyes or mouth when handling raw meat, and they must be washed thoroughly afterward. Kitchen surfaces should be cleaned carefully. Fruits and vegetables may have oocysts on their surfaces and should be washed or peeled before being eaten (149). Prenatal health education programs can bring about changes in personal behavior that reduce a susceptible woman's risk of acquiring toxoplasmosis by as much as two-thirds (175).

Secondary prevention entails the identification and treatment of pregnant women who are acutely infected. Because about 90% of patients with acute toxoplasmosis have minimal or no symptoms, a systematic serologic screening program would be needed. A national prevention program for congenital toxoplasmosis that mandates monthly serologic screening of all seronegative pregnant women has been in place since 1976 in France (176). A comparable policy for routine screening does not exist in the United States, as it generally is regarded as not being cost effective and can lead to adverse pregnancy outcomes (because of the difficulties associated with interpreting serologic test results), not the least of which is the termination of several pregnancies with uninfected fetuses per case prevented (177–179).

Women found to be seronegative early in pregnancy should be advised to follow the hygienic measures outlined earlier. Retesting at 18 to 22 weeks of gestation can identify women who seroconverted during the first one-half of their pregnancy, affording them the opportunity to consider options such as maternal chemotherapy, prenatal diagnostic procedures, or elective pregnancy termination (180,181). Seronegative women gain from testing at the end of pregnancy; this helps to identify asymptomatic newborns with toxoplasmosis who may derive benefit from treatment during the first year of life.

Women found to be seropositive early in gestation should be evaluated further to exclude a recent *Toxoplasma* infection. As a group, infants born to seropositive pregnant women with IHA titers of 1:256 to 1:512 have double the predicted frequency of deafness, a 60% increase in microcephaly, and a 30% increase in the occurrence of intelligence quotients less than 70 (126).

Fetal infections after reactivation of latent toxoplasmosis in immunosuppressed pregnant women or following reinfection of immunocompetent seropositive women are known to occur but are very rare (182–184).

Congenital Toxoplasmosis

Epidemiology

The true incidence of congenital toxoplasmosis is unknown. Reported figures underestimate its occurrence. Published rates vary by locale, but they range from 0 to 10 per 1,000 live births. Representative incidence estimates per 1,000 live births include New York City with 0.7, Birmingham, Alabama, with 0.12, Mexico City with 2, Paris with 3, and Austria with 8.3 (125). Prospectively collected data from Massachusetts and New Hampshire, where all heelstick blood specimens adsorbed onto a filterpaper card for routine neonatal screening for metabolic and endocrine disorders also are tested for intrauterine *T. gondii* infection using an IgM capture immunoassay, have shown the rate of congenital toxoplasmosis to be about 1 per 10,000 newborns (185).

As treatment of acutely infected pregnant women becomes more commonplace, the occurrence of congenital toxoplasmosis should decline. Trimester-specific *T. gondii* transmission rates have been shown to decrease with proper maternal chemotherapy from 25% to 8% for the first trimester, from 54% to 19% for the second trimester, and from 65% to 44% for the third trimester (125).

Clinical Manifestations

At least two-thirds of infants with congenital toxoplasmosis have inapparent disease at birth; however, one-third of all asymptomatic neonates who undergo detailed examinations are found to have abnormalities such as CSF pleocytosis or elevated protein content (20%), chorioretinitis (15%), or intracranial calcifications (10%) (125,185). Several weeks or months later, untreated infants develop signs or symptoms of disease.

Symptomatic *Toxoplasma* infection of the newborn can be mild, moderate, or severe. It can involve multiple organ systems or present as isolated abnormalities such as hydrocephalus, hepatosplenomegaly, or prolonged hyperbilirubinemia. Approximately 25% to 50% of symptomatic infants are delivered prematurely. Only 10% of infected infants have severe disease at birth. Systemic manifestations such as fever, jaundice, anemia, hepatomegaly, splenomegaly, or chorioretinitis may predominate in some infants, and neurologic abnormalities such as encephalitis, seizures, hydrocephalus, or intracranial calcifications may be prominent in others. About 10% of congenitally infected infants who have severe disease die, and most surviving infants are left with major neurologic sequelae, such as mental retardation, seizures, spasticity, and visual deficits (13).

CNS involvement is common. Parenchymal lesions may extend to surrounding blood vessels, leading to vasculitis with thrombosis and infarction. Substantial destruction of brain parenchyma can lead to obstruction of the aqueduct of Sylvius with resultant secondary enlargements of the third and lateral ventricles and, ultimately, hydrocephalus. Hydrocephalus can be the sole manifestation of congenital toxoplasmosis. It may be present at birth or develop later in infancy, and it may be static or gradually worsen to the point of requiring shunt placement. Diffuse intracranial calcifications occur in 10% to 20% of infants with congenital toxoplasmosis, but they can be found in 30% to 70% of those with symptomatic disease at birth (Fig. 47–2) (125,185,186). They may increase in number and size over time. However, about 75% of these intracranial calcifications decrease or resolve within 1 year in adequately treated infants (186). Other neurologic findings encountered in this infection include bulging anterior fontanelle, encephalitis, hydranencephaly, hypotonia or paralysis, spasticity, microcephaly, opisthotonus, swallowing difficulties, or proteinorachia (187). Radiologic CNS findings may be consistent with an old insult (e.g., hydrocephalus, porencephaly, encephalomalacia, cortical atrophy) or, less commonly, with an acute process (e.g., single or multiple hypodense lesions with contrast ring enhancement) (188,189).

Manifestations of active congenital ocular toxoplasmosis may include chorioretinal scars, chorioretinitis, iritis, leukocoria, microphthalmia, nystagmus, optic atrophy, optic coloboma, retinal folds and traction detachments, granulomas in the posterior pole, strabismus, small cornea, and cataracts (13,190–192). Chorioretinal scars are the most common eye findings and are most likely to be found in the periphery. Macular scars are noted in 75% of untreated infants and are bilateral in about 23%; visual acuity can be markedly reduced in these patients (192). On ophthalmoscopy, the typical findings are single or multiple yellow-white, fluffy necrotic lesions with indistinct margins that arise at the borders of preexisting, healed, hyperpigmented retinochoroidal scars (Fig. 47–3). Other findings may include retinal hemorrhages, iridocyclitis, vitreous haziness, papillitis, and papilledema. Untreated infants who were asymptomatic at birth are at great risk of subsequent development of chorioretinitis (about 50% for patients older than 10 years) (13).

Sensorineural hearing loss may occur in 15% to 25% of congenitally infected infants, and educationally significant hearing loss afflicts 10% to 15% of infected infants (193). *T. gondii* has been found in the mastoid and middle ear at autopsy of some infants. Gastrointestinal disturbances such as feeding difficulties, diarrhea, and vomiting are common. The liver and spleen may be enlarged, and hepatic calcifications may be found. Conjugated hyperbilirubinemia sometimes takes months to subside. Biliary atresia associated with congenital toxoplasmosis has been reported (194). Myocarditis, nephrotic syndrome, hydrops fetalis, interstitial pneumonia, and skeletal metaphyseal lucencies occur infrequently. Cutaneous

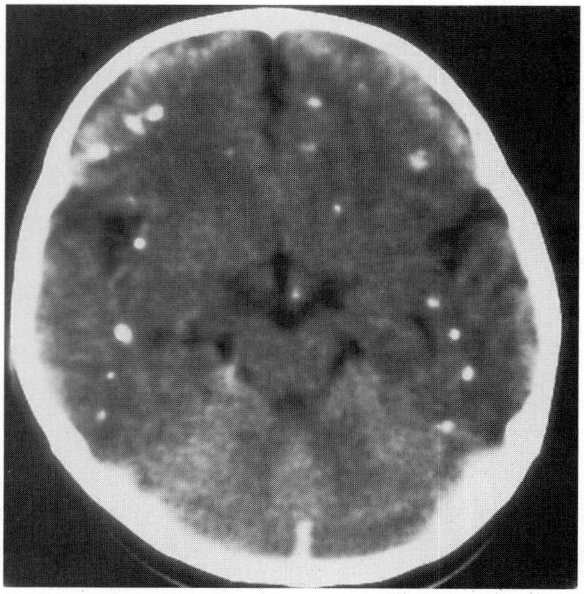

FIG. 47–2. Computerized axial head tomogram of a 5-month-old girl with congenital toxoplasmosis. Notice the diffuse parenchymal calcifications and the prominent subarachnoid space bilaterally.

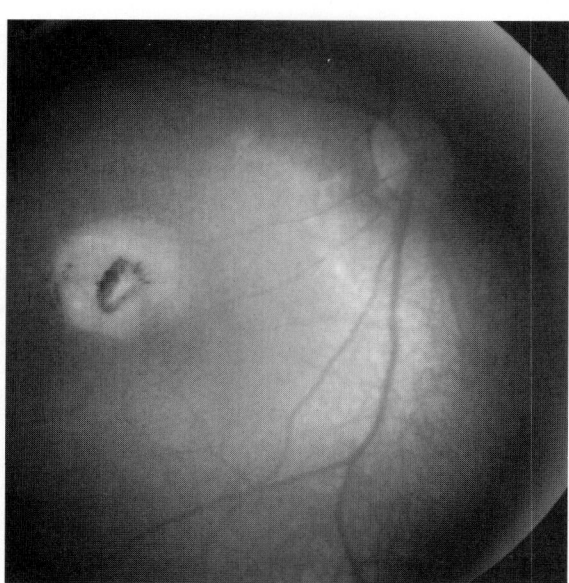

FIG. 47–3. Active chorioretinitis in a 5-month-old boy with untreated congenital toxoplasmosis.

lesions include ecchymoses, petechiae, purpura, and maculopapular rashes.

Hematologic abnormalities include anemia, eosinophilia, and thrombocytopenia (125). Transient quantitative (e.g., neutropenia) and qualitative (e.g., enlarged, vacuolated lymphocytes) changes in the leukocytes are common (195). Total CD4 lymphocyte counts and CD4-to-CD8 ratios usually are depressed (196). Compared with adults, infants with congenital toxoplasmosis have no or reduced lymphocyte blastogenic responses on exposure to *Toxoplasma* lysate antigens, with failure to produce interferon-γ or interleukin-2; however, they do respond normally to nonspecific stimulators such as concanavalin A (197). The severe organ damage seen in congenital toxoplasmosis may be due to specific deficits in cell-mediated immune responses to *Toxoplasma* antigens.

Diagnosis

Congenital toxoplasmosis is diagnosed if the parasite is recovered from the placenta. *T. gondii* can be isolated from the blood of asymptomatic or symptomatic infants; isolation rates peak at 71% during the first week of life and then decline to 33% at 2 to 4 weeks of age. Attempts at recovering the parasite from the blood of older infants generally are fruitless. The detection of *Toxoplasma* antigens or DNA in body fluids such as urine, CSF, or serum is considered diagnostic (13,198,199).

Specific IgM antibodies can be detected in the serum of 25% of congenitally infected infants with the IFA method and in as many as 75% with the DS-IgM-ELISA technique (125). The sensitivity of the IgM-ISAGA test probably is even greater (200). Passively transferred maternal anti-*Toxoplasma* IgG antibodies can suppress an infant's specific IgM response. Gross and colleagues (198,201) have shown that about 5% of sera have strain-specific immune responses. Unless antigens from more than one *T. gondii* strain are used in the assay, the sera would have no detectable specific antibodies in one test but be positive in another (201). IgM antibodies can persist for more than 1 year when measured by very sensitive assays (200). Rarely, intrathecal production of anti-*Toxoplasma* IgM is demonstrable despite the absence of specific antibodies in the serum of congenitally infected infants with CNS involvement (198).

Levels of anti-*Toxoplasma* IgG antibodies of maternal origin typically drop at a rate of 50% per month in the infant's serum, but they may continue to be detectable for about 1 year. Active congenital infection should be suspected if specific IgG titers do not show the anticipated decline or if they increase. Untreated infants begin synthesizing their own anti-*Toxoplasma* IgG antibodies by 3 months of age. The intrathecal production of specific IgG is demonstrable in about 2% of infants with CNS involvement (125).

Toxoplasma-specific serum IgA antibodies are detectable in most congenitally infected infants, significantly more often than IgM antibodies (147). Specific IgA antibodies were found in the CSF of the few infants in whom it had been measured (202). Specific serum IgE antibodies can be measured from birth in some patients, especially infants with complications such as hydrocephalus or chorioretinitis (163). Research is ongoing to refine existing serologic methods for the diagnosis of congenital toxoplasmosis. Newer techniques that are still considered investigational include IgG and IgM immunoblotting and serial measurements of IgG avidity to *Toxoplasma* antigens in sera of infants (203,204).

Transformation of lymphocytes on exposure to *Toxoplasma* antigens is a sensitive and specific indicator of congenital infection if performed on symptomatic or asymptomatic infants 3 months of age or older (13,205). The observed blastogenic response is lower in infants than in infected adults (197).

Treatment

Controlled trials examining the benefits of various treatment protocols are lacking. Drug regimens have been arrived at empirically, and conclusions about their efficacies are based on comparisons with historic data.

The treatment of symptomatic infants during the first 6 months of life usually consists of a combination of pyrimethamine, sulfadiazine, and leucovorin supplements. Pyrimethamine (1 mg/kg orally; maximum 25 mg) in one or two divided doses is given daily or every other day. A 75 mg/kg/d loading dose of sulfadiazine (maximum 4 g/d) in two divided oral doses is given for the first 2 days, followed by 100 mg/kg/d (maximum 8 g/d) in two divided oral doses administered daily thereafter. Leucovorin (5 mg) is injected intramuscularly every 3 days; the dose can be increased to 10 mg or more every 3 days in infants with bone marrow toxicities (125). After the first 6 months of treatment are completed, the regimen is modified to include 1-month courses of spiramycin alternating with 1-month courses of pyrimethamine, sulfadiazine, and leucovorin supplements for an additional 6 months. Spiramycin is given daily at a dose of 100 mg/kg/d in two divided oral doses. An alternative treatment regimen is to treat with pyrimethamine, sulfadiazine, and leucovorin for 1 year without using spiramycin; pyrimethamine at 1 mg/kg can be given on an every-other-day basis after 2 to 6 months of daily administration (206,207).

Corticosteroids such as prednisone or methylprednisolone (1.0–1.5 mg/kg/d orally in two divided doses) are used in infants with chorioretinitis or CSF protein elevations (≥1 g/dL) to reduce the inflammatory response (125,208). They should be used concurrently with anti-*Toxoplasma* drugs.

Infants with asymptomatic congenital toxoplasmosis are treated for 1 year. They receive an initial 6-week course of pyrimethamine, sulfadiazine, and leucovorin supplements, followed by alternating courses of spiramycin for 6 weeks and the pyrimethamine, sulfadiazine, and leucovorin combination for 4 weeks.

Healthy infants born to mothers with gestational toxoplasmosis and for whom serologic tests have not provided definitive answers as to the presence or absence of infection can be treated with a 4-week course of pyrimethamine, sulfadiazine, and leucovorin followed by 4 to 6 weeks of spiramycin. If the diagnosis of congenital toxoplasmosis is later established, chemotherapy is continued as delineated earlier for infants with subclinical *T. gondii* infection. For healthy infants born to mothers with high Sabin–Feldman dye test titers and undetermined timing of maternal infection, a 1-month course of spiramycin usually is prescribed. Therapy is extended if clinical or laboratory evidence of congenital toxoplasmosis is uncovered (13).

Pyrimethamine serum levels do not vary significantly with age during infancy; they are comparable for infants receiving the drug daily or every other day. Pyrimethamine serum concentrations and half-life may be reduced in infants concomitantly treated with phenobarbital. The drug achieves CSF concentrations that are 10% to 25% of concurrently measured serum levels. Seizures have been observed in patients with pyrimethamine overdosage (209).

Clindamycin has been used effectively for the treatment of ocular toxoplasmosis in older patients because of its tendency to concentrate in the choroid (208). There are no data on its efficacy in congenital infection. Photocoagulation of active lesions and of normal retinal tissues immediately bordering chorioretinal scars may be helpful in reducing recurrences (210). Trimethoprim-sulfamethoxazole has been reported to be equally as effective as the combination of pyrimethamine and sulfadiazine or of clindamycin and sulfadiazine in the treatment of ocular toxoplasmosis (211). Treatment with pyrimethamine, sulfadiazine, and leucovorin (with corticosteroids during the phase of active inflammation) currently is preferred for ocular toxoplasmosis, primarily because of the limited body of data on the efficacy of alternative regimens. Therapy should be continued for 2 weeks after resolution of active ocular inflammation (207). Active lesions usually become quiescent after 10 to 14 days of therapy (192).

Infants treated with pyrimethamine and sulfadiazine should be closely monitored. One or two blood and platelet counts should be done every week for the early detection of pyrimethamine-related adverse effects. The frequency of monitoring can be reduced to one or two times per month for infants receiving pyrimethamine on an every-other-day basis. The leucovorin dose is increased if the absolute neutrophil count falls below 1,000 cells/μL. If the absolute neutrophil count falls below 500 cells/μL, pyrimethamine also should be withheld temporarily until the neutropenia resolves (207).

Prognosis

Most infants with severe symptomatic congenital toxoplasmosis who survive beyond the neonatal period suffer from serious long-term residual problems, such as mental retardation and blindness (13,127). The majority of those born with subclinical infection who are not treated develop eye problems, and about half will suffer neurologic sequelae (13).

Short-term follow-up studies indicate that maternal therapy during gestation, followed postnatally by treatment of all congenitally infected infants, improves prognosis by reducing the frequency and severity of late-appearing disease sequelae. In the study by Hohlfeld and colleagues (137), congenital infection remained subclinical in 76%. Almost all treated infants developed normally and were neurologically normal (137). Peripheral chorioretinitis that did not impair vision developed in about 10% between 5 and 17 months of age. In another study, early institution of anti-*Toxoplasma* therapy may have prevented the occurrence of sensorineural hearing loss in congenitally infected infants (193). Guerina and colleagues (185) reported that only one of 46 congenitally infected but treated infants identified through their neonatal screening program had a neurologic deficit (hemiplegia), and 10% of those followed for 1 to 6 years had eye lesions.

Long-term follow-up studies of infants with symptomatic or subclinical congenital toxoplasmosis suggest that most patients develop chorioretinitis or chorioretinal scars by 10 to 20 years of age, but treatment may reduce the frequency and severity of adverse sequelae (212–215). The prognosis of infants with symptomatic congenital toxoplasmosis treated for 1 year with the pyrimethamine, sulfadiazine, and leucovorin regimen appears to be much better than that of historic untreated controls (186,192,206,216). All untreated patients develop chorioretinal scars, but this is seen in only 75% of those treated for 1 year. Among treated patients, peripheral chorioretinal scars and macular scarring are seen in 58% and 54%, respectively (compared with 82% and 76%, respectively, of untreated historic controls). Thirteen percent of treated infants and 44% of controls later have recurrences of ocular toxoplasmosis. The median time to ocular recurrence is 5 years (range 3 to 10) in treated infants; new lesions can occur in previously normal-appearing retina as well as contiguous to old scars (192).

Neurologic and developmental outcomes of 36 infants with treated congenital toxoplasmosis was assessed by Roizen and colleagues (216). Tone and motor abnormalities were present on the initial examinations of 20 infants, and these resolved in 12 of them by 1 year of age. Six infants had perinatal seizures; four could be taken off their anticonvulsant medications within a few months. Low cognitive functioning as measured by a score of less than 50 was found in 21%. Seven children with a score above 50 on the Mental Developmental Index were compared to their siblings who served as controls; patients scored lower than their uninfected siblings (87 vs. 112). Sequential IQ tests done at intervals of at least 1.5 years showed no deterioration over time for congenitally infected children. Seventeen of 18 patients without hydrocephalus, and six of eight children with obstructive hydrocephalus that responded to shunt placement, were neurodevelopmentally normal or near normal; those with more severe CNS involvement did not fare as well. Intracranial calcifications in treated infants may diminish or disappear in as many as 75% and remain unchanged in the rest (186).

RUBELLA

Rubella (i.e., German measles, third disease) typically is a subclinical or mild exanthematous infection of children and adults. Gestational rubella can have deleterious effects on the fetus. The infant may have physical and mental abnormalities, such as cataracts, congenital heart disease, deafness, microcephaly, or psychomotor retardation, or present with severe neonatal disease that may include thrombocytopenia, bleeding, hepatosplenomegaly, pneumonia, and myocarditis. Some manifestations of congenital rubella infection may not appear until years or decades later, even among patients asymptomatic at birth (7).

The rubella virus is an enveloped, single-stranded ribonucleic acid (RNA) virus that is spherical and has spike-like projections containing hemagglutinin. Only one antigenic type of the virus is known. Man is the only natural host for rubella virus, but some animals such as primates, rabbits, and ferrets can be infected under experimental conditions. Rubella virus has three structural polypeptides; two are envelope acylated glycoproteins (i.e., E1 and E2), and one is a nonglycosylated RNA-associated capsid protein (i.e., C). E1 contains the domains responsible for binding to host cell receptors and for hemagglutination. The function of E2 is not well defined, but it may carry strain-specific antigens as well as one weak neutralizing domain associated with virus infectivity. The C protein may be involved in the transfer of viral RNA into host cell cytoplasm (217,218). Molecular techniques such as PCR and nucleotide sequencing allow the differentiation between rubella virus strains. This is useful in the analysis of the molecular epidemiology of the virus as well as in differentiating between wild-type virus and the RA 27/3 vaccine strain when rubella virus is isolated from individuals with possible vaccine-related adverse effects (219,220).

Person-to-person transmission usually occurs by airborne spread of infected respiratory secretions, and direct contact with virus-containing urine or feces is a less likely route of infection. Although rubella virus can be recovered from the genital tract of infected women, verti-

cal transmission during pregnancy is believed to occur almost exclusively through the placenta (221,222).

On entry into the body in cases of postnatal infection, the rubella virus multiplies in nasopharyngeal epithelial cells and in local lymph nodes. This is followed by a period of viremia and shedding from the throat. It is during this maternal viremic phase that placental and fetal infection occurs. The frequency and nature of fetal involvement depends on the mother's immune status against the virus and the timing during gestation of maternal rubella (7).

The mechanisms by which the virus ravages the fetus are not clearly understood. Necrotic placental vascular endothelial cells can serve as a source of virus-infected emboli. Damage to endothelial cells can lead to thrombosis of small blood vessels, resulting in hypoxic tissue damage (223,224). Rubella-infected cells have diminished mitotic activity due to chromosomal breaks, the production of a growth-inhibiting protein, or damaging effects of the virus on the cytoskeletal microtubular system (225). Focal lysis of infected cells can be seen in some organs, but inflammation is not a salient feature of congenital rubella (223). Growth-retarded infants have reduced cell numbers on histopathologic examination (226). Moreover, the virus can modify cell receptors for specific growth factors (227). Late-onset manifestations of congenital rubella may be due to viral persistence with ongoing cell destruction or to organ damage by means of a number of immune mechanisms such as circulating rubella-specific immune complexes, defective cytotoxic effector cell function, or the development of autoimmunity (228–232). The rubella virus E1 and E2 proteins, but not the C nucleoprotein, appear to be responsible for autoantibody induction (233).

Long-lasting immunity normally develops after recovery from postnatal rubella. Reinfections can occur in persons with low antibody titers, but these are usually asymptomatic (222). Persons with low antibody levels after rubella vaccination are more prone to reinfections than persons with similarly low titers after natural infection (222).

Circulating antibodies and cell-mediated immune responses are generated after rubella infection. Rubella-specific IgM, IgG, IgA, IgD, and IgE antibodies are induced in response to postnatal infection (234). IgM antibodies appear early and are short lived. They usually disappear 5 to 8 weeks after onset of illness, although rubella-specific IgM antibodies rarely can persist for months or years (235). The IgM response after rubella vaccination or natural reinfection generally is weak and of brief duration (236–238). Moreover, rubella-specific IgM antibodies can be detected in acute infections by viruses such as parvovirus B19 and Epstein–Barr virus (239). Specific IgD and IgE antibodies appear early and then decline more slowly than specific IgM antibodies (234). Specific IgA antibodies generally emerge within the first 10 days of illness, and they may continue to be measurable for periods ranging from 3 weeks to several years (234,240). Rubella-specific IgG antibodies increase rapidly and persist throughout life; rubella-specific IgG1 has been shown to be the principal IgG subclass (222,241). The most vigorous antibody and lymphocyte proliferative responses in postnatal rubella are directed against glycoprotein E1 (242,243). The avidity of specific IgG to rubella antigens increases with time after primary infection; a low avidity index (less than 40%) can be seen up to 6 weeks after onset of the rubella rash, whereas a high avidity index (greater than 60%) is not seen until after 13 weeks (239). Measurement of rubella IgG avidity can be useful in women with positive rubella-specific IgM reactions, as it can help distinguish primary infections from unusually prolonged IgM persistence or from reinfection. Rubella-specific IgG also can be detected in the urine, and the results correlate well with serum IgG measurements (244). Men and women appear to differ in the nature and magnitude of their antibody responses to rubella virus structural proteins (245). Men never produce anti-E2 IgA and generate significantly lower levels of IgG antibodies directed against E2 than women. Anti-E1 IgM and IgG antibodies appear earlier in male patients, but female patients have higher levels of rubella-specific IgG antibodies after recovery from the illness. The observed gender differences in antibody responses to viral proteins may be under genetic or hormonal influences and may be related to the increased susceptibility of women to the joint complications of rubella (245).

Immune responses in congenitally infected infants differ from those observed in adults with rubella. Fetal IgM production usually begins after 16 weeks of gestation. Rubella-specific IgM antibodies are detectable until 6 to 12 months of age. Specific IgG antibody levels decrease over time; as many as 20% of affected children have no measurable antibody titers by 5 years of age (222). Circulating antirubella antibodies in infants with intrauterine infection have lower affinities to rubella antigen than antibodies from adults with natural infection (246,247). Serum antibodies to the E2 glycoprotein are quantitatively more abundant than those directed against E1 in some patients with congenital rubella, particularly among older infants. Antibody reactivities against the C protein are poor (242,248). Infants with congenital rubella have diminished cell-mediated immune responses on exposure to rubella antigens compared with children or adults with postnatal infection, and the responses are weakest for infants infected earlier during gestation. The reduction in response is mainly seen with the E1 protein (243,249).

Maternal Rubella

Epidemiology

Major epidemics of rubella formerly occurred at 6- to 9-year intervals in the United States. The last major pandemic took place between 1964 and 1965, at which time 20,000 cases of congenital rubella occurred. Rubella did not become a notifiable disease in the United States until 1966. From 1966 through 1971, between 45,000 and 58,000 cases of postnatal rubella were reported to the CDC each year (14). Since licensure of the rubella vaccine in 1969, the number of postnatal rubella and congenital rubella syndrome (CRS) cases declined by 99.6% and 97.4%, respectively. A modest resurgence of rubella occurred between 1989 and 1991. The number of reported postnatal rubella cases between 1992 through 1996 reached a historic low, with an average of 183 cases annually. Of 567 postnatal rubella cases reported between 1994 and 1996, 85% occurred in persons 15 years of age or older; 171 (30.5%) were women 15 to 44 years of age, five of whom were pregnant at the time of their infection. For the time period from 1994 to 1996, there were six outbreaks (each with five or more cases), but the three largest accounted for 44% of all reported cases; 12 infants with CRS were born. The mothers of seven of the 12 CRS cases acquired their infections in the United States; four other cases were imported and one was unknown (250).

Outbreaks of infection occur mostly in unimmunized populations such as inner city children and adults, illegal aliens, prison inmates, and religious groups that refuse vaccination (e.g., Amish communities) (17,251–254). Medical students and other health professionals serve as vectors for rubella infection, placing susceptible pregnant women to whom they are exposed in a medical setting at significant risk (255). In a study of one hospital system in St. Louis, Missouri, 5.3% of about 6,000 new employees were found to be seronegative for rubella; unfortunately, only 14% were subsequently vaccinated by their Employee Health Service (256).

Approximately 10% to 20% of women of child-bearing age (15 to 44 years of age) are susceptible to rubella, and more than 70% of cases occur among persons in this age group (257). Women delivering infants with CRS tend to be younger than the national average for mothers giving birth in the United States; a disproportionate number of these mothers are African-American or Hispanic (251). Rubella susceptibility rates for women of child-bearing age in European countries generally are comparable to those found in the United States, but lower seropositivity rates are encountered among island populations such as those in Hawaii and Jamaica and in certain tropical African countries (222,258–263). Significant regional differences have been found in large countries, such as India and China (264,265).

Clinical Manifestations

More than 30% of postnatal rubella infections are subclinical (257). Illness occurs 14 to 21 days (mean 18) after exposure. A prodrome consisting of malaise, low-grade fever that rarely lasts beyond the first day of the exanthem, headache, and conjunctivitis precede the rash by 1 to 5 days. The exanthem consists of discrete macules or papules that initially appear on the face and behind the ears, spread downward over 1 to 2 days, and usually disappear over 3 to 5 days; rubella virus can be isolated from these skin lesions (266). Postauricular, suboccipital, and posterior cervical lymphadenopathy is common and may persist for several weeks. Complications of rubella develop more frequently in adults. Transient arthralgias may occur in as many as one-third of infected women, but arthritis is uncommon (7). Other complications are rare and include thrombocytopenic purpura, hemolytic anemia, hepatitis, Guillain–Barré syndrome, encephalitis, progressive panencephalitis, myelitis, peripheral neuritis, myocarditis, and pericarditis (7,267–269).

Pregnancy has no effect on the natural course of rubella infection. However, rubella is associated with an increased risk of miscarriages, spontaneous abortions, and stillbirths (7).

Laboratory Diagnosis

The diagnosis of rubella on clinical grounds alone is unreliable, because similar illnesses may be produced by enteroviruses, measles virus, or parvovirus B19. Laboratory confirmation by virus isolation or serologic testing thus is essential in pregnant women, for whom an accurate diagnosis of gestational rubella is critical. Shirley and colleagues (270) investigated 627 patients clinically suspected of having rubella, but they could confirm this diagnosis in only 229 (37%). Human parvovirus B19 infection accounted for 7%, measles for 1%, and other infectious agents for 1%; the causes for the remaining 54% could not be determined.

Rubella virus is shed from the nasopharynx for 1 week before and 1 week after onset of the rash. The virus is present in blood and urine during the week preceding the exanthem but disappears thereafter. Rubella virus isolation is impractical for diagnostic purposes because it is expensive, labor intensive, and frequently unavailable to the clinician.

Serologic techniques are the most useful methods for diagnosing rubella infection. Available tests include hemagglutination inhibition, ELISA, immunofluorescence, radioimmunoassay, hemolysis in gel, complement fixation, passive hemagglutination, and latex agglutination tests (238,271). Serum specimens obtained as soon as feasible after the appearance of the exanthem and again 2 weeks later can prove the diagnosis if seroconversion or a fourfold or greater rise in rubella-specific antibody titers can be documented. Paired sera are best tested in unison because of the variability in results of assays done on separate days or by different personnel. If measured by ELISA, hemagglutination inhibition, or radioimmunoassay, rubella-specific IgG antibodies can be found as early as 1 to 2 days before the emergence of the rash; if assayed by the less readily available passive hemagglutination method, these antibodies are not detected until 15 to 50 days after onset of the exanthem and peak approximately 6 to 7 months later. The detection of rubella-specific IgM antibodies within 28 days of the appearance of the rash usually is diagnostic, the caveats being that IgM responses sometimes can persist for prolonged periods after a primary infection and that they also can be detected in some patients with rubella reinfection (272). Newer tests that can be used for the diagnosis of acute postnatal rubella include avidity ELISA, in which acutely infected persons have low IgG avidity compared with persons previously immune to rubella who exhibit greater IgG avidity (239). IgG produced in response to rubella vaccination shows low avidity to rubella antigens during the first 2 months after immunization, but this increases significantly over the ensuing months and remains at high levels thereafter (273). Immunoblot techniques have been developed for the sensitive detection of rubella-specific IgG, IgM, and IgA antibodies (274).

Rubella reinfections are confirmed by a fourfold or greater rise in the titer of preexisting rubella-specific IgG antibodies. The specific IgM response is absent or weak, but it is sometimes high enough to be within the range deemed sufficient for the diagnosis of primary rubella (238).

False-positive IgM reactions can occur in sera containing rheumatoid factor, although the IgM capture assay appears to be unaffected by its presence (238). Cross-reactions between rubella and human parvovirus B19, Epstein–Barr virus, or CMV infections in specific IgM tests necessitate caution in interpreting low or equivocal levels of rubella-specific IgM antibodies (239,275).

Rubella virus RNA can be detected in clinical specimens using a reverse transcription nested PCR assay. This molecular technique has been used on pharyngeal swabs, chorionic villi, amniotic fluid, fetal blood, and lens aspirates (276–278).

Treatment

Therapy of postnatal rubella is symptomatic. Patients with rubella shed the virus from the nasopharynx for 1 week after appearance of the rash; therefore, these patients should avoid contact with susceptible persons until the exanthem has vanished.

Prevention

The principal goal of rubella immunization programs is the elimination of CRS. The vaccine used in the United States is the RA 27/3 attenuated live rubella virus vaccine (257). It is available in a monovalent form (i.e., rubella only) and in combination with measles and mumps (i.e., measles–mumps–rubella) (279). The vaccine induces antirubella antibodies in more than 95% of recipients 12 months of age or older, and its protective efficacy is greater than 90% for at least 15 years (257). Immunizing children whose pregnant mothers are susceptible to rubella does not pose a threat to the mother or her fetus. The vaccine is recommended for all susceptible persons 12 months of age or older and usually is given at 15 months of age; a second booster dose is given to children at the time of school entry.

A clinical diagnosis of rubella is considered unreliable and cannot be considered proof of immunity. Persons are deemed protected if they have serologic evidence of immunity or previously had been vaccinated on or after their first birthday. Birth before 1957 is not acceptable evidence of rubella immunity for women who could become pregnant (279).

Pregnant women whose rubella-immune status is not known should be tested for the presence of antirubella antibodies during their first prenatal visit. If a previously unimmunized pregnant woman with unknown antibody status is exposed to rubella, a blood sample should be immediately obtained for rubella antibody testing. If antibody to rubella is found, the woman is considered immune (280). The risk of rubella reinfection after natural disease or vaccination is small, but it is more likely to occur in women with low specific IgG titers (281). Rubella reinfections do not seem to be related to a lack of neutralizing antibodies or to an impaired rubella-specific lymphocyte transformation response (282). Significant fetal pathology after reinfection occurs infrequently, despite rubella virus transmission to the fetus (283–291).

Susceptible women exposed to rubella should be informed of the risks to the fetus if maternal infection occurs. If the woman develops fever, lymphadenopathy, or a rash within the expected incubation period, serum for rubella-specific IgM measurement should be obtained. If a clinical illness does not occur, serum should be obtained 6 to 8 weeks after exposure to exclude a subclinical infection. For women who seroconvert or become positive for rubella-specific IgM, the rate of fetal infection is 81% after maternal rubella during the first 12 weeks of gestation, 54% at 13 to 16 weeks, 36% at 17 to 22 weeks, 30% at 23 to 30 weeks, 60% at 31 to 36 weeks, and 100% at more than 36 weeks of pregnancy (292). Infants infected before 11 weeks of gestation usually develop congenital defects, most often cardiac anomalies and deafness, but only 35% of infants infected at 13 to 16 weeks of gestation have abnormalities at birth, usually deafness (292). In a study of 106 infants with confirmed CRS in whom the timing of maternal infection was known with reasonable accuracy, Munro and colleagues (293) found deafness in 58% of patients, and it was the sole abnormality in 40% of all infants; infants with congenital cardiac, ocular, or CNS defects almost always were deaf as well. The risk of deafness is small if maternal infection occurs at 17 weeks of gestation or later (292,293). Other investigators have con-

firmed that rubella virus can be transmitted to the fetus at any stage of pregnancy, and that the earlier the maternal infection during pregnancy, the greater is the severity of congenital defects (294–296).

If maternal rubella occurs during the first 5 months of pregnancy, the option of therapeutic pregnancy termination can be considered. Infections occurring after this time do not produce congenital defects. If available, an attempt at prenatal diagnosis can be made, because fetal involvement after maternal rubella is not universal. The virus has been isolated from amniotic fluid by culture or directly visualized using electron microscopy in a few cases (297,298). The low sensitivities of these methods limits their usefulness. Amniotic fluid cells in rubella-infected patients are abnormal when examined with a transmission and scanning electron microscope (lack of chromatin, disappearance of electron-dense cytoplasmic layer, membrane damage expressed by a decrease in the size and number of microvilli) (299). Daffos and colleagues (300) studied 18 pregnancies complicated by maternal rubella; fetal blood was obtained at 20 to 26 weeks of gestation, and rubella-specific IgM was detected in 12 fetuses. Contamination of fetal blood specimens by maternal blood was excluded. Of the six fetuses without detectable rubella-specific IgM antibodies, one was found to be infected at birth (300). In another study, investigators were able to detect rubella-specific IgM and IgA as early as 22 weeks of pregnancy (240). Hwa and colleagues (301) performed fetal blood sampling at 22 to 30 weeks gestation (at least 2 weeks after appearance of the rash) on 93 rubella-specific IgM positive pregnant women. Of six infants infected *in utero*, five had rubella-specific IgM in cord blood (301). The drawbacks of this method are that the fetus does not synthesize IgM until the fifth month of gestation, and the quantity produced initially may be meager and below the limits of detection of the assay. Despite these disadvantages, the technique still is helpful in the management of pregnancies complicated by maternal rubella (302).

Terry and associates (303) detected rubella antigens and RNA sequences in a chorionic villus biopsy specimen obtained at 11 weeks of gestation from a woman with rubella in early pregnancy, and this led to pregnancy termination at week 13 of gestation. Infection was verified in the aborted fetus and placenta by virus isolation, immunoblotting, and hybridization methods (303). However, the detection of rubella virus in chorionic villus samples may not always predict fetal infection (277). PCR has been used successfully to detect rubella virus RNA in fetal and placental tissues, amniotic fluid, chorionic villus samples, and fetal blood (298,304–306). Positive results can be obtained within 24 to 48 hours with PCR, several days to a few weeks earlier than is possible with virus culture methods (277,278,306).

The administration of immunoglobulin to susceptible pregnant women who are exposed to rubella does not prevent maternal or fetal infection. Its use is confined to women who would not contemplate pregnancy termination under any circumstances (257).

Pregnant women who do not have rubella antibody should be immunized in the immediate postpartum period. However, reports by a group of investigators from Canada have suggested that acute arthritis can occur in as many as 8% of women receiving the rubella RA 27/3 vaccine in the postpartum period, and that some subsequently develop chronic arthropathy, neurologic abnormalities such as the carpal tunnel syndrome or paresthesias, and chronic rubella viremia. These women tend to transmit rubella virus to some of their infants through breast-feeding, and a few infected infants go on to develop chronic rubella viremia (307,308). More recently, the same research group conducted a prospective, placebo-controlled, double-blind trial of postpartum rubella immunization (using the RA 27/3 vaccine) in 543 seronegative women and showed a higher incidence of acute joint problems, but only a marginally increased risk of chronic or recurrent arthralgias, in vaccine recipients (309). Data from the United States and elsewhere indicate that such complications are rare with the RA 27/3 live rubella vaccine (257,310,311). The mechanisms of rubella vaccine-induced joint disease are poorly understood, but they may include infection of the synovial membrane by vaccine virus or the deposition of rubella antigen-containing immune complexes in the synovium (312,313). Certain human leukocyte antigen class II (HLA-DR) phenotypes may be associated with an increased risk of postpartum arthropathy following rubella vaccination. The relative risk of arthropathy is eightfold higher for persons with both DR1 and DR4 and sevenfold higher for those with both DR4 and DR6 (314). It is advised that all susceptible pregnant women be vaccinated against rubella before hospital discharge (257). An estimated 40% to 55% of CRS cases could be prevented with implementation of postpartum rubella immunization of susceptible women (251,253). Although rubella vaccine virus can be shed in breast milk, breast-feeding is not a contraindication to maternal immunization (257,315).

The rubella vaccine should not be knowingly administered during pregnancy because of its small risk of teratogenicity. Data from the CDC for the period 1979 to 1988 indicate that none of 562 infants born to 683 women inadvertently immunized with the RA 27/3 vaccine within 3 months of conception in the United States had malformations compatible with CRS (316). Between January 1971 and April 1989, 321 known rubella-susceptible women who had been immunized against rubella within 3 months before or after their estimated date of conception with the RA 27/3 or earlier vaccines (Cendehill, HPV-77) were followed by the CDC; none of the 324 infants born to these women had defects consistent with the CRS (257). The RA 27/3 rubella vaccine virus, how-

ever, does cross the placenta and produces a subclinical infection in about 3% of infants; the rate of fetal infection was considerably higher (20%) for the earlier rubella vaccines (316). The possible risk of serious congenital defects after accidental rubella vaccination has been calculated by the CDC to be 0% to 1.6%; the observed risk has been zero (257). This risk is considerably lower than the 20% or greater risk of CRS after maternal gestational infection, and it is comparable to the 2% to 3% rate of major birth defects observed in the absence of rubella vaccine exposure (316).

Congenital Rubella

Epidemiology

The incidence of congenital rubella has shown a consistent decline since the introduction of rubella vaccination programs in the United States. For the period 1985 through 1996, the CDC received reports of 106 confirmed cases of CRS and 16 others that were probable CRS; three CRS clusters from New York, southern California, and the Amish in Pennsylvania accounted for 42% of all cases. The median age of the mothers was 23 years. Forty-four percent of infants with CRS were born to Hispanic mothers compared with 15% for all births in the United States (relative risk of 2.9). Rubella was acquired in the United States in 78% of mothers; 33% stated that they had been previously vaccinated for rubella (317). Because of the passive nature of the CRS reporting system, it is estimated that the reported number of infants with CRS represents only 20% to 30% of actual cases (18).

CRS continues to be a problem in other parts of the world (258,318,319); however, rubella immunization programs have been successful in reducing the occurrence of CRS wherever implemented (320,321). As an example, the incidence of CRS declined from 3.5 per 100,000 live births in 1980 to 0.41 per 100,000 live births in 1986 in 19 European birth defects registries (320).

Clinical Manifestations

More than one-half of all newborns with congenital rubella are asymptomatic at birth, but most later manifest with one or more signs and symptoms of disease. The most common abnormalities encountered in CRS listed in order of decreasing frequency are sensorineural hearing loss, mental retardation, cardiac malformations, and ocular defects (322). Table 47–3 is a summary of the clinical abnormalities encountered in congenital rubella (225,226,229,230,267,293,317,323–357).

If the findings of mental retardation and infection of neurosensory organs such as the eyes or ears are combined, then CNS involvement occurs in more than 80% of CRS patients (267). Vascular abnormalities, prominent

TABLE 47–3. *Clinical abnormalities in infants with symptomatic congenital rubella*

Clinical abnormality	Remarks
General	
Intrauterine growth retardation	Common (50%–85%); usually have other manifestations of congenital infection; may be due to reduced number of body cells (226)
Postnatal growth retardation	Retarded growth is most severe in infants with multiple congenital defects; long-term follow-up studies indicate that most will have subnormal growth (323,324)
Cardiovascular system	
Patent ductus arteriosus	Most frequently encountered structural defect (30%); may occur with other heart lesions, especially pulmonary valvular or artery stenosis (293)
Pulmonary artery stenosis	Second most common heart defect; results from intimal proliferation (325)
Miscellaneous defects	Individually uncommon; include coarctation of the aorta, atrial and ventricular septal defects, myocarditis, tetralogy of Fallot, and ventricular aneurysm
Hearing loss	The most common congenital defect; almost always present in infants with other malformations; uncommon if maternal rubella occurs at ≥17 weeks of gestation; usually bilateral; may be present at birth or develop later; can be progressive (7,326)
Ocular abnormalities	
Cataract	Found in about 35% of infants; can be unilateral or bilateral; noted at birth or early infancy; virus can be isolated from lens; spontaneous reabsorption of cataracts has been described in rare cases (327–330)
Retinopathy	Common (35%–60%); may be present at birth or appear later in life; often unilateral; salt-and-pepper appearance; does not affect visual acuity (331–334)
Cloudy cornea	Rare; usually present at birth; may coexist with glaucoma; resolves spontaneously; rarely persists (335)
Glaucoma	Occurs in ≤10%; may be bilateral; can be found at birth or appear later in life; leads to blindness if not treated (7,334)
Microphthalmia	Common in infants with cataract; concomitant glaucoma common (7,334)
Miscellaneous abnormalities	Uncommon; includes iris hypoplasia, strabismus, and iridocyclitis
Interstitial pneumonia	Occurs in about 5%; probably immunologically mediated; may be acute, subacute, or chronic (229)
Central nervous system	
Meningoencephalitis	Occurs in as many as 20%; manifests with bulging anterior fontanelle, hypotonia, irritability, and seizures; cerebrospinal fluid findings include elevated protein concentration, mononuclear pleocytosis, and rubella virus isolation in 30%; transient; most infants have neurodevelopmental deficits; progressive rubella panencephalitis is a delayed manifestation of chronic infection that begins ≥10 years after the primary infection characterized by fibrinoid necrosis, severe neuronal loss and demyelination, and old microinfarcts (225,267,336,337)
Microcephaly	Uncommon; may be associated with normal intelligence
Intracranial calcifications	May be present in early infancy (338,339)
Electroencephalographic abnormalities	Occurs in 36%; usually resolves by 1 year of age (267)
Mental retardation	Occurs in 10%–20%; associated with other stigmata of congenital rubella
Speech defects	Uncommon in absence of hearing impairment
Behavioral disorders	Common; occurs primarily in deaf patients (336,340)
Miscellaneous problems	Autism; central language disorders; spastic quadriparesis; hydrocephalus; cerebral arterial stenosis
Skin	
Bluberry-muffin spots	Transient; infrequent (5%); represents dermal erythropoiesis (341)
Chronic rashes	Generalized; persists for weeks; appears in infancy; virus can be isolated from skin (342,343)
Dermatoglyphic abnormalities	May serve as marker for viral teratogenicity (344)
Miscellaneous abnormalities	Skin dimples, seborrhea, cutis marmorata, patchy pigmentation (343)
Genitourinary system	Cryptorchidism; testicular agenesis; scrotal calcifications; polycystic kidneys; renal agenesis; renal artery stenosis with hypertension; hypospadias; hydroureter; hydronephrosis; ureteral duplication (345–349)
Skeletal system	
Metaphyseal radiolucencies	Occurs in 10%–20%; most common in distal femur and proximal tibia; usually normalizes by 3 months of age; due to a direct inhibitory effect of rubella virus on bone and cartilage cells (350–354)
Large anterior fontanelle	Found in the most severely affected infants (350)
Miscellaneous problems	Micrognathia; pathologic fractures; myositis
Gastrointestinal system	
Hepatosplenomegaly	Common (>50%); transient
Hepatitis	Occurs in 5%–10%; may not be associated with jaundice
Obstructive jaundice	Infrequent (5%)
Miscellaneous problems	Esophageal, jejunal, or rectal atresia; pancreatitis; chronic diarrhea; intraabdominal calcifications (349)
Blood	
Thrombocytopenic purpura	Occurs in 5%–10%; associated with severe disease; transient (350,355)
Anemia	Transient (355)
Miscellaneous abnormalities	Hemolytic anemia; altered blood group expression (356)
Immune system	
Hypogammaglobulinemia	Rare; transient
Thymic hypoplasia	Rare; fatal
Endocrine glands	Diabetes mellitus; hypothyroidism; hyperthyroidism; thyroiditis; growth hormone deficiency; precocious puberty (7,230,357)

pathologic characteristic of congenital rubella, contribute to the neuropathology by causing ischemic necrosis of adjacent tissues. Microcephaly may be due to the generalized organ hypocellularity seen with rubella infection (226).

The development of late-onset CRS manifestations that were inapparent in early infancy may be related to persistence or reactivation of rubella virus infection, the body's immune responses to the infection, or vascular damage. Insulin-dependent diabetes mellitus occurs in about 20% of patients by 35 years of age (357). Rubella virus can infect human fetal pancreatic islet cells and can reduce secretion of insulin (358). About 20% of CRS patients and 50% to 80% of those with glucose intolerance have circulating pancreatic islet cell cytotoxic or surface antibodies (359). These autoantibodies are triggered by rubella virus and cause destruction of pancreatic cells, unmasking the person with a genetic susceptibility to diabetes mellitus (360). Thyroid abnormalities develop in about 5%; thyroid microsomal or thyroglobulin antibodies are found more frequently in deaf CRS patients than in those who are hearing impaired from other causes (230). Rare cases of growth hormone deficiency of hypothalamic origin have been described (361). About 10% of CRS patients incur additional forms of late-appearing ocular insults, such as glaucoma, keratoconus, corneal hydrops, and spontaneous lens absorption. Permanent damage to the vascular endothelium can induce the formation of obstructive lesions of major vessels such as the pulmonary and renal arteries. Choroidal neovascularization with significant visual loss can complicate CRS

retinopathy. Autism and behavioral problems usually are delayed in appearance and can be progressive. Progressive rubella panencephalitis is a rare but ultimately fatal CNS manifestation of CRS that appears late, usually in the second decade of life (357).

Diagnosis

The CDC has established clinical and laboratory criteria for the classification of CRS cases to allow better CRS surveillance (Table 47–4) (362).

The diagnosis of CRS usually is suspected on the basis of the maternal history and the clinical findings. A definitive diagnosis can be achieved by isolating the virus from pharyngeal washings or, less commonly, from urine, CSF, conjunctivae, or available organs such as the lens at surgery or autopsy. Although nasopharyngeal shedding of rubella virus may continue for 6 to 12 months, the frequency of its isolation declines from about 85% during the first month of life to approximately 10% at 9 to 12 months of age (363). In children with congenital rubella encephalitis, the virus can be isolated from the CSF for months or even years (336). However, viral isolation seldom is used in clinical practice because of its difficulty, expense, and limited availability. Rubella virus RNA can be detected in clinical specimens using PCR, and the results become available sooner than with traditional culture methods; these assays are not widely available at present (276).

Rubella-specific IgM usually is present in congenitally infected infants and may persist for 6 to 12 months. It can

TABLE 47–4. *Outline of the Centers for Disease Control and Prevention criteria for the classification of congenital rubella syndrome cases*

I. Congenital rubella syndrome confirmed
   Defects present and at least one of the following:
      Isolation of rubella virus
      Detection of rubella-specific IgM antibodies
      Persistence of rubella-specific HI titer beyond the period expected from that of passively transferred maternal antibodies
II. Congenital rubella syndrome compatible
   Incomplete laboratory data for confirmation of diagnosis and any two complications from A or one from A and one from B:
      A. Cataracts or congenital glaucoma, congenital heart disease, hearing loss, pigmentary retinopathy
      B. Purpura, splenomegaly, jaundice, bone radiolucencies, meningoencephalitis, microcephaly, mental retardation
III. Congenital rubella syndrome possible
   Some compatible clinical findings but insufficient criteria for the confirmed or compatible categories
IV. Congenital rubella infection only
   No defects, but laboratory evidence of infection is found
V. Stillbirths
   Stillbirths believed to be a consequence of maternal rubella infection
VI. Congenital rubella syndrome excluded
   At least one of the following inconsistent laboratory findings in a child without evidence of an immunodeficiency disease:
      Absence of rubella-specific HI titer in a child ≤24 months of age
      Absence of rubella-specific HI titer in the mother
      Decrease of rubella-specific HI titer in an infant in a manner consistent with that expected from passively transferred maternal antibodies (i.e., a twofold dilution drop per month)

HI, hemagglutination inhibition.
Adapted from ref. 362.

be used to make a definitive diagnosis of congenital rubella infection; false-positive results may be encountered in sera containing rheumatoid factor. Delays in obtaining serum for IgM measurements can introduce interpretation difficulties because of the possibility that the infant may have acquired rubella infection postnatally. Persistence of rubella-specific IgG antibodies at 6 to 12 months of age, especially in high titers, provides presumptive evidence of congenital or early postnatal infection.

Other techniques for establishing the diagnosis of congenital rubella include negative virus-specific lymphocyte transformation responses in seropositive children younger than 3 years of age, detection of rubella-specific IgM in CSF or saliva, demonstration of low-avidity rubella-specific IgG in seropositive infants, or immunoblotting (246,247,364–367).

Treatment

There is no specific therapy for CRS. A few patients have been treated with amantadine or interferon-α with minimal or no clinical improvement (231,368–370). Susceptible pregnant women should avoid contact with CRS patients during their first year of life. The appearance of delayed manifestations of CRS that were not present early in life underscores the importance of close follow-up. CRS patients often require surgical correction of heart or genitourinary defects, removal of dense cataracts, hearing aids, and special schooling.

HEPATITIS B

HBV afflicts nearly 330,000 persons in the United States each year, about 5% of whom become chronic HBV carriers (371,372). Estimates from the CDC place the number of chronic, infectious HBV carriers in the United States at about 1 to 1.25 million (373). Globally, the World Health Organization estimates that the number of chronic carriers will reach 400 million by the year 2000, and that as many as 1 million people die each year from HBV-related acute and chronic hepatic disease (374). More than one-fourth of all carriers develop HBV-related chronic active hepatitis, liver cirrhosis, or hepatocellular carcinoma (373). Chronic carriers of this virus can transmit HBV to their offspring during pregnancy; as many as 70% to 90% of perinatally infected infants become chronic carriers themselves (375).

The complete HBV is known as the Dane particle and consists of an outer lipid-containing envelope and an inner core or nucleocapsid. On the surface of the outer coat is the hepatitis B surface antigen (HBsAg), an antigenically complex glycoprotein. HBsAg has many antigenic epitopes that permit the identification of several HBV subtypes; the subtyping scheme is valuable as an epidemiologic tool, but it has no correlation with disease severity. The surface envelope contains three proteins (i.e., major, middle, and large S proteins) coded for by the HBV DNA genome. Variations in the major protein account for the subtype determinants, and the middle and large proteins are implicated in receptor-mediated virus uptake by hepatocytes (374).

The virus inner core consists of hepatitis B core antigen (HBcAg), hepatitis B e antigen (HBeAg), hepatitis B x antigen (HBxAg), a partially double-stranded DNA molecule, DNA-dependent DNA polymerase enzyme with reverse transcription activity, and a protein kinase. HBcAg is found primarily in the nuclei of infected hepatocytes. In serum, HBcAg is found only as a component of circulating Dane particles, but it is never found in free form. HBeAg is a prematurely terminated polypeptide product of the same gene that codes for HBcAg; its presence in serum indicates infectivity. HBxAg is probably an independent marker of infectivity. HBV DNA is a partially double-stranded DNA, and HBV DNA polymerase repairs the single-stranded HBV DNA region to form a complete double-stranded molecule (374).

With very sensitive assays, HBsAg can be detected in the blood within 1 to 2 weeks of exposure to HBV. However, clinical disease usually occurs 1 to 3 months, and occasionally 6 months, after exposure. HBeAg can be detected late in the incubation period, usually coinciding with or within days of HBsAg appearance. HBV DNA polymerase and HBV DNA are measurable at this stage and generally peak by the latter part of the incubation period. Their concentrations fall with onset of liver disease. In patients who recover, HBsAg usually can no longer be detected at about the time of clinical resolution (376).

The earliest antibodies to appear are those directed against HBcAg (anti-HBc), typically 2 to 4 weeks after HBsAg is first detected. Anti-HBc titers increase during the acute stage of infection and persist for many years. Antibodies to HBeAg (anti-HBe) appear immediately after or within several weeks of HBeAg clearance and usually while HBsAg is still present. A window period that occasionally can be as long as 20 weeks follows HBsAg clearance from the circulation, during which neither HBsAg nor anti-HBs are detectable. However, specific IgM and IgG anti-HBc antibodies usually are present. The patient is contagious during this period. After anti-HBs antibodies become measurable, their titers continue to increase for approximately 6 to 12 months (374,376). About 18% of patients have detectable HBV DNA in their serum for 3 to 6 months after first appearance of anti-HBs antibodies; this can persist for as long as 5 years in some patients (377,378). Anti-HBs antibodies persist for life and protect against future HBV reinfections. Antibodies to HBxAg (anti-HBx) can be detected in only 17% of patients with acute HBV infection and usually appear 3 to 4 weeks after onset of clinical symptoms; their clinical significance is not yet defined (379).

Patients who continue to have detectable serum HBsAg for 20 weeks or longer, HBeAg for 10 weeks or longer, or HBV DNA for 4 weeks or longer are likely to become chronic HBsAg carriers. Their serum anti-HBc titers usually are high, and IgM anti-HBc tends to persist for a long time. Approximately 25% to 50% of chronic carriers are HBeAg positive, and the remainder have anti-HBe. Persons who are positive for HBeAg, HBV DNA polymerase, or HBV DNA are highly contagious. Chronically infected patients clear HBV particles from their plasma with a half-life of about 1 day, and about 10^{11} virus particles are released daily into the periphery from HBV-infected cells (380). Most chronic carriers remain HBV infected for life, but 1.5% to 2% of carriers spontaneously lose their HBsAg each year.

Young age is an important risk factor for developing the chronic carrier state; 70% to 90% of infected newborns become carriers, compared with 25% to 50% of children infected before their fifth birthday and 5% (range less than 1% to 12%) of adults. Other risk factors include a positive HIV-1 antibody status, hemodialysis, other immunodeficiency, Down syndrome, and male gender (8,371). Reactivation of chronic HBV infection can occur during pregnancy, but this is rare (381).

Clinical Manifestations

Most HBV infections are subclinical, particularly in children. Symptomatic infections can be mild and anicteric or be severe enough to produce encephalopathy, coagulopathy, and death. Fulminant hepatitis is more common in adults than in children and in those infected with certain mutant HBV strains or coinfected with the hepatitis C or D viruses (374,382–384). Extrahepatic disease may manifest as a serum sickness-type illness in patients with acute infections, polyarteritis nodosa, membranous glomerulonephritis, cryoglobulinemia, or infantile papular acrodermatitis (374,385).

Approximately two-thirds of chronic HBsAg carriers develop chronic persistent hepatitis. They usually are healthy but have persistent or recurrent serum transaminase elevations. The remaining third eventually develop chronic active hepatitis, a progressive disorder that ultimately results in postnecrotic liver cirrhosis. Primary hepatocellular carcinoma, a common malignant tumor in certain parts of the world such as southeast Asia, Japan, Greece, and Italy, may be as much as 300 times more common in HBsAg-positive men than in their HBsAg-negative counterparts. Primary hepatocellular carcinoma develops after an average of 35 years of HBsAg carriage; coexisting cirrhosis is found in 60% to 90%.

Most neonates and infants who acquire HBV from their mothers remain asymptomatic; those with symptoms typically have benign illnesses. Fulminant disease is rare. Most infected infants become chronic carriers and have a 25% or greater lifetime chance of dying of primary hepatocellular carcinoma or liver cirrhosis.

Modes of Transmission

HBsAg has been found in blood, blood products, urine, feces, bile, saliva, tears, sweat, semen, vaginal secretions, gastric contents of newborns, breast milk, cord blood, CSF, synovial fluid, and wound exudate (8). Many routes for HBV spread are possible, but the most significant are percutaneous or permucosal exposure to infected blood or body fluids during birth or sexual intercourse or by contaminated needles.

HBV-infected blood can enter the body through contaminated needles shared by drug users, if health care providers mistakenly puncture themselves, or if other persons reuse unsterilized devices in medical or dental offices, acupuncture clinics, or tattooing parlors. Contaminated blood can be introduced through mucous membranes, open wounds, and abrasions. Screening of blood and blood products for HBsAg has almost eradicated transfusion-acquired HBV infection.

HBV can spread to sexual partners of chronic HBsAg carriers or patients with acute hepatitis B. HBV infection is more likely in persons with multiple sex partners, more years of sexual activity, and histories of other sexually transmitted diseases. Heterosexual transmission now accounts for 25% of new HBV cases in the United States, a 38% increase from the early 1980s. It is the most important risk factor for women, with parenteral drug abuse in second place. Close, long-term contact with chronic carriers, as happens in households or institutions for the developmentally disabled, is a risk factor. Intrafamilial nonsexual transmission accounts for 2% of new HBV infections in the United States each year. Transplanted organs are uncommon vehicles of HBV spread to susceptible recipients. About 30% to 40% of all patients have no identifiable risk factors (386).

Perinatal Epidemiology

About 0.2% of American Caucasians and 0.9% of African-Americans are HBsAg positive. The prevalence is notably higher in certain high-risk groups, such as immigrants from areas of high HBV endemicity (13%), Alaskan natives or Pacific Islanders (5% to 15%), clients in institutions for the developmentally disabled (10% to 20%), users of illicit parenteral drugs (7%), household contacts of an HBV carrier (3% to 6%), health care workers with frequent blood contact (1% to 2%), and heterosexuals with multiple partners (0.5%) (387).

The rate of vertical transmission from mother to infant hinges on several factors. For women with acute HBV infection, the risk is about 76% if infection occurs during the third trimester or shortly after delivery, but it is only about 10% if it takes place during the first or second trimester. For HBsAg carrier mothers, the risk of mother-to-infant transmission depends on their HBeAg/anti-HBe status. The rate is estimated to be 70% to 90% for those who are HBeAg positive, 31% for those who are negative for HBeAg and anti-HBe, and 10% or less for those who are positive for anti-HBe. About one-third of HBsAg-positive pregnant women in the United States also are HBeAg positive. Other variables that enhance vertical transmission are high maternal HBsAg and anti-HBc titers and a high HBV DNA concentration (8). In one study of HBsAg-positive pregnant Taiwanese women, the odds ratio of having a persistently infected infant climbed from 1.0 to 147 as the maternal serum HBV DNA level increased from less than 0.005 to ≥1.4 ng/mL (388). Carrier mothers can transmit HBV to infants born after sequential pregnancies.

Mother-to-infant transmission occurs during delivery in most cases through transplacental microhemorrhages or from ingestion of contaminated maternal secretions. Intrauterine infection is uncommon but may account for 5% to 15% of cases for HBeAg-positive mothers (375). HBsAg is found in about 71% of breast milk samples from carrier mothers, but no differences in antigenemia rates have been found between breast-fed and bottle-fed infants born to infected mothers.

Unimmunized infants who acquire HBV infection from their mothers usually have no detectable serum HBsAg until 1 to 4 months later. Passively acquired low levels of HBsAg may be detected in the peripheral blood of some neonates, and they do not necessarily imply HBV infection. Cord blood should not be used for HBsAg testing because it can be contaminated with maternal blood.

Immunoprophylaxis

Two preparations have been used for passive immunization against HBV: immune serum globulin and hepatitis B immunoglobulin (HBIG). Immune serum globulin has anti-HBs titers of 1:16 to 1:1,000. HBIG, a hyperimmunoglobulin product, has anti-HBs titers of 1:100,000 to 1:250,000. HBIG is prepared from plasma obtained from HIV antibody-negative donors with a high anti-HBs titer, and its administration does not interfere with the host's immune response to hepatitis B vaccines.

Plasma-derived and recombinant hepatitis B vaccines are used for active immunization. The plasma-derived vaccine, Heptavax-B, is no longer manufactured in the United States. Two recombinant hepatitis B vaccines are available: Recombivax HB and Engerix-B. These vaccines are prepared by insertion of a plasmid containing the HBsAg gene into common baker's yeast, followed by lysis of yeast cells after the intracellular production, assembly, and accumulation of HBsAg polypeptides. HBsAg is later separated from disrupted yeast cell components; less than 5% of the final product is yeast-derived protein. Recombivax HB contains 10 μg of HBsAg protein per milliliter, and Engerix-B contains 20 μg/mL (389).

The usual regimen for primary hepatitis B vaccination consists of three intramuscular doses given at 0, 1, and 6 months. The three-dose schedule induces a good antibody response in more than 90% of healthy adults and more than 95% of pediatric patients (i.e., newborn through 19 years of age). Hepatitis B vaccines have a protective efficacy of 80% to 95% when given to susceptible recipients. About 30% to 50% of vaccinees have no detectable anti-HBs titer after 7 years; it is not known whether booster doses are needed for such persons (389).

Susceptible pregnant women with accidental percutaneous or permucosal exposure to HBV-infected blood or who had sexual contact with a chronic HBV carrier or an acutely infected man should receive immunoprophylaxis. Regimens using multiple HBIG doses or vaccine alone are only 70% to 85% effective in preventing HBV infection if used for postexposure prophylaxis of otherwise healthy persons (389).

Pregnancy is not a contraindication to hepatitis B vaccination. However, vaccine manufacturers advise against their use during pregnancy for liability reasons. Avoidance of vaccination in early pregnancy (i.e., period of embryogenesis) is recommended by some experts. No fetal or maternal risks from hepatitis B vaccination are known, and the limited available data suggest that its use in early or late pregnancy is safe (390,391).

Immunoprophylaxis after exposure to HBV-contaminated blood should consist of two doses of HBIG (0.06 mL/kg given intramuscularly; maximum 5 mL). The first dose of HBIG should be given as soon as possible or within 24 hours of exposure; its effectiveness when given after 7 days of exposure is unknown. The second dose is given 1 month later. This regimen has not been specifically evaluated in pregnant women, but it is about 75% effective in preventing infection in healthy persons. If the physician decides to use the hepatitis B vaccine, which is the preferred approach, only one HBIG dose needs to be given. The vaccine should be administered intramuscularly at a site different from that used for HBIG, and the first dose can be given concomitantly with HBIG or within 7 days of exposure. For sexual HBV exposure, the prophylactic regimen is similar, except that immunization can begin within 14 days of the last sexual encounter.

Prevention of Perinatal Hepatitis B Virus Transmission

The CDC estimates that 22,000 births per year occur to HBsAg-positive women in the United States and, unless immunoprophylaxis is given at birth, about 6,000 of these newborns would become chronic HBV carriers (8). The administration of HBIG and the initiation of hepatitis B vaccination is 85% to 95% effective in preventing the development of the chronic carrier state in these infants (375).

The CDC initially recommended that all high-risk women be screened for HBsAg during pregnancy. However, targeting women in high-risk groups identifies only about 35% to 65% of HBsAg carriers. The guidelines were later revised, and universal prenatal screening for HBsAg is now recommended (392). All pregnant women should be routinely screened for HBsAg during an early prenatal visit. HBsAg-negative women at high risk of infection (e.g., those with other sexually transmitted diseases or illicit drug users) should be retested late in pregnancy. Screening of all pregnant women and reporting of the results to health care providers is not complete in many geographic areas, and perinatal screening for women who do not have screening results is not consistently practiced. This can lead to failure to identify HBsAg-positive women and to administer appropriate immunoprophylaxis to their newborns (393,394). In one survey of obstetricians in the San Francisco, California, area, 79% of respondents believed that the hepatitis B vaccine should be given to all infants, but only 53% provided education on the subject to their expectant mothers (395).

Infants born to HBsAg-positive mothers should be bathed as soon as possible to remove HBV-infected blood and other secretions. Suctioning of the stomach contents, if needed, should be performed gently to avoid mucosal trauma that could promote HBV entry into the blood. Delivery by elective cesarean section has been advocated by some as a way to reduce maternal-to-infant HBV transmission; this approach is not recommended because of the lack of evidence to support the practice and because of the efficacy of immunoprophylaxis.

HBIG at a dose of 0.5 mL intramuscularly should be given as soon as possible after birth and no later than 12 hours of life. An HBIG dose given at 12 to 48 hours of life probably is effective, but this has not been proved. The first vaccine dose should be given within the first week of life, preferably within the first 12 hours; the intramuscular dose is 0.5 mL (5 μg of Recombivax HB or 10 μg of Engerix-B). Later doses are given at 1 and 6 months of age. Breast-feeding should be allowed for infants who have started immunoprophylaxis.

The CDC and the American Academy of Pediatrics have recommend universal hepatitis B vaccination of all infants, regardless of the maternal HBsAg status (373,396). Infants born to HBsAg-positive women are given HBIG and the vaccine as outlined earlier. Infants born to women admitted in labor and whose HBsAg status is unknown should receive the first dose of the vaccine within 12 hours of birth; maternal HBsAg testing should be immediately performed and, if positive, the infant should receive HBIG (0.5 mL) as soon as feasible after birth and no later than 7 days of age. The second and third vaccine doses are given at 1 to 2 months and at 6 months of age, respectively. Household contacts and sex partners of HBsAg-positive women should be vaccinated

against hepatitis B; prevaccination susceptibility testing should be done in adults whenever possible, but is not required in children because of low rates of HBV infection in that age group and the lower costs of smaller individual vaccine doses.

Infants born to HBsAg-negative mothers do not need HBIG administration. They can receive their first dose of vaccine at birth or within the first 2 months of life at routine health maintenance visits. Hepatitis B virus vaccines can be given concurrently but in different syringes with diphtheria-tetanus-pertussis, measles–mumps–rubella, poliomyelitis, or *Haemophilus influenzae* type b conjugate vaccines.

Preterm infants generally will respond well to the hepatitis B vaccines if the first dose is given at 1 month of age or at hospital discharge. Anti-HBs titers tend to be lower than those elicited in vaccinated term infants. Very-low-birth-weight infants (≤1,500 g) who receive their first dose of vaccine within the first 72 hours of life are less likely to have protective anti-HBs levels after the third dose of the vaccine is given than infants of similar weight and gestation who receive their first vaccine dose at 1 month of age (397–399).

Infants who become chronic HBV carriers despite correct immunoprophylaxis may have been infected *in utero*, or their mothers may have had a high virus load or were infected with vaccine-escape virus mutants (400–402). Infants who fail immunoprophylaxis do not become HBsAg positive until 6 to 9 months of age. Immunized infants born to HBsAg-positive mothers should be tested at the age of 9 months or later for HBsAg and anti-HBs. Those who test negative for both should receive a fourth vaccine dose and be tested again 1 month later, and infants found to be HBsAg positive should be monitored closely to determine whether a chronic carrier state has developed (375).

HEPATITIS C

Hepatitis C is currently the most common chronic bloodborne infection in the United States. There were 36,000 new cases in 1996, which is much lower than the estimated 230,000 cases per year that were seen in the 1980s before the causative agent was identified and serologic tests became available for screening the blood supply (19). About 4 million Americans are chronically infected with HCV, representing 1.8% of the population of the United States (19). Higher rates of infection are found in certain parts of eastern Europe and Africa (especially Egypt, where 15% of the population is seropositive for HCV) (403).

HCV is a single-stranded RNA virus whose genome encodes for both structural and nonstructural proteins. The structural proteins include two envelope proteins (i.e., E1 and E2), which contain neutralizing epitopes and a nucleocapsid core protein (i.e., C). The nonstructural proteins are essential for viral multiplication and include a viral protease, helicase, and an RNA-dependent RNA polymerase. There are at least six known HCV genotypes, which are divided further into more than 90 subtypes; 70% of HCV-infected persons in the United States are infected with genotype 1 (with subtype 1a predominating) (19,403,404). Viruses circulating within an individual may show nucleotide variability (quasispecies). Quasispecies arise as a result of ongoing host immune surveillance and mutations occurring during viral replication (404). Antibodies elicited by one virus type may not recognize another HCV type; therefore, patients are not protected against reinfection by either the same or different HCV genotypes (405). A consequence of the genetic diversity of HCV is its ability to escape host immune surveillance leading to a high rate (greater than 80%) of chronic infections.

Epidemiology

The highest incidence of acute HCV infection occurs in persons 20 to 39 years of age. There is great variation in the seroprevalence of HCV within the United States. The highest rates are found in persons with repeated or large percutaneous exposure to blood, such as injecting drug users (72% to 86%) or persons with hemophilia treated with products made before 1987 (74% to 90%). Lower rates are found in other groups, such as chronic hemodialysis patients (10%), persons receiving blood transfusions before 1990 (6%), and persons with a history of a sexually transmitted disease (6%) (19). About 1% to 2% of pregnant women in the United States are HCV positive, about 5% of whom pass the virus to their newborns (405).

HCV also can spread via organ transplantation from HCV-infected donors, tattoos, body piercing, sexual activity with an infected person, and nonsexual household contact. These sources account for a very small fraction of all HCV infections in the United States. Only 10% of patients have no identifiable source of infection (19,406). Although HCV RNA has been detected in breast milk from infected mothers, there have been no cases of infection acquired through breast-feeding.

Clinical Manifestations

The incubation period of hepatitis C infection is 6 to 7 weeks on average, with a range of 2 weeks to 6 months. Acute HCV is mostly asymptomatic. Jaundice is seen in 25%, and fulminant hepatitis is rare (405).

Most patients (85%) develop chronic HCV infection. Symptoms are vague and nonspecific (arthralgias, fatigue). Serum aminotransferase levels are either persistently or intermittently elevated. Aminotransferase levels correlate poorly with the degree of liver injury. Extrahepatic manifestations include mixed cryoglobulinemia,

glomerulonephritis, and porphyria cutanea tarda. Cirrhosis develops in as many as 20% within 10 to 20 years of infection. One to four percent of HCV-infected patients are at risk of developing hepatocellular carcinoma (403).

Diagnosis

Serologic tests permit the detection of antibodies to HCV (anti-HCV) but do not allow differentiation among acute, chronic, or resolved infections. The enzyme immunoassay (EIA) is used for screening and has a sensitivity of more than 97%. Repeatedly positive results on EIA require confirmation with a supplemental test such as the recombinant immunoblot assay (RIBA). Both tests detect IgG anti-HCV; no specific IgM test is available (19,407). The performance of these assays has improved with the recent introduction of third-generation tests (EIA-3, RIBA-3).

Very sensitive RNA detection tests are now commercially available, but none are approved by the Food and Drug Administration. Qualitative tests such as the reverse transcriptase PCR (RT-PCR) detect the presence of circulating HCV RNA. These tests are positive as early as 1 to 2 weeks after exposure. Their threshold for detection of virus is usually 100 to 1,000 viral genome copies per milliliter. Some HCV-infected patients are only intermittently HCV RNA positive, and a single negative test result is not considered conclusive. False-positive and false-negative results can occur with this test. Quantitative assays for measuring HCV RNA titers also are available from commercial laboratories. The two most commonly used assays are the quantitative RT-PCR (threshold 500 viral genome copies per milliliter) and a branched DNA signal amplification assay (threshold 200,000 genome equivalents per milliliter); both are less sensitive than the qualitative RT-PCR. Patients with chronic hepatitis C infection usually have from 10^5 to 10^7 genome copies per milliliter of circulating virus. The quantitative tests generally have been used to assess the response of chronically infected patients to antiviral therapy (19,408).

It is also possible to group HCV by genotype and subtype using commercially available assays. The clinical utility of these assays is limited at present to possibly altering the length of antiviral therapy, depending on a person's specific HCV genotype (19).

Vertical Transmission

The risk of HCV infection for infants born to women with anti-HCV has been assessed in numerous studies (19,409–415). The average transmission rate for HCV-infected but HIV-negative women is 5%, with a range from 0% to 25%. The presence of HCV RNA in the mother at delivery is the most consistent factor associated with vertical transmission. Limited data suggest that women with higher HCV RNA titers at delivery may be more likely to infect their newborns (19,416). Infants tend to have less HCV nucleotide variability than their mothers, thus suggesting that not all clones of a quasispecies are vertically transmitted. With time, nucleotide variability in infants increases, but the evolution differs from what occurs in their mothers (417,418).

The average infection rate for infants born to women coinfected with HCV and HIV-1 is higher and estimated at 14%, with a range from 5% to 36% (19). Limited data suggest that the delivery route (i.e., vaginal or by cesarean section) has no impact on the risk of HCV infection for infants, regardless of maternal HIV-1 status.

Perinatal Management

Routine screening of all pregnant women for HCV infection currently is not recommended. Testing should be limited to women who have high-risk exposure histories.

Postexposure prophylaxis with immune globulin preparations or antiviral agents for infants born to HCV-infected mothers also is not recommended. Because passively acquired transplacental IgG antibodies against HCV can persist for several months, it is recommended that infants not be tested for anti-HCV before 12 months of age (19,405). If earlier diagnosis is needed, RT-PCR for HCV RNA can be performed after the first month of life; HCV RNA detected in the first month of life may reflect only transient carriage (419). Cord blood should not be used for HCV diagnosis because of the potential for its contamination with maternal blood. Infants and children found to be infected with HCV require periodic monitoring because of their increased risk of serious liver disease.

HERPES SIMPLEX VIRUS INFECTIONS

Infections caused by HSV are common. Conservative estimates indicate that, in the United States, each year almost 500,000 people have their first episode of genital herpes, and another 10 million have recurring genital lesions (420). Neonatal HSV infection occurs in at least 700 to 1,000 newborns, and approximately 720,000 cesarean sections are performed annually for the purpose of preventing neonatal herpetic infection (16,420). The optimal management of women with active or suspected genital HSV infections during pregnancy or at labor is not well defined (421).

HSV is a double-stranded DNA virus that can infect a broad range of hosts. The virus enters the body through mucosal surfaces or abraded skin, and it multiplies in cells of the epidermis or dermis. Sensory or autonomic nerve endings in its vicinity become infected, and the virus travels intraaxonally in a retrograde fashion to the ganglia. HSV then can continue its multiplication in the ganglia and later spread to other skin and mucous membrane areas through anterograde travel along peripheral sensory nerves, or it can enter a phase of latency in the ganglia. The virus intermittently reactivates and travels to the body surface, where it can produce clinical disease. Exposure to ultraviolet light, trauma to skin, or immunosuppression can provoke HSV reactivation. Antibody- and cell-mediated immune reactions are generated in response to HSV, both of which are important for control of the infection (16,422,423).

The various HSV strains found in the general population can be grouped into two serologic subtypes, HSV-1 and HSV-2. The two subtypes can be differentiated on the basis of their cell culture range, restriction endonuclease analysis, monoclonal antibody-based serologic assays, or PCR (424,425).

Seven HSV glycoproteins (g) have been characterized; three (B, D, H) are essential for HSV replication, and four (C, E, G, I) are not essential for viral multiplication but may play a role in the pathogenesis and spread of HSV (426). One of the glycoproteins, gG-2, is a highly type-specific antigen and has been found to be helpful in differentiating HSV-1 from HSV-2 antibody responses.

Maternal Infection

Epidemiology

Serologic surveys conducted in the United States reveal that the prevalence of antibodies to HSV increases with age, and that it is higher in persons from lower socioeconomic strata and in groups with greater levels of sexual activity. Antibodies to HSV-1 may be present in 90% or more of adults from lower socioeconomic groups but in only about 30% of college students. Antibodies to HSV-2 are present in approximately 21.9% of the United States population 12 years of age or older, and in 27.2% of persons 30 to 49 years of age. African-Americans are more likely to have antibodies against HSV-2 than Caucasians or Mexican-Americans (45.9%, 17.6%, and 22.3%, respectively). Among African-Americans, women are more likely than men to be seropositive for this virus (55.1% vs. 34.7%, respectively) (427). However, only 2.6% of adults report ever having genital herpes. The seroprevalence of HSV-2 has increased by about 30% during the period from 1988 to 1994 as compared with the years 1976 to 1980 (427). HSV-2 seropositivity is significantly correlated with being female, African-American, or Hispanic, having a low educational level, income below the poverty line, having ever used cocaine, and the number of lifetime sexual partners (427,428).

Two percent or more of susceptible pregnant women become seropositive for HSV during pregnancy, but only one-third of them will have symptoms consistent with a herpes infection. Seroconversion that is completed by the time of onset of labor was not associated with increased neonatal morbidity or cases of congenital herpes infection in one recent study; however, infants born to mothers who acquired HSV infection shortly before delivery had an almost 50% chance of developing neonatal herpes (429).

By measuring type-specific antibodies against HSV-2 gG in a group of 190 pregnant women and their husbands, Kulhanjian and colleagues (430) found that 73% of the couples were concordant with respect to their HSV-2 serologies (i.e., both partners were seronegative or seropositive). However, about 9.5% of the pregnant women were seronegative but had seropositive spouses, and therefore they were at risk of gestational primary HSV-2 infection; 56% of these husbands had no history of previous genital HSV infection. Approximately 5% of pregnant women in this particular study were susceptible to HSV-2 infection but were unaware of their risk of acquiring the virus from their seropositive spouses, who gave no history of prior genital herpes (430).

Asymptomatic shedding of HSV occurs in 0.2% to 7.4% of pregnant women and in 0.2% to 4% of those at or near term. Most HSV infections during pregnancy represent recurrent disease. The frequency of asymptomatic shedding increases as pregnancy advances (10).

Clinical Manifestations

Many primary HSV infections are subclinical. Symptomatic primary HSV disease can include gingivostomatitis, genital herpes, herpetic whitlow, keratitis, chorioretinitis, encephalitis, esophagitis, pneumonia, and hepatitis (10,422).

The most common manifestations of primary HSV-1 infections are gingivostomatitis and pharyngitis (431,432). HSV-1 causes 7% to 50% of primary genital herpes infections (433). Recurrent episodes of herpes labialis are common, and HSV-1 may be recovered from the pharynx of as many as 5% of asymptomatic healthy persons (10).

The most common clinical illness caused by HSV-2 is genital herpes. Most initial HSV-2 infections are subclinical or mild. Symptomatic patients can have extensive, painful, vesicular or ulcerative genital lesions with or without associated systemic manifestations (434,435). Women with recurrent disease typically have mild or subclinical infections. Serious complications of HSV infections include pneumonia, hepatitis, and encephalitis (436–439). The likelihood of reactivation of HSV infection is greater for genital than oral–labial disease and for HSV-2 than for HSV-1 (440,441). One-fifth of all patients with primary genital herpes subsequently will have nongenital recurrences; this is most likely to occur on the hands and face for HSV-1 and on the buttocks and legs for HSV-2. Buttock recurrences occur less frequently but last longer than genital lesions (442). Asymptomatic HSV-2 shedding occurs more often during the first 3 months after the primary genital HSV-2 infection than during subsequent periods (441). For women with recurrent genital herpes, 55% of those with HSV-2 and 29% of those with HSV-1 had recurrences during a median follow-up of 105 days in one study (443). HSV-2 shedding (detected by culture) occurred on 2% of all days and usually lasted for 36 hours per recurrence; however, 5.5% of women shed HSV-2 for 4 days or longer. Subclinical shedding is more common in women with frequent symptomatic recurrences (443).

Genital herpes infections are categorized according to HSV subtype, serologic evidence of past HSV-1 or HSV-2 infection, and the presence or absence of symptoms. This classification scheme is useful when examining the impact of gestational HSV infection on pregnancy outcome according to the type of maternal genital infection. First episode, primary HSV-1 or HSV-2 infection is considered if the virus is isolated from the genital tract of a symptomatic or asymptomatic woman who has no serologic evidence of prior infection with HSV-1 or HSV-2 in the acute phase serum, but she subsequently has antibodies to the same HSV subtype when convalescent serum is tested. If the acute-phase serum contains antibodies to the other HSV subtype (e.g., HSV-1 antibodies in a woman with an HSV-2 genital isolate), first episode, nonprimary genital infection is considered present. Recurrent HSV-1 or HSV-2 infection is diagnosed if the patient has antibodies to the same HSV subtype isolated from the genital tract in the acute- and convalescent-phase sera (421). To illustrate the value of this classification scheme, Hensleigh and colleagues (444) evaluated 23 women whose clinical illnesses were consistent with the diagnosis of primary genital herpes. The diagnosis was verified serologically in only one woman with primary HSV-1 infection, whereas three others had nonprimary HSV-2 infection; the remaining 19 women proved to have recurrent disease (444).

Diagnosis

The diagnosis can be made by isolating the virus from tissue cultures of clinical specimens. The best specimen is usually vesicle fluid obtained within 3 days of its appearance (424). Positive culture results may be obtained within 16 hours to 7 days, depending on the viral load in the clinical specimen. Shell vial cultures may become positive within 16 to 48 hours (424). Direct detection of HSV antigens in exfoliated cells using a DFA stain can yield a positive result within 45 minutes. The Tzanck smear is a rapid and inexpensive method, but it is only 60% sensitive for HSV infections (445). It involves scraping the base of a fresh vesicle with a scalpel and spreading the cells and debris on a glass slide. The adherent cells are stained with Giemsa, Sedi, or Wright stain. The slide is examined for the presence of virus-induced cytopathic abnormalities, such as multinucleated giant cells, atypical keratinocytes with large nuclei, and ground-glass cytoplasm (445). A positive Tzanck smear cannot differentiate between VZV and HSV lesions.

Serologic diagnosis is used infrequently for the diagnosis of acute HSV infections. HSV-specific IgM may be detected within 3 to 10 days of onset of infection, and it persists for 6 to 8 weeks (424). Demonstration of seroconversion or a fourfold rise in HSV-specific IgG titers is significant.

Molecular biological techniques have been applied for the diagnosis of HSV infection through the detection of viral DNA in clinical specimens (445–448). The PCR continues to detect HSV DNA in clinical specimens for several days after the culture becomes negative. The test is relatively rapid and can be completed within a few hours. The clinical relevance of culture-negative, PCR-positive results from genital specimens remains to be elucidated. PCR detection of HSV DNA in CSF specimens helps in the diagnosis of herpes encephalitis (449). Because the PCR technique is sensitive to even minuscule amounts of HSV, contamination from external sources, such as laboratory personnel, physicians, or nurses who may be shedding the virus, can yield false-positive results. Extreme care should be taken while handling the CSF specimen to avoid making an erroneous diagnosis of herpes encephalitis and possibly missing the true culprit (449,450).

Treatment

Acyclovir is the drug of choice for primary and symptomatic recurrent genital HSV infection (451). The drug inhibits the replication of HSV-1, HSV-2, and VZV. Acyclovir is converted in the body to its active triphosphate form, initially through the action of viral thymidine kinase to the monophosphate form and later by cellular enzymes to the diphosphate and triphosphate forms. Acyclovir triphosphate concentrations are 40 to 100 times higher in HSV-infected cells than in uninfected cells. The active form of the drug competes with deoxyguanosine triphosphate as a substrate for viral DNA polymerase and, once incorporated into viral DNA, leads to termination of HSV DNA synthesis (451).

The use of acyclovir during pregnancy is not approved by the Food and Drug Administration and generally is reserved for life-threatening or severe HSV infections such as pneumonia. Maternal antiviral therapy may fail to prevent fetal infection with HSV (452). Acyclovir is teratogenic in rats (453). It crosses the placenta, concentrates in amniotic fluid, and can accumulate in human breast milk (454,455).

A registry of acyclovir use in pregnancy was established on June 1, 1984. As of June 30, 1993, 601 acyclovir-exposed pregnancies from 18 countries had been reported and followed (456). Of 425 exposures that took place during the first trimester, outcomes included 47 spontaneous fetal losses, 67 legal induced abortions, 298 live births without congenital malformations, and 13 with congenital anomalies. Among 176 second- and third-trimester exposures, three infants were born with anomalies. The reported birth defects were heterogeneous and without a specific pattern. These findings were not different from what was expected for the general population of pregnant women. The size of the cohort in the registry is adequate to detect a teratogenic risk that is twofold higher than expected, but is not large enough to detect smaller increases in risk of birth defects should they exist (456).

Acyclovir-resistant HSV strains are uncommon, except in patients with AIDS. The mechanism of resistance appears to be a mutation that renders the virus deficient in thymidine kinase (451). Infections caused by these acyclovir-resistant HSV strains can be treated with foscarnet or vidarabine; neither drug is approved by the Food and Drug Administration for use during pregnancy (457).

Two new drugs, valacyclovir and famciclovir, are active against HSV and have been approved for the management of genital herpes in nonpregnant adults. Valacyclovir is the L-valyl ester of acyclovir; it is rapidly absorbed and hydrolyzed in the body to acyclovir and results in much greater bioavailability of the active drug (425). Famciclovir is a prodrug of the antiviral compound penciclovir (458). Acyclovir-resistant HSV mutants usually are resistant to these two drugs as well, although penciclovir may be active against some of these strains (457). Both drugs are classified by the Food and Drug Administration as being in pregnancy category B. The manufacturer of famciclovir, SmithKline Beecham, maintains a pregnancy registry for this antiviral drug similar to what was previously done for acyclovir.

Fetal and Neonatal Infection

Epidemiology

Most neonatal HSV infections are acquired during passage through an infected birth canal. Transplacental spread occurs occasionally, with major deleterious fetal effects. About 40% of newborns with herpes are delivered before week 36 of pregnancy (10).

Intrapartum transmission is more likely to occur with primary maternal HSV genital infection. Other risk factors for HSV acquisition by the infant are cervical HSV infection, multiple genital lesions, prematurity, prolonged rupture of maternal membranes, intrauterine instrumentation (e.g., scalp electrodes), and absent or low titers of transplacentally acquired neutralizing HSV antibodies. The risk of vertical transmission is about 40% to 50% for mothers with primary herpes and about 5% for those with recurrent infections (10). Postpartum HSV spread to newborns occurs infrequently (423).

Clinical Manifestations

Asymptomatic HSV infections are rare in the newborn. Disease manifestations may be localized or widely disseminated. About 60% to 80% of infants with HSV infections are born to women who are asymptomatic at the time of delivery and who have no history of genital herpes (459). Infants born to asymptomatic women shedding HSV in early labor are ten times more likely to develop neonatal HSV infection if the mother had recently experienced a first episode genital herpes than neonates born to women whose HSV shedding is secondary to reactivated infection (460).

Intrauterine HSV infection is uncommon and accounts for about 5% of all neonatal herpes cases (423,461,462). Its hallmarks are a vesicular rash that is present at birth or appears shortly thereafter. Associated abnormalities include microcephaly (60%), chorioretinitis (40% to 50%), and microphthalmia (25%). The rash is more likely to be generalized than localized. Other skin lesions include bullae and cutaneous scars in 10% to 15% of patients. The intracranial calcifications seen in 15% may be present at birth or evolve later in infancy. Lesions indicative of brain damage, such as hydranencephaly, cerebral necrosis, and brain atrophy, can be seen on computed tomographic (CT) scans of the head. Other findings can include radiographic bone lucencies, intrauterine growth retardation, hepatosplenomegaly, cloudy corneas, and cataracts. About 30% have seizures during the neonatal period. The mortality rate is 40%, and about one-half of the survivors are expected to have significant long-term residual problems, such as psychomotor retardation, seizure disorders, spasticity, blindness, or deafness (462). Most cases are caused by HSV-2.

About one-fourth of infants with neonatal HSV infection become sick within the first day of life, and about two-thirds are ill by the end of the first week (423). Because of the nonspecific nature of the initial symptoms, the average time from disease onset to diagnosis is 4 to 5 days (423). Thus, a high index of suspicion is needed so that HSV-infected infants can be identified and treated earlier to reduce the risk of progression to more serious disease manifestations. Infections resulting from the intrapartum acquisition of HSV may not manifest until about 10 to 11 days of age, with disease localized to the skin, eyes, or oral cavity (10). Cutaneous lesions include discrete vesicles, large bullae, or denuded skin (Fig. 47–4). Recurrent mucocutaneous herpes develops in some of these infants. Ulcerative mouth lesions without skin disease may sometimes occur. Eye disease includes keratoconjunctivitis and chorioretinitis. Neurologic abnormalities eventually develop in 25% of these infants, even though CNS involvement may not have been evident during the acute illness.

A second group of infants may present at 15 to 17 days of age with localized CNS involvement, with or without skin, mouth, or ocular lesions. The mortality rate for this group is about 17%, and 40% to 50% of survivors suffer long-term sequelae.

A third group presents at 9 to 11 days of age with disseminated disease. CNS involvement is found in about two-thirds of these infants. Other organs that are severely affected are the adrenal glands, gastrointestinal tract, liver, heart, pancreas, and kidneys. Without appropriate therapy, about 80% die. With acyclovir therapy, the mortality rate is about 55%, and 40% to 55% of the survivors have severe neurologic impairments.

The National Institute of Allergy and Infectious Diseases Collaborative Antiviral Study Group (NIAID

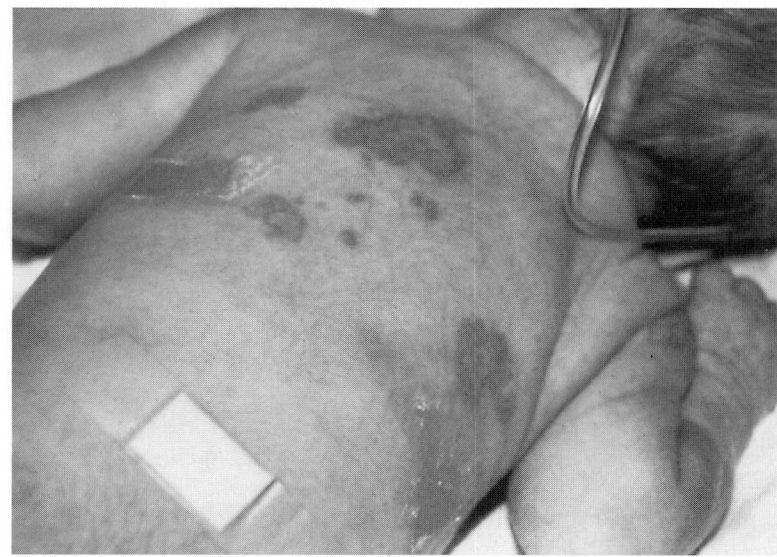

FIG. 47–4. Localized cutaneous herpes simplex virus type 2 infection in a neonate. Notice the coalescing vesicular lesions on the back and right arm. The vesicles are surrounded by an erythematous border.

CASG) studied 202 infants younger than 1 month of age with HSV infection (463–465). About 4% of infants had congenital HSV infection, and 40% had disease confined to the skin, eyes, or mouth. CNS disease occurred in 34%, and 22% had disseminated infections. Two-thirds of the isolates were HSV-2.

The clinical manifestations of herpes encephalitis in the newborn includes focal or generalized seizures, lethargy, apnea, and pyramidal tract signs. Eventual loss of gag and suck reflexes is common. Involvement of other organs is frequent. Skin vesicles may be absent in about 40% of infants. CSF analysis reveals mononuclear pleocytosis and elevated protein concentrations (as high as 1,000 mg/dL). Rarely, the CSF may show a predominance of neutrophils or be completely normal (16,466). Focal or generalized electroencephalographic abnormalities are common (467). About 8% of surviving infants have CNS relapse within 1 month of completing therapy (463).

Ocular herpetic infection may be an isolated problem, but it is more likely to occur in infants with CNS disease. Eye abnormalities include keratitis, conjunctivitis, chorioretinitis, necrotizing retinitis, optic atrophy, and cataracts. Long-term follow-up studies of survivors of neonatal HSV infection indicate that 40% (94% in patients with neurologic impairment; 20% in patients who are neurologically normal) have persistent abnormalities, such as cataracts, corneal scars, optic atrophy, and chorioretinal scars. About 44% have disturbed oculomotor control (468,469).

HSV pneumonia usually presents between days 3 and 14 of life with gradually worsening respiratory distress (470–473). Chest roentgenograms reveal perihilar infiltrates that gradually progress into severe diffuse interstitial and alveolar disease (i.e., "white-out" lungs) (474). Other findings include thrombocytopenia, neutropenia, jaundice, and hyperammonemia (475). The mortality rate of neonatal HSV pneumonia is about 80%, and almost 100% in infants with pneumonia and disseminated intravascular coagulopathy (464).

Diagnosis

Neonatal HSV infections are best diagnosed by isolating the virus from a vesicular lesion. The virus can be recovered from 25% to 40% of CSF specimens obtained from infants with CNS disease. Cultures of urine, feces, blood, nasopharyngeal secretions, and conjunctivae may yield the virus in some patients. Serology is not useful in neonatal HSV infections. Direct fluorescent antibody staining of scrapings from the base of fresh vesicles may reveal HSV antigens (423,476).

PCR assays for the detection of HSV DNA are valuable diagnostic tools and are fast becoming the gold standard for the diagnosis of HSV encephalitis (465,477). In the NIAID CASG trials, HSV DNA was detected in the CSF of 26 (76%) of 34 infants with CNS disease, in 13 (93%) of 14 infants with disseminated infection, and in 7 (24%) of 29 infants with disease seemingly limited to the skin, eyes, or mouth. One of seven PCR-positive patients with disease limited to the skin, eyes, or mouth later developed severe neurologic impairment (478). PCR assays on serum and CSF may remain positive for 1 to 2 weeks after starting antiviral therapy (479).

Treatment

Antiviral therapy with acyclovir or vidarabine is the mainstay of treatment. In the NIAID CASG reports, infants treated with acyclovir or vidarabine had comparable morbidity and mortality rates (463). No deaths occurred among 85 infants with localized skin, eyes, or mouth disease; about 94% seemed developmentally normal after 1 year. The mortality rates for the encephalitis and the disseminated HSV groups were 14% and 54%, respectively, and 40% to 70% of the survivors were neurologically impaired. Factors influencing mortality included level of consciousness at the start of treatment, prematurity, disease classification, pneumonia, and disseminated intravascular coagulopathy (464). Cutaneous HSV recurrences occurred in 46% of survivors by 6 months after the end of therapy, and the rates were similar for infants treated with acyclovir or vidarabine. Seventy-five percent of survivors with disease caused by HSV-2 were impaired compared with 27% of infants with HSV-1 infection. This is explained partially by the greater *in vitro* susceptibility of HSV-1 to acyclovir (451).

Infants receiving acyclovir shed lower virus titers than those on vidarabine. Given the ease of administration of acyclovir compared with vidarabine, its fairly benign toxicity profile, and its efficacy against HSV, acyclovir (15 mg/kg/dose given every 8 hours intravenously) is preferred as initial therapy of suspected or proven neonatal HSV infections. Dosage reductions are needed for infants with renal or hepatic dysfunction (480). The optimal duration of therapy is unknown, but it appears that 14 to 21 days may be preferable to the 10-day course; higher dosage regimens (about 60 mg/kg/d) are being evaluated (465). Neonatal infections caused by acyclovir-resistant HSV strains have been encountered, but are very rare (481). Topical antiviral agents, such as the ophthalmic preparations of trifluorothymidine, vidarabine, or iododeoxyuridine, should be used in newborns with ocular involvement. The use of commercial intravenous gammaglobulin preparations for HSV postexposure prophylaxis or treatment of neonates is not recommended, although evidence gleaned from animal studies suggests that the administration of monoclonal or polyclonal neutralizing antibodies given as late as 3 days after HSV infection can decrease mortality and morbidity (482,483).

Given the frequency of cutaneous or CNS recurrences after completion of antiviral therapy, some investigators have tried using oral acyclovir for posttreatment prophylaxis (484,485). The NIAID CASG conducted a phase I/II trial of oral acyclovir prophylactic therapy at a dose of 300 mg/m^2/dose given two or three times daily for 6 months to newborns recovering from HSV-2 infections limited to the skin, eyes, or mouth. Of 16 infants taking the thrice daily acyclovir regimen, 13 (81%) had no recurrences over the ensuing 6 months. This compared favorably with the 54% rate observed for historic control patients. The number of infants on the twice daily regimen was too small to permit any meaningful conclusions on its effectiveness as prophylaxis. Although acyclovir suppressive therapy appears able to limit cutaneous recurrences, its effectiveness in improving neurologic outcome for these infants is not known. Half the infants became neutropenic (absolute neutrophil counts less than 1,000 cells/μL) while on acyclovir therapy. One infant had an acyclovir-resistant HSV mutant isolated from a skin recurrence that occurred 36 hours after the conclusion of the 6-month suppressive regimen (485).

Prevention

Because of the enormous morbidity and mortality rates of neonatal HSV infections despite the early initiation of antiviral therapy, the focus of many research groups has been the development of effective prevention strategies. In a detailed decision analysis study, Libman and colleagues (486) used published data to theoretically evaluate nine different obstetric approaches for the prevention of neonatal HSV disease. The investigators concluded that, given the state of technology, physical examination at the time of labor was the most reasonable strategy. This tactic would be expected to reduce the number of neonatal HSV cases by 36% while increasing the rate of cesarean sections by only 3%. The strategy of obtaining genital HSV cultures at weekly intervals from women with a history of recurrent genital herpes and then delivering by cesarean section those whose most recent culture results were positive by onset of labor would result in 547 additional cesarean sections performed to prevent less than one case of neonatal HSV infection (rates per 100,000 deliveries) (486). Studies on women with histories of recurrent genital herpes have demonstrated that weekly antepartum cultures fail to predict the risks to their infants of HSV exposure at delivery and that most infants exposed to asymptomatic HSV shedding at delivery are born to women without a history of recurrent genital herpes infection (487,488). Roberts and colleagues (489) were able to reduce the HSV-related cesarean section rate at their institution by 37% (without adverse neonatal consequences) by questioning women in labor about prodromal symptoms of genital HSV infection followed by careful visual inspection of the lower genital tract. Previously, the strategy at their institution had incorporated the use of weekly HSV cultures beginning at 34 weeks of gestation and delivering by cesarean section those whose last genital cultures were positive or unavailable (489).

Cesarean section should be performed on women with signs and symptoms suggesting genital HSV infection at the onset of labor. It is not known whether cesarean delivery can reduce the risk of neonatal herpes when the membranes have been ruptured for longer than 4 to 6 hours. Infants delivered through an infected birth canal should be isolated to protect other infants in the nursery. The risk of invasive HSV infection is small for infants delivered vaginally to women with recurrent genital herpes who are asymptomatic but shedding the virus at the time of labor (490,491). Cultures of exposed mucous membranes (e.g., eyes, nasopharynx) should be obtained at 24 to 48 hours of life. Earlier positive cultures may reflect transient contamination and not true infection. If the cultures are positive for HSV, antiviral therapy should be started, even if the infant is asymptomatic. Animal data suggest that acyclovir therapy concomitant with HSV inoculation could inhibit acute viral replication and decrease the number of neurons with latent infection (492).

A number of studies have assessed the potential benefits of suppressive acyclovir therapy for pregnant women with recurrent genital herpes. Various acyclovir doses were tried and started at 36 weeks of gestation. The results of these trials were not in complete agreement, but all showed a decrease in clinical recurrences and a probable decline in the cesarean section rates for these women (493–495).

Numerous HSV candidate vaccines are currently in various stages of development. None are available commercially (425).

CYTOMEGALOVIRUS INFECTIONS

CMV is the most common congenital viral infection of humans in the United States and is one of the most important opportunistic pathogens causing serious illness and death in immunocompromised patients (496–498). CMV infections are benign for most adults. However, when CMV infection occurs during pregnancy, the virus can be transmitted to the fetus and result in symptomatic neonatal disease or subclinical congenital infection that may later manifest with hearing loss or learning disabilities.

CMV is an enveloped, double-stranded DNA virus that belongs to the herpes family of viruses (497). CMV is not eradicated after resolution of the primary infection. It persists in the body in a low-grade chronic infection form or in a latent state with periodic reactivations (499). CMV transmission occurs primarily by direct or indirect person-to-person spread of infected oropharyngeal secretions, sexual intercourse, blood transfusions, or transplacental spread from mother to fetus.

Maternal Infection

Serologic surveys in the United States and Great Britain have shown that about 40% to 60% of adults of middle or upper socioeconomic status have antibodies to CMV. The seropositivity rate is about 80% for adults of lower socioeconomic status (500). The higher the prevalence of maternal CMV antibody in a population, the greater is the rate of congenital CMV infection (500). Factors correlating with CMV seropositivity in pregnant women include non-Caucasian race, unmarried status, lower educational and income levels, and increasing parity (501,502). Sexual activity is an important risk factor for CMV infection in adolescents and young adults, and coinfection with bacterial vaginosis, trichomoniasis, or gonorrhea increases the odds of intrauterine CMV transmission (503–505).

Intrafamilial CMV transmission from young children to their seronegative pregnant mothers can occur. The risk of CMV seroconversion for a seronegative mother with an infected child is estimated at 10% to 30% per year and is even higher if the child is younger than 20 months of age (500,506). Annual seroconversion rates for seronegative day care providers is about 8% to 12% (507,508). Health care workers with CMV-infected patient contact do not appear to be at increased risk of CMV acquisition compared with persons without patient contact (509).

About 0.7% to 4.1% of susceptible women acquire primary CMV infection during pregnancy, a risk comparable to that of nonpregnant women (510). Seropositive women can reactivate their latent CMV infection during pregnancy or, less commonly, become reinfected by an exogenous CMV strain. Cervical and urinary CMV excretion increases as pregnancy advances from the first to the third trimester (511). Pregnant women may shed CMV from the cervix (8%), urinary tract (4%), throat (2%), and breast milk in the postpartum period (14%) (10).

Primary and recurrent maternal CMV infection can result in transmission of the virus to the fetus. This occurs in about 40% (range 24% to 75%) of pregnancies complicated by primary CMV infection (509). The presence of maternal antibodies to CMV in women with recurrent infection does not prevent viral transmission to the fetus, but it does protect against major fetal damage by CMV (512). Severe congenital CMV after maternal reactivation or reinfection by other strains can occur, but is rare (513–516).

Most women (90%) with primary CMV infection are asymptomatic. The remainder usually have illnesses resembling infectious mononucleosis. Other manifestations are rare but include interstitial pneumonia, myocarditis, aseptic meningitis, hepatitis, colitis, thrombocytopenia, and hemolytic anemia. Primary CMV infection during the first trimester of pregnancy does not cause fetal loss (517).

Infection can be documented by isolating the virus from urine, saliva, buffy coat, or cervical secretions. Viral isolation, however, does not differentiate between primary and recurrent CMV infections. Measurement of CMV-specific IgM antibodies is useful for the diagnosis of primary infection, but this antibody can persist in serum for 4 to 8 months (518). CMV-specific IgG antibody levels are helpful if seroconversion or a fourfold titer rise can be demonstrated. The IFA and ELISA are the most practical and reliable methods for detecting CMV antibodies. CMV-specific IgG avidity is low (mean 30%) when measured within the first 14 weeks after seroconversion, and it increases over time (mean 88% for patients with remote infections). This assay may prove helpful in the diagnosis of primary CMV infection during pregnancy (519). Rapid diagnosis of CMV infection is possible using newly developed antigen assays or molecular biological techniques such as the PCR (520). One needs to be aware that interlaboratory variability exists in the results of CMV PCR assays, especially for specimens containing lesser quantities of viral DNA (521).

Ganciclovir, an acyclic nucleoside analog of acyclovir, has excellent inhibitory activity against CMV (522). It has been extensively evaluated in immunocompromised patients (e.g., AIDS, organ transplant recipients) with serious CMV infections such as pneumonia or retinitis, but its use in immunocompetent persons has not been examined. Ganciclovir is both mutagenic and teratogenic in pregnant experimental animals. The drug crosses the placenta into the fetal compartment passively and without being metabolized (523). Foscarnet (phosphonoformate), another anti-CMV drug, inhibits the DNA polymerase of CMV. Like ganciclovir, foscarnet is used only in the immunosuppressed patient with CMV disease (522). Cidofovir is a nucleotide analogue that inhibits viral DNA polymerase. It has a long intracellular half-life, which allows its administration to adults once every 1 to 2 weeks. Its use currently is limited to immunocompromised adults, especially those with CMV retinitis (524).

Congenital Infection

Congenital infection with CMV occurs in 0.4% to 2.3% of all live births (500). About 10% are symptomatic, and the rest have subclinical infections. Infants with symptomatic congenital CMV have a mortality rate of 15% to 30%, and most survivors have long-term sequelae (10,525–528). Petechiae, jaundice, and hepatosplenomegaly are found in two-thirds of patients; conjugated hyperbilirubinemia and thrombocytopenia are found in about 80% of cases (512,525). Neurologic abnormalities such as seizures and hypotonia are common, and microcephaly occurs in about 50% to 75% of infants. Intracranial calcifications are seen on the CT scans of one-half of the patients. At autopsy, evidence of multiorgan involvement is apparent (525). Neuropathologic findings include periventricular necrosis, calcifications, cerebellar hypoplasia, periventricular leukomalacia, hydrocephalus, and porencephalic cyst (528). Hearing loss and neurologic impairment (e.g., psychomotor and mental retardation) develop in one-half of the survivors (526,527). Infants whose cranial CT scans are abnormal at birth have a 90% risk of developing at least one long-term sequela such as mental or psychomotor retardation, seizures, cerebral palsy, or hearing loss. In contrast, only 29% of infants with symptomatic congenital CMV infection and normal cranial CT scans at birth have similar long-term residual problems (529).

Chorioretinitis is the most frequent eye abnormality, followed by optic atrophy. Microphthalmia, cloudy cornea, optic nerve hypoplasia, nystagmus, and strabismus also occur. Eye abnormalities are common in infants with intracranial calcifications (10).

Unilateral or bilateral sensorineural hearing loss that can vary from mild to profound develops in about 30% of infants with symptoms at birth, and in 7% to 13% of those with subclinical infections. Hearing loss may be present at birth in otherwise asymptomatic infants, and it subsequently deteriorates in more than one-half of the patients with a median age at first progression of 18 months (range 2 to 70) (530–532). Some patients have normal hearing for the first several years of life, but they subsequently develop sudden or fluctuating hearing loss (532,533).

Intellectual deficits are common, particularly in infants with symptomatic congenital CMV. Many infants with subclinical disease may develop mental or behavioral problems. However, it appears that children with asymptomatic congenital CMV who are developmentally normal at 1 year of age are unlikely to be at increased risk of subsequent neurodevelopmental or intellectual impairments (534).

Dental defects can be found in 40% of the survivors of symptomatic neonatal disease but in only 5% of asymptomatic cases (535). A variety of other congenital anomalies have been described in infants with congenital CMV infection, but these probably reflect coincidental associations rather than true cause-and-effect relationships (536). Reported associations include atrial and ventricular septal defects, tetralogy of Fallot, congenital mitral stenosis, congenital lobar emphysema, Mondini deformity of the temporal bone (congenital anomaly of osseous and membranous labyrinth characterized by aplastic cochlea, and deformity of the vestibule and semicircular canal with partial or complete loss of auditory or vestibular function), stuck twin syndrome, renal agenesis, diabetes insipidus, inguinal hernia, hip dislocation, clubfoot, esophageal atresia, megacolon, and extrahepatic biliary atresia (10,537–543).

Maternal CMV antibodies protect the fetus against major CMV-related pathology. Fowler and colleagues (512) found that 18% of 125 infants born to women with primary CMV during pregnancy had symptomatic neonatal disease compared with none of 64 infants born to women with reactivated CMV infection. After a 5-year follow-up period, 13% of infants born to mothers with primary infection had mental impairment (i.e., intelligence quotient ≤70) compared with none in the recurrent infection group. Sensorineural hearing loss was found in 15% and 5% of infants born to mothers with primary and recurrent CMV infections, respectively (512). Bilateral hearing loss occurred only in the primary infection group.

Discordant fetal outcomes are possible after primary maternal CMV infection in twin pregnancies. CMV usually affects both twins if they are monozygotic with a monochorionic placenta. In dizygotic twins with a dichorionic placenta, one twin can be severely affected whereas the other completely escapes infection (544). In one report of a quadruplet pregnancy complicated by primary maternal CMV infection, one infected fetus died antenatally, another died at 3 months of liver failure, one had hearing loss and developmental delay, and the fourth infected infant was normal at his last evaluation at age 18 months (545).

Congenital infection can be diagnosed by isolation of CMV from the urine or saliva within the first 2 weeks of life. Positive cultures from specimens obtained at 3 weeks or later may reflect perinatal CMV acquisition. Congenitally infected infants shed CMV in their urine for many years. The use of shell vial cultures hastens viral isolation. CMV can be detected in the urine by electron microscopy or ELISA. CMV DNA can be detected in a variety of clinical specimens using sensitive hybridization or PCR methods. CMV-specific IgM is detected in many of the infected newborns. IgM detection by radioimmunoassay or ELISA is superior to immunofluorescence (500,546–549).

Ganciclovir is being evaluated as treatment for symptomatic congenital CMV infection. Ganciclovir suppresses viral replication in immunocompromised patients with serious CMV infections. Several problems are associated with ganciclovir use, including the resumption of viral replication upon discontinuation of therapy, emergence of ganciclovir-resistant CMV strains after prolonged use in immunosuppressed patients, and drug toxicity (e.g., neutropenia, thrombocytopenia) (550). Information on the utility of ganciclovir for infants with symptomatic congenital CMV infection comes from individual case reports, small case series, and uncontrolled trials utilizing more than one dosage regimen for the drug (500,551–561). From these studies, it appears that ganciclovir can lessen or stop viral multiplication and inhibit its shedding; however, viruria resumes upon discontinuation of therapy. Regimens that used higher individual doses (7.5 instead of 5 mg/kg) given twice daily and for longer periods (6 to 12 weeks or longer instead of 2 to 3 weeks) were associated with improved outcomes. Drug-related hematologic toxicities (e.g., neutropenia, thrombocytopenia) develop in the majority of treated infants. A controlled trial of ganciclovir versus no therapy for 6 weeks with a follow-up of 5 years has been underway in the United States, and this may provide more precise information on the value of, or lack thereof, ganciclovir therapy in CMV-infected symptomatic infants (559). Intrauterine therapy for CMV infection was attempted for one fetus at 27 weeks of gestation by infusing ganciclovir once daily into the umbilical vein for 12 days (562). There was initial improvement in the fetal platelet count and liver enzyme concentrations, as well as a reduction in the amount of virus in the amniotic fluid and fetal urine, and clearance of CMV from fetal blood. However, viral replication promptly resumed upon discontinuation of the drug, and the fetus died *in utero* at 32 weeks of gestation. Disseminated CMV was demonstrated at autopsy (562). CMV hyperimmune globulin used in conjunction with ganciclovir has improved the survival of bone marrow transplant recipients with CMV pneumonia. The combination was not beneficial in one infant in whom it was tried (553). CMV hyperimmune globulin was injected into the abdominal cavity of a CMV-infected fetus with ascites at 28 and again at 29 weeks of gestation (563). The fetus was delivered at 34 weeks because of fetal distress. The ascites was still evident at that time but disappeared by the fourth day of life. The need for more effective anti-CMV chemotherapeutic agents is evident. There is no experience with foscarnet or cidofovir in the treatment of congenitally infected infants.

Perinatal Infection

Infants can acquire CMV during passage through an infected birth canal or by ingestion of CMV-positive breast milk (564). CMV is found in the milk of 20% to 70% of seropositive mothers for up to 12 weeks postpartum, and 60% to 80% of infants receiving CMV-containing milk will become infected. One of the components of human milk, sialyllactose, has been found to consistently increase the titer of CMV in tissue culture systems at concentrations found in milk. The addition of another component of breast milk, lactoferrin, negates the effects of sialyllactose on CMV growth (565,566).

In contrast to congenital disease, perinatally acquired CMV infection usually is benign. Most infections are subclinical. A self-limited, infantile pneumonitis is the clinical abnormality encountered most commonly among symptomatic term infants. Premature infants may have severe illness, including pneumonia, hepatitis, anemia, thrombocytopenia, and neutropenia. Those born to CMV-seronegative mothers are at risk of acquiring CMV through blood transfusions from CMV-positive donors (567). The long-term prognosis for intellectual abilities and intact hearing for patients with perinatal CMV infection is excellent (568).

Prevention

Termination of the pregnancy can be considered for women who develop a primary CMV infection during gestation. With primary infection, the overall risk of delivering an infant with symptomatic congenital infection is only about 5%.

Prenatal diagnosis of fetal CMV infection is feasible and has been accomplished by a variety of invasive methods such as cordocentesis and amniocentesis. Fetal blood can be cultured and PCR assays for CMV DNA can be performed. In addition, it can be analyzed for the presence of CMV-specific fetal IgM, fetal liver enzyme elevations, anemia, and thrombocytopenia. Amniotic fluid can be tested by culture and PCR assays for evidence of CMV infection. More than 300 pregnant women with primary CMV infection in whom prenatal diagnosis was attempted have been described in the literature (569–582). In the aggregate, these studies revealed that fetal blood testing is not as sensitive as amniocentesis in establishing the diagnosis of fetal CMV infection and that it need not be performed. Patients with positive results with the CMV-specific IgM assay, fetal blood culture, or fetal blood PCR testing also are positive when their amniotic fluid is examined, but the reverse is not true. Fetal blood testing for CMV infection no longer is warranted, because amniocentesis is easier to perform and carries less risk to the mother and her baby. These studies also showed that neither culture methods nor PCR assays on amniotic fluid are 100% sensitive, and that false-negative results are more likely to be encountered if testing is done shortly after the diagnosis of primary CMV infection is made in the mother (579). Most disturbing is the recognition that positive PCR results on amniotic fluid do not necessarily reflect fetal infection. In one study of 82 women with primary CMV infection, PCR detected viral DNA in the amniotic fluid of 27; in only 12 was a congenital infection documented after birth (positive predictive value of 48%) (582). Isolation of CMV from the amniotic fluid by culture implies intrauterine infection but does not provide information regarding the severity of fetal disease (579). A false-positive amniotic fluid culture or PCR result is possible if contamination with maternal blood occurs. PCR assays have been used to detect CMV DNA in chorionic villi, but the sensitivity, specificity, and positive and negative predictive values of the method are not known (583).

Fetal abnormalities detected by ultrasonography in women with gestational primary or recurrent CMV infection generally indicate more severe fetal disease. A variety of sonographic findings have been reported, including microcephaly, ventricular dilation, ascites, hepatosplenomegaly, hyperechogenic fetal bowel, hydrops, pleural and pericardial effusions, oligohydramnios, intrauterine growth retardation, and intracranial and abdominal calcifications (510,569,581,584–587).

CMV vaccines are not yet available in the United States, but they are being tested in special populations (588). Routine CMV serologic screening of pregnant women is not cost effective (510).

Because blood from seropositive donors contains leukocytes that are latently infected with CMV, many blood banks now screen the blood for CMV antibodies (68%), use leukocyte filters, or use washed erythrocytes. The practice of giving only CMV-negative blood or blood products to ill neonates has greatly reduced or eliminated the occurrence of transfusion-acquired CMV infections in many nurseries. Disseminated CMV infection after extracorporeal membrane oxygenation has been described. CMV screening of blood had not been done (589).

VARICELLA

Varicella (i.e., chickenpox) and herpes zoster (i.e., shingles) are caused by VZV. VZV is an enveloped, double-stranded DNA virus. Only one serotype is known.

Maternal Infection

In the United States, about 95% of women of childbearing age have serologic evidence of past VZV infection. The proportion of seropositive women is smaller in those from tropical or semitropical countries (590).

Varicella is a highly communicable and usually benign disease of childhood. Children younger than 15 years of age account for more than 90% of cases. Fewer than 2% of reported cases occur in those 20 years of age or older (591). The estimated incidence of gestational varicella is 1 to 7 per 10,000 pregnancies (592,593). Zoster results from reactivation of latent VZV and is encountered more frequently in elderly or immunosuppressed patients. Its incidence in pregnancy is unknown, but it is probably lower than that of varicella. One estimate places the incidence at about 0.5 per 10,000 pregnancies (592).

Less than 5% of primary VZV infections are subclinical (594). Varicella usually becomes clinically evident 10 to 20 days after exposure of susceptible persons to VZV. The typical illness consists of fever, malaise, and a pruritic rash. The exanthem is mostly truncal in distribution and is characterized by crops of maculopapules that rapidly evolve into vesicles. The vesicles gradually crust over. New lesions continue to appear for 3 to 5 days, producing the distinctive finding of cutaneous lesions in various stages of evolution. Complications of varicella include pneumonia, encephalitis, arthritis, bacterial cellulitis, and bleeding diathesis. The risk of incurring complications from varicella in otherwise normal adults may be up to 25-fold greater than that for normal children (591). Pregnancy is not a risk factor for maternal complications. Immunity after varicella is usually long lasting, but recurrent VZV infections can occur rarely in immunocompetent persons (595,596).

Zoster is characterized by pain localized to the area of distribution of one or more sensory nerve roots. The rash is unilateral in most patients and follows the same evolutionary pattern seen in varicella except for its restricted distribution.

Varicella and herpes zoster usually are diagnosed clinically, and laboratory confirmation is needed infrequently. The virus can be isolated from vesicular fluid by inoculating freshly collected specimens onto human diploid cell lines. The VZV-specific antigens can be detected in vesicular fluid by immunofluorescence staining of smears of cell scrapings collected from the base of fresh vesicles (597). VZV DNA can be detected in vesicle samples, including most crusted lesions, by PCR methodologies (598,599).

Several serologic assays are available for the detection of antibodies to VZV. These include complement fixation, neutralization, IHA, immune adherence hemagglutination, radioimmunoassay, immunoblot, latex agglutination, fluorescent antibody against membrane antigen (FAMA), IFA, and ELISA. These tests can be used to diagnose VZV infections or to ascertain the susceptibility status of an individual (600).

Complement fixation antibodies develop within 10 days of onset of varicella and peak at 2 to 3 weeks. These antibodies appear earlier in herpes zoster. Complement fixation antibodies tend to disappear with time. By 1 year after infection, about two-thirds of persons do not have detectable complement fixation antibody titers. The complement fixation test is relatively insensitive compared with FAMA or ELISA, and it is now rarely used in clinical laboratories. The FAMA test is very sensitive and is considered to be the gold standard for VZV antibody measurements. However, FAMA is arduous to perform and is not readily available. The ELISA test is being used increasingly for VZV antibody measurements. The IFA methods have been shown to be as sensitive as FAMA (424).

Two serum samples collected 1 to 2 weeks apart can provide a retrospective diagnosis of VZV infection if a fourfold or greater rise in antibody titer is demonstrated. If the first sample is collected late in the course of the illness, a single high titer indicates a recent primary or a reactivated VZV infection.

Measurement of VZV-specific IgM antibodies is useful for documenting a recent infection with this virus. The VZV-specific IgM antibodies can be detected in serum for several weeks after varicella and may be transiently found after herpes zoster.

For uncomplicated varicella, symptomatic treatment with antipruritics and cleansing of lesions is adequate. Analgesics are needed for pain control in herpes zoster. Early therapy of varicella within the first day of illness with oral acyclovir (800 mg given orally five times per day for 7 days) hastens resolution of fever and shortens the time period to complete crusting of the lesions

(601,602). Acyclovir is not recommended for use during pregnancy, but it can be given for the treatment of severe or life-threatening VZV complications such as pneumonia.

There have been several reports of pregnant women with varicella pneumonia who were treated with acyclovir (603–609). The drug was used at doses ranging from 5 to 18 mg/kg every 8 hours, and the treatment results generally have been favorable.

Transmission to the Fetus

VZV transmission to the fetus occurs primarily through the transplacental route. Congenital malformations after maternal infection during the first half of pregnancy occur infrequently. VZV antigens and its DNA have been detected in fetal tissues from pregnancies complicated by varicella using immunohistochemical staining methods and PCR, respectively (610–612).

About one-fourth of newborns delivered to mothers who contract varicella during the last 3 weeks of pregnancy develop clinical infection (609). Paryani and Arvin (613) used several clinical and immunologic criteria to document intrauterine transmission of VZV in 43 pregnancies complicated by varicella and 14 others complicated by herpes zoster. These criteria included malformations consistent with the congenital varicella syndrome, acute varicella of the newborn, detection of VZV-specific IgM in the neonatal period, specific lymphocyte transformation to VZV antigen, persistence of anti-VZV IgG, and the occurrence of herpes zoster in infancy. The rate of intrauterine transmission was 24% after maternal varicella and 0% after maternal herpes zoster (613).

Fetal Infection

Varicella during pregnancy is not associated with an increased incidence of prematurity or fetal death (613–615). Chromosomal abnormalities have occurred after VZV infections in experimentally infected human diploid fibroblasts and in the peripheral leukocytes of patients with acute varicella (616,617). Leukocyte chromosomal breaks were described in one child whose mother had gestational varicella (618). An increased risk of leukemia in the offspring of women with gestational varicella has been found by some investigators, but the numbers are too small to confirm the association (619).

Numerous case reports published over the past 51 years have described the occurrence of congenital malformations in the progeny of women who acquire chickenpox during pregnancy (614,620–659). With the exception of a few infants with congenital anomalies after maternal varicella at 25.5 to 32 weeks of gestation, these infections usually occurred during the first half of gestation, and mostly between weeks 8 and 20 of pregnancy (660–662). Abnormalities are primarily cutaneous, musculoskeletal, neurologic, and ocular (Table 47–5).

The risk of fetal or congenital varicella syndrome after maternal chickenpox during pregnancy is low. Pastuszak and colleagues (663) studied 106 women with varicella in their first 20 weeks of pregnancy and found a 1.2% risk (95% confidence interval [CI] of 0% to 2.4%) of varicella embryopathy. Enders and associates (664) studied 1,373 women with gestational varicella between 1980 and 1993 and found the risk of fetal varicella syndrome to be 0.4% (95% CI of 0.05% to 1.5%) for infections occurring between weeks 0 to 12 of pregnancy, and 2% (95% CI of 0.8% to 4.1%) for those occurring between weeks 13 to 20 of pregnancy. Jones and colleagues (665) found that 2 of 146 infants born to women with gestational varicella had abnormalities consistent with the fetal varicella syndrome; four others had a single major malformation. No infants were born with the fetal varicella syndrome to 57 women described in two other similar studies (666,667).

Cicatricial lesions are the most common skin abnormalities (Fig. 47–5). Cutaneous scars usually occur on hypoplastic extremities, but they can extend to the trunk or opposite extremity. Limb hypoplasia usually is unilateral and most commonly involves the leg. The arm, mandible, or hemithorax can be affected. Rudimentary digits are common on hypoplastic extremities. Detailed clinical and histopathologic studies of some patients suggest that limb abnormalities after intrauterine VZV infection probably are due to a neuropathy resulting from damage to dorsal ganglia and anterior columns of the spinal cord (645,647).

TABLE 47–5. *Abnormalities in newborns after maternal gestational varicella*

Timing of maternal varicella	Neonatal clinical abnormalities
0–20 weeks of pregnancy	Cicatricial skin lesions, denuded skin, herpes zoster, limb hypoplasia, rudimentary digits, muscle atrophy, intrauterine growth retardation, psychomotor retardation, microcephaly, cerebellar and cortical atrophy, seizures, intracranial calcifications, sensory deficits, Horner syndrome, spinal cord atrophy, anal sphincter dysfunction, dysphagia, intestinal atresia, neurogenic bladder, recurrent aspiration pneumonia, clubfoot, microphthalmia, optic atrophy, hypoplasia of optic disc, chorioretinitis, chorioretinal scars, cataract, nystagmus
Last 5 days of pregnancy–2 days postpartum	Fever, vesicular exanthem, hemorrhagic rash, respiratory distress, cyanosis, pneumonia, widespread necrotic lesions of the viscera (in fatal cases)

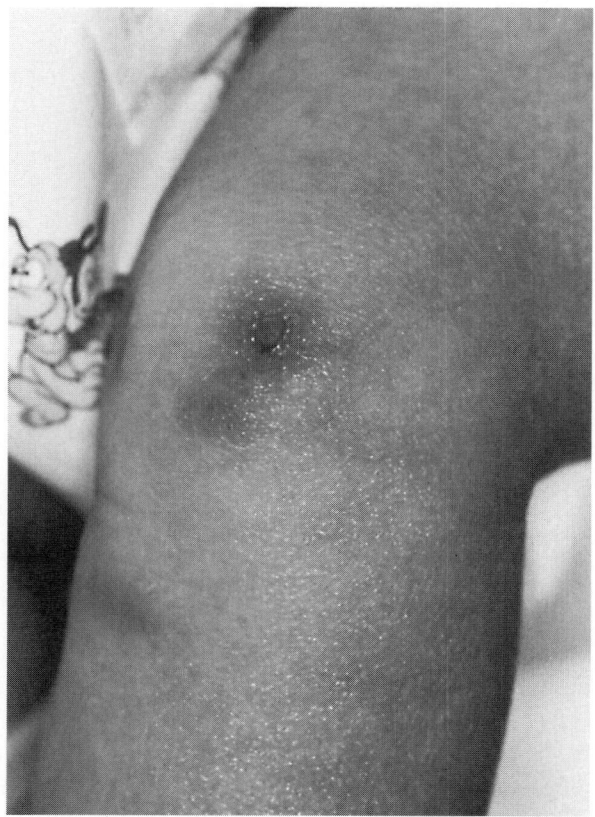

FIG. 47–5. Newborn with congenital varicella after maternal infection at about week 13 of pregnancy. Notice the ulcerated area with surrounding scars over the knee; a second scar is visible distally, over the tibia. Despite an otherwise normal physical examination, computerized tomography of the head revealed multiple areas of cerebral infarction and diffuse intracranial calcifications.

CNS pathology is common and includes microcephaly, cortical and cerebellar atrophy, psychomotor retardation, seizures, and focal brain calcifications. Autonomic dysfunction, manifested by loss of bowel and urinary sphincter control, dysphagia, intestinal obstruction, and Horner syndrome, is observed in some patients. Unilateral or bilateral ocular anomalies are common; the eye may be the only organ affected in fetal VZV infection.

The literature contains references to a few infants born with congenital malformations after maternal herpes zoster during pregnancy (668–671). Reported birth defects include microcephaly, microphthalmia, cataracts, and talipes equinovarus. These rare cases probably represent chance occurrences rather than true associations. Paryani and Arvin (613) prospectively followed 14 pregnancies complicated by herpes zoster and were unable to uncover any clinical or immunologic evidence of intrauterine VZV infection. Enders and associates (664) found no evidence of intrauterine VZV infection in infants of 366 women who developed herpes zoster during the first 36 weeks of pregnancy.

Neonatal Infection

About 25% of newborns become infected when maternal varicella occurs during the last 3 weeks of pregnancy (609). The most important determinant of the severity of neonatal disease is the time of onset of maternal varicella relative to delivery. If maternal infection occurs within 5 days before and 2 days after delivery, varicella lesions in neonates usually appear at 5 to 10 days of age. The illness may be mild, with only a few cutaneous lesions, or may become severe, with fever, hemorrhagic rash, and generalized visceral involvement (see Table 47–5). The mortality rate is about 30%, and death usually is caused by severe pulmonary disease. If maternal varicella occurs 5 to 21 days before delivery, lesions in newborns typically appear in the first 4 days of life and the prognosis is good, with no associated mortality. The mild course probably is due to the production and transplacental passage of maternal antibodies, which modify the course of the illness in newborns. Passive transfer of maternal VZV antibodies across the placenta at titers considered to be protective can occur as early as 24 to 28 weeks of gestation (672).

The diagnosis can be confirmed by viral isolation or VZV antigen detection. Infected newborns may have VZV-specific IgM, but these usually disappear shortly after birth. Newborns with varicella should be kept in strict isolation if they require hospitalization. Acyclovir can be used for infants with severe disease (559,673). If started early in the illness, acyclovir usually leads to more rapid resolution of disease symptoms and signs. Varicella-zoster immune globulin (VZIG) is not beneficial after clinical disease has developed.

Prevention

Management of persons exposed to VZV is critical because varicella is a highly communicable infection that can adversely affect pregnant women and their offspring. Exposed susceptible persons can be protected by passive immunization with VZIG. VZIG is prepared from plasma of normal blood donors found to have high IgG antibody titers to VZV. VZIG can prevent or modify clinical varicella in susceptible persons if given shortly after exposure.

Pregnant women exposed to varicella who have negative or uncertain prior histories of this infection should be tested for VZV susceptibility if sensitive assays are available and the results can be obtained rapidly. About 80% to 95% of these women are immune to varicella, as indicated by positive FAMA, IFA, or ELISA test results (591,674).

If a pregnant woman has significant exposure to varicella and is susceptible or if the laboratory test result cannot be obtained in a timely fashion, VZIG should be administered for the purpose of preventing or modifying the infection in the mother to avoid complications. It is not known whether passive maternal immunization can prevent fetal VZV infection (591). VZIG is most efficacious when given as soon after exposure as is feasible, but not later than 96 hours.

A history of previous varicella infection is not always reliable. In a recent study of 184 military personnel with acute varicella, 20 (10.8%) reported a prior history of chickenpox. Sera from 19 of these individuals collected 3 days to 34 months earlier and stored at -70°C were available for testing; none had VZV-specific IgG (675).

Discordant results with respect to fetal infections are possible in multiple gestation pregnancies. Borzyskowski and collaborators (624) reported a set of female identical twins sharing a single placenta whose mother developed varicella at 10 weeks of gestation. The first twin was normal, and the second had congenital defects consistent with intrauterine VZV infection.

Prenatal diagnosis by detection of VZV-specific IgM in fetal blood was successful in one fetus evaluated at about 32 weeks of gestation, approximately 12 weeks after his mother developed chickenpox (628). Anti-VZV IgM could not be detected in another fetus whose mother developed chickenpox at 12.5 weeks of gestation; cord blood samples were obtained at 27 and 35 weeks of gestation (later testing of stored amniotic fluid was positive for VZV DNA by PCR) (676). Isada and colleagues (677) attempted to diagnose intrauterine VZV infection in two patients by chorionic villus sampling and PCR. Tissues from both mothers were PCR positive but culture negative. One mother elected to terminate her pregnancy at 23 weeks; examination of the fetal brain by Southern blot hybridization was negative. The second woman continued her pregnancy to term, and her newborn infant was clinically normal. Tests for VZV-specific IgM in cord blood and viral placental cultures were negative. Thus, the detection of VZV DNA sequences in chorionic villus samples did not equate with fetal infection (677). Amniotic fluid viral culture done at 22 weeks of gestation (11 weeks after maternal varicella) confirmed the diagnosis in another infected fetus; concomitant testing of fetal blood failed to detect VZV-specific IgM (678). Amniotic fluid testing using PCR confirmed the diagnosis of fetal varicella infection in 9 of 107 women who had chickenpox before week 24 of gestation; none had detectable VZV-specific IgM in fetal blood (679).

A variety of antenatal sonographic abnormalities have been described for VZV-infected fetuses. These include hypoplastic extremities, clubfoot, flexed limbs, ventriculomegaly, porencephalic cyst, oligohydramnios, polyhydramnios, hydrops, ascites, and calcifications of the lungs, myocardium, liver, and spleen (679–682).

Children born to mothers who develop varicella within 5 days before and 2 days after delivery should receive 125 U of VZIG as soon as possible. VZIG does not reduce the clinical attack rate in treated newborns, but these infants generally contract milder infections than untreated neonates (591,683). Because severe varicella can develop in newborns despite timely administration of VZIG, some clinicians have advocated the use of acyclovir prophylaxis in these infants (684,685).

Although a few cases of severe neonatal varicella after exposure to mothers who developed the infection more than 2 days after delivery have been described, routine VZIG administration is not recommended, because this group of infants is not regarded as being at increased risk of varicella complications (591,686).

Pregnant women with varicella at the time of delivery should be isolated from their newborns until all vesicles have crusted. Neonates with varicella lesions should be isolated from other infants but not from their mothers.

A live, attenuated varicella vaccine (VARIVAX) was licensed in the United States in March 1995. The vaccine should not knowingly be administered to susceptible pregnant women. The vaccine manufacturer, Merck and Company, has established a VARIVAX Pregnancy Registry (telephone number 1-800-986-8999) to collect data on the pregnancy outcomes of inadvertently immunized women (593).

Screening of pregnant women for varicella susceptibility is not recommended at the present time. Some obstetricians routinely screen their gravid patients who have negative or uncertain histories of past varicella infections, but this approach is felt not to be cost effective (687). A recent cost-effectiveness analysis concluded that serologic testing of women without prior history of chickenpox, if coupled with postpartum vaccination of susceptibles, could prevent about 43% of adult varicella and at a reasonable cost to the health care system (688). These analyses notwithstanding, the varicella vaccine is expected to have a profound impact on the epidemiology of VZV infections in the United States, which inevitably will modify our current approaches to the management of this problem in pregnant women and their infants.

PARVOVIRUS B19 INFECTIONS

Human parvovirus B19 was discovered fortuitously in the mid-1970s by British scientists who had been evaluating new laboratory methods for the improved detection of HBsAg in blood donor sera (689). Since then, B19 has been etiologically linked to a variety of conditions, including erythema infectiosum (i.e., fifth disease), aplastic crises in sickle-cell anemia and other hemolytic diseases, chronic anemia in immunocompromised patients, acute arthritis, and fetal hydrops. Less commonly recognized B19-related conditions are myocarditis, hepatitis, aseptic meningitis, and virus-associated hemophagocytosis (690).

B19 is a small, nonenveloped, single-stranded DNA virus. Despite its many genotypes, only one B19 antigenic type is recognized at present (690). The virus does not grow in conventional cell lines, but it can be propagated in erythropoietin-stimulated bone marrow explant cultures, fetal liver cells of erythroid lineage, a novel cell line with megakaryocytic phenotype, human umbilical cord blood, and erythroid progenitor cells generated *in vitro* from peripheral human blood in the presence of recombinant erythropoietin and interleukin-3 (691).

B19 causes a lytic infection of human erythroid progenitor cells. The erythroid tropism of B19 is due to the tissue distribution of globoside (blood group P antigen), its major cellular receptor. Globoside is a neutral glycophospholipid of red blood cell membranes. Persons who do not have P on their erythrocytes (i.e., p phenotype) are naturally resistant to infection with B19. The frequency of the p phenotype is 1 per 200,000 persons (692). Globoside also can be found on megakaryocytes, endothelial cells, placenta, fetal liver, and heart cells. B19 binds not only to globoside but also to several tissue-specific neutral glycophospholipids, such as those found in granulocytes, kidneys, liver, and bowel tissue (693).

Cessation of erythrocyte production, manifesting as reticulocytopenia, does not cause symptomatic anemia in otherwise healthy persons. However, patients who have reduced erythrocyte lifespans (e.g., sickle-cell anemia, thalassemia major) may develop transient aplastic crises. Patients with congenital or acquired immunodeficiency disorders may fail to clear the acute infection; a persistent B19 infection ensues, which results in chronic anemia (690). Establishment of a persistent infection sometimes can occur in persons without recognized immune deficiency disorders. A qualitatively or quantitatively aberrant immune response is thought to be responsible for this phenomenon (694). The rash and arthropathy seen in B19 infections are immune-mediated manifestations and are not directly related to the lytic infection of erythrocyte progenitor cells.

Maternal Infection

Serologic surveys have found that 30% to 60% of adults in the United States have serum antibodies against B19, indicating prior infection (695,696). B19 seroprevalence rates among pregnant women in other countries is variable; rates of 35% are reported from Barcelona, Spain, and 81% from Stockholm, Sweden (697,698). The virus is transmitted primarily by B19-infected respiratory secretions. Transmission through transfusions of blood or blood products is uncommon. One in 3,000 units of blood contains detectable amounts of B19 DNA when screened by PCR assays, but the rate can be higher during epidemic years (699). The incubation period is 4 to 14 days, but it can be as long as 20 days.

About 1% of susceptible pregnant women without known exposure to B19-infected persons seroconvert each year in the United States. Rates of 3.7% to 6.8% for acute gestational B19 infections have been reported from other countries (697,698,700). During a large erythema infectiosum outbreak in Connecticut, pregnant women were tested for serologic evidence of recent B19 infection. The highest infection rates among exposed susceptible pregnant women were for school teachers (16%), day care workers (9%), and homemakers (9%) (701). Attack rates of 36% to 38% have been documented among susceptible nursing staff who were exposed to patients with sickle-cell anemia and aplastic crisis at a children's hospital (702). However, another study of health care workers under similar circumstances showed no transmission of B19 from patients to susceptible staff members (703).

About 20% of acute B19 infections are subclinical. Erythema infectiosum is the most commonly identified B19-related condition. This illness is seen primarily in children, and its most characteristic feature is a facial exanthem (i.e., slapped-cheek appearance). The rash is lacy or reticulated, spreads to the trunk and extremities, and fades within 2 weeks. Recrudescence of the rash is observed with stimuli such as temperature changes, sunlight, or emotional stress. Pruritic, petechial, purpuric, vesicular, or erythema multiforme types of rashes are possible with acute B19 infection (690,704,705).

In addition to erythema infectiosum, acute B19 infections in otherwise healthy adults can manifest with influenza-type illnesses and symmetric polyarthropathies (e.g., polyarthralgias, polyarthritis). B19-associated joint disease is more common in women (706). Rheumatoid factor may be positive transiently; therefore the illness could be misdiagnosed as early rheumatoid arthritis (707). B19 infections in compromised patients can result in transient aplastic crises, chronic anemia, and viral-induced hemophagocytic syndrome (690).

A diagnosis of acute or recent B19 infection can be made by detecting B19-specific IgM using enzyme immunoassays. These antibodies are present in the serum of more than 90% of patients by the third day of illness. B19-specific IgM can persist for 4 months or longer in more than 75% of patients, rendering the distinction between acute or recent B19 infection on serologic grounds alone difficult (708). B19-specific IgG usually is formed by the end of the first week of the illness, and it persists for life. The detection of B19-specific antibodies of the IgG class with negative IgM test results is considered evidence of past infection and, probably, immunity to B19 reinfections. However, B19 reinfection of women known to be previously seropositive for this virus, with transmission to the fetus, leading to hydrops fetalis and fetal demise rarely have been described (709).

B19 DNA can be detected in serum and tissues by nucleic acid hybridization techniques and PCR assays (690). B19 DNA can be found in serum for 2 to 6 months after the onset of illness, but it can persist for months or years in a few patients (708,710). B19 antigens can be detected by immunofluorescence, immunoperoxidase, or enzyme immunoassays, but these methods are not widely available (711).

There is no specific treatment for B19-associated illnesses. Immunosuppressed patients with chronic anemia secondary to persistent B19 infections have benefitted from immunoglobulin intravenous (IGIV) administration (690). Scant evidence suggests that high-dose IGIV may be beneficial in preeclamptic B19-infected women with hydropic fetuses (712). Patients with erythema infectiosum are not contagious to others after the rash is evident, but those with aplastic crises continue shedding their viruses during the first few days of their hospitalization and require contact isolation.

Fetal Infection

Maternal B19 infection during pregnancy can have an adverse effect on pregnancy outcome, but most fetuses escape infection. Fetal infection can lead to hydrops fetalis or death. B19 is responsible for 8% to 18% of nonimmune hydrops cases (695,713–715). The histopathology of fetal B19 infection consists principally of infected erythroblasts with eosinophilic intranuclear inclusions, which are found mostly in the liver, spleen, and bone marrow (713,716).

Gestational B19 infections are associated with a less than 10% risk of pregnancy loss from spontaneous abortion, stillbirth, or delivery of a hydropic infant. In a British prospective study of 190 pregnant women found to be positive for B19-specific IgM during the period 1985 to 1988, the B19-related fetal death rate was estimated at 9% (717). A follow-up study of 274 pregnant women diagnosed between 1992 and 1995 again found the excess rate of B19-related fetal loss to be about 9%, but this risk was confined to the first 20 weeks of gestation; the risk of fetal hydrops in this study was 2.9% (95% CI of 1.2% to 5.9%) (718). In a case control study conducted in the United States, it was shown that B19 was not a common cause of fetal death in the general population (719).

B19 suppresses fetal bone marrow erythrocyte production, leading to chronic anemia. This is not well tolerated by the fetus because of its rapidly expanding cell volume and its immature immune system, which fails to rapidly contain the B19 infection. Congestive heart failure ensues, usually secondary to the severe anemia. Direct infection of cardiac muscles by B19 can occur and may contribute to cardiac dysfunction (720).

Koch and colleagues (721) reported on 43 pregnant women with primary B19 infection who were followed to delivery. None of the infants was hydropic. Twenty-two (51%) of the 43 infants had evidence of congenital infection as determined by finding B19 DNA, B19-specific IgM, or B19-specific IgA; one infant tested negative at birth but became positive on all three assays at 6 weeks of age. A 20% rate of intrauterine infection among asymptomatic newborns was noted by Miller and co-workers (718). Thus, it appears that intrauterine B19 infection after primary B19 infection in the mother occurs commonly, but that serious complications such as fetal

hydrops or stillbirth are infrequent. Congenital anemia and transient erythroblastopenia of the newborn are uncommon manifestations of congenital B19 infection (722,723). A few reports of twin pregnancies complicated by maternal B19 infection indicate that it is possible for one fetus to be severely affected by the virus while the other fetus can remain asymptomatic or escape infection altogether (724,725).

Congenital malformations after intrauterine B19 infection rarely have been described, and they may represent chance occurrences rather than a true teratogenic effect of B19. Hartwig and colleagues (726) described a 9-week-old embryo whose tissues were positive for B19 DNA and who had abnormalities of the eyes and damage to skeletal and smooth muscles. Rodis and associates (727) described an electively terminated pregnancy in which the B19-infected fetus had anencephaly. Tiessen and co-workers (728) found B19 DNA in several fetal tissues by PCR in an aborted fetus with cleft lip and palate, micrognathia, webbed joints, and multifocal degenerative changes of skeletal and smooth muscles. Katz and colleagues (729) described two infants with congenital malformations after maternal B19 infection. One infant had myocardial infarction, hepatic and splenic calcifications, and mild hydrocephalus, whereas the second infant had moderate hydrocephalus with dysplasia of the cerebral cortex and glial overgrowth. If B19 is a true teratogen, the associated risk must be small. One case report described a hydropic fetus that died at 24 weeks of gestation after his mother had developed primary B19 infection (730). The fetus had a flat nose and low implanted deformed ears. Upon detailed examination, these dysmorphic features were found to be due to a partial trisomy 3q and a partial monosomy 11q resulting from a balanced translocation between chromosomes 3 and 11 in the mother. This report suggests that some of the rare congenital malformations noted in the offspring of B19-infected women may be related to small chromosomal abnormalities that can be missed unless a careful evaluation is undertaken. Some infants without obvious dysmorphic features had ileal stenosis or atresia with resultant meconium peritonitis after maternal B19 infection (724,731).

The diagnosis of intrauterine B19 infection in a newly born infant is difficult and rests on detection of B19-specific IgM in serum or B19 DNA in the fetal blood or tissues. Parvovirus particles can be observed in tissues by electron microscopy (715,732–734).

Management of hydropic newborns is supportive and almost invariably includes packed erythrocyte transfusions. There are no recognized long-term sequelae for healthy infants born to mothers with gestational B19 infection (718,735).

Prevention

Pregnant women who sustain a significant exposure to a B19-associated illness at home (e.g., erythema infectiosum in a child) and whose B19 antibody status is unknown can be informed that their overall risk of fetal death is at most 2.5%. This figure can be arrived at by multiplying the rate of susceptibility (about 50%), the rate at which exposed susceptible persons acquire B19 infection (maximum of 50%), and the estimated rate of death in documented infection (9%). Had the exposure taken place in a school or day care setting, the risk would decline to less than 1.5%.

Some investigators have suggested the use of IGIV for postexposure prophylaxis of B19-susceptible pregnant women (736). Commercial IGIV preparations contain anti-B19 IgG antibodies, and they have been shown to be helpful in the treatment of immunosuppressed patients with B19-induced chronic anemia. There are no data to support or refute the use of IGIV for the prevention or amelioration of B19 infection.

If acute or recent B19 infection is confirmed in the pregnant woman by a positive B19-specific IgM assay, serial ultrasound examinations should be performed for the detection of early signs indicative of fetal hydrops or, rarely, meconium peritonitis (724,731,737). Maternal serum alpha-fetoprotein elevations have been observed in pregnancies with B19-related adverse fetal outcomes such as hydrops, but this has been an inconsistent finding (738,739).

Limited published experience suggests that the prenatal diagnosis of fetal B19 infection is possible and accurate (740–746). B19 can be demonstrated in fetal blood by electron microscopy, molecular biological techniques, or detection of B19-specific IgM antibodies. Török and colleagues (743) used the sensitive PCR assay to detect B19 DNA in amniotic fluid and fetal blood. Fifteen mothers who were positive for B19-specific IgM were evaluated. Eight of 15 fetuses were positive for B19 DNA only, and the other seven were positive for B19 DNA and B19-specific IgM. Nine (60%) fetuses had hydrops. Ten infants were born healthy, including four found to have hydrops at 17 to 23 weeks of gestation, which resolved without specific intervention. PCR detected B19 DNA in the sera of 20% of mothers with negative B19-specific IgM assay results, with or without B19-specific IgG; one-half of the fetal specimens corresponding to this group of mothers were B19 DNA positive by PCR (743).

Zerbini and associates (746) studied 18 fetuses with B19-related hydrops fetalis and could detect B19 DNA by nested PCR in nine maternal sera. The less sensitive dot blot hybridization assay failed to detect B19 DNA in any of these specimens. For the 18 hydropic fetuses, B19 DNA was detected in blood obtained at cordocentesis in 62% by PCR and 40% by dot blot hybridization. However, 100% of cell smears prepared from fetal blood were positive for B19 DNA using *in situ* hybridization. In contrast, only 15% of fetal blood samples were positive for B19-specific IgM. When amniotic fluid was tested for B19 DNA, 83% were found to be positive by PCR, 20%

by dot blot hybridization, and 70% by *in situ* hybridization (746). Thus, a combination of virologic and serologic tests may be needed to ensure an accurate diagnosis of intrauterine B19 infection.

Some B19-infected pregnant women may remain negative for B19-specific IgM and IgG antibodies, despite the detection of B19 particles in serum and saliva using electron microscopy or the detection of B19 DNA using PCR or other techniques (743,747). B19 infection of their newborns may or may not be symptomatic.

Fetal therapy with intrauterine blood transfusions or digitalization has been attempted in some infants (695,740–742,748–750). The indications for intrauterine transfusion are not well defined (751). Fetal hydrops can resolve spontaneously before birth in as many as one-third of patients without specific intervention (752–754). All of these infants remained well after birth and during several months of follow-up (743,752–754). This indicates that fetal hydrops is not uniformly fatal if not treated and that some fetuses are capable of eventually resolving their B19 infection and reversing the observed pathophysiologic abnormalities.

Candidate B19 vaccines are in development or in early trials. A commercially available product is not expected for several years to come (690).

HUMAN IMMUNODEFICIENCY VIRUS TYPE 1 INFECTION

In 1997, HIV-1 infections accounted for 32% of deaths due to infectious diseases (a decline of 62% from 1995 rates) and 0.7% of deaths from all causes in the United States (5.9 deaths per 100,000 population) (755). A similar trend of declining AIDS-related mortality was observed across Europe for the period from March 1995 to March 1998. The mortality rate (expressed as deaths per 100 person-years of follow-up) was 65.4, 7.5, and 3.4 for persons on no antiretroviral therapy, dual-drug therapy, or triple-combination therapy, respectively (756).

The global impact of HIV-1 infection is staggering. It is estimated that HIV-1 had infected 30 million people by the end of 1996, 11 million of whom were women and 3 million of whom were children. Ninety-four percent of these infections occurred in developing countries, and 70% of adult infections were the result of heterosexual transmission (757). By the year 2000, the World Health Organization estimates that there will be 40 million people around the world living with HIV-1 (758). Perinatal HIV-1 infection killed 2.7 million children under 15 years of age between 1982 and 1997. In 1997 alone, approximately 590,000 children acquired this infection, 460,000 died from AIDS, and 1.1 million children were still living with various stages of their HIV-1 infection. Moreover, about 8.2 million children were orphaned by HIV-1 infection (758). Globally, half of all new cases of HIV-1 are being reported in women compared with a rate of 22% for the United States (14,757).

Perinatal HIV-1 infection in the United States has accounted for 7,310 (1%) of the 626,334 total AIDS cases reported to the CDC as of September 30, 1997 (15). New York, Florida, New Jersey, California, and Puerto Rico accounted for 64% of these cases. A disproportionate number of perinatally infected infants were non-Hispanic black (61%), 24% were Hispanic, and 14% were non-Hispanic white. The median age at diagnosis was 17 months, with 40% being diagnosed during infancy (15). The number of children with newly diagnosed perinatal AIDS declined by 43% between 1992 and 1996, most likely the result of increased use of zidovudine to prevent vertical transmission of HIV-1.

HIV-1 is one of several known human retroviruses. It is a single stranded, enveloped RNA virus that is composed of inner core proteins (p18, p24, and p27), surface proteins (gp120, gp41), genomic RNA, and enzymes such as reverse transcriptase and protease. The virion contains three structural genes (*gag, pol,* and *env*) and regulatory-genes (*tat, vif, nef, vpu, vpr,* and *rev*). HIV-1 requires a cell-surface glycoprotein known as CD4 for viral entry into cells. CD4 is found on the subset of T lymphocytes referred to as helper T cells, as well as on macrophages and other cell types (e.g., placenta, CNS cells). Other cell surface molecules (chemokine receptors) serve as coreceptors for HIV-1 entry into cells. Genetic variants of HIV-1 may preferentially bind to different coreceptors. For example, HIV-1 variants that induce syncytium formation depend on the receptor molecule CXCR4, whereas the nonsyncytium-inducing variants use CCR5 coreceptors (759–761). The absence of CCR5 in about 1% of Caucasians, due to homozygosity for a 32-nucleotide deletion in the coding region (*CCR5Δ32* allele), protects against HIV-1 transmission. Heterozygosity for this allele delays disease progression (762). More recently, other chemokine receptors used by HIV-1 have been described (e.g., *CCR-2b, CCR-3,* and *CCR-8*) (761,763). Patients considered to be long-term nonprogressors also tend to have lower amounts of circulating HIV-1 RNA, and their activated CD8 lymphocytes may help suppress viral replication through the release of inhibitory chemokines such as RANTES, MIP-1α, and MIP-1β (761). HIV-1 infection leads to gradual but progressive CD4 T-cell depletion, which renders patients susceptible to a variety of opportunistic infections and malignancies.

Major strides have been made in the prevention of perinatal HIV-1 infection in the last few years. The most pivotal has been the demonstration that the risk of vertical transmission can be reduced significantly by administration of zidovudine during pregnancy, at delivery, and to newborns (764). The CDC subsequently recommended use of zidovudine to reduce perinatal transmission of the virus (765). Use of PCR assays has allowed the diagnosis of HIV-1 infection in early infancy, and the availability of antiviral drugs active at various sites in the viral replication cycle has allowed more potent drug combinations to be provided to infected patients. Viral load monitoring now provides a measure of how successful our therapeutic regimens are in suppressing viral replication for the individual patient, and HIV-1 strains can be examined for mutations associated with resistance to specific antiretroviral agents (766–768).

Maternal Infection

Women accounted for about 22% of AIDS cases reported to the CDC in 1997 (14). It is projected that more than 100,000 women aged 15 to 44 years were living with HIV-1 infection in the United States in 1994, and that only 15% had developed AIDS (769). The HIV-1 seroprevalence among women of child-bearing age varies by state. It ranges from a low of about 0 per 1,000 in Wyoming to highs of 6.9 and 5.2 per 1,000 for the District of Columbia and New York State, respectively. Five states (New York, Florida, California, New Jersey, and Texas) accounted for 60% of all births to HIV-1-infected women in 1994. The overall seroprevalence for this group of American women has remained stable at 1.5 to 1.7 per 1,000 between 1989 and 1994; however, it had decreased significantly in the northeast (from 4.1 to 3.2 per 1,000 women) and increased in the south (from 1.6 to 2.0 per 1,000 women) during that period. Seroprevalence rates for African-American women are 15- to 20-fold higher than for white women, with intermediate rates noted for Hispanic women (769). African-American and Hispanic women account for 77% of all HIV-1 infections among women of child-bearing age (770). Most women acquire HIV-1 infection during sexual intercourse with infected men who themselves had acquired the virus either sexually or from injecting drug use. Injecting drug use among women is another route of HIV-1 infection, and it had been their leading mode of transmission before 1993 (770). The odds of HIV-1 infection increase, depending on the high-risk behaviors practiced: use of crack cocaine, multiple sexual partners, sexual intercourse with a high-risk partner, presence of other sexually transmitted diseases, and low level of condom use (771,772).

HIV-1 screening programs targeted at patients who acknowledge high-risk behavior generally fail to identify most HIV-1–infected pregnant women (773,774). Screening should be offered to all pregnant women. With proper education, the majority of women offered antenatal HIV-1 testing agree to being screened for this virus (775). With nondirective counseling about options for terminating or continuing pregnancy, 85% of HIV-1–infected women elect to continue their pregnancies (773,776).

Many studies have examined for any consequences that HIV-1 infection might have on pregnancy outcome, and most have found no significant effects. Maternal HIV-1 infection may increase the rate of spontaneous fetal loss, but the prevalence of premature delivery, fetal growth retardation, and early neonatal disease is comparable to that of infants born to HIV-1–uninfected mothers (760,777). Pregnancy itself has a marginal effect, if any, on accelerating the progression of HIV-1 infection in women (760,778–780). In one study of 160 HIV-1–infected women, HIV-1 RNA viral loads did not change significantly during the pregnancy (780).

Mother-to-Infant Transmission

Vertical transmission of HIV-1 can occur *in utero*, intrapartum, or postpartum (through breast-feeding). Most infants in the United States acquire HIV-1 infection at the time of delivery (3).

Intrauterine transmission accounts for about one-third of all vertically infected infants. Although the frequency of transmission by trimester of pregnancy is not known, most *in utero* infections occur less than 2 months before delivery (3). Second-trimester fetal blood sampling performed on HIV-1–infected women scheduled for elective pregnancy termination confirmed the low rate of early *in utero* HIV-1 fetal infections (781,782).

Many studies have examined maternal and obstetric factors that increase the risk of vertical HIV-1 transmission. Not all risk factors have been identified consistently as such in every study, but there are definite patterns that have been observed. Maternal factors that enhance the risk of HIV-1 transmission to infants include advanced stage of maternal infection, low CD4 absolute cell count or percentage, elevated CD8 cell count or percentage, high viral load, p24 antigenemia, illicit drug use, coinfection by other sexually transmitted diseases, low titers or avidity of maternal HIV-1 antibodies, and infection by certain HIV-1 genotypes or phenotypes. Maternal vitamin A deficiency is a risk factor for vertical HIV-1 transmission in developing countries. Obstetric factors favoring HIV-1 vertical transmission include premature delivery, vaginal delivery, cervicovaginal HIV-1 viral load, maternofetal blood transfusions, longer (more than 4 hours) durations of membrane rupture, chorioamnionitis, and use of invasive fetal monitoring devices (783—792). For twins born to HIV-1–infected mothers, the first infant delivered, whether vaginally or by cesarean section, is at least twice as likely to be infected as the second-born twin (793). This may be due to more intense exposure of the first born to HIV-infected genital secretions. de Martino and associates (794) could not confirm these observations in their studies of twins born to HIV-1–infected mothers. They did observe that, if the first-born twin became infected, 42% of their second-born siblings were infected. If the first-born twin escaped HIV-1 infection, only 13% of their second-born siblings were infected (794).

An infant is considered to have early (i.e., *in utero*) infection if the HIV-1 genome is detected by PCR or if HIV-1 is isolated from blood within 48 hours of birth. Positive results should be confirmed with at least one sample obtained after the neonatal period. An infant is considered to have late (i.e., intrapartum) infection if diagnostic studies (e.g., HIV-1 isolation, PCR, serum p24 antigen assays) are negative in blood samples obtained during the first week of life but become positive during the period from day 7 to 90, and the infant has not been breast-fed. Care should be exercised to avoid contaminating cord blood with maternal blood (795).

In the United States, breast-feeding of infants by infected mothers is not recommended. Postnatal HIV-1 transmission rates by breast-feeding are 8% to 18%, but can be as high as 13% to 39% (mean 26%) when mothers acquire their HIV-1 infection while lactating (796). Both HIV-1–infected cells as well as cell-free virus are found in breast milk (796,797). Cell-free virus more commonly is found in mature milk than in colostrum (797). In 1998, the World Health Organization recommended that HIV-1–infected women in developing countries be provided information about the benefits and risks of breast-feeding so that they can make an informed decision regarding nutrition for their infants.

Vertical HIV transmission has been reported to occur at various rates in different areas of the world. A report by the 19-center European Collaborative Study provided a rate of 14.4% among a cohort of 721 children followed for 18 months or longer (798). A similar rate of 14% to 20% was observed in a nationwide study of a cohort of 286 children born to HIV-1–positive mothers in Switzerland (799). The rate is about 25% to 30% in the United States for women not receiving zidovudine prophylaxis (764,800). Rates as high as 50% have been reported from African countries such as Zaire and Kenya (801).

Multiple HIV-1 variants exist in infected persons. These variants arise through errors in reverse transcription and by recombination during retroviral replication. Because of the high turnover rate in the HIV-1 population (more than 10 billion virions are generated daily) and the high error frequency during replication (estimated at 3.4×10^{-5}), a large number of variants is generated. These variants subsequently undergo selective pressure from cellular tropism, host immune responses, and antiretroviral therapy. Only a small subset of the HIV-1 variants is transmitted from the mother to her infant, but it can include HIV-1 strains that carry specific drug-resistance mutations (802–805).

Treatment

Women should receive antiretroviral therapy appropriate for their stage of infection without regard to whether or not they are pregnant. However, the potential impact of such therapy on the fetus is largely unknown. Women who are in their first trimester of pregnancy and who are not already receiving antiretroviral agents may consider delaying initiation of therapy until after 10 to 12 weeks of gestation (806).

Available antiretroviral drugs are classified by the Food and Drug Administration as being in Pregnancy Category B (didanosine, saquinavir, ritonavir, and nelfinavir) or Pregnancy Category C (zidovudine, zalcitabine, stavudine, abacavir, indinavir, nevirapine, delavirdine, and efavirenz). Information on transplacental passage in humans is available for zidovudine, didanosine, lamivudine, and nevirapine. Cord blood concentrations of zidovudine, lamivudine, and nevirapine are similar to those observed in maternal blood at delivery. In primate studies, didanosine and zalcitabine have significantly less placental transfer than zidovudine, stavudine, or lamivudine (806). Single-dose studies of nevirapine (a nonnucleoside reverse transcriptase inhibitor that can prevent HIV-1 infection in experimentally challenged chimpanzees) in HIV-1–infected women in labor and their newborns show that one 200-mg dose of the drug given to the mother results in very high cord blood levels. If a single 2 mg/kg dose is given to their infants at 48 to 72 hours of life, then the high serum concentrations can be maintained through 7 days of life without any apparent adverse effects (807).

Zidovudine is the only antiretroviral agent to date that has been shown to reduce the risk of perinatal HIV-1 transmission. If the maternal antiretroviral treatment regimen does not include zidovudine, then the drug should be added whenever possible. If the mother is on stavudine, then zidovudine should not be given antenatally but it should still be administered intravenously intrapartum and subsequently given to the newborn infant (806).

The safety and efficacy of zidovudine as a chemoprophylactic agent against the vertical transmission of HIV-1 was demonstrated in a double-blind, placebo-controlled trial known as the Pediatric AIDS Clinical Trials Group (PACTG) Protocol 076 (764,808). Pregnant women who were HIV-1 positive and whose CD4 T-lymphocyte counts were higher than 200 cells per cubic millimeter were enrolled if they had no other indication for antiretroviral therapy and were between 14 and 34 weeks of gestation. Zidovudine (or matching placebo) was given antenatally at a dose of 100 mg orally five times daily followed by intravenous zidovudine during labor (2 mg/kg of body weight given over 1 hour, followed by 1 mg/kg/h until delivery). The newborns received zidovudine at a dose of 2 mg/kg orally every 6 hours beginning at 8 to 12 hours of age, which was continued for 6 weeks. The final analysis of this study included 402 mother–infant pairs. The rate of HIV-1 transmission was 7.6% (95% CI of 4.3% to 12.3%) with zidovudine treatment and 22.6% (95% CI of 17% to 29%) with placebo. The difference was very significant statistically (808). The study noted that women in the placebo group with large viral burdens were more likely to transmit HIV-1 to their newborns (41% risk for those with more than 15,700 HIV-1 RNA copies per milliliter using the RT-PCR assay or more than 7,530 HIV-1 RNA copies per milliliter using a second-generation branched-chain DNA signal amplification assay). The rate of transmission in the zidovudine-treated cohort was lower than that for the placebo group for women with comparable HIV-1 RNA viral load measurements. Interestingly, the reduced vertical transmission noted with zidovudine was found not be due to a reduction of viral RNA from baseline to delivery (808).

This study raised several important and practical questions. What part of the treatment protocol (antenatal, intrapartum, or postpartum) was most critical for reducing HIV-1 transmission to newborns? Could similar results be obtained using shorter (and thus less expensive) protocols that could be implemented in developing countries with scarce resources and with the bulk of the global HIV-1 burden? Could similar results be obtained in women with more advanced HIV-1 infections? Would the regimen work in women who harbor zidovudine-resistant HIV-1 strains? Would other antiretroviral agents work as well, or perhaps better? Would combination antiretroviral therapy be more efficacious in reducing HIV-1 transmission to newborns?

Since the results of PACTG 076 became available, several studies have documented increased zidovudine use during pregnancy and in newborns (809,810). Other studies have confirmed that pregnant women receiving zidovudine were less likely to transmit HIV-1 to their offspring (809–814).

The New York State Department of Health examined the risks of perinatal HIV-1 transmission for 939 exposed infants whose mothers received abbreviated zidovudine treatment regimens during pregnancy. The study found that the risk of HIV-1 infection for infants whose mothers received no zidovudine was 26.6% (95% CI of 21.1% to 32.7%). When treatment was started antenatally, the risk of perinatal HIV-1 transmission dropped to 6.1% (95% CI of 4.1% to 8.9%). When started intrapartum, the rate increased to 10% (95% CI of 3.3% to 21.8%). When started within the first 48 hours of life, the rate was 9.3% (95% CI of 4.1% to 17.5%); and when started at 72 hours of life or later, the rate was 18.4% (95% CI of 7.7% to 34.3%) (815). Therefore, zidovudine should be given during labor or the early neonatal period even to women who received no antenatal therapy.

A randomized, placebo-controlled trial of zidovudine prophylaxis for the prevention of perinatal HIV-1 infection was performed in Thailand using a simpler and less expensive protocol. Pregnant women received zidovudine at a dose of 300 mg orally twice daily beginning at 36 weeks of gestation until onset of labor, followed by 300 mg orally every 3 hours from onset of labor to delivery. Women were advised not to breast-feed their infants. Interim analysis of the data on 397 women revealed that the risk of perinatal HIV-1 transmission was 18.6% (95% CI of 13% to 24%) in the placebo recipients compared with 9.2% (95% CI of 5% to 13.5%) in the zidovudine-treated mothers, representing a 51% decrease in HIV-1 transmission (816).

Other approaches to the prevention of perinatal HIV-1 transmission are being explored. These include the administration of hyperimmune anti–HIV-1 immunoglobulin to infected mothers and their newborns, the use of lamivudine alone or in combination with zidovudine during pregnancy, and the use of nevirapine beginning at 38 weeks of gestation (765,817,818). The combined use of elective cesarean delivery and zidovudine may provide additive protective effects (819).

The CDC currently recommends that all HIV-1–infected pregnant women be offered antenatal and intrapartum zidovudine prophylaxis and that their newborns be treated for 6 weeks, using the dosage regimens utilized in PACTG 076 as outlined earlier (765). Women who do not receive antenatal zidovudine because of non-life-threatening serious drug-related toxicity or personal choice still should receive the drug intrapartum and their newborns should be treated (806). Zidovudine dosing for premature newborns (less than 34 weeks of gestation) has not been determined, but the CDC is evaluating a regimen of 1.5 mg/kg given orally or intravenously every 12 hours for the first 2 weeks of life, followed by a dose of 2 mg/kg every 8 hours for infants 2 to 6 weeks of age (765). The newborns should have a complete blood count done before zidovudine initiation and again at 6 weeks of age at the minimum. If anemia develops, a repeat hemoglobin measurement at 12 weeks of age usually shows resolution of zidovudine-related hematologic toxicity. Infants should begin *Pneumocystis carinii* prophylaxis at 6 weeks of life, upon completion of zidovudine therapy, using trimethoprim-sulfamethoxazole (given at a dose of 150 mg/M^2/d of the trimethoprim component in two divided doses, and administered three times per week on consecutive days) (820). The daily dose of trimethoprim-sulfamethoxazole also can be given as a single dose (instead of two divided doses), or it can be given 7 days per week (instead of on three consecutive days each week), or it can be given in two divided daily doses but administered three times per week on alternate days (820). Dapsone at a dose of 2 mg/kg can be given once daily to infants intolerant of trimethoprim-sulfamethoxazole. This is continued until the diagnosis of perinatal HIV-1 infection is excluded.

Fetal and Neonatal Infection

Congenitally infected infants usually are asymptomatic during the neonatal period, although detectable subtle signs such as lymphadenopathy and hepatosplenomegaly have been observed in 2% to 8% of cases, and some infants have been born with evidence of cerebral atrophy (821,822). Kaposi sarcoma presenting within the first month of life has been described rarely in HIV-1–infected infants (823). The clinical latency period to development of AIDS is shorter than that for adults; the median age at perinatal AIDS diagnosis was 17 months for the 7,310 children reported to the CDC through September 30, 1997 (15). About one-fourth of all perinatally infected infants develop AIDS by 1 year of age, and 40% to 50% do so by age 3 to 4 years; 33% of all perinatally infected patients remain free of AIDS by 13 years of age. About 10% of all HIV-1–infected infants die by age 1 year, and 25% to 30% by age 5 years (824–826). Higher HIV-1 viral loads have been shown to correlate with more rapid progression to AIDS. The slowest progression occurs in infants with low viral loads (plasma RNA levels of less than 10,000 copies per milliliter) and high CD4 counts (827–830). Infants with intrauterine HIV-1 infection are 2.5-fold (95% CI of 1.1 to 5.8) more likely to progress to AIDS or death than those with intrapartum HIV-1 infection (830a).

The diagnosis of HIV-1 infection during the neonatal period or early infancy is difficult (831,832). Measurement of HIV-1–specific IgG is not useful because of passive transplacental passage of this antibody and its persistence for several months. The median age to clearance of passively acquired HIV-1 antibodies is 13 months (range 10 to 16) (833). Positive HIV-1 antibody test results in those younger than 18 months of age indicate maternal infection but cannot diagnose infection in the infant (834). Although positive HIV-1 antibody test results in toddlers 18 months of age or older generally are considered indicative of infection, the reverse may not be true. Some infants with virologic evidence of HIV-1 infection can have negative or indeterminate serologic test results at 18 to 24 months of age (835). A few infants who serorevert to an HIV-1–seronegative status in early infancy may actually be HIV-1 infected, and close follow-up is required (836,837). Virus coculture methods, p24 antigen detection, immune complex dissociation, and HIV-1–specific IgM and IgA measurements are all hampered by low sensitivities in the first weeks of life (838–842). Assays for HIV-1–specific IgA during the first month of life detect fewer than 10% of HIV-1–infected infants, but their sensitivities increase to 60% for 3-month-old infants and to 77% to 100% at 6 months of age or older (840,841).

The early diagnosis of HIV-1 infection can be accomplished by using a DNA PCR assay (843,844). The sensitivity and specificity of PCR is somewhat higher in older infants than in neonates (844). For infants at low risk of perinatal HIV-1 transmission, the positive predictive value for PCR is about 56% for neonates and 83% for older infants. Approximately 30% to 50% of HIV-1–infected infants are DNA PCR positive at birth, which suggests intrauterine infection, and about 50% to 70% of infected infants have negative DNA PCR results at birth but become positive after 7 days of age, which suggests intrapartum transmission of the virus (845). Plasma HIV-1 RNA assays seem to be more sensitive and are positive earlier in the newborn period than DNA PCR assays (846). The PCR can be falsely positive if contamination with maternal blood occurs or if there is cross contamination from other blood specimens in the laboratory.

Infants exposed to HIV-1 should be tested by PCR or viral cultures at birth and again at 1 to 2 months of age. If either test result is positive for HIV-1, it should be repeated immediately for confirmation. If results of tests taken at birth and at 1 to 2 months are negative and the infant remains asymptomatic, the PCR or viral culture should be repeated at 4 months of age. A negative test result at 4 months of age or later provides more than 95% assurance that the infant is not infected with HIV-1. Continued follow-up serologic testing should be performed until disappearance of passively transferred maternal antibodies. An exposed infant is considered uninfected when there are no physical findings suggestive of HIV-1 infection, virologic test results are negative, immunologic test results (CD4 count and percentage) are normal, and, after the infant is 12 months of age or older, two or more HIV-1 antibody test results are negative (834). Follow-up of HIV-1–uninfected infants who were exposed *in utero* to maternal zidovudine prophylactic therapy have shown no drug-related ill effects 3 to 5.6 years later (846a).

Antiretroviral treatment should be started in all HIV-1–infected infants younger than 1 year of age as soon as the diagnosis is confirmed, regardless of clinical or immunologic status or viral load results, because they are considered to be at high risk of disease progression. Treatment with three drugs (preferably two nucleoside reverse transcriptase inhibitors and one protease inhibitor) is recommended, as this affords the infected infant the best opportunity to preserve immune function and delay disease progression by maximally suppressing viral replication (to undetectable levels, if possible) (820). A variety of alternative antiretroviral drug regimens can be prescribed, but the cumulative experience with their use in infants is limited.

The most common AIDS-defining conditions in pediatric patients are *P. carinii* pneumonia, lymphoid interstitial hyperplasia, recurrent bacterial infections, HIV-1 wasting syndrome, candidiasis, and HIV-1 encephalopathy (824,826), Other problems may include *Mycobacterium avium-intracellulare* infections, tuberculosis, CMV retinitis, disseminated HSV infection, herpes zoster, toxoplasmosis, extrapulmonary cryptococcosis, and cryptosporidiosis. *P. carinii* pneumonia can occur at any age, but it is diagnosed most commonly in young infants not receiving appropriate prophylaxis. Lymphoid interstitial hyperplasia is a chronic lung disease that results from the proliferation of lymphoid tissue in the interstitium of the lungs leading to tachypnea, hypoxia, and digital clubbing (847). Progressive encephalopathy can be the first manifestation of HIV-1 infection in 10% to 15% of patients, and can range in severity from minor developmental delays to severe CNS involvement. Ventricular enlargement is the most common finding, followed by cortical atrophy, attenuation of periventricular white matter, and cerebral calcifications (848). Impaired linear growth occurs early and appears to be more pronounced in infants with higher viral loads (849,850). Parotitis occurs in one-third of children surviving for 5 years or longer (851). Infusions of IGIV every 4 weeks can reduce the risk of serious and minor viral and bacterial infections (852). HIV-1–infected infants should receive all childhood immunizations with the exception of the oral poliomyelitis vaccine (inactivated poliomyelitis vaccine should be given instead) and the varicella vaccine. The live, attenuated measles–mumps–rubella vaccine can be given to HIV-1–infected infants who are not severely immunodeficient based on their absolute CD4 cell count or percentage. The influenza vaccine should be given every season for infants 6 months of age or older (834).

REFERENCES

1. Atmar RL, Englund JA, Hammill H. Complications of measles during pregnancy. *Clin Infect Dis* 1992;14:217.
2. Zeichner SL, Plotkin SA. Mechanisms and pathways of congenital infections. *Clin Perinatol* 1988;15:163.
3. Newell M-L. Mechanisms and timing of mother-to-child transmission of HIV-1. *AIDS* 1998;12:831.
4. Tseng C-J, Liang C-C, Soong Y-K, Pao C-C. Perinatal transmission of human papillomavirus in infants: relationship between infection rate and mode of delivery. *Obstet Gynecol* 1998;91:92.
5. Hershow RC, Riester KA, Lew J, et al. Increased vertical transmission of human immunodeficiency virus from hepatitis C virus-coinfected mothers. *J Infect Dis* 1997;176:414.
6. Freij BJ, Sever JL. Congenital viral infections. *Curr Opin Infect Dis* 1992;5:558.
7. Freij BJ, South MA, Sever JL. Maternal rubella and the congenital rubella syndrome. *Clin Perinatol* 1988;15:247.
8. Shapiro CN, Margolis HS. Impact of hepatitis B virus infection on women and children. *Infect Dis Clin North Am* 1992;6:75.
9. Bortolotti F, Resti M, Giacchino R, et al. Hepatitis C virus infection and related liver disease in children of mothers with antibodies to the virus. *J Pediatr* 1997;130:990.
10. Freij BJ, Sever JL. Herpesvirus infections in pregnancy: risks to embryo, fetus, and neonate. *Clin Perinatol* 1988;15:203.
11. Sánchez PJ. Congenital syphilis. *Adv Pediatr Infect Dis* 1992;7:161.
12. Dobbins JG, Stewart JA, Demmler GJ, and the Collaborating Registry Group. Surveillance of congenital cytomegalovirus disease, 1990–1991. *MMWR* 1992;41(SS-2):35.
13. Remington JS, McLeod R, Desmonts G. Toxoplasmosis. In: Remington JS, Klein JO, eds. *Infectious diseases of the fetus and newborn infant*, 4th ed. Philadelphia: WB Saunders, 1995:140.
14. Centers for Disease Control and Prevention. Summary of notifiable diseases, United States, 1997. *MMWR* 1997;46(54):1.
15. Centers for Disease Control and Prevention. Update: perinatally acquired HIV/AIDS—United States, 1997. *MMWR* 1997;46:1086.
16. Whitley RJ, Arvin AM. Herpes simplex virus infections. In: Remington JS, Klein JO, eds. *Infectious diseases of the fetus and newborn infant*, 4th ed. Philadelphia: WB Saunders, 1995:354.
17. Lindegren ML, Fehrs LJ, Hadler SC, Hinman AR. Update: rubella and congenital rubella syndrome, 1980–1990. *Epidemiol Rev* 1991;13:341.
18. Cochi SL, Edmonds LE, Dyer K, et al. Congenital rubella syndrome in the United States, 1970–1985: on the verge of elimination. *Am J Epidemiol* 1989;129:349.
19. Centers for Disease Control and Prevention. Recommendations for prevention and control of hepatitis C virus (HCV) infection and HCV-related chronic disease. *MMWR* 1998;47(RR-19):1.
20. Kinney JS, Kumar ML. Should we expand the TORCH complex? A description of clinical and diagnostic aspects of selected old and new agents. *Clin Perinatol* 1988;15:727.
21. Alpert G, Plotkin SA. A practical guide to the diagnosis of congenital infections in the newborn infant. *Pediatr Clin North Am* 1986;33:465.
22. Greenough A. The TORCH screen and intrauterine infections. *Arch Dis Child Fetal Neonatal Ed* 1994;70:F163.

23. Cullen A, Brown S, Cafferkey M, et al. Current use of the TORCH screen in the diagnosis of congenital infection. *J Infect* 1998;36:185.

24. Gutman LT. The spirochetes. In: Joklik WK, Willett HP, Amos DB, Wilfert CM, eds. *Zinsser microbiology*, 20th ed. Norwalk: Appleton & Lange, 1992:657.

25. Blanco DR, Miller JN, Lovett MA. Surface antigens of the syphilis spirochete and their potential as virulence determinants. *Emerg Infect Dis* 1997;3:11.

26. Hook EW III, Marra CM. Acquired syphilis in adults. *N Engl J Med* 1992;326:1060.

27. Baughn RE. Role of fibronectin in the pathogenesis of syphilis. *Rev Infect Dis* 1987;9:S372.

28. Nelson KE, Vlahov D, Cohn S, et al. Sexually transmitted diseases in a population of intravenous drug users: association with seropositivity to the human immunodeficiency virus (HIV). *J Infect Dis* 1991;164:457.

29. Sánchez PJ, Wendel GD. Syphilis in pregnancy. *Clin Perinatol* 1997; 24:71.

30. Dobson SRM, Taber LH, Baughn RE. Recognition of Treponema pallidum antigens by IgM and IgG antibodies in congenitally infected newborns and their mothers. *J Infect Dis* 1988;157:903.

31. Wicher V, Zabek J, Wicher K. Pathogen-specific humoral response in Treponema pallidum-infected humans, rabbits, and guinea pigs. *J Infect Dis* 1991;163:830.

32. Sánchez PJ, McCracken GH Jr, Wendel GD, et al. Molecular analysis of the fetal IgM response to Treponema pallidum antigens: implications for improved serodiagnosis of congenital syphilis. *J Infect Dis* 1989;159:508.

33. Lewis LL, Taber LH, Baughn RE. Evaluation of immunoglobulin M Western blot analysis in the diagnosis of congenital syphilis. *J Clin Microbiol* 1990;28:296.

34. Larsen SA, Steiner BM, Rudolph AH. Laboratory diagnosis and interpretation of tests for syphilis. *Clin Microbiol Rev* 1995;8:1.

35. Borenstein LA, Selsted ME, Lehrer RI, Miller JN. Antimicrobial activity of rabbit leukocyte defensins against Treponema pallidum subsp. pallidum. *Infect Immun* 1991;59:1359.

36. Borenstein LA, Ganz T, Sell S, et al. Contribution of rabbit leukocyte defensins to the host response in experimental syphilis. *Infect Immun* 1991;59:1368.

37. Fitzgerald TJ. The Th$_1$/Th$_2$-like switch in syphilitic infection: is it detrimental? *Infect Immun* 1992;60:3475.

38. Baker-Zander SA, Lukehart SA. Macrophage-mediated killing of opsonized Treponema pallidum. *J Infect Dis* 1992;165:69.

39. Baughn RE, Jiang A, Abraham R, et al. Molecular mimicry between an immunodominant amino acid motif on the 47-kDa lipoprotein of Treponema pallidum (Tpp47) and multiple repeats of analogous sequences in fibronectin. *J Immunol* 1996;157:720.

40. Wicher K, Abbruscato F, Wicher V, et al. Identification of persistent infection in experimental syphilis by PCR. *Infect Immun* 1998;66:2509.

41. Nakashima AK, Rolfs RT, Flock ML, et al. Epidemiology of syphilis in the United States, 1941–1993. *Sex Transm Dis* 1996;23:16.

42. St. Louis ME, Wasserheit JN. Elimination of syphilis in the United States. *Science* 1998;281:353.

43. Centers for Disease Control and Prevention. Epidemic of congenital syphilis—Baltimore, 1996–1997. *MMWR* 1998;47:904.

44. Rolfs RT, Goldberg M, Sharrar RG. Risk factors for syphilis: cocaine use and prostitution. *Am J Public Health* 1990;80:853.

45. Andrus JK, Fleming DW, Harger DR, et al. Partner notification: can it control epidemic syphilis? *Ann Intern Med* 1990;112:539.

46. Webber MP, Lambert G, Bateman DA, Hauser WA. Maternal risk factors for congenital syphilis: a case-control study. *Am J Epidemiol* 1993;137:415.

47. Coles FB, Hipp SS, Silberstein GS, Chen J-H. Congenital syphilis surveillance in upstate New York, 1989–1992: implications for prevention and clinical management. *J Infect Dis* 1995;171:732.

48. Sison CG, Ostrea EM Jr, Reyes MP, Salari V. The resurgence of congenital syphilis: a cocaine-related problem. *J Pediatr* 1997;130:289.

49. Mascola L, Pelosi R, Blount JH, et al. Congenital syphilis: why is it still occurring? *JAMA* 1984;252:1719.

50. Ricci JM, Fojaco RM, O'Sullivan MJ. Congenital syphilis: the University of Miami/Jackson Memorial Medical Center experience, 1986–1988. *Obstet Gynecol* 1989;74:687.

51. Ong KR, Rubin S, Brome-Bunting M, Labes K. Congenital syphilis in New York City: 1985–1990. *N Y State J Med* 1991;91:531.

52. Tseng CK, Hughes MA, Hsu P-L, et al. Syphilis superinfection activates expression of human immunodeficiency virus 1 in latently infected rabbits. *Am J Pathol* 1991;138:1149.

53. Marra CM, Handsfield HH, Kuller L, et al. Alterations in the course of experimental syphilis associated with concurrent simian immunodeficiency virus infection. *J Infect Dis* 1992;165:1020.

54. Schulz KF, Murphy FK, Patamasucon P, Meheus AZ. Congenital syphilis. In: Holmes KK, Mårdh P-A, Sparling PF, et al, eds. *Sexually transmitted diseases*, 2nd ed. New York: McGraw-Hill, 1990:821.

55. Lewis LL. Congenital syphilis: serologic diagnosis in the young infant. *Infect Dis Clin North Am* 1992;6:31.

56. Romanowski B, Sutherland R, Fick GH, et al. Serologic response to treatment of infectious syphilis. *Ann Intern Med* 1991;114:1005.

57. Rompalo AM, Cannon RO, Quinn TC, Hook EW III. Association of biologic false-positive reactions for syphilis with human immunodeficiency virus infection. *J Infect Dis* 1992;165:1124.

58. Berkowitz K, Baxi L, Fox HE. False-negative syphilis screening: the prozone phenomenon, nonimmune hydrops, and diagnosis of syphilis during pregnancy. *Am J Obstet Gynecol* 1990;163:975.

59. Levine Z, Sherer DM, Jacobs A, Rotenberg O. Nonimmune hydrops fetalis due to congenital syphilis associated with negative intrapartum maternal serology screening. *Am J Perinatol* 1998;15:233.

60. Centers for Disease Control and Prevention. 1998 Guidelines for treatment of sexually transmitted diseases. *MMWR* 1998;47(RR-1):1.

61. Myles TD, Elam G, Park-Hwang E, Nguyen T. The Jarisch-Herxheimer reaction and fetal monitoring changes in pregnant women treated for syphilis. *Obstet Gynecol* 1998;92:859.

62. Rawstron SA, Bromberg K. Failure of recommended maternal therapy to prevent congenital syphilis. *Sex Transm Dis* 1991;18:102.

63. Fenton LJ, Light IJ. Congenital syphilis after maternal treatment with erythromycin. *Obstet Gynecol* 1976;47:492.

64. Rein MF. Biopharmacology of syphilotherapy. *J Am Vener Dis Assoc* 1976;3:109.

65. Marra CM, Slatter V, Tartaglione TA, et al. Evaluation of aqueous penicillin G and ceftriaxone for experimental neurosyphilis. *J Infect Dis* 1992;165:396.

66. Wendel GD Jr, Stark BJ, Jamison RB, et al. Penicillin allergy and desensitization in serious infections during pregnancy. *N Engl J Med* 1985;312:1229.

67. Chisholm CA, Katz VL, McDonald TL, Bowes WA Jr. Penicillin desensitization in the treatment of syphilis during pregnancy. *Am J Perinatol* 1997;14:553.

68. Quinn TC, Cannon RO, Glasser D, et al. The association of syphilis with risk of human immunodeficiency virus infection in patients attending sexually transmitted disease clinics. *Arch Intern Med* 1990; 150:1297.

69. McFarlin BL, Bottoms SF. Maternal syphilis: the next pregnancy. *Am J Perinatol* 1996;13:513.

70. Zenker PN, Berman SM. Congenital syphilis: trends and recommendations for evaluation and management. *Pediatr Infect Dis J* 1991; 10:516.

71. Centers for Disease Control and Prevention. Congenital syphilis—New York City, 1986–1988. *MMWR* 1989;38:825.

72. Zenker PN, Berman SM. Congenital syphilis: reporting and reality. *Am J Public Health* 1990;80:271.

73. Risser WL, Hwang L-Y. Problems in the current case definitions of congenital syphilis. *J Pediatr* 1996;129:499.

74. Cohen DA, Boyd D, Prabhudas I, Mascola L. The effects of case definition in maternal screening and reporting criteria on rates of congenital syphilis. *Am J Public Health* 1990;80:316.

75. Fitzgerald TJ, Froberg MK. Congenital syphilis in newborn rabbits: immune functions and susceptibility to challenge infection at 2 and 5 weeks of age. *Infect Immun* 1991;59:1869.

76. Wicher K, Baughn RE, Wicher V, Nakeeb S. Experimental congenital syphilis: guinea pig model. *Infect Immun* 1992;60:271.

77. Wicher V, Baughn RE, Wicher K. Congenital and neonatal syphilis in guinea-pigs show a different pattern of immune response. *Immunology* 1994;82:404.

78. Fox H. *Pathology of the placenta*, 2nd ed. Philadelphia: WB Saunders, 1997:307.

79. Genest DR, Choi-Hong SR, Tate JE, et al. Diagnosis of congenital syphilis from placental examination: comparison of histopathology, Steiner stain, and polymerase chain reaction for Treponema pallidum DNA. *Hum Pathol* 1996;27:366.

80. Lucas MJ, Theriot SK, Wendel GD Jr. Doppler systolic-diastolic ratios in pregnancies complicated by syphilis. *Obstet Gynecol* 1991;77:217.

81. Fojaco RM, Hensley GT, Moskowitz L. Congenital syphilis and necrotizing funisitis. *JAMA* 1989;261:1788.

82. Schwartz DA, Larsen SA, Beck-Sague C, et al. Pathology of the umbilical cord in congenital syphilis: analysis of 25 specimens using histochemistry and immunofluorescent antibody to Treponema pallidum. *Hum Pathol* 1995;26:784.

83. Boot JM, Oranje AP, Menke HE, et al. Congenital syphilis in The Netherlands: diagnosis and clinical features. *Genitourin Med* 1989;65:300.

84. Dorfman DH, Glaser JH. Congenital syphilis presenting in infants after the newborn period. *N Engl J Med* 1990;323:1299.

85. Wright MS, Tecklenburg FW. Critical illness in congenital syphilis after the newborn period. *Clin Pediatr (Phila)* 1992;31:247.

86. Pieper CH, van Gelderen WFC, Smith J, et al. Chest radiographs of neonates with respiratory failure caused by congenital syphilis. *Pediatr Radiol* 1995;25:198.

87. Liu C-C, So WCM, Lin C-H, Yeh T-F. Congenital syphilis: clinical manifestations in premature infants. *Scand J Infect Dis* 1993;25:741.

88. Naeye RL. Fetal growth with congenital syphilis: a quantitative study. *Am J Clin Pathol* 1971;55:228.

89. Long WA, Ulshen MH, Lawson EE. Clinical manifestations of congenital syphilitic hepatitis: implications for pathogenesis. *J Pediatr Gastroenterol Nutr* 1984;3:551.

90. Venter A, Pettifor JM, Duursma J, et al. Liver function in early congenital syphilis: does penicillin cause a deterioration? *J Pediatr Gastroenterol Nutr* 1991;12:310.

91. Herman TE. Extensive hepatic calcification secondary to fulminant neonatal syphilitic hepatitis. *Pediatr Radiol* 1995;25:120.

92. Noseda G, Roy C, Phan P, et al. Acute hepatic failure in an infant with congenital syphilis. *Arch Fr Pediatr* 1990;47:445.

93. Berry MC, Dajani AS. Resurgence of congenital syphilis. *Infect Dis Clin North Am* 1992;6:19.

94. Hira SK, Bhat GJ, Patel JB, et al. Early congenital syphilis: clinico-radiologic features in 202 patients. *Sex Transm Dis* 1985;12:177.

95. Rasool MN, Govender S. The skeletal manifestations of congenital syphilis: a review of 197 cases. *J Bone Joint Surg [Br]* 1989;71:752.

96. Brion LP, Manuli M, Rai B, et al. Long-bone radiographic abnormalities as a sign of active congenital syphilis in asymptomatic newborns. *Pediatrics* 1991;88:1037.

97. Greenberg SB, Bernal DV. Are long bone radiographs necessary in neonates suspected of having congenital syphilis? *Radiology* 1992;182:637.

98. Moyer VA, Schneider V, Yetman R, et al. Contribution of long-bone radiographs to the management of congenital syphilis in the newborn infant. *Arch Pediatr Adolesc Med* 1998;152:353.

99. Lim HK, Smith WL, Sato Y, Choi J. Congenital syphilis mimicking child abuse. *Pediatr Radiol* 1995;25:560.

100. Kocher MS, Caniza M. Parrot pseudoparalysis of the upper extremities. *J Bone Joint Surg Am* 1996;78:284.

101. Wolf B, Kalangu K. Congenital neurosyphilis revisited. *Eur J Pediatr* 1993;152:493.

102. Austin R, Melhem RE. Pulmonary changes in congenital syphilis. *Pediatr Radiol* 1991;21:404.

103. Hill LL, Singer DB, Falletta J, Stasney R. The nephrotic syndrome in congenital syphilis: an immunopathy. *Pediatrics* 1972;49:260.

104. Daaboul JJ, Kartchner W, Jones KL. Neonatal hypoglycemia caused by hypopituitarism in infants with congenital syphilis. *J Pediatr* 1993;123:983.

105. Fiumara NJ, Lessell S. Manifestations of late congenital syphilis: an analysis of 271 patients. *Arch Dermatol* 1970;102:78.

106. Hendershot EL. Luetic deafness. *Otolaryngol Clin North Am* 1978;11:43.

107. Wendel GD Jr, Sánchez PJ, Peters MT, et al. Identification of Treponema pallidum in amniotic fluid and fetal blood from pregnancies complicated by congenital syphilis. *Obstet Gynecol* 1991;78:890.

108. Hill LM, Maloney JB. An unusual constellation of sonographic findings associated with congenital syphilis. *Obstet Gynecol* 1991;78:895.

109. Satin AJ, Twickler DM, Wendel GD Jr. Congenital syphilis associated with dilation of fetal small bowel: a case report. *J Ultrasound Med* 1992;11:49.

110. Hallak M, Peipert JF, Ludomirsky A, Byers J. Nonimmune hydrops fetalis and fetal congenital syphilis: a case report. *J Reprod Med* 1992;37:173.

111. Nathan L, Twickler DM, Peters MT, et al. Fetal syphilis: correlation of sonographic findings and rabbit infectivity testing of amniotic fluid. *J Ultrasound Med* 1993;12:97.

112. Raafat NA, Birch AA, Altieri LA, et al. Sonographic osseous manifestations of fetal syphilis: a case report. *J Ultrasound Med* 1993;12:783.

113. Glover DD, Winter CA, Charles D, Larsen B. Diagnostic considerations in intra-amniotic syphilis. *Sex Transm Dis* 1985;12:145.

114. Grimprel E, Sanchez PJ, Wendel GD, et al. Use of polymerase chain reaction and rabbit infectivity testing to detect Treponema pallidum in amniotic fluid, fetal and neonatal sera, and cerebrospinal fluid. *J Clin Microbiol* 1991;29:1711.

115. Nathan L, Bohman VR, Sanchez PJ, et al. In utero infection with Treponema pallidum in early pregnancy. *Prenat Diagn* 1997;17:119.

116. Rawstron SA, Bromberg K. Comparison of maternal and newborn serologic tests for syphilis. *Am J Dis Child* 1991;145:1383.

117. Chhabra RK, Brion LP, Castro M, et al. Comparison of maternal sera, cord blood, and neonatal sera for detecting presumptive congenital syphilis: relationship with maternal treatment. *Pediatrics* 1993;91:88.

118. Bromberg K, Rawstron S, Tannis G. Diagnosis of congenital syphilis by combining Treponema pallidum-specific IgM detection with immunofluorescent antigen detection for T. pallidum. *J Infect Dis* 1993;168:238.

119. Meyer MP, Eddy T, Baughn RE. Analysis of Western blotting (immunoblotting) technique in diagnosis of congenital syphilis. *J Clin Microbiol* 1994;32:629.

120. Beeram MR, Chopde N, Dawood Y, et al. Lumbar puncture in the evaluation of possible asymptomatic congenital syphilis in neonates. *J Pediatr* 1996;128:125.

121. Sánchez PJ, Wendel GD Jr, Grimprel E, et al. Evaluation of molecular methodologies and rabbit infectivity testing for the diagnosis of congenital syphilis and neonatal central nervous system invasion by Treponema pallidum. *J Infect Dis* 1993;167:148.

122. Chang SN, Chung K-Y, Lee M-G, Lee JB. Seroreversion of the serological tests for syphilis in the newborns born to treated syphilitic mothers. *Genitourin Med* 1995;71:68.

123. Jackson MH, Hutchison WM. The prevalence and source of Toxoplasma infection in the environment. *Adv Parasitol* 1989;28:55.

124. Wong S-Y, Remington JS. Biology of Toxoplasma gondii. *AIDS* 1993;7:299.

125. Freij BJ, Sever JL. Toxoplasmosis. *Pediatr Rev* 1991;12:227.

126. Sever JL, Ellenberg JH, Ley AC, et al. Toxoplasmosis: maternal and pediatric findings in 23,000 pregnancies. *Pediatrics* 1988;82:181.

127. Couvreur J, Desmonts G. Toxoplasmosis. In: MacLeod CL, ed. *Parasitic infections in pregnancy and the newborn.* Oxford: Oxford University Press, 1988:112.

128. Lappalainen M, Koskela P, Hedman K, et al. Incidence of primary Toxoplasma infections during pregnancy in Southern Finland: a prospective cohort study. *Scand J Infect Dis* 1992;24:97.

129. Buffolano W, Gilbert RE, Holland FJ, et al. Risk factors for recent Toxoplasma infection in pregnant women in Naples. *Epidemiol Infect* 1996;116:347.

130. Kapperud G, Jenum PA, Stray-Pedersen B, et al. Risk factors for Toxoplasma gondii in pregnancy: results of a prospective case-control study in Norway. *Am J Epidemiol* 1996;144:405.

131. Wong S-Y, Remington JS. Toxoplasmosis in pregnancy. *Clin Infect Dis* 1994;18:853.

132. Sayre MR, Jehle D. Elevated Toxoplasma IgG antibody in patients tested for infectious mononucleosis in an urban emergency department. *Ann Emerg Med* 1989;18:383.

133. Katholm M, Johnsen NJ, Siim C, Willumsen L. Bilateral sudden deafness and acute acquired toxoplasmosis. *J Laryngol Otol* 1991;105:115.

134. Evans TG, Schwartzman JD. Pulmonary toxoplasmosis. *Semin Respir Infect* 1991;6:51.

135. Holliman RE. Toxoplasmosis, behaviour and personality. *J Infect* 1997;35:105.

136. Rabaud C, May T, Amiel C, et al. Extracerebral toxoplasmosis in patients infected with HIV: a French national survey. *Medicine (Baltimore)* 1994;73:306.

137. Hohlfeld P, Daffos F, Thulliez P, et al. Fetal toxoplasmosis: outcome of pregnancy and infant follow-up after in utero treatment. *J Pediatr* 1989;115:765.

138. Ghidini A, Sirtori M, Spelta A, Vergani P. Results of a preventive program for congenital toxoplasmosis. *J Reprod Med* 1991;36:270.

139. Freij BJ, Wiedbrauk DL, Sever JL. Immunologic assessment of infectious diseases. *Immunol Allergy Clin North Am* 1994;14:451.

140. Hafid J, Tran Manh Sung R, Raberin H, et al. Detection of circulating antigens of Toxoplasma gondii in human infection. *Am J Trop Med Hyg* 1995;52:336.

141. Weiss JB. DNA probes and PCR for diagnosis of parasitic infections. *Clin Microbiol Rev* 1995;8:113.

142. Dupon M, Cazenave J, Pellegrin J-L, et al. Detection of Toxoplasma gondii by PCR and tissue culture in cerebrospinal fluid and blood of human immunodeficiency virus-seropositive patients. *J Clin Microbiol* 1995;33:2421.

143. Nguyen TD, de Kesel M, Bigaignon G, et al. Detection of Toxoplasma gondii tachyzoites and bradyzoites in blood, urine, and brains of infected mice. *Clin Diagn Lab Immunol* 1996;3:635.

144. Huskinson J, Stepick-Biek PN, Araujo FG, et al. Toxoplasma antigens recognized by immunoglobulin G subclasses during acute and chronic infection. *J Clin Microbiol* 1989;27:2031.

145. Jenum PA, Stray-Pedersen B, Gundersen A-G. Improved diagnosis of primary Toxoplasma gondii infection in early pregnancy by determination of antitoxoplasma immunoglobulin G avidity. *J Clin Microbiol* 1997;35:1972.

146. Cozon GJN, Ferrandiz J, Nebhi H, et al. Estimation of the avidity of immunoglobulin G for routine diagnosis of chronic Toxoplasma gondii infection in pregnant women. *Eur J Clin Microbiol Infect Dis* 1998;17:32.

147. Decoster A. Detection of IgA anti-P30 (SAG1) antibodies in acquired and congenital toxoplasmosis. *Curr Top Microbiol Immunol* 1996; 219:199.

148. Beazley DM, Egerman RS. Toxoplasmosis. *Semin Perinatol* 1998; 22:332.

149. Alger LS. Toxoplasmosis and parvovirus B19. *Infect Dis Clin North Am* 1997;11:55.

150. Bobić B, Šibalić D, Djurković-Djaković O. High levels of IgM antibodies specific for Toxoplasma gondii in pregnancy 12 years after primary Toxoplasma infection: case report. *Gynecol Obstet Invest* 1991;31:182.

151. Gross U, Keksel O, Dardé ML. Value of detecting immunoglobulin E antibodies for the serological diagnosis of Toxoplasma gondii infection. *Clin Diagn Lab Immunol* 1997;4:247.

152. Nicoll S, Burns SM, Brettle RP, Leen CSL. A comparison of two methods of gene amplification for the diagnosis of Toxoplasma gondii in AIDS. *J Infect* 1996;33:177.

153. Haentjens M, Sacré L, Demeuter F. Congenital toxoplasmosis after maternal infection before or slightly after conception. *Acta Paediatr Scand* 1986;75:343.

154. Pons JC, Sigrand C, Grangeot-Keros L, et al. Toxoplasmose congénitale: transmission au foetus d'une infection maternelle antéconceptionnelle. *Presse Med* 1995;24:179.

155. Lynfield R, Eaton RB. Teratogen update: congenital toxoplasmosis. *Teratology* 1995;52:176.

156. Abboud P, Harika G, Saniez D, et al. Signes échographiques de la foetopathie toxoplasmique: revue de la littérature. *J Gynecol Obstet Biol Reprod (Paris)* 1995;24:733.

157. Daffos F, Forestier F, Capella-Pavlovsky M, et al. Prenatal management of 746 pregnancies at risk for congenital toxoplasmosis. *N Engl J Med* 1988;318:271.

158. Holliman RE, Johnson JD, Constantine G, et al. Difficulties in the diagnosis of congenital toxoplasmosis by cordocentesis: case report. *Br J Obstet Gynaecol* 1991;98:832.

159. Fricker-Hidalgo H, Pelloux H, Muet F, et al. Prenatal diagnosis of congenital toxoplasmosis: comparative value of fetal blood and amniotic fluid using serological techniques and cultures. *Prenat Diagn* 1997; 17:831.

160. Decoster A, Darcy F, Caron A, et al. Anti-P30 IgA antibodies as prenatal markers for congenital Toxoplasma infection. *Clin Exp Immunol* 1992;87:310.

161. Pratlong F, Boulot P, Villena I, et al. Antenatal diagnosis of congenital toxoplasmosis: evaluation of the biological parameters in a cohort of 286 patients. *Br J Obstet Gynaecol* 1996;103:552.

162. Cotty F, Descamps P, Body G, Richard-Lenoble D. Prenatal diagnosis of congenital toxoplasmosis: the role of Toxoplasma IgA antibodies in amniotic fluid. *J Infect Dis* 1995;171:1384.

163. Pinon JM, Toubas D, Marx C, et al. Detection of specific immunoglobulin E in patients with toxoplasmosis. *J Clin Microbiol* 1990;28:1739.

164. Grover CM, Thulliez P, Remington JS, Boothroyd JC. Rapid prenatal diagnosis of congenital Toxoplasma infection by using polymerase chain reaction and amniotic fluid. *J Clin Microbiol* 1990;28:2297.

165. Cazenave J, Forestier F, Bessieres MH, et al. Contribution of a new PCR assay to the prenatal diagnosis of congenital toxoplasmosis. *Prenat Diagn* 1992;12:119.

166. Dupouy-Camet J, Bougnoux ME, Lavareda de Souza S, et al. Comparative value of polymerase chain reaction and conventional biological tests for the prenatal diagnosis of congenital toxoplasmosis. *Ann Biol Clin (Paris)* 1992;50:315.

167. Hohlfeld P, Daffos F, Costa J-M, et al. Prenatal diagnosis of congenital toxoplasmosis with a polymerase-chain-reaction test on amniotic fluid. *N Engl J Med* 1994;331:695.

168. Li S, Ding Z, Liang Y, et al. A preliminary study on the antenatal diagnosis and prevention of the fetus toxoplasmosis infection. *Chung Hua Fu Chan Ko Tsa Chih* 1995;30:200.

169. Knerer B, Hayde M, Gratz G, et al. Direkter Nachweis von Toxoplasma gondii mit Polymerase-Kettenreaktion zur Diagnostik einer fetalen Toxoplasma-Infektion. *Wien Klin Wochenschr* 1995;107:137.

170. Guy EC, Pelloux H, Lappalainen M, et al. Interlaboratory comparison of polymerase chain reaction for the detection of Toxoplasma gondii DNA added to samples of amniotic fluid. *Eur J Clin Microbiol Infect Dis* 1996;15:836.

171. Couvreur J, Desmonts G, Thulliez P. Prophylaxis of congenital toxoplasmosis: effects of spiramycin on placental infection. *J Antimicrob Chemother* 1988;22[Suppl B]:193.

172. St. Georgiev V. Management of toxoplasmosis. *Drugs* 1994;48:179.

173. Pajor A. Pancytopenia in a patient given pyrimethamine and sulphamethoxidiazine during pregnancy. *Arch Gynecol Obstet* 1990;247: 215.

174. Schoondermark-van de Ven E, Vree T, Melchers W, et al. In vitro effects of sulfadiazine and its metabolites alone and in combination with pyrimethamine on Toxoplasma gondii. *Antimicrob Agents Chemother* 1995;39:763.

175. Foulon W, Naessens A, Derde MP. Evaluation of the possibilities for preventing congenital toxoplasmosis. *Am J Perinatol* 1994;11:57.

176. Jeannel D, Costagliola D, Niel G, et al. What is known about the prevention of congenital toxoplasmosis? *Lancet* 1990;336:359.

177. American College of Obstetricians and Gynecologists. Perinatal viral and parasitic infections: ACOG Technical Bulletin Number 177-February 1993. *Int J Gynaecol Obstet* 1993;42:300.

178. Eskild A, Oxman A, Magnus P, et al. Screening for toxoplasmosis in pregnancy: what is the evidence of reducing a health problem? *J Med Screen* 1996;3:188.

179. Bader TJ, Macones GA, Asch DA. Prenatal screening for toxoplasmosis. *Obstet Gynecol* 1997;90:457.

180. Berrebi A, Kobuch WE, Bessieres MH, et al. Termination of pregnancy for maternal toxoplasmosis. *Lancet* 1994;344:36.

181. Szénási Z, Ozsvár Z, Nagy E, et al. Prevention of congenital toxoplasmosis in Szeged, Hungary. *Int J Epidemiol* 1997;26:428.

182. D'Ercole C, Boubli L, Franck J, et al. Recurrent congenital toxoplasmosis in a woman with lupus erythematosus. *Prenat Diagn* 1995;15:1171.

183. Biedermann K, Flepp M, Fierz W, et al. Pregnancy, immunosuppression and reactivation of latent toxoplasmosis. *J Perinat Med* 1995;23: 191.

184. Gavinet MF, Robert F, Firtion G, et al. Congenital toxoplasmosis due to maternal reinfection during pregnancy. *J Clin Microbiol* 1997;35:1276.

185. Guerina NG, Hsu H-W, Meissner HC, et al. Neonatal serologic screening and early treatment for congenital Toxoplasma gondii infection. *N Engl J Med* 1994;330:1858.

186. Patel DV, Holfels EM, Vogel NP, et al. Resolution of intracranial calcifications in infants with treated congenital toxoplasmosis. *Radiology* 1996;199:433.

187. Wallon M, Caudie C, Rubio S, et al. Value of cerebrospinal fluid cytochemical examination for the diagnosis of congenital toxoplasmosis at birth in France. *Pediatr Infect Dis J* 1998;17:705.

188. Taccone A, Fondelli MP, Ferrea G, Marzoli A. An unusual CT presentation of congenital cerebral toxoplasmosis in an 8-month-old boy with AIDS. *Pediatr Radiol* 1992;22:68.

189. Virkola K, Lappalainen M, Valanne L, Koskiniemi M. Radiological signs in newborns exposed to primary Toxoplasma infection in utero. *Pediatr Radiol* 1997;27:133.

190. de Jong PTVM. Ocular toxoplasmosis; common and rare symptoms and signs. *Int Ophthalmol* 1989;13:391.

191. Brézin AP, Kasner L, Thulliez P, et al. Ocular toxoplasmosis in the fetus: immunohistochemistry analysis and DNA amplification. *Retina* 1994;14:19.

192. Mets MB, Holfels E, Boyer KM, et al. Eye manifestations of congenital toxoplasmosis. *Am J Ophthalmol* 1996;122:309.

193. McGee T, Wolters C, Stein L, et al. Absence of sensorineural hearing loss in treated infants and children with congenital toxoplasmosis. *Otolaryngol Head Neck Surg* 1992;106:75.

194. Glassman MS, Dellalzedah S, Beneck D, Seashore JH. Coincidence of congenital toxoplasmosis and biliary atresia in an infant. *J Pediatr Gastroenterol Nutr* 1991;13:298.

195. Rajantie J, Siimes MA, Taskinen E, et al. White blood cells in infants with congenital toxoplasmosis: transient appearance of cALL antigen on reactive marrow lymphocytes. *Scand J Infect Dis* 1992;24:227.

196. Hohlfeld P, Forestier F, Marion S, et al. Toxoplasma gondii infection during pregnancy: T lymphocyte subpopulations in mothers and fetuses. *Pediatr Infect Dis J* 1990;9:878.

197. McLeod R, Mack DG, Boyer K, et al. Phenotypes and functions of lymphocytes in congenital toxoplasmosis. *J Lab Clin Med* 1990;116:623.

198. Gross U, Müller J, Roos T, et al. Possible reasons for failure of conventional tests for diagnosis of fatal congenital toxoplasmosis: report of a case diagnosed by PCR and immunoblot. *Infection* 1992;20:149.

199. Fuentes I, Rodriguez M, Domingo CJ, et al. Urine sample used for congenital toxoplasmosis diagnosis by PCR. *J Clin Microbiol* 1996;34:2368.

200. Skinner LJ, Chatterton JMW, Joss AWL, et al. The use of an IgM immunosorbent agglutination assay to diagnose congenital toxoplasmosis. *J Med Microbiol* 1989;28:125.

201. Gross U, Roos T, Appoldt D, Heesemann J. Improved serological diagnosis of Toxoplasma gondii infection by detection of immunoglobulin A (IgA) and IgM antibodies against P30 by using the immunoblot technique. *J Clin Microbiol* 1992;30:1436.

202. Stepick-Biek P, Thulliez P, Araujo FG, Remington JS. IgA antibodies for diagnosis of acute congenital and acquired toxoplasmosis. *J Infect Dis* 1990;162:270.

203. Holliman RE, Raymond R, Renton N, Johnson JD. The diagnosis of toxoplasmosis using IgG avidity. *Epidemiol Infect* 1994;112:399.

204. Chumpitazi BFF, Boussaid A, Pelloux H, et al. Diagnosis of congenital toxoplasmosis by immunoblotting and relationship with other methods. *J Clin Microbiol* 1995;33:1479.

205. Wilson CB, Desmonts G, Couvreur J, Remington JS. Lymphocyte transformation in the diagnosis of congenital Toxoplasma infection. *N Engl J Med* 1980;302:785.

206. McAuley J, Boyer KM, Patel D, et al. Early and longitudinal evaluations of treated infants and children and untreated historical patients with congenital toxoplasmosis: The Chicago Collaborative Treatment Trial. *Clin Infect Dis* 1994;18:38.

207. Lynfield R, Guerina NG. Toxoplasmosis. *Pediatr Rev* 1997;18:75.

208. Wilson CB. Treatment of congenital toxoplasmosis. *Pediatr Infect Dis J* 1990;9:682.

209. McLeod R, Mack D, Foss R, et al. Levels of pyrimethamine in sera and cerebrospinal and ventricular fluids from infants treated for congenital toxoplasmosis. *Antimicrob Agents Chemother* 1992;36:1040.

210. Dutton GN. Recent developments in the prevention and treatment of congenital toxoplasmosis. *Int Ophthalmol* 1989;13:407.

211. Rothova A, Meenken C, Buitenhuis HJ, et al. Therapy for ocular toxoplasmosis. *Am J Ophthalmol* 1993;115:517.

212. Wilson CB, Remington JS, Stagno S, Reynolds DW. Development of adverse sequelae in children born with subclinical congenital Toxoplasma infection. *Pediatrics* 1980;66:767.

213. Koppe JG, Loewer-Sieger DH, de Roever-Bonnet H. Results of 20-year follow-up of congenital toxoplasmosis. *Lancet* 1986;1:254.

214. Koppe JG, Rothova A. Congenital toxoplasmosis: a long-term follow-up of 20 years. *Int Ophthalmol* 1989;13:387.

215. Meenken C, Assies J, van Nieuwenhuizen O, et al. Long term ocular and neurological involvement in severe congenital toxoplasmosis. *Br J Ophthalmol* 1995;79:581.

216. Roizen N, Swisher CN, Stein MA, et al. Neurologic and developmental outcome in treated congenital toxoplasmosis. *Pediatrics* 1995;95:11.

217. Mauracher CA, Mitchell LA, Tingle AJ. Selective tolerance to the E1 protein of rubella virus in congenital rubella syndrome. *J Immunol* 1993;151:2041.

218. Wolinsky JS. Rubella. In: Fields BN, Knipe DM, Howley PM, et al, eds. *Fields virology*, 3rd ed. Philadelphia: Lippincott-Raven Publishers, 1996:899.

219. Katow S, Minahara H, Fukushima M, Yamaguchi Y. Molecular epidemiology of rubella by nucleotide sequences of the rubella virus E1 gene in three East Asian countries. *J Infect Dis* 1997;176:602.

220. Frey TK, Abernathy ES, Bosma TJ, et al. Molecular analysis of rubella virus epidemiology across three continents, North America, Europe, and Asia, 1961–1997. *J Infect Dis* 1998;178:642.

221. Seppälä M, Vaheri A. Natural rubella infection of the female genital tract. *Lancet* 1974;1:46.

222. Holmes SJ, Orenstein WA. Rubella. In: Evans AS, Kaslow RA, eds. *Viral infections of humans: epidemiology and control,* 4th ed. New York: Plenum Publishing Corporation, 1997:839.

223. Töndury G, Smith DW. Fetal rubella pathology. *J Pediatr* 1966;68:867.

224. Garcia AGP, Marques RLS, Lobato YY, et al. Placental pathology in congenital rubella. *Placenta* 1985;6:281.

225. Webster WS. Teratogen update: congenital rubella. *Teratology* 1998;58:13.

226. Naeye RL, Blanc W. Pathogenesis of congenital rubella. *JAMA* 1965;194:1277.

227. Yoneda T, Urade M, Sakuda M, Miyazaki T. Altered growth, differentiation, and responsiveness to epidermal growth factor of human embryonic mesenchymal cells of palate by persistent rubella virus infection. *J Clin Invest* 1986;77:1613.

228. Coyle PK, Wolinsky JS, Buimovici-Klein E, et al. Rubella-specific immune complexes after congenital infection and vaccination. *Infect Immun* 1982;36:498.

229. Boner A, Wilmott RW, Dinwiddie R, et al. Desquamative interstitial pneumonia and antigen-antibody complexes in two infants with congenital rubella. *Pediatrics* 1983;72:835.

230. Clarke WL, Shaver KA, Bright GM, et al. Autoimmunity in congenital rubella syndrome. *J Pediatr* 1984;104:370.

231. Verder H, Dickmeiss E, Haahr S, et al. Late-onset rubella syndrome: coexistence of immune complex disease and defective cytotoxic effector cell function. *Clin Exp Immunol* 1986;63:367.

232. Williams LL, Shannon BT, Leguire LE, Fillman R. Persistently altered T cell immunity in high school students with the congenital rubella syndrome and profound hearing loss. *Pediatr Infect Dis J* 1993;12:831.

233. Yoon J-W, Choi D-S, Liang H-C, et al. Induction of an organ-specific autoimmune disease, lymphocytic hypophysitis, in hamsters by recombinant rubella virus glycoprotein and prevention of disease by neonatal thymectomy. *J Virol* 1992;66:1210.

234. Salonen E-M, Hovi T, Meurman O, et al. Kinetics of specific IgA, IgD, IgE, IgG, and IgM antibody responses in rubella. *J Med Virol* 1985;16:1.

235. Al-Nakib W, Best JM, Banatvala JE. Rubella-specific serum and nasopharyngeal immunoglobulin responses following naturally acquired and vaccine-induced infection: prolonged persistence of virus-specific IgM. *Lancet* 1975;1:182.

236. Banatvala JE, Best JM, O'Shea S, Dudgeon JA. Persistence of rubella antibodies after vaccination: detection after experimental challenge. *Rev Infect Dis* 1985;7:S86.

237. Zolti M, Ben-Rafael Z, Bider D, et al. Rubella-specific IgM in reinfection and risk to the fetus. *Gynecol Obstet Invest* 1990;30:184.

238. Cradock-Watson JE. Laboratory diagnosis of rubella: past, present and future. *Epidemiol Infect* 1991;107:1.

239. Böttiger B, Jensen IP. Maturation of rubella IgG avidity over time after acute rubella infection. *Clin Diagn Virol* 1997;8:105.

240. Grangeot-Keros L, Pillot J, Daffos F, Forestier F. Prenatal and postnatal production of IgM and IgA antibodies to rubella virus studied by antibody capture immunoassay. *J Infect Dis* 1988;158:138.

241. Stokes A, Mims CA, Grahame R. Subclass distribution of IgG and IgA responses to rubella virus in man. *J Med Microbiol* 1986;21:283.

242. Katow S, Sugiura A. Antibody response to individual rubella virus proteins in congenital and other rubella virus infections. *J Clin Microbiol* 1985;21:449.

243. Chaye HH, Mauracher CA, Tingle A, Gillam S. Cellular and humoral immune responses to rubella virus structural proteins E1, E2, and C. *J Clin Microbiol* 1992;30:2323.

244. Takahashi S, Machikawa F, Noda A, et al. Detection of immunoglobulin G and A antibodies to rubella virus in urine and antibody

responses to vaccine-induced infection. *Clin Diagn Lab Immunol* 1998;5:24.

245. Mitchell LA, Zhang T, Tingle AJ. Differential antibody responses to rubella virus infection in males and females. *J Infect Dis* 1992;166:1258.

246. Fitzgerald MG, Pullen GR, Hosking CS. Low affinity antibody to rubella antigen in patients after rubella infection in utero. *Pediatrics* 1988;81:812.

247. Herne V, Hedman K, Reedik P. Immunoglobulin G avidity in the serodiagnosis of congenital rubella syndrome. *Eur J Clin Microbiol Infect Dis* 1997;16:763.

248. de Mazancourt A, Waxham MN, Nicolas JC, Wolinsky JS. Antibody response to the rubella virus structural proteins in infants with the congenital rubella syndrome. *J Med Virol* 1986;19:111.

249. Buimovici-Klein E, Cooper LZ. Cell-mediated immune response in rubella infections. *Rev Infect Dis* 1985;7:S123.

250. Centers for Disease Control and Prevention. Rubella and congenital rubella syndrome—United States, 1994–1997. *MMWR* 1997;46:350.

251. Kaplan KM, Cochi SL, Edmonds LD, et al. A profile of mothers giving birth to infants with congenital rubella syndrome: an assessment of risk factors. *Am J Dis Child* 1990;144:118.

252. Centers for Disease Control and Prevention. Outbreaks of rubella among the Amish—United States, 1991. *MMWR* 1991;40:264.

253. Lee SH, Ewert DP, Frederick PD, Mascola L. Resurgence of congenital rubella syndrome in the 1990s: report on missed opportunities and failed prevention policies among women of childbearing age. *JAMA* 1992;267:2616.

254. Mellinger AK, Cragan JD, Atkinson WL, et al. High incidence of congenital rubella syndrome after a rubella outbreak. *Pediatr Infect Dis J* 1995;14:573.

255. Poland GA, Nichol KL. Medical students as sources of rubella and measles outbreaks. *Arch Intern Med* 1990;150:44.

256. Fraser V, Spitznagel E, Medoff G, Dunagan WC. Results of a rubella screening program for hospital employees: a five-year review (1986–1990). *Am J Epidemiol* 1993;138:756.

257. Centers for Disease Control and Prevention. Rubella prevention: recommendations of the Immunization Practices Advisory Committee (ACIP). *MMWR* 1990;39(RR-15):1.

258. Assaad F, Ljungars-Esteves K. Rubella—world impact. *Rev Infect Dis* 1985;7:S29.

259. Lever AML, Ross MGR, Baboonian C, Griffiths PD. Immunity to rubella among women of child-bearing age. *Br J Obstet Gynaecol* 1987;94:208.

260. Mingle JAA. Frequency of rubella antibodies in the population of some tropical African countries. *Rev Infect Dis* 1985;7:S68.

261. Prabhakar P, Bailey A, Smikle MF, et al. Seroprevalence of Toxoplasma gondii, rubella virus, cytomegalovirus, herpes simplex virus (TORCH) and syphilis in Jamaican pregnant women. *West Indian Med J* 1991;40:166.

262. Zufferey J, Jacquier P, Chappuis S, et al. Seroprevalence of rubella among women of childbearing age in Switzerland. *Eur J Clin Microbiol Infect Dis* 1995;14:691.

263. Ukkonen P. Rubella immunity and morbidity: impact of different vaccination programs in Finland 1979–1992. *Scand J Infect Dis* 1996;28:31.

264. Seth P, Manjunath N, Balaya S. Rubella infection: the Indian scene. *Rev Infect Dis* 1985;7:S64.

265. Wannian S. Rubella in the People's Republic of China. *Rev Infect Dis* 1985;7:S72.

266. Heggie AD. Pathogenesis of the rubella exanthem: isolation of rubella virus from the skin. *N Engl J Med* 1971;285:664.

267. Waxham MN, Wolinsky JS. Rubella virus and its effects on the central nervous system. *Neurol Clin* 1984;2:367.

268. Onji M, Kumon I, Kanaoka M, et al. Intrahepatic lymphocyte subpopulations in acute hepatitis in an adult with rubella. *Am J Gastroenterol* 1988;83:320.

269. Thanopoulos BD, Rokas S, Frimas CA, et al. Cardiac involvement in postnatal rubella. *Acta Paediatr Scand* 1989;78:141.

270. Shirley JA, Revill S, Cohen BJ, Buckley MM. Serological study of rubella-like illnesses. *J Med Virol* 1987;21:369.

271. Mahony JB, Chernesky MA. Rubella virus. In: Rose NR, de Macario EC, Fahey JL, Friedman H, Penn GM, eds. *Manual of clinical laboratory immunology*, 4th ed. Washington, DC: American Society for Microbiology, 1992:600.

272. Katow S, Sugiura A, Janejai N. Single-serum diagnosis of recent rubella infection with the use of hemagglutination inhibition test and enzyme-linked immunosorbent assays. *Microbiol Immunol* 1989;33:141.

273. Hedman K, Hietala J, Tiilikainen A, et al. Maturation of immunoglobulin G avidity after rubella vaccination studied by an enzyme linked immunosorbent assay (avidity-ELISA) and by haemolysis typing. *J Med Virol* 1989;27:293.

274. Zhang T, Mauracher CA, Mitchell LA, Tingle AJ. Detection of rubella virus-specific immunoglobulin G (IgG), IgM, and IgA antibodies by immunoblot assays. *J Clin Microbiol* 1992;30:824.

275. Kurtz JB, Anderson MJ. Cross-reactions in rubella and parvovirus specific IgM tests. *Lancet* 1985;2:1356.

276. Bosma TJ, Corbett KM, O'Shea S, et al. PCR for detection of rubella virus RNA in clinical samples. *J Clin Microbiol* 1995;33:1075.

277. Bosma TJ, Corbett KM, Eckstein MB, et al. Use of PCR for prenatal and postnatal diagnosis of congenital rubella. *J Clin Microbiol* 1995;33:2881.

278. Tanemura M, Suzumori K, Yagami Y, Katow S. Diagnosis of fetal rubella infection with reverse transcription and nested polymerase chain reaction: a study of 34 cases diagnosed in fetuses. *Am J Obstet Gynecol* 1996;174:578.

279. Centers for Disease Control and Prevention. Measles, mumps, and rubella—vaccine use and strategies for elimination of measles, rubella, and congenital rubella syndrome and control of mumps: recommendations of the Advisory Committee on Immunization Practices (ACIP). *MMWR* 1998;47(RR-8):1.

280. American College of Obstetricians and Gynecologists. Rubella and pregnancy: ACOG Technical Bulletin Number 171-August 1992. *Int J Gynaecol Obstet* 1993;42:60.

281. Wolf JE, Eisen JE, Fraimow HS. Symptomatic rubella reinfection in an immune contact of a rubella vaccine recipient. *South Med J* 1993;86:91.

282. O'Shea S, Corbett KM, Barrow SM, et al. Rubella reinfection; role of neutralising antibodies and cell-mediated immunity. *Clin Diagn Virol* 1994;2:349.

283. Levine JB, Berkowitz CD, St Geme JW Jr. Rubella virus reinfection during pregnancy leading to late-onset congenital rubella syndrome. *J Pediatr* 1982;100:589.

284. Grangeot-Keros L, Nicolas JC, Bricout F, Pillot J. Rubella reinfection and the fetus. *N Engl J Med* 1985;313:1547.

285. Best JM, Banatvala JE, Morgan-Capner P, Miller E. Fetal infection after maternal reinfection with rubella: criteria for defining reinfection. *BMJ* 1989;299:773.

286. Condon R, Bower C. Congenital rubella after previous maternal vaccination. *Med J Aust* 1992;156:882.

287. Robinson J, Lemay M, Vaudry WL. Congenital rubella after anticipated maternal immunity: two cases and a review of the literature. *Pediatr Infect Dis J* 1994;13:812.

288. Weber B, Enders G, Schlößer R, et al. Congenital rubella syndrome after maternal reinfection. *Infection* 1993;21:118.

289. Braun C, Kampa D, Fressle R, et al. Congenital rubella syndrome despite repeated vaccination of the mother: a coincidence of vaccine failure with failure to vaccinate. *Acta Paediatr* 1994;83:674.

290. Barfield W, Gardner R, Lett S, Johnsen C. Congenital rubella reinfection in a mother with anti-cardiolipin and anti-platelet antibodies. *Pediatr Infect Dis J* 1997;16:249.

291. Aboudy Y, Fogel A, Barnea B, et al. Subclinical rubella reinfection during pregnancy followed by transmission of virus to the fetus. *J Infect* 1997;34:273.

292. Miller E, Cradock-Watson JE, Pollock TM. Consequences of confirmed maternal rubella at successive stages of pregnancy. *Lancet* 1982;2:781.

293. Munro ND, Sheppard S, Smithells RW, et al. Temporal relations between maternal rubella and congenital defects. *Lancet* 1987;2:201.

294. Grillner L, Forsgren M, Barr B, et al. Outcome of rubella during pregnancy with special reference to the 17th–24th weeks of gestation. *Scand J Infect Dis* 1983;15:321.

295. Bitsch M. Rubella in pregnant Danish women 1975–1984. *Dan Med Bull* 1987;34:46.

296. Enders G, Nickerl-Pacher U, Miller E, Cradock-Watson JE. Outcome of confirmed periconceptional maternal rubella. *Lancet* 1988;1:1445.

297. Segondy M, Boulot J, N'Dakortamanda N, et al. Detection of rubella virus in amniotic fluid by electron microscopy. *Eur J Obstet Gynecol Reprod Biol* 1990;37:77.

298. Sandow D, Rosmus K, Karnahl K, et al. Ein Beitrag zur pränatalen Rötelndiagnostik. *Z Geburtshilfe Perinatol* 1991;195:95.

299. Straussberg R, Amir J, Harel L, Djaldetti M. Ultrastructural alterations of the amniocytes in 2 patients with rubella during the first trimester of pregnancy. *Fetal Diagn Ther* 1995;10:60.

300. Daffos F, Forestier F, Grangeot-Keros L, et al. Prenatal diagnosis of congenital rubella. *Lancet* 1984;2:1.

301. Hwa H-L, Shyu M-K, Lee C-N, et al. Prenatal diagnosis of congenital rubella infection from maternal rubella in Taiwan. *Obstet Gynecol* 1994;84:415.

302. Enders G, Jonatha W. Prenatal diagnosis of intrauterine rubella. *Infection* 1987;15:162.

303. Terry GM, Ho-Terry L, Warren RC, et al. First trimester prenatal diagnosis of congenital rubella: a laboratory investigation. *BMJ* 1986; 292:930.

304. Cradock-Watson JE, Miller E, Ridehalgh MKS, et al. Detection of rubella virus in fetal and placental tissues and in the throats of neonates after serologically confirmed rubella in pregnancy. *Prenat Diagn* 1989;9:91.

305. Ho-Terry L, Terry GM, Londesborough P. Diagnosis of foetal rubella virus infection by polymerase chain reaction. *J Gen Virol* 1990;71:1607.

306. Revello MG, Baldanti F, Sarasini A, et al. Prenatal diagnosis of rubella virus infection by direct detection and semiquantitation of viral RNA in clinical samples by reverse transcription-PCR. *J Clin Microbiol* 1997;35:708.

307. Tingle AJ, Chantler JK, Pot KH, et al. Postpartum rubella immunization: association with development of prolonged arthritis, neurological sequelae, and chronic rubella viremia. *J Infect Dis* 1985;152:606.

308. Losonsky GA, Fishaut JM, Strussenberg J, Ogra PL. Effect of immunization against rubella on lactation products. II. Maternal-neonatal interactions. *J Infect Dis* 1982;145:661.

309. Tingle AJ, Mitchell LA, Grace M, et al. Randomised double-blind placebo-controlled study on adverse effects of rubella immunisation in seronegative women. *Lancet* 1997;349:1277.

310. Ray P, Black S, Shinefield H, et al. Risk of chronic arthropathy among women after rubella vaccination. *JAMA* 1997;278:551.

311. Slater PE. Chronic arthropathy after rubella vaccination in women: false alarm? *JAMA* 1997;278:594.

312. Howson CP, Katz M, Johnston RB Jr, Fineberg HV. Chronic arthritis after rubella vaccination. *Clin Infect Dis* 1992;15:307.

313. Bosma TJ, Etherington J, O'Shea S, et al. Rubella virus and chronic joint disease: is there an association? *J Clin Microbiol* 1998;36:3524.

314. Mitchell LA, Tingle AJ, MacWilliam L, et al. HLA-DR class II associations with rubella vaccine-induced joint manifestations. *J Infect Dis* 1998;177:5.

315. Landes RD, Bass JW, Millunchick EW, Oetgen WJ. Neonatal rubella following postpartum maternal immunization. *J Pediatr* 1980;97:465.

316. Centers for Disease Control and Prevention. Rubella vaccination during pregnancy—United States, 1971–1988. *MMWR* 1989;38:289.

317. Schluter WW, Reef SE, Redd SC, Dykewicz CA. Changing epidemiology of congenital rubella syndrome in the United States. *J Infect Dis* 1998;178:636.

318. De Owens CS, De Espino RT. Rubella in Panama: still a problem. *Pediatr Infect Dis J* 1989;8:110.

319. Banatvala JE. Rubella—could do better. *Lancet* 1998;351:849.

320. De la Mata I, De Wals P, Dolk H, et al. Incidence of congenital rubella syndrome in 19 regions of Europe in 1980–1986. *Eur J Epidemiol* 1989;5:106.

321. Cheffins T, Chan A, Keane RJ, et al. The impact of rubella immunisation on the incidence of rubella, congenital rubella syndrome and rubella-related terminations of pregnancy in South Australia. *Br J Obstet Gynaecol* 1998;105:998.

322. South MA, Sever JL. Teratogen update: the congenital rubella syndrome. *Teratology* 1985;31:297.

323. Tokugawa K, Ueda K, Fukushige J, et al. Congenital rubella syndrome and physical growth: a 17-year, prospective, longitudinal follow-up in the Ryukyu Islands. *Rev Infect Dis* 1986;8:874.

324. Chiriboga-Klein S, Oberfield SE, Casullo AM, et al. Growth in congenital rubella syndrome and correlation with clinical manifestations. *J Pediatr* 1989;115:251.

325. Campbell PE. Vascular abnormalities following maternal rubella. *Br Heart J* 1965;27:134.

326. Peckham CS. Clinical and laboratory study of children exposed in utero to maternal rubella. *Arch Dis Child* 1972;47:571.

327. Gregg NM. Congenital cataract following German measles in the mother. *Trans Ophthalmol Soc Aust* 1941;3:35.

328. Romano A, Weinberg M, Bar-Izhak R, et al. Rate and various aspects of eye infection resulting from congenital rubella. *J Pediatr Ophthalmol Strabismus* 1979;16:26.

329. Kanra G, Firat T. Isolation of rubella virus from lens material in cases of congenital cataracts. *J Pediatr Ophthalmol Strabismus* 1979;16:31.

330. Smith GTH, Shun-Shin GA, Bron AJ. Spontaneous reabsorption of a rubella cataract. *Br J Ophthalmol* 1990;74:564.

331. Kresky B, Nauheim JS. Rubella retinitis. *Am J Dis Child* 1967;113: 305.

332. Geltzer AI, Guber D, Sears ML. Ocular manifestations of the 1964–65 rubella epidemic. *Am J Ophthalmol* 1967;63:221.

333. Collis WJ, Cohen DN. Rubella retinopathy: a progressive disorder. *Arch Ophthalmol* 1970;84:33.

334. Givens KT, Lee DA, Jones T, Ilstrup DM. Congenital rubella syndrome: ophthalmic manifestations and associated systemic disorders. *Br J Ophthalmol* 1993;77:358.

335. Deluise VP, Cobo LM, Chandler D. Persistent corneal edema in the congenital rubella syndrome. *Ophthalmology* 1983;90:835.

336. Desmond MM, Fisher ES, Vorderman AL, et al. The longitudinal course of congenital rubella encephalitis in nonretarded children. *J Pediatr* 1978;93:584.

337. Carey BM, Arthur RJ, Houlsby WT. Ventriculitis in congenital rubella: ultrasound demonstration. *Pediatr Radiol* 1987;17:415.

338. Yamashita Y, Matsuishi T, Murakami Y, et al. Neuroimaging findings (ultrasonography, CT, MRI) in 3 infants with congenital rubella syndrome. *Pediatr Radiol* 1991;21:547.

339. Chang Y-C, Huang C-C, Liu C-C. Frequency of linear hyperechogenicity over the basal ganglia in young infants with congenital rubella syndrome. *Clin Infect Dis* 1996;22:569.

340. Lim KO, Beal M, Harvey RL Jr, et al. Brain dysmorphology in adults with congenital rubella plus schizophrenialike symptoms. *Biol Psychiatry* 1995;37:764.

341. Hendricks WM, Hu C-H. Blueberry muffin syndrome: cutaneous erythropoiesis and possible intrauterine viral infection. *Cutis* 1984;34: 549.

342. Marshall WC, Trompeter RS, Risdon RA. Chronic rashes in congenital rubella: isolation of virus from skin. *Lancet* 1975;1:1349.

343. Ostlere LS, Harris D, Stevens HP, et al. Chronic rash associated with congenital rubella. *J R Soc Med* 1994;87:242.

344. Alter M, Schulenberg R. Dermatoglyphics in the rubella syndrome. *JAMA* 1966;197:685.

345. Menser MA, Dorman DC, Reye RDK, Reid RR. Renal-artery stenosis in the rubella syndrome. *Lancet* 1966;1:790.

346. Menser MA, Robertson SEJ, Dorman DC, et al. Renal lesions in congenital rubella. *Pediatrics* 1967;40:901.

347. Forrest JM, Menser MA. Congenital rubella in schoolchildren and adolescents. *Arch Dis Child* 1970;45:63.

348. Kaplan GW, McLaughlin AP III. Urogenital anomalies and congenital rubella syndrome. *Urology* 1973;2:148.

349. Radner M, Vergesslich KA, Weninger M, et al. Meconium peritonitis: a new finding in rubella syndrome. *J Clin Ultrasound* 1993;21:346.

350. Rudolph AJ, Singleton EB, Rosenberg HS, et al. Osseous manifestations of the congenital rubella syndrome. *Am J Dis Child* 1965;110: 428.

351. Reed GB Jr. Rubella bone lesions. *J Pediatr* 1969;74:208.

352. London WT, Fuccillo DA, Anderson B, Sever JL. Concentration of rubella virus antigen in chondrocytes of congenitally infected rabbits. *Nature* 1970;226:172.

353. Sekeles E, Ornoy A. Osseous manifestations of gestational rubella in young human fetuses. *Am J Obstet Gynecol* 1975;122:307.

354. Heggie AD. Growth inhibition of human embryonic and fetal rat bones in organ culture by rubella virus. *Teratology* 1977;15:47.

355. Zinkham WH, Medearis DN Jr, Osborn JE. Blood and bone-marrow findings in congenital rubella. *J Pediatr* 1967;71:512.

356. Sherman LA, Silberstein LE, Berkman EM. Altered blood group expression in a patient with congenital rubella infection. *Transfusion* 1984;24:267.

357. Sever JL, South MA, Shaver KA. Delayed manifestations of congenital rubella. *Rev Infect Dis* 1985;7:S164.

358. Numazaki K, Goldman H, Wong I, Wainberg MA. Infection of cultured human fetal pancreatic islet cells by rubella virus. *Am J Clin Pathol* 1989;91:446.

359. Ginsberg-Fellner F, Witt ME, Fedun B, et al. Diabetes mellitus and autoimmunity in patients with the congenital rubella syndrome. *Rev Infect Dis* 1985;7:S170.

360. McEvoy RC, Fedun B, Cooper LZ, et al. Children at high risk of diabetes mellitus: New York studies of families with diabetes and of children with congenital rubella syndrome. *Adv Exp Med Biol* 1988;246:221.

361. Preece MA, Kearney PJ, Marshall WC. Growth-hormone deficiency in congenital rubella. *Lancet* 1977;2:842.

362. Centers for Disease Control and Prevention. Rubella and congenital rubella syndrome—New York City. *MMWR* 1986;35:770.

363. Cooper LZ, Krugman S. Clinical manifestations of postnatal and congenital rubella. *Arch Ophthalmol* 1967;77:434.

364. O'Shea S, Best J, Banatvala JE. A lymphocyte transformation assay for the diagnosis of congenital rubella. *J Virol Methods* 1992;37:139.

365. Vesikari T, Meurman OH, Mäki R. Persistent rubella-specific IgM-antibody in the cerebrospinal fluid of a child with congenital rubella. *Arch Dis Child* 1980;55:46.

366. Meitsch K, Enders G, Wolinsky JS, et al. The role of Rubella-Immunoblot and Rubella-Peptide-EIA for the diagnosis of the congenital rubella syndrome during the prenatal and newborn periods. *J Med Virol* 1997;51:280.

367. Eckstein MB, Brown DWG, Foster A, et al. Congenital rubella in south India: diagnosis using saliva from infants with cataract. *BMJ* 1996;312:161.

368. Plotkin SA, Klaus RM, Whitely JP. Hypogammaglobulinemia in an infant with congenital rubella syndrome; failure of l-adamantanamine to stop virus excretion. *J Pediatr* 1966;69:1085.

369. Larsson A, Forsgren M, Hård af Segerstad S, et al. Administration of interferon to an infant with congenital rubella syndrome involving persistent viremia and cutaneous vasculitis. *Acta Paediatr Scand* 1976;65:105.

370. Arvin AM, Schmidt NJ, Cantell K, Merigan TC. Alpha interferon administration to infants with congenital rubella. *Antimicrob Agents Chemother* 1982;21:259.

371. Hyams KC. Risks of chronicity following acute hepatitis B virus infection: a review. *Clin Infect Dis* 1995;20:992.

372. Coleman PJ, McQuillan GM, Moyer LA, et al. Incidence of hepatitis B virus infection in the United States, 1976–1994: estimates from the National Health and Nutrition Examination Surveys. *J Infect Dis* 1998;178:954.

373. Centers for Disease Control and Prevention. Hepatitis B virus: a comprehensive strategy for eliminating transmission in the United States through universal childhood vaccination. Recommendations of the Immunization Practices Advisory Committee (ACIP). *MMWR* 1991; 40(RR-13):1.

374. Lee WM. Hepatitis B virus infection. *N Engl J Med* 1997;337:1733.

375. Stevens CE. Immunoprophylaxis of hepatitis B virus infection. *Semin Pediatr Infect Dis* 1991;2:135.

376. Hoofnagle JH, Di Bisceglie AM. Serologic diagnosis of acute and chronic viral hepatitis. *Semin Liver Dis* 1991;11:73.

377. Baker BL, Di Bisceglie AM, Kaneko S, et al. Determination of hepatitis B virus DNA in serum using the polymerase chain reaction: clinical significance and correlation with serological and biochemical markers. *Hepatology* 1991;13:632.

378. Michalak TI, Pasquinelli C, Guilhot S, Chisari FV. Hepatitis B virus persistence after recovery from acute viral hepatitis. *J Clin Invest* 1994;93:230.

379. Levrero M, Stemler M, Pasquinelli C, et al. Significance of anti-HBx antibodies in hepatitis B virus infection. *Hepatology* 1991;13:143.

380. Nowak MA, Bonhoeffer S, Hill AM, et al. Viral dynamics in hepatitis B virus infection. *Proc Natl Acad Sci U S A* 1996;93:4398.

381. Rawal BK, Parida S, Watkins RPF, et al. Symptomatic reactivation of hepatitis B in pregnancy. *Lancet* 1991;337:364.

382. Omata M, Ehata T, Yokosuka O, et al. Mutations in the precore region of hepatitis B virus DNA in patients with fulminant and severe hepatitis. *N Engl J Med* 1991;324:1699.

383. Liang TJ, Hasegawa K, Rimon N, et al. A hepatitis B virus mutant associated with an epidemic of fulminant hepatitis. *N Engl J Med* 1991;324:1705.

384. Romero R, Lavine JE. Viral hepatitis in children. *Semin Liver Dis* 1994;14:289.

385. Aach RD. Viral hepatitis due to hepatitis viruses A-E and GB virus. In: Feigin RD, Cherry JD, eds. *Textbook of pediatric infectious diseases*, 4th ed. Philadelphia: WB Saunders, 1998:612.

386. Alter MJ, Hadler SC, Margolis HS, et al. The changing epidemiology of hepatitis B in the United States: need for alternative vaccination strategies. *JAMA* 1990;263:1218.

387. Centers for Disease Control and Prevention. Protection against viral hepatitis: recommendations of the Immunization Practices Advisory Committee (ACIP). *MMWR* 1990;39(S-2):1.

388. Burk RD, Hwang L-Y, Ho GYF, et al. Outcome of perinatal hepatitis B virus exposure is dependent on maternal virus load. *J Infect Dis* 1994;170:1418.

389. Hadler SC, Margolis HS. Hepatitis B immunization: vaccine types, efficacy, and indications for immunization. In: Remington JS, Swartz MN, eds. *Current clinical topics in infectious diseases,* vol 12. Boston: Blackwell Scientific Publications, 1992:282.

390. Levy M, Koren G. Hepatitis B vaccine in pregnancy: maternal and fetal safety. *Am J Perinatol* 1991;8:227.

391. Grosheide PM, Schalm SW, van Os HC, et al. Immune response to hepatitis B vaccine in pregnant women receiving post-exposure prophylaxis. *Eur J Obstet Gynecol Reprod Biol* 1993;50:53.

392. Centers for Disease Control and Prevention. Prevention of perinatal transmission of hepatitis B virus: prenatal screening of all pregnant women for hepatitis B surface antigen. *MMWR* 1988;37:341.

393. Centers for Disease Control and Prevention. Maternal hepatitis B screening practices—California, Connecticut, Kansas, and United States, 1992–1993. *MMWR* 1994;43:311.

394. Petermann S, Ernest JM. Intrapartum hepatitis B screening. *Am J Obstet Gynecol* 1995;173:369.

395. Zola J, Smith N, Goldman S, Woodruff BA. Attitudes and educational practices of obstetric providers regarding infant hepatitis B vaccination. *Obstet Gynecol* 1997;89:61.

396. American Academy of Pediatrics. Committee on Infectious Diseases. Universal hepatitis B immunization. *Pediatrics* 1992;89:795.

397. Kim SC, Chung EK, Hodinka RL, et al. Immunogenicity of hepatitis B vaccine in preterm infants. *Pediatrics* 1997;99:534.

398. Patel DM, Butler J, Feldman S, et al. Immunogenicity of hepatitis B vaccine in healthy very low birth weight infants. *J Pediatr* 1997; 130:641.

399. Blondheim O, Bader D, Abend M, et al. Immunogenicity of hepatitis B vaccine in preterm infants. *Arch Dis Child Fetal Neonat Ed* 1998; 79:F206.

400. Marion SA, Pastore MT, Pi DW, Mathias RG. Long-term follow-up of hepatitis B vaccine in infants of carrier mothers. *Am J Epidemiol* 1994;140:734.

401. Tang J-R, Hsu H-Y, Lin H-H, et al. Hepatitis B surface antigenemia at birth: a long-term follow-up study. *J Pediatr* 1998;133:374.

402. Ngui SL, Andrews NJ, Underhill GS, et al. Failed postnatal immuno-prophylaxis for hepatitis B: characteristics of maternal hepatitis B virus as risk factors. *Clin Infect Dis* 1998;27:100.

403. Di Bisceglie AM. Hepatitis C. *Lancet* 1998;351:351.

404. Purcell R. The hepatitis C virus: overview. *Hepatology* 1997;26[Suppl 1]:11S.

405. American Academy of Pediatrics, Committee on Infectious Diseases. Hepatitis C virus infection. *Pediatrics* 1998;101:481.

406. Hunt CM, Carson KL, Sharara AI. Hepatitis C in pregnancy. *Obstet Gynecol* 1997;89:883.

407. Lok ASF, Gunaratnam NT. Diagnosis of hepatitis C. *Hepatology* 1997;26[Suppl 1]:48S.

408. Pawlotsky J-M. Measuring hepatitis C viremia in clinical samples: can we trust the assays? *Hepatology* 1997;26:1.

409. Fioredda F, Ranieri E, Lorusso C, et al. Vertical transmission of hepatitis C. *Pediatr Infect Dis J* 1996;15:642.

410. Sabatino G, Ramenghi LA, di Marzio M, Pizzigallo E. Vertical transmission of hepatitis C virus: an epidemiological study on 2,980 pregnant women in Italy. *Eur J Epidemiol* 1996;12:443.

411. Polywka S, Feucht H, Zöllner B, Laufs R. Hepatitis C virus infection in pregnancy and the risk of mother-to-child transmission. *Eur J Clin Microbiol Infect Dis* 1997;16:121.

412. Croxson M, Couper A, Voss L, et al. Vertical transmission of hepatitis C virus in New Zealand. *N Z Med J* 1997;110:165.

413. Tanzi M, Bellelli E, Benaglia G, et al. The prevalence of HCV infection in a cohort of pregnant women, the related risk factors and the possibility of vertical transmission. *Eur J Epidemiol* 1997;13:517.

414. La Torre A, Biadaioli R, Capobianco T, et al. Vertical transmission of HCV. *Acta Obstet Gynecol Scand* 1998;77:889.

415. Granovsky MO, Minkoff HL, Tess BH, et al. Hepatitis C virus infec-

tion in the Mothers and Infants Cohort Study. *Pediatrics* 1998;102: 355.

416. Ohto H, Terazawa S, Sasaki N, et al. Transmission of hepatitis C virus from mothers to infants. *N Engl J Med* 1994;330:744.

417. Aizaki H, Saito A, Kusakawa I, et al. Mother-to-child transmission of a hepatitis C virus variant with an insertional mutation in its hypervariable region. *J Hepatol* 1996;25:608.

418. Ni Y-H, Chang M-H, Chen P-J, et al. Evolution of hepatitis C virus quasispecies in infants and mothers infected through mother-to-infant transmission. *J Hepatol* 1997;26:967.

419. Sasaki N, Matsui A, Momoi M, et al. Loss of circulating hepatitis C virus in children who developed a persistent carrier state after mother-to-baby transmission. *Pediatr Res* 1997;42:263.

420. Roizman B. Introduction: objectives of herpes simplex virus vaccines seen from a historical perspective. *Rev Infect Dis* 1991;13:S892.

421. Prober CG, Corey L, Brown ZA, et al. The management of pregnancies complicated by genital infections with herpes simplex virus. *Clin Infect Dis* 1992;15:1031.

422. Annunziato PW, Gershon A. Herpes simplex virus infections. *Pediatr Rev* 1996;17:415.

423. Kohl S. Neonatal herpes simplex virus infection. *Clin Perinatol* 1997; 24:129.

424. Wiedbrauk DL, Johnston SL. *Manual of clinical virology.* New York: Raven Press, 1993.

425. Riley LE. Herpes simplex virus. *Semin Perinatol* 1998;22:284.

426. Courtney RJ. Membrane-associated antigens of herpes simplex virus. *Rev Infect Dis* 1991;13:S917.

427. Fleming DT, McQuillan GM, Johnson RE, et al. Herpes simplex virus type 2 in the United States, 1976 to 1994. *N Engl J Med* 1997;337: 1105.

428. Siegel D, Golden E, Washington AE, et al. Prevalence and correlates of herpes simplex infections: the population-based AIDS in Multiethnic Neighborhoods Study. *JAMA* 1992;268:1702.

429. Brown ZA, Selke S, Zeh J, et al. The acquisition of herpes simplex virus during pregnancy. *N Engl J Med* 1997;337:509.

430. Kulhanjian JA, Soroush V, Au DS, et al. Identification of women at unsuspected risk of primary infection with herpes simplex virus type 2 during pregnancy. *N Engl J Med* 1992;326:916.

431. Taieb A, Body S, Astar I, et al. Clinical epidemiology of symptomatic primary herpetic infection in children: a study of 50 cases. *Acta Paediatr Scand* 1987;76:128.

432. Kuzushima K, Kimura H, Kino Y, et al. Clinical manifestations of primary herpes simplex virus type 1 infection in a closed community. *Pediatrics* 1991;87:152.

433. Straus SE, Rooney JF, Sever JL, et al. Herpes simplex virus infection: biology, treatment, and prevention. *Ann Intern Med* 1985;103:404.

434. Breinig MK, Kingsley LA, Armstrong JA, et al. Epidemiology of genital herpes in Pittsburgh: serologic, sexual, and racial correlates of apparent and inapparent herpes simplex infections. *J Infect Dis* 1990;162:299.

435. Koutsky LA, Stevens CE, Holmes KK, et al. Underdiagnosis of genital herpes by current clinical and viral-isolation procedures. *N Engl J Med* 1992;326:1533.

436. Whitley RJ. Herpes simplex virus infections of the central nervous system: encephalitis and neonatal herpes. *Drugs* 1991;42:406.

437. Jacques SM, Qureshi F. Herpes simplex virus hepatitis in pregnancy: a clinicopathologic study of three cases. *Hum Pathol* 1992;23:183.

438. Mudido P, Marshall GS, Howell RS, et al. Disseminated herpes simplex virus infection during pregnancy: a case report. *J Reprod Med* 1993;38:964.

439. Glorioso DV, Molloy PJ, Van Thiel DH, Kania RJ. Successful empiric treatment of HSV hepatitis in pregnancy: case report and review of the literature. *Dig Dis Sci* 1996;41:1273.

440. Lafferty WE, Coombs RW, Benedetti J, et al. Recurrences after oral and genital herpes simplex virus infection: influence of site of infection and viral type. *N Engl J Med* 1987;316:1444.

441. Koelle DM, Benedetti J, Langenberg A, Corey L. Asymptomatic reactivation of herpes simplex virus in women after the first episode of genital herpes. *Ann Intern Med* 1992;116:433.

442. Benedetti JK, Zeh J, Selke S, Corey L. Frequency and reactivation of nongenital lesions among patients with genital herpes simplex virus. *Am J Med* 1995;98:237.

443. Wald A, Zeh J, Selke S, et al. Virologic characteristics of subclinical and symptomatic genital herpes infections. *N Engl J Med* 1995;333: 770.

444. Hensleigh PA, Andrews WW, Brown Z, et al. Genital herpes during pregnancy: inability to distinguish primary and recurrent infections clinically. *Obstet Gynecol* 1997;89:891.

445. Nahass GT, Goldstein BA, Zhu WY, et al. Comparison of Tzanck smear, viral culture, and DNA diagnostic methods in detection of herpes simplex and varicella-zoster infection. *JAMA* 1992;268:2541.

446. Cone RW, Hobson AC, Palmer J, et al. Extended duration of herpes simplex virus DNA in genital lesions detected by the polymerase chain reaction. *J Infect Dis* 1991;164:757.

447. Rogers BB, Josephson SL, Mak SK, Sweeney PJ. Polymerase chain reaction amplification of herpes simplex virus DNA from clinical samples. *Obstet Gynecol* 1992;79:464.

448. Cone RW, Hobson AC, Brown Z, et al. Frequent detection of genital herpes simplex virus DNA by polymerase chain reaction among pregnant women. *JAMA* 1994;272:792.

449. Linde A, Klapper PE, Monteyne P, et al. Specific diagnostic methods for herpesvirus infections of the central nervous system: a consensus review by the European Union Concerted Action on Virus Meningitis and Encephalitis. *Clin Diagn Virol* 1997;8:83.

450. Whitley RJ, Cobbs CG, Alford CA Jr, et al. Diseases that mimic herpes simplex encephalitis: diagnosis, presentation, and outcome. *JAMA* 1989;262:234.

451. Whitley RJ, Gnann JW Jr. Acyclovir: a decade later. *N Engl J Med* 1992;327:782.

452. Berger SA, Weinberg M, Treves T, et al. Herpes encephalitis during pregnancy: failure of acyclovir and adenine arabinoside to prevent neonatal herpes. *Isr J Med Sci* 1986;22:41.

453. Stahlmann R, Klug S, Lewandowski C, et al. Teratogenicity of acyclovir in rats. *Infection* 1987;15:261.

454. Frenkel LM, Brown ZA, Bryson YJ, et al. Pharmacokinetics of acyclovir in the term human pregnancy and neonate. *Am J Obstet Gynecol* 1991;164:569.

455. Lau RJ, Emery MG, Galinsky RE. Unexpected accumulation of acyclovir in breast milk with estimation of infant exposure. *Obstet Gynecol* 1987;69:468.

456. Centers for Disease Control and Prevention. Pregnancy outcomes following systemic prenatal acyclovir exposure—June 1, 1984–June 30, 1993. *MMWR* 1993;42:806.

457. Hodinka RL. What clinicians need to know about antiviral drugs and viral resistance. *Infect Dis Clin North Am* 1997;11:945.

458. LaRussa PS. Famciclovir. *Semin Pediatr Infect Dis* 1996;7:138.

459. Stone KM, Brooks CA, Guinan ME, Alexander ER. National surveillance for neonatal herpes simplex virus infections. *Sex Transm Dis* 1989;16:152.

460. Brown ZA, Benedetti J, Ashley R, et al. Neonatal herpes simplex virus infection in relation to asymptomatic maternal infection at the time of labor. *N Engl J Med* 1991;324:1247.

461. Baldwin S, Whitley RJ. Teratogen update: intrauterine herpes simplex virus infection. *Teratology* 1989;39:1.

462. Freij BJ, Sever JL. Fetal herpes simplex virus infection. In: Buyse ML, ed. *Birth defects encyclopedia.* Boston: Blackwell Scientific Publications, 1990:713.

463. Whitley R, Arvin A, Prober C, et al. A controlled trial comparing vidarabine with acyclovir in neonatal herpes simplex virus infection. *N Engl J Med* 1991;324:444.

464. Whitley R, Arvin A, Prober C, et al. Predictors of morbidity and mortality in neonates with herpes simplex virus infections. *N Engl J Med* 1991;324:450.

465. Jacobs RF. Neonatal herpes simplex virus infections. *Semin Perinatol* 1998;22:64.

466. Silverman MS, Gartner JG, Halliday WC, et al. Persistent cerebrospinal fluid neutrophilia in delayed-onset neonatal encephalitis caused by herpes simplex virus type 2. *J Pediatr* 1992;120:567.

467. Cameron PD, Wallace SJ, Munro J. Herpes simplex virus encephalitis: problems in diagnosis. *Dev Med Child Neurol* 1992;34:134.

468. el-Azazi M, Malm G, Forsgren M. Late ophthalmologic manifestations of neonatal herpes simplex virus infection. *Am J Ophthalmol* 1990;109:1.

469. Mansour AM, Nichols MM. Congenital diffuse necrotizing herpetic retinitis. *Graefes Arch Clin Exp Ophthalmol* 1993;231:95.

470. Andersen RD. Herpes simplex virus infection of the neonatal respiratory tract. *Am J Dis Child* 1987;141:274.

471. Hubbell C, Dominguez R, Kohl S. Neonatal herpes simplex pneumonitis. *Rev Infect Dis* 1988;10:431.

472. Barker JA, McLean SD, Jordan GD, et al. Primary neonatal herpes simplex virus pneumonia. *Pediatr Infect Dis J* 1990;9:285.

473. Stewart DL, Cook LN, Rabalais GP. Successful use of extracorporeal membrane oxygenation in a newborn with herpes simplex virus pneumonia. *Pediatr Infect Dis J* 1993;12:161.

474. Dominguez R, Rivero H, Gaisie G, et al. Neonatal herpes simplex pneumonia: radiographic findings. *Radiology* 1984;153:395.

475. Schutze GE, Edwards MS, Adham BI, Belmont JW. Hyperammonemia and neonatal herpes simplex pneumonitis. *Pediatr Infect Dis J* 1990;9:749.

476. Stanberry LR, Floyd-Reising SA, Connelly BL, et al. Herpes simplex viremia: report of eight pediatric cases and review of the literature. *Clin Infect Dis* 1994;18:401.

477. Mitchell PS, Espy MJ, Smith TF, et al. Laboratory diagnosis of central nervous system infections with herpes simplex virus by PCR performed with cerebrospinal fluid specimens. *J Clin Microbiol* 1997;35: 2873.

478. Kimberlin DW, Lakeman FD, Arvin AM, et al. Application of the polymerase chain reaction to the diagnosis and management of neonatal herpes simplex virus disease. *J Infect Dis* 1996;174:1162.

479. Kimura H, Futamura M, Kito H, et al. Detection of viral DNA in neonatal herpes simplex virus infections: frequent and prolonged presence in serum and cerebrospinal fluid. *J Infect Dis* 1991;164:289.

480. Englund JA, Fletcher CV, Balfour HH Jr. Acyclovir therapy in neonates. *J Pediatr* 1991;119:129.

481. Nyquist A-C, Rotbart HA, Cotton M, et al. Acyclovir-resistant neonatal herpes simplex virus infection of the larynx. *J Pediatr* 1994;124: 967.

482. Toltzis P. Current issues in neonatal herpes simplex virus infection. *Clin Perinatol* 1991;18:193.

483. Whitley RJ. Neonatal herpes simplex virus infections: is there a role for immunoglobulin in disease prevention and therapy? *Pediatr Infect Dis J* 1994;13:432.

484. Rudd C, Rivadeneira ED, Gutman LT. Dosing considerations for oral acyclovir following neonatal herpes disease. *Acta Paediatr* 1994;83: 1237.

485. Kimberlin D, Powell D, Gruber W, et al. Administration of oral acyclovir suppressive therapy after neonatal herpes simplex virus disease limited to the skin, eyes and mouth: results of a Phase I/II trial. *Pediatr Infect Dis J* 1996;15:247.

486. Libman MD, Dascal A, Kramer MS, Mendelson J. Strategies for the prevention of neonatal infection with herpes simplex virus: a decision analysis. *Rev Infect Dis* 1991;13:1093.

487. Arvin AM, Hensleigh PA, Prober CG, et al. Failure of antepartum maternal cultures to predict the infant's risk of exposure to herpes simplex virus at delivery. *N Engl J Med* 1986;315:796.

488. Prober CG, Hensleigh PA, Boucher FD, et al. Use of routine viral cultures at delivery to identify neonates exposed to herpes simplex virus. *N Engl J Med* 1988;318:887.

489. Roberts SW, Cox SM, Dax J, et al. Genital herpes during pregnancy: no lesions, no cesarean. *Obstet Gynecol* 1995;85:261.

490. Prober CG, Sullender WM, Yasukawa LL, et al. Low risk of herpes simplex virus infections in neonates exposed to the virus at the time of vaginal delivery to mothers with recurrent genital herpes simplex virus infections. *N Engl J Med* 1987;316:240.

491. Arvin AM. Relationships between maternal immunity to herpes simplex virus and the risk of neonatal herpesvirus infection. *Rev Infect Dis* 1991;13:S953.

492. Dobson AT, Little BB, Scott LL. Prevention of herpes simplex virus infection and latency by prophylactic treatment with acyclovir in a weanling mouse model. *Am J Obstet Gynecol* 1998;179:527.

493. Scott LL, Sanchez PJ, Jackson GL, et al. Acyclovir suppression to prevent cesarean delivery after first-episode genital herpes. *Obstet Gynecol* 1996;87:69.

494. Scott LL, Alexander J. Cost-effectiveness of acyclovir suppression to prevent recurrent genital herpes in term pregnancy. *Am J Perinatol* 1998;15:57.

495. Brocklehurst P, Kinghorn G, Carney O, et al. A randomised placebo controlled trial of suppressive acyclovir in late pregnancy in women with recurrent genital herpes infection. *Br J Obstet Gynaecol* 1998;105:275.

496. Alford CA, Stagno S, Pass RF, Britt WJ. Congenital and perinatal cytomegalovirus infections. *Rev Infect Dis* 1990;12:S745.

497. Gehrz RC. Human cytomegalovirus: biology and clinical perspectives. *Adv Pediatr* 1991;38:203.

498. Arribas JR, Storch GA, Clifford DB, Tselis AC. Cytomegalovirus encephalitis. *Ann Intern Med* 1996;125:577.

499. Grundy JE. Virologic and pathogenetic aspects of cytomegalovirus infection. *Rev Infect Dis* 1990;12:S711.

500. Demmler GJ. Summary of a workshop on surveillance for congenital cytomegalovirus disease. *Rev Infect Dis* 1991;13:315.

501. Walmus BF, Yow MD, Lester JW, et al. Factors predictive of cytomegalovirus immune status in pregnant women. *J Infect Dis* 1988; 157:172.

502. Tookey PA, Ades AE, Peckham CS. Cytomegalovirus prevalence in pregnant women: the influence of parity. *Arch Dis Child* 1992;67:779.

503. Sohn YM, Oh MK, Balcarek KB, et al. Cytomegalovirus infection in sexually active adolescents. *J Infect Dis* 1991;163:460.

504. Fowler KB, Pass RF. Sexually transmitted diseases in mothers of neonates with congenital cytomegalovirus infection. *J Infect Dis* 1991;164:259.

505. Coonrod D, Collier AC, Ashley R, et al. Association between cytomegalovirus seroconversion and upper genital tract infection among women attending a sexually transmitted disease clinic: a prospective study. *J Infect Dis* 1998;177:1188.

506. Adler SP. Cytomegalovirus and child day care: risk factors for maternal infection. *Pediatr Infect Dis J* 1991;10:590.

507. Murph JR, Baron JC, Brown CK, et al. The occupational risk of cytomegalovirus infection among day-care providers. *JAMA* 1991;265: 603.

508. Ford-Jones EL, Kitai I, Davis L, et al. Cytomegalovirus infections in Toronto child-care centers: a prospective study of viral excretion in children and seroconversion among day-care providers. *Pediatr Infect Dis J* 1996;15:507.

509. Nelson CT, Demmler GJ. Cytomegalovirus infection in the pregnant mother, fetus, and newborn infant. *Clin Perinatol* 1997;24:151.

510. Brown HL, Abernathy MP. Cytomegalovirus infection. *Semin Perinatol* 1998;22:260.

511. Shen C-Y, Chang S-F, Yen M-S, et al. Cytomegalovirus excretion in pregnant and nonpregnant women. *J Clin Microbiol* 1993;31:1635.

512. Fowler KB, Stagno S, Pass RF, et al. The outcome of congenital cytomegalovirus infection in relation to maternal antibody status. *N Engl J Med* 1992;326:663.

513. Nigro G, Clerico A, Mondaini C. Symptomatic congenital cytomegalovirus infection in two consecutive sisters. *Arch Dis Child* 1993;69:527.

514. Bratcher DF, Bourne N, Bravo FJ, et al. Effect of passive antibody on congenital cytomegalovirus infection in guinea pigs. *J Infect Dis* 1995;172:944.

515. Portolani M, Cermelli C, Sabbatini AMT, et al. A fatal case of congenital cytomegalic inclusion disease following recurrent maternal infection. *New Microbiol* 1995;18:427.

516. Schwebke K, Henry K, Balfour HH Jr, et al. Congenital cytomegalovirus infection as a result of nonprimary cytomegalovirus disease in a mother with acquired immunodeficiency syndrome. *J Pediatr* 1995;126:293.

517. Putland RA, Ford J, Korban G, et al. Investigation of spontaneously aborted concepti for microbial DNA: investigation for cytomegalovirus DNA using polymerase chain reaction. *Aust N Z J Obstet Gynaecol* 1990;30:248.

518. Griffiths PD, Stagno S, Pass RF, et al. Infection with cytomegalovirus during pregnancy: specific IgM antibodies as a marker of recent primary infection. *J Infect Dis* 1982;145:647.

519. Grangeot-Keros L, Mayaux MJ, Lebon P, et al. Value of cytomegalovirus (CMV) IgG avidity index for the diagnosis of primary CMV infection in pregnant women. *J Infect Dis* 1997;175:944.

520. Ehrnst A. The clinical relevance of different laboratory tests in CMV diagnosis. *Scand J Infect Dis Suppl* 1996;100:64.

521. Grundy JE, Ehrnst A, Einsele H, et al. A three-center European external quality control study of PCR for detection of cytomegalovirus DNA in blood. *J Clin Microbiol* 1996;34:1166.

522. Drew WL. Cytomegalovirus infection in patients with AIDS. *Clin Infect Dis* 1992;14:608.

523. Henderson GI, Hu ZQ, Yang Y, et al. Ganciclovir transfer by human placenta and its effects on rat fetal cells. *Am J Med Sci* 1993;306:151.

524. Lea AP, Bryson HM. Cidofovir. *Drugs* 1996;52:225.

525. Boppana SB, Pass RF, Britt WJ, et al. Symptomatic congenital cytomegalovirus infection: neonatal morbidity and mortality. *Pediatr Infect Dis J* 1992;11:93.

526. Bale JF Jr, Blackman JA, Sato Y. Outcome in children with symptomatic congenital cytomegalovirus infection. *J Child Neurol* 1990;5:131.

527. Ramsay MEB, Miller E, Peckham CS. Outcome of confirmed symptomatic congenital cytomegalovirus infection. *Arch Dis Child* 1991;66:1068.

528. Perlman JM, Argyle C. Lethal cytomegalovirus infection in preterm infants: clinical, radiological, and neuropathological findings. *Ann Neurol* 1992;31:64.

529. Boppana SB, Fowler KB, Vaid Y, et al. Neuroradiographic findings in the newborn period and long-term outcome in children with symptomatic congenital cytomegalovirus infection. *Pediatrics* 1997;99:409.

530. Williamson WD, Demmler GJ, Percy AK, Catlin FI. Progressive hearing loss in infants with asymptomatic congenital cytomegalovirus infection. *Pediatrics* 1992;90:862.

531. Fowler K, McCollister F, Pass R, et al. Childhood deafness: the importance of congenital cytomegalovirus screening. *Am J Epidemiol* 1992;136:954(abst).

532. Fowler KB, McCollister FP, Dahle AJ, et al. Progressive and fluctuating sensorineural hearing loss in children with asymptomatic congenital cytomegalovirus infection. *J Pediatr* 1997;130:624.

533. Huygen PLM, Admiral RJC. Audiovestibular sequelae of congenital cytomegalovirus infection in 3 children presumably representing 3 symptomatically different types of delayed endolymphatic hydrops. *Int J Pediatr Otorhinolaryngol* 1996;35:143.

534. Ivarsson S-A, Lernmark B, Svanberg L. Ten-year clinical, developmental, and intellectual follow-up of children with congenital cytomegalovirus infection without neurologic symptoms at one year of age. *Pediatrics* 1997;99:800.

535. Stagno S, Pass RF, Thomas JP, et al. Defects of tooth structure in congenital cytomegalovirus infection. *Pediatrics* 1982;69:646.

536. Morris DJ. Epidemiological evidence is crucial as proof of causation in cytomegalovirus disease. *J Infect* 1991;23:233.

537. Hart MH, Kaufman SS, Vanderhoof JA, et al. Neonatal hepatitis and extrahepatic biliary atresia associated with cytomegalovirus infection in twins. *Am J Dis Child* 1991;145:302.

538. Mena W, Royal S, Pass RF, et al. Diabetes insipidus associated with symptomatic congenital cytomegalovirus infection. *J Pediatr* 1993;122:911.

539. Comas C, Martinez Crespo JM, Puerto B, et al. Bilateral renal agenesis and cytomegalovirus infection in a case of Fraser syndrome. *Fetal Diagn Ther* 1993;8:285.

540. Baker ER, Eberhardt H, Brown ZA. "Stuck twin" syndrome associated with congenital cytomegalovirus infection. *Am J Perinatol* 1993;10:81.

541. Bauman NM, Kirby-Keyser LJ, Dolan KD, et al. Mondini dysplasia and congenital cytomegalovirus infection. *J Pediatr* 1994;124:71.

542. Tarr PI, Haas JE, Christie DL. Biliary atresia, cytomegalovirus, and age at referral. *Pediatrics* 1996;97:828.

543. Carrol ED, Campbell ME, Shaw BNJ, Pilling DW. Congenital lobar emphysema in congenital cytomegalovirus infection. *Pediatr Radiol* 1996;26:900.

544. Ahlfors K, Ivarsson S-A, Nilsson H. On the unpredictable development of congenital cytomegalovirus infection: a study in twins. *Early Hum Dev* 1988;18:125.

545. Schneeberger PM, Groenendaal F, de Vries LS, et al. Variable outcome of a congenital cytomegalovirus infection in a quadruplet after primary infection of the mother during pregnancy. *Acta Paediatr* 1994;83:986.

546. Jenson HB, Robert MF. Congenital cytomegalovirus infection with osteolytic lesions: use of DNA hybridization in diagnosis. *Clin Pediatr (Phila)* 1987;26:448.

547. Warren WP, Balcarek K, Smith R, Pass RF. Comparison of rapid methods of detection of cytomegalovirus in saliva with virus isolation in tissue culture. *J Clin Microbiol* 1992;30:786.

548. Chang M-H, Huang H-H, Huang E-S, et al. Polymerase chain reaction to detect human cytomegalovirus in livers of infants with neonatal hepatitis. *Gastroenterology* 1992;103:1022.

549. Nelson CT, Istas AS, Wilkerson MK, Demmler GJ. PCR detection of cytomegalovirus DNA in serum as a diagnostic test for congenital cytomegalovirus infection. *J Clin Microbiol* 1995;33:3317.

550. Drew WL, Miner RC, Busch DF, et al. Prevalence of resistance in patients receiving ganciclovir for serious cytomegalovirus infection. *J Infect Dis* 1991;163:716.

551. Zhou X-J, Gruber W, Demmler G, et al. Population pharmacokinetics of ganciclovir in newborns with congenital cytomegalovirus infections. *Antimicrob Agents Chemother* 1996;40:2202.

552. Hocker JR, Cook LN, Adams G, Rabalais GP. Ganciclovir therapy of congenital cytomegalovirus pneumonia. *Pediatr Infect Dis J* 1990;9:743.

553. Evans DGR, Lyon AJ. Fatal congenital cytomegalovirus infection acquired by an intra-uterine transfusion. *Eur J Pediatr* 1991;150:780.

554. Reigstad H, Bjerknes R, Markestad T, Myrmel H. Ganciclovir therapy of congenital cytomegalovirus disease. *Acta Paediatr* 1992;81:707.

555. Attard-Montalto SP, English MC, Stimmler L, Snodgrass GJ. Ganciclovir treatment of congenital cytomegalovirus infection: a report of two cases. *Scand J Infect Dis* 1993;25:385.

556. Stronati M, Revello MG, Cerbo RM, et al. Ganciclovir therapy of congenital human cytomegalovirus hepatitis. *Acta Paediatr* 1995;84:340.

557. Halwachs G, Kutschera J, Tiran A, et al. Antiviral treatment of congenitally infected children with a positive cytomegalovirus polymerase chain reaction in the cerebrospinal fluid. *Scand J Infect Dis Suppl* 1995;99:89.

558. Nigro G, Scholz H, Bartmann U. Ganciclovir therapy for symptomatic congenital cytomegalovirus infection in infants: a two-regimen experience. *J Pediatr* 1994;124:318.

559. Whitley RJ, Kimberlin DW. Treatment of viral infections during pregnancy and the neonatal period. *Clin Perinatol* 1997;24:267.

560. Nigro G, Krzysztofiak A, Bartmann U, et al. Ganciclovir therapy for cytomegalovirus-associated liver disease in immunocompetent or immunocompromised children. *Arch Virol* 1997;142:573.

561. Whitley RJ, Cloud G, Gruber W, et al. Ganciclovir treatment of symptomatic congenital cytomegalovirus infection: results of a phase II study. *J Infect Dis* 1997;175:1080.

562. Revello MG, Percivalle E, Baldanti F, et al. Prenatal treatment of congenital human cytomegalovirus infection by fetal intravascular administration of ganciclovir. *Clin Diagn Virol* 1993;1:61.

563. Negishi H, Yamada H, Hirayama E, et al. Intraperitoneal administration of cytomegalovirus hyperimmunoglobulin to the cytomegalovirus-infected fetus. *J Perinatol* 1998;18:466.

564. Alford C. Breast milk transmission of cytomegalovirus (CMV) infection. *Adv Exp Med Biol* 1991;310:293.

565. Portelli J, Gordon A, May JT. Effect of human milk sialyllactose on cytomegalovirus. *Eur J Clin Microbiol Infect Dis* 1998;17:66.

566. Portelli J, Gordon A, May JT. Effect of compounds with antibacterial activities in human milk on respiratory syncytial virus and cytomegalovirus in vitro. *J Med Microbiol* 1998;47:1015.

567. de Cates CR, Gray J, Roberton NRC, Walker J. Acquisition of cytomegalovirus infection by premature neonates. *J Infect* 1994;28:25.

568. Gentile MA, Boll TJ, Stagno S, Pass RF. Intellectual ability of children after perinatal cytomegalovirus infection. *Dev Med Child Neurol* 1989;31:782.

569. Lynch L, Daffos F, Emanuel D, et al. Prenatal diagnosis of fetal cytomegalovirus infection. *Am J Obstet Gynecol* 1991;165:714.

570. Hohlfeld P, Vial Y, Maillard-Brignon C, et al. Cytomegalovirus fetal infection: prenatal diagnosis. *Obstet Gynecol* 1991;78:615.

571. Lamy ME, Mulongo KN, Gadisseux J-F, et al. Prenatal diagnosis of fetal cytomegalovirus infection. *Am J Obstet Gynecol* 1992;166:91.

572. Weber B, Opp M, Born HJ, et al. Laboratory diagnosis of congenital human cytomegalovirus infection using polymerase chain reaction and shell vial culture. *Infection* 1992;20:155.

573. Hogge WA, Buffone GJ, Hogge JS. Prenatal diagnosis of cytomegalovirus (CMV) infection: a preliminary report. *Prenat Diagn* 1993;13:131.

574. Catanzarite V, Dankner WM. Prenatal diagnosis of congenital cytomegalovirus infection: false-negative amniocentesis at 20 weeks gestation. *Prenat Diagn* 1993;13:1021.

575. Donner C, Liesnard C, Content J, et al. Prenatal diagnosis of 52 pregnancies at risk for congenital cytomegalovirus infection. *Obstet Gynecol* 1993;82:481.

576. Achiron R, Pinhas-Hamiel O, Lipitz S, et al. Prenatal ultrasonographic diagnosis of fetal cerebral ventriculitis associated with asymptomatic maternal cytomegalovirus infection. *Prenat Diagn* 1994;14:523.

577. Nicolini U, Kustermann A, Tassis B, et al. Prenatal diagnosis of congenital human cytomegalovirus infection. *Prenat Diagn* 1994;14:903.

578. Watt-Morse ML, Laifer SA, Hill LM. The natural history of fetal cytomegalovirus infection as assessed by serial ultrasound and fetal blood sampling: a case report. *Prenat Diagn* 1995;15:567.

579. Revello MG, Baldanti F, Furione M, et al. Polymerase chain reaction for prenatal diagnosis of congenital human cytomegalovirus infection. *J Med Virol* 1995;47:462.

580. Kyriazopoulou V, Bondis J, Frantzidou F, et al. Prenatal diagnosis of fetal cytomegalovirus infection in seropositive pregnant women. *Eur J Obstet Gynecol Reprod Biol* 1996;69:91.

581. Lipitz S, Yagel S, Shalev E, et al. Prenatal diagnosis of fetal primary cytomegalovirus infection. *Obstet Gynecol* 1997;89:763.

582. Lazzarotto T, Guerra B, Spezzacatena P, et al. Prenatal diagnosis of congenital cytomegalovirus infection. *J Clin Microbiol* 1998;36:3540.

583. Dong Z-W, Yan C, Yi W, Cui Y-Q. Detection of congenital cytomegalovirus infection by using chorionic villi of the early pregnancy and polymerase chain reaction. *Int J Gynaecol Obstet* 1994;44:229.

584. Pletcher BA, Williams MK, Mulivor RA, et al. Intrauterine cytomegalovirus infection presenting as fetal meconium peritonitis. *Obstet Gynecol* 1991;78:903.

585. Mazeron M-C, Cordovi-Voulgaropoulos L, Pérol Y. Transient hydrops fetalis associated with intrauterine cytomegalovirus infection: prenatal diagnosis. *Obstet Gynecol* 1994;84:692.

586. Dogra VK, Menon PA, Poblete J, Smeltzer JS. Neurosonographic imaging of small-for-gestational-age neonates exposed and not exposed to cocaine and cytomegalovirus. *J Clin Ultrasound* 1994;22: 93.

587. Muller F, Dommergues M, Aubry M-C, et al. Hyperechogenic fetal bowel: an ultrasonographic marker for adverse fetal and neonatal outcome. *Am J Obstet Gynecol* 1995;173:508.

588. Adler SP. Current prospects for immunization against cytomegaloviral disease. *Infect Agent Dis* 1996;5:29.

589. Tierney AJ, Higa TE, Finer NN. Disseminated cytomegalovirus infection after extracorporeal membrane oxygenation. *Pediatr Infect Dis J* 1992;11:241.

590. Wharton M. The epidemiology of varicella-zoster virus infections. *Infect Dis Clin North Am* 1996;10:571.

591. Centers for Disease Control and Prevention. Varicella-zoster immune globulin for the prevention of chickenpox. *MMWR* 1984;33:84.

592. Sever JL, Ellenberg JH, Ley A, Edmonds D. Incidence of clinical infections in a defined population of pregnant women. In: Marois M, ed. *Prevention of physical and mental congenital defects. Part B:* epidemiology, early detection and therapy, and environmental factors. New York: Alan R. Liss, 1985:317.

593. Chapman SJ. Varicella in pregnancy. *Semin Perinatol* 1998;22:339.

594. Ross AH. Modification of chicken pox in family contacts by administration of gamma globulin. *N Engl J Med* 1962;267:369.

595. Junker AK, Angus E, Thomas EE. Recurrent varicella-zoster virus infections in apparently immunocompetent children. *Pediatr Infect Dis J* 1991;10:569.

596. Martin KA, Junker AK, Thomas EE, et al. Occurrence of chickenpox during pregnancy in women seropositive for varicella-zoster virus. *J Infect Dis* 1994;170:991.

597. Enders G. Varicella-zoster virus infection in pregnancy. *Prog Med Virol* 1984;29:166.

598. Kido S, Ozaki T, Asada H, et al. Detection of varicella-zoster virus (VZV) DNA in clinical samples from patients with VZV by the polymerase chain reaction. *J Clin Microbiol* 1991;29:76.

599. Koropchak CM, Graham G, Palmer J, et al. Investigation of varicella-zoster virus infection by polymerase chain reaction in the immunocompetent host with acute varicella. *J Infect Dis* 1991;163:1016.

600. Krah DL. Assays for antibodies to varicella-zoster virus. *Infect Dis Clin North Am* 1996;10:507.

601. Rothe MJ, Feder HM Jr, Grant-Kels JM. Oral acyclovir therapy for varicella and zoster infections in pediatric and pregnant patients: a brief review. *Pediatr Dermatol* 1991;8:236.

602. Wallace MR, Bowler WA, Murray NB, et al. Treatment of adult varicella with oral acyclovir: a randomized, placebo-controlled trial. *Ann Intern Med* 1992;117:358.

603. Broussard RC, Payne DK, George RB. Treatment with acyclovir of varicella pneumonia in pregnancy. *Chest* 1991;99:1045.

604. Esmonde TF, Herdman G, Anderson G. Chickenpox pneumonia: an association with pregnancy. *Thorax* 1989;44:812.

605. Cox SM, Cunningham FG, Luby J. Management of varicella pneumonia complicating pregnancy. *Am J Perinatol* 1990;7:300.

606. Lotshaw RR, Keegan JM, Gordon HR. Parenteral and oral acyclovir for management of varicella pneumonia in pregnancy: a case report with review of literature. *W V Med J* 1991;87:204.

607. Smego RA Jr, Asperilla MO. Use of acyclovir for varicella pneumonia during pregnancy. *Obstet Gynecol* 1991;78:1112.

608. Katz VL, Kuller JA, McMahon MJ, et al. Varicella during pregnancy: maternal and fetal effects. *West J Med* 1995;163:446.

609. Nathwani D, Maclean A, Conway S, Carrington D. Varicella infections in pregnancy and the newborn: a review prepared for the UK Advisory Group on Chickenpox on behalf of the British Society for the Study of Infection. *J Infect* 1998;36[Suppl 1]:59.

610. Puchhammer-Stöckl E, Kunz C, Wagner G, Enders G. Detection of varicella zoster virus (VZV) DNA in fetal tissue by polymerase chain reaction. *J Perinat Med* 1994;22:65.

611. Sauerbrei A, Müller D, Eichhorn U, Wutzler P. Detection of varicella-zoster virus in congenital varicella syndrome: a case report. *Obstet Gynecol* 1996;88:687.

612. Oyer CE, Cai R, Coughlin JJ, Singer DB. First trimester pregnancy loss associated with varicella zoster virus infection: histological definition of a case. *Hum Pathol* 1998;29:94.

613. Paryani SG, Arvin AM. Intrauterine infection with varicella-zoster virus after maternal varicella. *N Engl J Med* 1986;314:1542.

614. Siegel M, Fuerst HT. Low birth weight and maternal virus diseases: a prospective study of rubella, measles, mumps, chickenpox, and hepatitis. *JAMA* 1966;197:680.

615. Siegel M, Fuerst HT, Peress NS. Comparative fetal mortality in maternal virus diseases: a prospective study on rubella, measles, mumps, chicken pox and hepatitis. *N Engl J Med* 1966;274:768.

616. Benyesh-Melnick M, Stich HF, Rapp F, Hsu TC. Viruses and mammalian chromosomes. III. Effect of herpes zoster virus on human embryonal lung cultures. *Proc Soc Exp Biol Med* 1964;117:546.

617. Aula P. Chromosomes and viral infections. *Lancet* 1964;1:720.

618. Massimo L, Vianello MG, Dagna-Bricarelli F, Tortorolo G. Chickenpox and chromosome aberrations. *BMJ* 1965;2:172.

619. Muñoz N. Perinatal viral infections and the risk of certain cancers. *Prog Biochem Pharmacol* 1978;14:104.

620. Alexander I. Congenital varicella. *BMJ* 1979;2:1074.

621. Alkalay AL, Pomerance JJ, Rimoin DL. Fetal varicella syndrome. *J Pediatr* 1987;111:320.

622. Andreou A, Basiakos H, Hatzikoumi I, Lazarides A. Fetal varicella syndrome with manifestations limited to the eye. *Am J Perinatol* 1995; 12:347.

623. Bennet R, Forsgren M, Herin P. Herpes zoster in a 2-week-old premature infant with possible congenital varicella encephalitis. *Acta Paediatr Scand* 1985;74:979.

624. Borzyskowski M, Harris RF, Jones RWA. The congenital varicella syndrome. *Eur J Pediatr* 1981;137:335.

625. Brice JEH. Congenital varicella resulting from infection during second trimester of pregnancy. *Arch Dis Child* 1976;51:474.

626. Charles NC, Bennett TW, Margolis S. Ocular pathology of the congenital varicella syndrome. *Arch Ophthalmol* 1977;95:2034.

627. Cotlier E. Congenital varicella cataract. *Am J Ophthalmol* 1978;86: 627.

628. Cuthbertson G, Weiner CP, Giller RH, Grose C. Prenatal diagnosis of second-trimester congenital varicella syndrome by virus-specific immunoglobulin M. *J Pediatr* 1987;111:592.

629. Dodion-Fransen J, Dekegel D, Thiry L. Congenital varicella-zoster infection related to maternal disease in early pregnancy. *Scand J Infect Dis* 1973;5:149.

630. Essex-Cater A, Heggarty H. Fatal congenital varicella syndrome. *J Infect* 1983;7:77.

631. Frey HM, Bialkin G, Gershon AA. Congenital varicella: case report of a serologically proved long-term survivor. *Pediatrics* 1977;59:110.

632. Friedman RM, Wood VE. Varicella gangrenosa in the newborn upper extremity: a case report. *J Hand Surg [Am]* 1996;21:487.

633. Hajdi G, Mészner Z, Nyerges G, et al. Congenital varicella syndrome. *Infection* 1986;14:177.

634. Harding B, Baumer JA. Congenital varicella-zoster: a serologically proven case with necrotizing encephalitis and malformation. *Acta Neuropathol (Berl)* 1988;76:311.

635. Higa K, Dan K, Manabe H. Varicella-zoster virus infections during pregnancy: hypothesis concerning the mechanisms of congenital malformations. *Obstet Gynecol* 1987;69:214.

636. Hitchcock R, Birthistle K, Carrington D, et al. Colonic atresia and spinal cord atrophy associated with a case of fetal varicella syndrome. *J Pediatr Surg* 1995;30:1344.

637. Huang Y-C, Lin T-Y, Wong K-S, Chiu C-H. Congenital anomalies fol-

lowing maternal varicella infection during early pregnancy. *J Formos Med Assoc* 1996;95:393.

638. König R, Gutjahr P, Kruel R, et al. Konnatale Varizellen-Embryo-Fetopathie. *Helv Paediatr Acta* 1985;40:391.

639. Kotchmar GS Jr, Grose C, Brunell PA. Complete spectrum of the varicella congenital defects syndrome in 5-year-old child. *Pediatr Infect Dis* 1984;3:142.

640. LaForet EG, Lynch CL Jr. Multiple congenital defects following maternal varicella: report of a case. *N Engl J Med* 1947;236:534.

641. McKendry JBJ, Bailey JD. Congenital varicella associated with multiple defects. *Can Med Assoc J* 1973;108:66.

642. Randel RC, Kearns DB, Nespeca MP, et al. Vocal cord paralysis as a presentation of intrauterine infection with varicella-zoster virus. *Pediatrics* 1996;97:127.

643. Rigsby CK, Donnelly LF. Fetal varicella syndrome: association with multiple hepatic calcifications and intestinal atresia. *Pediatr Radiol* 1997;27:779.

644. Rinvik R. Congenital varicella encephalomyelitis in surviving newborn. *Am J Dis Child* 1969;117:231.

645. Savage MO, Moosa A, Gordon RR. Maternal varicella infection as a cause of fetal malformations. *Lancet* 1973;1:352.

646. Siegel M. Congenital malformations following chickenpox, measles, mumps, and hepatitis: results of a cohort study. *JAMA* 1973;226:1521.

647. Srabstein JC, Morris N, Bryce Larke RP, et al. Is there a congenital varicella syndrome? *J Pediatr* 1974;84:239.

648. Taranger J, Blomberg J, Strannegård Ö. Intrauterine varicella: a report of two cases associated with hyper-A-immunoglobulinemia. *Scand J Infect Dis* 1981;13:297.

649. Trlifajová J, Benda R, Beneš Č. Effect of maternal varicella-zoster virus infection on the outcome of pregnancy and the analysis of transplacental virus transmission. *Acta Virol (Praha)* 1986;30:249.

650. Tudehope DI. Two lethal cases of congenital varicella syndrome. *J Paediatr Child Health* 1995;31:259.

651. Unger-Köppel J, Kilcher P, Tönz O. Varizellenfetopathie. *Helv Paediatr Acta* 1985;40:399.

652. Wheatley R, Morton RE, Nicholson J. Chickenpox in mid-trimester pregnancy: always innocent? *Dev Med Child Neurol* 1996;38:462.

653. Williamson AP. The varicella-zoster virus in the etiology of severe congenital defects: a survey of eleven reported instances. *Clin Pediatr (Phila)* 1975;14:553.

654. Lambert SR, Taylor D, Kriss A, et al. Ocular manifestations of the congenital varicella syndrome. *Arch Ophthalmol* 1989;107:52.

655. Lloyd KM, Dunne JL. Skin lesions as the sole manifestation of the fetal varicella syndrome. *Arch Dermatol* 1990;126:546.

656. Scharf A, Scherr O, Enders G, Helftenbein E. Virus detection in the fetal tissue of a premature delivery with a congenital varicella syndrome: a case report. *J Perinat Med* 1990;18:317.

657. Da Silva O, Hammerberg O, Chance GW. Fetal varicella syndrome. *Pediatr Infect Dis J* 1990;9:854.

658. Scheffer IE, Baraitser M, Brett EM. Severe microcephaly associated with congenital varicella infection. *Dev Med Child Neurol* 1991;33:916.

659. Magliocco AM, Demetrick DJ, Sarnat HB, Hwang WS. Varicella embryopathy. *Arch Pathol Lab Med* 1992;116:181.

660. Asha Bai PV, John TJ. Congenital skin ulcers following varicella in late pregnancy. *J Pediatr* 1979;94:65.

661. Salzman MB, Sood SK. Congenital anomalies resulting from maternal varicella at 25½ weeks of gestation. *Pediatr Infect Dis J* 1992;11:504.

662. Al-Qattan MM, Thomson HG. Congenital varicella of the upper limb: a preventable disaster. *J Hand Surg [Br]* 1995;20:115.

663. Pastuszak AL, Levy M, Schick B, et al. Outcome after maternal varicella infection in the first 20 weeks of pregnancy. *N Engl J Med* 1994;330:901.

664. Enders G, Miller E, Cradock-Watson J, et al. Consequences of varicella and herpes zoster in pregnancy: prospective study of 1739 cases. *Lancet* 1994;343:1547.

665. Jones KL, Johnson KA, Chambers CD. Offspring of women infected with varicella during pregnancy: a prospective study. *Teratology* 1994;49:29.

666. Figueroa-Damian R, Arredondo-Garcia JL. Perinatal outcome of pregnancies complicated with varicella infection during the first 20 weeks of gestation. *Am J Perinatol* 1997;14:411.

667. Balducci J, Rodis JF, Rosengren S, et al. Pregnancy outcome following first-trimester varicella infection. *Obstet Gynecol* 1992;79:5.

668. Brazin SA, Simkovich JW, Johnson WT. Herpes zoster during pregnancy. *Obstet Gynecol* 1979;53:175.

669. Duehr PA. Herpes zoster as a cause of congenital cataract. *Am J Ophthalmol* 1955;39:157.

670. Klauber GT, Flynn FJ Jr, Altman BD. Congenital varicella syndrome with genitourinary anomalies. *Urology* 1976;8:153.

671. Webster MH, Smith CS. Congenital abnormalities and maternal herpes zoster. *BMJ* 1977;2:1193.

672. Mendez DB, Sinclair MB, Garcia S, et al. Transplacental immunity to varicella-zoster virus in extremely low birthweight infants. *Am J Perinatol* 1992;9:236.

673. Williams H, Latif A, Morgan J, Ansari BM. Acyclovir in the treatment of neonatal varicella. *J Infect* 1987;15:65.

674. McGregor JA, Mark S, Crawford GP, Levin MJ. Varicella zoster antibody testing in the care of pregnant women exposed to varicella. *Am J Obstet Gynecol* 1987;157:281.

675. Wallace MR, Chamberlin CJ, Zerboni L, et al. Reliability of a history of previous varicella infection in adults. *JAMA* 1997;278:1520.

676. Lécuru F, Taurelle R, Bernard J-P, et al. Varicella zoster virus infection during pregnancy: the limits of prenatal diagnosis. *Eur J Obstet Gynecol Reprod Biol* 1994;56:67.

677. Isada NB, Paar DP, Johnson MP, et al. In utero diagnosis of congenital varicella zoster virus infection by chorionic villus sampling and polymerase chain reaction. *Am J Obstet Gynecol* 1991;165:1727.

678. Pons J-C, Rozenberg F, Imbert M-C, et al. Prenatal diagnosis of second-trimester congenital varicella syndrome. *Prenat Diagn* 1992;12:975.

679. Mouly F, Mirlesse V, Méritet JF, et al. Prenatal diagnosis of fetal varicella-zoster virus infection with polymerase chain reaction of amniotic fluid in 107 cases. *Am J Obstet Gynecol* 1997;177:894.

680. Pretorius DH, Hayward I, Jones KL, Stamm E. Sonographic evaluation of pregnancies with maternal varicella infection. *J Ultrasound Med* 1992;11:459.

681. Hofmeyr GJ, Moolla S, Lawrie T. Prenatal sonographic diagnosis of congenital varicella infection—a case report. *Prenat Diagn* 1996;16:1148.

682. Ong C-L, Daniel ML. Antenatal diagnosis of a porencephalic cyst in congenital varicella-zoster virus infection. *Pediatr Radiol* 1998;28:94.

683. Hanngren KAJ, Grandien M, Granström G. Effect of zoster immunoglobulin for varicella prophylaxis in the newborn. *Scand J Infect Dis* 1985;17:343.

684. Bakshi SS, Miller TC, Kaplan M, et al. Failure of varicella-zoster immunoglobulin in modification of severe congenital varicella. *Pediatr Infect Dis* 1986;5:699.

685. Haddad J, Simeoni U, Messer J, Willard D. Acyclovir in prophylaxis and perinatal varicella. *Lancet* 1987;1:161.

686. Rubin L, Leggiadro R, Elie MT, Lipsitz P. Disseminated varicella in a neonate: implications for immunoprophylaxis of neonates postnatally exposed to varicella. *Pediatr Infect Dis* 1986;5:100.

687. Glantz JC, Mushlin AI. Cost-effectiveness of routine antenatal varicella screening. *Obstet Gynecol* 1998;91:519.

688. Smith WJ, Jackson LA, Watts DH, Koepsell TD. Prevention of chickenpox in reproductive-age women: cost-effectiveness of routine prenatal screening with postpartum vaccination of susceptibles. *Obstet Gynecol* 1998;92:535.

689. Cossart YE, Field AM, Cant B, Widdows D. Parvovirus-like particles in human sera. *Lancet* 1975;1:72.

690. Brown KE, Young NS. Human parvovirus B19 infections in infants and children. *Adv Pediatr Infect Dis* 1998;13:101.

691. Kerr JR. Parvovirus B19 infection. *Eur J Clin Microbiol Infect Dis* 1996;15:10.

692. Brown KE, Hibbs JR, Gallinella G, et al. Resistance to parvovirus B19 infection due to lack of virus receptor (erythrocyte P antigen). *N Engl J Med* 1994;330:1192.

693. Cooling LLW, Koerner TAW, Naides SJ. Multiple glycosphingolipids determine the tissue tropism of parvovirus B19. *J Infect Dis* 1995;172:1198.

694. von Poblotzki A, Hemauer A, Gigler A, et al. Antibodies to the nonstructural protein of parvovirus B19 in persistently infected patients: implications for pathogenesis. *J Infect Dis* 1995;172:1356.

695. Centers for Disease Control and Prevention. Risks associated with human parvovirus B19 infection. *MMWR* 1989;38:81.

696. Harger JH, Adler SP, Koch WC, Harger GF. Prospective evaluation of 618 pregnant women exposed to parvovirus B19: risks and symptoms. *Obstet Gynecol* 1998;91:413.

697. Gratacós E, Torres P-J, Vidal J, et al. The incidence of human parvovirus B19 infection during pregnancy and its impact on perinatal outcome. *J Infect Dis* 1995;171:1360.

698. Skjöldebrand-Sparre L, Fridell E, Nyman M, Wahren B. A prospective study of antibodies against parvovirus B19 in pregnancy. *Acta Obstet Gynecol Scand* 1996;75:336.

699. Markenson GR, Yancey MK. Parvovirus B19 infections in pregnancy. *Semin Perinatol* 1998;22:309.

700. Koch WC, Adler SP. Human parvovirus B19 infections in women of childbearing age and within families. *Pediatr Infect Dis J* 1989;8:83.

701. Cartter ML, Farley TA, Rosengren S, et al. Occupational risk factors for infection with parvovirus B19 among pregnant women. *J Infect Dis* 1991;163:282.

702. Bell LM, Naides SJ, Stoffman P, et al. Human parvovirus B19 infection among hospital staff members after contact with infected patients. *N Engl J Med* 1989;321:485.

703. Ray SM, Erdman DD, Berschling JD, et al. Nosocomial exposure to parvovirus B19: low risk of transmission to healthcare workers. *Infect Control Hosp Epidemiol* 1997;18:109.

704. Lobkowicz F, Ring J, Schwarz TF, Roggendorf M. Erythema multiforme in a patient with acute human parvovirus B19 infection. *J Am Acad Dermatol* 1989;20:849.

705. Zerbini M, Musiani M, Venturoli S, et al. Different syndromes associated with B19 parvovirus viraemia in paediatric patients: report of four cases. *Eur J Pediatr* 1992;151:815.

706. Woolf AD, Campion GV, Chishick A, et al. Clinical manifestations of human parvovirus B19 in adults. *Arch Intern Med* 1989;149:1153.

707. Naides SJ, Field EH. Transient rheumatoid factor positivity in acute human parvovirus B19 infection. *Arch Intern Med* 1988;148:2587.

708. Erdman DD, Usher MJ, Tsou C, et al. Human parvovirus B19 specific IgG, IgA, and IgM antibodies and DNA in serum specimens from persons with erythema infectiosum. *J Med Virol* 1991;35:110.

709. Cassinotti P, Schultze D, Wieczorek K, et al. Parvovirus B19 infection during pregnancy and development of hydrops fetalis despite the evidence for preexisting anti-B19 antibody: how reliable are serological results? *Clin Diagn Virol* 1994;2:87.

710. Musiani M, Zerbini M, Gentilomi G, et al. Parvovirus B19 clearance from peripheral blood after acute infection. *J Infect Dis* 1995;172:1360.

711. Gentilomi G, Musiani M, Zerbini M, et al. Dot immunoperoxidase assay for detection of parvovirus B19 antigens in serum samples. *J Clin Microbiol* 1997;35:1575.

712. Selbing A, Josefsson A, Dahle LO, Lindgren R. Parvovirus B19 infection during pregnancy treated with high-dose intravenous gammaglobulin. *Lancet* 1995;345:660.

713. Rogers BB, Mark Y, Oyer CE. Diagnosis and incidence of fetal parvovirus infection in an autopsy series: I. Histology. *Pediatr Pathol* 1993;13:371.

714. Yaegashi N, Okamura K, Yajima A, et al. The frequency of human parvovirus B19 infection in nonimmune hydrops fetalis. *J Perinat Med* 1994;22:159.

715. Jordan JA. Identification of human parvovirus B19 infection in idiopathic nonimmune hydrops fetalis. *Am J Obstet Gynecol* 1996;174:37.

716. Schwarz TF, Nerlich A, Hottenträger B, et al. Parvovirus B19 infection of the fetus: histology and in situ hybridization. *Am J Clin Pathol* 1991;96:121.

717. Public Health Laboratory Service Working Party on Fifth Disease. Prospective study of human parvovirus (B19) infection in pregnancy. *BMJ* 1990;300:1166.

718. Miller E, Fairley CK, Cohen BJ, Seng C. Immediate and long term outcome of human parvovirus B19 infection in pregnancy. *Br J Obstet Gynaecol* 1998;105:174.

719. Kinney JS, Anderson LJ, Farrar J, et al. Risk of adverse outcomes of pregnancy after human parvovirus B19 infection. *J Infect Dis* 1988;157:663.

720. Porter HJ, Quantrill AM, Fleming KA. B19 parvovirus infection of myocardial cells. *Lancet* 1988;1:535.

721. Koch WC, Harger JH, Barnstein B, Adler SP. Serologic and virologic evidence for frequent intrauterine transmission of human parvovirus B19 with a primary maternal infection during pregnancy. *Pediatr Infect Dis J* 1998;17:489.

722. Brown KE, Green SW, de Mayolo JA, et al. Congenital anaemia after transplacental B19 parvovirus infection. *Lancet* 1994;343:895.

723. Tugal O, Pallant B, Shebarek N, Jayabose S. Transient erythroblastopenia of the newborn caused by human parvovirus. *Am J Pediatr Hematol Oncol* 1994;16:352.

724. Zerbini M, Musiani M, Gentilomi G, et al. Symptomatic parvovirus B19 infection of one fetus in a twin pregnancy. *Clin Infect Dis* 1993;17:262.

725. Pustilnik TB, Cohen AW. Parvovirus B19 infection in a twin pregnancy. *Obstet Gynecol* 1994;83:834.

726. Hartwig NG, Vermeij-Keers C, van Elsacker-Niele AMW, Fleuren GJ. Embryonic malformations in a case of intrauterine parvovirus B19 infection. *Teratology* 1989;39:295.

727. Rodis JF, Hovick TJ Jr, Quinn DL, et al. Human parvovirus infection in pregnancy. *Obstet Gynecol* 1988;72:733.

728. Tiessen RG, van Elsacker-Niele AMW, Vermeij-Keers C, et al. A fetus with a parvovirus B19 infection and congenital anomalies. *Prenat Diagn* 1994;14:173.

729. Katz VL, McCoy MC, Kuller JA, Hansen WF. An association between fetal parvovirus B19 infection and fetal anomalies: a report of two cases. *Am J Perinatol* 1996;13:43.

730. Willekes C, Roumen FJME, van Elsacker-Niele AMW, et al. Human parvovirus B19 infection and unbalanced translocation in a case of hydrops fetalis. *Prenat Diagn* 1994;14:181.

731. Zerbini M, Gentilomi GA, Gallinella G, et al. Intra-uterine parvovirus B19 infection and meconium peritonitis. *Prenat Diagn* 1998;18:599.

732. Clewley JP, Cohen BJ, Field AM. Detection of parvovirus B19 DNA, antigen, and particles in the human fetus. *J Med Virol* 1987;23:367.

733. Field AM, Cohen BJ, Brown KE, et al. Detection of B19 parvovirus in human fetal tissues by electron microscopy. *J Med Virol* 1991;35:85.

734. Yamakawa Y, Oka H, Hori S, et al. Detection of human parvovirus B19 DNA by nested polymerase chain reaction. *Obstet Gynecol* 1995;86:126.

735. Rodis JF, Rodner C, Hansen AA, et al. Long-term outcome of children following maternal human parvovirus B19 infection. *Obstet Gynecol* 1998;91:125.

736. Schwarz TF, Roggendorf M, Hottenträger B, et al. Immunoglobulins in the prophylaxis of parvovirus B19 infection. *J Infect Dis* 1990;162:1214.

737. Bloom MC, Rolland M, Bernard JD, et al. Materno-fetal infection by parvovirus associated with antenatal meconium peritonitis. *Arch Fr Pediatr* 1990;47:437.

738. Carrington D, Gilmore DH, Whittle MJ, et al. Maternal serum alphafetoprotein—a marker of fetal aplastic crisis during intrauterine human parvovirus infection. *Lancet* 1987;1:433.

739. Saller DN Jr, Rogers BB, Canick JA. Maternal serum biochemical markers in pregnancies with fetal parvovirus B19 infection. *Prenat Diagn* 1993;13:467.

740. Naides SJ, Weiner CP. Antenatal diagnosis and palliative treatment of non-immune hydrops fetalis secondary to fetal parvovirus B19 infection. *Prenat Diagn* 1989;9:105.

741. Peters MT, Nicolaides KH. Cordocentesis for the diagnosis and treatment of human fetal parvovirus infection. *Obstet Gynecol* 1990;75:501.

742. Sahakian V, Weiner CP, Naides SJ, et al. Intrauterine transfusion treatment of nonimmune hydrops fetalis secondary to human parvovirus B19 infection. *Am J Obstet Gynecol* 1991;164:1090.

743. Török TJ, Wang Q-Y, Gary GW Jr, et al. Prenatal diagnosis of intrauterine infection with parvovirus B19 by the polymerase chain reaction technique. *Clin Infect Dis* 1992;14:149.

744. Iwa N, Yutani C. Cytodiagnosis of parvovirus B19 infection from ascites fluid of hydrops fetalis: report of a case. *Diagn Cytopathol* 1995;13:139.

745. Nikkari S, Ekblad U. A rapid and safe method to detect fetal parvovirus B19 infection in amniotic fluid by polymerase chain reaction: report of a case. *Am J Perinatol* 1995;12:447.

746. Zerbini M, Musiani M, Gentilomi G, et al. Comparative evaluation of virological and serological methods in prenatal diagnosis of parvovirus B19 fetal hydrops. *J Clin Microbiol* 1996;34:603.

747. Weiner CP, Naides SJ. Fetal survival after human parvovirus B19 infection: spectrum of intrauterine response in a twin gestation. *Am J Perinatol* 1992;9:66.

748. Odibo AO, Campbell WA, Feldman D, et al. Resolution of human parvovirus B19-induced nonimmune hydrops after intrauterine transfusion. *J Ultrasound Med* 1998;17:547.

749. Fairley CK, Smoleniec JS, Caul OE, Miller E. Observational study of effect of intrauterine transfusions on outcome of fetal hydrops after parvovirus B19 infection. *Lancet* 1995;346:1335.

750. Duthie SJ, Walkinshaw SA. Parvovirus associated fetal hydrops: reversal of pregnancy induced proteinuric hypertension by in utero fetal transfusion. *Br J Obstet Gynaecol* 1995;102:1011.

751. Levy R, Weissman A, Blomberg G, Hagay ZJ. Infection by parvovirus B 19 during pregnancy: a review. *Obstet Gynecol Surv* 1997;52:254.

752. Morey AL, Nicolini U, Welch CR, et al. Parvovirus B19 infection and transient fetal hydrops. *Lancet* 1991;337:496.

753. Bhal PS, Davies NJ, Westmoreland D, Jones A. Spontaneous resolution of non-immune hydrops fetalis secondary to transplacental parvovirus B19 infection. *Ultrasound Obstet Gynecol* 1996;7:55.

754. Rodis JF, Borgida AF, Wilson M, et al. Management of parvovirus infection in pregnancy and outcomes of hydrops: a survey of members of the Society of Perinatal Obstetricians. *Am J Obstet Gynecol* 1998; 179:985.

755. Guyer B, MacDorman MF, Martin JA, et al. Annual summary of vital statistics—1997. *Pediatrics* 1998;102:1333.

756. Mocroft A, Vella S, Benfield TL, et al. Changing patterns of mortality across Europe in patients infected with HIV-1. *Lancet* 1998;352:1725.

757. Fowler MG, Melnick SL, Mathieson BJ. Women and HIV: epidemiology and global overview. *Obstet Gynecol Clin North Am* 1997;24:705.

758. Wilfert CM. Perinatal HIV transmission—a global problem: controversy and protection of the next generation. *Semin Pediatr Infect Dis* 1998;9:339.

759. Landers DV, Martínez de Tejada B, Coyne BA. Immunology of HIV and pregnancy: the effects of each on the other. *Obstet Gynecol Clin North Am* 1997;24:821.

760. Minkoff HL. Human immunodeficiency virus infection in pregnancy. *Semin Perinatol* 1998;22:293.

761. Garzino-Demo A, Devico AL, Gallo RC. Chemokine receptors and chemokines in HIV infection. *J Clin Immunol* 1998;18:243.

762. Misrahi M, Teglas J-P, N'Go N, et al. CCR5 chemokine receptor variant in HIV-1 mother-to-child transmission and disease progression in children. *JAMA* 1998;279:277.

763. Kostrikis LG, Huang Y, Moore JP, et al. A chemokine receptor CCR2 allele delays HIV-1 disease progression and is associated with a CCR5 promoter mutation. *Nat Med* 1998;4:350.

764. Connor EM, Sperling RS, Gelber R, et al. Reduction of maternal-infant transmission of human immunodeficiency virus type 1 with zidovudine treatment. *N Engl J Med* 1994;331:1173.

765. Centers for Disease Control and Prevention. Public Health Service task force recommendations for the use of antiretroviral drugs in pregnant women infected with HIV-1 for maternal health and for reducing perinatal HIV-1 transmission in the United States. *MMWR* 1998; 47(RR-2):1.

766. Moyle GJ. Current knowledge of HIV-1 reverse transcriptase mutations selected during nucleoside analogue therapy: the potential to use resistance data to guide clinical decisions. *J Antimicrob Chemother* 1997;40:765.

767. Hodinka RL. The clinical utility of viral quantitation using molecular methods. *Clin Diagn Virol* 1998;10:25.

768. Cavert W. In vivo detection and quantitation of HIV in blood and tissues. *AIDS* 1998;12[Suppl A]:S27.

769. Davis SF, Rosen DH, Steinberg S, et al. Trends in HIV prevalence among childbearing women in the United States, 1989–1994. *J Acquir Immune Defic Syndr Hum Retrovirol* 1998;19:158.

770. Cohen M. Natural history of HIV infection in women. *Obstet Gynecol Clin North Am* 1997;24:743.

771. Ellerbrock TV, Lieb S, Harrington PE, et al. Heterosexually transmitted human immunodeficiency virus infection among pregnant women in a rural Florida community. *N Engl J Med* 1992;327:1704.

772. Catania JA, Coates TJ, Stall R, et al. Prevalence of AIDS-related risk factors and condom use in the United States. *Science* 1992;258:1101.

773. Lindsay MK, Peterson HB, Willis S, et al. Incidence and prevalence of human immunodeficiency virus infection in a prenatal population undergoing routine voluntary human immunodeficiency virus screening, July 1987 to June 1990. *Am J Obstet Gynecol* 1991;165:961.

774. Puro V, D'Ubaldo C, Aloisi MS, Ippolito G. Women attending human immunodeficiency virus counselling and testing site because of pregnancy, and prevalence of newly diagnosed infections. *Eur J Obstet Gynecol Reprod Biol* 1998;79:51.

775. Carusi D, Learman LA, Posner SF. Human immunodeficiency virus test refusal in pregnancy: a challenge to voluntary testing. *Obstet Gynecol* 1998;91:540.

776. Stratton P, Mofenson LM, Willoughby AD. Human immunodeficiency virus infection in pregnant women under care at AIDS clinical trials centers in the United States. *Obstet Gynecol* 1992;79:364.

777. Langston C, Lewis DE, Hammill HA, et al. Excess intrauterine fetal demise associated with maternal human immunodeficiency virus infection. *J Infect Dis* 1995;172:1451.

778. Bessinger R, Clark R, Kissinger P, et al. Pregnancy is not associated with the progression of HIV disease in women attending an HIV outpatient program. *Am J Epidemiol* 1998;147:434.

779. Weisser M, Rudin C, Battegay M, et al. Does pregnancy influence the course of HIV infection? Evidence from two large Swiss cohort studies. *J Acquir Immune Defic Syndr Hum Retrovirol* 1998;17:404.

780. Burns DN, Landesman S, Minkoff H, et al. The influence of pregnancy on human immunodeficiency virus type 1 infection: antepartum and postpartum changes in human immunodeficiency virus type 1 viral load. *Am J Obstet Gynecol* 1998;178:355.

781. Viscarello RR, Cullen MT, DeGennaro NJ, Hobbins JC. Fetal blood sampling in human immunodeficiency virus-seropositive women before elective midtrimester termination of pregnancy. *Am J Obstet Gynecol* 1992;167:1075.

782. Mandelbrot L, Brossard Y, Aubin J-T, et al. Testing for in utero human immunodeficiency virus infection with fetal blood sampling. *Am J Obstet Gynecol* 1996;175:489.

783. Dickover RE, Garratty EM, Herman SA, et al. Identification of levels of maternal HIV-1 RNA associated with risk of perinatal transmission: effect of maternal zidovudine treatment on viral laod. *JAMA* 1996; 275:599.

784. Landesman SH, Kalish LA, Burns DN, et al. Obstetrical factors and the transmission of human immunodeficiency virus type 1 from mother to child. *N Engl J Med* 1996;334:1617.

785. Mandelbrot L, Mayaux M-J, Bongain A, et al. Obstetric factors and mother-to-child transmission of human immunodeficiency virus type 1: the French perinatal cohorts. *Am J Obstet Gynecol* 1996;175: 661.

786. The European Collaborative Study. Vertical transmission of HIV-1: maternal immune status and obstetric factors. *AIDS* 1996;10:1675.

787. Coll O, Hernandez M, Boucher CAB, et al. Vertical HIV-1 transmission correlates with a high maternal viral load at delivery. *J Acquir Immune Defic Syndr Hum Retrovirol* 1997;14:26.

788. John GC, Nduati RW, Mbori-Ngacha D, et al. Genital shedding of human immunodeficiency virus type 1 DNA during pregnancy: association with immunosuppression, abnormal cervical or vaginal discharge, and severe vitamin A deficiency. *J Infect Dis* 1997;175:57.

789. Ugen KE, Srikantan V, Goedert JJ, et al. Vertical transmission of human immunodeficiency virus type 1: seroreactivity by maternal antibodies to the carboxy region of the gp41 envelope glycoprotein. *J Infect Dis* 1997;175:63.

790. Mayaux MJ, Dussaix E, Isopet J, et al. Maternal virus load during pregnancy and mother-to-child transmission of human immunodeficiency virus type 1: the French perinatal cohort studies. *J Infect Dis* 1997;175:172.

791. Mostad SB, Overbaugh J, DeVange DM, et al. Hormonal contraception, vitamin A deficiency, and other risk factors for shedding of HIV-1 infected cells from the cervix and vagina. *Lancet* 1997;350:922.

792. Mofenson LM. Mother-child HIV-1 transmission: timing and determinants. *Obstet Gynecol Clin North Am* 1997;24:759.

793. Goedert JJ, Duliège A-M, Amos CI, et al. High risk of HIV-1 infection for first-born twins. *Lancet* 1991;338:1471.

794. de Martino M, Tovo P-A, Galli L, et al. HIV-I infection in perinatally exposed siblings and twins. *Arch Dis Child* 1991;66:1235.

795. Bryson YJ, Luzuriaga K, Sullivan JL, Wara DW. Proposed definitions for in utero versus intrapartum transmission of HIV-1. *N Engl J Med* 1992;327:1246.

796. Van de Perre P. Postnatal transmission of human immunodeficiency virus type 1: the breast-feeding dilemma. *Am J Obstet Gynecol* 1995; 173:483.

797. Lewis P, Nduati R, Kreiss JK, et al. Cell-free human immunodeficiency virus type 1 in breast milk. *J Infect Dis* 1998;177:34.

798. European Collaborative Study. Risk factors for mother-to-child transmission of HIV-1. *Lancet* 1992;339:1007.

799. Kind C, Brändle B, Wyler C-A, et al. Epidemiology of vertically transmitted HIV-1 infection in Switzerland: results of a nationwide prospective study. *Eur J Pediatr* 1992;151:442.

800. Hutto C, Parks WP, Lai S, et al. A hospital-based prospective study of

perinatal infection with human immunodeficiency virus type 1. *J Pediatr* 1991;118:347.

801. Van de Perre P, Simonon A, Msellati P, et al. Postnatal transmission of human immunodeficiency virus type 1 from mother to infant: a prospective cohort study in Kigali, Rwanda. *N Engl J Med* 1991;325:593.

802. Wolinsky SM, Wike CM, Korber BTM, et al. Selective transmission of human immunodeficiency virus type-1 variants from mothers to infants. *Science* 1992;255:1134.

803. Lamers SL, Sleasman JW, She JX, et al. Persistence of multiple maternal genotypes of human immunodeficiency virus type 1 in infants infected by vertical transmission. *J Clin Invest* 1994;93:380.

804. Colgrove RC, Pitt J, Chung PH, et al. Selective vertical transmission of HIV-1 antiretroviral resistance mutations. *AIDS* 1998;12:2281.

805. Pasquier C, Cayrou C, Blancher A, et al. Molecular evidence for mother-to-child transmission of multiple variants by analysis of RNA and DNA sequences of human immunodeficiency virus type 1. *J Virol* 1998;72:8493.

806. Centers for Disease Control and Prevention. Report of the NIH Panel to Define Principles of Therapy of HIV Infection and Guidelines for the Use of Antiretroviral Agents in HIV-Infected Adults and Adolescents. *MMWR* 1998;47(RR-5):43.

807. Mirochnick M, Fenton T, Gagnier P, et al. Pharmacokinetics of nevirapine in human immunodeficiency virus type 1-infected pregnant women and their neonates. *J Infect Dis* 1998;178:368.

808. Sperling RS, Shapiro DE, Coombs RW, et al. Maternal viral load, zidovudine treatment, and the risk of transmission of human immunodeficiency virus type 1 from mother to infant. *N Engl J Med* 1996;335:1621.

809. Fiscus SA, Adimora AA, Schoenbach VJ, et al. Perinatal HIV infection and the effect of zidovudine therapy on transmission in rural and urban counties. *JAMA* 1996;275:1483.

810. Lansky A, Jones JL, Wan P-CT, et al. Trends in zidovudine prescription for pregnant women infected with HIV. *J Acquir Immune Defic Syndr Hum Retrovirol* 1998;18:289.

811. Phuapradit W, Chaturachinda K, Taneepanichskul S, et al. Vertical transmission of HIV-1 in mid-trimester gestation. *Aust N Z J Obstet Gynaecol* 1995;35:427.

812. Matheson PB, Abrams EJ, Thomas PA, et al. Efficacy of antenatal zidovudine in reducing perinatal transmission of human immunodeficiency virus type 1. *J Infect Dis* 1995;172:353.

813. Cooper ER, Nugent RP, Diaz C, et al. After AIDS Clinical Trial 076: the changing pattern of zidovudine use during pregnancy, and the subsequent reduction in the vertical transmission of human immunodeficiency virus in a cohort of infected women and their infants. *J Infect Dis* 1996;174:1207.

814. Simonds RJ, Steketee R, Nesheim S, et al. Impact of zidovudine use on risk and risk factors for perinatal transmission of HIV. *AIDS* 1998;12:301.

815. Wade NA, Birkhead GS, Warren BL, et al. Abbreviated regimens of zidovudine prophylaxis and perinatal transmission of the human immunodeficiency virus. *N Engl J Med* 1998;339:1409.

816. Centers for Disease Control and Prevention. Administration of zidovudine during late pregnancy and delivery to prevent perinatal HIV transmission—Thailand, 1996–1998. *MMWR* 1998;47:151.

817. Stiehm ER, Lambert JS, Mofenson LM, et al. Efficacy of zidovudine and human immunodeficiency virus (HIV) hyperimmune immunoglobulin for reducing perinatal HIV transmission from HIV-infected women with advanced disease: results of Pediatric AIDS Clinical Trials Group Protocol 185. *J Infect Dis* 1999;179:567.

818. Moodley J, Moodley D, Pillay K, et al. Pharmacokinetics and antiretroviral activity of lamivudine alone or when coadministered with zidovudine in human immunodeficiency virus type 1-infected pregnant women and their offspring. *J Infect Dis* 1998;178:1327.

819. Kind C, Rudin C, Siegrist C-A, et al. Prevention of vertical HIV transmission: additive protective effect of elective cesarean section and zidovudine prophylaxis. Swiss Neonatal HIV Study Group. *AIDS* 1998;12:205.

820. Centers for Disease Control and Prevention. 1995 Revised guidelines for prophylaxis against Pneumocystis carinii pneumonia for children infected or perinatally exposed to human immunodeficiency virus. *MMWR* 1995;44(RR-4):1.

821. Galli L, de Martino M, Tovo P-A, et al. Onset of clinical signs in children with HIV-1 perinatal infection. *AIDS* 1995;9:455.

822. Mayaux M-J, Burgard M, Teglas J-P, et al. Neonatal characteristics in rapidly progressive perinatally acquired HIV-1 disease. *JAMA* 1996;275:606.

823. McCarty KA, Bungu Z. Kaposi's sarcoma in a two week old infant born to a mother with Kaposi's sarcoma/AIDS. *Cent Afr J Med* 1995;41:330.

824. The European Collaborative Study. Natural history of vertically acquired human immunodeficiency virus-1 infection. *Pediatrics* 1994;94:815.

825. Barnhart HX, Caldwell MB, Thomas P, et al. Natural history of human immunodeficiency virus disease in perinatally infected children: an analysis from the Pediatric Spectrum of Disease project. *Pediatrics* 1996;97:710.

826. Pliner V, Weedon J, Thomas PA, et al. Incubation period of HIV-1 in perinatally infected children. *AIDS* 1998;12:759.

827. Shearer WT, Quinn TC, LaRussa P, et al. Viral load and disease progression in infants infected with human immunodeficiency virus type 1. *N Engl J Med* 1997;336:1337.

828. Zaknun D, Orav J, Kornegay J, et al. Correlation of ribonucleic acid polymerase chain reaction, acid dissociated p24 antigen, and neopterin with progression of disease: a retrospective, longitudinal study of vertically acquired human immunodeficiency virus type 1 infection in children. *J Pediatr* 1997;130:898.

829. Palumbo PE, Raskino C, Fiscus S, et al. Predictive value of quantitative plasma HIV RNA and CD4$^+$ lymphocyte count in HIV-infected infants and children. *JAMA* 1998;279:756.

830. Dickover RE, Dillon M, Leung K-M, et al. Early prognostic indicators in primary perinatal human immunodeficiency virus type 1 infection: importance of viral RNA and the timing of transmission on long-term outcome. *J Infect Dis* 1998;178:375.

830a. Kuhn L, Steketee RW, Weedon J, et al. Distinct risk factors for intrauterine and intrapartum human immunodeficiency virus transmission and consequences for disease progression in infected children. *J Infec Dis* 1999;179:52.

831. Sison AV, Campos JM. Laboratory methods for early detection of human immunodeficiency virus type 1 in newborns and infants. *Clin Microbiol Rev* 1992;5:238.

832. Long SS, Lischner HW. Early and accurate detection of infection with human immunodeficiency virus type 1 in vertically exposed infants. *J Pediatr* 1996;129:189.

833. Palasanthiran P, Robertson P, Ziegler JB, Graham GG. Decay of transplacental human immunodeficiency virus type 1 antibodies in neonates and infants. *J Infect Dis* 1994;170:1593.

834. American Academy of Pediatrics, Committee on Pediatric AIDS. Evaluation and treatment of the HIV-exposed infant. *Pediatrics* 1997;99:909.

835. McIntosh K, FitzGerald G, Pitt J, et al. A comparison of peripheral blood coculture versus 18- or 24-month serology in the diagnosis of human immunodeficiency virus infection in the offspring of infected mothers. *J Infect Dis* 1998;178:560.

836. Borkowsky W, Krasinski K, Pollack H, et al. Early diagnosis of human immunodeficiency virus infection in children <6 months of age: comparison of polymerase chain reaction, culture, and plasma antigen capture techniques. *J Infect Dis* 1992;166:616.

837. Lepage P, Van de Perre P, Simonon A, et al. Transient seroreversion in children born to human immunodeficiency virus 1-infected mothers. *Pediatr Infect Dis J* 1992;11:892.

838. Burgard M, Mayaux M-J, Blanche S, et al. The use of viral culture and p24 antigen testing to diagnose human immunodeficiency virus infection in neonates. *N Engl J Med* 1992;327:1192.

839. Palomba E, Gay V, de Martino M, et al. Early diagnosis of human immunodeficiency virus infection in infants by detection of free and complexed p24 antigen. *J Infect Dis* 1992;165:394.

840. Landesman S, Weiblen B, Mendez H, et al. Clinical utility of HIV-IgA immunoblot assay in the early diagnosis of perinatal HIV infection. *JAMA* 1991;266:3443.

841. Quinn TC, Kline RL, Halsey N, et al. Early diagnosis of perinatal HIV infection by detection of viral-specific IgA antibodies. *JAMA* 1991;266:2439.

842. Miles SA, Balden E, Magpantay L, et al. Rapid serologic testing with immune-complex-dissociated HIV p24 antigen for early detection of HIV infection in neonates. *N Engl J Med* 1993;328:297.

843. Bremer JW, Lew JF, Cooper E, et al. Diagnosis of infection with human immunodeficiency virus type 1 by a DNA polymerase chain reaction assay among infants enrolled in the Women and Infants' Transmission Study. *J Pediatr* 1996;129:198.

844. Owens DK, Holodniy M, McDonald TW, et al. A meta-analytic evaluation of the polymerase chain reaction for the diagnosis of HIV infection in infants. *JAMA* 1996;275:1342.

845. Luzuriaga K, Sullivan JL. DNA polymerase chain reaction for the diagnosis of vertical HIV infection. *JAMA* 1996;275:1360.

846. Steketee RW, Abrams EJ, Thea DM, et al. Early detection of perinatal human immunodeficiency virus (HIV) type 1 infection using HIV RNA amplification and detection. *J Infect Dis* 1997;175:707.

846a.Culnane M, Fowler MG, Lee SS, et al. Lack of long-term effects of *in utero* exposure to zidovudine among uninfected children born to HIV-infected women. *JAMA* 1999;281:151.

847. Scarlatti G. Paediatric HIV infection. *Lancet* 1996;348:863.

848. Exhenry C, Nadal D. Vertical human immunodeficiency virus-1 infection: involvement of the central nervous system and treatment. *Eur J Pediatr* 1996;155:839.

849. Pollack H, Glasberg H, Lee E, et al. Impaired early growth of infants perinatally infected with human immunodeficiency virus: correlation with viral load. *J Pediatr* 1997;130:915.

850. Carey VJ, Yong FH, Frenkel LM, McKinney RE Jr. Pediatric AIDS prognosis using somatic growth velocity. *AIDS* 1998;12:1361.

851. Italian Register for HIV Infection in Children. Features of children perinatally infected with HIV-1 surviving longer than 5 years. *Lancet* 1994;343:191.

852. Mofenson LM, Moye J Jr, Bethel J, et al. Prophylactic intravenous immunoglobulin in HIV-infected children with CD4$^+$ counts of 0.20×10^9/L or more: effect on viral, opportunistic, and bacterial infections. *JAMA* 1992;268:483.

CHAPTER 48

Acute Infections

Bishara J. Freij and George H. McCracken, Jr.

Infections are significant causes of mortality and long-term morbidity in neonates, especially for premature infants of very low birth weight (1–4). Temporal and geographic differences in the relative frequencies of various neonatal pathogens are well recognized (5,6). In North America in the 1930s and 1940s, gram-positive cocci such as group A β-hemolytic streptococci and *Staphylococcus aureus* were the most common bacterial isolates from neonates with sepsis, with *Escherichia coli* accounting for most of the remaining cases. *S. aureus* and *E. coli* became the major pathogens in the 1950s, but since the late 1960s, group B β-hemolytic streptococci and *E. coli* have predominated. Coagulase-negative staphylococci emerged in the 1980s and have surpassed *S. aureus* and gram-negative enteric bacilli as the bacteria most frequently associated with nosocomial infections in many neonatal intensive care units, and several *Candida* species have increased in frequency to become major neonatal pathogens in the 1990s. This has largely been a consequence of the survival of very-low-birth-weight infants who require lengthy hospitalizations and considerable mechanical and nutritional support (7,8).

The outcome of neonatal infections can be improved if illness is recognized early and appropriate antimicrobial agents are administered promptly. This chapter presents pertinent epidemiologic and pathogenetic concepts of specific infections, clinical manifestations, and diagnostic evaluations of patients with these diseases, with a rational approach to therapy and control of neonatal infections.

B. J. Freij: Division of Infectious Diseases, Department of Pediatrics, William Beaumont Hospital, Royal Oak; Department of Pediatrics, Wayne State University School of Medicine, Detroit, Michigan

G. H. McCracken, Jr.: Department of Pediatrics, University of Texas, Southwestern Medical Center; and Children's Medical Center, Dallas, Texas

PHARMACOLOGIC BASIS OF ANTIMICROBIAL THERAPY

Selection of antimicrobial therapy for neonatal infections must be based on pharmacokinetic properties of antibiotics in newborn infants of different gestational and postnatal ages, antimicrobial susceptibilities of commonly encountered pathogens within each nursery, and the natural history of the infectious disease being treated (9).

Combining two or more antibiotics is the usual clinical practice when initiating therapy for presumed systemic bacterial disease (e.g., ampicillin and an aminoglycoside are combined to treat suspected early-onset septicemia or meningitis before identification of the pathogen). After a bacterium has been identified and its susceptibility to various antimicrobial agents is determined, a single appropriate antibiotic usually is satisfactory for treating most infections.

Although antibiotics are used commonly to prevent infection, they are effective prophylactically only if directed against a single pathogen. For example, a single dose of penicillin G given intramuscularly at birth reduces the colonization rate and incidence of early-onset group B streptococcal (GBS) disease, except in infants who acquire the infection *in utero* (10). However, if antibiotics are used as broad-spectrum coverage against many potential pathogens, they rarely are effective. This umbrella method of chemoprophylaxis encourages the emergence of resistant strains among previously susceptible bacteria and alters the normal flora of the gastrointestinal and respiratory tracts with overgrowth of potentially virulent organisms. Broad-coverage prophylaxis may partially suppress a bacterium, masking the development of clinical disease and causing neglect of important surgical measures or serious delay in administering more effective therapy.

EPIDEMIOLOGY

The two principal sources of newborn infection are the mother and the nursery environment. Infection is acquired from the mother transplacentally, at the time of delivery, or in the postnatal period. The infant may acquire infection postnatally from environmental sources, such as nursery personnel, respiratory equipment, sinks, contaminated total parenteral nutrition solutions or medication vials, and incubators. Infections manifesting within the first week of life are usually the result of exposure to microorganisms of maternal origin, but infections presenting later can have a maternal or environmental source.

Myriad aerobic and anaerobic bacteria, mycoplasmas, chlamydiae, fungi, viruses, and protozoa can be found in the maternal genital tract. Some of these organisms pose little threat to the newborn infant (e.g., *Lactobacillus,* α-hemolytic streptococci, *Veillonella*), and others are infrequent causes of neonatal disease (e.g., *Streptococcus pneumoniae, Neisseria meningitidis*) (11–13). More commonly, organisms such as groups A and B β-hemolytic streptococci, *E. coli, Listeria monocytogenes, Haemophilus influenzae, Neisseria gonorrhoeae,* cytomegalovirus, and herpes simplex virus are responsible for serious neonatal infections (3,4).

Within a few days after birth, α-hemolytic streptococci, *Staphylococcus epidermidis,* and gram-negative enteric bacilli colonize the throat, nose, umbilicus, and stool (14). The gastrointestinal tract of newborns becomes heavily colonized by lactobacilli. Infants in neonatal intensive care units tend to have delayed colonization, which probably is related to early antimicrobial therapy for possible sepsis, and are more likely to acquire nosocomial strains of gram-negative bacilli such as *Klebsiella, Enterobacter, Citrobacter,* and *E. coli* (14–16). Colonization of the scalp, axilla, and groin by coagulase-negative staphylococci is universal by 48 hours of age (7). In a prospective study of 18 premature infants admitted to a neonatal intensive care unit, *S. epidermidis* as the only coagulase-negative staphylococcal species isolated from the axilla, ear, nasopharynx, and rectum was found in about 11% of infants during their first day of life; this increased to 100% by 4 weeks of age. None of these infants had a predominant *S. epidermidis* biotype on the first day compared with 89% by 4 weeks of age. The prevalence of slime production and multidrug resistance among isolates rose from 68% to 95% and from 32% to 82%, respectively, during the 4-week study period (17).

Postnatal fungal colonization is more likely to occur in low-birth-weight infants. An estimated 10% of term infants have gastrointestinal *Candida* colonization within the first 5 days of life; infants weighing less than 1,500 g have colonization rates of about 25%. Early colonization (less than 2 weeks of age) is more common, involves the gastrointestinal and respiratory tracts, and is with *Candida albicans* or *Candida tropicalis,* unlike late colonization (≥2 weeks of age), which usually involves the skin and is more likely to be with *Candida parapsilosis* (18). *C. albicans* colonization of infants is usually of maternal origin, whereas *C. parapsilosis* colonization is acquired from exogenous sources such as the hands of nursery personnel (19). Cutaneous colonization with *Malassezia (Pityrosporum) furfur,* a lipophilic yeast best known as the cause of tinea versicolor, is common and is found in as many as two-thirds of all critically ill newborns; fewer than 3% of healthy newborns and young infants have skin colonization by this fungus (20–22). The use of water-in-oil emollient creams (e.g., Eucerin Creme) as a moisturizer for premature infants does not alter colonization patterns or rates by bacteria or fungi (23).

The vagina or cervix of asymptomatic, sexually active women is colonized by *Ureaplasma urealyticum* in 40% to 80% and by *Mycoplasma hominis* in 21% to 53%. Vertical transmission rates from 45% to 66% for preterm and term neonates have been reported for *U. urealyticum* (24). By 3 months of age, about 33% to 68% of these infants continue to have detectable pharyngeal, ocular, or vaginal colonization (25). Vertical transmission rates for infants born to women with cervical *Chlamydia trachomatis* infections have been estimated at 40% to 70%; about 35% of untreated infants continue to be infected at one or more sites (e.g., conjunctiva, nasopharynx, oropharynx, rectum, vagina) at 12 months of age (26–28).

The incidence of neonatal sepsis is from 1 to 8 cases per 1,000 live births (29). The average national incidence rate for nursery-acquired infections is about 1.4%, but figures reported for neonatal intensive care units are considerably higher and range from 5% to 30% (3,30–33). The most important risk factors for acquiring a nosocomial infection are low birth weight and gestational age; others include prolonged hospitalization, invasive procedures, placement of indwelling devices such as central venous catheters or ventriculoperitoneal shunts, bacterial or fungal colonization, and overcrowded nurseries.

INFECTION CONTROL IN THE NURSERY

Microorganisms can be transmitted to infants through direct contact with infected or colonized persons (e.g., mother, hospital personnel), indirect contact with a contaminated object (e.g., resuscitation equipment, pressure monitoring transducers), droplet contact (e.g., coughing or sneezing by infected caretakers), and contaminated products (e.g., milk, lipid emulsions, blood). Transmission of bacteria and yeast by the hands of hospital personnel is the most important mode of circulation within nurseries (30).

Prevention of nosocomial infection depends on recognizing and correcting environmental risk factors. Personnel should wash their hands thoroughly with a scrub brush and an antibacterial cleaning agent before and between the handling of patients. Overcrowding in nurseries and a high infant-to-nurse ratio have increased the risk of nosocomial infections by 5- to 15-fold (30). Continuous surveillance through review of patient and microbiologic records helps to identify changing colonization patterns, to detect newly introduced virulent organisms in the nursery environment, and to recognize changes in the antibiotic susceptibility patterns of the predominant pathogens. Repeated treatment with broad-spectrum antimicrobials encourages colonization of infants by *Candida* and multiresistant bacteria. Routine neonatal surveillance cultures usually are inadequate predictors of future infection of newborns by their colonizing microorganisms, but they are useful during outbreaks because they allow cohorting of infants within the nursery to minimize spread of an epidemic viral or bacterial strain to uninfected patients. Invasive procedures, such as endotracheal intubation, placement of fetal scalp electrodes, and insertion of ventriculoperitoneal shunts, are well-recognized risk factors for hospital-acquired infections.

Umbilical and peripheral arterial and venous indwelling catheters are important sources of nosocomial bacteremia (34,35). As many as 60% of umbilical catheters become colonized by bacteria, but the prevalence of umbilical catheter-related sepsis has been estimated at 3% to 16%. The most common causative agents are coagulase-negative staphylococci, followed by *S. aureus*; gram-negative bacilli and fungi account for about one-third of all cases. Risk factors for umbilical arterial catheter-related sepsis include very low birth weight and duration of antibiotic therapy. Umbilical venous catheter-related sepsis occurs most often in larger infants receiving infusions of hyperalimentation solutions (35).

There is increasing use of central venous catheters in seriously ill infants for providing prolonged, dependable vascular access for the administration of intravenous fluids, hyperalimentation solutions, and medications. About 30% to 50% of critically ill infants with central venous catheters develop catheter-related sepsis (36,37). Central venous catheter infections can be caused by contaminated infusates, hematogenous seeding from distant sites of infection, or contamination of the catheter hub. The most important source appears to be organisms found on an infant's skin, such as coagulase-negative staphylococci, that travel along the central venous catheter track to the catheter tip, where colonization takes place (38).

Preventive measures designed to reduce the incidence of central venous catheter-related infections generally aim at decreasing the number of organisms at catheter exit sites. Disinfection of central venous catheter exit sites by repeatedly applying topical antiseptics is viewed as one of the most important ways of reducing the frequency of catheter-related sepsis. Two percent aqueous chlorhexidine has been more efficacious than 10% povidone-iodine or 70% alcohol for this purpose when used in adults (39). Chlorhexidine is nontoxic to newborns, and its absorption through neonatal skin is minimal (40,41). The popular semipermeable transparent dressings that are applied to central venous catheter exit sites produce significantly heavier bacterial growth on the underlying skin compared with gauze dressings and result in a higher incidence of central venous catheter contamination (42). The use of silver-impregnated collagen cuffs that can be attached to central venous catheters has reduced the incidence of catheter-related sepsis in adults, but the antiinfective effect is short lived because the collagen to which the silver ions are chelated is biodegraded (38). The use of central venous catheters that are coated on the external surface with antibiotics or antiseptics can reduce the rate of catheter colonization and catheter-related sepsis, but this approach has not been studied in neonates (38). The prophylactic infusion of low doses of vancomycin administered with either heparin flushes or total parenteral nutrition solutions, or as separate infusions, is effective in preventing catheter-related bacteremias with vancomycin-susceptible organisms such as coagulase-negative staphylococci or *S. aureus* (43). However, this practice may promote the emergence of vancomycin-resistant strains of a variety of gram-positive bacteria such as enterococci, *S. aureus,* or coagulase-negative staphylococci in neonatal intensive care units.

Nosocomial Bacterial Outbreaks

When an infectious disease caused by the same organism appears in several infants from the same nursery in a short period, a nosocomial outbreak should be suspected. The sick infants should be isolated and cultured to identify the pathogen. If a specific pathogen is responsible for the outbreak, epidemiologic investigations to determine the source of infection must be initiated, and measures should be taken to prevent further colonization and disease. Specific typing of organisms, using techniques such as phage typing for *S. aureus,* determination of antibiotic susceptibility and biochemical profiles for *S. epidermidis,* and pyocin typing for *Pseudomonas* have been replaced largely by the more powerful tools of molecular biology. Plasmid fingerprinting, restriction endonuclease analysis of plasmid and genomic deoxyribonucleic acid (DNA), immunoblotting, ribosomal ribonucleic acid typing, pulsed-field gel electrophoresis, and polymerase chain reactions now are used commonly in the analysis of nosocomial epidemics (44).

Staphylococcus aureus *Infection*

In the late 1950s and early 1960s, phage group I *S. aureus* (i.e., phage types 29, 52, 52A, 79, 80, and 81) caused significant hospital disease, ranging from pustules and cellulitis to pneumonia, septicemia, and meningitis. Although most infants are colonized with the epidemic strain during outbreaks, staphylococcal disease occurs in only a small fraction of those infants. Disease caused by phage group I staphylococci has diminished in the past decade. Theories to explain this decline are unsatisfactory but include changes in the virulence of the organism, implementation of infection control techniques in nurseries, and introduction of the semisynthetic β-lactamase–resistant penicillins.

Disease caused by phage group II *S. aureus* (i.e., phage types 3A, 3B, 3C, 55, and 71) in newborn and young infants may be encountered. Clinical manifestations caused by these organisms have been classified broadly as the expanded scalded skin syndrome (45–47). Nursery epidemics of bullous impetigo, toxic epidermal necrolysis, or both caused by group II staphylococci have been reported (47,48). Outbreaks are usually a result of lapses in infection control techniques and spread of the organism to other infants through hand carriage by nursery personnel. A staphylococcal nasal carrier among the nursery staff only rarely is the source.

Methicillin-resistant *S. aureus* (MRSA) strains have become important nosocomial pathogens in the United States since 1975 (49). The major route by which MRSA is spread is through hand carriage by transiently colonized personnel (50). Nasal MRSA carriage rates for hospital personnel caring for colonized patients are from 1% to 6% (49). Outbreaks of disease caused by multiresistant *S. aureus* strains have been reported from several nurseries in North America (51,52). These organisms are resistant to the antistaphylococcal penicillins, cephalosporins, lincomycin, and aminoglycosides but are susceptible to vancomycin, rifampin, and trimethoprim-sulfamethoxazole. Vancomycin is the preferred therapy. About 14% of newborns colonized with MRSA continued to harbor the organism by 1 year of age in one study (53).

When staphylococcal disease occurs in a nursery, the extent of infection must be determined. Cultures are obtained from all infants and personnel associated with the index patient and a random sampling of the other infants. Culture sites include the nasopharynx and umbilicus for infants, and the anterior nares and hands for personnel. Several measures commonly are used to control a nursery epidemic:

Increase emphasis on hand washing by all personnel (54).

Isolate all symptomatic and asymptomatic infants colonized with the virulent staphylococcal strain, with cohorting of all exposed but not colonized infants and all new admissions to the nursery and cohorting of caretakers. Maintain infant cohorts until discharge from the nursery.

Use parenteral antistaphylococcal therapy to treat systemic disease, with application of topical agents such as triple dye (i.e, mixture of brilliant green, crystal violet, and proflavine hemisulfate), bacitracin ointment, sulfadiazine cream, isopropyl alcohol, iodophor, chlorhexidine, or mupirocin to the umbilical stump of infants to delay or reduce colonization (55–57).

Initiate routine bathing with antistaphylococcal cleansing agents such as chlorhexidine. Iodophor detergents are not recommended because of cutaneous staining and the potential for transdermal absorption of iodine, with resultant suppression of neonatal thyroid function (30). Hexachlorophene is neurotoxic and should not be used routinely. This agent remains an option for difficult-to-contain epidemics, but it should be used in a 1:4 or 1:5 dilution in water and only in full-term infants (55).

Colonize the umbilical stump of infants with a less virulent *Staphylococcus* species, such as the 502A strain of *S. aureus* (i.e., bacterial interference) (55). Although associated with low risk if properly performed, this procedure is used rarely and should be undertaken only after other control techniques have failed.

Close the nursery to new admissions if an outbreak is difficult to control.

Enteropathogenic Escherichia coli

Because diarrhea caused by enteropathogenic strains of *E. coli* occurs rarely during the first week of life, nosocomial disease usually is confined to intensive and special care nurseries. The mother is frequently the source of infection for the index case; subsequent cases usually are transmitted from infant to infant by nursery personnel. The epidemiology, symptoms, treatment, and control measures for enteropathogenic *E. coli* diarrhea are considered later.

Group A Streptococcal Infection

Group A β-hemolytic streptococci were a common cause of puerperal and neonatal sepsis in the 1930s and early 1940s. With the advent of penicillin and its frequent use in maternity and nursery units, neonatal infections caused by this organism have become relatively uncommon (58,59). The primary source of group A streptococci in nursery outbreaks is a nurse or physician working in the unit or the mother. After group A streptococci are introduced into a nursery, many infants become colonized, but few develop clinical disease. The most common clinical manifestation is a low-grade granulating omphalitis that fails to heal despite local measures. However, more significant disease may occur, including extensive cellulitis, pneumonia, septicemia, and meningitis.

One neonate with group A streptococcal colonization is enough to warrant investigation of the nursery for a potential source of disease. All infants in close contact with the index case, a random sampling of other infants, and nursery personnel should be cultured. Nasopharyngeal and umbilical cultures from infants and nasopharyngeal, skin, and rectal cultures from personnel should be obtained. The epidemiologic workup should be coordinated with the obstetric service of the hospital.

Infants with streptococcal disease should be treated with aqueous penicillin G. During nosocomial outbreaks, all asymptomatic infants colonized with group A strepto-cocci should receive penicillin. The prophylactic use of penicillin for new admissions to the nursery may be indicated. Benzathine penicillin G had been used effectively as prophylaxis against group A streptococcal infection in nursery outbreaks; however, it failed to eradicate the organism in any colonized infant in a recent neonatal intensive care unit outbreak in Houston, Texas, where intravenous clindamycin subsequently was used successfully for that purpose (59).

Gram-Negative Bacillary Infections

Routine nasopharyngeal and rectal cultures from normal newborn infants usually reveal one or several coliform organisms. These bacteria and others represent the normal flora of the neonate's gastrointestinal tract. It is likely that the gastrointestinal tract is a source of systemic neonatal infections caused by coliform and other gram-negative bacteria (14,60).

Several nursery outbreaks caused by specific gram-negative bacteria have been described (61–74). Among the organisms incriminated were *Flavobacterium meningosepticum*, *Klebsiella pneumoniae*, *Serratia marcescens*, *Pseudomonas aeruginosa*, *Proteus mirabilis*, *Acinetobacter* spp, *Citrobacter diversus* (now *C. koseri*), *Enterobacter* spp, *Salmonella* spp, and *E. coli*. A common feature of these outbreaks was that most colonized infants were asymptomatic, and those who developed disease usually had pneumonia, septicemia, or meningitis.

Infected fomites represent the single most common source of nursery outbreaks caused by gram-negative bacteria. Contaminated faucet aerators, sink traps, drains, suction equipment, bottles containing distilled water, cleansing solutions, humidification apparatus, incubators, aerosols, and air conditioners have been incriminated. Contaminated formula and breast milk are infrequent sources (75). Colonized infants may act as a source of infection, and the organism is transmitted from infant to infant by the hands or gowns of personnel. During epidemics, the rate of asymptomatic colonization of infants with the specific pathogen ranges from 0% to 90%.

The general approach to nursery outbreaks caused by gram-negative organisms is similar to that for outbreaks caused by *S. aureus*. Identification of an infant in a nursery or intensive care unit with a potentially virulent pathogen such as *P. aeruginosa* should serve as a warning. This infant should be segregated, preferably outside the nursery, from the other infants and managed appropriately. All infants in the same unit should be cultured. If additional infants are discovered to be asymptomatic carriers of the organism, they should be segregated from other infants in the nursery, and an epidemiologic investigation should be initiated. Resuscitation and inhalation equipment, cleansing solutions, washing facilities, and other objects in the patient's environment are cultured so that the source of nosocomial infection can be identified. It may become necessary to close the nursery to new admissions until the source of infection is identified and appropriate measures have been taken to prevent new cases. A review of empiric antibiotic treatment regimens in use in the nursery should be undertaken, and sometimes it is necessary to change these regimens before the circulation of a particular multiresistant bacterial strain can be stopped (72).

Nosocomial Viral Outbreaks

Several viral agents have been incriminated in nursery outbreaks of infection (76,77). Most viral nosocomial outbreaks tend to parallel the activity of the agent in the community. The original source of infection is frequently the mother, who transmits the viral agent transplacentally or by direct contact postnatally. A second common source of nosocomial viral disease is infected nursery personnel. Although the mechanisms accounting for spread of virus from infant to infant are not well defined, it appears likely that respiratory viruses such as influenza and parainfluenza are spread by the airborne route, whereas respiratory syncytial virus (RSV) is spread primarily by infected hands of personnel. Viruses causing diarrhea may be transferred from infant to infant by the hand-to-mouth route through intermediary nursery personnel. Viruses excreted in the urine in high concentrations may be aerosolized when diapers or sheets are changed.

During a nursery outbreak of viral infection, most infected infants are asymptomatic and serve as reservoirs for perpetuation of infection. Even more important, infants with minimal symptoms and signs of disease such as sneezing, stuffy nose, or several loose stools may contribute significantly to transmission of virus by airborne or fecal-oral routes.

Coxsackieviruses

Coxsackievirus A is rarely incriminated in nursery epidemics. In one outbreak at a regular nursery in Bangkok, 48 of 598 infants developed herpangina in the first week of life (78). Several infants had coxsackievirus A5 isolated from their throat or rectum or developed rising antibody titers to the virus.

There have been several well-documented nursery outbreaks of the encephalomyocarditis syndrome associated with coxsackieviruses of the B group (79,80). Coxsackieviruses B1 through B5 have been associated etiologically with this illness, and the virus has been isolated from multiple organs, including the myocardium, lungs, brain, blood, kidneys, and liver. The severe involvement found in many infants explains the relatively high mortality rate of this condition. The clinical picture is one of abrupt onset of fever, listlessness, and feeding difficulty. Respiratory distress and cyanosis are found frequently, and cardiac signs such as tachycardia, cardiomegaly, murmurs, and gallop rhythm are present in most patients (81). Hepatosplenomegaly is common, and signs and symptoms referable to central nervous system involvement affect one-third of patients. The newborn apparently can acquire coxsackievirus infection *in utero* or after birth. The postnatally acquired disease has been traced to direct contact with the mother or an infected attendant.

Echoviruses

Several echovirus types cause illness in premature and term infants (81–89). Although echovirus 9 is the most prevalent type, it is echovirus 11 that has been responsible for most nursery outbreaks caused by this group of viruses (76). Reported neonatal secondary attack rates during hospital outbreaks have been as high as 50% (77).

Mother-to-infant vertical transmission appears to be the major route of infection. The virus spreads to other newborns through the contaminated hands of nursery personnel, especially to infants requiring mouth care and gavage feeding. Echovirus infections acquired from the mother tend to be more serious than those acquired through secondary nosocomial spread; this may be because of the lack of passively transferred protective maternal neutralizing antibodies against the offending agent in infants born to women infected at or near the time of delivery (87,90).

The clinical manifestations of echovirus infection range from mild diarrhea to overwhelming hepatic necrosis. Separate nursery outbreaks caused by the same echovirus type may produce different clinical diseases. For example, in a premature nursery outbreak, echovirus type 19 produced respiratory illness associated with roentgenographic findings of cystic emphysema (81). In a separate outbreak of echovirus type 19, the initial clinical picture was strikingly similar to that of sepsis neonatorum and was characterized by overwhelming infection and hepatic necrosis (84). This disparity in the clinical diseases that characterize individual nosocomial outbreaks also has been observed for echovirus type 11 (86).

During nursery outbreaks, infection control measures should include cohorting of cases and increased emphasis on hand washing (77,91). The use of gloves and gowns is helpful, especially when handling secretions and feces (77). Closure of the nursery to new admissions sometimes is needed. The administration of immune globulin intramuscular (IGIM) or intravenous (IGIV) may attenuate the infection in some recipients, whereas other newborns may develop an asymptomatic infections with these viruses (92).

Hepatitis A

There have been several reported outbreaks of hepatitis A in neonatal intensive care units (93–96). The virus is transmitted primarily by person-to-person contact through fecal contamination and oral ingestion (97). Approximately 16% to 30% of an inoculum of hepatitis A virus can be recovered from infected hands after 4 hours (98). Indirect person-to-person transmission of infectious virus also can occur through contact with inanimate objects, such as hard surfaces (98). In some of the nursery outbreaks, the initial infection occurred through transfusion of neonates with blood or fresh frozen plasma from donors with hepatitis A viremia during the prodromal phase of their illness (94–96).

Hepatitis A virus is highly communicable. In one nursery outbreak, 20% of infants, 24% of nurses, and several nonnursing staff and household contacts were affected (95). Fecal excretion of hepatitis A virus may persist for 4 to 5 months (95). Risk factors for spread of hepatitis A to other infants and nursery personnel include asymptomatic infection, prolonged fecal shedding of the virus, frequent contact with soiled diapers, and breaks in infection control measures. One study found that having long fingernails, not wearing gloves for certain procedures, smoking, and drinking beverages in the nursery facilitated direct hand-to-mouth contact (95). The use of IGIM for postexposure prophylaxis may be helpful in controlling hospital outbreaks. To be most effective, IGIM in a dosage of 0.02 mL/kg of body weight should be given as soon as possible after the last exposure and within a period not exceeding 2 weeks.

Adenoviruses

Neonatal adenoviral infections are infrequent but can be severe (99–101). Nursery outbreaks have been caused by adenovirus serotypes 1, 2, 3, 7, 7a, 8, and 21 (102–104). Manifestations of nosocomial adenovirus infection can include pseudomembranous conjunctivitis, apnea, bradycardia, tachypnea, wheezing, coryza, respiratory failure, fever, hypothermia, feeding intolerance, and diarrhea. Deaths during nosocomial outbreaks have been described (102). Adenoviruses can spread by means of contaminated hands and fomites; fecal-oral and small-particle aerosol spread also is possible (77). Conjunctival shedding of the virus persists for 7 to 10 days; rectal shedding is intermittent and more prolonged (102). Adenoviruses remain stable on environmental surfaces for long periods; this property enhances their ability to spread to susceptible infants and personnel.

Outbreak control can be achieved through cohorting of infected infants, exclusion of ill personnel from the workplace, hand washing, and wearing of gloves and masks; the use of goggles is advocated by some investigators. The use of immune serum globulins was ineffective in preventing or modifying adenoviral infection in one nursery outbreak, and the administered preparation had minimal neutralizing activity against the specific serotype responsible for that outbreak (103).

Respiratory Syncytial Virus

Community outbreaks of RSV infection occur in winter and early spring. The virus is highly contagious; as many as 50% of personnel on pediatric wards become infected during nosocomial RSV outbreaks. Shedding of RSV in respiratory secretions of infants usually lasts from 1 to 21 days (mean 7) but can continue for 6 or more weeks in immunosuppressed patients (77).

RSV has caused nursery outbreaks of bronchiolitis and pneumonia (105–109). Infants initially demonstrate coryza and cough lasting several days, followed by the acute onset of dyspnea associated with roentgenographic evidence of pneumonia in most patients (105). During a community outbreak in Rochester, New York, 35% of infants in a nursery acquired RSV infection (106). Illness often was atypical, especially in infants younger than 3 weeks of age, in whom lower respiratory tract involvement was less common. Four infants died; two infants died unexpectedly after the acute illness had subsided. Infection was acquired by 34% of the nursery staff, who appeared to be important in the spread of RSV within the nursery. Infected infants are at risk of respiratory arrest due to RSV-related apnea (110,111). Bradycardia is a common presenting feature in RSV-infected premature newborns (112). Patients with pulmonary disease, congenital heart disease, or immunodeficiency are at highest risk of severe and potentially fatal RSV infections (113). Infection with group A RSV may be more severe than that caused by group B RSV (114). Simultaneous outbreaks of viral respiratory disease caused by RSV and rhinovirus or parainfluenza virus type 3 have been described in newborn nurseries (107,108).

Control of nosocomial RSV infection should emphasize diligent hand washing before and after handling infants, cohorting of RSV-infected neonates, and not allowing nursery personnel to care for infected and uninfected infants at the same time. Gowns and masks are generally ineffective in reducing nosocomial RSV spread (77). The use of eye-nose goggles has reduced the rates of nosocomial RSV infections among infants and personnel (115,116). Occasionally it is necessary to close the nursery to admissions if new cases of disease continue to occur despite the strict infection control measures.

RSV immune globulin intravenous (RSV-IGIV) was licensed by the Food and Drug Administration in 1996 for the prevention of severe RSV lower respiratory tract disease in infants and children younger than 2 years of age with bronchopulmonary dysplasia or a history of premature birth (≤35 weeks of gestation) (117). A randomized, double-blind, placebo-controlled trial conducted at 54 medical centers in the United States showed that the monthly infusion of 750 mg/kg of RSV-IGIV to infants with bronchopulmonary dysplasia or prematurity during the RSV season reduced hospitalizations by 41%, the number of hospital days by 53%, the number of hospital

days with increased oxygen requirements by 60%, and the number of RSV-related hospital days with moderate or severe lower respiratory tract illness by 54% (118). The efficacy of RSV-IGIV during a nursery outbreak of RSV has not been documented (117). Infants with cyanotic congenital heart disease should not receive RSV-IGIV because of a higher frequency of cyanotic episodes and poor outcomes after surgery among those receiving the product compared with similar infants not receiving RSV immunoprophylaxis (119). The Food and Drug Administration approved a second product, palivizumab, for RSV prophylaxis in 1998. Palivizumab is a humanized monoclonal immunoglobulin G1 antibody that binds to the F-protein of RSV and is active against groups A and B of the virus. Palivizumab is given at a dose of 15 mg/kg intramuscularly once a month during the RSV season. Indications for its use are similar to those for RSV-IGIV (120–122). Its efficacy in controlling nursery outbreaks of RSV has not been studied (Table 48–1).

The use of aerosolized ribavirin for the treatment of RSV infection in high-risk infants may be considered (123,124). When given early in the course of an RSV

TABLE 48–1. *Summary of the American Academy of Pediatrics recommendations for the use of respiratory syncytial virus immune globulin intravenous or palivizumab for prevention of respiratory syncytial virus infection in high-risk infants*

- Target population
  Definite: Infants and children younger than 2 years of age with BPD who currently are on oxygen or have received oxygen during the 6 months before the start of the RSV season; infants with severe BPD may benefit from prophylaxis for 2 RSV seasons.
  Possible: Infants born at ≤28 weeks of gestation without BPD who are younger than 1 year of age at onset of RSV season, and infants born at 29–32 weeks of gestation without BPD and who are 6 months of age or younger at start of RSV season.
- Do not use in infants with CHD, especially cyanotic CHD (not approved by the Food and Drug Administration); however, patients with BPD and asymptomatic, acyanotic CHD (e.g., patent ductus arteriosus, ventricular septal defect) may benefit from RSV prophylaxis.
- Start prophylaxis before onset of RSV season (usually October to December) and stop at the end of the RSV season (usually March to May); regional differences should determine optimal start and finish dates.
- The dose for RSV-IGIV is 750 mg/kg once a month, and the dose of palivizumab is 15 mg/kg given intramuscularly once a month.
- Defer the measles–mumps–rubella and varicella vaccines for 9 months after the last RSV-IGIV dose is given; other vaccines can be given at their scheduled times. No immunization schedule adjustments are needed with palivizumab.

BPD, bronchopulmonary dysplasia; CHD, congenital heart disease; RSV, respiratory syncytial virus; RSV-IGIV, respiratory syncytial virus immune globulin intravenous.
Adapted from ref. 117.

infection, ribavirin can reduce the amount and duration of viral shedding, lead to more rapid resolution of the illness, and lower mortality rates. Ribavirin can be administered safely to mechanically ventilated infants if careful attention is paid to correcting problems resulting from drug precipitation in the respirator tubing and around the expiratory valves of ventilators (125).

Influenza

Epidemics of usually mild respiratory illness caused by influenza A virus have been described in newborn infants (126,127). Clinical findings are nonspecific and can be indistinguishable from bacterial sepsis. Apnea, lethargy, nasal congestion, and poor feeding have been observed. Interstitial pneumonia may be seen on chest radiographs (127).

SEPSIS NEONATORUM

The term sepsis neonatorum is used to describe a disease of infants who are younger than 1 month of age, are clinically ill, and have positive blood cultures. The presence of clinical manifestations differentiates this condition from the transient bacteremia observed in some healthy neonates.

The bacteria responsible for neonatal sepsis vary geographically. GBS predominates in the United States, whereas *S. aureus* and gram-negative bacilli are much more common in developing countries (6). At Parkland Memorial Hospital, Dallas, Texas, a total of 964 infants had neonatal sepsis with or without meningitis between January 1, 1987 and July 31, 1997; GBS accounted for 307 (31.8%) of these cases. Other pathogens included *S. aureus* 10.9% (two-thirds of which were methicillin-resistant strains), coagulase-negative staphylococci 27%, enterococci 4%, *E. coli* 7.7%, *Klebsiella* 2.3%, *Enterobacter* 2%, *H. influenzae* 1.5%, *Serratia* 0.7%, *Pseudomonas* 0.4%, and fungi 2.1% (Jane D. Siegel, M.D., *personal communication,* 1997).

The bacterial etiology of sepsis also varies by the postnatal age of the infant. In a study of a cohort of 7,861 very-low-birth-weight infants (401 to 1,500 g) admitted to 12 medical centers in the United States during a 32-month period between 1991 and 1993, the incidence of early-onset sepsis (occurring during the first 72 hours of life) was 1.9% and that of late-onset sepsis (occurring after 3 days of age) was 25%. The nature of the pathogens associated with the early-onset and late-onset infections differed markedly, with GBS predominating in the former and coagulase-negative staphylococci in the latter (Table 48–2) (3,4).

Pathogenesis

Maternal, environmental, and host factors determine which infants exposed to a potentially pathogenic organ-

TABLE 48–2. *Distribution of pathogens in a cohort of 7,861 very-low-birth-weight infants (401–1,500 g) in the United States from May 1, 1991 to December 31, 1993*

Organism	Early-onset sepsis (N = 147)	Late-onset sepsis (N = 2,355)
Gram-positive bacteria		
Group B streptococci	45 (31)	53 (2)
Streptococcus viridans	13 (9)	NS
Other streptococci	10 (7)	NS
Enterococcus/group D streptococci	NS	111 (5)
Coagulase-negative staphylococci	11 (7)	1,288 (55)
Staphylococcus aureus	4 (3)	209 (9)
Other	0 (0)	52 (2)
Gram-negative bacteria		
Escherichia coli	24 (16)	101 (4)
Haemophilus influenzae	17 (11)	NS
Klebsiella	7 (5)	85 (4)
Pseudomonas	NS	53 (2)
Enterobacter	NS	102 (4)
Other	15 (10)	82 (4)
Fungi		
Candida albicans	1 (1)	111 (5)
Candida parapsilosis	0 (0)	57 (2)
Other	0 (0)	51 (2)

Values are given as number (percent).
NS, not specified.

ism will develop sepsis, meningitis, or other serious invasive infections.

Many prepartum and intrapartum obstetric complications have been associated with increased risk of infection in the newborn, the most significant of which are premature onset of labor, prolonged rupture of fetal membranes, chorioamnionitis, and maternal fever. In one study of 963 pregnancies complicated by premature rupture of membranes, the incidence of clinical sepsis increased from 2% among infants born within 23 hours of membrane rupture to 7% and 11% among those delivered 24 to 47 hours and 48 to 71 hours after rupture, respectively. The risk was highest for the premature, low-birth-weight infants (128). The incidence of infection has been estimated at 8.7% for infants born to mothers with prolonged rupture of membranes (≥24 hours) and clinical chorioamnionitis (129). Intraamniotic infection is associated with a higher incidence of sepsis among infants weighing less than 2,500 g at birth compared with those weighing 2,500 g or more (16% and 4%, respectively). Death from sepsis is greater in the low-birth-weight group (11% and 0%, respectively) (130). Isolation of bacteria from the chorioamnion has been associated with an increased risk of neonatal death among preterm infants (131). Maternal urinary tract infections, low parity, and the use of internal monitoring devices are risk factors for chorioamnionitis (132). Concurrent maternal and neonatal bacteremia has been documented for many microorganisms (133–135).

With improved supportive care of the sick neonate has come increased opportunity for microorganisms of relatively low virulence to cause systemic disease. The use of arterial and venous umbilical catheters, central venous catheters, indwelling urinary catheters, and endotracheal tubes provides access to the debilitated infant for organisms in the respiratory, gastrointestinal, or genitourinary tract, on the skin, or in respiratory support equipment.

Bacterial colonization of the skin and mucosal surfaces precedes invasive disease in most infants with sepsis. Type III strains of GBS, the ones most commonly associated with early-onset septicemia and with meningitis at any age in early infancy, adhere better to vaginal and neonatal buccal epithelial cells *in vitro* than do other GBS strains (136,137). Bloodstream invasion generally follows local multiplication of the organism at sites of colonization. Aspiration of infected amniotic fluid is another proposed route for fetal infection among infants born to mothers with chorioamnionitis.

Animals have been used to define the host–bacteria interactions that determine pathogenesis of disease. Bloodstream infection in infant rats or mice caused by *E. coli* K1 or any of the GBS serotypes can be prevented by pretreatment with type-specific capsular polysaccharide antibody (138,139). The orogastric route for *E. coli* K1 in the infant rat and the intratracheal installation of GBS in the rhesus monkey or rat produce illnesses that closely parallel the human syndromes (140–142).

Several investigations of the host–parasite association of humans with GBS have focused on measurement of specific antibody in the serum of infected and colonized persons. Protective concentrations of antibody to GBS serotype III were found in 73% of women whose newborn infants were well but in only 17% of women whose neonates developed sepsis or meningitis caused by this organism (143). The amount of antibody to GBS serotype III was considerably lower in ill infants than in healthy neonates born to mothers with vaginal colonization (143). Levels of GBS serotype III antibodies correlate with *in vitro* opsonic activity and *in vivo* protection of animals experimentally infected with these strains (144,145). The administration of standard intravenous immunoglobulin preparations with activities against GBS, of human GBS monoclonal antibodies, or of GBS hyperimmune polyclonal antibodies provides significant protection to animals experimentally infected with this pathogen (146,147). Asymptomatic colonization also is associated with antibody formation (148,149). Although less extensively studied, similar observations have been made for other GBS serotypes (147,150–153).

Evidence suggests that antibodies to the K1 *E. coli* antigen are protective against infection by this organism, but this is not firmly established (154). Neonatal serum has been shown to be inefficient in killing *E. coli* because of a deficiency of non-immunoglobulin G serum components, such as complement factor 9 (155,156).

Physiologic deficiencies of the classic and alternative pathways of complement activation in neonates contribute to inefficient bacterial opsonization (157,158). Organisms such as GBS and *E. coli* that have a high capsular sialic acid content tend to be poor activators of the alternative complement pathway (159).

Fibronectin is a multifunctional glycoprotein found in the plasma and on the surface of certain epithelial cells, basement membranes, and connective tissues. In plasma, fibronectin acts as a nonspecific opsonin that enhances clearance of invading bacteria (160). Fibronectin is deficient in neonatal plasma, and its concentration varies inversely with gestational age (160,161). Septic infants have been shown to have significantly lower plasma concentrations of this glycoprotein than healthy, age-matched controls (162). The soluble form of fibronectin binds poorly to GBS (163). Fibronectin enhances phagocyte function in *vitro and in vivo* (160).

Quantitative and qualitative deficiencies in neonatal neutrophils contribute to the immaturity of the immune system of newborns. The abnormalities become most pronounced at times of stress or during infections and include impaired chemotaxis, decreased deformability, reduced C3bi receptor expression, depressed bacterial killing by phagocytes, and oxidative metabolic abnormalities. The neutrophil storage pool of neonates is markedly depleted compared with that of adults. Stem cell proliferative rates are at near maximal capacity and cannot increase appreciably in response to infection (164).

Clinical Manifestations

Most infants with septicemia present with nonspecific signs and symptoms that usually are observed first by the nurse or mother rather than by the physician. The most common of these vague signs are temperature instability, lethargy, apnea, and poor feeding (165). Although hypothermia is more common, a temperature elevation above 37.8°C is significant in the neonate and frequently associated with bacterial infections, especially with temperatures higher than 39°C (166). The signs and symptoms in some infants may suggest respiratory or gastrointestinal disease (e.g., tachypnea and cyanosis or vomiting, diarrhea, and abdominal distention). Septicemia must always be included in the differential diagnosis when evaluating an infant with these findings (165).

Clinical manifestations of sepsis in very-low-birthweight infants (501 to 1,500 g) include increasing apnea (55%), feeding intolerance, abdominal distension, or guaiac-positive stools (43%), increased respiratory support (29%), and lethargy and hypotonia (23%). Abnormal white blood cell count, unexplained metabolic acidosis, and hyperglycemia are noted in 46%, 11%, and 10%, respectively (33).

Although it is tempting to recommend a workup for septicemia in all infants with nonspecific clinical manifestations, this is impractical and unnecessary in many cases. A complete history and physical examination, coupled with clinical experience, are the best guides in determining the extent of the workup. If doubt exists, a blood culture should be obtained. Hepatosplenomegaly, jaundice, and petechiae are classic signs of neonatal infection but represent late manifestations.

Streptococcal Disease

Group B β-hemolytic streptococci are the most common gram-positive bacteria isolated from blood of infants with septicemia in North America (167). In 1990, an estimated 7,600 invasive GBS infections occurred among infants ≤90 days of age (1.8 per 1,000 live births) in the United States, with 310 deaths; early-onset infections accounted for 80% of all cases (168). The annual number of neonatal GBS cases is expected to decline with wider implementation of prevention strategies recommended by the Centers for Disease Control and Prevention and the American College of Obstetricians and Gynecologists (10). The epidemiology, pathogenesis, and clinical features of GBS disease have been defined (169). The organism is a common inhabitant of the female genital tract and can be isolated from vaginal and anorectal cultures of as many as 35% of asymptomatic pregnant women (169–172). Risk factors for maternal GBS colonization include lower parity, higher frequency of intercourse, multiple sexual partners, and concurrent colonization with *Candida* spp (171). Peripartum GBS colonization of the lower urogenital tract has been associated with several maternal complications including preterm labor, premature rupture of membranes, endometritis, chorioamnionitis, urinary tract infection, intrapartum or postpartum fever, late abortions, and invasive infections, such as bacteremia or meningitis (135,173). The identical serotype can be isolated frequently from urethral cultures of the sexual partners of these culture-positive women (174). Although most infected pregnant women have normal, healthy infants, 1% to 2% of pregnancies involving maternal infection result in stillbirths or infants with neonatal disease. Vertical transmission of group B organisms occurs in approximately 50% to 70% of mother–infant pairs, resulting in neonatal colonization rates of from 8% to 25%. Transmission is most likely to occur among infants born to heavily colonized mothers (175).

The early-onset GBS syndrome occurs within the first 72 hours of life (mean age of onset 20 hours), and 65% of reported cases involve premature infants. There is often a history of other maternal obstetric complications (Table 48–3) (173). Onset is sudden and follows a fulminant course, with the primary focus of inflammation in the lungs, although meningitis can develop. Respiratory distress is the most common initial sign among infants with early-onset meningitis (176). Apnea, hypotension, and disseminated intravascular coagulation cause rapid dete-

TABLE 48–3. *Risk factors for early-onset group B streptococcal disease*

Premature delivery
Low birth weight
Increased interval between membrane rupture and delivery
Rupture of membranes before labor onset
Amnionitis and intrapartum fever
Maternal group B streptococcal rectovaginal colonization
  (especially heavy colonization)
African American race
Young (<20 yr) maternal age
Group B streptococcal bacteriuria during current pregnancy
Low level of capsular polysaccharide type-specific
  antibodies
Previous stillbirth or spontaneous abortion
Multiple gestation
Previous delivery of infant with group B streptococcal
  disease
Prolonged duration of intrauterine monitoring

Adapted from ref. 173.

rioration and often lead to the patient's demise within 24 hours. It is difficult to identify the infant with respiratory distress caused by GBS infection, because in 60% of infected patients, the chest radiograph shows a reticulogranular pattern with air bronchograms indistinguishable from that seen with uncomplicated hyaline membrane disease. The mortality rate is approximately 6% and is inversely correlated with birth weight (168,177). All five GBS serotypes have been incriminated in early-onset disease in roughly similar proportions. A similar syndrome has been associated with groups D and G streptococci (178,179).

A late-onset syndrome caused by GBS or *L. monocytogenes* occurs most frequently at 2 to 4 weeks of age, but it may be seen as late as 16 weeks. The onset is insidious; poor feeding and fever are the most frequent presenting symptoms. A fulminant illness with rapid onset and progressive deterioration occasionally is encountered (180). Meningitis is seen in approximately 60% of infants with the late-onset syndrome, and GBS serotype III accounts for about 95% of these cases (169). Rarely, infants with late-onset meningitis caused by GBS present with hydrocephalus. These infants may appear to have uncomplicated hydrocephalus with normal lumbar cerebrospinal fluid (CSF). Examination of ventricular fluid reveals pleocytosis, and the organism is recovered on culture. Spinal fluid cultures of infants with meningitis caused by gram-positive organisms usually are sterile within 24 to 36 hours of therapy, and the mortality rate is 10% to 15%.

Approximately 20% of neonatal infections caused by GBS do not fit into the early- or late-onset syndromes and extend over a broad clinical spectrum involving many different organ systems. Several manifestations have been observed (169,181,182):

- Cellulitis
- Scalp abscess

- Impetigo
- Fasciitis
- Breast abscess
- Adenitis
- Supraglottitis
- Conjunctivitis
- Orbital cellulitis
- Ethmoiditis
- Otitis media
- Pneumonia complicated by empyema
- Myocarditis
- Endocarditis
- Hepatitis
- Septic arthritis
- Osteomyelitis
- Bursitis
- Urinary tract infection
- Omphalitis
- Peritonitis
- Asymptomatic transient bacteremia.

The transient bacteremia is remarkable because these infants appear clinically well and are cultured because of a history of maternal obstetric complications. A repeat blood culture before the institution of antibiotic therapy frequently is sterile.

Both relapses and reinfections can occur after invasive GBS infections (169). Reasons for relapse may include an inadequate penicillin dose, a short duration of therapy of the initial episode, or unrecognized foci of infection (e.g., endocarditis, brain abscess). Reinfection can occur because of maternal GBS mastitis (183). Rifampin (20 mg/kg/d for 4 to 7 days) has been used to eradicate GBS carriage in infants with recurrent disease and is given after completion of systemic penicillin therapy (183).

Coagulase-Positive Staphylococcal Disease

The phage group I *S. aureus*, which was common in the late 1950s, still exists in some nurseries and occasionally causes serious systemic neonatal disease. The pathogenicity of this organism is based on its ability to invade the skin and musculoskeletal system, producing furuncles, breast abscesses, adenitis, and osteomyelitis. Septicemia usually is secondary to local invasion. After *S. aureus* is recovered from blood cultures of neonates, a careful search should be made for a primary focus. Some group I *S. aureus* strains produce toxic shock syndrome toxin-1, formerly known as enterotoxin F or pyrogenic toxin C, and have caused toxic shock syndrome in older neonates (184,185). Clinical characteristics of this disease include the sudden onset of fever, diarrhea, shock, mucous membrane hyperemia, and a diffuse erythematous macular rash with subsequent desquamation of the hands and feet, commencing on about the fifth or sixth day of illness.

In the early 1970s, phage group II coagulase-positive staphylococci emerged as a common cause of neonatal infection. Although this organism may be invasive, pathogenicity depends principally on production of exotoxins (i.e., exfolatiative or epidermolytic toxins A and B). Common areas of primary infection include the umbilical stump, conjunctiva, and throat; infection of a surgical wound has been described (186). The exfoliative toxins act on the zona granulosa of the epidermis and cause epidermal splitting through activity of the toxins on the desmosomes (187). Clinical disease may take one of several forms, including bullous impetigo, toxic epidermal necrolysis (i.e., Ritter disease), and nonstreptococcal scarlatina. Collectively, these diseases have been referred to as the expanded scalded skin syndrome (Fig. 48–1) (45).

The initial finding in Ritter disease is generalized erythema associated with edema and tenderness on palpation, usually noticed between days 3 and 16 of life (188). After several days, a distinctive desquamation of large sheets of epidermis occurs, which is different from the fine desquamation observed in the second and third weeks of streptococcal scarlet fever. Large flaccid bullae commonly observed in Ritter disease will, on rupture, leave a tender, weeping erythematous base. Some infants may appear quite toxic with the generalized form of disease. A rare, congenital form of staphylococcal scalded skin syndrome has been described (189). Spread within a

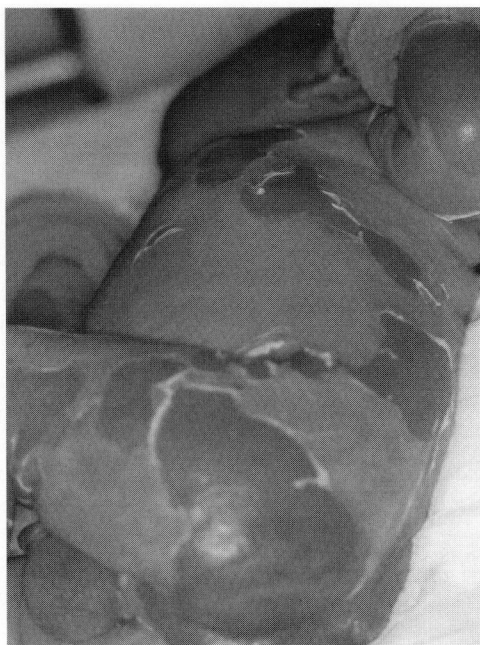

FIG. 48–1. A 10-day-old Caucasian boy with staphylococcal scalded skin syndrome. He was treated with fluids, oral dicloxacillin, and wound care. His skin healed completely and without scarring within 2 weeks of this photograph being taken.

nursery can occur, and its recognition warrants the prompt institution of infection control measures to limit the spread of the toxigenic strain of *S. aureus* (190).

Umbilical venous or arterial catheters and central venous lines are well-recognized risk factors for staphylococcal bacteremia. *S. aureus* is second only to coagulase-negative staphylococci as a cause of catheter-related infections (35).

The mortality rate for neonates with *S. aureus* bacteremia is about 20%. Low-birth-weight infants are at highest risk of death from this infection (191).

Coagulase-Negative Staphylococcal Disease

The isolation of coagulase-negative staphylococci from blood, CSF, or urine of newborns with signs and symptoms of sepsis can be significant, and these bacteria should not be dismissed as contaminants. Of the at least 30 recognized coagulase-negative staphylococcal species, *S. epidermidis* is clinically the most significant for neonates (192–194). Experience indicates that these bacteria are responsible for about 10% to 27% of all cases of sepsis in neonatal intensive care units, but can account for as many as 55% of late-onset sepsis cases in very-low-birth weight infants (3,167,195). Coagulase-negative staphylococcal infections are nosocomial in origin and result in substantially longer hospitalizations for affected infants (196,197). Risk of infection with these organisms increases with decreasing gestational age and birth weight (198–201).

Clinical manifestations of coagulase-negative staphylococcal infections are similar to those caused by other pathogens and include apnea, bradycardia, temperature instability (e.g., hypothermia, hyperthermia), respiratory distress (e.g., tachypnea, retractions, cyanosis), gastrointestinal manifestations (e.g., poor feeding, abdominal distention, bloody stools), lethargy, and metabolic acidosis (7,193). Clinical illnesses include septicemia, meningitis with or without CSF abnormalities, necrotizing enterocolitis, pneumonia, omphalitis, soft tissue abscesses associated with persistent bacteremia, endocarditis, and scalp abscesses and osteomyelitis at insertion sites of fetal monitoring electrodes (198–209).

Risk factors for coagulase-negative staphylococcal infections include the presence of foreign bodies, such as central venous lines, ventriculoperitoneal shunts, or peritoneal dialysis catheters, prior antibiotic therapy, and intravenous infusion of lipid emulsions for nutritional support (193,210,211). The organisms travel along catheter tracks from colonization sites. They eventually adhere to, and proliferate on, certain biosynthetic materials and later cause local or systemic reactions. The mechanism by which adherence occurs appears initially to involve hydrophobic and electrostatic interactions between the bacteria and the biopolymers (193). Once attached, a viscous exopolysaccharide referred to as slime is formed. Slime covers the bacteria to form a surface biofilm that protects them from such environmental factors as antibiotics and host defenses while allowing continued access to nutrition (193). The density of the biofilm may be increased if the organisms are exposed to subinhibitory concentrations of antibiotics to which they are susceptible (e.g., vancomycin) (212). Slime appears to inhibit neutrophil chemotaxis and phagocytosis and the lymphoproliferative responses of mononuclear cells to mitogens (213,214). Slime-producing strains account for most coagulase-negative staphylococci isolated from infants with invasive infections (200). Ineffective opsonophagocytosis due to intrinsic deficiencies in neonatal host defenses contributes to the increased susceptibility of low-birth-weight infants to infection with these organisms (215,216).

Coagulase-negative staphylococci produce a variety of toxins that may serve as virulence factors, including hemolysins, proteases, urease, and fibrinolysin (7). Most fecal isolates produce a hemolysin that functionally and immunologically is identical to the delta toxin produced by *S. aureus* (217). This toxin causes severe mucosal necrosis and hemorrhage when injected into ligated infant rat bowel loops and may play a role in the pathogenesis of neonatal necrotizing enterocolitis (218,219).

Listeria monocytogenes *Disease*

The incidence of perinatal listeriosis decreased by about 51% between 1989 and 1993, from 17.4 to 8.6 per 100,000 persons younger than 1 year of age (220). This reduction was related temporally with industry, regulatory, and educational efforts to aggressively enforce food monitoring policies.

The pathogenesis of clinical diseases caused by *L. monocytogenes* is similar to those caused by GBS. A fulminant, disseminated disease (i.e., granulomatosis infantiseptica) may occur during the first several days of life. The pathogen is acquired transplacentally or by aspiration at the time of vaginal delivery, and multiple organ systems (e.g., liver, spleen, kidneys, lungs, brain, and skin) are involved; 35% to 55% of infants die of their infection (221,222). The infant frequently presents with hypothermia, lethargy, and poor feeding. Early passage of meconium in a premature infant suggests *Listeria* infection (223). A characteristic rash consisting of small, salmon-colored papules scattered primarily on the trunk can be observed in some infants. The chest roentgenogram shows parenchymal infiltrates suggestive of aspiration pneumonitis in most infants. A miliary-type of bronchopneumonia can be seen in some cases. *Listeria* serotypes Ia, Ib, and IVb produce the early-onset disease, whereas serotype IVb is the predominant type in late-onset meningitic disease (224).

A delayed form of neonatal listeriosis occurs during the second through fifth weeks of life and primarily involves the meninges (224,225). The infected infant usually is the full-term product of an uncomplicated labor and delivery. Onset of symptoms and signs is relatively insidious and indistinguishable from those observed with meningitis caused by other pathogens. The source of the organism in late-onset disease is unclear. Although acquisition of *Listeria* may occur during passage through an infected birth canal, it appears that most cases result from postpartum horizontal spread. In favor of the latter route of infection are several reported clusters of neonatal listeriosis and the demonstration of cross-infections between newborns using enzyme electrophoretic typing and DNA fingerprinting (221,226–228).

The peripheral leukocyte count usually shows a brisk leukocytosis, with a predominance of polymorphonuclear leukocytes in the differential count (229). A significant elevation in the number of monocytes, to 7% to 21% of the total leukocyte count, has been documented on admission laboratory evaluation of infected infants. A monocytosis of this magnitude can be demonstrated in most remaining infants on repetitive testing of the peripheral leukocyte count, but monocytes typically are not found in the spinal fluid of infants infected with *L. monocytogenes*. Polymorphonuclear leukocytes predominate in about 75% of cases, with a relative lymphocytosis in the remaining 25%. In contrast, adults with *Listeria* meningoencephalitis may have CSF monocytosis of 80% to 90% (222). As with other pyogenic meningitides, hypoglycorrhachia and elevated protein concentrations are frequent findings. Examination of the stained smear of spinal fluid has not been rewarding in more than 50% of cases. This is a reflection of the relatively low concentrations of organisms in the fluid. The bacteriology laboratory should be forewarned of the clinical suspicion of *Listeria* meningitis, because these microorganisms occasionally are discarded as contaminants because of their tinctorial and morphologic similarities with diphtheroids. Overnight refrigeration of spinal fluid specimens frequently enhances growth of this organism.

Enterococcal Infection

Group D streptococci were formerly divided into enterococcal and nonenterococcal types. The enterococci are now included in the new genus *Enterococcus*; most neonatal infections are caused by *Enterococcus faecalis* and, to a lesser extent, by *E. faecium* (230–232).

Early-onset enterococcal disease (less than 7 days of age) is relatively mild and presents clinically with respiratory distress or diarrhea. No associations with underlying conditions, invasive procedures, or maternal obstetric complications have been observed (233). Late-onset disease (≥7 days of age) most commonly afflicts low-birth-weight infants with complicated clinical problems that often require surgical procedures (e.g., bowel resection), central venous catheters, or prior treatment with antimi-

crobials. Clinical manifestations of late-onset disease include apnea, bradycardia, circulatory failure, meningitis, pneumonia, scalp abscesses, catheter-related bacteremia, and necrotizing enterocolitis-associated septicemia (233). About 20% of enterococcal blood isolates represent skin contamination; clinical correlation is needed to differentiate contamination from true infection (231).

Enterococci can spread rapidly within a nursery (234). Nosocomial outbreaks of enterococcal septicemia in neonatal intensive care units are well documented (232,235). The mortality rate is estimated at 6% to 11%, but it can be as high as 17% in infants with necrotizing enterocolitis-associated septicemia (231,233).

The importance of identifying *Enterococcus* as the etiologic agent in septicemia primarily relates to selection of proper antimicrobial agents. The enterococci are moderately resistant to penicillin alone, due to certain properties of their penicillin-binding proteins (231,236). Some enterococcal strains have acquired new mechanisms of antibiotic resistance that include β-lactamase production and high-level aminoglycoside resistance (i.e., minimal inhibitory concentrations [MIC] ≥2,000 µg/mL) (234,237,238). Strains resistant to the glycopeptides vancomycin and teicoplanin (glycopeptide-resistant enterococci) were first described in 1987 and since have emerged as major nosocomial pathogens (239,240). Nonenterococcal group D streptococci continue to be highly susceptible to penicillin (231).

Gram-Negative Bacterial Infection

In North America, *E. coli* is the most common gram-negative organism causing septicemia during the neonatal period. *Klebsiella* and *Enterobacter* strains are second (167). In contradistinction to illness caused by GBS and *L. monocytogenes*, *E. coli* infections do not fit into distinct clinical syndromes of early- and late-onset disease. Approximately 40% of *E. coli* strains causing septicemia possess K1 capsular antigen, and strains identical with those isolated from blood cultures usually can be identified in the patient's nasopharynx or rectal cultures. The clinical features of *E. coli* sepsis generally are similar to those observed in infants with disease caused by other pathogens. Respiratory distress is noted in about 73% with *E. coli* sepsis occurring during the first week of life (241). Localized *E. coli* infections have included breast abscess, cellulitis, pneumonia, lung abscess, empyema, osteomyelitis, septic arthritis, urinary tract infection, ascending cholangitis, and otitis media.

An increase in the proportion of neonatal *E. coli* sepsis cases caused by ampicillin-resistant strains has been noted by some investigators (241,242). This shift occurred as maternal intrapartum prophylaxis for the prevention of early-onset GBS sepsis was being implemented more widely by obstetricians at these medical centers. Most deaths were seen in neonates infected with ampicillin-resistant *E. coli* strains.

Pseudomonas septicemia may present with a characteristic violaceous papular lesion or lesions that, after several days, develop central necrosis. Although these skin lesions most commonly are seen in *Pseudomonas* infection, they may be associated with other organisms (243). Pseudomonas typically is encountered in late-onset sepsis, although occasional newborns with an early-onset form of this infection have been reported.

Neonatal infections caused by *H. influenzae* biotype IV have increased in frequency in the last 20 years and currently account for about 11% of early-onset sepsis in very-low-birth-weight infants (401–1,500 g) (4,244). These strains are nontypeable, have a distinct multilocus enzyme genotype revealed by clonal analysis, express peritrichous fimbriae and a variant P6 outer membrane protein, and have a characteristic outer membrane electrophoretic profile. Genetic analysis suggests that these strains represent a cryptic genospecies only distantly related to *H. influenzae* or *Haemophilus haemolyticum* (244,245).

Anaerobic Infections

Anaerobes have accounted for 1% to 25% of all bacteria isolated from blood cultures of neonates with suspected septicemia in various studies (246–249). *Bacteroides* spp, primarily *Bacteroides fragilis*, and clostridia are most commonly recovered (248). *Peptostreptococcus* spp, *Veillonella* spp, *Propionibacterium acnes, Eubacterium* spp, and *Fusobacterium* spp occur relatively infrequently. Anaerobes are found mixed in cultures with aerobic bacteria in about one-third of cases. Clinical illnesses include transient bacteremia, fulminant septicemia, postoperative infections, and intrauterine death associated with septic abortion (246). Localized diseases such as omphalitis, cellulitis, and necrotizing fasciitis are seen commonly with clostridia (250). Conditions predisposing to anaerobic septicemia include prolonged rupture of membranes, chorioamnionitis, prematurity, and gastrointestinal disease.

Anaerobes isolated from blood within the first 2 days of life are usually gram-positive and penicillin G-susceptible, but those isolated from older newborns tend to be gram-negative and penicillin G-resistant (247). Gram-positive anaerobes are more likely to be recovered from blood of infants with sepsis associated with chorioamnionitis, whereas gram-negative anaerobes predominate in necrotizing enterocolitis-associated bacteremia (247). The mortality rates for reported cases of anaerobic septicemia are about 35% for illnesses caused by *Bacteroides* spp and 12% for other anaerobes (248).

Genital Mycoplasmas

M. hominis and *U. urealyticum* occasionally are isolated from the blood of neonates with sepsis. Cassell and colleagues (24) observed concomitant bacteremia in 40% and 26% of preterm infants with positive endotracheal cultures for *M. hominis* and *U. urealyticum*, respectively. Other investigators were unable to recover genital mycoplasmas from the blood or CSF of neonates with suspected sepsis (251,252). An association between persistent pulmonary hypertension and *U. urealyticum* sepsis and pneumonia has been observed (253).

Fungal Infections

Fungal sepsis occurs in as many as 10% of low-birth-weight infants (3). Most cases are due to *Candida* spp, particularly *C. albicans* (254–256). *C. tropicalis, C. parapsilosis, Candida lusitaniae,* and *Candida glabrata* also cause systemic candidiasis (256). Congenital candidiasis is uncommon and results from ascending infection through intact membranes. It usually manifests with early skin lesions (e.g., maculopapular rash, pustules, vesicles, desquamation, skin abscesses), but disseminated and life-threatening infections can occur (257,258).

The incidence of candidemia in neonatal intensive care units is increasing steadily. In one such unit in Norfolk, Virginia, the rate of candidemia increased over 11-fold in the 15-year period between 1981 and 1995. In addition, *C. parapsilosis* was responsible for 60% of all candidemias during the last 5 years of the study period (259).

Risk factors for late-onset systemic candidiasis include prematurity, low birth weight, use of broad-spectrum antimicrobial agents, steroid therapy, central vascular catheters, parenteral hyperalimentation, intralipid infusions, prolonged endotracheal intubation, necrotizing enterocolitis, and immunologic immaturity (254,260). The most important of these factors appears to be the number of prior antibiotics and the duration of therapy (261,262). Low-birth-weight infants in whom mucocutaneous candidiasis develops are at considerable risk of subsequent invasive disease (261,263). Infants with invasive candidiasis caused by *C. albicans* are more likely to have antecedent candidal thrush or perineal dermatitis and to die of their infection than neonates with severe *C. parapsilosis* infections (259,264). Clinical manifestations vary and are indistinguishable from those caused by other pathogens. A fungal cause for sepsis should be considered strongly in an infant weighing less than 1,500 g who has been hospitalized for a prolonged period, is receiving parenteral hyperalimentation through a central vascular catheter, and previously has been treated with multiple antibiotics; a history of gastrointestinal disease or surgery adds to the clinical suspicion. Diseases caused by *Candida* spp include, but are not limited to, pneumonia, endocarditis, endophthalmitis, meningitis, cerebral abscesses, pyelonephritis, fungal balls in the kidney and bladder, peritonitis, hepatosplenic abscesses, arthritis, and osteomyelitis (254,265–272).

Malassezia furfur causes invasive neonatal fungal disease. Most infections involve chronically ill premature infants who are receiving lipid emulsions through a central venous catheter (273). The most commonly reported presenting symptoms and signs include fever (50%) and respiratory distress (50%). Pathologic analysis reveals mycotic thrombi around catheter tips, endocardial vegetations, and lung lesions that include mycotic emboli with occlusion of pulmonary arteries, septic thrombi, pulmonary vasculitis, and alveolitis (273). Involvement of other organs is uncommon. *Malassezia pachydermatis* is a recently recognized human pathogen that has been incriminated in neonatal intensive care unit outbreaks of bloodstream, urinary tract, and central nervous system infections. In one recently reported outbreak, the source of *M. pachydermatis* was the contaminated hands of health care workers who were colonized from their pet dogs at home (274). Systemic infections due to other fungi such as *Torulopsis glabrata, Hansenula anomala, Aspergillus* spp, *Cryptococcus neoformans, Coccidioides immitis, Blastomyces* spp, and *Trichosporon beigelii* are rare (256,275–278).

Laboratory Tests and Findings

Since the early 1970s, several screening tests and scoring systems have been described that are purported to aid the physician in making the diagnosis of neonatal infection. Although a few are helpful in identifying the infant at high risk of developing infection, the diagnosis of septicemia can be made only by recovery of the organism from blood cultures or other normally sterile body fluids (29,279). It is imperative that these cultures be obtained by strict aseptic technique. Blood should be obtained from a peripheral vein rather than from the umbilical vessels, the outer several millimeters of which are contaminated frequently with bacteria. Femoral vein aspiration may result in cultures contaminated with coliform organisms from the perineum. Heelstick samples have low sensitivities. The skin above the vein to be punctured should be cleansed with an antiseptic solution, such as an iodophor, and allowed to dry for maximal antiseptic effect. The amount of blood drawn is critical; 1 to 2 mL of blood is required for optimal results (280). The sensitivity of a single blood culture in identifying septicemia is only 80% (279). Obtaining blood cultures from multiple sites may enhance the yield and aid in identifying false-positive results (281). Quantitative blood cultures, if available, are helpful in differentiating true pathogens from culture contaminants (282,283). If *M. furfur* is a suspected pathogen, the microbiology laboratory should be alerted so that blood can be inoculated onto special media that provide for the organism's absolute nutritional requirement for medium-chain fatty acids; routine culture media do not support its growth (256).

It frequently is helpful to obtain cultures of other sites before initiating antimicrobial therapy. For example, percutaneous bladder aspiration of urine for culture can be helpful in identifying the urinary tract as the focus of infection. This is particularly true for illness occurring after the third day of life. Nasopharyngeal, skin, umbilical cord, gastric, and rectal cultures frequently are positive in the early septicemic form of listeriosis and GBS disease. However, these colonization sites are not predictive of the cause of bloodstream infection and should not be used to guide antimicrobial therapy (284). All clinically stable infants with suspected septicemia should have CSF obtained for examination and culture before therapy. This practice has been challenged for infants younger than 7 days of age because of its low yield; the yield from a lumbar puncture is much higher when performed on infants older than 1 week of age (29,285–291). Practitioners opting to forego performing a lumbar puncture for infants with suspected early-onset sepsis should anticipate that, on occasion, the diagnosis of meningitis will be delayed or missed because not all newborns with bacterial meningitis have positive blood culture results (290).

The peripheral leukocyte count is the most useful of the indirect indicators of bacterial infection. After correction for the nucleated erythrocyte count, the total absolute neutrophil count and the ratio of immature to total neutrophilic forms are compared with normal standard values for age. In the absence of maternal hypertension, severe asphyxia, periventricular hemorrhage, maternal fever, or hemolytic disease, absolute total neutropenia and an elevated ratio of immature to total neutrophilic forms strongly suggest bacterial infection (292,293). Infants born in high-altitude areas have higher total and immature neutrophil counts (294). Wide interreader differences in band neutrophil identification have been observed, thereby limiting the utility of the immature to total neutrophil ratio in actual clinical practice (295). Repeating complete blood counts within 24 hours of birth has been shown to enhance the value of the test as a screen for sepsis (296).

Gastric aspirate stains and culture, erythrocyte sedimentation rate, C-reactive protein (CRP), and the nitroblue tetrazolium test have not proved useful as indicators of bacterial infection, although in combination these tests may offer some guidance (29). CRP values appear not to be influenced by perinatal asphyxia, hyperbilirubinemia, periventricular hemorrhage, or respiratory distress syndrome (297). Serial CRP measurements may be helpful in identifying infants not likely to be infected and in whom antibiotics can be safely stopped (298). The detection of interleukin-6 (IL-6) in serum, especially in conjunction with an elevated CRP measurement, may be useful in the early diagnosis of neonatal infection (299–302). The levels of granulocyte colony-stimulating factor, neutrophil CD11b expression, circulating intracellular adhesion molecule-1, interleukin-1 receptor antagonist (IL-1ra), serum procalcitonin, and interleukin-8 are all elevated in newborns with sepsis, but how these laboratory findings can best be utilized for the diagnosis of neonatal sepsis is yet to be defined (299,301–304). In one study, IL-1ra and IL-6 levels were found to be elevated (a 15-fold median maximal increase) 2 days before a diagnosis of sepsis was made (302).

Detection of the soluble antigens of *E. coli* K1, GBS, *H. influenzae* type b, *N. meningitidis,* and *S. pneumoniae* by latex particle agglutination (LPA) is useful for identifying the infant infected with these pathogens. The absence of antigen does not rule out infection by these organisms. Substantial sensitivity differences have been found among the commercially available LPA assays for GBS antigen (305). False-positive LPA test results for GBS in urine specimens can result from contamination of bag specimens with these bacteria from perineal and rectal colonization, cross-reacting antigens, or absorption of antigen from the gastrointestinal tract (306,307). Similar false-positive test results may be obtained for the other bacteria. Rapid diagnosis of invasive *Candida* infection by detection of its circulating cell wall (e.g., mannan), cytoplasmic (e.g., enolase), or heat-labile antigens is possible, although the reliability of these tests is yet to be proved (308).

Therapy

After septicemia is suspected, suitable cultures should be obtained and therapy with ampicillin and an aminoglycoside started immediately. If meningitis has been excluded, ampicillin is administered intravenously or intramuscularly in a dosage of 50 mg/kg/d divided in two doses for infants younger than 1 week of age and 100 to 150 mg/kg/d divided in three or four doses for infants 1 to 4 weeks of age. The selection of the aminoglycoside antibiotic should be based on antimicrobial susceptibilities of enteric organisms isolated from infants in each nursery. Gentamicin is the drug of choice for treatment of infections caused by susceptible gram-negative organisms and is administered intravenously or intramuscularly in a dosage of 5 to 7.5 mg/kg/d divided in two or three doses, depending on the infant's age.

Aminoglycoside-resistant *E. coli* have been encountered in some nurseries in North America. In these nurseries or in an infant from whom an isolate is shown to be resistant to kanamycin or gentamicin, amikacin or cefotaxime should be used. Studies have demonstrated no significant ototoxicity in infants and children who were treated in the neonatal period with kanamycin or gentamicin (9). However, in premature infants and in those receiving these drugs for prolonged periods, brainstem evoked response audiometry should be performed whenever possible. Serum concentrations of the aminoglycosides should be monitored in low-birth-weight premature infants because of erratic absorption and elimination of the drugs in these infants. Although cefotaxime should not be used routinely for initial empiric therapy of neonatal sepsis, it is an effective agent when used alone or combined with an aminoglycoside for infections caused by coliform bacilli.

When the type of skin lesions or historic experience suggests the possibility of *Pseudomonas* infection, ceftazidime or ticarcillin with or without an aminoglycoside is the therapy of choice. Although not approved for use in neonates by the Food and Drug Administration, we have successfully used ticarcillin-clavulanate for treatment of sepsis caused by multiresistant gram-negative enteric bacilli, *Pseudomonas*, and anaerobic bacteria.

If *S. aureus* sepsis is suspected but not proved, parenteral methicillin or nafcillin should be substituted for penicillin or ampicillin, because approximately 80% of these staphylococci will be penicillin-resistant. Although gentamicin and kanamycin possess activity against most staphylococci, these agents cannot be recommended because there are no studies of their efficacy in neonatal staphylococcal disease. For disease caused by coagulase-negative staphylococci or multiresistant *S. aureus* strains, vancomycin is the preferred therapy. Peak and trough serum vancomycin concentrations should be monitored because of the drug's narrow therapeutic index.

After the pathogen is identified and its antimicrobial susceptibilities are known, the most appropriate drug or drugs should be selected. As a general rule, gentamicin alone or in combination with ampicillin, or cefotaxime alone or in combination with an aminoglycoside, should be used for susceptible *E. coli, Klebsiella* spp, and *Enterobacter* spp; amikacin alone or in combination with cefotaxime for gentamicin-resistant coliform bacteria; ceftazidime, ticarcillin, or ticarcillin-clavulanate, with or without an aminoglycoside, for *Pseudomonas*; ampicillin alone or in combination with an aminoglycoside for *P. mirabilis*, enterococci, and *L. monocytogenes;* and penicillin for other gram-positive organisms, except for penicillin-resistant *S. aureus,* for which methicillin or nafcillin is the drug of choice. Vancomycin is used for coagulase-negative staphylococci and MRSA. Rarely, coagulase-negative staphylococcal strains that are resistant to vancomycin can emerge during treatment with this agent (309). *S. aureus* strains with reduced susceptibility to vancomycin (glycopeptide-intermediate *S. aureus* [GISA]) have been isolated from a few patients with a variety of infections. The first such clinical isolate was described in a 4-month-old Japanese infant with a nosocomial surgical site infection (310,311). No GISA strains have been identified in newborns to date. Treatment of GISA-related infections generally requires the use of drugs considered investigational for newborns. The MIC and minimal bactericidal concentration (MBC) of penicillin and ampicillin should be determined for GBS because a small percentage of these organisms are tolerant (i.e., have an MBC to MIC ratio greater than 32) to these antibiotics (312). These strains are best treated with a penicillin-aminoglycoside combination. Penicillin-resistant and vancomycin-tolerant pneumococci have not yet emerged as neonatal pathogens. The therapeutic options for vancomycin-resistant enterococcal infections in neonates are seriously limited. Some strains may be susceptible to a combination of penicillin or ampicillin and an aminoglycoside. Chloramphenicol or tetracyclines may be effective against some strains, but these drugs have serious toxicities for neonates. Nitrofurantoin is active against many vancomycin-resistant enterococcal strains and has been used to treat enterococcal urinary tract infections in adults. Dalfopristin-quinupristin recently was approved for use in adults, but there are no data on its use in infants. Several investigational ketolides, oxazolidinones, glycylcyclines, and even newer semisynthetic glycopeptides with *in vitro* activities against vancomycin-resistant enterococci are being evaluated (313). *U. urealyticum* infections are treated with erythromycin (314).

The drug of choice for systemic fungal infections is amphotericin B, with or without flucytosine (254,315). The half-life and serum concentrations of amphotericin B are highly variable during the neonatal period (316). The drug appears to be better tolerated by infants than older children and adults, but renal and hepatic functions should be monitored carefully (254,317). The optimal daily dosage of amphotericin B is not universally agreed on. The most commonly used dosage regimen is to begin with 0.5 mg/kg of the drug on the first day and, if tolerated, to increase the daily dosage to 1.0 mg/kg by the second or third day of treatment. The cumulative dosage of amphotericin B needed for the adequate treatment of systemic *Candida* infection is not well defined, but it is estimated to be 20 to 30 mg/kg (254). Resistance to amphotericin B among *Candida* species is not a major clinical problem (318). Amphotericin B frequently is combined with flucytosine for the treatment of central nervous system fungal infection because of flucytosine's excellent CSF penetration and the *in vitro* synergy of this drug combination against *Candida*. Gastrointestinal intolerance, myelosuppression, and hepatotoxicity are common side effects of flucytosine (254).

Experience with the use of liposomal amphotericin B preparations in newborns is limited (319–321). Weitkamp and colleagues (320) from Germany reported on their experience with liposomal amphotericin B (AmBisome) in 21 infants with birth weights less than 1,500 g who had systemic candidiasis. The median age at the start of therapy was 13 days (range 1 to 49). The dose of the drug was 1 to 5 mg/kg/d and was given for 11 to 79 days (median 28). All treated infants recovered, and no definite drug-related toxicity was observed (320). Scarcella and co-workers (321) from Italy also used AmBisome in 40 preterm and 4 term infants with severe fungal infections, 70% of which were due to *C. albicans*.

The duration of therapy ranged from 7 to 49 days, and the cumulative drug dose given during therapy ranged from 7 to 138.8 mg/kg. The drug was effective in 73% of infants, including 5 of 6 with meningitis. No drug-related adverse effects were noted (321). Lipid formulations of amphotericin B are not more efficacious than conventional amphotericin B deoxycholate, and their use should be limited to patients who are either refractory to, or intolerant of, the regular amphotericin B preparation (322).

The use of fluconazole for the treatment of neonatal candidiasis is increasing slowly, but the cumulative published experience is meager (323–325). Huttova and associates (324) from the Slovak Republic treated 40 newborns with fluconazole, 28 of whom weighed less than 1,500 g at birth. All infants had fungemia with *C. albicans*. Fluconazole was administered as a single daily intravenous dose of 6 mg/kg for a total of 6 to 48 days. A cure rate of 80% was achieved; 10% died as a direct consequence of their infection. Mild elevations of liver enzyme concentrations were noted in 5% of neonates. Wenzl and colleagues (325) successfully treated three premature infants (gestational ages 24 to 29 weeks) with *C. albicans* sepsis using oral fluconazole at doses of 4.5 to 6 mg/kg once daily for 4 to 6 weeks.

Guidelines for determining duration of therapy in the neonatal period often are lacking, because objective evidence of illness may be minimal. Culture of the blood should be repeated 24 to 48 hours after initiation of therapy; if positive, alteration of therapy may be necessary. In the absence of deep tissue involvement or abscess formation, treatment usually is continued 5 to 7 days after clinical improvement. If multiple organs are involved or clinical response is slow, treatment may need to be continued for 2 to 3 weeks.

Suspected central venous catheter-related bacterial sepsis can be managed initially with the intraluminal infusion of vancomycin combined with ceftazidime or an aminoglycoside. After infection is confirmed and the pathogen identified, single-drug therapy usually is sufficient. Reported cure rates with antibiotics alone without catheter removal have ranged from 50% to more than 90% for pediatric patients. Persistently positive blood cultures after 2 to 4 days of appropriate antimicrobial therapy warrants catheter removal. A continuous infusion of a low dose of urokinase for 24 hours may help in clearing catheter-related infections in some infants who fail conventional antibiotic therapy (326). Patients responding to antibiotic therapy should be treated for 2 to 3 weeks or at least for 10 days from the time of the first negative blood culture. Catheter-related fungal infections rarely are cured without catheter removal (38).

Immunotherapy of neonatal sepsis is discussed in Chapter 46. Extracorporeal membrane oxygenation for newborns with persistent pulmonary hypertension due to overwhelming early-onset GBS sepsis may improve their survival (327).

Prevention

The identification of high-risk GBS-carrier mothers and the subsequent interruption of vertical transmission by intrapartum maternal chemotherapy can prevent many cases of early-onset neonatal GBS disease (10,168). Many approaches have been suggested and some have been tested. They range from giving penicillin prophylaxis to all newborns or ceftriaxone prophylaxis to all women in labor, to screening all pregnant women for GBS carriage at one or more points in pregnancy and treating antepartum or intrapartum with penicillin or ampicillin, to only offering intrapartum antibiotics to women who meet certain criteria that place them at high risk of delivering an infant with early-onset GBS disease.

The Centers for Disease Control and Prevention issued guidelines aimed at identifying and treating most GBS carriers while minimizing the number of women receiving unnecessary intrapartum antibiotics (Table 48–4). Two approaches are endorsed. The first is based on

TABLE 48–4. *Summary of Centers for Disease Control and Prevention recommendations for the prevention of neonatal early-onset group B streptococcal sepsis*

- Screening-based approach
  1. Women who had previously delivered an infant with invasive GBS disease, had GBS bacteriuria during the current pregnancy, and those delivering before 37 weeks of gestation should be given IAP.
  2. All other women should have a rectovaginal swab for GBS culture performed at 35 to 37 weeks of gestation.
     A. If culture is positive for GBS, offer IAP.
     B. If culture is not done or result is not available, give IAP if she develops intrapartum fever (≥100.4°F or ≥38.0°C) or has membrane rupture for ≥18 h.
     C. If culture is negative for GBS, or if it is not done or is incomplete at the time of delivery but the mother has no intrapartum fever or prolonged rupture of membranes, then no IAP is needed.
- Risk factor-based approach
  1. No antenatal cultures for GBS are obtained.
  2. Women with any of the following risk factors should be given IAP: previously delivered an infant who had invasive GBS disease; GBS bacteriuria during the current pregnancy; delivery at <37 weeks of gestation; duration of ruptured membranes ≥18 h; intrapartum temperature ≥100.4°F (≥38.0°C).
- Recommended IAP regimens
  1. Penicillin G, 5 mU IV loading dose, and then 2.5 mU IV every 4 h until delivery *or* ampicillin, 2 g IV loading dose, then 1 g IV every 4 h until delivery.
  2. For penicillin-allergic patients, use either clindamycin 900 mg IV every 8 h or erythromycin 500 mg IV every 6 h, until delivery.

GBS, group B *Streptococcus;* IAP, intrapartum antibiotic prophylaxis.
Adapted from ref. 168.

obtaining rectovaginal cultures for GBS at 35 to 37 weeks of gestation and treating only GBS carriers thus identified. The concordance between culture results at 35 to 37 weeks and those obtained intrapartum approaches 100%. In contrast, a positive GBS culture at 26 to 28 weeks of gestation will still be positive at delivery in only 67% of women; conversely, 7.4% of women with negative GBS cultures at 26 to 28 weeks of gestation will be found to be GBS positive at delivery. The second approach, and the one favored by the American College of Obstetricians and Gynecologists, foregoes antepartum testing in favor of intrapartum therapy for women with certain high-risk characteristics that can be assessed at the time of delivery. It is estimated that with the prenatal culture approach, approximately 80% of early-onset GBS disease can be prevented and that one-fourth of all women in labor would receive intrapartum antibiotics. With the risk factors-based approach, 69% of early-onset GBS cases would be prevented and 18% of women would receive intrapartum antibiotics (168). However, a risk factors-based approach would have detected only 10% of women whose term newborns contracted early-onset GBS sepsis in one study (328).

Another suggested approach involves screening pregnant women for anogenital GBS carriage at 26 to 28 weeks of gestation. Latex agglutination tests can be used at the time of delivery for women with no prenatal care. Culture-positive women with onset of labor or rupture of membranes before 37 weeks of gestation, fever during labor, rupture of membranes for more than 12 hours, a history of GBS bacteriuria during pregnancy, or a history of having previously delivered an infant with GBS disease would be treated intravenously with ampicillin until delivery. This approach prevents only 51% of all early-onset GBS disease, but only 3.4% of pregnant women would receive intrapartum antibiotics (168). This approach to prevention was favored by 81% of pregnant women, 65% of pediatricians, and only 15% of obstetricians in one published survey (329).

Intrapartum antibiotic prophylaxis-related adverse effects include the small but real risk of death from anaphylaxis for women (estimated risk of 0.001%) and an increase in the proportion of infants with sepsis caused by ampicillin-resistant bacteria. A recent study examined the susceptibility profile of 119 colonizing and 8 invasive GBS strains collected from two hospitals in Birmingham, Alabama, between January 1996 and September 1997 from predominantly vaginally delivered term newborns and found that the GBS isolates almost universally were penicillin susceptible, with only a small minority of the strains showing moderate penicillin or ampicillin susceptibility (330). However, between 16% to 21% of GBS isolates are erythromycin resistant and 4% to 15% are clindamycin resistant, which raises concerns about the possible inadequacy of currently recommended alternatives for penicillin-allergic women (330,331).

The rectovaginal swabs for GBS cultures should be placed in a transport medium that will maintain GBS viability, unless direct inoculation into a selective broth medium is possible. One study suggests that rectovaginal swabs placed in standard transport media can be used as long as the specimens subsequently are transferred to selective growth media within 2 hours of collection (332).

The management of infants born to women given intrapartum antimicrobial prophylaxis depends on their clinical status. If signs or symptoms suggestive of sepsis are present, then a full diagnostic evaluation is performed and empiric antibiotic therapy is started. If the neonate is asymptomatic at birth but is less than 35 weeks of gestation, or if the infant is ≥35 weeks of gestation but intrapartum antibiotic prophylaxis was given 4 hours or less before delivery, then a complete blood count and differential and a blood culture should be done and the infant should be observed for at least 48 hours. If sepsis subsequently is suspected, then a full diagnostic workup and empiric therapy are initiated. No evaluation or therapy is needed for asymptomatic neonates born at ≥35 weeks of gestation and whose mothers had received intrapartum antibiotic prophylaxis more than 4 hours before delivery, but the infant should be observed for at least 48 hours for signs or symptoms suggestive of sepsis (168). The timing of intrapartum penicillin or ampicillin administration is important. In one study from Spain, the rate of GBS colonization of neonates born to carrier mothers was 46%, 29%, 2.9%, and 1.2% when ampicillin was given less than 1 hour, 1 to 2 hours, 2 to 4 hours, and more than 4 hours before delivery, respectively (333).

Immunologic approaches to prevention include passive or active immunization of mothers, with transplacental passage of protective antibodies to the fetus. Immunoprophylaxis is not a clinically available option at the present time.

MENINGITIS

Bacterial Meningitis

The incidence of bacterial meningitis is 0.4 per 1,000 live births, but rates as high as 1 per 1,000 live births have been reported in a few nurseries (165). The disease is seen more commonly in premature infants, male infants, and infants born to mothers with complicated pregnancies or deliveries.

Etiology

The bacteria causing neonatal meningitis are similar to those causing sepsis neonatorum. Group B β-hemolytic streptococci and E. coli presently account for approximately 75% of all cases. The next most common etiologic agent is L. monocytogenes (334).

Pathology

The pathologic findings in cases of neonatal meningitis are similar, regardless of the bacterial agent. The most consistent finding at necropsy is a purulent exudate coating the meninges and ependymal surfaces of the ventricles (335). Perivascular inflammation is observed. The inflammatory response of neonates is similar to that in adults with meningitis, with the exception that babies show a relative sparsity of plasma cells and lymphocytes during the subacute stage of meningeal reactions. Hydrocephalus and a noninfectious encephalopathy can be demonstrated in approximately 50% of infants dying of meningitis. Subdural effusions occur rarely in neonates. Various degrees of phlebitis and arteritis of intracranial vessels can be found in all infants. Thrombophlebitis with occlusions of veins may occur in the subependymal zone. Ventriculitis can be demonstrated in virtually all infants dying of meningitis and in approximately 75% of infants at the time of diagnosis.

Clinical Manifestations

The signs and symptoms of central nervous system infection frequently are indistinguishable from those associated with neonatal septicemia. Lethargy, feeding problems, and altered temperature are the most frequent presenting complaints, and respiratory distress, vomiting, diarrhea, and abdominal distention are common findings. Seizures are observed frequently and may be caused by direct central nervous system inflammation or may be associated with hypoglycemia or hypocalcemia. Signs suggesting meningeal involvement, such as a bulging anterior fontanelle, neck stiffness, or opisthotonus, are infrequent.

Pathogenesis

Most cases of meningitis result from bacteremia; spread from a contiguous infected focus is rare. Although there are more than 100 K types of E. coli, the K1 type accounts for more than 70% of E. coli meningitis cases (138). Most pathogenic E. coli carry both the capsular antigen K1 and S fimbria adhesins; the latter promote adherence of E. coli to epithelial cells in the choroid plexus and brain ventricles, and to vascular endothelial cells (336). The extracellular polysaccharide capsule allows the organism to avoid host clearance mechanisms. The outer membrane lipopolysaccharide (i.e., endotoxin) is released from dying bacteria and initiates an intense inflammatory reaction. Endotoxin stimulates the production of tumor necrosis factor, interleukin-1β (IL-1β), and other mediators by monocyte-macrophage cells. Tumor necrosis factor and IL-1β induce phospholipase A_2 activity, production of other mediators, and receptor–ligand interactions between leukocytes and endothelia. Phospholipase A_2 then acts on membrane phospholipids to produce a variety of lipid proinflammatory substances such as platelet-activating factor, leukotrienes, prostaglandins, and thromboxanes. The inflammatory changes result in vascular injury and alterations in the permeability of the blood–brain barrier, with resultant vasogenic edema. The cytokines activate adhesion-promoting receptors on cerebral vascular endothelial cells, which leads to recruitment of leukocytes to sites of stimulation. These polymorphonuclear leukocytes subsequently enter the subarachnoid space, release toxic substances, and cause cytotoxic edema (337). The net pathophysiologic effect is the development of increased intracranial pressure and severe brain edema. Cerebral edema, increased intracranial pressure, systemic hypotension, decreased cerebral perfusion pressure, and a variety of vascular changes result in global or regional reductions of cerebral blood flow and can lead to brain ischemia (338). The pathophysiologic aberrations ultimately cause focal or diffuse neuronal injury, which may be irreversible.

Among the five GBS serotypes, the BIII organisms account for more than 80% of cases of neonatal GBS meningitis. The presence of type-specific antibodies enhances opsonization of the organism in the presence of complement. Cell wall components of the organism can stimulate the inflammatory cascade in a manner similar to that described for endotoxins.

Laboratory Findings

Interpretation of CSF values in newborn infants may be difficult (Table 48–5). The upper limits of "normal" for infants with birth weights of 1,500 g or less are even higher than those for term newborns (339–341).

TABLE 48–5. *Cerebrospinal fluid values of noninfected term newborns*

CSF parameter	Age (d)	Mean	SD	Median	Range
WBC count/mm^3	0–7	15.3	30.3	6	1–130
	8–14	5.4	4.4	6	0–18
	15–21	7.7	12.1	4	0–62
	22–30	4.8	3.4	4	0–18
ANC/mm^3	0–7	4.4	15.2	0	0–65
	8–14	0.1	0.3	0	0–1
	15–21	0.2	0.5	0	0–2
	22–30	0.1	0.2	0	0–1
Protein (mg/dL)	0–7	80.8	30.8	NA	NA
	8–14	69	22.6	NA	NA
	15–21	59.8	23.4	NA	NA
	22–30	54.1	16.2	NA	NA
Glucose (mg/dL)	0–7	45.9	7.5	NA	NA
	8–14	54.3	17	NA	NA
	15–21	46.8	8.8	NA	NA
	22–30	54.1	16.2	NA	NA

ANC, absolute neutrophil count; CSF, cerebrospinal fluid; NA, not available; SD, standard deviation; WBC, white blood cells.
Adapted from ref. 339.

It is important to examine carefully a stained smear of the CSF of every infant with suspected meningitis. In babies with meningitis caused by GBS or coliform bacteria, each oil-immersion field usually contains several to many bacteria. This is because there are 10^4 to 10^8 colony-forming units (CFU) per 1 mL of spinal fluid (average 10^7 CFU/mL) present at the time of diagnosis. *Listeria* organisms often are difficult to identify on stained smears because the bacterial counts frequently are on the order of 10^3 CFU/mL. Bacterial antigens can be detected by LPA for GBS, *E. coli* K1, *H. influenzae* type b, *S. pneumoniae,* and non-type B meningococci. Polymerase chain reaction assays for the detection of bacterial DNA in CSF specimens are being developed (342,343). Nonculture methods of diagnosis are most useful for newborns who receive antibiotics before a lumbar puncture is performed.

Blood and urine cultures should be obtained from every infant suspected of meningitis. As many as 15% of infants with positive CSF cultures have sterile blood cultures (285).

Treatment

Considerable data have been gathered on the pharmacokinetic properties of antibiotics in neonates with meningitis (344,345). After an intramuscular dose of 2.5 mg/kg of gentamicin, peak levels in lumbar CSF and ventricular fluid are approximately 1 to 2 µg/mL. If lumbar intrathecal gentamicin is added to this regimen, values of 20 to 40 µg/mL or greater several hours after instillation may be observed in the lumbar area. Intraventricular administration of 2.5 mg results in ventricular fluid levels of 20 to 80 µg/mL and in lumbar spinal fluid values of 10 to 50 µg/mL 1 to 4 hours later. With kanamycin, peak CSF values of 6 to 10 µg/mL are observed 4 to 6 hours after an intramuscular dose of 7.5 mg/kg. Peak values of 10 to 30 µg/mL are demonstrated in CSF approximately 2 to 4 hours after a 50 to 70 mg/kg dose of ampicillin.

For the aminoglycosides, the MIC values for the common pathogens frequently are greater than the antibiotic levels achieved in CSF. For example, an *E. coli* with a gentamicin MIC value of 2.5 or 5 µg/mL is considered susceptible when bloodstream infection is being treated but may be considered resistant when therapy is for meningitis. This is because peak cerebrospinal and ventricular fluid gentamicin levels after parenteral therapy usually are lower than this MIC value. Alternative therapeutic regimens must be considered, such as adding a second antibiotic, selecting a different antibiotic class, or changing the route of administration. In experimental models of *E. coli* meningitis, the administration of the total daily gentamicin dose undivided results in CSF concentrations of the drug that are threefold higher than those achieved in animals receiving conventional dosing, and the rate of bacterial killing is greater early on in animals receiving once-daily gentamicin (346).

Ampicillin and gentamicin or ampicillin and cefotaxime are recommended for initial empiric therapy of neonatal meningitis. The dosage of ampicillin or cefotaxime is 100 mg/kg/d in two divided doses during the first week of life and 200 mg/kg/d in three or four divided doses thereafter. The gentamicin dosage is the same as that used for septicemia. All infants should have repeat spinal fluid examinations and cultures at 48 hours after initiation of therapy. If organisms are seen on a Gram stain of the fluid, the patient should be reevaluated completely with regard to making alterations in antimicrobial therapy and to obtaining computed tomography of the head. The radiologic procedures may demonstrate the presence of a subdural empyema, brain abscess, or ventriculitis that requires neurosurgical intervention.

Cefotaxime, with or without an aminoglycoside, can be used for therapy of neonatal meningitis due to susceptible gram-negative enteric organisms (347). Although there are no large controlled trials of cefotaxime in neonates, accumulated experience from open studies indicates that this cephalosporin is effective for therapy of neonatal sepsis and meningitis.

The Neonatal Meningitis Cooperative Study group reported that there is no beneficial effect of lumbar intrathecal or intraventricular instillation of gentamicin in the therapy of meningitis caused by gram-negative organism (345). The mortality rate in infants given intraventricular gentamicin was threefold greater than that in infants treated with systemic therapy only. The mean and peak ventricular CSF concentrations of endotoxin and IL-1β were significantly higher for infants treated with intraventricular gentamicin than those receiving intravenous antibiotics alone (348). This difference may have resulted from the enhanced bacterial killing achieved through higher ventricular CSF gentamicin concentrations, with the consequent increased release of damaging inflammatory mediators, which resulted in greater periventricular inflammation.

Therapy for meningitis is continued for a minimum of 2 weeks after sterilization of CSF cultures. This equates to 14 days of therapy for meningitis caused by gram-positive organisms and a minimum of 21 days of therapy for meningitis caused by gram-negative pathogens.

Treatment for *Candida* meningitis is with amphotericin B and flucytosine for a period of 3 to 6 weeks (256). Fluconazole has been used to treat neonatal candidal meningitis, but the optimal dose is not known and the published experience is very limited (324). In an experimental model of *C. albicans* meningitis, amphotericin B was more effective than fluconazole in clearing the infection at the dosage levels that were used (349).

Attention to general supportive therapy is essential in caring for infants with meningitis and is the single most important factor that accounts for the improved outcome during recent years. Disturbances of fluid and electrolyte balance are common, particularly in the first several days of illness when inappropriate antidiuretic hormone secretion may lead to fluid retention and hyponatremia. Hypoglycemia, hypocalcemia, and hyperbilirubinemia are frequent complications. Ventilatory assistance frequently is necessary, and blood pressure should be monitored carefully. During the course of illness, hemoglobin and hematocrit values should be checked frequently because infection may exaggerate and prolong the anemias of infancy, particularly in premature infants. Because of the frequent occurrence of bleeding diathesis, platelet counts, prothrombin time, and partial thromboplastin time should be followed. Neurosurgical evaluation is needed for neonates with a brain abscess to determine the need for abscess decompression.

Prognosis

The mortality from neonatal meningitis is considerable. The overall mortality rate is approximately 10% to 30%, but this varies with etiologic agent, infant population, and the nursery or intensive care unit.

Short- and long-term sequelae of neonatal meningitis are frequent. The acute complications include communicating or noncommunicating hydrocephalus, subdural effusions, ventriculitis, and blindness (350). In 70% of infants with *Citrobacter koseri* (formerly *diversus*) meningitis, there is associated brain abscess (Fig. 48–2)

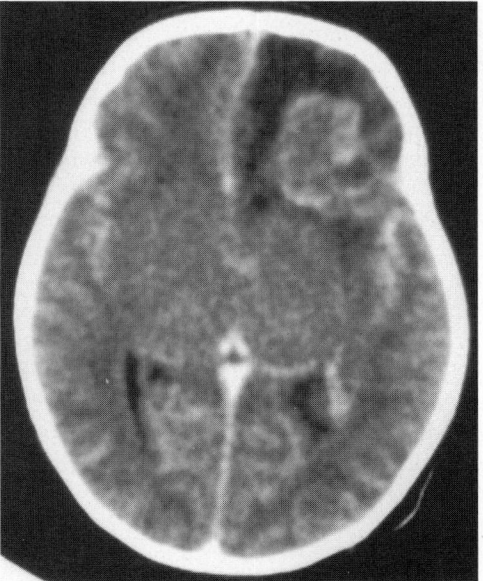

FIG. 48–2. Contrast-enhanced computed tomographic scan of the head of a 25-day-old African-American girl with *Citrobacter koseri* infection of the central nervous system. Note the cavitating enhancing lesion abutting the lateral ventricle on the left, with surrounding vasogenic edema.

(344,345,351,352). With computed tomographic scanning of the head, abnormalities can be identified in approximately 70% of neonates with coliform meningitis. Gross retardation may be obvious immediately, but many infants appear relatively normal at the time of discharge. It is only after prolonged and careful follow-up that perceptual difficulties, reading problems, or minimal brain damage is apparent. It is estimated that 30% to 50% of survivors have some evidence of neurologic damage (176,353–355). Recurrence of gram-negative bacillary meningitis may occur in as many as 10% of patients (350).

Aseptic Meningitis

Aseptic meningitis is an acute nonbacterial inflammatory disease of the meninges that is caused principally by viral agents. The illness occurs frequently in older infants and children and is uncommon in newborn infants. Disease in young infants is sporadic or occurs in sharply defined epidemics. It is important to differentiate aseptic from bacterial meningitis of infancy, because the therapy and prognosis are different in the two conditions.

It frequently is difficult to make a clinical distinction between aseptic meningitis and encephalitis in young infants. The cause of viral central nervous system disease depends, in part, on seasonal variation, age, and immune status of the host. In older infants and children, the enteroviruses (e.g., coxsackievirus B, echoviruses) account for most cases of aseptic meningitis during the summer months, and mumps, lymphocytic choriomeningitis, and other viruses are more common during the other seasons. During epidemics of encephalitis, such as those caused by St. Louis encephalitis virus, a mild aseptic meningitis may be seen in young infants and occasionally in neonates. The mild nature of the disease in early life may be due, in part, to passively transferred antibodies from immune mothers and the relatively isolated status of young infants during community outbreaks.

Certain viruses appear to cause significant disease in the very young, such as encephalomyocarditis caused by type B coxsackieviruses. In this disease, brain, myocardium, blood, kidney, and liver are involved. In one nursery outbreak, coxsackievirus type B5 caused aseptic meningitis only (356). Echovirus 2 has been etiologically associated with a nursery epidemic of aseptic meningitis, and sporadic cases have been caused by echoviruses 1, 2, 3, 5, 9, 11, 14, 16, 17, 18, 19, 24, 25, 30, 31, and 71 (357).

Encephalitis, with or without involvement of the meninges, may occur in young infants and is caused by the aforementioned viral agents and by other arboviruses, principally Eastern equine encephalomyelitis virus and Western equine encephalomyelitis virus. St. Louis encephalomyelitis is rare in newborn infants. Congenital cytomegalovirus, herpes simplex virus types 1 and 2, rubella, and varicella-zoster viruses produce encephalitis in some infants (discussed in Chap. 47).

Symptoms

Poor temperature control, lethargy, irritability, loose stools, vomiting, diminished appetite, and "failure to thrive" are the most common symptoms (358). In some infants, a shock-like syndrome occurs that is associated with seizures. It may be difficult to differentiate this clinical illness from that of bacterial meningitis. In a few patients, an erythematous maculopapular eruption, with or without petechiae, may suggest a viral cause.

Diagnosis

Aseptic meningitis should be suspected if several infants in a nursery develop illness over a short period or if illness is detected in an infant during a community outbreak of aseptic meningitis. Although the outbreak is caused by a single etiologic agent, the clinical manifestations may differ among infected infants. While one infant manifests respiratory symptoms primarily, another may have gastrointestinal illness, and all may have findings indicating involvement of the meninges. Aseptic meningitis is diagnosed in these infants by failure to demonstrate bacteria on stained smears and cultures of CSF. Whereas the CSF leukocyte count usually is lower than that observed in bacterial meningitis, high counts with predominance of polymorphonuclear cells may be observed early in aseptic meningitis. The CSF protein and sugar content usually are within normal limits. A definitive diagnosis is made by isolation of a viral agent from cultures of CSF or from the throat or rectum, accompanied by a significant rise in serum antibody titer to the specific agent. Polymerase chain reaction assays using primers complementary to highly conserved regions of the genome of enteroviruses can provide rapid and accurate diagnosis of enteroviral meningitis when CSF is tested (359).

With the exception of meningoencephalitis caused by herpes simplex, there is no specific antiviral therapy for postnatally acquired viral aseptic meningitis. Intensive supportive care frequently is necessary, with particular attention to maintenance of pH and electrolyte balance, respiratory assistance, and adequate nutrition. It is possible, although unproved, that intravenous immunoglobulins may be beneficial in some infants with persistent viral central nervous system disease, especially that caused by the enteroviruses. If an infant develops illness in a newborn nursery, every effort should be made to define the cause and source of infection. The affected infants should be isolated and treated as cohorts until discharge. Survivors may be at risk of developing neurologic sequelae, especially if they had seizures during their illness (360–362).

OSTEOMYELITIS AND SEPTIC ARTHRITIS

Because of the unique nature of the vascular supply of the neonatal skeletal system, osteomyelitis and septic arthritis frequently occur concomitantly. During the first 12 months of life, capillaries perforate the epiphyseal plate of long bones and provide a communication between the metaphysis and the joint space (363). Infections originating in one anatomic location easily spread to the other. This is not true after approximately 1 year of age, when the perforating capillaries disappear.

The capsules of the hip and shoulder attach below the metaphysis of the femur and humerus, respectively. Infection of the epiphyseal cartilage may rupture through the periosteum and enter the joint space, producing purulent arthritis. Because of the capsular articulation of the hip and shoulder, osteomyelitis and septic arthritis may coexist, making the origin of infection difficult to determine.

Infections of the musculoskeletal system are uncommon in the neonate, but incidence figures are not available.

Etiology and Pathogenesis

The infecting organisms in osteomyelitis and septic arthritis vary, but the predominant ones are GBS, *S. aureus,* and gram-negative enteric organisms such as *Klebsiella* spp, *Proteus* spp, and *E. coli.* Although gonococcal arthritis and tenosynovitis were encountered commonly in previous decades, they are seen only occasionally today. Other etiologic agents associated with newborn bone and joint infection are *Salmonella* spp, *Pseudomonas* spp, *H. influenzae, S. pneumoniae,* and *C. albicans* (364–367). Hospital-acquired MRSA osteomyelitis and septic arthritis can develop in sick premature infants after catheter-associated septicemia (368).

Osteomyelitis and arthritis have been reported after several invasive procedures in newborns, including heel puncture, femoral venipuncture, exchange transfusions, fetal monitoring electrode placement, and umbilical artery catheterization (208,364). Osteomyelitis of cranial bones has complicated infected cephalhematomas. In most cases, the origin is unknown and is presumed to be hematogenous.

Clinical Presentation

Nonspecific symptoms of infection, such as lethargy, irritability and poor feeding, may be the initial manifestations of neonatal musculoskeletal infection. Diminished movement of the affected limb, unrelated temporally to birth trauma, is a common clinical sign (369). Heat, ery-

thema, and swelling are late manifestations. The long bones are affected most commonly. Occasionally, the diagnosis is made unsuspectingly when purulent material is obtained on attempted aspiration of the femoral vein and the needle enters the swollen hip capsule. GBS osteomyelitis is indolent and usually involves a single bone, most commonly the proximal humerus, but can involve the vertebral spine as well (363,370).

Although blood cultures frequently are positive, the infants usually are not clinically toxic. The exception is group A β-hemolytic streptococcal infection, in which the infant may appear gravely ill.

Laboratory Tests and Findings

Blood cultures should be obtained from all infants with suspected infection of the musculoskeletal system. A diagnostic aspiration of the joint or subperiosteal space should be attempted in all patients, and the material obtained should be treated with Gram stain and cultured. Identification of the organism is particularly important, because it may be necessary to treat with more than one potentially nephrotoxic drug until the causative bacterium has been isolated.

The peripheral leukocyte count frequently is elevated, and juvenile forms may be seen. There is little information regarding the erythrocyte sedimentation rate during the neonatal period. In older infants and children, the sedimentation rate is accelerated in osteomyelitis; its return toward normal is a rough indicator of therapeutic success.

Radiographs of the affected bone or joint taken early in illness may be normal or show widening of the articular space. Later in the course of disease, subluxation and destruction of the joint are common. If osteomyelitis is present, the normal fat markings on roentgenograms of the deep tissues may be obliterated, indicating inflammation. Lifting of the periosteum from the bone may be observed, but cortical destruction is unusual before the second week of illness. A complete skeletal survey should be performed because of frequent involvement of multiple sites (369,371). Resolution of bone changes is considerably slower than clinical improvement. Although radioisotope scans (e.g., technetium, gallium) of bone are useful in early diagnosis of osteomyelitis in older infants and children, they may be normal in newborns with proven infection (364). Nevertheless, bone scintigraphy remains more sensitive than plain radiography for the early diagnosis of osteomyelitis (372).

Therapy

Selection of initial antimicrobial therapy should be based on results of the Gram stain of aspirated purulent material and associated clinical findings, such as furuncles or cellulitis. If gram-positive cocci are observed on stained smears, methicillin or nafcillin should be started. Vancomycin may be preferable in nurseries with multiresistant *S. aureus* strains. Cefotaxime or gentamicin is indicated if gram-negative organisms are observed. If no organisms are identified on stained smears, a combination of an antistaphylococcal drug and an aminoglycoside is used. After the organism has been identified and susceptibility studies are available, the most appropriate antibiotic or combination of antibiotics should be used. Direct instillation of an antimicrobial agent into the joint space is unnecessary because most antibiotics penetrate the inflamed synovium, and adequate concentrations are achieved in purulent material (373). This also applies to treatment of osteomyelitis; direct instillation of antibiotics into infected bone is unwarranted.

As a general rule, infection of the joint space and bone should be drained by repeated aspiration or by surgery. Suppurative arthritis of the hip and shoulder is best treated with incision and drainage to prevent vascular compromise or extension of infection into the metaphysis. Orthopedic consultation must be obtained for all patients.

Antimicrobial therapy of neonatal musculoskeletal infections caused by *S. aureus* or coliform organisms should be continued for approximately 3 weeks and, in some patients, for a longer period. For gonococcal or streptococcal infections, 10 days of therapy generally are sufficient with adequate surgical drainage. The duration of therapy must be individualized. In general, systemic symptoms disappear within several days of initiation of therapy and drainage, but local signs such as heat, erythema and swelling may persist for 4 to 7 days. Full range of motion of the involved limb may not return for several months, and physical therapy should be instituted early to prevent contractures. Complete resolution of roentgenographic changes may take several months. The use of large oral dosages of antibiotics for outpatient therapy of neonatal musculoskeletal infections has not been studied systematically and should be undertaken with caution (374).

Prognosis

Death from these diseases is unusual. However, morbidity may be considerable, particularly if weight-bearing joints such as the hip are involved. Bone deformations or shortening, contractures, or muscle damage can be permanent (364,375–377).

CUTANEOUS INFECTIONS

Most infections of the skin and subcutaneous tissues in neonates are caused by *S. aureus*. There are three major presentations of superficial staphylococcal disease. The first and most common are pustules and furuncles, which may be solitary or appear in clusters during the neonatal period. Pustules are frequently in the periumbilical and diaper areas, and they may coalesce gradually and spread to other areas of the body. Bloodstream or organ invasion is unusual unless the cutaneous infection involves extensive areas. Omphalitis usually is caused by staphylococci or streptococci, and infected circumcisions are usually caused by *S. aureus*.

The occurrence of staphylococcal skin infections in several infants from the same nursery should alert the physician to the possibility of nosocomial infection caused by a single, virulent strain of *S. aureus*. If infections are caused by the same strain of *Staphylococcus*, prompt measures should be instituted so that the source of infection can be determined and further colonization and disease can be prevented.

Therapy of cutaneous staphylococcal disease depends on the extent of the lesions and the general condition of the infant. Small, isolated pustules can be managed by local care with a mild cleansing agent or an antiseptic agent such as hexachlorophene or povidone-iodine. Infants with more extensive cutaneous involvement, systemic signs and symptoms of infection, or both should be treated with parenteral antimicrobial agents. The selection of the proper penicillin is based on historic experience and antimicrobial susceptibility studies of staphylococci isolated from the nursery unit.

The second form of neonatal staphylococcal disease has been described as the expanded scalded skin syndrome (45). This group of illnesses includes bullous impetigo, toxic epidermal necrolysis (i.e., Ritter disease), and nonstreptococcal scarlatina, usually caused by phage group II staphylococci. The pathogenesis of these entities appears to be related to release of exotoxins (i.e., epidermolytic toxins A and B) that act primarily on the stratum granulosa of the epidermis, causing a generalized erythema, edema, and tenderness, frequently progressing to desquamation and formation of flaccid bullae. The usual sites of staphylococcal infection are conjunctivae, throat, and umbilicus. Infants usually are afebrile. Cultures of blood, nasopharynx, eyes, and other areas should be obtained before therapy. Because phage group II staphylococci frequently are resistant to penicillin, methicillin is the initial drug of choice. Vancomycin should be used for multiresistant strains. *Pseudomonas putida* sepsis presenting as scalded skin syndrome has been described recently in a 9-day-old newborn (378).

The third form of staphylococcal disease is necrotizing fasciitis, which also can be caused by streptococci, *E. coli*, *Klebsiella*, and anaerobes (379–385). Necrotizing fasciitis, an unusual disease of newborns, is associated with surgical procedures, circumcision, birth trauma, or cutaneous infections. In this condition, subcutaneous tissues, including muscle layers, are invaded, and the organism spreads along the fascial planes. Overlying skin may appear violaceous, and the borders of the lesion usually are indistinct. Extensive surgery to resect the destroyed tissue is imperative in treating necrotizing fasciitis. Blood and tissue cultures should be obtained, and the patient started on methicillin or nafcillin and an aminoglycoside until culture results are available. If necrotizing fasciitis involves the abdomen or perineum, then either clindamycin or metronidazole should be added (384). The necrotic fatty tissue may combine with calcium, resulting in tetany and convulsions. Vigorous fluid resuscitation and correction of electrolyte imbalances are critical.

Breast abscesses most commonly are caused by *S. aureus*, but gram-negative enteric organisms can be causative (386). Anaerobes can be recovered from as many as 40% of samples, one-half of which are in mixed cultures with aerobic bacteria (387). Bacteremia is rare. The physician should attempt to establish an etiologic diagnosis by expressing fluid from the nipple after thorough cleaning or by needle aspiration of the abscess. Treatment is with methicillin, with or without an aminoglycoside, depending on the results of the Gram stain and culture, and it should be continued for 5 to 7 days. For mild infections, antibiotic therapy is adequate; with more severe inflammation, incision and drainage of the abscess are required. Long-term follow-up studies suggest that some girls will have diminished tissue in the affected breast.

Scalp abscesses occur most commonly as a complication of fetal monitoring in which scalp electrodes are used and may occur as localized manifestations of systemic disease (e.g., enterococcal sepsis) (233,388). Etiologic agents include staphylococci, enterococci, gram-negative enteric bacteria, and gonococci (233,388,389). Polymicrobial flora, including anaerobes, are commonly isolated. Treatment consists of incision and drainage. If there is an associated cellulitis, antibiotics are given and continued for 5 to 7 days.

Fungal infections of the neonatal skin can range from localized or widespread candidal dermatitis, to localized, discrete follicular pustules, plaques, or nodules caused by *Trichophyton tonsurans*, to rapidly progressive ulceration and necrosis requiring surgical debridement seen with mucormycosis (390–392). The characteristic pathology of mucormycosis is invasion of blood vessels by fungal hyphae resulting in ischemia and infarction of areas supplied by these vessels. Predisposing factors for serious cutaneous fungal disease includes prematurity, disruption of the barrier function of newborn skin associated with adhesive removal, multiple antibiotic treatment courses, and postnatal steroid therapy (390,393). In one study, wooden tongue depressors used to make splints were identified as the source of *Rhizopus microsporus* invasive infection in premature infants (390). The choice of antifungal agent for therapy depends on the specific infection being treated: griseofulvin for superficial dermatophyte infections, topical nystatin for mild-to-moderate candidal dermatitis, fluconazole or amphotericin B for extensive candidal dermatitis, and amphotericin B for mucormycosis.

URINARY TRACT INFECTION

Improved methods for obtaining sterile specimens have made it possible for investigators to define more accurately the incidence of neonatal urinary tract infection. Bacteriuria may be demonstrated in 0.5% to 1.0% of full-term infants and as many as 3% of premature infants in studies using the bladder aspiration technique (394). Urinary tract infections are more common in babies born to bacteriuric mothers and in male neonates, in contrast to the predominance of female infants beyond this period of life.

Etiology

E. coli is the most common etiologic agent of urinary tract infection, as found in older patients. Approximately 50% of causative *E. coli* strains belong to one of eight common O antigen groups. Several polysaccharide capsular antigens (e.g., K1, K2, K12, K13) are found more often in infants with upper tract disease. This particularly pertains to the K1 antigen (395). Fimbriated *E. coli* can attach to specific receptors on uroepithelial cells. Glycolipids of the P blood group constitute a specific receptor that is believed to be associated with pyelonephritis in patients who do not have reflux. *Klebsiella* and *Pseudomonas* species are encountered less frequently. Gram-positive bacteria, with the exception of enterococci, are rare causes of urinary tract infections. Fungal cystitis and pyelonephritis are encountered in chronically ill premature infants previously treated with multiple broad-spectrum antibiotics and are associated with mucocutaneous candidiasis or invasive disease (254,396).

Clinical Manifestations

Many infants with significant bacteriuria are asymptomatic (397). If clinical signs are present, they usually are nonspecific and consist of poor weight gain, altered temperature, cyanosis or gray skin color, abdominal distention, malodorous urine, and poor feeding. In a few patients, jaundice and hepatomegaly may be the presenting features of urinary tract infection (398,399). Thrombocytopenic purpura is found in some of these infants. Localizing signs suggesting urinary tract involvement are unusual; they usually consist of a weak urinary stream or an abdominal tumor from bladder distention or hydronephrosis (399). Gross hematuria has been described as the only presenting symptom, but this is rare (400). The most important predisposing factor is vesicoureteral reflux, which allows easy access for bacteria to ascend to the kidneys and leads to residual urine in the bladder (399,401). Circumcised infants have a lower risk of acquiring a urinary tract infection compared with those who are uncircumcised (402).

Diagnosis

The diagnosis of urinary tract infection is confirmed by examination and culture of urine. The result of these tests depends largely on the method of urine collection. Most pediatricians obtain urine with a sterile, plastic receptacle applied to the cleansed perineum. However, urine obtained by this method may have an elevated cell count because of recent circumcision, vaginal reflux of urine, or contamination from the perineum. Neonatal asphyxia may increase the urinary cell count. Leukocytes must be differentiated from round epithelial cells that appear in the urine in appreciable numbers during the early days of life. Although pyuria commonly accompanies significant bacteriuria, cells can be few or absent in the presence of bacteriuria in as many as one-half of the patients (403). Direct microscopic examination of uncentrifuged, fresh urine is useful. If bacteria are seen readily in each oil-immersion field, there are generally more than 10^5 CFU/mL. Glitter cells are believed by many to be diagnostic of urinary tract infections.

Quantitative urine cultures from infants with documented disease contain more than 50,000 CFU/mL (usually ≥100,000 CFU/mL), but a smaller number of organisms can be found in as many as 20% of patients (404). Any number of bacteria in a urine specimen obtained by percutaneous needle puncture of the bladder should be considered significant. This latter procedure is the single best source of urine for culture and is safe in most newborn infants. Its primary complication is transient gross hematuria lasting less than 24 hours in 0.6% of patients (399,405). Very rare complications of suprapubic bladder aspirations include bowel perforation, peritonitis, hematoma, abdominal wall abscess, and bacteremia (405).

Treatment

There are several approaches to the treatment of neonatal urinary tract infections. Antimicrobial agents initially should be administered parenterally, because septicemia is found in 15% to 30% of infants, and absorption after oral administration may be erratic in neonates (406). The physician should assume that there is infection of renal parenchyma resulting from hematogenous spread.

Antibiotic selection should be based on results of antimicrobial susceptibility studies. Gentamicin is effective against the commonly encountered coliform bacteria. Because urinary concentrations of these drugs are considerably higher than those seen in serum, the usual dosages may be halved. For gentamicin, 2 to 3 mg/kg/d is satisfactory, provided the initial blood cultures are sterile. Ampicillin and gentamicin should be administered to symptomatic infants with pyuria before results of culture and susceptibility tests. Renal candidiasis should be

treated systemically with amphotericin B. Bladder irrigation with amphotericin B for infants with uncomplicated *Candida* cystitis has not been properly evaluated, and its use cannot be recommended (407).

A repeat urine culture should be sterile 36 to 48 hours after initiation of appropriate therapy. Infants with persistent bacteriuria must be evaluated for possible abscess formation, with or without urinary obstruction. In the uncomplicated patient, therapy usually is continued for a period of approximately 10 days. Blood urea nitrogen and serum creatinine levels should be determined at the initiation of therapy. If there is evidence of renal compromise, dosage and frequency of administration of the drugs, particularly the aminoglycosides, may need to be reduced. Approximately 1 week after therapy is discontinued, a repeat urine culture is obtained. If the culture is positive, therapy is reinstituted and a thorough investigation of the urinary tract is made to rule out obstruction or abscess formation.

All infants with documented urinary tract infections should have radiologic evaluation of the urinary tract. A renal scan or ultrasound examination is obtained some time during therapy so that the possibility of gross congenital abnormalities of the urinary system can be excluded. Technetium 99m dimercaptosuccinic acid cortical scintigraphy is more sensitive than ultrasound examinations and is abnormal in as many as 73% of infants with pyelonephritis (Fig. 48–3) (408). If obstruction is

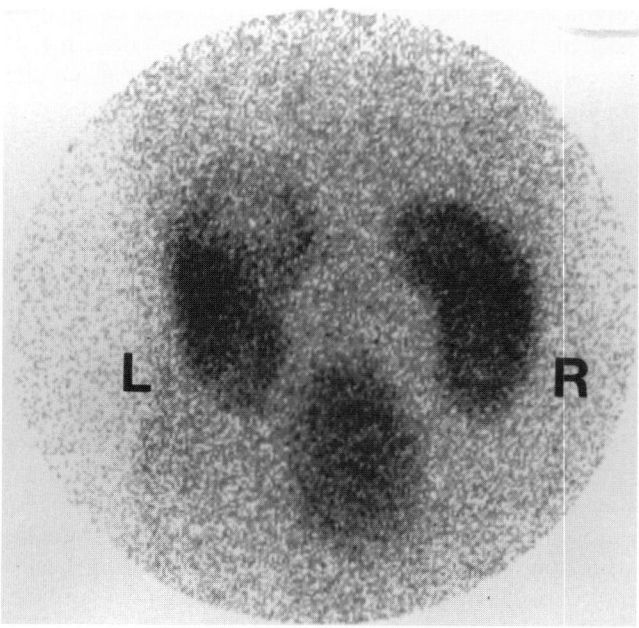

FIG. 48–3. Technetium 99m dimercaptosuccinic acid (DMSA) cortical scintigraphy study done on an 11-day-old Caucasian boy with ampicillin-resistant *Escherichia coli* pyelonephritis. This posterior image of the renal beds shows that the left kidney is larger than the right and has a large cold defect involving its superior half.

demonstrated, urologic procedures to ensure proper drainage are mandatory if therapy is to be successful. A voiding cystourethrogram usually is obtained several weeks after therapy has been completed. Radiologic abnormalities, such as vesicoureteral reflux, obstructive uropathy, and renal scars, are found in approximately 45% of infants, especially in girls (399,406,409).

Prognosis

It is the physician's responsibility to be certain that neonates with documented urinary tract infections do not have congenital abnormalities of the urinary system. In such patients, recurrent urinary tract infections are common, and physical growth may be retarded until definitive surgery for stage IV or V vesicoureteral reflux has been performed (410). Renal growth retardation is common after neonatal urinary tract infections, even in patients without reflux (411). Patients with recurrent urinary tract infections may be at increased risk of hypertension or renal insufficiency, but the magnitude of this threat is poorly defined (412). Every patient must have careful long-term follow-up studies to detect recurrent infections, many of which are asymptomatic. Prophylactic antibiotics such as trimethoprim-sulfamethoxazole or nitrofurantoin should be provided for infants with clinically significant reflux to avoid new scar formation and to ensure normal renal growth. Siblings of infants with urinary tract infection and vesicoureteral reflux should be screened with a voiding cystourethrogram because their risk of having vesicoureteral reflux is 27% to 45% (413).

NEONATAL OPHTHALMIA

Infections of the eye of the newborn may be caused by a variety of microorganisms, including *N. gonorrhoeae, C. trachomatis, S. aureus,* and *P. aeruginosa.* From a review of 302 cases of eye infections diagnosed in newborns at Grady Memorial Hospital in Atlanta, Georgia, between 1967 and 1973 it was determined that 29% were caused by chlamydiae, 14% by gonococci, 10% by staphylococci, 2% by chemical reactions, and 1% by mixed gonococcal and chlamydial infections (414). The causes of the remaining 44% were uncertain. This frequency distribution of etiologic agents was typical of the experience at large urban general hospitals.

The incidence of ophthalmia neonatorum has not paralleled the significant increase in gonococcal disease rates among adolescents and young adults (415). This almost certainly is a result of universal neonatal gonococcal prophylaxis. The invasive, destructive ophthalmitis described so vividly in old literature rarely is seen today. Several agents have been effective prophylactically against gonococci: 1% silver nitrate, erythromycin or tetracycline ophthalmic ointments, one dose of ceftriax-

one administered intramuscularly, and 2.5% solution of povidone-iodine (416–418).

Clinical Manifestations

Gonococcal ophthalmia usually becomes apparent within the first 5 days of life and initially is characterized by a clear, watery discharge. Conjunctival hyperemia and chemosis are associated with a copious discharge of thick, white, purulent material. Both eyes usually are involved but not necessarily to the same degree. Untreated gonococcal ophthalmia may extend to involve the cornea (i.e., keratitis) and the anterior chamber of the eye. Corneal perforation and blindness may occur. Before the introduction of adequate prophylactic measures, ophthalmia neonatorum was the most frequent cause of acquired blindness in the United States.

Differential Diagnosis

Any infant presenting with a conjunctival discharge should be evaluated carefully to determine the cause. Three tests should be performed:

1. Gram stain of the exudate
2. Culture of the exudate
3. Direct immunofluorescent chlamydial stain of scrapings made from the lower palpebral conjunctiva after exudate has been wiped away (419).

Appropriate therapy should be instituted on the basis of the results of the stained smears.

Conjunctivitis occurring in the first days of life can be chemical or bacterial. Chemical irritants, such as silver nitrate, cause transient conjunctival hyperemia and a watery discharge that rarely turns purulent.

If gram-negative rods are seen in the stained exudate, the greatest concern is *P. aeruginosa* because of the virulent, necrotizing endophthalmitis that can result. In this condition, a relatively mild conjunctivitis can progress to infection of the entire globe within 12 to 24 hours. Systemic complications such as bacteremia, meningitis, and brain abscess can occur without evidence of invasive eye disease, especially in very-low-birth-weight infants (420). Prompt diagnosis and immediate institution of appropriate antimicrobial therapy are mandatory (421). A blood culture should be obtained before antibiotics are started (420).

Conjunctivitis during the second or third week of life may be caused by viral, bacterial, or chlamydial agents. Viral conjunctivitis frequently is associated with other symptoms of respiratory tract disease, such as rhinorrhea, cough, and rash. Several persons in the family or nursery simultaneously may have the disease. The discharge in viral conjunctivitis is watery or mucopurulent but rarely purulent. Preauricular adenopathy is common. Staphylococci, streptococci, *H. influenzae, Moraxella catarrhalis,* and occasionally gonococci cause conjunctivitis in this age group. A smear of purulent material offers some help in differentiating between these bacterial agents. However, the presence of bacteria on a gram-stained smear of exudate is not necessarily related etiologically to the conjunctivitis. Normal inhabitants of the skin and mucous membranes, such as *Staphylococcus*, diphtheroids, and *Neisseria* species may be observed.

Chlamydial eye infection may begin in the first days of life, but it usually does not come to the attention of the physician until the second or third week (422). Clinical manifestations of chlamydial infection vary from mild conjunctivitis to intense inflammation and swelling of the lids, associated with copious purulent discharge. Pseudomembrane formation and a diffuse injection of the tarsal conjunctiva are common. The cornea rarely is affected, and preauricular adenopathy is unusual. In the early stages of disease, one eye may appear more swollen and inflamed than the other, but both eyes usually are involved. The physician establishes the diagnosis by scraping the tarsal conjunctiva and looking for typical cytoplasmic inclusions within epithelial cells or by direct immunofluorescent staining for chlamydial antigens. The scrapings also can be cultured or tested for chlamydial antigens by enzyme immunoassays. Polymerase chain reaction assays for the detection of *C. trachomatis* in ocular and nasopharyngeal specimens appear to be equally specific and more sensitive than culture methods, but the tests are not yet approved by the Food and Drug Administration for diagnosis of chlamydial conjunctivitis (423,424). There is no information on the use of the ligase chain reaction for the diagnosis of chlamydial conjunctivitis.

Therapy

Initial therapy is based on the results of stained smears of exudate and epithelial cells. If gonococci are seen, a single dose of ceftriaxone (25 to 50 mg/kg, maximum 125 mg) is given intramuscularly or intravenously (425). If staphylococci are seen, methicillin or another penicillinase-resistant penicillin analog is used. Topical antibiotics are unnecessary, because ample antibiotic to inhibit bacteria exists in the eye secretions (425).

Pseudomonas eye infection should always be treated with parenteral therapy consisting of ceftazidime or ticarcillin and gentamicin. Gentamicin ophthalmic drops are used for simple *Pseudomonas* conjunctivitis, and subconjunctival or sub-Tenon space injections of gentamicin may be needed for endophthalmitis (426).

Ophthalmic solutions containing 1% tetracycline, erythromycin, or sulfacetamide are inferior to oral erythromycin in the treatment of chlamydial conjunctivitis. Topical therapy suppresses chlamydial growth, whereas oral erythromycin eradicates the organism from the eyes and nasopharynx in most infants (427). Erythromycin is used at a dose of 50 mg/kg/d orally divided into four doses daily for 10 to 14 days. Erythromycin therapy is associated with a 20% to 30% failure rate, which may require second and third courses of therapy. A shorter course of the new azalide antibiotic, azithromycin, may be effective in the treatment of neonatal conjunctivitis, but the optimal dosage and duration of therapy have yet to be determined (428).

Patients with gonococcal ophthalmia should be segregated, and strict hand-washing techniques should be used because of the highly contagious nature of the exudate. The eyes should be irrigated with saline to remove the purulent material. Follow-up examination of infants treated for gonococcal ophthalmia is important to treat subsequent *C. trachomatis* ophthalmia, which can manifest after completion of therapy for gonococcal infection.

DIARRHEAL DISEASE

Although diarrheal disease during the neonatal period usually is brief and self-limited, it can cause significant morbidity in some infants and represents a potential danger to other infants in the nursery unit.

Etiology and Pathogenesis

The most common cause of diarrhea in young infants is alteration of diet and feeding practices, rather than specific bacterial or viral pathogens. Of the infectious causes of diarrhea, rotaviruses are important agents. Both sporadic infections and nursery epidemics have been described. Rotavirus is stable on environmental surfaces and is difficult to eradicate using the usual disinfectants. As a result, it can remain endemic in a nursery for as long as 2 years once established (429). One study from France indicated that 32% of neonates shed rotavirus in their stools; however, of the neonates shedding the virus, 71% had no associated diarrhea (430). Reasons for the asymptomatic nature of most neonatal rotavirus infections are not clear but may include passive protection from transplacentally acquired maternal rotavirus antibodies, the presence of rotavirus antibodies and trypsin inhibitors in breast milk, immaturity of the pancreatic enzymes which may not allow the VP4 protein of the virus to be cleaved (an important step that allows the virus to infect intestinal epithelial cells), and the possibility that rotaviruses that circulate in nurseries may represent attenuated strains of the virus (429). However, neonatal rotavirus diarrhea can be severe and associated with dehydration, hypocalcemia, seizures, and increased frequencies of apnea and bradycardia episodes. It also has been associated with the development of necrotizing enterocolitis (429,431,432). The finding of rotavirus in the stools of a neonate with diarrhea may be coincidental and not represent the true etiologic agent.

Diarrhea caused by *E. coli* can be mediated through several mechanisms. Some strains are enterotoxigenic (elaborate heat-labile and/or heat-stable toxins), whereas others are enteropathogenic (cause effacement of microvilli and show intimate adherence between the bacterium and the epithelial cell membrane in localized areas), enterohemorrhagic (produce Shiga-like toxin), enteroaggregative (adhere diffusely to intestinal epithelial cells), or enteroinvasive (invade the colonic epithelium and cause ulceration). Enteropathogenic *E. coli* serotypes once were considered the most common bacterial agents responsible for diarrhea in young infants (433). Enterotoxigenic strains of *E. coli* have been identified in nursery outbreaks of diarrheal disease (434). These organisms inhabit the small bowel, where they attach to, but do not invade, the intestinal mucosa. The enterotoxin produced by these organisms stimulates cyclic adenosine monophosphate, which inhibits sodium and chloride transport across the intestinal wall. These salts are lost into the lumen of the upper bowel, followed passively by water, causing a net loss of stools high in electrolyte content. *Vibrio cholerae, Vibrio parahaemolyticus, Aeromonas,* and some strains of *Campylobacter* and *Yersinia* are examples of other bacteria that cause diarrhea by this mechanism.

Toxigenic and nontoxigenic *Clostridium difficile* strains commonly are recovered from stool cultures of newborn infants (435). Their significance, however, is unknown because most culture-positive or toxin-positive infants are asymptomatic.

Shigella causes diarrhea through invasion of the intestinal mucosa. Colonic invasion, with subsequent destruction of the mucosa, causes an outpouring of polymorphonuclear cells and mucus. The resultant diarrhea usually is bloody and contains mucus and pus (436). Other organisms causing bloody diarrhea are *Campylobacter, Yersinia,* and *Aeromonas* species (437–440). *Salmonella* species also invade the intestinal mucosa, but extensive destruction does not occur. The epithelial lining is left intact and the organisms reach the lamina propria, where an inflammatory response is elicited.

Epidemiologic Control

Serotyping of *E. coli* for identification of the traditional enteropathogenic strains no longer is practiced in most hospitals. After an index case of enteropathogenic *E. coli* diarrhea is recognized in a nursery, secondary cases are likely to ensue. This applies to the other etiologic agents of diarrhea in neonates. Any nursery infant with diarrhea should be suspected of having a potentially communicable disease. Ill and healthy colonized infants should be segregated. Infants with diarrhea caused by noninvasive strains of *E. coli* can be treated with nonabsorbable drugs such as oral neomycin (100 mg/kg/d in four divided doses) or colistin sulfate (15 mg/kg/d in

three divided doses) for 5 days. Neomycin causes rapid disappearance of the organism and abbreviates the period of diarrhea, but approximately 20% of infants revert to the asymptomatic carrier state after treatment (441). Repeated surveillance of infants is necessary until the pathogenic strain has been eliminated from the nursery.

Clinical Manifestations

The cause of diarrhea cannot be differentiated on clinical grounds in newborn infants. Diarrhea caused by enteropathogenic strains of *E. coli* is insidious in onset, is associated with seven to ten green, watery stools daily, and usually is without blood or mucus. The infants do not appear acutely ill. Complications are rare and are related primarily to dehydration and electrolyte disturbances. *Shigella* infection is uncommon, usually episodic in neonates, and does not spread within nurseries. Shigellosis in the newborn may present as a diarrheic or dysenteric syndrome or may be evidenced only by a septic or toxic infant (436). Suppurative complications are rare, but dehydration and electrolyte disturbances are common and need immediate and constant attention. *Campylobacter* species can cause bloody diarrhea in otherwise asymptomatic infants (442). Enteritis is the most common manifestation of neonatal *Campylobacter* infection, but more serious disease such as sepsis or meningitis can occur, albeit infrequently (443,444).

Rotavirus infection may be asymptomatic or associated with vomiting and diarrhea. The infants usually are afebrile, but temperature elevation as high as 39°C can occur. Most patients vomit, and the diarrhea is characterized by watery stools containing mucus and no blood. Moderate or severe dehydration may occur, which results in significant electrolyte disturbance in some infants. Fatal disease has been described in a small number of infants. In one report, an outbreak of necrotizing enterocolitis was associated with rotavirus infection (445).

Other viruses can cause neonatal diarrhea. These include enteric adenoviruses, enteroviruses, small round viruses, and coronavirus. The clinical symptoms associated with enteroviruses can vary from a self-limited gastrointestinal illness to more severe systemic manifestations such as fever, rash, aseptic meningitis, apnea, or myocarditis (444).

Therapy

The most important aspect of therapy for diarrheal disease of newborn infants is maintenance of hydration and electrolyte balance. Parenteral solutions containing appropriate electrolytes should be administered during the time of active diarrhea, and the infant should be examined and weighed frequently so that proper rehydration and prevention of complications are ensured. Estimation of fluid loss from diarrhea and vomiting should be recorded carefully and used as a basis for replacement therapy.

Selection of appropriate antimicrobial therapy depends, in part, on the mechanism of diarrhea. An absorbable antibiotic, such as ampicillin or trimethoprim-sulfamethoxazole, is indicated for disease caused by invasive bacteria (i.e., shigellosis), but orally administered nonabsorbable drugs, such as neomycin or colistin sulfate, are used for noninvasive organisms that produce enterotoxin (e.g., strains of *E. coli*).

Antimicrobial therapy for *Salmonella* gastroenteritis is controversial. Antibiotics do not alter the course of illness and usually prolong intestinal carriage of the organism. Clinical relapse is more common in antibiotic-treated infants. We do not recommend antibiotic therapy for uncomplicated *Salmonella* gastroenteritis if it occurs in older infants and children. Therapy probably is indicated for those with prolonged illness or evidence of colitis, for all neonates, and for infants with systemic symptoms suggesting bloodstream invasion. Ampicillin or amoxicillin usually is satisfactory, as are trimethoprim-sulfamethoxazole, cefotaxime, and ceftriaxone.

Ampicillin was formerly the antibiotic of choice for shigellosis, but significant resistance to this agent has been observed in many areas of the country in recent years. Most strains are susceptible *in vitro* to trimethoprim-sulfamethoxazole, and infants respond clinically and bacteriologically to a regimen of 10 mg of trimethoprim with 50 mg/kg/d sulfamethoxazole in two divided doses given for 5 days. However, we have limited experience with this agent in newborn infants, and the drug should not be used in those with jaundice. For multiresistant *Shigella* strains, ceftriaxone or cefixime may be effective. Erythromycin is the preferred drug for the treatment of symptomatic *Campylobacter* infections.

Any infant with diarrhea must be isolated from other babies in the nursery. Surveillance of all infants in contact with the index case and adoption of strict infection control measures are mandatory.

A live, attenuated, orally administered, tetravalent rhesus reassortment rotavirus vaccine was approved in 1998 for infant immunizations. Three doses are given at 2, 4, and 6 months of age. The vaccine is about 80% effective in the prevention of severe rotavirus disease. Although the data are limited, premature infants may receive the first dose of this vaccine at or after discharge from the hospital nursery if they have achieved a chronologic age of at least 6 weeks (446).

LOWER RESPIRATORY TRACT INFECTION

Lower respiratory tract infection is an important cause of morbidity in the neonate and is demonstrable on postmortem examination in approximately 20% of neonatal deaths.

Pneumonias can be divided into three categories on the basis of route of acquisition and age at presentation. The first is transplacental pneumonitis, which is acquired *in utero* and presents clinically in the early hours of life. Pneumonia may be part of a generalized congenital infection caused by cytomegalovirus, herpesvirus, rubella virus, *Toxoplasma gondii*, or *L. monocytogenes*. *Treponema pallidum* produces a severe, usually fatal pneumonitis (i.e., pneumonia alba), and genital mycoplasmas can cause congenital pneumonia. These infants usually have many organ systems involved, and the pneumonitis may be obscured. Clinical findings may include hepatosplenomegaly, cutaneous manifestations such as rash or petechiae, neurologic abnormalities, and teratogenic effects.

The second category, aspiration pneumonia, is acquired in the immediate perinatal period, and onset of illness occurs within the first hours to days of life. Pathogenesis is by aspiration of amniotic fluid or material from the maternal cervix during the period immediately before or during delivery. Most infants with roentgenographic evidence of aspiration have not swallowed infected material and do not require antimicrobial therapy. This is also true of meconium aspiration, in which the pneumonitis is chemical. The bacterial pathogens most commonly encountered are the group B β-hemolytic streptococci and coliform organisms. Infants with these infections may present in the first 12 hours of life with acute respiratory distress, with or without shock. Mortality is considerable in this condition, even if appropriate antimicrobial therapy is instituted early.

The third category consists of pneumonias acquired during delivery or in the postpartum period, usually beyond the first week of life. Acquired pneumonitis may be caused by viral, chlamydial, or bacterial agents and most frequently is bronchopneumonic or interstitial. RSV is the most important pathogen causing lower respiratory tract disease in young infants (447). The parainfluenza viruses, enteroviruses, rhinoviruses, and adenoviruses cause bronchiolitis and pneumonia during early infancy. Herpes simplex virus infection can be acquired at the time of delivery and present in the first week of life. Bronchiolitis, pneumonia, or both usually occur in epidemics among premature and full-term nursery infants or in the community.

Documented nursery outbreaks of lower respiratory tract disease have been associated with RSV, adenovirus, echovirus type 22, influenza A and B viruses, and parainfluenza virus infections. During these outbreaks, many infants are colonized with the epidemic virus strains, but only a few manifest clinical disease.

S. aureus and coliform organisms are the most common bacterial pathogens causing postnatally acquired pneumonia. Disease caused by *S. aureus* and *K. pneumoniae* may occur sporadically or in epidemic fashion during the neonatal period. Pyogenic complications, such as septicemia, osteomyelitis, and meningitis, frequently are associated with the epidemic form of these infections.

Acquisition of *C. trachomatis* in the intrapartum period may result in conjunctivitis (i.e., inclusion blennorrhea) or in pneumonia that usually presents between the fourth and twelfth weeks of life. The pneumonia is associated with a staccato cough, often terminating in vomiting or cyanosis, and with tachypnea; the infants usually are afebrile (448). Rales are heard, and there may be a history of the infant having conjunctivitis in the newborn period. Eosinophilia is seen in approximately half the patients. Chlamydial pneumonia occasionally can occur in the early neonatal period (first 2 weeks of life) (449,450). *C. trachomatis* can cause severe and chronic pneumonia in low-birth-weight infants (451,452). *C. trachomatis* pneumonia in otherwise healthy infants has been associated with long-term pulmonary function abnormalities (453).

A considerable body of data indicates that *U. urealyticum* colonization of low-birth-weight infants is associated with the subsequent development of chronic lung disease (454–458). *Ureaplasma*-positive infants have much higher ratios of IL-1β to IL-6 and tumor necrosis factor to IL-6 in their tracheal aspirates than do *Ureaplasma*-negative infants (459). Thus, in the preterm lung, *U. urealyticum* may contribute to early injury by inducing the release of inflammatory cytokines. *Pneumocystis carinii* is an uncommon cause of pneumonia in the neonatal period; susceptible infants include malnourished premature newborns living in endemic geographic areas, infants with congenital immunodeficiencies (e.g., severe combined immunodeficiency), and neonates infected with the human immunodeficiency virus type 1 (460–462). *Legionella* pneumonia is uncommon but has been described in newborns, most of whom had underlying problems such as prematurity, chronic lung disease, congenital heart disease, steroid treatment, or hypoxic–ischemic encephalopathy. *Legionella* can cause a range of respiratory symptoms from a mild influenza-like illness to severe cavitary pneumonia and death (463,464). *Bordetella pertussis* infection continues to occur and should be suspected in newborns with paroxysmal cough and a parent or sibling with a persistent cough.

Clinical Manifestations

The early signs of lower respiratory tract disease in the neonate and young infant frequently are nonspecific and include change in feeding status, listlessness or irritability, and poor color. More specific findings that may not be present at the onset of illness are tachypnea, dyspnea, cyanosis, hypothermia, cough, and grunting. Accentuation of the normal irregularity of breathing is a common finding in neonates.

The physical findings of pneumonia vary. Flaring of the alae nasi, rapid respirations, and sternal and subcostal retractions frequently are observed. A cough is indicative of lower respiratory tract involvement; a brassy cough frequently is found in viral disease. Percussion dullness is difficult to demonstrate, but it is indicative of consolidation, effusion, or both. Auscultation may reveal diminished breath sounds over the affected area. Rales, wheezes, or both usually can be heard on deep inspiration or when the baby is crying, but may be absent early in the illness. The clinician frequently is surprised by the meager clinical signs in the face of clearly demonstrable and sometimes extensive roentgenographic findings of pneumonia.

Infants with pertussis usually become ill between weeks 2 and 6 of life. The characteristic whoop seen in older infants and children usually is absent. Paroxysmal cough, excessive mucous, and apneic spells are common in these infants. Complications of pertussis are many and include secondary bacterial pneumonia, atelectasis, and asphyxia.

Diagnosis

The leukocyte count can sometimes help to differentiate viral from bacterial pneumonia. Infants with early-onset bacterial pneumonia with sepsis may have leukopenia with an increased number of band forms. Chorioamnionitis has been demonstrated in the mothers of some infants with congenital pneumonia.

Cultures of blood and material from the trachea frequently help to define the etiologic agent of neonatal pneumonia. However, results of cultures from the ear canal, throat, and other external sites are not helpful and may be misleading in newborn and young infants. Thoracentesis or lung puncture should be considered in infants with pleural effusion or consolidated pneumonia, respectively, if the cause is unknown or the infant fails to respond to conventional antimicrobial therapy. Material obtained at puncture should be Gram stained for direct visualization of bacteria and cultured. Chlamydial pneumonia is best diagnosed by direct immunofluorescent staining and culture of nasopharyngeal secretions (465). Under ceratin circumstances, the tracheal aspirates or fluid obtained after bronchoalveolar lavage can be examined for *P. carinii* cysts, cultured for viruses, fungi, mycoplasmas, *B. pertussis,* acid-fast bacteria, and *Legionella*, and examined by polymerase chain reaction assays for a variety of infectious agents including *U. urealyticum, B. pertussis,* and viruses such as hepres simplex virus and cytomegalovirus (462,464, 466,467).

A chest radiograph may reveal roentgenographic evidence of pneumonia despite the absence of physical findings. Although it usually is not possible to determine the cause of neonatal pneumonia from chest radiographs, certain roentgenographic patterns may be associated with specific diseases. A consolidating bronchopneumonia with pneumatoceles, with or without empyema, suggests staphylococcal disease. This is particularly true when the radiologic findings advance markedly in a few hours. If a lobar infiltrate is associated with bulging fissures on the radiograph, *K. pneumoniae* infection should be considered. A miliary-type of bronchopneumonia in a septic neonate is characteristic of listeriosis. GBS pneumonia frequently is indistinguishable radiographically from hyaline membrane disease.

A bronchopneumonic infiltrate is encountered most commonly in the first month of life (468). This can be caused by aspiration of sterile or infected amniotic fluid or by viral, chlamydial, or bacterial pathogens, or it can represent patchy atelectasis.

Staphylococcal pneumonia is found most commonly in young infants; 30% of patients are younger than 3 months of age, and 70% are younger than 1 year of age. Epidemics of staphylococcal disease caused by phage group I organisms are encountered infrequently.

Staphylococci cause a confluent bronchopneumonia characterized by extensive areas of hemorrhagic necrosis and irregular areas of cavitation. The pleural surface usually is covered by a thick layer of fibrinopurulent exudate. Multiple small abscesses are scattered throughout the lungs. Rupture of a small subpleural abscess may result in a pyopneumothorax, which may erode into a bronchus, producing a bronchopleural fistula.

The onset of illness in staphylococcal pneumonia is abrupt, with fever, cough, and respiratory distress as the major manifestations. Tachypnea, grunting respirations, retractions, cyanosis, and anxiety usually are observed. Severe dyspnea and a shock-like state may occur. Rapid progression of symptoms is characteristic. Moist, scattered rales, diminished breath sounds, and rhonchi may be heard early in the illness. With the development of pleural effusion, dullness on percussion is associated with diminished breath sounds.

Most patients with staphylococcal pneumonia have roentgenographic evidence of bronchopneumonia early in the illness. The infiltrate may be patchy and limited in extent or be dense and homogeneous, involving an entire lobe or hemithorax. Pleural effusions or empyema are found in most infants (469). Pneumatoceles of various sizes are common. Although no radiographic change can be considered diagnostic, progression over a few hours from bronchopneumonia to effusion or pyopneumothorax with or without pneumatoceles is highly suggestive of staphylococcal pneumonia.

Treatment

All diagnostic procedures and cultures should be obtained before initiation of therapy. Methicillin is the initial drug of choice for staphylococcal pneumonia and should be administered parenterally in a dosage of 75 mg/kg/d divided in two or three doses for infants younger than 1 week of age and in a dosage of 100 mg/kg/d divided in four doses for older infants.

If infection extends to the pleural surfaces, surgical intervention usually becomes necessary. With small amounts of effusion, repeated pleural taps may be successful in removing fluid, but empyema is best treated by closed drainage with a chest tube of the largest possible caliber.

Vancomycin is preferred for disease due to MRSA. For pneumonia caused by *K. pneumoniae* or other coliforms, kanamycin or gentamicin should be used in a total dosage of 15 mg/kg/d or 5 to 7.5 mg/kg/d, respectively. Alternatively, a third-generation cephalosporin, such as cefotaxime, can be used. Treatment for *Listeria* pneumonia is parenteral ampicillin in a dosage of 50 to 100 mg/kg/d divided in two doses for infants younger than 1 week of age and 100 to 150 mg/kg/d divided in three doses for older neonates. Infants with GBS septicemia and pneumonia should be given penicillin in a dosage of 50,000 U/kg/d divided in two doses for infants younger than 1 week of age and 75,000 to 100,000 U/kg/d divided in three or four doses for older infants. Larger doses are required for meningitis. Ampicillin or cefotaxime may be used in place of penicillin.

Pertussis and chlamydial and ureaplasmal pneumonias probably are treated best with orally or intravenously administered erythromycin, depending on the infant's clinical status. This agent has been shown to shorten the course of illness and to eradicate shedding of the organisms from the nasopharynx. *Legionella* pneumonia also is treated with erythromycin; rifampin sometimes is added (464). Trimethoprim-sulfamethoxazole is the initial drug of choice for *P. carinii* pneumonia; pentamidine and trimetrexate are reserved for treatment failures.

Pneumonia may be one manifestation of generalized congenital viral infections. It is important to differentiate these infections from congenital syphilis and bacterial pneumonias resulting from aspiration. Ganciclovir can be used for cytomegalovirus pneumonia, but infants may worsen again upon discontinuation of the drug. Vidarabine or acyclovir is effective if given early in disease caused by herpes simplex virus.

Most infants with aspiration pneumonia do not require antimicrobial therapy. It frequently is difficult to differentiate infants with aspiration of sterile amniotic fluid from those aspirating infected materials. If doubt exists, therapy with penicillin and kanamycin or gentamicin should be initiated and continued until results of cultures are available.

OTITIS MEDIA

Otitis media is a frequent finding in premature infants receiving intensive care and an almost universal finding in autopsy studies of infants who died after a period of intensive care (470–473). A principal predisposing factor for otitis media in the newborn is nasotracheal intubation that results in ipsilateral obstruction of the eustachian tube, establishing the conditions eventuating in middle ear infection. The diagnosis is missed frequently because pneumatic otoscopy is not performed routinely in neonates.

The exact incidence of this condition is unknown. In one prospective study of 70 term infants followed from birth, 34% developed their first episode of otitis media before 2 months of age (474). Symptoms are nonspecific and include irritability, lethargy, fever, cough, diarrhea, vomiting, tachypnea, and anorexia (475). An associated conjunctivitis, pneumonia, or meningitis may be found in as many as half the patients. The diagnosis usually is made by pneumatic otoscopy. Tympanometry is unreliable in neonates.

Pathogenic organisms include *S. pneumoniae, H. influenzae, S. aureus, M. catarrhalis, P. aeruginosa,* and coliforms. The predominant isolates vary in different study populations (470,473,475–478).

Tympanocentesis should be performed on all newborns with otitis media who develop illness while in the nursery or intensive care unit (479). This may yield an etiologic agent when cultures of other sites are sterile. Some infants have positive blood cultures (478). The choice of antibiotic therapy can be based on the results of the Gram stain and culture of the aspirated middle ear effusion. If no organisms are seen on the smear, treatment should be with methicillin and an aminoglycoside until additional information is available. Infants with otitis media who are seen in the clinic or office usually do not require tympanocentesis for etiologic diagnosis if the illness is mild and can be managed at home. In these infants, a second-generation cephalosporin or Augmentin (amoxicillin and clavulanate) is preferred for therapy, and the patients should be reexamined 2 or 3 days after initiation of therapy to ascertain improvement. Infants with onset of otitis media before 2 months of age may need as long as 3 months to clear the effusion, and 33% of them develop chronic otitis media (474).

PERITONITIS

Spontaneous bacterial (i.e., primary) peritonitis without an evident intraabdominal source is rare during the neonatal period (480). It is postulated that bacteria can reach the peritoneal cavity by means of hematogenous, lymphatic, genital, or transmural (i.e., across the gut wall) routes of spread (481). A concurrent omphalitis is common (482). Gram-positive bacteria (e.g., *S. pneumoniae,* groups A and B streptococci) are the predominant pathogens, but gram-negative bacilli such as *Pseudomonas* or *Klebsiella* are responsible for some cases.

Most infants develop peritonitis after perforation of an abdominal viscus, usually as a complication of necrotizing enterocolitis. Other predisposing conditions include spontaneous focal gastrointestinal perforations, wound infections after abdominal surgery, traumatic perforations (e.g., feeding tube, rectal thermometer), ruptured omphalocele, and meconium peritonitis with subsequent bacterial contamination. Organisms isolated from peritoneal fluid cultures generally mirror the infant's gut flora and include *E. coli, Klebsiella* spp, *Enterobacter* spp, *Pseudomonas,* coagulase-positive and coagulase-negative staphylococci, streptococci, enterococci, anaerobic bacteria (e.g., clostridia, *Bacteroides* spp), and *Candida* (483–486).

Clinical signs of peritonitis include vomiting, abdominal distention, abdominal wall edema or discoloration, constipation, diarrhea, grunting, temperature instability (i.e., usually hypothermia), shock, and scrotal or vulvar swelling (487). Abdominal radiographs may reveal free air in the peritoneal cavity, indicating intestinal perforation, or patterns suggesting necrotizing enterocolitis (e.g., pneumatosis intestinalis) or intestinal obstruction. Abdominal ultrasound is helpful in visualizing peritoneal fluid. An abdominal paracentesis may yield pus or reveal a different cause for the illness (e.g., hemoperitoneum, bile peritonitis). Aerobic and anaerobic cultures of the peritoneal fluid and of the blood should be obtained in all cases.

The management of peritonitis consists of supportive measures aimed at reversing hypovolemia, shock, and electrolyte imbalances; surgical correction of underlying conditions; and administration of broad-spectrum antimicrobial agents. Acceptable initial antibiotic regimens include ampicillin, gentamicin and clindamycin, Timentin and an aminoglycoside, or vancomycin, ceftazidime, and metronidazole. The broadest antibacterial coverage is attained by the vancomycin, ceftazidime, and metronidazole combination. Treatment can be simplified after the blood and peritoneal fluid culture results become available. Antibiotics usually are continued for 10 days. The prognosis depends on several factors, including birth weight and precipitating conditions, and fatality rates range from 10% to 50% (480).

REFERENCES

1. Jason JM. Infectious disease-related deaths of low birth weight infants, United States, 1968 to 1982. *Pediatrics* 1989;84:296.
2. Msall ME, Buck GM, Rogers BT, et al. Risk factors for major neurodevelopmental impairments and need for special education resources in extremely premature infants. *J Pediatr* 1991;119:606.
3. Stoll BJ, Gordon T, Korones SB, et al. Late-onset sepsis in very low birth weight neonates: a report from the National Institute of Child Health and Human Development Neonatal Research Network. *J Pediatr* 1996;129:63.
4. Stoll BJ, Gordon T, Korones SB, et al. Early-onset sepsis in very low birth weight neonates: a report from the National Institute of Child Health and Human Development Neonatal Research Network. *J Pediatr* 1996;129:72.
5. Freedman RM, Ingram DL, Gross I, et al. A half century of neonatal sepsis at Yale: 1928 to 1978. *Am J Dis Child* 1981;135:140.
6. Stoll BJ. The global impact of neonatal infection. *Clin Perinatol* 1997;24:1.

7. St. Geme JW III, Harris MC. Coagulase-negative staphylococcal infection in the neonate. *Clin Perinatol* 1991;18:281.

8. Gaynes RP, Edwards JR, Jarvis WR, et al. Nosocomial infections among neonates in high-risk nurseries in the United States. *Pediatrics* 1996;98:357.

9. Sáez-Llorens X, McCracken GH Jr. Clinical pharmacology of antibacterial agents. In: Remington JS, Klein JO, eds. *Infectious diseases of the fetus and newborn infant*, 4th ed. Philadelphia: WB Saunders, 1995:1287.

10. Boyer KM, Gotoff SP. Alternative algorithms for prevention of perinatal group B streptococcal infections. *Pediatr Infect Dis J* 1998;17:973.

11. Bortolussi R, Thompson TR, Ferrieri P. Early-onset pneumococcal sepsis in newborn infants. *Pediatrics* 1977;60:352.

12. Kaplan M, Rudensky B, Beck A. Perinatal infections with *Streptococcus pneumoniae*. *Am J Perinatol* 1993;10:1.

13. Chugh K, Bhalla CK, Joshi KK. Meningococcal brain abscess and meningitis in a neonate. *Pediatr Infect Dis J* 1988;7:136.

14. Goldmann DA. Bacterial colonization and infection in the neonate. *Am J Med* 1981;70:417.

15. Fryklund B, Tullus K, Burman LG. Epidemiology of enteric bacteria in neonatal unit—influence of procedures and patient variables. *J Hosp Infect* 1991;18:15.

16. Goering RV, Ehrenkranz NJ, Sanders CC, Sanders WE Jr. Long term epidemiological analysis of *Citrobacter diversus* in a neonatal intensive care unit. *Pediatr Infect Dis J* 1992;11:99.

17. D'Angio CT, McGowan KL, Baumgart S, et al. Surface colonization with coagulase-negative staphylococci in premature neonates. *J Pediatr* 1989;114:1029.

18. Baley JE, Kliegman RM, Boxerbaum B, Fanaroff AA. Fungal colonization in the very low birth weight infant. *Pediatrics* 1986;78:225.

19. Waggoner-Fountain LA, Walker MW, Hollis RJ, et al. Vertical and horizontal transmission of unique Candida species to premature newborns. *Clin Infect Dis* 1996;22:803.

20. Aschner JL, Punsalang A Jr, Maniscalco WM, Menegus MA. Percutaneous central venous catheter colonization with *Malassezia furfur*: incidence and clinical significance. *Pediatrics* 1987;80:535.

21. Bell LM, Alpert G, Slight PH, Campos JM. *Malassezia furfur* skin colonization in infancy. *Infect Control Hosp Epidemiol* 1988;9:151.

22. Stuart SM, Lane AT. Candida and Malassezia as nursery pathogens. *Semin Dermatol* 1992;11:19.

23. Lane AT, Drost SS. Effect of repeated application of emollient cream to premature neonates' skin. *Pediatrics* 1993;92:415.

24. Cassell GH, Waites KB, Crouse DT. Perinatal mycoplasmal infections. *Clin Perinatol* 1991;18:241.

25. Syrogiannopoulos GA, Kapatais-Zoumbos K, Decavalas GO, et al. *Ureaplasma urealyticum* colonization of full term infants: perinatal acquisition and persistence during early infancy. *Pediatr Infect Dis J* 1990;9:236.

26. Hammerschlag MR, Anderka M, Semine DZ, et al. Prospective study of maternal and infantile infection with *Chlamydia trachomatis*. *Pediatrics* 1979;64:142.

27. Schachter J, Grossman M, Sweet RL, et al. Prospective study of perinatal transmission of *Chlamydia trachomatis*. *JAMA* 1986;255:3374.

28. Bell TA, Stamm WE, Wang SP, et al. Chronic *Chlamydia trachomatis* infections in infants. *JAMA* 1992;267:400.

29. Kaftan H, Kinney JS. Early onset neonatal bacterial infections. *Semin Perinatol* 1998;22:15.

30. Peter G, Cashore WJ. Infections acquired in the nursery: epidemiology and control. In: Remington JS, Klein JO, eds. *Infectious diseases of the fetus and newborn infant*, 4th ed. Philadelphia: WB Saunders, 1995:1264.

31. Thompson PJ, Greenough A, Hird MF, et al. Nosocomial bacterial infections in very low birth weight infants. *Eur J Pediatr* 1992;151:451.

32. Moro ML, De Toni A, Stolfi I, et al. Risk factors for nosocomial sepsis in newborn intensive and intermediate care units. *Eur J Pediatr* 1996;155:315.

33. Fanaroff AA, Korones SB, Wright LL, et al. Incidence, presenting features, risk factors and significance of late onset septicemia in very low birth weight infants. *Pediatr Infect Dis J* 1998;17:593.

34. Adams JM, Speer ME, Rudolph AJ. Bacterial colonization of radial artery catheters. *Pediatrics* 1980;65:94.

35. Landers S, Moise AA, Fraley JK, et al. Factors associated with umbilical catheter-related sepsis in neonates. *Am J Dis Child* 1991;145:675.

36. Hruszkewycz V, Holtrop PC, Batton DG, et al. Complications associated with central venous catheters inserted in critically ill neonates. *Infect Control Hosp Epidemiol* 1991;12:544.

37. Maas A, Flament P, Pardou A, et al. Central venous catheter-related bacteraemia in critically ill neonates: risk factors and impact of a prevention programme. *J Hosp Infect* 1998;40:211.

38. Raad I. Intravascular-catheter-related infections. *Lancet* 1998;351:893.

39. Elliott TSJ, Tebbs SE. Prevention of central venous catheter-related infection. *J Hosp Infect* 1998;40:193.

40. Cowen J, Ellis SH, McAinsh J. Absorption of chlorhexidine from the intact skin of newborn infants. *Arch Dis Child* 1979;54:379.

41. Meberg A, Schøyen R. Bacterial colonization and neonatal infections: effects of skin and umbilical disinfection in the nursery. *Acta Paediatr Scand* 1985;74:366.

42. Hoffmann KK, Weber DJ, Samsa GP, Rutala WA. Transparent polyurethane film as an intravenous catheter dressing: a meta-analysis of the infection risks. *JAMA* 1992;267:2072.

43. Salzman MB, Rubin LG. Intravenous catheter-related infections. *Adv Pediatr Infect Dis* 1995;10:337.

44. John JF Jr. Molecular analysis of nosocomial epidemics. *Infect Dis Clin North Am* 1989;3:683.

45. Melish ME, Glasgow LA, Turner MD. The staphylococcal scalded-skin syndrome: isolation and partial characterization of the exfoliative toxin. *J Infect Dis* 1972;125:129.

46. Curran JP, Al-Salihi FL. Neonatal staphylococcal scalded skin syndrome: massive outbreak due to an unusual phage type. *Pediatrics* 1980;66:285.

47. Mackenzie A, Johnson W, Heyes B, et al. A prolonged outbreak of exfoliative toxin A-producing *Staphylococcus aureus* in a newborn nursery. *Diagn Microbiol Infect Dis* 1995;21:69.

48. Albert S, Baldwin R, Czekajewski S, et al. Bullous impetigo due to group II *Staphylococcus aureus*: an epidemic in a normal newborn nursery. *Am J Dis Child* 1970;120:10.

49. Boyce JM. Methicillin-resistant *Staphylococcus aureus*: detection, epidemiology, and control measures. *Infect Dis Clin North Am* 1989;3:901.

50. Boyce JM. Should we vigorously try to contain and control methicillin-resistant *Staphylococcus aureus*? *Infect Control Hosp Epidemiol* 1991;12:46.

51. Graham DR, Correa-Villasenor A, Anderson RL, et al. Epidemic neonatal gentamicin-methicillin-resistant *Staphylococcus aureus* infection associated with nonspecific topical use of gentamicin. *J Pediatr* 1980;97:972.

52. Dunkle LM, Naqvi SH, McCallum R, Lofgren JP. Eradication of epidemic methicillin-gentamicin-resistant *Staphylococcus aureus* in an intensive care nursery. *Am J Med* 1981;70:455.

53. Mitsuda T, Arai K, Fujita S, Yokota S. Epidemiological analysis of strains of methicillin-resistant *Staphylococcus aureus* (MRSA) infection in the nursery; prognosis of MRSA carrier infants. *J Hosp Infect* 1995;31:123.

54. Raju TNK, Kobler C. Improving handwashing habits in the newborn nurseries. *Am J Med Sci* 1991;302:355.

55. Goldmann DA. Prevention and management of neonatal infections. *Infect Dis Clin North Am* 1989;3:779.

56. Rosenfeld CR, Laptook AR, Jeffery J. Limited effectiveness of triple dye in preventing colonization with methicillin-resistant *Staphylococcus aureus* in a special care nursery. *Pediatr Infect Dis J* 1990;9:290.

57. Davies EA, Emmerson AM, Hogg GM, et al. An outbreak of infection with a methicillin-resistant *Staphylococcus aureus* in a special care baby unit: value of topical mupirocin and of traditional methods of infection control. *J Hosp Infect* 1987;10:120.

58. Geil CC, Castle WK, Mortimer EA Jr. Group A streptococcal infections in newborn nurseries. *Pediatrics* 1970;46:849.

59. Campbell JR, Arango CA, Garcia-Prats JA, Baker CJ. An outbreak of M serotype 1 group A Streptococcus in a neonatal intensive care unit. *J Pediatr* 1996;129:396.

60. Lambert-Zechovsky N, Bingen E, Denamur E, et al. Molecular analysis provides evidence for the endogenous origin of bacteremia and meningitis due to *Enterobacter cloacae* in an infant. *Clin Infect Dis* 1992;15:30.

61. Eidelman AI, Reynolds J. Gentamicin-resistant Klebsiella infections in a neonatal intensive care unit. *Am J Dis Child* 1978;132:421.

62. Eisen D, Russell EG, Tymms M, et al. Random amplified polymor-

phic DNA and plasmid analyses used in investigation of an outbreak of multiresistant *Klebsiella pneumoniae*. *J Clin Microbiol* 1995;33: 713.

63. Abrahamsen TG, Finne PH, Lingaas E. *Flavobacterium meningosepticum* infections in a neonatal intensive care unit. *Acta Paediatr Scand* 1989;78:51.

64. Smith PJ, Brookfield DSK, Shaw DA, Gray J. An outbreak of *Serratia marcescens* infection in a neonatal unit. *Lancet* 1984;1:151.

65. Muyldermans G, de Smet F, Pierard D, et al. Neonatal infections with *Pseudomonas aeruginosa* associated with a water-bath used to thaw fresh frozen plasma. *J Hosp Infect* 1998;39:309.

66. Archibald LK, Ramos M, Arduino MJ, et al. *Enterobacter cloacae* and *Pseudomonas aeruginosa* polymicrobial bloodstream infections traced to extrinsic contamination of a dextrose multidose vial. *J Pediatr* 1998;133:640.

67. Burke JP, Ingall D, Klein JO, et al. *Proteus mirabilis* infections in a hospital nursery traced to a human carrier. *N Engl J Med* 1971;284: 115.

68. Horrevorts A, Bergman K, Kollée L, et al. Clinical and epidemiological investigations of *Acinetobacter genomospecies* 3 in a neonatal intensive care unit. *J Clin Microbiol* 1995;33:1567.

69. McDonald LC, Walker M, Carson L, et al. Outbreak of *Acinetobacter* spp. bloodstream infections in a nursery associated with contaminated aerosols and air conditioners. *Pediatr Infect Dis J* 1998;17:716.

70. Parry MF, Hutchinson JH, Brown NA, et al. Gram-negative sepsis in neonates: a nursery outbreak due to hand carriage of *Citrobacter diversus*. *Pediatrics* 1980;65:1105.

71. Modi N, Damjanovic V, Cooke RWI. Outbreak of cephalosporin resistant *Enterobacter cloacae* infection in a neonatal intensive care unit. *Arch Dis Child* 1987;62:148.

72. Finnström O, Isaksson B, Hæggman S, Burman LG. Control of an outbreak of a highly beta-lactam-resistant *Enterobacter cloacae* strain in a neonatal special care unit. *Acta Paediatr* 1998;87:1070.

73. Khan MA, Abdur-Rab M, Israr N, et al. Transmission of *Salmonella worthington* by oropharyngeal suction in hospital neonatal unit. *Pediatr Infect Dis J* 1991;10:668.

74. Cook LN, Davis RS, Stover BH. Outbreak of amikacin-resistant *Enterobacteriaceae* in an intensive care nursery. *Pediatrics* 1980;65: 264.

75. Biering G, Karlsson S, Clark NC, et al. Three cases of neonatal meningitis caused by *Enterobacter sakazakii* in powdered milk. *J Clin Microbiol* 1989;27:2054.

76. Modlin JF. Perinatal echovirus and group B coxsackievirus infections. *Clin Perinatol* 1988;15:233.

77. Graman PS, Hall CB. Epidemiology and control of nosocomial viral infections. *Infect Dis Clin North Am* 1989;3:815.

78. Chawareewong S, Kiangsiri S, Lokaphadhana K, et al. Neonatal herpangina caused by coxsackie A-5 virus. *J Pediatr* 1978;93:492.

79. Javett SN, Heymann S, Mundel B, et al. Myocarditis in the newborn infant: a study of an outbreak associated with coxsackie group B virus infection in a maternity home in Johannesburg. *J Pediatr* 1956;48:1.

80. Swender PT, Shott RJ, Williams ML. A community and intensive care nursery outbreak of coxsackievirus B5 meningitis. *Am J Dis Child* 1974;127:42.

81. Butterfield J, Moscovici C, Berry C, Kempe CH. Cystic emphysema in premature infants: a report of an outbreak with the isolation of type 19 ECHO virus in one case. *N Engl J Med* 1963;268:18.

82. McDonald LL, St. Geme JW Jr, Arnold BH. Nosocomial infection with ECHO virus type 31 in a neonatal intensive care unit. *Pediatrics* 1971;47:995.

83. Lapinleimu K, Hakulinen A. A hospital outbreak caused by ECHO virus type 11 among newborn infants. *Ann Clin Res* 1972;4:183.

84. Philip AGS, Larson EJ. Overwhelming neonatal infection with ECHO 19 virus. *J Pediatr* 1973;82:391.

85. Purdham DR, Purdham PA, Wood BSB, et al. Severe echo 19 virus infection in a neonatal unit. *Arch Dis Child* 1976;51:634.

86. Davies DP, Hughes CA, MacVicar J, et al. Echovirus-11 infection in a special-care baby unit. *Lancet* 1979;1:96.

87. Modlin JF, Polk BF, Horton P, et al. Perinatal echovirus infection: risk of transmission during a community outbreak. *N Engl J Med* 1981;305:368.

88. Rabkin CS, Telzak EE, Ho M-S, et al. Outbreak of echovirus 11 infection in hospitalized neonates. *Pediatr Infect Dis J* 1988;7:186.

89. Birenbaum E, Handsher R, Kuint J, et al. Echovirus type 22 outbreak associated with gastro-intestinal disease in a neonatal intensive care unit. *Am J Perinatol* 1997;14:469.

90. Reyes MP, Ostrea EM Jr, Roskamp J, Lerner AM. Disseminated neonatal echovirus 11 disease following antenatal maternal infection with a virus-positive cervix and virus-negative gastrointestinal tract. *J Med Virol* 1983;12:155.

91. Larson E. A causal link between handwashing and risk of infection? Examination of the evidence. *Infect Control Hosp Epidemiol* 1988;9: 28.

92. Pasic S, Jankovic B, Abinun M, Kanjuh B. Intravenous immunoglobulin prophylaxis in an echovirus 6 and echovirus 4 nursery outbreak. *Pediatr Infect Dis J* 1997;16:718.

93. Klein BS, Michaels JA, Rytel MW, et al. Nosocomial hepatitis A: a multinursery outbreak in Wisconsin. *JAMA* 1984;252:2716.

94. Azimi PH, Roberto RR, Guralnik J, et al. Transfusion-acquired hepatitis A in a premature infant with secondary nosocomial spread in an intensive care nursery. *Am J Dis Child* 1986;140:23.

95. Rosenblum LS, Villarino ME, Nainan OV, et al. Hepatitis A outbreak in a neonatal intensive care unit: risk factors for transmission and evidence of prolonged viral excretion among preterm infants. *J Infect Dis* 1991;164:476.

96. Lee KK, Vargo LR, Lê CT, Fernando L. Transfusion-acquired hepatitis A outbreak from fresh frozen plasma in a neonatal intensive care unit. *Pediatr Infect Dis J* 1992;11:122.

97. Centers for Disease Control and Prevention. Protection against viral hepatitis: recommendations of the Immunization Practices Advisory Committee (ACIP). *MMWR* 1990;39(S-2):1.

98. Mbithi JN, Springthorpe VS, Boulet JR, Sattar SA. Survival of hepatitis A virus on human hands and its transfer on contact with animate and inanimate surfaces. *J Clin Microbiol* 1992;30:757.

99. Abzug MJ, Levin MJ. Neonatal adenovirus infection: four patients and review of the literature. *Pediatrics* 1991;87:890.

100. Brown M, Rossier E, Carpenter B, Anand CM. Fatal adenovirus type 35 infection in newborns. *Pediatr Infect Dis J* 1991;10:955.

101. Aebi C, Headrick CL, McCracken GH Jr, Lindsay CA. Intravenous ribavirin therapy in a neonate with disseminated adenovirus infection undergoing extracorporeal membrane oxygenation: pharmacokinetics and clearance by hemofiltration. *J Pediatr* 1997;130:612.

102. Finn A, Anday E, Talbot GH. An epidemic of adenovirus 7a infection in a neonatal nursery: course, morbidity, and management. *Infect Control Hosp Epidemiol* 1988;9:398.

103. Piedra PA, Kasel JA, Norton HJ, et al. Evaluation of an intravenous immunoglobulin preparation for the prevention of viral infection among hospitalized low birth weight infants. *Pediatr Infect Dis J* 1990;9:470.

104. Piedra PA, Kasel JA, Norton HJ, et al. Description of an adenovirus type 8 outbreak in hospitalized neonates born prematurely. *Pediatr Infect Dis J* 1992;11:460.

105. Berkovich S. Acute respiratory illness in the premature nursery associated with respiratory syncytial virus infections. *Pediatrics* 1964;34: 753.

106. Hall CB, Kopelman AE, Douglas RG Jr, et al. Neonatal respiratory syncytial virus infection. *N Engl J Med* 1979;300:393.

107. Valenti WM, Clarke TA, Hall CB, et al. Concurrent outbreaks of rhinovirus and respiratory syncytial virus in an intensive care nursery: epidemiology and associated risk factors. *J Pediatr* 1982;100:722.

108. Meissner HC, Murray SA, Kiernan MA, et al. A simultaneous outbreak of respiratory syncytial virus and parainfluenza virus type 3 in a newborn nursery. *J Pediatr* 1984;104:680.

109. Snydman DR, Greer C, Meissner HC, McIntosh K. Prevention of nosocomial transmission of respiratory syncytial virus in a newborn nursery. *Infect Control Hosp Epidemiol* 1988;9:105.

110. Church NR, Anas NG, Hall CB, Brooks JG. Respiratory syncytial virus-related apnea in infants: demographics and outcome. *Am J Dis Child* 1984;138:247.

111. Kneyber MCJ, Brandenburg AH, de Groot R, et al. Risk factors for respiratory syncytial virus associated apnoea. *Eur J Pediatr* 1998;157:331.

112. Forster J, Schumacher RF. The clinical picture presented by premature neonates infected with the respiratory syncytial virus. *Eur J Pediatr* 1995;154:901.

113. MacDonald NE, Hall CB, Suffin SC, et al. Respiratory syncytial viral infection in infants with congenital heart disease. *N Engl J Med* 1982;307:397.

114. Walsh EE, McConnochie KM, Long CE, Hall CB. Severity of respiratory syncytial virus infection is related to virus strain. *J Infect Dis* 1997;175:814.

115. Gala CL, Hall CB, Schnabel KC, et al. The use of eye-nose goggles to control nosocomial respiratory syncytial virus infection. *JAMA* 1986; 256:2706.

116. Agah R, Cherry JD, Garakian AJ, Chapin M. Respiratory syncytial virus (RSV) infection rate in personnel caring for children with RSV infections: routine isolation procedure vs routine procedure supplemented by use of masks and goggles. *Am J Dis Child* 1987;141:695.

117. American Academy of Pediatrics, Committee on Infectious Diseases, Committee on Fetus and Newborn. Respiratory syncytial virus immune globulin intravenous: indications for use. *Pediatrics* 1997;99: 645.

118. The PREVENT Study Group. Reduction of respiratory syncytial virus hospitalization among premature infants and infants with bronchopulmonary dysplasia using respiratory syncytial virus immune globulin prophylaxis. *Pediatrics* 1997;99:93.

119. Simoes EAF, Sondheimer HM, Top FH Jr, et al. Respiratory syncytial virus immune globulin for prophylaxis against respiratory syncytial virus disease in infants and children with congenital heart disease. *J Pediatr* 1998;133:492.

120. Johnson S, Oliver C, Prince GA, et al. Development of a humanized monoclonal antibody (MEDI-493) with potent in vitro and in vivo activity against respiratory syncytial virus. *J Infect Dis* 1997;176: 1215.

121. The IMpact-RSV Study Group. Palivizumab, a humanized respiratory syncytial virus monoclonal antibody, reduces hospitalization from respiratory syncytial virus infection in high-risk infants. *Pediatrics* 1998; 102:531.

122. Storch GA. Humanized monoclonal antibody for prevention of respiratory syncytial virus infection. *Pediatrics* 1998;102:648.

123. Lau YR, Whitley RJ. Evaluation of ribavirin for treatment of respiratory syncytial virus. *Semin Pediatr Infect Dis* 1991;2:279.

124. American Academy of Pediatrics, Committee on Infectious Diseases. Reassessment of the indications for ribavirin therapy in respiratory syncytial virus infections. *Pediatrics* 1996;97:137.

125. Smith DW, Frankel LR, Mathers LH, et al. A controlled trial of aerosolized ribavirin in infants receiving mechanical ventilation for severe respiratory syncytial virus infection. *N Engl J Med* 1991;325: 24.

126. Bauer CR, Elie K, Spence L, Stern L. Hong Kong influenza in a neonatal unit. *JAMA* 1973;223:1233.

127. Meibalane R, Sedmak GV, Sasidharan P, et al. Outbreak of influenza in a neonatal intensive care unit. *J Pediatr* 1977;91:974.

128. Bada HS, Alojipan LC, Andrews BF. Premature rupture of membranes and its effect on the newborn. *Pediatr Clin North Am* 1977;24:491.

129. St. Geme JW Jr, Murray DL, Carter JA, et al. Perinatal bacterial infection after prolonged rupture of amniotic membranes: an analysis of risk and management. *J Pediatr* 1984;104:608.

130. Sperling RS, Newton E, Gibbs RS. Intraamniotic infection in low-birth-weight infants. *J Infect Dis* 1988;157:113.

131. Hillier SL, Krohn MA, Kiviat NB, et al. Microbiologic causes and neonatal outcomes associated with chorioamnion infection. *Am J Obstet Gynecol* 1991;165:955.

132. Belady PH, Farkouh LJ, Gibbs RS. Intra-amniotic infection and premature rupture of the membranes. *Clin Perinatol* 1997;24:43.

133. Marston G, Wald ER. *Hemophilus influenzae* type b sepsis in infant and mother. *Pediatrics* 1976;58:863.

134. Simpson JM, Patel JS, Ispahani P. *Streptococcus pneumoniae* invasive disease in the neonatal period: an increasing problem? *Eur J Pediatr* 1995;154:563.

135. Grossman J, Tompkins RL. *Group B beta-hemolytic streptococcal* meningitis in mother and infant. *N Engl J Med* 1974;290:387.

136. Botta GA. Hormonal and type-dependent adhesion of *group B streptococci* to human vaginal cells. *Infect Immun* 1979;25:1084.

137. Broughton RA, Baker CJ. Role of adherence in the pathogenesis of neonatal *group B streptococcal* infection. *Infect Immun* 1983;39:837.

138. Robbins JB, McCracken GH Jr, Gotschlich EC, et al. *Escherichia coli* K1 capsular polysaccharide associated with neonatal meningitis. *N Engl J Med* 1974;290:1216.

139. Givner LB, Baker CJ. Pooled human IgG hyperimmune for type III *group B streptococci*: evaluation against multiple strains in vitro and in experimental disease. *J Infect Dis* 1991;163:1141.

140. Glode MP, Sutton A, Moxon ER, Robbins JB. Pathogenesis of neonatal *Escherichia coli* meningitis: induction of bacteremia and meningitis in infant rats fed E. coli K1. *Infect Immun* 1977;16:75.

141. Larsen JW Jr, London WT, Palmer AE, et al. Experimental *group B streptococcal* infection in the rhesus monkey. I. Disease production in the neonate. *Am J Obstet Gynecol* 1978;132:686.

142. Martin TR, Ruzinski JT, Rubens CE, et al. The effect of type-specific polysaccharide capsule on the clearance of *group B streptococci* from the lungs of infant and adult rats. *J Infect Dis* 1992;165:306.

143. Baker CJ, Edwards MS, Kasper DL. Role of antibody to native type III polysaccharide of *group B streptococcus* in infant protection. *Pediatrics* 1981;68:544.

144. Anderson DC, Edwards MS, Baker CJ. Luminol-enhanced chemiluminescence for evaluation of type III *group B streptococcal* opsonins in human sera. *J Infect Dis* 1980;141:370.

145. Vogel LC, Kretschmer RR, Boyer KM, et al. Human immunity to *group B streptococci* measured by indirect immunofluorescence: correlation with protection in chick embryos. *J Infect Dis* 1979;140:682.

146. Fischer GW, Hemming VG, Hunter KW Jr, et al. Intravenous immunoglobulin in the treatment of neonatal sepsis: therapeutic strategies and laboratory studies. *Pediatr Infect Dis* 1986;5:S171.

147. Hill HR, Gonzales LA, Knappe WA, et al. Comparative protective activity of human monoclonal and hyperimmune polyclonal antibody against *group B streptococci*. *J Infect Dis* 1991;163:792.

148. Baker CJ, Webb BJ, Kasper DL, et al. The natural history of *group B streptococcal* colonization in the pregnant woman and her offspring. II. Determination of serum antibody to capsular polysaccharide from type III, *group B streptococcus*. *Am J Obstet Gynecol* 1980;137:39.

149. Anthony BF, Concepcion NF, Concepcion KF. Human antibody to the group-specific polysaccharide of *group B streptococcus*. *J Infect Dis* 1985;151:221.

150. Klegerman ME, Boyer KM, Papierniak CK, Gotoff SP. Estimation of the protective level of human IgG antibody to the type-specific polysaccharide of *group B streptococcus* type Ia. *J Infect Dis* 1983;148: 648.

151. Boyer KM, Kendall LS, Papierniak CK, et al. Protective levels of human immunoglobulin G antibody to *group B streptococcus* type Ib. *Infect Immun* 1984;45:618.

152. Gotoff SP, Papierniak CK, Klegerman ME, Boyer KM. Quantitation of IgG antibody to the type-specific polysaccharide of *group B streptococcus* type 1b in pregnant women and infected infants. *J Pediatr* 1984;105:628.

153. Gray BM, Pritchard DG, Dillon HC Jr. Seroepidemiological studies of *group B streptococcus* type II. *J Infect Dis* 1985;151:1073.

154. Anthony BF. The role of specific antibody in neonatal bacterial infections: an overview. *Pediatr Infect Dis* 1986;5:S164.

155. Lassiter HA, Tanner JE, Miller RD. Inefficient bacteriolysis of *Escherichia coli* by serum from human neonates. *J Infect Dis* 1992; 165:290.

156. Lassiter HA, Watson SW, Seifring ML, Tanner JE. Complement factor 9 deficiency in serum of human neonates. *J Infect Dis* 1992;166: 53.

157. Edwards MS, Buffone GJ, Fuselier PA, et al. Deficient classical complement pathway activity in newborn sera. *Pediatr Res* 1983;17:685.

158. Máródi L, Leijh PCJ, Braat A, et al. Opsonic activity of cord blood sera against various species of microorganism. *Pediatr Res* 1985;19: 433.

159. Edwards MS, Kasper DL, Jennings HJ, et al. Capsular sialic acid prevents activation of the alternative complement pathway by type III, *group B streptococci*. *J Immunol* 1982;128:1278.

160. Yoder MC. Therapeutic administration of fibronectin: current uses and potential applications. *Clin Perinatol* 1991;18:325.

161. Gerdes JS, Yoder MC, Douglas SD, Polin RA. Decreased plasma fibronectin in neonatal sepsis. *Pediatrics* 1983;72:877.

162. Domula M, Bykowska K, Wegrzynowicz Z, et al. Plasma fibronectin concentrations in healthy and septic infants. *Eur J Pediatr* 1985;144: 49.

163. Butler KM, Baker CJ, Edwards MS. Interaction of soluble fibronectin with *group B streptococci*. *Infect Immun* 1987;55:2404.

164. Cairo MS. Neonatal neutrophil host defense: prospects for immunologic enhancement during neonatal sepsis. *Am J Dis Child* 1989;143:40.

165. Klein JO, Marcy SM. Bacterial sepsis and meningitis. In: Remington JS, Klein JO, eds. *Infectious diseases of the fetus and newborn infant,* 4th ed. Philadelphia: WB Saunders, 1995:835.

166. Voora S, Srinivasan G, Lilien LD, et al. Fever in full-term newborns in the first four days of life. *Pediatrics* 1982;69:40.

167. Gladstone IM, Ehrenkranz RA, Edberg SC, Baltimore RS. A ten-year review of neonatal sepsis and comparison with the previous fifty-year experience. *Pediatr Infect Dis J* 1990;9:819.

168. Centers for Disease Control and Prevention. Prevention of perinatal *group B streptococcal* disease: a public health perspective. *MMWR* 1996;45(RR-7):1.

169. Baker CJ, Edwards MS. *Group B streptococcal* infections. In: Remington JS, Klein JO, eds. *Infectious diseases of the fetus and newborn infant*, 4th ed. Philadelphia: WB Saunders, 1995:980.

170. Dillon HC Jr, Khare S, Gray BM. *Group B streptococcal* carriage and disease: a 6-year prospective study. *J Pediatr* 1987;110:31.

171. Regan JA, Klebanoff MA, Nugent RP, for the Vaginal Infections and Prematurity Study Group. The epidemiology of *group B streptococcal* colonization in pregnancy. *Obstet Gynecol* 1991;77:604.

172. Stoll BJ, Schuchat A. Maternal carriage of *group B streptococci* in developing countries. *Pediatr Infect Dis J* 1998;17:499.

173. Schuchat A. Epidemiology of *group B streptococcal* disease in the United States: shifting paradigms. *Clin Microbiol Rev* 1998;11:497.

174. Gardner SE, Yow MD, Leeds LJ, et al. Failure of penicillin to eradicate *group B streptococcal* colonization in the pregnant woman: a couple study. *Am J Obstet Gynecol* 1979;135:1062.

175. Jones DE, Kanarek KS, Lim DV. *Group B streptococcal* colonization patterns in mothers and their infants. *J Clin Microbiol* 1984;20:438.

176. Chin KC, Fitzhardinge PM. Sequelae of early-onset *group B hemolytic streptococcal* neonatal meningitis. *J Pediatr* 1985;106:819.

177. Pyati SP, Pildes RS, Ramamurthy RS, Jacobs N. Decreasing mortality in neonates with early-onset *group B streptococcal* infection: reality or artifact. *J Pediatr* 1981;98:625.

178. Siegel JD, McCracken GH Jr. *Group D streptococcal infections. J Pediatr* 1978;93:542.

179. Dyson AE, Read SE. *Group G streptococcal* colonization and sepsis in neonates. *J Pediatr* 1981;99:944.

180. Isaacman SH, Heroman WM, Lightsey AL. Purpura fulminans following late-onset *group B β-hemolytic streptococcal* sepsis. *Am J Dis Child* 1984;138:915.

181. Howard JB, McCracken GH Jr. The spectrum of *group B streptococcal* infections in infancy. *Am J Dis Child* 1974;128:815.

182. Yagupsky P, Menegus MA, Powell KR. The changing spectrum of *group B streptococcal* disease in infants: an eleven-year experience in a tertiary care hospital. *Pediatr Infect Dis J* 1991;10:801.

183. Atkins JT, Heresi GP, Coque TM, Baker CJ. Recurrent *group B streptococcal* disease in infants: who should receive rifampin? *J Pediatr* 1998;132:537.

184. Whitley CB, Thompson LR, Osterholm MT, et al. Toxic shock syndrome in a newborn infant. *Pediatr Res* 1982;16:254A(abst).

185. Chesney PJ, Jaucian RC, McDonald RA, et al. *Exfoliative dermatitis* in an infant: association with enterotoxin F-producing staphylococci. *Am J Dis Child* 1983;137:899.

186. Peters B, Hentschel J, Mau H, et al. Staphylococcal scalded-skin syndrome complicating wound infection in a preterm infant with postoperative chylothorax. *J Clin Microbiol* 1998;36:3057.

187. Ladhani S, Evans RW. Staphylococcal scalded skin syndrome. *Arch Dis Child* 1998;78:85.

188. Dancer SJ, Simmons NA, Poston SM, Noble WC. Outbreak of staphylococcal scalded skin syndrome among neonates. *J Infect* 1988;16:87.

189. Loughead JL. Congenital staphylococcal scalded skin syndrome: report of a case. *Pediatr Infect Dis J* 1992;11:413.

190. Saiman L, Jakob K, Holmes KW, et al. Molecular epidemiology of staphylococcal scalded skin syndrome in premature infants. *Pediatr Infect Dis J* 1998;17:329.

191. Espersen F, Frimodt-Møller N, Rosdahl VT, Jessen O. *Staphylococcus aureus* bacteraemia in children below the age of one year: a review of 407 cases. *Acta Paediatr Scand* 1989;78:56.

192. Pfaller MA, Herwaldt LA. Laboratory, clinical, and epidemiological aspects of coagulase-negative staphylococci. *Clin Microbiol Rev* 1988;1:281.

193. Patrick CC. Coagulase-negative staphylococci: pathogens with increasing clinical significance. *J Pediatr* 1990;116:497.

194. Neumeister B, Kastner S, Conrad S, et al. Characterization of coagulase-negative staphylococci causing nosocomial infections in preterm infants. *Eur J Clin Microbiol Infect Dis* 1995;14:856.

195. Vesikari T, Isolauri E, Tuppurainen N, et al. Neonatal septicaemia in Finland 1981–85: predominance of *group B streptococcal* infections with very early onset. *Acta Paediatr Scand* 1989;78:44.

196. Sidebottom DG, Freeman J, Platt R, et al. Fifteen-year experience with bloodstream isolates of coagulase-negative staphylococci in neonatal intensive care. *J Clin Microbiol* 1988;26:713.

197. Freeman J, Epstein MF, Smith NE, et al. Extra hospital stay and antibiotic usage with nosocomial coagulase-negative staphylococcal bacteremia in two neonatal intensive care unit populations. *Am J Dis Child* 1990;144:324.

198. Baumgart S, Hall SE, Campos JM, Polin RA. Sepsis with coagulase-negative staphylococci in critically ill newborns. *Am J Dis Child* 1983;137:461.

199. Noel GJ, Edelson PJ. *Staphylococcus epidermidis* bacteremia in neonates: further observations and the occurrence of focal infection. *Pediatrics* 1984;74:832.

200. Hall RT, Hall SL, Barnes WG, et al. Characteristics of coagulase-negative staphylococci from infants with bacteremia. *Pediatr Infect Dis J* 1987;6:377.

201. Yeung C-Y, Lee H-C, Huang F-Y, Wang C-S. Sepsis during total parenteral nutrition: exploration of risk factors and determination of the effectiveness of peripherally inserted central venous catheters. *Pediatr Infect Dis J* 1998;17:135.

202. Gruskay J, Harris MC, Costarino AT, et al. Neonatal *Staphylococcus epidermidis* meningitis with unremarkable CSF examination results. *Am J Dis Child* 1989;143:580.

203. Gruskay JA, Abbasi S, Anday E, et al. *Staphylococcus epidermidis*-associated enterocolitis. *J Pediatr* 1986;109:520.

204. Mollitt DL, Tepas JJ, Talbert JL. The role of coagulase-negative Staphylococcus in neonatal necrotizing enterocolitis. *J Pediatr Surg* 1988;23:60.

205. Patrick CC, Kaplan SL, Baker CJ, et al. Persistent bacteremia due to coagulase-negative staphylococci in low birth weight neonates. *Pediatrics* 1989;84:977.

206. Noel GJ, O'Loughlin JE, Edelson PJ. Neonatal *Staphylococcus epidermidis* right-sided endocarditis: description of five catheterized infants. *Pediatrics* 1988;82:234.

207. Wagener MM, Rycheck RR, Yee RB, et al. Septic dermatitis of the neonatal scalp and maternal endomyometritis with intrapartum internal fetal monitoring. *Pediatrics* 1984;74:81.

208. Overturf GD, Balfour G. Osteomyelitis and sepsis: severe complications of fetal monitoring. *Pediatrics* 1975;55:244.

209. Spellerberg B, Steidel K, Lütticken R, Haase G. Isolation of *Staphylococcus caprae* from blood cultures of a neonate with congenital heart disease. *Eur J Clin Microbiol Infect Dis* 1998;17:61.

210. Freeman J, Goldmann DA, Smith NE, et al. Association of intravenous lipid emulsion and coagulase-negative staphylococcal bacteremia in neonatal intensive care units. *N Engl J Med* 1990;323:301.

211. Matrai-Kovalskis Y, Greenberg D, Shinwell ES, et al. Positive blood cultures for coagulase-negative staphylococci in neonates: does highly selective vancomycin usage affect outcome? *Infection* 1998;26:85.

212. Dunne WM Jr. Effects of subinhibitory concentrations of vancomycin or cefamandole on biofilm production by coagulase-negative staphylococci. *Antimicrob Agents Chemother* 1990;34:390.

213. Gray ED, Peters G, Verstegen M, Regelmann WE. Effect of extracellular slime substance from *Staphylococcus epidermidis* on the human cellular immune response. *Lancet* 1984;1:365.

214. Johnson GM, Lee DA, Regelmann WE, et al. Interference with granulocyte function by *Staphylococcus epidermidis* slime. *Infect Immun* 1986;54:13.

215. Fleer A, Gerards LJ, Aerts P, et al. Opsonic defense to *Staphylococcus epidermidis* in the premature neonate. *J Infect Dis* 1985;152:930.

216. Schutze GE, Hall MA, Baker CJ, Edwards MS. Role of neutrophil receptors in opsonophagocytosis of coagulase-negative staphylococci. *Infect Immun* 1991;59:2573.

217. Scheifele DW, Bjornson GL. Delta toxin activity in coagulase-negative staphylococci from the bowels of neonates. *J Clin Microbiol* 1988;26:279.

218. Scheifele DW, Bjornson GL, Dyer RA, Dimmick JE. Delta-like toxin produced by coagulase-negative staphylococci is associated with neonatal necrotizing enterocolitis. *Infect Immun* 1987;55:2268.

219. Scheifele DW. Role of bacterial toxins in neonatal necrotizing enterocolitis. *J Pediatr* 1990;117:S44.

220. Tappero JW, Schuchat A, Deaver KA, et al. Reduction in the incidence

of human listeriosis in the United States: effectiveness of prevention efforts? *JAMA* 1995;273:1118.

221. Gellin BG, Broome CV. Listeriosis. *JAMA* 1989;261:1313.

222. Southwick FS, Purich DL. Intracellular pathogenesis of listeriosis. *N Engl J Med* 1996;334:770.

223. Becroft DMO, Farmer K, Seddon RJ, et al. Epidemic listeriosis in the newborn. *BMJ* 1971;3:747.

224. Mulder CJJ, Zanen HC. *Listeria monocytogenes* neonatal meningitis in The Netherlands. *Eur J Pediatr* 1986;145:60.

225. Kessler SL, Dajani AS. Listeria meningitis in infants and children. *Pediatr Infect Dis J* 1990;9:61.

226. Schuchat A, Lizano C, Broome CV, et al. Outbreak of neonatal listeriosis associated with mineral oil. *Pediatr Infect Dis J* 1991;10:183.

227. Facinelli B, Varaldo PE, Casolari C, Fabio U. Cross-infection with *Listeria monocytogenes* confirmed by DNA fingerprinting. *Lancet* 1988;2:1247.

228. Farber JM, Peterkin PI, Carter AO, et al. Neonatal listeriosis due to cross-infection confirmed by isoenzyme typing and DNA fingerprinting. *J Infect Dis* 1991;163:927.

229. Visintine AM, Oleske JM, Nahmias AJ. *Listeria monocytogenes* infection in infants and children. *Am J Dis Child* 1977;131:393.

230. Bavikatte K, Schreiner RL, Lemons JA, Gresham EL. *Group D streptococcal* septicemia in the neonate. *Am J Dis Child* 1979;133:493.

231. Boulanger JM, Ford-Jones EL, Matlow AG. Enterococcal bacteremia in a pediatric institution: a four-year review. *Rev Infect Dis* 1991;13:847.

232. Coudron PE, Mayhall CG, Facklam RR, et al. *Streptococcus faecium* outbreak in a neonatal intensive care unit. *J Clin Microbiol* 1984;20:1044.

233. Dobson SRM, Baker CJ. Enterococcal sepsis in neonates: features by age at onset and occurrence of focal infection. *Pediatrics* 1990;85:165.

234. Rhinehart E, Smith NE, Wennersten C, et al. Rapid dissemination of β-lactamase-producing, aminoglycoside-resistant *Enterococcus faecalis* among patients and staff on an infant-toddler surgical ward. *N Engl J Med* 1990;323:1814.

235. Luginbuhl LM, Rotbart HA, Facklam RR, et al. Neonatal enterococcal sepsis: case-control study and description of an outbreak. *Pediatr Infect Dis J* 1987;6:1022.

236. Klare I, Rodloff AC, Wagner J, et al. Overproduction of a penicillin-binding protein is not the only mechanism of penicillin resistance in *Enterococcus faecium*. *Antimicrob Agents Chemother* 1992;36:783.

237. Patterson JE, Singh KV, Murray BE. Epidemiology of an endemic strain of β-lactamase-producing *Enterococcus faecalis*. *J Clin Microbiol* 1991;29:2513.

238. Sahm DF, Boonlayangoor S, Schulz JE. Detection of high-level aminoglycoside resistance in enterococci other than *Enterococcus faecalis*. *J Clin Microbiol* 1991;29:2595.

239. Kaplan AH, Gilligan PH, Facklam RR. Recovery of resistant enterococci during vancomycin prophylaxis. *J Clin Microbiol* 1988;26:1216.

240. Woodford N. Glycopeptide-resistant enterococci: a decade of experience. *J Med Microbiol* 1998;47:849.

241. Joseph TA, Pyati SP, Jacobs N. Neonatal early-onset *Escherichia coli* disease: the effect of intrapartum ampicillin. *Arch Pediatr Adolesc Med* 1998;152:35.

242. Towers CV, Carr MH, Padilla G, Asrat T. Potential consequences of widespread antepartal use of ampicillin. *Am J Obstet Gynecol* 1998;179:879.

243. Ghosal SP, Gupta PCS, Mukherjee AK, et al. Noma neonatorum: its aetiopathogenesis. *Lancet* 1978;2:289.

244. Quentin R, Martin C, Musser JM, et al. Genetic characterization of a cryptic genospecies of *Haemophilus* causing urogenital and neonatal infections. *J Clin Microbiol* 1993;31:1111.

245. Quentin R, Ruimy R, Rosenau A, et al. Genetic identification of cryptic genospecies of *Haemophilus* causing urogenital and neonatal infections by PCR using specific primers targeting genes coding for 16S rRNA. *J Clin Microbiol* 1996;34:1380.

246. Chow AW, Leake RD, Yamauchi T, et al. The significance of anaerobes in neonatal bacteremia: analysis of 23 cases and review of the literature. *Pediatrics* 1974;54:736.

247. Noel GJ, Laufer DA, Edelson PJ. Anaerobic bacteremia in a neonatal intensive care unit: an eighteen-year experience. *Pediatr Infect Dis J* 1988;7:858.

248. Brook I. *Pediatric anaerobic infection: diagnosis and management,* 2nd ed. St. Louis: CV Mosby, 1989:65.

249. Rønnestad A, Abrahamsen TG, Gaustad P, Finne PH. Blood culture isolates during 6 years in a tertiary neonatal intensive care unit. *Scand J Infect Dis* 1998;30:245.

250. Spark RP, Wike DA. Nontetanus clostridal neonatal fatality after home delivery. *Arizona Med* 1983;40:697.

251. Likitnukul S, Kusmiesz H, Nelson JD, McCracken GH Jr. Role of genital mycoplasmas in young infants with suspected sepsis. *J Pediatr* 1986;109:971.

252. Izraeli S, Samra Z, Sirota L, et al. Genital mycoplasmas in preterm infants: prevalence and clinical significance. *Eur J Pediatr* 1991;150:804.

253. Waites KB, Crouse DT, Philips JB III, et al. Ureaplasmal pneumonia and sepsis associated with persistent pulmonary hypertension of the newborn. *Pediatrics* 1989;83:79.

254. Baley JE. Neonatal candidiasis: the current challenge. *Clin Perinatol* 1991;18:263.

255. Sharp AM, Odds FC, Evans EGV. Candida strains from neonates in a special care baby unit. *Arch Dis Child* 1992;67:48.

256. Ng PC. Systemic fungal infections in neonates. *Arch Dis Child* 1994;71:F130.

257. Schwartz DA, Reef S. *Candida albicans* placentitis and *funisitis*: early diagnosis of congenital candidemia by histopathologic examination of umbilical cord vessels. *Pediatr Infect Dis J* 1990;9:661.

258. Santos LA, Beceiro J, Hernandez R, et al. Congenital cutaneous candidiasis: report of four cases and review of the literature. *Eur J Pediatr* 1991;150:336.

259. Kossoff EH, Buescher ES, Karlowicz MG. Candidemia in a neonatal intensive care unit: trends during fifteen years and clinical features of 111 cases. *Pediatr Infect Dis J* 1998;17:504.

260. Lee BE, Cheung P-Y, Robinson JL, et al. Comparative study of mortality and morbidity in premature infants (birth weight, <1,250 g) with candidemia or candidal meningitis. *Clin Infect Dis* 1998;27:559.

261. Faix RG, Kovarik SM, Shaw TR, Johnson RV. Mucocutaneous and invasive candidiasis among very low birth weight (<1,500 grams) infants in intensive care nurseries: a prospective study. *Pediatrics* 1989;83:101.

262. Wey SB, Mori M, Pfaller MA, et al. Risk factors for hospital-acquired candidemia: a matched case-control study. *Arch Intern Med* 1989;149:2349.

263. Rowen JL, Atkins JT, Levy ML, et al. Invasive fungal dermatitis in the ≤1000-gram neonate. *Pediatrics* 1995;95:682.

264. Faix RG. Invasive neonatal candidiasis: comparison of albicans and parapsilosis infection. *Pediatr Infect Dis J* 1992;11:88.

265. Sánchez PJ, Siegel JD, Fishbein J. Candida endocarditis: successful medical management in three preterm infants and review of the literature. *Pediatr Infect Dis J* 1991;10:239.

266. Zenker PN, Rosenberg EM, Van Dyke RB, et al. Successful medical treatment of presumed Candida endocarditis in critically ill infants. *J Pediatr* 1991;119:472.

267. Annable WL, Kachmer ML, DiMarco M, DeSantis D. Long-term follow-up of *Candida endophthalmitis* in the premature infant. *J Pediatr Ophthalmol Strabismus* 1990;27:103.

268. Goldsmith LS, Rubenstein SD, Wolfson BJ, et al. Cerebral calcifications in a neonate with candidiasis. *Pediatr Infect Dis J* 1990;9:451.

269. Baetz-Greenwalt B, Debaz B, Kumar ML. Bladder fungus ball: a reversible cause of neonatal obstructive uropathy. *Pediatrics* 1988;81:826.

270. Rehan VK, Davidson DC. Neonatal renal candidal bezoar. *Arch Dis Child* 1992;67:63.

271. Butler KM, Rench MA, Baker CJ. Amphotericin B as a single agent in the treatment of systemic candidiasis in neonates. *Pediatr Infect Dis J* 1990;9:51.

272. Ward RM, Sattler FR, Dalton AS Jr. Assessment of antifungal therapy in an 800-gram infant with candidal arthritis and osteomyelitis. *Pediatrics* 1983;72:234.

273. Marcon MJ, Powell DA. Human infections due to Malassezia spp. *Clin Microbiol Rev* 1992;5:101.

274. Chang HJ, Miller HL, Watkins N, et al. An epidemic of *Malassezia pachydermatis* in an intensive care nursery associated with colonization of health care workers' pet dogs. *N Engl J Med* 1998;338:706.

275. Henwick S, Henrickson K, Storgion SA, Leggiadro RJ. Disseminated neonatal Trichosporon beigelii. *Pediatr Infect Dis J* 1992;11:50.

276. Reich JD, Huddleston K, Jorgensen D, Berkowitz FE. Neonatal Torulopsis glabrata fungemia. *South Med J* 1997;90:246.

277. Sweet D, Reid M. Disseminated neonatal *Trichosporon beigelii* infection: successful treatment with liposomal amphotericin B. *J Infect* 1998;36:120.

278. Meessen NEL, Oberndorff KMEJ, Jacobs JA. Disseminated aspergillosis in a premature neonate. *J Hosp Infect* 1998;40:249.

279. Gerdes JS. Clinicopathologic approach to the diagnosis of neonatal sepsis. *Clin Perinatol* 1991;18:361.

280. Schelonka RL, Chai MK, Yoder BA, et al. Volume of blood required to detect common neonatal pathogens. *J Pediatr* 1996;129:275.

281. Wiswell TE, Hachey WE. Multiple site blood cultures in the initial evaluation for neonatal sepsis during the first week of life. *Pediatr Infect Dis J* 1991;10:365.

282. Phillips SE, Bradley JS. Bacteremia detected by lysis direct plating in a neonatal intensive care unit. *J Clin Microbiol* 1990;28:1.

283. St. Geme JW III, Bell LM, Baumgart S, et al. Distinguishing sepsis from blood culture contamination in young infants with blood cultures growing coagulase-negative staphylococci. *Pediatrics* 1990;86:157.

284. Evans ME, Schaffner W, Federspiel CF, et al. Sensitivity, specificity, and predictive value of body surface cultures in a neonatal intensive care unit. *JAMA* 1988;259:248.

285. Visser VE, Hall RT. Lumbar puncture in the evaluation of suspected neonatal sepsis. *J Pediatr* 1980;96:1063.

286. Fielkow S, Reuter S, Gotoff SP. Cerebrospinal fluid examination in symptom-free infants with risk factors for infection. *J Pediatr* 1991;119:971.

287. Weiss MG, Ionides SP, Anderson CL. Meningitis in premature infants with respiratory distress: role of admission lumbar puncture. *J Pediatr* 1991;119:973.

288. Schwersenski J, McIntyre L, Bauer CR. Lumbar puncture frequency and cerebrospinal fluid analysis in the neonate. *Am J Dis Child* 1991;145:54.

289. Kumar P, Sarkar S, Narang A. Role of routine lumbar puncture in neonatal sepsis. *J Paediatr Child Health* 1995;31:8.

290. Wiswell TE, Baumgart S, Gannon CM, Spitzer AR. No lumbar puncture in the evaluation for early neonatal sepsis: will meningitis be missed? *Pediatrics* 1995;95:803.

291. Joshi P, Barr P. The use of lumbar puncture and laboratory tests for sepsis by Australian neonatologists. *J Paediatr Child Health* 1998;34:74.

292. Manroe BL, Weinberg AG, Rosenfeld CR, Browne R. The neonatal blood count in health and disease. I. Reference values for neutrophilic cells. *J Pediatr* 1979;95:89.

293. Benuck I, David RJ. Sensitivity of published neutrophil indexes in identifying newborn infants with sepsis. *J Pediatr* 1983;103:961.

294. Carballo C, Foucar K, Swanson P, et al. Effect of high altitude on neutrophil counts in newborn infants. *J Pediatr* 1991;119:464.

295. Schelonka RL, Yoder BA, Hall RB, et al. Differentiation of segmented and band neutrophils during the early newborn period. *J Pediatr* 1995;127:298.

296. Greenberg DN, Yoder BA. Changes in the differential white blood cell count in screening for *group B streptococcal* sepsis. *Pediatr Infect Dis J* 1990;9:886.

297. Schouten-Van Meeteren NYN, Rietveld A, Moolenaar AJ, Van Bel F. Influence of perinatal conditions on C-reactive protein production. *J Pediatr* 1992;120:621.

298. Ehl S, Gering B, Bartmann P, et al. C-reactive protein is a useful marker for guiding duration of antibiotic therapy in suspected neonatal bacterial infection. *Pediatrics* 1997;99:216.

299. Lehrnbecher T, Schrod L, Rutsch P, et al. Immunologic parameters in cord blood indicating early-onset sepsis. *Biol Neonate* 1996;70:206.

300. Doellner H, Arntzen KJ, Haereid PE, et al. Interleukin-6 concentrations in neonates evaluated for sepsis. *J Pediatr* 1998;132:295.

301. Weimann E, Rutkowski S, Reisbach G. G-CSF, GM-CSF and IL-6 levels in cord blood: diminished increase of G-CSF and IL-6 in preterms with perinatal infection compared to term neonates. *J Perinat Med* 1998;26:211.

302. Küster H, Weiss M, Willeitner AE, et al. Interleukin-1 receptor antagonist and interleukin-6 for early diagnosis of neonatal sepsis 2 days before clinical manifestation. *Lancet* 1998;352:1271.

303. Chiesa C, Panero A, Rossi N, et al. Reliability of procalcitonin concentrations for the diagnosis of sepsis in critically ill neonates. *Clin Infect Dis* 1998;26:664.

304. Weirich E, Rabin RL, Maldonado Y, et al. Neutrophil CD11b expression as a diagnostic marker for early-onset neonatal infection. *J Pediatr* 1998;132:445.

305. Ascher DP, Wilson S, Fischer GW. Comparison of commercially available *group B streptococcal* latex agglutination assays. *J Clin Microbiol* 1991;29:2895.

306. Sánchez PJ, Siegel JD, Cushion NB, Threlkeld N. Significance of a positive urine *group B streptococcal* latex agglutination test in neonates. *J Pediatr* 1990;116:601.

307. Ascher DP, Wilson S, Mendiola J, Fischer GW. *Group B streptococcal* latex agglutination testing in neonates. *J Pediatr* 1991;119:458.

308. Mitsutake K, Miyazaki T, Tashiro T, et al. Enolase antigen, mannan antigen, Cand-Tec antigen, and β-glucan in patients with candidemia. *J Clin Microbiol* 1996;34:1918.

309. Schwalbe RS, Stapleton JT, Gilligan PH. Emergence of vancomycin resistance in coagulase-negative staphylococci. *N Engl J Med* 1987;316:927.

310. Tenover FC, Lancaster MV, Hill BC, et al. Characterization of staphylococci with reduced susceptibilities to vancomycin and other glycopeptides. *J Clin Microbiol* 1998;36:1020.

311. Smith TL, Pearson ML, Wilcox KR, et al. Emergence of vancomycin resistance in *Staphylococcus aureus*. *N Engl J Med* 1999;340:493.

312. Siegel JD, Shannon KM, DePasse BM. Recurrent infection associated with penicillin-tolerant *group B streptococci*: a report of two cases. *J Pediatr* 1981;99:920.

313. Eliopoulos GM. Vancomycin-resistant enterococci: mechanism and clinical relevance. *Infect Dis Clin North Am* 1997;11:851.

314. Waites KB, Crouse DT, Cassell GH. Antibiotic susceptibilities and therapeutic options for *Ureaplasma urealyticum* infections in neonates. *Pediatr Infect Dis J* 1992;11:23.

315. Rowen JL, Tate JM, for the Neonatal Candidiasis Study Group. Management of neonatal candidiasis. *Pediatr Infect Dis J* 1998;17:1007.

316. Baley JE, Meyers C, Kliegman RM, et al. Pharmacokinetics, outcome of treatment, and toxic effects of amphotericin B and 5-fluorocytosine in neonates. *J Pediatr* 1990;116:791.

317. Koren G, Lau A, Klein J, et al. Pharmacokinetics and adverse effects of amphotericin B in infants and children. *J Pediatr* 1988;113:559.

318. Conly J, Rennie R, Johnson J, et al. Disseminated candidiasis due to amphotericin B-resistant *Candida albicans*. *J Infect Dis* 1992;165:761.

319. Lackner H, Schwinger W, Urban C, et al. Liposomal amphotericin-B (AmBisome) for treatment of disseminated fungal infections in two infants of very low birth weight. *Pediatrics* 1992;89:1259.

320. Weitkamp J-H, Poets CF, Sievers R, et al. Candida infection in very low birth-weight infants: outcome and nephrotoxicity of treatment with liposomal amphotericin B (AmBisome®). *Infection* 1998;26:11.

321. Scarcella A, Pasquariello MB, Giugliano B, et al. Liposomal amphotericin B treatment for neonatal fungal infections. *Pediatr Infect Dis J* 1998;17:146.

322. Wong-Beringer A, Jacobs RA, Guglielmo BJ. Lipid formulations of amphotericin B: clinical efficacy and toxicities. *Clin Infect Dis* 1998;27:603.

323. Wiest DB, Fowler SL, Garner SS, Simons DR. Fluconazole in neonatal disseminated candidiasis. *Arch Dis Child* 1991;66:1002.

324. Huttova M, Hartmanova I, Kralinsky K, et al. *Candida fungemia* in neonates treated with fluconazole: report of forty cases, including eight with meningitis. *Pediatr Infect Dis J* 1998;17:1012.

325. Wenzl TG, Schefels J, Hörnchen H, Skopnik H. Pharmacokinetics of oral fluconazole in premature infants. *Eur J Pediatr* 1998;157:661.

326. Fishbein JD, Friedman HS, Bennett BB, Falletta JM. Catheter-related sepsis refractory to antibiotics treated successfully with adjunctive urokinase infusion. *Pediatr Infect Dis J* 1990;9:676.

327. Hocker JR, Simpson PM, Rabalais GP, et al. Extracorporeal membrane oxygenation and early-onset *group B streptococcal* sepsis. *Pediatrics* 1992;89:1.

328. McLaren RA, Chauhan SP, Gross TL. Intrapartum factors in early-onset *group B streptococcal* sepsis in term neonates: a case-control study. *Am J Obstet Gynecol* 1996;174:1934.

329. Peralta-Carcelen M, Fargason CA Jr, Coston D, Dolan JG. Preferences of pregnant women and physicians for 2 strategies for prevention of early-onset *group B streptococcal* sepsis in neonates. *Arch Pediatr Adolesc Med* 1997;151:712.

330. Rouse DJ, Andrews WW, Lin F-YC, et al. Antibiotic susceptibility profile of *group B Streptococcus* acquired vertically. *Obstet Gynecol* 1998;92:931.

331. Pearlman MD, Pierson CL, Faix RG. Frequent resistance of clinical *group B streptococci* isolates to clindamycin and erythromycin. *Obstet Gynecol* 1998;92:258.

332. Crisp BJ, Yancey MK, Uyehara C, Nauschuetz WF. Effect of delayed inoculation of selective media in antenatal detection of *group B streptococci*. *Obstet Gynecol* 1998;92:923.

333. de Cueto M, Sanchez M-J, Sampedro A, et al. Timing of intrapartum ampicillin and prevention of vertical transmission of *group B Streptococcus*. *Obstet Gynecol* 1998;91:112.

334. Smith AL. Neonatal bacterial meningitis. In: Scheld WM, Whitley RJ, Durack DT, eds. *Infections of the central nervous system*, 2nd ed. Philadelphia: Lippincott-Raven Publishers, 1997:313.

335. Bell WE, McGuinness GA. Suppurative central nervous system infections in the neonate. *Semin Perinatol* 1982;6:1.

336. Bingen E, Bonacorsi S, Brahimi N, et al. Virulence patterns of *Escherichia coli* K1 strains associated with neonatal meningitis. *J Clin Microbiol* 1997;35:2981.

337. Sáez-Llorens X, Ramilo O, Mustafa MM, et al. Molecular pathophysiology of bacterial meningitis: current concepts and therapeutic implications. *J Pediatr* 1990;116:671.

338. Ashwal S, Tomasi L, Schneider S, et al. Bacterial meningitis in children: pathophysiology and treatment. *Neurology* 1992;42:739.

339. Ahmed A, Hickey SM, Ehrett S, et al. Cerebrospinal fluid values in the term neonate. *Pediatr Infect Dis J* 1996;15:298.

340. Sarff LD, Platt LH, McCracken GH Jr. Cerebrospinal fluid evaluation in neonates: comparison of high-risk infants with and without meningitis. *J Pediatr* 1976;88:473.

341. Rodriguez AF, Kaplan SL, Mason EO Jr. Cerebrospinal fluid values in the very low birth weight infant. *J Pediatr* 1990;116:971.

342. Hall LMC, Duke B, Urwin G. An approach to the identification of the pathogens of bacterial meningitis by the polymerase chain reaction. *Eur J Clin Microbiol Infect Dis* 1995;14:1090.

343. Cherian T, Lalitha MK, Manoharan A, et al. PCR-enzyme immunoassay for detection of *Streptococcus pneumoniae* DNA in cerebrospinal fluid samples from patients with culture-negative meningitis. *J Clin Microbiol* 1998;36:3605.

344. McCracken GH Jr, Mize SG. A controlled study of intrathecal antibiotic therapy in gram-negative enteric meningitis of infancy: report of the Neonatal Meningitis Cooperative Study Group. *J Pediatr* 1976;89:66.

345. McCracken GH Jr, Mize SG, Threlkeld N. Intraventricular gentamicin therapy in gram-negative bacillary meningitis of infancy: report of the Second Neonatal Meningitis Cooperative Study Group. *Lancet* 1980;1:787.

346. Ahmed A, París MM, Trujillo M, et al. Once-daily gentamicin for experimental *Escherichia coli* meningitis. *Antimicrob Agents Chemother* 1997;41:49.

347. Kaplan SL, Patrick CC. Cefotaxime and aminoglycoside treatment of meningitis caused by gram-negative enteric organisms. *Pediatr Infect Dis J* 1990;9:810.

348. Mustafa MM, Mertsola J, Ramilo O, et al. Increased endotoxin and interleukin-1β concentrations in cerebrospinal fluid of infants with coliform meningitis and ventriculitis associated with intraventricular gentamicin therapy. *J Infect Dis* 1989;160:891.

349. Jafari HS, Sáez-Llorens X, Severien C, et al. Effects of antifungal therapy on inflammation, sterilization, and histology in experimental *Candida albicans* meningitis. *Antimicrob Agents Chemother* 1994;38:83.

350. Unhanand M, Mustafa MM, McCracken GH Jr, Nelson JD. Gram-negative enteric bacillary meningitis: a twenty-one-year experience. *J Pediatr* 1993;122:15.

351. Graham DR, Anderson RL, Ariel FE, et al. Epidemic nosocomial meningitis due to *Citrobacter diversus* in neonates. *J Infect Dis* 1981;144:203.

352. Foreman SD, Smith EE, Ryan NJ, Hogan GR. Neonatal *Citrobacter* meningitis: pathogenesis of cerebral abscess formation. *Ann Neurol* 1984;16:655.

353. Edwards MS, Rench MA, Haffar AAM, et al. Long-term sequelae of *group B streptococcal* meningitis in infants. *J Pediatr* 1985;106:717.

354. Wald ER, Bergman I, Taylor HG, et al. Long-term outcome of *group B streptococcal* meningitis. *Pediatrics* 1986;77:217.

355. Franco SM, Cornelius VE, Andrews BF. Long-term outcome of neonatal meningitis. *Am J Dis Child* 1992;146:567.

356. Brightman VJ, McNair Scott TF, Westphal M, Boggs TR. An outbreak of coxsackie B-5 virus infection in a newborn nursery. *J Pediatr* 1966;69:179.

357. Miller DG, Gabrielson MO, Bart KJ, et al. An epidemic of aseptic meningitis, primarily among infants, caused by echovirus 11-prime. *Pediatrics* 1968;41:77.

358. Dagan R, Jenista JA, Menegus MA. Association of clinical presentation, laboratory findings, and virus serotypes with the presence of meningitis in hospitalized infants with enterovirus infection. *J Pediatr* 1988;113:975.

359. Ahmed A, Brito F, Goto C, et al. Clinical utility of the polymerase chain reaction for diagnosis of enteroviral meningitis in infancy. *J Pediatr* 1997;131:393.

360. Sells CJ, Carpenter RL, Ray CG. Sequelae of central-nervous-system enterovirus infections. *N Engl J Med* 1975;293:1.

361. Wilfert CM, Thompson RJ Jr, Sunder TR, et al. Longitudinal assessment of children with enteroviral meningitis during the first three months of life. *Pediatrics* 1981;67:811.

362. Baker RC, Kummer AW, Schultz JR, et al. Neurodevelopmental outcome of infants with viral meningitis in the first three months of life. *Clin Pediatr (Phila)* 1996;35:295.

363. Ogden JA. Pathophysiology of neonatal osteomyelitis and septic arthritis. In: Polin RA, Fox WM, eds. *Fetal and neonatal physiology*, 2nd ed. Philadelphia: WB Saunders, 1998:2382.

364. Asmar BI. Osteomyelitis in the neonate. *Infect Dis Clin North Am* 1992;6:117.

365. Williams R, Kirkbride V, Corcoran GD. Neonatal osteomyelitis in Down's syndrome due to non-encapsulated *Haemophilus* influenzae. *J Infect* 1994;29:203.

366. Evdoridou J, Roilides E, Bibashi E, Kremenopoulos G. Multifocal osteoarthritis due to *Candida albicans* in a neonate: serum level monitoring of liposomal amphotericin B and literature review. *Infection* 1997;25:112.

367. Eisenstein EM, Gesundheit B. Neonatal hand abscess, osteomyelitis and meningitis caused by *Streptococcus pneumoniae*. *Pediatr Infect Dis J* 1998;17:760.

368. Ish-Horowicz MR, McIntyre P, Nade S. Bone and joint infections caused by multiply resistant *Staphylococcus aureus* in a neonatal intensive care unit. *Pediatr Infect Dis J* 1992;11:82.

369. Fox L, Sprunt K. Neonatal osteomyelitis. *Pediatrics* 1978;62:535.

370. Barton LL, Villar RG, Rice SA. Neonatal *group B streptococcal* vertebral osteomyelitis. *Pediatrics* 1996;98:459.

371. Mok PM, Reilly BJ, Ash JM. Osteomyelitis in the neonate. *Radiology* 1982;145:677.

372. Aigner RM, Fueger GF, Ritter G. Results of three-phase bone scintigraphy and radiography in 20 cases of neonatal osteomyelitis. *Nucl Med Commun* 1996;17:20.

373. Nelson JD. Antibiotic concentrations in septic joint effusions. *N Engl J Med* 1971;284:349.

374. Perkins MD, Edwards KM, Heller RM, Green NE. Neonatal *group B streptococcal* osteomyelitis and suppurative arthritis: outpatient therapy. *Clin Pediatr (Phila)* 1989;28:229.

375. Wopperer JM, White JJ, Gillespie R, Obletz BE. Long-term follow-up of infantile hip sepsis. *J Pediatr Orthop* 1988;8:322.

376. De Smet L, Gunst P, Fabry G. Acquired ulnar clubhand resulting from neonatal osteomyelitis. *J Pediatr Orthop B* 1998;7:77.

377. Bos CFA, Mol LJCD, Obermann WR, Tjin a Ton ER. Late sequelae of neonatal septic arthritis of the shoulder. *J Bone Joint Surg Br* 1998;80:645.

378. Ladhani S, Bhutta ZA. Neonatal Pseudomonas putida infection presenting as staphylococcal scalded skin syndrome. *Eur J Clin Microbiol Infect Dis* 1998;17:642.

379. Weinberger M, Haynes RE, Morse TS. Necrotizing fasciitis in a neonate. *Am J Dis Child* 1972;123:591.

380. Ramamurthy RS, Srinivasan G, Jacobs NM. Necrotizing fasciitis and necrotizing cellulitis due to *group B streptococcus*. *Am J Dis Child* 1977;131:1169.

381. Wilson HD, Haltalin KC. Acute necrotizing fasciitis in childhood: report of 11 cases. *Am J Dis Child* 1973;125:591.

382. Bliss DP, Healey PJ, Waldhausen JHT. Necrotizing fasciitis after Plastibell circumcision. *J Pediatr* 1997;131:459.

383. Bodemer C, Panhans A, Chretien-Marquet B, et al. Staphylococcal necrotizing fasciitis in the mammary region in childhood: a report of five cases. *J Pediatr* 1997;131:466.

384. Quinonez JM, Steele RW. Necrotizing fasciitis. *Semin Pediatr Infect Dis* 1997;8:207.

385. Chen JW, Broadbent RS, Thomson IA. Staphylococcal neonatal

necrotising fasciitis: survival without radical debridement. *N Z Med J* 1998;111:251.

386. Rudoy RC, Nelson JD. Breast abscess during the neonatal period: a review. *Am J Dis Child* 1975;129:1031.

387. Brook I. The aerobic and anaerobic microbiology of neonatal breast abscess. *Pediatr Infect Dis J* 1991;10:785.

388. Plavidal FJ, Werch A. Fetal scalp abscess secondary to intrauterine monitoring. *Am J Obstet Gynecol* 1976;125:65.

389. Plavidal FJ, Werch A. Gonococcal fetal scalp abscess: a case report. *Am J Obstet Gynecol* 1977;127:437.

390. Mitchell SJ, Gray J, Morgan MEI, et al. Nosocomial infection with Rhizopus microsporus in preterm infants: association with wooden tongue depressors. *Lancet* 1996;348:441.

391. Linder N, Keller N, Huri C, et al. Primary cutaneous mucormycosis in a premature infant: case report and review of the literature. *Am J Perinatol* 1998;15:35.

392. Weston WL, Morelli JG. Neonatal tinea capitis. *Pediatr Infect Dis J* 1998;17:257.

393. Lund CH, Nonato LB, Kuller JM, et al. Disruption of barrier function in neonatal skin associated with adhesive removal. *J Pediatr* 1997; 131:367.

394. Nelson JD, Peters PC. Suprapubic aspiration of urine in premature and term infants. *Pediatrics* 1965;36:132.

395. Israele V, Darabi A, McCracken GH Jr. The role of bacterial virulence factors and Tamm-Horsfall protein in the pathogenesis of *Escherichia coli* urinary tract infection in infants. *Am J Dis Child* 1987;141:1230.

396. Hitchcock RJI, Pallett A, Hall MA, Malone PSJ. Urinary tract candidiasis in neonates and infants. *Br J Urol* 1995;76:252.

397. Nebigil I, Tümer N. Asymptomatic urinary tract infection in childhood. *Eur J Pediatr* 1992;151:308.

398. Bergström T, Larson H, Lincoln K, Winberg J. Studies of urinary tract infections in infancy and childhood. XII. Eighty consecutive patients with neonatal infection. *J Pediatr* 1972;80:858.

399. Leung AKC, Robson WLM. Urinary tract infection in infancy and childhood. *Adv Pediatr* 1991;38:257.

400. Verma RP, Pizzica A. Early neonatal urinary tract infection: a case report and review. *J Perinatol* 1998;18:480.

401. Anderson PAM, Rickwood AMK. Features of primary vesicoureteric reflux detected by prenatal sonography. *Br J Urol* 1991;67:267.

402. Roberts JA. Neonatal circumcision: an end to the controversy? *South Med J* 1996;89:167.

403. Crain EF, Gershel JC. Urinary tract infections in febrile infants younger than 8 weeks of age. *Pediatrics* 1990;86:363.

404. Hansson S, Brandström P, Jodal U, Larsson P. Low bacterial counts in infants with urinary tract infection. *J Pediatr* 1998;132:180.

405. Barkemeyer BM. Suprapubic aspiration of urine in very low birth weight infants. *Pediatrics* 1993;92:457.

406. Ginsburg CM, McCracken GH Jr. Urinary tract infections in young infants. *Pediatrics* 1982;69:409.

407. Wong-Beringer A, Jacobs RA, Guglielmo J. Treatment of funguria. *JAMA* 1992;267:2780.

408. Benador D, Benador N, Slosman DO, et al. Cortical scintigraphy in the evaluation of renal parenchymal changes in children with pyelonephritis. *J Pediatr* 1994;124:17.

409. Bourchier D, Abbott GD, Maling TMJ. Radiological abnormalities in infants with urinary tract infections. *Arch Dis Child* 1984;59:620.

410. Feld LG, Greenfield SP, Ogra PL. Urinary tract infections in infants and children. *Pediatr Rev* 1989;11:71.

411. Hellström M, Jacobsson B, Jodal U, et al. Renal growth after neonatal urinary tract infection. *Pediatr Nephrol* 1987;1:269.

412. Dick PT, Feldman W. Routine diagnostic imaging for childhood urinary tract infections: a systematic overview. *J Pediatr* 1996;128:15.

413. Devriendt K, Groenen P, Van Esch H, et al. Vesico-ureteral reflux: a genetic condition? *Eur J Pediatr* 1998;157:265.

414. Armstrong JH, Zacarias F, Rein MF. Ophthalmia neonatorum: a chart review. *Pediatrics* 1976;57:884.

415. Centers for Disease Control and Prevention. Increasing incidence of gonorrhea-Minnesota, 1994. *MMWR* 1995;44:282.

416. Laga M, Naamara W, Brunham RC, et al. Single-dose therapy of gonococcal ophthalmia neonatorum with ceftriaxone. *N Engl J Med* 1986;315:1382.

417. Bell TA, Grayston JT, Krohn MA, et al. Randomized trial of silver nitrate, erythromycin, and no eye prophylaxis for the prevention of conjunctivitis among newborns not at risk for gonococcal ophthalmitis. *Pediatrics* 1993;92:755.

418. Isenberg SJ, Apt L, Wood M. A controlled trial of povidone-iodine as prophylaxis against ophthalmia neonatorum. *N Engl J Med* 1995; 332:562.

419. Rapoza PA, Quinn TC, Kiessling LA, et al. Assessment of neonatal conjunctivitis with a direct immunofluorescent monoclonal antibody stain for *Chlamydia*. *JAMA* 1986;255:3369.

420. Shah SS, Gallagher PG. Complications of conjunctivitis caused by *Pseudomonas aeruginosa* in a newborn intensive care unit. *Pediatr Infect Dis J* 1998;17:97.

421. Burns RP, Rhodes DH Jr. Pseudomonas eye infection as a cause of death in premature infants. *Arch Ophthalmol* 1961;65:517.

422. Rowe DS, Aicardi EZ, Dawson CR, Schachter J. Purulent ocular discharge in neonates: significance of *Chlamydia trachomatis*. *Pediatrics* 1979;63:628.

423. Talley AR, Garcia-Ferrer F, Laycock KA, et al. Comparative diagnosis of neonatal chlamydial conjunctivitis by polymerase chain reaction and McCoy cell culture. *Am J Ophthalmol* 1994;117:50.

424. Hammerschlag MR, Roblin PM, Gelling M, et al. Use of polymerase chain reaction for the detection of *Chlamydia trachomatis* in ocular and nasopharyngeal specimens from infants with conjunctivitis. *Pediatr Infect Dis J* 1997;16:293.

425. Centers for Disease Control and Prevention. 1998 Guidelines for treatment of sexually transmitted diseases. *MMWR* 1998;47(RR-1):65.

426. Golden B. SubTenon injection of gentamicin for bacterial infections of the eye. *J Infect Dis* 1971;124:S271.

427. Patamasucon P, Rettig PJ, Faust KL, et al. Oral v topical erythromycin therapies for chlamydial conjunctivitis. *Am J Dis Child* 1982;136:817.

428. Hammerschlag MR, Gelling M, Roblin PM, et al. Treatment of neonatal chlamydial conjunctivitis with azithromycin. *Pediatr Infect Dis J* 1998;17:1049.

429. Haffejee IE. The epidemiology of rotavirus infections: a global perspective. *J Pediatr Gastroenterol Nutr* 1995;20:275.

430. Champsaur H, Questiaux E, Prevot J, et al. Rotavirus carriage, asymptomatic infection, and disease in the first two years of life. I. Virus shedding. *J Infect Dis* 1984;149:667.

431. Riedel F, Kroener T, Stein K, et al. Rotavirus infection and bradycardia-apnoea-episodes in the neonate. *Eur J Pediatr* 1996;155:36.

432. Foldenauer A, Voβbeck S, Pohlandt F. Neonatal hypocalcaemia associated with rotavirus diarrhoea. *Eur J Pediatr* 1998;157:838.

433. Nataro JP, Kaper JB. Diarrheagenic *Escherichia coli*. *Clin Microbiol Rev* 1998;11:142.

434. Boyer KM, Petersen NJ, Farzaneh I, et al. An outbreak of gastroenteritis due to *E. coli* 0142 in a neonatal nursery. *J Pediatr* 1975;86:919.

435. Lyerly DM, Krivan HC, Wilkins TD. Clostridium difficile: its disease and toxins. *Clin Microbiol Rev* 1988;1:1.

436. Haltalin KC. Neonatal shigellosis: report of 16 cases and review of the literature. *Am J Dis Child* 1967;114:603.

437. Wong S-N, Tam AY-C, Yuen K-Y. Campylobacter infection in the neonate: case report and review of the literature. *Pediatr Infect Dis J* 1990;9:665.

438. Reina J, Borrell N, Fiol M. Rectal bleeding caused by *Campylobacter jejuni* in a neonate. *Pediatr Infect Dis J* 1992;11:500.

439. Paisley JW, Lauer BA. Neonatal *Yersinia enterocolitica* enteritis. *Pediatr Infect Dis J* 1992;11:331.

440. Freij BJ. Aeromonas: biology of the organism and diseases in children. *Pediatr Infect Dis* 1984;3:164.

441. Nelson JD. Duration of neomycin therapy for enteropathogenic *Escherichia coli* diarrheal disease: a comparative study of 113 cases. *Pediatrics* 1971;48:248.

442. DiNicola AF. *Campylobacter jejuni* diarrhea in a 3-day-old male neonate. *Am J Dis Child* 1986;140:191.

443. Berger A, Salzer HR, Weninger M, et al. Septicaemia in an Austrian neonatal intensive care unit: a 7-year analysis. *Acta Paediatr* 1998;87:1066.

444. Kinney JS, Eiden JJ. Enteric infectious disease in neonates: epidemiology, pathogenesis, and a practical approach to evaluation and therapy. *Clin Perinatol* 1994;21:317.

445. Rotbart HA, Levin MJ, Yolken RH, et al. An outbreak of rotavirus-associated neonatal necrotizing enterocolitis. *J Pediatr* 1983;103:454.

446. American Academy of Pediatrics, Committee on Infectious Diseases. Prevention of rotavirus disease: guidelines for use of rotavirus vaccine. *Pediatrics* 1998;102:1483.

447. Abzug MJ, Beam AC, Gyorkos EA, Levin MJ. Viral pneumonia in the first month of life. *Pediatr Infect Dis J* 1990;9:881.
448. Tipple MA, Beem MO, Saxon EM. Clinical characteristics of the afebrile pneumonia associated with *Chlamydia trachomatis* infection in infants less than 6 months of age. *Pediatrics* 1979;63:192.
449. Colarizi P, Chiesa C, Pacifico L, et al. *Chlamydia trachomatis*-associated respiratory disease in the very early neonatal period. *Acta Paediatr* 1996;85:991.
450. Niida Y, Numazaki K, Ikehata M, et al. Two full-term infants with *Chlamydia trachomatis* pneumonia in the early neonatal period. *Eur J Pediatr* 1998;157:950.
451. Attenburrow AA, Barker CM. Chlamydial pneumonia in the low birthweight neonate. *Arch Dis Child* 1985;60:1169.
452. Numazaki K, Chiba S, Kogawa K, et al. Chronic respiratory disease in premature infants caused by *Chlamydia trachomatis*. *J Clin Pathol* 1986;39:84.
453. Weiss SG, Newcomb RW, Beem MO. Pulmonary assessment of children after chlamydial pneumonia of infancy. *J Pediatr* 1986;108:659.
454. Walsh WF, Stanley S, Lally KP, et al. *Ureaplasma urealyticum* demonstrated by open lung biopsy in newborns with chronic lung disease. *Pediatr Infect Dis J* 1991;10:823.
455. Wang EEL, Ohlsson A, Kellner JD. Association of *Ureaplasma urealyticum* colonization with chronic lung disease of prematurity: results of a metaanalysis. *J Pediatr* 1995;127:640.
456. Alfa MJ, Embree JE, Degagne P, et al. Transmission of *Ureaplasma urealyticum* from mothers to full and preterm infants. *Pediatr Infect Dis J* 1995;14:341.
457. Pacifico L, Panero A, Roggini M, et al. *Ureaplasma urealyticum* and pulmonary outcome in a neonatal intensive care population. *Pediatr Infect Dis J* 1997;16:579.
458. Bhandari V, Hussain N, Rosenkrantz T, Kresch M. Respiratory tract colonization with mycoplasma species increases the severity of bronchopulmonary dysplasia. *J Perinat Med* 1998;26:37.
459. Patterson AM, Taciak V, Lovchik J, et al. *Ureaplasma urealyticum* respiratory tract colonization is associated with an increase in interleukin 1-beta and tumor necrosis factor alpha relative to interleukin 6 in tracheal aspirates of preterm infants. *Pediatr Infect Dis J* 1998;17:321.
460. Gajdusek DC. *Pneumocystis carinii*—etiologic agent of interstitial plasma cell pneumonia of premature and young infants. *Pediatrics* 1957;19:543.
461. Beach RS, Garcia ER, Sosa R, Good RA. *Pneumocystis carinii* pneumonia in a human immunodeficiency virus 1-infected neonate with meconium aspiration. *Pediatr Infect Dis J* 1991;10:953.
462. Panero A, Roggini M, Papoff P, et al. *Pneumocystis carinii* pneumonia in preterm infants: report of two cases successfully diagnosed by non-bronchoscopic bronchoalveolar lavage. *Acta Paediatr* 1995;84:1309.
463. Famiglietti RF, Bakerman PR, Saubolle MA, Rudinsky M. Cavitary legionellosis in two immunocompetent infants. *Pediatrics* 1997;99: 899.
464. Levy I, Rubin LG. *Legionella pneumonia* in neonates: a literature review. *J Perinatol* 1998;18:287.
465. Paisley JW, Lauer BA, Melinkovich P, et al. Rapid diagnosis of *Chlamydia trachomatis* pneumonia in infants by direct immunofluorescence microscopy of nasopharyngeal secretions. *J Pediatr* 1986; 109:653.
466. Abele-Horn M, Wolff C, Dressel P, et al. Polymerase chain reaction versus culture for detection of *Ureaplasma urealyticum* and *Mycoplasma hominis* in the urogenital tract of adults and the respiratory tract of newborns. *Eur J Clin Microbiol Infect Dis* 1996;15: 595.
467. Matlow AG, Nelson S, Wray R, Cox P. Nosocomial acquisition of pertussis diagnosed by polymerase chain reaction. *Infect Control Hosp Epidemiol* 1997;18:715.
468. Haney PJ, Bohlman M, Sun C-CJ. Radiographic findings in neonatal pneumonia. *AJR* 1984;143:23.
469. Freij BJ, Kusmiesz H, Nelson JD, McCracken GH Jr. Parapneumonic effusions and empyema in hospitalized children: a retrospective review of 227 cases. *Pediatr Infect Dis* 1984;3:578.
470. Berman SA, Balkany TJ, Simmons MA. Otitis media in the neonatal intensive care unit. *Pediatrics* 1978;62:198.
471. deSa DJ. Mucosal metaplasia and chronic inflammation in the middle ear of infants receiving intensive care in the neonatal period. *Arch Dis Child* 1983;58:24.
472. Eavey RD. Abnormalities of the neonatal ear: otoscopic observations, histologic observations, and a model for contamination of the middle ear by cellular contents of amniotic fluid. *Laryngoscope* 1993;103[1 Pt 2 Suppl 58]:1.
473. Burton DM, Seid AB, Kearns DB, Pransky SM. Neonatal otitis media: an update. *Arch Otolaryngol Head Neck Surg* 1993;119:672.
474. Marchant CD, Shurin PA, Turczyk VA, et al. Course and outcome of otitis media in early infancy: a prospective study. *J Pediatr* 1984;104: 826.
475. Tetzlaff TR, Ashworth C, Nelson JD. Otitis media in children less than 12 weeks of age. *Pediatrics* 1977;59:827.
476. Bland RD. Otitis media in the first six weeks of life: diagnosis, bacteriology, and management. *Pediatrics* 1972;49:187.
477. Shurin PA, Howie VM, Pelton SI, et al. Bacterial etiology of otitis media during the first six weeks of life. *J Pediatr* 1978;92:893.
478. Parker PC, Boles RG. *Pseudomonas otitis* media and bacteremia following a water birth. *Pediatrics* 1997;99:653.
479. Arriaga MA, Bluestone CD, Stool SE. The role of tympanocentesis in the management of infants with sepsis. *Laryngoscope* 1989;99:1048.
480. Bell MJ. Peritonitis in the newborn—current concepts. *Pediatr Clin North Am* 1985;32:1181.
481. Freij BJ, Votteler TP, McCracken GH Jr. Primary peritonitis in previously healthy children. *Am J Dis Child* 1984;138:1058.
482. Duggan MB, Khwaja MS. Neonatal primary peritonitis in Nigeria. *Arch Dis Child* 1975;50:130.
483. Genta VM, Gilligan PH, McCarthy LR. *Clostridium difficile* peritonitis in a neonate: a case report. *Arch Pathol Lab Med* 1984;108:82.
484. Aronoff SC, Olson MM, Gauderer MWL, et al. *Pseudomonas aeruginosa* as a primary pathogen in children with bacterial peritonitis. *J Pediatr Surg* 1987;22:861.
485. Mollitt DL, Tepas JJ III, Talbert JL. The microbiology of neonatal peritonitis. *Arch Surg* 1988;123:176.
486. Kaplan M, Eidelman AI, Dollberg L, Abu-Dalu K. Necrotizing bowel disease with *Candida peritonitis* following severe neonatal hypothermia. *Acta Paediatr Scand* 1990;79:876.
487. Fonkalsrud EW, Ellis DG, Clatworthy HW Jr. Neonatal peritonitis. *J Pediatr Surg* 1966;1:227.

CHAPTER 49

Neurological and Neuromuscular Disorders

Alan Hill and Joseph J. Volpe

In the context of dramatic improvements in obstetric care and in the treatment of neonatal respiratory disorders and infection, neurologic problems remain a major cause of morbidity and mortality in the newborn. In this chapter, an approach to the neurologic assessment of the newborn is outlined, and practical aspects of diagnosis and management of the most common neurologic and neuromuscular problems of the newborn are reviewed (e.g., seizures, hypoxic–ischemic cerebral injury, intracranial hemorrhage, traumatic birth injury, spinal muscular atrophy, muscular dystrophies and myopathies). Major bacterial and viral infections, metabolic derangements that affect the central nervous system, and cerebral dysgenesis are discussed in other chapters.

NEUROLOGIC EVALUATION OF THE NEWBORN

History and Physical Examination

The importance of a detailed history and neurologic examination for assessment of the newborn with suspected neurologic problems cannot be overemphasized (1). Such history must include details of the family history and complications encountered during pregnancy, labor, and delivery, because many neurologic abnormalities that present during the neonatal period actually originate antenatally. Detailed discussion of advances in the fetal assessment are outside the scope of this chapter and have been reviewed elsewhere (2).

The format of the neurologic examination in the newborn is similar to that used in older patients. However, observations must be interpreted in the context of the

A. Hill: Department of Pediatrics, University of British Columbia; and Division of Neurology, Department of Pediatrics, British Columbia's Children Hospital, Vancouver, British Columbia, Canada

J. J. Volpe: Department of Neurology, Harvard Medical School; and Children's Hospital, Boston, Massachusetts

level of cerebral maturation at different gestational ages. The examination should not be prolonged unnecessarily in order to avoid hypoxemia and fluctuations in arterial blood pressure that may be associated even with routine handling, especially in premature newborns.

Neurologic observations also are influenced considerably by the level of alertness of the infant. After 28 weeks of gestation, infants are able to awaken spontaneously or may be roused for several minutes by stimulation. Distinct sleep–wake patterns may be recognized by 40 weeks of gestation.

In an examination of the cranial nerves, pupillary constriction to light and the blink reflex may be elicited as early as 28 weeks of gestation. Pupillary responses are consistent by 31 to 32 weeks. Consistent visual tracking of a bright light and opticokinetic nystagmus can be elicited consistently in the awake infant at term. Fundoscopy may reveal retinal hemorrhages in 20% to 50% of newborns following vaginal delivery, but these rarely indicate significant central nervous system injury. Dysconjugate and jerky eye movements are common in premature infants and may persist to some extent for several months after term. Full extraocular eye movements to doll's-head maneuver or to caloric stimulation may be elicited after 32 weeks of gestation. Facial muscle weakness may be of central or peripheral origin. Hearing may be difficult to assess, although infants startle to loud noises as early as 28 weeks of gestation. The act of feeding requires coordination of breathing, sucking, and swallowing, which involve principally cranial nerves V, VII, IX, X, and XII.

The major features of the motor examination include evaluation of limb posture, spontaneous and elicited movements, muscle power, tendon reflexes, and primitive neonatal reflexes. Muscle tone may be assessed by careful observation of the infant's resting posture during various maneuvers of passive manipulation. With increasing gestational age, there is development of predominance of flexor tone in all limbs. Asymmetry of muscle tone and spontaneous limb movements may indicate focal cerebral lesions or peripheral injury, e.g., brachial plexus injury. Tendon reflexes are elicited readily in the term newborn. Undue emphasis should not be placed on brisk tendon reflexes, ankle clonus, or crossed adductor responses in the absence of other corroborative abnormal neurologic signs.

Careful evaluation of sensory function is particularly important in the evaluation of spinal cord or peripheral nerve injury. A useful aspect of sensory evaluation is determining habituation, i.e., the normal dampening of responses to multiple (e.g., 5 to 10) stimulations. Habituation indicates a high level of response that appears to require input from cerebral hemispheres. It is characteristically absent in anencephalic infants.

Neurodiagnostic Techniques

Because the neurologic examination is often limited by concomitant systemic illness and the requirement for complex life-support systems, especially in premature infants, a variety of noninvasive neurodiagnostic techniques often are used as adjunctive methods for the evaluation of neurologic problems. The clinical applications of various techniques will be discussed in the context of specific neurologic conditions.

NEONATAL SEIZURES

Seizures are a common manifestation of serious central nervous system disease in the newborn. Prompt diagnosis and intervention are indicated because seizures indicate serious underlying disease and may interfere with supportive care, e.g., ventilation and alimentation (1,3). Experimental animal studies suggest that neonatal seizures may have a deleterious effect on the developing brain, depleting cerebral glucose levels, which, in turn, may interfere with DNA synthesis, glial proliferation, differentiation, and myelination (4,5). Although the relevance of data from experimental animal studies to the human newborn is not entirely clear, the significance of

neonatal seizures has been corroborated by *in vivo* studies with magnetic resonance spectroscopy (MRS) (6). In terms of management, the possible detrimental effects of neonatal seizures must be balanced against the potentially deleterious effects of anticonvulsants on behavior and learning in the developing brain (7).

Clinical Features

Neonatal seizures differ considerably from seizures observed in older children, principally because the immature brain is less capable of propagating generalized or organized electrical discharges. The principal types of neonatal seizures are summarized in Table 49–1 (8). Although individual seizure types are not indicative of specific varieties of brain injury, certain seizure types are associated more commonly with some conditions. For example, generalized tonic seizures, which may represent brainstem release phenomena or posturing, have been observed with major germinal matrix hemorrhage/intraventricular hemorrhage (GMH/IVH) (9). Focal clonic seizures may be associated with focal cerebral infarction or traumatic cerebral contusion.

Differentiation of seizures from nonepileptic movements may be difficult in the newborn. Clonic seizures may be particularly difficult to differentiate clinically from jitterinesss or tremulousness, particularly because both occur frequently in similar clinical contexts, e.g., hypoxic–ischemic encephalopathy, metabolic derangements, and drug withdrawal. However, jitteriness is classified as a movement disorder that may be associated with good outcome. Benign jitteriness often resolves within weeks. The distinction between jitteriness and seizures may be made clinically as follows:

- Jitteriness is not accompanied by abnormal eye movements.
- Jitteriness may be spontaneous or stimulus sensitive.
- The flexion and extension phases of the tremor are equal in amplitude compared to the unequal phases observed with clonic seizure movements.

TABLE 49–1. *Clinical features of neonatal seizures*

Seizure type	Major clinical manifestations
Subtle	Repetitive blinking, eye deviation, staring
	Repetitive mouth or tongue movements
	Apnea
	Bicycling–rowing movements
Tonic (i.e., generalized or focal)	Tonic extension of limb or limbs
	Tonic flexion of upper limbs, extension of lower limbs
Clonic (i.e., multifocal or focal)	Multifocal, synchronous, or asynchronous limb movements
	Repetitive, jerky limb movements
	Nonordered progression
	Localized repetitive clonic limb movements with preservation of consciousness
Myoclonic (i.e., generalized, focal, multifocal)	Single or several flexion jerks of upper limbs (common) and lower limbs (rare)

- Jitteriness may be stopped by passive flexion or repositioning of the affected body part.

Benign neonatal sleep myoclonus occurs during active sleep in healthy premature and term newborns. Myoclonus may be florid and consists of either bilateral synchronous or asynchronous or asymmetric movements that are not stimulus sensitive, but which cease on arousal from sleep. They are not associated with epileptiform or background disturbances on the electroencephalogram (EEG). Benign sleep myoclonus usually resolves over several months (10).

Infants with severe dysfunction of the central nervous system may have stimulus-sensitive myoclonus, which may be associated with spike or sharp wave discharges on the EEG (9).

Simultaneous video and EEG monitoring has raised major issues concerning the incidence, classification, pathophysiology, and management of neonatal seizures. Some stereotypic, paroxysmal clinical phenomena, e.g., oral-buccal-lingual movements, generalized tonic, or extensor posturing are not associated consistently with epileptiform discharges on EEG recordings performed using surface electrodes. Subtle clinical phenomena correlate more frequently with simultaneous abnormal EEG discharges in premature than in term newborns (3,9, 11,12).

Etiology

Neonatal seizures are rarely idiopathic in origin. Thus, when neonatal seizures occur, immediate attention must be directed toward the identification of an underlying etiology in order to permit rapid and appropriate intervention (when available) as well as meaningful prediction of outcome. Although neonatal seizures may be due to numerous underlying causes, most result from a relatively few causes, e.g., hypoxic–ischemic cerebral injury, intracranial hemorrhage, or metabolic derangements. The most important causes of neonatal seizures and their prognostic significance are listed in order of relative frequency in Table 49–2.

Seizures are a distinctly uncommon manifestation of withdrawal from passive addiction to narcotics, e.g., heroin, methadone, or barbiturates. In contrast, maternal cocaine abuse may be associated more commonly with epileptiform EEG abnormalities or seizures in newborns exposed *in utero* or by breast-feeding. This may relate to direct neuronal excitotoxicity, teratogenic effects, or destructive ischemic and hemorrhagic lesions (1).

Rarely, intoxication with local anaesthetic may result in severe but self-limited neonatal seizures, after inadvertent injection into the infant's scalp during placement of pudendal, paracervical, or epidural blocks (13). Characteristically, severe, tonic seizures begin during the first hours of life, associated with apnea and severe hypoventilation, bradycardia, hypotonia, fixed and dilated pupils, and absence of extraocular movements in response to the doll's-head maneuver. The latter two features are useful for distinguishing anaesthetic intoxication from hypoxic–ischemic encephalopathy. Evaluation involves careful inspection of the scalp for evidence of injection. Management consists of vigorous support and removal of the drug by diuresis.

In addition to the underlying etiologies listed in Table 49–2, there are at least four recognized epilepsy syndromes that may present during the newborn period. These include two benign syndromes, i.e., "fifth day fits" and benign familial neonatal seizures. The latter often present as frequent seizures on the third day of life and usually are linked to autosomal dominant gene loci on chromosomes 20 or 8 (14,15). In addition, there are two severe epilepsy syndromes. Early myoclonic encephalopathy presents within hours of birth with severe, fragmentary, refractory myoclonus, which often is worsened by handling or stimulation. Infants often have a high-arched palate. The initial neuroimaging is normal, but diffuse cerebral atrophy develops and affected infants fre-

TABLE 49–2. *Etiology and prognosis of neonatal seizures*

Etiology	Gestational age		Time of onset (d of age)		Outcome normal (%)
	Premature	Term	0–3	4–10	
Hypoxic–ischemic encephalopathy	+	+	+		50
Intracranial hemorrhage					
Intraventricular hemorrhage	+	−	+		<10
Subarachnoid hemorrhage	−	+	+		90
Hypoglycemia	+	+	+		50
Infection	+	+		+	<50
Cerebral dysgenesis	+	+		+	0
Hypocalcemia					
Early onset	+	+	+		50
Late onset	−	+		+	100

+, common; −, rare.
Adapted from ref. 1.

quently die in the first 2 years of life. Another entity, early infantile epileptic encephalopathy, also termed "Ohtahara's syndrome," may present with structural cerebral lesions (dysgenesis or destruction) and a severe burst-suppression pattern on the EEG.

Diagnosis

Diagnostic evaluation must begin with a careful history and physical examination. Obtaining maternal history of possible drug abuse, intrauterine infection, and genetic or metabolic conditions is critical, and it should be obtained directly from the mother whenever possible.

Although the EEG may be useful for confirmation of suspected seizures and for establishment of prognosis, it is rarely helpful for the identification of a specific etiology. Continuous EEG monitoring may be of value for identifying seizures in patients who are paralyzed pharmacologically or those who have electrographic seizures only.

Initial laboratory investigations should address potentially treatable causes (e.g., hypoglycemia, hypocalcemia, hypomagnesemia). Lumbar puncture may identify intracranial infection or hemorrhage. If the initial screening investigations fail to identify a specific etiology, additional studies should be considered, including neuroimaging, metabolic investigations, e.g., serum amino acids, lactate, ammonia, urine organic acids, screening for drugs, and investigation for congenital viral infections. In many instances, several underlying factors may be operative in the same patient.

Treatment

Treatment of neonatal seizures is directed toward minimizing physiologic and metabolic derangements and preventing the recurrence of seizures. This should involve immediate support of ventilation and perfusion, if required, as well as correction of hypoglycemia, hypocalcemia, or other metabolic derangements. If seizures persist, a single loading dose of phenobarbital (20 mg/kg) should be administered intravenously, which may be followed by additional doses of 5 mg/kg to a total of 40 mg/kg (including loading dose) as required, if there is no cardiac decompensation. If seizures are still uncontrolled, a single loading dose of phenytoin (20 mg/kg) may be administered slowly with concomitant careful monitoring of cardiac function. If seizures remain refractory to therapy, the use of a benzodiazepine may be considered, e.g., diazepam, lorazepam, or midazolam. In addition, there are anecdotal reports concerning the use of other anticonvulsants, such as primidone, carbamazepine, lamotrigine, and thiopentone.

Several major issues regarding the treatment of seizures remain unresolved. These include the optimal maintenance doses and therapeutic ranges of serum levels of anticonvulsants, the importance of eliminating electrographic seizures, and the optimal duration of anticonvulsant therapy. The duration of therapy should be guided by the underlying etiology and the risk of seizure recurrence. Clearly, unnecessary prolongation of therapy should be avoided because of unresolved concerns about possible deleterious effects of anticonvulsants on the immature nervous system (7).

Prognosis

The mortality rate for clinical seizures has decreased in recent years; it has been reported to be approximately 15%. The incidence of neurologic sequelae, especially mental retardation and motor deficits (e.g., cerebral palsy), has been estimated to be between 35% and 55% (1).

Of course, the most important determinant of outcome is the underlying neurologic disease (Table 49–2). In addition, the early onset of seizures, frequent or prolonged seizures, and seizures that are refractory to multiple anticonvulsants often are associated with poor prognosis. Clearly, these features reflect the severity of the underlying cerebral abnormality. Furthermore, in term newborns, a normal, interictal EEG is reported to result in normal development in more than 85% of patients, whereas a suppressed, periodic, interictal recording is associated with only approximately 8% probability of normal outcome (16). However, in a significant proportion of newborns, the EEG is borderline, equivocal, or contains less marked abnormalities that are associated with an uncertain prognosis.

HYPOXIC–ISCHEMIC CEREBRAL INJURY

Hypoxic–ischemic cerebral injury results from a combination of hypoxemia and ischemia, which often is associated with impaired cerebrovascular autoregulation and probably exacerbated by diminished cerebral glucose substrates, lactic acidosis, the accumulation of free radicals and excitotoxic amino acids (especially glutamate), and other metabolic derangements. The extent and distribution of perinatal hypoxic–ischemic cerebral injury is determined principally by the maturity of the brain at the time of insult and the severity and duration of the insult (1,17,18).

Although the importance of antepartum and intrapartum factors have been recognized since 1862, when Little initially described a relationship between perinatal complications and cerebral palsy, data from large, epidemiologic studies, including the National Collaborative Perinatal Project and the Western Australian Cerebral Palsy Register, suggest that the etiologic role of antepartum factors may have been underestimated previously (19–21). Review of these large populations of children with cerebral palsy indicate that the incidence of cerebral palsy related to intrapartum asphyxia may not exceed 20% when all factors are considered. Moreover, approximately one-third of these patients had at least one congenital anomaly unrelated to the central nervous system. This observation raises the possibility that an insult that originated much earlier during gestation may predispose some infants to subsequent hypoxic–ischemic insult at the time of delivery. Nevertheless, there is extensive experimental, clinical, and neuroimaging data that provide compelling evidence that acute, intrapartum hypoxic–ischemic insult is an important etiologic factor for brain injury, especially in the term newborn (22).

Diagnosis

Clinical Features

Infants who sustain hypoxic–ischemic cerebral injury earlier in gestation may be asymptomatic during the neonatal period. However, term newborns who sustain sufficient intrapartum insult to result in long-term sequelae invariably demonstrate clinical evidence of acute encephalopathy during the first days of life. It is important to consider that the clinical features of hypoxic–ischemic encephalopathy are nonspecific, and similar clinical features may occur in the context of other types of brain abnormalities, e.g., metabolic derangements, cerebral dysgenesis, and infection. Several complications of labor and delivery have been used as clinical markers of possible hypoxic–ischemic insult, e.g., prolonged fetal bradycardia or repetitive late decelerations of the fetal heart rate, low fetal scalp or cord pH, and low extended Apgar scores after 5 minutes of age. However, no single factor or combination of factors can predict accurately the severity or duration of the hypoxic–ischemic insult or long-term sequelae. However, in the term newborn, the clinical features and the EEG and neuropathologic patterns of cerebral injury, which may be identified by neuroimaging, may permit determination of outcome with a reasonable degree of accuracy.

Although there is a complete spectrum of hypoxic–ischemic encephalopathy in the term newborn, classification of the severity of encephalopathy (Table 49–3) is useful for prognostic purposes (23–26). Mild encephalopathy is characterized by hyperalertness, jitteriness, exaggerated tendon reflexes and Moro response that last only approximately 24 hours and generally are not associated with long-term neurologic sequelae. Moderate encephalopathy is associated with lethargy and stupor, hypotonia, and suppressed tendon reflexes. Seizures may occur. Abnormal long-term outcome has been reported in 20% to 40% of affected infants. Severe encephalopathy is associated invariably with coma, seizures, brainstem and autonomic dysfunction, and, in some cases, elevated intracranial pressure (27–29). All infants with severe encephalopathy either die or develop major neurologic sequelae, e.g., microcephaly, spastic quadriplegia, and seizures. In severe encephalopathy, the clinical features characteristically worsen during the first 3 days of life. Death occurs most commonly between 24 and 72 hours of life, which corresponds to the time of maximal cerebral edema (27). Autopsy studies of patients with elevated intracranial pressure demonstrate extensive cerebral necrosis. It appears that elevated intracranial pressure is a consequence rather than a cause of extensive brain injury, and intervention with antiedema agents may reduce the intracranial pressure but does not appear to improve the ultimate neurologic outcome (27,30–32).

Seizures occur in approximately 50% of asphyxiated infants and are indicative of at least moderate or severe encephalopathy. Seizures, which most commonly are subtle and multifocal clonic, usually begin during the first 24 hours of life. In severe cases, they often occur within hours of delivery and are refractory to anticonvulsant therapy. Infants with hypoxic–ischemic encephalopathy who survive beyond 3 or 4 days of age generally demonstrate an improving level of consciousness and gradual resolution of seizures, although impairment of feeding, abnormal muscle tone, and developmental delay may persist.

In addition to the neurologic dysfunction, there is often evidence of acute hypoxic–ischemic insult to organs other than brain, e.g., kidneys and myocardium (33–35). Such involvement of systemic organs is often transient and reversible, even in the context of severe encephalopathy. Although the extent of systemic abnormalities

TABLE 49–3. *Severity and outcome of hypoxic–ischemic encephalopathy in the full-term neonate*

Severity	Level of consciousness	Seizures	Primitive reflexes	Brain stem dysfunction	Elevated intracranial pressure	Duration	Poor outcome[a] (%)
Mild	Increased irritability, hyperalertness	–, Jitteriness	Exaggerated	–	–	<24 h	0
Moderate	Lethargy	Variable	Suppressed	–	–	>24 h (variable)	20–40
Severe	Stupor or coma	+	Absent	+	Variable	>5 d	100

[a]Poor outcome is defined as the presence of mental retardation, cerebral palsy, or seizures.
+, common; –, rare.

appears to correlate with the severity of encephalopathy, in some instances, there may be no evidence of injury to organs other than the brain.

Neuroimaging

In addition to the clinical examination, neuroimaging techniques often permit the delineation of specific neuropathologic patterns and the extent of cerebral injury (36).

Cranial Ultrasound

Features in term newborns with severe hypoxic–ischemic injury include diffuse increased echogenicity of parenchyma and effacement of cortical sulci by cerebral edema. Unfortunately, if abnormalities are diffuse, detection may be difficult. This accounts for a disappointing correlation between sonographic findings and neurologic outcome in term newborns (36,37). Ultrasound has better predictive value in the assessment of premature infants, in whom increased periventricular echoes in the first days of life may herald the development of cystic changes (cavitation) in these regions during the ensuing 2 to 3 weeks (38–40). If the phase of cyst formation is not doc-

umented by serial ultrasound examinations, a later sonogram may show only *ex vacuo* enlargement of the ventricles with irregular margins.

Computed Tomography

In the term newborn, computed tomography (CT) scanning during the newborn period has excellent prognostic value and may demonstrate diffuse or focal cerebral injury. Optimal timing of CT scans to demonstrate the maximal extent of decreased tissue attenuation is between 2 and 5 days of age approximately, which corresponds to the timing of maximal extent of cerebral edema (Fig. 49–1*A*) (27). Accurate interpretation of tissue attenuation on CT requires careful attention to scanning technique (41). CT scans performed later in childhood may demonstrate focal or generalized cerebral atrophy, often with multicystic encephalomelacia (Fig. 49–1*B*). More recently, we have documented that a pattern of low attenuation in thalami and basal ganglia on the CT scan at 2 to 5 days of life, with relative preservation of cortex and subcortical white matter, is consistent with acute, total hypoxic–ischemic insult and poor outcome (18). In contrast to the term newborn, CT is of limited value for assessment of acute hypoxic–ischemic injury in the pre-

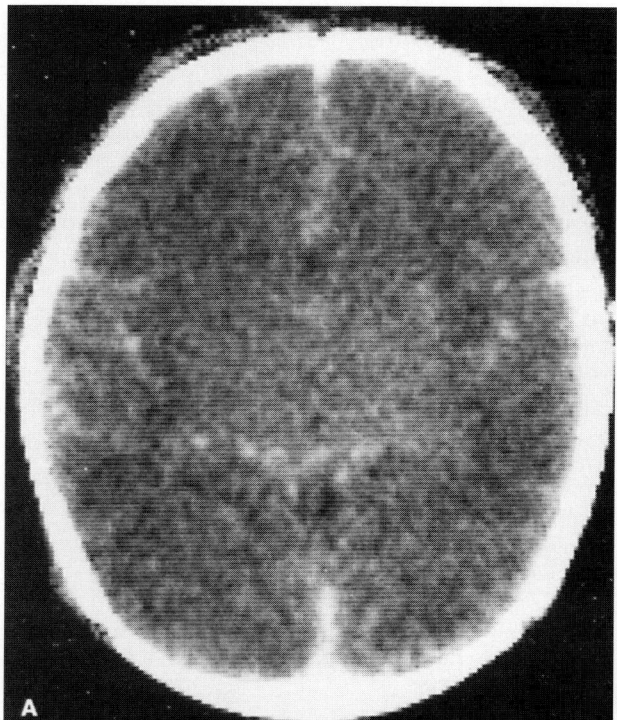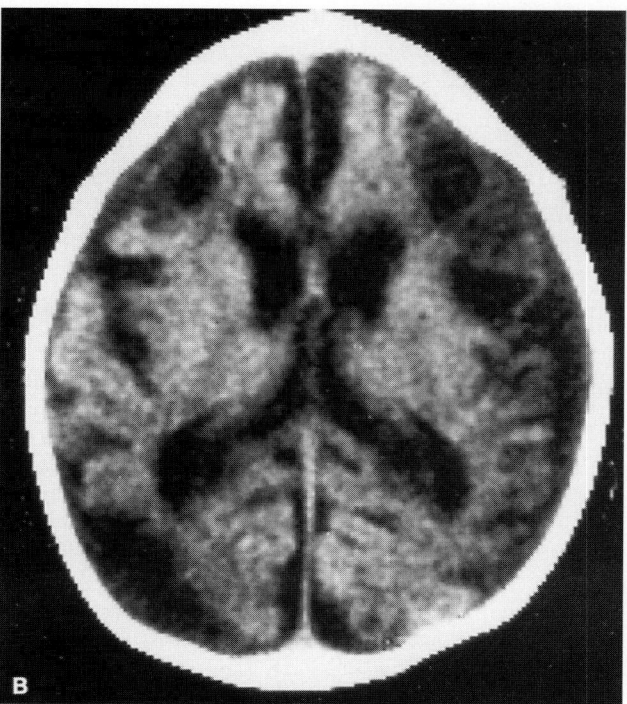

FIG. 49–1. A: Computed tomographic scan of a full-term newborn with severe, acute hypoxic–ischemic encephalopathy shows generalized, decreased tissue attenuation throughout both cerebral hemispheres. **B:** Computed tomographic scan performed at 4 months of age after hypoxic–ischemic cerebral injury at term demonstrates multicystic encephalomalacia and cerebral atrophy.

mature newborn, because the high water content of the immature brain results in normally low tissue attenuation. However, CT may demonstrate characteristic features of end-stage periventricular leukomalacia, which include (a) ventricular dilation with irregular margins of the body and trigone of the lateral ventricles, (b) decreased volume of periventricular white matter, and (c) deep sulci that abut directly on the lateral walls of the ventricles (42).

Magnetic Resonance Imaging

There is increasing evidence that magnetic resonance imaging (MRI) has the capability to demonstrate specific patterns of injury in term newborns that may not be visualized by other imaging techniques (18,36,43–46). Thus, T2 prolongation resulting from edema (which may be transient or permanent) may appear as early as 12 to 18 hours after injury, and T1 shortening (high signal on T1-weighted images) appears in injured areas after approximately 3 days (36). Diffusion-weighted MRI appears to be even more sensitive than standard MRI during the first hours following hypoxic–ischemic injury (47). However, technical difficulties, such as the prolonged scanning time and difficulty with monitoring the sick newborn in the scanner, still limit the clinical application of MRI in the context of acute hypoxic–ischemic encephalopathy.

Radionuclide Scanning

O'Brien and associates (48) have demonstrated the value of technetium scanning for documentation of patterns of hypoxic–ischemic cerebral injury. More recently, experimental techniques, e.g., positron emission tomography (49) and single photon emission CT (50), which utilize radionuclides that have the capacity to cross the intact blood–brain barrier, can provide insights into regional abnormalities of cerebral perfusion.

Magnetic Resonance Spectroscopy

In severely affected infants studied by phosphorus and proton MRS, a consistent observation has been the development of delayed derangements in cerebral energy metabolism between 12 and 48 hours after resuscitation, despite the maintenance of cardiovascular and respiratory homeostasis, which, in turn, correlates closely with poor neurologic outcome (51,52). However, because of its complexity and expense, MRS remains an experimental technique that is available only on a limited basis at a few research centers.

Near-Infrared Spectroscopy

Near-infrared spectroscopy (NIRS), a noninvasive technique that may be used at the bedside, has the capability of providing information concerning cerebral oxyhemoglobin delivery and intracellular oxygen availability (51). However, the technical limitations of the equipment and complexity of the data analysis have limited its application to clinical studies on critically ill infants. In a small number of infants, significant cerebral vasodilation and vasoparalysis have been observed using NIRS (52).

Electrodiagnostic Techniques

Electrodiagnostic techniques have been used in the evaluation of hypoxic–ischemic cerebral injury, especially in term newborns. EEG recordings that demonstrate a discontinuous pattern with voltage suppression and rapid bursts of sharp and slow waves generally are associated with poor outcome. In contrast, rapid resolution of EEG abnormalities and a normal interictal EEG pattern are associated with a good outcome (23).

Evoked responses, e.g., brainstem evoked responses, visual evoked responses, and somatosensory evoked responses. also may have prognostic value (53,54). However, their routine clinical application has been limited by technical difficulties.

Biochemical Markers

Several enzymes and metabolites (e.g., creatine kinase BB isozyme, hypoxanthine, lactate) in blood or cerebrospinal fluid (CSF) are of value as indicators of hypoxic–ischemic cerebral injury (1). In this regard, the measurement of lactic acid levels in CSF appears to be most promising (55). Furthermore, metabolic derangements that are considered secondary to the hypoxic injury, e.g., acidosis, hypoglycemia, and hyponatremia due inappropriate secretion of antidiuretic hormone, may contribute to the cerebral injury.

Pathogenesis and Neuropathology

The pathogenetic mechanisms that determine the major neuropathologic patterns of injury may be explained by a combination of regional circulatory and metabolic factors of the affected brain, especially the regional distribution of excitatory amino acid synapses (e.g., glutamate receptors) as well as the severity and duration of the hypoxic–ischemic insult. The major neuropathologic patterns of hypoxic–ischemic cerebral injury are listed in Table 49–4.

Circulatory Factors

The initial circulatory response to perinatal asphyxia involves the redistribution of cardiac output with increased perfusion of vital organs such as brain, heart, and adrenals and concomitant decreased blood flow to other organs, such as the lungs, kidneys, and gastrointestinal tract. Prolonged hypoxic–ischemic insult results

TABLE 49–4. *Major neuropathologic patterns*

| Pattern of injury | Gestational age | | Anatomic distribution |
	Full term	Premature	
Selective neuronal necrosis	+	+	Cerebral and cerebellar cortex, thalamus, brainstem, hippocampus
Parasagittal	+	–	Parasagittal cortex, subcortical white matter
Status marmoratus of basal ganglia and thalamus	+	–	Thalamus, basal ganglia, cerebral cortex
Focal or multifocal necrosis	+	+	Unilateral or bilateral cerebral cortex
Periventricular leukomalacia	–	+	Periventricular white matter

+, common; –, rare.

in systemic hypotension. The potential significance of hypotension is potentiated by impairment of cerebrovascular autoregulation, which has been reported even after relatively moderate hypoxic–ischemic insult (56,57). Cerebrovascular autoregulation is a homeostatic mechanism that maintains relatively constant cerebral perfusion over a wide range of systemic arterial blood pressures by means of cerebral arteriolar constriction or dilation. Due to a deficiency in the muscular lining of cerebral arterioles in the immature brain, the frequent association of hypercarbia or hypoxemia, or because the normal blood pressure of the newborn is close to the downslope of the normal autoregulatory curve, or on account of a combination of these factors, this protective mechanism may be disrupted. Impaired cerebrovascular autoregulation results in a direct, linear correlation between cerebral perfusion and systemic blood pressure.

Systemic hypotension associated with moderate decreases in cerebral perfusion may result in injury that is confined principally to the watershed zones of arterial supply. In the term newborn, the watershed zones between the anterior, middle. and posterior cerebral arteries are located in the parasagittal regions of the cerebral cortex. In the premature newborn, the most vulnerable watershed zone is located in the periventricular white matter.

Metabolic Factors

Regional differences in the rate of energy metabolism, lactate accumulation, calcium influx, and free-radical formation may explain the increased susceptibility of specific regions, e.g., thalamus, basal ganglia, and brainstem, to acute hypoxic–ischemic insult. In addition, selective vulnerability may reflect the active myelination in these regions during the newborn period.

There is compelling experimental evidence that excitatory amino acids, especially glutamate, play a critical role in the expression of hypoxic–ischemic neuronal injury. For example, death of hippocampal neurons in tissue culture or in an experimental rat model following exposure to anoxia can be prevented by specific glutamate receptor blockers or antagonists, e.g., magnesium and MK-801

(58–60). Furthermore, there appears to be a relationship between the distribution of glutamatergic synapses in the mammalian brain and the common neuropathologic patterns of hypoxic–ischemic cerebral injury (58,61). Currently, there is ongoing research into the potential clinical applications of glutamate antagonists (62,63).

Major Neuropathologic Patterns of Injury

Selective Neuronal Necrosis

Selective neuronal necrosis of neurons involves specific regions of the cortex, e.g., the Sommer sector of the hippocampus, thalamus, brainstem, cerebellum, and anterior horn cells of the spinal cord. Major pathogenetic factors include circulatory factors as well as the severity and duration of the insult. Thus, in both experimental animal models (64–66) and human term newborns (18,67), "prolonged, partial" hypoxic–ischemic insult results in cerebral injury involving principally the cortex and subcortical white matter. In contrast, "acute, total" asphyxia, which may occur in the context of events such as umbilical cord prolapse or uterine rupture, results in a pattern of injury affecting predominantly thalami, basal ganglia, and brainstem with relative preservation of cortex and subcortical white matter. This regional vulnerability relates principally to the varying rates of metabolism and myelination as well as the stage of maturation of different sites within the affected brain, including the anatomic distribution of glutamatergic synapses (1,66).

The clinical manifestations in the newborn relate to the specific sites of injury. For example, infants with extensive cortical/subcortical injury may have seizures and possibly raised intracranial pressure, whereas infants who have predominantly thalamic, basal ganglia and brainstem involvement have characteristic features of irritability, tonic posturing, and lower cranial nerve dysfunction (18,67).

The late neuropathologic sequelae of selective neuronal necrosis are cerebral atrophy and multicystic encephalomalacia (Fig. 49–1B). Clinical features in older children include varying degrees of cerebral palsy, mental retardation, microcephaly, and possibly seizures.

Parasagittal Cerebral Injury

In the term newborn, the parasagittal cortex and subcortical white matter are located in the watershed zone of arterial supply between the anterior, middle, and posterior cerebral arteries, an area that is vulnerable to ischemic injury (Fig. 49–2).

Clinical features of parasagittal injury during the newborn period include hypotonia and weakness, which are more prominent in the proximal upper extremities than in the lower limbs.

Status Marmoratus of Basal Ganglia and Thalamus

Neuronal necrosis, gliosis, and hypermyelination in basal ganglia, thalamus, and cerebral cortex may result in a striking, marbled appearance of these structures (Fig. 49–3). This pattern actually may represent one specific pattern of selective neuronal necrosis (see previous) (18,64,67). This neuropathologic pattern may relate to the type of hypoxic–ischemic insult (i.e., "acute, total asphyxia") as well as the transient, dense glutamatergic innervation of the basal ganglia in the newborn and the increased metabolic demands of the actively differentiating neurons in these regions (65,66).

The clinical neurologic abnormalities in the newborn that are associated with this pattern of injury have not been established with certainty. Late sequelae include choreoathetoid cerebral palsy.

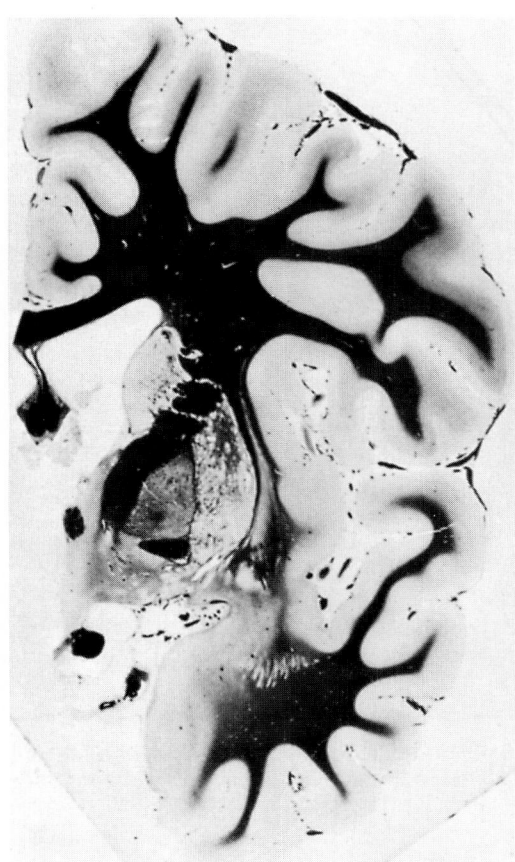

FIG. 49–3. Status marmoratus of basal ganglia is demonstrated in a coronal section of cerebral hemisphere, stained for myelin, from a patient who died years after the insult. The marbled appearance is especially striking in the putamen. (Courtesy of E. P. Richardson, Jr., M.D.)

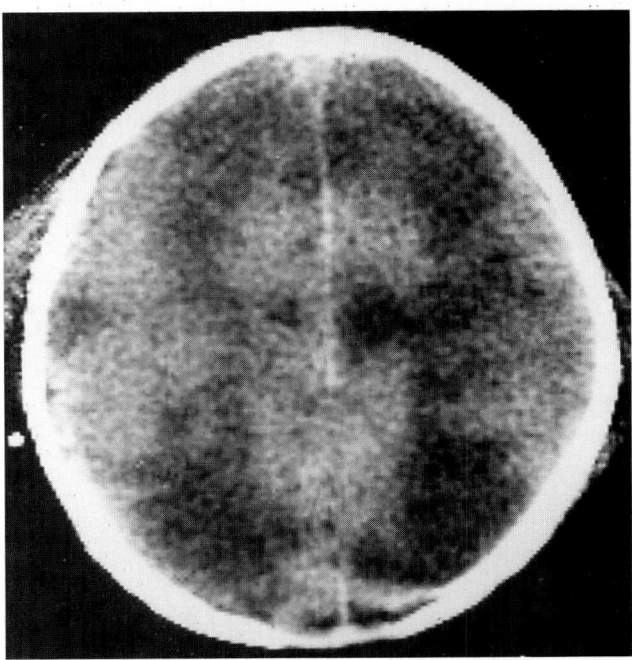

FIG. 49–2. Computed tomographic scan of a full-term newborn demonstrates decreased tissue attenuation in the parasagittal watershed zones.

Focal and Multifocal Cerebral Necrosis

Focal arterial occlusion by embolus or thrombus is well recognized in the newborn (Fig. 49–4). In premature newborns, such infarction is often multifocal. In the majority of cases, no specific cause can be identified. However, conditions that may predispose to focal ischemic necrosis include coagulation disturbances, e.g., polycythemia, disseminated intravascular coagulation, protein C or S deficiency, antithrombin III deficiency, maternal isoimmune thrombocytopenia, as well as intrauterine cocaine exposure, vascular maldevelopment, and emboli from punctured or catheterized vessels or involuting placental vessels.

Newborn infants who develop focal arterial infarction most commonly present with unilateral, focal seizures. Alternatively, infants may be asymptomatic or display asymmetric motor function. Long-term sequelae include cerebral palsy (often hemiparesis), seizures, and intellectual impairment.

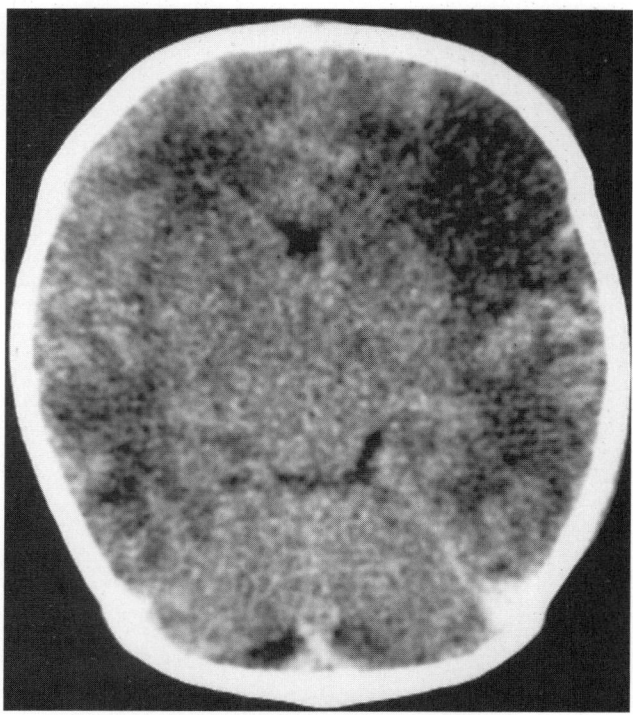

FIG. 49–4. Computed tomographic scan of a full-term newborn with acute, focal infarction involving the territory of the middle cerebral artery.

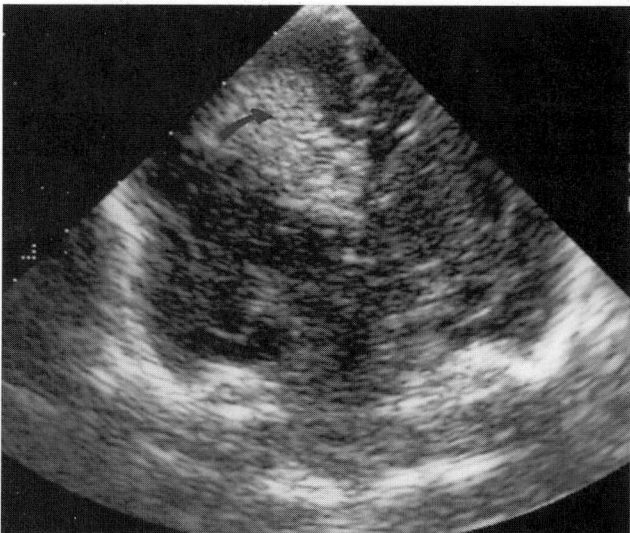

FIG. 49–5. Coronal ultrasound scan delineates the periventricular hemorrhagic infarction (*arrow*) in a premature newborn with intraventricular hemorrhage.

Venous sinus thrombosis in the newborn has been diagnosed more frequently since MRI has become more readily available. Predisposing conditions include coagulation disturbances, dehydration, and sepsis (68,69). Clinical features in the newborn include lethargy and seizures that are not necessarily focal. The long-term sequelae are not well defined. Approximately one-third of affected children have developmental delay.

Periventricular Leukomalacia

This hypoxic–ischemic lesion involves the arterial end zones within the periventricular white matter in the premature brain (70–72). More diffuse periventricular white matter injury has been termed "telencephalic leukoencephalopathy" (73,74). There is increasing evidence that such white matter injury relates to a combination of intrinsic vulnerability of early differentiating oligodendroglial precursors to free radicals associated with hypoxic–ischemic insult or endotoxemia (74–76). Secondary hemorrhage, albeit often of mild severity, has been reported in approximately 25% of autopsy studies in patients with periventricular leukomalacia (77) as well as in survivors (78).

Hemorrhagic periventricular leukomalacia must be distinguished from periventricular hemorrhagic infarction, which is usually unilateral (Fig. 49–5) or strikingly asymmetric (79). This lesion is associated with large GMH or IVH, and it is considered to represent venous infarction resulting from obstruction of the terminal vein by a large GMH (80,81). The severity of white matter injury ranges from small focal areas of gliosis or necrosis to diffuse involvement that may develop into cavitations (Fig. 49–6). Severe lesions may be visualized *in vivo* by cranial ultrasonography as areas of increased echogenicity in periventricular white matter during the first days of life, which subsequently evolve into cystic lesions after approximately 2 to 3 weeks (39,40,82).

The clinical features of periventricular leukomalacia in the premature newborn may be subtle and include weakness or altered muscle tone involving predominantly the lower extremities. Long-term sequelae include spastic diplegia and, occasionally, visual and auditory impairment related to involvement of the optic and auditory radiations (1,83). In addition, periventricular leukomalacia may have a role in the genesis of derangements of cerebral cortical organization because of injury to subplate neurons or interference with late migrating astrocytes, which, in turn, may have an impact on cognitive function (84–86).

Management

There is no consensus concerning the optimal management of hypoxic–ischemic cerebral injury in the newborn (31,63). Awareness of the risk factors during the intrauterine period has promoted prevention of cerebral injury by early diagnosis and close monitoring of the high-risk fetus and consideration of urgent delivery in the event of persistant fetal distress. Furthermore, an asphyxiated newborn requires immediate and close surveillance to minimize

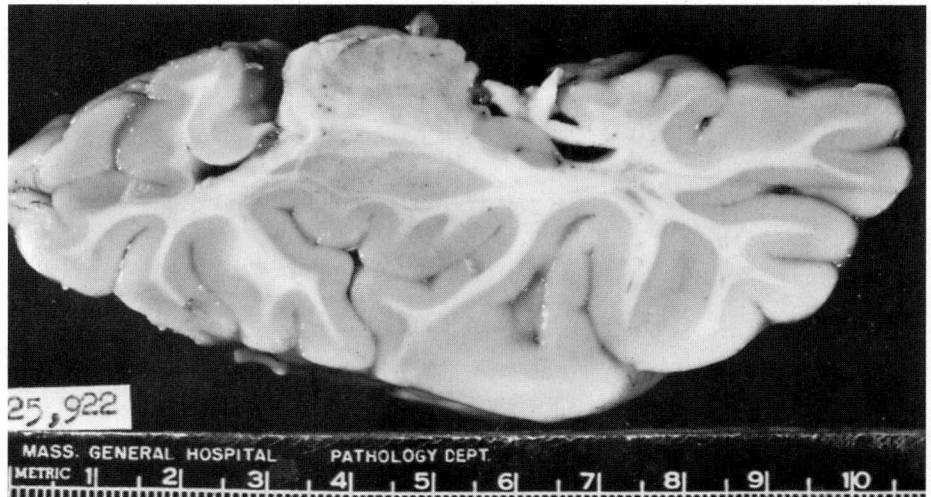

FIG. 49–6. Periventricular leukomalacia is demonstrated in the coronal section of cerebral hemisphere from a 20-month-old child who was the product of a 35-week pregnancy and experienced cardiorespiratory difficulties in the neonatal period. Small, cavitated lesions can be seen approximately 5 mm from the external angle of the lateral ventricle of the parietal lobe. (From DeReuck J, Chattha AS, Richardson EP Jr. Pathogenesis and evolution of periventricular leukomalacia in infancy. *Arch Neurol* 1972; 27:229.)

additional postnatal injury. Provision of adequate ventilation and perfusion, maintenance of normal blood pressure and normoglycemia, and control of seizures are of critical importance. There is a high incidence of dysfunction of other organ systems, e.g., heart, kidneys, and gastrointestinal tract, which must be monitored carefully.

Adequate ventilation and the avoidance of postnatal hypoxemia may be difficult to achieve because of the cardiorespiratory problems associated with severe hyaline membrane disease in the premature newborn and persistent fetal circulation and pulmonary hypertension in the term newborn. Administration of surfactant, extracorporeal membrane oxygenation and high-frequency ventilation are newer treatment modalities. Because hypoxemic episodes in the premature newborn may be associated with events such as suctioning or spontaneous crying, minimal handling is recommended for these infants. On the other hand, hyperoxia should be avoided because of the possibility of developing pontosubicular necrosis and retrolental fibroplasia (87).

Because impaired cerebrovascular autoregulation has been documented in the context of moderate hypoxic–ischemic encephalopathy, maintenance of normal systemic arterial blood pressure and adequate cerebral perfusion are essential. This may require volume replacement and the use of inotropic agents (e.g., dopamine) if there is evidence of myocardial dysfunction. In the premature newborn, systemic hypotension may occur in the context of patent ductus arteriosus and recurrent apnea of prematurity. On the other hand, systemic hypertension must be avoided, especially in the premature newborn,

because it may predispose to GMH/IVH originating within the fragile vasculature of the germinal matrix.

Seizures that occur in the context of acute hypoxic–ischemic encephalopathy may be refractory to anticonvulsant therapy. Nevertheless, treatment is indicated to minimize associated apnea, hypertension, and metabolic derangements, such as depletion of brain glucose and high-energy phosphate compounds.

The optimal levels of blood glucose that should be maintained after hypoxic–ischemic insult have not been established. Maintenance of normoglycemia is recommended. Inappropriate antidiuretic hormone secretion following major hypoxic–ischemic cerebral injury may result in hyponatremia and decreased osmolality, with a consequent risk of cerebral edema and seizures. Fluid overload should be avoided.

Data from human and experimental animal studies suggest that elevated intracranial pressure associated with hypoxic–ischemic encephalopathy in the term newborn reflects extensive cerebral necrosis, which represents a consequence rather than a cause of hypoxic–ischemic brain injury. Maximal elevations of intracranial pressure are observed between 36 and 96 hours after the initial insult and are associated with a poor outcome (27). Although it is possible to reduce elevated intracranial pressure by antiedema agents (e.g., mannitol and diuretics), there is no evidence that such intervention improves long-term neurologic outcome (28,30–32).

Several management strategies are currently under investigation. These include antenatal administration of phenobarbital, the use of glutamate receptor antagonists (e.g., dextromethorphan, ketamine, MK-801, magnesium), calcium channel blockers (e.g., flunarizine), and free-radical scavengers (e.g., vitamin E, indomethacin, allopurinol) (63).

Prognosis

In our experience in the term newborn, the severity and duration of the clinical hypoxic–ischemic encephalopathy, combined with the extent of decreased tissue attenuation visualized on CT scans performed between 2 and 5 days after the original insult, permit reasonably accurate prediction of poor outcome. The prediction of outcome in the asphyxiated premature newborn is more difficult.

INTRACRANIAL HEMORRHAGE

The incidence of GMH/IVH in premature newborns is estimated between 20% and 40% (1). Although there has been a significant reduction in incidence during recent years, GMH/IVH remains a major concern, principally because of the improved survival rates of very-low-birth-weight infants who are at highest risk for the development of GMH/IVH. In the premature newborn, GMH/IVH originates principally from rupture of fragile vessels in the subependymal germinal matrix (Fig. 49–7). In approximately 80% of cases, there is associated IVH, and in approximately 15% there is associated parenchymal hemorrhagic infarction. Serial cranial ultrasonography has demonstrated that 50% of cases of GMH/IVH originate during the first day of life and 90% occur before 4 days of age. In 20% to 40%, the hemorrhage may extend during the first week of life.

Diagnosis

Neuroimaging

Cranial ultrasonography is considered the neuroimaging modality of choice for the diagnosis of GMH/IVH because of its portability, high resolution, and lack of ionizing radiation. Nevertheless, CT and MRI remain superior for the diagnosis of other types of intracranial hemorrhage, including primary subarachnoid, convexity, and posterior fossa subdural or epidural hematomas and for differentiating between hemorrhagic and ischemic parenchymal infarction. Figure 49–8 illustrates the appearance of GMH/IVH on CT scan.

Because of the relatively high risk of GMH/IVH, routine cranial ultrasonography is recommended at 4 to 5 days of age for high-risk infants younger than 32 weeks of gestation. Ultrasonography should be performed earlier if there are specific clinical concerns. Because there may be extension in the size of the hemorrhage, ultrasound scans should be repeated after the first week of life to establish the maximal extent of the lesion. Subsequently, serial scans may be performed every 1 to 2 weeks after major GMH/IVH for surveillance of ventricular size and possible development of posthemorrhagic hydrocephalus (Fig. 49–9). This is particularly important because of the high degree of compliance of the premature brain and cranium and the relatively large subarachnoid spaces that permit considerable increase in ventricular size prior to the onset of excessive head growth.

Clinical Features

The diagnosis of GMH/IVH may be suspected on the basis of clinical signs alone only in approximately 50% of

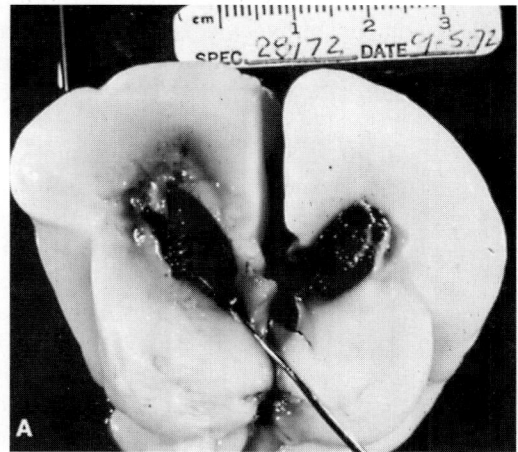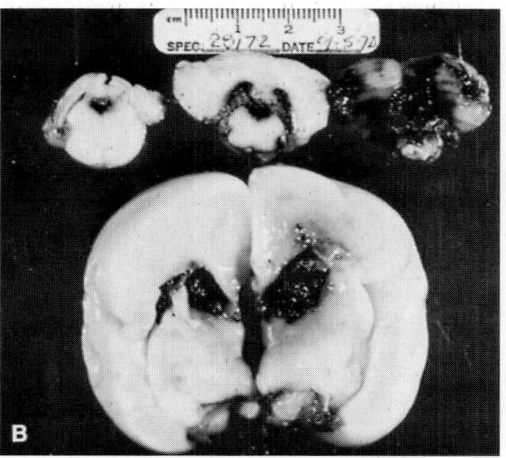

FIG. 49–7. A: Periventricular hemorrhage with intraventricular rupture at the level of the foramen of Monro. Blood fills both lateral ventricles. The site of rupture of the hemorrhage from the right subependymal region can be seen. **B:** Extension of intraventricular hemorrhage, same case as shown in (A). Hemorrhage can be seen in the lateral ventricles, the aqueduct of Sylvius, the fourth ventricle, and the subarachnoid space around the cerebellum and base of the brain. (Courtesy of John Axley, M.D.)

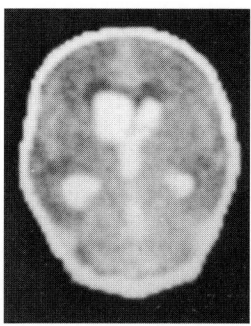

FIG. 49–8. Computed tomographic scan of marked intraventricular hemorrhage demonstrates blood in the frontal horns, third ventricle, and occipital horns.

patients (88). The severity of clinical features ranges from an asymptomatic state through a saltatory neurologic deterioration over several days to a catastrophic presentation with coma, apnea, tonic extensor posturing, brainstem dysfunction, and flaccid quadriparesis. Associated

systemic abnormalities may include hypotension, metabolic acidosis, bradycardia, and disturbances of serum glucose and electrolytes. Bloody or xanthochromic CSF supports a diagnosis of intracranial hemorrhage.

Pathogenesis

The pathogenesis of GMH/IVH is multifactorial and consists of a combination of intravascular, vascular, and extravascular factors (Table 49–5). The importance of individual factors may vary in different situations. Consideration of these major pathogenetic mechanisms provides a framework for the selection of appropriate interventional strategies.

Intravascular factors involve principally the regulation of cerebral perfusion (i.e., cerebral blood flow and pressure) within the fragile vasculature of the germinal matrix and platelet–capillary interactions and coagulation disturbances. Vascular pathogenetic factors include the fragility of vessels in the germinal matrix and their vulnerability to hypoxic–ischemic insult. Extravascular factors relate

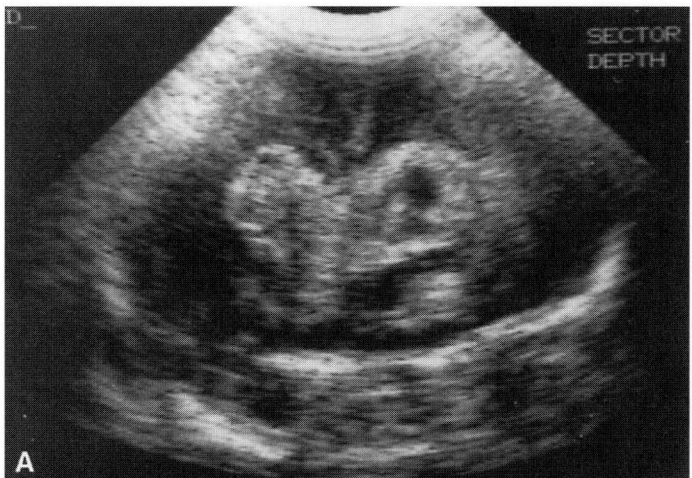

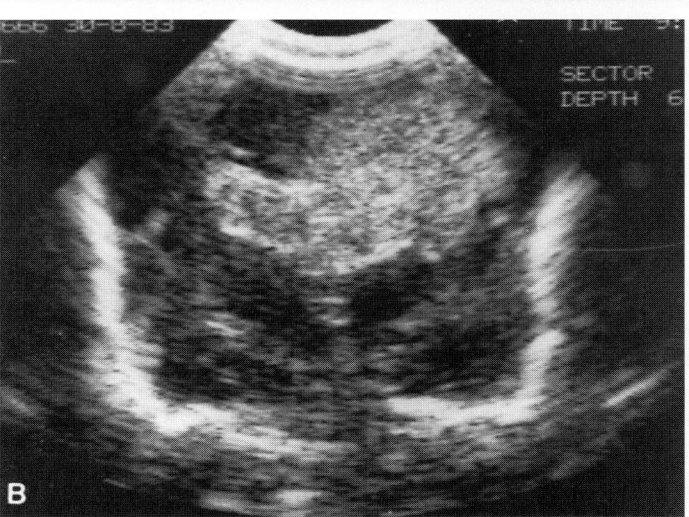

FIG. 49–9. A: Ultrasonographic scan in the coronal plane of marked intraventricular hemorrhage delineates blood in the dilated frontal horns of the lateral ventricles and central clearing of the hematoma (*left*). **B:** Ultrasonographic scan in the coronal plane of marked intraventricular hemorrhage shows blood in the dilated frontal horns of lateral ventricles and intraparenchymal hematoma (*left*).

TABLE 49–5. *Pathogenesis and management of germinal matrix–intraventricular hemorrhage*

Pathogenic factor	Management
Intravascular	
Alterations in cerebral blood flow	Avoidance of systemic hypertension or hypotension; paralysis of ventilated infants
Alterations in cerebral venous pressure	Avoidance of prolonged labor and difficult vaginal delivery; avoidance of pneumothorax, minimal handling
Coagulation disturbances	Avoidance of hypoxic–ischemic insult; prophylactic infusion of fresh-frozen plasma (?); platelet infusion (?)
Vascular	
Fragility of vessels in subependymal germinal matrix	Ethamsylate (?), vitamin E (?)
Extravascular	
Poor vascular support of germinal matrix	Tranexamic acid (?)
Decrease in tissue pressure (?)	

to the characteristics of the supporting tissues, excessive fibrinolytic activity, and a possible decrease in tissue pressure postnatally.

Posthemorrhagic hydrocephalus and periventricular hemorrhagic infarction are the major complications of GMH/IVH. Other mechanisms involved in cerebral injury associated with GMH/IVH include concomitant or preceding hypoxic–ischemic cerebral injury (e.g., periventricular leukomalacia, neuronal necrosis of the brainstem), acute increase in intracranial pressure associated with major hemorrhage, and destruction of the germinal matrix with its glial precursors.

Ventriculomegaly and hydrocephalus occur commonly after major GMH/IVH (Table 49–6). Massive GMH/IVH may be associated with ventriculomegaly. Communicating hydrocephalus is often a consequence of impaired CSF reabsorption secondary to an obliterative arachnoiditis in the posterior fossa. A second potential mechanism involves the blockage of CSF resorption at the small arachnoid villi by particulate debris floating in CSF after GMH/IVH. Obstructive hydrocephalus may occur secondary to blockage of the flow of CSF at the level of the aqueduct of Sylvius by blood clot or other intraventricular debris (1,89).

The characteristic clinical signs of hydrocephalus (e.g., abnormally rapid increase in head circumference, bulging anterior fontanel, suture diastasis) may be delayed for days or weeks after the onset of ventricular dilation is observed on serial ultrasound scans (1).

The delay in clinical manifestation of increased intracranial pressure is related to the high compliance of periventricular tissue in the immature brain, especially after hypoxic–ischemic injury, the relatively generous subarachnoid space in the premature infant, and the distensible cranium, all of which allow increase in ventricular size without expansion of head circumference.

Ventriculomegaly after GMH/IVH may become static or resolve spontaneously after days or weeks in approximately 65% of cases (1,89). In the remainder, amelioration of increased intracranial pressure by temporary or permanent drainage of CSF or medical intervention to decrease CSF production is required. In approximately 5% of cases, progressive posthemorrhagic hydrocephalus may be delayed for many months, which necessitates ongoing surveillance of ventricular size by serial cranial ultrasonography during the first year of life (90).

Periventricular hemorrhagic infarction has been documented in approximately 15% of infants with major GMH/IVH. These parenchymal lesions are a major determinant of long-term neurologic sequelae (79). Neuropathologic studies indicate that such fan-shaped parenchymal hemorrhage results from venous infarction, usually with secondary hemorrhage related to obstruction of the medullary and terminal veins by large GMH (80,81). This pathogenesis differs from that of hemorrhagic periventricular leukomalacia, which represents an arterial ischemic lesion with secondary hemorrhage.

Management

Clearly, the primary goal is prevention of GMH/IVH. Prevention of premature labor and delivery may be considered to be the optimal management strategy. Alternatively, interventions should address the major pathogenetic mechanisms as outlined previously.

TABLE 49–6. *Major complications of germinal matrix–intraventricular hemorrhage*

- Ventriculomegaly, posthemorrhagic hydrocephalus
- Periventricular hemorrhagic cerebral infarction
- Acute increased intracranial pressure with major intraventricular hemorrhage
- Destruction of germinal matrix glial precursors
- Focal ischemia (?)
- Concomitant hypoxic–ischemic cerebral injury (i.e., periventricular leukomalacia)

Antenatal Interventions

Prevention of premature labor and delivery may be attempted with maternal tocolytic therapy with beta-sympathomimetics, indomethacin, or magnesium sulfate. Unfortunately, these medications often succeed in delaying labor for only several days, although even such brief delay may be sufficient to permit administration of a course of antenatal steroids, to induce fetal lung maturation, thereby reducing the likelihood of GMH/IVH. Unfortunately, both beta-sympathomimetic medications and indomethacin may have adverse hemodynamic effects in the fetus, which, in turn, may increase the risk of hemorrhagic and ischemic cerebral injury and outweigh any potential benefits (91,92). In contrast, magnesium sulfate may provide a protective effect against cerebral injury (93). Furthermore, antenatal corticosteroids that induce fetal lung maturation, as well as resolution of the germinal matrix, definitely reduce the overall incidence and severity of GMH/IVH (94–98). Because even an incomplete course of antenatal corticosteroid has some benefit, prompt treatment is indicated for most women who are at imminent risk for premature delivery. In addition, transfer of the high-risk mother to a tertiary perinatal center prior to delivery is recommended.

Intrapartum Management

There is increasing evidence that the occurrence of vaginal delivery, duration of labor longer than 12 hours, regardless of the mode of delivery, and a trial of labor before cesarian section all increase the probability of GMH/IVH (98,99). Administration of phenobarbital antenatally may dampen fluctuations in arterial blood pressure and, hence, fluctuations in cerebral blood flow, thereby decreasing the risk of overall incidence and severity of GMH/IVH (100–102). Although preliminary data are encouraging, antenatal phenobarbital is not recommended routinely pending further confirmatory trials.

Antenatal administration of vitamin K to improve coagulation abnormalities has been reported to be of possible benefit. However, data again remain inconclusive (103).

Postnatal Management

Correction or prevention of major hemodynamic disturances, including fluctuating cerebral blood flow, systemic hypotension and hypertension, and increases in cerebral venous pressure, may reduce the overall incidence and severity of GMH/IVH. Because of the impaired cerebrovascular autoregulation in the sick premature newborn, alterations in systemic blood pressure are reflected directly in changes in cerebral blood flow. Care must be taken to prevent systemic hypertension associated with excessive handling, suctioning, and rapid infusions of blood or colloid. In addition, adequate ventilation must be maintained to avoid apnea, pneumothorax, and hypercapnia.

In mechanically ventilated infants, muscle paralysis with pancuronium bromide is highly effective for transforming a fluctuating pattern of cerebral blood flow into a stable pattern, resulting in an impressive decrease in all grades of GMH/IVH (104,105).

Abnormalities of coagulation or platelet–capillary interactions may play a role in the pathogenesis of GMH/IVH in some patients. However, to date, there is no conclusive evidence that administration of fresh-frozen plasma or other coagulation factors reduces the incidence of GMH/IVH. On the other hand, there are reports that heparinization of umbilical catheters may be associated with increased risk of GMH/IVH (106).

Two pharmacologic agents, ethamsylate and vitamin E, theoretically are of value for the stabilization of the fragile germinal matrix vessels. Several studies have demonstrated a reduction in the overall incidence and severity of GMH/IVH following administration of ethamsylate (107,108). However, there is concern that this treatment may cause cerebral ischemia, and additional studies are needed to evaluate the risks and benefits of this therapy, which is not available in the United States. Vitamin E has antioxidant properties and may function as a free-radical scavenger to protect endothelial cells of the germinal matrix from hypoxic injury. There are conflicting data about the use of vitamin E for prevention of GMH/IVH. Potential detrimental effects of vitamin E therapy include an increased risk of infection, necrotizing enterocolitis, liver and renal toxicity, thrombocytopenia, and death (109). Additional data are required.

Posthemorrhagic Hydrocephalus

Ventriculomegaly has been reported to occur in approximately 35% of infants with GMH/IVH. However, it may arrest or resolve spontaneously in approximately 65% usually within several weeks. In the remainder, several treatment modalities may be of benefit. These include either intermittent or permanent mechanical drainage of CSF, or medications, such as osmotic agents or agents that decrease CSF production. The optimal timing of intervention or the selection of specific treatment modalities has not been established. Our practice in infants with slowly progressive, moderate ventriculomegaly without signs of increased intracranial pressure initially involves frequent (often daily) lumbar punctures. Due to the significant rate of technical failure with this procedure, we often proceed to the early use of a ventricular catheter with a subcutaneous reservoir (McComb reservoir), which may be tapped as necessary. Another temporizing measure, prior to definitive therapy by placement of a permanent ventriculoperitoneal shunt, is the use of a ventriculosubgaleal shunt, where fluid is drained from the ventricles into the subgaleal space.

The use of medical therapy, e.g., carbonic anhydrase inhibitors (acetozolamide, furosemide) to decrease CSF production and osmotic agents (isosorbide, glycerol), is limited by complications of electrolyte imbalance, nephrocalcinosis, and concern about potential toxic effects on myelination (89).

Prognosis

The short-term outcome of GMH/IVH is related principally to the size of the hemorrhage and may be considered in terms of mortality or hydrocephalus among survivors. The short-term outcome of the infant with GMH/IVH appears to have improved because of detection by routine cranial ultrasonography of small lesions that are silent clinically and of little practical consequence. Improvements in neonatal intensive care have contributed to a decrease in mortality rate during the newborn period for infants with larger lesions. For infants with small GMH/IVH, survival without ventricular dilation is the rule. With moderate-sized hemorrhage, mortality is low (approximately 10%), and progressive hydrocephalus occurs in fewer than 20%. However, large hemorrhage has a high mortality rate (50% to 60%), and posthemorrhagic hydrocephalus develops frequently (65% to 100%) (1). Of course, the most critical determinant of long-term outcome is the extent of parenchymal involvement. Major GMH/IVH occurs frequently in the context of hypoxic–ischemic cerebral insult, and long-term neurologic outcome depends on a concomitant or preceding hemorrhagic or nonhemorrhagic hypoxic–ischemic cerebral injury.

There is also a high risk of major neurologic sequelae in infants with posthemorrhagic hydrocephalus, especially those who had placement of a ventriculoperitoneal shunt. In one study, approximately 35% died and 50% had moderate or severe neurologic impairment at 5 years of age (110). In another multicenter, randomized controlled trial of 157 cases of posthemorrhagic hydrocephalus, 20% died and 76% had major motor impairment. Furthermore, early drainage of CSF did not improve outcome significantly compared with controls (111).

SUBDURAL HEMORRHAGE

Improvements in obstetric practice and a decrease in mechanical birth trauma have reduced considerably the incidence of severe subdural hemorrhage. This type of hemorrhage accounts for less than 5% to 10% of intracranial hemorrhage in the newborn (112). However, the data must be interpreted with the recognition that mild subdural hemorrhage may have few associated clinical abnormalities and may remain undiagnosed.

Subdural hemorrhage occurs in premature and term infants and results from laceration of the major veins and sinuses, usually associated with a tear of the dura or dural reflections (e.g., falx, tentorium) overlying the cerebral hemispheres or cerebellum. Excessive molding of the head may play a role in the genesis of subdural hemorrhage. Clinical features include a decreased level of consciousness, seizures, or asymmetry of motor function. Clinical outcome is determined in large part by the extent of associated hypoxic–ischemic injury.

Diagnosis

CT is the technique of choice for the identification of subdural hemorrhage. Differentiating subdural from intracerebellar hemorrhage may be difficult in infants who have evidence of hemorrhage in the posterior fossa on CT scans. Intracerebellar hemorrhage appears to be more common in premature infants, and posterior fossa subdural hemorrhage is more common in term newborns (1).

The diagnosis of posterior fossa hemorrhage and small lesions located over the cerebral convexities may be difficult using cranial ultrasonography alone. However, large convexity subdural hemorrhage, especially if associated with lateral displacement of midline structures, can be detected by this technique.

Occipital diastasis and skull fractures are demonstrated best by skull radiographs.

Management

Convexity subdural hemorrhage, particularly if associated with displacement of the midline, should be evacuated by subdural tap or craniotomy, especially if there is clinical deterioration with signs of transtentorial hernia-tion. Massive subdural hemorrhage located in the posterior fossa may require surgical evacuation. Surgical intervention may not significantly improve the long-term outcome if there are no major neurologic signs (1).

Prognosis

The prognosis for infants with major lacerations of the tentorium or falx is poor. The mortality rate is approximately 45%, and survivors frequently develop hydrocephalus and other sequelae. More than 50% of survivors who sustain lesser degrees of hemorrhage are neurologically normal at follow-up. Concomitant hypoxic–ischemic cerebral injury is often the critical factor in determining outcome.

PRIMARY SUBARACHNOID HEMORRHAGE

Primary subarachnoid hemorrhage, which is located most prominently in the subarachnoid space over the cerebral convexities and in the posterior fossa, refers to hemorrhage within the subarachnoid space that is not secondary to extension of subdural hemorrhage, IVH, or cerebellar hemorrhage. Unlike the dramatic arterial hemorrhage in adults, subarachnoid hemorrhage in the newborn is usually self-limited and of venous origin, originating from small vessels in the leptomeningeal plexus or in bridging veins within the subarachnoid space (1). Trauma or hypoxic events may be important antecedents of major degrees of primary subarachnoid hemorrhage, although the pathogenesis usually is uncertain. Long-term sequelae are uncommon. Rarely, hydrocephalus may develop secondary to adhesions at the outflow of the fourth ventricle or over the cerebral convexities.

Clinical Features

Definition of the clinical features related solely to primary subarachnoid hemorrhage has been made difficult by its association with trauma, hypoxic insult, and other forms of intracerebral hemorrhage that produce abnormal neurologic signs. Nevertheless, three syndromes of primary subarachnoid hemorrhage are recognized (1). The first syndrome of minimal or no clinical features is the most common. In the second syndrome, seizures occur most commonly on the second day of life, and the infant is usually well between seizures. The third syndrome, associated with massive subarachnoid hemorrhage, consists of rapid neurologic deterioration and is uncommon. The infant usually has sustained severe hypoxic–ischemic cerebral injury, with or without trauma, or has a major vascular abnormality, such as arteriovenous malformation or aneurysm.

Diagnosis

The diagnosis of primary subarachnoid hemorrhage is based on the finding of uniformly blood-stained CSF on lumbar puncture in an infant in whom other forms of intracranial hemorrhage have been excluded by CT. With primary subarachnoid hemorrhage, CT usually demonstrates blood in the superior longitudinal fissure and in sulci.

Management

Seizures are treated with anticonvulsant medication. Hydrocephalus is managed as described previously in this chapter.

Prognosis

In the absence of preceding severe trauma, hypoxic–ischemic cerebral injury, or ruptured vascular lesion, the outcome is favorable. Outcome correlates well with the neonatal clinical syndrome. In infants with minimal or no clinical signs, the prognosis is excellent. In term infants with seizures, 90% are normal at follow-up. In the rare instance of massive subarachnoid hemorrhage with catastrophic deterioration, death and hydrocephalus are common.

INTRACEREBELLAR HEMORRHAGE

Postmortem studies suggest that primary hemorrhage into the cerebellum is a relatively common lesion, reported in 15% to 25% of infants who are less than 32 weeks of gestation or of birth weight less than 1,500 g (113), as well as in term newborns. The routine use of cranial ultrasonography in premature infants has confirmed that this lesion is much less common in surviving infants than was considered previously.

Neuropathology

Causes of cerebellar hemorrhage include traumatic laceration of the cerebellum or sinuses, venous infarction, or extension of IVH or massive subarachnoid hemorrhage into the cerebellum. Pathogenetic factors include tenuous vascular integrity, skull deformation, occipital diastasis, impaired cerebrovascular autoregulation with hypoxic–ischemic insult, and bleeding from fragile vessels of the germinal external granule cell layer of the cerebellum.

Clinical Features

Most reports of intracerebellar hemorrhage in premature infants are based on autopsy studies. Clinical details are based on retrospective analyses. There is usually a history of hypoxic–ischemic insult or an association with severe respiratory distress syndrome. In most instances, there is a catastrophic deterioration with apnea, bradycardia, and a decrease in hematocrit. Clinical signs appear usually in the first 3 weeks of life, with most beginning within the first 2 days of life. In term infants, there is usually a history of difficult breech delivery, with subsequent development of neurologic signs referable to brainstem compression, e.g., stupor or coma, cranial nerve abnormalities, apnea, bradycardia, and opisthotonus.

Diagnosis

The lesion is suspected on the basis of the history and physical features described previously. Definitive diagnosis is made by CT or MRI (114). In some instances, cranial ultrasonography may demonstrate intracerebellar hemorrhage.

Management

Early detection by CT, MRI, or ultrasound scans is essential. Decisions concerning surgical or conservative management are based on the size of the lesion and the clinical state of the infant. Recovery without surgical intervention has been reported. Fishman and colleagues (115) reported successful conservative management of four full-term infants with intracerebellar hemorrhage and recommend that, if the clinical picture is stable and there is no increase in intracranial pressure, supportive care and serial CT examinations may be all that is necessary. Our experience with nonsurgical management of selected cases supports this notion.

Prognosis

Most reports of intracerebellar hemorrhage in the premature infant are based on autopsy studies. For the infant with severe intracerebellar hemorrhage, the prognosis is poor. In a study of 700 newborns diagnosed using CT scans, Scotti and associates (114) observed eight cases of intracerebellar hemorrhage. Four premature infants had concomitant IVH and died. In the four term infants, the intracerebellar hemorrhages were evacuated. All these infants survived, but all had significant motor and cognitive impairment.

NEUROMUSCULAR DISORDERS

Neuromuscular disease implies dysfunction of the motor system at a level between the motor cortex and muscle.

Diagnosis

Lower motor neuron disorders should be considered whenever an alert newborn presents with hypotonia and weakness. However, in many instances, e.g., congenital muscular dystrophy, myotonic dystrophy, and mitochondrial cytopathies, there may be associated central nervous system involvement. Furthermore, infants with neuromuscular disease may sustain secondary hypoxic–ischemic brain injury related to respiratory muscle weakness or pulmonary hypoplasia.

Because most neuromuscular disorders are inherited and some, e.g., Duchenne muscular dystrophy, may be asymptomatic in the newborn period, a detailed family history is of critical importance. Specific complications of pregnancy, e.g., decreased fetal movements, polyhydramnios, and breech presentation, are a common occurrence. In addition to assessment of muscle bulk, tone, and power, examination for presence of muscle fasciculations, facial diplegia, or ptosis support a diagnosis of neonatal neuromuscular disease.

Laboratory investigations in older children with muscle disease often include elevation of serum creatine phosphokinase levels. Unfortunately, this screening test is of limited value in the newborn, because levels may be increased up to tenfold following normal vaginal delivery. Chest x-ray may demonstrate thin ribs related to decreased fetal respiratory efforts (116) or cardiac enlargement suggestive of cardiomyopathy. Nerve conduction velocities and electromyography may establish the level of involvement of the motor system, but the technical performance and interpretation of data are difficult in the newborn age group (117–119). Although imaging techniques, e.g., ultrasonography, CT, and MRI, have some role in the investigation of muscle disease, there is little experience in the newborn. Muscle biopsy, either by open, surgical, or needle biopsy technique, is technically feasible. However, problems with histologic interpretation may arise during the newborn period, due to nonspecific abnormalities that exist in the early stages of progressive muscular dystrophies.

Molecular genetic techniques clearly are revolutionizing the diagnosis and classification of neuromuscular disease as well as decreasing the need for invasive investigations. However, clinical assessment must direct these costly genetic investigations.

Major Neuromuscular Conditions

Anterior Horn Cell Disease

Anterior horn cell disorders, e.g., type I spinal muscular atrophy (Werdnig–Hoffman disease), type II glycogen storage disease (Pompe's disease), neurogenic arthrogryposis multiplex congenita, and neonatal poliomyelitis, account for approximately 35% of all cases of neonatal hypotonia of neuromuscular origin. Characteristically, infants are alert but profoundly hypotonic and weak. with absent tendon reflexes, paradoxical diaphragmatic respiratory movements, and the majority have prominent fasciculations of the tongue. Electrical studies and muscle biopsy demonstrate severe acute and chronic denervation. The genetic defect of autosomal recessive type I spinal muscular atrophy has been identified on chromosome 5q, which enables molecular diagnostic tests and prenatal testing. Although muscle strength may remain relatively static, overall deterioration and decreased survival result from repeated respiratory infections and aspiration, prolonged immobility, and hospitalization.

Peripheral Nerve Disorders

Disorders of peripheral nerves rarely present in the newborn period. The clinical course is variable and may even be nonprogressive or reversible (1). Diagnosis may be confirmed by nerve conduction studies. Adjunctive investigations include measurement of CSF protein, lactate levels, and sural nerve biopsy.

Disorders of the Neuromuscular Junction

These conditions present with fluctuating muscle weakness, variable ptosis, ophthalmoplegia, facial weakness, impaired feeding, hypoventilation, and autonomic disturbances. Major categories include myasthenia gravis (transient or congenital) and toxic-metabolic problems, e.g., hypermagnesemia, aminoglycoside toxicity, and infantile botulism.

Transient myasthenia gravis, related to circulating maternal antiacetylcholine receptor antibodies, occurs in approximately 20% of infants of mothers with myasthenia. The diagnosis may be confirmed by evaluating the infant's response to neostigmine. Management includes supportive treatment, anticholinesterase therapy, and possibly exchange transfusion until symptoms resolve after several weeks. Congenital myasthenia relates to anatomic defects of the neuromuscular junction, which have variable response to pyridostigmine.

Early diagnosis of disorders of neuromuscular transmission is critical because many of these conditions respond to treatment, and timely intervention may prevent serious complications.

Primary Muscle Disorders

Generalized muscle disorders include the genetically determined progressive muscular dystrophies, which have nonspecific histologic features of muscle necrosis, regeneration, fibrosis, and nonprogressive congenital myopathies, which are characterized by distinctive histologic abnormalities.

The major muscular dystrophies that present in the newborn include congenital myotonic dystrophy and congenital muscular dystrophy. Congenital myotonic dystrophy is inherited exclusively from the mother, so the diagnosis may be confirmed by molecular genetic studies in either the mother or the affected newborn, i.e., demonstration of an increase in trinucleotide repeats (CTG) at the myotonic dystrophy gene locus at chromosome 19q (120). Affected infants present with hypotonia, weakness, hypoventilation, impaired sucking and swallowing, facial diplegia, ptosis, and arthrogryposis. In addition, there is usually significant cognitive impairment, which may be associated with abnormalities on neuroimaging. The mortality rate is high and the long-term clinical course is variable (121).

Congenital muscular dystrophy comprises several disorders that have an autosomal recessive inheritance pattern and may be classified according to whether there is isolated muscular dystrophy or a combination of central nervous system and skeletal muscle involvement. Central nervous system involvement may include cerebral dysgenesis, cerebral white matter, and ocular abnormalities. It may be suspected on the basis of seizures, glaucoma, optic nerve abnormalities, or cataracts. The clinical course of patients with central nervous system involvement is often progressive with decreased survival, whereas in infants who have myopathy alone, muscle weakness is often static and affected individuals may even attain ambulation (121,122).

Investigations include normal or moderate elevation of creatine kinase levels and dystrophic abnormalities on muscle biopsy. Results of neuroimaging studies may be abnormal. In cases with central nervous system abnormalities, immunocytochemical analysis of the muscle biopsy may reveal deficiency of merosin, an extracellular protein that is associated closely with the muscle membrane. The merosin protein is thought to play a significant pathogenetic role in congenital muscular dystrophy.

In addition to the muscular dystrophies, there are numerous congenital myopathies that are classified according to their specific histologic abnormalities. With the exception of nemaline myopathy and X-linked myotubular myopathy, which may present with respiratory failure in early infancy, hypotonia and weakness often are relatively mild and static.

Metabolic Myopathies

With the availability of electron microscopy, muscle enzyme assays, and MRS, muscle conditions that have primary derangements of energy metabolism, e.g., mitochondrial cytopathies, carnitine deficiency, and disorders of lipid and glycogen, are being recognized with increasing frequency. Clinical features include hypotonia, weakness, failure to thrive, encephalopathy, hypoglycemia, and cardiomyopathy. Muscle histology and enzyme abnormalities usually are diagnostic. Clearly, detailed discussion of the biochemical aspects of metabolic myopathies is beyond the scope of this chapter.

Management

The management of neuromuscular disorders in the newborn often is associated with major genetic and ethical dilemmas, especially with regard to a reasonable approach to mechanical ventilatory support. Unfortunately, few scientific guidelines exist. Other supportive management strategies include oxygen therapy, nasogastric feeding, and aggressive physiotherapy to minimize joint contractures. Specific therapies exist for some conditions, e.g., pyridostigmine for myasthenia gravis.

Clearly, the prognosis of neuromuscular conditions is variable and depends principally on the specific disorder involved.

REFERENCES

1. Volpe JJ. *Neurology of the newborn.* Philadelphia: WB Saunders, 1995.
2. Hill A, Volpe JJ, eds. *Fetal neurology. International review of child neurology series.* New York: Raven Press, 1989.
3. Clancy RR. The management of neonatal seizures. In: Stevenson K, Sunshine P, eds. *Fetal & neonatal brain injury—mechanisms, management and the risks of practice.* Oxford: Oxford University Press, 1997:432.
4. Wasterlain CG, Vert P, eds. *Neonatal seizures.* New York: Raven Press, 1990.
5. Yager JY, Shuaib A, Thornhill J. The effect of age on susceptibility to brain damage in a model of global hemisphere hypoxia–ischemia. *Dev Brain Res* 1996;93:143.

6. Younkin DP, Delivoria-Papadopoulos M, Maris J, Donlon E, Clancy R, Chance B. Cerebral metabolic effects of neonatal seizures measured with *in vivo* ^{31}P NMR spectroscopy. *Ann Neurol* 1986;20:513.

7. Holmes GL. Epilepsy in the developing brain: lessons from the laboratory and clinic. *Epilepsia* 1997;38:12.

8. Volpe JJ. Neonatal seizures: current concepts and revised classification. *Pediatrics* 1989;84:422.

9. Sher MS. Seizures in the newborn: diagnosis, treatment, and outcome. *Clin Perinatol* 1997;24:735.

10. Daoust-Ray J, Seshia SS. Benign neonatal sleep myoclonus—a differential diagnosis of neonatal seizures. *Am J Dis Child* 1992;146:1236.

11. Sher MS. Neonatal seizures. Seizures in special clinical settings In: Wyllie E, ed. *The treatment of epilepsy. Principles and practice*, 2nd ed. Baltimore: Williams & Wilkins, 1997, p 243.

12. Mizrahi EM, Kellaway P. Characterization and classification of neonatal seizures. *Neurology* 1987;37:1837.

13. Hillman L, Hillman R, Dodson WE. Diagnosis, treatment and follow-up of neonatal mepivacaine intoxication secondary to paracervical and pudendal blocks during labor. *J Pediatr* 1979;95:472.

14. Steinlein O, Haussler M, Fischer C, Schuster V. Benign familial neonatal convulsions: confirmation of genetic heterogeneity and further evidence for a second locus on chromosome 8g. *Hum Genet* 1995;95:411.

15. Berkovic SF, Nicholson GA, Hwang PA, Scheffer IE, Howell RA, Kennerson ML. Phenotypic expression of benign familial neonatal convulsions linked to chromosome 20. *Arch Neurol* 1994;51:1125.

16. Rose AL, Lombroso CT. Neonatal seizure states. A study of clinical, pathological and electroencephalographic features in 137 full-term babies with long-term follow-up. *Pediatrics* 1972;45:404.

17. Roland EH, Hill A. Clinical aspects of perinatal hypoxic–ischemic brain injury. *Semin Pediatr Neurol* 1995;2:57.

18. Roland EH, Poskitt K, Rodriguez E, Lupton BA, Hill A. Perinatal hypoxic–ischemic thalamic injury: clinical features and neuroimaging. *Ann Neurol* 1998;44:161.

19. Nelson KB, Ellenberg JH. Antecedents of cerebral palsy: multivariate analysis of risk. *N Engl J Med* 1986;315:81.

20. Nelson KB, Emery III ES. Birth asphyxia and the neonatal brain: what do we know and when do we know it? *Clin Perinatol* 1993;20:327.

21. Blair E, Stanley FJ. Intrapartum asphyxia: a rare cause of cerebral palsy. *J Pediatr* 1988;112:515.

22. Roland EH, Hill A. How important is perinatal asphyxia in the causation of brain injury? *MRDD Res Rev* 1997;3:22.

23. Sarnat HB, Sarnat MS. Neonatal encephalopathy following fetal distress. *Arch Dis Child* 1976;33:696.

24. Robertson CMT, Finer NN. Term infants with hypoxic–ischemic encephalopathy: outcome at 3.5 years. *Dev Med Child Neurol* 1985;27:473.

25. Robertson CMT, Finer NN. Longterm follow-up of term neonates with perinatal asphyxia. *Clin Perinatol* 1993;20:483.

26. Robertson CMT, Grace MGA. Validation of prediction of kindergarten-age-school readiness scores of non-disabled survivors of moderate neonatal encephalopathy in term infants. *Can J Public Health* 1992;83[Suppl]:51.

27. Lupton BA, Hill A, Roland EH, Whitfield MF, Flodmark O. Brain-swelling in the asphyxiated term newborn: pathogenesis and outcome. *Pediatrics* 1988;82:139.

28. Levene MI, Evans DH, Forde A, et al. Value of intracranial pressure monitoring of asphyxiated newborn infants. *Dev Med Child Neurol* 1987;29:311.

29. Clancy R, Legido A, Newell R, et al. Continuous intracranial pressure monitoring and serial electroencephalographic recordings in severely asphyxiated term newborns. *Am J Dis Child* 1988;142:740.

30. Whitelaw A. Intervention after birth asphyxia. *Arch Dis Child* 1989;64:66.

31. Vannucci RC. Current and potentially new management strategies for perinatal hypoxic–ischemic encephalopathy. *Pediatrics* 1990;85:961.

32. Adhikari M, Moodley M, Desai PK. Mannitol in neonatal cerebral oedema. *Brain Dev* 1990;23:349.

33. Perlman JM, Tack ED, Martin T, et al. Acute systemic organ injury in the term infant after asphyxia. *Am J Dis Child* 1989;143:617.

34. Cordes I, Roland EH, Lupton BA, et al. Systemic organ involvement and hypoxic–ischemic encephalopathy in the term newborn. *Ann Neurol* 1992;32:462A.

35. Martin-Ancel A, Garcia-Alix A, Gaya F, et al. Multiple organ involvement in perinatal asphyxia. *J Pediatr* 1995;127:786.

36. Barkovich AJ, Hallam D. Neuroimaging in perinatal hypoxic–ischemic injury. *MRDD Res Rev* 1997;3:28.

37. Stark JE, Seibert JJ. Cerebral artery Doppler ultrasonography for prediction of outcome after perinatal asphyxia. *J Ultrasound Med* 1994;13:595.

38. Fuzzi E, Orcesi S, Caffi L, et al. Neuro developmental outcome of 5–7 years in preterm infants with periventricular leukomalacia. *Neuropediatrics* 1994;25:134.

39. deVries LS, Eken P, Dubowitz LMS. The spectrum of leukomalacia using cranial ultrasound. *Behav Brain Res* 1992;49:1.

40. Goldstein RB, Filly RA, Hechts, et al. Noncystic increased periventricular echogenicity and other mild cranial ultrasonographic abnormalities: predictors of outcome in low birthweight infants. *J Clin Ultrasound* 1989;17:553.

41. Flodmark O. The neonatal brain. In: *Syllabus:* a categorical course in diagnostic radiology–neuroradiology. Oak Brook, 1987:43.

42. Flodmark O, Roland EH, Hill A, et al. Periventricular leukomalacia: radiologic diagnosis. *Radiology* 1987;162:119.

43. Baenziger OE, Martin E, Steinlin M. Early pattern recognition in severe perinatal asphyxia: a prospective MRI study. *Neuroradiology* 1993;35:437.

44. Kuenzle C, Baenziger O, Martin E, et al. Prognostic value of early MR imaging in term infants with severe perinatal asphyxia. *Neuropediatrics* 1994;25:191.

45. Rutherford MA, Pennock JM, Schwieso JE, et al. Hypoxic–ischemic encephalopathy: early magnetic resonance imaging findings and their evolution. *Neuropediatrics* 1995;26:183.

46. Barkovich AJ, Westmark KD, Ferreiro D, et al. Perinatal asphyxia: MR findings in the firstt 10 days. *AJNR* 1995;16:427.

47. Cowan FM, Pennock JM, Hanrahon JD et al. Early detection of cerebral infarction and hypoxic–ischemic encephaloptahy in neonates using diffusion weighted magnetic resonance imaging. *Neuropediatrics* 1994;25:172.

48. O'Brien MJ, Ash JM, Gilday DL. Radionuclide brain scanning in perinatal hypoxia–ischemia. *Dev Med Child Neurol* 1979;21:161.

49. Volpe JJ, Herscovitch P, Perlman JM, et al. Positron emission tomography in the asphyxiated term newborn: parasagittal impairment of cerebral blood flow. *Ann Neurol* 1985;17:287.

50. Denays R, Pachterbeke TV, Tondeur M, et al. Brain single photon emission computed tomography in neonates. *J Nucl Med* 1989;30:1337.

51. Wyatt JS. Magnetic resonance spectroscopy and near-infrared spectroscopy in the assessment of the asphyxiated term infant. *MRDD Res Rev* 1997;3:42.

52. Wyatt JS. Near infrared spectroscopy in asphyxial brain injury. *Clin Perinatol* 1993;20:329.

53. Whyte HE, Taylor MJ, Menzies R, Chin KC, MacMillan LJ. Prognostic utility of visual evoked potentials in term asphyxiated neonates. *Pediatr Neurol* 1986;2:220.

54. Stockard JE, Stockard JJ, Kleinberg F, Westmoreland BF. Prognostic value of brainstem auditory evoked potentials in neonate. *Arch Neurol* 1983;40:360.

55. Groenendaal F, Veenhoven RH, van der Grond J, et al. Cerebral lactate and N-acetyl aspartate/choline ratios in asphyxiated full-term neonates demonstrated *in vivo* using proton magnetic resonance spectroscopy. *Pediatr Res* 1994;35:148.

56. Pryds O, Greisen G, Lou H, et al. Vasoparalysis is associated with brain damage in asphyxiated term infants. *J Pediatr* 1990;117:119.

57. Greisen G. Cerebral blood flow and energy metabolism in the newborn. *Clin Perinatol* 1997;24:531.

58. McDonald JW, Johnston MV. Physiological and pathophysiological roles of excitatory amino acids during central nervous system development. *Brain Res Rev* 1990;15:41.

59. McDonald JW, Silverstein FS, Johnston MV. Magnesium reduces N-methyl-D-aspartate (NMDA)-mediated brain injury in perinatal rats. *Neurosci Lett* 1990;109:234.

60. Hagberg H, Gillard E, Diemer N-H, et al. Hypoxia–ischemia in the neonatal rat brain: histopathology after post-treatment with NMDA and non-NMDA receptor antagonists. *Biol Neonate* 1994;66:205.

61. Greenamyre JT, Penney JB, Young AB, et al. Evidence for transient perinatal glutamatergic innervation of globus pallidus. *J Neurosci* 1987;7:1022.

62. Albers G, Goldberg MP, Choi DW. N-methyl-D-aspartate antagonists: ready for clinical trial in brain ischemia? *Ann Neurol* 1989;25:398.

63. Vannucci RC, Perlman JM. Interventions for perinatal hypoxic–ischemic encephalopathy. *Pediatrics* 1997;100:1.

64. Myers RE. Four patterns of perinatal brain damage and their conditions of occurrence in primates. *Adv Neurol* 1975;10:223.

65. Martin LJ, Brambrink AM, Koehler RC, et al. Primary sensory forebrain motor systems in the newborn brain are preferentially damaged by hypoxia–ischemia. *J Comp Neurol* 1997;377:262.

66. Martin LJ, Brambrink AM, Lehmann C, et al. Hypoxia–ischemia causes abnormalities in glutamate transporters and death of astroglia and neurons in newborn striatum. *Ann Neurol* 1997;42:335.

67. Roland EH, Hill A, Norman MG, Flodmark O, MacNab AJ. Selective brain stem injury in an asphyxiated newborn. *Ann Neurol* 1988;23:89.

68. Rivkin MJ, Anderson ML, Kaye EM. Neonatal idiopathic cerebral venous thrombosis: an unrecognized cause of transient seizures or lethargy. *Ann Neurol* 1992;32:51.

69. Baram TZ, Butler IJ, Nelson MD Jr, et al. Transverse sinus thrombosis in newborns: clinical and magnetic resonance imaging findings. *Ann Neurol* 1988;24:792.

70. DeReuck JL. Cerebral angioarchitecture and perinatal brain lesions in premature and full-term infants. *Acta Neurol Scand* 1984;70:391.

71. Takashima S, Tanaka K. Development of cerebrovascular architecture and its relationshiop to periventricular leukomalacia. *Arch Neurol* 1978;35:11.

72. Takashima S, Mito T, Houdou S, et al. Relationship between periventricular hemorrhage, leukomalacia and brainstem lesions in prematurely born infants. *Brain Dev* 1989;11:121.

73. Leviton A, Gilles FH. Acquired perinatal leukoencephalopathy. *Ann Neurol* 1984;16:1.

74. Volpe JJ. Brain injury in the premature infant: neuropathology, clinical aspects and pathogenesis. *MRDD Res Rev* 1997;3:3.

75. Back SA, Volpe JJ. Cellular and molecular pathogenesis of periventricular white matter injury. *MRDD Res Rev* 1997;3:96.

76. Yoon BH, Romero R, Yang SH, et al. Interleukin-6 concentrations in umbilical cord plasma are elevated in neonates with white matter lesions associated with periventricular leukomalacia. *Am J Obstet Gynecol* 1996;174:1433.

77. Armstrong D, Norman MG. Periventricular leukomalacia in neonates: complications and sequelae. *Arch Dis Child* 1974;99:367.

78. Trounce JQ, Rutter N, Levene MI. Periventricular leukomalacia and intraventricular haemorrhage in the preterm neonate. *Arch Dis Child* 1986;61:1196.

79. Guzzetta F, Shackelford GD, Volpe S, et al. Periventricular intraparenchymal echodensities in the premature newborn: critical determinant of neurological status. *Pediatrics* 1986;78:995.

80. Gould SJ, Howard S, Hope PL, et al. Periventricular intraparenchymal cerebral haemorrhage in preterm infants: the role of venous infarction. *J Pathol* 1987;151:197.

81. Takashima S, Mito T, Ando Y. Pathogenesis of periventricular white matter hemorrhages in preterm infants. *Brain Dev* 1986;8:25.

82. Dubowitz LMS, Bydder GM, Mushin J. Developmental sequence of periventricular leukomalacia *Arch Dis Child* 1985;60:349.

83. Roland EH, Jan JE, Hill A, et al. Cortical visual impairment following birth asphyxia. *Pediatr Neurol* 1986;2:133.

84. Volpe JJ. Subplate neurons—missing link in brain injury of the premature infant? *Pediatrics* 1996;97:112.

85. Evrard P, Gressens P, Volpe JJ. New concepts to understand the neurological consequences of subcortical lesions in the premature brain [Editorial]. *Biol Neonate* 1992;61:1.

86. Kostovic I, Lukinovic N, Judas M, et al. Structural basis of the developmental plasticity in the human cerebral cortex: the role of the transient subplate zone. *Metab Brain Dis* 1989;4:17.

87. Barmada MA, Moosy J, Painter M. Pontosubicular necrosis and hyperoxemia *Pediatrics* 1980;68:840.

88. Lazzara A, Ahmann P, Dykes F, Brann AW, Schwartz J. Clinical predictability of intraventricular hemorrhage in preterm infants. *Pediatrics* 1980;65:30.

89. Roland EH, Hill A. Intraventricular hemorrhage and posthemorrhagic

90. Perlman JM, Lynch B, Volpe JJ. Late hydrocephalus after arrest and resolution of neonatal posthemorrhagic hydrocephalus. *Dev Med Child Neurol* 1990; 32:725.

91. Norton ME, Merrill J, Cooper BAB, et al. Neonatal complications after administration of indomethacin for preterm labor. *N Engl J Med* 1993;329:1602.

92. Groome, LJ, Goldenberg RL, Cliver SP. Neonatal periventricular-intraventricular hemorrhage after maternal beta-sympathomimetic tocolysis. *Am J Obstet Gynecol* 1992;167:873.

93. Nelson KB, Grether JK. Can magnesium sulfate reduce the risk of cerebral palsy in very low birthweight infants? *Pediatrics* 1995;95:263.

94. Shankaran S, Bauer CR, Bain R, Wright LL, Zachary J, for the NICHD Neonatal Research Network. Prenatal and perinatal risk and protective factors for neonatal intracranial hemorrhage. *Arch Pediatr Adolesc Med* 1996;150:491.

95. Horbar JD. Prevention of periventricular-intraventricular hemorrhage. In: Sinclair JC, Bracken MB, eds. *Effective care of the newborn infant.* New York: Oxford University Press 1992:562.

96. Horbar JD, et al. Antenatal corticosteroid treatment and neonatal outcomes for infants 501 to 1500 g in the Vermont-Oxford Trials Network. *Am J Obstet Gynecol* 1995;173:275.

97. Wright LL, Verter J, Younes N, et al. Antenatal corticosteroid administration and neonatal outcome in very low birthweight infants: The NICHD Neonatal Research Network. *Am J Obstet Gynecol* 1995;173:269.

98. Ment LR, Oh W, Ehrenkranz RA, et al. Antenatal steroids, delivery mode and intraventricular hemorrhage in preterm infants. *Am J Obstet Gynecol* 1995;172:795.

99. Leviton A, Fenton T, Kuban KC, et al. Labor and delivery characteristics and the risk of germinal matrix hemorrhage in low birthweight infants. *J Child Neurol* 1991;6:35.

100. Kaempf JW, Porreco R, Moline R, et al. Antenatal phenobarbital for the prevention of periventricular and intraventricular hemorrhage: a double-blind, randomized, placebo-controlled multihospital trial. *Pediatrics* 1990;117:933.

101. Shankaran S, Cepeda E, Muran G, et al. Antenatal phenobartial therapy and neonatal outcome. I. Effect on intracranial hemorrhage. *Pediatrics* 1996;97:644.

102. Shankaran S, Soldt E, Nelson J, et al. Antenatal phenobarbital therapy and neonatal outcome. II. Neurodevelopmental outcome at 36 months. *Pediatrics* 1996;97:649.

103. Thorp JA, Parriot J, Ferrette-Smith D, et al. Antepartum vitamin K and phenobarbital for preventing intraventricular hemorrhage in the premature newborn: a randomized, double-blind, placebo-controlled trial. *Obstet Gynecol* 1994;83:70.

104. Perlman JM, McMenamin JB, Volpe JJ. Fluctuating cerebral blood flow velocity in respiratory distress syndrome: relation to the development of intraventricular hemorrhage. *N Engl J Med* 1983;309:204.

105. Perlman JM, Goodman S, Kreusser K, et al. Reduction in intraventricular hemorrhage by elimination of fluctuating cerebral blood-flow velocity in preterm infants with respiratory distress syndrome. *N Engl J Med* 1985;312:1353.

106. Lesko SM, Mitchell AA, Epstein MF, et al. Heparin use as a risk factor for intraventricular hemorrhage in low-birthweight infants. *N Engl J Med* 1986;314:1156.

107. Cooke RWI, Morgan MEI. Prophylactic ethamsylate for periventricular hemorrhage. *Arch Dis Child* 1984;59:82.

108. Benson JWT, Drayton MR, Hayward C, et al. Multicentre trial of ethamsylate for prevention of periventricular haemorrhage in very low birthweight infants. *Lancet* 1986;2:1297.

109. Arrowsmith JB, Faich GA, Tomita DK, et al. Morbidity and mortality among low birthweight infants exposed to an intravenous vitamin E product. *Pediatrics* 1989;83:244.

110. Resch B, Gedermann A, Maurer U, et al. Neurodevelopmental outcome of hydrocephalus following intra/periventricular hemorrhage in preterm infants: short and longterm results. *Child Nerv Syst* 1996;12:27.

111. Ventriculomegaly Trial Group. Randomized trial of early tapping in neonatal posthemorrhagic ventricular dilation: results at 30 months. *Arch Dis Child* 1994;70:F129.

hydrocephalus: current and potential future interventions. *Clin Perinatol* 1997;24:589.

112. Bergman I, Bauer RE, Barmada MA, et al. Intracerebral hemorrhage in the full-term neonatal infant. *Pediatrics* 1985;74:488.
113. Grunnet ML, Shields WO. Cerebellar hemorrhage in the premature infant. *J Pediatr* 1975;88:605.
114. Scotti G, Flodmark O, Harwood-Nash DC, Humphries RP. Posterior fossa hemorrhages in the newborn. *J Comput Assist Tomogr* 1981; 5:68.
115. Fishman MA, Percy AK, Cheek WR, Speer ME. Successful conservative management of cerebellar hematomas in term neonates. *J Pediatr* 1981;98:466.
116. Osborne JP, Murphy EG, Hill A. Thin ribs on chest X-ray: a useful sign in the differential diagnosis of the floppy newborn. *Dev Med Child Neurol* 1983;25:343.
117. Jones HR. Pediatric electromyography. In: Brown WF, Bolton CF, eds. *Clinical electromyography*. Boston: Butterworth-Heinemann, 1993, p 161.
118. Packer RJ, Brown MJ, Bermann PH. The diagnostic value of electromyography in infantile hypotonia. *Am J Dis Child* 1982;54:331.
119. David WS, Jones HR. Electromyography and biopsy correlation with suggested protocol for evaluation of the floppy infant. *Muscle Nerve* 1994;17:424.
120. Shelbourne P, Davies J, Buxton J, et al. Direct diagnosis of myotonic dystrophy with a disease-specific DNA marker. *N Engl J Med* 1993; 328:471.
121. Dubowitz V. *Muscle disorders in childhood*, 2nd ed. London: WB Saunders, 1995.

CHAPTER 50

Neurosurgery of the Newborn

Joseph R. Madsen and David M. Frim

Treatment of structural and functional abnormalities of the neonatal central nervous system (CNS) provides unique challenges to both the neurosurgeon and the neonatologist caring for the newborn infant. Considerations of several interrelated pathophysiologic processes can lead to an understanding of the nature of the abnormality and the goal of treatment. This understanding forms the basis for a successful interdisciplinary team approach to the management of these infants.

NEONATAL NEUROSURGICAL PATHOPHYSIOLOGY

What is unique about the neurosurgeon's contribution to the care of the neonatal CNS? The neurosurgeon brings to the neonate a series of technical interventions, which include (i) drainage or diversion of fluids, (ii) closure of openings (including neural tube defects), (iii) removal of tissue (including neoplasms and anomalous masses), and (iv) opening of fusions (such as craniosynostoses). Other neonatal nervous system problems, such as vascular disorders, do not yet have a workable neurosurgical intervention. In the management of many newborn patients, two or more of these techniques may be necessary, but almost all neurosurgical interventions in the neonate can be discussed in terms of these categories.

When applying these techniques to neonatal care, their use must be guided by pathophysiologic mechanisms unique to the neonate, such as (i) the biomechanics of neonatal brain tissue and a distensible skull, (ii) recognized and unrecognized congenital anomalies (microscopic and macroscopic), and (iii) the plasticity of neonatal CNS tissue and its effects on response to injury. Recent advances in antenatal diagnosis allow unprecedented opportunity to manage these processes even before birth. Frequently, solutions to a neonatal neurosurgical problem must address combinations, or complex interactions, of these pathophysiologic mechanisms.

The biomechanical nature of neonatal brain tissue and a distensible skull accounts for one of the best known cardinal signs of neurosurgical difficulty in the neonate, abnormal head growth. The prodigious ability of the skull to grow and the sutures to widen can allow some of the most severe cases of hydrocephalus to result in relatively few pressure effects, even with an obvious need for cerebrospinal fluid (CSF) shunting for long-term management. These same considerations in the type and nature of response of the tissues to abnormal fluid buildup can result in dramatic difficulties structurally once the pressure is relieved. The certainty that the brain and skull biomechanics will change over time adds particular challenge to management of these problems.

Obvious congenital anomalies, especially those involving open neural tube defects and exposed CNS tissue, may require urgent neurosurgical intervention. A complicating aspect is the potential occurrence of concurrent microscopic abnormalities, such as congenital problems with the wiring of the nervous system at the synaptic level. In many cases, neurologic deficits may be present in a patient with macroscopic structural abnormalities, but major neurologic disability may come from less obvious problems with tissue development, currently not treatable by neurosurgical means.

The specific vulnerability of the neonatal CNS is discussed by Hill and Volpe (Chap. 49). It is well known that the ability to recover function after CNS injury is age-dependent and seems to be better in younger individuals. Interaction between the age-dependent changes in vulnerability in CNS tissue and age-dependent differences in plasticity and ability to recover in CNS tissue make the

J. R. Madsen: Department of Surgery, Harvard Medical School; and Department of Neurosurgery, Children's Hospital, Boston, Massachusetts

D. M. Frim: Department of Surgery and Pediatrics, The University of Chicago; and Section of Pediatric Neurosurgery, The University of Chicago Children's Hospital, Chicago, Illinois

task of estimating prognosis after an injury or neurosurgical intervention extremely difficult.

The possibility of antenatal diagnosis has changed aspects of obstetric management, especially in cases of neural tube defect. In addition, the psychological issues around the time of neurosurgical therapy of the newborn are altered, as the child's family now has the opportunity to meet the neurosurgeon prenatally and fully discuss any contemplated care plan before birth.

FLUID COLLECTIONS AND THEIR MANAGEMENT

Disorders of Cerebrospinal Fluid Accumulation

The most common neurosurgical consultation on newborn patients involves evaluation and treatment of enlargement of the ventricular system. The clinical signs of progressive enlargement of the ventricular system are well known. They include excessive increase in the head circumference, fullness in the anterior fontanelle (especially evident when the patient is upright and the expected venous and fontanelle pressures should be low), episodic apnea and bradycardia, general lethargy, and ocular movement abnormalities, especially restricted upgaze. These findings are nonspecific and can be found with hydrocephalus of any etiology. At a practical level, the most important distinction is between progressive and static abnormalities in ventricular volume. This is relatively easy to determine using serial intracranial ultrasound examinations (Fig. 50–1). The recent addition of resistive index measurements adds a physiologic dimension to the anatomic images gathered by ultrasonography (1). In our experience, the presence of dramatic changes in the Doppler-measured flow signals in the anterior cerebral artery with gentle, brief compression of the anterior fontanelle correlates extremely well with the intracranial pressure by measurement and the probability of eventual need for a ventriculoperitoneal shunt (1).

The vast majority of cases of hydrocephalus seen in neonates are a result of abnormal resorption of CSF. After intraventricular hemorrhage (Fig. 50–1), this is likely a result of partial occlusion of the normal resorptive pathways of the CSF through the arachnoid villae. It has long been known that resorption of CSF is a function of the pressure differential between the CSF space and the venous pressure. Presumably, relative blockade of CSF absorption would raise the steady state to a relatively higher pressure. In the neonate with open sutures, this results in a steady state with a larger intracranial volume. It also follows that there would be some cases of mild increase in resistance to absorption of fluid that would not require specific treatment, where higher grades of failure to absorb fluid would cause dramatic increases in pressure, leading to neurologic symptoms if treatment is not instituted. The fact that hydrocephalus is a quantitative physiologic abnormality, which may occur within a variety of different parameters, implies that the need and indications for diversion of CSF may change over the child's lifetime.

Placement of a shunt in borderline cases may result in atrophy of physiologic resorption systems and, therefore, cause more permanent obstruction to resorption of CSF. This is conceptualized as atrophy of arachnoid granulations or failure to develop normal resorptive pathways, but the detailed pathology is not well known. A related paradox of shunt physiology, particularly applicable to neonates, is that it is impossible to distinguish with current available hardware a well-functioning shunt from a nonfunctioning shunt in a patient who is no longer shunt

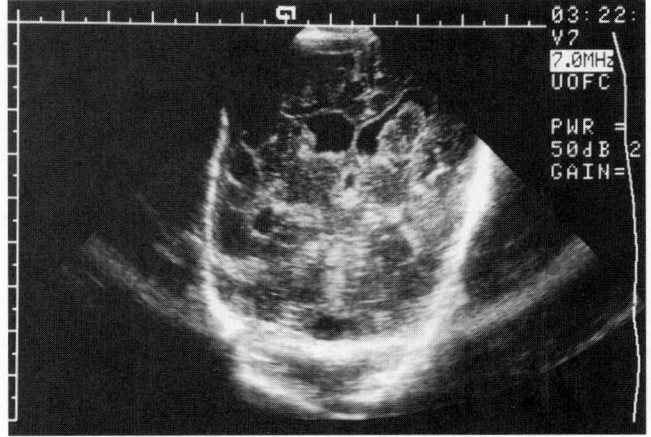 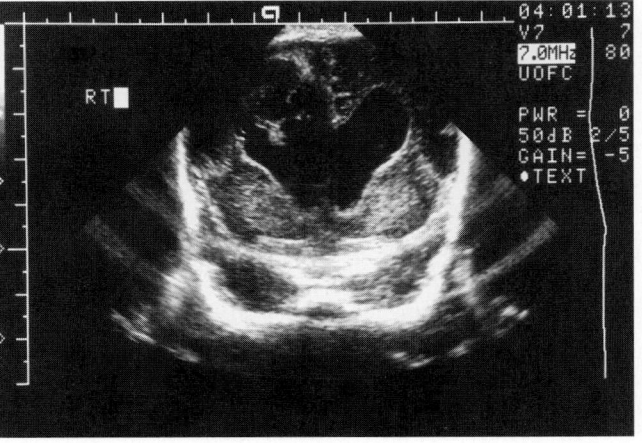

A   B

FIG. 50–1. Cranial ultrasonography of intraventricular hemorrhage in the coronal plane. **A:** Head ultrasound performed within the first week of life depicts a clot in the left lateral ventricle with mildly dilated ventricles. **B:** Ultrasonography performed 1 month later shows no residual clot, but significant enlargement of the ventricular system, consistent with posthemorrhagic hydrocephalus.

dependent. Technologies that accurately measure the flow through the shunt, or through some physiologic pathway such as the aqueduct of Sylvius, or a ratio of these two numbers, could be a reliable descriptor of shunt dependence. It is theoretically possible that such measurements could be made from dynamic magnetic resonance imaging (MRI) studies. So far, such a technique has not been applied reliably.

One of the problems with assessing the growth of ventricular size in the neonate is the possibility that the enlargement of the ventricles may reflect loss of tissue in the brain, rather than increase in pressure. This can become a very complicated situation, as prolonged hydrocephalus itself certainly can cause loss of tissue bulk (2), and the value of shunt placement may be more difficult to determine when the tissue loss is not obviously the result of high pressure. The specific loss of myelination, called periventricular leukomalacia, is discussed in Chapter 49. The relationship between periventricular leukomalacia and hydrocephalus is of particular concern in neurosurgical decision-making. When a preterm infant, especially one who has sustained an intracranial hemorrhage, shows lateral ventricular enlargement, it is difficult to determine to what extent this is a result of impaired CSF flow or absorption versus what is a result of diffuse white matter damage or inadequate density of axons. In general, the absence of macrocephaly is an indicator of the atrophy. More specific strategies to rescue white matter in such damages probably will evolve and may diminish the call for shunts in some of these patients (3). Nevertheless, assessing when macrocephaly is present is complicated by the changing growth rate in the normal neonatal head. In the first week after birth, the typical rate of growth is 0.6 cm per week, in the second week 0.5 cm, and in the third week 0.75 cm, with approximately 1 cm per week thereafter (4).

Fluid in the subarachnoid space outside the brain, sometimes termed "benign external hydrocephalus," is probably a normal variant. The increased collection of extraaxial fluid is, generally, in the frontal regions. The diagnosis of subdural hygroma frequently has been applied to these cases, and, if it is intended to imply a pathologic collection benefiting from drainage, this diagnosis must be applied with great caution (5).

Treatment of Neonatal Hydrocephalus

Due to the disadvantages and complications of ventriculoperitoneal shunting, the decision to place a shunt necessarily must follow all other nonsurgical attempts to manage the situation. The fact that the CSF resorption may change with time, and indeed may improve, gives a rationale for conservatism.

Children born with hydrocephalus due to nonhemorrhagic causes, such as aqueductal stenosis, posterior fossa cysts, holoprosencephaly, or hydranencephaly, can be shunted within 1 to 2 days of birth, pending evaluation of general medical status. Although affected infants usually are born at or near term, a presurgical weight of approximately 1,500 to 2,000 g will predict adequate size to support peritoneal drainage of ventricular CSF (6). There are ethical issues that should be raised before placing a ventriculoperitoneal shunt in a child suffering from hydrocephalus with significantly reduced brain function from either an *in utero* event or a developmental anomaly. Certainly, frank discussion with the child's parents regarding prognosis is in order. Shunting for affected children without other severe anomalies is certainly reasonable for the purposes of controlling head size in the growing infant. With maximal interventive therapy, most of these children are expected to live beyond a few weeks, and such day-to-day issues as whether the child's head will fit in an infant car seat need to be considered. Shunting at birth is a relatively low-risk method of preventing massive head enlargement and allowing other factors aside from congenital hydrocephalus to determine the child's outcome (7).

Nearly all acquired hydrocephalus in the premature neonate is posthemorrhagic (Fig. 50–1). In these cases, infants have not achieved adequate weight for placement of permanent shunts, and the final determination of lifelong hydrocephalus has not been made. In this situation, the use of repeated lumbar punctures is a common technique for the management of hydrocephalus, as are the nonsurgical approaches of carbonic anhydrase inhibitors and loop diuretics such as furosemide (8). The use of these maneuvers is discussed in Chapter 49. An additional approach that has been tried for posthemorrhagic hydrocephalus (PHH) is the introduction of fibrinolytic therapy directly into the ventricular system. Enzymes such as streptokinase, urokinase, and tissue plasminogen activator all have been proposed and tested with variable success. Some centers have suggested that some ventriculoperitoneal shunts can be avoided using this technique (9). Hansen et al. (10) and Luciano et al. (11) have been unable to show a decrease in the need for ventriculoperitoneal shunting with this maneuver. It is possible that the trials that found no helpful effect from fibrinolytic therapy had less favorable results because of patient selection, with a trend toward accepting into the protocols the most severe and potentially intractable cases. At any rate, this cannot be considered standard therapy at the current time.

Another intervention that has been suggested is the use of ventriculoscopic removal of clot, but this has not been demonstrated to avert the need for ventriculoperitoneal shunts, although there is little published experience. Another new technique, using the fiberoptic ventriculoscope, is the treatment of hydrocephalus caused by obstruction of the aqueduct of Sylvius by placement of a fenestration in the floor of the third ventricle, which allows escape of CSF into the subarachnoid space.

Indeed, even in such cases of aqueductal stenosis, where eventual therapy using the ventriculoscope works well in older children, most surgeons currently find that the defect in the floor of the third ventricle in the neonate tends to close at a very high rate (12).

Many of the obvious problems of CSF diversion can be managed with simple surgical tricks. For example, the problem that shunts tend to clog with very high protein concentrations may be avoided by putting in an externally draining system or a ventricular catheter with a tapping reservoir first (Fig. 50–2), to be changed at a latter time to a ventriculoperitoneal shunt if the infant still requires permanent diversion (13). This has been our general strategy as well (7). The other problem is the frequent need to lengthen the shunt. The general solution accepted in many centers now is to place a very long catheter into the peritoneum, even in a small baby. In our experience, catheters up to 90 cm in length are well tolerated, even by neonates. Prospective studies have not shown any increase in complications, even with tubing up to 120 cm in length (14). Longer tubing certainly eliminates the need to periodically lengthen the peritoneal catheter because of growth.

Although serial lumbar punctures may be useful in many cases, they often fail because of abnormalities within the spinal system that block CSF flow, particularly common after intraventricular hemorrhage. These have been documented with spinal ultrasound (15).

There are many published management protocols for children who have PHH (6,7,16,17). We use a four-level grading system, although other grading systems have been described (16): grade I, subependymal hemorrhage only; grade II, intraventricular hemorrhage without ventriculomegaly and low risk of PHH; grade III, intraventricular hemorrhage with ventriculomegaly and moderate risk of PHH; and grade IV, intraventricular hemorrhage with intraparenchymal extent and very high risk of need for ventriculoperitoneal shunting. After neurosurgical consultation, our workup includes an ultrasound of the head to assess the size of the ventricles and a lumbar puncture to measure CSF pressure.

Our interventions are tailored to maintain the lumbar or ventricular CSF pressure at approximately 5 cm of water while evaluating for permanent shunt placement. The medical approaches to this problem have been described (8). Acetazolamide (Diamox) is of value in reducing CSF production, and mechanical CSF drainage by serial lumbar puncture or direct ventricular access is the mainstay of our treatment of elevated intracranial pressure while awaiting the appropriate time for ventriculoperitoneal shunt insertion. As we have described, to determine the frequency of CSF drainage procedures, we have measured "opening" CSF pressures on all lumbar taps and tried to maintain each opening pressure below 10 cm of water with serial CSF drainage (7). For example, if an every third day tapping schedule allows the CSF pressure to rise to greater than 11 cm of water, we would recommend increasing the frequency of CSF withdrawal to every other day. Certainly, fontanelle tenseness, head circumference, and ultrasonographic resistive indexes also are acceptable indications of intracranial pressure (1). While draining CSF, we remove approximately 10 cc per kilogram of CSF in order to leave the CSF pressure as low as is feasible, usually less than 3 cm of water. This approach is based on cerebral perfusion management rather than measures of head circumference or ultrasonographic documentation of ventricular size.

Of course, head circumference, ultrasonographic criteria, and other physical examination criteria are reasonable guides to CSF drainage therapy. These approaches are acceptable, as long as the protocol seeks to maximize the potential for neuronal development in an environment of low intracranial pressure and minimal periventricular axonal stretch.

Acetazolamide treatment and serial episodes of CSF drainage are carried out until the patient reaches a weight of approximately 1,750 g. At that time, in our experience, the infant's size will permit implantation of a permanent ventriculoperitoneal shunt with minimal complication. During the period of serial CSF drainage procedure, the requirement for CSF drainage will either accelerate or decrease. This is ascertained by continuing to measure CSF pressures. If there is no increase in pressure between taps, then it is likely the CSF is being reabsorbed internally. In this situation, the ultrasound image of the ventricles as well as the head circumference measurements are helpful in confirming that the reabsorptive surface is functioning adequately. If, after long intervals between CSF taps, the pressure is unchanged and the ventricles are not enlarging, it is reasonable to continue to follow

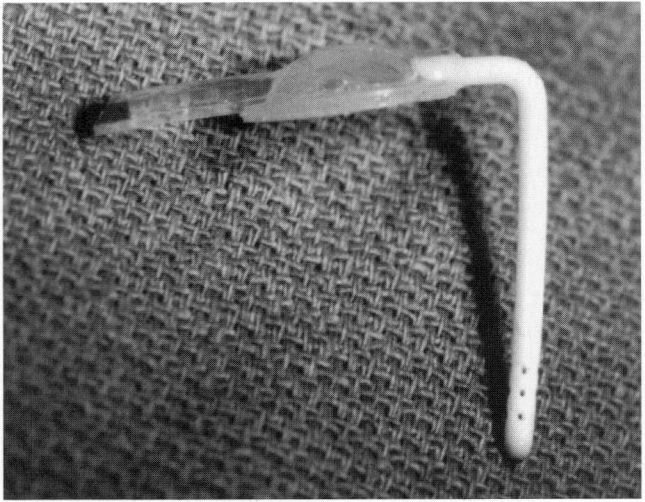

Fig. 50–2. Ventricular access device with 30-mm catheter. Implantation allows easy percutaneous access to ventricular fluid.

ventricular size by ultrasound alone. At that point, aceta-zolamide treatment is weaned, although generally this is done after resolution of all other medical problems. If the need for CSF drainage remains unchanged or accelerates as the patient approaches a weight of 1,750 g, then the diagnosis of uncompensated hydrocephalus is made and a ventriculoperitoneal shunt is inserted.

We consider implantation of devices that allow easier intermittent CSF drainage (Fig. 50–2), or continuous CSF drainage, when the need for CSF drainage acceler-ates to the point where the neonatal intensivist or the neu-rosurgeon is performing lumbar punctures daily or with such frequency as to endanger a child's medical stability. Similarly, serial lumbar puncture can cause arachnoid scarring and lead to an inability to obtain adequate CSF drainage from a lumbar approach. In those cases also, direct approach to the ventricles either by percutaneous tap or an implanted access device is required.

Percutaneous ventricular tap in a neonate is a simple procedure. A 20-gauge intravenous catheter is introduced perpendicular to a plane tangential to the scalp at the lat-eral edge of the anterior fontanelle. After penetrating the dura with the inner needle, the soft catheter is advanced over the needle into the ventricle. Drainage then proceeds as with lumbar puncture. As needed, we also have surgi-cally placed ventricular access devices (Fig. 50–2). This device allows direct percutaneous access to the ventricle via the subcutaneous reservoir. The protocol for CSF drainage is identical to that for lumber puncture. We have had very little difficulty with infection of these devices despite frequent percutaneous access. Ventricular access devices can be rigged for continuous drainage by place-ment of a Heuber needle into the reservoir, which is con-nected to a ventricular drainage bag. This maneuver is performed when serial taps are required more than once a day. During periods of continuous drainage, we have treated infants with prophylactic intravenous antibiotics.

There are contraindications to implantation of a perma-nent ventriculoperitoneal shunt. They are similar to those found in older children: evidence of CSF infection, signif-icantly elevated CSF protein or presence of a high CSF red blood cell count, which may mechanically obstruct the shunt, or peritoneal inflammation or infection, such as necrotizing enterocolitis. These problems necessitate a delay in implantation until the child is healthy. We have had experience with CSF glucose parameters being quite low (less than 20 mg/dL) in neonates with PHH, in the absence of infection. The significance of this finding is unclear; however, we do not note an increase in shunt infection in these patients. Similarly, intraventricular hemorrhage patients, whether adult or neonatal, can manifest fever, per-haps from the presence of blood in the CSF. In the absence of positive culture data, we have not delayed shunt place-ment. The exact cause of this increased temperature in the neonate is unclear, but without positive bacteriologic data, it is unlikely to be infection.

Complications of Ventriculoperitoneal Shunting

The neonate is particularly susceptible to shunt infection and shunt malfunction, which are the most important com-plications of ventriculoperitoneal shunting at any age. Fac-tors such as the relatively thin skin, nutritional difficulties with delayed wound healing, and tendency for the fluid to be proteinaceous all tend to increase the complication risk. Plastic hardware items such as shunts are particularly sus-ceptible to infection, because a small pathogen inoculation, with a relatively nonpathogenic bacterium, can avoid nor-mal immune surveillance due to the presence of the plas-tic. In several series, the rate of infection correlated signif-icantly with age and often with little else (18).

Another problem with ventriculoperitoneal shunting sometimes seen in infants, although rarely seen in older individuals, is injury to bowel or other abdominal viscera. This is a result of the fragility of these tissues (19). In addition, migration of the catheter within the infant has been seen. Penetration into an abdominal viscus and into the pleural cavity (Fig. 50–3) have been seen (19). Migra-tion into the heart has been documented for ventriculoa-trial shunts (20).

Especially with very large ventricles, rapid decompres-sion of the ventricular system can cause bleeding into the subdural space, ventricles, or into the parenchyma of the brain (Fig. 50–4). For this reason, we typically remove only moderate amounts of CSF at the time of surgery, and keep the patients flat for the immediate postoperative period, titrating the elevation of the head gradually and monitoring this by checks of the anterior fontanelle. The head can be raised as long as there is not extreme con-cavity or "ashtray deformity" of the fontanelle. Other authors have suggested the use of higher pressure valves with very large ventricles (21).

Ventricular asymmetry has been seen frequently. Deliberate placement of catheters across the midline, so that openings on either side of the septum can drain both ventricles, has been shown in a randomized trial to decrease this problem (22). We have seen spontaneous resolution of ventricular asymmetry and generally have been somewhat conservative in following it unless there is an associated asymmetric physical examination.

Intracranial Cystic Spaces in the Neonate

Interhemispheric, temporal fossa, posterior fossa, and other arachnoid cysts frequently can complicate the treat-ment of hydrocephalus. A variety of techniques for dealing with these entities is possible, including fenestration using either open technique or ventriculoscopy, direct shunting of the cyst, or combined shunting of the cyst and ventricle. Interhemispheric cysts can become quite large, and gener-ally large arachnoid cysts require treatment. Fenestration of the cyst may be the best way to avoid the need for an addi-tional catheter (23). Large interhemispheric cysts can be

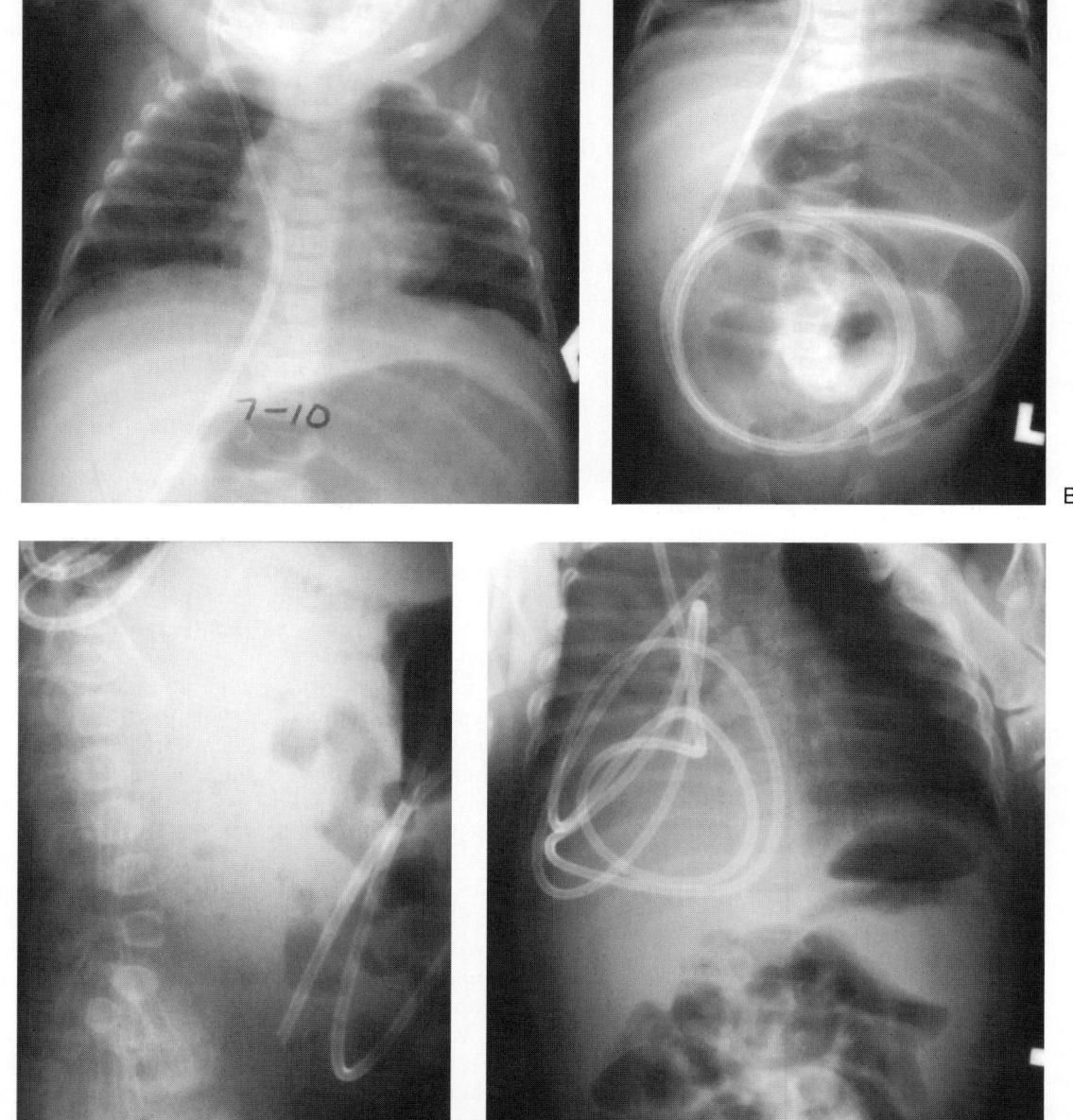

FIG. 50–3. Example of an unusual infection-related shunt complication related to placement at a very early age—erosion through the chest wall into the pleural cavity. **A,B:** This ventriculoperitoneal shunt was placed in a 1,300-g neonate after treatment of posthemorrhagic hydrocephalous with a ventricular access device and serial taps. Several months later, an umbilical hernia appeared to enlarge, and plain radiographs were obtained of the abdomen. The loops of shunt tubing, which had already migrated into the chest cavity, were not appreciated at that point. Panel **(C)** was obtained only 3 days prior to panel **(D)**. The patient was discharged and returned with a suddenly sunken anterior fontanelle and diminished breath sounds on the right. A plain x-ray demonstrated migration of the shunt tubing into the right pleural cavity **(D)**. The fluid in the chest proved to be purulent. A functioning shunt ultimately was replaced in the peritoneum after removal of hardware, external drainage, and treatment with antibiotics. Presumably a distal catheter infection, although not presenting with sepsis, resulted in fluid along the shunt, which erupted into the pleural space, allowing the tubing to retract and coil there with movement of the patient.

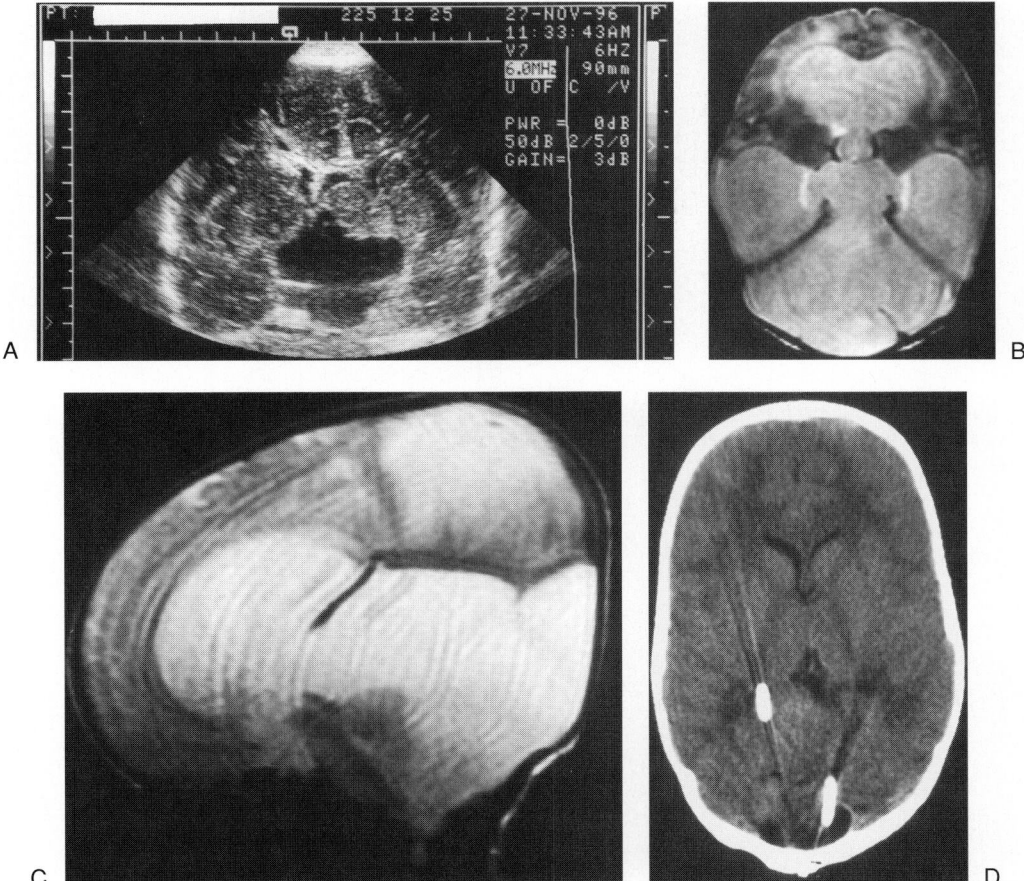

FIG. 50–4. Intracranial cysts in the neonate. **A:** Coronal ultrasonography of a suprasellar cyst in a newborn. **B,C:** An intrahemispheric cyst may mimic fluid collections in the posterior fossa, allowing them to be confused with Dandy–Walker malformations. This patient was born with a very severe craniomegaly and compression of brain tissue, and ultimately required a catheter in both the cystic space and in the residual ventricular system. With these two catheters, the brain configuration eventually returned much more to normal **(D)**, and the patient has had normal developmental milestones subsequently.

confused with a lobar holoprosencephaly, with a considerably better neurologic prognosis for the patients with a large cyst. Frequently, these require placement of a specific shunt catheter (Fig. 50–4) (24). The isolated fourth ventricle is a particularly difficult surgical problem, in part because the posterior fossa is a somewhat more technically difficult area into which to place a catheter that will continue to work over a long period of time, and because the neurologic risks are quite high if the catheter draining such a cyst has a momentary failure. This can result in emergent brainstem symptoms, such as apnea and bradycardia. The risks of fourth ventricular cysts and the specific placement of shunts into the cysts to drain them have been documented in several reports (25,26).

MANAGEMENT OF THE INFANT WITH AN OPEN DEFECT OF THE NEURAL AXIS

Abnormal developmental folding of the neural tube and anterior neuropore can result in a spectrum of abnor-malities as benign as spina bifida occulta—a bifid spinal arch seen in up to 30% of the general population with no neurologic sequelae—or as severe as anencephaly or craniospinal raschisis—complete absence of neural tube closure. The general guideline that we have followed is to defer urgent repair of these defects if they are small and truly skin covered, i.e., lipomyelomeningocele. Open defects, such as myelomeningocele, or defects that leak CSF or interfere with airway patency, such as large nasofrontal encephaloceles, require repair within a few days of birth, or sooner. Enlarging lesions, such as occipital encephaloceles, may need to be addressed during the short period of intended observation for the child to achieve adequate weight to minimize surgical risks.

Neurosurgeons frequently are called upon to evaluate a variety of midline "lumps, bumps, and dimples" along the neural axis from nose to coccyx (Figs. 50–5 through 50–7). These lesions often represent myelodysplasia that will require repair. However, we have found that, in the stable newborn, evaluation and treatment can be deferred

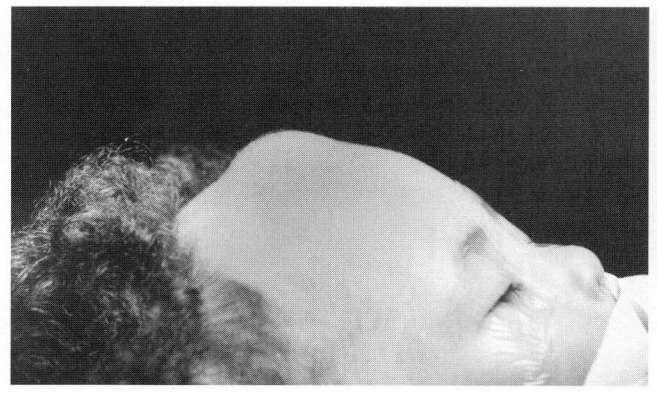

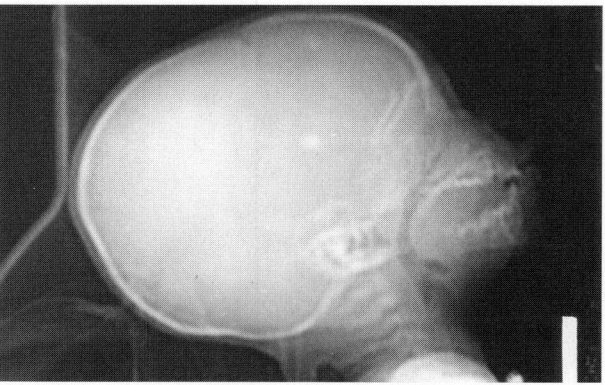

FIG. 50–5. Dermoid cyst. External view **(A)** and lateral topogram **(B)** of dermoid cyst arising from the anterior fontanelle. The lesion had eroded the bone around the fontanelle but was removed easily in its entirety.

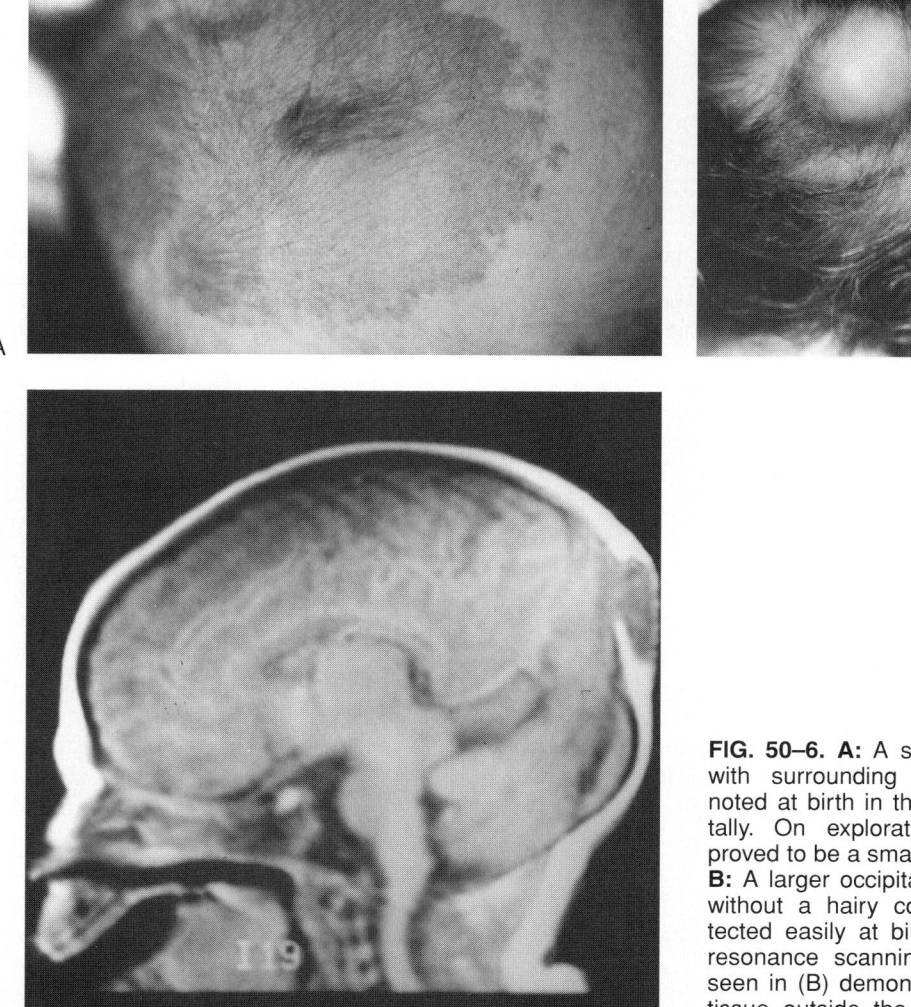

FIG. 50–6. A: A small hairy patch with surrounding discolored skin noted at birth in the midline occipitally. On exploration, this lesion proved to be a small encephalocele. **B:** A larger occipital encephalocele without a hairy covering was detected easily at birth. **C:** Magnetic resonance scanning of the lesion seen in (B) demonstrates the brain tissue outside the confines of the skull as well as anomalous hindbrain anatomy.

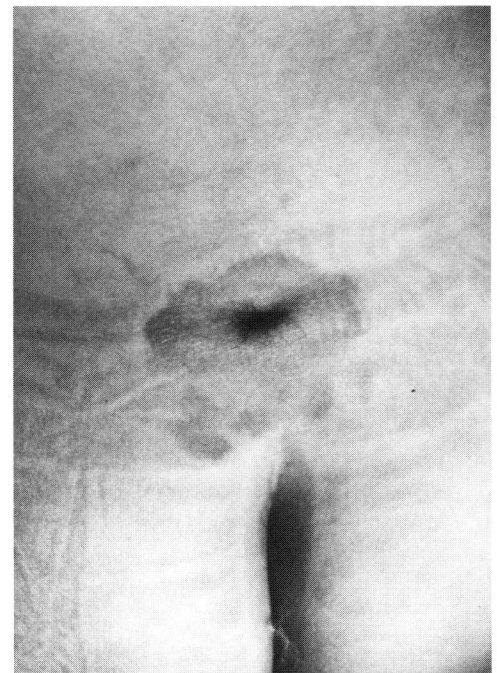

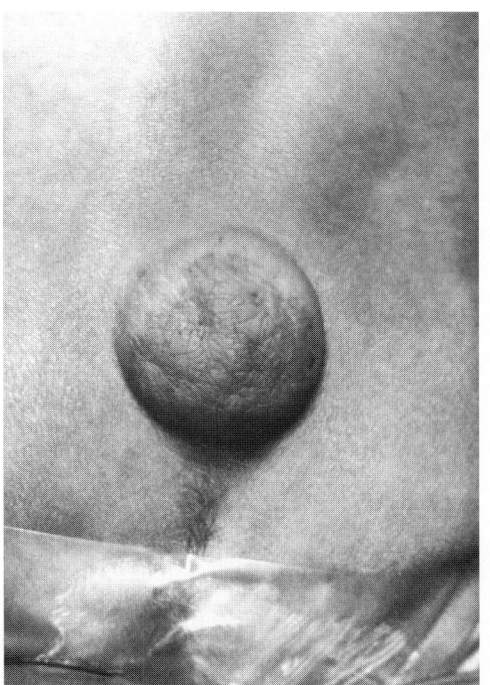

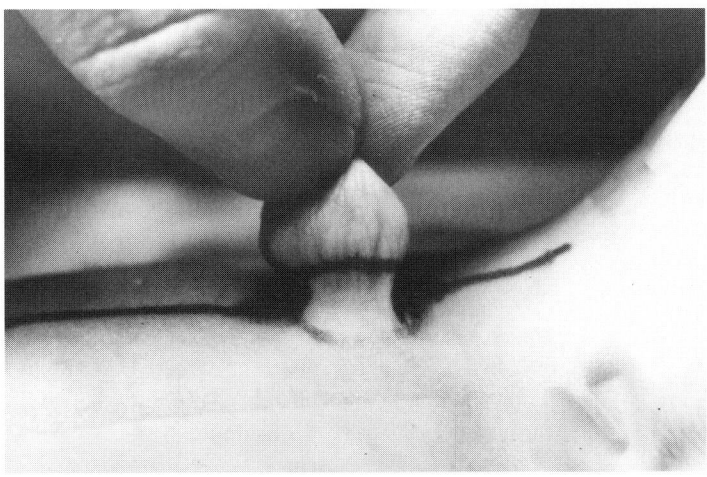

FIG. 50-7. **A:** This small sacral dimple, with encircling reddened patch, was noted at birth. At surgery, it was found to be a dermal sinus tract into the spinal cord. The gluteal cleft is seen below. **B:** This skin-covered lesion noted at birth was found to be an anatomically identifiable myelomeningocele with intact placode and associated meningocele sac. The child had no neurologic deficits at birth. **C:** The skin tag being held up at the cervical area was noted at birth but not referred for evaluation until 3 months of life. Upon surgical exploration, a dermal sinus tract was identified and followed directly into the central canal of the spinal cord. The child had no preoperative or postoperative neurologic deficits.

until after 3 months of age, when surgical intervention is medically safer. Even MRI evaluation can be deferred until that time in order to obtain a more technically clear study. We have found head and spine ultrasound to be useful in the neonatal period for screening these lesions, but we have noted a high false-negative rate. The MRI scan remains the standard for preoperative planning of these occult lesions.

Myelomeningocele

A major change in the management of patients with myelomeningoceles has resulted from the availability of antenatal diagnosis. The vast majority of patients with this deformity in our practice now have had prenatal diag-

nosis on the basis of an elevated serum alpha-fetoprotein, generally followed by an ultrasound study and sometimes an antenatal MRI scan (27,28). The study by Luthy et al. (29) in the Seattle area documented the advantage of obstetric management of myelomeningocele patients with cesarean section, avoiding the onset of labor. Specifically, this study demonstrated an improvement in the functional outcome relative to the anatomic level of the myelomeningocele level. We recommend elective cesarean section for such patients as soon as the fetal lungs are known to be sufficiently mature. The technical considerations have been well outlined for the past 10 years by McCullough and Johnson (30). Because of the associated type II Chiari malformation, as well as some potential obstruction to flow of CSF around the incisura and the subarachnoid space, well over 90% of these patients require placement of a ventriculoperitoneal shunt. Most commonly, the shunt does not have to be placed at the time of the initial closure. Our practice in recent years has been to delay placement of the ventriculoperitoneal shunt for at least several days, so that the CSF coming in contact with the shunt has not recently been in contact with the open defect. In some series, the patients with myelomeningocele manifested high incidences of shunt malfunction within the first year, some in excess of 40% (23). In general, the more severe the ventricular dilatation, the higher the incidence of complications, which also may be a measure of the degree of shunt dependence of individual patients.

Surgery for repair of a myelomeningocele has been described by McCullough and Johnson (30) and McLone (31). The specific surgery is an attempt to reconstruct the terminal end of the neuraxis and approximate the topologic relationships that would have occurred if complete closure of the neural tube had occurred. The neural placode itself usually is plainly visible beneath, or associated with, translucent abnormal tissue stretching from the edge of the skin defect inward to the small island of pinkish tissue, which represents the termination of the spinal cord. It is flat with a groove down the middle. With surgical dissection, it is found to have nerve roots projecting both ventrally through the remnants of the sacrum and lumbar bony elements, as well as some nerve roots projecting more aberrantly out into the soft tissue and skin. Because of the tendency of this placode tissue to dry out in the hours prior to closure, dressing with a sterile gauze kept continuously moist with sterile saline is crucial. We administer antibiotics as prophylaxis against meningitis until the skin defect is closed.

Once in the operating room, handling and management of the patient is designed to avoid any further trauma to the placode. Intubation usually is accomplished with the patient in the lateral or in the supine position, with very careful padding arranged to avoid any pressure on the meningocele sac or placode.

The dissection begins with a circumferential division of the abnormal, thinly epithelialized translucent tissue, which joins the placode to the surrounding skin from the normal skin itself. The surgeon must carefully remove from the space any remaining dermal elements that may end up inside the dura. Such elements later can cause dermoid tumors that require resection and chronic inflammatory conditions that make later spinal cord untethering difficult.

The tissue of the placode itself is trimmed. Magnification with operating loupes or the operating microscope is extremely helpful in preserving all of the neural tissue but removing any possible dermal remnant. The placode then can be rolled into a tubular structure if its shape permits, with anchoring of pia to pia using very fine sutures. It is important at this stage of the procedure to examine both above and below the placode for other intraspinal pathology, such as a fatty filum or diastematomyelia. Sometimes removal of one lumbar level above the area of exposure is necessary to permit full exploration.

Spinal Dysrhaphism other than Myelomeningocele

Although myelomeningocele is the easiest spinal cord defect to identify, other patients who will show signs of tethered cord syndrome or spinal lipomas, or other related closed malformations, can be diagnosed as neonates. In general, patients who have hemangiomas, hairly patches, fatty lumps, or deep sinus tracts in the area of the lumbosacral spine deserve investigation within the first few months of life. Spinal ultrasound can be an excellent screening test for determining the level of the conus medullaris, as well as the respiratory excursions of the nerve roots, and is useful in cases of dimples without any other associated findings. As mentioned previously, in the absence of a truly open defect or a draining sinus that increases risk of early meningitis or other infection, there is no urgent need to surgically correct these deformities. We typically allow the patients to reach 3 months of age or older to diminish the risk of surgical complication before performing elective repair of tethered spinal cords. Urodynamic studies with electromyographic studies of sphincter function can be useful in comparing the preoperative to postoperative bladder functions in patients too young to be toilet trained. Although MRI is extremely helpful for preoperative study of such patients, the quality of the study will be better if deferred until closer to surgery at several months of age, when the characteristics of the tissue allow better anatomic definition of structures. It is now a generally recommended pediatric neurosurgical practice that all tethered spinal cords be untethered at an early age to prevent the neurologic deterioration that may occur later in life.

Encephaloceles

The cranial analog of the open myelomeningocele is the encephalocele (Fig. 50–8). Clinically, these vary from small lesions that may cause relatively little disruption of brain structure to large lesions with massive amounts of brain tissue extruded through the cranial opening. Again, the availability of ultrasound and MRI scanning antenatally has allowed improvements in the planning and advice given to prospective parents of babies with these problems. As with open myelomeningocele defects, open cranial defects require acute closure, generally within 24 hours of birth, to diminish the risk of meningitis. Closed lesions can be managed in a variety of ways. If the lesion is large, could potentially cause airway obstruction, or is enlarging, early repair will be required. As with occult spinal dysraphic states, repair of small lesions can be

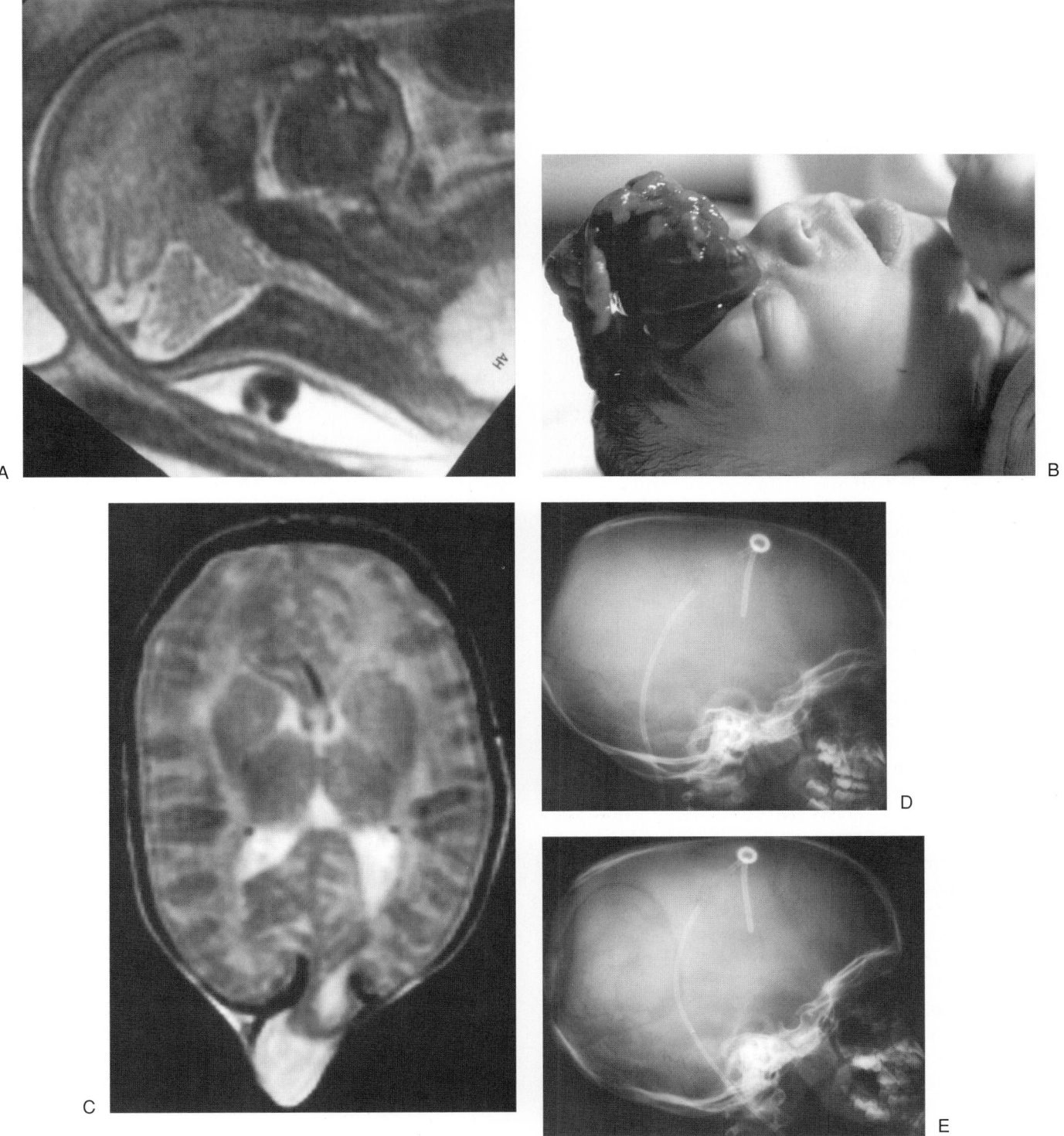

FIG. 50–8. Encephaloceles, or open defects of the cranial end of the neuraxis, span a broad range of clinical presentations. A frontal encephalocele with a large extrusion of brain tissue frontally. This was demonstrated on an antenatal magnetic resonance imaging scan **(A)**, which accurately predicted the appearance of the mass at birth **(B)**. A smaller occipital encephalocele **(C)** had much less central nervous system tissue within it and was almost entirely cystic. This required a skull reconstruction to patch the cranial defect **(D,E)**, which healed without any bony defects 1 year after surgery in a neurologically normal child.

deferred until radiologic imaging quality is maximized and the child can more safely undergo surgery.

The surgical repair of an encephalocele is very much analogous to myelomeningocele repair. The encephalocele sac is entered and explored for nervous tissue. Generally, extracranial tissue is truncated and discarded because it is nonfunctional. The remainder of the repair is devoted to reconstructing a barrier between brain and subcutaneous tissue by repairing the dural lining and forming a reinforced barrier to CSF leakage at the skin.

The normal skin around the margin of the encephalocele is inspected and trimmed to yield a skin edge that eventually can be closed. There is typically a defect in the cranium as well as in the normal dura. As with myelomeningoceles, there is typically a gradual change from normal tissue to abnormal scar tissue around the edges of the lesion. If the encephalocele is quite large, it is often essentially pedunculated glial material, and it becomes necessary to amputate the excess neural tissue to allow any possibility of a closure. The edges of relatively normal dura are identified and then either closed primarily or with a patched graft, which can be taken from pericranium in some cases, or commercially available dural substitute materials can be used. After a watertight seal is obtained, the scalp over the dural closure is approximated. In some cases, relaxing incisions or rotational flaps have to be made to allow for a satisfactory closure. Careful observation of the patients postoperatively for the development of symptomatic hydrocephalus, which may have been masked by a gradual leakage of fluid out of the encephalocele, must be undertaken. Some encephalocele patients require shunts, but the majority in our experience do not.

Outcome from children born with encephaloceles, either frontal or occipital, can be variable. In general, frontal nasal encephaloceles that involve the frontal cortex or are purely fluid filled can be resected and repaired with good neurologic and cosmetic outcome. A high percentage of these children will go on to have normal cognitive function. Hydrocephalus is common but certainly not the rule in these children. Occipital encephaloceles, particularly those that involve a significant amount of herniated brain tissue, are predictive of a less robust cognitive outcome. These children have a very high percentage of hydrocephalus and often will grow to have developmental delay and other cognitive difficulties.

REMOVAL OF EXCESS INTRACRANIAL MASS

Increased intracranial pressure in the newborn easily can be caused by an increase in the contents of the cranial vault other than CSF. This harks back to the distensibility of the neonatal skull and the fact that intracranial mass may not present with neurologic symptoms. The fontanelle remains an available intracranial pressure monitor for constant assessment. Head trauma and con-

genital CNS tumors are pathophysiologic categories that cause an increase in intracranial contents relevant to neurosurgical intervention.

Head Trauma in the Neonate

Mechanical injury to the CNS or the peripheral nervous system in the neonate generally is a result of conditions immediately surrounding birth itself. These injuries are dramatically less frequent than they were only a decade or two ago, largely a result of improvements in monitoring and imaging that have improved the level of obstetric care. There are clearly many more injuries, some of them trivial, than are recognized. The ratio of birth injuries to neonatal deaths due to trauma is estimated at 20 to 1, although the true incidence of less severe head injury is not known (32,33). Isolated spinal cord or brainstem injury has been observed in 3% to 10% of neonatal autopsies (34).

Extracranial injuries resulting in blood collections in the neonate can be important because of the low circulating blood volume and the relatively large capacity for sequestration of blood in infants of this size. An important example is subgaleal hemorrhage, where blood collects below the galea and, therefore, is not bounded by suture lines, so that dramatic blood loss can occur. Occasionally, these require aspiration of nonclotted blood, and coagulopathies should be excluded.

Cephalohematoma, on the other hand, is the collection of blood below the pericranium of the outer surface of the skull, which means that it does not cross suture lines, is unilateral, and is almost always over parietal areas. Underlying skull fractures can be identified in one tenth to one fourth of these cases, but it is likely that less clinically evident fractures, which spontaneously reduce, were present in many of the remaining cases. These clots resolve spontaneously over time. We generally avoid aspirating these clots because of risk of introducing infection into a space in a self-limited problem. Occasionally, cephalohematomas require surgical intervention when the lesions calcify and cause an obvious cosmetic deformity.

Minimally depressed fractures of the parietal bones, generally greenstick in nature, often are called "ping-pong" fractures. Some of these may vanish spontaneously or occasionally can be elevated by a limited and careful digital manipulation. The major surgical question is whether to elevate a minimally depressed skull fracture. An argument for early surgery in borderline cases is that a very simple operation can be done, which involves making a small hole and passing an instrument below a ping-pong–type fracture to pop it back into place.

Leptomeningeal cysts, also called growing skull fractures, are usually the result of an underlying brain injury and failure of normal CSF reabsorption, with communication of the leptomeninges through the subarachnoid space. Most frequently, they communicate with the ventricular system through a porencephalic cyst and may be associated with hydrocephalus. In cases of more significant brain injury, it is important to identify these lesions to effect primary closure of the dura, or at least to follow these children closely to determine that this secondary condition does not occur.

With respect to intracranial injuries, the full range of epidural, subdural, subarachnoid, and parenchymal hemorrhages is possible in the neonate, although they only rarely require surgical exploration or treatment. An important sign frequently seen on scans is the accumulation of blood within the leaves of the tentorium, which may mimic a tentorial subdural hematoma. It is important to identify this condition because it may look quite dramatic on computed tomographic scan, but surgical exploration can lead to disastrous, uncontrolled bleeding, essentially from the communication of this intradural space with the sinuses. The distensibility of the head and the open sutures and fontanelle provides unique direct access to the intracranial space for the neurosurgeon. Percutaneous aspiration of subdural hematoma or intraparenchymal clot is possible in the neonatal head in a fashion impossible in older children. In many cases, percutaneous aspiration of subdural clot is the procedure of choice for the injured neonate (35).

Spinal Cord Injury

Ligaments in the pediatric patient generally, and particularly in the neonatal infant, are lax. It is possible to stretch the spinal cord beyond its elasticity to the point of injury. Damage can cause neurologic syndromes, ranging from no observable abnormality to quadriplegia. An extensive lesion of the lower cervical cord would be expected to cause partial dysfunction in the upper extremities, impaired diaphragmatic respiration, and paraplegia. The presence or absence of Horner's syndrome or failure of sympathetic innervation to the pupil and face on one side can be an important clue to the structural integrity of the roots emerging from the cervical spinal cord.

Congenital Tumors of the Central Nervous System

Congenital CNS tumors (Fig. 50–9) are rare and of several types, and variable biological behavior depends on location and histology (36). Important types of tumors to consider include choroid plexus papillomas (37), teratomas (38,39), anaplastic lesions such as astrocytomas (40), glioblastoma (41), primary neuroblastoma (42), and astroblastoma (43). Asymptomatic antenatal tumors have even been noted, with one very large intracranial teratoma that caused maternal pain (44).

Although these tumors are extraordinarily rare, their diagnosis is generally rather straightforward because the

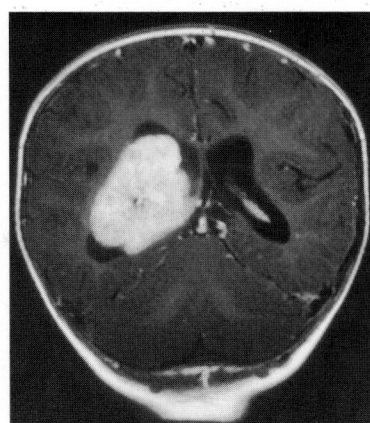

FIG. 50–9. Congenital tumors are quite rare and actual diagnosis during the neonatal period is particularly unusual. This patient proved to have a choroid plexus papilloma, which presented at 4 months of age with a large mass and growing head circumference, although it almost surely was present at birth.

masses themselves may show up on antenatal ultrasound or postnatal ultrasound for macrocranium. The initial management of the tumor almost always is neurosurgical, requiring biopsy and generally decompression of tissue, both to establish prognosis and to initiate therapy.

OPENING PREMATURE FUSIONS IN THE NEONATE

Craniofacial Anomalies

With the exception of severe synostosis of all of the sutures (Fig. 50–10), treatment of craniosynostosis is designed to allow development of a more spherically shaped skull, but has minimal, if any effect, on ultimate neurologic outcome. Generally, the earlier synostosis is treated, the less severe the surgery needed to treat it. The most common isolated synostosis is sagittal synostosis (Fig. 50–11), which produces a long, narrow cranium, often with a ridge and a characteristic lack of movement in the sagittal suture on physical examination. A variety of procedures have been proposed for this condition, but we favor wide sagittal craniectomy early on, within the first few months of life. We find that, for this condition, the rounding effect of brain growth is adequate for restoring excellent contours. For more complex deformities, particularly the syndromic categories of Crouzon, Apert, and Pfeiffer syndromes, all of which have associated abnormalities of the extremities and other congenital defects, we tend to defer treatment of the brachycephaly for several months beyond the neonatal period so that a more definitive and planned craniofacial approach can be done with frontal advancement and orbital reshaping, if necessary.

Treatment of the cloverleaf deformity, when all sutures are congenitally closed, is the only craniosynostotic syn-

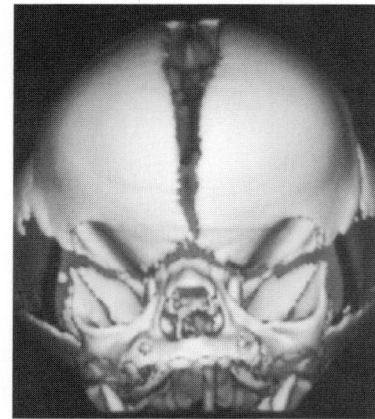

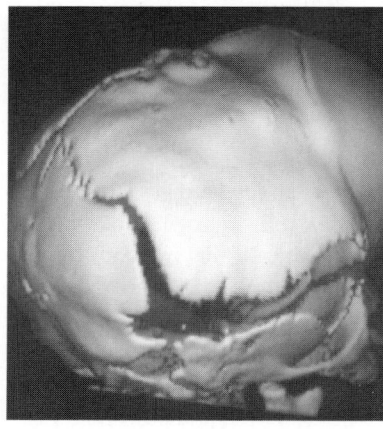

FIG. 50–10. Closed sutures. Cranial synostosis is a condition that usually is managed several months after birth, but certain conditions, such as kleeblattschädel **(A,B)**, require earlier decompression to diminish the risk of increased intracranial pressure.

drome requiring neonatal treatment. Such multisuture synostosis requires early craniectomy, which may involve almost complete removal of the cranial vault to allow early growth. It generally requires one or more frontal advancements, starting several months later to achieve an acceptable cranial shape.

CEREBROVASCULAR ANOMALIES OF THE NEWBORN

Although adult-type aneurysms have been demonstrated in children and even neonates, the most common of vascular lesions are arteriovenous malformations (45). The characteristic neonatal presentation of an arteriovenous malformation derives from its deep drainage into the vein of Galen system. It can cause a very large dilatation of the vein of Galen, called a vein of Galen aneurysm. Such lesions frequently present as cardiac failure in the neonate, due to the very high flow shunting that occurs. These lesions have a very high mortality. However, there are many lesions with less severe flow, which can be managed with postnatal interventional angiographic techniques with occlusion of a fistula. The arteriovenous malformations themselves may be identified and respond to resection. Some of these patients do quite well (46).

Burrows and Robertson (47) have reviewed the angiographic diagnosis and interventional radiographic treatment of arteriovenous malformations, fistulas, and other associated lesions in the neonate. These lesions can be subgrouped according to the morphology of the channels that make them up (e.g., venous vs. arteriovenous), flow characteristics (low vs. high), and location (galenic, parenchymal, pial, or dural). They point out that antenatal diagnosis has significantly altered the thinking about some of these lesions. Furthermore, the point is made that

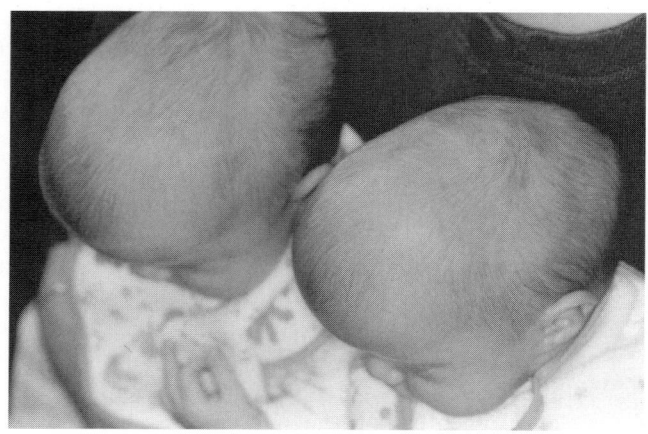

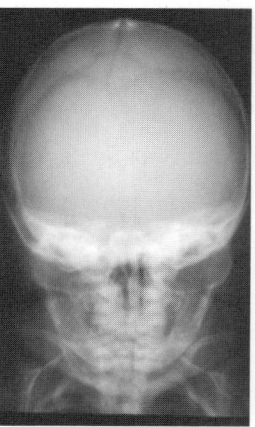

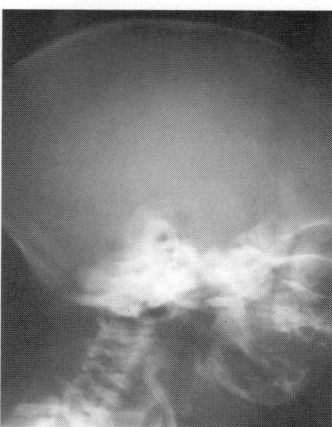

FIG. 50–11. Sagittal synostosis, a far more common type of craniosynostosis, can be detected in the nursery and referred for neurosurgical intervention. Definitive treatment may be delayed for several months.

for high-flow lesions, the flow itself becomes the major symptom, with systemic signs of high-output cardiac state and, in severe cases, cardiac failure with multiple organ dysfunction. Smaller lesions with lower flow may present as macrocephaly and hydrocephalus related to the increased venous pressure and subsequent functional diminution in absorption of CSF. Furthermore, progressive cerebral atrophy may develop.

Vein of Galen aneurysms are believed to occur between 6 and 11 weeks of gestation as a result of arterial communications with the embryologic precursor of the vein of Galen. Essentially, the aneurysm itself becomes symptomatic of the venous hypertension, which results from the abnormal communication.

Transcatheter occlusion of galenic arteriovenous shunts can be done by either a transarterial or transvenous route. Although the transarterial modality is preferred by many endovascular centers, a transvenous approach involving access to the venous drainage by transtorcular, tranfemoral, or transjugular catheterization can result in subtotal occlusion of the venous drainage, thereby reducing the shunt volume and cardiac failure. Ultimate cure by thrombosis potentially can be seen in either type of therapy. In cases of severe cardiac failure, however, the prognosis from the cardiac problem itself is poor enough that the outcome is guarded. If possible, these patients should be managed in centers where interventional radiology is available, and the availability of antenatal diagnosis makes such evaluation considerably more feasible.

The management of other arteriovenous malformations and fistulas away from the vein of Galen also can be undertaken with endovascular or open surgical treatment.

PROGNOSIS AND LONG-TERM OUTLOOK FOR THE NEUROSURGICAL NEONATE

An understanding of the long-term prognosis after any particular type of injury is crucial for planning and evaluating therapeutic strategies and for counseling the parents. In patients for whom neurosurgical interventions begin to be discussed with the parents, the long-term prognostic issues always weigh heavily on their decision-making. Unfortunately, the best they can be given currently is a general set of guidelines relevant to all patients, which cannot be considered predictive for an individual, single baby. DuPlessis and Volpe (48) have outlined a rational sequence of considerations to use when discussing prognosis in these cases. They emphasize the importance of establishing the etiology of a disease process, as the most important predictor. Thus, a particular degree of ventriculomegaly may be associated with a significantly worse cognitive prognosis in Dandy–Walker malformation or aqueductal stenosis than in myelomeningocele or communicating hydrocephalus posthemorrhage. Such differences can be understood on the basis of major contributions from associated cerebral

dysgenesis: what we called earlier the microanatomic malformation or "wiring" abnormalities. In addition, hydrocephalus resulting from infection will depend, to a very large degree, on the nature of the infection at the cellular level, and this will be more predictive of developmental outcome than the degree of ventriculomegaly resulting from the infection. From the neurosurgical point of view, it is important to separate the portion of the projected disability which is on the basis of the hydrodynamic or other neurosurgically solvable problem from that which is intrinsic to the neurons themselves and not remediable by the treating modalities of the neurosurgeon. In counseling parents, we often make this distinction quite explicit and state that the disease process involves at least two types of processes: those that can be treated with the shunt (or other neurosurgical intervention) and those that cannot be so treated. This gives the neurosurgeon the freedom to be able to say that, for example, a shunt may be absolutely necessary to treat a particular infant's condition, but whether it will be sufficient to correct the overall neurologic problems is a matter that only time can tell. In effect, this defers part of the issue of prognosis back to the medical and neurologic teams, while enforcing the importance of the proposed physical intervention. Nevertheless, the general implications of recent literature on the outcome of patients with common neurosurgical conditions should be well understood by neurosurgeons and other clinicians involved at the time of this family counseling.

For the particular case of progressive hydrocephalus after germinal matrix hemorrhage in preterm infants, a recent statistical study of outcomes by Levy et al. (49) found highly significant predictors for mortality and neurologic outcome on the basis of factors that intuitively are consistent with clinical experience. Mortality was best predicted in this study by the extent of intracranial hemorrhage, the number of shunt revisions, and birth weight, in that order, with a very high degree of statistical correlation. The grade of hemorrhage, weight at birth, and presence of seizure activity were the most important determinants of motor outcome. The grade of hemorrhage itself proved to be the most important variable determining cognitive outcome, motor function, and seizure activity. The need for more than five shunt revisions also turned out to be a negative predictor of survival. Of note, these investigators used a modified rating of the degree of hemorrhage, such that very mild invasions into parenchyma, although technically grade IV, were not scored as grade IV.

The issue of prognosis in neonatal patients requiring neurosurgical intervention remains one of the most vexing issues for neurosurgeons and neonatologists alike in the management of these patients. It is likely to remain so: as prospective long-term outcome studies yield results on neurologic outcome of prior practice, techniques and practices advance forward, altering (hopefully for the better) the prognosis of *today's* infants. Clear communication between neurosurgeons and neonatologists will remain a cornerstone of treatment for these small patients.

REFERENCES

1. Taylor GA, Madsen JR. Neonatal hydrocephalus: hemodynamic response to fontanelle compression—correlation with intracranial pressure and need for shunt placement. *Radiology* 1996;201:685.
2. McAllister JP, Chovan P. Neonatal hydrocephalus: mechanisms and consequences. *Neurosurg Clin N Am* 1998;9:73.
3. Leviton A, Gilles F. Ventriculomegaly, delayed myelination, white matter hypoplasia, and "periventricular" leukomalacia: how are they related? *Pediatr Neurol* 1996;15:127.
4. Gross SJ, Eckerman CO. Normative early head growth in very low birth weight infants. *J Pediatr* 1983;103:946.
5. Fan YF, Chong VF, Tan KP. Subarachnoid spaces in infants and young children. *Ann Acad Med Singapore* 1993;22:732.
6. Gurtner P, Bass T, Gudeman SK. Surgical management of posthemorrhagic hydrocephalus in 22 low birth weight infants. *Childs Nerv Syst* 1992;8:198.
7. Frim DM, Scott MR, Madsen JR. Surgical management of neonatal hydrocephalus. *Neurosurg Clin N Am* 1998;9:105.
8. Hansen AR, Snyder EY. Medical management of neonatal posthemorrhagic hydrocephalus. *Neurosurg Clin N Am* 1998;9:95.
9. Hudgins RJ, Boydston WR, Hudgins PA, Adler SR. Treatment of intraventricular hemorrhage in the premature infant with urokinase. A preliminary report. *Pediatr Neurosurg* 1994;20:190.
10. Hansen AR, Volpe JJ, Goumnerova LC, Madsen JR. Intraventricular urokinase for the treatment of posthemorrhagic hydrocephalus. *Pediatr Neurol* 1997;17:213.
11. Luciano R, Velardi F, Romagnoli C, Papacci P, De SV, Tortorolo G. Failure of fibrinolytic endoventricular treatment to prevent neonatal post-haemorrhagic hydrocephalus. A case-control trial. *Childs Nerv Syst* 1997;13:73.
12. Wilcock DJ, Jaspan T, Punt J. CSF flow through third ventriculostomy demonstrated with colour Doppler ultrasonography. *Clin Radiol* 1996;51:127.
13. Morimoto K, Hayakawa T, Yoshimine T, Wakayama A, Kuroda R. Two-step procedure for early neonatal surgery of fetal hydrocephalus. *Neurol Med Chir* 1993;33:158.
14. Couldwell WT, LeMay DR, McComb JG. Experience with use of extended length peritoneal shunt catheters. *J Neurosurg* 1996;85:425.
15. Rudas G, Almassy Z, Varga E, Somogyvary Z, Taylor GA. Alterations in spinal fluid drainage in infants with hydrocephalus. *Pediatr Radiol* 1997;27:580.
16. Holt PJ. Posthemorrhagic hydrocephalus. *J Child Neurol* 1989;4:523.
17. Marlin AE, Gaskill SJ. The etiology and management of hydrocephalus in the preterm infant. *Concept Neurosurg* 1990;3:67.
18. Dallacasa P, Dappozzo A, Galassi E, Sandri F, Cocchi G, Masi M. Cerebrospinal fluid shunt infections in infants. *Childs Nerv Syst* 1995;11:643.
19. Alonso VM, Alvarez JL, Delgado L, Mendizabal R, Jimenez JL, Sanchez CJ. Gastric perforation due to ventriculo-peritoneal shunt. *Pediatr Neurosurg* 1994;21:192.
20. Kang JK, Jeun SS, Chung DS, Lee IW, Sung WH. Unusual proximal migration of ventriculoperitoneal shunt into the heart. *Childs Nerv Syst* 1996;12:176.
21. Bass T, White LE, Wood RD, Werner AL, Schinco FP. Rapid decompression of congenital hydrocephalus associated with parenchymal hemorrhage. *J Neuroimag* 1995;5:249.
22. Steinbok P, Poskitt KJ, Cochrane DD, Kestle JR. Prevention of post-shunting ventricular asymmetry by transseptal placement of ventricular catheters. A randomized study. *Pediatr Neurosurg* 1994;21:59.
23. Caldarelli M, Di Rocco C. Surgical options in the treatment of interhemispheric arachnoid cysts. *Surg Neurol* 1996;46:212.
24. Lena G, van Calenberg F, Genitori L, Choux M. Supratentorial inter-hemispheric cysts associated with callosal agenesis: surgical treatment and outcome in 16 children. *Childs Nerv Syst* 1995;11:568.
25. Eder HG, Leber KA, Gruber W. Complications after shunting isolated IV ventricles. *Childs Nerv Syst* 1997;13:13.
26. Rademaker KJ, Govaert P, Vandertop WP, Gooskens R, Meiners LC, de Vries L. Rapidly progressive enlargement of the fourth ventricle in the preterm infant with post-haemorrhagic ventricular dilatation. *Acta Paediatr* 1995;84:1193.
27. Levine D, Barnes PD, Madsen JR, Li W, Edelman RR. HASTE MR imaging improves sonographic diagnosis of fetal CNS anomalies. *Am J Radiol* 1997;204:635.
28. Madsen JR, Estroff J, Levine D. Prenatal neurosurgical diagnosis and counseling. *Neurosurg Clin N Am* 1998;9:49.
29. Luthy DA, Wardinsky T, Shurtleff DB, et al. Cesarean section before the onset of labor and subsequent motor function in infants with meningomyelocele diagnosed antenatally. *N Engl J Med* 1991;324:662.
30. McCullough DC, Johnson DL. Myelomeningocele repair: technical considerations and complications. 1988 [Classical article]. *Pediatr Neurosurg* 1994;21:83.
31. McLone DG. Care of the neonate with a myelomeningocele. *Neurosurg Clin N Am* 1998;9:111.
32. DiRocco C, Verlandi F. Epidemiology and etiology of craniocerebral trauma in the first two years of life. In: Raimondi AJ, Choux M, Di Rocco CD, eds. *Head injuries in the newborn and infant.* New York: Springer-Verlag, 1986:125.
33. Hovind K. Traumatic birth injuries. In: Raimondi AJ, Choux M, Di Rocco CD, eds. *Head injuries in the newborn and infant.* New York: Springer-Verlag, 1986:87.
34. Morota N, Sakamoto K, Kobayashi N. Traumatic cervical sytingomyelia related to birth injury. *Childs Nerv Syst* 1992;8:234.
35. Macdonald RL, Hoffman HJ, Kestle JR, Rutka JT, Weinstein G. Needle aspiration of acute subdural hematomas in infancy. *Pediatr Neurosurg* 1994;20:73.
36. Fort DW, Rushing EJ. Congenital central nervous system tumors. *J Child Neurol* 1997;12:157.
37. Tacconi L, Delfini R, Cantore G. Choroid plexus papillomas: consideration of a surgical series of 33 cases. *Acta Neurochir* 1996;138:802.
38. Ferreira J, Eviatar L, Schneider S, Grossman R. Prenatal diagnosis of intracranial teratoma. Prolonged survival after resection of a malignant teratoma diagnosed prenatally by ultrasound: a case report and literature review. *Pediatr Neurosurg* 1993;19:84.
39. Storr U, Rupprecht T, Bornemann A, et al. Congenital intracerebral teratoma: a rare differential diagnosis in newborn hydrocephalus. *Pediatr Radiol* 1997;27:262.
40. Heckel S, Favre R, Gasser B, Christmann D. Prenatal diagnosis of a congenital astrocytoma: a case report and literature review. *Ultrasound Obstet Gynecol* 1995;5:63.
41. Mazzone D, Magro G, Lucenti A, Grasso S. Report of a case of congenital glioblastoma multiforme: an immunohistochemical study. *Childs Nerv Syst* 1995;11:311.
42. Mondkar J, Kalgutkar A, Nalavade Y, Fernandez A. Congenital primary cerebral neuroblastoma. *Indian Pediatr* 1994;31:698.
43. Pizer BL, Moss T, Oakhill A, Webb D, Coakham HB. Congenital astroblastoma: an immunohistochemical study. Case report. *J Neurosurg* 1995;83:550.
44. Soares FA, Fischer SE, Reis MA, Soares EG. Massive intracranial immature teratoma. Report of a case with polyhidramnios and intense pelvic pain. *Arq Neuropsiquiatr* 1996;54:309.
45. Hosotani K, Tokuriki Y, Takebe Y, Kawaguchi K, Tsuji A, Kubota T. Ruptured aneurysm of the distal posterior inferior cerebellar artery in a neonate—case report. *Neurol Med Chir* 1995;35:892.
46. Tekkok IH, Ventureyra EC. Spontaneous intracranial hemorrhage of structural origin during the first year of life. *Childs Nerv Syst* 1997;13:154.
47. Burrows PE, Robertson RL. Neonatal central nervous system vascular disorders. *Neurosurg Clin N Am* 1998;9:155.
48. DuPlessis A, Volpe JJ. Prognosis for development in the newborn requiring neurosurgical intervention. *Neurosurg Clin N Am* 1998;9:187.
49. Levy ML, Masri LS, McComb JG. Outcome for preterm infants with germinal matrix hemorrhage and progressive hydrocephalus. *Neurosurgery* 1997;41:1111.

CHAPTER 51

Orthopedics

Paul P. Griffin and William W. Robertson, Jr.

The orthopedic or musculoskeletal examination of the newborn is a significant part of the evaluation of the neonate. Normal variations in contour, size, relationships, and range of motion of joints are influenced by genetic factors and by position *in utero*. These normal variations must be distinguished from congenital anomalies and traumatic lesions. The basic principle, that the earlier appropriate treatment is started, the better the correction, makes it incumbent on those caring for the neonate to make an early diagnosis and to obtain appropriate consultation promptly.

PHYSICAL EXAMINATION

The clinician examines the musculoskeletal system first by inspection, looking for abnormalities in contour, size, and position and observing the spontaneous and reflex movements of the infant, and second by palpation and manipulation to determine whether there are abnormalities of passive motion. This is followed by stimulation, where indicated, so that active motion can be noted. All observations include comparison between opposite extremities where indicated. A routine for examining a newborn should be developed so that each examination will be complete. This routine may vary among physicians, but each part of the musculoskeletal system should be examined systematically.

Head and Neck

The neck is examined passively for rotation, lateral flexion, anterior flexion, and extension. Rotation of 80 degrees and lateral flexion of 40 degrees should be present. Both

P. P. Griffin: Department of Orthopedic Surgery, Medical University of South Carolina; and Department of Orthopedic Surgery, University Hospital, Charleston, South Carolina

W. W. Robertson, Jr.: Departments of Orthopaedic Surgery and Pediatrics, The George Washington University School of Medicine; and Department of Pediatric Orthopaedic Surgery, Children's National Medical Center, Washington, D.C.

these motions are normally symmetric to the right and left. Extension and flexion are difficult to measure, but in flexion the chin should touch or nearly touch the chest wall. Extension should be at least 45 degrees from neutral. When rotation or lateral flexion is asymmetric or when motion is limited, radiographs of the neck should be made.

Upper Extremities

The clavicle and shoulder girdle, including the scapula and proximal humerus, elbow, forearm, and hand, are inspected and palpated, with any anomalies in contour, size, and postural attitudes noted. Range of motion of the shoulder girdle is evaluated. Flexion and abduction of the shoulder are 175 degrees to 180 degrees. Extension, internal rotation, and external rotation of the shoulder should be at least 25 degrees, 80 degrees, and 45 degrees, respectively.

The elbow is inspected next, and its motion is evaluated. Normally, the newborn's elbow lacks 10 degrees to 15 degrees from going to full extension and flexes 145 degrees. The forearm should pronate and supinate at least 80 degrees. Limitation of these two motions can be missed easily. Supination and pronation are tested by holding the humerus at the side of the trunk with the elbow held flexed 90 degrees with one hand while checking supination and pronation with the other. The wrist flexes 75 degrees to 80 degrees and extends 65 degrees to 75 degrees. The normally clenched fist of the newborn should have full passive extension of the thumb and all fingers. Active finger extension may be elicited if necessary by a pinprick to the palm. Extension should be to 0 degrees at the metacarpophalangeal joint, but active extension of the interphalangeal joint usually lacks 5 degrees to 15 degrees from going to 0 degrees.

Spine

In the newborn, congenital anomalies of the spine are not readily detectable on physical examination; however, gross anomalies frequently can be recognized by inspection of the spine. Passive flexion and extension and lateral bending of the spine should show smooth contours. Lateral flexion may be slightly asymmetric, secondary to position *in utero*. A hairy tuft, cutaneous vascular pattern, or lipomatous mass frequently signals underlying axial anomalies.

Lower Extremities

The lower extremities are observed for symmetry and variations in contour, position, and size. The hips of a newborn will flex 145 degrees and generally have flexion contractures, as shown by the Thomas test. This test is performed by fully flexing the infant's hips, then extending the hip being tested while holding the opposite hip in flexion to lock the pelvis. The number of degrees that the extended thigh lacks from going to 0-degree extension is the degree of flexion contracture present in that hip. It is normal for the newborn to have a 25- to 30-degree flexion contracture. The hip flexion contracture gradually diminishes during the first 12 weeks after birth, but occasionally will be present longer than 3 months. When hip extension is asymmetric, the more extended hip may be unstable. The stability of the hip always must be evaluated by an Ortolani test (Fig. 51–1) or the oppositely directed provocative Barlow test. When there is a difference in the extension of the hips or a positive Ortolani or Barlow test, additional evaluation of the hip by radiography or, preferably, sonography is indicated. The timing of this imaging is discussed later in this chapter.

Internal and external rotation of the newborn's hip will range between 40 degrees and 80 degrees, abduction is between 45 degrees and 75 degrees, and normal abduction is between 10 degrees and 20 degrees. Any asymmetry of motion should be investigated to determine the cause.

Infants who were not in a frank breech fetal position generally will have a knee flexion contracture of 10 degrees to 25 degrees, with additional ability to flex to 120 degrees to 145 degrees. In those positioned in frank breech, the knees usually will hyperextend 10 degrees to 15 degrees and have limitation of flexion.

Examination of the ankles and feet includes observation of resting positions and range of active motion, stimulated by stroking the sole and the dorsal, medial, and lateral sides of the foot. The rane of passive motion of the ankle in both dorsiflexion and plantarflexion varies depending on the fetal position. Dorsiflexion to above neutral always should be present. Plantarflexion of less than 10 degrees below neutral generally is abnormal. Abduction and adduction of the forefoot is at least 10 degrees to 15 degrees, and the hindfoot has 5 degrees to 10 degrees or more of motion in both varus and valgus.

MUSCULOSKELETAL ANOMALIES

It is not within the scope of this text to discuss all the congenital and acquired abnormalities of the musculoskeletal system seen in the neonate; this chapter does, however, cover most of the more common abnormalities.

Neck

Klippel–Feil syndrome is a defect in segmentation of the cervical vertebrae. There is both a decrease in the number of vertebrae and a fusion of two or more vertebrae. The neck appears shorter than normal, and motion is limited in all directions. The limitation of motion depends on the number of fused segments and frequently is asymmetric in both rotation and lateral flexion. The asymmetric motion may simulate muscular torticollis, but radiographic examination of the neck can confirm the presence of the Klippel–Feil deformity. Treatment started

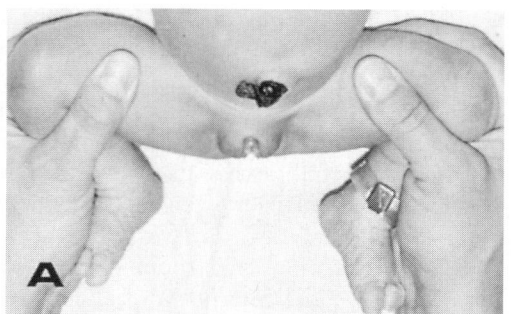
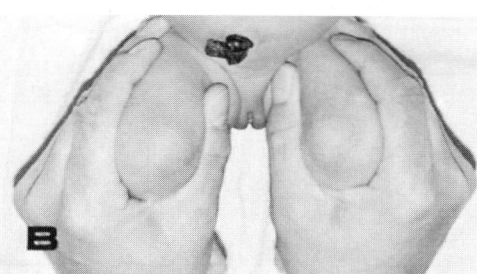

FIG. 51–1. A: Ortolani sign. The fingers are on the trochanter and the thumbs grip the femurs as shown. The femurs are lifted forward as the thighs are abducted. If the head was dislocated, it can be felt to reduce. **B:** Barlow maneuver. The thighs are adducted. If the head dislocates, it will be both felt and seen as it suddenly jerks over the acetabulum.

early, done several times a day, and consisting of passive stretching of the neck to improve rotation, lateral bending, and flexion–extension, may improve the range of motion of the neck.

Torticollis of the neonate may be one of several types. The typical muscular torticollis (Fig. 51–2A) involves a mass from an intramuscular hematoma that appears in the sternocleidomastoideus at 2 weeks of age and gradually disappears during the next 8 to 10 weeks. This mass may go unnoticed, and the torticollis unrecognized until there is facial asymmetry and limited motion of the neck. The physical findings of muscular torticollis are limited rotation of the neck toward the side of the lesion (Figs. 51–2B and 51–2C) and limited lateral flexion away from the lesion. In well-established, persistent torticollis, there is flattening of the maxillary and frontal bones on the side of the lesion and of the occiput on the opposite side. The asymmetry is not present in the newborn, but may

become apparent as early as 2 or 3 weeks and is progressive until the tightness is corrected. Torticollis associated with intrauterine deformation may be apparent at birth.

Initial treatment of muscular torticollis is by passive exercise and appropriate positioning of the infant in bed. The neck should be gently but firmly stretched, four or five times each day, toward the direction of limited rotation and lateral flexion. Sandbags or some similar objects may be used to position the baby's head to prevent it from assuming the position that the tight muscle encourages.

There is a type of congenital torticollis that is associated with neither a mass in the sternocleidomastoideus nor cervical spine abnormalities. In these infants, there is a myostatic contracture of the sternocleidomastoideus, probably secondary to *in utero* position or compression. This type of torticollis often is associated with scoliosis and abductor contracture of one hip and adductor tightness of the opposite hip. The adducted hip may show

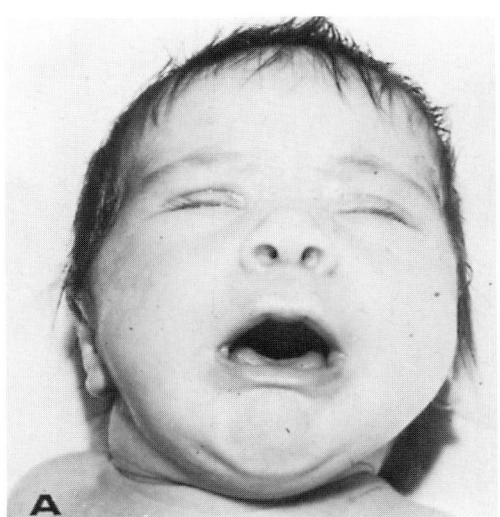

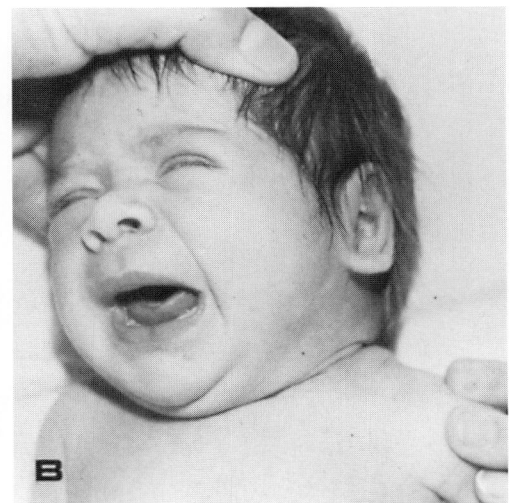

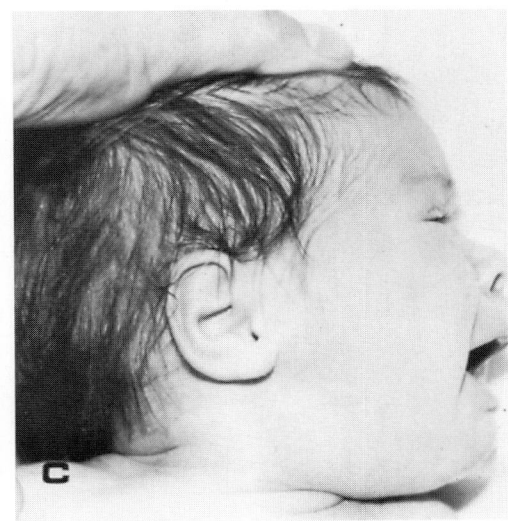

FIG. 51–2. A: Congenital muscular torticollis. There is a fibrous mass in the right sternocleidomastoideus muscle. **B:** Rotation toward the right is limited by the tightness in the right sternocleidomastoideus muscle. **C:** Rotation toward the left is normal.

acetabular dysplasia (Fig. 51–3). The abductor contracture may not be detectable until the normally present tightness of hip flexors spontaneously has diminished enough that the hip can be extended. Whereas this type of torticollis corrects with little or no treatment, the associated hip contractions require stretching. The tight hip abductor needs particular attention, with passive stretching and abduction devices such as multiple diaper layers. Rarely, the associated acetabular dysplasia progresses to dislocation.

Spine

Scoliosis

Congenital scoliosis is difficult to recognize at birth, unless there is asymmetric movement, a cutaneous lesion (such as aplasia, flat hemangioma, hairy tuft), or a lipomatous mass. In the newborn infant, scoliosis is caused by an isolated defect in vertebral body formation or by failure of segmentation. There is little evidence that it is an inherited anomaly, except when it occurs as part of a genetically transmitted syndrome. Because spinal orthoses seldom are of benefit, congenital scoliosis initially is followed only by observation. If a curve is progressive, spinal fusion will be needed and should be done before the curve becomes cosmetically or functionally significant (1). Fusion of a short segment may be done as early as necessary. Congenital scoliosis is associated with a high incidence of related genitourinary anomalies, so the function and anatomy of the genitourinary system should be evaluated by renal ultrasound (2).

Myelomeningocele

Diagnosis of a myelomeningocele generally poses little problem when there is a skin defect. Because the skin over myelomeningoceles is not always defective, any soft

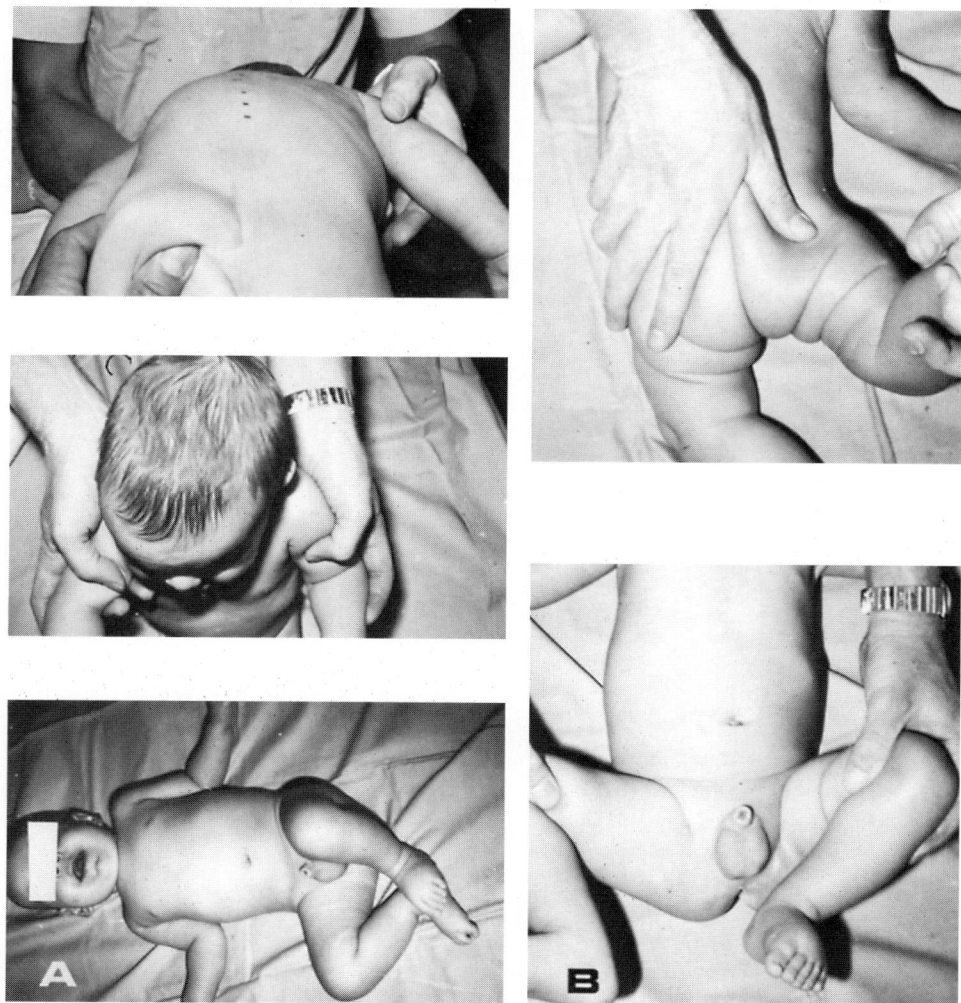

FIG. 51–3. A: A 6-month-old infant with left torticollis, left scoliosis, right abductor contracture, and left adductor tightness. **B:** The right abductor and left adductor are tight.

mass in or off the midline must be examined closely to determine its composition. Lipomas always have good skin coverage and tend to be off the midline.

The care of an infant born with myelomeningocele is complex and requires input from several specialties (see Chap. 50). It is important to determine immediately after birth the level of involvement by inspection of the back, careful examination of the muscle function of the lower extremities, and radiographic examination before surgical closure.

The most common abnormalities of the lower extremities associated with myelomeningocele are deformations of the feet, indicating lack of normal fetal muscle activity. Initial treatment of the deformed foot is with plaster cast correction, followed, if necessary, by surgical releases and transfer of muscle insertions to maintain the correction. These surgeries may be done at almost any age.

Flexion or extension deformities of the knee are treated by gentle passive exercising and progressive splinting. New splints need to be made frequently as the deformity improves.

Treatment of a dislocated hip in the patient with myelomeningocele is controversial. There is general agreement that in those children with intact hip musculature, the dislocated hip, as in an otherwise normal newborn, reduces easily in flexion and abduction. For those lesions below L2, hip abduction therapy will help in developing a more stable hip. The flexed, abducted, and externally rotated position achieved in a Pavlik harness should not be used when the lesion is above L2, because this position may lead to development of contractures that prevent the hip from extending and adducting.

Infants with high lumbar or low thoracic myelomeningoceles have very high mortality and morbidity. The degree of disability correlates well with the level of defect, the presence and degree of hydrocephalus, and the presence of a bony kyphosis. A lesion above L1 associated with hydrocephalus and kyphosis indicates, almost without exception, significant mental and motor disability.

Upper Extremities

Duplication and Reduction

Supernumerary parts, absence or reduction anomalies of the extremities, and segmentation defects of the limb should offer no problem in diagnosis. These orthopedic anomalies seldom need immediate attention, but they should be seen early by the orthopedist to plan appropriate therapy and discuss prognosis with the family. This is true for anomalies of both the upper and lower extremities.

Syndactylism, or fusion of any portion of two or more digits, is a common anomaly that is transmitted through an autosomal dominant gene with varying expressivity. Surgical treatment should be within the first year, with its timing dependent on the completeness of the syndactyly and the fingers involved. The thumb and index finger should be separated at 6 months of age and the little and ring finger separated at 1 year. It is important to determine by radiography if there is a synostosis between fingers, because this should be divided by 1 year of age. A delay in surgical separation in synostosis will result in a bowing of the longer finger due to differential growth.

Polydactyly is correctable by surgery, with timing dependent on the extent of duplication. When the duplication does not contain bone or cartilage, it should be removed in infancy. When there is a question about function, surgical correction should be delayed until the degree of function present in each of the duplicated digits can be ascertained.

Absence of the radius, commonly called radial clubhand, is easily recognized (Fig. 51–4). The wrist and hand are deviated 90 degrees or more. Absence of the radius may be bilateral or unilateral, and the thumb may be present, absent, or hypoplastic. The clubhand is caused by damage to the apical ectoderm or to the deeper mesenchymal tissue of the limb bud (3). It is not genetically transmitted in the otherwise normal child, but it is associated with several genetically transmitted syndromes and frequently is accompanied by aplastic anemia. Early treatment by corrective splints may be sufficient to correct the radial deviation and prepare the extremity for surgery at a later date.

Congenital absence of the thumb occurs as an isolated anomaly or may be associated with a radial clubhand. When unilateral, little or no treatment is needed, but when the absence is bilateral, pollicization of the index finger of the dominant hand will improve function. When the thumb is rudimentary and nonfunctional, treatment is controversial.

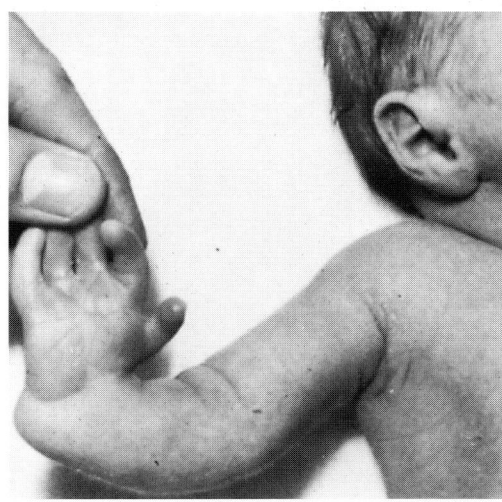

FIG. 51–4. Congenital absence of the radius.

Shoulder Girdle

The Sprengel deformity of congenital elevated scapula is one of the more common congenital anomalies of the shoulder girdle. The deformity may be bilateral or unilateral, and usually it is associated with other abnormalities, such as Klippel–Feil syndrome, congenital anomalies of the upper thoracic vertebrae, or anomalies of the ribs. Asymmetry of the shoulders in unilateral involvement makes recognition easier. On palpation, the affected scapula is high and rotated outward and downward so that its vertebral border lies superiorly and more horizontally than normal. Shoulder abduction and flexion usually, but not always, are limited. The early, conservative treatment is passive range of motion. Surgical correction at 3 to 4 years or up to 16 years of age generally improves appearance and function, with the overall improvement from surgery better in the younger child.

The clavicle has two congenital malformations: congenital pseudarthrosis and congenital absence of part or all of the clavicle. The physical signs on palpation of congenital pseudarthrosis are angulation of the clavicle and a painless, bulbar mass in the midclavicular area (Fig. 51–5). The shoulder girdle is hypermobile, with motion in the clavicle at the pseudarthrosis. Early treatment is not needed before surgical grafting of the defect at 3 to 4 years of age. Because the need for any intervention is controversial, therapy should be individualized. Congenital pseudarthrosis of the clavicle can be differentiated from perinatal fracture of the clavicle because of abundant callus formation in the healing fracture within 2 to 3 weeks after birth.

Partial or complete absence of the clavicle may be recognized by palpation and by the presence of excessive scapulothoracic motion (Fig. 51–6). The completely absent clavicle usually is associated with cranial dysostosis or a widened pubic symphysis. There are no symptoms, and no treatment is needed in complete absence. With partial absence, the end of the clavicle may irritate the brachial plexus, necessitating excision of the fragment. Whereas congenital pseudarthrosis tends to be an isolated anomaly, partial absence of the clavicle almost always accompanies an axial or appendageal skeletal anomaly.

Defects of Limb Segmentation

Synostosis of the elbow and synostosis of the radius and ulna are two of the more common skeletal anomalies of limb segmentation. Elbow synostosis is easily recognized by the lack of motion and significantly smaller size of the affected extremity. Synostosis of the radius and ulna seldom is diagnosed in the nursery and, commonly, not for several years. This is particularly true if the defect is bilateral, because the child himself will not appreciate a difference in his arms. Supinating and pronating the forearm in the initial examination of the newborn should demonstrate this anomaly by lack of range of motion.

Lower Extremities

Variations in contours and postural attitudes of the lower extremities, in general, and the feet, in particular, are frequent causes of concern. *In utero*, the feet seldom rest in a neutral position, being dorsiflexed or plantarflexed, inverted or everted, or in a combination of these positions. At times, it may be difficult to determine

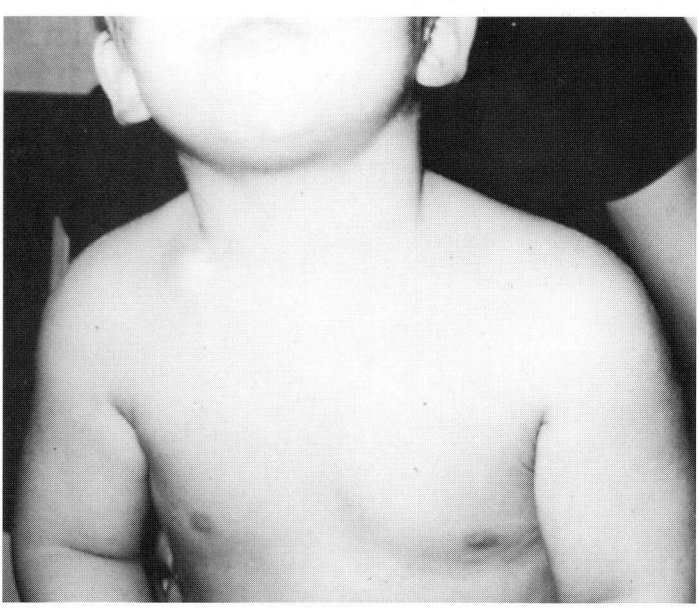

FIG. 51–5. A 2-year-old child with pseudarthrosis of the right clavicle.

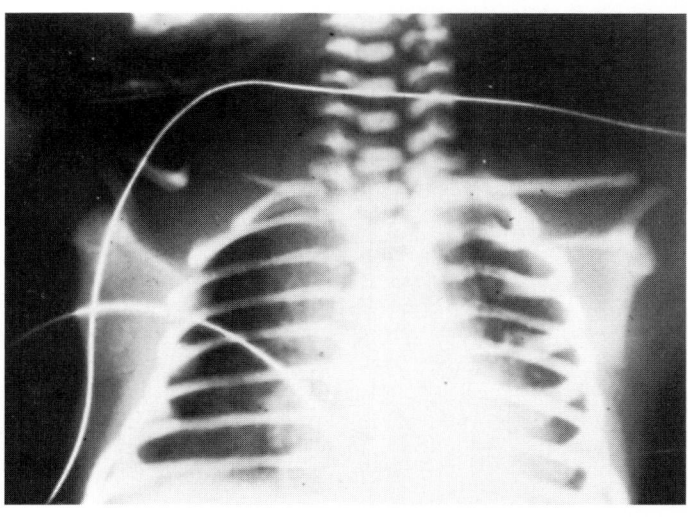

FIG. 51–6. Partial absence of the right clavicle.

whether there is a structural abnormality or only a temporary positional deformation.

Feet

Metatarsus adductus (Fig. 51–7) may be either a positional deformity with no bony abnormality or a structural defect, and it is not always easy to distinguish between the two. The distinction becomes easier with time, because a positional metatarsus adductus corrects fairly rapidly by passive exercises or even without treatment. A structural deformity does not spontaneously correct completely, becoming more rigid with time.

The differentiation between postural and structural metatarsus adductus is made mostly by physical examination. In structural metatarsus adductus (Fig. 51–7A), the base of the fifth metatarsus and the cuboid are prominent, creating an impressive, well-defined skin crease on the medial side of the foot at the first metatarsal–cuneiform joint. In a positional metatarsus adductus, the lateral and medial borders of the foot are curved more gently than in the structural deformity. The most significant physical finding, however, is the presence or absence of rigidity of the forefoot, as determined by its resistance to abduction. In structural deformity, the forefoot usually cannot be abducted beyond the midline (Fig. 51–7B), whereas in positional deformity the forefoot is more flexible and can be abducted (Fig. 51–7C). The heel of the structural metatarsus adductus foot usually is in valgus, and in positional deformity it is likely to be in varus or at neutral. The valgus position of the hindfoot can be seen on clinical evaluation and, if necessary, confirmed by radiographic studies.

Treatment of the flexible positional deformity is either observation for spontaneous resolution or passive stretching of the forefoot into abduction with the foot held as shown in Fig. 51–7B. Structural metatarsus adductus generally needs treatment with repeated cast changes. Surgical treatment may be necessary in the case of more severe structural abnormalities, such as a skew foot.

Talipes calcaneovalgus is not a structural deformity, but rather a reflection of the foot's position *in utero* (Fig. 51–8). The sole lies against the uterine wall, and the foot is dorsiflexed so that its dorsal skin lies against the anterior surface of the tibia. The fibula is prominent and appears to be dislocated posteriorly, being pushed backward by the excessive dorsiflexion. There is a depression over the sinus tarsus. The calcaneovalgus foot is flexible and passively plantarflexes at least to neutral and, in most instances, to 5 degrees to 10 degrees beyond neutral.

Treatment of the calcaneovalgus foot is by either passive exercises or corrective plaster cast, depending on to the severity of the deformity. Mild cases are treated with exercises that stretch the foot into equinus and varus 15 to 20 times at four to five sessions daily.

The more severely resistant deformities, those that flex only to neutral plantarflexion, are treated by repeated applications of plaster casts for 8 weeks. Casts are changed as needed with growth, and, at each change, the foot is placed in equinus and varus with a mold placed in the arch to relax the plantar ligaments and posterior tibialis muscle. The goal of treatment is to obtain a plantarflexed, varus position to allow the plantar ligaments and posterior tibialis tendon that have been stretched *in utero* to shorten.

It is important that the positional calcaneovalgus foot not be confused with congenital vertical talus, a rare but serious anomaly. In congenital vertical talus, the forefoot is dorsiflexed, and the hindfoot is in equinus (Fig. 51–9). The talus is rigidly fixed in plantarflexion, and if the examiner places one thumb on the talus, and with the other hand dorsiflexes and plantarflexes the foot, the talus will remain almost stationary as the forefoot moves around it. The forefoot cannot be plantarflexed as much

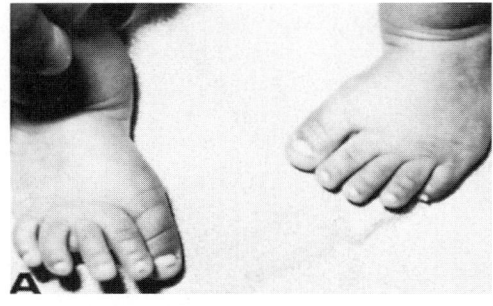

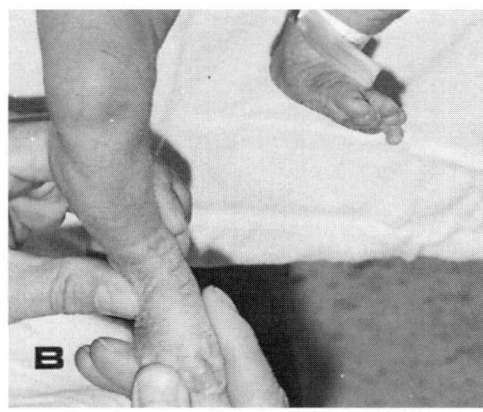

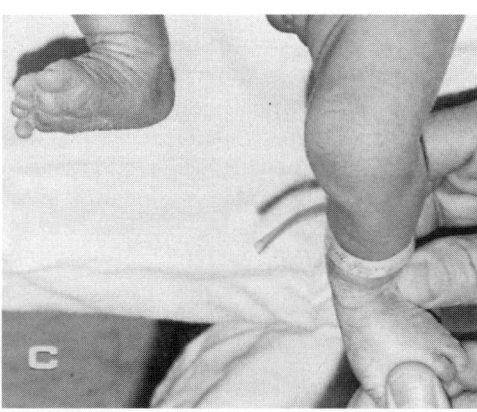

FIG. 51–7. A: Structural metatarsus adductus. **B:** Structural metatarsus adductus. The forefoot does not abduct beyond neutral. **C:** Positional metatarsus. The forefoot abducts beyond the midline.

as the calcaneovalgus foot, and seldom can it be plantarflexed more than 5 degrees beyond neutral. A radiographic examination of the foot will demonstrate the hindfoot equinus and forefoot dorsiflexion plus the other radiographic characteristics of this anomaly. Serial casting rarely results in correction of this deformity. Although treatment will not create a normal foot, the results are far better when started in the first year of life.

The classic clubfoot is a developmental anomaly of the entire foot (Fig. 51–10). There is varus of the hindfoot, varus and adduction of the forefoot, and equinus that is not apparent until the varus and adduction are corrected

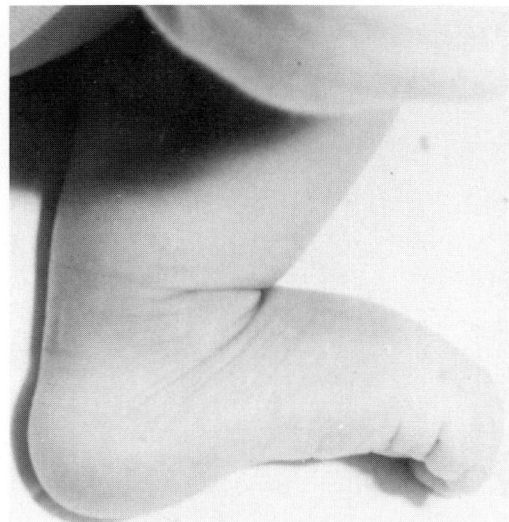

FIG. 51–8. Talipes calcaneovalgus.

to neutral. This is a structural deformity and resists correction; it is easily recognized by its rigidity. There is a positional equinovarus foot that may resemble the true clubfoot, but it is flexible and can be corrected beyond neutral with little difficulty. Treatment of the structural clubfoot is by repeated manipulation and strapping or by manipulation and application of a cast. Although early treatment usually is instituted, no studies have demonstrated clearly the advantage of casting the newborn as opposed to the infant. When conservative measures are unsuccessful in correcting the foot, surgical correction is necessary.

Tibia and Fibula

Significant deformities of the tibia and fibula occur infrequently and are not difficult to detect. Congenital absence of the tibia or fibula, congenital amputation, and congenital bowing all are easily recognized. When the tibia is absent, the foot is in varus; when the fibula is absent, the foot has an equinovalgus deformity. These deformities should be seen early by the orthopedist, because conservative and supervised treatment of the foot

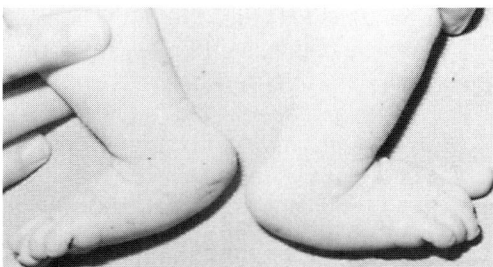

FIG. 51–9. Congenital vertical talus.

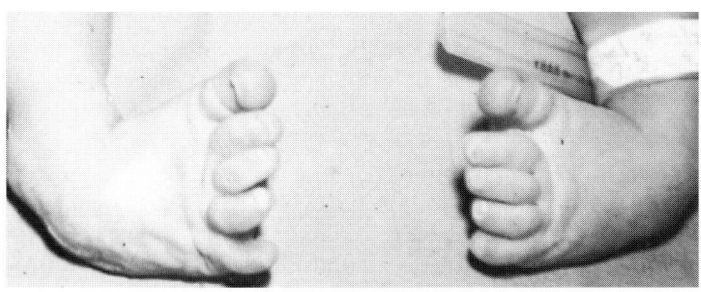

FIG. 51–10. Talipes equinocavovarus foot (i.e., club-foot).

deformities is indicated in some of these children, whereas in others early amputation is the treatment of choice (4–6). With newer techniques and knowledge of the biology of bone elongation, more of these limbs are being salvaged.

Anterior bowing of the tibia is a serious deformity (Fig. 51–11). The bone of the tibia is of poor quality, and in most cases it either is sclerotic with partial or complete obliteration of the intermedullary space or has cystic areas that contain material similar to that in fibrous dysplasia. Pseudarthrosis may be present at birth, or always following a fracture, which is likely within the first 2 years of life. Protection of the tibia by casts and braces is important and may be sufficient to prevent a fracture. Although the case shown in Fig. 51–11 is mild, there is a narrow intramedullary canal, and the bone needs protection, for it is unlikely to heal should it fracture. There is no tendency for these cases of anterior bowing to improve spontaneously.

Conversely, a tibia that is posteriorly bowed corrects spontaneously. Any rare fractures in this condition should heal. The posteriorly bowed tibia needs only to be observed. There can be subsequent leg length discrepancy as a residual of this deformity.

Most neonates have an inward or medial torsion of the leg distal to the knee and outward rotation above the knee. The medial torsion below the knee may occur in the knee, tibia, ankle, or a combination of these, and, except in extreme cases, no treatment is necessary because alignment will improve progressively. The exception to this may be in relatively immobile, premature infants who lie in the same position most of the time.

Knee

Significant deformities of the knee are very rare. Genu recurvatum, a relatively frequent positional deformity associated with a frank breech position, is not serious and will respond to gentle exercising. The positional recurvatum must be differentiated from the more serious subluxation or dislocation of the knee. When there is doubt as to whether or not a recurvatum represents a subluxation or a dislocation, a radiograph should be made. In subluxation, the tibia is forward on the femur but is not completely dislocated, whereas in dislocation, the tibia will be completely anterior to the femur. In congenital dislocation, the knee can be hyperextended but not flexed beyond neutral, and the tibia is anteriorly displaced on palpation. Both subluxation and dislocation of the knee can be treated with early serial casting. Care must be taken to follow the reduction of the aticular surfaces with x-rays. The subluxed knee reduces with casting, but a dislocated knee may require open reduction.

Congenital fibrosis of part of the quadriceps is an anomaly that prevents knee flexion, causing a more extended posture than normal in neonates. Active and passive flexion is limited and seldom is more than 40 degrees. Treatment is by surgical excision of the fibrous mass.

Hip

Developmental Dysplasia of the Hip

The most common of the neonatal hip abnormalities is developmental dysplasia. This hip is embryologically

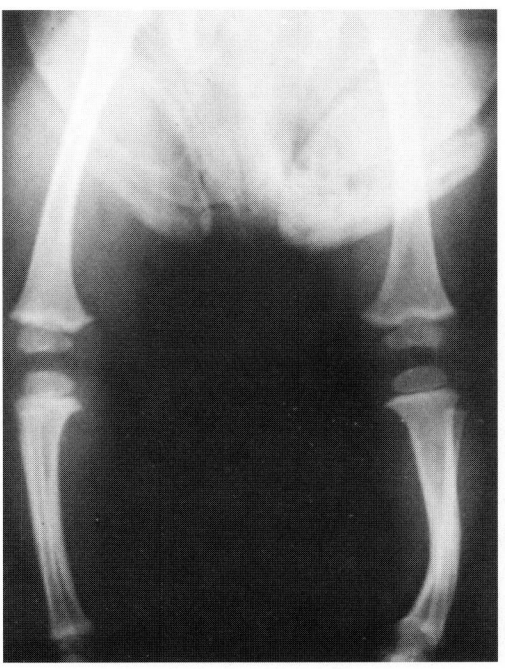

FIG. 51–11. Anterior bowed tibia.

normal but, as a result of mechanical forces *in utero* and maternal hormones that relax tissues in preparation for parturition, it is dislocated or dislocatable in the perinatal period. The less common type is a teratogenic hip that probably dislocates in the embryologic period of gestation and is associated with malformation of the pelvis and femur.

Developmental dysplasia of the hips occurs more frequently in female infants who present in breech position at term gestation and who have a positive family history. The dysplasia more often is unilateral, with the left hip more frequently affected, but it may be bilateral.

In the newborn, the typical dislocated hip may not have the classically described signs of dislocation, such as asymmetric skin folds, limited abduction, and shorter-appearing femur (i.e., Galeazzi sign). These signs are secondary and may not develop until the end of 6 weeks of life, as the dislocated hip migrates laterally and superiorly. The clinician diagnoses this condition in the newborn by demonstrating that the femoral head can be lifted into the acetabulum as the thigh is abducted in flexion (i.e., Ortolani maneuver; Fig. 51–1A) and that it dislocates as the hip is flexed, adducted, and pushed posteriorly (i.e., Barlow maneuver; Fig. 51–1B). The Ortolani test is positive in the dislocated hip until 6 to 8 weeks of age, sometimes longer. In addition to feeling the dislocation as the thigh is adducted, the examiner should reduce the hip by abduction in flexion and, while maintaining the same degree of abduction, extend the thigh to dislocate the hip. In each instance, whether dislocation is obtained by adducting or by extending the thigh, the examiner not only can feel the hip dislocate and relocate but also can see the sudden jerk that occurs as the femoral head rides in and out of the acetabulum.

Hip dislocation usually can be recognized clinically in the first few days of life. However, a large number of hips that are unstable at birth may become stable once the intrauterine environment, both positional and hormonal, is eliminated (7). Those unstable hips most at risk for development of dysplasia are those with evidence of uterine packing problems (e.g., first born, breech presentation, torticollis, or metatarsus adductus), female sex, and a positive family history of hip dysplasia. The widespread use of hip ultrasound to evaluate and confirm hip dysplasia makes the quantification of the problem much easier. The question arises as to when to treat an abnormal hip. Some authors advocate the initiation of treatment as soon as any abnormality is discovered (8,9). Other authors feel that this approach may cause overtreatment of as many as one in three hips that would stabilize within 1 month of birth without treatment (10–12). Early treatment is easier on the family and child, with results that are far better than when treatment is started several months or years later.

Hip displacement almost always is reduced in flexion and abduction. The hip is usually, but not always, stable if held flexed 90 degrees or more and then abducted. In the newborn, radiographs of the hip are not necessarily diagnostic, although in some, the hip appears laterally displaced in the anteroposterior projection (Fig. 51–12). Sonography, if well done, is the method of choice in the neonate, both to confirm the diagnosis of hip dysplasia and to follow the progress of acetabular development during treatment (13). The greatest advantage of the hip ultrasound is the ability to view the hip when it is stressed in a Barlow-like maneuver.

When sonograms are not available, hip radiographs in both the anteroposterior and horizontal planes should be taken, with the infant in the splint to determine that the

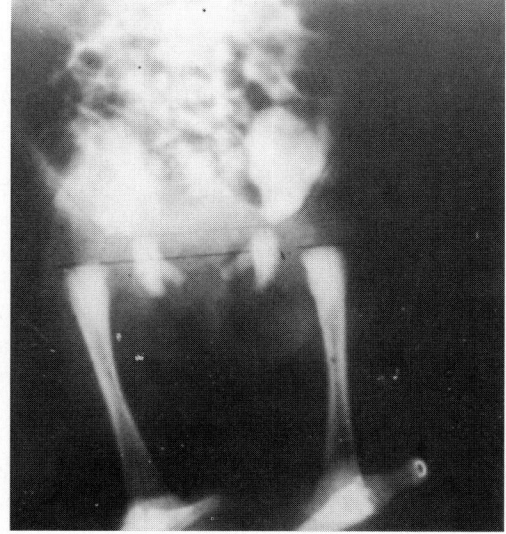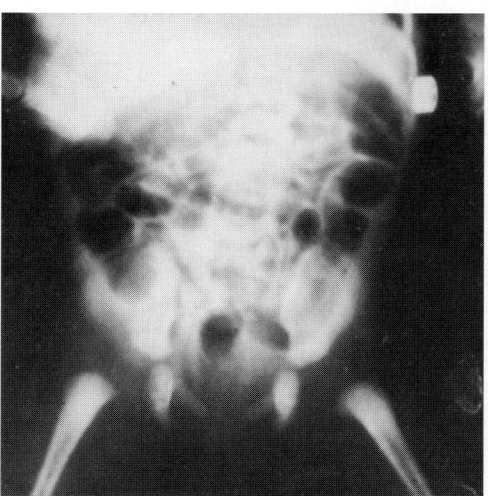

FIG. 51–12. Bilateral congenital dislocation of the hip. The metaphyseal–acetabulum distance is wide.

hip is held reduced. Rarely, the hip dislocates posteriorly in the splint, but appears to be reduced in the anteroposterior view; only the horizontal view will show the dislocation in this instance.

The Pavlik harness is the splint of choice from birth to 6 months of age, but it must be applied properly. Excessive abduction from tight posterior straps can cause avascular necrosis (14).

All infants should have follow-up hip examinations at well-baby checks the first 3 months. The Ortolani test may be positive for 6 to 12 weeks, but, more commonly, the late physical signs of dislocation are the following:

- Asymmetric folds in unilateral dislocation
- An apparent discrepancy of leg length caused by pelvic obliquity and a high-riding femoral head
- High trochanter
- Limited abduction
- A palpable defect in the anterior groin where the femoral head normally lies
- A piston or telescoping motion

These signs are sufficient to make the diagnosis, but sonography or radiography will confirm it. After the development of the ossific nucleus of the femoral head (at 3 to 6 months), the ultrasound no longer is useful, so plain radiographic views are indicated to demonstrate hip displacement.

Developmental hip dislocation is probably the most important condition in the musculoskeletal system in which a delay in diagnosis and treatment has a profound effect on the outcome. The results of treatment in the neonate are far superior to those at any other time, so special care in diagnosing this condition is warranted.

Teratologic Hip Dislocation

Teratogenic hip dislocation presents with different findings. The hip, which has dislocated early in fetal life, ordinarily will not reduce by flexion and abduction because the femoral head is displaced proximally. Therefore, the Ortolani sign is not present in the teratogenic dislocation. If the dislocation is unilateral, there is asymmetry of abduction of the hips. The dislocated hip will have more extension than the opposite hip and may have limited rotation. When the dislocation is bilateral, the diagnosis is more difficult because there is no asymmetry. Abduction of both hips is limited, the thighs appear short in relation to the lower legs, and the perineum appears wider than normal. Although the diagnosis can be confirmed by ultrasound, plain radiographic examination is always abnormal in teratogenic hip dislocation.

Proximal Femoral Focal Deficiency

Proximal femoral focal deficiency is an anomaly of serious magnitude that may be either unilateral or bilateral. The degree of deficiency is variable and ranges from absence of the diaphysis, upper metaphysis, and femoral head to a very short femur, with coxa vara of the neck and head. It is not uncommon as well for the fibula to be absent and the foot deformed in the more severely affected infant with proximal femoral focal deficiency. The shortness of the femur is obvious on inspection. Motion of the hip may be limited. Early referral to the orthopedist, who will give the definitive treatment, is important. Initial treatment may include stretching exercises or traction, or both, for correction of contractures about the hip, although these have proven to be of limited value. Definitive surgical management depends on the potential for function in the extremity and ranges from measures to correct leg length discrepancy to fusion of the knee and amputation of the foot to create a stump for an above-knee prosthesis.

GENERALIZED MUSCULOSKELETAL ANOMALIES

The many syndromes that primarily involve the epiphysis, epiphyseal plate, metaphysis, or diaphysis are, with few exceptions, easily recognized by their phenotypes. There are similarities in all of the chondrodystrophies, but there are important differences in prognoses. Because classification of the various types is made by the radiographic appearance of the skeleton, radiographs of the spine, skull, and extremities should be examined before a diagnosis is made and the prognosis is discussed with the parent (15). There is little to be done for most of these syndromes, but, when there is a deformity, treatment should be initiated early.

Achondroplasia, chondroectodermal dysplasia (i.e., Ellis–van Creveld disease), and epiphyseal dysostosis (i.e., diastrophic dwarfism) are three of the more common congenital, generalized skeletal affectations recognizable at birth that are associated with dwarfism. Children with large heads, short extremities, excessive or restricted motion of joints, unusual-appearing facies, and short, stubby phalanges suggest that a skeletal dysplasia is present that usually can be identified by radiographs of the skull, spine, and extremities (16). Infants affected by certain skeletal dysplasias or by metabolic skeletal abnormalities, however, appear normal at birth, with the skeletal anomalies appearing later in infancy and childhood.

Osteogenesis imperfecta is a generalized disturbance of the skeleton manifested by soft, fragile bone. If severe, it is very obvious at birth, but it may be mild enough to go undiagnosed until the child is several years old. Osteogenesis imperfecta involves primarily the skeleton, but also affects the skin, ligaments, tendons, sclera, nose, ear, platelet function, and probably other systems (17–19).

The diagnosis of osteogenesis imperfecta is not difficult when there are multiple fractures, a very soft skull, paradoxic respirations indicating rib fractures, and bluish-gray sclera. For those who survive the delivery, gentle handling to prevent additional injuries and skin traction to align the extremities are important considerations. It is possible to align all four extremities simultaneously with traction. The fractures heal rapidly, and by 9 or 10 days the traction usually can be discontinued (20). An important key to the treatment of fractures of osteogenesis imperfecta is to avoid increasing bone fragility with prolonged immobilization.

There are several classifications of osteogenesis imperfecta according to the severity of involvement. The classification of Sillence appears to be the most helpful in prognosis and genetic counseling (19).

Arthrogryposis multiplex congenita (Fig. 51–13) is an uncommon but easily recognizable syndrome of the musculoskeletal system. All four extremities and the trunk may be affected, or the abnormalities may be limited to the arms or legs. The hallmark of this entity is the lack of active and passive motion in the affected extremities.

The microscopic picture of the muscle in arthrogryposis shows changes of denervation and fibrofatty replacement. Secondary to the muscle weakness and dysfunction, there is distortion of the joints, as well as limitation of motion. Frequently, these infants have dislocation of the hips, knees, or radial heads, or combinations of the three. In addition, they may have either clubfeet or vertical talus, both of which are more resistant to treatment than those not associated with arthrogryposis. Treatment

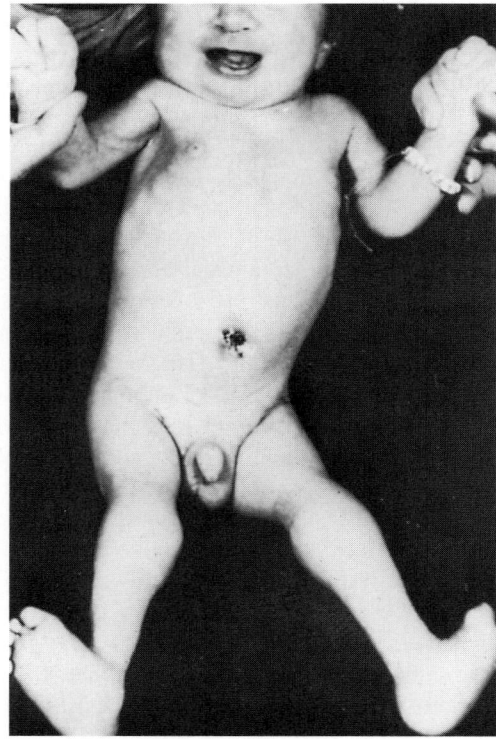

FIG. 51–13. Arthrogryposis multiplex congenita.

should begin in the nursery and is directed at increasing the motion of all affected joints by passive exercises done six to eight times each day. Joint dislocation and the hand and foot deformities should be treated early with appropriate plaster splints or casts or with traction.

BIRTH FRACTURES

Long, difficult labor—particularly with a breech position, a large infant, or fetal distress requiring rapid extraction—makes birth injuries in otherwise normal infants more likely. Birth fractures almost always involve clavicle, humerus, or femur. It is rare for birth fractures in a normal infant to occur below the elbow or below the knee. The fracture is more likely to be through either the diaphysis or the epiphyseal plate, so that the epiphysis and epiphyseal plate are separated from the metaphysis. At times, the fractures are not noted, because pain may be minimal and a deformity may not be apparent. Diagnosis in such cases is made incidental to a radiograph taken for unrelated indications. In other infants, the fracture is painful and is a cause of pseudoparalysis, with the limb lying limp and not moving on stimulation.

Diaphyseal Fractures

Fractures of the diaphysis of the humerus generally are diagnosed by the obstetrician, who hears and feels the snap when the humerus breaks as the baby is being extracted. The same can be said about fractures of the femoral shaft and clavicle. A radiograph confirms the fracture.

Fracture of the shaft of the humerus is treated by immobilization of the arm by the side. Soft padding is placed between the arm and the chest, and the elbow is held at 90 degrees flexion.

Fractures of the femoral shaft can be held with a posterior splint that extends from below the knee to over the buttock and is held in place with an elastic bandage for 10 to 14 days.

Fractures of the clavicle may be asymptomatic if undisplaced and need no treatment except care in handling the infant. If the fracture is displaced, it usually is painful. The fracture can be treated either by strapping the arms to the chest, with padding placed in the axilla and the elbow flexed 90 degrees, or by using a figure-of-eight bandage made of stockinette to immobilize the fracture. In 8 to 10 days, the callus is sufficient for immobilization to be discontinued.

Epiphyseal Injuries

An epiphyseal separation or fracture occurs through the hypertrophied layer of cartilage cells in the epiphysis. A fracture through the proximal epiphyseal plate of the humerus is one of the more common skeletal injuries associated with a difficult delivery. The diagnosis has to be made primarily on the clinical findings of swelling about the shoulder and crepitus and pain when the shoulder is moved. Motion is painful, and the arm lies limply. The proximal humeral epiphysis is not ossified at birth and, therefore, is not visible on radiograph. This makes diagnosis by radiography very difficult. If there is complete or almost complete separation of the epiphysis, the metaphysis appears displaced in relation to the glenoid of the scapula, but usually the separation is minimal and there are no radiographic changes noted except soft tissue swelling. After 8 to 10 days, callus appears and is visible on radiographs. Ultrasonic evaluation of suspected epiphyseal injuries is gaining popularity, because nonossified epiphyses and hematomas, as well as bony structures, are visible (21).

Treatment for a fracture of the proximal epiphysis of the humerus is immobilization of the arm by the side, with soft padding in the axilla for 8 to 10 days. Healing is rapid, and remodeling is such that even a striking angulation will improve progressively to where the contour appears normal. If a complete separation is present, reduction by gentle traction probably should be attempted before immobilization.

A fracture separation of the distal humeral epiphysis is very rare. It is difficult to diagnose radiographically because this epiphysis, like the proximal epiphysis, is completely cartilaginous. When an injury is present, there will be swelling about the elbow with pain and crepitus on passive motion. If the epiphysis is displaced, the anteroposterior radiograph will show that the olecranon is placed medially or laterally in its relationship with the long axis of the humerus. A fracture of the distal epiphysis is more likely to have a significant residual deformity than is a fracture of the proximal humeral epiphysis. Skin traction on the forearm for 9 to 10 days is an option to treat this injury.

Fracture of the proximal femoral epiphysis is an uncommon problem but one that can be confused with a congenital dislocation or with acute pyarthrosis. The epiphyseal plate of the proximal femur is a crescent-shaped line extending from the greater to the lesser trochanter and includes the cartilaginous epiphysis of the trochanter, neck, and femoral head. Swelling about the hip is difficult to appreciate, and suspicion of the presence of this injury should be aroused when the baby does not move the extremity on stimulation. This is confirmed by the presence of pain and crepitus when the hip is moved passively. The radiograph of the hip will show the upper end of the femoral metaphysis to be displaced laterally, and, if the separation is complete, the metaphysis is likely to be displaced above the center of the acetabulum as well as displaced laterally. Ultrasonic evaluation will confirm the position of the cartilaginous femoral head in relation to the acetabulum and femoral metaphysis. After several days of incomplete separation, the hip will no longer be

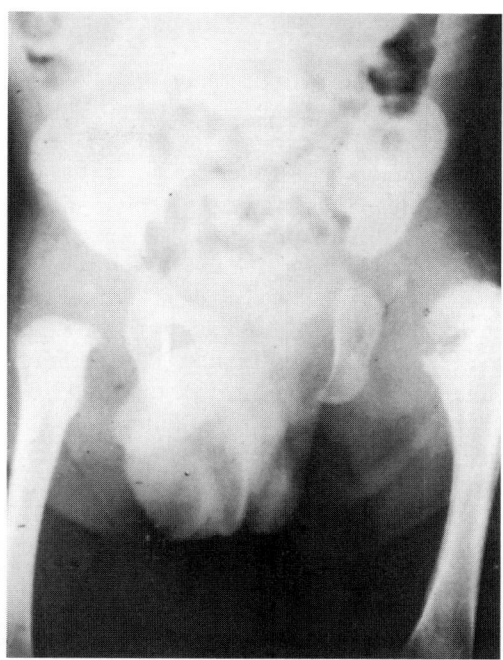

FIG. 51–14. A 3-week-old infant with a birth fracture of the proximal epiphysis of the femur.

painful, and, most of these will be recognized only after callus formation is seen on an incidental radiograph or after a large callus presents as a firm mass in the groin or upper thigh (Fig. 51–14). If the diagnosis is recognized before healing is underway, the hip should be manipulated gently and immobilized in flexion and abduction for 10 to 14 days.

If ultrasound is not available, aspiration of the joint will help differentiate a fracture from congenital dislocation and acute pyarthrosis. If a fracture is present, blood should be found in the joint.

Diagnosis of a fracture separation of the distal femoral epiphysis can be made by radiographic studies. Ossification of the distal femoral epiphysis is present at birth, and even slight displacement and angulation can be recognized. If there is swelling around the knee and pain on passive motion, a radiograph will confirm the diagnosis. Treatment is by immobilization in plaster for 10 to 14 days, if displacement is not severe. When displacement or angulation is excessive, reduction by manipulation should be done and the extremity immobilized in plaster for 14 days.

OBSTETRIC PALSY

Traumatic neuropathy of the brachial plexus is one of the more common birth injuries. It is caused most usually by traction and lateral flexion of the neck. In vertex presentations, it occurs by traction and lateral flexion applied to deliver the shoulder in large babies, and in breech presentations by traction and lateral flexion to deliver the head.

The clinical picture is easily recognized by the absence of active motion of the involved extremity in the Moro reflex. There may be supraclavicular swelling and an associated fractured clavicle.

There are three types of obstetric palsy, and the clinical findings are different in each. The upper plexus type is called Erb–Duchenne (Fig. 51–15), in which the C5 and C6 nerve roots are affected, and C7 roots are less involved. In the lower plexus type, known as Klumpke palsy, the C8 and T1 roots are involved. The third type is a total involvement of all roots that make up the plexus. If the C5 and C6 roots are affected, the shoulder is held internally rotated with the forearm supinated and the elbow extended and the wrist and fingers flexed. A grasp may be present, whereas traction will be absent. When the lower roots, C8 and T1, are involved, the hand is flaccid, with little or no control. When the entire plexus is affected, the total extremity is flaccid.

The early treatment of obstetric palsy is conservative. Myelography and surgical exploration have little to offer initially in the management of this problem. Recovery of function depends, of course, on the degree of injury. When the injury is a neurapraxia, complete recovery over several weeks usually takes place. When there is a neurotmesis or complete avulsion, no recovery takes place. Loss of sensory function suggests a more severe involvement. Because it is not possible to say which degree of injury is present, all should be treated by prevention of additional injury to the plexus by gentle handling. The arm needs protection for the first 4 to 5 days, until swelling has subsided. After this period, the joints of the arm may be carried through a passive range of motion several times each day for maintenance of flexibility. The paralyzed muscles should be supported in a position of relaxation for part of each day, with care being taken that a contraction of the protected muscles does not occur. Denervated muscles undergo fibrosis, which can become contracted, producing a fixed deformity. Most obstetric plexus palsy patients recover within 3 months (22). The return of function of the deltoid and biceps are the best clinical parameters to follow recovery. If these have not shown some recovery by 3 months, return of function is unlikely. When the lesion is limited to the C5 and C6 nerve roots without recovery at 3 months, surgical intervention should be considered (23).

In those patients with residual paralysis, passive exercises and progressive active exercises should be continued for months and years, as long as there is some progressive improvement. At 3 to 5 years, certain residual deformities can be improved surgically. Brachial plexus injuries are discussed further in Chapter 49.

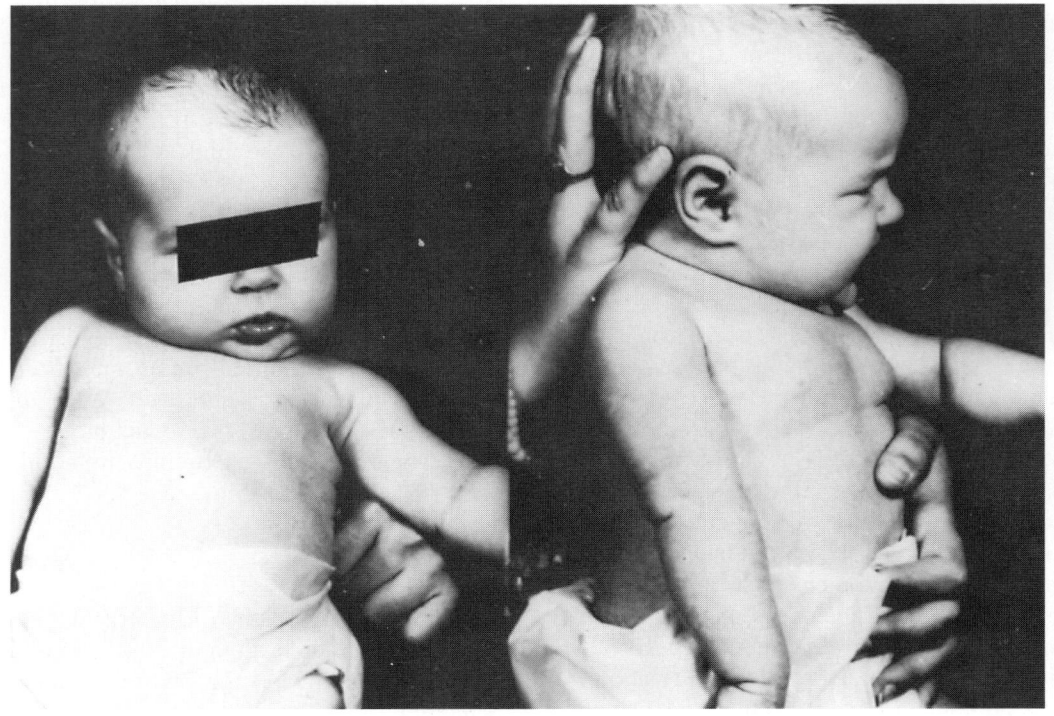

FIG. 51–15. An Erb–Duchenne type of brachial plexus injury.

BONE AND JOINT INFECTIONS

Osteomyelitis and acute septic arthritis occur in the neonate, although not as frequently as in older infants. Additionally, changes in obstetric and neonatal practices have contributed to a decreased incidence of bony infections in the neonatal period. Infants with altered immune function or the presence of indwelling vascular lines remain at particular risk for these unusual infections. The priorities of treatment are different in osteomyelitis and septic arthritis, and the differences are of paramount importance.

Osteomyelitis almost always occurs by hematogenous spread, from either a cutaneous or oral lesion, or from other sources such as omphalitis or an indwelling arterial line. *Staphylococcus* and *Streptococcus* species are the most frequent causative organisms, with group B β-hemolytic streptococcus and gram-negative organisms increasing in frequency more recently.

Osteomyelitis begins in the metaphyses of long bones. Bacteria reach the metaphysis through the nutrient artery, which terminates in the sinusoids adjacent to the epiphyseal plate (24,25). The rate of flow in the sinusoid is slower, creating an ideal situation for bacterial stasis and multiplication. Edema, vascular engorgement, and cellulitis are followed by thrombosis and abscess formation, with destruction and absorption of trabeculae. The purulent exudate in the metaphysis spreads by way of Volkmann canals to the periosteal space and elevates the loosely attached periosteum, which responds by laying down new bone over the original cortex. The new bone is the involucrum. In infants, unlike in older children, the exudate perforates the cortex of the metaphysis early and does not spread down the diaphysis, sparing the endosteal and haversian vessels and, therefore, does not cause massive sequestrum in infants as readily as in older children.

In children beyond infancy, the epiphyseal plate acts as a barrier against spread to the epiphysis. In the infant, Trueta (24) has shown that vessels cross the epiphyseal plate, so that infection of the metaphysis may spread to the epiphysis and cause irreparable damage to the secondary center of the ossification and the epiphyseal plate. For this reason, early diagnosis and treatment are very important to prevent destruction of the metaphysis and epiphysis.

The neonate with hematogenous osteomyelitis presents with varied complaints and findings. Movement of the affected part may provoke crying. There may be loss of active motion of the affected extremity (i.e., pseudoparalysis), or the baby may have unexplained fever. Palpable swelling of the extremity appears early after the onset of bone infection and is visible in a soft tissue radiograph. In the newborn, this swelling may be massive, including the entire extremity, before visual changes in the bone are apparent on radiographic evaluation. In a newborn with extensive swelling of an extremity, osteomyelitis must be strongly considered as the diagnosis, until proven otherwise. Alternatively, the infant may be so overwhelmed by infection that he or she responds very little to stimulation and even may be afebrile. In any infant who is seriously ill or who is failing to thrive, careful examination of the extremities should be done, with observation for any evidence of tenderness, pain, and swelling that may indicate the presence of osteomyelitis.

The symptoms of osteomyelitis due to group B β-hemolytic streptococcus are unusual. There may be minimal systemic response and little or no local swelling, with a pseudoparalysis or pain on motion as the only symptom of osteomyelitis. When the proximal humerus is involved, the infant holds the affected arm in the same position as does the infant with an obstetric palsy.

Early treatment with appropriate antibiotics and immobilization usually will control the osteomyelitis. If treatment is started too late, abscesses may form that will require surgical drainage.

Acute septic arthritis has even greater urgency of treatment than osteomyelitis in the neonate, although delay in either may cause irreparable damage to the secondary centers of ossification. Joint infection is primarily by hematogenous spread, although the hip may be infected by needle inoculation during attempted femoral vein puncture.

The neonate with septic arthritis generally is very ill, but may be so overwhelmed that there are few specific signs. Failure to thrive, as in osteomyelitis, may be the reason for admission. Pseudoparalysis, pain on passive motion, swelling, and increased warmth are the usual physical findings. Diagnosis is difficult when the hip is affected, because visible swelling and palpable warmth are minimal, except when there is osteomyelitis associated with the arthritis. Radiographic examination will show a joint effusion and distention, with widening of the joint space. The hip frequently will be subluxated, and, if diagnosis is delayed several days, the intraarticular pressure will cause dislocation of the hip. When dislocation occurs secondary to pyarthrosis, the joint usually is severely and permanently damaged.

Treatment of an infected joint in an infant should be by joint cleaning to remove debris as soon as the diagnosis is confirmed. If the hip is infected, there is no acceptable alternative to arthrotomy for decompression and debridement. A delay in surgical decompression may cause the hip to dislocate by the increasing accumulation of joint fluid. The blood supply to the femoral head is vulnerable both to the increased pressure and to the products of the infection, and delay in adequate debridement may cause occlusion of the vessels, which will result in further deterioration of the femoral head. Both these complications can be prevented by early diagnosis, treatment with appropriate antibiotics, and surgical decompression. In other joints, repeated needle aspiration and irrigation may sufficiently debride, but the clinician never knows whether there is pannus covering the joint surface that must be removed to prevent further destruction of the articular cartilage. Because of this, open surgical decompression with debridement is a more reliable method than needle aspiration (26). If the hip is affected, traction should pull the thigh into abduction, and moderate flexion should be applied with the traction force just sufficient to overcome muscle spasm. Great care should be taken not to overpull the hip so as to cause further distraction. If the hip joint is tending to dislocate, immobilization in abduction and flexion in a spica cast may be needed to maintain reduction of the hip.

REFERENCES

1. McMaster MJ, Ohtsuka K. The natural history of congenital scoliosis: a study of two hundred and fifty-one patients. *J Bone Joint Surg Am* 1982;64:1128.
2. Drvaric DM, Ruderman RJ, Conrad RW, et al. Congenital scoliosis and urinary tract abnormalities: are intravenous pyelograms necessary? *J Pediatr Orthop* 1987;7:441.
3. Lamb DW. Radial clubhand, a continuing study of sixty-eight patients with one hundred and seventeen clubhands. *J Bone Joint Surg Am* 1977; 59:1.
4. Brown FW. Construction of a knee joint in congenital total absence of the tibia. *J Bone Joint Surg Am* 1965;47:695.
5. Farmer AW, Laurin CA. Congenital absence of the fibula. *J Bone Joint Surg Am* 1960;42:1.
6. Wood WL, Zlolsky N, Westin GW. Congenital absence of the fibula: treatment by Syme amputation—indications and technique. *J Bone Joint Surg Am* 1965;47:1159.
7. Barlow TG. Early diagnosis and treatment of congenital dislocation of the hip. *J Bone Joint Surg Am* 1962;44:292.
8. Hernandez RJ, Cornell RG, Hensinger RH. Ultrasound diagnosis of neonatal congenital dislocation of the hip. *J Bone Joint Surg Br* 1994; 76:539.
9. Herring JA. Conservative treatment of congenital dislocation of the hip in the newborn and infant. *Clin Orthop* 1992;28:41.
10. Boeree NR, Clarke NMP. Ultrasound imaging and secondary screening for congenital dislocation of the hip. *J Bone Joint Surg Br* 1994;76:525.
11. Castelain RM, Sauter AJM, de Vlieger M, et al. Natural history of ultrasound hip abnormalities in clinically normal newborns. *J Pediatr Orthop* 1992;12:423.
12. Robertson WW. *Treatment of developmental dysplasia of the hip in infancy.* Presented at the 1st Balkan Congress of Orthopaedics, Thessaloniki, Greece, 1997.
13. Hangen DH, Kassen JR, Emans JB, et al. The Pavlik harness and developmental dysplasia of the hip: has ultrasound changed treatment patterns? *J Pediatr Orthop* 1995;15:729.
14. Mubarak S, Garfins S, Vance R, et al. Pitfalls in the use of the Pavlik harness for treatment of congenital dysplasia, subluxation and dislocation of the hip. *J Bone Joint Surg Am* 1981;63:1239.
15. Ruben P. *Dynamic classification of bone dysplasia.* Chicago: Year Book, 1964.
16. Fairbank HAT. *An atlas of general affectation of the skeleton.* Edinburgh: E & S Livingstone, 1951.
17. McKusick VA. *Heritable disorders of the connective tissue*, 3rd ed. St. Louis: CV Mosby, 1966.
18. Weber M. Osteogenesis imperfecta congenita: a study of its histopathogenesis. *Arch Pathol* 1930;9:984.
19. Sillence D. Osteogenesis imperfecta: an expanding panorama of variants. *Clin Orthop* 1981;159:11.
20. Sofield HA, Miller EA. Fragmentation, realignment and intramedullary rod fixation of deformities of long bones of children. *J Bone Joint Surg Am* 1959;41:1371.
21. Davidson RS, Markowitz RI, Dormans J, et al. Ultrasonic evaluation of the elbow in infants and young children after suspected trauma. *J Bone Joint Surg Am* 1994;76:1804.
22. Jackson ST, Hoffer MM, Parrish N. Brachial plexus palsy in the newborn. *J Bone Joint Surg Am* 1988;70:1217.
23. Waters PM. Obstetrical brachial plexus injuries: evaluation and management. *JAAOS* 1997;5:205.
24. Trueta J. The three types of acute hematogenous osteomyelitis: a clinical and vascular study. *J Bone Joint Surg Br* 1959;41:671.
25. Trueta J. The normal vascular anatomy of the human femoral head during growth. *J Bone Joint Surg Br* 1972;39:358.
26. Griffin PP. Bone and joint infections in children. *Pediatr Clin North Am* 1967;3:533.

CHAPTER 52

Eye Disorders

Sherwin J. Isenberg

The eye is possibly the fastest developing organ in the body. As soon as 4 to 6 months after birth, some ocular functions are permanently set and, if impaired, cannot be fully restored to normalcy. The neonate with a serious ophthalmic disorder may be compared to a time bomb. It is not adequate to simply reverse or cure the problem. The treatment must be conducted rapidly and effectively. Thus, the neonatologist has some responsibility to recognize ocular abnormalities and quickly begin the process of healing.

GENERAL CONSIDERATIONS

Amblyopia

Amblyopia can be defined as a reduction in vision in the absence of, or beyond that explained by, an apparent organic cause. Amblyopia can be divided into a few etiologic classes. Strabismic amblyopia results from a child preferring one eye when the visual axes are misaligned. Reversal, generally with occlusion of the preferred eye, can only be achieved by age 7 to 9 years; the earlier the better. Refractive amblyopia generally results from significant inequality of the refractive errors in each eye. This form of amblyopia also should be reversed by 7 to 9 years of age, with treatment usually consisting of spectacles (or contact lenses) and occlusion of the sound eye. Either of these two forms of amblyopia can begin within the first few postnatal months.

The form of amblyopia that is most feared in infants is deprivation amblyopia. It usually arises before 3 months of age. The cause is blockage of a clear image from reaching the retina. It may be unilateral or bilateral and may be caused by a cataract, corneal opacity, or severe eyelid ptosis. There is considerable urgency in reversing this form of amblyopia, because good vision can only be attained

within the first 3 to 6 months after birth. This time table coincides with the "critical period" of ocular development in humans (1). Thus, for example, if a significant unilateral congenital cataract is discovered after 6 months of age, one would not expect excellent visual recovery, even after surgery and optical (usually contact lens) therapy.

Growth and Development of the Eye

At birth, the sagittal (axial) diameter of the eye is 16 mm in full-term neonates (2). It is less in preterm infants at birth. In the next year, this dimension grows 3.8 mm, with half the expected lifetime increase achieved by 12 months of age. With this information, one can appreciate the early anatomic maturity of the eye.

The corneal diameter often is used as an indicator of the size of the entire eye. At term, the corneal diameter averages 10.0 mm. The diagnosis of microcornea (less than 9 mm) or megalocornea (greater than 11 mm) suggests a similar abnormality in size of the entire globe, which should lead to an appropriate workup (see following). Ultrasonography can be utilized to determine precisely the size of the entire eye.

Three developmental markers exist in the preterm eye that can help the neonatologist define a neonate's postconceptional age. The tunica vasculosa lentis is a plexus of vessels, which is visible prior to 32 to 34 weeks postconception, crossing the pupil anterior to the lens. The lens surface is covered by these vessels at 27 to 28 weeks postconception, at which time they begin to disintegrate (3). Except for a few vessels at the lens periphery, they should be gone by 34 weeks (Fig. 52–1).

The status of the pupil follows a relatively predictable developmental pattern (Fig. 52–2) (4). At 26 to 31 weeks postconception, the pupillary diameter in relative darkness is quite large (up to 5.0 mm), and the pupil does not respond to light. By 31 weeks, the pupil diameter has decreased to a stable size of 3.5 mm, and the pupil begins

S. J. Isenberg: Department of Ophthalmology, Jules Stein Eye Institute, Harbor–UCLA Medical Center, Los Angeles, California

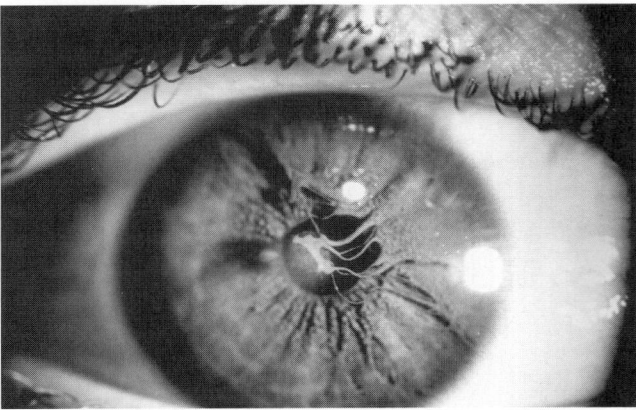

FIG. 52–1. Persistent pupillary membranes, remaining from tunica vasculosa lentis vessels, are the most common embryonic remnants found in adults.

to react to light. The light reaction increases in magnitude until reaching stability at term.

The appearance of the macula in the retina is easily appreciated with the ophthalmoscope after the pupil is dilated. The examiner can indicate the infant's postconceptional age by observing the development of three landmarks in the macula: pigmentation, annular reflex, and foveola (Table 52–1) (5).

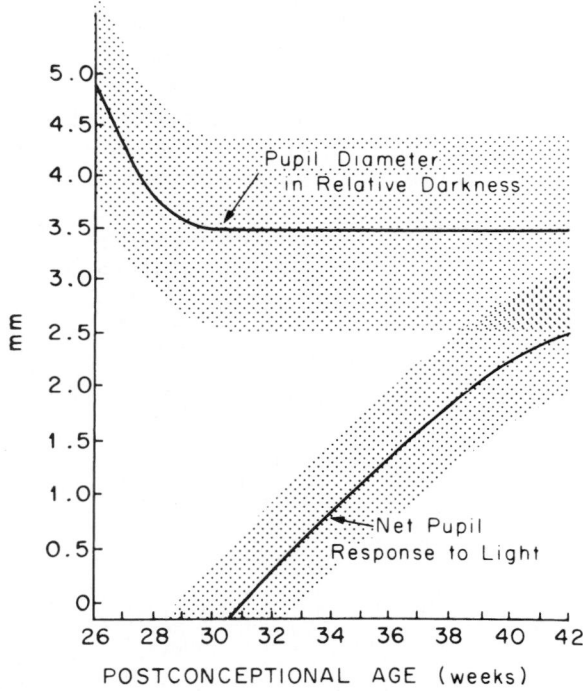

FIG. 52–2. Diameter of the pupil (mean ± standard deviation) in term and preterm neonates in relative darkness (less than 10 ft-c) and after light stimulation (600 ft-c). (From Isenberg SJ. Examination methods. In: Isenberg SJ, ed. *The eye in infancy,* 2nd ed. St. Louis: Mosby-Year Book, 1994:47.)

TABLE 52–1. *Development of the macula*

Observations in the macula	Postconceptional age (wk)
No pigmentation exists	31.5 ± 1.5
Dark red pigmentation appears	34.8 ± 1.0
Part of the annular reflex is evident	34.7 ± 2.4
Annular reflex is complete	36.3 ± 2.2
Foveolar pit is difficult to appreciate	37.6 ± 3.3
Foveolar light reflex is easily observed	41.7 ± 4.0

From ref. 5.

With these three anatomic findings, a neonate's postconceptional age can be estimated from 27 weeks postconception to term.

EXAMINATION TECHNIQUES

Visual Acuity

In the neonatal period, there is seldom a reason to even attempt to determine the infant's visual acuity. In the first 2 months after birth, the visual acuity is no better than 20/400 because of immaturity of the retina. The retinal periphery, however, can be stimulated with horizontal optokinetic targets to produce nystagmus. This will prove that the infant is developing some vision. Vertical nystagmus responses develop later. Laboratory techniques can be utilized, if necessary, to determine more precisely visual acuity. These techniques include preferential forced looking and pattern electroretinograms. A blink response to light confirms the presence of light perception.

Anterior Segment

The anterior segment can be examined using a strong penlight, with magnification as provided with loupes. Alternatively, a direct ophthalmoscope with a setting of about +5 can be utilized. The examiner should observe the eyelids, conjunctiva, cornea, iris, and lens. The corneal diameter can be measured. As described previously, the pupil diameter initially should be observed with a dim light, followed by evaluation of the reactivity to a bright light.

Posterior Segment

Prior to examining the vitreous and retina, it is usually necessary to dilate the pupil. The choice of dilating agents is important, because retinal examinations often are indicated in low-weight preterm infants to rule out retinopathy of prematurity (ROP). Sympathomimetic eyedrops can raise a low-weight neonate's blood pressure (6), whereas anticholinergic eyedrops that are thought to be of low concentration can significantly increase gastric acid (7). A safe and effective combination mydriatic eyedrop is Cyclomydril (Alcon Laboratories, Inc., Fort

Worth, TX). It consists of 1.0% phenylephrine and 0.2% cyclopentolate. One drop should be applied to both eyes and then repeated 5 to 10 minutes later. A third set occasionally may be required if the iris is darkly pigmented.

Although the eyelids can be held open by an assistant if the examination will be brief, usually an eyelid speculum specifically designed for neonatal use is utilized after application of an anesthetic eyedrop. When manipulating the eye, infants have been shown to display an oculocardiac reflex, defined as any dysrhythmia or a bradycardia of 10% or more, as frequently as in 31% of cases (8). Therefore, the assistant, often the nurse, should monitor the baby, as well as the eye, as the retinal examination progresses. During the retinal examination, the cornea tends to become dry and opacify somewhat because of the heat of the light, exposure, evaporation, and the recent finding that neonates, especially preterm infants, produce both basal and reflex tears at a reduced rate (9). Thus, while ensuring the stability of the speculum, the assistant also will need to lubricate the cornea.

CONGENITAL ANOMALIES

Ocular Size and Shape

Enlarged Eyes

An enlarged eye is suspected when the corneal diameter exceeds 11.0 mm in a term newborn. For confirmation, an A-scan ultrasound can be obtained easily to measure the ocular axial length, which is normally 16 mm at birth (2). If the eye is enlarged, infantile glaucoma caused by an elevated intraocular pressure should be suspected immediately. Infantile glaucoma also often will present with tearing, squinting, photosensitivity, and a cloudy cornea (Fig. 52–3). The cornea often is found to have horizontal lines called Haab's striae, which result from a disruption of Descemet's membrane. The optic nerve is noted to have an enlarged cup on fundus examination. To differentiate the tearing of glaucoma from that of the much more common nasolacrimal duct obstruction, the examiner should look at, or into, the nostrils. If tears emanate from the nostrils, the nasolacrimal apparatus is patent and glaucoma is possible. If no tears are found in the nostril, a nasolacrimal duct obstruction is likely.

The treatment of glaucoma is fairly urgent, because uncontrolled infantile glaucoma will cause the cornea to opacify, the eye to enlarge, create significant myopia, and damage the optic nerve. If unilateral, the myopia engendered can cause amblyopia, even if the cornea is fairly clear. The corneal opacification can cause deprivation amblyopia.

The infant must be examined while under anesthesia to confirm the diagnosis. After confirmation, the treatment is surgical. The ophthalmologist must open the trabecular meshwork filtration system either internally (goniotomy) or externally (trabeculotomy). If those approaches fail, the ophthalmologist may create an external filtration area (trabeculectomy) or implant an artificial drainage device.

Infantile glaucoma has been associated with other ocular problems, such as aniridia, goniodysgeneses (or mesodermal dysgeneses), which include Axenfeld's and Rieger's syndromes, and persistent fetal vasculature (see following). It has been associated with a number of systemic disorders and syndromes, including Sturge–Weber, neurofibromatosis, Marfan, Pierre Robin, homocystinuria, Lowe, rubella, Rubenstein–Taybi, and chromosomal abnormalities.

The cornea also may be enlarged on a structural basis without glaucoma. However, in this case, the rest of the eye has a normal shape, as can be demonstrated by ultrasonographic examination. Megalocornea is uncommon and usually has an X-linked inheritance pattern.

Small Eyes

A small eye will present with a corneal diameter less than 9 mm in a term birth. Confirmation of an axial length less than the normal 16 mm, as shown by ultrasound, is desirable. Microphthalmos can range from an eye that is slightly smaller than normal, but otherwise intact, to an eye that is so small, it cannot be found on routine examination (anophthalmos). In cases of anophthalmos, a small, often cystic, eye sometimes can be demonstrated by magnetic resonance imaging, computed tomography, or ultrasound. It may be associated with Klinefelter syndrome or trisomy 13.

There are two, not infrequent, ophthalmic disorders associated with microphthalmos. A coloboma is a developmental gap generally located inferiorly in the eye. It can be recognized externally as an inferior notch in the pupil caused by missing iris tissue, which by itself does not affect vision. More ominously, the defect also can include the optic nerve, macula, and other parts of the retina, which can result in legal blindness (Fig. 52–4).

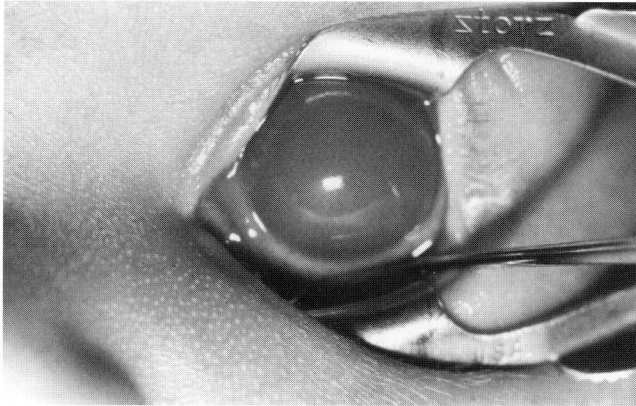

FIG. 52–3. This cornea is diffusely opacified and enlarged from infantile glaucoma.

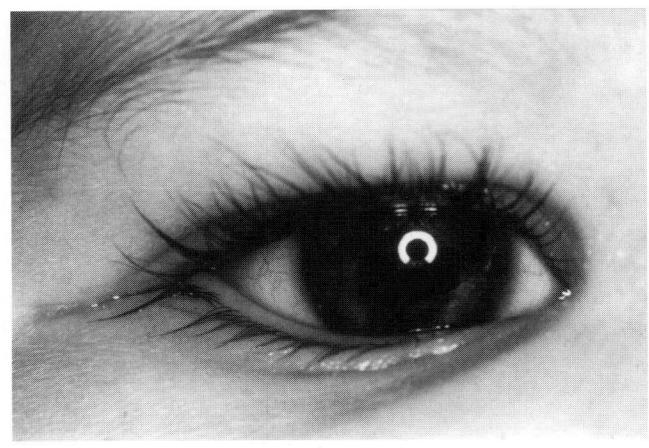

A

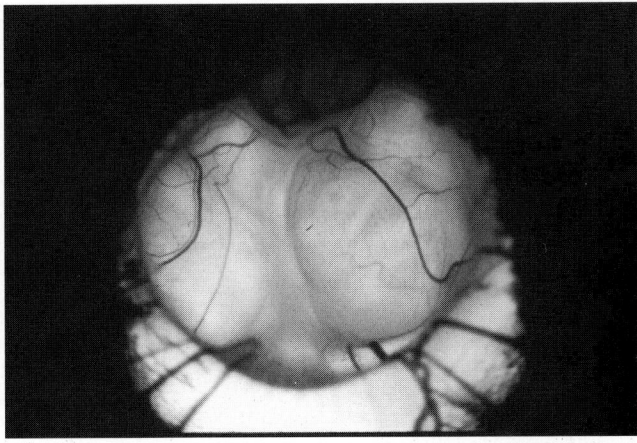

B

FIG. 52–4. **A:** The inferior iris defect, which resembles a keyhole, does not by itself affect vision. **B:** In this coloboma of the posterior pole of the fundus, the optic nerve is seen at the **top**. This large a defect will compromise vision, especially if fibers to the macula are deficient.

With experience, ophthalmologists now are recognizing the frequent combination of systemic findings called the CHARGE association. It consists of coloboma (C), heart defects (H), atresia choanae (A), retarded growth and development (R), genital hypoplasia (G), and ear anomalies and deafness (E). Facial palsy also is common. At least four of these findings must be present to make the diagnosis.

A second ophthalmic disorder commonly associated with microphthalmos is persistent hyperplastic primary vitreous. It has recently been renamed persistent fetal vasculature, a more encompassing name (10). This disorder often is associated with microphthalmos and hypoplasia of the fovea, as it represents an arrest of ocular development. Many of the sequelae result from abnormal vessels in the vitreous, anterior lens, and equator, causing persistent pupillary membranes, pigmented star-shaped structures on the anterior lens capsule, fibrovascular remnants on the optic nerve (Bergmeister papilla), and nonattachment of the retina. Serious secondary events can ensue, including cataract, glaucoma, lens subluxation, corneal opacities, intraocular hemorrhages, retinal detachments, and chronic inflammation. Because some of these manifestations are treatable, the neonatologist should seek an ophthalmic consultation for any infant with a small eye.

Eyelid Abnormalities

Congenital eyelid ptosis is readily apparent to the parents and all who observe a baby. Therefore, its presence often generates an examination within a few weeks of birth. Although the ptosis can be surgically corrected at any time in the baby's life, two considerations will indicate the proper timing of surgery. If the ptosis threatens the infant's vision, it should be corrected early—even

within the first few postnatal months. The vision can be threatened in two ways. If the ptosis is total or near total, the visual axis will be obstructed and the child may develop deprivation amblyopia. This is unusual, because the ptosis is seldom total, which allows the child, once head control is established, to elevate the chin to see under the ptotic eyelid. A more likely mechanism of potential visual loss is by an astigmatism induced by the ptotic eyelid applying subtle pressure to the cornea. This unilateral astigmatism can cause refractive amblyopia, even in a young infant. If vision is not threatened, the surgery can be deferred until 4 or 5 years of age.

A number of eyelid tumors can present at birth. Most frequent is the capillary hemangioma (Fig. 52–5). It generally continues to grow after birth. The skin overlying

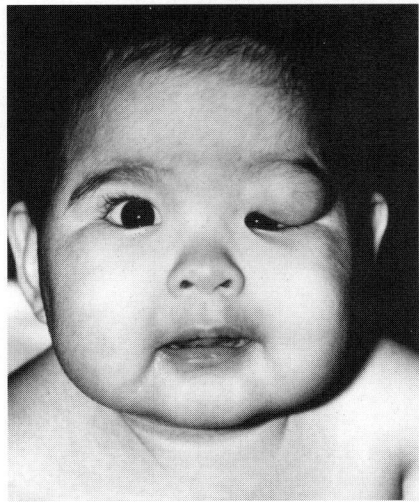

FIG. 52–5. A hemangioma of the eyelid may not affect vision, even if it is large.

the mass can be dimpled and red, resembling a strawberry, or assume a diffuse purple color if the lesion is deeper. The lesion does not transilluminate and feels spongy. Left untreated, most of these tumors will spontaneously involute after 1 to 2 years of age. Treatment is indicated if vision is threatened by obstruction of the visual axis or induction of astigmatism, as noted previously. Treatment is by injection of a combination of corticosteroids directly into the tumor or by systemic corticosteroids. The direct route may be safer. Favorable results recently have been reported with subcutaneous injections of interferon alfa-2b (11). Lymphangiomas and dermoid cysts of the eyelid also can present at birth.

Corneal Opacities

A number of congenital anomalies can cause corneal opacities at birth. Congenital glaucoma and persistent fetal vasculature have been discussed and must always be ruled out; however other diagnoses also should be considered.

Birth trauma, usually induced by a forceps placed at or near the eye during delivery, can cause opacities of the cornea. These opacities usually clear within a few days, but may leave corneal scars. The corneal damage can leave scarring in the visual axis or induce significant refractive error, which can result in poor vision.

Sclerocornea is a nonprogressive, usually bilateral, anomaly in which the cornea is replaced by opaque sclera-like tissue. Central or total sclerocornea usually is devastating to a child's vision.

Dermoid tumors of the cornea may affect vision similarly if located centrally. A peripheral corneal tumor can affect vision by inducing refractive error. The tumor may be isolated or part of Goldenhar's syndrome.

Peter's anomaly, characterized by a central corneal opacity and variable iris–corneal or lens–corneal adhesions, is uncommon, but a frequent cause of corneal transplant in infants (Fig. 52–6). The periphery of the cornea usually is normal. It has been associated with fetal alcohol syndrome. Corneal surgery often is reserved for bilateral cases, because the prognosis for good vision following even initially successful corneal transplantation is guarded. In unilateral cases, poor vision is almost inevitable because of amblyopia in the affected eye. The amblyopia may result from a number of causes, including a possible graft rejection, significant refractive errors, recurrent opacities, and secondary glaucoma.

Aniridia

Aniridia, in which much or even all of the iris visible to the examiner is missing, can be compatible with good vision (Fig. 52–7). However, vision can be quite compromised by other ocular associations, including cataracts, peripheral corneal opacities, foveal hypoplasia, and glaucoma. If the vision is quite reduced in infancy, nystagmus usually is found.

These children must be followed closely, because some of the problems, such as glaucoma and central corneal pannus, may arise later in childhood. The glaucoma is particularly difficult to treat, because it often is refractory to medical management. Surgical treatment of the glaucoma can induce a cataract, because there may be no iris to protect the lens during and after the operation.

Wilms tumor has been reported to occur in up to one third of all sporadic aniridia cases. Therefore, periodic abdominal ultrasonography of children with aniridia is justified. An 11p deletion has been associated with the complex of aniridia, ambiguous genitalia, and mental retardation (AGR). Wilms tumor also may occur with this deletion.

Cataracts

Lens opacities in infants may be isolated or associated with a systemic condition. The morphology of infantile cataracts often is distinctive, which differentiates the infantile from other forms of cataract (Fig. 52–8). The

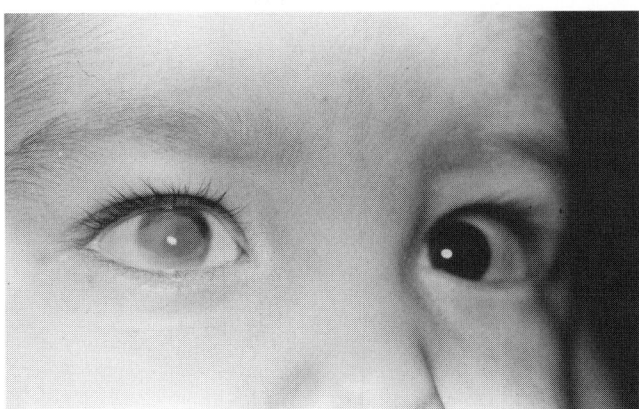

FIG. 52–6. In this unilateral case of Peter's anomaly, the cornea is opaque centrally and clear peripherally.

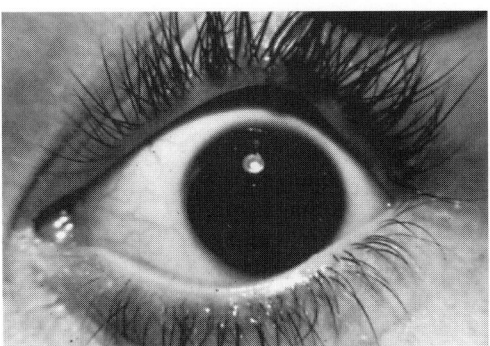

FIG. 52–7. Aniridia is evident by the largely missing iris.

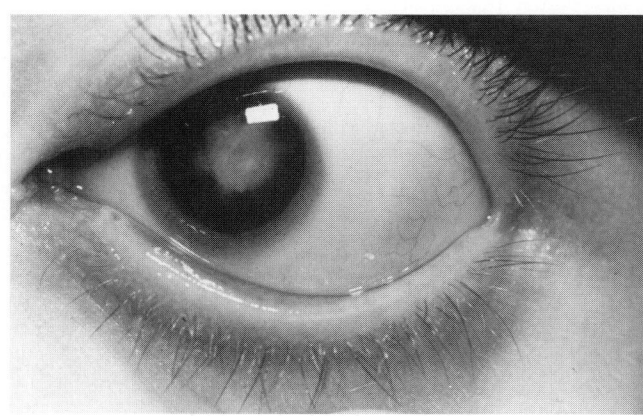
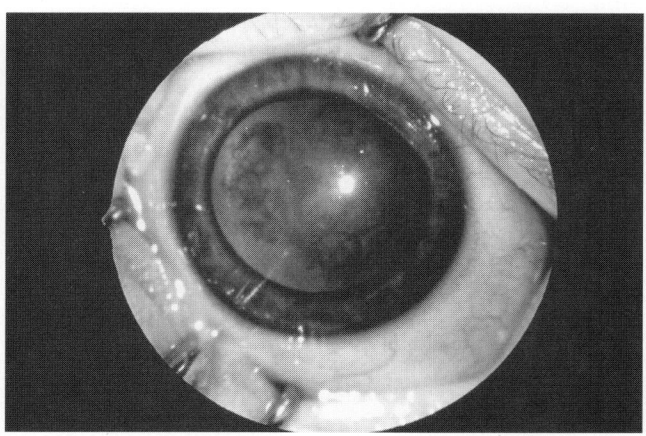

FIG. 52–8. A: This zonular (or lamellar) lens opacity occupies a central area of the lens with small satellite opacities. **B:** The red retinal light reflex is disrupted by a cataract.

location of the opacity within the baby's lens permits a classification of polar, zonular (or lamellar), nuclear, sutural, or total cataract.

About 25% of infantile cataracts are hereditary, especially if bilateral. Therefore, in the workup of infantile cataracts, it is important to examine the parents and siblings. If an asymptomatic cataract that resembles an infantile cataract is found in a family member, the etiology is attributed to heredity and an extensive workup can be avoided. The most frequent mode of inheritance is autosomal dominant with variable expressivity, but almost complete penetrance.

Metabolic problems have been noted to cause cataracts in infants. Among these are hypoglycemia, mannosiderosis, hypoparathyroidism, maternal diabetes, and galactosemia. Galactosemia, inherited as autosomal recessive trait, should be diagnosed on neonatal screening of urinary reducing substances. But a child with a galactosemia cataract may still present to the pediatrician if he or she was born abroad or has the galactokinase deficiency type, which usually presents after 5 months of age. The cataract resembles a typical oil droplet. Early intervention with a lactose-free diet may reduce the lens level of dulcitol and reverse some or all of the lens opacity. Medications, such as corticosteroids, may cause cataracts, but not in neonates.

A number of systemic conditions are associated with cataracts. In rubella, cataracts are characteristically total or near total opacities in a smaller than normal lens. In addition, the eye in rubella often is small, has abnormalities of the retinal pigment epithelium (noted as "salt and pepper" changes), and may be glaucomatous. Live rubella virus can survive in the lens for years. Therefore, at surgery, care should be taken with the lens aspirates, especially if personnel in the operating room may be pregnant. Cataracts have been described in other congenital infections, including herpes simplex and varicella.

The presence of a cataract should initiate an appropriate workup with the many causes and associations in mind. The list of other conditions associated with infantile cataract is very long and have been discussed elsewhere (12). To rule out familial cataract, both a family history, including any consanguinity, and an examination of the lenses of the parents and siblings should be undertaken. The history should include questions regarding low birth weight, ROP, hypoglycemia, serum calcium abnormalities, syndromes, or any systemic disorders. A maternal history of infections while pregnant, diabetes, drug ingestion, and toxin exposure should be sought. Laboratory evaluation should include serum for glucose, BUN, calcium, phosphorus, galactose, and "TORCH" titers (toxoplasmosis, rubella, cytomegalovirus, varicella, and herpes simplex). Urine should be sent for amino acid levels and hematuria. Other tests should be ordered, as indicated by the nonocular findings.

An ophthalmologist should judge if the cataract(s) are vision threatening. If so, and the child is less than about 4 months old in unilateral cases or 4 to 6 months old in bilateral cases, surgery is urgent to avoid legal blindness from deprivation amblyopia. The surgeon will remove the cataract using an intraocular suction-cutting device (lensectomy) and remove the anterior vitreous (vitrectomy) to avoid the postoperative development of posterior opacified membranes. It should be emphasized that many of the techniques used for cataract surgery in adults are not applicable to children. Compared with adults, a baby's sclera is more elastic, which can allow an eye to collapse during surgery, the lens itself is softer, the lens capsule is stiffer, and the vitreous is more solid. For these reasons, special training and experience is desirable prior to operating on the cataracts of babies.

The end of the surgery is far from the end of the infant's visual rehabilitation. An optical device must be used to provide focus after loss of the lens. Spectacles could work, but few infants will keep spectacles in place while in the crib or toddling later. Intraocular lenses, as commonly utilized in adults, generally are not used in infants in developed countries. Current intraocular lenses have one fixed power (focal length), which the surgeon must choose at the time of surgery. The refractive power of the baby's eye will decrease up to eight diopters by 12 months of age and decrease even more later 13). Thus, a lens properly powered for a 1-month-old infant will make the baby highly myopic by 1 year of age. Conversely, a lens placed in an infant's eye with a power appropriate for later in life will leave him quite hyperopic in infancy, when good focus is crucial to developing vision and avoiding amblyopia. For these reasons, and because of the concern of leaving a "plastic" lens in an eye for perhaps more than 80 years, intraocular lenses generally are not used by ophthalmologists in infants, unless under a special protocol. It is hoped that an appropriate intraocular device will be developed in the future to aid these infants. In underdeveloped countries where no alternative exists, intraocular lenses are being implanted in infants.

The current method of choice to rehabilitate infant's eyes after cataract surgery is contact lenses. The parents are taught to insert the lens in the morning and remove it in the evening. Certain types of contact lenses may be left in overnight, but some ophthalmologists avoid them because of the increased risk of ocular infection. With contact lenses, the eye doctor can easily change the power as the eye grows and the hyperopic prescription decreases.

In all unilateral cases and some bilateral cases, the optical rehabilitation must be accompanied by occlusion of the better seeing eye to reverse amblyopia. Whether to occlude many hours a day to best improve visual acuity or fewer hours to maximize binocularity is a controversial subject (14).

Optic Nerve Hypoplasia

This disorder is a frequent cause of unsuspected visual loss. It results in a diminished number of axons in the optic nerve. The number can be low enough to cause legal or complete blindness, or reduced sufficiently to cause peripheral field loss with a normal visual acuity. The appearance of the nerve can vary from a subtle reduction in size in one segment to a grossly small nerve surrounded by a pigment ring and yellow halo known as the "double ring sign" (Fig. 52–9). If bilateral and vision reducing, this entity often will cause nystagmus in infancy. If unilateral and vision reducing, it usually will present as a unilateral strabismus in the first 5 years of life. The diagnosis can be made with the direct ophthalmoscope by comparing features of the two optic nerves or with other instruments.

Although this disorder is associated with a number of other entities, two deserve the special interest of neonatologists. Fetal alcohol syndrome appears to be a major

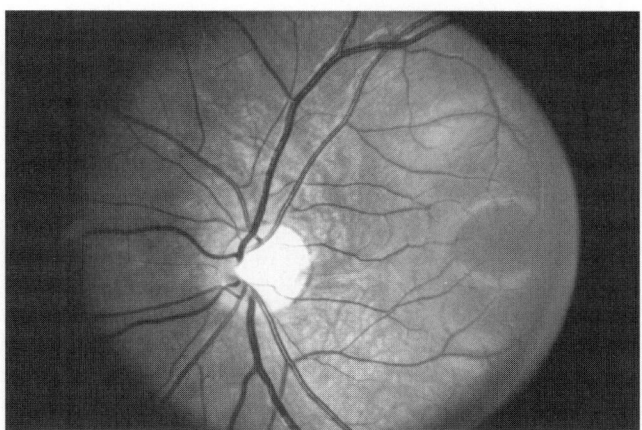

FIG. 52–9. Although not extremely small, the diagnosis of optic nerve hypoplasia is revealed by the rings of white representing sclera and pigmentation representing retinal pigment epithelium.

cause of optic nerve hypoplasia. In Scandinavia, optic nerve hypoplasia was found to occur in almost half the cases of fetal alcohol syndrome (15). It may be the most frequently encountered ocular teratogenic event. Another association with optic nerve hypoplasia is septooptic dysplasia (DeMorsier syndrome), in which the child has a number of midline central nervous disorders, such as absence of the septum pellucidum, agenesis of the corpus callosum, and dysplasia of the third ventricle. Hypopituitarism, most commonly evident by dwarfism, occurs frequently. Hypothyroidism, neonatal hypoglycemia, sexual infantilism or precocity, hypoadrenalism, hyperprolactinemia, and diabetes insipidus also have been reported. This diagnosis, suggested by the presence of optic nerve hypoplasia, can lead to early treatment to modify these endocrinopathies.

Strabismus

In the first few months after birth, infants usually display a variable intermittent exotropia. This divergence decreases with time, as visual acuity and binocularity develop until the eyes are generally straight by 3 to 6 months of age. Even infants who develop infantile esotropia are initially exotropic after birth (16). Unless the eye position is constantly abnormal in the first 3 postnatal months, observation is appropriate until the baby is 4 months old. A constant unilateral strabismus may not only suggest an examination for the strabismus, but the presence of amblyopia, possibly caused by an organic lesion such as retinoblastoma. Neonatologists and pediatricians should examine the posterior fundus of any child with unilateral constant strabismus to rule out a retinoblastoma, because an early diagnosis can be life saving.

ACQUIRED DISORDERS

Infections

Ophthalmia Neonatorum

This infection arises in the first postnatal month by microorganisms entering the eye during the birth process. The most feared infection is caused by Neisseria gonorrheae. In the nineteenth century, neonatal gonococcal conjunctivitis was the major cause of blindness in European children. An extremely marked inflammation characterized by eyelid swelling, conjunctival edema, and copious amounts of purulent discharge usually arises at postnatal day 4 to 6 (Fig. 52–10). The cornea can be perforated within days, which can lead to loss of the eye or, if mild, corneal scarring and possible blindness. The majority of cases are bilateral. As the incidence of adult gonococcal infections has increased in recent decades, so has the incidence of neonatal gonococcal conjunctivitis. Treatment is with ceftriaxone 50 mg per kg intravenously or intramuscularly with proper toilet for the eye to prevent conjunctival membranes.

Chlamydia trachomatis infection is the most common form of ophthalmia neonatorum today, occurring in up to 1% of births in developed countries. The infection produces a mild and chronic conjunctivitis, with pseudomembrane formation and corneal scarring. The signs first appear between 4 and 12 days of age. After a few months, follicles appear in the conjunctiva. Because these infants also can develop pneumonitis, systemic treatment is necessary with erythromycin (usually as an oral syrup), as well as ocular treatment with erythromycin or sulfacetamide ointment.

Other organisms, such as *Staphylococcus and Streptococcus,* also can cause ophthalmia neonatorum. The onset of infection usually is later—often after 1 week of age. Some of these organisms may have been acquired postnatally. Treatment is with a broad-spectrum ocular antibiotic ointment, such as sulfacetamide or a polymyxin B–bacitracin combination.

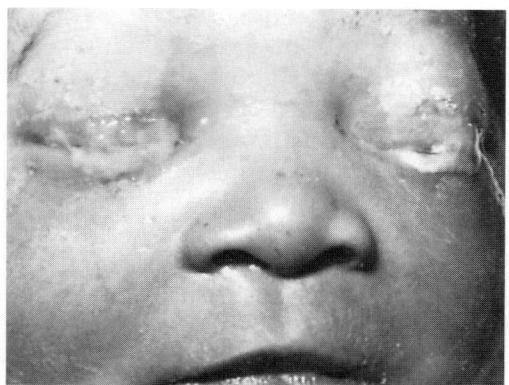

FIG. 52–10. Gonococcal ophthalmia neonatorum.

Chemical conjunctivitis must always be ruled out. This is a noninfectious inflammation caused by the toxic effects of some prophylactic eye medications on the sensitive conjunctiva of newborns. The inflammation almost always is gone by 24 to 48 hours after birth. It is especially frequent after application of silver nitrate to the eyes.

Prophylaxis against ophthalmia neonatorum began in 1881 by Credé in Leipzig. Using 2% silver nitrate solution placed in the eyes at birth, he reduced the incidence of ophthalmia neonatorum in his hospital from 10% to 0.3%. Today, prophylaxis is required in the United States and most developed countries. Silver nitrate is no longer manufactured in the United States and many other countries. Tetracycline ointment can be useful, but has lost popularity because of the frequency of tetracycline-resistant gonococci. Erythromycin ointment may be used (17), but it is better at reducing than eliminating organisms (18). A new prophylactic agent, povidone–iodine 2.5% ophthalmic solution, has proven to be very effective and inexpensive in a large clinical trial in Kenya when compared with silver nitrate and erythromycin (19). It now is being used in underdeveloped countries and may become the medication of choice for ophthalmia neonatorum prophylaxis.

Workup for a neonate with an inflamed eye includes a history obtained from each parent about genital discharge, genital vesicles, and a history of any sexually transmitted diseases. Laboratory analysis includes conjunctival scrapings for Gram and Giemsa stains. Chlamydia is assessed by culture or direct fluorescent antibody assay. Cultures should be sent using Thayer–Martin and blood agar media. More specific tests can be ordered if herpes or other organisms are considered.

Nasolacrimal Obstructions

The distal end of the nasolacrimal duct frequently is imperforate at birth. Subsequent infection of the nasolacrimal sac is evidenced by a purulent discharge from the puncta and tearing in the presence of a relatively white eye. In most cases, the infection is alleviated by opening of the occluded duct by 7 months of age (20). The opening may occur spontaneously or be induced by conservative treatment, which consists of digital massage over the duct followed by application of an antibiotic eyedrop, if a discharge is observed. Ointments may only further occlude the duct.

When the symptoms persist beyond 6 to 7 months of age, a probing of the duct usually is indicated. The success rate of a probing procedure is greater than 90%. For persistent obstruction, the probing can be repeated, the turbinate bone can be infractured, or the entire nasolacrimal system can be intubated with silicone tubing. The tubes are removed in 3 to 6 months.

Systemic Infections

Acquired Immunodeficiency Syndrome

Most infants with human immunodeficiency virus (HIV) infection are asymptomatic. Young HIV-positive children have been reported to have retinal vascular sheathing, optic atrophy, and dry eye syndrome, but these are unusual. They may have a mildly increased risk to develop strabismus and amblyopia. Opportunistic infections of the eye, such as ocular toxoplasmosis and cytomegalovirus retinitis, are less common than in adults and often develop later in childhood. Bacterial infections of the ocular adnexa may be more common than in adults (21).

Rubella

Ocular manifestations of the congenital rubella syndrome include pigmentary retinopathy, cataracts, glaucoma, shallowing of the anterior chamber, anterior uveitis, microphthalmos, and corneal clouding with or without glaucoma. About half of all children with rubella will have ocular symptoms, which are bilateral in 70% of cases.

Rubella retinopathy, characterized by pigmentary changes secondary to damage to the retinal pigment epithelium, may be the most common ocular manifestation. The appearance has led to the term "salt and pepper" retinopathy. It usually is concentrated in the posterior pole and can be seen with the direct ophthalmoscope if the media are clear. Despite the appearance, visual acuity is seldom affected by the retinal involvement alone.

Cataracts occur in 30% to 75% of cases (Fig. 52–11). The morphology of the cataract is fairly typical, being either a total opacification or dense nuclear opacities. About half of the cataracts develop and worsen after birth. Because live virus can still be cultured from the lens up to 3 years after birth, it is wise to exclude from the surgical suite during lensectomy any surgical personnel who could potentially be pregnant, even if rubella is only suspected. The surgeon must obsessively remove all the lens protein and much of the capsule. Residual lens particles in rubella can cause a severe inflammation that itself can lead to blindness.

Cytomegalovirus

The cytomegaloviruus reaches the eye hematogenously. It essentially affects only the retina and choroid. The retinopathy presents as patches of retinal whitening, generally in the periphery. The borders of the lesions are indistinct, and retinal hemorrhages with vascular sheathing may be found. The retinopathy occurs in about 5% of infected infants either at birth or later.

Toxoplasmosis

Seventy-five percent of all patients with congenital toxoplasmosis will have ocular involvement. In 10%, the ocular lesions will be present with no evidence of infection in other organs. *Toxoplasma gondii* causes a focally destructive retinal lesion, with severe inflammation that also affects the choroid. The overlying vitreous becomes hazy with inflammatory cells and exudate. The infection often is unappreciated when it is acute, but is recognized later as a discrete yellow-white atrophic scar with hyperpigmented borders and smaller satellite scars (Fig. 52–12). The macula, which is involved in 46% of cases, will not only reduce vision, but may cause a secondary strabismus (22). Peripheral retinal lesions are generally asymptomatic. Although lesions may look quiescent, live organisms may survive within them for years. This is probably the cause of recurrent inflammation in children and adults.

Local treatment with subconjunctival corticosteroid injections usually is reserved for severely inflamed eyes in conjunction with systemic therapy, as with

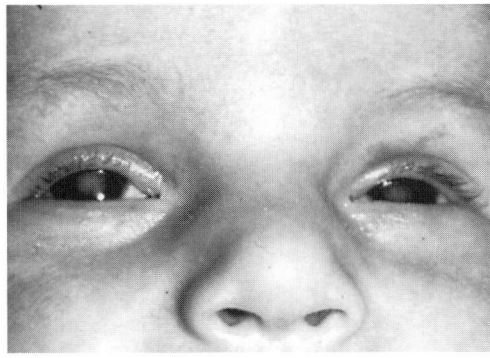

FIG. 52–11. Rubella cataracts in a 7-week-old infant.

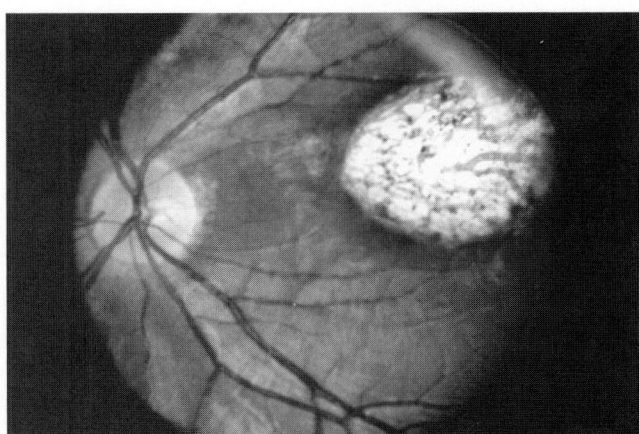

FIG. 52–12. A large chorioretinal scar has destroyed the fovea in this child with toxoplasmosis.

pyrimethamine and sulfonamides (23). Treatment may not prevent late recurrence.

TRAUMA

Birth Trauma

Any portion of the eye or adnexa can be injured in the birth process in up to 50% of difficult deliveries. The eyelids can be swollen and ecchymotic. Rarely, the eyelids can be everted totally, with the conjunctiva exposed to the environment. If everted, the exposed surfaces should be kept moist with lubricants until reversion is achieved spontaneously or with manual or surgical measures.

The eyeball has been subluxated, usually by delivery forceps. Orbital fractures and hemorrhages have been reported. The conjunctiva may have hemorrhages in at least 13% of births.

A cloudy cornea may result form forceps injury. It almost always is unilateral. Glaucoma, which also presents with a cloudy cornea, must be ruled out (see glaucoma section). Following birth, the cornea trauma often is accompanied by eyelid edema and ecchymosis, as well as conjuncti-val hemorrhage. Corneal examination may reveal linear opacities, usually oriented vertically, caused by Descemet's membrane rupture. Although the overall corneal opacity clears within 2 weeks, healing of the Descemet's membrane rupture can create a severe astigmatism or myopia, which can lead to amblyopia and strabismus.

A hyphema (hemorrhage within the anterior chamber) may result from forceps delivery, especially if residual fetal vessels are present. These hyphemas clear in a few weeks with no specific treatment. Vitreous hemorrhages, however, can persist to cause amblyopia and myopia. They have been associated with protein C deficiency. Vit-rectomy ultimately may be necessary if the hemorrhage does not spontaneously clear. Compression of the head in the course of a vaginal delivery often results in retinal hemorrhages (Fig. 52–13). The incidence has been reported to be 40% within 1 hour of birth, which decreases to 11% by 72 hours (24). They can occur in any area or layer of the retina. Retinal hemorrhages in the nerve fiber layer appear flame shaped, in the inner plexiform layer are dot shaped, and those beneath the internal limiting membrane resemble domes. The domes may look like Roth spots, with a white center surrounded by an elevated red hemorrhage. Even extensive hemorrhage will resorb within 6 weeks after birth. Rarely, hemor-rhages in the fovea have resorbed slower, resulting in amblyopia in a normal-appearing eye.

Nonaccidental Trauma

Amniocentesis has been reported to damage eyes, usually in the midtrimester of pregnancy. Although most cases have resulted in blindness with frequent loss of the

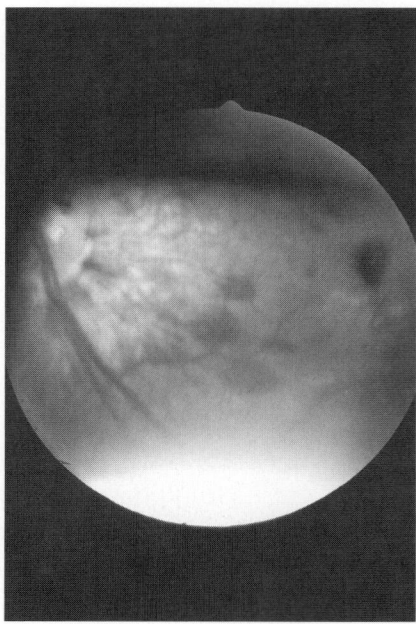

FIG. 52–13. Retinal hemorrhages in an infant 1 day after birth.

eye, early repair may salvage vision (25). The presence of segmental edema of the conjunctiva or corneal edema in a neonate should raise the possibility of an amniocentesis injury.

Child abuse often will affect the eye. There are many possible ocular effects of abuse, but intraocular hemor-rhage is the most specific sign. Buys et al. (26) reported no retinal hemorrhages in a series of 75 children with documented accidental head trauma. However, their nonaccidental trauma cases all had retinal hemorrhages. Thus, any case of suspected child abuse should have an ophthalmology consultation.

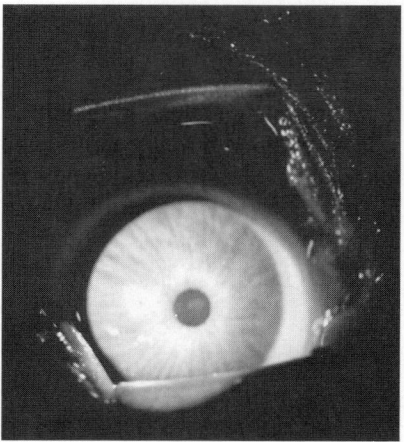

FIG. 52–14. Tortuous and dilated iris vessels run peripher-ally to and from the pupil in this cocaine-intoxicated newborn.

A different sort of "child abuse" also should be considered. The self-abusing mother may affect ocular development. The most frequent teratogenic effect is probably optic nerve hypoplasia in the fetal alcohol syndrome, as described previously. Cocaine abuse has been noted to affect the eye by inducing hypervascularization of the iris (Fig. 52–14) (27). The dilated and tortuous vessels, which run from the pupil to the periphery, usually are gone 1 week after birth. If these vessels are noted shortly after birth, a toxicity screen, which includes cocaine, is indicated.

PHOTOTHERAPY FOR HYPERBILIRUBINEMIA

Light has the ability to photooxidize bilirubin from the skin and subcutaneous tissue. Although useful to reduce hyperbilirubinemia, animal studies have shown that very intense light damages the outer retinal layers irreversibly. In human infants, however, there has been little evidence of long-term damage from these lights (28). Nonetheless, it is prudent to occlude both eyes with an opaque mask or eye patches during this therapy. To prevent the possibility of amblyopia, both eyes should be occluded equally and securely.

RETINOPATHY OF PREMATURITY

In developed countries, ROP is one of the major causes of blindness in infants. This disorder of abnormal vascularization of the retina, formerly called retrolental fibroplasis (RLF), tends to occur in low-weight neonates often exposed to large amounts of oxygen. The more premature the child, the more likely the disease. Of infants with a birth weight under 1 kg, 82% will develop ROP, with 9.3% progressing to vision-threatening sequelae (29). Of infants with a birth weight between 1 and 1.5 kg, 47% will develop ROP, and 2% will be in danger of losing vision.

Prevention

Infants who develop ROP often have other morbidities of the very preterm infant, as well as a complicated hospital course. This makes clinical correlations between ROP and other clinical entities difficult to interpret. Nonetheless, measures have been taken to prevent ROP. Oxygen use is often minimized, because hyperoxemia has been shown to be associated or causative in many, but not all, studies (30). Although it has been recommended to keep arterial oxygen levels between 50 and 80 mm Hg, studies have not definitely determined that this range is safe. Pulse oximetry can be useful, but when the percent saturation reaches 98 or 99, the arterial oxygen tension can be very elevated, which may be conducive to the development of ROP.

A number of studies have investigated the use of vitamin E to prevent ROP. Despite early enthusiasm, especially in infants born beyond 27 postconceptional weeks (31), more recent studies have been less supportive. Any benefit from high doses of vitamin E has been overshadowed by the morbidity it has produced in clinical trials, including sepsis, necrotizing enterocolitis, intraventricular hemorrhage, and increased mortality (32–34).

The bright lights often found in nurseries have been considered as possibly contributing to ROP. Glass et al. (35) found less ROP in two nurseries utilizing lower ambient light levels. However, problems with controls, randomization, and masking in this study have left the topic of bright lights still in doubt. Studies in humans and animals have yielded conflicting results regarding the effects of bright lights on ROP (36). A multicenter clinical trial is now underway to investigate this issue.

Pathogenesis

The pathogenesis of ROP is thought to begin from a combination of prematurity, supplemental oxygen, and other possible factors causing vasoconstriction of immature retinal vessels. This vasoconstriction interrupts the normal developmental migration of the blood vessels from the optic nerve peripherally to the ora serrata. Vascular closure may cause localized ischemia. Endothelial proliferation adjacent to the vessels extends within the retina and into the vitreous. Fibrous and glial tissue grow, producing hemorrhage, traction, and retinal detachment.

Others feel that the neovascularization is induced by oxidative insult to spindle cells, resulting in gap junctions. If correct, antioxidants would help prevent the disease. The lack of strong evidence for the role of antioxidants, as tocopherol (vitamin E), has limited the acceptance of this theory.

Examination

The decision of which babies to screen is somewhat controversial. Most nurseries desire an examination of any infant with a birth weight below 1,250 g, whereas others use a weight as high as 1,600 g. A Pittsburgh study found that, above a birth weight of 1,500 g, ROP developed only in infants exposed to at least 6 weeks of continuous oxygen (37).

The examination should be performed as soon as the media is clear enough to permit ophthalmoscopy and the neonate can tolerate the "trauma" of a retinal examination. The use of proper dilating eye drops was discussed previously. A number of centers advise the first examination be performed 6 weeks after birth. Because vision-threatening ROP has been shown to arise at 33 to 41 weeks postconception, it would be wise to time the first examination at approximately 32 weeks, if possible. The larger preterm newborns may need their first examination sooner after birth than the smaller ones.

The subsequent examinations should be conducted as indicated by the findings of the first examination. If no ROP is found but the retina is still being vascularized, the examination should be repeated every 1 to 2 weeks. If ROP is found, the examinations should be repeated weekly. If "plus disease" (tortuosity and dilation of the blood vessels in the posterior pole of the fundus) is noted, the disease may be progressing faster, justifying a repeat evaluation in 3 to 4 days. The examinations are continued until the retinal vascularization has reached zone III (see following), the threshold for treatment (see following) is achieved, or the disease has definitely regressed. There are some rare cases in which regression was followed by reactivation.

Classification

The internationally established classification of acute ROP is meant to characterize accurately the extent of the disorder in a particular eye. Three dimensions or criteria are used—stage, location (anterior to posterior), and extent.

The staging scheme is presented in Table 52–2. In stage 1, the normal progression of vascularization of the retina toward the periphery is halted at a thin demarcation line found by an abrupt change in color of the retina. The line divides the vascularized from the nonvascularized retina. Importantly, the vessels multibranch or arcade at the line. The latter appearance differentiates early ROP from normal vascularization because, in the normal state, the advancing vessels usually bifurcate and do not break into an arcade. In stage 2, the demarcation line extends up out of the retinal plane toward the vitreous. This ridge may change color from white or tan to red. In stage 3, extraretinal fibrovascular tissue grows either on the top of the ridge, yielding a ragged appearance, or just posterior. As it grows, it reaches into the vitreous (Fig. 52–15). Stage 4 is reached when the retina begins to detach from traction exerted by the extraretinal fibrovascular tissue condensing (analogous to a purse string) or, less commonly, from serous fluid elevating the retina. The macula still is spared from detachment in stage 4A, and the visual prognosis is still hopeful. The visual prognosis decreases markedly in stage 4B as the macula detaches. In stage 5, the retinal detachment is total and shaped like a funnel or

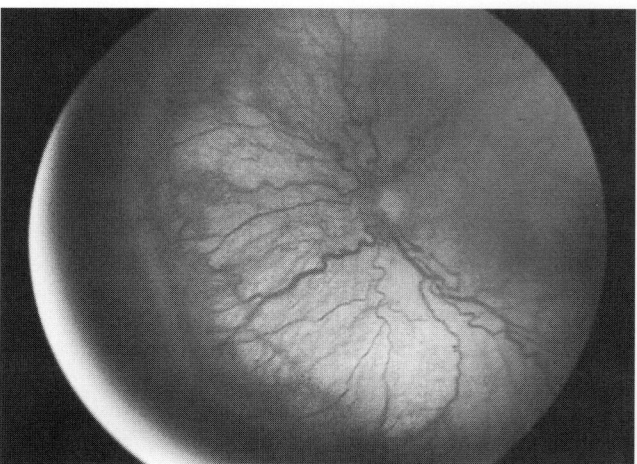

FIG. 52–15. In stage 3 retinopathy of prematurity, laser or cryotherapy is applied when all criteria are met. Note the dilation and tortuosity of the retinal vessels in "plus disease."

tulip. In describing the stage, one also should indicate if "plus disease" is present. "Plus disease" is the presence of tortuosity and dilation of the blood vessels in the posterior pole of the fundus. These posterior vascular changes usually indicate that an arteriovenous shunt is occurring in the extraretinal fibrovascular tissue on top of the ridge. "Plus disease" is a worse prognostic sign and may indicate that the disease is progressing faster.

The location is described in zones (Fig. 52–16). Zone I, the most posterior, is a circle centered on the optic nerve, with a radius twice the distance from the optic nerve to the fovea. Zone II extends from the edge of zone I all the way to the ora serrata on the nasal side and, on the temporal side, to the anatomic equator. This leaves zone III, which is a peripheral crescent on the temporal side. ROP in zone I is potentially the most dangerous, whereas disease in zone III is seldom of any concern. The circumferential extent of the disease is noted in clock hours, with an entire eye composed of 12 clock hours. One clock hour equals 30 degrees.

This classification pertains to the acute changes of ROP. There also are cicatricial changes that should be considered. Classification of the cicatricial changes is not yet universally accepted. Usually, these changes arise in eyes that reached acute stage 3, but did not progress to a significant retinal detachment. In these eyes, the vessels are drawn to the lateral side by cicatrization distorting the optic nerve and dragging the fovea laterally (Fig. 52–17). A retinal fold may form. These developments often reduce vision significantly.

Treatment

Many eyes that develop ROP will improve without treatment, to the point that few or no remnants of the disorder are evident later. The point at which the prognosis

TABLE 52–2. *Stages of retinopathy of prematurity*

Stage	Character
1	Demarcation line
2	Ridge
3	Extraretinal fibrovascular proliferation
4A	Partial retinal detachment, macula still attached
4B	Partial retinal detachment, macula detached
5	Total retinal detachment
Plus	Dilation and tortuosity of posterior retinal vessels

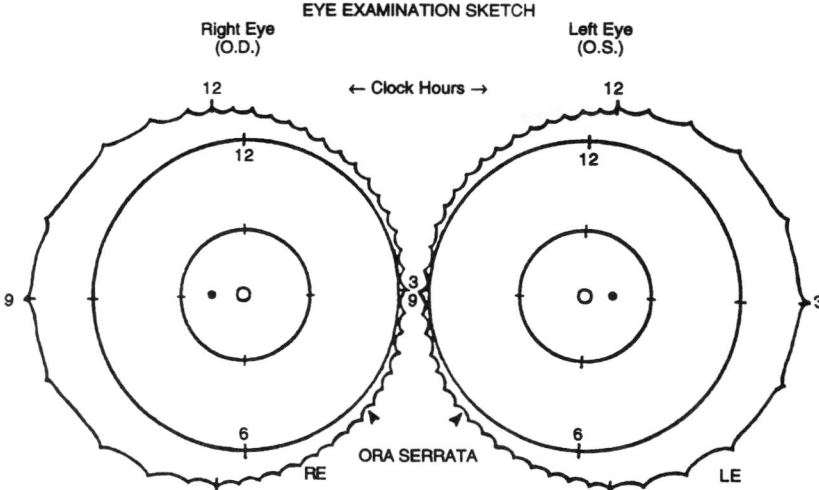

EYE EXAMINATION SKETCH

FIG. 52–16. The scheme of zones and clock hours in the classification of acute retinopathy of prematurity.

for regression is below 50% is considered the threshold level for treatment. The multicenter trial of cryotherapy defined the threshold level as stage 3 in five adjacent or eight cumulative clock hours in combination with plus disease (38). This definition has proven appropriate for disease in zone II. But the results of treatment using this threshold have not been as favorable for disease in zone I. It is very likely that a lower threshold for treatment will be established for zone I disease in the next few years.

The rationale behind this treatment is to ablate the peripheral avascular retina for 360 degrees in the affected eye(s). This approach has been shown in numerous studies to improve diabetic retinopathy, presumably by reducing or eliminating the signal from the ischemic or avascular tissue to the retina to produce neovascular vessels. Initially, cryotherapy was used to destroy areas of the peripheral retina by freezing. Cryotherapy had a number of both trivial and important complications, including

subconjunctival hematoma, vitreous hemorrhage, bradycardia or dysrythmia, and conjunctival laceration.

Currently, cryotherapy has been replaced for most applications by the use of lasers, which usually are mounted on an indirect ophthalmoscope worn on the head of the surgeon (39). There are some specific instances in which cryotherapy is still the method of choice. Laser therapy has a number of advantages over cryotreatment. Laser surgery can be performed in the nursery with mild sedation and only topical anesthesia, because it probably causes less pain than cryotherapy. The treatment session is faster with laser. The eyelids, conjunctiva, and cornea look normal after laser, whereas, after cryotherapy, they easily become edematous and inflamed. The latter consideration often is important to parents concerned about the fate of their premature child. With laser, the incidence of subconjunctival hematoma, conjunctival laceration, and other complications seen with cryotherapy has been reduced to almost zero. However, cataracts have been reported to occur after laser treatment in less than 1% of cases.

The beneficial effects demonstrated by cryotherapy in the large multicenter trial mentioned previously also have been found in a number of smaller trials studying the use of laser therapy. Essentially, the frequency of the potentially blinding ROP sequelae of retinal detachment and retinal fold was reduced by half after cryotherapy (40). At about 6 years of age, poor visual acuity (20/200 or worse) was found in 62% of untreated eyes compared with 47% of treated eyes (41). Despite the destruction of parts of the peripheral retina by cryotherapy, long-term follow-up has found only a six-degree loss of peripheral visual field (42). Whether treating with laser or cryotherapy, the parents must be informed that, although the treatment will reduce the possibility of blindness, blindness may still result despite treatment. Too often, parents assume that, with treatment, blindness definitely will be avoided.

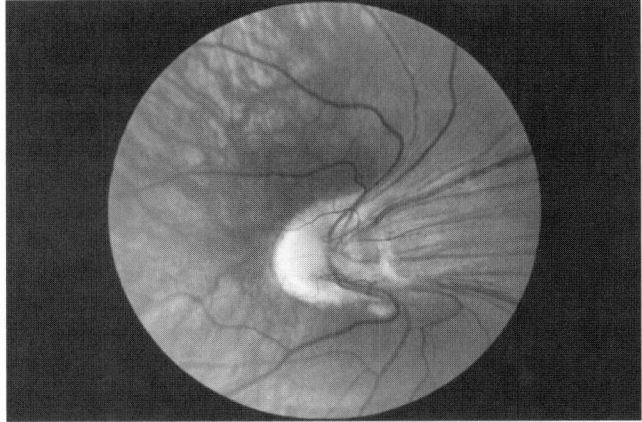

FIG. 52–17. The macula is dragged laterally amidst the retinal folds in cicatricial retinopathy of prematurity.

If a retinal detachment occurs, all is not lost. Modern vitreo–retinal surgery can reattach a detached retina with ROP more than 30% of the time. Once the macula detaches, however, the visual prognosis decreases markedly, even if the retina is reattached successfully. For stage 4A, visual acuity results as good as 20/20 have been reported with the macula still attached. Stage 4B results have been in the 20/80 to 20/200 range. With a total detachment (stage 5), the results decrease considerably to the 20/600 to 20/1600 range or even lower (43). This low level of vision may allow the child to ambulate independently and certainly is better than the blindness that would occur without surgery.

Long-Term Problems

Aside from the problems of poor vision from a detached retina or retinal folds that occur to the more unfortunate children with ROP, there are other sequelae that can arise in the eyes of infants with regressed ROP. Even with an attached retina and an intact macula, children with regressed ROP have been shown to be more susceptible to a number of visual disorders, including myopia, amblyopia, strabismus, and nystagmus. Children who developed cicatricial retinal changes, even with good vision, are at risk for future retinal problems, including detachment. Therefore, these children should be examined at least annually throughout their life, or at least until they are mature and literate enough to rule out amblyopia and strabismus.

COMMON DIFFERENTIAL DIAGNOSTIC PROBLEMS

Leukokoria

When faced with an infant with a white pupil or unusual retinal light reflex, the neonatologist or pediatrician should consider the differential diagnosis and begin a workup (Fig. 52–18). The first obligation is to rule out the potentially fatal retinoblastoma, even in a neonate (Fig. 52–19). The most common lesions that may, to some extent, simulate a retinoblastoma by presenting with leukokoria in infancy include cataract, persistent fetal vasculature, Coats' disease, large retinal coloboma, and a retinal detachment resulting from ROP. Toxocariasis is not a disease of infants. Coats' disease is caused by anomalous telangiectatic retinal vessels that cause massive exudation and retinal detachment. It is important to realize that behind an opaque cataract can lie other problems, such as retinal detachment or a mass.

The history should reveal the presence of prematurity, oxygen use, illnesses during pregnancy (such as rubella, toxoplasmosis, and cytomegalovirus), possible child abuse, or a traumatic birth. The nonocular history may help. Deafness suggests the possibility of rubella or Nor-

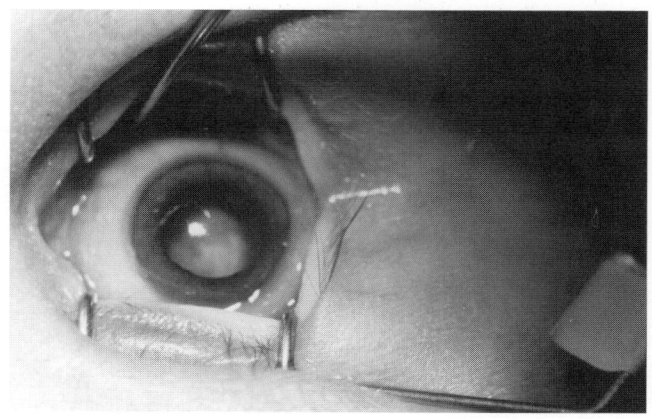

FIG. 52–18. Bilateral leukokoria was found in this neonate. A family history of Norrie's disease simplified the diagnosis.

rie's disease (cataract with retinal detachment). Toxoplasmosis or tuberous sclerosis may present with seizures. Incontinentia pigmenti or tuberous sclerosis may have skin lesions. Bilateral leukokoria would favor the diagnoses of ROP, Norrie's disease, child abuse, and retinal dysplasias. Unilateral leukokoria is more consistent with Coats' disease, persistent fetal vasculature, and intraocular foreign body. Although Norrie's disease and Coats' disease are more common in males, incontinentia pigmenti is more frequent in females.

The examination may actually begin with the eyes of the parents. We have found parents to have an asymptomatic congenital cataract, regressed retinoblastoma, an unappreciated coloboma, and the findings of familial exudative retinopathy, which closely resembles ROP. Any of these findings in a parent, who usually will cooperate better with the examination, generally will make the diagnosis for the baby. Examination of the child may reveal microphthalmos, which would be consistent with

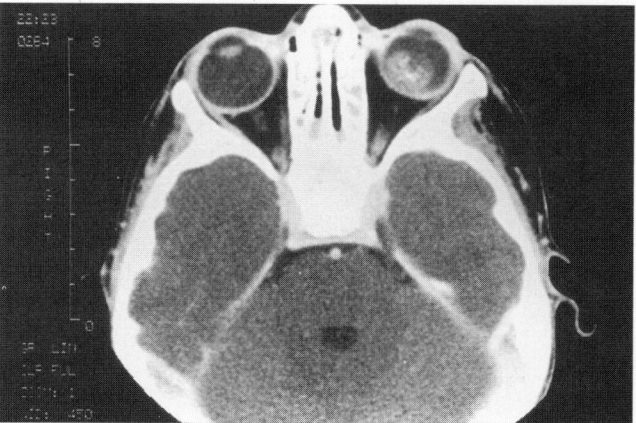

FIG. 52–19. A calcified intraocular mass in an infant with retinoblastoma.

coloboma or persistent fetal vasculature. The level of the opacity may be evident with a light or portable slit lamp. If there is a defect in the inferior iris, coloboma should be considered. Lens opacity would, of course, constitute a cataract, but additional examination, perhaps with ultrasound or radiologic tests, may reveal pathology in the vitreous or retina. A detailed retinal examination is crucial, if the media are sufficiently clear, to diagnose many entities that present with leukokoria.

Cloudy Cornea

Profound amblyopia will result from an opacified cornea, especially if it is unilateral. Although some opacities will clear with time, others will remain. The history, associated findings, and examination will clarify the prognosis.

The history should include illnesses during pregnancy to rule out rubella, syphilis, and herpes, which can cause keratitis. Delivery by forceps of a large neonate suggests birth trauma (Fig. 52–20). Systemic physical abnormalities may imply an etiology as an umbilical hernia suggests glaucoma associated with Reiger's syndrome. Glaucoma also is suggested by a history of photosensitivity and tearing. Family history is important.

On examination, the eyelids may reveal evidence of phakomatoses as the angiomatosis of Sturge–Weber syndrome or a neurofibroma. Conjunctival hemorrhages suggest a traumatic etiology. The presence of conjunctival inflammation implies infection or pupillary block glaucoma as an etiology.

Most important is the corneal examination. The corneal diameter should be measured as accurately as possible. An enlarged cornea strongly indicates glaucoma, whereas a small opacified cornea may result from sclerocornea, microphthalmos, trisomy 13, or rubella. Striae in the cornea are often helpful. Horizontally oriented striae are compatible with glaucoma, whereas vertical or oblique ones often result from birth trauma. A mass overlying the cornea may be a dermoid tumor.

Measurement of the intraocular pressure in these cases often is imperative to rule in glaucoma. Examination of the iris may reveal adhesions to the cornea. This can result from trauma or may indicate a mesodermal dysgenesis syndrome. This syndrome encompasses a number of developmental disorders, such as Peter's anomaly—the most frequent reason to perform corneal transplants in infants. A cataractous lens behind an opacified cornea may be caused by rubella, birth trauma, Lowe syndrome, or a mesodermal dysgenesis. If the eye and the intraocular pressure are otherwise normal, the opacified cornea may result from a hereditary corneal dystrophy.

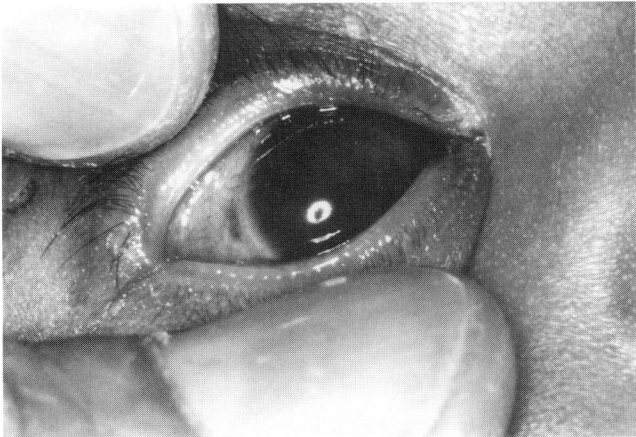

FIG. 52–20. One week after birth, the corneal opacity caused by a forceps injury is fading.

REFERENCES

1. Rakic P. Development of visual centers in the primate brain depends on binocular competition before birth. *Science* 1981;214:928.
2. Isenberg S, Neumann D, Cheong P, Ling Y, McCall L, Ziffer A. Growth of the internal and external eye in term and preterm infants. *Ophthalmology* 1995;102:827.
3. Hittner HM, Hirsch NJ, Rudolph AJ. Assessment of gestational age by examination of the anterior vascular capsule of the lens. *J Pediatr* 1977;91:455.
4. Isenberg SJ. Clinical application of the pupil examination in neonates. *J Pediatr* 1991;118:650.
5. Isenberg SJ. Macular development in the premature infant. *Am J Ophthalmol* 1986;101:74.
6. Isenberg SJ, Everett S. Cardiovascular effect of mydriatics in low-weight infants. *J Pediatr* 1984; 105:111.
7. Isenberg SJ, Hyman P, Abrams C. Effect of cyclopentolate eyedrops on gastric secretory function in pre-term infants. *Ophthalmology* 1985;92:698.
8. Clarke WN, Hodges E, Noel LP, Roberts D, Coneys M. The oculocardiac reflex during ophthalmoscopy in premature infants. *Am J Ophthalmol* 1985;99:649.
9. Isenberg SJ, Apt L, McCarty JA, Cooper LL, Lim L, Del Signore M. The development of tearing in preterm and term neonates. *Arch Ophthalmol* 1998;116:773.
10. Goldberg MF. Persistent fetal vasculature (PFV): an integrated interpretation of signs and symptoms associated with persistent hyperplastic vitreous (PHPV). *Am J Ophthalmol* 1997;124:587.
11. Hastings MM, Milot J, Barsoum-Homsy M, Hershon L, Dubois J, Leclerc J-M. Recombinant interferon alfa-2b in the treatment of vision-threatening capillary hemangiomas in childhood. *J Am Assoc Pediatr Ophthalmol Strabismus* 1997;1:226.
12. Hiles DA, Kilty LA. Disorders of the lens. In: Isenberg SJ, ed. *The eye in infancy,* 2nd ed. St. Louis: Mosby-Year Book, 1994:336.
13. Neumann D, Weissman B, Isenberg SJ, Rosenbaum AL, Bateman JB. The effectiveness of daily wear contact lenses for the correction of infantile aphakia. *Arch Ophthalmol* 1993;111:927.
14. Wright KW. Pediatric cataracts. *Curr Opin Ophthalmol* 1997;8:50.
15. Stromland K. Ocular abnormalities in the fetal alcohol syndrome. *Acta Ophthalmol Scan Suppl* 1985;171:1.
16. Archer SM, Sondhi N, Helveston EM. Strabismus in infancy. *Ophthalmology* 1989;96:133.
17. Hammerschlag MR, Cummings C, Roblin PM, Williams TH, Delke I. Efficacy of neonatal ocular prophylaxis for the prevention of chlamydial and gonococcal conjunctivitis. *N Engl J Med* 1989;320:769.
18. Isenberg SJ, Apt L, Yoshimori R, Leake RD, Rich R. The use of povidone–iodine for ophthalmia neonatorum prophylaxis. *Am J Ophthalmol* 1994;118:701.
19. Isenberg SJ, Apt L, Wood M. A clinical trial of povidone–iodine as prophylaxis against ophthalmia neonatorum. *N Engl J Med* 1995;32:562.
20. Petersen RA, Robb RM. The natural course of congenital obstruction of the nasolacrimal duct. *J Pediatr Ophthalmol Strabismus* 1978;15:246.
21. Dennehy PJ, Warman R, Flynn JT, Scott GB, Mastrucci MT. Ocular

manifestations in pediatric patients with acquired immunodeficiency syndrome. *Arch Ophthalmol* 1989;107:978-982.

22. Hogan MJ, Kimura SJ, O'Connor GR. Ocular toxoplasmosis. *Arch Ophthalmol* 1964;72:592.

23. Engstrom RE, Holland GN, Nussenblatt RB, Jabs DA. Current practices in the management of ocular toxoplasmosis. *Am J Ophthalmol* 1991;111:601.

24. Jain IS, Singh YP, Grupta SL, Gupta A. Ocular hazards during birth. *J Pediatr Ophthalmol Strabismus* 1980;17:14.

25. Naylor G, Roper JP, Willshaw HE. Ophthalmic complications of amniocentesis. *Eye* 1990;4:845.

26. Buys YM, Levin AV, Enzenauer RW, et al. Retinal findings after head trauma in infants and young children. *Ophthalmology* 1992;99:1718.

27. Isenberg SJ, Spierer A, Inkelis SH. Ocular signs of cocaine intoxication in neonates. *Am J Ophthalmol* 1987;103:211.

28. Kalina RE, Forrest GL. Ocular hazards of phototherapy for hyperbilirubinemia. *J Pediatr Ophthalmol* 1971;8:116.

29. Palmer EA, Flynn JT, Hardy RJ, et al. Incidence and early course of retinopathy of prematurity. *Ophthalmology* 1991;98:1628.

30. Flynn JT, Bancalari E, Snyder ES, et al. A cohort study of transcutaneous oxygen tension and the incidence and severity of retinopathy of prematurity. *N Engl J Med* 1992;326:1050.

31. Phelps DL. Vitamin E and retinopathy of prematurity. In: Silverman WA, Flynn JT, eds. *Contemporary issues in fetal and neonatal medicine 2:* retinopathy of prematurity. Boston: Blackwell, 1985, p 181.

32. Johnson L, Bowen FW Jr, Abassi S, et al. Relationship of prolonged pharmacologic serum levels of vitamin E to incidence of sepsis and necrotizing enterocolitis in infants with birth weights 1,500 grams or less. *Pediatrics* 1985;75:619.

33. Martone WJ, Williams WW, Mortensen ML, et al. Illness with fatalities in premature infants: association with an intravenous vitamin E preparation, E-Ferol. *Pediatrics* 1986;78:591.

34. Phelps DL, Rosenbaum AL, Isenberg SJ, Leake RD, Dorey FJ. Tocopherol efficacy and safety for preventing retinopathy of prematurity: a randomized, controlled, double-masked trial. *Pediatrics* 1987;79: 489.

35. Glass P, Avery GB, Kolinjavadi N, et al. Effect of bright light in the hospital nursery on the incidence of retinopathy of prematurity. *N Engl J Med* 1985;313:401.

36. Ackerman B, Sherwonit E, Williams J. Reduced incidental light exposure: effect on the development of retinopathy of prematurity in low birth weight infants. *Pediatrics* 1989;83:958.

37. Brown DR, Biglan AW, Stretavsky MAM. Screening criteria for the detection of retinopathy of prematurity in patients in a neonatal intensive care unit. *J Pediatr Ophthalmol Strabismus* 1987;24:212.

38. Cryotherapy for Retinopathy of Prematurity Cooperative Group. Multicenter trial of cryotherapy for retinopathy of prematurity: preliminary results. *Arch Ophthalmol* 1988;106:471.

39. Hunter DG, Repka MX. Diode laser photocoagulation for threshold retinopathy of prematurity. A randomized study. *Ophthalmology* 1993; 100:238.

40. Cryotherapy for Retinopathy of Prematurity Cooperative Group. Multicenter trial of cryotherapy for retinopathy of prematurity: one year outcome—structure and function. *Arch Ophthalmol* 1990;108: 1408.

41. Cryotherapy for Retinopathy of Prematurity Cooperative Group. Multicenter trial of cryotherapy for retinopathy of prematurity: Snellen acuity and structural outcome at 5½ years. *Arch Ophthalmol* 1996;114:417.

42. Quinn GR, Dobson V, Hardy RJ, et al. Visual fields measured with double-arc perimetry in eyes with threshold retinopathy of prematurity from the cryotherapy for retinopathy of prematurity trial. *Ophthalmology* 1996;103:1432.

43. Maguire AM, Trese MT. Visual results of lens-sparing vitreoretinal surgery in infants. *J Pediatr Ophthalmol Strabismus* 1993;30:28.

CHAPTER 53

Neoplasia

Robert J. Arceci and Howard J. Weinstein

Although neoplasia in infancy is quite rare, it presents important and unique biologic, diagnostic, and therapeutic problems. Such neoplasms show peculiarities that distinguish them from those occurring later. Many tumors in early life are composed of persistent embryonal or fetal tissues, suggesting a failure of proper maturation or cytodifferentiation during intrauterine or postnatal life. Indeed, the failure of proper maturation of fetal tissue may be difficult to distinguish from neoplasia. In addition, an unexpectedly large number of neoplasms of early life are associated with growth disturbances and congenital anomalies. Spontaneous regression and cytodifferentiation also occur most frequently in tumors of early life.

The application of new technologies, such as ultrasonic imaging and intrauterine surgery, has provided potentially valuable opportunities for prenatal detection and partial resection of tumors, such as in large congenital sacrococcygeal teratomas. The unique physiology of the developing neonate provides the clinician with special problems in terms of therapeutic interventions and their long-term sequelae. The neonatal period can be considered one in which various types of treatment and exposures may affect the long-term risk of secondary malignancies.

EPIDEMIOLOGY

From the data in The Third National Cancer Survey (1969 to 1971), Bader and Miller (1) reported that, in the United States, the annual incidence of malignant neoplasms in infants younger than 1 year of age was 183.4 per 1 million live births and within the first 28 days of life was 36.5 per 1 million live births. They further estimated that approximately 653 infants per year in the United

States are diagnosed with cancer and that about 130 (20%) of these patients are neonates. In a more recent study from Denmark, the incidence of neonatal cancer was calculated to be between 1.88 to 2.98 cases per 100,000 births (2). Approximately one-half of the neonatal malignancies are noted on the first day of life (3). The incidence of childhood cancers also has been observed to show regional differences over time and, over the past 20 years, an absolute increase in childhood cancer has been reported (4,5).

When incidence for all malignancies is compared with mortality as determined from death certificates, the incidence in patients younger than 1 year is 3.5 times greater than mortality, whereas the incidence in patients younger than 29 days old is 4.8 times greater than mortality (1,6). These figures offer an interesting comparison to those reported in children up to 15 years of age, among whom the incidence of malignancy is only about 1.3 to 1.8 times greater than mortality. When individual diseases are considered, there are marked differences in incidence versus mortality. For example, in neonates, the incidence of neuroblastoma is 10 times greater than the mortality, whereas the incidence of leukemia is only 1.8 times the mortality. The distribution of the types of malignancies found in infants younger than 1 year of age differs from that found in later childhood. In infants younger than 1 year of age, neuroblastoma is the most common malignancy and accounts for about 50% of malignancies in the neonatal period; it is followed by leukemia, renal tumors, sarcomas, central nervous system (CNS) tumors, and hepatic malignancy (2,3,7). However, when one considers the total spectrum of neoplastic disorders of infancy, teratoma usually is reported as the most frequently encountered neoplasm, followed by hemangiomas, lymphangiomas, and small nevi lesions (8). In older children younger than 15 years of age, leukemia is the most common malignancy (about 30%), followed by CNS tumors, lymphoma, neuroblastoma, sarcoma, and renal tumors.

R. J. Arceci and H. J. Weinstein: Division of Hematology and Oncology, Children's Hospital Medical Center, Cincinnati, Ohio; and Massachusetts General Hospital, Boston, Massachusetts

GROWTH DISTURBANCES, GENETIC ABERRATIONS, AND CANCER PATHOGENESIS

Primary, inherited, cytogenetic syndromes usually occur as a result of chromosomal aneuploidy, deletions, translocations, or increased fragility, which represent the end result of germline chromosomal defects. An example of aneuploidy is Down syndrome (trisomy 21), in which the frequency of acute leukemia is approximately 15 times the normal. In addition, an increased incidence of solid tumors has been reported for persons with trisomy 8, 9, 13, and 18 (9). Deletion of part of the long arm of chromosome 13 is associated with psychomotor retardation, microcephaly, cardiac and skeletal defects, and the early development of retinoblastoma. The deletion of the short arm of chromosome 11 results in mental retardation, microcephaly, aniridia, ear and genital anomalies, and an increased incidence of Wilms tumor (WAGR syndrome). These syndromes provided support for the assignment of a retinoblastoma locus to chromosome 13q14 and a Wilms tumor locus (WT1) to 11p13. These mutant alleles (i.e., loci) are heterozygous in constitutional cells and homozygous in retinoblastoma and Wilms tumor cells, respectively. The actual development of the tumor appears to require that each allele be abnormal. WAGR syndrome results from loss of several genes from the 11p13 region. Deletion of one copy of PAX 6 is responsible for aniridia, and loss of one WT1 allele results in genitourinary anomalies. Deletion of the WT1 gene in patients with WAGR syndrome is thought to be the first hit in the genesis of a Wilms tumor. The function of WT1 is not clear, but it may play a role in the control of a cell's entry into the S phase of the cell cycle. Homozygosity at the "Wilms tumor locus" on chromosome 11 has been found in embryonal rhabdomyosarcomas (RMS) and hepatoblastomas, suggesting a common pathogenesis for these embryonal tumors (10). The specific loss of constitutional heterozygosity and its relationship to oncogenesis has been confirmed in studies of transgenic mice that lack a functional tumor suppressor gene, p53. This phenotype is characterized by a higher incidence of embryopathy, as well as an increased incidence of malignancies developing early in life (11–14).

A number of inherited syndromes, including Bloom syndrome, Fanconi Anemia, ataxia–telangiectasia, xeroderma pigmentosum, and Werner's syndrome, are characterized by developmental abnormalities and increased incidence of various types of cancer (15,16). These syndromes also demonstrate increased defects in DNA recombination, increased sensitivity to genotoxic agents, increased chromosomal fragility, and abnormal DNA repair (17–19). Of particular interest is that these syndromes now are known to be caused by defects in genes encoding several novel proteins involved in DNA/RNA recombination and repair, such as the DEAD-box helicase of Bloom syndrome or excision repair enzymes associated with some of the complementation groups of xeroderma pigmentosum (17–20). It is intriguing that when these defective genes are inherited through the germline, patients show both developmental abnormalities as well as an increased incidence of cancer. It will be important to determine whether somatic cell mutations of such genes will increase the chances of a cell becoming malignant.

Malformation syndromes without obvious cytogenetic abnormalities include hemihypertrophy and Beckwith–Wiedemann syndrome (BWS), which consists of mental retardation, gigantism, macroglossia, omphalocele, and organomegaly; both of these disorders are associated with the development of Wilms tumor, hepatoblastoma, and adrenocortical carcinoma. BWS, which occurs in approximately 1 in 13,000 births, usually is sporadic, although an autosomal dominant inheritance pattern with incomplete penetrance also has been proposed. Patients with BWS have an approximately 7.5% to 10% risk of developing a tumor (21). Sacrococcygeal teratomas and teratocarcinomas are associated with anomalies of the lower spine and urogenital region.

Hamartomas are benign proliferations of cells in their normal anatomic location. Hamartomas in which malignant neoplasms arise include congenital melanotic nevi, which can progress to melanoma, and familial polyposis, which may evolve into colonic carcinoma. Examples of malignancies developing from persistent fetal rests include craniopharyngioma arising from tissue derived embryologically from the Rathke pouch, and persistent neuroblastic cellularity leading to adrenal neuroblastoma.

Naturally occurring DNA sequences homologous to transforming viral oncogenes exist in normal, untransformed cells of all metazoa. Such DNA sequences are called cellular oncogenes and are used in normal cells during growth, development, and differentiation in precise temporal and tissue-specific patterns (22–24). Some of their products function as potent cell growth and death (apoptosis) regulators. The protein products of some cellular oncogenes are quite similar to the products from the homologous viral oncogenes. Because of their expression during normal development, inherited or acquired mutations affecting cellular oncogene expression might lead to a variety of developmental abnormalities and congenital defects, such as hemihypertrophy syndromes and hamartomas. In addition, the persistent expression beyond birth of certain growth-related oncogenes may play a role in such proliferative states as the transient myeloproliferative disorder associated with Down syndrome and stage IV-S neuroblastoma found in infants, which both are characterized by subsequent regression.

Such predisposing conditions share at least one common element: an inherited or developmental disturbance of cellular growth and/or cell survival, which may be linked to the molecular pathways regulating these genetically determined cellular responses. The finding of these different classes of genes helps to define the molecular links between conditions of abnormal development (i.e., teratogenesis) and neoplastic transformation (25,26).

EXPOSURE TO MATERNAL MALIGNANCY

In addition to the susceptibility of the fetus to adverse effects of chemotherapy during pregnancy, there also is the possibility that the maternal cancer will metastasize to the placenta and fetus. Although many anecdotal reports have documented such involvement, it occurs only very rarely. The types of tumors shown to be transmitted from the mother to the placenta or fetus are quite varied, with melanoma most commonly cited (27,28). Although lymphoma and leukemia may involve the placenta, they have not been found to be transmitted to the fetus.

TUMORS OF NEUROEPITHELIAL ORIGIN

Neuroectodermal cells of the neural tube differentiate to neuroblasts, which become nervous system tissue and melanocytes; free spongioblasts, which become either astrocytes or oligodendroglia cells; and ependymal spongioblasts, which become ependymal cells. These primitive neuroectodermal cells may be the target for neoplasia, giving rise to a group of morphologically similar tumors in central and peripheral sites of the nervous system. Neonatal tumors originating from neuroectodermal cells include neuroblastoma, retinoblastoma, peripheral nerve tumors (i.e., neuroepithelioma), medulloblastoma, choroid plexus papilloma, ependymoblastoma, and melanotic neuroectodermal tumors. These tumors show varying degrees of cellular differentiation, have similar histologic features (e.g., small, primitive cells with rosettes or pseudorosettes), and tend to spread along cerebrospinal fluid pathways.

Neuroblastoma

Neuroblastoma is the most common malignant tumor in neonates. It originates from neural crest cells that normally give rise to the adrenal medulla and sympathetic ganglia. Its reported occurrence in siblings and other family members suggests that some cases are hereditary (29). In such cases, the tumors usually are diagnosed at an earlier age and often are characterized by having multifocal primary tumors (30). An interesting syndrome has been reported in several women who delivered infants diagnosed as having neuroblastoma during the first few months of life (31). The mothers had sweating, pallor, headaches, palpitations, hypertension, and tingling in their hands and feet during the last trimester of pregnancy. These symptoms were relieved after the birth of the affected infants. The authors of that study postulated that this symptom complex is caused by the introduction

of fetal tumor catecholamines into the maternal circulation. Neuroblastoma may present as a tumor mass anywhere that sympathetic neural tissue normally occurs (32).

Although at least half of infants present with an abdominal mass from tumors arising in the adrenal medulla or retroperitoneal sympathetic ganglia, neuroblastoma may arise anywhere along the sympathetic nervous system as well as present with disseminated disease. An abdominal sonogram or computed tomography (CT) scan demonstrates displacement of the kidney without distortion of the calyceal system. The neoplasm also may originate in the posterior mediastinum, neck, or pelvis. Cervical sympathetic ganglion involvement in the neck may result in Horner's syndrome; posterior mediastinal tumors may cause respiratory distress; paravertebral tumors tend to grow through the intervertebral foramina and cause symptoms of spinal cord compression; and presacral neuroblastomas may mimic presacral teratomas. Neuroblastoma also has been detected prenatally by ultrasonography, showing a solid and sometimes cystic suprarenal mass (33–35). Two unusual presentations of neuroblastoma are intractable diarrhea secondary to release of vasoactive intestinal peptide, and the syndrome of opsoclonus, myoclonus, and truncal ataxia (36,37), the etiology of which remains an enigma. The diarrhea secondary to vasoactive intestinal peptide abates after removal of the neuroblastoma. In contrast is the unpredictable improvement after the removal or treatment of neuroblastoma associated with opsoclonus–myoclonus. Nevertheless, survival for children with this syndrome is excellent.

Metastatic lesions are common presenting findings of neuroblastoma, especially in the neonate (38). The primary tumor often cannot be found in infants younger than 6 months of age. These infants present with bluish subcutaneous nodules and extensive hepatomegaly. The liver may be studded with tumor nodules and be so large that it causes respiratory distress secondary to abdominal distention. Clumps of tumor cells often are found in the bone marrow aspirates. Metastases to bones, skull, and orbit, which present as periorbital ecchymoses, are rare in the neonate. The unique metastatic pattern to liver, bone marrow, and skin in infants is classified as stage IV-S neuroblastoma (39,40).

The differential diagnosis for neuroblastoma is limited. The subcutaneous nodules appear similar to those found in congenital leukemia cutis and several congenital infections. The leukoerythroblastosis secondary to bone marrow metastases from neuroblastoma also is observed with congenital infection, severe hemolytic disease, and leukemia. More than 90% of children with neuroblastoma will have elevated urinary excretion of catecholamine metabolites, vanillylmandelic acid or homovanillic acid, or both (41). The diagnosis of neuroblastoma is made by biopsy of the primary tumor or metastatic lesions. The most histologically primitive lesion is neuroblastoma without differentiation and is composed of small, round cells with scant cytoplasm. The ganglioneuroma, its benign counterpart, is composed of large, mature ganglion cells. Ganglioneuroblastoma is intermediate in its degree of cellular differentiation. In the absence of a tissue specimen, the findings of elevated urinary catecholamines and tumor pseudorosettes in a bone marrow specimen usually are sufficient to make a definitive diagnosis.

The prognosis for children with neuroblastoma is inversely correlated to the age of the child at diagnosis as well as the extent of disease. The infant with stage IV-S disease has a better chance of survival than does the older child with less advanced disease. Evans et al. (39) proposed a clinical staging system for children with neuroblastoma that was prognostically useful (32,40,42). This system has evolved into an International Staging System, which takes into account many of these basic concepts (40).

Infants with stage IV-S have had spontaneous regression of disease, and in other patients malignant neuroblastomas apparently have undergone maturation into mature ganglioneuromas (43). The incidence of spontaneous regression of neuroblastoma may be more common than is clinically evident. Primitive sympathetic neuroblasts, which are derived from neural crest ectoderm, migrate in early embryonic life into the adrenal primordium, where they arrange themselves in nodules before differentiation into adrenomedullary tissue. These nodules are present in all fetal adrenal glands at 14 to 18 weeks of gestation (44). Beckwith and Perrin (45) detected the presence of microscopic clusters of neuroblastoma cells (i.e., neuroblastoma *in situ*) in the adrenal glands in a number of autopsies from infants younger than age 3 months who had no clinical evidence of tumor. They estimated that neuroblastoma *in situ* occurs in 1 of 250 stillborn infants and infants younger than 3 months of age. Clinically detectable neuroblastoma is noted in only 1 of 10,000 live births. Also pertinent to these data are the observations of the catecholamine screening programs done on 3-week-old and 6-month-old infants in Japan and Canada (46–48). These programs demonstrated that this type of screening resulted in an increased incidence of early stage neuroblastoma that, most likely, would not have presented as clinically detectable disease.

These observations raise the interesting question as to whether stage IV-S neuroblastoma is not a true malignancy. If stage IV-S neuroblastoma is a classic malignant neoplasm, it should be clonally derived. One such example of clonality in stage IV-S neuroblastoma tumor specimens has been demonstrated by cytogenetic analysis. Although no consistent and specific chromosomal alteration has been found in all stage IV-S specimens, there are increasing numbers of examples of cytogenetic clonality. In addition, it is becoming clear that stage IV-S neuroblastoma is characterized by usually being hyperdiploid and lacking the 1p deletion as well as N-*myc* amplification (49,50). The reason(s) for spontaneous regression of stage IV-S disease remains a mystery.

The extent of treatment for neuroblastoma depends on the stage of the disease as well as biological factors such as histology, N-*myc* amplification, and DNA ploidy. The infant with stage IV-S disease should be observed for a period of weeks to months before treatment is initiated because of the reasonable likelihood of spontaneous regression (42,51). Respiratory difficulties, blood vessel (usually vena cava) obstruction, and gastrointestinal compression secondary to rapid tumor expansion can develop and should be considered a medical emergency, with more than 50% mortality in some reports (52). Hsu et al. (53) have described a monitoring and scoring system to follow these patients and predict when, and if, therapeutic interventions should be initiated. This scoring system is based on the presence of the severity of several clinical symptoms, including respiratory compromise, renal insufficiency, extent of lower extremity edema, disseminated intravascular coagulopathy, and the rate of increasing abdominal girth (53). Although both chemotherapy (often single-agent cyclophosphamide) or radiation therapy have been used to effect symptomatic relief for such patients, more recent reports suggest that 200 to 600 cGy delivered tangentially to the liver in order to avoid other organs, such as kidneys and gonads, provides for the most rapid response and ultimately the best outcome (53,54).

Complete surgical removal of neuroblastoma usually is accomplished in infants with stage I or II disease. Postoperative treatment generally is not indicated for these patients, and their long-term survival is excellent (50,55). For infants with stage III disease in whom gross residual tumor remains after surgery, postoperative chemotherapy, radiotherapy, or both are indicated. Chemotherapy is the treatment of choice for infants with stage IV disease (50,56). The active chemotherapeutic agents against neuroblastoma include alkylating compounds (e.g., cisplatinum, cyclophosphamide, dacarbazine, nitrogen mustard), vincristine, and doxorubicin. Combinations of several of these agents administered for 6 months to 1 year have resulted in greater than 50% long-term survival for children younger than 1 year of age with stage IV neuroblastoma. This is in contrast to the dismal prognosis for similarly staged children who are older than 1 year of age at diagnosis and in whom bone marrow transplantation trials are being investigated.

Retinoblastoma

Retinoblastoma is a congenital malignant tumor arising from the nuclear layer of the retina. Although an extremely rare tumor, it is the most common ocular tumor of childhood. The median age at presentation is 18 months, or 14 months for bilateral cases, but a small percentage of infants are diagnosed during the first few months of life (57). Approximately 10% of children with retinoblastoma have a family history of the disease. Approximately 30% with bilateral or multifocal unilateral tumors have a negative family history (58,59). These two groups are capable of transmitting the disease to their offspring in an autosomal dominant fashion. This hereditary tendency is governed by a genetic locus on the long arm of chromosome 13 (i.e., band 13q14), which includes the retinoblastoma (rb) tumor suppressor gene. If there is a family history of retinoblastoma, an experienced ophthalmologist should examine the eyes of unaffected siblings regularly while they are under general anesthesia to detect cases early.

The most common initial signs of retinoblastoma include an abnormal white pupil (i.e., leukocoria), known as a cat's-eye reflex and a squint or strabismus. A clinical picture resembling retinoblastoma may result from granulomatosis uveitis, congenital defects, and severe retrolental fibroplasia. Once the diagnosis of retinoblastoma is suspected, both eyes should be examined with the infant under general anesthesia. A bone marrow aspiration and spinal tap for malignant cells should be performed for staging. A staging system for retinoblastoma is based on the size, location, number of tumors in each eye, and distant hematogenous metastases. Vitreous seeding, tumors extending anteriorly to the ora serrata, tumors invading over one-half of the retina, residual orbital disease, and optic nerve or distant metastases are adverse prognostic features.

Retinoblastoma usually is curable when diagnosed early; vision often need not be sacrificed even when bilateral disease is present. Radiotherapy always should be considered if the eye has a chance for useful vision. More recent treatment approaches using cryosurgery in combination with chemotherapy and/or radiation therapy are being developed with the hope of preserving vision and reducing the risk of subsequent in-field radiation-induced secondary malignancies. In addition, stereotactic and proton beam radiation methods are being tested in order to reduce the amount of normal tissue irradiated and the risk of radiation-induced secondary malignancies (60–63). Patients with adverse prognosis features often require enucleation. Children with very advanced and metastatic disease require aggressive chemotherapy regimens (63–66).

Brain Tumors and Other Neuroectodermal Tumors

Intracranial tumors presenting in the first year of life are uncommon. In a review from the Hospital for Sick Children in London, 107 of 1,296 children with brain tumors had symptoms before the age of 1 year; 17 were symptomatic within 2 months of birth (67,68). Brain tumors in children in this age group tend to be supratentorial, in contrast to those in older children, which tend to be infratentorial. In infants, the most common presenting symptom is macrocrania, with a bulging fontanelle secondary either to hydrocephalus or tumor volume. Seizures, vomiting, failure to thrive, abnormal eye movement, and irritability also are frequent. CNS tumors have been reported to be associated with the presence of a bifid epiglottis (69). The histologic diagnoses of the neuroectodermal tumors are similar to those of tumors in later childhood, with gliomas accounting for most. Of particular interest, a majority of intracranial tumors in neonates have been reported to be teratomas (70). There is also a high frequency of choroid plexus papillomas in this age group (71). An association of choroid plexus papillomas and the presence of SV40 viral DNA has been reported (72).

Desmoplastic infantile gangliogliomas are rare, but massive, cystic tumors that usually occur supratentorially in the neonatal period (73). They present most commonly with signs of increased intracranial pressure, including seizures. Therapy has included surgery and chemotherapy, but without radiation therapy. For patients who have a complete surgical resection, additional therapy may not be required (74). Prognosis may be better than that observed with other tumors, such as high-grade astrocytoma. In contrast, pineoblastomas are malignant tumors with an extremely poor outcome, even when treated with surgery, chemotherapy. and radiation therapy. Part of the reason for the poor outcome in these infants may be the propensity of pineoblastoma to involve the leptomeninges as well as extraneural spread (74).

Treatment of infants with brain tumors historically included surgical removal or biopsy followed by radiotherapy (75–77). Operative mortality has been high, and few infants survived for longer than 1 year. In these few, brain radiotherapy resulted in severe intellectual and psychomotor retardation. In attempts to avoid the adverse effects of radiotherapy on the developing brain, more recent therapeutic approaches have evaluated surgery followed by preradiation chemotherapy (78–81).

Primitive neuroectodermal tumors of peripheral nerve represent a group of soft tissue tumors known as neuroepitheliomas, medulloepitheliomas, and peripheral neuroblastomas (82,83). They are associated with major branches of peripheral nerves (i.e., tumor of the chest wall arising from intercostal nerve). These are extremely rare tumors, quite aggressive in their biologic behavior, with frequently occurring distant metastases, including to the CNS. Treatment approaches include wide excision, if possible, and chemotherapy modeled after either neuroblastoma or brain tumor protocols.

The melanotic neuroectodermal tumor of infancy has its origin in the neural crest population. Most of these tumors are diagnosed between 1 and 8 months of age and occur in the maxilla, although extremely rare cases have been reported in other sites such as the epididymis (84,85). They are considered a benign neoplasm, with a local recurrence rate of about 15%. These tumors originate from pluripotential neural crest cells that give rise to both melanoblasts and neuroblasts. The rate of malignancy for this tumor is reported to be approximately 5%. Recommended treatment is wide local excision.

CONGENITAL LEUKEMIA

Leukemia in the newborn is extremely rare (86–88). It has been customary to categorize leukemia as congenital when it is diagnosed within a few days after birth and as neonatal when it manifests itself during the first 4 to 6 weeks of life. The kinetics of leukemic cell growth and the estimated leukemic cell burden at the time of diagnosis make it reasonable to assume that clinically detectable leukemia during the first 4 weeks of life originated *in utero*. However, recent data indicate a prenatal initiation of acute lymphoblastic leukemia (ALL), specifically the t(4,11) subtype, in children diagnosed in infancy within the first 2 years (89). In the following discussion, congenital leukemia is considered as leukemia diagnosed from birth to 4 weeks of age.

The etiology and pathogenesis of congenital leukemia, as well as other leukemias, are unknown. The strongest evidence for a genetic predisposition to acute leukemia is its occurrence in identical twins (90). If leukemia develops in one of a set of identical twins before 6 years of age, the risk of disease in the other twin is 20%. Leukemia usually develops in the other twin within months of the first case. In some of these cases, the intrauterine exchange of leukemic cells from one twin to the other has been strongly suggested by the identity of molecular and genetic changes observed postnatally in the leukemias from each twin (91). For fraternal twins and siblings, the risk of development of leukemia is two and four times higher, respectively, than in the general population. Congenital leukemia has been associated with trisomy 9, trisomy 13, Turner syndrome, and Down syndrome (92–96).

More than 95% of the childhood leukemias, including congenital leukemia, are classified as acute, because they are characterized by a predominance of immature lymphoid or myeloid precursors. In children, the proportion of cases of ALL to acute myelogenous leukemia (AML) is approximately 4 to 1, but this ratio is less skewed in the congenital leukemias (86,87). Whereas lymphoblasts from most children with ALL express the common acute lymphoblastic leukemia antigen (CALLA or CD10) on the cell surface and express markers of early B-cell differentiation (e.g., cytoplasmic immunoglobulin or Ig gene rearrangement), the lymphoblasts of congenital and infant ALL often are pre-B but CD10-negative (97,98). These infants have a higher incidence of CNS leukemia at diagnosis, a higher leukocyte count, increased frequency of hepatosplenomegaly, and a poorer prognosis than older children with ALL. A translocation of the long arms of chromosomes 4 and 11, t(4;11), involving the MLL gene at 11q23 is commonly observed in infant leukemia. This translocation is associated with greater than 80% of ALL in infancy and carries a poor prognosis (99–104).

The most common subtype of AML in the neonate is acute monocytic leukemia, which accounts for only 20% of AML in older children (105). It is associated with a high incidence of extramedullary leukemia, especially in the CNS. Translocations involving chromosome 11q23 with MLL gene rearrangements are associated with this subtype of AML, but usually involve different partner genes than in ALL (106).

Cutaneous manifestations are the most frequent clinical findings noted at birth. In addition to petechiae and purpura, leukemic skin nodules (i.e., leukemia cutis) have been observed in approximately 50% of cases (107–109). These skin nodules may vary in size from a few millimeters to a few centimeters, are bluish to slate gray in color, may appear in all sites, and are palpated as firm tumors of the deep skin (Fig. 53–1). Neonatal leukemia cutis may undergo a spontaneous, temporary regression, but tends to recur in a more generalized form within a few weeks to months (105).

Hepatosplenomegaly is common, but lymphadenopathy is not. Respiratory distress, secondary to leukostasis

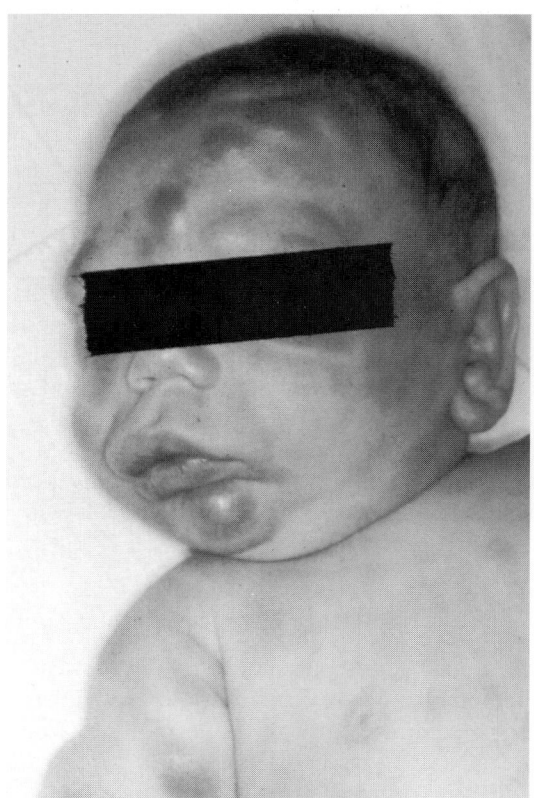

FIG. 53–1. Congenital acute monocytic leukemia with skin nodules.

within the pulmonary vasculature, may complicate the clinical course. Other nonspecific symptoms of neonatal leukemia include lethargy, pallor, poor feeding, and umbilical, gastrointestinal, or genitourinary bleeding.

In the report of congenital leukemia by Pierce (86), the mean hemoglobin concentration at birth was normal, with a wide range of values (7 to 20 g/dL); the mean leukocyte counts were 150,000 per mm^3 (range 2,000 to 850,000); and mean platelet counts were 70,000 per mm^3 (range 6,000 to 300,000). The diagnosis of leukemia is confirmed by examination of a bone marrow aspirate obtained from the posterior iliac crest.

A variety of disorders in the newborn imitate leukemia. The newborn bone marrow response to infection, hypoxemia, or severe hemolysis commonly is a leukemoid reaction and an increase in circulating nucleated erythrocytes. This frequently has been confused with congenital leukemia.

An enigmatic myeloproliferative disorder described as transient acute leukemia, or ineffective regulation of granulopoiesis masquerading as congenital leukemia, occurs in about 10% of infants with Down syndrome (92,110,111). This syndrome, noted during the first few days of life, mimics AML. Peripheral leukocyte counts can range from 25,000 to several hundred thousand; bone marrow aspirates reveal 30% to 70% blasts. Hepatosplenomegaly and thrombocytopenia also are common findings. The hematologic status of these neonates usually returns to normal in 1 to 4 months, with only supportive therapy. Several of these children who subsequently died of cardiac or pulmonary disease years after the resolution of their transient myeloproliferative syndrome showed no evidence of leukemia at autopsy. This syndrome has been observed in neonates with stigmata of Down syndrome and in phenotypically normal infants who have trisomy 21 mosaicism in their hematopoietic cells or skin fibroblasts (112).

In approximately 25% of these infants, acute leukemia requiring systemic chemotherapy will develop within the first 4 years of life. This leukemia is nearly always acute megakaryoblastic leukemia (M7 subtype). In the setting of constitutional trisomy 21, acute megakaryoblastic leukemia usually has an excellent prognosis, even with less intense therapy than observed for non-Down syndrome children with the same subtype of leukemia (111,113–117).

An infant with Down syndrome has an equal likelihood of having either a transient myeloproliferative syndrome or congenital leukemia (111). Although time is still the most definitive indicator of transiency, serial cytogenetic studies may be of value. If there is a chromosome marker in addition to trisomy 21 in spontaneously dividing bone marrow cells, a more aggressive leukemic clone is likely to be present.

Congenital ALL is fatal if untreated and should be managed with systemic chemotherapy. Several national trials are ongoing to improve the outcome of these infants with this poor prognosis leukemia. Age has been an important prognostic variable in childhood ALL, with the most favorable prognosis for patients between 2 and 9 years of age. Prognosis for young infants with ALL remains poor (98,103,118). Because untreated congenital AML also is fatal, aggressive combination chemotherapy in an institution with maximal supportive services is mandatory. One report has described the successful treatment of several neonates with acute monocytic leukemia with either VP-16 or VM-26, but this experience has not been confirmed (105). Aggressive AML treatment regimens have met with considerable success in achieving long-term disease-free survival in neonates with AML (119–121).

NEOPLASMS OF THE KIDNEY

Mesoblastic Nephroma

Most abdominal masses presenting in infancy are renal in origin, and most can be accounted for by cystic disease of the kidney and congenital malformations of the urinary tract leading to hydronephrosis. Although neoplasms of the kidney are rare in infancy, that they do occur and have important prognostic implications makes it mandatory that they be included in the evaluation of abdominal masses.

The most common renal tumor found in infants is the mesoblastic nephroma, which accounts for nearly 80% of renal tumors in the neonatal period. It also has been called fetal renal hamartoma, mesenchymal hamartoma of infancy, and leiomyomatous hamartoma (122). Mesoblastic nephroma commonly presents as an asymptomatic, enlarging abdominal mass during the first few months of life (123). It is not associated with congenital anomalies and has no race predilection. Of note is the more frequent occurrence of polyhydramnios and premature labor in women whose infants have mesoblastic nephroma (124). The differential diagnosis includes renal cystic disease, congenital malformations of the urinary tract resulting in hydronephrosis, and Wilms tumor. Molecular studies have demonstrated that mesoblastic nephroma shares with most Wilms tumors the expression of insulin-like growth factor II (IGF-II), but, unlike Wilms tumor, does not express the WT1 gene and shows no loss of heterozygosity at 11p13 or 11p15 (125). The bi-allelic expression of the IGF-II has shown that there is a relaxation of the normal imprinting pattern of this gene (i.e., the paternal allele is normally expressed with the maternal allele silent) (126).

Most patients with mesoblastic nephroma are cured by surgical excision without adjuvant chemotherapy or radiotherapy (127). The addition of chemotherapy has resulted in increased morbidity and, in some instances, fatal complications. In rare cases, such as older infants presenting with metastatic disease or when there is tumor rupture and spillage, chemotherapeutic intervention with regimens containing actinomycin D, vincristine, cyclophosphamide, and doxorubicin have been used effectively. Similar regimens have been used in the rare recurrences (128–130). Radiotherapy also has shown efficacy in patients with local recurrence.

Persistent Renal Blastema, Nephroblastomatosis, and Wilms Tumor

The adult or metanephric kidney arises from a complex, inductive interaction between the evaginating uteric bud and its bifurcations with the metanephric, mesodermally derived blastema. By 36 weeks of gestation, normal nephrogenesis is complete, with no residual metanephric blastema. When these metanephric blastemal elements persist, they usually are characterized by microscopic clusters of primitive blastema and occasionally some tubular differentiation (i.e., persistent metanephric blastema). If these fetal rests proliferate, they may develop along several different histologic pathways, each of which has particular relevance to the evolution of Wilms tumor (128–133). Nephroblastomatosis represents the persistence and cellular expansion of metanephric blastema beyond the cessation of nephrogenesis. The proliferation may occur in characteristic patterns, either multifocal or diffuse.

Multifocal nephroblastomatosis refers to the widespread proliferation of blastemal cells, most prominently in the subcapsular cortex as well as along the penetrating columns of Bertin. Nephromegaly is not always evident. Unlike mesoblastic nephroma, multifocal nephroblastomatosis is associated with congenital malformation syndromes and chromosomal abnormalities. Within the category of multifocal nephroblastomatosis, there are several characteristic lesions. When persistent blastema proliferate in small 100- to 300-μm foci separated by normal renal parenchyma, they are referred to as nodular renal blastema. Nodular renal blastema may regress or evolve into what has been called sclerosing metanephric hamartoma as well as into Wilms tumorlets, which are 0.3 to 3.5 cm in diameter, noninfiltrating, often multiple, neoplastic tumors separated by normal renal parenchyma. They usually consist of blastema with a monomorphous epithelial pattern of differentiation. Although they resemble true Wilms tumor, they are distinguishable by their smaller size and their noninfiltrating behavior.

A second type of nephroblastomatosis, which is quite rare but found more commonly in infants and young children, is diffuse nephroblastomatosis. The blastemal proliferation may be pannephric or superficial, with the latter lesion encasing a normal cortex and medulla. Diffuse nephroblastomatosis presents as bilateral, palpable nephromegaly in association with congenital malformations. Radiographic examination by intravenous pyelo-gram reveals distortion and elongation of the calyceal system without obstruction (134). On gross inspection, there is an exaggerated pattern of fetal lobulation of the enlarged kidneys.

That these various histologic lesions are related to one another and to the evolution of frank Wilms tumor has been strongly suggested by case studies as well as by epidemiologic and pathologic correlations (135–137). In about one-third of cases of Wilms tumor, there is suggestive pathologic evidence for the association of nodular renal blastema, nephroblastomatosis, Wilms tumorlets, and Wilms tumor; in bilateral Wilms tumor, this association is nearly always present (138–140).

Management of nephroblastomatosis involves surgery and sometimes chemotherapy, depending on the extent of disease. Radiation therapy is not very effective. If only one kidney is involved, surgical resection is sufficient, but exploration and biopsy of the contralateral kidney are critical. When both kidneys are extensively involved, nephroblastomatosis usually will respond to the combination chemotherapy used in Wilms tumor (i.e., vincristine and actinomycin). The goal of such treatment is to cause regression of the nephroblastomatosis or cause its evolution to an end-stage hamartoma. The duration of treatment is based on clinical response. Close follow-up with both radiographic and second-look operations is important in that patients still may progress to the development of true Wilms tumor despite therapy.

True Wilms tumor rarely is seen in the neonatal period (123). It generally presents as an asymptomatic abdominal mass that does not cross the midline but, occasionally, the mass is large enough to cause dystocia at the time of delivery. It is rarely associated with gross hematuria, hypertension, or polycythemia secondary to increased erythropoietin levels. The most common congenital abnormalities associated with Wilms tumor are genitourinary and musculoskeletal anomalies, hemihypertrophy, aniridia, and hamartomas (e.g., hemangiomas, nevi, cafe-au-lait spots). In addition, there is the Wilms tumor–aniridia syndrome with its associated deletion of part of the short arm of chromosome 11. CT scan and particularly magnetic resonance imaging (MRI), along with renal ultrasonography, can help define the extent of the tumor.

Pathologically, classic Wilms tumor consists of neoplastic blastemal elements with epithelial and stromal components. In the neonate, Wilms tumor is predominantly epithelial and localized, displaying little invasiveness or metastatic potential. The primary prognostic variables include histology, extent of disease, and age (128,141,142).

The management of a patient with Wilms tumor depends primarily on staging. In the neonate, most patients will be classified as stage I, in that the tumors usually are relatively small (i.e., less than 550 g), localized, noninvasive, and completely resectable. Neonatal

Wilms tumor commonly shows favorable histology and appears to metastasize infrequently. At the time of surgery, a frozen section diagnosis is important in ascertaining whether or not nephroblastomatosis also is present. If it is present, wedge biopsy of the contralateral kidney is indicated, even if it is grossly normal. The management of bilateral Wilms tumor must often be individualized, with the intent of trying to spare as much normal renal parenchyma as possible (143,144). Careful follow-up in such cases is critical.

For patients with stage I disease, the National Wilms Tumor Study group has recommended 6 months of combination chemotherapy with vincristine and actinomycin; radiation therapy is not given. Disease-free, long-term survival has been greater than 90%. More recent information has indicated, however, that in infants with localized, noninvasive, nonmetastatic, histologically favorable tumors weighing less than 550 g, reduced courses of chemotherapy or even no further therapy apart from radical nephrectomy is all that is required (145–147). For advanced stages and for tumors with unfavorable histology, more aggressive therapy, including radiation and intensive chemotherapy, is used (148).

Renal Neoplasms Not Associated with Wilms Tumor

Malignant rhabdoid tumor of the kidney, which represents about 2% of primary renal malignancies in childhood and for which the mean age at diagnosis is 13 months, was first described as a rhabdomyosarcomatoid variant of Wilms tumor. Subsequent studies have suggested that this tumor is neuroepithelial in origin, possibly from neural crest, and therefore is unrelated to Wilms tumor (149–153). This tumor also may be primary in the liver, chest wall, or paravertebral area. There is an association with posterior fossa brain tumors and a predilection for metastasizing to the brain (154). In addition, another potential association with the development of rhabdoid tumor is the presence of dermal neurovascular hamartomas (155). Despite aggressive therapy, this tumor is associated with a very poor prognosis.

The clear cell sarcoma of the kidney, also originally described as a Wilms tumor variant, is now considered a separate entity (156–158). It represents about 2% to 5% of all childhood malignant tumors of the kidney. Age at presentation is similar to that in Wilms tumor. Clear cell renal sarcoma demonstrates a predilection to metastasize to bone. It carries a poor prognosis, with at least a 50% mortality even with aggressive therapy.

TUMORS OF GERM CELL ORIGIN

Germ cell tumors are derived from the stem cells of the embryo that ultimately are determined to differentiate into spermatocytes or ova. Such cells are totipotent and, therefore, are capable of giving rise to tumors containing any fetal, embryonal, or adult tissue. In addition, their spatial distribution and migration pattern during embryogenesis help explain the various anatomic sites in which such tumors may develop. For example, human primordial germ cells can be recognized first in the 4-week embryo as large cells embedded in a restricted area of the yolk sac. During the fifth week of gestation, the germ cells migrate from the yolk sac to the hindgut wall and along the mesentery to the gonadal ridge, where they encounter the gonadal anlage. From there they descend into the pelvis or scrotal sac. During their migration from the yolk sac to the definitive gonad, germ cells may be left behind or they may migrate too far along the dorsal wall of the embryo near the midline. Thus, aside from the gonads, germ cell-derived tumors quite commonly arise in locations at or near the midline, anywhere from the sacrum to the head. Depending on their viability, embryonic stage, and anatomic location, they may differentiate along a variety of different cell lineages.

For example, germinomas arise from primitive but developmentally restricted germ cells. When they occur in the testis, they are referred to as seminomas; when they are found in the ovary, they are called dysgerminomas. These neoplasms also may be found outside the gonads, particularly in the mediastinal and pineal regions, and in such cases are referred to as extragonadal germinomas. Germinomas occur only rarely during infancy and develop almost exclusively in older children and adults.

Embryonal carcinoma, which occurs most commonly in individuals from 4 to 28 years of age (median age 15 years), represents a highly malignant tumor of the multipotential germ cells that has the capacity to differentiate further into either extraembryonal or embryonal tissue lineages. Because of this capacity, embryonal carcinoma is considered to arise in the stem cells that can give rise to endodermal sinus (i.e., yolk sac) tumor or choriocarcinoma, both of which are extraembryonal in origin, as well as to teratomas, which are embryonal in origin.

Endodermal Sinus or Yolk Sac Tumors

The endodermal sinus, or yolk sac, tumor represents the most common testicular malignancy occurring in children under the age of 4 years. This tumor also has been called embryonal adenocarcinoma, mesoblastoma, orchioblastoma, and choroid teratoma. At times, it has been confused with embryonal carcinoma. These tumors characteristically form a histologic picture reminiscent of the yolk sac. They may metastasize to the retroperitoneal lymph nodes, which constitute the drainage pathway from the testis, to the liver, to the lung, and to bone, although metastatic disease in the infant is unusual (159,160). Biochemically, yolk sac tumors usually are associated with elevated levels of alpha-fetoprotein, which serves as a useful marker in diagnosis, assessment of treatment response, or of relapse.

The assessment of a patient with the possibility of a germ cell tumor of the testis should include an assay for both alpha-fetoprotein and human chorionic gonadotropin levels; the latter, if positive, suggests a mixed tumor with choriocarcinomatous elements. Radiographic workup should include a chest radiograph, chest CT scan, and abdominal CT scan or MRI. A radionuclide scan may be helpful in detecting spread to bone.

After the workup, the operation of choice is a radical orchiectomy with high ligation of the spermatic cord at the level of the internal inguinal ring. A transscrotal approach is contraindicated because of the risk of seeding the scrotal sac with tumor cells. Whether or not all children with testicular yolk sac tumors should undergo retroperitoneal dissection as part of further staging remains controversial. Some studies suggest that in infants younger than 12 months of age, only orchiectomy is needed, with close follow-up including radiographic studies, monitoring of alpha-fetoprotein levels, and physical examination (160—162). In other studies, however, approximately 40% of children younger than age 2 years treated only with orchiectomy die from metastatic disease, compared to only 12% treated with retroperitoneal node dissection and radiation therapy with or without chemotherapy (163,164). These reports suggest that management should include orchiectomy, lymph node dissection, combination chemotherapy, and radiation therapy for those patients with retroperitoneal nodes positive for metastatic disease. Endodermal sinus tumors also may arise in the ovary, usually at a median age of 19 years, as well as in extragonadal sites such as the pineal body, mediastinum, sacrococcyx, and the infant vagina.

The extraembryonal cell lineage pathway also may lead to a trophoblastic-derived tumor called choriocarcinoma. Although this neoplasm is extremely rare, when it occurs in infants younger than 12 months of age, it usually is a result of transmission of a placental choriocarcinoma. Patients usually present with pallor, hepatomegaly, and a history of gastrointestinal bleeding with hemoptysis or hematuria. There may be endocrinologic manifestations, with breast enlargement and pubic hair. Chest radiographs may reveal pulmonary metastases; human chorionic gonadotropin levels most often are elevated. Such gestational-related choriocarcinomas are particularly responsive to treatment with methotrexate (165).

Teratomas

When germ cell tumors arise from the embryonal compartment, they form teratomas. These are neoplasms that contain cellular or tissue derivatives of more than one of the three primary embryonal germ layers and that are foreign to the anatomic region in which they arise. The name teratoma is derived from the Greek *teratos,* which literally means monster, plus the ending "-oma," which is used to denote a neoplasm. This name derived from cases in which these tumors contained tissue elements so well organized as to resemble a deformed fetus.

In early childhood, teratomas primarily occur as extragonadal masses located along the midline axis; about 40% to 50% occur in the sacrococcygeal region, with head and neck, brain, mediastinum, retroperitoneum, abdomen, spinal cord, and other soft tissue locations accounting for 1% to 5% each (166). Gonadal teratomas occur more frequently after puberty, particularly in the ovary. About 80% to 90% of early childhood teratomas are benign; malignant teratomas usually are characterized histologically by areas containing embryonal carcinoma or endodermal sinus tumor. Such malignant lesions most often arise in the sacrococcygeal region.

Sacrococcygeal teratoma is the most common teratoma in infancy, with about 67% diagnosed by the age of 1 year. These tumors occur at a rate of 1 in 25,000 to 1 in 40,000 live births and display a significant gender predilection, with girls being affected more than 75% of the time (167,168).

Clinically, these tumors present as a mass protruding between the coccyx and the rectum (Fig. 53–2). They nearly always arise from the tip of the coccyx and vary greatly in the amount of their internal versus external tissue extensions (167). Some lesions can be diagnosed only by rectal examination; however, this examination should be done with extreme care in the neonate to avoid any traumatic damage. The differential diagnosis of a sacrococcygeal teratoma includes meningomyelocele, rectal abscess, pilonidal cyst, bladder neck obstruction, rectal prolapse, duplications of the rectum, imperforate anus, dermoid cyst, angioma, lymphangioma, lipoma, neurogenic tumors of the pelvis and perineum, giant cell tumor of the sacrum, and soft tissue sarcoma.

Benign teratomas usually will produce no functional problems other than obstruction, whereas the presence of bowel or bladder dysfunction suggests a malignant lesion. Evidence for venous or lymphatic obstruction or lower leg paralysis is found more commonly in malignant tumors. Approximately 15% of patients with sacrococcygeal teratomas have associated congenital anomalies, including imperforate anus, sacral bone defects, genitourinary abnormalities such as duplication of the uterus or vagina, and occasionally spina bifida and meningomyelocele (169). Radiographic evaluation of the spine can be informative in that meningomyeloceles are associated with characteristic vertebral abnormalities. Abdominal and pelvic ultrasonography along with CT or MRI scanning are useful in assessing the internal extension of the mass. Barium enema may distinguish between a bowel duplication and displacement caused by a tumor mass. Chest radiographs and liver–spleen scans may indicate evidence of metastatic disease. Serum alpha-fetoprotein and human chorionic gonadotropin levels may be elevated in those teratomas with mixed cellular elements.

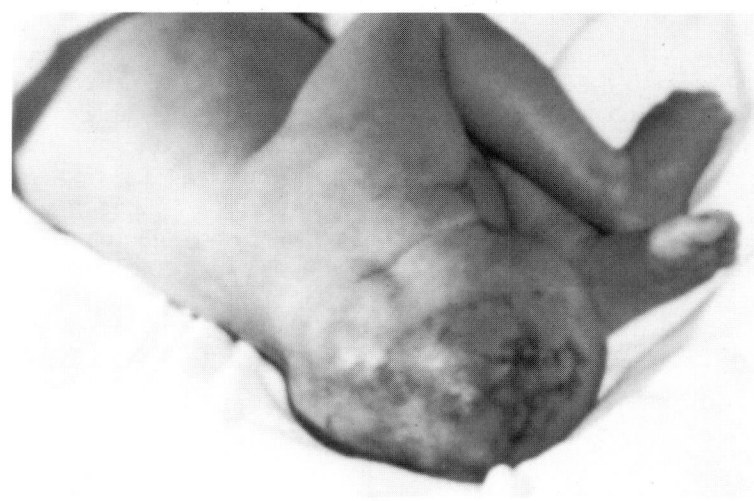

FIG. 53–2. Large sacrococcygeal teratoma in a newborn infant.

The prognosis for a patient with a sacrococcygeal teratoma depends primarily on whether the lesion is benign or malignant (170). For benign lesions, disease-free survival is greater than 90%, whereas for those tumors with malignant components, such as anaplasia or yolk sac histology, associated mortality secondary to tumor may be greater than 90%. The age of the patient at diagnosis appears to be extremely important in determining the likelihood of malignancy. For example, the incidence of malignancy is only 7% to 10% for tumors diagnosed at younger than 2 months of age, whereas this figure increases to about 37% at age 1 year and to 50% by age 2 years. In addition, there is a significantly higher incidence of malignancy in lesions that show mostly internal tissue extension (167).

The management of a patient with a benign sacrococcygeal teratoma is primarily surgical and includes removal of the coccyx, the site where the tumor arises. Leaving the coccyx is associated with a 30% to 40% incidence of recurrence, many of which are malignant (171). Patients with malignant teratomas are managed after surgery with irradiation, if residual disease is present, and always with combination chemotherapy. Some regimens include vincristine, actinomycin D, and cyclophosphamide; others use vinblastine, bleomycin, and *cis*-platinum (172,173). Regardless of intensive therapy, the prognosis in such patients is poor. The average interval between diagnosis and death usually is less than 10 months, with metastatic disease occurring in lungs, bone, liver, lymph nodes, and peritoneum (167,174,175). Not surprisingly, survival is extremely rare among patients who develop metastatic disease.

PRIMARY HEPATIC NEOPLASMS

The differential diagnosis of a right upper quadrant mass with hepatomegaly in infants is extensive and includes nonneoplastic lesions as well as a variety of benign and malignant tumors (176,177). Hemangioendothelioma is the most common tumor found in neonates. Hepatomegaly associated with malignant disease in the infant is secondary much more commonly to leukemia or disseminated neuroblastoma than to a primary hepatic cancer.

Hepatocellular carcinoma, often associated with chronic underlying liver disease, rarely occurs in infancy. This tumor usually is massive, multifocal, and rapid growing, all contributing factors to its frequent unresectability. In spite of aggressive combined modality treatment, such patients have a poor prognosis, with up to 90% mortality (178,179).

Hepatoblastoma occurs primarily but not exclusively in children younger than age 3 years, with a mean age of 18 months; it also has been reported in neonates (180–182). There have been anecdotal reports of patients with hepatoblastoma associated with the maternal use of oral contraceptives or with the fetal alcohol syndrome (183,184). Low birth weight also has been associated with the development of hepatoblastoma (185,186). Familial cases of hepatoblastoma have been documented, suggesting an environmental or genetic contribution in some instances (187,188). Hepatoblastoma also has been associated with a variety of congenital anomalies, most notably hemihypertrophy and renal abnormalities, but also with macroglossia, Meckel's diverticulum, tetralogy of Fallot, diaphragmatic hernia, talipes equinovarus, and digital clubbing (188). Wilms tumor and adrenal cortical neoplasms also have been found in patients with hepatoblastoma (189).

Hepatoblastoma presents in most cases with abdominal enlargement and hepatomegaly. In approximately 25% of patients, there also will be associated anorexia, weight loss, pallor, and pain. Less common are vomiting and jaundice. Diarrhea, fever, and precocious puberty are rare. Laboratory studies reveal a mild anemia, a thrombocytosis with bone marrow megakaryocytosis, and, occasionally, thrombocytopenia secondary to platelet trapping (190,191). Increased levels of liver enzyme transaminases and alkaline phosphatase are variable, but mild elevation of bilirubin may be present in up to 15% of cases with hepatoblastoma. Alpha-fetoprotein is elevated manyfold in nearly 70% of patients with hepatoblastoma (192). Although not specific for hepatoblastoma, this protein marker, with a half-life of 4 to 6 days, is useful in the assessment of the response to therapy and of tumor recurrence. It should be noted, however, that not all recurring metastatic lesions are positive for alpha-fetoprotein, even though the primary tumor was positive. All values for alpha-fetoprotein should be compared to age-matched values, because levels normally are elevated in the neonatal period and may normalize to adult values for up to 9 months (193,194).

Abdominal radiographs show enlargement of the liver, with the right lobe more commonly involved. Areas of calcification occur in up to 20% of cases. Chest radiographs may reveal pulmonary metastases, present in about 10% of cases at diagnosis. Abdominal CT or MRI scanning and hepatic angiography are useful in determining tumor size and surgical resectability. Radioisotopic liver scans demonstrate the tumor by its decreased ability to take up the isotope; it appears as a cold lesion when compared with the surrounding, normal hepatic tissue.

The prognosis for patients with hepatoblastoma appears to depend primarily on the lesion's surgical resectability and on histology. Complete surgical excision is possible in 40% to 75% of patients, although perioperative mortality may be as high as 10% to 25%. Local and metastatic recurrences after surgical resection appear within 36 months, although there have been recurrences as late as 8 years after surgery (181,195).

The histopathology of hepatoblastoma can be viewed as occurring in two major patterns. The first is the pure fetal epithelial type. Several studies have strongly suggested that this type of tumor is associated with a better outcome (179,196–198). The second type, composed of both epithelial and mesenchymal elements, usually is referred to as a mixed hepatoblastoma and has been associated with a poorer prognosis. In addition, some hepatoblastomas may have anaplastic or sarcomatous elements that portend a poor prognosis.

Although some reports have demonstrated that approximately 30% to 60% of patients can be cured with complete surgical resection alone, others have shown that adjuvant chemotherapy after tumor resection significantly reduces the risk of development of distant metastases. Chemotherapy should begin about 4 weeks after resection to allow for the adequate regeneration of normal hepatic tissue. For those children with unresectable primary tumors, preoperative irradiation or combination chemotherapy or both may reduce tumor size to allow resection (199–204). Radiation therapy has a limited role, in part because normal liver has a relatively low tolerance to irradiation. The response of both the primary tumor and metastatic disease to chemotherapeutic agents has been best when such agents have been used in combination; they include vincristine, actinomycin D, cyclophosphamide, 5-fluorouracil, doxorubicin, cis-platinum, and methotrexate (205–208). Chemotherapy not only has caused regression of primary tumors, but it also has been associated with a few long-term remissions in patients with pulmonary metastases. For situations where the tumor cannot be resected, even after cytoreductive therapy, liver transplantation has been used.

SOFT TISSUE SARCOMAS

Soft tissue tumors represent a diverse group of neoplasms, all of which share a common cellular origin from mesenchymal elements. In the infant, the spectrum of soft tissue tumor types includes fibrosarcomas, RMS, non-RMS soft tissue sarcomas, and fibrous proliferative neoplasms as well as the rhabdoid tumor (see section on neoplasms of the kidney) (209–212).

RMS accounts for about one-half of soft tissue sarcomas, but is extraordinarily rare in the neonate (213). It may present as an orbital, nasopharyngeal, or sinus tumor; as a truncal or extremity lesion; as a genitourinary tract tumor, usually arising from bladder, prostate, or vagina; or as a paratesticular mass. At the time of diagnosis, about 20% to 40% of patients have evident metastatic disease, usually to lung, lymph nodes, liver, bone marrow, bone, and brain (214,215).

After appropriate assessment of the primary tumor and possible metastatic sites, complete surgical resection with clean margins should be attempted if this can be accomplished with acceptable morbidity. Adjuvant chemotherapy with vincristine, actinomycin D, and cyclophosphamide significantly prolongs disease-free survival. If there is residual microscopic disease as evidenced by involved surgical margins, irradiation usually is used in older children, but should be modified for the neonate or infant because of long-term toxicities (216).

The prognosis for patients with RMS depends on the stage at presentation and histology. In children with the embryonal subtype and early-stage tumors, disease-free survival is greater than 80%, whereas in those with more extensive disease or alveolar histology, prognosis remains poor (211,212,214,215,217–219).

Fibrosarcoma represents about 10% of soft tissue sarcomas in patients younger than age 15 years, and more than one-half occur in children younger than age 5 years, with about one-third of these appearing at or shortly after birth (220,221). Congenital infantile fibrosarcoma is a cellular, mitotically active neoplasm with a paradoxically limited biologic potential in most children in contrast to fibrosarcomas in older children (222,223). Fibrosarcoma most commonly arises in the extremities, with the remaining cases involving the back, retroperitoneum, sacrococcyx, and the head and neck, as well as occurring as an intracardiac lesion (220,221,224,225).

For extremity lesions, complete surgical resection is curative in more than 90% of cases, even though local recurrences are common, appearing about 20% to 40% of the time. Occasionally, amputation may be required. Metastatic disease occurs only rarely. For tumors that are not amenable to surgical resection because of size or location, or both, there is some evidence that combination chemotherapy may be quite effective (222,226). Overall survival for infants with fibrosarcoma, RMS, or non-RMS neoplasms has been estimated to be about 60% (209). Results with radiation therapy have been poor (220,221).

Possibly related to fibrosarcoma, but nevertheless distinguishable pathologically, is a group of fibroblastic proliferative disorders that may be seen in the infant and newborn. The digital fibroma is usually found as a soft tissue mass on the medial side of digits, with the exclusion of the thumbs and great toes. As with fibrosarcoma, surgical resection is curative, although recurrence rates may be as high as 75% to 90%. Congenital (i.e., infantile) fibromatosis may occur as solitary or multiple soft tissue lesions (227,228). The solitary lesions occur nearly anywhere on the body. The lesions can involve a wide variety of skeletal sites, and be the cause of significant bone pain in the neonate (229–234). When present as multiple lesions, they involve subcutaneous tissue, muscle, and bones; in some cases, the lesions may become more generalized, producing significant morbidity and mortality from visceral organ involvement (235,236). These tumors are pathologically benign in appearance. The solitary and multiple lesions are histologically similar, and it has been proposed that they are related to congenital fibrosarcoma and congenital hemangiopericytoma (237).

Treatment of solitary lesions is surgical and curative. There have been several reports of patients with multiple congenital fibromatosis in which spontaneous regression has occurred (238–240). After a diagnosis is made, treatment has been primarily supportive, with an excellent prognosis for multiple lesions involving subcutaneous tissue, muscle, and bone, and a poor prognosis when visceral organ involvement is extensive (235,236). There is little proven benefit from the use of chemotherapy in cases of fibromatosis, although a report of use of a combination of vincristine, actinomycin D, and cyclophosphamide in an infant with unresectable neck fibromatosis showed an apparently good response (241).

VASCULAR NEOPLASMS AND MALFORMATIONS

Hemangiomas are the most common tumors found in infancy and childhood (242,243). They usually appear during late fetal or early neonatal life and affect girls more commonly than boys. Skin is the most frequent site of involvement, although they may arise in any organ and often occur in multiple locations. They are soft, compressible, bright red to blue lesions found on a level with, or slightly above, the surface of the skin. They range in size from a few millimeters to quite massive, occupying large areas of the skin or internal organs.

Their natural course is characterized by rapid growth for the first 4 to 6 months of life, followed by stabilization, then gradual involution over several years. They may be considered true neoplasms in that, during the proliferative phase, they show greatly increased endothelial cell proliferation. They should be distinguished from vascular malformations such as arteriovenous fistulas, which represent anomalous vascular development and do not demonstrate endothelial cell proliferation. Such lesions nearly always are present at birth and increase in size along with the patient, without the usual phase of involution. Lymphatic lesions, such as lymphangioma, are best considered malformations rather than neoplastic growths (244–246).

The clinical complications that arise from hemangiomas are secondary to their size, site of origin, and physiology. They may compromise vision by encroaching on the eye; cause respiratory distress by impinging on the trachea; cause severe and even fatal congestive heart failure when they are very large, as in some liver lesions; cause gastrointestinal or CNS hemorrhage; or cause a consumptive coagulopathy from platelet and fibrinogen trapping, as in Kasabach–Merritt syndrome. Lesions responsible for Kasabach–Merritt syndrome may be a mixture of a proliferative endothelial neoplasm as well as a malformation sometimes involving lymphatic channels (247).

The first principle of treatment should be to do no harm, because most of these lesions eventually will regress on their own. Nevertheless, when they are the cause of significant morbidity, intervention may be necessary. Corticosteroids probably are an effective treatment and may accelerate regression (246,248,249). Radiotherapy may cause undesirable side effects, such as cutaneous scarring, dermatitis, growth disturbances, and possible second tumors (250–252). Surgery may be difficult for large lesions and may result in unsightly scarring (253). For large lesions of the liver, hepatic artery ligation or embolization occasionally has been successful in controlling high-output cardiac failure, but liver necrosis, renal failure, and other embolic complications may result (254–256). One study has used the intralesional injection of bleomycin to effect regression of complex cutaneous hemangiomas (257). In cases of Kasabach–Merritt syndrome, heparin or aspirin plus dipyridamole, pentoxifylline, and steroids plus ε-aminocaproic acid have proved useful in treating the associated consumptive coagulopathy (258–261). Laser therapy also has been used effectively (262). Subglottic hemangiomas may be life threatening secondary to airway compromise; their treatment has involved laser therapy and surgery, as well as steroids and α-interferon (263,264). The use of α-interferon has demonstrated promising results in cases resistant to corticosteroids (264). MRI can be an effective tool for imaging hemangiomas as well as assessing their response to therapy (265).

Malignant tumors arising from vascular endothelium, such as hemangioendothelioma, hemangiopericytoma, and angiosarcoma, are extremely rare but have been reported in infants (266,267). More information on vascular neoplasms and malformations is given in Chapter 54.

HISTIOCYTOSES

The histiocytoses of childhood represent a heterogeneous group of disorders involving bone marrow derived antigen-presenting cells (268–271). In the late 1980s, the histiocytoses were classified into three separate classes, in part based on the type of histiocyte believed to be pathologically involved (272). This classification schema separated these disorders into: class I—Langerhans cell histiocytosis (LCH); class II—non-LCH; and class III—malignant histiocytosis. Although this classification system has proven useful in delineating these complex disorders, particularly for treatment study purposes, improved understanding of the biology of these diseases will undoubtedly change the manner in which they are defined, grouped, and treated.

Class I, or the Langehrhans cell histiocytoses, includes disorders historically referred to as eosinophilic granuloma, Hand–Christian–Schuller disease, and Letterer–Siwe disease. The diagnosis of the class I histiocytoses is made by biopsy showing characteristic pathologic changes, which include a histologically mixed, reactive infiltrate of cells including eosinophils, neutrophils, lymphocytes, multinucleated giant cells, and proliferation of Langerhans cell histiocytes. Langerhans cell histiocytes are identified by their expression of S-100 and CD1a surface antigens and/or the presence of cytoplasmic Birbeck granules. Birbeck granules most probably represent internalized membrane components and have a characteristic racquet appearance under the electron microscope. Several studies have demonstrated that LCH is a clonal neoplastic disorder (273–277).

Eosinophilic granuloma is found predominantly in older children, teenagers, and young adults, usually presenting as solitary or multiple lytic lesions of bone. Surgical curettage alone is usually curative. The prognosis is excellent. Local recurrences rarely need additional surgery and often can be treated with local injection of steroids if in an easily accessible site (278), local radiation therapy with doses in the 400- to 800-cGy range, or even oral, nonsteroidal antiinflammatory agents such as indomethacin (279,280).

Hand–Schuller–Christian disease occurs in younger children from ages 2 to 5 years and often presents with multifocal, lytic bone lesions, particularly of the skull; exophthalmia; oral soft tissue involvement; eczematoid rash; and, sometimes, diabetes insipidus secondary to hypothalamic infiltration. The clinical course is chronic, with multiple recurrences over several years. Therapeutic interventions are indicated for disease that is symptomatic, potentially disfiguring, or likely to result in loss of function, such as loss of vision with proptosis, loss of hearing with extensive mastoid involvement, or paralysis secondary to cord compression (281–286). For localized lesions, surgical curettage, lesional injection of steroids, or low-dose radiation therapy is effective. When there are multifocal bone lesions or multisystem disease, chemotherapy is indicated (281–287). Vinblastine or steroids alone or in combination has been shown to be quite effective (284,287,288). An international randomized trial compared vinblastine plus steroid with etoposide plus steroid and demonstrated no difference in efficacy of one regimen over the other (286). More intensive, combination chemotherapy is being studied for patients with extensive disease in an attempt to reduce the incidence of recurring disease and long-term sequelae due to the disease (285).

Letterer–Siwe disease is the most severe and life-threatening form of LCH. It most commonly presents within the first year of life and occasionally in neonates. Cases have been reported among siblings as well as in twins (289,290). Infants present with scaly, seborrheic, eczematoid, and sometimes maculopapular rashes involving the scalp, face, ear canals, abdomen, and intertriginous areas. Hepatosplenomegaly is common, and there may be signs of hepatic dysfunction with hypoproteinemia and coagulopathy. Draining ears, lymphadenopathy, cough, and tachypnea are common. These infants are irritable and fail to thrive, secondary either to chronic disease and liver dysfunction, or to malabsorption due to gastrointestinal infiltration. Lytic bone lesions often are present.

The prognosis for severe Letterer–Siwe disease with liver, lung, or hematopoietic organ dysfunction is poor despite intensive combination chemotherapy, with mortality reaching 50% (270,271,284,287,288,291,292). Hematologic studies reveal anemia, a variable leukocytosis, and thrombocytopenia, with the latter finding frequently predicting a fatal outcome. As in the case of Hand–Schuller–Christian disease, vinblastine with prednisone has been shown to be a relatively effective combination, although a more intensive combination chemotherapy regimen is being tested in an international trial (284–286,293,294). Anecdotal cases using cyclosporine A have been reported (295–297). In refractory cases, allogeneic bone marrow transplantation has been effective, but the overall results have been disappointing (298–303). Low-dose hemi-body or whole-body radiation therapy has been used, but without prolonged efficacy (304). New agents such as nucleoside inhibitors and more potent immunosuppressive agents are being tested (305–311).

Class II represents the non-Langerhans cell histiocytoses and primarily includes the hemophagocytic lymphohistiocytic disorders also referred to as familial erythrophagocytic lymphohistiocytosis (FEL) and infection-associated hemophagocytic syndrome. FEL, which presents in early infancy, is inherited as an autosomal recessive condition (312–318). Infants present with failure to thrive, anorexia, fever, and irritability. Seizures and spastic weakness of the limbs may occur secondary to CNS involvement (319,320). Hepatosplenomegaly usually is prominent. Skin, bones, and lymph nodes, although often affected, are less involved than in Letterer–Siwe disease. Laboratory data characteristically show a hypofibrinogenemia as well as a distinctive hyperlipidemia, with increased triglycerides and decreased high-density lipoproteins (315,321–323). Pancytopenia develops, and bleeding often becomes a major concern for these critically ill patients. These patients usually have very low to absent natural killer lymphocyte function, suggesting that these disorders may be due to an underlying immune defect (317,324). It currently is not possible, however, to detect the carrier status for this disease with absolute certainty, although it is intriguing that otherwise normal parents or siblings of these patients also may show severely depressed natural killer lymphocyte function (317,324, 325). Pathologically, there is extensive lymphohistiocytic infiltration associated with erythrophagocytosis in the visceral organs and leptomeninges, with ultimate depletion of lymphoid tissue.

Prognosis is poor, and most infants will die within weeks of diagnosis from sepsis or hemorrhage, or both. Plasmapheresis, repeated blood exchange, and high-dose intravenous immunoglobulin have been reported to produce temporary remissions (326). Treatment with the epipodophyllotoxin, VP-16, along with high-dose steroids and intrathecal methotrexate, is an effective regimen that can achieve a temporary remission of disease (327,328). Following the induction of a remission, however, allogeneic stem cell transplantation is the only know curative therapy (298,329,330).

Some infants may present with a picture of histiocytosis localized primarily to the skin and occasionally bone. They usually have a rash that shows hard, red to dark blue nodules, which occasionally may crust over. This disorder, which undergoes spontaneous resolution within weeks to months, requires no therapy. It is referred to as congenital self-healing histiocytosis, or self-healing reticulohistiocytosis (331–333).

Class III includes malignant disorders of the histiocyte, such as malignant histiocytosis and histiocytic sarcoma, neither of which occurs in the neonatal period (272). In addition, it is now appreciated that most cases described as malignant histiocytosis are really anaplastic large cell lymphomas, which rarely, if ever, appear in infants (314, 334,335).

THERAPEUTIC ISSUES AND LATE EFFECTS OF THERAPY

The issues surrounding the treatment of cancer in infants and young children are unique. Because of their very young age, the balance between therapy and long-term side effects becomes especially important. A close collaboration and coordination by subspecialists is critical.

Surgical management must consider the distinctive aspects of neonatal biology (336). Some tumors, such as hemangiomas and stage IV-S neuroblastoma, frequently involute or regress on their own, obviating surgical intervention. With other tumors, such as localized neuroblastomas, a complete resection may be unnecessary, whereas in cases of hepatoblastoma, an incomplete resection may portend a fatal outcome.

The detrimental effects of irradiation to infants are profoundly demonstrated in the treatment of patients with brain tumors, resulting in a high incidence and degree of mental retardation. Skeletal growth also may be severely affected, with deformities of limbs and scoliosis. Liver, lung, and kidney are major organs whose short- and long-term function can be compromised (337). In addition, the late appearance of second tumors may be significantly increased as a result of the mutagenic effects of irradiation (338).

For many solid tumors, chemotherapy has been effective in the treatment of micrometastatic disease as well as residual disease after incomplete resection. In cases of disease that is disseminated at the time of diagnosis, such as in leukemia or advanced neuroblastoma, systemic chemotherapy is imperative. The use of chemotherapy in the newborn is complicated by unique differences in absorption, distribution, metabolism, and excretion of such drugs (339,340). In addition, these characteristics are constantly changing, as the infant undergoes rapid developmental changes. Dose adjustments are required for certain chemotherapeutic drugs to avoid untoward complications in situations where decreased drug metabolism occurs, as well as in cases of increased drug metabolism in order to achieve effective antitumor drug levels (341,342). Some of the signs and symptoms of drug toxicity may be subtle and must be related to the behavioral repertoire of the infant. Survivors of the successful treatment of malignancy in infancy should be followed closely for long-term sequelae (343,344).

REFERENCES

1. Bader J, Miller R. US Cancer incidence and mortality in the first year of life. *Am J Dis Child* 1979;133:157.

2. Borch K, Jacobsen T, Olsen JH, Hirsch FR, Hertz H. Neonatal cancer in Denmark 1943–1985. *Ugeskr Laeger* 1994;156:176.

3. Parkes S, Muir K, Southern L, et al. Neonatal tumours: a thirty-year population-based study. *Med Pediatr Oncol* 1994;22:309.

4. Ross JA, Severson RK, Pollock BH, Robison LL. Childhood cancer in the United States. A geographical analysis of cases from the Pediatric Cooperative Clinical Trials groups. *Cancer* 1996;77:201.

5. Gurney JG, Davis S, Severson RK, Fang JY, Ross JA, Robison LL. Trends in cancer incidence among children in the U.S. *Cancer* 1996; 78:532.

6. Fraumeni JF Jr, Miller RW. Cancer deaths in the newborn. *Am J Dis Child* 1969;117:186.

7. Xue H, Horwitz J, Smith M, et al. Malignant solid tumors in neonates: a 40-year review. *J Pediatr Surg* 1995;30:543.

8. Martinez-Climent J, Cavalle T, Ferris-Tortajada J. Non-malignant tumors that can mimic cancer during the neonatal period. *Eur J Pediatr Surg* 1995;5:156.

9. Satge D, Van Den Berghe H. Aspects of the neoplasms observed in patients with constitutional autosomal trisomy. *Cancer Genet Cytogenet* 1996;87:63.

10. Koufos A, Hansen M, Coperland N, Jenkins NA, Lampkin BC, Cavenee WK. Loss of heterozygosity in three embryonal tumors suggests a common pathogenetic mechanism. *Nature* 1985;316:330.

11. Donehower LA, Harvey M, Slagle BL, et al. Mice deficient for p53 are developmentally normal but susceptible to spontaneous tumours. *Nature* 1992;356:215.

12. Hansen R, Oren M. p53; from inductive signal to cellular effect. *Curr Opin Genet Dev* 1997;7:46.

13. Haupt Y, Oren M. p53-mediated apoptosis: mechanisms and regulation. *Behring Inst Mitt* 1996;97:32.

14. Oren M. Lonely no more: p53 finds its kin in a tumor suppressor haven. *Cell* 1997;90:829.

15. Reardon JT, Bessho T, Kung HC, Bolton PH, Sancar A. In vitro repair of oxidative DNA damage by human nucleotide excision repair system: possible explanation for neurodegeneration in xeroderma pigmentosum patients. *Proc Natl Acad Sci U S A* 1997;94:9463.

16. Ellis NA. DNA helicases in inherited human disorders. *Curr Opin Genet Dev* 1997;7:354.

17. Rothstein R, Gangloff S. Hyper-recombination and Bloom's syndrome: microbes again provide clues about cancer. *Genome Res* 1995; 5:421.

18. Kunkel TA, Resnick MA, Gordenin DA. Mutator specificity and disease: looking over the FENce. *Cell* 1997;88:155.

19. Kolodner RD. Mismatch repair: mechanisms and relationship to cancer susceptibility. *Trends Biochem Sci* 1995;20:397.

20. D'Andrea AD, Grompe M. Molecular biology of Fanconi anemia: implications for diagnosis and therapy. *Blood* 1997;90:1725.

21. Quesnel S, Malkin D. Genetic predisposition to cancer and familial and familial cancer syndromes. *Pediatr Oncol* 1997;44:791.

22. Slamon DJ, Cline MJ. Expression of cellular oncogenes during embryonic and fetal development of the mouse. *Proc Natl Acad Sci U S A* 1984;81:7141.

23. Forrester LM, Brunkow M, Bernstein A. Proto-oncogenes in mammalian development. *Curr Opin Genet Dev* 1992;2:38.

24. Pavelic K, Slaus, NP, Spaventi R. Growth factors and proto-oncogenes in early mouse embryogenesis and tumorigenesis. *Int J Dev Biol* 1991;35:209.

25. Clarke AR. The role of the tumor suppressor genes p53 and Rb-1 in development and cell death. *Birth Defects* 1996;30:261.

26. Kruslin B, Hrascan R, Manojlovic S, Pavelic K. Oncoproteins and tumor suppressor proteins in congenital sacrococcygeal teratomas. *Pediatr Pathol Lab Med* 1997;17:43.

27. Donegan WL. Cancer and pregnancy. *CA Can J Clin* 1983;33:194.

28. Baergen R, Johnson D, Moore T, Benirschke K. Maternal melanoma metastatic to the placenta: a case report and review of the literature. *Arch Pathol Lab Med* 1997;121:508.

29. Chatten J, Voorhess M. Familial neuroblastoma. Report of a kindred with multiple disorders, including neuroblastomas in four siblings. *N Engl J Med* 1967;277:1230.

30. Mario JM, Brodeur GM. Are certain children more likely to develop neuroblastoma? *J Pediatr* 1997;131:656.

31. Voute P, Wadman S, van Putten W. Congenital neuroblastoma: symptoms in the mother during pregnancy. *Clin Pediatr* 1970;9:206.

32. Jaffe N. Neuroblastoma: review of the literature and an examination of the factors contributing to its enigmatic character. *Cancer Treat Rev* 1976;3:61.

33. Giulian BB, Chang CCN, Yoss BS. Prenatal ultrasonographic diagnosis of fetal adrenal neuroblastoma. *J Clin Ultrasound* 1986;14:225.

34. Forman HP, Leonidas JC, Berdon WE, Slovis TL, Wood BP, Samudrala R. Congenital neuroblastoma: evaluation with multimodality imaging. *Radiology* 1990;175:365.

35. Ho PT, Estroff JA, Kozakewich H, et al. Prenatal detection of neuroblastoma: a ten-year experience from the Dana-Farber Cancer Institute and Children's Hospital. *Pediatrics* 1993;92:358.

36. Iida Y, Nose O, Kai H. Watery diarrhea with vasoactive intestinal peptide-producing ganglioneuroblastoma. *Arch Dis Child* 1980;55:929.

37. Delalieux C, Ebinger G, Maurus R, Sliwoski H. Myoclonic encephalopathy and neuroblastoma. *N Engl J Med* 1975;292:46.

38. D'Angio G, Evans A, Koop C. Special pattern of widespread neuroblastoma with a favorable prognosis. *Lancet* 1971;1:1046.

39. Evans A, D'Angio G, Randolph J. A proposed staging for children with neuroblastoma. *Cancer* 1971;27:374.

40. Brodeur G, Pritchard J, Berthold F, et al. Revisions of the international criteria for neuroblastoma diagnosis, staging and response to treatment. *J Clin Oncol* 1993;11:1466.

41. Laug W, Seigel S, Shaw K, Landing B, Baptista J, Gutenstein M. Initial urinary catecholamine metabolite concentrations and prognosis in neuroblastoma. *Pediatrics* 1978;62:77.

42. van Noesel MM, Hahlen K, Hakvoort-Cammel FG, Egeler RM. Neuroblastoma 4S: a heterogeneous disease with variable risk factors and treatment strategies. *Cancer* 1997;80:834.

43. Schwartz A, Dadash-Zadeh M, Lee H, Swaney J. Spontaneous regression of disseminated neuroblastoma. *J Pediatr* 1974;85:760.

44. Ikeda Y, Lister J, Bouton J, Buyukpamukcu M. Congenital neuroblastoma *in situ* and the normal fetal development of the adrenal. *J Pediatr Surg* 1981;16:636.

45. Beckwith J, Perrin E. In situ neuroblastomas: a contribution to the natural history of neural crest tumors. *Am J Pathol* 1963;43:1089.

46. Esteve J, Parker L, Roy P, et al. Is neuroblastoma screening evaluation needed and feasible? *Br J Cancer* 1995;72:1125.

47. Woods W, Tuchman M, Robison L, et al. The utility of screening for neuroblastoma: a population based study. *Lancet* 1996;348:1682.

48. Law C. Neuroblastoma screening test may do more harm than good. *J Natl Cancer Inst* 1997;89:276.

49. Brodeur GM. Neuroblastoma: clinical significance of genetic abnormalities. *Cancer Surv* 1990;9:673.

50. Castleberry RP. Biology and treatment of neuroblastoma. *Pediatr Clin North Am* 1997;44:919.

51. Evans A, Chatten J, D'Angio G, Gerson JM, Robinson J, Schnaufer L. A review of 17 IV-S neuroblastoma patients at Children's Hospital of Philadelphia. *Cancer* 1980;45:833.

52. Hain R, Rayner L, Weitzman S, Lorenzana A. Acute tumor lysis syndrome complicating treatment of stage IVS neuroblastoma in infants under 6 months old. *Med Pediatr Oncol* 1994;23:136.

53. Hsu L, Evans A, D'Angio G. Hepatomegaly in neuroblastoma stage 4s: criteria for treatment of the vulnerable neonate. *Med Pediatr Oncol* 1996;27:521.

54. Blatt J, Deutsch M, Wollman M. Results of therapy in stage IVs neuroblastoma with massive hepatomegaly. *Int J Radiat Oncol Biol Phys* 1987;13:1467.

55. Hosoda Y, Miyano T, Kimura K, et al. Characteristics and management of patients with fetal neuroblastoma. *J Pediatr Surg* 1992;27: 623.

56. Saito T, Tsunematsu Y, Saeki M, et al. Trends of survival in neuroblastoma and independent risk factors for survival at a single institution. *Med Pediatr Oncol* 1997;29:197.

57. Ellsworth RM. Current concepts in the treatment of retinoblastoma. In: Peyman GA, Apple DJ, Sanders DR, eds. *Intraocular tumors*. New York: Appleton-Century-Crofts, 1977:335.

58. Murphree A, Benedict W. Retinoblastoma: clues to human oncogenes. *Science* 1984;223:1028.

59. Knudson A. Retinoblastoma: a prototypic hereditary neoplasm. *Semin Oncol* 1978;5:57.

60. Sauerwein W, Hopping W, Bornfeld N. Radiotherapy for retinoblastoma. Treatment strategies. *Front Radiat Ther Oncol* 1997;30:93.

61. Pradhan DG, Sandridge AL, Mullaney P, et al. Radiation therapy for retinoblastoma: a retrospective review of 120 patients. *Int J Radiat Oncol Biol Phys* 1997;39:3.

62. Wong FL, Boice JD Jr, Abramson DH, et al. Cancer incidence after retinoblastoma. Radiation dose and sarcoma risk. *JAMA* 1997;278:1262.

63. Gallie BL, Budning A, DeBoer G, et al. Chemotherapy with focal therapy can cure intraocular retinoblastoma without radiotherapy. *Arch Ophthalmol* 1996;114:1321.

64. O'Brien JM, Smith BJ. Chemotherapy in the treatment of retinoblastoma. *Int Ophthalmol Clin* 1996;36:11.

65. Shields CL, De Potter P, Himelstein BP, Shields JA, Meadows AT, Maris JM. Chemoreduction in the initial management of intraocular retinoblastoma. *Arch Ophthalmol* 1996;114:1330.

66. Murphree AL, Villablanca JG, Deegan WF, et al. Chemotherapy plus local treatment in the management of intraocular retinoblastoma. *Arch Ophthalmol* 1996;114:1348.

67. Jooma R, Kendall BE. Intracranial tumours in the first year of life. *Neuroradiology* 1982;23:267.

68. Jooma R, Kendall B, Hayward R. Intracranial tumors: a report of seventeen cases. *Surg Neurol* 1984;21:165.

69. Goldenberg J, Holinger L, Bressler F, Hutchinson L. Bifid epiglottis. *Ann Otol Rhinol Laryngol* 1996;105:2.

70. Takaku A, Kodama N, Ohara H, Hori S. Brain tumor in newborn babies. *Childs Brain* 1978;4:365.

71. Matson DD. Hydrocephalus in a premature infant caused by papilloma of the choroid plexus. *J Neurosurg* 1953;10:416.

72. Bergsagel DJ, Finegold MJ, Butel JS, Kupsky WJ, Garcea RL. DNA sequences similar to those of Simian virus 40 in ependymomas and choroid plexus tumors of childhood. *N Engl J Med* 1992;326:988.

73. Duffner P, Burger P, Cohen M, et al. Desmoplastic infantile gangliogliomas: an approach to therapy. *Neurosurgery* 1994;34:583.

74. Duffner P, Cohen M, Sanford R, et al. Lack of efficacy of postoperative chemotherapy and delayed radiation in very young children with pinoblastoma. Pediatric Oncology Group. *Med Pediatr Oncol* 1995;25:38.

75. Allen JC, Siffert J. Contemporary issues in the management of childhood brain tumors. *Curr Opin Neurol* 1997;10:137.

76. Kun LE. Brain tumors. Challenges and directions. *Pediatr Clin North Am* 1997;44:907.

77. Kuttesch JF Jr. Advances and controversies in the management of childhood brain tumors. *Curr Opin Oncol* 1997;9:235.

78. van Eys J, Cangir A, Coody D, Smith B. MOPP regimen as primary chemotherapy for brain tumors in infants. *J Neurol Oncol* 1985;3:237.

79. Geyer JR, Finlay JL, Boyett JM, et al. Survival of infants with malignant astrocytomas. A report from the Childrens Cancer Group. *Cancer* 1995;75:1045.

80. Duffner PK, Krischer JP, Burger PC, et al. Treatment of infants with malignant gliomas: the Pediatric Oncology Group experience. *J Neurooncol* 1996;28:245.

81. Ater JL, van Eys J, Woo SY, Moore BR, Copeland DR, Bruner J. MOPP chemotherapy without irradiation as primary postsurgical therapy for brain tumors in infants and young children. *J Neurooncol* 1997;32:243.

82. Das L, Chang C, Cushing B, Jewell P. Congenital primitive neuroectodermal tumor (neuroepithelioma) of the chest wall. *Med Pediatr Oncol* 1982;10:349.

83. Seemayer T, Themo W, Bolande R, Wiglesworth F. Peripheral neuroectodermal tumors. *Perspect Pediatr Pathol* 1975;2:151.

84. Cutler L, Chaudhry A, Topazian R. Melanotic neuroectodermal tumor of infancy: an ultrastructural study, literature reviews, and re-evaluation. *Cancer* 1981;48:257.

85. Jurincic-Winkler C, Metz K, Klippel K. Melanotic neuroectodermal tumor of infancy (MNTI) in the epididymis. A case report with immunohistological studies and special consideration of malignant features. *Zentralbl Pathol* 1994;140:181.

86. Pierce MI. Leukemia in the newborn infant. *J Pediatr* 1959;54:691.

87. Ross JA, Davies SM, Potter JD, Robison LL. Epidemiology of childhood leukemia, with a focus on infants. *Epidemiol Rev* 1994;16:243.

88. Shu XO. Epidemiology of childhood leukemia. *Curr Opin Hematol* 1997;4:227.

89. Gale KB, Ford AM, Repp R, et al. Backtracking leukemia to birth: identification of clonotypic gene fusion sequences in neonatal blood spots. *Proc Natl Acad Sci U S A* 1997;94:13950.

90. MacMachon B, Levy MA. Prenatal origin of childhood leukemia: evidence from twins. *N Engl J Med* 1964;270:1082.

91. Mahmoud HH, Ridge SA, Behm FG, et al. Intrauterine monoclonal origin of neonatal concordant acute lymphoblastic leukemia in monozygotic twins. *Med Pediatr Oncol* 1995;24:77.

92. Rosner F, Lee SL. Down's syndrome and acute leukemia: myeloblastic or lymphoblastic? Report of forty-three cases and review of the literature. *Am J Med* 1972;53:203.

93. Krivit W, Good RA. Simultaneous occurrence of leukemia and mongolism. Report of a nationwide survey. *Am J Dis Child* 1957;94:289.

94. Djernes BW, Soukup SW, Bove KE, Wong KY. Congenital leukemia associated with mosaic trisomy 9. *J Pediatr* 1976;88:596.

95. Miller RW. Neoplasia and Down's syndrome. *Ann N Y Acad Sci* 1970;171:637.

96. Miller RW. Persons with exceptionally high risk of leukemia. *Cancer Res* 1967;27:2420.

97. Spier C, Kjeldsberg G, O'Brien R, Marty J. Pre-B cell acute lymphoblastic leukemia in the newborn. *Blood* 1984;64:1064.

98. Crist W, Puller J, Boyett J. Clinical and biologic features predict a poor prognosis in acute lymphoid leukemias in infants: a pediatric oncology groups study. *Blood* 1986;67:135.

99. Abe R, Ryan D, Cecalupo A, Cohen H, Sandberg A. Cytogenetic findings in congenital leukemia: case report and review of the literature. *Cancer Genet Cytogenet* 1983;9:139.

100. de Alarcon PA, Patil S, Golberg J, Allen JB, Shaw S. Infants with Down's Syndrome. Use of cytogenetic studies and in vitro colony assay for granulocyte progenitor to distinguish acute nonlymphocytic leukemia from a transient myeloproliferative disorder. *Cancer* 1987;60:987.

101. Heerema N, Arthur D, Sather H, et al. Cytogenetic features of infants less than 12 months of age at diagnosis of acute lymphoblastic leukemia: impact of the 11q23 breakpoint on outcome: a report of the Children's Cancer Group. *Blood* 1994;83:2274.

102. Behm FG, Raimondi SC, Frestedt JL, et al. Rearrangement of the MLL gene confers a poor prognosis in childhood acute lymphoblastic leukemia, regardless of presenting age. *Blood* 1996;87:2870.

103. Pui CH, Kane JR, Crist WM. Biology and treatment of infant leukemias. *Leukemia* 1995;9:762.

104. Hilden JM, Smith FO, Frestedt JL, et al. MLL gene rearrangement, cytogenetic 11q23 abnormalities, and expression of the NG2 molecule in infant acute myeloid leukemia. *Blood* 1997;89:3801.

105. Odom L, Gordon E. Acute monoblastic leukemia in infancy and early childhood: successful treatment with an epipodophyllotoxin. *Blood* 1984;4:876.

106. Berger R, Bernheim A, Weh H. Cytogenetic studies on acute monocytic leukemia. *Leuk Res* 1980;4:119.

107. Reimann D, Clemmens R, Pillsbury W. Congenital leukemia. Skin nodules a first diagnostic sign. *J Pediatr* 1955;46:415.

108. Yen A, Sanchez R, Oblender M, Raimer S. Leukemia cutis: Darier's sign in a neonate with acute lymphoblastic leukemia. *J Am Acad Dermatol* 1996;34:375.

109. Millot F, Robert A, Bertrand Y, et al. Cutaneous involvement in children with acute lymphoblastic leukemia or lymphoblastic lymphoma. The Children's Leukemia Cooperative Group of the European Organization of Research and Treatment of Cancer (EORTC). *Pediatrics* 1997;100:60.

110. Engel RR, Hammond D, Eitzman D, Pearson H, Krivit W. Transient congenital leukemia in 7 infants with mongolism. *J Pediatr* 1964;65:303.

111. Zipursky A, Brown E, Christensen H, Sutherland R, Doyle J. Leukemia and/or myeloproliferative syndrome in neonates with Down syndrome. *Semin Perinatol* 1997;21:97.

112. Brodeur G, Dahl G, Williams D, Tipton RE, Kalwinsky DK. Transient leukemoid reaction and trisomy 21 mosaicism in a phenotypically normal newborn. *Blood* 1980;55:691.

113. Drabkin HA, Erickson P. Down syndrome and leukemia, an update. *Prog Clin Biol Res* 1995;393:169.

114. Kojima S, Kato K, Matsuyama T, Yoshikawa T, Horibe K. Favorable treatment outcome in children with acute myeloid leukemia and Down syndrome. *Blood* 1993;81:3164.

115. Zipusky A. The treatment of children with acute megakaryoblastic leukemia who have Down syndrome. *J Pediatr Hematol Oncol* 1996;18:10.

116. Tchernia G, Lejeune F, Boccara JF, Denavit MF, Dommergues JP, Bernaudin F. Erythroblastic and/or megakaryoblastic leukemia in Down syndrome: treatment with low-dose arabinosyl cytosine. *J Pediatr Hematol Oncol* 1996;18:59.

117. Slavc I, Urban C, Haas OA, Kroisel PM, Koller U. Acute megakaryocytic leukemia in children. Clinical, immunologic, and cytogenetic findings in two patients. *Cancer* 1991;68:2266.

118. Frankel LS, Ochs J, Shuster et al. Therapeutic trial for infant acute lymphoblastic leukemia: the Pediatric Oncology Group experience (POG 8493). *J Pediatr Hematol Oncol* 1997;19:35.

119. Creutzig U, Ritter J, Ludwig WD, et al. Acute myeloid leukemia in children with Down syndrome. *Klin Padiatr* 1995;207:136.

120. Ebb DH, Weinstein HJ. Diagnosis and treatment of childhood acute myelogenous leukemia. *Pediatr Clin North Am* 1997;44:847.

121. Vormoor J, Boos J, Stahnke K, Jurgens H, Ritter J, Creutzig U. Therapy of childhood acute myelogenous leukemias. *Ann Hematol* 1996; 73:11.

122. Bolande RP, Brough AJ, Izant RJ. Congenital mesoblastic nephroma of infancy: a report of eight cases and the relationship to Wilms' tumor. *Pediatrics* 1967;40:272.

123. Hrabovsky EE, Othersen HB Jr, deLorimier A, Kelalis P, Beckwith JB, Takashima J. Wilms' tumor in the neonate: a report from the National Wilms' Tumor Study. *J Pediatr Surg* 1986;21:385.

124. Blank E, Nerhout RC, Burry RA. Congenital mesoblastic nephroma and polyhydramnios. *JAMA* 1978;240:1504.

125. Tomlinson G, Argyle J, Velasco S, Nisen P. Molecular characterization of congenital mesoblastic nephroma and its distinction from Wilms' tumor. *Cancer* 1992;70:2358.

126. Becroft D, Mauger D, Skeen J, Ogawa O, Reeve A. Good prognosis of cellular mesoblastic nephroma with hyperdiploidy and relaxation of imprinting of the maternal IGF2 gene. *Pediatr Pathol Lab Med* 1995;15:679.

127. Howell CG, Othersen HB, Kiviat NE. Therapy and outcome in 51 children with mesoblastic nephroma: a report of the National Wilms' Tumor Study. *J Pediatr Surg* 1982;17:826.

128. D'Angio GJ, Evans A, Breslow N. The treatment of Wilms' tumor: results of the second National Wilms' Tumor Study. *Cancer* 1981; 47:2302.

129. Gonzales-Crussi F, Sotelo-Avila C, Kidd JM. Malignant mesenchymal nephroma of infancy: a report of a case with pulmonary metastases. *Am J Surg Pathol* 1980;4:185.

130. Varsa EW, McConnell TS, Dressler LG, Duncan M. Atypical congenital mesoblastic nephroma. Report of a case with karyotypic and flow cytometric analysis. *Arch Pathol Lab Med* 1989;113:1078.

131. Machin GA. Part II: significance of nephroblastomatosis in the genesis of Wilms' tumor. *Am J Pediatr Hematol Oncol* 1980;2:253.

132. Machin GA. Part III: clinical aspects of nephroblastomatosis. *Am J Pediatr Hematol Oncol* 1980;2:353.

133. Machin GA. Persistant renal blastema (nephroblastomatosis) as a frequent precursor of Wilms' tumor: a pathological and clinical review. Part I: Nephroblastomatosis in the context of embryology and genetics. *Am J Pediatr Hematol Oncol* 1980;2:165.

134. Gylys-Morin V, Hoffer FA, Kozakewich H, Shamberger RC. Wilms tumor and nephroblastomatosis: imaging characteristics at gadolinium-enhanced MR imaging. *Radiology* 1993;188:517.

135. Kulkarni R, Bailie MD, Bernsetin J, Newton B. Progression of nephroblastomatosis to Wilms' tumor. *J Pediatr* 1980;96:178.

136. Bennington JL, Beckwith JB. Tumors of the kidney, renal pelvis and ureter. In: Bennington JL, Beckwith JB, eds. *Atlas of tumor pathology, 2nd series, Fascicle 12, vol 12, series 2*. Washington, DC: Armed Forces Institute of Pathology, 1975:32

137. Bove DE, McAdams AJ. The nephroblastomatosis complex and its relationship to Wilms' tumor: a clinicopathologic treatise. In: Rosenberg HS, Bolande RP, eds. *Perspectives in pediatric pathology*, vol 3. Chicago: Year Book Medical Publishers, 1976:185.

138. Dimmick JE, Johnson HW, Coleman GU, Carter M. Wilms tumorlet, nodular renal blastema and multicystic renal dysplasia. *J Urol* 1989; 142:484.

139. Steenman M, Redeker B, de Meulemeester M, et al. Comparative genomic hybridization analysis of Wilms tumors. *Cytogenet Cell Genet* 1997;77:296.

140. Beckwith JB. Precursor lesions of Wilms tumor: clinical and biological implications. *Med Pediatr Oncol* 1993;21:158.

141. Beckwith JB. Wilms' tumor and other renal tumors of childhood. *Hum Pathol* 1983;14:481.

142. Cassady JR, Tefft M, Filler RM. Considerations in the radiation therapy of Wilms' tumor. *Cancer* 1973;32:298.

143. Regalado JJ, Rodriguez MM, Toledano S. Bilaterally multicentric synchronous Wilms' tumor: successful conservative treatment despite persistence of nephrogenic rests. *Med Pediatr Oncol* 1997;28:420.

144. Delgado G, Viluce C, Fletcher E, de Espinosa H, Del Rio B, Chen LN. Bilateral Wilms' tumor. Current treatment. *Rev Med Panama* 1996; 21:93.

145. Green DM. Treatment of stage I Wilms' tumor. *J Clin Oncol* 1995;13: 1530.

146. Green DM, Thomas PR, Shochat S. The treatment of Wilms tumor. Results of the National Wilms Tumor Studies. *Hematol Oncol Clin North Am* 1995;9:1267.

147. Green DM, D'Angio GJ, Beckwith JB, et al. Wilms tumor. *CA Cancer J Clin* 1996;46:46.

148. Green DM, Breslow NE, Evans I, Moksness J, D'Angio GJ. Treatment of children with stage IV favorable histology Wilms tumor: a report from the National Wilms Tumor Study Group. *Med Pediatr Oncol* 1996;26:147.

149. Beckwith JB, Palmer NF. Histopathology and prognosis of Wilms' tumor: results from the First National Wilms' Tumor Study. *Cancer* 1978;41:1937.

150. Haas JE, Palmer NF, Weinberg AG, Beckwith JB. Ultrastructure of the rhabdoid tumor of kidney. A distinctive renal tumor of children. *Hum Pathol* 1981;12:646.

151. Palmer NF, Sutlow W. Clinical aspects of the rhabdoid tumor of the kidney: a report of The National Wilms' Tumor Study Group. *Med Pediatr Oncol* 1983;11:242.

152. Lynch HT, Shwim SB, Dahms BB. Paravertebral malignant rhabdoid tumor in infancy. *Cancer* 1983;52:290.

153. Agrons GA, Kingsman KD, Wagner BJ, Sotelo-Avila C. Rhabdoid tumor of the kidney in children: a comparative study of 21 cases. *AJR Am J Roentgenol* 1997;168:447.

154. Bonnin JM, Rubinstein LJ, Palmer NF, Beckwith JB. The association of embryonal tumors originating in the kidney and in the brain. *Cancer* 1984;54:2137.

155. Perez-Atayde A, Newbury R, Fletcher J, Barnhill R, Gellis S. Congenital "neurovascular harmartoma" of the skin. A possible marker of malignant rhabdoid tumor. *Am J Surg Pathol* 1994;18:1030.

156. Gonzalez-Crussi F, Baum ES. Renal sarcomas of childhood. A clinicopathologic and ultrastructural study. *Cancer* 1983;51:898.

157. Carcassonne C, Raybaud C, Lebreuil G. Clear cell sarcoma of the kidney in children: a distinct entity. *J Pediatr Surg* 1983;16:645.

158. Newbould MJ, Kelsey AM. Clear cell sarcoma of the kidney in a 4-month-old infant: a case report. *Med Pediatr Oncol* 1993;21:525.

159. Ise T, Ohtsuki H, Matsumoto K, Sana R. Management of malignant testicular tumors in children. *Cancer* 1976;37:1539.

160. Exelby PR. Testis cancer in children. *Semin Oncol* 1979;6:116.

161. Jeffs RD. Management of embryonal adenocarcinoma of the testis in childhood: an analysis of 164 cases. In: Gooden JA, ed. *Cancer in childhood*. New York: Plenum Press, 1973:68.

162. Brosman SA. Testicular tumors in prepubertal children. *Urology* 1979;13:581.

163. Drago JR, Nelson RP, Palmer JM. Childhood embryonal carcinoma of testes. *Urology* 1978;12:499.

164. Colodny A, Hopkins TB. Testicular tumors in infants and children. *Urol Clin North Am* 1977;4:347.

165. Witzleben CH, Bruninga G. Infantile choriocarcinoma: a characteristic syndrome. *J Pediatr* 1968;73:374.

166. Tapper D, Lack E. Teratomas in infancy and childhood. A 54-year experience at The Children's Hospital Medical Center. *Ann Surg* 1983; 198:398.

167. Altman RP, Randolph JG, Lilly JR. Sacrococcygeal teratoma: American Academy of Pediatrics Surgical Section Survey. *J Pediatr Surg* 1974;9:389.

168. Damjanov II, Knowles BB, Solter D. *The human teratomas:* experimental and clinical biology. Clifton, NJ: Humana Press, 1983.

169. Fraumeni JF, Li FP, Dalager S. Teratomas in children: epidemiologic features. *J Natl Cancer Inst* 1973;51:1425.

170. Hawkins E, Issacs H, Cushing B, Rogers P. Occult malignancy in neonatal sacrococcygeal teratomas. A report from a Combined Pediatric Oncology Group and Children's Cancer Group study. *Am J Pediatr Hematol Oncol* 1993;15:406.

171. Donnellan WA, Swenson O. Benign and malignant sacrococcygeal teratomas. *Surgery* 1968;64:834.

172. Raney RB Jr, Chatten J, Littman P. Treatment strategies for infants with malignant sacrococcygeal teratoma. *J Pediatr Surg* 1981;16:573.

173. Einhorn H, Donohue J. *Cis*-diaminedichloroplatinum vinblastine, bleomycin combination chemotherapy in disseminated testicular cancer. *Ann Intern Med* 1977;87:293.

174. Noseworthy J, Lack EE, Kozakewich HPW. Sacrococcygeal germ cell tumors in childhood. An updated experience with 118 patients. *J Pediatr Surg* 1981;16:258.

175. Valdiserri RO, Yunis EJ. Sacrococcygeal teratomas: a review of 68 cases. *Cancer* 1981;48:217.

176. Edmondson HA. Differential diagnosis of tumors and tumor-like lesions of liver in infancy and childhood. *Am J Dis Child* 1956;91:168.

177. von Schweinitz D, Gluer S, Mildenberger H. Liver tumors in neonates and very young infants: diagnostic pitfalls and therapeutic problems. *Eur J Pediatr Surg* 1995;5:72.

178. Lack EE, Neave C, Vawte GF. Hepatocellular carcinoma. Review of 32 cases in childhood and adolescence. *Cancer* 1983;52:1510.

179. Weinberg AG, Finegold MJ. Primary hepatic tumors of childhood. *Hum Pathol* 1983;14:512.

180. Randolph JG, Altman RP, Arensman RM. Liver resection in children with hepatic neoplasms. *Ann Surg* 1978;187:599.

181. Ein SH, Stephens CA. Malignant liver tumors in children. *J Pediatr Surg* 1974;9:491.

182. Clatworthy HW, Schiller M, Grosfeld JL. Primary liver tumors in infancy and childhood: 41 cases variously treated. *Arch Surg* 1974;109:143.

183. Khan A, Bader JL, Hoy GR, Sinks LF. Hepatoblastoma in child with fetal alcohol syndrome. *Lancet* 1979;i:1403.

184. Otten J, Smets R, de Jager R, Gerard A, Maurus R. Hepatoblastoma in an infant after contraceptive intake during pregnancy. *N Engl J Med* 1977;297:222.

185. Ikeda H, Matsuyama S, Tanimura M. Association between hepatoblastoma and very low birth weight: a trend or a chance? *J Pediatr* 1997;130:557.

186. Ross JA. Hepatoblastoma and birth weight: too little, too big, or just right? *J Pediatr* 1997;130:516.

187. Napoli V, Campbell W Jr. Hepatoblastoma in infant sister and brother. *Cancer* 1977;39:2647.

188. Berry CL, Keeling J, Hilton C. Coincidence of congenital malformation and embryonic tumors in childhood. *Arch Dis Child* 1970;45:229.

189. Fraumeni JF Jr, Miller RW. Adrenocortical neoplasms with hemihypertrophy, brain tumors, and other disorders. *J Pediatr* 1967;70:129.

190. Nickerson HJ, Silberman TL, McDonald TP. Hepatoblastoma, thrombocytosis and increased thrombopoietin. *Cancer* 1980;45:315.

191. Yamaguchi H, Ishii E, Hayashida Y, Hirata Y, Sakai R, Miyazaki S. Mechanism of thrombocytosis in hepatoblastoma: a case report. *Pediatr Hematol Oncol* 1996;13:539.

192. Exelby PR, Filler RM, Grosfeld JL. Liver tumors in children in particular reference to hepatoblastoma and hepatocellular carcinoma: American Academy of Pediatrics Surgical Section Survey. *J Pediatr Surg* 1975;10:329.

193. Tsuchida Y, Endo Y, Saito S, et al. Evaluation of alpha-fetoprotein in early infancy. *J Pediatr Surg* 1978;13:155.

194. Tsuchida Y, Honna T, Fukui M, Sakaguchi H, Ishiguro T. The ratio of fucosylation of alpha-fetoprotein in hepatoblastoma. *Cancer* 1989;63:2174.

195. Moazam F, Talbert JL, Rodgers BM. Primary tumors of the liver in infancy and childhood. *J Fla Med Assoc* 1982;69:991.

196. Lack EE, Neave C, Vawter FG. Hepatoblastoma: a clinical and pathologic study of 54 cases. *Am J Surg Pathol* 1982;6:693.

197. Kasai M, Watanabe I. Histologic classification of liver cell carcinoma in infancy and childhood and its clinical evaluation: a study of 70 cases collected in Japan. *Cancer* 1970;25:551.

198. Gonzalez-Crussi F, Upton PM, Macurer SH. Hepatoblastoma: attempt at characterization of histologic subtypes. *Am J Surg Pathol* 1982;6:599.

199. Forouhar FA, Quinn JJ, Cooke R, Foster JH. The effect of chemotherapy on hepatoblastoma. *Arch Pathol Lab Med* 1984;108:311.

200. Weinblatt ME, Siegel SE, Siegal MM. Preoperative chemotherpay for unresectable primary hepatic malignancies in childhood. *Cancer* 1982;50:1061.

201. Reynolds M. Conversion of unresectable to resectable hepatoblastoma and long-term follow-up study. *World J Surg* 1995;19:814.

202. Bowman LC, Riely CA. Management of pediatric liver tumors. *Surg Oncol Clin N Am* 1996;5:451.

203. Geiger JD. Surgery for hepatoblastoma in children. *Curr Opin Pediatr* 1996;8:276.

204. Achilleos OA, Buist LJ, Kelly DA, et al. Unresectable hepatic tumors in childhood and the role of liver transplantation. *J Pediatr Surg* 1996;31:1563.

205. Evans AE, Land VJ, Newton WA. Combination chemotherapy (vincristine, adriamycin, cyclophosphamide, and 5-fluorouracil) in the treatment of children with malignant hepatoma. *Cancer* 1982;50:821.

206. Holton CP, Burrington JD, Hatch EI. A multiple chemotherapeutic approach to the management of hepatoblastoma. *Cancer* 1975;35:1083.

207. van Hoff J, Grier HE, Douglass EC, Green DM. Etoposide, ifosfamide, and cisplatin therapy for refractory childhood solid tumors. Response and toxicity. *Cancer* 1995;75:2966.

208. von Schweinitz D, Byrd DJ, Hecker H, et al. Efficiency and toxicity of ifosfamide, cisplatin and doxorubicin in the treatment of childhood hepatoblastoma. Study Committee of the Cooperative Paediatric Liver Tumour Study HB89 of the German Society for Paediatric Oncology and Haematology. *Eur J Cancer* 1997;33:1243.

209. Dillon P, Whalen T, Azizkhan R, et al. Neonatal soft tissue sarcomas: the influence of pathology on treatment and survival. Children's Cancer Group Surgical Committee. *J Pediatr Surg* 1995;30:1038.

210. Filston HC. Common lumps and bumps of the head and neck in infants and children. *Pediatr Ann* 1989;18:180.

211. Koscielniak E, Harms D, Schmidt D, et al. Soft tissue sarcomas in infants younger than 1 year of age: a report of the German Soft Tissue Sarcoma Study Group (CWS-81). *Med Pediatr Oncol* 1989;17:105.

212. Salloum E, Flamant F, Rey A, et al. Rhabdomyosarcoma in infants under one year of age: experience of the Institut Gustave-Roussy. *Med Pediatr Oncol* 1989;17:424.

213. Ragab AH, Heyn R, Tefft M, Hays DN, Newton W Jr, Beltangady M. Infants younger than 1 year of age with rhabdomyosarcoma. *Cancer* 1986;58:2606.

214. King DR, Clatworthy HW Jr. The pediatric patient with sarcoma. *Semin Oncol* 1981;8:215.

215. Grosfeld JL, Weber TR, Weetman RM, Baehner RL. Rhabdomyosarcoma in childhood: analysis of survival in 98 cases. *J Pediatr Surg* 1983;18:141.

216. Piver MS, Rose PG. Long-term follow-up and complications of infants with vulvovaginal embryonal rhabdomyosarcoma treated with surgery, radiation therapy, and chemotherapy. *Obstet Gynecol* 1988;71:435.

217. Coffin CM, Dehner LP. Soft tissue tumors in the first year of life: a report of 190 cases. *Pediatr Pathol* 1990;10:509.

218. Alvarez Silvan AM, Garcia Canton JA, Pineda Cuevas G, Alfuro Gutierrez J. Successful treatment of orbital rhabdomyosarcoma in two infants using chemotherapy alone. *Med Pediatr Oncol* 1996;26:186.

219. Nag S, Martinez-Monge R, Ruymann F, Jamil A, Bauer C. Innovation in the management of soft tissue sarcomas in infants and young children: high-dose-rate brachytherapy. *J Clin Oncol* 1997;15:3075.

220. Chung EB, Enzinger FM. Infantile fibrosarcoma. *Cancer* 1976;38:729.

221. Soule EH, Pritchard DJ. Fibrosarcoma in infants and children: a review of 110 cases. *Cancer* 1977;40:1711.

222. Kynaston JA, Malcolm AJ, Craft AW, et al. Chemotherapy in the management of infantile fibrosarcoma. *Med Pediatr Oncol* 1993;21:488.

223. Coffin CM, Jaszcz W, O'Shea PA, Dehner LP. So-called congenital-infantile fibrosarcoma: does it exist and what is it? *Pediatr Pathol* 1994;14:133.

224. Takach TJ, Reul GJ, Ott DA, Cooley DA. Primary cardiac tumors in infants and children: immediate and long-term operative results. *Ann Thorac Surg* 1996;62:559.

225. Boon LM, Fishman SJ, Lund DP, Mulliken JB. Congenital fibrosarcoma masquerading as congenital hemangioma: report of two cases. *J Pediatr Surg* 1995;30:1378.

226. Cofer BR, Vescio PJ, Wiener ES. Infantile fibrosarcoma: complete excision is the appropriate treatment. *Ann Surg Oncol* 1996;3:159.

227. Parker RK, Mallory SB, Baker GF. Infantile myofibromatosis. *Pediatr Dermatol* 1991;8:129.

228. Hartig G, Koopmann C Jr, Esclamado R. Infantile myofibromatosis: a commonly misdiagnosed entity. *Otolaryngol Head Neck Surg* 1993;109:753.

229. Duffy MT, Harris M, Hornblass A. Infantile myofibromatosis of orbital bone. A case report with computed tomography, magnetic res-

onance imaging, and histologic findings. *Ophthalmology* 1997;104:1471.

230. Linder JS, Harris GJ, Segura AD. Periorbital infantile myofibromatosis. *Arch Ophthalmol* 1996;114:219.

231. Atar D, Tenenbaum Y, Lehman WB, Grant AD. Hip dislocation caused by infantile myofibromatosis. *Am J Orthop* 1995;24:774.

232. Queralt JA, Poirier VC. Solitary infantile myofibromatosis of the skull. *AJNR Am J Neuroradiol* 1995;16:476.

233. Dautenhahn L, Blaser SI, Weitzman S, Crysdale WS. Infantile myofibromatosis: a cause of vertebra plana. *AJNR Am J Neuroradiol* 1995;16:828.

234. Jenkins EA, Cawley MI. Infantile myofibromatosis: a cause of severe bone pain in a neonate. *Br J Rheumatol* 1993;32:849.

235. Chung EB, Enzinger FM. Infantile myofibromatosis. *Cancer* 1981;48:1807.

236. Briselli MF, Soule EH, Gilchrist GS. Congenital fibromatosis: report of 18 cases of solitary and 4 cases of multiple tumors. *Mayo Clin Proc* 1980;55:554.

237. Variend S, Bax NM, van Gorp J. Are infantile myofibromatosis, congenital fibrosarcoma and congenital haemangiopericytoma histogenetically related? *Histopathology* 1995;26:57.

238. Kauffman SL, Stout AP. Congenital mesenchymal tumors. *Cancer* 1965;18:460.

239. Schaffzin EA, Chung SMK, Kaye R. Congenital generalized fibromatosis with complete spontaneous regression: a case report. *J Bone Joint Surg Am* 1972;54:657.

240. Teng P, Warden MJ, Cohn WL. Congenital generalized fibromatosis (renal and skeletal) with complete spontaneous remission. *J Pediatr* 1963;62:748.

241. Stein R. Chemotherapeutic responses in fibromatosis of the neck. *J Pediatr* 1977;90:482.

242. Silverman RA. Hemangiomas and vascular malformations. *Pediatr Clin North Am* 1991;38:811.

243. Esterly NB. Hemangiomas in infants and children: clinical observations. *Pediatr Dermatol* 1992;9:353.

244. Mulliken JB, Glowacki J. Hemangiomas and vascular malformations in infants and children: a classification based on endothelial characteristics. *Plast Reconstr Surg* 1982;69:412.

245. Edgerton MT, Hiebert JM. Vascular and lymphatic tumors in infancy, childhood and adulthood: challenge of diagnosis and treatment. *Curr Probl Cancer* 1978;2:1.

246. Williams HB. Vascular neoplasms. *Clin Plast Surg* 1980;7:397.

247. Enjolras O, Wassef M, Mazoyer E, et al. Infants with Kasabach–Merritt syndrome do not have "true" hemangiomas. *J Pediatr* 1997;130:631.

248. Pereyra R, Andrassy RJ, Mahow GH. Management of massive hepatic hemangiomas in infants and children: a review of 13 cases. *Pediatrics* 1982;70:254.

249. Padalkar JA, Bapat VS, Phadke MA, Ujjainwalla F. Successful treatment of hepatic hemangiomas with corticosteroids. *Indian Pediatr* 1992;29:769.

250. Park WC, Phillips R. The role of radiation therapy in the management of hemangiomas of the liver. *JAMA* 1970;212:1496.

251. Bennett RG, Keller JW, Ditty JF Jr. Hemangiosarcoma subsequent to radiotherapy for a hemangioma in infancy. *J Dermatol Surg Oncol* 1978;4:881.

252. Schild SE, Buskirk SJ, Frick LM, Cupps RE. Radiotherapy for large symptomatic hemangiomas. *Int J Radiat Oncol Biol Phys* 1991;21:729.

253. Belli L, DeCarlis L, Beati C, et al. Surgical treatment of symptomatic giant hemangiomas of the liver. *Surg Gynecol Obstet* 1992;174:474.

254. Flint LM, Polk HC. Selective hepatic artery ligation: limitations and failure. *J Trauma* 1979;19:319.

255. Williams MD, Pearson MH, Thomas FD. Arterial embolization of a facial haemangioma. *Br Dent J* 1992;173:102.

256. Boon LM, Burrows PE, Paltiel HJ, et al. Hepatic vascular anomalies in infancy: a twenty-seven-year experience. *J Pediatr* 1996;129:346.

257. Sarihan H, Mocan H, Yildiz K, Abes M, Akyazici R. A new treatment with bleomycin for complicated cutaneous hemangioma in children. *Eur J Pediatr Surg* 1997;7:158.

258. Carnelli V, Bellini F, Ferrari M. Giant hemangioma with consumption coagulopathy: sustained response to heparin and radiotherapy. *J Pediatr* 1977;91:504.

259. Koerper MA, Addiego JE Jr, Delorimier AA. Use of aspirin and dipyridamole in children with platelet trapping syndromes. *J Pediatr* 1983;102:311.

260. de-Prost Y, Teillac D, Bodemer C, Enjolras O, Nihoul-Fekete C, de-

261. Prost D. Successful treatment of Kasabach-Merritt syndrome with pentoxifylline. *J Am Acad Dermatol* 1991;25:854.

262. Dresse MF, David M, Hume H, et al. Successful treatment of Kasabach–Merritt syndrome with prednisone and epsilon-aminocaproic acid. *Pediatr Hematol Oncol* 1991;8:329.

262. Lemarchand-Venecie F. Indications for laser in the treatment of capillary hemangioma. *J Mal Vasc* 1992;17:41.

263. Froehlich P, Seid AB, Morgon A. Contrasting strategic approaches to the management of subglottic hemangiomas. *Int J Pediatr Otorhinolaryngol* 1996;36:137.

264. Ezekowitz RA, Mulliken JB, Folkman J. Interferon α-2a therapy for life-threatening hemangiomas of infancy. *N Engl J Med* 1992;326:1456.

265. Chung T, Hoffer FA, Burrows PE, Paltiel HJ. MR imaging of hepatic hemangiomas of infancy and changes seen with interferon alpha-2a treatment. *Pediatr Radiol* 1996;26:341.

266. Falk H, Herbert JT, Edmonds L. Review of four cases of childhood hepatic angiosarcoma—elevated environmental arsenic exposure in one case. *Cancer* 1981;47:382.

267. Bedos AA, Munson J, Toomey FE. Hemangioendothelioma presenting as posterior mediastinal mass in a child. *Cancer* 1980;46:801.

268. Osband ME, Pochedly C. *Histiocytosis X:* Hematology/Oncology Clinics of North America, vol 1. Philadelphia: WB Saunders, 1987.

269. Ladisch S, Jaffe ES. The histiocytoses. In: Pizzo PA, Poplack DG, eds. *Principles and practice of pediatric oncology,* 2nd ed. Philadelphia: JB Lippincott Co., 1993:617

270. Egeler RM, Nesbit ME. Langerhans cell histiocytosis and other disorders of monocyte-histiocyte lineage. *Crit Rev Oncol Hematol* 1995;18:9.

271. Egeler RM, D'Angio GJ. Langerhans cell histiocytosis. *J Pediatr* 1995;127:1.

272. Chu T, D'Angio G, Favara B, et al. Histiocytosis syndromes in children. *Lancet* 1987;1:208.

273. Willman C. Detection of clonal histiocytes in Langerhans cell histiocytosis: biology and clinical significance. *Br J Cancer* 1994;23 [Suppl]:S29.

274. Egeler RM. Clonality in Langerhan's cell histiocytosis. *Br Med J* 1995;310:804.

275. Cotter FE, Pritchard J. Clonality in Langerhans' cell histiocytosis. *Br Med J* 1995;310:74.

276. Willman CL. Detection of clonal histiocytes in Langerhans cell histiocytosis: biology and clinical significance. *Br J Cancer* 1994;23 [Suppl]:S29.

277. Yu RC, Chu C, Buluwela L, Chu AC. Clonal proliferation of Langerhans cells in Langerhans cell histiocytosis. *Lancet* 1994;343:767.

278. Bernstrand C, Bjork O, Ahstrom L, Henter JI. Intralesional steroids in Langerhans cell histiocytosis of bone. *Acta Paediatr* 1996;85:502.

279. Cassady JR. Current role of radiation therapy in the management of histiocytosis-X. *Hematol Oncol Clin North Am* 1987;1:123.

280. Libicher M, Roeren T, Troger J. Localized Langerhans cell histiocytosis of bone: treatment and follow-up in children. *Pediatr Radiol* 1995;25:S134.

281. Webb DK. Histiocyte disorders. *Br Med Bull* 1996;52:818.

282. Davids JR. Treatment of Langerhans-cell histiocytosis in children. Experience at the Children's Hospital of Nancy. *J Bone Joint Surg Am* 1996;78:472.

283. Anonymous. A multicentre retrospective survey of Langerhans' cell histiocytosis: 348 cases observed between 1983 and 1993. The French Langerhans' Cell Histiocytosis Study Group. *Arch Dis Child* 1996;75:17.

284. Ladisch S, Gadner H. Treatment of Langerhans cell histiocytosis—evolution and current approaches. *Br J Cancer* 1994;23[Suppl]:S41.

285. Gadner H, Heitger A, Grois N, Gatterer-Menz I, Ladisch S. Treatment strategy for disseminated Langerhans cell histiocytosis. DAL HX-83 Study Group. *Med Pediatr Oncol* 1994;23:72.

286. Ladisch S, Gadner H, Arico M, et al. LCH-I: a randomized trial of etoposide vs. vinblastine in disseminated Langerhans cell histiocytosis. The Histiocyte Society. *Med Pediatr Oncol* 1994;23:107.

287. Starling KA. Chemotherapy for histiocytosis-X. *Hematol Oncol Clin North Am* 1987;1:119.

288. Arceci R. Histiocytoses and disorders of the reticuloendothelial system. In: Handin RI, Lux SE, Stossel TP, eds. *BLOOD:* principles and practice of hematology. Philadelphia: JB Lippincott Co., 1995:915.

289. Glass AG, Miller RW. U.S. mortality from Letterer–Siwe disease 1900–1964. *Pediatrics* 1968;42:364.

290. Jugberg RC, Kloepfer HW, Oberman HA. Genetic determination of

acute disseminated histiocytosis X (Letterer–Siwe syndrome). *Pediatrics* 1970;45:753.

291. Matus-Ridley M, Raney RB, Thawerani H, Meadows AT. Histiocytosis X in children: patterns of disease and results of treatment. *Med Pediatr Oncol* 1983;11:99.

292. Greenberger JS, Crocker AC, Vawter G. Results of treatment of 127 patients with systemic histiocytosis (Letterer–Siwe syndrome, Schuller–Christian syndrome and multifocal eosinophilic granuloma). *Medicine* 1981;60:331.

293. Urbano-Marquez A, Estruch R, Fernandez-Huerta JM, et al. Etoposide in the treatment of multifocal eosinophilic granuloma. *Cancer Treat Rep* 1985;69:238.

294. Ceci A, deTerlizzi M, Colella R, et al. Etoposide in recurrent childhood Langerhans' cell histiocytosis: an Italian cooperative study. *Cancer* 1988;62:2528.

295. Mahmoud H, Wang WC, Murphy SB. Cyclosporine therapy for advanced Langerhans cell Histiocytosis. *Blood* 1991;77:721.

296. Forssman T, Fluhr J, Djawari D, Gloor M, Rumpelt HJ. Treatment of Langerhans-cell histiocytosis by oral cyclosporin A and topical nitrogen mustard. *Ann Dermatol Venereol* 1994;121:734.

297. Sawamura M, Yamaguchi S, Marayama K, et al. Cyclosporine therapy for Langerhans cell histiocytosis. *Br J Haematol* 1993;83:178.

298. Fischer A, Cerf-Bensussan N, Blanche S. Allogeneic bone marrow transplantation for erythrophagocytic lymphohistiocytosis. *J Pediatr* 1986;108:267.

299. Ringden O, Ahstrom L, Lonnqvist B, Baryd I, Svedmyr E, Gahrton G. Allogeneic bone marrow transplantation in a patient with chemotherapy-resistant progressive histiocytosis X. *N Engl J Med* 1987;316:733.

300. Stoll M, Freund M, Schmid H, et al. Allogeneic bone marrow transplantation for Langerhans' cell histiocytosis. *Cancer* 1990;66:284.

301. Newell KA, Alonso EM, Kelly SM, Rubin CM, Thistlethwaite JR Jr, Whitington PF. Association between liver transplantation for Langerhans cell histiocytosis, rejection, and development of posttransplant lymphoproliferative disease in children. *J Pediatr* 1997;131:98.

302. Conter V, Reciputo A, Arrigo C, Bozzato N, Sala A, Arico M. Bone marrow transplantation for refractory Langerhans' cell histiocytosis. *Haematologica* 1996;81:468.

303. Morgan G. Myeloablative therapy and bone marrow transplantation for Langerhans' cell histiocytosis. *Br J Cancer* 1994;23[Suppl]:S52.

304. Richter MP, D'Angio GJ. The role of radiation therapy in the management of children with histiocytosis X. *Am J Pediatr Hematol Oncol* 1981;3:161.

305. Stine KC, Saylors RL, Williams LL, Becton DL. 2-Chlorodeoxyadenosine (2-CDA) for the treatment of refractory or recurrent Langerhans cell histiocytosis (LCH) in pediatric patients. *Med Pediatr Oncol* 1997;29:288.

306. Dimopoulos MA, Theodorakis M, Kostis E, Papadimitris C, Moulopoulos LA, Anastasiou-Nana M. Treatment of Langerhans cell histiocytosis with 2 chlorodeoxyadenosine. *Leuk Lymphoma* 1997;25:187.

307. Daoud MS, Dahl PR, Dicken CH, Phyliky RL. Indeterminate cell histiocytosis treated successfully with 2-chlorodeoxyadenosine. *Cutis* 1997;59:27.

308. Saven A, Foon KA, Piro LD. 2-Chlorodeoxyadenosine-induced complete remissions in Langerhans-cell histiocytosis. *Ann Intern Med* 1994;121:430.

309. Saven A, Figueroa ML, Piro LD, Rosenblatt JD. 2-Chlorodeoxyadenosine to treat refractory histiocytosis X. *N Engl J Med* 1993;329:734.

310. Misery L, Larbre B, Lyonnet S, Faure M, Thivolet J. Remission of Langerhans cell histiocytosis with thalidomide treatment. *Clin Exp Dermatol* 1993;18:487.

311. Thomas L, Ducros B, Secchi T, Balme B, Moulin G. Successful treatment of adult's Langerhans cell histiocytosis with thalidomide. Report of two cases and literature review. *Arch Dermatol* 1993;129:1261.

312. Farguhar J, Claireaux A. Familial haemophagocytic reticulosis. *Arch Dis Child* 1952;27:519.

313. MacMahon HE, Bedizel M, Ellis CA. Familial erythrophagocytic lymphohistiocytosis. *Pediatrics* 1963;32:868.

314. Favara BE, Feller AC, Pauli M, et al. Contemporary classification of histiocytic disorders. The WHO Committee On Histiocytic/Reticulum Cell Proliferations. Reclassification Working Group of the Histiocyte Society. *Med Pediatr Oncol* 1997;29:157.

315. Henter JI, Nennesmo I. Neuropathologic findings and neurologic symptoms in twenty-three children with hemophagocytic lymphohistiocytosis. *J Pediatr* 1997;130:358.

316. Imashuku S, Hlbi S, Todo S. Hemophagocytic lymphohistiocytosis in infancy and childhood. *J Pediatr* 1997;130:352.

317. Filipovich AH. Hemophagocytic lymphohistiocytosis: a lethal disorder of immune regulation. *J Pediatr* 1997;130:337.

318. Tsuda H. Hemophagocytic syndrome (HPS) in children and adults. *Int J Hematol* 1997;65:215.

319. Wong KF, Chan JK, Ha SY, Wong HW. Reactive hemophagocytic syndrome in childhood—frequent occurrence of atypical mononuclear cells. *Hematol Oncol* 1994;12:67.

320. Favara BE. Hemophagocytic lymphohistiocytosis: a hemophagocytic syndrome. *Semin Diagn Pathol* 1992;9:63.

321. Ansbacher LG, Singsen BH, Hosler MW, Grimminger H, Herbert PN. Familial erythrophagocytic lymphohistiocytosis: an association with serum lipid abnormalities. *J Pediatr* 1983;102:270.

322. Arico M, Janka G, Fischer A, et al. Hemophagocytic lymphohistiocytosis. Report of 122 children from the International Registry. FHL Study Group of the Histiocyte Society. *Leukemia* 1996;10:197.

323. Henter JI, Ehrnst A, Andersson J, Elinder G. Familial hemophagocytic lymphohistiocytosis and viral infections. *Acta Paediatr* 1993;82:369.

324. Egeler RM, Shapiro R, Loechelt B, Filipovich A. Characteristic immune abnormalities in hemophagocytic lymphohistiocytosis. *J Pediatr Hematol Oncol* 1996;18:340.

325. Osugi Y, Hara J, Tagawa S, et al. Cytokine production regulating Th1 and Th2 cytokines in hemophagocytic lymphohistiocytosis. *Blood* 1997;89:4100.

326. Ladisch S, Ho W, Matheson D, Pilkington R, Hartman G. Immunologic and clinical effects of repeated blood exchange in familial erythrophagocytic lymphohistiocytosis. *Blood* 1982;60:814.

327. Henter JI, Elinder G, Finkel Y, Soder O. Successful induction with chemotherapy including teniposide in familial erythrophagocytic lymphohistiocytosis. *Lancet* 1986;13:1402.

328. Henter JI, Arico M, Egeler RM, et al. HLH-94: a treatment protocol for hemophagocytic lymphohistiocytosis. HLH study Group of the Histiocyte Society. *Med Pediatr Oncol* 1997;28:342.

329. Baker KS, DeLaat CA, Steinbuch M, et al. Successful correction of hemophagocytic lymphohistiocytosis with related or unrelated bone marrow transplantation. *Blood* 1997;89:3857.

330. Adachi S, Kubota M, Akiyama Y, Kato T, Kitoh T, Furusho K. Successful bone marrow transplantation from an HLA-identical unrelated donor in a patient with hemophagocytic lymphohistiocytosis. *Bone Marrow Transplant* 1997;19:183.

331. Hashimoto K, Griffin D, Kohsbaki M. Self-healing reticulohistiocytosis: a clinical, histologic, and ultrastructural study of the fourth case in the literature. *Cancer* 1982;49:331.

332. Hashimoto K, Pritzker M. Electron microscopic study of reticulohistiocytoma. *Arch Dermatol* 1973;107:263.

333. Marsh WI, Lew SW, Heath VC, Lightsey AL. Congenital self-healing histiocytosis-X. *Am J Pediatr Hematol Oncol* 1983;5:227.

334. Egeler RM, Schmitz L, Sonneveld P, Mannival C, Nesbit ME. Malignant histiocytosis: a reassessment of cases formerly classified as histiocytic neoplasms and review of the literature. *Med Pediatr Oncol* 1995;25:1.

335. Akiyama M, Inamoto N, Kakamura K. Malignant histiocytosis presenting as multiple erythematous plaques and cutaneous depigmentation. *Am J Dermatopathol* 1997;19:299.

336. deLorimier AA, Harrison MR. Surgical treatment of tumors in the newborn. *Am J Pediatr Hematol Oncol* 1981;3:271.

337. Littman P, D'Angio GJ. Radiation therapy in the neonate. *Am J Pediatr Hematol Oncol* 1981;3:279.

338. Pastore G, Antonelli R, Fine W. Late effects of treatment of cancer in infancy. *Med Pediatr Oncol* 1982;10:369.

339. Morselli P. Clinical pharmacokinetics in neonates. *Clin Pharmacokinet* 1976;1:81.

340. Siegel SE, Moran RG. Problems in the chemotherapy of cancer in the neonate. *Am J Pediatr Hematol Oncol* 1981;3:287.

341. McLeod H, Relling M, Crom W, et al. Disposition of neoplastic agents in the very young child. *Br J Cancer* 1992;66:S23.

342. Woods W, O'Leary M, Nesbit M. Life-threatening neuropathy and hepatotoxicity in infants during induction therapy for acute lymphoblastic leukemia. *J Pediatr* 1981;98:642.

343. Mulhern RK, Kovnar E, Langston J, et al. Long-term survivors of leukemia treated in infancy: factors associated with neuropsychologic status. *J Clin Oncol* 1992;10:1095.

344. Meadows AT, Gallagher-Fenton J. Secondary cancers in pediatric patients: assessing the risks. *Contemp Oncol* 1992;2:47.

CHAPTER 54

Dermatologic Conditions

Andrew M. Margileth

Careful assessment of skin in the healthy or sick newborn frequently provides clues for a presumptive diagnosis of a primary cutaneous disease, a systemic disease, or both. During the initial examination, an exact dermatologic diagnosis often is difficult to make. The diagnosis evolves, however, by analysis of the descriptive morphology, configuration, and distribution of the skin lesions. Close observation with a bright light and small magnifying glass identifies the type of primary and secondary cutaneous lesions (see the following outline). In the well newborn, there are many skin lesions that are normal and transient but require differentiation from those that are permanent, pathologic, or indicative of underlying conditions. Many of the skin lesions present in neonates require little or no therapy but, because of their visibility, are of concern to the parents. These conditions are summarized in Table 54–1. The following is an outline of the classification of skin lesions.

Primary cutaneous lesions
    Lesions ≤ 5 mm
        Papule
            Comedo
            Vesicle
        Lesions > 5 mm
            Patch
            Plaque
            Nodule (5 to 10 mm)
            Tumor (> 1 cm)
            Bulla
    Lesions of varying sizes
        Cyst
        Pustule
        Wheal

        Macule
        Burrow
        Telangiectasia
Secondary skin lesions
    Atrophy
    Crusts
    Eczema
    Erosion
    Excoriation
    Fissure
    Pigmentation
    Scar
    Scale
    Ulcer

Configuration refers to patterning of lesions (e.g., annular, circinate, serpiginous or gyrate, linear, iris, zosteriform, along lines of cleavage, marbled, multiform). Distribution refers to the body area, sites of predilection, and whether symmetric, localized or circumscribed, scattered, generalized, single or multiple, and discrete or confluent. With a good history, including that of family and medications, presence or absence of pruritus, and a descriptive analysis of the lesions, common dermatologic entities are identified. Finally, if the diagnosis is not clear after a short period of observation with a few selected tests, dermatologic consultation is indicated (1–7).

Skin consists of epidermis, a relatively impermeable membrane, and dermis, which constitutes the bulk of skin. Dermis consists of minimally cellular fibrous tissue containing collagen and elastic fibers embedded in a gel continuum of mucopolysaccharides. This fibrous complex contains mast cells, blood and lymph vessels, neural structures, eccrine and apocrine sweat glands, hair follicles, sebaceous glands, and smooth muscle. The epidermis is an avascular, cellular structure composed chiefly of keratinocytes stratified into five layers (1,3,4). Prenatal and postnatal epidermal changes and the functional components of skin are discussed in detail (6).

A. M. Margileth: Department of Pediatrics, Mercer University School of Medicine, Hilton Head, South Carolina; and Department of Pediatrics and Dermatology, Backus Children's Hospital, Savannah, Georgia

TABLE 54–1. Neonatal skin lesions requiring minimal or no therapy[a]

Lesion	Frequency	Location and usual course	Associated conditions
Hemangioma, macular stain, salmon patch	Caucasian, 75%; black, 60%	Eyelids clear by 6 to 12 months of age; neck and glabella persist for 5–6 years or longer	Over 36 syndromes
Milia	40%; Caucasian, 64%	Cheeks, forehead, nasolabial folds; ears few weeks to 2 months of age	Gorlin and orofaciodigital syndromes
		Palate; Epstein pearls	
Sebaceous gland hyperplasia	Common in full-term infants	Nose, upper lip, malar areas; clear by 6 months of age	None
Acne neonatorum	Occurs more often in boys than girls	Face, chest, back, groin; papules, comodones, occasionally pustules by 2 to 4 weeks of age, clear by 1 to 2 years of age; keratolytic gel is prescribed for extensive cases	Beckwith–Wiedemann, Apert, and XYY syndromes
Cutis marmorata	Uncommon	Extremities, trunk; fade by adulthood	Adams–Oliver, De Lange, Down, KTW, and trisomy 18 and 21 syndromes
Harlequin color change	Rare in low-birth-weight infants	Dependent one-half of body, deep red color for 15 to 20 min	None
Miliaria rubra, crystallina	Common in warm environment	Forehead, neck, intertriginous areas; resolve rapidly in cool environment; dry, cool environment is prescribed	Consider secondary infection if pustules occur
Erythema toxicum	50% of full-term infants, less in premature infants	Body except palms and soles; onset 24–28 hours of age, resolving in few hours to 10 days of age	Eosinophils in vesicle or pustule, blood eosinophilia 20%
Transient neonatal pustular melanosis	Relatively common, African-American infants	Generalized, including palms and soles; pustules resolve by 5 days of age; hyperpigmented macules resolve by 3 months of age	Pustule aspirate shows predominance of neutrophils
Mongolian spot	Black, oriental, Indian, 90%; Caucasian, 5%	Buttocks, flanks, shoulders, extremities; fades in late infancy to adulthood	Seen in six rare syndromes
Caput succedaneum	Common	Presenting part, usually scalp; resolves by 7 days of age	Prolonged labor
Sucking blisters	Uncommon	Thumb, finger, wrists; lip; resolve in a few days	None
Subcutaneous fat necrosis	Uncommon	Cheeks, buttocks, arms, thighs; begins in the first 2 weeks of age; resolves in weeks to months	Well infant, hypercalcemia
Aplasia cutis congenita	Rare (i.e., 1 per 3,000 live births)	Scalp, commonly; trunk, face or proximal extremities with healing in several months, leaving a scar	Cleft palate, lip; absent digits, syndactyly; congenital heart disease; trisomy 13; dystrophic EB
Hemangioma: raised, strawberry, or cavernous	5% to 10% neonates, increased in premature infants	Generalized; spontaneous involution 5 to 10 years steroids prescribed if vital orifice affected, platelet trapping occurs, or cardiac failure occurs	More than 15 syndromes
Incontinentia pigmenti	Rare; female–male ratio 9:1	Extremities; trunk with vesicles resolves in first 3 months of age to warty linear lesion, then to linear hyperpigmented swirls after 1 year of age	Dental, hair, ocular, CNS, osseous defects occur in 30%
Urticaria pigmentosa, mastocytosis	Rare	Trunk, face, head, extremities as single or multiple lesions; resolve by adolescence	Urtication sign (i.e., Darier); dermatographism
Juvenile xanthogranuloma	Rare	Generalized: head, neck, upper trunk, extremities; spontaneous involution occurs by 6 months to 2 years of age	Ocular, pulmonary, testicular, renal lesions are rare

[a]CNS, central nervous system; EB, epidermolysis bullosa; KTW, Klippel–Trenauney–Weber.

PHYSIOLOGIC AND GENETIC VARIATIONS

The appearance of the newborn skin depends primarily on gestational maturation, state of nutrition, racial origin, and amount of vernix caseosa. Activity, distribution and amount of fat, hemoglobin and bilirubin levels, and the type and intensity of available light produce variations in the skin appearance. The premature infant has thin, taut skin, whereas the dysmature infant has loose, wrinkled skin (4).

Keratinization

The degree of desquamation, part of the keratinization process, varies with maturity, nutritional state, and presence of cutaneous disease. Normally, term infants show little or no desquamation until 1 or 2 days of age; peeling is complete after a few days with no treatment necessary. Desquamation occurs later in premature infants and may be quite severe in very immature infants. Desquamation is abnormal if present at birth but may indicate dysmaturity, intrauterine asphyxia, or, rarely, congenital ichthyosiform dermatosis.

Macular Hemangiomas

Macular stains of the nape, eyelids, and glabella are found in 50% of newborns. These salmon patches (i.e., nevus simplex or flammeus) have diffuse borders and become pinker when the infant cries; most eyelid lesions fade by 1 year of age. The nuchal and glabellar lesions persist longer and may appear transiently in the older child or adult when angered. Unna nevus is a persistent nuchal salmon patch (3). No therapy is indicated (4–6).

Cutis Marmorata

Cutis marmorata is a physiologic, generalized marbling effect in infants who become chilled. The netlike pattern (mottling) is caused by dilation of the capillaries and venules. It usually disappears with rewarming and is uncommon after several months of age unless there is prolonged exposure to low environmental temperatures. Persistent cutis marmorata is frequent in trisomies 18 and 21 and De Lange syndrome (5–8). Localized marbling or reticulation with atrophy of skin and larger depressed blue venous malformations is called "cutis marmorata telangiectatica congenita" (8). This vascular ectasia involves both capillaries and veins. Lesions become less noticeable by adulthood. If the condition persists or is extensive, the patient should be evaluated for skull, tooth, ocular, and skeletal malformations (3,8,9).

Harlequin Color Change

Harlequin color change is a rare phenomenon observed only in neonates, especially low-birth-weight infants. A sharply demarcated deep red color develops in the dependent one-half of the body when the infant is side lying, compared to the pale, superior half. The color change lasts from 1 to 30 minutes and reverses sides if the infant is rotated to the opposite side. The harlequin sign, observed in well and sick infants, is of no pathologic significance (3,4,6).

Milia

Epidermal inclusion cysts, or milia, are multiple yellow or white 1-mm papules noted over the cheeks, nasal bridge, forehead, nasolabial folds, hard palate, and alveolar ridges (i.e., Epstein pearls). Epstein pearls, seen in 85% of newborns, usually rupture soon after birth. Milia, observed in 40% of term infants as grouped, noninflamed papules, disappear within a few weeks to 2 months (3–6).

Sebaceous Gland Hyperplasia

In contrast to milia are innumerable tiny (<0.5 mm) yellow to flesh-colored spots involving the pilosebaceous follicles of the nose, upper lip, and malar areas. These hyperplastic sebaceous glands, rare in preterm infants, spontaneously become smaller and disappear by 2 to 6 months of age (4,6).

Acne Neonatorum

This disorder, seen more often in boys, occasionally develops during the first or second postnatal months, particularly in breast-fed infants (Fig. 54–1). Characteristically, erythematous comodones and papules are seen; pustules, nodules, and cystic lesions are rare. Lesions occur over the cheeks primarily, but also on the chin and forehead. Most lesions disappear by 1 or 2 years of age; rarely, they may persist to puberty. Most patients require no therapy except daily cleansing with a mild soap. Petrolatum, baby oils, and lotions should be avoided. Keratolytic agents or 4% benzoyl peroxide gel may be needed for more severe cases after the neonatal period (3,4,6).

Miliaria

Retention of sweat as a result of keratinous plugging of eccrine ducts causes four types of miliaria (m.): m. rubrum (i.e., prickly heat), m. crystallina (i.e., sudamina), m. pustulosa, and m. profunda (2,3). The last two conditions are rarely seen in temperate climates. Miliaria rubrum, small groups of erythematous papules and papulovesicles, is observed commonly in infants but rarely in neonates unless environmental temperature and humidity are excessively high. Miliaria crystallina, 1- to 2-mm superficial vesicles that are clear and uninflamed, is observed commonly over the forehead, neck, and intertriginous areas, and occasionally in the diaper area (Fig.

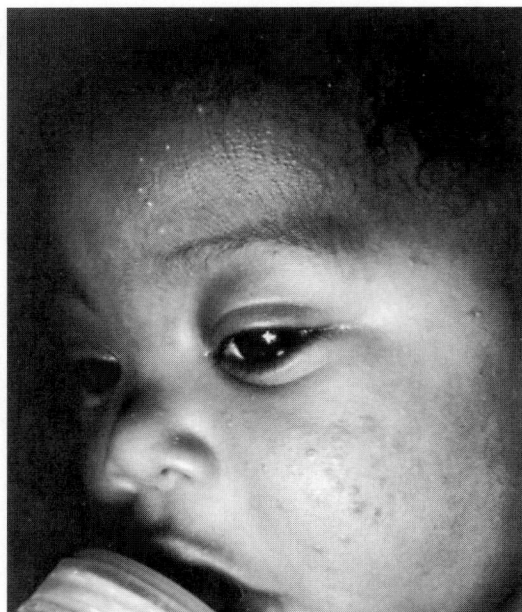

FIG. 54–1. Acne neonatorum of the cheeks in a 4-month-old boy; comedones developed at 4 weeks of age. Six miliaria pustulosa lesions are present on the forehead. There was much improvement 1 month after petrolatum was discontinued.

54–2). They may be seen at birth, particularly if there has been maternal fever. The distribution and grouping of vesicles that contain no eosinophils distinguish m. crystallina from erythema toxicum. The lesions disappear rapidly in a cooler environment and reappear in heat and humidity. Miliaria pustulosa, with leukocytic infiltration of the vesicles, is rare but may be distinguished from staphylococcal impetigo by a negative Gram stain or culture and by its rapid resolution in a cool, dry environment (3,5–7).

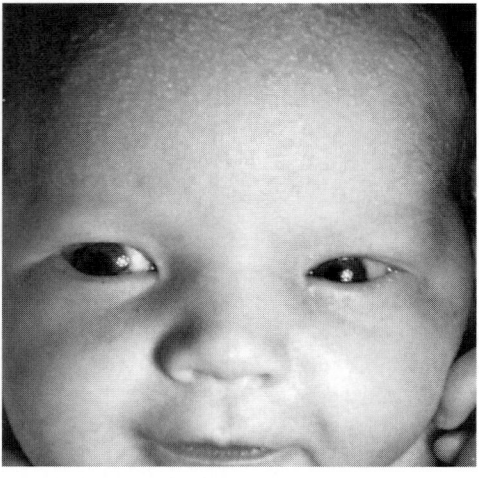

FIG. 54–2. Miliaria crystallina in a 5-day-old infant. Cooling resulted in disappearance of the lesions overnight.

Erythema Toxicum

This benign, self-limiting, perifollicular eruption, observed in 30% to 70% of healthy term infants, usually is seen at birth or shortly thereafter. Its peak incidence is at 24 to 48 hours of life, but it may appear until 1 or 2 weeks of age. The lesion starts as a red macule that quickly becomes smaller and fades as it develops into a firm, 1- to 3-mm white or pale yellow papule or pustule with a small erythematous base (Fig. 54–3). Occasionally, only erythematous macules 3 cm or smaller are seen. These may become confluent, especially over the trunk, but any body area may be involved except the palms and soles. The lesions usually fade spontaneously in a few hours or by age 10 days. Diagnosis can be confirmed by resolution within hours or by a smear of the pustule aspirate showing numerous eosinophils but no bacteria. The etiology is unknown, and treatment is unnecessary (3,6,7).

Transient Neonatal Pustular Melanosis

Transient vesicopustular melanosis or transient pustulosis occurs often in the healthy newborn (3). Over 90% of infants with this dermatosis are black. Three stages of lesions may be observed: noninflammatory pustules, ruptured vesicopustules with a collarette of scale usually surrounding a central hyperpigmented macule (Fig. 54–4),

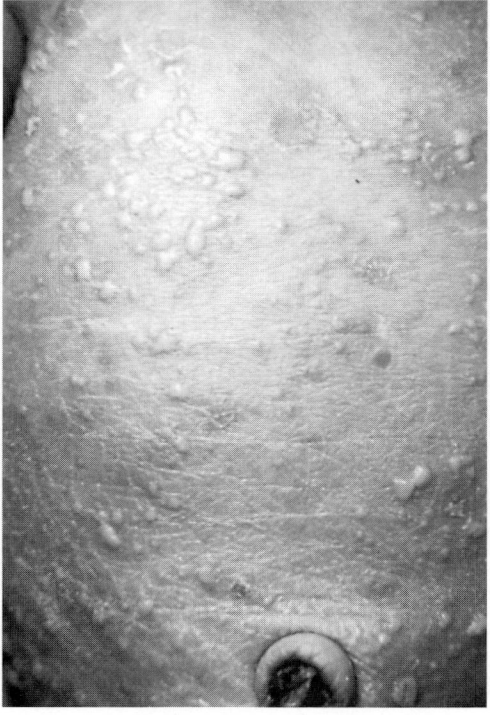

FIG. 54–3. Erythema toxicum in a 12-hour-old healthy full-term infant. At birth, many sterile pustules were present and continued to form. Wright stain of aspirate showed numerous eosinophils. The skin cleared spontaneously in 1 week.

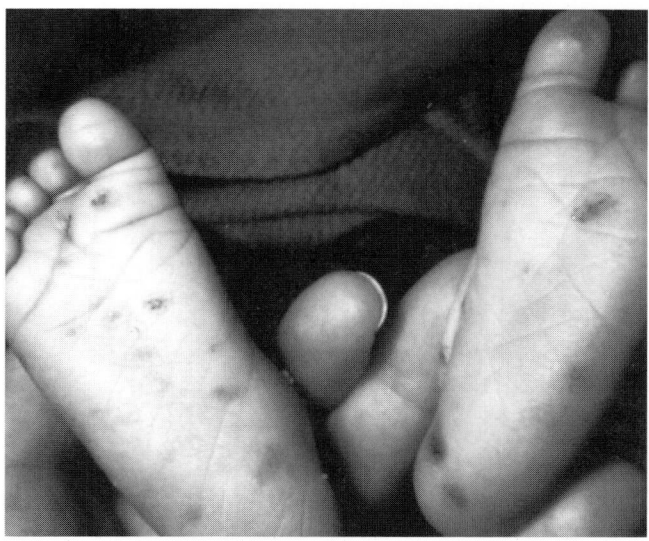

FIG. 54–4. Transient neonatal pustular melanosis in a 6-day-old African-American infant. Vesicles that were noted over the entire body at birth began scaling at 24 hours of age. A few vesicopustules developed. Note collarette of scales surrounding the hyperpigmented macules, which were very prominent by 1 month of age. TORCHES studies were negative.

and hyperpigmented macules that may persist for up to 3 months of age. Cultures are sterile; aspirated pus shows neutrophils, rare or no eosinophils, and cellular debris. The pustules, lasting 1 to 5 days, may never be observed because they ruptured before birth or with the first bath, leaving only the collarette or hyperpigmented macule. It is self-limited and requires no treatment. Differential diagnosis of vesicopustules is discussed later (3,4,7,10).

Infantile Acropustulosis

Acropustulosis of infancy presents in a healthy infant, birth to 12 months of age, with vesicopustules on the palms and soles. Erythematous papules occur initially with rapid (24-hour) development of very pruritic vesicles and pustules. The infant is often fretful or irritable, especially with recurrent crops of lesions. The pustules resolve in 7 to 14 days, leaving a scale. Occasionally papules or pustules occur on other areas of the body. A new outbreak may recur after 2 to 4 weeks, and a cyclic pattern may continue during infancy. Oral antihistamines such as diphenhydramine HCl, 5 mg/kg/day, are usually effective. Reassessment with a continued suspician of scabies is indicated. In equivocal cases a therapeutic trial of a scabicide is warranted (2,5–7,11).

Pigmented Lesions

Mongolian Spot

Mongolian spot, the most common pigmented lesion seen at birth, is present in 90% of black, Indian, and Asian infants. It occurs in 5% of Caucasian infants. These large (2–10 cm or more), macular, slate blue or gray lesions, usually seen over the lumbosacral area, also may be observed over buttocks, flanks, shoulders, and extremities. Lesions may be single or multiple and are caused by

deep infiltration of melanocytes in the dermis. The spots usually fade during late infancy but may persist into adulthood (2–6).

Café-au-Lait Spots

Café-au-lait spots, which are oval, tan, or brown macules, are seen occasionally in newborns, may develop during infancy, and are more likely in black infants (120/1,000 live births) than Caucasian infants (3/1,000) (6). Single lesions under 3 cm in length are found in 19% of normal children. An infant with five or fewer Café-au-lait spots smaller than 0.5 cm and a negative family history for von Recklinghausen disease probably is normal. Subsequently, if six or more spots larger than 1.5 cm develop postpuberty, a diagnosis of cutaneous neurofibromatosis, Proteus or Albright syndrome, or tuberous sclerosis should be considered and the patient followed closely (2–6).

Melanocytic Nevi

Melanocytic nevi (flat, junctional nevi) are pigmented lesions noted in 1% to 2% of neonates (7). These nevi are brown or black and vary from 0.1 cm to several centimeters. Usually, very few lesions are present at birth, with their number increasing with age. They may be associated with neurofibromatosis, tuberous sclerosis, bathing trunk nevi, lentiginosis, or xeroderma pigmentosum. Therapy rarely is necessary except that lesions larger than 1.5 cm should be followed closely with measurements and photographs to document any change or dysplasia, particularly if there is a family history of malignant melanoma (2–4,6).

Diffuse Hyperpigmentation

Diffuse hyperpigmentation in the newborn is unusual. The degree and location of hyperpigmentation must be considered in view of the infant's racial and genetic background (2–6,12). Diffuse hyperpigmentation may be postinflammatory or be caused by congenital Addison disease, nutritional disorders (e.g., pellagra, sprue), hepatitis or biliary atresia, hereditary disorders (e.g., lentiginosis, melanism), metabolic disease (e.g., Hartnup disease, porphyria), or be the result of bronze discoloration in Niemann–Pick disease. Androgens may produce hyperpigmentation of the labial folds with clitoral hypertrophy as a result of transplacental passage during pregnancy. Therapy depends on the basic disorder. I observed a newborn boy with slate gray melanosis at birth secondary to maternal malignant melanoma with placental metastases. The mother died 6 weeks postpartum; the infant survived without treatment and was well at 10 years of age. Although his deciduous teeth were brown, his permanent teeth were normal. Linear and whorled nevoid hypermelanosis recently reported is a benign congenital dermatoses (12).

Hypopigmentation

Hypopigmentation, a diffuse or localized loss of pigment in the neonate, may be the result of genetic (e.g., piebaldism, vitiligo, tuberous sclerosis, albinism), metabolic (e.g., phenylketonuria), endocrine (e.g., Addison disease), traumatic, or postinflammatory causes (2–7). The melanocytes may be absent or sparse.

Hypomelanosis of Ito

Hypomelanosis of Ito, a neurocutaneous syndrome, may be associated with seizures, delayed development, and ocular and/or skeletal anomalies. Usually unilateral, the skin lesions resemble those of incontinentia pigmenti, but as a negative image, i.e., bizarre hypopigmented swirls that follow Blaschko's lines (3,4,6,13).

Albinism

Albinism, an autosomal recessive disorder, occurs in all races. There are four classes of ocular cutaneous albinism (6). The infant shows markedly reduced pigmentation, yellow or white hair, pink pupils, blue irides, and photophobia with photosensitivity. Nystagmus with reduced vision is common. Small stature, mental retardation, and deafness may occur. Protection from ultraviolet light is necessary to prevent actinic keratoses and squamous cell carcinomas (2–7).

Piebaldism or Partial Albinism

Piebaldism, or partial albinism, an autosomal dominant disorder present at birth, is detected easily in the dark-skinned infant. Usually amelanotic (i.e., off-white) macules involve the scalp, widow's peak, and forehead, with extension to the base of the nose, chin, trunk, and extremities. Because an isolated white forelock may be the only manifestation, with deafness developing much later, Klein–Waardenburg syndrome must be considered (2–7,14). Differential diagnoses in the newborn are vitiligo, nevus anemicus, Addison disease, and white macules of tuberous sclerosis. Most of these entities may be excluded by the characteristic distribution of the hypomelanotic areas in piebaldism, which contain normal pigmented islands (i.e., 1- to 5-cm macules). Vitiligo (i.e., pure white macules) usually develops after 6 months of age (2–7). When illuminated with a Wood's light, these amelanotic areas exhibit a brilliant whiteness.

Nevus Achromicus or Depigmentosus

Nevus achromicus or depigmentosus, present at birth, appears as irregularly shaped, long, linear streaks of hypomelanosis that may be very small or may cover one-half of the body (Fig. 54–5). The area of hypopigmentation is uniform in color and usually unilateral. The lesion, when rubbed, shows a normal vasodilation response, in contrast to nevus anemicus, which is unresponsive and remains pale compared to normal adjacent vasodilated skin. Therapy is not necessary for either lesion because both usually occur in covered areas (2,3,5–7).

White Macules

White macules (i.e., leukoderma, hypopigmented spots), detected in 90% of infants with tuberous sclerosis

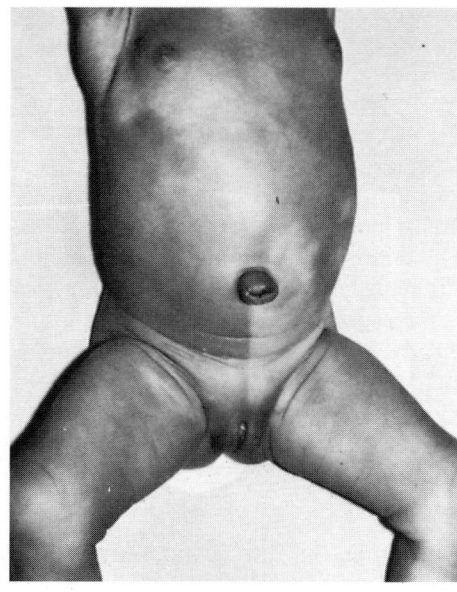

FIG. 54–5. Nevus achromicus of the right chest, left abdomen, and leg in a healthy 3-week-old premature infant. Hypopigmentation was noted at 10 days of age. A normal flare response developed after rubbing. Family history was negative for hypopigmented lesions. (Courtesy of M. Renfield, M.D. and F. Bowen, M.D.)

(epiloia), may be present at birth. These spots may be missed in light-skinned infants unless a Wood's lamp is used. The macules are about the size of a thumbprint or mountain ash leaf, vary in number from four to more than 100, usually are seen over the trunk or buttocks, and have a normal physiologic response to stroking. All infants with otherwise unexplained seizures should be examined carefully for these macules with a Wood's lamp. Most hypopigmented macules seen at birth are not associated with epiloia. In one study, only one of 35 hypopigmented macules seen in 4,641 newborns was caused by tuberous sclerosis. The other macules may be normal or associated with nevus anemicus, neurofibromatosis, or a developing hemangioma. Because other cutaneous features of epiloia (e.g., angiofibromas, shagreen patch, periungual fibroma) take years to develop, careful follow-up is essential (2–5,7,13).

Purpuric Light Eruption

Purpuric light eruption is a newly recognized transient, benign cutaneous eruption in transfused neonates who received phototherapy for hyperbilirubinemia. Transfusions were given and phototherapy instituted within 24 hours of birth in six neonates. Five had erythroblastosis fetalis. The photodistributed purpura appeared within 4 days of light therapy and cleared within one week of cessation of phototherapy (15).

TRAUMA

Caput Succedaneum

A diffuse, edematous, occasionally hemorrhagic swelling of the presenting part occurs secondary to compression of local vessels associated with prolonged labor. The scalp, scrotum, labia majora, or an extremity (Fig. 54–6) may be involved. Edema recedes in a few days; ecchymoses, if present, clear in several weeks. No therapy is needed, and sequelae are not reported (2,4–7,14).

Sucking Blisters

Occasionally, a few intact or ruptured 1-cm bullae may be noted on the thumb, index finger, wrist, or lip where the infant sucked vigorously *in utero* (2,4–7). The blisters contain sterile, serous fluid and resolve spontaneously.

Skin Trauma

Abrasions, ulcerations, ecchymoses, lacerations, or areas of pressure necrosis of the presenting part may be seen after prolonged labor, vacuum extraction, application of forceps or scalp electrodes, or fetal blood sampling. Cephalohematoma, a subperiosteal collection of blood bounded by the suture lines of the skull, often feels

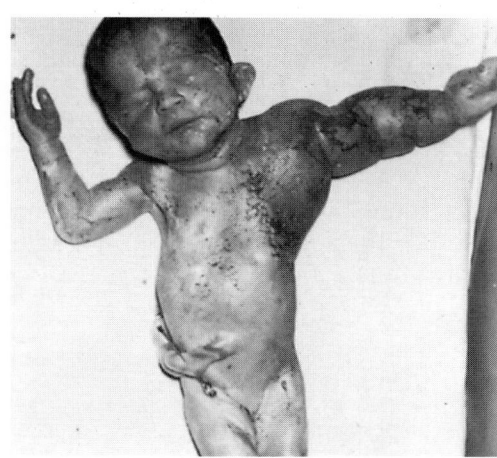

FIG. 54–6. Caput succedaneum edema and ecchymoses of the presenting part in a 1-day-old premature infant. Labor was prolonged; a cesarean section was necessary. Swelling disappeared spontaneously in 1 week; the arm functioned normally.

fluctuant. Rarely secondary bacterial infection may occur (2–7). Ulcerated areas should be kept clean and dry, especially if a deep ulcer develops from pressure necrosis. If serous drainage occurs, application of water or normal saline dressings, changed every 4 hours, for 1 to 2 days will minimize exudate formation and infection. Application of local antibiotic ointment will be effective for secondary superficial infection. Subconjunctival hemorrhage or petechiae usually are inconsequential and spontaneously disappear within a few weeks.

Fat Necrosis

Fat necrosis, an uncommon, sharply circumscribed, red-purple, indurated subcutaneous nodule or plaque appearing on the extremities, trunk, or buttocks during the first weeks of life, has been attributed to trauma, shock, cold, and asphyxia. It appears most commonly under the area of forceps application if a fat cheek has been compressed against the zygoma. The lesion is nonpitting and hard, may be painful, and may have a deep reddish or purplish discoloration. The infant is healthy and nurses vigorously. As the lesions resolve, some rarely may undergo liquefaction and appear as a sterile abscess but should not be drained. All lesions resolve spontaneously over weeks to months. Residual atrophy and scarring are unusual. Hypercalcemia occurs rarely (2–7).

Sclerema Neonatorum

Sclerema neonatorum more commonly affects the preterm or severely debilitated infant. It may have the same etiology and adipose tissue abnormality in the subcutaneous tissues as noted in fat necrosis (3,6). Low environmental temperature alone can produce the injury. A diffuse hardening of subcutaneous tissue develops with cold, stony hard, nonpitting induration. The extremities may be involved at first, but generalized involvement occurs within 3 to 4 days. Most infants are severely ill, but, if they survive, the sclerematous changes rarely persist beyond 2 weeks. Differential diagnosis includes edema neonatorum, Milroy and Turner syndromes, and panniculitis (1). Therapy is based on the underlying systemic disease, restoration of body temperature, and adequate nutrition (2,4).

DIAPER DERMATITIS

Napkin or diaper dermatitis is a common, transient, erythematous eruption localized to the diaper area. Maceration and scaling are common; eventually, nodular ulcerations develop after improper care. Neonatal skin is more permeable and susceptible to irritation. Predisposing factors are inheritance of a reactive skin with a seborrheic or atopic diathesis; systemic disease such as syphilis, acrodermatitis enteropathica, or Letterer–Siwe disease; activating factors such as occlusive moist heat or retention of sweat; secondary infection caused by pyogenic invaders, viruses, or yeasts; mechanical irritation; contact factors (e.g., retained urine or stool, especially diarrhea); and parental factors such as overcleaning or inability to carry out proper skin care or therapeutic directions (2–7).

Contact Diaper Dermatitis

Primary irritant or contact dermatitis, a common problem, often is caused by direct application of harsh soaps, detergents, lanolin, and sensitizers (e.g., neomycin, nystatin, parabens, ethylenediamine, sulfur) or is secondary to recurrent diarrhea, especially with alkaline stools. Petrolatum or mineral oil, tolerated in older infants or young black infants, may cause maceration with sweat retention in Caucasian infants. When the intertriginous areas are clear and the eruption involves the mons pubis,

scrotum, penis, medial thighs, and buttocks, a clinical diagnosis of contact dermatitis is likely (Fig. 54–7) (2–7).

Therapy consists of frequent diaper changes; keeping the area clean, dry, and cool; and elimination of the offending irritant (e.g., stool and urine). Impermeable plastic pants foster heat and sweat retention and are to be avoided. In the acute stage, rapid healing will occur if no diapers are used for 24 to 72 hours. Irritation will be diminished by application of a zinc oxide paste with each new diaper. Warm water only or with a mild soap (Dove) should be used for cleansing. Aveeno or starch baths are soothing. Alternatively, multiple cotton diapers laundered in a mild soap and carefully rinsed with a vinegar solution may be used. Loosely applied paper diapers with wicking materials to keep moisture away from the skin and without added perfumes are effective if changed frequently.

Intertrigo

Intertrigo, a symmetric red, moist, macerated eruption in skin folds and creases, is secondary to excessive sweating and close approximation of opposing gluteal or inguinal surfaces. It is managed in the same way as contact diaper dermatitis; exposure to dry air is most helpful. Ointments must be avoided. Because secondary yeast or bacterial infection usually occurs within a few days, cultures or smears should be considered. A light application of 0.5% to 1% hydrocortisone cream after each diaper change for a few days may be helpful.

Monilial Diaper Dermatitis

Diaper dermatitis occasionally is caused by or associated with *Candida* species. Over several days, a vesiculopustular eruption becomes confluent to form a moist, bright red, macerated rash. Diagnosis is suspected by the presence of many 0.5- to 1-cm superficial satellite erosions or moist patches and pustules outside the diaper rash (Fig. 54–8) or perianal eruption. *Candida albicans*

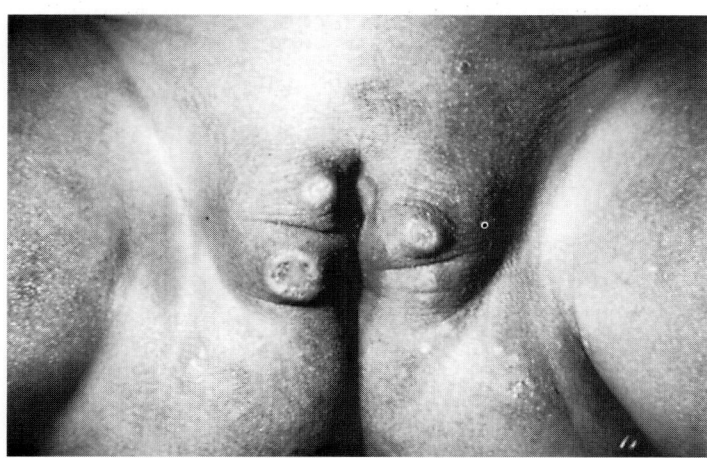

FIG. 54–7. Chronic ulceronodular contact diaper dermatitis and secondary staphylococcal infection in a 1-month-old infant. The rolled edges of the ulcers are characteristic. Note the absence of skin involvement in the thigh folds.

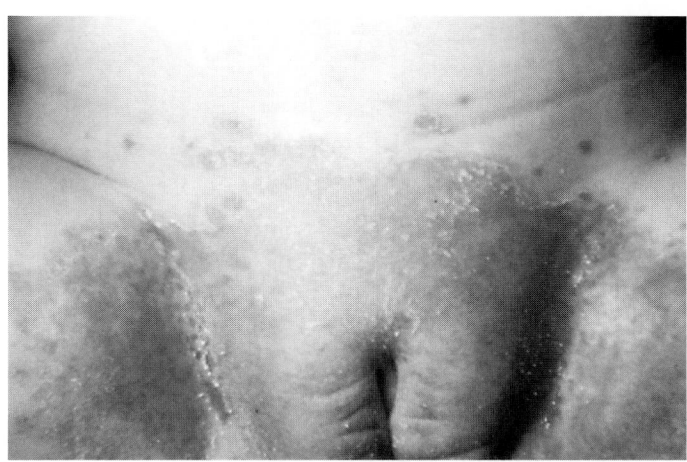

FIG. 54–8. Monilial diaper rash persisted for 3 weeks in a 6-week-old infant. There was no response to nystatin ointment. However, gentian violet, 1% aqueous, applied three times a day for 3 days was effective. Note the presence of satellite lesions.

can be identified quickly by Gram stain of scrapings. Oral thrush with white plaques over the tongue and soft and hard palates usually is seen after the second week of life, whereas cutaneous lesions may occur at any age. A generalized rash may develop in untreated infants, especially if an endocrinopathy or immunologic deficiency exists or the infant is very premature. Prolonged antibiotic therapy, diabetes mellitus, and excessive sweating are predisposing factors. Candidal diaper dermatitis is treated with proper cleansing followed by nystatin cream (100,000 U/g) applied three or four times a day for 7 to 10 days. If erythema is intense, a 1% hydrocortisone ointment applied three times daily can be helpful. When there is failure of nystatin (see Fig. 54–8), 1% aqueous gentian violet, applied three times a day for 3 days, is recommended. A repeat 3-day course of therapy occasionally is necessary after a 3-day lapse. It is essential that the diaper area remain clean and dry (2–7).

Seborrheic Diaper Dermatitis

Seborrhea of the diaper area, rarely seen in the absence of scalp or truncal involvement (see Seborrheic Dermatitis), is characterized by patchy redness, fissuring, scaling, and occasional weeping, especially in intertriginous (e.g., gluteal) folds. The scalp and postauricular regions should be examined for an oily, scaly, minimally erythematous eruption, which is diagnostic. Scraping the scales and rubbing them between the fingers produces a soapy sensation. The eruption, rarely seen during the first week of life, may become widespread (i.e., truncal) by 1 or 2 months of age. The principal therapy consists of a selenium sulfide shampoo to the scalp every night for 1 to 2 weeks. Application of 2% ketoconazole cream to the scalp once daily is an alternative therapy. Application of 1% hydrocortisone cream three times a day for 4 to 7 days to the diaper or other inflamed areas may promote healing. If secondary candidal infection exists, nystatin cream applied three times a day for 7 to 10 days is recommended (2,3,5–7).

Subacute and Chronic Secondary Diaper Dermatitis

Diaper rash may occur in association with cutaneous or systemic bacterial, viral, or fungal infections; diarrhea; atopic eczema; or prolonged use of fluorinated topical steroids (2,3). Secondary staphylococcal infection superimposed on eczematous diaper dermatitis can produce an erosive nodular eruption (see Fig. 54–7) that can be resistant to local therapy. Elimination of the primary irritant and of allergic and physical agents (e.g., cold, heat) as well as use of a systemic antibiotic effective against staphylococci will clear the infection. Hydrocortisone, 1% in zinc oxide ointment, or zinc oxide paste alone will provide protection from irritants in infants with atopic dermatitis. Mild, nonalkaline soaps are necessary to keep the skin clean without irritation. Education of the parent is essential to avoid recurrence (2,3,5–7).

MISCELLANEOUS SKIN LESIONS

Redundant Skin

Loose skin folds are observed over the neck posteriorly in Turner, Down, and trisomy 13 syndromes. Redundant skin in a more generalized distribution is seen in infants with trisomy 18 and combined immunodeficiency syndrome with dwarfism and alopecia. Dermatomegaly or cutis laxa and cutis hyperelastica (i.e., Ehlers–Danlos syndrome), although rare, must be differentiated. The diagnostic features may not be evident in the neonatal period (1–8,13).

Congenital Fistulas

Auricular, branchiogenic, and thyroglossal fistulas and cysts are relatively common and easily detected in the ear, lower lip, and anterolateral neck. Most fistulas may be

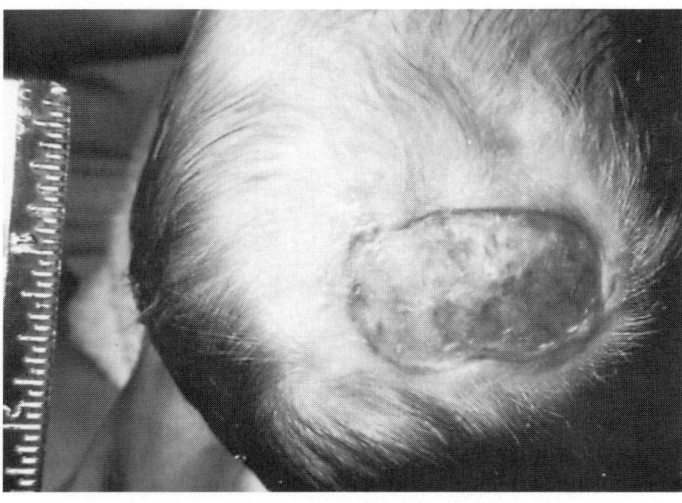

FIG. 54–9. Cutis aplasia of the scalp in a 1-month-old infant with trisomy 13. Healing occurred spontaneously by 4 months of age.

noted in the neonatal period; cysts develop in later infancy or childhood, particularly when secondary infection develops. Surgical excision is the definitive treatment (2,3,5).

Umbilical Anomalies

After the cord has separated, a small (3- to 7-mm), dull red, dry, velvety granuloma may slowly develop. Purulent exudate caused by secondary infection may occur. Daily application of a silver nitrate stick effectively will cauterize the granuloma and cause it to recede, whereas the rare umbilical polyp (i.e., persistent remnant of the omphalomesenteric duct or urachus) will not. The latter lesions require surgical excision (1).

Aplasia Cutis Congenita

Congenital absence of skin, not uncommon, may present as a localized, midline posterior scalp defect or as several small or one large defect involving the extremities and occasionally the trunk. The typical scalp lesion is a 2- to 3-cm, circular, sharply marginated area (Fig. 54–9). At birth, the lesion usually is covered by a smooth membrane that often desquamates, leaving a dry ulcer. These lesions heal slowly over several months by reepithelialization, leaving a hypertrophic (Fig. 54–10) or atrophic scar. Infection is rare. Other embryologic malformations, cleft lip and palate, defects of hands and feet, and trisomy 13 or 4p syndrome may be associated. Extensive congenital defects of the skin present at birth (Fig. 54–11A) usually are multiple and heal spontaneously by epithelial growth from the borders. The end result is an acceptable thin scar (Fig. 54–11B). Histologically, these areas show an absence of epidermis, few appendageal structures, and decreased dermal elastic tissue. Infection should be prevented by handling with gloves, with local cleansing, and through application of antibiotic ointment TID. Extensive aplasia cutis may be associated with epidermolysis bullosa (EB) (1–3,5–7,16). In either case, skin grafting should be avoided.

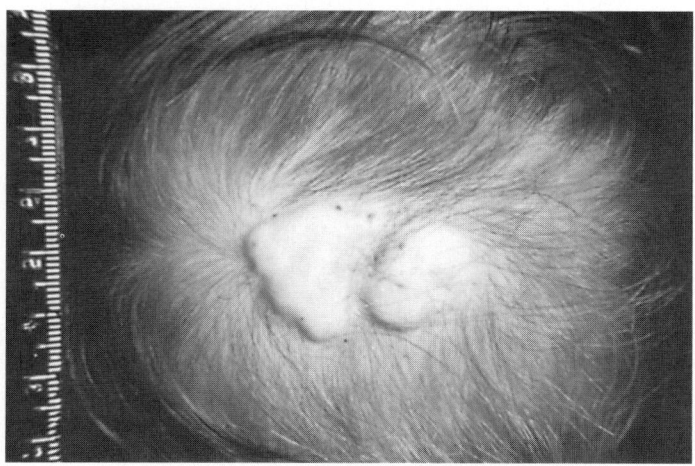

FIG. 54–10. Keloid of the scalp of a normal 1-year-old child who had an isolated posterior scalp defect at birth. A hypertrophic scar developed spontaneously during the first 3 months of life.

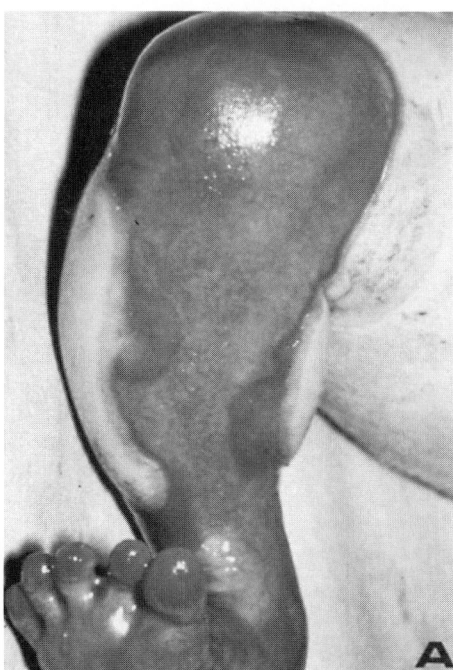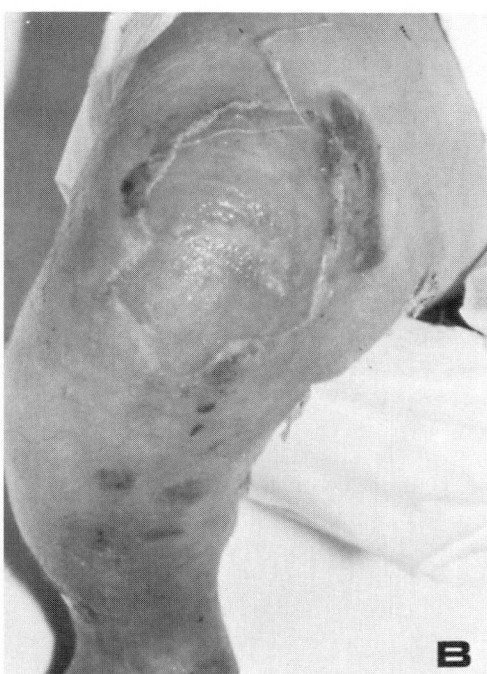

FIG. 54–11. A: Cutis aplasia and epidermolysis bullosa simplex in a 4-day-old infant with absent epidermis of the leg. Note bullae on the toes. **B:** The same patient with spontaneous healing at 6 weeks of age. (Courtesy of K. A. Gill, Jr., M.D.)

Hypoplasias

Focal dermal hypoplasia (Goltz syndrome) is characterized by linear areas of thinning or absence of dermis with herniation of fat through surrounding skin. The areas resemble red or yellowish brown deflated balloons. Atrophic scars, aplasia cutis, telangiectasias, intense whealing after stroking, and red papillomas (e.g., perioral, intraoral, perianal, vulvar) may be found. Additional cutaneous (e.g., alopecia, nail), skeletal, ocular, dental, aural, and mental defects may be present (2,3,5–8,13). Therapy is symptomatic and based on the major findings. Genetic counseling is recommended (13).

NAIL, SWEAT, AND HAIR DISORDERS

Nail Disorders

Hypoplastic Nails

Total absence (i.e., anonychia), partial absence, or dysplasia of nails occurs in 25 known disorders (1–8, 13). Well-known entities include anhidrotic ectodermal dysplasia and Apert, Ellis–van Creveld, trisomy, and nail–patella syndromes. Many of these conditions will be apparent in the neonatal period; a large number are familial (Fig. 54–12). In general, etiology and pathogenesis are poorly understood; therapy is not available or needed.

Hypertrophic Nails

Hypertrophic nails, rarely observed in the neonate, may occur as familial onychogryposis, as congenital onychauxis, or in association with congenital hemihypertrophy or the pachyonychia congenita syndrome (1–8,13). Treatment is relatively ineffective; amputation may be necessary for restoration of function.

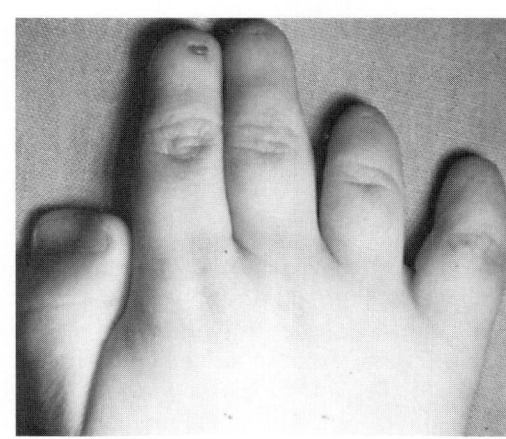

FIG. 54–12. Anonychia and hypoplasia of the nails in an infant who was otherwise normal. Similar nail defects with broad thumbs were present in five siblings and family members for five generations.

Sweat Disorders

Anhidrotic or Hypohidrotic Sweating

Anhidrotic (i.e., absent) or hypohidrotic (i.e., decreased) sweating occurs in several disorders (2,4,5). Anhidrotic ectodermal dysplasia with hypotrichosis and defective dentition is the most striking disorder and may be recognized during early infancy by absence of the eyebrow and eyelashes (1–8). By 1 year of age, facies are distinctive with frontal bossing, flattened nasal bridge, depressed central face, and absent eyebrows. Alopecia occurs later. The skin is dry, hypopigmented, and thin with prominent vessels. Absence of sweat can be detected after 6 weeks of age by pilocarpine iontophoresis. Hyperpyrexia with fever of undetermined origin, caused by marked heat intolerance, often is the first major clue that brings the infant to a physician's attention. Therapy consists of a cool environment and application of wet towels during warm weather. Deficient lacrimation can be palliated by use of artificial tears; a wig will conceal severe alopecia. Genetic counseling is indicated. The disease is inherited in an X-linked recessive pattern linked to Xq 12q13.1 region; over 90% are male (1–8,13).

Hair Disorders

Hair disorders rarely present as isolated defects. Hypertrichosis, hypotrichosis, and abnormal morphology (e.g., twisted, ringed, beaded, node-like hair) usually are not appreciated until after the neonatal period. Exceptions are hypertrichosis of the Cornelia de Lange syndrome, trisomy 18, and localized hairiness seen in congenital hemihypertrophy and diastematomyelia. Hypertrichosis occurs in normal Hispanic infants. Alopecia totalis congenita may occur alone or with hidrotic ectodermal dysplasia. Changes in hair color, caliber, and fragility may suggest a specific diagnosis. The best test is to perform dissecting microscopic examination of the hair shaft. Therapy is based on the specific diagnosis because many systemic disorders are associated with hair disorders (1–8,13).

NEVI AND TUMORS

Many nevi and cutaneous tumors are not present at birth but develop during the early months of life. A nevus is a localized, highly differentiated, proliferative malformation arising from keratinocytes, melanocytes, or appendageal (i.e., organoid) or vascular structures (3). Two distinct forms of nevi are congenital and acquired moles. The type of nevus is described best by its origin or location, such as melanocytic nevus, sebaceous nevus, or systematized nevus.

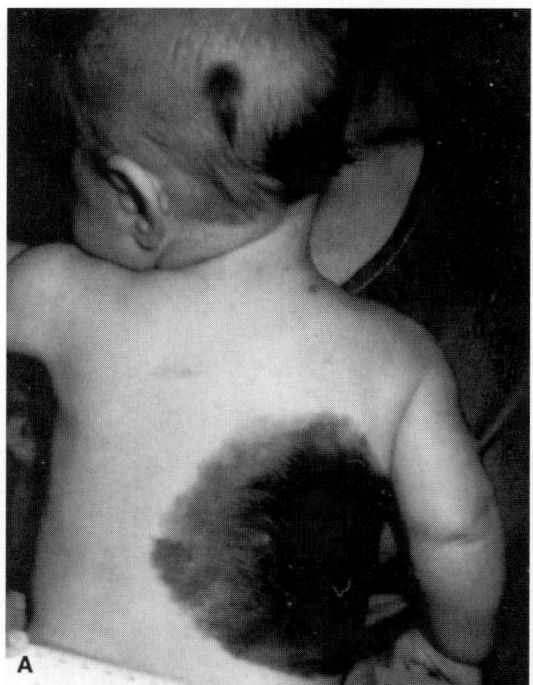

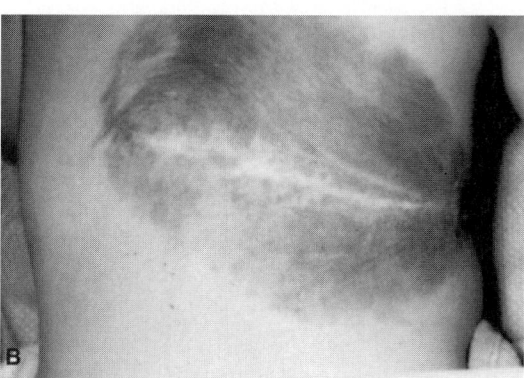

FIG. 54–13. A: Giant hairy nevus in a 9-week-old healthy infant. Multiple smaller hairy nevi were present. **B:** Same infant at 20 months of age after first wedge resection of the center of the nevus. Note the much lighter color of the entire nevus. (Courtesy of M. Boyajian, M.D., Children's National Medical Center, Washington, DC.)

The following is an outline of a classification of nevi (3):

    Dermal: congenital and acquired
        Melanocytic: nevocellular or pigmented (1–7)
            Junctional
            Intradermal
            Compound
            Giant hairy, congenital
            Blue: common, cellular
        Vascular
        Nervous tissue

Epidermal (1–7)
  Keratinocytic
    Nevus unius lateris
    Verrucoid: small, systematized
    Systematized
    Epidermal nevus syndrome
  Appendageal (i.e., organoid)
    Nevus comedonicus (3,5,6)
    Sebaceous
    Hair follicle
    Apocrine duct
  Connective tissue (1,3,6)
    Solitary nodular calcification (6)
    Osteoma cutis (3)

Melanocytic Nevi

Junctional, compound, and intradermal nevi rarely are encountered at birth. They are classified histologically as follows: in junctional nevi, all melanocytes are above the basement membrane; in compound nevi, all melanocytes are in the epidermis and dermis; and in intradermal nevi, all melanocytes are in the dermis. In one study, pigmented nevi occurred in 3% of Caucasian newborns and 16% of black infants (3). In another, 1.1% of 4,641 newborn infants had these lesions (3).

Blue Nevi

Blue nevi in neonates present in two forms: the common, large (1- to 3-cm) congenital Mongolian spot (i.e., cellular dermal melanocytic) discussed previously, and the small, dermal melanocytoma (i.e., blue nevus) rarely noted at birth. The latter presents as a grayish or steel blue 0.3- to 1.0-cm papule or nodule that remains static. Found on the buttocks and upper body, these nevi may be difficult to differentiate clinically from vascular lesions. If diagnosed clinically, routine follow-up is sufficient. Otherwise, simple complete elliptic excision with histologic diagnosis is curative (1–7).

Giant Hairy Nevi

Giant hairy nevi [i.e., congenital raised melanocytic nevi, nevocellular nevi (NCN), larger than 10 to 20 cm, are present at birth in four of 4,641 newborns and may be found anywhere on the body. Less commonly found lesions on the neck and scalp may be associated with lep-

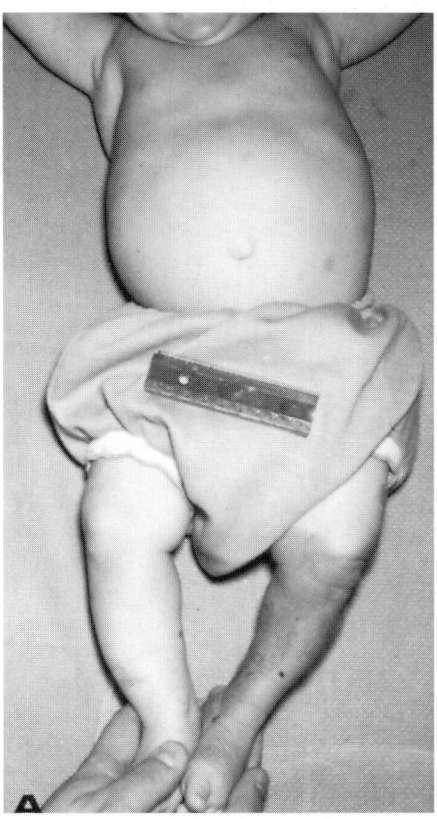
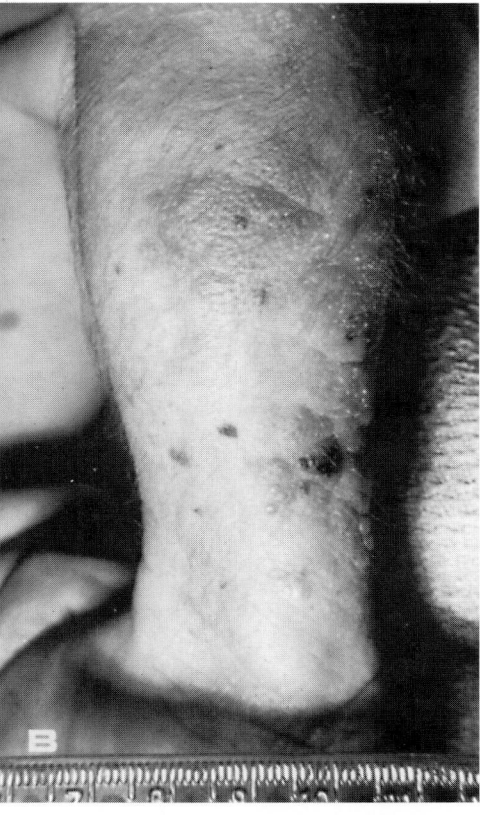

FIG. 54–14. A: Mixed nevus with atrophy of the leg in a 3-month-old child. More than six café-au-lait spots larger than 1.5 cm are present. **B:** Elements of lymphangioma circumscriptum (i.e., angioma cystica), hairy pigmentation, and shagreen plaques are present.

tomeningeal melanocytosis and epilepsy or signs of focal neurologic abnormalities (17). Complete excision (Fig. 54–13) with plastic reconstruction should be considered by 15 years of age because the lesions may be associated with a 1% to 15% lifetime risk of melanoma (17). Depilation alone of associated small (<2 cm), hairy, intradermal nevi may produce a cosmetically acceptable result. Shave excision and electrodesiccation of hairy nevi in special areas (e.g., eyebrow) may be more desirable than total excision with skin grafting (1–7).

Nervous Tissue Nevi

Nevi of neural origin, found in neurofibromatosis, rarely are observed in the newborn. Occasionally, these nevi may be part of a mixed cutaneous malformation with osseous defects (Fig. 54–14A). These congenital lesions may consist of hemangioma or lymphangioma tissue, nevus pigmentosus et pilosus, and plexiform neuromas. Localized hypertrophy with or without elephantiasis of tissues usually is seen; rarely, atrophy of the affected part is observed (Fig. 54–14B). In selected cases, surgical resection will improve function and appearance (Fig. 54–15). Fortunately, these lesions change very slowly over many years (4,9,13).

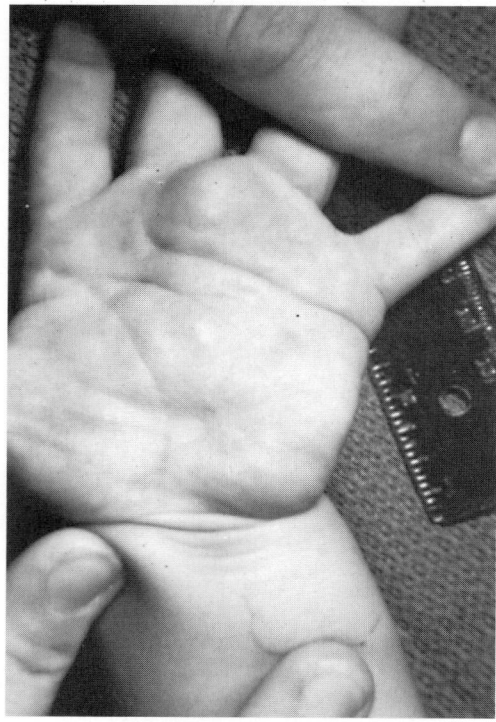

FIG. 54–15. Neurofibroma of the left wrist and hand in an infant. The larger left hand and swelling were noted at 9 months of age. Resection of a painful plexiform neuroma of the palmar area was performed at 2 and 6 years of age, resulting in improved function.

Tumors

Malignant skin tumors rarely are observed in the newborn period (17). The following congenital skin tumors and cysts may occur (1–7):

- Dermoids
- Digital fibroma
- Epithelial cysts
- Fibrosarcoma, rhabdomyosarcoma
- Lipomas
- Mastocytomas
- Neuroblastomas
- Neurofibromas
- Teratomas
- Xanthogranulomas

Because of concern about malignant potential of a congenital nevi or a tumor, consultation is indicated (3,17). Potential precursors of cutaneous melanoma in children include giant congenital NCN, seen in 1% of newborns, and dysplastic melanocytic nevi, usually seen during adolescence. Most small (<2 cm) NCN require no therapy. After a detailed history is obtained, the lesion should be examined carefully with a magnifying lens; it should be palpated and measured accurately. A photograph is invaluable for subsequent reference. Repeated assessment of the lesion every 6 to 12 months will help the parents and physician decide whether excisional therapy is needed (18). Excision of NCN or congenital tumors should be considered in the following situations: for cosmetic reasons, particularly if the lesion is a large hairy nevus; repeated trauma or changes in the lesion morphology, color, size, surface, or borders; if the lesion is pruritic, bleeding, or painful; if the lesion appears atypical (e.g., very dark, irregular pigmentation); or there is a positive family history of cutaneous melanoma, dysplastic nevi, or tumors. Histopathologic examination of all tissue removed is mandatory (1–7,18).

EPIDERMAL NEVI

Verrucoid nevi commonly seen in the neonate are local or systematized nevi and nevus unius lateris (Fig. 54–16). The latter lesion consists of linear or spiral, unilateral, hypertrophic papules or warty lesions in a continuous or interrupted pattern in single or multiple sites. They usually are found over the neck, trunk, or an extremity at a single site. Pruritus and inflammation may occur. Rarely, one-half of the body is involved and shows signs identical with those seen in congenital ichthyosiform erythroderma. Widespread linear, systematized, verrucous lesions may involve the oral mucosa, ocular conjunctiva, or scalp (1–8). Cases involving epidermal nevi, skeletal defects, vascular anomalies, and severe mental retardation, convulsions, or both (Fig. 54–17) were designated the epidermal nevus syndrome (8).

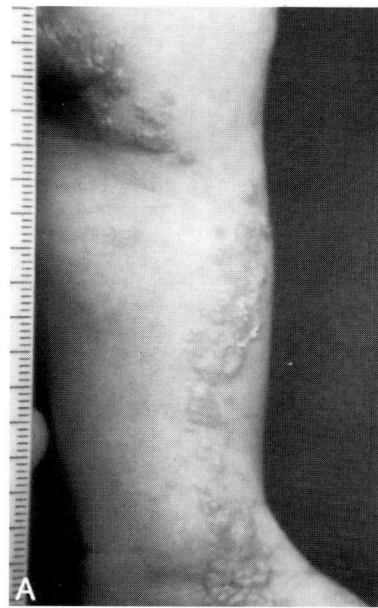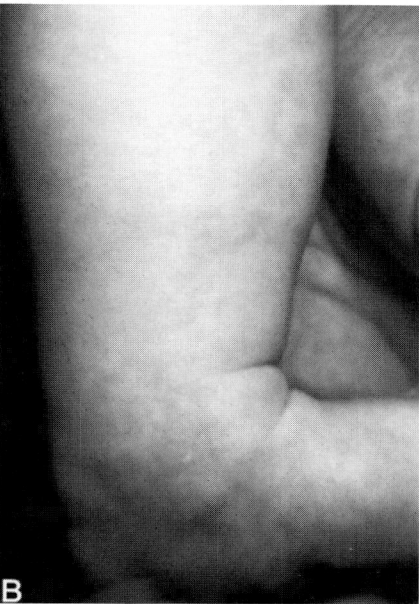

FIG. 54–16. Nevus unius lateris. **A:** Left leg of a 13-day-old healthy infant with linear hypertrophic papules and warty lesions noted at birth. **B:** Same infant at 3 months of age had spontaneous clearing of most of the lesions.

Management consists of repeated observation and application of Eucerin or Eucerine Plus cream after bathing to soften the lesions. Spontaneous improvement of the nevus unius lateris has been noted. Eventually, the verrucous epidermal nevus should be removed by full-thickness excision during late childhood (1–3,5–7).

Sebaceous Nevi

This lesion, observed in the newborn over the scalp (Fig. 54–18) or forehead, is a discrete yellowish to yellowish brown or orange, cobblestoned, oval, hairless plaque. It may occur on the face, ears, or neck. Untreated, these

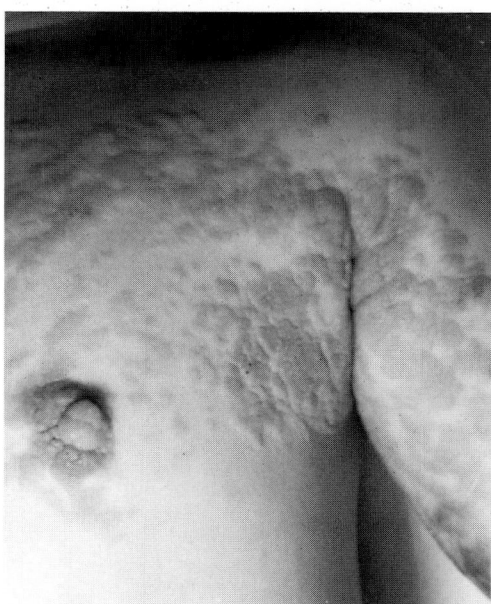

FIG. 54–17. Epidermal nevus syndrome. The left chest of a 5-month-old infant who had a large epidermal nevus that covered the left scalp, forehead, face, and upper chest at birth. Infantile spasms and severe mental retardation occurred at 2 months of age.

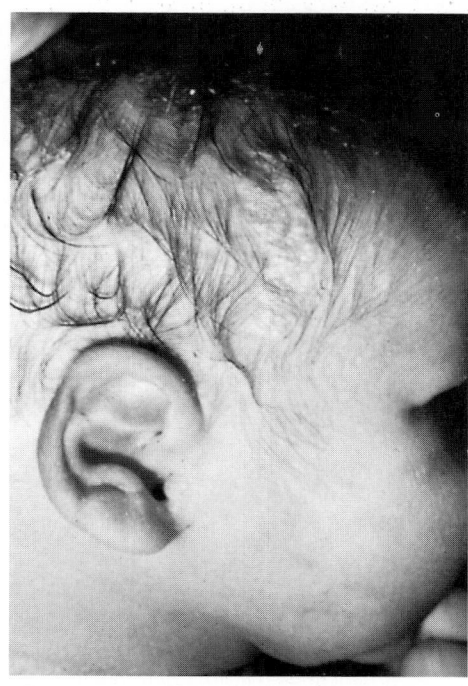

FIG. 54–18. Nevus sebaceous in a newborn infant's scalp. The cobblestone yellowish lesion remained unchanged after several years.

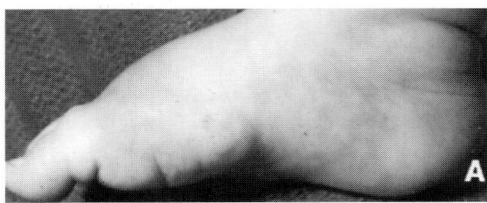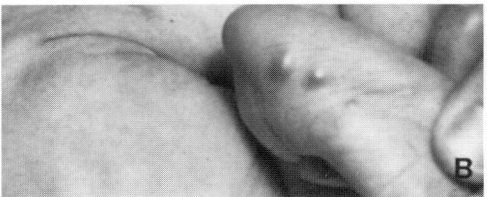

FIG. 54–19. A: Neuroblastoma. Thirty cutaneous nodules and hepatosplenomegaly occurred in a 1-month-old infant. The nodules regressed after surgical removal of a retroperitoneal neuroblastoma and cyclophosphamide therapy for 1 year. The patient was well at 4 years of age. (Courtesy of S. Leikin, M.D., Children's National Medical Center, Washington, DC.) **B:** A 2-month-old infant had 13 violaceous nodules; excision of eight of the nodules revealed neuroblastoma. No primary tumor was found; no treatment was given. The nodules involuted by 6 months of age; the patient was well at 3 years of age. (Courtesy of J. L. Kennedy, Jr., M.D., Saint Elizabeth Hospital, Boston, MA.)

lesions change little, if at all, for years. About 15% eventually transform into basal cell carcinoma; therefore, simple excision during early puberty is advised. Juvenile xanthogranuloma and syringocystadenoma papilliferum must be considered differentially in the young infant (1–8).

Congenital Tumors

Dermoids

Dermoids (i.e., epidermal inclusion cysts), which present at birth or soon thereafter, are round or ovoid 1- to 15-cm subcutaneous tumors of soft or rubbery consistency. They are encapsulated and contain sebaceous material and hair and often are located at the outer ends of eyebrows or on the neck, sternum, scrotum, perineal raphe, or sacrum. In one study, they were found in 58% of 775 superficial lumps (18). Simple surgical excision is effective. Midline pits or cysts need investigation for a possible intracranial connection (1–7).

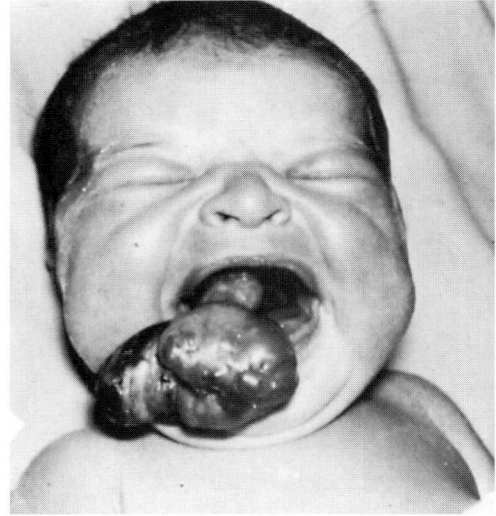

FIG. 54–20. Epignathi arising from a hard palate in a newborn infant. Surgical removal took place at 1 day of age; no recurrence was seen at 1 year of age. (Courtesy of W. Bason, M.D., and M. Museles, M.D.)

Neuroblastoma

Neuroblastoma, the most common cutaneous cancer at birth, is detected in one-third of affected infants by the presence of five to 30 small (2- to 20-mm), bluish or pale blue nontender nodules (Fig. 54–19). Stroking results in blanching and a red halo (1,3,5,7). Hepatomegaly and a retroperitoneal primary neuroblastoma frequently are present. Prognosis in this age group is excellent (90%) with low-stage disease plus surgery and chemotherapy.

Teratomas

Teratomas present as neck, intraoral, or sacrococcygeal tumors. They are large (3 to 10 cm), firm, nontender, and fixed to underlying tissue. Multiple calcifications often are seen on radiographs. Epignathi (i.e., intraoral teratomas) contain structures resembling fetal parts (Fig. 54–20). Prompt surgical excision is necessary for functional and cosmetic reasons. After the patient is 5 months of age, these tumors tend to reveal embryonal carcinomatous elements. Recurrences, if they appear, will do so within 2 years after removal. Epulis, a fibrous tumor of the gums, tends to resolve spontaneously (5).

DEVELOPMENTAL VASCULAR ABNORMALITIES

Angiomas, or vascular nevi, are common cutaneous congenital malformations seen in 10% of infants but in only 2% of newborns. Two major groups seen in children are the involuting and noninvoluting vascular lesions, which may be flat (i.e., macular or telangiectatic) or raised (i.e., hemangiomatous). The following is an outline of these abnormalities (1–7,19–21):

Hemangiomas: involuting
    Macular stains
        Salmon patch
        Erythema nuchae
        Cutis marmorata congenita
    Angiomatous nevi
        Superficial strawberry (i.e., capillary–endothelial)

Mixed capillary–cavernous, combined type
Deep cavernous–subcutaneous types
Hemangioendothelioma (spindle cell)
Benign diffuse neonatal hemangiomatosis
Vascular malformations: noninvoluting, present at birth (20)
    Port-wine nevus (i.e., nevus flammeus)
      Sturge–Weber syndrome
      Hemangioendothelioma, giant, Kaposiform, or tufted, thrombocytopenia (Kasabach–Merritt syndrome) (19)
    Congenital multiple systemic hemangiomatosis
      Cutis marmorata telangiectasia congenita– congenital phlebectasia
      Telangiectatic congenital erythema (Bloom syndrome)
      Angiokeratoma circumscriptum (hyperkeratotic, capillary)
      Nevus vasculosis hypertrophicus: Klippel–Trenaunay–Weber
    Venous malformation (with/without nodule)
      Blue rubber bleb nevus syndrome
      Arteriovenous fistula
Lymphatics: vasoformative and noninvoluting lymphangiomas and lymphedema
    Simple lymphangioma: solitary nodules
    Lymphangioma circumscriptum: vesicles (angioma cystica)
    Cystic hygroma
    Lymphedema, congenital, hereditary (Turners, Milroys) (3)

Studies of the common involuting types (i.e., erythema nuchae, salmon patch, spider nevi or telangiectases, superficial strawberry, mixed, deep cavernous) have shown that no active therapy is necessary and that problems occur only when improper intervention is attempted. The natural pattern for the strawberry or cavernous hemangioma is rapid growth (i.e., to double or triple in size) within several weeks or months during early infancy. At birth, the skin usually appears normal or shows a macular lesion that has a pink flush or off-white color. Rarely, a tumor will be present at birth (Fig. 54–21) (21). By 2 months of age, the strawberry lesion is bright red, or blue if cavernous type, in about 90% of infants. When maximal size is attained, usually between 9 and 12 months of age, the color becomes a dark red.

At this time the hemangioma remains quiescent; its growth rate is the same as that of the infant. By 12 to 18 months, often earlier, spontaneous involution begins. The color gradually fades to a grayish pink; a grayish white hue appears in the center of the lesion and spreads until the whole area becomes white or pink. There is a decrease in tenseness as involution progresses. Although the bulk of the lesion diminishes, the area of discoloration decreases very slowly over several years (1–7,20,21).

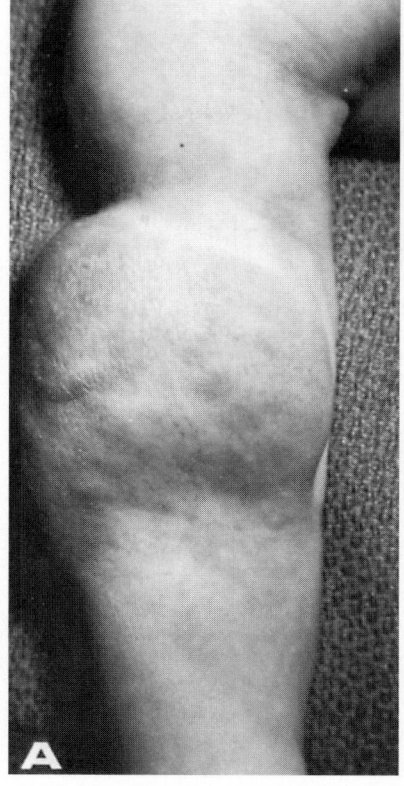
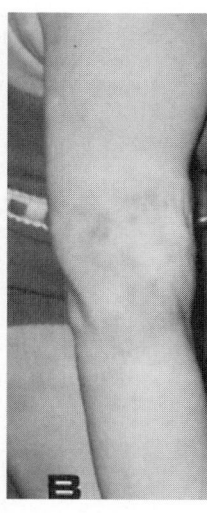

FIG. 54–21. A: A cavernous hemangioma of the arm in a 6-day-old infant. The mass, which was 6 × 10 cm × 1 cm elevated, was compressible (50%) and blanched and felt like a bag of worms. **B:** The same patient at 15 months of age; no therapy was used. (Courtesy of E. Kraybill, M.D., University of North Carolina, Chapel Hill, NC.)

Macular Stains and Telangiectatic Nevi

Involuting nevi, the salmon patch (i.e., erythema nuchae), and cutis marmorata congenita, have been discussed previously.

Angiomatous Involuting Nevi or Raised Lesions

Superficial Strawberry Hemangioma

Strawberry hemangioma is a capillary hemangioma, usually bright red or purplish red with well defined margins. Rarely present at birth, it usually appears within a few days or weeks as a pink or red macule, resulting from a myriad of tiny capillaries. The lesion enlarges during the first 5 to 6 months. The strawberry nevus blanches incompletely with pressure, and on palpation is a firm, rubbery mass that compresses minimally. It is found on any part of the cutis and rarely involves mucous membranes. One or two are common; rarely, 20 or 30 lesions may be observed in an infant (Fig. 54–22).

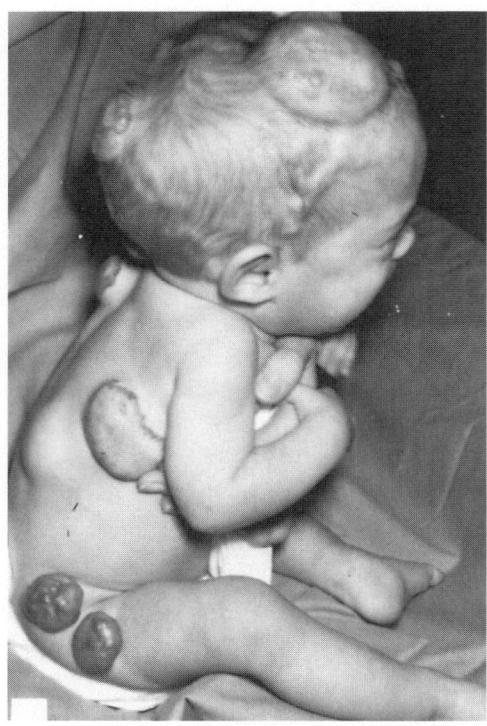

FIG. 54–22. A 7-month-old infant with 21 strawberry, cavernous, and mixed hemangiomas. No lesions were seen until 1 month of age. Between 7 and 8 months of age, one new lesion developed. Nine hemangiomas are visible over the scalp, back, and thigh. By 6 years of age, only three involuting lesions remained; these were gone by 12 years of age.

Deep Cavernous Hemangioma

The cavernous hemangioma arises deeper in the dermis, usually with poorly defined borders (see Fig. 54–21A), but may be well circumscribed and elevated (see Fig. 54–21B). The tumor, composed primarily of large venous channels lined by mature endothelial cells, usually imparts a reddish blue discoloration to the overlying normal skin. On palpation, these lesions often are cystic and feel like a bag of worms. The swelling usually compresses to one-half of the original size and quickly resumes its usual size on release of pressure. When the infant strains and cries, the tumor often becomes larger and darker blue. The mixed (capillary–caverous, combined) hemangioma consists of a cavernous lesion with an overlying strawberry component (Fig. 54–23).

Natural Course

The natural growth pattern of strawberry, cavernous, and mixed hemangiomas is a noticeable increase in size during the first 3 to 6 months of life, a stationary period of several months during which the hemangioma grows at the same rate as the patient, and then spontaneous involution. Based on the size of the hemangioma at 1 to 3 months, 80% of 420 hemangiomas observed in 308 children grew less than double in size. About 5% tripled and 2% quadrupled their size. Because hemangiomas are benign, and diagnosis is made easily by careful evaluation and repeated observation, a biopsy is not indicated (1–7,22). In a 20-year study, the strawberry, cavernous, and mixed hemangiomas regressed spontaneously and at similar rates during an 8- to 10-year period (22). By 5 years of age, one-half of these had involuted spontaneously. One infant I observed had over 200 hemangiomas that involuted spontaneously by 3 years of age.

Treatment

Superficial vascular nevi located in exposed areas often cause great parental concern because of their cosmetic impact. Parental anxiety increases as the hemangioma grows and causes deformities, especially in the breast, lip, ear, or eye. Additional concern develops when

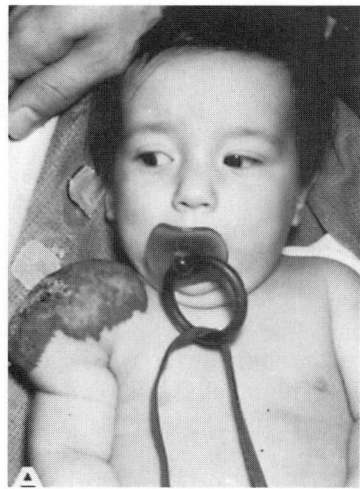
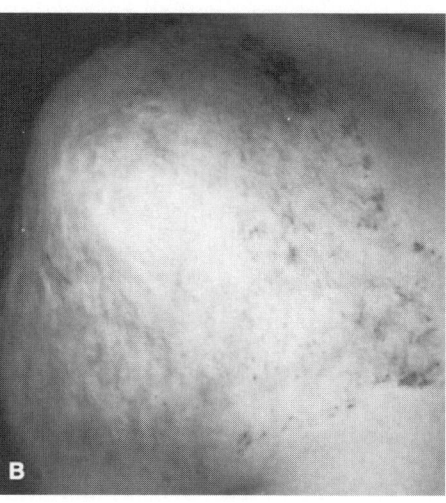

FIG. 54–23. A: A combined hemangioma in a 4-month-old infant was first noted at 1 month of age. Rapid growth occurred until 2½ months of age. Ulceration developed at 3 months. The volume was 284 cm³. **B:** When the patient was 9 years and 10 months of age, the volume was 20 cm³; this is a spontaneous reduction of 90%. The lesion disappeared by 11.5 years of age.

ulceration or bleeding occurs from trauma, maceration, or infection (20–22).

Complications following unnecessary therapy occurred in 12 of 20 of my patients treated elsewhere. Radiation and injection therapy caused greater morbidity and resulted in more extensive scarring than did surgery or dry ice. By contrast, complications during spontaneous involution are infrequent. In decreasing frequency, these are ulceration, bleeding, and infection. Therapy after breakdown includes local saline compresses, gentle cleansing, and an antibiotic ointment. Bleeding and secondary infection appear to be natural processes that hasten spontaneous involution. Residual scarring after complete involution is uncommon and rarely unsightly. Minimal bleeding, controlled by direct local pressure, occurs in about 5% of children.

Active treatment rarely is needed (20–22). Education of parents is essential. Reassurance with close observation for several years is necessary. Color photographs should be taken of exposed lesions to document the nat-ural pattern of involution (22). For the parent who wishes a more active yet conservative treatment, local massage or application of a compression bandage for 23 hours changed twice daily may be effective (Fig. 54–24) (22).

In rare instances in which the diagnosis is uncertain (e.g., atypical growth or no evidence of a vascular lesion), excisional biopsy may be required. In a patient in whom a hemangioma enlarges rapidly (i.e., within a few weeks) and vital structures are compromised (Fig. 54–25) so that tissue destruction results, prednisone may be effective. Prednisone, 2 to 5 mg/kg per day for 3 to 4 weeks, was beneficial in 24 of 28 patients with hemangiomas obstructing the nares, auditory canal, or vision (20–22). If signs of involution (Fig. 54–26) occur after several weeks, prednisone should be continued as alternate-day therapy for an additional 4 weeks. After 8 weeks, the prednisone should be tapered, and the lesion observed for recurrence. Regrowth may occur; it was not noted in 26 of my 28 patients (see Fig. 54–26). A second course of prednisone may be effective when necessary. The use of

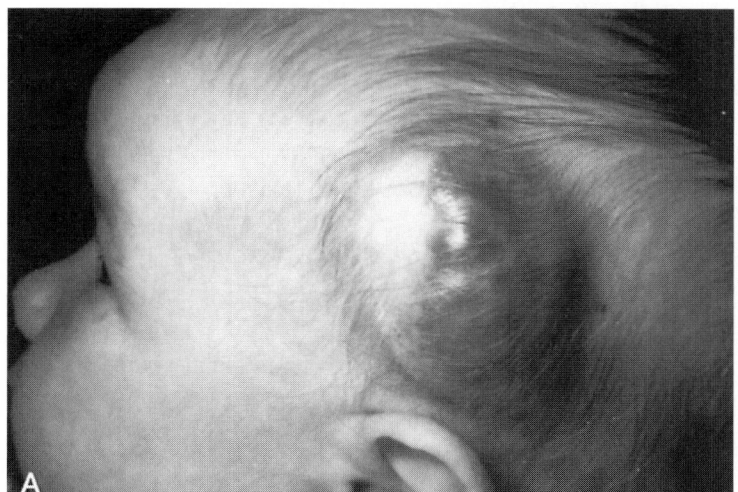

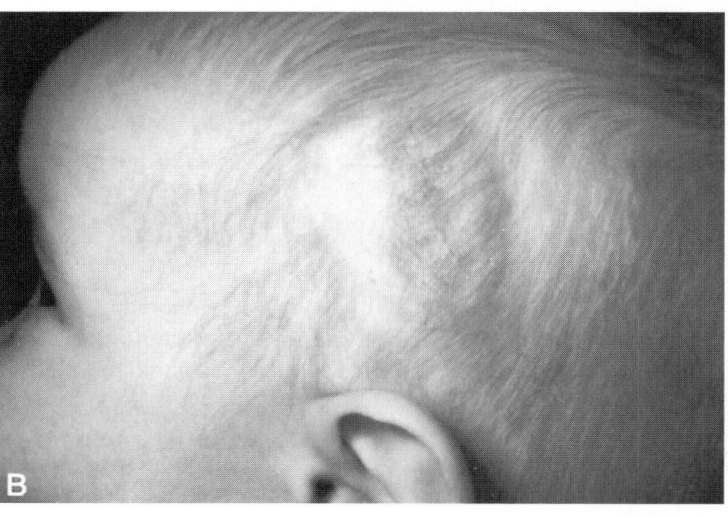

FIG. 54–24. A: A cavernous strawberry hemangioma grew rapidly since birth in a healthy 5-week-old infant; the volume of the lesion was 42 cm³. **B:** At 4.5 months of age, the lesion was 90% involuted because of active daily compression and massage by the infant's mother 100 times per day.

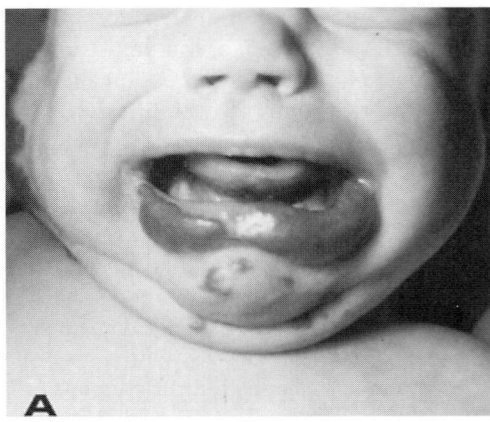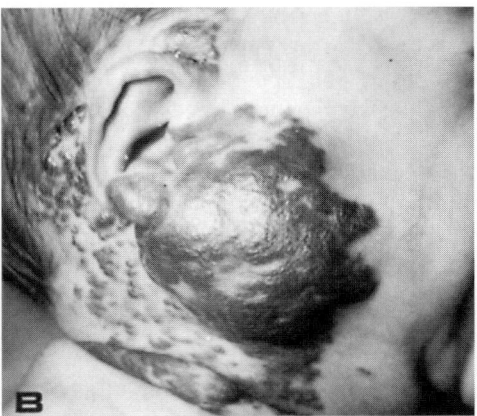

FIG. 54–25. A: Strawberry hemangiomas of the lip and chin. **B:** A combined dermal and right parotid hemangioma in a 6-week-old infant. The lesions were first noted at 5 days of age and continued to enlarge; new strawberry hemangiomas appeared on the neck and chin.

intralesional corticosteroid injections has proved effective in treating capillary hemangiomas of the eyelid; however, visual loss may occur after injection (3,23). Plastic surgery may be necessary for redundant tissue persisting after spontaneous regression or in an older child whose lesion has not regressed.

Congenital Vascular Malformations

These noninvoluting nevi are the capillary port-wine nevus or stain, the telangiectatic, hypertrophic capillary, venous, arteriovenous, and lymphatic malformations (2,5–8,20,24). A few of the more common lesions are discussed.

Port-Wine Nevus

The port-wine nevus (nevus flammeus), present at birth, is a mature capillary angioma. The lesion is flat, sharply delineated, shows stable growth with the child, and blanches minimally. It may be very small (i.e., a few millimeters) or cover almost one-half of the body. In black infants, these nevi appear jet black. The characteristic red or reddish purple color intensifies when the infant cries. Unfortunately, facial lesions are common. Involvement of the lower and upper eyelids (i.e., first and second branches of trigeminal nerve) with associated seizures, mental retardation, contralateral hemiplegia, or intracortical calcification suggests the Sturge–Weber syndrome (1–8,13). Patients with upper eyelid port-wine stains alone had no eye or CNS complications. Most port-wine nevi occur as isolated defects (24). They may occur in trisomy 13, Rubenstein–Taybi, Beckwith–Wiedemann, and Klippel–Trenauney–Weber syndromes (8,13). In a few children, the lesions may become lighter with age; however, they rarely disappear. A water-repellent cosmetic cream (e.g., Covermark, Retouch) will conceal the mark effectively. Pulsed dye laser therapy is cosmetically effective and can safely be started by age 2 weeks (6,25).

Giant hemangioendothelioma with thrombocytopenia (i.e., Kasabach–Merritt syndrome) occurs during the first 3 months of life. The hemangioma may be small, 5 to 6 cm, or consist of smaller multiple hemangiomas involving dermal or internal organs (19). Thrombocytopenia (2 to 40,000/mm^3) with or without hemorrhagic manifestations caused by platelet entrapment occurs after several weeks or months. The hemangioma itself may suddenly enlarge as a result of bleeding. Because of severe thrombocytopenia, consumption of fibrinogen, anemia, spleno-

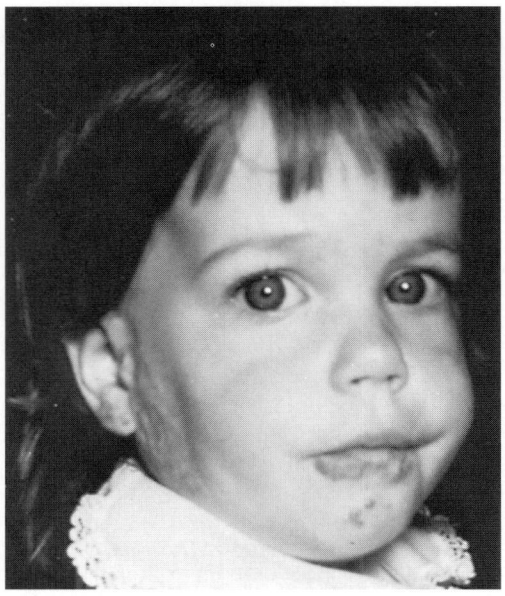

FIG. 54–26. The same patient shown in Fig. 54–25 at 18 months of age. There was no recurrence after a 3-month course of prednisone, 10 mg, on alternate days.

megaly, and purpura, close observation and appropriate hematologic studies are necessary (19). Spontaneous resolution has been reported in some patients who were treated conservatively. Oral prednisone, 2 to 5 mg/kg per day for 1 to 2 months, may be effective treatment. If feasible, compression of the tumor by an elastic bandage 22 to 23 hours daily may reduce its size within a few weeks (22). Death may occur from infection or hemorrhage.

Congenital Multiple Systemic Hemangiomatosis

Diffuse neonatal hemangiomatosis, a very rare condition, may result in an early death in infants from cardiac failure, gastrointestinal hemorrhage, infection, or hydrocephalus from aqueductal compression by hemangioma. Criterion for diagnosis is the recognition by magnetic resonance imaging (MRI) of nonmalignant visceral hemangiomas in one to several organ systems; cutaneous hemangiomas in varying numbers (one to 100 or more) are found concomitantly (2–7,20).

Therapy is supportive. A trial of oral prednisone in large doses (5 to 10 mg/kg daily) should be tried initially in seriously ill infants. Diffuse neonatal hemangiomatosis should be differentiated from the Riley–Smith and blue rubber bleb syndromes (3,5,8).

Other Vascular Nevi and Cutaneous Vascular Tumors

Phlebectasia, or venous ectasia, a rare vascular lesion consisting of dilated mature vessels in the dermis and subcutaneous tissues, presents in two forms in the newborn or young infant. Single or multiple tumors resembling cavernous hemangiomas grow slowly and may be associated with hypertrophy of the extremity. I observed three children with neck varicosities and four with unilateral leg or forearm lesions (22). The other form, cutis marmorata telangiectatica with generalized phlebectasia, is apparent at birth and involves underdevelopment of subcutaneous and osseous tissues and other associated anomalies in 25% to 50% of patients. In both types, therapy rarely is necessary because steady improvement occurs with growth (2–7).

Hemangiectatic hypertrophy (i.e., Klippel–Trenaunay–Weber syndrome) of a limb associated with an extensive cutaneous nevus and a developmental hypertrophy of underlying bone and soft structures (i.e., osteohypertrophic varicose nevus) is a rare congenital abnormality. It is seen more frequently in boys than in girls. The three major clinical features—hypertrophy of an extremity, vascular nevus, and venous varicosity—are not necessarily proportionate in extent and severity (2,3,5–7,26). The nevus may be unilateral and the hypertrophy bilateral; minimal hypertrophy may be associated with an extensive nevus. Varicosity of the superficial veins with deep subcutaneous involvement may be a conspicuous feature noted at birth (Fig. 54–27). The nevus may be flat, strawberry, or cavernous with thick-

ening and deformity of subcutaneous tissues. Occasionally, atrophy of bone, muscle, and soft tissue develops and, in fact, did occur in one of my eight patients. Selective amputation of a grossly malformed digit and orthopedic measures to prevent limb hypertrophy will improve appearance and function (see Fig. 54–27). When lymphedema is extensive with gross deformity of an extremity, treatment with a sequential linear compression device 8 to 12 hours daily may be helpful (3,27). Education of parents in care is essential (6,26).

Lymphangiomas

Tumors of lymphatic origin, less common than hemangiomas, are hamartomatous malformations consisting of dilated lymph channels of various sizes lined by normal endothelium. Of four major types observed, three may be present at birth. All four usually develop during infancy or before age 5 years (1–8). Generally, these tumors grow slowly or not at all.

Simple lymphangioma, the least common, presents as a solitary, well-defined, skin-colored dermal subcutaneous tumor on the face or neck. Mucous membranes rarely are involved. Simple surgical excision usually is satisfactory.

Lymphangioma circumscriptum, observed most commonly, consists of small, thick-walled vesicles in the skin resembling frog spawn (Fig. 54–28). Sites commonly involved are axillary folds, neck, shoulder, proximal limbs (see Fig. 54–28A), perineum, tongue, and buccal mucous membrane (28). Usually localized, such lesions may be extensive. Often a hemangiomatous component is present, including blood-filled vesicles (see Fig. 54–28B). Rarely, after several years of observation during which the lesion remains unchanged, the tumor will enlarge suddenly because of spontaneous bleeding or trauma. Spontaneous involution is uncommon, occurring in only one of ten patients in my series. Satisfactory results will follow complete surgical excision, which is difficult but necessary to avoid recurrence (2–5,7).

Cystic Lymphangioma or Hygroma

Cystic lymphangioma, or hygroma, occurs most often in the neck (i.e., hygroma colli) and axilla, but it may also occur in inguinal, popliteal, and retroperitoneal regions and as mesenteric cysts. These are usually large unilocular cysts, but they may also be multilocular, especially in the neck. Transillumination will be present unless bleeding occurs. Because these lesions may grow rapidly with infiltration of vessels and nerves, surgical excision should be considered, but results are often unsatisfactory. Rarely, spontaneous regression may occur (3).

Lymphedema

Congenital lymphedema occurs in two forms: as primary lymphedema, which mainly involves the lower

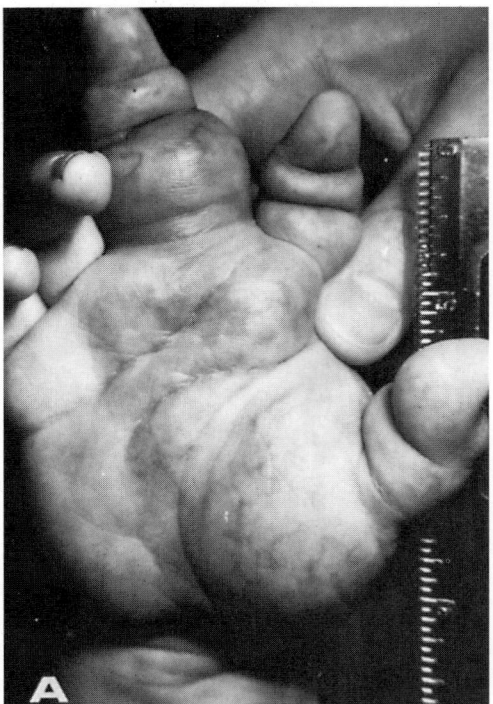
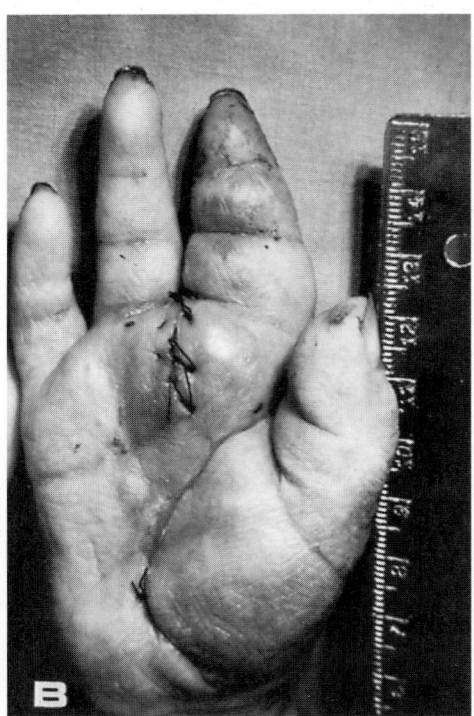

FIG. 54–27. A: Hemangiectatic venous hypertrophy of the hand, arm, and shoulder of a 3-year-old child. The lesion was present at birth and enlarged slowly during the first 6 months of life. There was no growth in the following 2 years, but the hand functioned poorly. B: The same patient at 3.5 years of age, 7 days after amputation of the middle finger. Subsequently, useful function of the hand returned.

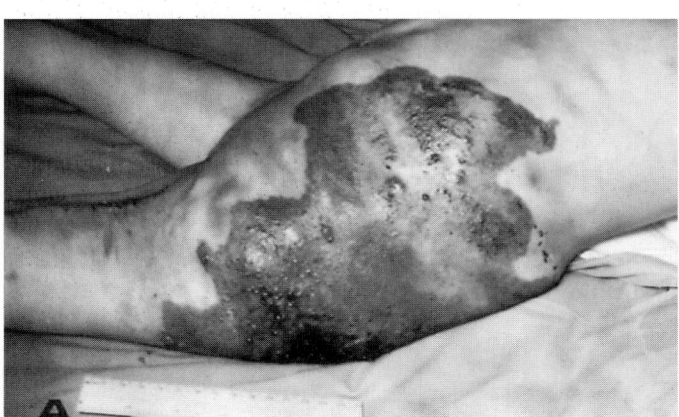

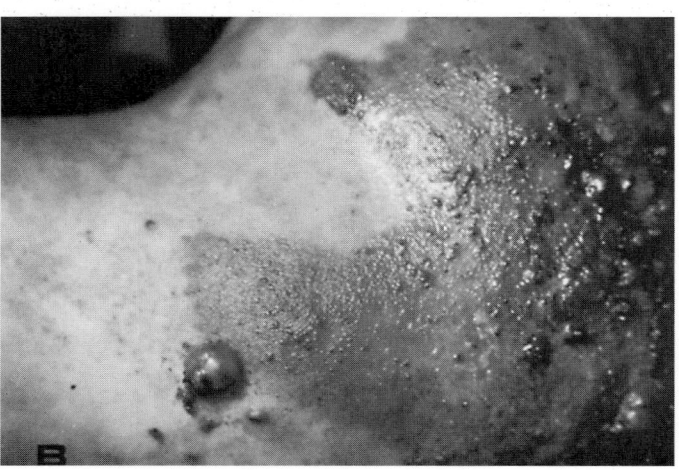

FIG. 54–28. A: A giant hemolymphangioma involving the upper thigh, flank, and retroperitoneal areas was present since birth. Radical extirpation was necessary to drain a staphylococcal abscess within the mass. B: Lymphangioma circumscriptum in the same patient shows thick-walled vesicles (i.e., frog spawn) overlying the tumor.

extremities and occurs mostly in girls; and as Turners or Milroy disease (i.e., hereditary lymphedema), which is almost always confined to the legs and feet. In Milroy disease, the edema is firm, and the temperature of overlying skin is elevated. Its pathogenesis is unclear; treatment during infancy is unnecessary. In both conditions, upper extremities and genitalia may be involved (1–8).

Rarely, chylothorax and chylous ascites may develop in infants with congenital lymphedema. The brawny edema that becomes permanent as progressive tissue fibrosis occurs may respond to compression therapy 8 to 12 hours daily with a sequential linear compression device (27). Antibiotics are effective for secondary streptococcal and staphylococcal infections. Reconstructive surgery may be helpful.

INFECTIONS OF THE SKIN

Blistering disorders in the neonate frequently result from infection of bacterial, fungal, or viral origin. The following is an outline of some of these eruptions (2–7,10,11).

Bacterial
  Impetigo caused by *Staphylococcus* sp., group A
    streptococci, or group B streptococci
  Haemophilus influenzae
  Listeria monocytogenes
  Pseudomonas aeruginosa
  Staphylococcus aureus causing staphylococcal
    scalded-skin syndrome (SSSS) or toxic epidermal
    necrolysis (TEN; i.e., Ritter disease)
Fungal
  Oral candidiasis (i.e., thrush)
  Paronychial infection
  Mucocutaneous candidiasis
  Aspergillus flavus
  Spirochetal
  Congenital syphilis
  Lyme disease
Viral
  Cytomegalovirus (CMV)
  Enteroviruses
  Herpes simplex (HSV)
  Herpes zoster
  Varicella

Blistering has not been reported in congenital rubella or toxoplasmosis. Maculopapular eruptions, usually without purpura, occur in the neonate as a result of fungal, parasitic, and viral infections. When purpuric or petechial maculopapular eruptions are seen, the clinician must look for bacterial sepsis, hematologic disorders, histiocytosis X, or viral (e.g., rubella) infections.(2) The following is an outline of various nonpurpuric and purpuric or petechial eruptions.

Nonpurpuric
  Aspergillosis
  Coccidiodomycosis
  Congenital syphilis (purpura may occur)
  Lyme disease
  Molluscum contagiosum
  Toxoplasmosis (purpura may occur)
  Warts
Purpuric or petechial
  Autoimmune neonatal lupus erythematosis (NLE)
  CMV disease
  Enterovirus
  Hematologic disorders
  Histiocytosis X
  Listeriosis
  Rubella syndrome
  Septicemia: group A and B streptococci,
    gram-negative bacilli

The clinical history and the morphologic characteristics of the cutaneous lesion (e.g., maculopapular, with or without purpura, vesicobullous) suggest the differential diagnosis of a specific eruption (2–7,10,11). Although a skin biopsy may delineate the cutaneous level of blister formation or histologic nature of the eruption, it rarely is necessary. Diagnosis may be obtained by routine or special cultures (e.g., fungal, viral), stained smears, scraping using 10% KOH solution, or a Tzanck smear to detect multinucleated giant epithelial cells caused by HSV and varicella–zoster virus (1,10). Antibody titers, coupled with the history and morphologic findings, will provide a diagnosis in most infants (2–7,11).

Vesicobullous Eruptions

The following is a partial list of noninfectious disorders that produce vesicobullous eruptions (2,3,5–7,10,11, 13):

Acrodermatitis enteropathica
Acropustulosis of infancy
Arthropod-induced blisters (i.e., scabies)
Bullous ichthyosiform erythroderma
Epidermolysis bullosa
Erythema toxicum neonatorum
Erythropoietic porphyria
Eosinophilic pustular folliculitis
Graft-versus-host disease (GVHD)
Histiocytosis X, congenital selfhealing
Incontinentia pigmenti
Miliaria pustulosa
Protein C deficiency
Transient neonatal pustular melanosis
Urticaria pigmentosa (i.e., mastocytosis)

Bullous impetigo of the newborn, a superficial vesicopurulent pyoderma involving the stratum corneum, commonly occurs in the neonate and infant and usually is caused by staphylococci. The blisters vary from small vesicles to large, flaccid bullae filled with clear or straw-colored fluid. These rupture quickly and leave a red, moist denuded area (Fig. 54–29). Lesions may be widely dispersed and vary from a few single ones to large denuded areas. Because of thick stratum corneum, blisters over the palms and soles are less likely to rupture. Regional lymphadenopathy is rare unless ecthyma or secondary infection occurs with insect bites, eczema, scabies, herpetic lesions, or varicella.

Coagulase-positive *S. aureus* frequently are cultured on aspiration of bullae. Rarely, β-hemolytic streptococci or a gram-negative bacteria will be isolated. Group A streptococci usually produce omphalitis, paronychia, erysipelas, perianal cellulitis, or sepsis (1–7,10,11). Skin abscesses or umbilical lesions can occur as a result of group B streptococci, although this is unusual. Blood cultures should be done if sepsis is suspected. Aseptic technique is essential to prevention in the hospital nursery. Infected infants should be isolated, with universal precautions carefully followed.

Topical therapy consists of cleansing the lesions with povidone–iodine (Betadine) skin cleanser three to four times daily for 5 to 7 days until no new lesions appear. Concomitantly, a bacitracin or 2% mupirocin ointment should be applied locally. For extensive lesions or symptoms compatible with sepsis, systemic antibiotics specific to the isolated organism are indicated.

Staphylococcal Scalded-Skin Syndrome

Staphylococcal scalded-skin syndrome (SSSS) occurs primarily in children younger than 10 years of age, whereas toxic epidermolysis bullosa (TEN) (Ritter–Lyell disease), seen in adults, appears to be a hypersensitivity disease triggered by drugs, infection, vaccination, and malignancy (1–7). Staphylococcal scalded-skin syndrome begins with an acute, painful, generalized erythema, followed rapidly by spreading bullous eruption and intraepidermal peeling, which closely resembles scalded skin. The skin is shed in sheets with minimal trauma (i.e., Nikolsky sign). In my series of 46 children with SSSS, five infants younger than 6 months of age were observed: three had Ritter disease, two had bullous impetigo. Characteristically, the skin was tender, and edema was noted about the mouth and eyes; low-grade fever (38°C; 101°F) occurred in 56% of 35 children. Within 24 hours of onset, vesicobullae were filled with clear, sterile fluid. Conjunctivitis, often purulent, developed with prominent perioral wrinkling of the skin (Fig. 54–30). Within 1 or 2 days, most bullae ruptured spontaneously with large, red, moist, denuded areas that became dry and tan or bronze. Within 48 hours of onset, the infants were less toxic, and exfoliation with large sheets of epidermis was widespread. Within 3 to 5 days, desquamation involved most of the erythematous areas, and by days 6 to 12, desquamation was complete. Cultures were positive for coagulase-positive *S. aureus* in all five of infants seen at Childrens National Medical Center.

This syndrome includes Ritter disease, scarletiniform eruption, staphylococcal scarlet fever, and bullous impetigo of infancy (2–6,29). The first three disorders have generalized cutaneous involvement; bullous impetigo usually is localized. In each disorder, *S. aureus* can be isolated from the nose, throat, conjunctivae, or skin. Bullae most often are sterile because they result from a epidermolysin toxin produced by *S. aureus*. The staphylococci usually are phage type 71, group II, and penicillin resistant.

Differential diagnosis may include syphilis, listeriosis, EB, bullous erythema multiforme, and GVHD (1–7). Erythema multiforme, extremely rare in young infants, is recognized easily by the typical target or iris lesions. Cultures and smears or dark-field examination would exclude bacterial or spirochetal infection. Family history

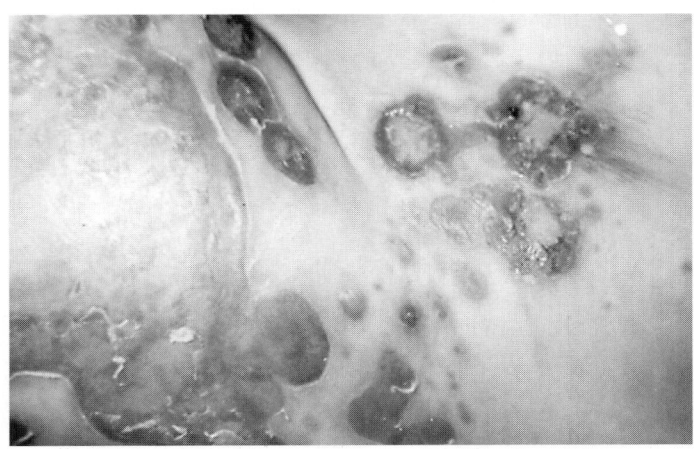

FIG. 54–29. Bullous impetigo in the groin of an infant. Note a collarette of scales around the red, superficial, ruptured pustules caused by *Staphylococcus aureus*.

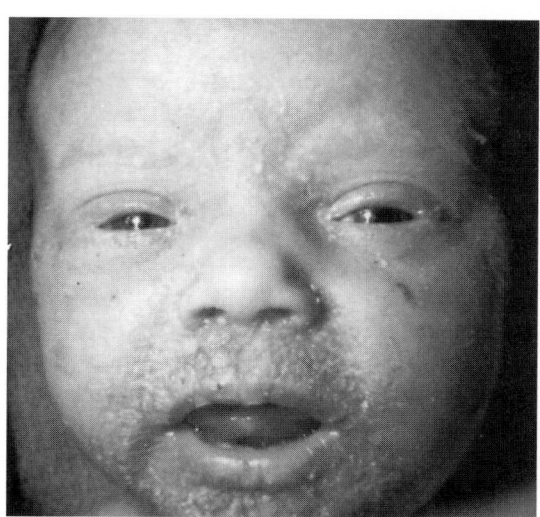

FIG. 54–30. Staphylococcal scaled-skin syndrome. This neonate had fever, exfoliative dermatitis, and positive *Staphylococcus aureus* blood culture for 2 days. Note the intraepidermal peeling with perioral crusting and rhagades of vermillion borders; *S. aureus* was cultured from purulent conjunctivitis.

and close observation over several days should exclude EB. Erythema multiforme major and TEN may be distinguished from the SSSS and acute GVHD by skin biopsy (2,3,5–7).

Management of the rare, mild case of SSSS in an older infant consists of gentle washing of lesions with Betadine skin cleanser three times daily, followed by bacitracin or 2% mupirocin ointment and close observation. Younger infants require hospitalization, reverse isolation, and systemic antistaphylococcal antibiotics. Steroids are contraindicated. Fluids, electrolytes, and temperature should be monitored carefully. If denudation is extensive, compresses of sterile water or normal saline, to which 0.1% silver nitrate has been added, are effective. In the healing phase, tepid baths twice daily followed by application of Aquaphore ointment or Eucerin cream are necessary to avoid dry skin. Sulfacetamide sodium eye drops or ointment is effective for conjunctivitis. Recovery in most cases is complete in 9 or 10 days. Prognosis is excellent for patients younger than 5 years of age.

Ecthyma or Phagedenic Ulcers

Phagedenic or ecthyma ulcers are small, circumscribed ulcers with black necrotic centers and erythematous areolas complicating preexisting lesions (e.g., varicella, puncture wounds). Severe debilitating disease, dysgammaglobulinemia, leukemia, or prematurity may be predisposing factors (1–7). The umbilicus may serve as a portal of entry. Initially, the lesions appear as grouped erythematous opalescent vesicles that rapidly become green or black and pustular and hemorrhagic at times. Because tissue is destroyed beyond the epithelium, ecthyma usually is followed by scars. *P. aeruginosa* is most frequently cultured from deep necrotic, punched-out ulcers with bright red areolae. Occasionally, *S. aureus*, β-streptococci, or *Aeromonas hydrophila* may be isolated (2,10). Treatment with systemic ceftazidime and gentamicin should be prompt and vigorous because of the likelihood of severe sepsis. For local lesions, silver nitrate 0.5% soak or silver sulfadiazine cream may be effective, applied 1 to 2 hours three times daily for 7 to 10 days.

If the clinical course is rapidly progressive with associated toxicity and involvement of the fascial planes overlying muscle, necrotizing fasciitis, a severe soft tissue infection, must be considered and treated vigorously (5,30).

Listeriosis

Listeriosis, caused by *L. monocytogenes,* may produce serious infection (e.g., sepsis, meningitis) or disseminated miliary granulomatosis in the neonate. A small percentage of infants show gray papules or papulopustules that resemble miliary abscesses at times. These may be widespread or localized to the back, oropharynx, or conjunctiva, where they appear as small, white foci. Occasionally, generalized erythema, maculopapular, or petechial–purpuric eruptions have been reported. The organism may be isolated from the pustule, blood, or spinal fluid. It is a gram-positive bacillus that produces hemolysis on blood agar. Treatment is intravenous ampicillin and gentamicin (4,5,7,10,29).

Fungal Infection

Fungal infection of skin in the full-term newborn is uncommon except for candidal vesicopustular diaper rash and thrush. Persistent oral or diaper candidal infection or systemic candidiasis occurs in premature or very-low-birth-weight (VLBW) infants, especially those infected with human immunodeficiency virus (HIV) (1–7,11). The clinical features, diagnosis, and therapy of severe fungal infections in 22 VLBW infants have been reviewed (30). The mean age of onset of infection was 24 days. In 13 (59%) infants the fungal infection was eradicated with amphotericim B and/or fluconazole (30). Congenital candidiasis is rare. Skin lesions are present at birth or within 12 hours of delivery (1–6,10,29,30).

Paronychial Infections

Paronychial infection, onychomycosis, rarely seen in neonates, is most often secondary to thumbsucking or local injury. Continuous wetness and sucking result in maceration and secondary candidal infection. *Staphylococcus aureus* or *P. aeruginosa* may be cultured. Red, swollen skin at the nail base with purulent discharge suggests a bacterial infection. Exudate rarely is seen with candidal infection. After cultures are taken, a finger cot partially filled with Betadine (7.5%) cleanser, is taped over the finger for 7 to 10 days. The cot should be changed every 24 hours. Drainage is facilitated, and infection usually resolves without need for systemic antibiotics or surgical incision. Alternatively, candidal paronychia usually responds to topical application of nystatin or Lotrimin cream, 2 or 3 times daily, with a cotton applicator to fill the gap between the nail plate and posterior nail fold. The finger must be kept perfectly dry (1–7).

Congenital Syphilis

Congenital syphilis, if untreated, will produce a maculopapular or bullous skin eruption in about 50% of infants between 2 and 6 weeks of life. Bullae and maculopapular or maculosquamous lesions occasionally are seen at birth on the palms and soles; infants with these lesions tend to have a more severe disease—hydrops fetalis. These vesicles are of irregular size and contain a cloudy fluid teeming with spirochetes that can be seen by dark-field examination (Fig. 54–31). When the lesions rupture, the denuded area dries and crusts or macerates if moisture is present. The most common eruption of secondary lues consists of erythematous or copper-colored maculopapular ovoid lesions of the palms and soles, which may spread over the entire body. Mucocutaneous lesions about the mouth, anus, and genitalia and snuffles with a highly infectious nasal discharge may be the first clinical manifestations of the disease, occurring in one-third of infants (1–7,29). Fissures may develop in these moist areas and, on healing, result in fine periorofacial scars (i.e., rhagades). Raised, flat, moist lesions, condylomata lata, may appear at angles of the mouth, nares, or anogenital region. Mucus patches may be seen on the lips, tongue, and palate. If untreated, the skin lesions regress spontaneously in 1 to 3 months, leaving residual hyperpigmentation or hypopigmentation.

The routine VDRL on the mother invariably is positive. If the infant is infected, the serology will be positive in 85% of infants at 1 month of age, 95% at 2 months of

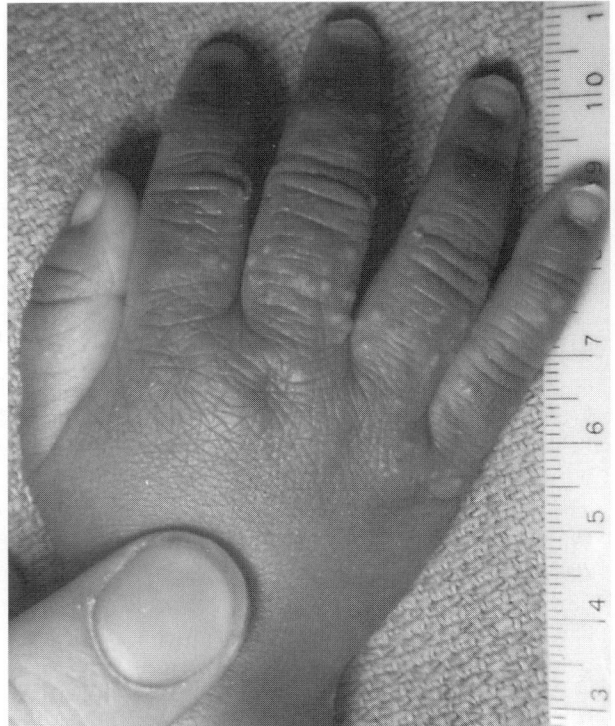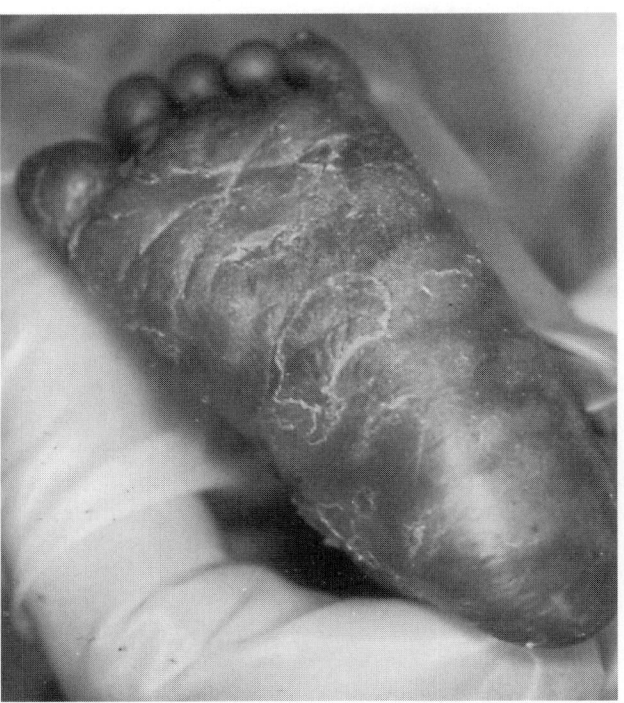

A   B

FIG. 54–31. A: Pustules on both hands and feet in a 4.5-month-old infant who had sniffles and respiratory congestion for 3 weeks, was VDRL positive and had VDRL-positive parents, and showed periosteal new bone formation in radiographs of long bones. Dark-field aspirate of pustules showed many spirochetes. **B:** Full-term girl born at 41 weeks of gestation to a 24-year-old quadripara with a history of drug abuse. Examination of the infant was negative except for marked hepatosplenomegaly and extensive exfoliation of skin, especially palms and soles. RPR was 1:256; CSF FTA 2+. Radiographs of the knees showed new bone periosteal formation of the femurs. Penicillin therapy was effective. (Courtesy of Joseph L. Kennedy, Jr., M.D., Saint Elizabeth Hospital, Boston, MA.)

age, and 100% by 3 months of age. An infant's serologic titer higher than four times the maternal titer is diagnostic (29). Other clinical features are reviewed elsewhere (see Chapter 48). Therapy consists of intramuscular aqueous crystalline penicillin, 100,000 to 150,000 U/kg per 24 hours in two divided daily doses over 10 to 14 days (29). Monitoring should continue with the infant having a nontreponemal quantitative titer at 3, 6, and 12 months, so that adequate therapeutic response is ensured. Serologic reversal usually is expected in 1 year. An examination of cerebrospinal fluid is recommended before therapy and at 6-month intervals until the CSF examination is normal (29). All physicians should be alert for this disease because of its increased incidence (3,6,29).

Viral Epidermal Lesions

Viral epidermal lesions usually present in the neonate or young infant with a characteristic morphologic picture (2–7,29,31). Vesicles are seen in varicella, herpes simplex, and herpes zoster; the virus may be isolated from early lesions. These diseases manifest in unusual and severe forms in infants with acquired immunodeficiency syndrome (AIDS). Multinucleated balloon cells and eosinophilic mononuclear cells may be seen on a (Wright, Giemsa) Tzanck smear from scrapings of the base of a fresh vesicle in the herpes group (e.g., simplex, varicella–zoster) (7,11). Petechial–purpuric lesions occurred in CMV inclusion disease and congenital rubella. Papular eruptions are characteristic of molluscum contagiosum and warts.

Herpesvirus Hominis Simplex

Herpesvirus hominis simplex infection is one of the most potentially serious viral diseases in infants. Cutaneous lesions are uncommon at birth unless intrauterine infection occurred (29). Lesions develop at any time up to 21 days (mean 6 days) in 60% of affected infants. They vary from a few scattered depressed scars or a local boggy swelling to one (Fig. 54–32) or many discrete groups of vesicles. A zosteriform distribution may occur. Vesicles may coalesce and become erosive. Cutaneous lesions can recur up to 5 years of age at the original site or in different areas (4,5,29). Concomitantly, erythema multiforme may occur in some infants. Acyclovir should be started as soon as this infection is suspected because the prognosis is guarded (4,5,29,31). Two-thirds of infants in whom encephalitis develops either die or live with mental retardation or hemiparesis (4,32).

Varicella–Zoster

Varicella–zoster, a rare transplacental infection, is one of the least threatening infections to the fetus and newborn. Varicella occurring in the first 10 days of life prob-

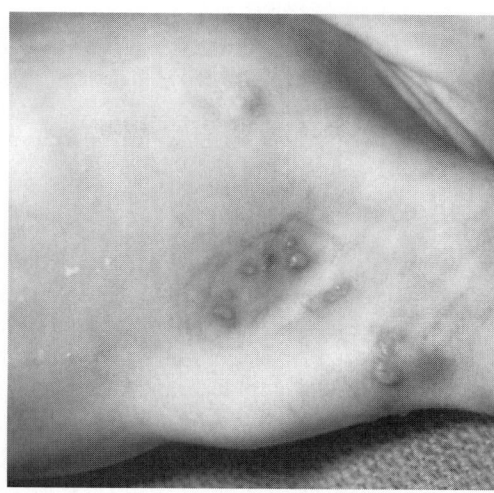

FIG. 54–32. Herpes simplex vesicles in the axilla of a 12-day-old infant with severe type 2 herpes encephalitis of 3 days' duration. The lesions cleared in 12 days. Severe mental retardation developed.

ably has been acquired *in utero* because the incubation period is 10 to 21 days. The vesicular eruption, lesions, and course of disease are identical with the signs of varicella at any age. Although a mortality of 30% has been reported, the course of neonatal varicella has been mild in most patients (29). In two of my patients, depressed white scars were observed at birth; each mother had varicella during the first trimester. Scars in a zosteriform distribution have been seen (4,5). Rarely, neonates with congenital varicella will have visceral involvement (3). Acyclovir may be effective if given within 24 hours of the onset of rash; intravenous varicella–zoster immune globulin (VZIG) may modify the course of disease if given shortly after exposure (6,10,29).

Vaccinia virus and variola infections have not occurred since 1977. Congenital vaccinia may be associated with cutaneous scars, ocular damage, and hypoplastic bony defects (3).

Petechial, Purpuric, and Maculopapular Eruptions with Infection

Cytomegalovirus Inclusion Disease

Cytomegalovirus inclusion disease usually is recognized in a small-for-dates infant with jaundice, lethargy, pallor, petechiae, or purpura with hepatosplenomegaly and chorioretinitis (3–5,29). Thrombocytopenia accounts for the purpuric lesions. In a few infants, generalized dark blue and magenta papules or nodules occur as a result of collections of extramedullary dermal erythropoiesis. These regress in 2 to 3 weeks, leaving dark red to pale gray macules. Differential diagnosis includes sepsis, toxoplasmosis, rubella, syphilis, and herpes simplex infections. Isolation of CMV from urine, pharynx, saliva, buffy coat, or tissue biopsy with a fourfold rise in IgM CMV specific antibody titer will confirm the diagnosis (3,29). Treatment with intravenous ganciclovir and CMV immune globulin may be beneficial for retinitis, but experience in neonates is limited (29).

Rubella

Rubella infection acquired in the first trimester of pregnancy may result in rubella embryopathy in the neonate. Petechiae and purpura often are seen at birth; new lesions rarely develop after several days of age unless thrombocytopenia is severe. Most lesions have faded by the second week and are gone by 4 to 6 weeks of age. The most unusual cutaneous finding is the blueberry-muffin lesion noted at birth in severely affected infants. These firm, bluish red papules, 2 to 8 mm in diameter, occur over the head, trunk, and extremities (3,4). They are caused by dermal erythropoiesis and resolve spontaneously in 3 to 6 weeks unless death occurs. Cutis marmorata, slate blue discoloration of dependent extremities and capillary flushing, has been reported (3). Isolation of these infants from susceptible personnel is mandatory because the virus is excreted for months to years (29). Septicemia caused by streptococci or gram-negative bacilli, toxoplasmosis, CMV, and syphilis should be considered in the differential diagnosis. Therapy is supportive (6,29).

Molluscum Contagiosum

Molluscum contagiosum, very rarely seen in neonates, is caused by a poxvirus (3,4,6,29). The benign lesions are characterized by discrete, waxy papules with a pink, tan, or ivory hue and central umbilication. Size varies from 1 mm to 1 cm, and lesions are found anywhere. Hundreds of lesions should raise suspicion of AIDS. Treatment consists of topical application of 0.7% cantharidin in collodion, used in minute quantities under an occlusive plastic tape for 12 to 24 hours to enhance blister formation (3,5,6,29). Examination of a curetted plug after clearing debris with 10% KOH will reveal the typical intracytoplasmic inclusions.

Warts

Warts, extremely uncommon in the newborn or young infant, are caused by a virus of the papova group. Mucous membrane warts (i.e., condylomata acuminata) occasionally are seen in older infants on moist mucosa of the anus, genitalia, or mouth (2,4–6,29,33). A VDRL always should be done. Anogenital warts can be acquired through direct contact with maternal lesions at delivery or by nonsexual contact with family members (33,34). The treatment of choice is 20% podophyllin in compound tincture of benzoin, applied carefully to the lesion for 4 to 6 hours and then washed off. Applications are repeated weekly for several weeks or until warts have cleared.

Toxoplasmosis

Toxoplasmosis, relatively uncommon in neonates, is caused by an intracellular parasite, *Toxoplasma gondii*. It is a transplacental infection with features simulating those found in erythroblastosis fetalis, rubella syndrome, CMV infection, or bacterial sepsis. A generalized maculopapular rash has been seen in 25% of infants, with hepatosplenomegaly, jaundice, fever, and anemia. The rash tends to spare the scalp, palms, and soles and rarely persists longer than 2 weeks. Desquamation and hyperpigmentation have followed severe eruptions (3–5). Diagnosis is made by a capture-EIA for IgM antibodies. Detection of toxoplasma-specific IgA are useful in congenital infections. Therapy is with pyrimethamine and sulfadiazine (29).

Both coccidioidomycosis and aspergillosis, extremely rare in the neonate, may produce maculopapular nonspecific eruptions (3,4). Vesicopustules have been reported in aspergillosis, and vesicles have occurred in the former disease. Systemic or disseminated disease is more likely in patients with AIDS. Clinical features and therapy with amphotericin B are discussed elsewhere (3,4,6,29).

NONINFECTIOUS BLISTERING DISEASES

Acrodermatitis Enteropathica

The classic tetrad of diarrhea, periorofacial and acral vesicobullous dermatitis, alopecia, and apathy is diagnostic of this rare disorder. Acrodermatitis enteropathica, an autosomal recessive trait, usually presents during the first year (2 weeks to 9 months) and is characterized by remissions and exacerbations. Premature infants and those with AIDS may have severe disease (1–3,5–7). Acrodermatitis enteropathica may occur in breast-fed infants, especially prematures (6). Symmetric vesicopustules, which usually evolve into chronic, persistent, erythematous eczematous patches, may be seen over the trunk and extremities. Low plasma zinc levels (≤ 65 μg/dL) should establish the diagnosis. Zinc gluconate or sulfate therapy, given twice a day, 5 mg/kg per day, is very effective with a dramatic response in 2 to 4 days and may prevent death (1–3,5–7). Biotin deficiency may produce a similiar cutaneous dermatitis (7).

Arthropod-Induced Blister

Bites and stings, although uncommon in the young infant, may product erythema, blisters, wheals, and rarely a gangrenous slough. Lesions tend to be localized or in a linear arrangement. Spiders (e.g., brown recluse) and scorpions can produce severe reactions locally and systemically (1–3,5–7). Intense erythema rapidly progresses through a blister, sometimes hemorrhagic, to sloughing of skin. The blister beetle may produce a subepidermal blister. Papular urticaria, caused by flea, fly, mosquito, bedbug, moth, wasp, or bee stings, characteristically develops on the distal extremities in a symmetric pattern. Lesions may become purpuric and occasionally develop over the trunk and face if repeated bites occur. Pruritus with secondary excoriations often is seen in an irritable infant. Local therapy consists of cool tapwater compresses or baths, diphenhydramine HCl (Benadryl), 5 to 10 mg/kg per 24 hours, and caladryl lotion. Hydrocortisone ointment applied three times a day after bathing may be helpful. Oral steroids rarely are necessary.

Mite infestations (i.e., scabies) may be considered, especially if the parent, sibling, or family pet has a pruritic rash (1–7,10,11). The gray or flesh-colored burrows vary in length up to 1.5 cm and commonly occur on the palms, soles, head, axillae, and neck. Papulovesicular and nodular lesions often appear at the end of the burrow. Because of the intense pruritus, excoriations, eczematous changes, and secondary infection are common. Diagnosis is confirmed by the presence of ova, mites, or fecal concretions seen microscopically from scrapings of burrows. Mineral oil is placed on a glass slide and on the tip of a no. 15 scalpel blade. The skin lesion or underside of the fingernail is scraped, and the material obtained is placed back into the drop of oil. A coverslip is applied, and the specimen is examined microscopically (1–3,5–7,10,11). Larvae of *Diptera* sp. may be similarly identified (4). A very effective treatment for the entire family with scabies is 5% permethrin cream (Elimite). The cream or lotion is applied from the neck down on dry skin for 8 to 14 hours. The skin is then bathed. Parents are advised that itching may persist for several weeks; diphenhydramine (Benadryl), 5 to 10 mg/kg per 24 hours, may be needed. A second application of Elimite for 8 hours only may be necessary in 1 week if new burrows, vesicopustules, or papulonodular lesions occur (1–3,5–7,10,11). Bacitracin or mupirocin ointment applied three times a day will be effective for secondary infection.

Epidermolysis Bullosa

Pearson has classified this rare hereditary mechanobullous disease into two major clinical subgroups: non-

scarring and scarring EB. Eight of the subtypes (Table 54–2) may occur at birth or in early infancy (1–7). The disorder is identified further by location of blister formation in the intraepidermal, junctional, or subepidermal layers produced as a result of minor trauma. At least 18 distinct hereditary types of EB have been described (1–3,6,7,13). Diagnosis depends on clinical features, histopathology, and molecular biological markers (1–7,35,36).

Nonscarring Epidermolysis Bullosa

Nonscarring EB presents in five forms: junctional autosomal recessive, epidermolysis bullosa letalis (EBL), and mitis, both extremely rare, and autosomal dominant epidermolysis bullosa simplex (EBS), generalized with discrete or grouped lesions and superficialis types. Characteristically in EBS, the legs, feet, and scalp show erosions or peeling skin that heal slowly without scars. Blisters can be produced within a few hours by gentle rubbing, as in most forms of EB. Bullae may contain blood (Fig. 54–33). Skilled nursing care will provide protection from minor trauma and pyogenic infection. Clean, soft cotton or fleece dressings may be helpful over pressure points. Bacitracin or 2% mupirocin ointment should be used after Betadine skin cleanser two or three times daily for secondary infection. Maceration must be avoided. Emollients (e.g., Aquaphor ointment) will prevent dry skin. Prognosis for EBS is good, with a tendency to improve by adolescence. Education of parents is essential (2,3,5–7).

Sheets of epidermis loosen with minimal trauma (i.e., dermal–epidermal separation) in EBL. The oral mucosa is severely affected. The resulting moist erosions become infected, ulcerate, and develop nonhealing granulomas. Multiorgan involvement, septicemia, growth retardation, and anemia are common (2,3,5–7). The prognosis is poor when large, denuded areas continually develop. In a few patients, lesions heal spontaneously and completely. Treatment is protective, palliative, and supportive, particularly with good nutritional supplements (2,35). Heat should be avoided; cool water compresses to traumatized skin and air conditioning are helpful. Local and systemic antibiotics are indicated for secondary infection (1–5,7).

TABLE 54–2. *Neonatal epidermolysis bullosa*

Type	Inheritance
Nonscarring: Intraepidermal and junctional separation	
Epidermolysis bullosa simplex, generalized and superficialis	Autosomal dominant
Junctional epidermolysis bullosa letalis	Autosomal recessive
Scarring: Dermolytic subepidermal separation	
Dominant dystrophic	Autosomal dominant
Albulopapuloid	Autosomal dominant
Recessive dystrophic (i.e., polydysplastic)	Autosomal recessive

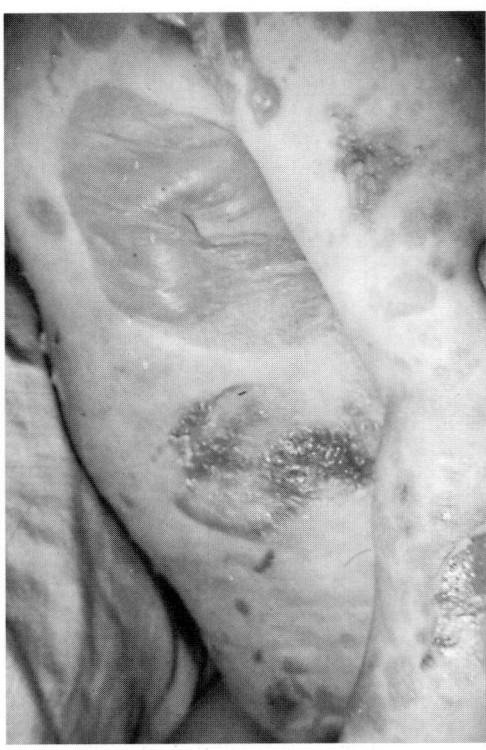

FIG. 54–33. Nonscarring epidermolysis bullosa (EB) in a 4-month-old infant whose sister died in infancy of EB lethalis. The vesiculobullae noted at birth recurred often until the patient was 2 years of age, when improvement began. The patient was much improved at 17 years of age.

Dominant Dystrophic Epidermolysis Bullosa

Dominant dystrophic EB, seen uncommonly in the newborn, is less severe than the recessive type of scarring EB (see Table 54–2). Lesions usually appear well after birth on the hands, feet, and sacrum secondary to minimal trauma. Nails may be lost, but deforming scars and contractures are infrequent. Mucous membrane lesions occur but are mild. Hypopigmentation and hyperpigmentation with soft, wrinkled scars are observed with healing. Therapy is the same as noted previously for EBS. Disposable diapers should be used. Adhesive tape should never be used on the skin. Once blistering has occurred, unroofing the bullae, compressing their contents, applying cool wet soaks for 5 minutes, and then applying 2% mupirocin ointment or silver sulfadiazine (Silvadene) cream and Telfa pad dressings encourage wound healing (1–3,5–7).

Recessive Scarring Dermolytic and Dystrophic Epidermolysis Bullosa

Recessive scarring and dystrophic EB initially may appear to be benign, but it is the most incapacitating form of EB. Rarely it may present with congenital localized absence of skin (i.e., Bart syndrome; see Fig. 54–11) (35). Eventually, after many months, the toe and finger blisters heal with pseudowebbing of the digits and loss of nails (Fig. 54–34A). Finally, over several years, the hands and arms become fixed in a flexed position with contractures. A positive family history helps differentiate this type from EBS and dominant scarring EB. Genetic counseling is advised (13). During early infancy, a skin biopsy

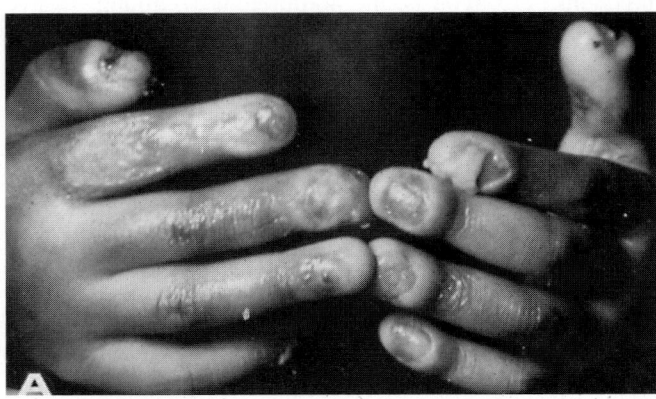
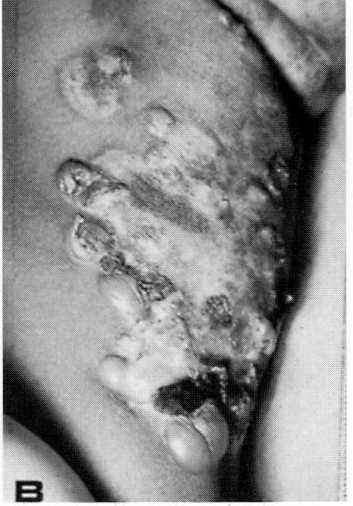

FIG. 54–34. Dystrophic scarring epidermolysis bullosa in a 3.5-year-old boy whose fingernails and toenails were absent at birth. At 1 week of age, recurrent clear and hemorrhagic blisters developed after minor trauma. **A:** Atrophic scarring of the fingertips occurred. **B:** The thigh showed blisters and dystrophic scars at 18 months of age.

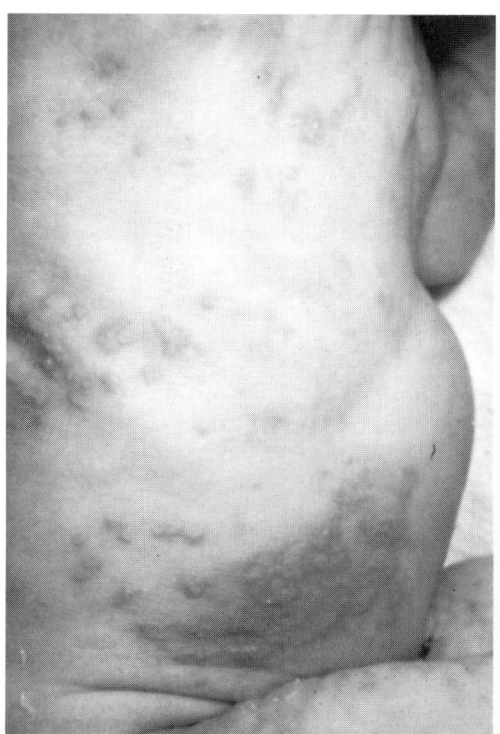

FIG. 54–35. Incontinentia pigmenti in a 1-week-old infant. Erythematous vesicles and papules developed at 4 days of age and progressed to pigmented whorls by 6 months of age. No other defects were present. The mother had similar pigmented linear macules on the thigh.

to localize depth of blister formation (Fig. 54–34B) may differentiate the severe scarring and nonscarring types (1–3,5–7). Therapy is similar to that for other forms of EB. For large nonhealing erosions, wound dressings (e.g., Vigilon, Second Skin, Duo Derm) may be useful (1–3,5–7). Painting the hands and feet two or three times a week with tincture of benzoin compound or Tuff-Skin spray may be helpful. Oral phenytoin (Dilantin) therapy has been helpful in some patients with recessive dystrophic EB (13).

Erythropoietic Porphyria Congenita

This rare autosomal recessive disease, caused by a defect in heme synthesis, may be seen in the newborn. Because of severe photosensitivity, usually in late infancy, burning, pruritus, erythema, and vesicobullous eruptions develop on sun exposure. Ulcerations and secondary infection are common. Scarring and loss of nails, digit, and cartilage of the ears and nose develop later. The urine may be pink or red. Teeth are stained pinkish brown and have a red fluorescence, as do the nails under ultraviolet illumination. Systemic and cutaneous manifestations are progressive, and there is a decreased life expectancy. Excess uroporphyrin I and orange-red fluorescence of erythrocytes are diagnostic. Therapy includes protection from light, wavelength < 510 μm, with application of wide-spectrum sunscreen creams, protective clothing, and appropriate management of hemolytic anemia and infection (1–3,5–7,13).

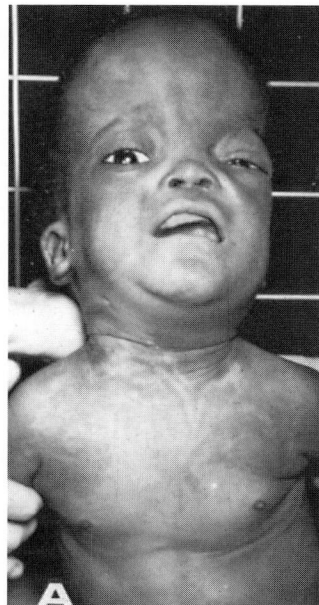
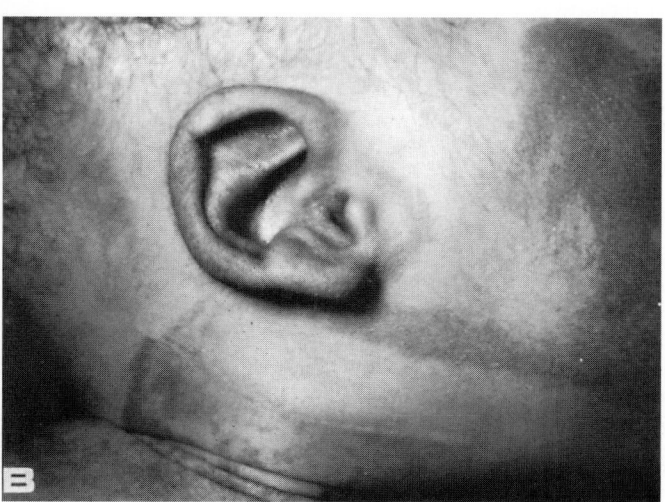

FIG. 54–36. A: Bloch–Sulzberger syndrome in a 6-month-old infant who demonstrated incontinentia pigmenti, ocular pseudogliomas, mental retardation, hydrocephalus, and heart disease. **B:** Note the typical pigmented brown brush strokes on the face.

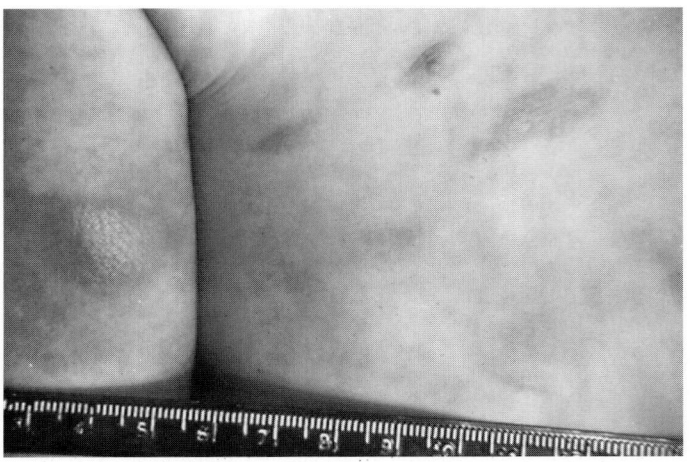

FIG. 54–37. Urticaria pigmentosa (i.e., mastocytosis) in a healthy infant with 30 maculopapular truncal lesions. Note the positive Darier sign on the arm, produced after a similar lesion was stroked ten times.

Incontinentia Pigmenti

Incontinentia pigmenti, an uncommon skin disorder, is an X-linked dominant condition and prenatally lethal to boys. Gene locus is X p11.21. Extracutaneous defects of the eyes, central nervous system, teeth, heart, and bones often are seen after the neonatal period and denote the Bloch–Sulzberger syndrome, which occurs in 30% of patients (1–8,13). The girl–boy ratio is 9:1 or greater. At birth or shortly thereafter, inflammatory vesicobullae and papules (Fig. 54–35) erupt in linear crops over the trunk or limbs. After several months, pigmented hypertrophic or verrucous lesions appear and gradually resolve, usually by 1 year of age, forming macular pigmented whorls and brush-stroke lines (Fig. 54–36). These marbled, brown or slate gray macules are diagnostic and should alert the physician to watch for retarded development, microcephaly, seizures, ocular pseudotumors, pegged teeth, and cardiac defects. Eosinophilia (65%) is present during the vesicular stage; the subcorneal vesicles are filled with eosinophils. No therapy is required for the skin. Genetic counseling is advisable (8,13,36). Approximately 50% of patients with incontinentia pigmenti achromians, or hypomelanosis of Ito (see Pigmentary Lesions), have similiar associated abnormalities (2–8,13,36).

Urticaria Pigmentosa

Cutaneous Mastocytosis

Cutaneous mastocytosis (i.e., mast cell disease), rarely observed in the newborn, is not uncommon during infancy. In young infants, the lesions may be single or multiple nodules and/or sterile bullae, appearing primarily on the trunk, limbs, or scalp. A single 2- to 6-cm mastocytoma may be seen. In older infants, disseminated maculopapular or nodular eruptions occur. As many as 20 to 400 tan to light brown lesions may develop. Minimal rubbing may produce urtication (i.e., Darier sign; Fig. 54–37) within a few minutes. This diagnostic reaction occurs in 90% of patients. Spontaneous resolution of lesions occurs over several years. Diphenhydramine (Benadryl), 5 mg/kg per day, will control flushing episodes caused by histamine release. Residual hyperpigmentation may persist through puberty (2–7).

Systemic Mastocytosis

Systemic mastocytosis, extremely rare in infants, occurs in 2% of patients with mastocytosis (2–7). Diffuse mast cell proliferation occurs in the skin, bone, liver, nodes, spleen, and bone marrow. In addition to presenting with multiple blisters (Fig. 54–38), these infants manifest episodes of flushing, irritability, tachycardia, respiratory distress, hypotension, pruritus, diarrhea, and abdominal pain. Cutaneous biopsy may be diagnostic. Therapy, rarely necessary for cutaneous lesions, is difficult in

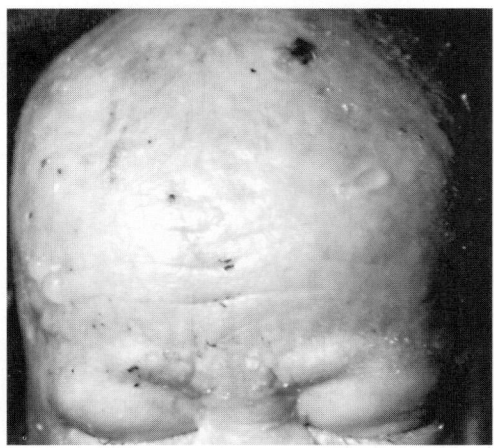

FIG. 54–38. Systemic mastocytosis in a 2-month-old infant. At 2 days of age, bright red macules that urticated and vesiculated with trauma were noted. Episodes of flushing and severe diarrhea occurred. Hepatosplenomegaly, pulmonary infiltrates, and anemia were present. (Courtesy of N. Movassaghi, M.D., Children's National Medical Center, Washington, DC.)

infants with extensive lesions. Cyproheptadine hydrochloride (Periactin), not to exceed 0.5 mg/kg per 24 hours in four divided doses, or diphenhydramine (Benadryl), 5 to 10 mg/kg per 24 hours in three or four doses orally, will alleviate pruritus and irritability. Rubbing of skin and hot water must be avoided. Aspirin, codeine, opiates, and procaine are contraindicated because severe reactions may occur after histamine release from mast cell granules. Prognosis is good for cutaneous mastocytosis but poor for systemic mastocytosis (2–7,37).

SCALING DISORDERS

Desquamation of skin occurs in 75% of newborns. It is observed commonly in infants of 40 to 42 weeks of gestation and rarely, if ever, in those under 35 weeks of gestation. Maximum shedding is observed by the end of the first week of life. Differential diagnosis of the scaly infant includes physiologic desquamation, dysmaturity, and the rare ichthyosiform dermatoses. Three of the four major types of ichthyosis (Table 54–3) may be present at birth (4,7,13). These are X-linked ichthyosis, nonbullous congenital ichthyosiform erythroderma, and bullous congenital ichthyosiform erythroderma. Ichthyosis vulgaris, the most common and benign form, rarely is observed before the third month. The well-known terms harlequin fetus and collodion baby are descriptive only and not separate types of ichthyosis (see Table 54–3). Very rare syndromes (e.g., Netherton, Sjögren–Larsson, KID, CHILD, Rud, Conradi, Refsum, Tay) have been reviewed elsewhere (1–8,13,36).

X-Linked Ichthyosis

This relatively mild disorder occurs in boys only; however, in female heterozygotes, scaling of the arms and lower legs may be present. In boys, the entire body is involved except palms and soles, midface, and flexural areas. Scales are large, yellow to dark brown, and thick (Fig. 54–39). At birth, the infant may present as a collodion baby or simply as a scaly infant. In one series, 36% were affected at birth; only 6% were unaffected by 3 months of age. An associated steroid sulfatase deficiency is reported (38). Prognosis is good, and therapy (see Management) is simple.

Lamellar Ichthyosis or Nonbullous Congenital Ichthyosiform Erythroderma

At birth, this autosomal recessive disorder may present in a healthy infant with generalized brilliant erythema or as the rare collodion baby (Fig. 54–40). Desquamation is universal, and with drying, the skin assumes a parchment-like appearance. In general, infants with a milder erythrodermic variant do well. After the neonatal period, scales develop that vary from a yellow to brownish black color and eventually form warty excrescences or thick

TABLE 54–3. *Types of ichthyosis in infants*

Condition	Incidence	Age at onset	Inheritance	Clinical features	Associated features
Ichthyosis vulgaris (i.e., ichthyosis simplex)	Common (1:250)	Usually after 3 months of life	Autosomal dominant	Scales: fine, branny, white Forehead and cheeks involved Extensor extremities and back involved Flexures always spared Increased palmar and plantar markings	Localized shiny hyperkeratosis of knees and elbows Atopic dermatitis common (50%) Family history positive for atopy Keratosis pilaris common
Sex-linked ichthyosis	Uncommon (1:6,000)	Birth to 3 months of age	X-linked recessive; female–male transmission	Scales: thick, dark brown, large, tightly adherent Lateral face, neck, and scalp most severely affected Abdomen involved more than back Limbs: total involvement common Flexures variably affected Palms and soles normal	Dirty appearance of scales Only boys affected Occasionally, collodion membrane at birth Deep corneal dystrophy by slit lamp Normal cellular kinetics
Lamellar ichthyosis (i.e., nonbullous congenital ichthyosiform erythroderma)	Rare (1:300,000)	Birth (i.e., collodion baby)	Autosomal recessive	Scales: flat, dark, large, coarse Upper face more than lower face Uniform generalized hyperkeratosis of trunk Limbs: generalized involvement Flexures always affected (dry) Palms and soles thickened	Universal erythroderma Prematurity common Collodion membrane possible Harlequin fetus, the most rare and severe Ectropion present and progressive Increased epidermal mitotic
Epidermolytic hyperkeratosis (e.g., bullous congenital ichthyosiform erythroderma, ichthyosis hystrix)	Rare (<1:100,000)	Birth to 6 months of age	Autosomal dominant	Scales: hard, verrucous, small Face relatively spared Limbs and trunk variably affected Flexures always affected (moist) Palms and soles usually affected	Variable erythroderma Bullae, recurrent during infancy and childhood Increased epidermal mitotic rate

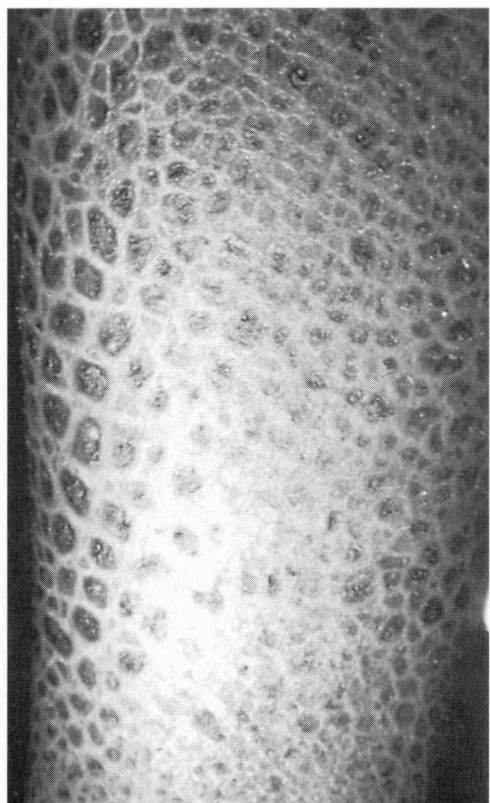

FIG. 54–39. X-linked ichthyosis on the leg of a 5-year-old boy. Five other male members of the family were affected. Note the large, thick, dark scales.

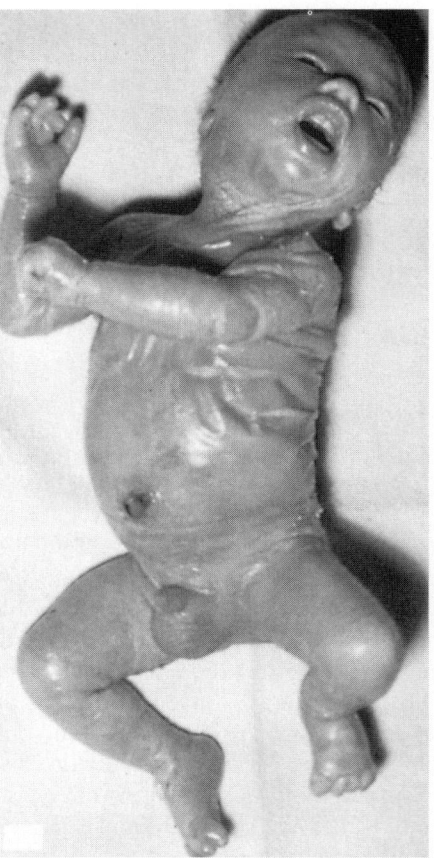

FIG. 54–40. A collodion baby, shortly after birth. By 3 days of age, the yellow collodion membrane peeled and shed in sheets, leaving large, coarse, lamellar scales. The older sister of this infant had dry, minimally scaly, hyperkeratotic skin and a similar appearance at birth.

horny plates covering large body areas in childhood. Secondary infection may occur if the skin becomes macerated, especially in intertriginous areas. Prognosis generally is good except for the extremely rare harlequin fetus with classic lamellar ichthyosis, for whom therapy is ineffective; death usually occurs from sepsis during the neonatal period (Fig. 54–41) (1–8).

Epidermolytic Hyperkeratosis or Bullous Congenital Ichthyosiform Erythroderma

Infants born with this disorder have widespread (0.5 to 30 cm) erythema and dry, peeling skin. The bullae, commonly appearing in crops during childhood, differentiate this disease from nonbullous congenital ichthyosiform erythroderma. In the newborn, extensive denudation with secondary infection and sepsis occurs often because of β-hemolytic streptococci or staphylococci. By age 3 months, hyperkeratosis may remain generalized or localized to flexural areas. Scales are small, hard, and coarse and shed in large quantities. Normal bacteria in the thickened horny layers produce a putrid odor, as in lamellar ichthyosis. Bacterial population may be decreased with antiseptic cleansers or Clorox added to the bath. It is

common to find several affected family members because this is an autosomal dominant disorder linked to chromosome 12q and 17q—Keratin K1, K10 gene (13).

Management

Management of ichthyosis primarily consists of daily hydration and lubrication of the skin. Two baths are given daily, followed by application of a Eucerin Plus cream or Aquaphor ointment. In severely affected areas, use of 12% ammonium lactate lotion (Lac-Hydrin), lactic or citric acid (5%), or urea (10% to 20%) in an ointment base may be effective (1–7). It is is most important to avoid dry indoor heat and detergent soaps that are drying and irritating. Alleviation of scaliness and associated pruritis is necessary.

Topical retinoids and keratolytics may be effective. In my experience, oral 13-*cis*-retinoic acid has been beneficial to older children with lamellar ichthyosis and epidermolytic hyperkeratosis (2). Genetic counseling is essential to these patients and their families (8,13,36).

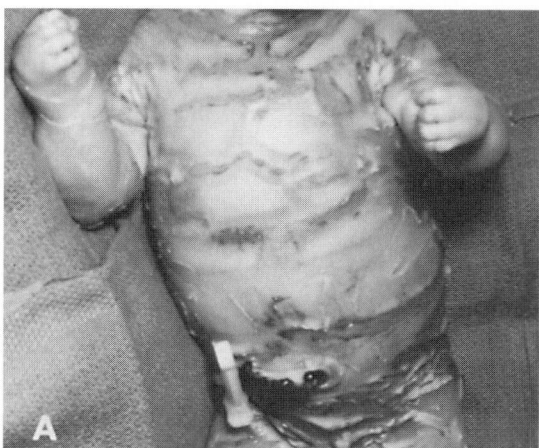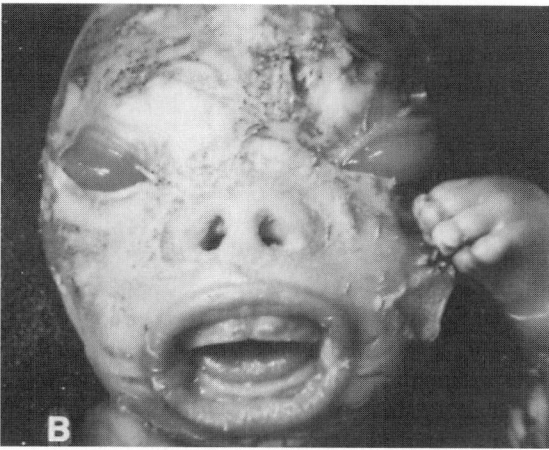

FIG. 54–41. A, B: Nonbullous ichthyosiform erythroderma is present in a harlequin fetus, 1 day of age, with severe ectropion, eclabium, and fissures; scaling; and deformity of hands, feet, and ears. Death resulted from sepsis and extensive bacterial abscesses at 1 month of age. Patient was the offspring of a primipara, and family history was negative. (Courtesy of A. Fletcher, M.D., Children's National Medical Center, Washington, DC.)

ECZEMA

Eczema, from the Greek *eksein*, meaning to boil out, is a common problem in the infant older than 2 months of age. However, it may begin in the neonatal period. It is a difficult management problem. Two of the common types of dermatitis are discussed. Several have been reviewed here and elsewhere (1–3,5–7). Eczema/dermatitis may be associated with the rare disorders seen in the neonatal period listed below:

Exogenous
    Contact primary irritant dermatitis
    Allergic, contact, or drug dermatitis
    Infectious eczematoid dermatitis
    Physical (e.g., light, cold, heat dermatitis)
Endogenous
    Atopic infantile dermatitis
    HIV
    Ichthyosis
    Seborrheic dermatitis
    Systemic diseases with dermatitis
        Acrodermatitis enteropathica
        Histidinemia
        Anhidrotic ectodermal dysplasia
    Histiocytosis X
        Leiner disease (i.e., C5 dysfunction)
        Phenylketonuria
        Wiskott–Aldrich syndrome
    Psoriasis

The four phases of eczema usually are seen simultaneously in the same patient. Pruritus, the major symptom, occurs in all phases. Initially, acute erythema proceeds rapidly to microvesicles with weeping. A burst of epidermal mitotic activity leads to scaling and finally to licheni-

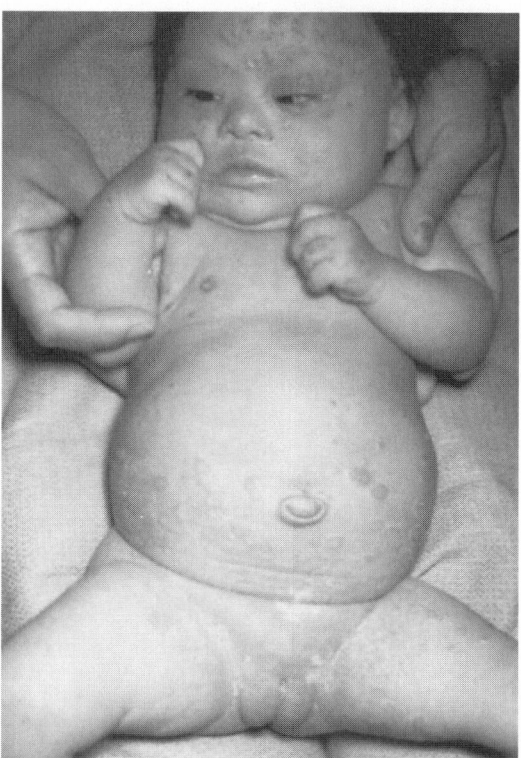

FIG. 54–42. Seborrheic dermatitis and Down syndrome occurred in a 6-week-old, otherwise healthy infant. Diaper rash with secondary monilial infection was present for 1 week; multiple scaly, greasy, crusted lesions involving the body, extremities, and scalp were present for 3 weeks.

fication (i.e., thickened skin with prominent dermal markings). Hypopigmentation or hyperpigmentation eventually develops. Some exogenous and endogenous types of diaper dermatitis observed during early infancy have been discussed. Allergic, contact, and drug dermatitis are extremely rare in neonates (1–3,5–7).

Atopic Dermatitis

Atopic, or infantile, eczema is the most common type of eczematous dermatitis that may develop in the first 2 months of life. Its etiology is unknown. Diagnostic features are a healthy child with a highly pruritic, erythematous, oozing, symmetric eruption of the cheeks, extensor surfaces of limbs, and diaper area and patchy lesions of the scalp and trunk; family history of allergy; rapid response to topical therapy and environmental measures; and recurrent exacerbations with a chronic (1- to 3-year) course. Elimination of exogenous causes (heat, humidity, dry skin, stress, bacterial infection) and consideration of other systemic disorders that may be excluded by time, course of the patient's disease,

and possibly a phenylalanine blood test for phenylketonuria make atopic dermatitis the likely diagnosis. Management consists of skin hydration, emollients, topical steroids, elimination of pruritus, and harsh soaps (1–3,5–7,39).

Seborrheic Dermatitis

This is the most difficult entity to differentiate from atopic dermatitis. In seborrheic dermatitis, the eruption usually begins on the scalp and is found most often behind the ears and in skin folds of the neck, axillae, and inguinal regions. Diaper area involvement is common. If the eruption becomes generalized, it is known as exfoliative erythroderma or Leiner disease. The scales are greasy, and, with drying, potato-chip scales may develop (Fig. 54–42). Patchy redness with weeping and fissuring may develop. Pruritus is minimal or absent, in contrast to atopic dermatitis. Rarely, eczema may occur simultaneously in the same patient. In most infants, several visits with careful observation and assessment of the therapeutic response will decide the proper diagnosis.

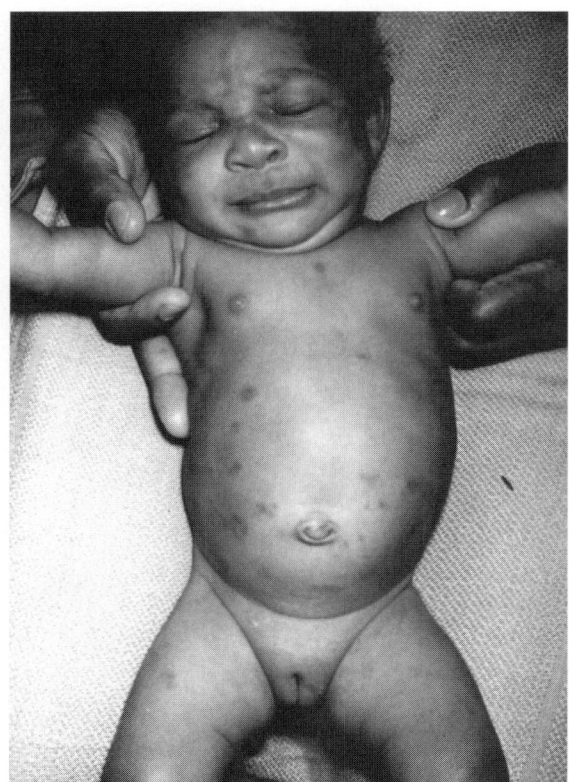 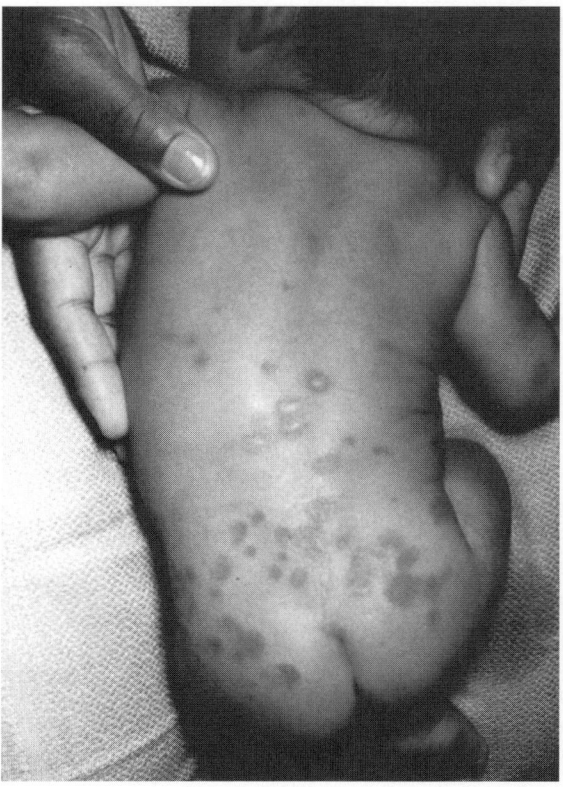

FIG. 54–43. A, B: Neonatal lupus erythematosus in a 6-week-old healthy infant. A discoid lupus rash present 3 weeks showed discrete, erythematous, annular, purpuric plaques with central hypopigmented atrophy over face, trunk, and proximal extremities. Cardiac status was normal. Splenomegaly was present with seborrhea of scalp, eyebrows, and diaper area. Family history showed parents and four siblings to be well; CBC, TORCHES, and sickle cell tests were normal or negative. Sedimentation rate was 36; an ANA was >1:160 (nl < 1:80). Topical steroid applied; rash resolved in 6 months. Infant was well with normal examination at age 19 months.

Cradle cap or seborrheic dermatitis may be treated with Selsun blue or Sebutone shampoo or 2% ketoconazole shampoo nightly. Ten to 14 daily shampoos are necessary, and then twice weekly thereafter. Application of 1% hydrocortisone cream three times daily to inflamed areas may be helpful. This disorder usually clears in a few months; recurrences are rare. Persistent severe atopic or seborrheic dermatitis may be associated with HIV infection.

Management of eczematous dermatoses must be individualized. Detailed written instructions for each infant must be given to nurses or parents to avoid confusion (39). Environmental factors, clothing, hygiene, and socioeconomic aspects must be reviewed during each visit. The details of management include parental reassurance, elimination of pruritus, topical medications, baths, avoidance of dry heat and skin irritants, and treatment of secondary infections (1–3,5,7,39).

IDIOPATHIC DERMATOSES

Histiocytosis X

The term Langerhans cell histiocytosis (LCH) includes the diseases previously called histiocytosis X. The benign, congenital, self-healing reticulohistiocytosis is observed at birth or during the first year of life (1–7). The cutaneous features that may precede systemic signs (e.g., fever, hepatosplenomegaly, lymphadenopathy, anemia) are valuable clues to the diagnosis of the less common severe form. In LCH, the initial lesions may be crusted, scaling dermatitis of scalp, postauricular, perineal, and axillary areas. The presence of red-brown purpuric papules and nodules within or peripheral to the seborrheic eruption suggests LCH. Skin biopsy will reveal histiocytic infiltration and establish the diagnosis. Topical therapy is limited to emollients or steroid cream or both for eczematous lesions. For the severe form, systemic steroids, alkylating agents, or cytokines are effective (1–7).

Neonatal Lupus Erythematosus

Neonatal lupus erythematosus (NLE), an autoimmune disease, presents with annular papulosquamous skin lesions and/or congenital heart block in newborns of both affected and unaffected mothers. These infants usually are not ill and have a discoid lupus rash (i.e., sharply demarcated, erythematous annular plaques or central atropic macules with peripheral scaling) that is predominant over the head, neck, and periorbital areas (Fig. 54–43) (1–7). Biopsy of an active lesion shows a patchy accumulation of lymphocytes around dermal blood vessels and hair follicles. Rarely, (<5%) NLE with systemic involvement occurs in newborns (40).

One-third of mothers who give birth to infants with NLE have systemic lupus erythematosus (40). These infants must be followed closely for cardiac involvement (e.g., primarily congenital complete heart block) because the mortality with heart block is significant (36,40). Otherwise, the prognosis is very good, with most manifestations disappearing by 1 year of age. Transplacental passage of anti–Ro Sjögren syndrome A (ss–A) (Ro) antibody is a diagnostic marker found in 98% of infants with NLE (5,36,40).

Therapy consists of avoidance of sunlight, physical trauma to skin, and protective clothing with regular use of sunscreens. Topical use of steroid creams twice daily is effective for skin lesions. Various treatment modalities are discussed (40). However, with the exception of cardiac involvement, NLE usually resolves spontaneously.

Juvenile Xanthogranuloma

This benign, self-limiting disorder often is seen at birth or shortly thereafter. The typical lesion, often located in the head, neck, upper trunk, or extremities, is a firm, nontender, yellowish-brown, orangish-brown, or reddish papule, plaque, or nodule. Size varies from 0.3 to 4 cm in diameter (Fig. 54–44). Almost half of the lesions are solitary, but multiple (five to several hundred) widely scattered or closely grouped lesions may be seen. Biopsy is diagnostic, showing a dense infiltrate of histiocytic cells throughout the dermis in early lesions and Touton giant cells in mature lesions. Spontaneous regression usually occurs within 6 months to several years (2–7,41).

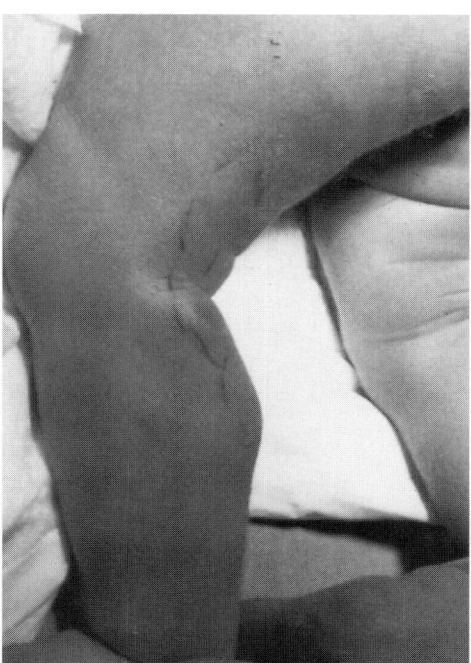

FIG. 54–44. Juvenile xanthogranuloma was noted at birth in a 2-week-old healthy neonate. Six nontender nodules slowly increased in size. Biopsy confirmed the diagnosis. Lesions involuted spontaneously by 15 months of age.

Of major importance is that ocular, pulmonary, testicular, and pericardial lesions may occur. The ocular infiltrates may involve the iris, ciliary body, or orbit and may predate the onset of skin nodules (41). Before ocular surgery is done, an infant should be examined thoroughly for skin tumors. Thus, a major ophthalmologic procedure may be avoided.

REFERENCES

1. Cohen BA. *Atlas of pediatric dermatology.* London: Wolfe, Mosby Europe, 1993.
2. Darmstadt GL, Lane AT. The skin. In Behrman RE, Kliegman RM, Arvin A, eds. *Nelson textbook of pediatrics,* 15th ed. Philadelphia: WB Saunders, 1996:1827–1914.
3. Hurwitz S. *Clinical pediatric dermatology,* 2nd ed. Philadelphia: WB Saunders, 1993.
4. Rudolph AJ. *Atlas of the newborn: dermatology and perinatal infection,* Vol 4. Hamilton, ON: BC Decker, 1997.
5. Schachner LA, Hansen RC. *Pediatric dermatology,* 2nd ed. New York: Churchill-Livingston, 1995.
6. Weston WL, Lane AT, Morelli JG. *Color textbook of pediatric dermatology,* 2nd ed. St Louis: Mosby Year Book, 1996.
7. Williams ML. The skin. In Rudolph AN, Hoffman JIE, Rudolph CD, eds. *Pediatrics,* 20th ed. Stamford, CT: Appleton and Lange, 1996: 879–938.
8. Wiedemann H-R, Kunze J. *Clinical syndromes,* 3rd ed. London: Mosby-Wolfe, 1997.
9. Karlsson JP, Telang GH, Tunnessen WW Jr. Cutis mamorata telangiectatica congenita. *Arch Pediatr Adolesc Med* 1997;151:949–950.
10. Van Praag MCG, Van Rooij RWG, Folkers E, Spritzer R, Menke HE, Oranje AP. Diagnosis and treatment of pustular disorders in the neonate. *Pediatr Dermatol* 1997;14:131–143.
11. Johr RH, Schachner LA. Neonatal dermatologic challenges. *Pediatr Rev* 1997;18:86–94.
12. Quecedo E, Febrer I, Aliaga A. Linear and whorled nevoid hypermelanosis. *Pediatr Dermatol* 1997;14:247–248.
13. Spitz JL. *Genodermatoses.* Baltimore: Williams & Wilkins, 1996.
14. Simon NP, Simon MW, Tunnessen WW Jr. White forelock of hair in a newborn. *Arch Pediatr Adolesc Med* 1995;149:1031–1032.
15. Paller AS, Eramo LR, Farrell EE, Millard DD, Honig PJ, Cunningham BB. Purpuric phototherapy-induced eruption in transfused neonates: relation to transient porphyrinemia. *Pediatrics* 1997;100:360–364.
16. Lambert J, Govaert P, Naeyaert JM. Aplasia cutis congenita. *Pediatr Dermatol* 1997;14:330–332.
17. DeDavid M, Orlow SJ, Provost N, et al. Neurocutaneus melanosis: clinical features of large melanocytic nevi in patients with manifest CNS melanosis. *J Am Acad Dermatol* 1996;35:529–538.
18. Knight PJ, Reiner CB. Superficial lumps in children: what, when and why? *Pediatrics* 1983;72:147.
19. Enjolras O, Wassef M, Mazoyer E, et al. Infants with Kasabach–Merritt syndrome do not have true hemangiomas. *J Pediatr* 1997;130:631–640.
20. Enjolras O, Gelbert F. Superficial hemangiomas: associations and management. *Pediatr Dermatol* 1997;14:173–179.
21. Frieden IJ, Enjolras O, Mulliken JB, et al. Management of hemangiomas symposium. *Pediatr Dermatol* 1997;14:57–83.
22. Margileth AM. Hemangiomas: a before and after look. *Contemp Pediatr* 1986;3:14–26.
23. Johns KJ, Chandra SR. Visual loss following intranasal corticosteroid injection. *JAMA* 1989;261:2413.
24. Burns AJ, Kaplan LS, Mulliken JB. Is there an association between hemangiomas and syndromes with dysmorphic features? *Pediatrics* 1991;88:1257–1267.
25. Ashinoff R, Geronemus RG. Flash-lamp-pumped-pulsed dye laser. *Pediatr Dermatol* 1993;10:77–80.
26. Meine JG, Schwartz RA, Jenninger CK. Klippel–Trenaunay–Weber syndrome. *Cutis* 1997;60:127–132.
27. Goldsmith MF. A granddaughter's distress leads to lymphedema aid. *JAMA* 1984;251:1002.
28. Darmstadt GL. Perianal lymphangioma circumscriptum mistaken for genital warts. *Pediatrics* 1996;98:461–463.
29. American Academy of Pediatrics. In Peter G, ed. *1997 Red Book: Report of the Committee on Infectious Diseases,* 24th ed. Elk Grove Village, IL: AAP, 1997.
30. Jeffries I, Soler M, Schwarty M, Fregeolle C. Fungal infections in the neonatal intensive care unit. *Int Pediatr* 1997;12:133–135.
31. Whitley R, Arvin A, Prober C, et al. A controlled trial comparing vidarabine with acyclovir in neonatal herpes simplex virus infection. *N Engl J Med* 1991;324:444–449.
32. Brown AZ, Selke S, Zeh J, et al. The acquisition of herpes simplex virus during pregnancy. *N Engl J Med* 1997;337:509–515.
33. Obalek S, Misiewicz J, Jablonska S, Favre M, Orth G. Childhood condyloma acuminatum: association with genital and cutaneous warts. *Pediatr Dermatol* 1993;10:101–106.
34. Handley J, Hanks E, Armstrong K, et al. Common association of HPV 2 with anogenital warts in prepubertal children. *Pediatr Dermatol* 1997;14:339–343.
35. Puvabanditsin S, Garrow E, Samransamraujkit R, Lopez LA, Lambert WC. Epidermolysis bullosa associated with congenital localized absence of skin, fetal abdominal mass and pyloric atresia. *Pediatr Dermatol* 1997;14:359–362.
36. Sybert VP. *Genetic skin disorders.* New York: Oxford University Press, 1997.
37. Stern RL, Manders SM, Buttress SH, Heymann WR. Urticaria pigmentosa presenting with massive peripheral eosinophilia. *Pediatr Dermatol* 1997;14:284–286.
38. Castano Suarez E, Rodriquez AS, Tapia AG, Simon de las Heras R, Lopes-Rios F, Rosell MJC. Ichthyosis: the skin manifestation of multiple sulfatase deficiency. *Pediatr Dermatol* 1997;14:369–372.
39. Halbert AR. The practical management of atopic dermatitis in children. *Pediatr Ann* 1996;25:72–78.
40. Borrego L, Rodrequez J, Soler E, Jimenez A, Hernandez B. Neonatal lupus erythematosus related to maternal leukocytoclastic vasculitis. *Pediatr Dermatol* 1997;14:221–225.
41. Resnick SD, Woosley J, Azizkhan RG. Giant juvenile xanthogranuloma: exophytic and endophytic variants. *Pediatr Dermatol* 1990;7: 185–187.

PART SIX

Pharmacology

CHAPTER 55

Drug Therapy in the Newborn

Robert M. Ward and Ralph A. Lugo

The developmental uniqueness of the neonate has tremendous impact on drug therapy. This uniqueness and the potential for dramatic and rapid developmental changes beginning shortly after birth defy accurate generalizations and illustrate the need for age-specific studies in the increasingly premature patients surviving today. These developmental changes affect all aspects of drug action, from absorption and protein binding to receptor interaction and elimination. The impact of these developmental changes on drug action and the use of pharmacokinetics to adjust drug dosages are outlined to guide the clinician between the Charybdis of ineffective therapy and the Scylla of drug overdose and toxicity.

PRINCIPLES OF PHARMACOLOGY APPLIED TO NEONATES

Free-Drug Theory and Protein Binding

Most clinical drug assays measure both bound and unbound drug; however, it is only the non–protein-bound or free drug molecules that are active (i.e., cross membranes, bind to receptors to exert pharmacologic action, undergo metabolism and excretion) (1–4). Serum protein binding usually is a rapidly reversible process, and additional drug is released to replace the unbound drug removed by distribution into tissue or by elimination. The rate of release from serum protein binding usually is much faster than the rate of transfer across membranes. Seldom is the rate of release from serum proteins so slow that it limits the availability of drug molecules for transfer across membranes to exert pharmacologic effects.

For most drugs in premature infants, the percentage of unbound drug in the circulation is greater than that in

R. M. Ward: Department of Pediatrics, University of Utah, Salt Lake City, Utah

R. A. Lugo: College of Pharmacy; and Department of Pediatrics, University of Utah, Salt Lake City, Utah

adults because both the amount and the binding affinity of circulating proteins are decreased (5). For example, the albumin of term newborns, compared to that of adults, binds less theophylline, warfarin, and sulfonamides but similar amounts of diazepam (6,7). Because the effects of a drug are related to the amount of unbound drug reaching the site of action, some drug effects in newborns may be explained by measuring circulating concentrations of free drug alone. Furthermore, circulating total drug concentrations that are in the therapeutic range for adults or older children may represent free-drug concentrations that are in a toxic range in the premature neonate (7).

Absorption

In drug treatment, absorption refers to the transfer of drug from the site of administration into the circulation. The rates of drug absorption are related to several factors, beginning with the route of administration and including the same characteristics that influence transfer of any substance across lipid bilayers: degree of ionization, molecular weight, lipid solubility, concentration gradient, and active transport.

Enteral

Enteral drug treatment of neonates may not produce reliable and reproducible circulating drug concentrations for a variety of reasons. Although most studies of enteral drug therapy have been conducted in adults, many of the problems of enteral drug administration identified from these studies are likely to occur in neonates.

Intestinal villi and microvilli increase the surface area of the gastrointestinal tract, so that rates of drug absorption are much greater from the intestine than from the stomach. Delayed gastric emptying slows passage of drug into the intestine, which prolongs the absorption phase of many drugs. Elimination begins during this absorption phase, so that delayed gastric emptying reduces the area under the curve (AUC) for circulating drug concentration versus time. This reduces the desired therapeutic effect for many drugs whose effects are directly proportional to the AUC. Gastroesophageal reflux is common in neonates and may be associated with delayed gastric emptying that reduces the therapeutic effects of drugs administered orally. Few studies have addressed this aspect of drug treatment of newborns (8).

Additional problems, unique to the immature patient, may affect enteral drug treatment of newborns. Neonates, especially premature neonates, malabsorb fat, which may alter enteral drug absorption. Elevated right atrial pressure, leading to passive congestion of hepatic and mesenteric circulations, often reduces enteral drug absorption in adults. Prolonged enteral drug administration often is necessary for treatment of infants with chronic disorders. These include bronchopulmonary dysplasia (BPD) and congestive heart failure, which may increase right atrial pressure and cause intestinal venous congestion that decreases enteral drug absorption and bioavailability. Therefore, larger doses may be required to achieve the desired therapeutic response. This phenomenon has been reported with furosemide in an infant with BPD, who required a sixfold higher enteral dose to reach plasma concentrations comparable to those produced by a 1 mg/kg dose administered intravenously (IV) (8).

Intramuscular

Intramuscular drug absorption is directly proportional to blood flow and to the surface area of the drug deposited in the muscle (9). Although intramuscular drug administration is often considered more reliable than enteral, the sick or hypothermic neonate with limited muscle mass and poor perfusion of muscle may not absorb intramuscular doses adequately. Because of limited amounts of muscle, injections intended for the muscle may enter subcutaneous tissue, from which absorption is slow and unpredictable. Caustic drugs (e.g., phenytoin, pH 12) damage surrounding tissues and isolate the dose of drug from blood flow, or precipitate to a chemical form that is absorbed very slowly in what has been described as a depot effect (10). Intramuscular injection sites in neonates may leave sterile abscesses that later require surgical repair. In general, prolonged intramuscular administration of drugs in neonates should be avoided.

Intravenous

Intravenous drug administration is most likely to ensure effective drug therapy in neonates. Although this route of drug treatment is the most reliable, certain problems must be recognized that are unique to neonates. The infusion rate for IV fluids in extremely small neonates is so slow that drug doses injected distant from where the IV enters the vessel or up the IV tubing away from the patient, may not reach the circulation for several hours (11).

The most reliable method for administering medications intravenously to neonates is to use a small-volume syringe pump and microbore tubing connected as close to the patient as possible. If the syringe is prepared to contain the exact dose, the tubing must be flushed following drug administration to ensure complete drug delivery. Alternatively, it may be preferable to include overfill in the syringe so that the tubing may be primed before drug administration. Thus, once the drug is infused, the tubing will contain extra drug that may be discarded without the necessity of flushing.

Distribution

Distribution is the partitioning of drug from the circulation into various body fluids, organs, and tissues (12, 13). At equilibrium, this distribution is related to organ blood flow; pH and composition of body fluids and tissues; physical and chemical properties of the drug including lipid solubility, polarity, and size; and the extent of binding to plasma and tissue proteins.

Dramatic developmental changes in body composition of newborns influence the distribution of polar and nonpolar drugs within the body. At 24 weeks of gestation, water comprises about 89% of body weight, and 0.1% to 0.5% is fat (14,15). Thus, water-soluble drugs that distribute primarily into extracellular fluid have larger distribution volumes in premature neonates. By 40 weeks of gestation, the body is approximately 75% water and 15% fat, compared to adults in whom the body is about 65% water and the fat content is variable. The low fat content of the brain of the extremely premature newborn may affect the distribution and effects of centrally active drugs such as barbiturates and gaseous anesthetics (16).

Metabolism

Many drugs require biotransformation to more polar forms before they can be eliminated from the body. Biotransformation reactions are designated as either phase I reactions, which make the drug more polar through oxidation, reduction, or hydrolysis, or phase II reactions, which include conjugation reactions such as glucuronidation, sulfation, and acetylation (12,13). The liver is the primary site for biotransformation; however, other organs are also involved. As early as 9 to 22 weeks of gestation, metabolic enzyme activities of the fetal liver vary from 2% to 36% of adult activity (17). This variation precludes broad generalizations regarding hepatic drug metabolism in premature newborns. Over the past decade, intense research into the biochemistry of drug metabolism has revealed multiple forms of cytochrome P450 with different substrate specificities. Clinicians should have an understanding of P450 nomenclature in addition to understanding which isoforms are responsible for metabolism of commonly used drugs. Both induction and inhibition of specific isoforms may require more frequent therapeutic drug monitoring and dosage adjustments.

Cytochromes P450

Quantitatively, the most important of the phase I enzymes are the cytochromes P450, a superfamily of heme-containing proteins that catalyze the metabolism of many lipophilic substances. The cytochrome P450 isozymes are designated as CYP followed in order by (a) an Arabic number representing the gene family; (b) a letter that indicates the subfamily of highly related genes; and (c) sequential numbering of the P450 enzymes in each subfamily (18). Isozymes that are important in human drug metabolism are found in the CYP1, CYP2, and CYP3 gene families. Table 55–1 outlines the P450 isozymes and their common substrates in the newborn.

Research in the early 1970s revealed that newborn infants have significantly reduced total quantities of cytochrome P450 in liver microsomes (19). This hemoprotein increases with gestational age but reaches only 50% of adult values at term (19). Reduced cytochrome P450 in neonates explains the low clearance and significantly prolonged half-lives of theophylline, caffeine, diazepam, phenytoin, phenobarbital and other substances that are metabolized via cytochrome P450 (7,20–23).

Although newborns are poor metabolizers of many xenobiotics, specific P450 cytochromes exhibit unique developmental patterns during gestation and postnatal life that invalidate broad generalizations about drug metabolism. Table 55–1 outlines important developmental patterns for each enzyme.

Ontogeny of Important P450 Cytochromes

Cytochrome P4501A2 is extensively involved in the metabolism of caffeine (1,3,7-trimethylxanthine) (24,25) and theophylline (1,3-dimethylxanthine) (26,27), drugs that are commonly used to treat neonatal apnea and bradycardia (see Methylxanthines). CYP1A2 is not significantly expressed in human fetal liver, and expression is very low in neonates (28). Metabolically, this results in limited N3- and N7-demethylation of caffeine in the newborn period (25). Caffeine elimination in both preterm and term infants is significantly prolonged (29). Maturation of this pathway to adult levels occurs between 4 and 6 months postnatally (30,31). A similar pharmacokinetic trend is noted with theophylline, where 3-demethylation and 8-hydroxylation are catalyzed by CYP1A2 (26,27). Clinically, theophylline clearance and urine metabolite patterns reach adult values by 55 weeks of postconceptional age or approximately 4 to 5 months postnatally (32).

TABLE 55–1. *Developmental patterns for important cytochrome P450 enzymes in the neonate*

Enzymes	Selected Substrates	Developmental Pattern
CYP1A2	Acetaminophen, caffeine, theophylline, warfarin	Not present to an appreciable extent in human fetal liver. Adult levels reached by 4 months of age and may be exceeded in children 1 to 2 years of age. Inhibited by cimetidine and erythromycin. Induced by cigarette smoke, phenobarbital, and phenytoin.
CYP2C9 CYP2C19	Phenytoin, torsemide,[a] S-warfarin Phenytoin, diazepam, omeprazole, propranolol	Not apparent in fetal liver. Inferential data using phenytoin disposition as a nonspecific pharmacologic probe suggest low activity during first week of life, with adult activity reached by 6 months of age and peak activity reached by 3–4 years of age. Metabolism induced by rifampin and phenobarbital and inhibited by cimetidine.
CYP2D6	Captopril, codeine, propranolol, ondansetron	Low to absent in fetal liver but uniformly present at 1-week postnatal age. Poor activity (approximately 20% of adult) at 1 month postnatal age. Adult competence reached by approximately 3 to 5 years of age. Metabolism inhibited by cimetidine.
CYP3A4 CYP3A7	Acetaminophen, alfentanil, amiodarone, budesonide, carbamazepine, diazepam, erythromycin, lidocaine, midazolam, nifedipine, omeprazole, cisapride, theophylline, verapamil, R-warfarin Dehydroepiandrosterone, ethinylestradiol, various dihydropyridines.	CYP3A4 has low activity in the first month of life, with approach toward adult levels by 6 to 12 months postnatally. CYP3A7 is functionally active in fetus; approximately 30% to 75% of adult levels of CYP3A4. Induced by carbamazepine, dexamethasone, phenobarbital, phenytoin, and rifampin. Enzyme inhibitors include azole antifungals, erythromycin, and cimetidine.

[a]Torsemide is a pyrodine–sulfonylurea diuretic.
Adapted from ref. 18.

Other P450 enzymes that appear to be reduced or absent in the fetus include CYP2D6 and CYP2C9 (33–35). The former is responsible for the metabolism of numerous important therapeutic compounds including β-blockers, antiarrhythmics, antidepressants, antipsychotics, and codeine. Although CYP2D6 is absent in the fetal liver and appears to be expressed postnatally (34), activity remains low for an extended period (see Table 55–1) (36). In contrast to the slow development of CYP1A2 and CYP2D6, other enzymes such as CYP2C9 (responsible for the metabolism of nonsteroidal antiinflammatory drugs, warfarin, and phenytoin) develop more rapidly after birth. For example, although CYP2C9 is not significantly present during fetal life (33), phenytoin pharmacokinetic data in newborns suggest rapid enzyme maturation within the first weeks of life (22,37).

For drug metabolism, the most important of the cytochromes P450 is CYP3A because of the large number of therapeutic substrates for this subfamily of enzymes (see Table 55–1). In addition, CYP3A accounts for the majority of P450 cytochromes present in the adult human liver. Unlike most of the other important cytochromes, CYP3A is functionally present during embryogenesis, primarily as CYP3A7 (28). CYP3A activity is detectable in large amounts as early as 17 weeks of gestation and reaches 75% of adult activity at 30 weeks of gestation (34). *In vivo*, CYP3A activity appears to be mature at birth (38). Postnatally, there is a poorly understood transition from the fetal CYP3A7 to the predominant adult isoform CYP3A4.

Phase II Reactions

The phase II reactions are known as synthetic or conjugation reactions and function to increase the hydrophilicity of drug molecules, which facilitates renal elimination (12,13). The phase II enzymes include glucuronosyltransferase, sulfotransferase, N-acetyltransferase, glutathione S-transferase, and methyltransferase. Although the ontogeny of phase II reactions as a group is not well studied, developmental changes during infancy influence drug clearance (see Table 55–2).

Most conjugation reactions show low activity in the fetus (39). One of the most common synthetic reactions involves conjugation with uridine diphosphoglucuronosyltransferases (UDP-GT). This enzyme system, which is comprised of numerous isoforms, is also responsible for glucuronidation of endogenous compounds such as bilirubin (39). Although UDP-GT activity for bilirubin develops relatively rapidly after birth (40), the ability of the infant to glucuronidate xenobiotics is significantly limited during the newborn period. Thus, without dosage adjustments, drug toxicity may develop during the newborn period. A tragic example occurred in the early 1960s when newborns received standard pediatric doses of chloramphenicol and developed fatal circulatory collapse, a condition known as gray baby syndrome (41–43). The clearance of chloramphenicol is low during the neonatal period, and dosage adjustments are necessary in preterm and full-term infants to avoid chloramphenicol toxicity (44).

Other drugs used in the newborn period that undergo glucuronidation include morphine, acetaminophen, and lorazepam. The major metabolic pathway of morphine in children and adults is glucuronidation in the 3 and 6 positions (45,46). However, neonates have limited ability to glucuronidate morphine and thus require dosage adjustment (47–49). Morphine clearance (48,50), in particular 3- and 6-glucuronide formation, is depressed at birth and increases with birth weight (49), gestational age (51), and postnatal age (45,47). Studies indicate that morphine's clearance and half-life begin to approach adult values after

TABLE 55–2. *Developmental patterns for important conjugation reactions in the neonate*

Enzymes	Selected substrates	Developmental pattern
Uridine diphosphoglucoronosyltransferase (UDP-GT)	Chloramphenicol, morphine, acetaminophen, valproic acid, lorazepam	Ontogeny is isoform specific. In general, adult activity is achieved by 6 to 18 months of age. May be induced by cigarette smoke and phenobarbital.
Sulfotransferase	Bile acids, acetaminophen, cholesterol, polyethylene glycols, dopamine, chloramphenicol	Ontogeny seems to be more rapid than UDP-GT; however, it is substrate specific. Activity for some isoforms may exceed adult values (e.g., that responsible for acetaminophen metabolism) during infancy and childhood
N-Acetyltransferase 2	Hydralazine, procainamide, clonazepam, caffeine, sulfamethoxazole	Some fetal activity present by 16 weeks. Virtually 100% of infants between birth and 2 months of age exhibit the slow-metabolizer phenotype. Adult activity present by approximately 1 to 3 years of age.

Adapted from ref. 18.

the age of 1 month (47,52), although other reports indicate that adult values are not reached until at least 5 to 6 months (48,53). Overall, the maturation of glucuronosyltransferase enzymes is isoform specific; however, adult activity is usually achieved by 6 to 18 months of age (18).

In contrast to glucuronosyltransferase, the sulfotransferase enzyme system is well developed in the newborn and may compensate for limited glucuronidation, as is the case with the metabolism of acetaminophen. Although acetaminophen is primarily glucuronidated in adults, the half-life of acetaminophen is only moderately prolonged in newborns as compared to older infants and adults (54–56). In the neonate, this is explained by a relatively large formation rate constant for the acetaminophen sulfate, leading to a greater percentage of the dose excreted as the acetaminophen sulfate conjugate (55,56). Preferential sulfation of acetaminophen continues into childhood (55,57).

Alterations in Biotransformation

Biotransformation reactions, especially those involving certain forms of cytochrome P450, are often inducible before birth through maternal exposure to drugs, cigarette smoke, or other inducing agents. Biotransformation reactions may also be induced by postnatal drug exposure (see Tables 55–1 and 55–2) and may be slowed postnatally by hypoxia/asphyxia, organ damage, and/or critical illness. Additional postnatal changes in hepatic blood flow, protein binding, and/or biliary function may also significantly alter drug elimination. Additional studies in premature neonates are required to generate the population pharmacokinetic data necessary to design safe and effective pharmacotherapeutic regimens.

Excretion

Excretion involves elimination of drug from the body by several potential routes, including the biliary tract, lungs, and kidneys. Both unchanged and metabolized forms of drug may be excreted, but only unbound drug undergoes filtration and tubular transport. Glomerular and tubular functions are decreased at birth, both in absolute terms and after normalization to body mass (58,59). Glomerular filtration of newborns averages 30% of the adult rate after normalization to body surface area. Birth accelerates maturation of glomerular filtration through an increase in cardiac output, decreased renal vascular resistance, redistribution of intrarenal blood flow, and changes in the intrinsic function of the glomerular basement membrane (58). Renal tubular maturation seems to proceed more slowly than glomerular maturation after birth (58). This produces an imbalance in glomerular and tubular function that persists for several months. Because most low-molecular-weight, unbound molecules are filtered, tubular reabsorption exerts a profound influence on the elimination rate for many drugs. In addition, hypoxemia,

nephrotoxic drugs, and underperfusion may alter renal function of newborns, which prevents accurate prediction of the rates of drug elimination after birth.

PHARMACOKINETICS

Pharmacokinetics describes the changes in drug concentrations within the body with time. These concepts are presented as a general overview to assist the clinician with dose adjustments and practical interpretation of therapeutic drug monitoring (12,13,60–62). The more rigorous mathematical intricacies of pharmacokinetics are covered elsewhere (63–66). Although a drug may penetrate several body fluids and tissues at different rates, the change in its circulating concentration is used to characterize its kinetics and to guide dosages. The rate of removal of drug from the circulation usually fits either first-order or zero-order exponential mathematical equations. These two types of equations describe two different processes that have important implications for dosage regimes.

Rates and Distribution

First-Order Kinetics

Most drugs are cleared from the body with first-order exponential rates. Exponential clearance indicates that a constant fraction or constant proportion of drug is removed per unit of time. This means that the higher the concentration, the greater the amount of drug removed from the body. Such changes in concentration fit exponential equations of the following form:

$$C = C_0 e^{-kt} \qquad [1]$$

where C is the concentration at a particular time t, C_0 is the starting concentration, which is a constant, and k is the elimination rate constant with units of 1/time. First-order indicates that the exponent is raised to the first power ($-kt$ in Eq. 1). First-order exponential equations, such as Eq. 1, may be solved by taking the natural logarithm of both sides.

$$\ln C = \ln C_0 + -kt \qquad [2]$$

This transforms the equation to that of a straight line ($y = mx + b$). If the natural logarithm of C ($\ln C$) is graphed versus time, the slope is $-k$, and the intercept is $\ln C_0$. If the common logarithm of C ($\log C$) is graphed versus time, the slope is $-k/2.303$ because $\ln x$ equals $2.303 \log x$. When graphed on linear–linear axes, exponential rates are curvilinear, and on semilogarithmic axes, they produce a straight line.

Half-Life

One of the more familiar exponential rates used clinically is the half-life, i.e., the time for a drug concentration to decrease by one-half. Half-life is a first-order kinetic process because the same proportion or fraction of the drug is removed during equal time periods. At higher concentrations, a greater amount is removed during a single half-life than when the concentration is lower. For example a drug concentration may decrease by 200 from 400 to 200 in one half-life, and decrease by 100 from 200 to 100 in the next half-life (Fig. 55–1).

Half-life can be determined by several methods. If concentration is converted to the natural logarithm of concentration and graphed versus time, as described in Eq. 2, the slope of this graph is the elimination rate constant, k. Usually at least three concentration–time points are needed to determine the slope accurately; however, in clinical practice, k is often determined from just two concentrations obtained during the terminal elimination phase. To increase the accuracy of the latter, at least one half-life should elapse between concentration–time points. With multiple data points, the slope of ln$C$ versus time may be calculated easily by least-squares linear regression analysis. Half-life ($t_{1/2}$) may be calculated from the elimination rate constant k (1/time) as follows:

$$t_{1/2} = \ln(2)/k = 0.693/k \qquad [3]$$

Half-life may be determined graphically from a series of drug concentrations graphed on semilogarithmic axes. With multiple data points, the best-fit line is determined either visually or by linear regression analysis. The times corresponding to carefully chosen concentrations are then used to estimate the interval required for the concentration to decrease by one-half. In Fig. 55–1, this is illustrated by the times corresponding to concentrations of 400, 200, and 100, estimated by the horizontal broken line intercepts with the concentration line and the intercepts with the time axis indicated by the vertical broken lines. Note that the concentrations decrease by 50% every 60 minutes, so that $t_{1/2}$ equals 60 minutes.

First-Order Single-Compartment Kinetics

The number of compartments refers to the number of exponential equations required to describe the observed changes in concentration. Although multiple transfers of drug among tissues and body fluids may be occurring, a drug's clearance may fit first-order, single-compartment kinetics if it distributes rapidly and homogeneously within the circulation from which it is removed through metabolism or excretion. This may be judged visually, if a semilogarithmic graph of a series of concentrations fits a single straight line. Kinetics may falsely appear to be single-compartment if drug concentrations are not measured quickly enough after IV administration to detect the initial distribution phase.

First-Order Multicompartment Kinetics

If drug clearance from the circulation is studied carefully, with measurement of concentration several times within the first 15 to 30 minutes after IV administration as well as during the next several hours, two or more rates of clearance often are detected by a change in slope of a semilogarithmic graph of concentration versus time (Fig. 55–2). The number and nature of the compartments for the clearance of a drug do not necessarily correspond to specific body fluids or tissues. When two first-order exponential equations are required to describe the clearance of drug from the circulation, the kinetics are designated first-order and two-compartment (i.e., central and peripheral compartments) and are represented by the following equation (60):

$$C = Ae^{-\alpha t} + Be^{-\beta t} \qquad [4]$$

In Eq. 4, C is concentration, t is time after the dose, A is the concentration at time 0 for the distribution rate represented by the broken line graph with the steepest slope,

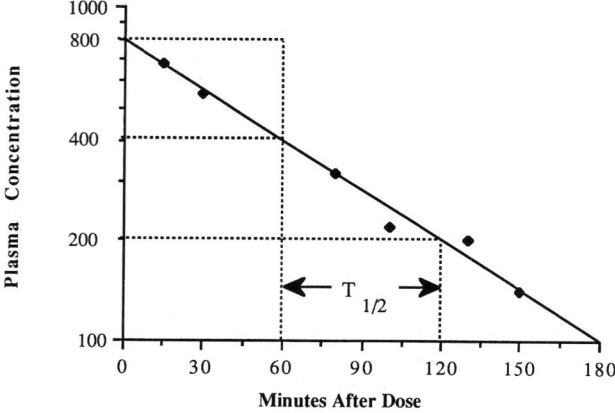

FIG. 55–1. Graph method for estimation of half-life. (From Ward RM. Pharmacologic principles and practicalities. In: Taeusch HW, Ballard RA, Avery ME, eds. *Shaffer and Avery's diseases of the newborn,* 6th ed. Philadelphia: WB Saunders, 1991:289.)

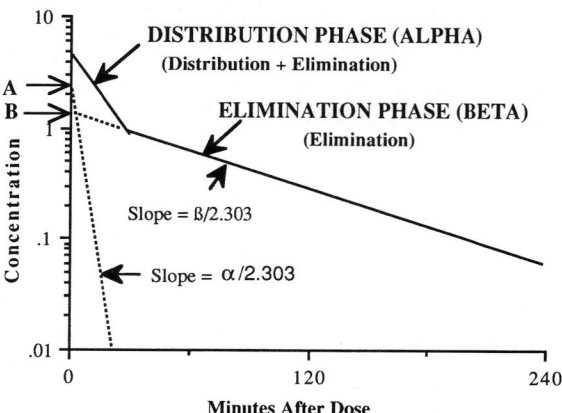

FIG. 55–2. Multicompartment first-order exponential kinetics. (From Ward RM. Pharmacologic principles and practicalities. In: Taeusch HW, Ballard RA, Avery ME, eds. *Schaffer and Avery's diseases of the newborn.* 6th ed. Philadelphia: WB Saunders, 1991:289.)

α is the rate constant for distribution, B is the concentration at time 0 for the terminal elimination rate, and β is the rate constant for terminal elimination. Rate constants indicate the rate of change in concentration and correspond to the slope of the line divided by 2.303 for logarithm concentration versus time.

Such biphasic kinetics are commonly observed for drugs that rapidly distribute out of the central compartment (blood volume plus extracellular fluid of highly perfused organs) after IV administration (60). For such drugs, the initial rapid decrease in concentration is referred to as the α distribution phase and primarily represents distribution to the peripheral (tissue) compartments in addition to drug elimination. After the inflection point in the slope and during the terminal (β) phase of the curve, elimination accounts for most of the change in drug concentration. The α distribution rate constant (see Fig. 55–2) can be determined from the slope of the line generated by subtracting concentrations from the β elimination phase from those during the α distribution phase. A more detailed mathematical discussion may be found elsewhere (60,63).

Although many drugs demonstrate multicompartment kinetics, the intensive blood sampling required to fit data to more than one compartment is not clinically feasible, particularly in newborns. Furthermore, the mathematical complexity of two-compartment models makes this kinetic approach clinically impractical. To minimize cost and simplify pharmacokinetic calculations, only two plasma concentrations (peak and trough) are usually obtained for therapeutic monitoring of commonly used drugs, e.g., gentamicin and vancomycin. Accordingly, a one-compartment model is assumed, and the elimination rate constant (k) is determined from the slope of these points plotted on semilogarithmic scale. Because the elimination rate constant should be determined from the terminal elimination phase, it is important that peak concentrations of multicompartment drugs not be drawn prematurely, that is, during the initial distribution phase. If drawn too early, the concentrations will be higher than those during the terminal elimination phase (see Fig. 55–2), which will overestimate the slope and the terminal elimination rate constant. Clinically, this is not usually problematic with gentamicin because the initial distribution phase commonly occurs during the 30- to 60-minute infusion (67). Thus, a peak concentration obtained 30 to 60 minutes after the end of infusion usually reflects the terminal phase of elimination. However, with vancomycin, the half-life of the initial distribution phase is approximately 0.5 hours (68). Thus, a peak vancomycin concentration drawn prematurely may lead to error in estimating the pharmacokinetic parameters.

Zero-Order Kinetics

Some drugs are eliminated by a constant amount per unit time rather than a constant fraction. Such rates are zero-order, and the following equation can be used to calculate the change in the amount of drug in the body (63):

$$-dA/dt = k_0 \qquad [5]$$

where dA is the change in the amount of drug in the body (mg), dt is the change in time, and k_0 is the elimination rate constant with units of amount per time. After solving this equation, it has the following form:

$$A = A_0 - k_0 t \qquad [6]$$

where A_0 is the initial amount in body, and A is the amount of drug in the body (mg) at time t.

Zero-order kinetics also is referred to as saturation kinetics because it may occur when excess amounts of drug saturate the capacity of metabolic enzymes or transport systems so that only a constant amount of drug is metabolized or transported per unit of time. This may be detected graphically from a serum concentration-versus-time plot where zero-order elimination is linear on linear–linear axes and is curved when graphed on logarithmic–linear (i.e., semilogarithmic) axes. Clinically, zero-order elimination may be observed after administration of excessive doses or during dysfunction of the organ of elimination without a decrease in dosage. Certain drugs administered to newborns exhibit zero-order kinetics at therapeutic doses and may accumulate to excessive concentrations (Table 55–3). Some drugs, such as phenytoin, may exhibit Michaelis–Menten kinetics: first-order at low concentrations and zero-order after enzymes are saturated at higher concentrations. For these drugs, a small increment in dose may cause disproportionately large increments in serum concentrations (Fig. 55–3).

Apparent Volume of Distribution

Volume of distribution does not necessarily correspond to a physiologic body fluid or tissue volume, hence the designation "apparent." The apparent volume of distribution (V_d) is a mathematical term that relates the dose to the circulating concentration observed immediately after intravenous administration. It might be viewed as the vol-

TABLE 55–3. *Drugs that demonstrate zero-order (saturation) kinetics with therapeutic doses in newborns*

Caffeine
Chloramphenicol
Diazepam
Furosemide
Indomethacin
Phenytoin

From Ward RM. Pharmacologic principles and practicalities. In: Taeusch HW, Ballard RA, Avery ME, eds. *Schaffer and Avery's diseases of the newborn*, 6th ed. Philadelphia: WB Saunders, 1991:285, with permission.

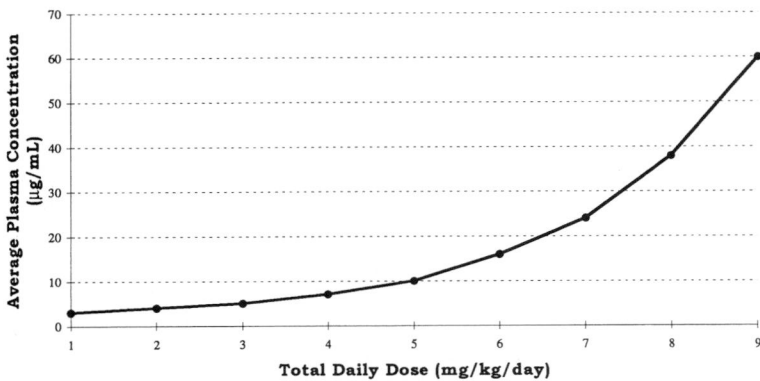

FIG. 55–3. Nonlinear (Michaelis–Menten) kinetics illustrated for a hypothetical drug. As dosage increases above 3 mg/kg/day, there is a disproportionate increase in average plasma concentration as elimination changes from a first-order to a zero-order process.

ume of dilution. For drugs such as digoxin, V_d in neonates may reach 10 L/kg, a physical impossibility. Such a large V_d occurs when drug concentrates outside of the plasma compartment, for example, bound to red blood cells or in tissue. This emphasizes the mathematical nature of V_d. The units used to express concentration are amount per volume and may help to remind the reader of the following equation, which expresses the relationship between dose (amount/kilogram) and the V_d (volume/kilogram) that dilutes the dose to produce the concentration:

Concentration change (mg/L)
$$= \text{Dose (mg/kg)}/V_d \text{ (L/kg)} \quad [7]$$

To facilitate canceling units, concentration is expressed with the unconventional units of milligrams per liter rather than micrograms per milliliter; they are equivalent. This equation serves as the basis for most of the pharmacokinetic calculations because it is easily rearranged to solve for V_d and dose. It is also important to note that this equation represents the change in concentration following a rapidly administered intravenous dose. Following a miniinfusion with, for example, vancomycin or gentamicin, a more complex exponential equation may be required to account for drug elimination during the time of infusion (63). However, such equations are needed only when the drug is rapidly eliminated, that is, when the duration of infusion approaches the drug's half-life. In neonates, who have relatively slow drug elimination, only a small fraction of drug is eliminated during the time of infusion, and such adjustments can be omitted. Accordingly, we may use the simpler and more practical equation to estimate pharmacokinetic parameters.

Knowledge of the apparent distribution volume is essential for dosage adjustments. V_d may be calculated by rearranging Eq. 7.

V_d (L/kg)
$$= \text{Dose (mg/kg)}/[C \text{ (postdose)} - C \text{ (predose)(mg/L)}] \quad [8]$$

The concentration after drug infusion, C (postdose), must be measured after the distribution phase to avoid overestimating the peak concentration that would result

in an erroneously low V_d. For the first dose, the predose concentration is 0.

PHARMACOKINETIC EXAMPLE

To illustrate the practical application of the principles outlined above, we recommend a simple four-step approach: (a) calculate V_d; (b) calculate half-life; (c) calculate a new dose and dosing interval based on a desired peak and trough; (d) check the peak and trough of the new dosage regimen.

For example, gentamicin, 2.5 mg/kg every 12 hours, was administered IV over 30 minutes. The following plasma concentrations were measured on the third day of treatment (presumed steady state). The predose or trough concentration was 1.8 mg/L; the peak concentration, measured 30 minutes after the end of the infusion, was 4.8 mg/L.

Step 1: Substituting the data into Eq. 8, we calculate V_d.

$$V_d \text{ (L/kg)} = (2.5 \text{ mg/kg})/(4.8 \text{ mg/L} - 1.8 \text{ mg/L})$$
$$= (2.5 \text{ mg/kg})/(3.0 \text{ mg/L})$$
$$= 0.83 \text{ L/kg}$$

Step 2: At steady state, trough concentrations remain unchanged from one dose to the next. Therefore, for the purpose of these calculations, steady-state trough concentration may be understood to follow the peak concentration. Thus, the time between the peak and trough concentrations is 11 hours, i.e., 12 hours minus 0.5 hour infusion, minus 0.5 hour to peak concentration. The plasma concentration decreased from 4.8 to 2.4 mg/L in one half-life, and then from 2.4 to 1.2 mg/L in a second half-life. The trough of 1.8 was reached approximately half way between the first and second half-lives. Since 1.5 half-lives elapsed during the 11 hours between the peak and trough, the half-life is approximately 11 hours/1.5 half-lives, or 7.3 hours.

Step 3: A new dosage regimen must be calculated if the concentrations are unsatisfactory. Accordingly, one must decide on desired peak and trough concentrations. If, for example, the desired gentamicin peak and trough concentrations were 6.5 mg/L (5 to 10 mg/L) and 1.5 mg/L (1 to 2 mg/L), respectively, then Eq. 8 may be rearranged to solve for the new dose.

$$\text{Dose (mg/kg)} = V_d \text{ (L/kg)} \times [C(\text{peak desired})$$
$$- C(\text{trough desired}) \text{ (mg/L)}]$$
$$\text{Dose (mg/kg)} = 0.83 \text{ L/kg} \times (6.5 \text{ mg/L} - 1.5 \text{ mg/L})$$
$$\text{Dose (mg/kg)} = 4.15 \text{ mg/kg} \qquad [9]$$

Increasing the dose to 4.15 mg/kg (66% increase) will lead to a higher trough if the dosage interval is kept at 12 hours. Because trough concentrations above 2 mg/L are associated with ototoxicity and nephrotoxicity, the dosage interval needs to be increased. Aminoglycosides, in general, are dosed every 2 to 2.5 half-lives for neonates. However, to reduce the risk of administration errors, one should choose a conventional dosage interval that approximates 2 to 2.5 half-lives, that is, every 8, 12, 18, 24, or 36 hours. In the above example, dosing every two half-lives would require a 15-hour dosage interval, which might lead to administration errors. Thus, the dosage interval should be increased to 18 hours, an interval that corresponds to approximately 2.5 half-lives.

Step 4: Mathematically estimating peak and trough concentrations with the new regimen provides a good double check against a math error. Because 18 hours was chosen as the new interval, waiting 18 hours after the previous dose to begin the new regimen is reasonable. At that time, approximately 2.5 half-lives after the measured peak of 4.8 mg/L, we would expect the trough concentration to be approximately 0.9 mg/L (half-life 1, 4.8 mg/L → 2.4 mg/L; half-life 2, 2.4 mg/L → 1.2 mg/L; half-life 3, 1.2 mg/L → 0.6 mg/L, with half of this third half-life occurring at 0.9 mg/L).[1]

Using Eq. 7, we calculate that the plasma concentration will increase by 5 mg/L after each 4.15 mg/kg dose. Accordingly, the peak concentration will be 5.9 mg/L after the first dose and will decrease to 1.1 mg/L over the next 2.5 half-lives (5.9 mg/L → 2.95 mg/L → 1.48 mg/L → 0.74 mg/L in 3 half-lives, or → 1.1 mg/L in 2.5 half-lives). After the second dose of 4.15 mg/kg, the peak concentration will be 6.1 mg/L and will decrease to 1.15 mg/L in 2.5 half-lives. Because the trough has not changed from the previous trough, one can conclude that this dosage schedule will meet the desired therapeutic levels.

Therapeutic Drug Monitoring

Circulating concentrations of drugs should be measured primarily to ensure that the treatment regimen achieves concentrations that are effective in clinical situations where drug treatment is critical, response is not immediately apparent (e.g., for culture-proven sepsis), and a good correlation exists between circulating drug concentration and desired effect. Drug concentrations should be measured to avoid toxicity when they clearly correlate with toxicity in newborns (e.g., for chloramphenicol), to verify toxicity when symptoms correspond to a known drug toxicity, or to investigate symptoms that are unexplained by the disease process. Extrapolation of toxic and therapeutic ranges from adults to neonates has led to some recommendations about therapeutic drug monitoring in newborns (e.g., for gentamicin) that are not well supported by subsequent experience (69).

Several basic requirements must be met to justify therapeutic drug monitoring in newborns and to modify drug treatment accurately based on measured circulating drug concentrations (70).

Drug analysis using small blood volumes must be accurate.

Circulating drug concentrations must correlate with both effective and toxic pharmacologic effects. This implies that the circulating total (i.e., free plus protein-bound) drug concentration correlates with the free-drug concentration at the site of drug action, such as the drug receptor or tissue site.

The therapeutic index, the concentration range between efficacy and toxicity, should be narrow.

Clinical studies should have established a concentration range for efficacy and toxicity in the population being monitored.

It should be recognized that pharmacokinetics are variable and unpredictable in newborns.

In the extremely premature newborn, decreased protein binding may significantly affect therapeutic drug monitoring. Because of unpredictable decreases in protein binding associated with organ dysfunction or immaturity, free-drug concentrations may be much higher than would be predicted from the total drug concentration that usually is measured clinically. Higher percentages of free drug in the newborn may account for signs of toxicity or adequate therapeutic response at paradoxically low total drug concentrations. When therapeutic concentration ranges have been established, as for phenytoin, measurement of free-drug concentrations may be helpful in newborns demonstrating signs of drug toxicity with therapeutic or subtherapeutic circulating total drug concentrations.

Effective drug therapy is measured by response, not by achievement of a particular circulating drug concentration. Concentration ranges described as therapeutic are statistical ranges for drug levels that usually are effective and nontoxic. Individual patients may require drug concentrations outside these ranges to achieve optimal drug treatment.

---

[1]Estimation of concentrations after a fraction of a half-life assumes a linear rather than logarithmic decline in concentrations and is not mathematically correct for first-order, exponential rates in which the amount of drug eliminated decreases as the concentration decreases. However, this approach is suitable for clinical applications, where only a reasonable estimate of plasma concentration is needed for dosage adjustments.

Repetitive Dosing and Drug Accumulation

During most courses of repetitive drug therapy, each dose is administered before complete elimination of the previous one. This leads to accumulation of drug, with increasing peak and trough concentrations, until a steady-state concentration is reached (Fig. 55–4). The average C_{ss} can be calculated as follows (61):

$$\text{Avg } C_{ss} = (1/\text{Clearance}) \times f \times D/\tau \qquad [10]$$

$$= [1/(k \times V_d\text{area})] \times f \times D/\tau$$

$$= (1.44 \times t_{1/2}/V_d\text{area}) \times f \times D/\tau \qquad [11]$$

In Eqs. 10 and 11, f is the fraction of the dose that is absorbed, D is the dose, τ is the dosing interval in the same units of time as the elimination half-life, k is the elimination rate constant, and 1.44 equals 1/0.693 (see Eq. 3). The magnitude of the average C_{ss} is directly proportional to a ratio of $t_{1/2}/\tau$ and D (61).

Steady State

Steady state occurs when the amount of drug removed from the body between doses equals the dose (62,66). Five half-lives are usually required for drug elimination and distribution among tissue and fluid compartments to reach an equilibrium. When all tissues are at equilibrium, that is, at steady state, the peak and trough concentrations are the same after each dose. However, before this time, constant peak and trough concentrations after intermittent doses, or constant concentrations during drug infusions, do not prove that a steady state has been achieved because drug may still be entering and leaving deep tissue compart-

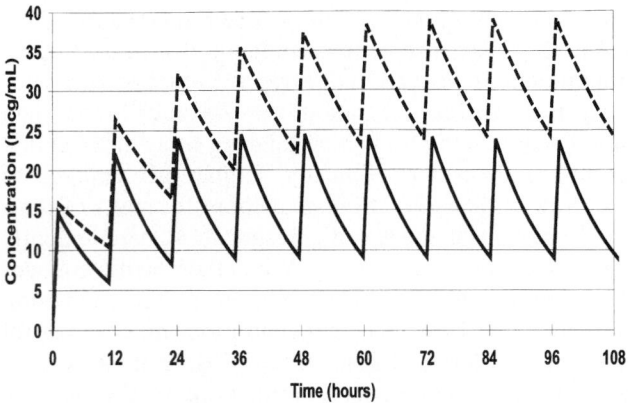

FIG. 55–4. The effect of two different half-lives on the steady-state concentrations of vancomycin during repetitive dosing with the same dose (15 mg/kg and a V_d of 0.9 L/kg). The *solid line* represents a half-life of 8 hours, and the *broken line* represents a half-life of 16 hours. Peak and trough concentrations increase until steady state is achieved. Apparent steady state is achieved by the fourth dose (36 hours) with the 8-hour half-life but not until the seventh dose (72 hours) with the 16-hour half-life.

ments. During continuous infusion, the fraction of steady-state concentration that has been reached can be calculated in terms of multiples of the drug's half-life (61). After 3 half-lives, the concentration is 88% of that at steady state. The effect of dosage changes on drug concentrations during chronic treatment usually should not be rechecked until several half-lives have elapsed, unless elimination is impaired or toxic symptoms occur. Drug concentrations may not need to be checked if symptoms improve.

Loading Dose

If the time to reach a constant concentration by continuous or intermittent dosing is too long, a loading dose may be used to reach a higher constant concentration more quickly. This frequently is applied to initial treatment with digoxin, which has a 35- to 69-hour half-life in term neonates and an even longer half-life in preterm newborns (71). Use of a loading dose produces a higher circulating drug concentration earlier in the therapeutic course, but the equilibration to reach a true steady-state still requires treatment for five or more half-lives. Loading doses must be used cautiously because they increase the likelihood of drug toxicity, as has been observed with digoxin digitalizing doses (71).

Special Considerations for Neonates

Intravenous Administration

Intravenous administration of drugs is considered the most reliable route. In neonates, especially those who weigh 500 to 1,000 g and receive small volumes of IV fluids, IV drug administration may not reliably deliver the dose into the circulation (11,72). Because some types of IV tubing may contain 12 to 15 mL of fluid, and the IV infusion rates for 500- to 1,000-g neonates may be 1.5 to 2.5 mL/hr, infusion of a drug into the IV tubing several centimeters from the patient will markedly delay drug administration. This may confound therapeutic drug monitoring by causing the peak concentration to be less than the trough, because the dose has not reached the patient. For this reason, microbore tubing, which has a volume of 0.5 mL, should be used whenever possible and should be connected to the port closest to the patient. Slow delivery of drug to the circulation may prevent the attainment of an adequate peak concentration to enhance drug diffusion into tissue down a concentration gradient. Last, filters present a potential obstacle to effective IV drug treatment. Drugs may adsorb to the filter or settle to the bottom of a reservoir in the filter, out of the main flow of the infusing solution (73).

Exchange Transfusion

Because few studies have evaluated the amount of drug actually removed from neonates during an exchange transfusion, theoretical estimates have been developed

(72,74). The amounts removed vary with the individual drug's volume of distribution, rate of distribution, and circulating concentration at the time of the exchange as well as with the volume of blood exchanged and the rate of the exchange.

CLINICAL TOXICOLOGY

Newborn infants, both full-term and premature, present an alarmingly wide spectrum of susceptibilities to unanticipated adverse effects from exposure to exogenous chemicals. New drugs, together with unrecognized chemicals ranging from tape remover to plasticizers, are introduced into the care of neonates each year. Prescription drug exposure of the extremely preterm neonate is extensive. In the late 1970s, neonates admitted to a NICU received up to 26 drugs, averaging 6.2 drugs per infant (75). This drug exposure was not innocuous: 30% of infants in the NICU manifested an adverse drug reaction, of which 15% were considered fatal or life-threatening (76). Similar drug exposure of newborns was documented in Boston from 1974 to 1977, where infants in the intensive care nursery received more drugs (10.4/patient) than any other hospitalized children (77).

Several factors increase the susceptibility of newborns and preterm newborns to chemical toxicities. Immaturity of liver and renal function frequently delays drug elimination, which prolongs the exposure of the newborn to a drug and predisposes to drug accumulation during repeated administration. New therapeutic agents often are introduced into treatment of critically ill neonates when all other therapy has failed, although pharmacokinetic data to guide dose and dosing intervals may be lacking. Without the guide of pharmacokinetic or concentration–response studies, treatment failure may be considered an indication to increase the dose rather than a result of administering excess amounts of the drug (78).

Specific enzyme immaturities of the newborn also may place them at risk. Inadequate function of the glucuronosyltransferase system predisposes the newborn to inadequate elimination of chemicals requiring glucuronide conjugation, such as bilirubin. Circulating albumin binds bilirubin at the levels encountered in physiologic jaundice and protects the newborn from bilirubin encephalopathy as long as the blood–brain barrier remains intact (79,80). Failure to recognize the competition of drugs for bilirubin's albumin-binding sites has led to displacement of bound bilirubin and kernicterus (81–83). Large doses of chloramphenicol were associated with unexplained cardiovascular collapse in infants in 1959 (42). That same year, a randomized, controlled study of antibiotics for neonatal sepsis revealed that the groups treated with chloramphenicol alone or in combination had a 60% mortality, threefold higher than neonates receiving no antibiotics (43). The no-treatment control group, however, showed the same survival as the alternate antibiotic treatment group. Inadequate glucuronide conjugation of chloramphenicol and decreased tubular secretion of conjugated chloramphenicol combined to reduce chloramphenicol elimination and led to accumulation to toxic concentrations (41). Acute intoxication with high serum chloramphenicol concentrations manifested with jaundice, vomiting, anorexia, respiratory distress, abdominal distention, cyanosis, green stools, lethargy, and ashen color (43).

The preservative benzyl alcohol has been implicated in a fatal syndrome in premature infants of cardiovascular collapse and death associated with metabolic acidosis, gasping respirations, thrombocytopenia, hepatic and renal failure, and progressive central nervous system (CNS) depression (84). The minimal intake to produce toxicity was estimated at 130 mg/kg/day (84). Removal of benzyl alcohol as a preservative in the fluid frequently used to flush IV catheters in neonates has essentially eliminated this problem. Although many nurseries and pharmacies have excluded all solutions and medications containing benzyl alcohol, the major problem seemed to lie with IV solutions and flush solutions. In view of the dose estimated for toxicity, exposure to the small amounts in medications (which can be estimated from the benzyl alcohol concentration and dosing volume) might pose an acceptable risk compared to the benefit of the drug treatment. Propylene glycol, a solvent frequently used with water-insoluble drugs, has also been associated with toxicity in neonates (85,86). At high doses, propylene glycol (PG) is partly metabolized to lactic acid and may cause serum hyperosmolality with a marked osmolar gap, lactic acidosis, seizures, and cardiac arrhythmias (85–89). Because up to 45% of PG is eliminated renally, patients with poor renal function (including preterm neonates) may be predisposed to PG toxicity. Lorazepam, which is commonly used in neonates, contains propylene glycol, and caution must be exercised in prescribing large scheduled doses of lorazepam for sedation of sick neonates.

Dermal exposure to a variety of chemical agents, including isopropyl alcohol, may be hazardous to the newborn (90,91). Toxic epidermal necrolysis was reported in a neonate after prolonged exposure to a commonly used distillate-containing adhesive remover (92). Unintended percutaneous absorption of toxic substances through the permeable skin of neonates has recurred with several substances. This has led to toxicity from methanol (93), isopropanol (94,95), hexachlorophene (96), iodine-containing topical disinfectants, (97,98), aniline dye in diapers (99), and topical antibiotics such as neomycin (100). Advantageous and disadvantageous transcutaneous drug absorption by newborns has been reviewed (101). Chemical intoxication of the fetus and newborn has been reviewed in detail (102).

Inadvertent exposure of the neonate to a variety of chemicals may occur with little notice. Phthalate plasticizers accumulate in the myocardial and gastrointestinal tissue of neonates with umbilical catheters and those who receive blood products (103). Although phthalates probably produce minimal acute toxicity, they accumulate in tissues and may exert effects that are not recognized. Since the report by Hillman and colleagues (103), the extent of exposure of NICU patients to plastic products appears to have increased, causing greater exposure to soluble chemicals in the plastic, such as phthalates.

SPECIFIC CLASSES OF DRUGS

Antiarrhythmics

Treatment of cardiac arrhythmias has advanced with increased understanding of the transmembrane ion currents that control both normal and abnormal myocardial depolarization (104–106). Developmental changes in these channels are described using both electrophysiologic techniques and molecular biological means of investigation (107). Careful interpretation of various studies is needed, however, because of species differences in the timing of innervation and in the development of various channels (107,108).

Antiarrhythmic drugs have been classified and reclassified according to the mechanisms responsible for arrhythmias, including effects on ion channels, duration of repolarization, and receptor interaction (Table 55–4) (106,109–111). A discussion of the various subtypes of ion channels is beyond the scope of this chapter (104–106,112,113). Such classification systems help with analysis of the effects of individual antiarrhythmic drugs and selection of treatment for specific arrhythmias,

but drugs and their metabolites may interact with multiple ion channels and more than one antiarrhythmic mechanism (111,114). Drugs within a given class, however, may differ in their effectiveness for an individual patient's arrhythmia. Dosages for drugs used frequently for resuscitation of newborns are listed (see Table 55–5) (115).

Drug selection for treatment of arrhythmias should be guided, whenever possible, by more precise identification of the type of arrhythmia. The most frequent arrhythmia requiring management in neonates is supraventricular tachycardia (SVT) (116). In general, SVT arises from either an aberrant conduction pathway or abnormal automaticity in a discrete focus that captures the ventricle (116). Reentrant mechanisms are the most common cause of SVT in neonates and usually involve retrograde conduction from the ventricle via the accessory conduction pathway to the atrium, which then depolarizes prematurely. This has been designated orthodromic reciprocating tachycardia (ORT). A variant of ORT arises from a posterior accessory conducting pathway that causes a slower but incessant form of SVT, permanent junctional reciprocating tachycardia (PJRT). Left untreated, PJRT may cause a cardiomyopathy and CHF. In the Wolff–Parkinson–White syndrome (WPW), the accessory conduction pathway can be identified during sinus rhythm from early depolarization that creates a beginning shoulder (delta wave) on the QRS complex with a shortened PR interval (116). Unfortunately, almost 50% of reentrant SVT in infants does not show preexcitation overtly during sinus rhythm. When the depolarization returns from the ventricle through the atrioventricular node to cause SVT, it is termed antidromic

TABLE 55–4. *Antiarrhythmic drugs by mechanism of action*

Class	Action/structure	Drugs
IA	Sodium ± potassium channel blockade Phase 0 *dV/dt*, slowed Conduction slowed (prolonged PR, QRS, and QT) Repolarization usually delayed Anticholinergic	Quinidine Procainamide Dysopyramide
IB	Sodium channel blockade Phase 0 *dV/dt*, minimal change Repolarization usually shortened (QT shortened) Fibrillation thresholds elevated	Lidocaine Mexilitine
IC	Sodium channel blockade Phase 0 *dV/dt*, markedly slowed Repolarization minimally changed, PR and QRS markedly prolonged	Flecainide Propafenone
II.	β-Adenergic blockade, variable selectivity	Propranolol Atenolol Esmolol
III.	Repolarization and action potential prolonged	Amiodarone Sotalol
IV.	Calcium channel blockade	Verapamil
V.	Digitalis glycosides	Digoxin Ouabain
VI.	Purinergic agonists	Adenosine

Adapted from refs. 106, 111, with permission.

TABLE 55–5. *Drugs for newborn resuscitation and acute treatment of arrhythmias*

Drug and formulation	Final concentration	Dose (Amount/kg)	Dose (mL/kg)
Adenosine, 6 mg/2 mL	3 mg/mL	Start: 50 µg/kg rapid IV push, followed by flush of IV catheter; if no response within 0.5 to 2 minutes, increase dose by 50 µg/kg and repeat until conversion of SVT or AV block, to maximum single dose of 250–500 µg/kg	Dilute 0.5 ml with 2.5 ml saline; infuse 0.1 mL/kg IV for every 50 µg/kg dose
Atropine, 1 mg/10 mL	0.1 mg/mL	IV dosage: 0.01 to 0.02 mg/kg; may repeat in 10 min to maximum of 0.04 mg/kg; IT* dosage: 0.02 to 0.04 mg/kg	0.1 to 0.2 mL/kg IV; 0.2–0.4 mL/kg IT[a]
Bicarbonate, 4.2%	0.5 mEq/mL	1 to 2 mEq/kg; treat measured metabolic acidosis; avoid 1.0 mEq/mL formulation in newborns; maintain ventilation	2 to 4 mL/kg IV
Calcium gluconate, 10%	100 mg/mL (9.3 mg Ca^{2+}/mL)	60 mg/kg infused slowly and stop infusion for symptomatic bradycardia; repeat as needed for clinical effect; extravasation causes tissue necrosis	0.6 mL/kg IV
Calcium chloride, 10%	100 mg/mL (27 mg Ca^{2+}/mL)	20 mg/kg infused slowly and stop infusion for symptomatic bradycardia; repeat as needed for clinical effect; extravasation causes tissue necrosis	0.2 mL/kg IV
Direct current defibrillation		1 watt-sec/kg; increase by 1 Watt-sec/kg if unsuccessful	
Epinephrine, 1:10,000	0.1 mg/mL	0.01 to 0.03 mg/kg IV or IO; 0.1 mg/kg IT[a]	0.1 to 0.3 mL/kg IV, IO; 1 mL/kg IT[a]
Glucose, 10%	100 mg/mL	200 to 500 mg/kg	2 to 5 mL/kg IV
Lidocaine, 2%	20 mg/mL	0.5 to 1.0 mg/kg; repeat every 5 to 10 minutes to maximum of mg/kg	Dilute 0.5 mL + 9.5 mL D5W; infuse: 0.5 to 1.0 mL/kg IV, IT[a]
Naloxone, 0.4 mg/mL	0.4 mg/mL	0.1 mg/kg, repeat every 10 to 15 minutes to clinical effect	0.25 mL/kg IV, IM
Procainamide, 100 mg/mL	100 mg/mL	3 to 6 mg/kg over 5 minutes, repeat to a titrated maximum of 15 mg/kg loading dose, infuse slowly with myocardial dysfunction	Dilute 1 mL + 9 mL D5W; infuse: 0.3–0.6 mL/kg IV

[a]IT, through endotracheal tube; dose should be diluted in saline or tube flushed with saline after dose.
Adapted from refs. 115 (with permission of the American Academy of Pediatrics) and 126, and from Roberts RJ. Drug therapy in infants. *Pharmacologic principles and clinical experience*. Philadelphia: WB Saunders, 1984.

reentrant tachycardia and causes a wide complex tachycardia. Reentrant tachycardias, either overt or concealed, can be identified during electrophysiologic studies by their ability to be initiated and terminated by atrial or ventricular extrastimulation (114,116).

Nonreentrant SVT is rare in infancy and difficult to treat pharmacologically. A SVT caused by a non–sinus-node focus of abnormal automaticity is designated automatic atrial tachycardia (AAT) and is difficult to treat medically (114). An AAT must be distinguished from sinus tachycardia because the heart rate may gradually speed up and slow down. The P-wave morphology during AAT differs from that during sinus rhythm, and the PR interval of conducted beats may lengthen, rather than shorten, as the rate increases (114). A SVT may also arise from a site of abnormal automaticity within or near the AV node; this syndrome is designated junctional ectopic tachycardia (JET) (114) and is also quite difficult to treat with the usual antiarrhythmics (117,118). Treatment of SVT may be required in two situations, acute termination of a symptomatic tachycardia and chronic suppression of SVT that has recurred or is likely to recur. Synchronized direct current electrocardioversion terminated SVT in about 50% of cases but was more successful if P waves were not present (119). Vagal maneuvers, such as stimulation of the diving reflex through ice applied to the face, are still frequently used for the acute termination of SVT, although bilateral carotid massage or pressure on the eyes should be avoided.

For the acute treatment of SVT, adenosine has been used with moderate success. Adenosine slows spontaneous heart rate, prolongs the PR interval, and decreases the slope of phase 4 repolarization through activation of A_1-purinoceptors coupled to sarcolemmal potassium channels. In one report, electroconversion was not required for conversion of infant-onset SVT during the 6 years after the introduction of adenosine (120). The ventricle is minimally affected by adenosine, whose action begins within seconds of administration. With a 9-second half-life, it must be administered as a rapid IV infusion over seconds, but it has been administered successfully by intraosseus infusion (121). Its short half-life limits its usefulness to the acute treatment of SVT. Adenosine treatment may be started with 50 to 150 μg/kg doses, with increases in the dose by 50 μg/kg every minute to a maximum of 300 to 350 μg/kg (111,122,123). Because theophylline is a competitive antagonist of adenosine (124), higher adenosine dosages may be required in infants treated with theophylline (125). Adenosine may precipitate bronchoconstriction and wheezing as well as hypotension as a result of vasodilation (126).

Supraventricular tachycardia that has not responded to adenosine may be managed with an infusion of procainamide, a class 1A drug that blocks both sodium and potassium channels (111). Rapid infusion may precipitate hypotension, whereas chronic treatment produces antinuclear antibodies in 50% to 90% of patients associated with a systemic lupus erythematosus–type syndrome (111,126). High concentrations of procainamide may depress myocardial contractility and predispose to congestive heart failure (111). Although more than half of a procainamide dose is excreted unchanged, it is metabolized in the liver to N-acetylprocainamide (NAPA), an active metabolite that acts through a different (class III) antiarrhythmic mechanism (111). Acetylation to NAPA involves the N-acetyltransferase enzyme system, which is involved in the metabolism of isoniazid. Adults may be phenotyped as fast or slow acetylators (127); however, infants between birth and 2 months of age are uniformly slow acetylators because of the immaturity of the enzyme system (18). Both NAPA and procainamide accumulate with renal insufficiency. Procainamide levels of 4 to 8 μg/ml are generally effective for control of arrhythmias.

Lidocaine, a class 1B antiarrhythmic, primarily blocks the fast inward sodium channel, like other local anesthetic antiarrhythmic drugs (111,126). Its effects are much greater on the conducting system and the ventricular muscle than on the atrium. It has active metabolites that also block the sodium channel. Plasma concentrations should be maintained between 2 and 5 μg/mL because concentrations exceeding 6 μg/mL may produce

seizures or respiratory arrest (111,126). Drugs known to decrease hepatic blood flow, such as cimetidine, will decrease hepatic clearance of lidocaine and increase concentrations unless the dose is reduced.

Chronic treatment of SVT is not needed in every patient (114). If episodes of SVT are rare, not associated with cardiovascular compromise, and easily terminated with vagal maneuvers, chronic treatment may not be required provided that the child can be monitored adequately at home (114). The presence of WPW, however, is a significant predictor of recurrence of SVT after stopping medications (128). Digoxin treatment of WPW is controversial because it has been associated with sudden death in 1% to 5% of patients (114,129). In another series of patients with SVT, digoxin treatment was successful in 65% regardless of whether or not they showed preexcitation (120). A review of patients treated for SVT at Texas Children's Hospital revealed no difference in the success rate for treatment of SVT with digitalis among patients with and without WPW (119).

Propranolol is frequently used to treat neonates with SVT if digoxin is contraindicated because of the presence of WPW (111). It has special pharmacokinetic features that must be considered in its administration. When administered enterally, propranolol is cleared largely through first-pass extraction by the liver. It is metabolized extensively to an active metabolite, 4-hydroxypropranolol (130). During repetitive doses, hepatic extraction decreases, and plasma concentrations may vary widely at steady state. If administered IV, the propranolol dose must be reduced at least tenfold because it bypasses hepatic extraction and produces a dose- and concentration-related decrease in heart rate and cardiac contractility. Propranolol has been used most frequently to treat supraventricular and ventricular arrhythmias. It also has a role in treatment of sinus tachycardia related to hypermetabolic states such as thyrotoxicosis (126). Data on dosing, kinetics, and efficacy in neonates for other β-adrenergic blocking drugs such as atenolol, nadolol, sotalol, and esmolol are limited.

Verapamil has been used for treatment of SVT with moderate success, but its use in infants younger than 12 months of age has been discouraged (111,131). Because of its negative inotropic activity and ability to decrease sinus function, verapamil should not be used with β-adrenergic blocking drugs in infants and children (126). They have been used together successfully in adults.

Amiodarone is a benzofuran compound with structural similarity to thyroxine that was originally synthesized in 1962 and released in the United States in 1985. Because of the associated toxicities, it was approved as a last-resort drug that should be reserved for refractory, life-threatening arrhythmias (132). During the last few years, much more information has accumulated about both its efficacy and its toxicity. Amiodarone illustrates the limitations of a classification system for antiarrhythmics. It inhibits both the fast sodium channel and the slow calcium channel, has noncompetitive antisympathetic effects, and modulates thyroid function (133). In addition, its acute effects differ from those during chronic treatment. Acutely, it slows AV node conduction with little effect on the QTc, but during chronic therapy, it lengthens QTc and prolongs the refractory period (133). Although reports are limited in neonates, the following adverse effects have been observed after amiodarone treatment of infants and children: photosensitivity (134,135), corneal deposits (134), gray skin color (134), abnormal liver function tests (134), hypothyroidism (134,135), hyperthyroidism (134,135), accelerated bone maturation (135), delayed longitudinal growth (135), excess weight gain (135), headaches (135), pulmonary infiltrates (136), and sleep disturbances (134). Amiodarone increases the concentration of several drugs, usually by decreasing clearance and volume of distribution, including digoxin, quinidine, procainamide, phenytoin, and flecainide. Decreased clearance of warfarin by amiodarone may precipitate hemorrhage. Overall, the frequency of adverse effects is greater in adults than in children and greater in older children than in infants.

Amiodarone treatment of refractory and serious arrhythmias in infants and children has been successful with limited acute toxicity. In a multicenter trial, Perry reported a 93% rate of improvement with the compassionate use of amiodarone for life-threatening arrhythmias in 40 patients from eight centers (137). Several serious and refractory arrhythmias have been successfully treated with amiodarone, including multifocal atrial tachycardia (chaotic atrial tachycardia) (138,139), ventricular tachycardia secondary to intracardiac tumor (140), and refractory SVT (141,142).

Dosages of amiodarone have varied widely from study to study. Initial treatment with amiodarone usually begins with a loading dose, but the dosages range from 5 mg/kg followed by an infusion of 10 to 15 mg/kg/day (137) to 7.5 to 13.5 mg/kg/day for 9 to 10 days (143). Larger dosages were required for infants less than 1 year of age in one study (134). Oral treatment alone has been successful in some studies (134). This prolonged loading dose likely relates to amiodarone's extremely long half-life, which has been estimated to exceed 50 days in adults (132). Levels of amiodarone are kept between 0.8 and 2.0 mg/L in adults (134), but there is no clear relationship between levels of amiodarone or its metabolite desethylamiodarone and toxicity or efficacy (144,145).

Newborns with fetal arrhythmias may be treated with amiodarone and require evaluation of potential adverse effects in the nursery. A healthy fetus whose mother was treated with amiodarone for sick sinus syndrome delivered and breast-fed with no changes in thyroid function (146). Both neonatal hyperthyroidism and hypothyroidism with or without a goiter have been observed after fetal exposure to amiodarone (147–150).

Anticonvulsants

Seizures remain a frequent therapeutic problem for newborns. They may be caused by a variety of disorders such as meningitis, inadequate pyridoxal-5-phosphate binding (i.e., pyridoxine dependency), hypoglycemia, hypocalcemia, inborn errors of metabolism, neonatal abstinence from narcotics, or intracranial hemorrhage (151). Because treatment differs according to etiology, causes for seizures outside the brain should always be considered and evaluated. Some noncerebral causes of seizures may produce recurrent seizures that require prolonged anticonvulsant drug treatment in addition to treatment of the primary metabolic or infectious disorder. Because prolonged seizures per se may harm the brain, treatment should not be delayed (151).

Phenobarbital remains the mainstay of seizure therapy in neonates (152). Although seizures are controlled in some patients with phenobarbital levels of 15 µg/mL, the minimal effective therapeutic concentration should be regarded as 20 µg/mL, and many patients may require concentrations as high as 40 µg/mL to achieve seizure control (153). Because phenobarbital has a volume of distribution of approximately 0.9 L/kg in neonates, a loading dose of 15 to 20 mg/kg is required to reach a minimum concentration of 20 µg/mL (154). To maximize efficacy and minimize adverse effects, neonatal seizures should be treated with a single drug to its maximal dose before a second drug is added or the patient is changed to a second drug. With this approach and a maximum dose of 40 µg/kg of phenobarbital, 85% of neonatal seizures could be controlled with phenobarbital alone (155).

The half-life of phenobarbital is prolonged at birth, ranging from 43 to 217 hours (156). Consequently, lower doses of phenobarbital (2 to 3 mg/kg/day) should be used during the first week of life. Phenobarbital clearance increases significantly during the neonatal period, and the half-life decreases to approximately 45 hours at 28 days of life (154). Thus, maintenance doses will often need to be increased within the first several weeks after birth (3 to 5 mg/kg/day). A good correlation has been demonstrated between plasma and brain concentrations of both phenobarbital and phenytoin, so that increasing plasma concentrations should increase the anticonvulsant concentration at the site of action (16).

Concerns have increased about the effects of long-term phenobarbital treatment on cognitive development. When phenobarbital was compared to placebo in two randomized groups of children treated for 2 years for febrile seizures, the phenobarbital-treated group had significantly lower IQs (157). In a randomized, crossover trial of three anticonvulsants, phenobarbital produced more impairment of neuropsychological performance than did carbamazepine or phenytoin (158). The American Academy of Pediatrics Committee on Drugs summarized concerns about the cognitive effects of phenobarbital (159).

Phenytoin has served as the second-line anticonvulsant for neonates. Disadvantages of phenytoin are its highly variable and nonlinear pharmacokinetics; that is, exponential elimination decreases with increasing serum concentrations. The latter phenomenon requires considerable caution because small increases in maintenance dose may result in disproportionately large increases in plasma concentrations. The initially prolonged half-life of phenytoin decreases rapidly during the neonatal period from 57.3 ± 48.2 hours during the first days of life to 19.7 ± 1.3 hours during the fourth week (37). In term infants between 2 and 21 weeks of age, the half-life ranged from 6.6 hours to 15.1 hours (22). However, preterm infants often exhibit prolonged half-lives (15.6 to 160 hours) up to 18 days after birth (22).

Phenytoin is a water-insoluble base, and the commercially available injection formulation is prepared using 40% propylene glycol at a final pH of 12. The accepted therapeutic serum concentration range for phenytoin is 10 to 20 µg/mL, and a loading dose of 15 to 20 mg/kg will achieve a therapeutic concentration (160). To avoid hypotension, arrhythmias, and precipitation during administration, phenytoin should be administered slowly (maximum 0.5 to 1 mg/kg/min) into an IV line containing only saline. Because the drug is caustic to tissues, intramuscular administration should be avoided, and intravenous doses should be infused through as large a vein as is available, with care taken to avoid extravasation.

Interpretation of phenytoin plasma concentrations requires consideration of protein binding. In adults, the unbound concentration of phenytoin is approximately 10% of the total concentration (161). Thus, the therapeutic range for unbound (free) phenytoin is 1 to 2 µg/mL. Because plasma protein concentrations and binding affinity of albumin are low in newborns, plasma protein binding of phenytoin is reduced in infants. In normobilirubinemic newborns, the free (unbound) fraction of phenytoin is 15% to 20%, and in hyperbilirubinemic infants, the free fraction may reach 30% (22,162,163). Thus, despite apparent subtherapeutic total concentrations (<10 µg/mL), free concentrations may be within the therapeutic range of 1 to 2 µg/mL. Monitoring free phenytoin concentrations may be useful in this circumstance to determine if concentrations are within the therapeutic range. If free concentrations of phenytoin are not available, targeting total concentrations to 6 to 14 µg/mL is appropriate in the immediate neonatal period (22). However, as protein binding normalizes in the weeks to months after birth, the therapeutic range will require readjustment to 10 to 20 µg/mL.

Because of the significant variability in pharmacokinetics during the first weeks of life, a standard dose of phenytoin cannot be recommended, and plasma concentrations must be monitored. During the first week of life, doses of 4 to 8 mg/kg/day may be required (22). However, chronic oral phenytoin therapy in infants often requires much higher doses (160). By the second week after birth, most infants will require at least 8 mg/kg/day divided every 6 to 8 hours (22); however, oral doses as high as 17.7 ± 4.3 mg/kg/day and intravenous doses of 25 mg/kg/day have been required to maintain therapeutic concentrations (160,164). Some have attributed these dose requirements to poor absorption of the oral formulation (160), but high doses are also required after intravenous administration (164). Other investigators have demonstrated complete absorption in infants receiving oral doses (165). High oral dosage requirements in infants likely reflect several pharmacokinetic events, including poor and erratic absorption, increased phenytoin metabolism during the first year of life, and hepatic enzyme induction by concomitant treatment with phenobarbital (160,164,165).

Recently, the introduction of fosphenytoin has significantly reduced the potential for the adverse effects usually associated with phenytoin, including pain on administration, extravasation injury, propylene glycol–associated hyperosmolality (85), central nervous system changes (87,88), acidosis (89), and cardiovascular compromise (166) following rapid intravenous injection. Fosphenytoin is a water-soluble prodrug that is rapidly hydrolyzed to phenytoin via blood and tissue phosphatases (167). Because it is an aqueous solution and contains no propylene glycol, it has few pharmaceutical compatibility problems and may be administered by intravenous injection or by intramuscular injection (167). Because fosphenytoin is converted to phenytoin, issues regarding protein binding, therapeutic concentrations, and drug interactions associated with phenytoin must still be considered. Studies must be conducted in newborns before its routine use in this population is recommended.

Benzodiazepines can be used for additional drug therapy beyond phenobarbital and phenytoin to control seizures in the newborn. Diazepam has been used to treat refractory seizures in neonates, but its efficacy is limited by its short duration of action, respiratory depression, prolonged half-life, and metabolism to active metabolites (168). Lorazepam, in a dose of 0.05 to 0.1 mg/kg, has been effective for controlling refractory seizures in neonates and has a duration of action up to 24 hours (86,168). Total doses up to 0.15 mg/kg may be necessary to control neonatal seizures that are refractory to phenobarbital (169). Because metabolism of lorazepam requires glucuronidation, which is poorly developed in newborns, the half-life of lorazepam in newborns is prolonged (mean 40 hours) and correlates with gestational age (170). The dose of benzyl alcohol associated with the IV preparation of lorazepam, which contains PG as a solubilizing agent and benzyl alcohol as a preservative, is low enough not to represent a risk for toxicity (102). Some have reported seizure-like stereotypic movements after lorazepam administration (171,172). The cause of this movement disorder is not known.

Recently midazolam has been used in adults and children for treatment of epileptic episodes of various types, including status epilepticus (173,174). A study was conducted in six neonates (aged 1 to 9 days; gestation 30 to 41 weeks) with persistent seizures despite a mean phenobarbital concentration of 50.5 mg/L (175). Seizures were controlled in all patients within 1 hour of administering a continuous intravenous infusion of midazolam (0.1 to 0.4 mg/kg/hr). Because neonatal seizures are sometimes refractory to high-dose phenobarbital, midazolam may be a valuable adjunctive therapy (175). Care must be taken to avoid rapid bolus doses of midazolam over 1 to 2 minutes that may cause hypotension in infants receiving fentanyl infusions (176) or tonic–clonic movements similar to those reported in older children following lorazepam (177).

The decision to continue or to stop treatment with anticonvulsant medications before discharge from the NICU remains controversial. Scher and Painter suggest that anticonvulsants may be discontinued for infants who show no abnormalities of the brain on imaging studies, have an age-appropriate neurologic examination, and have a normal interictal electroencephalogram (178). Up to 30% of neonates with seizures later have epilepsy, but frequently the later seizure pattern takes the form of infantile spasms or minor motor seizures that are not very responsive to phenobarbital and phenytoin (178).

Antihypertensives

Drug treatment of hypertension in pediatric patients should follow a stepped treatment regimen in which a single drug's effects are optimized before another is added (179,180). When this approach is extended to the newborn, treatment may begin with diuretics, and centrally acting agents such as methyldopa or β-receptor blockers such as propranolol are then added if needed. A vasodilator, such as hydralazine, may be substituted or added to β-adrenergic blockers. Recently, calcium channel blockers such as nifedipine, verapamil, and diltiazem have emerged as effective antihypertensives (181). Vasodilators often need to be used with a diuretic to avoid fluid retention. Calcium channel blockers, usually, do not cause fluid retention and are roughly equivalent to α-adrenergic antagonists or diuretics for the treatment of hypertension (181).

Angiotensin-converting enzyme inhibitors (e.g., captopril) have a special role in the treatment of neonatal renovascular hypertension that is caused by markedly elevated renin and angiotensin (182). Aortic catheters may distribute microemboli to the kidneys, which increase secretion of renin and angiotensin in response to focal underperfusion. Although captopril may be relatively specific treatment for many cases of renovascular hypertension in neonates, dosage adjustments are difficult because a liquid dosage form is not commercially available. Dosage adjustments require the pharmacy to grind tablets and weigh individual doses, or the parents to for-

mulate tablets into suspensions for each dose. An extemporaneously compounded dosage form containing ascorbate has been shown to be stable for 14 days at room temperature (183). Captopril treatment of neonates should start with doses of 0.01 mg/kg rather than the earlier recommendations of 0.1 to 0.3 mg/kg/dose to avoid hypotension and acute renal insufficiency (184). Doses should be increased daily if hypertension persists. Initial captopril treatment may cause a triphasic reaction of hypotension with renal failure, managed by dose reduction, followed by a rise in blood pressure despite increasing doses above the original dose (185). At the start of captopril treatment, hypotension is exaggerated in salt- and water-depleted patients (186). As in adults, captopril may be useful for afterload reduction in the treatment of chronic congestive heart failure in newborns (186).

Hypertensive emergencies are infrequent in neonates but can be treated with sodium nitroprusside if renal function is normal or with diazoxide if renal function is inadequate (180). As observed in older patients, thiocyanate and cyanide may accumulate during sodium nitroprusside treatment, and hyperglycemia may occur with diazoxide infusions.

Antimicrobials

β-Lactams

Ampicillin and an aminoglycoside have been the mainstay for treatment of presumed sepsis and meningitis in the newborn (187). The advantages of this combination include low cost, relatively few problems with resistance (188,189), and a combined spectrum of activity that covers the majority of neonatal pathogens, including group B *Streptococcus, E. coli,* and *Listeria monocytogenes* (187). In select circumstances, ampicillin and cefotaxime may be a preferred alternative. Cefotaxime has excellent gram-negative activity (including gentamicin-resistant isolates) (190), does not cause nephro- or ototoxicity, and does not require plasma concentration monitoring. There has been concern, however, that extensive use of cefotaxime may result in rapid development of multidrug resistance (191,192), and most experts have favored a regimen of a penicillin and aminoglycoside for primary therapy of suspected sepsis (193).

The ureidopenicillins, ticarcillin and piperacillin, provide broader gram-negative coverage than ampicillin (194). For treatment of *Pseudomonas* sp. infections, piperacillin is more active *in vitro* than ticarcillin and may be combined with an aminoglycoside for synergy and to decrease the emergence of resistant organisms (195–197). When piperacillin is combined with an aminoglycoside such as gentamicin, the combination provides excellent activity against aerobic and anaerobic bacteria encountered after intestinal perforation. Piperacillin dosage requirements are based on both gestational and postnatal age (198).

The most common mechanism for resistance to β-lactam antibiotics is production of inactivating β-lactamases (199). β-Lactamase inhibitors, including clavulanate and tazobactam, were developed to bind irreversibly to enzyme substrate, thereby blocking this mode of resistance and preserving activity of the penicillins against many organisms. As a result, ticarcillin–clavulanate and piperacillin–tazobactam have significantly improved spectra of activity, including β-lactamase-producing strains of gram-positive organisms, methicillin-sensitive *Staphylococcus aureus,* many Enterobacteriaceae, fastidious gram-negative bacteria such as *H. influenzae* and *M. catarrhalis,* and many anaerobes (200–202). Generally, piperacillin–tazobactam is more active than ticarcillin–clavulanate against *Enterococcus faecalis* and gram-negative bacilli, including *Pseudomonas aeruginosa* (200). Piperacillin–tazobactam may be a useful combination in the treatment of *Klebsiella pneumoniae* infections in neonates (203).

The antistaphylococcal penicillin, nafcillin, has largely replaced methicillin for the treatment of *Staphylococcus aureus* infections because it has a lower risk of adverse reactions. Nafcillin is eliminated primarily through biliary excretion, which may be impaired in neonates as a result of cholestasis related to prolonged hyperalimentation (204). To reduce vancomycin resistance in hospitals, the antistaphylococcal penicillins should be used whenever possible.

The use of third-generation cephalosporins (e.g., cefotaxime, ceftriaxone, and ceftazidime) continues to proliferate, primarily because of their broad gram-negative activity (including *Klebsiella* sp.), excellent penetration into cerebrospinal fluid, and minimal nephrotoxicity. The choice of these agents over an aminoglycoside will depend on institutional susceptibility patterns. Except during outbreaks of aminoglycoside-resistant bacteria, their widespread use as empirical therapy has been discouraged because of growing threats of resistance (187, 192,205). When *Listeria monocytogenes* or Enterococci are potential causes of infection, initial empirical therapy with third-generation cephalosporins must be combined with ampicillin because the cephalosporins are not active against these pathogens.

Among the cephalosporins, there is considerable experience using cefotaxime in severe neonatal infections (206). Cefotaxime has often replaced gentamicin for coverage of gram-negative bacilli during outbreaks of sepsis caused by gentamicin-resistant gram-negative bacteria (192,207). Although this combination may increase the relative number of enterobacter isolates and perhaps their resistance (191,192,207,208), the incidence of serious gram-negative infections decreased during a 5-year period when cefotaxime was substituted for gentamicin (207). Ceftriaxone has a spectrum of activity very similar to that of cefotaxime, with the primary difference being its pharmacokinetic profile. Ceftriaxone was recently studied in 80 neonates (mean gestational age 34 weeks), and it was well tolerated. Six patients had sonographic findings consistent with biliary sludge that resolved spontaneously within 2 weeks (209). It is believed that ceftriaxone forms a complex with calcium that is poorly soluble in bile, resulting in biliary sludge, which appears to be a transient phenomenon (210). Recent studies have also called to attention ceftriaxone's potential to displace bilirubin from albumin binding sites (211,212). An *in vivo* study demonstrated the potential significance of this interaction, and the investigators recommended that ceftriaxone be withheld from jaundiced neonates or premature newborns with acidosis, hypoxia, or sepsis, who are at increased risk for developing bilirubin encephalopathy (211).

Certain cephalosporins have unique properties that fit clinical problems encountered frequently in neonates; for example, ceftazidime is considered the drug of choice to treat Pseudomonas infections. It should be used with an aminoglycoside for synergy and to avoid emergence of resistant strains (213,214). A recent study of 1,316 cases of suspected sepsis in the newborn (median age ≤3 days) found that ceftazidime in combination with ampicillin had a significantly higher cure rate (97%) than ampicillin and an aminoglycoside (66%) (215). No problems with ceftazidime resistance were encountered. Recent pharmacokinetic data in preterm infants indicate that the ceftazidime dose during the first 2 weeks of life should be based on gestational age and postnatal age-related changes in glomerular filtration rate (216,217). In addition, exposure of preterm infants to indomethacin or asphyxia in term infants may reduce ceftazidime's clearance and dosage requirements (217,218).

Enterobacter cloacae, Enterococcus sp., and *Klebsiella pneumoniae* are emerging in neonatal patients as multiply resistant organisms, possibly as a result of the increased use of cephalosporin antibiotics in NICUs (192,219–221). This growing problem of bacterial resistance requires that new classes of antibacterial agents be evaluated for the treatment of severe infections in neonates. Because these potent and broad-spectrum antibiotics have received less study in neonates, they should be used judiciously and with guidance from a specialist in infectious diseases.

The carbapenems, imipenem–cilastatin and meropenem, have an extremely broad spectrum of activity, including gram-positive, gram-negative, and anaerobic organisms (222). Both agents are β-lactamase stable and have activity against penicillin-resistant pneumococci, *Enterococcus faecalis, Listeria monocytogenes, Pseudomonas aeruginosa,* and multiresistant strains of gram-negative organisms (223). Imipenem is combined with cilastatin, a renal dehydropeptidase I inhibitor, which prevents metabolic activation of imipenem to a nephrotoxic compound. Meropenem is more active against gram-negative bacilli and less active against gram-positive cocci (including *Enterococcus* sp.) than is imipenem (223). Both agents penetrate into cerebrospinal fluid in the presence of inflammation associated with meningitis (224). Meropenem and cefotaxime were equally efficacious in the treatment of meningitis in 190 children (median age 1 year) (225).

Carbapenems, through epileptogenic activity, are potentially more neurotoxic than the penicillins and cephalosporins (226). A study of imipenem–cilastatin treatment of bacterial meningitis in 21 infants and children was terminated when 33% developed seizures after antibiotic administration (227). Seizures with imipenem have often been associated with high plasma concentrations associated with renal dysfunction and high doses, or increased susceptibility, such as underlying central nervous system abnormality (223). An additive risk with concomitant theophylline treatment has been reported (228). The safety margin of meropenem appears to be higher, and meropenem can be used at higher doses than imipenem–cilastatin (226). More than 1,200 children (ages 3 months to 12 years) have been treated in prospective, randomized, clinical trials of meropenem (222). A promising finding is that meropenem does not cause seizures with greater frequency than other antibiotics used to treat meningitis (222,229).

The published experience of imipenem in neonates and in particular in preterm neonates is limited. Nalin et al. assessed the safety of imipenem in 61 children up to 6 months old and noted that 15% developed seizures; however, neonates weighing < 750 g or those who were critically ill were excluded (230). Stuart and colleagues investigated the safety of imipenem (20 to 80 mg/kg/day) in 80 neonates at 32 weeks of postconceptional age and noted that only two patients developed seizures (2.5%), both of whom had documented seizures before commencing imipenem (231). Overall, adverse effects were minimal, and no neonate was withdrawn because of toxicity. There are currently no studies evaluating the efficacy or safety of meropenem in neonates.

Both imipenem and meropenem are primarily excreted in the urine (223). Both agents demonstrate age-related pharmacokinetics; thus, the longest half-lives are in premature neonates (232). The carbapenems are administered every 6 to 8 hours in adults, but plasma concentrations in neonates should exceed the MICs for most organisms for 12 hours after a single dose, suggesting that twice-a-day dosing may be appropriate; however, additional studies are required to determine the optimal dose and interval (232).

Aztreonam is a monobactam and shows excellent activity against aerobic gram-negative bacilli, including *Pseudomonas aeruginosa,* but it is devoid of activity against gram-positive or anaerobic bacteria (233). A limited evaluation of its efficacy and pharmacokinetics has been conducted in neonates (234,235). Ampicillin plus aztreonam was compared to ampicillin plus amikacin in 147 neonates, 60 with documented gram-negative bacterial infections (235). Clinical response was noted in 90%

of those who received aztreonam as compared with 72% of those who received amikacin. Because aztreonam does not have the nephrotoxic potential of aminoglycosides, it may be considered as an alternative in the treatment of serious gram-negative infections, particularly when there is a concern regarding concomitant treatment with several nephrotoxic agents.

Vancomycin

Patterns of antimicrobial use in neonatology have evolved with the changing spectrum of infections and development of new antimicrobial agents. Emergence of infections with β-lactam-resistant *Staphylococcus epidermidis, Staphylococcus aureus,* and *Enterococcus* sp. has led to the frequent use of vancomycin in neonates. Recent reports of the increasing prevalence of enterococcal infections in newborns is of significant concern (236), particularly in view of the nationwide 20-fold increase in the percentage of nosocomial enterococci resistant to vancomycin (237). Among vancomycin-resistant strains of enterococci isolated in a pediatric center, the prevalence of *Enterococcus faecium* has increased dramatically (238). Forty-two percent of isolates were from the NICU (238). This trend suggests that future enterococcal infections in neonates may become far more difficult to treat. Although recent studies in newborns demonstrate that prophylactically administered vancomycin reduces infections with coagulase-negative Staphylococcus (239,240), clinicians must be cognizant of the dangers of overusing (and misusing) antibiotics, particularly vancomycin. In response to the increasing prevalence of vancomycin-resistant Enterococcus (VRE), the Hospital Infection Control Practices Advisory Committee of the CDC drafted guidelines to prevent the spread of VRE. These guidelines address, among other things, the appropriate use of vancomycin (241). To minimize the pressure for selecting antibiotic-resistant organisms, vancomycin should generally be reserved for methicillin-resistant staphylococci and ampicillin-resistant enterococcal infections (241).

There appears to be a widely held belief that vancomycin is a nephrotoxin. Consequently, significant resources are allocated to monitoring serum vancomycin concentrations. Although early preparations of vancomycin were impure, and high peaks and troughs were associated with nephro- and ototoxicity (242), these toxicities are now relatively uncommon; however, concomitant administration with aminoglycosides or other nephrotoxins may increase this risk (243,244). Despite a poor correlation between vancomycin plasma concentrations and efficacy and toxicity, medical care has evolved to include the monitoring of vancomycin concentrations. The currently accepted therapeutic range for vancomycin was not derived from rigorous scientific evaluation. Because MICs for most *Staphylococcus* sp. were ≤5 μg/mL or lower, and early toxicities most often occurred at serum concentrations over 30 to 40 µg/mL, desired trough concentrations were designated as 5 to 10 µg/mL, and peak concentrations 20 to 40 µg/mL (245). These somewhat arbitrary ranges have become the standard for therapeutic vancomycin concentrations; however, there is a paucity of data to substantiate these recommendations (246). In the last decade, clinicians have questioned the utility and cost-effectiveness of measuring peak and trough concentrations (246–249). Because the association between peak concentrations and toxicity is poor, some have recommended measuring trough concentrations only (250), but others have suggested not measuring any concentrations in the majority of children with normal renal function (249). However, in critically ill neonates, one must consider the inherently poor glomerular filtration rate associated with prematurity and compromised cardiovascular function as well as the large intrapatient variation in the pharmacokinetics of vancomycin (251). Accordingly, it remains prudent to measure both peak and trough concentrations, particularly in those with poor or changing renal function and those receiving multiple nephrotoxic agents.

Vancomycin clearance in premature infants is directly proportional to postconceptional age, body weight, and surface area (252). Its half-life and volume of distribution range from 3 hours and 0.38 L/kg, respectively, in infants whose postconceptional age is over 43 weeks to 9.8 hours and 0.74 L/kg in premature infants at 32 weeks of gestation (253,254). The reader is referred to a recent review for a more in-depth discussion of vancomycin pharmacokinetics and dosage recommendations (255).

Adverse effects of vancomycin include thrombophlebitis and infusion-related histamine release, hypotension, and red-man syndrome. Doses of vancomycin should be infused over at least 1 hour, and never in a rapid IV bolus dose, to avoid this reaction (256).

Aminoglycosides

Aminoglycosides continue to play an important role in the treatment of severe gram-negative sepsis. Clearance of aminoglycosides is directly related to the glomerular filtration rate, which is quite low and variable in premature and sick newborns; thus, plasma concentration monitoring is essential to maximizing efficacy and minimizing toxicity. Desired peak gentamicin concentrations are between 5 to 10 µg/mL, and trough concentrations should be kept between 1 and 2 µg/mL (67,257). Therapeutic drug monitoring may be unnecessary during the first 2 to 3 days of therapy while cultures are pending, unless the patient exhibits overt renal dysfunction (69). To reach appropriate peak concentrations, larger initial doses are necessary in premature infants than in infants and children. This is because aminoglycosides distribute primarily into the extracellular fluid compartment, which is larger in premature infants. Accordingly, a 4 mg/kg gen-

tamicin loading dose has been recommended to reach therapeutic peaks more expeditiously (258). Although gentamicin trough concentrations should always be kept below 2 µg/mL, gentamicin-induced renal toxicity and ototoxicity are uniquely less frequent in neonates than in adults (69).

In recent years, the use of a single, large, daily dose of an aminoglycoside (once-daily aminoglycosides) has increased in frequency, both in adult medicine and in pediatrics. The rationale for this regimen is based on concentration-dependent bactericidal activity of aminoglycosides (259,260). Thus, a peak concentration:MIC ratio of at least 8:1 to 10:1 optimizes bactericidal activity (261). Secondly, the postantibiotic effect (PAE) of aminoglycosides against gram-negative bacteria is longer at increasingly higher serum concentrations (262,263). PAE refers to the continued suppression of bacterial growth after antibiotic exposure, thus permitting trough concentrations to fall below the MIC with reduced risk of bacterial regrowth (262). Aminoglycosides demonstrate a PAE of 1-8 hours when tested against gram-negative organisms at concentrations of 2–10 times the MIC (257). Third, longer dosing intervals permit drug-free periods, which may limit the development of adaptive resistance, a phenomenon that occurs when an organism is constantly exposed to aminoglycosides (261). Last, the uptake of aminoglycoside into the renal cortex is saturable, resulting in reduced renal accumulation and a ceiling effect with regard to nephrotoxicity (257,264).

Over 30 studies, primarily in adults, have evaluated the efficacy and toxicity of once-daily aminoglycoside. Approximately 60% of studies demonstrate no difference in efficacy or toxicity between dosage regimens (257). The remainder suggest that once-daily aminoglycosides are superior in either efficacy or toxicity. The reader is referred to extensive reviews and meta-analyses on the subject (257,261,265).

The use of the phrase "once-daily gentamicin" is potentially confusing because preterm newborns often receive gentamicin every 24 hours, albeit at a much lower dose than the usual 4.5 to 7 mg/kg reported for once-daily dosing of gentamicin. Thus, it may be less confusing to use the phrase "extended-interval dosing" to refer to the single, large, daily dose of aminoglycoside. Nonetheless, this principle has not been well studied in neonates or infants. In a recent study, which compared 4 mg/kg as a single daily dose to 2 mg/kg every 12 hours in 20 term newborns, peak concentrations ranged from 8.5 to 13 µg/mL and 5.2 to 10.1 µg/mL, respectively. Mean trough concentrations were 0.8 µg/mL and 1.2 µg/mL for the two groups, respectively. *In vitro*, the 4 µg/kg once daily dose was significantly superior in bactericidal activity against isolates with high MICs, including *Pseudomonas aeruginosa, Enterococcus faecalis,* and *Listeria monocytogenes.* In another study of 302 term infants, 3.5 to 4 mg/kg administered once daily produced peak concentrations over 6 μg/mL in 100% of infants as compared with only 45% of those who received 2 to 2.5 mg/kg every 12 hours (266). In the single-daily-dose group, only one patient (1.2%) had a trough concentration above 2 μg/mL, as compared to 4.5% of those receiving the twice-daily regimen. In a study of gentamicin, 5 mg/kg, in predominantly term infants, peak and trough concentrations averaged 10.7 μg/mL and 1.7 μg/mL, respectively (267). As compared to peak concentrations achieved with conventional aminoglycoside dosing, the peak concentrations in this study were more suitable for optimizing bactericidal activity. However, the mean trough concentration was higher than that reported in most adult studies (<1 μg/mL). Because patients with renal dysfunction were excluded from most clinical studies of once-daily aminoglycosides, the toxic effects of these higher troughs are unknown. Furthermore, it is not known whether these trough concentrations are low enough to prevent the development of adaptive resistance.

Premature neonates have significantly larger aminoglycoside distribution volumes and longer half-lives than infants and children. Thus, achieving serum concentration–time curves consistent with once-daily gentamicin in adults, that is, peak concentrations over 10 to 15 μg/mL and trough concentrations below 1 μg/mL in a 24-hour period, is impossible in most preterm infants. This was demonstrated in a study of predominantly preterm infants (gestational age of 14 of 21 infants not over 34 weeks) who received netilmicin, 6 mg/kg per day (268). One-third of the infants had 24-hour trough concentrations that exceeded 2 μg/mL, and only two of 21 infants had trough concentrations below 1 μg/mL (268). These high trough concentrations may increase the potential for nephrotoxicity, and increasing the dosing interval to 36 or 48 hours has not been adequately studied in children or adults. Furthermore, it is not known whether the postantibiotic effect would be long enough to permit such a long dosing interval.

In summary, bactericidal activity may be improved in term infants with normal renal function by administering gentamicin, 4 mg/kg, as a single daily dose rather than as divided doses. However, more studies must be conducted in preterm infants and those with renal dysfunction to determine the optimal dosage regimen. Until then, it is prudent to administer a loading dose of 4 mg/kg followed by conventional dosing and plasma concentration monitoring.

Antireflux Medications

The relationship of gastroesophageal reflux (GER) in newborns to apnea and chronic lung disease remains controversial. Certain infants with BPD clearly reflux, aspirate, and have apnea (269–271). Many other infants regurgitate feeds without a clear association with symptoms of chronic lung disease or apnea (272). Gastroe-

sophageal reflux is more frequent in more premature neonates (273) and correlates with reduced lower esophageal sphincter tone and inadequate lower esophageal clearance (274,275). Some of the controversy may relate to measurement of GER by pH probe and the buffering effect of formula on gastric acid, which would prevent detection of reflux by a drop in pH. A recent study using impedance found that 34% of reflux episodes were not detected by pH probe measurements (276). Although gastric emptying may be delayed in premature infants, it does not correlate with GER (277).

Despite the debate about whether clinical signs such as gagging and bradycardia and apnea relate to GER, treatment for GER in neonates is frequent in NICUs (270, 278,279). Drug treatment has included cholinomimetics such as bethanechol, prokinetic drugs such as metoclopramide and cisapride, and drugs to reduce gastric acid such as ranitidine, cimetidine, and omeprazole. Side effects have limited the use of these drugs at times.

A blinded, placebo-controlled, crossover trial evaluated bethanechol treatment of GER in 30 infants aged 3 weeks to 12 months with careful manometric measurements (280). Bethanechol improved lower esophageal sphincter tone, decreased vomiting, decreased the number and duration of reflux episodes, and improved weight gain. One study confirmed these observations (281), but another study did not (282). As a cholinomimetic, bethanechol may increase bronchial secretions as well as bronchoconstriction. Reactive airway disease is a relative contraindication to treatment with bethanechol (280).

Metoclopramide, a derivative of procainamide that antagonizes dopamine, stimulates gastrointestinal motility (283) and has been used to treat GER in preterm neonates (284). Through its cholinergic effects, metoclopramide increases gastric fundal and lower esophageal sphincter tone as well as peristalsis in the esophagus, gastric antrum, and small intestine (283). Consistent with its central dopamine antagonist activities, it may precipitate extrapyramidal symptoms and stimulate prolactin secretion. Facial spasms, opisthotonos, and oculogyric crisis have been observed in children treated with metoclopramide (283). In an uncontrolled study of six preterm infants with signs of GER and impaired gastric emptying, metoclopramide (0.1 mg/kg/day) decreased gastric residual volume, improved feeding tolerance, and improved weight gain without dystonic reactions (284). When compared to placebo in a well-designed, prospective, blinded, crossover trial, metoclopramide decreased the length of time that the esophageal pH was less than 4.0 without changing the total number of reflux episodes or the number of prolonged episodes (285). A significant placebo effect was observed on symptom scores reported by parents. Greater efficacy was observed in infants older than 3 months. In a dosage of 0.1 mg/kg/dose four times daily, no side effects were noted (285). In dosages of 0.5 mg/kg/day divided into four doses, metoclopramide actually increased the number of reflux episodes and the time during which the esophageal pH was less than 4 (286). Hyams and colleagues suggested that infants (mean 3.2 months) with GER may require metoclopramide dose escalation to 1.2 mg/kg/day (287). Although these higher dosages improved efficacy in some studies (287), higher dosages caused more irritability to the point of patients dropping out of the study (286). These higher doses must be used very cautiously, if at all, in preterm infants. Kearns and colleagues found that 30% of preterm infants (31 to 40 weeks postconceptional age) had delayed metoclopramide clearance (288). Thus, high doses may result in unacceptable toxicity in some preterm infants. Although clearance did not correlate with age, the investigators recommended that oral metoclopramide therapy be initiated at a dose of 0.15 mg/kg every 6 hours in preterm infants beyond 31 weeks of postconceptional age (288).

Cisapride, a benzamide that is structurally related to metoclopramide, is widely recommended for treatment of neonatal GER (278,289–291). Cisapride increases lower esophageal sphincter tone, force of gastric contractions, and small intestinal propulsion by release of acetylcholine following binding to 5-hydroxytryptamine₄ receptors (291,292). It lacks the antidopaminergic effects of metoclopramide that contribute to agitation and extrapyramidal effects (291,292). Although cisapride has been viewed as a safer and more effective drug than metoclopramide (290–292), recent reports have demonstrated bradycardic arrhythmias in neonates who were at risk for having high cisapride concentrations through delayed metabolism or excessive dosages (279,293). Older infants (294) and adults develop a prolonged cardiac refractory period associated with a prolonged QTc interval that predisposes them to torsade de pointes arrhythmias that may be fatal (295–297). This occurs through inhibition of the rapid component of the myocardial delayed rectifying K^+ (I_{kr}) current, which then lengthens the action potential, an adverse effect of class III antiarrhythmic drugs (105,298). Similar mechanisms account for some cases of congenital long-QT syndrome (105). Cisapride is metabolized by CYP3A4, which can be inhibited by several drugs, in particular erythromycin and ketoconazole (see Table 55–1). This leads to increased cisapride concentrations, which may prolong QTc and predispose to arrhythmias. In a survey of adverse effects associated with cisapride use in preterm neonates, the only arrhythmias reported occurred following tenfold overdoses or cotreatment with erythromycin (279). Erythromycin itself can block the I_{kr} current and lengthen the time of repolarization (299). These reports culminated in publication of a letter to physicians warning them about potential risks of excessive cisapride concentrations from high dosages and cotreatment with a long list of inhibitors of its metabolism. Among drugs commonly used in neonates, this list included macrolide antibiotics and azole antifungal drugs (300). Cisapride

should be avoided in neonates with congenital prolonged-QT syndrome, probably best defined as a QTc over 440 nanoseconds (301). The most frequent dosages used in neonates from a survey of over 11,000 preterm infants treated with cisapride were 0.1 to 0.2 mg/kg/dose every 6 to 8 hours (279). More detailed kinetic studies are needed, especially in the ELBW population.

In summary, there is no single optimal treatment for GER. Potentially significant side effects are associated with pharmacologic treatment, and debate persists about the efficacy and indications for drug treatment of gastroesophageal reflux.

Bronchodilators

The use of bronchodilators has increased with the survival of more immature newborns with greater susceptibility to development of BPD. Histologic studies in infants with BPD confirm bronchiolar smooth muscle hypertrophy, which can lead to airway narrowing (302). Consistent with these anatomic changes, infants with BPD demonstrate bronchodilation, increased dynamic airway compliance, and reduction in airway resistance in response to β-adrenergic agents and ipratropium, an anticholinergic drug (303–316). Airway responsiveness to bronchodilators develops by 2 weeks of postnatal age in most neonates requiring mechanical ventilation and as early as 26 weeks postconceptional age (317). Consequently, bronchodilator treatment is frequently used in the management of BPD in preterm neonates.

The method of administering bronchodilators may influence efficacy. Aerosolized albuterol may be administered by either nebulizer or metered dose inhaler (MDI) and spacer. Until recently, the former was commonly used in mechanically ventilated patients. Nebulized albuterol (2.5 mg) increased respiratory system compliance (C_{rs}/kg) by 35.3% as compared with a 2.8% improvement following saline placebo ($p < 0.001$) in ventilator-dependent ELBW infants as early as 5 to 31 days after birth (315). A significant decrease in PCO_2 (> 10 mm Hg) was noted in 47% of measurements. As expected, heart rate increased an average of 17.5 beats/min and persisted for 30 to 120 minutes after albuterol administration. In a study by Wilkie and colleagues, both nebulized salbutamol (albuterol) and ipratropium bromide improved lung mechanics in ventilator-dependent neonates who were progressing into chronic lung disease (313). These infants, whose gestational ages ranged from 25 to 29 weeks with birth weights of 560 to 1,050 g, demonstrated bronchodilation as early as 19 days after birth. These findings were confirmed in ventilator-dependent preterm infants who demonstrated dose-related bronchodilation to nebulized ipratropium alone and in combination with salbutamol (albuterol) by 18 to 34 days after birth (318). No synergistic bronchodilation in neonates between an anticholinergic agent and albuterol has been reported (316). Oral administration of albuterol has also been noted to improve lung function in infants with BPD (307,319).

Nebulization of albuterol has several undesirable effects, including cooling of the inspired gas, higher cost of administration as compared with metered-dose inhaler (MDI), loss of drug by continuous flow, and inefficient delivery. Previous studies in ventilator models revealed that only 1% to 3% of nebulized drug is delivered to the patient (320–322). Our data in a neonatal ventilator model indicate that only 0.2% of nebulized albuterol is delivered to the lungs of the ventilated neonate (323). Delivery of aerosolized albuterol is markedly improved when it is administered by MDI and spacer (323). When administered by MDI and spacer, both 72 μg of ipratropium and 400 μg of albuterol improved oxygenation and ventilation in 1-week-old 880-g neonates by 30 minutes after administration and increased heart rate an average of 23 beasts/min (306). In 2-week-old, average 28-week gestation, ventilator-dependent newborns, albuterol improved pulmonary mechanics in nine of ten patients (308). Seven of ten patients responded after one MDI actuation (100 μg), and two of the remaining three patients after 200 μg (308). Improvement in pulmonary resistance was maximal at 30 minutes and lasted 3 hours. Albuterol treatment was associated with a significant tachycardia (mean 180 beats/min).

Beta-agonists also improve pulmonary function of nonventilated infants with BPD. Nebulized isoproterenol markedly improved airway resistance and specific airway conductance in nonventilated infants with BPD at 41 weeks of postconceptional age (310). Today, albuterol is the preferred agent over isoproterenol because of its greater selectivity for β2 receptors. Gappa and colleagues reported a significant reduction in airway resistance following albuterol administration by either nebulizer or MDI in spontaneously breathing infants (postconceptional age 37.1 ± 2.3 weeks) with BPD (305). Administration of the latter was facilitated by attaching the MDI to a holding chamber and face mask and allowing the infant to breathe for 30 seconds between puffs.

Choosing between albuterol delivery by nebulizer and by MDI requires careful consideration of the differences in delivery efficiency, convenience and ease of use, disturbance to the patient, and adverse effect profile. In most cases, MDIs are the preferred method of administration because of their greater efficiency in drug delivery (305), short delivery time, and reduced administration costs. In addition, MDIs obviate the need to change ventilator flow rates and do not cause potentially troublesome cooling of ventilator gas. On the other hand, MDI dosages can be changed only in fixed increments.

Diuretics

Several classes of diuretic drugs are available, including osmotic agents such as mannitol, carbonic anhydrase inhibitors such as acetazolamide, thiazides such as chlorothiazide, high-ceiling or loop diuretics such as furosemide, and potassium-sparing diuretics such as spironolactone (324). The last three classes are used frequently in the treatment of neonates, both for acute fluid overload and for chronic therapy of BPD and congestive heart failure. Distinct differences in mechanisms of action and potency should guide selection of specific drugs (325,326).

Thiazides are sulfonamide diuretics whose major action is to block sodium and chloride cotransport in the first portion of the distal tubule, which causes a natriuresis (324–326). Thiazide-induced diuresis produces a greater loss of sodium and potassium per urine volume than does a diuresis induced by loop diuretics, although only a moderate amount of sodium is excreted (324). Among diuretics, thiazides are distinctive in that they decrease the renal excretion of calcium, although magnesium excretion is increased. In high doses, thiazides may inhibit carbonic anhydrase with a potency equal to that of acetazolamide. They also may induce hypoglycemia, hypercholesterolemia, and hypertriglyceridemia (324). Thiazide elimination occurs through the renal tubular organic acid transport system and may be inhibited by other organic acids such as probenecid. The diuretic action of thiazides depends on secretion into the renal tubular fluid, so that competitive inhibition of the transport of a thiazide by another organic acid may blunt its diuretic effect.

Spironolactone, the potassium-sparing diuretic most frequently used for treatment of newborns, is a 17-spironolactone steroid that competitively antagonizes mineralocorticoids, predominantly aldosterone (324, 325). Because aldosterone increases sodium reabsorption and potassium secretion, increased aldosterone secretion may be suspected by the ratio of urine sodium to potassium. Similarly, effective antagonism of aldosterone by spironolactone may be detected by an increasing urine sodium-to-potassium ratio. The appropriate dose of spironolactone relates to the concentration of aldosterone because it acts through competitive inhibition. Spironolactone is available only for enteral administration and undergoes extensive first-pass hepatic metabolism to an active metabolite, canrenone.

The most serious toxicity of spironolactone is hyperkalemia during cotreatment with potassium supplements (325). Spironolactone increases calcium excretion and, in older men, may produce gynecomastia through an antiandrogen effect. In rats exposed to high doses of spironolactone for prolonged periods, tumors may develop, but this has not been reported in humans to date (324). Other side effects include rashes, diarrhea, and vomiting.

Alternate potassium-sparing diuretics that do not work through aldosterone inhibition, such as triamterene and amiloride, rarely are administered to neonates. Their potassium-sparing action probably occurs through inhibition of the electrogenic sodium transport in the distal nephron (324).

Among the three loop diuretics in clinical use in the United States, bumetanide, ethacrynic acid, and furosemide, furosemide is the best studied in neonates. All three are organic acids, but furosemide and bumetanide are sulfonamides. All three diuretics induce diuresis by inhibiting the chloride pump in the ascending limb of the loop of Henle. Their diuretic effects require secretion into the tubular fluid by the organic acid transport system that may be competitively inhibited by other organic acids such as probenecid or penicillin (326,327). Because of these similarities in action, there is almost no reason to use two loop diuretics simultaneously. Patients who are resistant to furosemide, however, may still respond to bumetanide, likely because of its greater potency (325). Loop diuretics produce excretion of dilute urine, with an increase in free-water excretion compared to sodium excretion (328).

Calcium excretion is increased by furosemide (325). This contributes to renal parenchymal calcification, nephrolithiasis, and osteopenia during chronic treatment of neonates with furosemide. Cholelithiasis has also been observed during chronic furosemide treatment. Although furosemide is highly protein bound, it appears unlikely that doses administered to neonates produce high enough concentrations to displace bilirubin (326).

As might be expected for a drug eliminated by renal tubular secretion, the half-life of furosemide in neonates is long and variable, ranging from 4.7 to 44.9 hours (329). During repetitive dosing, Vert and colleagues demonstrated an inverse relationship between postconceptional age and furosemide half-life. Petersen and colleagues have confirmed this prolonged half-life for furosemide in preterm neonates during the first few weeks after birth (8). They also noted that some neonates have poor absorption of orally administered furosemide, leading to an inadequate diuretic response. The prolonged half-life does not support the current clinical practice of administering furosemide every 6 to 8 hours in neonates.

The effects of furosemide on lung function, both acutely and chronically, have been studied in neonates with BPD (330) and in neonates recovering from hyaline membrane disease (331). In patients with BPD, pulmonary compliance improved after a single dose of furosemide. Prolonged treatment improved pulmonary compliance, pulmonary resistance, and oxygenation without an effect on transcutaneous PCO_2 (330). In a controlled study of preterm neonates recovering from hyaline membrane disease, furosemide improved pulmonary compliance by 2 hours after administration (331). This improvement persisted for 4 hours and then returned to baseline by 6 hours. Chronic furosemide treatment for 4 days produced a further improvement in alveolar–arterial difference in partial pressure of oxygen ($AaDO_2$).

One prospective, controlled study of newborns has found that furosemide treatment increases the frequency of patent ductus arteriosus, presumably through release of prostaglandin (PG) E_2 that accompanies diuresis (332). Other investigators have administered furosemide with indomethacin to blunt the oliguric response to indomethacin without loss of indomethacin-induced ductal closure (333). Indomethacin blocks the natriuretic response to furosemide as well as the increase in renal blood flow that furosemide produces (334).

Both furosemide and ethacrynic acid may produce ototoxicity (324). Furosemide-induced hearing loss occurs after large doses (1,000 mg in adults) administered IV, especially to patients with renal failure who would be expected to have poor clearance of the drug (335). This transient ototoxicity correlates with changes in electrolyte concentrations in the inner ear fluids, endolymph and perilymph, that reduce endocochlear potentials (335). Compared to furosemide, bumetanide caused a similar frequency of adverse effects, except for ototoxicity, which appeared to be less with bumetanide (336).

Both thiazides and furosemide may produce allergic interstitial nephritis (324). The most frequent adverse effects associated with treatment of newborns with loop diuretics reflect their actions that frequently lead to hypochloremic, hypokalemic alkalosis. Electrolyte monitoring is needed at the start of treatment to detect excessive sodium depletion to serum values less than 120 mEq/L.

Although seldom used as a diuretic, methylxanthines may produce significant diuresis, natriuresis, and choliuresis (337).

Histamine₂ Receptor Antagonists

Acid suppressant therapy is commonly used in critically ill patients to prevent acute gastric mucosal damage (AGMD) and its severe complications, such as hemorrhage or perforation (338–340). Studies evaluating the risk of AGMD in critically ill infants and children are few in number and discrepant in results, thus making the issue of stress ulcer prophylaxis controversial (341,342). A small study in critically ill preterm infants (median gestational age 29.7 weeks) endoscopically demonstrated a high prevalence (94%) of asymptomatic esophageal and gastric lesions, including macroscopic esophagitis and gastritis together with ulceration (343). In children, a histamine₂ antagonist, ranitidine, has been the agent of choice to treat these lesions and prevent the development of gastric hemorrhage (344).

Histamine₂ receptor antagonists inhibit histamine-induced gastric acid secretion (345). A series of structurally related compounds have been developed to block the H₂ receptor, including cimetidine, ranitidine, and famotidine. Although all of these drugs are used clinically, patients report adverse effects more often with cimetidine than ranitidine (346). Adverse effects most commonly reported by adults include diarrhea, nausea, vomiting, and constipation. In newborns, the most important undesired effect of cimetidine is its inhibition of the elimination of numerous drugs metabolized by CYP isoenzymes, including those metabolized by CYP1A2, CYP2C9, and CYP2D6 (347). Cimetidine, like other drugs with an imidazole structure, such as ketoconazole and metronidazole, binds to cytochrome P450 and reduces its activity (348). In newborns, one of the most frequently encountered and troublesome drug–drug interactions during cimetidine therapy is its inhibition of theophylline metabolism (CYP1A2) (349). This drug interaction requires vigilance and careful monitoring of theophylline concentrations to prevent toxicity. Other potential interactions include decreased clearance of propranolol, phenytoin, lidocaine, nifedipine, and diazepam (348). Drugs such as lorazepam, which require conjugation for elimination, are not affected by cimetidine treatment. Ranitidine, in which the imidazole ring is replaced with a furan ring, binds to liver microsomes and cytochrome P450, with approximately one-tenth the affinity of cimetidine (348). Because of its greater potency and longer duration of effect, ranitidine is administered less frequently than cimetidine. Because ranitidine has at least three to four times the molar potency of cimetidine, it has minimal effects on cytochrome P450 in usual clinical doses. Accordingly, it is often the preferred agent in newborns and infants for suppression of histamine$_2$ receptor-mediated acid secretion.

In a randomized, controlled study of 23 mechanically ventilated, preterm and full-term newborns (mean gestational age 32 weeks), 5 mg/kg/day of ranitidine markedly decreased the risk for endoscopically proven gastric mucosal lesions (344). In a case report, ranitidine provided effective treatment for a preterm neonate with a life-threatening upper gastrointestinal hemorrhage after indomethacin (352). In this preterm newborn, an infusion of 0.2 mg/kg/hr resulted in high concentrations with a half-life of approximately 5.5 hours, which is greater than twice the elimination half-life reported in older children (353).

To determine the optimal dosage requirement of ranitidine, many investigators have used gastric pH as a surrogate endpoint. The validity of this endpoint is based on adult data that demonstrate that maintaining gastric pH above 4 reduces the risk of stress ulceration and gastric hemorrhage in critically ill patients (354). Kelly et al. found that ranitidine infused at 0.0625 mg/kg/hr was sufficient to increase and maintain gastric pH above 4 in ten premature neonates (median gestational age 27.5 weeks) who were receiving dexamethasone (355). Mallet and associates examined ranitidine kinetics and therapeutic responses in 11 infants with reflux esophagitis or near-miss sudden infant death syndrome (356). They noted that gastric pH could be maintained above 4 as long as the plasma ranitidine concentration remained above 100 ng/mL. Fontana et al. studied the pharmacokinetics of ranitidine in 27 term infants during the first day after birth and reported that concentrations greater than 100 ng/mL and 200 ng/mL could be expected for at least 12 hours after a single intravenous bolus dose of 1.6 mg/kg and 3.3 mg/kg, respectively (357). The same average concentration could be maintained at steady state with an intravenous infusion rate between 0.03 and 0.06 mg/kg/hr based on their reported mean half-life of 207 minutes (357).

Famotidine is a relatively new H$_2$ antagonist that is not well studied in neonates and infants. Advantages over ranitidine and cimetidine include its potency, relatively longer elimination half-life, and lack of interaction with the cytochrome P450 isoforms. Pharmacokinetic and efficacy studies have been conducted in children (358); however, no data have been reported in neonates.

Inotropes

Although inotropy refers to myocardial contractility, inotropic drugs improve cardiac contractility, increase cardiac rate, and alter vascular tone (359,360). The inotrope should be selected according to the specific cardiovascular disorder to be corrected. Because cardiac output is determined by preload, contractility, and afterload, these pharmacologic properties of various inotropes are described and may be used to select the optimal drug for a specific clinical situation. Despite frequent administration of inotropes to newborns, they have received limited study in young infants.

TABLE 55–6. *Relative cardiovascular receptor interactions of inotropes and the associated effects*

	Cardiovascular receptor interactions and effects					
Catecholmine	α_1 vasoconstriction; ↑cardiac contractility	α_2 vasoconstriction; ↓norepinephrine release	β_1 ↑contractility, ↑conduction velocity	β_2 vasodilation bronchodilation	Dopamine D$_1$ renal, mesenteric and coronary vasodilation	Indirect release of endogenous norepinephrine
Dobutamine	1+	0	3+	1+	0	0
Dopamine	0 to 3+	1+	2+ to 3+	2+	3+	1+
Epinephrine	2+	2+	3+	3+	0	0
Isoproterenol	0	0	3+	3+	0	0

0, lowest; 3+, highest interaction.
Adapted from ref. 361, and from Lefkowitz RJ, Hoffman BB, Taylor P. Neurotransmission. The autonomic and somatic motor nervous systems. In: Hardman JG, Limbird LE, Molinoff PB, Ruddon RW, Goodman-Gilman AG, eds. *Goodman & Gilman's the pharmacological basis of therapeutics,* 9th ed. New York: McGraw-Hill, 1996:105–139.

Shock occurs when blood flow and oxygen supply are inadequate to meet tissue demands. The same principles apply to the myocardium. Increasing cardiac wall stiffness increases myocardial oxygen consumption and may decrease flow during diastole. Inotropic drug treatment for the failing heart must balance increasing myocardial oxygen consumption against the increase in cardiac output that provides more oxygenated blood through the coronary circulation to the myocardium. Disproportionate increases in myocardial wall stiffness may impede coronary flow and worsen myocardial ischemia. Similarly, excess peripheral vasodilation may reduce the blood pressure to a level where there is too little pressure to maintain coronary flow during diastole.

Specific receptor interactions of inotropic drugs should guide their clinical use (Table 55–6) (360–362). Dosages for drugs used frequently in newborn resuscitation are indicated in Table 55–5. Isoproterenol is a direct-acting, potent, pure β-adrenergic agonist whose usefulness is limited by tachycardia and peripheral vasodilation. Tachycardia and diversion of blood flow to the extensive vasculature in muscle may steal perfusion away from more vital organs and extend myocardial infarction (363). Isoproterenol is most effective for raising heart rate, for instance, in the treatment of complete heart block.

Epinephrine stimulates all adrenergic receptors directly, but its vascular effects vary among organs, with $β_2$ stimulation usually exceeding $α_1$ vasoconstriction so that peripheral vascular resistance usually falls (362). Blood pressure rises as a result of increases in cardiac contractility and cardiac output.

Dopamine, the immediate precursor of norepinephrine, is unique among inotropes because it dilates renal, coronary, and mesenteric vascular beds at low doses through activation of the D_1-dopaminergic receptors. At high concentrations, its $α_1$ receptor activity causes vasoconstriction to predominate in all circulations (359). Studies of renal vascular resistance in newborn animals infused with 32 to 50 μg/kg/min of dopamine have not detected this effect (364,365). Interestingly, similar high-dose (30 to 50 μg/kg/min) infusions in oliguric, hypotensive, near-term newborns improved urine output, suggesting that the $α_1$ vasoconstrictor effects that are expected at high dosages may not predominate and reduce renal perfusion in all newborns (366).

Dopamine exerts some of its effects through release of endogenous norepinephrine, which may become depleted during prolonged infusions (362). Peripheral infusions of dopamine do not cross the blood–brain barrier to interact with CNS dopamine receptors. Extravasation of dopamine may cause severe ischemic tissue damage, which may be treated by local infiltration of diluted phentolamine (367).

The lower portion of dopamine's dose–response relationship has been studied in a small number of hypotensive neonates with hyaline membrane disease who did not respond to volume expansion with 5% albumin (368).

Dopamine doses of 2 μg/kg/min increased systolic blood pressure alone. With doses of 4 μg/kg/min, both systolic and diastolic blood pressures increased significantly. At 8 μg/kg/min, both systolic and diastolic blood pressures increased further, and heart rate increased significantly.

Dobutamine is the product of directed structural manipulation of dopamine and isoproterenol to produce hydroxyphenyl-isobutyl-dopamine (dobutamine), an inotrope designed to increase contractility with a minimum of tachycardia and vasodilation (369). Initially, dobutamine was thought to possess balanced vascular $α_1$ and $β_2$ activities. Later study demonstrated that dobutamine exists in two enantiomorphic forms with different receptor activities (370). The (-) isomer is a potent $α_1$ agonist that increases cardiac contractility, whereas the (+) isomer is a potent $α_2$ antagonist. The (+) isomer is severalfold more potent for β receptors than the (−) isomer. Overall, dobutamine is more selective for $β_1$ than for $β_2$ receptors. With infusions at less than 20 μg/kg/min, dobutamine increases cardiac output and contractility with minimal changes in peripheral resistance and modest increases in heart rate (362). In neonates, dosages of 5 and 7.5 μg/kg/min increased cardiac output without changing heart rate or blood pressure (371). The lack of vasoconstriction may limit dobutamine's usefulness in patients with severe hypotension but may be useful in patients with cardiogenic failure in whom cardiac function may worsen with increased afterload.

Dobutamine and dopamine have been compared for treatment of hypotensive, preterm neonates with hyaline membrane disease (372,373). Although the study designs differed somewhat, both studies demonstrated that dopamine improved blood pressure more often and at lower doses than did dobutamine. The dopamine-treated group in each study achieved the desired blood pressure with dosages no greater than 10 μg/kg/min except for one infant. Tachycardia (>180 beats/min) occurred equally with dopamine and dobutamine (373). These differences may reflect the differences in vascular receptor effects between dopamine and dobutamine because studies in young animals show that dopamine tends to vasoconstrict and dobutamine tends to vasodilate (365). Dobutamine augments cardiac contractility more than it increases blood pressure in preterm and term newborns (371,374,375).

Digoxin remains a useful drug for the chronic enteral treatment of congestive heart failure. The efficacy of digitalis for the treatment of congestive heart failure varies according to myocardial dynamics (376). In a study of 21 infants with congestive heart failure from ventricular septal defects, digoxin improved 12 clinically, but only six improved by echocardiographic measurements (377). The digoxin serum half-life averages 35 hours (range 17 to 52 hours) in term newborns and 57 hours (range 38 to 88 hours) in premature (birth weight range of 1,150 to 2,230 g) newborns (378). This likely reflects the dependence on renal excretion for most of the elimination of digoxin (379) and suggests that premature neonates require a smaller digoxin maintenance dose (380).

Digoxin toxicity, like efficacy, is defined not by a specific concentration but by signs and symptoms such as emesis, arrhythmias, or conduction abnormalities such as complete heart block (381). Various drugs may increase digoxin concentrations: antibiotics that reduce inactivation by gut flora (382); spironolactone, which reduces its clearance (383); and amiodarone, which may either reduce the clearance or increase the bioavailability of digoxin (132). Life-threatening arrhythmias from excessive digitalis concentrations may be treated successfully with antidigoxin Fab antibody fragments (384).

Older assays for therapeutic monitoring of digoxin cross-reacted with an endogenous molecule, digoxin-like immunoreactive substance (DLIS), which was increased in the circulation of preterm newborns, pregnant women, and patients with renal failure (385,386). DLIS has been identified as having both the structure (387) and function of ouabain (388). The cross-reactivity of the newer assays has been eliminated.

Methylxanthines

Methylxanthines, including caffeine, theophylline, and aminophylline (an ethylenediamine complex of theophylline), are commonly administered to preterm neonates to treat apnea of prematurity and to aid in weaning from mechanical ventilation. The proposed mechanisms of actions of methylxanthines include (389) (a) increased central neural drive; (b) adenosine receptor blockade, which inhibits adenosine's potent respiratory depressant effects (390); (c) improved respiratory muscle function, particularly diaphragmatic contraction (391); and (d) natriuresis. The often-cited mechanism of increased cAMP through phosphodiesterase inhibition does not explain the *in vivo* effects of theophylline because this mechanism requires concentrations that are usually toxic (>20 µg/mL) (392). Other factors that may contribute to the action of methylxanthines include catecholamine release, which increases cardiac output and improves oxygenation, and increased blood glucose, which may reduce the frequency of apneic spells (389).

Theophylline

The effectiveness of theophylline in the treatment of neonatal apnea was first documented over two decades ago (393–395). Theophylline increases minute ventilation, reduces $PaCO_2$, increases central respiratory drive, and significantly reduces the frequency of apnea (389,394,396–398). In addition, theophylline may promote extubation of infants recovering from respiratory distress syndrome (399).

The desired plasma concentration of theophylline in the treatment of apnea is approximately 5 to 15 µg/mL

(400), although concentrations as low as 2.8 to 3.9 µg/mL have been reported to be effective (401). To achieve and maintain therapeutic concentrations, a loading dose of 5 to 6 mg/kg of theophylline is administered, followed by a maintenance dose of 2 to 4 mg/kg/day in two to four divided doses (389). Note that the therapeutic range to treat apnea is lower than the commonly accepted therapeutic range to treat asthma in older patients (10 to 20 µg/mL). This is caused by reduced protein binding and higher free concentrations of theophylline in neonates as compared to adults (7). Because the unbound fraction of drug in plasma is considered pharmacologically active, a greater response may be expected in the newborn than in the adult, despite the same plasma concentrations. For example, at a total theophylline plasma concentration of 17 µg/mL, approximately 44% is unbound and pharmacologically active in the adult as compared to 64% in the full-term infant (7). Thus, 17 µg/mL of theophylline in a newborn would be equivalent to 24.7 µg/mL total theophylline concentration in the adult. Despite achieving therapeutic concentrations of theophylline, about 25% of infants with apnea may not respond (389).

Metabolism of theophylline (1,3-dimethylxanthine) and caffeine (1,3,7-trimethylxanthine) via demethylation is primarily mediated by cytochrome P4501A2 (CYP1A2) (24–27). However, because expression of CYP1A2 is low in neonates, clearance of these agents is significantly reduced, especially in preterm infants (25,28). Newborns, unlike adults, are able to hepatically methylate theophylline to caffeine, and plasma caffeine/theophylline ratios may reach 0.3 to 0.4 at steady state (402–404). Thus, both compounds may contribute to theophylline's therapeutic effects (403,405). Changes in theophylline kinetics during maturation of infants born at gestations of 25 to 30 weeks were studied with stable isotopes (406). This technique allows more accurate determination of the elimination phase by monitoring concentrations for prolonged periods while continuing administration of the unlabeled medication. Theophylline half-life correlated best with postnatal age rather than postconceptional age. As would be expected, the theophylline half-life varied inversely with postnatal age as follows:

$$\log t_{1/2} \text{ (hours)} = 1.72 - 0.00565$$
$$\times \text{ postnatal age (days)} \quad [12]$$

Clinically, theophylline clearance and urine metabolite patterns reach adult values by 55 weeks of postconceptional age or approximately 4 to 5 months after birth (32). Because of the significant interindividual variability in clearance and protein binding, theophylline plasma concentrations should be monitored, and doses should be adjusted to maintain therapeutic concentrations.

When monitoring theophylline concentrations, one must consider factors that alter theophylline clearance. Theophylline's metabolism is increased and its half-life shortened by inducing agents, such as anticonvulsants (407). Metabolism is delayed by viral infections, such as influenza (408), and numerous interacting drugs, including erythromycin and cimetidine (409). Ranitidine was also noted to reduce theophylline clearance, although this interaction is less significant and less predictable than that with cimetidine (410,411).

Adverse effects of theophylline include irritability, sleeplessness, natriuresis, hyperglycemia, hyperreflexia, tremor, seizures, hypertension, tachycardia, and cardiac arrhythmias (412,413). Tachycardia is the most common side effect associated with aminophylline. Theophylline relaxes the gastroesophageal sphincter of adults and probably has the same effect in newborns. If apnea is caused by gastroesophageal reflux, theophylline treatment may worsen this problem.

Caffeine

Caffeine and theophylline have similar efficacy in treating or preventing apnea and bradycardia in premature infants (414–416). However, caffeine has fewer associated adverse effects and a more favorable therapeutic index than aminophylline (412,413,417). In addition, caffeine has a longer half-life, thus permitting a convenient once- or twice-daily dosage schedule.

Apnea was reduced by administering caffeine citrate, 20 mg/kg, followed by 5 to 10 mg/kg/day once or twice daily to 18 preterm infants with a mean gestational age of 27.5 weeks (418). The average number of episodes was reduced from 13.6 to 2.1 episodes per day. Note that caffeine citrate doubles the weight of the administered drug, so that 20 mg/kg is equivalent to 10 mg/kg of caffeine base. Subsequent pharmacokinetic studies from the same group led to the current dosing recommendation of 10 mg/kg of caffeine base, followed by a maintenance dose of 2.5 mg/kg/day given as a single daily dose (29). More recently, Scanlon et al. reported that high-dose caffeine (50 mg/kg caffeine citrate loading dose followed by 12 mg/kg/day) improved apnea more rapidly than the standard dose (25 mg/kg loading dose followed by 6 mg/kg/day) without increasing adverse effects (419).

Effective caffeine concentrations for the treatment of apnea of prematurity range from 5 to 25 µg/mL (413). Previous reports suggest that caffeine plasma concentrations of up to 50 µg/mL may be tolerated without significant adverse effects (29,419). Caffeine is noted to have minimal metabolic effects in the newborn infant (420). In a study of 12 premature neonates, 20 mg/kg caffeine citrate did not increase excretion of electrolytes or catecholamine metabolites; however, glucose concentrations were lower in formula-fed infants after caffeine administration (420). Infants who received continuous glucose infusions had no change in plasma glucose concentrations. Caffeine's wide therapeutic index reduces the necessity for the close plasma concentration monitoring

that is required with theophylline. Similar to theophylline, approximately one-third of patients do not respond to treatment with caffeine (389).

Because of its limited biotransformation, caffeine elimination in the neonate is dependent on renal clearance. Unchanged caffeine comprised about 86% of the methylated xanthines and methyluric acids in the urine of infants less than 1 month of age (412). As a consequence of limited biotransformation, the half-life of caffeine is significantly prolonged and may exceed 200 hours in preterm infants (29). Similar to theophylline, the half-life of caffeine in preterm infants decreases after birth (421, 422). In 34 preterm infants 25 to 32 weeks of gestational age, with a mean postnatal age of 4.8 ± 0.7 days, the half-life of caffeine was markedly reduced from 129.8 hours to 93.5 hours ($p < 0.005$) by treatment day 7 (422). Even full-term infants, who were exposed to caffeine transplacentally, have prolonged half-lives, ranging from 31 to 132 hours (423). In general, adult values for the caffeine half-life are reached at approximately 60 weeks postconception or 4 to 6 months postnatally (30,31).

Muscle Relaxants

Muscle relaxants are commonly administered to neonates during mechanical ventilation and anesthesia for surgical procedures (424). Nondepolarizing muscle relaxants, which competitively inhibit acetylcholine at the motor end plate, have become the mainstay for neuromuscular (NM) blockade in the NICU. Although pancuronium has been used extensively in treatment of neonates, the use of the shorter-acting nondepolarizing agents vecuronium and atracurium has increased in recent years.

Pancuronium is a long-acting neuromuscular blocker with an average duration of action in neonates of 60 to 120 minutes following a 0.05 mg/kg dose (424). Pancuronium is primarily excreted by the kidney (60% to 80%) with approximately 15% hepatically metabolized to an active metabolite (425). Its predominant renal elimination requires that caution be used to avoid accumulation in premature neonates or infants with poor renal function. Pancuronium does not cause histamine release; however, tachycardia and increased systolic blood pressure from vagal blockade are characteristic (426,427).

Pancuronium dosage requirements for neonates increase with postnatal age and decrease with prematurity (428). Treatment during the first week after birth required a dose of 0.03 mg/kg, compared to 0.09 mg/kg by 2 to 4 weeks after birth. Dose reductions were required not only for prematurity, but also for acidosis and hypothermia. By monitoring muscle twitch to determine neuromuscular blockade, others have shown that newborns have widely variable dosage requirements for pancuronium (429). Generally, larger doses of pancuronium are required for muscle relaxation in infants than in adults, presumably because of a larger volume of distribution. Repeated administration of pancuronium to neonates may lead to prolonged neuromuscular blockade, possibly as a result of its pharmacologically active metabolite and long half-life, which is related to immaturity of liver and renal function.

Vecuronium and atracurium are intermediate-acting neuromuscular blockers with a shorter duration of effect than pancuronium. In contrast to pancuronium, vecuronium and, in large part, atracurium have little to no cardiovascular effects (426). In neonates, 0.03 mg/kg of vecuronium produces a 30- to 40-minute duration of action as compared to 20 to 30 minutes after 0.15 to 0.3 mg/kg of atracurium (424). Vecuronium's effects are much longer in neonates and infants than in children and adolescents (430). A 0.1 mg/kg dose maintained neuromuscular blockade, as analyzed by muscle twitch, for more than 58 minutes in infants and 18 minutes in children aged 3 to 10 years (430).

Vecuronium is 20% excreted renally unchanged, and the remainder is excreted in the bile (431). Vecuronium's limited renal excretion has often led to its choice in patients with renal dysfunction; however, its active metabolite (3-desacetylvecuronium) may accumulate in renal failure and produce prolonged neuromuscular blockade (427). Although repeated administration of vecuronium carries a lower risk than pancuronium of prolonged neuromuscular blockade, this phenomenon has been reported in neonates both with and without renal failure (432,433). The latter occurred in a 2-month-old infant as a result of vecuronium accumulation at doses of 1.67 µg/kg/min for 5 days followed by 0.83 µg/kg/min for 2 days. The infant required 48 hours to regain full neuromuscular function. Lower doses may be required in some neonates and infants, and monitoring of the neuromuscular junction may reduce the use of excessive doses.

Atracurium does not rely on renal or hepatic elimination and undergoes a spontaneous, nonenzymatic, ester hydrolysis at the pH of body fluids (Hoffmann elimination). The breakdown products are not pharmacologically active, making this an excellent agent for use in patients with renal and/or hepatic dysfunction (434). Unlike pancuronium and vecuronium, atracurium has the potential for histamine release that may result in cutaneous flushing and/or hypotension. Neonates appear to be more sensitive to atracurium than older children (435), and infusion requirements are approximately 25% lower than in older children to maintain 90% to 95% neuromuscular blockade (436).

Neuromuscular blockade for several days may produce prolonged muscle weakness. Several metabolic factors and other drugs may enhance neuromuscular blockade, including acidosis and hypokalemia, as well as treatment with magnesium and aminoglycoside antibiotics (424). The contribution of drug accumulation at the myoneural junction or alteration of the myoneural junction requires more study. Monitoring of muscle fiber twitch during prolonged paralysis may be helpful for evaluating and avoiding this side effect.

Prostaglandins and Prostaglandin Inhibitors

During the last 25 years, understanding of the pharmacology and physiology of the eicosanoids has expanded dramatically from PGE_1 and $PGF_{1\alpha}$ to thromboxane and prostacyclin, products of the cyclooxygenase pathway, and leukotrienes, noncyclized products of the lipoxygenase pathway. Better understanding of leukotrienes has helped to account for previously recognized biological mediators such as slow-reacting substance A, which is the same as leukotriene C. Despite the enormous variety of functions mediated through the eicosanoids, PGE_1 and PGE_2 are the most frequently used eicosanoids in newborn medicine (437). They have been used primarily to maintain patency of the ductus arteriosus and occasionally for pulmonary vasodilation in the treatment of persistent pulmonary hypertension of the newborn (PPHN). The effectiveness of PGE_1 for maintaining ductal patency has been confirmed in various studies, including a multicenter collaborative investigation (438).

Prostaglandin E_1 usually has been administered only by continuous venous or arterial infusion (439). Dosages generally have started at 0.1 µg/kg/min and have been associated with a variety of adverse reactions, including cutaneous vasodilation, edema, hypotension, apnea, fever, irritability, seizures, hypoglycemia, diarrhea, disseminated intravascular coagulation, osteolysis, hypercalcemia, and thrombocytopenia (439). By reducing starting dosages to 0.05 µg/kg/min, side effects, in particular apnea, are reduced. If oxygenation is maintained, dosages can be tapered to 0.01 µg/kg/min (440).

Prolonged treatment with PGE_2 is needed for patients with ductal-dependent cardiac malformations awaiting transplantation. Oral PGE_2 also is effective for maintaining ductal patency and oxygenation (440). Patients who were changed from the IV to the oral route, however, did have a significant decrease in PaO_2. Oral treatment utilized doses of 35 to 65 µg/kg/hr by gastric drip, with a slow increase in dosing intervals from 1 to 4 hours during the second and third weeks of treatment. This is consistent with recent reports of treatment of adults with PGE analogs for healing of ulcers (441).

Closure of the patent ductus arteriosus with cyclooxygenase inhibitors also is an integral part of neonatal pharmacology. Ductal patency after birth is maintained by PGE_2, the secretion of which is inhibited by rising oxygen tension (437). Ductal closure was first achieved with oral indomethacin in large dosages (2.5 to 5 mg/kg) (442). Since that report, indomethacin has been formulated in an IV preparation and used in a multicenter collaborative trial that demonstrated the efficacy of treatment with a 0.2 mg/kg loading dose, followed by 0.1 to 0.25 mg/kg doses every 12 hours for a total of three doses (443). This study also illustrated the side effects of cyclooxygenase inhibition in neonates, including oliguria, increased serum creatinine, and transient mild bleeding.

Infants with intracranial hemorrhage were excluded from the collaborative study (443). Subsequent studies have found that early indomethacin treatment actually decreases the risk of intracranial hemorrhage (444). When the presence of an intracranial hemorrhage was not a contraindication to indomethacin treatment, it has not been shown to cause extension of intracranial hemorrhages (445,446). These studies do not indicate that intracranial hemorrhage should be a contraindication for indomethacin treatment, although some physicians follow the approach used in the multicenter collaborative trial and avoid administration of indomethacin to neonates with intracranial hemorrhages (443).

Developmental changes in the pharmacokinetics of indomethacin have been defined for preterm infants (447). Lower average indomethacin concentrations were noted in patients who did not sustain ductal closure after treatment with indomethacin. Indomethacin clearance increased with both postnatal age and body weight. A correlation between individual indomethacin levels and ductal closure was not found, however, possibly as a result of variation in rates of PGE_2 production among patients.

The optimal duration of indomethacin treatment for low-birth-weight neonates has not been settled. After initial treatment with three doses of indomethacin, once-daily doses of indomethacin have been continued for an additional 5 days in 22 infants with birth weight under 1,500 g (448). The group that was treated for a sustained period of time had no patent ductus 3 days after ending treatment and fewer intraventricular hemorrhages. The ductus reopened eventually in almost one-half of this group, but at a much older age. Longer courses of indomethacin need more study but may be more effective for ductal closure.

The neonate who is several weeks old and has a symptomatic patent ductus arteriosus presents a therapeutic dilemma. McCarthy and colleagues reported failure of ductal closure in infants who were 37 to 40 weeks of postconceptional age at the time of indomethacin treatment (449). Efforts to maintain effective indomethacin concentrations in older patients with patent ductus arteriosus, by higher doses administered more frequently, have not ensured ductal closure (450).

The renal effects of indomethacin in premature infants are quite similar to those observed in symptomatic adults (451). In premature infants, indomethacin decreases urine flow, glomerular filtration rate, and free-water clearance, which combine to decrease renal electrolyte excretion (452). Oliguria during indomethacin treatment of premature infants has been improved with dopamine (453) and with furosemide (331). In adults, salt depletion and hypovolemia accentuate the adverse effects of non-steroidal antiinflammatory drugs on renal function (451,454,455). Seri and colleagues found that dopamine prevented a decrease in urine flow and increased sodium excretion (453).

The rate of indomethacin infusion has a significant effect on its cardiovascular effects. When indomethacin was infused over 0.2 to 4 minutes, cerebral blood flow velocity decreased 48% to 75% (456). When indomethacin was infused over 20 minutes, cerebral blood flow velocity was not reduced (457). A similar reduction in mesenteric blood flow occurs when indomethacin is administered over 20 seconds or less, and this can be prevented by slow infusion over 30 to 35 minutes (458). It is too early to determine whether the common practice of discontinuation of feeds during indomethacin treatment is unnecessary when doses are administered more slowly.

Pulmonary Vasodilators

Because the pulmonary vasculature of many neonates is in parallel with the systemic vasculature through patency of the ductus arteriosus and foramen ovale, an effective pulmonary vasodilator must dilate the pulmonary vasculature more than the systemic vasculature (459). Endothelium-derived relaxing factor (EDRF) was shown to be involved in control of the perinatal pulmonary circulation as it dilates after birth (460,461). EDRF was shown to have the same properties as nitric oxide (NO) (462). Over the last few years, NO has been demonstrated to selectively dilate pulmonary arteries through release of cyclic guanosine monophosphate (cGMP) (463,464). Infants with persistent pulmonary hypertension of the newborn (PPHN) have lower circulating cGMP, likely secondary to inadequate NO production needed to dilate the pulmonary vasculature after birth (465). The selectivity of NO for the pulmonary vasculature derives from its administration by inhalation and inactivation by binding to hemoglobin as soon as it enters the bloodstream. This same binding, however, may induce methemoglobinemia at higher doses of NO (466).

Nitric oxide is currently available only as an experimental drug, in part because it is a highly reactive compound whose dose must be carefully monitored to avoid potentially severe or even lethal toxicity (463). Improved oxygenation and a reduced need for ECMO have been demonstrated in randomized, controlled trials of NO treatment of near-term neonates with respiratory failure (467–470). Although NO has been used to treat a variety of disorders (471), when respiratory failure is accompanied by pulmonary disease and severe infiltrates, NO treatment is less successful, possibly because inhalational delivery does not reach the pulmonary vasculature (472). Dose–response studies indicate that neonates achieve maximum improvement in oxygenation at 20 ppm (473) to 40 ppm (474,475). Prolonged treatment longer than 10 days has been associated with pulmonary toxicity, demonstrated by detection of nitrotyrosine (476). Platelet function has been reduced during NO treatment of adults, likely through increased cGMP, and this may represent a risk for neonates (477). In this critically ill population treated with NO, follow-up has been reported at Denver for 32 infants seen at both 1 and 2 years after discharge (478). Reactive airway disease was reported in 30%, weight less than the fifth percentile in 21%, and severe neurodevelopmental delay in 12%. Modest improvement in development and growth was observed between years 1 and 2.

As long as NO remains under investigational new drug control and unavailable at many sites, infants with respiratory failure and PPHN will require alternate treatment, including ECMO. Among the other drugs that have been used, with mixed success, for treatment of PPHN are tolazoline, PGE_1, PGI_2, PGD_2, acetylcholine, isoproterenol, chlorpromazine, and nitroprusside (479). None of these has proven to be selective for the pulmonary vasculature. Although tolazoline has been reported to improve oxygenation in approximately 60% of patients, high mortality persisted, and adverse effects occurred at an unacceptably high rate (78). Inappropriately high doses of tolazoline, used without the guidance of kinetic studies, may have contributed to the high rate of adverse effects associated with tolazoline treatment (78). In a study of tolazoline kinetics in newborns, a 1.0 mg/kg bolus loading dose followed by a low-dose infusion of 0.2 mg/kg/hr prevented accumulation to potentially toxic concentrations (480).

Investigations of the mechanisms through which NO controls neonatal pulmonary vascular tone and that control NO production in the pulmonary vasculature point to potential new alternatives for treatment of PPHN (461,463). For now, inhaled NO remains the only selective pulmonary vasodilator and is most effective in patients without prominent pulmonary infiltrates that may prevent it from reaching the site of action. Its toxicities require close monitoring. Alternative drug treatment may still be successful at improving pulmonary perfusion in patients with PPHN, especially when systemic hypotension is adequately treated.

Respiratory Stimulants

Doxapram has been administered to newborns both IV and orally to treat apnea that was unresponsive to methylxanthines (see Methylxanthines) (481). Doxapram is a general stimulant of the CNS respiratory center along with the entire cerebrospinal axis. Originally, doxapram was administered by continuous IV infusion for treatment of apnea of prematurity (482,483). When doxapram is administered enterally, only 10% to 12% of the dose is absorbed (484). Despite its poor enteral absorption, doxapram decreases apnea of the newborn (485). Side effects observed during enteral administration included occult blood in stools, necrotizing enterocolitis, and premature

tooth buds. Seizures have been associated with high circulating concentrations, although Alpan and colleagues suggest that the ratio of effective to convulsive concentration is 1:70 (482). Seizures have been observed in two neonates treated with doxapram, but these were thought most likely to reflect intraventricular hemorrhages (483).

Steroids

The use of dexamethasone for the prevention and treatment of BPD in ventilator-dependent neonates has increased dramatically in recent years (486). This strategy is based on efforts to reduce pulmonary inflammation associated with the pathogenesis of chronic lung disease (487–491). Dexamethasone is a pure glucocorticoid without mineralocorticoid activity and is approximately 30 times more potent than hydrocortisone (492). Randomized, placebo-controlled studies have documented that dexamethasone reduces ventilator settings and oxygen requirement and facilitates extubation of ventilator-dependent neonates at 14 to 35 days of age (493–498). The most common dosage regimen is 0.5 mg/kg/day divided into two daily doses and tapered over a period of 7 to 42 days (493–496,498). Although there is uncertainty about the optimal duration of treatment, Cummings et al. reported that a 42-day tapered dexamethasone regimen resulted in more rapid weaning from mechanical ventilation and fewer days on supplemental oxygen than an 18-day regimen or placebo (495). Despite short-term improvements noted with dexamethasone, none of these initial studies demonstrated a significant reduction in BPD, mortality, or any other major endpoints. Follow-up studies have also failed to demonstrate that dexamethasone produced any long-term improvements in pulmonary function (499,500).

Because respiratory distress syndrome is associated with inflammation, it has been hypothesized that a long delay in antiinflammatory therapy may lead to a critical degree of lung injury. In support of this hypothesis, treatment with steroids shortly after birth has reduced the duration of mechanical ventilation and need for oxygen supplementation (501–503). Rastogi and colleagues reported that a 12-day course of dexamethasone begun within 12 hours of birth reduced the incidence of BPD at 28 days and eliminated BPD at 36 weeks of postconceptional age (502). Others reported no difference in BPD between placebo and dexamethasone treatment during the first 3 days after birth, perhaps suggesting that a longer treatment duration is required to suppress pulmonary inflammation and reduce the incidence of BPD (504). No study has attempted to compare early versus late dexamethasone; thus, optimal timing of steroids still remains unclear. However, a recent study by Papile et al. reported no benefit when steroids were initiated at 14 days of age versus 28 days of age (505). It is noteworthy that the earlier treatment was associated with an increased incidence of nosocomial bacteremia and hyperglycemia.

Adverse effects of dexamethasone include poor growth and weight gain during treatment (494,498,502,505–508), hypertension (501–505,509,510), hypothalamic–pituitary–adrenal (HPA) axis suppression (511–516), hypertrophic cardiomyopathy (517–520), gastrointestinal hemorrhage and perforation (504,521,522), and hyperglycemia (503–505). Many adverse effects are reversible on drug discontinuation; however, some may be severe or even life-threatening. Some degree of HPA-axis suppression is often evident following dexamethasone regimens of 14 to 42 days (511–516). Adrenal suppression may persist for months, so this population may require a prolonged steroid taper (512). During this period, Byyny found that stresses such as surgery or infection require temporary administration of exogenous glucocorticoids at two to three times the maintenance dose (523). The effect of a short course of dexamethasone on the HPA axis is more controversial. Some investigators reported that 7 days of dexamethasone had no effect on adrenal responsiveness to ACTH (524,525). Others reported hyporesponsiveness to both ACTH and corticotropin-releasing hormone following a 7-day course of dexamethasone (526–528), although this effect appears short-lived and not clinically significant (527).

It is of concern that, in a recent multicenter trial, rate of head growth was reduced during dexamethasone therapy (505). Animal studies have also raised the concern that prolonged dexamethasone treatment may adversely affect brain growth (529–531). Only a few studies have evaluated long-term neurologic outcome in infants who received dexamethasone postnatally. Cummings et al. reported an improved neurologic outcome with a 42-day dexamethasone regimen as compared with an 18-day treatment regimen or placebo (495). One-year and 3-year follow-up studies have not demonstrated any long-term neurologic benefits or adverse effects associated with steroid treatment during infancy (499,500). In a preliminary report of a 2-year follow-up study, a higher percentage of infants treated with dexamethasone had a significant delay in developmental outcome and abnormal neuromotor function as compared with infants who receive placebo (532). Further study is needed to evaluate the long-term risks and benefits of treating neonates with potent systemic steroids.

Inhaled Steroids

Concern for the adverse effects associated with intravenous dexamethasone has prompted recent interest in treating BPD with aerosolized topical corticosteroids such as beclomethasone. In theory, administration of topical steroids to the lung may minimize systemic drug exposure, thus reducing the potential for systemic adverse effects. Although data are still lacking, recent studies in small numbers of patients suggest modest benefit in ventilator-dependent neonates. In a retrospective review of 32 ventilator-dependent infants treated with beclomethasone (84 μg administered every 4 to 6 hours via metered-dose inhaler into the ventilator circuit), Gal et al. reported that 78% of infants responded to treatment as defined by a reduced oxygen requirement and subsequent extubation (533). The endotracheal tube was removed within a mean 10.5 days in responders versus 40.8 days in nonresponders. In a prospective study, LaForce and colleagues randomized 13 oxygen- and ventilator-dependent infants to receive nebulized beclomethasone (50 μg every 8 hours) or saline placebo for 28 days (534). Beclomethasone-treated infants had a significant reduction in airway resistance by week 2 and an increased dynamic lung compliance by week 3, as compared to placebo ($p < 0.05$). The incidence of infection was similar in both groups, and no immediate adverse effects were noted during administration of beclomethasone or placebo. In a recent placebo-controlled study, 7 days of inhaled budesonide (600 mg twice daily) reduced ventilator settings and Aa oxygen gradient without complications (535).

Clinically, it appears that pulmonary function among neonates with BPD improves more slowly during inhaled steroid treatment than during treatment with intravenous dexamethasone (536). However, a high-dose beclomethasone dosage regimen (1,000 μg/kg/day in three divided doses for 7 days) may shorten the time to improvement without suppressing the HPA axis or increasing infections (537). Larger studies must be conducted to determine efficacy, optimal dose, and safety of inhaled steroids. Although no study has demonstrated significant systemic effects from inhaled steroids in ventilated neonates, this may not be true at higher, more efficacious doses. Potential toxicities from chlorofluorocarbon propellants, including bronchospasm and cardiac toxicity, must be evaluated at higher dosages (538–540).

Vitamin E

Vitamin E refers to several chemically related compounds, differing in degrees of methylation, desaturation, and oxygen content, classified generically as tocopherols (541). The oxygen molecules and aromatic ring conjugation allow interconversion between hydroxyl and quinone forms, so that vitamin E functions as an antioxidant. α-tocopherol is the primary, naturally occurring member of this group.

The clinical administration of vitamin E to premature neonates is based on its antioxidant activity, low vitamin E concentrations in many preterm neonates at birth, and animal studies suggesting that vitamin E protects against oxidant injury to the lung and eye. Initial favorable effects of vitamin E on BPD (542) were not confirmed in a subsequent randomized, double-blind study by the same investigators (543).

For prevention of retinopathy of prematurity (ROP), a prospective, double-blind, randomized trial reported that 100 mg of vitamin E per day reduced the severity, but not frequency, of ROP (544). Studies of tocopherol in a kitten model of ROP, in doses of 50 to 1,000 mg/kg/day, revealed a high frequency of mortality with lethargy, weight loss, and seizures (545). Livers were enlarged and extensively vacuolated with fat in the vitamin E-treated animals.

In 1984, the Centers for Disease Control and Bodenstein separately described infants with a new symptom complex that included pulmonary deterioration, thrombocytopenia, liver failure, ascites, and renal failure leading to death in some cases (546,547). These symptoms were attributed to a specific brand of α-tocopherol acetate, E-Ferol, which had begun to be administered IV to prevent oxidant injury to eyes and lungs. This syndrome ceased after the use of E-Ferol was discontinued. It was never completely clear whether the toxicity resided in the α-tocopherol, the polysorbate emulsifiers, or an unknown contaminant (548,549). Sepsis, necrotizing enterocolitis, and intraventricular hemorrhage also have been attributed to treatment of neonates with vitamin E (541). The American Academy of Pediatrics Committee on Fetus and Newborn (COFN) concluded that pharmacologic doses of vitamin E should be regarded as experimental and not routinely indicated for infants weighing under 1,500 g (550). The COFN recommends 5 to 10 IU of vitamin E per day for preterm infants, provided through supplemented formulas or supplemental vitamins (236).

DRUG EXCRETION IN BREAST MILK

Over 50% of newborn infants are breast-feeding at the time of discharge (551). Although almost all drugs and chemicals present in the maternal circulation may enter human milk, the extent of transfer is quite variable. Maternal intake of prescription medications, over-the-counter medications, illicit drugs, and exposure to a multitude of environmental substances may expose the breast-feeding infant to a complex mixture of potentially harmful chemicals.

The nature of human milk influences its drug content. Human milk has been described as a suspension of fat in a protein–mineral–carbohydrate solution (552). The lactose secreted in milk is synthesized from glucose by the alveolar cells of the breast in a process that requires α-lactalbumin. Milk contains a variety of proteins, including α-lactalbumin, lactoferrin albumin, lysozyme, and immunoglobulin A, all of which may bind drugs during transport into milk (552). The lipid within milk is maintained in the aqueous phase in milkfat globules surrounded by lipoprotein membranes. Milk is isosmotic to plasma, with an average pH of 7.2.

Several factors affect drug transfer into milk, including molecular weight, lipid solubility, maternal plasma pro-

tein binding, and extent of ionization. These are similar factors to those that influence transfer of molecules across any lipid bilayer membrane. Because milk usually is acidic to maternal plasma, and non–protein-bound, nonionized molecules are free to cross membranes, the Henderson–Hasselbach equation may be used to estimate drug distribution between maternal plasma and milk (553). This predicts that organic bases ($pK_a < 7.4$) will reach a higher concentration in milk than in maternal serum. Many quantitative studies of human milk drug excretion have estimated that approximately 1% to 2% of a maternal drug dose will appear in milk (554).

These data on human milk drug excretion have been reviewed with respect to specific recommendations about continuing or discontinuing breast-feeding during specific drug intake by the mother (see Appendix H1) (551).

ACKNOWLEDGMENT

We are grateful to Sharon Gough for assistance with the preparation of this manuscript.

REFERENCES

1. Koch-Weser J, Sellers EM. Binding of drugs to serum albumin (first of two parts). *N Engl J Med* 1976;294:311–316.
2. Svensson CK, Woodruff MN, Lalka D. Influence of protein binding and use of unbound (free) drug concentrations. In: Evans WE, Schentag JJ, Jusko WJ, eds. *Applied therapeutics. Principles of therapeutic drug monitoring,* 2nd ed. Spokane: *Applied Therapeutics,* 1986: 187–219.
3. Oellerich M. Influence of protein binding commentary. In: Evans WE, Schentag JJ, Jusko WJ, eds. *Applied pharmacokinetics,* 2nd ed. Spokane: Applied Therapeutics, 1986:220–228.
4. Somogyi A. Clinical pharmacokinetics and dosing schedules. In: Brody TM, Larner J, Minneman KP, eds. *Human pharmacology molecular to clinical,* 3rd ed. St Louis: Mosby-Year Book, 1998:47–64.
5. Boreus LO. *Principles of pediatric pharmacology.* New York: Churchill-Livingston, 1982.
6. Brodersen R, Honore B. Drug binding properties of neonatal albumin. *Acta Paediatr Scand* 1989;78:342–346.
7. Aranda JV, Sitar DS, Parsons WD, Loughnan PM, Neims AH. Pharmacokinetic aspects of theophylline in premature newborns. *N Engl J Med* 1976;295:413–416.
8. Peterson RG, Simmons MA, Rumack BH, Levine RL, Brooks JG. Pharmacology of furosemide in the premature newborn infant. *J Pediatr* 1980;97:139–143.
9. Evans EF, Proctor JD, Fratkin MJ, Velandia J, Wasserman AJ. Blood flow in muscle groups and drug absorption. *Clin Pharmacol Ther* 1975;17:44–47.
10. Kostenbauder HB, Rapp RP, McGovren JP, et al. Bioavailability and single-dose pharmacokinetics of intramuscular phenytoin. *Clin Pharmacol Ther* 1975;18:449–456.
11. Leff RD, Roberts RJ. Methods for intravenous drug administration in the pediatric patient. *J Pediatr* 1981;98:631–635.
12. Benet LZ, Kroetz DL, Sheiner LB. Pharmacokinetics: The dynamics of drug absorption, distribution, and elimination. In: Hardman JG, Limbird LE, Molinoff PB, Ruddon RW, Goodman-Gilman A, eds. *Goodman & Gilman's the pharmacological basis of therapeutics,* 9th ed. New York: McGraw-Hill, 1996:3–27.
13. Hollenberg PF, Brody TM. Absorption, distribution, metabolism, and elimination. In: Brody TM, Larner J, Minneman KP, eds. *Human pharmacology molecular to clinical,* 3 ed. St Louis: Mosby-Year Book, 1998:35–46.
14. Friis-Hansen B. Body composition during growth *in vivo* measurements and biochemical data correlated to differential anatomical growth. *Pediatrics* 1971;47:264–274.

15. Ziegler EE, O'Donnell AM, Nelson SE, Fomon SJ. Body composition of the reference fetus. *Growth* 1976;40:329–341.
16. Painter MJ, Pippenger C, Wasterlain C, et al. Phenobarbital and phenytoin in neonatal seizures: metabolism and tissue distribution. *Neurology* 1981;31:1107–1112.
17. Pelkonen O, Kaltiala EH, Larmi TKI, Karki NT. Comparison of activities of drug-metabolizing enzymes in human fetal and adult livers. *Clin Pharmacol Ther* 1973;14:840–846.
18. Leeder JS, Kearns GL. Pharmacogenetics in pediatrics. Implications for practice. *Pediatr Clin North Am* 1997;44:55–77.
19. Aranda JV, MacLeod SM, Renton KW, Eade NR. Hepatic microsomal drug oxidation and electron transport in newborn infants. *Pediatr Pharmacol Ther* 1974;85:534–542.
20. Aldridge A, Aranda JV, Neims AH. Caffeine metabolism in the newborn. *Clin Pharmacol Ther* 1979;25:447–453.
21. Morselli PL, Principi N, Tognoni G, et al. Diazepam elimination in premature and full term infants, and children. *J Perinatol Med* 1973;1:133–141.
22. Loughnan PM, Greenwald A, Purton WW, Aranda JV, Watters G, Neims AH. Pharmacokinetic observations of phenytoin disposition in the newborn and young infant. *Arch Dis Child* 1977;52:302–309.
23. Pitlick W, Painter M, Pippenger C. Phenobarbital pharmacokinetics in neonates. *Clin Pharmacol Ther* 1978;23:346–350.
24. Kalow W, Tang BK. The use of caffeine for enzyme assays: A critical appraisal. *Clin Pharmacol Ther* 1993;53:503–514.
25. Cazeneuve C, Pons G, Rey E, et al. Biotransformation of caffeine in human liver microsomes from foetuses, neonates, infants and adults. *Br J Clin Pharmacol* 1994;37:405–412.
26. Zhang ZY, Kaminsky LS. Characterization of human cytochromes P450 involved in theophylline 8-hydroxylation. *Biochem Pharmacol* 1995;50:205–211.
27. Ha HR, Chen J, Freiburghaus AU, Follath F. Metabolism of theophylline by cDNA-expressed human cytochromes P-450. *Br J Clin Pharmacol* 1995;39:321–326.
28. Yang HY, Lee QP, Rettie AE, Juchau MR. Functional cytochrome P4503A isoforms in human embryonic tissues: expression during organogenesis. *Mol Pharmacol* 1994;46:922–928.
29. Aranda JV, Cook CE, Gorman W, et al. Pharmacokinetic profile of caffeine in the premature newborn infant with apnea. *J Pediatr* 1979;94:663–668.
30. Carrier O, Pons G, Rey E, et al. Maturation of caffeine metabolic pathways in infancy. *Clin Pharmacol Ther* 1988;44:145–151.
31. Pons G, Carrier O, Richard MO, et al. Developmental changes in caffeine elimination in infancy. *Dev Pharmacol Ther* 1988;11:258–264.
32. Kraus DM, Fischer JH, Reitz SJ, et al. Alterations in theophylline metabolism during the first year of life. *Clin Pharmacol Ther* 1993;54:351–359.
33. Shimada T, Yamazaki H, Mimura M, et al. Characterization of microsomal cytochrome P450 enzymes involved in the oxidation of xenobiotic chemicals in human fetal livers and adult lungs. *Drug Metab Dispos* 1996;24:515–522.
34. Jacqz-Aigrain E, Cresteil T. Cytochrome P450-dependent metabolism of dextromethorphan: fetal and adult studies. *Dev Pharmacol Ther* 1992;18:161–168.
35. Ladona MG, Lindström B, Thyr C, Dun-Ren P, Rane A. Differential foetal development of the O- and N-demethylation of codeine and dextromethorphan in man. *Br J Clin Pharmacol* 1991;32:295–302.
36. Treluyer JM, Jacqz-Aigrain E, Alvarez F, Cresteil T. Expression of CYP2D6 in developing human liver. *Eur J Biochem* 1991;202:583–588.
37. Bourgeois BF, Dodson WE. Phenytoin elimination in newborns. *Neurology* 1983;33:173–178.
38. Vauzelle-Kervroedan F, Rey E, Pariente-Khayat A, et al. Noninvasive *in vivo* study of the maturation of CYP IIIA in neonates and infants. *Eur J Clin Pharmacol* 1996;51:69–72.
39. Radde IC, Kalow W. Drug biotransformation and its development. In: Radde I, MacLeod S, eds. *Pediatric pharmacology & therapeutics,* 2nd ed. St. Louis: Mosby-Year Book, 1993:57–86.
40. Coughtrie MW, Burchell B, Leakey JE, Hume R. The inadequacy of perinatal glucuronidation: Immunoblot analysis of the developmental expression of individual UDP-Glucuronosyltransferase isoenzymes in rat and human liver microsomes. *Mol Pharmacol* 1988;34:729–735.
41. Weiss CF, Glazko AJ, Weston JK. Chloramphenicol in the newborn infant: A physiologic explanation of its toxicity when given in excessive doses. *N Engl J Med* 1960;262:787–794.

42. Sutherland JM. Fatal cardiovascular collapse of infants receiving large amounts of chloramphenicol. *Am J Dis Child* 1959;97:761–767.
43. Burns LE, Hodgeman JE, Cass AB. Fatal and circulatory collapse in premature infants receiving chloramphenicol. *N Engl J Med* 1959;261:1318–1321.
44. Mulhall A, Berry DJ, de Louvois J. Chloramphenicol in paediatrics: Current prescribing practice and the need to monitor. *Eur J Pediatr* 1988;147:574–578.
45. Choonara LA, McKay P, Hain R, Rane A. Morphine metabolism in children. *Br J Clin Pharmacol* 1989;28:599–604.
46. Säwe J, Kager L, Eng JO, Rane A. Oral morphine in cancer patients: *in vivo* kinetics and *in vitro* hepatic glucuronidation. *Br J Clin Pharmacol* 1985;19:495–501.
47. Pokela ML, Olkkola KT, Seppälä T, Koivisto M. Age-related morphine kinetics in infants. *Dev Pharmacol Ther* 1993;20:26–34.
48. McRorie TI, Lynn AM, Nespeca MK, Opheim KE, Slattery JT. The maturation of morphine clearance and metabolism. *Am J Dis Child* 1992;146:972–976,1305.
49. Hartley R, Green M, Quinn MW, Rushforth JA, Levene MI. Development of morphine glucuronidation in premature neonates. *Biol Neonate* 1994;66:1–9.
50. Mikkelsen S, Feilberg VL, Christensen CB, Lundstrom KE. Morphine pharmacokinetics in premature and mature newborn infants. *Acta Paediatr* 1994;83:1025–1028.
51. Bhat R, Chari G, Gulati A, Aldana O, Velamati R, Bhargava H. Pharmacokinetics of a single dose of morphine in preterm infants during the first week of life. *J Pediatr* 1990;117:477–481.
52. Lynn AM, Slattery JT. Morphine pharmacokinetics in infancy. *Anesthesiology* 1987;66:136–139.
53. Olkkola KT, Maunuksela EL, Korpela R, Rosenberg PH. Kinetics and dynamics of postoperative intravenous morphine in children. *Clin Pharmacol Ther* 1988;44:128–136.
54. Autret E, Dutertre JP, Breteau M, Jonville AP, Furet Y, Laugier J. Pharmacokinetics of paracetamol in the neonate and infant after administration of propacetamol chlorhydrate. *Dev Pharmacol Ther* 1993;20:129–134.
55. Miller RP, Roberts RJ, Fischer LJ. Acetaminophen elimination kinetics in neonates, children, and adults. *Clin Pharmacol Ther* 1976;19:284–294.
56. Levy G, Khanna NN, Soda DM, Tsuzuki O, Stern L. Pharmacokinetics of acetaminophen in the human neonate: Formation of acetaminophen glucuronide and sulfate in relation to plasma bilirubin concentration and D-glucaric acid excretion. *Pediatrics* 1975;55:818–825.
57. Alam SN, Roberts RJ, Fischer LJ. Age-related differences in salicylamide and acetaminophen conjugation in man. *J Pediatr* 1977;90:130–135.
58. Aperia A, Broberger O, Elinder G, Herin P, Zetterstrom R. Postnatal development of renal function in pre-term and full-term neonates. *Acta Paediatr Scand* 1981;70:183–187.
59. Engle WD. Evaluation of renal function and acute renal failure in the neonate. *Pediatr Clin North Am* 1986;33:129–151.
60. Greenblatt DJ, Koch-Weser J. Clinical pharmacokinetics (first of two parts). *N Engl J Med* 1975;293:702–705.
61. Greenblatt DJ, Koch-Weser J. Clinical pharmacokinetics (second of two parts). *N Engl J Med* 1975;293:964–970.
62. Roberts RJ. Pharmacokinetics: basic principles and clinical applications. In: *Drug therapy in infants. Pharmacologic principles and clinical experience.* Philadelphia: WB Saunders, 1984:13–24.
63. Galinsky RE, Svvensson CK. Basic pharmacokinetics. In: Gennaro AR, Chase GD, Mardersonian AD, et al, eds. *Remington: The science and practice of pharmacy,* 19th ed. Easton: Mack Publishing, 1995:724–760.
64. Gibaldi M, Perrier D. *Pharmacokinetics,* 2nd ed. New York: Marcel Dekker, 1982.
65. Jusko WJ. Guidelines for collection and analysis of pharmacokinetic data. In: Evans WE, Schentag JJ, Jusko WJ, eds. *Applied therapeutics. Principles of therapeutic drug monitoring,* 2nd ed. Spokane: Applied Therapeutics, 1986:9–54.
66. Notari RE. *Principles of pharmacokinetics. Biopharmaceutics and Clinical Pharmacology,* 3rd ed. New York: Marcel Dekker, 1980:45–106.
67. Zaske DE. Aminoglycosides. In: Evans WE, Schentag JJ, Jusko WJ, eds. *Applied pharmacokinetics: Principles of therapeutic drug monitoring,* 3rd ed, Chap 14. Vancouver: Applied Therapeutics, 1992:1–47.

68. Matzke G. Vancomycin. In: Evans W, Schentag J, Jusko W, eds. *Applied pharmacokinetics: Principles of therapeutic drug monitoring,* 3rd ed, Chap 15. Vancouver, WA: Applied Therapeutics, 1992:1–31.

69. McCracken GH Jr. Aminoglycoside toxicity in infants and children. *Am J Med* 1986;80(Suppl 6B):172–178.

70. Spector R, Park GD, Johnson GF, Vesell ES. Therapeutic drug monitoring. *Clin Pharmacol Ther* 1988;43:345–353.

71. Roberts RJ. Cardiovascular drugs. In: *Drug therapy in infants. Pharmacologic principles and clinical experience.* Philadelphia: WB Saunders, 1984:138–225.

72. Roberts RJ. Special considerations in drug therapy in infants. In: *Drug therapy in infants. Pharmacologic principles and clinical experience.* Philadelphia: WB Saunders, 1984:25–34.

73. Wagman GH, Bailey JV, Weinstein MJ. Binding of aminoglycoside antibiotics to filtration materials. *Antimicrob Agents Chemother* 1975; 7:316–319.

74. Lackner TE. Dose replacement following exchange transfusion. *J Pediatr* 1982;100:811–814.

75. Aranda JV, Collinge JM, Clarkson S. Epidemiologic aspects of drug utilization in a newborn intensive care unit. *Semin Perinatol* 1982;6: 148–154.

76. Aranda JV, Portuguez-Malavasi A, Collinge JM, Germanson T, Outerbridge EW. Epidemiology of adverse drug reactions in the newborn. *Dev Pharmacol Ther* 1982;5:173–184.

77. Mitchell AA, Goldman P, Shapiro S, Slone D. Drug utilization and reported adverse reactions in hospitalized children. *Am J Epidemiol* 1979;110:196–204.

78. Ward RM. Pharmacology of tolazoline. *Clin Perinatol* 1984;11: 703–713.

79. Hansen TWR, Bratlid D. Bilirubin and brain toxicity. *Acta Paediatr Scand* 1986;75:513–522.

80. Maisels MJ. Jaundice. In: Avery GB, Fletcher MA, MacDonald MG, eds. *Neonatology. Pathophysiology and management of the newborn,* 4th ed. Philadelphia: JB Lippincott, 1994:630–725.

81. Silverman WA, Andersen DH, Blanc WA, Crozier DN. A difference in mortality rate and incidence of kernicterus among premature infants allotted to two prophylactic antibacterial regiments. *Pediatrics* 1956; 18:614–624.

82. Odell GB. The distribution and toxicity of bilirubin. E. Mead Johnson address 1969. *Pediatrics* 1970;46:16–24.

83. Rose AL, Wisniewski H. Acute bilirubin encephalopathy induced with sulfadimethoxine in Gunn rats. *J Neuropathol Exp Neurol* 1979;38: 152–164.

84. Brown WJ, Buist NR, Gipson HT, Huston RK, Kennaway NG. Fatal benzyl alcohol poisoning in a neonatal intensive care unit. *Lancet* 1982;1:1250.

85. Glasgow AM, Boeckx RL, Miller MK, MacDonald MG, August GP, Goodman SI. Hyperosmolality in small infants due to propylene glycol. *Pediatrics* 1983;72:353–355.

86. MacDonald MG, Getson PR, Glasgow AM, Miller MK, Boeckx RL, Johnson EL. Propylene glycol: Increased incidence of seizures in low birth weight infants. *Pediatrics* 1987;79:622–625.

87. Arulanantham K, Genel M. Central nervous system toxicity associated with ingestion of propylene glycol. *J Pediatr* 1978;93:515–516.

88. Martin G, Finberg L. Propylene glycol: a potentially toxic vehicle in liquid dosage form. *J Pediatr* 1970;77:877–878.

89. Cate JC 4th, Hedrick R. Propylene glycol intoxication and lactic acidosis (letter). *N Engl J Med* 1980;303:1237.

90. Weintraub Z, Iancu TC. Isopropyl alcohol burns (letter). *Pediatrics* 1982;69:506.

91. Schick JB, Milstein JM. Burn hazard of isopropyl alcohol in a neonate. *Pediatrics* 1981;68:587–588.

92. Ittmann PI, Bozynski ME. Toxic epidermal necrolysis in a newborn infant after exposure to adhesive remover. *J Perinatol* 1993;13: 476–477.

93. Wenzl JE, Mills SD, McCall JT. Methanol poisoning in an infant. Successful treatment with peritoneal dialysis. *Am J Dis Child* 1968;116: 445–447.

94. Vicas IM, Beck R. Fatal inhalational isopropyl alcohol poisoning in a neonate. *Clin Toxicol* 1993;31:473–481.

95. Moss MH. Alcohol-induced hyperglycemia and coma caused by alcohol sponging. *Pediatrics* 1970;46:445–447.

96. Shuman RM, Leech RW, Alvord EC Jr. Neurotoxicity of hexachlorophene in humans: II. A clinical pathological study of 46 premature infants. *Arch Neurol* 1975;32:320–325.

97. l'Allemand D, Gruters A, Heidemann P, Schurnbrand P. Iodine-induced alterations of thyroid function in newborn infants after prenatal and perinatal exposure to povidone iodine. *J Pediatr* 1983;102: 935–938.

98. Linder N, Davidovitch N, Reichman B, et al. Topical iodine-containing antiseptics and subclinical hypothyroidism in preterm infants. *J Pediatr* 1997;131:434–439.

99. Fisch RO, Beglund EB, Bridge AG, Finley PR, Quie PG, Raile R. Methemoglobinemia in a hospital nursery. *JAMA* 1963;185:760–763.

100. Morrell P, Hey E, Mackee IW, Rutter N, Lewis M. Deafness in a preterm baby associated with topical antibiotic spray containing neomycin. *Lancet* 1985;1:1167–1168.

101. Rutter N. Percutaneous drug absorption in the newborn: hazards and uses. *Clin Perinatol* 1987;14:911–930.

102. Roberts RJ. Fetal and infant intoxication. In: *Drug therapy in infants. Pharmacologic principles and clinical experience.* Philadelphia: WB Saunders, 1984:322–383.

103. Hillman LS, Goodwin SL, Sherman WR. Identification and measurement of plasticizer in neonatal tissues after umbilical catheters and blood products. *N Engl J Med* 1975;292:381–386.

104. Whalley DW, Wendt DJ, Grant AO. Basic concepts in cellular cardiac electrophysiology: Part I: Ion channels, membrane currents, and the action potential. *Pacing Clin Electrophysiol* 1995;18:1556–1574.

105. Roden DM, George AL Jr. The cardiac ion channels: Relevance to management of arrhythmias. *Annu Rev Med* 1996;47:135–148.

106. Grant AO. Mechanisms of action of antiarrhythmic drugs: From ion channel blockage to arrhythmia termination. *Pacing Clin Electrophysiol* 1997;20(Pt II):432–444.

107. Wetzel GT, Klitzner TS. Developmental cardiac electrophysiology recent advances in cellular physiology. *Cardiovasc Res* 1996;31: E52–E60.

108. Robinson RB. Autonomic receptor-effector coupling during post-natal development. *Cardiovasc Res* 1996;31:E68–E76.

109. Vaughan Williams EM. Classification of antiarrhythmic drugs. In: Sandoe E, Flensted-Jensen E, Olesen KH, eds. *Symposium on cardiac arrhythmias.* Sodertalje, Sweden: Astra, 1970:449–501.

110. Task Force of the Working Group on Arrhythmias of the European Society of Cardiology. The Sicilian Gambit. A new approach to the classification of antiarrhythmic drugs based on their actions on arrhythmogenic mechanisms. *Circulation* 1991;84:1831–1851.

111. Perry JC. Pharmacologic therapy of arrhythmias. In: Deal BJ, Wolff G, Gelband H, eds. *Current concepts in diagnosis and management of arrhythmias in infants and children.* Armonk, NY: Futura Publishing, 1998:267–305.

112. Deal KK, England SK, Tamkun MM. Molecular physiology of cardiac potassium channels. *Physiol Rev* 1996;76:49–67.

113. Barry DM, Nerbonne JM. Myocardial potassium channels: Electrophysiological and molecular diversity. *Annu Rev Physiol* 1996;58: 363–394.

114. Young M-L, Deal BJ, Wolff GS. Supraventricular tachycardia—electrophysiologic evaluation and treatment. In: Deal BJ, Wolff G, Gelband H, eds. *Current concepts in diagnosis and management of arrhythmias in infants and children.* Armonk, NY: Futura Publishing, 1998:145–179.

115. American Academy of Pediatrics Committee on Drugs. Drugs for pediatric emergencies. *Pediatrics* 1998;101:e13.

116. Deal BJ. Supraventricular tachycardia mechanisms and natural history. In: Deal BJ, Wolff G, Gelband H, eds. *Current concepts in diagnosis and management of arrhythmias in infants and children.* Armonk, NY: Futura Publishing, 1998:117–143.

117. Cilliers AM, du Plessis JP, Clur S-AB, Dateling F, Levin SE. Junctional ectopic tachycardia in six paediatric patients. *Heart* 1997;78: 413–415.

118. Garson A Jr, Gillette PC. Junctional ectopic tachycardia in children: Electrocardiography, electrophysiology and pharmacologic response. *Am J Cardiol* 1979;44:298–302.

119. Ludomirsky A, Garson A Jr. Supraventricular tachycardia. In: Gillette PC, Garson A Jr, eds. *Pediatric arrhythmias: Electrophysiology and pacing.* Philadelphia: WB Saunders, 1990;380–426.

120. Pfammatter J-P, Stocker FP. Re-entrant supraventricular tachycardia in infancy: Current role of prophylactic digoxin treatment. *Eur J Pediatr* 1998;157:101–106.

121. Friedman FD. Intraosseus adenosine for the termination of supraventricular tachycardia in an infant. *Ann Emerg Med* 1996;28:356–358.

122. Luedtke SA, Kuhn RJ, McCaffrey FM. Pharmacologic management of supraventricular tachycardias in children. Part 2: Atrial flutter, atrial fibrillation, and atrial ectopic tachycardia. *Ann Pharmacother* 1997;31:1347–1359.

123. Paret G, Steinmetz D, Kuint J, Hegesh J, Frand M, Barzilay Z. Adenosine for the treatment of paroxysmal supraventricular tachycardia in full-term and preterm newborn infants. *Am J Perinatol* 1996;13:343–346.

124. Smits P, Lenders JW, T T. Caffeine and theophylline attenuate adenosine-induced vasodilation in humans. *Clin Pharmacol Ther* 1990;48:410–418.

125. Berul CI. Higher adenosine dosage required for supraventricular tachycardia in infants treated with theophylline. *Clin Pediatr* 1993;32:167–168.

126. Moak JP. Pharmacology and electrophysiology of antiarrhythmic drugs. In: Gillette PC, Garson A Jr, eds. *Pediatric arrhythmias: Electrophysiology and pacing.* Philadelphia: WB Saunders, 1990:37–115.

127. Reidenberg MM, Drayer DE, Levy M, Warner H. Polymorphic acetylation of procainamide in man. *Clin Pharmacol Ther* 1975;17:722–730.

128. Lemner MS, Schaffer MS. Neonatal supraventricular tachycardia: Predictors of successful treatment withdrawal. *Am Heart J* 1997;133:130–131.

129. Byrum CJ, Wahl RA, Behrendt DM, MacDonald D. Ventricular fibrillation associated with the use of digitalis in the newborn infant with Wolff–Parkinson–White syndrome. *J Pediatr* 1982;101:400–403.

130. Niese AS, Shand DG. Clinical pharmacology of propranolol. *Circulation* 1975;52:6–15.

131. Epstein ML, Kiel EA, Victorica BE. Cardiac decompensation following verapamil therapy in infants with supraventricular tachycardia. *Pediatrics* 1985;75:737–740.

132. Mason JW. Amiodarone. *N Engl J Med* 1987;316:455–466.

133. Kodama I, Kamiya K, Toyama J. Cellular electropharmacology of amiodarone. *Cardiovasc Res* 1997;35:13–29.

134. Keeton BR, Bucknall CA, Curry PVL, Joseph MC, Sutherland GR, Holt DW. Use of amiodarone in childhood. *Br J Clin Pract* 1986;44(Suppl):115–120.

135. Ardura J, Hermoso F, Bermejo J. Effect on growth of children with cardiac dysrhythmias treated with amiodarone. *Pediatr Cardiol* 1988;9:33–36.

136. Daniels CJ, Schutte DA, Hammond S, Franklin WH. Acute pulmonary toxicity in an infant from intravenous amiodarone. *Am J Cardiol* 1997;80:1113–1116.

137. Perry JC, Fenrich AL, Hulse JE, Triedman JK, Friedman RA, Lamberti JJ. Pediatric use of intravenous amiodarone: Efficacy and safety in critically ill patients from a multicenter protocol. *J Am Coll Cardiol* 1996;27:1246–1250.

138. Dodo H, Gow RM, Hamilton RM, Freedom RM. Chaotic atrial rhythm in children. *Am Heart J* 1995;129:990–995.

139. Fish FA, Mehta AV, Johns JA. Characteristics and management of chaotic atrial tachycardia of infancy. *Am J Cardiol* 1996;78:1052–1055.

140. Bouillon T, Schiffmann H, Bartmus D, Gundert-Remy U. Amiodarone in a newborn with ventricular tachycardia and an intracardiac tumor: Adjusting the dose according to an individualized dosing regimen. *Pediatr Cardiol* 1996;17:112–114.

141. Rosenberg EM, Elbl F, Solinger RE, Palakurthy P, Rees AH. Neonatal refractory supraventricular tachycardia: Successful treatment with amiodarone. *South Med J* 1988;81:539–540.

142. Chen RP-C, Ignaszewski AP, Robertson MA. Successful treatment of supraventricular tachycardia-induced cardiomyopathy with amiodarone: Case report and review of literature. *Can J Cardiol* 1995;11:918–922.

143. Fenrich AL Jr, Perry JC, Friedman RA. Flecainide and amiodarone: Combined therapy for refractory tachyarrhythmias in infancy. *J Am Coll Cardiol* 1995;25:1195–1198.

144. Vrobel TR, Miller PE, Mostow ND, Rakita L. A general overview of amiodarone toxicity: Its prevention, detection, and management. *Prog Cardiovasc Dis* 1989;31:393–426.

145. Kannan R, Yabek SM, Garson A Jr, Miller S, McVey P, Singh BN. Amiodarone efficacy in a young population: Relationship to serum amiodarone and desethylamiodarone levels. *Am Heart J* 1987;114:283–287.

146. Strunge P, Frandsen J, Andreasen F. Amiodarone during pregnancy. *Eur Heart J* 1988;9:106–109.

147. Magee LA, Downar E, Sermer M, Boulton BC, Allen LC, Koren G. Pregnancy outcome after gestational exposure to amiodarone in Canada. *Am J Obstet Gynecol* 1995;172:1307–1311.

148. De Wolf D, De Schepper J, Verhaaren H, Deneyer M, Smitz J, Sacre-Smits L. Congenital hypothyroid goiter and amiodarone. *Acta Paediatr Scand* 1988;77:616–618.

149. Tubman R, Jenkins J, Lim J. Neonatal hyperthyroxinaemia associated with maternal amiodarone therapy: Case report. *Ir J Med Sci* 1988;157:243.

150. Laurent M, Betremieux P, Biron Y, LeHelloco A. Neonatal hypothyroidism after treatment by amiodarone during pregnancy (letter). *Am J Cardiol* 1987;60:942.

151. Volpe JJ. Neonatal seizures. *Neurology of the newborn,* 2nd ed. Philadelphia: WB Saunders, 1987:129–157.

152. Pellock JM. Efficacy and adverse effects of antiepileptic drugs. *Pediatr Clin North Am* 1989;36:435–448.

153. Gilman JT, Gal P, Duchowny MS, Weaver RL, Ransom JL. Rapid sequential phenobarbital treatment of neonatal seizures. *Pediatrics* 1989;83:674–678.

154. Painter MJ, Pippenger C, McDonald H, Pitlick W. Phenobarbital and diphenylhydantoin levels in neonates with seizures. *J Pediatr* 1978;92:315–319.

155. Gal P, Toback J, Boer HR, Erkan NV, Wells TJ. Efficacy of phenobarbital monotherapy treatment of neonatal seizures—relationship to blood levels. *Neurology* 1982;32:1401–1404.

156. Fischer JH, Lockman LA, Zaske D, Kriel R. Phenobarbital maintenance dose requirements in treating neonatal seizures. *Neurology* 1981;31:1042–1044.

157. Farwell J, Lee Y, Hirtz D, Sulzbacher S, Ellenberg J, Nelson K. Phenobarbital for febrile seizures—effects on intelligence and on seizure recurrence. *N Engl J Med* 1990;322:364–369.

158. Meador KJ, Loring DW, Huh K, Gallagher BB, King DW. Comparative cognitive effects of anticonvulsants. *Neurology* 1990;40:391–394.

159. American Academy of Pediatrics Committee on Drugs. Behavioral and cognitive effects of anticonvulsant therapy. *Pediatrics* 1985;76:644–647.

160. Albani M, Wernicke I. Oral phenytoin in infancy: Dose requirement, absorption, and elimination. *Pediatr Pharmacol* 1983;3:229–236.

161. Tozer TN, Winter ME. Phenytoin. In: Evans W, Schentag J, Jusko W, eds. *Applied pharmacokinetics: Principles of therapeutic drug monitoring,* 3rd ed, vol 25. Vancouver: Applied Therapeutics, 1992:1–44.

162. Ehrnebo M, Agurell S, Jalling B, Boreus LO. Age differences in drug binding by plasma proteins: Studies on human foetuses, neonates, and adults. *Eur J Clin Pharmacol* 1971;3:189–193.

163. Fredholm BB, Rane A, Persson B. Diphenylhydantoin binding to proteins in plasma and its dependence on free fatty acid and bilirubin concentration in dogs and newborn infants. *Pediatr Res* 1975;9:26–30.

164. Whelan HT, Hendeles L, Haberkern CM, Neims AH. High intravenous phenytoin dosage requirement in a newborn infant. *Neurology* 1983;33:106–108.

165. Leff RD, Fischer LJ, Roberts RJ. Phenytoin metabolism in infants following intravenous and oral administration. *Dev Pharmacol Ther* 1986;9:217–223.

166. Louis S, Kutt H, McDowell F. The cardiovascular changes caused by intravenous Dilantin and its solvent. *Am Heart J* 1967;74:523–529.

167. Fierro LS, Savulich DH, Benezra DA. Safety of fosphenytoin sodium. *Am J Health–Syst Pharm* 1996;53:2707–2712.

168. Deshmukh A, Wittert W, Schnitzler E, Mangurten HH. Lorazepam in the treatment of refractory neonatal seizures. A pilot study. *Am J Dis Child* 1986;140:1042–1044.

169. Maytal J, Novak GP, King KC. Lorazepam in the treatment of refractory neonatal seizures. *J Child Neurol* 1991;6:319–323.

170. McDermott CA, Kowalczyk AL, Schnitzler ER, Mangurten HH, Rodvold KA, Metrick S. Pharmacokinetics of lorazepam in critically ill neonates with seizures. *J Pediatr* 1992;120:479–483.

171. Sexson WR, Thigpen J, Stajich GV. Stereotypic movements after lorazepam administration in premature neonates: A series and review of the literature. *J Perinatol* 1995;15:146–149.

172. Chess PR, D'Angio CT. Clonic movements following lorazepam administration in full-term infants. *Arch Pediatr Adolesc Med* 1998;152:98–99.

173. Kumar A, Bleck TP. Intravenous midazolam for the treatment of refractory status epilepticus. *Crit Care Med* 1992;20:483–488.

174. Lahat E, Aladjem M, Eshel G, Bistritzer T, Katz Y. Midazolam in treatment of epileptic seizures. *Pediatr Neurol* 1992;8:215–216.

175. Sheth RD, Buckley DJ, Gutierrez AR, Gingold M, Bodensteiner JB, Penney S. Midazolam in the treatment of refractory neonatal seizures. *Clin Neuropharmacol* 1996;19:165–170.

176. Jacqz-Aigrain E, Daoud P, Burtin P, Maherzi S, Beaufils F. Pharmacokinetics of midazolam during continuous infusion in critically ill neonates. *Eur J Clin Pharmacol* 1992;42:329–332.

177. Grawe G, Ward RM. Seizure-like activity following bolus administration of midazolam to neonates. *Clin Res* 1994;42:16A.

178. Scher MS, Painter MJ. Controversies concerning neonatal seizures. *Pediatr Clin North Am* 1989;36:281–310.

179. Sinaiko AR, Mirkin BL. Clinical pharmacology of antihypertensive drugs in children. *Pediatr Clin North Am* 1978;25:137–157.

180. Task Force on Blood Pressure Control in Children. Report of the second task force on blood pressure control in children—1987. *Pediatrics* 1987;79:1–25.

181. Inouye IK, Massie BM, Benowitz N, Simpson P, Loge D. Antihypertensive therapy with diltiazem and comparison with hydrochlorothiazide. *Am J Cardiol* 1984;53:1588–1592.

182. Bauer SB, Feldman SM, Gellis SS, Retik AB. Neonatal hypertension. A complication of umbilical-artery catheterization. *N Engl J Med* 1975;293:1032–1033.

183. Nahata MC, Morosco RS, Hipple TF. Stability of captopril in three liquid dosage forms. *Am J Hosp Pharm* 1994;51:95–96.

184. O'Dea RF, Mirkin BL, Alward CT, Sinaiko AR. Treatment of neonatal hypertension with captopril. *J Pediatr* 1988;113:403–406.

185. Tack ED, Perlman JM. Renal failure in sick hypertensive premature infants receiving captopril therapy. *J Pediatr* 1988;112:805–810.

186. Romankiewicz JA, Brogden RN, Heel RC, Speight TM, Avery GS. Captopril: an update review of its pharmacological properties and therapeutic efficacy in congestive heart failure. *Drugs* 1983;25:6–40.

187. Starr SE. Antimicrobial therapy of bacterial sepsis in the newborn infant. *J Pediatr* 1985;106:1043–1048.

188. Powell KR, Pincus PH. Five years of experience with the exclusive use of amikacin in a neonatal intensive care unit. *Pediatr Infect Dis J* 1987;6:461–466.

189. Krediet TG, Fleer A, Gerards LJ. Development of resistance to aminoglycosides among coagulase-negative staphylococci and enterobacteriaceae in a neonatal intensive care unit. *J Hosp Infect* 1993;24:39–46.

190. Braveny I, Dickert H. *In vitro* activity of cefotaxime against gentamicin and mezlocillin resistant strains. *Lancet* 1979;2:1023–1024.

191. Modi N, Damjanovic V, Cooke RWI. Outbreak of cephalosporin resistant *Enterobacter cloacae* infection in a neonatal intensive care unit. *Arch Dis Child* 1987;62:148–151.

192. Bryan CS, John JF Jr, Pai MS, Austin TL. Gentamicin vs. cefotaxime for therapy of neonatal sepsis. Relationship to drug resistance. *Am J Dis Child* 1985;139:1086–1089.

193. Word BM, Klein JO. Therapy of bacterial sepsis and meningitis in infants and children: 1989 poll of directors of programs in pediatric infectious diseases. *Pediatr Infect Dis J* 1989;8:635–637.

194. Placzek M, Whitelaw A, Want S, Sahathevan M, Darrell J. Piperacillin in early neonatal infection. *Arch Dis Child* 1983;58:1006–1009.

195. Eichenwald HF. Antimicrobial therapy in infants and children: Update 1976–1985. Part II. *J Pediatr* 1985;107:337–345.

196. Jones RN, Thornsberry C, Barry AL, Fuchs PC, Gavan TL, Gerlach EH. Piperacillin (T-1220), a new semisynthetic penicillin. *In vitro* antimicrobial activity comparison with carbenicillin, ticarcillin, ampicillin, cephalothin, cefamandole, and cefoxitin. *J Antibiot* 1977;30:1107–1114.

197. Jones RN, Packer RR, Barry AL, Badal RE, Thornsbery C, Baker C. Piperacillin (T-1220), a new semisynthetic penicillin. II. *In vitro* antimicrobial activity and synergy comparison with carbenicillin and gentamicin. *J Antibiot* 1979;32:29–35.

198. Kacet N, Roussel-Delvallez M, Gremillet C, Dubos JP, Storme L, Lequien P. Pharmacokinetic study of piperacillin in newborns relating to gestational and postnatal age. *Pediatr Infect Dis J* 1992;11:365–369.

199. Sanders CC. Beta-lactamases of gram-negative bacteria: New challenges for new drugs. *Clin Infect Dis* 1992;14:1089–1099.

200. Sanders WE Jr, Sanders CC. Piperacillin/tazobactam: A critical review of the evolving clinical literature. *Clin Infect Dis* 1996;22:107–123.

201. Hickey SM, McCracken GH Jr. Antibacterial therapeutic agents. In: Feigin RD, Cherry JD, eds. *Textbook of pediatric infectious diseases*, 4th ed. Philadelphia: WB Saunders, 1998.

202. Clark AM, Zemcov SJ. Clavulanic acid in combination with ticarcillin: An *in vitro* comparison with other beta-lactams. *J Antimicrob Chemother* 1984;13:121–128.

203. Pillay T, Pillay DG, Adhikari M, Sturm AW. Piperacillin/tazobactam in the treatment of *Klebsiella pneumoniae* infections in neonates. *Am J Perinatol* 1998;15:47–51.

204. Banner WJ Jr, Gooch WM III, Burckart G, Korones SB. Pharmacokinetics of nafcillin in infants with low birth weights. *Antimicrob Agents Chemother* 1980;17:691–694.

205. McCracken GH Jr. Use of third-generation cephalosporins for treatment of neonatal infections (editorial). *Am J Dis Child* 1985;139:1079–1080.

206. Kafetzis DA, Brater DC, Kapiki AN, Papas CV, Dellagramaticas H, Papadatos CJ. Treatment of severe neonatal infections with cefotaxime: Efficacy and pharmacokinetics. *J Pediatr* 1982;100:483–489.

207. Spritzer R, van der Kamp HJ, Dzoljic G, Sauer PJ. Five years of cefotaxime use in a neonatal intensive care unit. *Pediatr Infect Dis J* 1990;9:92–96.

208. Heusser MF, Patterson JE, Kuritza AP, Edberg SC, Baltimore RS. Emergence of resistance to multiple beta-lactams in *Enterbacter cloacae* during treatment for neonatal meningitis with cefotaxime. *Pediatr Infect Dis* 1990;9:509–512.

209. Van Reempts PJ, Van Overmeire B, Mahieu LM, Vanacker KJ. Clinical experience with ceftriaxone treatment in the neonate. *Chemotherapy* 1995;41:316–322.

210. Schaad UB. Transient transformation of precipitations in the gallbladder associated with ceftriaxone therapy. *Pediatr Infect Dis J* 1986;5:708–710.

211. Martin E, Fanconi S, Kälin P, et al. Ceftriaxone–bilirubin–albumin interactions in the neonate: An *in vivo* study. *Eur J Pediatr* 1993;152:530–534.

212. Gulian JM, Gonard V, Dalmasso C, Palix C. Bilirubin displacement by ceftriaxone in neonates: Evaluation by determination of "free" bilirubin and erythrocyte-bound bilirubin. *J Antimicrob Chemother* 1987;19:823–829.

213. Barriere SL. Bacterial resistance to beta-lactams, and its prevention with combination antimicrobial therapy. *Pharmacotherapy* 1992;12:397–402.

214. Gerceker AA, Gürler B. *In vitro* activities of various antibiotics, alone and in combination with amikacin against *Pseudomonas aeruginosa*. *J Antimicrob Chemother* 1995;36:707–711.

215. de Louvois J, Dagan R, Tessin I. A comparison of ceftazidime and aminoglycoside based regimen as empirical treatment in 1316 cases of suspected sepsis in the newborn. European Society for Paediatric Infectious Diseases–Neonatal Sepsis Study Group. *Eur J Pediatr* 1992;151:876–884.

216. van den Anker JN, Schoemaker RC, Hop WCJ, et al. Ceftazidime pharmacokinetics in preterm infants: Effects of renal function and gestational age. *Clin Pharmacol Ther* 1995;58:650–659.

217. van den Anker JN, Hop WCJ, Shoemaker RC, van der Heijden BJ, Neijens HJ, deGroot R. Ceftazidime pharmacokinetics in preterm infants: Effect of postnatal age and postnatal exposure to indomethacin. *Br J Clin Pharmacol* 1995;40:439–443.

218. van den Anker JN, van der Heijden BJ, Hop WCJ, et al. The effect of asphyxia on the pharmacokinetics of ceftazidime in the term newborn. *Pediatr Res* 1995;38:808–811.

219. Snelling S, Hart CA, Cooke RWI. Ceftazidime or gentamicin plus benzylpenicillin in neonates less than forty-eight hours old. *J Antimicrob Chemother* 1983;12(Suppl A):353–356.

220. Reish O, Ashkenazi S, Naor N, Samra Z, Merlob P. An outbreak of multiresistant *Klebsiella* in a neonatal intensive care unit. *J Hosp Infect* 1993;25:287–291.

221. Weinstein RA. Endemic emergence of cephalosporin-resistant *Enterobacter:* Relation to prior therapy. *Infect Control* 1986;7:120–123.

222. Bradley JS. Meropenem: A new, extremely broad spectrum beta-lactam antibiotic for serious infections in pediatrics. *Pediatr Infect Dis J* 1997;16:263–268.

223. Craig WA. The pharmacology of meropenem, a new carbapenem antibiotic. *Clin Infect Dis* 1997;24(Suppl 2):S266–S275.

224. Klugman KP, Dagan R. Carbapenem treatment of meningitis. *Scand J Infect Dis [Suppl]* 1995;96:45–48.

225. Klugman KP, Dagan R. Randomized comparison of meropenem with cefotaxime for treatment of bacterial meningitis. Meropenem Meningitis Study Group. *Antimicrob Agents Chemother* 1995;39:1140–1146.

226. Norrby SR. Neurotoxicity of carbapenem antibacterials. *Drug Safety* 1996;15:87–90.

227. Wong VK, Wright H Jr, Ross LA, Mason WH, Inderlied CB, Kim KS. Imipenem/cilastatin treatment of bacterial meningitis in children. *Pediatr Infect Dis J* 1991;10:122–125.

228. Semel JD, Allen N. Seizures in patients simultaneously receiving theophylline and imipenem or ciprofloxacin or metronidazole. *South Med J* 1991;84:465–468.

229. Arrieta A. Use of meropenem in the treatment of serious infections in children: Review of the current literature. *Clin Infect Dis* 1998;24 (Suppl 2):S207–S212.

230. Nalin DR, Jacobsen CA. Imipenem/cilastatin therapy for serious infections in neonates and infants. *Scand J Infect Dis [Suppl]* 1987;52:46–55.

231. Stuart RL, Turnidge J, Grayson ML. Safety of imipenem in neonates. *Pediatr Infect Dis J* 1995;14:804–805.

232. Blumer JL. Pharmacokinetic derminants of carbapenem therapy in neonates and children. *Pediatr Infect Dis J* 1996;15:733–737.

233. Stutman HR. Clinical experience with aztreonam for treatment of infections in children. *Rev Infect Dis* 1991;13(Suppl 7):S582–S585.

234. Cuzzolin L, Fanos V, Zambreri D, Padovani EM, Benoni G. Pharmacokinetics and renal tolerance of aztreonam in premature infants. *Antimicrob Agents Chemother* 1991;35:1726–1728.

235. Umaña MA, Odio CM, Castro E, Salas JL, McCracken GH Jr. Evaluation of aztreonam and ampicillin v. amikacin and ampicillin for treatment of neonatal bacterial infections. *Pediatr Infect Dis J* 1990;9:175–180.

236. McNeeley DF, Saint-Louis F, Noel GJ. Neonatal enterococcal bacteremia: An increasingly frequent event with potentially untreatable pathogens. *Pediatr Infect Dis J* 1996;15:800–805.

237. Centers for Disease Control and Prevention. Nosocomial enterococci resistant to vancomycin-United States, 1989–1993. *MMWR* 1993;42:597–599.

238. McNeeley DF, Brown AE, Noel GJ, Chung M, De Lencastre H. An investigation of vancomycin-resistant *Enterococcus faecium* within the pediatric service of a large urban medical center. *Pediatr Infect Dis J* 1998;17:184–188.

239. Möller JC, Nachtrodt G, Richter A, Tegtmeyer FK. Prophylactic vancomycin to prevent staphylococcal septicaemia in very-low-birth-weight infants (letter). *Lancet* 1992;340:424.

240. Baier RJ, Bocchini JA Jr, Brown EG. Selective use of vancomycin to prevent coagulase-negative staphylococcal nosocomial bacteremia in high risk very low birth weight infants. *Pediatr Infect Dis J* 1998;17:179–183.

241. Centers for Disease Control and Prevention. Recommendations for preventing the spread of vancomycin resistance. *MMWR* 1995;44:1–19.

242. Bailie GR, Neal D. Vancomycin ototoxicity and nephrotoxicity. A review. *Med Toxicol Adv Drug Exp* 1988;3:376–386.

243. Rybak MJ, Albrecht LM, Boike SC, Chandrasekar PH. Nephrotoxicity of vancomycin, alone and with an aminoglycoside. *J Antimicrob Chemother* 1990;25:679–687.

244. Farber BF, Moellering RC Jr. Retrospective study of the toxicity of preparations of vancomycin from 1974 to 1981. *Antimicrob Agents Chemother* 1983;23:138–141.

245. Wilhelm MP. Vancomycin. *Mayo Clin Proc* 1991;66:1165–1170.

246. Freeman CD, Quintiliani R, Nightingale CH. Vancomycin therapeutic drug monitoring: Is it necessary? *Ann Pharmacother* 1993;27:594–598.

247. Moellering RC Jr. Monitoring serum vancomycin levels: Climbing the mountain because it is there? (editorial). *Clin Infect Dis* 1994;18:544–546.

248. Cantú TG, Yamanaka-Yuen NA, Lietman PS. Serum vancomycin concentrations: Reappraisal of their clinical value. *Clin Infect Dis* 1994;18:533–543.

249. Thomas MP, Steele RW. Monitoring serum vancomycin concentrations in children: Is it necessary? *Pediatr Infect Dis J* 1998;17:351–352.

250. Saunders NJ. Why monitor peak vancomycin concentrations? *Lancet* 1994;344:1748–1750.

251. Gous AGS, Dance MD, Lipman J, Luyt DK, Mathivha R, Scribante J. Changes in vancomycin pharmacokinetics in critically ill infants. *Anaesth Intens Care* 1995;23:678–682.

252. Reed MD, Kliegman RM, Weiner JS, Huang M, Yamashita TS, Blumer JL. The clinical pharmacology of vancomycin in seriously ill preterm infants. *Pediatr Res* 1987;22:360–363.

253. Schaad UB, McCraken GH Jr, Nelson JD. Clinical pharmacology and efficacy of vancomycin in pediatric patients. *J Pediatr* 1980;96:119–126.

254. Naqvi SH, Keenan WJ, Reichley RM, Fortune KP. Vancomycin pharmacokinetics in small, seriously ill infants. *Am J Dis Child* 1986;140:107–110.

255. Wandstrat TL, Phelps SJ. Vancomycin dosing in neonatal patients: The controversy continues. *Neonat Netw* 1994;13:33–39.

256. Levy M, Koren G, Dupuis L, Read SE. Vancomycin-induced red man syndrome. *Pediatrics* 1990;86:572–580.

257. Barclay ML, Begg EJ, Hickling KG. What is the evidence for once-daily aminoglycoside therapy? *Clin Pharmacokinet* 1994;27:32–48.

258. Isemann BT, Kotagal UR, Mashni SM, Luckhaupt EJ, Johnson CJ. Optimal gentamicin therapy in preterm neonates includes loading doses and early monitoring. *Ther Drug Monit* 1996;18:549–555.

259. Kapusnik JE, Hackbarth CJ, Chambers HF, Carpenter T, Sande MA. Single, large, daily dosing versus intermittent dosing of tobramycin for treating experimental pseudomonas pneumonia. *J Infect Dis* 1988;158:7–12.

260. Vogelman B, Craig WA. Kinetics of antimicrobial activity. *J Pediatr* 1986;108:835–840.

261. Freeman CD, Nicolau DP, Belliveau PP, Nightingale CH. Once-daily dosing of aminoglycosides: Review and recommendations for clinical practice. *J Antimicrob Chemother* 1997;39:677–686.

262. Zhanel GG, Craig WA. Pharmacokinetic contributions to postantibiotic effects: Focus on aminoglycosides. *Clin Pharmacokinet* 1994;27:377–392.

263. Isaksson B, Nilsson L, Maller R, Sörén L. Postantibiotic effect of aminoglycosides on gram-negative bacteria evaluated by a new method. *J Antimicrob Chemother* 1988;22:23–33.

264. Verpooten GA, Giuliano RA, Verbist L, Eestermans G, De Broe ME. Once-daily dosing decreases renal accumulation of gentamicin and netilmicin. *Clin Pharmacol Ther* 1989;45:22–27.

265. Munckhof WJ, Grayson ML, Turnidge JD. A meta-analysis of studies on the safety and efficacy of aminoglycosides given either once daily or as divided doses. *J Antimicrob Chemother* 1996;37:645–663.

266. Skopnik H, Heimann G. Once daily aminoglycoside dosing in full term neonates. *Pediatr Infect Dis J* 1995;14:71–72.

267. Hayani KC, Hatzopoulos FK, Frank AL, et al. Pharmacokinetics of once-daily dosing of gentamicin in neonates. *J Pediatr* 1997;131:76–80.

268. Ettlinger JJ, Bedford KA, Lovering AM, Reeves DS, Speidel BD, MacGowan AP. Pharmacokinetics of once-a-day netilmicin (6 mg/kg) in neonates. *J Antimicrob Chemother* 1996;38:499–505.

269. Leape LL, Holder TM, Franklin JD, Amoury RA, Ashcraft KW. Respiratory arrest in infants secondary to gastroesophageal reflux. *Pediatrics* 1977;60:924–928.

270. Hampton FJ, MacFadyen UM, Beardsmore CS, Simpson H. Gastro-oesophageal reflux and respiratory function in infants with respiratory symptoms. *Arch Dis Child* 1991;66:848–853.

271. Spitzer AR, Boyle JT, Tuchman DN, Fox WW. Awake apnea associated with gastroesophageal reflux: A specific clinical syndrome. *J Pediatr* 1984;194:200–205.

272. Paton JY, Macfadyen U, Williams A, Simpson H. Gastro-oesophageal reflux and apnoeic pauses during sleep in infancy—no direct relation. *Eur J Pediatr* 1990;149:680–686.

273. Sutphen JL, Dillard VL. Effects of maturation and gastric acidity on gastroesophageal reflux in infants. *Am J Dis Child* 1986;140:1062–1064.

274. Weihrauch TR. Gastro-oesophageal reflux—pathogenesis and clinical implications. *Eur J Pediatr* 1985;144:215–218.

275. Cucchiara S, Staiano A, Di Lorenzo C, De Luca G, della Rocca A, Auricchio S. Pathophysiology of gastroesophageal reflux and distal esophageal motility in children with gastroesophageal reflux disease. *J Pediatr Gastrenterol Nutr* 1988;7:830–836.

276. Skopnik H, Silny J, Heiber O, Schulz J, Rau G, Heimann G. Gastro-sophageal reflux in infants: Evaluation of a new intraluminal impedance technique. *J Pediatr Gastroenterol Nutr* 1996;23:591–598.

277. Ewer AK, Durbin GM, Morgan MEI, Booth IW. Gastric emptying and gastro-oesophageal reflux in preterm infants. *Arch Dis Child* 1996;75:F117–F121.

278. Marcon MA. Advances in the diagnosis and treatment of gastroesophageal reflux disease. *Curr Opin Pediatr* 1997;9:490–493.

279. Ward RM, Lemons JA, Molteni RA. Cisapride: A survey of frequency of use and adverse events in premature newborns. *Pediatrics* 1999;103:469–472.

280. Euler AR. Use of bethanechol for the treatment of gastroesophageal reflux. *J Pediatr* 1980;96:321–324.

281. Strickland AD, Chang JHT. Results of treatment of gastroesophageal reflux with bethanechol. *J Pediatr* 1983;103:311–315.

282. Sondheimer JM, Mintz HL, Michaels M. Bethanechol treatment of gastroesophageal reflux in infants: Effect on continuous esophageal pH records. *J Pediatr* 1984;104:128–131.

283. Schulze-Delrieu K. Metoclopramide. *N Engl J Med* 1981;305:28–33.

284. Sankaran K, Yeboah E, Bingham WT, Ninan A. Use of metoclopramide in preterm infants. *Dev Pharmacol Ther* 1982;5:114–119.

285. Tolia V, Calhoun J, Kuhns L, Kauffman RE. Randomized, prospective double-blind trial of metoclopramide and placebo for gastroesophageal reflux in infants. *J Pediatr* 1989;115:141–145.

286. Machida HM, Forbes DA, Gall DG, Scott RB. Metoclopramide in gastroesophageal reflux in infancy. *J Pediatr* 1988;112:483–487.

287. Hyams JS, Leichtner AM, Zamett LO, Walters JK. Effect of metoclopramide on prolonged intraesophageal pH testing in infants with gastroesophageal reflux. *J Pediatr Gastroenterol* 1986;5:716–720.

288. Kearns GL, van den Anker JN, Reed MD, Blumer JL. Pharmacokinetics of metoclopramide in neonates. *J Clin Pharmacol* 1998;38:122–128.

289. Vandenplas Y, Ashkenazi A, Belli D, et al. A proposition for the diagnosis and treatment of gastro-oesophageal reflux disease in children: a report from a working group on gastro-oesophageal reflux disease. *Eur J Pediatr* 1993;152:704–711.

290. Vandenplas Y, Belli D, Benhamou P-H, et al. Current concepts and issues in the management of regurgitation of infants: A reappraisal. *Acta Paediatr* 1996;85:531–534.

291. Cucchiara S. Cisapride therapy for gastrointestinal disease. *J Pediatr Gastroenterol Nutr* 1996;22:259–269.

292. Wiseman LR, Faulds D. Cisapride: an updated review of its pharmacology and therapeutic efficacy as a prokinetic agent in gastrointestinal motility disorders. *Drugs* 1994;47:116–152.

293. Lewin MB, Bryant RM, Fenrich AL, Grifka RG. Cisapride-induced long QT interval. *J Pediatr* 1996;128:279–281.

294. Hill SL, Evangelista JK, Pizzi AM, Mobassaleh M, Fulton DR, Berul CI. Proarrhythmia associated with cisapride in children. *Pediatrics* 1998;101:1053–1056.

295. Napolitano C, Priori SG, Schwartz PJ. Torsade de pointes mechanisms and management. *Drugs* 1994;47:51–65.

296. Bran S, Murray WA, Hirsch IB, Palmer JP. Long QT syndrome during high-dose cisapride. *Arch Intern Med* 1995;155:765–768.

297. Tan HL, Hou CJY, Lauer MR, Sung RJ. Electrophysiologic mechanisms of the long QT interval syndromes and torsade de pointes. *Ann Intern Med* 1995;122:701–714.

298. Carlsson L, Amos GJ, Andersson B, Drews L, Duker G, Wadstedt G. Electrophysiological characterization of the prokinetic agents cisapride and mosapride *in vivo* and *in vitro*: implications for proarrhythmic potential? *J Pharmacol Exp Ther* 1997;282:220–227.

299. Daleau P, Lessard E, Groleau M-F, Turgeon J. Erythromycin blocks the rapid component of the delayed rectifier potassium current and lengthens repolarization of guinea pig ventricular myocytes. *Circulation* 1995;91:3010–3016.

300. Klausner M. *Dear Doctor. Important safety and efficacy information.* Janssen Pharmaceutica Research Foundation, June 26, 1998.

301. Schwartz PJ, Stramba-Badiale M, Segantini A, et al. Prolongation of the QT interval and the sudden infant death syndrome. *N Engl J Med* 1998;338:1709–1714.

302. Bonikos DI, Bensch KG, Northway WH Jr, Edwards DK. Bronchopulmonary dysplasia: the pulmonary pathologic sequelae of necrotizing bronchiolitis and pulmonary fibrosis. *Hum Pathol* 1976;7:643–666.

303. Yuksel B, Greenough A. Effect of nebulized salbutamol in preterm infants during the first year of life. *Eur Respir J* 1991;4:1088–1092.

304. Pfenninger J, Aebi C. Respiratory response to salbutamol (albuterol) in ventilator-dependent infants with chronic lung disease: Pressurized aerosol delivery versus intravenous injection. *Intens Care Med* 1993;19:251–255.

305. Gappa M, Gärtner M, Poets CF, von der Hardt H. Effects of salbutamol delivery from a metered dose inhaler versus jet nebulizer on dynamic lung mechanics in very preterm infants with chronic lung disease. *Pediatr Pulmonol* 1997;23:442–448.

306. Lee H, Arnon S, Silverman M. Bronchodilator aerosol administered by metered dose inhaler and spacer in subacute neonatal respiratory distress syndrome. *Arch Dis Child* 1994;70:F218–F222.

307. Stefano JL, Bhutani VK, Fox WW. A randomized placebo-controlled study to evaluate the effects of oral albuterol on pulmonary mechanics in ventilator-dependent infants at risk of developing BPD. *Pediatr Pulmonol* 1991;10:183–190.

308. Denjean A, Guimaraes H, Migdal M, Miramand JL, Dehan M, Gaultier C. Dose-related bronchodilator response to aerosolized salbutamol (albuterol) in ventilator-dependent premature infants. *J Pediatr* 1992;120:974–979.

309. Kirpalani H, Koren G, Schmidt B, Tan Y, Santos R, Soldin S. Respiratory response and pharmacokinetics of intravenous salbutamol in infants with bronchopulmonary dysplasia. *Crit Care Med* 1990;18:1374–1377.

310. Kao LC, Warburton D, Platzker ACG, Keens TG. Effect of isoproterenol inhalation on airway resistance in chronic bronchopulmonary dysplasia. *Pediatrics* 1984;73:509–514.

311. Sosulski R, Abbasi S, Bhutani VK, Fox WW. Physiologic effects of terbutaline on pulmonary function of infants with bronchopulmonary dysplasia. *Pediatr Pulmonol* 1986;2:269–273.

312. Gomez-Del Rio M, Gerhadt T, Hehre D, Feller R, Bancalari E. Effect of a beta-agonist nebulization on lung function in neonates with increased pulmonary resistance. *Pediatr Pulmonol* 1986;2:287–291.

313. Wilkie RA, Bryan MH. Effect of bronchodilators on airway resistance in ventilator-dependent neonates with chronic lung disease. *J Pediatr* 1987;111:278–282.

314. Cabal LA, Larrazabal C, Ramanathan R, et al. Effects of metaproterenol on pulmonary mechanics, oxygenation, and ventilation in infants with chronic lung disease. *J Pediatr* 1987;110:116–119.

315. Rotschild A, Solimano A, Puterman M, Smyth J, Sharma A, Albersheim S. Increased compliance in response to salbutamol in premature infants with developing bronchopulmonary dysplasia. *J Pediatr* 1989;115:984–991.

316. Kao LC, Durand DJ, Nickerson BG. Effects of inhaled metaproterenol and atropine on the pulmonary mechanics of infants with bronchopulmonary dysplasia. *Pediatr Pulmonol* 1989;6:74–80.

317. Motoyama EK, Fort MD, Klesh KW, Mutich RL, Guthrie RD. Early onset of airway reactivity in premature infants with bronchopulmonary dysplasia. *Am Rev Respir Dis* 1987;136:50–57.

318. Brundage KL, Mohsini KG, Froese AB, Fisher JT. Bronchodilator response to ipratropium bromide in infants with bronchopulmonary dysplasia. *Am Rev Respir Dis* 1990;142:1137–1142.

319. Kraemer R, Birrer P, Schöni MH. Dose–response relationships and time course of the response to systemic beta adrenoreceptor agonists in infants with bronchopulmonary dysplasia. *Thorax* 1988;43:770–776.

320. Grigg J, Arnon S, Jones T, Clarke A, Silverman M. Delivery of therapeutic aerosols to intubated babies. *Arch Dis Child* 1992;67:25–30.

321. Fuller HD, Dolovich MB, Posmituck G, Pack WW, Newhouse MT. Pressurized aerosol versus jet aerosol delivery to mechanically ventilated patients. Comparison of dose to the lungs. *Am Rev Respir Dis* 1990;141:440–444.

322. MacIntyre NR, Silver RM, Miller CW, Schuler F, Coleman RE. Aerosol delivery in intubated, mechanically ventilated patients. *Crit Care Med* 1985;13:81–84.

323. Lugo RA, Kenney JK, Keenan J, Salyer JW, Ballard J, Ward RM. Albuterol delivery in a neonatal ventilator–lung model. *Pediatrics* 1998;102(Suppl Pt 2):703.

324. Jackson EK. Diuretics. In: Hardman JG, Limbird LE, Molinoff PB, Ruddon RW, Goodman-Gilman A, eds. *Goodman and Gilman's the pharmacological basis of therapeutics,* 9th ed. New York: McGraw-Hill, 1996:685–713.

325. Green T. The pharmacologic basis of diuretic therapy in the newborn. *Clin Perinatol* 1987;14:951–964.

326. Chemtob S, Kaplan BS, Sherbotie JR, Aranda JV. Pharmacology of diuretics in the newborn. *Pediatr Clin North Am* 1989;36:1231–1250.

327. Brater DC. Determinants of the overall response to furosemide: pharmacokinetics and pharmacodynamics. *Fed Proc* 1983;42:1711–1713.

328. Schrier RW, Lehman D, Zacherele B, Earley LE. Effect of furosemide on free water excretion in edematous patients with hyponatremia. *Kidney Int* 1973;3:30–34.

329. Vert P, Broquaire M, Legagneur M, Morselli PL. Pharmacokinetics of furosemide in neonates. *Eur J Clin Pharmacol* 1982;22:39–45.

330. Englehardt B, Elliott S, Hazinski TA. Short- and long-term effects of furosemide on lung function in infants with bronchopulmonary dysplasia. *J Pediatr* 1986;109:1034–1039.

331. Najak ZD, Harris EM, Lazzara A Jr, Pruitt AW. Pulmonary effects of furosemide in preterm infants with lung disease. *J Pediatr* 1983;102:758–763.

332. Green TP, Thompson TR, Johnson DE, Lock JE. Furosemide promotes patent ductus arteriosus in premature infants with the respiratory-distress syndrome. *N Engl J Med* 1983;308:743–748.

333. Yeh TF, Wilks A, Singh J, Betkerur M, Lilien L, Pildes RS. Furosemide prevents the renal side effects of indomethacin therapy in premature infants with patent ductus arteriosus. *J Pediatr* 1982;101:433–437.

334. Brater DC. Resistance to loop diuretics: why it happens and what to do about it. *Drugs* 1985;30:427–443.

335. Rybak LP. Furosemide ototoxicity: Clinical and experimental aspects. *Laryngoscope* 1985;95(Part II, Suppl 38):1–14.

336. Flamenbaum W, Friedman R. Pharmacology, therapeutic efficacy, and adverse effects of bumetanide, a new "loop" diuretic. *Pharmacotherapy* 1982;2:213–222.

337. Shannon DC, Gotay F. Effects of theophylline on serum and urine electrolytes in preterm infants with apnea. *J Pediatr* 1979;94:963–965.

338. Cook DJ, Witt LG, Cook RJ, Guyatt GH. Stress ulcer prophylaxis in the critically ill: A meta-analysis. *Am J Med* 1991;91:519–527.

339. Cook DJ, Fuller HD, Guyatt GH, et al. Risk factors for gastrointestinal bleeding in critically ill patients. *N Engl J Med* 1994;330:377–381.

340. Cook D, Guyatt G, Marshall J, et al. A comparison of sucralfate and ranitidine for the prevention of upper gastrointestinal bleeding in patients requiring mechanical ventilation. Canadian Critical Care Trials Group. *N Engl J Med* 1998;338:791–797.

341. Lopez-Herce J, Dorao P, Elola P, Delgado MA, Ruza F, Madero SR. Frequency and prophylaxis of upper gastrointestinal hemorrhage in critically ill children: A prospective study comparing the efficacy of almagate, ranitidine, and sucralfate. The Gastrointestinal Hemorrhage Study Group. *Crit Care Med* 1992;20:1082–1089.

342. Lacroix J, Nadeau D, Laberge S, Gauthier M, Lapierre G, Farrell CA. Frequency of upper gastrointestinal bleeding in a pediatric intensive care unit. *Crit Care Med* 1992;20:35–42.

343. Mäki M, Ruuska T, Kuusela AL, Karikoski-Leo R, Ikonen RS. High prevalence of asymptomatic esophageal and gastric lesions in preterm infants in intensive care. *Crit Care Med* 1993;21:1863–1867.

344. Kuusela AL, Ruuska T, Karikoski R, et al. A randomized, controlled study of prophylactic ranitidine in preventing stress-induced gastric mucosal lesions in neonatal intensive care unit patients. *Crit Care Med* 1997;25:346–351.

345. Black JW, Duncan WA, Durant CJ, Ganellin CR, Parsons EM. Definition and antagonism of histamine H₂-receptors. *Nature* 1972;236:385–390.

346. Smith K, Crisp C. Clinical comparison of H₂-antagonists. *Conn Med* 1986;50:815–817.

347. Hansten PD. *Drug interactions and updates.* Vancouver: Applied Therapeutics, 1990.

348. Powell JR, Donn KH. Histamine H₂-antagonist drug interactions in perspective: Mechanistic concepts and clinical implications. *Am J Med* 1984;77(Suppl 5B):57–84.

349. Fenje PC, Isles AF, Baltodano A, MacLeod SM, Soldin S. Interaction of cimetidine and theophylline in two infants. *Can Med Assoc J* 1982;126:1178.

350. Peterson WL, Richardson CT. Intravenous cimetidine or two regimens of ranitidine to reduce fasting gastric acidity. *Ann Intern Med* 1986;104:505–507.

351. Zeldis JB, Friedman LS, Isselbacher KJ. Ranitidine: A new H₂-receptor antagonist. *N Engl J Med* 1983;309:1368–1373.

352. Rosenthal M, Miller PW. Ranitidine in the newborn. *Arch Dis Child* 1988;63:88–89.

353. Blumer JL, Rothstein FC, Kaplan BS, et al. Pharmacokinetic determination of ranitidine pharmacodynamics in pediatric ulcer disease. *J Pediatr* 1985;107:301–306.

354. Zinner MJ, Zuidema GD, Smith PL, Mignosa M. The prevention of upper gastrointestinal tract bleeding in patients in an intensive care unit. *Surg Gynecol Obstet* 1981;153:214–220.

355. Kelly EJ, Chatfield SL, Brownlee KG, et al. The effect of intravenous ranitidine on the intragastric pH of preterm infants receiving dexamethasone. *Arch Dis Child* 1993;69:37–39.

356. Mallet E, Mouterde O, Dubois F, Flipo JL, Moore N. Use of ranitidine in young infants with gastro-oesophageal reflux. *Eur J Clin Pharmacol* 1989;36:641–642.

357. Fontana M, Massironi E, Rossi A, et al. Ranitidine pharmacokinetics in newborn infants. *Arch Dis Child* 1993;68:602–603.

358. James LP, Kearns GL. Pharmacokinetics and pharmacodynamics of famotidine in paediatric patients. *Clin Pharmacokinet* 1996;31:103–110.

359. Driscoll DJ. Use of inotropic and chronotropic agents in neonates. *Clin Perinatol* 1987;14:931–941.

360. Lefkowitz RJ, Hoffman BB, Taylor P. Neurotransmission: The autonomic and somatic motor nervous systems. In: Hardman JG, Limbird LE, Molinoff PB, Ruddon RW, Goodman-Gilman A, eds. *Goodman and Gilman's the pharmacological basis of therapeutics,* 9th ed. McGraw Hill;1996:105–139.

361. Zaritsky A, Chernow B. Use of catecholamines in pediatrics. *J Pediatr* 1984;105:341–350.

362. Hoffman BB, Lefkowitz RJ. Catecholamines and sympathomimetic drugs, and adrenergic receptor antagonists. In: Hardman JG, Limbird LE, Molinoff PB, Ruddon RW, Goodman-Gilman A, eds. *Goodman and Gilman's the pharmacological basis of therapeutics,* 9th ed. New York: McGraw-Hill, 1996:199–248.

363. Rude RE, Bush LR, Izquierdo C, Buja LM, Willerson JT. Effects of inotropic and chronotropic stimuli on acute myocardial ischemic injury. III. Influence of basal heart rate. *Am J Cardiol* 1984;53:1688–1694.

364. Driscoll DJ, Gillette PC, Lewis RM, Hartley CJ, Schwartz A. Comparative hemodynamic effects of isoproterenol, dopamine, and dobutamine in the newborn dog. *Pediatr Res* 1979;13:1006–1009.

365. Fiser DH, Fewell JE, Hill DE, Brown AL. Cardiovascular and renal effects of dopamine and dobutamine in healthy, conscious piglets. *Crit Care Med* 1988;16:340–345.

366. Perez CA, Reimer JM, Schreiber MD, Warburton D, Gregory GA. Effect of high-dose dopamine on urine output in newborn infants. *Crit Care Med* 1986;14:1045–1049.

367. Siwy BK, Sadove AM. Acute management of dopamine infiltration injury with Regitine. *Plast Reconstr Surg* 1987;80:610–612.

368. Seri I, Tulassay T, Kiszel J, Machay T, Csomor S. Cardiovascular response to dopamine in hypotensive preterm neonates with severe hyaline membrane disease. *Eur J Pediatr* 1984;142:3–9.

369. Tuttle RR, Mills J. Dobutamine: Development of a new catecholamine to selectively increase cardiac contractility. *Circ Res* 1975;36:185–196.

370. Ruffolo RR Jr, Yaden EL. Vascular effects of the stereoisomers of dobutamine. *J Pharmacol Exp Ther* 1983;224:46–50.

371. Martinez AM, Padbury JF, Thio S. Dobutamine pharmacokinetics and cardiovascular responses in critically ill neonates. *Pediatrics* 1992;89:47–51.

372. Greenough A, Emery EF. Randomized trial comparing dopamine and dobutamine in preterm infants. *Eur J Pediatr* 1993;152:925–927.

373. Klarr JM, Faix RG, Pryce CJE, Bhatt-Mehta V. Randomized, blind trial of dopamine versus dobutamine for treatment of hypotension in preterm infants with respiratory distress syndrome. *J Pediatr* 1994;125:117–122.

374. Stopfkuchen H, Schranz D, Huth R, Jungst B-K. Effects of dobutamine on left ventricular performance in newborns as determined by systolic time intervals. *Eur J Pediatr* 1987;146:135–139.

375. Stopfkuchen H, Queisser-Luft A, Vogel K. Cardiovascular responses to dobutamine determined by systolic time intervals in preterm infants. *Crit Care Med* 1990;18:722–724.

376. Smith TW. Digitalis. Mechanisms of action and clinical use. *N Engl J Med* 1988;318:358–365.

377. Berman W, Yabek SM, Dillon T, Niland C, Carlew S, Christensen D. Effects of digoxin in infants with a congested circulatory state due to a ventricular septal defect. *N Engl J Med* 1983;308:363–366.

378. Lang D, von Bernuth G. Serum concentration and serum half-life of digoxin in premature and mature newborns. *Pediatrics* 1977;59:902–906.

379. Steiness E. Renal tubular secretion of digoxin. *Circulation* 1974;50:103–107.

380. Hastreiter AR, van der Horst RL, Voda C, Chow-Tung E. Maintenance digoxin dosage and steady-state plasma concentration in infants and children. *J Pediatr* 1985;107:140–146.

381. Ingelfinger JA, Goldman P. The serum digitalis concentration—does it diagnose digitalis toxicity? *N Engl J Med* 1976;294:867–870.

382. Lindenbaum J, Rund DG, Butler VP Jr, Tse-Eng D, Saha JR. Inactivation of digoxin by the gut flora: Reversal by antibiotic therapy. *N Engl J Med* 1981;305:789–794.

383. Waldorff S, Andersen JD, Heeboll-Nielsen N, et al. Spironolactone-induced changes in digoxin kinetics. *Clin Pharmacol Ther* 1978;24:162–167.

384. Smith TW, Butler VP, Haber E, et al. Treatment of life-threatening digitalis intoxication with digoxin-specific Fab antibody fragments: experience in 26 cases. *N Engl J Med* 1982;307:1357–1362.

385. Seccombe DW, Pudek MR, Whitfield MF, Jacobson BE, Wittmann BK, King JF. Perinatal changes in a digoxin-like immunoreactive substance. *Pediatr Res* 1984;18:1097–1099.

386. Valdes R Jr. Endogenous digoxin-immunoreactive factor in human subjects. *Fed Proc* 1985;44:2800–2805.

387. Mathews WR, DuCharme DW, Hamlyn JM, et al. Mass spectral characterization of an endogenous digitalislike factor from human plasma. *Hypertension* 1991;17:930–935.

388. Bova S, Blaustein MP, Ludens JH, Harris DW, DuCharme DW, Hamlyn JM. Effects of an oubainlike compound on heart and aorta. *Hypertension* 1991;17:944–950.

389. Aranda JV, Lopes JM, Blanchard P, Eyal F, Alpan G. Drug treatment of neonatal apnea. In: Yaffe SJ, Aranda JV, eds. *Pediatric pharmacology: therapeutic principles in practice,* 2nd ed. Philadelphia: WB Saunders, 1992:193–204.

390. Runold M, Lagercrantz H, Fredholm BB. Ventilatory effect of an adenosine analogue in unanesthetized rabbits during development. *J Appl Physiol* 1986;61:255–259.

391. Aubier M, De Troyer A, Sampson M, Macklem PT, Roussos C. Aminophylline improves diaphragmatic contractility. *N Engl J Med* 1981;305:249–252.

392. Serafin WE. Drugs used in the treatment of asthma. In: Hardman JG, Limbird LE, Molinoff PB, Ruddon RW, Goodman-Gilman A, eds. *Goodman & Gilman's the pharmacological basis of therapeutics,* 9th ed. New York: McGraw-Hill, 1996:659–682.

393. Kuzemko JA, Paala J. Apnoeic attacks in the newborn treated with aminophylline. *Arch Dis Child* 1973;48:404–406.

394. Shannon DC, Gotay F, Stein IM, Rogers MC, Todres ID, Moylan FM. Prevention of apnea and bradycardia in low-birthweight infants. *Pediatrics* 1975;55:589–594.

395. Uauy R, Shapiro DL, Smith B, Warshaw JB. Treatment of severe apnea in prematures with orally adminstered theophylline. *Pediatrics* 1975;55:595–598.

396. Cordoba E, Gerhardt T, Rojas M, Duara S, Bancalari E. Comparison of the effects of acetazolamide and aminophylline on apnea incidence and on ventilatory response to CO_2 in preterm infants. *Pediatr Pulmonol* 1994;17:291–295.

397. Barrington KJ, Finer NN. A randomized, controlled trial of aminophylline in ventilatory weaning of premature infants. *Crit Care Med* 1993;21:846–850.

398. Roberts JL, Mathew OP, Thach BT. The efficacy of theophylline in premature infants with mixed and obstructive apnea associated with pulmonary and neurologic disease. *J Pediatr* 1982;100:968–970.

399. Harris MC, Baumgart S, Rooklin AR, Fox WW. Successful extubation of infants with respiratory distress syndrome using aminophylline. *J Pediatr* 1983;103:303–305.

400. Peabody JL, Neese AL, Philip AG, Lucey JF, Soyka LF. Transcutaneous oxygen monitoring in aminophylline treated apneic infants. *Pediatrics* 1978;62:698–701.

401. Myers TF, Milsap RL, Krauss AN, Auld PA, Reidenberg MM. Low-dose theophylline therapy in idiopathic apnea of prematurity. *J Pediatr* 1980;96:99–103.

402. Aranda JV, Louridas AT, Vitullo B, Thom P, Aldridge A, Haber R. Metabolism of theophylline to caffeine in human fetal liver. *Science* 1979;206:1319–1321.

403. Bory C, Baltassat P, Porthault M, Bethenod M, Frederich A, Aranda JV. Metabolism of theophylline to caffeine in premature newborn infants. *J Pediatr* 1979;94:988–993.

404. Bada HS, Khanna NN, Somani SM, Tin AA. Interconversion of theophylline and caffeine in newborn infants. *J Pediatr* 1979;94:993–995.

405. Boutroy MJ, Vert P, Royer RJ, Monin P, Royer-Morrot MJ. Caffeine, a metabolite of theophylline during the treatment of apnea in the premature infant. *J Pediatr* 1979;94:996–998.

406. Dothey CI, Tserng KY, Kaw S, King KC. Maturational changes of theophylline pharmacokinetics in preterm infants. *Clin Pharmacol Ther* 1989;45:461–468.

407. Marquis JF, Carruthers SG, Spence JD, Brownstone YS, Toogood JH. Phenytoin–theophylline interaction. *N Engl J Med* 1982;307:1189–1190.

408. Kraemer MJ, Furukawa CT, Koup JR, Shapiro GG, Pierson WE, Bierman CW. Altered theophylline clearance during an influenza B outbreak. *Pediatrics* 1982;69:476–480.

409. Prince RA, Wing DS, Weinberger MM, Hendeles LS, Riegelman S. Effect of erythromycin on theophylline kinetics. *J Allergy Clin Immunol* 1981;68:427–431.

410. Fernandes E, Melewicz FM. Ranitidine and theophylline (letter). *Ann Intern Med* 1984;100:459.

411. Gardner ME, Sikorski GW. Ranitidine and theophylline (letter). *Ann Intern Med* 1985;102:559.

412. Aranda JV, Grondin D, Sasyniuk B. Pharmacologic considerations in the therapy of neonatal apnea. *Pediatr Clin North Am* 1981;28:113–133.

413. Roberts RJ. Methylxanthine therapy: Caffeine and theophylline. In: *Drug therapy in infants. Pharmacologic principles and clinical experience.* Philadelphia: WB Saunders, 1984:119–137.

414. Bairam A, Boutroy MJ, Badonnel Y, Vert P. Theophylline versus caffeine: Comparative effects in treatment of idiopathic apnea in the preterm infants. *J Pediatr* 1987;110:636–639.

415. Brouard C, Moriette G, Murat I, et al. Comparative efficacy of theophylline and caffeine in the treatment of idiopathic apnea in premature infants. *Am J Dis Child* 1985;139:698–700.

416. Larsen PB, Brendstrup L, Skov L, Flachs H. Aminophylline versus caffeine for apnea and bradycardia prophylaxis in premature neonates. *Acta Paediatr* 1995;84:360–364.

417. Raval DS, Yeh TF. Apnea. In: Yeh T, ed. *Drug therapy in the neonate and small infant.* Chicago: Year Book Medical Publishers, 1985:57–71.

418. Aranda JV, Gorman W, Bergsteinsson H, Gunn T. Efficacy of caffeine in treatment of apnea in the low-birth-weight infant. *J Pediatr* 1977;90:467–472.

419. Scanlon JE, Chin KC, Morgan ME, Durbin GM, Hale KA, Brown SS. Caffeine or theophylline for neonatal apnoea? *Arch Dis Child* 1992;67:425–428.

420. Rothberg AD, Marks KH, Ward RM, Maisels MJ. The metabolic effects of caffeine in the newborn infant. *Pediatr Pharmacol* 1981;1:181–186.

421. Le Guennec J-C, Billon B, Pare C. Maturational changes of caffeine concentrations and disposition in infancy during maintenance therapy for apnea of prematurity: Influence of gestational age, hepatic disease, and breast-feeding. *Pediatrics* 1985;76:834–840.

422. Wakamatsu A, Umetsu M, Motoya H, Nakao T. Change of plasma half-life of caffeine during therapy for apnea in premature infants. *Acta Paediatr Jpn* 1987;29:595–599.

423. Parsons WD, Neims AH. Prolonged half-life of caffeine in healthy term newborn infants. *J Pediatr* 1981;98:640–641.

424. Costarino AT, Polin RA. Neuromuscular relaxants in the neonate. *Clin Perinatol* 1987;14:965–989.

425. Larijani GE, Gratz I, Silverberg M, Jakobi AG. Clinical pharmacology of the neuromuscular blocking agents. *Ann Pharmacother* 1991;25:54–56.

426. Miller RD, Rupp SM, Fisher DM, Cronnelly R, Fahey MR, Sohn YJ. Clinical pharmacology of vecuronium and atracurium. *Anesthesiology* 1984;61:444–453.

427. Gronert BJ, Brandom BW. Neuromuscular blocking drugs in infants and children. *Pediatr Clin North Am* 1994;41:73–91.

428. Bennett EJ, Ramamurthy S, Dalal FY, Salem MR. Pancuronium and the neonate. *Br J Anaesth* 1975;47:75–78.

429. Goudsouzian NG, Crone RK, Todres ID. Recovery from pancuronium blockade in the neonatal intensive care unit. *Br J Anaesth* 1981;53:1303–1309.

430. Meretoja OA. Is vecuronium a long-acting neuromuscular blocking agent in neonates and infants? *Br J Anaesth* 1989;62:184–187.

431. Bencini AF, Scaf AH, Sohn YJ, et al. Disposition and urinary excretion of vecuronium bromide in anesthetized patients with normal renal function or renal failure. *Anesth Analg* 1986;65:245–251.

432. Haynes SR, Morton NS. Prolonged neuromuscular blockade with vecuronium in a neonate with renal failure. *Anaesthesia* 1990;45:743–745.

433. Sinclair JF, Malcolm GA, Stephenson JB, Halworth D. Prolonged neuromuscular blockade in an infant. *Anaesthesia* 1987;49:1020.

434. Hilgenberg JC. Comparison of the pharmacology of vecuronium and atracurium with that of other currently available muscle relaxants. *Anesth Analg* 1983;62:524–531.

435. Meakin G, Shaw EA, Baker RD, Morris P. Comparison of atracurium-induced neuromuscular blockade in neonates, infants and children. *Br J Anaesth* 1988;60:171–175.

436. Kalli I, Meretoja OA. Infusion of atracurium in neonates, infants, and children. *Br J Anaesth* 1988;60:651–654.

437. Coceani F, Olley PM. Role of prostaglandins, prostacyclin, and thromboxanes in the control of prenatal patency and postnatal closure of the ductus arteriosus. *Semin Perinatol* 1980;4:109–113.

438. Freed MD, Heymann MA, Lewis AB, Roehl SL, Kensey RC. Prostaglandin E₁ in infants with ductus arteriosus-dependent congenital heart disease. *Circulation* 1981;64:899–905.

439. Lewis AB, Takahashi M, Lurie PR. Administration of prostaglandin E₁ in neonates with critical congenital cardiac defects. *J Pediatr* 1978;93:481–485.

440. Thanopoulos BD, Andreou A, Frimas C. Prostaglandin E₂ administration in infants with ductus-dependent cyanotic congenital heart disease. *Eur J Pediatr* 1987;146:279–282.

441. Monk JP, Clissold SP. Misoprostol: A preliminary review of its pharmacodynamic and pharmacokinetic properties, and therapeutic efficacy in the treatment of peptic ulcer disease. *Drugs* 1987;33:1–30.

442. Friedman WF, Hirschklau MJ, Printz MP, Pitlick PT, Kirkpatrick SE. Pharmacologic closure of patent ductus arteriosus in the premature infant. *N Engl J Med* 1976;295:526–529.

443. Gersony WM, Peckham GH, Ellison RC, Miettinen OS, Nadas AS. Effects of indomethacin in premature infants with patent ductus arteriosus: Results of a national collaborative study. *J Pediatr* 1983;102:895–906.

444. Bandstra ES, Mantalvo BM, Goldberg RN, et al. Prophylactic indomethacin for prevention of intraventricular hemorrhage in premature infants. *Pediatrics* 1988;82:533.

445. Merritt TA, Bejar R, Corazza M, Ikonen RS, Davis R, Rosenberg M. Clinical trials of intravenous indomethacin for closure of the patent ductus arteriosus. *Pediatr Cardiol* 1983;4(Suppl II):71–79.

446. Maher P, Lane B, Ballard R, Piecuch R, Clyman RI. Does indomethacin cause extension of intracranial hemorrhages: A preliminary study. *Pediatrics* 1985;75:497–500.

447. Wiest DB, Pinson JB, Gal PS, et al. Population pharmacokinetics of intravenous indomethacin in neonates with symptomatic patent ductus arteriosus. *Clin Pharmacol Ther* 1991;49:550–557.

448. Rhodes PG, Ferguson MG, Reddy NS, Joransen JA, Gibson J. Effects of prolonged versus acute indomethacin therapy in very low birth-weight infants with patent ductus arteriosus. *Eur J Pediatr* 1988;147:481–484.

449. McCarthy JS, Zies LG, Gelband H. Age-dependent closure of the patent ductus arteriosus by indomethacin. *Pediatrics* 1978;62:706–712.

450. Achanti B, Pyati S, Yeh TF. Indomethacin therapy in premature infants of advanced postnatal age. *J Perinatol* 1987;7:235–237.

451. Dibona GF. Prostaglandins and nonsteroidal anti-inflammatory drugs: Effects on renal hemodynamics. *Am J Med* 1986;80(Suppl 1A):12–21.

452. Cifuentes RF, Olley PM, Balfe JW, Radde IC, Soldin SJ. Indomethacin and renal function in premature infants with persistent patent ductus arteriosus. *J Pediatr* 1979;95:583–587.

453. Seri I, Tulassay T, Kiszel J, Csomor S. The use of dopamine for the prevention of the renal side effects of indomethacin in premature infants with patent ductus arteriosus. *Int J Pediatr Nephrol* 1984;5:209–214.

454. Walsh JJ, Venuto RC. Acute oliguric renal failure induced by indomethacin: Possible mechanism. *Ann Intern Med* 1979;91:47–49.

455. Clive DM, Stoff JS. Renal syndromes associated with nonsteroidal antiinflammatory drugs. *N Engl J Med* 1984;310:563–572.

456. Cowan F. Indomethacin, patent ductus arteriosus, and cerebral blood flow. *J Pediatr* 1986;109:341–344.

457. Colditz P, Murphy D, Rulfe P, Wilkinson AR. Effect of infusion rate of indomethacin on cerebral vascular responses in premature neonates. *Arch Dis Child* 1989;64:8–12.

458. Coombs RC, Morgan MEI, Durbin GM. Gut blood flow velocities in the newborn: Effects of patent ductus arteriosus and parenteral indomethacin. *Arch Dis Child* 1990;65:1067–1071.

459. Ward RM. Persistent pulmonary hypertension. In: Nelson NM, ed. *Current therapy in neonatal–perinatal medicine–2.* Toronto: BC Decker, 1990:331–338.

460. Abman SH, Chatfield BA, Hall SL, McMurtry IF. Role of endothelium-derived relaxing factor during transition of pulmonary circulation at birth. *Am J Physiol* 1990;259:H1921–H1927.

461. Shaul P. Ontogeny of nitric oxide in the pulmonary vasculature. *Semin Perinatol* 1997;21:381–392.

462. Palmer RMJ, Ferrige AG, Moncada S. Nitric oxide release accounts for the biological activity of endothelium-derived relaxing factor. *Nature* 1987;327:524–526.

463. McAndrew J, Patel RP, Jo H, et al. The interplay of nitric oxide and peroxynitrite with signal transduction pathways: Implications for disease. *Semin Perinatol* 1997;21:351–366.

464. Steinhorn RH, Morin FC III, Fineman JR. Models of persistent pulmonary hypertension of the newborn (PPHN) and the role of cyclic guanosine monophosphate (GMP) in pulmonary vasorelaxation. *Semin Perinatol* 1997;21:393–408.

465. Christou H, Adatia I, Van Marter LJ, et al. Effect of inhaled nitric oxide on endothelin-1 and cyclic guanosine 5'-monophosphate plasma concentrations in newborn infants with persistent pulmonary hypertension. *J Pediatr* 1997;130:603–611.

466. Nakajima W, Ishida A, Arai H, Takada G. Methaemoglobinaemia after inhalation of nitric oxide in infant with pulmonary hypertension. *Lancet* 1997;350:1002–1003.

467. Roberts JD Jr, Fineman JR, Morin FC III, et al. Inhaled nitric oxide and persistent pulmonary hypertension of the newborn. *N Engl J Med* 1997;336:605–610.

468. The Neonatal Inhaled Nitric Oxide Study Group. Inhaled nitric oxide in full-term and nearly full-term infants with hypoxic respiratory failure. *N Engl J Med* 1997;336:597–604.

469. Kinsella JP, Truog WE, Walsh WF, et al. Randomized, multicenter trial of inhaled nitric oxide and high-frequency oscillatory ventilation in severe, persistent pulmonary hypertension of the newborn. *J Pediatr* 1997;131:55–62.

470. Finer NN, Barrington KJ. Nitric oxide in respiratory failure in the newborn infant. *Semin Perinatol* 1997;21:426–440.

471. Nelin LD, Hoffman GM. The use of inhaled nitric oxide in a wide variety of clinical problems. *Pediatr Clin North Am* 1998;45:531–548.

472. Day RW, Lynch JM, White KS, Ward RM. Acute response to inhaled nitric oxide in newborns with respiratory failure and pulmonary hypertension. *Pediatrics* 1996;98:698–705.

473. Demirakca S, Dotsch J, Knothe C, et al. Inhaled nitric oxide in neonatal and pediatric acute respiratory distress syndrome: Dose response, prolonged inhalation and weaning. *Crit Care Med* 1996;24:1913–1919.

474. Nakagawa TA, Morris A, Gomez RJ, Johnston SJ, Sharkey PT, Zaritsky AL. Dose response to inhaled nitric oxide in pediatric patients with pulmonary hypertension and acute respiratory distress syndrome. *J Pediatr* 1997;131:63–69.

475. Lonnqvist PA. Inhaled nitric oxide in newborn and paediatric patients with pulmonary hypertension and moderate to severe impaired oxygenation: Effects of doses of 3–100 parts per million. *Intens Care Med* 1997;23:773–779.

476. Hallman M, Bry K, Turbow R, Waffarn F, Lappalainen U. Pulmonary toxicity associated with nitric oxide in term infants with severe respiratory failure. *J Pediatr* 1998;132:827–829.

477. Cheung P-Y, Salas E, Schulz R, Radomski MW. Nitric oxide and platelet function: Implications for neonatology. *Semin Perinatol* 1997;21:409–417.

478. Rosenberg AA, Kennaugh JM, Moreland SG, et al. Longitudinal follow-up of a cohort of newborn infants treated with inhaled nitric oxide for persistent pulmonary hypertension. *J Pediatr* 1997;131:70–75.

479. Kulik TJ, Lock JE. Pulmonary vasodilator therapy in persistent pulmonary hypertension of the newborn. *Clin Perinatol* 1984;11:693–701.

480. Ward RM, Green TP. Developmental pharmacology and toxicology: Principles of study design and problems of methodology. *Pharmacol Ther* 1988;36:309–334.

481. Peliowski A, Finer NN. A blinded, randomized, placebo-controlled trial to compare theophylline and doxapram for the treatment of apnea of prematurity. *J Pediatr* 1990;116:648–653.

482. Alpan G, Eyal F, Sagi E, Springer C, Patz D, Goder K. Doxapram in the treatment of idiopathic apnea of prematurity unresponsive to aminophylline. *J Pediatr* 1984;104:634–637.

483. Barrington KJ, Finer NN, Peters KL, Barton J. Physiologic effects of doxapram in idiopathic apnea of prematurity. *J Pediatr* 1986;108:124–129.

484. Bairam A, Akramoff-Gershan L, Beharry K, Laudiognon N, Papageorgiou A, Aranda JV. Gastrointestinal absorption of doxapram in neonates. *Am J Perinatol* 1991;8:110–113.

485. Tay-Uyboco J, Kwiatkowski K, Cates DB, Seifert B, Hasan SU, Rigatto H. Clinical and physiological responses to prolonged nasogastric administration of doxapram for apnea of prematurity. *Biol Neonate* 1991;59:190–200.

486. Bull DH, Wakeley A, Sola A. Current use of steroids in newborns with lung disease: Results of a national survey. *Pediatr Res* 1993;33:205A.

487. Merritt TA, Cochrane CG, Holcomb K, et al. Elastase and α_1-proteinase inhibitor activity in tracheal aspirates during respiratory distress syndrome: Role of inflammation in the pathogenesis of bronchopulmonary dysplasia. *J Clin Invest* 1983;72:656–666.

488. Groneck P, Götze-Speer B, Opperman M, Eiffert H, Speer C. Association of pulmonary inflammation and increased microvascular permeability during the development of bronchopulmonary dysplasia: a sequential analysis of inflammatory mediators in respiratory fluids of high-risk preterm neonates. *Pediatrics* 1994;93:712–718.

489. Groneck P, Götze-Speer B, Speer CP. Inflammatory bronchopulmonary response of preterm infants with microbial colonisation of the airways at birth. *Arch Dis Child* 1996;74:F51–F55.

490. Bagchi A, Viscardi RM, Taciak V, Ensor JE, McCrea KA, Hasday JD. Increased activity of interleukin-6 but not tumor necrosis factor-α in lung lavage of premature infants is associated with the development of bronchopulmonary dysplasia. *Pediatr Res* 1994;36:244–252.

491. Ogden BE, Murphy SA, Saunders GC, Pathak D, Johnson JD. Neonatal lung neutrophils and elastase/proteinase inhibitor imbalance. *Am Rev Respir Dis* 1984;130:817–821.

492. Schimmer BP, Parker KL. Adrenocorticotropic hormone; adrenocortical steroids and their synthetic analogs; inhibitors of the synthesis and actions of the adrenocortical hormones. In: Hardman JG, Limbird LE, Molinoff PB, Ruddon RW, Goodman-Gilman A, eds. *Goodman and Gilman's the pharmacological basis of therapeutics,* 9th ed. New York: McGraw-Hill, 1996:1459–1485.

493. Avery GB, Fletcher AB, Kaplan M, Brudno DS. Controlled trial of dexamethasone in respirator-dependent infants with bronchopulmonary dysplasia. *Pediatrics* 1985;75:106–111.

494. Harkavy KL, Scanlon JW, Chowdhry PK, Grylack LJ. Dexamethasone therapy for chronic lung disease in ventilator- and oxygen-dependent infants: A controlled trial. *J Pediatr* 1989;115:979–983.

495. Cummings JJ, D'Eugenio DB, Gross SJ. A controlled trial of dexamethasone in preterm infants at high risk for bronchopulmonary dysplasia. *N Engl J Med* 1989;320:1505–1510.

496. Kazzi NJ, Brans YW, Poland RL. Dexamethasone effects on the hospital course of infants with bronchopulmonary dysplasia who are dependent on artificial ventilation. *Pediatrics* 1990;86:722–727.

497. Collaborative Dexamethasone Trial Group. Dexamethasone therapy in neonatal chronic lung disease: an international placebo-controlled trial. *Pediatrics* 1991;88:421–427.

498. Ohlsson A, Calvert S, Hosking M, Shennan AT. Randomized controlled trial of dexamethasone treatment in very-low-birth-weight infants with ventilator-dependent chronic lung disease. *Acta Paediatr* 1992;81:751–756.

499. Jones R, Wincott E, Elbourne D, Grant A. Controlled trial of dexamethasone in neonatal chronic lung disease: A 3-year follow-up. *Pediatrics* 1995;96:897–906.

500. O'Shea TM, Kothadia JM, Klinepeter KL, Goldstein DJ, Jackson B, Dillard RG. Follow-up of preterm infants treated with dexamethasone for chronic lung disease. *Am J Dis Child* 1993;147:658–661.

501. Sanders RJ, Cox C, Phelps DL, Sinkin RA. Two doses of early intravenous dexamethasone for the prevention of bronchopulmonary dysplasia in babies with respiratory distress syndrome. *Pediatr Res* 1994;36:122–128.

502. Rastogi A, Akintorin SM, Bez ML, Morales P, Pildes RS. A controlled trial of dexamethasone to prevent bronchopulmonary dysplasia in surfactant-treated infants. *Pediatrics* 1996;98:204–210.

503. Durand M, Sardesai S, McEvoy C. Effects of early dexamethasone therapy on pulmonary mechanics and chronic lung disease in very low birth weight infants: a randomized, controlled trial. *Pediatrics* 1995;95:584–590.

504. Shinwell ES, Karplus M, Reich D, et al. Failure of early postnatal dex-

505. amethasone to prevent chronic lung disease in infants with respiratory distress syndrome. *Arch Dis Child* 1996;74:F33–F37.

505. Papile L, Tyson JE, Stoll BJ, et al. A multicenter trial of two dexamethasone regimens in ventilator-dependent premature infants. *N Engl J Med* 1998;338:1112–1118.

506. Yeh TF, Torre JA, Rastogi A, Anyebuno MA, Pildes RS. Early postnatal dexamethasone therapy in premature infants with severe respiratory distress syndrome: a double-blind, controlled study. *J Pediatr* 1990;117:273–282.

507. Noble-Jamieson CM, Regev R, Silverman M. Dexamethasone in neonatal chronic lung disease: pulmonary effects and intracranial complications. *Eur J Pediatr* 1989;148:365–367.

508. Skinner AM, Battin M, Solimano A, Daaboul J, Kitson HF. Growth and growth factors in premature infants receiving dexamethasone for bronchopulmonary dysplasia. *Am J Perinatol* 1997;14:539–546.

509. Smets K, Vanhaesebrouck P. Dexamethasone associated systemic hypertension in low birth weight babies with chronic lung disease. *Eur J Pediatr* 1996;155:573–575.

510. Marinelli KA, Burke GS, Herson VC. Effects of dexamethasone on blood pressure in premature infants with bronchopulmonary dysplasia. *J Pediatr* 1997;130:594–602.

511. Ng PC, Blackburn ME, Brownlee KG, Buckler JM, Dear PR. Adrenal response in very low birthweight babies after dexamethasone treatment for bronchopulmonary dysplasia. *Arch Dis Child* 1989;64:1721–1726.

512. Alkalay AL, Pomerance JJ, Puri AR, et al. Hypothalamic–pituitary–adrenal axis function in very low birth weight infants treated with dexamethasone. *Pediatrics* 1990;86:204–210.

513. Arnold JD, Leslie GI, Williams G, Rack P, Silink M. Adrenocortical responsiveness in neonates weaned from the ventilator with dexamethasone. *Aust Paediatr J* 1987;23:227–229.

514. Ford LR, Willi SM, Hollis BW, Wright NM. Suppression and recovery of the neonatal hypothalamic–pituitary–adrenal axis after prolonged dexamethasone therapy. *J Pediatr* 1997;131:722–726.

515. Ng PC, Wong GW, Lam CW, et al. Pituitary–adrenal suppression and recovery in preterm very low birth weight infants after dexamethasone treatment for bronchopulmonary dysplasia. *J Clin Endocrinol Metab* 1997;82:2429–2432.

516. Sauder SE, Powers WF, Wise JE. Suppression of pituitary–adrenal axis in very low birth weight infants after dexamethasone therapy for bronchopulmonary dysplasia (abstract). *Clin Res* 1987;35:913A.

517. Brand PL, van-Lingen RA, Brus F, Talsma MD, Elzenga NJ. Hypertrophic obstructive cardiomyopathy as a side effect of dexamethasone treatment for bronchopulmonary dysplasia. *Acta Paediatr* 1993;82:614–617.

518. Ohning BL, Fyfe DA, Riedel PA. Reversible obstructive hypertrophic cardiomyopathy after dexamethasone therapy for bronchopulmonary dysplasia. *Am Heart J* 1993;125:253–256.

519. Werner JC, Sicard RE, Hansen TW, Solomon E, Cowett RM, Oh W. Hypertrophic cardiomyopathy associated with dexamethasone therapy for bronchopulmonary dysplasia. *J Pediatr* 1992;120:286–291.

520. Israel BA, Sherman FS, Guthrie RD. Hypertrophic cardiomyopathy associated with dexamethasone therapy for chronic lung disease in preterm infants. *Am J Perinatol* 1993;10:307–310.

521. Ng PC, Fok TF, So KW, Wong W, Yip PK, Liu K. Lower gastrointestinal tract perforation in preterm infants treated with dexamethasone for bronchopulmonary dysplasia. *Pediatr Surg Int* 1997;12:211–212.

522. O'Neil EA, Chwals WJ, O'Shea MD, Turner CS. Dexamethasone treatment during ventilator dependency: Possible life threatening gastrointestinal complications. *Arch Dis Child* 1992;67:10–11.

523. Byyny RL. Withdrawal from glucocorticoid therapy. *N Engl J Med* 1976;295:30–32.

524. Brundage KL, Mohsini KG, Froese AB, Walker CR, Fisher JT. Dexamethasone therapy for bronchopulmonary dysplasia: improved respiratory mechanics without adrenal suppression. *Pediatr Pulmonol* 1992;12:162–169.

525. Wilson DM, Baldwin RB, Ariagno RL. A randomized, placebo-controlled trial of effects of dexamethasone on hypothalamic–pituitary–adrenal axis in preterm infants. *J Pediatr* 1988;113:764–768.

526. Rizvi ZB, Aniol HS, Myers TF, Zeller WP, Fisher SG, Anderson CL. Effects of dexamethasone on the hypothalamic–pituitary–adrenal axis in preterm infants. *J Pediatr* 1992;120:961–965.

527. Kari MA, Heinonen K, Ikonen RS, Koivisto M, Raivio KO. Dexam-

ethasone treatment in preterm infants at risk for bronchopulmonary dysplasia. *Arch Dis Child* 1993;68:566–569.

528. Kari MA, Raivio KO, Stenman UH, Voutilainen R. Serum cortisol, dehydroepiandrosterone sulfate, and steroid-binding globulins in preterm neonates: Effect of gestational age and dexamethasone therapy. *Pediatr Res* 1996;40:319–324.

529. Gumbinas M, Oda M, Huttenlocher P. The effects of corticosteroids on myelination of the developing rat brain. *Biol Neonate* 1973;22:355–366.

530. Cotterrell M, Balázs R, Johnson A. Effects of corticosteroids on the biochemical maturation of rat brain: postnatal cell formation. *J Neurochem* 1972;19:2151–2167.

531. Weichsel M Jr. The therapeutic use of glucocorticoid hormones in the perinatal period: Potential neurological hazards. *Ann Neurol* 1977;2:364–366.

532. Yeh TF, Lin YJ, Lin CH, et al. Early postnatal (<12 hours) dexamethasone therapy for prevention of BPD in preterm infants with RDS—A two year follow-up study. *Pediatr Res* 1997;41:188A.

533. Gal P, Diaz PR, Ransom JL, Carlos RQ, Thorson DW. Beclomethasone for treating premature infants with bronchopulmonary dysplasia (letter). *J Pediatr* 1993;123:490–491.

534. LaForce WR, Brudno DS. Controlled trial of beclomethasone dipropionate by nebulization in oxygen- and ventilator-dependent infants. *J Pediatr* 1993;122:285–288.

535. Arnon S, Grigg J, Silverman M. Effectiveness of budesonide aerosol in ventilator-dependent preterm babies: A preliminary report. *Pediatr Pulmonol* 1996;21:231–235.

536. Dimitriou G, Greenough A, Giffin FJ, Kavadia V. Inhaled versus systemic steroids in chronic oxygen dependency of preterm infants. *Eur J Pediatr* 1997;156:51–55.

537. Giep T, Raibble P, Zuerlein T, Schwartz ID. Trial of beclomethasone dipropionate by metered-dose inhaler in ventilator-dependent neonates less than 1500 grams. *Am J Perinatol* 1996;13:5–9.

538. Yarbrough J, Mansfield LE, Ting S. Metered dose inhaler induced bronchospasm in asthmatic patients. *Ann Allergy* 1985;55:25–27.

539. Graff-Lonnevig V. Diurnal expiratory flow after inhalation of freons and fenoterol in childhood asthma. *J Allergy Clin Immunol* 1979;64:534–538.

540. Taylor GJ, Harris WS. Cardiac toxicity of aerosol propellants. *JAMA* 1970;214:81–85.

541. Roberts RJ, Knight ME. Pharmacology of vitamin E in the newborn. *Clin Perinatol* 1987;14:843–855.

542. Ehrenkranz RA, Bonta BW, Ablow RC, Warshaw JB. Amelioration of bronchopulmonary dysplasia after vitamin E administration. A preliminary report. *N Engl J Med* 1978;299:564–569.

543. Ehrenkranz RA, Ablow RC, Warshaw JB. Prevention of bronchopulmonary dysplasia with vitamin E administration during the acute stages of respiratory distress syndrome. *J Pediatr* 1979;95:873–878.

544. Hittner HM, Godio LB, Rudolph AJ, Adams JM, Garcia-Prats JA, Friedman Z. Retrolental fibroplasia: efficacy of vitamin E in a double-blind clinical study of preterm infants. *N Engl J Med* 1981;305:1365–1371.

545. Phelps DL. Local and systemic reactions to the parenteral administration of vitamin E. *Dev Pharmacol Ther* 1981;2:156–171.

546. Centers for Disease Control. Unusual syndrome with fatalities among premature infants: association with a new intravenous vitamin E product. *MMWR* 1984;33:198–199.

547. Bodenstein CJ. Intravenous vitamin E and deaths in the intensive care unit (letter). *Pediatrics* 1984;73:733.

548. Balistreri WF, Farrell MK, Bove KE. Lessons from the E-Ferol tragedy. *Pediatrics* 1986;78:503–506.

549. Martone WJ, Williams WW, Mortensen ML, et al. Illness with fatalities in premature infants: Association with an intravenous vitamin-E preparation, E-Ferol. *Pediatrics* 1986;78:591–600.

550. American Academy of Pediatrics Committee on Fetus and Newborn. Vitamin E and the prevention of retinopathy of prematurity. *Pediatrics* 1985;76:315–316.

551. American Academy of Pediatrics Committee on Drugs. Transfer of drugs and other chemicals into human milk. *Pediatrics* 1994;93:137–150.

552. Berlin CM Jr. Pharmacologic considerations of drug use in the lactating mother. *Obstet Gynecol* 1981;58(Suppl):17S–23S.

553. Berlin CM Jr. The excretion of drugs in human milk. *Prog Clin Biol Res* 1980;36:115–127.

554. Berlin CM Jr. Drugs and chemicals: exposure of the nursing mother. *Pediatr Clin North Am* 1989;36:1089–1097.

CHAPTER 56

The Infant of the Drug-Dependent Mother

Enrique M. Ostrea, Jr., J. Edgar C. Posecion, and Maria Esterlita T. Villanueva

The problem of drug abuse has reached epidemic proportions during the past two decades, with increases not only in the number of drug users but also in the types of drugs abused. Equally alarming is the increase in the proportion of drugs users who are women of childbearing age or who are pregnant because the effects of drugs on the pregnancy and fetus can be significant. In this chapter, the latter are addressed; existing information in the literature on the maternal, neonatal, and long-term complications in infants of drug use during pregnancy is consolidated, and a brief historical and epidemiologic perspective on the problem is given. There are many instances in which the data presented are conflicting. This reflects the limitations of studies on the human population, because the confounding effects of many factors such as types of drugs used, socioeconomic status, environmental factors, parent education, and the like are difficult to identify accurately and control for.

EPIDEMIOLOGY

In 1996, the National Household Survey on Drug Abuse (1) estimated that approximately 13 million Americans were current illicit drug users (defined as the use of illicit drug in the month preceding the interview), which represents 6.1% of the population 12 years of age and older (Table 56–1). A decline in the incidence of drug use was observed over the past two decades. The rate of illicit drug use was highest in 1979 (15.4 million, 14.1%), declined in 1992 (12 million, 5.8%), and has remained at approximately the same level (6.1%) up to 1996. Among

E. M. Ostrea, Jr.: Department of Pediatrics, Wayne State University School of Medicine; and Department of Pediatrics, Hutzel Hospital, Detroit, Michigan

J. E. C. Posecion and M. E. T. Villanueva: Division of Neonatal–Perinatal Medicine, Department of Pediatrics, Wayne State University School of Medicine, Hutzel Hospital; and Children's Hospital of Michigan, Detroit, Michigan

the illicit drugs abused, marijuana used alone was the most common (54%), whereas use of marijuana and some other illicit drugs was 23%, and use of other illicit drugs without marijuana was 23%.

The rate of drug use varied substantially by age. It was 2.2% among youths aged 12 to 13 and was highest among young people 16 to 17 years old (15.6%) and 18 to 20 years old (20%). The rate of current illicit drug use was higher for blacks (7.5%) than for whites (6.1%) and Hispanics (5.2%), However, among the youths, the rate of use was the same for the three groups. As in prior years, men continue to have a higher rate of current illicit drug use than women (8.1% versus 4.2%). Illicit drug use remains highly correlated with educational status and employment. Those who did not complete a high school education had the highest rate of use (16.8%) compared to college graduates (6.9%). Similarly, the rate of illicit drug use was 12.5% among unemployed adults (18 years or older) compared to 6.2% of full-time employed adults.

Among women of childbearing age (15 to 44 years), it is estimated that about 4.1 million are current illicit drug users. Among women aged 14 to 44 years with no children who are not pregnant, 10% are current illicit drug users compared to 3.2% among pregnant women. This suggests that most women may reduce their drug use when pregnant. However, there is a resumption of illicit drug use after giving birth. Similar patterns are seen for alcohol and cigarette use. Among pregnant women, rates of substance use generally vary as they do among nonpregnant women (1.6% for marijuana, 0.5% for cocaine or crack, 0.2% for hallucinogens, 0.3% for heroin, 0.2% for stimulants, 16.1% for alcohol, and 20.3% for cigarettes). These rates were obtained exclusively from maternal interviews and are therefore highly underestimated. Rates are higher among women aged 15 to 25 years than among those 26 to 44 years, and they are higher among unmarried women than among married women. One exception to this pattern is in smoking rates by age. Non-

TABLE 56–1. *Estimated number and percentage of current illicit drug use in the United States population aged 12 years and older*[a]

Drug use	1979 ($N = 180,343$)[b]	1992 ($N = 205,713$)	1996 ($N = 214,532$)
1. Any illicit drug	14.1%	5.8%	6.1%
2. Marijuana	13.2%	4.7%	4.7%
3. Cocaine	2.6%	0.7%	0.7%
4. Hallucinogens	1.9%	0.4%	0.6%
5. PCP	—	0.0%	0.1%
6. Heroin	0.1%	0.1%	0.1%
7. Sedatives	—	0.2%	0.2%
8. Alcohol	63.2%	52.2%	51.0%
9. Cigarettes	—	31.9%	28.9%

[a]From the National Household Survey on Drug Abuse, 1996.
[b]In thousands.

pregnant women aged 15 to 25 years and those aged 26 to 44 years had about the same rates of smoking. However, among pregnant women, those aged 26 to 44 had a significantly lower past-month smoking rate than those aged 15 to 25 years, suggesting that older women smokers are more likely to reduce their smoking during pregnancy than are younger women smokers.

The true prevalence of illicit drug use among pregnant women is difficult to determine because of significant underreporting of drug use by these women. One study, based on a survey of predominantly urban hospitals, gave an estimate of drug use among pregnant women as 0.4% to 27%; cocaine use ranged from 0.2% to 17%. Drug detection was obtained by maternal history, urine toxicology, or both. With the use of a more sensitive drug-screening method (a meconium drug test), a 44% prevalence of illicit drug use in pregnant women in one high-risk center was found, in contrast to 11% by maternal self-report, and 30% of the infants were also positive for cocaine (2).

NARCOTICS

The term "opiate" or "narcotic" refers to any natural or synthetic drug that has morphine-like pharmacologic actions. The natural opiates include morphine and codeine, whereas the synthetic opiates include heroin, methadone, propoxyphene (Darvon), pentazocine (Talwin), meperidine (Demerol), oxycodone (Percodan, Tylox, Vecodine, Percocet), morphinone (Dilaudid), and fentanyl (Immovar, Sublimaze). Chronic use of narcotics, even in therapeutic doses, results in addiction, which is characterized by psychological as well as physical dependence on the drug.

History

Opium use probably dates back about 6,000 years (3). One of the earliest references to opiate complications in the perinatal period was made by Hippocrates, who mentioned "uterine suffocation" as possibly secondary to opium use (4). By the late 19th and early 20th centuries, reference to the passively addicted neonate is evident from reports describing the diffusion through the placenta and transmission through the breast milk of morphine (5).

The naturally occurring opiates, morphine and codeine, are derived from the seeds of the unripe poppy plant, *Papaver somniferum,* and were consumed for their narcotic and analgesic properties. Heroin (diacetylmorphine), a semisynthetic opioid, was first introduced in 1874. It became popular because of the rapid onset of its central nervous system (CNS) effects. By 1950, heroin had supplanted morphine as the drug of choice among abusers (6). It is available illicitly in bags containing up to 40 to 50 mg of the active ingredient, cut or diluted variably with quinine, lactose, starch, lidocaine, or even powdered milk. Methadone was first synthesized in 1945. It is longer-acting than heroin and can be administered orally. These properties render it the drug of choice for replacement–substitution therapy of heroin addicts undergoing detoxification. Since Dole and Nyswander advocated the use of methadone in maintenance treatment programs (7), it has become the most widely used and studied opiate in pregnancy.

Almost all narcotic drugs ingested by the female addict during pregnancy cross the placenta and enter the fetal circulation. Thus, the fetus is chronically exposed to these drugs and encounters problems *in utero* and after birth. Although the development of passive addiction to narcotic agents is the most widely known of these fetal complications, other major problems also are encountered (Table 56–2).

Antenatal Problems

Intrauterine asphyxia is perhaps the single greatest risk to the fetus of a drug-dependent woman. This is based on findings within this group of infants of a high incidence of stillbirths, meconium-stained amniotic fluid, fetal distress, low Apgar scores, and neonatal aspiration pneumonia (8–14). The predisposition of the fetus to asphyxia

TABLE 56–2. *Perinatal and long-term problems associated with abuse of narcotics during pregnancy*

Antenatal problems
    Intrauterine asphyxia
    Meconium-stained amniotic fluid
    Infection
    Abruptio placenta or placenta praevia
Neonatal problems
    Prematurity
    Low birth weight
    Small head circumference
    Small for gestational age
    Low Apgar score
    Jaundice
    Aspiration pneumonia
    Meconium aspiration syndrome
    Persistent pulmonary circulation of the newborn
    Transient tachypnea
    Hyaline membrane disease
    Congenital malformation
    Infection
    Thrombocytosis
    Abnormal auditory brainstem evoked response
    Abnormal sleep patterns
    Abnormal heart rate and breathing patterns
    Neurobehavioral effects
    Abstinence syndrome
Longterm outcome
    Persistence of withdrawal
    Sudden infant death syndrome
    Child abuse
    Small head circumference
    Behavioral problems, e.g., hyperactivity, impulsiveness, lack of inhibition and concentration
    School problems, e.g., truancy, school suspension

underscores the need for repeated evaluation of fetal well-being during the course of the pregnancy. Fetal asphyxia in the pregnant addict may be secondary to a number of factors. Studies using methadone in a fetal lamb model suggest that opiates affect both quiet and rapid-eye-movement (REM) sleep, which is associated with a hyperactive state that causes a 20% increase in fetal oxygen consumption (15). Sleep disturbances consisting of more REM and less quiet sleep have been demonstrated in newborn infants chronically exposed *in utero* to low doses of methadone with or without concomitant heroin usage (16,17). Another possible cause of fetal asphyxia is fetal withdrawal, which usually coincides with the mother's withdrawal. Because fetal withdrawal results in hyperactivity and increase in catecholamines, this increases the oxygen consumption of the fetus, which, if not adequately compensated for, leads to fetal asphyxia (18). In a fetal lamb model, withdrawal has been induced in the morphine-exposed lamb fetus by the administration of naloxone, an opiate antagonist. Manifestations included immediate bradycardia associated with transient increases in systolic and diastolic blood pressure; rapid, continuous deep breathing movements;

increased total body movements, eye movements, and neck tone; and desynchronization of electrocortical activity (17). The high incidence of preeclampsia, abruptio placentae, and placenta previa in the pregnant addict also predisposes to placental insufficiency and fetal distress (14).

Meconium-stained amniotic fluid frequently is encountered in the pregnant addict and is a manifestation of fetal distress (14). Aspiration of meconium during fetal distress may account for the increased frequency of meconium aspiration syndrome and persistent pulmonary hypertension of the newborn after birth.

Intrauterine infection is another risk in the fetus of a drug addict. The lifestyle of the pregnant addict predisposes her to infection, particularly venereal disease, hepatitis, and acquired immunodeficiency syndrome (AIDS), which also may affect her fetus (14,19–22). During delivery or before labor, the increased incidence of premature membrane rupture in the pregnant addict further exposes the fetus to the risk of nonspecific infections (14). Opiates may also compromise immune functions through their effect on both cell-mediated and humoral immune responses (23,24).

Neonatal Problems

Prematurity and Low Birth Weight

Infants born to mothers on heroin have a higher incidence of prematurity, twinning, low birth weight, small size for gestation, and small head circumference (i.e., between the third and fifth percentile) than drug-free control subjects (24–31). Birth weights of infants of mothers on methadone programs, on the other hand, have variably been reported as higher (32,33) or lower (27,28) than those infants of untreated pregnant addicts or not significantly different from the general newborn population (26). This may reflect the better prenatal care that the women receive while on the program. Studies on pregnant rats exposed to methadone have shown their offspring to have significantly lower body weight, length, head diameter, and organ weight (34) and impaired brain development (35) and thermoregulation (36) relative to non–methadone-exposed pups.

Low Apgar Score

There is a high incidence of low Apgar score in infants of drug-dependent mothers. This may be related to intrauterine asphyxia or to the effects of narcotics that the mother received before delivery. Not infrequently, the pregnant addict will obtain a heroin fix before entering the hospital, which can depress the infant. Significantly large amounts of morphine have been found in the urine and cord blood of infants born to these women (33). Caution must therefore be exercised with the use of narcotic antagonists to reverse the respiratory depression in drug-dependent infants because the narcotic antagonists can precipitate an acute withdrawal in the infant.

Other Problems

In addition to withdrawal, other problems are seen with increased frequency in the infant of a drug-dependent mother: jaundice, aspiration pneumonia and meconium aspiration, persistent pulmonary hypertension of the newborn, transient tachypnea, hyaline membrane disease, congenital malformations, and infections (14). These problems are important because they are the principal causes of death in these infants.

Aspiration pneumonia, hyaline membrane disease, and transient tachypnea are the leading pulmonary problems in the infant of the drug-dependent mother. About 30% of aspiration pneumonia results from meconium aspiration (14). Transient tachypnea may be secondary to the inhibitory effects of narcotics on the reflex clearing of fluid by the lungs (37). The high incidence of hyaline membrane disease among infants of drug-dependent mothers is secondary to prematurity. What has been reported as a protection of premature drug-dependent infants against hyaline membrane disease is related primarily to the increased incidence of small-for-gestational-age infants in this group (14,38). Thus, the factors that cause a fetus to be small for gestational age are probably more important determinants of the infant's risk for development of hyaline membrane disease than is the direct action of narcotics (e.g., heroin) in accelerating pulmonary maturation (39–41). Meconium aspiration, persistent pulmonary hypertension of the newborn, and hyaline membrane disease account for more than 50% of the deaths among infants of drug-dependent mothers (14).

In general, the opiates are not believed to be teratogenic to the fetus. Most reports do not show an increase in the frequency of congenital anomalies (9,13,19,23,42, 43), and in one study, although an increased frequency of malformations was found (14), no consistent pattern of malformation was observed. Animal studies, however, have shown a dose-related teratogenic effect of narcotics on the CNS of the developing hamster, which was blocked by narcotic antagonists (44). *In vitro* studies have also shown opiates to impair DNA repair and to cause chromosome aberration with hyperdiploidy (45).

There is an altered sleep pattern in these infants characterized by more rapid eye movement sleep than quiet sleep (16,46). In term infants exposed to opiates, abnormal auditory brainstem evoked responses show decreased conductance time for waves I–III (47,48). Abnormal heart rate and breathing patterns have also been observed (49). The respiratory rates are higher, with low end-tidal volume PCO_2 and a shift to the left of the breathing response to CO_2 (50). These abnormalities have been suggested to increase their predisposition to the sudden infant death syndrome.

There is an increased incidence of jaundice in the infants of drug-dependent mothers, which may be related to the high incidence of prematurity in this group (14). In animals, induction of liver enzymes by morphine has been demonstrated (51), although the dose of morphine used was exceedingly high (250 mg/kg), a situation unlikely to be paralleled in a clinical setting.

A significant thrombocytosis, occasionally exceeding 1,000,000 platelets/mm^3, has been reported in infants of mothers receiving maintenance doses of 40 to 90 mg of methadone per day. Onset was by the second week of life, with counts remaining high for over 16 weeks. The thrombocytosis and associated increased circulating platelet aggregates may play a role in the development of the focal cerebral infarctions and germinal matrix and subarachnoid hemorrhages encountered in postmortem examinations of some of these infants (52). The incidence of intraventricular hemorrhage in the opiate-exposed infant is not increased (53). Cranial ultrasound has shown slit-like ventricles and a small intracranial diameter (54,55).

Along with the high incidence of infection in the pregnant addict is a correspondingly high incidence of infection in her infant. Although a number of the neonatal infections are nonspecific in nature, such as sepsis, omphalitis, necrotizing enterocolitis, and gastroenteritis, some of the infections are related to the antenatal lifestyle and problems of the mother. The latter include hepatitis and venereal diseases (e.g., syphilis, gonorrhea, herpes simplex), group B streptococcal infections, and HIV infection (14,19–22).

Neonatal Narcotic Withdrawal or Abstinence Syndrome

The onset of withdrawal usually occurs within the first 72 hours after birth, commonly within the first 24 to 48 hours. In a few instances, the onset may appear soon after birth, if the mother has already begun to experience withdrawal before delivery. Reports of withdrawal occurring after the first or second week may be secondary to withdrawal from other drugs, e.g., phenobarbital, beside the narcotics (56). Many factors, such as maternal drug dosage, timing of the last dose before delivery, character of the labor, type and amount of anesthesia or analgesia given to the mother, and the maturity and nutritional status of the infant, influence the onset of withdrawal (33).

Withdrawal in the infant usually peaks by about the third day of postnatal life and decreases in intensity by the fifth to seventh day. The duration of withdrawal is related to its severity. When drugs are used to treat the withdrawal, relapse may occur if treatment is discontinued abruptly. The withdrawal manifestations, although they subside within a week, do not completely disappear until about 8 to 16 weeks of age (see Long-Term Outcome).

The severity of the withdrawal is influenced by several factors. It is less severe in preterm infants, probably secondary to their neurologic immaturity or reduced total exposure to narcotics (57). Withdrawal is significantly related to the amount of narcotics that the mother has used during pregnancy. With methadone, a high maternal methadone maintenance dose during pregnancy or the dose at the last methadone intake is associated with more intense withdrawal (33,58–62). Neither the infant's gender, race, or Apgar score nor the mother's age, parity, or duration of heroin intake correlate with the severity of withdrawal (33). Similarly, manipulation of the environment such as reducing the amount of light or noise in the nursery does not ameliorate the severity of withdrawal in the infants (33). Adults experience abdominal cramps, palpitation, nausea, and other discomforts while undergoing withdrawal. It is possible that similar discomforts also are experienced by the infant, and these may nullify any potential benefits from light or noise reduction in the nursery.

Neonatal narcotic withdrawal is associated with noradrenergic hyperactivity (63), and the manifestations involve the CNS and respiratory, gastrointestinal, vasomotor, and cutaneous systems (Table 56–3) (64).

TABLE 56–3. *Manifestations of neonatal narcotic withdrawal*[a]

Central nervous system
  Hyperactivity
  Hyperirritability: excess crying, high-pitched outcry
  Increased muscle tone
  Exaggerated reflexes
  Tremors
  Sneezing, hiccups, yawning
  Short, nonquiet sleep
  Fever
Respiratory system
  Tachypnea
  Excess secretions
Gastrointestinal system
  Disorganized sucking with reduced pressure
  Vomiting
  Drooling
  Sensitive gag
  Hyperphagia
  Diarrhea
  Abdominal cramps
Vasomotor system
  Stuffy nose
  Flushing
  Sweating
  Sudden circumoral pallor
Cutaneous system
  Excoriated buttocks
  Facial scratches
  Pressure-point abrasions

[a]From Ostrea EM, Chavez CJ, Stryker JS. *The care of the drug-dependent woman and her infant.* Lansing, MI: Michigan Department of Public Health, 1978:30.

Central Nervous System Signs

Neurologic signs predominate and appear early. Findings are those of CNS excitability, such as hyperactivity, irritability, tremors, and hypertonicity. Occasionally, fever may accompany these increased neuromuscular activities.

Hyperactivity manifests as almost incessant movements of the extremities. When the infant is supine and unrestrained, movements assume a jerky, purposeless, *en masse* nature, apparently perpetuated by unchecked proprioceptive stimuli. When the infant is placed in the prone position, the motor behavior becomes more organized. There are crawling movements, which may actually lead to the infant's displacement from the crib, and other motions such as chin lifting, head movement from side to side, chest elevation, and hand-to-mouth facility. The latter usually quiets the infant, indicating the usefulness of pacifiers. Hyperirritability manifests as an almost incessant crying with shrill, high-pitched outcries. The infant's muscle tone is exaggerated; sometimes an opisthotonic position is assumed. This makes the infant difficult to hold because of its failure to mold to the body of the holder. Sleep is also disturbed. Tremors and myoclonic jerks are frequent and sometimes are sustained. To distinguish from seizures, tremors can be abolished by restraint of the tremulous extremities. The reflexes of the infant (i.e., Moro, traction response, weight bearing, placing, stepping, crawling, and Landau) are all exaggerated. The infant's response to stimuli, such as sound and light, also is increased disproportionately. In premature infants, the neural hyperexcitability is more episodic. The infants appear restless and overactive for short periods and then lapse into periods of lethargy and inactivity. Sustained tremors usually are not seen in premature infants until they mature to a point when sufficient tone is present in the upper and lower extremities.

Electroencephalographic (EEG) tracings on the addicted neonate may be abnormal and show high-frequency asynchronous activity suggestive of CNS irritability.

Respiratory Signs

Infants who are withdrawing may be tachypneic, with irregular respirations. Alkalosis may result from hyperventilation. Fluid loss also may be increased.

Gastrointestinal Signs

The suck of the infant is disorganized, reduced in rate and sucking pressure (65), and poorly coordinated with swallowing. Consequently, milk frequently drools around the corners of the infant's mouth. The infant appears incessantly hungry, which, when unfulfilled, leads to mounting agitation, persistent crying, hyperactivity, and exhaustion. Proper positioning of the infant to enhance hand-to-mouth facility may be extremely soothing. Vomiting and diarrhea also are often observed. This can lead to dehydration, electrolyte imbalance, and excoriations around the buttocks (see Complications).

Vasomotor Signs

Significant vasomotor instability manifests as stuffy nose, flushing, mottling, sweating, and episodes of sudden circumoral pallor.

Cutaneous Signs

Because of hyperactivity, facial scratches and abrasions on pressure points may be observed on the infant's skin. Excoriations of the buttocks may occur if diarrhea is present.

Complications

The complications associated with neonatal drug withdrawal are related to its severity. Alterations in the serum electrolytes and pH and dehydration may occur secondary to vomiting and diarrhea. Weight loss may be profound, not only from excess fluid losses but also from poor and ineffective oral intake. Aspiration pneumonia may occur secondary to vomiting and incoordinated sucking and swallowing. Respiratory alkalosis can result from tachypnea in the infant. In rare cases, convulsions may be observed. It should be noted that convulsions are a more frequent manifestation of nonnarcotic than of narcotic withdrawal (see Nonnarcotic Abstinence Syndrome).

Mortality

The mortality rate among infants born to drug-dependent mothers used to be as high as 50%. With early recognition and treatment of the withdrawal syndrome and prevention of its complications, the mortality from neonatal withdrawal has become negligible. Nonetheless, mortality, in general, in infants of drug-dependent mothers remains high. In one report, mortality rate was 27 per 1,000 live births compared to 12 per 1,000 live births in the general population (14). The causes of death were related to immaturity, prematurity, hyaline membrane disease, meconium aspiration, persistent pulmonary hypertension of the newborn (PPHN), and major congenital malformations. Pulmonary problems (e.g., meconium aspiration, PPHN, hyaline membrane disease) accounted for more than 50% of the deaths.

Neonatal Neurobehavioral Abnormalities

By the use of the Brazelton Neonatal Assessment Scale, the manifestations of neonatal withdrawal such as

hypertonicity, hyperirritability, hyperactivity, and increased hand-to-mouth facility can be demonstrated. Some other fine behavioral abnormalities are also found that could affect early infant–caregiver interactions (66–69). For instance, congenital addiction seems to affect those behavior systems that are associated with arousal and the early development of mother–infant bonding. Although the addicted infant is more likely to elicit caregiver consolation because he cries more often, he is less easy to cuddle because of increased tone. He also is less readily maintained in an alert state through the course of handling and becomes increasingly less responsive to stimuli, particularly visual, although auditory evoked responses are better integrated. Because cuddliness, alertness, and visual regard are the primary means by which the infant initiates and maintains social interaction with his or her mother, the impairment of these behavior patterns may have a profound effect on the early infant–mother interaction.

Long-Term Outcome

Persistence of Withdrawal

Infants who manifest narcotic withdrawal will show a persistence of the withdrawal for as long as 8 to 16 weeks (70,71). The prolonged manifestations are usually milder than the initial and consist of irritability, tremors, hypertonicity, sneezing, hiccups, and regurgitation. The persistence of withdrawal is related directly to its initial severity and is more prolonged in those who had severe withdrawal. Infants who were treated with drugs for withdrawal also show prolonged withdrawal. Thus, drug treatment may ameliorate the manifestations of withdrawal but does not shorten its duration. It is important that the mother be made aware of the persistence of the infant's withdrawal when the infant is discharged from the nursery. Otherwise, she may become alarmed when the infant continues to manifest some withdrawal at home. The unwarned mother may also misinterpret the infant's irritability as hunger, and overfeed the infant. This can lead to diarrhea and vomiting. The mother also should be instructed on how to reduce the infant's discomfort by swaddling and cuddling the infant. In addition, she should be reassured that the infant's withdrawal will subside eventually without the use of medications. In most instances, the mother who is well informed can cope with the situation successfully.

Child Abuse and Sudden Infant Death Syndrome

The high incidence of child abuse and neglect constitutes one of the serious medical problems in the infant of the drug-addicted woman. Thermal burns, usually from cigarettes, traumatic ecchymoses, and hematomas have been observed in 8% of infants during the first 8 months of life (64). During the same period, about 8.3% of the infants had to be placed in alternative care because of maternal neglect or abandonment or maternal death. Many factors contribute to the risk of abuse. The persistence of the withdrawal, feeding problems, abnormal sleep patterns, and periods of restlessness in the infant can generate undue tension in the mother, whose tolerance for frustration is already low. Thus, the mother, unable to cope with the situation, may simply withdraw from her infant and avoid any contact, or she may abandon or injure the infant. Similarly, the home situation may be adverse to appropriate infant rearing. Problems include arrest or incarceration of the mother or parents and their treatment for emotional disorders (72,73). The mother also frequently needs assistance in parenting and is more socially isolated and less likely to pursue vocational or educational attainment (74). It is therefore important that someone is available at home to help the mother in the care of her child and that the visiting or public health nurse and the social and protective service workers actively participate in the follow-up of these infants.

There is a four- to fivefold increase in the incidence of sudden death syndrome in infants of opiate-dependent mothers (75,76). This is observed whether the infant is cared for by the mother or in an extended family or foster home. The cause is not known, although its occurrence is significantly higher in those infants who had moderate to severe withdrawal after birth (75,76). Abnormal breathing pattern, control of breathing, and exposure of the infant to maternal smoking have been implicated as contributory causes (50,77).

Growth and Psychomotor Development

In general, the physical growth of the opiate-exposed infant has shown a catch-up in growth when adjusted for sex, race, maternal education, and smoking. At 12 months of age, the growth in terms of weight, head circumference, and length of the infants has been observed to fall within the tenth to the 90th percentile on the growth chart. Similarly, the percentage of addicted infants whose growth parameters were below the tenth percentile did not differ significantly from the nonaddict group (78). However, some studies have reported retardation in the weight, length, and head circumference at age 3 to 6 years (79–82). A high incidence of transient or minor motor deficits, poor motor coordination, as well as abnormal eye findings such as nystagmus and strabismus have also been observed in these infants in the first year of life (81,83–85).

The mental and cognitive performance of the opiate-exposed infants has been shown to be comparable to the control, non–drug-exposed group (71,78,86,87). Within the first year of life, the infants of narcotic addicts have been shown to manifest some difficulty in regulating their behavior but otherwise had normal developmental scores (79–81). At preschool age, compared to controls (i.e., children at similar environmental risk and sociodemographic background), the addicted children performed less well in terms of perception, short-term memory, and organization but did just as well on objective tests of activity and attention (80).

Behavioral problems have been observed among the opiate-exposed infants and have persisted even in late childhood. These consist of hyperactivity, aggressiveness, inattention, impulsiveness, short attention span, and lack of concentration and inhibition (71,88–91). These problems have been related to environmental and emotional deprivation of the infant rather than to the effects of *in utero* drug exposure. In school, this leads to learning problems, truancy, and school suspension (72).

NONNARCOTIC HYPNOSEDATIVES

Nonnarcotic Abstinence Syndrome

Infants born to women who have used nonnarcotic hypnosedatives during pregnancy (Table 56–4) also manifest addiction and withdrawal from these drugs. The manifestations of nonnarcotic withdrawal in the neonate are similar to those of narcotic withdrawal (92). In a few instances (e.g., with barbiturate withdrawal or ethchlorvynol withdrawal), hyperphagia has been described as a prominent manifestation.

Although the manifestations of withdrawal from narcotic and nonnarcotic drugs are similar, major differences exist (64):

In adults, the rate of developing physical dependence to the nonnarcotic hypnosedatives does not increase with the drug dose, as it does with narcotics. Rather, prolonged and continuous administration of large and partially incapacitating doses is necessary, over months or years, to produce addiction to nonnarcotics, especially if the drugs are taken orally. The situation is different in the newborn infant. Passive addiction in the fetus and infant has been observed even when therapeutic doses of nonnarcotic drugs are used by the mother during pregnancy. Thus, a pregnant woman who is treated

TABLE 56–4. *Nonnarcotic drugs*

Hypnosedatives
  Barbiturate
  Nonbarbiturate sedatives and tranquilizers
  Bromide
  Chloral hydrate
  Chlordiazepoxide (Librium)
  Diazepam (Valium)
  Ethchlorvynol (Placidyl)
  Glutethimide (Doriden)
Alcohol
  Ethanol

with phenobarbital for epilepsy can cause addiction in her fetus, although she may not be addicted to the drug (56).

The manifestations of the nonnarcotic abstinence syndrome are more frequently intense and life-threatening compared to narcotic withdrawal. The occurrence of convulsions is also more frequent.

Most of the withdrawal from narcotics is seen within the first 3 days of postnatal life because of the relatively short half-life of the narcotics. In contrast, withdrawal from the nonnarcotics, such as phenobarbital, may be observed at 7 to 10 days after birth because of the slow clearance of the drug in the infant.

Unlike the narcotics, neonatal addiction to many of the nonnarcotic hypnosedatives has been induced by physicians who prescribed the drug to the mother while totally unaware that the drugs are addicting to her fetus (64).

Barbiturates

Although barbiturates have been used in clinical medicine for many years, their addiction potential was recognized only recently. The frequent association in the adult of barbiturate use with alcohol may have contributed to the delayed recognition of the addicting potential of the barbiturates because of the ability of barbiturates to control the withdrawal from alcohol (93,94).

Barbiturates are classified on the basis of the duration of their action as ultrashort, intermediate, and long acting. The intermediate-acting barbiturates are the most frequently abused [e.g., secobarbital (Seconal), pentobarbital (Nembutal), amobarbital (Amytal), butabarbital (Butisol)]. The abuse of the long-acting barbiturates (e.g., phenobarbital) is not as common as the abuse of the shorter-acting forms. Phenobarbital, however, is more frequently involved in withdrawal syndrome in the newborn because it is used frequently in the mother for insomnia, for the relief of anxiety, as an anticonvulsant, or for sedation when toxemia of pregnancy occurs.

Passive addiction of the fetus to barbiturates can occur after prolonged intrauterine exposure to the drug (56,95). Barbiturates cross the placenta readily and establish high levels in both the maternal and cord blood. Relatively high levels of barbiturates have been found in the fetal brain, liver, and adrenal glands (96). The manifestations of barbiturate withdrawal in the neonate are similar, regardless of the type of barbiturate used by the mother; however, the onset of withdrawal may differ. Withdrawal typically occurs within a day after birth with intermediate-acting barbiturates(97) and from 3 to 7 days after birth with the long-acting barbiturates (66,95).

Barbiturates are metabolized principally by the liver, although a significant portion may be excreted unchanged by the kidney. In adults, up to 30% of the total dose of phenobarbital ingested is excreted unchanged in the urine (98).

The half-life of phenobarbital prenatally administered to infants is almost twice that in the adult and varies inversely with the extent of the prenatal exposure to phenobarbital (99). Phenobarbital levels in the arterial cord blood have ranged from 77% to 100% of maternal levels depending on the duration of maternal treatment, gestational age, and cord pH in the infant (100).

The signs of withdrawal from barbiturates in neonates are similar to those described in adults. The infants are overactive and restless, with excessive crying, twitching, hyperactive reflexes, and hypertonicity. They also manifest diarrhea, vomiting, and poor sucking ability. When tonic–clonic convulsions occur, the EEG patterns show diffuse, paroxysmal, high-voltage, slow-wave bursts not unlike those seen in adults (95). A subacute phase of hyperphagia, episodes of prolonged crying, episodic irritability, hyperacusis, and sweating have been described (66). These manifestations may last from 2 to 6 months.

Recognition of the abstinence syndrome is essential to the adequate management of the infant. An awareness of the possibility of a late onset of withdrawal, especially after exposure to long-acting barbiturates, should alert the clinician to follow these infants closely during the first 2 weeks of life.

Bromide and Chloral Hydrate

Bromides and chloral hydrate were popular hypnosedative drugs for many years, until they gradually were replaced by the barbiturates and other hypnosedative agents. Addiction to chloral hydrate has been described in adults (101). Many cases of bromide intoxication could have been caused partly by chloral hydrate because combination use of the two drugs was not unusual (101). A withdrawal syndrome and growth retardation have been reported in newborn infants after the use of bromides by the mother during pregnancy (102,103). In one report, the mother took a large amount of bromide, in the form of Relaxa tablets, to relieve anxiety. The infant was born at term but was small for gestational age and heavily meconium stained. Soon after birth the infant manifested extreme irritability, a high-pitched cry, and feeding difficulties, which lasted for 9 weeks (103). Studies on rat pups whose dams were given sodium bromide *ad libitum* showed significant delay in postnatal development, permanent deficits in body weight, brain weight, and protein content of brain tissue, but with an increased size of the olfactory glomeruli (104).

Chlordiazepoxide and Diazepam

Chlordiazepoxide (Librium) and diazepam (Valium) are widely used for their hypnosedative effects (105). Abuse of these drugs and dependence on them both have been reported in adults. During pregnancy, benzodiazepines cross the placenta with relative ease, resulting in significant levels of the drug in the serum and tissue of the fetus

(106). Placental transfer of diazepam can occur from the sixth week of gestation, and the drug can accumulate in the fetal tissues during organogenesis (107). Mean levels of diazepam were found to be markedly higher in the umbilical cord serum than in the maternal serum after a single intravenous injection of 10 mg diazepam (108).

An acute withdrawal syndrome from chlordiazepoxide or diazepam has been observed in the newborn infant (109,110). A presumptive diagnosis of chlordiazepoxide withdrawal was made in a set of twins born to a mother who used chlordiazepoxide, 20 mg per 24 hours, during the second and third trimesters of her pregnancy (109). The withdrawal occurred on day 21 of life and consisted of severe irritability and coarse tremors. Three cases of presumptive neonatal withdrawal from diazepam have also been noted (110). The onset of withdrawal occurred within 2.5 to 6 hours after birth and consisted of tremors, irritability, hypertonicity, vigorous sucking, vomiting, and diarrhea. The dose of diazepam taken by the mother during pregnancy and up to the time of birth ranged from 15 to 20 mg per 24 hours. In all three cases, phenobarbital was effective in controlling the withdrawal in the infant, although the drug had to be administered for a prolonged period (13 to 25 days). A report on narcotic withdrawal in two neonates that was complicated by concomitant prenatal exposure to high doses of diazepam revealed an initial good response of the infants to therapy for narcotic withdrawal but intensification of withdrawal manifestations at 7 to 14 days of life. The late withdrawal was attributed to prenatal diazepam exposure (111). Late third-trimester use and exposure to diazepam during labor have also been associated with the floppy infant syndrome or marked neonatal withdrawal. The manifestations varied from mild sedation, hypotonia, and reluctance to suck to apneic spells, cyanosis, and impaired metabolic responses to cold stress. These signs may persist from a few hours to months after birth (112). High-dose intravenous administration or prolonged duration of diazepam therapy in mothers has also caused significant depression in the newborn with poor muscle tone (108,113). Most studies involving first-trimester use of benzodiazepines have shown the majority of infants to be normal at birth and to have normal postnatal development (112). There is a report of an omphalo-coele–exstrophy–imperforate anus–spina bifida complex that occurred in an infant whose mother took 30 mg of diazepam daily for an affective disorder during the entire pregnancy (114). Offspring of rats who were treated with chlordiazepoxide during the critical period of neural development showed significant deficits in learning acquisition and retention (115).

Ethchlorvynol

Ethchlorvynol (Placidyl) was introduced in 1955 as a nonbarbiturate hypnotic for the treatment of insomnia. Like other nonbarbiturate sedatives, there were claims regarding its nonaddictive property (116–118). The drug was used to relieve anxiety and as a sleep-inducing medication (119). As in the cases of the barbiturate and non-barbiturate sedatives, tolerance to the drug develops, and increasing doses are needed to attain the desired effect. Reports of addiction to ethchlorvynol subsequently have been reported (120–124).

Ethchlorvynol crosses the placenta readily, and studies in animals indicate that the drug achieves rapid equilibration between the maternal and fetal blood. It also can be detected in the chorionic and amniotic fluids (125).

An abstinence syndrome in a newborn infant secondary to withdrawal from ethchlorvynol has been reported (126). Extreme jitteriness, irritability, and hyperphagia were noted in the infant on the second day of life. The mother took the drug (500 mg/24 hours) for 3 months before giving birth. This dose was within the recommended therapeutic range for adults. The onset of withdrawal in the infant occurred during the second day of life. No convulsions were noted because the infant received phenobarbital treatment early in the course of the abstinence syndrome.

Glutethimide

Glutethimide (Doriden) was first introduced in 1954 as a nonbarbiturate hypnosedative, allegedly free of addicting properties. As was the case with the other nonbarbiturate hypnosedatives, this led to its widespread use, particularly as a substitute drug for the treatment of alcohol addiction (127). Since that time, there have been numerous reports of acute and sometimes fatal intoxication with the drug in adults and the occurrence of physical dependence (128–130).

Glutethimide is structurally related to phenobarbital and to the teratogenic sedative thalidomide. It is metabolized in the liver to a hydroxylated product, as is phenobarbital. There are, however, no reports of teratogenicity after the use of glutethimide during pregnancy.

A possible case of neonatal withdrawal from glutethimide has been observed (131). The mother was a heroin addict who supplemented her habit with 2 to 3 g of glutethimide three or four times a week to get the desired euphoric effect. Within 8 hours of birth, the infant had shown initial signs of withdrawal from narcotics that were readily controlled with chlorpromazine. On the tenth day of life, however, while on tapering doses of chlorpromazine, the infant suddenly manifested diarrhea, fever, tachypnea, irritability, hypertonicity, and diaphoresis. It was presumed that the unusual recurrence of withdrawal on the tenth day of life may have been secondary to withdrawal from glutethimide.

Differential Diagnosis

Withdrawal from the narcotic and nonnarcotic drugs should be distinguished from clinical conditions such as hypoglycemia, hypocalcemia, hypomagnesemia, sepsis, meningitis, subarachnoid hemorrhage, infectious diarrhea, and intestinal obstruction. Blood chemistry, cerebrospinal fluid examination, radiographic examination, and cultures should be performed as indicated by the clinical circumstances.

Infants whose mothers had taken tricyclic antidepressants and lithium during pregnancy for psychiatric conditions may manifest toxicity similar to withdrawal, such as irritability, tachycardia, respiratory distress, sweating, and convulsions (132–136). Likewise, maternal intake of phenothiazines (e.g., chlorpromazine) may induce extrapyramidal dysfunctions in the newborn infant, such as tremors, facial grimacing, increased muscle tone, cogwheel rigidity, increased reflexes, and torticollis, all of which can resemble the withdrawal syndrome (137,138). The prenatal history and the identification of the corresponding drug in the infant's serum or urine are necessary to establish the diagnosis.

COCAINE

Types

Cocaine is an alkaloid that is extracted from the leaves of the *Erythroxylon coca* bush. Its chemical name is methylbenzoylecgonine, and it is the only known local anesthetic that is found naturally. The pure cocaine substance was first extracted and identified by the German chemist Albert Nieman in 1860. The drug is extracted from the leaves of the coca plant by a series of solvent extractions. Coca paste is the first extraction product of cocaine and contains about 80% cocaine (100). The paste can be smoked after being applied to tobacco or marijuana. Cocaine hydrochloride is the most common available form of cocaine. In its acid state, cocaine HCl is a white powder that is soluble in water and can be snorted or injected. Cocaine HCl usually is adulterated with starch, glucose, phencyclidine (PCP), heroin, or amphetamines, and its purity ranges from 20% to 80% (139,140).

An alkaloidal base of cocaine can be obtained from cocaine HCl (i.e., free-basing) by alkalizing the aqueous solution of cocaine HCl and then extracting the cocaine alkaloid base using volatile organic solvents, such as ether. The gummy cocaine residue, called rock, has a lower melting point than cocaine HCl and can be smoked using a special pipe. Crack cocaine is the most popular abused form of the drug. Crack cocaine is produced when cocaine HCl is mixed with ammonia, water, and baking soda and heated. The resulting paste, once dried, forms a hard, rocklike substance that can be smoked. The term "crack" is derived from the crackling sound that is produced when crack cocaine is prepared or smoked.

When taken orally, cocaine HCl has a peak effect at between 45 minutes and 90 minutes. Intranasal adminis-

tration of cocaine (i.e., snorting) has a peak effect in 15 to 30 minutes and lasts from 60 to 90 minutes. Smoking cocaine (i.e., free-basing) provides the most rapid delivery of the drug to the body. Peak effect is within 60 to 90 seconds, but the high lasts only for about 5 to 10 minutes. The intense high is followed by a down period as the effect of the drug wears off. The down period may be so unpleasant that more of the drug is used to reexperience the high, or other drugs, such as alcohol, are used. Thus, cocaine use promotes the abuse of other drugs (139).

Cocaine is metabolized by plasma and hepatic esterases into three major water-soluble metabolites, ecgonine methyl ester, benzoylecgonine, and ecgonine, although other minor metabolites are also present. The half-life of the drug in adults depends on the route of administration—an average of 0.6 hour after intravenous administration, 0.9 hour after oral use, and 1.3 hours after intranasal use. The metabolites can be found in the urine 72 hours after administration. In infants, metabolites can be found for up to 2 weeks after administration (141).

Pharmacology

The neuropharmacologic effect of cocaine is secondary to its effect on three neurotransmitters: norepinephrine, dopamine, and serotonin. Cocaine inhibits the reuptake of norepinephrine and dopamine (142), which accumulate at the synaptic cleft, leading to prolonged stimulation of their corresponding receptors. Therefore, the effects of norepinephrine stimulation (e.g., tachycardia, hypertension, arrhythmia, diaphoresis, tremors) and dopamine stimulation (e.g., increased alertness, euphoria or enhanced feeling of well-being, sexual excitement, heightened energy) are experienced. Cocaine also decreases the uptake of tryptophan, which affects serotonin biosynthesis. A diminished serotonin level is associated with diminished need for sleep because serotonin regulates the sleep–wake cycle (140).

Adverse Effects on Pregnancy

Studies in pregnant sheep have shown that maternal blood pressure becomes elevated within 5 minutes after cocaine infusion (143–145), coupled with an increase in uterine vascular resistance and a decrease in uterine blood flow. Fetal heart rate and blood pressure also increase, but fetal PO_2 and O_2 content decrease as a consequence of the reduced uterine blood flow. Thus, oxygen availability to the fetus is impaired (Table 56–5).

The cocaine-induced uterine vasoconstriction is mediated solely by α-adrenergic stimulation because α-adrenergic blockade by phentolamine does not ablate the response. Pregnancy can potentiate the toxic effects of cocaine because progesterone can increase the α-adrenergic sensitivity of the receptors or delay cocaine metabolism (146).

TABLE 56–5. *Perinatal and long-term problems associated with cocaine use during pregnancy*

Obstetric problems
  Spontaneous abortion
  Stillbirth
  Uterine ischemia
  Abruptio placenta
  Premature labor
  Precipitous delivery
  Meconium stained amniotic fluid
  Infections, including syphilis, HIV infection
Neonatal problems
  Fetal distress
  Low Apgar score
  Prematurity
  Low birth weight
  Small length and head circumference
  Small for gestation
  Congenital malformation?
  Neurobehavioral effects
Longterm problems
  Child abuse
  Sudden infant death syndrome
  Strabismus
  High blood pressure
  Hypertonicity
  Difficulty in early language development
  Low verbal comprehension and reasoning
  Poor recognition memory and information processing
  Behavioral problems, such as attention deficit and easy
    distractability

At serum levels found in humans, cocaine per se has no effect on human and animal umbilical arteries; however, cocaine enhances the umbilical artery vasoconstrictor action of catecholamines and serotonin, presumably by increasing the sensitivity of the α-adrenergic receptors of arterial smooth muscle (147).

Overall, the cardiovascular effect of cocaine on the maternofetal circulation is maternal hypertension, increase in uterine vascular resistance, decrease in uterine blood flow, decrease in oxygen transport to the fetus, and fetal hypoxemia.

Obstetric Effects

A characteristic profile has been observed in the pregnant woman who abuses cocaine: a multigravid, multiparous, service patient with little to no prenatal care (2). The lifestyle of prostitution, with little attention to personal health care, contributes to these attributes. In addition, the pregnant addict is generally of poor health due to poor nutrition and vitamin deficiency, and is at high risk for infection, particularly hepatitis, syphilis and HIV infection (147,148). Cocaine use and HIV infection have also noted as significant risk factors for maternal pneumonia (149).

Maternal use of cocaine has been associated with a number of obstetric complications (Table 56–5). Sponta-neous abortion occurs in 25% to 38% of pregnancies of cocaine-using women (150–152). The rate of stillbirth is five to ten times higher among pregnant women who continue to use cocaine late in the third trimester. This has been ascribed to abruptio placentae, placental infarcts, or hemorrhage (150,153). Use of other drugs is high among cocaine users (1). Fetal anuria, anasarca, and neonatal gastrointestinal hemorrhage have been reported in association with use of cocaine and indomethacin during pregnancy (154).

Cocaine use during pregnancy has been associated with up to a tenfold increase in the incidence of abruptio placentae (150–153,156). This has been attributed to an increased incidence of hypertension in these women. Other studies, however, do not show an association between cocaine use and placental abruption (2,157,158). One of these was a study based on a large obstetric population and the use of a more sensitive test to detect widespread cocaine exposure in the infants (2).

The increased occurrence of premature labor and premature rupture of the membranes has been observed among women who use cocaine (150,159–161). There is a belief among them that cocaine will shorten the duration of their labor. Although one study has refuted this belief (162), another has shown a significant decrease in the duration of labor in women who used cocaine compared to nonusers or those who used only opiates during their pregnancy (2).

There has not been an observed increase in the incidence of amnionitis, abnormal presentation, eclampsia, preeclampsia, or placenta praevia in pregnant women who abuse cocaine (150).

Placental Transfer

Because of its low molecular weight and high lipid solubility, cocaine crosses the placenta by simple diffusion (152); however, the fetal concentration of cocaine is only one-fourth to one-ninth that of the mother. Nonetheless, the elimination of cocaine and its metabolites is much slower in the fetus than in the mother; thus, the risk of cocaine toxicity in the fetus is increased.

Effects on the Neonate

The cocaine-exposed infant is at risk for a number of complications (Table 56–5). Cocaine decreases placental perfusion, which leads to poor gas exchange and fetal oxygenation (143–145). Fetal hypoxemia in turn leads to fetal distress, meconium staining of the amniotic fluid, and low Apgar scores. Meconium staining has been observed in 23% of births in cocaine-abusing women—approximately twice the incidence among nondrug users (2,150).

Premature birth has occurred in approximately 25% (150,159,160,163–168), and intrauterine growth retardation in about 21%, of the pregnancies of cocaine users (152,158,161,164,169). These rates are three to four times higher than in nonusers. Studies also report lower birth weights and smaller body length and head circumference in the infants (152,155,160,163,164,166,167,170–172). However, duration and amount of cocaine used during pregnancy (165,173), maternal smoking, alcohol and opiate use (174), and lead exposure (175) are important contributing factors or confounders for these reduced growth parameters.

Cocaine use during pregnancy has been associated with an increased incidence of the congenital malformations in animals (150,156,161,176). It is suggested that fetal vascular disruption secondary to vasoconstriction may lead to these defects (177). No specific pattern of organ involvement has been observed. The reported increase in genitourinary malformations in infants was not substantiated in a routine renal ultrasound study of 100 term infants exposed to cocaine during pregnancy (178). Likewise, polydrug abuse, including alcohol abuse, is not uncommon among cocaine users (2). Thus, the potential of cocaine alone as a teratogen is difficult to establish in these clinical settings. Nonetheless, studies in the offspring of rats that have received cocaine during pregnancy have shown teratogenic effects such as neural tube defects, skeletal deficits (e.g., camptodactyly, bradydactyly), and hydrocephalus (150).

In utero cocaine exposure of the human fetus also has been associated with a number of multiorgan effects (179) (Table 56–6). Neurologic abnormalities have been described, including seizures (180), transient dystonia (181), hypertonia/hyperreflexia and tremors (182–184), and transient abnormal EEG suggestive of central nervous system irritability (185). The infant's cry is characterized as few, short, and less crying in the hyperphonation mode (186). The sleep pattern shows more wakefulness, more frequent arousals, and a higher proportion of active compared to quiet sleep (187–189). The infant's auditory brainstem evoked response shows prolonged interpeak and absolute latencies (190,191). The incidence of intraventricular hemorrhage among preterm infants is not increased (192). Abnormal cranial ultrasound studies have been reported, consisting of echolucencies in the basal ganglia and caudate nucleus, ventricle dilation, and germinal matrix cysts (193). Although high-resolution single-photon emission computed tomographic (SPECT) scans have shown normal cerebral blood flow in 21 infants with confirmed cocaine exposure (194), cerebral infarction and hemorrhage have been reported in an infant whose mother had taken a large amount of cocaine during the intrapartum period. Similarly, a Mobius syndrome was observed in an infant born to a mother with heavy use of cocaine and alcohol. It is speculated that cocaine-induced vasoconstriction at a critical time of cerebrovascular development produced a vascular disruption sequence leading to the syndrome

TABLE 56–6. *Reported complications involving specific organ systems in cocaine exposed infants*

Central nervous system
  Cerebral infarction
  Mobius syndrome
  Seizures, tremors
  Hypertonicity/hyperreflexia and transient dystonia
  Abnormal head ultrasound, such as echolucencies in basal ganglia, ventricles, periventricular and germinal matrix cysts
  Abnormal EEG
  Abnormal sleep pattern
  Abnormal cry
Sensory organs
  Abnormal brainstem auditory evoked response
  Increased auditory startle response
  Retinal hemorrhage and tortuosity and dilation of iris vessels
Cardiovascular system
  Transient tachycardia
  Hypertension and diminished stroke volume and cardiac output
  Atrial and ventricular arrythythmia
Respiratory system
  Apnea
  Abnormal breathing pattern, such as periodic breathing
Genitourinary system
  Renal ectopia

(195). Thus, the vasoconstrictive effect of cocaine on the cerebral circulation may be evident *in utero* because the fetus is directly exposed to the effects of the drug. Postnatally, this may no longer be observed because of the waning effects of cocaine as evidenced by a significant drop in arterial blood pressure and cerebral blood flow velocities in the second compared to the first day of life (196). Unlike in opiate exposure, an abstinence syndrome has not been commonly observed with cocaine exposure. Reports of withdrawal-like manifestations with cocaine may be related to polydrug abuse, particularly opiates.

In the respiratory system, abnormal breathing patterns have been observed in the cocaine-exposed infants, such as higher respiratory rate, decreased end-tidal PCO_2, and a shift to the left of the breathing response curve to CO_2 (50). Increased apnea density and periodic breathing have also been described (165,197). In the cardiovascular system, decreased cardiac output and stroke volume and increased arterial blood pressure have been reported (196,198) as well as atrial and ventricular arrhythmias (199).

Other neonatal findings have included elevation in serum myoglobin and creatine kinase secondary to tremors (200) and decreased jaundice because cocaine is a strong inducer of the glutathione-S- transferase family of enzymes that is closely associated with bilirubin transport (ligandin) in the liver (201). Reports of eye findings have consisted of retinal hemorrhages (202) and dilated and tortuous iris vessels (203).

On neurobehavioral assessments using the Neonatal Brazelton Assessment Scale, cocaine-exposed newborns have shown significantly depressed performance on the habituation clusters, including lower state regulation and greater depression. During sleep–wake behavior observations, the infants showed difficulty in maintaining alert states and self-regulating their behavior, spent more time in indeterminate sleep, had decreased periods of quiet sleep and increased levels of agitated behavior, including tremulousness, mouthing, multiple limb movements, and clenched fists (204–206). High urinary norepinephrine, dopamine, and cortisol levels were noted under these conditions (206). A significant negative correlation was observed between serum norepinephrine concentration and orientation cluster score for the cocaine-exposed newborns (207). Similarly, a significant negative effect was observed between cocaine concentration in meconium and the cluster scores on motor and regulation state (208). There is also an increase in the infant's auditory startle response (172,209). Two neurobehavioral syndromes have been described in these infants: an excitable state, which may result from the direct neurotoxic effects of the drug, and a depressed state that may be indirect effects of placental deficiency (210).

Cocaine use during pregnancy has not only caused significant medical problems in the infant but has also been an economic burden. Increased hospitalization costs have resulted from prematurity and adverse birth outcomes, prolonged stay while awaiting home and social evaluation of foster care placement, and laboratory fees (211–216).

Long-Term Outcome

There are many confounding factors, besides prenatal cocaine exposure, that influence the long-term outcome of cocaine-exposed infants. These include poverty (217–219), maternal polydrug abuse, particularly alcohol (220), and a chaotic child-rearing environment (221). Controlling for these confounding factors has demonstrated that the outcome of cocaine-exposed infants is better than was previously predicted.

In physical growth and development, the infants show catch-up in weight and length (222), although head circumference tends to remain smaller (223,218) than that in control infants. Strabismus, high blood pressure, and hypertonicity have been noted in the infants, particularly during the first year (182,224,225). Difficulties in early language development, lower verbal comprehension and reasoning, and poor recognition memory and information processing have been more consistently reported (222,223,226–230). Cocaine exposure is not associated with differences in play behavior of the infant at 18 and 24 months (231) despite a previous report to the contrary (232). However, behavior problems dealing with attention deficits and distractability have been noted (233).

As in the opiate-exposed infant, there is increased risk of SIDS and child abuse with prenatal cocaine exposure (187). The chaotic home environment and a high incidence of depression, emotional and physical neglect, inadequate skills, and poor self-esteem in the mother are important contributing factors for the latter (221). Perinatal drug abuse including cocaine, opiates, and cannabinoid has not been associated with increased infant mortality within the first 2 years of life (234).

Cocaine Exposure During Infancy and Childhood

The harmful effects of cocaine in the infant do not result solely from prenatal exposure to the drug. There may be ongoing exposure to cocaine through breast-feeding, intentional administration, accidental ingestion of cocaine or cocaine-contaminated household dust via normal hand-to-mouth activity, or passive inhalation of crack vapors during freebasing by adults (235). Cocaine and benzoylecgonine have been found in the hair, saliva, skin, and urine of these children (224,236). Morbidity from postnatal cocaine exposure has included seizures, drowsiness, unsteady gait, diarrhea, and shock from intoxication and, sometimes, death (237–240). Two major age-related patterns have been seen in postnatal cocaine exposure: in children under 5 years of age, seizures (focal or generalized) and obtundation, and in older children, delirium, dizziness, drooling, and lethargy (241). Thus, the differential diagnosis of afebrile seizures in infants and young children should include cocaine intoxication.

ALCOHOL

The use or abuse of alcohol during pregnancy has serious effects on the fetus and newborn. The adverse effects of alcohol on the offspring have been observed for centuries, although the fetal alcohol syndrome (FAS) was not defined as a medical entity until 1973 (242,243). Children born to alcoholic parents were observed to have a higher than expected incidence of delayed growth and development and of neurologic disorders (244,245). Since 1973, numerous reports on the mild or severe effects of maternal alcohol use on the fetus and newborn have been reported. Excellent reviews on the subject also have been written (246–248).

Epidemiology

Drinking during pregnancy has decreased dramatically, with a 20% to 32% decline in the overall rate of alcohol use during pregnancy over a 3-year period from 1985 to 1988 (249). From 1991 to 1995, rates of alcohol use during pregnancy increased, especially for frequent drinking, underscoring the need for renewed attention to advising pregnant women to abstain from alcohol use. In 1995, 4.7% of women aged 18 to 44 years reported being pregnant at the time of the interview. Of these, 16.3% reported any drinking during the preceding month, compared with 12.4% in 1991. The rate of frequent drinking among pregnant women was approximately four times higher in 1995 than in 1991 (3.5% versus 0.8%; $p < 0.01$). This difference persisted after controlling for selected sociodemographic characteristics (i.e., age, household income, marital status, employment status, educational level, smoking status, and race). Among all women of childbearing age in 1995, 50.6% reported any drinking, and 12.6% reported frequent drinking prevalences similar to those found in 1991 (1).

Metabolism and Placental Transfer

Ethanol is an anxiolytic analgesic with a depressant effect on the CNS (247). It is absorbed rapidly by diffusion across the mucosa of the stomach (20%) and intestines (80%). The absorption rate is not affected by pregnancy, but blood alcohol levels may be higher in pregnancy (246). Alcohol usually is cleared from the bloodstream within 1 hour in adults and 2 hours in newborns. Approximately 95% is metabolized by the liver, and 5% is eliminated by the kidneys and lungs. Ethanol is metabolized to acetaldehyde, then to acetate. Acetaldehyde is more toxic than ethanol itself. There is an unimpeded bidirectional placental transfer of ethanol during pregnancy. Alcohol is distributed rapidly and nearly equally in maternal and fetal tissues (250). Fetal ethanol is eliminated by maternal hepatic biotransformation. Ethanol has been detected in amniotic fluid, a reservoir for additional fetal exposure (247,251).

Ethanol has been implicated in the impairment of normal placental function. It affects or interferes with the transport of amino acids across the placenta to the fetus (252). Ethanol has also been found to inhibit DNA synthesis, protein synthesis (253), inhibit phospholipase A_2 (254), decrease prostaglandin I_2 (PGI_2) production (255), and increase human chorionic gonadotropin (hCG) production in the placenta (256).

Effects on Pregnancy

Increased incidences of spontaneous abortion, abruptio placentae, and breech presentation have been observed among women who abuse alcohol during pregnancy.

The incidence of spontaneous abortion among alcoholic pregnant women is high, ranging from 18.8% to 52% of pregnancies (246). In a large prospective study of 12,127 pregnant women, alcoholic women were found to have a 2.3 times higher incidence of three or more spontaneous abortions than nonalcoholics (257). The single variable that correlated highly with spontaneous abortion was an extremely heavy episode of drinking during the early first trimester. Other reports, however, do not show an association of alcohol consumption with an increased risk for spontaneous abortions in nonheavy drinkers

(258). Studies in nonhuman primates showed that an increase in spontaneous abortion occurred only when blood alcohol levels reached approximately 200 mg/dL (259–264).

An increase in the frequency of aneuploidy was found in abortuses of women who consumed two or more drinks per week (263). Although in mice, preovulatory alcohol exposure did not increase the incidence of abortion (264) or aneuploidy (265), alcohol administration shortly after ovulation resulted in a 7.5% incidence of aneuploidy. Ingestion shortly after mating also resulted in a 15% incidence of aneuploidy (266). Alcohol administration to mating female mice 2 hours after ovulation resulted in a significant increase in fetal death associated with aneuploidy. Another study showed that successful fertilization of such eggs after a single "binge" consequently resulted in the production of aneuploid embryos, which have a very high chance of being spontaneously aborted during the first trimester. Those relatively few aneuploid conceptuses that survived to term invariably showed moderate to severe degress of mental retardation, craniofacial and other abnormalities, as well as having a significantly reduced life expectancy (267). These studies raise the possibility that the high rate of spontaneous abortions among alcoholic women may be related to a single episode of heavy drinking around the time of conception (268).

An increased risk of stillbirths has not been shown with alcohol use during pregnancy, even among women classified as problem or heavy drinkers (257,258, 269,270). However, the risk of abruptio placentae is increased (271,272).

Fetal alcohol syndrome is strongly associated with breech presentation. Seventy percent of infants with FAS were breech births (246). In other studies, nine of 23 (39%) infants born to heavy drinkers were delivered as breech (273); however, only three of 59 infants of moderate drinkers had breech presentations (274). Thus, it appears that heavy consumption of alcohol increases the incidence of breech births.

Effects on the Fetus

Animal studies have shown that *in utero* alcohol exposure may cause fetal malnutrition and chronic fetal hypoxia by inducing hypoglycemia at high blood alcohol levels (247). Alcohol decreases adrenergic receptors on the hepatic plasma membrane, resulting in reduced epinephrine-induced stimulation of glycogen phosphorylase activity and interference with carbohydrate metabolism and prenatal and postnatal growth. Low concentrations of somatomedin C and high growth hormone levels have been noted in infants of alcoholic mothers (275). A dose-dependent contraction of the human umbilical cord *in vitro* as well as decreased fetal placental flow *in vivo* have been demonstrated with alcohol exposure and may further contribute to fetal hypoxia (276). Abnormal fetal heart patterns (277), decreased fetal breathing (278), and decreased fetal movements (279) have also been described with alcohol use during pregnancy. There also is a reduction in the neurotransmitters in the human brain, a decrease in the myelination process, and decreases in fetal hippocampal nitric oxide synthase activity (280–285).

Effects on the Newborn Infant

Prematurity

The incidence of prematurity ranges from 46% to 52% in infants with FAS (284,286). The relationship between alcohol exposure and preterm birth in which FAS is not a factor is not as clear. Several reports indicate increased preterm delivery in alcohol abusers (287,288). This may result from an associated increase in congenital anomalies rather than directly from alcohol itself. Nonetheless, heavy alcohol consumption during pregnancy (i.e., six or more drinks per day) has been associated with an approximately threefold increased risk of preterm delivery (289).

Growth and Morphology

Maternal alcohol consumption has been associated with an increased risk for infants with low birth weight and with length and head circumference below the tenth percentile, if the mother's drinking took place during the early first trimester of pregnancy (248,291). Similarly, birth weight, length, and head circumference have been reported to be significantly reduced in the offspring of women who drank continuously throughout pregnancy (292,293). Abnormalities in fetal brain development have also been described (294,295). The low birth weight was influenced by both dose and duration of alcohol exposure. Moderate or light drinking also has been associated with a decrease in the birth weight of the infants (246). The birth weights, however, are within the range of normal, have no biological significance, and often cease to achieve statistical significance when other risk factors, such as smoking, are taken into account. On the other hand, there are reports that show no association between alcohol use and the infant's birth weight. In a group of healthy, full-term infants, no growth difference was noted between those exposed and those not exposed to alcohol (296–298). Some minor morphologic malformations in the infant have been observed with alcohol use during pregnancy (297–301). In contrast, other reports have failed to demonstrate this (296,302–304). In a large prospective birth defects study involving 32,870 women, light and moderate drinkers were not found to have an increased rate of malformations in their offspring relative to nondrinkers (305).

Newborn Withdrawal

Withdrawal from alcohol occurs in infants but rarely is noted because the withdrawal may be confused with nar-

cotic or other drug withdrawal. The withdrawal from ethanol has been described to occur within 12 hours of birth and may manifest as abdominal distention, opisthotonus, convulsions, tremors, hypertonia, apnea, and cyanosis. The infants are irritable, have restless sleep, and engage in exaggerated mouthing behavior (306,307).

Neurobehavioral Effects

Alcohol-exposed infants have been found to habituate less well to aversive stimuli as measured by the Neonatal Behavioral Assessment Scale (308,309), exhibit changes in their reflexive behavior, state control, and motor behavior (296,310), and have increased irritability (311) and depressed range of state (312). These effects, however, have not been universally observed (297,301).

Sleep cycling and arousal have been studied as a measure of neurophysiologic development, integrity, and maturation. Infants of mothers who drank heavily throughout pregnancy showed a greater amount of restless sleep and more bodily movements (313,314). Electroencephalographic power spectrum analyses of the infants showed hypersynchrony of the EEG as well as an increase in the integrated power in all sleep states, particularly with active sleep (315,316). Electroencephalographic maturation also was affected by maternal binge drinking (317).

Breast-Feeding and Alcohol

Alcohol is distributed into breast milk; however, the amount ingested by the infant is only a small fraction of that consumed by the mother (246). Short-term alcohol consumption by lactating women has an immediate effect on the odor of their milk and the feeding behavior of their infant (318). The infants sucked more frequently during the first minute after their mothers had consumed alcohol but consumed significantly less milk. The postnatal growth was not affected in breast-fed infants whose mothers consumed alcohol during lactation (319). In animal studies, ethanol has been shown to block the secretion of oxytocin, thereby preventing milk ejection (320). A similar effect was found in normal women (321). A slight but significant negative effect on motor development as measured by the psychomotor developmental index (PDI) but not on the mental developmental index was observed, using the Bayley scales, in infants who ingested ethanol through breast milk (322).

Long-Term Effects of Prenatal Alcohol Use

Growth

Growth deficits were found in infants at 8 and 18 months of age and were related to alcohol use during the second and third trimesters of pregnancy (323). These children continued to be smaller in weight, length, and head circumference at 3 years of age, even after controlling for nutrition, current environment, exposure to alcohol during lactation, and other significant covariates. Variations in growth retardation have been observed. Growth retardation at 8 months of age but not at subsequent evaluations (324) and significant effects on height and head circumference in children at 6 years of age have been reported (301). Some catch-up growth after 8 months of age has been observed whether the children were exposed to alcohol in the first and second trimesters or throughout gestation (325–327). However, head circumference remained smaller among children who were exposed throughout pregnancy (328). On the other hand, there are reports that show no effects of prenatal alcohol exposure on the infants' growth at 1 and 2 years of age (329,330).

Behavioral and Cognitive Effects

Infants of mothers who drank throughout pregnancy showed less improvement in reflexes and autonomic regulation over the first month of life than infants of women who stopped drinking or who never drank (331). At 6 to 8 months of age, these infants had significantly lower Bayley mental and motor scores (332–334), slower reaction time, longer fixation time, lower scores in elicited play, and longer periods of toy exploration, which may indicate slower cognitive processing (335,336). At 13 months of age, infants of women who drank during pregnancy did less well on the mental index and on the verbal comprehension and spoken language cluster scores derived from the Bayley Scales (329,337,338). In contrast, others have found that prenatal alcohol use did not significantly predict Bayley mental or motor scores at either 8 or 18 months of age (339).

Alcohol use during pregnancy was associated negatively with IQ at 4 years of age (340). At 4 years of age, children who were exposed prenatally to moderate drinking were less attentive and more active during naturalistic observations at home (341) and were less attentive and had longer reaction times on a vigilance task in a laboratory setting (342). Prepregnancy alcohol exposure also was related to increased fine motor errors, increased time to correct the errors, and poorer gross motor balance (343). Preschool children who were exposed to alcohol throughout gestation (with a range of two to nine drinks per day) were more likely to show hyperactivity, language problems, and motor deficits than those whose mothers stopped drinking by the second trimester (344). In children evaluated between 2 and 12 years of age, alcohol exposure during any part of pregnancy appears to be associated with poorer academic achievement, although exposure during the third trimester appears to be associated with lower aptitude scores (328). Attention, distraction, and reaction time on a continuous performance task at 7 years of age continued to be negatively related to alcohol exposure during pregnancy (345). Intelligence quotient effects persisted at 7.5 years, with a decrement of 7 IQ points with exposure to more than 1 ounce of alcohol per day during pregnancy (346). Achievement scores were related to binge drinking before pregnancy. Evaluation during adolescence shows difficulties in tasks that involve manipulation of information, goal management (347), attention, memory (326), calculation, and estimation tests with intact reading and writing ability (348). Fried and Watkinson found that infants exposed to alcohol prenatally evidenced no deficits at 12 months of age (349). However, at 24 months of age, they performed more poorly than non–alcohol-exposed controls on the Bayley Mental Scale and the Reynell Language Scale. At 36 months of age, the language development of the exposed children continued to be affected, but at 48 months of age no significant relationships were found (350).

These inconsistencies regarding the long-term effects of prenatal alcohol exposure on the child's development may lie in the difficulty in separating the teratogenic effects of alcohol from the effects of the disordered environments, both interpersonal and structural, that often accompany alcohol and drug use (351).

Fetal Alcohol Syndrome

The Fetal Alcohol Study Group of the Research Society on Alcoholism defined three specific criteria for the diagnosis of FAS (246). An infant must exhibit an abnormality from each category to qualify for a diagnosis of FAS:

Prenatal or postnatal growth retardation (i.e., weight, length, or head circumference below the 10th percentile when corrected for gestational age).

CNS involvement, which includes signs of neurologic abnormalities (e.g., irritability in infancy, hyperactivity during childhood), developmental delay, hypotonia, or intellectual impairment (e.g., mental retardation).

Characteristic facial dysmorphology (at least two of the three must be present).
  Microcephaly (i.e., head circumference below the third percentile).
  Microphthalmia or short palpebral fissures.
  Poorly developed philtrum, thin upper lip (i.e., vermillion border), and flattening of the maxilla.

Physical findings of smooth philtrum, thin upper lip, and short palpebral fissure have a 100% sensitivity in diagnosing FAS (352,353). Presence of some, but not all, of these features is defined as alcohol-related birth defects (ARBD), or fetal alcohol effects (Table 56–7). Current criteria for diagnosis of FAS depend on recognition of subtle physical anomalies, growth retardation, and nonspecific developmental aberrations, which may change with time, as well as varying degrees of severity which are affected by patient's age or racial background. Underdiagnosis may usually occur when complete patterns of abnormalities cannot be substantiated or clinicians fear stigmatizing the mother and child (354).

Incidence

The incidence of FAS in the world is approximately 1.9 per 1,000 live births. The reported rate in the United States is 2.2 per 1,000 live births (246). Prevalence estimates vary, depending on geographic location and specific population studied (355). The highest reported incidence of FAS occurs in the Native American and black population and those with low socioeconomic status. Sokol and colleagues, in a prospective study of 8,331 pregnancies, identified 25 cases of FAS (356). Four significant prenatal risk factors were identified: black race, high parity, percentage drinking days, and positive Michigan Alcoholism Screening Test. In the absence of any of these factors, the probability of a child being afflicted with FAS was 2%; in the presence of all four, the probability was 85.2%.

Among alcohol-abusing women, the incidence of FAS in the world literature is 71 per 1,000 live births, and in the United States, from 24 to 42 per 1,000 live births (246). The National Institute on Drug Abuse (NIDA) estimates that 7.62 million babies (18.6%) were exposed to alcohol during gestation (357). One factor that has been associated with an increase in the risk of FAS is the history of previous siblings with FAS in the family. It has been estimated that the risk of a younger sibling having FAS, given an older sibling diagnosed as having FAS, is increased by 406 times, so that the incidence of FAS occurring in this group is 771 per 1,000 live births (146). Older siblings are not as likely to be severely affected as younger siblings (246). There is a higher risk of FAS with increasing maternal age and parity. This may be because of an increased maternal body fat-to-water ratio and a faster rate of alcohol metabolism in chronic drinking women (358).

Alcohol has the most teratogenic effect during organogenesis and development of nervous system (359). Teratogenesis is grossly dose related (309,360), although the threshold dose is still not known. Estimates of 21 ounces of absolute alcohol per week around the time of conception may be a critical dose (334,360).

Alcohol-Related Birth Defects

Alcohol-related birth defects may account for as many as 5% of all congenital anomalies (247). Alcohol-related birth defects result from variable dose exposures at variable gestational times and are offset by the genetic background. These determinants place the fetus at a higher risk for possible adverse outcome. The frequency of ARBD is three to five per 1,000 live births. Table 56–7 shows the various dysmorphic features that may be observed in the infant after prenatal alcohol exposure.

Follow-Up of Infants with Fetal Alcohol Syndrome

Postnatal growth retardation and retarded motor performance are hallmarks of prenatal alcohol exposure, especially of FAS. A 10-year follow-up of patients diagnosed to have FAS showed that the children continued to be growth retarded with respect to weight, height, and head circumference. Weight for height was especially decreased (361,362). Long-term study of children with FAS show that the characteristic craniofacial malformations of FAS diminish with time but that the microcephaly and, to a lesser degree, short stature and underweight persist in boys; in female adolescents, body weight normalizes (363,364). However, mental retardation persists, ranging from near normal to severe (365,366). Significant adaptive behavior defects in adolescents and adults with FAS and fetal alcohol effect (FAE), particularly in areas of socialization and communicative skills, also persist (364). Behavioral problems include general spatial memory deficit and distorted spatial arrangement (367), profound verbal and learning deficits (368), stereotyped behaviors, irritability, hyperactivity, attention deficits, tremulousness, and hyperdistractibility (286,366–372). Speech may be delayed or impaired, which may be related in part to hearing impairments (370–376).

Slow growth of the head circumference indicates slow brain growth in children with moderate to severe FAS (354). Neurologic findings by MRI showed significant reduction in the cerebellar vermis (377), cerebral vault, basal ganglia, and diencephalon. The basal ganglia changes may relate to behavioral findings seen in these children (378). Another study has shown mildline anomalies such as complete callosal agenesis, hypoplastic corpus callosum, cavum septum pellucidum, and cavum vergae, which is associated with a greater number of facial anomalies (320,379).

Ophthalmologic abnormalities are also found in children with FAS. These consist primarily of fundus anomalies and optic nerve hypoplasia (381–383). These defects have been attributed to competition of ethanol with retinol at the same ADH-binding sites (384). Other eye findings include strabismus, blepharoptosis, epicanthus, cataract, glaucoma, persistent hyperplastic primary vision, and increased tortuosity of retinal vessels with reduced vascular branching (381,383).

Four types of hearing disorders are associated with FAS: (a) developmental delay in auditory maturation, (b) sensorineural hearing loss, (c) intermittent conductive hearing loss from recurrent serous otitis media, and (d) central hearing loss (385). Seventy-seven percent of children with FAS have conductive hearing loss secondary to recurrent serous otitis media. Twenty-seven percent have

TABLE 56–7. Alcohol and fetal dysmorphogenesis[c]

Central nervous system	
Neurobehavioral	Intellectual impairment (i.e., mild to moderate mental retardation),[a] low IQ (65–70), hypotonia,[b] developmental delay, poor coordination, cognitive and sensory deficits, attention deficits, hyperactivity and irritability in infancy, hyperactivity in childhood,[c] language disabilities and sleep–wake cycle disturbances, electroencephalogram hypersynchrony, delayed or deficient myelination, corpus callosum hypoplasia, echolalia, cerebral palsy
Craniofacial	
Head	Microcephaly,[a] Dandy–Walker malformation, anencephaly, porencephaly, meningomyelocele, spasmus nutans
Eyes	Ocular retinal tortuosity, ptosis, strabismus, epicanthal folds, myopia, retinal coloboma, astigmatism, steep corneal curvature, anterior chamber anomalies, sensorineural hearing loss
Ears	Poorly formed conchae and posterior rotation of the ear and eustachian tube
Nose	Short, upturned[b] hypoplastic philtrum[a]
Mouth	Dental malalignments, small teeth with faulty enamel, retrognathia in infancy[a] or relative prognathia in adolescence, cleft lip or cleft palate, malocclusions, prominent palatine ridges, thinned upper vermillion,[a] poor suck reflex
Maxilla	Hypoplastic[b]
Cardiovascular	
Heart	All cardiac defects (57%), particularly ventricular septal defect, atrial septal defects, murmurs, tetralogy of Fallot, double-outlet right ventricle, dextrocardia, patent ductus arteriosus, and great vessel anomalies
Pulmonary	
Chest	Pectus excavatum, bifid xiphoid
Lungs	Pulmonary atresia, atelectasis, upper respiratory infections
Gastrointestinal	
Abdomen	Inguinal and abdominal hernias, diastasis recti, gastroschisis, hepatic fibrosis, childhood cirrhosis, extrahepatic biliary atresia, hyperbilirubinemia in childhood
Urogenital	
Renal	Hydronephrosis; small rotated kidneys; aplastic, dysplastic, or hypoplastic kidneys; horseshoe kidneys; ureteral duplications; megaloureter, cystic diverticula; vesicovaginal fistula; pyelonephritis
Dermatologic	
Dermatogliphic	Aberrant fingerprint and palmar creases, hemangiomas in one-half of the cases, disproportionately diminished adipose tissue,[b] abnormal whorls on scalp, hirsutism in infancy, nail hypoplasia, poor proprioception
Orthopedic	
Skeletal	Polydactyly, radioulnar synostosis, talipes equinovarus, dislocated hip, scoliosis, Klippel–Feil syndrome, limited joint movement, lumbosacral lipoma, shortened fifth digit, syndactyly, camptodactyly, clinodactyly, flexion contractures
Endocrinology	
Congenital	DiGeorge syndrome

[a]Feature seen in 80% of patients.
[b]Feature seen in more than 50% of patients.
[c]From Pietrantoni M, Knuppel RA. Alcohol in pregnancy. *Clin Perinatol* 1991;18:93.

sensorineural hearing loss, and 100% have central hearing function injuries. A majority of the patients have associated speech pathology, expressive language defects, and receptive language defects (386). The craniofacial abnormalities may also increase the susceptibility to peripheral hearing disorders (387).

MARIJUANA

Marijuana is the most widely used illicit drug among women of childbearing age in the United States (388). In 1996, an estimated 10.1 million Americans were current (past month) marijuana or hashish users, which represents 8.6% of the population 12 years or older. Among pregnant women, 1.6% were current users of marijuana (1,389).

Terminology pertaining to marijuana includes the following: (a) cannabis refers to the crude material from the plant *Cannabis sativa;* (b) marijuana refers to a mixture of crushed leaves, twigs, seeds, and sometimes flowers of the plant; (c) sinsemilla is a variety of high-potency marijuana originally grown in northern California; and (d) hashish is a resin obtained by pressing, scraping, and shaking the plant in hash oil to produce a potent extract (390,391). Cannabis contains more than 400 chemicals; 61 are unique to cannabis and are referred to collectively as cannabinoids. The primary psychoactive component is Δ^9-tetrahydrocannabinol (THC). Other cannabinoids, however, such as cannabidiol and cannabinol, also have biological activity and potentially can affect the fetus (392,393).

Placental Transfer

Tetrahydrocannabinol is highly bound to the lipoprotein fraction in the blood. Studies using radiolabeled THC have shown that tissues with high blood flow show a rapid uptake of the drug (246). Tetrahydrocannabinol crosses the placenta within minutes of administration; however, the placenta may retard THC passage to the fetus. In rats, the placenta contained ten times more radiolabeled THC than fetal serum (394), and fetal rat THC serum levels were well below the maternal serum levels (395). In humans, however, the concentrations of THC in maternal and fetal sera essentially are identical (396).

Effects on Pregnancy

Based on the report of a large perinatal center study, no significant differences were observed between marijuana users and control subjects who were matched in terms of alcohol consumption, cigarette use, and family income with regard to several birth outcome measures such as miscarriage rate, presentation at birth, Apgar status, and the frequency of complications at birth (397,398). Another prospective, multicenter cohort study also showed no significant association between marijuana use during pregnancy and preterm delivery or abruptio placentae (399) (Table 56–8).

Effects on the Fetus and Newborn Infant

A reduction by 0.8 weeks was observed in the gestational age of infants of heavy marijuana users (six or more times/week) compared to infants of nonusers, although in some studies, 25% had premature infants (398,400). However, this effect was not consistently observed (401–403).

Most studies have not reported an increase in the incidence of major or minor malformations in the offspring with prenatal marijuana exposure (403–405). In the few reported cases of malformations, the confounding variables of poor nutrition, little prenatal care, low socioeconomic status, and other factors that may have interacted to produce these abnormalities were not controlled for (406).

There seems to be an increase in the gender ratio of live male–female offspring in marijuana users. In animals, litters from dams fed 50 mg/kg of THC showed a significant increase in the proportion of male offspring, ranging from 57% to 61% (407,408). In a study of women who smoked marijuana during pregnancy, heavy use similarly was associated with a significant increase in male over female births (402).

Most studies do not show a significant effect of prenatal marijuana use on fetal growth weight. In animal studies, reduced birth weights among the drug-exposed offspring were observed (395) but appeared to have resulted

TABLE 56–8. *Complications associated with cannabinoid, nicotine, PCP, amphetamine, methamphetamine, and caffeine use during pregnancy*

	Antenatal	Intrapartum	Neonatal	Long-term
Marijuana	IUGR	Premature delivery	LBW Abnormal neurobehavioral outcome Fine tremors Exaggerated and prolonged startles Poor visual habituation Less ability to regulate state and disrupted sleep patterns	Poor abstract/visual reasoning at 36 months Poor memory and verbal outcome at 48 months of age
Nicotine	Late fetal death	Spontaneous abortion Abruptio placenta Preterm labor	SIDS	Poor performance in tests of cognitive, psychomotor, language, and general academic achievement
PCP	IUGR	Precipitate labor Meconium-stained amniotic fluid Premature delivery	Neonatal drug withdrawal/intoxication Abnormal neurobehavioral outcome Irritability, tremors, hypertonicity, poor attention, bizarre eye movements	Temperament and sleep problems at 12 months
Amphetamine/ methamphetamine	IUGR	Premature delivery Retroplacental hemorrhage	LBW IVH Necrosis in basal ganglia, frontal lobes and posterior fossa Neonatal drug withdrawal	Increased illness and accident rates Low IQ at 4 years Aggressive behavior and peer-related problems
Caffeine	IUGR Fetal arrhythmia		LBW Neonatal withdrawal Cardiac arrhythmia	

largely from the reduced maternal food and water intake rather than the effect of the drug (409).

There is an equivocal relationship between prenatal marijuana use and neurobehavioral outcome of the offspring (410). Prenatal marijuana exposure has been associated with increased fine tremors in the infant, accompanied by exaggerated and prolonged startles, both spontaneous and in response to mild stimuli; poorer visual but not auditory stimuli habituation (410); and decreased ability to regulate state and disrupted sleep patterns (411). Elevated serum norepinephrine levels have been observed among these infants (412). Other reports have found no altered neurobehavioral patterns in marijuana-exposed offspring (313,402,413).

Long-Term Outcome

After controlling for confounding variables, prenatal marijuana use was found to be associated with increased infant weight at 12 months and increased height at 24 months of age (349). One report, however, found no effect on infant growth at 12 months of age (402). In general, there has been no observed effect of marijuana use on infant motor and mental development at 12 months of age, as determined by the Bayley Scales of Infant Development (349,402). However, women who used marijuana prenatally were found to be less involved with their children at 24 months of age and provided less stimulating home environments. From a preschool sample, no effect of prenatal marijuana use on IQ scores was found at 4 years of age. However, there are reports that have shown, in infants at age 36 to 48 months, poor abstract/visual reasoning and poor memory and verbal outcome in association with heavy prenatal marijuana use (223,349,350,410).

NICOTINE AND SMOKING

Cigarette smoke contains about 4,000 chemical compounds. Most of these chemical agents are in the gas phase of cigarette smoke and include carbon monoxide, carbon dioxide, nitrogen oxides, ammonia, hydrogen cyanide, and other compounds. A smaller number of these undesirable compounds are in the particulate phase of cigarette smoke (i.e., nicotine and tar). Tar is what remains after the moisture and nicotine are subtracted. It consists primarily of polycyclic aromatic hydrocarbons (e.g., nitrosamines, aromatic amines, polycyclic hydrocarbons) and numerous other compounds, including metallic ions and radioactive compounds (414).

Absorption and Metabolism

Nicotine is the most studied substance in cigarette smoke and is considered the compound primarily responsible for the pharmacologic effects of smoking. It is absorbed readily from the lungs, almost with the same efficiency as by intravenous administration. Blood nicotine levels vary depending on the amount of nicotine delivered. The amount of nicotine delivered depends on the duration and intensity of inhalation, the number of inhalations per cigarette, the presence or absence of filters, the brand of the cigarette (which affects the composition of the tobacco), how densely the tobacco is packed, and the length of the column of tobacco (414).

Nicotine is distributed rapidly throughout the body. It reaches the brain within 8 seconds after inhalation. Peak concentrations of nicotine in plasma after a cigarette is smoked are typically 25 to 50 ng/mL. The course of elimination of nicotine is multiexponential. After a single cigarette, concentrations decline rapidly (i.e., over 5 to 10 minutes), primarily reflecting distribution. After long-term smoking, the elimination half-life of nicotine is approximately 2 hours (414).

Nicotine is metabolized mainly in the liver but also in the kidneys and lungs. The two main metabolites are cotinine and nicotine-1'-N-oxide. Cotinine has few or no cardiovascular or subjective effects. It is cleared more slowly than nicotine, with a half-life of about 19 hours. Cotinine concentrations in the plasma and milk of mothers and in the urine of their infants have been reported to reflect the smoking habits of the mothers during pregnancy (415). Thus, it is a better measure of overall intake than nicotine itself. Nicotine crosses the placenta and also is excreted in the milk of lactating women (414). There is a close correlation between nicotine concentration in the mother's plasma and milk after smoking (415).

Incidence

An estimated 62 million Americans were current smokers in 1996, representing a smoking rate of 29% for the population age 12 and older (1). Tobacco is still widely used by women of childbearing age. Data from the 1995 and 1996 National Household Survey on Drug Abuse show that 63.1% of pregnant women had smoked tobacco in their lifetime, 29% had smoked tobacco in the past year, and 20.3% were current smokers. Most of those who smoked during pregnancy were Caucasian women. About 23.6% of current smokers smoked during the first trimester, 23.8% continued to smoke during the second trimester, and 17% up to third trimester. Most of the current smokers were 26 to 44 years old (1,389).

Spontaneous Abortion

The relationship between cigarette smoking and spontaneous abortion has been documented in both animal and human studies. When other risk factors are controlled, women who smoke cigarettes during pregnancy are 1.2 to 2 times more likely to have a spontaneous abortion than those who do not smoke (416). The higher rate of abortion was noted in women who smoke one-half of a pack per day compared to nonsmokers. The mechanism for this association has not been completely elucidated, although studies support the theory that this may be related to the vasoactive effects of nicotine on the umbilical arteries (417). Nicotine decreases prostacyclin production in the umbilical artery and reduces its capacity for vasodilation, thereby affecting fetal nutrition and oxygen transport, especially in conditions causing asphyxia (418). Other studies attribute the higher rate of abortion to abnormalities in placental development as well as to dysfunction of hormones that sustain pregnancy (419,420).

Placental Effects

An increased incidence of placental abruption and an increase in fetal death from abruption were seen among women who smoke more than ten cigarettes per day (421). Maternal smoking was associated with the finding of decidual necrosis on pathologic examination. Extensive placental calcification occurred significantly more often in smokers than in nonsmokers (46% versus 14%) (419). Intervillous blood flow was reported to be reduced acutely during smoking and for 15 minutes afterward (420).

Apgar Scores

Several studies have noted that maternal cigarette smoking during pregnancy is associated with low Apgar scores; however, other risk factors were not controlled for in the analysis (422). When potentially confounding factors were controlled for, no significant independent association was noted between cigarette smoking and Apgar scores (423).

Preterm Birth

Maternal smoking has been reported to be a risk factor for preterm labor. The incidence of preterm labor increases with the number of cigarettes smoked per day (424,425). However, other studies have shown no effect of smoking on length of gestation (426).

Sudden Infant Death Syndrome

Several studies have reported that maternal cigarette smoking significantly increases the likelihood of sudden infant death syndrome (427). It is proposed that nicotine affects catecholamine metabolism in the brain, causing an attenuated response to hypoxia, which later causes disturbances in respiratory and cardiovascular control mechanisms (428). Maternal smoking has also been associated with increased incidence of central apnea among infants

(429). Mothers of infants who died from the sudden infant death syndrome were more likely to smoke cigarettes either during pregnancy or after their baby was born.

Fetal Death and Neonatal Mortality

Epidemiologic studies have noted a significant effect of smoking on late fetal death and neonatal mortality. Among first-born infants in mothers who smoked, there was a 25% greater risk for fetal death and neonatal mortality for less than one-pack-per-day smokers and a 56% greater risk for more than one-pack-per-day smokers, compared to the nonsmokers (430). For second or higher births, a 30% greater risk of late fetal death and neonatal mortality was noted in maternal smokers compared to nonsmokers. Maternal smoking had a relative risk for late fetal death of 1.4 and a relative risk for early neonatal mortality of 1.2 (431).

Growth and Development

Several studies have examined the association between smoking before or during pregnancy and birth weight. These studies have consistently demonstrated a decrease in birth weight of approximately 200 g as well as an increased percentage of low-birth-weight (LBW) infants (335,425,432–434). In addition, a dose–response relationship has been demonstrated between the number of cigarettes smoked and the decrease in birth weight (435,436) and the percentage of LBW infants (437). These findings remain consistent when confounding variables are controlled for (335). For Caucasian mothers, the incidence of LBW babies ranges from 4.8% for women who do not smoke to 8% for women who smoke one to ten cigarettes per day and to 13.4% for women who smoke more than 20 cigarettes per day. For black women, the incidence of LBW babies ranges from 8.3% for women who do not smoke to 13.5% for women who smoke one to ten cigarettes per day to 22.7% for women who smoke more than 20 cigarettes per day (437). One study demonstrated that serum nicotine levels were more strongly correlated with reduced birth weight than with smoking history (438). This indicates the importance of using biochemical markers in studies of pregnancy outcome.

Studies comparing infant birth weights show that mothers who quit smoking during pregnancy have infants with higher birth weights than do mothers who continue to smoke during pregnancy, although the birth weight is still about 179 g lower than that of infants of nonsmoking mothers (436). The difference in birth weight was highly significant when smoking was discontinued by as late as 16 weeks of gestation, compared to persistent smokers. However, even beyond 16 weeks of gestation, cessation of smoking was still found to be associated with infants with higher birth weights than the offspring of persistent smokers (435). Passive smoking does not seem to cause significant reduction in corrected birth weight (434).

The nature of the growth deficit, in terms of newborn body composition, was assessed by examining the anthropometric indices of subcutaneous fat deposition and lean body mass in infants of smokers and nonsmokers. There was no difference between the two groups of infants in the skinfold measurements or in the calculated cross-sectional fat area of the upper arm. These results suggest that the reduction in birth weight of infants whose mothers smoke resides primarily in a decrease in the lean body mass of the newborn, whereas deposition of subcutaneous fat is relatively unaffected (439). Besides birth weight, length and head circumference were also found to be smaller for infants of smoking mothers (433), especially among those who continued to smoke to the third trimester (440).

Various studies assessing the association between cigarette smoking during pregnancy and congenital malformations have shown conflicting results. The British Perinatal Mortality Survey, in a study of 17,418 subjects, demonstrated that maternal smoking was associated with congenital heart defects, even after maternal age, parity, and social class were controlled for (441). The United States Collaborative Perinatal Project, in a study of 50,282 subjects, did not demonstrate this association (442,443). The inconsistency of reports suggests that cigarette smoking per se may not be a cause of congenital malformations in infants (444).

Neurobehavioral Effects

Several studies have investigated the impact of cigarette smoking during pregnancy on newborn behavior and on later child development (445,446). Offspring of mothers who smoked during pregnancy have been observed to perform less well on the Brazelton Neonatal Behavioral Assessment Score in items such as habituating to sound or orienting to a voice, compared to offspring of nonsmoking mothers. Other studies indicate poorer performance with head turning and sucking; lower visual alertness; more crying, tremors, and startles; and increased lability of color. Most of the studies, however, do not demonstrate a clinically significant effect on neonatal behavior that can be attributed independently to maternal cigarette smoking alone.

Long-term follow-up evaluation of children's cognitive and developmental functions seems to indicate that when sociodemographic factors are controlled for, children exposed to cigarette smoke *in utero* do less well in tests of cognitive, psychomotor, language, and general academic achievement, including reading and mathematics. Although differences are statistically significant between the two groups, they are small compared to other factors that affect the children's performance (447–450).

PHENCYCLIDINE

Phencyclidine was first introduced as a dissociative anesthetic in 1957. Despite its wide margin of safety in humans, its clinical use was discontinued after reports of adverse effects that include agitation, confusion, delirium, and persistent hallucinations. Other untoward effects noted with its use were feelings of paranoia, impending death, outbursts of bizarre, agitated, or violent behavior, and a psychosis mimicking schizophrenia. It remains popular as a drug of abuse because of its sedative and hallucinogenic effects, its synthesis from readily available precursors, low cost, and variety of routes of administration. Most users smoke PCP; others sniff or snort the powder, drink the liquid form mixed with lemonade or alcohol, or inject it intravenously (451–454).

Placental Transfer and Metabolism

Placental transfer of PCP has been studied in the pig, mouse, rabbit, and humans. In piglets, serum levels of PCP were ten times higher than in the sow (455,456); in fetal rabbits, similar high serum levels were found that reached a peak 2 hours after parenteral administration of the drug to the doe (457). In the mouse, there was almost a tenfold higher concentration of PCP in fetal tissue than in maternal blood (457), and PCP appeared in the pup's brain as early as 15 minutes after subcutaneous injection to the dam (452). Phencyclidine also has been detected in amniotic fluid and umbilical cord blood at high concentrations (458).

Phencyclidine appears rapidly in breast milk, appearing within 15 minutes of maternal administration. By 3 hours, the ratio of its level in milk to that in plasma is approximately ten to one (457).

Phencyclidine is lipophilic. It is stored in body fat and in the CNS for a prolonged period and is released slowly into the bloodstream. The major routes of elimination involve metabolism of PCP in the liver and excretion in the urine and feces (459). The half-life of the drug in the body usually is about 3 days, although it has been found in the urine as long as 8 days after last use (460). The half-life of PCP in the fetus is approximately twice that in the mother (457).

Mode of Action

Phencyclidine has strong centrally mediated effects in animals and humans and influences many different neuronal systems. It inhibits the uptake and increases the release of monoamines in the brain, interacts with cholinergic and serotonergic systems, and antagonizes the neuronal stimulation caused by the excitatory amino acid, N-methyl aspartate (451). Phencyclidine may produce a general enhancement of neurotransmitter release by blocking voltage-sensitive potassium channels, and thus might act at several different loci (461).

Incidence

The abuse of PCP first occurred in 1970, peaked in 1979, and then declined by 1981 (462). National surveys, however, since have indicated that PCP abuse is again on the rise, especially in large urban areas.

The prevalence of PCP abuse during pregnancy has not been firmly established because most reports have come from urban areas and could not be generalized to a national level. Between 1981 and 1982 in Cleveland, 7.5% of 2,327 pregnant women gave a history of PCP use, although only 0.8% could be confirmed by maternal urine screening (463,464). In 1983, a study from Los Angeles reported that 12% of a random sample of 200 newborns had measurable quantities of PCP in their cord blood (458). In 1995 and 1996, about 2.6% of pregnant women admitted having used PCP in their lifetime, and 0.2% admitted having used it in the past year (389).

Growth and Morphology

Animal studies indicate that maternal weight gain is lower in PCP-exposed mice. The birth weights of exposed pups were approximately 7% lower than those of nonexposed pups (452). In humans, no significant difference in birth weight or length or head circumference was observed in PCP-exposed newborns compared to matched controls (465). In another study, two of five preterm and none of seven term PCP-exposed newborns were small for gestational age. All 12 newborns were normocephalic (466). In one study, however, intrauterine growth retardation, precipitate labor, neonatal drug withdrawal/intoxication, and longer hospital stay were observed among PCP-exposed newborns, which were comparable to, if not less pronounced (467) than, cocaine effects (468).

There was also a higher incidence of meconium-stained amniotic fluid and less incidence of premature delivery (468). In both animal and human studies, PCP has not been shown to be teratogenic, and no reports of congenital malformations attributable to PCP have as yet been made.

Neurobehavioral Effects

Early case reports of PCP-exposed newborns showed abnormal neurobehavioral findings in the infants. These included irritability, tremors, hypertonicity, poor attention, bizarre eye movements, staring spells, hypertonic ankle reflexes, and depressed grasp and rooting reflexes (464,465,469). One of the most characteristic features in infants is a sudden and rapid change in level of consciousness, with lethargy alternating with irritability. The behavioral outcome of these newborns has been attributed to PCP intoxication rather than to withdrawal (467). The very low threshold of stimulation, coarse, flapping tremors, and rapid changes in state are similar to behavior reported in children and adults intoxicated with PCP (465).

Long-Term Outcome

The Bayley psychomotor and mental development indices of PCP-exposed infants at 3 months and at 1 year (470) of age were not statistically different from those of controls (465). In one study, however, temperament and sleep problems were noted at 12 months of age (470). At 9 and 18 months of age, fine motor development, adaptive or playing behavior, language skills, and personal–social development as determined by the Gesell Developmental Evaluation were within normal range. Phencyclidine exposure reportedly does not affect Bayley scores during the first 2 years of life (471). These findings are consistent with the interpretation that the observed PCP effects on infants at birth result from acute intoxication rather than from morphologic CNS damage.

AMPHETAMINES

The amphetamines are a group of chemically related sympathomimetic amines that have both CNS stimulant and peripheral α and β actions (472). Since their synthesis in the 1880s, therapeutic uses have included the treatment of exogenous obesity, narcolepsy, hyperkinesis, and depression. There is a very strong abuse potential because of their psychic effects, which include a decreased sense of fatigue, wakefulness, alertness, mood elevation, self-confidence, and often euphoria and elation.

Epidemiology

After initial epidemics of abuse of speed in the 1950s and 1960s, there was a decline in the abuse of amphetamines with the emergence of other drugs of abuse (e.g., heroin, crack cocaine). Lately, a resurgence of amphetamine use in epidemic proportions has occurred, particularly in Japan and parts of Asia, Hawaii, and areas of the West Coast. The incidence of stimulant use during pregnancy has been reported as 1.8% for past-year users and 0.6% for current users during 1995 and 1996 (389).

Methamphetamine

Methamphetamine is the methylated derivative of amphetamine and is prepared through the reduction of ephedrine or pseudoephedrine. The ease of its synthesis, its availability and affordability, and a prolonged high have made it an increasingly popular drug of abuse. Ice, the smokable form of methamphetamine, is claimed to produce an intense euphoria. High doses may cause aggressive behavior, arrhythmias, severe anxiety, seizures, shock, and death. Chronic use can produce paranoid psychosis.

Effects on Pregnancy

Outcomes of pregnancies in 52 self-reported intravenous methamphetamine abusers were studied; these patients used other drugs as well (473). The infants had significantly lower birth weight, length, and head circumference than infants of non–drug users. There was no significant difference, however, in the frequency of pregnancy complications such as pregnancy-induced hypertension, peripartum hemorrhage, chorioamnionitis, syphilis, and hepatitis.

No significant increase in the frequency of major congenital anomalies has been associated with methamphetamine use during pregnancy (473,474).

Higher incidences of prematurity, intrauterine growth retardation, and smaller head circumference have been reported in infants of mothers who abused cocaine and methamphetamine (464,476). A higher incidence of retroplacental hemorrhage also was noted (475).

Effects on Neonates

An infant of a known amphetamine addict manifested after birth with diaphoresis, episodes of agitation alternating with lassitude, miosis, and vomiting (477). Infants exposed to both cocaine and methamphetamine were described as having abnormal sleep patterns, tremors, poor feeding, hypertonia, sneezing, a high-pitched cry, frantic fist sucking, tachypnea, loose stools, fever, yawning, hyperreflexia, and excoriation (475). Cranial ultrasound performed on term neonates exposed to cocaine, methamphetamine, or cocaine and a narcotic showed a higher incidence of cranial abnormalities similar to the incidence of infants at risk for hypoxic ischemic injury. The abnormalities include intraventricular hemorrhage, cavitary lesions, echo densities associated with necrosis, mostly in basal ganglia, frontal lobes, and posterior fossa. This is probably related to the vasoconstrictive property of these drugs (478).

Long-Term Effects

Long-term, prospective follow-up of 65 children of women who abused amphetamines and also used alcohol and smoked cigarettes during pregnancy revealed that, at 1 year of age, somatic growth was normal, although illness and accident rates were increased (479). At 4 and 8 years of age, somatic growth and general health remained normal (480,481). Prenatal amphetamine and or cocaine exposure has been reported as a risk factor for later subtle neurologic abnormalities (233). Developmental screening at 4 years of age, using the Terman Merrill method, revealed significantly lower IQs (480), but IQ and psychomotor development were within normal limits by 8 years of age (481). Aggressive behavior and peer-related problems also were noted (481).

CAFFEINE

Caffeine (1,3,7-trimethylxanthine) is a mild CNS stimulant that is the most widely used psychoactive drug in the world. It is found in coffee (the most important source of caffeine in the American diet), tea, chocolate, cocoa, and in numerous prescription and over-the-counter medications (482).

Caffeine is readily absorbed from the digestive tract and is rapidly distributed to all tissues. It easily crosses the placenta and is found in breast milk. Caffeine has several proposed mechanisms of action. One is that it inhibits phosphodiesterase, thereby causing intracellular accumulation of cAMP. It may also block adenosine receptors and cause increased release of calcium ions from the terminal cisternae of the sarcoplasmic reticulum (483). The major effects of caffeine, as with other xanthine derivatives, are CNS stimulation, emesis, cardiovascular effects, diuresis, and smooth muscle effects leading to vasodilation or bronchodilation (483).

Teratogenicity, Spontaneous Abortion, and Prematurity

Caffeine is teratogenic when given in high concentrations to experimental animals, causing limb and facial anomalies. However, no correlation exists between caffeine consumption in humans and birth defects (484). In rodents, caffeine causes malformations, usually at high doses, not seen in humans. Maternal caffeine consumption during gestation affects the hematologic parameters in both rat and human infants (485). Overwhelming evidence indicates that caffeine is not a human teratogen and that caffeine appears to have no effect on preterm labor and delivery (426,486,487).

Growth and Development

Most of the reported effects of maternal caffeine consumption on fetal growth and development describe a negative effect on birth weight and a higher incidence of IUGR. Caffeine ingested in large amounts (over seven cups of coffee/day or more than 300 g of caffeine/day) during pregnancy causes a dose-dependent decrease in birth weight of about 6.5% (485–490). The risk for low birth weight is further increased by concomitant use of alcohol, nicotine, and illicit drugs (489). Other studies, however, have reported no adverse effects, especially with moderate maternal consumption (491) or when other confounding variables such as maternal smoking (492), cannabis (330), alcohol (493), and socioeconomic factors are controlled for. Pregnant mothers are therefore advised to consume coffee or caffeinated beverages in moderation.

Neurobehavioral Effects

Maternal caffeine consumption has been reported to induce long-term effects on sleep, locomotion, learning abilities, emotivity, and anxiety among experimental animals. More studies are needed to confirm these observations among human infants (485). Other effects reported include cardiac arrhythmias (494,495) and a possible withdrawal syndrome characterized by jitteriness, irritability, and vomiting (496). It is postulated that these withdrawal signs are caused by a tripling of the half-life of caffeine during the last two trimesters of pregnancy, resulting in much higher caffeine blood levels in both the mother and the fetus. This is further aggravated by the neonate's relative inability to metabolize caffeine (485,497).

DIAGNOSIS OF DRUG EXPOSURE

Methods to Detect Drug Exposure in the Mother and Infant

The identification of drug exposure in the mother or her neonate is not easy. Mothers rarely spontaneously admit to the use of drugs because of fear of the consequences stemming from such an admission. Even with maternal cooperation, information on the type and extent of drug use often is inaccurate (14). Similarly, many of the drugs to which the fetus is exposed *in utero* do not produce immediate or recognizable effects in neonates (498). There are a number of methods used to detect prenatal drug exposure.

Methods to detect substance abuse in a pregnant woman or intrauterine drug exposure in a neonate ideally should address not only the types of drug abused but also the amount, frequency, and duration of drug exposure. Two general methods are used to achieve this: maternal interview and laboratory tests.

Maternal Interview

Maternal interview has the greatest potential for providing comprehensive information on the type, amount, frequency, and duration of drug use. Two types of maternal interview generally are used.

Routine Interview

The routine interview forms an integral part of the obstetric history, which is obtained either prenatally or when a woman is admitted in labor. The accuracy of the data obtained by this method depends on the attention devoted to the interview. A cursory interview often results in underreporting of drug use, whereas the incidence increases threefold to fivefold if a more organized protocol is used (499). There are many elements inherent to routine history taking that affect its accuracy. Maternal fear of the consequences of admission, underestimation of drug use even by those who admit to the use of drugs, and physical discomfort experienced by the woman, particularly if in labor, all influence the accuracy of her self-report (14). Under these circumstances, the reporting of

drug abuse by the mother can be as low as one-fourth of the true incidence (2).

Structured Interview

A structured interview is a highly organized interview, frequently using a standard questionnaire. Examples of this are the Khavari Alcohol Test (300,501) or its modification (25) and the Cahalan Volume Variability Scale (502). The structured interview is more accurate because more time is spent with the patient and the interview frequently is conducted in a more favorable environment than is the routine interview (i.e., it is not conducted when the mother is in labor). Structured interviews frequently are used as research tools. On the other hand, structured interviews are expensive and time-consuming to conduct and are not practical for routine clinical use when dealing with patients who present in labor and have received little or no prenatal care.

Laboratory Tests

Most of the laboratory tests for drug detection are used simply for screening purposes. Confirmation with the use of another, unrelated procedure usually is needed if results are to withstand further scrutiny. It is apparent that as more confirmatory tests are done, the testing process becomes more expensive. Thus, the extent to which further tests are carried out after the initial screen is determined by the reasons that initiated the test.

Various analytic procedures are used for drug detection: thin-layer chromatography and immunoassays for screening; high-performance liquid chromatography (HPLC), gas chromatography, and gas chromatography–mass spectrometry (GCMS)for confirmation. A good review of the use and limitations of these procedures has been published (503).

Specimens for Drug Testing

Urine. The testing for drugs in biological fluids is by far the most common method used to detect drug abuse in a pregnant woman or intrauterine drug exposure in a neonate. There are several limitations to this method, however. Identification of drugs in biological fluids will only differentiate those who have been exposed to drugs from those who were not. The test cannot provide information on the amount, frequency, duration, or the time of last drug use. Among the biological fluids, urine has been most often tested because of several advantages (504): urine collection is easy and noninvasive; drug metabolites in urine usually are found in higher concentrations than in serum, as a result of the concentrating ability of the kidneys; large volumes of urine can be collected; urine is easier to analyze than blood because it usually is devoid of protein and other cellular constituents; the metabolites in urine usually are stable, especially if frozen; and urine is amenable to all of the drug-testing methods described earlier.

There are several drawbacks to the use of urine for testing, however. Foremost is the high rate of false-negative results (14,505). In the mother, unless collection is watched closely, urine easily can be substituted with a clean specimen. Urine samples can be tampered with by dilution or by the addition of ions, such as salt, which may interfere with the testing methods. Drug metabolites in urine also reflect only very recent use of the drug, so that negative results may occur if the woman abstains from the use of the drug for a few days before testing (504). In the infant, the incidence of false-negative urine tests also is high, ranging from 32% to 63% (506–508). Urine specimens must be obtained as close to birth as possible to reflect the intrauterine exposure of the infant to drugs. The longer after birth that urine is collected and tested, the higher is the likelihood of a false-negative test. Collection of the requisite volume of urine for both the screening test and the confirmatory test from an extremely small or very sick infant may prove impossible. The cutoff concentration for positivity used by the laboratory also may influence the detection rate (509). Recent abstention by the mother from the use of drugs may result in a negative urine test in the infant. The detection rate for drugs in the urine can be improved if a battery rather than a single test is used (508).

Meconium. The concept behind meconium drug testing was based on studies in pregnant rhesus monkeys that received morphine throughout gestation; high concentrations of morphine and its metabolites were found in the gastrointestinal tracts or "meconium" of their fetuses (510). It was postulated that the drug accumulated in meconium as a consequence of fetal swallowing of amniotic fluid that contained drugs originating from fetal urine or from the excretion of drug metabolites through the bile. Subsequent studies in pregnant rats further showed that the concentration of morphine and cocaine in meconium was related to the dose, timing, and duration of drug administration to the dam (511,512).

Meconium drug testing has been adapted to various analytic methods, which include radioimmunoassay, EMIT, FPIA, HPLC, and GCMS (513). The original analysis of meconium for drugs was by radioimmunoassay and the recovery of morphine and benzoylecgonine that were spiked in meconium ranged from 84% to 97% and 70% to 100%, respectively (514). The use of radioimmunoassays that can detect both parent drug and its metabolites, e.g., Coat-a-Count (DPC, Los Angeles, CA) will result in a higher detection rate than those that are specific only for the metabolites. A radioimmunoassay-based meconium drug-testing kit, Mectest (Meco Industries, Walnut, CA), has recently been approved by the FDA for the testing of cocaine, opiate, and cannabinoid in meconium. Mectest exhibits very high sensitivity and specificity; the detection limit was 7.62 ng/mL for

cocaine, 27.8 ng/mL for opiate, and 5.3% ng/mL for cannabinoid. Intraassay precision showed a coefficient of variation of 5.9% for cocaine, 4.5% for opiate, and 11.9% for cannabinoid and interassay precision of 8.4% for cocaine, 1.1% for opiate, and 8.9% for cannabinoid. Endogenous compounds in meconium, such as bilirubin, blood, and protein, did not interfere with the analysis of cocaine, morphine, and cannabinoid, and minimal (0% to 0.2%) cross-reactivity to other drugs was found.

The concentration of drugs in meconium will change if meconium is left at room temperature for 24 hours: 25% decrease in cocaine, 62% increase in morphine, and 30% decrease in cannabinoid. The increase in morphine results from the endogenous hydrolysis of morphine glucuronide into morphine in meconium from the action of β-glucuronidase and the higher sensitivity of the radioimmunoassay for morphine compared to its glucuronide. On the other hand, drugs are stable in meconium, if frozen, for as long as 9 months.

Meconium drug testing has also been adapted to EMIT and FPIA (515). However, relative to radioimmunoassay, the sensitivity of enzyme immunoassay for cocaine, opiate, and cannabinoid was decreased at low drug concentrations in meconium, although the specificity was 100%. With EMIT and FPIA, the cutoff concentrations for meconium drug testing were 50 ng/ml for cocaine, 100 ng/ml for morphine, and 25 ng/ml for cannabinoid (515). Meconium has also been tested for methamphetamine and phencyclidine using EMIT. The detection limits were 730 and 100 ng/g meconium, respectively (516). Meconium drug testing has been adapted to HPLC (516–519) and GCMS analysis (520–524). The detection limit by HPLC was 50 ng/g meconium for benzoylecgonine and 500 ng/g meconium for morphine and amphetamine. By GCMS, the limit of detection was 11 ng/ml for cocaine and its metabolites, 5 ng/g meconium for morphine, codeine, hydromorphine, and hydrocodone, and 2 ng/g meconium for cannabinoids. Fatty acid esters of ethanol have been analyzed in meconium by GCMS, and their concentrations correlated to maternal alcohol use during pregnancy (525). Likewise, nicotine metabolites (cotinine and *trans*-3′-hydroxycotinine) have been measured in meconium by radioimmunoassay and GCMS (526).

A number of clinical studies using the meconium drug test have demonstrated major advantages of meconium drug testing over urine testing in newborn infants. These included the ease and noninvasiveness of meconium collection, which was particularly useful in an anonymous drug prevalence study; high sensitivity and specificity of the test; large window for detecting intrauterine drug exposure to as early as the 16th week of gestation, reliability of testing meconium samples even for those obtained beyond 24 hours after birth, and positive correlation between concentration of drugs in meconium and the amount of drug use by the mother during gestation (512,527–532,535). However, one study found that when a sufficiently sensitive method, such as GCMS, was used for drug analysis, maternal urine, infant urine, and meconium analysis yielded equivalent results (533). The main disadvantage of meconium drug testing is the nonhomogeniety of meconium, which requires preparative procedures to produce the analyte.

Hair. Hair analysis is one of the most recent additions to drug testing (534). The test is based on the principle that illicit substances and their metabolic products in the patient's blood become incorporated into the hair follicle and grow into the cuticle and hair shaft. The drug, once deposited in the hair shaft, remains for an indefinite period. As the hair grows at the rate of 1 to 2 cm month, the deposited drugs follow the growth of the hair shaft. The section of the hair closest to the scalp is the most recently exposed portion. Sectional analysis can be performed by month to provide information on the duration and time of drug use. The information on the chronicity of drug use makes hair analysis advantageous compared with urine or other body fluid testing. Furthermore, quantitative detection of drugs in hair has been correlated with the amount of drug use in the past.

Hair has been analyzed successfully to detect opiates (535), cocaine (536), PCP (537), methamphetamine, antidepressants, and nicotine (538). The analytic procedures that have been used include radioimmunoassay (534), gas chromatography–mass spectrometry (539), HPLC (540), and collisional spectroscopy (541).

The validity of hair analysis for drug detection has been demonstrated in both the mother and her neonate (542). Although hair analysis has some exciting potential, there are some significant drawbacks to the use of hair for testing in women (543). Patients who are not chronic drug users may not be detected by this technique because drug deposition in hair relies on serum levels during hair growth. The expense of the test mounts with the number of drugs being screened for, and this has limited its usefulness in prenatal clinics. The quantity of hair necessary to perform the drug screen (i.e., a pencil-sized diameter plug of hair from the posterior scalp) may be difficult to collect in some newborns. Use of hair dye, bleach, and other cosmetic agents by the woman may modify the quantity of drug found in hair but should not totally eliminate its presence because the drug is incorporated into the hair shaft. Some ethnic groups weave hair from other individuals into their own hair, and this creates the potential for false test results. Because of misconceptions about cosmetic effects, some patients may refuse hair testing. Hair can also be passively exposed to drugs that can be smoked (e.g., cocaine, marijuana).

Other Specimens

Other types of specimens have been tested for drugs. These include perspiration, nail clippings, menstrual blood, semen, and saliva (544,545). The use of these specimens for drug detection has been uncommon, however.

TREATMENT

Initial management of the infant is directed to the antenatal and neonatal complications associated with maternal drug abuse such as asphyxia, fetal distress, prematurity, meconium aspiration, and congenital malformation. In addition, the infant should routinely receive serologic tests for syphilis, HIV disease, and hepatitis B; be assessed for signs of drug withdrawal; undergo a drug screen; and receive social service referral.

Narcotic Withdrawal

The infant of an opiate-dependent mother should be observed closely for withdrawal. The severity of the withdrawal can be assessed by several clinical scoring systems (546,547). We use a system that evaluates the infant specifically on manifestations that are life-threatening: vomiting, diarrhea, weight loss, irritability, tremors, and tachypnea (Table 56–9). With this system, drugs are used to treat the withdrawal if there is moderate vomiting, diarrhea, or weight loss; or any severe criterion.

Both narcotic and nonnarcotic drugs have been used to treat narcotic withdrawal (Table 56–10). Narcotics are preferred, however, because their action is more physiologic for an abstinence state. The neurologic manifestations of withdrawal may be controlled successfully by nonnarcotic drugs, but the narcotics are more effective in relieving the non-CNS manifestations (e.g., diarrhea). Withdrawal has been treated successfully with barbiturate.

Among the narcotic drugs, paregoric, laudanum, and sometimes methadone are used. We prefer to use tincture of opium or laudanum, United States Pharmacopeia (USP), rather than paregoric because paregoric contains camphor, a CNS stimulant. Laudanum USP is available in a standard 10% solution, contains 1.0% morphine, and must be used with caution. Laudanum USP must be diluted 25-fold to a concentration of 0.4% to reduce its morphine content to a level equivalent to that present in paregoric. Laudanum USP 0.4% can be given at the same dose as paregoric (i.e., 3–6 drops every 4–6 hours).

The aim of treatment with drugs is to render the infant comfortable but not obtunded. Thus, the drug should be titrated, starting with the smallest recommended dose and increased accordingly until the desired effect is achieved. Once the infant is asymptomatic, the drug can be tapered slowly until it is completely discontinued. This usually takes from 4 to 6 days. The infant should be observed for a day or two after discontinuance of the drug for possible recurrence of the symptoms (i.e., rebound phenomenon). When the infant is discharged from the nursery, the mother should be instructed to anticipate some mild jitteriness and irritability that may persist in the infant for 8 to 16 weeks, depending on the initial severity of the withdrawal.

In view of their hyperirritability, infants manifesting withdrawal should be swaddled, placed in a prone posi-

TABLE 56–9. *Assessment of the clinical severity of neonatal narcotic withdrawal*

Sign	Mild	Moderate	Severe
Vomiting	Spitting up	Extensive vomiting for three successive feedings	Vomiting associated with imbalance of serum electrolytes
Diarrhea	Watery stools <four times per day	Watery stools five to six times per day for 3 days; no electrolyte imbalance	Diarrhea associated with imbalance of serum electrolytes
Weight loss	<10% of birth weight	10% to 15% of birth weight	>15 % of birth weight
Irritability	Minimal	Marked but relieved by cuddling or feeding	Unrelieved by cuddling or feeding
Tremors or twitching	Mild tremors when stimulated	Marked tremors	Convulsions and/or twitching when stimulated
Tachypnea	60–80 breaths/min	80–100 breaths/min	>100 breaths/min; associated with respiratory alkalosis

tion, and cuddled more often. Swaddling, particularly with the infant's extremities flexed and hands placed in front of its mouth, enhances the infant's hand-to-mouth facility, which is soothing. A similar soothing action can be achieved with a pacifier.

The frequency of diarrhea and vomiting should be noted, and the infant's weight checked at least every 8 hours. Temperature, heart rate, and respiratory rates should be recorded every 4 hours. Laboratory examinations to detect serum electrolyte or pH imbalance should be done as indicated.

Nonnarcotic Withdrawal

A cross-reaction exists between the different drugs belonging to the alcohol–hypnosedative group (see Table 56–4). Each drug is therefore effective in treating withdrawal from any of the drugs belonging to this group. Thus, barbiturates can be used to treat withdrawal from nonbarbiturates, including alcohol, or vice versa.

The two drugs that have been used commonly during the neonatal period for this purpose are phenobarbital, 3 to 5 mg/kg per day in divided doses every 6 hours, and chlorpromazine, 1 to 2 mg intramuscularly every 8 hours. Chlorpromazine also has been used successfully at a dose of 2 to 3 mg/kg per day in divided doses every 6 hours (14). Although chlorpromazine does not belong to the group of nonnarcotic drugs that can cause withdrawal manifestations, its ability to ameliorate the signs and symptoms of withdrawal may be secondary to its capacity to suppress REM sleep, which is exaggerated during the state of withdrawal (16).

TABLE 56–10. *Treatment of neonatal withdrawal syndrome*

Drug	Dosage
Paregoric	3–6 drops every 4 to 6 hours PO
Laudanum (0.4%)	3–6 drops every 4 to 6 hours PO
Chlorpromazine	2–3 mg/kg/day every 6 hours PO
Phenobarbital	3–5 mg/kg/day every 6 hours PO

During the treatment of withdrawal, attention also should be focused on the nutrition and the fluid and electrolyte balance of the infants, particularly if vomiting, diarrhea, hyperpyrexia, and hyperhidrosis occur. Appropriate intravenous fluids may be required to correct deficits or prevent the occurrence of imbalances in some patients.

Maternal Support

The addicted woman has some serious impediments to a successful mothering role. She has meager past mothering experience to rely on; often there is little or no support from a father or husband because frequently she is single; and, finally, the neurobehavioral abnormalities and withdrawal in her infant may hamper the gratifying feedback that she wishes to experience from her infant.

Thus, the mother and child should have early and repeated contacts. A staff member also should have repeated and relatively brief contacts with the mother, to describe the status of the child and to reassure her that, with the disappearance of withdrawal, the infant will feed more vigorously and will respond better to maternal ministrations.

On the other hand, should it be decided that the infant will be placed in a foster care home, it should be remembered that the infant will need human contact for its normal growth and development. As part of its care in the nursery, the child should be stimulated appropriately through frequent handling or fondling by the staff professionals.

Breast-Feeding

Most drugs taken by the mother will cross into her breast milk. The concentration of illicit drug in the breast milk will depend on the amount and time of drug intake by the mother. There also is the danger of transmission of HIV through the breast milk. In general, breast-feeding is not recommended if the mother has been shown to abuse drugs continuously during pregnancy or is HIV antibody-positive.

Drug-Addicted Women as Infant Caregivers

The ability of the drug-addicted woman to perform her functions as a mother and provide adequate care for her infant has been seriously questioned on many occasions. Frequently, these women have been denied their maternal rights and responsibilities soon after the infant's birth on the basis of their unstable homes, lifestyles, and emotional and psychological weaknesses. Evidence suggests that this practice may be unnecessary and counterproductive in many cases. A study that determined outcome of infants on the basis of the type of caregiver showed that the outcome, measured by growth, development, frequency of medical illnesses, and child abuse, for infants cared for by the mother with the help of a caregiver (i.e., either a husband or relative) was better than the outcome for infants in foster home care (83). Thus, with proper guidance and supervision, the addict mother may be capable of providing adequate care for her infant, particularly because most of these women desire to fulfill their mothering functions. Similarly, although a high incidence of problems suggestive of child abuse (e.g., cigarette burns, hematoma) were noted in infants who were cared for exclusively by the mother, very few of these complications were noted in infants whose mother had help available. Thus, it is important that, when the mother is allowed to care for her infant, someone should help her at home to ensure better care and protection of the infant.

Social Service Referral

All infants of drug-dependent mothers should have a social service referral to assess the adequacy of parenting and care at home. The discharge of the infant to the mother's care is the primary objective unless serious conditions dictate otherwise. The care of the infant by the mother, with the help of a support person, usually a grandmother or other relative, has, in our experience, been the best arrangement for a favorable outcome for the infant. The discharge of the infant to a person other than the mother (i.e., foster parent) or an agency should be resorted to only when it is apparent that the infant will be neglected, poorly cared for, or abused. Most mothers hesitate to admit to the use of drugs during pregnancy because of fear that their infants will be taken away from them. They should be assured otherwise; in fact, they should be encouraged to be responsible for the primary care of their infants. The social worker and physician also should advise the mother about available medical and social services in the community, such as substance abuse counseling and family planning services.

Potential Child Abuse

As part of child protection laws that are operative in many states, infants born to drug-dependent mothers are considered as potentially abused and are required by law to be reported to child protection agencies. Many of these agencies require a positive drug screen on the infant before they will take action on the reports. The precautionary measure of referring the infant to the child protection agencies is useful if the intent is to ensure the adequacy of care of the infant at home. It is when punitive measures are taken against the mother that the outcome may become counterproductive.

Follow-Up

The infant of the drug-dependent mother is at risk for many long-term problems. These include child abuse, delays in physical, mental, and motor development, and learning disabilities. The infant also is at risk for ongoing exposure to the drugs in the household as a result of accidental ingestion or passive exposure, particularly to crack cocaine. Follow-up of these infants should be planned not only to assess their medical well-being but to ascertain the occurrence of such complications and to initiate appropriate interventions.

ACKNOWLEDGMENTS

We would like to acknowledge Mr. Victor Morales for his help in the preparation of the manuscript and Ms. Sara Anderson for her invaluable secretarial help.

REFERENCES

1. Substance Abuse and Mental Health Services Administration. *National Household Survey on Drug Abuse: Main Findings 1995.* DHHS Pub no. (SMA) 95-3127. Washington, DC: US Government Printing Office, 1997.
2. Ostrea EM, Brady M, Gause S, et al. Drug screening of newborn infants by meconium analysis: a large scale prospective, epidemiologic study. *Pediatrics* 1992;89:107.
3. Blum RH. A history of opium. In Blum RH, ed. *Society and drugs: I. Social and cultural observations.* San Francisco: Jossey-Bass, 1969:45.
4. Martin E. L'opium ses abus, mangeurs et fumerus d'opium morphinomenes. Paris: 1893.
5. Zagon IS. Opioids and development: new lessons from old problems. *NIDA Res Monogr Ser* 1985;60:58.
6. Goodfriend MJ, Shey IA, Klein MD. The effect of maternal narcotic addiction on the newborn. *Am J Obstet Gynecol* 1956;71:29.
7. Dole VP, Nyswander MA. Medical treatment for diacetyl-morphine (heroin) addiction. *JAMA* 1965;193:646.
8. Connaughton JF, Finnegan LP, Schur J, et al. Current concepts in the management of the pregnant opiate addict. *Addict Dis* 1975;2:21.
9. Naeye RL, Blanc W, Leblanc W, et al. Fetal complications of maternal heroin addiction: abnormal growth, infections, and episodes of stress. *J Pediatr* 1973;83:1055.
10. Zelson C. Infant of the addicted mother. *N Engl J Med* 1973;288:1393.
11. Strauss ME, Andresko M, Stryker JC, et al. Methadone maintenance during pregnancy, birth and neonatal course. *Am J Obstet Gynecol* 1974;120:895.

12. Kandall SR, Album S, Dreyer E, et al. Differential effects of heroin and morphine on birth weights. *Addict Dis* 1975;2:347.

13. Little BB, Snell LM, Klein VR, et al. Maternal and fetal effects of heroin addiction during pregnancy. *J Reprod Med* 1990;35:159.

14. Ostrea EM, Chavez CJ. Perinatal problems (excluding neonatal withdrawal) in maternal drug addiction: a study of 830 cases. *J Pediatr* 1979;94:292.

15. Szeto HH. Effects of narcotic drugs on fetal behavioral activity: acute methadone exposure. *Am J Obstet Gynecol* 1983;146:211.

16. Dinges DF, Davis MM, Glass P. Fetal exposure to narcotics: neonatal sleep as a measure of nervous system disturbance. *Science* 1980;209:619.

17. Umans JG, Szeto HH. Precipitated opiate abstinence *in utero*. *Am J Obstet Gynecol* 1985;151:441.

18. Zuspan FB, Gumpel JA, Mejia-Zelaya A, et al. Fetal stress from methadone withdrawal. *Am J Obstet Gynecol* 1975;122:43.

19. Stone M, Salerno LJ, Green M, et al. Narcotic addiction in pregnancy. *Am J Obstet Gynecol* 1971;109:716.

20. Finnegan LP. Narcotic dependence in pregnancy. *J Psychedelic Drugs* 1975;7:299.

21. Perlmutter JF. Heroin addiction and pregnancy. *Obstet Gynecol Surv* 1974;29:439.

22. Rementeria JL, Lotongkhum K. The fetus of the drug-addicted woman: conception fetal wastage and complications. In Rementeria JL, ed. *Drug abuse in pregnancy and neonatal effects*. St Louis: CV Mosby, 1977:1.

23. Donahoe R. Opiates as immunocompromising drugs: the evidence and possible mechanisms. *NIDA Res Monogr Ser* 1988;90:105.

24. Shafer DA, Falek A, Donahoe RM, Madden JJ. Biogenetic effects of opiates. *Int J Addict* 1990–1991;25:1.

25. Harper RG, Solish GI, Purow HM, et al. The effect of a methadone treatment program upon pregnant heroin addicts and their newborn infants. *Pediatrics* 1974;54:300.

26. Chasnoff I, Hatcher R, Burns WJ. Early growth patterns in methadone-addicted infants. *Am J Dis Child* 1980;134:1049.

27. Chasnoff I, Hatcher R, Burns WJ. Polydrug and methadone addicted newborns: a continuum of impairment. *Pediatrics* 1982;70:210.

28. Kaltenbach K, Finnegan LP. Children exposed to methadone *in utero*. *Ann NY Acad Sci* 1989;562:360.

29. Doberczak TM, Thornton JC, Bernstein J, Kandall SR. Impact of maternal drug dependency on birth weight and head circumference of offspring. *Am J Dis Child* 1987;141:1163.

30. Rementeria JL, Janakammal S, Hollander M. Multiple births in drug-addicted women. *Am J Obstet Gynecol* 1975;122:958.

31. Wittmann BK, Segal S. A comparison of the effects of single- and split-dose methadone administration on the fetus: ultrasound evaluation. *Int J Addict* 1991;26:213.

32. Rosen TS, Johnson A. Children of methadone-maintained mothers: follow-up to 18 months of age. *J Pediatr* 1982;101:192.

33. Ostrea EM, Chavez CJ, Strauss ME. A study of the factors that influence the severity of neonatal narcotic withdrawal. *J Pediatr* 1976;88:642.

34. McLaughlin PJ, Zagon IS, White WJ. Perinatal methadone exposure in rats: effects on body and organ development. *Biol Neonate* 1978;34:48.

35. Zagon IS, McLaughlin PJ. Effect of chronic maternal methadone exposure on perinatal development. *Biol Neonate* 1977;31:271.

36. Thompson CI, Zagon IS. Long-term thermoregulatory changes following perinatal methadone exposure in rats. *Pharmacol Biochem Behav* 1980;14:653.

37. Sundell H, Garrot J, Blakenship WJ, et al. Studies on infants with type II respiratory distress syndrome. *J Pediatr* 1971;78:754.

38. Glass L, Rajegowda BK, Evans HE. Absence of respiratory distress syndrome in premature infants of heroin-addicted mothers. *Lancet* 1971;2:685.

39. Gluck L, Kulovich MV. Lecithin/sphingomyelin ratios in amniotic fluid in normal and abnormal pregnancy. *Am J Obstet Gynecol* 1973;115:539.

40. Taeusch HM Jr, Carson SH, Wang NS, et al. Heroin induction of lung maturation and growth retardation in fetal rabbits. *J Pediatr* 1973;82:869.

41. Smith BT, Torday JS. Factors affecting lecithin synthesis by fetal lung cells in culture. *Pediatr Res* 1974;8:848.

42. Rothstein P, Gould JB. Born with a habit: infants of drug-addicted mothers. *Pediatr Clin North Am* 1974;21:307.

43. Stimmell B, Adams K. Narcotic dependency in pregnancy: methadone maintenance compared to use of street drugs. *JAMA* 1976;235:1121.

44. Geber WF, Schramm LC. Congenital malformations of the central nervous system produced by narcotic analgesics in the hamster. *Am J Obstet Gynecol* 1975;123:705.

45. Amarose AP. Chromosome aberrations in the mother and the newborn from drug-addiction pregnancies. *J Reprod Med* 1978;20:323.

46. Pinto F, Torrioli MG, Casella G, Tempesta E, Fundaro C. Sleep in babies born to chronically heroin addicted mothers. A follow up study. *Drug Alcohol Depend* 1988;21:43.

47. McPherson DL, Madden JD, Payne TF. Auditory brainstem-evoked potentials in term infants born to mothers addicted to opiates. *J Perinatol* 1989;9:262.

48. Trammer RM, Aust G, Koster K, Obladen M. Narcotic and nicotine effects on the neonatal auditory system. *Acta Paediatr* 1992;81:962.

49. Ostrea EM Jr, Kresbach P, Knapp DK, Simkowski K. Abnormal heart rate tracings and serum creatine phosphokinase in addicted neonates. *Neurotoxicol Teratol* 1987;9:305.

50. McCann EM, Lewis K. Control of breathing in babies of narcotic- and cocaine-abusing mothers. *Early Hum Dev* 1991;27:175.

51. Nathenson G, Cohen M, Litt I, et al. The effect of maternal heroin addiction on neonatal jaundice. *J Pediatr* 1972;81:899.

52. Burstein Y, Giardina PJV, Rausen AR, et al. Thrombocytosis and increased circulating platelet aggregates in newborn infants of poly-drug users. *J Pediatr* 1979;94:895.

53. Cepeda EE, Lee MI, Mehdizadeh B. Decreased incidence of intraventricular hemorrhage in infants of opiate dependent mothers. *Acta Paediatr* 1987;76:16.

54. Pasto ME, Graziani LJ, Tunis SL, et al. Ventricular configuration and cerebral growth in infants born to drug-dependent mothers. *Pediatr Radiol* 1985;15:77.

55. Kaltenbach KA, Finnegan LP. Prenatal narcotic exposure perinatal and developmental effects. *Neurotoxicology* 1989;10(3):597.

56. Desmond MM, Schwanecke RP, Wilson GS, et al. Maternal barbiturate utilization and neonatal withdrawal symptomatology. *J Pediatr* 1972;80:190.

57. Doberczak TM, Kandal SR, Wilets I. Neonatal opiate abstinence syndrome in term and preterm infants. *J Pediatr* 1991;118(6):933.

58. Hagopian GS, Wolfe HM, Sokol RJ, Ager JW, Wardell JN, Cepeda EE. Neonatal outcome following methadone exposure *in utero*. *J Matern Fetal Med* 1996;5:348.

59. Offidani C, Chiarotti M, De Giovanni N, Falasconi AM. Methadone in pregnancy: clinical-toxicological aspects. *J Toxicol Clin Toxicol* 1986;24:295.

60. Harper RG, Solish G, Feingold E, Gersten-Woolf NB, Sokal MM. Maternal ingested methadone, body fluid methadone, and the neonatal withdrawal syndrome. *Am J Obstet Gynecol* 1977;129:417.

61. Strauss ME, Andresko M, Stryker JC, Wardell JN. Relationship of neonatal withdrawal to maternal methadone dose. *Am J Drug Alcohol Abuse* 1976;3:339.

62. Rosen TS, Pippenger CE. Pharmacologic observations on the neonatal withdrawal syndrome. *J Pediatr* 1976;88:1044.

63. Little BB, Wilson GN, Jackson G. Is there a cocaine syndrome? Dysmorphic and anthropometric assessment of infants exposed to cocaine. *Teratology* 1996;54:145.

64. Ostrea EM, Chavez CJ, Stryker JS. *The care of the drug dependent woman and her infant*. Lansing, MI: Michigan Department of Public Health, 1978:28.

65. Kron RE, Finnegan LP, Kaplan SL, Litt M, Phoenix MD. The assessment of behavioral change in infants undergoing narcotic withdrawal: comparative data from clinical and objective methods. *Addict Dis* 1975;2:257.

66. Strauss ME, Lessen-Firestone JK, Starr RH, et al. Behavior of narcotic addicted newborns. *Child Dev* 1975;46:887.

67. Soule AB, Standley K, Cpoans SA, et al. Clinical uses of the Brazelton Neonatal Scale. *Pediatrics* 1974;54:583.

68. Lodge A, Marcus MM, Ramer CM. Behavioral and electrophysical characteristics of the addicted neonate. *Addict Dis* 1975;2:235.

69. Coppolillo HP. Drug impediments to mothering behavior. *Addict Dis Int J* 1975;2:201.

70. Chavez CJ, Ostrea EM, Strauss ME, et al. Prognosis of infants born to drug dependent mothers: its relation to the severity of the withdrawal during the neonatal period. *Pediatr Res* 1976;10:328A.

71. Hutchings DE. Methadone and heroin during pregnancy: a review of

behavioral effects in human and animal offspring. *Neurobehav Toxicol* 1982;4:429.

72. Kolar AF, Brown BS, Haertzen CA, Michaelson BS. Children of substance abusers: the life experiences of children of opiate addicts in methadone maintenance. *Am J Drug Alcohol Abuse* 1994;20:159.

73. Casado-Flores J, Bano-Rodrigo A, Romero E. Social and medical problems in children of heroin-addicted parents. A study of 75 patients. *Am J Dis Child* 1990;144:977.

74. Fiks KB, Johnson HL, Rosen TS. Methadone-maintained mothers: 3-year follow-up of parental functioning. *Int J Addict* 1985;20:651.

75. Chavez CJ, Ostrea EM, Stryker JS, et al. Sudden infant death syndrome among infants of drug dependent mothers. *J Pediatr* 1979;95:407.

76. Pierson PS, Howard P, Kleber HD. Sudden deaths in infants born to methadone maintained addicts. *JAMA* 1972;220:1933.

77. Kandall SR. Perinatal effects of cocaine and amphetamine use during pregnancy. *Bull NY Acad Med* 1991;67:240.

78. Strauss ME, Starr RH, Ostrea EM, et al. Behavior concomitants of prenatal addiction to narcotics. *J Pediatr* 1976;89:842.

79. Wilson GS, Desmond MM, Verniaud WW. Early development of infants of heroin addicted mothers. *Am J Dis Child* 1973;126:457.

80. Wilson, GS, McCreary R, Kean J, et al. The development of preschool children of heroin-addicted mothers: a controlled trial study. *Pediatrics* 1979;63:135.

81. Wilson GS, Desmond MM, Wait RB. Follow-up of methadone-treated and untreated narcotic-dependent women and their infants: health, developmental and social implications. *J Pediatr* 1981;98:716.

82. Rosen TS, Johnson HL. Children of methadone-maintained mothers: follow-up to 18 months of age. *J Pediatr* 1982;101:192.

83. Chavez CJ, Ostrea EM. Outcome of infants of drug dependent mothers based on the type of caregiver (abstract). *Pediatr Res* 1977;11:375A.

84. Nelson LB, Ehrlich S, Calhoun JH, Matteucci T, Finnegan LP. Occurrence of strabismus in infants born to drug-dependent women. *Am J Dis Child* 1987;141:175.

85. Marcus J, Hans SL, Jeremy RJ. A longitudinal study of offspring born to methadone-maintained women. III. Effects of multiple risk factors on development at 4, 8, and 12 months. *Am J Drug Alcohol Abuse* 1984;10:195.

86. Kaltenbach K, Finnegan LP. Perinatal and developmental outcome of infants exposed to methadone *in-utero*. *Neurotoxicol Teratol* 1987;9:311.

87. Strauss ME, Lessen-Firestone JK, Chavez CJ, Stryker JC. Children of methadone-treated women at five years of age. *Pharmacol Biochem Behav* 1979;11(Suppl):3.

88. Herjanic BM, Barredo VH, Herjanic M, et al. Children of heroin addicts. *Int J Addict* 1979;14:919.

89. Marcus J, Hans SL, Jeremy RJ. Differential motor and state functioning in newborns of women on methadone. *Neurobehav Toxicol* 1982;4:459.

90. Ornoy A, Michailevskaya V, Lukashov I, Bar-Hamburger R, Harel S. The developmental outcome of children born to heroin-dependent mothers, raised at home or adopted. *Child Abuse Neglect* 1996;20:385.

91. Olofsson M, Buckley W, Andersen GE, Friis-Hansen B. Investigation of 89 children born by drug-dependent mothers. I. Neonatal course. *Acta Paediatr* 1983;72:403.

92. Levy M, Spino M. Neonatal withdrawal syndrome: associated drugs and pharmacologic management. *Pharmacotherapy* 1993;13:202.

93. Essig CF. Addiction to barbiturate and nonbarbiturate sedative drugs. *Res Publ Assoc Res Nerv Ment Dis* 1968;46:188.

94. Isbell H. Addiction to barbiturates and the barbiturate abstinence syndrome. *Ann Intern Med* 1950;33:108.

95. Bleyer W, Marshall RE. Barbiturate withdrawal syndrome in a passively addicted infant. *JAMA* 1972;221:185.

96. Ploman L, Persson BH. On the transfer of barbiturates to the human fetus and their accumulation in some of its vital organs. *Br J Obstet Gynaecol* 1957;64:706.

97. Ostrea EM Jr. Neonatal withdrawal from intrauterine exposure to butalbital. *Am J Obstet Gynecol* 1982;143:597.

98. Harvey SC. Hypnotics and sedatives: barbiturates. In Gilman A, Rall TW, Goodman LS, et al, eds. *Goodman and Gilman's the pharmacological basis of therapeutics,* 8th ed. New York: Pergamon Press, 1990:358.

99. Jalling B, Boreus LO, Kallberg N, et al. Disappearance from the newborn of circulating prenatally administered phenobarbital. *Eur J Clin Pharmacol* 1973;6:234.

100. De Carolis MP, Romagnoli C, Frezza S, et al. Placental transfer of phenobarbital: what is new? *Dev Pharmacol Ther* 1992;19:19.

101. Margetts EL. Chloral delirium. *Psychiatry* 1950;24:278.

102. Opitz JM, Grosse FR, Heneberg B. Congenital effects of bromism. *Lancet* 1972;1:91.

103. Rossiter EJR, Rendle-Short TJ. Congenital effects of bromism. *Lancet* 1972;2:705.

104. Disse M, Joo F, Schulz H, Wolff JR. Prenatal exposure to sodium bromide affects the postnatal growth and brain development. *J Hirnforsch* 1996;37(1):127.

105. Marchetti F, Romero M, Bonati M, Tognoni G. Use of psychotropic drugs during pregancy. A report of the international co-operative drug use in pregnancy (DUP) study. Collaborative Group on Drug Use in Pregnancy (CGDUP). *Eur J Clin Pharmacol* 1993;45(6):495.

106. Erkkola R, Kangas L, Pekkarinen A. The transfer of diazepam across the placenta during labour. *Acta Obstet Gynaecol Scand* 1973;52:167.

107. Jauniaux E, Jurjovic D, Lees C, Campbell S, Gulbis B. *In vivo* study of diazepam transfer across the first trimester human placenta. *Hum Reprod* 1996;11(4):8899.

108. Pan B, Lu Y, Wang D. Determination of diazepam concentration in maternal and fetal serum after intravenous administration during active phase of labor and its effects in neonates [Chinese]. *Chinese J Obstet Gynecol* 1995;30(12):707.

109. Athinarayanan P, Pierog SH, Nigam SK, et al. Chlordiazepoxide withdrawal in the neonate. *Am J Obstet Gynecol* 1976;124:212.

110. Rementeria JL, Bhatt K. Withdrawal symptoms in neonates from intrauterine exposure to diazepam. *J Pediatr* 1977;90:123.

111. Sutton LR, Hinderliter SA. Diazepam abuse in pregnant women on methadone maintenance. Implications for the neonate. *Clin Pediatr* 1990;29:108.

112. McElhatton PR. The effects of benzodiazepine use during pregancy and lactation. *Reprod Toxicol* 1994;8(6):461.

113. Kanjilal S, Pan NR, Chakraborty DP, Mukherjee N. Cord blood diazepam: clinical effects in neonates of eclamptic mothers. *Indian J Pediatr* 1993;60:257.

114. Liscano-Gil LA, Garcia-Cruz D, Sanchez-Corona J. Omphalocele–exstrophy–imperforate-anus–spina bifida (OEIS) complex in a male prenatally exposed to diazepam [letter]. *Arch Med Res* 1995;26:95.

115. Jaiswal AK, Bhattacharya SK. Effect of gestational undernutrition and chlordiazepoxide treatment on black/white discrimination learning and retention in young rats. *Indian J Exp Biol* 1884;32(3):184.

116. Cuthbert KJR. Two hypnotics. *Practitioner* 1963;190:509.

117. Tsapogas MJC, Modle J, Wheeler T. A comparison between two hypnotics: ethchlorvynol and dichloralphenazone. *Br J Clin Pract* 1963;17:407.

118. Wood-Walker RB. A clinical evaluation of a nonbarbiturate hypnotic. Ethchlorvynol. *Br J Clin Pract* 1963;17:201.

119. Garetz FD. Ethchlorvynol: addiction hazard. *Minn Med* 1969;52:1131.

120. Magness JL. Ethchlorvynol intoxication and severe abstinence reaction. *Lancet* 1965;1:80.

121. Harenko A. On special traits of acute ethchlorvynol poisoning. *Acta Neurol Scand* 1967;43:141.

122. Aycrigg JB. Two cases of withdrawal from ethchlorvynol. *Am J Psychiatry* 1964;120:1201.

123. Flemenbaum A, Gunby B. Ethchlorvynol (placidyl) abuse and withdrawal. *Dis Nerv Syst* 1971;32:188.

124. Hudson HS, Walker HI. Withdrawal symptoms following ethchlorvynol dependence. *Am J Psychiatry* 1961;118:361.

125. Hume AS, Williams JM, Douglas BG. Disposition of ethchlorvynol in maternal blood, amniotic fluid and chorionic fluid. *J Reprod Med* 1971;6:229.

126. Rumack BH, Walravens PA. Neonatal withdrawal following maternal ingestion of ethchlorvynol (Placidyl). *Pediatrics* 1973;52:714.

127. Sadwin A, Glen RS. Addiction to glutethimide (Doriden). *Am J Psychiatry* 1958;115:469.

128. Eidelman JR. Doriden intoxication. *Mol Med* 1956;53:194.

129. Kanter DM. The acute toxicity of Doriden overdosage. *Conn Med J* 1957;21:314.

130. McBay AJ, Katsas GG. Glutethimide poisoning: a report of four fatal cases. *N Engl J Med* 1957;257:97.

131. Pildes RS. Neonatal withdrawal symptoms associated with glu-

thetimide (Doriden) addiction in the mother during pregnancy. *Clin Pediatr* 1977;16:424.

132. Eggermont E. The adverse influence of imipramine on the adaptation of the newborn infant to extrauterine life. *Acta Pediatr Belg* 1972;26:197.

133. Sothers J. Lithium toxicity in the newborn. *Br Med J* 1973;3:233.

134. Tunnessen W. Toxic effects of lithium in newborn infants. *J Pediatr* 1972;81:804.

135. Webster PAC. Withdrawal symptoms in neonates associated with maternal antidepressant therapy. *Lancet* 1973;2:318.

136. Wilbanks B. Toxic effects of lithium carbonate in a mother and newborn infant. *JAMA* 1970;213:865.

137. Hill RM, Desmond MM, Kay JL. Extrapyramidal dysfunction in an infant of a schizophrenic mother. *J Pediatr* 1966;69:589.

138. Levy W, Wisniewski K. Chlorpromazine causing extrapyramidal dysfunction in newborn infant of psychotic mother. *NY State J Med* 1974;74:684.

139. Krug S. Cocaine abuse: historical epidemiologic and clinical perspectives for pediatricians. *Adv Pediatr* 1989;36:369.

140. Farrar HC, Kearns GL. Cocaine: clinical pharmacology and toxicology. *J Pediatr* 1989;115:665.

141. Udell B. Crack cocaine: crack vs. cocaine. In *Special currents: cocaine babies.* Columbus, OH: Ross Laboratories, 1989:5.

142. Tarr JE, Macklin M. Cocaine. *Pediatr Clin North Am* 1987;34:319.

143. Woods JR, Plessinger MA, Clark KE. Effect of cocaine on uterine blood flow and fetal oxygenation. *JAMA* 1987;257:957.

144. Moore TR, Sorg J, Miller L, et al. Hemodynamic effects of intravenous cocaine on the pregnant ewe and fetus. *Am J Obstet Gynecol* 1986;155:883.

145. Woods JR, Plessinger MA. Pregnancy increases cardiovascular toxicity to cocaine. *Am J Obstet Gynecol* 1990;162:529.

146. Cejtin HE, Parsons MT, Wilson L. Cocaine use and its effects on umbilical artery prostacyclin production. *Prostaglandins* 1990;40:249.

147. Sison CG, Ostrea EM Jr, Reyes MP, Salari V. The resurgence of congenital syphilis: a cocaine-related problem. *J Pediatr* 1997;130:289.

148. Rodriguez EM, Mofenson LM, Chang BH, et al. Association of maternal drug use during pregnancy with maternal HIV culture positivity and perinatal HIV transmission. *AIDS* 1997;10:273.

149. Berkowitz K, LaSala A. Risk factors associated with the increasing prevalence of pneumonia during pregnancy. *Am J Obstet Gynecol* 1990;163(3):981.

150. Church MW, Kaufmann RA, Keenan JA, et al. Effect of prenatal cocaine exposure. In Watson R, ed. *Biochemistry and physiology of substance abuse,* vol 3. Boca Raton, FL: CRC Press, 1990:179.

151. Chasnoff IJ, Burns WJ, Schnoll SH, et al. Cocaine use in pregnancy. *N Engl J Med* 1985;313:666.

152. Hadeed AJ, Siegel SR. Maternal cocaine use during pregnancy: effect on the newborn infant. *Pediatrics* 1989;84:205.

153. Meeker JE, Reynolds PC. Fetal and newborn death associated with maternal cocaine use. *J Anal Toxicol* 1990;14:379.

154. Carlan SJ, Stromquist C, Angel JL, Harris M, O'Brien WF. Cocaine and indomethacin: fetal anuria, neonatal edema, and gastrointestinal bleeding. *Obstet Gynecol* 1991;78:501.

155. Bingol N, Fuchs M, Diaz V, et al. Teratogenicity of cocaine in humans. *J Pediatr* 1987;110:93.

156. Chasnoff IJ, Burns KA, Burns WJ. Cocaine use in pregnancy: perinatal morbidity and mortality. *Neurotoxicol Teratol* 1987;9:291.

157. Chouteau M, Namerow PB, Leppert P. The effect of cocaine abuse on birth weight and gestational age. *Obstet Gynecol* 1988;72:351.

158. Doberczak TM, Shanzer S, Senie RT, et al. Neonatal neurologic and electroencephalographic effects of intrauterine cocaine exposure. *J Pediatr* 1988;133:354.

159. Neerhof M, MacGregor S, Retzky S, et al. Cocaine abuse during pregnancy: peripartum prevalence and perinatal outcome. *Am J Obstet Gynecol* 1989;161:633.

160. Cerukuri R, Minkoff H, Feldman J, et al. A cohort study of alkaloidal cocaine ("crack") in pregnancy. *Obstet Gynecol* 1988;72:147.

161. Fulroth R, Phillips B, Durand D. Perinatal outcome of infants exposed to cocaine and or heroin *in utero. Am J Dis Child* 1989;143:905.

162. Dombrowski MP, Wolfe HM, Welch RA, et al. Cocaine abuse is associated with abruptio placentae and decreased birth weight, but not shorter labor. *Obstet Gynecol* 1991;77:139.

163. Little B, Snell L, Klein V, et al. Cocaine abuse during pregnancy: maternal and fetal complications. *Obstet Gynecol* 1989;73:157.

164. Oro A, Dixon S. Perinatal cocaine and methamphetamine exposure: maternal and neonatal correlates. *J Pediatr* 1987;117:571.

165. Chasnoff I, Griffith D, MacGregor S, et al. Temporal patterns of cocaine use in pregnancy. *JAMA* 1989;261:1741.

166. Leblar P, Parekh A, Naso B, et al. Effects of intrauterine exposure to alkaloidal cocaine (crack). *Am J Dis Child* 1987;141:937.

167. Zuckerman B, Frank D, Hingson R, et al. Effects of maternal marijuana and cocaine use on fetal growth. *N Engl J Med* 1989;320:762.

168. Kliegman RM, Madura D, Kiwi R, Eisenberg I, Yamashita T. Relation of maternal cocaine use to the risks of prematurity and low birth weight. *J Pediatr* 1994;124:751.

169. Hume R Jr, O'Donnell K, Stanger C, et al. *In utero* cocaine exposure: observations of fetal behavioral state may predict neonatal outcome. *Am J Obstet Gynecol* 1989;161:685.

170. Ryan L, Ehrlich S, Finnegan L. Cocaine abuse in pregnancy: effects on the fetus and newborn. *Neurotoxicol Teratol* 1987;9:295.

171. Chouteau M, Namerow P, Leppert P. The effects of cocaine abuse on birth weight and gestational age. *Obstet Gynecol* 1988;72:351.

172. Anday E, Cohen M, Kelly N, et al. Effect of in utero cocaine exposure on startle and its modifications. *Dev Pharmacol Ther* 1989;12:137.

173. Mirochnick M, Frank DA, Cabral H, Turner A, Zuckerman B. Relation between meconium concentration of the cocaine metabolite benzoylecgonine and fetal growth. *J Pediatr* 1995;126:636.

174. Jacobson JL, Jacobson SW, Sokol RJ. Effects of prenatal exposure to alcohol, smoking, and illicit drugs on postpartum somatic growth. *Alcohol Clin Exp Res* 1994;18:317.

175. Neuspiel DR, Markowitz M, Drucker E. Intrauterine cocaine, lead, and nicotine exposure and fetal growth. *Am J Public Health* 1994;84:1492.

176. Chasnoff I, Chisum G, Kaplan W. Maternal cocaine use and genitourinary tract malformations. *Teratology* 1988;37:201.

177. Hoyme HE, Jones KL, Dixon SD, et al. Prenatal cocaine exposure and fetal vascular disruption. *Pediatrics* 1990;85:743.

178. Rosenstein BJ, Wheeler JS, Heid PL. Congenital renal abnormalities in infants with *in utero* cocaine exposure. *J Urol* 1990;144:110.

179. Bandstra E, Burkett G. Maternal–fetal and neonatal effects of *in utero* cocaine exposure. *Semin Perinatol* 1991;15:288.

180. Kramer LD, Locke GE, Ogunyemi A, Nelson L. Neonatal cocaine-related seizures. *J Child Neurol* 1990;5(1):60.

181. Beltran RS, Coker SB. Transient dystonia of infancy, a result of intrauterine cocaine exposure? *Pediatr Neurol* 1995;12:354.

182. Chiriboga CA, Vibbert M, Malouf R, et al. Neurological correlates of fetal cocaine exposure: transient hypertonia of infancy and early childhood. *Pediatrics* 1995;96:1070.

183. Chiriboga CA, Bateman DA, Brust JC, Hauser WA. Neurologic findings in neonates with intrauterine cocaine exposure. *Pediatr Neurol* 1993;9:115.

184. Tsay CH, Partridge JC, Villarreal SF, Good WV, Ferriero DM. Neurologic and ophthalmologic findings in children exposed to cocaine in utero. *J Child Neurol* 1996;11(1):25.

185. Doberczak TM, Shanzer S, Senie RT, Kandall SR. Neonatal neurologic and electroencephalographic effects of intrauterine cocaine exposure. *J Pediatr* 1988;113:354.

186. Corwin MJ, Lester BM, Sepkoski C, McLaughlin S, Kayne H, Golub HL. Effects of *in utero* cocaine exposure on newborn acoustical cry characteristics. *Pediatrics* 1992;89:1199.

187. Chasnoff IJ, Hunt CE, Kletter R, et al. Prenatal cocaine exposure is associated with respiratory pattern abnormalities. *Am J Dis Child* 1989;143:583.

188. Gingras JL, Feibel JB, Dalley LB, Muelenaer A, Knight CG. Maternal polydrug use including cocaine and postnatal infant sleep architecture: preliminary observations and implications for respiratory control and behavior. *Early Hum Dev* 1995;43:197.

189. Karmel BZ, Gardner JM. Prenatal cocaine exposure effects on arousal-modulated attention during the neonatal period. *Dev Psychobiol* 1996;29:463.

190. Salamy A, Eldredge L. Risk for ABR abnormalities in the nursery. *Electroencephalogr Clin Neurophysiol* 1994;92:392.

191. Shih L, Cone-Wesson B, Reddix B. Effects of maternal cocaine abuse on the neonatal auditory system. *Int J Pediatr Otorhinolaryngol* 1988;15:245.

192. McLenan DA, Ajayi PA, Rydmn RJ, Pildes RS. Evaluation of the rela-

tionship between cocaine and intraventricular hemorrhage. *J Natl Med Assoc* 1994;86(4):281.

193. Dogra VS, Shyken JM, Menon PA, Poblete J, Lewis D, Smeltzer JS. Neurosonographic abnormalities associated with maternal history of cocaine use in neonates of appropriate size for their gestational age. *Am J Neuroradiol* 1994;15:697.

194. Konkol RJ, Tikofsky RS, Wells R, et al. Normal high-resolution cerebral ⁹⁹ᵐTc-HMPAO SPECT scans in symptomatic neonates exposed to cocaine. *J Child Neurol* 1994;9:278.

195. Kankirawatana P, Tennison MB, D'Cruz O, Greenwood RS. Mobius syndrome in infant exposed to cocaine *in utero*. *Pediatr Neurol* 1993;9:71.

196. van de Bor M, Walther FJ, Sims ME. Increased cerebral blood flow velocity in infants of mothers who abuse cocaine. *Pediatrics* 1990;85:733.

197. Silvestri JM, Long JM, Weese-Mayer DE, Barkov GA. Effect of prenatal cocaine on respiration, heart rate, and sudden infant death syndrome. *Pediatr Pulmonol* 1991;11:328.

198. Horn PT. Persistent hypertension after prenatal cocaine exposure. *J Pediatr* 1992;121:288.

199. Mayes LC, Carroll KM. Neonatal withdrawal syndrome in infants exposed to cocaine and methadone. *Subst Use Misuse* 1996;31:241.

200. Roby PV, Glenn CM, Watkins SL, et al. Association of elevated umbilical cord blood creatine kinase and myoglobin levels with the presence of cocaine metabolites in maternal urine. *Am J Perinatol* 1996;13:453.

201. Wennberg RP, Yin J, Miller M, Maynard A. Fetal cocaine exposure and neonatal bilirubinemia. *J Pediatr* 1994;125:613.

202. Silva-Araujo A, Tavares MA, Patacao MH, Carolino RM. Retinal hemorrhages associated with in utero exposure to cocaine. Experimental and clinical findings. *Retina* 1996;16:411.

203. Isenberg SJ, Spierer A, Inkelis SH. Ocular signs of cocaine intoxication in neonates. *Am J Ophthalmol* 1987;103(2):211.

204. Mayes LC, Granger RH, Frank MA, Schottenfeld R, Bornstein MH. Neurobehavioral profiles of neonates exposed to cocaine prenatally. *Pediatrics* 1993;91:778.

205. Eisen LN, Field TM, Bandstra ES, et al. Perinatal cocaine effects on neonatal stress behavior and performance on the Brazelton Scale. *Pediatrics* 1991;88:477.

206. Scafidi FA, Field TM, Wheeden A, et al. Cocaine-exposed preterm neonates show behavioral and hormonal differences. *Pediatrics* 1996; 97:851.

207. Mirochnick M, Meyer J, Cole J, Herren T, Zuckerman B. Circulating catecholamine concentrations in cocaine-exposed neonates: a pilot study. *Pediatrics* 1991;88:481.

208. Delaney-Black V, Covington C, Ostrea E Jr, et al. Prenatal cocaine and neonatal outcome: evaluation of dose–response relationship. *Pediatrics* 1996;98:735.

209. Anday E, Cohen M, Kelly N, et al. Effect of *in utero* cocaine exposure on startle and its modificaions. *Dev Pharmacol Ther* 1989;12:137.

210. Lester BM, Corwin MJ, Sepkoski C, et al. Neurobehavioral syndromes in cocaine-exposed newborn infants. *Child Dev* 1991;62:694.

211. Chiu TT, Vaughn AJ, Carzoli RP. Hospital costs for cocaine-exposed infants. *J Fla Med Assoc* 1990;77(10):897

212. Joyce T, Racine AD, McCalla S, Wehbeh H. The impact of prenatal exposure to cocaine on newborn costs and length of stay. *Health Serv Res* 1995;30(2):341.

213. Phibbs CS, Bateman DA. Schwartz RM. The neonatal costs of maternal cocaine use. *JAMA* 1991;266(11):1521.

214. Calhoun BC, Watson PT. The cost of maternal cocaine abuse: I. Perinatal cost. *Obstet Gynecol* 1991;78(5 Pt 1):731.

215. Ostrea EM Jr, Lizardo E, Tanafranca M. The prevalence of illicit drug exposure in infants in the NICU as determined by meconium drug screen: Its medical and economic impact. *Pediatr Res* 1992;31:215A.

216. Behnke M, Eyler FD, Conlon M, Casanova OQ, Woods NS. How fetal cocaine exposure increases neonatal hospital costs. *Pediatrics* 1997; 99:204.

217. Fetters L, Tronick EZ. Neuromotor development of cocaine-exposed and control infants from birth through 15 months: poor and poorer performance. *Pediatrics* 1996;98:938.

218. Hurt H, Brodsky NL, Braitman LE, Giannetta J. Natal status of infants of cocaine users and control subjects: a prospective comparison. *J Perinatol* 1995;15:297.

219. Azuma SD, Chasnoff IJ. Outcome of children prenatally exposed to cocaine and other drugs: a path analysis of three-year data. *Pediatrics* 1993;92(3):396.

220. Jacobson SW, Jacobson JL, Sokol RJ. Effects of fetal alcohol exposure on infant reaction time. *Alcohol Clin Exp Res* 1994;18:1125.

221. Hawley TL, Halle TG, Drasin RE, Thomas NG. Children of addicted mothers: effects of the "crack epidemic" on the caregiving environment and the development of preschoolers. *Am J Orthopsychiatry* 1995;65(3):364.

222. Nulman I, Rovet J, Altmann D, Bradley C, Einarson T, Koren G. Neurodevelopment of adopted children exposed *in utero* to cocaine. The neonatal costs of maternal cocaine use. *JAMA* 1991;266(11): 1521–1526. *Can Med Assoc J* 1994;151(11):1591.

223. Griffith DR, Azuma SD, Chasnoff IJ. Three-year outcome of children exposed prenatally to drugs. *J Am Acad Child Psychiatry* 1994;33:20.

224. Rosenberg NM, Meert KL, Marino D, Yee H, Kauffman RE. Occult cocaine and opiate exposure in children and associated physical findings. *Pediatr Emerg Care* 1995;11(3):167.

225. Block SS, Moore BD, Scharre JE. Visual anomalies in young children exposed to cocaine. *Optom Vis Sci* 1997;74(1):28.

226. van Baar A. Development of infants of drug dependent mothers. *J Child Psychol Psychiatry* 1990;31(6):911.

227. Mentis M, Lundgren K. Effects of prenatal exposure to cocaine and associated risk factors on language development. *J Speech Hear Res* 1995;38(6):1303.

228. Bender SL, Word CO, DiClemente RJ, Crittenden MR, Persaud NA, Ponton LE. The developmental implications of prenatal and/or postnatal crack cocaine exposure in preschool children: a preliminary report. *J Dev Behav Pediatr* 1995;16(6):418–425.

229. Angelilli ML, Fischer H, Delaney-Black V, Rubinstein M, Ager JW, Sokol RJ. History of *in utero* cocaine exposure in language-delayed children. *Clin Pediatr* 1994;33(9):514.

230. Jacobson SW, Jacobson JL, Sokol RJ, Martier SS, Chiodo LM. New evidence for neurobehavioral effects of in utero cocaine exposure. *J Pediatr* 1996;129:581.

231. Hurt H, Brodsky NL, Betancourt L, Braitman LE, Belsky J, Giannetta J. Play behavior in toddlers with *in utero* cocaine exposure: a prospective, masked, controlled study. *J Dev Behav Pediatr* 1996;17:373.

232. Rodning C, Beckwith L, Howards J. Characteristics of attachment organization and play organization in prenatally drug exposed toddlers. *Dev Psychopathol* 1990;1:277.

233. Struthers JM, Hansen RL. Visual recognition memory in drug-exposed infants. *J Dev Behav Pediatr* 1992;13:108.

234. Ostrea EM Jr, Ostrea AR, Simpson PM. Mortality within the first 2 years in infants exposed to cocaine, opiate, or cannabinoid during gestation. *Pediatrics* 1997;100:79.

235. Kharasch SJ, Glotzer D, Vinci R, Weitzman M, Sargent J. Unsuspected cocaine exposure in young children. *Am J Dis Child* 1991;145:204.

236. Smith FP, Kidwell DA. Cocaine in hair, saliva, skin swabs, and urine of cocaine users children. *Forensic Sci Int* 1996;83;179.

237. Bateman DA, Heagarty MC. Passive freebase cocaine ("crack") inhalation by infants and toddlers. *Am J Dis Child* 1989;143:25.

238. Riggs D, Weibley RE. Acute hemorrhagic diarrhea and cardiovascular collapse in a young child owing to environmentally acquired cocaine. *Pediatr Emerg Care* 1991;7:154.

239. Ernst AA, Sanders WM. Unexpected cocaine intoxication presenting as seizures in children. *Ann Emerg Med* 1989;18:774.

240. Mirchandani HG, Mirchandani IH, Hellman F, English-Rider R, Rosen S, Laposata EA. Passive inhalation of free-base cocaine ("crack") smoke by infants. *Arch Pathol Lab Med* 1991;115:494.

241. Mott SH, Packer RJ, Soldin SJ. Neurologic manifestations of cocaine exposure in childhood. *Pediatrics* 1994;93(4):557.

242. Jones KL, Smith DW. Recognition of the fetal alcohol syndrome in early infancy. *Lancet* 1973;2:999.

243. Jones KL, Smith DW, Ulleland CN, Streissguth AP. Pattern of malformation in offspring of chronic alcoholic mothers. *Lancet* 1973;1: 1267.

244. Christiaens L, Mizon JP, Delmarie G. Sur la descendance des alcooliques (On the offspring of alcoholics). *Ann Pediatr* 1960;36:37.

245. Heuyer H, Mises R, Dereux JF. La descendance les alcooliques (The offspring of alcoholics). *Nouv Presse Med (Paris)* 1957;29:657.

246. Abel EL. *Fetal alcohol syndrome*. Oradell, NJ: Medical Economics, 1990.

247. Pietrantoni M, Knuppel RA. Alcohol in pregnancy. *Clin Perinatol* 1991;18:93.

248. Day NL, Richardson GA. Prenatal alcohol exposure: a continuum of effects. *Semin Perinatol* 1991;15:271.

249. Day NL, Richardson GA, Geva D, Robles N. Alcohol, marijuana and tobacco: effects of prenatal exposure on offspring growth and morphology at age six. *Alcohol Clin Exp Res* 1994;18:786

250. Brien JF, Loomis CW, Trammer J, McGrath M. Disposition of ethanol in human maternal venous blood and amniotic fluid. *Am J Obstet Gynecol* 1983;146(2):181.

251. Brien J, Clark D, Smith G, et al. Disposition of acute, multiple-dose ethanol in the near-term pregnant ewe. *Am J Obstet Gynecol* 1987; 157:204.

252. Fisher ES. Selective fetal malnutrition: the fetal alcohol syndrome. *J Am Coll Nutr* 1988;7:101.

253. Weston WM, Greene RM, Uberti M, Pisano MM. Etahnol effects on embryonic craniofacial growth and development: implications for study of the fetal alcohol syndrome. *Alcohol Clin Exp Res* 1994;18(1): 177.

254. Ylikorkala O, Halmesmaki E, Viinikka L. Effect of ethanol on thromboxane and prostacyclin synthesis by fetal platelets and umbilical artery. *Life Sci* 1987;41:371.

255. Randall CL, Saulnier JL. Effect of ethanol on prostacyclin, thromboxane, and prostaglandin E production in human umbilical veins. *Alcohol Clin Exp Res* 1995;19:741.

256. Karl PI, Harvey B, Fisher SE. Ethanol and mitotic inhibitors promote differentiation of trophoblastic cells. *Alcohol Clin Exp Res* 1996;20: 1269.

257. Sokol RJ, Miller SI, Reed G. Alcohol abuse during pregnancy: an epidemiologic study. *Alcohol Clin Exp Res* 1980;4:135.

258. Plant M. *Women, drinking and pregnancy.* London: Tavistock Publications, 1985.

259. Clarren SK. Fetal alcohol syndrome: a new primate model for binge drinking and its relevance to human ethanol teratogenesis. *J Pediatr* 1982;101:819.

260. Scott WJ, Fradkin R. The effects of prenatal ethanol in cynomolgus monkeys *Macaca fascicularis. Teratology* 1984;29:49.

261. Altshuler HL, Shippenberg TS. A subhuman primate model for fetal alcohol syndrome research. *Neurotoxicol Teratol* 1981;3:121.

262. Abel EL. Maternal alcohol consumption and spontaneous abortion. *Alcohol Alcoholism* 1997;32(3):211.

263. Kline J, Shrout P, Stein Z, et al. Drinking during pregnancy and spontaneous abortion. *Lancet* 1980;2:176.

264. Machemer L, Lorke D. Experiences with the dominant lethal test in female mice: effects of alkylating agents and artificial sweeteners on pre-ovulatory oocyte stages. *Mutat Res* 1975;29:209.

265. Koike M. Cytogenetic effects of maternal alcohol uptake on F1 mouse fetuses. *Jpn J Hyg* 1985;40:575.

266. Kaufman MH. Ethanol-induced chromosomal abnormalities at conception. *Nature* 1983;302:258.

267. Kaufman MH. The teratogenic effects of alcohol following exposure during pregnancy, and its influence on the chromosome constitution of the pre-ovulatory egg. *Alcohol Alcoholism* 1997;32(2):113.

268. Washington WJ, Cain KT, Cacheiro NLA, et al. Ethanol-induced late fetal death in mice exposed around the time of fertilization. *Mutat Res* 1985;147:205.

269. Marbury MC, Linn S, Monson RP, et al. The association of alcohol consumption with outcome of pregnancy. *Am J Public Health* 1983; 73:1165.

270. Prager K, Malin H, Graves C, et al. Maternal smoking and drinking behavior before and during pregnancy. In *Health and prevention profile.* Hyattsville, MD: US Department of Health and Human Services, National Center for Health Statistics, 1983:19.

271. National Institute on Alcohol Abuse and Alcoholism. *Program strategies for preventing fetal alcohol syndrome and alcohol-related birth defects.* Washington, DC: US Department of Health and Human Services, Public Health Service, Alcohol, Drug Abuse, and Mental Health Administration, 1986.

272. Randall CL, Taylor WJ, Walker DW. Ethanol-induced malformations in mice. *Alcohol Clin Exp Res* 1977;1:219.

273. Halliday HC, MacReid M, MacClure G. Results of heavy drinking in pregnancy. *Br J Obstet Gynaecol* 1982;89:892.

274. Staisey N, Fried P. Relationships between moderate maternal alcohol consumption during pregnancy and infant neurological development. *J Stud Alcohol* 1983;44:262.

275. Halmesmaki E, Valimaki M, Karonen S. Low somatomedin C and high growth hormone levels in newborns damaged by maternal alcohol abuse. *Obstet Gynecol* 1989;74:366.

276. Savoy-Moore RT, Dombrowski MP, Cheng A, Abel EA, Sokol RJ. Low dose alcohol contracts the human umbilical artery *in vitro. Alcohol Clin Exp Res* 1989;13:40.

277. Silva PD, Miller KD, Madden J, Keegan KA Jr. Abnormal fetal heart rate pattern associated with severe intrapartum maternal ethanol intoxication. A case report. *J Reprod Med* 1987;32:144.

278. Akay M, Mulder EJ. Investigating the effect of maternal alcohol intake on human fetal breathing rate using adaptive time-frequency analysis methods. *Early Hum Dev* 1996;46:153.

279. McLeod WJ, Brien C, Loomis L, Carmichael L, Probert C, Patrick J. Effect of maternal ingestion on fetal breathing movements, gross body movements and heart rate at 37 to 40 weeks gestational age. *Am J Obstet Gynecol* 1983;145:251.

280. Druse MJ, Hoffeig JH. The effect of chronic maternal alcohol consumption on the development of the central nervous system myelin subfractions in rat offspring. *Drug Alcohol Depend* 1977;2:421.

281. Hoff S. Synaptogenesis in the hippocampal dentate gyrus: effects of *in utero* ethanol exposure. *Brain Res Bull* 1988;21:47.

282. Kennedy LA. The pathogenesis of brain abnormalities in the fetal alcohol syndrome: an intergrading hypothesis. *Teratology* 1984;29:263.

283. Shoemaker WJ, Baetge G, Azad R, et al. Effects of prenatal alcohol exposure on amine and peptide neurotransmitter systems. *Monogr Neural Sci* 1983;9:130.

284. Dehaene PH, Crepin G, Delahousse G, et al. Aspects epidemiologiques du syndrome d'alcoolisme foetal: 45 observations en 3 ans (Epidemiological aspects of the foetal alcoholism syndrome: 45 cases). *Nouv Presse Med* 1981;10:2639.

285. Kimura KA, Parr AM, Brien JF. Effect of chronic maternal ethanol administration on nitric oxide synthase activity in the hippocampus of the mature fetal guinea pig. *Alcohol Clin Exp Res* 1996;20:948.

286. Ollegard R, Sabel K, Aronsson M, et al. Effects on the child of alcohol abuse during pregnancy: retrospective and prospective studies. *Acta Paediatr Scand* 1979;275:112.

287. Dehaene PH, Samaille-Villette CH, Samaille P, et al. Le syndrome d'alcoolisme foetal dans le nord de la France (The fetal alcohol syndrome in the north of France). *Rev Alcoolisme (Paris)* 1977;23:145.

288. Ouellette EM, Rosett HL, Rosman NP, et al. Adverse effects on offspring of maternal alcohol abuse during pregnancy. *N Engl J Med* 1977;297:528.

289. Wilsnack SC, Klassen AD, Wilsnack RW. Drinking and reproductive dysfunction among women in a 1981 national survey. *Alcohol Clin Exp Res* 1984;8:451.

290. Berkowitz GS. An epidemiologic study of preterm delivery. *Am J Epidemiol* 1981;113:81.

291. Day NL, Jasperse D, Richardson G, et al. Prenatal exposure to alcohol: effect on infant growth and morphologic characteristics. *Pediatrics* 1989;84:536.

292. Smith IE, Coles CD, Lancaster J, et al. The effect of volume and duration of prenatal ethanol exposure on neonatal physical and behavioral development. *Neurotoxicol Teratol* 1986;8:375.

293. Coles CD, Platzman KA, Rashkind-Hood CL, Brown RT, Falek A, Smith IE. A comparison of children affected by prenatal alcohol exposure and attention deficit, hyperactivity disorder. *Alcohol Clin Exp Res* 1997;21(1):150.

294. Konovalov, HV, Kovetsky NS, Bobryshev YV, Ashwell KW. Disorders in brain development in the progeny of mothers who use alcohol during pregnancy. *Early Hum Dev* 1997;48(1–2):153.

295. Holzman C, Paneth N, Little R, Pinto-Martin J. Perinatal brain injury in premature infants born to mothers using alcohol in pregnancy. Neonatal Brain Hemorrhage Study Team. *Pediatrics* 1995;95:66.

296. Coles CD, Smith I, Fernhoff PM, et al. Neonatal neurobehavioral characteristics as correlates of maternal alcohol use during gestation. *Alcohol Clin Exp Res* 1985;9:454.

297. Ernhart CB, Wolf AW, Linn PL, et al. Alcohol-related birth defects: syndromal anomalies, intrauterine growth retardation, and neonatal behavioral assessment. *Alcohol Clin Exp Res* 1985;9:447.

298. Anderson RC, Anderson KE. The effects of alcohol consumption during pregnancy. *AAOHN J* 1986;34(2):88.

299. Sokol RJ, Miller SI, Debanne S, et al. The Cleveland NIAAA prospective alcohol-in-pregnancy study: the first year. *Neurotoxicol Teratol* 1981;3:203.

300. Hanson J, Streissguth AP, Smith D. The effects of moderate alcohol consumption during pregnancy on fetal growth and morphogenesis. *J Pediatr* 1978;92:457.

301. Russell M. Clinical implications of recent research on the fetal alcohol syndrome. *Bull NY Acad Med* 1991;67:207.

302. Kaminski M, Rumeau C, Schwartz D. Alcohol consumption in pregnant women and the outcome of pregnancy. *Alcohol Clin Exp Res* 1978;2:155.

303. Tennes K, Blackard C. Maternal alcohol consumption, birth weight and minor physical anomalies. *Am J Obstet Gynecol* 1980;138:774.

304. Hingson R, Alpert J, Day NL, et al. Effects of maternal drinking and marijuana use on fetal growth and development. *Pediatrics* 1982;70:539.

305. Mills JL, Graubard BI. Is moderate drinking during pregnancy associated with an increased rate of malformations? *Pediatrics* 1987;80:309.

306. Robe LB, Gromisch DS, Iosub S. Symptoms of neonatal ethanol withdrawal. *Curr Alcohol* 1981;8:485.

307. Coles CD, Smith I, Fernhoff PM, et al. Neonatal ethanol withdrawal: characteristics in clinically normal, nondysmorphic neonates. *J Pediatr* 1984;105:445.

308. Streissguth A, Barr H, Martin D. Maternal alcohol use and neonatal habituation assessed with the Brazelton Scale. *Child Dev* 1983;545:1109.

309. Streissguth AP, Sampson PD, Barr HM, Clarren SK, Martin DC. Studying alcohol teratogenesis from the perspective of the fetal alcohol syndrome: methodological and statistical issues. *Ann NY Acad Sci* 1986;477:63.

310. Smith IE, Coles CD, Lancaster J, Fernhoff PM, Falek A. The effect of volume and duration of prenatal ethanol exposure on neonatal physical and behavioral development. *Neurobehav Toxicol Teratol* 1986;8:375.

311. Fried PA, Makin JE. Neonatal behavioral correlates of prenatal exposure to marijuana cigarettes and alcohol in a low-risk population. *Neurotoxicol Teratol* 1987;9:1.

312. Jacobson SW, Fein GG, Jacobson JL, et al. Neonatal correlates of prenatal exposure to smoking, caffeine, and alcohol. *Infant Behav Dev* 1984;7:253.

313. Richardson GA, Day NL, Taylor P. The effect of prenatal alcohol, marijuana and tobacco exposure on neonatal behavior. *Infant Behav Dev* 1989;12:199.

314. Rosett H, Snyder P, Sander LW, et al. Effects of maternal drinking on neonate state regulation. *Dev Med Child Neurol* 1979;21:464.

315. Chernick V, Childiaeva R, Ioffe S. Effects of maternal alcohol intake and smoking on neonatal electroencephalogram and anthropometric measurements. *Am J Obstet Gynecol* 1983;146:41.

316. Ioffe S, Childiaeva R, Chernick V. Prolonged effects of maternal alcohol ingestion on the neonatal encephalogram. *Pediatrics* 1984;74:330.

317. Ioffe S, Chernick V. Development of the EEG between 30 and 40 weeks gestation in normal and alcohol-exposed infants. *Dev Med Child Neurol* 1988;30:797.

318. Mennella JA, Beauchamp GK. The transfer of alcohol to human milk. *N Engl J Med* 1991;325:981.

319. Flores-Huerta S, Hernandez-Montes H, Argote RM, Villalpando S. Effects of ethanol consumption during pregnancy and lactation on the outcome and postnatal growth of the offspring. *Ann Nutr Metab* 1992;36:121.

320. Kiessling KH, Pilstrom L. Effects of ethanol on rat liver: the influence of vitamins, electrolytes and amino acids on the structure and function of mitochondria from rats receiving ethanol. *Br J Nutr* 1967;21:547.

321. Cobo E. Effect of different doses of ethanol on the milk-ejecting reflex in lactating women. *Am J Obstet Gynecol* 1973;115:817.

322. Little RE, Anderson KW, Ervin CH, et al. Maternal alcohol use during breast-feeding and infant mental and motor development at one year. *N Engl J Med* 1989;321:425.

323. Day NL, Robles N, Richardson G, et al. The effects of prenatal alcohol use on the growth of children at three years of age. *Alcohol Clin Exp Res* 1991;15:67.

324. Barr HM, Streissguth AP, Martin DC, et al. Infant size at 8 months of age: relationships to maternal use of alcohol, nicotine and caffeine during pregnancy. *Pediatrics* 1984;74:336.

325. Sampson PD, Bookstein FL, Barr HM, Streissguth AP. Prenatal alcohol exposure, birthweight, and measures of child size from birth to age 14 years. *Am J Public Health* 1994;84:1421.

326. Streissguth AP, Barr HM, Olson HC, Sampson PD, Bookstein FL, Burgess DM. Drinking during pregnancy decreases word attack and arithmetic scores on standardized tests: adolescent data from a population-based prospective study. *Alcohol Clin Exp Res* 1994;18:248.

327. Greene T, Ernhart CB, Sokol RJ, et al. Prenatal alcohol exposure and preschool physical growth: a longitudinal analysis. *Alcohol Clin Exp Res* 1991;15:905.

328. Coles CD, Brown RT, Smith LE, Platzman KA, Erickson S, Falek A. Effects of prenatal alcohol exposure at school age: I. Physical and cognitive development. *Curr Alcohol* 1991;13(4):1.

329. O'Connor MJ, Brill NJ, Sigman M. Alcohol use in primiparous women older than 30 years of age: relation to infant development. *Pediatrics* 1986;78:444.

330. Fried PA, O'Connell CM. A comparison of effects of prenatal exposure to tobacco, alcohol, cannabis and caffeine on birth size and subsequent growth. *Neurotoxicol Teratol* 1987;9:79.

331. Coles CD, Smith IE, Lancaster JS, et al. Persistence over the first month of neurobehavioral differences in infants exposed to alcohol prenatally. *Infant Behav Dev* 1987;10:23.

332. Coles CD, Smith IE, Falek A. Prenatal alcohol exposure and infant behavior: immediate effects and implications for later development. In Bean-Bayog M, ed. *Children of alcoholics.* New York: Hayworth Press, 1987:87.

333. Streissguth AP, Barr HM, Martin DC, et al. Effects of maternal alcohol, nicotine and caffeine use during pregnancy on infant mental and motor development at eight months. *Alcohol Clin Exp Res* 1980;4:152.

334. Jacobson JL, Jacobson SW, Sokol RJ, Martier SS, Ager JW, Kaplan-Estrin MG. Teratogenic effects of alcohol on infant development. *Alcohol Clin Exp Res* 1993;17:174.

335. Jacobson JL, Jacobson SW, Sokol RJ, Martier SS, Ager JW, Shankaran S. Effects of alcohol use, smoking, and illicit drug use on fetal growth in black infants. *J Pediatr* 1994;124:757.

336. Jacobson SW, Jacobson JL, Sokol RJ, Martier SS, Ager JW. Prenatal alcohol exposure and infant information processing ability. *Child Dev* 1993;64:1706.

337. Gusella J, Fried P. Effects of maternal social drinking and smoking on offspring at 13 months. *Neurotoxicol Teratol* 1984;6:13.

338. O'Connor MJ, Brill NJ, Sigman M. Alcohol use in primiparous women older than 30 years of age: relation to infant development. *Pediatrics* 1986;78:444.

339. Richardson GA, Day NL. *Prenatal exposure to alcohol, marijuana and tobacco: effect on infant mental and motor development.* Paper presented at the meeting of the Society for Research in Child Development, Seattle, Washington, April 1991.

340. Streissguth AP, Barr HM, Sampson PD, et al. IQ at age 4 in relation to maternal alcohol use and smoking during pregnancy. *Dev Psychol* 1989;25:3.

341. Landesman-Dwyer S, Ragozin A, Little R. Behavioral correlates of prenatal alcohol exposure: a four-year follow-up study *Neurotoxicol Teratol* 1981;3:187.

342. Streissguth AP, Martin DC, Barr HM, et al. Intrauterine alcohol and nicotine exposure: attention and reaction time in 4-year-old children. *Dev Psychol* 1984;20:533.

343. Barr HM, Streissguth AP, Darby BL, et al. Prenatal exposure to alcohol, caffeine, tobacco and aspirin: effects on fine and gross motor performance in 4-year-old children. *Dev Psychol* 1990;26:339.

344. Larsson G, Bohlin A-B, Tunnell R. Prospective study of children exposed to variable amounts of alcohol *in utero*. *Arch Dis Child* 1985;60:315.

345. Streissguth AP, Barr HM, Sampson PD, et al. Attention distraction and reaction time at seven years and prenatal alcohol exposure. *Neurotoxicol Teratol* 1986;8:717.

346. Streissguth AP, Barr HM, Sampson PD. Moderate prenatal alcohol exposure: effects on child IQ and learning problems at age 7½ years. *Alcohol Clin Exp Res* 1990;14:662.

347. Kodituwakku PW, Handmaker NS, Cutler SK, Weathersby EKM, Handmaker SD. Specific impairments in self-regulation in children exposed to alcohol prenatally. *Alcohol Clin Exp Res* 1995;19(6):1558.

348. Kopera-Frye K, Dehaene S, Streissguth AP. Impairments of number processing induced by prental alcohol exposure. *Neuropsychologia* 1996;32(12):1187.

349. Fried PA, Watkinson B. 12- and 24-month neurobehavioral follow-up of children prenatally exposed to marijuana, cigarettes and alcohol. *Neurotoxicol Teratol* 1988;10:305.

350. Fried PA, Watkinson B. 36- and 48-month neurobehavioral follow-up of children prenatally exposed to marijuana, cigarettes and alcohol. *J Dev Behav Pediatr* 1990;11:49.

351. Kolata GB. Fetal alcohol advisory debated. *Science* 1981;214:642.

352. Astley SJ, Clarren SK. A fetal alcohol syndrome screening tool. *Alcohol Clin Exp Res* 1995;19(6):1565.

353. Astley SJ, Clarren SK. A case definition and photographic screening tool for the facial phenotype of fetal alcohol syndrome. *J Pediatr* 1996;129(1):33.

354. Aase JM. Clinical recognition of FAS: difficulties of detection and diagnosis. *Alcohol World* 1994;18(1):5.

355. Spagnolo A. Teratogenesis of alcohol. *Ann Ist Super Sanita* 1993;29:89.

356. Sokol RJ, Ager J, Martier S, et al. Significant determinants of susceptibility to alcohol teratogenicity. *Ann NY Acad Sci* 1986;77:87.

357. Young NK. Effects of alcohol and other drugs on children. *J Psychoact Drugs* 1997;29(1):23.

358. Jacobson JL, Jacobson SW, Sokol RJ. Increased vulnerability to alcohol-related birth defects in the offspring of mothers over 30. *Alcohol Clin Exp Res* 1996;20(2):359–63.

359. Armant DR. Saunders DE. Exposure of embryonic cells to alcohol: contrasting effects during preimplantation and postimplantation development. *Semin Perinatol* 1996;20(2):127.

360. Ernhart CB, Sokol RJ, Martier S, et al. Alcohol teratogenicity in the human: a detailed assessment of specificity, critical period, and threshold. *Am J Obstet Gynecol* 1987;156:33.

361. Streissguth AP, Clarren SK, Jones KL. Natural history of the fetal alcohol syndrome: a ten-year follow-up of eleven patients. *Lancet* 1985;2:85.

362. Kyllerman M, Aronson M, Sabel KG, et al. Children of alcoholic mothers (growth and motor performance compared to matched controls). *Acta Paediatr Scand* 1985;70:20.

363. Spohr HL, Willms J, Steinhahusen HC. Prenatal alcohol exposure and long-term developmental consequences. *Lancet* 1993;341:907.

364. Streissguth AP. Fetal alcohol syndrome in older patients. *Alcohol Alcohol Suppl* 1993;2:209.

365. Landesman-Dwyer S. The relationship of children's behavior to maternal alcohol consumption. In Abel EL, ed. *Fetal alcohol syndrome: human studies*, vol 2. Boca Raton, FL: CRC Press, 1982:127.

366. Streissguth AP, Herman C, Smith D. Stability of intelligence in the fetal alcohol syndrome: a preliminary report. *Alcohol Clin Exp Res* 1978;2:165.

367. Ueker A. Nadel L. Spatial locations gone awry: object and spatial memory deficits in children with fetal alcohol syndrome. *Neuropsychologia* 1996;34(3):209.

368. Mattson SN, Riley EP, Delis DC, Stern C, Jones KL. Verbal learning and memory in children with fetal alcohol syndrome. *Alcohol Clin Exp Res* 1996;20(5):810.

369. Shaywitz S, Cohen D, Shaywitz B. Behavior and learning difficulties in children of normal intelligence born to alcoholic mothers. *J Pediatr* 1980;96:978.

370. Steinhausen HC, Nestler V, Spohr HL. Development and psychopathology of children with the fetal alcohol syndrome. *J Dev Behav Pediatr* 1982;3:49.

371. Caruso K, ten Bensel R. Fetal alcohol syndrome and fetal alcohol effects. The University of Minnesota experience. *Minn Med* 1993;76(4):25.

372. Coles CD, Platzman KA, Rashkind-Hood CL, Brown RT, Falek A, Smith IE. A comparison of children affected by prenatal alcohol exposure and attention deficit, hyperactivity disorder. *Alcohol Clin Exp Res* 1997;21(1):150.

373. Church MW, Gerkin KP. Hearing disorders in children with fetal alcohol syndrome: findings from case reports. *Pediatrics* 1988;82:147.

374. Flint EF. Severe childhood deafness in Glasgow, 1965–1979. *J Laryngol Otol* 1983;97:421.

375. Thiringer K, Kankkunen A, Liden G, et al. Perinatal risk factors in the etiology of hearing loss in preschool children. *Dev Med Child Neurol* 1984;26:799.

376. Aronson M, Kyllerman M, Sabel KG, et al. Children of alcoholic mothers (developmental, perceptual and behavioral characteristics as compared to matched controls). *Acta Paediatr* 1985;74:27.

377. Sowell ER, Jernigan TL, Mattson SN, Sobel DF, Jones KL. Abnormal development of the cerebellar vermis in children prenatally exposed to alcohol size reduction in lobules I–V. *Alcohol Clin Exp Res* 1996;20(1):31.

378. Mattson SN, Riley EP, Delis DC, Stern C, Jones KL. Verbal learning and memory in children with fetal alcohol syndrome. *Alcohol Clin Exp Res* 1996;20(5):810.

379. Swayze VW 2nd, Johnson VP, Hanson JW, et al.Piven J, Sato Y, Giedd JN, Mosnik D, Andreasen NC. Magnetic resonance imaging of brain anomalies in fetal alcohol syndrome. *Pediatrics* 1997;99(2):232.

380. Johnson VP, Swayze VW 2nd, Sato Y, Andreasen NC. Fetal alcohol syndrome: craniofacial and central nervous system manifestations. *Am J Med Genet* 1996;61(4):329–339.

381. Hellstrom A, Chen Y, Stromland K. Fundus morphology assessed by digital analysis in children with fetal alcohol syndrome. *J Pediatr Ophthalmol Strabismus* 1997;34(1):17.

382. Stromland K. Hellstrom A. Fetal alcohol syndrome—an ophthalmologic and socioeducational prospective study. *Pediatrics* 1996;97 (6 Pt 1):845.

383. Stromland K, Pinazo-Duran MD. Optic nerve hypoplasia: Comparative effects in children and rats exposed to alcohol during preganancy. *Teratology* 1994;50(2):100.

384. Duester G. Retinoids and the alcohol dehydrogenase gene family. *EXS* 1994;71:279.

385. Church MW, Eldis F, Blakley BW, Bawle EV. Hearing, language, speech, vestibular and dentofacial disorders in fetal alcohol syndrome. *Alcohol Clin Exp Res* 1997;21(2):227.

386. Church MW, Kaltenbach JA. Hearing, speech, language and vestibular disorders in the fetal alcohol syndrome: A literature review. *Alcohol Clin Exp Res* 1997;21:495.

387. Rossig C. Wasser S, Oppermann P. Audiologic manifestations in fetal alcohol syndrome assessed by brainstem auditory-evoked potentials. *Neuropaediatrie* 1994;25(5):245.

388. Khalsa Jh, Gfroerer JC. Epidemiology and health consequences of drug abuse among pregnant women. *Semin Perinatol* 1991;15:265.

389. Substance Abuse and Mental Health Services Administration. *National household survey on drug abuse: Population estimates, 1996.* DHHS Pub. No. (SMA) 97-3137. Washington, DC: Superintendent of Documents, US Government Printing Office, 1997.

390. Abel EL. *Marijuana, the first twelve thousand years.* New York: Plenum Press, 1980.

391. *Marijuana and Health. Report of a study by the Committee of the Institute of Medicine, Division of Health Sciences Policy.* Washington, DC: National Academy Press, 1982.

392. Dewey WL. Cannabinoid pharmacology. *Pharmacol Rev* 1986;38:151.

393. Martin BR. Cellular effects of cannabinoids. *Pharmacol Rev* 1986;38:45.

394. Harbison RD, Mantilla-Plata B. Prenatal, toxicity, maternal distribution and placental transfer of tetrahydrocannabinol. *J Pharmacol Exp Ther* 1972;180:446.

395. Abel EL, Rockwood GA, Riley EP. The effects of early marijuana exposure. In Riley EP, Vorhees CV, eds. *Handbook of behavioral teratology.* New York: Plenum Press, 1986:267.

396. Ostrea EM, Subramanian MG, Abel EL. Placental transfer of cannabinoids in humans: comparison between meconium, maternal and cord blood sera. In Chesner G, Consroe P, Musty R, eds. *Marijuana: an international research report: proceedings of the Melbourne Symposium on Cannabis,* Series 7. Canberra: Australian Government Publishing Service, 1987:103.

397. Fried PA, Buckingham M, Von Kulmiz P. Marijuana use during pregnancy and perinatal risk factors. *Am J Obstet Gynecol* 1983;144:22.

398. Fried PA, Watkinson B, Willan A. Marijuana use during pregnancy and decreased length of gestation. *Am J Obstet Gynecol* 1984;150:23.

399. Shiono PH, Klebanoff MA, Nugent RP, et al. The impact of cocaine and marijuana use on low birth weight and preterm birth: a multicenter study. *Am J Obstet Gynecol* 1995;172:19.

400. Gibson GT, Baghurst PA, Colley DP. Maternal alcohol, tobacco and cannabis consumption and the outcome of pregnancy. *Aust NZ J Obstet Gynaecol* 1983;23:15.

401. Day NL, Richardson GA. Prenatal marijuana use: epidemiology, methodologic issues, and infant outcome. *Clin Perinatol* 1991;18:77.

402. Tennes K, Avitable N, Blackard C, et al. Marijuana: prenatal and postnatal exposure in the human. *NIDA Res Monogr Ser* 1985;59:48.

403. Linn S, Schoenbaum S, Monson R, et al. The association of marijuana use with outcome of pregnancy. *Am J Public Health* 1983;73:1161.

404. Zuckerman B, Frank D, Hingson R, et al. Effects of maternal marijuana and cocaine use on fetal growth. *N Engl J Med* 1989;320:762.

405. O'Connell CM, Fried PA. An investigation of prenatal cannabis exposure and minor physical anomalies in a low risk population. *Neurotoxicol Teratol* 1984;6:345.

406. Qazi QH, Mariano E, Milman DH, et al. Abnormalities in offspring associated with prenatal marijuana exposure. *Dev Pharmacol Ther* 1985;8:141.

407. Hutchings DE, Morgan B, Brake SC, et al. Delta-9-tetrahydrocannabinol during pregnancy in the rat: I. Differential effects on maternal nutrition, embryotoxicity and growth in the offspring. *Neurotoxicol Teratol* 1987;9:39.

408. Morgan B, Brake SC, Hutchings DE, et al. Delta-9-tetrahydrocannabinol during pregnancy in the rat: effects on development of RNA, DNA, and protein in offspring brain. *Pharmacol Biochem Behav* 1988;31:365.

409. Hutchings DE, Dow-Edwards D. Animal models of opiate, cocaine and cannabis use. *Clin Perinatol* 1991;18:1.

410. Fried PA. Marijuana use during pregnancy: consequences for the offspring. *Semin Perinatol* 1991;15:280.

411. Scher MS, Richardson GA, Coble PA, et al. The effects of prenatal alcohol and marijuana exposure: disturbances in neonatal sleep cycling and arousal. *Pediatr Res* 1988;24:101.

412. Mirochnick M, Meyer J, Frank DA, Cabral H, Tronick EZ, Zuckerman B. Elevated plasma norepinephrine after *in utero* exposure to cocaine and marijuana. *Pediatrics* 1997;99:555–559.

413. Hayes JS, Dreher MC, Nugent JK. Newborn outcomes with maternal marijuana use in Jamaican women. *Pediatr Nurs* 1988;14:107.

414. Taylor P. Agents acting at the neuromuscular junction and autonomic ganglia: nicotine. In Gilman A, Goodman LS, Rall TW, et al, eds. *Goodman and Gilman's the pharmacologic basis of therapeutics,* 8th ed. New York: Pergamon Press, 1990:180.

415. Dahlstrom A, Lundell B, Curvall M, Thapper L. Nicotine and cotinine concentrations in the nursing mother and her infant. *Acta Paediatr* 1990;79:142.

416. Kline J, Stein ZA, Susser M. Smoking as a risk factor for spontaneous abortion. *N Engl J Med* 1977;297:793.

417. Milart P, Kauffels W, Schneider J. Vasoactive effects of nicotine in human umbilical arteries. *Zentralbl Gynakol* 1994;116:217.

418. Ahlsten G, Ewald U, Tuvemo T. Maternal smoking reduces prostacyclin formation in human umbilical arteries. A study on strictly selected pregnancies. *Acta Obstet Gynecol Scand* 1986;65:645.

419. Brown HL, Miller JM, Khawli O, et al. Premature placental calcification in maternal cigarette smokers. *Obstet Gynecol* 1988;71:914.

420. Lehtovirta P, Forss M. The acute effect of smoking on intervillous blood flow of the placenta. *Br J Obstet Gynaecol* 1978;85:729.

421. Naeye RL, Harkness WL, Utts J. Abruptio placentae and perinatal death: a prospective study. *Am J Obstet Gynecol* 1977;128:740.

422. Garn SM, Johnson M, Ridella SA, et al. Effects of maternal cigarette smoking on Apgar scores. *Am J Dis Child* 1981;135:503.

423. Hingson R, Gould JR, Morelock S, et al. Maternal cigarette smoking, psychoactive substance use and infant Apgar scores. *Am J Obstet Gynecol* 1982;144:959.

424. Meyer MB, Tonascia JA. Maternal smoking, pregnancy complications, and perinatal mortality. *Am J Obstet Gynecol* 1977;128:494.

425. Wen SW, Goldenberg RL, Cutter GR, et al. Smoking, maternal age, fetal growth, and gestational age at delivery. *Am J Obstet Gynecol* 1990;162:53.

426. Peacock JL, Bland JM, Anderson HR. Preterm delivery: effects of socioeconomic factors, psychological stress, smoking, alcohol, and caffeine. *Br Med J* 1995;311:531.

427. Bergman AB, Wiesner LA. Relationship of passive cigarette smoking to sudden infant death syndrome. *Pediatrics* 1976;58:665.

428. Milerad J, Sundell H. Nicotine exposure and the risk of SIDS. *Acta Paediatr [Suppl]* 1993;389:70.

429. Toubas PL, Duke JC, McCaffree MA, Mattice CD, Bendell D, Orr WC. Effects of maternal smoking and caffeine habits on infantile apnea: a retrospective study. *Pediatrics* 1986;78:159.

430. Kleinman JC, Pierre MB, Madans JS, et al. The effects of maternal smoking on fetal and infant mortality. *Am J Epidemiol* 1988;127:274.

431. Cnattingius S, Haglund B, Meirik O. Cigarette smoking as risk factor for late fetal and early neonatal death. *Br Med J* 1988;297:258.

432. Miller HC, Hassanein K. Maternal smoking and fetal growth of full term infants. *Pediatr Res* 1974;8:960.

433. Beaulac-Baillargeon L, Desrosiers C. Caffeine–cigarette interaction on fetal growth. *Am J Obstet Gynecol* 1987;157:1236.

434. Brooke OG, Anderson HR, Bland JM, Peacock JL, Stewart CM. Effects on birth weight of smoking, alcohol, caffeine, socioeconomic factors, and psychosocial stress. *Br Med J* 1989;298:795.

435. MacArthur C, Knox EG. Smoking in pregnancy: effects of stopping at different stages. *Br J Obstet Gynaecol* 1988;95:551.

436. Shu XO, Hatch MC, Mills J, Clemens J, Susser M. Maternal smoking, alcohol drinking, caffeine consumption, and fetal growth: results from a prospective study. *Epidemiology* 1995;6:115.

437. Abel EL. *Marijuana, tobacco, alcohol and reproduction.* Boca Raton, FL: CRC Press, 1983.

438. Haddow JE, Knight GJ, Palomaki GE, et al. Cigarette consumption and serum cotinine in relation to birth weight. *Br J Obstet Gynaecol* 1987;94:678.

439. Harrison GG, Ranson RS, Vaugher YE. Association of maternal smoking with body composition of the newborn. *Am J Clin Nutr* 1983;38:757.

440. Fried PA, O'Connell CM. A comparison of the effects of prenatal exposure to tobacco, alcohol, cannabis and caffeine on birth size and subsequent growth. *Neurotoxicol Teratol* 1987;9:79.

441. Fedick J, Alberman E, Goldstein H. Possible teratogenic effect of cigarette smoking. *Nature* 1971;231:530.

442. Heinonen OP. Risk factors for congenital heart disease: a prospective study. In Kelly S, Hook EB, Janerich DT, eds. *Birth defects: risks and consequences.* New York: Academic Press, 1976:221.

443. Martin JC, Martin DC, Lund C. Maternal alcohol ingestion and cigarette smoking and their effect upon newborn conditioning. *Alcohol Clin Exp Res* 1973;1:243.

444. Chiriboga CA. Fetal effects. *Neurol Clin* 1993;11:707.

445. Saxton DW. The behavior of infants whose mothers smoke in pregnancy. *Early Hum Dev* 1978;2:363.

446. Landesman-Dwyer S, Keller LS, Streissguth AP. Naturalistic observations of newborns: effects of maternal alcohol intake. *Alcohol Clin Exp Res* 1978;2:171.

447. Woodson EM, DaCosta P, Woodson RH. *Maternal smoking and newborn behavior.* Paper presented at the International Conference on Infant Studies, New Haven, CT, 1980.

448. Butler NR, Goldstein H. Smoking in pregnancy and subsequent child development. *Br Med J* 1973;4:573.

449. Dunn HG, McBurney AK, Ingram S, et al. Maternal cigarette smoking during pregnancy and the child's subsequent development: II. Neurological and intellectual maturation to the age of 6.5 years. *Can J Public Health* 1977;68:43.

450. Zuckerman B. Marijuana and cigarette smoking during pregnancy: neonatal effects. In Chasnoff IJ, ed. *Drugs, alcohol, pregnancy and parenting.* Lancaster, UK: Kluwer Academic Publishers, 1988:73.

451. Johnston M, Evans V, Baigel S. Phencyclidine. *Br J Anaesth* 1959;31:433.

452. Marwah J, Pitts DK. Psychopharmacology of phencyclidine. *NIDA Res Monogr Ser* 1986;64:127.

453. Fico TA, Vanderwende C. Phencyclidine during pregnancy: behavioral and neurochemical effects in the offspring. *Ann NY Acad Sci* 1989;562:319.

454. McCarron M. Phencyclidine intoxication. *NIDA Res Monogr Ser* 1986;64:209.

455. Cummings AJ. Transplacental disposition of phencyclidine in the pig. *Xenobiotica* 1979;9:447.

456. Cooper JE, Cummings AJ, Jones H. The placental transfer of phencyclidine in the pig, plasma levels in the sow and its piglets. *J Physiol* 1977;267:17.

457. Nicholas JM, Lipshitz J, Schreiber E. Phencyclidine: its transfer across the placenta as well as into breast milk. *Am J Obstet Gynecol* 1982;143:143.

458. Kaufman KR, Petrucha RA, Pitts FN, et al. Phencyclidine in umbilical cord blood: preliminary data. *Am J Psychiatry* 1983;140:450.

459. Aniline O, Pitts FN. Phencyclidine (PCP): a review and perspectives. *Crit Rev Toxicol* 1982;10:145.

460. Domino ET, Wilson AE. Effects of urine acidification on plasma and urine phencyclidine levels in overdosage. *Clin Pharmacol Ther* 1977;22:421.

461. Blaustein MP, Bartschat DK, Sorensen RG. Phencyclidine (PCP) selectively blocks certain presynaptic potassium channels. *NIDA Res Monogr Ser* 1986;64:37.

462. Crider R. Phencyclidine: changing abuse patterns. *NIDA Res Monogr Ser* 1986;64:163.

463. Golden NL, Kuhnert BR, Sokol RJ, et al. Phencyclidine use during pregnancy. *Am J Obstet Gynecol* 1984;148:254.

464. Golden NL, Kuhnert BR, Sokol RJ, et al. Neonatal manifestations of maternal phencyclidine exposure. *J Perinat Med* 1987;15:185.

465. Chasnoff IJ, Burns WJ, Hatcher RP, et al. Phencyclidine: effects on the fetus and neonate. *Dev Pharmacol Ther* 1983;6:404.

466. Howard J, Kropenske V, Tyler R. The long-term effects on neurodevelopment in infants exposed prenatally to PCP. *NIDA Res Monogr Ser* 1986;64:237.

467. Rahbar F, Fomufod A, White D, Westney LS. Impact of intrauterine exposure to phencyclidine (PCP) and cocaine on neonates. *J Natl Med Assoc* 1993;85:349.

468. Tabor BL, Smith-Wallace T, Yonekura ML. Perinatal outcome associated with PCP versus cocaine use. *Am J Drug Alcohol Abuse* 1990;16:337.

469. Strauss AA, Modanlou D, Bosu SK. Neonatal manifestations of maternal phencyclidine (PCP) abuse. *Pediatrics* 1981;68:550.

470. Wachsman L, Schuetz S, Chan LS, Wingert WA. What happens to babies exposed to phencyclidine (PCP) *in utero? Am J Drug Alcohol Abuse* 1989;15:31.

471. Chasnoff IJ, Burns KA, Burns WJ, Schnoll SH. Prenatal drug exposure: effects on neonatal and infant growth and development. *Neurobehav Toxicol Teratol* 1986;8:357.

472. Hoffman BB, Lefkowitz RJ. Catecholamines and sympathomimetics. In Gilman AG, Rall TW, Nies AS, et al, eds. *Goodman and Gilman's the pharmacological basis of therapeutics,* 8th ed. New York: Pergamon Press, 1990:187.

473. Little BB, Snell LM, Gilstrap LC III. Methamphetamine abuse during pregnancy: outcome and fetal effects. *Obstet Gynecol* 1988;72:541.

474. Milkovich L, Van den Berg BJ. Effects of antenatal exposure to anorectic drugs. *Am J Obstet Gynecol* 1977;129:637.

475. Oro AS, Dixon SD. Perinatal cocaine and methamphetamine exposure: maternal and neonatal correlates. *J Pediatr* 1987;111:571.

476. Dixon SD. Effects of transplacental exposure to cocaine and methamphetamine on the neonate. *West J Med* 1989;150:436.

477. Ramer CM. The case history of an infant born to an amphetamine-addicted mother. *Clin Pediatr* 1974;13:596.

478. Dixon SD, Bejar R. Echoencephalographic findings in neonates associated with maternal cocaine and methamphetamine use: incidence and clinical correlates. *J Pediatr* 1989;115:770.

479. Eriksson M, Larsson G, Winbladh B, et al. The influence of amphetamine addiction on pregnancy and the newborn infant. *Acta Paediatr Scand* 1978;67:95.

480. Billing L, Eriksson M, Steneroth G, et al. Pre-school children of amphetamine-addicted mothers: I. Somatic and psychomotor development. *Acta Paediatr Scand* 1985;74:179.

481. Eriksson M, Billing L, Steneroth G, et al. Health and development of 8 year-old children whose mother abused amphetamines during pregnancy. *Acta Paediatr Scand* 1989;78:944.

482. O Brien CP. Drug Addiction and Drug Abuse. In Gilman AG, Hardman JG, et al, eds. *Goodman and Gilman's the pharmacologic basis of therapeutics,* 9th ed. New York: McGraw Hill, 1996:557.

483. Rall TW. CNS stimulants: the methylxanthenes. In Gilman AG, Goodman LS, Rall TW, et al, eds. *Goodman and Gilman's the pharmacological basis of therapeutics,* 7th ed. New York: Macmillan Press, 1985:589.

484. Schardein JL. Current status of drugs as teratogens in man. *Prog Clin Biol Res* 1985;163C:181.

485. Nehlig A, Debry G. Potential teratogenic and neurodevelopmental consequences of coffee and caffeine exposure: A review of human and animal data. *Neurotoxicol Teratol* 1994;16:531.

486. Martin TR, Bracken MB. The association between low birth weight and caffeine consumption during pregnancy. *Am J Epidemiol* 1987;126:813.

487. Fenster L, Eskenazi B, Windham GC, Swan SH. Caffeine consumption during pregnancy and fetal growth. *Am J Public Health* 1991;81:458.

488. Caan BJ, Goldhaber MK. Caffeinated beverages and low birthweight: a case-control study. *Am J Public Health* 1989;79:1299.

489. Bland JM, Anderson HR. Effects on birthweight of alcohol and caffeine consumption in smoking women. *J Epidemiol Commun Health* 1991;45(2):159.

490. Fortier I, Marcoux S, Beaulac-Baillargeon L. Relation of caffeine intake during pregnancy to intrauterine growth retardation and preterm birth. *Am J Epidemiol* 1993;137:931.

491. Leviton A. Caffeine consumption and the risk of reproductive hazards. *J Reprod Med* 1988;33:175.

492. Larroque B, Kaminski M, Lelong N, Subtil D, Dehaene P. Effects of birth weight of alcohol and caffeine consumption during pregnancy. *Am J Epidemiol* 1993;137(9):941.

493. Shu XO, Hatch MC, Mills J, Clemens J, Susser M. Maternal smoking, alcohol drinking, caffeine consumption, and fetal growth: results from a prospective study. *Epidemiology* 1995;6:115.

494. Hadeed A, Siegel S. Newborn cardiac arrhythmias associated with maternal caffeine use during pregnancy. *Clin Pediatr* 1993;32:45.

495. Oei SG, Vosters RP, van der Hagen NL. Fetal arrhythmia caused by excessive intake of caffeine by pregnant women. *Br Med J* 1989;298:568.

496. McGowan JD, Altman RE, Kanto WP Jr. Neonatal withdrawal symptoms after chronic maternal ingestion of caffeine. *South Med J* 1988;81:1092.

497. McKim EM. Caffeine and its effects on pregnancy and the neonate. *J Nurse Midwifery* 1991;36:226.

498. Kandall SR, Gartner LM. Late presentation of drug withdrawal symptoms in newborns. *Am J Dis Child* 1974;127:58.

499. Chasnoff IJ. Drug use and women: establishing a standard of care. *Ann NY Acad Sci* 1989;562:208.

500. Khavari K, Farber P. A profile instrument for the quantification and assessment of alcohol consumption. *J Stud Alcohol* 1978;39:1525.

501. Khavari KA, Douglass FM. The drug use profile (DUP): an instrument for clinical and research evaluations for drug use patterns. *Drug Alcohol Depend* 1981;8:119.

502. Cahalan D, Cisin I, Crossley H. *American drinking practices.* Monograph No. 6. New Brunswick, NJ: Rutgers Center of Alcohol Studies, 1969.

503. Ostrea EM Jr, Welch RR. Detection of prenatal drug exposure in the pregnant woman and her newborn infant. *Clin Perinatol* 1991;18:629.

504. Schonberg SK, Blasinsky M, eds. *Substance abuse: a guide for health professionals.* Chicago, IL: American Academy of Pediatrics Center for Advanced Heath Studies, 1988:48.

505. Ostrea EM, Martier S, Welch R, et al. Sensitivity of meconium drug screen in detecting intrauterine drug exposure of infants. *Pediatr Res* 1990;27:219A.

506. Ostrea EM, Brady MJ, Parks PM, et al. Drug screening of meconium in infants of drug dependent mothers: an alternative to urine testing. *J Pediatr* 1989;115:474.

507. Halstead AC, Godolphin W, Lockitch G, et al. Timing of specimens is crucial in urine screening of drug dependent mothers and infants. *Clin Biochem* 1988;21:59.

508. Osterloh JD, Lee BL. Urine drug screening in mothers and infants. *Am J Dis Child* 1989;143:791.

509. Hicks JM, Morales A, Soldin SJ. Drugs of abuse in a pediatric outpatient population. *Clin Chem* 1990;36:1256.

510. Ostrea EM, Lynn SN, Wayne RH, et al. Tissue distribution of morphine in the newborns of addicted monkeys and humans. *Dev Pharmacol Ther* 1980;1:163.

511. Silvestre MA, Lucena J, Ostrea EM. The effect of timing, dosage and duration or morphine intake during pregnancy on the amount of morphine in meconium in a rat model. *Pediatr Res* 1991;29:66A.

512. Ostrea EM Jr, Romero A, Knapp DK, Ostrea AR, Utarnachitt RB. Postmortem analysis of meconium in early gestation human fetuses exposed to cocaine: Clinical implications. *J Pediatr* 1994;124:477.

513. Ostrea EM. Detection of prenatal drug exposure in the pregnant woman and her newborn infant. In Kilbey MM, Asghar K, eds. *Methodological issues in epidemiological, prevention and treatment research on drug exposed women and their children.* Washington, DC: US Department of Health and Human Services, NIDA Research Monograph Series 1992;96–121.

514. Ostrea EM, Parks P, Brady M. Rapid isolation and detection of drugs in meconium of infants of drug dependent mothers. *Clin Chem* 1988;34:2372.

515. Ostrea EM Jr, Romero A, Yee H. Adaptation of the meconium drug test for mass screening. *J Pediatr* 1993;122:152.

516. Mac E, Matias O, Ostrea EM, Mazhar M. Clinical adaptation of HPLC to meconium drug testing. *Pediatr Res* 1995;37:221A.

517. Murphey LJ, Olsen GD, Konkol RJ. Quantitation of benzoylecgonine and other cocaine metabolites in meconium by high-performance liquid chromatography. *J Chromatogr* 1993;12:330.

518. Browne SP, Moore CM, Negrusz A, Tebbett IR, Covert R, Dusick A. Detection of cocaine norcocaine and cocaethylene in the meconium of premature neonates. *J Forens Sci* 1994;39:1515.

519. Browne SP, Tebbett IR, Moore CM, Dusick A, Covert R, Yee GT. Analysis of meconium for cocaine in neonates. *J Chromatogr* 1992;75(1):158.

520. Montes N, Romero A, Ostrea EM, Ostrea MR. Improved method of GC/MS analysis of meconium for opiate, cocaine and cannabinoid. *Pediatr Res* 1993;33:66A.

521. Wingert WE, Feldman MS, Kim MH, et al. A comparison of meconium, maternal urine and neonatal urine for detection of maternal drug use during pregnancy. *J Forens Sci* 1994;39:150.

522. Moriya F, Chan KM, Noguchi TT, Wu PY. Testing for drugs of abuse in meconium of newborn infants. *J Anal Toxicol* 1994;18:41.

523. Clark GD, Rosenweig B, Raisys VA. Analysis of cocaine and benzoylecgonine in meconium of infants born to cocaine dependent mothers. *Clin Chem* 1990;36:1022A.

524. Lombardero N, Casanova O, Behnke M, Eyler FD, Bertholf RL. Measurement of cocaine and metabolites in urine, meconium, and diapers by gas chromatography/mass spectrometry. *Ann Clin Lab Sci* 1993; 23:385.

525. Mac E, Pacis M, Garcia G, Ostrea EM. A marker of fetal exposure to alcohol by meconium analysis. *Pediatr Res* 1994;35:238A.

526. Ostrea EM, Knapp DK, Romero A, Montes M, Ostrea AR. Meconium analysis to assess fetal exposure to access fetal exposure to active and passive maternal smoking. *J Pediatr* 1994;15:474.

527. Ostrea EM, Brady MJ, Parks PM, Asensio DC, Naluz A. Drug screening of meconium in infants of drug-dependent mothers: An alternative to urine testing. *J Pediatr* 1989;15:474.

528. Ryan RM, Wagner CL, Schultz JM, et al. Meconium analysis for improved identification of infants exposed to cocaine *in utero. J Pediatr* 1994;125:435.

529. Maynard E, Amoroso LP, Oh W. Osteopathic hospitals. Meconium for drug testing. *Am J Dis Child* 1991;45:650.

530. Callahan CM, Grant TM, Phipps P, et al. Measurement of gestational cocaine exposure: Sensitivity of newborn hair, meconium, and urine. *J Pediatr* 1992;120:763.

531. Lewis DE, Moore CM, Leikin JB, Koller A. Meconium analysis for cocaine: A validation study and comparison with paired urine analysis. *J Anal Toxicol* 1995;19:148.

532. Bandstra E, Steele B, Chitwood D. Detection of *in utero* cocaine exposure: A comparative methodologic study. *Pediatr Res* 1992;31,58A.

533. Casanova OQ, Lombardero N, Behnke M, Eyler FD, Conlon M, Bertholf RL. Detection of cocaine exposure in the neonate. Analyses of urine, meconium, and amniotic fluid from mothers and infants exposed to cocaine. *Arch Pathol Lab Med* 1994;118(10):988.

534. Baumgartner A, Jones P, Black C. Detection of phencyclidine in hair. *J Forens Sci* 1981;26:576.

535. Baumgartner A, Jones P, Baumgartner W, et al. Radioimmunoassay of hair for determining opiate abuse histories. *J Nucl Med* 1979; 2:748.

536. Baumgartner W, Black C, Jones P, et al. Radioimmunoassay of cocaine in hair: a concise communication. *J Nucl Med* 1982;23:790.

537. Baumgartner A, Jones P, Black C. Detection of phencyclidine in hair. *J Forens Sci* 1981;26:576.

538. Ishiyama I. Detection of basic drugs (methamphetamine, antidepressants and nicotine) from human hair. *J Forens Sci* 1983;28:380.

539. Balabanova S, Homoki J. Determination of cocaine in human hair by gas chromatography/mass spectrometry. *Z Rechtsmed* 1987;98: 235.

540. Marigo M, Tagliaro F, Poiesi C, et al. Determination of morphine in the hair of heroin addicts by high performance liquid chromatography with fluorimetric detection. *J Anal Toxicol* 1986;10:158.

541. Pelli B, Traldi P, Tagliaro F, et al. Collisional spectroscopy for unequivocal and rapid determination of morphine at ppb level in the hair of heroin addicts. *Biomed Environ Mass Spectrum* 1987;14:63.

542. Graham K, Koren G, Klein J, et al. Determination of gestational cocaine exposure by hair analysis. *JAMA* 1989;262:3328.

543. Bailey DN. Drug screening in an unconventional matrix: hair analysis. *JAMA* 1989;262:3331.

544. Smith FP, Liu RH. Detection of cocaine metabolites in perspiration stain, menstrual bloodstain and hair. *J Forens Sci* 1986;31:1269.

545. Smith FP. Detection of phenobarbital in bloodstains, semen, seminal stains, saliva stains, saliva, perspiration stains and hair. *J Forens Sci* 1981;26:582.

546. Finnegan LP. Neonatal abstinence. In Nelson NM, ed. *Current therapy in neonatal perinatal medicine.* Philadelphia: BC Decker, 1990: 314.

547. Lipsitz PJ. A proposed narcotic withdrawal score for use with newborn infants. *Clin Pediatr* 1975;14:592.

CHAPTER 57

Anesthesia and Analgesia

Anthony J. Camerota and John H. Arnold

Despite the widespread use of potent analgesic agents in adult patients and older children, it is remarkable that, until recently, systemic analgesia and sedation were rarely administered to neonates. An analysis of neonatal anesthetic practice published in 1985 revealed that only 23% of preterm infants undergoing patent ductus arteriosus ligation received adequate intraoperative anesthesia (1). In a retrospective survey of opioid use in a single institution, only 14% of 933 neonates received opioid analgesia after a variety of surgical procedures (2). However, in a 1995 questionnaire, all neonates received either systemic opioids and/or regional anesthesia for major surgery (3). Although adequate anesthesia and analgesia were not given to neonates in the past because of the belief that they could not feel pain, there is overwhelming evidence that pain perception and physiologic responses to stress occur in neonates of all gestational ages (4). It is broadly accepted that anesthesia and analgesia in the neonatal population have important clinical and physiologic consequences and may have long-term psychological impact. Control of the stress response in the perioperative period may improve the outcome of infants after cardiac surgery (5,6).

As these data are assimilated and accepted, there is often a discrepancy between the growing understanding of neonatal pain and actual clinical practice. A survey of British pediatric anesthetists found that only 5% routinely prescribed systemic opioids to neonates postoperatively, although 80% of the respondents believed that neonates feel pain (7). There are probably several reasons for the lag in changing clinical practice to match current knowledge, but a crucial element may be the lack of standard guidelines for the use of drugs, doses, and schedules that

can be applied to various clinical situations by the practitioner at the bedside.

This chapter reviews the rapidly developing field of neonatal anesthesia and analgesia, summarizes the relevant pharmacokinetic and pharmacodynamic data, and highlights practical considerations for the most commonly used agents.

PAIN PERCEPTION

In addition to the ethical arguments for preventing needless human suffering, the risks and benefits of using anesthesia and analgesia to prevent pain and stress must be physiologically evaluated. Pivotal aspects of this physiologic rationale are based on one question: Does the neonate feel pain?

Components of the pain system may be traced from sensory receptors in the skin to sensory areas in the cerebral cortex and used as a framework to study its development (4). The density of nociceptive nerve endings in newborn skin, the labeling of specific proteins (e.g., GAP-43) produced by axonal growth cones, the reflex activity and receptive fields of primary afferent neurons, and the development of synapses between primary afferents and interneurons in the dorsal horn of the spinal cord indicate the anatomic and functional maturity of the peripheral pain system during fetal life (8,9). Cellular and subcellular organization in the dorsal horn, with maturation of primary afferent terminations, occur during later gestation and postnatally (10,11). In the dorsal horn, various neurotransmitter and neuromodulator substances associated with pain (e.g., substance P, somatostatin, calcitonin gene-related peptide, vasoactive intestinal peptide, met-enkephalin, glutamate) appear during early gestation (12).

Lack of myelination in neonatal nerves or central nerve tracts is offset completely by the shorter interneuronal and neuromuscular distances traveled by the impulse. Quantitative neuroanatomic data show that nociceptive

A. J. Camerota: Department of Critical Care Medicine, Naval Regional Center, Portsmouth, Virginia

J. H. Arnold: Department of Anaesthesia (Pediatrics), Harvard Medical School; and Multidisciplinary Intensive Care Unit, Children's Hospital, Boston, Massachusetts

nerve tracts in the spinal cord and central nervous system undergo complete myelination during the second and third trimesters of gestation (4). Subcortical foci associated with nociception are characterized by a high density of opioid receptors during the middle of gestation, with a differential reduction in binding capacities during the third trimester (13). Development of the fetal neocortex begins at 8 weeks of gestation; by 20 weeks, each cortex has a full complement of 109 neurons. Arborization of dendritic processes in the cortical neurons is followed by synaptogenesis with incoming thalamocortical fibers by 24 to 26 weeks of gestation. Functional maturity of the cerebral cortex is suggested by fetal and neonatal electroencephalographic patterns, cortical somatosensory evoked potentials, studies of regional cerebral metabolism, early behavioral development, and the specific behavioral responses of neonates to painful stimuli (4,14).

Endorphinergic cells in the anterior pituitary are responsive to corticotrophin-releasing factor stimulation *in vitro* and show increased β-endorphin production during fetal and neonatal life. Endogenous opioids and other hormones (e.g., catecholamines, steroid hormones, glucagon, growth hormone) are secreted by the human fetus in response to stress, leading to catabolism and other complications (6,15). Significant changes in cardiovascular parameters, transcutaneous partial pressure of oxygen (PO_2), and palmar sweating have been observed in neonates undergoing painful clinical procedures. These physiologic changes are closely associated with behavioral responses of newborns to pain. Neonatal behavioral responses are characterized by simple motor responses, precise changes in facial expression associated with pain, highly specific patterns of crying activity, and a variety of complex behavioral changes. These neonatal responses suggest integrated emotional and behavioral changes correlated with pain, and they are retained in memory long enough to modify subsequent behavior patterns (4).

The surgical stress responses of neonates can be inhibited by potent anesthesia, as demonstrated by randomized trials of halothane anesthesia in term neonates, fentanyl anesthesia in preterm neonates, and sufentanil anesthesia in neonates undergoing cardiac surgery (6,16,17). These results imply that the nociceptive stimuli during surgery are at least partially responsible for the marked stress responses of neonates and are prevented by the provision of adequate anesthesia. In these trials, the reduction in surgical stress responses was associated with significant improvements in clinical outcome, supporting the use of potent anesthetic agents for newborns undergoing surgery.

In recent years, the concept of blunting the pain response in neonates to improve physiologic parameters has been extended from the operating room to the intensive care unit. High-dose narcotic anesthesia for the first postoperative night after complex cardiac surgery reduces mortality (18–20). Using narcotics during painful procedures, such as tracheal suctioning, has been shown to reduce concomitant hypoxemia (21).

ANESTHESIA

Anesthesia is classically defined as a drug-induced state that includes analgesia, amnesia, and muscle relaxation. The provision of anesthesia to infants undergoing surgical procedures has undergone a remarkable transition coincident with the development of new intravenous agents and more sophisticated monitoring techniques. As recently as 1985, there was considerable debate about whether neonates feel pain, and sophisticated researchers advocated the use of minimal anesthesia in neonates undergoing surgical procedures, citing the dangers of anesthetic administration to this population (22–24). Beginning with the landmark paper of Robinson and Gregory (25), practitioners of neonatal and pediatric anesthesia have proclaimed the importance of providing adequate anesthesia, particularly to ill preterm infants (25,26). In modern anesthetic practice, adequate anesthetic depth and control of the neonatal stress response can be achieved without undue risk to the infant.

The appropriate anesthetic technique is dictated by the preoperative condition of the patient, the planned surgical procedure, and the skills of the anesthetist. The encounter between the anesthesiologist and the neonate usually occurs in the setting of a surgical emergency, and a general anesthetic with control of the airway is most often the technique of choice. General anesthesia is provided using a combination of inhaled and intravenous agents and muscle relaxants. The inhaled agents include an inorganic gas (e.g., nitrous oxide) and the volatile liquids (e.g., halothane, enflurane, isoflurane, sevoflurane, and desflurane). Delivery of potent inhaled agents by means of the respiratory system offers a reliable route of administration and excretion with the ability to rapidly alter anesthetic concentrations in the central nervous system.

Inhaled Anesthetics

Each of the inhaled anesthetic agents has unique effects on the cardiovascular, respiratory, and central nervous systems, which are not exhaustively reviewed here (Table 57–1). The volatile anesthetics produce dose-dependent decreases in mean arterial blood pressure, particularly in premature infants, due to direct myocardial depression and decreases in systemic vascular resistance due to exaggerated depression of the baroreceptor reflex (27–29). Nitrous oxide produces minimal alterations in myocardial performance or systemic vascular resistance, due in part to direct stimulation of the sympathetic nervous system (30). However, if combined with a potent volatile agent or opioids, nitrous oxide significantly depresses myocardial contractility (31). If ventilation is

TABLE 57–1. *Systemic effects of inhaled anesthetics*

	Myocardial function	Heart rate	Systemic vascular resistance	Cerebral blood flow
Halothane	––	–	+/–	++
Enflurane	–	+	–	+
Isoflurane	–	++	––	+/–[a]
N$_2$O	+/–	+/–	–/–	+/–
Desflurane	–	++	––	+/–[a]
Sevoflurane	–	+/–	+/–	+/–[a]

[a]In doses <1.0 minimum alveolar concentration.

++, greatly increased; +, moderately increased; +/– no consistent effect; –, moderately decreased; ––, greatly decreased.

carefully controlled, nitrous oxide has insignificant effects on pulmonary vascular resistance (32).

All inhaled agents increase the respiratory rate, reduce tidal volume and functional residual capacity, decrease the ventilatory responses to hypoxemia and hypercapnia, and decrease bronchial smooth muscle reactivity. These agents produce a dose-dependent increase in cerebral blood flow despite simultaneous depression of cerebral metabolic oxygen requirement. At high concentrations, isoflurane and desflurane induce an isoelectric electroencephalographic pattern; this property is not shared by the other inhaled anesthetic agents.

Although halothane is most frequently associated with perioperative hepatic dysfunction, other inhaled agents and intravenous anesthetics may result in hepatic necrosis (33). True halothane-induced hepatitis is a rare event, occurring in approximately 1 of 30,000 patients. It is seen most commonly after repeated administration and is probably mediated by an immune mechanism involving an intermediate oxidative metabolite (34,35). The inhaled agents produce dose-related decreases in renal blood flow and urine output due to effects on cardiac output and systemic vascular resistance. Fluoride-induced nephrotoxicity is a potential complication of prolonged exposure to the fluorinated hydrocarbons (e.g., enflurane, isoflurane), although it is of practical concern only during prolonged administration of enflurane and sevoflurane (36,37).

Two newer inhaled anesthetics are gaining popularity due to their low lipid solubility, sevoflurane and desflurane (38). This property allows for rapid induction of anesthesia as well as a short recovery time. Sevoflurane has the advantage of providing a smooth, less irritating induction of anesthesia that rivals that of halothane, with less risk of hepatitis and fewer hemodynamic effects (39). The drawbacks are the biotransformation of sevoflurane into potentially toxic Compound A and the accumulation of fluoride ions (40,41). Desflurane does not undergo biodegradation *in vivo* or *in vitro*, but its irritating effects on the airway prevent its role as an induction agent (42,43).

Opioid Anesthesia

Morphine and the synthetic opioids have been a consistent adjunct to the volatile agents throughout the his-

tory of anesthesia. High-dose opioids have become the preferred anesthetic technique for cardiac surgical procedures in adults and children (44,45). The virtues of opioids include minimal effects on myocardial performance, ablation of pulmonary vascular responses to nociceptive stimuli, and preservation of hypoxic pulmonary vasoconstriction (46–48).

Because of their wide margin of safety in ill infants with congenital heart disease, opioid anesthesia is often effective in ill preterm infants with cardiopulmonary instability undergoing surgical stress. Fentanyl, sufentanil, and remifentanil are the most popular agents due to their negligible effect on cardiovascular function, but if combined with other anesthetic agents, these opioids may be associated with significant hemodynamic instability. Morphine anesthesia may increase plasma histamine concentrations and decrease vascular resistance, and it is not recommended as a primary anesthetic for ill neonates (49).

The elimination half-lives (T$_{1/2}\beta$) of the opioids are significantly prolonged in the neonate (Table 57–2) and may be further prolonged by any compromise of hepatic blood flow (50–55). In addition, there is considerable variabilty in their elimination half-lives (T$_{1/2}\beta$) in the neonate. Prolonged postoperative respiratory depression may occur if these important pharmacokinetic variables are ignored in the perioperative period.

Regional, Neuraxial, and Local Anesthesia

Regional anesthetic techniques have become increasingly popular in the pediatric and neonatal populations (56). General anesthesia may be associated with an

TABLE 57–2. *Elimination half-lives of opioids*

Opioid	Relative dose	T$_{1/2}\beta$ (h) Neonate	Child
Morphine	0.1 mg	6.8	2.2
Fentanyl	1–5 µg	4.2	3.5
Sufentanil	0.2–1 µg	12.3	2.3
Alfentanil	5–25 µg	8.8	1.4
Remifentanil	0.25–1 µg	8–48	8–48

increased incidence of postoperative apnea in the preterm infant (57). This may be a particularly difficult issue in the day-surgery setting, where former preterm neonates commonly present for minor surgical procedures (e.g., circumcision, herniorrhaphy). It is in this population that regional or local anesthetic techniques may be particularly advantageous. Preliminary experience suggests that the use of spinal anesthesia may reduce the risk of postoperative apnea in former preterm infants (58).

Spinal anesthesia consists of injection of an anesthetic agent into the subarachnoid space. The technique is easy to perform and safe (59). The most frequent local anesthetic agents are hyperbaric lidocaine, tetracaine, and bupivacaine. Side effects of spinal anesthesia, such as dural puncture headaches and hemodynamic compromise, are common in adults but surprisingly uncommon in infants or children (59,60).

Epidural anesthesia consists of injection of an anesthetic agent into the potential space between the dura mater and the ligamentum flavum by a single injection or repeated injections through an epidural catheter. The advantage epidural has over spinal anesthesia is the potential for long-term, continuous, or intermittent administration of anesthetics. Although the epidural space can be approached at any level, for most infants, a lumbar or caudal epidural blockade is used. Caudal epidural blockade with bupivacaine is used most frequently for postoperative pain relief after lower abdominal and lower extremity procedures. Compared with older children and adults, infants and toddlers require higher doses of local anesthetic and demonstrate a shorter duration of effect. Combining local anesthetics with an epidural opioid (fentanyl, hydromorphone), clonidine, or ketamine prolongs the duration of analgesia (61). Caudal anesthesia has been sufficient as the sole anesthetic technique for lower abdominal procedures (62). Caudal epidural blockade may be used in combination with general anesthesia in infants during abdominal procedures. Rarely, complications result from improper placement of the needle and injection of the anesthetic agent into a vein, the dura, the subarachnoid space, or sacral marrow.

Local anesthetics may be used to block peripheral nerves in infants undergoing limited surgical procedures (e.g., orchiopexy, herniorrhaphy, circumcision). These techniques are simple to perform, have limited complications, and significantly decrease the need for postoperative analgesia (63–65).

Local anesthetic toxicity is manifested by effects on the cardiovascular system (e.g., myocardial depression, arrhythmias) and the central nervous system (e.g., delirium, seizures) (66,67). In premature infants, the subtle behavioral changes that precede cardiovascular collapse and generalized seizures may be difficult to recognize. The reduced protein binding and prolonged elimination of local anesthetics in this population make the neonate susceptible to toxic effects at lower doses, decreasing the

therapeutic index. Careful attention to total administered dose (particularly with field blocks) and monitoring of cardiovascular parameters during the administration of any local anesthetic are essential.

The topical anesthetic EMLA, a eutectic mixture of 2.5% lidocaine and 2.5% prilocaine, has shown efficacy in neonatal circumcisions, but not in reducing pain with heelsticks (68,69). Its incidental vasoconstriction may require more vigorous squeezing in obtaining a blood sample. Although methemoglobinemia is a potential side effect of EMLA, it appears to be safe, even in preterm infants (70,71). A newer topical agent, amethocaine, in a 4% gel, not only avoids the possibility of methemoglobinemia, but its vasodilatory effects on the skin may facilitate blood sampling (72).

Propofol

Propofol, as a loading dose of 2 to 4 mg/kg, acts as a complete anesthetic with a short recovery period, similar to, or even briefer than, the lipid-soluble pentothal. A continuous infusion of 50 to 100 mg/kg/min maintains anesthesia and may, when discontinued, have a shorter recovery time than that of inhalation agents. However, prolonged infusions lead to lipid deposition and persistent anesthetic effects of propofol, even with discontinuation. Postoperative emesis and analgesic requirements may be reduced versus pentothal–halothane. Pain at the infusion site has limited the enthusiasm for propofol. Pain can be alleviated by adding 0.2 mg/kg of lidocaine for every 3 mg/kg of propofol. The incidence of hypotension is comparable to similar agents. Prolonged propofol infusion (3 to 5 days) has been linked to metabolic acidosis, heart failure, and death in critically ill children. Associated with these have been lipemic serum and fatty infiltration of the liver (73). Although propofol may be used during the course of some anesthetics, the drug is not recommended for use in children below the age of 3 years, for sedation in children, or for sedation in the pediatric intensive care unit because its safety and efficacy have not been established.

ANALGESIA

Opioids

The provision of adequate analgesia for painful diseases and procedures should be of utmost concern to the neonatologist (74). Despite widespread misgivings about their potential side effects, systemic therapy with opioid analgesics remains the mainstay of treatment for severe pain in neonates. The administration of opioids produces profound analgesia and sedation through specific activity on μ_1, δ, and other opioid receptors in the brain and spinal cord (75).

The dosage and mode of administration of opioids should be carefully titrated to avoid undertreatment of pain or oversedation (Fig. 57–1). Continuous intravenous

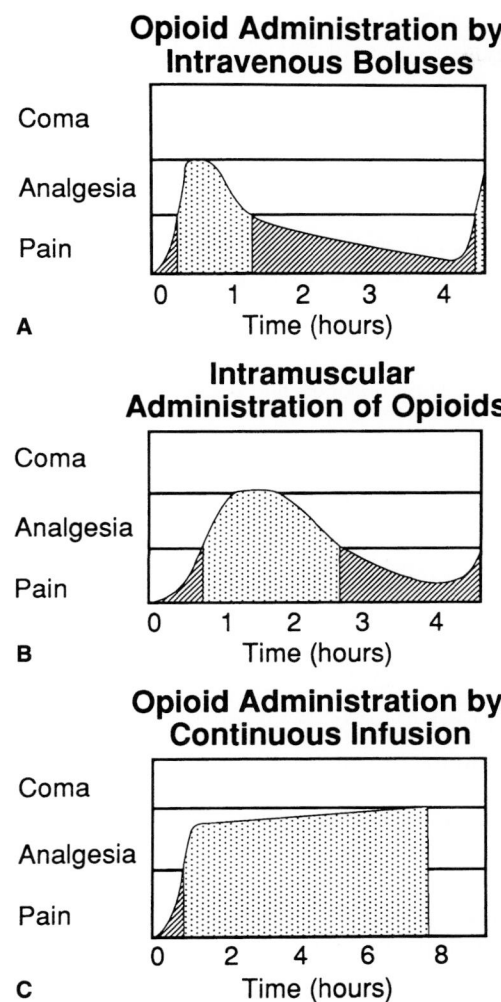

Opioid Administration by Intravenous Boluses

Coma

Analgesia

Pain

0   1   2   3   4

A   Time (hours)

Intramuscular Administration of Opioids

Coma

Analgesia

Pain

0   1   2   3   4

B   Time (hours)

Opioid Administration by Continuous Infusion

Coma

Analgesia

Pain

0   2   4   6   8

C   Time (hours)

FIG. 57–1. Modes of opioid administration. **A:** Patients given intermittent intravenous boluses every 4 hours experience deep sedative effects at peak levels after a dose, with prolonged periods of pain between doses. **B:** Patients given intramuscular injections experience less fluctuation in opioid effects but undergo alternate periods of pain and analgesia. **C:** Patients receiving continuous infusions of opioids experience constant analgesia but are at risk for a slow build-up in plasma levels resulting in sedation or toxicity. (Adapted from Berde CB. Pediatric postoperative pain management. *Pediatr Clin North Am* 1989;36:926.)

infusion of opioids provides an effective alternative to intermittent intravenous doses, with constant blood levels and minimal fluctuations in analgesia. All opioids have prolonged half-lives in neonates (see Table 57–2), and continuous infusions can result in a slow accumulation of the drug over time, with high blood levels that may not be considered or detected immediately. In addition, morphine has an active metabolite that can accumulate in renal insufficiency, compounding the narcotic effect. Despite this disadvantage, continuous intravenous infusion is ideal for providing a constant level of analgesia if appropriate precautions are observed.

A newer agent, remifentanil, is quickly degraded by red cell and tissue esterases, giving it an elimination half-life ($T_{1/2}\beta$) of about 3 minutes. Unlike the other opioids, its brief duration of action is maintained, even after prolonged continuous infusions (76). There is little experience using remifentanil in neonates.

Alternative modes of administration are rarely indicated in neonates. Subcutaneous morphine or fentanyl, given as a lozenge or transdermally, is not routinely used in neonates, because precise documentation of their efficacy and safety is not available. The transdermal route may be an attractive future alternative to intravenous infusions in premature neonates, particularly because the permeability of preterm skin is 102 to 103 times greater than the skin of term neonates (77). Oral or rectal opioids can be used in the neonate, but only if the same close monitoring provided for intravenous opioid analgesia can be given to these patients. The oral bioavailabilities of commonly used opioids are listed in Table 57–3, although these data have been derived mostly from older children and adults. The pharmacokinetics of oral opioids have not been studied in neonates, but the onset and duration of action are likely to be delayed, and close monitoring should continue for at least 24 hours after the last dose.

Opioid side effects include respiratory depression, tolerance and dependence, alterations in chest wall compliance, decreased gastrointestinal motility, and nausea. Exogenously administered opioids may alter endogenous opioid receptor physiology and possibly influence subsequent behavioral development (13,78,79). Chronic opioid administration also has immunosuppressive effects through both direct (immune cell receptors) and indirect (centrally mediated) mechanisms (80). However, these agents are probably the most suitable and effective analgesics currently available for treatment of severe pain in neonates.

All opioids produce dose-related respiratory depression characterized by decreased ventilatory and behavioral responses to hypoxemia and hypercarbia. The CO_2 response curve is displaced to the right and resting PCO_2 rises. Clinically, the respiratory rate decreases with an incomplete compensatory increase in tidal volume. It is not widely appreciated that standard doses of morphine (0.1 mg/kg) almost abolish the ventilatory response to hypoxemia. In patients with airway obstruction or atelectasis after surgery, blunting of hypoxic drive can lead to dangerous hypoventilation. Opioid-induced respiratory depression can be reversed with naloxone, but the effect of this drug diminishes within 30 minutes, and repeated dosing may be required, particularly after the use of morphine or methadone (81). It was long believed that newborn infants were more prone than older children or adults to opioid-induced respiratory depression, perhaps because of an immature blood–brain barrier (82). It has been shown that opioid-induced apnea is less common in neonates than in older infants and children at similar

TABLE 57–3. *Recommended dosages and oral–parenteral ratios for opioids*

Drug	Routes of administration	Parental dosage (mg/kg)	Frequency (parenteral)	Oral–parenteral ratio	Frequency (oral/rectal)
Morphine	IM, IV,[a] SQ, PO, PR, neuraxial[b]	0.05–0.2	q 1–2 h IV q 2–4 h IM or SQ	3–6	q 4–6 h[c] q 8–12 h[d]
Meperidine	IM, IV, SQ, PO	0.5–1.5	q 1–2 h IV q 2–4 h IM or SQ	4	q 4–6 h
Codeine	IM, IV,[a] SQ, PO	0.5–1.0	q 2–4 h	1.5–2	q 4–6 h
Hydromorphone	IM, IV, SQ, PO, PR	0.02–0.04	q 2–4 h	2–4	q 4–6 h PO q 6–8 h PR
Methadone	IM, IV, SQ, PO	0.05–0.2	q 12–24 h	2	q 24 h
Fentanyl	IM, IV, TM/TD,[e] neuraxial[b]	0.001–0.005	q 1–2 h		

[a]IV administration may be associated with significant histamine release and possible hypotension.

[b]Neuraxial (i.e., epidural, subarachnoid) administration can be performed only by qualified and experienced anesthesiologists.

[c]Pertains to regular oral preparations (e.g., MSIR, Roxanal; tablets and oral solutions).

[d]Pertains to slow-release oral or rectal preparations (e.g., MS Contin, Duramorph, Roxanol SR).

[e]Transmucosal/transdermal (TM/TD) preparations have not been standardized for use in full-term or preterm neonates.

plasma concentrations (83,84). Neonates conjugate morphine into morphine 6-glucuronide and morphine 3-glucuronide. Compared with infants and older children, however, the neonate produces less of the 6-glucoronide-metabolite. Morphine 6-glucuronide is a more potent analgesic than morphine itself, and it induces less apnea. The more plentiful metabolite in the neonate, morphine 3-glucoronide, may actually antagonize the effects of its parent molecule, morphine (85,86). This may partially explain the susceptibility of the neonate to morphine-induced apnea.

Tolerance occurs if there is a reduction in the clinical effects of a drug with repeated administration. The rate of development of tolerance to the analgesic effects of opioids is extremely variable. There is evidence that tolerance may develop more rapidly in the absence of nociceptive stimulation (87). Dependence is the requirement for continued drug administration to prevent withdrawal symptoms, including agitation, dysphoria, tachycardia, tachypnea, piloerection, nasal congestion, temperature instability, and feeding intolerance. Tolerance and dependence have been described in neonatal and pediatric patients during the therapeutic use of opioids (88–91). Although tolerance to opioids may appear to develop more rapidly in neonates than at other ages, it is likely that tolerance to the sedative and cardiovascular effects of opioids may precede a tolerance to their analgesic effects (92). Infusions of higher potency analgesics (e.g., fentanyl) may produce less tolerance compared to lower potency opioids, such as morphine. The development of physical dependence is quite variable, and withdrawal symptoms have been observed in infants in whom opioid administration was discontinued abruptly after periods of administration as short as 5 days (90). Fear of precipitating the abstinence syndrome should not inhibit the appropriate administration of opioids, because withdrawal

symptoms can be effectively managed by gradually tapering the opioid dosage over 5 to 7 days (Fig. 57–2).

Dependence is a set of physiologic responses that should be differentiated from addiction, which is a behavioral syndrome of compulsive drug seeking. Addiction is extremely rare in patients of all ages receiving opioids for pain or sedation, and fear of addiction should not affect the appropriate treatment of acute pain or agitation in neonatal intensive care.

Opioids increase airway resistance, and there is much debate about the effect of histamine release on bronchial smooth muscle and whether histamine-releasing agents such as morphine are contraindicated in patients with reactive airway disease (93). Although intravenous morphine releases greater amounts of histamine than fentanyl, precipitation of bronchospasm has not been reported after the administration of morphine (49). Intravenous morphine has been used frequently in patients with severe asthma requiring mechanical ventilation, based on evidence that it might inhibit bronchoconstriction and mucous hypersecretion (94–96).

Chest wall rigidity is a well-described complication of opioid administration and has been documented in patients receiving large doses of fentanyl, sufentanil, or alfentanil (31,97,98). The administration of 30 μg/kg of fentanyl in tracheostomized patients produced a minor increase in total lung compliance, suggesting that inability to maintain a mask airway during fentanyl administration is due to supraglottic obstruction and not chest wall rigidity (99,100). Rigidity has occurred at an average dose of 15 to 17 μg/kg of fentanyl (99,100). There are no controlled data available in term or preterm neonates receiving fentanyl. However, clinical experience indicates that chest wall rigidity may occur at significantly lower opioid doses in the neonate. The mechanism that mediates this phenomenon may involve μ_1-opioid receptor

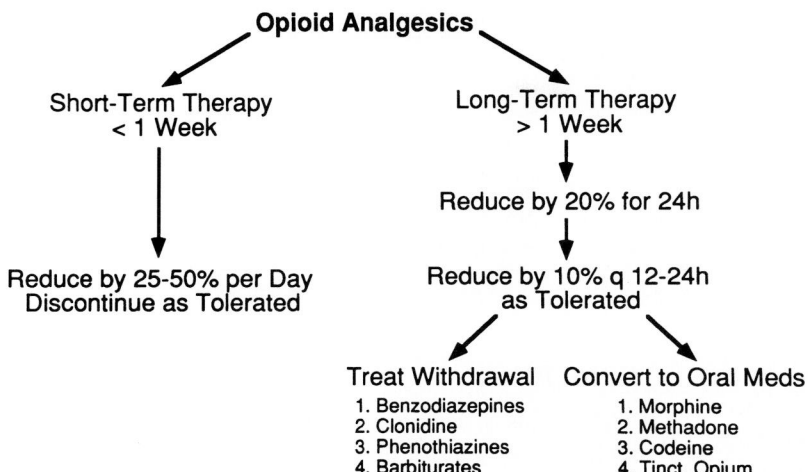

Opioid Analgesics

Short-Term Therapy
< 1 Week

Long-Term Therapy
> 1 Week

Reduce by 20% for 24h

Reduce by 25-50% per Day
Discontinue as Tolerated

Reduce by 10% q 12-24h
as Tolerated

Treat Withdrawal
1. Benzodiazepines
2. Clonidine
3. Phenothiazines
4. Barbiturates

Convert to Oral Meds
1. Morphine
2. Methadone
3. Codeine
4. Tinct. Opium

FIG. 57–2. Suggested algorithm for weaning a patient from opioid analgesics after short-term and long-term therapy. These pharmacologic approaches can be applied in conjunction with nonpharmacologic therapies to decrease the duration of therapy for the opioid abstinence syndrome.

modulation of gamma-aminobutyric acid pathways in the spinal cord. Rigidity on induction of anesthesia is avoided by pretreatment with a subrelaxant dose of pancuronium (0.01 to 0.02 mg/kg) and by slow intravenous infusion of the opioid (97,101,102).

All opioids delay gastric emptying, decrease intestinal motility, produce nausea by direct stimulation of the chemoreceptor trigger zone, and increase the common bile duct pressure. Impaired absorption of enteral nutrients is undesirable in neonates, and opiate-induced ileus may increase the risk of regurgitation and aspiration of gastric contents. One case report described a newborn given morphine who developed a reversible and nonobstructive dilation of the common hepatic duct that resolved after morphine was discontinued (103). Although such side effects are mediated by means of μ_2-opioid receptors, they may occur with high doses of opioids devoid of μ_2-activity (e.g., fentanyl) as a result of nonspecific effects on all opioid receptors.

Nonopioid Agents

There are many nonopioid agents available for the treatment of mild pain or use as adjuvants for decreasing the doses and potential side effects of opioid drugs. Various other analgesic agents can be used systemically for providing sedation or in combination with regional and topical analgesia to produce effective analgesia while minimizing the side effects of any single agent.

Acetaminophen

Acetaminophen (N-acetyl-p-aminophenol) is used commonly in all age groups as an antipyretic and analgesic. Its use in neonates has been limited by misconceptions about its metabolism and excretion and about its potential for hepatotoxicity. Experimental data and clinical experience have supported the relative safety and

analgesic efficacy of acetaminophen in newborn infants, without the significant side effects on platelet aggregation, the ductus arteriosus, or the gastric mucosa, commonly seen with aspirin or other nonsteroidal antiinflammatory drugs (NSAIDs) (104).

The hepatic metabolism of acetaminophen occurs primarily by sulfation or glucuronidation, but a small fraction is oxidized by the cytochrome P450 mixed-function oxidase system into an arene compound (i.e., a reactive metabolite), which is conjugated with glutathione before excretion (105,106). In acute toxicity, the hepatic stores of glutathione are depleted rapidly, and this reactive metabolite binds irreversibly to membrane proteins, leading to liver cell necrosis. In the newborn or fetal liver, this metabolic pathway is seven to ten times slower than in the adult liver and occurs well after the development of glutathione synthesis, mediating a protective effect in fetal hepatocytes (107). These experimental data have been substantiated by the absence of hepatic dysfunction in clinical reports of neonatal poisoning with acetaminophen (108,109). The clinical use of acetaminophen in term or preterm neonates should not be overly restrained by concerns about its potential hepatotoxicity.

Acetaminophen has many potential advantages as an analgesic in neonates. It has approximately the same analgesic efficacy as 0.5 to 1.0 mg/kg of codeine, and the analgesia is additive to that provided by opioids. It produces no respiratory depression, and tolerance to acetaminophen-induced analgesia has not been reported. It can be given rectally in doses of 20 to 25 mg/kg, avoiding the need for intravenous lines in infants who cannot be given oral medications.

Nonsteroidal Antiinflammatory Drugs

The NSAIDs are a group of drugs with many actions, including potent analgesic and antiinflammatory properties. The antiinflammatory effects are mediated through

TABLE 57–4. *Recommended doses for nonsteroidal antiinflammatory drugs*

Drug	Dosage (mg/kg)	Routes of administration	Frequency
Acetaminophen	10–20	PO, PR	q 4–6 h
Aspirin	10–15	PO	q 4 h
Choline-magnesium trisalicylate	10–15	PO	q 6–8 h
Ibuprofen	5–15	PO, PR	q 6–8 h
Naprosyn	5–7	PO	q 8–12 h
Tolectin	5–7	PO	q 8–12 h
Ketorolac tromethamine	0.3–0.6	PO, IM, IV	q 6–8 h

inhibition of prostaglandin synthesis by means of the cyclooxygenase pathway. Several NSAIDs have been used in pediatric patients, although data pertaining to neonates are scarce and come from uncontrolled clinical reports (110). Indomethacin and ibuprofen are the most commonly prescribed NSAIDs, but drugs such as ketorolac tromethamine, tolmetin (Tolectin), and naproxen (Naprosyn) are being used with increasing frequency.

The toxicity of NSAIDs limits their potency and clinical usefulness as analgesics (111). Major toxicity is related to gastrointestinal bleeding, hepatotoxicity, blood dyscrasias, decreased renal and splanchnic perfusion, and severe skin reactions. Because of their chemical diversity, adverse reactions to a particular NSAID does not predict similar reactions to other NSAIDs. Significant advantages include the low incidence of side effects in judicious analgesic doses (Table 57–4), the absence of respiratory depression or sedative effects, the relatively long duration of analgesia, and the lack of tolerance or potential for abuse.

NONPHARMACOLOGIC TECHNIQUES

Neonatal pain may be reduced by using a variety of nonpharmacologic methods. The analgesic properties of intraoral sucrose are suggested by its ability to reduce spontaneous crying and crying associated with circumcisions and heelstick and arm venipuncture (112–114). The antinociceptive effects of sucrose appear to be opioid receptor mediated. Its antinociceptive properties in rats can be reversed with naltrexone administration (115). However, neonates born to mothers on methadone do not appear to derive analgesic benefits from sucrose (116). Infant formula and its components (protein, fat, sucrose, but not lactose) also have shown antinociceptive properties (117).

Facilitated tucking, by holding the the neonate's extremities flexed and close to the trunk, lowered the heart rate and produced less crying (118). Nonnutritive sucking, enhanced by the use of a pacifier, reduces the physiologic response to circumcision pain (119). Clearly, nonpharmacologic techniques to reduce pain should be sought whenever possible, because of their effectiveness coupled with a rarity of side effects.

SEDATION

The goals of sedation in the intensive care unit include analgesia for painful diseases and procedures and compliance with controlled ventilation and routine care. The ideal agent would not have hemodynamic or pulmonary side effects and would not be associated with the production or accumulation of toxic metabolites. It would have a short duration of action and a high therapeutic index. The wide variety of medications and combinations of agents that have been used suggests that no single agent meets this ideal standard. Opioids have become exceeding popular due to their relatively high toxic-to-therapeutic ratio, reported lack of side effects, and their potent analgesic properties. Although opioids are considered the mainstay of sedation in the intensive care setting, tolerance to their sedating effects may occur rapidly, and adequate sedation for prolonged periods can be ensured only by administration of adjuvant sedative agents (90,120).

Benzodiazepines

The benzodiazepines have a variety of desirable clinical effects that include hypnosis, anxiolysis, anticonvulsant activity, anterograde amnesia, and muscle relaxation. The amnestic properties of benzodiazepines may be affected by the clinical status of the patient before administration. In the presence of a painful stimulus, the benzodiazepines may produce hyperalgesia and agitation (120–123). These problems usually do not occur if benzodiazepines are combined with opioids.

Benzodiazepines act on specific receptors, located mainly in the cerebral cortex, hypothalamus, cerebellum, corpus striatum, and medulla oblongata, which are coupled to gamma-aminobutyric acid receptors by means of a common chloride channel in synaptic membranes (124). Early pharmacokinetic data showed that the half-life of diazepam and its active metabolites was markedly prolonged in neonates (125). Diazepam is used commonly for sedation in neonates, with doses of 0.1 to 0.3 mg/kg given every 4 to 6 hours. Doses as high as 50 mg/kg/d have been used to treat neonatal tetanus, with a low incidence of side effects (126). Diazepam has no analgesic effects, and it causes respiratory depression and mild hypotension, both of which are potentiated by opioids and other sedatives. Prolonged use may produce tolerance and withdrawal. In preterm neonates, doses as high as 0.5 mg/kg were associated with cardiovascular stability and no alteration in cerebral blood flow (127).

Lorazepam is five to ten times more potent than diazepam. In doses of 0.05 to 0.1 mg/kg, therapeutic levels may persist for 24 to 48 hours. Oral administration results in reliable absorption, with maximal plasma concentrations in 2 to 4 hours. Although lorazepam is insoluble unless combined with an organic solvent, it is suitable for intramuscular or intravenous injection and causes much less tissue irritation than diazepam (128). Lorazepam is glucuronidated to form inactive metabolites. Its elimination half-life is 10 to 20 hours, but clinical effects may be prolonged because of its pharmacodynamic differences from the other benzodiazepines. The cardiovascular and respiratory effects of lorazepam are similar to those of diazepam. Lorazepam should be used judiciously for sedation in the intensive care setting because of prolonged effects on mental status and respiratory drive. Unlike the other benzodiazepines, it contains polyethylene glycol, which produces nephrotoxicity when large amounts of lorazepam are given (129). There have been case reports of lorazepam triggering myoclonus and seizures in neonates (130).

Midazolam, a water-soluble and shorter-acting benzodiazepine, has been used in neonates requiring sedation, alone or combined with opioid analgesics such as fentanyl. Loading doses of 0.2 mg/kg and continuous infusions of 0.4 µg/kg/min of midazolam were used in patients weighing as little as 3 kg and provided good sedation without any apparent adverse effects (131). At the benzodiazepine receptor, midazolam has twice the binding affinity of diazepam and inhibits gamma-aminobutyric acid reuptake. The pharmacokinetics of midazolam in neonates are characterized by rapid redistribution, a plasma clearance of 6.9 mL/kg/min, and an elimination half-life of 6.5 hours, which is significantly longer than the elimination half-life reported for older infants and children (132,133).

After prolonged intravenous therapy with midazolam, a withdrawal syndrome has been described in infants, which is characterized by agitation, poor visual tracking, constant choreoathetoid and dyskinetic movements of the face, tongue, and limbs, and depression of consciousness (134–136). Midazolam may be used intermittently as premedication for specific invasive procedures in doses of 0.05 to 0.2 mg/kg, or for short-term sedation by continuous infusion (less than 12 hours) at rates of 25 to 50 µg/kg/h. The respiratory depression and hypotension caused by benzodiazepines are synergistic with the similar effects of potent opioids. Midazolam and fentanyl given by rapid intravenous injection may cause severe, life-threatening hypotension and cardiorespiratory arrest (137). This combination should be used with extreme caution in neonates and only with close monitoring in an intensive care unit.

Flumazenil, a short-acting benzodiazepine antagonist, can be used as a bolus of 10 µg/kg followed by an infusion (5 µg/kg/min) to reverse the effects of the benzodiazepines. Rapid reversal of the benzodiazepines can trigger seizures in susceptible patients.

Barbiturates

Phenobarbital has long been used as an anticonvulsant in newborns and children, although its routine use for sedation has been discouraged because of several drawbacks. Phenobarbital has hyperalgesic effects and may increase the requirement for analgesia, and rapid tolerance to its sedative action invariably occurs (138). It has a prolonged elimination half-life in neonates (5 to 6 days), and it may increase the risk of intraventricular hemorrhage in premature neonates (139,140). Phenobarbital has no specific antagonist, and prolonged use is associated with microsomal induction of hepatic enzymes and with a withdrawal syndrome. Its advantages in neonates include increased bilirubin metabolism, relatively mild cardiovascular and respiratory depression, and familiarity with its usage in preterm and term neonates. In ventilated preterm neonates, the changes in mean arterial pressure and intracranial pressure associated with endotracheal suctioning were blunted with phenobarbital therapy (141). A neonatal dose–response study found increasing degrees of sedation and feeding difficulties with increasing serum phenobarbital concentrations. These responses were greater in preterm neonates than in term neonates (142). Loading doses of 5 to 10 mg/kg and maintenance doses of 2.5 mg/kg every 12 hours, given orally or intravenously, are generally used for sedation.

Chloral Hydrate

Chloral hydrate is used frequently as a sedative in doses of 25 to 50 mg/kg or as a hypnotic in doses of 50 to 100 mg/kg for short procedures in neonates and for infants with chronic lung disease (143). Higher doses may be required after repeated use in neonates because of the slow development of tolerance. The advantages of chloral hydrate include ease of administration (e.g., oral syrup, rectal suppositories), although repeated doses can be irritating to the enteral mucosa; lack of respiratory depression; lack of other side effects (e.g., emesis, changes in vital signs or behavior) with usual therapeutic doses; and familiarity with its use in newborns and older infants (144,145). However, an infant who received 165 mg/kg of chloral hydrate over 16 hours developed the toxic reactions of respiratory depression and lethargy (146). Other reports have documented complications such as direct hyperbilirubinemia, decreased tidal volume, hypertriglyceridemia, acute laryngeal edema, and cardiac arrhythmias (e.g., supraventricular tachycardia) in neonates and infants (147–151). One of its metabolites, trichloroethylene, has been described as carcinogenic with chronic exposure (152).

The sedative action of chloral hydrate may be mediated by generalized neuronal depression, similar to other halogenated hydrocarbons. A precise mechanism of action is unknown, and there is no specific antagonist. The pharmacokinetics of chloral hydrate are not clearly defined in neonates. Onset of clinical effects after oral dosage occurs at 30 minutes, and its duration of action is usually 2 to 4 hours, depending on the exact doses used.

Ketamine

Ketamine is a dissociative anesthetic that has been used as an induction agent for anesthesia, an analgesic for conscious sedation, a premedication before induction of anesthesia, and a sedative for critically ill patients. There is a broad range of experience with this agent in older patients, but limited experience in infants and newborns (153,154). Ketamine has been used to provide anesthesia in the spontaneously breathing, nonintubated newborn and causes less neonatal neurobehavioral depression than thiopental after maternal administration for vaginal delivery (155,156). Ketamine produces reliable serum levels within 1 minute when administered intravenously or within 5 minutes when administered intramuscularly, and it is rapidly redistributed, with awakening occurring in 10 to 15 minutes. In neonates, the elimination half-life is significantly longer than 130 minutes, which has been reported in older children and adults (157,158). Extensive hepatic biotransformation necessitates higher doses when administered orally or rectally.

Tolerance and hepatic enzyme induction have been demonstrated during chronic administration of ketamine. Cross tolerance with opiates has been demonstrated in animals, but convincing evidence from human studies is lacking (159,160). The precise site of action of ketamine is unknown, despite suggestions that ketamine may interfere with excitatory transmission by means of N-methyl-D-aspartate receptors (161). The anesthetic effects of ketamine have been attributed to electrophysiologic dissociation between the thalamoneocortical and limbic systems. Other clinical effects at anesthetic plasma concentrations include catalepsy, nystagmus, hypertonicity, and nonpurposeful movements. Ketamine is a potent stimulator of the cardiovascular system, presumably by means of central sympathetic effects and inhibition of catecholamine reuptake (162). Compared with isoflurane, halothane, and fentanyl, ketamine had the least effects on mean arterial pressure in ill preterm neonates undergoing surgery (163). Pulmonary vascular resistance does not appear to be altered in infants with or without preexisting pulmonary hypertension (164). For critically ill patients with moderate hypovolemia, low doses of ketamine (i.e., 0.5 to 1 mg/kg) are safer than barbiturates as rapid induction agents before tracheal intubation.

SUMMARY

The proper approach to sedation includes an individualized regimen, which ensures analgesia with careful consideration of the important pharmacokinetic and pharmacodynamic differences in the neonatal population. Analgesia and sedation is needed for neonates undergoing stressful or painful procedures required for essential monitoring and therapy in intensive care. Safe and effective techniques are available that can be used in a variety of clinical circumstances. We strongly urge the reader to follow the guidelines proposed by the American Academy of Pediatrics (165) and later endorsed by the American Society of Anesthesiologists (166):

> ... local or systemic pharmacologic agents are now available to permit relatively safe administration of anesthesia and analgesia to neonates undergoing surgical procedures, and ... such administration is indicated according to the usual guidelines.... The decision to withhold such medication should be based on the same medical criteria used for older patients.

REFERENCES

1. Anand KJ, Aynsley Green A. Metabolic and endocrine effects of surgical ligation of patent ductus arteriosus in the human preterm neonate: are there implications for improvement of postoperative outcome? *Mod Probl Pediatr* 1985;23:143.
2. Purcell-Jones G, Dormon F, Sumner E. The use of opioids in neonates. A retrospective study of 933 cases. *Anaesthesia* 1987;42:1316.
3. de Lima J, Lloyd-Thomas AR, Quinn, TM, et al. Anesthetists perceptions and prescribing patterns. *Br Med J* 1996;313:787.
4. Anand KJ, Hickey PR. Pain and its effects in the human neonate and fetus. *N Engl J Med* 1987;317:1321.
5. Anand KJ, Hansen DD, Hickey PR. Hormonal-metabolic stress responses in neonates undergoing cardiac surgery. *Anesthesiology* 1990;73:661.
6. Anand KJ, Hickey PR. Stress responses and clinical outcome in neonatal cardiac surgery: randomized trial of high dose sufentanil vs. halothane-morphine anesthesia. *N Engl J Med* 1992;326:1.
7. Purcell-Jones G, Dormon F, Sumner E. Paediatric anaesthetists' perceptions of neonatal and infant pain. *Pain* 1988;33:181.
8. Reynolds ML, Fitzgerald M, Benowitz LI. GAP-43 expression in developing cutaneous and muscle nerves in the rat hind limb. *Neuroscience* 1991;41:201.
9. Fitzgerald M. A physiological study of the prenatal development of cutaneous sensory inputs to dorsal horn cells in the rat. *J Physiol (Lond)* 1991;432:473.
10. Rizvi TA, Wadhwa S, Mehra RD, Bijlani V. Ultrastructure of marginal zone during prenatal development of human spinal cord. *Exp Brain Res* 1986;64:483.
11. Pignatelli D, Ribeiro da Silva A, Coimbra A. Postnatal maturation of primary afferent terminations in the substantia gelatinosa of the rat spinal cord. An electron microscopic study. *Brain Res* 1989;491:33.
12. Anand KJ, Carr DB. The neuroanatomy, neurophysiology, and neurochemistry of pain, stress, and analgesia in newborns and children. *Pediatr Clin North Am* 1989;36:795.
13. Kinney HC, Ottoson CK, White WF. Three-dimensional distribution of 3H-naloxone binding to opiate receptors in the human fetal and infant brainstem. *J Comp Neurol* 1990;291:55.
14. Klimach VJ, Cooke RW. Maturation of the neonatal somatosensory evoked response in preterm infants. *Dev Med Child Neurol* 1988;30:208.
15. Anand KJ. Hormonal and metabolic functions of neonates and infants undergoing surgery. *Curr Opin Cardiol* 1986;1:681.
16. Anand KJ, Sippell WG, Schofield NM, Aynsley Green A. Does halothane anaesthesia decrease the metabolic and endocrine stress responses of newborn infants undergoing operation? *Br Med J* 1988;296:668.

17. Anand KJ, Sippell WG, Aynsley Green A. Randomised trial of fentanyl anaesthesia in preterm babies undergoing surgery: effects on the stress response. *Lancet* 1987;1:62.
18. Anand KJS, Hickey PR. Halothane-morphine compared with high-dose sufentanil for anesthesia and postoperative analgesia in neonatal cardiac surgery. *N Engl J Med* 1992;326:1.
19. Newburger JW, Jonas RA, Wernovsky G, et al. A comparison of the perioperative neurological effects of hypothermic circulatory arrest versus low-flow cardiopulmonary bypass in infant heart surgery. *N Engl J Med* 1993;329:1119.
20. Wessel, DL. Hemodynamic responses to perioperative pain and stress in infants. *Crit Care Med* 1993;21[S]:361.
21. Pokela ML. Pain relief can reduce hypoxemia in distressed neonates during routine treatment procedures. *Pediatrics* 1994;93:379.
22. Richards T. Can a fetus feel pain? *Br Med J* 1985;291:1220.
23. Lippmann M, Nelson RJ, Emmanouilides GC, et al. Ligation of patent ductus arteriosus in premature infants. *Br J Anaesth* 1976;48:365.
24. Shearer MH. Surgery on the paralyzed, unanesthetized newborn. *Birth* 1986;13:79.
25. Robinson S, Gregory GA. Fentanyl-air-oxygen anesthesia for ligation of patent ductus arteriosus in preterm infants. *Anesth Analg* 1981;60:331.
26. Yaster M. Analgesia and anesthesia in neonates. *J Pediatr* 1987;111:394.
27. Friesen RH, Lichtor JL. Cardiovascular effects of inhalation induction with isoflurane in infants. *Anesth Analg* 1983;62:411.
28. Friesen RH, Lichtor JL. Cardiovascular depression during halothane anesthesia in infants: study of three induction techniques. *Anesth Analg* 1982;61:42.
29. Gregory GA. The baroresponses of preterm infants during halothane anaesthesia. *Can Anaesth Soc J* 1982;29:105.
30. Eisele JH, Smith NT. Cardiovascular effects of 40 percent nitrous oxide in man. *Anesth Analg* 1972;51:956.
31. Lunn JK, Stanley TH, Eisele J, et al. High dose fentanyl anesthesia for coronary artery surgery: plasma fentanyl concentrations and influence of nitrous oxide on cardiovascular responses. *Anesth Analg* 1979;58:390.
32. Hickey PR, Hansen DD, Strafford M, et al. Pulmonary and systemic hemodynamic effects of nitrous oxide in infants with normal and elevated pulmonary vascular resistance. *Anesthesiology* 1986;65:374.
33. Shingu K, Eger EI II, Johnson BH, et al. Effect of oxygen concentration, hyperthermia, and choice of vendor on anesthetic-induced hepatic injury in rats. *Anesth Analg* 1983;62:146.
34. Summary of the National Halothane Study. Possible association between halothane anesthesia and postoperative hepatic necrosis. *JAMA* 1966;197:775.
35. Hubbard AK, Roth TP, Gandolfi AJ, et al. Halothane hepatitis patients generate an antibody response toward a covalently bound metabolite of halothane. *Anesthesiology* 1988;68:791.
36. Mazze RI, Calverley RK, Smith NT. Inorganic fluoride nephrotoxicity: prolonged enflurane and halothane anesthesia in volunteers. *Anesthesiology* 1977;46:265.
37. Conzen PH, Nuscheler M, Peter K, et al. Renal function and serum fluoride concentrations in patients with stable renal insufficiency after anesthesia with sevoflurane or enflurane. *Anesth Analg* 1995;81:569.
38. Young CJ, Apfelbaum JL. Inhalational anesthetics: desflurane and sevoflurane. *J Clin Anesth* 1995;7:564.
39. Harkin CP, Pagel PS, Warltier DC, et al. Direct negative inotropic and lusitropic effects of sevoflurane. *Anesthesiology* 1994;81:156.
40. Holaday DA, Smith FR. Clinical characteristics and biotransformation of sevoflurane in healthy human volunteers. *Anesthesiology* 1981;54:100.
41. Kharasch ED, Karol MD, Lanni C, Sawchuk W. Clinical sevoflurane metabolism and disposition: I. Sevoflurane and metabolite pharmacokinetics. *Anesthesiology* 1995;82:1369.
42. Eger EI. Desflurane animal and human pharmacology: aspects of kinetics, safety, and MAC. *Anesth Analg* 1992;75[S]:3.
43. Walker TJ, Chakrabarti MK, Lockwood GG. Uptake of desflurane during anesthesia. *Anaesthesia* 1996;51:33.
44. Bovill JG, Sebel PS, Stanley TH. Opioid analgesics in anesthesia: with special reference to their use in cardiovascular anesthesia. *Anesthesiology* 1984;61:731.
45. Koren G, Goresky G, Crean P, et al. Pediatric fentanyl dosing based on pharmacokinetics during cardiac surgery. *Anesth Analg* 1984;63:577.

46. Hickey PR, Hansen DD, Wessel DL, et al. Pulmonary and systemic hemodynamic responses to fentanyl in infants. *Anesth Analg* 1985;64:483.
47. Hickey PR, Hansen DD, Wessel DL, et al. Blunting of stress responses in the pulmonary circulation of infants by fentanyl. *Anesth Analg* 1985;64:1137.
48. Bjertnaes L, Hauge A, Kriz M. Hypoxia-induced pulmonary vasoconstriction: effects of fentanyl following different routes of administration. *Acta Anaesthesiol Scand* 1980;24:53.
49. Rosow CE, Moss J, Philbin DM, Savarese JJ. Histamine release during morphine and fentanyl anesthesia. *Anesthesiology* 1982;56:93.
50. Lynn AM, Slattery JT. Morphine pharmacokinetics in early infancy. *Anesthesiology* 1987;66:136.
51. Gauntlett IS, Fisher DM, Hertzka RE, et al. Pharmacokinetics of fentanyl in neonatal humans and lambs: effects of age. *Anesthesiology* 1988;69:683.
52. Greeley WJ, de Bruijn NP, Davis DP. Sufentanil pharmacokinetics in pediatric cardiovascular patients. *Anesth Analg* 1987;66:1067.
53. Greeley WJ, de Bruijn NP. Changes in sufentanil pharmacokinetics within the neonatal period. *Anesth Analg* 1988;67:86.
54. Killian A, Davis PJ, Stiller RL, et al. Influence of gestational age on pharmacokinetics of alfentanil in neonates. *Dev Pharmacol Ther* 1991;15:82.
55. Mather LE. Clinical pharmacokinetics of fentanyl and its newer derivatives. *Clin Pharmacokinet* 1983;8:422.
56. Dalens B. Regional anesthesia in children. *Anesth Analg* 1989;68:654.
57. Liu LM, Cote CJ, Goudsouzian NG, et al. Life-threatening apnea in infants recovering from anesthesia. *Anesthesiology* 1983;59:506.
58. Welborn LG, Rice LJ, Hannallah RS, et al. Postoperative apnea in former preterm infants: prospective comparison of spinal and general anesthesia. *Anesthesiology* 1990;72:838.
59. Abajian JC, Mellish RW, Browne AF, et al. Spinal anesthesia for surgery in the high-risk infant. *Anesth Analg* 1984;63:359.
60. Mahe V, Ecoffey C. Spinal anesthesia with isobaric bupivacaine in infants. *Anesthesiology* 1988;68:601.
61. Cook B, Doyle E. The use of additives to local anesthetic solutions for caudal epidural blockade. *Paediatr Anaesth* 1996;6:353.
62. Spear RM, Deshpande JK, Maxwell LG. Caudal anesthesia in the awake, high-risk infant. *Anesthesiology* 1988;69:407.
63. Shandling B, Steward DJ. Regional analgesia for postoperative pain in pediatric outpatient surgery. *J Pediatr Surg* 1980;15:477.
64. Broadman LM, Hannallah RS, Belman AB, et al. Post-circumcision analgesia—a prospective evaluation of subcutaneous ring block of the penis. *Anesthesiology* 1987;67:399.
65. Hannallah RS, Broadman LM, Belman AB, et al. Comparison of caudal and ilioinguinal/iliohypogastric nerve blocks for control of post-orchiopexy pain in pediatric ambulatory surgery. *Anesthesiology* 1987;66:832.
66. Reiz S, Nath S. Cardiotoxicity of local anaesthetic agents. *Br J Anaesth* 1986;58:736.
67. Scott DB. Toxic effects of local anaesthetic agents on the central nervous system. *Br J Anaesth* 1986;58:732.
68. Benini F, Johnston C, Faucher D, Aranda J. Topical anesthesia during circumcision in newborn infants. *JAMA* 1993;270:850.
69. McIntosh N, van Veen L, Bramayer H. Alleviation of the pain of heelstick in preterm infants. *Arch Dis Child* 1994;70:F177.
70. Taddio A, Shennan AT, Koren G, et al. Safety of lidocaine-prilocaine cream in the treatment of preterm neonates. *J Pediatr* 1995;127:1002.
71. Gourrier E, Karoubi A, el Hanache S, Merbouche S, Mouchnino G, Leraillez J. Safety of EMLA cream in a department of neonatology. *Pain* 1996;68:431.
72. Lawson RA, Smart NG, Gudgeon AC, Morton NS. Evaluation of an amethocaine gel preparation for percutaneous analgesia before venous cannulation in children. *Br J Anaesth* 1995;75:282.
73. Parke TJ, Stevens JE, Verghese C, et al. Metabolic acidosis and fatal myocardial failure after propofol infusion in children: five case reports. *Br Med J* 1992;305:613.
74. Truog R, Anand KJ. Management of pain in the postoperative neonate. *Clin Perinatol* 1989;16:61.
75. Callahan P, Pasternak GW. Opiates, opioid peptides, and their receptors. *J Cardiothorac Anesth* 1987;569:576.
76. Davis PJ, Ross A, Stiller R, et al. Pharmacokinetics of remifentanil in anesthetized children 2–12 years of age. *Anesth Analg* 1995;80:S93.
77. Barker N, Hadgraft J, Rutter N. Skin permeability in the newborn. *J Invest Dermatol* 1987;88:409.

78. Hess GD, Zagon IS. Endogenous opioid systems and neural development: ultrastructural studies in the cerebellar cortex of infant and weanling rats. *Brain Res Bull* 1988;20:473.

79. Bardo MT, Hughes RA. Single-dose tolerance to morphine-induced analgesic and hypoactive effects in infant rats. *Dev Psychobiol* 1981;14:415.

80. Roy S, Loh HH. Effects of opioids on the immune system. *Neurochem Res* 1996;21:1375.

81. Evans JM, Hogg MIJ, Rosen M. Reversal of narcotic depression in the neonate by naloxone. *Br Med J* 1976;2:1098.

82. Way WL, Costley EC, Way EL. Respiratory sensitivity of the newborn infant to meperidine and morphine. *Clin Pharmacol Ther* 1965;6:454.

83. Hertzka RE, Gauntlett IS, Fisher DM, Spellman MJ. Fentanyl-induced ventilatory depression: effects of age. *Anesthesiology* 1989;70:213.

84. Olkkola KT, Maunuksela E-L, Korpela R, Rosenberg PH. Kinetics and dynamics of postoperative intravenous morphine in children. *Clin Pharmacol Ther* 1991;44:128.

85. Chay PC, Duffy BJ, Walker JS. Pharmacokinetic-pharmacodynamic relationships of morphine in neonates. *Clin Pharmacol Ther* 1992;51:334.

86. Hartley R, Green M, Levene MI, et al. Development of morphine glucuronidation in premature neonates. *Biol Neonate* 1994;66:1.

87. Colpaert FC, Niemegeers CJ, Janssen PA, Maroli AN. The effects of prior fentanyl administration and of pain on fentanyl analgesia: tolerance to and enhancement of narcotic analgesia. *J Pharmacol Exp Ther* 1980;213:418.

88. Hasday JD, Weintraub M. Propoxyphene in children with iatrogenic morphine dependence. *Am J Dis Child* 1983;137:745.

89. Miser AW, Chayt KJ, Sandlund JT, et al. Narcotic withdrawal syndrome in young adults after the therapeutic use of opiates. *Am J Dis Child* 1986;140:603.

90. Arnold JH, Truog RD, Orav EJ, et al. Tolerance and dependence in neonates sedated with fentanyl during extracorporeal membrane oxygenation. *Anesthesiology* 1990;73:1136.

91. Tobias JD, Schleien CL, Haun SE. Methadone as treatment for iatrogenic narcotic dependency in pediatric intensive care unit patients. *Crit Care Med* 1990;18:1292.

92. Arnold JH, Truog RD, Scavone JM, Fenton T. Changes in the pharmacodynamic response to fentanyl in neonates during continuous infusion. *J Pediatr* 1991;119:639.

93. Yasuda I, Hirano T, Yusa T, Satoh M. Tracheal constriction by morphine and by fentanyl in man. *Anesthesiology* 1978;49:117.

94. Soleymani Y, Weiss NS, Sinnott EC, Goldzier S II. Management of life-threatening asthma in children. A preliminary study of the use of morphine in respiratory failure. *Am J Dis Child* 1972;123:533.

95. Eschenbacher WL, Bethel RA, Boushey HA, Sheppard D. Morphine sulfate inhibits bronchoconstriction in subjects with mild asthma whose responses are inhibited by atropine. *Am Rev Respir Dis* 1984;130:363.

96. Rogers DF, Barnes PJ. Opioid inhibition of neurally mediated mucus secretion in human bronchi. *Lancet* 1989;1:930.

97. Comstock MK, Carter JG, Moyers JR, Stevens WC. Rigidity and hypercarbia associated with high dose fentanyl induction of anesthesia [Letter]. *Anesth Analg* 1981;60:362.

98. Kentor ML, Schwalb AJ, Lieberman RW. Rapid high-dose fentanyl induction for CABG. *Anesthesiology* 1980;53:S95.

99. Scamman FL. Fentanyl-O$_2$-N$_2$O rigidity and pulmonary compliance. *Anesth Analg* 1983;62:332.

100. Hill AB, Nahrwold ML, de Rosayro AM, et al. Prevention of rigidity during fentanyl–oxygen induction of anesthesia. *Anesthesiology* 1981;55:452.

101. Bailey PL, Wilbrink J, Zwanikken P, et al. Anesthetic induction with fentanyl. *Anesth Analg* 1985;64:48.

102. Freye E, Hartung E, Buhl R. Lung compliance in man is impaired by the rapid injection of alfentanil. *Anaesthetist* 1986;35:543.

103. Schlesinger AE, Null DM. Enlarged common hepatic duct secondary to morphine in a neonate. *Pediatr Radiol* 1988;18:235.

104. Peterson RG. Consequences associated with nonnarcotic analgesics in the fetus and newborn. *Fed Proc* 1985;44:2309.

105. Levy G, Khanna NN, Soda DM, et al. Pharmacokinetics of acetaminophen in the human neonate: formation of acetaminophen glucuronide and sulfate in relation to plasma bilirubin concentration and D-glucaric acid excretion. *Pediatrics* 1975;55:818.

106. Miller RP, Roberts RJ, Fischer LJ. Acetaminophen elimination kinetics in neonates, children, and adults. *Clin Pharm* 1976;19:284.

107. Collins E. Maternal and fetal effects of acetaminophen and salicylates in pregnancy. *Obstet Gynecol* 1981;58[Suppl]:57.

108. Beattie JO, Chen CP, MacDonald TH. Neonatal distalgesic poisoning. *Lancet* 1981;2:49.

109. Roberts I, Robinson MJ, Mughal MZ, et al. Paracetamol metabolites in the neonate following maternal overdose. *Br J Clin Pharm* 1984;18:201.

110. Stiehm ER. Nonsteroidal anti-inflammatory drugs in pediatric patients. *Am J Dis Child* 1988;142:1281.

111. Brogden RN. Nonsteroidal anti-inflammatory analgesics other than salicylates. *Drugs* 1986;4:27.

112. Butcher H, Moser T, Duc G, et al. Sucrose reduces pain reaction to heel lancing in preterm infants: a placebo-controlled randomized and masked study. *Pediatr Res* 1995;38:332.

113. Haouari N, Wood C, Griffiths G, Levene MI. The analgesic effect of sucrose in full term infants: a randomized controlled trial. *Br Med J* 1995;310:1498.

114. Blass EM, Shah A. Pain-reducing properties of sucrose in human newborns. *Chem Senses* 1995;20:29.

115. Shide DJ, Blass EM. Opioid like effects of intraoral infusions of corn oil and polycose on stress reactions in 10-day-old rats. *Behav Neurosci* 1989;103:1168.

116. Chasnoff IJ, Hatcher R, Burns WJ. Early growth patterns of methadone-addicted infants. *Am J Dis Child* 1980;134:1049.

117. Blass EM. Milk-induced hypoalgesia in human newborns. *Pediatrics* 1997;99:825.

118. Corff K, Seideman R, Venkataraman P, et al. Facilitated tucking: a nonpharmacological comfort measure for pain in preterm neonates. *J Obstet Gynecol Neonatal Nurs* 1995;24:143.

119. Stevens B. Management of painful procedures in the newborn. *Cure Opin Pediatr* 1996;8:102.

120. Norton SJ. Aftereffects of morphine and fentanyl analgesia: a retrospective study. *Neonatal Network* 1988;7:25.

121. Desai N, Taylor Davies A, Barnett DB. The effects of diazepam and oxprenolol on short term memory in individuals of high and low state anxiety. *Br J Clin Pharmacol* 1983;15:197.

122. Niv D, Davidovich S, Geller E, Urca G. Analgesic and hyperalgesic effects of midazolam: dependence on route of administration. *Anesth Analg* 1988;67:1169.

123. Rattan AK, McDonald JS, Tejwani GA. Differential effects of intrathecal midazolam on morphine-induced antinociception in the rat: role of spinal opioid receptors. *Anesth Analg* 1991;73:124.

124. Reves JG, Fragen RJ, Vinik HR, Greenblatt DJ. Midazolam: pharmacology and uses. *Anesthesiology* 1985;62:310.

125. Morselli PL, Principi N, Tognoni G. Diazepam elimination in premature and full term infants, and children. *J Perinatol* 1973;1:133.

126. Tekur U, Gupta A, Tayal G, Agrawal KK. Blood concentrations of diazepam and its metabolites in children and neonates with tetanus. *J Pediatr* 1983;102:145.

127. Jorch G, Rabe H, Rickers E, et al. Cerebral blood flow velocity assessed by Doppler technique after intravenous application of diazepam in very low birth weight infants. *Dev Pharmacol Ther* 1989;14:102.

128. Hegarty JE, Dundee JW. Sequelae after the intravenous injection of three benzodiazepines—diazepam, lorazepam, and flunitrazepam. *Br Med J* 1977;2:1384.

129. Laine GA, Hossain SM, Solis RT, Adams SC. Polyethylene glycol nephrotoxicity secondary to prolonged high-dose intravenous lorazepam. *Ann Pharmacother* 1995;29:1110.

130. Lee DS, Wong HA, Knoppert DC. Myoclonus associated with lorazepam therapy in very-low-birth-weight infants. *Biol Neonate* 1994;66:311.

131. Silvasi DL, Rosen DA, Rosen KR. Continuous intravenous midazolam infusion for sedation in the pediatric intensive care unit. *Anesth Analg* 1988;67:286.

132. Jacqz-Aigrain E, Wood C, Robieux I. Pharmacokinetics of midazolam in critically ill neonates. *Eur J Clin Pharmacol* 1990;39:191.

133. Byatt CM, Lewis LD, Dawling S, Cochrane GM. Accumulation of midazolam after repeated dosage in patients receiving mechanical ventilation in an intensive care unit. *Br Med J* 1984;289:799.

134. Boisse NR, Quaglietta N, Samoriski GM, Guarino JJ. Tolerance and physical dependence to a short-acting benzodiazepine, midazolam. *J Pharmacol Exp Ther* 1990;252:1125.

135. McLellan I, Douglas E. Midazolam withdrawal syndrome. *Anaesthesia* 1991;46:420.

136. Bergman I, Steeves M, Burckart G, Thompson A. Reversible neurologic abnormalities associated with prolonged intravenous midazolam and fentanyl administration. *J Pediatr* 1991;119:644.

137. Burtin P, Daoud P, Jacqz-Aigrain E, et al. Hypotension with midazolam and fentanyl in the newborn. *Lancet* 1991;337:1545.

138. Kissin I, Mason JO, Bradley EL Jr. Morphine and fentanyl interactions with thiopental in relation to movement response to noxious stimulation. *Anesth Analg* 1986;65:1149.

139. Grasela TH, Donn SM. Neonatal population pharmacokinetics of phenobarbital derived from routine clinical data. *Dev Pharmacol Ther* 1985;8:374.

140. Kuban KCK, Leviton A, Krishnamoorthy KS. Neonatal intracranial hemorrhage and phenobarbital. *Pediatrics* 1986;77:443.

141. Ninan A, O'Donnell M, Hamilton K, et al. Physiologic changes induced by endotracheal instillation and suctioning in critically ill preterm infants with and without sedation. *Am J Perinatol* 1986;3:94.

142. Gilman JT, Gal P, Duchowny MS, et al. Rapid sequential phenobarbital treatment of neonatal seizures. *Pediatrics* 1989;83:674.

143. Franck LS. A national survey of the assessment and treatment of pain and agitation in the neonatal intensive care unit. *J Obstet Gynecol Neonatal Nurs* 1987;16:387.

144. Lees MH, Olsen GD, McGilliard KL, et al. Chloral hydrate and the carbon dioxide chemoreceptor response: a study of puppies and infants. *Pediatrics* 1982;70:447.

145. Rumm PD, Takao RT, Fox DJ, Atkinson SW. Efficacy of sedation of children with chloral hydrate. *South Med J* 1990;83:1040.

146. Laptook AR, Rosenfeld CR. Chloral hydrate toxicity in a preterm infant. *Pediatr Pharmacol* 1984;4:161.

147. Lambert GH, Muraskas J, Anderson CL, Myers TF. Direct hyperbilirubinemia associated with chloral hydrate administration in the newborn. *Pediatrics* 1990;86:277.

148. Turner DJ, Morgan SE, Landau LI, LeSouef PN. Methodological aspects of flow-volume studies in infants. *Pediatr Pulmonol* 1990;8:289.

149. Gonzalez JL, Lambert GH, Muraskas J, Anderson CL. Hypertriglyceridemia in infants with bronchopulmonary dysplasia [Letter]. *J Pediatr* 1989;115:506.

150. Farber B, Abramow A. Acute laryngeal edema due to chloral hydrate. *Isr J Med Sci* 1985;21:858.

151. Hirsch IA, Zauder HL. Chloral hydrate: a potential cause of arrhythmias. *Anesth Analg* 1986;65:691.

152. Salmon AG, Kizer KW, Smith MT, et al. Potential carcinogenicity of chloral hydrate—a review. *Clin Tox* 1995;33:115.

153. Reich DL, Silvay G. Ketamine: an update on the first twenty-five years of clinical experience. *Can J Anaesth* 1989;36:186.

154. Tashiro C, Matsui Y, Nakano S, et al. Respiratory outcome in extremely premature infants following ketamine anaesthesia. *Can J Anaesth* 1991;38:287.

155. Chatterjee SC, Syed A. Ketamine and infants [Letter]. *Anaesthesia* 1983;38:1007.

156. Hodgkinson R, Marx GF, Kim SS, Miclat NM. Neonatal neurobehavioral tests following vaginal delivery under ketamine, thiopental, and extradural anesthesia. *Anesth Analg* 1977;56:548.

157. Grant IS, Nimmo WS, McNicol LR, Clements JA. Ketamine disposition in children and adults. *Br J Anaesth* 1983;55:1107.

158. Cook DR. Newborn anaesthesia: pharmacological considerations. *Can Anaesth Soc J* 1986;33:S38.

159. Winters WD, Hance AJ, Cadd GG, et al. Ketamine- and morphine-induced analgesia and catalepsy. I. Tolerance, cross-tolerance, potentiation, residual morphine levels and naloxone action in the rat. *J Pharmacol Exp Ther* 1988;244:51.

160. Finck AD, Samaniego E, Ngai SH. Morphine tolerance decreases the analgesic effects of ketamine in mice. *Anesthesiology* 1988;68:397.

161. Thomson AM, West DC, Lodge D. An N-methylaspartate receptor-mediated synapse in rat cerebral cortex: a site of action of ketamine. *Nature* 1985;313:479.

162. Lundy PM, Lockwood PA, Thompson G, Frew R. Differential effects of ketamine isomers on neuronal and extraneuronal catecholamine uptake mechanisms. *Anesthesiology* 1986;64:359.

163. Friesen RH, Henry DB. Cardiovascular changes in preterm neonates receiving isoflurane, halothane, fentanyl, and ketamine. *Anesthesiology* 1986;64:238.

164. Hickey PR, Hansen DD, Cramolini GM, et al. Pulmonary and systemic hemodynamic responses to ketamine in infants with normal and elevated pulmonary vascular resistance. *Anesthesiology* 1985;62:287.

165. American Academy of Pediatrics, Committee on Fetus and Newborn, Committee on Drugs, Section on Anesthesiology, Section on Surgery. Neonatal anesthesia. *Pediatrics* 1987;80:446.

166. American Society of Anesthesiologists. Neonatal anesthesia. *ASA Newsletter* 1987;51:12.

PART SEVEN

Beyond the Nursery

CHAPTER 58

Medical Care after Discharge

Judy C. Bernbaum

Once the high-risk infant is discharged from the hospital, his or her many special care needs do not cease. Although they still require well-child care, many of these infants have needs that are far from routine. Special attention must be given to their growth and nutrition, immunizations, vision and hearing, and sequelae of illnesses experienced during the neonatal period. Premature infants have a higher likelihood for long-term sequelae and continuing medical problems than term infants do, but many of the issues discussed specifically about prematurity apply to term infants as well.

EXPECTATIONS OF GROWTH

Growth patterns are a valuable indicator of an infant's well-being. Aberrant growth may reflect the presence of chronic illness, feeding difficulties, inadequate nutrition, or social–emotional difficulties. Preterm infants are at particular risk for growth disorders. Many infants with chronic illness, while at an age when rapid growth is expected, have high caloric requirements but are unable to meet them because they have impaired feeding abilities. It is crucial to monitor nutritional intake closely and to interpret growth rates with a complete understanding of the infant's past history, current problems, and expectations for growth.

Many factors affect the growth of a preterm infant, including gestational age, birth weight, severity of neonatal illness, caloric intake, current illnesses, environmental factors in the home, and heredity. Caloric requirements for a healthy preterm infant generally exceed those of a term, normal-birth-weight infant, especially during rapid catch-up growth (1). Chronic illnesses that increase caloric expenditure add to an infant's daily requirements.

J. C. Bernbaum: Department of Pediatrics, University of Pennsylvania School of Medicine; and Neonatal Follow-Up Program, The Children's Hospital of Philadelphia, Philadelphia, Pennsylvania

Malabsorption after necrotizing enterocolitis (NEC) or chronic emesis from gastroesophageal reflux (GER) may impair growth through increased losses. In contrast, decreased intake may be caused by fatigue, hypoxemia, oral motor dysfunction, or reflux esophagitis. Finally, infants with intrauterine growth retardation caused by congenital infections, chromosomal abnormalities, or other syndromes may never achieve normal growth.

Patterns of Growth

When the growth of a low-birth-weight (LBW) infant is evaluated, the gestational age should be considered. Growth parameters should be plotted on growth curves that have been developed using low-birth-weight preterm infants exclusively (2). Measurements should be plotted according to the infant's adjusted age until approximately 2.5 years of age, when the age difference becomes insignificant. Various patterns of growth emerge from different groups of patients.

Healthy, LBW, appropriate-for-gestational-age (AGA) infants generally experience catch-up growth during the first 2 years of life, with maximal growth rates between 36 and 40 weeks of gestational age. Little catch-up growth occurs after 3 years of age. Head circumference usually is the first parameter to demonstrate catch-up growth and often plots at a higher percentile than do weight and length. Increases in weight are followed within several weeks by increases in length. Rapid catch-up head growth must be distinguished from pathologic growth associated with hydrocephalus. An imaging study may be indicated if the infant's history or symptoms suggest hydrocephalus. Insufficient brain growth, a head circumference falling more than two standard deviations below the mean, indicates that the infant is at risk for significant developmental disability.

Growth velocities for weight and height vary considerably. Some preterm infants show growth on curves between the 75th and 97th percentiles by 3 months adjusted age, whereas others remain on low curves well beyond the child's first year. It is helpful to evaluate an infant's weight gain in comparison to gains in length. Low weight for length or a decline in all growth parameters suggests inadequate nutrition. Weight percentiles significantly greater than length percentiles indicate obesity. Obesity may occur in a preterm infant whose parents overfeed their previously underweight baby. It is common to see an infant who was formerly failing to thrive rather abruptly become obese when the medical problems resolve but the diet remains high in calories.

Growth of the small-for-gestational-age (SGA) infant is influenced strongly by the cause of the intrauterine growth retardation. Overall, LBW–SGA infants demonstrate less catch-up growth than LBW–AGA infants, but if they do, acceleration starts by 8 to 12 months of adjusted age. Approximately 50% of LBW–SGA infants are below average in weight at 3 years of age, whereas only 15% of LBW–AGA infants remain below average weight at the same age (3). Symmetric SGA infants with birth head circumference similar in percentile to birth weight are less likely to demonstrate catch-up growth than are those asymmetric SGA infants whose birth head circumference was at a significantly higher percentile than their weight. As with AGA infants, head circumference is normally the first parameter to demonstrate catch-up, followed by weight and then by length.

Because of the wide range of growth that is considered normal during the first several years of life, it is best to analyze trends in growth rather than make assumptions based on single measurements. When abnormalities are noted in growth trends, investigation of the infant's nutritional status during hospitalization, the results of cranial sonography studies, and the status of continuing illnesses should be undertaken to identify a possible cause.

Nutritional Requirements

Traditionally, although somewhat controversial, the goal for preterm infants is to achieve a growth rate approximating that expected had they not been born prematurely (1). Because weight gain is suboptimal during acute illness, all efforts should be made to promote catch-up growth once the medical condition is stable. The nutritional needs of the preterm infant during the first few months of life exceed those of a term neonate and may continue for the entire first year of life even if there are no exceptional medical or feeding problems. Appropriate choices for many preterm infants include breast milk and routine infant formulas, but because many preterm infants continue to have increased caloric requirements, breast milk and routine formulas often need to be supplemented with either carbohydrates or fats. Formulas can be concentrated somewhat to increase their caloric density, allowing the infant to consume more calories per unit volume. There are now commercially available formulas tailored to address the unique protein and caloric needs of the growing preterm infant for the first year of life (4). Most infants do not tolerate feedings with caloric densities greater than 30 kcal/oz. Infants given feedings concentrated beyond 24 kcal/oz should be monitored for symptoms of intolerance such as vomiting and diarrhea and for hyperosmolar dehydration secondary to insufficient free water intake. Whole cow's milk is poorly tolerated and should be avoided. When caloric additives or concentrated formulas are used, care should be taken to maintain an appropriate caloric distribution of nutrients with a ratio among carbohydrates–fats–protein of approximately 40–50–10.

Caloric requirements for adequate growth vary. Healthy preterm infants generally require 110 to 130 kcal/kg per day, but some infants with chronic disease may require up to 150 to 180 kcal/kg per day. Caloric intake should be increased as tolerated until weight gain is satisfactory. Caloric requirements needed for catch-up growth can be calculated for infants older than 40 weeks corrected gestational age by using the following formula (5):

$$\text{kcal/kg required} = 120 \text{ kcal/kg} \times [(\text{ideal weight for actual height})/(\text{actual weight})]$$

Often infants with ongoing illness or those just recovering from their long hospitalization will be unable to consume the volume of formula or breast milk needed to provide them with the calories they need for catch-up or even maintenance of their ideal growth rate. It is not uncommon to suggest offering up to one-half of their daily calculated needs by continuous feedings (by tube) through the night and allowing them to feed orally during the day. Taking that approach often decreases the pressure to get in a large volume per oral feeding and allows the infant to increase volumes as tolerated during the day, after which nighttime volumes can begin to be decreased.

FEEDING PROBLEMS

Although unusual in term infants, feeding disorders are relatively common in preterm infants. Most feeding problems occur in the neonatal period, but many infants demonstrate recurrent or chronic problems with sucking and swallowing (6). Unrecognized, these problems may lead to significantly impaired nutritional intake and negatively affect the parent–infant relationship. Infants at risk for development of feeding problems include those with oral feedings delayed during the neonatal period and those with immature oral motor skills related to prematurity. In addition, those with transient neurologic immaturity or more permanent neurologic deficits are at highest risk. Additional risk factors for development of feeding dysfunction include chronic lung disease, tracheostomy, gastroesophageal reflux, and repeated exposure to noxious, albeit life-sustaining, equipment secured around the area of the nose and mouth including suction catheters, endotracheal tubes, naso- or orogastric tubes, and oxygen cannulas.

Oral reflexes that allow normal feeding and protect the airway from aspiration may be hypoactive or hyperactive in preterm infants. Abnormal reflexes such as an abnormal tongue thrust or hyperactive gag can further complicate successful and pleasurable feeding. A hyperactive gag is particularly troublesome because the infant may manifest oral hypersensitivity and be unable to tolerate the nipple or spoon on the tongue and resist any oral stimulation. Other causes of hypersensitivity or tactile defensiveness include the noxious stimuli mentioned above.

The evaluation of a possible feeding disorder includes a detailed history of feeding behaviors and nutritional intake, a physical examination with assessment of oral motor reflexes, and observation of a feeding. If an infant with chronic lung disease desaturates during feeding, increasing the supplemental oxygen during feeding can improve feeding behavior (7). Evaluation of the type of nipple and the size of its hole may show that the hole is too small, causing fatigue, or too large, making it difficult to control the flow. Indications for radiologic evaluation include suspected aspiration during feeding or an anatomic abnormality such as a tracheoesophageal fistula.

All of these conditions are amenable to therapy if identified early. Treatment of underlying medical problems often helps ameliorate the feeding problems. A pediatric speech pathologist or occupational therapist trained in feeding techniques can assess an infant and develop an appropriate feeding program once a problem has been defined.

Feeding an infant is normally a relaxing, nurturing act that plays a role in parent–infant bonding. In the presence of a feeding disorder, feedings may become a major source of stress, frustration, and anxiety for the infant, parents, and physicians.

IMMUNIZATIONS

Most preterm infants should receive the same immunizations as the term infant and on similar schedules (8). Measles, mumps, rubella, *Haemophilus influenzae* type B, and hepatitis B vaccines should be given at the same chronologic age as recommended for full-term infants.

Diphtheria, Tetanus, Pertussis

The American Academy of Pediatrics (AAP) recommends that full doses of DTaP vaccine be administered to prematurely born infants at the appropriate postnatal (i.e., chronologic) age. A large percentage of preterm infants demonstrate inadequate protection if given a reduced dosage of DTaP vaccine at the routine intervals. Fewer side effects occur in preterm infants who receive full-

dose vaccine than in their full-term counterparts, and the use of acellular pertussis vaccine should obviate any concerns in this regard. The same contraindications to immunizing full-term infants against pertussis apply to preterm infants. Most important, infants with bronchopulmonary dysplasia (BPD) are at highest risk for serious sequelae if they contract pertussis. Therefore, the pertussis component of this vaccine should not be withheld because of their chronic disease. Similarly, the pertussis component should be given to any child with cerebral palsy or other muscle tone abnormalities as long as there is no underlying seizure disorder.

Polio

The AAP Committee on Immunization Practices recommends that full-dose oral (OPV) or inactivated, enhanced potency polio vaccine (IPV) or oral (OPV) be administered at the appropriate chronologic age. If using OPV, it should be used only after discharge from the hospital because of the potential hazards that excretion of a live virus after vaccination may have on other patients. A full course of inactivated polio vaccine, enhanced potency, can be used in any infant but should always be considered for use in the child who either remains hospitalized beyond 2 months of age, is immunocompromised, or lives with an immunodeficient person.

Influenza

Infants with chronic pulmonary disease (e.g., BPD) or cardiac disease with pulmonary vascular congestion are at high risk for the development of serious illness if infected with an influenza virus (8,9). Infants with influenza have presented with symptoms of sepsis, apnea, and lower airways disease. To protect vulnerable infants, immunization with influenza vaccine is indicated for household contacts, including siblings, primary caretakers, and home care nurses as well as hospital personnel. For infants older than 6 months of age, two doses of split virus vaccine should be given 1 month apart between October and December, followed by an annual dose if necessary. Older siblings under 9 years of age also require two doses initially; however, adults and older siblings with natural immunity or who have received previous immunizations need only one yearly dose.

Respiratory Syncytial Virus

Preterm infants, especially those with underlying chronic lung disease, are particularly at high risk for serious sequelae after becoming infected with respiratory syncytial virus (RSV) during the late fall and winter months. Many will require rehospitalization and reintubation for respiratory failure and are often left with worsening lung disease requiring increased support with supplemental oxygen, bronchodilators, or and/or diuretics.

Attempts at developing a vaccine to protect against RSV have been unsuccessful; however, an anti-RSV clonal antibody (Synagis®) has been approved for use in high-risk infants. Monthly intramuscular infusions are necessary to provide passive protection throughout the RSV season. Synagis® is expensive; thus, its use should be limited to those infants most at risk. According to the guidelines set forth by the American Academy of Pediatrics (8), those who should be considered to receive monthly injections include the following:

Children under 24 months with BPD who require
    Supplemental oxygen
    Have required oxygen within 6 months of RSV season
    Are currently requiring mechanical ventilation
    Are being treated with bronchodilators or diuretics
Premature infants without BPD may benefit if gestational age is:
    Between 29 and 32 weeks until they are 6 months of age
    ≤28 weeks until they are 12 months of age.

Additional criteria placing these children at risk for serious sequelae include parental smoking, older siblings (especially if in day care or school), and living in crowded conditions.

Hepatitis B

For infants with birth weights below 2,000 g born to hepatitis B surface antigen–negative women, it is advised to delay the initiation of hepatitis B vaccine until just before initial hospital discharge, provided the infant weighs more than 2,000 g or until 2 months of age when other immunizations are given.

SPECIALIZED CARE

In addition to routine well-child care, the preterm infant may require specialized follow-up for the monitoring, detection, and management of sequelae from neonatal problems. The remainder of this chapter is devoted to a discussion of these special needs.

Retinopathy of Prematurity

Retinopathy of prematurity (ROP; see Chap. 52) is a disorder that interrupts the normal vascularization of the developing retina. Although it has been reported in term infants, ROP is mainly a disease associated with prematurity. The incidence and severity of ROP increase with decreasing gestational age. Most cases of ROP resolve spontaneously, but even with complete resolution, scarring of the retina may occur. Generally, the more severe the disease, the longer it takes for resolution. An infant who has had ROP, however, is at a ten times greater risk for visual sequelae than one who has not (10).

According to recommendations in the *AAP Guidelines for Perinatal Care* (1), all infants delivered at less than 35 weeks of gestation or under 1,800 g who received oxygen therapy, and all infants younger than 28 weeks of gestational age or weighing less than 1,500 g, regardless of oxygen exposure, should have an ophthalmologic examination for ROP. The initial examination should not take place before 4 to 6 weeks in the younger infants because a vitreous haze may interfere with visualization of the retina, and the yield for identifying ROP is low. If only one examination is possible, it should be at 7 to 9 weeks of age to catch the peak period of occurrence. A schedule of follow-up visits is based on the retinal findings. All infants with immature fundi or any stage of ROP require close monitoring until the eyes have matured or the ROP has completely resolved. Thereafter, follow-up to assess for refractive errors should be at 1 year of age and before kindergarten, or earlier for clinical signs. Infants with resolving ROP need careful follow-up because some revert to severe active disease.

Sequelae of ROP depend largely on the extent of retinal scarring. As much as 80% of stage 3 ROP resolves spontaneously without significant scarring, but, even in infants with fully regressed ROP, there may be subtle retinal changes resulting in refractive errors, strabismus, or amblyopia. In addition, an infant left with moderate scarring can experience retinal tears, late retinal detachment, nystagmus, glaucoma, cataracts, vitreous hemorrhage or membranes, and severe scarring that can lead to blindness (11).

Services for visually impaired children are available on county and state levels. Early identification of a child with visual handicaps to such programs is essential to provide the child and family with the services and resources they need.

Hearing Problems

The incidence of sensorineural hearing loss in preterm infants is generally reported to be between 1% and 3% (12). Several factors place these infants at particular risk for hearing loss, including hypoxia, hyperbilirubinemia, infections, unstable blood pressure, environmental noise, and ototoxic drugs. According to the Joint Committee on Infant Hearing, infants with any of the criteria listed should receive auditory screening, preferably by brainstem auditory evoked response, before 3 months of age.

The factors that identify neonates (i.e., infants from birth to 28 days of age) who are at risk for sensorineural hearing impairment include the following:

- Family history of congenital or delayed onset of sensorineural impairment in childhood.
- Congenital infection known or suspected to be associated with sensorineural hearing impairment (e.g., toxoplasmosis, syphilis, rubella, cytomegalovirus, herpes).

- Craniofacial anomalies (e.g., morphologic abnormalities of the pinna and ear canal, absent philtrum).
- Birth weight < 1,500 g (3.3 lb).
- Hyperbilirubinemia at a level exceeding indication for exchange transfusion.
- Ototoxic medications, including but not limited to the aminoglycosides (e.g., gentamicin, tobramycin, kanamycin, streptomycin), used for more than 5 days, and loop diuretics used in combination with aminoglycosides.
- Bacterial meningitis.
- Severe depression at birth, which may include infants with Apgar scores of 0 to 3 at 5 minutes after birth, those who fail to initiate spontaneous respiration by 10 minutes after birth, or those with hypotonia persisting to 2 hours of age.
- Prolonged mechanical ventilation for longer than 10 days (e.g., persistent pulmonary hypertension).
- Stigmata or other findings associated with a syndrome known to include sensorineural hearing loss (e.g., Waardenburg syndrome, Usher syndrome).

Passing an initial hearing screening does not preclude the possibility of a later, acquired hearing loss. Absent or abnormal responses to auditory stimulation, delays in speech development, poor articulation, or inattentiveness should raise the suspicion of a hearing loss that requires a more thorough evaluation. All infants who fail an initial hearing screen should be referred to an audiologist for further testing and intervention. In general, an infant with a sensorineural hearing loss should have a repeat audiologic evaluation performed every 3 months for 1 year after initial diagnosis, every 6 months during the preschool period, and yearly while in school.

In hearing tests, zero-decibel (dB) represents the level at which response to a sound should occur 50% of the time. If sound is not heard at this level, the decibel level is raised until the sound is audible 50% of the time. Responses above 15 dB are indicative of some degree of hearing loss (Table 58–1).

Children with moderate to profound hearing loss are at high risk for delayed onset of language, problems with articulation, language impairment, and alterations in voice quality. Cognitive delays may be encountered as a result of a loss of auditory input or a language delay.

TABLE 58–1. *Classification of hearing loss*

Hearing Loss (dB)	Description
0–15	Normal
16–25	Borderline–mild
26–40	Mild
41–55	Mild–moderate
56–70	Moderate–severe
71–90	Severe
91 and above	Profound

Behavior problems often are experienced and include inattentiveness, overactive or aggressive behaviors, and immature peer relations.

Hearing aids can be fitted early in infancy to avoid acoustic deprivation. With auditory stimulation being provided, language acquisition may proceed more normally. Along with hearing amplification, language stimulation therapy should be provided.

For those children whose hearing loss cannot be improved by hearing aids, different modes of communication are necessary. These include sign language, alternate methods of gesturing or word spelling, language boards, or computer-assisted communication devices. The latter two methods are particularly useful for a child with cerebral palsy.

Necrotizing Enterocolitis

Survivors of NEC, especially those who required surgical intervention, may have problems after discharge. The most common complications include strictures or adhesions and short bowel syndrome (SBS).

Strictures or adhesions of the small or large intestines may develop within 2 weeks to 2 months after the acute episode of NEC. Symptoms of complete or, more commonly, partial intestinal obstruction include vomiting, abdominal distention, constipation or obstipation, or hematochezia. Lower gastrointestinal bleeding may be the only symptom of stricture formation without any associated symptoms of obstruction evident. Intermittent or persistent problems with constipation or obstipation are the more common symptoms that an infant may experience well into the first year of life. Management of significant strictures or adhesions generally involves surgical resection, but those with minimal symptoms may be treated conservatively. Stool softeners are useful in preventing obstipation or constipation.

Short bowel syndrome often results from decreased intestinal length or function. Necrotizing enterocolitis requiring significant bowel resection is one of the most common causes of SBS. The associated symptoms are caused by decreased digestion and absorption of nutrients by a smaller intestinal surface area and a more rapid transit time. Most often, evidence is seen of carbohydrate, protein, fat, vitamin, and mineral malabsorption and an increase in colonic water secretion. Occasionally, SBS is associated with a decreased enterohepatic circulation and gallstones. The resultant problems of SBS constitute a syndrome of chronic diarrhea, malabsorption, growth retardation, and vitamin and mineral deficiencies (13). The prognosis of SBS is reasonably good if more than 25 cm of small bowel without an ileocecal valve, or more than 15 cm of small bowel with an ileocecal valve, remains after surgery. If long-term total parenteral nutrition (TPN) is needed, complications with its use will affect the child's prognosis.

Gastroesophageal Reflux

Gastroesophageal reflux (GER) refers to a condition in which gastric contents reflux into the esophagus and cause subtle or overt signs and symptoms. Although it can develop in full-term infants, GER occurs more commonly in preterm infants. Symptoms develop from incompetence of the lower esophageal sphincter often complicated by poor stomach emptying. Recurrent, nonprojectile emesis is the most common presenting symptom of GER. Usually, infants vomit within 1 to 2 hours after a feeding. An infant may experience several small-volume emeses after a feeding or only one or two large-volume emeses. Some children, however, have no significant emesis but reflux into the esophagus or mouth and then reswallow. Infants also may present with Sandifer syndrome, a condition in which an infant cranes his or her neck in various directions, attempting to stretch the esophagus and reduce the discomfort associated with reflux. An infant with this presentation may be misdiagnosed as having dystonia or a neurologic abnormality.

Failure to thrive or dehydration may result from chronic vomiting. In addition, many of these infants avoid or refuse feedings because they quickly learn to associate feeding with the discomfort of GER and its related esophagitis.

Apnea and bradycardia are complications of GER. Often, GER will worsen if an attempt is made to treat apnea and bradycardia with theophylline because this medication tends to decrease lower esophageal tone, exacerbating symptoms of GER. The physician should consider an evaluation for GER in an infant when his or her apnea or bradycardia worsens, fails to respond to traditional therapy such as caffeine, other causes are ruled out, or if symptoms persist beyond 44 weeks of adjusted age (14).

Aspiration pneumonia is a serious sequela of GER. If acute in onset, symptoms are overt, so GER-related aspiration is more likely to be suspected and diagnosed. If chronic, unrecognized aspiration may cause or exacerbate underlying reactive airway disease. The possibility of GER should be considered in infants with BPD whose disease worsens or fails to improve even in the absence of other signs and symptoms of GER (15).

The evaluation of GER should be individualized. A clinical assessment is sufficient if the history and observation of a feeding present a classic picture of reflux. A technetium-labeled milk scan is helpful to document suspected aspiration and will be able to assess gastric emptying. A pH–thermistor study is useful to document the amount and the degree of acid reflux and any associated apnea or bradycardia. Because of the high false-positive and false-negative rates, a barium swallow and upper gastrointestinal series are of limited value except for documenting underlying anatomic abnormalities (15).

Management of GER depends on the severity of the reflux and its associated symptoms. Simple medical management, successful in 80% of patients, includes thickening formula with cereal, keeping the infant in a semi-upright position after meals, and avoiding any increase in abdominal pressure such as may occur when the infant is placed in an infant seat after meals. Medications may be considered for infants who do not respond to conservative management or who have more severe symptoms. Medications are used to increase lower esophageal sphincter tone and improve gastric emptying. These include metoclopramide (Reglan) and bethanechol (Urecholine). Bethanechol should be used with caution in infants with chronic lung disease because it may induce or worsen bronchospasm. Another agent, cisapride (Propulsid), is a prokinetic agent that increases transit time throughout the entire GI tract. The latter must be used with caution in a child with prolonged QT interval. Antacids or the histamine H$_2$-receptor antagonists cimetidine or ranitidine can be used as adjunct therapy to treat or prevent secondary esophagitis.

Surgical management, most often a Nissen fundoplication, is necessary in about 10% of patients with GER. Surgery should be reserved for infants who either fail to respond to medical management or manifest recurrent pulmonary infections from suspected chronic aspiration pneumonia, chronic esophagitis, unremitting apnea, or failure to thrive despite aggressive medical management.

Intraventricular Hemorrhage

Intraventricular hemorrhage (IVH) is one of the most serious neurologic events encountered by neonates. It occurs in up to 50% of infants born weighing under 1,500 g (16). There is an inverse relationship between gestational age and the incidence of hemorrhage. With the increase in survival of infants at lower gestational ages, an increase in the number of infants with IVH may be expected as well. Follow-up imaging studies should be performed to demonstrate resolution of hemorrhage and to diagnose any anatomic sequelae. The most common complications of IVH include hemorrhagic infarction, posthemorrhagic hydrocephalus, porencephalic cyst, and ventriculomegaly without hydrocephalus (i.e., hydrocephalus *ex vacuo*).

In clinical practice, a common problem when an infant's head circumference crosses percentiles is distinguishing the onset of hydrocephalus from catch-up head growth. Clinically, all premature infants with and without IVH should be monitored with at least monthly measurements of head circumference and documentation of neurodevelopmental progress. If a child has a weekly increase in head circumference greater than 2 cm or demonstrates any symptoms of increased intracranial pressure or a change in neurologic status, hydrocephalus should be considered and evaluated by cranial imaging studies (3). In general, most ventriculomegaly following

IVH occurs within 2 weeks of the initial insult, and radiographic appearance rarely changes after 3 months unless a shunt was required.

Most often, when a ventriculoperitoneal shunt is placed for progressive hydrocephalus, it continues to work without complication according to the principle of volume dependence. If complications occur, they usually are caused by mechanical malfunction or infection. Mechanical malfunctions may result from disconnections at any point along the shunt apparatus or from an obstruction either proximally, along the length of the tubing, or distally within the peritoneum. Signs of malfunction are those associated with an increase in intracranial pressure.

If symptoms suggest malfunction, ultrasonography or a computed tomographic (CT) scan is recommended to evaluate the size of the ventricles compared to baseline, as is a simple roentgenogram of the entire length of shunt tubing to determine its integrity. Pumping the reservoir, if one is present, should be performed only by a physician familiar with the procedure. The information obtained can help determine the location of a blockage but could be misinterpreted by those unfamiliar with the technique. An obstructed or malfunctioning shunt dictates immediate neurosurgical evaluation.

Symptoms of an infected shunt include signs of increased intraventricular pressure associated with an obstruction plus fever and irritability. Shunt infections result in ventriculitis more often than meningitis. Infection may represent colonization of the apparatus only. Diagnosis is made by performing a needle aspiration of cerebrospinal fluid (CSF) from the reservoir using aseptic technique and obtaining a Gram stain and culture. Treatment usually includes appropriate intravenous antibiotics. Removing or externalizing the shunt tubing may also be required. If it is still felt to be necessary, the shunt tubing can be replaced once the CSF remains sterile for at least 72 hours (17).

If a shunt functions properly, follow-up usually is based on the individual neurosurgeon's recommendations. A routine imaging study for baseline usually is obtained when the infant is medically stable before hospital discharge. The clinician following the infant as an outpatient should use the same imaging technique so that a comparison can be made with the baseline study for any change suggestive of an obstruction. If the brain appears normal, and no symptoms of obstruction or infection develop, a follow-up scan may be avoided.

Periventricular Leukomalacia

Periventricular leukomalacia (PVL) is caused by ischemic infarction of the white matter adjacent to the lateral ventricles. A weakening in the integrity of the white matter in this area occurs, followed by either repair or the development of cysts. The reported incidence of PVL in infants with birth weights under 1,500 g varies from 2%

to 22% (18–20). Infants at risk for PVL are those whose perinatal course was complicated by severe hypoxia, ischemia, or both. Infants of early gestational age are particularly susceptible to the development of PVL because of their poorly developed cerebral vascular system, especially after sepsis, seizures, meningitis, IVH, cardiorespiratory (CR) arrest, or life-threatening apnea.

In the weeks that follow a major insult leading to PVL, phagocytosis of the necrotic material occurs with development of fluid-filled periventricular cysts. Periventricular leukomalacia and, subsequently, the presence and size of cysts can be determined using cranial ultrasonography, CT, or magnetic resonance imaging scan. Resolution of the cysts is highly variable, and some never completely resolve.

Beyond the neonatal period, screening for the presence of PVL should be considered in any child with cerebral palsy without an apparent cause (21). Because there are no symptoms specific for PVL, it can easily be missed during the neonatal period if routine screening is not performed.

If PVL is associated with the loss of vital areas of neural tissue as with the formation of cysts greater than 3 mm in diameter, the infant so affected is at increased risk for cerebral palsy, developmental delay, and visual or auditory impairments. If PVL is not associated with residual cysts, few if any sequelae develop. When cysts persist, an infant's motor development is most affected. Cerebral palsy, manifested as moderate to severe quadriplegia or diplegia, is reported to develop in 90% to 100% of children with cystic residua after PVL. The intellectual capacities of children with PVL and cyst formation are more variable. Mental retardation is more common in infants with residual cysts but ranges from mild to severe. If the cysts develop in the occipital region, visual impairment may result (21).

All infants with PVL, especially with cysts, should be monitored closely for neurodevelopmental sequelae. Periodic cranial imaging studies, preferably head ultrasonography, will determine stability or resolution of the cysts. Parents of infants with PVL should be counseled on the importance of periodic neurodevelopmental assessments for early detection of any sequelae and intervention when appropriate.

Seizures

Seizures during the newborn period may be subtle or overt and may occur singly or repetitively. Diagnosis usually is made while the infant still is hospitalized. Medical staff often document motor activity or behavioral changes consistent with seizure activity that can then be confirmed by electroencephalography (EEG). Although the normal immature cortex has a relatively high seizure threshold, cortical injury enhances the brain's susceptibility to seizures. Most neonatal seizures are provoked by a significant neurologic insult such as intracranial hemorrhage, hypoxic–ischemic insult (i.e., asphyxia), metabolic disturbances, or central nervous system (CNS) infections (22).

The primary determinant of the outcome of neonatal seizures is correlated closely with the underlying cause. Infants with relatively harmless conditions such as hypocalcemia do well with appropriate treatment of the underlying disturbance. Those with an intracranial hemorrhage or an anoxic insult experience greater morbidity. Infants with seizures associated with asphyxia that were noted at younger than 24 hours of age have a poorer outcome than those with later onset of seizures (22). Similarly, those with more severe seizures (e.g., status epilepticus, frequent seizures) fare worse.

The decision to treat seizures with anticonvulsants usually is made early in the evolution of the infant's evaluation. If a transient metabolic abnormality is identified and corrected, seizure activity should cease, usually without anticonvulsant therapy. Recommendations regarding the duration of long-term anticonvulsant therapy for neonatal seizures vary. In some cases, medications may be discontinued before initial hospital discharge. Most often, however, once seizures are well controlled, a seizure-free interval of at least 3 months passes before anticonvulsants are withdrawn. Before making a decision to withdraw medications, the physician should make certain that the infant has no further clinical seizure activity and no epileptiform discharges on EEG. A neurologist should evaluate any infant with seizures that persist, to help in their long-term management.

APNEA AND BRADYCARDIA

Infants may continue to experience episodes of apnea or bradycardia after initial hospital discharge. The incidence of apnea and bradycardia and its chronicity are inversely proportional to the gestational age of the infant and parallel the severity of problems the infant had during the neonatal period. Although CNS immaturity is the most common cause for apnea in preterm infants, it is important to rule out medical problems that may cause apnea even after hospital discharge. If clinically indicated, the symptomatic infant with apnea should be evaluated for the possibility of underlying anemia (23), sepsis, meningitis or other infections, seizures, upper airway obstruction, GER, hypoxia, or bronchospasm as possible inciting factors.

Once it has been determined that no remediable factors exist, a decision should be made whether to monitor a child at home (24). The need for home CR monitoring with or without medication is determined before hospital discharge based on clinical judgment or results of specialized evaluations. The use of CR monitoring remains somewhat controversial. The 1986 National Institutes of Health Consensus Panel on Apnea, Sudden Infant Death Syndrome (SIDS), and Home Monitoring established medical indications for use of CR monitoring (25):

- One or more severe apparent life-threatening events requiring vigorous stimulation or mouth-to-mouth resuscitation
- Symptomatic premature infants documented by parental report or observation by trained personnel
- Documentation of episodes of apnea or increased periodic breathing by means of a thermistor–pneumocardiogram
- Siblings in families in which two or more infants have died from SIDS
- Infants with diseases such as central hypoventilation

Alarm settings usually are placed at a low heart rate of 80 beats per minute with a maximum respiratory pause of 20 seconds. These may be changed depending on the infant's age or specific clinical circumstances. In most infants, resting heart rate decreases with increasing age.

Often, preterm infants require either theophylline or caffeine in addition to or in lieu of home monitoring (26). Unless dosage is adjusted as the infant gains weight, the blood level of medication gradually will fall, but it rarely is necessary to recheck levels after discharge as long as apneic episodes are infrequent. If episodes continue or increase in frequency despite therapeutic xanthine levels, an evaluation for other possible causes is indicated.

In most cases, the infant should be allowed to outgrow and discontinue the medication when there are no more episodes of apnea for 2 months either clinically or by CR monitor or pneumogram. If, however, the infant is receiving theophylline as a bronchodilator for BPD, it should not be discontinued until symptoms associated with underlying bronchospasm have resolved. Parents should be counseled as to the signs of toxicity of these and all medications.

Most infants initially requiring methylxanthines may be permitted to outgrow the medication while on CR monitors. Many institutions send infants receiving a methylxanthine alone home with no CR monitor and allow them to outgrow this medication. Once they are at least 40 weeks of corrected gestational age, true apnea of prematurity should no longer be significant, although some infants have prolonged need for xanthine therapy in the absence of other causes. As infants mature, their resting heart rate decreases. This may result in an increase in frequency of false alarms if the lower alarm limit is too high. If the infant is otherwise healthy and without accompanying apnea, the monitor company should lower the heart rate alarm by 10 beats per minute to as low as 60 to 70 beats per minute. If bradycardia persists when awake, or heart rate is documented at less than 60 to 70 beats per minute, further evaluation may be warranted.

Once the infant is symptom-free for 2 months, medication most often can be safely stopped. If no subsequent episodes are identified by the monitor, a home pneumocardiogram recording can be performed several days after stopping the medication to determine the need for continued monitoring. If no further episodes are documented, the monitor can be safely discontinued (Fig. 58–1).

Chronic Lung Disease

Bronchopulmonary dysplasia is the most frequently diagnosed chronic lung disease in preterm infants. Usually it develops as a sequel to the acute lung injury experienced during the first few weeks of life. The definition of BPD has changed over the years. A traditional diagnosis covered lung disease resulting from respiratory distress shortly after birth that required more than 28 days of oxygen exposure with representative findings noted on chest roentgenogram (27). Because many infants with a gestational age younger than 30 weeks require oxygen for more than 28 days without developing chronic lung disease, a more restrictive definition of BPD is more appropriate: BPD in a preterm infant less than 30 weeks of ges-

tation is now defined as lung disease for which supplemental oxygen is still required beyond 36 weeks corrected gestational age (7).

Although the diagnosis of BPD is given before initial hospital discharge, some infants with mild or minimal residual lung disease may come to the primary care provider's attention with their first viral respiratory tract infection. Those with more severe disease often will be discharged with medications, nebulizer treatments, and supplemental oxygen. Clinical manifestations are similar to those in the nursery and include tachypnea, tachycardia, retractions, rhonchi, bronchospasm, and poor air movement into the lungs bilaterally. More subtle signs of chronic respiratory distress include poor weight gain, feeding intolerance, decreased activity, and a reduced tolerance of exercise. Medical management of infants with BPD often includes any combination of the following: fluid restriction, diuretic therapy, bronchodilator medications, steroids, and supplemental oxygen, even after initial hospital discharge. These therapies are altered

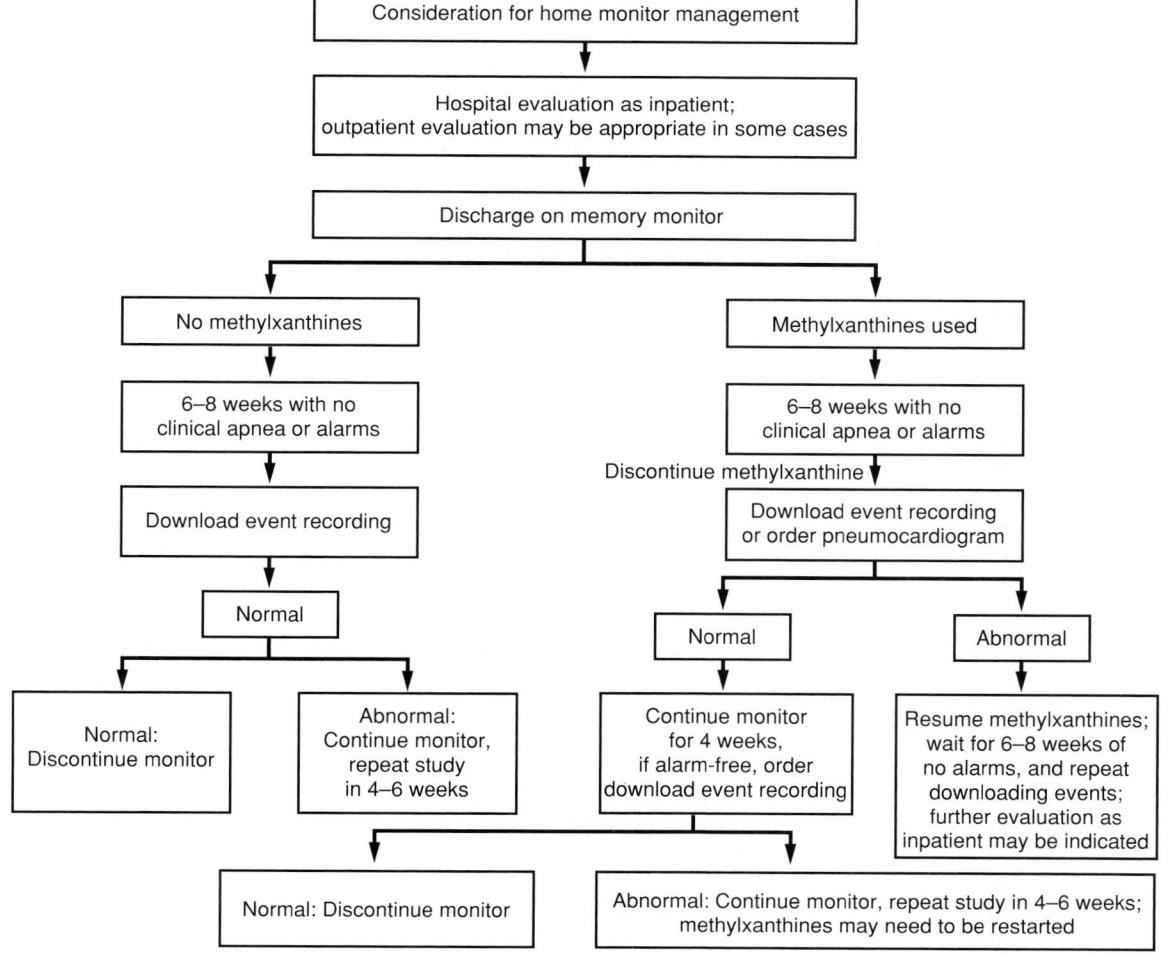

FIG. 58–1. Schema for home monitor management. (From ref. 24.)

depending on the infant's clinical status and eventually withdrawn as the infant matures and improves. How early withdrawal can begin depends on both the severity of lung disease at the time of discharge and its resolution over time. Additionally, BPD may continue to worsen after discharge so that infants who tolerated either no medication or lower doses may begin to require aggressive intervention after discharge. This occurs most often if the infant contracts a serious respiratory tract infection such as RSV pneumonia or less serious but more frequent intercurrent respiratory-related illnesses.

Diuretics

Most often diuretic therapy supplements fluid restriction in an attempt to decrease the fluid retention typical of BPD. Although rarely initiated after discharge, diuretic usage requires monitoring of oral intake, urine output, weight gain, and, less frequently, electrolytes. Normally, one spot-check of serum electrolytes a few weeks after discharge is sufficient and, if normal, need not be rechecked as long as the infant remains medically stable with no significant dietary changes. Infants can outgrow their diuretic doses if there is no worsening of respiratory distress, evidence of peripheral or pulmonary edema, or clinical signs or symptoms of right ventricular strain or failure.

Bronchodilators

Many infants with BPD are discharged on maintenance bronchodilator medications. Unlike diuretics, these medications may need to be modified and continued as part of an aggressive medical regimen. Bronchodilators are used for outpatient therapy of BPD primarily to help maintain the infant's airways maximally dilated and in a bronchospasm-free state. They are used either as maintenance therapy or during intercurrent illnesses. Although the mechanisms of action of the different medications

vary, all cause bronchodilation by relaxation of the smooth muscles of the small airways, allowing better oxygenation and prevention of recurrent bronchospasm. Common bronchodilators used in BPD are described in Appendix H–4 (8).

When xanthines are used as bronchodilators, the dosage needs adjustment for weight gain. This is particularly true if there continues to be a supplemental oxygen requirement or if there is intermittent exacerbation of underlying bronchospasm, tachypnea, increased work of breathing, or a poor activity level. If the infant remains stable or improves, bronchodilators can be weaned by allowing the child to outgrow the medication. Many clinicians have been prescribing inhaled, aerosolized bronchodilators with increasing frequency because of its ease of administration and its direct effect on small airways without much in the way of systemic effect. Bronchodilators can be withdrawn if there has been adequate weight gain, medical stability, good activity level and continued developmental progress, and no exacerbation of underlying bronchospasm. Usually, weaning is not attempted until the infant is off supplemental oxygen. Systemic or inhaled bronchodilators may be needed either as maintenance therapy or intermittently for acute intercurrent illnesses that precipitate bronchospasm (Table 58–2; see Intercurrent Illnesses).

Supplemental Oxygen

The decision to continue an infant on supplemental oxygen relates to the severity of underlying lung disease; however, the need for supplemental oxygen that can be administered via a nasal cannula should not necessarily interfere with hospital discharge. Some of the more common indications for the use of supplemental oxygen include the following: evidence of desaturation while breathing room air, poor oral feeding because of air hunger, apnea, or bradycardia associated with hypoxia, poor growth associated with borderline hypoxia, poor

TABLE 58–2. *Examples of medication changes for infants with chronic lung disease who have increased bronchospasm associated with acute illness*[a]

Maintenance regimen	During acute illness with bronchospasm[b]
No medication	Add theophylline PO, β_2 agonist, or both
Theophylline	Add β_2 agonist (PO or by inhalation)
β_2 Agonist	Add theophylline, a second β_2 agonist (by inhalation), or both
Theophylline and β_2 agonist	Change to β_2 agonist given by nebulizer if not already being given by this route; increase frequency of nebulizer treatments and consider a short course of adrenocortical steroids
β_2 Agonist and cromolyn inhalation	Change to β_2 agonist given by nebulizer if not already being given by this route; increase frequency of nebulizer treatments and consider a short course of adrenocortical steroids

[a]Modified from Bernbaum JC, Hoffman-Williamson M. *Primary care of the preterm infant.* St. Louis: Mosby Year Book, 1991:110.
[b]Consider β_2 agonist treatment nebulizer treatment in office for immediate stabilization before initiating supplemental therapy. Consider increasing inspired oxygen as needed.

exercise tolerance, lethargy, and tachycardia or tachypnea that improves with the use of supplemental oxygen. If possible, it is best to determine the adequacy of oxygenation during sleep, feedings, and periods of activity. Pulse oximetry should indicate saturations of at least 95%. This level of saturation has been shown to result in a significant increase in pulmonary vasodilation, which may preclude the development of pulmonary hypertension and resultant right heart strain (28). Although many centers begin weaning infants with lower oxygen saturations, studies have shown that infants with chronic lung disease who are optimally oxygenated demonstrate better weight gain, attain corrected age-appropriate milestones more readily, and have fewer intercurrent respiratory illnesses than do infants with lower saturations (7).

Before an infant is weaned from supplemental oxygen, its medical stability must be assured, as must adequacy of weight gain, exercise tolerance, and caloric intake. It is preferable to wean a child off oxygen slowly and in a stepwise fashion (9). A period of several weeks to a month should pass during which the infant remains medically stable, gains adequate weight, demonstrates good exercise tolerance, and maintains adequate oxygen saturations before a move to the next step is considered (Table 58–3). Many home care services can perform intermittent oximetry in the home to assist in making management decisions. It is easier to wean an infant off oxygen if he or she is kept maximally bronchodilated with supplemental medications. During an illness, it is common to have to increase the amount of supplemental oxygen or to restart it temporarily if the child has been recently weaned.

To compensate for increased energy expenditures, the infant with BPD often requires a high caloric intake, between 120 and 150 kcal/kg per day (29). Increased caloric needs complicated by poor nutritional intake often result in poor growth. Poor nutritional intake in this population may be caused by hypoxemia, anorexia, tachypnea, exercise intolerance, oral motor dysfunction, or GER. In addition, it often is difficult to maximize caloric intake in the face of fluid restriction and exercise intolerance related to feeding. Caloric intake can be maximized by adding supplements, concentrating formulas, or using isocaloric formulas (Table 58–4).

Even when supplemental calories are provided, there are times when growth is not adequate because the infant either tires easily or refuses any additional increased oral intake. It is then that supplemental nasogastric feedings should be considered, to be given either after each bottle feeding or continuously during the night. Each method has its own advantages and disadvantages and must be considered within the context of individual family and patient needs. It is crucial to offer sucking opportunities routinely to any child who is tube-fed to stimulate the development of the sucking reflex (6). A feeding therapist may need to begin working early with an infant with BPD who demonstrates feeding difficulties to prevent the poor quality suck/swallow coordination frequently encountered in these children.

Intercurrent Illnesses

Bronchospasm with viral or bacterial respiratory illnesses will develop in many infants with BPD (Table 58–5). When the infant is not already on maintenance therapy, bronchodilators can be initiated during acute illnesses (Table 58–2). If the infant is on maintenance bronchodilator therapy, synergistic medications can be added during acute exacerbations and withdrawn as the acute symptoms resolve, returning to maintenance therapy. The modes of action of the common bronchodilators and supplemental medications are detailed in Appendix H-4.

Minimizing the exposure of infants with BPD to environmental irritants and communicable diseases will help decrease the frequency of intercurrent episodes of bronchospasm and allow more time for the lung to heal. Some environmental irritants include cigarette or fireplace smoke, pet fur or dander, kerosene heaters, perfumes, paint, and infectious agents. The less irritation the lung is exposed to, the quicker the recovery process will be.

Rehospitalization is a common occurrence in children with BPD, especially during the first year of life. Parents of these infants should be advised of this possibility before the initial hospital discharge. Every effort should be made to treat intercurrent illnesses and associated bronchospasm on an outpatient basis, but if the infant does not respond readily, hospitalization is appropriate for more aggressive treatment. If, however, the child requires an elective surgical procedure such as a hernia repair, admission should be avoided during epidemics of respiratory-related illnesses.

Managing infants with BPD is one of the greatest clinical challenges for the practicing physician. The many facets of their care require a complete understanding of how their lung disease affects their physical well-being. Fortunately, most of their medical problems occur during

TABLE 58–3. *Weaning a patient from supplemental oxygen*

Time	Amount of oxygen per minute
At hospital discharge	0.5 L at all times
1 month after discharge[a]	0.5 L during feedings and sleep; 0.25 L when awake
2 months after discharge[a]	0.25 L at all times
3 months after discharge[a]	0.25 L during feedings and sleep; room air when awake
4 months after discharge[a]	Room air at all times

[a]Assumes clinical stability, appropriate weight gain, and documentation of adequate oxygen saturation. Intervals may vary depending on such criteria.

From Bernbaum JC, Hoffman-Williamson M. *Primary care of the preterm infant.* St. Louis: Mosby Year Book, 1991:102.

TABLE 58–4. *Selected caloric supplements*

Supplement	Caloric density	Advantages	Disadvantages
Polycose[a]	2 kcal/mL	Well tolerated	Low caloric density
Karo syrup[a]	4 kcal/mL	Well tolerated; readily available; inexpensive	May cause loose stools
Microlipids[b]	4.5 kcal/mL	Well tolerated	Limited availability; high cost
Medium-chain triglyceride oil[b]	7.6 kcal/mL	High caloric density; usually well tolerated	May cause diarrhea; does not mix well with formula
Vegetable oil[b]	9 kcal/mL	Easily available and low cost	Does not mix well with formula
Avocado (pureed; ½ avocado/26 oz formula)[c]			
California variety, brown	Adds 7.4 kcal/oz	High caloric density; well tolerated	Season availability; expensive; more preparation needed
Florida variety, green	Adds 5.7 kcal/oz		
Dry baby cereal	10 kcal/Tbsp	Readily available; inexpensive; may help with gastroesophageal reflux	Low caloric density; may cause constipation
Powdered skim milk	27 kcal/Tbsp	Readily available; mixes well with formula	

[a]Often not used as a supplementation for infants with bronchopulmonary dysplasia because those infants have been shown to have increased work of breathing when receiving a high carbohydrate load, compared to those supplemented with fat.

[b]Use of oil supplements is contraindicated in cases where aspiration is suspected.

[c]May be pureed in large batches and frozen in half-avocado portions.

From Bernbaum JC, Hoffman-Williamson M. *Primary care of the preterm infant.* St. Louis: Mosby Year Book, 1991:105.

TABLE 58–5. *Signs and symptoms suggestive of lower airway disease[a]*

Signs and symptoms	Likely causes	Best treatment
Cough	Underlying bronchospasm	Bronchodilator(s)
	Inflamed and irritated airways	Bronchodilator(s)
	Increased secretions from upper respiratory infection	Consider antihistamine
Tachypnea	Same as for cough	Same as for cough
	Partial obstruction of nasal passages by increased secretions	Suctioning and saline nose drops
	Borderline hypoxia	Consider adding or increasing supplemental oxygen
	Fever	Antipyretics
	Cor pulmonale	Diuretics; digoxin (controversial) Treatment directed at improving hypoxia and bronchospasm
Fever	Underlying inflammatory reaction (unlikely to be bacterial etiology); otitis media can often cause respiratory exacerbation	Antipyretics
Wheezing	Underlying bronchospasm and prolonged expiration	Bronchodilators
Desaturation	Poor oxygen exchange because of tachypnea and wheezing	Consider treatments for cough, tachypnea, fever, and wheezing plus supplemental oxygen
Infiltrate on chest roentgenogram	Pneumonia	Consider antibiotic only if certain of diagnosis
	Partial atelectasis common in chronic lung disease	Chest percussion
	Residual chronic changes that were present since time of initial hospital discharge	Supportive treatment only

[a]From Bernbaum JC, Hoffman-Williamson M. *Primary care of the preterm infant,* St. Louis: Mosby Year Book, 1991:109.

the first year or two of life, and improvement can be expected in each subsequent year.

DISCHARGE PLANNING

Discharge of the intensive care graduate either to home or back to the referral hospital is frequently viewed as one of the most challenging tasks for the hospital staff and can be equally stressful and time-consuming for the family and the child's primary care physician. This transition can be made more smoothly and with less stress if a method is established for an organized discharge planning process. Discharge planning is a method whereby the needs of the patient and family are identified and a plan of care is designed and communicated to the appropriate people who will be providing care to the infant and family in the community. The process is intended to lessen the impact on the family of having to care for an infant without the support of the NICU staff on whom they have come to rely 24 hours a day. The discharge planning team usually consists of the physician caring for the infant, the patient's primary care nurse, social worker, therapist(s), and discharge planner (involved in obtaining home nursing, equipment and therapy needs, and coordinating this with insurance provider). Once a plan is determined, it must be communicated with the community agencies that will be involved in providing care. It is crucial that a primary care physician be identified well in advance of discharge not only so that they can continue to be updated on the child's progress while in the hospital but also that the discharge plan is reviewed to insure a seamless transition to home.

Preparation of the child for discharge begins with a thorough assessment of all aspects of the child's management with the goal of minimizing the disruption in the level of care being provided in the transition from hospital to home. One must first determine the feasibility for discharge. The following criteria should be met:

- Medical stability must be present, with minimal fluctuation in the day-to-day level of care.
- The child must tolerate a nutritional regimen that can be provided in a home setting, resulting in consistent weight gain.
- Level of care needed is practical for home.
- Parents are emotionally and technically competent in providing medical care themselves and appropriate support systems are identified when necessary.
- Funding must be available for equipment, medications, formula, and support services.
- Alternative discharge sites (chronic care facility, foster care, or relatives) should be considered for infants whose families are unable to provide the necessary care.

A thorough chart review close to the time of discharge will assist in the determination of outstanding issues. In particular, a list can be generated of pending medical test results, evaluations that are necessary before or after discharge, the types of equipment, medications, and nutritional supplements that will be needed for home care, and any unmet parental teaching needs. In addition, a list of predischarge tests should be developed at each institution and should be reviewed before each child's discharge. Guidelines may vary from institution to institution, and the tests performed should be individualized based on the patient's history and clinical course. Tests listed in Table 58–6 can function as a guideline for the predischarge examination.

When it is decided that discharge is medically feasible, all aspects of the child's care should be assessed for ways to minimize home care needs. Attempts should be made to withdraw medications that are in the subtherapeutic range based on weight or blood levels. Medications that are no longer needed should be discontinued. Once the medication needs are established, dosage should be adjusted to an amount appropriate for the infant's weight with a buffer for weight gain included. Repeat blood levels at the new dosage should be obtained when appropriate to confirm therapeutic adequacy (e.g., phenobarbital, caffeine, or theophylline). In addition, medication schedules should be streamlined to avoid middle-of-the-night doses and to decrease the frequency of administration when possible. Many pediatric medications are difficult to obtain in some communities. To minimize these difficulties, prescriptions should be written and given to the parents several days before discharge to allow time for the local pharmacy to obtain the medications. To avoid confusion, the concentration and dosage of each medication should be written. Parents should be encouraged to bring the filled prescriptions to the hospital before discharge for a final medication teaching session.

Determination of postdischarge nutritional needs should be based on the following:

- Expected as opposed to actual rate of growth:
- The infant's tolerance of the present feeding regimen just before discharge
- The infant's ability to feed orally or the need for supplemental NG feedings
- The presence of underlying illness that may increase metabolic demands, require fluid restriction, predispose to malabsorption, or require special nutritional formulations

When possible, fluid intake should be liberalized several days before discharge to assess the child's ability to feed orally and tolerate larger volumes of formula. If possible several days before discharge, the child should be switched to a commercially available formula that can be concentrated or have supplements added when additional calories are needed to assess tolerance of the formulation and rate of growth. If a special formula or nutritional supplements are needed, arrangements must be made far enough in advance of discharge to allow for procurement of these items. The infant who is a borderline oral feeder

TABLE 58–6. *Suggested tests in preparation for discharge after complicated neonatal course*

Test	<1,000	<1,500	>1,500 g	Other considerations
Ophthalmologic exam	Yes	Yes	See other	1. <35 Weeks of gestation or birth weight 1,500–1,800 and received supplemental oxygen 2. ECMO
Audiologic evaluation	Yes	Yes	See other	1. Congenital infection 2. Anatomic malformation of head/neck 3. Family history of childhood hearing impairment 4. Hyperbilirubinemia at exchange levels 5. Bacterial meningitis 6. Severe with asphyxia 7. Syndrome with known risk for hearing loss 8. Ototoxic drugs 9. Prolonged ventilation (including for PPHN) 10. ECMO or high frequency
Thermistor pneumogram	See other	See other	See other	Perform if clinically indicated; consider if 1. recent clinical A's and B's 2. receiving methylxanthines 3. reflux
Evaluation of oxygen saturation while in car seat	Yes	Yes	<36 weeks	1. First hospital discharge 2. At risk of apnea or oxygen desaturation
CBC with reticulocyte count	See other	See other	See other	All infants approaching discharge
Drug levels	See other	See other	See other	All infants receiving medications requiring monitoring or blood levels
Rickets screening	Yes	See other	See other	1. Prolonged use of TPN 2. GI malabsorption 3. Cholestatic liver disease
Nephrocalcinosis screening	Yes	See other	See other	Any preterm infant receiving chronic furosemide therapy
ECG	See other	See other	See other	All infants with significant chronic lung disease. Should be obtained baseline and every 6 months.
Chest radiograph	See other	See other	See other	A recent chest radiograph should be obtained for those with chronic lung disease and a copy provided to the family to keep with infant records.

may avoid the need for nasogastric supplementation after discharge through the use of concentrated formula or nutritional supplements.

A careful assessment of appointments that are needed after discharge can avoid fragmentation of care. A thorough chart review can identify any services that have been involved during the hospitalization, and some of these services may have suggested continued involvement immediately before or after discharge. These appointments should be set up before discharge, and attempts made to coordinate as many as possible on the same day without overstressing the child. Remind parents that some insurance policies do not cover many of the outpatient visits or they may need a referral for the visit from the infant's primary care physician. If the child requires oxygen, CPAP, or mechanical ventilation, these needs should be identified so that support can be provided during the outpatient visit.

A comprehensive discharge summary aids in providing continuity of care between the hospital and the primary care provider. The summary should include the following:

- Birth weight, gestational age, Apgar scores, and date of birth
- Significant prenatal and delivery history
- Summary of hospital course, including
    Severity of respiratory illness
    Type and length of ventilatory support
    Significant neurologic insults
    Any surgical procedures
    Complete list of diagnoses
- Results of screening tests
- Immunizations given and dates
- List of problems remaining at the time of discharge
- Discharge medications and dosages and recent blood levels when applicable
- Relevant social history
- Need for therapeutic interventions (physical, occupational, speech/feeding, or educational services)
- Home equipment needs
- Need for specialized nursing interventions

Careful planning and coordination of all aspects of an infant's care form the most challenging part of a successful discharge. When health care providers anticipate postdischarge needs and work in collaboration with the child's family to meet those needs, the quality of care should remain unchanged during the transition from hospital to home.

REFERENCES

1. Screening examination of premature infants for retinopathy of prematurity. Joint Statement. *Pediatrics* 1997;100:273–274.
2. Casey P, Bernbaum JC, Kraemer HC, et al. *Growth curves for preterm infants.* Columbus, OH: Ross Products Division, Abbott Laboratories, 1995.
3. Friedman SA, Bernbaum JC. Growth outcome of critically-ill neonates. In Polin RA, Fox WW, eds. *Fetal and neonatal physiology,* 2nd ed, vol 1. Philadelphia: WB Saunders, 1998:394–400.
4. Van Beck RH, Carnielli VP, Sauer PJ. Nutrition in the neonate. *Curr Opin Pediatr* 1995;7(2):146–151.
5. Maclean WC, LeRomana GL, Masse E, et al. Nutritional management of chronic diarrhea and malnutrition: primary reliance on oral feeding. *J Pediatr* 1980;97:316.
6. Bernbaum JC, Pererra GR, Watkins JB, et al. Non-nutritive sucking during gavage feeding enhances growth and maturation in premature infants. *Pediatrics* 1983;71:41.
7. Shennan AT, Dunn MS, Ohlsson A, et al. Abnormal pulmonary outcomes in premature infants: prediction from oxygen requirement in the neonatal period. *Pediatrics* 1988;82:327.
8. American Academy of Pediatrics, Committee on Infectious Diseases. In Peter G, ed. *1997 Redbook: Report of the Committee on Infectious Diseases,* 25th ed. Elk Grove Village, IL. American Academy of Pediatrics, 1997.
9. Bernbaum J, Hoffman-Williamson M. *Primary care of the preterm infant.* St Louis: Mosby Year Book, 1991.
10. Gobel W, Richard G. Retinopathy of prematurity—diagnosis and management. *Eur J Pediatr* 1993;152(4):286–290.
11. Screening examination of premature infants for retinopathy of prematurity. A joint statement of the American Academy of Pediatrics, American Academy of Ophthalmology and Strabismus, and the American Academy of Ophthalmology. *Pediatrics* 1997;100:273.
12. Early identification of hearing impairment in infants and young children. *NIH Consensus Statement* 1993;11:1–24.
13. Ricketts RR. Surgical treatment of necrotizing enterocolitis and the short bowel syndrome. Clin Perinatol 1994;21(29):365–387.
14. Gorrotxategi I, Eizaguirre A, Saenz de Ugarte MJ, et al. Contintinuous esophageal pH-metering in infants with gastroesophageal reflux and apparent life threatening events. *Neonat Intens Care* 1997;Jan/Feb:29–31.
15. Sondheimer JM. Gastroesophageal reflux: update on pathogenesis and diagnosis. *Pediatr Clin North Am* 1988;35:103.
16. Allen MC, Donohue PK, Dusman AE. The limits of viability–neonatal outcome of infants born at 22–25 weeks gestation. *N Engl J Med* 1993;329(22):1597–1601.
17. Hanekom WA, Yageu R. Cerebrospinal fluid shunt infections. *Adv Pediatr Infect Dis* 1994;11:29–54.
18. Wilkinson I, Bear J, Smith J, et al. Neurological outcome of severe cystic periventricular leukomalacia. *J Pediatr Child Health* 1996;32(5):445–449.
19. Olsen P, Paakko E, Vainlopa L, Pyhtinen J, Jarvelin MR. MRI imaging of periventricular leukomalacia and its clinical correlation in children. *Ann Neurol* 1997;41(6):754–761.
20. Vohr B, Ment LR. Intraventricular hemorrrhage in the preterm infant. *Early Hum Dev* 1996;44(1):1–16.
21. Graziani LJ, Pasto M, Stanley C, et al. Neonatal neurosonographic correlates of cerebral palsy in preterm infants. *Pediatrics* 1986;78:88.
22. Clancy RR. Neonatal seizures. In Stevenson DL, Sunshine P, eds. *Fetal and neonatal brain injury: mechanisms, management and the risk of practice.* Philadelphia: BC Decker, 1989:123.
23. DeMaio JG, Harris MC, Deuber C, et al. Effect of blood transfusion on apnea frequency in growing premature infants. *J Pediatr* 1989;114:1039.
24. Spitzer AR, Gibson E. Considerations for home monitor management. *Clin Perinatol* 1992;19:907.
25. NIH Consensus Development Conference Statement. Infantile apnea and home monitoring. *NIH Consensus Statement* 1986;6(6):1–10.
26. Larsen PB, Brendstrup L, Skov L, Flachs H. Aminophylline versus caffeine citrate for apnea and bradycardia prophylaxis in premature neonates. *Acta Paediatr* 1995;84(4):360–364.
27. Avery ME, Tooley WH, Keller JB, et al. Is chronic lung disease in LBW infants preventable? A survey of 8 centers. *Pediatrics* 1987;79:26.
28. Abman SH, Woolfe RR, Acccurso FJ, et al. Pulmonary vascular response to oxygen in infants with severe BPD. *Pediatrics* 1985;75:80.
29. Yeh TF, McClenan DA, Ajayi OA, et al. Metabolic rate and energy balance in infants with BPD. *J Pediatr* 1989;114:448.

CHAPTER 59

Developmental Outcome

Forrest C. Bennett

More than 250,000 low-birth-weight infants (LBW; ≤2,500 g) are born each year in the United States, constituting approximately 7% of all live births. Of these infants, approximately 50,000 annually are of very low birth weight (VLBW; ≤1,500 g), constituting approximately 1.5% of all births. Because the estimated LBW incidence has remained relatively stable over the past 40 years (Fig. 59–1), contemporary reductions in neonatal mortality are steadily increasing the prevalence of biologically vulnerable infants and children in the overall population (1).

Although much medical, legal, ethical, and economic debate continues to occur over the effects of neonatal intensive care on the long-term developmental status of LBW survivors, most investigators are in agreement that the single clearest outcome of this technically enhanced care has been a dramatic and continuing reduction in neonatal mortality since the early 1960s, particularly for VLBW infants since the mid-1970s (see Fig. 59–1) (2,3). With current standards of practice in the neonatal intensive care unit (NICU), many more LBW, premature infants are surviving to be discharged home after extended hospitalizations than was the case even 5 to 10 years ago. The major factors responsible for this increased survival include the technical ability to provide assisted mechanical ventilation to the smallest of LBW infants; the regionalization of perinatal–neonatal care, with greater numbers of maternal transports to and infants born in tertiary centers; and the widespread use of exogenous surfactant.

Remarkable improvements in the birth-weight–specific mortality rates accounted for 90% of the overall decline in neonatal mortality between 1960 and 1980 (4). During these two decades, decreases in the mortality rates of infants weighing between 1,500 and 2,500 g contributed

more than any other weight group because of both greater proportional decreases and higher absolute declines in mortality; however, there has been steady and statistically significant reduction in mortality rates among VLBW infants throughout the last 15 to 20 years. Mortality for infants with birth weights of 1,001 to 1,500 g has fallen from more than 50% in 1961 to less than 10% today. Moreover, the most substantial improvement of the 1980s over the 1970s in neonatal mortality rates was in the 751 to 1,000 g birth weight group, where today's infants have greater than an 80% chance of surviving if they are admitted to an NICU (5). Finally, in the 1990s, 40% to more than 60% survival for infants between 500 and 750 g birth weight is being accomplished (6–8). The intact survival of a 380-g infant has been described (9).

Although survival continues to increase in all LBW categories, the greatest impact of neonatal intensive care technology clearly has been on the smallest, sickest, and

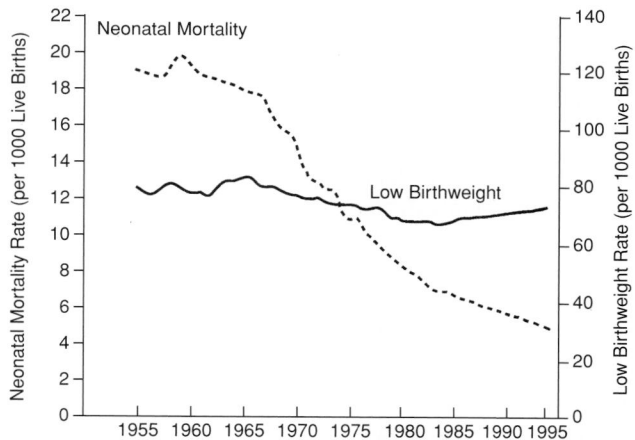

FIG. 59–1. United States annual rates of neonatal mortality and low-birth-weight births from 1955 to 1995. (Adapted from Lee KS, Paneth N, Gartner LM, et al. Neonatal mortality: an analysis of the recent improvement in the United States. *Am J Public Health* 1980;70:15, with permission.)

F. C. Bennett: Department of Pediatrics, University of Washington, Seattle, Washington most medically fragile infants. The success in achieving these improved survival rates for LBW, premature infants raises obvious concerns about the subsequent development of such vulnerable infants. It mandates an organized neurodevelopmental follow-up approach to carefully and continuously monitor the quality of survival of the NICU graduate.

ORGANIZATION OF A HIGH-RISK INFANT FOLLOW-UP PROGRAM

Objectives

There are a number of compelling reasons for conducting longitudinal neurodevelopmental surveillance of survivors of neonatal intensive care. There also are practical problems encountered in providing comprehensive follow-up services. Individual follow-up programs must clearly define their own goals and objectives and then organize their roles and activities accordingly. A community hospital's follow-up efforts likely will be determined by a different set of expectations than those of a university-affiliated tertiary care center. Furthermore, ideal follow-up care in the United States frequently is constrained by limited resources. In general, follow-up programs are designed to meet one or more of the following objectives.

Quality Control

Regular, periodic follow-up of a large proportion of survivors can provide one type of audit of an individual NICU's performance. Because intensive care nurseries differ in such critical management areas as neonatal resuscitation, modes of assisted ventilation, treatment of ventriculomegaly, and use of parenteral nutrition, and also in such neonatal outcomes as mortality and prevalence of medical complications [e.g., bronchopulmonary dysplasia (BPD), intracranial hemorrhage], units may wish to compare their neurodevelopmental morbidity with the contemporary experience of similar nurseries (10). They also may wish to monitor their major disabling morbidities from year to year to detect any significant differences that might accompany further reductions in mortality or the introduction of new intensive care procedures or treatments. It must be recognized that follow-up at 1 or 2 years of age, although providing much useful information about the prevalence of major neurosensory impairment among survivors, is of insufficient duration to identify changes over time in more subtle aspects of brain function such as learning and behavior.

Developmental Services

Neurodevelopmental follow-up can provide important ongoing subspecialty care to at-risk children and families. Follow-up clinic personnel with a multidisciplinary approach will likely have the most experience and expertise in a given community concerning the unique developmental patterns of LBW, premature infants. In general, the follow-up program will complement and serve as secondary or tertiary developmental consultants to the primary health care providers. The program will encourage and facilitate the establishment of a community-based medical home (e.g., private practitioner, public health clinic) for every medically complex survivor. Experience with biologically and environmentally vulnerable indigent populations, however, suggests that actual provision of primary health care, in addition to evaluation and case management services, may be necessary in some situations to prevent attrition and maintain contact with those children and families at greatest long-term risk (11). Although the appropriate approach to this issue of role definition is likely to vary with different populations and access to medical care in different settings, it obviously is of fundamental importance to the organization of follow-up clinics and also to the maintenance of mutual trust relationships with the primary care community.

The specific objectives of follow-up neurodevelopmental assessment activities may be grouped conveniently as follows: to provide cautious reassurance to anxious parents; to ensure early identification and intervention for persistent developmental abnormalities; and to recognize the natural history of transient developmental abnormalities and thereby avoid unnecessary, costly interventions. Maintaining an appropriate balance of diagnostic and reassurance functions is one of the greatest challenges for the contemporary high-risk follow-up program.

Developmental Training

The follow-up clinic provides a marvelous setting for interdisciplinary developmental training. It is a clinical laboratory for the observation of the gradual recovery and normalization over time of most at-risk infants and, in other cases, the gradual evolution of a wide variety of permanent neurodevelopmental dysfunctions. Thus, the at-risk population offers a longitudinal training experience that spans the normal–abnormal development continuum. In many pediatric training programs, the follow-up clinic is the sole opportunity for pediatric residents to observe the outcomes of their own intensive care efforts. It would seem virtually impossible for physicians to be informed adequately about the ethical debates and dilemmas surrounding neonatal intensive care without a first-hand follow-up experience. Likewise, other child development professionals (e.g., psychologists, physical therapists, communication disorders specialists) can use the follow-up clinic profitably as a diverse training base, particularly to broaden the range of normative development for their students. Obviously, these training objectives will apply primarily to university-affiliated tertiary care centers, with their numerous and varied trainee availability.

Outcome Research

The university-affiliated follow-up program should be engaged actively in clinical research that contributes to the understanding of the neurodevelopmental and neurobehavioral outcomes of children who experienced neonatal intensive care. These studies may take the form of either descriptive observational reports or clinical trials of specific perinatal–neonatal interventions. For example, the University of Washington's High Risk Infant follow-up Program has published studies describing the outcome of infants weighing less than 800 g at birth (12–14) as well as studies evaluating the utility of procedures such as electronic fetal monitoring of premature labor and delivery (15) and treatments such as high-frequency mechanical ventilation (16). Although tremendous variability exists in the target populations, methodologies, and general scientific quality of the accumulated high-risk follow-up research, a growing consensus of valid outcome observations gradually has emerged over the last 30 years, and informative summary conclusions can be synthesized. Even though the ideal, population-based, non–risk-controlled, longitudinal to school age study rarely is accomplished for a variety of practical reasons (e.g., cost, subject mobility, investigator discontinuity), individual follow-up investigations, carefully performed albeit with a limited scope, continue to modify and refine overall knowledge and, in some cases, challenge assumptions.

This is not to say that broad, well-funded, collaborative follow-up efforts should not be pursued vigorously on both regional and national, and even international, levels. A recognized need for uniform population descriptions, standardized assessment protocols, common disability definitions, and adequate numbers of pooled subjects still exists. Threats to the interpretability and generalizability of small, local studies include population demographic bias, neonatal treatment differences, attrition of highest-risk (i.e., doubly vulnerable) subjects, and cross-sectional data analysis combining multiple age endpoints. A great deal has been learned about the short- and long-term prognoses of NICU survivors from hundreds of independent follow-up studies, but much more has yet to be clarified by enhanced research approaches (17).

Personnel

The size and complexity of the neurodevelopmental follow-up team depend on the scope of the program and the size of the patient population. For example, a level II to III community hospital with primarily developmental service objectives will likely employ a smaller team, follow for a shorter period of time, and administer fewer standardized measures than a university-affiliated tertiary care center with training and research responsibilities. In either case, certain key tasks must be accomplished. Probably the most critical role in terms of maximizing follow-up compliance and minimizing attrition is that of the follow-up coordinator, usually a program nurse. This person is the liaison between the NICU and the follow-up clinic. The nurse coordinator can identify and meet eligible infants and families before they leave the nursery, participate in the discharge conference and transition plans, and, in some cases, make preliminary contact with the family by means of a home visit before the initial follow-up evaluation. This liaison function is particularly important in those programs that conduct high-risk follow-up at a separate site away from the intensive care nursery and in which none of the follow-up personnel is actively involved in the NICU.

Overall program direction is typically provided by a physician or psychologist. This person ultimately is responsible both for meeting the broad programmatic objectives and also for day-to-day operations. The director of a university-affiliated follow-up program frequently must balance competing service, training, and research obligations while eclectically maintaining sufficient funding sources to ensure long-term program viability. The director certainly should be knowledgeable in terms of current follow-up literature and contemporary models of program structure and function.

Other follow-up roles of the interdisciplinary team include the following:

Medical–neurologic assessment. This may be provided by a neonatologist, developmental pediatrician, or child neurologist. In some programs a pediatric nurse practitioner or the nurse coordinator may provide health, nutritional, and behavioral guidance pertaining especially to such issues as feeding, sleeping, temperament, and discipline.

Developmental–intellectual–academic achievement assessment. This often will be performed by a physical therapist during infancy and by a clinical psychologist or psychometrist thereafter. Some tertiary centers may use a neuropsychologist at school age. In some programs, an early childhood educator or infant developmental specialist participates in early assessments.

Neuromotor assessment. This usually will be done by a physical therapist during the first years of life when gross motor concerns are paramount, and then by an occupational therapist during the preschool and school years when fine motor concerns predominate.

Language–speech assessment. In many follow-up programs, this responsibility is assumed by the psychologist. Some programs have the necessary personnel and funding resources to use a communication disorders specialist on a regular basis.

Family assessment. The increasingly important task of evaluating and monitoring the home parenting environment may be performed by a social worker, a clinical nurse specialist, or both. As the number of dysfunctional families in the NICU setting steadily increases because of such prevalent influences as poverty, single parenthood, and prenatal substance abuse, so does the requirement of follow-up programs increase for qualified psychosocial personnel.

Hearing assessment. The adequate ability to assess hearing at any age by a clinical audiologist is imperative for tertiary follow-up programs. Both electrophysiologic and behavioral audiometric procedures should be available.

Visual assessment. A pediatric ophthalmologist should be readily accessible by consultation to the follow-up program, particularly for extremely low-birth-weight (ELBW; ≤1,000 g birth weight) infants.

Patient Selection

Once again, the goals, objectives, personnel, and resources of an individual follow-up program will combine to determine the proportion and nature of at-risk survivors that can be served. Since it usually is impossible for a program to follow all infants receiving neonatal intensive care, somewhat arbitrary risk criteria generally are established to provide broad follow-up guidelines (18). In light of the variation and imperfection of assigned risk factors in accurately predicting neurodevelopmental outcome, a follow-up program is wise to adopt a flexible, rather than rigid, approach to the issue of eligibility. In general, a follow-up program will target the smallest and sickest NICU graduates to maximize the likely necessity of its services. Different levels of follow-up priority (e.g., high, medium, low) frequently are used to structure the selection and longitudinal monitoring process. University-affiliated follow-up programs conducting specific clinical research will tailor patient selection according to study requirements.

Common risk criteria for follow-up include the following factors:

- VLBW. In smaller programs with limited personnel and resources, the birth weight criterion may, by necessity, be arbitrarily lowered to 1,250, 1,200, or even 1,000 g. This category also generally will incorporate those infants of 32 weeks of gestational age or younger.
- Small for gestational age (SGA). Most programs strive to include infants whose weight or head circumference at birth was more than two standard deviations below the mean for gestational age.
- BPD. Programs will vary on the required duration of mechanical ventilation and oxygen administration.
- Neuroimaging abnormalities. This criterion typically will include such findings as severe intracranial hemorrhage (e.g., large intraventricular hemorrhage, intraparenchymal hemorrhage), severe ventriculomegaly, or extensive cystic periventricular leukomalacia.
- Prolonged seizures or other abnormal neurologic behavior. This would include those infants who continue to demonstrate an atypical neurologic examination at the time of nursery discharge.
- Central nervous system infection. The targeted infection may have occurred during the intrauterine, intrapartum, or neonatal time period.
- Miscellaneous perinatal–neonatal events of potential neurodevelopmental significance. Most programs will prioritize infants who have experienced to a severe degree such complications as asphyxia, hyperbilirubinemia, hypoglycemia, or polycythemia. Specific threshold determinations will vary from program to program. Table 59–1 quantifies the major neurodevelopmental risk associated with many of these follow-up inclusion criteria.

Many states use or are developing some type of comprehensive high-risk tracking or screening system to monitor the growth and development of biologically vulnerable infants (19). In some states (e.g., Iowa, North Carolina, Washington), this broadly based tracking system serves as an initial screen to identify those infants and toddlers who merit complete, tertiary developmental assessment. This coordinated approach to follow-up offers the advantages of tracking many more at-risk infants and families while also increasing the efficiency and appropriate use of the formal follow-up clinic.

Clinic Schedule

The schedule of evaluations conducted by the University of Washington's High Risk Infant Follow-up Program is

TABLE 59–1. *Risk factors for major neurologic and cognitive sequelae in surviving infants requiring neonatal intensive care*

Birth weight (g)	Category	Risk factor (%)
>2,500	All admissions	<5
	Respiratory distress syndrome	5
	Postasphyxia seizure	30–50
	Meningitis	30–50
1,501–2,500	All admissions	10
	Small for gestation age	<10
	Respiratory distress syndrome	<10
	Bronchopulmonary dysplasia	20–30
	Postasphyxia seizure	30–50
	Meningitis	30–50
≤1,500	All admissions	10–30
	Appropriate for gestational age, nonventilated	10–15
	Appropriate for gestational age, ventilated	30–40
	small for gestational age	30–50
	Seizures, decerebrate posture	75–80
≤1,000	All admissions	10–40

Adapted from Fitzhardinge PM. Follow-up studies of the high-risk newborn. In: Avery Gb, ed. *Neonatology: pathophysiology and management of the newborn,* 2nd ed. Philadelphia: JB Lippincott, 1981:353.

outlined in Table 59–2. This plan is illustrated as an example of a follow-up program with combined clinical service, training, and research objectives. Smaller hospital-based programs without training or research requirements often will be able to meet their clinical needs with different formats, shorter duration of follow-up, and fewer standardized assessments. Basic monitoring concepts applicable to all follow-up programs, however, include special attention to neuromotor development the first year, language and cognitive development the second and third years, school readiness skills between 4 and 5 years of age, and academic achievement during the early school years. In addition, attention to family function ideally should be an integral part of each clinic visit. With this developmental sequence of evaluations, timely identification of delays and dysfunctions as well as appropriate referral to community-based intervention services are optimized (20).

A frequent topic of debate concerns the calculation of assessment age for premature infants (21). Whereas most follow-up programs plan their clinic visit schedule and score their evaluation measures on the basis of fully corrected age (i.e., chronologic age minus the number of weeks premature), a number of others continue to use unadjusted chronologic age or even, in a few cases, one-half correction (i.e., chronologic age minus one-half the number of weeks premature). The reluctance to use full gestational age correction stems from a concern over the

potential artificial inflation of developmental test scores and coincident underuse of early intervention services during the first several years of life. Although these are valid clinical concerns to consider when providing parental feedback and making referral decisions, the weight of the evidence in terms of the neuromaturation of premature infants favors the practice of gestational age correction, at least to 3 years of age, when monitoring the growth and development of NICU survivors.

Regardless of the scheduling mode used, all follow-up personnel must appreciate the imprecisions and variabilities of early developmental assessment. Low-birth-weight, premature infants may demonstrate improving developmental performance during the first years of life as they recover from perinatal–neonatal insults and chronic health impairments (e.g., BPD, necrotizing enterocolitis). Conversely, they also may demonstrate additional developmental dysfunction over time as more subtle disabilities become increasingly apparent and testable. In light of these patterns of development, health and developmental professionals who work with premature infants and their families must be aware of the hazards implicit in the high-risk concept. Parents may permanently regard their child as vulnerable, once so labeled, and contribute to a self-fulfilling prophecy. There can be an overzealous tendency in well-intended follow-up programs to presume the presence of abnormality rather than normality, despite the evidence of more optimistic outcome data to the contrary. In fact, most high-risk infants do not develop the conditions for which they are at increased statistical risk, and there frequently is a poor correlation between the severity of the neonatal course and specific neurodevelopmental outcomes for individual premature infants. There is a need for monitoring of this population with a keen awareness of, but not an expectation of, adverse sequelae. Documented developmental dysfunction certainly should not be ignored, but an initial follow-up posture of cautious optimism is appropriate in most cases.

NEURODEVELOPMENTAL OUTCOME OF LOW-BIRTH-WEIGHT PREMATURE INFANTS

Despite contemporary reductions in LBW morbidity compared to disability rates before the introduction of neonatal intensive care, permanent neurodevelopmental problems are seen in many survivors. Such problems include major neurosensory impairments, cognitive and language delays, specific neuromotor deficits, neurobehavioral and socioemotional abnormalities, and school dysfunction (22).

Major Neurosensory Impairments

The major neurosensory impairments associated with prematurity are cerebral palsy, particularly of the

TABLE 59–2. *High-risk infant follow-up clinic schedule*

Corrected age	Test
4 mo	BSID[a]
	MAI
	Physical and Neurologic Examination
8 mo[b]	BSID
	MAI
	Audiologic Evaluation by Visual Reinforcement Audiometry
	Physical and Neurologic Examination
12 mo	BSID
	Physical and Neurologic Examination
24 mo	BSID
	Physical and Neurologic Examination
36 mo	Stanford–Binet Intelligence Scale
	Peabody Picture Vocabulary Test
	Expressive Language Sample
	Physical and Neurologic Examination
4.5 years	Wechsler Preschool and Primary Scale of Intelligence
	Peabody Developmental Motor Scales
	Physical and Neurologic Examination
6 and 8 years	Wechsler Intelligence Scale for Children
	Peabody Individual Achievement Test
	Physical and Neurologic Examination

[a]BSID, Bayley Scales of Infant Development; MAI, Movement Assessment of Infants.
[b]Scheduled selectively for those infants with possible neuromotor abnormalities at 4 months of age.

spastic diplegia type; mental retardation [i.e., intelligence quotient (IQ) more than two standard deviations below the standardized test mean]; sensorineural hearing loss; and visual impairment, primarily the consequences of retinopathy of prematurity (ROP) (23). These major developmental disabilities may occur together in the same child and occasionally are complicated by progressive hydrocephalus or a chronic seizure disorder. They usually are clinically apparent by 2 years of age and vary in severity from mild to profound. Children with one or more of these major impairments generally require special educational programming and individual therapeutic intervention throughout childhood. These conditions occur two to five times more frequently in LBW compared to full-birth-weight (FBW) infants. As a group, their prevalence increases with decreasing birth weight and gestational age; the disability rate in boys consistently exceeds that in girls (24). Table 59–3 provides combined prevalence estimates and ranges by birth weight group for these chronic neurosensory impairments. The actual numbers represent a synthesis from reporting tertiary care centers in the United States, Canada, Australia, and Western Europe.

Such major morbidity statistics may be viewed either positively or negatively, or both. On the one hand, the occurrence of these major sequelae is far less than initially predicted at the beginning of the NICU era, and many more nondisabled than disabled survivors (approximately 8:1) are being added to the population (25). Conversely, epidemiologic investigations appear to document that reductions in LBW major morbidity have not paralleled or kept pace with reductions in LBW mortality and that the major impairment rate has changed little over the past 20 to 25 years. Actual increases in both the incidence and prevalence of major disabilities among the smallest and sickest survivors have been reported by some (26,27). Others, however, have reported a stable major morbidity rate for infants weighing less than 800 g at birth (Table 59–4), a subgroup whose survival has dramatically increased during this time period (12–14). This encouraging observation that the overall incidence of serious neurodevelopmental deficits is remaining stable while survival continues to increase has been repeatedly corroborated even for those ELBW infants who weighed less than 750 g at birth (8,28–30).

TABLE 59–3. *Low-birth-weight infants who survive with one or more major impairments*

Birth weight (g)	Percent with major impairments (range)
1,501–2,500	8 (5–20)
1,001–1,500	15 (5–30)
≤1,000	25 (8–40)

TABLE 59–4. *Prevalence of major impairments in survivors weighing less than 800 g at birth at the University of Washington*

	Major impairment (%)
1986–1990	17/78 (22)
1983–1985	8/38 (21)
1977–1980	3/16 (19)

From LaPine TR, Jackson JC, Bennett FC. Outcome of infants weighing less than 800 grams at birth: 15 years' experience. *Pediatrics* 1995;96:479.

Cerebral Palsy

Cerebral palsy, of varying types and severities, remains the most prevalent major developmental disability encountered in premature infants; the prevalence in VLBW infants varies between 6% and 10%, and approximately 40% of all children with cerebral palsy were born prematurely (i.e., <37 weeks of gestation) (31). Although both spastic (i.e., pyramidal) and athetoid (i.e., extrapyramidal) types of cerebral palsy may be encountered in NICU graduates, the spastic cerebral palsy syndromes (i.e., diplegia, hemiplegia, and quadriplegia) are the neuromuscular disorders most commonly seen in LBW infants. One specific type, spastic diplegia, in which the legs are much more affected than arms, is so strongly associated with prematurity (i.e., at least twothirds of all children with this disorder are born before 37 weeks of gestation) that for over a century it has been referred to as "the disease of immaturity" (31a). Figure 59–2 illustrates the relationship between spastic diplegia and gestational age. Most cases occur in a window of vulnerability in infants born between 28 and 34 weeks of gestation.

Despite the long consistency of the spastic diplegia–prematurity association, the exact etiologic factors involved often have been elusive and difficult to identify precisely prospectively (32). Neither the severity of perinatal–neonatal illness nor the presence or the severity of intracranial

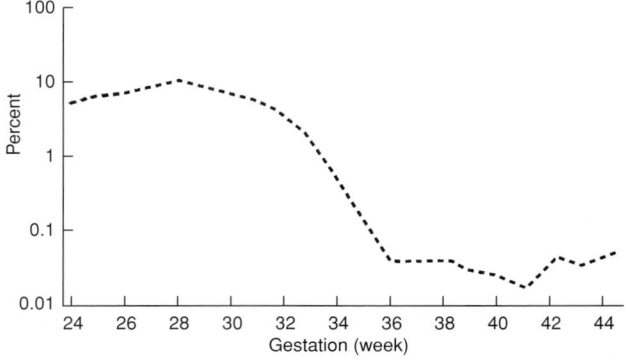

FIG. 59–2. Occurrence of spastic diplegia as related to gestational age.

hemorrhage reliably predicts spastic diplegia. Data derived primarily from studies correlating ultrasonographic, neuropathologic, and clinical information led to the conclusion that spastic diplegia is the clinical expression of periventricular leukomalacia and its variants (33). Periventricular leukomalacia appears to be caused, in large part, by hypoxic–ischemic injury to the periventricular white matter. The demonstration on serial cranial ultrasounds of initial extensive periventricular echodensities followed in days to weeks by large, bilateral cyst formation (i.e., periventricular white matter infarction) is highly predictive (80% to 85%) of permanent cerebral palsy, especially the spastic diplegia type (34,35). Many cases of symmetric cystic periventricular leukomalacia occur in infants with relatively benign clinical courses and are detected only by routine ultrasound screening. Premature infants born to mothers with prolonged rupture of membranes and/or chorioamnionitis seem to be at an increased risk (36). Several investigators have implicated prenatal factors (e.g., intrauterine growth retardation) in the etiology of some cases of spastic diplegia. Hagberg has postulated that the complex interaction of prenatal abnormalities (i.e., "fetal deprivation of supply") with perinatal difficulties in the birth process and the adjustment to the extrauterine environment may constitute a common pathogenetic mechanism of spastic diplegia (37). Accordingly, the etiology of spastic diplegia frequently is multifactorial, and all LBW infants merit close neuromotor monitoring during the first 2 years of life, regardless of the severity of their nursery course.

In contrast, development of the more severe spastic quadriplegia type of cerebral palsy, in which all four extremities are equally affected, often can be predicted better in NICU graduates on the basis of specific perinatal or neonatal events, including asphyxia, marked bilateral intraventricular hemorrhage with ventriculomegaly, prolonged neonatal seizures, and central nervous system infection. Although most premature children with spastic diplegia have average or near-average mental abilities, children with spastic quadriplegia are far more likely also to have serious cognitive impairments. Spastic hemiplegia, in which only one side is affected, with the arm usually more than the leg, often is heralded by the ultrasonographic appearance of a unilateral, periventricular hemorrhagic infarction with subsequent cystic transformation that occurs in association with and presumably as a result of substantial asymmetric intraventricular hemorrhage (33).

Cerebral palsy typically presents over time in a developmental manner. Thus, very early neurologic signs and symptoms may prove to be transient in nature and not indicative of eventual cerebral palsy. Conversely, infants may initially appear asymptomatic with a relatively normal neurologic examination at the time of nursery discharge and even for several months thereafter, particularly in the cases of spastic diplegia and spastic hemiplegia, only to manifest clearly evident cerebral palsy by 1 year of age. Premature infants with evolving cerebral palsy reveal increasing neuromotor abnormalities of muscle tone, movement, posture, and reflex activity, particularly between 6 and 18 months of corrected age, in combination with increasingly delayed motor milestones.

Mental Retardation

Mental retardation, as defined by a standardized intelligence or developmental quotient consistently more than two standard deviations below the test mean for corrected age, often occurs in conjunction with one or more of the other major handicaps, especially cerebral palsy. In fact, severe mental retardation and severe cerebral palsy share associated perinatal–neonatal risk factors. Evidence suggests some increase in the prevalence of severely multihandicapped children after increased VLBW survival (27). Mental retardation occurs in 4% to 5% of VLBW infants followed longitudinally to school age. Isolated mental retardation, without cerebral palsy, is a reported consequence of severe BPD, particularly in cases of greatly prolonged duration of mechanical ventilation and oxygen administration (38,39).

Hearing Impairment

Neonatal intensive care unit graduates are at increased risk for both sensorineural and conductive hearing loss. Although the risk of sensorineural loss sufficient to require hearing aids, special education, and nonvocal communication strategies (60 to 100 dB) usually is estimated to be 2% to 3% for VLBW infants, some investigators have reported prevalence estimates between 5% and 9% coincident with the increased survival of more vulnerable infants (40). Exposure to ototoxic drugs, infections, hypoxia/ischemia, and hyperbilirubinemia are among the interacting and cumulative factors contributing to the risk of sensorineural loss. The duration and extent of hyperbilirubinemia in VLBW infants has been examined carefully. DeVries and colleagues found bilirubin levels in excess of 14 mg/dL to be associated with a high risk of deafness in VLBW infants but not in healthy premature infants with a birth weight greater than 1,500 g (41). Others also have emphasized the potential ototoxicity of hyperbilirubinemia in VLBW infants in combination with hypoxia, acidosis, and prolonged administration of multiple ototoxic medications such as the aminoglycoside antibiotics and furosemide. These investigators conclude that the additive effects of protracted illness plus its associated treatments, independent of specific diagnostic categories, constitute important risk factors for permanent hearing loss in this population (42).

There is ample evidence that infants of all birth weights who sustain severe persistent pulmonary hypertension of the newborn comprise a particularly high-risk subgroup for sensorineural hearing loss, with prevalence estimates ranging from 20% to 40% (43). In some cases, the loss is progressive during the first 3 years of life. The exact mechanism of insult remains unclear in this population of infants who typically experience prolonged hypoxia, severe acute and chronic lung disease, and multiple aggressive interventions. Another concern has been the potential deleterious effect of prolonged incubator noise on hearing function. Abramovich and associates found no evidence for this hypothesis in VLBW infants (44). Many of the risk factors associated with hearing impairment also are associated with cerebral palsy, and these two disabilities often occur together in the same child.

Mild and moderate (25 to 59 dB) sensorineural hearing losses, sufficient to contribute to delayed language development but compatible with oral communication, also occur with increased frequency (6% to 8%) in LBW infants. Previously unrecognized unilateral sensorineural hearing losses, with adverse language and learning consequences, may become apparent in the older child (45). A high prevalence (20% to 30%) of chronic otitis media with middle ear effusion and fluctuating, conductive hearing loss greater than 25 dB is reported in LBW, premature infants (46). Suggested mechanisms for this relationship focus on probable eustachian tube dysfunction initiated by a combination of dolichocephalic head shape, muscular hypotonia, and prolonged nasotracheal intubation.

There have been important advances in the hearing assessment of LBW infants. Two techniques in particular, electrophysiologic auditory brain stem response (ABR) audiometry and behavioral visual reinforcement audiometry, have made early, reliable detection of hearing loss in the NICU graduate clinically feasible. Centers that routinely screen high-risk, LBW infants with ABR before nursery discharge report a false-positive rate of 8% to 10% compared to follow-up testing at 4 months of age (47). Conversely, the unanticipated appearance of severe sensorineural hearing loss in high-risk survivors of neonatal intensive care after having passed an initial ABR screening test in the newborn period has been reported (48). It also must be recognized that ABR tests only the high sound frequencies (i.e., 2,000 Hz and above) and will not detect hearing losses confined to the lower frequencies. Thus, clinicians must remember that determinations of the adequacy of hearing made only with ABR test data before nursery discharge are subject to error. Visual reinforcement audiometry is an operant conditioning technique that reliably can provide auditory thresholds for infants who are functioning at a developmental age of approximately 6 months or older. It has great utility in the high-risk follow-up clinic. A third and newer audiologic procedure, evoked otoacoustic emissions, offers promise to be of use in newborn screening in conjunction with ABR.

Visual Impairment

The major cause of visual loss in LBW infants is retrolental fibroplasia, now included under the rubric of ROP. With controlled oxygen administration, ROP was relatively rare until the last 15 years or so, when significant numbers of extremely premature infants began to survive. The name ROP recognizes that immaturity at birth is the single largest risk factor for this disease. For all practical purposes, this is a disorder of the VLBW infant. Virtually no retinal detachment and little retinal scarring is described in larger premature infants. For the entire VLBW population, current prevalence estimates range from 20% to 25% with early-stage, regressed ROP; 5% to 10% with more advanced-stage, scarred ROP; and 2% to 4% with major visual impairments, including legal blindness, requiring special educational assistance. The distribution of visually impaired infants, however, is skewed heavily toward those weighing 1,000 g or less at birth. In these ELBW infants, regressed ROP occurs in 40% to 50% of survivors, scarred ROP in 10% to 25%, and major visual impairments in 5% to 10%. Figure 59–3 shows the overall prevalence of ROP by birth weight.

Alteration of normal retinal vascular development is the hallmark of ROP. Although a great deal of effort has been invested in clinical and animal studies of ROP, there remains an etiologic maze in which no single factor stands alone (49). It appears that the embryonic retina of the small premature, developing outside the uterus, is vulnerable to many sources of disturbance that can disrupt orderly differentiation and vascularization. In addition to the well-known impact of hyperoxia, it seems that hypoxia, variations in $PaCO_2$, pH, retinal oxygen consumption, light exposure, and other factors that affect retinal perfusion all may play a role. A formula for ROP could be: immaturity (always) + oxygen (often) + other factors (variably) = ROP (50). Simply stated, the smallest

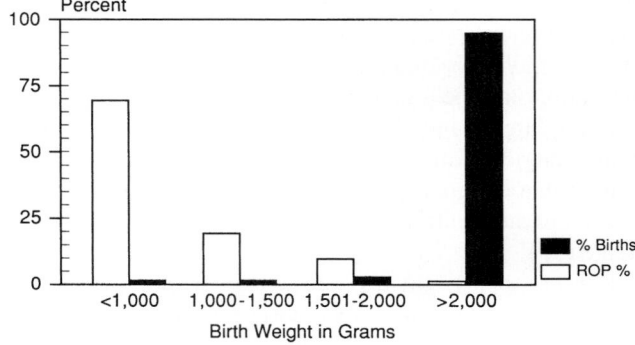

FIG. 59–3. Percentage of retinopathy of prematurity (ROP) by birth weight versus proportion of births by birth weight. (From Glass P, Avery GB, Subramanian KNS, et al. Effect of bright light in the hospital nursery on the incidence of retinopathy of prematurity. *N Engl J Med* 1985;313:401, with permission.)

and sickest newborns have the most complications that potentially can impede retinal function, and they also have the most ROP.

Even regressed ROP is associated with an increased risk for refractive errors, amblyopia, and strabismus. "Myopia of prematurity," even without ROP, has been described to occur in approximately one-third of surviving ELBW infants (51). It is considered to be mostly lenticular in origin and to improve slowly, but not completely, throughout childhood, with slight visual acuity differences still apparent in early adulthood. Strabismus may represent an isolated problem or, in some cases, may be an initial indication of a generalized neuromotor problem such as cerebral palsy. Visual and hearing impairments may coexist, and prematurity is the leading cause of children with both deficits. Monitoring of eye muscle balance and alignment and visual acuity should be part of routine follow-up of the premature infant, particularly during the preschool years. Required interventions may include eye muscle surgery, antisuppression patching, or corrective lenses.

Progressive Hydrocephalus

Depending on the reporting center, between 20% and 40% of VLBW infants have neonatal ultrasonographic evidence of intracranial hemorrhage, frequently including intraventricular hemorrhage with ventriculomegaly (10). Whereas older reports indicated discouragingly high rates of posthemorrhagic hydrocephalus, recent reports are much more hopeful in describing a very low prevalence (2% to 4%) of progressive hydrocephalus requiring ventriculoperitoneal shunting in VLBW infants (52,53). Serial scanning with cranial ultrasonography has revealed that most cases of early ventriculomegaly either spontaneously resolve or arrest. The necessity of medical intervention (e.g., repeated lumbar puncture, diuresis) to prevent the transition from relatively asymptomatic ventriculomegaly to progressive hydrocephalus remains unclear. Surgical ventriculostomy drainage is frequently employed as a temporizing procedure in more advanced cases.

For the infant in whom posthemorrhagic progressive hydrocephalus does develop, it generally becomes clinically evident between 2 and 8 weeks of age; however, appearance during late infancy occasionally has been reported. Vigilance in measurement of the head circumference at each follow-up examination of the infant is important, and obtaining a cranial ultrasound if head growth becomes substantially out of proportion to the other growth parameters may be indicated. Although the initial months of life are the time when progressive hydrocephalus is most likely to develop in premature infants, it also is the period of time when the normal phenomenon of catch-up head growth in these recovering infants becomes most apparent. Thus, increase in head circumference relative to weight and length usually is an anticipated sign rather than a pathologic one, and such awareness should guide clinical investigative decisions. When progressive hydrocephalus does occur, neurodevelopmental outcome is frequently, although not invariably, abnormal, complicated by one or more of the major disabilities (e.g., cerebral palsy, mental retardation, sensory impairments) (54).

Minor Impairments

Although major disabling sequelae are by far the easiest to quantify and report, a large and persuasive body of long-term follow-up studies clearly indicates that a broad spectrum of cognitive, behavioral, and other minor neurodevelopmental and neurobehavioral sequelae are substantially more prevalent in surviving LBW, premature infants. These morbidities become increasingly apparent in a variety of clinical manifestations with increasing age, particularly during the first 6 years of life. These early, often subtle, developmental and behavioral delays and differences are not necessarily outgrown but frequently portend future school dysfunction and may therefore become major impediments to normal academic and social progress. Collectively, these problems often are referred to as the "new morbidity" of prematurity, reflecting their more insidious nature and more intense scrutiny in recent years (23).

Specific types of developmental morbidities described in LBW cohorts include cognitive delays (i.e., lower IQ), speech and language disorders, persistent neuromotor abnormalities, including difficulties with balance and coordination, and perceptual problems. Specific areas of suboptimal behavioral style and performance include neonatal behavior, infant and toddler temperament, emotional maturity, social competence, and selective attention. As with major impairments, the overall prevalence of these minor sequelae increases with decreasing birth weight and gestational age and also is greater in male survivors. Prevalence estimates in VLBW infants vary between 15% and 25%. Accordingly, when the 15% to 20% major disability rate is combined, between 35% and 45% of VLBW survivors demonstrate a residual developmental or behavioral problem that compromises their anticipated function (55). Recent estimates for ELBW infants are in excess of 50% (56). As with major impairments, most of the minor developmental morbidities associated with LBW and prematurity also are related to the severity of perinatal–neonatal illness. That is, LBW infants who experience a prolonged hospital course with many medical complications have an increased likelihood of development of some type of developmental dysfunction. Thus, the smallest and sickest infants, particularly those ELBW new survivors of the 1990s, are the most vulnerable to experience these problems.

In the hundreds of outcome studies across multiple developmental and behavioral domains, a consistent finding is that, regardless of the measures used, groups of premature children are less competent and score less well than groups of full-term children (25). However, this does not mean that individual premature children will invariably be less capable than individual full-term children. Despite the large number of significant group associations in follow-up studies, individual developmental outcome remains very difficult to predict prospectively with accuracy in the NICU, and infants with apparently similar neonatal courses may develop entirely differently.

Cognitive and Perceptual Development

Consistent deficits in performance on intelligence measures repeatedly have been observed and reported in LBW, premature children compared to FBW, full-term children (57,58). Furthermore, these differences in cognitive development become apparent in the first years of life and then persist and increase during the preschool and early school years even when the single most powerful predictor of IQ—socioeconomic status—is adequately controlled. In other words, significant deficits in cognitive and perceptual function occur frequently even in middle to upper-middle social class children born prematurely, particularly compared to their full-term peers. This important and academically relevant group difference exists despite the fact that most LBW children will have measured IQs within the average range (22).

Cognitive developmental differences between premature and full-term infants have been reported in early infancy. Rose investigated the effect of increasing familiarization time on the visual recognition memory of 6- and 12-month-old premature and full-term infants (59). Whereas the older infants showed evidence of recognition memory after less familiarization time than the younger ones, at both ages premature infants required considerably longer familiarization times (i.e., more practice) than did full-term infants. These results suggest that there are persistent differences between premature and full-term infants throughout at least the first year of life in a very fundamental aspect of cognition, namely, visual information processing.

Because manipulative exploration of objects may be important to the infant's perception and conceptualization of objects, Ruff and colleagues studied this developmental function in both premature and full-term 9-month-old infants by means of coded and scored videotapes (60). The videotapes were scored for behaviors such as looking, handling, mouthing, turning the object around, transferring the object from hand to hand, and banging. A high-risk subgroup of premature infants based on neonatal complications manipulated the objects significantly less than either the low-risk prematures or the full-term infants. There was a relationship between manipulative exploration at 9 months and later cognitive functioning at 24 months.

Low-birth-weight cognitive deficits have been described from the earliest days of neonatal intensive care and even before. Using a sample of approximately 600 children born in two Edinburgh, Scotland, hospitals in 1953 to 1955, Drillien demonstrated that IQ scores decline with decreasing birth weight in the first 4 years of life (61). The percentage of children with IQ scores below 80 at 4 years was 29% for those under 4 lb 8 oz, 13% for those between 4 lb 8 oz and 5 lb 8 oz, and 4% for those above 5 lb 8 oz. Wiener and colleagues, reporting on a sample of 417 8- to 10-year-old LBW children who had been tested with the Wechsler Intelligence Scale for Children, found that the verbal IQ, which consists of predominantly cognitive and language items, performance IQ, which consists of predominantly motor–perceptual items, and full-scale IQ, which consists of a combination of the verbal and performance scales, all showed increasing impairment with decreasing birth weight even though all subtest means remained within the average range of intelligence (62). Moreover, approximately twice as large a proportion of LBW children as FBW control children fell into the borderline IQ category (70 to 84), which usually is associated with special educational needs. Visual–motor–perceptual skills, as measured independently by the Bender Gestalt Test, also varied directly with birth weight. Hunt and colleagues reported the following cognitive outcome proportions in a cohort of 108 VLBW children at 8 years of age: 4.6% had a very low IQ (<70), 13.9% had a low IQ (70 to 84), and, for those with an IQ greater than 84, 12.0% had language disability, 12.0% had performance disability, 21.4% had visual–motor disability, and 36.1% were apparently normal (63).

In a Vancouver, British Columbia, study of 501 LBW and 203 FBW children born between 1958 and 1965, the IQ difference between LBW and FBW groups on the Stanford–Binet Intelligence Scale was 9 points at 30 months of age and 15 points at 48 months, even after exclusion of children with major cerebral deficit or IQ scores under 50 or significant visual problems (57). In both the Edinburgh and Vancouver studies, the poor functioning of LBW children is convincingly exacerbated in socioeconomically disadvantaged subgroups. Table 59–5 illustrates this interaction of both biological and environmental risk factors in the determination of measured IQ of the Vancouver study children. At both 2.5 and 4 years of age, FBW, highest-social-class children earned the highest subgroup mean IQ score, whereas LBW, lowest-social-class children earned the lowest. Both FBW and LBW groups demonstrated an IQ score continuum from the highest social class, which had the highest mean IQ, to the lowest social class, which had the lowest mean IQ, with the FBW subgroup always higher than the LBW regardless of social class; at 4 years of age, even FBW, lowest-social-class children scored higher than their LBW, highest-social-class peers.

TABLE 59–5. *Comparison of intelligence quotient means for low-birth-weight children versus normal-birth-weight controls within social class groups*

Hollingshead social class	Statistic	30 Months of age		48 Months of age	
		IQ	Number	IQ	Number
I, II, III	LBW[a] mean±SD	97.0±15.1	48	99.5±13.7	67
	Control mean±SD	108.8±8.2	19	118.3±11.4	26
	Difference±SE	11.8±2.9		18.8±2.8	
	p	<0.001		<0.001	
IV	LBW mean±SD	91.7±10.7	59	94.3±11.3	100
	Control mean±SD	102.9±12.6	43	110.0±16.8	58
	Difference±SE	11.2±2.4		15.7±2.5	
	p	<0.001		<0.001	
V	LBW mean±SD	89.5±13.9	52	90.6±15.8	79
	Control mean±SD	96.0±9.7	32	102.3±12.9	42
	Difference±SE	6.5±2.6		11.7±2.7	
	p	<0.01		<0.001	

[a]LBW, low birth weight; FBW, full birth weight; IQ determined from Stanford–Binet tests.
Adapted from McBurney AK, Eaves LC. Evolution of developmental and psychological test scores. In: Dunn HG, ed. *Sequelae of low birthweight: the Vancouver Study.* Philadelphia: JB Lippincott, 1986:61.

The cognitive performance of ELBW preschool children has been the subject of more recent attention. Halsey and colleagues compared predominantly white, middle-class ELBW 4-year olds to matched full-term children and also to matched LBW children (1,500 to 2,500 g birth weight) and found both comparison groups to be two-and-a-half times more likely to have optimal development (64). Comparison children had mean cognitive scores 15 to 18 points higher than ELBW children. The investigators concluded that weaker performance on all study measures (i.e., language, motor, memory, visual–motor, perceptual) exists before school entry among nondisabled ELBW children compared with their peers. Breslau and colleagues confirmed these cognitive concerns for ELBW survivors in describing a gradient relationship between LBW and IQ at age 6 years (65). They found the largest deficit in full-scale IQ in those children born weighing 1,500 g or less, an intermediate deficit in those born weighing 1,501 through 2,000 g, and the least pronounced deficit in those born weighing 2,001 through 2,500 g.

Language Development

Communication skills involving auditory and visual perception, the learning and conceptualizing of a verbal symbol system (i.e., language), and the actual production of speech are critical to academic learning and social adjustment. Several investigations have focused exclusively on this important area of development in premature infants. Zarin-Ackerman and colleagues noted both receptive and expressive language deficiencies at 2 years of age in a group of children born as at-risk (i.e., predominantly premature) infants compared to others born as healthy, full-term infants (66). They emphasized that

these deficits could not be a function of social class, which is a major factor influencing language development, because this variable was controlled. In Switzerland, Largo and associates compared 114 premature children to 97 healthy, full-term children throughout the first 5 years of life (67). Most stages of language development occurred at slightly later ages among the premature children than among those born at term. Birth weight and gestational age were negatively correlated with language development at all ages. Perinatal–neonatal complications also were significantly negatively correlated with the ages at which the stages of language development were reached, and also with final language performance at 5 years of age. There were no significant differences in socioeconomic status between the premature and full-term groups. The particular demographics of this unique study allowed the authors to conclude that biomedical factors exert a considerable effect on the early language development of premature children and that this effect is greater than previously had been recognized (67).

Several smaller studies have confirmed the existence of linguistic dysfunctions among premature children, particularly those with complicated neonatal courses (68,69). On the basis of a wide variety of measures, inferior performance has been reported consistently in receptive language or comprehension, expressive language parameters such as vocabulary and word finding, and speech qualities such as articulation and fluency.

Motor Development

Numerous studies from several continents repeatedly have documented that the neuromotor development of LBW, premature infants during the first 2 years of life is different, more delayed, and generally more worrisome than that of healthy, full-term infants. Not only are premature developmental scores, using such measures as the Bayley Scales of Infant Development, consistently and significantly below those of full-term infants at 12 months of corrected age but premature motor scores also usually are 10 to 15 points (i.e., practically one standard deviation) below premature mental scores at this age (70).

This phenomenon of transiently abnormal neuromotor signs in the first years of life was described initially by Drillien, in a 1972 report from Scotland, as "transient dystonia of low birth weight infants" (71). Drillien reported that its prevalence during the first one-half of infancy varied inversely with birth weight, involving approximately 35% of infants weighing 1,501 to 2,000 g at birth and 60% to 70% of infants weighing 1,500 g or less at birth, and that its prevalence also varied directly with perinatal–neonatal complications (i.e., more frequent among sick premature infants). Transient dystonia includes such neurologic findings as increased or decreased muscle tone, diminished volitional movement, retention and accentuation of primitive reflex patterns, delayed appearance of normal infantile automatic reactions, and asymmetric neuromotor development. Because these neuromotor signs also are the very signs seen in infants in whom cerebral palsy is developing, it is not surprising that a reliable diagnosis of cerebral palsy is quite difficult in most premature infants throughout early infancy. As described by Amiel-Tison, however, by 8 to 10 months of corrected age, most LBW infants with transient dystonia are gradually and spontaneously normalizing on examination, whereas those relatively few infants in whom permanent cerebral palsy is developing appear increasingly abnormal (72). With the knowledge of this common evolution of neuromotor signs, every VLBW infant can be assigned to one of three diagnostic and prognostic groups at 12 months of age: those who were always neurologically normal throughout infancy (25% to 30%); those who showed transient dystonia with subsequent normalization (65% to 70%); and those with cerebral palsy (5% to 10%).

Coolman and colleagues and others have extended these observations to 24 months of age, albeit most neuromotor changes occur in the first year of life (73). They found that some infants with transient dystonia retained subtle, persistent neuromotor differences that would not be labeled as cerebral palsy but that represented qualitative deviations from the norm. Longitudinal studies indicate that infants who have experienced transient dystonia are far more likely to have language, learning, and behavioral problems (i.e., minimal brain dysfunction) in later childhood than are infants who never demonstrated these abnormalities (74,75). This would indicate that although transient dystonia largely resolves, these neuromotor signs in early infancy may be predictive markers for later manifestations of central nervous system disorganization.

Differences in the motor development of premature infants throughout the preschool years have been reported. Burns and Bullock found premature children at

5 years of age to be significantly different from their full-term peers in terms of tremulous involuntary hand movements, less competent gross motor ability, and difficulties in postural control and balance (76). Crowe and associates described ELBW infants as a group to have significantly inferior skills in all motor functions at 4 years of age (77). Symptomatic intracranial hemorrhage was associated with poorer motor performance.

Neurobehavioral Development

As LBW, premature survivors are assessed more critically and at older ages, a variety of potential behavioral dysfunctions throughout infancy and childhood become evident. Numerous studies have compared the neonatal neurobehavioral performance of LBW infants to that of FBW infants. These studies typically compare premature infants at their corrected age and also tend to use premature infants with relatively uncomplicated neonatal courses. Nevertheless, despite these sampling features that might obscure group differences, premature infants consistently perform less optimally than healthy, full-term infants on these early measures.

Ferrari and colleagues compared low-risk premature infants to healthy, full-term infants using the Brazelton Neonatal Behavioral Assessment Scale (78). They found the premature infants to be significantly inferior in sensory orientation, regulation of behavioral state (i.e., quiet–active status), and autonomic regulation. Additionally, the clustering of neurobehavioral items was more heterogeneous among premature infants. The authors concluded that prematurity itself is associated with a behavioral repertoire that is different, more variable, and on the average less competent than that of full-term infants (78). Friedman and colleagues, also comparing low-risk premature infants and healthy, full-term infants, found that the premature infants fussed and cried more, were less soothable, and tended to change behavioral state more frequently (79). They suggested that these neonatal neurobehavioral differences are potential contributors to suboptimal interaction between premature infants and their caregivers. Aylward and colleagues, in a report from the National Institutes of Health (NIH) Collaborative Study on Antenatal Steroid Therapy, reported significant effects of both gestational age and severity of perinatal–neonatal illness on the neurobehavioral responses of premature infants (80). Specifically, at 40 weeks of corrected age, premature infants born at younger gestational ages and with greater medical complications demonstrated altered behavior in terms of diminished spontaneous activity and vigor, inability to maintain and modulate responses, and poorer visual orientation capabilities.

A number of studies using a wide variety of electrophysiologic techniques have supported the results of these clinical behavioral investigations. Compared to full-term infants, premature infants have been shown to have delayed maturation of both cortical and brainstem auditory evoked potentials, more variable and labile behavioral state organization as measured by time-lapse videosomnography, and decreased resting heart rate variability and vagal tone (i.e., an indirect measure of overall autonomic nervous system activity) (81–84). Several of these functions, particularly state organization and autonomic regulation, have been related positively to longer-term developmental outcome (85,86).

Several studies have explored the related behavioral areas of temperament, social interaction and competence, and emotional expression and affect. Most of these studies have examined mother–infant interactions, and there is an overall consensus of findings that indicates an imbalance in LBW, premature dyads compared to FBW, full-term dyads, with LBW infants typically less responsive and low in communicative signaling behavior, and their mothers compensating for this relative inactivity by displaying high levels of stimulating and engaging activity. Investigations of LBW infants with complicated perinatal–neonatal courses have indicated that these infants exhibit high levels of gaze aversion, avoidance of interaction, and low levels of vocalizing and playing (87–89). Field has reported these interactional differences in depth and succinctly summarizes the problem: "High risk infants and their parents 'have less fun' than normal infants and their parents during their early interactions together" (90). In a study comparing premature–mother dyads with full-term–mother dyads at approximately 4 months of corrected age, Field found the premature infants to be less alert and attentive, less responsive, less interested in game playing, less contingent, less smiling and content, and more affectively negative and irritable than the matched full-term infants. Correspondingly, the mothers of prematures exhibited fewer happy expressions than the mothers of full-terms but were more vocal as they attempted to elicit social and communicative responses from their infants.

Crnic and associates (91) and Malatesta and colleagues (92) have replicated and extended these observations throughout the entire first year of life; LBWFBW differences in expressive behavior and affect were persistent and continued to affect maternal behavior. Malatesta and colleagues emphasized that in their primarily middle to upper-middle social class sample, these differences were seen even in the absence of confounding neonatal medical complications. They speculate that the observed LBWFBW differences probably are even more pronounced with less advantaged, more stressed, or sicker premature infants. Of long-term importance and concern is the increasing evidence of continuity between early interactional disturbances and later behavioral dysfunctions.

School Function

Finally, as increasing numbers of studies have followed LBW, premature infants into the school years, the full spectrum of these children's learning and behavioral performance is emerging and becoming clearer. Although prevalence estimates of school problems vary between reports, almost all investigators agree that LBW survivors have a distinctly increased risk for school dysfunction in some form (23). The most recent reports have focused on school-age ELBW children and consistently describe the most problematic school function of all. Again, these new survivors, although relatively small in overall number, are disproportionately represented in regard to academic and social failure. There also is general agreement that although this substantial risk exists independently of socioeconomic status, the combination and interaction of biologic and environmental risks produces an especially worrisome doubly vulnerable milieu and a highly appropriate target population for early developmental intervention efforts because of the documented importance of psychosocial variables in the ultimate prognosis for LBW, premature infants (93).

Dunn and colleagues, in one of the most extensive longitudinal follow-up studies published, reported minimal cerebral dysfunction (i.e., minor developmental and behavioral abnormalities) to be the single most prevalent (20%) disabling syndrome at school age in a population of over 300 LBW, premature children (94). Furthermore, the authors stress the difficulty in adequately predicting or identifying such dysfunctions before school entry at the age of 5 years (94). This important group of sequelae consequently is liable to be missed when the outcome of NICU graduates is assessed before that age. Figure 59–4 illustrates this diagnostic evolution and increase in developmental–behavioral problems over time. As in other studies, this study found a disproportionate number of boys compared to girls who experienced school dysfunction and required remedial assistance. This investigation was continued into adolescence (95). Although several of the LBW children with earlier problems no longer were demonstrating all of them, an almost equal number of previously unrecognized children had manifested academic and social problems, thus resulting in a relatively stable number of such problems over time. Additionally, whereas behaviors such as overactivity, temper tantrums, and perseveration had greatly subsided, symptoms of neuropsychiatric disturbance, including distractibility, irritability, unhappiness, low frustration tolerance, fears, disobedience, poor motivation, and sleep difficulties, persisted or increased.

Other studies have confirmed these observations in VLBW children at 8 to 15 years of age and have documented, in such areas as verbal expression, academic achievement, social competence, and emotional maturity, continued problems that cannot be attributed primarily to social class or differences in the quality of parenting (96,97). Nickel and colleagues evaluated the school performance at a mean age of 10 years of 25 ELBW children who were cared for at a time (1960–1972) when only very

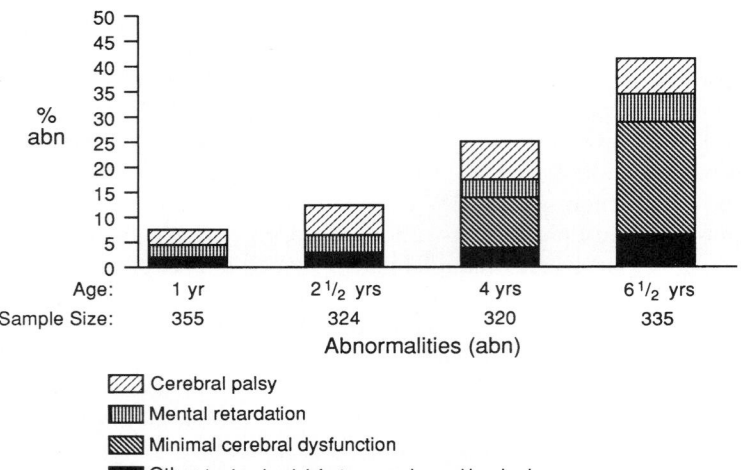

FIG. 59–4. Evolution of developmental dysfunction in low-birth-weight, premature children. (Adapted from ref. 94, with permission.)

premature infants who had little or no neonatal illness survived (98). Despite an overall mean IQ of 90 (range 50 to 141), 16 (64%) of these children had been or currently were in special educational programs. Only seven (28%) were rated by their teachers to be achieving at or above grade level. Arithmetic reasoning, mathematics achievement, reading comprehension, balance, fine motor coordination, and perceptual function were specific and common weaknesses for these children.

Klein and associates compared 65 9-year-old children born in Cleveland, Ohio, in 1976, who were VLBW and who were free of neurologic impairment, to 65 FBW children who had been matched for age, gender, race, and social class on measures of IQ, visual–motor and fine motor abilities, and academic achievement (99). The following were the major findings:

- The VLBW children scored significantly lower than the FBW children on tests that measure general intelligence, even though both group means were within the average range.
- The VLBW children scored significantly lower than the FBW children on tests that measure academic achievement.
- The VLBW children had particular deficits in mathematics achievement.
- The VLBW children had particular deficits on tests that involve visual or spatial skills.
- These results were independent of social class.

In a similarly controlled and longitudinal New York City study, Ross and colleagues showed that a much higher proportion of 8-year-old VLBW children required special educational interventions (48%) than either FBW children (15%) or the New York State public elementary school population (10%) (100). Very-low-birth-weight children scored significantly lower than FBW children on tests of IQ, verbal ability, academic achievement, and auditory memory. There was an interaction of prematurity and social class on IQ, verbal tests, academic achievement, and attention, with premature children of lower socioeconomic status scoring lowest on these measures.

A number of more recent reports emphasize the school problems of ELBW children. From an analysis by birth weight subgroups, Klebanov and colleagues indicated that as birth weight decreases, the prevalence of grade failure, placement in special classes, and classification as impaired increases, even when maternal education and neonatal length of stay are controlled for (101). The ELBW children scored lower than all other birth-weight groups on math and reading achievement tests. Even among children with IQ scores above 85, ELBW children still obtained lower math scores than the other children. Even with optimal socioeconomic environments, approximately one of every two ELBW children requires special educational services (102). In a Scottish population-based sample of 8-year-old children, ELBW children placed heavy demands on regular schools, with 52% requiring learning support compared with 16% of FBW comparison children (103). Hack and colleagues have delineated school-age outcomes in ELBW children with birth weights under 750 g (Fig. 59–5) (56). Compared with VLBW children weighing 750 to 1,499 g at birth and also to FBW children, these markedly ELBW children were inferior in cognitive ability, psychomotor skills, and academic achievement. They had poorer social skills and adaptive behavior and more behavioral and attention problems. In all assessed areas, the functioning of VLBW children was intermediate between that of ELBW and FBW children.

Although data on the prevalence of behavior problems in older LBW children are somewhat sparse, it is likely that the prevalence is substantially higher than in FBW children. For example, Escalona found that 30% of a primarily disadvantaged premature sample exhibited major

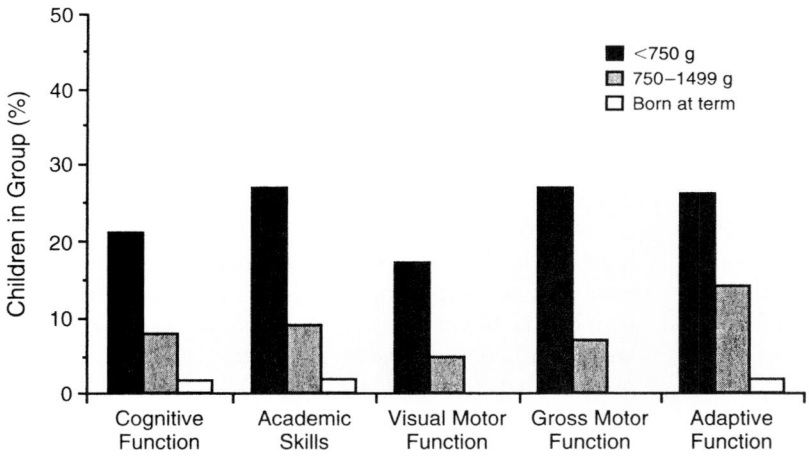

FIG. 59–5. Percentage of children in each study group with subnormal functioning. (From ref. 56, with permission.)

behavior problems before the age of 4 years (104). The most comprehensive investigation of long-term behavioral function in this population comes from the same Cleveland, Ohio cohort described in terms of academic achievement (99). Breslau and colleagues compared 65 9-year-old VLBW children to 65 FBW children, matched for age, gender, race, social class, and school, on parents' ratings on the Child Behavior Checklist and teachers' ratings on the Teacher's Report Form (105). Results from parents and teachers converged on key findings. The major findings were the following:

The VLBW boys manifested significantly more behavioral disturbance and poorer social competence than FBW boys.

The excess in behavior problems in VLBW boys spanned over a wide range of behavioral domains, including both internalizing (e.g., depressive–anxious) and externalizing (e.g., hyperactive, aggressive, conduct problems) syndromes.

The effect of VLBW on behavior problems and social adjustment in boys was not a function of IQ.

These results were independent of social class.

Although VLBW girls did not differ significantly from FBW girls, suggestive trends in the same direction as the boys may indicate that there is an increased risk for behavior problems in both genders but that these sequelae become evident at an earlier age in boys than in girls.

As in other neurodevelopmental and neurobehavioral domains, Klebanov and colleagues found that ELBW children had lower attention, language skills, overall social competence, scholastic competence, and athletic ability than all other birth-weight groups (very low, low, and normal) as measured by classroom teachers, even when neonatal length of stay, child's gender and ethnicity, and maternal education were controlled for (106). The classroom behavior of ELBW children was rated by teachers as poor, even for children who had not failed a grade.

SPECIFIC PERINATAL–NEONATAL COMPLICATIONS IN HIGH-RISK INFANTS

Intrauterine Growth Retardation

The SGA infant has a higher mortality rate, a higher incidence of perinatal–neonatal complications, and a higher prevalence of chronic neurologic impairments than the appropriate-for-gestational-age (AGA) infant of similar gestational age (107). The diagnosis of SGA is useful in identifying a high-risk population needing careful follow-up; however, the population of SGA infants is a heterogeneous one with multiple etiologies. Intrauterine growth pattern, associated congenital anomalies, mortality rate, risk of perinatal–neonatal complications, and long-term outcome reflect not only the nature of the insult but the timing as well. Drillien and colleagues have stressed the need to differentiate early-pregnancy-onset SGA infants, many of whom demonstrate intrinsic defects such as congenital anomalies, from late-pregnancy-onset SGA infants, who may have antenatal histories of placental insufficiency or maternal chronic illness (74). Long-term developmental prognosis, in terms of major and minor impairments and school function, is significantly worse for early-pregnancy-onset SGA infants.

Most SGA outcome studies also distinguish between full-term and premature SGA infants because of marked differences in mortality and morbidity rates, both of which are significantly higher for premature SGA infants. For both groups of SGA infants, great variability among outcome studies is the norm, again reflecting the inevitable heterogeneity of the SGA diagnosis. Many studies report few major neurologic disabilities in full-term SGA infants followed from birth. In 96 full-term SGA infants followed to the age of 5 years, Fitzhardinge and Stevens reported only a 1% prevalence of cerebral palsy and a 6% prevalence of seizures (108). In a cerebral-palsied population in Sweden, full-term SGA infants had a somewhat higher risk for cerebral palsy than full-term AGA infants but a much lower risk than premature AGA and premature SGA infants (37). Most full-term SGA infants are of average intelligence, whether tested during the preschool or school years, even though the mean IQ of the SGA population usually has been somewhat lower than that of control groups (109). Fitzhardinge and Stevens, however, found that, despite average intelligence, 50% of the SGA boys and 36% of the SGA girls were doing poorly in school. One-third of the SGA children with IQs above 100 were failing consistently at school. A history of perinatal asphyxia was an important contributing risk factor. Other studies provide good evidence of an increased prevalence of speech and language problems, minor neurologic findings, and attention deficits in this subgroup (110).

Relatively few studies evaluate the outcome of premature SGA infants, and the results are contradictory. The prevalence of reported impairments varies from nearly 50% to as low as 10%. Commey and Fitzhardinge found that 15% of premature SGA infants had cerebral palsy at the age of 2 years, twice the prevalence encountered in premature AGA infants (111). In the Swedish cerebral palsy study, premature SGA infants had the highest risk for cerebral palsy, 15 times greater than full-term AGA infants and significantly more than full-term SGA and premature AGA infants (37). Commey and Fitzhardinge found a high prevalence of subnormal intelligence in premature SGA infants tested at the age of 2 years. Drillien reported that, in all birth-weight subgroups, fewer premature SGA infants were average cognitively, and more had borderline intelligence or mental retardation, especially those born to parents of low socioeconomic status (112).

There is little specific information about school function in this subgroup, but premature SGA infants certainly must be presumed to be at substantial risk in this area as well. A recent report compared the cognitive and neurologic outcomes of 129 premature SGA infants with 300 premature AGA infants through 6 years of age (113). The SGA infants had significantly poorer cognitive scores at each assessment age than AGA infants of similar gestational ages. Normal neurologic status was more likely at all assessments for the AGA than for SGA infants of comparable gestational age. Nevertheless, there was a significant effect of SGA on cognitive outcome at school age independent of neurologic status.

Asphyxia

Hypoxic–ischemic brain injury is the single most important neurologic problem occurring in the perinatal period (114). This variety of brain injury accounts for many, although not the majority, of the severe, nonprogressive neurologic deficits seen in children. This is particularly the case for full-term infants but also is of etiologic significance for premature infants. The neurodevelopmental deficits of concern are principally the triad of cerebral palsy, mental retardation, and epilepsy, often occurring together in varying degrees. In addition, more subtle developmental and behavioral dysfunctions in the areas of language, fine motor coordination, socioemotional competence, attention, and school learning are increasingly recognized in the relatively few studies designed to investigate these long-term sequelae. The common denominator of this form of brain injury is deprivation of the supply of oxygen to the central nervous system. The developing brain can be deprived of oxygen by two major pathogenetic mechanisms—hypoxemia (i.e., diminished amount of oxygen in the blood supply) or ischemia (i.e., diminished amount of blood perfusing the tissue). These two overlapping mechanisms typically coexist clinically, are virtually impossible to isolate and delineate precisely in the individual infant, and together constitute the basis of the syndrome of asphyxia (115).

As noted by Paneth and Stark, the fundamental problem in assessing the exact relationship between asphyxia and subsequent neurodevelopmental outcome has been the difficulty in assessing the degree of asphyxia (116). Various techniques have been used to identify the asphyxiated infant, including the time to initiate spontaneous respiration (<1 minute), the time that positive-pressure ventilation was required to sustain the infant (<1 minute), and the use of the neonatal scoring system developed by Virginia Apgar (117). This scoring system originally was created to identify infants who were physiologically depressed at birth and who required resuscitative efforts. It has been shown to have limited utility in premature infants (118). Although Apgar did not design the scoring system to be used as a tool to predict long-term neurologic status, it has been used by many for correlation with ultimate outcome because of the paucity of alternative asphyxial markers. Fetal scalp blood and umbilical cord blood sampling for pH and other acid–base parameters have been recommended as potentially providing more objective perinatal data.

Although the Apgar scoring system is not perfect, it continues to be the standard by which almost all neonates are evaluated immediately after birth, and, as such, was the perinatal measure used in the NIH National Collaborative Perinatal Project between 1959 and 1966. This multisite prospective study of more than 50,000 pregnant woman and their children remains the largest single resource for investigating the associations between perinatal asphyxia and neurodevelopmental outcome, particularly cerebral palsy. Several main conclusions emerge (119):

Cerebral palsy does not develop in most (95%) asphyxiated full-term infants with an Apgar score ≤3 at 5 minutes.

As the duration of severe asphyxia increases from 5 to 20 minutes, the likelihood of neonatal death or permanent cerebral palsy also increases in parallel fashion; approximately 60% cerebral palsy prevalence exists in full-term survivors with Apgar scores of ≤3 at 20 minutes.

The more premature the infant, the greater the incidence (i.e., approximately 30% at 28 weeks of gestational age), severity, and mortality associated with perinatal asphyxia.

Most infants in whom cerebral palsy develops were not asphyxiated at birth.

Although perinatal asphyxia certainly is an important cause of severe psychomotor retardation, especially during the intrapartum period, its relative contribution to these adverse outcomes has, in the past, frequently been overstated. It is estimated that between 10% and 20% of all cases of cerebral palsy are attributable to intrapartum asphyxia. Many of these cases are complicated by mental retardation of variable severity. Freeman and Nelson correctly emphasize the four necessary criteria to link causally intrapartum asphyxia and neurodevelopmental disability in full-term infants (120):

1. Intrapartum abnormalities (e.g., nonreassuring fetal heart rate patterns, passage of meconium, hemorrhage)
2. Depression at birth (e.g., low Apgar scores, need for resuscitation)
3. Neonatal hypoxicischemic encephalopathy (e.g., seizures in the first 48 hours, hypotonia and lethargy, metabolic acidosis, apnea)
4. Anticipated outcomes (e.g., cerebral palsy with associated deficits, not severe mental retardation or epilepsy by themselves).

Outcome studies in full-term infants have identified the neonatal factors most predictive of neurodevelopmental disability after an episode of intrapartum asphyxia. The key predictors include failure to establish spontaneous respiration by 5 minutes, onset of seizures within the first 12 hours and refractory to treatment, prolonged deep encephalopathy (i.e., Sarnat stage 3) (121), failure of the electroencephalogram to normalize by 5 to 7 days, and inability to establish adequate oral feedings by 1 week of age (122). Fitzhardinge and colleagues described the predictive utility of the computed tomography scan between 1 and 2 weeks after birth (123). The most ominous findings were diffuse hypodensities throughout both the white and gray matter and extensive intraparenchymal or intraventricular hemorrhage. Byrne and associates reported that 8 months of age appears to be the earliest time at which magnetic resonance imaging findings (e.g., delayed myelination, acquired structural abnormalities) correlate well with later adverse neurodevelopmental outcome in this populatio (124). Finally, Robertson and colleagues compared 145 asphyxiated full-term children who had experienced neonatal encephalopathy with a similar number of nonasphyxiated peer children at 8 years of age (125). The prevalence of major impairment, which included cerebral palsy, mental retardation, epilepsy, cortical blindness, and severe hearing loss, was

16%. Intellectual, visualmotor integration, and receptive vocabulary scores, as well as reading, spelling, and arithmetic grade levels for those children with moderate or severe encephalopathy were significantly below those in the mild encephalopathy or peer comparison groups. Thus, children who survive moderate or severe neonatal asphyxial encephalopathy are at increased risk for both major neurosensory impairment and reduced school performance.

REFERENCES

1. McCormick MC. The contribution of low birthweight to infant mortality and childhood morbidity. *N Engl J Med* 1985;312:82.
2. Philip AGS, Little GA, Polivy DR, et al. Neonatal mortality risk for the 80s: the importance of birthweight/gestational age groups. *Pediatrics* 1981;68:122.
3. Paneth N, Kiely JL, Wallenstein S, et al. Newborn intensive care and neonatal mortality in low birthweight infants: a population study. *N Engl J Med* 1982;307:149.
4. Buehler JW, Kleinman JC, Hogue CJR. Birthweight-specific infant mortality, United States, 1960 and 1980. *Public Health Rep* 1987; 102:151.
5. Herdman RC, Behney CJ, Wagner JL, et al. *Neonatal intensive care for low birthweight infants: costs and effectiveness. Health Technology Case Study 38, Publication OTA-HCS-38.* Washington, DC: Office of Technology Assessment, 1987.
6. Hack M, Fanaroff AA. Outcomes of extremely low birthweight infants between 1982 and 1988. *N Engl J Med* 1989;321:1642.
7. Phelps DL, Brown DR, Tung B, et al. 28-day survival rates of 6,676 neonates with birthweights of 1250 grams or less. *Pediatrics* 1991; 87:7.
8. Hack M, Friedman H, Fanaroff AA. Outcomes of extremely low birth weight infants. *Pediatrics* 1996;98:931.
9. Ginsberg HG, Goldsmith JP, Stedman CM. Intact survival and 20month follow-up of a 380-gram infant. *J Perinatol* 1990;10:330.
10. Hack M, Horbar JD, Malloy MH, et al. Very low birthweight outcomes of the National Institute of Child Health and Human Development Neonatal Network. *Pediatrics* 1991;87:587.
11. Lasky RE, Tyson JE, Rosenfeld CR, et al. Disappointing follow-up findings for indigent high-risk newborns. *Am J Dis Child* 1987; 147:100.
12. Bennett FC, Robinson NM, Sells CJ. Growth and development of infants weighing less than 800 grams at birth. *Pediatrics* 1983;71:319.
13. Hoffman EL, Bennett FC. Birthweight less than 800 grams: changing outcomes and influences of gender and gestation number. *Pediatrics* 1990;86:27.
14. LaPine TR, Jackson JC, Bennett FC. Outcome of infants weighing less than 800 grams at birth: 15 years experience. *Pediatrics* 1995;96:479.
15. Shy KK, Luthy DA, Bennett FC, et al. Effects of electronic fetal heart rate monitoring, as compared with periodic auscultation, on the neurologic development of premature infants. *N Engl J Med* 1990;322:588.
16. The HIFI Study Group. High-frequency oscillatory ventilation compared with conventional intermittent mechanical ventilation in the treatment of respiratory failure in preterm infants: neurodevelopmental status at 16 to 24 months of postterm age. *J Pediatr* 1990;117:939.
17. Aylward GP, Pfeiffer SI, Wright A, et al. Outcome studies of low birthweight infants published in the last decade: a metaanalysis. *J Pediatr* 1989;115:515.
18. Blackman J. *Warning signals: basic criteria for tracking at-risk infants and toddlers.* Washington, DC: National Center for Clinical Infant Programs, 1986.
19. Blackman JA, Hein HA. Iowa's system for screening and tracking high-risk infants. *Am J Dis Child* 1985;139:826.
20. TeKolste KA, Bennett FC. The high risk infant: transitions in health, development, and family during the first years of life. *J Perinatol* 1987;7:368.
21. Barrera ME, Rosenbaum PL, Cunningham CE. Corrected and uncorrected Bayley scores: longitudinal developmental patterns in low and high birthweight infants. *Infant Behav Dev* 1987;10:337.

22. McCormick MC. long-term follow-up of infants discharged from neonatal intensive care units. *JAMA* 1989;261:1767.

23. Bennett FC. Neurodevelopmental outcome in low birthweight infants: the role of developmental intervention. *Clin Crit Care Med* 1988; 13:221.

24. Brothwood M, Wolke D, Gamsu H, et al. Prognosis of the very low birthweight baby in relation to gender. *Arch Dis Child* 1986;61:559.

25. Bennett FC, Scott DT. Long-term perspective on premature infant outcome and contemporary intervention issues. *Semin Perinatol* 1997; 21:190.

26. Paneth N, Kiely JL, Stein Z, et al. Cerebral palsy and newborn care: III. Estimated prevalence rates of cerebral palsy under differing rates of mortality and impairment of low birthweight infants. *Dev Med Child Neurol* 1981;23:801.

27. Hagberg B, Hagberg G, Olow I, et al. The changing panorama of cerebral palsy in Sweden: V. The birth year period 1979–82. *Acta Paediatr Scand* 1989;78:283.

28. Blaymore-Bier J, Pezzullo J, Kim E, et al. Outcome of extremely low-birth-weight infants: 1980–1990. *Acta Paediatr* 1994;83:1244.

29. Robertson CMT, Hrynchyshyn GJ, Etches PC, et al. Population-based study of the incidence, complexity, and severity of neurologic disability among survivors weighing 500 through 1250 grams at birth: A comparison of two birth cohorts. *Pediatrics* 1992;90:750.

30. O Shea TM, Klinepeter KL, Goldstein DJ, et al. Survival and developmental disability in infants with birth weights of 501 to 800 grams, born between 1979 and 1994. *Pediatrics* 1997;100:982.

31. Pharoah PO, Cooke T, Cooke RW, et al. Birthweight specific trends in cerebral palsy. *Arch Dis Child* 1990;65:602.

31a. Freud S. *Infantile cerebral paralysis.* Russin LA, trans. Coral Gables, FL: University of Miami Press, 1968.

32. Bennett FC, Chandler LS, Robinson NM, et al. Spastic diplegia in premature infants: etiologic and diagnostic considerations. *Am J Dis Child* 1981;135:732.

33. Volpe JJ. Cognitive deficits in premature infants. *N Engl J Med* 1991; 325:276.

34. Graziani LJ, Pasto M, Stanley C, et al. Neonatal neurosonographic correlates of cerebral palsy in preterm infants. *Pediatrics* 1986;78:88.

35. Bozynski ME, Nelson MN, Genaze D, et al. Cranial ultrasonography and the prediction of cerebral palsy in infants weighing ≤ 1200 grams at birth. *Dev Med Child Neurol* 1988;30:342.

36. Perlman JM, Risser R, Broyles RS. Bilateral cystic periventricular leukomalacia in the premature infant: Associated risk factors. *Pediatrics* 1996;97:822.

37. Hagberg B. Epidemiological and preventive aspects of cerebral palsy and severe mental retardation in Sweden. *Eur J Pediatr* 1979;130:71.

38. Gibson RL, Jackson JC, Twiggs GA, et al. Bronchopulmonary dysplasia: survival after prolonged mechanical ventilation. *Am J Dis Child* 1988;142:721.

39. Singer L, Yamashita T, Lilien L, et al. A longitudinal study of developmental outcome of infants with bronchopulmonary dysplasia and very low birth weight. *Pediatrics* 1997;100:987.

40. Bradford BC, Baudin J, Conway MJ, et al. Identification of sensory neural hearing loss in very preterm infants by brainstem auditory evoked potentials. *Arch Dis Child* 1985;60:105.

41. de Vries LS, Lary S, Dubowitz LMS. Relationship of serum bilirubin levels to ototoxicity and deafness in high-risk low birthweight infants. *Pediatrics* 1985;76:351.

42. Salamy A, Eldredge L, Tooley WH. Neonatal status and hearing loss in high-risk infants. *J Pediatr* 1989;114:847.

43. Leavitt AM, Watchko JF, Bennett FC, et al. Neurodevelopmental outcome following persistent pulmonary hypertension of the neonate. *J Perinatol* 1987;7:288.

44. Abramovich SJ, Gregory S, Slemick M, et al. Hearing loss in very low birthweight infants treated with neonatal intensive care. *Arch Dis Child* 1979;54:421.

45. Bess FH, Tharpe AM. Unilateral hearing impairment in children. *Pediatrics* 1984;74:206.

46. Thompson G, Folsom R. Hearing assessment of at-risk infants. *Clin Pediatr* 1981;20:257.

47. Marshall RE, Reichert TJ, Kerley SV, et al. Auditory function in newborn intensive care unit patients revealed by auditory brainstem potentials. *J Pediatr* 1980;96:731.

48. Nield TA, Schrier S, Ramos AD, et al. Unexpected hearing loss in high-risk infants. *Pediatrics* 1986;78:417.

49. Avery GB, Glass P. Retinopathy of prematurity: progress report. *Pediatr Ann* 1988;17:528.

50. Avery GB, Glass P. Retinopathy of prematurity: what causes it? *Clin Perinatol* 1988;15:917.

51. Scharf J, Zonis S, Zeltzer M. Refraction in premature babies: a prospective study. *J Pediatr Ophthalmol Strabismus* 1978;15:48.

52. Camfield PR, Camfield CS, Allen AC, et al. Progressive hydrocephalus in infants with birthweights less than 1500 grams. *Arch Neurol* 1981;38:653.

53. Shinnar S, Molteni RA, Gammon K, et al. Intraventricular hemorrhage in the premature infant. *N Engl J Med* 1982;306:1464.

54. Chaplin ER, Goldstein GW, Myerberg DZ, et al. Posthemorrhagic hydrocephalus in the preterm infant. *Pediatrics* 1980;65:901.

55. Saigal S, Rosenbaum P, Stoskopf B, et al. follow-up of infants 501 to 1500 gm birthweight delivered to residents of a geographically defined region with perinatal intensive care facilities. *J Pediatr* 1982;100:606.

56. Hack M, Taylor HG, Klein N, et al. School-age outcomes in children with birth weights under 750 g. *N Engl J Med* 1994;331:753.

57. McBurney AK, Eaves LC. Evolution of developmental and psychological test scores. In Dunn HG, ed. *Sequelae of low birthweight: the Vancouver study.* Philadelphia: JB Lippincott, 1986.

58. Hoy EA, Bill JM, Sykes DH. Very low birthweight: a long-term developmental impairment? *Int J Behav Dev* 1988;11:37.

59. Rose SA. Differential rates of visual information processing in full-term and preterm infants. *Child Dev* 1983;54:1189.

60. Ruff HA, McCarton C, Kurtzberg D, et al. Preterm infants' manipulative exploration of objects. *Child Dev* 1984;55:1166.

61. Drillien CM. *The growth and development of the prematurely born infant.* Edinburgh: Livingstone, 1964.

62. Wiener G, Rider RV, Oppel WC, et al. Correlates of low birthweight: psychological status at eight to ten years of age. *Pediatr Res* 1968; 2:110.

63. Hunt JV, Cooper BAB, Tooley WH. Very low birthweight infants at 8 and 11 years of age: role of neonatal illness and family status. *Pediatrics* 1988;82:596.

64. Halsey CL, Collin MF, Anderson CL. Extremely low birth weight children and their peers: A comparison of preschool performance. *Pediatrics* 1993;91:807.

65. Breslau N, DelDotto JE, Brown GG, et al. A gradient relationship between low birth weight and IQ at age 6 years. *Arch Pediatr Adolesc Med* 1994;148:377.

66. Zarin-Ackerman J, Lewis M, Driscoll JM. Language development in 2-year-old normal and risk infants. *Pediatrics* 1977;59:982.

67. Largo RH, Molinari L, Comenale-Pinto L, et al. Language development of term and preterm children during the first five years of life. *Dev Med Child Neurol* 1986;28:333.

68. Michelsson K, Noronen M. Neurological, psychological and articulatory impairment in fiveyearold children with a birthweight of 2000 g or less. *Eur J Pediatr* 1983;137:96.

69. Hubatch LM, Johnson CJ, Kistler DJ, et al. Early language abilities of high-risk infants. *J Speech Hear Disord* 1985;50:195.

70. Bennett FC, Robinson NM, Sells CJ. Hyaline membrane disease, birthweight, and gestational age: effects on development in the first two years. *Am J Dis Child* 1982;136:888.

71. Drillien CM. Abnormal neurologic signs in the first year of life in low birthweight infants: possible prognostic significance. *Dev Med Child Neurol* 1972;14:575.

72. Amiel-Tison C. A method for neurologic evaluation within the first year of life. *Curr Prob Pediatr* 1976;7:1.

73. Coolman RB, Bennett FC, Sells CJ, et al. Neuromotor development of graduates of the neonatal intensive care unit: patterns encountered in the first two years of life. *J Dev Behav Pediatr* 1985;6:327.

74. Drillien CM, Thomson AJM, Burgoyne K. Low birthweight children at early school age: a longitudinal study. *Dev Med Child Neurol* 1980;22:26.

75. Ross G, Lipper EG, Auld PAM. Consistency and change in the development of premature infants weighing less than 1501 grams at birth. *Pediatrics* 1985;76:885.

76. Burns YR, Bullock MI. Comparison of abilities of preterm and mature born children at 5 years of age. *Aust Paediatr J* 1985;21:31.

77. Crowe TK, Deitz JC, Bennett FC, et al. Preschool motor skills of children born prematurely and not diagnosed as having cerebral palsy. *J Dev Behav Pediatr* 1988;9:189.

78. Ferrari F, Grosoli MV, Fontana G, et al. Neurobehavioral comparison

of low-risk preterm and full-term infants at term conceptional age. *Dev Med Child Neurol* 1983;25:450.

79. Freidman SL, Jacobs BS, Werthmann MW. Preterms of low medical risk: spontaneous behaviors and soothability at expected date of birth. *Infant Behav Dev* 1982;5:3.

80. Aylward GP, Hatcher RP, Leavitt LA, et al. Factors affecting neurobehavioral responses of preterm infants at term conceptional age. *Child Dev* 1984;55:1155.

81. Kurtzberg D, Hilpert PL, Kreuzer JA, et al. Differential maturation of cortical auditory evoked potentials to speech sounds in normal full-term and very low birthweight infants. *Dev Med Child Neurol* 1984;26:466.

82. Anders TF, Keener M. Developmental coarse of nighttime sleep–wake patterns in full-term and premature infants during the first year of life: I. *Sleep* 1985;8:173.

83. Fox NA, Porges SW. The relation between neonatal heart period patterns and developmental outcome. *Child Dev* 1985;56:28.

84. Kaga K, Hashira S, Marsh RR. Auditory brainstem responses and behavioral responses in preterm infants. *Br J Audiol* 1986;20:121.

85. Anders TF, Keener M, Kraemer H. Sleep–wake state organization, neonatal assessment and development in premature infants during the first year of life: II. *Sleep* 1985;8:193.

86. Cohen SE, Parmelee AH, Beckwith L, et al. Cognitive development in preterm infants: birth to eight years. *J Dev Behav Pediatr* 1986;7:102.

87. DiVitto B, Goldberg S. The effects of newborn medical status on early parent–infant interactions. In Field TM, ed. *Infants born at risk.* New York: Spectrum, 1979:311.

88. Field TM. Interaction patterns of preterm and term infants. In Field TM, ed. *Infants born at risk.* New York: Spectrum, 1979:333.

89. Watt J. Interaction and development in the first year: I. The effects of prematurity. *Early Hum Dev* 1986;13:195.

90. Field TM. High-risk infants "have less fun" during early interactions. *Top Early Child Spec Educ* 1983;3(1):77.

91. Crnic KA, Ragozin AS, Greenberg MT, et al. Social interaction and developmental competence of preterm and full-term infants during the first year of life. *Child Dev* 1983;54:1199.

92. Malatesta CZ, Grigoryev P, Lamb C, et al. Emotion socialization and expressive development in preterm and full-term infants. *Child Dev* 1986;57:316.

93. Kopp CB. Risk factors in development. In Haith MM, Campos JJ, eds. *Handbook of child psychology,* vol 2. *Infancy and developmental psychobiology.* New York: John Wiley & Sons, 1983:1081.

94. Dunn HG, Crichton JU, Grunau RVE, et al. Neurological, psychological and educational sequelae of low birthweight. *Brain Dev* 1980;2:57.

95. Dunn HG, ed. Sequelae of low birthweight: the Vancouver Study. *Clin Dev Med* 1986;95:96.

96. Wright FH, Blough RR, Chamberlin A, et al. A controlled follow-up study of small prematures born from 1952 through 1956. *Am J Dis Child* 1972;124:506.

97. Caputo DV, Goldstein KM, Taub HB. The development of prematurely born children through middle childhood. In Field TM, ed. *Infants born at risk.* New York: Spectrum, 1979:219.

98. Nickel RE, Bennett FC, Lamson FN. School performance of children with birthweights of 1000 g or less. *Am J Dis Child* 1982;136:105.

99. Klein NK, Hack M, Breslau N. Children who were very low birthweight: development and academic achievement at nine years of age. *J Dev Behav Pediatr* 1989;10:32.

100. Ross G, Lipper EG, Auld PAM. Educational status and schoolrelated abilities of very low birthweight premature children. *Pediatrics* 1991;88:1125.

101. Klebanov PK, Brooks-Gunn J, McCormick MC. School achievement and failure in very low birth weight children. *J Dev Behav Pediatr* 1994;15:248.

102. Halsey CL, Collin MF, Anderson CL. Extremely low-birth-weight children and their peers: A comparison of school-age outcomes. *Arch Pediatr Adolesc Med* 1996;150:790.

103. Hall A, McLeod A, Counsell C, et al. School attainment, cognitive ability and motor function in a total Scottish very-low-birthweight population at eight years: A controlled study. *Dev Med Child Neurol* 1995;37:1037.

104. Escalona SK. Babies at double hazard: early development of infants at biologic and social risk. *Pediatrics* 1982;70:670.

105. Breslau N, Klein N, Allen L. Very low birthweight: behavioral sequelae at nine years of age. *J Am Acad Child Adolesc Psychiatry* 1988;27:605.

106. Klebanov PK, Brooks-Gunn J, McCormick MC. Classroom behavior of very low birth weight elementary school children. *Pediatrics* 1994;94:700.

107. Allen MC. Developmental outcome and follow-up of the small for gestational age infant. *Semin Perinatol* 1984;8:123.

108. Fitzhardinge PM, Stevens EM. The small-for-date infant: II. Neurological and intellectual sequelae. *Pediatrics* 1972;50:50.

109. Westwood M, Kramer MS, Munz D, et al. Growth and development of full-term nonasphyxiated small-for-gestational-age newborns: follow-up through adolescence. *Pediatrics* 1983;71:376.

110. Neligan GA, Kolvin I, Scott DM, et al. Born too soon or born too small: a follow-up study to seven years of age. *Clin Dev Med* 1976;61:81.

111. Commey JO, Fitzhardinge PM. Handicap in the preterm small-for-gestational-age infant. *J Pediatr* 1979;94:779.

112. Drillien CM. Aetiology and outcome in low birthweight infants. *Dev Med Child Neurol* 1972;14:563.

113. McCarton CM, Wallace IF, Divon M, et al. Cognitive and neurologic development of the premature, small for gestational age infant through age 6: Comparison by birth weight and gestational age. *Pediatrics* 1996;98:1167.

114. Shaywitz BA. The sequelae of hypoxicischemic encephalopathy. *Semin Perinatol* 1987;11:180.

115. Volpe JJ. Perinatal hypoxicischemic brain injury. *Pediatr Clin North Am* 1976;23:383.

116. Paneth N, Stark RI. Cerebral palsy and mental retardation in relation to indicators of perinatal asphyxia: an epidemiologic overview. *Am J Obstet Gynecol* 1983;147:960.

117. Apgar V, James LS. Further observations on the newborn scoring system. *Am J Dis Child* 1962;104:419.

118. Hegyi T, Carbone T, Anwar M, et al. The Apgar score and its components in the preterm infant. *Pediatrics* 1998;101:77.

119. Nelson KB, Ellenberg JH. Apgar scores as predictors of chronic neurologic disability. *Pediatrics* 1981;68:36.

120. Freeman JM, Nelson KB. Intrapartum asphyxia and cerebral palsy. *Pediatrics* 1988;82:240.

121. Sarnat HB, Sarnat MS. Neonatal encephalopathy following fetal distress: a clinical and electroencephalographic study. *Arch Neurol* 1976;33:696.

122. Finer NN, Robertson CM, Richards RT, et al. Hypoxicischemic encephalopathy in term neonates: perinatal factors and outcome. *J Pediatr* 1981;98:112.

123. Fitzhardinge PM, Flodmark O, Fitz CR, et al. The prognostic value of computed tomography as an adjunct to assessment of the term infant with postasphyxial encephalopathy. *J Pediatr* 1981;99:777.

124. Byrne P, Welch R, Johnson MA, et al. Serial magnetic resonance imaging in neonatal hypoxicischemic encephalopathy. *J Pediatr* 1990;117:694.

125. Robertson CM, Finer NN, Grace MG. School performance of survivors of neonatal encephalopathy associated with birth asphyxia at term. *J Pediatr* 1989;114:753.

APPENDICES

Contents

1499

APPENDIX A

Selected Laboratory Values

1. BLOOD

APPENDIX A–1a. *Normal blood chemistry values, term infants*

Determination	0–1 wk	1 wk–1 mo	1–6 mo	>1 yr
Sodium (mM/L)	133–146	134–144	134–142	134–143
Potassium (mM/L)	3.2–5.5	3.4–6.0	3.5–5.6	3.3–4.6
Chloride (mM/L)	96–111	96–110	96–110	96–109
Calcium (mg/dl)	7.9–10.7	8.5–10.6	8.7–10.5	8.7–9.8
Calcium (ionized)	3.9–6.0		3.7–5.9	
Phosphorus (mg/dl)	4.0–4.1	3.6–6.6		3.2–6.0
Blood urea (mg/dl)	2–13	2–16	2–12	3–12
Total protein (g/dL)	4.1–6.3		4.7–6.7	5.7–8.0
Glucose (mg/dL)	55–115		55–117	
Lactate (mM/L)	1.1–2.3			0.8–1.5

Data from Soldin SJ, Brugnara C, Gunter KC, Hicks JM, eds. *Pediatric reference ranges,* 2nd ed. Washington: AACC Press, 1997.

APPENDIX A–1b. *Normal blood chemistry values, low-birth-weight infants, capillary blood, first day*

Determination	<1000 g	1001–1500 g	1501–2000 g	2001–2500 g
Sodium (mM/L)	138	133	135	134
Potassium (mM/L)	6.4	6.0	5.4	5.6
Chloride (mM/L)	100	101	105	104
Total CO_2 (mM/L)	19	20	20	20
Urea (mg/dL)	22	21	16	16
Total protein (g/dL)	4.8	4.8	5.2	5.3

Pincus JB, et al. *Pediatrics* 1956;18:39. Copyright © American Academy of Pediatrics, 1956.

APPENDIX A–1c. *Blood chemistry values during the first 7 weeks of life in premature infants with birth weights of 1500 to 1750 g*

Determination	1 wk of age			3 wk of age			5 wk of age			7 wk of age		
	Mean	SD	Range	Mean	SD	Range	Mean	SD	Range	Mean	SD	Range
Na (mM/L)	139.6	±3.2	133–146	136.3	±2.9	129–142	136.8	±2.5	133–148	137.2	±1.8	133–142
K (mM/L)	5.6	±0.5	4.6–6.7	5.8	±0.6	4.5–7.1	5.5	±0.6	4.5–6.6	5.7	±0.5	4.6–7.1
Cl (mM/L)	108.2	±3.7	100–117	108.3	±3.9	102–116	107	±3.5	100–115	107	±3.3	101–115
CO_2 (mM/L)	20.3	±2.8	13.8–27.1	18.4	±3.5	12.4–26.2	20.4	±3.4	12.5–26.1	20.6	±3.1	13.7–26.9
Ca (mg/dL)	9.2	±1.1	6.1–11.6	9.6	±0.5	8.1–11	9.4	±0.5	8.6–10.5	9.5	±0.7	8.6–10.8
P (mg/dL)	7.6	±1.1	5.4–10.9	7.5	±0.7	6.2–8.7	7	±0.6	5.6–7.9	6.8	±0.8	4.2–8.2
BUN (mg/dL)	9.3	±5.2	3.1–25.5	13.3	±7.8	2.1–31.4	13.3	±7.1	2–26.5	13.4	±6.7	2.5–30.5
Total protein (g/dL)	5.49	±0.42	4.4–6.26	5.38	±0.48	4.28–6.7	4.98	±0.5	4.14–6.9	4.93	±0.61	4.02–5.86
Albumin (g/dL)	3.85	±0.3	3.28–4.5	3.92	±0.42	3.16–5.26	3.73	±0.34	3.2–4.34	3.89	±0.53	3.4–4.6
Globulin (g/dL)	1.58	±0.33	0.88–2.2	1.44	±0.63	0.62–2.9	1.17	±0.49	0.48–1.48	1.12	±0.33	0.5–2.6
Hemoglobin (g/dL)	17.8	±2.7	11.4–24.8	14.7	±2.1	9–19.4	11.5	±2	7.2–18.6	10	±1.3	7.5–13.9

BUN, blood urea nitrogen; SD, standard deviation.
Adapted from Thomas JL, Reichelderfer TE. Premature infants: analysis of serum during the first seven weeks. *Clin Chem* 1968;14:272.

APPENDIX A–1d. *Other serum values[a]*

Ammonia nitrogen, newborn (μm/L)	21–95
Amylase (U/L)	0–6
Copper, 0–6 mo (μg/dL)	9–46
Ceruloplasmin (mg/L)	50–260
Zinc (μg/dL)	65–140
Serum enzymes	
Alkaline phosphatase (U/L)	77–375
CPK (U/L)	
1 d	Up to 500
2 d–2 wk	Up to 440
LDH (37°C; U/L)	160–1800
AST, newborn (U/L)	Up to 100
ALT, newborn (IU/L)	Up to 45
Triglyceride, fasting (mg/dL)	Up to 125
Magnesium (mg/dL)	1.7–2.5
Osmolality (mOsmol/kg)	275–300
Phenylalanine, newborn (nmol/L)	Up to 200
α_1-Antitrypsin (mg/dL)	143–490
Vitamin A (retinol; μg/dL)	
0–1 y	14–52
Vitamin E (μg/dL)	1.0–3.5
IgG (g/L)	
Birth	2.5–10.3
1–3 mo	1.9–7.0
4–6 mo	1.8–9.7
IgA (g/L)	
Birth	None detected
1–3 mo	0.05–0.59
4–6 mo	0.09–1.0
IgM (g/L)	
Birth	0.12–1.17
1–3 mo	0.27–1.6
4–6 mo	0.41–2.0
Transferrin (g/L)	
≤3 mo	0.9–2.5

[a]Normal values depend on method used.

ALT, alanine aminotransferase, formerly SGPT; AST, aspartate aminotransferase, formerly SGOT; CPK, creatine phosphokinase; LDH, lactate dehydrogenase.

Data from Soldin SJ, Brugnara C, Gunter KC, Hicks JM, eds. *Pediatric reference ranges,* 2nd ed. Washington: AACC Press, 1997.

APPENDIX A–1e. *Amino acid concentration in plasma or serum (micromolar)*

Amino acid	Neonates (Mean ± SD)	Infants (Mean ± SD)
Taurine	141 ± 40	
Hydroxyproline	32	
Aspartic acid	8 ± 4	19 ± 2
Threonine	217 ± 21	177 ± 36[a]
Serine	163 ± 34	131 ± 27
Asparagine and glutamine[b]	759 ± 136	
Proline	183 ± 32	193 ± 52
Glutamic acid	52 ± 25	
Glycine	343 ± 69	213 ± 35
Alanine	329 ± 55	292 ± 53
Valine	136 ± 39	161 ± 38
Half cystine	62 ± 13	42 ± 9
Methionine	29 ± 8	18 ± 3
Isoleucine	39 ± 8	39 ± 8
Leucine	72 ± 17	77 ± 21
Tyrosine	69 ± 16	54 ± 21
Phenylalanine	78 ± 14	55 ± 10
Ornithine	91 ± 25	50 ± 11
Lysine	200 ± 46	135 ± 28
Histidine	77 ± 16	78 ± 14
Arginine	54 ± 17	62 ± 9
Tryptophan	32 ± 17	
β-Alanine	14.5	

All data obtained by elution chromatography on ion exchange resin columns.

[a]Includes asparagine.

[b]Stands for asparagine and glutamine as combined amounts.

SD, standard deviation.

Adapted from Hicks J, Boeckx RL. *Pediatric clinical chemistry.* Philadelphia: WB Saunders, 1984:684.

2. URINE

APPENDIX A–2. *Urinary values*

Determination	17-Ketosteroids	17-Hydroxycorticoids	Pregnanetriol
Adrenal steroids (mg/d)			
Newborn–1 wk	2–2.5	0.05–0.3	0.01
1 wk–3 mo	0.5	0.05–0.5	0.01
3 mo–1 yr	0.5	0.1–0.5	0.01

Determination	Values
Electrolytes (depends on intake)	
Sodium (mM/L)	18–60
Potassium (mM/L)	10–40
Chloride (mM/kg/d)	1.7–8.5
Bicarbonate (mM/L)	1.5–2
Calcium (mM/kg/d)	<2
Other urinary values	
Ammonia (μM/min/m^2)	
Infants 2–11.5 mo	4–40
Older children	5.9–16.5
Creatinine (mg/kg/d)	
Premature, 2–12 wk	8.3–19.9
Full-term, 1–7 wk	10–15.5
Older child, 2–3 yr	6.4–21.9
Glucose (mg/L)	50
Osmolality (infant; mOsm/kg)	50–600
VMA (infant; μg/mg creatinine)	5–19 (<1 mg/24 h)
HVA (μg/mg creatinine)	3–16
Protein	Trace
Urea nitrogen (depends on intake; mg/L)	300–3000
Titratable acidity (μM/minute/m^2)	Minus bicarbonate
Premature	0–12
Term	0–11

HVA, homovanillic acid; VMA, vanillylmandelic acid.

Data from Normal values for pediatric clinical chemistry, Special Committee on Pediatric Clinical Chemistry, American Association of Clinical Chemists, August 1974.

3. CEREBROSPINAL FLUID

APPENDIX A–3a. *Cerebrospinal fluid examination in high-risk neonates without meningitis*

Determination	Term	Preterm
WBC count (cells/mm^3)		
Number of infants	87	30
Mean	8.2	9.0
Median	5	6
SD	7.1	8.2
Range	0–32	0–29
±2 SD	0–22.4	0–25.4
Percentage PMN	61.3%	57.2%
Protein (mg/dL)		
Number of infants	35	17
Mean	90	115
Range	20–170	65–150
Glucose (mg/dL)		
Number of infants	51	23
Mean	52	50
Range	34–119	24–63
CSF/blood glucose (%)		
Number of infants	51	23
Mean	81	74
Range	44–248	55–105

CSF, cerebrospinal fluid; PMN, polymorphonuclear cells; SD, standard deviation; WBC, leukocyte.

From Sarff LD, et al. Cerebrospinal fluid evaluation in neonates: comparison of high-risk infants with and without meningitis. *J Pediatr* 1976;88:474.

APPENDIX A–3b. *Comparison of leukocyte counts in cerebrospinal fluid in neonates with or without meningitis*

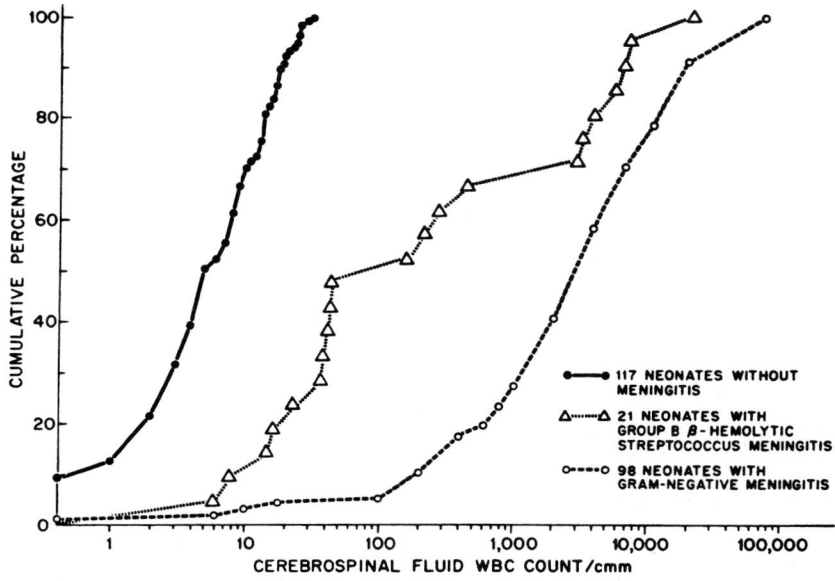

From Sarff LD, et al. Cerebrospinal fluid evaluation in neonates: comparison of high-risk infants with and without meningitis. *J Pediatr* 1976;88(3):475.

4. ANALYTE CONVERSION

APPENDIX A–4. *SI unit conversion table*

Analyte	Present unit	Conversion factor	SI unit
Acetaminophen	mg/dL	66.16	μmol/L
Acetoacetic acid	mg/dL	97.95	μmol/L
Adrenocorticotropin	pg/mL	0.2202	pmol/L
Alanine aminotransferase	U/L	1.0	U/L
	Karmen units/mL	0.482	U/L
Albumin	g/dL	10.0	g/L
Aldolase	U/L	1.0	U/L
	Sibley–Lehninger units/mL	0.7440	U/L
Aldosterone (serum)	ng/dL	27.74	pmol/L
Aldosterone (urine)	μg/24 h	2.774	nmol/d
α_1-Antitrypsin	mg/dL	0.01	g/L
α_2-Macroglobulin	mg/dL	0.01	g/L
Aminolevulinic acid	mg/24 h	7.626	μmol/d
Ammonia			
As ammonia	μg/dL	0.5872	μmol/L
As ammonium ion	μg/dL	0.5543	μmol/L
As ammonia nitrogen	μg/dL	0.7139	μmol/L
Amylase	U/L	1.00	U/L
	Somogyi units/dL	1.850	U/L
	Dye units/dL	1.59	U/L
	Street Close units/dL	5.7	U/L
Androstenedione	μg/L	3.492	nmol/L
Aspartate aminotransferase	U/L	1.00	U/L
	Karmen units/mL	0.482	U/L
β-Hydroxybutyric acid	mg/dL	96.05	μmol/L
β_2-Microglobulin (serum)	mg/L	84.75	nmol/L
β_2-Microglobulin (urine)	μg/24 h	0.08475	nmol/L
Bilirubin	mg/dL	17.10	μmol/L
Calcium	mg/dL	0.2495	mmol/L
Calcium, ionized	mEq/L	0.500	mmol/L
Calcium (urine)	mg/24 h	0.02495	mmol/d
Carbon dioxide (total)	mEq/L	1.00	mmol/L
Ceruloplasmin	mg/dL	10.0	mg/L
Chloride	mEq/L	1.00	mmol/L
Cholesterol	mg/dL	0.02586	mmol/L
Chorionic gonadotropin	mIU/mL	1.00	IU/L
Complement, C3	mg/dL	0.01	g/L
Complement, C4	mg/dL	0.01	g/L
Copper (serum)	μg/dL	0.1574	μmol/L
Copper (urine)	μg/24 h	0.01574	μmol/d
Coproporphyrins	μg/24 h	1.527	nmol/d
Cortisol (free, urine)	μg/24 h	2.759	nmol/d
Cortisol (serum)	μg/dL	27.59	nmol/L
Creatine kinase	U/L	1.00	U/L
Creatinine (serum)	mg/dL	88.40	μmol/L
Creatinine (urine)	g/24 h	8.840	mmol/d
Creatinine clearance	mL/min	0.01667	mL/s
Dehydroepiandrosterone	μg/L	3.467	nmol/L
Dehydroepiandrosterone sulfate	ng/mL	0.002714	μmol/L
11-Deoxycortisol	μg/dL	28.86	nmol/L
Diazepam	mg/L	3512	nmol/L
Digoxin	ng/mL	1.281	nmol/L
Epinephrine	pg/mL	5.458	pmol/L
Estradiol	pg/mL	3.671	pmol/L
Estriol (urine)	μg/24 h	3.468	nmol/d
Estrone (plasma)	pg/ml	3.699	pmol/L
Estrone (urine)	μg/24 h	3.699	nmol/d
Ethanol	mg/dL	0.2171	mmol/L
Fat (fecal), as stearic acid	g/24 h	3.515	mmol/d
Ferritin	ng/mL	1.00	μg/L
Folate	ng/mL	2.226	nmol/L
Follicle stimulating hormone	mIU/mL	1.00	IU/L

APPENDIX A–4. *Continued.*

Analyte	Present unit	Conversion factor	SI unit
Galactose	mg/dL	0.05551	mmol/L
τ-Glutamyltransferase	U/L	1.00	U/L
Gases			
PO$_2$	mm Hg	0.1333	kPa
PCO$_2$	mm Hg	0.1333	kPa
Gastrin	pg/mL	1	ng/L
Glucose	mg/dL	0.05551	mmol/L
Growth hormone	ng/mL	1.00	μg/L
Haptoglobin	mg/dL	0.01	g/L
Homovanillic acid	mg/24 h	5.489	μmol/d
5-Hydroxyindoleacetic acid	mg/24 h	5.230	μmol/d
17-Hydroxyprogesterone	μg/L	3.026	nmol/L
Immunoglobulins			
IgA	mg/dL	0.01	g/L
IgD	mg/dL	10	mg/L
IgE	U/mL	2.4	μg/L
IgG	mg/dL	0.01	g/L
IgM	mg/dL	0.01	g/L
Insulin	mU/L	7.175	pmol/L
Iron	μg/dL	0.1791	μmol/L
Iron-binding capacity	μg/dL	0.1791	μmol/L
Lactate, as lactic acid	mEq/L	1.00	mmol/L
	mg/dL	0.1110	mmol/L
Lactate dehydrogenase	U/L	1.00	U/L
Wrobleski units/mL	0.482	U/L	
Lipase	U/L	1.00	U/L
	Cherry Crandall units	278	U/L
Lipoproteins			
Low density as cholesterol	mg/dL	0.02586	mmol/L
High density as cholesterol	mg/dL	0.02586	mmol/L
Lithium	mEq/L	1.00	mmol/L
Luteinizing hormone (LH)	mIU/mL	1.00	IU/L
Magnesium	mg/dL	0.4114	mmol/L
	mEq/L	0.500	mmol/L
Metanephrines	mg/24 h	5.458	μmol/d
Methanol	mg/dL	0.3121	mmol/L
Methotrexate	mg/L	2.200	μmol/L
Norepinephrine	pg/mL	0.005911	nmol/L
Osmolality	mOsm/kg	1.00	mmol/kg
Oxalate	mg/24 h	11.11	μmol/d
Pentobarbital	mg/L	4.419	μmol/L
Phenobarbital	mg/L	4.306	μmol/L
Phenytoin	mg/L	3.964	μmol/L
Phosphatase, acid	King Armstrong units/dL	1.77	U/L
	Bodansky units/dL	5.37	U/L
	Kind–King units/dL	1.77	U/L
	Bessey–Lowry–Brock units/dL	16.67	U/L
Phosphatase, alkaline	U/L	1.00	U/L
	Bodansky units/dL	5.37	U/L
	King Armstrong units/dL	7.1	U/L
	Bessey–Lowry–Brock units/dL	16.67	U/L
Phosphate, as inorganic phosphorus	mg/dL	0.3229	mmol/L
Porphobilinogen	mg/24 h	4.420	μmol/d
Potassium	mEq/L	1.00	mmol/L
Pregnanediol	mg/24 h	3.120	μmol/d
Pregnanetriol	mg/24 h	2.972	μmol/d
Primidone	mg/L	4.582	μmol/L
Procainamide	mg/L	4.249	μmol/L
N-Acetylprocainamide	mg/L	3.606	μmol/L
Progesterone	ng/mL	3.180	nmol/L
Prolactin	ng/mL	1.00	μg/L
Propranolol	ng/mL	3.856	nmol/L
Protein (total, cerebrospinal fluid)	mg/dL	0.01	g/L

(continued)

APPENDIX A–4. *Continued.*

Analyte	Present unit	Conversion factor	SI unit
Protein (total, serum)	g/dL	10.0	g/L
Protein (total, urine)	mg/24 h	0.001	g/d
Protoporphyrin (erythrocyte)	μg/dL	0.0177	μmol/L
Pyruvate, as pyruvic acid	mg/dL	113.6	μmol/L
Quinidine	mg/L	3.082	μmol/L
Renin	ng/mL/h	0.2778	ng/L/s
Salicylate, as salicylic acid	mg/dL	0.07240	mmol/L
Serotonin	μg/dL	0.05675	μmol/L
Sodium	mEq/L	1.00	mmol/L
Testosterone	ng/mL	3.467	nmol/L
Theophylline	mg/L	5.550	μmol/L
Thiocyanate	mg/dL	0.1722	mmol/L
Thiopental	mg/L	4.126	μmol/L
Thyroid stimulating hormone	μU/mL	1.00	mU/L
Thyroxine (T4)	μg/dL	12.87	nmol/L
Thyroxine, free	ng/dL	12.87	pmol/L
Thyroxine binding globulin, as T4	μg/dL	12.87	nmol/L
Transferrin	mg/dL	0.01	g/L
Triglycerides	mg/dL	0.01129	mmol/L
Triiodothyronine (T3)	ng/dL	0.01536	nmol/L
T3 uptake	%	0.01	1
Urate, as uric acid	mg/dL	59.48	μmol/L
Urea nitrogen	mg/dL	0.3570	mmol/L urea
Urobilinogen	mg/24 h	1.693	μmol/d
Uroporphyrin	μg/24 h	1.204	nmol/d
Valproic acid	mg/L	6.934	μmol/L
Vanillylmandelic acid	mg/24 h	5.046	μmol/d
Vitamin A	μg/dL	0.03491	μmol/L
Vitamin B_{12}	ng/dL	7.378	pmol/L
Vitamin D_3 (25-OH-cholecalciferol)	ng/mL	2.496	nmol/L
Vitamin E	mg/dL	23.22	μmol/L
Zinc (serum)	μg/dL	0.1530	μmol/L
Zinc (urine)	μg/24 h	0.0153	μmol/d

Adapted from the *SI manual in health care,* 2nd ed. Ottawa: Metric Commission of Canada, 1982.

APPENDIX B

Hematologic Values

1. ERYTHROCYTES

APPENDIX B–1a. *Erythrocyte values at various ages: mean and lower limit of normal (±2 SD)*

Age	Hemoglobin (g/dL)		Hematocrit (%)		Erythrocyte count (RBC × 10⁻⁶)		MCV (fl)		MCH (pg)		MCHC (g/dL)	
	Mean	±2 SD	Mean	±2 SD	Mean	±2 SD	Mean	±2 SD	Mean	±2 SD	Mean	±2 SD
Birth (cord blood)	16.5	13.5	51	42	4.7	3.9	108	98	34	31	33	30
1–3 d (capillary)	18.5	14.5	56	45	5.3	4.0	108	95	34	31	33	29
1 wk	17.5	13.5	54	42	5.1	3.9	107	88	34	28	33	28
2 wk	16.5	12.5	51	39	4.9	3.6	105	86	34	28	33	28
1 mo	14	10	43	31	4.2	3	104	85	34	28	33	29
2 mo	11.5	9	35	28	3.8	2.7	96	77	30	26	33	29
3–6 mo	11.5	9.5	35	29	3.8	3.1	91	74	30	25	33	30
0.5–2 yr	12	10.5	36	33	4.5	3.7	78	70	27	23	33	30
2–6 yr	12.5	11.5	37	34	4.6	3.9	81	75	27	24	34	31
6–12 yr	13.5	11.5	40	35	4.6	4	86	77	29	25	34	31
12–18 yr												
Female	14	12	41	36	4.6	4.1	90	78	30	25	34	31
Male	14.5	13	43	37	4.9	4.5	88	78	30	25	34	31
18–49 yr												
Female	14	12	41	36	4.6	4	90	80	30	26	34	31
Male	15.5	13.5	47	41	5.2	4.5	90	80	30	26	34	31

These data were compiled from several sources. Emphasis is placed on studies using electronic counters and on the selection of populations that are likely to exclude individuals with iron deficiency. The mean ±2 SD can be expected to include 95% of the observations in a normal population.

MCH, mean corpuscular hemoglobin; MCHC, mean corpuscular hemoglobin concentration; MCV, mean corpuscular volume; SD, standard deviation.

From Dallman PR. In: Rudolph A, ed. *Pediatrics,* 16th ed. New York: Appleton-Century-Crofts, 1977;1111.

APPENDIX B–1b. *The relative concentration of fetal hemoglobin in infants and its variation with age*

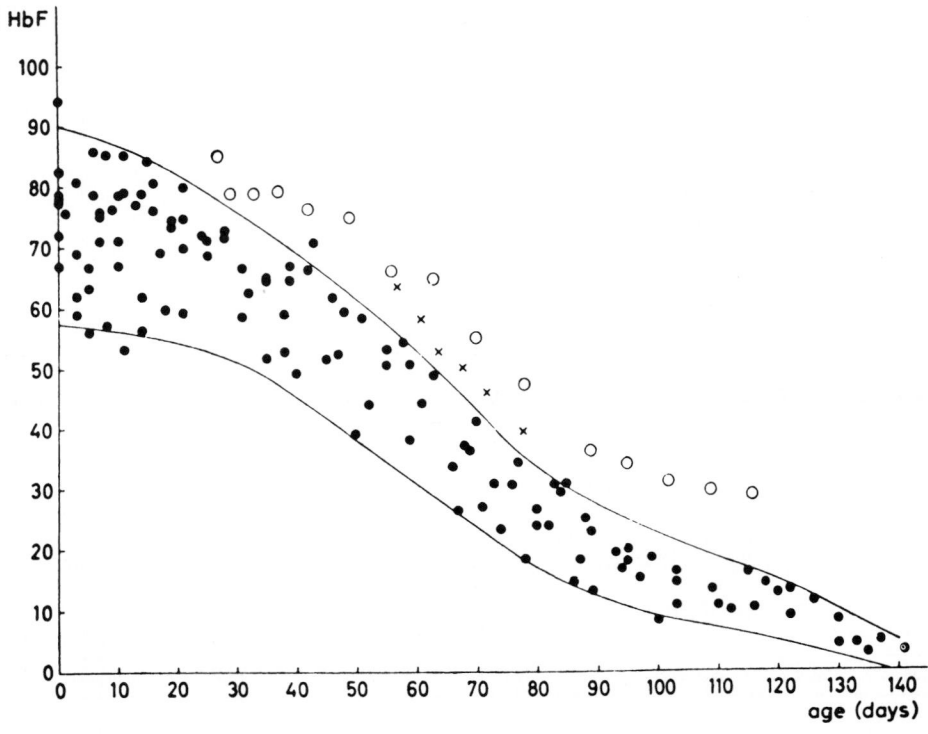

The region between the curved lines contains 120 observations in 17 normal children. HbF, fetal hemoglobin.
From Garby L, Sjolin S. *Acta Paediatr* 1962;51:245.

2. LEUKOCYTES

APPENDIX B–2a. *The leukocyte count and differential count during the first 2 weeks of life (number/mm³)*

Age	Leukocytes	Neutrophils			Eosinophils	Basophils	Lymphocytes	Monocytes
		Total	Segmented	Band				
Birth								
Mean	18,100	11,000	9400	1600	400	100	5500	1050
Range	9,000–30,000	6,000–26,000			20–850	0–640	2,000–11,000	400–3,100
Mean (%)	100	61	52	9	2.2	0.6	31	5.8
7 d								
Mean	12,200	5500	4700	830	500	50	5000	1100
Range	5,000–21,000	1,500–10,000			70–1100	0–250	2,000–17,000	300–2.700
Mean (%)	100	45	39	6	4.1	0.4	41	9.1
14 d								
Mean	11,400	4500	3900	630	350	50	5500	1000
Range	5,000–20,000	1,000–9,500			70–1000	0–230	2,000–17,000	200–2,400
Mean (%)	100	40	34	5.5	3.1	0.4	48	8.8

APPENDIX B–2b. *Total neutrophil count in the first 60 hours of life*

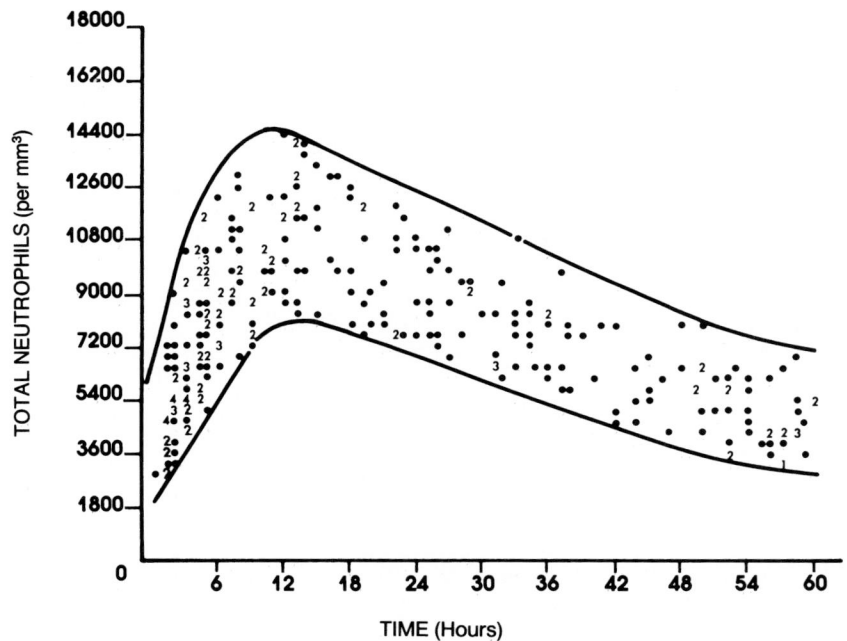

• Single value; number, number of values at the same point; ———, envelope banding the data.
From Monroe BL, et al. *J Pediatr* 1979;95:91.

3. PLATELETS

APPENDIX B–3a. *Venous platelet counts[a] in normal low-birth-weight infants*

Day	Number of Infants	Mean (mm³)	Range (×10,000)
0	60	203,000	80–356
3	47	207,000	61–335
5	14	233,000	100–502
7	52	319,000	124–678
10	40	399,000	172–680
14	50	386,000	147–670
21	47	388,000	201–720
28	40	384,000	212–625

[a]Manual method.
From Appleyard WJ, Bunton WA. *Biol Neonate* 1971;17:30.

APPENDIX B–3b. *Platelet counts in full-term infants*

	Mean	Range (×1,000)
Cord	200,000	100–280
1 d	192,000	100–260
3 d	213,000	80–320
7 d	248,000	100–300
14 d	252,000	

From Behrman R, ed. *Neonatology: diseases of the fetus and infant.* St. Louis: CV Mosby, 1973.

4. BONE MARROW

APPENDIX B–4. *Bone marrow differential counts: mean percent changes with age (range)*

	1 wk	1 mo	3 mo	6 mo	12 mo	Adult
Myeloblasts	0.3 (0–1)	1.2 (0.4–1.9)	2.5	0.4	0.7	0.9 (0.75–1.1)
Promyelocytes	1 (0.5–1.5)	1.8 (1–2.5)	4.5	1.6	2.6	1.9 (1.8–2.1)
Myelocytes	1.6 (0.6–2.4)	4.3 (2.5–7.2)	5.4	1.5	4.8	10.5 (2.4–18.7)
Metamyclocytes	2 (0.7–3)	5.5 (3.1–9.1)	6.9	2	6.2	13.4 (3.1–23.8)
Bands	19 (13–23)	22.9 (17–32)	33.2 (14–52)	8.3	15.7	13.9 (7–20)
Segmented neutrophils	23.3 (9.6–39)	22 (8.7–30.2)	5.8 (4–7.6)	8.1 (3.7–11.5)	10.6	13.9 (9.7–14.6)
Eosinophils	1.3 (1–3)	2.9 (1.9–5.3)	6	3.9	3.2	4 (5–7)
Basophils	<0.1 (0–0.2)	<0.1 (0–0.2)	2.5 (0–5)	0.1	0.2	0.2 (0.2–1.8)
Pronormoblasts	1.6 (0.4–2.5)	0.8 (0.4–1.1)	1.3	0.3	0.2	1 (0.2–2.5)
Normoblasts	37.8 (21–54)	19.1 (12–25)	13.9	18.4 (13–24)	10.4	23.4 (19–29)
Lymphocytes	6.1 (3.7–8)	14.5 (9.5–19)	12.1 (4–20)	51	37.2	24.3 (14–28)
Monocytes	5.3 (2–7.3)	5.2 (3–10)	6.8	5	8	6.3 (2–12)
Plasma cells		0.2 (0–0.2)			0.2	0.8 (0.6–0.9)
M:E ratio	1.24	2.91	3.83	1.4	3.83	2.71

From Miller DR, et al. *Blood diseases of infancy and childhood,* 5th ed. St. Louis: CV Mosby, 1984:27.
See also Rosse C, et al. *J Lab Clin Med* 1977;89:1225; Mauer AM. *Pediatric hematology.* New York: McGraw-Hill, 1969; Jandl JH. *Blood: textbook of hematology.* Boston: Little, Brown & Co., 1987.

5. SERUM IRON AND IRON-BINDING CAPACITY

APPENDIX B–5. *Values of serum iron, total iron-binding capacity, and transferrin saturation in infants during the first year of life*

	0.5 mo of age	1 mo of age	2 mo of age	4 mo of age	6 mo of age	9 mo of age	12 mo of age
SI (median 95% range)							
μM/L	22 (11–36)	22 (10–31)	16 (3–29)	15 (3–29)	14 (5–24)	15 (6–24)	14 (6–28)
μg/dL	120 (63–201)	125 (58–172)	87 (15–159)	84 (18–164)	77 (28–135)	84 (34–135)	78 (35–155)
TIBC (mean ± SD)							
μM/L	34 ± 8	36 ± 8	44 ± 10	54 ± 7	58 ± 9	61 ± 7	64 ± 7
μg/dL	191 ± 43	199 ± 43	246 ± 55	300 ± 39	321 ± 51	341 ± 42	358 ± 38
S% (median 95% range)	68 (30–99)	63 (35–94)	34 (21–63)	27 (7–53)	23 (10–43)	25 (10–39)	23 (10–47)

These data were obtained from a group of healthy, full-term infants who were born at the Helsinki University Central Hospital. Infants received from supplementation in formula and cereal throughout the 12-month period. Infants with hemoglobin below 110 g/dL, mean corpuscular volume of red blood cells below 71 μ^3, or serum ferritin below 10 ng/mL were excluded from the study. The 95% range of the transferrin saturation values indicates that the lower limit of normal is about 10% after 4 months of age.
S%, transferrin saturation; SD, standard deviation; SI, serum iron; TIBC, total iron-binding capacity.
From Saarien UM, Slimes MA. *J Pediatr* 1977;91:876.

6. COAGULATION

APPENDIX B–6a. *Reference values for coagulation tests in healthy premature infants (30 to 36 weeks of gestation) during the first 6 months of life and in the adult*

Tests	Day 1 Mean	Day 1 Boundaries	Day 5 Mean	Day 5 Boundaries	Day 30 Mean	Day 30 Boundaries	Day 90 Mean	Day 90 Boundaries	Day 180 Mean	Day 180 Boundaries	Adult Mean	Adult Boundaries
PT (s)	13.0	(10.6–16.2)[a]	12.5	(10.0–15.3)[a,b]	11.8	(10.0–13.6)[c]	12.3	(10.0–14.6)[c]	12.5	(10.0–15.0)[c]	12.4	(10.8–13.9)
APTT (s)	53.6	(27.5–79.4)[c]	50.5	(26.9–74.1)[c]	44.7	(26.9–62.5)	39.5	(28.3–50.7)	37.5	(21.7–53.3)[c]	33.5	(26.6–40.3)
TCT (s)	24.8	(19.2–30.4)[a]	24.1	(18.8–29.4)[a]	24.4	(18.8–29.9)[a]	25.1	(19.4–30.8)[a]	26.2	(18.9–31.5)[a]	25.0	(19.7–30.3)
Fibrinogen (g/L)	2.43	(1.50–3.73)[a,b,c]	2.80	(1.60–4.18)[a,b,c]	2.54	(1.50–4.14)[a,b]	2.46	(1.50–3.52)[a,b]	2.28	(1.50–3.60)[b]	2.78	(1.56–4.00)
H (u/mL)	0.45	(0.20–0.77)[b]	0.57	(0.29–0.85)[c]	0.57	(0.36–0.95)[b,c]	0.68	(0.30–1.06)	0.87	(0.51–1.23)	1.08	(0.70–1.46)
V (U/mL)	0.88	(0.41–1.44)[a,b,c]	1.00	(0.46–1.54)	1.02	(0.48–1.56)	0.99	(0.59–1.39)	1.02	(0.58–1.46)	1.06	(0.62–1.50)
VII (U/mL)	0.67	(0.21–1.13)	0.84	(0.30–1.38)	0.83	(0.21–1.45)	0.87	(0.31–1.43)	0.99	(0.47–1.51)[a]	1.05	(0.67–1.43)
VIII (U/mL)	1.11	(0.50–2.13)[a,b]	1.15	(0.53–2.05)[a,b,c]	1.11	(0.50–1.99)[a,b,c]	1.06	(0.58–1.88)[a,b,c]	0.99	(0.50–1.87)[a,b,c]	0.99	(0.50–1.49)
vWF (U/mL)	1.36	(0.78–2.10)[b]	1.33	(0.72–2.19)[b]	1.36	(0.66–2.19)[b]	1.12	(0.75–1.84)[a]	0.98	(0.54–1.58)[a,b]	0.92	(0.50–1.58)
IX (U/mL)	0.35	(0.19–0.65)[b,c]	0.42	(0.14–0.74)[b,c]	0.44	(0.13–0.80)[b]	0.59	(0.25–0.93)	0.81	(0.50–1.20)[b]	1.09	(0.55–1.63)
X (U/mL)	0.41	(0.11–0.71)	0.51	(0.19–0.83)	0.56	(0.20–0.92)	0.67	(0.35–0.99)	0.77	(0.35–1.19)	1.06	(0.70–1.52)
XI (U/mL)	0.30	(0.08–0.52)[b,c]	0.41	(0.13–0.69)[c]	0.43	(0.15–0.71)[c]	0.59	(0.25–0.93)[c]	0.78	(0.46–1.10)	0.97	(0.67–1.27)
XII (U/mL)	0.38	(0.10–0.66)[c]	0.39	(0.09–0.69)[c]	0.43	(0.11–0.75)	0.61	(0.15–1.07)	0.82	(0.22–1.42)	1.08	(0.52–1.64)
PK (U/mL)	0.33	(0.09–0.57)	0.45	(0.26–0.75)[b]	0.59	(0.31–0.87)	0.79	(0.37–1.21)	0.78	(0.40–1.16)	1.12	(0.62–1.62)
HMWK (U/mL)	0.49	(0.09–0.89)	0.62	(0.24–1.00)[c]	0.64	(0.16–1.12)[c]	0.78	(0.32–1.24)	0.83	(0.41–1.25)[a]	0.92	(0.50–1.36)
XIIIa (U/mL)	0.70	(0.32–1.08)	1.01	(0.57–1.45)[a]	0.99	(0.51–1.47)[a]	1.13	(0.71–1.55)[a]	1.13	(0.65–1.61)[a]	1.05	(0.55–1.55)
XIIIb (U/mL)	0.81	(0.35–1.27)	1.10	(0.68–1.58)[a]	1.07	(0.57–1.57)[a]	1.21	(0.75–1.67)	1.15	(0.67–1.63)	0.97	(0.57–1.37)
Plasminogen (CTA, U/mL)	1.70	(1.12–2.48)[b,c]	1.91	(1.21–2.61)[c]	1.81	(1.09–2.53)	2.38	(1.58–3.18)	2.75	(1.91–3.59)[c]	3.36	(2.48–4.24)

All factors except fibrinogen and plasminogen are expressed as U/mL, where pooled plasma contains 1.0 U/mL. Plasminogen units are those recommended by the Committee on Thrombolytic Agents (CTA). All values are given as a mean followed by the lower and upper boundaries encompassing 95% of the population. Between 40 and 96 samples were assayed for each value for newborns.

[a]Values indistinguishable from those of adults.

[b]Measurements are skewed owing to a disproportionate number of high values. Lower limit, which excludes the lower 2.5% of the population, is given.

[c]Values different from those of full-term infants.

APTT, activated partial thromboplastin time; H, biotin; HMWK, high-molecular-weight kininogen; PK, pyruvate kinase; PT, prothrombin time; TCT, thrombin clotting time; VIII, factor VIII coagulant; vWF, von Willebrand factor.

From Andrew M, et al. Development of the coagulation system in the healthy premature infant. *Blood* 1988;72:1653.

APPENDIX B–6b. *Reference values for coagulation inhibitors in healthy premature infants during the first 6 months of life and in the adult*

Tests	Day 1		Day 5		Day 30		Day 90		Day 180		Adult	
	Mean	Boundaries	Mean	Boundaries	Mean	Boundaries	Mean	Boundaries	Mean	Boundaries	Mean	Boundaries
AT-III (U/mL)	0.38	(0.14–0.62)[c]	0.56	(0.30–0.82)[a]	0.59	(0.37–0.81)[c]	0.83	(0.45–1.21)[c]	0.90	(0.52–1.28)[c]	1.05	(0.79–1.31)
α_2M (U/mL)	1.10	(0.56–1.82)[b,c]	1.25	(0.71–1.77)[a]	1.38	(0.72–2.04)	1.80	(1.20–2.66)[b]	2.09	(1.10–3.21)[b]	0.86	(0.52–1.20)
α_2AP (U/mL)	0.78	(0.40–1.16)	0.81	(0.49–1.13)[a]	0.89	(0.55–1.23)[c]	1.06	(0.64–1.48)[a]	1.15	(0.77–1.53)	1.02	(0.68–1.36)
C_1INH (U/mL)	0.65	(0.31–0.99)	0.83	(0.45–1.21)	0.74	(0.40–1.24)[b,c]	1.14	(0.60–1.68)[a]	1.40	(0.96–2.04)[b]	1.01	(0.71–1.31)
α_2AT (U/mL)	0.90	(0.36–1.44)[a]	0.94	(0.42–1.46)[c]	0.76	(0.38–1.12)[c]	0.81	(0.49–1.13)[a,c]	0.82	(0.48–1.16)[a]	0.93	(0.55–1.31)
HCII (U/mL)	0.32	(0.00–0.60)[c]	0.34	(0.00–0.69)[a]	0.43	(0.15–0.71)	0.61	(0.20–1.11)[b]	0.89	(0.45–1.40)[a,b,c]	0.96	(0.66–1.26)
Protein C (U/mL)	0.28	(0.12–0.44)[a,c]	0.31	(0.11–0.51)[a]	0.37	(0.15–0.59)[c]	0.45	(0.23–0.67)[c]	0.57	(0.31–0.83)	0.96	(0.64–1.28)
Protein S (U/mL)	0.26	(0.14–0.38)[c]	0.37	(0.13–0.61)[a]	0.56	(0.22–0.90)	0.76	(0.40–1.12)[c]	0.82	(0.44–1.20)	0.92	(0.60–1.24)

All values are expressed in U/mL, where pooled plasma contains 1.0 U/mL. All values are given as a mean followed by the lower and upper boundaries encompassing 95% of the population. Between 40 and 75 samples were assayed for each value for newborns.

[a]Values indistinguishable from those of adults.

[b]Measurements are skewed owing to a disproportionate number of high values. Lower limit, which excludes the lower 2.5% of the population, is given.

[c]Values different from those of full-term infants.

α_2AP, α_2-antiplasmin; α_2AT, α_2-antitrypsin; α_2M, α_2-macroglobulin; AT-III, antithrombin-III; C_1INH, C_1 esterase inhibitor; HCII, heparin cofactor II.

From Andrew M, et al. Development of the coagulation system in the healthy premature infant. *Blood* 1988;72:1653.

APPENDIX B–6c. *Reference values for coagulation tests in the healthy full-term infant during the first 6 months of life and in the adult*

Tests	Day 1	Day 5	Day 30	Day 90	Day 180	Adult
PT (s)	13.0 ± 1.43 (61)[a]	12.4 ± 1.46 (77)[a,b]	11.8 ± 1.25 (67)[a,b]	11.9 ± 1.15 (62)[b]	12.3 ± 0.79 (47)[a]	12.4 ± 0.78 (29)
APTT (s)	42.9 ± 5.80 (61)	42.6 ± 8.62 (76)	40.4 ± 7.42 (67)	37.1 ± 6.52 (62)[b]	35.5 ± 3.71 (47)[a]	33.5 ± 3.44 (29)
TCT (s)	23.5 ± 2.38 (58)[a]	23.1 ± 3.07 (64)[b]	24.3 ± 2.44 (53)[a]	25.1 ± 2.32 (52)[a]	25.5 ± 2.86 (41)[a]	25.0 ± 2.66 (19)
Fibrinogen (g/L)	2.83 ± 0.58 (61)[a]	3.12 ± 0.75 (77)[a]	2.70 ± 0.54 (67)[a]	2.43 ± 0.68 (60)[a,b]	2.51 ± 0.68 (47)[a,b]	2.78 ± 0.61 (29)
II (U/mL)	0.48 ± 0.11 (61)	0.63 ± 0.15 (76)	0.68 ± 0.17 (67)	0.75 ± 0.15 (62)	0.88 ± 0.14 (47)	1.08 ± 0.19 (29)
V (U/mL)	0.72 ± 0.18 (61)	0.95 ± 0.25 (76)	0.98 ± 0.18 (67)	0.90 ± 0.21 (62)	0.91 ± 0.18 (47)	1.06 ± 0.22 (29)
VII (U/mL)	0.66 ± 0.19 (60)	0.89 ± 0.27 (75)	0.90 ± 0.24 (67)	0.91 ± 0.26 (62)	0.87 ± 0.20 (47)	1.05 ± 0.19 (29)
VIII (U/mL)	1.00 ± 0.39 (60)[a,b]	0.88 ± 0.33 (75)[a,b]	0.91 ± 0.33 (67)[a,b]	0.79 ± 0.23 (62)[a,b]	0.73 ± 0.18 (47)[b]	0.99 ± 0.25 (29)
vWF (U/mL)	1.53 ± 0.67 (40)[b]	1.40 ± 0.57 (43)[b]	1.28 ± 0.59 (40)[b]	1.18 ± 0.44 (40)[b]	1.07 ± 0.45 (46)[b]	0.92 ± 0.33 (29)[b]
IX (U/mL)	0.53 ± 0.19 (59)	0.53 ± 0.19 (75)	0.51 ± 0.15 (67)	0.67 ± 0.23 (62)	0.86 ± 0.25 (47)	1.09 ± 0.27 (29)
X (U/mL)	0.40 ± 0.14 (60)	0.49 ± 0.15 (76)	0.59 ± 0.14 (67)	0.71 ± 0.18 (62)	0.78 ± 0.20 (47)	1.06 ± 0.23 (29)
XI (U/mL)	0.38 ± 0.14 (60)	0.55 ± 0.16 (74)	0.53 ± 0.13 (67)	0.69 ± 0.14 (62)	0.86 ± 0.24 (47)	0.97 ± 0.15 (29)
XII (U/mL)	0.53 ± 0.20 (60)	0.47 ± 0.18 (75)	0.49 ± 0.16 (67)	0.67 ± 0.21 (62)	0.77 ± 0.19 (47)	1.08 ± 0.28 (29)
PK (U/mL)	0.37 ± 0.16 (45)[b]	0.48 ± 0.14 (51)	0.57 ± 0.17 (48)	0.73 ± 0.16 (46)	0.86 ± 0.15 (43)	1.12 ± 0.25 (29)
HMWK (U/mL)	0.54 ± 0.24 (47)	0.74 ± 0.28 (63)	0.77 ± 0.22 (50)[a]	0.82 ± 032 (46)[b]	0.82 ± 0.23 (48)[a]	0.92 ± 0.22 (29)
XIIIa (U/mL)	0.79 ± 0.26 (44)	0.94 ± 0.25 (49)[a]	0.93 ± 0.27 (44)[a]	1.04 ± 0.34 (44)[a]	1.04 ± 0.29 (41)[a]	1.05 ± 0.25 (29)
XIIIb (U/mL)	0.76 ± 0.23 (44)	1.06 ± 0.37 (47)[a]	1.11 ± 0.36 (45)[a]	1.16 ± 0.34 (44)[a]	1.10 ± 0.30 (41)[a]	0.97 ± 0.20 (29)
Plasminogen (CTA, U/mL)	1.95 ± 0.35 (44)	2.17 ± 0.38 (60)	1.98 ± 0.36 (52)	2.48 ± 0.37 (44)	3.01 ± 0.40 (47)	3.36 ± 0.44 (29)

All factors except fibrinogen and plasminogen are expressed as U/mL, where pooled plasma contains 1.0 U/mL. Plasminogen units are those recommended by the Committee on Thrombolytic Agents (CTA).
All values are expressed as mean ±1 SD.

[a]Values that do not differ statistically from the adult values.

[b]These measurements are skewed because of a disproportionate number of high values. The lower limit, which excludes the lower 2.5th percentile of the population, has been given in the respective figures. The lower limit for factor VIII was 0.50 U/mL at all times points for the infant.

APTT, activated partial thromboplastin time; HMWK, high-molecular-weight kininogen; PK, pyruvate kinase; PT, prothrombin time; TCT, thrombin clotting time; vWF, von Willebrand factor.

From Andrew M, et al. Development of the human coagulation system in the full-term infant. *Blood* 187; 70:166.

APPENDIX B–6d. *Reference values for the inhibition of coagulation in the healthy full-term infant during the first 6 months of life and in the adult*

Tests	Day 1	Day 5	Day 30	Day 90	Day 180	Adult
AT-III	0.63 ± 0.12 (58)	0.67 ± 0.13 (74)	0.78 ± 0.15 (66)	0.97 ± 0.12 (60)[a]	1.04 ± 0.10 (56)[a]	1.05 ± 0.13 (28)
α₂M	1.39 ± 0.22 (54)	1.48 ± 0.25 (73)	1.50 ± 0.22 (61)	1.76 ± 0.25 (55)	1.91 ± 0.21 (55)	0.86 ± 0.17 (29)
α₂AP	0.85 ± 0.15 (55)	1.00 ± 0.15 (75)[a]	1.00 ± 0.12 (62)[a]	1.08 ± 0.16 (55)[a]	1.11 ± 0.14 (53)[a]	1.02 ± 0.17 (29)
C₁INH	0.72 ± 0.18 (59)	0.90 ± 0.15 (76)[a]	0.89 ± 0.21 (63)	1.15 ± 0.22 (55)	1.41 ± 0.26 (55)	1.01 ± 0.15 (29)
α₁AT	0.83 ± 0.22 (57)[a]	0.89 ± 0.20 (75)[a]	0.62 ± 0.13 (61)	0.72 ± 0.15 (56)	0.77 ± 0.15 (55)	0.93 ± 0.19 (29)
HCII	0.43 ± 0.25 (56)	0.48 ± 0.24 (72)	0.47 ± 0.20 (58)	0.72 ± 0.37 (58)	1.20 ± 0.35 (55)	0.96 ± 0.15 (29)
Protein C	0.35 ± 0.09 (41)	0.42 ± 0.11 (44)	0.43 ± 0.11 (43)	0.54 ± 0.13 (44)	0.59 ± 0.11 (52)	0.96 ± 0.16 (28)
Protein S	0.36 ± 0.12 (40)	0.50 ± 0.14 (48)	0.63 ± 0.15 (41)	0.86 ± 0.16 (46)[a]	0.87 ± 0.16 (49)[a]	0.92 ± 0.16 (29)

All values are expressed in U/mL as the mean ±1 SD.

[a]Values that do not differ statistically from the adult values.

α₂AP, α₂-antiplasmin; α₁AT, α₁-antitrypsin; α₂M, α₂ macroglobulin; AT-III, antithrombin III; C₁INH, C₁ esterase inhibitor; HCII, heparin cofactor II.

From Andrew M, et al. Development of the coagulation system in the full-term infant. *Blood* 1987;70:167.

APPENDIX C

Physiologic Values

1. BLOOD PRESSURE AND HYPERTENSION

APPENDIX C–1a. *Average systolic, diastolic, and mean blood pressures during the first 12 hours of life in normal newborn infants grouped according to birth weight*

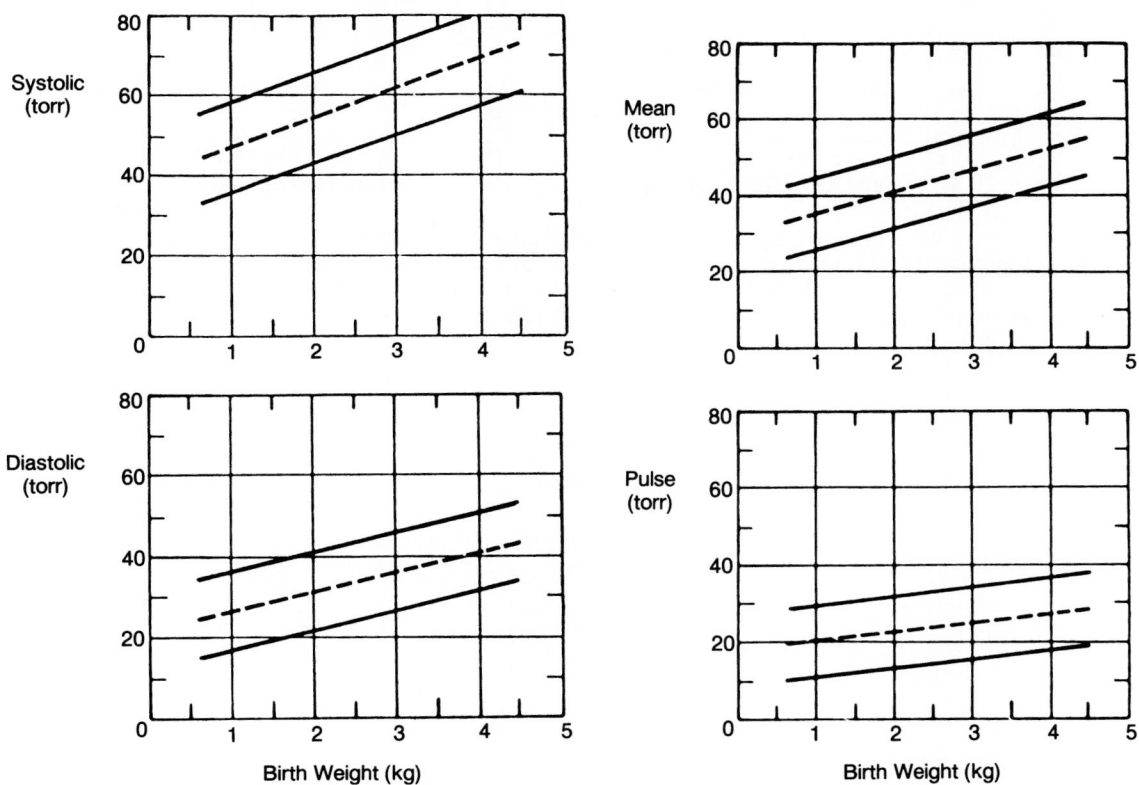

Pressures were obtained by direct measurement through umbilical artery catheter in healthy newborn infants during the first 12 hours of life. Broken lines represent linear regressions; solid lines represent 95% confidence limits.

From Versmold HT, Kitterman JA, Phibbs RH, et al. Aortic blood pressure during the first 12 hours of life in infants with birth weight 610 to 4220 grams. *Pediatrics* 1981;67(5):611. Copyright © American Academy of Pediatrics, 1981.

APPENDIX C–1b. *Evolution of systolic blood pressure during the first month of life in premature infants*

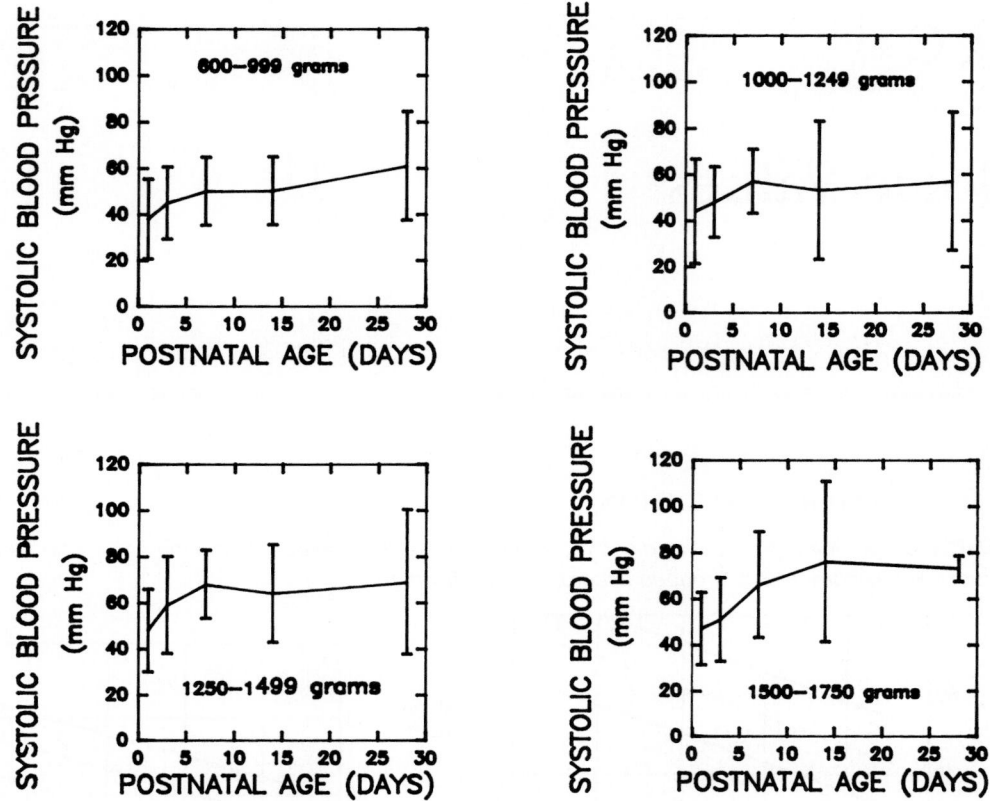

These values were obtained by Doppler or by oscillometric technique (i. e., Dinamap) in well infants (i. e., in the absence of respiratory distress syndrome, sepsis, or heart failure.) Each point represents the mean ± 2 standard deviations for systolic or diastolic blood pressure from 5 to 18 infants.
Adapted from Ingelfinger J, et al. *Pediatr Res* 1983;17:319.

APPENDIX C–1c. *Evolution of mean blood pressure in premature infants*

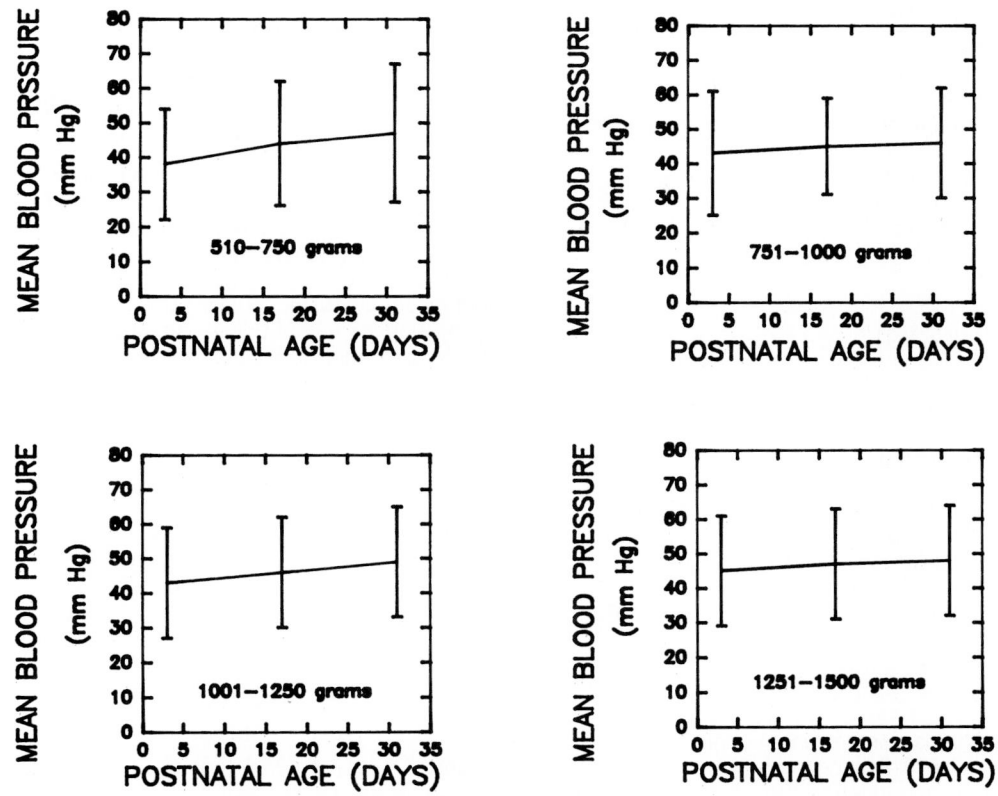

These values were obtained by oscillometric technique (i. e., Dinamap) in 896 infants. Each point represents the mean ± 2 standard deviations. The mean GA in these 4 groups was 25.6, 27.3, 29.0, and 30.3 weeks, respectively.

Adapted from Fanaroff AA, et al. *Pediatr Res* 1990;27:205

APPENDIX C–1d. *Evolution of systolic blood pressure in full-term infants*

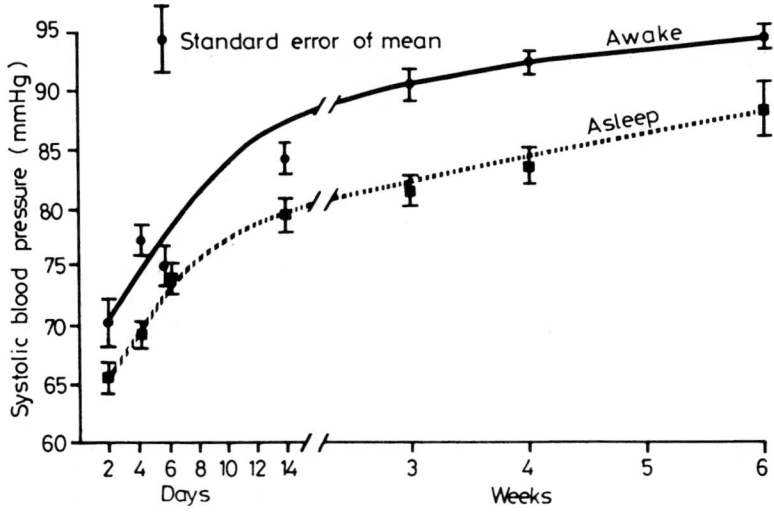

Systolic blood pressure was measured in 99 full-term infants (gestational age ≥ 38 weeks) using a Doppler technique, first in the maternity ward and then at home. Each value was the average of 3 successive measurements. Values represent the mean ± the standard error of mean. Note the difference between the measurements awake (*top*) and asleep (*bottom*).

From Earley A, et al. *Arch Dis Child* 1980;55:755.

APPENDIX C–1e. *Causes of neonatal or infantile hypertension and specific therapy*

Diagnosis	Specific treatment/approach
Inaccurate Diagnosis	
Agitation, crying, pain, procedure	Local or general anesthesia; consider sedation
Indirect measurement: too small cuff	Cuff width: limb circumference ratio should be 0.45–0.55
Direct measurement: poor transducer calibration	Calibrate routinely
Iatrogenic	
Excessive sodium or fluid intake	Diuretics, fluid restriction, PD, hemofiltration
Aminophylline, theophylline	Hold, check level, decrease dose, consider D/C
Adrenergic agents by mouth, IV, aerosols, or eye drops	Decrease dose, use a more selective agonist, or D/C
Cortocosteroids	Decrease dose, consider D/C, or treat symptomatically
Vitamin D	Hold vitamin D, correct hypercalcemia if any
Doxapram	Hold, decrease dose, consider D/C
Pancuronium	Try infusion instead of bolus; use other medication
ECMO	Check fluid intake; induce diuresis
Surgical repair of omphalocele or gastroschisis	Symptomatic therapy
Bronchopulmonary dysplasia	
Pneumothorax (initially)	Most often needs test tube
Renovascular Hypertension	
Thrombus or embolism of the aorta and/or renal artery	Heparin, urokinase, or PTA, surgery if refractory hypertension
Stenosis or hypoplasia of the renal artery and aorta	Surgery
Segmental intimal hyperplasia	Surgery
Idiopathic arterial calcification of infancy	Biphosphonate, flunarizine
Intramural hematoma of the renal artery	Surgery
Extrinsic compression: urinoma, hematoma, adrenal hemorrhage	Surgery
Renal vein thrombosis	Surgery if refractory hypertension
Renal	
Acquired	
Acute tubular necrosis, interstitial nephritis	
Renal medullary or cortical necrosis	Surgery if refractory hypertension
Renal tumor: Wilms, congenital mesoblastic nephroma	Chemotherapy and surgery
Postoperative: urinary tract obstruction	Surgery
Neurofibromatosis	
Congenital	
Dysplasia, hypoplasia, glomerular dysgenesis	Surgery if refractory hypertension
Polycystic or multicystic kidney disease	Surgery if refractory hypertension
Cockayne syndrome	
Gordon syndrome	Thiazide
Liddle's syndrome (pseudoaldosteronism)	KCl and aldosterone-independent K-sparing diuretic
Acquired or congenital	
Urinary tract obstruction	Surgery
Nephrolithiasis, nephrocalcinosis	Replace furosemide by thiazide, if possible
Acute or chronic renal failure	Consider peritoneal dialysis or hemofiltration
Coarctation of the Aorta	Prostaglandin E_1 for initial stabilization; surgery
Neurologic	
Pain	Appropriate pain medicine
Drug withdrawal: narcotics	Phenobarbital, diazepam, paregoric, or methadone
Drug intoxication through placenta or breast milk: cocaine	
Intracranial hypertension	Hyperventilation or surgery
Seizures	Phenobarbital, dilantin, lorazepam
Familial dysautonomia	
Endocrine	
Congenital adrenal hyperplasia	
11β-Hydroxylase deficiency	Cortisol
17α-Hydroxylase deficiency	Cortisol
11β-Hydroxysteroid dehydrogenase deficiency	Cortisol
Dexamethasone-suppressible hyperaldosteronism	Dexamethasone
Primary hyperaldosteronism	Surgery (tumor)
Cushing disease	Surgery (tumor)
Hyperthyroidism	Lugol; propylthiouracil or methimazole
Neural crest tumors	
Neuroblastoma	Radiotherapy, chemotherapy, and surgery
ganglioneuroma, pheochromocytoma	Surgery with several antihypertension medications

continue; ECMO: extracorporeal membrane oxygenation; PD, peritoneal dialysis; PTA, plasma
astin antecedent.

APPENDIX C–1f. *Work-up of neonatal hypertension*

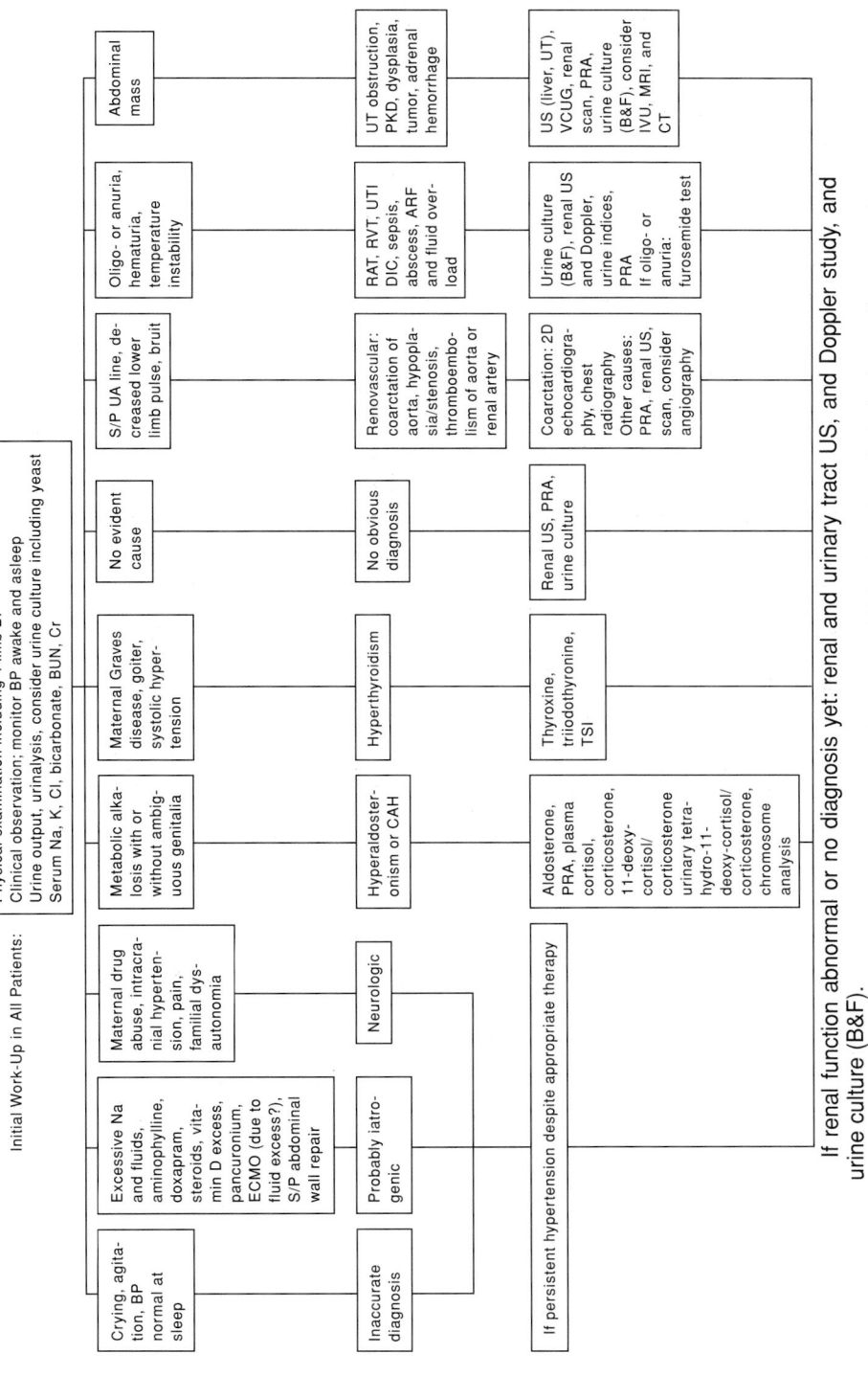

If renal function abnormal or no diagnosis yet: renal and urinary tract US, and Doppler study, and urine culture (B&F).

If no diagnosis yet, consider: plasma aldosterone, PRA, thyroxin, triiodothyrine, urinary catecholamines and metabolites, urine aldosterone, renal vein PRA, long bone radiographs, plain abdomen radiograph, IVU, MRI, CT.

If severe or persistent hypertension; chest radiograph, 2D echocardiography, ECG, eye fungus.

After the initial work-up, the patient should be classified according to the most pertinent features (*top*); this leads to a series of presumptive diagnoses (*middle*) and to further diagnostic tests (*bottom*).

2D, two-dimensional; ARF, acute renal failure; B&F, bacterial and fungal; BP, blood pressure; BUN, blood urea nitrogen; CAH, congenital adrenal hyperplasia; CT, computed tomography; DIC, disseminated intravascular coagulation; ECG, echocardiography; ECMO, extracorporeal membrane oxygenation; IVU, intravenous urography; MRI, magnetic resonance imaging; Pcr, plasma creatinine concentration; PKD, polycystic kidney disease; PRA, plasma renin activity; RAT, renal artery thrombosis; RVT, renal vein thrombosis; S/P, status post; TSI, thyroid stimulating immunoglobulin; UA, umbilical artery; US ultrasonography; UT, urinary tract; UTI, urinary tract infection; VCUG, voiding cystourethrogram.

2. SIGGAARD-ANDERSEN NOMOGRAM

APPENDIX C–2. *Siggaard-Andersen nomogram*

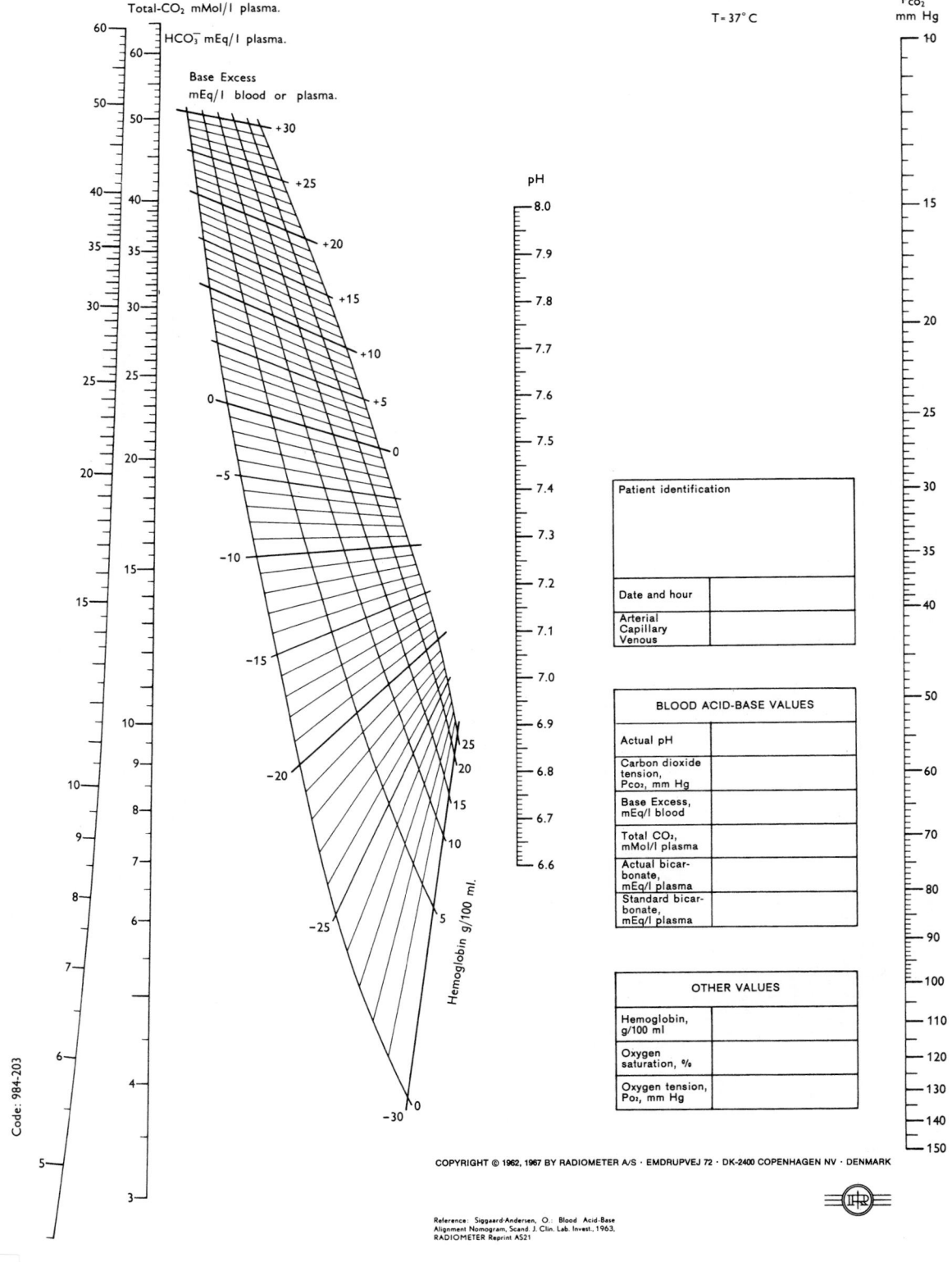

From Siggaard-Andersen O. Blood acid-base alignment nomogram. *Scand J Clin Lab Invest* 1963; *Radiometer* reprint AS21.

3. RIGHT-TO-LEFT SHUNT CURVES

APPENDIX C–3. *Right-to-left shunt curves*

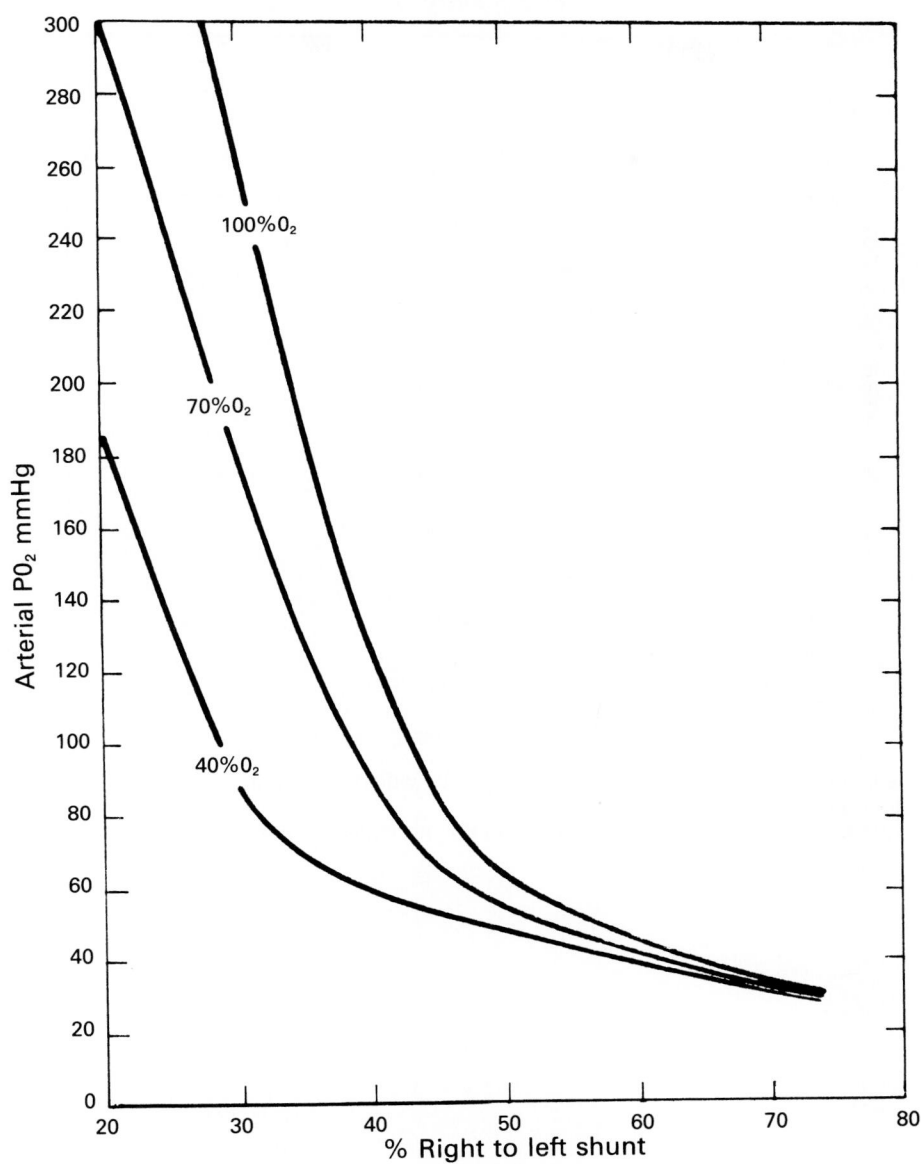

Arterial oxygen tensions at different right-to-left shunts, breathing 40%, 70%, and 100% oxygen. Calculations assumed hemoglobin 16 g/dl, arterial pH 7.4, temperature 37°C, constant arteriovenous saturation difference 13.8%, and no change in cardiac output or oxygen consumption.

From Barnett H. Pediatrics. 15th ed. Englewood Cliffs, NJ: Appleton-Century-Crofts, 1972.

4. HEMOGLOBIN–OXYGEN DISSOCIATION CURVES

APPENDIX C-4. *Oxygen dissociation curves of fetal and adult hemoglobins at a pH of 7.4 and temperature of 37°C*

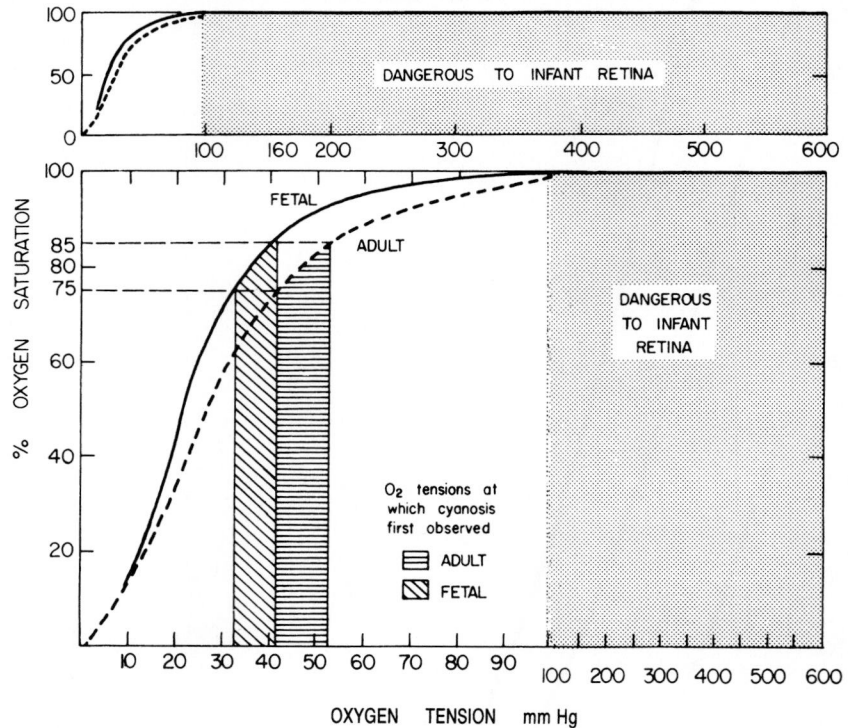

Cyanosis is observed at 5 g unsaturated hemoglobin, which corresponds to different arterial tensions in the adult and the infant.

From Klaus MH, Fanaroff AA. Care of the high risk neonate. Philadelphia: WB Saunders, 1973.

5. BLOOD VOLUMES

5. Blood Volumes / 1525

APPENDIX C–5. *Estimated blood volumes*

Age	Plasma volume (mL/kg)	Erythrocyte mass (mL/kg)	Total blood volume (mL/kg)	
			From plasma volume	From erythrocyte mass
Newborn	41.3	43.1	82.1	86.1
	46		78	84.7
1–7 d	51–54		82–86	
		37.9		77.8
1–12 mo	46.1		78.1	
		25.5		72.8
1–3 yr	44.4		73.8	
	47.2		81.8	
		24.9		69.1
4–6 yr	48.5		80	
	49.6		85.6	
		25.5		67.5
7–9 yr	52.2		87.6	
	49		86.1	
		24.3		67.5
10–12 yr	51.9		87.6	
	46.2		83.2	
		26.3		67.4
13–15 yr	51.2		88.3	
16–18 yr	50.1		90.2	
Adult	39–44	25–30	68–88	55–75

From Price DC, Ries C. In: Handmaker H, Lowenstein JM, eds. *Nuclear medicine in clinical pediatrics.* New York: Society of Nuclear Medicine, 1975.

APPENDIX D

Growth Parameters

1. INTRAUTERINE GROWTH CURVES

APPENDIX D–1. *The Colorado intrauterine growth charts*

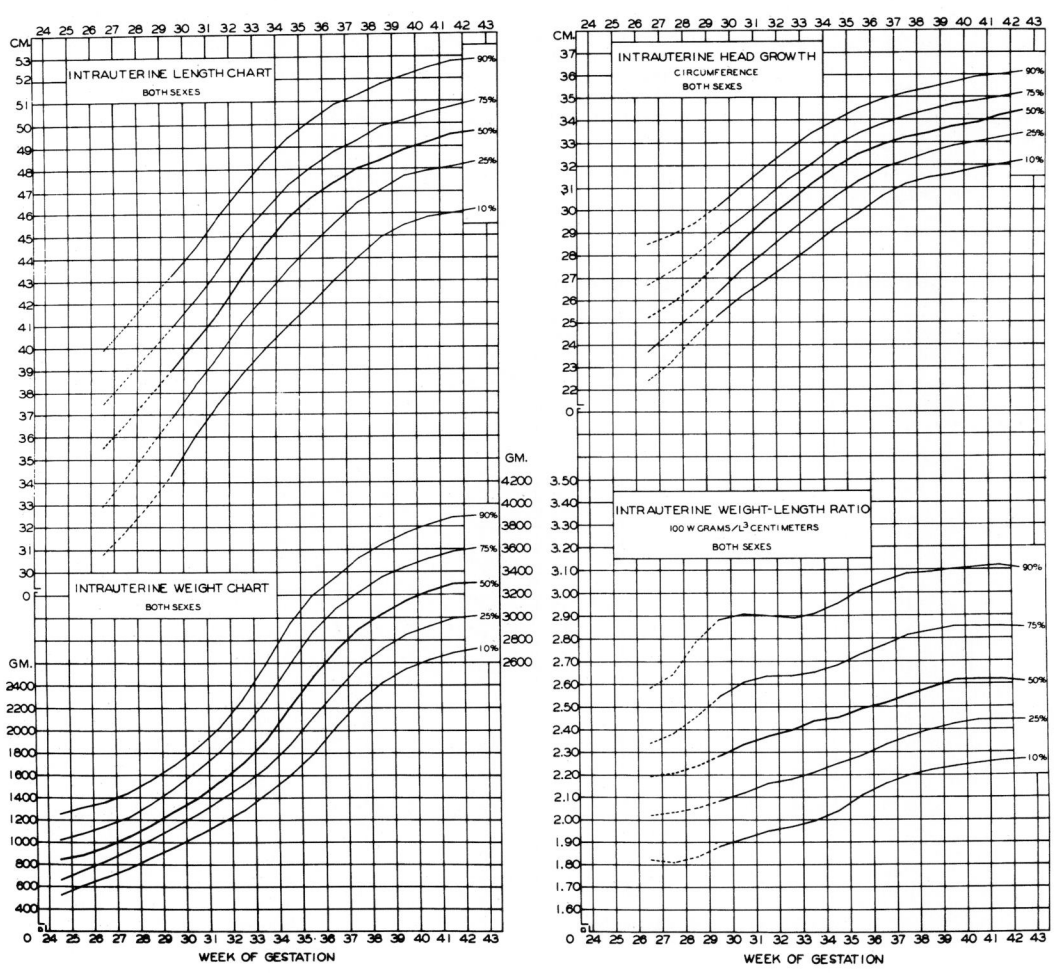

The Colorado curves give percentiles of intrauterine growth for weight, length, and head circumference.

From Lubchenco LO, Hansman C, Boyd E. *Pediatrics* 1966;37:403. Copyright © American Academy of Pediatrics, 1966.

2. INTRAUTERINE GROWTH CURVES FOR TWINS

APPENDIX D–2a. *Intrauterine growth chart for monochorionic twins, both genders*

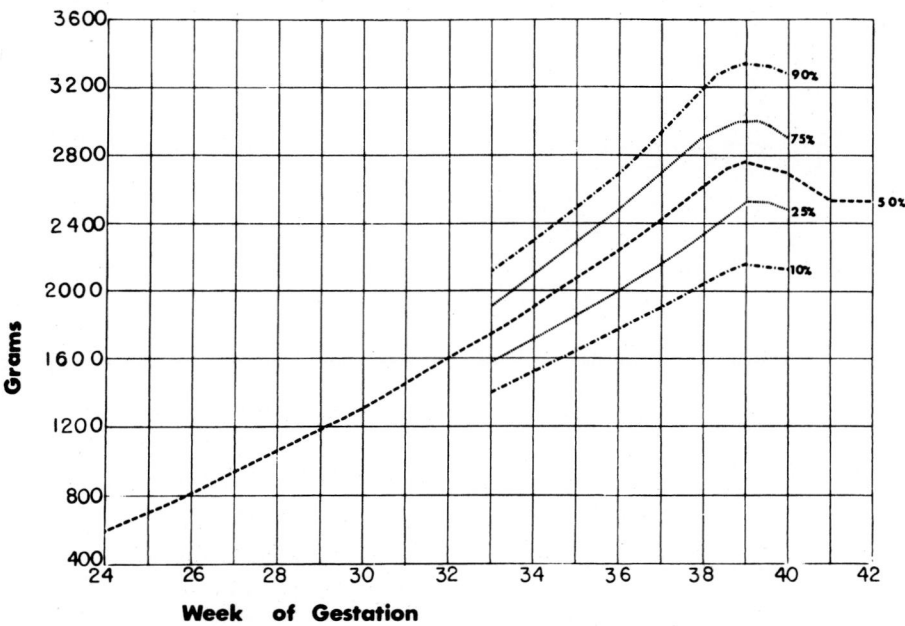

The weights of liveborn monochorionic twins at 24 to 42 weeks gestational ages are graphed as percentages.

From Naeye R, Bernirschke K, Hagstrom J, et al. *Pediatrics* 1966;37:409. Copyright © American Academy of Pediatrics, 1966.

APPENDIX D–2b. *Intrauterine growth chart for dichorionic twins, both genders*

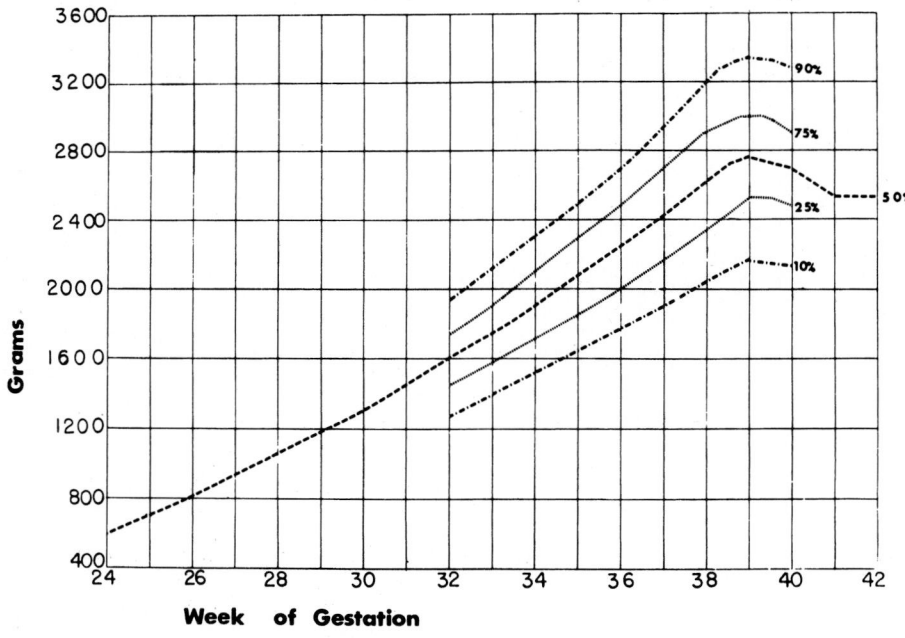

From Naeye R, Bernirschke K, Hagstrom J, et al. *Pediatrics* 1966;37:409. Copyright © American Academy of Pediatrics, 1966.

3. POSTNATAL GROWTH CURVES FOR FULL-TERM INFANTS

APPENDIX D–3a. *Postnatal growth curves, boys*

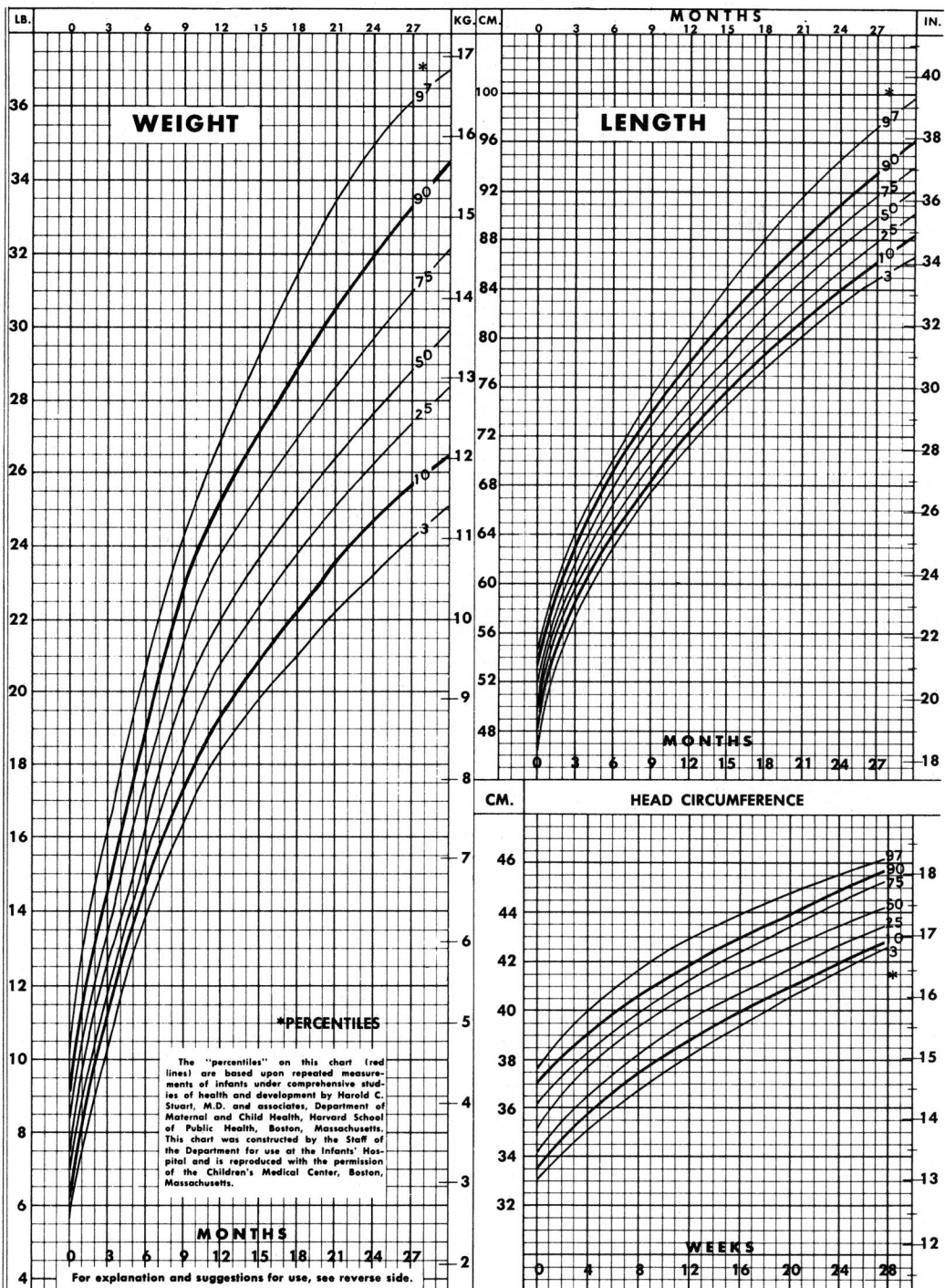

Courtesy of The Children's Medical Center, Boston, MA.

APPENDIX D–3b. *Postnatal growth curves, girls*

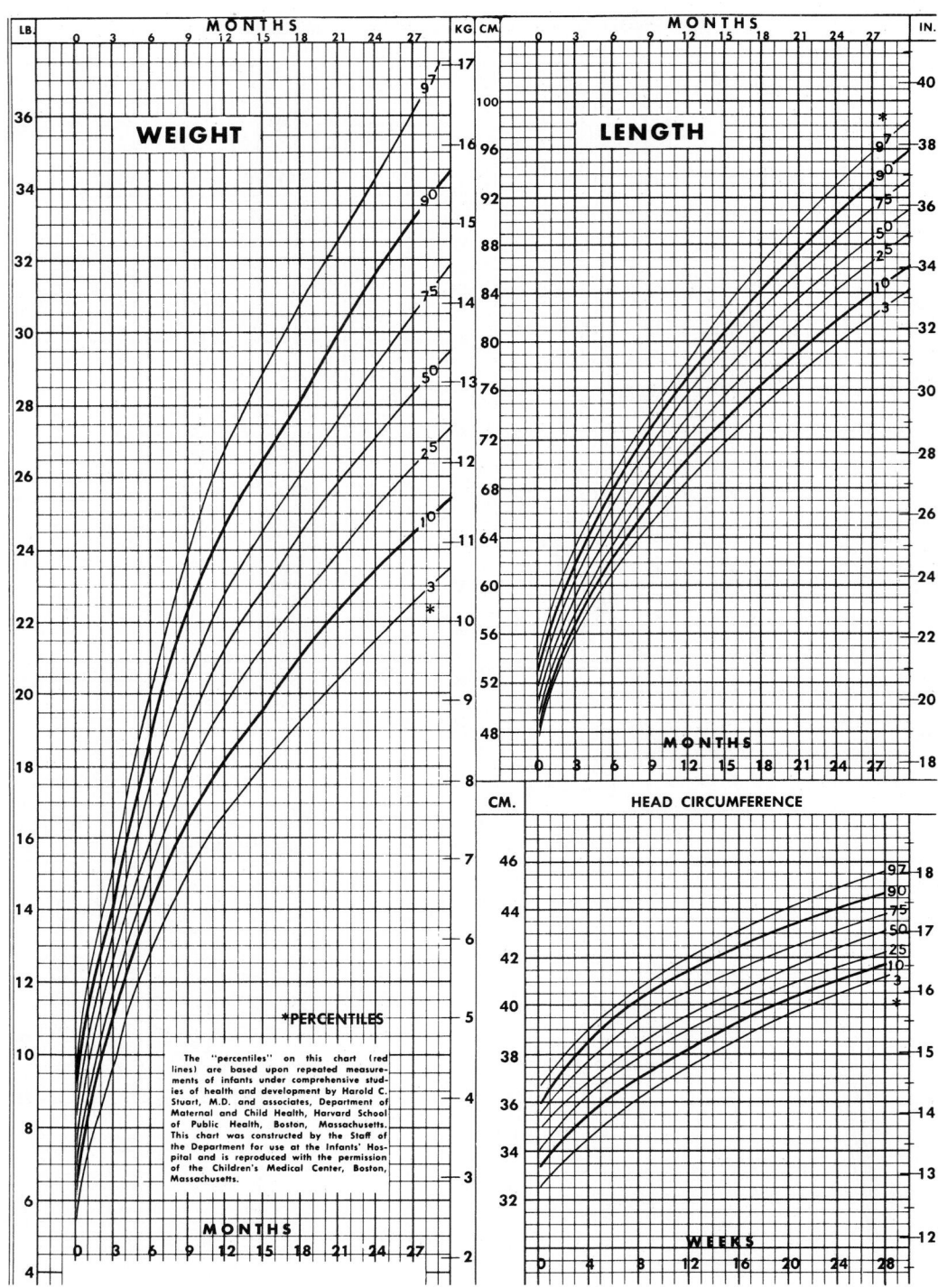

Courtesy of The Children's Medical Center, Boston, MA.

4. HEAD CIRCUMFERENCE

APPENDIX D–4a. *Head circumference, boys*

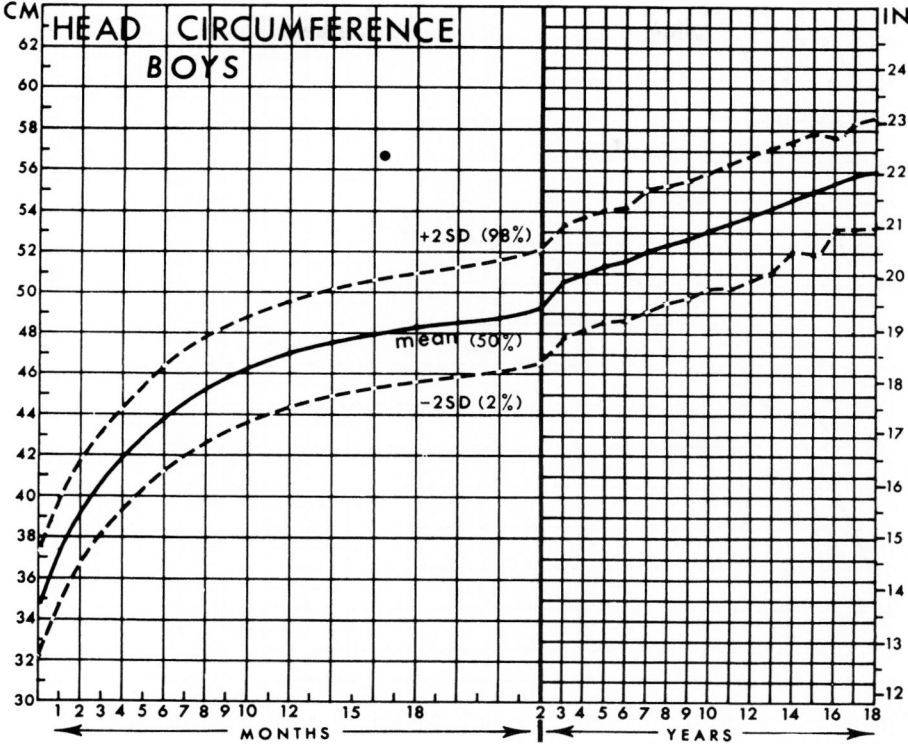

From Nellhaus G. Head circumference from birth to eighteen years: practical composite international and interracial graphs. *Pediatrics* 1968;41:106.

APPENDIX D–4b. *Head circumference, girls*

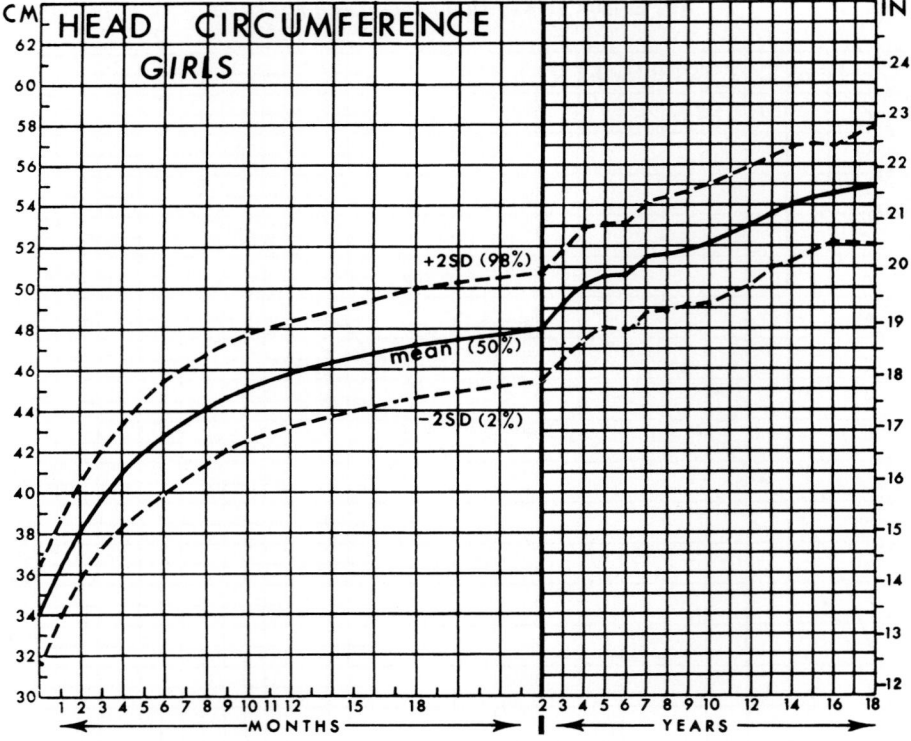

From Nellhaus G. Head circumference from birth to eighteen years: practical composite international and interracial graphs. *Pediatrics* 1968;41:106

5. WEIGHT CONVERSION

APPENDIX D–5. Conversions of pounds and ounces to grams

Pounds	Ounces															
	0	1	2	3	4	5	6	7	8	9	10	11	12	13	14	15
0		28	57	85	113	142	170	198	227	255	283	312	340	369	397	425
1	454	482	510	539	567	595	624	652	680	709	737	765	794	822	850	879
2	907	936	964	992	1021	1049	1077	1106	1134	1162	1191	1219	1247	1276	1304	1332
3	1361	1389	1417	1446	1474	1503	1531	1559	1588	1616	1644	1673	1701	1729	1758	1786
4	1814	1843	1871	1899	1928	1956	1984	2013	2041	2070	2098	2126	2155	2183	2211	2240
5	2268	2296	2325	2353	2381	2410	2438	2466	2495	2523	2551	2580	2608	2637	2665	2693
6	2722	2750	2778	2807	2835	2863	2892	2920	2948	2977	3005	3033	3062	3090	3118	3147
7	3175	3203	3232	3260	3289	3317	3345	3374	3402	3430	3459	3487	3515	3544	3572	3600
8	3629	3657	3685	3714	3742	3770	3799	3827	3856	3884	3912	3941	3969	3997	4026	4054
9	4082	4111	4139	4167	4196	4224	4252	4281	4309	4337	4366	4394	4423	4451	4479	4508
10	4536	4564	4593	4621	4649	4678	4706	4734	4763	4791	4819	4848	4876	4904	4933	4961
11	4990	5018	5046	5075	5103	5131	5160	5188	5216	5245	5273	5301	5330	5358	5386	5415
12	5443	5471	5500	5528	5557	5585	5613	5642	5670	5698	5727	5755	5783	5812	5840	5868
13	5897	5925	5953	5982	6010	6038	6067	6095	6123	6152	6180	6209	6237	6265	6294	6322
14	6350	6379	6407	6435	6464	6492	6520	6549	6577	6605	6634	6662	6690	6719	6747	6776
15	6804	6832	6860	6889	6917	6945	6973	7002	7030	7059	7087	7115	7144	7172	7201	7228
16	7257	7286	7313	7342	7371	7399	7427	7456	7484	7512	7541	7569	7597	7626	7654	7682
17	7711	7739	7768	7796	7824	7853	7881	7909	7938	7966	7994	8023	8051	8079	8108	8136
18	8165	8192	8221	8249	8278	8306	8335	8363	8391	8420	8448	8476	8504	8533	8561	8590
19	8618	8646	8675	8703	8731	8760	8788	8816	8845	8873	8902	8930	8958	8987	9015	9043
20	9072	9100	9128	9157	9185	9213	9242	9270	9298	9327	9355	9383	9412	9440	9469	9497
21	9525	9554	9582	9610	9639	9667	9695	9724	9752	9780	9809	9837	9865	9894	9922	9950
22	9979	10007	10036	10064	10092	10120	10149	10177	10206	10234	10262	10291	10319	10347	10376	10404

APPENDIX E

Nutritional Values

1. BASIC REQUIREMENTS

APPENDIX E-1. Recommended dietary allowances[a]

Age (yr) or condition	Weight[b] (kg)	Weight[b] (lb)	Height[b] (cm)	Height[b] (in)	Protein (g)	Fat-Soluble Vitamins Vitamin A (µg RE)[c]	Vitamin D (µg)[d]	Vitamin E (mg α-TE)[e]	Vitamin K (µg)	Water-Soluble Vitamins Vitamin C (mg)	Thiamin (mg)	Riboflavin (mg)	Niacin (mg NE)[f]	Vitamin B6 (mg)	Folate (µg)	Vitamin B12 (µg)	Minerals Calcium (mg)	Phosphorus (mg)	Magnesium (mg)	Iron (mg)	Zinc (mg)	Iodine (µg)	Selenium (µg)
Infants																							
0.0–0.5	6	13	60	24	13	375	7.5	3	5	30	0.3	0.4	5	0.3	25	0.3	400	300	40	6	5	40	10
0.5–1.0	9	20	71	28	14	375	10	4	10	35	0.4	0.5	6	0.6	35	0.5	600	500	60	10	5	50	15
Children																							
1–3	13	29	90	35	16	400	10	6	15	40	0.7	0.8	9	1.0	50	0.7	800	800	80	10	10	70	20
4–6	20	44	112	44	24	500	10	7	20	45	0.9	1.1	12	1.1	75	1.0	800	800	120	10	10	90	20
7–10	28	62	132	52	28	700	10	7	30	45	1.0	1.2	13	1.4	100	1.4	800	800	170	10	10	120	30
Males																							
11–14	45	99	157	62	45	1000	10	10	45	50	1.3	1.5	17	1.7	150	2.0	1200	1200	270	12	15	150	40
15–18	66	145	176	69	59	1000	10	10	65	60	1.5	1.8	20	2.0	200	2.0	1200	1200	400	12	15	150	50
19–24	72	160	177	70	58	1000	10	10	70	60	1.5	1.7	19	2.0	200	2.0	1200	1200	350	10	15	150	70
25–50	79	174	176	70	63	1000	5	10	80	60	1.5	1.7	19	2.0	200	2.0	800	800	350	10	15	150	70
51+	77	170	173	68	63	1000	5	10	80	60	1.2	1.4	15	2.0	200	2.0	800	800	350	10	15	150	70
Females																							
11–14	46	101	157	62	46	800	10	8	45	50	1.1	1.3	15	1.4	150	2.0	1200	1200	280	15	12	150	45
15–18	55	120	163	64	44	800	10	8	55	60	1.1	1.3	15	1.5	180	2.0	1200	1200	300	15	12	150	50
19–24	58	128	164	65	46	800	10	8	60	60	1.1	1.3	15	1.6	180	2.0	1200	1200	280	15	12	150	55
25–50	63	138	163	64	50	800	5	8	65	60	1.1	1.3	15	1.6	180	2.0	800	800	280	15	12	150	55
51+	65	143	160	63	50	800	5	8	65	60	1.0	1.2	13	1.6	180	2.0	800	800	280	10	12	150	55
Pregnant					60	800	10	10	65	70	1.5	1.6	17	2.2	400	2.2	1200	1200	320	30	15	175	65
Lactating First 6 mo					65	1300	10	12	65	95	1.6	1.8	20	2.1	280	2.6	1200	1200	355	15	19	200	75
Second 6 mo					62	1200	10	11	65	90	1.6	1.7	20	2.1	260	2.6	1200	1200	340	15	16	200	75

[a]The allowances, expressed as average daily intakes over time, are intended to provide for individual variations among most normal persons as they live in the United States under usual environmental stresses. Diets should be based on a variety of common foods in order to provide other nutrients for which human requirements have been less well defined.

[b]Weights and heights of reference adults are actual medians for the United States population of the designated ages, as reported by NHANES II. The median weights and heights of those under 19 years of age were taken from Hamill PUV, Drizd TA, Johnson CL, et al. Physical growth: National Center for Health Statistics percentiles. *Am J Clin Nutr* 1979;32:607. The use of these figures does not imply that the height-to-weight ratios are ideal.

[c]Retinol equivalents. 1 retinal equivalent = 1 mg retinol or 6 mg β-carotene.

[d]As cholecalciferol. 10 mg cholecalciferol = 400 IU of vitamin D.

[e]α-Tocopherol equivalents. 1 mg d-α tocopherol = 1 α-TE.

[f]Niacin equivalents. 1 NE = 1 mg of niacin or 60 mg of dietary tryptophan.

From *Recommended dietary allowances*, 10th ed. Washington, DC: National Academy Press, 1969.

2. SELECTED VITAMIN AND MINERAL REQUIREMENTS

APPENDIX E–2. *Estimated safe and adequate daily dietary intakes of selected vitamins and minerals*

Category	Age (yr)	Vitamins		Trace elements[a]				
		Biotin (µg)	Pantothenic acid (mg)	Copper (mg)	Manganese (mg)	Fluoride (mg)	Chromium (µg)	Molybdenum (µg)
Infants	0–0.5	10	2	0.4–0.6	0.3–0.6	0.1–0.5	10–40	15–30
	0.5–1	15	3	0.6–0.7	0.6–1.0	0.2–1.0	20–60	20–40
Children and adolescents	1–3	20	3	0.7–1.0	1.0–1.5	0.5–1.5	20–80	25–50
	4–6	25	3–4	1.0–1.5	1.5–2.0	1.0–2.5	30–120	30–75
	7–10	30	4–5	1.0–2.0	2.0–3.0	1.5–2.5	50–200	50–150
	11+	30–100	4–7	1.5–2.5	2.0–5.0	1.5–2.5	50–200	75–250
Adults		30–100	4–7	1.5–3.0	2.0–5.0	1.5–4.0	50–200	75–250

[a]Because the toxic levels for many trace elements may be only several times usual intakes, the upper levels for the trace elements given in this table should not be habitually exceeded.

From *Recommended dietary allowances,* 10th ed. Washington, DC: National Academy Press, 1989.

3. ENERGY REQUIREMENTS

APPENDIX E–3. Median heights and weights and recommended energy intake

Category	Age (yr) or condition	Weight		Height		REE[a] (kcal/d)	Average energy allowance (kcal)[b]		
		(kg)	(lb)	(cm)	(in)		Multiples of REE	Per kg	Per day[c]
Infants	0.0–0.5	6	13	60	24	320		108	650
	0.5–1.0	9	20	71	28	500		98	850
Children	1–3	13	29	90	35	740		102	1300
	4–6	20	44	112	44	950		90	1800
	7–10	28	62	132	52	1130		70	2000
Males	11–14	45	99	157	62	1440	1.70	55	2500
	15–18	66	145	176	69	1760	1.67	45	3000
	19–24	72	160	177	70	1780	1.67	40	2900
	25–50	79	174	176	70	1800	1.60	37	2900
	51+	77	170	173	68	1530	1.50	30	2300
Females	11–14	46	101	157	62	1310	1.67	47	2200
	15–18	55	120	163	64	1370	1.60	40	2200
	19–24	58	128	164	65	1350	1.60	38	2200
	25–50	63	138	163	64	1380	1.55	36	2200
	51+	65	143	160	63	1280	1.50	30	1900
Pregnant	First trimester								+0
	Second trimester								+300
	Third trimester								+300
Lactating	First 6 months								+500
	Second 6 months								+500

[a]Calculation based on the World Health Organization equations, then rounded.

[b]In the range of light to moderate activity, the coefficient of variation is ±20%.

[c]Figure is rounded.

REE, resting energy expenditure.

From *Recommended dietary allowances,* 10th ed. Washington, DC: National Academy Press, 1989.

4. COMMERCIAL FORMULAS AND FOODS

APPENDIX E–4a. *Formulas for metabolic disorders*

Indicated use	Product
Phenylketonuria	Lofenalac[a], Phenyl-Free[a]
PKU, infant	PKU 1[a], Analog XP[b]
PKU, child	PKU 2[a], Maxamaid XP[b]
PKU, adult	PKU 3[a], Maxamaid XP[b]
Maple Syrup Urine Disease	MSUD[a]
MSUD, infant	MSUD 1[a], Analog MSUD[b]
MSUD, child	MSUD 2[a], Maxamaid MSUD[b]
MUSD, adult	Maximum MSUD[b]
Tyrosinemia	LowPhenylTyr (3200AB)[a], Analog XPHEN, TYR, MET[b]
Tyrosinemia, infant	TYR 1[a]
Tyrosinemia, child	TYR 2[a], Maxamaid XPHEN, TYR[b]
Homocystinuria	Low methionine (3200K)[a], Maxamaid XMET[b]
Homocystinuria, infant	Hominex-1[a]
Homocystinuria, child	Hominex-2[a]
Histinemia, infant	Hist 1[a]
Histinemia, child	Hist 2[a]
Hyperlysinemia, infant	LYS 1[a]
Hyperlysinemia, child	LYS 2[a]
I proprionic acidemia methylmalonic aciduria	OS 1[a]
C proprionic acidemia methylmalonic aciduria	OS 2[a]
Methylmalonic acidemia	Analog XMET, TYR, MET[b]; or Maxamaid XMET, THRE, VAL, ISLEU[b]
Hyperammonemia, infant	UCD 1[a]
Hyperammonemia, child	UCD 2[a]
Disaccharidase deficiency	Monosaccharide and Disaccharide-Free Diet Powder (3232A)[a]

[a]Mead Johnson Laboratories, Evansville, IN; Ross Laboratories, Columbus, OH.
[b]Ross Products Division, Abbott Laboratories, Columbus, OH.
MSUD, maple syrup urine disease; PKU, phenylketonuria.

APPENDIX E–4b. *Composition of human milk, standard infant formulas, and some specialized formulas*

Formula type	Calorie distribution	Carbohydrate type	Protein type	Fat type	Osmolality (mOsm)
		Human milk and standard infant formulas			
Human milk	Carbohydrate, 38% Protein, 7% Fat, 55%	Lactose	Whey, 80% Casein, 20%	Human milk fat	300
Enfamil[a]	Carbohydrate, 43% Protein, 9% Fat, 48%	Lactose	Nonfat cow's milk Demineralized whey Whey, 60% Casein, 40%	Coconut, soy or oleo, or both, safflower	300
Similac[b]	Carbohydrate, 43% Protein, 9% Fat, 48%	Lactose	Nonfat cow's milk Casein, 82% Whey, 18%	Coconut, soy	300
Gerber[c]	Carbohydrate, 43% Protein, 10% Fat, 46%	Lactose	Nonfat cow's milk Casein, 82% Whey, 18%	Palm olein Soy Coconut Sunflower	320
Good Start[d]	Carbohydrate, 44% Protein, 10% Fat, 50%	Lactose, 70% Maltodextrin, 30%	Whey protein 42% hydrolyzed Soy Coconut Sunflower	Palm olein	265
Similac PM[b] 60/40	Carbohydrate, 41% Protein, 10% Fat, 50%	Lactose	Nonfat cow's milk Demineralized whey Whey, 60% Casein, 40%	Soy, coconut	280
	Formulas free of lactose and or cow's milk protein and special milk-based (casien-hydrolysate) formulas				
Lactofree[a]	Carbohydrate, 42% Protein, 9% Fat, 49%	Corn syrup solids	Milk protein isolate	Palm olein Soy Coconut Sunflower	200
Soy Isomil[b] Isomil DF[b] Nursoy Alsoy[d] Gerber Soy[c] Soy (sucrose free)	Carbohydrate, 40% Protein, 11–13% Fat, 47–49%	Corn syrup solids or sucrose, or both	Soy isolate	Soy or coconut, or both, corn, oleo, safflower	250–296
Isomil SF[b] Prosobee[a]	Carbohydrate, 40% Protein, 12% Fat, 48%	Corn syrup solids	Soy isolate	Soy, coconut, palm olein, sunflower	180–200
Neocate infant w/ iron	Carbohydrate, 47% Protein, 12% Fat, 41%	Corn syrup solids Refined vegetable oil (coconut, soy)	Amino acids	Safflower	342
Nutramigen[a]	Carbohydrate, 44% Protein, 12% Fat, 45%	Corn syrup solids, modified corn starch	Casein hydrolysate	Palm olein, soy, coconut	320
Alimentum[b]	Carbohydrate, 41% Protein, 11% Fat, 48%	Sucrose, modified tapioca starch	Casein hydrolysate	MCT, 50%; safflower, soy	370
Pregestimil[a]	Carbohydrate, 41% Protein, 11% Fat, 48%	Corn syrup solids, modified corn starch, dextrose	Casein hydrolysate with L-cysteine, L-tryptophan, L-tyrosine	MCT, 55%; corn, 20%; safflower, 12.5%; soy, 12.5%	300
RCF[b] (Ross carbohydrate free)	Carbohydrate, 40% Protein, 12% Fat, 48%	Type desired 52 g and 12 oz H_2O with 13 oz RCF-full strength	Soy isolate	Soy, coconut	Varies with source of carbohydrate

(continued)

APPENDIX E–4b. Continued.

Formula type	Calorie distribution	Carbohydrate type	Protein type	Fat type	Osmolality (mOsm)
Formulas with altered fat, protein, and carbohydrates						

Formulas with altered fat, protein, and carbohydrates

Formula type	Calorie distribution	Carbohydrate type	Protein type	Fat type	Osmolality (mOsm)
Fat alterations Portagen[a]	Carbohydrate, 46% Protein, 14% Fat, 40%	Corn syrup solids, sucrose	Sodium caseinate	MCT, 85%; corn, 12.5%; lecithin, 2.5%	220
Progestimil[a]	See above				
Alimentum[b]	See above				
Elemental Neocate One[e]	Carbohydrate, 58.5% Protein, 10% Fat, 31.5%	Maltodexterin, 68%; sucrose, 32%	Amino acids	Safflower, 65%, MCT, 35%	835, liquid, 1 cal/ml; 610, powder, 1 cal/ml
Peptamen Jr[f]	Carbohydrate, 55% Protein, 12% Fat, 33%	Maltodexterin, starch	Hydrolyzed whey	MCT, 60%; soy; canola	260, unflavored, 1 cal/ml; 365, vanilla, 1 cal/ml
Vivonex[g] Pediatric	Carbohydrate, 62% Protein, 12% Fat, 26%	Maltodexterin, modified starch	Amino acids	MCT, 68%; soy, 32%	360, 0.8 cal/ml
Preterm formulas						
Enfamil Premature[a]	Carbohydrate, 44% Protein, 12% Fat, 44%	Lactose, 40%; corn syrup solids, 60%	Nonfat cow's milk Demineralized whey Whey, 60% Casein, 40%	MCTs, 40%; corn, 40%; coconut, 20%	300
Similac Special Care[b]	Carbohydrate, 42% Protein, 11% Fat, 47%	Lactose, 50%; hydrolyzed corn starch, 50%	Nonfat cow's milk Demineralized whey Whey, 60% Casein, 40%	MCTs, 50%; corn, 30%; coconut, 20%	300
Similac NeoCare[b]	Carbohydrate, 41% Protein, 10% Fat, 49%	Lactose, 50%; corn syrup solids, 50%	Nonfat cow's milk Demineralized whey Whey, 50% Casein, 50%	MCT, 25%; coconut, 30% or 20% powder only; soy, 45% or 28% powder only; safflower, 27% powder only	290

[a]Mead Johnson Product Division, Evansville, IN.
[b]Ross Product Division, Abbott Laboratories, Columbus, OH.
[c]Gerber Products Comapany, Fremont, MI.
[d]Carnation Nutritional Products, Los Angeles, CA.
[e]Adequate sodium, potassium, and chloride must also be supplied.
[f]Clintec Nutrition Company, Deerfield, IL.
[g]Sandoz Nutrition Corporation, Minneapolis, MN.
MCT, medium-chain triglycerides.

APPENDIX E-4c. *Iron and caloric content of commercially prepared strained and junior foods*

Food	Mean iron content (mg/100 g)	Caloric content (kcal/100 g)
Dry Cereals		
1 tbsp = 2.4 g	73.8	378
Mixed 1:6 with milk	12.3	110
Cereal with Fruit, Strained Rice	6.6	79
Strained Food		
Juices	0.5	40–72
Fruits	0.2	37–83
Plain vegetables	0.3	25–59
Creamed vegetables	0.3	37–56
Meats	1.5	99–113
Egg yolks	2.6	203
High-meat dinners	0.76	74–85
Soups and dinners	1.4	47–87
Desserts	0.2	60–80
Junior Foods[a]		
Meat sticks	1.4	185

[a]Other foods similar to strained foods.

From Pennington, JAT. *Bowes and Church's food values of portions commonly used,* 16th ed. Philadelphia: JB Lippincott, 1994.

APPENDIX F

Technical Procedures

1. LOCATION OF ABDOMINAL AORTIC BRANCHES

APPENDIX F–1. *Distribution of the major aortic branches in fifteen infants*

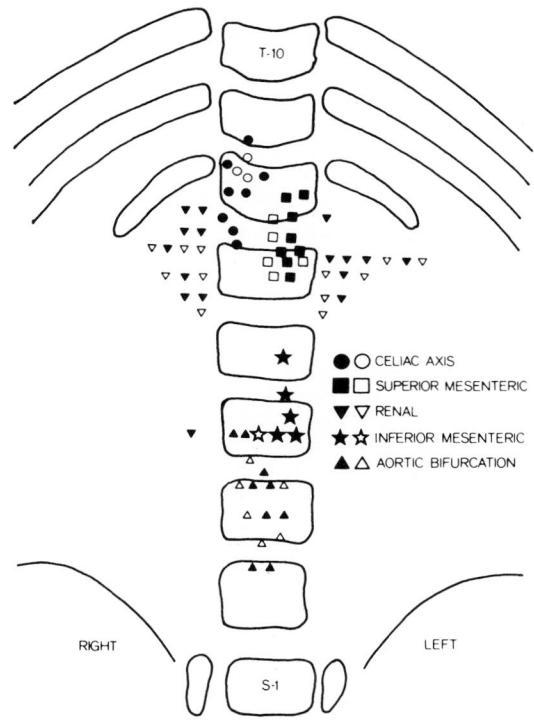

Solid symbols, infants with cardiac and/or renal anomalies; open symbols, infants without these abnormalities.

From Phelps DL, Lachman RS, Leake RD, Oh W. *J Pediatr* 1972;81:337.

2. PLACEMENT OF UMBILICAL CATHETERS

APPENDIX F–2a. *The length of catheter inserted into the umbilical artery in order to reach the bifurcation of the aorta, the diaphragm, or the aortic valves versus the total body length of an infant*

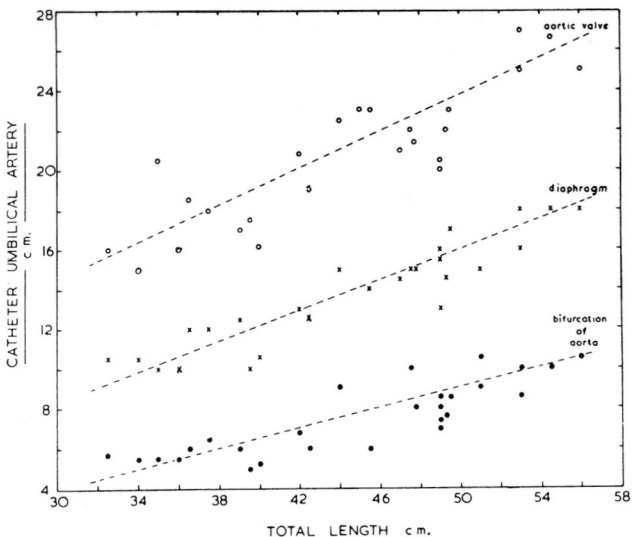

From Dunn PM. *Arch Dis Child* 1966;41:71.

APPENDIX F–2b. *The length of catheter inserted into the umbilical vein in order to reach the diaphragm (x) and the left atrium (o) versus the shoulder–umbilicus length of an infant*

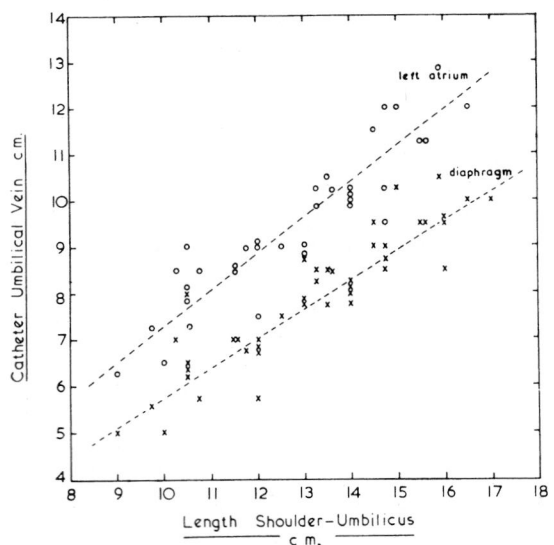

From Dunn PM. *Arch Dis Child* 1966;41:71.

APPENDIX F–2c. *Distance of catheter insertion from the umbilical ring for L3, L5, and aortic bifurcation*

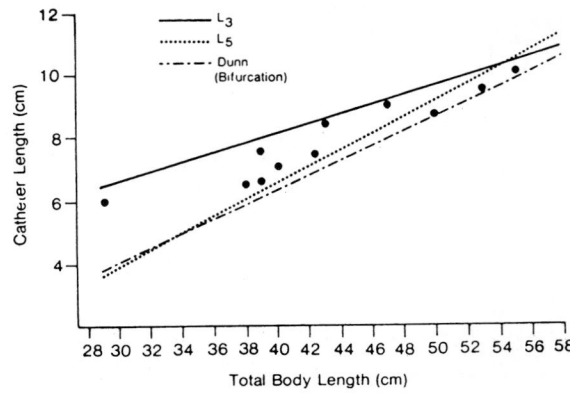

•, catheters positioned at L4. From Rosenfeld W, Estrada R, Jhaveri R, et al. Evaluation of graphs for insertion of umbilical artery catheters below the diaphragm. *J Pediatr* 1981;98:628.

APPENDIX F-2d. *Catheter insertion to level of T8 using the total body length of the infant*

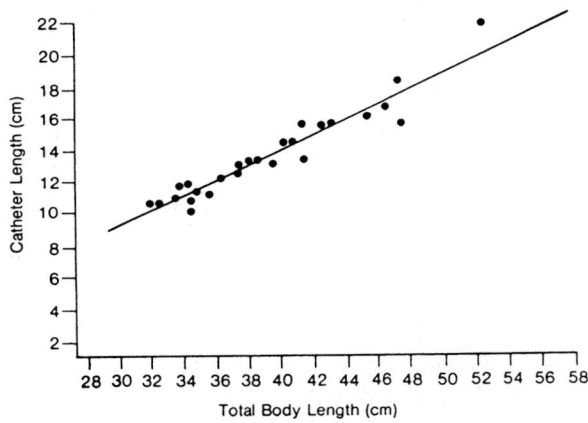

From Rosenfeld W, Biagtan J, Schaeffer H, et al. Evaluation of graphs for insertion of umbilical artery catheters below the diaphragm. *J Pediatr* 1981;98:628.

APPENDIX F–2e. *Estimates of insertional length of umbilical catheters based on birth weight, with 95% confidence intervals*

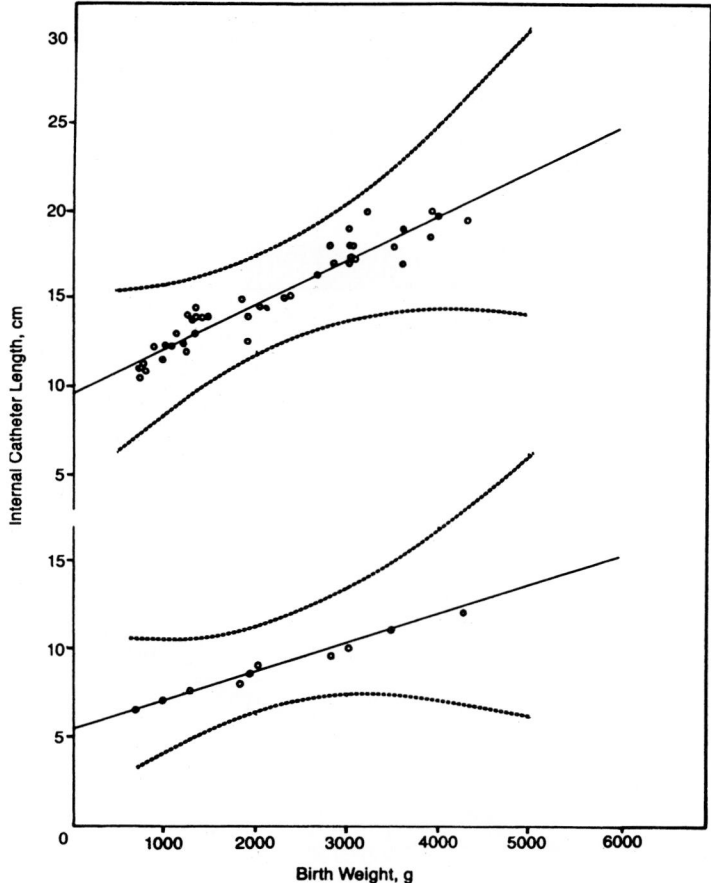

Umbilical artery catheter tip inserted between T6 and T10; umbilical vein catheter tip inserted above diaphragm in inferior vena cava near the right atrium. Modified estimating equations using birth weight (BW) are as follows: umbilical artery length = 2.5 x BW + 9.7 (top) and umbilical vein length = 1.5 x BW + 5.6 (*bottom*), where BW is measured in kilograms and lengths in centimeters.

From Shukla H, Ferrara A. *Am J Dis Child* 1986;140:786.

3. DETERMINING ENDOTRACHEAL TUBE SIZE

APPENDIX F–3. *Endotracheal tube size*

Infant weight (g)	Tube Diameter	
	Inside	Outside
<1000	2.5 mm	12 Fr
1000–1500	3 mm	14 Fr
1500–2200	3.5 mm	16 Fr
2200+	4 mm	18 Fr

4. DETERMINING OROTRACHEAL TUBE SIZE AND LENGTH

APPENDIX F–4. *Orotracheal tube size and distance versus body weight*

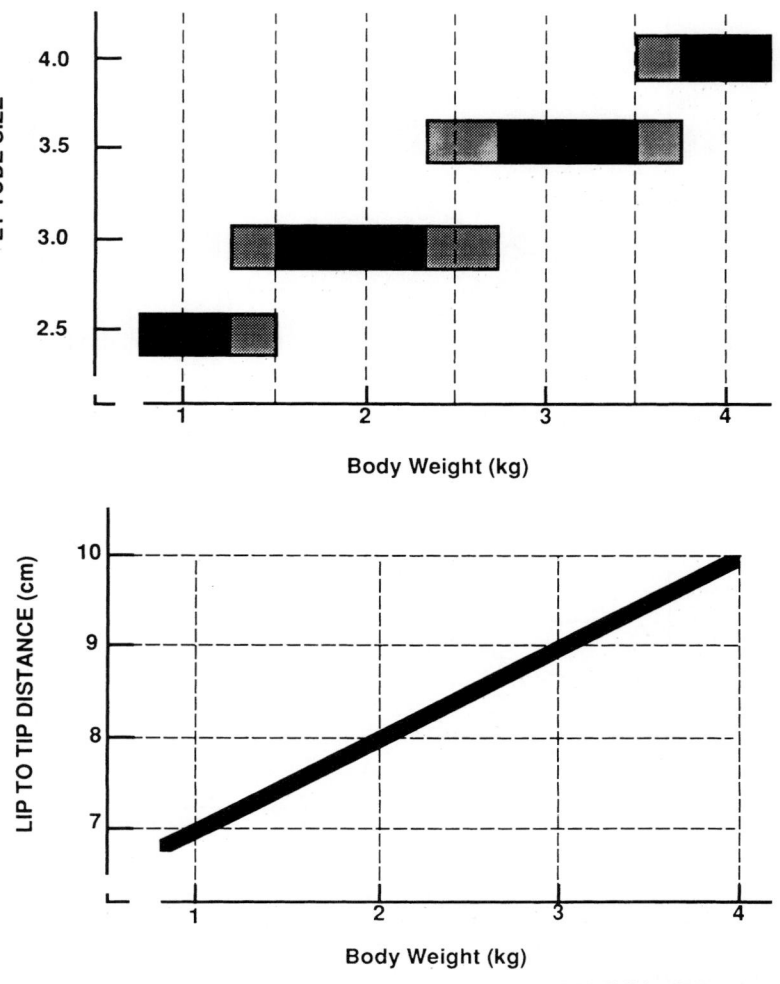

R.H. Phibbs, M.D. 1992

Top: solid bars, usual size of tube to be used for infants of the corresponding birth weight; shaded bars, range of bigger and smaller infants in which that size of tube may be needed on occasion.

Bottom: Distance from the infant's lip to the tip of the tube when the tip is in the midtrachea. Most endotracheal tubes have numbered centimeter marks on the sides indicating the distance to the tip. The appropriate number should be even with the infant's lip.

These are guidelines. There will be some variation among infants.

APPENDIX G

Developmental Screening

1. DENVER II DEVELOPMENTAL SCREENING TEST

APPENDIX G–1. *Denver II Developmental Screening Test*

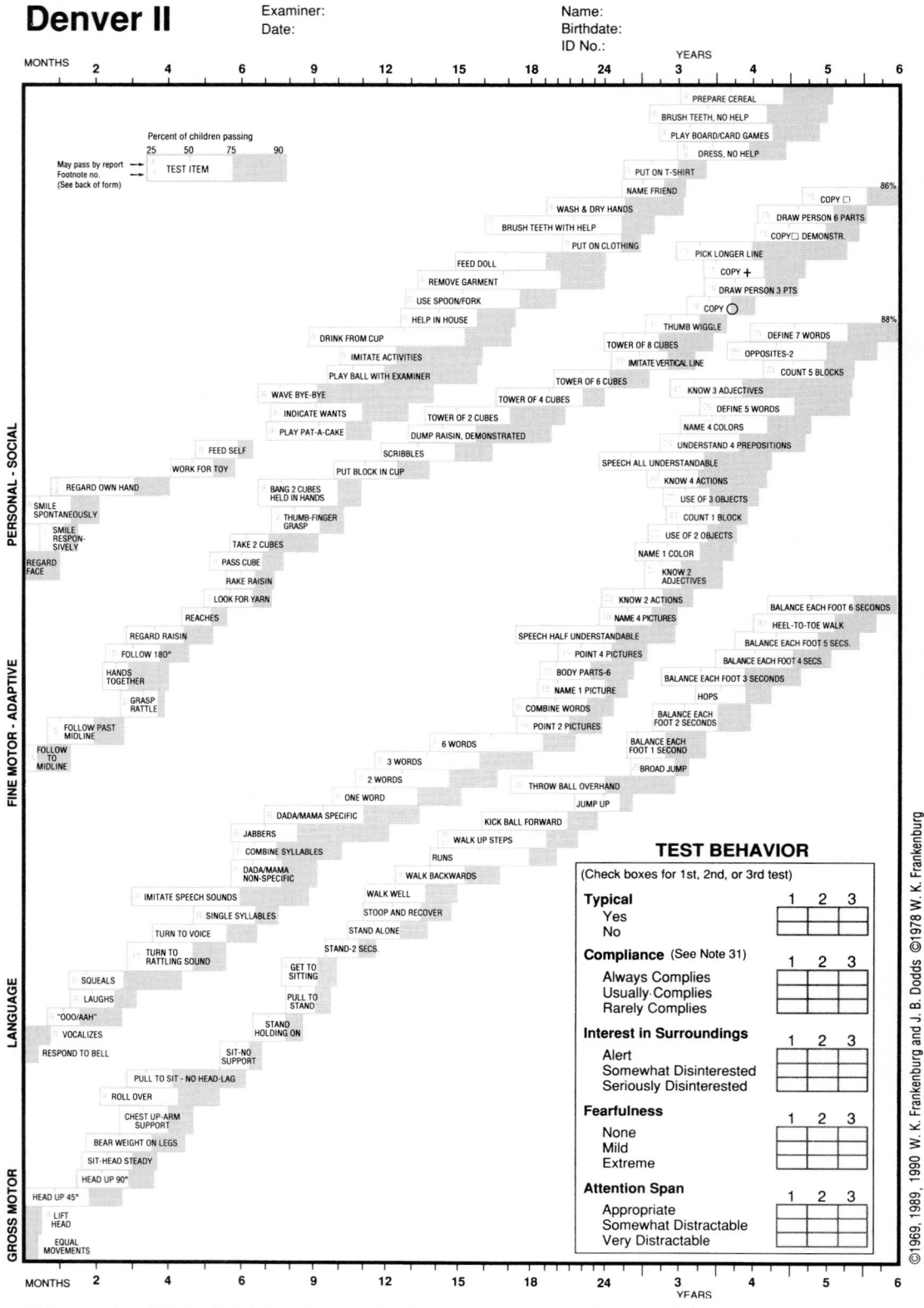

This test should be administered and scored in accordance with the guidelines in the Denver II Technical Manual. Accurate interpretation of the screening results requires consideration of the entire clinical picture. Its purpose is to serve as a screening tool to indicate infants who require further testing. It is not intended to be either diagnostic or predictive.

From Frankenburg WK, Dodds JB. University of Colorado Medical Center and Denver Developmental Materials, Inc.

Drugs

1. MEDICATIONS IN BREAST MILK

APPENDIX H–1a. *Drugs that are contraindicated during breast-feeding*

Drug	Reason for concern
Bromocriptine	Suppresses lactation; may be hazardous to the mother
Cocaine	Cocaine intoxication
Cyclophosphamide	Possible immune suppression; unknown effect on growth or association with carcinogenesis; neutropenia
Cyclosporine	Possible immune suppression; unknown effect on growth or association with carcinogenesis
Doxorubicin[a]	Possible immune suppression; unknown effect on growth or association with carcinogenesis
Ergotamine	Vomiting, diarrhea, convulsions (doses used in migraine medications)
Lithium	One-third to one-half therapeutic blood concentration in infants
Methotrexate	Possible immune suppression; unknown effect on growth or association with carcinogenesis; neutropenia
Phencyclidine (PCP)	Potent hallucinogen
Phenindione	Anticoagulant: increased prothrombin and partial thromboplastin time in one infant; not used in the United States

[a]Drug is concentrated in human milk.

APPENDIX H–1b. *Drugs of abuse that are contraindicated during breast-feeding*

Drug	Reported effect or reason for concern
Amphetamine	Irritability, poor sleeping pattern
Cocaine	Cocaine intoxication
Heroin	Tremors, restlessness, vomiting, poor feeding
Marijuana	Only one report in literature; no effect mentioned
Nicotine (smoking)	Shock, vomiting, diarrhea, rapid heart rate, restlessness; decreased milk production
Phencyclidine (PCP)	Potent hallucinogen

APPENDIX H–1c. *Radioactive compounds that require temporary cessation of breast-feeding*

Drug	Recommended time for cessation of breast-feeding
Copper 64 (^{64}Cu)	Radioactivity in milk present at 50 h
Gallium 67 (^{67}Ga)	Radioactivity in milk present for 2 wk
Indium 111 (^{111}In)	Very small amount present at 20 h
Iodine 123 (^{125}I)	Radioactivity in milk present up to 36 h
Iodine 125 (^{125}I)	Radioactivity in milk present for 12 d
Iodine 131 (^{131}I)	Radioactivity in milk present 2–14 d, depending on study
Radioactive sodium	Radioactivity in milk present 96 h
Technetium 99m (^{99m}Tc), ^{99m}Rc macroaggregates, ^{99m}Tc O4	Radioactivity in milk present at 15 h to 3 d

APPENDIX H–1d. *Drugs whose effect on nursing infants is unknown, but may be of concern*

Drug	Drug precaution during breast-feeding
Antianxiety agents	
Diazepam	None
Lorazepam	None
Midazolam	....
Perphenazine	None
Prazepam[a]	None
Quazepam	None
Temazepam	....
Antidepressants	
Amitriptyline	None
Amoxapine	None
Desipramine	None
Dothiepin	None
Doxepin	None
Fluoxetine	....
Fluvoxamine	....
Imipramine	None
Trazodone	None
Antipsychotics	
Chlorpromazine	Galactorrhea in adult; drowsiness and lethargy in infant
Chlorprothixene	None
Haloperidol	None
Mesoridazine	None
Chloramphenicol	Possible idiosyncratic bone marrow suppression
Metoclopramide[a]	None described; dopaminergic blocking agent
Metronidazole	*In vitro* mutagen; may discontinue breast-feeding 12–24 h to allow excretion of dose when single-dose therapy given to mother
Tinidazole	See metronidazole

[a]Drug is concentrated in human milk.

APPENDIX H–1e. *Drugs that have been associated with significant effects on some nursing infants and should be given to nursing mothers with caution[a]*

Drug	Drug precaution during breast-feeding
5-Aminosalicyclic acid	Diarrhea (one case)
Aspirin (salicylates)	Metabolic acidosis (one case)
Clemastine	Drowsiness, irritability; refusal to feed, high-pitched cry, neck stiffness (one case)
Phenobarbital	Sedation; infantile spasms after weaning from milk containing phenobarbital, methemoglobinemia (one case)
Primidone	Sedation, feeding problem
Salicylazosulfapyridine (sulfasalazine)	Bloody diarrhea (one case)

[a]Measure blood concentration in the infant when possible.

Modified from American Academy of Pediatrics, Committee on Drugs. Transfer of drugs and other chemicals into human milk. *Pediatrics* 1994;93:137–150.

2. PHARMACOPOEIA

APPENDIX H–2. *Pharmacopoeia*

Drug	Dose/kg	Route and frequency	Comments
Abelcet®	See Amphotericin B lipid complex		
Acetazolamide	Diuretic: 5 mg	PO, IV, qd	• May cause acidosis, hypokalemia, and GI irritation
	Hydrocephalus: 5 mg (titrate to max of 20 mg)	q6h	
Acyclovir	Neonatal HSV 10 mg	IV; over 1 h Term, normal renal function: q8h	• Treat for 14–21 d
		<30 wk or mod. ↓ renal function: q12h ↓ renal function and ↓ u/o (Cr > 1.2): q24h	• Adequate hydration required to avoid crystalline nephropathy
Adenosine	0.05 mg	IVP Titrate dose in increments of 0.05 mg/kg every 2 min to a max of 0.25 mg/kg or until termination of PSVT (max single dose: 12 mg)	• Push over 1 to 2 seconds flush with NS • Higher doses may be needed for peripheral administration vs, central administration
Albumin 5%	0.5–1 g (1 g/20 mL)	IV over 2–4 h	• Contains 0.13–0.16 mEq of Na+ per mL • Avoid circulatory overload
Albuterol	0.05–0.25 mg per dose	Inhalation for bronchodilation q2h to q6h	• Tachycardia, arrhythmias, tremor, hypokalemia, and irritable behavior have been reported
Amikacin	7.5 mg	IM, IV; over 30 min to 1 h <7 d <28 wk: q24h 28–34 wk: q18h Term: q12h >7 d <28 wk: q18h 28–34 wk: q12h Term: q8h	• Therapeutic levels: Pk = 20–30 µg/mL Tr = 5–10 µg/mL • Dose adjustment required in renal dysfunction • Risk of ototoxicity increases when given concurrently with loop diuretics
Aminophylline	Loading dose: 4–6 mg	IV once	• Therapeutic levels: Bronchospasm: 10–20 µ/mL Neonatal apnea: 6–13 µg/mL
	Maintenance dose: 1–2 mg	IV q8h–q12h Give first maintenance dose 8–12 hr after the loading dose	• Signs of toxicity include irritability, GI upset and arrhythmias • When switching to theophylline, remember that aminophylline is 80% theophylline
Ammonium chloride	Metabolic alkalosis: 1–2 mEq	PO, IV × 1	• GI irritation • Hyperventilation • Pain at site of injection if infused too rapidly
	Urinary acidification: 0.25–0.37 mEq	PO, IV q6h	• Maximum concentration for injection = 0.4 mEq/mL. Infusion rate should not exceed 1 mEq/kg/h
Amoxicillin	7–13 mg	PO q8h	• See comments for Ampicillin
Amphotericin B	Test dose for infants and children: 0.1 mg (Maximum total dose: 1 mg) test dose is optional in the neonate	IV once. Infuse over 1 h On the first day of treatment, subtract the test dose from the initial dose and give the remainder over 3 h if there is no adverse reaction	• Total dose: Disseminated infection: 25–30 mg/kg Catheter-associated infection: 10–15 mg/kg
	Initial dose: 0.5 mg		• Max. concentration: 0.1 mg/mL • Max. dextrose concentration: 20%
	Maintenance dose: 0.5–1 mg (increase dose in increments of 0.25 mg/kg/d)	IV qd over 2–4 h	• Incompatible with saline solution and TPN • Monitor electrolytes, renal and hematological status • Avoid additional nephrotoxic drugs

(continued)

APPENDIX H–2. *Continued.*

Drug	Dose/kg	Route and frequency	Comments
Amphotericin B lipid complex	1–5 mg (increase dose daily in 1 mg/kg increments)	Infuse over 2 h	• Use higher doses for meningitis, osteoarthritis, cryptococcal infections, and aspergillosis • Mix to a 1–2 m/mL dilution with D5W only • Do not mix with saline or any other drug • Flush line with D5W
Ampicillin	Sepsis: 50–100 mg (max daily dose 200 mg/kg) Meningitis: 75–100 mg (max daily dose 400 mg/kg)	IM, IV <7 d q12h >7 d q6h–q8h q6h–q8h	• May cause rash, interstitial nephritis hemolytic anemia, and pseudomembranous colitis • Lengthen interval in renal dysfunction
Atracurium	Initial dose: 0.3–0.5 mg Maintenance dose: 0.08–0.1 mg	IV; once Every 20–45 min to maintain paralysis	• Hypertension associated with histamine release • Ventilatory rate may need to be adjusted to compensate for loss of spontaneous ventilation • Aminoglycoside antibiotics prolong duration of action • Contains 9 mg benzyl alcohol/mL • Elimination not substantially altered by renal or hepatic dysfunction
Atropine	Bradycardia: 0.02 mg Bronchospasm: 0.03–0.05 mg	IV over 1 min; min single dose 0.1 mg, max single dose 0.5 mg May repeat every 5 min to a maximum *total* dose of 1 mg or 0.04 mg/kg Via inhalation q8h–q6h; min single dose 0.25 mg, max single dose 1 mg	• May cause hyperthermia, urinary retentio, tachycardia, and elevated WBC count • Antidote: physostigmine
Bumetanide	0.01–0.05 mg	IV, IM, PO qod–qd	• Push IV doses over 1–2 min • 40 times more potent than furosemide • Monitor serum electrolytes • Ototoxic
Caffeine Base	Loading dose: 10–15 mg Maintenance daily dose: 2.5–3 mg	IV, PO once qd or divided q12h Administer first maintenance dose 24 h after the loading dose	• DO NOT SKIP SCHEDULED DOSES WHEN GIVING A BOLUS • Therapeutic levels: 15–25 µg/mL • Toxicity (CV, neurological and GI) rarely occurs at levels <50 µg/ml
Calcium chloride 10% (27 mg elemental Ca^{2+}/mL)	Hypocalcemia: 10–20 mg elemental CA Cardiac arrest: 5 mg elemental Ca	IV PO q6h IV slow push over 10 min	• Use IV solution with extreme caution. Severe tissue necrosis occurs in extravasation. • Monitor serum calcium levels • Use with caution in digitalized patients • Give prior to feeds for best absorption
Calcium Glubionate (Neo-Calglucon®) (23 mg elemental Ca^{2+}/mL)	Hypocalcemia: 10–20 mg elemental Ca	PO q6h	• High osmotic load; large doses may cause diarrhea. Dilute 1:1 with sterile water to halve osmolarity. • Monitor serum Ca levels
Calcium Gluconate 10% (9.4 10% mg elemental Ca^{2+}/mL)	Hypocalcemia: 10–20 mg elemental Ca Cardiac arrest: 10 mg elemental Ca	IV, PO q6–q12h IV may repeat every 10 min	• May cause bradycardia and potentiation of digitalis • Extravasation causes necrosis of subcutaneous tissues • Do not use scalp veins • Precipitates with NaBicard and phosphate salts • Monitor serum Ca levels
Captopril	0.05–0.1 mg; may titrate up to 0.5 mg	PO q6h–q24h	• Give 1 h prior to feeds • Adjust dose in renal dysfunction • Monitor blood pressure; severe hypotension may occur in patients who are Na^+ or volume depleted • May cause rash, proteinuria, neutropenia

APPENDIX H–2. *Continued.*

Drug	Dose/kg	Route and frequency	Comments
Cefazolin	25 mg	IV, IM ≤ 7 d: q12h > 7 d, ≤ 2 Kg: q12h > 7 d >2 Kg: q8h	• First generation cephalosporin • Adjust dose and/or interval in renal dysfunction • May cause rash and elevated liver enzymes
Cefotaxime	50 mg	IV, IM < 1.2 Kg, < 7 d: q12h ≥ 1.2 Kg, > 7 d: q8h	• Third-generation cephalosporin • Good CNS penetration • Adjust dose and/or interval in renal dysfunction • Rash
Ceftazidime	30–50 mg	IV, IM <1.2 Kg 0–4 wk: q12h >1.2 Kg <7 d: q12h >1.2 Kg >7 d: q8h	• Third-generation cephalosporin • Adjust dose and/or interval in renal impairment • Rash, false positive Coomb's test
Ceftriaxone	50 mg	IV, IM ≤ 7 d: q24h >7 d <2 kg: q24h	• Third-generation cephalosporin • No adjustment necessary in renal impairment
	50–75 mg	>7 d >2 kg: qd or may divide into two daily doses	• Painful IM injection. The use of lidocaine for reconstitution of ceftriaxone doses for very small babies is not recommended due to possible lidocaine-related cardiac adverse effects.
	Meningitis: LD 75–100 MG MD 50 mg or LD 100 mg MD 800 mg	IV × 1 IV q12h Begin maintenance dose 12–24 h after loading dose IV × 1 IV, q24h	• Not recommended for use in neonates with hyperbilirubinemia
Cefuroxime	10–25 mg	IV, IM q12h	• Second-generation cephalosporin • Adjust dose in renal dysfunction • May cause transient elevation in BUN/Cr, pseudomembranous colitis and rash
Chloral Hydrate	Sedative: 10–15 mg Hypnotic: 25–50 mg	PO, PR q6–q8h prn PO, PR once	• May cause paradoxical excitement and accumulation of toxic metabolites • Use with caution in hepatic and/or renal failure • May cause GI distress and indirect hyperbilirubinemia
Chlorampenicol	25 mg	IV PO >2 Kg: qd >2 Kg <7 d: qd >2 Kg <7 d: q12h	• Therapeutic levels: 10–25 µg/mL • "Gray baby" syndrome with levels >50 µg/mL • May cause bone marrow depression • Increases phenytoin blood levels
Chlorothiazide	10–20 mg	IV PO q12h	• Use with caution in liver and severe renal failures • May cause fluid and electrolyte imbalance, hyperbilirubinemia, and hyperglycemia
Cholestyramine	80 mg of the active resin	PO tid with feeds	• May cause constipation, diarrhea, malabsorption of fat-soluble vitamins, and metabolic acidosis • Alters absorption of drugs when given concurrently. Give oral meds 1 h prior to, or 4–6 h after, cholestyramine
Clindamycin	5 mg	IV, IM <2 kg < 1 mo: q12h >2 kg < 1 mo: q6h–q8h	• Not indicated in meningitis • GI disturbance • Pseudomembraneous colitis (rare in children)
	5–10 mg	>1 mo: q6h	
Cimetidine	2.5–5 mg	IV, IM PO Q6h	• May cause diarrhea, rash, neutropenia, and gynecomastia • Increases blood levels of theophylline, phenytoin, and other drugs • Decrease dose in renal dysfunction

(continued)

APPENDIX H–2. *Continued.*

Drug	Dose/kg	Route and frequency	Comments
Cisapride	0.15–0.3 mg	PO tid–qid, 15–30 min prior to feeds	• May cause diarrhea, nausea, and vomiting • Do not administer with ketoconazole, itraconazole, miconazole, and troleandomycin due to possible occurrence of cardiac arrhythmias
Cromolyn	20 mg/dose	Inhalation q6h–q8h	• Bronchospasm, cough, nasal congestion, and pharyngeal irritation have been reported
Dexamethasone	Antiinflammatory: 0.025–0.05 mg	IV, IM, PO q6–q12h	• May increase risk of infection • May cause hypertension, salt retention, adrenal suppression, hyperglycemia, and leukocytosis • Consider steroid coverage for periods of stress after therapy for BPD, and in intercurrent illness (see BPD section) • Give hydrocortisone stress doses for surgery up to 6 mo after stopping taper • See Hydrocortisone for stress dosing guidelines • All calculations must use the same body weight
	Airway edema: 0.25 mg	IV, IM, PO q6h pm For extubation: Give first dose 4 h prior to extubation. Then repeat 4 and 12 h after extubation	
	BPD	IV, IM, PO Taper:	

Taper schedule:

Day	Daily dose	Frequency
1–3	0.5 mg/kg	+q12h
4–6	0.3 mg/kg	+q12h
7–9	0.27 mg/kg	+q12h
10–12	0.24 mg/kg	+q12h
13–15	0.22 mg/kg	+q12h
16–18	0.2 mg/kg	+q12h
19–21	0.18 mg/kg	+q12h
22–24	0.16 mg/kg	+q12h
25–27	0.14 mg/kg	+q12h
28–30	0.12 mg/kg	+q12h
31–38	0.1 mg/kg	qd
40, 42	0.1 mg/kg	qd

Drug	Dose/kg	Route and frequency	Comments
Diazepam	Status epilepticus: 0.1–0.5 mg	Slow IV push (over 3 min) every 15–30 or two to three doses; may repeat in 4 h to a max of 2 mg per 24 h	• Not a first-line agent for neonates • Lorazepam is a better choice for maintenance therapy • May cause hypotension and respiratory depression • Displacement of bilirubin by sodium benzoate may occur
	Sedation: 0.04–0.3 mg	IV q6h–q8h prn Maximum of 0.6 mg/kg within an 8-h period	
Diazoxide	Hypertension: 1–3 mg	IV push every 5–15 min until blood pressure is controlled, then q4h–q24h	• May cause hyperglycemia, ketoacidosis, GI irritation, salt and water retention, hypotension
	Hypoglycemia: 2–5 mg	PO q8h–q12h	
Digoxin	Total digitalizing dose (TDD) oral: Premie: 20–30 µg Term: 3–3.75 µg 1–24 mo: 35–60 µg Oral maintenance dose (25% of TDD): Premie: 2.5–3.75 µg Term: 3–3.75 µg 1–24 mo: 4–7.5 µg TDD injectable: Premie: 15–25 µg Term: 20–30 µg 1–24 mo: 30–50 µg Injectable maintenance dose (25% of TDD): Premie: 2–3 µg Term: 2.5–3.75 µg 1–24 mo: 3.75–6 µg	Give 1/2 of the TDD initially, then 1/4 of the TDD q8h–q24h × 2 doses q12 IV, IM Follow same guidelines as for oral administration IV, IM q12h	• May cause bradycardia, PVCs, vomiting, poor feeding, and arrhythmias • Check ECG trace during digitalization and periodically • Adjust dose per clinical response and renal function • Bioavailability of elixir is 70%–85% of the injectable preparation

APPENDIX H–2. *Continued.*

Drug	Dose/kg	Route and frequency	Comments
Dobutamine	2.5–20 µg/min; max dose: 40 µg/min	IV infusion	• Titrate according to patient's response • Use same precautions as with dopamine
Dopamine	2–5 µg/min	IV infusion, mostly dopaminergic effect and some beta-adrenergic	• Monitor blood and pulse pressures
	5–15 µg/min	Mostly beta-adrenergic; some dopaminergic effect at lower end of this range: some alpha-adrenergic at higher end of dosage range	• Observe for pulmonary hypertension • Tissue necrosis may occur with extravasation
	>20 µg/min; max dose: 50 µg/min	Mostly alpha-adrenergic effect	• May cause ectopic beats
Doxapram	Loading dose: 3 mg Maintenance dose: 1–2.5 mg/kg/h	IV infusion over 1 h Continuous IV infusion; start at 1 mg/kg/h and titrate up to minimum effective dose maximum conc: 2 mg/mL	• Maintain therapeutic caffeine or theophylline levels while on doxapram • Taper drug to avoid rebound apneic episodes • Increases oxygen consumption and may cause hypertension, tachycardia, and seizures
Edrophonium	Myasthenia gravis test: Neonates: 0.1 mg (single dose, not per Kg) Infants: 0.04 mg/kg/dose × 1 (max of 1 mg for body weigh ≤34 kg)	IV once If no IV access available, may give IM or SC	• Keep atropine and resuscitation equipment available • Antidote: • Atropine 0.01–0.04 mg/kg/dose
Enalapril (PO)	0.05–0.1 mg	PO qd titrate to maximum of 0.5 mg/kg	• Adjust dose in renal impairment: • CrCl 10–50 mL/min: give 75% of dose
Enalaprilat (IV)	5–10 µg	IV q8h–q24h administer over 5 min	• CrCl <10 mL/min: give 50% of dose • May cause hypoglycemia, hyperkalemia, neutropenia, anemia, and deterioration of renal function
Epinephrine 1:10,000	0.1–0.3 mL	IV, SC, intratracheal Every 3–5 min as needed	• IV drip used for hypotension refractory to dopamine and dobutamine
	0.1 µg/kg/min	Continuous IV infusion; titrate up as needed	• Higher end of dosage range used for cardiac resuscitation; intracardiac route should be last resort • Dilute intratracheal doses to 1–2 mL with saline soln
Epinephrine (racemic) 2.25% solution	0.25 mL total dose	Inhalation via nebulizer over 15 min q4hr prn Dilute with NS to total volume of 2.5–3 mL	• May cause tachycardia and arrhythmias
Epoetin	(see Erythropoietin)		
Erythromycin	antiinfective: 10 mg	IV, PO ≤7 d: q12h >7 d <1.2 kg: q12h >7 d >1.2 kg: q8h	• Decreases clearance of theophylline, digoxin, carbamazepine, and others • Causes GI distress
	prokinetic agent: 3 mg 5 mg	IV q6h; infuse over 60 min PO q6h	
Erythropoietin	Anemia of prematurity: 50–100 U or 200 U	SC three times weekly Titrate dose up based on clinical response IV/SC qd–qod for 2–6 wk	• Must give iron supplementation • Monitor hematocrit, retics, serum Fe, smear, and ferritin levels • Contraindicated in newborns with neutropenia
Exosurf	(see Surfactant)		

(continued)

APPENDIX H–2. *Continued.*

Drug	Dose/kg	Route and frequency	Comments
Fentanyl	1–3 µg	IV, IM q2h–q4h prn pain	• Causes muscle rigidity, respiratory depression and dependence; causes less CV effects than morphine
	1 µg/kg/h	Continuous IV infusion; titrate up	
Ferrous sulfate	Iron deficiency anemia: 2–3 mg elemental Fe	PO q12h	• Do not give concurrently with antacids, milk, or cereal
	With Erythropoietin: 3–6 mg elemental Fe	PO q12h–q8h Max 12 mg/kg/d	• Cimetidine decreases absorption of iron
	Premature supplement: 1 mg	PO q12h or give formula with Fe	• May cause GI irritation; colors stools black
Fluconazole	3–6 mg	IV q24h Infuse over 1–2 h	• Monitor renal and liver functions • Renal dosing: CrCl 21–50 mL/min: 50% of dose CrCl 11–20 mL/min: 25% of dose
Flucytosine	20–40 mg	PO q6h	• May cause GI irritation, bone marrow depression, elevated liver enzymes, elevated BUN, and creatinine • Used in combination with amphotericin B or fluconazole
Furosemide	1–2 mg	IV, IM q12h–q24h	• Causes sodium and potassium depletion; dehydration
	2–4 mg	PO q12h–q24h	• Additive ototoxicity with aminoglycosides
Gentamicin	Loading dose: 5 mg	IV, IM once	• Monitor renal function • Ototoxicity is related to length of therapy
	Maintenance dose: 4 mg	24 h after loading dose ≥37 wk ≥2500 g: q24h	• Therapeutic levels:
	2.5 mg	<37 wk <2500 g: q24h	• Pk = 5–12 µg/mL
	Alternate regimen: 2.5 mg	<28 wk: q24h 28–34 wk: q18h >34 wk: q12h >14 postnatal d, adjust dosing interval up one level	• Tr = <2 µg/mL
Gentian violet	1% topical solution	Dilute to 0.5% solution 3–4 drops under the tongue or apply to lesions after feedings bid–tid	• Stains skin and clothing; apply with cotton tip applicator • Do not apply to face
Glucagon	Hypoglycemia or insulin shock: 0.03–0.3 mg Max dose: 1 mg/dose	IV push, SC, IM Every 30min prn	• 1 unit = 1 mg • May cause rebound hypoglycemia
Heparin	For maintenance of central catheters: 0.5–2 U/mL of IV fluid	IV	• See protamine sulfate for treatment of overdosage
	Anticoagulation: bolus 50 U/kg	IV once	• Monitor clotting time; titrate dose to achieve 1.5–2.5 times normal physiologic values
	Maintenance: 10–25 U/kg/h	IV continuous infusion titrate up based on APTT/PTT	
	Intermittent dosing: 50–100 U/kg/dose	IV q4h	
Hydralazine	Parenteral: Initial: 0.1–0.8 titrate up not to exceed 2 mg/kg/dose Oral:	IV, IM q4h–q6h	• Adjust dose in renal impairment: CrCl = 10–50 mL/min: give q8h CrCl <10 mL/min: give q12–q24h
	Initial: 0.2–0.3 mg titrate up Max *daily* dose: 5 mg/kg	PO, NG q8h–q12h	• May cause tachycardia and sodium and water retention
Hydrocortisone	Congenital adrenal hyperplasia: Initial: 20–35 mg/m²/d Maintenance: 12.5–37.5 mg/m²/d	PO divided as follows: 1/4 dose in morning and at noon, 1/2 dose at night	• Increases chance of infection • May cause hypertension, salt and water retention, adrenal suppression, and hyperglycemia

APPENDIX H–2. *Continued.*

Drug	Dose/kg	Route and frequency	Comments

Hydrocortisone	Shock:
	Initial: 35–50 mg/kg
	Maintenance:
	  12.5–37.5 mg/kg
	
	Stress dose:
	50 mg/m^2/d
		IV, once
		
		IV q6h × 48–72
		
		IV, IM
		  divided q12h–q6h
			• Approximate weight to body surface area conversion table:
			Weight (kg) M^2
			  0.5 0.05
			  1 0.1
			  2 0.15
			  3 0.2
			  4 0.25

Indomethacin	Doses (mg/kg)
	No. 1 No. 2 No. 3
	  0.2 0.1 0.1
	  0.2 0.2 0.2
	  0.2 0.25 0.25
	Extended treatment: 0.2 mg
		IV q8h–q12h × 3 doses:
		  <48 h of life
		  2–7 d
		  >7 d
		IV qd × 5 days following
		  standard three-dose regimen
		  with extended 1× may
		  decrease recurrence of PDA
		Prevention of IVH: 0.1 mg/kg
		  q24h for three doses, beginning
		  at 6–12 h of age
			• Decreases GFR
			
			• Decreases platelet aggregation

Insulin	Hyperglycemia: Initial: 0.1 U Maintenance: 0.02–0.1 U/h Intermittent: 0.1–0.2 U Hyperkalemia: 0.3 U/g of glucose	IV once, over 15–20 min IV, continuous infusion SC, q6h–q12h IV with dextrose 500 mg/kg/dose	• Monitor blood glucose and titrate dose accordingly; may cause rebound hyperglycemia if discontinued abruptly • Use only human regular insulin for IV infusions
Iron	(see Ferrous sulfate)		
Isoniazid	10–20 mg	PO, IM	• May cause vitamin B$_6$ (pyridoxine) depletion; monitor liver function
Isoproterenol	0.05–0.2 µg/min	IV infusion conc: 2–10 µg/mL	• May cause hypotension, ventricular arrhythmias, and tachycardia
Kayexalate® (sodium polystyrene)	1 g	PO, PR q6h prn	• Hyperosmotic; monitor serum • Electrolytes

Labetalol	Bolus: 0.25 mg
	
	Maintenance:
	0.25–1 mg
	1.5–2 mg
	0.25–1.5 mg/kg/h
		IV over 2 min
		Dose can be doubled and
		  repeated every 10 min until
		  desired clinical response or
		  total dose of 4 mg/kg is
		  reached
		
		IV q4h
		PO q12h
		Continuous IV infusion
		max conc 1 mg/mL
			• Absolute contraindications: CHF, heart block, sinus tachycardia
			
			• May cause bradycardia, edema, and bronchospasm

Levothyroxine	5–8 µg 8–14 µg Alternate dose: 25–50 µg *total*	IV push over 30–60 sec; q24h PO q24h PO q24h	• Monitor serum T4 and TSH levels • Do not mix with any other IV fluids; mix immediately prior to administration • Increases effects of oral anticoagulants
Lidocaine	0.5–1 mg 10–50 µg/min	IV every 5–10 min × 2 doses Continuous IV infusion max conc 8 mg/mL	• May cause bradycardia and hypotension; decrease dose in CHF;contraindicated in severe heart block • Therapeutic levels: 1.5–5 mg/mL
Lorazepam	Status epilepticus: 0.05 mg Sedation: 0.05–0.1 mg	IV may repeat every 15–20 min × 2 doses IV q4h–q8h Maximum dose: 2 mg	• Contains benzyl alcohol; may cause respiratory depression, hypotension, and bradycardia • Do not give intraarterially

(continued)

APPENDIX H–2. *Continued.*

Drug	Dose/kg	Route and frequency	Comments
Magnesium SO$_4$	Hypomagnesemia: 0.2–0.4 mEq	IV, IM 2–3 doses q8h–q12h	• Monitor serum levels • May cause hypotension and respiratory depression
Mannitol	0.25–1 g (15%–20% solution) Oliguria test dose: 0.2 g	IV once over 2–6 h IV over 3–5 min	• Always use a 5-μm filter • May cause rebound edema and circulatory overload
Methylene blue	1–2 mg	IV slow push over 5 min (1% soln) May repeat in 1 h	• Methylene blue is a reducing agent; it may decrease hemoglobin O$_2$ capacity
Metoclopramide	0.1–0.2 mg Renal dose adjustment: C/Cr % of dose 20–50 75 <40 50 <10 25–50	IV, IM, PO q6h	• Dilute to 0.2 mg/mL and infuse over 15–30 min • May cause extrapyramidal symptoms with higher doses; may lower seizure threshold
Metolazone	0.2 mg	PO q12h–q24h	• May cause metabolic alkalosis and hyperuricemia; monitor serum electrolytes
Metronidazole	7.5 mg 15 mg	IV, PO 0–4 wk <1.2 kg: q24h ≤7 d >1.2 kg: q12h >7 d 1.2–2 kg: q12h >7 d >2 kg: q12h	• Penetrates effectively into the CSF; may cause leukopenia, rash, phlebitis, and seizures • Low cost is an advantage over other agents with similar antimicrobial range
Midazolam	0.03–0.1 mg 0.05 mg/h	IV, IM q2h–q4h prn Continuous IV infusion; titrate up based on clinical response	• May cause respiratory depression, hypotension, and dependence
Morphine	0.05–0.1 mg 10–20 μg/h	IV, IM, SC q2h–q4h prn Continuous IV infusion; titrate up based on clinical response	• May cause respiratory and CNS depression, hypotension, and dependence • Naloxone (Narcan®) reverses acute overdose
Nafcillin	25 mg	IV, IM <1.2 kg <1 mo: q12h 1.2–2 kg ≤7 d: q12h >2 kg ≤7 d: q8h 1.2–2 kg >7 d: q8h >2 kg >7 d: q6h	• Consider changing dosing interval in patients with hepatic dysfunction • Cases of granulocytopenia or agranulocytosis have been reported
Naloxone	Maternal opiate exposure 0.1 mg Reversal of opiate analgesia 0.01 mg	IV, IM, SC, endotracheally Every 2–3 min prn	• For ET administration dilute to 1–2 mL with NS • Max conc for IV infusion: 4 μg/mL; undiluted drug may be pushed over 30 sec • May precipitate withdrawal symptoms in patients with physical dependence
Neo-calglucon®	See Calcium glubionate		
Neomycin	12.5–25 mg	PO q6h	• May cause nephrotoxicity and ototoxicity
Neostigmine	Myasthenia gravis test: 0.025–0.04 mg Treatment: 0.01–0.04 mg 0.25–0.3 mg	IM once IV, IM, SC q2h–q4h prn PO q3h–q4h prn	• May cause cholinergic crisis • Antidote: atropine 0.01–0.04 mg/kg
Nitroprusside	Initial: 0.3–0.5 μg/min Maintenance: 3–4 μg/min Max 8–10 μg/min	IV continuous infusion	• Monitor for cyanide toxicity • May cause hypotension and tachyphylaxis • Protect from light
Nystatin	100,000–200,000 U *Total* dose	PO q6h Apply ½ of the dose to each side of the mouth for oral thrush	• Poor oral absorption

APPENDIX H–2. *Continued.*

Drug	Dose/kg	Route and frequency	Comments
Octreotide	1–10 μg	IV, SC q12h–q24h	• Start treatment using lower end of dosage range • Causes growth hormone suppression
Oxacillin		IV, IM	• Contraindicated in patients allergic to penicillins
	25 mg	≤2 kg ≤7 d: q12h	• May cause thrombophlebitis and *clostridium difficile* colitis
	33 mg	≤2 kg >7 d: q8h	
	25 mg	>2 kg ≤7 d: q8h	• Monitor liver function
	37.5 mg	>2 kg >7 d: q6h	
Palivizumab	See Synagis		
Pancuronium	0.04–0.1 mg	IV q1h–q4h prn movement	• Short half-life; titrate dose based on clinical response • Aminoglycosides increase the action of pancuronium
Paraldehyde	0.3 mL (1g/mL solution)	PR q4h–q6h	• CNS depression may occur if patient is overdosed; do not use discolored solution: Do not use plastic equipment
	Max single dose: 5 mL	Dilute 1:1 with mineral oil for rectal administration	
Paregoric	Initial dose:		• Monitor for CNS depression
	0.2–0.3 mL *total* dose	PO q3h–q4h	• Give with feeds to minimize GI irritation; same adverse effects as morphine
	Subsequent doses: increase by 0.05 mL up to max of 0.7 mL *total* dose		
Penicillin-G K	Congenital syphilis: 50,000 U	IV, IM ≤7 d: q12h >7 d: q8h	• May cause hypersensitivity reactions, thrombophlebitis, and acute interstitial nephritis
	Meningitis/group B strep: 75,000–100,000 U	IV, IM ≤2 kg ≤7 d: q12h	
	Other infections: 25,000–50,000 U	≤2 kg >7 d: q8h >2 kg ≤7 d: q8h >2 kg >7 d: q6h	
Phenobarbital	Loading dose: 20 mg	IV, IM once	• Induces the metabolism of other drugs; may cause respiratory and CNS depression at higher doses
	Maintenance dose: 2.5 mg	IV, IM, PO q12h	
	1.5–2 mg	q12h in asphyxiated infants and in liver dysfunction	• Therapeutic levels: seizures: 20–40 μg/mL
		Monitor levels weekly or as clinically indicated	• hyperbilirubinemia: 15 μg/mL
Phenytoin	Loading dose: 20 mg	IV once	• Rapid infusion may precipitate cardiovascular collapse; do not exceed 0.5 mg/kg/min infusion
	Maintenance dose: 2–4 mg	IV, PO q12h Some patients may need q8h intervals	• Toxicity may lead to seizures and CNS depression • Therapeutic range: 15–20 μg/mL • Toxicity may lead to seizures and CNS depression
Phytonadione	Neonatal hemorrhagic disease: Prophylaxis: 0.5–1 mg *total* dose	IM, SC once within 1 hour of birth; may repeat 6–8 h later	• IV route should be used only when other routes are not available: infuse rate at a max rate of 1 mg/min; severe reactions resembling anaphylaxis may occur with IV administration
	Treatment: 1–2 mg *total* dose	IV, SC once	
Piperacillin		IV	• Used in combination with aminoglycosides
	50 mg	≤7 d: q8h >7 d: q6h	• Eosinophilia, hyperbilirubinemia, elevations in ALT, AST, BUN, and serum creatinine have been observed.
Prednisolone	Antiinflammatory: 0.5–1 mg	PO q12h	• May cause hypertension, GI irritation, and adrenal suppression
Propranolol	0.01–0.1 mg maximum dose: 1 mg	IV push over 10 min q6h–q8h	• May cause hypotension, bronchospasm, and heart block
	0.25 mg	PO q6h–q8h titrate up to maximum of 5 mg/kg/day	

(continued)

APPENDIX H–2. *Continued.*

Drug	Dose/kg	Route and frequency	Comments
Prostaglandin E₁	0.05–0.4 µg/min	IV continuous infusion; use lowest effective dose	• May cause apnea, fever, hypotension, and cutaneous vasodilation
Protamine	Dose of protamine in mg to neutralize 100 U of heparin	Protamine — Time elapsed 1–1.5 — Immediate 0.5–0.75 — 30–60 min 0.25–0.375 — >2 h	• May cause hypotension and bradycardia • Max conc: 10 mg/mL
Pyridoxine (vitamin B₆)	Deficiency: 5–10 mg total dose B₆-dependent seizure: 50–100 mg total dose	PO, IV, IM q24h PO, IV, IM q24h	• Decreases serum levels of phenobarbital, phenytoin, and folic acid; may cause hypersensitivity reactions, respiratory distress, and burning at site of injection
Pyrimethamine	Toxoplasmosis: LD 2 mg MD 1 mg	PO; qd for 2 d PO; qd for 2–6 months, then 3× per week to complete 12 months treatment	• Supplementation with folic acid is recommended • May cause glossitis, seizures, and rash
Ranitidine	0.75–1.5 mg 1.25–2.5 mg	IV, IM q6h–q8h max 6 mg/kg/d PO q12h CNMC GI recommendation for GER: 6–12 mg/kg/d + q6h–q8h	• Renal dosing: CrCl <50 mL/min oral: give q24h IV, IM: give q18h–q24h Monitor serum creatinine
RSV immune globulin	750 mg (15 mL)	IV, monthly during RSV season Administration guidelines: 1.5 mL/kg/h × 15 min 3 mL/kg/h × 15 min 6 mL/kg/h until finished	• Not recommended for use in patients with cyanotic heart disease • Some patients may develop respiratorydistress due to excessive fluid • Live vaccines should be delayed for 9 mo after administration
Spironolactone	0.5–1.5 mg	PO q8h–q12h	• Avoid in hyperkalemia; may cause rash, vomiting, and diarrhea; contraindicated in renal failure
Surfactant	Survanta® (beractant) 4 mL	Endotracheal rescue treatment: One dose as soon as RDS diagnosis is confirmed. May repeat q6h to a total of four doses Prophylaxis: First dose given as soon as possible after birth; may give a total of four doses during first 48 h of life, no more frequently than 6 h apart	• Adverse effects include pulmonary hemorrhage, apnea, and mucous plugging • Adjust ventilatory parameters to prevent hyperoxia and hypocarbia • May open ductus
	Exosurf® (colfosceril) 5 mL	Endoctracheal rescue treatment: One dose as soon as RDS diagnosis is confirmed. May repeat 12 h after first dose if baby is still ventilator dependent Prophylaxis: First dose given as soon as possible after birth; a second and third dose may be given 12 and 24 h after the first dose	
Survanta	See Surfactant		
Synagis®	15 mg	IM; monthly during RSV season	• Typically RSV season begins in November and lasts through April • Inject in the anterolateral aspect of the thigh. Gluteal injections may damage the sciatic nerve
Tham®	See Tromethamine		

APPENDIX H–2. *Continued.*

Drug	Dose/kg	Route and frequency	Comments
Ticarcillin + clavulanic acid (Timentin®)	75 mg	IV, IM ≤2 kg 0–7 d: q12h ≤2 kg >7 d: q8h >2 kg 0–7 d: q8h >2 kg >7 d: q6h	• May cause hypersensitivity reactions, phlebitis, pseudomembranous colitis, hypernatremia, and inhibition of platelet aggregation
Tobramycin	2.5 mg	IV, IM <28 wk: q24h 28–34 wk: q18h >34 wk: q12h >14 postnatal d, adjust dosing interval up one level	• Monitor renal function • Therapeutic range: Pk: 5–10 µg/mL Tr: <2 µg/mL
Tolazoline	Test dose: 1–2 mg Maintenance dose: 1–2 mg/h	IV over 10 min IV continuous infusion	• May cause hypotension and GI and pulmonary hemorrhage; for severe hypotension resistant to volume expansion use ephedrine to increase peripheral resistance, not epinephrine or norepinephrine. The latter cause rebound hypotension.
Tromethamine	3 mL	IV slow infusion Max rate: 1 ml/h	• 1 mL = 0.3 mEq; 1 mM = 1 mEq • Infuse preferably in large blood vessel; may cause hypoglycemia, hyperkalemia, apnea, and fluid overload
Vancomycin	15 mg 24 mg 18 mg 22.5 mg 15 mg *Clostridium difficile:* 10 mg	IV infused over 60 min <28 wk: q24h 28–30 wk: q24h 31–36 wk: q12h–q18h ≥37 wk: q12h Term and 30 d: q8h PO q6h	• Therapeutic range: Pk: 20–40 µg/mL Tr: <10 µg/mL • May cause renal and ototoxicity, red-man syndrome may occur with rapid IV infusion; some patients may require a 2-h infusion period
Vasopressin (aqueous)	2.5–10 U total dose	IM, SC q12h–q16h	• May cause bronchoconstriction, diarrhea and electrolyte imbalance
Vecuronium	0.03–0.15 mg 0.05–0.1 mg/h	IV q1h–2h prn movement IV continuous infusion Max conc: 1 mg/mL	• Neuromuscular effects may be prolonged after continuous infusion and when aminoglycosides are administered concurrently
Vitamin K₁	See Phytonadione		

Dosages in this table are single dose per kilogram (U/kg per dose) unless otherwise noted. Frequency is suggested in the third column, but may vary with maturity and rate of metabolism. In most cases, the most conservative dosage is given.

AV, atrioventricular; BP, blood pressure; BUN, blood urea nitrogen; CNS, central nervous system; CSF, cerebrospinal fluid; ECG, electrocardiogram; ET, endotracheal; GI, gastrointestinal; HSV, herpes simplex virus; IT, intrathecal; LD, loading dose; MD, maintenance dose; NS, normal saline; Pk, peak; PO, by mouth; PR, per rectum; prn, as needed; PSVT, paroxysmal supraventricular virus; PVC, premature ventricular contraction; RSV, repiratory syncytial virus; SC, subcutaneous; TDD, total digitalizing dose; Tr, trough; TSH, thyroid stimulating hormone; WBC, leucocyte.

Reviewed and updated by Karl Gumpper, R.Ph., B.C.N.S.P., Clinical Coordinator, and Luisa Kelly, R.Ph., Neonatology, Pharmacy Information System Coordinator, Children's National Medical Center, Washington, D.C.

3. ANTIDYSRHYTHMIC AGENTS

APPENDIX H–3. *Neonatal antiarrhythmic agents*

Drug/class	Currently commonly used	Route of metabolism/ excretion	Oral dose	IV dose	Therapeutic level	Indications	Contraindications	Oral dose toxicity level
Adenosine	Yes	Red blood cells, and vascular endothelium		0.075–0.10mg/kg rapid IV push, PRN↑ to 0.15–0.25mg/kg after 1 min		Rx-Re-Entry SVT, Dx, Atrial flutter		Transient AV block, ↓HR, ↓BP, and flushing rare atrial fibrillation
Digoxin	Yes	Renal	Load: 20–30μ g/kg/divided in 3 doses, Maintenance: 3–5 μg/kg/ 12 hours↓ w/renal hepatic dysfunction	80% of oral dose	0.8–2.2 ng/ml	SVT, Atrial flutter	AV block, VT, many WPW	AV block, ↓HR, tachyarrhythmias, vomiting, use w/caution w/renal failure, toxicity with hypocalcemia
Quinidine IA	Yes	Hepatic	4–15 mg/kg/6 hours,↓ w/renal hepatic dysfunction		2–5 μg/ml	SVT, WPW w/ propranolol, PVC, VT	Long QT, known sensitivity, IV use, conduction block, myasthenia gravis	↓Contractility, ↑QT, VT, conduction block, vomiting, diarrhea, rash, blood dyscrasias, ↑HR w/atrial flutter w/o digoxin, ↑digoxin level, need to ↓digoxin dose by ½
Procainamide IA	Yes	Renal, hepatic	2.5–8 mg/kg/4 hours	7 mg/kg over 1 hour, Infusion: 20–60 μg/kg/min	Procainamide[a] 4–10μg/ml	SVT, WPW, PVC, VT	Conduction block, myasthenia gravis	Similar to Quinidine, ↓BP, lupus-like reaction, no effect on digoxin level
Disopyramide IA	No	Hepatic, renal	3.5–7.5 mg/kg/6 hours		2–5μg/ml	SVT, WPW, PVC, VT	Conduction block myasthenia gravis	Similar to Quinidine, ↓ contractility, anticholinergic, hypoglycemia, no effect on digoxin level
Lidocaine IB	Yes	Hepatic		Bolus: 1 mg/kg/5–10 min Infusion: 20–50 μg/kg/min, ↓ with cyanosis or hepatic dysfunction	2–5 μg/ml	PVC, VT	Conduction block ↓ junctional and ventricular escape rate	CNS reactions, seizure, ↓BP, ↓respiratory drive
Phenytoin IB	No	Renal, hepatic	2–3 mg/kg/12 hours, ↓ w/hepatic dysfunction	Load: 10 mg/kg maintenance: same as oral	10–20μg/ml	PVC, VT, Digitalis intoxication	Not FDA approved for VT	CNS reactions, ↓BP, blood dyscrasias, hepatic dysfunction, hypertrichosis, gingival hyperplasia, coarse facies, rash

Drug	Active metabolite	Elimination	Oral dose	IV dose	Serum level	Indications	Contraindications	Adverse effects
Flecainide IC	No	Renal, hepatic	1–2.5 mg/kg/8 hours, ↓ w/renal, hepatic dysfunction		0.2–1.0 µg/ml	Refractory life-threatening SVT, PJRT, PVC, VT	Conduction block, hepatic dysfunction, myocardial dysfunction, not FDA approved for children	Occasional ↑SVT frequency w/WPW, ↑ pacing threshold and conduction block, VT, nausea, ↓ contractility
Propranolol II	Yes	Hepatic	0.3–1.0 mg/kg/6 hours, ↓ w/chronic cyanosis, renal, hepatic dysfunction	0.02–0.10 mg/kg over 20 min		SVT, WPW, PVC, VT, hypertrophic cardiomyopathy, Long QT	Use w/verapamil, bronchospasm, conduction block, CHF	↓ HR, conduction block, bronchospasm, ↓BP, hypoglycemia, depression, ↓ cardiac reflexes w/anesthesia
Sotalol II/III	No	Renal	25–70 mg/M2BSA/8hours	Not available		SVT, WPW & VT with structurally normal heart	Use with verapamil, bronchospasm conduction block, unknown with structural heart disease	As per β-blockers plus proarrhythmias
Amiodarone III	No	Hepatic	5mg/kg/12 hours x 1 week then 5 mg/kg/day, ↓ w/hepatic dysfunction	Load: 5mg/kg over 15–30 min Infusion: 10–20µg/kg/min	1–2 mg/L	Refractory, life-threatening, SVT, VT, recurrent VF	Conduction block; not FDA approved for children	Extremely long half-life, corneal deposits, thyroid and hepatic dysfunction, pulmonary fibrosis may ↑ conduction block and Digoxin and Quinidine levels, need to ↓ Digoxin by 1/2
Bretylium III	No	Renal		Load: 5 mg/kg over 15 min Infusion: 20–50 µg/kg/min		Refractory VT, VF	Not FDA approved for children	Transient ↑BP, arrhythmia, then ↓ BP
Verapamil IV	No	Hepatic	2–4 mg/kg/8 hours, ↓ with hepatic, renal dysfunction, neuromuscular disease			Refractory SVT, hypertrophic cardiomyopathy, some PVC, VT	IV use, conduction dysfunction, CHF, many WPW, propranolol, muscular dystrophy, use w/Quinidine	↓ BP, ↓ HR, conduction block, myocardial depression, constipation, may ↑ digoxin level, need to ↓ digoxin dose 1/3 to 1/2

Continuous echocardiographic monitoring should be done during initiation of antidysrhythmic therapy and with IV administration because of potential prodysrhythmia and conduction block.

[a]To differentiate from metabolite measured by some laboratories.

AV, atrioventricular; BSA, body surface area; CHF, congestive heart failure; CNS, central nervous system; Dx, diagnosis; FDA, Federal Drug Administration; HR, heart rate; IV, intravenous; PJRT, permanent junctional reciprocating tachycardia; PVC, premature ventricular contractions; Rx, prescription; SVT, supraventricular tachycardia; VF, ventricular fibrillation; VT, ventricular tachycardia; w/, with; WPW, Wolff-Parkinson-White syndrome.

Courtesy of M.F. Flanagan, M.D. and D.C. Fyler, M.D.

4. EFFECT OF DRUGS USED IN NEONATOLOGY ON BILIRUBIN–ALBUMIN BINDING

APPENDIX H–4. *Effect of drugs used in neonatology on bilirubin–albumin binding*

Agent	δ	Agent	δ
Anticonvulsants		Moxalactam	1.63
Diazepam	1.00	Nafcillin	1.05
Phenobarbital	1.04	Oxacillin	1.07
Phenytoin	1.02	Penicillin G	1.06
Valproate	1.09	Piperacillin	1.03
Testing not required: lorazepam		Polymyxin B	1.00
Antihypertensive Agents		Quinine	?
Diazoxide	?	Spiramycin	1.00
Testing not required: hydralazine, methyldopa,		Streptomycin	1.00
nitroprusside, reserpine		Sulfadiazine	1.18
Cardiac Drugs		Sulfamethoxazole	1.69
Lidocaine	1.00	Sulfisoxazole	2.43
Procainamide	1.00	Tazobactam	1.00
Testing not required: bretylium tosylate, digoxin,		Ticarcillin	1.27
disopyramide, quinidine, verapamil		Trimethoprim	1.01
Diuretics		Vancomycin	1.01
Acetazolamide	1.10	Vidarabine	1.00
Bumetanide	1.00	Testing not required: amphotericin B,	
Chlorothiazide	1.03	ciprofloxacin, erythromycin, isoniazid,	
Ethacrynic acid	1.27	miconazole, netilmicin, pyrimethamine,	
Furosemide	1.07	tobramycin	
Hydrochlorothiazide	1.04	**Miscellaneous**	
Testing not required: spironolactone		Calcium chloride	1.00
Infectious Disease Agents		Calcium gluconate	1.00
Acyclovir	1.00	Calcium lactate	1.00
Amdinocillin	1.00	Carnitine	1.00
Ampicillin	1.08	Clofibrate	1.00
Azlocillin	1.33	Diatrizoate	1.24
Atreonam	1.12	Indomethacin	1.00
Carbenicillin	1.35	Magnesium sulfate	1.00
Cefamandole	1.07	Mannitol	1.00
Cefazolin	1.17	Tin protoporphyrin	?
Cefmenoxime	1.10	Tolazoline	1.00
Cefmetazole	2.01	Tromethamine	1.00
Cefonicid	1.71	Testing not required: bicarbonate, cimetidine,	
Cefoperazone	1.18	dextran, enalapril, flumecinol, heparin,	
Ceforanide	1.04	ketamine, metoclopramide, naloxone,	
Cefotaxime	1.05	nicardipine, prostaglandin E_1	
Cefotetan	1.74	**Neuromuscular Junction Agents**	
Cefoxitin	?	Pancuronium	1.01
Ceftazidime	1.02	Testing not required: atracurium besylate,	
Ceftizoxime	1.03	neostigmine, tubocurarine, vecuronium	
Ceftriaxone	3.00	**Sedative and Analgesic Agents**	
Cefuroxime	1.02	Chloral hydrate	1.00
Cephalothin	1.03	Paraldehyde	1.00
Cephapirin	1.03	Pentobarbital	1.03
Cephradine	1.02	Thiopental	1.04
Chloramphenicol	1.02	Testing not required: alfentanil, chlorpromazine,	
Chloroquine	1.00	fentanyl, meperidine, midazolam, morphine	
Cilastatin	1.00	**Stimulants**	
Clindamycin	1.00	Aminophylline	1.24
Fusidate	1.00	Doxapram	1.00
Imipenem	1.00	**Sympathetic and Parasympathetic Agents**	
Lincomycin	1.00	Edrophonium chloride	1.00
Methicillin	1.17	Testing not required: atropine dobutamine,	
Metronidazole	1.00	dopamine, epinephrine, isoproterenol,	
Mezlocillin	1.11	propranolol	

Drugs are listed according to the category of their use. The symbol δ represents the maximal displacement factor. If δ = 1.2, there is a 20% increase in free-bilirubin concentration following drug administration. Drugs listed as not requiring testing have low protein binding or low mean peak serum concentrations. A question mark indicates that the drug requires testing but that the peroxidase technique is not applicable.

From Robertson A, Carp W, Brodersen R. Bilirubin displacing effect of drugs used in neonatology. *Acta Paediatr Scand* 1991;80:1119.

APPENDIX I

Renal Anomalies

1. ASSOCIATIONS WITH OTHER STRUCTURAL DEFECTS

APPENDIX I–1. *Associations between renal-urinary tract anomalies and other structural defects*

Diagnosis (mode of genetic transmission)	Frequency of anomalies	Renal anomalies	Urologic anomalies	Other associations
Hereditary associations				
Acrorenal syndrome, or radial ray aplasia and renal anomalies (AD)	100%	Agenesis, ectopia		Absence of radius and thumb
Acrorenocular syndrome (AD/sporadic)	100%	Malrotation, ectopia	VUR, bladder diverticula	Thumb hypoplasia preaxial polydactyly, coloboma, ptosis
Acrorenomandibular syndrome (AR)	Frequent	Agenesis, ectopia		Split hand/split foot, cataracts ear and genital anomalies
Adams-Oliver syndrome (AD)	Occasional		Duplicated collecting system	Aplasia cutis congenita, terminal transverse defects of limbs
Alport syndrome (AD, but fully expressed only in males; X-linked)	Frequent	Nephritis; recurrent hematuria		Deafness cataracts, myopia lenticonus
Antley-Bixler syndrome (AR?)	Occasional	Displaced kidney, accessory renal artery		Craniosynostosis, choanal atresia, radiohumeral synostosis
Arthrogryposis multiplex congenita with renal and hepatic abnormalities (AR/X-linked?)	100%	Glycosuria, polyuria, nephrocalcinosis hypercalciuria, hyperposphaturia		Arthrogryposis multiplex congenita, rarefaction of motor neurons in anterior horn, cholestasis, all reported patients died before 4 months of age
Baller-Gerold syndrome, or Craniosynostosis-radial aplasia syndrome (AR)	Occasional	Pelvic kidney		MR (50%), growth deficiency, craniosynostosis, radial aplasia, CHD
Branchiootoureteral) syndrome (AD	50%	Bifid renal pelvis	Bifid ureters	Preauricular pit/tag, bilateral hearing loss
Campomelic dysplasia (AR)	30%	Usually hydronephrosis, MKD		Bowed tibiae, hypoplastic scapulae, flat facies growth deficiency, CNS disorganization, most die of respiratory failure as neonates or in infancy
Carpenter syndrome (AR)	Occasional		Ureteral dilatation	Acrocephaly, polydactyly—syndactyly of feet, lateral displacement of inner canthi, hypogenitalism
CHILD syndrome (X-linked?, lethal in hemizygotic male)	Occasional	Unilateral agenesis		Unilateral hypomelia, ichthyosis, CHD, mild SGA

(continued)

APPENDIX I–1. *Continued.*

Diagnosis (mode of genetic transmission)	Frequency of anomalies	Renal anomalies	Urologic anomalies	Other associations
COFS syndrome (AR)	Occasional	Agenesis		Neurogenic arthrogryposis, microcephaly, microphthalmia/cataract/blepharophimosis, large ear pinnae, prominent nasal bridge, no growth, usually die before 5 years of age
Cohen syndrome (AR)	Occasional		UPJ obstruction	Hypotonia, obesity, prominent incisors, moderate MR
Deal syndrome (AR)	100%	Fanconi syndrome		Ichthyosis, jaundice, musculoskeletal deformities, diarrhea, failure to thrive, death in infancy
Digitorenocerebral syndrome (AR)	Frequent	Agenesis, hypoplasia, dysplasia		Facial dysmorphism, seizures, malformed fingers and toes
EEC syndrome (AD, variable penetrance)	Occasional	Agenesis, hydronephrosis medullary dysplasia	Ureterocele	Ectrodactyly, ectodermal dysplasia, cleft lip/palate, defective lacrimal duct
Fanconi-pancytopenia syndrome (AR)	Frequent	Hypoplastic/malformed	Hypospadias, ureter duplication	Radial hypoplasia, hyperpigmentation, pancytopenia, short stature, microcephaly, MR
FG syndrome (X-linked R)	Occasional		Dilation	Prominent forehead, hypotonia, MR, imperforate anus
Fraser or cryptophthalmos syndrome (AR)	Frequent	Agenesis or hypoplasia		Cryptophthalmos, ear anomalies, genital anomaly, laryngeal stenosis/atresia, anal atresia, CHD
Frontometaphyseal dysplasia (X-linked, severe in male)	Occasional		Obstruction	Coarse facies, prominent supraorbital ridges, joint limitations, splayed metaphyses
Hereditary renal aplasia (AD, 50%–90% penetrance)	50%–90%	Unilateral or bilateral agenesis		Potter (oligohydramnios) sequence if bilateral agenesis, uterine anomaly
Jarcho-Levin syndrome, or spondylothoracic dysplasia (AR)	Occasional	Hydronephrosis	Urethral atresia Ureteral obstruction, bilobate bladder	Prominent occiput, short neck, most die in infancy due to lung hypoplasia, short thorax, diminished ribs, vertebral defects, most Puerto Rican origin
Johanson-Blizzard syndrome (AR)	Frequent	Caliectasis, hydronephrosis		Hypoplasia alae nasi, hypothyroidism, deafness
LEOPARD syndrome, or multiple lentigines syndrome (AD)	Occasional	Agenesis or hypoplasia		Lentigines, hypertelorism, deafness, pulmonary stenosis, obstructive cardiomyopathy, mild growth failure, variable expression in individual patient
Lethal multiple pterygium syndrome (AR)	Occasional	Hydronephrosis	Megaureter	SGA, hypertelorism, epicanthal folds, joint contractures, pterygia, early death due to lung hypoplasia
Levy-Hollister syndrome, or lacrimo-auriculo-dento-digital syndrome (AD)	Occasional	Agenesis, nephrosclerosis		Nasolacrimal duct obstruction, ear anomalies, hearing loss, variable anomalies of upper limbs
Melnick-Fraser syndrome, or branchio-oto-renal syndrome (AD)	Frequent	Dysplasia, hypoplasia, agenesis, ectopia		Hearing loss, preauricular pits, anomalous pinna, branchial fistula

APPENDIX I–1. *Continued.*

Diagnosis (mode of genetic transmission)	Frequency of anomalies	Renal anomalies	Urologic anomalies	Other associations
Melnick-Needles syndrome (AD?; lethal in male or X-linked)	Occasional	Hydronephrosis	Ureteral stenosis	Prominent eyes, bowing of long bones, ribbonlike ribs
Neu-Laxova syndrome (AR)	Occasional	Agenesis		Microcephaly, lissencephaly, exophthalmos, syndactyly and edema, polyhydramnios, short umbilical cord, early death
Opitz-Frias syndrome, G syndrome, or hypertelorism-hypospadias syndrome (AD)	Occasional	Renal defect	Hypospadias, cryptorchidism, bifid scrotum	Hypertelorism, swallowing difficulties
Perlman syndrome (AR?)		Nephromegaly, nephroblastomatosis	Cryptorchidism, hypospadias	Macrosomia, visceromegaly, polyhydramnios, diaphragmatic hernia, interrupted aortic arch, polysplenia
Rutledge syndrome (AR?)	100%	Oligopapillary renal hypoplasia	Urethral anomalies	Joint contractures, cerebellar hypoplasia, tongue cysts, short limbs, eye and ear anomalies, CHD, gallbladder agenesis
Saethre-Chotzen syndrome (AD)	Occasional	Renal anomaly		Craniosynostosis, brachycephaly, maxillary hypoplasia, abnormal ear, syndactyly
Schinzel-Giedion syndrome (AR)	Frequent	Hydronephrosis	Hydroureter, hypospadias	Severe growth failure, profound MR, midface retraction, cardiac and skeletal anomalies
TAR syndrome (AR)	Occasional	Ectopia, dysplasia	Hypospadias	Thrombocytopenia, granulocytosis, eosinophilia, anemia, radial absence or hypoplasia with thumbs present, CHD
Townes syndrome (AD)	Frequent	Hypoplasia	Ureterovesical reflux, urethral valves	Thumb, ear, and anal anomalies
Weyers oligodactyly syndrome (AR)	Frequent	Bilateral hydronephrosis		Deficient ulnar and fibular rays, oligodactyly
Chromosomal anomalies				
4p—syndrome	Occasional	Agenesis		Hypertelorism, broad or beaked nose, microcephaly, cranial asymmetry, low-set ears, dimple, CHD, severe MR, seizures
5p—syndrome, or cri du chat syndrome	Occasional	Agenesis		SGA, slow growth, catlike cry, MR, hypotonia, CHD, microcephaly, downslanting palpebral fissures, hypertelorism, round face, epicanthal folds, strabismus, low set ears
9p—syndrome	Occasional	Hydronephrosis		Craniostenosis, trigonocephaly, upslanting palpebral fissures, hypoplastic supraorbital ridges
13q—syndrome	Occasional	Agenesis or hypoplasia, PKD, hydronephrosis		Microcephaly, high nasal bridge, MR, CHD, hypertelorism, coloboma, microphthalmia, retinoblastoma
18q—syndrome	Occasional	Horseshoe kidney		Poor growth, microcephaly, hypotonia, midfacial hypoplasia, abnormal ears, cleft palate, thumb hypoplasia

(continued)

APPENDIX I–1. *Continued.*

Diagnosis (mode of genetic transmission)	Frequency of anomalies	Renal anomalies	Urologic anomalies	Other associations
Cat-eye syndrome[a]	Frequent	Horseshoe kidney, agenesis, hydronephrosis		Coloboma of the iris, downslanting palpebral fissures, anal atresia
Partial trisomy 10q syndrome	Frequent			Ptosis, short palpebral fissures, campodactyly, marked MR
Penta X syndrome, or XXXXX syndrome	Occasional	Dysplasia		Microcephaly, growth deficiency, upward slanting palpebral fissures, low nasal bridge, short neck, small hands, clinodactyly of fifth fingers, PDA
Triploidy syndrome	Frequent	Cystic kidney, hydronephrosis, dysplasia		Large placenta and hydatiform changes; poor growth; brain, facies, and cardiac anomalies; syndactyly
Trisomy 4p syndrome	Occasional	Atresia, horseshoe kidney, hypoplasia, hydronephrosis	VUR	Microcephaly, severe MR, hypertonia in infancy, seizures, SGA, bulbous nose, prominent forehead, clinodactyly
Trisomy 8 syndrome, or mosaic syndrome	Occasional	Hydronephrosis, horseshoe kidney, agenesis	Bifid pelvis	Prominent forehead and ears, deep-set eyes, hypertelorism, micrognathia, MR, CHD, vertebral anomalies, campodactyly
Trisomy 9 mosaic syndrome	Frequent			Joint contractures; heart, CNS, and ear anomalies
Trisomy 9p syndrome	Occasional	Malformations		SGA, macrocephaly, hypertelorism, downslanting palpebral fissures, distal phalangeal hypoplasia, skeletal anomalies
Trisomy 13 syndrome	Occasional	PKD, glomerular cysts, duplication	Ureter duplication, hydroureter	Holoprosencephaly, occipital scalp defect, polydactyly, microphthalmia, narrow hyperconvex fingernails
Trisomy 18 syndrome	Frequent	Horseshoe kidney, ectopic, PKD, hypoplasia or agenesis, duplication	Ureter duplication	Polyhydramnios, single UA, poor growth, prominent occiput, clenched hand
Trisomy 20p syndrome	Occasional	Malformations		Blepharophimosis, brachycephaly, large ears, MR, cubitus valgus, vertebral defects, CHD
Turner syndrome, or XO syndrome	60%	Horseshoe kidney, hypertension	Double or cleft pelvis	Short broad chest, widely spaced nipples, lymphedema, webbed neck, cubitus valgus
Sporadic associations				
Aniridia-Wilms tumor association[b]	50%	Bilateral Wilms tumor		Microcephaly, growth deficiency, MR, prominent lips, cataracts, ptosis, nystagmus, ambiguous genitalia
Beckwith-Wiedemann syndrome, or exomphalos-"macroglossia-gigantism syndrome	Frequent	Large kidneys, medullary dysplasia	Hypospadias	Omphalocele, macroglossia, gigantism, ear creases, polyhydramnios, prematurity, hypoglycemia, polycythemia, apnea
Caudal dysplasia sequence, or caudal regression sequence	Occasional	Agenesis	Neurogenic bladder	Abnormal vertebrae and lower limbs, neurologic defects, R/O maternal diabetes, imperforate anus

APPENDIX I–1. *Continued.*

Diagnosis (mode of genetic transmission)	Frequency of anomalies	Renal anomalies	Urologic anomalies	Other associations
CHARGE association	5%	Agenesis, hypoplasia, hydronephrosis, heterotopic kidneys		Coloboma (iris, retina, anophthalmos), CHD, choanal atresia, growth retardation (postnatal), mental deficiency, genital hypoplasia (in males), ear anomalies, deafness
Goldenhar syndrome, facioauriculovertebral spectrum, first and second branchial arch syndrome	Occasional	Renal anomalies		Hemifacial microsomia, hemivertebrae, occasional abnormal ears and eyes, deafness, CHD, MR, SGA
Klippel-Feil syndrome	Frequent	Renal anomalies		Short neck, abnormal cervical vertebrae, deafness, CHD
Laterality sequences Ivemark syndrome, or bilateral right-sidedness	Frequent	Renal anomalies		Situs inversus, asplenia, CHD and vessel anomalies,
Bilateral left-sidedness	Occasional	Renal anomalies		Situs inversus, CHD, polysplenia
Meningomyelocele, spina bifida and occult spinal dysraphism sequence	Frequent	Hydronephrosis, UTI, renal failure, horseshoe kidney, hypoplasia, agenesis, ectopia, duplication	Neurogenic bladder	Neurologic defect, hydrocephalus
Megacystis-microcolon-intestinal hypoperistalsis syndrome	100%	Hydronephrosis	Massive bladder distention (100%), VUR	Neonatal bowel obstruction, hypoperistalsis, microcolon, frequently early death
Müllerian aplasia, Rokitansky sequence, or Rokitansky-Kustner-Hauser syndrome	30%–50%	Unilateral renal aplasia, hypoplasia, ectopia	Ureter duplication	Vaginal atresia, rudimentary uterus
MURCS association	>50%	Agenesis or ectopia (88%)		Absence of vagina, hypoplasia of uterus, abnormal cervico-thoracic vertebrae
Monozygote twinning	Occasional		Exstrophy of the cloaca	Sacrococcygeal teratoma, sirenomelia, VATER, holo-prosencephaly, anencephaly
Pallister-Hall syndrome	Frequent	Dysplasia		Hypothalamic hamartoblastoma, hypopituitarism, imperforate anus, polydactyly
Poland anomaly	Occasional	Renal anomaly		Variable unilateral features: absence of pectoralis muscle, upper limb hypoplasia, syndactyly
Potter sequence, or oligohydramnios sequence	100%	Hypoplasia, aplasia, agenesis, PKD, dysplasia	Urethral valves	Amnion nodosum, oligohydramnios, lung hypoplasia, limb malposition, facies compression
Prune-belly syndrome, or early urethral obstruction sequence	100%	Dysplasia, hypoplasia, horseshoe kidney, hydronephrosis	Urethral valves, persistent urachus, bladder agenesis, ectopic ureter	Prune belly, cryptorchidism, abnormal genitalia, Potter GI malformation (anal, hepatobiliary, mesentery, esophageal, pancreas), talipes equinovarus, scoliosis, thorax deformities, cardiac anomalies, iliac vessel compression
Rubinstein-Taybi syndrome	Frequent	Duplication	Ureter duplication	Broad thumbs and toes, hypoplastic maxilla, MR, slanted palpebral fissures
Sirenomelia sequence	Frequent	Agenesis, dysplasia	Bladder agenesis	Fusion of lower limbs, single UA, absence of genitalia except gonads, absence of sacrum and rectum, imperforate anus

(continued)

APPENDIX I–1. *Continued.*

Diagnosis (mode of genetic transmission)	Frequency of anomalies	Renal anomalies	Urologic anomalies	Other associations
Thanatophoric dysplasia	Occasional	Horseshoe kidney, hydronephrosis		Short limbs, flat vertebrae, large cranium, low nasal bridge, severe SGA, hypotonia, polyhydramnios, lung hypoplasia, early death
Tracheal agenesis association[c]	50%	Agenesis, hydronephrosis, dysplasia	Duplication	Laryngeal/tracheal atresia, GI) anomalies (e.g., duodenal atresia), CHD, limb reduction defect (i.e., radial hypoplasia
VATER/VACTERL association	50%–74%	Agenesis, hydronephrosis, cystic dysplasia	Duplication, urethral atresia	TEF, vertebral and anal atresia, CHD, limb anomalies (i.e., radial dysplasia)
Renal cystic disease[d]				
Alagille syndrome, or arteriohepatic dysplasia (AD)	Occasional	Cystic tubular dilatations, CRF, tubulointerstitial disease		Facies: deep-set eyes, prominent forehead, cholestasis, PPS, butterfly vertebrae
Apert syndrome, or acrocephalosyndactyly (AD; fresh mutation common)	Occasional	MKD, hydronephrosis		Craniosynostosis, midfacial hypoplasia, syndactyly, broad distal phalanx (i.e., thumb and big toe), occasional CHD, GI tract and lung anomalies
Congenital nephrotic syndrome, Finnish type (AR)	100%	CNF, tubular cystic dilatations		Polyhydramnios, elevated α-fetoprotein in amniotic fluid
Cystic hamartomata of lung and kidney	100%	Multilocular cysts		Hamartomatous pulmonary cysts
Dandy-Walker malformation	Occasional	MKD		Congenital hepatic fibrosis
Ehler-Danlos syndrome (AD, AR, X-linked)	Occasional	RTA		Skin and joint hyperextensibility, poor wound healing
Elejalde syndrome (AR)		Cystic dysplasia		Short-limb dwarfism, acrocephaly, polysyndactyly, subcutaneous hypertrophy, cholestasis, pancreatic dysplasia
Ellis-van Creveld syndrome, or chondroectodermal dysplasia (AR)	Occasional	Agenesis, cystic/medullary dysplasia	Epispadias	Short distal extremities, polydactyly, nail hypoplasia CHD (50%), SGA and short eventual stature, cholestasis
Familial juvenile nephronophthisis with hepatic fibrosis (AR)	Frequent	Glomerular cysts		Congenital hepatic fibrosis
Familial renal-retinal dystrophy (AR)	Common	Nephronophthisis-medullary cystic kidney disease		Pigmentary retinal dystrophy
Femoral hypoplasia-unusual facies syndrome		PKD, agenesis	Abnormal collecting system	Femoral hypoplasia, short nose, cleft palate
Fryns syndrome (AR)	50%	MKD, cortical cysts		Facial dysmorphism, microretrognathia, diaphragm defects, lung hypoplasia, neonatal death, bicornuate uterus or scrotum anomaly, distal limb hypoplasia
Glutaric aciduria syndrome, type II, or multiple acyl-coA dehydrogenase deficiency (AR)	Frequent	Cystic dysplasia, ultrastructural anomaly of glomerular basement membrane		Cerebral dysplasia, macrocephaly, facial dysmorphism, fatty liver, genital defects, hypoglycemia, metabolic acidosis
Ivemark syndrome, or renal-hepatic-pancreatic dysplasia (AR)	Frequent	Glomerular cysts, cystic dysplasia		Hepatic and pancreatic dysplasia, occasional splenic anomalies, may be associated with homogenous syndrome (Bernstein)

APPENDIX I–1. *Continued.*

Diagnosis (mode of genetic transmission)	Frequency of anomalies	Renal anomalies	Urologic anomalies	Other associations
Jeune asphyxiating thoracic dystrophy (AR)	Frequent	Glomerular sclerosis, tubular cysts, renal failure		Small chest, lung hypoplasia, short limbs, cholestasis
Lowe syndrome, or oculocerebrorenal syndrome (X-linked)	100% (male)	Fanconi syndrome, CRF		Cataracts, mental deficiency, hypotonia
Meckel-Gruber syndrome, or dysencephalia splanchnocystica (AR)	100%	MKD, PKD, dysplasia, hypoplasia		Encephalocele, holoprosencephaly, polydactyly, Potter sequence, cholestasis
Nail-patella syndrome, or hereditary osteoonychodystrophy	Frequent	Proteinuria, hematuria, casts, CRF, PKD	Ureter duplication	Nail dysplasia, patella hypoplasia, iliac spurs
Orofacial digital syndrome, type 1 (D, lethal in male)	Frequent	Glomerular cysts		Oral frenula and clefts, hypoplasia of alae nasi, digital asymmetry
Roberts-SC phocomelia syndrome, hypomelia-hypotrichosis-facial hemangioma syndrome, or pseudothalidomide (AR)	Occasional	MKD, horseshoe kidney		Hypomelia, midfacial defect, cleft palate and lip, severe growth deficiency, cholestasis
Short-rib polydactyly, type I (Saldino-Noonan type)	Frequent	MKD, hypoplastic		Short-limb dwarfism, severe lung hypoplasia, early death, short ribs, with or without polydactyly, CHD, imperforate anus
Short rib-polydactyly syndrome, type II (Majewski type) (AR)	Frequent	Glomerular cysts, focal dilatation of distal tubules		Short-limb dwarfism, severe lung hypoplasia, early death, short ribs, with or without polydactyly, CHD, ambiguous genitalia
Smith-Lemli-Opitz syndrome (AR)	Occasional	MKD		MR, growth retardation, microcephaly, micrognathia, anteverted nostrils, ptosis of eyelids, syndactyly of second-third toes, ambiguous genitalia
Tuberous sclerosis (AD)	50%–80%	Glomerular and tubular cysts (rarely neonatal), angiomyolipomas, CRF		Seizures, skin lesions, tumors
Von Hippel-Lindau syndrome (AD)	Occasional	PKD		Retinal angioma, cerebellar hemangioblastoma
Zellweger syndrome, or cerebrohepatorenal syndrome (AR)	100%	Glomerular cysts, albuminuria		Hypotonia, abnormal brain, seizures, flat facies, peroxisomal deficiency, cholestasis
Metabolic diseases				
Hyperoxaluria type I, or oxalosis (AR)	100%	Nephrocalcinosis/ lithiasis, CRF		Anorexia, failure to thrive, vomiting, dehydration and fever, liver failure, acidosis
Galactose-1-phosphate uridyl transferase deficiency, or galactosemia (AR)	Frequent	Fanconi syndrome		Hypoglycemia, anorexia, liver failure, sepsis, cataracts, MR
Hereditary fructose intolerance, fructose-1-phosphate aldolase deficiency (AR)	Frequent	Fanconi syndrome		Hypoglycemia, anorexia, liver failure, failure to thrive
Tyrosinemia type I, tyrosinosis, or hepatorenal tyrosinemia (AR)	Frequent	Fanconi syndrome		Growth failure, cabbagelike odor, vomiting, diarrhea, metabolic acidosis, liver failure, edema, fever
Glycogenosis with Fanconi syndrome, or Fanconi-Bickel syndrome (AR)	100%	Fanconi syndrome		Fever, vomiting, growth failure, rickets, hypoglycemia, hepatomegaly

(continued)

APPENDIX I–1. *Continued.*

Diagnosis (mode of genetic transmission)	Frequency of anomalies	Renal anomalies	Urologic anomalies	Other associations
Cystinosis (AR)	100%	Fanconi syndrome		Light skin and hair, failure to thrive, anorexia, fussiness, episodes of acidosis, dehydration and fever, rickets
Teratogens				
Fetal alcohol syndrome	18%	Renal agenesis, hypoplasia, hydronephrosis	Ureteral duplication	SGA, microcephaly, facial dysmorphism, MR
Fetal hydantoin syndrome	Occasional	Various malformations		Poor growth; microcephaly; craniofacial dysmorphism; brain, limb, and GI anomalies; CHD
Thalidomide embryopathy	Occasional	Various malformations		Phocomelia; polydactyly; syndactyly; hydrocephalus; facial capillary hemangioma; CHD; ear, eye, and GI anomalies
Fetal trimethadione syndrome	Occasional	Various malformations		Poor growth, craniofacial anomalies, CHD
Angiotensin converting enzyme inhibitors	Frequent(?)	Nephron dysgenesis		Hypocalvaria
Congenital infections				
Congenital syphilis	Occasional	Nephrotic syndrome		Snuffles, meningitis, bone changes
Congenital toxoplasmosis	Rare	Nephrotic syndrome		Microcephaly, deafness, chorioretinitis, SGA
Renal failure[e]				
Bardet-Biedl syndrome, or Laurence-Moon-Biedl syndrome (AR)	Frequent	Dysplasia, nephrosclerosis, interstitial scarring, cyst, HTN	Hydroureter	Retinitis pigmentosa, obesity, polydactyly
Drash syndrome, or nephropathy associated with gonadal dysgenesis and Wilms tumor	100%	Glomerulonephritis, interstitial changes, nephrotic syndrome, hematuria, HTN, ESRD, often Wilms tumor		Ambiguous genitalia (often male pseudohermaphroditism)
Fabry syndrome, or angiokeratoma corporis diffusum (X-linked)	Frequent	Proteinuria, hematuria, casts, leukocyturia		Dark nodular angiectases, corneal opacities, seizures, CNS symptoms
Russell-Silver syndrome (AD)	Sporadic	Wilms syndrome	Posterior urethral valves, hypospadias	Small stature, skeletal asymmetry, small fifth finger, small triangular facies
Williams syndrome	Occasional	Hypertension	Bladder diverticula	Decreased growth, hypercalcemia, subaortic stenosis, prominent lips, hoarse voice

This table has been made by selecting well-defined associations, described in at least three patients, in whom renal manifestations may develop before 1 year of age.

[a]Extra chromosome corresponding to segments of chromosome 22.

[b]May have partial deletion of chromosome 1p.

[c]Overlaps with VATER association.

[d]See also trisomy 13 and 18, VATER, cocaine, and other subheadings (i.e., renal dysplasia).

[e]See also other headings.

AD, autosomal dominant; AR, autosomal recessive; CHD, congenital heart disease; CHARGE, coloboma, heart disease, atresia of the choanae, retarded mental development and growth, genital hypoplasia, ear anomalies; CHILD, congenital hemidysplasia with ichthyosiform erythroderma and limb defects; COFS, cerebrooculofacioskeletal; CNS; central nervous system; CRF, chronic renal failure; D, dominant; EEC, ectrodactyly-ectodermal dysplasia-clefting; EKG, electrocardiogram; ESRD, end-stage renal disease; GI, gastrointestinal; HTN, hypertension; LEOPARD, lentigenes, EKG anomalies, ocular anomalies, pulmonary stenosis, abnormal genitalia, retardation of growth, and deafness; MKD, multicystic kidney disease; MR, mental retardation; MURCS, Müllerian duct, renal, cervical somite; PDA, patent ductus arteriosus; PKD, polycystic kidney disease; PPS, peripheral pulmonic stenosis; R, recessive; R/O, rule out; RTA, renal tubular acidosis; SGA, small for gestational age; TAR, radial aplasia-thrombocytopenia; TEF, tracheoesophageal fistula; UA, umbilical artery; UPJ, ureteropelvic junction; UTI, urinary tract infection; VACTERL, vertebrae, anus, cardiac, tracheoesophageal, renal, limb; VATER, vertebrae, anus, tracheoesophageal, renal; VUR, vesicoureteral reflux.

2. SINGLE SIGNS OF RENAL–URINARY TRACT MALFORMATIONS

APPENDIX I–2. *Relationship between single signs and renal–urinary tract malformations*

Sign	Criteria for entry into the study	Method used to detect renal-urinary tract malformations	Type of malformations	Minimum incidence[a] of patients with renal-urinary tract anomalies	Incidence of patients with renal-urinary tract anomalies who had no evidence of other malformations at birth[b]
Abnormal Vertebrae					
Kohler 1982 (1)	Abnormal vertebrae or vertebrae	IVU	Agenesis, ectopic, horseshoe kidney, duplication	8/46 (17%)	NA
Macewen 1972 (2)	Congenital scoliosis, without suspicion of neurogenic bladder	IVU	Agenesis, duplication, ectopia, obstruction, VUR, horseshoe kidney	42/231 (18%)	NA
Anorectal Anomalies					
Munn 1983 (3)	Imperforation or atresia	IVU	Agenesis, duplication, VUR, hypospadias, UPJ obstruction, neurogenic bladder	20/28 (71%)	NA
Hoekstra 1983 (4)[c]	Congenital anomalies	Autopsy; IVU excess in 3/126	VUR, agenesis, hypoplasia, ectopia, PKD UPJ obstruction, horseshoe kidney, hypospadias	95/150 (63%)	NA
Khuri 1981 (5)[d]	Imperforate anus and hypospadias	IVU	NA (part of study on hypospadias)	6/13 (46%)	NA
Congenital Diaphragmatic Hernia					
Siebert 1990 (6)	Autopsy	Autopsy	Agenesis, dysplasia or hypoplasia, UPJ/ureterovesical obstruction	16/27 (59%)	4/16 (25%)
Cunniff 1990 (7)	Chart review	Surgery or autopsy	Agenesis, hydronephrosis, cysts, ectopic or duplicated ureter	5/103 (5%)	0%
Hypospadias					
Khuri 1981 (5)	Hypospadias	IVU in 460/1076	Agenesis, UPJ obstruction, VUR, Wilms, PKD, ectopic kidney, horseshoe kidney	48/1076 (4%)	15/48 (31%)[e]
Shelton 1985 (8)	Asymptomatic hypospadias	IVU, VCUG	Agenesis, duplication, pelvic kidney, VUR	27/102 (27%)	0%
Pulmonary Hypoplasia					
Page 1982 (9)	Neonatal autopsy	Autopsy	Agenesis, dysgenesis, dysplasia, PKD	16/77 (21%)	NA
Single Umbilical Artery					
Bourke (10)	Isolated single UA, examination of umbilical cord	US with VCUG if persistently abnormal	VUR, megaureter, agenesis, dilation of collecting system	8/112 (7%)	8/112 (7%)
Spontaneous Air Leak Syndrome					
Bashour 1977 (11)	Symptomatic pneumothorax	IVU	hypoplasia or agenesis, PKD, dysplasia, urethral valves, Potter facies (n = 3)	12/47 (26%)	3/12 (25%)

(continued)

APPENDIX I–2. *Continued.*

Sign	Criteria for entry into the study	Method used to detect renal-urinary tract malformations	Type of malformations	Minimum incidence[a] of patients with renal-urinary tract anomalies	Incidence of patients with renal-urinary tract anomalies who had no evidence of other malformations at birth[b]
Supernumerary Nipples					
Mehes 1983 (12)	Hospitalized	Clinical examination and IVU	Hydronephrosis, megaureter, duplication	9/37 (24%)	NA
Mimouni 1983 (13)	Neonatal (Israel)	Physical examination US (11/42)		0/43 (0%)	0%
Varsano 1984 (14)	ER/pediatric clinic (Israel)	IVU	PKD, hydronephrosis (UPJ obstruction), duplicated ureter, ureteral prolapse	6/26 (23%)	6/6 (100%)[g]
Robertson 1986 (15)	Neonatal (African-Americans)	US		0/32 (0%)	0%
Hersh 1987 (16)	Genetic/developmental clinic; 10 controls (United States, mostly Caucasian)	US or IVU	MKD, agenesis, hydronephrosis, horseshoe kidney	7/65 (11%)	2/7 (29%)[h]
Urbani 1996 (17)	Adult subjects	US, urinalysis	ADPKD, unilateral renal agenesis MKD, familial cysts, UPJ stenosis	NA	NA

[a]Hypospadias excluded.
[b]Except for minor anomalies such as pes equinovarus.
[c]Eighty-one of 150 patients in the study had no congenital abnormalities of the other organs (54%).
[d]Among patients with first-degree hypospadias, the incidence of upper urinary tract malformations was 1.3%.
[e]Also 3 patients with undescended testes.
[f]One patient had epilepsy; two patients had pyloric stenosis.
[g]One patient had Niemann-Pick disease.
[h]Three patients had anomalies.
ER, emergency room; IVU, intravenous urography; MKD, multicystic kidney dysplasia; NA, not available; PKD, polycystic kidney disease; UA, umbilical artery, UPJ/UV, ureteropelvic junction-ureterovesical; US, ultrasound; VUR, vesicoureteral reflex.

REFERENCES

1. Kohler R, Dodat H, Charollais Y. Malformations congénitales vertébrales et urinaires. Fréquence de leur association et conduite à tenir. *Pédiatrie* 1982;37:91.
2. Macewen GD, Winter RB, Hardy JH. Evaluation of kidney anomalies in congenital scoliosis. *J Bone Joint Surg* 1972;54:1451.
3. Munn R, Schillinger JF. Urologic abnormalities found with imperforate anus. *Urol* 1983;21:260.
4. Hoekstra WJ, Scholtmeijer RJ, Molenar JC, Schreeve RH, Schroeder FH. Urogenital tract abnormalities associated with congenital anorectal anomalies. *J Urol* 1983;130:962.
5. Khuri FJ, Hardy BE, Churchill BM. Urologic anomalies associated with hypospadias. *Urol Clin North Am* 1981;8:565.
6. Siebert JR, Benjamin DR, Juul S, Glick PL. Urinary tract anomalies associated with congenital diaphragmatic defects. *Am J Med Genet* 1990;37:1.
7. Cunniff C, Jones KL, Jones MC. Patterns of malformation in children with congenital diaphragmatic defects. *J Pediatr* 1990;116:258.
8. Shelton TB, Noe HN. The role of excretory urography in patients with hypospadias. *J Urol* 1985;134:97.
9. Page DV, Stocker JT. Anomalies associated with pulmonary hypoplasia. *Am Rev Resp Dis* 1982;125:216.
10. Bourke WG, Clarke TA, Mathews TG, O'Halpin D, Donoghue VB. Isolated single umbilical artery—the case for routine renal screening. *Arch Dis Child* 1993;68(5Spec No):600.
11. Bashour BN, Balfe JW. Urinary tract anomalies in neonates with spontaneous pneumothorax and/or pneumomediastinum. *Pediatr* 1977;59 (Suppl):1048.
12. Méhes K. Association of supernumerary nipples with other anomalies (letter). *J Pediatr* 1983;102:161.
13. Mimouni F, Merlob P, Reisner SH. Occurrence of supernumerary nipples in newborns. *Am J Dis Child* 1983;137:952.
14. Varsano IB, Jaber L, Garty BZ, Mukamel MM, Grünebaum M. Urinary tract abnormalities in children with supernumerary nipples. *Pediatrics* 1984;73:103.
15. Robertson A, Sale P, Sathyanarayan. Lack of association of supernumerary nipples with renal anomalies in black infants. *J Pediatr* 1986;109:502.
16. Hersh JH, Bloom AS, Cromer AO, Harrison HL, Weisskopf B. Does a supernumerary nipple/renal field defect exist? *Am J Dis Child* 1987;141:989.
17. Urbani, CE, Betti R. Accessory mammary tissue associated with congenital and hereditary nephrourinary malformations. *Int J Dermatol* 1996;35:349.

3. CLASSIFICATION OF CYSTIC KIDNEY DISEASE

APPENDIX I–3. *Classification of cystic kidney disease*

Genetic Diseases
AR polycystic kidney disease: associated with congenital hepatic fibrosis
AD polycystic kidney disease: associated with central nervous system aneurysms
Juvenile nephronophthisis—medullary cystic disease complex
    Juvenile nephronophthisis with hepatic fibrosis (AR)
    Medullary cystic disease complex (AD)
Glomerulocystic kidney disease:
    AD glomerulocystic kidney disease
    Familial hypoplastic glomerulocystic kidney disease (AD)
Malformation syndromes
    Multicystic kidney disease
        Apert syndrome, or acrocephalosyndactyly (AD, fresh mutation common)
        Elejalde syndrome (AR)
        Ellis-van Creveld syndrome, or chondroectodermal dysplasia (AR)
        Fryns syndrome (AR)
        Meckel-Gruber syndrome, or dysencephalia splanchnocystica (AR)
        Roberts phocomelia, hypomelia—hypotrichosis—facial hemangioma syndrome, or
          pseudothalidomide syndrome (AR)
        Short rib-polydactyly syndrome, Saldino-Noonan type (AR)
        Smith-Lemli-Optiz syndrome (AR)
    Glomerulocystic disease
        Short rib-polydactyly syndrome, Majewski type (AR)
        Tuberous sclerosis (AD): glomerular and tubular cysts
        Zellweger cerebrohepatorenal syndrome (AR)
        Ivemark syndrome, or renal-hepatic-pancreatic dysplasia (AR): cystic dysplasia
        Orofacial digital syndrome, type 1 (D, lethal in male infants)
    Nephronophthisis-medullary cystic disease
        Familial renal-retinal dystrophy (AR)
    Other
        Von Hippel-Lindau syndrome (AD)
        Jeune syndrome, or asphyxiating thoracic dystrophy (AR)
        Alagille syndrome, or arteriohepatic dysplasia (AD)
        Trisomy D (13)
        Trisomy E (18)
        Ehlers-Danlos syndrome (AD, AR, X-linked)
        Glutaric aciduria syndrome, type II, or multiple acyl-coA dehydrogenase deficiency (AR)
        Lowe syndrome, or oculo-cerebro-renal syndrome (X-linked)
        Nail-patella syndrome, or hereditary osteoonychodystrophy (AD)
Congenital hypernephronic nephromegaly with tubular dysgenesis syndrome (AR)
Congenital nephrotic syndrome, Finnish type, or infantile microcystic disease (AR)
Sporadic and Acquired Diseases
Multicystic kidney disease, or multicystic dysplasia
    Dandy-Walker malformation
Sporadic glomerulocystic kidney disease
Nephron dysgenesis: glomerular or tubular immaturity
Brachymesomelia-renal syndrome (only one case described)
Femoral hypoplasia-unusual facies syndrome
Multilocular cystic nephroma, or cystadenoma
Simple cyst (benign)
Medullary sponge kidney (<5% inherited; no renal failure)
Cystic hamartoma of lung and kidney (multilocular cysts)
Acquired renal cystic disease in chronic hemodialysis patients
Caliceal diverticulum, or pyelogenic cyst

AD, autosomal dominant; AR, autosomal recessive; D, dominant.
See Appendix I–1 for description of associated malformations.

Subject Index